AF861316

evolve

ELSEVIER

YOU'VE JUST PURCHASED MORE THAN A TEXTBOOK!

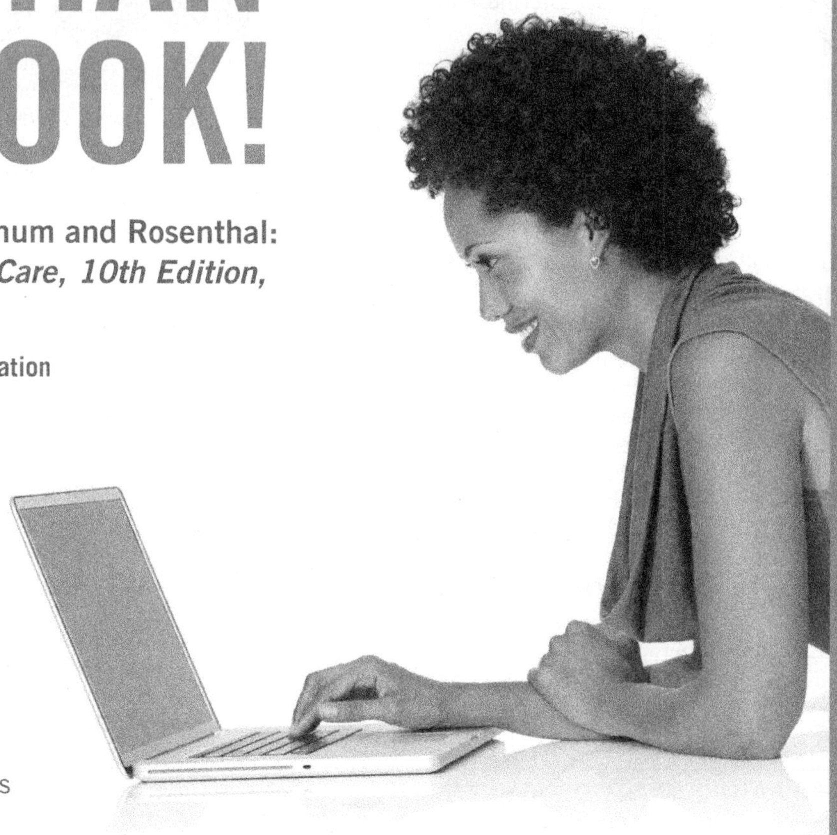

Evolve Student Resources for Burchum and Rosenthal: *Lehne's Pharmacology for Nursing Care, 10th Edition,* include the following:

- **Review Questions for the NCLEX® Examination**
  NCLEX® Examination–style Review Questions for every chapter offer practice in preparing for licensure examinations.
- **Downloadable Key Points**
  Key Points for every chapter are available as downloadable files so you can review essential chapter content anywhere.
- **Interactive Unfolding Case Studies**
  Case Studies offer an engaging way to apply important pharmacology concepts to true-to-life patient scenarios.
- **Additional Resources**
  Additional resources include animations, videos, and periodic content updates!

Activate the complete learning experience that comes with each textbook purchase by registering at

http://evolve.elsevier.com/Lehne

REGISTER TODAY!

You can now purchase Elsevier products on Evolve!
Go to evolve.elsevier.com/html/shop-promo.html to search and browse for products.

2015v1.0

Lehne's
PHARMACOLOGY
for NURSING CARE

10TH EDITION

Lehne's
PHARMACOLOGY
for NURSING CARE

Jacqueline Rosenjack Burchum, DNSc, FNP-BC, CNE
Associate Professor, College of Nursing
Department of Advanced Practice and Doctoral Studies
University of Tennessee Health Science Center
Memphis, Tennessee

Laura D. Rosenthal, RN, DNP, ACNP-BC, FAANP
Associate Professor, College of Nursing
University of Colorado, Anschutz Medical Campus
Denver, Colorado

ELSEVIER

ELSEVIER

3251 Riverport Lane
St. Louis, Missouri 63043

LEHNE'S PHARMACOLOGY FOR NURSING CARE, TENTH EDITION ISBN 978-0-323-51227-5

Previous editions copyrighted 2016, 2013, 2010, 2007, 2004, 2001, 1998, 1994, 1990.

International Standard Book Number: 978-0-323-51227-5

Executive Content Strategist: Sonya Seigafuse
Senior Content Development Manager: Luke Held
Content Development Specialist: Jennifer Wade
Publishing Services Manager: Jeff Patterson
Senior Project Manager: Jodi M. Willard
Design Direction: Paula Catalano

Printed in the United States of America

Last digit is the print number: 9 8 7 6 5 4 3 2 1

To my son, Jade Charmagan, BSN, RN. Congratulations, and welcome to the world of nursing!
JRB

For Ashley, Christine, Courtney, Erica, Laura B., Laura P., and Stacy—my official support team in life.
LDR

About the Authors

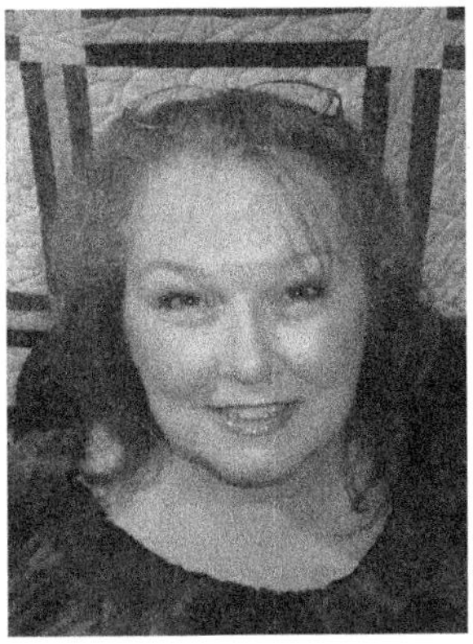

Jacqueline Rosenjack Burchum, DNSc, FNP-BC, CNE, has been a registered nurse since 1981 and a family nurse practitioner since 1996. She completed her Doctor of Nursing Science degree in 2002.

Dr. Burchum currently serves as an associate professor for the University of Tennessee Health Science Center (UTHSC) College of Nursing. She is credentialed as a certified nurse educator (CNE) by the National League for Nursing. She is a two-time recipient of the UTHSC Student Government Association's Excellence in Teaching Award and a recipient of the 2014 UT Alumni Association's Outstanding Teacher Award. Dr. Burchum was also the 2016–2017 Faculty Innovation Scholar for the UTHSC Teaching and Learning Center.

Dr. Burchum has a special interest in online teaching and program quality. To this end, she serves as an on-site evaluator for the Commission on Collegiate Nursing Education (CCNE), a national agency that accredits nursing education programs. In addition, she is a peer reviewer for Quality Matters, a program that certifies the quality of online courses.

As a nurse practitioner, Dr. Burchum's primary interests have centered on addressing the needs of vulnerable populations. She is a member of the National Organization for Nurse Practitioner Faculties, Sigma Theta Tau International Honor Society, the American and Tennessee Nurses Associations, and the National League for Nursing.

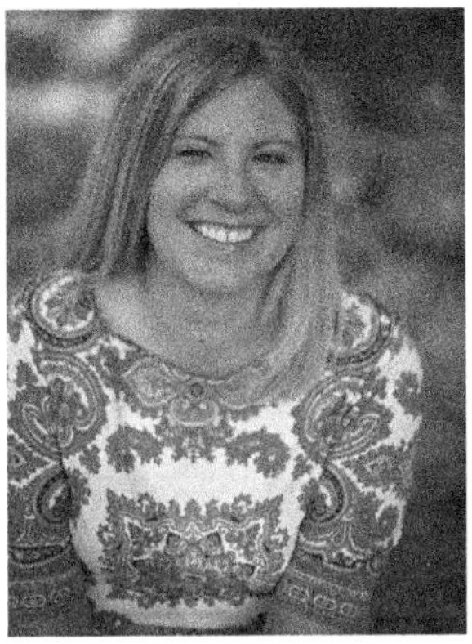

Laura D. Rosenthal, RN, DNP, ACNP-BC, FAANP, has been a registered nurse since graduating with her Bachelor of Science in Nursing degree from the University of Michigan in 2000. She completed her Master of Science in Nursing degree in 2006 at Case Western Reserve University in Cleveland, Ohio. She finished her nursing education at the University of Colorado, College of Nursing, graduating with her Doctor of Nursing Practice degree in 2011. Her background includes practice in acute care and inpatient medicine. While working as a nurse practitioner at the University of Colorado Hospital, she assisted in developing one of the first fellowships for advanced practice clinicians in hospital medicine.

Dr. Rosenthal serves as an associate professor at the University of Colorado, College of Nursing, where she teaches within the undergraduate and graduate programs. She received the Dean's Award for Excellence in Teaching in 2013. She serves on the board of the Colorado Nurses Association, remains a member of the NP/PA committee for the Society of Hospital Medicine, and volunteers as a Health Services RN for the Red Cross. In her spare time, Dr. Rosenthal enjoys running, skiing, and fostering retired greyhounds for Colorado Greyhound Adoption.

Contributors and Reviewers

CONTRIBUTOR

Joshua J. Neumiller, PharmD, CDE, FASCP
Assistant Professor of Pharmacotherapy
Washington State University
Spokane, Washington
Chapter 57

REVIEWERS

Laura Brennan, MS, RN
Assistant Professor
Elmhurst College
Elmhurst, Illinois

Joan Parker Frizzell, PhD, CRNP, ANP-BC
Associate Professor
School of Nursing and Health Sciences
La Salle University;
Nurse Practitioner
Roxborough Memorial Hospital
Philadelphia, Pennsylvania

James Graves, PharmD
Clinical Pharmacist
University of Missouri Inpatient Pharmacy
Columbia, Missouri

Ellen Ketcherside, RN, MA
Nursing Professor
Allied Health Department
Mineral Area College
Park Hills, Missouri

Lisa Miklush, PhD, RNC, CNS
Adjunct Faculty
Nursing Department
Gonzaga University
Spokane, Washington

Janet Czermak Russell MA, MS, APN-BC
Associate Professor of Nursing
Nursing Department
Essex County College
Newark, New Jersey

Carin Tripodina, EdD, MS, RN, CPN, CNE
Assistant Professor of Nursing
Nursing Department
American International College
Springfield, Massachusetts

Jennifer J. Yeager, PhD, RN
Assistant Professor
Department of Nursing
Tarleton State University
Stephenville, Texas

Preface

Pharmacology pervades all phases of nursing practice and relates directly to patient care and education. Yet despite its importance, many students—and even some teachers—are often uncomfortable with the subject. Why? Because traditional texts have stressed *memorizing* rather than *understanding*. In this text, the guiding principle is to establish a basic understanding of drugs, after which secondary details can be learned as needed.

This text has two major objectives: (1) to help you, the nursing student, establish a knowledge base in the basic science of drugs, and (2) to show you how that knowledge can be applied in clinical practice. The methods by which these goals are achieved are described in the following sections.

LAYING FOUNDATIONS IN BASIC PRINCIPLES

To understand drugs, you need a solid foundation in basic pharmacologic principles. To help you establish that foundation, this text has major chapters on the following topics: basic principles that apply to all drugs (Chapters 4 through 8), basic principles of drug therapy across the life span (Chapters 9 through 11), basic principles of neuropharmacology (Chapter 12), basic principles of antimicrobial therapy (Chapter 83), and basic principles of cancer chemotherapy (Chapter 101).

REVIEWING PHYSIOLOGY AND PATHOPHYSIOLOGY

To understand the actions of a drug, it is useful to understand the biologic systems influenced by the drug. Accordingly, for all major drug families, relevant physiology and pathophysiology are reviewed. In almost all cases, these reviews are presented at the beginning of each chapter rather than in a systems review at the beginning of a unit. This juxtaposition of pharmacology, physiology, and pathophysiology is designed to help you understand how these topics interrelate.

TEACHING THROUGH PROTOTYPES

Within each drug family we can usually identify a prototype—a drug that embodies the characteristics shared by all members of the group. Because other family members are similar to the prototype, to know the prototype is to know the basic properties of all family members.

The benefits of teaching through prototypes can be appreciated with an example. Let's consider the nonsteroidal anti-inflammatory drugs (NSAIDs), a family that includes aspirin, ibuprofen [Motrin], naproxen [Aleve], celecoxib [Celebrex], and more than 20 other drugs. Traditionally, information on these drugs is presented in a series of paragraphs describing each drug in turn. When attempting to study from such a list, you are likely to learn many drug names and little else; the important concept of similarity among family members is easily lost. In this text, the family prototype—aspirin—is discussed first and in depth. After this, the small ways in which individual NSAIDs differ from aspirin are pointed out. Not only is this approach more efficient than the traditional approach, it is also more effective in that similarities among family members are emphasized.

LARGE PRINT AND SMALL PRINT: A WAY TO FOCUS ON ESSENTIALS

Pharmacology is exceptionally rich in detail. There are many drug families, each with multiple members and each member with its own catalog of indications, contraindications, adverse effects, and drug interactions. This abundance of detail confronts teachers with the difficult question of what to teach and confronts students with the equally difficult question of what to study. Attempting to answer these questions can frustrate teachers and students alike. Even worse, basic concepts can be obscured in the presence of myriad details.

To help you focus on essentials, two sizes of type are used in this text. Large type is intended to say, "On your first exposure to this topic, this is the core of information you should learn." Small type is intended to say, "Here is additional information that you may want to learn after mastering the material in large type." As a rule, we reserve large print for prototypes, basic principles of pharmacology, and reviews of physiology and pathophysiology. We use small print for secondary information about the prototypes and for the discussion of drugs that are not prototypes. This technique allows the book to contain a large body of detail without having that detail cloud the big picture. Furthermore, because the technique highlights essentials, it minimizes questions about what to teach and what to study.

The use of large and small print is especially valuable for discussing adverse effects and drug interactions. Most drugs are associated with many adverse effects and interactions. As a rule, however, only a few of these are noteworthy. In traditional texts, practically all adverse effects and interactions are presented, creating long and tedious lists. In this text, we use large print to highlight the few adverse effects and interactions that are especially characteristic; the rest are noted briefly in small print. Rather than overwhelming you with long and forbidding lists, this text delineates a moderate body of information that is truly important, thereby facilitating comprehension.

USING CLINICAL REALITY TO PRIORITIZE CONTENT

This book contains two broad categories of information: pharmacology (the basic science about drugs) and therapeutics (the clinical use of drugs). To ensure that content is clinically relevant, we use evidence-based treatment guidelines as a basis for deciding what to stress and what to play down. Unfortunately, clinical practice is a moving target. Guidelines change when effective new drugs are introduced and when clinical trials reveal new benefits or new risks of older drugs, and so we need to work hard to keep this book current. Despite our best efforts, the book and clinical reality may not always agree: Some treatments discussed here will be considered inappropriate before the 11th edition is published. Furthermore, in areas where controversy exists, the treatments discussed here may be considered inappropriate by some clinicians right now.

NURSING IMPLICATIONS: DEMONSTRATING THE APPLICATION OF PHARMACOLOGY IN NURSING PRACTICE

The principal reason for asking you to learn pharmacology is to enhance your ability to provide patient care and education. To show you how pharmacologic knowledge can be applied to nursing practice, nursing implications are integrated into the body of each chapter. That is, as specific drugs and drug families are discussed, the nursing implications inherent in the pharmacologic information are noted side-by-side with the basic science.

To facilitate access to nursing content, nursing implications are also summarized at the end of most chapters. These summaries serve to reinforce the information presented in the chapter body. These summaries have been omitted in chapters that are especially brief or that address drugs that are infrequently used. However, even in these chapters, nursing implications are incorporated into the main chapter text.

WHAT'S NEW IN THE BOOK?

Lehne's Pharmacology for Nursing Care has been revised cover to cover to ensure that the latest and most accurate information is presented. Three new features have been added to help promote our focus on the most useful and most critical information for nursing students:

- **Prototype Drugs:** This content, which appeared in an end-of-book appendix in previous editions, has been moved into the book's chapters as a new, easy-to-find feature.
- **Safety Alerts:** This eye-catching new feature draws the reader's attention to important safety concerns related to contraindications, adverse effects, pregnancy categories, and more.
- **Patient-Centered Care Across the Life Span:** New tables in many chapters highlight care concerns for patients throughout their lives, from infancy to older adulthood.

In addition, the popular **Special Interest Topics** of past editions have been thoroughly revised to allow for the most current research. **Canadian trade names** have been updated and continue to be identified by a **maple-leaf icon.**

LEARNING SUPPLEMENTS FOR STUDENTS

- Online Evolve Resources accompany this edition and include **Downloadable Key Points, Review Questions for the NCLEX® Examination, Unfolding Case Studies,** and more. These resources are available at http://evolve.elsevier.com/Lehne.
- **Pharmacology Online** for *Lehne's Pharmacology for Nursing Care,* tenth edition, is a dynamic online course resource that includes interactive self-study modules, a collection of interactive learning resources, and a media-rich library of supplemental resources.
- The ***Study Guide,*** which is keyed to the book, includes study questions; critical thinking, prioritization, and delegation questions; and case studies.

TEACHING SUPPLEMENTS FOR INSTRUCTORS

- The Instructor Resources for the tenth edition are available online and include **TEACH® for Nurses Lesson Plans,** a **Test Bank,** a **PowerPoint Collection,** and an **Image Collection.**

WAYS TO USE THIS TEXTBOOK

Thanks to its focus on essentials, this text is especially well suited to serve as the primary text for a course dedicated specifically to pharmacology. In addition, the focused approach makes it a valuable resource for pharmacologic instruction within an integrated curriculum and for self-directed learning by students, teachers, and practitioners.

How is this focus achieved? Four primary techniques are employed: (1) teaching through prototypes, (2) using standard print for essential information and small print for secondary information, (3) limiting discussion of adverse effects and drug interactions to information that matters most, and (4) using evidence-based clinical guidelines to determine what content to stress. To reinforce the relationship between pharmacologic knowledge and nursing practice, nursing implications are integrated into each chapter. To provide rapid access to nursing content, nursing implications are summarized at the end of most chapters using a nursing process format. In addition, key points are listed at the end of each chapter. As in previous editions, the tenth edition emphasizes conceptual material—reducing rote memorization, promoting comprehension, and increasing reader friendliness.

Pharmacology can be an unpopular subject due to the vast and rapidly changing area of content. Often, nursing students feel that pharmacology is one of the most difficult classes to master. We hope that this book makes the subject of pharmacology easier and more enjoyable for you to understand by allowing you to focus on the most important umbrella concepts of pharmacology as they relate to nursing care and the safety of patients.

ACKNOWLEDGMENTS

We would like to acknowledge the support of our colleagues at Elsevier, including Executive Content Strategist Sonya Seigafuse, Executive Content Strategist Lee Henderson, Content Development Specialist Jennifer Wade, and Senior Project Manager Jodi Willard.

Finally, we would like to express our gratitude to Richard A. Lehne for his dedication to this book for eight editions. We are honored to be able to continue his work.

Jacqueline Rosenjack Burchum
Laura D. Rosenthal

Lehne's
PHARMACOLOGY
for NURSING CARE

UNIT I INTRODUCTION

CHAPTER 1

Orientation to Pharmacology

By now you've been hitting the science books for many years and have probably asked yourself, "What's the purpose of all this education?" In the past your question may have lacked a satisfying answer. Happily, now you have one: Those courses have provided an excellent background for your studies in pharmacology!

There's good reason you haven't approached pharmacology before now. Pharmacology is a science that draws on information from multiple disciplines, among them anatomy, physiology, chemistry, microbiology, and psychology. Consequently, before you could study pharmacology, you had to become familiar with these other sciences. Now that you've established the requisite knowledge base, you're finally ready to learn about drugs.

FOUR BASIC TERMS

At this point, I'd like to define four basic terms: *drug, pharmacology, clinical pharmacology,* and *therapeutics.* As we consider these definitions, I will indicate the kinds of information that we will and will not discuss in this text.

Drug

A drug is defined as *any chemical that can affect living processes.* By this definition, virtually all chemicals can be considered drugs, since, when exposure is sufficiently high, all chemicals will have some effect on life. Clearly, it is beyond the scope of this text to address all compounds that fit the definition of a drug. Accordingly, rather than discussing all drugs, we will focus primarily on drugs that have therapeutic applications.

Pharmacology

Pharmacology can be defined as *the study of drugs and their interactions with living systems.* Under this definition, pharmacology encompasses the study of the physical and chemical properties of drugs as well as their biochemical and physiologic effects. In addition, pharmacology includes knowledge of the history, sources, and uses of drugs as well as knowledge of drug absorption, distribution, metabolism, and excretion. Because pharmacology encompasses such a broad spectrum of information, it would be impossible to address the entire scope of pharmacology in this text. Consequently, we limit consideration to information that is *clinically relevant.*

Clinical Pharmacology

Clinical pharmacology is defined as *the study of drugs in humans.* This discipline includes the study of drugs in *patients* as well as in *healthy volunteers* (during new drug development). Because clinical pharmacology encompasses all aspects of the interaction between drugs and people, and since our primary interest is the use of drugs to treat patients, clinical pharmacology includes some information that is outside the scope of this text.

Therapeutics

Therapeutics, also known as *pharmacotherapeutics,* is defined as *the use of drugs to diagnose, prevent, or treat disease or to prevent pregnancy.* Alternatively, therapeutics can be defined simply as *the medical use of drugs.*

In this text, therapeutics is our principal concern. Accordingly, much of our discussion focuses on the basic science that underlies the clinical use of drugs. This information is intended to help you understand how drugs produce their therapeutic and adverse (undesirable) effects, the reasons for giving a particular drug to a particular patient, and the rationale underlying selection of dosage, route, and schedule of administration. This information will also help you understand the strategies employed to promote beneficial drug effects and to minimize undesired effects. Armed with this knowledge, you will be well prepared to provide drug-related patient care and education. In addition, by making drugs less mysterious, this knowledge should make working with drugs more comfortable, and perhaps even more satisfying.

PROPERTIES OF AN IDEAL DRUG

If we were developing a new drug, we would want it to be the best drug possible. To approach perfection, our drug should have certain properties, such as effectiveness and safety. In the discussion that follows, we consider these two characteristics as well as others that an ideal drug might have. Please note, however, that the ideal medication exists in theory only: In reality, *there is no such thing as a perfect drug.* The truth of this statement will become apparent as we consider the properties that an ideal drug should have.

The Big Three: Effectiveness, Safety, and Selectivity

The three most important characteristics that any drug can have are effectiveness, safety, and selectivity.

Effectiveness

An effective drug is one that elicits the responses for which it is given. *Effectiveness is the most important property a drug can have.* Regardless of its other virtues, if a drug is not effective—that is, if it doesn't do what it is intended to do—there is no justification for giving it. Current U.S. law requires that all new drugs be proved effective prior to release for marketing.

Safety

A safe drug is defined as one that cannot produce harmful effects—even if administered in very high doses and for a very long time. All drugs have the ability to cause injury, especially with high doses and prolonged use. The chances of producing harmful effects can be reduced by proper drug selection and proper dosing. However, the risk of harmful effects can never be eliminated. The following examples illustrate this point:

- Certain anticancer drugs (e.g., cyclophosphamide, methotrexate), at usual therapeutic doses, always increase the risk of serious infection.
- Opioid analgesics (e.g., morphine, meperidine), at high therapeutic doses, can cause potentially fatal respiratory depression.
- Aspirin and related drugs, when taken long term in high therapeutic doses, can cause life-threatening gastric ulceration, perforation, and bleeding.

Clearly, drugs have both benefits and risks. This fact may explain why the Greeks used the word *pharmakon,* which can be translated as both *remedy* and *poison.*

Selectivity

A selective drug is defined as one that elicits *only* the response for which it is given. *There is no such thing as a wholly selective drug because all drugs cause side effects.* Common examples include the drowsiness that can be caused by many antihistamines; the peripheral edema that can be caused by calcium channel blockers; and the sexual dysfunction commonly caused by certain antidepressants.

Additional Properties of an Ideal Drug

Reversible Action

For most drugs, it is important that effects be reversible. That is, in most cases, we want drug actions to subside within an appropriate time. General anesthetics, for example, would be useless if patients never woke up. Likewise, it is unlikely that oral contraceptives would find wide acceptance if they caused permanent sterility. For a few drugs, however, reversibility is not desirable. With antibiotics, for example, we want toxicity to microbes to endure.

Predictability

It would be very helpful if, before drug administration, we could know with certainty just how a given patient will respond. Unfortunately, because each patient is unique, the accuracy of predictions cannot be guaranteed. Accordingly, to maximize the chances of eliciting desired responses, we must tailor therapy to the individual.

Ease of Administration

An ideal drug should be simple to administer: The route should be convenient, and the number of doses per day should be low. Patients with diabetes, who must inject insulin multiple times a day, are not likely to judge insulin ideal. Similarly, nurses who must set up and monitor many IV infusions are unlikely to consider intravenous drugs ideal.

In addition to convenience, ease of administration has two other benefits: (1) it can enhance patient adherence, and (2) it can decrease risk. Patients are more likely to adhere to a dosing schedule that consists of one daily dose rather than several doses a day. Furthermore, whenever skin integrity is broken, as is the case when drugs are given by injection, there is a risk of infection as well as injection-site pain and discomfort.

Freedom From Drug Interactions

When a patient is taking two or more drugs, those drugs can interact. These interactions may either augment or reduce drug responses. For example, respiratory depression caused by diazepam [Valium], which is normally minimal, can be greatly *intensified* by alcohol. Conversely, the antibacterial effects of tetracycline can be greatly *reduced* by taking the drug with iron or calcium supplements. Because of the potential for interaction among drugs, when a patient is taking more than one agent, the possible impact of drug interactions must be considered. An ideal drug would not interact with other agents. Unfortunately, few medicines are devoid of significant interactions.

Low Cost

An ideal drug would be easy to afford. The cost of drugs can be a substantial financial burden. As an example, treatment with adalimumab [Humira], a drug for rheumatoid arthritis and Crohn's disease, cost up to $65,000 or more per year in 2017. More commonly, expense becomes a significant factor when a medication must be taken chronically. For example, people with hypertension, arthritis, or diabetes may take medications every day for life. The cumulative expense of such treatment can be exorbitant—even for drugs of moderate price.

Chemical Stability

Some drugs lose effectiveness during storage. Others that may be stable on the shelf can rapidly lose effectiveness when put into solution (e.g., in preparation for infusion). These losses in efficacy result from chemical instability. Because of chemical instability, stocks of certain drugs must be periodically discarded. An ideal drug would retain its activity indefinitely.

Possession of a Simple Generic Name

Generic names of drugs are usually complex, and so they may be difficult to remember and pronounce. As a rule, the brand name for a drug is much simpler than its generic name. Examples of drugs that have complex generic names and simple brand names include acetaminophen [Tylenol], ciprofloxacin [Cipro], and simvastatin [Zocor]. Because generic names are preferable to brand names (for reasons discussed in Chapter 3), an ideal drug should have a generic name that is easy to recall and pronounce.

Because No Drug Is Ideal

From the preceding criteria for ideal drugs, we can see that available medications are not ideal. All drugs have the potential to produce side effects. Drug responses may be difficult to predict and may be altered by drug interactions. Drugs may be expensive, unstable, and hard to administer. Because medications are not ideal, all members of the healthcare team must exercise care to promote therapeutic effects and minimize drug-induced harm.

THE THERAPEUTIC OBJECTIVE

The therapeutic objective of drug therapy is to provide maximum benefit with minimal harm. If drugs were ideal, we could achieve this objective with relative ease. However, because drugs are not ideal, we must exercise skill and care if treatment is to result in more good than harm. As detailed in Chapter 2, you have a critical responsibility in achieving the therapeutic objective. To meet this responsibility, you must understand drugs. The primary purpose of this text is to help you achieve that understanding.

FACTORS THAT DETERMINE THE INTENSITY OF DRUG RESPONSES

Multiple factors determine how an individual will respond to a prescribed dose of a particular drug (Fig. 1.1). By understanding these factors, you will be able to think rationally about how drugs produce their effects. As a result, you will be able to contribute maximally to achieving the therapeutic objective.

Our ultimate concern when administering a drug is the intensity of the response. Working our way up from the bottom of Fig. 1.1, we can see that the intensity of the response is determined by the concentration of a drug at its sites of action. As the figure suggests, the primary determinant of this concentration is the administered dose. When administration is performed correctly, the dose that was given will be the same as the dose that was prescribed. The steps leading from prescribed dose to intensity of the response are considered in the sections that follow.

Administration

The drug dosage, route, and timing of administration are important determinants of drug responses. Accordingly, the prescriber will consider these variables with care. Unfortunately,

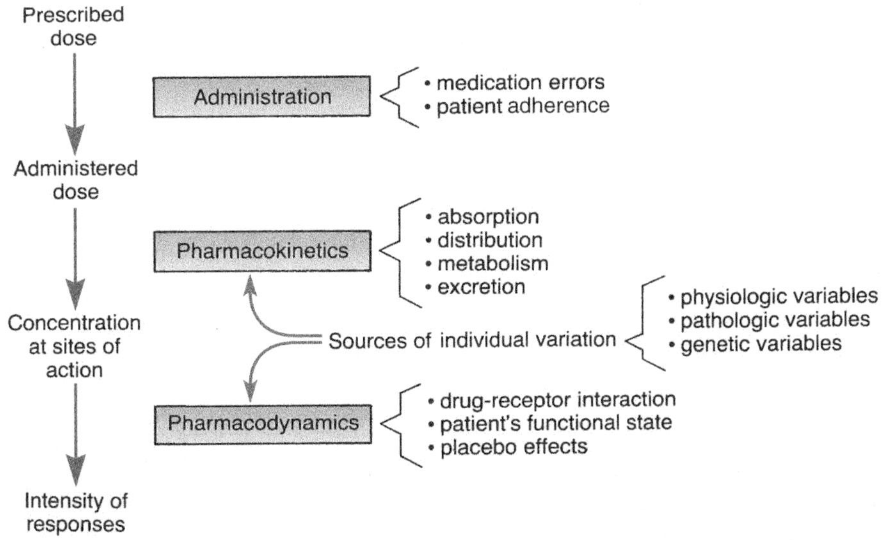

Fig. 1.1 ■ Factors that determine the intensity of drug responses.

drugs are not always taken or administered as prescribed. The result may be toxicity if the dosage is too high or treatment failure if the dosage is too low.

Sometimes patients do not take medicine as prescribed. This is called poor adherence. To help minimize errors caused by poor adherence, you should give patients complete instructions about their medication and how to take it.

Medication errors made by hospital staff may result in a drug being administered by the wrong route, in the wrong dose, or at the wrong time; the patient may even be given the wrong drug. These errors can be made by pharmacists, physicians, and nurses. Any of these errors will detract from achieving the therapeutic objective. Medication errors are discussed at length in Chapter 7.

Pharmacokinetics

Pharmacokinetic processes determine how much of an administered dose gets to its sites of action. There are four major pharmacokinetic processes: (1) drug absorption, (2) drug distribution, (3) drug metabolism, and (4) drug excretion. Collectively, these processes can be thought of as the *impact of the body on drugs.* These pharmacokinetic processes are discussed at length in Chapter 4.

Pharmacodynamics

Once a drug has reached its sites of action, pharmacodynamic processes determine the nature and intensity of the response. Pharmacodynamics can be thought of as the *impact of drugs on the body.* In most cases, the initial step leading to a response is the binding of a drug to its receptor. This drug-receptor interaction is followed by a sequence of events that ultimately results in a response. As indicated in Fig. 1.1, the patient's functional state can influence pharmacodynamic processes. For example, a patient who has developed tolerance to morphine will respond less intensely to a particular dose than will a patient who lacks tolerance. Placebo effects also help determine the responses that a drug elicits. Pharmacodynamics is discussed at length in Chapter 5.

Sources of Individual Variation

Characteristics unique to each patient can influence pharmacokinetic and pharmacodynamic processes and, by doing so, can help determine the patient's response to a drug. As indicated in Fig. 1.1, sources of individual variation include physiologic variables (e.g., age, gender, weight); pathologic variables (especially diminished function of the kidneys and liver, the major organs of drug elimination); and genetic variables. Genetic factors can alter the metabolism of drugs and can predispose the patient to unique drug reactions. Because individuals differ from one another, no two patients will respond identically to the same drug regimen. Accordingly, to achieve the therapeutic objective, we must tailor drug therapy to the individual. Individual variation in drug responses is the subject of Chapter 8.

KEY POINTS

- The most important properties of an ideal drug are effectiveness, safety, and selectivity.
- If a drug is not effective, it should not be used.
- Drugs have both benefits and risks.
- There is no such thing as a wholly selective drug: All drugs can cause side effects.
- The objective of drug therapy is to provide maximum benefit with minimum harm.
- Because all patients are unique, drug therapy must be tailored to each individual.

Please visit **http://evolve.elsevier.com/Lehne** for chapter-specific NCLEX® examination review questions.

CHAPTER

2 Application of Pharmacology in Nursing Practice

Our principal goal in this chapter is to answer the question "Why should a nursing student learn pharmacology?" By addressing this question, I want to give you some extra motivation to study. Why do I think you might need some motivation? Because pharmacology can be challenging and other topics in nursing are often more alluring. Hopefully, when you complete the chapter, you will be convinced that understanding drugs is essential for nursing practice and that putting time and effort into learning about drugs will be a good investment.

EVOLUTION OF NURSING RESPONSIBILITIES REGARDING DRUGS

In the past, a nurse's responsibility regarding medications focused on the *Five Rights of Drug Administration* (the Rights)—namely, give the *right drug* to the *right patient* in the *right dose* by the *right route* at the *right time.* More recently, various other rights—*right assessment, right documentation, right evaluation, the patient's rights to education,* and *the patient's right of refusal*—have been recommended for inclusion. Clearly, the original five Rights and their subsequent additions are important. However, although these basics are vital, much more is required to achieve the therapeutic objective. The Rights guarantee only that a drug will be administered as prescribed. Correct administration, without additional interventions, cannot ensure that treatment will result in maximum benefit and minimum harm.

The limitations of the Rights can be illustrated with this analogy: The nurse who sees his or her responsibility as being complete after correct drug administration would be like a major league baseball pitcher who felt that his responsibility was over once he had thrown the ball toward the batter. As the pitcher must be ready to respond to the consequences of the interaction between ball and bat, you must be ready to respond to the consequences of the interaction between drug and patient. Put another way, although both the nurse and the pitcher have a clear obligation to deliver their objects in the most appropriate fashion, proper delivery is only the beginning of their responsibilities: *Important events will take place after the object is delivered, and these must be responded to.* Like the pitcher, the nurse can respond rapidly and effectively only by anticipating what the possible reactions to the drug might be.

To anticipate possible reactions, both the nurse and the pitcher require certain kinds of knowledge. Just as the pitcher must understand the abilities of the opposing batter, you must understand the patient and the disorder for which the patient is being treated. As the pitcher must know the most appropriate pitch (e.g., fastball, slider) to deliver in specific circumstances, you must know what medications are appropriate for the patient and must check to ensure that the ordered medication is an appropriate medication. Conversely, as the pitcher must know what pitches *not* to throw at a particular batter, you must know what drugs are *contraindicated* for the patient. As the pitcher must know the most likely outcome after the ball and bat interact, you must know the probable consequences of the interaction between drug and patient.

Although this analogy is not perfect (the nurse and patient are on the same team, whereas the pitcher and batter are not), it does help us appreciate that the nurse's responsibility extends well beyond the Rights. Consequently, in addition to the limited information needed to administer drugs in accordance with the Rights, you must acquire a broad base of pharmacologic knowledge so as to contribute fully to achieving the therapeutic objective.

Nurses, together with healthcare providers and pharmacists, participate in a system of checks and balances designed to promote beneficial effects and minimize harm. Nurses are especially important in this system because it is the nurse who follows the patient's status most closely. As a result, you are likely to be the first member of the healthcare team to observe and evaluate drug responses, and to intervene if required. To observe and evaluate drug responses, and to intervene rapidly and appropriately, you must know *in advance* the responses that a medication is likely to elicit. The better your knowledge of pharmacology, the better you will be able to *anticipate* drug responses and not simply react to them after the fact.

Within our system of checks and balances, the nurse has an important role as patient advocate. It is your responsibility to detect mistakes made by pharmacists and prescribers. For example, the prescriber may overlook potential drug interactions, or may be unaware of alterations in the patient's status that would prohibit use of a particular drug, or may select the correct drug but may order an inappropriate dosage or route of administration. Because the nurse actually administers drugs, the nurse is the last person to check medications before they are given. Consequently, *you are the patient's last line of defense against medication errors.* It is ethically and legally unacceptable for you to administer a drug that is harmful to the patient—even though the medication has been prescribed by a licensed prescriber and dispensed by a licensed pharmacist. In serving as patient advocate, it is impossible to know too much about drugs.

The two major areas in which you can apply pharmacologic knowledge are patient care and patient education. The application of pharmacology in patient care and patient education is considered in the following two sections.

APPLICATION OF PHARMACOLOGY IN PATIENT CARE

In discussing the applications of pharmacology in patient care, we focus on eight aspects of drug therapy: (1) preadministration assessment, (2) dosage and administration, (3) promoting therapeutic effects, (4) minimizing adverse effects, (5) minimizing adverse interactions, (6) making "as needed" (PRN) decisions, (7) evaluating responses to medication, and (8) managing toxicity.

Preadministration Assessment

All drug therapy begins with assessment of the patient. Assessment has three basic goals: (1) collecting baseline data needed to evaluate therapeutic and adverse (i.e., undesired) responses, (2) identifying high-risk patients, and (3) assessing the patient's capacity for self-care. The first two goals are highly specific for each drug. Accordingly, we cannot achieve these goals without understanding pharmacology. The third goal applies generally to all drugs, and hence it does not usually require specific knowledge of the drug you are about to give. Preadministration assessment is discussed here and again under *Application of the Nursing Process in Drug Therapy.*

Collecting Baseline Data

Baseline data are needed to evaluate both therapeutic and adverse drug responses. Without these data, we would have no way of determining the effectiveness of our drug. For example, if we plan to give a drug to lower blood pressure, we must know the patient's blood pressure before treatment. Similarly, if we are planning to give a drug that can damage the liver, we need to assess baseline liver function to evaluate this potential toxicity. Obviously, to collect appropriate baseline data, we must first know the effects that a drug is likely to produce.

Identifying High-Risk Patients

Multiple factors can predispose an individual to adverse reactions from specific drugs. Important predisposing factors are pathophysiology (especially liver and kidney impairment), genetic factors, drug allergies, and life span considerations such as pregnancy or very young or advanced age.

Patients with penicillin allergy provide a dramatic example of those at risk because giving penicillin to such a patient can be fatal. Accordingly, whenever treatment with penicillin is under consideration, we must determine whether the patient has had an allergic reaction to a penicillin in the past, and details about the type of reaction. If there is a history of true penicillin allergy, an alternative antibiotic should be prescribed.

From the preceding example, we can see that, when planning drug therapy, we must identify patients who are at high risk of reacting adversely. To identify such patients, we use three principal tools: the patient history, physical examination, and laboratory data. Of course, if identification is to be successful, you must know what to look for (i.e., you must know the factors that can increase the risk of severe reactions to the drug in question). Once the high-risk patient has been identified, we can take steps to reduce the risk.

Dosage and Administration

Earlier we noted the Rights of Drug Administration and agreed on their importance. Although you can implement the Rights without a detailed knowledge of pharmacology, having this knowledge can help reduce your contribution to medication errors. The following examples illustrate this point:

- Certain drugs have more than one indication, and dosage may differ depending on which indication the drug is used for. Aspirin, for example, is given in low doses to relieve pain and in high doses to suppress inflammation. If you don't know about these differences, you might administer too much aspirin to the patient with pain or too little to the patient with inflammation.
- Many drugs can be administered by more than one route, and dosage may differ depending upon the route selected. Morphine, for example, may be administered by mouth or by injection. Oral doses are generally much larger than injected doses. Accordingly, if a large dose intended for oral use were to be mistakenly administered by injection, the resulting overdose could prove fatal. The nurse who understands the pharmacology of morphine is unlikely to make this error.
- Certain intravenous agents can cause severe local injury if the drug extravasates (seeps into the tissues surrounding the IV line). The infusion must be monitored closely, and if extravasation occurs, corrective steps must be taken immediately. The nurse who doesn't understand the dangers of these drugs will be unprepared to work with them safely.

The following guidelines can help ensure correct administration:

- Read the medication order carefully. If the order is unclear, verify it with the prescriber.
- Verify the identity of the patient by comparing the name on the wristband with the name on the drug order or medication administration record.
- Read the medication label carefully. Verify the identity of the drug, the amount of drug (per tablet, volume of liquid, etc.), and its suitability for administration by the intended route.
- Verify dosage calculations.
- Implement any special handling the drug may require.
- Don't administer any drug if you don't understand the reason for its use.

Measures to minimize medication errors are discussed further in Chapter 7.

Promoting Therapeutic Effects

Drug therapy can often be enhanced by nonpharmacologic measures. Examples include (1) enhancing drug therapy of asthma through breathing exercises, biofeedback, and emotional support; (2) enhancing drug therapy of arthritis through exercise, physical therapy, and rest; and (3) enhancing drug therapy of hypertension through weight reduction, smoking cessation, and sodium restriction.

Short-term interventions are also helpful. For instance, mild to moderate pain may be experienced more intensely by the patient who lies slumped down in an uncomfortable bed compared with the patient who is carefully positioned for maximum comfort. Similarly, the pediatric patient with mild to moderate pain who is in a nonstimulating environment may experience the pain more acutely than the patient for whom toys, games, or videos provide distraction.

As a nurse, you will have many opportunities to seek out creative solutions to promote therapeutic effects. You may provide these supportive measures directly or by coordinating the activities of other healthcare providers. Be sure to include these interventions in your patient education to empower patients and their families in optimal self-care.

Minimizing Adverse Effects

All drugs have the potential to produce undesired effects. Common examples include gastric erosion caused by aspirin, sedation caused by older antihistamines, hypoglycemia caused by insulin, and excessive fluid loss caused by diuretics. When drugs are employed properly, the incidence and severity of such events can be reduced. Measures to reduce adverse events include identifying high-risk patients, ensuring proper administration, and teaching patients to avoid activities that might precipitate an adverse event.

When untoward effects cannot be avoided, discomfort and injury can often be minimized by appropriate intervention. For example, timely administration of glucose will prevent brain damage from insulin-induced hypoglycemia. To help reduce adverse effects, you must know the following about the drugs you administer:

- The major adverse effects the drug can produce
- When these reactions are likely to occur
- Early signs that an adverse reaction is developing
- Interventions that can minimize discomfort and harm

Minimizing Adverse Interactions

When a patient is taking two or more drugs, those drugs may interact with one another to diminish therapeutic effects or intensify adverse effects. For example, the ability of oral contraceptives to protect against pregnancy can be reduced by concurrent therapy with carbamazepine (an antiseizure drug), and the risk of thromboembolism from oral contraceptives can be increased by smoking cigarettes.

As a nurse, you can help reduce the incidence and intensity of adverse interactions in several ways. These include taking a thorough drug history, advising the patient to avoid over-the-counter drugs that can interact with the prescribed medication, monitoring for adverse interactions *known* to occur between the drugs the patient is taking, and being alert to the possibility of *as-yet-unknown* interactions.

Making PRN Decisions

PRN stands for *pro re nata,* a Latin phrase meaning *as needed.* A PRN medication order is one in which the nurse has discretion regarding when to give a drug and, in some situations, how much drug to give. PRN orders are common for drugs that promote sleep, relieve pain, and reduce anxiety. To implement a PRN order rationally, you must know the reason the drug is prescribed and be able to assess the patient's medication needs. Clearly, the better your knowledge of pharmacology, the better your PRN decisions are likely to be.

Evaluating Responses to Medication

Evaluation is one of the most important aspects of drug therapy. After all, this is the process that tells us whether a drug is producing a benefit or is causing harm. Because the nurse follows the patient's status most closely, the nurse is in the best position to evaluate therapeutic responses.

To make an evaluation, you must know the rationale for treatment and the nature and time course of the intended response. When desired responses do *not* occur, it may be essential to identify the reason quickly so that timely implementation of alternative therapy may be ordered.

When evaluating responses to a drug that has more than one application, you can do so only if you know the specific indication for which the drug is being used. Nifedipine, for example, is given for both hypertension and angina pectoris. When the drug is used for hypertension, you should monitor for a reduction in blood pressure. In contrast, when this drug is used for angina, you should monitor for a reduction in chest pain. Clearly, if you are to make the proper evaluation, you must understand the reason for drug use.

Managing Toxicity

Some adverse drug reactions are extremely dangerous. If toxicity is not diagnosed early and responded to quickly, irreversible injury or death can result. To minimize harm, you must know the early signs of toxicity and the procedure for toxicity management.

APPLICATION OF PHARMACOLOGY IN PATIENT EDUCATION

Very often, the nurse is responsible for educating patients about medications. In your role as educator, you must give the patient the following information:

- Drug name and therapeutic category (e.g., penicillin: antibiotic)
- Dosage
- Dosing schedule
- Route and technique of administration
- Expected therapeutic response and when it should develop
- Nondrug measures to enhance therapeutic responses
- Duration of treatment
- Method of drug storage
- Symptoms of major adverse effects, and measures to minimize discomfort and harm
- Major adverse drug-drug and drug-food interactions
- Whom to contact in the event of therapeutic failure, severe adverse reactions, or severe adverse interactions

To communicate this information effectively and accurately, you must first understand it. That is, to be a good drug educator, you must know pharmacology.

In the following discussion, we consider the relationship between patient education and the following aspects of drug therapy: dosage and administration, promoting therapeutic effects, minimizing adverse effects, and minimizing adverse interactions.

Dosage and Administration

Drug Name

The patient should know the name of the medication he or she is taking. If the drug has been prescribed by brand name, the patient should be given its generic name, too. This information will reduce the risk of overdose that can result when a patient fails to realize that two prescriptions that bear different names actually contain the same medicine.

Dosage and Schedule of Administration

Patients must be told how much drug to take and when to take it. For some medications, dosage must be adjusted by the patient. Insulin is a good example. For insulin therapy to be most beneficial, the patient may need to adjust doses to accommodate changes in diet and subsequent glucose levels.

With PRN medications, the schedule of administration is not fixed. Rather, these drugs are taken as conditions require. For example, some people with asthma experience exercise-induced bronchospasm. To minimize such attacks, they can take supplementary medication before anticipated exertion. It is your responsibility to teach patients when PRN drugs should be taken.

The patient should know what to do if a dose is missed. With certain oral contraceptives, for example, if one dose is missed, the omitted dose should be taken together with the next scheduled dose. However, if three or more doses are missed, a new cycle of administration must be initiated.

Patient Adherence

Adherence—also known as compliance or concordance—may be defined as the extent to which a patient's behavior coincides with medical advice. If we are to achieve the therapeutic objective, adherence to the prescribed drug regimen is essential. Drugs that are self-administered in the wrong dose, by the wrong route, or at the wrong time cannot produce maximum benefit—and may even prove harmful. Obviously, successful therapy requires active and informed participation by the patient. By educating patients about the drugs they are taking, you can help elicit the required participation.

Some patients have difficulty remembering whether they have taken their medication. Possible causes include mental illness, advanced age, and complex regimens. To facilitate adherence for these patients, one solution is to provide the patient with a pill organizer that has separate compartments for each day of the week and then to teach the patient or family member to load the compartments weekly. To determine whether a dose of medication has been taken, patients and their families can simply check the day of the week in the pill organizer to see whether the drugs have been removed.

Technique of Administration

Patients must be taught how to administer their drugs. This is especially important for routes that may be unfamiliar (e.g., sublingual for nitroglycerin) and for techniques that can be difficult (e.g., subcutaneous injection of insulin). Patients taking oral medications may require special instructions. For example, some oral preparations must not be chewed or crushed; some should be taken with fluids; and some should be taken with meals, whereas others should be taken on an empty stomach. Careful attention must be paid to the patient who, because of disability (e.g., visual or intellectual impairment, limited manual dexterity), may find self-medication difficult.

Duration of Drug Use

Just as patients must know when to take their medicine, they must know when to stop. In some cases (e.g., treatment of acute pain), patients should discontinue drug use as soon as symptoms subside. In other cases (e.g., treatment of hypertension), patients should know that therapy will probably continue lifelong. For some conditions (e.g., gastric ulcers), medication may be prescribed for a specific time interval, after which the patient should return for reevaluation.

Drug Storage

Certain medications are chemically unstable and deteriorate rapidly if stored improperly. Patients who are using unstable drugs must be taught how to store them correctly (e.g., under refrigeration, in a lightproof container). All drugs should be stored where children can't reach them.

Promoting Therapeutic Effects

To participate fully in achieving the therapeutic objective, patients must know the nature and time course of expected beneficial effects. With this knowledge, patients can help evaluate the success or failure of treatment. By recognizing treatment failure, the informed patient will know to return to the healthcare provider for changes in therapy.

With some drugs, such as those used to treat depression and schizophrenia, beneficial effects may take several weeks to become maximal. Awareness that treatment may not produce immediate results allows the patient to have realistic expectations and helps reduce anxiety about therapeutic failure.

As noted, nondrug measures can complement drug therapy. For example, although drugs are useful in managing high cholesterol, exercise and diet are also important. Teaching the patient about nondrug measures can greatly increase the chances of success.

Minimizing Adverse Effects

Knowledge of adverse drug effects will enable the patient to avoid some adverse effects and minimize others through early detection. The following examples underscore the value of educating patients about the undesired effects of drugs:

- Insulin overdose can cause blood glucose levels to drop precipitously. Early signs of hypoglycemia include shakiness, perspiration, and anxiety. The patient who has been taught to recognize these early signs can respond by ingesting glucose or other fast-acting carbohydrate-rich foods, thereby restoring blood sugar to a safe level. In contrast, the patient who fails to recognize evolving hypoglycemia and does not ingest glucose or similar substances may become comatose, and may even die.
- Many anticancer drugs predispose patients to acquiring serious infections. The patient who is aware of this possibility can take steps to avoid contagion by avoiding contact with people who have an infection and by avoiding foods likely to contain pathogens. In addition, the informed patient is in a position to notify the prescriber at the first sign that an infection is developing, thereby allowing early treatment. In contrast, the patient who has not received adequate education is at increased risk of illness or death from an untreated infectious disease.
- Some side effects, although benign, can be disturbing if they occur without warning. For example, rifampin (a drug for tuberculosis) imparts a harmless red-orange color to urine, sweat, saliva, and tears. Your patient will appreciate knowing about this in advance.

Minimizing Adverse Interactions

Patient education can help avoid hazardous drug-drug and drug-food interactions. For example, phenelzine (an antidepressant) can cause dangerous elevations in blood pressure if taken in combination with certain drugs (e.g., amphetamines) or certain foods (e.g., sauerkraut, aged or smoked meats, most cheeses). Accordingly, it is essential that patients taking phenelzine be given specific and emphatic instructions regarding the drugs and foods they must avoid.

APPLICATION OF THE NURSING PROCESS IN DRUG THERAPY

The nursing process is a conceptual framework that nurses employ to guide healthcare delivery. In this section we consider how the nursing process can be applied in drug therapy.

Review of the Nursing Process

Before discussing the nursing process as it applies to drug therapy, we need to review the process itself. Because you are probably familiar with the process already, this review is brief.

In its simplest form, the nursing process can be viewed as a cyclic procedure that has five basic steps: (1) assessment, (2) analysis (including nursing diagnoses), (3) planning, (4) implementation, and (5) evaluation.

Assessment

Assessment consists of collecting data about the patient. These data are used to identify actual and potential health problems. The database established during assessment provides a foundation for subsequent steps in the process. Important methods of data collection are the patient interview, medical and drug-use histories, the physical examination, observation of the patient, and laboratory tests.

Analysis or Nursing Diagnoses

In this step, the nurse analyzes information in the database to determine actual and potential health problems. These problems may be physiologic, psychologic, or sociologic. Problems may be stated in the form of a *nursing diagnosis,*[a] which can be defined as an actual or potential health problem that nurses are qualified and licensed to treat.

A complete nursing diagnosis consists of three statements: (1) a statement of the patient's actual or potential health problem, followed by (2) a statement of the problem's probable cause or risk factors, and (3) the signs, symptoms, or other evidence of the problem. (This third component is omitted for potential problems.) Typically, the statements are separated by the phrases related to and as evidenced by, as in this example of a drug-associated nursing diagnosis: "noncompliance with the prescribed regimen [the problem] related to complex medication administration schedule [the cause] as evidenced by missed drug doses and patient's statement that the schedule is confusing [the evidence]."

Planning

In the planning step, the nurse delineates specific interventions directed at solving or preventing the problems identified in analysis. The plan must be individualized for each patient. When creating a care plan, the nurse must define goals, set priorities, identify nursing interventions, and establish criteria for evaluating success. In addition to nursing interventions, the plan should include interventions performed by other healthcare providers. Planning is an ongoing process that must be modified as new data are gathered and the patient's situation changes.

Implementation

Implementation begins with carrying out the interventions identified during planning. Some interventions are collaborative while others are independent. Collaborative interventions require a healthcare provider's order, whereas independent interventions do not. In addition to carrying out interventions, implementation involves coordinating actions of other members of the healthcare team. Implementation is completed by observing and documenting the outcomes of treatment.

Evaluation

Evaluation is performed to determine the degree to which treatment has succeeded. By evaluating the outcomes of

[a]Nursing diagnosis is not taught in some schools and colleges of nursing. Information is provided here for those programs that include this information.

treatment, nurses identify those interventions that should be continued, those that should be discontinued, and potential new interventions that may be implemented. Evaluation is accomplished by analyzing the data collected following implementation. This step completes the initial cycle of the nursing process and provides the basis for beginning the cycle anew.

Applying the Nursing Process in Drug Therapy

Having reviewed the nursing process itself, we can now discuss the process as it pertains to drug therapy. Recall that the overall objective in drug therapy is to produce maximum benefit with minimum harm.

Preadministration Assessment

Preadministration assessment establishes the baseline data needed to tailor drug therapy to the individual. By identifying the variables that can affect an individual's responses to drugs, we can adapt treatment so as to maximize benefits and minimize harm. Preadministration assessment has four basic goals:

- Collection of baseline data needed to evaluate therapeutic effects
- Collection of baseline data needed to evaluate adverse effects
- Identification of high-risk patients
- Assessment of the patient's capacity for self-care

The first three goals are specific to the particular drug being used. Accordingly, to achieve these goals, you must know the pharmacology of the drug under consideration. The fourth goal applies more or less equally to all drugs—although this goal may be more critical for some drugs than others.

Important methods of data collection include interviewing the patient and family, observing the patient, performing a physical examination, checking results of laboratory tests, and taking the patient's medical and drug histories. The drug history should include prescription drugs, over-the-counter drugs, herbal remedies, and drugs taken for nonmedical or recreational purposes (e.g., alcohol, nicotine, caffeine, and illegal drugs). Prior adverse drug reactions should be noted, including drug allergies and idiosyncratic reactions (i.e., reactions unique to the individual).

Baseline Data Needed to Evaluate Therapeutic Effects. Drugs are administered to achieve a desired response. To know whether we have produced that response, we need to establish baseline measurements of the parameter that therapy is directed at changing. For example, if we are giving a drug to lower blood pressure, we need to know what the patient's blood pressure was before treatment. Without this information, we have no basis for determining the effect of our drug.

Baseline Data Needed to Evaluate Adverse Effects. All drugs have the ability to produce undesired effects. In most cases, the adverse effects that a particular drug can produce are known. In many cases, development of an adverse effect will be completely obvious in the absence of any baseline data. For example, we don't need special baseline data to know that hair loss following cancer chemotherapy was caused by the drug. However, in other cases, baseline data are needed to determine whether an adverse effect has occurred. For example, some drugs can impair liver function. To know whether a drug has compromised liver function, we need to know the state of liver function before drug use. Without this information, we can't tell from later measurements whether liver dysfunction was preexisting or caused by the drug.

Identification of High-Risk Patients. Because of individual characteristics, a particular patient may be at high risk of experiencing an adverse response to a particular drug. Just which individual characteristics will predispose a patient to an adverse reaction depends on the drug under consideration. For example, if a drug is eliminated from the body primarily by renal excretion, an individual with impaired kidney function will be at risk of having this drug accumulate to a toxic level. Similarly, if a drug is eliminated by the liver, an individual with impaired liver function will be at risk of having that drug accumulate to a toxic level.

Multiple factors can increase the patient's risk of adverse reactions to a particular drug. Impaired liver and kidney function were just mentioned. Other factors include age, body composition, pregnancy, diet, genetic heritage, other drugs being used, and practically any pathophysiologic condition. These factors are discussed at length in Chapters 6 through 11.

When identifying factors that put the patient at risk, you should distinguish between factors that put the patient at extremely high risk versus factors that put the patient at moderate or low risk. The terms *contraindication* and *precaution* are used for this distinction. A *contraindication* is defined as a condition that prohibits use of a particular drug under all but the most critical of circumstances. For example, a previous severe allergic reaction to penicillin would be a contraindication to using penicillin again—unless the patient has a life-threatening infection that cannot be effectively treated with another antibiotic. In this situation, in which the patient *will* die if the drug *isn't* administered yet the patient *may* die if the drug *is* administered, the provider may decide to give the penicillin along with other drugs and measures to decrease the severity of the allergic reaction. A *precaution,* by contrast, can be defined as a condition that significantly increases the risk of an adverse reaction to a particular drug, but not to a degree that is life threatening. For example, sedating antihistamines pose a risk to elderly patients who are at risk of falling, which would constitute a precaution against using this drug in older adults. That is, the drug may be used, but greater than normal caution must be exercised. Preferably, an alternative nonsedating antihistamine would be selected.

Assessment of the Patient's Capacity for Self-Care. If drug therapy is to succeed, the outpatient must be willing and able to self-administer medication as prescribed. Accordingly, his or her capacity for self-care must be determined. If assessment reveals that the patient is incapable of self-medication, alternative care must be arranged.

Multiple factors can affect the capacity for self-care and the probability of adhering to the prescribed regimen. Patients with reduced visual acuity or limited manual dexterity may be unable to self-medicate, especially if the technique for administration is complex. Patients with limited intellectual ability may be incapable of understanding or remembering what they are supposed to do. Patients with severe mental illness (e.g., depression, schizophrenia) may lack the understanding or motivation needed to self-medicate. Some patients may lack the money to pay for drugs. Others may fail to take medications as prescribed because of individual or cultural attitudes toward drugs. For example, a common cause for failed self-medication is a belief that the drug was simply not needed in the dosage prescribed. A thorough assessment will identify all of these factors, thereby enabling you to account for them when formulating nursing diagnoses and the patient care plan.

Analysis and Nursing Diagnoses

With respect to drug therapy, the analysis phase of the nursing process has three objectives. First, you must judge the appropriateness of the prescribed regimen. Second, you must identify potential health problems that the drug might cause. Third, you must determine if your assessment of the patient's capacity for self-care identified an impaired ability for self-care.

As the last link in the patient's chain of defense against inappropriate drug therapy, you must analyze the data collected during assessment to determine whether the proposed treatment has a reasonable likelihood of being effective and safe. This judgment is made by considering the medical diagnosis, the known actions of the prescribed drug, the patient's prior responses to the drug, and the presence of contraindications to the drug. You should question the drug's appropriateness if (1) the drug has no actions that are known to benefit individuals with the patient's medical diagnosis, (2) the patient failed to respond to the drug in the past, (3) the patient had a serious adverse reaction to the drug in the past, or (4) the patient has a condition or is using a drug that contraindicates the prescribed drug. If any of these conditions apply, you should consult with the prescriber to determine whether the drug should be given.

Analysis must identify potential adverse effects and drug interactions. This is accomplished by integrating knowledge of the drug under consideration and the data collected during assessment. Knowledge of the drug itself will indicate adverse effects that practically all patients are likely to experience. Data on the individual patient will indicate additional adverse effects and interactions to which the particular patient is predisposed. Once potential adverse effects and interactions have been identified, pertinent nursing diagnoses can be formulated. For example, if treatment is likely to cause respiratory depression, an appropriate nursing diagnosis would be "risk for impaired gas exchange related to drug therapy." Table 2.1 presents additional examples of nursing diagnoses that can be readily derived from your knowledge of adverse effects and interactions that treatment may cause.

Analysis must characterize the patient's capacity for self-care. The analysis should indicate potential impediments to self-care (e.g., visual impairment, reduced manual dexterity, impaired cognitive function, insufficient understanding of the prescribed regimen) so that these factors can be addressed in the care plan. To varying degrees, nearly all patients will be unfamiliar with self-medication and the drug regimen. Accordingly, a nursing diagnosis applicable to almost every patient is "knowledge deficit related to the drug regimen."

Planning

Planning consists of defining goals, establishing priorities, identifying specific interventions, and establishing criteria for evaluating success. Good planning will allow you to promote beneficial drug effects. Of equal or greater importance, good planning will allow you to anticipate adverse effects—rather than react to them after the fact.

Defining Goals. In all cases, the goal of drug therapy is to produce maximum benefit with minimum harm. That is, we want to employ drugs in such a way as to maximize therapeutic responses while preventing or minimizing adverse reactions and interactions. The objective of planning is to formulate ways to achieve this goal.

Setting Priorities. Priority setting requires knowledge of the drug under consideration and the patient's unique characteristics—and even then, setting priorities can be difficult. Highest priority is given to life-threatening conditions (e.g., anaphylactic shock, ventricular fibrillation). These may be drug induced or the result of disease. High priority is also given to reactions that cause severe, acute discomfort and to reactions that can result in long-term harm. Because we cannot manage all problems simultaneously, less severe problems are relegated to lower positions when prioritizing care.

Identifying Interventions. The heart of planning is identification of nursing interventions. For medication purposes, these interventions can be divided into four major groups: (1)

TABLE 2.1 ▪ Examples of Nursing Diagnoses That Can Be Derived From Knowledge of Adverse Drug Effects

Drug	Adverse Effect	Related Nursing Diagnosis
Amphetamine	CNS stimulation	Disturbed sleep pattern related to drug-induced CNS excitation
Aspirin	Gastric erosion	Pain related to aspirin-induced gastric erosion
Atropine	Urinary retention	Urinary retention related to drug therapy
Bethanechol	Stimulation of GI smooth muscle	Bowel incontinence related to drug-induced increase in bowel motility
Cyclophosphamide	Reduction in white blood cell counts	Risk for infection related to drug-induced neutropenia
Digoxin	Dysrhythmias	Ineffective tissue perfusion related to drug-induced cardiac dysrhythmias
Furosemide	Excessive urine production	Deficient fluid volume related to drug-induced diuresis
Gentamicin	Damage to the eighth cranial nerve	Disturbed sensory perception: hearing impairment related to drug therapy
Glucocorticoids	Thinning of the skin	Impaired skin integrity related to drug therapy
Haloperidol	Involuntary movements	Low self-esteem related to drug-induced involuntary movements
Propranolol	Bradycardia	Decreased cardiac output related to drug-induced bradycardia
Warfarin	Bleeding	Risk for injury related to drug-induced bleeding

CNS, Central nervous system; *GI,* gastrointestinal.

drug administration, (2) interventions to enhance therapeutic effects, (3) interventions to minimize adverse effects and interactions, and (4) patient education (which encompasses information in the first three groups).

When planning drug administration, you must consider dosage and route of administration as well as less obvious factors, including timing of administration with respect to meals and with respect to administration of other drugs. Timing with respect to side effects is also important. For example, if a drug causes sedation, it may be desirable to give the drug at bedtime, rather than in the morning; conversely, a diuretic, which increases urination, is better given earlier in the morning rather than at bedtime.

Nondrug measures can help promote therapeutic effects and should be included in the plan. For example, drug therapy for hypertension can be combined with weight loss (in overweight patients), salt restriction, and smoking cessation.

Interventions to prevent or minimize adverse effects are of obvious importance. When planning these interventions, you should distinguish between reactions that develop quickly and reactions that are delayed. A few drugs can cause severe adverse reactions (e.g., anaphylactic shock) shortly after administration. When planning to administer such a drug, you should ensure that facilities for managing possible reactions are immediately available. Delayed reactions can often be minimized, if not avoided entirely. The plan should include interventions to do so.

Well-planned patient education is central to success. Patient education is discussed at length earlier in this chapter.

Establishing Criteria for Evaluation. The need for objective criteria by which to measure desired drug responses is obvious: Without such criteria we could not determine how well our drug achieved the therapeutic objective. As a result, we would have no rational basis for making dosage adjustments or for deciding whether a drug should be continued.

Criteria for evaluation vary depending on the drug and its purpose. For an analgesic, the criterion for evaluation is a decrease or resolution of pain. For the patient prescribed thyroid hormones for hypothyroidism, a criterion for evaluation is typically a laboratory test (e.g., thyroid stimulating hormone level and free thyroxine level within normal range). Conversely, for the patient prescribed an antihypertensive, a criterion for evaluation may be a target blood pressure goal. Often, there are several criteria for evaluation for a given drug.

If the drug is to be used on an outpatient basis, follow-up visits for evaluation should be planned. It is important to educate the patient on the importance of these visits even if the patient is feeling well.

Implementation

Implementation of the care plan in drug therapy has four major components: (1) drug administration, (2) patient education, (3) interventions to promote therapeutic effects, and (4) interventions to minimize adverse effects. These critical nursing activities are discussed at length in the previous section.

Evaluation

Over the course of drug therapy, the patient must be evaluated for (1) therapeutic responses, (2) adverse drug reactions and interactions, (3) adherence to the prescribed regimen, and (4) satisfaction with treatment. How frequently evaluations are performed depends on the expected time course of therapeutic and adverse effects. Like assessment, evaluation is based on laboratory tests, observation of the patient, physical examination, and patient interviews. The conclusions drawn during evaluation provide the basis for modifying nursing interventions and the drug regimen.

Therapeutic responses are evaluated by comparing the patient's current status with the baseline data. To evaluate treatment, you must know the reason for drug use, the criteria for evaluation, and the expected time course of responses (some drugs act within minutes, whereas others may take weeks to produce beneficial effects).

The need to anticipate and evaluate adverse effects is self-evident. To make these evaluations, you must know which adverse effects are likely to occur, how they manifest, and their probable time course. The method of monitoring is determined by the expected effect. For example, if hypotension is expected, blood pressure is monitored; if constipation is expected, bowel function is monitored. Because some adverse effects can be fatal in the absence of timely detection, it is impossible to overemphasize the importance of monitoring and being prepared for rapid intervention.

Evaluation of adherence is desirable in all patients—and is especially valuable when therapeutic failure occurs or when adverse effects are unexpectedly severe. Methods of evaluating adherence include measurement of plasma drug levels, interviewing the patient, and counting pills. The evaluation should determine whether the patient understands when to take medication, what dose to take, and the technique of administration as well as whether the patient is taking the drug(s) exactly as prescribed.

Patient satisfaction with drug therapy increases quality of life and promotes adherence. If the patient is dissatisfied, an otherwise effective regimen may not be taken as prescribed. Factors that can cause dissatisfaction include unacceptable side effects, inconvenient dosing schedule, difficulty of administration, and high cost. When evaluation reveals dissatisfaction, an attempt should be made to alter the regimen to make it more acceptable.

Use of a Modified Nursing Process Format to Summarize Nursing Implications

Throughout this text, nursing implications are *integrated into the body of each chapter.* The reason for integrating nursing information with basic science information is to reinforce the relationship between pharmacologic knowledge and nursing practice. In addition to being integrated, nursing implications are *summarized at the end of most chapters* under the heading "Summary of Major Nursing Implications." The purpose of these summaries is to provide a concise and readily accessible reference on patient care and patient education related to specific drugs and drug families.

The format employed for summarizing nursing implications reflects the nursing process (Table 2.2). Some headings have been modified to accommodate the needs of pharmacology instruction and to keep the summaries concise. The components of the format are as follows.

Preadministration Assessment

This section summarizes the information you should have before giving a drug. Each section begins by stating the reason for drug use. This is followed by a summary of the baseline data needed to evaluate therapeutic and adverse effects. After this, contraindications and precautions are summarized under the heading *Identifying High-Risk Patients.*

Implementation: Administration

This section summarizes routes of administration, guidelines for dosage adjustment, and special considerations in administration, such as timing with respect to meals, preparation of intravenous solutions, and unusual techniques of administration.

Implementation: Measures to Enhance Therapeutic Effects

This section addresses issues such as diet modification, measures to increase comfort, and ways to promote adherence to the prescribed regimen.

Ongoing Evaluation and Interventions

This section summarizes nursing implications that relate to both therapeutic and undesired drug responses. As indicated in Table 2.2, the section has five subsections: (1) summary of monitoring, (2) evaluating therapeutic effects, (3) minimizing adverse effects, (4) minimizing adverse interactions, and (5) managing toxicity. The monitoring section summarizes the physiologic and psychologic parameters that must be monitored to evaluate therapeutic and adverse responses. The section on therapeutic effects summarizes criteria and procedures for evaluating therapeutic responses. The section on adverse effects summarizes the major adverse reactions that should be monitored for and presents interventions to minimize harm. The section on adverse interactions summarizes the major drug interactions to be alert for and gives interventions to minimize them. The section on toxicity describes major symptoms of toxicity and treatment.

Patient Education

This topic does not have a section of its own. Rather, patient education is integrated into the other sections. That is, as we summarize the nursing implications that relate to a particular topic, such as drug administration or a specific adverse effect, patient education related to that topic is discussed concurrently.

TABLE 2.2 ■ Modified Nursing Process Format Used for Summaries of Major Nursing Implications

PREADMINISTRATION ASSESSMENT
Therapeutic Goal
Baseline Data
Identifying High-Risk Patients
IMPLEMENTATION: ADMINISTRATION
Routes
Administration
IMPLEMENTATION: MEASURES TO ENHANCE THERAPEUTIC EFFECTS
ONGOING EVALUATION AND INTERVENTIONS
Summary of Monitoring
Evaluating Therapeutic Effects
Minimizing Adverse Effects
Minimizing Adverse Interactions
Managing Toxicity

This integration is done to promote clarity and efficiency of communication. To help this important information stand out, it appears in blue type.

What About Diagnosis and Planning?

These headings are not used in the summaries. There are several reasons for the omission, the dominant one being efficiency of communication.

Nursing diagnoses have been left out primarily because they are highly individualized. When caring for patients, you will develop nursing diagnoses based on your analysis of assessment data.

Planning has not been used as a heading for three reasons. First, planning applies primarily to the overall management of the disorder for which a particular drug is being used—and much less to the drug itself. Second, because planning is discussed at length and more appropriately in nonpharmacologic nursing texts, such as those on medical-surgical nursing, there is no need to repeat this information here. Third, planning is reflected in interventions that are implemented.

KEY POINTS

- Nursing responsibilities with regard to drugs extend far beyond the Rights of Drug Administration.
- You are the patient's last line of defense against medication errors.
- Your knowledge of pharmacology has a wide variety of practical applications in patient care and patient education.
- By applying your knowledge of pharmacology, you will make a large contribution to achieving the therapeutic objective of maximum benefit with minimum harm.
- Application of the nursing process in drug therapy is directed at individualizing treatment, which is critical to achieving the therapeutic objective.
- The goal of preadministration assessment is to gather data needed for (1) evaluation of therapeutic and adverse effects, (2) identification of high-risk patients, and (3) assessment of the patient's capacity for self-care.
- The analysis and diagnosis phase of treatment is directed at (1) judging the appropriateness of the prescribed therapy, (2) identifying potential health problems treatment might cause, and (3) characterizing the patient's capacity for self-care.
- Planning is directed at (1) defining goals, (2) establishing priorities, and (3) establishing criteria for evaluating success.
- In the evaluation stage, the objective is to evaluate (1) therapeutic responses, (2) adverse reactions and interactions, (3) patient adherence, and (4) patient satisfaction with treatment.

Please visit http://evolve.elsevier.com/Lehne for chapter-specific NCLEX® examination review questions.

CHAPTER

3 Drug Regulation, Development, Names, and Information

In this chapter we complete our introduction to pharmacology by considering five diverse but important topics. These are (1) drug regulation, (2) new drug development, (3) the annoying problem of drug names, (4) over-the-counter drugs, and (5) sources of drug information.

LANDMARK DRUG LEGISLATION

The history of drug legislation in the United States reflects an evolution in our national posture toward regulating the pharmaceutical industry. That posture has changed from one of minimal control to one of extensive control. For the most part, increased regulation has been beneficial, resulting in safer and more effective drugs.

The first American law to regulate drugs was the *Federal Pure Food and Drug Act* of 1906. This law set standards for drug quality and purity in addition to strength. It specifically focused on product labeling and required that any variations from the standards be placed on the label.

The *Food, Drug and Cosmetic Act,* passed in 1938, was the first legislation to address drug safety. The motivation behind the law was a tragedy in which more than 100 people died following use of a new medication. The lethal preparation contained sulfanilamide, an antibiotic, plus diethylene glycol as a solubilizing agent. Tests showed that the solvent was the cause of death. (Diethylene glycol is commonly used as automotive antifreeze.) To reduce the chances of another such tragedy, Congress required that all new drugs undergo testing for safety. The results of these tests were to be reviewed by the *Food and Drug Administration* (FDA), and only those drugs judged safe would receive FDA approval for marketing.

In 1962, Congress passed the *Harris-Kefauver Amendments* to the Food, Drug and Cosmetic Act. This bill was created in response to the thalidomide tragedy that occurred in Europe in the early 1960s. Thalidomide is a sedative now known to cause birth defects and fetal death. Because the drug was used widely by pregnant patients, thousands of infants were born with phocomelia, a rare birth defect characterized by the gross malformation or complete absence of arms or legs. This tragedy was especially poignant in that it resulted from nonessential drug use: The women who took thalidomide could have managed their conditions without it. Thalidomide was not a problem in the United States because the drug never received approval by the FDA.

Because of the European experience with thalidomide, the Harris-Kefauver Amendments sought to strengthen all aspects of drug regulation. A major provision of the bill required that drugs be proved *effective* before marketing. Remarkably, this was the first law to demand that drugs actually offer some benefit. The new Act also required that all drugs that had been introduced between 1932 and 1962 undergo testing for effectiveness; any drug that failed to prove useful would be withdrawn. Lastly, the Harris-Kefauver Amendments established rigorous procedures for testing new drugs. These procedures are discussed later in this chapter under *New Drug Development.*

In 1970, Congress passed the *Controlled Substances Act* (Title II of the Comprehensive Drug Abuse Prevention and Control Act). This legislation set rules for the manufacture and distribution of drugs considered to have the potential for abuse. One provision of the law defines five categories of controlled substances, referred to as Schedules I, II, III, IV, and V. Drugs in Schedule I have no accepted medical use in the United States and are deemed to have a high potential for abuse. Examples include heroin, mescaline, and lysergic acid diethylamide (LSD). Drugs in Schedules II through V have accepted medical applications but also have a high potential for abuse. The abuse potential of these agents becomes progressively less as we proceed from Schedule II to Schedule V. The Controlled Substances Act is discussed further in Chapter 37.

In 1992, FDA regulations were changed to permit *accelerated approval* of drugs for acquired immunodeficiency syndrome (AIDS) and cancer. Under these guidelines, a drug could be approved for marketing before completion of Phase III trials (discussed later in the chapter), provided that rigorous follow-up studies (Phase IV trials) were performed. The rationale for this change was that (1) medications are needed, even if their benefits may be marginal, and (2) the unknown risks associated with early approval are balanced by the need for more effective drugs. Although accelerated approval seems like a good idea, in actual practice, it has two significant drawbacks. First, manufacturers often fail to conduct or complete the required follow-up studies. Second, if the follow-up studies—which are more rigorous than the original—fail to confirm a clinical benefit, the guidelines have no clear mechanism for removing the drug from the market.

The *Prescription Drug User Fee Act* (PDUFA), passed in 1992, was a response to complaints that the FDA takes too long to review applications for new drugs. Under the Act, drug sponsors pay the FDA fees that are used to fund additional reviewers. In return, the FDA must adhere to strict review timetables. Because of the PDUFA, new drugs now reach the market much sooner than in the past.

The *Food and Drug Administration Modernization Act* (FDAMA) of 1997—an extension of the Prescription Drug User Fee Act—called for widespread changes in FDA regulations. Implementation is in progress. For health professionals, four provisions of the Act are of particular interest:

- The fast-track system created for AIDS drugs and cancer drugs now includes drugs for other serious and life-threatening illnesses.
- Manufacturers who plan to stop making a drug must inform patients at least 6 months in advance, thereby giving them time to find another source.
- A clinical trial database was required for drugs directed at serious or life-threatening illnesses. These data allow clinicians and patients to make informed decisions about using experimental drugs.
- Drug companies can now give prescribers journal articles and certain other information regarding off-label uses of drugs. (An *off-label use* is a use that has not been evaluated by the FDA.) Before the new Act, clinicians were allowed to prescribe a drug for an off-label use, but the manufacturer was not allowed to promote the drug for that use—even if promotion was limited to providing potentially helpful information, including reprints of journal articles. In return for being allowed to give prescribers information regarding off-label uses, manufacturers must promise to do research to support the claims made in the articles.

Two laws—the *Best Pharmaceuticals for Children Act* (BPCA), passed in 2002, and the *Pediatric Research Equity Act* (PREA) of 2003—were designed to promote much-needed research on drug efficacy and safety in children. The BPCA offers a 6-month patent extension to manufacturers who evaluate a drug already on the market for its safety, efficacy, and dosage in children. The PREA gives the FDA the power, for the first time, to require drug companies to conduct pediatric clinical trials on new medications that might be used by children. (In the past, drugs were not tested in children, so there is a general lack of reliable information upon which to base therapeutic decisions.)

In 2007, Congress passed the *FDA Amendments Act* (FDAAA), the most important legislation on drug safety since the Harris-Kefauver Amendments of 1962. The FDAAA expands the mission of the FDA to include rigorous oversight of drug safety *after* a drug has been approved. (Before this Act, the FDA focused on drug efficacy and safety *prior* to approval, but had limited resources and authority to address drug safety after a drug was released for marketing.) Under the new law, the FDA has the legal authority to require postmarketing safety studies, to order changes in a drug's label to include new safety information, and to restrict distribution of a drug based on safety concerns. In addition, the FDA was required to establish an active postmarketing risk surveillance system, mandated to include 25 million patients by July 2010 and 100 million by July 2012. Because of the FDAAA, adverse effects that were not discovered before drug approval came to light much sooner than in the past, and the FDA now has the authority to take action (e.g., limit distribution of a drug) if postmarketing information shows a drug to be less safe than previously understood.

In 2009, Congress passed the *Family Smoking Prevention and Tobacco Control Act,* which, at long last, allows the FDA to regulate cigarettes, which are responsible for about one in five deaths in the United States each year. Under the Act, the FDA was given the authority to strengthen advertising restrictions, including a prohibition on marketing to youth; require revised and more prominent warning labels; require disclosure of all ingredients in tobacco products and restrict harmful additives; and monitor nicotine yields and mandate gradual reduction of nicotine to nonaddictive levels.

The *Comprehensive Addiction and Recovery Act of 2016* was signed into law by President Barack Obama in July 2016. The purpose of this law was to combat a nationwide opioid epidemic by addressing the crisis from multiple approaches. To that end, it provides grants to support efforts directed toward prevention, treatment, and rehabilitation/recovery; opioid overdose reversal by first responders, law enforcement officers, and families; law enforcement training and role expansion; and criminal justice reform that focuses on treatment over imprisonment. Implications for nursing are significant because nurses have important roles in the expanded drug education and other prevention programs and in drug addiction treatment and recovery programs. Additionally, nurses are often in roles in which they serve as first responders.

HAZARDOUS DRUG EXPOSURE

Exposure to certain drugs can be dangerous for nurses and other healthcare workers who handle them. It is imperative to ensure your own safety as well as the safety of your patients.

The National Institute for Occupational Safety and Health (NIOSH), established in 1970, has the responsibility to promote and enhance worker safety. Thus NIOSH identifies which of the thousands of drugs are hazardous for handling and publishes guidance on the safe handling of these drugs.

In their publication *NIOSH List of Antineoplastic and Other Hazardous Drugs in Healthcare Settings, 2016* (available online at www.cdc.gov/niosh/topics/antineoplastic/pdf/hazardous-drugs-list_2016-161.pdf), NIOSH identifies a drug as hazardous for handling if it meets one or more of the following criteria:

- Carcinogenicity
- Teratogenicity or developmental toxicity
- Reproductive toxicity
- Organ toxicity at low doses
- Genotoxicity
- New drugs with structure and toxicity profiles similar to drugs previously determined to be hazardous

It is probably not surprising to find that antineoplastic drugs (drugs that kill cancer cells) are included in the list. However, common drugs such as oral contraceptives (birth control pills) are also included. You will learn about these throughout the textbook, and the full listing is also available in the NIOSH publication.

NIOSH provides instructions on how nurses and other healthcare workers can use protective equipment and environmental controls to prevent potentially harmful effects associated with these drugs. These guidelines are provided in Table 3.1.

NEW DRUG DEVELOPMENT

The development and testing of new drugs is an expensive and lengthy process, requiring 10 to 15 years for completion. Of the thousands of compounds that undergo testing, only a few enter clinical trials, and of these, only 1 in 5 gains approval. According to an article in the May 2016 issue of the *Journal of Health Economics,* the cost of developing a new drug and gaining approval for marketing averages $2.558 billion for each approved drug.

Rigorous procedures for testing have been established so that newly released drugs might be both safe and effective. Unfortunately, although testing can determine effectiveness, it cannot guarantee that a new drug will be safe: Significant adverse effects may evade detection during testing, only to become apparent after a new drug has been released for general use.

The Randomized Controlled Trial

Randomized controlled trials (RCTs) are the most reliable way to objectively assess drug therapies. RCTs have three distinguishing features: use of controls, randomization, and blinding. All three serve to minimize the influence of personal bias on the results.

Use of Controls

When a new drug is under development, we want to know how it compares with a standard drug used for the same disorder, or perhaps how it compares with no treatment at all. To make these comparisons, some subjects in the RCT are given the new drug and some are given either (1) a standard treatment or (2) a placebo (i.e., an inactive compound formulated to look like the experimental drug). Subjects receiving either the standard drug or the placebo are referred to as *controls.* Controls are important because they help us determine whether the new treatment is more (or less) effective than standard treatments,

TABLE 3.1 ▪ Personal Protective Equipment and Engineering Controls for Working With Hazardous Drugs in Healthcare Settings

Formulation	Activity	Double Chemotherapy Gloves	Protective Gown	Eye-Face Protection	Respiratory Protection	Ventilated Engineering Control
All types of hazardous drugs	Administration from unit-dose package	No (single glove can be used)	No	No	No	NA
Intact tablet or capsule	Cutting, crushing, or manipulating tablets or capsules; handling uncoated tablets	Yes	Yes	No	Yes, if not done in a control device	Yes[a]
Tablets or capsules	Administration	No (single glove can be used)	No	Yes, if vomit or potential to spit up[b]	No	NA
Oral liquid drug or feeding tube	Compounding	Yes	Yes	Yes, if not done in a control device	Yes, if not done in a control device	Yes[a]
	Administration	Yes	Yes	Yes, if vomit or potential to spit up[b]	No	NA
Topical drug	Compounding	Yes	Yes	Yes, if not done in a control device	Yes, if not done in a control device	Yes,[a] BSC or CACI (Note: carmustine and mustargen are volatile)
	Administration	Yes	Yes	Yes, if liquid that could splash[b]	Yes, if inhalation potential	NA
Subcutaneous/ intramuscular injection from a vial	Preparation (withdrawing from vial)	Yes	Yes	Yes, if not done in a control device	Yes, if not done in a control device	Yes, BSC or CACI
	Administration from prepared syringe	Yes	Yes	Yes, if liquid that could splash[b]	No	NA

TABLE 3.1 ■ Personal Protective Equipment and Engineering Controls for Working With Hazardous Drugs in Healthcare Settings—cont'd

Formulation	Activity	Double Chemotherapy Gloves	Protective Gown	Eye-Face Protection	Respiratory Protection	Ventilated Engineering Control
Withdrawing and/or mixing intravenous or intramuscular solution from a vial or ampoule	Compounding	Yes[c]	Yes	No	No	Yes, BSC or CACI; use of CSTD recommended
	Administration of prepared solution	Yes	Yes	Yes; if liquid that could splash[b]	No	NA; CSTD required per USP 800 if the dosage form allows
Solution for irrigation	Compounding	Yes	Yes	Yes, if not done in a control device	Yes, if not done in a control device	Yes, BSC or CACI; use of CSTD recommended
	Administration (e.g., bladder, HIPEC, limb perfusion)	Yes	Yes	Yes	Yes	NA
Powder/solution for inhalation/ aerosol treatment	Compounding	Yes	Yes	Yes, if not done in a control device	Yes, if not done in a control device	Yes, BSC or CACI
	Aerosol administration	Yes	Yes	Yes	Yes	Yes, when applicable
	Administration	Yes	Yes	Yes, if liquid that could splash[b]	Yes, if inhalation potential	NA
Drugs and metabolites in body fluids	Disposal and cleaning	Yes	Yes	Yes, if liquid that could splash	Yes, if inhalation potential	NA
Drug-contaminated waste	Disposal and cleaning	Yes	Yes	Yes, if liquid that could splash	Yes, if inhalation potential	NA
Spills	Cleaning	Yes	Yes	Yes	Yes	NA

[a]For nonsterile preparations, a ventilated engineering control such as a fume hood or Class I BSC or a HEPA-filtered enclosure (such as a powder hood) is sufficient if the control device exhaust is HEPA filtered or appropriately exhausted to the outside of the building. It is recommended that these activities be carried out in a control device, but it is recognized that under some circumstances, it is not possible. If the activity is performed in a ventilated engineering control that is used for sterile intravenous preparations, a thorough cleaning is required following the activity.
[b]Required if patient may resist (infant, unruly patient, patient predisposed to spitting out, patient who has difficulty swallowing, veterinary patient) or if the formulation is hard to swallow.
[c]Sterile gloves are required for aseptic drug preparation in BSC or CACI.
BSC, Class II biological safety cabinet; *CACI,* compounding aseptic containment isolator; *CSTD,* closed system drug-transfer device; *HIPEC,* hyperthermic intraperitoneal chemotherapy; *NA,* not applicable.
Reproduced from *NIOSH List of Antineoplastic and Other Hazardous Drugs in Healthcare Settings,* 2016, pp. 32-34.

or at least whether the new treatment is better (or worse) than no treatment at all. Likewise, controls allow us to compare the safety of the new drug with that of the old drug, a placebo, or both.

Randomization

In an RCT, subjects are randomly assigned to either the control group or the experimental group (i.e., the group receiving the new drug). The purpose of randomization is to prevent allocation bias, which results when subjects in the experimental group are different from those in the control group. For example, in the absence of randomization, researchers could load the experimental group with patients who have mild disease and load the control group with patients who have severe disease. In this case, any differences in outcome may well be due to the severity of the disease rather than differences in treatment. And even if researchers try to avoid bias by purposely assigning subjects who appear similar to both groups, allocation bias can result from *unknown* factors that can influence outcome. By assigning subjects randomly to the control and experimental groups, all factors—known and unknown, important and unimportant—should be equally represented in both groups. As a result, the influences of these factors on outcome should tend to cancel each other out, leaving differences in the treatments as the best explanation for any differences in outcome.

Blinding

A blinded study is one in which the people involved do not know to which group—control or experimental—individual subjects have been randomized. If only the subjects have been "blinded," the trial is referred to as *single blind.* If the researchers as well as the subjects are kept in the dark, the trial is referred to as *double blind.* Of the two, double-blind trials are more objective. Blinding is accomplished by administering the experimental drug and the control compound (either placebo or comparison drug) in identical formulations (e.g., green capsules, purple pills) that bear a numeric code. At the end of the study, the code is accessed to reveal which subjects were controls and which received the experimental drug. When subjects and researchers are not blinded, their preconceptions about the benefits and risks of the new drug can readily bias the results. Hence, blinding is done to minimize the impact of personal bias.

Stages of New Drug Development

The testing of new drugs has two principal steps: *preclinical testing* and *clinical testing.* Preclinical tests are performed in animals. Clinical tests are done in humans. The steps in drug development are shown in Table 3.2.

Preclinical Testing

Preclinical testing is required before a new drug may be tested in humans. During preclinical testing, drugs are evaluated for *toxicities, pharmacokinetic properties,* and *potentially useful biologic effects.* Preclinical tests may take 1 to 5 years. When sufficient preclinical data have been gathered, the drug developer may apply to the FDA for permission to begin testing in humans. If the application is approved, the drug is awarded *Investigational New Drug* status and clinical trials may begin.

Clinical Testing

Clinical trials occur in four phases and may take 2 to 10 years to complete. The first three phases are done before a new drug is marketed. The fourth is done following FDA approval for marketing.

Phase I. Phase I trials are usually conducted in *healthy volunteers.* However, if a drug is likely to have severe side effects, as many anticancer drugs do, the trial is done in volunteer patients who have the disease under consideration. Phase I testing has three goals: to evaluate drug metabolism, pharmacokinetics, and biologic effects.

Phases II and III. In these trials, drugs are tested in *patients.* The objective is to determine therapeutic effects, dosage range, safety, and effectiveness. During Phase II and Phase III trials, 500 to 5000 patients receive the drug, and only a few hundred take it for more than 3 to 6 months. Upon completing Phase III, the drug manufacturer applies to the FDA for conditional approval of a *New Drug Application.* If conditional approval is granted, Phase IV may begin.

Phase IV: Postmarketing Surveillance. In Phase IV, the new drug is released for general use, permitting observation of its effects in a large population. Thanks to the FDAAA of 2007, postmarketing surveillance is now much more effective than in the past.

TABLE 3.2 ▪ Steps in New Drug Development

Preclinical Testing (in animals)

- **Toxicity**
- **Pharmacokinetics**
- **Possible Useful Effects**

↓

Investigational New Drug (IND) Status

↓

Clinical Testing (in humans)

Phase I
↓ *Subjects:* Healthy volunteers
Tests: Metabolism, pharmacokinetics, and biologic effects

Phase II
↓ *Subjects:* Patients
Tests: Therapeutic utility and dosage range

Phase III
↓ *Subjects:* Patients
Tests: Safety and effectiveness

Conditional Approval of New Drug Application (NDA)

↓

Phase IV: Postmarketing Surveillance

Limitations of the Testing Procedure

It is important for nurses and other healthcare professionals to appreciate the limitations of the drug development process. Two problems are of particular concern. First, until recently, information on drug use in women and children has been limited. Second, new drugs are likely to have adverse effects that were not detected during clinical trials.

Limited Information on Women and Children

Women. Very little drug testing was done in women before 2000. In almost all cases, women of childbearing age were excluded from early clinical trials out of concern for fetal safety. Unfortunately, FDA policy took this concern to an extreme, effectively barring *all* women of childbearing age from Phase I and Phase II trials—even if the women were not pregnant and were using adequate birth control. The only women allowed to participate in early clinical trials were those with a life-threatening illness that might respond to the drug under study.

Because of limited drug testing in women, we don't know with precision how women will respond to most drugs because most drugs in current use were developed before inclusiveness of women in trials was ensured. As a result, we don't know whether beneficial effects in women will be equivalent to those seen in men, nor do we know whether adverse effects will be equivalent to those in men. We don't know how timing of drug administration with respect to the menstrual cycle will affect beneficial and adverse responses. We don't know whether drug disposition (absorption, distribution, metabolism, and excretion) will be the same in women as in men. Furthermore, of the drugs that might be used to treat a particular illness, we don't know whether the drugs that are most effective in men will also be most effective in women. Lastly, we don't know about the safety of drug use during pregnancy.

During the late 1990s, the FDA issued a series of guidelines mandating participation of women (and minorities) in trials of new drugs. In addition, the FDA revoked a 1977 guideline that barred women from most trials. Because of these changes, the proportion of women in trials of most new drugs now equals the proportion of women in the population. The data generated since the implementation of the new guidelines have been reassuring: Most gender-related effects have been limited to pharmacokinetics. More importantly, for most drugs, gender has shown little impact on efficacy, safety, or dosage. However, although the new guidelines are an important step forward, even with them, it will take a long time to close the gender gap in our knowledge of drugs.

Children. Until recently, children, like women, had been excluded from clinical trials. As a result, information on dosage, therapeutic responses, and adverse effects in children has been limited. Because our knowledge of drug use in children is often derived from postmarketing surveillance, it will still be a long time before we have the information needed to use drugs safely and effectively in young patients.

Failure to Detect All Adverse Effects

Premarketing clinical trials cannot detect all adverse effects before a new drug is released. There are three reasons why: (1) during clinical trials, a relatively small number of patients are given the drug; (2) because these patients are carefully selected, they do not represent the full spectrum of individuals who will eventually take the drug; and (3) patients in trials take the drug for a relatively short time. Because of these unavoidable limitations in the testing process, effects that occur infrequently, effects that take a long time to develop, and effects that occur only in certain types of patients can go undetected. Hence, despite our best efforts, when a new drug is released, it may well have adverse effects of which we are as yet unaware. In fact, about half of the drugs that reach the market have serious adverse effects that were not detected until after they were released for general use.

The hidden dangers in new drugs are shown in Table 3.3, which presents information on eight drugs that were withdrawn from the U.S. market soon after receiving FDA approval. In all cases, the reason for withdrawal was a serious adverse effect that went undetected in clinical trials. Admittedly, only a few hidden adverse effects are as severe as the ones in the table. Hence, most do not necessitate drug withdrawal. Nonetheless, the drugs in the table should serve as a strong warning about the unknown dangers that a new drug may harbor.

Because adverse effects may go undetected, when caring for a patient who is prescribed a new drug, you should be especially watchful for previously unreported drug reactions. If a patient taking a new drug begins to show unusual symptoms, it is prudent to suspect that the new drug may be the cause—even though the symptoms are not yet mentioned in the literature.

Exercising Discretion Regarding New Drugs

When thinking about prescribing a new drug, clinicians would do well to follow this guideline: *Be neither the first to adopt the new nor the last to abandon the old.* Recall that the therapeutic objective is to produce maximum benefit with minimum harm. To achieve this objective, we must balance the potential benefits of a drug against its inherent risks. As a rule, new drugs have actions very similar to those of older agents. That is, it is rare for a new drug to be able to do something that an older drug can't accomplish. Consequently, the need to treat a particular disorder seldom constitutes a compelling reason to select a new drug over an agent that has been available for years. Furthermore, new drugs generally present greater risks than the old ones. As noted, at the time of its introduction, a new drug is likely to have adverse effects that have not yet been reported, and these effects may prove harmful for some patients. In contrast, older, more familiar drugs are less likely to cause unpleasant surprises. Consequently, when we weigh the benefits of a new drug against its risks, it is less likely that the benefits will be sufficient to justify the risks—especially when an older drug, whose properties are well known, is available. Accordingly, when it comes to the use of new drugs, it is important to be alert to the possibility that a new patient problem may be the manifestation of an as-yet-unknown adverse reaction.

DRUG NAMES

This topic is important because the names we employ affect our ability to communicate about medicines. The subject is

TABLE 3.3 ▪ Drugs That Were Withdrawn From the U.S. Market for Safety Reasons

Drug	Indication	Year Introduced/ Year Withdrawn	Months on the Market	Reason for Withdrawal
Niacin ER/lovastatin [Advicor] Niacin ER/simvastatin [Simcor]	Hypercholesterolemia	2008/2016	96	Risks exceed benefits
Peginesatide [Omontys]	Anemia	2012/2013	12	Life-threatening reactions
Rotigotine[a] [Neupro]	Parkinson disease	2007/2008	10	Patch formulation delivered erratic doses
Tegaserod[b] [Zelnorm]	Irritable bowel syndrome	2002/2007	60	Myocardial infarction, stroke
Natalizumab[b] [Tysabri]	Multiple sclerosis	2004/2005	3	Progressive multifocal leukoencephalopathy
Rapacuronium [Raplon]	Neuromuscular blockade	1999/2001	19	Bronchospasm, unexplained fatalities
Alosetron[b] [Lotronex]	Irritable bowel syndrome	2000/2000	9	Ischemic colitis, severe constipation; deaths have occurred
Troglitazone [Rezulin]	Type 2 diabetes	1999/2000	12	Fatal liver failure

[a]Note that rotigotine was withdrawn because the *formulation* was unsafe, not because the drug itself is inherently dangerous.
[b]Alosetron, natalizumab, and tegaserod were later returned to the market. With all three drugs, risk management guidelines must be followed. Tegaserod may only be prescribed with FDA authorization for emergency situations.

potentially confusing because we have evolved a system in which any drug can have a large number of names.

In approaching drug names, we begin by defining the types of names that drugs have. After that we consider (1) the complications that arise from assigning multiple names to a drug, and (2) the benefits of using just one name: the generic (nonproprietary) name.

The Three Types of Drug Names

Drugs have three types of names: (1) a chemical name, (2) a generic or nonproprietary name, and (3) a brand or proprietary name (Table 3.4). All of the names in the table are for the same drug, a compound most familiar to us under the brand name *Tylenol.*

TABLE 3.4 ▪ The Three Types of Drug Names[a]

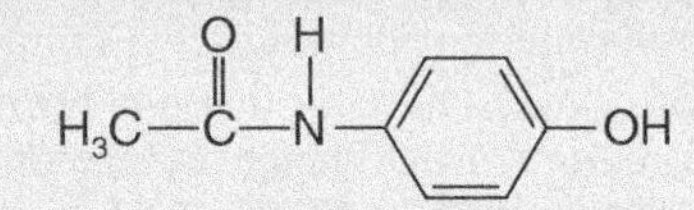

Type of Drug Name	Examples
Chemical Name	*N*-acetyl-*para*-aminophenol
Generic Name (nonproprietary name)	Acetaminophen
Brand Names (proprietary names)	Acephen; APAP; Aspirin Free Anacin Extra Strength; Cetafen; Excedrin Tension Headache; Feverall; Little Fevers; Mapap; Nortemp Children's; Ofirmev; Pain & Fever Children's; Pain Eze; Q-Pap; RapiMed; Silapap; Triaminic; Tylenol; Valorin

[a]The chemical, generic, and brand names listed are all names for the drug whose structure is pictured in this table. This drug is most familiar to us as Tylenol, one of its brand names.

Chemical Name

The chemical name constitutes a description of a drug using the nomenclature of chemistry. As you can see from Table 3.4, a drug's chemical name can be long and complex. Because of their complexity, chemical names are inappropriate for everyday use. For example, few people would communicate using the chemical term *N*-acetyl-*para*-aminophenol when a simple generic name (*acetaminophen*) or brand name (e.g., *Tylenol*) could be used.

Generic Name

The generic name of a drug is assigned by the United States Adopted Names Council. Each drug has only one generic name. The generic name is also known as the *nonproprietary* name. Generic names are less complex than chemical names.

In many cases, the final syllables of the generic name indicate a drug's pharmacologic class. For example, the syllables *-cillin* at the end of *amoxicillin* indicate that amoxicillin belongs to the penicillin class of antibiotics. Similarly, the syllables *-statin* at the end of *lovastatin* indicate that lovastatin is an HMG-CoA reductase inhibitor, our most effective class of drugs for lowering cholesterol. Table 3.5 presents additional examples of generic names whose final syllables indicate the class to which the drugs belong.

Brand Name

Brand names, also known as *proprietary* or *trade* names, are the names under which a drug is marketed. These names are created by drug companies with the intention that they be easy for nurses, physicians, pharmacists, and consumers to recall and pronounce. Because any drug can be marketed in different formulations and by multiple companies, a single drug may have a large number of brand names.

Brand names must be approved by the FDA. The review process tries to ensure that no two brand names are too similar. In addition, brand names are not supposed to imply efficacy—which may be why orlistat (a diet pill) is named

TABLE 3.5 ▪ Generic Drug Names Whose Final Syllables Indicate Pharmacologic Class

Representative Drugs	Class-Indicating Final Syllable(s)	Pharmacologic Class	Therapeutic Use
Amoxicillin, ticarcillin	-cillin	Penicillin antibiotic	Infection
Lovastatin, simvastatin	-statin	HMG-CoA reductase inhibitor	High cholesterol
Propranolol, metoprolol	-olol	Beta-adrenergic blocker	Hypertension, angina
Phenobarbital, secobarbital	-barbital	Barbiturate	Seizures, anxiety
Benazepril, captopril	-pril	Angiotensin-converting enzyme inhibitor	Hypertension, heart failure
Candesartan, valsartan	-sartan	Angiotensin II receptor blocker	Hypertension, heart failure
Nifedipine, amlodipine	-dipine	Dihydropyridine calcium channel blocker	Hypertension
Eletriptan, sumatriptan	-triptan	Serotonin$_{1B/1D}$ receptor agonist	Migraine
Dalteparin, enoxaparin	-parin	Low-molecular-weight heparin	Anticoagulation
Sildenafil, tadalafil	-afil	Phosphodiesterase type 5 inhibitor	Erectile dysfunction
Rosiglitazone, pioglitazone	-glitazone	Thiazolidinedione	Type 2 diabetes
Omeprazole, pantoprazole	-prazole	Proton pump inhibitor	Peptic ulcer disease
Alendronate, zoledronate	-dronate	Bisphosphonate	Osteoporosis
Ciprofloxacin, norfloxacin	-floxacin	Fluoroquinolone antibiotic	Infection

Xenical, rather than something more suggestive, like *Fat-B-Gone* or *PoundsOff.* However, despite the rule against suggestive names, some still slip by FDA scrutiny, like these two gems: *Flomax* (tamsulosin) and *Rapaflo* (silodosin). Can you guess what these drugs are used for? (Hint: It's an old guy malady.)

Which Name to Use, Generic or Brand?

Just as scientists use a common terminology to discuss scientific phenomena, we need a common terminology when discussing drugs. When large numbers of drug names are unfamiliar or not standardized, as is common with many brand names, it creates the potential for confusion. For this reason, many professionals advocate for the universal use of generic names.

Problems With Brand Names

A Single Drug Can Have Multiple Brand Names. The principal objection to brand names is their vast number. Although a drug can have only one generic name, it can have unlimited brand names. As the number of brand names for a single drug expands, the burden of name recognition becomes progressively heavier. By way of illustration, the drug whose generic name is acetaminophen has more than 15 brand names (see Table 3.4). Although most clinicians will recognize this drug's generic name, few are familiar with all the brand names.

Use of brand names can result in "double medication"—with potentially disastrous results. Because patients frequently see more than one healthcare provider, a patient may receive prescriptions for the same drug by two (or more) prescribers. If the provider refers to these drugs by their brand names, the patient may believe these are two different drugs. If these medications are taken as prescribed, excessive dosing will result.

Over-the-Counter (OTC) Products With the Same Brand Name May Have Different Active Ingredients. As indicated in Table 3.6, OTC products that have similar or identical brand names can actually contain different drugs. For example, although the two Lotrimin AF products have identical brand names, they actually contain two different drugs: miconazole and clotrimazole. Confusion would be avoided by labeling these products *miconazole spray* and *clotrimazole cream,* rather than labeling both Lotrimin AF.

The two 4-Way Nasal Spray products listed in Table 3.6 further illustrate the potential for confusion. For most drugs, the words "fast-acting" and "long-acting" indicate different formulations of the same drug; however, 4-Way Fast-Acting Nasal Spray is phenylephrine and 4-Way 12-Hour Nasal Spray is oxymetazoline.

Perhaps the most disturbing aspect of brand names is illustrated by the reformulation of *Kaopectate,* a well-known antidiarrheal product. In 2003, the manufacturer switched the active ingredient in Kaopectate from attapulgite (which had replaced kaolin and pectin in the late 1980s) to bismuth subsalicylate. However, although the active ingredient changed, the brand name did not. As a result, current formulations of Kaopectate pose a risk for patients who should not take salicylates, such as young children at risk for Reye's syndrome. This example illustrates an important point: Manufacturers of OTC drugs can reformulate brand-name products whenever they want—without changing the name at all. Hence, there is no guarantee that the brand-name product you buy today contains the same drug as the brand-name product you bought last week, last month, or last year.

In the spring of 1999, the FDA issued a ruling to help reduce the confusion created by OTC brand names. This ruling requires generic names for the drugs in OTC products to be clearly and prominently listed on the label. Unfortunately, this is of no help to patients who have long relied on brand names alone to guide OTC choices.

Brand Names Can Endanger International Travelers. For people who travel to other countries, brand names present two kinds of problems. First, the brand name used in one country may differ from the brand name used in another country. The second (and more disturbing) problem is this: Products with the *identical* brand name may have *different* active ingredients, depending on where you buy the drug (Table 3.7). As a result, when a prescription for a brand-name product is filled in another country, the patient may receive the wrong drug. For example, when visiting Mexico, Americans or Canadians with a prescription for *Vantin* will be given naproxen (an antiinflammatory drug) rather than the cefpodoxime (an antibiotic) that they were expecting. Not only can this lead to unnecessary side effects (possible kidney damage and GI ulceration), but the target infection will continue unabated. Hence, the patient is exposed to all the risks of medication without getting any of the benefits.

TABLE 3.6 ▪ Some OTC Products That Share the Same Brand Name

Product Name	Drugs in the Product
Lotrimin AF	Miconazole (spray)
Lotrimin AF	Clotrimazole (cream)
4-Way 12-Hour Nasal Spray	Oxymetazoline
4-Way Fast-Acting Nasal Spray	Phenylephrine
Kaopectate	Originally formulated as *kaolin + pectin* Reformulated to *attapulgite* in the late 1980s Reformulated to *bismuth subsalicylate* in 2003

OTC, Over-the-counter.

Generic Products Versus Brand-Name Products

To complete our discussion of drug names, we need to address two questions: (1) Do significant differences exist between different brands of the same drug? and (2) If such differences do exist, do they justify the use of brand names? The answer to both questions is NO!

Are Generic Products and Brand-Name Products Therapeutically Equivalent? When a new drug comes to market, it is sold under a brand name by the company that developed it. When that company's patent expires, other companies can produce the drug and market it under its generic name. (A list of FDA-approved generic equivalents is available online at www.accessdata.fda.gov/scripts/cder/ob/default.cfm.) Our question, then, is, "Are the generic formulations equivalent to the brand-name formulation produced by the original manufacturer?"

Because all equivalent products—generic or brand name—contain the same dose of the same drug, the only real concern with generic formulations is their rate and extent of absorption.

TABLE 3.7 ■ Products From the United States and Canada That Have the Same Brand Name but Different Active Ingredients in Other Countries

Brand Name	Country	Active Drug	Indication
Norpramin	United States, Canada	Desipramine	Depression
	Spain	Omeprazole	Peptic ulcer disease
Flomax	United States, Canada	Tamsulosin	Enlarged prostate
	Italy	Morniflumate	Inflammation
Allegra	United States, Canada	Fexofenadine	Allergies
	Germany	Frovatriptan	Migraine
Mobic	United States, Canada	Meloxicam	Inflammation, pain
	India	Amoxicillin	Bacterial infection
Avastin	United States, Canada	Bevacizumab	Cancer, macular degeneration
	India	Atorvastatin	High cholesterol
Vantin	United States, Canada	Cefpodoxime	Bacterial infection
	Mexico	Naproxen	Inflammation, pain

For a few drugs, a slight increase in absorption can result in toxicity, and a slight decrease can result in therapeutic failure. For example, when health plans in Minnesota required the substitution of generic for brand-name drugs, patients at MINCEP Epilepsy Care whose symptoms were previously controlled with Dilantin (phenytoin) began to have seizures after switching to a generic form of phenytoin. Hence, with agents for which a small difference in absorption can be important, decisions to stay with a brand name should be based on the evidence and made on a case-by-case basis.

Conclusions Regarding Generic Names and Brand Names

In the preceding discussion, we considered concerns associated with brand names and generic names. In this text, generic names are employed for routine discussion. Although brand names are presented, they are not emphasized.

OVER-THE-COUNTER DRUGS

OTC drugs are defined as drugs that can be purchased without a prescription. These agents are used for a wide variety of complaints, including mild pain, motion sickness, allergies, colds, constipation, and heartburn. Whether a drug is available by prescription or over the counter is ultimately determined by the FDA.

OTC drugs are an important part of healthcare. When used properly, these agents can provide relief from many ailments while saving consumers the expense and inconvenience of visiting a prescriber. The following facts underscore how important the OTC market is:

- Americans spend more than $30 billion annually on OTC drugs.
- OTC drugs account for 60% of all medications administered.
- Forty percent of Americans take at least one OTC drug every 2 days.
- Four times as many illnesses are treated by a consumer using an OTC drug as by a consumer visiting a prescriber.
- With most illnesses (60% to 95%), initial therapy consists of self-care, including self-medication with an OTC drug.
- The average home medicine cabinet contains 24 OTC preparations.

Some drugs that were originally sold only by prescription are now sold over the counter. Since the 1970s, more than 100 prescription drugs have been switched to OTC status. Because of this process, more and more highly effective drugs are becoming directly available to consumers. Unfortunately, most consumers lack the knowledge needed to choose the most appropriate drug from among the steadily increasing options.

In 2006, the FDA began to phase in new labeling requirements for OTC drugs. The goal is to standardize labels and to make them more informative and easy to understand. The labels, titled *Drug Facts,* are to be written in plain language, have a user-friendly format, and use type that is big enough to read. Active ingredients will be listed first, followed by uses, warnings, directions, and inactive ingredients. This information is designed to help consumers select drugs that can provide the most benefit with the least risk.

In contrast to some texts, which present all OTC drugs in a single chapter, this text presents OTC drugs throughout. This format allows discussion of OTC drugs in their proper pharmacologic and therapeutic contexts.

SOURCES OF DRUG INFORMATION

There is much more to pharmacology than we can address in this text. When you need additional information, the following sources may be helpful. They cover a broad range of topics, but in limited depth. Accordingly, these sources are most useful as initial sources of information. If more detail is needed, specialty publications should be consulted.

Newsletters

The Medical Letter on Drugs and Therapeutics is a bimonthly publication that gives current information on drugs. It is available both in print and online. A typical issue addresses two or three agents. Discussions consist of a summary of data from clinical trials plus a conclusion regarding the drug's therapeutic utility. The conclusions can be a valuable guide when deciding whether to use a new drug.

Prescriber's Letter is a monthly publication with very current information. Unlike *The Medical Letter,* which usually focuses on just two or three drugs, this newsletter addresses (briefly) most major drug-related developments—from new drugs to FDA warnings to new uses of older agents. Like *The Medical Letter,* it is available in both print and online versions.

Reference Books

The *Physicians' Desk Reference,* also known as the PDR, is a reference work financed by the pharmaceutical industry. The information on each drug is identical to the FDA-approved information on its package insert. In addition to textual content, the PDR has a pictorial section for product identification. The PDR is updated annually and is available online.

Drug Facts and Comparisons is a comprehensive reference that contains monographs on virtually every drug marketed in the United States. Information is provided on drug actions, indications, warnings, precautions, adverse reactions, dosage, and administration. In addition to describing the properties of single medications, the book lists the contents of most combination products sold in this country. Indexing is by generic name and brand name. *Drug Facts and Comparisons* is available in a loose-leaf format (updated monthly), an online format (updated monthly), and a hard-cover format (published annually).

A number of drug references have been compiled expressly for nurses. All address topics of special interest to nurses, including information on administration, assessment, evaluation, and patient education. Representative nursing drug references include *Saunders Nursing Drug Handbook* and *Mosby's Nursing Drug Reference,* both published annually.

The Internet

The Internet can be a valuable source of drug information. However, because anyone, regardless of qualifications, can post information, not everything you find will be accurate. Accordingly, you need to exercise discretion when searching for information.

KEY POINTS

- The Food, Drug and Cosmetic Act of 1938 was the first legislation to regulate drug safety.
- The Harris-Kefauver Amendments, passed in 1962, were the first legislation to demand that drugs actually be of some benefit.
- The Controlled Substances Act, passed in 1970, set rules for the manufacture and distribution of drugs considered to have potential for abuse.
- The FDA Amendments Act, passed in 2007, expanded the mission of the FDA to include rigorous oversight of drug safety *after* a drug has been released for marketing.
- The *Comprehensive Addiction and Recovery Act of 2016* provides funding to combat a nationwide opioid epidemic by addressing the crisis from multiple approaches.
- The National Institute for Occupational Safety and Health (NIOSH) identifies drugs that are hazardous for handling and provides instructions for use of protective equipment and environmental controls to protect nurses and other health care workers from harm due to exposure.
- Development of a new drug is a very expensive process that takes years to complete.
- The randomized controlled trial is the most reliable way to objectively assess drug efficacy and safety.
- Clinical trials occur in four phases. The first three phases are done before a new drug is marketed. The fourth is done following FDA approval for marketing.
- Drug testing in Phase II and Phase III clinical trials is limited to a relatively small number of patients, most of whom take the drug for a relatively short time.
- Because women and children have been excluded from drug trials in the past, our understanding of drug efficacy and safety in these groups is limited for many drugs.
- When a new drug is released for general use, it may well have adverse effects that have not yet been detected. Consequently, when working with a new drug, you should be especially watchful for previously unreported adverse events.
- Drugs have three types of names: a chemical name, a generic or nonproprietary name, and a brand or proprietary name.
- Each drug has only one generic name but can have many brand names.
- With over-the-counter (OTC) products, the same brand name may be used for more than one drug.
- Brand names for the same drug may differ from one country to another.
- Generic names facilitate communication better than brand names, which are potentially confusing.
- OTC drugs are drugs that can be purchased without a prescription.

Please visit **http://evolve.elsevier.com/Lehne** for chapter-specific NCLEX® examination review questions.

UNIT II BASIC PRINCIPLES OF PHARMACOLOGY

CHAPTER 4 Pharmacokinetics

The term *pharmacokinetics* is derived from two Greek words: *pharmakon* (drug or poison) and *kinesis* (motion). As this derivation implies, pharmacokinetics is the study of drug movement throughout the body. Pharmacokinetics also includes what happens to the drug as it makes this journey.

There are four basic pharmacokinetic processes: *absorption, distribution, metabolism,* and *excretion* (Fig. 4.1). Absorption is defined as the movement of a drug from its site of administration into the blood. Distribution is defined as drug movement from the blood to the interstitial space of tissues and from there into cells. Metabolism (biotransformation) is defined as enzymatically mediated alteration of drug structure. Excretion is the movement of drugs and their metabolites out of the body. The combination of metabolism plus excretion is called *elimination.* The four pharmacokinetic processes, acting in concert, determine the concentration of a drug at its sites of action.

APPLICATION OF PHARMACOKINETICS IN THERAPEUTICS

By applying knowledge of pharmacokinetics to drug therapy, we can help maximize beneficial effects and minimize harm. Recall that the intensity of the response to a drug is directly related to the concentration of the drug at its site of action. To maximize beneficial effects, a drug must achieve concentrations that are high enough to elicit desired responses; to minimize harm, we must avoid concentrations that are too high. This balance is achieved by selecting the most appropriate route, dosage, and dosing schedule.

As a nurse, you will have ample opportunity to apply knowledge of pharmacokinetics in clinical practice. For example, by understanding the reasons behind selection of route, dosage, and dosing schedule, you will be less likely to commit medication errors than will the nurse who, through lack of this knowledge, administers medications by blindly following prescribers' orders. Also, as noted in Chapter 2, prescribers do make mistakes. Accordingly, you will have occasion to question or even challenge prescribers regarding their selection of dosage, route, or schedule of administration. To alter a prescriber's decision, you will need logical rationale to support your position. To present your case, you will need to understand pharmacokinetics.

Knowledge of pharmacokinetics can increase job satisfaction. Working with medications is a significant component of nursing practice. If you lack knowledge of pharmacokinetics, drugs will always be somewhat mysterious and, as a result, will be a potential source of unease. By helping to demystify drug therapy, knowledge of pharmacokinetics can decrease some

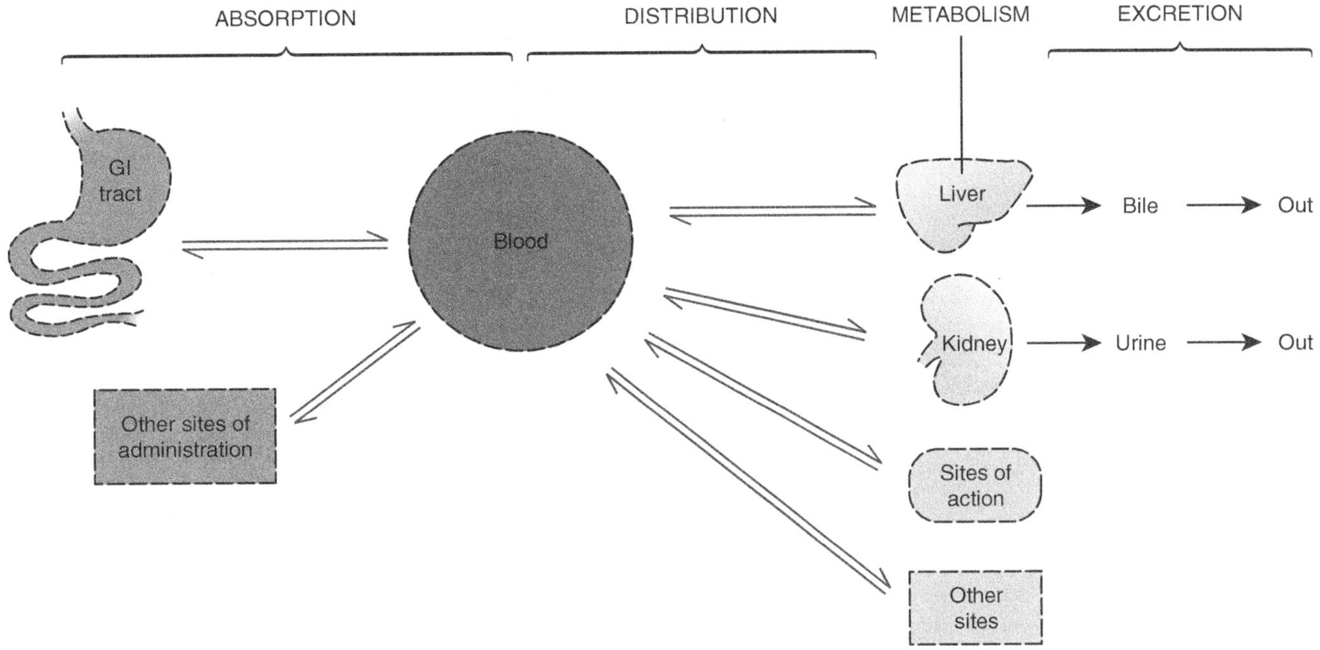

Fig. 4.1 ■ The four basic pharmacokinetic processes.
Dotted lines represent membranes that must be crossed as drugs move throughout the body.

of the stress of nursing practice and can increase intellectual and professional satisfaction.

A NOTE TO CHEMOPHOBES

Before we proceed, some advance notice (and encouragement) is in order for chemophobes (students who fear chemistry). Because drugs are chemicals, we cannot discuss pharmacology meaningfully without occasionally talking about chemistry. This chapter has some chemistry in it. Because the concepts addressed here are fundamental, and because they reappear frequently, all students, including chemophobes, are encouraged to learn this material now, regardless of the effort and anxiety involved.

I also want to comment on the chemical structures that appear in the book. Structures are presented only to illustrate and emphasize concepts. They are not intended for memorization, and they are certainly not intended for exams. So, relax, look at the pictures, and focus on the concepts.

PASSAGE OF DRUGS ACROSS MEMBRANES

All four phases of pharmacokinetics—absorption, distribution, metabolism, and excretion—involve drug movement. To move throughout the body, drugs must cross membranes. Drugs must cross membranes to enter the blood from their site of administration. Once in the blood, drugs must cross membranes to leave the vascular system and reach their sites of action. In addition, drugs must cross membranes to undergo metabolism and excretion. Accordingly, the factors that determine the passage of drugs across biologic membranes have a profound influence on all aspects of pharmacokinetics.

Membrane Structure

Biologic membranes are composed of layers of individual cells. The cells composing most membranes are very close to one another—so close, in fact, that drugs must usually pass *through* cells, rather than between them, to cross the membrane. Hence, the ability of a drug to cross a biologic membrane is determined primarily by its ability to pass through single cells. The major barrier to passage through a cell is the cytoplasmic membrane (the membrane that surrounds every cell).

The basic structure of the cell membrane is depicted in Fig. 4.2. As indicated, the membrane structure consists of a double layer of molecules known as *phospholipids.* Phospholipids are simply lipids (fats) that contain an atom of phosphate.

In Fig. 4.2, the phospholipid molecules are depicted as having a round head (the phosphate-containing component) and two tails (long-chain hydrocarbons). The large objects embedded in the membrane represent protein molecules, which serve a variety of functions.

Three Ways to Cross a Cell Membrane

The three most important ways by which drugs cross cell membranes are (1) passage through channels or pores, (2) passage with the aid of a transport system, and (3) direct penetration of the membrane itself. Of the three, direct penetration of the membrane is most common.

Channels and Pores

Very few drugs cross membranes via channels or pores. The channels in membranes are extremely small (approximately 4 angstroms or less), and are specific for certain molecules. Consequently, only the smallest of compounds (e.g., potassium or sodium) can pass through these channels, and then only if the channel is the right one.

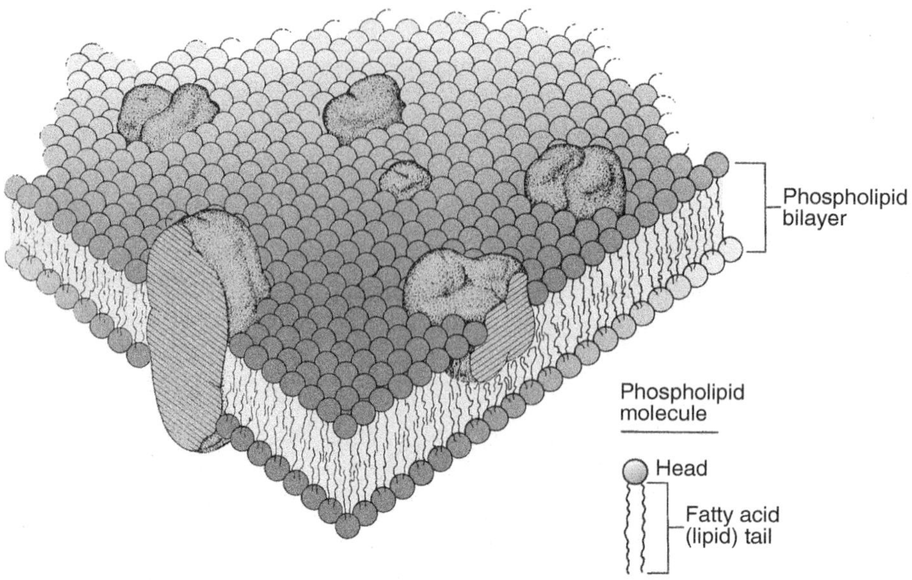

Fig. 4.2 ■ Structure of the cell membrane.
The cell membrane consists primarily of a double layer of phospholipid molecules. The large globular structures represent protein molecules embedded in the lipid bilayer. (Modified from Singer SJ, Nicolson GL: The fluid mosaic model of the structure of cell membranes, *Science* 175:720, 1972.)

Transport Systems

Transport systems are carriers that can move drugs from one side of the cell membrane to the other. Some transport systems require the expenditure of energy; others do not. All transport systems are selective: They will not carry just any drug. Whether a transporter will carry a particular drug depends on the drug's structure.

Transport systems are an important means of drug transit. For example, certain orally administered drugs could not be absorbed unless there were transport systems to move them across the membranes that separate the lumen of the intestine from the blood. A number of drugs could not reach intracellular sites of action without a transport system to move them across the cell membrane. Renal excretion of many drugs would be extremely slow were it not for transport systems in the kidney that can pump drugs from the blood into the renal tubules.

P-Glycoprotein. One transporter, known as *P-glycoprotein (PGP)* or *multidrug transporter protein,* deserves special mention. PGP is a transmembrane protein that transports a wide variety of drugs *out* of cells. This transporter is present in cells at many sites, including the liver, kidney, placenta, intestine, and capillaries of the brain. In the liver, P-glycoprotein transports drugs into the bile for elimination. In the kidney, it pumps drugs into the urine for excretion. In the placenta, it transports drugs back into the maternal blood, thereby reducing fetal drug exposure. In the intestine, it transports drugs into the intestinal lumen, and can thereby reduce drug absorption into the blood. And in brain capillaries, it pumps drugs into the blood, thereby limiting drug access to the brain.

Direct Penetration of the Membrane

For most drugs, movement throughout the body is dependent on the ability to penetrate membranes directly. Why? Because (1) most drugs are too large to pass through channels or pores, and (2) most drugs lack transport systems to help them cross all of the membranes that separate them from their sites of action, metabolism, and excretion.

A general rule in chemistry states that "like dissolves like." Membranes are composed primarily of lipids; therefore, to directly penetrate membranes, a drug must be *lipid soluble* (lipophilic).

Certain kinds of molecules are *not* lipid soluble and therefore cannot penetrate membranes. This group consists of *polar molecules* and *ions.*

Polar Molecules. Polar molecules are molecules with uneven distribution of electrical charge. That is, positive and negative charges within the molecule tend to congregate separately from one another. Water is the classic example. As depicted in Fig. 4.3A, the electrons (negative charges) in the water molecule spend more time in the vicinity of the oxygen atom than in the vicinity of the two hydrogen atoms. As a result, the area around the oxygen atom tends to be negatively charged, whereas the area around the hydrogen atoms tends to be positively charged. Gentamicin (Fig. 4.3B), an antibiotic, is an example of a polar drug. The hydroxyl groups, which attract electrons, give gentamicin its polar nature.

Although polar molecules have an uneven *distribution* of charge, they have no *net* charge. Polar molecules have an equal number of protons (which bear a single positive charge) and electrons (which bear a single negative charge). As a result, the positive and negative charges balance each other exactly, and the molecule as a whole has neither a net positive charge nor a net negative charge. Molecules that *do* bear a net charge are called *ions.* These are discussed in the following section.

In accord with the "like dissolves like" rule, polar molecules will dissolve in *polar* solvents (such as water) but not in *nonpolar* solvents (such as oil). Table sugar provides a common example. Sugar, a polar compound, readily dissolves in water but not in salad oil, butter, and other lipids, which are nonpolar

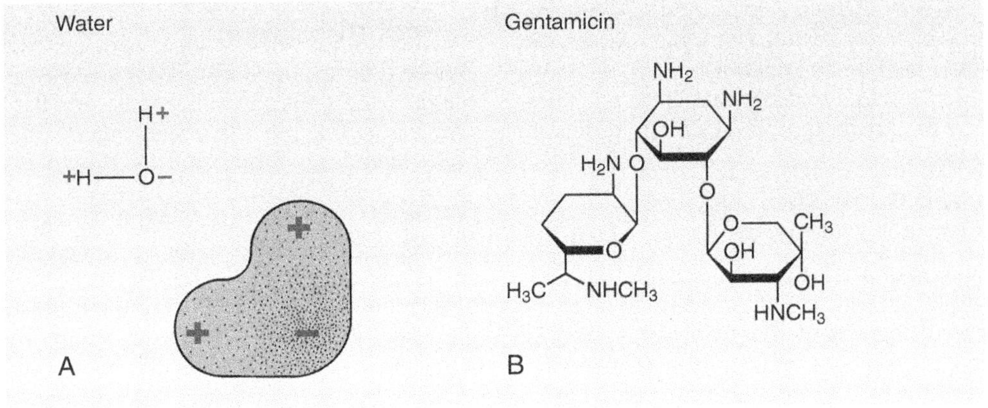

Fig. 4.3 ▪ Polar molecules.
A, Stippling shows the distribution of electrons within the water molecule. As indicated at the lower right, water's electrons spend more time near the oxygen atom than near the hydrogen atoms, making the area near the oxygen atom somewhat negative and the area near the hydrogen atoms more positive. **B,** Gentamicin is a polar drug. The two –OH groups of gentamicin attract electrons, thereby causing the area around these groups to be more negative than the rest of the molecule.

compounds. Just as sugar is unable to dissolve in lipids, polar drugs are unable to dissolve in the lipid bilayer of the cell membrane.

Ions. Ions are defined as molecules that have a *net electrical charge* (either positive or negative). Except for very small molecules, *ions are unable to cross membranes.*

Quaternary Ammonium Compounds

Quaternary ammonium compounds are molecules that contain at least one atom of nitrogen and *carry a positive charge at all times.* The constant charge on these compounds results from atypical bonding to the nitrogen. In most nitrogen-containing compounds, the nitrogen atom bears only three chemical bonds. In contrast, the nitrogen atoms of quaternary ammonium compounds have four chemical bonds. Because of the fourth bond, quaternary ammonium compounds always carry a positive charge. And because of the charge, these compounds are unable to cross most membranes.

Tubocurarine is a representative quaternary ammonium compound. Until recently, purified tubocurarine was employed as a muscle relaxant for surgery and other procedures. A crude preparation—curare—is used by South American Indians as an arrow poison. When employed for hunting, tubocurarine (curare) produces paralysis of the diaphragm and other skeletal muscles, causing death by asphyxiation. Interestingly, even though meat from animals killed with curare is laden with poison, it can be eaten with no ill effect. Why? Because tubocurarine, being a quaternary ammonium compound, cannot cross membranes, and therefore cannot be absorbed from the intestine; as long as it remains in the lumen of the intestine, curare can do no harm. As you might gather, when tubocurarine was used clinically, it could not be administered by mouth. Instead, it had to be injected. Once in the bloodstream, tubocurarine then had ready access to its sites of action on the surface of muscles.

pH-Dependent Ionization

Unlike quaternary ammonium compounds, which always carry a charge, many drugs are either weak organic acids or weak organic bases, which can exist in charged and uncharged forms. Whether a weak acid or base carries a charge is determined by the pH of the surrounding medium.

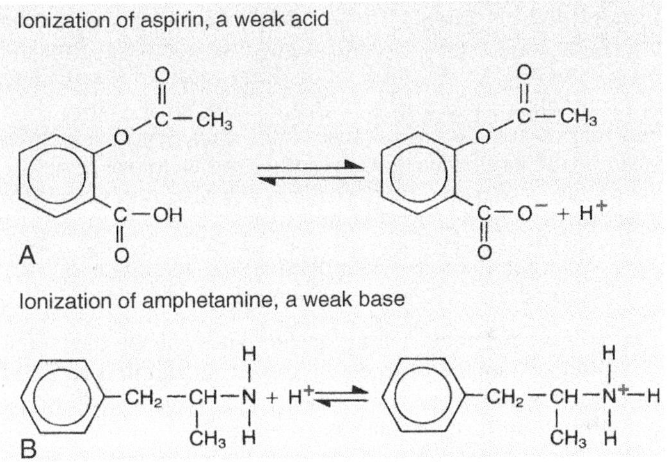

Fig. 4.4 ▪ Ionization of weak acids and weak bases.
The extent of ionization of weak acids **(A)** and weak bases **(B)** depends on the pH of their surroundings. The ionized (charged) forms of acids and bases are not lipid soluble and hence do not readily cross membranes. Note that acids ionize by giving up a proton and that bases ionize by taking on a proton.

A review of acid-base chemistry should help. An acid is defined as a compound that can give up a hydrogen ion (proton). Put another way, *an acid is a proton donor.* A base is defined as a compound that can take on a hydrogen ion. That is, *a base is a proton acceptor.* When an acid gives up its proton, which is positively charged, the acid itself becomes negatively charged. Conversely, when a base accepts a proton, the base becomes positively charged. These reactions are depicted in Fig. 4.4, which shows aspirin as a representative acid and amphetamine as a representative base. Because the process of an acid giving up a proton or a base accepting a proton converts the acid or base into a charged particle (ion), the process for either an acid or a base is termed *ionization.*

The extent to which a weak acid or weak base becomes ionized is determined in part by the pH of its environment. The following rules apply:

- Acids tend to ionize in basic (alkaline) media.
- Bases tend to ionize in acidic media.

To illustrate the importance of pH-dependent ionization, consider the ionization of aspirin. Aspirin, an acid, tends to give up its proton (become ionized) in basic media. Conversely, aspirin keeps its proton and remains nonionized in acidic media. Accordingly, when aspirin is in the stomach (an acidic environment), most of the aspirin molecules remain nonionized. Because aspirin molecules are nonionized in the stomach, they can be absorbed across the membranes that separate the stomach from the bloodstream. When aspirin molecules pass from the stomach into the small intestine, where the environment is relatively alkaline, they change to their ionized form. As a result, absorption of aspirin from the intestine is impeded.

Ion Trapping (pH Partitioning)

Because the ionization of drugs is pH dependent, when the pH of the fluid on one side of a membrane differs from the pH of the fluid on the other side, drug molecules will tend to accumulate on the side where the pH most favors their ionization. Accordingly, because acidic drugs tend to ionize in basic media and because basic drugs tend to ionize in acidic media, *when there is a pH gradient between two sides of a membrane,*

- Acidic drugs will accumulate on the alkaline side.
- Basic drugs will accumulate on the acidic side.

The process whereby a drug accumulates on the side of a membrane where the pH most favors its ionization is referred to as *ion trapping* or *pH partitioning.* Fig. 4.5 shows the steps of ion trapping using aspirin as an example.

Because ion trapping can influence the movement of drugs throughout the body, the process is not simply of academic interest. Rather, ion trapping has practical clinical implications. Knowledge of ion trapping helps us understand drug absorption as well as the movement of drugs to sites of action, metabolism, and excretion. Understanding of ion trapping can be put to practical use when we need to actively influence drug movement. Poisoning is the principal example: By manipulating urinary pH, we can employ ion trapping to draw toxic substances from the blood into the urine, thereby accelerating their removal.

ABSORPTION

Absorption is defined as *the movement of a drug from its site of administration into the blood.* The *rate* of absorption determines how *soon* effects will begin. The *amount* of absorption helps determine how *intense* effects will be.

Factors Affecting Drug Absorption

The rate at which a drug undergoes absorption is influenced by the physical and chemical properties of the drug itself and by physiologic and anatomic factors at the absorption site.

Rate of Dissolution

Before a drug can be absorbed, it must first dissolve. Hence, the rate of dissolution helps determine the rate of absorption. Drugs in formulations that allow rapid dissolution have a faster onset than drugs formulated for slow dissolution.

Surface Area

The surface area available for absorption is a major determinant of the rate of absorption. The larger the surface area, the faster absorption will be. For this reason, orally administered drugs are usually absorbed from the small intestine rather than from the stomach. (Recall that the small intestine, because of its lining of microvilli, has an extremely large surface area, whereas the surface area of the stomach is relatively small.)

Blood Flow

Drugs are absorbed most rapidly from sites where blood flow is high. Why? Because blood containing a newly absorbed drug will be replaced rapidly by drug-free blood, thereby maintaining a large gradient between the concentration of drug outside the blood and the concentration of drug in the blood. The greater the concentration gradient, the more rapid absorption will be.

Lipid Solubility

As a rule, highly lipid-soluble drugs are absorbed more rapidly than drugs whose lipid solubility is low. Why? Because lipid-soluble drugs can readily cross the membranes that separate them from the blood, whereas drugs of low lipid solubility cannot.

pH Partitioning

pH partitioning can influence drug absorption. Absorption will be enhanced when the difference between the pH of plasma and the pH at the site of administration is such that drug molecules will have a greater tendency to be ionized in the plasma.

Characteristics of Commonly Used Routes of Administration

The routes of administration that are used most commonly fall into two major groups: *enteral* (via the gastrointestinal [GI] tract) and *parenteral.* The literal definition of *parenteral* is *outside the GI tract.* However, in common parlance, the term *parenteral* is used to mean *by injection.* The principal parenteral routes are *intravenous, subcutaneous,* and *intramuscular.*

For each of the major routes of administration—oral (PO), intravenous (IV), intramuscular (IM), and subcutaneous (subQ)—the pattern of drug absorption (i.e., the rate and extent of absorption) is unique. Consequently, the route by which a drug is administered will significantly affect both the onset and the intensity of effects. Why do patterns of absorption differ between routes? Because the barriers to absorption associated with each route are different. In the discussion that follows, we examine these barriers and their influence on absorption pattern. In addition, as we discuss each major route, we will consider its clinical advantages and disadvantages. The distinguishing characteristics of the four major routes are summarized in Table 4.1.

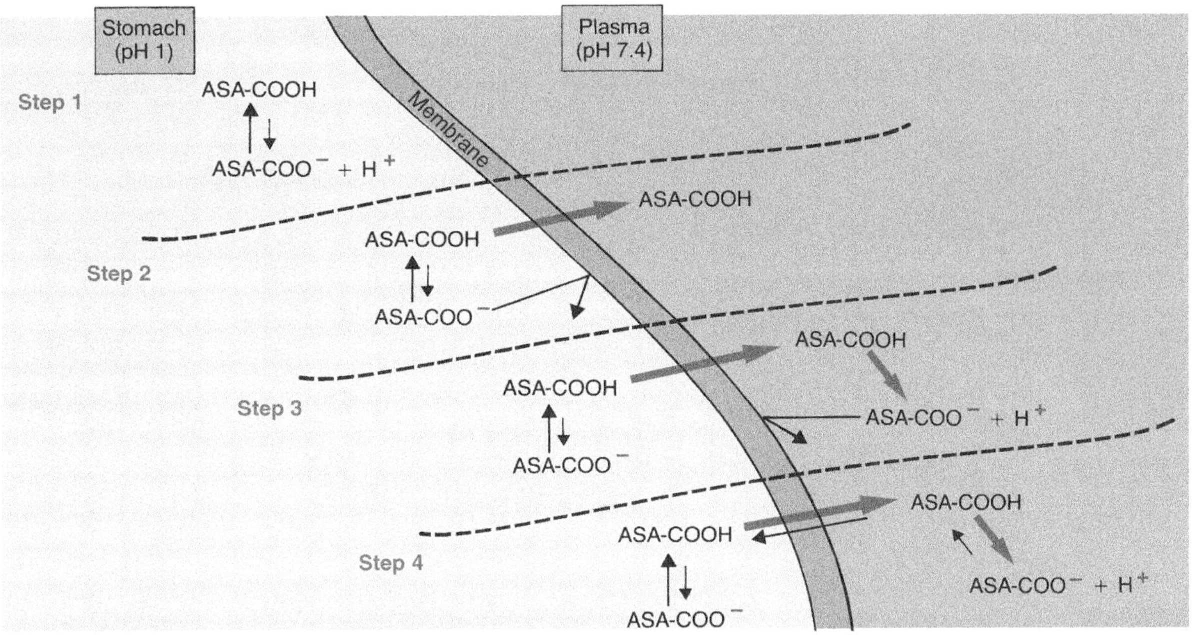

Fig. 4.5 ■ Ion trapping of drugs.
This figure demonstrates ion trapping using aspirin as an example. Because aspirin is an acidic drug, it will be nonionized in acid media and ionized in alkaline media. As indicated, ion trapping causes molecules of orally administered aspirin to move from the acidic (pH 1) environment of the stomach to the more alkaline (pH 7.4) environment of the plasma, thereby causing aspirin to accumulate in the blood. In the figure, aspirin (acetylsalicylic acid) is depicted as ASA with its COOH (carboxylic acid) group attached. ***Step 1:*** Once ingested, ASA dissolves in the stomach contents, after which some ASA molecules give up a proton and become ionized. However, most of the ASA in the stomach remains nonionized, because the stomach is acidic, and acidic drugs don't ionize in acidic media. ***Step 2:*** Because most ASA molecules in the stomach are nonionized (and therefore lipid soluble), most ASA molecules in the stomach can readily cross the membranes that separate the stomach lumen from the plasma. Because of the concentration gradient that exists between the stomach and the plasma, nonionized ASA molecules will begin moving into the plasma. (Note that, because of their charge, ionized ASA molecules cannot leave the stomach.) ***Step 3:*** As the nonionized ASA molecules enter the relatively alkaline environment of the plasma, most give up a proton (H^+) and become negatively charged ions. ASA molecules that become ionized in the plasma cannot diffuse back into the stomach. ***Step 4:*** As the nonionized ASA molecules in the plasma become ionized, more nonionized molecules will pass from the stomach to the plasma to replace them. This movement occurs because the laws of diffusion demand equal concentrations of diffusible substances on both sides of a membrane. Because only the nonionized form of ASA is able to diffuse across the membrane, it is this form that the laws of diffusion will attempt to equilibrate. Nonionized ASA will continue to move from the stomach to the plasma until the amount of ionized ASA in plasma has become large enough to prevent conversion of newly arrived nonionized molecules into the ionized form. Equilibrium will then be established between the plasma and the stomach. At equilibrium, there will be equal amounts of *nonionized* ASA in the stomach and plasma. However, on the plasma side, the amount of ionized ASA will be much larger than on the stomach side. Because there are equal concentrations of nonionized ASA on both sides of the membrane, but a much higher concentration of ionized ASA in the plasma, the total concentration of ASA in plasma will be much higher than that in the stomach.

Intravenous

Barriers to Absorption. When a drug is administered IV, there are no barriers to absorption. Why? Because, with IV administration, absorption is bypassed. Recall that absorption is defined as the movement of a drug from its site of administration into the blood. Because IV administration puts a drug directly into the bloodstream, all barriers are bypassed.

Absorption Pattern. Intravenous administration results in absorption that is both instantaneous and complete. Intravenous absorption is instantaneous in that drug enters the blood directly. Absorption is complete in that virtually all of the administered dose reaches the blood.

Advantages

Rapid Onset. Intravenous administration results in rapid onset of action. Although rapid onset is not always important, it has obvious benefit in emergencies.

Control. Because the entire dose is administered directly into the blood, the nurse has precise control over levels of

TABLE 4.1 ▪ Properties of Major Routes of Drug Administration

Route	Barriers to Absorption	Absorption Pattern	Advantages	Disadvantages
PARENTERAL				
Intravenous (IV)	None (absorption is bypassed)	Instantaneous	Rapid onset, and hence ideal for emergencies Precise control over drug levels Permits use of large fluid volumes Permits use of irritant drugs	Irreversible Expensive Inconvenient Difficult to do, and hence poorly suited for self-administration Risk of fluid overload, infection, and embolism Drug must be water soluble
Intramuscular (IM)	Capillary wall (easy to pass)	Rapid with water-soluble drugs Slow with poorly soluble drugs	Permits use of poorly soluble drugs Permits use of depot preparations	Possible discomfort Inconvenient Potential for injury
Subcutaneous (subQ)	Same as IM	Same as IM	Same as IM	Same as IM
ENTERAL				
Oral (PO)	Epithelial lining of GI tract; capillary wall	Slow and variable	Easy Convenient Inexpensive Ideal for self-medication Potentially reversible, and hence safer than parenteral routes	Variability Inactivation of some drugs by gastric acid and digestive enzymes Possible nausea and vomiting from local irritation Patient must be conscious and cooperative

drug in the blood. This contrasts with the other major routes of administration, and especially with oral administration, in which the amount absorbed is less predictable.

Permits Use of Large Fluid Volumes. The IV route is the only parenteral route that permits the use of large volumes of fluid. Some drugs that require parenteral administration are poorly soluble in water, and hence must be dissolved in a large volume. Because of the physical limitations presented by soft tissues (e.g., muscle, subcutaneous tissue), injection of large volumes at these sites is not feasible. In contrast, the amount of fluid that can be infused into a vein, although limited, is nonetheless relatively large.

Permits Use of Irritant Drugs. Certain drugs, because of their irritant properties, can only be given IV. A number of anticancer drugs, for example, are very chemically reactive. If present in high concentrations, these agents can cause severe local injury. However, when administered through a freely flowing IV line, these drugs are rapidly diluted in the blood, thereby minimizing the risk of injury.

Disadvantages

High Cost, Difficulty, and Inconvenience. Intravenous administration is expensive, difficult, and inconvenient. The cost of IV administration sets and their setup charges can be substantial. Also, setting up an IV line takes time and special training. Because of the difficulty involved, most patients are unable to self-administer IV drugs and therefore must depend on a healthcare professional. In contrast, oral administration is easy, convenient, and cheap.

Irreversibility. More important than cost or convenience, IV administration can be *dangerous.* Once a drug has been injected, there is no turning back: The drug is in the body and cannot be retrieved. Hence, if the dose is excessive, avoiding harm may be challenging or impossible.

To minimize risk, *most* IV drugs should be injected slowly (over 1 minute or more). Because all of the blood in the body is circulated about once every minute, by injecting a drug over a 1-minute interval, the drug is diluted in the largest volume of blood possible.

Performing IV injections slowly has the additional advantage of reducing the risk of toxicity to the central nervous system (CNS). When a drug is injected into the antecubital vein of the arm, it takes about 15 seconds to reach the brain. Consequently, if the dose is sufficient to cause CNS toxicity, signs of toxicity may become apparent 15 seconds after starting the injection. If the injection is being done slowly (e.g., over a 1-minute interval), only 25% of the total dose will have been administered when signs of toxicity appear. If administration is discontinued immediately, adverse effects will be much less than they would have been had the entire dose been given.

Fluid Overload. When drugs are administered in a large volume, fluid overload can occur. This can be a significant problem for patients with hypertension, kidney disease, or heart failure.

Infection. Infection can occur from injecting a contaminated drug or from improper technique. Fortunately, the risk of infection is much lower today than it was before the development of modern techniques for sterilizing drugs intended for IV use and the institution of strict standards for the administration of drugs that are given intravenously.

Embolism. Intravenous administration carries a risk of embolism (blood vessel blockage at a site distant from the point of administration). Embolism can be caused in several ways. First, insertion of an IV needle can injure the venous wall, leading to formation of a thrombus (clot); embolism can result if the clot breaks loose and becomes lodged in another vessel. Second, injection of hypotonic or hypertonic fluids can destroy red blood cells; the debris from these cells can produce embolism.

Finally, injection of drugs that are not fully dissolved can cause embolism. Particles of undissolved drug are like small grains of sand, which can become embedded in blood vessels and cause blockage. Because of the risk of embolism, you should check IV solutions before administration to ensure that drugs are in solution. If the fluid is cloudy or contains particles, the drug is not dissolved and must not be administered.

The Importance of Reading Labels. Not all formulations of the same drug are appropriate for IV administration. Accordingly, it is essential to read the label before giving a drug IV. Two examples illustrate why this is so important. The first is insulin. Several types of insulin are now available (e.g., insulin aspart, regular insulin, NPH insulin, insulin detemir). Some of these formulations can be given IV; others cannot. Aspart and regular insulin, for example, are safe for IV use. In contrast, NPH and detemir insulin are safe for subQ use, but they could be fatal if given IV. By checking the label, inadvertent IV injection of particulate insulin can be avoided.

Epinephrine provides our second example of why you should read the label before giving a drug IV. Epinephrine, which stimulates the cardiovascular system, can be injected by several routes (IM, IV, subQ, intracardiac, intraspinal). Be aware, however, that a solution prepared for use by one route will differ in concentration from a solution prepared for use by other routes. For example, whereas solutions intended for *subcutaneous* administration are *concentrated,* solutions intended for *intravenous* use are *dilute.* If a solution prepared for subQ use were to be inadvertently administered IV, the result could prove *fatal.* (Intravenous administration of concentrated epinephrine could overstimulate the heart and blood vessels, causing severe hypertension, cerebral hemorrhage, stroke, and death.) The take-home message is that simply giving the *right drug* is not sufficient; you must also be sure that the formulation and concentration are *appropriate for the intended route.*

Intramuscular

Barriers to Absorption. When a drug is injected IM, the only barrier to absorption is the *capillary wall.* In capillary beds that serve muscles and most other tissues, there are relatively large spaces between the cells that compose the capillary wall. Drugs can pass through these spaces with ease, and need not cross cell membranes to enter the bloodstream. Accordingly, like IV administration, IM administration presents no significant barrier to absorption.

Absorption Pattern. Drugs administered IM may be absorbed rapidly or slowly. The rate of absorption is determined largely by two factors: (1) water solubility of the drug, and (2) blood flow to the site of injection. Drugs that are highly soluble in water will be absorbed rapidly (within 10 to 30 minutes), whereas drugs that are poorly soluble will be absorbed slowly. Similarly, absorption will be rapid from sites where blood flow is high, and slow where blood flow is low.

Advantages. The IM route can be used for parenteral administration of *poorly soluble drugs.* Recall that drugs must be dissolved if they are to be administered IV. Consequently, the IV route cannot be used for poorly soluble compounds. In contrast, because little harm will come from depositing a suspension of undissolved drug in the interstitial space of muscle tissue, the IM route is acceptable for drugs whose water solubility is poor.

A second advantage of the IM route is that we can use it to administer *depot preparations* (preparations from which the drug is absorbed slowly over an extended time). Depending on the depot formulation, the effects of a single injection may persist for days, weeks, or even months. For example, *benzathine penicillin G,* a depot preparation of penicillin, can release therapeutically effective amounts of penicillin for a month following a single IM injection. In contrast, a single IM injection of penicillin G itself would be absorbed and excreted in less than 1 day. The obvious advantage of depot preparations is that they can greatly reduce the number of injections required during long-term therapy.

Disadvantages. The major drawbacks of IM administration are discomfort and inconvenience. Intramuscular injection of some preparations can be painful. Also, IM injections can cause local tissue injury and possibly nerve damage (if the injection is done improperly). Lastly, because of bleeding risk, IM injections cannot be used for patients receiving anticoagulant therapy. Like all other forms of parenteral administration, IM injections are less convenient than oral administration.

Subcutaneous

The pharmacokinetics of subQ administration are nearly identical to those of IM administration. As with IM administration, there are no significant barriers to absorption: Once a drug has been injected subQ, it readily enters the blood by passing through the spaces between cells of the capillary wall. As with IM administration, blood flow and drug solubility are the major determinants of how fast absorption takes place. Because of the similarities between subQ and IM administration, these routes have similar advantages (suitability for poorly soluble drugs and depot preparations) and similar drawbacks (discomfort, inconvenience, potential for injury).

Oral

In the discussion that follows, the abbreviation PO is used in reference to oral administration. This abbreviation stands for *per os,* a Latin phrase meaning *by way of the mouth.*

Barriers to Absorption. Following oral administration, drugs may be absorbed from the stomach, the intestine, or both. In either case, there are two barriers to cross: (1) the layer of *epithelial cells* that lines the GI tract, and (2) the *capillary wall.* Because the walls of the capillaries that serve the GI tract offer no significant resistance to absorption, the major barrier to absorption is the GI epithelium. To cross this layer of tightly packed cells, drugs must pass *through* cells rather than between them. For some drugs, intestinal absorption may be *reduced* by *P-glycoprotein,* a transporter that can pump certain drugs *out* of epithelial cells back into the intestinal lumen.

Absorption Pattern. Because of multiple factors, the rate and extent of drug absorption following oral administration can be *highly variable.* Factors that can influence absorption include (1) solubility and stability of the drug, (2) gastric and intestinal pH, (3) gastric emptying time, (4) food in the gut, (5) coadministration of other drugs, and (6) special coatings on the drug preparation.

Drug Movement Following Absorption. Before proceeding, we need to quickly review what happens to drugs following their absorption from the GI tract. As depicted in Fig. 4.6, drugs absorbed from all sites along the GI tract (except the oral mucosa and the distal segment of the rectum) must pass through the liver (via the portal blood) before they can

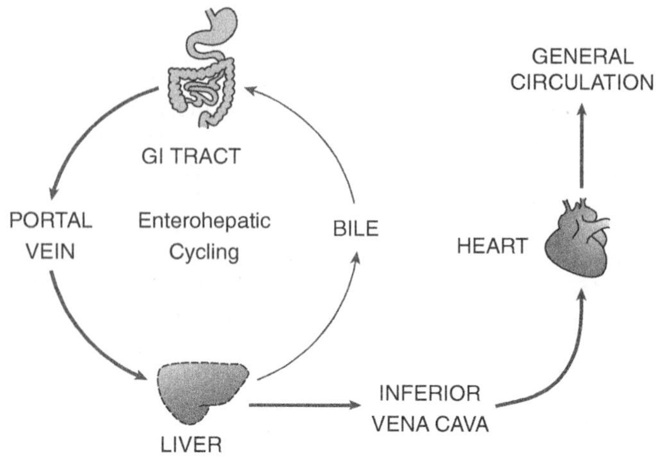

Fig. 4.6 ■ Movement of drugs following GI absorption. All drugs absorbed from sites along the GI tract—stomach, small intestine, and large intestine (but not the oral mucosa or distal rectum)—must go through the liver, via the portal vein, on their way to the heart and then the general circulation. For some drugs, passage is uneventful. Others undergo extensive hepatic metabolism. And still others undergo *enterohepatic recirculation,* a repeating cycle in which a drug moves from the liver into the duodenum (via the bile duct) and then back to the liver (via the portal blood). As discussed in the text under *Enterohepatic Recirculation,* the process is limited to drugs that have first undergone hepatic glucuronidation.

reach the general circulation. For many drugs, this passage is uneventful: They go through the liver, enter the inferior vena cava, and eventually reach the general circulation. Other drugs undergo extensive hepatic metabolism. And still others may undergo *enterohepatic recirculation,* a repeating cycle in which a drug moves from the liver into the duodenum (via the bile duct) and then back to the liver (via the portal blood). This cycle is discussed further under *Enterohepatic Recirculation.*

Advantages. Oral administration is easy and convenient. This makes it the preferred route for self-medication.

Although absorption of oral drugs can be highly variable, this route is still *safer than injection.* With oral administration, there is no risk of fluid overload, infection, or embolism. Furthermore, because oral administration is potentially reversible, whereas injections are not, oral administration is safer. Recall that with parenteral administration there is no turning back: Once a drug has been injected, there is little we can do to prevent absorption and subsequent effects. In contrast, if need be, there are steps we can take to prevent absorption following inappropriate oral administration. For example, we can decrease absorption by giving activated charcoal, a compound that adsorbs (soaks up) drugs while they are still in the GI tract. Once drugs are adsorbed onto the charcoal, they cannot be absorbed into the bloodstream. This ability to prevent the absorption of orally administered drugs gives PO medications a safety factor that is unavailable with drugs given by injection.

Disadvantages

Variability. The major disadvantage of PO therapy is that absorption can be highly variable. That is, a drug administered to patient A may be absorbed rapidly and completely, whereas the same drug given to patient B may be absorbed slowly and incompletely. This variability makes it difficult to control the concentration of a drug at its sites of action, and therefore makes it difficult to control the onset, intensity, and duration of responses.

Inactivation. Oral administration can lead to inactivation of certain drugs. Penicillin G, for example, can't be taken orally because it would be destroyed by stomach acid. Similarly, insulin can't be taken orally because it would be destroyed by digestive enzymes. Other drugs (e.g., nitroglycerin) undergo extensive inactivation as they pass through the liver, a phenomenon known as the *first-pass effect* (see *Special Considerations in Drug Metabolism*).

Patient Requirements. Oral drug administration requires a conscious, cooperative patient. Drugs cannot be administered PO to comatose individuals or to individuals who, for whatever reason (e.g., psychosis, seizure, obstinacy, nausea), are unable or unwilling to swallow medication.

Local Irritation. Some oral preparations cause local irritation of the GI tract, which can result in discomfort, nausea, and vomiting.

Comparing Oral Administration With Parenteral Administration

Because of ease, convenience, and relative safety, *oral administration is generally preferred to parenteral administration.* However, there *are* situations in which parenteral administration may be superior:

- Emergencies that require rapid onset of drug action.
- Situations in which plasma drug levels must be tightly controlled. (Because of variable absorption, oral administration does not permit tight control of drug levels.)
- Treatment with drugs that would be destroyed by gastric acidity, digestive enzymes, or hepatic enzymes if given orally (e.g., insulin, penicillin G, nitroglycerin).
- Treatment with drugs that would cause severe local injury if administered by mouth (e.g., certain anticancer agents).
- Treating a systemic disorder with drugs that cannot cross membranes (e.g., quaternary ammonium compounds).
- Treating conditions for which the prolonged effects of a depot preparation might be desirable.
- Treating patients who cannot or will not take drugs orally.

Pharmaceutical Preparations for Oral Administration

There are several kinds of "packages" (formulations) into which a drug can be put for oral administration. Three such formulations—*tablets, enteric-coated preparations,* and *sustained-release preparations*—are discussed in the sections that follow.

Before we discuss drug formulations, it will be helpful to define two terms: *chemical equivalence* and *bioavailability.* Drug preparations are considered *chemically equivalent* if they contain the same amount of the identical chemical compound (drug). Preparations are considered equal in *bioavailability* if the drug they contain is absorbed at the same rate and to the same extent. Please note that it is possible for two formulations of the same drug to be chemically equivalent while differing in bioavailability.

Tablets

A tablet is a mixture of a drug plus binders and fillers, all of which have been compressed together. Tablets made by different manufacturers may differ in their rates of disintegration and dissolution, causing differences in bioavailability. As a result, two tablets that contain the same amount of the same drug may differ with respect to onset and intensity of effects.

Enteric-Coated Preparations

Enteric-coated preparations consist of drugs that have been covered with a material designed to dissolve in the intestine but not the stomach. Materials used for enteric coatings include fatty acids, waxes, and shellac. Because enteric-coated preparations release their contents into the intestine and not the stomach, these preparations are employed for two general purposes: (1) to protect drugs from acid and pepsin in the stomach, and (2) to protect the stomach from drugs that can cause gastric discomfort.

The primary disadvantage of enteric-coated preparations is that absorption can be even more variable than with standard tablets. Because gastric emptying time can vary from minutes up to 12 hours, and because enteric-coated preparations cannot be absorbed until they leave the stomach, variations in gastric emptying time can alter time of onset. Furthermore, enteric coatings sometimes fail to dissolve, thereby allowing medication to pass through the GI tract without being absorbed at all.

Sustained-Release Preparations

Sustained-release formulations are capsules filled with tiny spheres that contain the actual drug; the individual spheres have coatings that dissolve at variable rates. Because some spheres dissolve more slowly than others, the drug is released steadily throughout the day. The primary advantage of sustained-release preparations is that they permit a reduction in the number of daily doses. These formulations have the additional advantage of producing relatively steady drug levels over an extended time (much like giving a drug by infusion). The major disadvantages of sustained-release formulations are high cost and the potential for variable absorption.

Additional Routes of Administration

Drugs can be administered by a number of routes in addition to those already discussed. Drugs can be applied *topically* for local therapy of the skin, eyes, ears, nose, mouth, rectum, and vagina. In a few cases, topical agents (e.g., nitroglycerin, nicotine, testosterone, estrogen) are formulated for *transdermal* absorption into the systemic circulation. Some drugs are *inhaled* to elicit local effects in the lungs, especially in the treatment of asthma. Other inhalational agents (e.g., volatile anesthetics, oxygen) are used for their systemic effects. *Rectal suppositories* may be employed for local effects or for effects throughout the body. *Vaginal suppositories* may be employed to treat local disorders. For management of some conditions, drugs must be given by *direct injection into a specific site* (e.g., heart, joints, nerves, CNS). The unique characteristics of these routes are addressed throughout the book as we discuss specific drugs that employ them.

DISTRIBUTION

Distribution is defined as drug movement from the blood to the interstitial space of tissues and from there into cells. Drug distribution is determined by three major factors: blood flow to tissues, the ability of a drug to exit the vascular system, and, to a lesser extent, the ability of a drug to enter cells.

Blood Flow to Tissues

In the first phase of distribution, drugs are carried by the blood to the tissues and organs of the body. The rate at which drugs are delivered to a particular tissue is determined by blood flow to that tissue. Because most tissues are well perfused, regional blood flow is rarely a limiting factor in drug distribution.

There are two pathologic conditions—abscesses and tumors—in which low regional blood flow can affect drug therapy. An abscess is a pus-filled pocket of infection that has no internal blood vessels. Because abscesses lack a blood supply, antibiotics cannot reach the bacteria within. Accordingly, if drug therapy is to be effective, the abscess must first be surgically drained.

Solid tumors have a limited blood supply. Although blood flow to the outer regions of tumors is relatively high, blood flow becomes progressively lower toward the core. As a result, it may not be possible to achieve high drug levels deep inside tumors. Limited blood flow is a major reason why solid tumors are resistant to drug therapy.

Exiting the Vascular System

After a drug has been delivered to an organ or tissue via the blood, the next step is to exit the vasculature. Because most drugs do not produce their effects within the blood, the ability to leave the vascular system is an important determinant of drug actions. Exiting the vascular system is also necessary for drugs to undergo metabolism and excretion. Drugs in the vascular system leave the blood at capillary beds.

Typical Capillary Beds

Most capillary beds offer no resistance to the departure of drugs. Why? Because, in most tissues, drugs can leave the vasculature simply by passing through pores in the capillary wall. Because drugs pass *between* capillary cells rather than *through* them, movement into the interstitial space is not impeded. The exit of drugs from a typical capillary bed is depicted in Fig. 4.7.

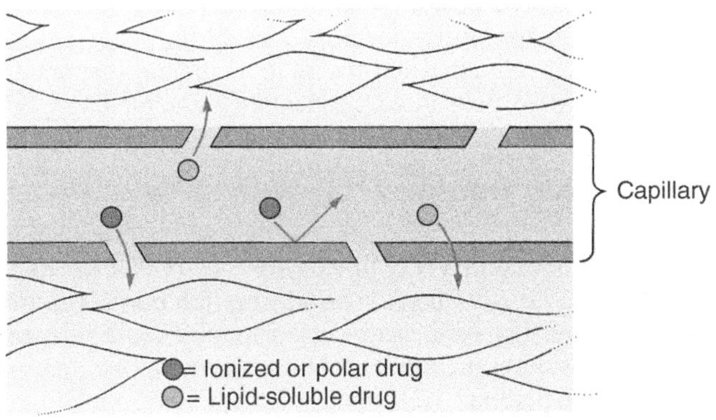

Fig. 4.7 ■ Drug movement at typical capillary beds. In most capillary beds, "large" gaps exist between the cells that compose the capillary wall. Drugs and other molecules can pass freely into and out of the bloodstream through these gaps. As illustrated, lipid-soluble compounds can also pass directly through the cells of the capillary wall.

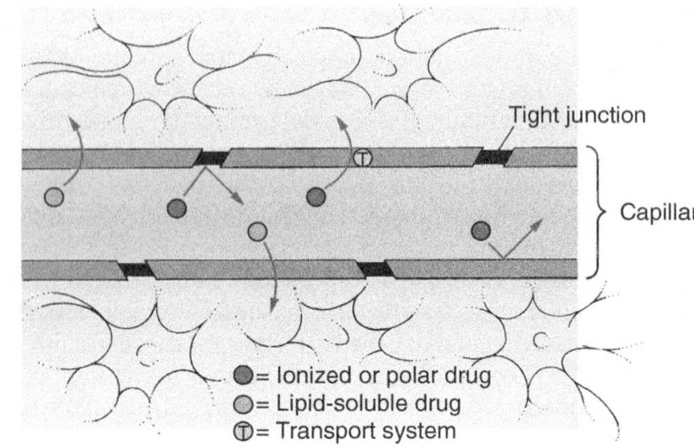

Fig. 4.8 ■ Drug movement across the blood-brain barrier. Tight junctions between cells that compose the walls of capillaries in the CNS prevent drugs from passing between cells to exit the vascular system. Consequently, to reach sites of action within the brain, a drug must pass directly through cells of the capillary wall. To do this, the drug must be lipid soluble or be able to use an existing transport system.

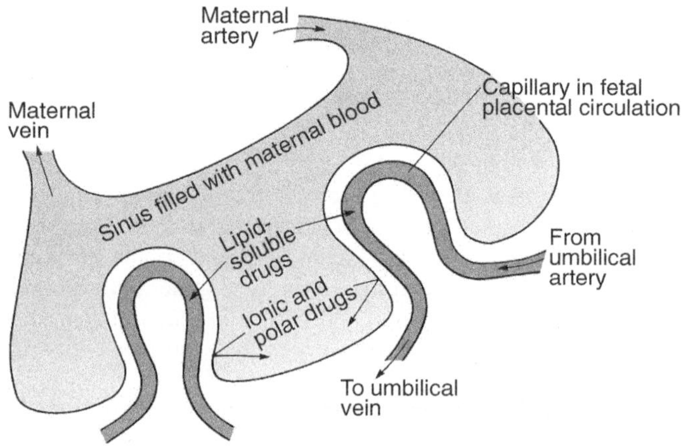

Fig. 4.9 ■ Placental drug transfer. To enter the fetal circulation, drugs must cross membranes of the maternal and fetal vascular systems. Lipid-soluble drugs can readily cross these membranes and enter the fetal blood, whereas ions and polar molecules are prevented from reaching the fetal blood.

The Blood-Brain Barrier

The term *blood-brain barrier* (BBB) refers to the unique anatomy of capillaries in the CNS. As shown in Fig. 4.8, there are *tight junctions* between the cells that compose the walls of most capillaries in the CNS. These junctions are so tight that they prevent drug passage. Consequently, to leave the blood and reach sites of action within the brain, a drug must be able to pass *through* cells of the capillary wall. Only drugs that are *lipid soluble* or have a *transport system* can cross the BBB to a significant degree.

Recent evidence indicates that, in addition to tight junctions, the BBB has another protective component: *P-glycoprotein.* As noted earlier, P-glycoprotein is a transporter that pumps a variety of drugs out of cells. In capillaries of the CNS, P-glycoprotein pumps drugs back into the blood, and thereby limits their access to the brain.

The presence of the BBB is a mixed blessing. The good news is that the barrier protects the brain from injury by potentially toxic substances. The bad news is that the barrier can be a significant obstacle to therapy of CNS disorders. The barrier can, for example, impede access of antibiotics to CNS infections.

The BBB is not fully developed at birth. As a result, newborns have heightened sensitivity to medicines that act on the brain. Likewise, neonates are especially vulnerable to CNS toxicity.

Placental Drug Transfer

The membranes of the placenta separate the maternal circulation from the fetal circulation (Fig. 4.9). *However, the membranes of the placenta do NOT constitute an absolute barrier to the passage of drugs.* The same factors that determine the movement of drugs across other membranes determine the movement of drugs across the placenta. Accordingly, lipid-soluble, nonionized compounds readily pass from the maternal bloodstream into the blood of the fetus. In contrast, compounds that are ionized, highly polar, or protein bound (see the following discussion) are largely excluded—as are drugs that are substrates for P-glycoprotein, a transporter that can pump a variety of drugs out of placental cells into the maternal blood.

Drugs that have the ability to cross the placenta can cause serious harm. Some compounds can cause birth defects, ranging from low birth weight to physical anomalies and alterations in mental aptitude. If a pregnant woman is a habitual user of opioids (e.g., heroin), her child will be born drug dependent, and hence will need treatment to prevent withdrawal. The use of respiratory depressants (anesthetics and analgesics) during delivery can depress respiration in the neonate. Accordingly, infants exposed to respiratory depressants must be monitored very closely until breathing has normalized.

Protein Binding

Drugs can form reversible bonds with various proteins in the body. Of all the proteins with which drugs can bind, *plasma albumin* is the most important, being the most abundant protein in plasma. Like other proteins, albumin is a large molecule, having a molecular weight of 69,000 daltons. Because of its size, *albumin always remains in the bloodstream.* Albumin is too large to squeeze through pores in the capillary wall, and no transport system exists by which it might leave.

Fig. 4.10A depicts the binding of drug molecules to albumin. Note that the drug molecules are much smaller than albumin. (The molecular mass of the average drug is about 300 to 500 daltons compared with 69,000 daltons for albumin.) As indicated by the two-way arrows, binding between albumin and drugs is *reversible.* Hence, drugs may be *bound* or *unbound* (free).

Even though a drug can bind albumin, only some molecules will be bound at any moment. The percentage of drug molecules that are bound is determined by the strength of the attraction between albumin and the drug. For example, the attraction between albumin and warfarin (an anticoagulant) is strong, causing nearly all (99%) of the warfarin molecules in plasma to be bound, leaving only 1% free. For gentamicin (an antibiotic), the ratio of bound to free is quite different; because the attraction between gentamicin and albumin is relatively weak, less than 10% of the gentamicin molecules in plasma are bound, leaving more than 90% free.

An important consequence of protein binding is restriction of drug distribution. Because albumin is too large to leave the

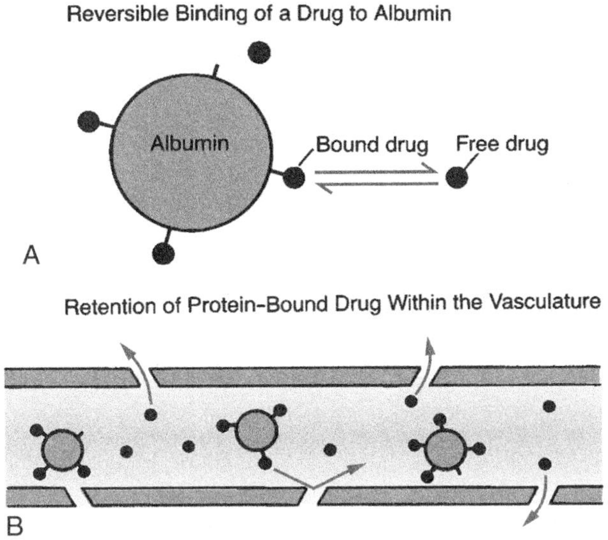

Fig. 4.10 ▪ Protein binding of drugs.
A, Albumin is the most prevalent protein in plasma and the most important of the proteins to which drugs bind. **B,** Only unbound (free) drug molecules can leave the vascular system. Bound molecules are too large to fit through the pores in the capillary wall.

bloodstream, drug molecules that are bound to albumin cannot leave either (Fig. 4.10B). As a result, bound molecules cannot reach their sites of action or undergo metabolism or excretion until the drug-protein bond is broken. This prolongs the distribution phase and increases the drug's half-life. (The concept of drug half-life is discussed later in this chapter.)

In addition to restricting drug distribution, protein binding can be a source of drug interactions. As suggested by Fig. 4.10A, each molecule of albumin has only a few sites to which drug molecules can bind. Because the number of binding sites is limited, drugs with the ability to bind albumin will compete with one another for those sites. As a result, one drug can displace another from albumin, causing the free concentration of the displaced drug to rise. By increasing levels of free drug, competition for binding can increase the intensity of drug responses. If plasma drug levels rise sufficiently, toxicity can result.

Entering Cells

Some drugs must enter cells to reach their sites of action, and practically all drugs must enter cells to undergo metabolism and excretion. The factors that determine the ability of a drug to cross cell membranes are the same factors that determine the passage of drugs across all other membranes, namely, lipid solubility, the presence of a transport system, or both.

As discussed in Chapter 5, many drugs produce their effects by binding with receptors located on the external surface of the cell membrane. Obviously, these drugs do not need to cross the cell membrane to act.

METABOLISM

Drug metabolism, also known as *biotransformation,* is defined as *the chemical alteration of drug structure.* Most drug metabolism takes place in the liver.

Hepatic Drug-Metabolizing Enzymes

Most drug metabolism that takes place in the liver is performed by the *hepatic microsomal enzyme system,* also known as the *P450 system.* The term *P450* refers to *cytochrome P450,* a key component of this enzyme system.

It is important to appreciate that cytochrome P450 is not a single molecular entity, but rather a group of 12 closely related enzyme families. Three of the cytochrome P450 (CYP) families—designated CYP1, CYP2, and CYP3—metabolize drugs. The other nine families metabolize endogenous compounds (e.g., steroids, fatty acids). Each of the three P450 families that metabolize drugs is itself composed of multiple forms, each of which metabolizes only certain drugs. To identify the individual forms of cytochrome P450, designations such as CYP1A2, CYP2D6, and CYP3A4 are used to indicate specific members of the CYP1, CYP2, and CYP3 families, respectively.

Hepatic microsomal enzymes are capable of catalyzing a wide variety of reactions. Some of these reactions are illustrated in Fig. 4.11. As these examples indicate, drug metabolism doesn't always result in the breakdown of drugs into smaller molecules; drug metabolism can also result in the synthesis of a molecule that is larger than the parent drug.

Therapeutic Consequences of Drug Metabolism

Drug metabolism has six possible consequences of therapeutic significance:

- Accelerated renal excretion of drugs
- Drug inactivation
- Increased therapeutic action
- Activation of "prodrugs"
- Increased toxicity
- Decreased toxicity

The reactions shown in Fig. 4.11 illustrate these outcomes.

Accelerated Renal Drug Excretion

The most important consequence of drug metabolism is promotion of renal drug excretion. As discussed under *Renal Drug Excretion* later in this chapter, the kidneys, which are the major organs of drug excretion, are unable to excrete drugs that are highly lipid soluble. Hence, by converting lipid-soluble drugs into more hydrophilic (water-soluble) forms, metabolic conversion can accelerate renal excretion of many agents. For certain highly lipid-soluble drugs (e.g., thiopental), complete renal excretion would take years were it not for their conversion into more hydrophilic forms.

What kinds of metabolic transformations enhance excretion? Two important mechanisms are shown in Fig. 4.11, panels *1A* and *1B.* In panel *1A,* a simple structural change (addition of a hydroxyl group) converts pentobarbital into a more polar (less lipid-soluble) form. In panel *1B,* a highly lipophilic drug (phenytoin) is converted into a highly hydrophilic form by undergoing *glucuronidation,* a process in which a hydrophilic glucose derivative (glucuronic acid) is attached to phenytoin. As a result of glucuronidation, phenytoin is rendered much more water soluble, and hence can be rapidly excreted by the kidneys.

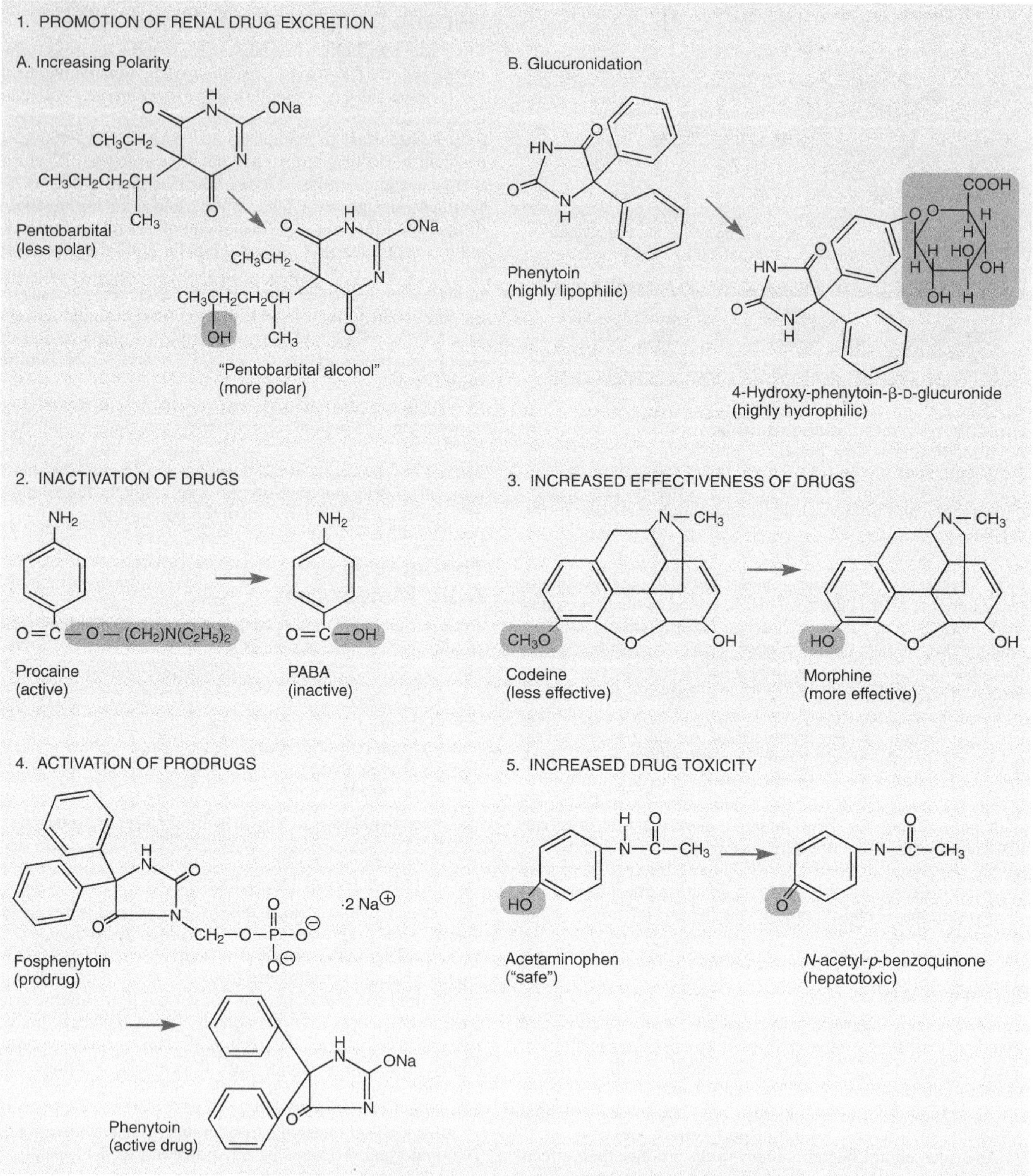

Fig. 4.11 ▪ Therapeutic consequences of drug metabolism.

It should be noted that not all glucuronides are excreted by the kidneys. In many cases, glucuronidated drugs are secreted into the bile and then transported to the duodenum (via the bile duct), after which they can undergo excretion in the feces. However, in some cases, secretion into the bile can result in *enterohepatic recirculation* (discussed later in this chapter).

Drug Inactivation

Drug metabolism can convert pharmacologically active compounds to inactive forms. This process is illustrated by the conversion of procaine (a local anesthetic) into *para*-aminobenzoic acid (PABA), an inactive metabolite (see Fig. 4.11, panel *2*).

Increased Therapeutic Action

Metabolism can increase the effectiveness of some drugs. This concept is illustrated by the conversion of codeine into morphine (see Fig. 4.11, panel *3*). The analgesic activity of morphine is so much greater than that of codeine that formation of morphine may account for virtually all the pain relief that occurs following codeine administration.

Activation of Prodrugs

A *prodrug* is a compound that is pharmacologically inactive as administered and then undergoes conversion to its active form via metabolism. Activation of a prodrug is illustrated by the metabolic conversion of fosphenytoin to phenytoin (see Fig. 4.11, panel *4*).

Increased or Decreased Toxicity

By converting drugs into inactive forms, metabolism can decrease toxicity. Conversely, metabolism can increase the potential for harm by converting relatively safe compounds into forms that are toxic. Increased toxicity is illustrated by the conversion of acetaminophen [Tylenol, others] into a hepatotoxic metabolite (see Fig. 4.11, panel *5*). It is this product of metabolism, and not acetaminophen itself, that causes injury when acetaminophen is taken in overdose.

Special Considerations in Drug Metabolism

Several factors can influence the rate at which drugs are metabolized. These must be accounted for in drug therapy.

Age

The drug-metabolizing capacity of infants is limited. The liver does not develop its full capacity to metabolize drugs until about 1 year after birth. During the time prior to hepatic maturation, infants are especially sensitive to drugs, and care must be taken to avoid injury. Similarly, the ability of older adults to metabolize drugs is commonly decreased. Drug dosages may need to be reduced to prevent drug toxicity.

Induction and Inhibition of Drug-Metabolizing Enzymes

Drugs may be P450 substrates, P450 enzyme inducers, or P450 enzyme inhibitors. Often a drug may have more than one property. For example, a drug may be both a substrate and an inducer.

Drugs that are metabolized by P450 hepatic enzymes are substrates. The rate at which substrates are metabolized is affected by drugs that act as P450 inducers or inhibitors.

Drugs that act on the liver to increase rates of drug metabolism are inducers. This process of stimulating enzyme synthesis is known as *induction*. As the rate of drug metabolism increases, plasma drug levels fall.

Induction of drug-metabolizing enzymes can have two therapeutic consequences. First, if the inducer is also a substrate, by stimulating the liver to produce more drug-metabolizing enzymes, the drug can increase the rate of its own metabolism, thereby necessitating an increase in its dosage to maintain therapeutic effects. Second, induction of drug-metabolizing enzymes can accelerate the metabolism of other substrates used concurrently, necessitating an increase in their dosages.

Drugs that act on the liver to decrease rates of drug metabolism are called *inhibitors*. This process is known as *inhibition*. These drugs also create therapeutic consequences because slower metabolism can cause an increase in active drug accumulation. This can lead to an increase in adverse effects and toxicity.

First-Pass Effect

The term *first-pass effect* refers to the rapid hepatic inactivation of certain oral drugs. When drugs are absorbed from the GI tract, they are carried directly to the liver via the hepatic portal vein. If the capacity of the liver to metabolize a drug is extremely high, that drug can be completely inactivated on its first pass through the liver. As a result, no therapeutic effects can occur. To circumvent the first-pass effect, a drug that undergoes rapid hepatic metabolism is often administered parenterally. This permits the drug to temporarily bypass the liver, thereby allowing it to reach therapeutic levels in the systemic circulation.

Nitroglycerin is the classic example of a drug that undergoes such rapid hepatic metabolism that it is largely without effect following oral administration. However, when administered sublingually (under the tongue), nitroglycerin is very active. Sublingual administration is effective because it permits nitroglycerin to be absorbed directly into the systemic circulation. Once in the circulation, the drug is carried to its sites of action before passage through the liver. Hence, therapeutic action can be exerted before the drug is exposed to hepatic enzymes.

Nutritional Status

Hepatic drug-metabolizing enzymes require a number of cofactors to function. In the malnourished patient, these cofactors may be deficient, causing drug metabolism to be compromised.

Competition Between Drugs

When two drugs are metabolized by the same metabolic pathway, they may compete with each other for metabolism, and may, thereby, decrease the rate at which one or both agents are metabolized. If metabolism is depressed enough, a drug can accumulate to dangerous levels.

Enterohepatic Recirculation

As noted earlier and depicted in Fig. 4.7, enterohepatic recirculation is a repeating cycle in which a drug is transported from the liver into the duodenum (via the bile duct) and then back to the liver (via the portal blood). It is important to note, however, that only certain drugs are affected. Specifically, the process is limited to drugs that have undergone *glucuronidation* (see Fig. 4.11, panel *1B*). Following glucuronidation, these drugs can enter the bile and then pass to the duodenum. Once there, they can be hydrolyzed by intestinal beta-glucuronidase, an enzyme that breaks the bond between the original drug and the glucuronide moiety, thereby releasing the free drug. Because the free drug is more lipid soluble than the glucuronidated form, the free drug can undergo reabsorption across the intestinal wall, followed by transport back to the liver, where the cycle can start again. Because of enterohepatic recycling, drugs can remain in the body much longer than they otherwise would.

Some glucuronidated drugs do not undergo extensive recycling. Glucuronidated drugs that are more stable to hydrolysis will be excreted intact in the feces, without significant recirculation.

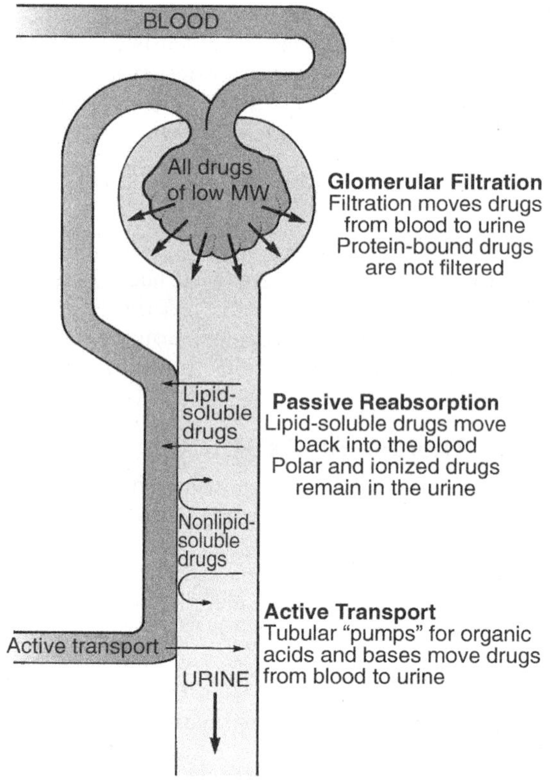

Fig. 4.12 ■ Renal drug excretion. *MW,* Molecular weight.

EXCRETION

Drug excretion is defined as *the removal of drugs from the body.* Drugs and their metabolites can exit the body in urine, bile, sweat, saliva, breast milk, and expired air. The most important organ for drug excretion is the kidney.

Renal Drug Excretion

The kidneys account for the majority of drug excretion. When the kidneys are healthy, they serve to limit the duration of action of many drugs. Conversely, if renal failure occurs, both the duration and intensity of drug responses may increase.

Steps in Renal Drug Excretion

Urinary excretion is the net result of three processes: (1) glomerular filtration, (2) passive tubular reabsorption, and (3) active tubular secretion (Fig. 4.12).

Glomerular Filtration. Renal excretion begins at the glomerulus of the kidney tubule. The glomerulus consists of a capillary network surrounded by Bowman's capsule; small pores perforate the capillary walls. As blood flows through the glomerular capillaries, fluids and small molecules—including drugs—are forced through the pores of the capillary wall. This process, called glomerular filtration, moves drugs from the blood into the tubular urine. Blood cells and large molecules (e.g., proteins) are too big to pass through the capillary pores and therefore do not undergo filtration. Because large molecules are not filtered, drugs bound to albumin remain behind in the blood.

Passive Tubular Reabsorption. As depicted in Fig. 4.12, the vessels that deliver blood to the glomerulus return to proximity with the renal tubule at a point distal to the glomerulus. At this distal site, drug concentrations in the blood are lower than drug concentrations in the tubule. This concentration gradient acts as a driving force to move drugs from the lumen of the tubule back into the blood. Because lipid-soluble drugs can readily cross the membranes that compose the tubular and vascular walls, *drugs that are lipid soluble undergo passive reabsorption from the tubule back into the blood.* In contrast, drugs that are not lipid soluble (ions and polar compounds) remain in the urine to be excreted. By converting lipid-soluble drugs into more polar forms, drug metabolism reduces passive reabsorption of drugs and thereby accelerates their excretion.

Active Tubular Secretion. There are active transport systems in the kidney tubules that pump drugs from the blood to the tubular urine. The tubules have two primary classes of pumps, one for organic acids and one for organic bases. In addition, tubule cells contain P-glycoprotein, which can pump a variety of drugs into the urine. These pumps have a relatively high capacity and play a significant role in excreting certain compounds.

Factors That Modify Renal Drug Excretion

pH-Dependent Ionization. The phenomenon of pH-dependent ionization can be used to accelerate renal excretion of drugs. Recall that passive tubular reabsorption is limited to lipid-soluble compounds. Because ions are not lipid soluble, drugs that are ionized at the pH of tubular urine will remain in the tubule and be excreted. Consequently, by manipulating urinary pH in such a way as to promote the ionization of a drug, we can decrease passive reabsorption back into the blood, and can thereby hasten the drug's elimination. This principle has been employed to promote the excretion of poisons as well as medications that have been taken in toxic doses.

The treatment of aspirin poisoning provides an example of how manipulation of urinary pH can be put to therapeutic advantage. When children have been exposed to toxic doses of aspirin, they can be treated, in part, by giving an agent that elevates urinary pH (i.e., makes the urine more basic). Because aspirin is an acidic drug and because acids tend to ionize in basic media, elevation of urinary pH causes more of the aspirin molecules in urine to become ionized. As a result, less drug is passively reabsorbed; therefore, more is excreted.

Competition for Active Tubular Transport. Competition between drugs for active tubular transport can delay renal excretion, thereby prolonging effects. The active transport systems of the renal tubules can be envisioned as motor-driven revolving doors that carry drugs from the plasma into the renal tubules. These "revolving doors" can carry only a limited number of drug molecules per unit of time. Accordingly, if there are too many molecules present, some must wait their turn. Because of competition, if we administer two drugs at the same time and if both use the same transport system, excretion of each will be delayed by the presence of the other.

Competition for transport has been employed clinically to prolong the effects of drugs that normally undergo rapid renal excretion. For example, when administered alone, penicillin is rapidly cleared from the blood by active tubular transport. Excretion of penicillin can be delayed by concurrent administration of probenecid, an agent that is removed from the blood by the same tubular transport system that pumps penicillin. Hence, if a large dose of probenecid is administered, renal excretion of penicillin will be delayed while the transport system is occupied with moving the probenecid. Years ago, when penicillin was expensive to produce, combined use with probenecid was common. Today penicillin is cheap. As a result, rather than using probenecid to preserve penicillin levels, penicillin is simply given in larger doses.

Age. The kidneys of newborns are not fully developed. Until their kidneys reach full capacity (a few months after birth), infants have a limited capacity to excrete drugs. This must be accounted for when medicating an infant.

In old age, renal function often declines. Older adults have smaller kidneys and fewer nephrons. The loss of nephrons results in decreased blood filtration. Additionally, vessel changes such as atherosclerosis reduce renal blood flow. As a result, renal excretion of drugs is decreased.

Nonrenal Routes of Drug Excretion

In most cases, excretion of drugs by nonrenal routes has minimal clinical significance. However, in certain situations, nonrenal excretion can have important therapeutic and toxicologic consequences.

Breast Milk

Drugs taken by breast-feeding women can undergo excretion into milk. As a result, breast-feeding can expose the nursing infant to drugs. The factors that influence the appearance of drugs in breast milk are the same factors that determine the passage of drugs across membranes. Accordingly, lipid-soluble drugs have ready access to breast milk, whereas drugs that are polar, ionized, or protein bound cannot enter in significant amounts. Because infants may be harmed by drugs excreted in breast milk, nursing mothers should avoid all unnecessary drugs. If a woman *must* take medication, she should consult with her prescriber to ensure that the drug will not reach concentrations in her milk high enough to harm her baby.

Other Nonrenal Routes of Excretion

The *bile* is an important route of excretion for certain drugs. Recall that bile is secreted into the small intestine and then leaves the body in the feces. In some cases, drugs entering the intestine in bile may undergo reabsorption back into the portal blood. This reabsorption, referred to as *enterohepatic recirculation,* can substantially prolong a drug's sojourn in the body (see *Enterohepatic Recirculation*, discussed previously).

The *lungs* are the major route by which volatile anesthetics are excreted.

Small amounts of drugs can appear in *sweat* and *saliva.* These routes have little therapeutic or toxicologic significance.

TIME COURSE OF DRUG RESPONSES

It is possible to regulate the time at which drug responses start, the time they are most intense, and the time they cease. Because the four pharmacokinetic processes—absorption, distribution, metabolism, and excretion—determine how much drug will be at its sites of action at any given time, these processes are the major determinants of the time course over which drug responses take place.

Plasma Drug Levels

In most cases, the time course of drug action bears a direct relationship to the concentration of a drug in the blood. Hence, before discussing the time course per se, we need to review several important concepts related to plasma drug levels.

Clinical Significance of Plasma Drug Levels

Clinicians frequently monitor plasma drug levels in efforts to regulate drug responses. When measurements indicate that drug levels are inappropriate, these levels can be adjusted up or down by changing dose size, dose timing, or both.

The practice of regulating plasma drug levels to control drug responses should seem a bit odd, given that (1) drug responses are related to drug concentrations at sites of action, and that (2) the site of action of most drugs is not in the blood. The question arises, "Why adjust plasma levels of a drug when what really matters is the concentration of that drug at its sites of action?" The answer begins with the following observation: More often than not, it is a practical impossibility to measure drug concentrations at sites of action. For example, when a patient with seizures takes phenytoin (an antiseizure agent), we cannot routinely draw samples from inside the brain to see whether levels of the medication are adequate for seizure control. Fortunately, in the case of phenytoin and most other drugs, it is not necessary to measure drug concentrations at actual sites of action to have an objective basis for adjusting dosage. Experience has shown that, for most drugs, *there is a direct correlation between therapeutic and toxic responses and the amount of drug present in plasma.* Therefore, although we can't usually measure drug concentrations at sites of action, we *can* determine plasma drug concentrations that, in turn, are highly predictive of therapeutic and toxic responses. Accordingly, the dosing objective is commonly spoken of in terms of achieving a specific plasma level of a drug.

Two Plasma Drug Levels Defined

Two plasma drug levels are of special importance: (1) the minimum effective concentration, and (2) the toxic concentration. These levels are depicted in Fig. 4.13 and defined in the following sections.

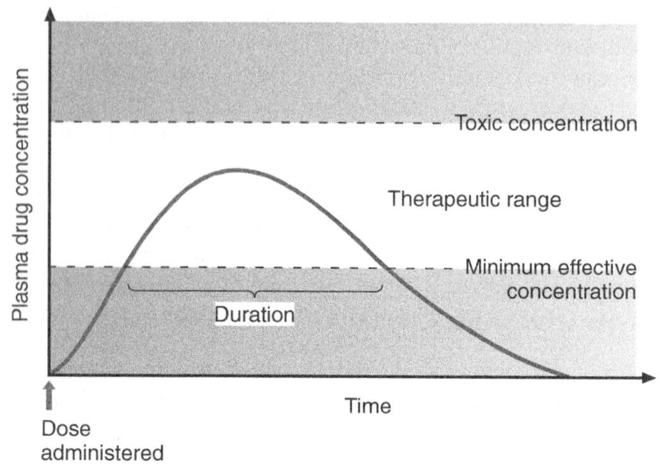

Fig. 4.13 ■ Single-dose time course.

Minimum Effective Concentration. The minimum effective concentration (MEC) is defined as *the plasma drug level below which therapeutic effects will not occur.* Hence, to be of benefit, a drug must be present in concentrations at or above the MEC.

Toxic Concentration. Toxicity occurs when plasma drug levels climb too high. The plasma level at which toxic effects begin is termed the *toxic concentration.* Doses must be kept small enough so that the toxic concentration is not reached.

Therapeutic Range

As indicated in Fig. 4.13, there is a range of plasma drug levels, falling between the MEC and the toxic concentration, that is termed the *therapeutic range.* When plasma levels are within the therapeutic range, there is enough drug present to produce therapeutic responses but not so much that toxicity results. *The objective of drug dosing is to maintain plasma drug levels within the therapeutic range.*

The width of the therapeutic range is a major determinant of the ease with which a drug can be used safely. Drugs that have a narrow therapeutic range are difficult to administer safely. Conversely, drugs that have a wide therapeutic range can be administered safely with relative ease. Acetaminophen, for example, has a relatively wide therapeutic range: The toxic concentration is about 30 times greater than the MEC. Because of this wide therapeutic range, the dosage does not need to be highly precise; a broad range of doses can be employed to produce plasma levels that will be above the MEC and below the toxic concentration. In contrast, lithium (used for bipolar disorder) has a very narrow therapeutic range: The toxic concentration is only 3 times greater than the MEC. Because toxicity can result from lithium levels that are not much greater than those needed for therapeutic effects, lithium dosing must be done carefully. If lithium had a wider therapeutic range, the drug would be much easier to use.

Understanding the concept of therapeutic range can facilitate patient care. Because drugs with a narrow therapeutic range are more dangerous than drugs with a wide therapeutic range, patients taking drugs with a narrow therapeutic range are the most likely to require intervention for drug-related complications. The nurse who is aware of this fact can focus additional attention on monitoring these patients for signs and symptoms of toxicity.

Single-Dose Time Course

Fig. 4.13 shows how plasma drug levels change over time after a single dose of an oral medication. Drug levels rise as the medicine undergoes absorption. Drug levels then decline as metabolism and excretion eliminate the drug from the body.

Because responses cannot occur until plasma drug levels have reached the MEC, there is a latent period between drug administration and onset of effects. The extent of this delay is determined by the rate of absorption.

The duration of effects is determined largely by the combination of metabolism and excretion. As long as drug levels remain above the MEC, therapeutic responses will be maintained; when levels fall below the MEC, benefits will cease. Since metabolism and excretion are the processes most responsible for causing plasma drug levels to fall, these processes are the primary determinants of how long drug effects will persist.

Drug Half-Life

Before proceeding to the topic of multiple dosing, we need to discuss the concept of half-life. When a patient ceases drug use, the combination of metabolism and excretion will cause the amount of drug in the body to decline. The half-life of a drug is an index of just how rapidly that decline occurs.

Drug half-life is defined as *the time required for the amount of drug in the body to decrease by 50%.* A few drugs have half-lives that are extremely short—on the order of minutes. In contrast, the half-lives of some drugs exceed 1 week. Drugs with short half-lives leave the body quickly. Drugs with long half-lives leave slowly.

Note that, in our definition of half-life, a *percentage*—not a specific *amount*—of drug is lost during one half-life. That is, the half-life does not specify, for example, that 2 gm or 18 mg will leave the body in a given time. Rather, the half-life tells us that, no matter what the amount of drug in the body may be, half (50%) will leave during a specified period of time (the half-life). The actual amount of drug that is lost during one half-life depends on just how much drug is present: The more drug that is in the body, the larger the amount lost during one half-life.

The concept of half-life is best understood through an example. Morphine provides a good illustration. The half-life of morphine is approximately 3 hours. By definition, this means that body stores of morphine will decrease by 50% every 3 hours—regardless of how much morphine is in the body. If there are 50 mg of morphine in the body, 25 mg (50% of 50 mg) will be lost in 3 hours; if there are only 2 mg of morphine in the body, only 1 mg (50% of 2 mg) will be lost in 3 hours. Note that, in both cases, morphine levels drop by 50% during an interval of one half-life. However, the actual *amount* lost is larger when total body stores of the drug are higher.

The half-life of a drug determines the dosing interval (i.e., how much time separates each dose). For drugs with a short half-life, the dosing interval must be correspondingly short. If a long dosing interval were used, drug levels would fall below the MEC between doses, and therapeutic effects would be lost. Conversely, if a drug has a long half-life, a long time can separate doses without loss of benefits.

Drug Levels Produced With Repeated Doses

Multiple dosing leads to drug accumulation. When a patient takes a single dose of a drug, plasma levels simply go up and then come back down. In contrast, when a patient takes repeated doses of a drug, the process is more complex and results in drug accumulation. The factors that determine the rate and extent of accumulation are considered in the following sections.

The Process by Which Plateau Drug Levels Are Achieved

Administering repeated doses will cause a drug to build up in the body until a *plateau* (steady level) has been achieved. What causes drug levels to reach plateau? If a second dose of a drug is administered before all of the prior dose has been eliminated, total body stores of that drug will be higher after the second dose than after the initial dose. As succeeding doses are administered, drug levels will climb even higher. The drug will continue to accumulate until a state has been achieved in which the amount of drug eliminated between doses equals the amount administered. *When the amount of drug eliminated between doses equals the dose administered, average drug levels will remain constant and plateau will have been reached.*

The process by which multiple dosing produces a plateau is illustrated in Fig. 4.14. The drug in this figure is a hypothetical agent with a half-life of exactly 1 day. The regimen consists of a 2-gm dose administered once daily. For the purpose of illustration, we assume that absorption takes place instantly. Upon giving the first 2-gm dose (day 1 in the figure), total body stores go from zero to 2 gm. Within one half-life (1 day), body stores drop by 50%—from 2 gm down to 1 gm. At the beginning of day 2, the second 2-gm dose is given, causing body stores to rise from 1 gm up to 3 gm. Over the next day (one half-life), body stores again drop by 50%, this time from 3 gm down to 1.5 gm. When the third dose is given, body stores go from 1.5 gm up to 3.5 gm. Over the next half-life, stores drop by 50% down to 1.75 gm. When the fourth dose is given, drug levels climb to 3.75 gm and, between doses, levels again drop by 50%, this time to approximately 1.9 gm.

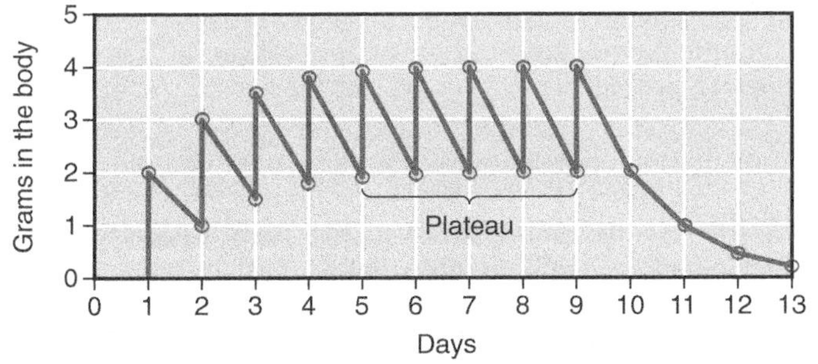

Fig. 4.14 ■ Drug accumulation with repeated administration.
The drug has a half-life of 1 day. The dosing schedule is 2 gm given once a day on days 1 through 9. Note that plateau is reached at about the beginning of day 5 (i.e., after four half-lives). Note also that, when administration is discontinued, it takes about 4 days (four half-lives) for most (94%) of the drug to leave the body.

When the fifth dose is given (at the beginning of day 5), drug levels go up to about 3.9 gm. This process of accumulation continues until body stores reach 4 gm. When total body stores of this drug are 4 gm, 2 gm will be lost each day (i.e., over one half-life). Since a 2-gm dose is being administered each day, when body stores reach 4 gm, the amount lost between doses will equal the dose administered. At this point, body stores will simply alternate between 4 gm and 2 gm; average body stores will be stable, and plateau will have been reached. Note that the reason that plateau is finally reached is that the actual amount of drug lost between doses gets larger each day. That is, although 50% of total body stores is lost each day, the *amount* in grams grows progressively larger because total body stores are getting larger day by day. Plateau is reached when the amount lost between doses grows to be as large as the amount administered.

Time to Plateau

When a drug is administered repeatedly in the same dose, *plateau will be reached in approximately four half-lives.* For the hypothetical agent illustrated in Fig. 4.14, total body stores approached their peak near the beginning of day 5, or approximately 4 full days after treatment began. Because the half-life of this drug is 1 day, reaching plateau in 4 days is equivalent to reaching plateau in four half-lives.

As long as dosage remains constant, the time required to reach plateau is independent of dosage size. Put another way, the time required to reach plateau when giving repeated large doses of a particular drug is identical to the time required to reach plateau when giving repeated small doses of that drug. Referring to the drug in Fig. 4.14, just as it took four half-lives (4 days) to reach plateau when a dose of 2 gm was administered daily, it would also take four half-lives to reach plateau if a dose of 4 gm were administered daily. It is true that the *height* of the plateau would be greater if a 4-gm dose were given, but the time required to reach plateau would not be altered by the increase in dosage. To confirm this statement, substitute a dose of 4 gm in the previous exercise and see when plateau is reached.

Techniques for Reducing Fluctuations in Drug Levels

As illustrated in Fig. 4.14, when a drug is administered repeatedly, its level will fluctuate between doses. The highest level is referred to as the *peak concentration,* and the lowest level is referred to as the *trough concentration.* The acceptable height of the peaks and troughs will depend upon the drug's therapeutic range: The peaks must be kept below the toxic concentration, and the troughs must be kept above the MEC. If there is not much difference between the toxic concentration and the MEC, then fluctuations must be kept to a minimum.

Three techniques can be employed to reduce fluctuations in drug levels. One technique is to *administer drugs by continuous infusion.* With this procedure, plasma levels can be kept nearly constant. Another is to *administer a depot preparation,* which releases the drug slowly and steadily. The third is to *reduce both the size of each dose and the dosing interval* (keeping the total daily dose constant). For example, rather than giving the drug from Fig. 4.14 in 2-gm doses once every 24 hours, we could give this drug in 1-gm doses every 12 hours. With this altered dosing schedule, the total daily dose would remain unchanged, as would total body stores at plateau.

However, instead of fluctuating over a range of 2 gm between doses, levels would fluctuate over a range of 1 gm.

Loading Doses Versus Maintenance Doses

As discussed earlier, if we administer a drug in repeated doses of *equal size,* an interval equivalent to about four half-lives is required to achieve plateau. For drugs whose half-lives are long, achieving plateau could take days or even weeks. When plateau must be achieved more quickly, a large initial dose can be administered. This large initial dose is called a *loading dose.* After high drug levels have been established with a loading dose, plateau can be maintained by giving smaller doses. These smaller doses are referred to as *maintenance doses.*

The claim that use of a loading dose will shorten the time to plateau may appear to contradict an earlier statement, which said that the time to plateau is not affected by dosage size. However, there is no contradiction. For any *specified dosage,* it will always take about four half-lives to reach plateau. When a loading dose is administered followed by maintenance doses, the plateau is not reached *for the loading dose.* Rather, we have simply used the loading dose to rapidly produce a drug level equivalent to the plateau level for a smaller dose. To achieve plateau level for the loading dose, it would be necessary to either administer repeated doses equivalent to the loading dose for a period of four half-lives or administer a dose even larger than the original loading dose.

Decline From Plateau

When drug administration is discontinued, most (94%) of the drug in the body will be eliminated over an interval equal to about four half-lives. This statement can be validated with simple arithmetic. Let's consider a patient who has been taking morphine. In addition, let's assume that, at the time dosing ceased, the total body store of morphine was 40 mg. Within one half-life after drug withdrawal, morphine stores will decline by 50%—down to 20 mg. During the second half-life, stores will again decline by 50%, dropping from 20 mg to 10 mg. During the third half-life, the level will decline once more by 50%—from 10 mg down to 5 mg. During the fourth half-life, the level will again decline by 50%—from 5 mg down to 2.5 mg. Hence, over a period of four half-lives, total body stores of morphine will drop from an initial level of 40 mg down to 2.5 mg, an overall decline of 94%. Most of the drug in the body will be cleared within four half-lives.

The time required for drugs to leave the body is important when toxicity develops. Let's consider the elimination of digitoxin (a drug once used for heart failure). Digitoxin, true to its name, is a potentially dangerous drug with a narrow therapeutic range. In addition, the half-life of digitoxin is prolonged—about 7 days. What will be the consequence of digitoxin overdose? Toxic levels of the drug will remain in the body for a long time: Because digitoxin has a half-life of 7 days and because four half-lives are required for most of the drug to be cleared from the body, it could take weeks for digitoxin stores to fall to a safe level. During the time that excess drug remains in the body, significant effort will be required to keep the patient alive. If digitoxin had a shorter half-life, body stores would decline more rapidly, thereby making management of overdose less difficult. (Because of its long half-life and potential for toxicity, digitoxin has been replaced by digoxin, a drug with identical actions but a much shorter half-life.)

It is important to note that the concept of half-life does not apply to the elimination of all drugs. A few agents, most notably ethanol (alcohol), leave the body at a *constant rate,* regardless of how much is present. The implications of this kind of decline for ethanol are discussed in Chapter 38.

KEY POINTS

- Pharmacokinetics consists of four basic processes: absorption, distribution, metabolism, and excretion.
- Pharmacokinetic processes determine the concentration of a drug at its sites of action, and thereby determine the intensity and time course of responses.
- To move around the body, drugs must cross membranes, either by (1) passing through pores, (2) undergoing transport, or (3) penetrating the membrane directly.
- P-glycoprotein—found in the liver, kidney, placenta, intestine, and brain capillaries—can transport a variety of drugs *out* of cells.
- To cross membranes, most drugs must dissolve directly into the lipid bilayer of the membrane. Accordingly, lipid-soluble drugs can cross membranes easily, whereas drugs that are polar or ionized cannot.
- Acidic drugs ionize in basic (alkaline) media, whereas basic drugs ionize in acidic media.
- Absorption is defined as the movement of a drug from its site of administration into the blood.
- Absorption is enhanced by rapid drug dissolution, high lipid solubility of the drug, a large surface area for absorption, and high blood flow at the site of administration.
- Intravenous administration has several advantages: rapid onset, precise control over the amount of drug entering the blood, suitability for use with large volumes of fluid, and suitability for irritant drugs.
- Intravenous administration has several disadvantages: high cost; difficulty; inconvenience; danger because of irreversibility; and the potential for fluid overload, infection, and embolism.
- Intramuscular administration has two advantages: suitability for insoluble drugs and suitability for depot preparations.
- Intramuscular administration has two disadvantages: inconvenience and the potential for discomfort.
- Subcutaneous administration has the same advantages and disadvantages as IM administration.
- Oral administration has the advantages of ease, convenience, economy, and safety.
- The principal disadvantages of oral administration are high variability and possible inactivation by stomach acid, digestive enzymes, and liver enzymes (because oral drugs must pass through the liver before reaching the general circulation).

- Enteric-coated oral formulations are designed to release their contents in the small intestine—not in the stomach.
- Sustained-release oral formulations are designed to release their contents slowly, thereby permitting a longer interval between doses.
- Distribution is defined as drug movement from the blood to the interstitial space of tissues and from there into cells.
- In most tissues, drugs can easily leave the vasculature through spaces between the cells that compose the capillary wall.
- The term *blood-brain barrier* refers to the presence of tight junctions between the cells that compose capillary walls in the CNS. Because of this barrier, drugs must pass through the cells of the capillary wall, rather than between them, to reach the CNS.
- The membranes of the placenta do not constitute an absolute barrier to the passage of drugs. The same factors that determine drug movements across all other membranes determine the movement of drugs across the placenta.
- Many drugs bind reversibly to plasma albumin. While bound to albumin, drug molecules cannot leave the vascular system.
- Drug metabolism (biotransformation) is defined as the chemical alteration of drug structure.
- Most drug metabolism takes place in the liver and is catalyzed by the cytochrome P450 system of enzymes.
- The most important consequence of drug metabolism is promotion of renal drug excretion by converting lipid-soluble drugs into more hydrophilic forms.
- Other consequences of drug metabolism are conversion of drugs to less active (or inactive) forms, conversion of drugs to more active forms, conversion of prodrugs to their active forms, and conversion of drugs to more toxic or less toxic forms.
- Drugs that are metabolized by P450 hepatic enzymes are called substrates. The rate at which substrates are metabolized is affected by drugs that act as P450 inducers or inhibitors.
- Drugs that act on the liver to increase rates of drug metabolism are inducers. This process of stimulating enzyme synthesis is known as *induction.* As the rate of drug metabolism increases, plasma drug levels fall.
- Drugs that act on the liver to decrease rates of drug metabolism are called *inhibitors.* This process is known as *inhibition.* These drugs also create therapeutic consequences because slower metabolism can cause an increase in active drug accumulation. This can lead to an increase in adverse effects and toxicity.
- The term *first-pass effect* refers to the rapid inactivation of some oral drugs as they pass through the liver after being absorbed.
- Enterohepatic recirculation is a repeating cycle in which a drug undergoes glucuronidation in the liver, transport to the duodenum via the bile, hydrolytic release of free drug by intestinal enzymes, followed by transport in the portal blood back to the liver, where the cycle can begin again.
- Most drugs are excreted by the kidneys.
- Renal drug excretion has three steps: glomerular filtration, passive tubular reabsorption, and active tubular secretion.
- Drugs that are highly lipid soluble undergo extensive passive reabsorption back into the blood, and therefore cannot be excreted by the kidney (until they are converted to more polar forms by the liver).
- Drugs can be excreted into breast milk, thereby posing a threat to the nursing infant.
- For most drugs, there is a direct correlation between the level of drug in plasma and the intensity of therapeutic and toxic effects.
- The minimum effective concentration (MEC) is defined as the plasma drug level below which therapeutic effects will not occur.
- The therapeutic range of a drug lies between the MEC and the toxic concentration.
- Drugs with a wide therapeutic range are relatively easy to use safely, whereas drugs with a narrow therapeutic range are difficult to use safely.
- The half-life of a drug is defined as the time required for the amount of drug in the body to decline by 50%.
- Drugs that have a short half-life must be administered more frequently than drugs that have a long half-life.
- When drugs are administered repeatedly, their levels will gradually rise and then reach a steady plateau.
- The time required to reach plateau is equivalent to about four half-lives.
- The time required to reach plateau is independent of dosage size, although the height of the plateau will be higher with larger doses.
- If plasma drug levels fluctuate too much between doses, the fluctuations could be reduced by (1) giving smaller doses at shorter intervals (keeping the total daily dose the same), (2) using a continuous infusion, or (3) using a depot preparation.
- For a drug with a long half-life, it may be necessary to use a loading dose to achieve plateau quickly.
- When drug administration is discontinued, most (94%) of the drug in the body will be eliminated over four half-lives.

Please visit **http://evolve.elsevier.com/Lehne** for chapter-specific NCLEX® examination review questions.

CHAPTER

5 Pharmacodynamics

Pharmacodynamics is defined as the study of the biochemical and physiologic effects of drugs on the body and the molecular mechanisms by which those effects are produced. In short, pharmacodynamics is the study of what drugs do to the body and how they do it.

To participate rationally in achieving the therapeutic objective, nurses need a basic understanding of pharmacodynamics. You must know about drug actions to educate patients about their medications, make PRN decisions, and evaluate patients for beneficial and harmful drug effects. You also need to understand drug actions when conferring with prescribers about drug therapy: If you believe a patient is receiving inappropriate medication or is being denied a required drug, you will need to support that conviction with discussions based, at least in part, on knowledge of pharmacodynamics.

DOSE-RESPONSE RELATIONSHIPS

The dose-response relationship (i.e., the relationship between the size of an administered dose and the intensity of the response produced) is a fundamental concern in therapeutics. Dose-response relationships determine the minimum amount of drug needed to elicit a response, the maximum response a drug can elicit, and how much to increase the dosage to produce the desired increase in response.

Basic Features of the Dose-Response Relationship

The basic characteristics of dose-response relationships are illustrated in Fig. 5.1. Part *A* shows dose-response data plotted on *linear* coordinates. Part *B* shows the same data plotted on *semilogarithmic* coordinates (i.e., the scale on which dosage is plotted is logarithmic rather than linear). The most obvious and important characteristic revealed by these curves is that the dose-response relationship is *graded.* That is, as the dosage increases, the response becomes progressively larger. Because drug responses are graded, therapeutic effects can be adjusted to fit the needs of each patient by raising or lowering the dosage until a response of the desired intensity is achieved.

As indicated in Fig. 5.1, the dose-response relationship can be viewed as having three phases. Phase 1 (Fig. 5.1B) occurs at low doses. The curve is flat during this phase because doses are too low to elicit a measurable response. During phase 2, an increase in dose elicits a corresponding increase in the response. This is the phase during which the dose-response relationship is graded. As the dose goes higher, eventually a point is reached at which an increase in dose is unable to elicit a further increase in response. At this point, the curve flattens out into phase 3.

Maximal Efficacy and Relative Potency

Dose-response curves reveal two characteristic properties of drugs: *maximal efficacy* and *relative potency.* Curves that reflect these properties are shown in Fig. 5.2.

Maximal Efficacy

Maximal efficacy is defined as *the largest effect that a drug can produce.* Maximal efficacy is indicated by the *height* of the dose-response curve.

The concept of maximal efficacy is illustrated by the dose-response curves for meperidine [Demerol] and pentazocine [Talwin], two morphine-like pain relievers (Fig. 5.2A). As you can see, the curve for pentazocine levels off at a maximum height below that of the curve for meperidine. This tells us that the maximum degree of pain relief we can achieve with pentazocine is smaller than the maximum degree of pain relief we can achieve with meperidine. Put another way, no matter how much pentazocine we administer, we can never produce the degree of pain relief that we can with meperidine. Accordingly, we would say that meperidine has greater maximal efficacy than pentazocine.

Despite what intuition might tell us, a drug with very high maximal efficacy is not always more desirable than a drug with lower efficacy. Recall that we want to match the intensity of the response to the patient's needs. This may be difficult to do with a drug that produces extremely intense responses. For example, certain diuretics (e.g., furosemide) have such high

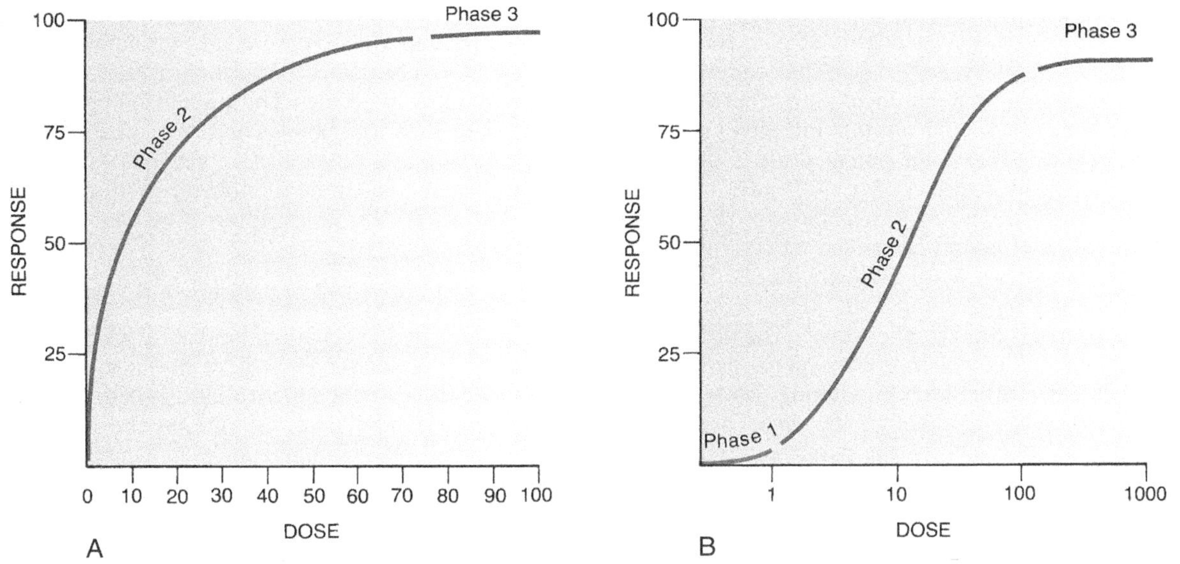

Fig. 5.1 ■ Basic components of the dose-response curve.
A, A dose-response curve with dose plotted on a linear scale. **B,** The same dose-response relationship shown in **A** but with the dose plotted on a logarithmic scale. Note the three phases of the dose-response curve: ***Phase 1,*** The curve is relatively flat; doses are too low to elicit a significant response. ***Phase 2,*** The curve climbs upward as bigger doses elicit correspondingly bigger responses. ***Phase 3,*** The curve levels off; bigger doses are unable to elicit a further increase in response. (Phase 1 is not indicated in **A** because very low doses cannot be shown on a linear scale.)

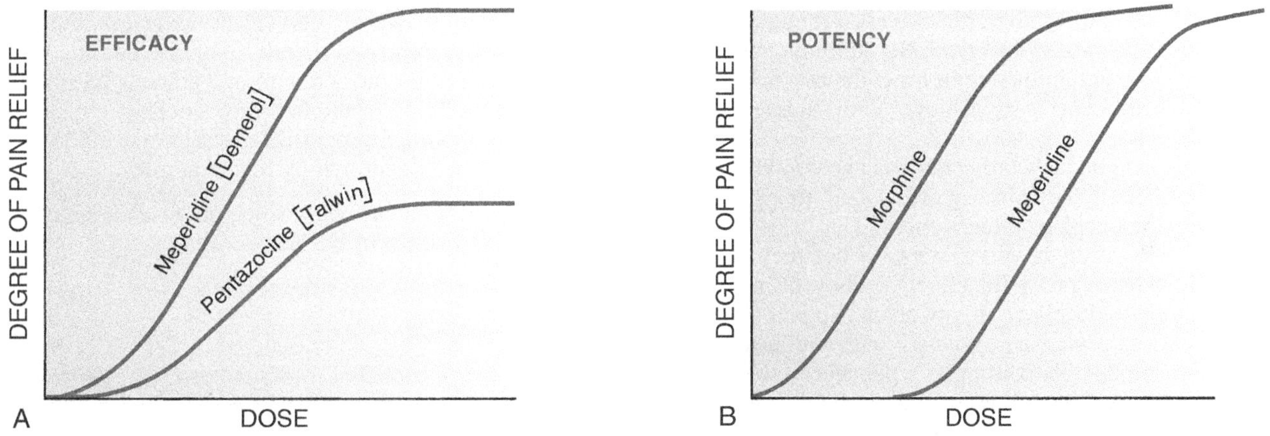

Fig. 5.2 ■ Dose-response curves demonstrating efficacy and potency.
A, Efficacy, or maximal efficacy, is an index of the maximal response a drug can produce. The efficacy of a drug is indicated by the height of its dose-response curve. In this example, meperidine has greater efficacy than pentazocine. Efficacy is an important quality in a drug. **B,** Potency is an index of how much drug must be administered to elicit a desired response. In this example, achieving pain relief with meperidine requires higher doses than with morphine. We would say that morphine is more potent than meperidine. Note that, if administered in sufficiently high doses, meperidine can produce just as much pain relief as morphine. Potency is usually not an important quality in a drug.

maximal efficacy that they can cause dehydration. If we only want to mobilize a modest volume of water, a diuretic with lower maximal efficacy (e.g., hydrochlorothiazide) would be preferred. Similarly, if a patient has a mild headache, we would not select a powerful analgesic (e.g., morphine) for relief. Rather, we would select an analgesic with lower maximal efficacy, such as aspirin.

Relative Potency

The term *potency* refers to the amount of drug we must give to elicit an effect. Potency is indicated by the relative position of the dose-response curve along the *x* (dose) axis.

The concept of potency is illustrated by the curves in Fig. 5.2B. These curves plot doses for two analgesics—morphine and meperidine—versus the degree of pain relief achieved. As you can see, for any particular degree of pain relief, the required dose of meperidine is larger than the required dose of morphine. Because morphine produces pain relief at lower doses than meperidine, we would say that morphine is more potent than meperidine. That is, a potent drug is one that produces its effects at low doses.

Potency is rarely an important characteristic of a drug. The fact that morphine is more potent than meperidine does not mean that morphine is a superior medicine. In fact, the only consequence of having greater potency is that a drug with greater potency can be given in smaller doses. The difference between providing pain relief with morphine versus meperidine is much like the difference between purchasing candy with a dime instead of two nickels; although the dime is smaller (more potent) than the two nickels, the purchasing power of the dime and the two nickels is identical.

Although potency is usually of no clinical concern, it can be important if a drug is so lacking in potency that doses become inconveniently large. For example, if a drug were of extremely low potency, we might need to administer that drug in huge doses multiple times a day to achieve beneficial effects. In this case, an alternative drug with higher potency would be desirable. Fortunately, it is rare for a drug to be so lacking in potency that doses of inconvenient magnitude need be given.

It is important to note that the potency of a drug implies nothing about its maximal efficacy! Potency and efficacy are completely independent qualities. Drug A can be more effective than drug B even though drug B may be more potent. Also, drugs A and B can be equally effective even though one may be more potent. As we saw in Fig. 5.2B, although meperidine happens to be less potent than morphine, the maximal degree of pain relief that we can achieve with these drugs is identical.

A final comment on the word *potency* is in order. In everyday parlance, people often use the word *potent* to express the pharmacologic concept of effectiveness. That is, when most people say, "This drug is very potent," what they mean is, "This drug produces powerful effects." They do not mean, "This drug produces its effects at low doses." In pharmacology, we use the words *potent* and *potency* with the specific and appropriate meanings. Accordingly, whenever you see those words in this book, they will refer only to the dosage needed to produce effects—never to the maximal effects a drug can produce.

DRUG-RECEPTOR INTERACTIONS

Introduction to Drug Receptors

Drugs are not "magic bullets"—they are simply chemicals. Being chemicals, the only way drugs can produce their effects is by interacting with other chemicals. Receptors are the special chemical sites in the body that most drugs interact with to produce effects.

We can define a receptor as *any functional macromolecule in a cell to which a drug binds to produce its effects.* Under this broad definition, many cellular components could be considered drug receptors, because drugs bind to many cellular components (e.g., enzymes, ribosomes, tubulin) to produce their effects. However, although the formal definition of a receptor encompasses all functional macromolecules, the term *receptor* is generally reserved for what is arguably the most important group of macromolecules through which drugs act: the body's own receptors for hormones, neurotransmitters, and other regulatory molecules. The other macromolecules to which drugs bind, such as enzymes and ribosomes, can be thought of simply as target molecules, rather than as true receptors.

The general equation for the interaction between drugs and their receptors is as follows (where D = drug and R = receptor):

$$D + R \rightleftharpoons \text{D-R COMPLEX} \rightarrow \text{RESPONSE}$$

As suggested by the equation, binding of a drug to its receptor is usually *reversible.*

A receptor is analogous to a light switch, in that it has two configurations: "ON" and "OFF." Like the switch, a receptor must be in the "ON" configuration to influence cellular function. Receptors are activated (turned on) by interaction with other molecules (Fig. 5.3). Under physiologic conditions, receptor activity is regulated by endogenous compounds (neurotransmitters, hormones, other regulatory molecules). When a drug binds to a receptor, all that it can do is mimic or block the actions of endogenous regulatory molecules. By doing so, the drug will either increase or decrease the rate of the physiologic activity normally controlled by that receptor.

As shown in Fig. 5.3, the same cardiac receptors whose function is regulated by endogenous norepinephrine (NE) can also serve as receptors for drugs. That is, just as endogenous molecules can bind to these receptors, so can chemicals that enter the body as drugs. The binding of drugs to these receptors can have one of two effects: (1) drugs can *mimic* the action of endogenous NE (and thereby increase cardiac output), or (2) drugs can *block* the action of endogenous NE (and thereby prevent stimulation of the heart by autonomic neurons).

Several important properties of receptors and drug-receptor interactions are illustrated by this example:

- The receptors through which drugs act are normal points of control of physiologic processes.

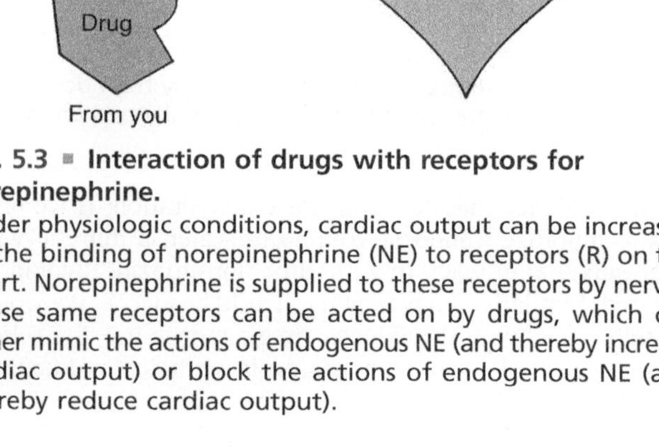

Fig. 5.3 ■ Interaction of drugs with receptors for norepinephrine.
Under physiologic conditions, cardiac output can be increased by the binding of norepinephrine (NE) to receptors (R) on the heart. Norepinephrine is supplied to these receptors by nerves. These same receptors can be acted on by drugs, which can either mimic the actions of endogenous NE (and thereby increase cardiac output) or block the actions of endogenous NE (and thereby reduce cardiac output).

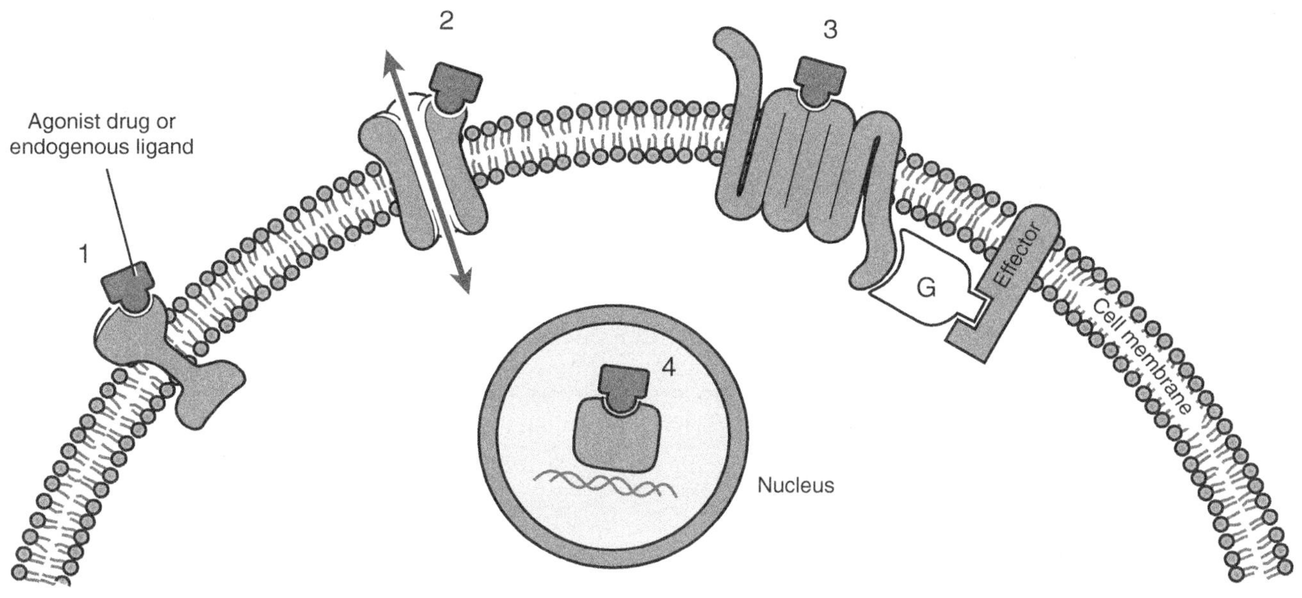

Fig. 5.4 ▪ The four primary receptor families.
1, Cell membrane–embedded enzyme. **2,** Ligand-gated ion channel. **3,** G protein–coupled receptor system (G, G protein). **4,** Transcription factor. (See text for details.)

- Under physiologic conditions, receptor function is regulated by molecules supplied by the body.
- All that drugs can do at receptors is mimic or block the action of the body's own regulatory molecules.
- Because drug action is limited to mimicking or blocking the body's own regulatory molecules, drugs cannot give cells new functions. Rather, drugs can only alter the rate of preexisting processes. In other words, drugs cannot make the body do anything that it is not already capable of doing.[a]
- Drugs produce their therapeutic effects by helping the body use its preexisting capabilities to the patient's best advantage. Put another way, medications simply help the body help itself.
- In theory, it should be possible to synthesize drugs that can alter the rate of any biologic process for which receptors exist.

The Four Primary Receptor Families

Although the body has many different receptors, they comprise only four primary families: cell membrane–embedded enzymes, ligand-gated ion channels, G protein–coupled receptor systems, and transcription factors. These families are depicted in Fig. 5.4. In the discussion that follows, the term *ligand-binding domain* refers to the specific region of the receptor where binding of drugs and endogenous regulatory molecules takes place.

Cell Membrane–Embedded Enzymes

As shown in Fig. 5.4, receptors of this type span the cell membrane. The ligand-binding domain is located on the cell surface, and the enzyme's catalytic site is inside. Binding of an endogenous regulatory molecule or agonist drug (one that mimics the action of the endogenous regulatory molecule) activates the enzyme, thereby increasing its catalytic activity. Responses to activation of these receptors occur in seconds. Insulin is a good example of an endogenous ligand that acts through this type of receptor.

Ligand-Gated Ion Channels

Like membrane-embedded enzymes, ligand-gated ion channels span the cell membrane. The function of these receptors is to regulate flow of ions into and out of cells. Each ligand-gated channel is specific for a particular ion (e.g., Na^+, Ca^{++}). As shown in Fig. 5.4, the ligand-binding domain is on the cell surface. When an endogenous ligand or agonist drug binds the receptor, the channel opens, allowing ions to flow inward or outward. (The direction of flow is determined by the concentration gradient of the ion across the membrane.) Responses to activation of a ligand-gated ion channel are extremely fast, usually occurring in milliseconds. Several neurotransmitters, including acetylcholine and gamma-aminobutyric acid (GABA), act through this type of receptor.

G Protein–Coupled Receptor Systems

G protein–coupled receptor systems have three components: the receptor itself, G protein (so named because it binds guanosine triphosphate [GTP]), and an effector (typically an ion channel or an enzyme). These systems work as follows: binding of an endogenous ligand or agonist drug activates the receptor, which in turn activates G protein, which in turn activates the effector. Responses to activation of this type of system develop rapidly. Numerous endogenous ligands—including NE, serotonin, histamine, and many peptide hormones—act through G protein–coupled receptor systems.

As shown in Fig. 5.4, the receptors that couple to G proteins are serpentine structures that traverse the cell membrane 7 times. For some of these receptors, the ligand-binding domain

[a]The only exception to this rule is gene therapy. By inserting genes into cells, we actually can make them do something they were previously incapable of doing.

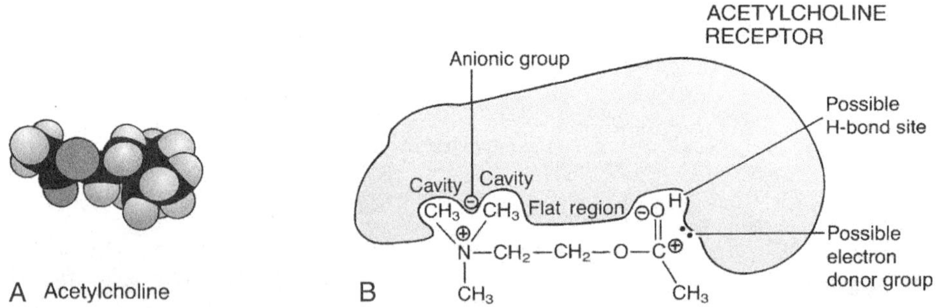

Fig. 5.5 ▪ Interaction of acetylcholine with its receptor.
A, Three-dimensional model of the acetylcholine molecule. **B,** Binding of acetylcholine to its receptor. Note how the shape of acetylcholine closely matches the shape of the receptor. Note also how the positive charges on acetylcholine align with the negative sites on the receptor.

is on the cell surface. For others, the ligand-binding domain is located in a pocket accessible from the cell surface.

Transcription Factors

Transcription factors differ from other receptors in two ways: (1) transcription factors are found *within* the cell rather than on the surface, and (2) responses to activation of these receptors are *delayed.* Transcription factors are situated on DNA in the cell nucleus. Their function is to regulate protein synthesis. Activation of these receptors by endogenous ligands or by agonist drugs stimulates transcription of messenger RNA molecules, which then act as templates for synthesis of specific proteins. The entire process—from activation of the transcription factor through completion of protein synthesis—may take hours or even days. Because transcription factors are intracellular, they can be activated only by ligands that are sufficiently lipid soluble to cross the cell membrane. Endogenous ligands that act through transcription factors include thyroid hormone and all of the steroid hormones (e.g., progesterone, testosterone, cortisol).

Receptors and Selectivity of Drug Action

In Chapter 1 we noted that selectivity, the ability to elicit only the response for which a drug is given, is a highly desirable characteristic of a drug because the more selective a drug is, the fewer side effects it will produce. Selective drug action is possible, in large part, because drugs act through specific receptors.

The body employs many different kinds of receptors to regulate its sundry physiologic activities. There are receptors for each neurotransmitter (e.g., NE, acetylcholine, dopamine); there are receptors for each hormone (e.g., progesterone, insulin, thyrotropin); and there are receptors for all of the other molecules the body uses to regulate physiologic processes (e.g., histamine, prostaglandins, leukotrienes). As a rule, each type of receptor participates in the regulation of just a few processes.

Selective drug action is made possible by the existence of many types of receptors, each regulating just a few processes. If a drug interacts with only one type of receptor, and if that receptor type regulates just a few processes, then the effects of the drug will be limited. Conversely, if a drug interacts with several different receptor types, then that drug is likely to elicit a wide variety of responses.

How can a drug interact with one receptor type and not with others? In some important ways, a receptor is analogous to a lock and a drug is analogous to a key for that lock: Just as only keys with the proper profile can fit a particular lock, only those drugs with the proper size, shape, and physical properties can bind to a particular receptor.

The binding of acetylcholine (a neurotransmitter) to its receptor illustrates the lock-and-key analogy (Fig. 5.5). To bind with its receptor, acetylcholine must have a shape that is complementary to the shape of the receptor. In addition, acetylcholine must possess positive charges that are positioned so as to permit their interaction with corresponding negative sites on the receptor. If acetylcholine lacked these properties, it would be unable to interact with the receptor.

Like the acetylcholine receptor, all other receptors impose specific requirements on the molecules with which they will interact. Because receptors have such specific requirements, it is possible to synthesize drugs that interact with just one receptor type preferentially over others. Such medications tend to elicit selective responses.

Even though a drug is selective for only one type of receptor, is it possible for that drug to produce nonselective effects? Yes: If a single receptor type is responsible for regulating several physiologic processes, then drugs that interact with that receptor will also influence several processes. For example, in addition to modulating perception of pain, opioid receptors help regulate other processes, including respiration and motility of the bowel. Consequently, although morphine is selective for one class of receptor, the drug can still produce a variety of effects. In clinical practice, it is common for morphine to cause respiratory depression and constipation along with reduction of pain. Note that morphine produces these varied effects not because it lacks receptor selectivity, but because the receptor for which morphine is selective helps regulate a variety of processes.

One final comment on selectivity: *Selectivity does not guarantee safety.* A compound can be highly selective for a particular receptor and still be dangerous. For example, although botulinum toxin is highly selective for one type of receptor, the compound is anything but safe: Botulinum toxin can cause paralysis of the muscles of respiration, resulting in death from respiratory arrest.

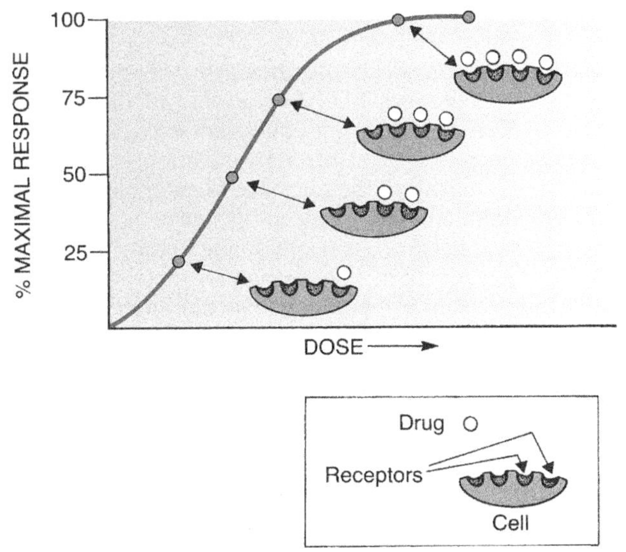

Fig. 5.6 ■ Model of simple occupancy theory.
The simple occupancy theory states that the intensity of response to a drug is proportional to the number of receptors occupied; maximal response is reached with 100% receptor occupancy. Because the hypothetical cell in this figure has only four receptors, maximal response is achieved when all four receptors are occupied. (***Note:*** Real cells have thousands of receptors.)

Theories of Drug-Receptor Interaction

In the discussion that follows, we consider two theories of drug-receptor interaction: (1) the simple occupancy theory and (2) the modified occupancy theory. These theories help explain dose-response relationships and the ability of drugs to mimic or block the actions of endogenous regulatory molecules.

Simple Occupancy Theory

The simple occupancy theory of drug-receptor interaction states that (1) the intensity of the response to a drug is proportional to the number of receptors occupied by that drug and that (2) a maximal response will occur when *all* available receptors have been occupied. This relationship between receptor occupancy and the intensity of the response is depicted in Fig. 5.6.

Although certain aspects of dose-response relationships can be explained by the simple occupancy theory, other important phenomena cannot. Specifically, there is nothing in this theory to explain why one drug should be more potent than another. In addition, this theory cannot explain how one drug can have higher maximal efficacy than another. That is, according to this theory, two drugs acting at the same receptor should produce the same maximal effect, providing that their dosages were high enough to produce 100% receptor occupancy. However, we have already seen this is not true. As illustrated in Fig. 5.2A, there is a dose of pentazocine above which no further increase in response can be elicited. Presumably, all receptors are occupied when the dose-response curve levels off. However, at 100% receptor occupancy, the response elicited by pentazocine is less than that elicited by meperidine. Simple occupancy theory cannot account for this difference.

Modified Occupancy Theory

The modified occupancy theory of drug-receptor interaction explains certain observations that cannot be accounted for with the simple occupancy theory. The simple occupancy theory assumes that all drugs acting at a particular receptor are identical with respect to (1) the ability to bind to the receptor and (2) the ability to influence receptor function once binding has taken place. The modified occupancy theory is based on different assumptions.

The modified theory ascribes two qualities to drugs: *affinity* and *intrinsic activity*. The term *affinity* refers to the strength of the attraction between a drug and its receptor. *Intrinsic activity* refers to the ability of a drug to activate the receptor following binding. *Affinity and intrinsic activity are independent properties.*

Affinity. As noted, the term *affinity* refers to the strength of the attraction between a drug and its receptor. Drugs with high affinity are strongly attracted to their receptors. Conversely, drugs with low affinity are weakly attracted.

The affinity of a drug for its receptor is reflected in its *potency*. Because they are strongly attracted to their receptors, drugs with high affinity can bind to their receptors when present in low concentrations. Because they bind to receptors at low concentrations, drugs with high affinity are effective in low doses. That is, *drugs with high affinity are very potent.* Conversely, drugs with low affinity must be present in high concentrations to bind to their receptors. Accordingly, these drugs are less potent.

Intrinsic Activity. The term *intrinsic activity* refers to the ability of a drug to activate a receptor upon binding. Drugs with high intrinsic activity cause intense receptor activation. Conversely, drugs with low intrinsic activity cause only slight activation.

The intrinsic activity of a drug is reflected in its *maximal efficacy*. Drugs with high intrinsic activity have high maximal efficacy. That is, by causing intense receptor activation, they are able to cause intense responses. Conversely, if intrinsic activity is low, maximal efficacy will be low as well.

It should be noted that, under the modified occupancy theory, the intensity of the response to a drug is still related to the number of receptors occupied. The wrinkle added by the modified theory is that intensity is also related to the ability of the drug to activate receptors once binding has occurred. Under the modified theory, two drugs can occupy the same number of receptors but produce effects of different intensity; the drug with greater intrinsic activity will produce the more intense response.

Agonists, Antagonists, and Partial Agonists

As previously noted, when drugs bind to receptors they can do one of two things: they can either *mimic* the action of endogenous regulatory molecules or they can *block* the action of endogenous regulatory molecules. Drugs that mimic the body's own regulatory molecules are called *agonists*. Drugs that block the actions of endogenous regulators are called *antagonists*. Like agonists, *partial agonists* also mimic the actions of endogenous regulatory molecules, but they produce responses of intermediate intensity.

Agonists

Agonists are molecules that activate receptors. Because neurotransmitters, hormones, and all other endogenous regulators of receptor function activate the receptors to which they bind, all of these compounds are considered agonists. When drugs act as agonists, they simply bind to receptors and mimic the actions of the body's own regulatory molecules.

In terms of the modified occupancy theory, an agonist is a drug that has both *affinity* and *high intrinsic activity.* Affinity allows the agonist to bind to receptors, while intrinsic activity allows the bound agonist to activate or turn on receptor function.

Many therapeutic agents produce their effects by functioning as agonists. Dobutamine, for example, is a drug that mimics the action of NE at receptors on the heart, thereby causing heart rate and force of contraction to increase. The insulin that we administer as a drug mimics the actions of endogenous insulin at receptors. Norethindrone, a component of many oral contraceptives, acts by turning on receptors for progesterone.

It is important to note that agonists do not necessarily make physiologic processes go faster; receptor activation by these compounds can also make a process go slower. For example, there are receptors on the heart that, when *activated* by acetylcholine (the body's own agonist for these receptors), will cause heart rate to *decrease.* Drugs that mimic the action of acetylcholine at these receptors will also decrease heart rate. Because such drugs produce their effects by causing receptor activation, they would be called agonists—even though they cause heart rate to decline.

Antagonists

Antagonists produce their effects by preventing receptor activation by endogenous regulatory molecules and drugs. Antagonists have virtually no effects of their own on receptor function.

In terms of the modified occupancy theory, an antagonist is a drug with affinity for a receptor but with no intrinsic activity. Affinity allows the antagonist to bind to receptors, but lack of intrinsic activity prevents the bound antagonist from causing receptor activation.

Although antagonists do not cause receptor activation, they most certainly *do* produce pharmacologic effects. Antagonists produce their effects by *preventing the activation of receptors by agonists.* Antagonists can produce beneficial effects by blocking the actions of endogenous regulatory molecules or by blocking the actions of drugs.

It is important to note that the response to an antagonist is determined by how much *agonist* is present. Because antagonists act by preventing receptor activation, *if there is no agonist present, administration of an antagonist will have no observable effect;* the drug will bind to its receptors but nothing will happen. On the other hand, if receptors are undergoing activation by agonists, administration of an antagonist will shut the process down, resulting in an observable response. This is an important concept, so please think about it.

Many therapeutic agents produce their effects by acting as receptor antagonists. Antihistamines, for example, suppress allergy symptoms by binding to receptors for histamine, thereby preventing activation of these receptors by histamine released in response to allergens. The use of antagonists to treat drug toxicity is illustrated by naloxone, an agent that blocks receptors for morphine and related opioids; by preventing activation of opioid receptors, naloxone can completely reverse all symptoms of opioid overdose.

Noncompetitive Versus Competitive Antagonists. Antagonists can be subdivided into two major classes: (1) noncompetitive antagonists and (2) competitive antagonists. Most antagonists are competitive.

Noncompetitive (Insurmountable) Antagonists. Noncompetitive antagonists bind *irreversibly* to receptors. The effect of irreversible binding is equivalent to reducing the total number of receptors available for activation by an agonist. Because the intensity of the response to an agonist is proportional to the total number of receptors occupied, and because noncompetitive antagonists decrease the number of receptors available for activation, noncompetitive antagonists *reduce the maximal response* that an agonist can elicit. If sufficient antagonist is present, agonist effects will be blocked completely. Dose-response curves illustrating inhibition by a noncompetitive antagonist are shown in Fig. 5.7A.

Because the binding of noncompetitive antagonists is irreversible, inhibition by these agents cannot be overcome, no matter how much agonist may be available. Because inhibition by noncompetitive antagonists cannot be reversed, these agents are rarely used therapeutically. (Recall from Chapter 1 that reversibility is one of the properties of an ideal drug.)

Although noncompetitive antagonists bind irreversibly, this does not mean that their effects last forever. Cells are constantly breaking down old receptors and synthesizing new ones. Consequently, the effects of noncompetitive antagonists wear off as the receptors to which they are bound are replaced. Because the life cycle of a receptor can be relatively short, the effects of noncompetitive antagonists may subside in a few days.

Competitive (Surmountable) Antagonists. Competitive antagonists bind *reversibly* to receptors. As their name implies, competitive antagonists produce receptor blockade by competing with agonists for receptor binding. If an agonist and a competitive antagonist have equal affinity for a particular receptor, then the receptor will be occupied by whichever agent—agonist or antagonist—is present in the highest concentration. If there are more antagonist molecules present than agonist molecules, antagonist molecules will occupy the receptors and receptor activation will be blocked. Conversely, if agonist molecules outnumber the antagonists, receptors will be occupied mainly by the agonist and little inhibition will occur.

Because competitive antagonists bind reversibly to receptors, the inhibition they cause is *surmountable.* In the presence of sufficiently high amounts of agonist, agonist molecules will occupy all receptors and inhibition will be completely overcome. The dose-response curves shown in Fig. 5.7B illustrate the process of overcoming the effects of a competitive antagonist with large doses of an agonist.

Partial Agonists

A partial agonist is an agonist that has only moderate intrinsic activity. As a result, *the maximal effect that a partial agonist can produce is lower than that of a full agonist.* Pentazocine is an example of a partial agonist. As the curves in Fig. 5.2A indicate, the degree of pain relief that can be achieved with pentazocine is much lower than the relief that can be achieved with meperidine (a full agonist).

Partial agonists are interesting in that they can act as *antagonists* as well as *agonists.* For this reason, they are sometimes referred to as agonists-antagonists. For example, when pentazocine is administered by itself, it occupies opioid receptors and produces moderate relief of pain. In this situation, the drug is acting as an agonist. However, if a patient is already

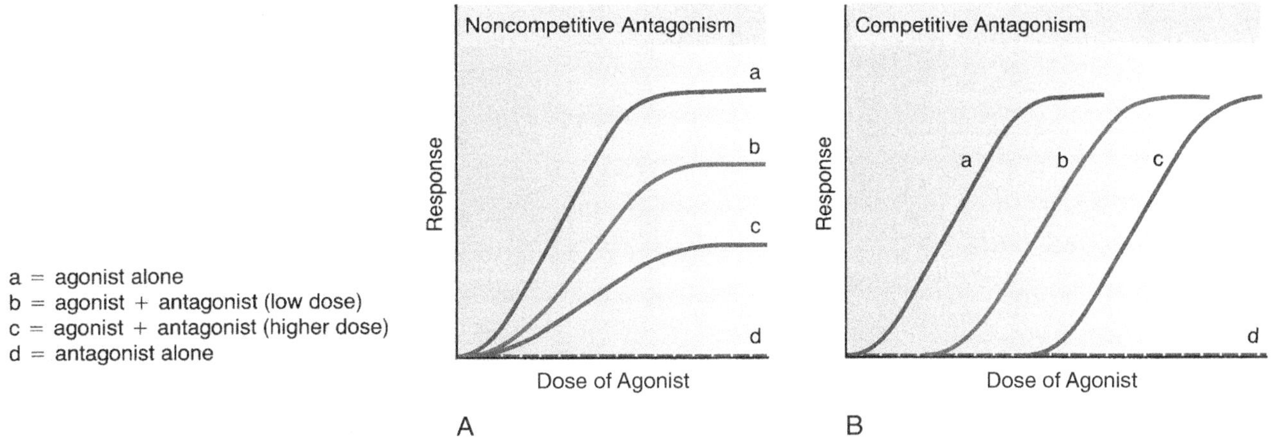

Fig. 5.7 ■ Dose-response curves in the presence of competitive and noncompetitive antagonists.
A, Effect of a noncompetitive antagonist on the dose-response curve of an agonist. Note that noncompetitive antagonists decrease the maximal response achievable with an agonist. **B,** Effect of a competitive antagonist on the dose-response curve of an agonist. Note that the maximal response achievable with the agonist is not reduced. Competitive antagonists simply increase the amount of agonist required to produce any given intensity of response.

taking meperidine (a full agonist at opioid receptors) and is then given a large dose of pentazocine, pentazocine will occupy the opioid receptors and prevent their full activation by meperidine. As a result, the patient cannot experience the high degree of pain relief that meperidine can produce. In this situation, pentazocine is acting as both an agonist (producing moderate pain relief) and an antagonist (blocking the higher degree of relief that could have been achieved with meperidine by itself).

Regulation of Receptor Sensitivity

Receptors are dynamic components of the cell. In response to continuous activation or continuous inhibition, the number of receptors on the cell surface can change, as can their sensitivity to agonist molecules (drugs and endogenous ligands). For example, when the receptors of a cell are continually exposed to an *agonist,* the cell usually becomes less responsive. When this occurs, the cell is said to be *desensitized* or *refractory,* or to have undergone *down-regulation.* Several mechanisms may be responsible, including destruction of receptors by the cell and modification of receptors such that they respond less fully. Continuous exposure to antagonists has the opposite effect, causing the cell to become *hypersensitive* (also referred to as *supersensitive*). One mechanism that can cause hypersensitivity is synthesis of more receptors.

DRUG RESPONSES THAT DO NOT INVOLVE RECEPTORS

Although the effects of most drugs result from drug-receptor interactions, some drugs do not act through receptors. Rather, they act through simple physical or chemical interactions with other small molecules.

Common examples of these drugs include antacids, antiseptics, saline laxatives, and chelating agents. Antacids neutralize gastric acidity by direct chemical interaction with stomach acid. The antiseptic action of ethyl alcohol results from precipitating bacterial proteins. Magnesium sulfate, a powerful laxative, acts by retaining water in the intestinal lumen through an osmotic effect. Dimercaprol, a chelating agent, prevents toxicity from heavy metals (e.g., arsenic, mercury) by forming complexes with these compounds. All of these pharmacologic effects are the result of simple physical or chemical interactions, and not interactions with cellular receptors.

INTERPATIENT VARIABILITY IN DRUG RESPONSES

The dose required to produce a therapeutic response can vary substantially from patient to patient because people differ from one another. In this section we consider interpatient variation as a general issue. The specific kinds of differences that underlie variability in drug responses are discussed in Chapter 8.

To promote the therapeutic objective, you must be alert to interpatient variation in drug responses. Because of interpatient variation, it is not possible to predict exactly how an individual patient will respond to medication. Hence, each patient must be evaluated to determine his or her actual response. The nurse who appreciates the reality of interpatient variability will be better prepared to anticipate, evaluate, and respond appropriately to each patient's therapeutic needs.

Measurement of Interpatient Variability

An example of how interpatient variability is measured will facilitate discussion. Assume we have just developed a drug that suppresses production of stomach acid, and now want to evaluate variability in patient responses. To make this evaluation, we must first define a specific *therapeutic objective* or *endpoint.*

Dose of Drug (mg)	Number of Subjects Responding at Each Dose
100	2
120	6
140	17
160	25
180	25
200	17
220	6
240	2

A

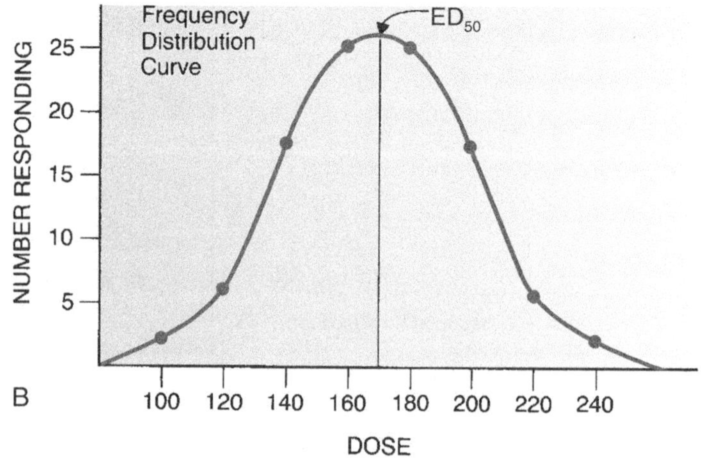

B

Fig. 5.8 ▪ Interpatient variation in drug responses.
A, Data from tests of a hypothetical acid suppressant in 100 patients. The goal of the study is to determine the dosage required by each patient to elevate gastric pH to 5. Note the wide variability in doses needed to produce the target response for the 100 subjects. **B,** Frequency distribution curve for the data in **A.** The dose at the middle of the curve is termed the ED_{50}—the dose that will produce a predefined intensity of response in 50% of the population.

Because our drug reduces gastric acidity, an appropriate endpoint is elevation of gastric pH to a value of 5.

Having defined a therapeutic endpoint, we can now perform our study. Subjects for the study are 100 people with gastric hyperacidity. We begin our experiment by giving each subject a low initial dose (100 mg) of our drug. Next we measure gastric pH to determine how many individuals achieved the therapeutic goal of pH 5. Let's assume that only two people responded to the initial dose. To the remaining 98 subjects, we give an additional 20-mg dose and again determine whose gastric pH rose to 5. Let's assume that six more responded to this dose (120 mg total). We continue the experiment, administering doses in 20-mg increments, until all 100 subjects have responded with the desired elevation in pH.

The data from our hypothetical experiment are plotted in Fig. 5.8. The plot is called a *frequency distribution curve.* We can see from the curve that a wide range of doses is required to produce the desired response in all subjects. For some subjects, a dose of only 100 mg was sufficient to produce the target response. For other subjects, the therapeutic endpoint was not achieved until the dose totaled 240 mg.

The ED_{50}

The dose at the middle of the frequency distribution curve is termed the *ED_{50}* (Fig. 5.8B). (ED_{50} is an abbreviation for *average effective dose.*) The ED_{50} is defined as *the dose that is required to produce a defined therapeutic response in 50% of the population.* In the case of the drug in our example, the ED_{50} was 170 mg—the dose needed to elevate gastric pH to a value of 5 in 50 of the 100 people tested.

The ED_{50} can be considered a standard dose and, as such, is frequently the dose selected for initial treatment. After evaluating a patient's response to this standard dose, we can then adjust subsequent doses up or down to meet the patient's needs.

Clinical Implications of Interpatient Variability

Interpatient variation has four important clinical consequences. As a nurse you should be aware of these implications:

- The initial dose of a drug is necessarily an approximation. Subsequent doses may need to be fine-tuned based on the patient's response. Because initial doses are approximations, it would be wise not to challenge the prescriber if the initial dose differs by a small amount (e.g., 10% to 20%) from recommended doses in a drug reference. Rather, you should administer the medication as prescribed and evaluate the response. Dosage adjustments can then be made as needed. Of course, if the prescriber's order calls for a dose that differs from the recommended dose by a large amount, that order should be clarified.
- When given an average effective dose (ED_{50}), some patients will be undertreated, whereas others will have received more drug than they need. Accordingly, when therapy is initiated with a dose equivalent to the ED_{50}, it is especially important to evaluate the response. Patients who fail to respond may need an increase in dosage. Conversely, patients who show signs of toxicity will need a dosage reduction.
- Because drug responses are not completely predictable, you must monitor the patient's response for both beneficial and harmful effects to determine whether too much or too little medication has been administered. In other words, dosage should be adjusted on the basis of the patient's response and not just on the basis of what some pharmacology reference says is supposed to work. For example, although many postoperative patients receive adequate pain relief with a standard dose of morphine, this dose is not appropriate for everyone: An average dose may be effective for some patients, ineffective for

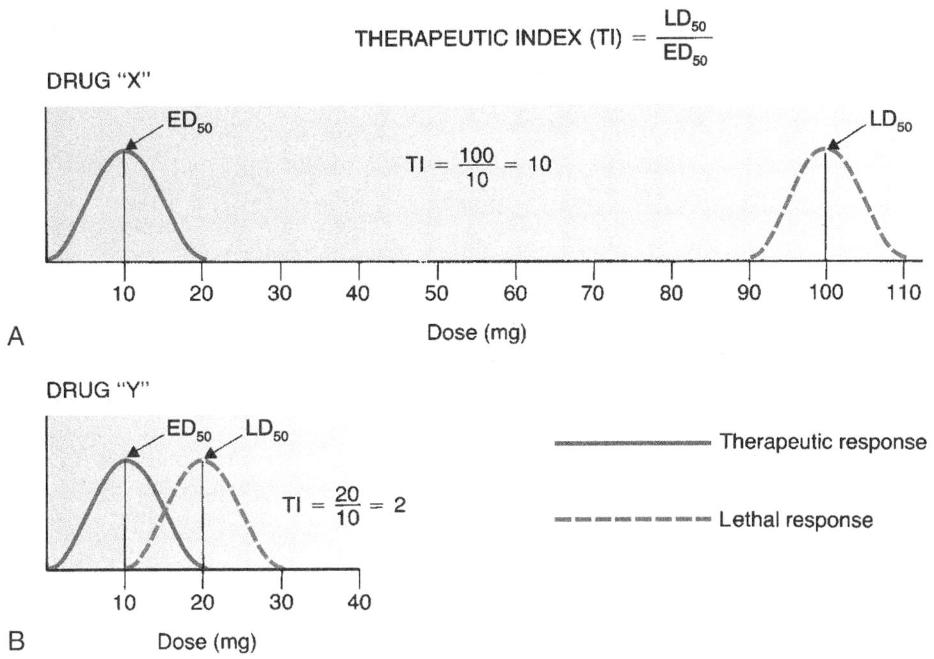

Fig. 5.9 ■ The therapeutic index.
A, Frequency distribution curves indicating the ED_{50} and LD_{50} for drug X. Because its LD_{50} is much greater than its ED_{50}, drug X is relatively safe. **B,** Frequency distribution curves indicating the ED_{50} and LD_{50} for drug Y. Because its LD_{50} is very close to its ED_{50}, drug Y is not very safe. Also note the overlap between the effective-dose curve and the lethal-dose curve.

others, and toxic for still others. Clearly, dosage must be adjusted on the basis of the patient's response, and must not be given in blind compliance with the dosage recommended in a book.

- Because of variability in responses, nurses, patients, and other concerned individuals must evaluate actual responses and be prepared to inform the prescriber about these responses so that proper adjustments in dosage can be made.

THE THERAPEUTIC INDEX

The therapeutic index is a measure of a drug's safety. The therapeutic index, determined using laboratory animals, is defined as *the ratio of a drug's LD_{50} to its ED_{50}*. (The LD_{50}, or average lethal dose, is the dose that is lethal to 50% of the animals treated.) A large (high or wide) therapeutic index indicates that a drug is relatively safe. Conversely, a small (low or narrow) therapeutic index indicates that a drug is relatively unsafe.

The concept of therapeutic index is illustrated by the frequency distribution curves in Fig. 5.9. Part *A* of the figure shows curves for therapeutic and lethal responses to drug X. Part *B* shows equivalent curves for drug Y. As you can see in Fig. 5.9A, the average lethal dose (100 mg) for drug X is much larger than the average therapeutic dose (10 mg). Because this drug's lethal dose is much larger than its therapeutic dose, common sense tells us that the drug should be relatively safe. The safety of this drug is reflected in its high therapeutic index, which is 10. In contrast, drug Y is unsafe. As shown in Fig. 5.9B, the average lethal dose for drug Y (20 mg) is only twice the average therapeutic dose (10 mg). Hence, for drug Y, a dose only twice the ED_{50} could be lethal to 50% of those treated. Clearly, drug Y is not safe. This lack of safety is reflected in its low therapeutic index.

The curves for drug Y illustrate a phenomenon that is even more important than the therapeutic index. As you can see, there is *overlap* between the curve for therapeutic effects and the curve for lethal effects. This overlap tells us that the high doses needed to produce therapeutic effects in some people may be large enough to cause death. The message here is that, if a drug is to be truly safe, the highest dose required to produce therapeutic effects must be substantially lower than the lowest dose required to produce death.

KEY POINTS

- Pharmacodynamics is the study of the biochemical and physiologic effects of drugs and the molecular mechanisms by which those effects are produced.
- For most drugs, the dose-response relationship is graded. That is, the response gets more intense with increasing dosage.
- Maximal efficacy is defined as the biggest effect a drug can produce.
- Although efficacy is important, there are situations in which a drug with relatively low efficacy is preferable to a drug with very high efficacy.
- A potent drug is simply a drug that produces its effects at low doses. As a rule, potency is not important.
- Potency and efficacy are independent qualities. Drug A can be more effective than drug B even though drug B may be more potent. Also, drugs A and B can be equally effective, although one may be more potent than the other.
- A receptor can be defined as any functional macromolecule in a cell to which a drug binds to produce its effects.
- Binding of drugs to their receptors is almost always reversible.
- The receptors through which drugs act are normal points of control for physiologic processes.
- Under physiologic conditions, receptor function is regulated by molecules supplied by the body.
- All that drugs can do at receptors is mimic or block the action of the body's own regulatory molecules.
- Because drug action is limited to mimicking or blocking the body's own regulatory molecules, drugs cannot give cells new functions. Rather, drugs can only alter the rate of preexisting processes.
- Receptors make selective drug action possible.
- There are four primary families of receptors: cell membrane–embedded enzymes, ligand-gated ion channels, G protein–coupled receptor systems, and transcription factors.
- If a drug interacts with only one type of receptor, and if that receptor type regulates just a few processes, then the effects of the drug will be relatively selective.
- If a drug interacts with only one type of receptor, but that receptor type regulates multiple processes, then the effects of the drug will be nonselective.
- If a drug interacts with multiple receptors, its effects will be nonselective.
- Selectivity does not guarantee safety.
- The term *affinity* refers to the strength of the attraction between a drug and its receptor.
- Drugs with high affinity have high relative potency.
- The term *intrinsic activity* refers to the ability of a drug to activate receptors.
- Drugs with high intrinsic activity have high maximal efficacy.
- Agonists are molecules that activate receptors.
- In terms of the modified occupancy theory, agonists have both affinity and high intrinsic activity. Affinity allows them to bind to receptors, while intrinsic activity allows them to activate the receptor after binding.
- Antagonists are drugs that prevent receptor activation by endogenous regulatory molecules and by other drugs.
- In terms of the modified occupancy theory, antagonists have affinity for receptors but no intrinsic activity. Affinity allows the antagonist to bind to receptors, but lack of intrinsic activity prevents the bound antagonist from causing receptor activation.
- Antagonists have no observable effects in the absence of agonists.
- Partial agonists have only moderate intrinsic activity. Hence their maximal efficacy is lower than that of full agonists.
- Partial agonists can act as agonists (if there is no full agonist present) and as antagonists (if a full agonist is present).
- Continuous exposure of cells to agonists can result in receptor desensitization (aka refractoriness or down-regulation), whereas continuous exposure to antagonists can result in hypersensitivity (aka supersensitivity).
- Some drugs act through simple physical or chemical interactions with other small molecules rather than through receptors.
- The ED_{50} is defined as the dose required to produce a defined therapeutic response in 50% of the population.
- An average effective dose (ED_{50}) is perfect for some people, insufficient for others, and excessive for still others.
- The initial dose of a drug is necessarily an approximation. Subsequent doses may need to be fine-tuned based on the patient's response.
- Because drug responses are not completely predictable, you must look at the patient (and not a reference book) to determine whether dosage is appropriate.
- The therapeutic index—defined as the $LD_{50}:ED_{50}$ ratio—is a measure of a drug's safety. Drugs with a high therapeutic index are safe. Drugs with a low therapeutic index are not safe.

Please visit **http://evolve.elsevier.com/Lehne** for chapter-specific NCLEX® examination review questions.

CHAPTER

6 Drug Interactions

In this chapter we consider the interactions of drugs with other drugs, with foods, and with dietary supplements. Our principal focus is on the mechanisms and clinical consequences of drug-drug interactions and drug-food interactions. Drug-supplement interactions are discussed briefly here and at greater length in Chapter 108.

DRUG-DRUG INTERACTIONS

Drug-drug interactions can occur whenever a patient takes two or more drugs. Some interactions are both intended and desired, as when we combine drugs to treat hypertension. In contrast, some interactions are both unintended and undesired, as when we precipitate malignant hyperthermia in a patient receiving succinylcholine. Some adverse interactions are well known, and hence generally avoidable. Others are yet to be documented.

Drug interactions occur because patients frequently take more than one drug. They may take multiple drugs to treat a single disorder. They may have multiple disorders that require treatment with different drugs. They may take over-the-counter drugs in addition to prescription medicines. And they may take caffeine, nicotine, alcohol, and other drugs that have nothing to do with illness.

Our objective in this chapter is to establish an overview of drug interactions, emphasizing the basic mechanisms by which drugs can interact. We will not attempt to catalog the huge number of specific interactions that are known. For information on interactions of specific drugs, you can refer to the chapters in which those drugs are discussed.

Consequences of Drug-Drug Interactions

When two drugs interact, there are three possible outcomes: (1) one drug may intensify the effects of the other, (2) one drug may reduce the effects of the other, or (3) the combination may produce a new response not seen with either drug alone.

Intensification of Effects

When a patient is taking two medications, one drug may intensify, or potentiate, the effects of the other. This type of interaction is often termed a *potentiative* interaction. Potentiative interactions may be beneficial or detrimental. Examples of beneficial and detrimental potentiative interactions follow.

Increased Therapeutic Effects. The interaction between sulbactam and ampicillin represents a beneficial potentiative interaction. When administered alone, ampicillin undergoes rapid inactivation by bacterial enzymes. Sulbactam inhibits those enzymes, and thereby prolongs and intensifies ampicillin's therapeutic effects.

Increased Adverse Effects. The interaction between aspirin and warfarin represents a potentially detrimental potentiative interaction. Both aspirin and warfarin suppress formation of blood clots. Aspirin does this through antiplatelet activity and warfarin does this through anticoagulant activity. As a result, if aspirin and warfarin are taken concurrently, the risk of bleeding is significantly increased. Clearly, potentiative interactions such as this are undesirable.

Reduction of Effects

Interactions that result in reduced drug effects are often termed *inhibitory* interactions. As with potentiative interactions, inhibitory interactions can be beneficial or detrimental. Inhibitory interactions that reduce toxicity are beneficial. Conversely, inhibitory interactions that reduce therapeutic effects are detrimental. Examples follow.

Reduced Therapeutic Effects. The interaction between propranolol and albuterol represents a detrimental inhibitory interaction. Albuterol is taken by people with asthma to dilate the bronchi. Propranolol, a drug for cardiovascular disorders, can act in the lung to block the effects of albuterol. Hence, if propranolol and albuterol are taken together, propranolol can reduce albuterol's therapeutic effects. Inhibitory actions such as this, which can result in therapeutic failure, are clearly detrimental.

Reduced Adverse Effects. The use of naloxone to treat morphine overdose is an excellent example of a beneficial inhibitory interaction. When administered in excessive dosage, morphine can produce coma and profound respiratory depression; death can result. Naloxone, a drug that blocks morphine's actions, can completely reverse all symptoms of toxicity. The benefits of such an inhibitory interaction are obvious.

Creation of a Unique Response

Rarely, the combination of two drugs produces a new response not seen with either agent alone. To illustrate, let's consider the combination of alcohol with disulfiram [Antabuse], a drug used to treat alcoholism. When alcohol and disulfiram are combined, a host of unpleasant and dangerous responses can result. These effects do not occur when disulfiram or alcohol is used alone.

Basic Mechanisms of Drug-Drug Interactions

Drugs can interact through four basic mechanisms: (1) direct chemical or physical interaction, (2) pharmacokinetic interaction, (3) pharmacodynamic interaction, and (4) combined toxicity.

Direct Chemical or Physical Interactions

Some drugs, because of their physical or chemical properties, can undergo direct interaction with other drugs. Direct physical and chemical interactions usually render both drugs inactive.

Direct interactions occur most commonly when drugs are combined in IV solutions. Frequently, but not always, the interaction produces a precipitate. If a precipitate appears when drugs are mixed together, that solution should be discarded. Keep in mind, however, that direct drug interactions may not always leave visible evidence. Hence, you cannot rely on simple inspection to reveal all direct interactions. Because drugs can interact in solution, *never combine two or more drugs in the same container unless it has been established that a direct interaction will not occur.*

The same kinds of interactions that can take place when drugs are mixed together in an IV solution can also occur when incompatible drugs are administered by other routes. However, because drugs are diluted in body water following administration, and because dilution decreases chemical interactions, significant interactions within the patient are much less likely than in IV solutions.

Pharmacokinetic Interactions

Drug interactions can affect all four of the basic pharmacokinetic processes. That is, when two drugs are taken together, one may alter the absorption, distribution, metabolism, or excretion of the other.

Altered Absorption. Drug absorption may be enhanced or reduced by drug interactions. In some cases, these interactions have great clinical significance. There are several mechanisms by which one drug can alter the absorption of another:

- By elevating gastric pH, antacids can decrease the ionization of basic drugs in the stomach, increasing the ability of basic drugs to cross membranes and be absorbed. Antacids have the opposite effect on acidic drugs.
- Laxatives can reduce absorption of other oral drugs by accelerating their passage through the intestine.
- Drugs that depress peristalsis (e.g., morphine, atropine) prolong drug transit time in the intestine, thereby increasing the time for absorption.
- Drugs that induce vomiting can decrease absorption of oral drugs.
- Drugs that are administered orally but do not undergo absorption (e.g., cholestyramine and certain other adsorbent drugs) can adsorb other drugs onto themselves, thereby preventing absorption of the other drugs into the blood.
- Drugs that reduce regional blood flow can reduce absorption of other drugs from that region. For example, when epinephrine is injected together with a local anesthetic (as is often done), the epinephrine causes local vasoconstriction, thereby reducing regional blood flow and delaying absorption of the anesthetic.

Altered Distribution. There are two principal mechanisms by which one drug can alter the distribution of another: (1) competition for protein binding and (2) alteration of extracellular pH.

Competition for Protein Binding. When two drugs bind to the same site on plasma albumin, coadministration of those drugs produces competition for binding. As a result, binding of one or both agents is reduced, causing plasma levels of free drug to rise. In theory, the increase in free drug can intensify effects. However, since the newly freed drug usually undergoes rapid elimination, the increase in plasma levels of free drug is rarely sustained or significant unless the patient has liver problems that interfere with drug metabolism, or renal problems that interfere with drug excretion.

Alteration of Extracellular pH. Because of the pH partitioning effect (see Chapter 4), a drug with the ability to change extracellular pH can alter the distribution of other drugs. For example, if a drug were to increase extracellular pH, that drug would increase the ionization of acidic drugs in extracellular fluids (i.e., plasma and interstitial fluid). As a result, acidic drugs would be drawn from within cells (where the pH was below that of the extracellular fluid) into the extracellular space. Hence, the alteration in pH would change drug distribution.

The ability of drugs to alter pH and thereby alter the distribution of other drugs can be put to practical use in the management of poisoning. For example, symptoms of aspirin toxicity can be reduced with sodium bicarbonate, a drug that elevates extracellular pH. By increasing the pH outside cells, bicarbonate causes aspirin to move from intracellular sites into the interstitial fluid and plasma, thereby minimizing injury to cells.

Altered Metabolism. Altered metabolism is one of the most important—and most complex—mechanisms by which drugs interact. Some drugs *increase* the metabolism of other drugs, and some drugs *decrease* the metabolism of other drugs. Drugs that increase the metabolism of other drugs do so by inducing synthesis of hepatic drug-metabolizing enzymes. Drugs that decrease the metabolism of other drugs do so by inhibiting those enzymes.

As discussed in Chapter 4, the majority of drug metabolism is catalyzed by the cytochrome (CYP) P450 enzymes, which are composed of isoenzyme families (e.g., CYP1, CYP2, CYP3). Of all the isoenzymes in the P450 group, five are responsible for the metabolism of most drugs. These five isoenzymes of CYP are designated CYP1A2, CYP2C9, CYP2C19, CYP2D6, and CYP3A4. Table 6.1 lists major drugs that are metabolized by each isoenzyme, and indicates drugs that can inhibit or induce those isoenzymes.

Induction of CYP Isoenzymes. Drugs that stimulate the synthesis of CYP isoenzymes are referred to as *inducing agents.* The classic example of an inducing agent is phenobarbital, a member of the barbiturate family. By increasing the synthesis of specific CYP isoenzymes, phenobarbital and other inducing agents can stimulate their own metabolism as well as that of other drugs.

Inducing agents can increase the rate of drug metabolism by as much as two- to threefold. This increase develops over 7 to 10 days. Rates of metabolism return to normal 7 to 10 days after the inducing agent has been withdrawn.

When an inducing agent is taken with another medicine, dosage of the other medicine may need adjustment. For example, if a woman taking oral contraceptives were to begin taking phenobarbital, induction of drug metabolism by phenobarbital would accelerate metabolism of the contraceptive, thereby lowering its level. If drug metabolism is increased enough, protection against pregnancy would be lost. To maintain contraceptive efficacy, dosage of the contraceptive should be increased. Conversely, when a patient *discontinues* an inducing agent, dosages of other drugs may need to be *lowered.* If dosage is not reduced, drug levels may climb dangerously high as rates of hepatic metabolism decline to their baseline (noninduced) values.

Inhibition of CYP Isoenzymes. If drug A inhibits the metabolism of drug B, then levels of drug B will rise. The result may be beneficial or harmful. The interaction of cobicistat (a strong CYP3A4 inhibitor) with atazanavir (an expensive drug used to treat HIV infection) provides an interesting case in point. Because cobicistat inhibits CYP3A4 (the CYP isoenzyme that metabolizes atazanavir), if cobicistat is combined with atazanavir, the plasma level of atazanavir will rise. Thus inhibition of CYP3A4 allows us to achieve therapeutic drug levels at lower doses, thereby greatly reducing the cost of treatment—a clearly beneficial result.

Although inhibition of drug metabolism can be beneficial, as a rule inhibition has undesirable results. That is, in most cases, when an inhibitor increases the level of another drug, the outcome is toxicity. To prevent this problem, when it is necessary to prescribe both an isoenzyme inhibitor along with a drug metabolized by the same isoenzymes (i.e., the substrate), the provider will prescribe the substrate at a lower dose. Still, because individual responses vary, you should be alert for possible adverse effects. Unfortunately, because the number of possible interactions of this type is large, keeping track is a challenge. The safest practice is to check for drug interactions in one of the reliable software applications that are widely available.

Altered Renal Excretion. Drugs can alter all three phases of renal excretion: filtration, reabsorption, and active secretion. By doing so, one drug can alter the renal excretion of another. Glomerular filtration can be decreased by drugs that reduce cardiac output: A reduction in cardiac output decreases renal perfusion (blood flow), which decreases drug filtration at the glomerulus, which in turn decreases the rate of drug excretion.

TABLE 6.1 ■ Drugs That Are Important Substrates, Inhibitors, or Inducers of Specific CYP Isoenzymes[a]

CYP	Substrates	Inhibitors		Inducers
CYP1A2	***CNS Drugs:*** amitriptyline, clomipramine, clozapine, desipramine, duloxetine, fluvoxamine, haloperidol, imipramine, methadone, ramelteon, rasagiline, ropinirole, tacrine ***Others:*** theophylline, tizanidine, warfarin	Acyclovir Ciprofloxacin Ethinyl estradiol Fluvoxamine Isoniazid Norfloxacin Oral contraceptives Zafirlukast Zileuton		Carbamazepine Phenobarbital Phenytoin Primidone Rifampin Ritonavir Tobacco St. John's wort
CYP2C9	Diazepam, phenytoin, ramelteon, voriconazole, warfarin	Amiodarone Azole antifungals Efavirenz Fenofibrate Fluorouracil Fluoxetine	Fluvastatin Fluvoxamine Gemfibrozil Isoniazid Leflunomide Zafirlukast	Aprepitant Carbamazepine Phenobarbital Phenytoin Primidone Rifampin Rifapentine Ritonavir St. John's wort
CYP2C19	Citalopram, clopidogrel, methadone, phenytoin, thioridazine, voriconazole	Chloramphenicol Cimetidine Esomeprazole Etravirine Felbamate Fluconazole Fluoxetine	Fluvoxamine Isoniazid Ketoconazole Lansoprazole Modafinil Omeprazole Ticlopidine Voriconazole	Carbamazepine Phenobarbital Phenytoin St. John's wort Tipranavir/ritonavir
CYP2D6	***CNS Drugs:*** amitriptyline, atomoxetine, clozapine, desipramine, donepezil, doxepin, duloxetine, fentanyl, haloperidol, iloperidone, imipramine, meperidine, nortriptyline, tetrabenazine, thioridazine, tramadol, trazodone ***Antidysrhythmic Drugs:*** flecainide, mexiletine, propafenone ***Beta Blocker:*** metoprolol ***Opioids:*** codeine, dextromethorphan, hydrocodone	Amiodarone Cimetidine Darifenacin Darunavir/ritonavir Duloxetine Fluoxetine Methadone	Paroxetine Propranolol Quinidine Ritonavir Sertraline Tipranavir/ritonavir	Not an inducible enzyme

Continued

TABLE 6.1 ■ Drugs That Are Important Substrates, Inhibitors, or Inducers of Specific CYP Isoenzymes[a]—cont'd

CYP	Substrates	Inhibitors		Inducers
CYP3A4	***Antibacterials/Antifungals:*** clarithromycin, erythromycin, ketoconazole, itraconazole, rifabutin, telithromycin, voriconazole ***Anticancer Drugs:*** busulfan, dasatinib, doxorubicin, erlotinib, etoposide, ixabepilone, lapatinib, paclitaxel, pazopanib, romidepsin, sunitinib, tamoxifen, vinblastine, vincristine ***Calcium Channel Blockers:*** amlodipine, felodipine, isradipine, nifedipine, nimodipine, nisoldipine, verapamil ***Drugs for HIV Infection:*** amprenavir, atazanavir, darunavir, etravirine, indinavir, maraviroc, nelfinavir, ritonavir, saquinavir, tipranavir ***Drugs for Erectile Dysfunction:*** sildenafil, tadalafil, vardenafil ***Drugs for Urge Incontinence:*** darifenacin, fesoterodine, solifenacin, tolterodine ***Immunosuppressants:*** cyclosporine, everolimus, sirolimus, tacrolimus ***Opioids:*** alfentanil, alfuzosin, fentanyl, methadone, oxycodone ***Sedative-Hypnotics:*** alprazolam, eszopiclone, midazolam, ramelteon, triazolam ***Statins:*** atorvastatin, lovastatin, simvastatin ***Antidysrhythmic Drugs:*** disopyramide, dronedarone, lidocaine, quinidine ***Others:*** aprepitant, bosentan, cinacalcet, cisapride, colchicine, conivaptan, dihydroergotamine, dronabinol, eplerenone, ergotamine, estrogens, ethosuximide, fluticasone, guanfacine, iloperidone, ondansetron, oral contraceptives, pimozide, ranolazine, rivaroxaban, saxagliptin, sertraline, silodosin, tiagabine, tolvaptan, trazodone, warfarin	Amiodarone Amprenavir Aprepitant Atazanavir Azole antifungals Chloramphenicol Cimetidine Clarithromycin Cobicistat Conivaptan Cyclosporine Darunavir/ritonavir Delavirdine Diltiazem Dronedarone Erythromycin Fluvoxamine Fosamprenavir Grapefruit juice	Indinavir Isoniazid Methylprednisolone Nefazodone Nelfinavir Nicardipine Nifedipine Norfloxacin Pazopanib Prednisone Protease inhibitors Quinine Quinupristin/dalfopristin Ritonavir Saquinavir Telithromycin Tipranavir/ritonavir Verapamil	Amprenavir Aprepitant Bosentan Carbamazepine Dexamethasone Efavirenz Ethosuximide Etravirine Garlic supplements Nevirapine Oxcarbazepine Phenobarbital Phenytoin Primidone Rifabutin Rifampin Rifapentine Ritonavir St. John's wort

CNS, Central nervous system; *HIV*, human immunodeficiency virus.
[a]This list is not comprehensive.

By altering urinary pH, one drug can alter the ionization of another and thereby increase or decrease the extent to which that drug undergoes passive tubular reabsorption. Finally, competition between two drugs for active tubular secretion can decrease the renal excretion of both agents.

Interactions That Involve P-Glycoprotein. As discussed in Chapter 4, P-glycoprotein (PGP) is a transmembrane protein that transports a wide variety of drugs *out* of cells, including cells of the intestinal epithelium, placenta, blood-brain barrier, liver, and kidney tubules. Like P450 isoenzymes, PGP is subject to induction and inhibition by drugs. In fact (and curiously), most of the drugs that induce or inhibit P450 have the same impact on PGP. Drugs that *induce* PGP can have the following impact on other drugs:

- *Reduced absorption*—by increasing drug export from cells of the intestinal epithelium into the intestinal lumen
- *Reduced fetal drug exposure*—by increasing drug export from placental cells into the maternal blood
- *Reduced brain drug exposure*—by increasing drug export from cells of brain capillaries into the blood
- *Increased drug elimination*—by increasing drug export from liver into the bile and from renal tubular cells into the urine

Drugs that inhibit PGP will have opposite effects.

Pharmacodynamic Interactions

By influencing pharmacodynamic processes, one drug can alter the effects of another. Pharmacodynamic interactions are of two basic types: (1) interactions in which the interacting drugs act at the *same* site and (2) interactions in which the interacting drugs act at *separate* sites. Pharmacodynamic interactions may be potentiative or inhibitory, and can be of great clinical significance.

Interactions at the Same Receptor. Interactions that occur at the same receptor are almost always *inhibitory.* Inhibition occurs when an antagonist drug blocks access of an agonist drug to its receptor. These agonist-antagonist interactions are described in Chapter 5. There are many agonist-antagonist interactions of clinical importance. Some reduce therapeutic effects and are therefore undesirable. Others reduce toxicity and are of obvious benefit. The interaction between naloxone and morphine noted earlier in this chapter is an example of a beneficial inhibitory interaction: By blocking access of morphine to its receptors, naloxone can reverse all symptoms of morphine overdose.

Interactions Resulting From Actions at Separate Sites. Even though two drugs have different mechanisms of action and act at separate sites, if both drugs influence the same physiologic process, then one drug can alter responses produced by the other. Interactions resulting from effects produced at different sites may be potentiative or inhibitory.

The interaction between morphine and diazepam [Valium] illustrates a potentiative interaction resulting from concurrent use of drugs that act at separate sites. Morphine and diazepam are central nervous system (CNS) depressants, but these drugs do not share the same mechanism of action. Hence, when these agents are administered together, the ability of each to depress CNS function reinforces the depressant effects of the other. This potentiative interaction can result in profound CNS depression.

The interaction between two diuretics—hydrochlorothiazide and spironolactone—illustrates how the effects of a drug acting at one site can *counteract* the effects of a second drug acting at a different site. Hydrochlorothiazide acts on the distal convoluted tubule of the nephron to *increase* excretion of potassium. Acting at a different site in the kidney, spironolactone works to *decrease* renal excretion of potassium. Consequently, when these two drugs are administered together, the potassium-sparing effects of spironolactone tend to balance the potassium-wasting effects of hydrochlorothiazide, leaving renal excretion of potassium at about the same level it would have been had no drugs been given at all.

Combined Toxicity

If drug A and drug B are both toxic to the same organ, then taking them together will cause more injury than if they were not combined. For example, when we treat tuberculosis with isoniazid and rifampin, both of which are hepatotoxic, the potential to cause liver injury is greater than it would be if we used just one of the drugs. As a rule, drugs with overlapping toxicity are not used together. Unfortunately, when treating tuberculosis, the combination is essential.

Clinical Significance of Drug-Drug Interactions

Clearly, drug interactions have the potential to affect the outcome of therapy. As a result of drug-drug interactions, the intensity of responses may be increased or reduced. Interactions that increase therapeutic effects or reduce toxicity are desirable. Conversely, interactions that reduce therapeutic effects or increase toxicity are detrimental.

The risk of a serious drug interaction is proportional to the number of drugs that a patient is taking. That is, the more drugs the patient receives, the greater the risk of a detrimental interaction. Because the average hospitalized patient receives 6 to 10 drugs, interactions are common. Be alert for them.

Interactions are especially important for drugs that have a narrow therapeutic range. For these agents, an interaction that produces a modest increase in drug levels can cause toxicity. Conversely, an interaction that produces a modest decrease in drug levels can cause therapeutic failure.

Although a large number of important interactions have been documented, many more are yet to be identified. Therefore, if a patient develops unusual symptoms, it is wise to suspect that a drug interaction may be the cause—especially since yet another drug might be given to control the new symptoms.

Minimizing Adverse Drug-Drug Interactions

We can minimize adverse interactions in several ways. The most obvious is to minimize the number of drugs a patient receives. A second and equally important way to avoid detrimental interactions is to take a thorough drug history. A history that identifies all drugs the patient is taking, including recreational drugs, over-the-counter drugs, and herbal supplements, allows the prescriber to adjust the regimen accordingly. Please note, however, that patients taking illicit drugs or over-the-counter preparations may fail to report such drug use unless you specifically ask about these (and, even then, some may not report illicit drugs for fear of criminal prosecution). You should be aware of this possibility and make a special effort to ensure that the patient's drug use profile includes drugs that are not prescribed as well as those that are. Additional measures for reducing adverse interactions include adjusting the dosage when an inducer of metabolism is added to or deleted from the regimen, adjusting the timing of administration to minimize interference with absorption, monitoring for early signs of toxicity when combinations of toxic agents cannot be avoided, and being especially vigilant when the patient is taking a drug with a narrow therapeutic range.

DRUG-FOOD INTERACTIONS

Drug-food interactions are both important and poorly understood. They are important because they can result in toxicity or therapeutic failure. They are poorly understood because research has been largely lacking.

Impact of Food on Drug Absorption

Decreased Absorption

Food frequently decreases the *rate* of drug absorption, and occasionally decreases the *extent* of absorption. Reducing the rate of absorption merely delays the onset of effects; peak effects are not lowered. In contrast, reducing the extent of absorption reduces the intensity of peak responses.

The interaction between calcium-containing foods and tetracycline antibiotics is a classic example of food reducing drug absorption. Tetracyclines bind with calcium to form an insoluble and nonabsorbable complex. Hence, if tetracyclines are administered with milk products or calcium supplements, absorption is reduced and antibacterial effects may be lost.

High-fiber foods can reduce absorption of some drugs. For example, absorption of digoxin [Lanoxin], used for cardiac disorders, is reduced significantly by wheat bran, rolled oats, and sunflower seeds. Because digoxin has a narrow therapeutic range, reduced absorption can result in therapeutic failure.

Increased Absorption

With some drugs, food increases the extent of absorption. When this occurs, peak effects are heightened. For example,

TABLE 6.2 ▪ Some Drugs Whose Levels Can Be Increased by Grapefruit Juice

Drug	Indications	Potential Consequences of Increased Drug Levels
Dihydropyridine CCBs: amlodipine, felodipine, nicardipine, nifedipine, nimodipine, nisoldipine	Hypertension; angina pectoris	Toxicity: flushing, headache, tachycardia, hypotension
Nondihydropyridine CCBs: diltiazem, verapamil	Hypertension; angina pectoris	Toxicity: bradycardia, AV heart block, hypotension, constipation
Statins: lovastatin, simvastatin (minimal effect on atorvastatin, fluvastatin, pravastatin, or rosuvastatin)	Cholesterol reduction	Toxicity: headache, GI disturbances, liver and muscle toxicity
Amiodarone	Cardiac dysrhythmias	Toxicity
Caffeine	Prevents sleepiness	Toxicity: restlessness, insomnia, convulsions, tachycardia
Carbamazepine	Seizures; bipolar disorder	Toxicity: ataxia, drowsiness, nausea, vomiting, tremor
Buspirone	Anxiety	Drowsiness, dysphoria
Triazolam	Anxiety; insomnia	Increased sedation
Midazolam	Induction of anesthesia; conscious sedation	Increased sedation
Saquinavir	HIV infection	Increased therapeutic effect
Cyclosporine	Prevents rejection of organ transplants	Increased therapeutic effects; if levels rise too high, renal and hepatic toxicity will occur
Sirolimus and tacrolimus	Prevent rejection of organ transplants	Toxicity
SSRIs: fluoxetine, fluvoxamine, sertraline	Depression	Toxicity: serotonin syndrome
Pimozide	Tourette's syndrome	Toxicity: QT prolongation resulting in a life-threatening ventricular dysrhythmia
Praziquantel	Schistosomiasis	Toxicity
Dextromethorphan	Cough	Toxicity
Sildenafil	Erectile dysfunction	Toxicity

AV, Atrioventricular; *CCBs,* calcium channel blockers; *GI,* gastrointestinal; *HIV,* human immunodeficiency virus; *SSRIs,* selective serotonin reuptake inhibitors.

a high-calorie meal more than doubles the absorption of saquinavir [Invirase], a drug for HIV infection. If saquinavir is taken without food, absorption may be insufficient for antiviral activity.

Impact of Food on Drug Metabolism: The Grapefruit Juice Effect

Grapefruit juice can inhibit the metabolism of certain drugs, thereby raising their blood levels. The effect is sometimes quite remarkable. In one study, coadministration of grapefruit juice produced a 406% increase in blood levels of felodipine [Plendil], a calcium channel blocker used for hypertension. In addition to felodipine and other calcium channel blockers, grapefruit juice can increase blood levels of lovastatin [Mevacor], cyclosporine [Sandimmune], midazolam [Versed], and many other drugs (Table 6.2). This effect is *not* seen with other citrus juices, including orange juice.

Grapefruit juice has four compounds[a] not found in other juices. These raise drug levels mainly by inhibiting CYP3A4 metabolism. CYP3A4 is an isoenzyme of cytochrome P450 found in the liver and the intestinal wall.

Inhibition of the *intestinal* isoenzyme is much greater than inhibition of the liver isoenzyme. By inhibiting CYP3A4, grapefruit juice decreases the intestinal metabolism of many drugs (see Table 6.2), and thereby increases the amount available for absorption. As a result, blood levels of these drugs rise, causing peak effects to be more intense. Because inhibition of CYP3A4 in the liver is minimal, grapefruit juice does not usually affect metabolism of drugs after they have been absorbed. Importantly, grapefruit juice has little or no effect

[a]Compounds contributing to the inhibitory effects of grapefruit juice are the furanocoumarins *bergapten* and *6′,7′-dihydroxybergamottin* and the flavonoids *naringin* and *naringenin*.

on drugs administered IV. Why? Because, with IV administration, intestinal metabolism is not involved.

Inhibition of CYP3A4 is dose dependent. The more grapefruit juice the patient drinks, the greater the inhibition.

Inhibition of CYP3A4 persists after grapefruit juice is consumed. Therefore, a drug need not be administered concurrently with grapefruit juice for an interaction to occur. Put another way, metabolism can still be inhibited even if a patient drinks grapefruit juice in the morning but waits until later in the day to take his or her medicine. In fact, when grapefruit juice is consumed on a regular basis, inhibition can persist up to 3 days after the last glass.

The effects of grapefruit juice vary considerably among patients because levels of CYP3A4 show great individual variation. In patients with very little CYP3A4, inhibition by grapefruit juice may be sufficient to stop metabolism completely. As a result, large increases in drug levels may occur. Conversely, in patients with an abundance of CYP3A4, metabolism may continue more or less normally, despite inhibition by grapefruit juice.

The clinical consequences of inhibition may be good or bad. As indicated in Table 6.2, by elevating levels of certain drugs, grapefruit juice can increase the risk of serious toxicity, an outcome that is obviously bad. On the other hand, by increasing levels of two drugs—saquinavir and cyclosporine—grapefruit juice can intensify therapeutic effects, an outcome that is clearly good.

What should patients do if the drugs they are taking can be affected by grapefruit juice? Unless a predictable effect is known, prudence dictates avoiding grapefruit juice entirely.

Impact of Food on Drug Toxicity

Drug-food interactions sometimes increase toxicity. The most dramatic example is the interaction between monoamine oxidase (MAO) inhibitors (a family of antidepressants) and foods rich in tyramine (e.g., aged cheeses, yeast extracts, Chianti wine). If an MAO inhibitor is combined with these foods, blood pressure can rise to a life-threatening level. To avoid disaster, patients taking MAO inhibitors must be warned about the consequences of consuming tyramine-rich foods and must be given a list of foods to strictly avoid (see Chapter 32). Other drug-food combinations that can increase toxicity include the following:

- Theophylline (an asthma medicine) plus caffeine, which can result in excessive CNS excitation
- Potassium-sparing diuretics (e.g., spironolactone) plus salt substitutes, which can result in dangerously high potassium levels
- Aluminum-containing antacids (e.g., Maalox) plus citrus beverages (e.g., orange juice), which can result in excessive absorption of aluminum

Impact of Food on Drug Action

Although most drug-food interactions concern drug absorption or drug metabolism, food may also (rarely) have a direct impact on drug action. For example, foods rich in vitamin K (e.g., broccoli, brussels sprouts, cabbage) can reduce the effects of warfarin, an anticoagulant. This occurs because warfarin inhibits vitamin K–dependent clotting factors. (See Chapter 52.) Accordingly, when vitamin K is more abundant, warfarin is less able to inhibit the clotting factors, and therapeutic effects decline.

Timing of Drug Administration With Respect to Meals

Administration of drugs at the appropriate time with respect to meals is an important part of drug therapy. As discussed, the absorption of some drugs can be significantly decreased by food, and hence these drugs should be administered on an empty stomach. Conversely, the absorption of other drugs can be increased by food, and hence these drugs should be administered with meals.

Many drugs cause stomach upset when taken without food. If food does not significantly reduce their absorption, then these drugs can be administered with meals. However, if food does reduce their absorption, then we have a difficult choice: We can administer them with food and thereby reduce stomach upset (good news), but also reduce absorption (bad news)—or, we can administer them without food and thereby improve absorption (good news), but also increase stomach upset (bad news). Unfortunately, the correct choice is not always obvious.

When the medication order says to administer a drug "with food" or "on an empty stomach," just what does this mean? To administer a drug with food means to administer it with or shortly after a meal. To administer a drug on an empty stomach means to administer it at least 1 hour before a meal or 2 hours after.

Medication orders frequently fail to indicate when a drug should be administered with respect to meals. As a result, inappropriate administration may occur.

DRUG-SUPPLEMENT INTERACTIONS

Dietary supplements (herbal medicines and other nonconventional remedies) are used widely, creating the potential for frequent and significant interactions with conventional drugs. Of greatest concern are interactions that reduce beneficial responses to conventional drugs and interactions that increase toxicity. These interactions occur through the same pharmacokinetic and pharmacodynamic mechanisms by which conventional drugs interact with each other. Unfortunately, reliable information about dietary supplements is largely lacking, including information on interactions with conventional agents. Interactions that *have* been well documented are discussed as appropriate throughout this text. Dietary supplements and their interactions are discussed at length in Chapter 108.

KEY POINTS

- Some drug-drug interactions are intended and beneficial; others are unintended and detrimental.
- Drug-drug interactions may result in intensified effects, diminished effects, or an entirely new effect.
- Potentiative interactions are beneficial when they increase therapeutic effects and detrimental when they increase adverse effects.
- Inhibitory interactions are beneficial when they decrease adverse effects and detrimental when they decrease beneficial effects.
- Because drugs can interact in solution, never combine two or more drugs in the same container unless you are certain that a direct interaction will not occur.
- Drug interactions can result in increased or decreased absorption.
- Competition for protein binding rarely results in a sustained or significant increase in plasma levels of free drug.
- Drugs that induce hepatic drug-metabolizing enzymes can accelerate the metabolism of other drugs.
- When an inducing agent is added to the regimen, it may be necessary to increase the dosages of other drugs. Conversely, when an inducing agent is discontinued, dosages of other drugs may need to be reduced.
- A drug that inhibits the metabolism of other drugs will increase their levels. Sometimes the result is beneficial, but usually it's detrimental.
- Drugs that act as antagonists at a particular receptor will diminish the effects of drugs that act as agonists at that receptor. The result may be beneficial (if the antagonist prevents toxic effects of the agonist) or detrimental (if the antagonist prevents therapeutic effects of the agonist).
- Drugs that are toxic to the same organ should not be combined (if at all possible).
- We can help reduce the risk of adverse interactions by minimizing the number of drugs the patient is given and by taking a thorough drug history.
- Food may reduce the rate or extent of drug absorption. Reducing the extent of absorption reduces peak therapeutic responses; reducing the rate of absorption merely delays the onset of effects.
- For some drugs, food may increase the extent of absorption.
- Grapefruit juice can inhibit the intestinal metabolism of certain drugs, thereby increasing their absorption, which in turn increases their blood levels.
- Foods may increase drug toxicity. The combination of an MAO inhibitor with tyramine-rich food is the classic example.
- When the medication order says to administer a drug on an empty stomach, this means administer it either 1 hour before a meal or 2 hours after.
- Conventional drugs can interact with dietary supplements. The biggest concerns are increased toxicity and reduced therapeutic effects of the conventional agent.

Please visit **http://evolve.elsevier.com/Lehne** for chapter-specific NCLEX® examination review questions.

CHAPTER

7 Adverse Drug Reactions and Medication Errors

In this chapter we discuss two related issues of drug safety: (1) adverse drug reactions (ADRs), also known as adverse drug events, and (2) medication errors, a major cause of ADRs. We begin with ADRs and then discuss medication errors.

ADVERSE DRUG REACTIONS

An ADR, as defined by the World Health Organization, is any noxious, unintended, and undesired effect that occurs at normal drug doses. Adverse reactions can range in intensity from mildly annoying to life threatening. Fortunately, when drugs are used properly, many ADRs can be avoided, or at least minimized.

Scope of the Problem

Drugs can adversely affect all body systems in varying degrees of intensity. Among the more mild reactions are drowsiness, nausea, mild itching, and minor rashes. Severe reactions include potential fatal conditions such as neutropenia, hepatocellular injury, cardiac dysrhythmias, anaphylaxis, and hemorrhage.

Although ADRs can occur in all patients, some patients are more vulnerable than others. Adverse events are most common in older adults and the very young. (Patients older than 65 years account for more than 50% of all ADR cases.) Severe illness also increases the risk of an ADR. Likewise, adverse events are more common in patients receiving multiple drugs than in patients taking just one drug.

Some data on ADRs will underscore their significance. A 2011 statistical brief by the Agency for Healthcare Research and Quality highlighted a dramatic rise in ADRs. Over 800,000 outpatients sought emergency treatment due to ADRs. Among hospitalized inpatients, 1,735,500 experienced adverse outcomes due to drug reactions and medication errors and, of these, over 53,800 patients died. Sadly, many of these incidents were preventable.

Definitions

Side Effect

A side effect is formally defined as *a nearly unavoidable secondary drug effect produced at therapeutic doses.* Common examples include drowsiness caused by traditional antihistamines and gastric irritation caused by aspirin. Side effects are generally predictable, and their intensity is dose dependent. Some side effects develop soon after drug use starts, whereas others may not appear until a drug has been taken for weeks or months.

Toxicity

The formal definition of toxicity is *the degree of detrimental physiologic effects caused by excessive drug dosing.* Examples include profound respiratory depression from an overdose of morphine and severe hypoglycemia from an overdose of insulin. Although the formal definition of toxicity includes only those severe reactions that occur when dosage is excessive, in everyday language the term *toxicity* has come to mean any severe ADR, regardless of the dose that caused it. For example, when administered in therapeutic doses, many anticancer drugs cause neutropenia (a severe decrease in neutrophilic white blood cells), thereby putting the patient at high risk of infection. This neutropenia may be called a toxicity even though it was produced when dosage was therapeutic.

Allergic Reaction

An allergic reaction is an immune response. For an allergic reaction to occur, there must be prior sensitization of the immune system. Once the immune system has been sensitized to a drug, reexposure to that drug can trigger an allergic response. The intensity of allergic reactions can range from mild itching to severe rash to anaphylaxis. (Anaphylaxis is a life-threatening response characterized by bronchospasm, laryngeal edema, and a precipitous drop in blood pressure.) Estimates suggest that less than 10% of ADRs are of the allergic type.

The intensity of an allergic reaction is determined primarily by the degree of sensitization of the immune system, not by drug dosage. Put another way, *the intensity of allergic reactions is largely independent of dosage.* As a result, a dose that elicits a very strong reaction in one allergic patient may elicit a very mild reaction in another. Furthermore, because a patient's sensitivity to a drug can change over time, a dose that elicits a mild reaction early in treatment may produce an intense reaction later on.

Very few medications cause severe allergic reactions. In fact, most serious reactions are caused by just one drug family—the *penicillins.* Other drugs noted for causing allergic reactions include the nonsteroidal anti-inflammatory drugs (e.g., aspirin) and the sulfonamide group of compounds, which includes certain diuretics, antibiotics, and oral hypoglycemic agents.

Idiosyncratic Effect

An idiosyncratic effect is defined as *an uncommon drug response resulting from a genetic predisposition.* A classic example of an idiosyncratic effect occurs in people with glucose-6-phosphate dehydrogenase (G6PD) deficiency. G6PD deficiency is an X-linked inherited condition that occurs primarily in people with African and Mediterranean ancestry. When people with G6PD deficiency take drugs such as sulfonamides or aspirin, they develop varying degrees of red blood cell hemolysis, which may become life threatening.

Paradoxical Effect

A paradoxical effect is the opposite of the intended drug response. A common example is the insomnia and excitement that may occur when some children and older adults are given benzodiazepines for sedation.

Iatrogenic Disease

An iatrogenic disease is a disease that occurs as the result of medical care or treatment. The term *iatrogenic disease* is also used to denote *a disease produced by drugs.*

Iatrogenic diseases are nearly identical to idiopathic (naturally occurring) diseases. For example, patients taking certain antipsychotic drugs may develop a syndrome whose symptoms closely resemble those of Parkinson disease. Because this syndrome is (1) drug induced and (2) essentially identical to a naturally occurring pathology, we would call the syndrome an iatrogenic disease.

Physical Dependence

Physical dependence is a state in which the body has adapted to drug exposure in such a way that an abstinence syndrome will result if drug use is discontinued. Physical dependence develops during long-term use of certain drugs, such as opioids, alcohol, barbiturates, and amphetamines. The precise nature of the abstinence syndrome is determined by the drug involved.

Although physical dependence is usually associated with "narcotics" (heroin, morphine, and other opioids), these are not the only dependence-inducing drugs. A variety of other centrally acting drugs (e.g., ethanol, barbiturates, amphetamines) can promote dependence. Furthermore, some drugs that work outside the central nervous system can cause physical dependence of a sort. Because a variety of drugs can cause physical dependence of one type or another, and because withdrawal reactions have the potential for harm, *patients should be warned against abrupt discontinuation of any medication without first consulting a health professional.*

Carcinogenic Effect

The term *carcinogenic effect* refers to the ability of certain medications and environmental chemicals to cause cancers. Fortunately, only a few therapeutic agents are carcinogenic. Ironically, several of the drugs used to *treat* cancer are among those with the greatest carcinogenic potential.

Evaluating drugs for the ability to cause cancer is extremely difficult. Evidence of neoplastic disease may not appear until 20 or more years after initial exposure to a cancer-causing compound. Consequently, it is nearly impossible to detect carcinogenic potential during preclinical and clinical trials. Accordingly, when a new drug is released for general marketing, the drug's carcinogenic potential is usually unknown.

Teratogenic Effect

A *teratogenic effect* is a drug-induced birth defect. Medicines and other chemicals capable of causing birth defects are called teratogens. Teratogenesis is discussed in Chapter 9.

Organ-Specific Toxicity

Many drugs are toxic to specific organs. Common examples include injury to the kidneys caused by amphotericin B (an antifungal drug), injury to the heart caused by doxorubicin (an anticancer drug), injury to the lungs caused by amiodarone (an antidysrhythmic drug), and injury to the inner ear caused by aminoglycoside antibiotics (e.g., gentamicin). Patients using such drugs should be monitored for signs of developing injury. In addition, patients should be educated about these signs and advised to seek medical attention if they appear.

Two types of organ-specific toxicity deserve special comment. These are (1) injury to the liver and (2) altered cardiac function, as evidenced by a prolonged QT interval on the electrocardiogram. Both are discussed in the sections that follow.

Hepatotoxic Drugs

As some drugs undergo metabolism by the liver, they are converted to toxic products that can injure liver cells. These drugs are called hepatotoxic drugs.

In the United States, drugs are the leading cause of acute liver failure, a rare condition that can rapidly prove fatal. Fortunately, liver failure from using known hepatotoxic drugs is rare, with an incidence of less than 1 in 50,000. (Drugs that cause liver failure more often than this are removed from the market—unless they are indicated for a life-threatening illness.) More than 50 drugs are known to be hepatotoxic. Some examples are listed in Table 7.1.

Combining a hepatotoxic drug with certain other drugs may increase the risk of liver damage. Acetaminophen (Tylenol) is a hepatotoxic drug that can damage the liver when taken in excessive doses. When taken in therapeutic doses, acetaminophen does not usually create a risk for liver injury; however, if the drug is taken with just two or three alcoholic beverages, severe liver injury can result.

Patients taking hepatotoxic drugs should undergo liver function tests (LFTs) at baseline and periodically thereafter. How do we assess liver function? By testing a blood sample for the presence of two liver enzymes: *aspartate aminotransferase* (AST, formerly known as SGOT) and *alanine aminotransferase* (ALT, formerly known as SGPT). Under normal conditions

TABLE 7.1 ▪ Some Hepatotoxic Drugs

STATINS AND OTHER LIPID-LOWERING DRUGS Atorvastatin [Lipitor] Fenofibrate [TriCor, Trilipix, Lipidil EZ 🍁] Fluvastatin [Lescol] Gemfibrozil [Lopid] Lovastatin [Mevacor] Niacin [Niaspan, others] Pitavastatin [Livalo] Pravastatin [Pravachol] Simvastatin [Zocor] **ORAL ANTIDIABETIC DRUGS** Acarbose [Precose, Glucobay 🍁] Pioglitazone [Actos] Rosiglitazone [Avandia] **ANTISEIZURE DRUGS** Carbamazepine [Tegretol] Felbamate [Felbatol] Phenytoin [Dilantin] Valproic acid [Depakene, others] **ANTIFUNGAL DRUGS** Fluconazole [Diflucan] Griseofulvin [Grifulvin V, Gris-PEG] Itraconazole [Sporanox] Ketoconazole [Nizoral] Terbinafine [Lamisil]	**ANTIGOUT DRUGS** Allopurinol [Zyloprim] Febuxostat [Uloric] **ANTIDEPRESSANT/ANTIPSYCHOTIC DRUGS** Buproprion [Wellbutrin, Zyban] Duloxetine [Cymbalta] Nefazodone Trazodone Tricyclic antidepressants **ANTIMICROBIAL DRUGS** Amoxicillin–clavulanic acid [Augmentin] Erythromycin Minocycline [Minocin] Nitrofurantoin [Macrodantin, Macrobid] Penicillin Trimethoprim-sulfamethoxazole [Septra, Bactrim] **DRUGS FOR TUBERCULOSIS** Isoniazid Pyrazinamide Rifampin [Rifadin] **IMMUNOSUPPRESSANTS** Azathioprine [Imuran] Leflunomide [Arava] Methotrexate [Rheumatrex]	**ANTIRETROVIRAL DRUGS** Nevirapine [Viramune] Ritonavir [Norvir] **OTHER DRUGS** Acetaminophen [Tylenol], but only when combined with alcohol or taken in excessive dose Amiodarone [Cordarone] Baclofen [Lioresal, Gablofen] Celecoxib [Celebrex] Diclofenac [Voltaren] Labetalol [Trandate] Lisinopril [Prinivil, Zestril] Losartan [Cozaar] Methyldopa [Aldomet] Omeprazole [Prilosec] Procainamide Tamoxifen [Nolvadex] Testosterone Zileuton [Zyflo]

blood levels of AST and ALT are low. However, when liver cells are injured, blood levels of these enzymes rise. LFTs are performed on a regular schedule (e.g., every 3 months) in hopes of detecting injury early. Because drug-induced liver injury can develop very quickly between scheduled tests, it is also important to monitor the patient for signs and symptoms of liver injury, such as jaundice (yellow skin and eyes), dark urine, light-colored stools, nausea, vomiting, malaise, abdominal discomfort, and loss of appetite. Additionally, patients receiving hepatotoxic drugs should be informed about these signs of liver injury and advised to seek medical attention if they develop.

QT Interval Drugs

The term *QT interval drugs*—or simply *QT drugs*—refers to the ability of some medications to prolong the QT interval on the electrocardiogram, thereby creating a risk of serious dysrhythmias. As discussed in Chapter 49, the QT interval is a measure of the time required for the ventricles to repolarize after each contraction. When the QT interval is prolonged (more than 470 msec for postpubertal males or more than 480 msec for postpubertal females), patients can develop a dysrhythmia known as *torsades de pointes,* which can progress to potentially fatal ventricular fibrillation.

More than 100 drugs are known to cause QT prolongation, torsades de pointes, or both. As shown in Table 7.2, QT drugs are found in many drug families. Several QT drugs have been withdrawn from the market because of deaths linked to their use, and use of another QT drug—cisapride—is now restricted. To reduce the risks from QT drugs, the Food and Drug Administration (FDA) now requires that all new drugs be tested for the ability to cause QT prolongation.

When QT drugs are used, care is needed to minimize the risk of dysrhythmias. These agents should be used with caution in patients predisposed to dysrhythmias. Among these are older adults and patients with bradycardia, heart failure, congenital QT prolongation, and low levels of potassium or magnesium. Women are at particular risk. Why? Because their normal QT interval is longer than the QT interval in men. Concurrent use of two or more QT drugs should be avoided, as should the concurrent use of a QT drug with another drug that can raise its blood level (e.g., by inhibiting its metabolism).

Identifying Adverse Drug Reactions

It can be very difficult to determine whether a specific drug is responsible for an observed adverse event. Why? Because other factors—especially the underlying illness and other drugs being taken—could be the actual cause. To help determine whether a particular drug is responsible, the following questions should be considered:

- Did symptoms appear shortly after the drug was first used?
- Did symptoms abate when the drug was discontinued?
- Did symptoms reappear when the drug was reinstituted?
- Is the illness itself sufficient to explain the event?
- Are other drugs in the regimen sufficient to explain the event?

TABLE 7.2 ▪ Drugs That Prolong the QT Interval, Induce Torsades De Pointes, or Both

CARDIOVASCULAR: ANTIDYSRHYTHMICS	Amiodarone [Cordarone] Disopyramide [Norpace] Dofetilide [Tikosyn] Dronedarone [Multaq] Flecainide [Tambocor] Ibutilide [Corvert] Mexiletine [Mexitil] Procainamide [Procan, Pronestyl] Quinidine Sotalol [Betapace]
CARDIOVASCULAR: ACE INHIBITORS/CCBs	Bepridil [Vascor] Isradipine [DynaCirc] Moexipril Nicardipine [Cardene]
ANTIBIOTICS	Azithromycin [Zithromax] Clarithromycin [Biaxin] Erythromycin Gemifloxacin [Factive] Levofloxacin [Levaquin] Moxifloxacin [Avelox] Ofloxacin [Floxin] Telithromycin [Ketek]
ANTIFUNGAL DRUGS	Fluconazole [Diflucan] Voriconazole [Vfend]
ANTIDEPRESSANTS	Amitriptyline [Elavil] Citalopram [Celexa] Desipramine [Norpramin] Doxepin [Sinequan] Escitalopram [Lexapro] Fluoxetine [Prozac] Imipramine [Tofranil] Mirtazepine [Remeron] Protriptyline [Pamelor, Aventyl] Sertraline [Zoloft] Trimipramine [Surmontil] Venlafaxine [Effexor]
ANTIPSYCHOTICS	Chlorpromazine [Thorazine] Clozapine [Clozaril] Haloperidol [Haldol] Iloperidone [Fanapt] Paliperidone [Invega] Pimozide [Orap] Quetiapine [Seroquel] Risperidone [Risperdal] Thioridazine [Mellaril] Ziprasidone [Geodon]
ANTIEMETICS/ANTINAUSEA DRUGS	Dolasetron [Anzemet] Domperidone 🍁 Droperidol [Inapsine] Granisetron [Kytril] Ondansetron [Zofran]
ANTICANCER DRUGS	Arsenic trioxide [Trisenox] Eribulin [Halaven] Lapatinib [Tykerb] Nilotinib [Tasigna] Sunitinib [Sutent] Tamoxifen [Nolvadex] Vandetanib [Caprelsa] Vorinostat [Zolinza]
DRUGS FOR ADHD	Amphetamine/dextroamphetamine [Adderall] Atomoxetine [Strattera] Dexmethylphenidate [Focalin] Dextroamphetamine [Dexedrine] Methylphenidate [Ritalin, Concerta]
NASAL DECONGESTANTS	Phenylephrine [Neo-Synephrine, Sudafed PE] Pseudoephedrine [Sudafed]
OTHER DRUGS	Alfuzosin [Uroxatral] Amantadine [Symmetrel] Chloroquine [Aralen] Cisapride [Propulsid][a] Cocaine Felbamate [Felbatol] Fingolimod [Gilenya] Foscarnet [Foscavir] Fosphenytoin [Cerebyx] Galantamine [Razadyne] Halofantrine [Halfan] Indapamide [Lozol] Lithium [Lithobid, Eskalith] Methadone [Dolophine] Midodrine [ProAmatine] Octreotide [Sandostatin] Pasireotide [Signifor] Pentamidine [Pentam, Nebupent] Phentermine [Fastin] Ranolazine [Ranexa] Ritodrine [Yutopar] Salmeterol [Serevent] Saquinavir [Invirase] Solifenacin [Vesicare] Tacrolimus [Prograf] Terbutaline Tizanidine [Zanaflex] Tolterodine [Detrol] Vardenafil [Levitra]

[a]Restricted availability.
ACE, Angiotensin-converting enzyme; *ADHD,* attention-deficit/hyperactivity disorder; *CCB,* calcium channel blocker.

If the answers reveal a temporal relationship between the presence of the drug and the adverse event, and if the event cannot be explained by the illness itself or by other drugs in the regimen, then there is a high probability that the drug under suspicion is indeed the culprit. Unfortunately, this process is limited. It can only identify adverse effects that occur while the drug is being used; it cannot identify adverse events that develop years after drug withdrawal. Nor can it identify effects that develop slowly over the course of prolonged drug use.

Adverse Reactions to New Drugs

As discussed in Chapter 3, preclinical and clinical trials of new drugs cannot detect all of the ADRs that a drug may be able to cause. In fact, about 50% of all new drugs have serious ADRs that are not revealed during Phase II and Phase III trials.

Because newly released drugs may have as-yet-unreported adverse effects, you should be alert for unusual responses when giving new drugs. If the patient develops new symptoms, it is wise to suspect that the drug may be responsible—even if the symptoms are not described in the literature. It is a good practice to initially check postmarketing drug evaluations at www.fda.gov/Drugs/GuidanceComplianceRegulatoryInformation/Surveillance/ucm204091.htm to see whether serious problems have been reported. If the drug is especially new, though, you may be the first clinician to have observed the effect. If you suspect a drug of causing a previously unknown adverse effect, you should report the effect to MEDWATCH, the FDA Medical Products Reporting Program. You can file your report online at www.fda.gov/medwatch. Because voluntary reporting by healthcare professionals is an important mechanism for bringing ADRs to light, you should report all suspected ADRs, even if absolute proof of the drug's complicity has not been established.

Ways to Minimize Adverse Drug Reactions

The responsibility for reducing ADRs lies with everyone associated with drug production and use. The pharmaceutical industry must strive to produce the safest medicines possible; the prescriber must select the least harmful medicine for a particular patient; the nurse must evaluate patients for ADRs and educate patients in ways to avoid or minimize harm; and patients and their families must watch for signs that a serious ADR may be developing and seek medical attention if one appears.

Anticipating ADRs can help minimize them. Nurses and patients should know the major ADRs that a drug can produce. This knowledge allows early identification of adverse effects, thereby permitting timely implementation of measures to minimize harm.

When patients are using drugs that are toxic to specific organs, function of the target organ should be monitored. The liver, kidneys, and bone marrow are important sites of drug toxicity. For drugs that are toxic to the liver, the patient should be monitored for signs and symptoms of liver damage (jaundice, dark urine, light-colored stools, nausea, vomiting, malaise, abdominal discomfort, loss of appetite), and periodic LFTs should be performed. For drugs that are toxic to the kidneys, the patient should undergo routine urinalysis and measurement of serum creatinine or creatinine clearance. For drugs that are toxic to bone marrow, periodic complete blood cell counts are required.

Adverse effects can be reduced by individualizing therapy. When choosing a drug for a particular patient, the prescriber must balance the drug's risks versus its benefits. Drugs that are likely to harm a specific patient should be avoided. For example, if a patient has a history of penicillin allergy, we can avoid a potentially severe reaction by withholding penicillin and contacting the prescriber to obtain an order for a suitable substitute. Similarly, when treating pregnant patients, we must withhold drugs that can injure the fetus (see Chapter 9). The only time a potentially harmful drug should be administered is when the benefits are much greater than the risk. Drugs that are used in treatment of cancer fall into this designation; they can have dangerous adverse effects, but they may be necessary to save the patient's life.

Patients with chronic disorders are especially vulnerable to ADRs. In this group are patients with hypertension, seizures, heart disease, and psychoses. When drugs must be used long term, the patient should be informed about the adverse effects that may develop over time and should be monitored for their appearance.

Medication Guides, Boxed Warnings, and REMS

In an effort to decrease harm associated with drugs that cause serious adverse effects, the FDA requires special alerts and management guidelines. These may take the form of a *Medication Guide* for patients, a *boxed warning* to alert prescribers, and/or a *Risk Evaluation and Mitigation Strategy* (REMS), which can involve patients, prescribers, and pharmacists.

Medication Guides

Medication Guides, commonly called MedGuides, are FDA-approved documents created to educate patients about how to minimize harm from potentially dangerous drugs. In addition, a MedGuide is required when the FDA has determined that (1) patient adherence to directions for drug use is essential for efficacy or (2) patients need to know about potentially serious effects when deciding to use a drug.

All MedGuides use a standard format that provides information under the following main headings:

- What is the most important information I should know about (*name of drug*)?
- What is (*name of drug*)? Including: a description of the drug and its indications.
- Who should not take (*name of drug*)?
- How should I take (*name of drug*)? Including: importance of adherence to dosing instructions, special instructions about administration, what to do in case of overdose, and what to do if a dose is missed.
- What should I avoid while taking (*name of drug*)? Including: activities (e.g., driving, sunbathing), other drugs, foods, pregnancy, breast-feeding.
- What are the possible or reasonably likely side effects of (*name of drug*)?
- General information about the safe and effective use of prescription drugs.

Additional headings may be added by the manufacturer as appropriate, with the approval of the FDA. MedGuides for all drug products that require one are available online at www.fda.gov/Drugs/DrugSafety/UCM085729.

The MedGuide should be provided whenever a prescription is filled, and even when drug samples are handed out. However, under special circumstances, the Guide can be withheld. For example, if the prescriber feels that the information in the Guide might deter a patient from taking a potentially lifesaving drug, the prescriber can ask the pharmacy to withhold the Guide. Nonetheless, if the patient asks for the information, the pharmacist must provide it, regardless of the request to withhold it.

Boxed Warnings

The *boxed warning,* also known as a *black box warning,* is the strongest safety warning a drug can carry and still remain on the market. Text for the warning is presented inside a box with a heavy black border. The FDA requires a boxed warning on drugs with serious or life-threatening risks. The purpose of the warning is to alert prescribers to (1) potentially severe side effects (e.g., life-threatening dysrhythmias, suicidality, major fetal harm) as well as (2) ways to prevent or reduce harm (e.g., avoiding a teratogenic drug during pregnancy). The boxed warning should provide a *concise summary* of the adverse effects of concern, not a detailed explanation. A boxed warning must appear prominently on the package insert, on the product label, and even in magazine advertising. Drugs that have a boxed warning must also have a MedGuide.

Risk Evaluation and Mitigation Strategies

An REMS is simply a plan to minimize drug-induced harm. For the majority of drugs that have an REMS, a MedGuide is all that is needed. For a few drugs, however, the REMS may have additional components. For example, the REMS for isotretinoin, a drug for severe acne, has provisions that pertain to the patient, prescriber, and pharmacist. This program, known as iPLEDGE, is needed because isotretinoin can cause serious birth defects. The iPLEDGE program was designed to ensure that patients who are pregnant, or may become pregnant, will not have access to the drug. Details of the iPLEDGE program are presented in Chapter 105. All REMS that have received FDA approval can be found online at www.fda.gov/Drugs/DrugSafety/PostmarketDrugSafetyInformationforPatientsandProviders/ucm111350.htm.

MEDICATION ERRORS

Medication errors are a major cause of morbidity and mortality. According to an FDA October 2016 update, medication errors injure approximately 1.3 million people each year. Researchers at Johns Hopkins estimated the 2016 death rate due to medication errors to be over 400,000 patients annually. They further noted that, if medication errors were listed on death certificates, these errors would comprise the third leading cause of death in the United States. The financial costs are staggering: Among hospitalized patients alone, treatment of drug-related injuries costs about $3.5 billion a year.

What Are Medication Errors and Who Makes Them?

The National Coordinating Council for Medication Error Reporting and Prevention (NCC MERP) defines a medication error as "any preventable event that may cause or lead to inappropriate medication use or patient harm while the medication is in the control of the healthcare professional, patient, or consumer. Such events may be related to professional practice, healthcare products, procedures, and systems, including prescribing; order communication; product labeling, packaging and nomenclature; compounding; dispensing; distribution; administration; education; monitoring; and use." Note that, by this definition, medication errors can be made by many people—beginning with workers in the pharmaceutical industry, followed by people in the healthcare delivery system, and ending with patients and their family members. In the hospital setting, a medication order must be processed by several people before it reaches the patient. The process typically begins when a healthcare provider enters the order into a computer. The pharmacist verifies it. The registered nurse (RN) removes it from an automated dispensing cabinet. Finally, the RN scans the order, the RN badge, the product, and the patient's armband. Once these steps have been taken, the RN administers the drug. Each of these people is in a position to make an error. Because the nurse is the last person who can catch mistakes made by others, and because no one is there to catch mistakes the nurse might make, the nurse bears a heavy responsibility for ensuring patient safety.

TABLE 7.3 ▪ Types of Medication Errors

Wrong patient
Wrong drug
Wrong route
Wrong time
Wrong dose
Omitted dose
Wrong dosage form
Wrong diluent
Wrong strength/concentration
Wrong infusion rate
Wrong technique (includes inappropriate crushing of tablets)
Deteriorated drug error (dispensing a drug after its expiration date)
Wrong duration of treatment (continuing too long or stopping too soon)

Types of Medication Errors

Medication errors fall into 13 major categories (Table 7.3). Some types of errors cause harm directly, and some cause harm indirectly. For example, giving an excessive dose can cause direct harm from dangerous toxic effects. Conversely, giving too little medication can lead to indirect harm through failure to adequately treat an illness. Among *fatal* medication errors involving drug administration, the most common types are giving an overdose (36.4%), giving the wrong drug (16.2%), and using the wrong route (9.5%).

Causes of Medication Errors

Medication errors can result from many causes. Among fatal medication errors, the IOM identifies three categories—human factors, communication mistakes, and name confusion—that account for 90% of all errors. Of the human factors that can cause errors, performance deficits (e.g., administering a drug IV instead of IM) are the most common (29.8%), followed by knowledge deficits (14.2%) and miscalculation of dosage (13%). These and other causes of medication errors are detailed in Table 7.4.

Miscommunication involving oral and written orders underlies 15.8% of fatal errors. Poor handwriting is an infamous cause of mistakes. When patients are admitted to the hospital, poor communication regarding medications they were taking at home can result in the wrong drug or wrong dosage being prescribed. Confusion over drug names underlies 15% of all reports to the Medication Errors Reporting (MER) Program. Many drugs have names that sound like or look like the names of other drugs. Table 7.5 lists some examples, such as *Anaspaz/Antispas* and *Nasarel/Nizoral.* Additionally, the Institute for Safe Medication Practices (ISMP) offers a more comprehensive list online at www.ismp.org/tools/confuseddrugnames.pdf. To reduce name-related medication errors, some hospitals are required to have a "read-back" system, in which verbal orders given to pharmacists or medical staff are transcribed and then read back to the prescriber.

Ways to Reduce Medication Errors

Organizations throughout the country are working to design and implement measures to reduce medication errors. A central

TABLE 7.4 ▪ Causes of Medication Errors

Cause	Examples
HUMAN FACTORS	
Performance deficit	Improper administration technique resulted in a drug intended for subcutaneous administration being given intramuscularly.
Knowledge deficit	Lack of knowledge regarding drug-drug interactions resulted in drug inactivation when incompatible drugs were administered simultaneously in the same IV line.
Miscalculation of dosage	Inaccurate placement of a decimal during drug calculation resulted in a drug overdose or underdose.
Drug preparation error	Failure to adequately dilute an intravenous medication resulted in severe phlebitis.
Computer error	Incorrect programming into the database resulted in improper drug labeling that caused a medication error.
Stocking error	Stocking otic drops instead of ophthalmic drops contributed to administration of the wrong drug formulation, which resulted in eye damage.
Transcription error	Substituting a "3" for an "8" when transcribing the original drug order to a computer resulted in the patient being prescribed a subtherapeutic drug dosage.
Stress	Inadequate time devoted to task due to higher-than-typical patient acuity contributed to failure to administer a scheduled drug.
Fatigue or lack of sleep	Decreased concentration on task resulted in inadequate safety checks that contributed to giving a drug overdose.
COMMUNICATION MISTAKES	
Written miscommunication	Illegible handwriting contributed to misinterpretation of a drug order, so the patient received the wrong drug.
Oral miscommunication	A verbal order for cefuroxime, a second-generation cephalosporin, was transcribed as cefotaxime, a third-generation cephalosporin.
NAME CONFUSION	
Brand name confusion	Celebrex, an analgesic to manage pain, was confused with Celexa, a drug used to manage depression.
Generic name confusion	Rifampin, a drug for treatment of tuberculosis, was given to the patient with traveler's diarrhea who was prescribed the less familiar drug rifaximin.
PACKAGING, FORMULATIONS, AND DELIVERY DEVICES	
Inappropriate packaging	Topical product packaged in sterile IV multidose vial.
Tablet or capsule confusion	Confusion because the tablet or capsule is similar in color, shape, or size to tablets or capsules that contain a different drug or a different strength of the same drug.
Delivery device problems	Malfunction; infusion pump problems; selection of wrong device.
LABELING AND REFERENCE MATERIALS	
Manufacturer's carton	Carton looks similar to other cartons from the same manufacturer or cartons from a different manufacturer.
Manufacturer's container label	Label looks similar to other labels from the same manufacturer or to labels from a different manufacturer.
Label of dispensed product	Wrong patient name; wrong drug name; wrong strength; wrong or incomplete directions.
Reference materials (package insert and other printed material, electronic material)	Inaccurate, incomplete, misleading, or outdated information.

theme in these efforts is to change institutional culture from one that focuses on "naming, shaming, and blaming" those who make mistakes to one focused on designing institution-wide processes and systems that can prevent errors from happening. Changes having the most dramatic effect have been those that focused on the IOM recommendations to (1) help and encourage patients and their families to be active, informed members of the healthcare team, and (2) give healthcare providers the tools and information needed to prescribe, dispense, and administer drugs as safely as possible.

Early work by the ISMP, in collaboration with the Regional Medication Safety Program for Hospitals (a consortium of hospitals in Pennsylvania) and the Emergency Care Research Institute (ECRI) identified 16 action goals divided into four major categories: institutional culture, infrastructure, clinical practice, and technology (Table 7.6). These general goals can

TABLE 7.5 ▪ Examples of Drugs With Names That Sound Alike or Look Alike[a]

Amicar	*Omacar*
Anaspaz	*Antispas*
Celebrex	*Cerebyx*
Clinoril	*Clozaril*
Cycloserine	Cyclosporine
Depo-Estradiol	*Depo-Testadiol*
Dioval	*Diovan*
Estratab	*Estratest*
Etidronate	Etretinate
Flomax	*Volmax*
Lamisil	*Lamictal*
Levoxine	*Levoxyl*
Lithobid	*Lithostat*
Lodine	Iodine
Naprelan	*Naprosyn*
Nasarel	*Nizoral*
Neoral	*Neosar*
Nicoderm	*Nitroderm*
Sarafem	*Serophene*
Serentil	*Seroquel*
Tamiflu	*Theraflu*
Tramadol	*Toradol*

[a]Brand names are italicized; generic names are not.

TABLE 7.6 ▪ Ways to Cut Medication Errors[a]

INSTITUTIONAL CULTURE
- Establish an organizational commitment to a culture of safety.
- Provide medication safety education for all new and existing professional employees.
- Maintain ongoing recognition of safety innovation.
- Create a nonpunitive environment that encourages identification of errors and the development of new patient safety systems.

INFRASTRUCTURE
- Designate a medication safety coordinator/officer and identify physician champions.
- Promote greater use of clinical pharmacists in high-risk areas.
- Establish area-specific guidelines for unit-stocked medications.
- Establish a mechanism to ensure availability of critical medication information to all members of the patient's care team.

CLINICAL PRACTICE
- Eliminate dangerous abbreviations and dose designations.
- Implement safety checklists for high-alert medications.
- Implement safety checklists for infusion pumps.
- Develop limitations and safeguards regarding verbal orders.
- Perform failure-mode analysis during procurement process.
- Implement triggers and markers to indicate potential adverse medication events.

TECHNOLOGY
- Eliminate the use of infusion pumps that lack free-flow protection.
- Implement use of computerized prescriber order entry systems.

[a]These strategies are recommended in the Regional Medication Safety Program for Hospitals (RMSPH), developed by a consortium of hospitals in southeastern Pennsylvania.

be adapted to meet individual institutional needs to decrease medication errors.

Some specific measures that have been widely implemented to reduce errors have had remarkable success, such as the following:

- Replacing handwritten medication orders with a computerized order entry system has reduced medication errors by 50%.
- Having a senior clinical pharmacist accompany physicians on rounds in ICUs has reduced medication errors by 66%.
- Using bar-code systems that match the patient's armband bar code to a drug bar code has decreased medication errors in some institutions by as much as 85%.
- Incorporating *medication reconciliation* (Box 7.1) has resulted in decreasing medication errors by 70% and reducing ADRs by 15%.

Many medication errors result from using error-prone abbreviations, symbols, and dose designations. To address this concern, the ISMP and the FDA together compiled a list of error-prone abbreviations, symbols, and dose designations (Table 7.7), and have recommended against their use. This list includes eight entries (at the top of Table 7.7) that have been *banned* by The Joint Commission (TJC). These banned abbreviations can no longer be used by hospitals and other organizations that require TJC accreditation. The full list is available online at www.ismp.org/tools/errorproneabbreviations.pdf.

A wealth of information is available on reducing medication errors. See Table 7.8 for some good places to start.

How to Report a Medication Error

You can report a medication error via the MER Program, a nationwide system run by the ISMP. All reporting is confidential and can be done by phone or through the Internet. Details on submitting a report are available at www.ismp.org/orderForms/reporterrortoISMP.asp. The MER Program encourages participation by all healthcare providers, including pharmacists, nurses, physicians, and students. The objective is not to establish blame, but to improve patient safety by increasing our knowledge of medication errors. All information gathered by the MER Program is forwarded to the FDA, the ISMP, and the product manufacturer.

si

BOX 7.1 ▪ SPECIAL INTEREST TOPIC

MEDICATION RECONCILIATION

The Joint Commission requires all hospitals to conduct medication reconciliations for all patients. The purpose is to reduce medication omissions, duplications, and dosing errors as well as adverse drug events and interactions.

What Is Medication Reconciliation and When Is It Done?

Medication reconciliation is the process of comparing a list of all medications that a patient is currently taking with a list of new medications that are about to be provided. Reconciliation is conducted whenever a patient undergoes a *transition in care* in which new medications may be ordered, or existing orders may be changed. Transitions in care include hospital admission, hospital discharge, moving to a different level of care within a hospital, transfer to another facility, or discharge home.

How Is Medication Reconciliation Conducted?

There are five steps:

Step 1. Create a list of current medications. For each drug, include the name, indication, route, dosage size, and dosing interval. For patients entering a hospital, the list would consist of all medications being taken at home, including vitamins, herbal products, and prescription and nonprescription drugs.

Step 2. Create a list of all medications to be prescribed in the new setting.

Step 3. Compare the medications on both lists.

Step 4. Adjust medications based on the comparison. For example, the prescriber would discontinue drugs that are duplicates or inappropriate, and would avoid drugs that can interact adversely.

Step 5. When the next transition in care occurs, provide the updated, reconciled list to the patient and the new provider. By consulting the list, the new provider will be less likely to omit a prescribed medication or commit a dosing error, and less likely to prescribe a new medication that might duplicate or negate the effects of a current medication, or interact with a current medication to cause a serious adverse event.

Every time a new transition in care occurs, reconciliation should be conducted again.

Does Medication Reconciliation Reduce Medication Errors?

Medication reconciliation is an important intervention to reduce medication errors. Roughly 60% of medication errors occur when patients undergo a transition in care. Medication reconciliation can eliminate most of these errors.

What Should Be Included in Medication Reconciliation at Discharge?

When patients leave a facility, they should receive a single clear, comprehensive list of *all* medications they will be taking after discharge. The list should include any medications ordered at the time of discharge, as well as any other medications the patient will be taking, including over-the-counter drugs, vitamins, and herbal products and other nutritional supplements. In addition, the list should include all prescription medications that the patient had been taking at home but that were temporarily discontinued during the episode of care. The discharge list should *not* include drugs that were used during the episode of care but are no longer needed. The patient and, with the patient's permission, the next provider of care should receive the discharge list so that the new provider will be able to continue the reconciliation process.

TABLE 7.7 ▪ Abbreviations, Symbols, and Dose Designations That Increase Risk for Medication Errors

Abbreviations, Symbols, or Dose Designations	Intended Meaning	Potential Misinterpretation	Preferred Alternative
ABBREVIATIONS AND NOTATIONS FOR WHICH THE ALTERNATIVE MUST BE USED (TJC MANDATED)			
U or u	Unit	Misread as 0 or 4 (e.g., 4 U seen as 40; 4 u seen as 44); mistaken to mean "cc" so dose given in volume instead of units (e.g., 4 u mistaken to mean 4 cc)	Write "unit"
IU	International unit	Misread as IV (intravenous) or "10"	Write "international unit"
q.d./Q.D.	Every day	Misread as q.i.d. (four times a day)	Write "daily"
q.o.d./Q.O.D.	Every other day	Misread as q.d. (daily) or q.i.d. (four times a day)	Write "every other day"
MS or MSO_4	Morphine sulfate	Mistaken as magnesium sulfate	Write "morphine sulfate"

Continued

TABLE 7.7 ■ Abbreviations, Symbols, and Dose Designations That Increase Risk for Medication Errors—cont'd

Abbreviations, Symbols, or Dose Designations	Intended Meaning	Potential Misinterpretation	Preferred Alternative
$MgSO_4$	Magnesium sulfate	Mistaken as morphine sulfate	Write "magnesium sulfate"
Trailing zero after final decimal point (e.g., 1.0 mg)	1 mg	Mistaken as 10 mg if the decimal point is missed	Never write a zero by itself after a decimal point
Leading decimal point not preceded by a zero (e.g., .5 mg)	0.5 mg	Mistaken as 5 mg if the decimal point is missed	Write "0" before a leading decimal point
SOME ABBREVIATIONS AND NOTATIONS FOR WHICH THE ALTERNATIVE IS RECOMMENDED (BUT NOT YET MANDATED BY TJC)			
µg	Microgram	Mistaken as "mg"	Write "mcg"
cc	Cubic centimeters	Mistaken as "u" (units)	Write "mL"
IN	Intranasal	Mistaken as "IM" or "IV"	Write "intranasal" or "NAS"
H.S.; hs	Half-strength; at bedtime	Mistaken as opposite of what was intended	Write "half-strength" or "at bedtime"
qhs	At bedtime	Mistaken as qhr (every hour)	Write "at bedtime"
q1d	Daily	Mistaken as q.i.d. (four times daily)	Write "daily"
q6PM, etc.	Nightly at 6 PM	Mistaken as every 6 hours	Write "nightly at 6 PM"
T.I.W.	Three times a week	Mistaken as three times a day or twice weekly	Write "three times weekly"
SC, SQ, sub q	Subcutaneous	SC mistaken as "SL" (sublingual); SQ mistaken as "5 every"; the "q" in "sub q" mistaken as "every" (e.g., a heparin dose ordered "sub q 2 hours before surgery" mistaken as "every 2 hours before surgery")	Write "subQ," "sub-Q," "subcut," or "subcutaneously"; write "every"
D/C	Discharge or discontinue	Premature discontinuation of medications if D/C (intended to mean "discharge") has been interpreted as "discontinued" when followed by a list of discharge medications	Write "discharge" or "discontinue"
AD, AS, AU	Right ear, left ear, each ear	Mistaken as OD, OS, OU (right eye, left eye, each eye)	Write "right ear," "left ear," or "each ear"
OD, OS, OU	Right eye, left eye, each eye	Mistaken as AD, AS, AU (right ear, left ear, each ear)	Write "right eye," "left eye," or "each eye"
Per os	By mouth, orally	The "os" can be mistaken as "left eye" (OS = oculus sinister)	Write "PO," "by mouth," or "orally"
> or <	Greater than or less than	Mistaken for the opposite	Write "greater than" or "less than"
AZT	Zidovudine [Retrovir]	Mistaken as azathioprine or aztreonam	Write complete drug name
CPZ	Prochlorperazine [Compazine]	Mistaken as chlorpromazine	Write complete drug name
ARA A	Vidarabine	Mistaken as cytarabine (ARA C)	Write complete drug name
HCT	Hydrocortisone	Mistaken as hydrochlorothiazide	Write complete drug name
HCTZ	Hydrochlorothiazide	Mistaken as hydrocortisone	Write complete drug name

Adapted from a list compiled by the Institute for Safe Medication Practices. The complete list is available at www.ismp.org/tools/errorproneabbreviations.pdf.
TJC, The Joint Commission.

TABLE 7.8 ■ Resources on Decreasing Medication Errors

Resource	Location
Agency for Healthcare Research and Quality's Patient Safety Network	https://psnet.ahrq.gov
Institute for Safe Medication Practices	www.ismp.org
Institute for Healthcare Improvement's Medication Reconciliation Information and Tools	www.ihi.org/topics/adesmedicationreconciliation/Pages/default.aspx
National Coordinating Council for Medication Error Reporting and Prevention	www.nccmerp.org
Preventing Medication Errors ("The IOM Report")	http://www.nationalacademies.org/hmd/Reports/2006/Preventing-Medication-Errors-Quality-Chasm-Series.aspx
The Joint Commission's Resources Related to Medication Errors	www.jointcommission.org/topics/default.aspx?k=660
U.S. Food and Drug Administration Medication Error Resources	www.fda.gov/Drugs/DrugSafety/MedicationErrors/default.htm

KEY POINTS

- An adverse drug reaction is any noxious, unintended, and undesired effect that occurs at normal drug doses.
- Patients at increased risk of adverse drug events include the very young, older adults, the very ill, and those taking multiple drugs.
- An iatrogenic disease is a disease that occurs as the result of medical care or treatment.
- An idiosyncratic effect is an adverse drug reaction based on a genetic predisposition.
- A paradoxical effect is the opposite of the intended drug effect.
- A carcinogenic effect is a drug-induced cancer.
- A teratogenic effect is a drug-induced birth defect.
- The intensity of an allergic drug reaction is based on the degree of immune system sensitization—not on drug dosage.
- Drugs are the most common cause of acute liver failure, and hepatotoxicity is the most common reason for removing drugs from the market.
- Drugs that prolong the QT interval pose a risk of torsades de pointes, a dysrhythmia that can progress to fatal ventricular fibrillation.
- At the time a new drug is released, it may well be able to cause adverse effects that are as yet unreported.
- Measures to minimize adverse drug events include avoiding drugs that are likely to harm a particular patient, monitoring the patient for signs and symptoms of likely adverse effects, educating the patient about possible adverse effects, and monitoring organs that are vulnerable to a particular drug.
- To reduce the risk of serious reactions to certain drugs, the FDA may require the manufacturer to create a MedGuide for patients, a boxed warning to alert prescribers, and/or a Risk Evaluation and Mitigation Strategy, which may involve patients, prescribers, and pharmacists.
- Medication errors are a major cause of morbidity and mortality.
- Medication errors can be made by many people, including pharmaceutical workers, pharmacists, prescribers, transcriptionists, nurses, and patients and their families.
- In a hospital, a medication order is processed by several people. Each is in a position to introduce errors, and each is in a position to catch errors made by others.
- The nurse is the patient's last line of defense against medication errors made by others—and the last person with the opportunity to introduce an error.
- Because the nurse is the last person who can catch mistakes made by others, and because no one is there to catch mistakes the nurse might make, the nurse bears a unique responsibility for ensuring patient safety.
- The three most common *types* of fatal medication errors are (1) giving an overdose, (2) giving the wrong drug, and (3) using the wrong route.
- The three most common *causes* of fatal medication errors are (1) human factors (e.g., performance or knowledge deficits), (2) miscommunication (e.g., because of illegible prescriber handwriting), and (3) confusion caused by similarities in drug names.
- At the heart of efforts to reduce medication errors is a change in institutional culture—from a punitive system focused on "naming, blaming, and shaming" to a nonpunitive system in which medication errors can be discussed openly, thereby facilitating the identification of errors and the development of new safety procedures.
- Effective measures for reducing medication errors include (1) using a safety checklist for high-alert drugs; (2) replacing handwritten medication orders with a computerized order-entry system; (3) having a clinical pharmacist accompany ICU physicians on rounds; (4) avoiding error-prone abbreviations; (5) helping and encouraging patients and their families to be active, informed participants in the healthcare team; (6) conducting a medication reconciliation whenever a patient undergoes a transition in care; and (7) using a computerized bar-code system that (a) identifies the administering nurse and (b) ensures that the drug is going to the right patient and that adverse interactions are unlikely.

Please visit **http://evolve.elsevier.com/Lehne** for chapter-specific NCLEX® examination review questions.

CHAPTER

8 Individual Variation in Drug Responses

Individual variation in drug responses has been a recurrent theme throughout earlier chapters. We noted that, because of individual variation, we must tailor drug therapy to each patient. In this chapter, we discuss the major factors that can cause one patient to respond to drugs differently from another. With this information, you will be better prepared to reduce individual variation in drug responses, thereby maximizing the benefits of treatment and reducing the potential for harm.

BODY WEIGHT AND COMPOSITION

Body size can be a significant determinant of drug effects. Recall that the intensity of the response to a drug is determined in large part by the concentration of the drug at its sites of action—the higher the concentration, the more intense the response. If we give the same dose to a small person and a large person, the drug will achieve a higher concentration in the small person and, therefore, will produce more intense effects. The potential consequences are that we will produce toxicity in the smaller person and undertreat the larger person. To compensate for this potential source of individual variation, providers consider the size of the patient when determining the dosage to prescribe.

When adjusting dosage to account for body weight, the prescriber may base the adjustment on body surface area rather than on weight per se. Why? Because surface area determinations account not only for the patient's weight but also for the patient's relative amount of body adiposity. Because percentage of body fat can change drug distribution and because altered distribution can change the concentration of a drug at its sites of action, dosage adjustments based on body surface area provide a more precise means of controlling drug responses than do adjustments based on weight alone.

AGE

Drug sensitivity varies with age. Infants and older adults are especially sensitive to drugs. In the very young patient, heightened drug sensitivity is the result of organ immaturity. In older adults, heightened sensitivity results largely from decline in organ function. Other factors that affect sensitivity in older adults are increased severity of illness, the presence of multiple comorbidities, and treatment with multiple drugs. The clinical challenge created by heightened drug sensitivity in very young or older-adult patients is the subject of Chapters 10 and 11, respectively.

PATHOPHYSIOLOGY

Physiologic alterations can modify drug responses. Four pathologic conditions, in particular, may have a profound effect on drug response: (1) kidney disease, (2) liver disease, (3) acid-base imbalance, and (4) altered electrolyte status.

Kidney Disease

Kidney disease can reduce drug excretion, causing drugs to accumulate in the body. If dosage is not lowered, drugs may accumulate to toxic levels. Accordingly, if a patient is taking a drug that is eliminated by the kidneys, and if renal function declines, dosage must be decreased.

The impact of kidney disease is illustrated in Fig. 8.1, which compares the decline in plasma levels of kanamycin (an antibiotic with exclusively renal elimination) following injection into a patient with healthy kidneys and a patient with renal

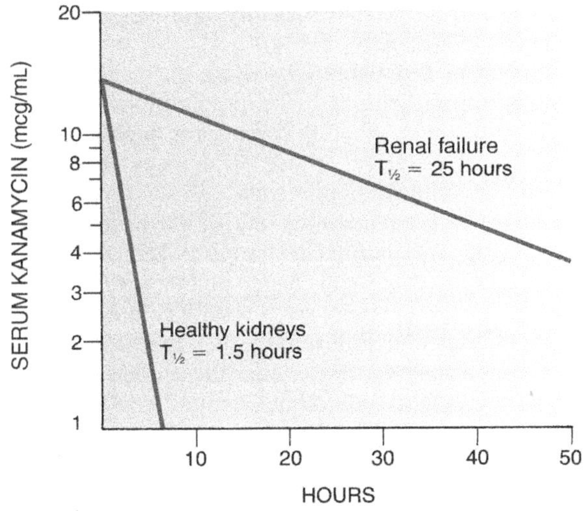

Fig. 8.1 ■ Effect of renal failure on kanamycin half-life. Kanamycin was administered at time "0" to two patients, one with healthy kidneys and one with renal failure. Note that drug levels declined very rapidly in the patient with healthy kidneys and extremely slowly in the patient with renal failure, indicating that renal failure greatly reduced the capacity to remove this drug from the body. ($T_{1/2}$, Half-life.)

failure. As indicated, kanamycin levels fall off rapidly in the patient with good kidney function. In this patient, the drug's half-life is brief—only 1.5 hours. In contrast, drug levels decline very slowly in the patient with renal failure. Because of kidney disease, the half-life of kanamycin has increased by nearly 17-fold—from 1.5 hours to 25 hours. Under these conditions, if dosage is not reduced, kanamycin will quickly accumulate to dangerous levels.

Liver Disease

Like kidney disease, liver disease can cause drugs to accumulate. This occurs because the liver is the major site of drug metabolism. Therefore, if liver function declines, the rate of metabolism will decline, causing drug levels to climb. Accordingly, to prevent accumulation to toxic levels, dosage of drugs eliminated via hepatic metabolism must be reduced or discontinued if liver disease develops.

Acid-Base Imbalance

By altering pH partitioning (see Chapter 4), changes in acid-base status can alter the absorption, distribution, metabolism, and excretion of drugs.

Recall that, because of pH partitioning, if there is a difference in pH on two sides of a membrane, a drug will accumulate on the side where the pH most favors its ionization. Because acidic drugs ionize in alkaline media, acidic drugs will accumulate on the alkaline side of the membrane. Conversely, basic drugs will accumulate on the acidic side.

Altered Electrolyte Status

Electrolytes (e.g., potassium, sodium, calcium, magnesium, phosphorus) have important roles in cell physiology. Consequently, when electrolyte levels become disturbed, multiple cellular processes can be disrupted. Excitable tissues (nerves and muscles) are especially sensitive to alterations in electrolyte status. Given that disturbances in electrolyte balance can have widespread effects on cell physiology, we might expect that electrolyte imbalances would cause profound and widespread effects on responses to drugs. However, this does not seem to be the case; examples in which electrolyte changes have a significant impact on drug responses are rare.

Digoxin, a drug for heart disease, provides an important example of an altered drug effect occurring in response to electrolyte imbalance. The most serious toxicity of digoxin is production of potentially fatal dysrhythmias. The tendency of digoxin to disturb cardiac rhythm is related to levels of potassium: When potassium levels are low, the ability of digoxin to induce dysrhythmias is greatly increased. Accordingly, all patients receiving digoxin must undergo regular measurement of serum potassium to ensure that levels remain within a safe range. Digoxin toxicity and its relationship to potassium levels are discussed in Chapter 48.

TOLERANCE

Tolerance is a *decreased responsiveness to a drug as a result of repeated drug administration.* Patients who are tolerant to a drug require higher doses to produce effects equivalent to those that could be achieved with lower doses before tolerance developed. There are three categories of drug tolerance: (1) pharmacodynamic tolerance, (2) metabolic tolerance, and (3) tachyphylaxis.

Pharmacodynamic Tolerance

The term *pharmacodynamic tolerance* refers to the familiar type of tolerance associated with long-term administration of drugs such as morphine and heroin. Pharmacodynamic tolerance is the result of adaptive processes that occur in response to chronic receptor occupation. Because increased drug levels are required to produce an effective response, the minimum effective concentration (MEC) of a drug becomes abnormally high.

Metabolic Tolerance

Metabolic tolerance is defined as tolerance resulting from accelerated drug metabolism. This form of tolerance may be brought about by the ability of certain drugs (e.g., barbiturates) to induce synthesis of hepatic drug-metabolizing enzymes, thereby causing rates of drug metabolism to increase. Because of increased metabolism, dosage must be increased to maintain therapeutic drug levels. Unlike pharmacodynamic tolerance, which causes the MEC to increase, metabolic tolerance does not affect the MEC.

Tachyphylaxis

Tachyphylaxis is a reduction in drug responsiveness brought on by repeated dosing over a short time. This is unlike pharmacodynamic and metabolic tolerance, which takes days or longer to develop. Tachyphylaxis is not a common mechanism of drug tolerance.

Transdermal nitroglycerin provides a good example of tachyphylaxis. When nitroglycerin is administered using a transdermal patch, effects are lost in less than 24 hours if the patch is left in place around the clock. As discussed in Chapter 51, the loss of effect results from depletion of a cofactor required for nitroglycerin to act. When nitroglycerin is administered on an intermittent schedule, rather than continuously, the cofactor can be replenished between doses and no loss of effect occurs.

PLACEBO EFFECT

A *placebo* is a preparation that is devoid of intrinsic pharmacologic activity. Any response that a patient may have to a placebo is believed to be based solely on the patient's psychologic reaction to the idea of taking a medication and not to any direct physiologic or biochemical action of the placebo itself. The primary use of the placebo is as a control preparation during clinical trials.

In pharmacology, the *placebo effect* is defined as that component of a drug response that is caused by psychologic factors and not by the biochemical or physiologic properties of the drug. Although it is impossible to assess with precision the contribution that psychologic factors make to the overall response to any particular drug, it is widely believed that, with practically all medications, some fraction of the total response results from a placebo effect. Although placebo effects are determined by psychologic factors and not physiologic responses to the inactive placebo, the presence of a placebo response does not imply that a patient's original pathology was imaginary.

Not all placebo responses are beneficial; placebo responses can also be negative. If a patient believes that a medication is going to be effective, then placebo responses are likely to help promote recovery. Conversely, if a patient is convinced that a particular medication is ineffective or perhaps even harmful, then placebo effects are likely to detract from the patient's progress.

Because the placebo effect depends on the patient's attitude toward medicine, fostering a positive attitude may help promote beneficial effects. In this regard, it is desirable that all members of the healthcare team present the patient with an optimistic (but realistic) assessment of the effects that therapy is likely to produce.

VARIABILITY IN ABSORPTION

Both the rate and extent of drug absorption can vary among patients. As a result, both the timing and intensity of responses can be changed. In Chapters 4 and 6 we discussed how differences in manufacturing, the presence or absence of food, and drug interactions can alter absorption. Individual variations also have an effect on drug response.

Bioavailability

The term *bioavailability* refers to the amount of active drug that reaches the systemic circulation from its site of administration. Different formulations of the same drug can vary in bioavailability. As discussed in Chapter 4, such factors as tablet disintegration time, enteric coatings, and sustained-release formulations can alter bioavailability, and can thereby make drug responses variable.

Differences in bioavailability occur primarily with oral preparations rather than parenteral preparations. Fortunately, even with oral agents, when differences in bioavailability do exist between preparations, those differences are usually so small as to lack clinical significance.

Differences in bioavailability are of greatest concern for drugs with a narrow therapeutic range. Why? Because with these agents, a relatively small change in drug level can produce a significant change in response: A small decline in drug level may cause therapeutic failure, whereas a small increase in drug level may cause toxicity. Under these conditions, differences in bioavailability could have a significant impact.

Individual Causes of Variable Absorption

Individual variations that affect the speed and degree of drug absorption affect bioavailability and can, thereby, lead to variations in drug responses. Alterations in gastric pH can affect absorption through the pH partitioning effect. For drugs that undergo absorption in the intestine, absorption will be delayed when gastric emptying time is prolonged. Diarrhea can reduce absorption by accelerating transport of drugs through the intestine. Conversely, constipation may enhance absorption of some drugs by prolonging the time available for absorption.

GENETICS AND PHARMACOGENOMICS

A patient's unique genetic makeup can lead to drug responses that are qualitatively and quantitatively different from those of the population at large. Adverse effects and therapeutic effects may be increased or reduced. Idiosyncratic responses to drugs may also occur.

Pharmacogenomics is the study of how genetic variations can affect individual responses to drugs. Although pharmacogenomics is a relatively young science, it has already produced clinically relevant information—information that can be used to enhance therapeutic effects and reduce harm. As a result, genetic testing is now done routinely for some drugs. In fact, for a few drugs, such as maraviroc [Selzentry] and trastuzumab [Herceptin], the Food and Drug Administration (FDA) now *requires* genetic testing before use, and for a few other drugs, including warfarin [Coumadin] and carbamazepine [Tegretol], genetic testing is recommended but not required. In the distant future, pharmacogenetic analysis of each patient may allow us to pick a drug and dosage that best fits his or her genotype, thereby reducing the risk of adverse reactions, increasing the likelihood of a strong therapeutic response, and decreasing the cost, inconvenience, and risks associated with prescribing a drug to which the patient is unlikely to respond.

In the discussion that follows, we look at ways in which genetic variations can influence an individual's responses to drugs, and then indicate how pharmacogenomic tests may be used to guide treatment (Table 8.1).

Genetic Variants That Alter Drug Metabolism

The most common mechanism by which genetic variants modify drug responses is by altering drug metabolism. These gene-based

TABLE 8.1 ▪ Examples of How Genetic Variations Can Affect Drug Responses

Genetic Variation	Drug Affected	Impact of the Genetic Variation	Explanation	FDA Stand on Genetic Testing
VARIANTS THAT ALTER DRUG METABOLISM				
CYP2D6 variants	Tamoxifen [Soltamox, Nolvadex-D ♣]	Reduced therapeutic effect	Women with inadequate CYP2D6 activity cannot convert tamoxifen to its active form; therefore, the drug cannot adequately protect them from breast cancer.	No recommendation
CYP2C19 variants	Clopidogrel [Plavix]	Reduced therapeutic effect	Patients with inadequate CYP2C19 activity cannot convert clopidogrel to its active form; therefore, the drug cannot protect them against cardiovascular events.	Recommended
CYP2C9 variants	Warfarin [Coumadin]	Increased toxicity	In patients with abnormal CYP2C9, warfarin may accumulate to a level that causes bleeding.	Recommended
TPMT variants	Thiopurines (e.g., thioguanine, mercaptopurine)	Increased toxicity	In patients with reduced TPMT activity, thiopurines can accumulate to levels that cause severe bone marrow toxicity.	Recommended
VARIANTS THAT ALTER DRUG TARGETS ON NORMAL CELLS				
ADRB1 variants	Metoprolol and other beta blockers	Increased therapeutic effect	$Beta_1$ receptors produced by ADRB1 variant genes respond more intensely to beta agonists, causing enhanced effects of blockade by beta antagonists.	No recommendation
VKORC1 variants	Warfarin [Coumadin]	Increased drug sensitivity	Variant VKORC1 is readily inhibited by warfarin, allowing anticoagulation with a reduced warfarin dosage.	Recommended
VARIANTS THAT ALTER DRUG TARGETS ON CANCER CELLS OR VIRUSES				
HER2 overexpression	Trastuzumab [Herceptin]	Increased therapeutic effect	Trastuzumab only acts against breast cancers that overexpress HER2.	Required
EGFR expression	Cetuximab [Erbitux]	Increased therapeutic effect	Cetuximab only works against colorectal cancers that express EGFR.	Required
CCR5 tropism	Maraviroc [Selzentry]	Increased therapeutic effect	Maraviroc only acts against HIV strains that express CCR5.	Required
VARIANTS THAT ALTER IMMUNE RESPONSES TO DRUGS				
HLA-B*1502	Carbamazepine [Tegretol, Carbatrol]	Increased toxicity	The HLA-B*1502 variant increases the risk of life-threatening skin reactions in patients taking carbamazepine.	Recommended for patients with Asian heritage
HLA-B*5701	Abacavir [Ziagen]	Increased toxicity	The HLA-B*5701 variant increases the risk of fatal hypersensitivity reactions in patients taking abacavir.	Recommended

ADRB1, $Beta_1$ adrenergic receptor; *CCR5,* chemokine receptor 5; *CYP2C9,* 2C9 isoenzyme of cytochrome P450 (CYP); *CYP2C19,* 2C19 isoenzyme of CYP; *CYP2D6,* 2D6 isoenzyme of CYP; *EGFR,* epidermal growth factor receptor; *HER2,* human epidermal growth factor receptor type 2; *HIV,* human immunodeficiency virus; *HLA-B*1502,* human leukocyte antigen B*1502; *HLA-B*5701,* human leukocyte antigen B*5701; *TPMT,* thiopurine methyltransferase; *VKORC1,* vitamin K epoxide reductase complex 1.

changes can either accelerate or slow the metabolism of many drugs. The usual consequence is either a reduction in benefits or an increase in toxicity.

For drugs that have a high therapeutic index (TI), altered rates of metabolism may have little effect on the clinical outcome. However, if the TI is low or narrow, then relatively small increases in drug levels can lead to toxicity, and relatively small decreases in drug levels can lead to therapeutic failure. In these cases, altered rates of metabolism can be significant.

The following examples show how a genetically determined variation in drug metabolism can *reduce the benefits* of therapy.

- Variants in the gene that codes for cytochrome P450-2D6 (CYP2D6) can greatly reduce the benefits of tamoxifen [Soltamox, Nolvadex-D ♣], a drug used to prevent breast cancer recurrence. Here's how. To work, tamoxifen must first be converted to its active form—endoxifen—by CYP2D6. Women with an inherited deficiency in the CYP2D6 gene cannot activate the drug well, so they get minimal benefit from treatment. In one study, the cancer recurrence rate in these poor metabolizers was 9.5 times higher than in good metabolizers. Who are the poor metabolizers? Between 8% and 10% of women of European ancestry have gene variants that prevent them from metabolizing tamoxifen to endoxifen. At this time, the FDA neither requires nor recommends testing for variants in the CYP2D6 gene. However, a test kit is available.
- Variants of the gene that codes for CYP2C19 can greatly reduce the benefits of clopidogrel [Plavix], a drug that prevents platelet aggregation. Like tamoxifen, clopidogrel is a prodrug that must undergo conversion to an active form. With clopidogrel, the conversion is catalyzed by CYP2C19. Unfortunately, about 25% of patients produce a variant form of the enzyme—CYP2C19*2. As a result, these people experience a weak antiplatelet response, which places them at increased risk of stroke, myocardial infarction, and other events. People with this genetic variation should use a different antiplatelet drug.
- Among Americans of European heritage, about 52% metabolize isoniazid (a drug for tuberculosis) slowly and 48% metabolize it rapidly. Why? Because, owing to genetic differences, these people produce two different forms of *N*-acetyltransferase-2, the enzyme that metabolizes isoniazid. If dosage is not adjusted for these differences, the rapid metabolizers may experience treatment failure and the slow metabolizers may experience toxicity.
- About 1 in 14 people of European heritage have a form of CYP2D6 that is unable to convert codeine into morphine, the active form of codeine. As a result, codeine cannot relieve pain in these people.

The following examples show how a genetically determined variation in drug metabolism can *increase drug toxicity:*

- Variants in the gene that codes for CYP2C9 can increase the risk of toxicity (bleeding) from *warfarin* [Coumadin], an anticoagulant with a narrow TI. Bleeding occurs because (1) warfarin is inactivated by CYP2D9 and (2) patients with altered CYP2D9 genes produce a form of the enzyme that metabolizes warfarin slowly, allowing it to accumulate to dangerous levels. To reduce bleeding risk, the FDA now recommends that patients be tested for variants of the CYP2C9 gene. It should be noted, however, that in this case outcomes using expensive genetic tests are no better than outcomes using cheaper traditional tests, which directly measure the impact of warfarin on coagulation.
- Variants in the gene that codes for *thiopurine methyltransferase* (TPMT) can reduce TPMT activity and can thereby delay the metabolic inactivation of two thiopurine anticancer drugs: *thioguanine* [generic only] and *mercaptopurine* [Purinethol]. As a result, in patients with inherited TPMT deficiency, standard doses of thioguanine or mercaptopurine can accumulate to high levels, posing a risk of potentially fatal bone marrow damage. To reduce risk, the FDA recommends testing for TPMT variants before using either drug. Patients who are found to be TPMT deficient should be given these drugs in reduced dosage.
- In the United States, about 1% of the population produces a form of *dihydropyrimidine dehydrogenase* that does a poor job of metabolizing *fluorouracil,* a drug used to treat cancer. Several people with this inherited difference, while receiving standard doses of fluorouracil, have died from central nervous system injury owing to accumulation of the drug to toxic levels.

Genetic Variants That Alter Drug Targets

Genetic variations can alter the structure of drug receptors and other target molecules and can thereby influence drug responses. These variants have been documented in normal cells and in cancer cells and viruses.

Genetic variants that affect drug targets on *normal cells* are illustrated by these two examples:

- Variants in the genes that code for the *beta$_1$-adrenergic receptor* (ADRB1) produce receptors that are hyperresponsive to activation, which can be a mixed blessing. The bad news is that, in people with hypertension, activation of these receptors may produce an exaggerated *increase* in blood pressure. The good news is that, in people with hypertension, blockade of these receptors will therefore produce an exaggerated *decrease* in blood pressure. Population studies indicate that variant ADRB1 receptors occur more often in people of European ancestry than in people of African ancestry, which may explain why *beta blockers* work better, on average, against hypertension in people with light skin than in people with dark skin.
- The anticoagulant *warfarin* works by inhibiting *vitamin K epoxide reductase complex 1* (VKORC1). Variant genes that code for VKORC1 produce a form of the enzyme that can be easily inhibited, and hence anticoagulation can be achieved with low warfarin doses. If normal doses are given, anticoagulation will be excessive, and bleeding could result. To reduce risk, the FDA recommends testing for variants in the VKORC1 gene before warfarin is used.

Genetic variants that affect drug targets on *cancer cells* and *viruses* are illustrated by these three examples:

- *Trastuzumab* [Herceptin], used for breast cancer, works only against tumors that overexpress *human epidermal growth factor receptor type 2* (HER2). The HER2 protein, which serves as a receptor for hormones that stimulate tumor growth, is overexpressed in about 25% of breast cancer patients. Overexpression of HER2 is associated with a poor prognosis, but also predicts a better response to trastuzumab. Accordingly, the FDA requires a positive test result for HER2 overexpression before trastuzumab is used.
- *Cetuximab* [Erbitux], used mainly for metastatic colorectal cancer, works only against tumors that express the *epidermal growth factor receptor* (EGFR). All other tumors are unresponsive. Accordingly, the FDA requires evidence of EGFR expression if the drug is to be used.
- *Maraviroc* [Selzentry], a drug for HIV infection, works by binding with a viral surface protein known as *chemokine receptor 5* (CCR5), which certain strains of HIV require for entry into immune cells. HIV strains that use CCR5 are known as being *CCR5 tropic.* If maraviroc is to be of benefit, patients must be infected with one of these strains. Accordingly, before maraviroc is used, the FDA requires that testing be done to confirm that the infecting strain is indeed CCR5 tropic.

Genetic Variants That Alter Immune Responses to Drugs

Genetic variants that affect the immune system can increase the risk of severe hypersensitivity reactions to certain drugs. Two examples follow.

- *Carbamazepine* [Tegretol, Carbatrol], used for epilepsy and bipolar disorder, can cause life-threatening skin reactions in some patients—specifically, patients of Asian ancestry who carry genes that code for an unusual *human leukocyte antigen* (HLA) known as *HLA-B*1502.* (HLA molecules are essential elements of the immune system.) Although the mechanism underlying toxicity is unclear, a good guess is that interaction between HLA-B*1502 molecules and carbamazepine (or a metabolite) may trigger a cellular immune response. To reduce risk, the FDA recommends that patients of Asian descent be screened for the HLA-B*1502 gene before carbamazepine is used. If the test is positive, carbamazepine should be avoided.
- *Abacavir* [Ziagen], used for HIV infection, can cause potentially fatal hypersensitivity reactions in patients who have a variant gene that codes for HLA-B*5701. Accordingly, the FDA recommends screening for the variant gene before using this drug. If the test is positive, abacavir should be avoided.

In the future, genomic analysis of each patient may allow us to engage in revolutionary personalized medicine that addresses the individual patient's genotype. For the present, though, while many advances have been made in pharmacogenomic knowledge, the science is still relatively new (as science goes). Still, the rapid expanse of knowledge in this area is astonishing. See Table 8.2 for resources to help you keep abreast of changes in this field.

GENDER- AND RACE-RELATED VARIATIONS

Gender- and race-related differences in drug responses are, ultimately, genetically based. Our discussion of pharmacogenomics continues with a focus on these important topics.

Gender

Men and women can respond differently to the same drug. A drug may be more effective in men than in women, or vice versa. Likewise, adverse effects may be more intense in men than in women, or vice versa. Unfortunately, for most drugs, we do not have adequate knowledge about gender-related differences. Why? Because before 1997, when the

TABLE 8.2 ▪ Pharmacogenomic Resources

Organization	Resource	Website
Food and Drug Administration	Table of Pharmacogenomic Biomarkers in Drug Labeling	http://www.fda.gov/drugs/scienceresearch/researchareas/pharmacogenetics/ucm083378.htm
Genetics/Genomics Competency Center (G2C2)	Genetics and genomics resource-specific search engine	http://genomicseducation.net
Personalized Medicine Coalition	Variety of resources, including a table that links drugs, biomarkers, and indications	http://www.personalizedmedicinecoalition.org http://www.personalizedmedicinecoalition.org/Userfiles/PMC-Corporate/file/pmc_personalized_medicine_drugs_genes.pdf
Pharmacogenomics Knowledgebase (PharmGKB)	A wealth of information, including a listing of drugs having labels with genetic information approved by the FDA and Health Canada (Santé Canada)	https://www.pharmgkb.org https://www.pharmgkb.org/view/drug-labels.do

FDA pressured drug companies to include women in trials of new drugs, essentially all drug research was done in men. Since that time, research has demonstrated that significant gender-related differences really do exist. Here are four examples:

- When used to treat heart failure, digoxin may *increase* mortality in women while having no effect on mortality in men.
- Alcohol is metabolized more slowly by women than by men. As a result, a woman who drinks the same amount as a man (on a weight-adjusted basis) will become more intoxicated.
- Certain opioid analgesics (e.g., pentazocine, nalbuphine) are much more effective in women than in men. As a result, pain relief can be achieved at lower doses in women.
- Quinidine causes greater QT interval prolongation in women than in men. As a result, women given the drug are more likely to develop torsades de pointes, a potentially fatal cardiac dysrhythmia.

While there is still a lack of adequate data related to drug effects in women, information generated by these drug trials, coupled with current and future trials, will permit drug therapy in women to be more rational than is possible today. In the meantime, clinicians must keep in mind that the information currently available may fail to accurately predict responses in female patients. Accordingly, clinicians should remain alert for treatment failures and unexpected adverse effects.

Race

In general, "race" is not very helpful as a basis for predicting individual variation in drug responses. To start with, race is nearly impossible to define. Do we define it by skin color and other superficial characteristics? Or do we define it by group genetics? If we define race by skin color, how dark must skin be, for example, to define a patient as "black"? On the other hand, if we define race by group genetics, how many black ancestors must an African American have to be considered genetically "black"? And what about most people, whose ancestry is ethnically heterogeneous? Latinos, for example, represent a mix of ethnic backgrounds from three continents.

What we really care about is not race per se, but rather the specific genetic and psychosocial factors—shared by many members of an ethnic group—that influence drug responses. Armed with this knowledge, we can identify group members who share those genetic and/or psychosocial factors and tailor drug therapy accordingly. Perhaps more importantly, application of this knowledge is not limited to members of the ethnic group from which the knowledge arose: We can use it in the management of *all* patients, regardless of ethnic background. How can this be? Owing to ethnic heterogeneity, these factors are not limited to members of any one race. Hence, once we know about a factor (e.g., a specific genetic variation), we can screen all patients for it and, if it's present, adjust drug therapy as indicated.

This discussion of race-based therapy would be incomplete without mentioning BiDil, a fixed-dose combination of two vasodilators: isosorbide dinitrate (ISDN) and hydralazine, both of which have been available separately for years. In 2005, BiDil became the first drug product approved by the FDA for treating members of just one race, specifically, African Americans. Approval was based on results of the African-American Heart Failure Trial (A-HeFT), which showed that, in self-described black patients, adding ISDN plus hydralazine to standard therapy of heart failure reduced 1-year mortality by 43%—a very impressive and welcome result. Does BiDil benefit African Americans more than other Americans? We do not know; only patients of African ancestry were enrolled in A-HeFT, so the comparison cannot be made. The bottom line? Even though BiDil is approved for treating a specific racial group, there is no proof that it would not work just as well (or even better) in some other group.

COMORBIDITIES AND DRUG INTERACTIONS

Individuals often have two or more medical conditions or disease processes. When this occurs, drugs taken to manage one condition may complicate management of the other condition. As an example, if a person who has both asthma and hypertension is prescribed a nonselective beta-adrenergic antagonist (beta blocker) to control blood pressure, this may worsen the patient's asthma symptoms if the dose is sufficient to cause airway constriction. This illustrates the necessity for the nurse to consider the whole patient, not only the disease treated, when examining drug therapy.

Because patients with comorbidities often take multiple medications, there is the increased likelihood of drug interactions. A drug interaction is a process in which one drug alters the effects of another. Drug interactions can be an important source of variability. The mechanisms by which one drug can alter the effects of another and the clinical consequences of drug interactions are discussed at length in Chapter 6.

DIET

Diet can affect responses to drugs, primarily by affecting the patient's general health status. A diet that promotes good health can enable drugs to elicit therapeutic responses and increase the patient's capacity to tolerate adverse effects. Poor nutrition can have the opposite effect.

Starvation can reduce protein binding of drugs (by decreasing the level of plasma albumin). Because of reduced binding, levels of free drug rise, thereby making drug responses more intense. For certain drugs (e.g., warfarin), the resultant increase in effects could be disastrous.

In some instances, a specific nutrient may affect the response to a specific drug. Perhaps the best example involves the monoamine oxidase (MAO) inhibitors, which are drugs used to treat depression. The most serious adverse effect of these drugs is malignant hypertension, which can be triggered by foods that contain tyramine, a breakdown product of the amino acid tyrosine. Accordingly, patients taking MAO inhibitors must rigidly avoid all tyramine-rich foods (e.g., beef liver, ripe cheeses, yeast products, Chianti wine). The interaction of tyramine-containing foods with MAO inhibitors is discussed at length in Chapter 32.

FAILURE TO TAKE MEDICINE AS PRESCRIBED

Failure to administer medication as prescribed is a common cause of variability in the response to a prescribed dose. Such failure may result from poor patient adherence or from medication errors.

Studies show that 30% to 60% of patients do not adhere to their prescribed medication regimen. Factors that can influence adherence include manual dexterity, visual acuity, intellectual capacity, psychologic state, attitude toward drugs, and the ability to pay for medication. Patient education that is both clear and convincing may help improve adherence, and may thereby help reduce variability.

Medication errors are another source of individual variation. Medication errors can originate with physicians, nurses, technicians, and pharmacists, or with processes. However, because the nurse is usually the last member of the healthcare team to check medications before administration, it is ultimately the nurse's responsibility to ensure that medication errors are avoided. Medication errors are discussed in Chapter 7.

KEY POINTS

- To maximize beneficial drug responses and minimize harm, we must adjust therapy to account for sources of individual variation.
- As a rule, small patients need smaller doses than large patients.
- Dosage adjustments made to account for size are often based on body surface area, rather than simply on body weight.
- Infants and older adults are more sensitive to drugs than are older children and younger adults.
- Kidney disease can decrease drug excretion, thereby causing drug levels to rise. To prevent toxicity, drugs that are eliminated by the kidneys should be given in reduced dosage.
- Liver disease can decrease drug metabolism, thereby causing levels to rise. To prevent toxicity, drugs that are eliminated by the liver should be given in reduced dosage.
- When a patient becomes tolerant to a drug, the dosage must be increased to maintain beneficial effects.
- Pharmacodynamic tolerance results from adaptive changes that occur in response to prolonged drug exposure. Pharmacodynamic tolerance increases the MEC of a drug.
- Pharmacokinetic tolerance results from accelerated drug metabolism. Pharmacokinetic tolerance does not increase the MEC.
- A placebo effect is defined as the component of a drug response that can be attributed to psychologic factors, rather than to direct physiologic or biochemical actions of the drug. Solid proof that most placebo effects are real is lacking.
- Bioavailability refers to the amount of active drug that reaches the systemic circulation from its site of administration.
- Differences in bioavailability matter most for drugs that have a narrow therapeutic range.
- Alterations in the genes that code for drug-metabolizing enzymes can result in increased or decreased metabolism of many drugs.
- Genetic variations can alter the structure of drug receptors and other target molecules, and can thereby influence drug responses.
- Genetic variations that alter immune reactions to drugs can result in severe injury, and even death.
- Therapeutic and adverse effects of drugs may differ between males and females. Unfortunately, for most drugs, data are insufficient to predict what the differences might be.
- Race is a poor predictor of drug responses. What really matters is not race, but rather the specific genetic variations and psychosocial factors (shared by some group members) that can influence drug responses.
- Poor patient adherence and medication errors are major sources of individual variation.

Please visit **http://evolve.elsevier.com/Lehne** for chapter-specific NCLEX® examination review questions.

UNIT III DRUG THERAPY ACROSS THE LIFE SPAN

CHAPTER 9

Drug Therapy During Pregnancy and Breast-Feeding

This chapter addresses drug therapy in women who are pregnant or breast-feeding. The clinical challenge is to provide effective treatment for the patient while avoiding harm to the fetus or nursing infant. Unfortunately, meeting this challenge is confounded by a shortage of reliable data on drug toxicity during pregnancy or breast-feeding.

DRUG THERAPY DURING PREGNANCY: BASIC CONSIDERATIONS

Drug use during pregnancy is common: About two-thirds of pregnant patients take at least one medication, and the majority take more. Some drugs are used to treat pregnancy-related conditions, such as nausea, constipation, and preeclampsia. Some are used to treat chronic disorders, such as hypertension, diabetes, and epilepsy. Still others are used for the management of invasive conditions such as infectious diseases or cancer. In addition to taking these therapeutic agents, pregnant patients may use drugs of abuse, such as alcohol, cocaine, and heroin.

Drug therapy in pregnancy presents a vexing dilemma. In pregnant patients, as in all other patients, the benefits of treatment must balance the risks. Of course, when drugs are used during pregnancy, risks apply to the fetus as well. Unfortunately, most drugs have not been tested during pregnancy. As a result, the risks for most drugs are unknown—hence the dilemma: The prescriber is obliged to balance risks versus benefits, without always knowing what the full risks really are.

Despite the imposing challenge of balancing risks versus benefits, drug therapy during pregnancy cannot and should not be avoided. Because the health of the fetus depends on the health of the mother, conditions that threaten the mother's health must be addressed. Chronic asthma is a good example. Uncontrolled maternal asthma is far more dangerous to the fetus than the drugs used to treat it. The incidence of stillbirth is doubled among those pregnant patients who do not take medications for asthma control.

One of the greatest challenges in identifying drug effects on a developing fetus has been the lack of clinical trials, which, by their nature, would put the developing fetus at risk. To address this challenge, in 2009, the Food and Drug Administration (FDA) launched the *Medication Exposure in Pregnancy Risk Evaluation Program* (MEPREP), a collaborative effort between the FDA, Kaiser Permanente, Vanderbilt University, and a consortium of health maintenance organizations (HMOs) called the HMO Research Network Center for Education and Research on Therapeutics. Through MEPREP, data were collected on 1,221,156 children born to 933,917 mothers who used drugs during pregnancy. Research based on these data sets has generated knowledge on drugs used to manage a large number of conditions, such as diabetes, depression, and fibromyalgia.

Other examples of studies that compared histories of women who took drugs during pregnancy is the National Birth Defects Prevention Study (http://www.nbdps.org), which examined births from 1997 to 2011, and the Birth Defects Study to Evaluate Pregnancy Exposures (http://www.cdc.gov/ncbddd/birthdefects/bd-steps.html), which began collecting data on children born January 2014 and beyond.

In addition to retrospective studies, there are a number of pregnancy registries that enroll women who need to take a drug while pregnant. These allow researchers to more closely monitor pregnancy outcomes associated with a drug. The FDA provides a list of pregnancy exposure registries at http://www.fda.gov/ScienceResearch/SpecialTopics/WomensHealthResearch/ucm134848.htm. While some are devoted to a single drug and its effect on pregnancy and the fetus, many of these study multiple drugs. This and continuing research will provide a body of evidence to guide safer selection of drugs to manage conditions during pregnancy.

Physiologic Changes During Pregnancy and Their Impact on Drug Disposition and Dosing

Pregnancy brings on physiologic changes that can alter drug disposition. Changes in the kidney, liver, and GI tract are of particular interest. Because of these changes, a compensatory change in dosage may be needed.

By the third trimester, renal blood flow is doubled, causing a large increase in glomerular filtration rate. As a result, there is accelerated clearance of drugs that are eliminated by glomerular filtration. Elimination of lithium, for example, is increased by 100%. To compensate for accelerated excretion, dosage must be increased.

For some drugs, hepatic metabolism increases during pregnancy. Three antiseizure drugs—phenytoin, carbamazepine, and valproic acid—provide examples.

Tone and motility of the bowel decrease in pregnancy, causing intestinal transit time to increase. Because of prolonged transit, there is more time for drugs to be absorbed. In theory, this could increase levels of drugs whose absorption is normally poor. Similarly, there is more time for reabsorption of drugs that undergo enterohepatic recirculation, possibly resulting in a prolongation of drug effects. In both cases, a reduction in dosage might be needed.

Placental Drug Transfer

Essentially all drugs can cross the placenta, although some cross more readily than others. The factors that determine drug passage across the membranes of the placenta are the same factors that determine drug passage across all other membranes. Accordingly, drugs that are lipid soluble cross the placenta easily, whereas drugs that are ionized, highly polar, or protein bound cross with difficulty. Nonetheless, for practical purposes, the clinician should assume that *any drug taken during pregnancy will reach the fetus.*

Adverse Reactions During Pregnancy

Not only are pregnant patients subject to the same adverse effects as nonpregnant patients, they may also suffer effects unique to pregnancy. For example, when heparin (an anticoagulant) is taken by pregnant patients, it can cause the patient to develop osteoporosis, which in turn can cause compression fractures of the spine. Use of aspirin increases the risk of serious bleeding during childbirth.

In addition to causing problems for the pregnant woman, drugs may also cause complications for the pregnancy, for the fetus, and for the neonate. For example, misoprostol, a drug taken to protect the stomach of people taking NSAIDs (nonsteroidal anti-inflammatory drugs), can cause a spontaneous abortion. The anticoagulant warfarin has been associated with fetal hemorrhage. Benzodiazepines taken late in pregnancy may cause hypoglycemia and respiratory complications in the neonate along with a hypotonic state that is commonly called floppy infant syndrome.

Regular use of dependence-producing drugs (e.g., heroin, barbiturates, alcohol) during pregnancy can result in the birth of a drug-dependent infant. If the infant's dependence is not supported with drugs following birth, a withdrawal syndrome will ensue. Symptoms include shrill crying, vomiting, and extreme irritability. The neonate should be weaned from dependence by giving progressively smaller doses of the drug on which he or she is dependent.

Opioid pain relievers (e.g., opioids) used during delivery can depress respiration in the neonate. The infant must be closely monitored until respiration is normal.

The drug effect of greatest concern is teratogenesis. This is the production of birth defects in the fetus.

DRUG THERAPY DURING PREGNANCY: TERATOGENESIS

The term *teratogenesis* is derived from *teras,* the Greek word for *monster.* Translated literally, teratogenesis means *to produce a monster.* Consistent with this derivation, we usually think of birth defects in terms of gross malformations, such as cleft palate, clubfoot, and hydrocephalus. However, birth defects are not limited to distortions of gross anatomy; they also include neurobehavioral and metabolic anomalies.

Incidence and Causes of Congenital Anomalies

The incidence of *major* structural abnormalities (e.g., abnormalities that are life threatening or require surgical correction) is between 1% and 3%. Half of these are obvious and are reported at birth. The other half involve internal organs (e.g., heart, liver, GI tract) and are not discovered until later in life or at autopsy. The incidence of minor structural abnormalities is unknown, as is the incidence of functional abnormalities (e.g., growth delay, intellectual disabilities).

Congenital anomalies have multiple causes, including genetic predisposition, environmental chemicals, and drugs. Genetic factors account for about 25% of all birth defects. Of the genetically based anomalies, Down's syndrome is the most common. Less than 1% of all birth defects are caused by drugs. For the majority of congenital anomalies, the cause is unknown.

Teratogenesis and Stage of Development

Fetal sensitivity to teratogens changes during development, thus the effect of a teratogen is highly dependent upon when the drug is given. As shown in Fig. 9.1, development occurs in three major stages: the *preimplantation/presomite period* (conception through week 2), the *embryonic period* (weeks 3 through 8), and the *fetal period* (week 9 through term). During the preimplantation/presomite period, teratogens act in an "all-or-nothing" fashion. That is, if the dose is sufficiently high, the result is death of the conceptus. Conversely, if the dose is sublethal, the conceptus is likely to recover fully.

Gross malformations are produced by exposure to teratogens during the *embryonic period* (roughly the first trimester). This is the time when the basic shape of internal organs and other structures is being established. Because the fetus is especially

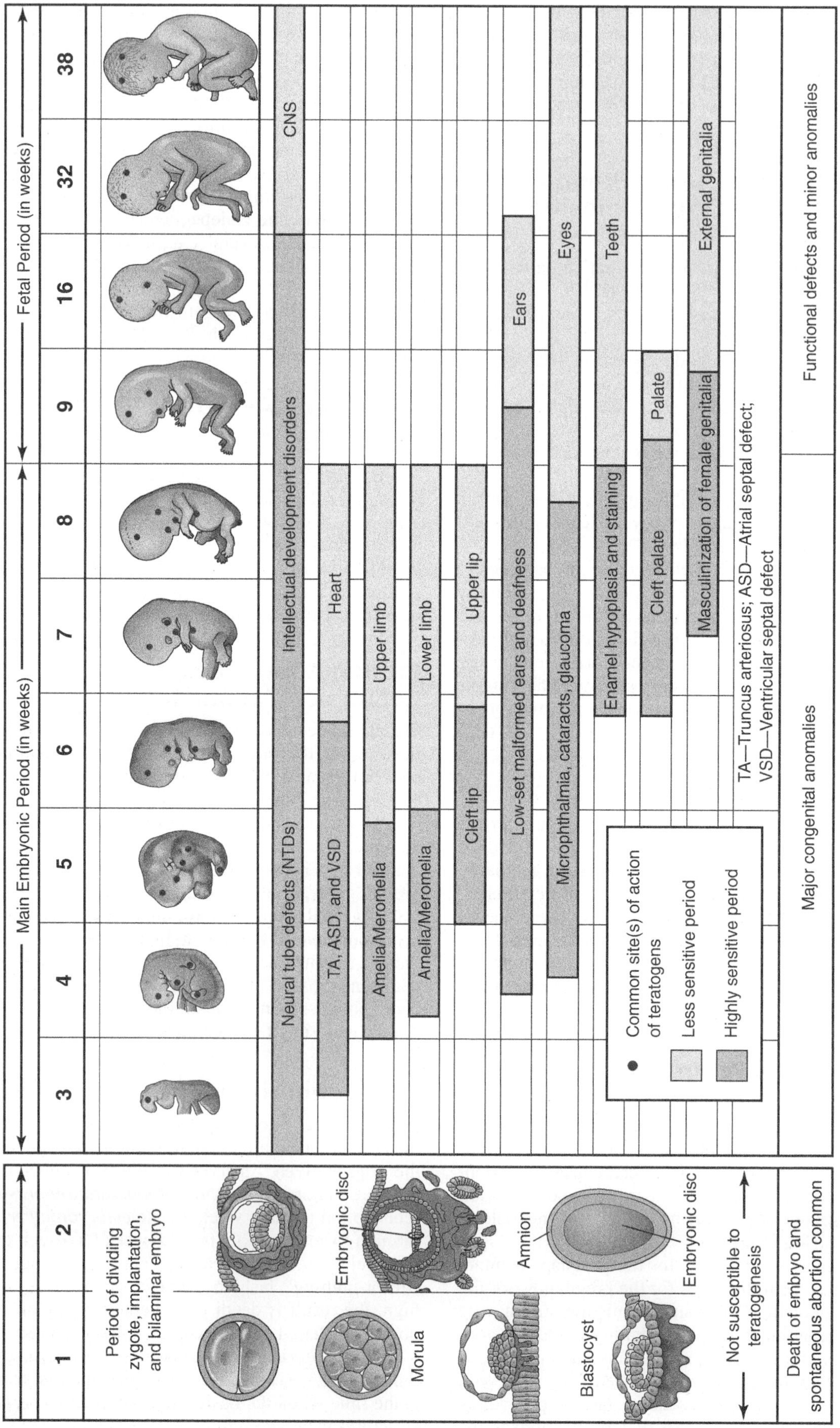

Fig. 9.1 ■ **Effects of teratogens at various stages of development of the fetus.**
(From Moore K, Persaud TVN, Torchia M: *The developing human: clinically oriented embryology*, ed 9, Philadelphia, 2012, Elsevier, with permission.)

vulnerable during the embryonic period, pregnant patients must take special care to avoid teratogen exposure during this time.

Teratogen exposure during the *fetal period* (i.e., the second and third trimesters) usually disrupts *function* rather than gross anatomy. Of the developmental processes that occur in the fetal period, growth and development of the brain are especially important. Disruption of brain development can result in learning deficits and behavioral abnormalities.

Identification of Teratogens

For the following reasons, human teratogens are extremely difficult to identify:

- The incidence of congenital anomalies is generally low.
- Animal tests may not be applicable to humans.
- Prolonged drug exposure may be required.
- Teratogenic effects may be delayed.
- Behavioral effects are difficult to document.
- Controlled experiments can't be done in humans.

As a result, only a few drugs are considered *proven* teratogens. Drugs whose teratogenicity has been documented (or at least is highly suspected) are listed in Table 9.1. It is important to note, however, that *lack of proof of teratogenicity does not mean that a drug is safe;* it only means that the available data are insufficient to make a definitive judgment. Conversely, *proof of teratogenicity does not mean that every exposure will result in a birth defect.* In fact, with most teratogens, the risk of malformation following exposure is only about 10%.

To prove that a drug is a teratogen, three criteria must be met:

- The drug must cause a characteristic set of malformations.
- It must act only during a specific window of vulnerability (e.g., weeks 4 through 7 of gestation).
- The incidence of malformations should increase with increasing dosage and duration of exposure.

Obviously, we cannot do experiments on humans to see whether a drug meets these criteria. The best we can do is to systematically collect and analyze data on drugs taken during pregnancy in the hope that useful information on teratogenicity will be revealed.

Studies in animals may be of limited value, in part because teratogenicity may be species-specific. That is, drugs that are teratogens in laboratory animals may be safe in humans. Conversely, and more importantly, drugs that fail to cause anomalies in animals may later prove teratogenic in humans. The most notorious example is thalidomide. In studies with pregnant animals, thalidomide was harmless; however, when thalidomide was taken by pregnant patients, about 30% had babies with severe malformations. The take-home message is this: *Lack of teratogenicity in animals is not proof of safety in humans.* Accordingly, we cannot assume that a new drug is safe for use in human pregnancy just because it has met FDA requirements, which are based on tests done in pregnant animals.

Some teratogens act quickly, whereas others require prolonged exposure. Thalidomide represents a fast-acting teratogen: a single dose can cause malformation. In contrast, alcohol (ethanol) must be taken repeatedly in high doses if gross malformation is to result. (Lower doses of alcohol may produce subtle anomalies.) Because a single exposure to a rapid-acting teratogen can produce obvious malformation, rapid-acting teratogens are easier to identify than slow-acting teratogens.

Teratogens that produce delayed effects are among the hardest to identify. The best example is diethylstilbestrol, an estrogenic substance that can cause vaginal cancer in female offspring 18 or so years after birth.

Teratogens that affect behavior may be nearly impossible to identify. Behavioral changes are often delayed and therefore may not become apparent until the child goes to school. By this time, it may be difficult to establish a correlation between drug use during pregnancy and the behavioral deficit. Furthermore, if the deficit is subtle, it may not even be recognized.

FDA Pregnancy Risk Categories and New Labeling Rules

In 1979, the FDA established a system for classifying drugs according to their probable risks to the fetus. According to this system, *drugs can be put into one of five risk categories: A, B, C, D,* and *X* (Table 9.2). Drugs in Risk Category A are the least dangerous; controlled studies have been done in pregnant patients and have failed to demonstrate a risk of fetal harm. In contrast, drugs in Category X are the most dangerous; these drugs are known to cause human fetal harm, and their risk to the fetus outweighs any possible therapeutic benefit. Drugs in Categories B, C, and D are progressively more dangerous than drugs in Category A and less dangerous than drugs in Category X. Although the current rating system is helpful, it is far from ideal.

In December 2014, the FDA issued the Pregnancy and Lactation Labeling Rule (PLLR), which provides new guidance for labeling. This rule, which phases out the Pregnancy Risk Categories, began implementation in 2015. By 2020, all drug manufacturers will cease using Pregnancy Risk Category labeling.

The PLLR requires three sections for labeling: (1) pregnancy, (2) lactation, and (3) females and males of reproductive potential. These are further divided into subsections containing specified content (Table 9.3). The full report is available at http://www.fda.gov/downloads/drugs/guidancecomplianceregulatoryinformation/guidances/ucm450636.pdf.

These changes put those of you studying pharmacology in a bit of a quandary. At the time of this writing (2017), most drugs still include Pregnancy Risk Categories in labeling and package inserts. We anticipate that most of you will graduate after 2020; therefore, these will no longer be in effect. Those of you in accelerated programs, however, may graduate at a time when these are still used. For these reasons, we have decided to maintain the categories for this edition while expanding on the reasons behind the categories and including additional information required by this new ruling.

Minimizing Drug Risk During Pregnancy

Common sense tells us that the best way to minimize drug risk is to minimize the use of drugs. If possible, pregnant patients should avoid unnecessary drugs entirely. Nurses and other health professionals should warn pregnant patients against the use of all nonessential drugs. If a high-risk drug will be prescribed to a woman of childbearing age, a pregnancy test should be performed if pregnancy status is unknown and there is a chance that the patient could be pregnant.

TABLE 9.1 ▪ Drugs With Proven or Strongly Suspected Teratogenicity[a]

Drug	Teratogenic Effect
ANTICANCER/IMMUNOSUPPRESSANT DRUGS	
Cyclophosphamide	CNS malformation, secondary cancer
Methotrexate	CNS and limb malformations
Thalidomide	Shortened limbs, internal organ defects
ANTISEIZURE DRUGS	
Carbamazepine	Neural tube defects, craniofacial defects, malformations of the heart, and hypospadias
Phenytoin	Growth delay, CNS defects
Topiramate	Growth delay, cleft lip with cleft palate
Valproic acid	Neural tube defects, craniofacial defects, malformations of the heart and extremities, and hypospadias
SEX HORMONES	
Androgens (e.g., danazol)	Masculinization of the female fetus
Diethylstilbestrol	Vaginal carcinoma in female offspring
Estrogens	Congenital defects of female reproductive organs
ANTIMICROBIALS	
Nitrofurantoin	Abnormally small or absent eyes, heart defects, cleft lip with cleft palate
Tetracycline	Tooth and bone anomalies
Trimethoprim-Sulfamethoxazole	Neural tube defects, cardiovascular malformations, cleft palate, club foot, and urinary tract abnormalities
OTHER DRUGS	
Alcohol	Fetal alcohol syndrome, stillbirth, spontaneous abortion, low birth weight, intellectual disabilities
5-Alpha-reductase inhibitors (e.g., dutasteride, finasteride)	Malformations of external genitalia in males
Angiotensin-converting enzyme inhibitors	Renal failure, renal tubular dysgenesis, skull hypoplasia (from exposure during the second and third trimesters)
Antithyroid drugs (propylthiouracil, methimazole)	Goiter and hypothyroidism
HMG-CoA reductase inhibitors (atorvastatin, simvastatin)	Facial malformations and CNS anomalies, including holoprosencephaly (single-lobed brain) and neural tube defects
Isotretinoin and other vitamin A derivatives (etretinate, megadoses of vitamin A)	Multiple defects (CNS, craniofacial, cardiovascular, others)
Lithium	Ebstein's anomaly (cardiac defects)
Nonsteroidal anti-inflammatory drugs (NSAIDs)	Premature closure of the ductus arteriosus
Oral hypoglycemic drugs (e.g., tolbutamide)	Neonatal hypoglycemia
Warfarin	Skeletal and CNS defects

[a]The absence of a drug from this table does not mean that the drug is not a teratogen. For most proven teratogens, the risk of a congenital anomaly is only 10%.
CNS, Central nervous system.

An essential intervention for decreasing risk during pregnancy is to review all prescription and over-the-counter drugs taken at every visit. It is crucial to also include herbal and nutritional supplements, as well as recreational drug use. Even vitamin A is dangerous when taken in excess. Vitamin A, which is designated Pregnancy Risk Factor X at the time of this writing, can cause craniofacial defects and CNS, cardiac, and thymus gland abnormalities.

As noted, some disease states (e.g., epilepsy, asthma, diabetes) pose a greater risk to fetal health than the drugs used for treating them. However, even with these disorders, in which drug therapy reduces the risk of disease-induced fetal harm, we must still take steps to minimize harm from drugs. Accordingly, drugs that pose a high risk of danger to the developing embryo or fetus should be discontinued and safer alternatives substituted.

Sometimes the use of a high-risk drug is unavoidable. A pregnant patient may have a disease that requires the use of drugs that have a high probability of causing harm. Some anticancer drugs, for example, are highly toxic to the developing fetus, yet cannot be ethically withheld from the pregnant patient. If a patient elects to use such drugs, termination of pregnancy should be considered.

Reducing the risk of teratogenesis also applies to female patients who are *not* pregnant, because about 50% of pregnancies are unintended. Accordingly, if a patient of reproductive age is taking a teratogenic drug, she should be educated about the risk as well as the necessity of using at least one reliable form of birth control.

Responding to Teratogen Exposure

When a pregnant patient has been exposed to a known teratogen, the first step is to determine exactly when the drug was taken and exactly when the pregnancy began. If drug exposure was not during the period of organogenesis (i.e., weeks 3 through 8), the patient should be reassured that the risk of drug-induced malformation is minimal. In addition, she should be reminded that 3% of all babies have some kind of conspicuous malformation independent of teratogen exposure. This is important because, otherwise, the drug is sure to be blamed if the baby is abnormal.

What should be done if the exposure *did* occur during organogenesis? First, an authoritative reference (e.g., FDA-approved prescribing information for the drug) should be consulted to determine the type of malformation expected. Next, at least two ultrasound scans should be done to assess the extent of injury. If the malformation is severe, termination

TABLE 9.2 ▪ FDA Pregnancy Risk Categories

Category	Category Description
A	*Remote Risk of Fetal Harm:* Controlled studies in women have been done and have failed to demonstrate a risk of fetal harm during the first trimester, and there is no evidence of risk in later trimesters.
B	*Slightly More Risk Than A:* Animal studies show no fetal risk, but controlled studies have not been done in women. or Animal studies do show a risk of fetal harm, but controlled studies in women have failed to demonstrate a risk during the first trimester, and there is no evidence of risk in later trimesters.
C	*Greater Risk Than B:* Animal studies show a risk of fetal harm, but no controlled studies have been done in women. or No studies have been done in women or animals.
D	*Proven Risk of Fetal Harm:* Studies in women show proof of fetal damage, but the potential benefits of use during pregnancy may be necessary despite the risks (e.g., treatment of life-threatening disease for which safer drugs are ineffective). A statement on risk will appear in the "WARNINGS" section of drug labeling.
X	*Proven Risk of Fetal Harm:* Studies in women or animals show definite risk of fetal abnormality. or Adverse reaction reports indicate evidence of fetal risk. The risks clearly outweigh any possible benefit. A statement on risk will appear in the "CONTRAINDICATIONS" section of drug labeling.

TABLE 9.3 ▪ FDA Pregnancy and Lactation Labeling Rule (PLLR) Requirements

Sections	Subsections	Headings and/or Content
Pregnancy	Pregnancy Exposure Registry (This subsection is omitted if there are no known pregnancy exposure registries for the drug.)	If a pregnancy exposure registry exists, the following sentence will be included: "There is a pregnancy exposure registry that monitors pregnancy outcomes in women exposed to (name of drug) during pregnancy." The statement is followed by registry enrollment information.
	Risk Summary (This subsection is required.)	Risk summaries are statements that summarize outcomes for the following content relative to drug dosage, length of time drug was taken, and weeks of gestation when the drug was taken as well as known pharmacologic mechanisms of action. a. Human data b. Animal data c. Pharmacology
	Clinical Considerations (This subsection is omitted if none of the headings are applicable.)	Information is provided for the following five headings: a. Disease-associated maternal and/or embryo/fetal risk b. Dose adjustments during pregnancy and the postpartum period c. Maternal adverse reactions d. Fetal/Neonatal adverse reactions e. Labor or delivery (Any heading that is not applicable is omitted.)
	Data (This subsection is omitted if none of the headings are applicable.)	This section describes research that served as a source of data for Risk Summaries. The following categories are included: a. Human data b. Animal data (Any heading that is not applicable is omitted.)

Continued

TABLE 9.3 ▪ FDA Pregnancy and Lactation Labeling Rule (PLLR) Requirements—cont'd

Sections	Subsections	Headings and/or Content
Lactation	Risk Summary (This subsection is required.)	Risk summaries are statements that summarize outcomes for the following content: a. Presence of drug in human milk b. Effects of drug on the breast-fed child c. Effects of drug on milk production/excretion d. Risk and benefit statement
	Clinical Considerations (This subsection is omitted if none of the headings are applicable.)	Information is provided for the following headings: a. Minimizing exposure b. Monitoring for adverse reactions (Any heading that is not applicable is omitted.)
	Data (This subsection is omitted if none of the headings are applicable.)	This section expands on the Risk Summary and Clinical Considerations subsections. There are no defined headings.
Females and Males of Reproductive Potential	(There is no defined subsection for this section.)	The following headings are included to address the need for pregnancy testing or contraception and adverse effects associated with preimplantation loss or adverse effects on fertility: a. Pregnancy testing b. Contraception c. Infertility (Any heading that is not applicable is omitted.)

Adapted from U.S. Department of Health and Human Services, Food and Drug Administration. Appendix A: *Organization and format for pregnancy, lactation, and females and males of reproductive potential subsections. Pregnancy, lactation, and reproductive potential: labeling for human prescription drug and biological products—content and format.* www.fda.gov/downloads/drugs/guidancecomplianceregulatoryinformation/guidances/ucm450636.pdf, June 2015.

of pregnancy should be considered. If the malformation is minor (e.g., cleft palate), it may be correctable by surgery, either shortly after birth or later in childhood.

DRUG THERAPY DURING BREAST-FEEDING

Drugs taken by lactating patients can be excreted in breast milk. If drug concentrations in milk are high enough, a pharmacologic effect can occur in the infant, raising the possibility of harm. Unfortunately, very little systematic research has been done on this issue. As a result, although a few drugs are known to be hazardous (Table 9.4), the possible danger posed by many others remains undetermined.

Although nearly all drugs can enter breast milk, the extent of entry varies greatly. The factors that determine entry into breast milk are the same factors that determine passage of drugs across membranes. Accordingly, drugs that are lipid soluble enter breast milk readily, whereas drugs that are ionized, highly polar, or protein bound tend to be excluded.

Most drugs can be detected in milk, but concentrations are usually too low to cause harm. While breast-feeding is usually safe, even though drugs are being taken, prudence is in order: If the nursing patient can avoid drugs, she should. Moreover, when drugs *must* be used, steps should be taken to minimize risk. These include:

- Dosing immediately *after* breast-feeding (to minimize drug concentrations in milk at the next feeding)
- Avoiding drugs that have a long half-life
- Avoiding sustained-release formulations
- Choosing drugs that tend to be excluded from milk
- Choosing drugs that are least likely to affect the infant (Table 9.5)
- Avoiding drugs that are known to be hazardous (see Table 9.4)
- Using the lowest effective dosage for the shortest possible time
- Abandoning plans to breast-feed if a necessary drug is known to be harmful to the child

TABLE 9.4 ▪ Drugs That Are Contraindicated During Breast-Feeding

CONTROLLED SUBSTANCES
Amphetamine
Cocaine
Heroin
Marijuana
Phencyclidine
ANTICANCER AGENTS/IMMUNOSUPPRESSANTS
Cyclophosphamide
Cyclosporine
Doxorubicin
Methotrexate
OTHERS
Atenolol
Bromocriptine
Ergotamine
Lithium
Nicotine
Radioactive compounds (temporary cessation)

TABLE 9.5 ▪ Drugs of Choice for Breast-Feeding Patients[a]

Drug Category	Drugs and Drug Groups of Choice	Comments
Analgesic drugs	Acetaminophen, ibuprofen, flurbiprofen, ketorolac, mefenamic acid, sumatriptan, morphine	Sumatriptan may be given for migraine. Morphine may be given for severe pain.
Anticoagulant drugs	Warfarin, acenocoumarol 🍁, heparin (unfractionated)	Among breast-fed infants whose mothers were taking warfarin, the drug was undetectable in plasma and bleeding time was not affected. The large molecular size of unfractionated heparin decreases amount excreted in breast milk. Furthermore, it is not bioavailable from the GI tract, so heparin in breast milk is not systemically absorbed.
Antidepressant drugs	Sertraline, paroxetine, tricyclic antidepressants (TCAs)	Fluoxetine [Prozac] may be given if other selective serotonin reuptake inhibitors (SSRIs) are ineffective; however, caution is needed because levels are higher in breast milk than levels of other SSRIs. Infant risk with TCAs cannot be ruled out; however, no significant adverse effects have been reported.
Antiepileptic drugs	Carbamazepine, phenytoin, valproic acid	The estimated level of exposure to these drugs in infants is less than 10% of the therapeutic dose standardized by weight.
Antihistamines (histamine$_1$ blockers)	Loratadine, fexofenadine	First-generation antihistamines are associated with irritability or sedation and may decrease milk supply.
Antimicrobial drugs	Penicillins, cephalosporins, aminoglycosides, macrolides	Avoid chloramphenicol and tetracycline.
Beta-adrenergic antagonists	Labetalol, metoprolol, propranolol	Angiotensin-converting enzyme inhibitors and calcium channel–blocking agents are also considered safe.
Endocrine drugs	Propylthiouracil, insulin, levothyroxine	The estimated level of exposure to propylthiouracil in breast-feeding infants is less than 1% of the therapeutic dose standardized by weight; thyroid function of the infant is not affected.
Glucocorticoids	Prednisolone and prednisone	The amount of prednisolone the infant would ingest in breast milk is less than 0.1% of the therapeutic dose standardized by weight.

[a]This list is not exhaustive. Cases of overdoses of these drugs must be assessed on an individual basis.

KEY POINTS

- Because hepatic metabolism and glomerular filtration increase during pregnancy, dosages of some drugs may need to be increased.
- Lipid-soluble drugs cross the placenta readily, whereas drugs that are ionized, polar, or protein bound cross with difficulty. Nonetheless, all drugs cross to some extent.
- When prescribing drugs during pregnancy, the clinician must try to balance the benefits of treatment versus the risks—often without knowing what the risks really are.
- About 3% of all babies are born with gross structural malformations without teratogenic drug exposure.
- Less than 1% of birth defects are caused by drugs.
- Teratogen-induced gross malformations result from exposure early in pregnancy (weeks 3 through 8 of gestation), the time of organogenesis.
- Functional impairments (e.g., intellectual disabilities) result from exposure to teratogens later in pregnancy.
- For most drugs, we lack reliable data on the risks of use during pregnancy.
- Lack of teratogenicity in animals is not proof of safety in humans.
- Some drugs (e.g., thalidomide) cause birth defects with just one dose, whereas others (e.g., alcohol) require prolonged exposure.
- FDA Pregnancy Risk Categories indicate relative risks of drug use. Drugs in Category X pose the highest risk of fetal harm and are contraindicated during pregnancy.
- Any female patient of reproductive age who is taking a known teratogen must be counseled about the teratogenic risk and the necessity of using at least one reliable form of birth control.
- Drugs that are lipid soluble readily enter breast milk, whereas drugs that are ionized, polar, or protein bound tend to be excluded. Nonetheless, all drugs enter to some extent.
- Although most drugs can be detected in breast milk, concentrations are usually too low to harm the nursing infant.
- If possible, drugs should be avoided during breast-feeding.
- If drugs cannot be avoided during breast-feeding, common sense dictates choosing drugs known to be safe and avoiding drugs known to be dangerous.

Please visit **http://evolve.elsevier.com/Lehne** for chapter-specific NCLEX® examination review questions.

CHAPTER

10 Drug Therapy in Pediatric Patients

Patients who are very young respond differently to drugs than do the rest of the population. Most differences are *quantitative.* Specifically, younger patients are more sensitive to drugs than adult patients, and they show greater individual variation. Drug sensitivity in the very young results largely from *organ system immaturity.* Because of heightened drug sensitivity, they are at increased risk of adverse drug reactions. In this chapter we discuss the physiologic factors that underlie heightened drug sensitivity in pediatric patients, as well as ways to promote safe and effective drug use.

Pediatrics covers all patients up to 16 years of age. Because of ongoing growth and development, pediatric patients in different age groups present different therapeutic challenges. Traditionally, the pediatric population is subdivided into six groups:

- Premature infants (less than 36 weeks' gestational age)
- Full-term infants (36 to 40 weeks' gestational age)
- Neonates (first 4 postnatal weeks)
- Infants (weeks 5 to 52 postnatal)
- Children (1 to 12 years)
- Adolescents (12 to 16 years)

Not surprisingly, as young patients grow older, they become more like adults physiologically, and hence more like adults with regard to drug therapy. Conversely, the very young—those under 1 year old and especially those under 1 month old—are very different from adults. If drug therapy in these patients is to be safe and effective, we must account for these differences.

Pediatric drug therapy is made even more difficult by insufficient drug information: Fully two-thirds of drugs used in pediatrics have never been tested in children. As a result, we often lack reliable information on dosing, pharmacokinetics, and both therapeutic and adverse effects. To help expand our knowledge, Congress enacted two important laws: the *Best Pharmaceuticals for Children Act* (BPCA), passed in 2002, and the *Pediatric Research Equity Act* (PREA) of 2003. Both were designed to promote drug research in children. Early studies revealed that

- About 20% of drugs were ineffective in children, even though they *were* effective in adults.
- About 30% of drugs caused unanticipated side effects, some of them potentially lethal.
- About 20% of the drugs studied required dosages different from those that had been extrapolated from dosages used in adults.

In 2012, the Institute of Medicine (IOM) published a synopsis of findings from research conducted under the BPCA and PREA. This report, available at http://nationalacademies.org/hmd/reports/2012/safe-and-effective-medicines-for-children.aspx, spoke not only to the importance of information derived from the research, but also to the need for continued research and additional studies addressing long-term safety and drug therapy in neonates. To this end, the BPCA and PREA were permanently reauthorized as part of the FDA Safety and Innovation Act (FDASIA) of 2012.

As more studies are done, the gaps in our knowledge will shrink. In the meantime, we must still treat children with drugs—even though we lack the information needed to prescribe rationally. Similar to drug therapy during pregnancy, prescribers must try to balance benefits versus risks, without precisely knowing what the benefits and risks really are.

PHARMACOKINETICS: NEONATES AND INFANTS

Pharmacokinetic factors determine the concentration of a drug at its sites of action, and hence determine the intensity and duration of responses. If drug levels are elevated, responses will be more intense. If drug elimination is delayed, responses will be prolonged. Because the organ systems that regulate drug levels are not fully developed in the very young, these patients are at risk of both possibilities: drug effects that are unusually intense *and* prolonged. By accounting for pharmacokinetic differences in the very young, we can increase the chances that drug therapy will be both effective and safe.

Fig. 10.1 illustrates how drug levels differ between infants and adults following administration of equivalent doses (i.e., doses adjusted for body weight). When a drug is administered *intravenously,* levels decline more slowly in the infant than in the adult. As a result, drug levels in the infant remain above the minimum effective concentration (MEC) longer than in the adult, thereby causing effects to be prolonged. When a drug is administered *subcutaneously,* not only do levels in the infant remain above the MEC *longer* than in the adult, but these levels also rise *higher,* causing effects to be more intense as well as prolonged. From these illustrations, it is clear that adjustment of dosage for infants on the basis of body size alone is not sufficient to achieve safe results.

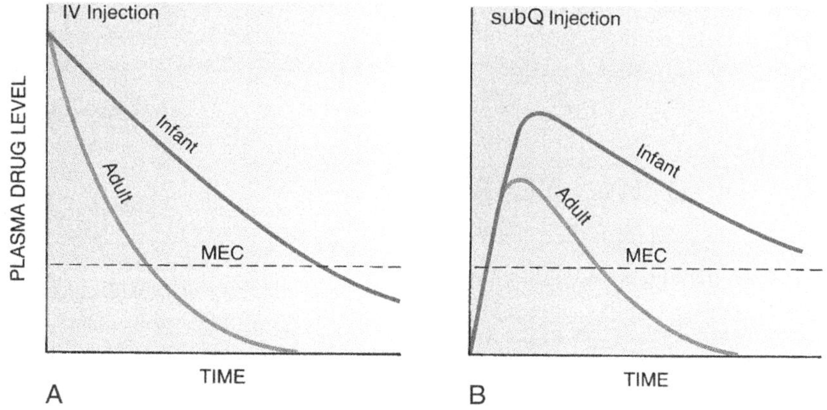

Fig. 10.1 ■ **Comparison of plasma drug levels in adults and infants.** **A,** Plasma drug levels following IV injection. Dosage was adjusted for body weight. Note that plasma levels remain above the minimum effective concentration (MEC) much longer in the infant. **B,** Plasma drug levels following subQ injection. Dosage was adjusted for body weight. Note that both the maximum drug level and the duration of action are greater in the infant.

If small body size is not the major reason for heightened drug sensitivity in infants, what is? The increased sensitivity of infants is due largely to the immature state of five pharmacokinetic processes: (1) drug absorption, (2) protein binding of drugs, (3) exclusion of drugs from the central nervous system (CNS) by the blood-brain barrier, (4) hepatic drug metabolism, and (5) renal drug excretion.

Absorption

Oral Administration

Gastrointestinal physiology in the infant is very different from that in the adult. As a result, drug absorption may be enhanced or impeded, depending on the physicochemical properties of the drug involved.

Gastric emptying time is both prolonged and irregular in early infancy, and then gradually reaches adult values by 6 to 8 months. For drugs that are absorbed primarily from the stomach, delayed gastric emptying enhances absorption. On the other hand, for drugs that are absorbed primarily from the intestine, absorption is delayed. Because gastric emptying time is irregular, the precise impact on absorption is not predictable.

Gastric acidity is very low 24 hours after birth and does not reach adult values for 2 years. Because of low acidity, absorption of acid-labile drugs is increased.

Intramuscular Administration

Drug absorption following IM injection in the *neonate* is *slow* and *erratic.* Delayed absorption is due in part to low blood flow through muscle during the first days of postnatal life. By early *infancy,* absorption of IM drugs becomes more *rapid* than in neonates and adults.

Transdermal Absorption

Drug absorption through the skin is more rapid and complete in infants than in older children and adults. The stratum corneum of the infant's skin is very thin, and blood flow to the skin is greater in infants than in older patients. Because of this enhanced absorption, infants are at increased risk of toxicity from topical drugs.

Distribution

Protein Binding

Binding of drugs to albumin and other plasma proteins is limited in the infant, because (1) the amount of serum albumin is relatively low and (2) endogenous compounds (e.g., fatty acids, bilirubin) compete with drugs for available binding sites. Consequently, drugs that ordinarily undergo extensive protein binding in adults undergo much less binding in infants. As a result, the concentration of *free* levels of such drugs is relatively high in the infant, thereby intensifying effects. To ensure that effects are not too intense, dosages in infants should be reduced. Protein-binding capacity reaches adult values within 10 to 12 months.

Blood-Brain Barrier

The blood-brain barrier is not fully developed at birth. As a result, drugs and other chemicals have relatively easy access to the CNS, making the infant especially sensitive to drugs that affect CNS function. Accordingly, all medicines employed for their CNS effects (e.g., morphine, phenobarbital) should be given in reduced dosage. Dosage should also be reduced for drugs used for actions *outside* the CNS if those drugs are capable of producing CNS toxicity as a side effect.

Hepatic Metabolism

The drug-metabolizing capacity of newborns is low. As a result, neonates are especially sensitive to drugs that are eliminated primarily by hepatic metabolism. When these drugs are used, dosages must be reduced. The capacity of the liver to metabolize many drugs increases rapidly about 1 month after birth, and approaches adult levels a few months later. Complete maturation of the liver develops by 1 year.

Renal Excretion

Renal drug excretion is significantly reduced at birth. Renal blood flow, glomerular filtration, and active tubular secretion are all low during infancy. Because the drug-excreting capacity of infants is limited, drugs that are eliminated primarily by renal excretion must be given in reduced dosage and/or at longer dosing intervals. Adult levels of renal function are achieved by 1 year.

PHARMACOKINETICS: CHILDREN 1 YEAR AND OLDER

By age 1 year, most pharmacokinetic parameters in children are similar to those in adults. Therefore, drug sensitivity in children older than 1 year is more like that of adults than that of the very young. Although pharmacokinetically similar to adults, children do differ in one important way: They metabolize drugs *faster* than adults. Drug-metabolizing capacity is markedly elevated until age 2 years, and then gradually declines. A further sharp decline takes place at puberty, when adult values are reached. Because of enhanced drug metabolism in children, an increase in dosage or a reduction in dosing interval may be needed for drugs that are eliminated by hepatic metabolism.

ADVERSE DRUG REACTIONS

Like adults, pediatric patients are subject to adverse reactions when drug levels rise too high. In addition, pediatric patients are vulnerable to unique adverse effects related to organ system immaturity and to ongoing growth and development. Among these age-related effects are growth suppression (caused by glucocorticoids), discoloration of developing teeth (caused by tetracyclines), and kernicterus (caused by sulfonamides). Table 10.1 presents a list of drugs that can cause unique adverse effects in pediatric patients of various ages. These drugs should be avoided in patients whose age puts them at risk.

TABLE 10.1 ■ Adverse Drug Reactions Unique to Pediatric Patients

Drug	Adverse Effect
Androgens	Premature puberty in males; reduced adult height from premature epiphyseal closure
Aspirin and other salicylates	Severe intoxication from acute overdose (acidosis, hyperthermia, respiratory depression); Reye's syndrome in children with chickenpox or influenza
Chloramphenicol	Gray syndrome (neonates and infants)
Fluoroquinolones	Tendon rupture
Glucocorticoids	Growth suppression with prolonged use
Hexachlorophene	Central nervous system toxicity (infants)
Nalidixic acid	Cartilage erosion
Phenothiazines	Sudden infant death syndrome
Promethazine	Pronounced respiratory depression in children under 2 years old
Sulfonamides	Kernicterus (neonates)
Tetracyclines	Staining of developing teeth

DOSAGE DETERMINATION

Because of the pharmacokinetic factors discussed previously, dosage selection for pediatric patients can be challenging. Selecting a dosage is especially difficult in the very young, as pharmacokinetic factors are undergoing rapid change.

Pediatric dosages have been established for a few drugs but not for most. For drugs that do not have an established pediatric dosage, the dosage can be extrapolated from adult dosages. The method of conversion employed most commonly is based on body surface area (BSA):

$$(\text{Child's BSA} \times \text{Adult dosage}) \div 1.73\ \text{m}^2 = \text{Pediatric dosage}$$

Please note that initial pediatric doses—whether based on established pediatric dosages or extrapolated from adult dosages—are at best an *approximation.* Subsequent doses must be adjusted on the basis of clinical outcome and plasma drug concentrations. These adjustments are especially important in neonates and younger infants. If dosage adjustments are to be optimal, it is essential that we monitor the patient for therapeutic and adverse responses.

PROMOTING ADHERENCE

Achieving accurate and timely dosing requires informed participation of the child's caregiver and, to the extent possible, active involvement of the child as well. Effective education is critical. The following issues should be addressed:

- Dosage size and timing
- Route and technique of administration
- Duration of treatment
- Drug storage
- The nature and time course of desired responses
- The nature and time course of adverse responses

Written instructions should be provided to reinforce verbal instructions. For techniques of administration that are difficult, a demonstration should be made, after which the child's caregivers should repeat the procedure to ensure that they understand. With young children, spills and spitting out are common causes of inaccurate dosing; parents should be taught to estimate the amount of drug lost and to readminister that amount, being careful not to overcompensate. When more than one person is helping to medicate a child, all participants should be warned against multiple dosing. Multiple dosing can be avoided by maintaining a drug administration chart. With some disorders—especially infections—symptoms may resolve before the prescribed course of treatment has been completed. Parents should be instructed to complete the full course nonetheless. Additional strategies to promote adherence are presented in Table 10.2.

TABLE 10.2 ▪ Strategies to Promote Medication Adherence in Children

STRATEGIES FOR CAREGIVERS

- Suggest medication reminders to avoid missed doses (e.g., pillboxes, calendars, computer alert systems).
- Recommend a reward system (e.g., stickers) to prompt the child to take medication.
- Provide pleasant-tasting medication when possible. If the medication is unpalatable:
  - Suggest keeping the medication refrigerated, even if refrigeration is not required for storage.
  - Administer with food to mask taste, unless contraindicated.
  - Have the child suck on a frozen treat to decrease taste sensation before administration.
  - Offer a treat to "get the taste out" immediately after taking the medication.
  - Praise the child for taking the medication well.

STRATEGIES FOR OLDER CHILDREN AND ADOLESCENTS

- Simplify medication regimens, when possible.
- Treat the patient with respect and develop trust.
- Teach and reinforce necessary skills (e.g., inhaler administration, insulin injection) to improve confidence.
- Provide developmentally appropriate information, games/software, and videos to reinforce teaching.
- Proactively address adverse effects when possible, and collaborate with the patient on preferred methods to manage them when they occur.
- Set up networks to connect the child/adolescent with others managing similar illnesses and medication regimens.
- Employ an interprofessional team approach for support and encouragement.

KEY POINTS

- The majority of drugs used in pediatrics have never been tested in children. As a result, we often lack reliable information on which to base drug selection or dosage.
- Because of organ system immaturity, very young patients are highly sensitive to drugs.
- In neonates and young infants, drug responses may be unusually intense and prolonged.
- Absorption of IM drugs in *neonates* is slower than in adults. In contrast, absorption of IM drugs in *infants* is more rapid than in adults.
- Protein-binding capacity is limited early in life, so free concentrations of some drugs may be especially high.
- The blood-brain barrier is not fully developed at birth. Therefore, neonates are especially sensitive to drugs that affect the CNS.
- The drug-metabolizing capacity of neonates is low, so neonates are especially sensitive to drugs that are eliminated primarily by hepatic metabolism.
- Renal excretion of drugs is low in neonates. Thus, drugs that are eliminated primarily by the kidney must be given in reduced dosage and/or at longer dosing intervals.
- In children 1 year of age and older, most pharmacokinetic parameters are similar to those in adults. Hence, drug sensitivity is more like that of adults than the very young.
- Children (1 to 12 years) differ pharmacokinetically from adults in that children metabolize drugs faster.
- Initial pediatric doses are at best an approximation. To ensure optimal dosing, subsequent doses must be adjusted on the basis of clinical outcome and plasma drug levels.

Please visit **http://evolve.elsevier.com/Lehne** for chapter-specific NCLEX® examination review questions.

CHAPTER

11 Drug Therapy in Older Adults

Drug use among older adults (those 65 years and older) is disproportionately high. Whereas older adults constitute only 12.8% of the U.S. population, they consume 33% of the nation's prescribed drugs. Reasons for this intensive use of drugs include increased severity of illness, multiple pathologies, and excessive prescribing.

Drug therapy in older adults represents a special therapeutic challenge. As a rule, older patients are more sensitive to drugs than are younger adults, and they show wider individual variation. In addition, older adults experience more adverse drug reactions and drug-drug interactions. The principal factors underlying these complications are (1) altered pharmacokinetics (secondary to organ system degeneration), (2) multiple and severe illnesses, (3) multidrug therapy, and (4) poor adherence. To help ensure that drug therapy is as safe and effective as possible, *individualization of treatment is essential: Each patient must be monitored for desired and adverse responses, and the regimen must be adjusted accordingly.* Because older adults typically suffer from chronic illnesses, the usual objective is to reduce symptoms and improve quality of life, because cure is generally impossible.

PHARMACOKINETIC CHANGES IN OLDER ADULTS

The aging process can affect all phases of pharmacokinetics. From early adulthood on, there is a gradual, progressive decline in organ function. This decline can alter the absorption, distribution, metabolism, and excretion of drugs. As a rule, these pharmacokinetic changes increase drug sensitivity (largely from reduced hepatic and renal drug elimination). It should be noted, however, that the extent of change varies greatly among patients: Pharmacokinetic changes may be minimal in patients who have remained physically fit, whereas they may be dramatic in patients who have aged less fortunately. Accordingly, you should keep in mind that age-related changes in pharmacokinetics are not only a potential source of increased sensitivity to drugs, they are also a potential source of increased variability. The physiologic changes that underlie alterations in pharmacokinetics are summarized in Table 11.1.

Absorption

Altered GI absorption is not a major factor in drug sensitivity in older adults. As a rule, the *percentage* of an oral dose that becomes absorbed does not usually change with age. However, the *rate* of absorption may be slowed (because of delayed gastric emptying and reduced splanchnic blood flow). As a result, drug responses may be somewhat delayed. Gastric acidity is reduced in older adults and may alter the absorption of certain drugs. For example, some drug formulations require high acidity to dissolve, and hence their absorption may be reduced.

Distribution

Four major factors can alter drug distribution in older adults: (1) increased percentage of body fat, (2) decreased percentage of lean body mass, (3) decreased total body water, and (4) reduced concentration of serum albumin. The increase in body fat seen in older adults provides a storage depot for *lipid-soluble* drugs (e.g., propranolol). As a result, plasma levels of these drugs are reduced, causing a reduction in responses. Because of the decline in lean body mass and total body water, *water-soluble* drugs (e.g., ethanol) become distributed in a smaller volume than in younger adults. As a result, the concentration of these drugs is increased, causing effects to be more intense. Although albumin levels are only slightly reduced in healthy older adults, these levels can be significantly reduced in older adults who are malnourished. Because of reduced albumin levels, sites for protein binding of drugs decrease, causing levels of free drug to rise. Accordingly, drug effects may be more intense.

Metabolism

Rates of hepatic drug metabolism tend to decline with age. Principal reasons are reduced hepatic blood flow, reduced liver mass, and decreased activity of some hepatic enzymes. Because liver function is diminished, the half-lives of certain drugs may be increased, thereby prolonging responses. Responses to oral drugs that ordinarily undergo extensive first-pass metabolism may be enhanced because fewer drugs are inactivated before entering the systemic circulation. Please note, however, that the degree of decline in drug metabolism varies greatly among individuals. As a result, we cannot predict whether drug responses will be significantly reduced in any particular patient.

TABLE 11.1 ■ Physiologic Changes That Can Affect Pharmacokinetics in Older Adults

ABSORPTION OF DRUGS
Increased gastric pH
Decreased absorptive surface area
Decreased splanchnic blood flow
Decreased GI motility
Delayed gastric emptying
DISTRIBUTION OF DRUGS
Increased body fat
Decreased lean body mass
Decreased total body water
Decreased serum albumin
Decreased cardiac output
METABOLISM OF DRUGS
Decreased hepatic blood flow
Decreased hepatic mass
Decreased activity of hepatic enzymes
EXCRETION OF DRUGS
Decreased renal blood flow
Decreased glomerular filtration rate
Decreased tubular secretion
Decreased number of nephrons

Excretion

Renal function, and hence renal drug excretion, undergoes progressive decline beginning in early adulthood. *Drug accumulation secondary to reduced renal excretion is the most important cause of adverse drug reactions in older adults.* The decline in renal function is the result of reductions in renal blood flow, glomerular filtration rate, active tubular secretion, and number of nephrons. Renal pathology can further compromise kidney function. The degree of decline in renal function varies greatly among individuals. Accordingly, when patients are taking drugs that are eliminated primarily by the kidneys, renal function should be assessed. In older adults, the proper index of renal function is *creatinine clearance,* not *serum creatinine levels.* Creatinine levels do not adequately reflect kidney function in older adults because the source of serum creatinine—lean muscle mass—declines in parallel with the decline in kidney function. As a result, creatinine levels may be normal even though renal function is greatly reduced.

PHARMACODYNAMIC CHANGES IN OLDER ADULTS

Alterations in receptor properties may underlie altered sensitivity to some drugs. However, information on such pharmacodynamic changes is limited. In support of the possibility of altered pharmacodynamics is the observation that beta-adrenergic blocking agents (drugs used primarily for cardiac disorders) are *less* effective in older adults than in younger adults, even when present in the same concentrations. Possible explanations for this observation include (1) a reduction in the number of beta receptors and (2) a reduction in the affinity of beta receptors for beta-receptor blocking agents. Other drugs (warfarin, certain central nervous system depressants) produce effects that are more intense in older adults, suggesting a possible increase in receptor number, receptor affinity, or both. Unfortunately, our knowledge of pharmacodynamic changes in older adults is restricted to a few families of drugs.

ADVERSE DRUG REACTIONS AND DRUG INTERACTIONS

Adverse drug reactions (ADRs) are seven times more common in older adults than in younger adults, accounting for about 16% of hospital admissions among older individuals and 50% of all medication-related deaths. The vast majority of these reactions are dose related, not idiosyncratic. Symptoms in older adults are often nonspecific (e.g., dizziness, cognitive impairment), making identification of ADRs difficult. Further, older adults may be less comfortable revealing alcohol or recreational drug use because of generational taboos in some segments of society. This can confound efforts to identify the source of a new ADR-related symptom.

Perhaps surprisingly, the increase in ADRs seen in older adults often is not the direct result of aging per se. Rather, multiple factors predispose older patients to ADRs. The most important are:

- Drug accumulation secondary to reduced renal function
- Polypharmacy (treatment with multiple drugs)
- Greater severity of illness
- The presence of comorbidities
- Use of drugs that have a low therapeutic index (e.g., digoxin, a drug for heart failure)
- Increased individual variation secondary to altered pharmacokinetics
- Inadequate supervision of long-term therapy
- Poor patient adherence

The majority of ADRs in older adults are avoidable. See Table 11.2 for measures that can reduce the incidence of ADRs.

Synthesizing information on disparate drugs that can cause harm has presented a challenge. A few lists have emerged over the years, but perhaps the most well known are the Beers list and START/STOPP criteria.

The *Beers list* identifies drugs with a high likelihood of causing adverse effects in older adults. Accordingly, drugs on this list should generally be avoided for adults over 65 except when a drug's benefits are significantly greater than the risks. A partial listing of these drugs appears in Table 11.3. The full list, updated in 2015, is available online at http://onlinelibrary.wiley.com/doi/10.1111/jgs.13702/pdf.

STOPP stands for Screening Tool of Older Persons' potentially inappropriate Prescriptions. Like the Beers list, STOPP criteria also identify drugs that may be dangerous if prescribed for older adults. It has an advantage of also considering the economic costs of drug therapy. Additionally, when combined with the Screening Tool to Alert doctors to Right Treatment (START), the set can be used to promote selection of appropriate treatment in addition to avoidance of inappropriate treatment. The current version is available at https://www.farmaka.be/frontend/files/publications/files/liste-start-stopp-version.pdf.

TABLE 11.2 ■ Measures to Reduce Adverse Drug Reactions in Older Adults

PROVIDER MEASURES

- Account for age-associated pharmacokinetic and pharmacodynamic alterations when making prescribing decisions.
- Initiate therapy at low doses ("Start low and go slow").
- Whenever possible, select drugs with a high therapeutic index.
- Use the *Screening Tool to Alert doctors to Right Treatment* (START) to guide appropriate treatment on older adults.
- Avoid prescribing drugs included in *Beers Criteria for Potentially Inappropriate Medication Use in Older Adults* (the Beers list) or in the *Screening Tool of Older People's potentially inappropriate Prescriptions* (STOPP).
- Before prescribing a new drug, check for interactions with current drugs the patient is taking.
- Use individual patient responses and laboratory studies to guide dosage adjustment.
- Do not increase a drug dosage due to inadequate response (e.g., continued high blood pressure) or subtherapeutic serum level without first verifying that the patient is taking the drug exactly as prescribed.
- Employ the simplest medication regimen possible.
- Monitor the need for continued therapy; discontinue medications when no longer necessary for care management.
- Before prescribing a drug for a new symptom or illness, always consider whether the symptom or illness could be iatrogenic due to drug therapy. The best treatment may be to discontinue a drug that is currently prescribed.

NURSE MEASURES

- Take a complete drug history at each new encounter (i.e., clinic visit, hospital admission, transfers to other units or facilities). Include not only what medications are prescribed, but also how the patient actually takes the medication to determine whether this matches what is prescribed.
- Check all drugs taken for drug interactions and common components (e.g., acetaminophen over-the-counter and acetaminophen with codeine prescribed) and report significant interactions or duplications to the prescriber.
- Use STOPP criteria or the Beers list to identify potentially inappropriate drugs.
- Monitor clinical responses and drugs and laboratory studies to identify potential ADRs early.
- Accommodate for age-related sensory issues, such as decreased vision or hearing, when providing patient education. Include a family member or significant other for patients with cognitive deficits.
- Encourage patients to dispose of all old drugs.

PROMOTING ADHERENCE

Between 26% and 59% of older adult patients fail to take their medicines as prescribed. Some patients never fill their prescriptions, some fail to refill their prescriptions, and some don't follow the prescribed dosing schedule. Nonadherence can result in therapeutic failure (from underdosing or erratic dosing) or toxicity (from overdosing). Of the two possibilities, underdosing with resulting therapeutic failure is by far (90%) the more common. Problems arising from nonadherence account for up to 10% of all hospital admissions, and their management may cost over $100 billion a year.

Multiple factors underlie nonadherence to the prescribed regimen (Table 11.4). Among these are forgetfulness; failure to comprehend instructions (because of intellectual, visual, or auditory impairment); inability to pay for medications; and use of complex regimens (several drugs taken several times a day). All of these factors can contribute to *unintentional* nonadherence. However, in the majority of cases (about 75%), nonadherence among older adults is *intentional.* The principal reason given for intentional nonadherence is the patient's conviction that the drug was simply not needed in the dosage prescribed. Unpleasant side effects and expense also contribute to intentional nonadherence.

Several measures can promote adherence, including:

- Simplifying the regimen so that the number of drugs and doses per day is as small as possible
- Explaining the treatment plan using clear, concise verbal and written instructions
- Choosing an appropriate dosage form (e.g., a liquid formulation if the patient has difficulty swallowing)
- Requesting that the pharmacist label drug containers using a large print size, and provide containers that are easy to open by patients with impaired dexterity (e.g., those with arthritis)
- Suggesting the use of a calendar, diary, or pill counter to record drug administration
- Asking the patient whether he or she has access to a pharmacy and can afford the medication
- Enlisting the aid of a friend, relative, or visiting healthcare professional
- Monitoring for therapeutic responses, adverse reactions, and plasma drug levels

It must be noted, however, that the benefits of these measures will be restricted primarily to patients whose nonadherence is *unintentional.* Unfortunately, these measures are generally inapplicable to the patient whose nonadherence is *intentional.* For these patients, intensive education may help.

CONSIDERATIONS FOR END-OF-LIFE CARE

End-of-life care poses a set of different concerns regarding the choice of drugs to best meet the needs of older patients. Priority treatment varies as goals shift from disease prevention and management to provision of comfort measures. Drugs that were once considered important in care (e.g., drugs for cholesterol management) may no longer be relevant and can be discontinued. Drugs that were once considered inappropriate due to patient age (e.g., sedatives) may need to become a predominant feature of care. Table 11.5 explores medication considerations and choices for the concerns that patients sometimes encounter near the end of life. Additional information is available at https://www.cancer.gov/about-cancer/advanced-cancer/caregivers/planning/last-days-hp-pdq#section/_7. The Institute of Medicine's report *Dying in America: Improving Quality and Honoring Individual Preferences Near the End of Life* addresses multiple concerns of dying patients and their families and is available at http://www.nap.edu/read/18748/chapter/1.

TABLE 11.3 ■ Some Drugs to Generally Avoid in Older Adults

Drug	Reason for Concern	Alternative Treatments
ANALGESICS		
Indomethacin [Indocin] Ketorolac [Toradol] Non–COX-2 selective NSAIDs (e.g., ibuprofen, aspirin >325 mg/day)	Risk of GI bleeding, especially with long-term use; some may contribute to heart failure Indomethacin is more prone to affect the CNS than other NSAIDs	Mild pain: acetaminophen, codeine, COX-2–selective inhibitors if no heart failure risk, *short-term* use of *low-dose* NSAIDs
Meperidine [Demerol]	Not effective at usual doses, risk of neurotoxicity, confusion, delirium	Moderate to severe pain: morphine, oxycodone, hydrocodone
TRICYCLIC ANTIDEPRESSANTS, FIRST GENERATION		
Amitriptyline Clomipramine [Anafranil] Doxepin (>6 mg/day) Imipramine [Tofranil]	Anticholinergic effects (constipation, urinary retention, blurred vision), risk of cognitive impairment, delirium, syncope	SSRIs with shorter half-life, SNRIs, or other antidepressants
ANTIHISTAMINES, FIRST GENERATION		
Chlorpheniramine [Chlor-Trimeton 🍁, Teldrin] Diphenhydramine [Benadryl] Hydroxyzine [Vistaril, Atarax 🍁] Promethazine [Phenergan]	Anticholinergic effects: constipation, urinary retention, blurred vision	Second-generation antihistamines, such as cetirizine [Zyrtec], fexofenadine [Allegra], or loratadine [Claritin]
ANTIHYPERTENSIVES, ALPHA-ADRENERGIC AGENTS		
Alpha$_1$ blockers (e.g., doxazosin [Cardura], prazosin [Minipress], terazosin [Hytrin])	High risk of orthostatic hypotension and falls; less dangerous drugs are available	Thiazide diuretic, ACE inhibitor, beta-adrenergic blocker, calcium channel blocker
Centrally acting alpha$_2$ agonists (e.g., clonidine [Catapres], methyldopa)	Risk of bradycardia, orthostatic hypotension, adverse CNS effects, depression, sedation	
SEDATIVE-HYPNOTICS		
Barbiturates	Physical dependence; compared with other hypnotics, higher risk of falls, confusion, cognitive impairment	Short-term zolpidem [Ambien], zaleplon [Sonata], or eszopiclone [Lunesta] Low-dose ramelteon [Rozerem] or doxepin Nonpharmacologic interventions (e.g., cognitive behavioral therapy)
Benzodiazepines, both short acting (e.g., alprazolam [Xanax], lorazepam [Ativan]) and long acting (e.g., chlordiazepoxide [Librium], diazepam [Valium])	Sedation, cognitive impairment, risk of falls, delirium risk	Low-dose ramelteon [Rozerem] or doxepin Nonpharmacologic interventions (e.g., cognitive behavioral therapy)
DRUGS FOR URGE INCONTINENCE		
Oxybutynin [Ditropan] Tolterodine [Detrol]	Anticholinergic effects, urinary retention, cognitive impairment, sedation	Behavioral therapy (e.g., bladder retraining, urge suppression)
MUSCLE RELAXANTS		
Carisoprodol [Soma] Cyclobenzaprine Metaxalone [Skelaxin] Methocarbamol [Robaxin]	Anticholinergic effects, sedation, cognitive impairment; may not be effective at tolerable dosage	Antispasmodics, such as baclofen [Lioresal] Nonpharmacologic interventions (e.g., exercises, proper body mechanics)
PROTON PUMP INHIBITORS		
Esomeprazole [Nexium] Lansoprazole [Prevacid] Omeprazole [Prilosec]	Increased risk of *C. difficile* infection, decreased bone integrity, and fractures	H_2 receptor antagonists (e.g., famotidine [Pepcid], ranitidine [Zantac]) Nonpharmacologic interventions (e.g., deleting foods that increase gastric acidity such as high-fat foods and deleting substances that lower esophageal sphincter pressure such as alcohol)

ACE, Angiotensin-converting enzyme; *CNS,* central nervous system; *COX-2,* cyclooxygenase-2; *GI,* gastrointestinal; *NSAIDs,* nonsteroidal anti-inflammatory drugs; *SNRI,* serotonin/norepinephrine reuptake inhibitor; *SSRI,* selective serotonin reuptake inhibitor.
Adapted from American Geriatrics Society 2015 updated Beers criteria for potentially inappropriate medication use in older adults, *J Am Geriatr Soc* 63:2227–2246, 2015. (*Note:* The original document lists many drugs in addition to those in this table.)

TABLE 11.4 ▪ Factors That Increase the Risk of Poor Adherence in Older Adults

- Multiple chronic disorders
- Multiple prescription medications
- Multiple doses per day for each medication
- Drug packaging that is difficult to open
- Multiple prescribers
- Changes in the regimen (addition of drugs, changes in dosage size or timing)
- Cognitive or physical impairment (reduction in memory, hearing, visual acuity, color discrimination, or manual dexterity)
- Living alone
- Recent discharge from hospital
- Low literacy
- Inability to pay for drugs
- Personal conviction that a drug is unnecessary or the dosage too high
- Presence of side effects

TABLE 11.5 ▪ Pharmacologic Considerations for End-of-Life Care

Problems	Considerations	Drug Choice
Constipation	Constipation may be opioid-induced; an order for opioids should be accompanied by an order to treat constipation. Stimulants typically cause some degree of abdominal cramping. Drugs specifically formulated for opioid-induced constipation (i.e., methylnaltrexone) are very expensive and may not be warranted if other interventions are effective. Increased fiber may cause constipation if there is insufficient fluid intake.	First-line choices are osmotic laxatives (e.g., lactulose, polyethylene glycol). Stimulants with stool softener (e.g., senna with docusate) are second-line if abdominal cramping is a concern; otherwise, they may be given as a first-line choice. For those who cannot swallow, bisacodyl rectal suppositories or enemas can provide relief. Methylnaltrexone may be used for refractory opioid-induced constipation.
Delirium	Delirium may be a manifestation of pain. Delirium may be a manifestation of opioid-induced neurotoxicity. Benzodiazepines may cause a paradoxical agitation but may be helpful if delirium is related to alcohol withdrawal or as an *adjunct* to antipsychotics. Underlying causes (constipation, urinary retention, infection) should be treated, if identified.	Treat with antipsychotics such as haloperidol or olanzapine. Benzodiazepines such as midazolam may be helpful short term to supplement antipsychotics for acute episodes of delirium. Consider adding analgesics (or evaluate adequacy of currently prescribed analgesics). For patients taking opioids (e.g., morphine), changing to a different opioid (e.g., fentanyl) has been helpful.
Dyspnea	Dyspnea may or may not be associated with hypoxemia. Management should consider severity of associated manifestations (e.g., profound fatigue exacerbated by respiratory effort). Bronchodilators may increase anxiety, which can further worsen sensation of shortness of breath.	Oxygen therapy is indicated if hypoxemia is present. Opioids are a first-line drug choice. Glucocorticoids are often helpful, if not contraindicated. Consider bronchodilators only if dyspnea is associated with bronchospasm.
Fatigue	Dexamphetamine has only short-term benefit due to tolerance; one study showed benefit did not extend past 8 days.	Methylphenidate has demonstrated improvement in some studies.
Nausea and Vomiting	Management should be tailored to the underlying cause.	Chemotherapy or radiation-induced N/V: 5-HT_3 receptor antagonists (e.g., ondansetron) or neurokinin$_1$ receptor antagonist (e.g., aprepitant) or glucocorticoid (e.g., dexamethasone). Metoclopramide is recommended first line for N/V due to gastroparesis, liver failure, and unknown causes. Haloperidol, a dopamine receptor antagonist, is often effective in relieving N/V of unknown causes and is first line for N/V due to bowel obstruction and renal failure. Glucocorticoids may be helpful in treating N/V secondary to brain tumors and bowel obstructions. For N/V of unknown cause, metoclopramide may be supplemented with 5-HT_3-receptor antagonists or dopamine receptor antagonists.

TABLE 11.5 ▪ Pharmacologic Considerations for End-of-Life Care—cont'd

Problems	Considerations	Drug Choice
Pain	Pain associated with conditions such as cancer is often intractable. Concerns about addiction are generally irrelevant at this stage of life, so highly addictive drugs may be employed. Opioids undergo hepatic metabolism and most undergo renal excretion. As organ failure occurs, opioids may accumulate to toxic levels. TCAs have adverse effects and drug-drug interactions that create complications when used for neuropathic pain.	Fentanyl is the drug of choice for severe pain in patients with renal and/or hepatic dysfunction. Methadone is a drug of choice for patients with renal dysfunction but without hepatic dysfunction. Schedule medication around-the-clock rather than PRN. Gabapentin or pregabalin is recommended for management of neuropathic pain. SSRIs and SNRIs may also be helpful.
Respiratory Secretions "Death Rattle"	Accumulation of secretions in the airway occurs as the patient nears death (within 2 weeks or less) and ineffective cough progresses to loss of cough reflex and pooling of secretions. Suctioning may be inadequate to relieve this problem. Expert opinion is divided regarding whether treatment is warranted. Many believe that the death rattle does not cause patient distress, but it is upsetting to families.	If drug therapy is desired, anticholinergics are often effective in decreasing secretions. Glycopyrrolate is the anticholinergic of choice due to decreased CNS adverse effects. Some studies have indicated that hyoscyamine is a good choice for this purpose.

CNS, Central nervous system; *N/V*, nausea and vomiting; *PRN*, as needed; *SSRI*, selective serotonin reuptake inhibitor; *SNRI*, serotonin-norepinephrine reuptake inhibitor; *TCA*, tricyclic antidepressants.

KEY POINTS

- Older patients are generally more sensitive to drugs than are younger adults, and they show wider individual variation.
- Individualization of therapy for older adults is essential. Each patient must be monitored for desired and adverse responses, and the regimen must be adjusted accordingly.
- Aging-related organ decline can change drug absorption, distribution, metabolism, and (especially) excretion.
- The *rate* of drug absorption may be slowed in older adults, although the *extent* of absorption is usually unchanged.
- Plasma concentrations of lipid-soluble drugs may be low in older adults, and concentrations of water-soluble drugs may be high.
- Reduced liver function may prolong drug effects.
- Reduced renal function, with resultant drug accumulation, is the most important cause of adverse drug reactions in older adults.
- Because the degree of renal impairment among older adults varies, creatinine clearance (a measure of renal function) should be determined for all patients taking drugs that are eliminated primarily by the kidneys.
- Adverse drug reactions are much more common in older adults than in younger adults.
- Factors underlying the increase in adverse reactions include polypharmacy, severe illness, comorbidities, and treatment with dangerous drugs.
- Tools such as the Beers list or START and STOPP criteria can be used to identify potentially inappropriate drug choices for elderly patients.
- Nonadherence is common among older adults.
- Reasons for *unintentional* nonadherence include complex regimens, awkward drug packaging, forgetfulness, side effects, low income, and failure to comprehend instructions.
- Most cases (75%) of nonadherence among older adults are *intentional*. Reasons include expense, side effects, and the patient's conviction that the drug is unnecessary or the dosage too high.
- Priority treatment varies as goals shift from disease prevention and management to provision of comfort measures.

Please visit **http://evolve.elsevier.com/Lehne** for chapter-specific NCLEX® examination review questions.

UNIT IV PERIPHERAL NERVOUS SYSTEM DRUGS

CHAPTER 12

Basic Principles of Neuropharmacology

Neuropharmacology can be defined as *the study of drugs that alter processes controlled by the nervous system.* Neuropharmacologic drugs produce effects equivalent to those produced by excitation or suppression of neuronal activity. Neuropharmacologic agents can be divided into two broad categories: (1) peripheral nervous system (PNS) drugs and (2) central nervous system (CNS) drugs.

The neuropharmacologic drugs constitute a large and important family of therapeutic agents. These drugs are used to treat conditions ranging from depression to epilepsy to hypertension to asthma. The clinical significance of these agents is reflected in the fact that over 25% of this text is dedicated to them.

Why do we have so many neuropharmacologic drugs? Because the nervous system participates in the regulation of practically all bodily processes, practically all bodily processes can be influenced by drugs that alter neuronal regulation. By mimicking or blocking neuronal regulation, neuropharmacologic drugs can modify such diverse processes as skeletal muscle contraction, cardiac output, vascular tone, respiration, GI function, uterine motility, glandular secretion, and functions unique to the CNS, such as ideation, mood, and perception of pain. Given the broad spectrum of processes that neuropharmacologic drugs can alter, and given the potential benefits to be gained by manipulating those processes, it should be no surprise that neuropharmacologic drugs have widespread clinical applications.

We begin our study of neuropharmacology by discussing PNS drugs (Chapters 14 through 19), after which we discuss CNS drugs (Chapters 20 through 36). The principal rationale for this order of presentation is that our understanding of PNS pharmacology is much clearer than our understanding of CNS pharmacology. Why? Because the PNS is less complex than the CNS, and more accessible to experimentation. By placing our initial focus on the PNS, we can establish a firm knowledge base in neuropharmacology before proceeding to the less definitive and vastly more complex realm of CNS pharmacology.

HOW NEURONS REGULATE PHYSIOLOGIC PROCESSES

As a rule, if we want to understand the effects of a drug on a particular physiologic process, we must first understand the process itself. Accordingly, if we wish to understand the impact of drugs on neuronal regulation of bodily function, we must first understand how neurons regulate bodily function when drugs are absent.

Fig. 12.1 illustrates the basic process by which neurons elicit responses from other cells. The figure depicts two cells: a neuron and a postsynaptic cell. The postsynaptic cell might be another neuron, a muscle cell, or a cell within a secretory gland. As indicated, there are two basic steps—*axonal conduction* and *synaptic transmission*—in the process by which the neuron influences the behavior of the postsynaptic cell. Axonal conduction is simply the process of conducting an action potential down the axon of the neuron. Synaptic transmission is the process by which information is carried across the gap between the neuron and the postsynaptic cell. As shown in the figure, synaptic transmission requires the release of neurotransmitter molecules from the axon terminal followed by binding of these molecules to receptors on the postsynaptic cell. As a result of transmitter-receptor binding, a series of events is initiated in the postsynaptic cell, leading to a change in its behavior. The precise nature of the change depends on the identity of the neurotransmitter and the type of cell involved. If the postsynaptic cell is another neuron, it may increase or decrease its firing rate; if the cell is part of a muscle, it may contract or relax; and if the cell is glandular, it may increase or decrease secretion.

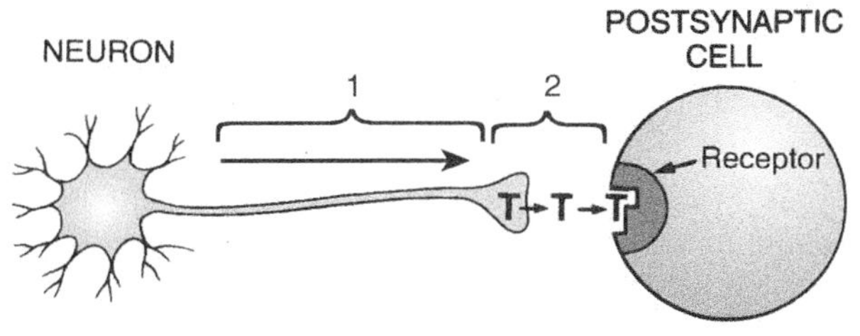

Fig. 12.1 ■ How neurons regulate other cells.
There are two basic steps in the process by which neurons elicit responses from other cells: (1) axonal conduction and (2) synaptic transmission. (*T*, Neurotransmitter.)

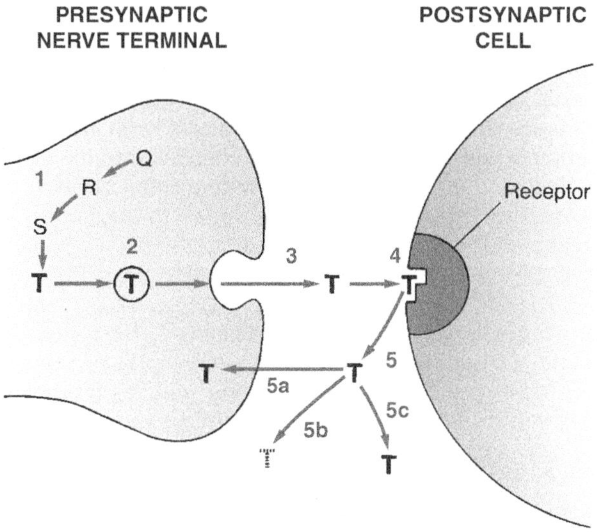

Fig. 12.2 ■ Steps in synaptic transmission.
Step 1, Synthesis of transmitter (T) from precursor molecules (Q, R, and S). *Step 2,* Storage of transmitter in vesicles. *Step 3,* Release of transmitter: In response to an action potential, vesicles fuse with the terminal membrane and discharge their contents into the synaptic gap. *Step 4,* Action at receptor: Transmitter binds (reversibly) to its receptor on the postsynaptic cell, causing a response in that cell. *Step 5,* Termination of transmission: Transmitter dissociates from its receptor and is then removed from the synaptic gap by (*a*) reuptake into the nerve terminal, (*b*) enzymatic degradation, or (*c*) diffusion away from the gap.

BASIC MECHANISMS BY WHICH NEUROPHARMACOLOGIC AGENTS ACT

Sites of Action: Axons Versus Synapses

To influence a process under neuronal control, a drug can alter one of two basic neuronal activities: axonal conduction or synaptic transmission. *Most neuropharmacologic agents act by altering synaptic transmission.* Only a few alter axonal conduction. This is to our advantage because drugs that alter synaptic transmission can produce effects that are much more *selective* than those produced by drugs that alter axonal conduction.

Axonal Conduction

Drugs that act by altering axonal conduction are not very selective. Recall that the process of conducting an impulse along an axon is essentially the same in all neurons. As a consequence, a drug that alters axonal conduction will affect conduction in all nerves to which it has access. Such a drug cannot produce selective effects.

Local anesthetics are drugs that work by altering (decreasing) axonal conduction. Because these agents produce nonselective inhibition of axonal conduction, they suppress transmission in any nerve they reach. Hence, although local anesthetics are certainly valuable, their indications are limited.

Synaptic Transmission

In contrast to drugs that alter axonal conduction, drugs that alter synaptic transmission can produce effects that are highly selective. This selectivity can occur because synapses, unlike axons, differ from one another. Synapses at different sites employ different transmitters. In addition, for most transmitters, the body employs more than one type of receptor. Hence, by using a drug that selectively influences a specific type of neurotransmitter or receptor, we can alter one neuronally regulated process while leaving most others unchanged. Because of their relative selectivity, drugs that alter synaptic transmission have many uses.

Receptors

The ability of a neuron to influence the behavior of another cell depends, ultimately, upon the ability of that neuron to alter receptor activity on the target cell. As discussed, neurons alter receptor activity by releasing transmitter molecules, which diffuse across the synaptic gap and bind to receptors on the postsynaptic cell. If the target cell lacked receptors for the transmitter that a neuron released, that neuron would be unable to affect the target cell.

The effects of neuropharmacologic drugs, like those of neurons, depend on altering receptor activity. That is, no matter what its precise mechanism of action, a neuropharmacologic drug ultimately works by influencing receptor activity on target cells. This commonsense concept is central to understanding the actions of neuropharmacologic drugs. In fact, this concept is so critical to our understanding of neuropharmacologic agents that I will repeat it: *The impact of a drug on a neuronally regulated process is dependent on the ability of that drug to directly or indirectly influence receptor activity on target cells.*

Steps in Synaptic Transmission

To understand how drugs alter receptor activity, we must first understand the steps by which synaptic transmission takes place—because it is by modifying these steps that neuropharmacologic drugs influence receptor function. The steps in synaptic transmission are shown in Fig. 12.2.

Step 1: Transmitter Synthesis

For synaptic transmission to take place, molecules of transmitter must be present in the nerve terminal. Hence, we can look upon transmitter synthesis as the first step in transmission. In the figure, the letters Q, R, and S represent the precursor molecules from which the transmitter (T) is made.

Step 2: Transmitter Storage

Once transmitter is synthesized, it must be stored until the time of its release. Transmitter storage takes place within vesicles—tiny packets present in the axon terminal. Each nerve terminal contains a large number of transmitter-filled vesicles.

Step 3: Transmitter Release

Release of transmitter is triggered by the arrival of an action potential at the axon terminal. The action potential initiates a process in which vesicles undergo fusion with the terminal membrane, causing release of their contents into the synaptic gap. Each action potential causes only a small fraction of all vesicles present in the axon terminal to discharge their contents.

Step 4: Receptor Binding

Following release, transmitter molecules diffuse across the synaptic gap and then undergo *reversible* binding to receptors on the postsynaptic cell. This binding initiates a cascade of events that result in altered behavior of the postsynaptic cell.

Step 5: Termination of Transmission

Transmission is terminated by dissociation of transmitter from its receptors, followed by removal of free transmitter from the synaptic gap. Transmitter can be removed from the synaptic gap by three processes: (1) reuptake, (2) enzymatic degradation, and (3) diffusion. In those synapses where transmission is terminated by reuptake, axon terminals contain "pumps" that transport transmitter molecules back into the neuron from which they were released (Step 5a in Fig. 12.2). Following reuptake, molecules of transmitter may be degraded, or they may be packaged in vesicles for reuse. In synapses where transmitter is cleared by enzymatic degradation (Step 5b), the synapse contains large quantities of transmitter-inactivating enzymes. Although simple diffusion away from the synaptic gap (Step 5c) is a potential means of terminating transmitter action, this process is very slow and generally of little significance.

Effects of Drugs on the Steps of Synaptic Transmission

As emphatically noted, all neuropharmacologic agents (except local anesthetics) produce their effects by directly or indirectly altering receptor activity. We also noted that the way in which drugs alter receptor activity is by interfering with synaptic transmission. Because synaptic transmission has multiple steps, the process offers a number of potential targets for drugs. In this section, we examine the specific ways in which drugs can alter the steps of synaptic transmission.

Before discussing specific mechanisms by which drugs can alter receptor activity, we need to understand what drugs are capable of doing to receptors in general terms. From the broadest perspective, when a drug influences receptor function, that drug can do just one of two things: it can enhance receptor activation, or it can reduce receptor activation. What do we mean by receptor activation? For our purposes, we can define *activation* as *an effect on receptor function equivalent to that produced by the natural neurotransmitter at a particular synapse*. Hence, a drug whose effects mimic the effects of a natural transmitter would be said to *increase* receptor activation. Conversely, a drug whose effects were equivalent to reducing the amount of natural transmitter available for receptor binding would be said to *decrease* receptor activation.

Please note that activation of a receptor does not necessarily mean that a physiologic process will go faster; receptor activation can also make a process go slower. For example, the heart rate will decline when the endogenous neurotransmitter acetylcholine activates cholinergic receptors on the heart; therefore, a drug that mimics acetylcholine at receptors on the heart will cause the heart to beat more slowly.

TABLE 12.1 ■ Effects of Drugs on Synaptic Transmission and the Resulting Impact on Receptor Activation

Step of Synaptic Transmission	Drug Action	Impact on Receptor Activation[a]
1. Synthesis of transmitter	Increased synthesis of T	Increase
	Decreased synthesis of T	Decrease
	Synthesis of "super" T	Increase
2. Storage of transmitter	Reduced storage of T	Decrease
3. Release of transmitter	Promotion of T release	Increase
	Inhibition of T release	Decrease
4. Binding to receptor	Direct receptor activation	Increase
	Enhanced response to T	Increase
	Blockade of T binding	Decrease
5. Termination of transmission	Blockade of T reuptake	Increase
	Inhibition of T breakdown	Increase

[a]Receptor activation is defined as producing an effect equivalent to that produced by the natural transmitter that acts on a particular receptor.
T, Transmitter.

Having defined receptor activation, we are ready to discuss the mechanisms by which drugs, acting on specific steps of synaptic transmission, can increase or decrease receptor activity (Table 12.1). As we consider these mechanisms one by one, their logical associations should become apparent.

Transmitter Synthesis

There are three different effects that drugs are known to have on transmitter synthesis. They can (1) increase transmitter synthesis, (2) decrease transmitter synthesis, or (3) cause the synthesis of transmitter molecules that are more effective than the natural transmitter itself.

Increased or decreased transmitter synthesis affects receptor activity. A drug that increases transmitter synthesis will cause receptor activation to increase. The process is this: As a result of increased transmitter synthesis, storage vesicles will contain transmitter in abnormally high amounts. Hence, when an action potential reaches the axon terminal, more transmitter will be released, and therefore more transmitter will be available to receptors on the postsynaptic cell, causing activation of those receptors to increase. Conversely, a drug that decreases transmitter synthesis will cause the transmitter content of vesicles to decline, resulting in reduced transmitter release and decreased receptor activation.

Some drugs can cause neurons to synthesize transmitter molecules whose structure is different from that of normal transmitter molecules. For example, by acting as substrates for enzymes in the axon terminal, drugs can be converted into "super" transmitters (molecules whose ability to activate receptors is greater than that of the naturally occurring transmitter at a particular site). Release of these supertransmitters will cause receptor activation to increase.

Transmitter Storage

Drugs that interfere with transmitter storage will cause receptor activation to decrease. This occurs because disruption of storage depletes vesicles of their transmitter content, thereby decreasing the amount of transmitter available for release.

Transmitter Release

Drugs can either *promote* or *inhibit* transmitter release. Drugs that promote release will increase receptor activation. Conversely, drugs that inhibit release will reduce receptor activation. The amphetamines (CNS stimulants) represent drugs that act by promoting transmitter release. Botulinum toxin, in contrast, acts by inhibiting transmitter release.

Receptor Binding

Many drugs act directly at receptors. These agents can either (1) bind to receptors and cause activation, (2) bind to receptors and thereby block receptor activation by other agents, or (3) bind to receptor components and thereby enhance receptor activation by the natural transmitter at the site.

In the terminology introduced in Chapter 5, drugs that directly activate receptors are called *agonists,* whereas drugs that prevent receptor activation are called *antagonists.* The direct-acting receptor agonists and antagonists constitute the largest and most important groups of neuropharmacologic drugs. (There is no single name or category for drugs that bind to receptors to enhance natural transmitter effects.)

Examples of drugs that act directly at receptors are numerous. Drugs that bind to receptors and cause *activation* include morphine (used for its effects on the CNS), epinephrine (used mainly for its effects on the cardiovascular system), and insulin (used for its effects in diabetes). Drugs that bind to and block receptors to *prevent* their activation include naloxone (used to treat overdose with morphine-like drugs), antihistamines (used to treat allergic disorders), and propranolol (used to treat hypertension, angina pectoris, and cardiac dysrhythmias). Benzodiazepines are the principal example of drugs that bind to receptors and thereby enhance the actions of a natural transmitter. Drugs in this family, which includes diazepam [Valium] and related agents, are used to treat anxiety, seizure disorders, and muscle spasm.

Termination of Transmitter Action

Drugs can interfere with the termination of transmitter action by two mechanisms: (1) blockade of transmitter reuptake and (2) inhibition of transmitter degradation. Drugs that act by either mechanism will increase transmitter availability, thereby causing receptor activation to increase.

MULTIPLE RECEPTOR TYPES AND SELECTIVITY OF DRUG ACTION

As we discussed in Chapter 1, selectivity is one of the most desirable qualities a drug can have. A selective drug is able to alter a specific disease process while leaving other physiologic processes largely unaffected.

Many neuropharmacologic agents display a high degree of selectivity. This selectivity is possible because the nervous system works through multiple types of receptors to regulate processes under its control. If neurons had only one or two types of receptors through which to act, selective effects by neuropharmacologic drugs could not be achieved.

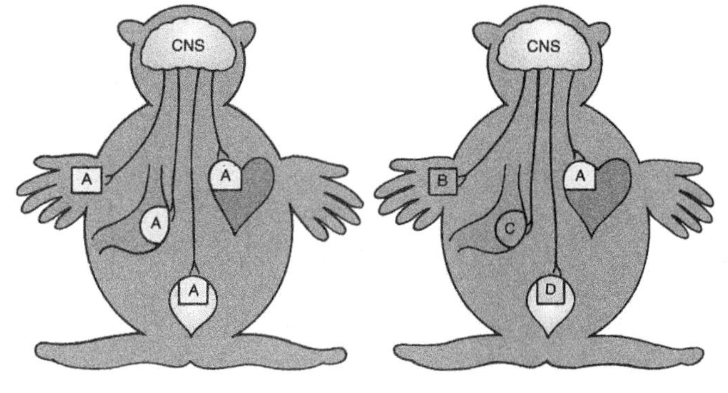

Fig. 12.3 ▪ Multiple drug receptors and selective drug action. All of **Mort's** organs are regulated through activation of type A receptors. Drugs that affect type A receptors on one organ will affect type A receptors on all other organs. Hence, selective drug action is impossible. **Merv** has four types of receptors (A, B, C, and D) to regulate his four organs. A drug that acts at one type of receptor will not affect the others. Hence, selective drug action is possible.

The relationship between multiple receptor types and selective drug action is illustrated by Mort and Merv, whose unique physiologies are depicted in Fig. 12.3. Let's begin with Mort. Mort can perform four functions: he can pump blood, digest food, shake hands, and empty his bladder. All four functions are under neuronal control, and, in all cases, that control is exerted by activation of the same type of receptor (designated A).

As long as Mort remains healthy, having only one type of receptor to regulate his various functions is no problem. Selective *physiologic* regulation can be achieved simply by sending impulses down the appropriate nerves. When there is a need to increase cardiac output, impulses are sent down the nerve to his heart; when digestion is needed, impulses are sent down the nerve to his stomach; and so forth.

Although having only one receptor type is no disadvantage when all is well, if Mort gets sick, having only one receptor type creates a therapeutic challenge. Let's assume he develops heart disease and we need to give a drug that will help increase cardiac output. To stimulate cardiac function, we need to administer a drug that will activate receptors on his heart. Unfortunately, since the receptors on his heart are the same as the receptors on his other organs, a drug that stimulates cardiac function will stimulate his other organs too. Consequently, any attempt to improve cardiac output with drugs will necessarily be accompanied by side effects. These will range from silly (compulsive handshaking) to embarrassing (enuresis) to hazardous (gastric ulcers). Please note that all of these undesirable effects are the direct result of Mort having a nervous system that works through just one type of receptor to regulate all organs. That is, the presence of only one receptor type has made selective drug action impossible.

Now let's consider Merv. Although Merv appears to be Mort's twin, Merv differs in one important way: Whereas all functions in Mort are regulated through just one type of receptor, Merv employs different receptors to control each of his four functions. Because of this simple but important difference, the selective drug action that was impossible with Mort can be achieved easily with Merv. We can, for example, selectively enhance cardiac function in Merv without risking the side effects to which Mort was predisposed. This can be done simply by administering an agonist agent that binds selectively to receptors on the heart (type A receptors). If this medication is sufficiently selective for type A receptors, it will not interact with receptor type B, C, or D. Hence, function in structures regulated by those receptors will be unaffected. Note that our ability to produce selective drug action in Merv is made possible because his nervous system works through different types of receptors to regulate function in his various organs. The message from this example is clear: *The more types of receptors we have to work with, the greater our chances of producing selective drug effects.*

AN APPROACH TO LEARNING ABOUT PERIPHERAL NERVOUS SYSTEM DRUGS

As discussed, to understand the ways in which drugs can alter a process under neuronal control, we must first understand how the nervous system itself regulates that process. Accordingly, when preparing to study PNS pharmacology, you must first establish a working knowledge of the PNS itself. In particular, you need to know two basic types of information about PNS function. First, you need to know the types of receptors through which the PNS works when influencing the function of a specific organ. Second, you need to know what the normal response to activation of those receptors is. All of the information you need about PNS function is reviewed in Chapter 13.

Once you understand the PNS itself, you can go on to learn about PNS drugs. To understand any particular PNS drug, you need three types of information: (1) the type (or types) of receptor through which the drug acts; (2) the normal response to activation of those receptors; and (3) what the drug in question does to receptor function (i.e., does it increase or decrease receptor activation). Armed with these three types of information, you can predict the major effects of any PNS drug.

An example will illustrate this process. Let's consider the drug *isoproterenol.* The first information we need is the identity of the receptors at which isoproterenol acts. Isoproterenol acts at two types of receptors, named $beta_1$ and $beta_2$ adrenergic receptors. Next, we need to know the normal responses to activation of these receptors. The most prominent responses to activation of $beta_1$ receptors are *increased heart rate* and *increased force of cardiac contraction.* The primary responses to activation of $beta_2$ receptors are *bronchial dilation* and *elevation of blood glucose levels.* Finally, we need to know whether isoproterenol increases or decreases the activation of $beta_1$ and $beta_2$ receptors. At both types of receptor, isoproterenol causes *activation.* Armed with these three primary pieces of information about isoproterenol, we can now predict the principal effects of this drug. By *activating* $beta_1$ and $beta_2$ receptors, isoproterenol can elicit three major responses: (1) increased cardiac output (by increasing heart rate and force of contraction); (2) dilation of the bronchi; and (3) elevation of blood glucose. Depending on the patient to whom this drug is given, these responses may be beneficial or detrimental.

From this example, you can see how easy it is to predict the effects of a PNS drug. Accordingly, I strongly encourage you to take the approach suggested when studying these agents. That is, for each PNS drug, you should learn (1) the identity of the receptors at which that drug acts, (2) the normal responses to activation of those receptors, and (3) whether the drug increases or decreases receptor activation.

KEY POINTS

- Except for local anesthetics, which suppress axonal conduction, all neuropharmacologic drugs act by altering synaptic transmission.
- Synaptic transmission consists of five basic steps: transmitter synthesis, transmitter storage, transmitter release, binding of transmitter to its receptors, and termination of transmitter action by dissociation of transmitter from the receptor followed by transmitter reuptake or degradation.
- Ultimately, the impact of a drug on a neuronally regulated process depends on that drug's ability to directly or indirectly alter receptor activity on target cells.
- Drugs can do one of two things to receptor function: they can increase receptor activation or they can decrease receptor activation.
- Drugs that increase transmitter synthesis increase receptor activation.
- Drugs that decrease transmitter synthesis decrease receptor activation.
- Drugs that promote synthesis of "super" transmitters increase receptor activation.
- Drugs that impede transmitter storage decrease receptor activation.
- Drugs that promote transmitter release increase receptor activation.
- Drugs that suppress transmitter release decrease receptor activation.
- Agonist drugs increase receptor activation.
- Antagonist drugs decrease receptor activation.
- Drugs that bind to receptors and enhance the actions of the natural transmitter at the receptor increase receptor activation.
- Drugs that block transmitter reuptake increase receptor activation.
- Drugs that inhibit transmitter degradation increase receptor activation.
- The presence of multiple receptor types increases our ability to produce selective drug effects.
- For each PNS drug that you study, you should learn the identity of the receptors at which the drug acts, the normal responses to activation of those receptors, and whether the drug increases or decreases receptor activation.

Please visit **http://evolve.elsevier.com/Lehne** for chapter-specific NCLEX® examination review questions.

CHAPTER

13 Physiology of the Peripheral Nervous System

To understand peripheral nervous system (PNS) drugs, we must first understand the PNS itself. The purpose of this chapter is to help you develop that understanding.

It's not uncommon for students to be at least slightly apprehensive about studying the PNS—especially the autonomic component. This book's approach to teaching the information is untraditional. Hopefully, it will make your work easier.

Because our ultimate goal concerns pharmacology—and not physiology—we do not address everything there is to know about the PNS. Rather, we limit the discussion to those aspects of PNS physiology that have a direct bearing on your ability to understand drugs.

DIVISIONS OF THE NERVOUS SYSTEM

The nervous system has two main divisions, the *central nervous system* (CNS) and the *PNS.* The PNS has two major subdivisions: (1) the *somatic motor system* and (2) the *autonomic nervous system.* The autonomic nervous system is further subdivided into the *parasympathetic nervous system* and the *sympathetic nervous system.* The somatic motor system controls voluntary movement of muscles. The two subdivisions of the autonomic nervous system regulate many involuntary processes.

The autonomic nervous system is the principal focus of this chapter. The somatic motor system is also considered, but discussion is brief.

OVERVIEW OF AUTONOMIC NERVOUS SYSTEM FUNCTIONS

The autonomic nervous system has three principal functions: (1) regulation of the *heart;* (2) regulation of *secretory glands* (salivary, gastric, sweat, and bronchial glands); and (3) regulation of *smooth muscles* (muscles of the bronchi, blood vessels, urogenital system, and GI tract). These regulatory activities are shared between the sympathetic and parasympathetic divisions of the autonomic nervous system.

Functions of the Parasympathetic Nervous System

The parasympathetic nervous system performs seven regulatory functions that have particular relevance to drugs. Specifically, stimulation of appropriate parasympathetic nerves causes

- Slowing of heart rate
- Increased gastric secretion
- Emptying of the bladder
- Emptying of the bowel
- Focusing the eye for near vision
- Constricting the pupil
- Contracting bronchial smooth muscle

Just how the parasympathetic nervous system elicits these responses is discussed later under *Functions of Cholinergic Receptor Subtypes.*

From the previous discussion we can see that the parasympathetic nervous system is concerned primarily with what might be called the "housekeeping" chores of the body (digestion of food and excretion of wastes). In addition, the system helps control vision and conserves energy by reducing cardiac work.

Therapeutic agents that alter parasympathetic nervous system function are used primarily for their effects on the GI tract, bladder, and eye. Occasionally, these drugs are also used for effects on the heart and lungs.

A variety of poisons act by mimicking or blocking effects of parasympathetic stimulation. Among these are insecticides, nerve gases, and toxic compounds found in certain mushrooms and plants.

Functions of the Sympathetic Nervous System

The sympathetic nervous system has three main functions:

- Regulating the cardiovascular system
- Regulating body temperature
- Implementing the acute stress response (commonly called a "fight-or-flight" reaction)

The sympathetic nervous system exerts multiple influences on the heart and blood vessels. Stimulation of sympathetic nerves to the heart increases cardiac output. Stimulation of sympathetic nerves to arterioles and veins causes vasoconstriction. Release of epinephrine from the adrenal medulla results in vasoconstriction in most vascular beds and vasodilation in certain others. By influencing the heart and blood vessels, the sympathetic nervous system can achieve three homeostatic objectives:

- Maintenance of blood flow to the brain
- Redistribution of blood flow during exercise
- Compensation for loss of blood, primarily by causing vasoconstriction

The sympathetic nervous system helps regulate body temperature in three ways: (1) By regulating blood flow to the skin, sympathetic nerves can increase or decrease heat loss. By *dilating* surface vessels, sympathetic nerves increase blood flow to the skin and thereby accelerate heat loss. Conversely, *constricting* cutaneous vessels conserves heat. (2) Sympathetic nerves to sweat glands promote secretion of sweat, thereby helping the body cool. (3) By inducing piloerection (erection of hair), sympathetic nerves can promote heat conservation.

When we are faced with an acute stress-inducing situation, the sympathetic nervous system orchestrates the fight-or-flight response, which consists of

- Increasing heart rate and blood pressure
- Shunting blood away from the skin and viscera and into skeletal muscles
- Dilating the bronchi to improve oxygenation
- Dilating the pupils (perhaps to enhance visual acuity)
- Mobilizing stored energy, thereby providing glucose for the brain and fatty acids for muscles

The sensation of being "cold with fear" is brought on by the shunting of blood away from the skin. The phrase "wide-eyed with fear" may be based on pupillary dilation.

Many therapeutic agents produce their effects by altering functions under sympathetic control. These drugs are used primarily for effects on the heart, blood vessels, and lungs. Agents that alter cardiovascular function are used to treat hypertension, heart failure, angina pectoris, and other disorders. Drugs affecting the lungs are used primarily for asthma.

BASIC MECHANISMS BY WHICH THE AUTONOMIC NERVOUS SYSTEM REGULATES PHYSIOLOGIC PROCESSES

To understand how drugs influence processes under autonomic control, we must first understand how the autonomic nervous system itself regulates those activities. The basic mechanisms by which the autonomic nervous system regulates physiologic processes are discussed in the following sections.

Patterns of Innervation and Control

Most structures under autonomic control are innervated by sympathetic nerves *and* parasympathetic nerves. The relative influence of sympathetic and parasympathetic nerves depends on the organ under consideration.

In many organs that receive dual innervation, the influence of sympathetic nerves *opposes* that of parasympathetic nerves. For example, in the heart, *sympathetic* nerves *increase* heart rate, whereas *parasympathetic* nerves *slow* heart rate (Fig. 13.1).

In some organs that receive nerves from both divisions of the autonomic nervous system, the effects of sympathetic and parasympathetic nerves are *complementary,* rather than opposite. For example, in the male reproductive system, erection is regulated by parasympathetic nerves while ejaculation is controlled by sympathetic nerves. If attempts at reproduction are to succeed, cooperative interaction of both systems is needed.

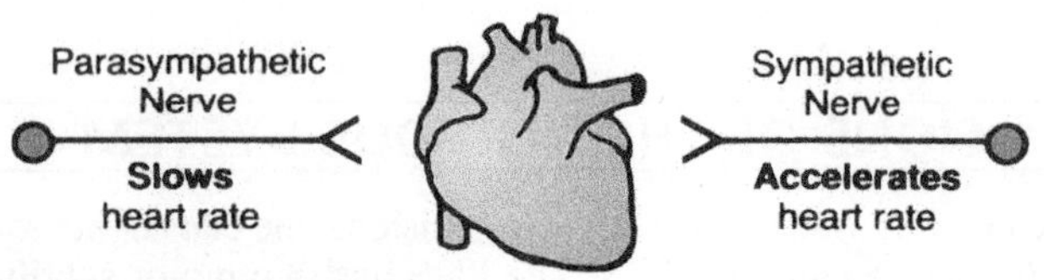

Fig. 13.1 ▪ Opposing effects of parasympathetic and sympathetic nerves.

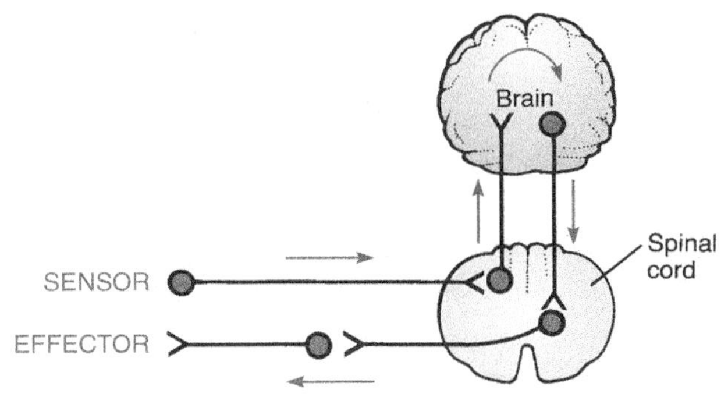

Fig. 13.2 ■ Feedback loop of the autonomic nervous system.

A few structures under autonomic control receive innervation from only one division. The principal example is blood vessels, which are innervated exclusively by sympathetic nerves.

In summary, there are three basic patterns of autonomic innervation and regulation:

- Innervation by *both* divisions of the autonomic nervous system in which the effects of the two divisions are *opposed*
- Innervation by *both* divisions of the autonomic nervous system in which the effects of the two divisions are *complementary*
- Innervation and regulation by *only one* division of the autonomic nervous system

Feedback Regulation

Feedback regulation is a process that allows a system to adjust itself by responding to incoming information. Practically all physiologic processes are regulated at least in part by feedback control.

Fig. 13.2 depicts a feedback loop typical of those used by the autonomic nervous system. The main elements of this loop are (1) a *sensor,* (2) an *effector,* and (3) neurons connecting the sensor to the effector. The purpose of the sensor is to monitor the status of a physiologic process. Information picked up by the sensor is sent to the CNS (spinal cord and brain), where it is integrated with other relevant information. Signals (instructions for change) are then sent from the CNS along nerves of the autonomic system to the effector. In response to these instructions, the effector makes appropriate adjustments in the process. The entire procedure is called a *reflex.*

Baroreceptor Reflex

From a pharmacologic perspective, the most important feedback loop of the autonomic nervous system is one that helps regulate blood pressure. This system is referred to as the *baroreceptor reflex.* (Baroreceptors are receptors that sense blood pressure.) This reflex is important to us because it frequently opposes our attempts to modify blood pressure with drugs.

Feedback (reflex) control of blood pressure is achieved as follows: (1) Baroreceptors located in the carotid sinus and aortic arch monitor changes in blood pressure and send this information to the brain. (2) In response, the brain sends impulses along nerves of the autonomic nervous system, instructing the heart and blood vessels to behave in a way that restores blood pressure to normal. Accordingly, when blood pressure *falls,* the baroreceptor reflex causes vasoconstriction and increases cardiac output. Both actions help bring blood pressure back up. Conversely, when blood pressure *rises* too high, the baroreceptor reflex causes vasodilation and reduces cardiac output, thereby causing blood pressure to drop. The baroreceptor reflex is discussed in greater detail in Chapter 43.

Autonomic Tone

Autonomic tone is the steady, day-to-day influence exerted by the autonomic nervous system on a particular organ or organ system. Autonomic tone provides a basal level of control over which reflex regulation is superimposed.

When an organ is innervated by both divisions of the autonomic nervous system, one division—either sympathetic or parasympathetic—provides most of the basal control, thereby obviating conflicting instruction. Recall that, when an organ receives nerves from both divisions of the autonomic nervous system, those nerves frequently exert opposing influences. If both divisions were to send impulses simultaneously, the resultant conflicting instructions would be counterproductive (like running heating and air conditioning simultaneously). By having only one division of the autonomic nervous system provide the basal control to an organ, conflicting signals are avoided.

The branch of the autonomic nervous system that controls organ function most of the time is said to provide the *predominant tone* to that organ. *In most organs, the parasympathetic nervous system provides the predominant tone.* The vascular system, which is regulated almost exclusively by the *sympathetic* nervous system, is the principal exception.

ANATOMIC CONSIDERATIONS

Although we know a great deal about the anatomy of the PNS, very little of this information helps us understand PNS drugs. The few details that *do* pertain to pharmacology are shown in Fig. 13.3.

Parasympathetic Nervous System

Pharmacologically relevant aspects of parasympathetic anatomy are shown in Fig. 13.3. Note that there are *two* neurons in the pathway leading from the spinal cord to organs innervated by parasympathetic nerves. The junction (synapse) between these two neurons occurs within a structure called a *ganglion.* (A ganglion is simply a mass of nerve cell bodies.) The neurons that go from the spinal cord to the parasympathetic ganglia are called *preganglionic neurons,* whereas the neurons that go from the ganglia to effector organs are called *postganglionic neurons.* The anatomy of the parasympathetic nervous system offers two general sites at which drugs can act: (1) the synapses between preganglionic neurons and postganglionic neurons and (2) the junctions between postganglionic neurons and their effector organs.

Sympathetic Nervous System

Pharmacologically relevant aspects of sympathetic nervous system anatomy are illustrated in Fig. 13.3. As you can see,

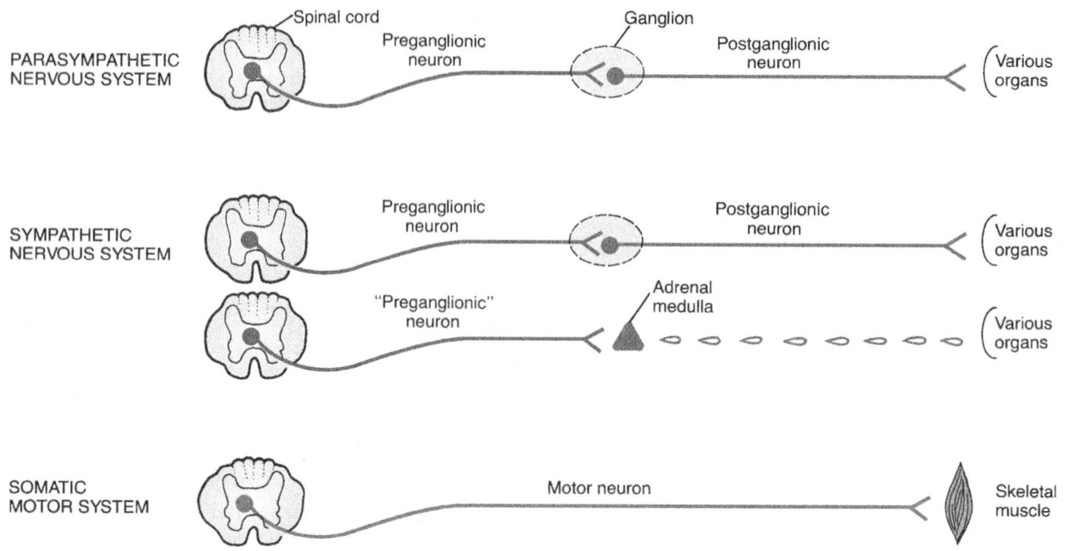

Fig. 13.3 ■ The basic anatomy of the parasympathetic and sympathetic nervous systems and the somatic motor system.

these features are nearly identical to those of the parasympathetic nervous system. Like the parasympathetic nervous system, the sympathetic nervous system employs two neurons in the pathways leading from the spinal cord to organs under its control. As with the parasympathetic nervous system, the junctions between those neurons are located in *ganglia.* Neurons leading from the spinal cord to the sympathetic ganglia are termed *preganglionic neurons,* and neurons leading from ganglia to effector organs are termed *postganglionic neurons.*

The *medulla of the adrenal gland* is a feature of the sympathetic nervous system that requires comment. Although not a neuron per se, the adrenal medulla can be looked on as the functional equivalent of a postganglionic neuron of the sympathetic nervous system. (The adrenal medulla influences the body by releasing epinephrine into the bloodstream, which then produces effects much like those that occur in response to stimulation of postganglionic sympathetic nerves.) Because the adrenal medulla is similar in function to a postganglionic neuron, the nerve leading from the spinal cord to the adrenal gland is commonly referred to as a preganglionic neuron, even though there is no ganglion in this pathway.

As with the parasympathetic nervous system, drugs that affect the sympathetic nervous system have two general sites of action: (1) the synapses between preganglionic and postganglionic neurons (including the adrenal medulla), and (2) the junctions between postganglionic neurons and their effector organs.

Somatic Motor System

Pharmacologically relevant anatomy of the somatic motor system is depicted in Fig. 13.3. Note that there is *only one* neuron in the pathway from the spinal cord to the muscles innervated by somatic motor nerves. Because this pathway contains only one neuron, peripherally acting drugs that affect somatic motor system function have only one site of action: the *neuromuscular junction* (i.e., the junction between the somatic motor nerve and the muscle).

INTRODUCTION TO TRANSMITTERS OF THE PERIPHERAL NERVOUS SYSTEM

The PNS employs three neurotransmitters: *acetylcholine, norepinephrine,* and *epinephrine.* Any given junction in the PNS uses only one of these transmitter substances. A fourth compound—*dopamine*—may also serve as a PNS transmitter, but this role has not been demonstrated conclusively.

To understand PNS pharmacology, it is necessary to know the identity of the transmitter employed at each of the junctions of the PNS. This information is shown in Fig. 13.4. As indicated, *acetylcholine* is the transmitter employed at most junctions of the PNS. Acetylcholine is the transmitter released by (1) all preganglionic neurons of the parasympathetic nervous system, (2) all preganglionic neurons of the sympathetic nervous system, (3) all postganglionic neurons of the parasympathetic nervous system, (4) all motor neurons to skeletal muscles, and (5) most postganglionic neurons of the sympathetic nervous system that go to sweat glands.

Norepinephrine is the transmitter released by practically all postganglionic neurons of the sympathetic nervous system. The only exceptions are the postganglionic sympathetic neurons that go to sweat glands, which employ acetylcholine as their transmitter.

Epinephrine is the major transmitter released by the adrenal medulla. (The adrenal medulla also releases some norepinephrine.)

Much of what follows in this chapter is based on the information in Fig. 13.4. Accordingly, we strongly urge you to learn this information now.

INTRODUCTION TO RECEPTORS OF THE PERIPHERAL NERVOUS SYSTEM

The PNS works through several different types of receptors. Understanding these receptors is central to understanding PNS

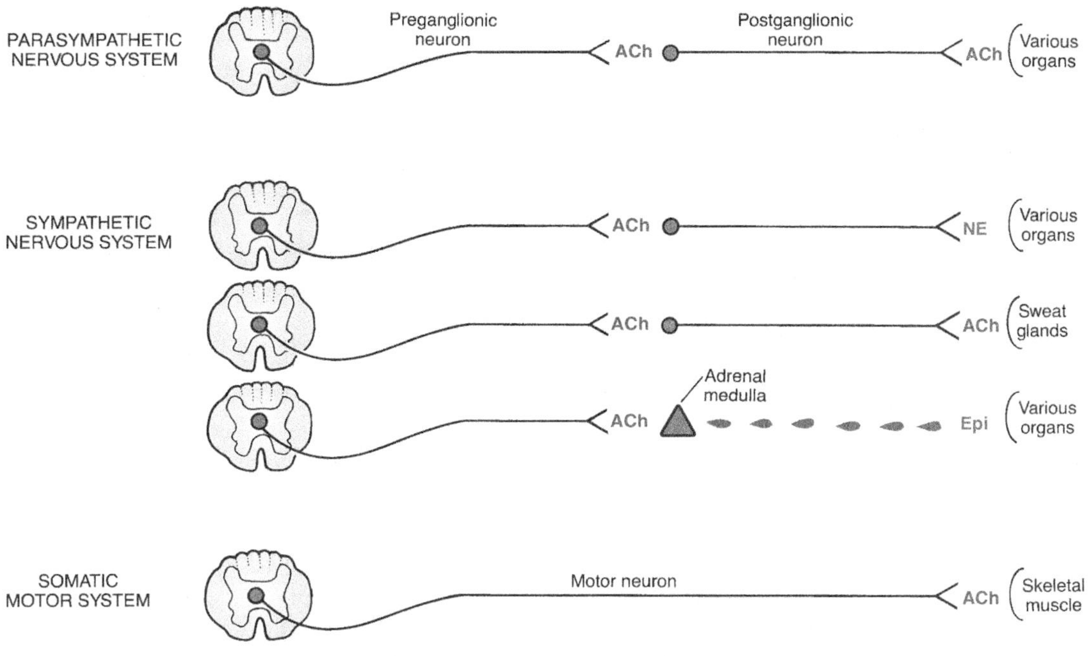

Fig. 13.4 ▪ Transmitters employed at specific junctions of the PNS.

1. *All preganglionic* neurons of the *parasympathetic* and *sympathetic* nervous systems release *acetylcholine* as their transmitter.
2. *All postganglionic* neurons of the *parasympathetic* nervous system release *acetylcholine* as their transmitter.
3. *Most postganglionic* neurons of the *sympathetic* nervous system release *norepinephrine* as their transmitter.
4. *Postganglionic* neurons of the sympathetic nervous system that innervate *sweat glands* release *acetylcholine* as their transmitter.
5. *Epinephrine* is the principal transmitter released by the *adrenal medulla.*
6. *All motor neurons* to *skeletal muscles* release *acetylcholine* as their transmitter.

pharmacology. All effort that you invest in learning about these receptors now will be rewarded as we discuss PNS drugs in later chapters.

Primary Receptor Types: Cholinergic Receptors and Adrenergic Receptors

There are two basic categories of receptors associated with the PNS: *cholinergic receptors* and *adrenergic receptors.* Cholinergic receptors are defined as receptors that mediate responses to acetylcholine. These receptors mediate responses at all junctions where acetylcholine is the transmitter. Adrenergic receptors are defined as receptors that mediate responses to epinephrine (adrenaline) and norepinephrine. These receptors mediate responses at all junctions where norepinephrine or epinephrine is the transmitter.

Subtypes of Cholinergic and Adrenergic Receptors

Not all cholinergic receptors are the same; likewise, not all adrenergic receptors are the same. For each of these two major receptor classes there are receptor subtypes. There are three major subtypes of cholinergic receptors, referred to as $nicotinic_N$, $nicotinic_M$, and muscarinic.[a] In addition, there are four major subtypes of adrenergic receptors, referred to as $alpha_1$, $alpha_2$, $beta_1$, and $beta_2$.

In addition to the four major subtypes of adrenergic receptors, there is another adrenergic receptor type, referred to as the *dopamine* receptor. Although dopamine receptors are classified as adrenergic, these receptors do not respond to epinephrine or norepinephrine. Rather, they respond only to dopamine, a neurotransmitter found primarily in the CNS.

EXPLORING THE CONCEPT OF RECEPTOR SUBTYPES

The concept of receptor subtypes is important and potentially confusing. In this section we discuss what a receptor subtype is and why receptor subtypes matter.

[a]Evidence indicates that muscarinic receptors, like nicotinic receptors, come in subtypes. Five have been identified. Of these, only three—designated M_1, M_2, and M_3—have clearly identified functions. At this time, practically all drugs that affect muscarinic receptors are nonselective. Accordingly, because our understanding of these receptors is limited, and because drugs that can selectively alter their function are few, we will not discuss muscarinic receptor subtypes further in this chapter. However, we will discuss them in Chapter 14 in the context of drugs for overactive bladder.

What Do We Mean By Receptor Subtype?

Receptors that respond to the same transmitter but nonetheless are different from one another are called receptor subtypes. For example, peripheral receptors that respond to acetylcholine can be found (1) in ganglia of the autonomic nervous system, (2) at neuromuscular junctions, and (3) on organs regulated by the parasympathetic nervous system. However, even though all of these receptors can be activated by acetylcholine, there is clear evidence that the receptors at these three sites are, in fact, different from one another. Hence, although all of these receptors belong to the same major receptor category (cholinergic), they are sufficiently different as to constitute distinct receptor subtypes.

How Do We Know That Receptor Subtypes Exist?

Historically, our knowledge of receptor subtypes came from observing responses to drugs. In fact, were it not for drugs, receptor subtypes might never have been discovered.

Table 13.1 illustrates the types of drug responses that led to the realization that receptor subtypes exist. These data summarize the results of an experiment designed to study the effects of a natural transmitter (acetylcholine) and a series of drugs (nicotine, muscarine, *d*-tubocurarine, and atropine) on two tissues: skeletal muscle and ciliary muscle. (The ciliary muscle is the muscle responsible for focusing the eye for near vision.) Although skeletal muscle and ciliary muscle both contract in response to acetylcholine, these tissues differ in their responses to drugs. In the discussion that follows, we examine the selective responses of these tissues to drugs and see how those responses reveal the existence of receptor subtypes.

At synapses on skeletal muscle and ciliary muscle, acetylcholine is the transmitter employed by neurons to elicit contraction. Because both types of muscle respond to acetylcholine, it is safe to conclude that both muscles have receptors for this substance. Because acetylcholine is the natural transmitter for these receptors, we would classify these receptors as *cholinergic.*

What do the effects of nicotine on skeletal muscle and ciliary muscle suggest? The effects of nicotine on these muscles suggest four possible conclusions: (1) Because skeletal muscle contracts in response to nicotine, we can conclude that skeletal muscle has receptors at which nicotine can act. (2) Because ciliary muscle does *not* respond to nicotine, we can tentatively conclude that ciliary muscle does not have receptors for nicotine. (3) Because nicotine mimics the effects of acetylcholine on skeletal muscle, we can conclude that nicotine may act at the same skeletal muscle receptors where acetylcholine acts. (4) Because both skeletal and ciliary muscles have receptors for acetylcholine, and because nicotine appears to act only at the acetylcholine receptors on skeletal muscle, we can tentatively conclude that the acetylcholine receptors on skeletal muscle are different from the acetylcholine receptors on ciliary muscle.

What do the responses to muscarine suggest? The conclusions that can be drawn regarding responses to muscarine are exactly parallel to those drawn for nicotine. These conclusions are: (1) ciliary muscle has receptors that respond to muscarine, (2) skeletal muscle may not have receptors for muscarine, (3) muscarine may be acting at the same receptors on ciliary muscle where acetylcholine acts, and (4) the receptors for acetylcholine on ciliary muscle may be different from the receptors for acetylcholine on skeletal muscle.

The responses of skeletal muscle and ciliary muscle to nicotine and muscarine suggest, but do not prove, that the cholinergic receptors on these two tissues are different. However, the responses of these two tissues to d-*tubocurarine* and *atropine,* both of which are receptor *blocking agents,* eliminate any doubts as to the presence of cholinergic receptor subtypes. When both types of muscle are pretreated with *d*-tubocurarine and then exposed to acetylcholine, the response to acetylcholine is blocked in skeletal muscle but not in ciliary muscle. *d*-Tubocurarine pretreatment does not reduce the ability of acetylcholine to stimulate ciliary muscle. Conversely, pretreatment with atropine selectively blocks the response to acetylcholine in ciliary muscle—but atropine does nothing to prevent acetylcholine from stimulating receptors on skeletal muscle. Because *d*-tubocurarine can selectively block cholinergic receptors in skeletal muscle, whereas atropine can selectively block cholinergic receptors in ciliary muscle, we can conclude with certainty that the receptors for acetylcholine in these two types of muscle must be different.

The data just discussed illustrate the essential role of drugs in revealing the presence of receptor subtypes. If acetylcholine were the only probe that we had, all that we would have been able to observe is that both skeletal muscle and ciliary muscle can respond to this agent. This simple observation would provide no basis for suspecting that the receptors for acetylcholine in these two tissues were different. It is only through the use of selectively acting drugs that the presence of receptor subtypes was initially revealed.

Today, the technology for identifying receptors and their subtypes is extremely sophisticated—not that studies like the one just discussed are no longer of value. In addition to performing traditional drug-based studies, scientists are now cloning receptors using DNA hybridization technology. As you can imagine, this allows us to understand receptors in ways that were unthinkable in the past.

TABLE 13.1 ▪ Responses of Skeletal Muscle and Ciliary Muscle to a Series of Drugs

	Response	
Drug	**Skeletal Muscle**	**Ciliary Muscle**
Acetylcholine	Contraction	Contraction
Nicotine	Contraction	No response
Muscarine	No response	Contraction
Acetylcholine		
After *d*-tubocurarine	No response	Contraction
After atropine	Contraction	No response

How Can Drugs Be More Selective Than Natural Transmitters at Receptor Subtypes?

Drugs achieve their selectivity for receptor subtypes by having structures that are different from those of natural transmitters.

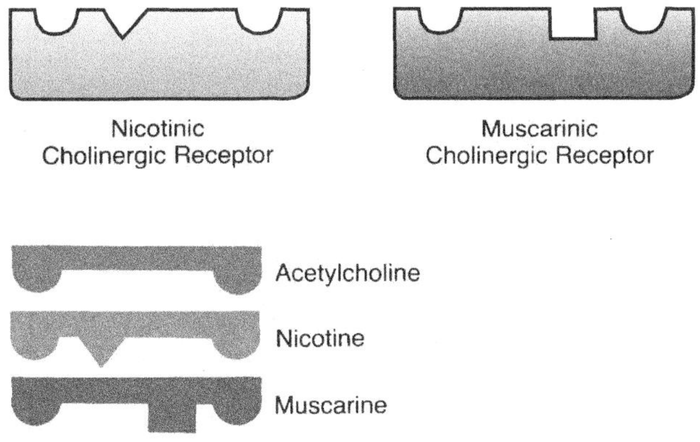

Fig. 13.5 ▪ Drug structure and receptor selectivity. The relationship between structure and receptor selectivity is shown. The structure of acetylcholine allows this transmitter to interact with both receptor subtypes. In contrast, because of their unique structures, nicotine and muscarine are selective for the cholinergic receptor subtypes whose structure complements their own.

The relationship between structure and receptor selectivity is illustrated in Fig. 13.5. Drawings are used to represent drugs (nicotine and muscarine), receptor subtypes (nicotinic and muscarinic), and acetylcholine (the natural transmitter at nicotinic and muscarinic receptors). From the structures shown, we can easily imagine how acetylcholine is able to interact with both kinds of receptor subtypes, whereas nicotine and muscarine can interact only with the receptor subtypes whose structure is complementary to their own. By synthesizing chemicals that are structurally related to natural transmitters, pharmaceutical chemists have been able to produce drugs that are more selective for specific receptor subtypes than are the natural transmitters that act at those sites.

Why Do Receptor Subtypes Exist, and Why Do They Matter?

The physiologic benefits of having multiple receptor subtypes for the same transmitter are not immediately obvious. In fact, as noted previously, were it not for drugs, we probably wouldn't know that receptor subtypes existed at all. Although receptor subtypes are of uncertain physiologic relevance, from the viewpoint of therapeutics, receptor subtypes are invaluable.

The presence of receptor subtypes makes possible a dramatic increase in drug selectivity. For example, thanks to the existence of subtypes of cholinergic receptors (and the development of drugs selective for those receptor subtypes), it is possible to influence the activity of certain cholinergic receptors (e.g., receptors of the neuromuscular junction) without altering the activity of all other cholinergic receptors (e.g., the cholinergic receptors found in all autonomic ganglia and all target organs of the parasympathetic nervous system). Were it not for the existence of receptor subtypes, a drug that acted on cholinergic receptors at one site would alter the activity of cholinergic receptors at all other sites. Clearly, the existence of receptor subtypes for a particular transmitter makes possible drug actions that are much more selective than could be achieved if all of the receptors for that transmitter were the same. (Recall our discussion of Mort and Merv in Chapter 12.)

LOCATIONS OF RECEPTOR SUBTYPES

Because many of the drugs discussed in later chapters are selective for specific receptor subtypes, knowledge of the sites at which specific receptor subtypes are located will help us predict which organs a drug will affect. Accordingly, in laying our foundation for studying PNS drugs, it is important to learn the sites at which the subtypes of adrenergic and cholinergic receptors are located. This information is shown in Fig. 13.6. You will find it helpful to master the content of this figure before proceeding. (In the interest of minimizing confusion, subtypes of adrenergic receptors in Fig. 13.6 are listed simply as alpha and beta rather than as $alpha_1$, $alpha_2$, $beta_1$, and $beta_2$. The locations of all four subtypes of adrenergic receptors are discussed in the section that follows.)

FUNCTIONS OF CHOLINERGIC AND ADRENERGIC RECEPTOR SUBTYPES

Knowledge of receptor function is essential for understanding PNS drugs. By knowing the receptors at which a drug acts, and by knowing what those receptors do, we can predict the major effects of any PNS drug.

Tables 13.2 and 13.3 show the pharmacologically relevant functions of PNS receptors. Table 13.2 summarizes responses elicited by activation of *cholinergic* receptor subtypes. Table 13.3 summarizes responses to activation of *adrenergic* receptor subtypes. You should master Table 13.2 before studying cholinergic drugs (Chapters 14, 15, and 16). And you should master Table 13.3 before studying adrenergic drugs (Chapters 17, 18, and 19). If you master these tables in preparation for learning about PNS drugs, you will find the process of learning the pharmacology relatively simple. Conversely, if you attempt to study the pharmacology without first mastering the appropriate table, you are likely to meet with frustration.

Functions of Cholinergic Receptor Subtypes

Table 13.2 shows the pharmacologically relevant responses to activation of the three major subtypes of cholinergic receptors: $nicotinic_N$, $nicotinic_M$, and muscarinic.

We can group responses to cholinergic receptor activation into three major categories based on the subtype of receptor involved:

- Activation of *$nicotinic_N$* (neuronal) receptors promotes *ganglionic transmission* at all ganglia of the sympathetic and parasympathetic nervous systems. In addition, activation of $nicotinic_N$ receptors promotes *release of epinephrine from the adrenal medulla.*
- Activation of *$nicotinic_M$* (muscle) receptors causes *contraction of skeletal muscle.*
- Activation of *muscarinic* receptors, which are located on target organs of the parasympathetic nervous system, elicits an appropriate response from the organ involved. Specifically, muscarinic activation causes (1) increased glandular secretions (from pulmonary, gastric, intestinal, and sweat glands); (2) contraction of smooth muscle in the bronchi and GI tract; (3) slowing of heart rate; (4) contraction of the sphincter muscle of the iris, resulting

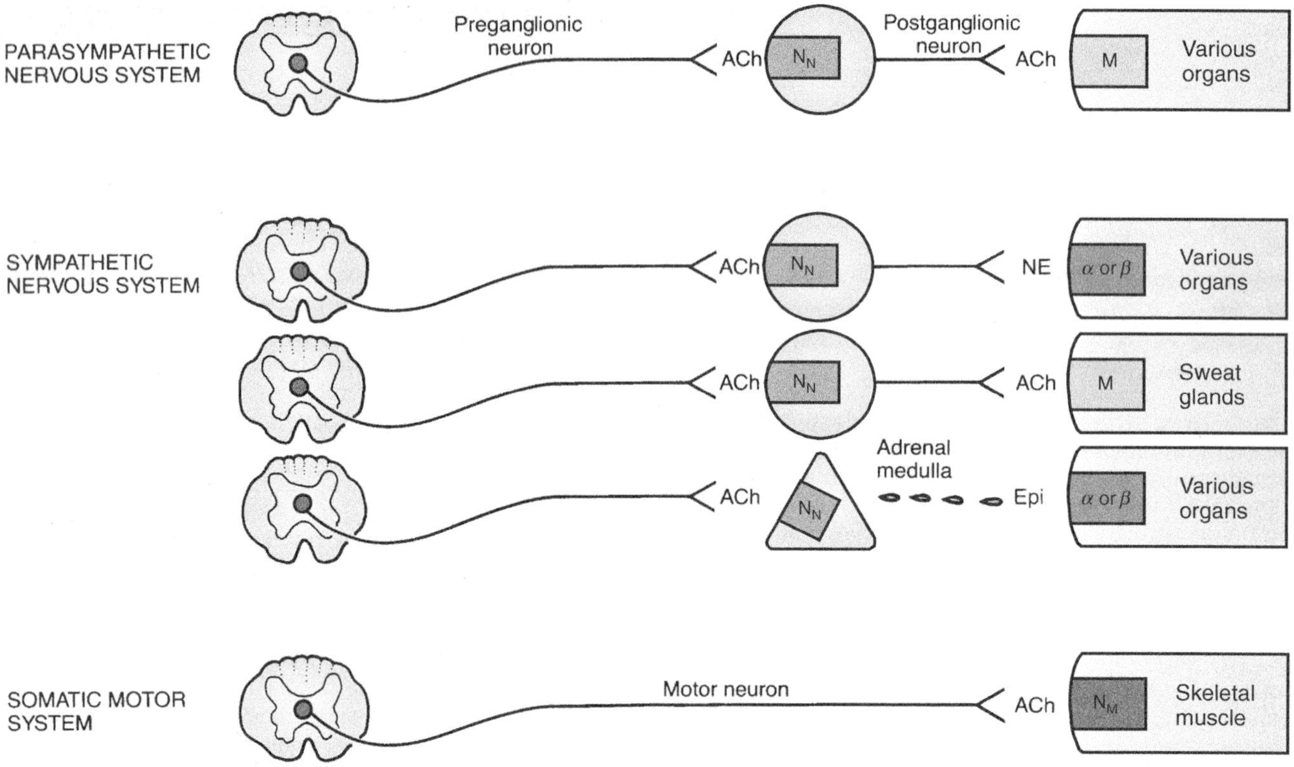

Cholinergic receptor subtypes: N_N = nicotinic$_N$, N_M = nicotinic$_M$, and M = muscarinic.
Adrenergic receptor subtypes: α = alpha and β = beta.

Fig. 13.6 ■ Locations of cholinergic and adrenergic receptor subtypes.

1. *Nicotinic$_N$* receptors are located on the *cell bodies of all postganglionic neurons* of the *parasympathetic* and *sympathetic* nervous systems. *Nicotinic$_N$* receptors are also located on cells of the *adrenal medulla.*
2. *Nicotinic$_M$* receptors are located on *skeletal muscle.*
3. *Muscarinic* receptors are located on *all organs* regulated by the *parasympathetic* nervous system (i.e., organs innervated by postganglionic parasympathetic nerves). *Muscarinic* receptors are also located on *sweat glands.*
4. *Adrenergic* receptors—*alpha, beta,* or both—are located on *all organs* (except sweat glands) regulated by the *sympathetic* nervous system (i.e., organs innervated by postganglionic sympathetic nerves). *Adrenergic* receptors are also located on organs regulated by epinephrine released from the *adrenal medulla.*

in miosis (reduction in pupillary diameter); (5) contraction of the ciliary muscle of the eye, causing the lens to focus for near vision; (6) dilation of blood vessels; and (7) voiding of the urinary bladder (by causing contraction of the detrusor muscle [which forms the bladder wall] and relaxation of the trigone and sphincter muscles [which block the bladder neck when contracted]).

Muscarinic cholinergic receptors on blood vessels require additional comment. These receptors are not associated with the nervous system in any way. That is, no autonomic nerves terminate at vascular muscarinic receptors. It is not at all clear as to how, or even if, these receptors are activated physiologically. However, regardless of their physiologic relevance, the cholinergic receptors on blood vessels do have *pharmacologic* significance, because drugs that are able to activate these receptors cause vasodilation, which in turn causes blood pressure to fall.

Functions of Adrenergic Receptor Subtypes

Adrenergic receptor subtypes and their functions are shown in Table 13.3.

Alpha$_1$ Receptors

Alpha$_1$ receptors are located in the eyes, blood vessels, male sex organs, prostatic capsule, and bladder (trigone and sphincter).

Ocular alpha$_1$ receptors are present on the radial muscle of the iris. Activation of these receptors leads to *mydriasis* (dilation of the pupil). As depicted in Table 13.3, the fibers of the radial muscle are arranged like the spokes of a wheel. Because of this configuration, contraction of the radial muscle causes the pupil to enlarge. (If you have difficulty remembering that *mydriasis* means pupillary enlargement, whereas *miosis* means pupillary constriction, just remember that mydriasis [dilation]

TABLE 13.2 ▪ Functions of Peripheral Cholinergic Receptor Subtypes

Receptor Subtype	Location	Response to Receptor Activation
Nicotinic$_N$	All autonomic nervous system ganglia and the adrenal medulla	Stimulation of parasympathetic and sympathetic postganglionic nerves and release of epinephrine from the adrenal medulla
Nicotinic$_M$	Neuromuscular junction	Contraction of skeletal muscle
Muscarinic	All parasympathetic target organs:	
	Eye	Contraction of the ciliary muscle focuses the lens for near vision Contraction of the iris sphincter muscle causes miosis (decreased pupil diameter)
	Heart	Decreased rate
	Lung	Constriction of bronchi Promotion of secretions
	Bladder	Contraction of detrusor increases bladder pressure Relaxation of trigone and sphincter allows urine to leave the bladder Coordinated contraction of detrusor and relaxation of trigone and sphincter causes voiding of the bladder
	GI tract	Salivation Increased gastric secretions Increased intestinal tone and motility Defecation
	Sweat glands[a]	Generalized sweating
	Sex organs	Erection
	Blood vessels[b]	Vasodilation

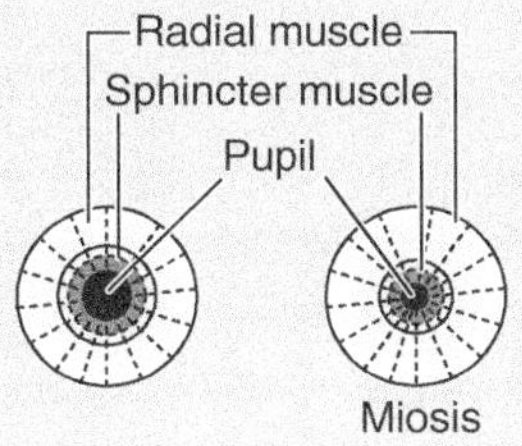

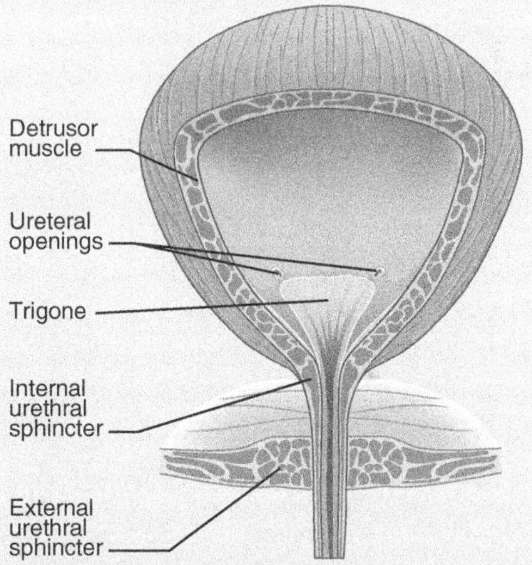

[a]Although sweating is due primarily to stimulation of muscarinic receptors by acetylcholine, the nerves that supply acetylcholine to sweat glands belong to the sympathetic nervous system rather than the parasympathetic nervous system.
[b]Cholinergic receptors on blood vessels are not associated with the nervous system.

TABLE 13.3 ▪ Functions of Peripheral Adrenergic Receptor Subtypes

Receptor Subtype	Location	Response to Receptor Activation
Alpha$_1$	Eye	Contraction of the radial muscle of the iris causes mydriasis (increased pupil size)

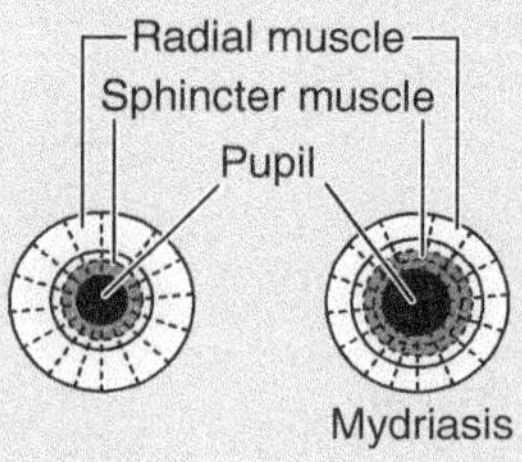

Receptor Subtype	Location	Response to Receptor Activation
	Arterioles Skin Viscera Mucous membranes	Constriction
	Veins	Constriction
	Sex organs, male	Ejaculation
	Prostatic capsule	Contraction
	Bladder	Contraction of trigone and sphincter

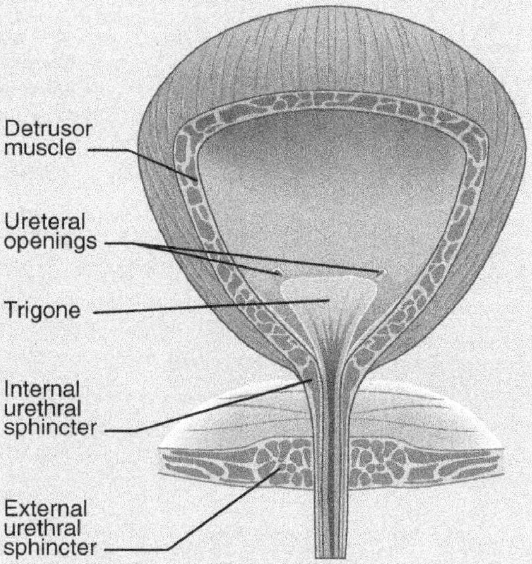

Receptor Subtype	Location	Response to Receptor Activation
Alpha$_2$	Presynaptic nerve terminals	Inhibition of transmitter release

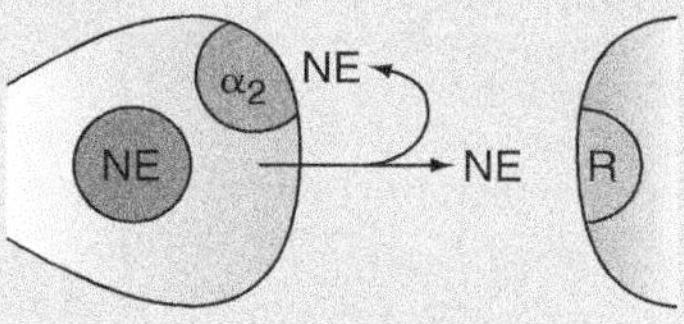

Receptor Subtype	Location	Response to Receptor Activation
Beta$_1$	Heart	Increased rate Increased force of contraction Increased AV conduction velocity
	Kidney	Release of renin
Beta$_2$	Arterioles Heart Lung Skeletal muscle	Dilation
	Bronchi	Dilation
	Uterus	Relaxation
	Liver	Glycogenolysis
	Skeletal muscle	Enhanced contraction, glycogenolysis
Dopamine	Kidney	Dilation of kidney vasculature

AV, Atrioventricular; *NE,* norepinephrine; *R,* receptor.

is a bigger word than miosis and that mydriasis contains a "d" for dilation.)

Alpha$_1$ receptors are present on veins and on arterioles in many capillary beds. Activation of alpha$_1$ receptors in blood vessels produces *vasoconstriction.*

Activation of alpha$_1$ receptors in the sexual apparatus of males causes *ejaculation.* Activation of alpha$_1$ receptors in smooth muscle of the bladder (trigone and sphincter) and prostatic capsule causes *contraction.*

Alpha$_2$ Receptors

Alpha$_2$ receptors of the PNS are located on nerve terminals (see Table 13.3) and not on the organs innervated by the autonomic nervous system. Because alpha$_2$ receptors are located on nerve terminals, these receptors are referred to as *presynaptic* or *prejunctional.* The function of these receptors is to *regulate transmitter release.* As depicted in Table 13.3, norepinephrine can bind to alpha$_2$ receptors located on the same neuron from which the norepinephrine was released. The consequence of this norepinephrine-receptor interaction is suppression of further norepinephrine release. Hence, presynaptic alpha$_2$ receptors can help reduce transmitter release when too much transmitter has accumulated in the synaptic gap. Drug effects resulting from activation of *peripheral* alpha$_2$ receptors are of minimal clinical significance.

Alpha$_2$ receptors are also present in the CNS. In contrast to peripheral alpha$_2$ receptors, central alpha$_2$ receptors are therapeutically relevant. We will consider these receptors in later chapters.

Beta$_1$ Receptors

Beta$_1$ receptors are located in the heart and the kidney. Cardiac beta$_1$ receptors have great therapeutic significance. Activation of these receptors *increases heart rate, force of contraction,* and *velocity of impulse conduction through the atrioventricular node.*

Activation of beta$_1$ receptors in the kidney causes *release of renin* into the blood. Because renin promotes synthesis of angiotensin, a powerful vasoconstrictor, activation of renal beta$_1$ receptors is a means by which the nervous system helps elevate blood pressure. (The role of renin in the regulation of blood pressure is discussed in depth in Chapter 44.)

Beta$_2$ Receptors

Beta$_2$ receptors mediate several important processes. Activation of beta$_2$ receptors in the lung leads to *bronchial dilation.* Activation of beta$_2$ receptors in the uterus causes *relaxation of uterine smooth muscle.* Activation of beta$_2$ receptors in arterioles of the heart, lungs, and skeletal muscles causes *vasodilation* (an effect opposite to that of alpha$_1$ activation). Activation of beta$_2$ receptors in the liver and skeletal muscle promotes *glycogenolysis* (breakdown of glycogen into glucose), thereby increasing blood levels of glucose. In addition, activation of beta$_2$ receptors in skeletal muscle enhances *contraction.*

Dopamine Receptors

In the periphery, the only dopamine receptors of clinical significance are located in the vasculature of the kidney. Activation of these receptors *dilates renal blood vessels,* enhancing renal perfusion.

In the CNS, receptors for dopamine are of great therapeutic significance. The functions of these receptors are discussed in Chapters 21 and 31.

Receptor Specificity of the Adrenergic Transmitters

The receptor specificity of adrenergic transmitters is more complex than the receptor specificity of acetylcholine. Whereas acetylcholine can activate all three subtypes of cholinergic receptors, not every adrenergic transmitter (epinephrine, norepinephrine, dopamine) can interact with each of the five subtypes of adrenergic receptors.

Receptor specificity of adrenergic transmitters is as follows: (1) *epinephrine* can activate all alpha and beta receptors, but not dopamine receptors; (2) *norepinephrine* can activate alpha$_1$, alpha$_2$, and beta$_1$ receptors, but not beta$_2$ or dopamine receptors; and (3) *dopamine* can activate alpha$_1$, beta$_1$, and dopamine receptors. (Note that dopamine itself is the only transmitter capable of activating dopamine receptors.) Receptor specificity of the adrenergic transmitters is shown in Table 13.4.

Knowing that epinephrine is the only transmitter that acts at beta$_2$ receptors can serve as an aid to remembering the functions of this receptor subtype. Recall that epinephrine is released from the adrenal medulla—not from neurons—and that the function of epinephrine is to prepare the body for fight or flight. Accordingly, because epinephrine is the only transmitter that activates beta$_2$ receptors and because epinephrine is released only in preparation for fight or flight, times of fight or flight will be the only occasions on which beta$_2$ receptors will undergo significant physiologic activation. As it turns out, the physiologic changes elicited by beta$_2$ activation are precisely those needed for success in the fight-or-flight response. Specifically, activation of beta$_2$ receptors will (1) dilate blood vessels in the heart, lungs, and skeletal muscles, thereby increasing blood flow to these organs; (2) dilate the bronchi, thereby increasing oxygenation; (3) increase glycogenolysis, thereby increasing available energy; and (4) relax uterine smooth muscle, thereby preventing delivery (a process that would be inconvenient for a pregnant woman preparing to fight or flee). Accordingly, if you think of the physiologic requirements for success during fight or flight, you will have a good picture of the responses that beta$_2$ activation can cause.

TRANSMITTER LIFE CYCLES

In this section we consider the life cycles of acetylcholine, norepinephrine, and epinephrine. Because a number of drugs produce their effects by interfering with specific phases of the

TABLE 13.4 ■ Receptor Specificity of Adrenergic Transmitters[a]

Transmitter	Alpha$_1$	Alpha$_2$	Beta$_1$	Beta$_2$	Dopamine
Epinephrine	←	—	—	→	
Norepinephrine	←	—	→		
Dopamine	↔		↔		↔

[a]Arrows indicate the range of receptors that the transmitters can activate.

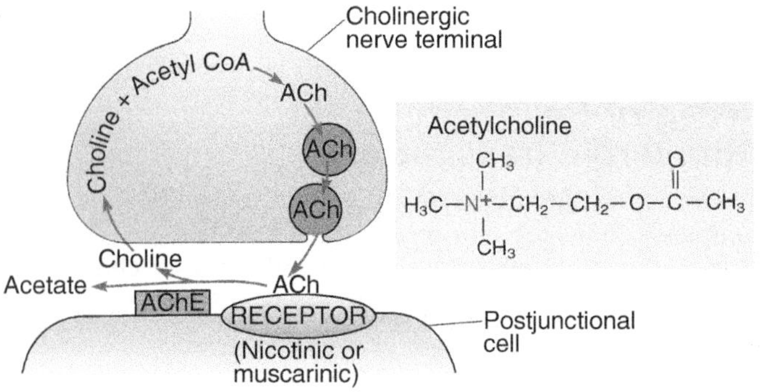

Fig. 13.7 ▪ **Life cycle of acetylcholine.**
Transmission is terminated by enzymatic degradation of ACh and not by uptake of intact ACh back into the nerve terminal. (*Acetyl CoA,* Acetylcoenzyme A; *ACh,* acetylcholine; *AChE,* acetylcholinesterase.)

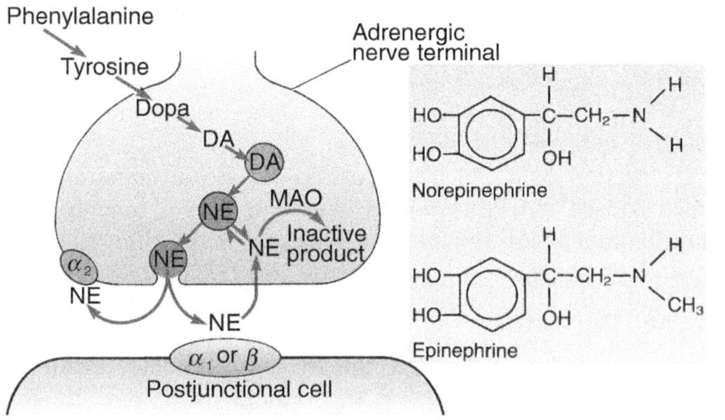

Fig. 13.8 ▪ **Life cycle of norepinephrine.**
Note that transmission mediated by NE is terminated by reuptake of NE into the nerve terminal, and not by enzymatic degradation. Be aware that, although postsynaptic cells may have alpha$_1$, beta$_1$, and beta$_2$ receptors, NE can activate only postsynaptic alpha$_1$ and beta$_1$ receptors; physiologic activation of beta$_2$ receptors is done by epinephrine. (*DA,* Dopamine; *MAO,* monoamine oxidase; *NE,* norepinephrine.)

transmitters' life cycles, knowledge of these cycles helps us understand drug actions.

Life Cycle of Acetylcholine

The life cycle of acetylcholine (ACh) is depicted in Fig. 13.7. The cycle begins with synthesis of ACh from two precursors: choline and acetylcoenzyme A. Following synthesis, ACh is stored in vesicles and later released in response to an action potential. Following release, ACh binds to receptors (nicotinic$_N$, nicotinic$_M$, or muscarinic) located on the postjunctional cell. Upon dissociating from its receptors, ACh is destroyed almost instantaneously by *acetylcholinesterase* (AChE), an enzyme present in abundance on the surface of the postjunctional cell. AChE degrades ACh into two inactive products: acetate and choline. Uptake of choline into the cholinergic nerve terminal completes the life cycle of ACh. Note that an inactive substance (choline), and not the active transmitter (ACh), is taken back up for reuse.

Therapeutic and toxic agents can interfere with the ACh life cycle at several points. Botulinum toxin inhibits ACh release. A number of medicines and poisons act at cholinergic receptors to mimic or block the actions of ACh. Several therapeutic and toxic agents act by inhibiting AChE, thereby causing ACh to accumulate in the junctional gap.

Life Cycle of Norepinephrine

The life cycle of norepinephrine is depicted in Fig. 13.8. As indicated, the cycle begins with synthesis of norepinephrine from a series of precursors. The final step of synthesis takes place within vesicles, where norepinephrine is then stored before release. Following release, norepinephrine binds to adrenergic receptors. Norepinephrine can interact with *postsynaptic* alpha$_1$ and beta$_1$ receptors (but not with beta$_2$ receptors) and with *presynaptic* alpha$_2$ receptors. Transmission is terminated by *reuptake* of norepinephrine back into the nerve terminal. (Note that the termination process for norepinephrine differs from that for ACh, whose effects are terminated by enzymatic degradation rather than reuptake.) Following reuptake, norepinephrine can undergo one of two fates: (1) uptake into vesicles for reuse or (2) inactivation by monoamine oxidase (MAO), an enzyme found in the nerve terminal.

Practically every step in the life cycle of norepinephrine can be altered by therapeutic agents. We have drugs that alter the synthesis, storage, and release of norepinephrine; we have drugs that act at adrenergic receptors to mimic or block the effects of norepinephrine; we have drugs, such as cocaine and tricyclic antidepressants, that inhibit the reuptake of norepinephrine (and thereby intensify transmission); and we have drugs that inhibit the breakdown of norepinephrine by MAO, causing an increase in the amount of transmitter available for release.

Life Cycle of Epinephrine

The life cycle of epinephrine is much like that of norepinephrine—although there are significant differences. The cycle begins with synthesis of epinephrine within chromaffin cells of the adrenal medulla. These cells produce epinephrine by first making norepinephrine, which is then converted enzymatically to epinephrine. (Because sympathetic neurons lack the enzyme needed to convert norepinephrine to epinephrine, epinephrine is not produced in sympathetic nerves.) Following synthesis, epinephrine is stored in vesicles to await release. Once released, epinephrine travels via the bloodstream to target organs throughout the body, where it can activate alpha$_1$, alpha$_2$, beta$_1$, and beta$_2$ receptors. Termination of epinephrine actions is accomplished primarily by hepatic metabolism, and not by uptake into nerves.

It's a lot of work, but there's really no way around it: You've got to incorporate this information into your personal database (i.e., memorize it).

KEY POINTS

- The PNS has two major divisions: the autonomic nervous system and the somatic motor system.
- The autonomic nervous system has two major divisions: the sympathetic nervous system and the parasympathetic nervous system.
- The parasympathetic nervous system has several functions relevant to pharmacology: it slows heart rate, increases gastric secretion, empties the bladder and bowel, focuses the eye for near vision, constricts the pupil, and contracts bronchial smooth muscle.
- Principal functions of the sympathetic nervous system are regulation of the cardiovascular system, regulation of body temperature, and implementation of the fight-or-flight response.
- In some organs (e.g., the heart), sympathetic and parasympathetic nerves have opposing effects. In other organs (e.g., male sex organs), the sympathetic and parasympathetic systems have complementary effects. And in still other organs (notably blood vessels), function is regulated by only one branch of the autonomic nervous system.
- The baroreceptor reflex helps regulate blood pressure.
- In most organs regulated by the autonomic nervous system, the parasympathetic nervous system provides the predominant tone.
- In blood vessels, the sympathetic nervous system provides the predominant tone.
- Pathways from the spinal cord to organs under sympathetic and parasympathetic control consist of two neurons: a preganglionic neuron and a postganglionic neuron.
- The adrenal medulla is the functional equivalent of a postganglionic sympathetic neuron.
- Somatic motor pathways from the spinal cord to skeletal muscles have only one neuron.
- The PNS employs three transmitters: acetylcholine, norepinephrine, and epinephrine.
- Acetylcholine is the transmitter released by all preganglionic neurons of the sympathetic nervous system, all preganglionic neurons of the parasympathetic nervous system, all postganglionic neurons of the parasympathetic nervous system, postganglionic neurons of the sympathetic nervous system that go to sweat glands, and all motor neurons.
- Norepinephrine is the transmitter released by all postganglionic neurons of the sympathetic nervous system, except those that go to sweat glands.
- Epinephrine is the major transmitter released by the adrenal medulla.
- There are three major subtypes of cholinergic receptors: $nicotinic_N$, $nicotinic_M$, and muscarinic.
- There are four major subtypes of adrenergic receptors: $alpha_1$, $alpha_2$, $beta_1$, and $beta_2$.
- Although receptor subtypes are of uncertain physiologic significance, they are of great pharmacologic significance.
- Activation of $nicotinic_N$ receptors promotes transmission at all autonomic ganglia, and promotes release of epinephrine from the adrenal medulla.
- Activation of $nicotinic_M$ receptors causes contraction of skeletal muscle.
- Activation of muscarinic receptors increases glandular secretion (from pulmonary, gastric, intestinal, and sweat glands); contracts smooth muscle in the bronchi and GI tract; slows heart rate; contracts the iris sphincter; contracts the ciliary muscle (thereby focusing the lens for near vision); dilates blood vessels; and promotes bladder voiding (by contracting the bladder detrusor muscle and relaxing the trigone and sphincter).
- Activation of $alpha_1$ receptors contracts the radial muscle of the eye (causing mydriasis), constricts veins and arterioles, promotes ejaculation, and contracts smooth muscle in the prostatic capsule and bladder (trigone and sphincter).
- Activation of *peripheral* $alpha_2$ receptors is of minimal pharmacologic significance.
- Activation of $beta_1$ receptors increases heart rate, force of myocardial contraction, and conduction velocity through the atrioventricular node, and promotes release of renin by the kidney.
- Activation of $beta_2$ receptors dilates the bronchi, relaxes uterine smooth muscle, increases glycogenolysis, enhances contraction of skeletal muscle, and dilates arterioles (in the heart, lungs, and skeletal muscle).
- Activation of dopamine receptors dilates blood vessels in the kidney.
- Norepinephrine can activate $alpha_1$, $alpha_2$, and $beta_1$ receptors, whereas epinephrine can activate $alpha_1$, $alpha_2$, $beta_1$, and $beta_2$ receptors.
- Neurotransmission at cholinergic junctions is terminated by degradation of acetylcholine by acetylcholinesterase.
- Neurotransmission at adrenergic junctions is terminated by reuptake of intact norepinephrine into nerve terminals.
- Following reuptake, norepinephrine may be stored in vesicles for reuse or destroyed by monoamine oxidase.

Please visit **http://evolve.elsevier.com/Lehne** for chapter-specific NCLEX® examination review questions.

CHAPTER

14 Muscarinic Agonists and Antagonists

INTRODUCTION TO CHOLINERGIC DRUGS

Cholinergic drugs are agents that influence the activity of cholinergic receptors. Most of these drugs act directly at cholinergic receptors, where they either mimic or block the actions of acetylcholine. The remainder—the cholinesterase inhibitors—influence cholinergic receptors indirectly by preventing the breakdown of acetylcholine. Cholinesterase inhibitors are discussed in Chapter 15.

The cholinergic drugs have both therapeutic and toxicologic significance. Therapeutic applications are limited but valuable. The toxicology of cholinergic drugs is extensive, encompassing such agents as nicotine, insecticides, and compounds designed for chemical warfare.

There are six categories of cholinergic drugs. These categories, along with representative agents, are shown in Table 14.1. The *muscarinic agonists,* represented by bethanechol, selectively mimic the effects of acetylcholine at muscarinic receptors. The *muscarinic antagonists,* represented by atropine, selectively block the effects of acetylcholine (and other muscarinic agonists) at muscarinic receptors. These two categories are discussed in this chapter.

Ganglionic stimulating agents, represented by nicotine itself, selectively mimic the effects of acetylcholine at $nicotinic_N$ receptors of autonomic ganglia. These drugs have little therapeutic value beyond the use of nicotine in smoking cessation programs (see Chapter 39). *Ganglionic blocking agents,* represented by mecamylamine, selectively block ganglionic $nicotinic_N$ receptors. *Neuromuscular blocking agents,* represented by *d*-tubocurarine and succinylcholine, selectively block the effects of acetylcholine at $nicotinic_M$ receptors at the neuromuscular junction. These three categories are discussed in Chapter 16.

The *cholinesterase inhibitors,* represented by neostigmine and physostigmine, prevent the breakdown of acetylcholine by acetylcholinesterase, and thereby increase the activation of all cholinergic receptors. This category is discussed in Chapter 15.

PATIENT-CENTERED CARE ACROSS THE LIFE SPAN

Cholinergic and Anticholinergic Drugs

Life Stage	Patient Care Concerns
Children	Anticholinergics have a prominent role in the management of respiratory conditions in childhood. Administration by inhalation decreases systemic effects. There is no contraindication to systemic use due to age, but due to numerous adverse effects, benefits should be weighed against risk.
Pregnant women	The Pregnancy Risk Category for cholinergic and anticholinergic drugs ranges from B (oxybutynin) to D (nicotine) with the remainder falling under category C.[a] Due to a lack of sufficient animal studies and clinical trials, the full risk is unknown. Caution is recommended with a strong consideration of whether benefits derived are worth potential risks.
Breast-feeding women	Anticholinergics may inhibit lactation in some women, resulting in decreased production of breast milk. Due to a lack of studies, full risks of breast-feeding are unknown. If decisions to breast-feed are made, monitor the infant to identify possible cholinergic or anticholinergic effects.
Older adults	Anticholinergic drugs have been designated as potentially inappropriate for use in geriatric patients. They can cause confusion, blurred vision, tachycardia, urinary retention, and constipation. Many of these complicate preexisting conditions (e.g., urinary retention secondary to benign prostatic hyperplasia) and increase the risk for other conditions (e.g., narrow-angle glaucoma risk secondary to pupil dilation and heat-related illness secondary to hyperthermia and impaired sweating mechanisms).

[a]As of 2020, the FDA will no longer use Pregnancy Risk Categories. Please refer to Chapter 9 for more information.

Table 14.2 is your key to understanding the cholinergic drugs. It lists the three major subtypes of cholinergic receptors (muscarinic, nicotinic$_N$, and nicotinic$_M$) and indicates for each receptor type: (1) location, (2) responses to activation, (3) drugs that produce activation (agonists), and (4) drugs that prevent activation (antagonists). This information, along with the detailed information on cholinergic receptor functions summarized in Table 13.2, is just about all you need to predict the actions of cholinergic drugs.

An example will demonstrate the combined value of Tables 14.2 and 13.2. Let's consider bethanechol. As shown in Table 14.2, bethanechol is a selective *agonist* at *muscarinic* cholinergic receptors. Referring to Table 13.2, we see that activation of muscarinic receptors can produce the following: ocular effects (miosis and ciliary muscle contraction), slowing of heart rate, bronchial constriction, urination, glandular secretion, stimulation of the gastrointestinal (GI) tract, and vasodilation. Because bethanechol *activates* muscarinic receptors, the drug is capable of eliciting all of these responses. Therefore, by knowing which receptors bethanechol activates (from Table 14.2), and by knowing what those receptors do (from Table 13.2), you can predict the kinds of responses you might expect bethanechol to produce.

In the chapters that follow, we will employ the approach just described. That is, for each cholinergic drug discussed, you will want to know (1) the receptors that the drug affects, (2) the normal responses to activation of those receptors, and (3) whether the drug in question increases or decreases receptor activation. All of this information is contained in Tables 14.2 and 13.2. If you learn this information now, you will be prepared to follow discussions in succeeding chapters with relative ease.

MUSCARINIC AGONISTS AND ANTAGONISTS

The muscarinic agonists and antagonists produce their effects through *direct* interaction with muscarinic receptors. The muscarinic agonists cause receptor activation; the antagonists produce receptor blockade. Like the muscarinic agonists, another group of drugs—the cholinesterase inhibitors—can also cause receptor activation, but they do so by an *indirect* mechanism. These drugs are discussed separately in Chapter 15.

MUSCARINIC AGONISTS

The muscarinic agonists bind to muscarinic receptors and thereby cause receptor activation. Because nearly all muscarinic receptors are associated with the parasympathetic nervous system, responses to muscarinic agonists closely resemble those produced by stimulation of parasympathetic nerves. Accordingly, muscarinic agonists are also known as *parasympathomimetic agents*.

TABLE 14.1 ▪ Categories of Cholinergic Drugs

Category	Representative Drugs
Muscarinic agonists	Bethanechol
Muscarinic antagonists	Atropine
Ganglionic stimulating agents	Nicotine
Ganglionic blocking agents	Mecamylamine
Neuromuscular blocking agents	*d*-Tubocurarine, succinylcholine
Cholinesterase inhibitors	Neostigmine, physostigmine

Prototype Drugs

CHOLINERGIC AGENTS

Muscarinic Agonists

Bethanechol [Urecholine, Duvoid 🍁]

Muscarinic Antagonists

Atropine [AtroPen, others]

TABLE 14.2 ▪ Cholinergic Drugs and Their Receptors

	Receptor Subtype		
	Muscarinic	**Nicotinic$_N$**	**Nicotinic$_M$**
Receptor Location	Sweat glands Blood vessels All organs regulated by the parasympathetic nervous system	All ganglia of the autonomic nervous system	Neuromuscular junctions (NMJs)
Effects of Receptor Activation	Many, including: ↓ Heart rate ↑ Gland secretion Smooth muscle contraction	Promotes ganglionic transmission	Skeletal muscle contraction
Receptor Agonists	Bethanechol	Nicotine	Nicotine[a]
Receptor Antagonists	Atropine	Mecamylamine	*d*-Tubocurarine, succinylcholine
Indirect-Acting Cholinomimetics	Cholinesterase inhibitors: Physostigmine, neostigmine, and other cholinesterase inhibitors can activate *all* cholinergic receptors (by causing accumulation of acetylcholine at cholinergic junctions)		

[a]The doses of nicotine needed to activate nicotinic$_M$ receptors of the NMJs are much higher than the doses needed to activate nicotinic$_N$ receptors in autonomic ganglia.

Bethanechol

Bethanechol [Urecholine, Duvoid ♣] embodies the properties that typify all muscarinic agonists and will serve as our prototype for the group.

Mechanism of Action

Bethanechol is a direct-acting muscarinic agonist. The drug binds reversibly to muscarinic cholinergic receptors to cause activation. At therapeutic doses, bethanechol acts selectively at muscarinic receptors yet has little or no effect on nicotinic receptors, either in ganglia or in skeletal muscle.

Pharmacologic Effects

Bethanechol can elicit all of the responses typical of muscarinic receptor activation. Accordingly, we can readily predict the effects of bethanechol by knowing the information on muscarinic responses summarized in Table 13.2.

The principal structures affected by muscarinic activation are the *heart, exocrine glands, smooth muscles,* and *eyes.* Muscarinic agonists act on the heart to cause bradycardia (decreased heart rate) and on exocrine glands to increase sweating, salivation, bronchial secretions, and secretion of gastric acid. In smooth muscles of the lungs and GI tract, muscarinic agonists promote contraction. The result is constriction of the bronchi and increased tone and motility of GI smooth muscle. In the bladder, muscarinic activation causes *contraction* of the detrusor muscle and *relaxation* of the trigone and sphincter; the result is bladder emptying. In vascular smooth muscle, these drugs cause relaxation; the resultant vasodilation can produce hypotension. Activation of muscarinic receptors in the eyes has two effects: (1) miosis (pupillary constriction); and (2) contraction of the ciliary muscle, resulting in accommodation for near vision. (The ciliary muscle, which is attached to the lens, focuses the eyes for near vision by altering lens curvature.)

Pharmacokinetics

Bethanechol is available for oral administration. Effects begin in 30 to 60 minutes and persist for about 1 hour. Because bethanechol is a quaternary ammonium compound (Fig. 14.1), the drug crosses membranes poorly. As a result, only a small fraction of each dose is absorbed.

Therapeutic Uses

Although bethanechol can produce a broad spectrum of pharmacologic effects, the drug is approved only for urinary retention.

Urinary Retention. Bethanechol relieves urinary retention by activating muscarinic receptors of the urinary tract. Muscarinic activation relaxes the trigone and sphincter muscles and increases voiding pressure (by contracting the detrusor muscle, which composes the bladder wall). It is approved to treat urinary retention in postoperative and postpartum patients and to treat retention secondary to neurogenic atony of the bladder. The drug should not be used to treat urinary retention caused by physical obstruction of the urinary tract because increased pressure in the tract in the presence of blockage could cause injury. When patients are treated with bethanechol, a bedpan or urinal should be readily available.

Investigational GI Uses. Bethanechol has been used off-label to treat *gastroesophageal reflux.* Benefits may result from increased esophageal motility and increased pressure in the lower esophageal sphincter.

Bethanechol can help treat disorders associated with GI paralysis. Benefits derive from increased tone and motility of GI smooth muscle. Specific applications are *adynamic ileus, gastric atony,* and *postoperative abdominal distention.* Bethanechol should not be given if physical obstruction of the GI tract is present because, in the presence of blockage, increased propulsive contractions might result in damage to the intestinal wall.

Adverse Effects

In theory, bethanechol can produce the full range of muscarinic responses as side effects. However, with oral dosing, side effects are relatively rare.

Cardiovascular System. Bethanechol can cause *hypotension* (secondary to vasodilation) and *bradycardia.* Accordingly, the drug is contraindicated for patients with low blood pressure or low cardiac output.

Gastrointestinal System. At usual therapeutic doses, bethanechol can cause *excessive salivation, increased secretion of gastric acid, abdominal cramps,* and *diarrhea.* Higher doses

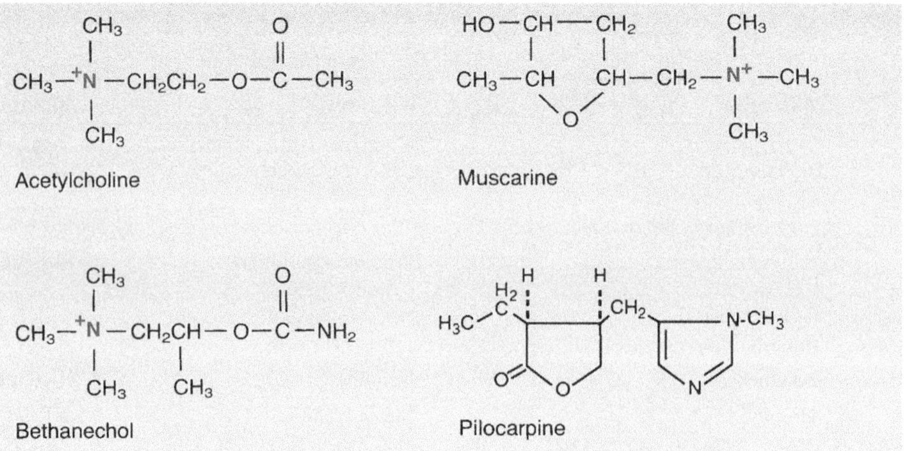

Fig. 14.1 ■ Structures of muscarinic agonists.
Note that, with the exception of pilocarpine, all of these agents are quaternary ammonium compounds and always carry a positive charge. Because of this charge, these compounds cross membranes poorly.

can cause involuntary defecation. Bethanechol is contraindicated in patients with gastric ulcers because stimulation of acid secretion could intensify gastric erosion, causing bleeding and possibly perforation. The drug is also contraindicated for patients with *intestinal obstruction* and for those recovering from recent *surgery of the bowel.* In both cases, the ability of bethanechol to increase the tone and motility of intestinal smooth muscle could result in rupture of the bowel wall.

Urinary Tract. Because of its ability to contract the bladder detrusor, and thereby *increase pressure within the urinary tract,* bethanechol can be hazardous to patients with urinary tract obstruction or weakness of the bladder wall. In both groups, elevation of pressure within the urinary tract could rupture the bladder. Accordingly, bethanechol is contraindicated for patients with either disorder.

Exacerbation of Asthma. By activating muscarinic receptors in the lungs, bethanechol can cause bronchoconstriction. Accordingly, the drug is contraindicated for patients with latent or active asthma.

Dysrhythmias in Hyperthyroid Patients. Bethanechol is contraindicated for people with hyperthyroidism. If given to patients with this condition, bethanechol may increase heart rate to the point of initiating a dysrhythmia. Note that increased heart rate is opposite to the effect that muscarinic agonists have in most patients. This alteration leads to dysrhythmia induction, as explained in the following paragraph.

When hyperthyroid patients are given bethanechol, their initial cardiovascular responses are like those of anyone else: bradycardia and hypotension. In reaction to hypotension, the baroreceptor reflex attempts to return blood pressure to normal. Part of this reflex involves the release of norepinephrine from sympathetic nerves that regulate heart rate. In patients who are not hyperthyroid, norepinephrine release serves to increase cardiac output, and thus helps restore blood pressure. However, in hyperthyroid patients, norepinephrine can induce cardiac dysrhythmias. The reason for this unusual response is that in hyperthyroid patients the heart is exquisitely sensitive to the effects of norepinephrine, and hence relatively small amounts can cause stimulation sufficient to elicit a dysrhythmia.

Preparations, Dosage, and Administration

Bethanechol [Urecholine] is available in tablets (5, 10, 25, and 50 mg) for oral therapy. For adults, the oral dosage ranges from 10 to 50 mg given 3 to 4 times a day. Administration with food can cause nausea and vomiting, so it should be administered 1 hour before meals or 2 hours after.

Other Muscarinic Agonists

Cevimeline

Actions and Uses. Cevimeline [Evoxac] is a derivative of acetylcholine with actions much like those of bethanechol. The drug is indicated for relief of xerostomia (dry mouth) in patients with *Sjögren's syndrome,* an autoimmune disorder characterized by xerostomia. Dry mouth results from extensive damage to salivary glands. Left untreated, dry mouth can lead to multiple complications, including periodontal disease, dental caries, altered taste, oral ulcers and candidiasis, and difficulty eating and speaking. Cevimeline relieves dry mouth by activating muscarinic receptors on residual healthy tissue in salivary glands, thereby promoting salivation. Because it stimulates salivation, cevimeline may also benefit patients with xerostomia induced by radiation therapy for head and neck cancer, although the drug is not approved for this use.

Cevimeline has also been used to manage *keratoconjunctivitis sicca* (dryness of the cornea and conjunctiva, commonly called dry eye). It is helpful in managing these conditions because it increases tear production.

Adverse Effects. Adverse effects result from activating muscarinic receptors, and hence are similar to those of bethanechol. The most common effects are *excessive sweating, nausea, rhinitis,* and *diarrhea.* To compensate for fluid loss caused by sweating and diarrhea, patients should increase fluid intake. Like bethanechol, cevimeline promotes *miosis* (constriction of the pupil) and may also cause *blurred vision.* Both actions can make driving dangerous, especially at night.

Activation of cardiac muscarinic receptors can reduce heart rate and slow cardiac conduction. Accordingly, cevimeline should be used with caution in patients with a history of heart disease.

Because muscarinic activation increases airway resistance, cevimeline is contraindicated for patients with uncontrolled asthma, and should be used with caution in patients with controlled asthma, chronic bronchitis, or chronic obstructive pulmonary disease (COPD).

Because miosis can exacerbate symptoms of both narrow-angle glaucoma and iritis (inflammation of the iris), cevimeline is contraindicated for people with these disorders.

Drug Interactions. Cevimeline can intensify cardiac depression caused by beta blockers because both drugs decrease heart rate and cardiac conduction.

Beneficial effects of cevimeline can be antagonized by drugs that block muscarinic receptors. Among these are atropine, tricyclic antidepressants (e.g., imipramine), antihistamines (e.g., diphenhydramine), and phenothiazine antipsychotics (e.g., chlorpromazine).

Preparations, Dosage, and Administration. See Table 14.3 for preparation, dosage, and administration of cevimeline and other muscarinic agonists.

Pilocarpine

Pilocarpine is a muscarinic agonist used mainly for topical therapy of glaucoma, an ophthalmic disorder characterized by elevated intraocular pressure with

TABLE 14.3 ▪ Preparation, Dosage, and Administration of Muscarinic Agonists

Drug	Preparation	Dosage	Administration
MUSCARINIC AGONISTS			
Bethanechol [Urecholine, Duvoid ♣]	Tablets: 5, 10, 25, 50 mg	10–50 mg 3–4 times/day	1 hr before meals or 2 hr after to prevent nausea and vomiting
Cevimeline [Evoxac]	Capsules: 30 mg	30 mg 3 times/day	May be given without regard to food. Food decreases the rate of absorption but not the amount absorbed.
Pilocarpine Ophthalmic [Isopto Carpine, Diocarpine ♣, Pilopine HS]	Solution: 1% in 15 mL, 2% in 15 mL, and 4% in 15 mL Gel: 4%	Solution: 1–2 gtts to affected eye up to 6 times/day Gel: apply a 0.5-in ribbon onto the lower conjunctival sac at hs	Apply pressure to lacrimal area for 1–2 min postadministration. If both solution and gel are needed, patient should apply the solution first and wait 5 min before applying the gel.
Pilocarpine Systemic [Salagen]	Tablets: 5, 7.5 mg	*Sjögren's syndrome:* 5 mg 4 times/day Postradiotherapy for cancer: 5 mg 3 times/day initially, may be titrated upward to 10 mg 3 times/day	Avoid administration with high-fat meals due to decreased rate of absorption.

subsequent injury to the optic nerve. The basic pharmacology of pilocarpine and its use in glaucoma are discussed in Chapter 104.

In addition to its use in glaucoma, oral pilocarpine is approved for treatment of dry mouth resulting from Sjögren's syndrome or from salivary gland damage caused by radiation therapy of head and neck cancer. For these applications, pilocarpine is available under the brand name *Salagen*. It may also be given to manage dry mouth secondary to head and neck cancer. At lower doses, the principal adverse effect is sweating. However, if dosage is excessive, pilocarpine can produce the full spectrum of muscarinic effects.

Acetylcholine

Clinical use of acetylcholine [Miochol-E] is limited primarily to producing rapid miosis (pupil constriction) following lens delivery in cataract surgery. Two factors explain the limited utility of this drug. First, acetylcholine lacks selectivity (in addition to activating muscarinic cholinergic receptors, acetylcholine can also activate all nicotinic cholinergic receptors). Second, because of rapid destruction by cholinesterase, acetylcholine has a half-life that is extremely short—too short for most clinical applications.

Muscarine

Although muscarine is not used clinically, this agent has historic and toxicologic significance. Muscarine is of historic interest because of its role in the discovery of cholinergic receptor subtypes. The drug has toxicologic significance because of its presence in certain poisonous mushrooms.

Toxicology of Muscarinic Agonists

Sources of Muscarinic Poisoning

Muscarinic poisoning can result from ingestion of certain mushrooms and from overdose with two kinds of medications: (1) direct-acting muscarinic agonists (e.g., bethanechol, pilocarpine), and (2) cholinesterase inhibitors (indirect-acting cholinomimetics).

Some poisonous mushrooms exert their effects through muscarinic activation. Mushrooms of the *Inocybe* and *Clitocybe* species have lots of muscarine, hence their ingestion can produce typical signs of muscarinic toxicity. Interestingly, *Amanita muscaria,* the mushroom from which muscarine was originally extracted, actually contains very little muscarine. Poisoning by this mushroom is due to toxins other than muscarinic agonists.

Symptoms

Manifestations of muscarinic poisoning result from excessive activation of muscarinic receptors. Prominent symptoms are profuse salivation, lacrimation (tearing), visual disturbances, bronchospasm, diarrhea, bradycardia, and hypotension. Severe poisoning can produce cardiovascular collapse.

Treatment

Management is direct and specific: administer *atropine* (a selective muscarinic blocking agent) and provide supportive therapy. By blocking access of muscarinic agonists to their receptors, atropine can reverse most signs of toxicity.

MUSCARINIC ANTAGONISTS (ANTICHOLINERGIC DRUGS)

Muscarinic antagonists competitively block the actions of acetylcholine at muscarinic receptors. Because the majority of muscarinic receptors are located on structures innervated by parasympathetic nerves, the muscarinic antagonists are also known as *parasympatholytic drugs.* Additional names for these agents are *antimuscarinic drugs, muscarinic blockers,* and *anticholinergic drugs.*

The term *anticholinergic* can be a source of confusion and requires comment. This term is unfortunate in that it implies blockade at *all* cholinergic receptors. However, as normally used, the term *anticholinergic* denotes blockade of only *muscarinic* receptors. Therefore, when a drug is characterized as being anticholinergic, you can take this to mean that it produces selective *muscarinic* blockade—and not blockade of all cholinergic receptors. In this chapter, the terms *muscarinic antagonist* and *anticholinergic agent* are used interchangeably.

Safety Alert

BEERS CRITERIA

Anticholinergic drugs have been designated as potentially inappropriate for use in geriatric patients.

Atropine

Atropine [AtroPen, others] is the best-known muscarinic antagonist and will serve as our prototype for the group. The actions of all other muscarinic blockers are much like those of this drug.

Atropine is found naturally in a variety of plants, including *Atropa belladonna* (deadly nightshade) and *Datura stramonium* (aka Jimson weed, stinkweed, and devil's apple). Because of its presence in *Atropa belladonna,* atropine is referred to as a *belladonna alkaloid.*

Mechanism of Action

Atropine produces its effects through competitive blockade at muscarinic receptors. Like all other receptor antagonists, atropine has no direct effects of its own. Rather, all responses to atropine result from *preventing receptor activation* by endogenous acetylcholine (or by drugs that act as muscarinic agonists).

At therapeutic doses, atropine produces selective blockade of muscarinic cholinergic receptors. However, if the dosage is sufficiently high, the drug will produce some blockade of nicotinic receptors too.

Pharmacologic Effects

Because atropine acts by causing muscarinic receptor blockade, its effects are opposite to those caused by muscarinic activation. Accordingly, we can readily predict the effects of atropine by knowing the normal responses to muscarinic receptor activation (see Table 13.2) and by knowing that atropine will reverse those responses. Like the muscarinic agonists, the muscarinic antagonists exert their influence primarily on the *heart, exocrine glands, smooth muscles,* and *eyes.*

Heart. Atropine *increases heart rate.* Because activation of cardiac muscarinic receptors decreases heart rate, blockade of these receptors will cause heart rate to increase.

Exocrine Glands. Atropine *decreases secretion* from salivary glands, bronchial glands, sweat glands, and the acid-secreting cells of the stomach. Note that these effects are opposite to those of muscarinic agonists, which increase secretion from exocrine glands.

Smooth Muscle. By preventing activation of muscarinic receptors on smooth muscle, atropine causes *relaxation of the bronchi, decreased tone of the urinary bladder detrusor,* and *decreased tone and motility of the GI tract.* In the absence of an exogenous muscarinic agonist (e.g., bethanechol), muscarinic blockade has no effect on vascular smooth muscle tone because there is no parasympathetic innervation to muscarinic receptors in blood vessels.

Eyes. Blockade of muscarinic receptors on the iris sphincter causes *mydriasis* (dilation of the pupil). Blockade of muscarinic receptors on the ciliary muscle produces *cycloplegia* (relaxation of the ciliary muscle), thereby focusing the lens for far vision.

Central Nervous System. At therapeutic doses, atropine can cause mild central nervous system (CNS) *excitation.* Toxic doses can cause *hallucinations* and *delirium,* which can resemble psychosis. Extremely high doses can result in coma, respiratory arrest, and death.

Dose Dependency of Muscarinic Blockade. It is important to note that not all muscarinic receptors are equally sensitive to blockade by atropine and most other anticholinergic drugs: At some sites, muscarinic receptors can be blocked with relatively low doses, whereas at other sites much higher doses are needed. Table 14.4 indicates the sequence in which specific muscarinic receptors are blocked as the dose of atropine is increased.

Differences in receptor sensitivity to muscarinic blockers are of clinical significance. As indicated in Table 14.4, the doses needed to block muscarinic receptors in the stomach and bronchial smooth muscle are higher than the doses needed to block muscarinic receptors at all other locations. Accordingly, if we want to use atropine to treat peptic ulcer disease (by suppressing gastric acid secretion) or asthma (by dilating the bronchi), we cannot do so without also affecting the heart, exocrine glands, many smooth muscles, and the eyes. Because of these obligatory side effects, atropine and most other muscarinic antagonists are not preferred drugs for treating peptic ulcers or asthma.

Pharmacokinetics

Atropine may be administered topically (to the eye) and parenterally (IM, IV, and subQ). The drug is rapidly absorbed following administration and distributes to all tissues, including the CNS. Elimination is by a combination of hepatic metabolism and urinary excretion. Atropine has a half-life of approximately 3 hours.

TABLE 14.4 ■ Relationship Between Dosage and Responses to Atropine

Dosage of Atropine	Response Produced
Low dose	Salivary glands—decreased secretion
↓	Sweat glands—decreased secretion
	Bronchial glands—decreased secretion
	Heart—increased rate
	Eyes—mydriasis, blurred vision
	Urinary tract—interference with voiding
	Intestines—decreased tone and motility
	Lungs—dilation of bronchi[a]
High dose	Stomach—decreased acid secretion[a]

[a]Doses of atropine that are high enough to dilate the bronchi or decrease gastric acid secretion will also affect all other structures under muscarinic control. As a result, atropine and most other muscarinic antagonists are not very desirable for treating peptic ulcer disease or asthma.

Therapeutic Uses

Preanesthetic Medication. The cardiac effects of atropine can help during surgery. Procedures that stimulate baroreceptors of the carotid body can initiate reflex slowing of the heart, resulting in profound bradycardia. Because this reflex is mediated by muscarinic receptors on the heart, pretreatment with atropine can prevent a dangerous reduction in heart rate.

Certain anesthetics irritate the respiratory tract, and thereby stimulate secretion from salivary, nasal, pharyngeal, and bronchial glands. If these secretions are sufficiently profuse, they can interfere with respiration. By blocking muscarinic receptors on secretory glands, atropine can help prevent excessive secretions. Fortunately, modern anesthetics are much less irritating. The availability of these new anesthetics has greatly reduced the use of atropine for this purpose during anesthesia.

Disorders of the Eyes. By blocking muscarinic receptors in the eyes, atropine can cause mydriasis and paralysis of the ciliary muscle. Both actions can be of help during eye examinations and ocular surgery. The ophthalmic uses of atropine and other muscarinic antagonists are discussed in Chapter 104.

Bradycardia. Atropine can accelerate heart rate in certain patients with bradycardia. Heart rate is increased because blockade of cardiac muscarinic receptors reverses parasympathetic slowing of the heart.

Intestinal Hypertonicity and Hypermotility. By blocking muscarinic receptors in the intestine, atropine can decrease both the tone and motility of intestinal smooth muscle. This can be beneficial in conditions characterized by excessive intestinal motility, such as mild dysentery and diverticulitis. When taken for these disorders, atropine can reduce both the frequency of bowel movements and associated abdominal cramps.

Muscarinic Agonist Poisoning. Atropine is a specific antidote to poisoning by agents that activate muscarinic receptors. By blocking muscarinic receptors, atropine can reverse all signs of muscarinic poisoning. As discussed previously, muscarinic poisoning can result from an overdose with medications that promote muscarinic activation (e.g., bethanechol, cholinesterase inhibitors) or from ingestion of certain mushrooms.

Peptic Ulcer Disease. Because it can suppress secretion of gastric acid, atropine has been used to treat peptic ulcer disease. Unfortunately, when administered in doses that are strong enough to block the muscarinic receptors that regulate secretion of gastric acid, atropine also blocks most other muscarinic receptors. Therefore, use of atropine in the treatment of ulcers is associated with a broad range of antimuscarinic side effects (e.g., dry mouth, blurred vision, urinary retention, constipation). Because of these side effects, atropine is not a first-choice drug for ulcer therapy. Rather, atropine is reserved for rare cases in which symptoms cannot be relieved with preferred medications (e.g., antibiotics, $histamine_2$ receptor antagonists, proton pump inhibitors).

Asthma. By blocking bronchial muscarinic receptors, atropine can promote bronchial dilation, thereby improving respiration in patients with asthma. Unfortunately, in addition to dilating the bronchi, atropine also causes drying and thickening of bronchial secretions, effects that can be harmful to patients with asthma. Furthermore, when given in the doses needed to dilate the bronchi, atropine causes a variety of antimuscarinic side effects. Because of the potential for harm and because superior medicines are available, atropine is rarely used for asthma.

Biliary Colic. Biliary colic is characterized by intense abdominal pain brought on by passage of a gallstone through the bile duct. In some cases, atropine may be combined with analgesics such as morphine to relax biliary tract smooth muscle, thereby helping alleviate discomfort.

Adverse Effects

Most adverse effects of atropine and other anticholinergic drugs are the direct result of muscarinic receptor blockade.

Accordingly, these effects can be predicted from your knowledge of muscarinic receptor function.

Xerostomia (Dry Mouth). Blockade of muscarinic receptors on salivary glands can inhibit salivation, thereby causing dry mouth. Not only is this uncomfortable, but it also can impede swallowing and can promote tooth decay, gum problems, and oral infections. Patients should be informed that dryness can be alleviated by sipping fluids, chewing sugar-free gum (e.g., Altoids Chewing Gum, Biotene Dry Mouth Gum), treating the mouth with a saliva substitute (e.g., Salivart, Biotene Gel), and using an alcohol-free mouthwash (Biotene mouthwash). Owing to increased risk of tooth decay, patients should avoid sugary gum and hard candy, which are commonly used to alleviate dry mouth.

Blurred Vision and Photophobia. Blockade of muscarinic receptors on the ciliary muscle and the sphincter of the iris can paralyze these muscles. Paralysis of the ciliary muscle focuses the eye for far vision, causing nearby objects to appear blurred. Patients should be forewarned about this effect and advised to avoid hazardous activities if vision is impaired.

Additionally, paralysis of the iris sphincter prevents constriction of the pupil, thereby rendering the eye unable to adapt to bright light. Patients should be advised to wear dark glasses if photophobia (intolerance to light) is a problem. Room lighting for hospitalized patients should be kept low.

Elevation of Intraocular Pressure. Paralysis of the iris sphincter can raise intraocular pressure (IOP) by a mechanism discussed in Chapter 104. Because they can increase IOP, anticholinergic drugs are contraindicated for patients with glaucoma, a disease characterized by abnormally high IOP. In addition, these drugs should be used with caution in patients who may not have glaucoma per se but for whom a predisposition to glaucoma may be present.

Urinary Retention. Blockade of muscarinic receptors in the urinary tract reduces pressure within the bladder and increases the tone of the urinary sphincter and trigone. These effects can produce urinary hesitancy or urinary retention. In the event of severe urinary retention, catheterization or treatment with a muscarinic agonist (e.g., bethanechol) may be required. Patients should be advised that urinary retention can be minimized by voiding just before taking their medication.

Constipation. Muscarinic blockade decreases the tone and motility of intestinal smooth muscle. The resultant delay in transit through the intestine can produce constipation. Patients should be informed that constipation can be minimized by increasing dietary fiber, fluids, and physical activity. A laxative may be needed if constipation is severe. Because of their ability to decrease smooth muscle tone, muscarinic antagonists are contraindicated for patients with intestinal atony, a condition in which intestinal tone is already low.

Anhidrosis. Blockade of muscarinic receptors on sweat glands can produce anhidrosis (a deficiency or absence of sweat). Because sweating is necessary for cooling, people who cannot sweat are at risk of hyperthermia. Patients should be warned of this possibility and advised to avoid activities that might lead to overheating (e.g., exercising on a hot day).

Tachycardia. Blockade of cardiac muscarinic receptors eliminates parasympathetic influence on the heart. By removing the "braking" influence of parasympathetic nerves, anticholinergic agents can cause tachycardia (excessive heart rate). Exercise caution in patients with preexisting tachycardia.

Asthma. In patients with asthma, antimuscarinic drugs can cause thickening and drying of bronchial secretions and can thereby cause bronchial plugging. Consequently, although muscarinic antagonists can be used to treat asthma, they can also do harm.

Drug Interactions

A number of drugs that are not classified as muscarinic antagonists can nonetheless produce significant muscarinic blockade. Among these are antihistamines, phenothiazine antipsychotics, and tricyclic antidepressants. Because of their prominent anticholinergic actions, these drugs can greatly enhance the antimuscarinic effects of atropine and other antimuscarinic agents. Accordingly, it is wise to avoid combined use of atropine with other drugs that can cause muscarinic blockade.

Preparations, Dosage, and Administration

General Systemic Therapy. Atropine sulfate is available in solution (0.05 to 1 mg/mL) for IM, IV, and subQ administration.

AtroPen for Cholinesterase Inhibitor Poisoning. The AtroPen is a prefilled auto-injector indicated for IM therapy of poisoning with an organophosphate cholinesterase inhibitor (nerve agent or insecticide, discussed in Chapter 15). Four strengths are available: 0.25 and 0.5 mg (for children weighing under 40 pounds), 1 mg (for children 40 to 90 pounds), and 2 mg (for adults and children over 90 pounds). The AtroPen should be used immediately on exposure or if exposure is strongly suspected. Injections are administered into the lateral thigh, directly through clothing if necessary.

Dosing is determined by symptom severity and weight. Dosage by weight is as follows:

- <6.8 kg (<15 lb): administer 0.25 mg/dose
- 6.8 to 18 kg (15 to 40 lb): administer 0.5 mg/dose
- 18 to 41 kg (40 to 90 lb): administer 1 mg/dose
- >41 kg (>90 lb): administer 2 mg/dose

Multiple doses are often required. If symptoms are severe, three weight-based doses should be administered rapidly. If symptoms are mild, one dose should be given; if severe symptoms develop afterward, additional doses can be given up to a maximum of three doses.

Ophthalmology. Formulations for ophthalmic use are discussed in Chapter 104.

Drugs for Overactive Bladder

Overactive Bladder: Characteristics and Overview of Treatment

Overactive bladder (OAB)—also known as urgency incontinence, detrusor instability, and sometimes "can't-hold-it-anymore" incontinence—is a disorder with four major symptoms: urinary urgency (a sudden, compelling desire to urinate), urinary frequency (voiding 8 or more times in 24 hours), nocturia (waking 2 or more times to void), and urge incontinence (involuntary urine leakage associated with a strong urge to void). In most cases, urge incontinence results from *involuntary contractions of the bladder detrusor* (the smooth muscle component of the bladder wall). These contractions are often referred to as detrusor instability or detrusor overactivity. Urge incontinence should not be confused with *stress incontinence,* defined as involuntary urine leakage caused by activities (e.g., exertion, sneezing, coughing, laughter) that increase pressure within the abdominal cavity, or *overflow incontinence*, which is the involuntary leakage of urine from an overly distended bladder.

OAB is a common disorder, affecting up to one-third of Americans. The condition can develop at any age, but is most prevalent in older populations. Among people 40 to 44 years of age, symptoms are reported by 3% of men and 9% of women. In comparison, among those 75 years and older, symptoms are reported by 42% of men and 31% of women. Because urine leakage, the most disturbing symptom, is both unpredictable and potentially embarrassing, many people with OAB curtail travel, social activities, and even work.

OAB has two primary modes of treatment: *behavioral therapy* and *drug therapy.* Behavioral therapy, which is at least as effective as drug therapy and lacks side effects, should be tried first. Behavioral interventions include scheduled voiding, timing fluid intake, doing Kegel exercises (to strengthen pelvic floor muscles), and avoiding caffeine, a diuretic that may also increase detrusor activity. As a rule, drugs should be reserved for patients who don't respond adequately to behavioral measures. If behavioral therapy and drugs are inadequate, a provider may offer specialized treatments (e.g., sacral neuromodulation, peripheral tibial nerve stimulation).

Introduction to Anticholinergic Therapy of OAB

When drug therapy *is* indicated, *anticholinergic agents* (e.g., oxybutynin, tolterodine) are indicated. These drugs block muscarinic receptors on the bladder detrusor and thereby inhibit bladder contractions and the urge to void.

Unfortunately, drugs that block muscarinic receptors in the bladder can also block muscarinic receptors elsewhere and cause the typical anticholinergic side effects previously described. Anticholinergic side effects can be reduced in at least three ways: (1) by using long-acting formulations, (2) by using drugs that don't cross the blood-brain barrier, and (3) by using drugs that are selective for muscarinic receptors in the bladder. Long-acting formulations (e.g., extended-release capsules, transdermal patches) reduce side effects by providing a steady but relatively low level of drug, thereby avoiding the high peak levels that can cause intense side effects. Drugs that can't cross the blood-brain barrier are unable to cause CNS effects.

What about drugs that are selective for muscarinic receptors in the bladder? To answer this question, we must first discuss muscarinic receptor subtypes. As noted in Chapter 13, there are five known muscarinic receptor subtypes. However, only three—designated M_1, M_2, and M_3—have clearly identified functions. Locations of these receptor subtypes, and responses to their activation and blockade, are shown in Table 14.5. As indicated, M_3 receptors are the most widely distributed, being found in salivary glands, the bladder detrusor, GI smooth muscle, and the eyes. M_2 receptors are found only in the heart, and M_1 receptors are found in salivary glands and the CNS. At each location, responses to receptor activation are the same as we discussed in Chapter 13—although, in that chapter, we didn't identify the receptors by subtype; rather, we called all of them *muscarinic.*

With this background, we can consider how receptor selectivity might decrease anticholinergic side effects of drugs for OAB. To be beneficial, an anticholinergic agent must block muscarinic receptors in the bladder detrusor. That is, it must block the M_3 receptor subtype. Because M_3 receptors are also found in GI smooth muscle, the eyes, and salivary glands, an M_3-selective blocker will still have some unwanted anticholinergic effects, namely, constipation (from reducing bowel motility), blurred vision and photophobia (from preventing contraction of the ciliary muscle and iris sphincter), dry eyes (from blocking tear production), and *some* degree of dry mouth (from blocking salivary gland M_3 receptors, while sparing salivary M_1 receptors). But an M_3-selective blocker will *not* cause tachycardia (because muscarinic receptors in the heart are the M_2 type) or impairment of CNS function (because muscarinic receptors in the brain are primarily the M_1 type).

Specific Anticholinergic Drugs for OAB

In the United States, six anticholinergic drugs are approved specifically for OAB (Table 14.6). All six work by M_3-muscarinic receptor blockade, although most block M_1 and M_2 receptors as well. With all of these drugs, we want sufficient M_3 blockade to reduce symptoms of OAB, but not so much as to cause urinary retention. You should be aware that responses to these agents are relatively modest and, for many patients, only slightly better than a placebo. None of the anticholinergics used for OAB is clearly superior to the others. However, if one anticholinergic fails to reduce symptoms, success may occur with a different anticholinergic approved for OAB. The newest drug in the OAB arsenal, mirabegron, is a beta$_3$ agonist rather than an anticholinergic drug. We include this in our discussion, even though it is in a different drug class, so that you have a common location for drugs used to treat OAB.

Oxybutynin. Oxybutynin [Ditropan XL, Gelnique, Oxytrol] is an anticholinergic agent that acts primarily at M_3 muscarinic receptors. The drug is approved only for OAB. Benefits derive from blocking M_3 receptors on the bladder detrusor.

Oxybutynin is rapidly absorbed from the GI tract, achieving peak plasma levels about 1 hour after dosing. However, despite rapid absorption, absolute bioavailability is low (about 6%) because oxybutynin undergoes extensive first-pass metabolism—both in the gut wall and liver—primarily by CYP3A4, the 3A4 isoenzyme of cytochrome P450. One metabolite—*N*-desethyloxybutynin—is highly active, especially against muscarinic receptors in the salivary glands. Oxybutynin is very lipid soluble; therefore, it can penetrate the blood-brain barrier. The drug has a short half-life (2 to 3 hours), and hence multiple daily doses are required.

TABLE 14.5 ▪ Muscarinic Receptor Subtypes

Muscarinic Subtype	Location	Response to Activation	Impact of Blockade
M_1	Salivary glands CNS	Salivation Enhanced cognition	Dry mouth Confusion, hallucinations
M_2	Heart	Bradycardia	Tachycardia
M_3	Salivary glands Bladder: detrusor GI smooth muscle Eyes: Iris sphincter Eyes: Ciliary muscle Eyes: Lacrimal gland	Salivation Contraction (increased pressure) Increased tone and motility Contraction (miosis) Contraction (accommodation) Tearing	Dry mouth Relaxation (decreased pressure) Decreased tone and motility (constipation) Relaxation (mydriasis) Relaxation (blurred vision) Dry eyes

CNS, Central nervous system; *GI,* gastrointestinal.

TABLE 14.6 ▪ Drugs for Overactive Bladder

Generic and Brand Names	Formulation[a]	Dosage: Initial	Dosage: Maximum	Administration
HIGHLY M_3 SELECTIVE ANTICHOLINERGICS				
Darifenacin				
Enablex	ER tablets: 7.5, 15 mg	7.5 mg once daily[b]	15 mg once daily	Swallow whole. May be taken with or without food.
PRIMARILY M_3 SELECTIVE ANTICHOLINERGICS				
Oxybutynin				
(generic only)	Syrup: 5 mg/5 mL	5 mg 2–3 times/day	5 mg 4 times/day	May be taken with or without food.
(generic only)	IR tablets: 5 mg	5 mg 2–3 times/day	5 mg 4 times/day	May be taken with or without food.
Ditropan XL	ER tablets: 5, 10, 15 mg	5 mg once daily	30 mg once daily[c]	Swallow whole. May be taken with or without food.
Oxytrol	Transdermal patch: 36 mg[d]	1 patch twice weekly (delivers 3.9 mg/day)	1 patch twice weekly	Apply to dry, intact skin of the abdomen, hip, or buttock. Rotate sites.
Gelnique	Topical gel pump: 3%/3 pumps Topical gel sachet: 10% (100 mg/gm packet)	*3%:* 3 pumps once daily *10%:* one 100-mg/1-gm gel packet once daily	100 mg once daily	Discard any gel dispensed when priming the pump. Apply to dry, intact, unshaven skin of the abdomen, upper arm, shoulder, or thigh. Rotate sites. Cover site to avoid drug transfer to others.
Solifenacin				
VESIcare	Tablets: 5, 10 mg	5 mg once daily[b]	10 mg once daily	Swallow whole. May be taken with or without food.
NONSELECTIVE ANTICHOLINERGICS				
Fesoterodine				
Toviaz	ER tablets: 4, 8 mg	4 mg once daily[b]	8 mg once daily	Swallow whole. May be taken with or without food.
Tolterodine				
Detrol	IR tablets: 1, 2 mg	2 mg twice daily If poorly tolerated, decrease to 1 mg twice daily[b]	2 mg twice daily	May be taken with or without food.
Detrol LA	ER capsules: 2, 4 mg	4 mg once daily If poorly tolerated, decrease to 2 mg daily	4 mg once daily	Swallow whole. May be taken with or without food.
Trospium				
(generic in U.S.), Trosec 🍁	Tablets: 20 mg	20 mg twice daily[e]	20 mg twice daily	Take 1 hour before meals or on an empty stomach.
(generic in U.S.), Sanctura XR 🍁	ER capsules: 60 mg	60 mg once daily	60 mg once daily	Take in the morning with a full glass of water at least 1 h before meals. Do not take within 2 h of consuming alcohol.
BETA-3 ADRENERGIC AGONISTS				
Mirabegron				
Myrbetriq	ER tablet: 25, 50 mg	25 mg once daily	50 mg once daily	Swallow whole. May be taken with or without food.

[a]*ER,* Extended release; *IR,* immediate release.
[b]Patients with moderate hepatic impairment or who are taking strong CYP3A4 inhibitors should not exceed lowest recommended dosage. Those with severe hepatic impairment should not take this drug.
[c]Titrate dose upward as needed and tolerated.
[d]The amount of drug in the patch is much higher than the amount delivered.
[e]Patients with a creatinine clearance less than 30 mL/min should not exceed 20 mg once daily at bedtime.

Anticholinergic side effects are common. The incidence of dry mouth is very high, in part because of muscarinic blockade by oxybutynin itself and in part because of blockade by *N*-desethyloxybutynin. Other common side effects include constipation, tachycardia, urinary hesitancy, urinary retention, mydriasis, blurred vision, and dry eyes. In the CNS, cholinergic blockade can result in confusion, hallucinations, insomnia, and nervousness. In postmarketing reports of CNS effects, hallucinations and agitation were prominent among reports involving pediatric patients, while hallucinations, confusion, and sedation were prominent among reports involving older adult patients. Combined use of oxybutynin with other anticholinergic agents (e.g., antihistamines, tricyclic antidepressants, phenothiazine antipsychotics) can intensify all anticholinergic side effects.

Drugs that inhibit or induce CYP3A4 may alter oxybutynin blood levels and may thereby either increase toxicity (inhibitors of CYP3A4) or reduce effectiveness (inducers of CYP3A4).

Oxybutynin is available in five formulations. Two are short acting (syrup and immediate-release [IR] tablets), and three are long acting (transdermal patch, topical gel, and extended-release [ER] tablets). Preparation, dosage, and administration of this and other drugs for OAB are presented in Table 14.6. Of note, oxybutynin ER tablets [Ditropan XL] are as effective as the IR tablets and somewhat better tolerated because the anticholinergic side effects are less intense with the long-acting products. The ER tablets have a small hole through which the medication leaks slowly once it is in the gastrointestinal tract. The tablet shell is insoluble; therefore, it is eliminated intact in the feces. Patients should be informed of this fact.

Transdermal Patch. The oxybutynin transdermal system [Oxytrol] provides an alternative method of dosing that is convenient for patients. Owing to its high lipid solubility, oxybutynin from the patch is readily absorbed directly through the skin. A new patch is applied twice weekly to dry, intact skin of the abdomen, hip, or buttock, rotating the site with each change. Reduction of OAB symptoms is about the same as with the ER tablets.

Pharmacokinetically, the patch is unique in two ways. First, absorption is both slow and steady, and hence the patch produces low but stable blood levels of the drug. Second, transdermal absorption bypasses metabolism in the intestinal wall and delays metabolism in the liver. As a result, levels of *N*-desethyloxybutynin, the active metabolite, are less than 20% of those achieved with oral therapy.

Transdermal oxybutynin is generally well tolerated. The most common side effect is application-site pruritus (itching). The incidence of dry mouth is much lower than with the oral formulations, presumably because (1) formation of *N*-desethyloxybutynin is low and (2) high peak levels of oxybutynin itself are avoided. Rates of constipation, blurred vision, and CNS effects are also low.

Topical Gel. Topical oxybutynin gel [Gelnique] is much like the transdermal patch. As with the patch, oxybutynin is absorbed directly through the skin. Stable blood levels are achieved following 10 days of daily application. The most common side effects are application-site reactions and dry mouth. Other reactions include dizziness, headache, and constipation. Gelnique should be applied to dry, intact skin of the abdomen, upper arm/shoulder, or thigh—but not to recently shaved skin—using a different site each day. Advise patients to wash their hands immediately after application and to avoid showering for at least 1 hour. Applying a sunscreen before or after dosing does not alter efficacy. Topical oxybutynin can be transferred to another person through direct contact. To avoid transfer, patients should cover the application site with clothing.

Darifenacin. Of the anticholinergic agents used for OAB, darifenacin [Enablex] displays the greatest degree of M_3 selectivity. As a result, the drug can reduce OAB symptoms while having no effect on M_1 receptors in the brain or M_2 receptors in the heart. However, darifenacin does block M_3 receptors outside the bladder, so it can still cause dry mouth, constipation, and other M_3-related effects.

Clinical benefits are similar to those of oxybutynin and tolterodine. On average, treatment reduces episodes of urge incontinence from 15/week down to 7/week (using 7.5 mg/day) and from 17/week down to 6/week (using 15 mg/day).

Darifenacin is administered orally in ER tablets. Absorption is adequate (15% to 19%), and not affected by food. In the blood, darifenacin is 98% protein bound. The drug undergoes extensive hepatic metabolism, primarily by CYP3A4. The resulting inactive metabolites are excreted in the urine (60%) and feces (40%). The drug's half-life is approximately 12 hours.

Darifenacin is relatively well tolerated. The most common side effect is dry mouth. Constipation is also common. Other adverse effects include dyspepsia, gastritis, and headache. Darifenacin has little or no effect on memory, reaction time, word recognition, or cognition. The drug does not increase heart rate.

Levels of darifenacin can be raised significantly by strong inhibitors of CYP3A4. Among these are azole antifungal drugs (e.g., ketoconazole, itraconazole), certain protease inhibitors used for HIV/AIDS (e.g., ritonavir, nelfinavir), and clarithromycin (a macrolide antibiotic). If darifenacin is combined with any of these, its dosage must be kept low. Low dosage is also important with moderate liver impairment. In patients with severe liver impairment, darifenacin should be avoided.

Solifenacin. Solifenacin [VESIcare] is very similar to darifenacin, although it's not quite as M_3 selective. In clinical trials, the drug reduced episodes of urge incontinence from 18/week down to 8/week (using 5 mg/day) and from 20/week down to 8/week (using 10 mg/day).

Solifenacin undergoes nearly complete absorption after oral dosing, achieving peak plasma levels in 3 to 6 hours. In the blood, the drug is highly (98%) protein bound. Like darifenacin, solifenacin undergoes extensive metabolism by hepatic CYP3A4. The resulting inactive metabolites are excreted in the urine (62%) and feces (23%). Solifenacin has a long half-life (about 50 hours), and hence can be administered just once a day.

The most common adverse effects are dry mouth, constipation, and blurred vision. Dyspepsia, urinary retention, headache, and nasal dryness occur infrequently. Rarely, solifenacin has caused potentially fatal angioedema of the face, lips, tongue, and/or larynx. At high doses, solifenacin can prolong the QT interval, thereby posing a risk of a fatal dysrhythmia. Accordingly, caution is needed in patients with a history of QT prolongation and in those taking other QT-prolonging drugs. As with darifenacin, levels of solifenacin can be increased by strong inhibitors of CYP3A4 (e.g., ketoconazole, ritonavir, clarithromycin). For patients taking a strong CYP3A4 inhibitor or for those with moderate hepatic impairment or severe renal impairment, dosage should be decreased. Patients with severe hepatic impairment should not take solifenacin.

Tolterodine. Tolterodine [Detrol, Detrol LA] is a nonselective muscarinic antagonist approved only for OAB. Like oxybutynin, tolterodine is available in short- and long-acting formulations. Anticholinergic side effects are less intense with the long-acting form.

Immediate-Release Tablets. In patients with OAB, tolterodine IR tablets [Detrol] can reduce the incidence of urge incontinence, urinary frequency, and urinary urgency. However, as with other drugs for OAB, benefits are modest.

Tolterodine is rapidly but variably absorbed from the GI tract. Plasma levels peak 1 to 2 hours after dosing. Following absorption, the drug undergoes conversion to 5-hydroxymethyl tolterodine, its active form. The active metabolite is later inactivated by CYP3A4 and CYP2D6 (the 2D6 isoenzyme of cytochrome P450). Parent drug and metabolites are eliminated in the urine (77%) and feces (17%). Tolterodine has a relatively short half-life.

Anticholinergic side effects with tolterodine affect fewer patients compared with other anticholinergics prescribed for OAB. For example, dry mouth occurs in 35% of patients taking IR tolterodine versus 70% with IR oxybutynin. At low doses, the most common side effects are dry mouth, constipation, and dry eyes. Effects on the CNS—somnolence, vertigo, dizziness—occur infrequently. The incidence of both tachycardia and urinary retention is less than 1%. Drugs that inhibit CYP3A4 (e.g., erythromycin, ketoconazole) can raise levels of tolterodine and can thereby intensify beneficial and adverse effects. *Accordingly, low doses should be prescribed for patients taking a strong inhibitor of CYP3A4. Dosage should also be low for those with significant hepatic or renal impairment.*

In addition to its anticholinergic effects, tolterodine can prolong the QT interval and can thereby promote serious cardiac dysrhythmias. Because of this risk, dosage should not exceed 4 mg/day.

Extended-Release Capsules. Tolterodine ER capsules [Detrol LA] are as effective as the IR tablets and cause less dry mouth. The incidence of other anticholinergic effects is about the same with both formulations. As with the IR tablets, a lower dosage should be used for patients with significant hepatic or renal impairment and for those taking an inhibitor of CYP3A4.

Fesoterodine. Fesoterodine [Toviaz] is a nonselective muscarinic antagonist very similar to tolterodine. Both agents are used only for OAB. Furthermore, both agents undergo conversion to the same active metabolite—5-hydroxymethyl tolterodine—which is later inactivated by CYP3A4 and CYP2D6. In patients taking a strong inhibitor of CYP3A4 (e.g., ketoconazole, clarithromycin), beneficial and adverse effects are increased. Conversely, in patients taking a strong inducer of CYP3A4 (e.g., carbamazepine, fosphenytoin), beneficial and adverse effects are reduced. In patients with severe renal impairment, and in those taking a strong inhibitor of CYP3A4, dosage should be reduced. However, in patients taking a strong inducer or inhibitor of CYP2D6, dosage adjustments are not recommended.

As with tolterodine, the most common side effect is dry mouth. Another common side effect is constipation. Less common side effects include dizziness, fatigue, and blurred vision. Unlike tolterodine, fesoterodine has not been associated with QT prolongation, and hence probably does not pose a risk of dysrhythmias.

Trospium. Trospium [Sanctura XR, Trosec 🍁] is a nonselective muscarinic blocker indicated only for OAB. Like oxybutynin and tolterodine, trospium is available in short- and long-acting formulations. Anticholinergic side effects are less intense with the long-acting form. Compared with other drugs for OAB, trospium is notable for its low bioavailability, lack of CNS effects, and lack of metabolism-related interactions with other drugs.

Immediate-Release Tablets. Trospium IR tablets [Trosec 🍁] reduce episodes of urge incontinence from 27/week down to 12/week (compared with 30/week down to 16/week with placebo). Reductions in urinary frequency are minimal.

Trospium is a quaternary ammonium compound (always carries a positive charge), so it crosses membranes poorly. Following oral dosing, absorption is poor (only 10%) on an empty stomach and is greatly reduced (70% to 80%) by food. Conversely, ethanol can cause an increase in peak serum levels. Plasma levels peak 3.5 to 6 hours after dosing and decline with a half-life of 18 hours. Trospium does not undergo hepatic metabolism and is eliminated unchanged in the urine.

Trospium IR tablets are generally well tolerated. The most common side effects are dry mouth and constipation. Rarely, the drug causes dry eyes and urinary retention. Owing to its positive charge, trospium cannot cross the blood-brain barrier and hence is devoid of CNS effects.

Few studies of drug interactions have been done. However, because trospium is eliminated by the kidneys, we can assume it may compete with other drugs that undergo renal tubular excretion. Among these are vancomycin (an antibiotic), metformin (used for diabetes), and digoxin and procainamide (both used for cardiac disorders). Because trospium is not metabolized, the drug is unlikely to influence hepatic metabolism of other agents.

Extended-Release Capsules. Trospium ER capsules [Sanctura XR 🍁] are as effective as the IR tablets and cause less dry mouth. The incidence of constipation and other side effects is about the same.

Mirabegron. Mirabegron [Myrbetriq] is not an anticholinergic. It is a selective $beta_3$ adrenergic agonist indicated only for management of OAB. $Beta_3$ receptor activation results in relaxation of detrusor muscle in the bladder. This in turn allows for increased filling, thus preventing urinary frequency and urgency.

The effects of mirabegron are modest; however, they provide an alternative therapy for patients who cannot tolerate the anticholinergic options. They may also be given in addition to the anticholinergic drugs.

As mentioned in Chapter 1, there is no such thing as a wholly selective drug. This is also true for mirabegron. While it is primarily selective for $beta_3$ receptors, other adrenergic receptors may be activated. While the effect is usually insignificant—most commonly a slight increase in blood pressure and heart rate—mirabegron should not be administered to patients with uncontrolled hypertension.

Mirabegron can increase digoxin levels, so digoxin dosage may need to be lowered for patients taking this drug. Mirabegron also inhibits CYP2D6 enzymes. This can result in increased levels of drugs that are CYP2D6 substrates.

Other Muscarinic Antagonists

Scopolamine

Scopolamine is an anticholinergic drug with actions much like those of atropine, but with two exceptions. First, whereas therapeutic doses of atropine produce mild CNS *excitation,* therapeutic doses of scopolamine produce *sedation.* And second, scopolamine *suppresses emesis and motion sickness,* whereas atropine does not. Principal uses for scopolamine are motion sickness (see Chapter 80), production of cycloplegia and mydriasis for ophthalmic procedures (see Chapter 104), and production of preanesthetic sedation and obstetric amnesia.

Ipratropium Bromide

Ipratropium [Atrovent] is an anticholinergic drug used to treat asthma, COPD, and rhinitis caused by allergies or the common cold. The drug is administered by inhalation for asthma and COPD and by nasal spray for rhinitis. Systemic absorption is minimal for both formulations. As a result, therapy is not associated with typical antimuscarinic side effects (e.g., dry mouth, blurred vision, urinary hesitancy, constipation). Ipratropium is discussed fully in Chapter 76.

Antisecretory Anticholinergics

Muscarinic blockers can be used to suppress gastric acid secretion in patients with peptic ulcer disease. However, because superior antiulcer drugs are available and because anticholinergic agents produce significant side effects, most of these drugs have been withdrawn. Today, only four agents—*glycopyrrolate* [Robinul, Cuvposa], *mepenzolate* [Cantil], *methscopolamine* [Pamine], and *propantheline* [generic]—remain on the market. All four are administered orally, and one—glycopyrrolate—may also be given IM and IV. Glycopyrrolate oral solution [Cuvposa] is also approved for reducing severe drooling in children with chronic severe neurologic disorders. The drug is also approved for reducing salivation caused by anesthesia. Though it was originally approved as an adjunct in treatment of peptic ulcer disease, it is no longer indicated for this purpose.

Dicyclomine

Dicyclomine [Bentyl, Bentylol 🍁] is indicated for irritable bowel syndrome (spastic colon, mucous colitis) and functional bowel disorders (diarrhea, hypermotility). Administration may be oral (20 to 40 mg 4 times a day) or by IM injection (10 to 20 mg 4 times a day for 1 to 2 days followed by conversion to oral therapy). It should not be administered IV.

Mydriatic Cycloplegics

Five muscarinic antagonists—*atropine, homatropine, scopolamine, cyclopentolate,* and *tropicamide*—are employed to produce mydriasis and cycloplegia in ophthalmic procedures. These applications are discussed in Chapter 104.

Centrally Acting Anticholinergics

Several anticholinergic drugs, including *benztropine* [Cogentin] and *trihexyphenidyl,* are used to treat Parkinson disease and drug-induced parkinsonism. Benefits derive from blockade of muscarinic receptors in the CNS. The centrally acting anticholinergics and their use in Parkinson disease are discussed in Chapter 21.

Toxicology of Muscarinic Antagonists

Sources of Antimuscarinic Poisoning

Sources of poisoning include natural products (e.g., *Atropa belladonna, Datura stramonium*), selective antimuscarinic drugs (e.g., atropine, scopolamine), and other drugs with pronounced antimuscarinic properties (e.g., antihistamines, phenothiazines, tricyclic antidepressants).

Symptoms

Symptoms of antimuscarinic poisoning, which are the direct result of excessive muscarinic blockade, include dry mouth, blurred vision, photophobia (secondary to mydriasis), hyperthermia, CNS effects (hallucinations, delirium), and skin that is hot, dry, and flushed. Death results from respiratory depression secondary to blockade of cholinergic receptors in the brain.

Treatment

Treatment consists of (1) minimizing intestinal absorption of the antimuscarinic agent and (2) administering an antidote. Minimizing absorption is accomplished by administering activated charcoal, which will adsorb the poison within the intestine, thereby preventing its absorption into the blood.

The most effective antidote to antimuscarinic poisoning is *physostigmine,* an inhibitor of acetylcholinesterase. By inhibiting cholinesterase, physostigmine causes acetylcholine to accumulate at all cholinergic junctions. As acetylcholine builds up, it competes with the antimuscarinic agent for receptor binding, thereby reversing excessive muscarinic blockade. The pharmacology of physostigmine is discussed in Chapter 15.

Warning

It is important to differentiate between antimuscarinic poisoning, which often resembles psychosis (hallucinations, delirium), and an actual psychotic episode. We need to make the differential diagnosis because some antipsychotic drugs have antimuscarinic properties of their own, and hence will intensify symptoms if given to a victim of antimuscarinic poisoning. Fortunately, because a true psychotic episode is not ordinarily associated with signs of excessive muscarinic blockade (e.g., dry mouth, hyperthermia, dry skin), differentiation is not usually difficult.

KEY POINTS

- Muscarinic agonists cause direct activation of muscarinic cholinergic receptors, and can thereby cause bradycardia; increased secretion from sweat, salivary, bronchial, and gastric glands; contraction of intestinal and bronchial smooth muscle; contraction of the bladder detrusor and relaxation of the bladder trigone and sphincter; and, in the eyes, miosis and accommodation for near vision.
- Bethanechol, the prototype of the muscarinic agonists, is used primarily to relieve urinary retention.
- Muscarinic agonist poisoning is characterized by profuse salivation, tearing, visual disturbances, bronchospasm, diarrhea, bradycardia, and hypotension.
- Muscarinic agonist poisoning is treated with atropine.
- Atropine, the prototype of the muscarinic antagonists (anticholinergic drugs), blocks the actions of acetylcholine (and all other muscarinic agonists) at muscarinic cholinergic receptors, and thereby (1) increases heart rate; (2) reduces secretion from sweat, salivary, bronchial, and gastric glands; (3) relaxes intestinal and bronchial smooth muscle; (4) causes urinary retention (by relaxing the bladder detrusor and contracting the trigone and sphincter); (5) acts in the eyes to cause mydriasis and cycloplegia; and (6) acts in the CNS to produce excitation (at low doses) and delirium and hallucinations (at toxic doses).
- Applications of anticholinergic drugs include preanesthetic medication, ophthalmic examinations, reversal of bradycardia, treatment of overactive bladder (OAB), and management of muscarinic agonist poisoning.
- Anticholinergic drugs that are selective for M_3 muscarinic receptors can still cause many anticholinergic side effects (e.g., dry mouth, constipation, impaired vision), but will not slow heart rate (which is mediated by cardiac M_2 receptors) and will be largely devoid of cognitive effects (which are mediated primarily by M_1 receptors).
- Classic adverse effects of anticholinergic drugs are dry mouth, blurred vision, photophobia, tachycardia, urinary retention, constipation, and anhidrosis (suppression of sweating).
- Certain drugs—especially antihistamines, tricyclic antidepressants, and phenothiazine antipsychotics—have prominent antimuscarinic actions. These should be used cautiously, if at all, in patients receiving atropine or other muscarinic antagonists.
- The anticholinergic drugs used for OAB are only moderately effective; for many patients they are only slightly better than a placebo. The short-acting anticholinergic drugs used for OAB cause more dry mouth and other anticholinergic side effects than do the long-acting drugs.
- Muscarinic antagonist poisoning is characterized by dry mouth, blurred vision, photophobia, hyperthermia, hallucinations and delirium, and skin that is hot, dry, and flushed.
- The best antidote for muscarinic antagonist poisoning is physostigmine, a cholinesterase inhibitor.

Please visit **http://evolve.elsevier.com/Lehne** for chapter-specific NCLEX® examination review questions.

Summary of Major Nursing Implications[a]

BETHANECHOL

Preadministration Assessment

Therapeutic Goal

Treatment of nonobstructive urinary retention.

Baseline Data

Record fluid intake and output.

Identifying High-Risk Patients

Bethanechol is *contraindicated* for patients with peptic ulcer disease, urinary tract obstruction, intestinal obstruction, coronary insufficiency, hypotension, asthma, and hyperthyroidism.

Implementation: Administration

Route

Oral.

Administration

Advise patients to take bethanechol 1 hour before meals or 2 hours after to reduce gastric upset.

Because effects on the intestine and urinary tract can be rapid and dramatic, ensure that a bedpan or bathroom is readily accessible.

Ongoing Evaluation and Interventions

Evaluating Therapeutic Effects

Monitor fluid intake and output to evaluate treatment of urinary retention.

Minimizing Adverse Effects

Excessive muscarinic activation can cause salivation, sweating, urinary urgency, bradycardia, and hypotension. Monitor blood pressure and pulse rate. Observe for signs of muscarinic excess and report these to the prescriber. **Inform patients about manifestations of muscarinic excess, and advise them to notify the prescriber if they occur.**

Management of Acute Toxicity

Overdose produces manifestations of excessive muscarinic stimulation (salivation, sweating, involuntary urination and defecation, bradycardia, severe hypotension). Treat with parenteral atropine and supportive measures.

Continued

Summary of Major Nursing Implications[a]—cont'd

ATROPINE AND OTHER MUSCARINIC ANTAGONISTS (ANTICHOLINERGIC DRUGS)

Preadministration Assessment

Therapeutic Goal

Atropine has many applications, including preanesthetic medication and treatment of bradycardia, biliary colic, intestinal hypertonicity and hypermotility, and muscarinic agonist poisoning.

Identifying High-Risk Patients

Atropine and other muscarinic antagonists are *contraindicated* for patients with glaucoma, intestinal atony, urinary tract obstruction, and tachycardia. Use with *caution* in patients with asthma.

Implementation: Administration

Routes

Atropine is administered PO, IV, IM, and subQ.

Administration

Dry mouth from muscarinic blockade may interfere with swallowing. **Advise patients to moisten the mouth by sipping water before oral administration.**

Ongoing Evaluation and Interventions

Minimizing Adverse Effects

Xerostomia (Dry Mouth). Decreased salivation can dry the mouth. **Teach patients that xerostomia can be relieved by sipping fluids, chewing sugar-free gum, treating the mouth with a saliva substitute, and using an alcohol-free mouthwash. Owing to increased risk of tooth decay, advise patients to avoid sugared gum, hard candy, and cough drops.**

Blurred Vision. Paralysis of the ciliary muscle may reduce visual acuity. **Warn patients to avoid hazardous activities if vision is impaired.**

Photophobia. Muscarinic blockade prevents the pupil from constricting in response to bright light. Keep room lighting low to reduce visual discomfort. **Advise patients to wear sunglasses outdoors.**

Urinary Retention. Muscarinic blockade in the urinary tract can cause urinary hesitancy or retention. **Advise patients that urinary retention can be minimized by voiding just before taking anticholinergic medication.** If urinary retention is severe, catheterization or treatment with bethanechol (a muscarinic agonist) may be required.

Constipation. Reduced tone and motility of the gut may cause constipation. **Advise patients that constipation can be reduced by increasing dietary fiber and fluids, and treated with a laxative if severe.**

Hyperthermia. Suppression of sweating may result in hyperthermia. **Advise patients to avoid vigorous exercise in warm environments.**

Tachycardia. Blockade of cardiac muscarinic receptors can accelerate heart rate. Monitor pulse and report significant increases.

Minimizing Adverse Interactions

Antihistamines, tricyclic antidepressants, and *phenothiazines* have prominent antimuscarinic actions. Combining these agents with atropine and other anticholinergic drugs can cause excessive muscarinic blockade.

Management of Acute Toxicity

Symptoms. Overdose produces dry mouth, blurred vision, photophobia, hyperthermia, hallucinations, and delirium; the skin becomes hot, dry, and flushed. Differentiate muscarinic antagonist poisoning from psychosis!

Treatment. Treatment centers on limiting absorption of ingested poison (e.g., by giving activated charcoal to adsorb the drug) and administering physostigmine, an inhibitor of acetylcholinesterase.

[a]Patient education information is highlighted as **blue text.**

CHAPTER

15 Cholinesterase Inhibitors and Their Use in Myasthenia Gravis

Cholinesterase inhibitors are drugs that prevent the degradation of acetylcholine by acetylcholinesterase (also known simply as cholinesterase). Cholinesterase inhibitors are also known as *anticholinesterase* drugs. By preventing the breakdown of acetylcholine, cholinesterase inhibitors increase the amount of acetylcholine available to activate receptors, thus enhancing cholinergic action. Because cholinesterase inhibitors do not bind directly with cholinergic receptors, they are viewed as indirect-acting cholinergic agonists. Because use of cholinesterase inhibitors results in transmission at all cholinergic junctions (muscarinic, ganglionic, and neuromuscular), these drugs can elicit a broad spectrum of responses. Because they lack selectivity, cholinesterase inhibitors have limited therapeutic applications.

There are two basic categories of cholinesterase inhibitors: (1) *reversible inhibitors* and (2) *irreversible inhibitors*. The reversible inhibitors produce effects of moderate duration, and the irreversible inhibitors produce effects of long duration.

Prototype Drugs

CHOLINESTERASE INHIBITORS

Reversible Cholinesterase Inhibitors

Neostigmine [Bloxiverz]

REVERSIBLE CHOLINESTERASE INHIBITORS

Neostigmine

Neostigmine [Bloxiverz] typifies the reversible cholinesterase inhibitors and will serve as our prototype for the group. Neostigmine has a role in the management of *myasthenia gravis*. Bloxiverz, a brand name product, is used to reverse the actions of nondepolarizing neuromuscular blockade following surgery.

Chemistry

As shown in Fig. 15.1, neostigmine contains a quaternary nitrogen atom, and hence always carries a positive charge. Because of this charge, neostigmine cannot readily cross membranes, including those of the GI tract, blood-brain barrier, and placenta. Consequently, neostigmine is absorbed poorly following oral administration and has minimal effects on the brain and fetus.

Mechanism of Action

Neostigmine and the other reversible cholinesterase inhibitors act as substrates for cholinesterase. As indicated in Fig. 15.2, the normal function of cholinesterase is to break down acetylcholine into choline and acetic acid. (This process is called a *hydrolysis reaction* because of the water molecule involved.) The overall reaction between acetylcholine and cholinesterase is extremely fast. As a result, one molecule of cholinesterase can break down a huge amount of acetylcholine in a very short time.

The reaction between neostigmine and cholinesterase is much like the reaction between acetylcholine and cholinesterase. The only difference is that cholinesterase splits neostigmine more slowly than it splits acetylcholine. Hence, once neostigmine becomes bound to cholinesterase, the drug remains in place for a relatively long time. Because cholinesterase remains bound until it finally succeeds in degrading neostigmine, less cholinesterase is available to catalyze the breakdown of acetylcholine. As a result, more acetylcholine is available to activate cholinergic receptors.

Pharmacologic Effects

By decreasing breakdown of acetylcholine, neostigmine and the other cholinesterase inhibitors make more acetylcholine available, and this can intensify transmission at virtually all junctions where acetylcholine is the transmitter. In sufficient doses, cholinesterase inhibitors can produce skeletal muscle stimulation, ganglionic stimulation, activation of peripheral muscarinic receptors, and activation of cholinergic receptors in the central nervous system (CNS). However, when used *therapeutically,* cholinesterase inhibitors usually affect only muscarinic receptors on organs and nicotinic receptors of the neuromuscular junction (NMJ). Ganglionic transmission and CNS function are usually unaltered.

Muscarinic Responses. Muscarinic effects of the cholinesterase inhibitors are identical to those of the direct-acting muscarinic agonists. By preventing breakdown of acetylcholine, cholinesterase inhibitors can cause bradycardia, bronchial constriction, urinary urgency, increased glandular secretions, increased tone and motility of GI smooth muscle, miosis, and focusing of the lens for near vision.

Neuromuscular Effects. The effects of cholinesterase inhibitors on skeletal muscle are dose dependent. At *therapeutic* doses, these drugs *increase* force of contraction. In contrast, *toxic* doses *reduce* force of contraction. Contractile force is reduced because excessive amounts of acetylcholine at the NMJ keep the motor end-plate in a state of constant depolarization, causing depolarizing neuromuscular blockade (see Chapter 16).

Central Nervous System. Effects on the CNS vary with drug concentration. *Therapeutic* levels can produce mild *stimulation,* whereas *toxic* levels *depress* the CNS, including the areas that regulate respiration. However, keep in mind that, for CNS effects to occur, the inhibitor must first penetrate the blood-brain barrier, which some cholinesterase inhibitors can do only when present in very high concentrations.

Pharmacokinetics

Neostigmine may be administered IM, IV, or by subQ injection. Because neostigmine carries a positive charge, the drug is poorly absorbed following oral administration. Consequently, oral formulations have been discontinued in the United States although they remain available in Canada and some other countries. Once absorbed, neostigmine can reach sites of action at the NMJ and peripheral muscarinic receptors, but cannot cross the blood-brain barrier to affect the CNS. Duration of action is 2 to 4 hours. Neostigmine is eliminated by enzymatic degradation by cholinesterase.

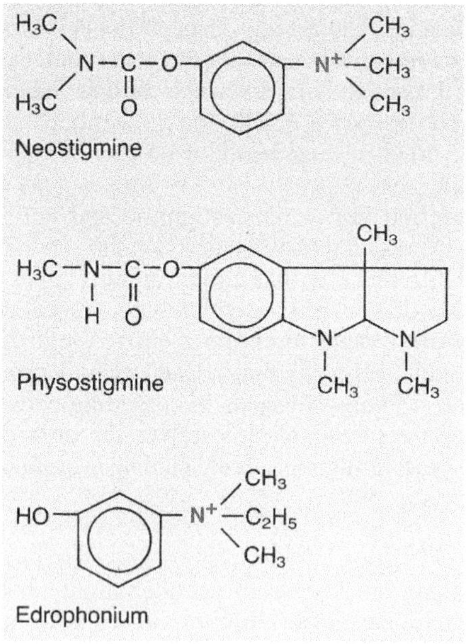

Fig. 15.1 ■ Structural formulas of reversible cholinesterase inhibitors.

Note that neostigmine and edrophonium are quaternary ammonium compounds, but physostigmine is not. What does this difference imply about the relative abilities of these drugs to cross membranes, including the blood-brain barrier?

Therapeutic Uses

Myasthenia Gravis. Myasthenia gravis is a major indication for neostigmine and some other reversible cholinesterase inhibitors. Treatment of myasthenia gravis is discussed later in this chapter.

Reversal of Competitive (Nondepolarizing) Neuromuscular Blockade. By causing accumulation of acetylcholine at the NMJ, cholinesterase inhibitors can reverse the effects of competitive neuromuscular blocking agents (e.g., pancuronium). This ability has two clinical applications: (1) reversal of neuromuscular blockade in postoperative patients and (2) treatment of overdose with a competitive neuromuscular blocker. When neostigmine is used to treat neuromuscular blocker overdose, artificial respiration must be maintained until muscle function has fully recovered. At the doses employed to reverse neuromuscular blockade, neostigmine is likely to elicit substantial muscarinic responses. If necessary, these can be reduced with atropine. It is important to note that cholinesterase inhibitors cannot be employed to counteract the effects of succinylcholine, a *depolarizing* neuromuscular blocker.

Adverse Effects

Excessive Muscarinic Stimulation. Accumulation of acetylcholine at muscarinic receptors can result in excessive salivation, increased gastric secretions, increased tone and motility of the GI tract, urinary urgency, bradycardia, sweating, miosis, and spasm of accommodation (the mechanism by which the lens focuses for near vision). If necessary, these responses can be suppressed with the anticholinergic drug atropine.

Neuromuscular Blockade. If administered in toxic doses, cholinesterase inhibitors can cause accumulation of acetylcholine in amounts sufficient to produce depolarizing neuromuscular blockade. Paralysis of the respiratory muscles can be fatal.

Precautions and Contraindications

Most of the precautions and contraindications regarding the cholinesterase inhibitors are the same as those for the direct-acting muscarinic agonists. These include obstruction of the GI tract, obstruction of the urinary tract, peptic ulcer disease, asthma, coronary insufficiency, and hyperthyroidism. The rationales underlying these precautions are discussed in Chapter 14. In addition to precautions related to muscarinic stimulation, cholinesterase inhibitors are contraindicated for patients receiving succinylcholine.

Drug Interactions

Muscarinic Antagonists. The effects of cholinesterase inhibitors at muscarinic receptors are opposite to those of

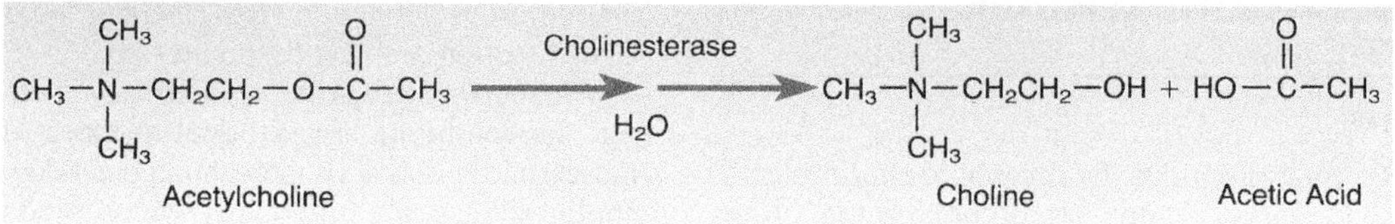

Fig. 15.2 ■ Hydrolysis of acetylcholine by cholinesterase.

atropine (and all other muscarinic antagonists). Consequently, cholinesterase inhibitors can be used to overcome excessive muscarinic blockade caused by atropine. Conversely, atropine can be used to reduce excessive muscarinic stimulation caused by cholinesterase inhibitors.

Competitive Neuromuscular Blockers. By causing accumulation of acetylcholine at the NMJ, cholinesterase inhibitors can reverse muscle relaxation or paralysis induced with pancuronium and other competitive neuromuscular blocking agents.

Depolarizing Neuromuscular Blockers. Cholinesterase inhibitors do not reverse the muscle-relaxant effects of succinylcholine, a depolarizing neuromuscular blocker. In fact, because cholinesterase inhibitors will decrease the breakdown of succinylcholine by cholinesterase, cholinesterase inhibitors will actually *intensify* neuromuscular blockade caused by succinylcholine.

Acute Toxicity

Symptoms. Overdose with cholinesterase inhibitors causes *excessive muscarinic stimulation* and *respiratory depression.* (Respiratory depression results from a combination of depolarizing neuromuscular blockade and CNS depression.) The state produced by cholinesterase inhibitor poisoning is sometimes referred to as *cholinergic crisis* (see Safety Alert).

Safety Alert

CHOLINERGIC CRISIS

Cholinesterase inhibitor toxicity can cause a life-threatening cholinergic crisis. Some common mnemonics can help you to identify these potentially dangerous conditions:

- **Mnemonic 1: SLUDGE and the Killer Bs:** *S*alivation, *L*acrimation, *U*rination, *D*iaphoresis/*D*iarrhea, *G*astrointestinal cramping, *E*mesis; *B*radycardia, *B*ronchospasm, *B*ronchorrhea
- **Mnemonic 2: DUMBELS:** *D*iaphoresis/*D*iarrhea; *U*rination; *M*iosis; *B*radycardia, *B*ronchospasm, *B*ronchorrhea; *E*mesis; *L*acrimation; *S*alivation

Treatment. Intravenous *atropine* can alleviate the muscarinic effects of cholinesterase inhibition. Respiratory depression from cholinesterase inhibitors cannot be managed with drugs. Rather, treatment consists of mechanical ventilation with oxygen. Suctioning may be necessary if atropine fails to suppress bronchial secretions.

Preparations, Dosage, and Administration

Preparations. Neostigmine [Bloxiverz, Prostigmin] is available as two salts: *neostigmine bromide* (for oral use) and *neostigmine methylsulfate* (for IM, IV, and subQ use). Neostigmine bromide is available in 15-mg tablets. Neostigmine methylsulfate is available in solution (0.5 and 1 mg/mL).

Dosage and Administration. Dosages of Prostigmin for *myasthenia gravis* are highly individualized, ranging from 15 to 375 mg/day administered PO in divided doses. The timing of doses is individualized to the patient and is often required around the clock to maintain adequate serum levels.

Bloxiverz is used to treat *poisoning by competitive neuromuscular blockers* or to *reverse nondepolarizing neuromuscular blockage after surgery.* The initial dose of Bloxiverz is 0.03 to 0.07 mg/kg administered by slow IV injection. Additional doses totaling a maximum of 5 mg may be given as required. A generic formulation of neostigmine is available and, when used for this purpose, the recommended dosing is 0.5 to 2 mg, repeated as needed up to a total of 5 mg.

Other Reversible Cholinesterase Inhibitors

Physostigmine

The basic pharmacology of physostigmine is identical to that of neostigmine—except that physostigmine readily crosses membranes, whereas neostigmine does not. This is possible because, in contrast to neostigmine, physostigmine is *not* a quaternary ammonium compound and hence does *not* carry a charge. Because physostigmine is uncharged, the drug crosses membranes with ease.

Physostigmine is the main cholinesterase inhibitor used to treat myasthenia gravis. It is also the drug of choice for treating *poisoning by atropine and other drugs that cause muscarinic blockade,* including antihistamines and phenothiazine antipsychotics—but *not* tricyclic antidepressants, owing to a risk of causing seizures and cardiotoxicity. Physostigmine counteracts antimuscarinic poisoning by causing acetylcholine to build up at muscarinic junctions. The accumulated acetylcholine competes with the muscarinic blocker for receptor binding, and thereby reverses receptor blockade. Physostigmine is preferred to neostigmine because, lacking a charge, physostigmine is able to cross the blood-brain barrier to reverse muscarinic blockade in the CNS. Information on preparation, dosage, and administration of this and other selected cholinesterase inhibitors is provided in Table 15.1.

Edrophonium and Pyridostigmine

Edrophonium [Enlon, Tensilon ♣] and pyridostigmine [Mestinon] have pharmacologic effects much like those of neostigmine. One of these drugs—edrophonium—is noteworthy for its very brief duration of action. Edrophonium is also unique in that it is indicated for *diagnosis, but not treatment,* of myasthenia gravis. In current practice, though, edrophonium is seldom used for this purpose because better and more accurate testing is now available. Routes of administration and indications are shown in Table 15.2.

Drugs for Alzheimer's Disease

Three cholinesterase inhibitors—*donepezil* [Aricept], *galantamine* [Razadyne], and *rivastigmine* [Exelon]—are approved for management of Alzheimer's disease, and one of them—rivastigmine—is also approved for dementia of Parkinson disease. With all three, benefits derive from inhibiting cholinesterase in the CNS. The pharmacology of these drugs is discussed in Chapter 22.

IRREVERSIBLE CHOLINESTERASE INHIBITORS

The irreversible cholinesterase inhibitors are highly toxic. These agents are employed primarily as *insecticides.* During World War II, huge quantities of irreversible cholinesterase inhibitors were produced for possible use as *nerve agents,* but were never deployed. Today, there is concern that these agents might be employed as weapons of terrorism. The only clinical indication for the irreversible inhibitors is *glaucoma.*

Basic Pharmacology

Chemistry

All irreversible cholinesterase inhibitors contain an atom of *phosphorus* (Fig. 15.3). Because of this phosphorus atom, the irreversible inhibitors are known as *organophosphate* cholinesterase inhibitors.

TABLE 15.1 ▪ Preparation, Dosage, and Administration of Selected Cholinesterase Inhibitors

Drug	Preparation	Dosage	Administration
Neostigmine [Bloxiverz, Prostigmin 🍁]	Tablets[a]: 15 mg Solution for injection: 0.5 mg/mL solution available in 1-mL and 10-mL vials Generic: 0.5 mg/mL and 1 mg/mL, both in 10-mL vials	**Myasthenia gravis treatment (highly individualized):** PO[a]: 15 mg 3 times/day initially, increased to typical dose of 150 mg/24 hr in divided doses. Solution: 0.5 mg IM or subQ initially with additional dosing based on patient response. Typical dosing is 15–375 mg/day in divided doses. **Neuromuscular blockade reversal:** Typical dose is 0.03–0.07 mg/kg.	Timing administration so that peak effects occur at mealtime may help with eating and swallowing.
Pyridostigmine [Mestinon, Regonol, Mestinon-SR 🍁]	Syrup: 60 mg/5 mL Tablet IR: 60 mg Tablet ER: 180 mg	**Myasthenia gravis treatment (highly individualized):** IR: 60–1500 mg/day. Typical dosing 600 mg/day divided into 5 doses. ER: 180–540 mg once or twice daily. It may be necessary to use both IR and ER dosing to sustain effects.	Take the ER tablets whole. Timing of syrup and IR tablets is spaced to provide optimal functioning.
Physostigmine	Solution for injection: 1 mg/mL in 2-mL vials	**Reversal of anticholinergic toxicity:** *Adults:* 0.5–2 mg IM or IV *Children:* 0.02 mg/kg Dose may be repeated every 10–30 minutes as needed.	Rapid IV administration can cause respiratory distress, bradycardia, and seizures. Limit rate to 1 mg/min in adults or 0.5 mg/min in children.

[a]Neostigmine oral formulation is not available in the United States.
IR, Immediate release; *ER,* extended release.

TABLE 15.2 ▪ Clinical Applications of Cholinesterase Inhibitors

		Myasthenia Gravis					
Drug	Routes	Diagnosis	Treatment	Glaucoma	Reversal of Competitive Neuromuscular Blockade	Antidote to Poisoning by Muscarinic Antagonists	Alzheimer's Disease
REVERSIBLE INHIBITORS							
Neostigmine [Bloxiverz, Prostigmin 🍁]	PO, IM, IV, subQ		✓		✓		
Pyridostigmine [Mestinon, Mestinon-SR 🍁]	PO		✓				
Edrophonium [Enlon]	IM, IV	✓			✓		
Physostigmine [generic]	IM, IV					✓	
Donepezil [Aricept][a]	PO						✓
Galantamine [Razadyne]	PO						✓
Rivastigmine [Exelon][a]	PO, Transdermal						✓
IRREVERSIBLE INHIBITOR							
Echothiophate [Phospholine Iodide]	Topical			✓			

[a]Also used for Parkinson disease dementia.

Almost all irreversible cholinesterase inhibitors are *highly lipid soluble.* As a result, these drugs are readily absorbed from all routes of administration. They can even be absorbed directly through the skin. Easy absorption, coupled with high toxicity, is what makes these drugs good insecticides—and gives them potential as agents of chemical warfare. Once absorbed, the organophosphate inhibitors have ready access to all tissues and organs, including the CNS.

Mechanism of Action

The irreversible cholinesterase inhibitors bind to the active center of cholinesterase, preventing the enzyme from hydrolyzing

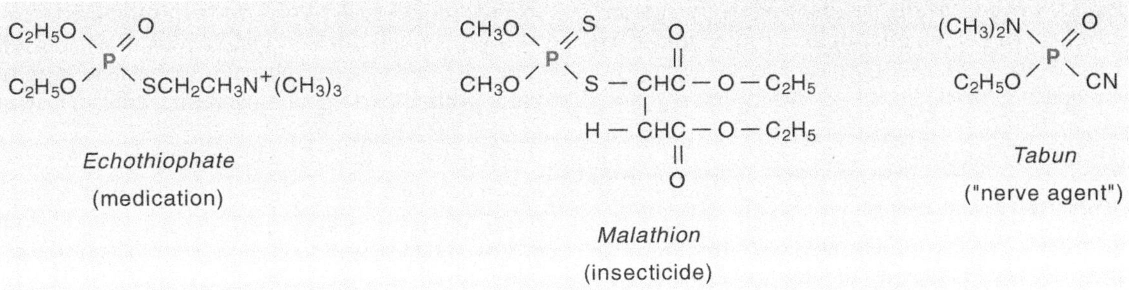

Fig. 15.3 ▪ Structural formulas of irreversible cholinesterase inhibitors.
Note that irreversible cholinesterase inhibitors contain an atom of phosphorus. Because of this atom, these drugs are known as organophosphate cholinesterase inhibitors. With the exception of echothiophate, all of these drugs are highly lipid soluble, and therefore move throughout the body with ease.

acetylcholine. Although these drugs can be split from cholinesterase, the splitting reaction takes place *extremely* slowly. Hence, under normal conditions, their binding to cholinesterase can be considered irreversible. Because binding is irreversible, effects persist until new molecules of cholinesterase can be synthesized.

Although we normally consider the bond between irreversible inhibitors and cholinesterase permanent, this bond can, in fact, be broken. To break the bond and reverse the inhibition of cholinesterase, we must administer *pralidoxime,* a cholinesterase reactivator.

Pharmacologic Effects

The irreversible cholinesterase inhibitors produce essentially the same spectrum of effects as the reversible inhibitors. The principal difference is that responses to irreversible inhibitors last a long time, whereas responses to reversible inhibitors are brief.

Therapeutic Uses

The irreversible cholinesterase inhibitors have only one indication: treatment of *glaucoma.* And for that indication, only one drug—echothiophate—is available. The limited indications for irreversible cholinesterase inhibitors should be no surprise given their potential for harm. The use of echothiophate for glaucoma is discussed in Chapter 104.

Toxicology

Sources of Poisoning

Poisoning by organophosphate cholinesterase inhibitors is a common occurrence. Agricultural workers have been poisoned by accidental ingestion of organophosphate insecticides and by absorption of these lipid-soluble compounds through the skin. In addition, because organophosphate insecticides are readily available to the general public, poisoning may occur accidentally or from attempted homicide or suicide. Exposure could also occur if these drugs were used as instruments of warfare or terrorism (see Chapter 110).

Symptoms

Toxic doses of irreversible cholinesterase inhibitors produce excessive muscarinic, nicotinic, and CNS effects. This condition, known as a *cholinergic crisis,* is characterized by *excessive muscarinic stimulation* and *depolarizing neuromuscular blockade.* Overstimulation of muscarinic receptors results in profuse secretions from salivary and bronchial glands, involuntary urination and defecation, laryngospasm, and bronchoconstriction. Prominent nicotinic effects reflect nicotinic activity at neuromuscular junctions resulting in muscle weakness, fasciculations, cramps, and twitching. CNS effects may range from anxiety and confusion to delirium. Neuromuscular blockade can result in paralysis, followed by death from apnea. Convulsions of CNS origin precede paralysis and apnea.

Treatment

Pharmacologic treatment involves giving *atropine* to reduce muscarinic stimulation and giving *pralidoxime* to reverse inhibition of cholinesterase (primarily at the NMJ), and giving a benzodiazepine such as *diazepam* to suppress convulsions. Respiratory depression from cholinesterase inhibitors cannot be managed with drugs. Rather, treatment consists of mechanical ventilation with oxygen.

Pralidoxime. Pralidoxime is a specific antidote to poisoning by the irreversible (organophosphate) cholinesterase inhibitors; the drug is *not* effective against poisoning by reversible cholinesterase inhibitors. In poisoning by irreversible inhibitors, benefits derive from causing the inhibitor to dissociate from the active center of cholinesterase. Reversal is most effective at the NMJ. Pralidoxime is much less effective at reversing cholinesterase inhibition at muscarinic and ganglionic sites. Furthermore, since pralidoxime is a quaternary ammonium compound, it cannot cross the blood-brain barrier and therefore cannot reverse cholinesterase inhibition in the CNS.

To be effective, pralidoxime must be administered soon after organophosphate poisoning has occurred. If too much time elapses, a process called *aging* takes place. In this process, the bond between the organophosphate inhibitor and cholinesterase increases in strength. Once aging has occurred, pralidoxime is unable to cause the inhibitor to dissociate from the enzyme. The time required for aging depends on the agent involved. For example, with a nerve agent called *soman,* aging occurs in just 2 minutes. In contrast, with a nerve agent called *tabun* (see Fig. 15.3), aging requires 13 hours.

The usual dose for pralidoxime is 1 to 2 gm administered IV or IM. Intravenous doses should be infused slowly (over 20 to 30 minutes) to avoid hypertension. Dosing intervals are individualized according to severity and persistence of symptoms. Pralidoxime is available alone under the brand name *Protopam,* and in combination with atropine under the brand names *DuoDote* and *ATNAA.*

MYASTHENIA GRAVIS

Pathophysiology

Myasthenia gravis (MG) is a neuromuscular disorder characterized by fluctuating muscle weakness and a predisposition to rapid fatigue. Common symptoms include ptosis (drooping eyelids), difficulty swallowing, and weakness of skeletal muscles. Patients with severe MG may have difficulty breathing owing to weakness of the muscles of respiration.

Symptoms of MG result from an autoimmune process in which the patient's immune system produces antibodies that attack $nicotinic_M$ receptors on skeletal muscle. As a result, the number of functional receptors at the NMJ is reduced by 70% to 90%, causing muscle weakness.

Treatment With Cholinesterase Inhibitors

Beneficial Effects

Reversible cholinesterase inhibitors (e.g., neostigmine) are the mainstay of therapy. By preventing acetylcholine inactivation, anticholinesterase agents can intensify the effects of acetylcholine released from motor neurons, increasing muscle strength. Cholinesterase inhibitors do not cure MG. Rather, they produce only symptomatic relief, so patients usually need therapy lifelong.

When working with a hospitalized patient with MG, keep in mind that muscle strength may be insufficient to permit swallowing. Accordingly, you should assess the ability to swallow before administering oral medications. Assessment is accomplished by giving the patient a few sips of water. If the patient is unable to swallow the water, parenteral medication must be substituted for oral medication.

Side Effects

Because cholinesterase inhibitors can inhibit acetylcholinesterase at any location, these drugs will cause acetylcholine to accumulate at muscarinic junctions as well as at NMJs. If muscarinic responses are excessive, atropine may be given to suppress them. However, atropine should not be employed *routinely* because the drug can mask the early signs (e.g., excessive salivation) of overdose with anticholinesterase agents.

Dosage Adjustment

In the treatment of MG, establishing an optimal dosage for cholinesterase inhibitors can be a challenge. Dosage determination is accomplished by administering a small initial dose followed by additional small doses until an optimal level of muscle function has been achieved. Important signs of improvement include increased ease of swallowing and increased ability to raise the eyelids. You can help establish a correct dosage by keeping records of (1) times of drug administration, (2) times at which fatigue occurs, (3) the state of muscle strength before and after drug administration, and (4) signs of excessive muscarinic stimulation.

To maintain optimal responses, patients must occasionally modify dosage themselves. To do this, they must be taught to recognize signs of undermedication (ptosis, difficulty in swallowing) and signs of overmedication (excessive salivation and other muscarinic responses). Patients may also need to modify dosage in anticipation of exertion. For example, they may find it necessary to take supplementary medication 30 to 60 minutes before activities such as eating or shopping.

Myasthenic Crisis and Cholinergic Crisis

Myasthenic Crisis. Patients who are inadequately medicated may experience myasthenic crisis, a state characterized by extreme muscle weakness caused by insufficient acetylcholine at the NMJ. Left untreated, myasthenic crisis can result in death from paralysis of the muscles of respiration. A cholinesterase inhibitor (e.g., neostigmine) is used to relieve the crisis.

Cholinergic Crisis. As noted previously, overdose with a cholinesterase inhibitor can produce cholinergic crisis. Like myasthenic crisis, cholinergic crisis is characterized by extreme muscle weakness or frank paralysis. In addition, cholinergic crisis is accompanied by signs of excessive muscarinic stimulation. Treatment consists of respiratory support plus atropine. The offending cholinesterase inhibitor should be withheld until muscle strength has returned.

Distinguishing Myasthenic Crisis From Cholinergic Crisis. Because myasthenic crisis and cholinergic crisis share similar symptoms (muscle weakness or paralysis), but are treated very differently, it is essential to distinguish between them. A history of medication use or signs of excessive muscarinic stimulation are usually sufficient to permit a differential diagnosis. If these clues are inadequate, the provider may elect to administer a challenging dose of *edrophonium,* an ultrashort-acting cholinesterase inhibitor. If edrophonium-induced elevation of acetylcholine levels alleviates symptoms, the crisis is myasthenic. Conversely, if edrophonium intensifies symptoms, the crisis is cholinergic. Because the symptoms of cholinergic crisis will be made even worse by edrophonium, and could be life threatening, atropine and oxygen should be immediately available whenever edrophonium is used for this test. For this reason, and because cholinergic crisis is relatively rare for patients with MG, the use of edrophonium for this purpose is controversial.

Medical Alert Identification. Because of the possibility of experiencing either myasthenic crisis or cholinergic crisis, and because both crises can be fatal, patients with MG should be encouraged to wear a Medic Alert bracelet or some other form of identification to inform emergency medical personnel of their condition.

KEY POINTS

- Cholinesterase inhibitors prevent breakdown of acetylcholine by acetylcholinesterase, causing acetylcholine to accumulate in synapses, which in turn causes activation of muscarinic receptors, nicotinic receptors in ganglia and the NMJ, and cholinergic receptors in the CNS.
- The major use of reversible cholinesterase inhibitors is treatment of myasthenia gravis. Benefits derive from accumulation of acetylcholine at the NMJ.
- Secondary uses for reversible cholinesterase inhibitors are reversal of competitive (nondepolarizing) neuromuscular blockade and treatment of glaucoma, Alzheimer's disease, Parkinson disease dementia, and poisoning by muscarinic antagonists.
- Because physostigmine crosses membranes easily, this drug is the preferred cholinesterase inhibitor for treating poisoning by muscarinic antagonists.
- Irreversible cholinesterase inhibitors, also known as organophosphate cholinesterase inhibitors, are used primarily as insecticides. The only indication for these potentially toxic drugs is glaucoma.
- Most organophosphate cholinesterase inhibitors are highly lipid soluble. As a result, they can be absorbed directly through the skin and distributed easily to all tissues and organs.
- Overdose with cholinesterase inhibitors produces cholinergic crisis, characterized by depolarizing neuromuscular blockade plus signs of excessive muscarinic stimulation (hypersalivation, tearing, sweating, bradycardia, involuntary urination and defecation, miosis, and spasm of accommodation). Death results from respiratory depression.
- Poisoning by *reversible* cholinesterase inhibitors is treated with atropine (to reverse muscarinic stimulation) plus mechanical ventilation.
- Poisoning by *organophosphate* cholinesterase inhibitors is treated with atropine, mechanical ventilation, pralidoxime (to reverse inhibition of cholinesterase, primarily at the NMJ), and diazepam (to suppress seizures).

Please visit **http://evolve.elsevier.com/Lehne** for chapter-specific NCLEX® examination review questions.

Summary of Major Nursing Implications[a]

REVERSIBLE CHOLINESTERASE INHIBITORS

Donepezil
Edrophonium
Galantamine
Neostigmine
Physostigmine
Pyridostigmine
Rivastigmine

Preadministration Assessment

Therapeutic Goal

Cholinesterase inhibitors are used to treat myasthenia gravis, glaucoma, Alzheimer's disease, Parkinson disease dementia, and poisoning by muscarinic antagonists, and to reverse competitive (nondepolarizing) neuromuscular blockade. Applications of individual agents are shown in Table 15.2.

Baseline Data

Myasthenia Gravis. Determine the extent of neuromuscular dysfunction by assessing muscle strength, fatigue, ptosis, and ability to swallow.

Identifying High-Risk Patients

Cholinesterase inhibitors are *contraindicated* for patients with mechanical obstruction of the intestine or urinary tract. Exercise *caution* in patients with peptic ulcer disease, bradycardia, asthma, or hyperthyroidism.

Implementation: Administration

Routes

These drugs are given orally, topically (transdermal, conjunctival), and parenterally (IM, IV, subQ). Routes for individual agents are shown in Table 15.2.

Administration and Dosage in Myasthenia Gravis

Administration. Assess the patient's ability to swallow before giving oral medication. If swallowing is impaired, substitute a parenteral medication.

Optimizing Dosage. Monitor for therapeutic responses and adjust the dosage accordingly. **Teach patients to distinguish between insufficient and excessive dosing so that they can participate effectively in dosage adjustment.**

Reversing Competitive (Nondepolarizing) Neuromuscular Blockade

To reverse toxicity from overdose with a competitive neuromuscular blocking agent (e.g., pancuronium), administer edrophonium IV. Support respiration until muscle strength has recovered fully.

Treating Muscarinic Antagonist Poisoning

Physostigmine is the drug of choice for this indication. The usual dose is 2 mg administered by IM or slow IV injection.

Continued

Summary of Major Nursing Implications[a]—cont'd

Implementation: Measures to Enhance Therapeutic Effects

Myasthenia Gravis

Promoting Compliance. **Inform patients that MG is not usually curable, so treatment is lifelong. Encourage patients to take their medication as prescribed and to play an active role in dosage adjustment.**

Using Identification. Because patients with MG are at risk of fatal complications (cholinergic crisis, myasthenic crisis), **encourage them to wear a Medic Alert bracelet or similar identification to inform emergency medical personnel of their condition.**

Ongoing Evaluation and Interventions

Evaluating Therapeutic Effects

Myasthenia Gravis. Monitor and record (1) times of drug administration; (2) times at which fatigue occurs; (3) state of muscle strength, ptosis, and ability to swallow; and (4) signs of excessive muscarinic stimulation. Dosage is increased or decreased based on these observations.

Monitor for *myasthenic crisis* (extreme muscle weakness, paralysis of respiratory muscles), which can occur when cholinesterase inhibitor dosage is insufficient. Manage with respiratory support and increased dosage.

Be certain to distinguish myasthenic crisis from cholinergic crisis. This is done by observing for signs of excessive muscarinic stimulation, which will accompany cholinergic crisis but not myasthenic crisis.

Minimizing Adverse Effects

Excessive Muscarinic Stimulation. Accumulation of acetylcholine at muscarinic receptors can cause profuse salivation, increased tone and motility of the gut, urinary urgency, sweating, miosis, spasm of accommodation, bronchoconstriction, and bradycardia. **Inform patients about signs of excessive muscarinic stimulation and advise them to notify the prescriber if these occur.** Excessive muscarinic responses can be managed with *atropine.*

Cholinergic Crisis. This condition results from cholinesterase inhibitor overdose. Manifestations are skeletal muscle paralysis (from depolarizing neuromuscular blockade) and signs of excessive muscarinic stimulation (e.g., salivation, sweating, miosis, bradycardia).

Manage with mechanical ventilation and atropine. Cholinergic crisis must be distinguished from myasthenic crisis.

[a]Patient education information is highlighted as **blue text.**

CHAPTER

16 Drugs That Block Nicotinic Cholinergic Transmission: Neuromuscular Blocking Agents

Neuromuscular blocking agents prevent acetylcholine from activating nicotinic$_M$ receptors on skeletal muscles, which results in muscle relaxation. These drugs are given to produce muscle relaxation during surgery, endotracheal intubation, mechanical ventilation, and other procedures. Based on mechanism of action, the neuromuscular blockers fall into two major groups: *competitive* (*nondepolarizing*) agents and *depolarizing* agents.

CONTROL OF MUSCLE CONTRACTION

Before we discuss the neuromuscular blockers, we need to review physiologic control of muscle contraction. In particular, we need to understand *excitation-contraction coupling,* the process by which an action potential in a motor neuron leads to contraction of a muscle.

Basic Concepts: Polarization, Depolarization, and Repolarization

The concepts of *polarization, depolarization,* and *repolarization* are important for understanding both muscle contraction and the neuromuscular blocking drugs. In *resting* muscle there is uneven distribution of electrical charge across the inner and outer surfaces of the cell membrane. As shown in Fig. 16.1, positive charges cover the outer surface of the membrane and negative charges cover the inner surface. Because of this uneven charge distribution, the resting membrane is said to be *polarized.*

When the membrane *depolarizes,* positive charges move from outside to inside. So many positive charges move inward that the inside of the membrane becomes more positive than the outside.

Under physiologic conditions, depolarization of the muscle membrane is followed almost instantaneously by *repolarization.* Repolarization is accomplished by pumping positively charged ions out of the cell. Repolarization restores the original resting membrane state, with positive charges on the outer surface and negative charges on the inner surface.

Steps in Muscle Contraction

The steps leading to muscle contraction are shown in Fig. 16.2. The process begins with the arrival of an action potential at the terminal of a motor neuron, causing release of acetylcholine into the subneural space. Acetylcholine then binds reversibly to nicotinic$_M$ receptors on the motor end-plate (a specialized region of the muscle membrane that contains the receptors for acetylcholine) and causes the end-plate to *depolarize.* This depolarization initiates a muscle action potential (i.e., a wave of depolarization that spreads rapidly over the entire muscle membrane), which in turn triggers the release of calcium from the sarcoplasmic reticulum (SR) of the muscle. This calcium permits the interaction of actin and myosin, thereby causing contraction. Very rapidly, acetylcholine dissociates from the motor end-plate, the motor end-plate repolarizes, the muscle membrane repolarizes, and calcium is taken back up into the SR. Because there is no longer any calcium available to support the interaction of actin and myosin, the muscle relaxes.

Sustained muscle contraction requires a continuous series of motor neuron action potentials. These action potentials cause repeated release of acetylcholine, which causes repeated activation of nicotinic receptors on the motor end-plate. As a result, the end-plate goes through repeating cycles of depolarization and repolarization, which results in sufficient release of calcium to sustain contraction. If for some reason the motor end-plate fails to repolarize—that is, if the end-plate remains in a *depolarized* state—the signal for calcium release will stop, calcium will undergo immediate reuptake into the SR, and contraction will cease.

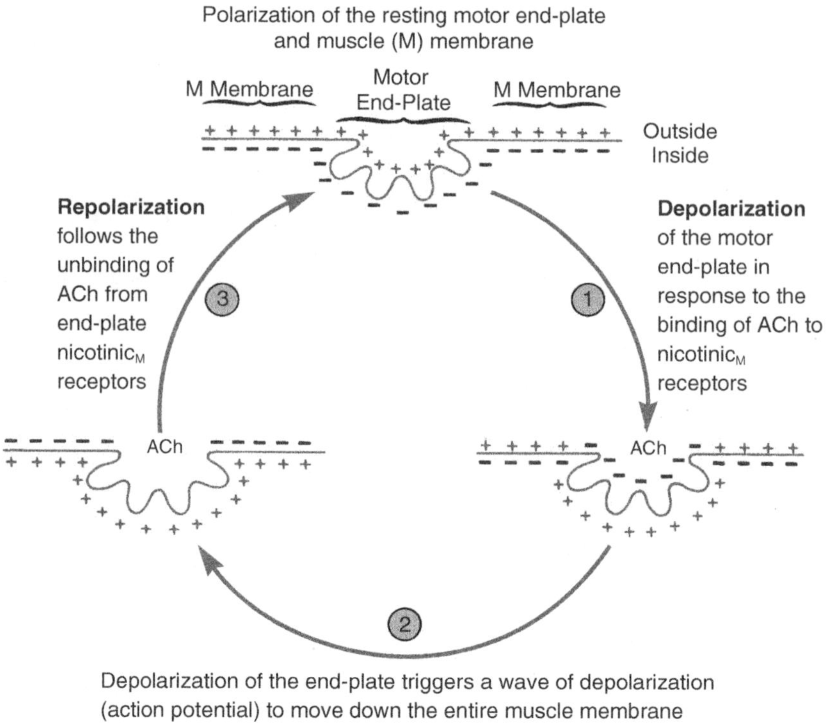

Fig. 16.1 ▪ The depolarization-repolarization cycle of the motor end-plate and muscle membrane.
(*ACh,* Acetylcholine.)

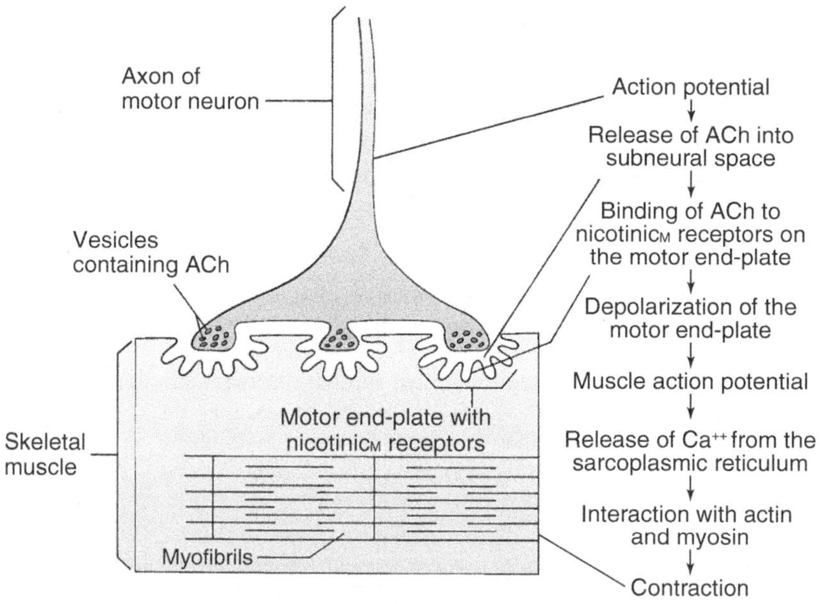

Fig. 16.2 ▪ Steps in excitation-contraction coupling.
(*ACh,* Acetylcholine.)

Safety Alert

NEUROMUSCULAR BLOCKING AGENTS

The Institute for Safe Medication Practices (ISMP) includes neuromuscular blocking agents among its list of high-alert medications. High-alert medications are those drugs that can cause devastating effects to patients in the event of a medication error.

COMPETITIVE (NONDEPOLARIZING) NEUROMUSCULAR BLOCKERS

Competitive neuromuscular blocking agents are drugs that compete with acetylcholine for binding to nicotinic$_M$ receptors. These drugs are also known as *nondepolarizing* neuromuscular blockers, because, unlike depolarizing neuromuscular blockers, they do not depolarize the motor end-plate.

The powers of *tubocurarine,* the oldest competitive neuromuscular blocker, were known to primitive hunters long before coming to the attention of modern scientists. Tubocurarine is one of several active principles found in *curare,* an arrow poison used for hunting by South American Indians. When shot into a small animal, curare-tipped arrows cause relaxation (paralysis) of skeletal muscles. Death results from paralyzing the muscles of respiration.

The clinical utility of the neuromuscular blockers is based on the same action that is useful in hunting: production of skeletal muscle relaxation. They are most commonly used as an adjunct to general anesthesia to aid in intubation and to maintain skeletal muscle relaxation during surgical procedures.

Basic Pharmacology of Competitive (Nondepolarizing) Neuromuscular Blockers

Chemistry

All of the neuromuscular blocking agents contain at least one *quaternary nitrogen* atom (Fig. 16.3). As a result, these drugs always carry a positive charge and therefore cannot readily cross membranes.

The inability to cross membranes has three clinical consequences. First, neuromuscular blockers cannot be absorbed from the gastrointestinal tract, so they cannot be administered orally. Instead, they must all be administered parenterally (almost always IV). Second, these drugs cannot cross the blood-brain barrier, and hence have no effect on the central nervous system (CNS). Third, neuromuscular blockers cannot readily cross the placenta, so they have little or no effect on the fetus.

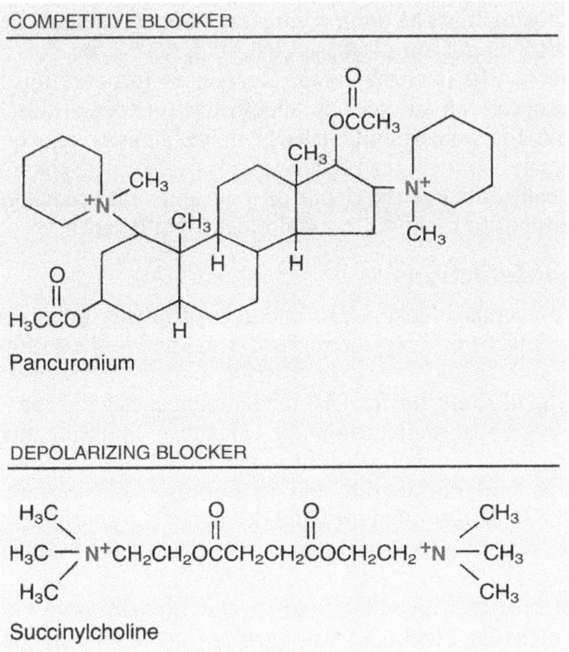

Fig. 16.3 ▪ Structural formulas of representative neuromuscular blocking agents.
Note that both agents contain a quaternary nitrogen atom and therefore cross membranes poorly. Consequently, they must be administered parenterally and have little effect on the central nervous system or the developing fetus.

Mechanism of Action

As their name implies, the competitive neuromuscular blockers compete with acetylcholine for binding to nicotinic$_M$ receptors on the motor end-plate (Fig. 16.4). However, unlike acetylcholine, these drugs do not cause receptor activation. When they bind to nicotinic$_M$ receptors, they block receptor activation by acetylcholine, causing the muscle to relax. Muscle relaxation persists as long as the amount of competitive neuromuscular blocker at the neuromuscular junction is sufficient to prevent receptor occupation by acetylcholine. Muscle function can be restored by eliminating the drug from the body or by increasing the amount of acetylcholine at the neuromuscular junction.

Pharmacologic Effects

Muscle Relaxation. The primary effect of neuromuscular blockers is relaxation of skeletal muscle, causing a state known as *flaccid paralysis.* Although these drugs can paralyze all skeletal muscles, not all muscles are affected at once. The first to become paralyzed are the levator muscle of the eyelid and the muscles of mastication. Paralysis occurs next in muscles of the limbs, abdomen, and glottis. The last muscles affected are the muscles of respiration—the intercostals and diaphragm.

Hypotension. Some neuromuscular blockers can lower blood pressure. Two mechanisms may be involved: (1) release of histamine from mast cells and (2) partial blockade of nicotinic$_N$ receptors in autonomic ganglia. Histamine lowers blood pressure by causing vasodilation. Partial ganglionic blockade lowers blood pressure by decreasing sympathetic tone to arterioles and veins.

Central Nervous System. As noted previously, the neuromuscular blockers cannot cross the blood-brain barrier. Consequently, these drugs have no effect on the CNS. Please note: *Neuromuscular blockers do not diminish consciousness or perception of pain—even when administered in doses that produce complete paralysis.* This is essential to understand because patients who receive neuromuscular blockers while

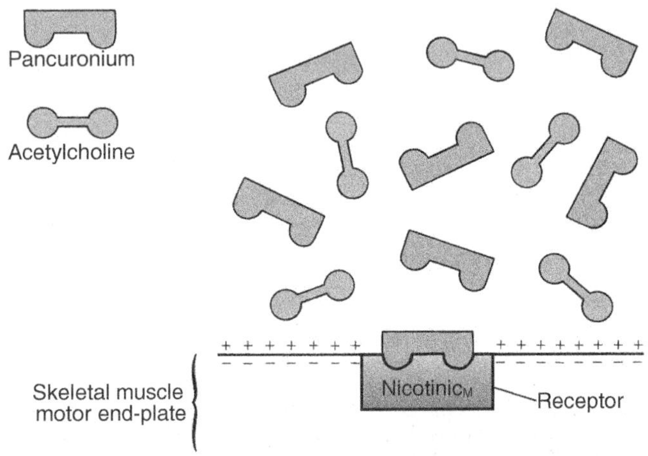

Fig. 16.4 ▪ Mechanism of competitive neuromuscular blockade.
Pancuronium, a competitive blocker, competes with acetylcholine (ACh) for binding to nicotinic$_M$ receptors on the motor end-plate. Binding of pancuronium does not depolarize the end-plate, and therefore does not cause contraction. At the same time, the presence of pancuronium prevents ACh from binding to the receptor, so contraction is prevented.

TABLE 16.1 ■ Properties of Competitive and Depolarizing Neuromuscular Blockers

		Time Course of Action[a]				
Drug	Route	Time to Maximum Paralysis (min)	Duration of Effective Paralysis (min)	Time to Nearly Full Spontaneous Recovery[b]	Promotes Histamine Release	Primary Mode of Elimination
COMPETITIVE AGENTS						
Atracurium	IV	2–5	20–35	60–70 min	Yes	Plasma cholinesterase[c]
Cisatracurium [Nimbex]	IV	2–5	20–35	—	Minimal	Spontaneous degradation
Mivacurium [Mivacron]	IV	2–5	15–20	20–35 min	Yes	Plasma cholinesterase[c]
Pancuronium	IV	3–4	35–45	60–70 min	No	Renal
Rocuronium [Zemuron 🍁]	IV	1–3	20–40	—	No	Hepatic/biliary
Vecuronium [Norcuron 🍁]	IV	3–5	25–30	45–60 min	No	Hepatic/biliary
DEPOLARIZING AGENT						
Succinylcholine [Anectine, Quelicin]	IV, IM[d]	1	4–6	—	Yes	Plasma cholinesterase[c]

[a]Time course of action can vary widely with dosage and route of administration. The values presented are for an average adult dose administered as a single IV injection.
[b]Because spontaneous recovery can take a long time, recovery from the *competitive* agents (all of the drugs listed except succinylcholine, which is a depolarizing agent) is often accelerated by giving a cholinesterase inhibitor.
[c]Plasma cholinesterase is also known as pseudocholinesterase to distinguish it from "true" cholinesterase, the enzyme found at synapses where acetylcholine is the transmitter.
[d]Intramuscular administration is rare.

on mechanical ventilators, for example, can be fully alert and in pain even though they are unable to communicate. Understandably, this can be a very frightening experience; therefore, sedatives and analgesics are commonly administered around the clock for these patients.

Pharmacokinetics

With the competitive neuromuscular blockers in use today, paralysis develops within minutes of IV injection. Peak effects persist 20 to 45 minutes and then decline. Complete recovery takes about 1 hour. As shown in Table 16.1, the mode of elimination—spontaneous degradation, degradation by plasma cholinesterase, renal excretion, or hepatic metabolism—depends on the agent involved.

Therapeutic Uses

The competitive neuromuscular blockers are used to provide muscle relaxation during surgery, mechanical ventilation, and endotracheal intubation. These applications are discussed further under *Therapeutic Uses of Neuromuscular Blockers.*

Adverse Effects

Respiratory Arrest. Paralysis of respiratory muscles can produce respiratory arrest. Because of this risk, facilities for artificial ventilation must be immediately available. Patients must be monitored closely and continuously. When neuromuscular blockers are withdrawn, vital signs must be monitored until muscle function fully recovers.

Hypotension. One competitive agent—atracurium—can release significant amounts of histamine. Hypotension can result.

Precautions and Contraindications

Myasthenia Gravis. Neuromuscular blocking agents must be used with special care in patients with myasthenia gravis, a condition characterized by skeletal muscle weakness. The cause of weakness is a reduction in the number of nicotinic$_M$ receptors on the motor end-plate. Because receptor number is reduced, neuromuscular blockade occurs readily. Also, doses that would have a minimal effect on other patients can produce complete paralysis in patients with myasthenia gravis. Accordingly, dosing must be done with great care. Myasthenia gravis and its treatment are discussed in Chapter 15.

Electrolyte Disturbances. Responses to neuromuscular blockers can be altered by electrolyte abnormalities. For example, low potassium levels can enhance paralysis, whereas high potassium levels can reduce paralysis. Because electrolyte status can influence the depth of neuromuscular blockade, it is important to maintain normal electrolyte balance.

Drug Interactions

Neuromuscular blockers can interact with many other drugs. Interactions of primary interest are discussed in the following sections.

General Anesthetics. All inhalational anesthetics produce some degree of skeletal muscle relaxation and can thereby enhance the actions of neuromuscular blockers. Consequently, when general anesthetics and neuromuscular blockers are combined (as they often are), the dosage of the neuromuscular blocker should be reduced to avoid excessive neuromuscular blockade.

Antibiotics. Several antibiotics can intensify responses to neuromuscular blockers. Among them are aminoglycosides (e.g., gentamicin), tetracyclines, and certain other nonpenicillin antibiotics.

Cholinesterase Inhibitors. Cholinesterase inhibitors can *decrease* the effects of *competitive* neuromuscular blockers. Cholinesterase degrades (breaks down) acetylcholine. By reducing the degradation of acetylcholine, cholinesterase inhibitors increase the amount of acetylcholine available to compete with the blocker. As more acetylcholine (and less of the blocker) occupies nicotinic$_M$ receptors on the motor end-plate, the degree of neuromuscular blockade declines.

The ability of cholinesterase inhibitors to decrease responses to competitive neuromuscular blockers has two clinical applications: (1) management of overdose with a competitive neuromuscular blocker and (2) reversal of neuromuscular blockade following surgery and other procedures.

As discussed later in the chapter, cholinesterase inhibitors *increase* responses to succinylcholine, a *depolarizing* neuromuscular blocker. Note that this is opposite to the effect that cholinesterase inhibitors have on competitive neuromuscular blockade.

Toxicity

When dosage is too high, all competitive neuromuscular blockers can produce *prolonged apnea.* Management consists of providing respiratory support plus a cholinesterase inhibitor (e.g., neostigmine) to reverse neuromuscular blockade. One competitive agent—atracurium—can cause hypotension secondary to release of histamine. Antihistamines can be given to counteract this effect.

Properties of Individual Agents

All competitive neuromuscular blockers share the same mechanism of action (blockade of acetylcholine binding to nicotinic$_M$ receptors), and they all have the same indications: production of muscle relaxation during intubation, general anesthesia, and mechanical ventilation. Differences among the drugs relate primarily to histamine release and mode of elimination (see Table 16.1). With all of these agents, respiratory depression secondary to neuromuscular blockade is the major concern. Respiratory depression can be reversed with a cholinesterase inhibitor.

Atracurium

Atracurium is approved for muscle relaxation during surgery, intubation, and mechanical ventilation. The drug can cause hypotension secondary to histamine release. Atracurium is eliminated primarily by plasma cholinesterase, not by the liver or kidneys. Hence, atracurium may be desirable for patients with renal or hepatic dysfunction, as these disorders will not prolong the drug's effects.

Cisatracurium

Cisatracurium [Nimbex], a close relative of atracurium, is approved for muscle relaxation during surgery, intubation, and mechanical ventilation. Elimination is by spontaneous degradation, not by hepatic metabolism or renal excretion. Hence, like atracurium, cisatracurium would seem desirable for patients with kidney or liver dysfunction. Histamine release is minimal.

Mivacurium

Mivacurium [Mivacron] is a short-acting skeletal muscle relaxant. It is approved for both inpatient and outpatient procedures requiring muscle relaxation for surgery, intubation, and mechanical ventilation. Histamine release is usually small. It is remarkable for its short duration of action, making it useful for short procedures. The underlying mechanism for the short duration is enzymatic hydrolysis by plasma cholinesterase.

Pancuronium

Pancuronium is approved for muscle relaxation during general anesthesia, intubation, and mechanical ventilation. The drug does not cause histamine release, ganglionic blockade, or hypotension. Vagolytic effects may produce tachycardia. Approximately 30% to 45% of the drug undergoes hepatic metabolism. Effects may be prolonged in patients with cirrhosis or other liver disease, requiring a decrease in dosage. Excretion occurs primarily through urine, with 55% to 70% excreted unchanged.

Prototype Drugs

NEUROMUSCULAR BLOCKING AGENTS

Competitive (Nondepolarizing)

Pancuronium

Depolarizing

Succinylcholine

Rocuronium

Rocuronium [Zemuron 🍁] is approved for muscle relaxation during intubation, surgery, and mechanical ventilation. Muscle relaxation begins in 1 to 3 minutes. The only neuromuscular blocker with a faster onset is succinylcholine, a depolarizing agent. In contrast to succinylcholine, whose effects fade relatively quickly, effects of rocuronium persist for 20 to 40 minutes before starting to decline. Rocuronium does not cause histamine release. Elimination is by hepatic metabolism.

Vecuronium

Vecuronium [Norcuron 🍁], an analog of pancuronium, is used for muscle relaxation during intubation, general anesthesia, and mechanical ventilation. The drug does not produce ganglionic or vagal block and does not release histamine. Consequently, cardiovascular effects are lessened. Vecuronium is excreted primarily in the bile; therefore, paralysis may be prolonged in patients with liver dysfunction or greater weight.

DEPOLARIZING NEUROMUSCULAR BLOCKERS: SUCCINYLCHOLINE

Succinylcholine [Anectine, Quelicin], an ultrashort-acting drug, is the only depolarizing neuromuscular blocker in clinical use in the United States. This drug differs from the competitive blockers with regard to time course, mechanism of action, mode of elimination, interaction with cholinesterase inhibitors, and management of toxicity.

Mechanism of Action

Succinylcholine produces a state known as *depolarizing neuromuscular blockade.* Like acetylcholine, succinylcholine binds to nicotinic$_M$ receptors on the motor end-plate and thereby causes depolarization. This depolarization produces transient muscle contractions (fasciculations). Then, instead of dissociating rapidly from the receptor, succinylcholine remains bound and thereby prevents the end-plate from repolarizing. That is, succinylcholine maintains the end-plate in a state of *constant depolarization.* Because the end-plate must repeatedly depolarize and repolarize to maintain muscle contraction, succinylcholine's ability to keep the end-plate depolarized causes paralysis (following the brief initial period of contraction). Paralysis persists until plasma levels of succinylcholine decline, thereby allowing the drug to dissociate from its receptors.

Pharmacologic Effects

Muscle Relaxation. The muscle-relaxant effects of succinylcholine are much like those of the competitive blockers in that both produce a state of flaccid paralysis. However, despite this similarity, there are two important differences: (1) paralysis from succinylcholine is preceded by transient contractions and (2) paralysis from succinylcholine abates much more rapidly.

Central Nervous System. Like the depolarizing blockers, succinylcholine has no effect on the CNS. The drug can produce complete paralysis without decreasing consciousness or the ability to feel pain.

Pharmacokinetics

Succinylcholine has an extremely short duration of action. Paralysis peaks about 1 minute after IV injection and fades completely 4 to 10 minutes later.

Paralysis is brief because succinylcholine is rapidly degraded by *pseudocholinesterase,* an enzyme present in plasma. (This enzyme is called pseudocholinesterase to distinguish it from "true" cholinesterase, the enzyme found at synapses where acetylcholine is the transmitter.) Because of its presence in plasma, pseudocholinesterase is also known as *plasma cholinesterase.* In most individuals, pseudocholinesterase is highly active and can eliminate succinylcholine in minutes.

Therapeutic Uses

Succinylcholine is used primarily for muscle relaxation during endotracheal intubation. Additionally, it is sometimes used off-label to decrease the strength of muscle contraction during electroconvulsive therapy. Because of its brief duration, succinylcholine is poorly suited for use in prolonged procedures, such as surgery, although it is approved for use in these situations.

Adverse Effects

Prolonged Apnea in Patients With Low Pseudocholinesterase Activity. A few people, because of their genetic makeup, produce a form of pseudocholinesterase that has extremely low activity. As a result, they are unable to degrade succinylcholine rapidly. If succinylcholine is given to these people, paralysis can persist for hours, rather than just a few minutes. Not surprisingly, succinylcholine is contraindicated for these individuals.

Patients suspected of having low pseudocholinesterase activity should be tested for this possibility before receiving a full succinylcholine dose. Pseudocholinesterase activity can be assessed by direct measurement of a blood sample or by administering a tiny test dose of succinylcholine. If the test dose produces muscle relaxation that is unexpectedly intense and prolonged, pseudocholinesterase activity is probably low.

Malignant Hyperthermia. Malignant hyperthermia is a rare and potentially fatal condition that can be triggered by succinylcholine. The condition is characterized by muscle rigidity associated with a profound elevation of body temperature—sometimes as high as 43°C. Temperature becomes elevated owing to excessive and uncontrolled metabolic activity in muscle, secondary to increased release of calcium from the SR. Other manifestations include cardiac dysrhythmias, unstable blood pressure, electrolyte derangements, and metabolic acidosis. Left untreated, the condition can rapidly prove fatal. Malignant hyperthermia is a genetically determined reaction that has an incidence of about 1 in 25,000. Individuals with a family history of the reaction should not receive succinylcholine.

Treatment of malignant hyperthermia includes (1) immediate discontinuation of succinylcholine, (2) cooling the patient with external ice packs and IV infusion of cold saline, and (3) administering IV *dantrolene,* a drug that stops heat generation by acting directly on skeletal muscle to reduce its metabolic activity. The pharmacology of dantrolene is discussed in Chapter 25.

Postoperative Muscle Pain. From 10% to 70% of patients receiving succinylcholine experience postoperative muscle pain, most commonly in the neck, shoulders, and back. Pain develops 12 to 24 hours after surgery and may persist several hours or even days. The cause may be the muscle contractions that occur during the initial phase of succinylcholine action.

Hyperkalemia. Succinylcholine promotes release of potassium from tissues. Rarely, potassium release is sufficient to cause severe hyperkalemia. Death from cardiac arrest has resulted. Significant hyperkalemia is most likely to occur in patients with major burns, multiple trauma, denervation of skeletal muscle, or upper motor neuron injury. Accordingly, the drug is contraindicated for these patients.

Drug Interactions

Cholinesterase Inhibitors. These drugs *potentiate* (intensify) the effects of succinylcholine. How? Cholinesterase inhibitors decrease the activity of pseudocholinesterase, the enzyme that inactivates succinylcholine. Note that the effect of cholinesterase inhibitors on succinylcholine is opposite to their effect on *competitive* neuromuscular blockers.

Antibiotics. The effects of succinylcholine can be intensified by certain antibiotics. Among these are aminoglycosides, tetracyclines, and certain other nonpenicillin antibiotics.

Toxicology

Overdose can produce prolonged apnea. Because there is no specific antidote to succinylcholine poisoning, management is purely supportive. Recall that paralysis from overdose with a competitive agent can be reversed with a cholinesterase inhibitor. Because cholinesterase inhibitors *delay* the degradation of succinylcholine, use of these agents would prolong—not reverse—succinylcholine toxicity.

Preparations, Dosage, and Administration

Succinylcholine chloride [Anectine, Quelicin] is available in solution. The drug is usually administered IV but can also be given IM.

Dosage must be individualized and depends on the specific application. A typical adult dose for a brief procedure such as intubation is 0.6 mg/kg, administered as a single IV injection. For rapid-sequence intubation, the dosage is 1 to 1.5 mg/kg IV.

THERAPEUTIC USES OF NEUROMUSCULAR BLOCKERS

The primary applications of the neuromuscular blocking agents center on their ability to provide significant muscle relaxation. All of the *competitive* agents in current use are indicated for muscle relaxation during general anesthesia, mechanical ventilation, and intubation. Succinylcholine is used primarily for muscle relaxation during intubation and electroconvulsive therapy, and rarely for other short procedures.

Muscle Relaxation During Surgery

Production of muscle relaxation during surgery offers two benefits. First, relaxation of skeletal muscles, especially those of the abdominal wall, makes the surgeon's work easier. Second, muscle relaxants allow us to decrease the dosage of the general anesthetic, thereby decreasing the risks associated with anesthesia. Before neuromuscular blockers became available, surgical muscle relaxation had to be achieved with the general anesthetic alone, often requiring high levels of anesthetic. By combining a neuromuscular blocker with the general anesthetic, we can achieve adequate surgical muscle relaxation with less anesthetic. By allowing a reduction in anesthetic levels, neuromuscular blockers have decreased the risk of complications from anesthesia and hastened recovery from anesthesia.

Whenever neuromuscular blockers are employed during surgery, it is very, very important that anesthesia be maintained at a level sufficient to produce unconsciousness. Recall that neuromuscular blockers do not enter the CNS and therefore have no effect on hearing, thinking, or the ability to feel pain; all these drugs do is produce paralysis. Neuromuscular blockers are obviously and definitely not a substitute for anesthesia. It does not require much imagination to appreciate the horror of the surgical patient who is completely paralyzed from neuromuscular blockade yet fully awake because of inadequate anesthesia. Does this really happen? Yes. In fact, it happens in from 0.1% to 0.2% of surgeries in which neuromuscular blockers are used. Clearly, full anesthesia must be provided whenever surgery is performed on a patient who is under neuromuscular blockade.

With the agents in current use, full recovery from surgical neuromuscular blockade takes about an hour. During the recovery period, patients must be monitored closely to ensure adequate ventilation. A patent airway should be maintained until the patient can swallow or speak. Recovery from the effects of *competitive* neuromuscular blockers (e.g., pancuronium) can be accelerated with a cholinesterase inhibitor.

Facilitation of Mechanical Ventilation

Some patients who require mechanical ventilation still have some spontaneous respiratory movements, which can fight the rhythm of the respirator. By suppressing these movements, neuromuscular blocking agents can reduce resistance to ventilation.

When neuromuscular blockers are used to facilitate mechanical ventilation, patients should be treated as if they were awake—even though they appear to be asleep. (Remember that the patient is paralyzed, and hence there is no way to assess state of consciousness.) Because the patient may be fully awake, steps should be taken to ensure comfort at all times. Furthermore, because neuromuscular blockade does not affect hearing, nothing should be said in the patient's presence that might be inappropriate for the patient to hear.

As you can imagine, being fully awake but completely paralyzed can be a stressful and horrific experience. Accordingly, many clinicians do not recommend routine use of neuromuscular blockers during prolonged mechanical ventilation in intensive care units.

Safety Alert

NEUROMUSCULAR BLOCKING AGENTS AND THE PATIENT'S STATE OF CONSCIOUSNESS

Patients who have been given neuromuscular blocking agents may appear unresponsive due to the drug-induced paralysis; however, they are fully alert and conscious and can feel pain. It is essential for the nurse to administer prescribed medications such as sedatives and/or analgesics on a regular basis to prevent undue suffering.

Endotracheal Intubation

An endotracheal tube is a large catheter that is inserted past the glottis and into the trachea to facilitate ventilation. Gag reflexes can fight tube insertion. By suppressing these reflexes, neuromuscular blockers can make intubation easier. Because of its short duration of action, succinylcholine is the preferred agent for this use, although all of the competitive agents are also approved for this use.

Adjunct to Electroconvulsive Therapy

Electroconvulsive therapy is an effective treatment for severe depression (see Chapter 32). Benefits derive strictly from the effects of electroshock on the brain; the convulsive movements that can accompany electroshock do not have a role in relieving depression. Because convulsions per se serve no useful purpose and because electroshock-induced convulsions can be harmful, a neuromuscular blocker is now used to prevent convulsive movements during electroshock therapy. Because of its short duration of action, succinylcholine is the preferred neuromuscular blocker for this application.

KEY POINTS

- Sustained contraction of skeletal muscle results from repetitive activation of nicotinic$_M$ receptors on the motor end-plate, causing the end-plate to go through repeating cycles of depolarization and repolarization.
- Neuromuscular blockers interfere with nicotinic$_M$ receptor activation, and thereby cause muscle relaxation.
- Competitive neuromuscular blockers act by competing with acetylcholine for binding to nicotinic$_M$ receptors.
- Succinylcholine, the only depolarizing neuromuscular blocker in use, binds to nicotinic$_M$ receptors, causing the end-plate to depolarize; the drug then remains bound, which keeps the end-plate from repolarizing.
- Neuromuscular blockers are used to produce muscle relaxation during surgery, endotracheal intubation, mechanical ventilation, and electroshock therapy.
- Neuromuscular blockers do not reduce consciousness or pain.

Continued

- The major adverse effect of neuromuscular blockers is respiratory depression.
- Cholinesterase inhibitors can reverse the effects of competitive neuromuscular blockers but will intensify the effects of succinylcholine.
- Succinylcholine can trigger malignant hyperthermia, a life-threatening condition.
- Succinylcholine is eliminated by plasma cholinesterase. Accordingly, effects are greatly prolonged in patients with low plasma cholinesterase activity.
- All of the neuromuscular blockers are quaternary ammonium compounds, and therefore must be administered parenterally (almost always IV).

Please visit **http://evolve.elsevier.com/Lehne** for chapter-specific NCLEX® examination review questions.

Summary of Major Nursing Implications[a]

NEUROMUSCULAR BLOCKING AGENTS

Atracurium
Cisatracurium
Mivacurium
Pancuronium
Rocuronium
Succinylcholine
Vecuronium

Except where noted, the implications summarized in this section apply to all neuromuscular blocking agents.

Preadministration Assessment

Therapeutic Goal

Provision of muscle relaxation during surgery, endotracheal intubation, mechanical ventilation, electroconvulsive therapy, and other procedures.

Identifying High-Risk Patients

Use all neuromuscular blockers with *caution* in patients with myasthenia gravis.

Succinylcholine is *contraindicated* for patients with low pseudocholinesterase activity, a personal or familial history of malignant hyperthermia, or conditions that predispose to hyperkalemia (major burns, multiple trauma, denervation of skeletal muscle, upper motor neuron injury).

Implementation: Administration

Routes

Intravenous. All neuromuscular blockers, including succinylcholine.

Intramuscular. Only *succinylcholine,* and only rarely.

Administration

Neuromuscular blockers should be administered by clinicians skilled in their use.

Implementation: Measures to Enhance Therapeutic Effects

Neuromuscular blockers do not affect consciousness or perception of pain. When used during surgery, these drugs must be accompanied by adequate anesthesia. When neuromuscular blockers are used for prolonged paralysis during mechanical ventilation, care should be taken to ensure comfort (e.g., positioning the patient comfortably, moistening the mouth periodically). Because patients may be awake (but won't appear to be), conversations held in their presence should convey only information appropriate for them to hear. It is important to inform family members of this.

Ongoing Evaluation and Interventions

Minimizing Adverse Effects

Apnea. All neuromuscular blockers can cause respiratory arrest. Facilities for intubation and mechanical ventilation should be immediately available.

Monitor respiration constantly during the period of peak drug action. When drug administration is discontinued, take vital signs frequently, according to policy, until recovery is complete. Typically this is carried out at least every 15 minutes.

A cholinesterase inhibitor can be used to reverse respiratory depression caused by *competitive* neuromuscular blockers, but not by succinylcholine, a *depolarizing* blocker.

Hypotension. *Atracurium* may cause hypotension by releasing histamine. Antihistamines can help counteract this effect.

Malignant Hyperthermia. Succinylcholine can trigger malignant hyperthermia. Predisposition to this reaction is genetic. Assess for a family history of the reaction. Management consists of stopping succinylcholine, cooling with ice packs and cold IV saline, and giving IV dantrolene.

Hyperkalemia With Cardiac Arrest. Succinylcholine can cause severe hyperkalemia resulting in cardiac arrest if given to patients with major burns, multiple trauma, denervation of skeletal muscle, or upper motor neuron injury. Accordingly, the drug is contraindicated for these people.

Muscle Pain. *Succinylcholine* may cause muscle pain. **Reassure the patient that this response, although unpleasant, is not unusual.**

Minimizing Adverse Interactions

Antibiotics. Certain antibiotics, including *aminoglycosides* and *tetracyclines,* can intensify neuromuscular blockade. Use them with caution.

Cholinesterase Inhibitors. These drugs delay inactivation of *succinylcholine,* thereby greatly prolonging paralysis. Accordingly, cholinesterase inhibitors are contraindicated for patients receiving succinylcholine.

[a]Patient education information is highlighted as **blue text.**

CHAPTER

17 Adrenergic Agonists

Adrenergic agonists produce their effects by activating adrenergic receptors. Since the sympathetic nervous system acts through these same receptors, responses to adrenergic agonists and responses to stimulation of the sympathetic nervous system are very similar. Because of this similarity, adrenergic agonists are often referred to as *sympathomimetics.* Adrenergic agonists have a broad spectrum of indications, ranging from heart failure to asthma to preterm labor.

Learning about adrenergic agonists can be a challenge. To facilitate the process, our approach to these drugs has four stages. We begin with the general mechanisms by which drugs can activate adrenergic receptors. Next we establish an overview of the major adrenergic agonists, focusing on their receptor specificity and chemical classification. After that, we address the adrenergic receptors themselves; for each receptor type—alpha$_1$, alpha$_2$, beta$_1$, beta$_2$, and dopamine—we discuss the beneficial and harmful effects that can result from receptor activation. Finally, we integrate all of this information by discussing the characteristic properties of representative sympathomimetic drugs.

This chapter is intended only as an *introduction* to the adrenergic agonists. Our objective is to discuss the basic properties of the sympathomimetic drugs and establish an overview of their applications and adverse effects. In later chapters, we will discuss the clinical applications of these agents in greater depth.

MECHANISMS OF ADRENERGIC RECEPTOR ACTIVATION

Drugs can activate adrenergic receptors by four basic mechanisms: (1) direct receptor binding, (2) promotion of norepinephrine (NE) release, (3) blockade of NE reuptake, and (4) inhibition of NE inactivation. Note that only the first mechanism is *direct.* With the other three, receptor activation occurs by an *indirect* process. Examples of drugs that act by these four mechanisms are presented in Table 17.1.

Direct Receptor Binding

Direct interaction with receptors is the most common mechanism by which drugs activate peripheral adrenergic receptors. The direct-acting receptor stimulants produce their effects by binding to adrenergic receptors and mimicking the actions of natural transmitters (NE, epinephrine, dopamine). In this chapter, all of the drugs discussed activate receptors directly.

Promotion of NE Release

By acting on terminals of sympathetic nerves to cause NE release, drugs can bring about indirect activation of adrenergic receptors. Agents that act by this mechanism include amphetamines and ephedrine. (Ephedrine can also activate adrenergic receptors directly.)

Inhibition of NE Reuptake

Recall that reuptake of NE into terminals of sympathetic nerves is the major mechanism for terminating adrenergic transmission. By blocking NE reuptake, drugs can cause NE to accumulate

TABLE 17.1 ■ Mechanisms of Adrenergic Receptor Activation

Mechanism of Stimulation	Examples
DIRECT MECHANISM	
Receptor activation through direct binding	Dopamine Epinephrine Isoproterenol Ephedrine[a]
INDIRECT MECHANISMS	
Promotion of NE release	Amphetamine Ephedrine[a]
Inhibition of NE reuptake	Cocaine Tricyclic antidepressants
Inhibition of MAO	MAO inhibitors

[a]Ephedrine is a mixed-acting drug that activates receptors directly and by promoting release of norepinephrine.
MAO, Monoamine oxidase; *NE,* norepinephrine.

within the synaptic gap, and can thereby increase receptor activation. Agents that act by this mechanism include cocaine and the tricyclic antidepressants.

Inhibition of NE Inactivation

As discussed in Chapter 13, some of the NE in terminals of adrenergic neurons is subject to inactivation by monoamine oxidase (MAO). Hence, drugs that inhibit MAO can increase the amount of NE available for release and enhance receptor activation. (In addition to being present in sympathetic nerves, MAO is present in the liver and the intestinal wall. The significance of MAO at these other sites is considered later.)

In this chapter, which focuses on *peripherally* acting sympathomimetics, nearly all of the drugs discussed act exclusively by *direct* receptor activation. The only exception is *ephedrine,* a drug that works by a combination of direct receptor activation and promotion of NE release.

Most of the indirect-acting adrenergic agonists are used for their ability to activate adrenergic receptors in the central nervous system (CNS)—not for their effects in the periphery. The indirect-acting sympathomimetics (e.g., amphetamine, cocaine) are mentioned here to emphasize that, although these agents are employed for effects on the brain, they can and will cause activation of adrenergic receptors in the periphery. Peripheral activation is responsible for certain toxicities of these drugs (e.g., cardiac dysrhythmias, hypertension).

OVERVIEW OF THE ADRENERGIC AGONISTS

Chemical Classification: Catecholamines Versus Noncatecholamines

The adrenergic agonists fall into two major chemical classes: catecholamines and noncatecholamines. As discussed below, the catecholamines and noncatecholamines differ in three important respects: (1) availability for oral use, (2) duration of action, and (3) ability to act in the CNS. Accordingly, if we know to which category a particular adrenergic agonist belongs, we will know three of its prominent features.

Catecholamines

The catecholamines are so named because they contain a *catechol* group and an *amine* group. A catechol group is simply a benzene ring that has hydroxyl groups on two adjacent carbons. The amine component of the catecholamines is *ethylamine.* Structural formulas for each of the major catecholamines—epinephrine, NE, isoproterenol, dopamine, and dobutamine—are shown in Fig. 17.1. Because of their chemistry, all catecholamines have three properties in common: (1) they cannot be used orally, (2) they have a brief duration of action, and (3) they cannot cross the blood-brain barrier.

The actions of two enzymes—*monoamine oxidase* and *catechol-O-methyltransferase* (COMT)—explain why the catecholamines have short half-lives and cannot be used orally. MAO and COMT are located in the liver and in the intestinal wall. Both enzymes are very active and quickly destroy catecholamines administered by any route. Because these enzymes are located in the liver and intestinal wall, catecholamines that are administered orally become inactivated before they can reach the systemic circulation. Hence, catecholamines are ineffective if given by mouth. Because of rapid inactivation by MAO and COMT, three catecholamines—NE, dopamine, and dobutamine—are effective only if administered by continuous infusion. Administration by other parenteral routes (e.g., subQ, IM) will not yield adequate blood levels, owing to rapid hepatic inactivation.

Catecholamines are polar molecules, so they cannot cross the blood-brain barrier. (Recall from Chapter 4 that polar compounds penetrate membranes poorly.) The polar nature of the catecholamines is due to the hydroxyl groups on the catechol portion of the molecule. Because they cannot cross the blood-brain barrier, catecholamines have minimal effects on the CNS.

Be aware that catecholamine-containing solutions, which are colorless when first prepared, turn pink or brown over time. This pigmentation is caused by oxidation of the catecholamine molecule. *Catecholamine solutions should be discarded as soon as discoloration develops.* The only exception is dobutamine, which can be used up to 24 hours after the solution was made, even if discoloration appears.

Noncatecholamines

The noncatecholamines have ethylamine in their structure (see Fig. 17.1), but do not contain the catechol moiety that characterizes the catecholamines. Here we discuss three noncatecholamines: ephedrine, albuterol, and phenylephrine.

The noncatecholamines differ from the catecholamines in three important respects. First, because they lack a catechol group, noncatecholamines are not substrates for COMT and are metabolized slowly by MAO. As a result, the half-lives of noncatecholamines are much longer than those of catecholamines. Second, because they do not undergo rapid degradation by MAO and COMT, noncatecholamines can be given orally, whereas catecholamines cannot. Third, noncatecholamines are considerably less polar than catecholamines, and hence are more able to cross the blood-brain barrier.

Receptor Specificity

To understand the actions of individual adrenergic agonists, we need to know their receptor specificity. Variability in receptor specificity among the adrenergic agonists can be illustrated

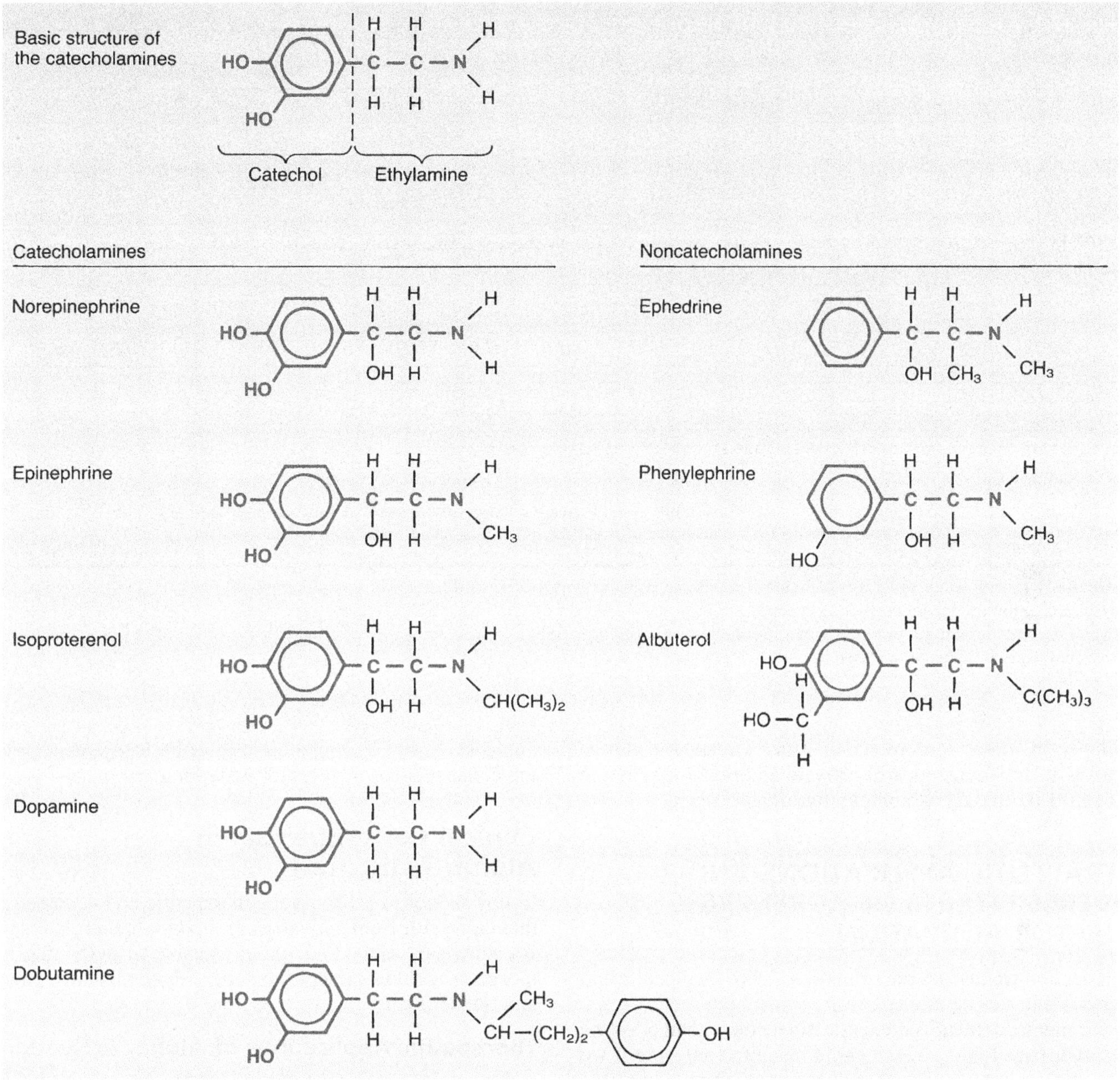

Fig. 17.1 ▪ Structures of representative catecholamines and noncatecholamines. *Catecholamines:* All of the catecholamines share the same basic chemical formula. Because of their biochemical properties, the catecholamines cannot be used orally, cannot cross the blood-brain barrier, and have short half-lives (owing to rapid inactivation by MAO and COMT). *Noncatecholamines:* Although structurally similar to catecholamines, noncatecholamines differ from catecholamines in three important ways: they can be used orally; they can cross the blood-brain barrier; and, because they are not rapidly metabolized by MAO or COMT, they have much longer half-lives.

with three drugs: albuterol, isoproterenol, and epinephrine. Albuterol is highly selective, acting at beta$_2$ receptors only. Isoproterenol is less selective, acting at beta$_1$ receptors and beta$_2$ receptors. Epinephrine is even less selective, acting at all four adrenergic receptor subtypes: alpha$_1$, alpha$_2$, beta$_1$, and beta$_2$.

The receptor specificities of the major adrenergic agonists are shown in Table 17.2. In the upper part of the table, receptor specificity is presented in tabular form. In the lower part, the same information is presented schematically. By learning this content, you will be well on your way to understanding the pharmacology of the sympathomimetic drugs.

Note that the concept of receptor specificity is relative, not absolute. The ability of a drug to selectively activate certain receptors to the exclusion of others depends on the dosage: at low doses, selectivity is maximal; as dosage increases, selectivity declines. For example, when albuterol is administered in low to moderate doses, the drug is highly selective for beta$_2$-adrenergic receptors. However, if the dosage is high, albuterol will activate beta$_1$ receptors as well. The information on receptor

TABLE 17.2 ▪ Receptor Specificity of Representative Adrenergic Agonists

Catecholamines		Noncatecholamines	
Drug	**Receptors Activated**	**Drug**	**Receptors Activated**
Epinephrine	α_1, α_2, β_1, β_2	Ephedrine[a]	α_1, α_2, β_1, β_2
Norepinephrine	α_1, α_2, β_1	Phenylephrine	α_1
Isoproterenol	β_1, β_2	Albuterol	β_2
Dobutamine	β_1		
Dopamine[b]	α_1, β_1, dopamine		

<table>
<tr><th colspan="5">Receptors Activated[c]</th></tr>
<tr><th>Alpha1</th><th>Alpha2</th><th>Beta1</th><th>Beta2</th><th>Dopamine</th></tr>
<tr><td colspan="4">← Epinephrine →</td><td></td></tr>
<tr><td colspan="4">← Ephedrine[a] →</td><td></td></tr>
<tr><td colspan="3">← Norepinephrine →</td><td></td><td></td></tr>
<tr><td>← Phenylephrine →</td><td></td><td colspan="2">← Isoproterenol →</td><td></td></tr>
<tr><td></td><td></td><td>← Dobutamine →</td><td>← Albuterol →</td><td></td></tr>
<tr><td>← Dopamine[b] →</td><td></td><td>← Dopamine[b] →</td><td></td><td>← Dopamine[b] →</td></tr>
</table>

[a]Ephedrine is a mixed-acting agent that causes NE release and also activates alpha and beta receptors directly.
[b]Receptor activation by dopamine is dose dependent.
[c]This chart presents in graphic form the same information on receptor specificity given above. *Arrows* indicate the range of receptors that the drugs can activate (at usual therapeutic doses).
α, Alpha; β, beta.

specificity in Table 17.2 refers to usual therapeutic doses. So-called selective agents will activate additional adrenergic receptors if the dosage is abnormally high.

THERAPEUTIC APPLICATIONS AND ADVERSE EFFECTS OF ADRENERGIC RECEPTOR ACTIVATION

In this section we discuss the responses—both therapeutic and adverse—that can be elicited with sympathomimetic drugs. Because many adrenergic agonists activate more than one type of receptor (see Table 17.2), it could be quite confusing if we were to talk about the effects of the sympathomimetics while employing specific drugs as examples. Consequently, rather than attempting to structure this presentation around representative drugs, we discuss the actions of the adrenergic agonists one receptor at a time. Our discussion begins with alpha$_1$ receptors, and then moves to alpha$_2$ receptors, beta$_1$ receptors, beta$_2$ receptors, and finally dopamine receptors. For each receptor type, we discuss both the therapeutic and adverse responses that can result from receptor activation.

To understand the effects of any specific adrenergic agonist, all you need is two types of information: (1) the identity of the receptor(s) at which the drug acts and (2) the effects produced by activating those receptors. Combining these two types of information will reveal a profile of drug action. This is the same approach to understanding neuropharmacologic agents that we discussed in Chapter 12.

Before you continue, I encourage you to review Table 13.3. We are about to discuss the clinical consequences of adrenergic receptor activation, and Table 13.3 shows the responses to activation of those receptors. If you choose not to memorize Table 13.3 now, be prepared to refer back to it as we discuss the consequences of receptor activation.

Clinical Consequences of Alpha$_1$ Activation

In this section we discuss the therapeutic and adverse effects that can result from activation of alpha$_1$-adrenergic receptors. As shown in Table 17.2, drugs capable of activating alpha$_1$ receptors include epinephrine, NE, phenylephrine, ephedrine, and dopamine.

Therapeutic Applications of Alpha$_1$ Activation

Activation of alpha$_1$ receptors elicits two responses that can be of therapeutic use: (1) *vasoconstriction* (in blood vessels of the skin, viscera, and mucous membranes), and (2) *mydriasis*. Of the two, vasoconstriction is the one for which alpha$_1$ agonists are used most often. Using these drugs for mydriasis is rare.

Safety Alert

IV ADRENERGIC AGONISTS AND ANTAGONISTS

The Institute for Safe Medication Practices (ISMP) includes all IV adrenergic agonists and adrenergic antagonists among its list of high-alert medications. High-alert medications are those drugs that can cause devastating effects to patients in the event of a medication error.

Hemostasis. Hemostasis is defined as the arrest of bleeding, which alpha$_1$ agonists support through vasoconstriction. Alpha$_1$

stimulants are given to stop bleeding primarily in the skin and mucous membranes. Epinephrine, applied topically, is the $alpha_1$ agonist used most for this purpose.

Nasal Decongestion. Nasal congestion results from dilation and engorgement of blood vessels in the nasal mucosa. Drugs can relieve congestion by causing $alpha_1$-mediated vasoconstriction. Specific $alpha_1$-activating agents employed as nasal decongestants include phenylephrine (administered topically) and pseudoephedrine (administered orally).

Adjunct to Local Anesthesia. $Alpha_1$ agonists are frequently combined with local anesthetics to delay systemic absorption. The mechanism is $alpha_1$-mediated vasoconstriction, which reduces blood flow to the site of anesthetic administration. Why delay anesthetic absorption? Because keeping the drug at the local site of action prolongs anesthesia, allows a reduction in anesthetic dosage, and reduces the systemic effects that a local anesthetic might produce. The drug used most frequently to delay anesthetic absorption is epinephrine.

Elevation of Blood Pressure. Because of their ability to cause vasoconstriction, $alpha_1$ agonists can elevate blood pressure in hypotensive patients. Please note, however, that $alpha_1$ agonists are not the primary therapy for hypotension. Rather, they are reserved for situations in which fluid replacement and other measures either are contraindicated or have failed to restore blood pressure to a satisfactory level.

Mydriasis. Activation of $alpha_1$ receptors on the radial muscle of the iris causes mydriasis (dilation of the pupil), which can facilitate eye examinations and ocular surgery. Note that producing mydriasis is the only clinical use of $alpha_1$ activation that is not based on vasoconstriction.

Adverse Effects of $Alpha_1$ Activation

All of the adverse effects caused by $alpha_1$ activation result directly or indirectly from vasoconstriction.

Hypertension. $Alpha_1$ agonists can produce hypertension by causing widespread vasoconstriction. Severe hypertension is most likely with parenteral dosing. Accordingly, when $alpha_1$ agonists are given parenterally, the patient's cardiac rhythm must be monitored continuously and other indicators of cardiovascular status and perfusion (e.g., blood pressure, peripheral pulses, urine output) should be assessed frequently.

Necrosis. If the IV line used to administer an $alpha_1$ agonist becomes extravasated, seepage of the drug into the surrounding tissues may result in necrosis (tissue death). The cause is lack of blood flow to the affected area secondary to intense local vasoconstriction. If extravasation occurs, the area should be infiltrated with an $alpha_1$-blocking agent (e.g., phentolamine), which will counteract $alpha_1$-mediated vasoconstriction and thereby help minimize injury.

Bradycardia. $Alpha_1$ agonists can cause reflex slowing of the heart. The mechanism is this: $Alpha_1$-mediated vasoconstriction elevates blood pressure, which triggers the baroreceptor reflex, causing heart rate to decline. In patients with marginal cardiac reserve, the decrease in cardiac output may compromise tissue perfusion.

Clinical Consequences of $Alpha_2$ Activation

$Alpha_2$ receptors in the periphery are located *presynaptically*, and their activation inhibits NE release. Several adrenergic agonists (e.g., epinephrine, NE) are capable of causing $alpha_2$ activation. However, their ability to activate $alpha_2$ receptors in the periphery has little clinical significance because there are no therapeutic applications related to activation of peripheral $alpha_2$ receptors. Furthermore, activation of these receptors rarely causes significant adverse effects.

In contrast to $alpha_2$ receptors in the *periphery*, $alpha_2$ receptors in the *CNS* are of great clinical significance. By activating central $alpha_2$ receptors, we can produce two useful effects: (1) *reduction* of sympathetic outflow to the heart and blood vessels and (2) relief of severe pain. The central $alpha_2$ agonists used for effects on the heart and blood vessels, and the agents used to relieve pain are discussed in Chapters 19 and 28, respectively.

Clinical Consequences of $Beta_1$ Activation

All of the clinically relevant responses to activation of $beta_1$ receptors result from activating $beta_1$ receptors in the *heart;* activation of renal $beta_1$ receptors is not associated with either beneficial or adverse effects. As indicated in Table 17.2, $beta_1$ receptors can be activated by epinephrine, NE, isoproterenol, dopamine, dobutamine, and ephedrine.

Therapeutic Applications of $Beta_1$ Activation

Heart Failure. Heart failure is characterized by a reduction in the force of myocardial contraction, resulting in insufficient cardiac output. Because activation of $beta_1$ receptors in the heart has a positive inotropic effect (i.e., increases the force of contraction), drugs that activate these receptors can improve cardiac performance.

Shock. This condition is characterized by profound hypotension and greatly reduced tissue perfusion. The primary goal of treatment is to maintain blood flow to vital organs. By increasing heart rate and force of contraction, $beta_1$ stimulants can increase cardiac output and can thereby improve tissue perfusion.

Atrioventricular Heart Block. Atrioventricular (AV) heart block is a condition in which impulse conduction from the atria to the ventricles is either impeded or blocked entirely. As a consequence, the ventricles are no longer driven at an appropriate rate. Because activation of cardiac $beta_1$ receptors can enhance impulse conduction through the AV node, $beta_1$ stimulants can help overcome AV block. It should be noted, however, that drugs are only a temporary form of treatment. For long-term management, a pacemaker is implanted.

Cardiac Arrest. By activating cardiac $beta_1$ receptors, drugs have a role in initiating contraction in a heart that has stopped beating. It should be noted, however, that drugs are not the preferred treatment. Initial management focuses on cardiopulmonary resuscitation, external pacing, or defibrillation (whichever is applicable), and identification and treatment of the underlying cause (e.g., hypoxia, severe acidosis, drug overdose). When a $beta_1$ agonist *is* indicated, epinephrine, administered IV, is the preferred drug. If IV access is not possible, epinephrine can be injected directly into the heart or endotracheally.

Adverse Effects of $Beta_1$ Activation

All of the adverse effects of $beta_1$ activation result from activating $beta_1$ receptors in the heart. Activating renal $beta_1$ receptors is not associated with untoward effects.

Altered Heart Rate or Rhythm. Overstimulation of cardiac $beta_1$ receptors can produce *tachycardia* (excessive heart rate) and *dysrhythmias* (irregular heartbeat).

Angina Pectoris. In some patients, drugs that activate $beta_1$ receptors can precipitate an attack of angina pectoris, a condition characterized by substernal pain in the region of the heart. Anginal pain occurs when cardiac oxygen supply (blood flow) is insufficient to meet cardiac oxygen needs. The most common cause of angina is coronary atherosclerosis (accumulation of lipids and other substances in coronary arteries). Because $beta_1$ agonists increase cardiac oxygen demand (by increasing heart rate and force of contraction), patients with compromised coronary circulation are at risk of an anginal attack.

Clinical Consequences of $Beta_2$ Activation

Applications of $beta_2$ activation are limited to the *lungs* and the *uterus*. Drugs used for their $beta_2$-activating ability include epinephrine, isoproterenol, and albuterol.

Therapeutic Applications of $Beta_2$ Activation

Asthma. Asthma is a chronic condition characterized by inflammation and bronchoconstriction occurring in response to a variety of stimuli. During a severe attack, the reduction in airflow can be life threatening. Because drugs that activate $beta_2$ receptors in the lungs promote bronchodilation, these drugs can help relieve or prevent asthma attacks.

For therapy of asthma, adrenergic agonists that are *selective for $beta_2$ receptors* (e.g., albuterol) are preferred to less selective agents (e.g., isoproterenol). This is especially true for patients who also suffer from *angina pectoris* or *tachycardia,* because drugs that can activate $beta_1$ receptors would aggravate these cardiac disorders.

Most $beta_2$ agonists used to treat asthma are administered by *inhalation.* This route is desirable in that it helps minimize adverse systemic effects. It should be noted, however, that inhalation does not guarantee safety: Serious systemic toxicity can result from overdosing with inhaled sympathomimetics, so patients must be warned against inhaling too much drug.

Delay of Preterm Labor. Activation of $beta_2$ receptors in the uterus relaxes uterine smooth muscle. This action can be employed to delay preterm labor.

Adverse Effects of $Beta_2$ Activation

Hyperglycemia. The most important adverse response to $beta_2$ activation is hyperglycemia (elevation of blood glucose). The mechanism is activation of $beta_2$ receptors in the liver and skeletal muscles, which promotes breakdown of glycogen into glucose. As a rule, $beta_2$ agonists cause hyperglycemia only in patients with *diabetes;* in patients with normal pancreatic function, insulin release will maintain blood glucose at an appropriate level. If hyperglycemia develops in the patient with diabetes, medications used for glucose control will need to be adjusted.

Tremor. Tremor is the most common side effect of $beta_2$ agonists. It occurs because activation of $beta_2$ receptors in skeletal muscle enhances contraction. This effect can be confounding for patients with diabetes because tremor is a common symptom of hypoglycemia; however, when due to $beta_2$ activation, it may be accompanied by hyperglycemia. Fortunately, the tremor generally fades over time and can be minimized by initiating therapy at low doses.

Clinical Consequences of Dopamine Receptor Activation

Activation of peripheral dopamine receptors causes dilation of the renal vasculature. This effect is employed in the treatment of *shock:* by dilating renal blood vessels, we can improve renal perfusion and can thereby reduce the risk of renal failure. *Dopamine* is the only drug available that can activate dopamine receptors. It should be noted that, when dopamine is given to treat shock, the drug also enhances cardiac performance because it activates $beta_1$ receptors in the heart.

Multiple Receptor Activation: Treatment of Anaphylactic Shock

Pathophysiology of Anaphylaxis

Anaphylactic shock is a manifestation of severe allergy. The reaction is characterized by *hypotension* (from widespread vasodilation), *bronchoconstriction,* and *edema of the glottis.* Although histamine contributes to these responses, symptoms are due largely to release of other mediators (e.g., leukotrienes). Anaphylaxis can be triggered by a variety of substances, including bee venom, wasp venom, latex rubber, certain foods (e.g., peanuts, shellfish), and certain drugs (e.g., penicillins).

Treatment

Epinephrine, injected IM or IV, is the treatment of choice for anaphylactic shock. Benefits derive from activating three types of adrenergic receptors: $alpha_1$, $beta_1$, and $beta_2$. By activating these receptors, epinephrine can reverse the most severe manifestations of the anaphylactic reaction. Activation of $beta_1$ receptors increases cardiac output, helping to elevate blood pressure. Blood pressure is also increased because epinephrine promotes $alpha_1$-mediated vasoconstriction. In addition to increasing blood pressure, vasoconstriction helps suppress glottal edema. By activating $beta_2$ receptors, epinephrine can counteract bronchoconstriction. Individuals who are prone to severe allergic responses should carry an epinephrine auto-injector (e.g., EpiPen) at all times. Antihistamines are not especially useful against anaphylaxis because histamine is only one of several contributors to the reaction.

PROPERTIES OF REPRESENTATIVE ADRENERGIC AGONISTS

Our aim in this section is to establish an overview of the adrenergic agonists. The information is presented in the form of short summaries that highlight characteristic features of representative sympathomimetic agents.

As noted, there are two keys to understanding individual adrenergic agonists: (1) knowledge of the receptors that the drug can activate and (2) knowledge of the therapeutic and adverse effects that receptor activation can elicit. By integrating these two types of information, you can easily predict the spectrum of effects that a particular drug can produce.

Unfortunately, knowing the effects that a drug is *capable* of producing does not always indicate how that drug is *actually used* in a clinical setting. Safer alternatives are often available. For example, NE can activate $alpha_1$ receptors and can therefore produce mydriasis, but safer drugs are available for this purpose. Similarly, although isoproterenol is capable of producing uterine relaxation through $beta_2$ activation, it is no longer used for this purpose because safer drugs are available. Because receptor specificity is not always a predictor of the therapeutic applications of a particular adrenergic agonist, for each of the drugs discussed below, approved clinical applications are indicated.

Prototype Drugs

ADRENERGIC AGONISTS

Adrenergic Agonists

Epinephrine [Adrenalin, others]

Beta-Selective Adrenergic Agonists

Isoproterenol [Isuprel]

Epinephrine

- *Receptor specificity:* $alpha_1$, $alpha_2$, $beta_1$, $beta_2$
- *Chemical classification:* catecholamine

Epinephrine [Adrenalin, others] was among the first adrenergic agonists employed clinically and can be considered the prototype of the sympathomimetic drugs. Because of its prototypic status, epinephrine is discussed in detail.

Therapeutic Uses

Epinephrine can activate all four subtypes of adrenergic receptors. As a consequence, the drug can produce a broad spectrum of beneficial sympathomimetic effects:

- Because it can cause $alpha_1$-mediated vasoconstriction, epinephrine is used to (1) delay absorption of local anesthetics, (2) control superficial bleeding, and (3) elevate blood pressure. In the past, epinephrine-induced vasoconstriction was also used for nasal decongestion.
- Because it can activate $beta_1$ receptors, epinephrine may be used to (1) overcome AV heart block and (2) restore cardiac function in patients in cardiac arrest experiencing ventricular fibrillation, pulseless ventricular tachycardia, pulseless electrical activity, or asystole.
- Activation of $beta_2$ receptors in the lung promotes bronchodilation, which can be useful in patients with asthma (although other drugs are preferred).
- Because it can activate a combination of alpha and beta receptors, epinephrine is the treatment of choice for anaphylactic shock. For patients with a history of severe allergic reaction who are at risk of exposure to the allergen (e.g., bee stings), automatic injectors may be prescribed. These are discussed in Box 17.1.

Pharmacokinetics

Absorption. Epinephrine may be administered topically or by injection. The drug cannot be given orally because epinephrine and other catecholamines undergo destruction by MAO and COMT before reaching the systemic circulation. Following subQ injection, absorption is slow, owing to epinephrine-induced local vasoconstriction. Absorption is more rapid following IM injection and is immediate with IV administration.

Inactivation. Epinephrine has a short half-life because of two processes: enzymatic inactivation and uptake into adrenergic nerves. The enzymes that inactivate epinephrine and other catecholamines are MAO and COMT.

Adverse Effects

Because it can activate the four major adrenergic receptor subtypes, epinephrine can produce multiple adverse effects.

Hypertensive Crisis. Vasoconstriction secondary to excessive $alpha_1$ activation can produce a dramatic increase in blood pressure. Cerebral hemorrhage can occur. Because of the potential for severe hypertension, patients receiving *parenteral* epinephrine must undergo continuous cardiovascular monitoring with frequent assessment of vital signs.

Dysrhythmias. Excessive activation of $beta_1$ receptors in the heart can produce dysrhythmias. Because of their sensitivity to catecholamines, hyperthyroid patients are at high risk for epinephrine-induced dysrhythmias.

Angina Pectoris. By activating $beta_1$ receptors in the heart, epinephrine can increase cardiac work and oxygen demand.

si

BOX 17.1 ■ SPECIAL INTEREST TOPIC

EPINEPHRINE AUTO-INJECTORS

Epinephrine is indicated for emergency treatment of anaphylaxis, a life-threatening allergic reaction caused by severe hypersensitivity to insect venoms (e.g., from bees), certain foods (e.g., peanuts, shellfish), and certain drugs (especially penicillins). Every year, anaphylaxis kills about 6000 Americans. Many of these deaths could have been avoided through immediate injection of epinephrine.

Anaphylaxis can develop within minutes of allergen exposure; therefore, anyone who has experienced a severe systemic allergic reaction should carry an epinephrine auto-injector.

Epinephrine auto-injectors [Adrenaclick, Auvi-Q, EpiPen, Twinject] feature a spring-activated needle, designed for IM injection of epinephrine. Because they are preloaded, they are available for rapid use. They are available only by prescription.

Epinephrine is sensitive to extreme heat and light, so auto-injectors should be stored at room temperature in a dark place. *This is not to infer that the device should be left in this environment until needed.* When the patient will be in an area where an encounter with an antigen is possible, it is essential to take the auto-injector along.

After epinephrine injection, it is still important to get immediate medical attention. The effects of epinephrine begin to fade in 10 to 20 minutes, and anaphylactic reactions can be biphasic and prolonged. To ensure a good outcome, hospitalization (up to 6 hours) is recommended.

If the increase in oxygen demand is significant, an anginal attack may ensue. Provocation of angina is especially likely in patients with coronary atherosclerosis.

Necrosis Following Extravasation. If an IV line containing epinephrine becomes extravasated, the ensuing localized vasoconstriction may result in necrosis. Because of this possibility, the IV site should be monitored closely. If extravasation occurs, injury can be minimized by local injection of phentolamine, an alpha-adrenergic antagonist.

Hyperglycemia. In patients with diabetes, epinephrine can cause hyperglycemia. How? By causing breakdown of glycogen secondary to activation of $beta_2$ receptors in liver and skeletal muscle. If hyperglycemia develops, dosage adjustments will need to be made for medications used to manage diabetes.

Drug Interactions

MAO Inhibitors. As their name implies, MAO inhibitors suppress the activity of MAO. These drugs are used primarily to treat depression (see Chapter 32). Because MAO is one of the enzymes that inactivate epinephrine and other catecholamines, inhibition of MAO will prolong and intensify epinephrine's effects. In most situations, patients receiving an MAO inhibitor should not receive epinephrine.

Tricyclic Antidepressants. Tricyclic antidepressants block the uptake of catecholamines into adrenergic neurons. Because neuronal uptake is one mechanism by which the actions of NE and other catecholamines are terminated, blocking uptake can intensify and prolong epinephrine's effects. Accordingly, patients receiving a tricyclic antidepressant may require a reduction in epinephrine dosage.

General Anesthetics. Several inhalational anesthetics render the myocardium hypersensitive to activation by $beta_1$ agonists. When the heart is in this hypersensitive state, exposure to epinephrine and other $beta_1$ agonists can cause tachydysrhythmias.

Alpha-Adrenergic Blocking Agents. Drugs that block alpha-adrenergic receptors can prevent alpha-adrenergic receptor activation by epinephrine. Alpha blockers (e.g., phentolamine) can be used to treat toxicity (e.g., hypertension, local vasoconstriction) caused by excessive epinephrine-induced alpha activation.

Beta-Adrenergic Blocking Agents. Drugs that block beta-adrenergic receptors can prevent beta-adrenergic receptor activation by epinephrine. Beta-blocking agents (e.g., metoprolol) can reduce adverse effects (e.g., dysrhythmias, anginal pain) caused by epinephrine and other $beta_1$ agonists.

Preparations, Dosage, and Administration

Epinephrine [Adrenalin, EpiPen, others] is supplied in solution for administration by several routes: IV, IM, subQ, intracardiac, intraspinal, inhalation, and topical. Solutions for injection are available in 0.1 mg/mL and 1 mg/mL.[a]

Patients receiving IV epinephrine should be monitored closely. They should be observed for signs of excessive cardiovascular activation (e.g., tachydysrhythmias, hypertension) and for possible extravasation of the IV line. If systemic toxicity develops, epinephrine should be discontinued; if indicated, an alpha-adrenergic blocker, a beta-adrenergic blocker, or both should be given to suppress symptoms. If an epinephrine-containing IV line becomes extravasated, administration should be discontinued and the region of extravasation infiltrated with an alpha-adrenergic blocker.

Treatment of anaphylaxis using an epinephrine auto-injector is discussed in Box 17.1.

[a]Prior to May 2016, labeling for epinephrine was based on ratios, so these drugs may remain in stock until they run out or expire. Equivalent strengths are 1:1000 equals 1 mg/mL and 1:10,000 equals 0.1 mg/mL.

PATIENT-CENTERED CARE ACROSS THE LIFE SPAN

Adrenergic Agonists

Life Stage	Considerations or Concerns
Children	These drugs are commonly used in emergency situations. There are no contraindications for children.
Pregnant women	Dobutamine is Pregnancy Risk Category B. The remaining adrenergic agonists are Pregnancy Risk Category C.[a] With epinephrine, norepinephrine, and dopamine, vasoconstriction in the uterus may decrease oxygenation to the fetus. Albuterol is associated with rare congenital anomalies. Albuterol also may decrease uterine contractility. Adequate animal studies have not been conducted for other drugs in this class. In any case, when used for emergencies in which the woman's life is at risk, treatment should not be withheld.
Breast-feeding women	Manufacturers recommend caution if breast-feeding because adequate studies are not available. Breast-feeding infants should be monitored for adrenergic effects.
Older adults	Older adult patients may be more disposed to the adverse effects of these drugs (e.g., blood pressure elevation, tachycardia, shakiness). Adrenergic agonists may also contribute to urinary retention.

[a]As of 2020, the FDA will no longer use Pregnancy Risk Categories. Please refer to Chapter 9 for more information.

Norepinephrine

- *Receptor specificity:* $alpha_1$, $alpha_2$, $beta_1$
- *Chemical classification:* catecholamine

Norepinephrine [Levophed] is similar to epinephrine in several respects. With regard to receptor specificity, NE differs from epinephrine only in that NE does not activate $beta_2$ receptors. Accordingly, NE can elicit all of the responses that epinephrine can, except those that are $beta_2$ mediated. Because NE is a catecholamine, the drug is subject to rapid inactivation by MAO and COMT, and hence cannot be given orally. Adverse effects are nearly identical to those of epinephrine: tachydysrhythmias, angina, hypertension, and local necrosis upon extravasation. In contrast to epinephrine, NE does not promote hyperglycemia, a response that is $beta_2$ mediated. As with epinephrine, responses to NE can be modified by MAO inhibitors, tricyclic antidepressants, general anesthetics, and adrenergic blocking agents.

Despite its similarity to epinephrine, NE has limited clinical applications. The only recognized indications are *hypotensive states* and *cardiac arrest.*

Norepinephrine is supplied in solution (1 mg/mL) for administration by IV infusion only. Monitor cardiovascular status continuously. Assess patient status frequently. Take care to avoid extravasation.

Isoproterenol

- *Receptor specificity:* $beta_1$ and $beta_2$
- *Chemical classification:* catecholamine

Isoproterenol [Isuprel] differs significantly from NE and epinephrine in that isoproterenol acts only at beta-adrenergic receptors. Isoproterenol was the first beta-selective agent employed clinically and will serve as our prototype of the beta-selective adrenergic agonists.

Therapeutic Uses

Cardiovascular. By activating $beta_1$ receptors in the heart, isoproterenol can benefit patients with cardiovascular disorders. Specifically, it is used to manage AV heart block, to improve outcomes in cardiac arrest, and to increase cardiac output during shock.

Adverse Effects

Because isoproterenol does not activate alpha-adrenergic receptors, it produces fewer adverse effects than NE or epinephrine. The major undesired responses, caused by activating $beta_1$ receptors in the heart, are *tachydysrhythmias* and *angina pectoris.* In patients with diabetes, isoproterenol can cause *hyperglycemia* by promoting $beta_2$-mediated glycogenolysis.

Drug Interactions

The major drug interactions of isoproterenol are nearly identical to those of epinephrine. Effects are enhanced by MAO inhibitors and tricyclic antidepressants and reduced by beta-adrenergic blocking agents. Like epinephrine, isoproterenol can cause dysrhythmias in patients receiving certain inhalational anesthetics.

Preparations and Administration

Isoproterenol hydrochloride is available in solution (0.2 mg/mL) for parenteral administration.

When used to *stimulate the heart,* isoproterenol can be administered IV and IM and by intracardiac injection. The dosage for IM administration is about 10 times greater than the dosage employed for the other two routes. The IM route would not be appropriate for use during cardiac arrest.

Dopamine

- *Receptor specificity:* dopamine, $beta_1$, and, at high doses, $alpha_1$
- *Chemical classification:* catecholamine

Receptor Specificity

Dopamine has *dose-dependent* receptor specificity. When administered in low therapeutic doses, dopamine acts on dopamine receptors only. At moderate therapeutic doses, dopamine activates $beta_1$ receptors in addition to dopamine receptors. And at very high doses, dopamine activates $alpha_1$ receptors along with $beta_1$ and dopamine receptors.

Therapeutic Uses

Shock. The major indication for dopamine is shock. Benefits derive from effects on the heart and renal blood vessels. By activating $beta_1$ receptors in the heart, dopamine can increase cardiac output, improving tissue perfusion. By activating dopamine receptors in the kidney, dopamine can dilate renal blood vessels, improving renal perfusion; however, studies indicate that it is not effective in preventing acute renal failure. Moreover, at very high doses that activate $alpha_1$ receptors, vasoconstriction may decrease renal perfusion, overriding the effects of dopamine activation. Therefore, monitoring urine output is an essential component of care for patients on this drug.

Heart Failure. Heart failure is characterized by reduced tissue perfusion secondary to reduced cardiac output. Dopamine can help alleviate symptoms by activating $beta_1$ receptors on the heart, which increases myocardial contractility and thereby increases cardiac output.

Adverse Effects

The most common adverse effects of dopamine—*tachycardia, dysrhythmias,* and *anginal pain*—result from activation of $beta_1$ receptors in the heart. Because of its cardiac actions, dopamine is contraindicated for patients with tachydysrhythmias or ventricular fibrillation. Because high concentrations of dopamine cause $alpha_1$ activation, extravasation may result in *necrosis* from localized vasoconstriction. Tissue injury can be minimized by local infiltration of phentolamine, an alpha-adrenergic antagonist.

Drug Interactions

MAO inhibitors can intensify the effects of dopamine on the heart and blood vessels. If a patient is receiving an MAO inhibitor, the dosage of dopamine must be reduced by at least 90%. Tricyclic antidepressants can also intensify dopamine's actions, but not to the extent seen with MAO inhibitors. Certain general anesthetics can sensitize the myocardium to stimulation by dopamine and other catecholamines, thereby increasing the risk of dysrhythmias. Diuretics can complement the beneficial effects of dopamine on the kidney.

Preparations, Dosage, and Administration

Preparations. Dopamine hydrochloride is supplied in aqueous solutions that range in concentration from 0.8 to 160 mg/mL.

Dosage. Concentrated solutions must be diluted before infusion. For treatment of shock, a concentration of 400 mcg/mL can be used. The recommended initial rate of infusion is 2 to 5 mcg/kg/min. If needed, the infusion rate can be gradually increased to a maximum of 20 to 50 mcg/kg/min.

Administration. Dopamine is administered IV. Because of extremely rapid inactivation by MAO and COMT, the drug must be given by *continuous infusion.* An infusion pump is needed to control flow rate. Cardiovascular status must be closely monitored. If extravasation occurs, the infusion should be stopped and the affected area infiltrated with an alpha-adrenergic antagonist (e.g., phentolamine).

Dobutamine

- *Receptor specificity:* $beta_1$
- *Chemical classification:* catecholamine

Actions and Uses

At therapeutic doses, dobutamine causes selective activation of $beta_1$-adrenergic receptors. The only indication for the drug is heart failure.

Adverse Effects

The major adverse effect is *tachycardia.* Blood pressure and the electrocardiogram (ECG) should be monitored closely.

Drug Interactions

Effects of dobutamine on the heart and blood vessels are intensified greatly by MAO inhibitors. Accordingly, in patients receiving an MAO inhibitor, dobutamine dosage must be reduced at least 90%. Concurrent use of tricyclic antidepressants may cause a moderate increase in the cardiovascular effects. Certain general anesthetics can sensitize the myocardium to stimulation by dobutamine, thereby increasing the risk of dysrhythmias.

Preparations, Dosage, and Administration

Dobutamine hydrochloride is supplied in concentrated and dilute solutions. The concentrated solution (12.5 mg/mL in 20- and 40-mL vials) must be diluted before use. The dilute solutions (1, 2, and 4 mg/mL in 250-mL single-use containers) can be used as is. Because of rapid inactivation by MAO and COMT, dobutamine is administered by continuous IV infusion. The usual rate is 2.5 to 10 mcg/kg/min.

Phenylephrine

- *Receptor specificity*: $alpha_1$
- *Chemical classification*: noncatecholamine

Phenylephrine [Neo-Synephrine, others] is a selective $alpha_1$ agonist. The drug can be administered locally to reduce nasal congestion and parenterally to elevate blood pressure. In addition, phenylephrine eye drops can be used to dilate the pupil. Also, phenylephrine can be coadministered with local anesthetics to delay anesthetic absorption.

Albuterol

- *Receptor specificity:* $beta_2$
- *Chemical classification:* noncatecholamine

Therapeutic Uses

Asthma. Albuterol [Ventolin, VoSpire, others] can reduce airway resistance in asthma by causing $beta_2$-mediated bronchodilation. Because albuterol is relatively selective for $beta_2$ receptors, it produces much less activation of cardiac $beta_1$ receptors than does isoproterenol. As a result, albuterol and other $beta_2$-selective agents have replaced isoproterenol for therapy of asthma. Remember, however, that receptor selectivity is only relative: If administered in large doses, albuterol will lose selectivity and activate $beta_1$ receptors as well as $beta_2$ receptors. Accordingly, patients should be warned not to exceed recommended doses, as doing so may cause undesired cardiac stimulation. Preparations and dosages for asthma are presented in Chapter 76.

Adverse Effects

Adverse effects are minimal at therapeutic doses. *Tremor* is most common. If dosage is excessive, albuterol can cause *tachycardia* by activating $beta_1$ receptors in the heart.

TABLE 17.3 ▪ Discussion of Adrenergic Agonists in Other Chapters

Drug Class	Discussion Topic	Chapter
$Alpha_1$ agonists	Nasal congestion	77
	Ophthalmology	104
$Alpha_2$ agonists	Cardiovascular effects	19
	Pain relief	28
	Hypertension	47
	Ophthalmology	104
$Beta_1$ agonists	Heart failure	48
$Beta_2$ agonists	Asthma	76
	Preterm labor	64
Amphetamines	Basic pharmacology	36
	Attention-deficit/hyperactivity disorder	36
	Drug abuse	40
	Appetite suppression	82

Ephedrine

- *Receptor specificity:* $alpha_1$, $alpha_2$, $beta_1$, $beta_2$
- *Chemical classification:* noncatecholamine

Ephedrine is referred to as a *mixed-acting drug,* because it activates adrenergic receptors by direct *and* indirect mechanisms. *Direct* activation results from binding of the drug to alpha and beta receptors. *Indirect* activation results from release of NE from adrenergic neurons.

Owing to the development of more selective adrenergic agonists, uses for ephedrine are limited. By promoting $beta_2$-mediated bronchodilation, ephedrine can benefit patients with *asthma.* By activating a combination of alpha and beta receptors, ephedrine can improve hemodynamic status in patients with *shock.* It may also be used to manage anesthesia-induced hypotension.

Because ephedrine activates the same receptors as epinephrine, both drugs share the same adverse effects: hypertension, dysrhythmias, angina, and hyperglycemia. In addition, because ephedrine can cross the blood-brain barrier, it can act in the CNS to cause insomnia.

All of the drugs presented here are also discussed in chapters that address specific applications (Table 17.3).

KEY POINTS

- Adrenergic agonists are also known as *sympathomimetics* because their effects mimic those caused by the sympathetic nervous system.
- Most adrenergic agonists act by direct activation of adrenergic receptors. A few act by indirect mechanisms: promotion of NE release, blockade of NE uptake, and inhibition of NE breakdown.
- Adrenergic agonists fall into two chemical classes: catecholamines and noncatecholamines.
- Agents in the catecholamine family cannot be taken orally (because of destruction by MAO and COMT), have a brief duration of action (because of destruction by MAO and COMT), and cannot cross the blood-brain barrier (because they are polar molecules).
- Adrenergic agonists that are noncatecholamines can be taken orally, have a longer duration than the catecholamines, and can cross the blood-brain barrier.
- Activation of $alpha_1$ receptors causes vasoconstriction and mydriasis.
- $Alpha_1$ agonists are used for hemostasis, nasal decongestion, and elevation of blood pressure, and as adjuncts to local anesthetics.
- Major adverse effects that can result from $alpha_1$ activation are hypertension and local necrosis (if extravasation occurs).
- Activation of $alpha_2$ receptors in the periphery is of minimal clinical significance. In contrast, drugs that activate $alpha_2$ receptors in the CNS produce useful effects, such as pain relief (see Chapters 19 and 28).
- All of the clinically relevant responses to activation of $beta_1$ receptors result from activating $beta_1$ receptors in the heart.
- Activation of cardiac $beta_1$ receptors increases heart rate, force of contraction, and conduction through the AV node.
- Drugs that activate $beta_1$ receptors can be used to treat heart failure, AV block, and cardiac arrest caused by asystole.
- Potential adverse effects from $beta_1$ activation are tachycardia, dysrhythmias, and angina.

- Drugs that activate $beta_2$ receptors are used primarily for asthma.
- Principal adverse effects from $beta_2$ activation are hyperglycemia (mainly in diabetic patients) and tremor.
- Activation of dopamine receptors dilates renal blood vessels, which helps maintain renal perfusion in shock.
- Epinephrine is a catecholamine that activates $alpha_1$, $alpha_2$, $beta_1$, and $beta_2$ receptors.
- Epinephrine is the drug of choice for treating anaphylactic shock: By activating $alpha_1$, $beta_1$, and $beta_2$ receptors, epinephrine can elevate blood pressure, suppress glottal edema, and counteract bronchoconstriction.
- Epinephrine can also be used to control superficial bleeding, restart the heart after cardiac arrest, and delay absorption of local anesthetics.
- Epinephrine should not be combined with MAO inhibitors, and should be used cautiously in patients taking tricyclic antidepressants.
- Isoproterenol is a catecholamine that activates $beta_1$ and $beta_2$ receptors.
- Isoproterenol can be used to enhance cardiac performance (by activating $beta_1$ receptors) and to treat bronchospasm (by activating $beta_2$ receptors).
- Dopamine is a catecholamine whose receptor specificity is highly dose dependent: at low therapeutic doses, dopamine acts on dopamine receptors only; at moderate doses, dopamine activates $beta_1$ receptors in addition to dopamine receptors; and at high doses, dopamine activates $alpha_1$ receptors along with $beta_1$ receptors and dopamine receptors.
- Albuterol is a noncatecholamine that produces selective activation of $beta_2$ receptors.
- Albuterol is used to treat asthma.
- Because albuterol is "selective" for $beta_2$ receptors, it produces much less stimulation of the heart than does isoproterenol. Accordingly, albuterol and related drugs have replaced isoproterenol for therapy of asthma.

Please visit **http://evolve.elsevier.com/Lehne** for chapter-specific NCLEX® examination review questions.

Summary of Major Nursing Implications

EPINEPHRINE

Preadministration Assessment

Therapeutic Goal

Epinephrine has multiple indications. The major use is treatment of *anaphylaxis.* Other uses include *control of superficial bleeding, delay of local anesthetic absorption,* and *management of cardiac arrest.*

Identifying High-Risk Patients

Epinephrine must be used with *great caution* in patients with hyperthyroidism, cardiac dysrhythmias, organic heart disease, or hypertension. *Caution* is also needed in patients with angina pectoris or diabetes and in those receiving MAO inhibitors, tricyclic antidepressants, or general anesthetics.

Implementation: Administration

Routes

Topical, inhalation, and parenteral (IV, IM, subQ, intracardiac, intraspinal). Rapid inactivation by MAO and COMT prohibits oral use.

Administration

Epinephrine solutions oxidize over time, causing them to turn pink or brown. Discard discolored solutions.

Ongoing Evaluation and Interventions

Evaluating Therapeutic Effects

In patients receiving IV epinephrine, monitor cardiovascular status continuously.

Minimizing Adverse Effects

Cardiovascular Effects. By stimulating the heart, epinephrine can cause *anginal pain, tachycardia,* and *dysrhythmias.* These responses can be reduced with a beta-adrenergic blocking agent (e.g., metoprolol).

By activating $alpha_1$ receptors on blood vessels, epinephrine can cause intense vasoconstriction, which can result in *severe hypertension.* Blood pressure can be lowered with an alpha-adrenergic blocking agent (e.g., phentolamine).

Necrosis. If an IV line delivering epinephrine becomes extravasated, necrosis may result. Exercise care to avoid extravasation. If extravasation occurs, infiltrate the region with phentolamine to minimize injury.

Hyperglycemia. Epinephrine may cause hyperglycemia in diabetic patients. If hyperglycemia develops, insulin dosage should be increased.

Minimizing Adverse Interactions

MAO Inhibitors and Tricyclic Antidepressants. These drugs prolong and intensify the actions of epinephrine. Patients taking these antidepressants require a reduction in epinephrine dosage.

General Anesthetics. When combined with certain general anesthetics, epinephrine can induce cardiac dysrhythmias. Dysrhythmias may respond to a $beta_1$-adrenergic blocker.

DOPAMINE

Preadministration Assessment

Therapeutic Goal

Dopamine is used to improve hemodynamic status in patients with *shock* or *heart failure.* Benefits derive from enhanced cardiac performance and increased renal perfusion.

Baseline Data

Full assessment of cardiac, hemodynamic, and renal status is needed.

Continued

Summary of Major Nursing Implications—cont'd

Identifying High-Risk Patients

Dopamine is *contraindicated* for patients with tachydysrhythmias or ventricular fibrillation. Use with *extreme caution* in patients with organic heart disease, hyperthyroidism, or hypertension, and in patients receiving MAO inhibitors. *Caution* is also needed in patients with angina pectoris and in those receiving tricyclic antidepressants or general anesthetics.

Implementation: Administration

Route

Intravenous.

Administration

Administer by continuous infusion, employing an infusion pump to control flow rate.

If extravasation occurs, stop the infusion immediately and infiltrate the region with an alpha-adrenergic antagonist (e.g., phentolamine).

Ongoing Evaluation and Interventions

Evaluating Therapeutic Effects

Monitor cardiovascular status continuously. Increased urine output is one index of success. Diuretics may complement the beneficial effects of dopamine on the kidney.

Minimizing Adverse Effects

Cardiovascular Effects. By stimulating the heart, dopamine may cause *anginal pain, tachycardia,* or *dysrhythmias.* These reactions can be decreased with a beta-adrenergic blocking agent (e.g., propranolol).

Necrosis. If the IV line delivering dopamine becomes extravasated, necrosis may result. Exercise care to avoid extravasation. If extravasation occurs, infiltrate the region with phentolamine.

Minimizing Adverse Interactions

MAO Inhibitors. Concurrent use of MAO inhibitors and dopamine can result in severe cardiovascular toxicity. If a patient is taking an MAO inhibitor, dopamine dosage must be reduced by at least 90%.

Tricyclic Antidepressants. These drugs prolong and intensify the actions of dopamine. Patients receiving them may require a reduction in dopamine dosage.

General Anesthetics. When combined with certain general anesthetics, dopamine can induce dysrhythmias. These may respond to a $beta_1$-adrenergic blocker.

DOBUTAMINE

Preadministration Assessment

Therapeutic Goal

Improvement of hemodynamic status in patients with heart failure.

Baseline Data

Full assessment of cardiac, renal, and hemodynamic status is needed.

Identifying High-Risk Patients

Use with *great caution* in patients with organic heart disease, hyperthyroidism, tachydysrhythmias, or hypertension and in those taking an MAO inhibitor. *Caution* is also needed in patients with angina pectoris and in those receiving tricyclic antidepressants or general anesthetics.

Implementation: Administration

Route

Intravenous.

Administration

Administer by continuous IV infusion. Dilute concentrated solutions before use. Infusion rates usually range from 2.5 to 10 mcg/kg/min. Adjust the infusion rate on the basis of the cardiovascular response.

Ongoing Evaluation and Interventions

Evaluating Therapeutic Effects

Monitor cardiac function (heart rate, ECG), blood pressure, and urine output. When possible, monitor central venous pressure and pulmonary wedge pressure.

Minimizing Adverse Effects

Major adverse effects are *tachycardia* and *dysrhythmias.* Monitor the ECG and blood pressure closely. Adverse cardiac effects can be reduced with a beta-adrenergic antagonist.

Minimizing Adverse Interactions

MAO Inhibitors. Concurrent use of an MAO inhibitor with dobutamine can cause severe cardiovascular toxicity. If a patient is taking an MAO inhibitor, dobutamine dosage must be reduced by at least 90%.

Tricyclic Antidepressants. These drugs can prolong and intensify the actions of dobutamine. Patients receiving them may require a reduction in dobutamine dosage.

General Anesthetics. When combined with certain general anesthetics, dobutamine can cause cardiac dysrhythmias. These may respond to a $beta_1$-adrenergic antagonist.

CHAPTER

18 Adrenergic Antagonists

The adrenergic antagonists cause direct blockade of adrenergic receptors. With one exception, all of the adrenergic antagonists produce *reversible* (competitive) blockade.

Unlike many adrenergic agonists, which act at alpha- *and* beta-adrenergic receptors, most adrenergic antagonists are more selective. As a result, the adrenergic antagonists can be neatly divided into two major groups (Table 18.1): (1) *alpha-adrenergic blocking agents* (drugs that produce selective blockade of alpha-adrenergic receptors); and (2) *beta-adrenergic blocking agents* (drugs that produce selective blockade of beta receptors).[a]

[a]Only two adrenergic antagonists—carvedilol and labetalol—act as alpha *and* beta receptors.

Our approach to the adrenergic antagonists mirrors the approach we took with the adrenergic agonists. We begin by discussing the therapeutic and adverse effects that can result from alpha- and beta-adrenergic blockade, after which we discuss the individual drugs that produce receptor blockade.

It is much easier to understand responses to the adrenergic drugs if you first understand the responses to activation of adrenergic receptors. Accordingly, if you have not yet mastered Table 13.3, you should do so now (or be prepared to consult the table as we proceed).

ALPHA-ADRENERGIC ANTAGONISTS

THERAPEUTIC AND ADVERSE RESPONSES TO ALPHA BLOCKADE

In this section we discuss the beneficial and adverse responses that can result from blockade of alpha-adrenergic receptors. Then, properties of individual alpha-blocking agents are discussed.

Therapeutic Applications of Alpha Blockade

Most clinically useful responses to alpha-adrenergic antagonists result from blockade of $alpha_1$ receptors on blood vessels. Blockade of $alpha_1$ receptors in the bladder and prostate can help those with benign prostatic hyperplasia (BPH). Blockade of $alpha_1$ receptors in the eyes and blockade of $alpha_2$ receptors have no recognized therapeutic applications.

Essential Hypertension

Hypertension (high blood pressure) can be treated with a variety of drugs, including the alpha-adrenergic antagonists. Alpha antagonists lower blood pressure by causing vasodilation by blocking $alpha_1$ receptors on arterioles and veins. Dilation of arterioles reduces arterial pressure directly. Dilation of veins lowers arterial pressure by an indirect process: In response to venous dilation, return of blood to the heart decreases, thereby decreasing cardiac output, which in turn reduces arterial pressure. The role of alpha-adrenergic blockers in essential hypertension is discussed further in Chapter 47.

Reversal of Toxicity From $Alpha_1$ Agonists

Overdose with an alpha-adrenergic agonist (e.g., epinephrine) can produce *hypertension* secondary to excessive activation of $alpha_1$ receptors on blood vessels. When this occurs, blood pressure can be lowered by reversing the vasoconstriction with an alpha-blocking agent.

TABLE 18.1 ■ Receptor Specificity of Adrenergic Antagonists

Category	Drugs	Receptors Blocked
ALPHA-ADRENERGIC BLOCKING AGENTS		
Nonselective Agents	Phenoxybenzamine	$alpha_1$, $alpha_2$
	Phentolamine	$alpha_1$, $alpha_2$
$Alpha_1$-Selective Agents	Alfuzosin	$alpha_1$
	Doxazosin	$alpha_1$
	Prazosin	$alpha_1$
	Silodosin	$alpha_1$
	Tamsulosin	$alpha_1$
	Terazosin	$alpha_1$
BETA-ADRENERGIC BLOCKING AGENTS		
Nonselective Agents	Carteolol	$beta_1$, $beta_2$
	Nadolol	$beta_1$, $beta_2$
	Pindolol	$beta_1$, $beta_2$
	Propranolol	$beta_1$, $beta_2$
	Sotalol	$beta_1$, $beta_2$
	Timolol	$beta_1$, $beta_2$
	Carvedilol	$beta_1$, $beta_2$, $alpha_1$
	Labetalol	$beta_1$, $beta_2$, $alpha_1$
$Beta_1$-Selective Agents	Acebutolol	$beta_1$
	Atenolol	$beta_1$
	Betaxolol	$beta_1$
	Bisoprolol	$beta_1$
	Esmolol	$beta_1$
	Metoprolol	$beta_1$
	Nebivolol	$beta_1$

If an IV line containing an alpha agonist extravasates (leaks out into the surrounding tissues), necrosis can occur secondary to intense local vasoconstriction. By infiltrating the region with phentolamine (an alpha-adrenergic antagonist), we can block the vasoconstriction and thereby prevent injury.

Safety Alert

INTRAVENOUS ADRENERGIC ANTAGONISTS

The Institute for Safe Medication Practices (ISMP) includes all IV adrenergic antagonists on its list of high-alert medications. High-alert medications can cause devastating effects to patients in the event of a medication error.

BPH

BPH results from proliferation of cells in the prostate gland. Symptoms include dysuria, increased frequency of daytime urination, nocturia, urinary hesitancy, urinary urgency, a sensation of incomplete voiding, and a reduction in the size and force of the urinary stream. All of these symptoms can be improved with drugs that block $alpha_1$ receptors. Benefits derive from reduced contraction of smooth muscle in the prostatic capsule and the bladder neck (trigone and sphincter). Please note that BPH and its treatment are discussed in Chapter 66.

Pheochromocytoma

A pheochromocytoma is a catecholamine-secreting tumor derived from cells of the sympathetic nervous system. These tumors are usually located in the adrenal medulla. If secretion of catecholamines (epinephrine, norepinephrine) is sufficiently great, persistent hypertension can result. The principal cause of hypertension is activation of $alpha_1$ receptors on blood vessels, although activation of $beta_1$ receptors on the heart can also contribute. The preferred treatment is surgical removal of the tumor, but alpha-adrenergic blockers may also be employed.

Alpha-blocking agents have two roles in managing pheochromocytoma. First, in patients with inoperable tumors, alpha blockers are given long term to suppress hypertension. Second, when surgery is indicated, alpha blockers are administered preoperatively to reduce the risk of acute hypertension during the procedure. This is necessary because the surgical patient is at risk because manipulation of the tumor can cause massive catecholamine release.

Raynaud's Disease

Raynaud's disease is a peripheral vascular disorder characterized by vasospasm in the toes and fingers. Prominent symptoms are local sensations of pain and cold. Alpha blockers can suppress symptoms by preventing alpha-mediated vasoconstriction. It should be noted, however, that although alpha blockers can relieve symptoms of Raynaud's disease, they are generally ineffective against other peripheral vascular disorders that involve inappropriate vasoconstriction.

Adverse Effects of Alpha Blockade

The most significant adverse effects of the alpha-adrenergic antagonists result from blockade of $alpha_1$ receptors. Detrimental effects associated with $alpha_2$ blockade are minor.

Adverse Effects of $Alpha_1$ Blockade

Orthostatic Hypotension. Orthostatic (postural) hypotension is the most serious adverse response to alpha-adrenergic blockade. This hypotension can reduce blood flow to the brain, causing dizziness, light-headedness, and even syncope (fainting).

The cause of orthostatic hypotension is blockade of alpha receptors on *veins,* which reduces muscle tone in the venous wall. Because of reduced venous tone, blood tends to pool (accumulate) in veins when the patient assumes an erect posture. As a result, return of blood to the heart is reduced, which decreases cardiac output, which in turn causes blood pressure to fall.

Patients should be informed about symptoms of orthostatic hypotension (light-headedness or dizziness on standing) and be advised to sit or lie down if these occur. In addition, patients should be informed that orthostatic hypotension can be minimized by avoiding abrupt transitions from a supine or sitting position to an erect posture.

Reflex Tachycardia. Alpha-adrenergic antagonists can increase heart rate by triggering the baroreceptor reflex. The mechanism is this: (1) blockade of vascular $alpha_1$ receptors causes vasodilation; (2) vasodilation reduces blood pressure; and (3) baroreceptors sense the reduction in blood pressure and, in an attempt to restore normal pressure, initiate a reflex increase in heart rate via the autonomic nervous system. If necessary, reflex tachycardia can be suppressed with a beta-adrenergic blocking agent.

Nasal Congestion. Alpha blockade can dilate the blood vessels of the nasal mucosa, producing nasal congestion.

Inhibition of Ejaculation. Because activation of $alpha_1$ receptors is required for ejaculation (see Table 13.3), blockade of these receptors can cause sexual dysfunction. This form of dysfunction is reversible and resolves when the alpha blocker is withdrawn. If a patient deems the adverse sexual effects of alpha blockade unacceptable, a change in medication will be required. Because males may be reluctant to discuss such concerns, a tactful interview may be needed to discern if drug-induced sexual dysfunction is discouraging drug use.

Sodium Retention and Increased Blood Volume. By reducing blood pressure, alpha blockers can promote renal retention of sodium and water, thereby causing blood volume to increase. The steps in this process are as follows: (1) by reducing blood pressure, $alpha_1$ blockers decrease renal blood flow; (2) in response to reduced renal perfusion, the kidney excretes less sodium and water; and (3) the resultant retention of sodium and water increases blood volume. As a result, blood pressure is elevated, blood flow to the kidney is increased, and, as far as the kidney is concerned, all is well. Unfortunately, when alpha blockers are used to treat hypertension (which they often are), this compensatory elevation in blood pressure can negate beneficial effects. To prevent the kidney from "neutralizing" hypotensive actions, alpha-blocking agents are usually combined with a diuretic when used in patients with hypertension.

Adverse Effects of $Alpha_2$ Blockade

The most significant adverse effect associated with $alpha_2$ blockade is *potentiation of the reflex tachycardia that can occur in response to blockade of $alpha_1$ receptors.* Why does $alpha_2$ blockade intensify reflex tachycardia? Recall that peripheral $alpha_2$ receptors are located presynaptically and that activation of these receptors inhibits norepinephrine release. Hence, if $alpha_2$ receptors are blocked, release of norepinephrine will increase. Because the reflex tachycardia caused by $alpha_1$ blockade is ultimately the result of increased firing of the sympathetic nerves to the heart, and because $alpha_2$ blockade will cause each nerve impulse to release a greater amount of norepinephrine, $alpha_2$ blockade will potentiate reflex tachycardia initiated by blockade of $alpha_1$ receptors. Accordingly, drugs such as phentolamine, which block $alpha_2$ as well as $alpha_1$ receptors, cause greater reflex tachycardia than do drugs that block $alpha_1$ receptors only.

Prototype Drugs

ADRENERGIC ANTAGONISTS

Selective ($Alpha_1$) Adrenergic Antagonist (Alpha Blocker)

Prazosin [Minipress]

Nonselective Beta Adrenergic Antagonist (Beta Blocker)

Propranolol [Inderal LA, InnoPran XL]

Selective ($Beta_1$) Adrenergic Antagonist (Beta Blocker)

Metoprolol [Lopressor, Toprol XL, Betaloc ♣]

PROPERTIES OF INDIVIDUAL ALPHA BLOCKERS

Eight alpha-adrenergic antagonists are employed clinically. Because the alpha blockers often cause postural hypotension, therapeutic uses are limited.

As indicated in Table 18.1, the alpha-adrenergic blocking agents can be subdivided into two major groups. One group, represented by *prazosin,* contains drugs that produce *selective $alpha_1$ blockade.* The second group, represented by *phentolamine,* consists of *nonselective alpha blockers,* which block $alpha_1$ *and* $alpha_2$ receptors.

PATIENT-CENTERED CARE ACROSS THE LIFE SPAN

Alpha-Adrenergic Antagonists

Life Stage	Patient Care Concerns
Children	Alpha blockers are not approved for use in children with the exceptions of OraVerse (the agent approved for reversal of local anesthesia following dental surgery) and phentolamine for prevention of tissue damage that can occur with extravasation of IV vasopressors. Phenoxybenzamine has been used off-label for the treatment of hypertension due to pheochromocytoma in children.
Pregnant women	Alfuzosin, silodosin, and tamsulosin are classified as Pregnancy Risk Category B; however, it is important to note that these three drugs are approved only for treatment of BPH. The remaining alpha-adrenergic blockers are classified as Pregnancy Risk Category C.[a]
Breast-feeding women	Manufacturers of phenoxybenzamine and phentolamine recommend that women taking this drug not breast-feed because of inadequate studies and potential risks. Labeling for the remaining drugs in this class recommends caution in breast-feeding.
Older adults	Older adults are especially vulnerable to the first-dose effects of alpha blockers. Alpha blockers are also associated with the worsening of urinary incontinence in women and increases of syncope in both genders. Beers Criteria specifically identifies the peripheral $alpha_1$ blockers doxazosin, prazosin, and terazosin as potentially inappropriate for older adults because of the high incidence of orthostatic hypotension. Commonly prescribed drugs such as diuretics and CNS depressants can cause additive adverse effects when given with alpha blockers.

[a]As of 2020, the FDA will no longer use Pregnancy Risk Categories. Please refer to Chapter 9 for more information.

Prazosin

Actions and Uses

Prazosin [Minipress], our prototype, is a competitive antagonist that produces selective blockade of $alpha_1$-adrenergic receptors. The result is dilation of arterioles and veins, and relaxation of smooth muscle in the bladder neck (trigone and sphincter) and prostatic capsule. Prazosin is approved only for hypertension, but it can also benefit men with BPH.

Pharmacokinetics

Prazosin is administered orally. Antihypertensive effects peak in 1 to 3 hours and persist for 10 hours. The drug undergoes extensive hepatic metabolism followed by excretion in the bile. Only 10% is eliminated in the urine. The half-life is 2 to 3 hours.

Adverse Effects

Blockade of $alpha_1$ receptors can cause *orthostatic hypotension, reflex tachycardia,* and *nasal congestion.* The most serious of these is hypotension. Patients should be educated about the symptoms of orthostatic hypotension and be advised to sit or lie down if they occur. Also, patients should be informed that orthostatic hypotension can be minimized by moving slowly when changing from a supine or sitting position to an upright position.

About 1% of patients lose consciousness 30 to 60 minutes after receiving their initial prazosin dose. This *first-dose effect* is the result of severe postural hypotension. To minimize the first-dose effect, the initial dose should be small (1 mg or less). Subsequent doses can be gradually increased with little risk of fainting. Patients who are starting treatment should be forewarned about the first-dose effect and advised to avoid driving and other hazardous activities for 12 to 24 hours. Administering the initial dose immediately before going to bed eliminates the risk of a first-dose effect.

Preparations, Dosage, and Administration

Prazosin hydrochloride [Minipress] is available in capsules (1, 2, and 5 mg) for oral use. The initial adult dosage for hypertension is 1 mg 2 or 3 times a day. The maintenance dosage is 2 to 20 mg/day taken in divided doses.

Terazosin

Actions and Uses

Like prazosin, terazosin [Hytrin 🍁] is a selective, competitive antagonist at $alpha_1$-adrenergic receptors. The drug is approved for hypertension and BPH.

Pharmacokinetics

Pharmacokinetics of terazosin and the remaining alpha blockers is available in Table 18.2.

Adverse Effects

Like other alpha-blocking agents, terazosin can cause *orthostatic hypotension, reflex tachycardia,* and *nasal congestion.* In addition, terazosin is associated with a high incidence (16%) of *headache.* As with prazosin, the first dose can cause profound hypotension. To minimize this first-dose effect, the initial dose should be administered at bedtime.

Preparations, Dosage, and Administration

Information on preparations, dosage, and administration of adrenergic antagonists is provided in Table 18.3.

Doxazosin

Actions and Uses

Doxazosin [Cardura, Cardura XL] is a selective, competitive inhibitor of $alpha_1$-adrenergic receptors. Immediate-release forms of this drug are indicated for hypertension and BPH. Extended-release doxazosin [Cardura XL] is approved for management of BPH only.

Adverse Effects

Like prazosin and terazosin, doxazosin can cause *orthostatic hypotension, reflex tachycardia,* and *nasal congestion.* As with prazosin and terazosin, the first dose can cause profound hypotension, which can be minimized by giving the initial dose at bedtime.

Tamsulosin

Actions and Uses

Tamsulosin [Flomax] is an $alpha_1$-adrenergic antagonist that causes "selective" blockade of $alpha_1$ receptors on smooth muscle of the bladder neck (trigone and sphincter), prostatic capsule, and prostatic urethra; blockade of vascular $alpha_1$ receptors is weak. The drug is approved only for BPH. It is not useful for hypertension. In men with BPH, tamsulosin increases urine flow rate and decreases residual urine volume. Maximum benefits develop within 2 weeks.

Adverse Effects

The most common adverse effects are *headache* and *dizziness.* From 8% to 18% of patients experience *abnormal ejaculation* (ejaculation failure, ejaculation decrease, retrograde ejaculation). In addition, the drug is associated with increased incidence of rhinitis.

Drug Interactions

Combined use with cimetidine increases tamsulosin serum levels, which may cause toxicity. Combined use with hypotensive drugs—including

TABLE 18.2 ■ Alpha-Adrenergic Antagonists: Pharmacokinetic Properties

Drug	Route	Peak	Half-Life	Metabolism[a]	Excretion
NONSELECTIVE AGENTS					
Phenoxybenzamine	PO, IV	PO: 4–6 hr	PO: unknown IV: 24 hr	Hepatic	Urine (primary), bile
Phentolamine	IM, IV, local infiltration	IM: 30–45 min IV: 1–2 min	IM: unknown IV: 20 min	Hepatic	Urine
$ALPHA_1$-SELECTIVE AGENTS					
Alfuzosin	PO	8 hr	10 hr[b]	Hepatic	Feces
Doxazosin	PO	2–3 hr	22 hr[c]	Hepatic	Bile
Prazosin	PO	1–3 hr	2–3 hr	Hepatic	Bile
Silodosin	PO	3–6 hr	13–24 hr[c]	Hepatic	Feces (primary), urine
Tamsulosin	PO	4–5 hr (with food) 6–7 hr (without food)	9–15 hr[c]	Hepatic	Urine (primary), feces
Terazosin	PO	1–2 hr	9–12 hr[c]	Hepatic	Bile (primary), urine

[a]Primary mechanism of metabolism.
[b]80–90% protein-bound.
[c]Greater than 90% protein-bound.

TABLE 18.3 ■ Alpha-Adrenergic Antagonists: Preparations, Dosage, and Administration

Drug	Preparations	Dosage	Administration
NONSELECTIVE AGENTS			
Phenoxybenzamine [Dibenzyline]	Tablet: 10 mg	10 mg twice daily up to 20–40 mg 2–3 times daily	NIOSH specifically stresses gloving before administration.
Phentolamine [OraVerse, Regitine ♣]	Sol: 5 mg/2 mL (concentrated) OraVerse: 0.4 mg/1.7 mL (Use of OraVerse is limited to reversal of anesthetic following dental surgery.)	*Infiltration post IV extravasation:* 5–10 mg diluted in 10 mL saline *To prevent hypertension during surgical excision of a pheochromocytoma:* 5 mg (IM or IV) given 1 to 2 hours before surgery	Infiltration post IV extravasation: Inject drug into extravasated region.
ALPHA$_1$-SELECTIVE AGENTS			
Alfuzosin (ER) [Uroxatral, Xatral ♣]	Tablet: 10 mg	10 mg/day	Administer 30 minutes after the same meal each day. Do not crush tablets.
Doxazosin (IR) [Cardura]	Tablets: 1, 2, 4, 8 mg	1–8 mg/day *Max:* 16 mg/day	Administer with or without food in either the morning or evening.
Doxazosin (ER) [Cardura XL]	Tablets: 4, 8 mg	4–8 mg/day	Administer with breakfast. Do not crush or cut tablets.
Prazosin [Minipress]	Tablets: 1, 2, 5 mg	1–2 mg 2–3 times daily up to 20 mg twice daily	Administer with or without food.
Silodosin [Rapaflo]	Capsules: 4, 8 mg	8 mg/day	Administer with meals. Capsules may be opened and contents sprinkled onto food, but do not crush or chew contents.
Tamsulosin [Flomax]	Capsules: 0.4 mg	0.4 mg/day	Administer 30 minutes after the same meal each day. Do not open or crush capsules.
Terazosin [Hytrin ♣]	Tablets: 1, 2, 5, 10 mg Capsules: 1, 2, 5, 10 mg	1–5 mg/day for hypertension 10 mg/day for BPH *Max:* 20 mg	Administer at the same time each day. Give the first dose at bedtime to minimize first-dose effect.

IR, Immediate release; *ER,* extended release; *max,* maximum dose; *sol,* solution; *NIOSH,* National Institute for Occupational Safety and Health.

phosphodiesterase type 5 (PDE-5) inhibitors such as sildenafil [Viagra]—may cause a significant reduction in blood pressure.

Alfuzosin

Actions and Uses

Like tamsulosin, alfuzosin [Uroxatral, Xatral ♣] is an alpha$_1$ blocker with selectivity for alpha$_1$ receptors in the prostate and urinary tract. At recommended doses, blockade of alpha$_1$ receptors on blood vessels is weak. Therefore, alfuzosin is indicated only for BPH.

Adverse Effects

Alfuzosin is generally well tolerated. The most common adverse effect is *dizziness.* Syncope and clinically significant hypotension are rare. Unlike tamsulosin, alfuzosin does not interfere with ejaculation.

Doses 4 times greater than recommended can prolong the QT interval, and might thereby pose a risk of ventricular dysrhythmias. In patients with moderate to severe hepatic impairment, alfuzosin levels increase three- to fourfold, thus increasing the likelihood of ventricular rhythm disturbances. The drug is contraindicated for these patients.

Drug Interactions

Levels of alfuzosin are markedly raised by powerful inhibitors of CYP3A4. Among these are erythromycin, clarithromycin, itraconazole, ketoconazole, nefazodone, and the HIV protease inhibitors, such as ritonavir. Concurrent use of alfuzosin with these drugs is contraindicated.

Although alfuzosin does not lower blood pressure much, combining it with other hypotensive agents could produce a more dramatic reduction. Accordingly, such combinations should be used with caution. Drugs of concern include organic nitrates, antihypertensive agents, and the PDE-5 inhibitors used for sexual dysfunction (e.g., sildenafil [Viagra]).

Silodosin

Actions and Uses

Silodosin [Rapaflo] is an alpha-adrenergic antagonist that selectively blocks alpha$_1$ receptors in the prostate, bladder, and urethra. Blockade of vascular alpha receptors is weak. The drug is indicated only for BPH.

Adverse Effects

Silodosin is generally well tolerated. However, like tamsulosin, silodosin can greatly reduce or eliminate release of semen during orgasm. This effect reverses when the drug is discontinued. Although blockade of vascular alpha receptors is usually minimal, silodosin *can* produce dizziness, light-headedness, and nasal congestion.

Phentolamine

Actions and Uses

Like prazosin, phentolamine [OraVerse, Regitine ♣] is a competitive adrenergic antagonist. However, in contrast to prazosin, phentolamine blocks alpha$_2$ receptors as well as alpha$_1$ receptors. Phentolamine has three approved applications: (1) diagnosis and treatment of pheochromocytoma; (2) prevention of tissue necrosis following extravasation of drugs that produce alpha$_1$-mediated vasoconstriction (e.g., norepinephrine); and (3) reversal of soft tissue anesthesia. (Local anesthetics are often combined with epinephrine, which prolongs anesthetic action by causing $alpha_1$-mediated vasoconstriction. Phentolamine blocks epinephrine-mediated vasoconstriction, and thereby increases local blood flow, which increases the rate of anesthetic removal.)

Adverse Effects

Like prazosin, phentolamine can produce the typical adverse effects associated with alpha-adrenergic blockade: *orthostatic hypotension, reflex tachycardia, nasal congestion,* and *inhibition of ejaculation.* Because it blocks $alpha_2$ receptors, *phentolamine produces greater reflex tachycardia than prazosin.* If reflex tachycardia is especially severe, heart rate can be reduced with a beta blocker. Because tachycardia can aggravate angina pectoris and myocardial infarction (MI), phentolamine is contraindicated for patients with either disorder.

Overdose can produce profound hypotension. If necessary, blood pressure can be elevated with *norepinephrine. Epinephrine* should *not* be used, because the drug can cause blood pressure to drop even further. In the presence of $alpha_1$ blockade, the ability of epinephrine to promote vasodilation (via activation of vascular $beta_2$ receptors) may outweigh the ability of epinephrine to cause vasoconstriction (via activation of vascular $alpha_1$ receptors). Further lowering of blood pressure is not a significant problem with norepinephrine because norepinephrine does not activate $beta_2$ receptors.

Phenoxybenzamine

Actions and Uses

Phenoxybenzamine [Dibenzyline] is an old drug that, like phentolamine, blocks $alpha_1$ and $alpha_2$ receptors. However, unlike all of the other alpha-adrenergic antagonists, phenoxybenzamine is a *noncompetitive* receptor antagonist. Hence, receptor blockade is *not reversible.* As a result, the effects of phenoxybenzamine are long lasting. (Responses to a single dose can persist for several days.) Effects subside as newly synthesized receptors replace the ones that have been irreversibly blocked. Phenoxybenzamine is approved only for *pheochromocytoma.*

Adverse Effects

Like the other alpha-adrenergic antagonists, phenoxybenzamine can produce *orthostatic hypotension, reflex tachycardia, nasal congestion,* and *inhibition of ejaculation.* Reflex tachycardia is greater than that caused by prazosin and about equal to that caused by phentolamine.

If dosage is excessive, phenoxybenzamine, like phentolamine, will cause profound hypotension. Furthermore, because hypotension is the result of *irreversible* $alpha_1$ blockade, it cannot be corrected with an $alpha_1$ agonist. To restore blood pressure, patients must be given IV fluids, which elevate blood pressure by increasing blood volume.

Phenoxybenzamine is classified by the National Institute for Occupational Safety and Health (NIOSH) as a Group 2 hazardous drug. Gloves should be worn when handling this drug; see Table 3.1 in Chapter 3 for administration and handling guidelines. Long-term use is not recommended due to a potential link to cancer development in patients who have taken this drug long term.

BETA-ADRENERGIC ANTAGONISTS

THERAPEUTIC AND ADVERSE RESPONSES TO BETA BLOCKADE

In this section we consider the beneficial and adverse responses that can result from blockade of beta-adrenergic receptors. Then we examine the properties of individual beta blockers.

Therapeutic Applications of Beta Blockade

Practically all of the therapeutic effects of the beta-adrenergic antagonists result from blockade of $beta_1$ receptors in the heart. The major consequences of blocking these receptors are (1) reduced heart rate, (2) reduced force of contraction, and (3) reduced velocity of impulse conduction through the atrioventricular (AV) node. Because of these effects, beta blockers are useful in a variety of cardiovascular disorders.

Angina Pectoris

Angina pectoris (cardiac pain due to ischemia) occurs when oxygen supplied to the heart via coronary circulation is insufficient to meet cardiac oxygen demand. Anginal attacks can be precipitated by exertion, intense emotion, and other factors. Beta-adrenergic blockers are a mainstay of antianginal therapy. By blocking $beta_1$ receptors in the heart, these drugs decrease cardiac workload. This reduces oxygen demand, bringing it back into balance with oxygen supply and thereby preventing ischemia and pain. Angina pectoris and its treatment are discussed in Chapter 51.

Hypertension

For years, beta blockers were considered drugs of choice for hypertension. However, more recent data indicate they are less beneficial than previously believed.

The exact mechanism by which beta blockers reduce blood pressure is not known. Older proposed mechanisms include reduction of cardiac output through blockade of $beta_1$ receptors in the heart and suppression of renin release through blockade of $beta_1$ receptors in the kidney (see Chapter 44 for a discussion of the role of renin in blood pressure control). More recently, we have learned that, with long-term use, beta blockers reduce peripheral vascular resistance, which could account for much of their antihypertensive effects. The role of beta-adrenergic blocking agents in hypertension is discussed in Chapter 47.

Cardiac Dysrhythmias

Beta-adrenergic blocking agents are especially useful for treating dysrhythmias that involve excessive electrical activity in the sinus node and atria. By blocking cardiac $beta_1$ receptors, these drugs can (1) decrease the rate of sinus nodal discharge and (2) suppress conduction of atrial impulses through the AV node, thereby preventing the ventricles from being driven at an excessive rate. The use of beta-adrenergic blockers to treat dysrhythmias is discussed in Chapter 49.

Myocardial Infarction

A myocardial infarction (MI) is a region of myocardial necrosis caused by localized interruption of blood flow to the heart wall. Treatment with a beta blocker can reduce pain, infarct size, mortality, and the risk of reinfarction. To be effective, therapy with a beta blocker must begin soon after an MI has occurred, and should be continued for several years. The role of beta blockers in treating MI is discussed in Chapter 53.

Reduction of Perioperative Mortality

Beta blockers may decrease the risk for mortality associated with noncardiac surgery in high-risk patients. In the DECREASE-IV trial, pretreatment with bisoprolol reduced the incidence of perioperative MI and death. However, for treatment to be both safe and effective, dosing should begin *early* (several days to weeks before surgery) and *doses should be low initially and then titrated up* (to achieve a resting heart rate of 60 to 80 beats/min). In addition, treatment should continue for 1 month after surgery. As shown in an earlier trial, known as POISE, if the beta blocker is started *late* (just before surgery), and if the doses are *large,* such treatment can actually *increase* the risk of perioperative mortality.

Heart Failure

Beta blockers are now considered standard therapy for heart failure. This application is relatively new and may come as a surprise to some readers because, until recently, heart failure was considered an absolute *contraindication* to beta blockers. At this time, only three beta blockers—carvedilol, bisoprolol, and metoprolol—have been shown effective for heart failure. Use of beta blockers for heart failure is discussed in Chapter 48.

Hyperthyroidism

Hyperthyroidism (excessive production of thyroid hormone) is associated with an increase in the sensitivity of the heart to catecholamines (e.g., norepinephrine, epinephrine). As a result, normal levels of sympathetic activity to the heart can generate tachydysrhythmias and angina pectoris. Blockade of cardiac $beta_1$ receptors suppresses these responses.

Migraine Prophylaxis

When taken prophylactically, beta-adrenergic blocking agents can reduce the frequency and intensity of migraine attacks. However, although beta blockers are effective as prophylaxis, these drugs are not able to abort a migraine headache once it has begun. The mechanism by which beta blockers prevent migraine is not known. Treatment of migraine and other headaches is discussed in Chapter 30.

Stage Fright

Public speakers and other performers sometimes experience "stage fright." Prominent symptoms are tachycardia, tremors, and sweating brought on by generalized discharge of the sympathetic nervous system. Some of you may experience similar symptoms when taking tests. Beta blockers help prevent stage fright—and test anxiety—by preventing $beta_1$-mediated tachycardia.

Pheochromocytoma

As discussed earlier in the chapter, a pheochromocytoma secretes large amounts of catecholamines, which can cause excessive stimulation of the heart resulting in life-threatening hypertension. Cardiac stimulation can be prevented by $beta_1$ blockade.

Glaucoma

Beta blockers are important drugs for treating glaucoma, a condition characterized by elevated intraocular pressure with subsequent injury to the optic nerve. The group of beta blockers used in glaucoma is different from the group of beta blockers discussed here. Glaucoma treatment is discussed in Chapter 104.

Adverse Effects of Beta Blockade

Although therapeutic responses to beta blockers are due almost entirely to blockade of $beta_1$ receptors, adverse effects involve both $beta_1$ and $beta_2$ blockade. Consequently, the nonselective beta-adrenergic blocking agents (drugs that block $beta_1$ *and* $beta_2$ receptors) produce a broader spectrum of adverse effects than do the cardioselective beta-adrenergic antagonists (drugs that block only $beta_1$ receptors at therapeutic doses).

Adverse Effects of $Beta_1$ Blockade

All of the adverse effects of $beta_1$ blockade are the result of blocking $beta_1$ receptors in the heart. Blockade of renal $beta_1$ receptors is not a concern.

Bradycardia. Blockade of cardiac $beta_1$ receptors can produce bradycardia (excessively slow heart rate). If necessary, heart rate can be increased using a beta-adrenergic agonist, such as isoproterenol, and atropine (a muscarinic antagonist). Isoproterenol competes with the beta blocker for cardiac $beta_1$ receptors, thereby promoting cardiac stimulation. By blocking muscarinic receptors on the heart, atropine prevents slowing of the heart by the parasympathetic nervous system.

Reduced Cardiac Output. $Beta_1$ blockade can reduce cardiac output by decreasing heart rate and the force of myocardial contraction. Because they can decrease cardiac output, *beta blockers must be used with great caution in patients with heart failure or reduced cardiac reserve.* In both cases, any further decrease in cardiac output could result in insufficient tissue perfusion.

Precipitation of Heart Failure. In some patients, suppression of cardiac function with a beta blocker can be so great as to cause heart failure. Patients should be informed about the early signs of heart failure (shortness of breath, night coughs, swelling of the extremities) and instructed to notify the prescriber if these occur. It is important to appreciate that, although beta blockers can precipitate heart failure, they are also used to *treat* heart failure.

AV Heart Block. Atrioventricular heart block is defined as a delay in the conduction of electrical impulses through the AV node. In its most severe form, AV block prevents *all* atrial impulses from reaching the ventricles. Because blockade of cardiac $beta_1$ receptors can suppress AV conduction, production of AV block is a potential complication of beta-blocker therapy. These drugs are contraindicated for patients with preexisting AV block.

Rebound Cardiac Excitation. Long-term use of beta blockers can sensitize the heart to catecholamines. As a result, if a beta blocker is withdrawn *abruptly,* anginal pain or ventricular dysrhythmias may develop. This phenomenon of increased cardiac activity in response to abrupt cessation of beta-blocker therapy is referred to as *rebound excitation.* The risk of rebound excitation can be minimized by withdrawing these drugs gradually (e.g., by tapering the dosage over a period of 1 to 2 weeks). If rebound excitation occurs, dosing should be temporarily resumed. Patients should be warned against abrupt cessation of treatment. Also, they should be advised to carry an adequate supply of their beta blocker when traveling.

Adverse Effects of $Beta_2$ Blockade

Bronchoconstriction. Blockade of $beta_2$ receptors in the lungs can cause constriction of the bronchi. (Recall that activation of these receptors promotes bronchodilation.) For most people, the degree of bronchoconstriction is insignificant. However, when bronchial $beta_2$ receptors are blocked in patients with asthma, the resulting increase in airway resistance can be life threatening. Accordingly, *drugs that block $beta_2$ receptors* are contraindicated for people with asthma. If these individuals must use a beta blocker, they should use an agent that is $beta_1$ selective (e.g., metoprolol).

Hypoglycemia From Inhibition of Glycogenolysis. Epinephrine, acting at $beta_2$ receptors in skeletal muscle and the liver, can stimulate glycogenolysis (breakdown of glycogen into glucose). $Beta_2$ blockade will inhibit this process, posing a risk of hypoglycemia in susceptible individuals. Although suppression of $beta_2$-mediated glycogenolysis is inconsequential for most people, interference with this process can be detrimental to patients with *diabetes.* These people are especially dependent on $beta_2$-mediated glycogenolysis as a way to overcome insulin-induced hypoglycemia. If the patient with diabetes requires a beta blocker, a $beta_1$-selective agent should be chosen.

Adverse Effects in Neonates From $Beta_1$ and $Beta_2$ Blockade

Use of beta blockers during pregnancy can have residual effects on the newborn infant. Specifically, because beta blockers can remain in the circulation for several days after birth, neonates may be at risk for bradycardia (from $beta_1$ blockade), respiratory distress (from $beta_2$ blockade), and hypoglycemia (from $beta_2$ blockade). Accordingly, for 3 to 5 days after birth, newborns should be closely monitored for these effects. Adverse neonatal effects have been observed with at least one beta blocker (betaxolol), and may be a risk with others as well.

PROPERTIES OF INDIVIDUAL BETA BLOCKERS

The beta-adrenergic antagonists can be subdivided into three groups:

- *First-generation (nonselective) beta blockers* (e.g., propranolol), which block $beta_1$ and $beta_2$ receptors
- *Second-generation (cardioselective) beta blockers* (e.g., metoprolol), which produce selective blockade of $beta_1$ receptors (at usual doses)
- *Third-generation (vasodilating) beta blockers* (e.g., carvedilol), which act on blood vessels to cause dilation, but may produce nonselective or cardioselective beta blockade

Our discussion of the individual beta blockers focuses on two prototypes: propranolol and metoprolol. Properties of these and other beta blockers are shown in Table 18.4.

Propranolol

Propranolol [Inderal LA, InnoPran XL], our prototype of the first-generation beta blockers, produces *nonselective* beta blockade. That is, this drug blocks both $beta_1$- *and* $beta_2$-adrenergic receptors. Propranolol was the first beta blocker to receive widespread clinical use and remains one of our most important beta-blocking agents.

Pharmacologic Effects

By blocking *cardiac* $beta_1$ receptors, propranolol can *reduce heart rate, decrease the force of ventricular contraction,* and *suppress impulse conduction through the AV node.* The net effect is a reduction in cardiac output.

By blocking *renal* $beta_1$ receptors, propranolol can *suppress secretion of renin.*

TABLE 18.4 ■ Beta-Adrenergic Antagonists: Pharmacokinetics and Pharmacologic Properties

Generic Name	ISA	Lipid Solubility	Peak	Half-Life (Adults)	Metabolism	Excretion
FIRST-GENERATION: NONSELECTIVE BETA BLOCKERS						
Nadolol	0	Low	3–4 hr	20–24 hr	Not metabolized	Urine (unchanged drug)
Pindolol	+++	Moderate	1 hr	3–4 hr	Hepatic	Urine
Propranolol	0	High	1–4 hr	3–5 hr	Hepatic	Urine
Sotalol	0	High	2.5–4 hr	12 hr	None	Urine (unchanged drug)
Timolol	0	Low	1–2 hr	4 hr	Hepatic	Urine
SECOND-GENERATION: CARDIOSELECTIVE BETA BLOCKERS						
Acebutolol	+	Moderate	2–4 hr	Drug: 3–4 hr Metabolite: 8–13 hr		Feces (primary), urine
Atenolol	0	Low	2–4 hr	6–9 hr	Hepatic	Feces (primary), urine
Betaxolol	0	Low	1.5–6 hr	14–22 hr	Hepatic	Urine
Bisoprolol	0	Moderate	2–4 hr	9–12 hr	Hepatic	Urine
Esmolol	0	Low	1–2 min	Drug: 9 min Metabolite: 3–4 hr	Red cell esterases	Urine
Metoprolol	0	High	IV: 20 min PO: 1–2 hr	3–7 hr	Hepatic	Urine
THIRD-GENERATION: BETA BLOCKERS WITH VASODILATING ACTIONS						
Carvedilol	0	Moderate	1–2 hr	5–11 hr	Hepatic	Feces (primary), urine
Labetalol	0	Low	IV: 5–15 min PO: 2–4 min	6–8 hr	Hepatic	Urine (primary), feces
Nebivolol	0	High	1.5–4 hr	12–19 hr	Hepatic	Urine (primary), feces

ISA, intrinsic sympathomimetic activity (partial agonist activity).

By blocking $beta_2$ receptors, propranolol can produce three major effects: (1) *bronchoconstriction* (through $beta_2$ blockade in the lungs), (2) *vasoconstriction* (through $beta_2$ blockade on certain blood vessels), and (3) *reduced glycogenolysis* (through $beta_2$ blockade in skeletal muscle and liver).

Pharmacokinetics

Propranolol is *highly lipid soluble* and therefore can readily cross membranes. The drug is well absorbed following oral administration, but because of extensive metabolism on its first pass through the liver, less than 30% of each dose reaches the systemic circulation. Because of its ability to cross membranes, propranolol is widely distributed to all tissues and organs, including the central nervous system (CNS). Propranolol undergoes hepatic metabolism followed by excretion in the urine.

Therapeutic Uses

Practically all of the applications of propranolol are based on blockade of $beta_1$ receptors in the heart. The most important indications are *hypertension, angina pectoris, cardiac dysrhythmias,* and *myocardial infarction.* The role of propranolol and other beta blockers in these disorders is discussed in Chapters 47, 49, 51, and 53. Additional indications include prevention of migraine headache and "stage fright."

Adverse Effects

The most serious adverse effects result from blockade of $beta_1$ receptors in the heart and blockade of $beta_2$ receptors in the lungs.

Bradycardia. $Beta_1$ blockade in the heart can cause bradycardia. Heart rate should be assessed before each dose. If the heart rate is below normal, the drug should be held and the prescriber should be notified. If necessary, heart rate can be increased by administering atropine and isoproterenol.

AV Heart Block. By slowing conduction of impulses through the AV node, propranolol can cause AV heart block. The drug is contraindicated for patients with preexisting AV block (if the block is greater than first degree).

Heart Failure. In patients with heart disease, suppression of myocardial contractility by propranolol can result in heart failure. Patients should be informed about the early signs of heart failure (shortness of breath on mild exertion or when lying supine, night coughs, swelling of the extremities, weight gain from fluid retention) and instructed to notify the prescriber if these occur. Propranolol is generally contraindicated for patients with preexisting heart failure (although other beta blockers are used to *treat* heart failure).

Rebound Cardiac Excitation. Abrupt withdrawal of propranolol can cause rebound excitation of the heart, resulting in tachycardia and ventricular dysrhythmias. This problem is especially dangerous for patients with preexisting cardiac ischemia. To avoid rebound excitation, propranolol should be withdrawn slowly by giving progressively smaller doses over 1 to 2 weeks. Patients should be warned against abrupt cessation of treatment. In addition, they should be advised to carry an adequate supply of propranolol when traveling.

Bronchoconstriction. Blockade of $beta_2$ receptors in the lungs can cause bronchoconstriction. As a rule, increased airway resistance is hazardous only to patients with asthma and other obstructive pulmonary disorders.

Inhibition of Glycogenolysis. Blockade of $beta_2$ receptors in skeletal muscle and the liver can inhibit glycogenolysis. This effect can be dangerous for people with diabetes, as discussed previously in this chapter.

CNS Effects. Because of its lipid solubility, propranolol can readily cross the blood-brain barrier, and hence has ready access to sites in the CNS. However, although propranolol is reputed to cause a variety of CNS reactions—depression, insomnia, nightmares, and hallucinations—these reactions are, in fact, very rare. Because of the possible risk of depression, prudence dictates avoiding propranolol in patients who already have this disorder.

Effects in Neonates. Propranolol crosses the placental barrier. Using propranolol and other beta blockers during pregnancy may put the neonate at risk of bradycardia, respiratory distress, and hypoglycemia. Neonates should be closely monitored for these effects.

Precautions, Warnings, and Contraindications

Severe Allergy. Propranolol should be avoided in patients with a history of severe allergic reactions (anaphylaxis). Recall that epinephrine, the drug of choice for anaphylaxis, relieves symptoms in large part by activating $beta_1$ receptors in the heart and $beta_2$ receptors in the lungs. If these receptors are blocked by propranolol, the ability of epinephrine to help will be impaired.

Diabetes. Propranolol can be detrimental to diabetic patients in two ways. First, by blocking $beta_2$ receptors in muscle and liver, propranolol can suppress glycogenolysis, thereby eliminating an important mechanism for correcting insulin-induced hypoglycemia. Second, by blocking $beta_1$ receptors, propranolol can suppress tachycardia, tremors, and perspiration, which normally serve as early warning signals that blood glucose levels are falling too low. (When glucose drops below a safe level, the sympathetic nervous system is activated, causing these symptoms.) By "masking" symptoms of hypoglycemia, propranolol can delay awareness of hypoglycemia, thereby compromising the patient's ability to correct the problem in a timely fashion. Patients with diabetes who take propranolol should be warned that these common symptoms may no longer be a reliable indicator of hypoglycemia. In addition, they should be taught to recognize alternative symptoms (hunger, fatigue, poor concentration) that blood glucose is falling perilously low.

Cardiac, Respiratory, and Psychiatric Disorders. Propranolol can exacerbate *heart failure, AV heart block, sinus bradycardia, asthma,* and *bronchospasm.* Accordingly, the drug is contraindicated for patients with these disorders. In addition, propranolol should be used with caution in patients with a history of *depression.*

Drug Interactions

Calcium Channel Blockers. The cardiac effects of two calcium channel blockers—verapamil and diltiazem—are identical to those of propranolol: reduction of heart rate, suppression of AV conduction, and suppression of myocardial contractility. When propranolol is combined with either of these drugs, excessive cardiosuppression may result.

Insulin. As discussed previously, propranolol can impede early recognition of insulin-induced hypoglycemia. In addition, propranolol can block glycogenolysis, the body's mechanism for correcting hypoglycemia.

Preparations, Dosage, and Administration

General Dosing Considerations. Establishing an effective propranolol dosage is difficult for two reasons: (1) patients vary widely in their requirements for propranolol and (2) there is a poor correlation between blood levels of propranolol and therapeutic responses. The explanation for these observations is that responses to propranolol are dependent on the activity of the sympathetic nervous system. If sympathetic activity is high, then the dose needed to reduce receptor activation will be high. Conversely, if sympathetic activity is low, then low doses will usually be sufficient to produce receptor blockade. Because sympathetic activity varies among patients, propranolol requirements vary also. Accordingly, the dosage must be adjusted by monitoring the patient's response, and not by relying on dosing information in a drug reference.

Preparations. Propranolol hydrochloride is available in three oral formulations: (1) IR tablets (10 to 80 mg) sold generically, (2) ER capsules (60 to 160 mg) sold as Inderal LA and InnoPran XL, and (3) oral solution (4 and 8 mg/mL) sold generically. The drug is also available in solution (1 mg/mL) for IV administration.

Dosage. For treatment of *hypertension,* the initial dosage is 40 mg twice a day (using IR tablets or oral solution) or 80 mg once a day (using ER capsules). Usual maintenance dosages are 120 to 240 mg/day in three or four divided doses (using IR tablets or oral solution) or 120 to 160 mg once a day (using ER capsules).

For *angina pectoris,* the initial dosage is 80 mg once a day (using ER capsules). The usual maintenance dosage is 160 mg once a day (using ER capsules) or 80 to 320 mg/day in two, three, or four divided doses (using IR tablets).

Intravenous administration of propranolol is not routinely done except in emergency situations or when a patient is under anesthesia. Dosing is 1 to 3 mg at a rate not exceeding 1 mg/min.

Metoprolol

Metoprolol [Lopressor, Toprol XL, Betaloc ♣], our prototype of the second-generation beta blockers, produces selective blockade of $beta_1$ receptors in the heart. At usual therapeutic doses, the drug does not cause $beta_2$ blockade. Please note, however, that selectivity for $beta_1$ receptors is not absolute: At higher doses, metoprolol and the other cardioselective agents will block $beta_2$ receptors as well. Because their effects on $beta_2$ receptors are normally minimal, cardioselective agents are not likely to cause bronchoconstriction or hypoglycemia. Accordingly, these drugs are preferred to the nonselective beta blockers for patients with asthma or diabetes.

Pharmacologic Effects

By blocking cardiac $beta_1$ receptors, metoprolol has the same impact on the heart as propranolol: it reduces heart rate, force of contraction, and conduction velocity through the AV node. Also like propranolol, metoprolol reduces secretion of renin by the kidney. In contrast to propranolol, metoprolol does not block bronchial $beta_2$ receptors at usual doses, and therefore does not increase airway resistance.

Pharmacokinetics

Metoprolol is very lipid soluble and well absorbed following oral administration. Like propranolol, metoprolol undergoes extensive metabolism on its first pass through the liver. As a result, only 40% of an oral dose reaches the systemic circulation. Elimination is by hepatic metabolism and renal excretion.

Therapeutic Uses

The primary indication for metoprolol is *hypertension.* The drug is also approved for *angina pectoris, heart failure,* and *myocardial infarction.* IV administration is reserved for treatment of myocardial infarction.

Adverse Effects

Major adverse effects involve the heart. Like propranolol, metoprolol can cause *bradycardia, reduced cardiac output, AV heart block,* and *rebound cardiac excitation following abrupt withdrawal.* Also, even though metoprolol is approved for *treating* heart failure, it can *cause* heart failure if used incautiously. In contrast to propranolol, metoprolol causes minimal bronchoconstriction and does not interfere with $beta_2$-mediated glycogenolysis.

Precautions, Warnings, and Contraindications

Like propranolol, metoprolol is contraindicated for patients with *sinus bradycardia* and *AV block greater than first degree.* In addition, it should be used with great care in patients with *heart failure.* Because metoprolol produces only minimal blockade of $beta_2$ receptors, the drug is safer than propranolol for patients with asthma or a history of severe allergic reactions. In addition, because metoprolol does not suppress $beta_2$-mediated glycogenolysis, it can be used more safely than propranolol by patients with diabetes. Please note, however, that metoprolol, like propranolol, will mask common signs and symptoms of hypoglycemia, thereby depriving the diabetic patient of an early indication that hypoglycemia is developing.

Preparations, Dosage, and Administration

Metoprolol is available in IR tablets (20, 50, and 100 mg) under the brand name Lopressor and in ER tablets (25, 50, 100, and 200 mg) under the brand name Toprol XL. The drug is also available in solution (1 mg/mL) for IV administration. Dosing depends on the reason the drug is prescribed and whether IR or ER drugs are used. For hypertension, initial dosage with IR metoprolol is 50 mg twice a day, while ER metoprolol is commonly started at 25 to 100 mg once daily. For angina, initial dosing is 50 mg twice daily of IR metoprolol or 100 mg once daily of the ER form. Dosages for maintenance therapy range from 50 to 400 mg/day in divided doses. Intravenous administration is reserved for *myocardial infarction.*

Other Beta-Adrenergic Blockers

In the United States, 16 beta blockers are approved for cardiovascular disorders (hypertension, angina pectoris, cardiac dysrhythmias, MI). Principal differences among these drugs concern receptor specificity, pharmacokinetics, indications, side effects, intrinsic sympathomimetic activity, and the ability to cause vasodilation.

In addition to the agents used for cardiovascular disorders, there is a group of beta blockers used for glaucoma (see Chapter 104).

Properties of the beta blockers employed for cardiovascular disorders are discussed in the sections that follow.

Receptor Specificity

With regard to receptor specificity, beta blockers fall into two groups: nonselective agents and cardioselective agents. The nonselective agents block $beta_1$ *and* $beta_2$ receptors, whereas the cardioselective agents block $beta_1$ receptors only when prescribed at usual doses. Because of their limited side effects, the cardioselective agents are preferred for patients with asthma or diabetes. Two beta blockers—*labetalol* and *carvedilol*—differ from all the others in that they block *alpha*-adrenergic receptors in addition to beta receptors. The receptor specificity of individual beta blockers is indicated in Table 18.1.

Pharmacokinetics

Pharmacokinetic properties of the beta blockers are shown in Table 18.4. The relative lipid solubility of these agents is of particular importance. The drugs with high solubility (e.g., propranolol, metoprolol) have two prominent features: (1) they penetrate the blood-brain barrier with ease and (2) they are eliminated primarily by hepatic metabolism. Conversely, the drugs with low lipid solubility (e.g., nadolol, atenolol) penetrate the blood-brain barrier poorly and are eliminated primarily by renal excretion.

PATIENT-CENTERED CARE ACROSS THE LIFE SPAN

Beta-Adrenergic Antagonists

Life Stage	Patient Care Concerns
Children	These drugs are commonly used in children. Typical monitoring for adverse effects is needed.
Pregnant women	Acebutolol, pindolol, and sotalol are classified as Pregnancy Risk Category B. Atenolol is classified as Pregnancy Risk Category D. All others are categorized as Pregnancy Risk Category C.[a] Beta blockers are associated with decreased intrauterine growth. They may cause decreased heart rate in both the fetus and neonate. Neonates born to women taking beta blockers may experience hypoglycemia. Close monitoring is warranted. Risks must be compared to benefits, which include that untreated dysrhythmias and hypertension also create risks for the fetus and neonate.
Breast-feeding women	Beta blockers may enter breast milk in varying amounts; those that are more lipid soluble can cross into breast milk in greater quantities. Betaxolol is more extensively excreted into breast milk than other beta blockers. There are no contraindications to breast-feeding; however, caution and close monitoring of infants are recommended.
Older adults	Beta blockers are commonly prescribed for older adults. As with most drugs for this age group, attention should be paid to hepatic and renal function; if function is decreased, impaired metabolism and elimination by these pathways may result in increased drug levels.

[a]As of 2020, the FDA will no longer use Pregnancy Risk Categories. Please refer to Chapter 9 for more information.

Therapeutic Uses

Principal indications for the beta-adrenergic blockers are *hypertension, angina pectoris,* and *cardiac dysrhythmias.* Other uses include prophylaxis of *migraine headache,* treatment of *myocardial infarction,* symptom suppression in individuals with *situational anxiety* (e.g., stage fright), and treatment of *heart failure* (see Chapter 48). Approved and investigational uses of beta blockers are shown in Table 18.5. Preparations, dosage, and administration are presented in Table 18.6.

Esmolol and *sotalol* differ from the other beta blockers in that they are not used for hypertension. Because of its very short half-life (15 minutes), *esmolol* is clearly unsuited for treating hypertension, which requires maintenance of blood levels throughout the day, every day, for an indefinite time. The only approved indication for esmolol is emergency IV therapy of *supraventricular tachycardia. Sotalol* is approved for *ventricular dysrhythmias* and for maintenance of normal sinus rhythm in patients who previously experienced symptomatic atrial fibrillation or atrial flutter. Esmolol and sotalol are discussed in Chapter 49.

Adverse Effects

By blocking $beta_1$ receptors in the heart, all of the beta blockers can cause *bradycardia, AV heart block,* and, rarely, *heart failure.* By blocking $beta_2$ receptors in the lung, the nonselective agents can cause significant *bronchoconstriction* in patients with asthma or chronic obstructive pulmonary disease. In addition, by blocking $beta_2$ receptors in the liver and skeletal muscle, the *nonselective* agents can *inhibit glycogenolysis,* compromising the ability of diabetic patients to compensate for insulin-induced hypoglycemia. Because of their ability to block alpha-adrenergic receptors, *carvedilol* and *labetalol* can cause *postural hypotension.*

Although *CNS effects* (insomnia, depression) can occur with all beta blockers, these effects are rare, and are most likely with the more lipid-soluble agents. Abrupt discontinuation of any beta blocker can produce *rebound cardiac excitation.* Accordingly, all beta blockers should be withdrawn slowly (by tapering the dosage over 1 to 2 weeks).

Intrinsic Sympathomimetic Activity (Partial Agonist Activity)

The term *intrinsic sympathomimetic activity* (ISA) refers to the ability of certain beta blockers—especially *pindolol*—to act as *partial agonists* at beta-adrenergic receptors. (A partial agonist is a drug that, when bound to a receptor, produces a limited degree of receptor activation while preventing strong agonists from binding to that receptor to cause full activation.)

In contrast to other beta blockers, agents with ISA have very little effect on resting heart rate and cardiac output. When patients are at rest, stimulation of the heart by the sympathetic nervous system is low. If an ordinary beta blocker is given, it will block sympathetic stimulation, causing heart rate and cardiac output to decline. However, if a beta blocker has ISA, its own ability to cause limited receptor activation will compensate for blocking receptor activation by the sympathetic nervous system; consequently, resting heart rate and cardiac output are not reduced. A comparison of ISA activity among beta blockers is provided in Table 18.4.

Because of their ability to provide a low level of cardiac stimulation, beta blockers with ISA are preferred to other beta blockers for use in patients with bradycardia. Conversely, these agents should not be given to patients with MI, because their ability to cause even limited cardiac stimulation can be detrimental.

Vasodilation

The third-generation beta blockers—*carvedilol, labetalol,* and *nebivolol*—can dilate blood vessels. Two mechanisms are employed: Carvedilol and labetalol block vascular $alpha_1$ receptors; nebivolol promotes synthesis and release of nitric oxide from the vascular epithelium. The exact clinical benefit of vasodilation by these drugs has not been clarified.

TABLE 18.5 ▪ Beta-Adrenergic Blocking Agents: Summary of Therapeutic Uses

	Hypertension	Angina Pectoris	Cardiac Dysrhythmias	Myocardial Infarction	Migraine Prophylaxis	Stage Fright	Heart Failure	Glaucoma
FIRST-GENERATION: NONSELECTIVE BETA BLOCKERS								
Carteolol		I						A
Nadolol	A	A	I		I	I		
Penbutolol	A							
Pindolol	A	I	I			I		
Propranolol	A	A	A	A	A	I		
Sotalol			A					
Timolol	A	I	I	A	A	I		
SECOND-GENERATION: CARDIOSELECTIVE BETA BLOCKERS								
Acebutolol	A	I	A	I				
Atenolol	A	A	I	A	I	I		
Betaxolol	A	I						
Bisoprolol	A	I	I				I	
Esmolol		I	A					
Metoprolol	A	A	I	A	I		A	
THIRD-GENERATION: BETA BLOCKERS WITH VASODILATING ACTIONS								
Carvedilol	A	I		A			A	
Labetalol	A	I						
Nebivolol	A						I	

A, U.S. Food and Drug Administration–approved use; *I,* investigational use.

TABLE 18.6 ▪ Beta-Adrenergic Antagonists: Preparations, Dosage, and Administration[a]

Drug	Preparations	Typical Dosage Range[b]	Administration
FIRST-GENERATION: NONSELECTIVE BETA BLOCKERS			
Nadolol [Corgard]	Tablets: 20, 40, 80 mg	40–80 mg/day; max 240 mg/day	Administer with or without food.
Pindolol [Visken 🍁]	Tablets: 5, 10, 15 mg	10–40 mg/day; max 60 mg/day	Administer with or without food.
Propranolol (IR) (generic only)	Tablets: 10, 20, 40, 60, 80 mg IV sol: 1 mg/mL	Tablets: 60–120 mg twice daily IV sol: highly individualized; typically begins at 1–3 mg	Administer oral doses on an empty stomach. IV: Do not exceed 1 mg/min.
Propranolol (ER) [Inderal LA, InnoPran XL]	Capsules: 60, 80, 120, 160 mg	80–120 mg/day; max 120 mg/day	Do not crush. May administer with or without food, but do the same for every dose.
Sotalol [Betapace, Betapace AF, Sorine]	Tablets: 80, 120, 160, 240 mg IV sol: 150 mg/10 mL	Tablets: 80–120 mg twice daily; max 160 mg twice daily IV sol: 112.5 mg twice daily; max 300 mg/day	Administer oral doses with or without food. IV: Administer diluted sol over 5 hr while monitoring for QT prolongation or ventricular arrhythmias.
Timolol [Blocadren]	Tablets: 5, 10, 20 mg	10–20 mg twice daily; max 60 mg/day	Administer with food.
SECOND-GENERATION: CARDIOSELECTIVE BETA BLOCKERS			
Acebutolol [Sectral]	Tablets: 100, 200, 400 mg	400–800 mg/day; max 1200 mg/day	Administer with or without food.
Atenolol [Tenormin]	Tablets: 25, 50, 100 mg	25–50 mg/day; max 100 mg/day	Administer with or without food.
Betaxolol [Kerlone]	Tablets: 10, 20 mg	10–20 mg/day; max 20 mg	Administer with or without food.
Bisoprolol [Zebeta]	Tablets: 5, 10 mg	5–10 mg/day	Administer with or without food.

TABLE 18.6 ■ Beta-Adrenergic Antagonists: Preparations, Dosage, and Administration[a]—cont'd

Drug	Preparations	Typical Dosage Range[b]	Administration
Esmolol [Brevibloc]	IV sol: 100 mg/10 mL; 200 mg/200 mL NaCl; 2500 mg/250 mL NaCl	Individualized	Administer initial bolus over 30–60 sec. Infuse only into large veins or ports to avoid thrombophlebitis.
Metoprolol (IR) [Lopressor, Betaloc ♣]	Tablets: 25, 37.5, 50, 75, 100 mg IV sol: 1 mg/mL in 5 mL, 5 mg/5 mL in 5 mL	Tablets: 50–100 mg/day; Max 200 mg/day IV sol: 1.25–5 mg 2–4 times daily	Administer with food. IV: Labeling advises 5-mg boluses administered 2 min apart.
Metoprolol (ER) [Toprol XL, Betaloc CR ♣]	Tablets: 25, 50, 100, 200 mg	100 mg/day; max 400 mg/day	Administer with or without food. Can split tablets at score but do not crush.
THIRD-GENERATION: BETA BLOCKERS WITH VASODILATING ACTIONS			
Carvedilol (IR) [Coreg]	Tablets: 3.125, 6.25, 12.5, 25 mg	6.5–25 mg twice daily; max 25 mg twice daily	Administer with food.
Carvedilol (ER) [Coreg CR]	Capsules: 10, 20, 40, 80 mg	20–40 mg/day; max 80 mg/day	Capsules may be opened and sprinkled on food, but do not crush capsule contents.
Labetalol [Trandate ♣]	Tablets: 100, 200, 300 mg IV sol: 5 mg/mL in 4, 20, 40 mL	100–300 mg twice daily	Administer with or without food, but do the same for every dose. IV bolus rate should not exceed 10 mg/min.
Nebivolol [Bystolic]	Tablets: 2.5, 5, 10, 20 mg	5–20 mg/day; max 40 mg/day	Administer with or without food.

[a]Ophthalmic preparations are covered in Chapter 104.
[b]Dosage may vary depending on treatment purpose.
ER, Extended release; *IR,* immediate release; *sol,* solution.

KEY POINTS

- Most beneficial responses to alpha blockers, including reduction of blood pressure in patients with hypertension, result from blockade of $alpha_1$ receptors on blood vessels.
- Alpha blockers reduce symptoms of BPH by blocking $alpha_1$ receptors in the bladder neck and prostatic capsule, which causes smooth muscle at those sites to relax.
- The major adverse effects of alpha blockers are *orthostatic hypotension* (caused by blocking $alpha_1$ receptors on veins); *reflex tachycardia* (caused by blocking $alpha_1$ receptors on arterioles); *nasal congestion* (caused by blocking $alpha_1$ receptors in blood vessels of the nasal mucosa); and *inhibition of ejaculation* (caused by blocking $alpha_1$ receptors in male sex organs).
- The first dose of an alpha blocker can cause fainting from profound orthostatic hypotension—the *first-dose effect.*
- The alpha blockers used most frequently—prazosin, doxazosin, and terazosin—produce selective blockade of $alpha_1$ receptors.
- Beta blockers produce most of their beneficial effects by blocking $beta_1$ receptors in the heart, thereby reducing heart rate, force of contraction, and AV conduction.
- Principal indications for the beta blockers are cardiovascular: hypertension, angina pectoris, heart failure, and supraventricular tachydysrhythmias.
- Potential adverse effects from $beta_1$ blockade are bradycardia, reduced cardiac output, AV block, and precipitation of heart failure (even though some beta blockers are used to *treat* heart failure).
- Potential adverse effects from $beta_2$ blockade are bronchoconstriction (a concern for people with asthma) and reduced glycogenolysis (a concern for people with diabetes).
- Beta blockers can be divided into three groups: (1) first-generation agents (i.e., nonselective beta blockers, such as propranolol, which block $beta_1$ and $beta_2$ receptors); (2) second-generation agents (i.e., cardioselective beta blockers, such as metoprolol, which block $beta_1$ receptors only at usual doses); and (3) third-generation agents (i.e., vasodilating beta blockers, which may be cardioselective or nonselective).
- Beta blockers can be hazardous to patients with severe allergies because they can block beneficial actions of epinephrine, the drug of choice for treating anaphylactic shock.
- Beta blockers can be detrimental to diabetic patients because they suppress glycogenolysis (an important mechanism for correcting insulin-induced hypoglycemia), and they suppress tachycardia, tremors, and perspiration, which normally serve as early warning signals that glucose levels are falling too low.
- Combining a beta blocker with a calcium channel blocker can produce excessive cardiosuppression.
- Cardioselective beta blockers are preferred to nonselective beta blockers for patients with asthma or diabetes.

Please visit **http://evolve.elsevier.com/Lehne** for chapter-specific NCLEX® examination review questions.

Summary of Major Nursing Implications[a]

ALPHA$_1$-ADRENERGIC ANTAGONISTS

Alfuzosin
Doxazosin
Prazosin
Silodosin
Tamsulosin
Terazosin

Preadministration Assessment

Therapeutic Goal

Doxazosin, Prazosin, Terazosin. Reduction of blood pressure in patients with *essential hypertension.*

Doxazosin, Terazosin, Alfuzosin, Silodosin, Tamsulosin. Reduction of symptoms in patients with BPH.

Baseline Data

Essential Hypertension. Determine blood pressure and heart rate.

BPH. Determine the degree of nocturia, daytime frequency, hesitance, intermittency, terminal dribbling (at the end of voiding), urgency, impairment of size and force of urinary stream, dysuria, and sensation of incomplete voiding.

Identifying High-Risk Patients

The only contraindication is hypersensitivity to these drugs.

Implementation: Administration

Route

Oral.

Administration

Instruct patients to take the initial dose at bedtime to minimize the first-dose effect. Except for *tamsulosin,* which is administered *after* eating, these drugs may be taken with food.

Ongoing Evaluation and Interventions

Evaluating Therapeutic Effects

Essential Hypertension. Evaluate by monitoring blood pressure.

BPH. Evaluate for improvement in the symptoms listed under *Baseline Data.*

Minimizing Adverse Effects

Orthostatic Hypotension. Alpha$_1$ blockade can cause postural hypotension. **Inform patients about the symptoms of orthostatic hypotension (dizziness or light-headedness on standing), and advise them to sit or lie down if these occur. Advise patients to move slowly when changing from a supine or sitting position to an upright posture.**

First-Dose Effect. The first dose may cause fainting from severe orthostatic hypotension. **Forewarn patients about first-dose hypotension, and advise them to avoid driving and other hazardous activities for 12 to 24 hours after the initial dose. To minimize risk, advise patients to take the first dose at bedtime.**

BETA-ADRENERGIC ANTAGONISTS

Acebutolol
Atenolol
Betaxolol
Bisoprolol
Carteolol
Carvedilol
Esmolol
Labetalol
Metoprolol
Nadolol
Nebivolol
Penbutolol
Pindolol
Propranolol
Sotalol
Timolol

Except where noted, the implications here apply to all beta-adrenergic blocking agents.

Preadministration Assessment

Therapeutic Goal

Principal indications are *hypertension, angina pectoris, heart failure,* and *cardiac dysrhythmias.* Indications for individual agents are shown in Table 18.5.

Baseline Data

All Patients. Determine heart rate.

Hypertension. Determine standing and supine blood pressure.

Angina Pectoris. Determine the incidence, severity, and circumstances of anginal attacks.

Cardiac Dysrhythmias. Obtain a baseline electrocardiogram (ECG).

Identifying High-Risk Patients

All beta blockers are *contraindicated* for patients with sinus bradycardia or AV heart block greater than first degree, and must be used with *great caution* in patients with heart failure. Use with *caution* (especially the nonselective agents) in patients with asthma, bronchospasm, diabetes, or a history of severe allergic reactions. Use all beta blockers with *caution* in patients with a history of depression and in those taking calcium channel blockers.

Implementation: Administration

Routes

Oral. All beta blockers listed previously except esmolol.

Intravenous. Atenolol, esmolol, labetalol, metoprolol, propranolol, and sotalol.

Administration

For maintenance therapy of hypertension, administer one or more times daily (see Table 18.6). **Warn patients against abrupt discontinuation of treatment.**

Summary of Major Nursing Implications[a]—cont'd

Ongoing Evaluation and Interventions

Evaluating Therapeutic Effects

Hypertension. Monitor blood pressure and heart rate before each dose. **Advise outpatients to monitor blood pressure and heart rate daily.**

Angina Pectoris. **Advise patients to record the incidence, circumstances, and severity of anginal attacks.**

Cardiac Dysrhythmias. Monitor for improvement in the ECG.

Minimizing Adverse Effects

Bradycardia. $Beta_1$ blockade can reduce heart rate. If bradycardia is severe, withhold medication and notify the physician. If necessary, administer atropine and isoproterenol to restore heart rate.

AV Heart Block. $Beta_1$ blockade can decrease AV conduction. Do not give beta blockers to patients with AV block greater than first degree.

Heart Failure. Suppression of myocardial contractility can cause heart failure. **Inform patients about early signs of heart failure (shortness of breath, night coughs, swelling of the extremities), and instruct them to notify the prescriber if these occur.**

Rebound Cardiac Excitation. Abrupt withdrawal of beta blockers can cause tachycardia and ventricular dysrhythmias. **Warn patients against abrupt discontinuation of drug use. Also, advise patients, when traveling, to carry an adequate supply of medication plus a copy of their prescription.**

Postural Hypotension. By blocking alpha-adrenergic receptors, *carvedilol* and *labetalol* can cause postural hypotension. **Inform patients about signs of hypotension (lightheadedness, dizziness) and advise them to sit or lie down if these develop. Advise patients to move slowly when changing from a supine or sitting position to an upright position.**

Bronchoconstriction. $Beta_2$ blockade can cause substantial airway constriction in patients with asthma. The risk of bronchoconstriction is much lower with the cardioselective agents than with the nonselective agents.

Effects in Diabetic Patients. $Beta_1$ blockade can mask early signs and symptoms of hypoglycemia by preventing common tachycardia, tremors, and perspiration. **Warn patients that tachycardia, tremors, and perspiration cannot be relied on as an indicator of impending hypoglycemia, and teach them to recognize other indicators (hunger, fatigue, poor concentration) that blood glucose is falling dangerously low.** $Beta_2$ blockade can prevent glycogenolysis, an emergency means of increasing blood glucose. Patients may need to reduce their insulin dosage. Cardioselective beta blockers are preferred to nonselective agents in patients with diabetes.

Effects in Neonates. Maternal use of *betaxolol* during pregnancy may cause bradycardia, respiratory distress, and hypoglycemia in the infant. Accordingly, for 3 to 5 days after birth, newborns should be closely monitored for these effects. Beta blockers other than betaxolol may pose a similar risk.

CNS Effects. Rarely, beta blockers cause depression, insomnia, and nightmares. If these occur, switching to a beta blocker with low lipid solubility may help (see Table 18.4).

Minimizing Adverse Interactions

Calcium Channel Blockers. Two calcium channel blockers—verapamil and diltiazem—can intensify the cardiosuppressant effects of the beta blockers. Use these combinations with caution.

Insulin. Beta blockers can prevent the compensatory glycogenolysis that normally occurs in response to insulin-induced hypoglycemia. Patients with diabetes may need to reduce their insulin dosage.

[a]Patient education information is highlighted as **blue text.**

CHAPTER

19 Indirect-Acting Antiadrenergic Agents

The indirect-acting antiadrenergic agents are drugs that prevent the activation of peripheral adrenergic receptors, but by mechanisms that do not involve direct interaction with peripheral receptors. There are two categories of indirect-acting antiadrenergic drugs. The first group—*centrally acting alpha$_2$ agonists*—consists of drugs that act within the central nervous system (CNS) to reduce the outflow of impulses along sympathetic neurons. The second group—*adrenergic neuron-blocking agents*—consists of drugs that act within the terminals of sympathetic neurons to decrease norepinephrine (NE) release. With both groups, the net result is reduced activation of peripheral adrenergic receptors. Hence, the pharmacologic effects of the indirect-acting adrenergic blocking agents are very similar to those of drugs that block adrenergic receptors directly.

Prototype Drugs

INDIRECT ACTING ANTIADRENERGIC AGENTS

Centrally Acting (Alpha$_2$) Adrenergic Agonists

Clonidine [Catapres, Catapres-TTS, Duraclon, Kapvay]

Adrenergic Neuron-Blocking Agents

Reserpine (generic)

CENTRALLY ACTING ALPHA$_2$ AGONISTS

The drugs discussed in this section act within the CNS to reduce the firing of sympathetic neurons. Their primary use is for hypertension.

Why are we discussing centrally acting drugs in a unit on peripheral nervous system pharmacology? Because the effects of these drugs are ultimately the result of decreased activation of alpha- and beta-adrenergic receptors in the periphery. That is, by inhibiting the firing of sympathetic neurons, the centrally acting agents decrease the release of NE from sympathetic nerves, and thereby decrease activation of peripheral adrenergic receptors. Hence, although these drugs act within the CNS, their effects are like those of the direct-acting adrenergic receptor blockers. Accordingly, it seems appropriate to discuss these agents in the context of peripheral nervous system pharmacology, rather than presenting them in the context of CNS drugs.

You may be wondering how an adrenergic *agonist* can act as an *antiadrenergic* agent. This occurs because alpha$_2$ receptors in the CNS are located on *presynaptic* nerve terminals. As NE accumulates in the synapse, it activates alpha$_2$ receptors. This activation signals that adequate NE is available. As a result, synthesis of NE is decreased. The decrease of available NE results in vasodilation, which in turn decreases blood pressure.

Clonidine

Clonidine [Catapres, Catapres-TTS, Duraclon, Kapvay] is a centrally acting alpha$_2$ agonist with three approved indications: *hypertension, severe pain,* and *attention-deficit/hyperactivity disorder (ADHD).* For treatment of hypertension, the drug is sold as *Catapres* and *Nexiclon XR.* For treatment of pain it's sold as *Duraclon* for epidural administration. For management of ADHD, *Kapvay* is used. Use for hypertension is discussed here. Use against pain is discussed in Chapter 28. Use in ADHD management is discussed in Chapter 36.

Clonidine is not used as often as many antihypertensive drugs; however, it has important indications in the management of severe hypertension. Except for rare instances of rebound hypertension, the drug is generally free of serious adverse effects. Dosing is done orally or by transdermal patch.

Mechanism of Antihypertensive Action

Clonidine is an alpha$_2$-adrenergic agonist that causes selective activation of alpha$_2$ receptors in the CNS—specifically, in brainstem areas associated with autonomic regulation of the cardiovascular system. By activating central alpha$_2$ receptors, clonidine reduces sympathetic outflow to blood vessels and to the heart.

Pharmacologic Effects

The most significant effects of clonidine concern the heart and vascular system. By suppressing the firing of sympathetic nerves to the heart, clonidine can cause *bradycardia* and *a decrease in cardiac output.* By suppressing sympathetic regulation of blood vessels, the drug promotes *vasodilation.* The net result of cardiac suppression and vasodilation is *decreased blood pressure.* Blood pressure is reduced in both supine and standing subjects. Because the hypotensive effects of clonidine are not posture dependent, orthostatic hypotension is minimal.

Pharmacokinetics

Clonidine is very lipid soluble. As a result, the drug is readily absorbed after oral dosing and is widely distributed throughout the body, including the CNS. Hypotensive responses begin 30 to 60 minutes after administration and peak in 4 hours. Effects of a single dose may persist as long as 1 day. Clonidine is eliminated by a combination of hepatic metabolism and renal excretion.

Therapeutic Uses

Clonidine has three *approved* applications: treatment of hypertension (its main use), relief of severe pain, and management of ADHD. It has been used off-label for managing opioid and methadone withdrawal, facilitating smoking cessation, treating conduct disorder and oppositional defiant disorder in children, and treating Tourette's syndrome, a CNS disease characterized by uncontrollable tics and verbal outbursts that are frequently obscene.

Adverse Effects

Drowsiness. CNS depression is common. About 35% of patients experience drowsiness; an additional 8% experience outright sedation. These responses become less intense with continued drug use. Patients in their early weeks of treatment should be advised to avoid hazardous activities if alertness is impaired.

Xerostomia. Xerostomia (dry mouth) is common, occurring in about 40% of patients. The reaction usually diminishes over the first 2 to 4 weeks of therapy. Although not dangerous, xerostomia can be annoying enough to discourage drug use. Patients should be advised that discomfort can be reduced by chewing gum, sucking hard candy, and taking frequent sips of fluids.

Rebound Hypertension. Rebound hypertension is characterized by a large increase in blood pressure occurring in response to abrupt clonidine withdrawal. This rare but serious reaction is caused by overactivity of the sympathetic nervous system, and can be accompanied by nervousness, tachycardia, and sweating. Left untreated, the reaction may persist for a week or more. If blood pressure climbs dangerously high, it should be lowered with a combination of alpha- and beta-adrenergic blocking agents. Rebound effects can be avoided by withdrawing clonidine slowly (over 2 to 4 days). Patients should be informed about rebound hypertension and warned not to discontinue clonidine without consulting the prescriber.

Use in Pregnancy. Clonidine is embryotoxic in animals. Because of the possibility of fetal harm, clonidine is not recommended for pregnant women. Pregnancy should be ruled out before clonidine is given.

Abuse. People who abuse cocaine, opioids (e.g., morphine, heroin), and other drugs frequently abuse clonidine as well. At high doses, clonidine can cause subjective effects—euphoria, sedation, hallucinations—that some individuals find desirable. In addition, clonidine can intensify the subjective effects of some abused drugs, including benzodiazepines, cocaine, and opioids. Because clonidine costs less than these drugs, the combination allows abusers to get high for less money.

Other Adverse Effects. Clonidine can cause a variety of adverse effects, including *constipation, impotence, gynecomastia,* and *adverse CNS effects* (e.g., vivid dreams, nightmares, anxiety, depression). *Localized skin reactions* are common with transdermal clonidine patches.

Preparations, Dosage, and Administration

Preparations. Clonidine hydrochloride is available in oral and transdermal formulations and as a solution for epidural administration. *Oral clonidine* is available in standard tablets (0.1, 0.2, and 0.3 mg) marketed as Catapres. *Transdermal clonidine* [Catapres-TTS] is available in 2.5-, 5-, and 7.5-mg patches that deliver 0.1, 0.2, and 0.3 mg/24 hr, respectively. *Duraclon* is supplied as 100-mcg/mL and 500-mcg/mL solutions for epidural administration. *Kapvay* and *Nexiclon XR* are extended-release preparations. Kapvay is available in 0.1-mg tablets. Nexiclon XR is supplied as 0.17- and 0.26-mg tablets.

Dosage and Administration

Oral. For treatment of hypertension, the initial adult dosage is 0.1 mg twice a day. The usual maintenance dosage is 0.1 to 0.8 mg/day, administered in divided doses. If an extended-release preparation is used, initial dosage is 0.17 mg daily. This may be increased up to 0.52 mg once a day. When immediate-release (twice-daily) dosing is used, taking the majority of the daily dose at bedtime can minimize daytime sedation. On the other hand, for ADHD, bedtime dosage is recommended: Kapvay is administered at an initial dose of 0.1 mg, which may be increased to a maximum of 0.4 mg/day.

Transdermal. Transdermal patches are applied to a region of hairless, intact skin on the upper arm or torso. A new patch is applied every 7 days.

Epidural. Duraclon is provided by continuous epidural administration for severe pain in patients with cancer who are inadequately relieved by opioids. It is particularly beneficial for neuropathic pain.

PATIENT-CENTERED CARE ACROSS THE LIFE SPAN

Centrally Acting Alpha$_2$ Agonists and Adrenergic Neuron-Blocking Agents

Life Stage	Patient Care Concerns
Children	Centrally acting agonists are approved for use in children 6 years and older, though clonidine has been used in children as young as 5 years old (for conduct/oppositional defiant disorders). While reserpine is sometimes given to children, it is not recommended unless other drugs fail.
Pregnant women	Guanfacine and methyldopa (noninjectable) are Pregnancy Risk Category B. Clonidine is Pregnancy Risk Category C.[a] Embryotoxicity in some animals raises concerns for administration of clonidine to pregnant women. Other drugs are preferable.
Breast-feeding women	Clonidine is excreted in relatively large amounts in breast milk. Breast-feeding is not recommended for women taking clonidine, especially if large doses are required, and should be avoided altogether if breast-feeding premature infants.
Older adults	Beers Criteria recommends the avoidance of centrally acting alpha blockers in patients age 65 and older. If reserpine, an adrenergic neuron-blocking drug, is required, Beers Criteria recommends maximum dosing at 0.1 mg/day.

[a]As of 2020, the FDA will no longer use Pregnancy Risk Categories. Please refer to Chapter 9 for more information.

Guanfacine

The pharmacology of guanfacine [Tenex] is very similar to that of clonidine. Like clonidine, guanfacine is indicated for hypertension. In addition, guanfacine, marketed as *Intuniv,* is used for ADHD. Benefits in hypertension derive from activating brainstem alpha$_2$-adrenergic receptors, an action that reduces sympathetic outflow to the heart and blood vessels. The result is a reduction in cardiac output and blood pressure. Both drugs have the same major adverse effects as clonidine: sedation and dry mouth. In addition, both can cause

TABLE 19.1 ■ Preparation, Dosage, and Administration of Indirect-Acting Antiadrenergic Agents

Drug	Preparation	Dosage	Administration
CENTRALLY ACTING ALPHA$_2$ AGONISTS			
Clonidine [Catapres, Catapres-TTS-1, Catapres-TTS-2, Catapres-TTS-3, Kapvay, Dixarit 🍁]	Tablets IR: 0.1, 0.2, 0.3 mg Tablets ER: 0.1, 0.2 mg Transdermal patch: 2.5-mg patch delivers 0.1 mg/24 hr 5-mg patch delivers 0.2 mg/24 hr 7.5-mg patch delivers 0.3 mg/24 hr	IR: 0.1 mg twice a day; typical maintenance dose 0.1–0.8 mg/day in divided doses ER: 0.1–0.4 mg/day Patches: 1 every 7 days	May be taken with or without food. When immediate-release (twice-daily) dosing is used, taking the majority of the daily dose at bedtime can minimize daytime sedation. Patches should be applied to hairless, intact skin on the upper arm or torso.
Guanfacine [Tenex, Intuniv XR[a]]	Tablets IR: 1, 2 mg Tablets ER: 1, 2, 3, 4 mg	Usual dose: 1 mg/day	Take IR tablets at bedtime to minimize daytime sedation. Do not administer with grapefruit juice.
Methyldopa	Tablets: 250, 500 mg	Initial dose: 250 mg 2–3 times/day Maintenance dose: 0.5–2 Gm in 2–4 divided doses	May be taken without regard to meals. If dosage is increased, scheduling the increase at bedtime can decrease daytime drowsiness.
ADRENERGIC NEURON-BLOCKING AGENTS			
Reserpine	Tablets: 0.1, 0.25 mg	0.5 mg/day for 1–2 weeks then increase as needed Maintenance dose: 0.1–0.25 mg daily	May be administered with food if GI upset occurs.

[a]Extended-release guanfacine (Intuniv XR) is approved only for treatment of ADHD.
ER, Extended release; *GI,* gastrointestinal; *IR,* immediate release.

rebound hypertension following abrupt withdrawal. Preparations, dosage, and administration of this and other drugs discussed in this chapter are provided in Table 19.1.

Safety Alert

OLDER ADULT PATIENTS

Centrally acting alpha agonists (clonidine, guanabenz, guanfacine, methyldopa) and the adrenergic neuron-blocking agent reserpine have been designated as potentially inappropriate for use in geriatric patients due to their high risk of adverse CNS effects, bradycardia, and hypotension. Other drugs are recommended for first-line hypertension management in older-adult patients.

Methyldopa and Methyldopate

Methyldopa is an oral antihypertensive agent that lowers blood pressure by acting at sites within the CNS. Two side effects—hemolytic anemia and hepatic necrosis—can be severe. Methyldopate, an intravenous agent, is nearly identical to methyldopa in structure and pharmacologic effects. In the discussion that follows, the term *methyldopa* is used in reference to both methyldopate and methyldopa itself.

Mechanism of Action

Methyldopa works much like clonidine. Like clonidine, methyldopa inhibits sympathetic outflow from the CNS by causing alpha$_2$ activation in the brain. However, methyldopa differs from clonidine in that methyldopa itself is not an alpha$_2$ agonist. Thus, before it can act, methyldopa must first be taken up into brainstem neurons, where it is converted to methylnorepinephrine, a compound that *is* an effective alpha$_2$ agonist. Release of methylnorepinephrine results in alpha$_2$ activation.

Pharmacologic Effects

The most prominent response to methyldopa is a drop in blood pressure. The principal mechanism is vasodilation, not cardiosuppression. Vasodilation occurs because of reduced sympathetic traffic to blood vessels. At usual therapeutic doses, methyldopa does not decrease heart rate or cardiac output. The hemodynamic effects of methyldopa are very much like those of clonidine: Both drugs lower blood pressure in supine and standing subjects, and both produce relatively little orthostatic hypotension.

Therapeutic Use

The only indication for methyldopa is *hypertension.* Studies regarding methyldopa use in pregnant patients have shown improved outcomes without fetal harm, so the American Congress of Obstetricians and Gynecologists has designated methyldopa as a preferred drug in management of hypertension during pregnancy.

Adverse Effects

Positive Coombs' Test and Hemolytic Anemia. A positive Coombs' test[a] develops in 10% to 20% of patients who take methyldopa chronically. A Coombs' test should be performed before treatment and 6 to 12 months later. Blood counts (hematocrit, hemoglobin, or red cell count) should also be

[a]The Coombs' test detects the presence of antibodies directed against the patient's own red blood cells. These antibodies can cause hemolysis (i.e., red blood cell lysis).

obtained before treatment and periodically thereafter. If the test turns positive, it usually occurs between 6 and 12 months of treatment. Of the patients who have a positive Coombs' test, about 5% develop hemolytic anemia. Coombs'-positive patients who do not develop hemolytic anemia may continue methyldopa treatment. However, if hemolytic anemia does develop, methyldopa should be withdrawn immediately. For most patients, hemolytic anemia quickly resolves following withdrawal, although the Coombs' test may remain positive for months.

Hepatotoxicity. Methyldopa has been associated with hepatitis, jaundice, and, rarely, fatal hepatic necrosis. All patients should undergo periodic assessment of liver function. If signs of hepatotoxicity appear, methyldopa should be discontinued immediately. Liver function usually normalizes after drug withdrawal.

Other Adverse Effects. Methyldopa can cause *xerostomia, sexual dysfunction, orthostatic hypotension,* and a variety of *CNS effects,* including drowsiness, reduced mental acuity, nightmares, and depression. These responses are not usually dangerous, but they can detract from adherence.

ADRENERGIC NEURON-BLOCKING AGENTS

The adrenergic neuron-blocking agents act presynaptically to reduce the release of NE from sympathetic neurons. These drugs have little or no effect on the release of epinephrine from the adrenal medulla. Reserpine is the only adrenergic neuron blocker available.[b]

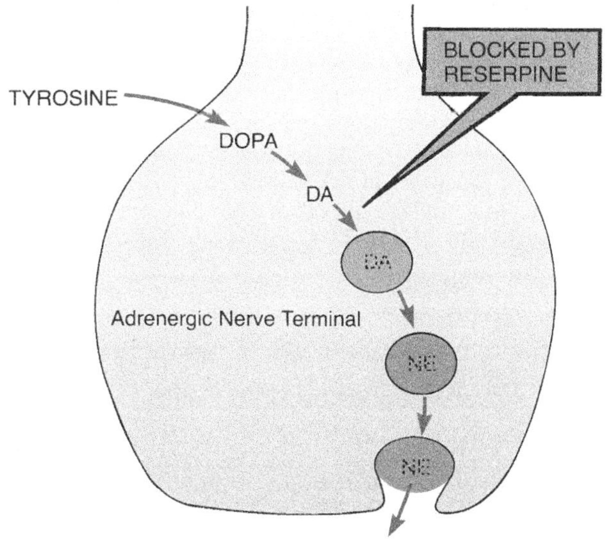

Fig. 19.1 ■ Mechanism of reserpine action.
Reserpine depletes neurons of norepinephrine (NE) by two mechanisms: (1) Reserpine blocks the uptake of dopamine (DA) into vesicles, preventing NE synthesis. (2) Reserpine also displaces NE from vesicles, thereby allowing degradation of NE by monoamine oxidase present in the nerve terminal (not shown).

Reserpine

Reserpine is a naturally occurring compound prepared from the root of *Rauwolfia serpentina,* a shrub indigenous to India. Because of its source, reserpine is classified as a *Rauwolfia alkaloid.* The primary indication for reserpine is hypertension. The side effect of greatest concern is severe depression.

Mechanism of Action

Reserpine causes *depletion of NE from postganglionic sympathetic neurons.* By doing so, the drug can decrease activation of practically all adrenergic receptors. Hence, the effects of reserpine closely resemble those produced by a combination of alpha- and beta-adrenergic blockade.

Reserpine depletes NE in two ways. First, the drug acts on vesicles within the nerve terminal to cause displacement of stored NE, thereby exposing the transmitter to destruction by monoamine oxidase. Second, reserpine suppresses NE synthesis by blocking the uptake of dopamine (the immediate precursor of NE) into presynaptic vesicles, which contain the enzymes needed to convert dopamine into NE (Fig. 19.1). A week or two may be required to produce maximal transmitter depletion.

In addition to its peripheral effects, reserpine can cause depletion of serotonin and catecholamines from neurons in the CNS. Depletion of these CNS transmitters underlies the most serious side effect of reserpine—deep emotional depression—and also explains the occasional use of reserpine in psychiatry.

Pharmacologic Effects

Peripheral Effects. By depleting sympathetic neurons of NE, reserpine decreases the activation of alpha- and beta-adrenergic receptors. Decreased activation of beta receptors slows heart rate and reduces cardiac output. Decreased alpha activation promotes vasodilation. All three effects cause a *decrease in blood pressure.*

Effects on the CNS. Reserpine produces sedation and a state of indifference to the environment. In addition, the drug can cause severe depression. These effects are thought to result from depletion of catecholamines and serotonin from neurons in the brain.

Therapeutic Uses

Hypertension. The principal indication for reserpine is hypertension. Benefits result from vasodilation and reduced cardiac workload. Because these effects occur secondary to depletion of NE and because transmitter depletion occurs slowly, full antihypertensive responses can take a week or more to develop. Conversely, when reserpine is discontinued, effects may persist for several weeks as the NE content of sympathetic neurons becomes replenished. Because its side effects can be severe and because more desirable drugs are available (see Chapter 47), reserpine is not a preferred drug for hypertension.

Psychotic States. Reserpine can be used to treat agitated psychotic patients, such as those suffering from certain forms of schizophrenia. However, because more effective drugs are available, reserpine is rarely employed in psychotherapy.

Adverse Effects

Depression. Reserpine can produce severe depression that may persist for months after the drug is withdrawn. Suicide has occurred. All patients should be informed about the risk of depression. Also, they should be educated about signs of depression (e.g., early morning insomnia, loss of appetite, change in mood) and instructed to notify the prescriber immediately if these develop. Because of the risk of suicide, patients who develop depression may require hospitalization. *Reserpine is contraindicated for patients with a history of depressive disorders.* The risk of depression can be minimized by keeping the dosage low (0.25 mg/day or less).

Cardiovascular Effects. Depletion of NE from sympathetic neurons can result in *bradycardia, orthostatic hypotension,* and *nasal congestion.* Bradycardia is caused by decreased activation of $beta_1$ receptors in the heart. Hypotension and nasal congestion result from vasodilation secondary to decreased activation of alpha receptors on blood vessels. Patients should be informed that orthostatic hypotension, the most serious cardiovascular effect, can be minimized by moving slowly when changing from a seated or supine position to an upright position. In addition, patients should be advised to sit or lie down if light-headedness or dizziness occurs.

GI Effects. By mechanisms that are not understood, reserpine can stimulate several aspects of GI function. The drug can increase secretion of gastric acid, which may result in *ulcer formation.* In addition, reserpine can increase the tone and motility of intestinal smooth muscle, causing *cramps* and *diarrhea.*

Preparations, Dosage, and Administration. Reserpine is available in 0.1- and 0.25-mg tablets, which may be administered with food if GI upset occurs. The usual initial dosage for hypertension in adults is 0.5 mg/day for 1 to 2 weeks. The usual maintenance dosage is 0.1 to 0.25 mg/day.

[b]By the time you read this, reserpine may have been discontinued, as well.

KEY POINTS

- All of the drugs discussed in this chapter reduce activation of peripheral alpha- and beta-adrenergic receptors, but they do so by mechanisms other than direct receptor blockade.
- The principal indication for these drugs is hypertension.
- Clonidine and methyldopa reduce sympathetic outflow to the heart and blood vessels by causing activation of $alpha_2$-adrenergic receptors in the brainstem.
- The principal adverse effects of clonidine are drowsiness and dry mouth. Rebound hypertension can occur if the drug is abruptly withdrawn.
- The principal adverse effects of methyldopa are hemolytic anemia and liver damage.
- Methyldopa is a preferred drug in management of hypertension during pregnancy.

Please visit **http://evolve.elsevier.com/Lehne** for chapter-specific NCLEX® examination review questions.

Summary of Major Nursing Implications[a]

CLONIDINE

Preadministration Assessment

Therapeutic Goal

Reduction of blood pressure in hypertensive patients.[b]

Baseline Data

Determine blood pressure and heart rate.

Identifying High-Risk Patients

Clonidine is embryotoxic to animals and should not be used during pregnancy. Rule out pregnancy before initiating treatment.

Implementation: Administration

Routes

Oral, transdermal.

Administration

Oral. **Advise the patient to take the major portion of the daily dose at bedtime to minimize daytime sedation.**

Transdermal. **Instruct the patient to apply transdermal patches to hairless, intact skin on the upper arm or torso, and to apply a new patch every 7 days.**

Ongoing Evaluation and Interventions

Evaluating Therapeutic Effects

Monitor blood pressure.

Minimizing Adverse Effects

Drowsiness and Sedation. **Inform patients about possible CNS depression and warn them to avoid hazardous activities if alertness is reduced.**

Xerostomia. Dry mouth is common. **Inform patients that discomfort can be reduced by chewing gum, sucking hard candy, and taking frequent sips of fluids.**

Rebound Hypertension. Severe hypertension occurs rarely following abrupt clonidine withdrawal. Treat with a combination of alpha- and beta-adrenergic blockers. To avoid rebound hypertension, withdraw clonidine slowly (over 2 to 4 days). **Inform patients about rebound hypertension and warn them against abrupt discontinuation of treatment.**

Abuse. People who abuse cocaine, opioids, and other drugs frequently abuse clonidine as well. Be alert for signs of clonidine abuse (e.g., questionable or frequent requests for a prescription).

METHYLDOPA

Preadministration Assessment

Therapeutic Goal

Reduction of blood pressure in hypertensive patients.

Baseline Data

Obtain baseline values for blood pressure, heart rate, blood counts (hematocrit, hemoglobin, or red cell count), Coombs' test, and liver function tests.

Identifying High-Risk Patients

Methyldopa is *contraindicated* for patients with active liver disease or a history of methyldopa-induced liver dysfunction.

Implementation: Administration

Routes

Oral. For routine management of hypertension.

Intravenous. For hypertensive emergencies.

Administration

Most patients on oral therapy require divided (two to four) daily doses. For some patients, blood pressure can be controlled with a single daily dose at bedtime.

Ongoing Evaluation and Interventions

Evaluating Therapeutic Effects

Monitor blood pressure.

Minimizing Adverse Effects

Hemolytic Anemia. If hemolysis occurs, withdraw methyldopa immediately; hemolytic anemia usually resolves soon. Obtain a Coombs' test before treatment and 6 to 12 months later. Obtain blood counts (hematocrit, hemoglobin, or red cell count) before treatment and periodically thereafter.

Hepatotoxicity. Methyldopa can cause hepatitis, jaundice, and fatal hepatic necrosis. Assess liver function before treatment and periodically thereafter. If liver dysfunction develops, discontinue methyldopa immediately. In most cases, liver function returns to normal soon.

[a]Patient education information is highlighted as **blue text.**

[b]Clonidine is also used to relieve severe pain and to manage ADHD.

UNIT V CENTRAL NERVOUS SYSTEM DRUGS

CHAPTER 20

Introduction to Central Nervous System Pharmacology

Central nervous system (CNS) drugs—agents that act on the brain and spinal cord—are used for medical and nonmedical purposes. Medical applications include relief of pain, suppression of seizures, production of anesthesia, and treatment of psychiatric disorders. CNS drugs are used nonmedically for their stimulant, depressant, euphoriant, and other "mind-altering" abilities.

Despite the widespread use of CNS drugs, knowledge of these agents is limited. Much of our ignorance stems from the anatomic and neurochemical complexity of the brain and spinal cord. (There are more than 50 billion neurons in the cerebral hemispheres alone.) We are a long way from fully understanding both the CNS and the drugs used to affect it.

TRANSMITTERS OF THE CNS

In contrast to the peripheral nervous system, in which only three compounds—acetylcholine, norepinephrine, and epinephrine—serve as neurotransmitters, the CNS contains at least 21 compounds that serve as neurotransmitters (Table 20.1). Furthermore, there are numerous sites within the CNS for which no transmitter has been identified, so it is clear that additional compounds, yet to be discovered, also mediate central neurotransmission.

None of the compounds believed to be CNS neurotransmitters have actually been *proved* to serve this function. The reason for uncertainty lies with the technical difficulties involved in CNS research. However, although absolute proof may be lacking, the evidence supporting a neurotransmitter role for several compounds (e.g., dopamine, norepinephrine, enkephalins) is completely convincing.

Although much is known about the actions of CNS transmitters at various sites in the brain and spinal cord, it is not usually possible to precisely relate these known actions to behavioral or psychologic processes. For example, we know the locations of specific CNS sites at which norepinephrine appears to act as a transmitter, and we know the effect of norepinephrine at most of these sites (suppression of neuronal excitability), but we do not know the precise relationship between suppression of neuronal excitability at each of these sites and the impact of that suppression on the overt function of the organism. This example shows the state of our knowledge of CNS transmitter function: We have a great deal of detailed information about the biochemistry and electrophysiology of CNS transmitters, but we are as yet unable to assemble those details into a completely meaningful picture.

THE BLOOD-BRAIN BARRIER

The blood-brain barrier impedes the entry of drugs into the brain. Passage across the barrier is limited to lipid-soluble agents and to drugs that cross by way of specific transport systems. Protein-bound drugs and highly ionized drugs cannot cross.

From a therapeutic perspective, the blood-brain barrier is a mixed blessing. The barrier protects the brain from injury by potentially toxic substances, but it can also be a significant obstacle to entry of therapeutic agents.

The blood-brain barrier is not fully developed at birth. Accordingly, infants are much more sensitive to CNS drugs than are older children and adults.

HOW DO CNS DRUGS PRODUCE THERAPEUTIC EFFECTS?

Although much is known about the biochemical and electrophysiologic effects of CNS drugs, in most cases we cannot state with certainty the relationship between these effects and

TABLE 20.1 ▪ Neurotransmitters of the CNS

MONOAMINES	**OPIOID PEPTIDES**
Dopamine	Dynorphins
Epinephrine	Endorphins
Norepinephrine	Enkephalins
Serotonin	
	NONOPIOID PEPTIDES
AMINO ACIDS	Neurotensin
Aspartate	Oxytocin
GABA	Somatostatin
Glutamate	Substance P
Glycine	Vasopressin
PURINES	**OTHERS**
Adenosine	Acetylcholine
Adenosine monophosphate	Histamine
Adenosine triphosphate	

GABA, Gamma-aminobutyric acid.

production of beneficial responses. Why? To fully understand how a drug alters symptoms, we need to understand, at the biochemical and physiologic levels, the pathophysiology of the disorder being treated. In the case of most CNS disorders, our knowledge is limited: We do not fully understand the brain in either health or disease. Therefore, we must exercise caution when attempting to assign a precise mechanism for a drug's therapeutic effects.

Although we can't state with certainty how CNS drugs act, we do have sufficient data to permit formulation of plausible hypotheses. Consequently, as we study CNS drugs, proposed mechanisms of action are presented. Keep in mind, however, that these mechanisms are tentative, representing our best guess based on available data. As we learn more, it is almost certain that these concepts will be modified, if not discarded.

ADAPTATION OF THE CNS TO PROLONGED DRUG EXPOSURE

When CNS drugs are taken chronically, their effects may differ from those produced during initial use. These altered effects are the result of adaptive changes that occur in the brain in response to prolonged drug exposure. The brain's ability to adapt to drugs can produce alterations in therapeutic effects and side effects. Adaptive changes are often beneficial, although they can also be detrimental.

Increased Therapeutic Effects

Certain drugs used in psychiatry—antipsychotics and antidepressants—must be taken for several weeks before full therapeutic effects develop. Beneficial responses may be delayed because they result from adaptive changes, not from direct effects of drugs on synaptic function. Hence, full therapeutic effects are not seen until the CNS has had time to modify itself in response to prolonged drug exposure.

Decreased Side Effects

When CNS drugs are taken long term, the intensity of side effects may decrease (while therapeutic effects remain undiminished). For example, phenobarbital (an antiseizure drug) produces sedation during the initial phase of therapy; however, with continued treatment, sedation declines while full protection from seizures is retained. Adaptations within the brain are believed to underlie this phenomenon.

Tolerance and Physical Dependence

Tolerance and physical dependence are special manifestations of CNS adaptation. *Tolerance* is a decreased response occurring in the course of prolonged drug use. *Physical dependence* is a state in which abrupt discontinuation of drug use will precipitate a withdrawal syndrome. The kinds of adaptive changes that underlie tolerance and dependence are such that, after they have taken place, continued drug use is required for the brain to function "normally." If drug use is stopped, the drug-adapted brain can no longer function properly, and withdrawal syndrome ensues. The withdrawal reaction continues until the adaptive changes have had time to revert, restoring the CNS to its pretreatment state.

DEVELOPMENT OF NEW PSYCHOTHERAPEUTIC DRUGS

Because of deficiencies in our knowledge of the neurochemical and physiologic changes that underlie mental disease, it is impossible to take a rational approach to the development of truly new (nonderivative) psychotherapeutic agents. History bears this out: Virtually all of the major advances in psychopharmacology have been serendipitous.

In addition to our relative ignorance about the neurochemical and physiologic correlates of mental illness, two other factors contribute to the difficulty in generating truly new psychotherapeutic agents. First, in contrast to many other diseases, we lack adequate animal models of mental illness. Accordingly, animal research is not likely to reveal new types of psychotherapeutic agents. Second, mentally healthy individuals cannot be used as subjects to assess potential psychotherapeutic agents, because most psychotherapeutic drugs either have no effect on healthy individuals or produce paradoxical effects.

After a new drug has been found, variations on that agent can be developed systematically: (1) structural analogs of the new agent are synthesized; (2) these analogs are run through biochemical and physiologic screening tests to determine whether they possess activity similar to that of the parent compound; and (3) after serious toxicity has been ruled out, promising agents are tested in humans for possible psychotherapeutic activity. Using this procedure, it is possible to develop drugs that have fewer side effects than the original drug and perhaps even superior therapeutic effects. However, although this procedure may produce small advances, it is not likely to yield a major therapeutic breakthrough.

APPROACHING THE STUDY OF CNS DRUGS

Because our understanding of the CNS is less complete than our understanding of the peripheral nervous system, our approach to studying CNS drugs differs from the approach we took with peripheral nervous system agents. When we studied the pharmacology of the peripheral nervous system, we emphasized the importance of understanding transmitters and their receptors before embarking on a study of drugs. Because our knowledge of CNS transmitters is insufficient to allow this approach, rather than making a detailed examination of CNS transmitters before we study CNS drugs, we will discuss drugs and transmitters concurrently. Hence, for now, all that you need to know about CNS transmitters is that (1) there are a lot of them, (2) their precise functional roles are not clear, and (3) their complexity makes it difficult for us to know with certainty just how CNS drugs produce their beneficial effects.

KEY POINTS

- In the CNS, at least 21 compounds appear to act as neurotransmitters.
- We do not understand with precision how CNS drugs produce their effects.
- The blood-brain barrier can protect the CNS from toxic substances, but can also block entry of medicines into the CNS.
- The CNS often undergoes adaptive changes during prolonged drug exposure. The result can be increased therapeutic effects, decreased side effects, tolerance, and physical dependence.

Please visit **http://evolve.elsevier.com/Lehne** for chapter-specific NCLEX® examination review questions.

CHAPTER

21 Drugs for Parkinson Disease

Parkinson disease (PD) is a slowly progressive neurodegenerative disorder that afflicts more than 1 million Americans, making it second only to Alzheimer's disease as the most common degenerative disease of neurons. Cardinal symptoms are tremor, rigidity, postural instability, and slowed movement. In addition to these motor symptoms, most patients also experience nonmotor symptoms, especially autonomic disturbances, sleep disturbances, depression, psychosis, and dementia. Years before functional impairment develops, patients may experience early symptoms of PD, including loss of smell, excessive salivation, clumsiness of the hands, worsening of handwriting, bothersome tremor, slower gait, and reduced voice volume. Symptoms first appear in middle age and progress relentlessly. The underlying cause of motor symptoms is loss of dopaminergic neurons in the substantia nigra. Although there is no cure for motor symptoms, drug therapy can maintain functional mobility for years, and can thereby substantially prolong quality of life and life expectancy.

PATHOPHYSIOLOGY THAT UNDERLIES MOTOR SYMPTOMS

Motor symptoms result from damage to the *extrapyramidal system,* a complex neuronal network that helps regulate movement. When extrapyramidal function is disrupted, *dyskinesias* (disorders of movement) result. The dyskinesias that characterize PD are tremor at rest, rigidity, postural instability, and bradykinesia (slowed movement). In severe PD, bradykinesia may progress to *akinesia*—complete absence of movement.

In people with PD, neurotransmission is disrupted primarily in the brain's *striatum.* A simplified model of striatal neurotransmission is depicted in Fig. 21.1A. As indicated, proper function of the striatum requires a balance between two neurotransmitters: *dopamine* and *acetylcholine.* Dopamine is an *inhibitory* transmitter; acetylcholine is *excitatory.* The neurons that release dopamine inhibit neurons that release gamma-aminobutyric acid (GABA), another inhibitory transmitter. In contrast, the neurons that release acetylcholine excite the neurons that release GABA. Movement is normal when the inhibitory influence of dopamine and the excitatory influence of acetylcholine are in balance. In PD there is an imbalance between dopamine and acetylcholine in the striatum (Fig. 21.1B). As noted, the imbalance results from *degeneration of the neurons in the substantia nigra that supply dopamine to the striatum.* In the absence of dopamine, the excitatory influence of acetylcholine goes unopposed, causing excessive stimulation of the neurons that release GABA. Overactivity of these GABAergic neurons contributes to the motor symptoms that characterize PD. That being said, from 70% to 80% of these neurons must be lost before PD becomes clinically recognizable. Because this loss takes place over 5 to 20 years, neuronal degeneration begins long before overt motor symptoms appear.

What causes degeneration of dopaminergic neurons? No one knows for sure. However, some evidence strongly implicates *alpha-synuclein*—a potentially toxic protein synthesized by dopaminergic neurons. Under normal conditions, alpha-synuclein is rapidly degraded. As a result, it doesn't accumulate and no harm occurs. Degradation of alpha-synuclein requires two other proteins: *parkin* and *ubiquitin.* (Parkin is an enzyme that catalyzes the binding of alpha-synuclein to ubiquitin. When bound to ubiquitin, alpha-synuclein can be degraded.) If any of these proteins—alpha-synuclein, parkin, or ubiquitin—is defective, degradation of alpha-synuclein cannot take place. When this occurs, alpha-synuclein accumulates inside the cell, forming neurotoxic fibrils. At autopsy, these fibrils are visible as so-called *Lewy bodies,* which are characteristic of PD pathology. Failure to degrade alpha-synuclein appears to result from two causes: genetic vulnerability and toxins in the environment. Defective genes coding for all three proteins have been found in families with inherited forms of PD. In people with PD that is not inherited, environmental toxins may explain the inability to degrade alpha-synuclein.

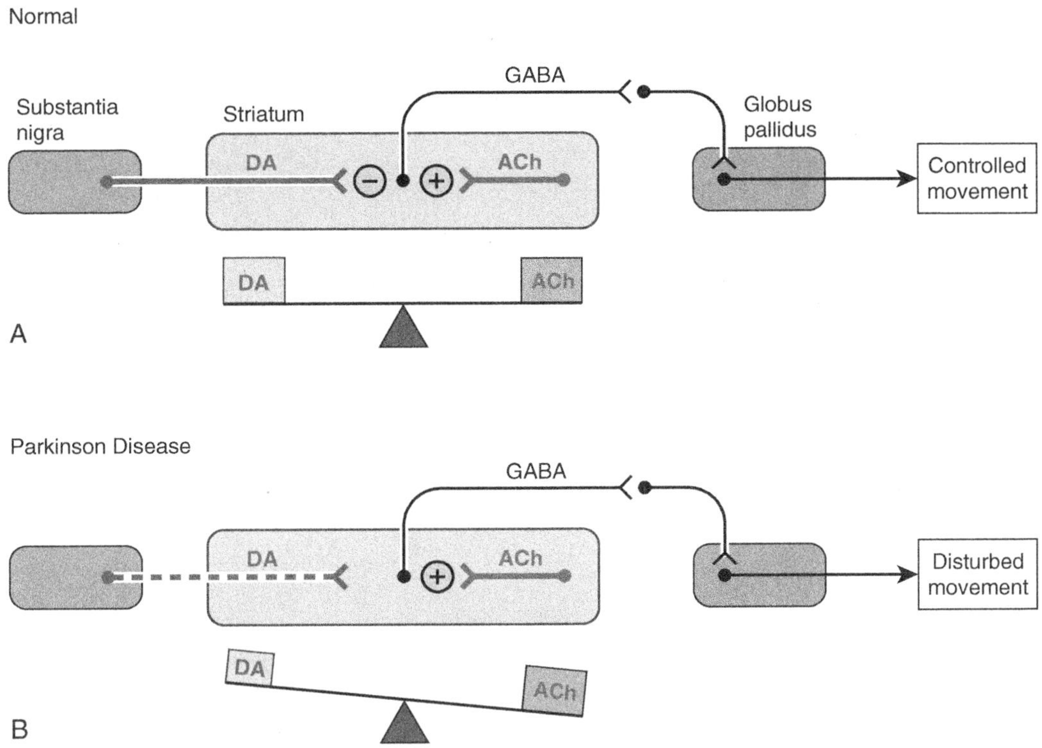

Fig. 21.1 ■ A model of neurotransmission in the healthy striatum and parkinsonian striatum.
A, In the healthy striatum, dopamine (DA) released from neurons originating in the substantia nigra *inhibits* the firing of neurons in the striatum that release gamma-aminobutyric acid (GABA). Conversely, neurons located within the striatum, which release acetylcholine (ACh), *excite* the GABAergic neurons. Therefore, under normal conditions, the inhibitory actions of DA are balanced by the excitatory actions of ACh, and controlled movement results. **B,** In Parkinson disease, the neurons that supply DA to the striatum degenerate. In the absence of sufficient DA, the excitatory effects of ACh go unopposed, and disturbed movement results.

As discussed in Chapter 31, movement disorders similar to those of PD can occur as side effects of antipsychotic drugs. These dyskinesias, which are referred to as *extrapyramidal side effects,* result from blockade of dopamine receptors in the striatum. This drug-induced parkinsonism can be managed with some of the drugs used to treat PD.

OVERVIEW OF MOTOR SYMPTOM MANAGEMENT

Therapeutic Goal

Ideally, treatment would reverse neuronal degeneration, or at least prevent further degeneration, and control symptoms. Unfortunately, the ideal treatment doesn't exist. We have no drugs that can prevent neuronal damage or reverse damage that has already occurred. Drugs can only provide symptomatic relief; they do not cure PD. Furthermore, there is no convincing proof that any current drug can delay disease progression. Hence, the goal of pharmacologic therapy is simply to improve the patient's ability to carry out activities of daily living. Drug selection and dosage are determined by the extent to which PD interferes with work, walking, dressing, eating, bathing, and other activities. Drugs benefit the patient primarily by improving bradykinesia, gait disturbance, and postural instability. Tremor and rigidity, although disturbing, are less disabling.

Drugs Employed

Given the neurochemical basis of parkinsonism—too little striatal dopamine and too much acetylcholine—the approach to treatment is obvious: Give drugs that can restore the functional balance between dopamine and acetylcholine. To accomplish this, two types of drugs are used: (1) *dopaminergic agents* (i.e., drugs that directly or indirectly activate dopamine receptors); and (2) *anticholinergic agents* (i.e., drugs that block receptors for acetylcholine). Of the two groups, dopaminergic agents are by far the more widely employed.

As shown in Table 21.1, dopaminergic drugs act by several mechanisms: Levodopa is converted to dopamine which activates dopamine receptors directly; inhibitors of monoamine oxidase-B (MAO-B) prevent dopamine breakdown; amantadine promotes dopamine release (and may also block dopamine reuptake); and the inhibitors of catechol-*O*-methyltransferase (COMT) enhance the effects of levodopa by blocking its degradation.

TABLE 21.1 ▪ Dopaminergic Agents for Parkinson Disease

Drug	Mechanism of Action	Therapeutic Role
DOPAMINE REPLACEMENT		
Levodopa/carbidopa	Levodopa undergoes conversion to DA in the brain and then activates DA receptors (carbidopa blocks destruction of levodopa in the periphery)	First-line drug, or supplement to a dopamine agonist.
DOPAMINE AGONISTS		
Nonergot Derivatives Apomorphine Pramipexole Ropinirole Rotigotine **Ergot Derivatives** Bromocriptine Cabergoline	Directly activate DA receptors	Pramipexole and ropinirole are first-line drugs, or supplements to levodopa. Apomorphine—a subQ nonergot agent—is reserved for rescue therapy during off times. Ergot derivatives are generally avoided.
COMT INHIBITORS		
Entacapone Tolcapone	Inhibit breakdown of levodopa by COMT	Adjunct to levodopa to decrease wearing off; entacapone is more effective and safer than tolcapone.
MAO-B INHIBITORS		
Rasagiline Selegiline	Inhibit breakdown of DA by MAO-B	Used in newly diagnosed patients and for managing off times during levodopa therapy.
DOPAMINE RELEASER		
Amantadine	Promotes release of DA from remaining DA neurons; may also block DA reuptake	May help reduce levodopa-induced dyskinesias.

COMT, Catechol-*O*-methyltransferase; *DA,* dopamine; *MAO-B,* type B monoamine oxidase.

PATIENT-CENTERED CARE ACROSS THE LIFE SPAN

Drugs for Parkinson Disease

Life Stage	Considerations or Concerns
Children	Juvenile PD in patients younger than 18 years is extremely rare; therefore, many drugs for PD have not been tested in children. Only amantadine, benztropine, and bromocriptine have approval for pediatric populations. Selegiline is contraindicated in children younger than 12 years old.
Pregnant women	Bromocriptine and cabergoline are FDA Pregnancy Risk Category B[a] (though the manufacturer recommends stopping them once pregnancy is determined). All other drugs in this chapter are FDA Pregnancy Risk Category C, owing to adverse events in animal studies. For ropinirole, in particular, animal studies demonstrated teratogenic effects and embryonic loss. Of note, it is rare for a woman of childbearing age to develop PD.
Breast-feeding women	Bromocriptine and cabergoline interfere with lactation. Anticholinergics such as benztropine can suppress lactation. Breast-feeding is not recommended for women taking other drugs in this chapter.
Older adults	The average age of PD diagnosis is 62 years; therefore, most prescriptions are written for older adults. Adverse effects tend to be more common and more serious in these patients. Beers Criteria designate anticholinergic drugs (e.g., benztropine and trihexyphenidyl) as potentially inappropriate for use in geriatric patients. As with all drugs, careful consideration must be given to drug choice, and benefits must be weighed against risks.

[a]As of 2020, the FDA will no longer use Pregnancy Risk Categories. Please refer to Chapter 9 for more information.

In contrast to the dopaminergic drugs, which act by multiple mechanisms, all of the anticholinergic agents share the same mechanism: blockade of muscarinic receptors in the striatum.

Clinical Guidelines

The American Academy of Neurology (AAN) has developed evidence-based guidelines for the treatment of PD. The recommendations that follow are based on these guidelines.

Drug Selection

Initial Treatment

For patients with mild symptoms, treatment can begin with selegiline, an MAO-B inhibitor that confers mild, symptomatic benefit. Rasagiline, an MAO-B inhibitor that was not available when the guidelines were published, would probably work just as well.

For patients with more severe symptoms, treatment should begin with either levodopa (combined with carbidopa) or a dopamine agonist. Levodopa is more effective than the dopamine agonists, but long-term use carries a higher risk for disabling dyskinesias. Hence, the choice must be tailored to the patient: If improving motor function is the primary objective, then levodopa is preferred. However, if drug-induced dyskinesias are a primary concern, then a dopamine agonist would be preferred.

Management of Motor Fluctuations

Long-term treatment with levodopa or dopamine agonists is associated with two types of motor fluctuations: *"off" times* (loss of symptom relief) and *drug-induced dyskinesias* (involuntary movements). Off times can be reduced with three types of drugs: dopamine agonists, COMT inhibitors, and MAO-B inhibitors. Evidence of efficacy is strongest for entacapone (a COMT inhibitor) and rasagiline (an MAO-B inhibitor). The only drug recommended for dyskinesias is amantadine.

Neuroprotection

To date, there is no definitive proof that any drug can protect dopaminergic neurons from progressive degeneration. However, although no drug has yet been proven to provide neuroprotective effects for people with PD, studies suggest that some drugs are promising. For example, MAO-B inhibitors have provided neuroprotective effects in animal studies. Similarly, dopamine agonists have demonstrated neuroprotective effects in laboratory studies. For both drug categories, however, clinical studies in humans have been inconclusive. A growing body of research with levodopa supports a likely role for neuroprotection; however, because some studies demonstrate toxic effects in patients with PD, the risks may outweigh the benefits when given for this purpose.

TABLE 21.2 ■ Drugs for Motor Complications of Levodopa Therapy

Drug	Drug Class
DRUGS FOR OFF TIMES	
Definitely Effective	
Entacapone	COMT inhibitor
Rasagiline	MAO-B inhibitor
Probably Effective	
Rotigotine	DA agonist
Pramipexole	DA agonist
Ropinirole	DA agonist
Tolcapone	COMT inhibitor
Possibly Effective	
Apomorphine	DA agonist
Cabergoline	DA agonist
Selegiline	MAO-B inhibitor
DRUG FOR LEVODOPA-INDUCED DYSKINESIAS	
Amantadine	DA-releasing agent

COMT, Catechol-*O*-methyltransferase; *DA,* dopamine; *MAO-B,* type B monoamine oxidase.

PHARMACOLOGY OF DRUGS USED FOR MOTOR SYMPTOMS

Levodopa

Levodopa was introduced in the 1960s, and has been a cornerstone of PD treatment ever since. Unfortunately, although the drug is highly effective, beneficial effects diminish over time. The most troubling adverse effects are dyskinesias.

Use in Parkinson Disease

Beneficial Effects. Levodopa is the most effective drug for PD. At the beginning of treatment, about 75% of patients experience a 50% reduction in symptom severity. Levodopa is so effective, in fact, that a diagnosis of PD should be questioned if the patient fails to respond.

Full therapeutic responses may take several months to develop. Consequently, although the effects of levodopa can be significant, patients should not expect immediate improvement. Rather, they should be informed that beneficial effects are likely to increase steadily over the first few months.

In contrast to the dramatic improvements seen during initial therapy, long-term therapy with levodopa has been disappointing. Although symptoms may be well controlled during the first 2 years of treatment, by the end of year 5 ability to function may deteriorate to pretreatment levels. This probably reflects disease progression and not development of tolerance to levodopa.

Acute Loss of Effect. Acute loss of effect occurs in two patterns: gradual loss and abrupt loss. Gradual loss—"wearing off"—develops near the end of the dosing interval, and simply indicates that drug levels have declined to a subtherapeutic value. Wearing off can be minimized in three ways: (1) shortening the dosing interval, (2) giving a drug (e.g., entacapone) that prolongs levodopa's plasma half-life, and (3) giving a direct-acting dopamine agonist.

Abrupt loss of effect, often referred to as the "on-off" phenomenon, can occur at any time during the dosing interval—even while drug levels are high. Off times may last from minutes to hours. Over the course of treatment, off periods are likely to increase in both intensity and frequency. Drugs that can help reduce off times are listed in Table 21.2. As discussed later in this chapter, avoiding high-protein meals may also help.

Mechanism of Action

Levodopa reduces symptoms by increasing dopamine synthesis in the striatum (Fig. 21.2). Levodopa enters the brain via an active transport system that carries it across the blood-brain barrier. Once in the brain, the drug undergoes uptake into the remaining dopaminergic nerve terminals that remain in the striatum. Following uptake, levodopa, which has no direct effects of its own, is converted to dopamine, its active form. As dopamine, levodopa helps restore a proper balance between dopamine and acetylcholine.

Conversion of levodopa to dopamine is depicted in Fig. 21.3. As indicated, the enzyme that catalyzes the reaction is called a *decarboxylase* (because it removes a carboxyl group from levodopa). The activity of decarboxylases is enhanced by *pyridoxine* (vitamin B_6).

Why is PD treated with levodopa and not with dopamine itself? There are two reasons. First, dopamine cannot cross the blood-brain barrier (see Fig. 21.2). As noted, levodopa

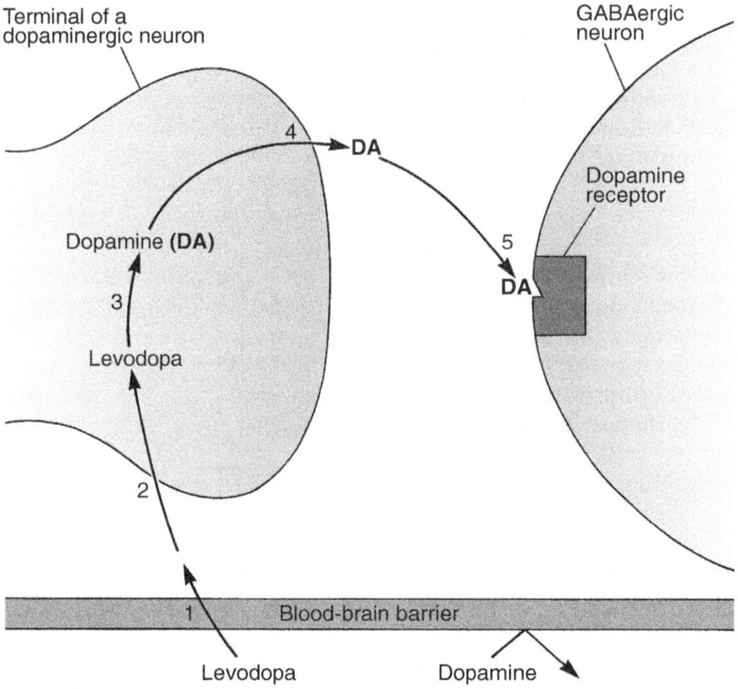

Fig. 21.2 ■ Steps leading to alteration of CNS function by levodopa.
To produce its beneficial effects in PD, levodopa must be (1) transported across the blood-brain barrier; (2) taken up by dopaminergic nerve terminals in the striatum; (3) converted into dopamine; (4) released into the synaptic space; and (5) bound to dopamine receptors on striatal GABAergic neurons, causing them to fire at a slower rate. Note that dopamine itself is unable to cross the blood-brain barrier, and hence cannot be used to treat PD.

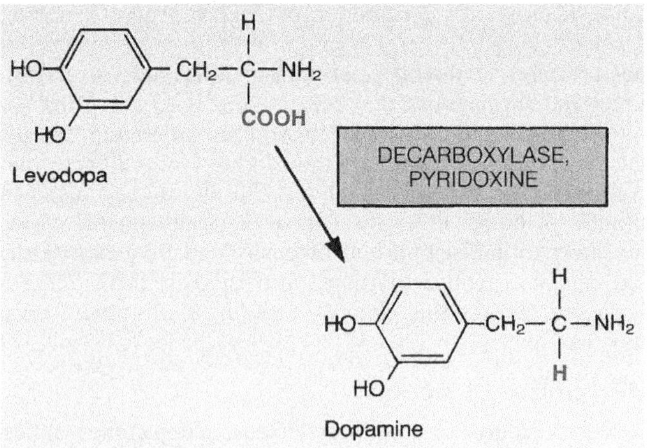

Fig. 21.3 ■ Conversion of levodopa to dopamine.
Decarboxylases present in the brain, liver, and intestine convert levodopa into dopamine. Pyridoxine (vitamin B_6) accelerates the reaction.

crosses the barrier by means of an active transport system, a system that does not transport dopamine. Second, dopamine has such a short half-life in the blood that it would be impractical to use even if it could cross the blood-brain barrier.

Pharmacokinetics

Levodopa is administered orally and undergoes rapid absorption from the small intestine. Food delays absorption by slowing gastric emptying. Furthermore, because neutral amino acids compete with levodopa for intestinal absorption (and for transport across the blood-brain barrier as well), high-protein foods will reduce therapeutic effects.

Only a small fraction of each dose reaches the brain. Most is metabolized in the periphery, primarily by *decarboxylase enzymes* and to a lesser extent by COMT. Peripheral decarboxylases convert levodopa into dopamine, an active metabolite. In contrast, COMT converts levodopa into an inactive metabolite. Like the enzymes that decarboxylate levodopa within the brain, peripheral decarboxylases work faster in the presence of pyridoxine. Because of peripheral metabolism, less than 2% of each dose enters the brain if levodopa is given alone. For this reason, levodopa is available only in combination preparations with either carbidopa or carbidopa and entacapone. These additional agents decrease the amount of decarboxylation in the periphery so that more of the drug can enter the CNS. This is discussed in greater detail later in the chapter.

Adverse Effects

Most side effects of levodopa are dose dependent. Older adult patients, who are the primary users of levodopa, are especially sensitive to adverse effects.

Nausea and Vomiting. Most patients experience nausea and vomiting early in treatment. The cause is activation of dopamine receptors in the chemoreceptor trigger zone (CTZ) of the medulla. Nausea and vomiting can be reduced by administering levodopa in low initial doses and with meals. (Food delays levodopa absorption, causing a decrease in peak plasma drug levels and a corresponding decrease in stimulation of the CTZ.) However, because administration with food can reduce therapeutic effects by decreasing levodopa absorption, administration with meals should be avoided if possible. Giving additional carbidopa (without levodopa) can help reduce nausea and vomiting. Why carbidopa helps is unknown.

Dyskinesias. Ironically, levodopa, which is given to *alleviate* movement disorders, actually *causes* movement disorders in many patients. About 80% develop involuntary movements within the first year. Some dyskinesias are just annoying (e.g., head bobbing, tics, grimacing), whereas others can be disabling (e.g., ballismus, a rapid involuntary jerking or flinging of proximal muscle groups, or choreoathetosis, a slow, involuntary writhing movement). These dyskinesias develop just before or soon after optimal levodopa dosage has been achieved. Dyskinesias can be managed in three ways. First, the dosage of levodopa can be reduced. However, dosage reduction may allow PD symptoms to re-emerge. Second, we can give amantadine (discussed later), which can reduce dyskinesias in some patients. If these measures fail, the remaining options are usually surgery and electrical stimulation.

Cardiovascular Effects. *Postural hypotension* is common early in treatment. The underlying mechanism is unknown. Hypotension can be reduced by increasing intake of salt and water. An alpha-adrenergic agonist can help too.

Conversion of levodopa to dopamine in the periphery can produce excessive activation of $beta_1$ receptors in the heart. *Dysrhythmias* can result, especially in patients with heart disease.

Psychosis. Psychosis develops in about 20% of patients. Prominent symptoms are visual hallucinations, vivid dreams or nightmares, and paranoid ideation (fears of personal endangerment, sense of persecution, feelings of being followed or spied on). Activation of dopamine receptors is in some way involved. Symptoms can be reduced by lowering levodopa dosage, but this will reduce beneficial effects, too.

Treatment of levodopa-induced psychosis with first-generation antipsychotics is problematic. Yes, these agents can decrease psychological symptoms. However, they will also *intensify* symptoms of PD because they block receptors for dopamine in the striatum. In fact, when first-generation antipsychotic agents are used for schizophrenia, the biggest problem is parkinsonian side effects, referred to as extrapyramidal symptoms (EPS).

Two second-generation antipsychotics—*clozapine* and *quetiapine*—have been used successfully to manage levodopa-induced psychosis. Unlike the first-generation antipsychotic drugs, clozapine and quetiapine cause little or no blockade of dopamine receptors in the striatum, so they do not cause EPS. In patients taking levodopa, these drugs can reduce psychotic symptoms without intensifying symptoms of PD. Interestingly, the dosage of clozapine used to treat PD-related psychosis is much lower than the dosage used for schizophrenia. Clozapine and quetiapine are discussed in Chapter 31.

Central Nervous System Effects. Levodopa may cause a number of central nervous system (CNS) effects. These range from anxiety and agitation to memory and cognitive impairment. Insomnia and nightmares are common. Some patients experience problems with impulse control, resulting in behavioral changes associated with promiscuity, gambling, binge eating, or alcohol abuse.

Other Adverse Effects. Levodopa may *darken sweat and urine;* patients should be informed about this harmless effect. Some studies suggest that levodopa can *activate malignant melanoma;* however, others have failed to support this finding. Until more is known, it is important to perform a careful skin assessment of patients who are prescribed levodopa.

Drug Interactions

Interactions between levodopa and other drugs can (1) increase beneficial effects of levodopa, (2) decrease beneficial effects of levodopa, and (3) increase toxicity from levodopa. Major interactions are shown in Table 21.3. Several important interactions are discussed later in this chapter.

First-Generation Antipsychotic Drugs. All of the first-generation antipsychotic drugs (e.g., chlorpromazine, haloperidol) block receptors for dopamine in the striatum. As a result, they can decrease therapeutic effects of levodopa. Accordingly, concurrent use of levodopa and these drugs should be avoided. As discussed previously, two second-generation agents—clozapine and quetiapine—do not block dopamine receptors in the striatum, so they can be used safely in patients with PD.

Monoamine Oxidase Inhibitors. Levodopa can cause a hypertensive crisis if administered to an individual taking a

TABLE 21.3 ■ Major Drug Interactions of Levodopa

Drug Category	Drug	Mechanism of Interaction
Drugs that *increase* beneficial effects of levodopa	Carbidopa	Inhibits peripheral decarboxylation of levodopa
	Entacapone, tolcapone	Inhibit destruction of levodopa by COMT in the intestine and peripheral tissues
	Rotigotine, apomorphine, bromocriptine, cabergoline, pramipexole, ropinirole	Stimulate dopamine receptors directly, and thereby add to the effects of dopamine derived from levodopa
	Amantadine	Promotes release of dopamine
	Anticholinergic drugs	Block cholinergic receptors in the CNS, and thereby help restore the balance between dopamine and ACh
Drugs that *decrease* beneficial effects of levodopa	Antipsychotic drugs[a]	Block dopamine receptors in the striatum
Drugs that *increase* levodopa toxicity	MAO inhibitors (especially *nonselective* MAO inhibitors)	Inhibition of MAO increases the risk of severe levodopa-induced hypertension

[a]First-generation antipsychotic agents block dopamine receptors in the striatum and can thereby nullify the therapeutic effects of levodopa. Two second-generation antipsychotics—clozapine [Clozaril] and quetiapine [Seroquel]—do not block dopamine receptors in the striatum, and thus do not nullify the therapeutic effects of levodopa.

ACh, Acetylcholine; *CNS,* central nervous system; *COMT,* catechol-*O*-methyltransferase; *MAO,* monoamine oxidase.

nonselective inhibitor of monoamine oxidase (MAO). The mechanism is as follows: (1) Levodopa elevates neuronal stores of dopamine and norepinephrine (NE) by promoting synthesis of both transmitters. (2) Because intraneuronal MAO serves to inactivate dopamine and NE, inhibition of MAO allows elevated neuronal stores of these transmitters to grow even larger. (3) Because both dopamine and NE promote vasoconstriction, release of these agents in supranormal amounts can lead to massive vasoconstriction, thereby causing blood pressure to rise dangerously high. To avoid hypertensive crisis, nonselective MAO inhibitors should be withdrawn at least 2 weeks before giving levodopa.

Anticholinergic Drugs. As discussed previously, excessive stimulation of cholinergic receptors contributes to the dyskinesias of PD. Therefore, by blocking these receptors, anticholinergic agents can enhance responses to levodopa.

Pyridoxine. You may read advice to limit pyridoxine (vitamin B_6) in patients taking this drug. It is true that pyridoxine accelerates decarboxylation of levodopa in the periphery; however, because levodopa is now always combined with carbidopa, a drug that suppresses decarboxylase activity, this potential interaction is no longer a clinical concern.

Food Interactions

High-protein meals can reduce therapeutic responses to levodopa. Neutral amino acids compete with levodopa for absorption from the intestine and for transport across the blood-brain barrier. Therefore, a high-protein meal can significantly reduce both the amount of levodopa absorbed and the amount transported into the brain. It has been suggested that a high-protein meal could trigger an abrupt loss of effect (i.e., an off episode). Accordingly, patients should be advised to spread their protein consumption evenly throughout the day.

Levodopa/Carbidopa and Levodopa/Carbidopa/Entacapone

At one time levodopa was available as a single drug. However, these single-drug preparations have been withdrawn from the market. Levodopa is now available only in combination preparations, either levodopa/carbidopa or levodopa/carbidopa/entacapone.

Mechanism of Action

Carbidopa has no therapeutic effects of its own; however, carbidopa inhibits decarboxylation of levodopa in the intestine and peripheral tissues, thereby making more levodopa available to the CNS. Carbidopa does not prevent the conversion of levodopa to dopamine by decarboxylases in the brain, because carbidopa is unable to cross the blood-brain barrier.

The effect of carbidopa is shown schematically in Fig. 21.4, which compares the fate of levodopa in the presence and absence of carbidopa. As mentioned previously, in the absence of carbidopa, about 98% of levodopa is lost in the periphery, leaving only 2% available to the brain. Why is levodopa lost? Primarily because decarboxylases in the gastrointestinal (GI) tract and peripheral tissues convert it to dopamine, which cannot cross the blood-brain barrier. When these decarboxylases are inhibited by carbidopa, only 90% of levodopa is lost in the periphery, leaving 10% for actions in the brain.

Advantages of Carbidopa

The combination of carbidopa plus levodopa is superior to levodopa alone in three ways:

- By increasing the fraction of levodopa available for actions in the CNS, carbidopa allows the dosage of levodopa to be reduced by about 75%. In the example in Fig. 21.4, to provide 10 mg of dopamine to the brain, we must administer 500 mg of levodopa if carbidopa is absent, but only 100 mg if carbidopa is present.
- By reducing production of dopamine in the periphery, carbidopa reduces cardiovascular responses to levodopa as well as nausea and vomiting.
- By causing direct inhibition of decarboxylase, carbidopa eliminates concerns about decreasing the effects of levodopa by taking a vitamin preparation that contains pyridoxine.

Disadvantages of Carbidopa

Carbidopa has no adverse effects of its own. Accordingly, any adverse responses from carbidopa/levodopa are the result of potentiating the effects of levodopa. When levodopa is combined with carbidopa, abnormal movements and psychiatric disturbances can occur sooner and be more intense than with levodopa alone.

Preparations, Dosage, and Administration

The combination of levodopa plus carbidopa is available under three brand names: Rytary, Sinemet, and Duopa. A triple-combination product—levodopa/carbidopa/entacapone—is discussed later in this chapter. As noted, levodopa without carbidopa is no longer available.

Levodopa/Carbidopa: Sinemet. The Sinemet brand of levodopa/carbidopa is available in immediate-release and extended-release tablets. The immediate-release tablets are available in three strengths: (1) 10 mg carbidopa/100 mg levodopa, (2) 25 mg carbidopa/100 mg levodopa, and (3) 25 mg carbidopa/250 mg levodopa. The extended-release tablets [Sinemet CR] are available in two strengths: 25 mg carbidopa/100 mg levodopa and 50 mg carbidopa/200 mg levodopa. With either the immediate- or extended-release formulation, dosage is low initially and then gradually increased. The usual maximum is 8 tablets a day, regardless of strength, administered in divided doses.

Preparation and dosage of the other combination products and nonprototype drugs are provided in Table 21.4. Administration guidelines are also included.

Carbidopa Alone. Carbidopa without levodopa, sold as Lodosyn, is available by special request. When carbidopa is added to levodopa/carbidopa, carbidopa can reduce levodopa-induced nausea and vomiting. It also allows smaller doses of levodopa to be used while promoting a more prompt response.

Dopamine Agonists

Dopamine agonists are first-line drugs for PD. Beneficial effects result from direct activation of dopamine receptors in the striatum. For patients with mild or moderate symptoms, dopamine agonists are drugs of first choice. Although dopamine agonists are less effective than levodopa, they still have advantages. Specifically, in contrast to levodopa, they aren't dependent on enzymatic conversion to become active, aren't converted to potentially toxic metabolites, and don't compete with dietary proteins for uptake from the intestine or transport across the blood-brain barrier. In addition, when used long term, dopamine agonists have a lower incidence of response failures and are less likely to cause disabling dyskinesias. However, dopamine agonists do cause serious side effects—especially hallucinations, daytime sleepiness, and postural hypotension. As a result, these drugs are usually reserved for younger patients, who tolerate their side effects better than do the older patients.

The dopamine agonists fall into two groups: derivatives of ergot (an alkaloid found in plants) and nonergot derivatives. The nonergot derivatives—*pramipexole, ropinirole,*

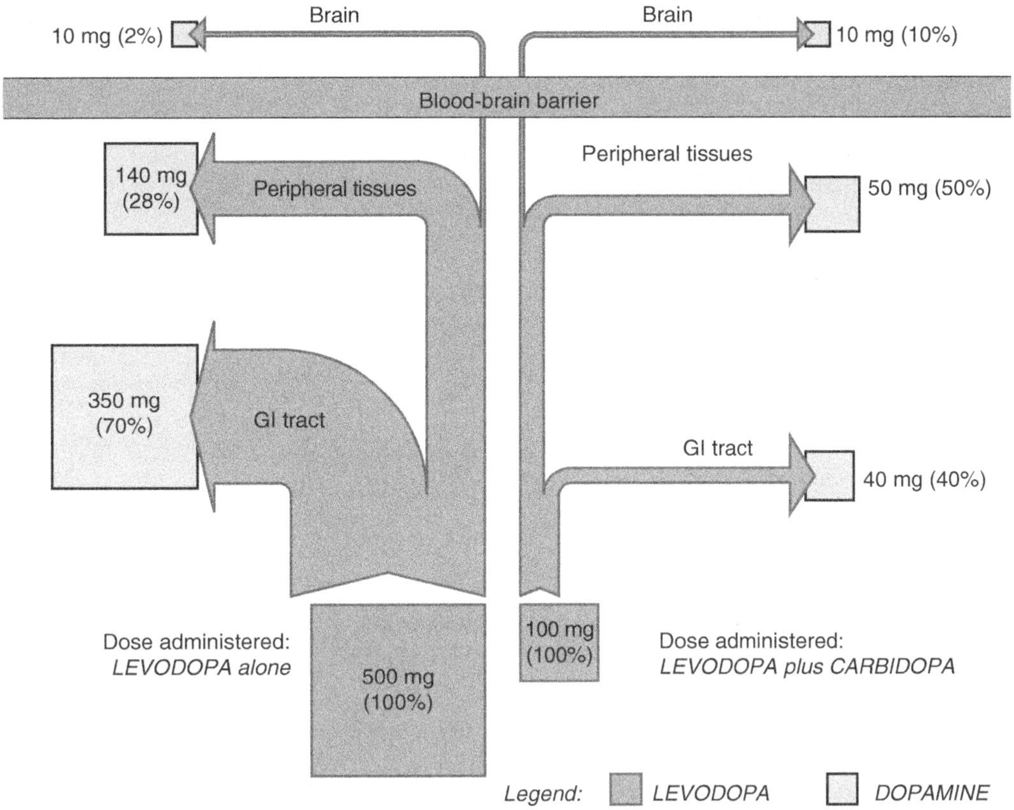

Fig. 21.4 ▪ Fate of levodopa in the presence and absence of carbidopa. In the absence of carbidopa, 98% of an administered dose of levodopa is metabolized in intestinal and peripheral tissues—either by decarboxylases or COMT—leaving only 2% for actions in the brain. Therefore, to deliver 10 mg of levodopa to the brain, the dose of levodopa must be large (500 mg). By inhibiting intestinal and peripheral decarboxylases, carbidopa increases the percentage of levodopa available to the brain. Thus, the dose needed to deliver 10 mg is greatly reduced (to 100 mg in this example). Because carbidopa cannot cross the blood-brain barrier, it does not suppress conversion of levodopa to dopamine in the brain. Furthermore, because carbidopa reduces peripheral production of dopamine (from 140 mg to 50 mg in this example), peripheral toxicity (nausea, cardiovascular effects) is greatly reduced.

rotigotine, and *apomorphine*—are highly selective for dopamine receptors. In contrast, the ergot derivatives—*bromocriptine* and *cabergoline*—are less selective: In addition to activating dopamine receptors, these drugs cause mild *blockage* of serotonergic and alpha-adrenergic receptors. Because of their selectivity, the nonergot derivatives cause fewer side effects than the ergot derivatives, and hence are preferred.

Prototype Drugs

Dopaminergic Drugs

Levodopa (increases dopamine [DA] synthesis)
Carbidopa (blocks levodopa destruction)
Pramipexole (DA receptor agonist)
Entacapone (inhibits catechol-*O*-methyltransferase)
Selegiline (inhibits monoamine oxidase-B)
Amantadine (promotes DA release)

Centrally Acting Anticholinergic Drugs

Benztropine

Nonergot Derivatives: Pramipexole, Ropinirole, Rotigotine, and Apomorphine

Pramipexole

Actions and Uses. Pramipexole [Mirapex] is a nonergot dopamine receptor agonist. The drug is used alone in early-stage PD, and is combined with levodopa in advanced-stage PD. Pramipexole binds selectively to dopamine-2 (D_2) and dopamine-3 (D_3) receptor subtypes. Binding to D_2 receptors underlies therapeutic effects. The significance of D_3 binding is unknown. When used as monotherapy in early PD, pramipexole can produce significant improvement in motor performance. When combined with levodopa in advanced PD, the drug can reduce fluctuations in motor control and may permit a reduction in levodopa dosage. In both cases, maximal benefits take several weeks to develop. Compared with levodopa, pramipexole is less effective at controlling motor symptoms of PD, but is also less likely to cause motor fluctuations.

In addition to its use in PD, pramipexole is approved for patients with moderate to severe *restless legs syndrome* (RLS), a sensorimotor disorder characterized by unpleasant leg sensations that create an urge to move the legs in an effort to ease

TABLE 21.4 ▪ Preparation, Dosage, and Administration of Drugs for Parkinson Disease

Drug	Preparation	Daily Dosage	Administration
LEVODOPA COMBINATIONS			
Levodopa/ Carbidopa [Sinemet, Rytary, Duopa, Duodopa 🍁]	Sinemet (IR): 10 mg carbidopa/100 mg levodopa; 25 mg carbidopa/100 mg levodopa; 25 mg carbidopa/250 mg levodopa Sinemet CR: 25 mg carbidopa/100 mg levodopa; 50 mg carbidopa/200 mg levodopa Rytary: carbidopa 23.75 mg/levodopa 95 mg; carbidopa 36.25 mg/levodopa 145 mg; carbidopa 48.75 mg/levodopa 195 mg; carbidopa 61.25 mg/levodopa 245 mg Duopa enteral suspension: carbidopa 4.63 mg/levodopa 20 mg/mL Duodopa 🍁 intestinal gel: carbidopa 5 mg/levodopa 20 mg/1 mL	Dosage is highly individualized. Typical dosage is one tablet daily or every other day initially and then gradually increased up to a maximum of 8 tablets a day, regardless of strength, administered in divided doses. Duopa and Duodopa are both highly individualized to the patient with dosage adjustments sometimes made on a daily basis.	Food reduces absorption; give on an empty stomach. Duopa enteral suspension and Duodopa intestinal gel are administered via PEG-J tube infusion.
Levodopa/ Carbidopa/ Entacapone [Stalevo]	Stalevo 50: carbidopa 12.5 mg/levodopa 50 mg/entacapone 200 mg Stalevo 75: carbidopa 18.75 mg/levodopa 75 mg/entacapone 200 mg Stalevo 100: carbidopa 25 mg/levodopa 100 mg/entacapone 200 mg Stalevo 125: carbidopa 31.25 mg/ levodopa 125 mg/entacapone 200 mg Stalevo 150: carbidopa 37.5 mg/levodopa 150 mg/entacapone 200 mg Stalevo 200: carbidopa 50 mg/levodopa 200 mg/entacapone 200 mg	Dosage is highly individualized. Typical dosage is 1 tablet of any strength at each dosing interval up to a maximum daily limit of 8 tablets of Stalevo 50 to Stalevo 150 or 6 tablets of Stalevo 200. Dosing intervals are determined by patient response.	May be given with or without food; however, foods that are high in fat may delay absorption. Tablets should be swallowed whole.
DOPAMINE AGONISTS: ERGOT DERIVATIVES			
Bromocriptine [Cycloset, Parlodel]	Cycloset: 0.8 mg tablet Parlodel: 5 mg capsule	Initial: 1.25 mg twice daily. Gradually increase dosage to achieve desired response or until side effects become intolerable. Maintenance: 30–100 mg/day.	Administer with food or meals to decrease GI symptoms. Cycloset should be administered within 2 hours of awakening.
Cabergoline [Dostinex 🍁, generic in U.S.]	0.5 mg tablet	Initial: 1 mg daily. Increase using 0.5–1 mg at 1–2 week intervals. Maintenance: 2–3 mg/day	Administer with food or meals to decrease GI symptoms.
DOPAMINE AGONISTS: NONERGOT DERIVATIVES			
Pramipexole [Mirapex, Mirapex ER]	IR tablets: 0.125, 0.25, 0.5, 0.75, 1, 1.5 mg ER tablets: 0.375, 0.75, 1.5, 2.25, 3, 4.5 mg	IR tablets: 0.125 mg 3 times/day initially, and then increased over 7 weeks to a maximum of 1.5 mg 3 times/day. ER tablets: 0.375 mg once daily initially, and then gradually increased to a maximum of 4.5 mg once daily. Reduced dosage for significant renal impairment.	May be taken with or without food; however, food decreases GI upset. ER formulation should be swallowed whole.
Ropinirole [Requip, Requip XL]	IR tablets: 0.25, 0.5, 1, 2, 3, 4, 5 mg ER tablets: 2, 4, 6, 8, 12 mg	IR tablets: 0.25 mg 3 times/day initially. Can increase over several months to a maximum of 8 mg 3 times/day. ER tablets: 2 mg once daily initially. Can increase over several months to a maximum of 24 mg once daily. Dosing for RLS: 0.25 mg 1–3 hours before bedtime	May be taken with or without food; however, food decreases GI upset. ER formulation should be swallowed whole.

TABLE 21.4 ▪ Preparation, Dosage, and Administration of Drugs for Parkinson Disease—cont'd

Drug	Preparation	Daily Dosage	Administration
Rotigotine [Neupro]	24-hour transdermal patch: 1, 2, 3, 4, 6, 8 mg	Early-stage PD: Usual starting dose is one 2-mg patch every 24 hours. Increase by 2 mg weekly until lowest effective dose is attained or until maximal dose of 6 mg/24 hr. Advanced-stage PD: Usual starting dose is one 4-mg patch every 24 hours. Increased by 2 mg weekly up to a maximum of 8 mg/24 hr. If it becomes necessary to discontinue treatment, withdrawal should be done at the same rate of 2 mg/week.	Apply to skin that is clean, dry, hairless, and free of abrasions or cuts. To decrease skin reactions, rotate site with each application. Allow at least a 2-week elapse before applying the patch to a site used previously.
Apomorphine [Apokyn]	10 mg/mL in 3-mL cartridges to be used with a multidose injector pen (provided)	2 to 6 mg (0.2 to 0.6 mL) subQ for each "off" episode. Maximum: 5 doses a day	Package labeling states that all patients should take an antiemetic (e.g., trimethobenzamide, 300 mg 3 times a day), starting 3 days before the first apomorphine dose.
COMT INHIBITORS			
Entacapone [Comtan]	200-mg tablets	Initial: 200 mg Can increase to a maximum of 8 doses (1600 mg) a day.	May be taken with or without food. Should be taken with each dose of levodopa/carbidopa.
Tolcapone [Tasmar]	100-mg tablets	100 mg 3 times a day. Increase to 200 mg 3 times/day, if needed.	May be taken with or without food. The first dose should be administered in the morning along with levodopa/carbidopa. The next two doses are taken 6 and 12 hours later.
MAO-B INHIBITORS			
Selegiline [Eldepryl, Zelapar]	Capsule (Eldepryl, generic): 5 mg Tablet (generic): 5 mg ODT (Zelapar): 1.25 mg (A 24-hour patch marketed as Emsam is available, but this is not approved for management of PD.)	5 mg taken with breakfast and lunch, for a total of 10 mg a day. This dosage produces complete inhibition of MAO-B, and hence larger doses are unnecessary. ODT: 1.25 mg once a day for 6 weeks. Can increase to a maximum dose of 2.5 mg daily, if needed.	ODT should be placed on top of tongue and allowed to dissolve. Take ODT before breakfast and allow at least 5 minutes before drinking or eating after administration.
Rasagiline [Azilect]	0.5-, 1-mg tablets	Monotherapy: usual dosage is 1 mg once daily or 0.5 mg daily for mild hepatic impairment Adjunctive therapy with levodopa: 0.5 mg daily initially. Increase to 1 mg daily, if needed.	May be taken with or without food.
ANTIVIRAL AGENT			
Amantadine [generic]	Tablet: 100 mg Capsules: 100 mg Syrup: 10 mg/mL	100 mg twice daily initially. May increase to 400 mg/day in divided doses. Dosage for patients taking high doses of other drugs for PD: 100 mg/day initially. May increase to 200 mg/day in divided doses.	May be taken with or without food; however, food decreases GI upset.

Continued

TABLE 21.4 ▪ Preparation, Dosage, and Administration of Drugs for Parkinson Disease—cont'd

Drug	Preparation	Daily Dosage	Administration
CENTRALLY ACTING ANTICHOLINERGIC DRUGS			
Benztropine [Cogentin]	Tablet: 0.5, 1, 2 mg Solution for injection: 1 mg/mL in 2-mL vials	Initial: 0.5 to 1 mg at bedtime. May increase by 0.5 mg every 5 to 6 days to a maximum dose of 6 mg/day.	May be taken with or without food. IM injection is preferable because, for PD, IV injection doesn't provide an advantage.
Trihexyphenidyl [generic]	Tablet: 2, 5 mg Elixir: 0.4 mg/mL	Initial: 1 mg once daily. May increase by 2 mg every 3 to 5 days to a maximum dose of 15 mg/day.	May be taken with or without food.

ER, Extended release; *IR,* immediate release; *ODT,* orally disintegrating tablets; *PD,* Parkinson disease; *PEG-J tube,* percutaneous endoscopic gastrostomy; *subQ,* subcutaneous.

discomfort. Symptoms are usually more intense in the evening and often disrupt sleep. People with severe RLS experience sleep loss, daytime exhaustion, and diminished quality of life.

Pharmacokinetics. Pramipexole is rapidly absorbed, and plasma levels peak in 1 to 2 hours. Food reduces the speed of absorption but not the extent. Cimetidine (a drug for peptic ulcer disease) can inhibit renal excretion of pramipexole, thereby increasing its blood level.

Pramipexole undergoes wide distribution and achieves a high concentration in red blood cells. The drug is eliminated unchanged in the urine.

Adverse Effects and Interactions. Pramipexole can produce a variety of adverse effects, primarily by activating dopamine receptors. The most common effects seen when pramipexole is used *alone* are nausea, dizziness, daytime somnolence, insomnia, constipation, weakness, and hallucinations. When the drug is *combined with levodopa,* about half of patients experience orthostatic hypotension and dyskinesias, which are not seen when the drug is used by itself. In addition, the incidence of hallucinations nearly doubles.

A few patients have reported *sleep attacks* (overwhelming and irresistible sleepiness that comes on without warning). Sleep attacks can be a real danger for people who are driving. Sleep attacks should not be equated with the normal sleepiness that occurs with dopaminergic agents. Patients who experience a sleep attack should inform their prescriber.

Pramipexole has been associated with *impulse control disorders,* including compulsive gambling, shopping, binge eating, and hypersexuality. These behaviors are dose related, begin about 9 months after starting pramipexole, and reverse when the drug is discontinued. Risk factors include younger adulthood, a family or personal history of alcohol abuse, and a personality trait called novelty seeking, characterized by impulsivity, a quick temper, and a low threshold for boredom. Before prescribing pramipexole, clinicians should screen patients for compulsive behaviors.

Preparations and Administration. Pramipexole is available in immediate release tablets sold as Mirapex, and in ER tablets sold as Mirapex XR. Dosing may be done with food to reduce nausea. To minimize adverse effects, dosage should be low initially and then gradually increased.

Dosage for Parkinson Disease. With the immediate-release tablets, dosage is 0.125 mg 3 times/day initially, and then increased over 7 weeks to a maximum of 1.5 mg 3 times/day. With the extended-release tablets, dosage is 0.375 mg once daily initially, and then gradually increased to a maximum of 4.5 mg once daily. With both formulations, dosage should be reduced in patients with significant renal impairment.

Dosage for Restless Legs Syndrome. Dosing is done once daily, 2 to 3 hours before bedtime, using the immediate-release tablets. The daily dosage is 0.125 mg initially, and can be gradually increased to a maximum of 0.5 mg.

Ropinirole

Actions, Uses, and Adverse Effects. Ropinirole [Requip], a nonergot dopamine agonist, is similar to pramipexole with respect to receptor specificity, mechanism of action, indications, and adverse effects. Like pramipexole, ropinirole is highly selective for D_2 and D_3 receptors, and both drugs share the same indications: PD and RLS. In patients with PD, ropinirole can be used as monotherapy (in early PD) and as an adjunct to levodopa (in advanced PD). In contrast to pramipexole, which is eliminated entirely by renal excretion, ropinirole is eliminated by hepatic metabolism. Some adverse effects are more common than with pramipexole. When ropinirole is used alone, the most common effects are nausea, dizziness, somnolence, and hallucinations. Rarely, sleep attacks occur. When ropinirole is combined with levodopa, the most important side effects are dyskinesias, hallucinations, and postural hypotension. Note that these occur less frequently than when pramipexole is combined with levodopa. Like pramipexole, ropinirole can promote compulsive gambling, shopping, eating, and hypersexuality. Animal tests indicate that ropinirole can harm the developing fetus. Accordingly, the drug should not be used during pregnancy.

Rotigotine

Actions and Uses. Rotigotine [Neupro] is a nonergot dopamine agonist that is specific for selected dopamine receptors. Although the exact mechanism of action is unknown, it is believed that rotigotine improves dopamine transmission by activating postsynaptic dopamine receptors in the substantia nigra. Rotigotine is approved for management of PD from early to advanced stages. It is also approved for management of moderate to severe primary RLS.

Pharmacokinetics. Because first-pass metabolism of rotigotine is extensive, oral formulations are not manufactured. Rotigotine is currently available as a transdermal patch. The time from application to peak is typically 15 to 18 hours but may range from 4 to 27 hours. Approximately 90% of the drug is protein bound. Rotigotine has a half-life of approximately 5 to 7 hours after patch removal. Excretion occurs in both urine (>70%) and feces.

Adverse Effects. The most common adverse effects are associated with the CNS and neuromuscular systems. These include a variety of sleep disorders, dizziness, headache, dose-related hallucinations, and dose-related dyskinesia. Orthostatic hypotension and peripheral edema may occur. Nausea and vomiting are common, especially when beginning the drug. Some patients develop skin reactions at the site of application, and hyperhidrosis (excessive perspiration) may occur.

Apomorphine

Actions and Therapeutic Use. Apomorphine [Apokyn] is a nonergot dopamine agonist approved for acute treatment of hypomobility during off episodes in patients with advanced PD. Unlike other dopamine agonists, the drug is not given by mouth (PO), and is not indicated for routine PD management. When tested in patients experiencing at least 2 hours of off time a day, apomorphine produced a 62% improvement in PD rating scores, compared with no improvement in patients receiving placebo. Benefits were sustained during 4 weeks of use. Apomorphine is a derivative of morphine, but is devoid of typical opioid effects (e.g., analgesia, euphoria, respiratory depression).

Pharmacokinetics. Apomorphine is highly lipophilic but undergoes extensive first-pass metabolism, and hence is ineffective when taken orally. After subcutaneous (subQ) injection, the drug undergoes rapid, complete absorption. Effects begin in 10 to 20 minutes and persist about 1 hour. The drug's half-life is about 40 minutes.

Adverse Effects. The most common adverse effects are injection-site reactions, hallucinations, yawning, drowsiness, dyskinesias, rhinorrhea, and nausea and vomiting. During clinical trials, there was a 4% incidence of serious cardiovascular events: angina, myocardial infarction, cardiac arrest, and/or sudden death. Postural hypotension and fainting occurred in 2% of patients. Like other dopamine agonists, apomorphine poses a risk for daytime sleep attacks. In addition, apomorphine can promote hypersexuality and enhanced erections (the drug is used in Europe to treat erectile dysfunction). Rarely, apomorphine causes priapism (sustained, painful erection), possibly requiring surgical intervention.

Combined Use With an Antiemetic. To prevent nausea and vomiting during clinical trials, nearly all patients were treated with an antiemetic, starting 3 days before the first dose of apomorphine. The antiemetic chosen was trimethobenzamide [Tigan, others]. Two classes of antiemetics cannot be used: serotonin receptor antagonists (e.g., ondansetron [Zofran]) and dopamine receptor antagonists (e.g., prochlorperazine [Compazine]). Serotonin receptor antagonists will increase the risk for postural hypotension while having no effect on the nausea, and dopamine receptor antagonists will decrease the effectiveness of apomorphine and most other drugs for PD. About half the trial participants discontinued the antiemetic at some point but continued taking apomorphine.

Ergot Derivatives: Bromocriptine and Cabergoline

Two ergot derivatives—bromocriptine and cabergoline—are used to manage PD. Bromocriptine is approved for PD; cabergoline is not. These drugs are poorly tolerated, so their use is limited. The side effect profile of the ergot derivatives differs from that of the nonergot agents because, in addition to activating dopamine receptors, the ergot drugs cause mild blockade of serotonergic and alpha-adrenergic receptors.

Bromocriptine. Bromocriptine [Cycloset, Parlodel], a derivative of ergot, is a direct-acting dopamine agonist. Beneficial effects derive from activating dopamine receptors in the striatum. Responses are equivalent to those seen with pramipexole and ropinirole. Bromocriptine is used alone in early PD and in combination with levodopa in advanced PD. When combined with levodopa, bromocriptine can prolong therapeutic responses and reduce motor fluctuations. In addition, because bromocriptine allows the dosage of levodopa to be reduced, the incidence of levodopa-induced dyskinesias may be reduced too.

Adverse effects are dose dependent and are seen in 30% to 50% of patients. Nausea is most common. The most common dose-limiting effects are psychological reactions (confusion, nightmares, agitation, hallucinations, paranoid delusions). These occur in about 30% of patients and are most likely when the dosage is high. Like levodopa, bromocriptine can cause dyskinesias and postural hypotension. Rarely, bromocriptine causes retroperitoneal fibrosis, pulmonary infiltrates, a Raynaud-like phenomenon, and erythromelalgia (vasodilation in the feet, and sometimes hands, resulting in swelling, redness, warmth, and burning pain). In addition, the ergot derivatives have been associated with valvular heart disease. The probable cause is activation of serotonin receptors on heart valves.

Bromocriptine is available in 5-mg capsules [Parlodel] and 2.5-mg tablets [Parlodel SnapTabs]. The initial dosage is 1.25 mg twice daily, administered with meals. Dosage is gradually increased until the desired response has been achieved, or until side effects become intolerable. Maintenance dosages range from 30 to 100 mg/day.

Cabergoline. Cabergoline, a drug approved for treatment of hyperprolactinemic disorders, is used occasionally in PD, although it is not approved by the U.S. Food and Drug Administration (FDA) for this disorder. According to the AAN guidelines, the drug is "possibly effective" for improving off times during levodopa therapy; however, the supporting evidence is weak. Consequently, cabergoline is rarely used unless other management attempts have failed. Common side effects are headaches, dizziness, nausea, and weakness. A more concerning adverse effect is the development of cardiac valve regurgitation and subsequent development of heart failure. Pulmonary and pericardial fibrosis have also occurred. The pharmacology of cabergoline, as well as its use in hyperprolactinemia, is discussed in Chapter 63.

Catechol-*O*-Methyltransferase Inhibitors

Two COMT inhibitors are available: entacapone and tolcapone. With both drugs, benefits derive from inhibiting metabolism of levodopa in the periphery; these drugs have no direct therapeutic effects of their own. Entacapone is safer and more effective than tolcapone, and hence is preferred.

Entacapone

Actions and Therapeutic Use. Entacapone [Comtan] is a selective, reversible inhibitor of COMT indicated only for use with levodopa. Like carbidopa, entacapone inhibits metabolism of levodopa in the intestine and peripheral tissues. However, the drugs inhibit different enzymes: carbidopa inhibits decarboxylases, whereas entacapone inhibits COMT. By inhibiting COMT, entacapone prolongs the plasma half-life of levodopa, and thereby prolongs the time that levodopa is available to the brain. In addition, entacapone increases levodopa availability by a second mechanism: By inhibiting COMT, entacapone decreases production of levodopa metabolites that compete with levodopa for transport across the blood-brain barrier. In clinical trials, entacapone increased the half-life of levodopa by 50% to 75%, and thereby caused levodopa blood levels to be more stable and sustained. As a result, entacapone is especially beneficial for patients who experience a wearing off of the effects of levodopa/carbidopa. Entacapone may also permit a reduction in levodopa dosage.

Pharmacokinetics. Entacapone is rapidly absorbed and reaches peak levels in 2 hours. Elimination is by hepatic metabolism followed by excretion in the feces and urine. The plasma half-life is 1.5 to 3.5 hours.

Adverse Effects. Most adverse effects result from increasing levodopa levels, though some are caused by entacapone itself. By increasing levodopa levels, entacapone can cause dyskinesias, orthostatic hypotension, nausea, hallucinations, sleep disturbances, and impulse control disorders (see *Pramipexole*). These can be managed by decreasing levodopa dosage. Entacopone should not be stopped abruptly, though. Doing so can result in a significant worsening of symptoms.

Entacapone itself is responsible for fewer adverse effects. The most common are vomiting, diarrhea, constipation, and yellow-orange discoloration of the urine.

Drug Interactions. Because it inhibits COMT, entacapone can, in theory, increase levels of other drugs metabolized by COMT. These include methyldopa (an antihypertensive agent), dobutamine (an adrenergic agonist), and isoproterenol (a beta-adrenergic agonist). If entacapone is combined with these drugs, a reduction in their dosages may be needed.

Preparations, Dosage, and Administration. Entacapone [Comtan] is available in 200-mg tablets. The recommended dosage is 200 mg taken with each dose of levodopa/carbidopa—to a maximum of 8 doses (1600 mg) a day. It is also available in fixed-dose combinations with levodopa/carbidopa under the brand name Stalevo (see *Levodopa/Carbidopa/Entacapone*).

Tolcapone

Actions and Therapeutic Use. Tolcapone [Tasmar] is a COMT inhibitor used only in conjunction with levodopa—and only if safer agents are ineffective or inappropriate. As with entacapone, benefits derive from inhibiting levodopa metabolism in the periphery, which prolongs levodopa availability. When given to patients taking levodopa, tolcapone improves motor function and may allow a reduction in levodopa dosage. When given to reduce the wearing-off effect that can occur with levodopa, it can extend levodopa on times by as much as 2.9 hours a day. Unfortunately, although tolcapone is effective, it is also potentially dangerous. Deaths from liver failure have occurred. Because it carries a serious risk, tolcapone should be reserved for patients who cannot be treated, or treated adequately, with safer drugs. When tolcapone is used, treatment should be limited to 3 weeks in the absence of a beneficial response.

Pharmacokinetics. Tolcapone is well absorbed after oral dosing. Plasma levels peak in 2 hours. In the blood, tolcapone is highly bound (>99.9%) to plasma proteins. The drug undergoes extensive hepatic metabolism followed by renal excretion. The plasma half-life is 2 to 3 hours.

Adverse Effects

Liver Failure. Tolcapone can cause severe hepatocellular injury, which is sometimes fatal. Before treatment, patients should be fully apprised of the risks. They also should be informed about signs of emergent liver dysfunction (persistent nausea, fatigue, lethargy, anorexia, jaundice, dark urine) and instructed to report these immediately. Patients with preexisting liver dysfunction should not take the drug. If liver injury is diagnosed, tolcapone should be discontinued and never used again.

Laboratory monitoring of liver enzymes is required. Tests for serum alanine aminotransferase (ALT) and aspartate aminotransferase (AST) should be conducted before treatment and then throughout treatment as follows: every 2 weeks for the first year, every 4 weeks for the next 6 months, and every 8 weeks thereafter. If ALT or AST levels exceed the upper limit of normal, tolcapone should be discontinued. Monitoring may not prevent liver injury, but early detection and immediate drug withdrawal can minimize harm.

Other Adverse Effects. By increasing the availability of levodopa, tolcapone can intensify levodopa-related effects, especially dyskinesias, orthostatic hypotension, nausea, hallucinations, sleep disturbances, and impulse control disorders (see *Pramipexole*); a reduction in levodopa dosage may be required. Tolcapone itself can cause diarrhea, hematuria, and yellow-orange discoloration of the urine. Abrupt withdrawal of tolcapone can produce symptoms that resemble neuroleptic malignant syndrome (fever, muscular rigidity, altered consciousness). In rats, large doses have caused renal tubular necrosis and tumors of the kidneys and uterus.

Levodopa/Carbidopa/Entacapone

Levodopa, carbidopa, and entacapone are now available in fixed-dose combinations sold as *Stalevo*. As discussed previously, both carbidopa and entacapone inhibit the enzymatic degradation of levodopa, and thereby enhance therapeutic effects. The triple combination is more convenient than taking levodopa/carbidopa and entacapone separately, and it costs a little less, too. Unfortunately, Stalevo is available only in immediate-release tablets. Patients who need more flexibility in their regimen cannot be treated with Stalevo, nor can patients who require a sustained-release formulation.

MAO-B Inhibitors

The MAO-B inhibitors—selegiline and rasagiline—are considered first-line drugs for PD even though benefits are modest. When combined with levodopa, they can reduce the wearing-off effect.

Selegiline

Selegiline [Eldepryl, Zelapar], also known as *deprenyl,* was the first MAO inhibitor approved for PD. The drug may be used alone or in combination with levodopa. In both cases, improvement of motor function is modest. There is some evidence suggesting that selegiline may delay neurodegeneration, and hence may delay disease progression. However, conclusive proof of neuroprotection is lacking. Nonetheless, current guidelines suggest trying selegiline in newly diagnosed patients, just in case the drug *does* confer some protection.

Actions and Use. Selegiline causes *selective, irreversible* inhibition of MAO-B, the enzyme that inactivates dopamine in the striatum. Another form of MAO, known as monoamine oxidase-A (MAO-A), inactivates NE and serotonin. As discussed in Chapter 32, nonselective inhibitors of MAO (i.e., drugs that inhibit MAO-A *and* MAO-B) are used to treat depression—and pose a risk for hypertensive crisis as a side effect. Because selegiline is a selective inhibitor of MAO-B, the drug is not an antidepressant and *at recommended doses* poses little or no risk for hypertensive crisis.

Selegiline appears to benefit patients with PD in two ways. First, when used as an adjunct to levodopa, selegiline can suppress destruction of dopamine derived from levodopa. The mechanism is inhibition of MAO-B. By helping preserve dopamine, selegiline can prolong the effects of levodopa, and can thereby decrease fluctuations in motor control. Unfortunately, these benefits decline dramatically within 12 to 24 months.

In addition to preserving dopamine, there is some hope that selegiline may delay the progression of PD. When used early in the disease, selegiline can delay the need for levodopa. This may reflect a delay in the progression of the disease, or it may simply reflect direct symptomatic relief from selegiline itself.

If selegiline does slow the progression of PD, what might be the mechanism? In experimental animals, selegiline can prevent development of parkinsonism after exposure to 1-methyl-4-phenyl-1,2,3,6-tetrahydropyridine (MPTP), a neurotoxin that causes selective degeneration of dopaminergic neurons. (Humans accidentally exposed to MPTP develop severe parkinsonism.) Neuronal degeneration is not caused by MPTP itself, but rather by a toxic metabolite. Formation of this metabolite is catalyzed by MAO-B. By inhibiting MAO-B, selegiline prevents formation of the toxic metabolite and thereby protects against neuronal injury. If selegiline delays progression of PD, this mechanism could explain the effect. That is, just as selegiline protects animals by suppressing formation of a neurotoxic metabolite of MPTP, the drug may delay progression of PD by suppressing formation of a neurotoxic metabolite of an as-yet-unidentified compound.

Pharmacokinetics. For treatment of PD, selegiline is available in two oral formulations (tablets and capsules) and in orally disintegrating tablets (ODTs).

Tablets and Capsules. Selegiline in tablets (generic only) and capsules [Eldepryl] undergoes rapid GI absorption, travels to the brain, and quickly penetrates the blood-brain barrier. Irreversible inhibition of MAO-B follows. Selegiline undergoes hepatic metabolism followed by renal excretion. Two metabolites—*l-amphetamine* and *l-methamphetamine*—are CNS stimulants. These metabolites, which do not appear to have therapeutic effects, can be harmful. Because selegiline causes irreversible inhibition of MAO-B, effects persist until more MAO-B can be synthesized.

Orally Disintegrating Tablets. Unlike selegiline in tablets and capsules, which is absorbed from the GI tract, selegiline in ODTs [Zelapar] is absorbed through the oral mucosa. As a result, bioavailability is higher than with tablets and capsules, and hence doses can be lower. Otherwise, the pharmacokinetics of selegiline in ODTs, tablets, and capsules are identical.

Adverse Effects. When selegiline is used alone, the principal adverse effect is insomnia, presumably because of CNS excitation by amphetamine and methamphetamine. Insomnia can be minimized by administering the last daily dose no later than noon. Other adverse effects include orthostatic hypotension, dizziness, and GI symptoms. Patients taking selegiline ODTs may experience irritation of the buccal mucosa.

Hypertensive Crisis. Although selegiline is selective for MAO-B, high doses can inhibit MAO-A, which creates a risk for hypertensive crisis, especially in younger patients. As discussed in Chapter 32, when a patient is taking an MAO inhibitor, hypertensive crisis can be triggered by ingesting foods that contain tyramine and by taking certain drugs, including sympathomimetics. Accordingly, patients should be instructed to avoid these foods and drugs, both while taking selegiline and for 2 weeks after stopping it.

Drug Interactions

Levodopa. When used with levodopa, selegiline can intensify adverse responses to levodopa-derived dopamine. These reactions—orthostatic hypotension, dyskinesias, and psychological disturbances (hallucinations, confusion)—can be reduced by decreasing the dosage of levodopa.

Meperidine. Like the nonselective MAO inhibitors, selegiline can cause a dangerous interaction with meperidine [Demerol]. Symptoms include stupor, rigidity, agitation, and hyperthermia. The combination should be avoided.

Selective Serotonin Reuptake Inhibitors (SSRIs). Selegiline should not be combined with SSRIs such as fluoxetine [Prozac]. The combination of an MAO-B inhibitor plus an SSRI can cause fatal serotonin syndrome. Accordingly, SSRIs should be withdrawn at least 5 weeks before giving selegiline.

Preparations, Dosage, and Administration

Tablets and Capsules. Selegiline is available in 5-mg tablets [generic only] and capsules sold as Eldepryl. For treatment of PD, the usual dosage is 5 mg taken with breakfast and lunch, for a total of 10 mg a day. This dosage produces complete inhibition of MAO-B, and hence larger doses are unnecessary.

Orally Disintegrating Tablets. Selegiline is available in 1.25-mg ODTs sold as *Zelapar*. For patients with PD, treatment begins with 1.25 mg once a day for 6 weeks. If needed and tolerated, the dosage can then be raised to 2.5 mg once a day. Note that the maximum daily dose (2.5 mg) is 4 times lower than the maximum daily dose with tablets and capsules. Dosing should be done in the morning before breakfast, without liquid. Tablets are placed on the tongue, where they dissolve in seconds. Selegiline is then absorbed through the oral mucosa.

Transdermal System. Selegiline is also available in a transdermal system, marketed as *Emsam*, for treatment of major depressive disorder. Transdermal selegiline is not used for PD.

Rasagiline

Actions and Therapeutic Use. Rasagiline [Azilect] is another MAO-B inhibitor for PD. Like selegiline, rasagiline is a selective, irreversible inhibitor of MAO-B. Benefits derive from preserving dopamine in the brain. The drug is approved for initial monotherapy of PD and for combined use with levodopa. Rasagiline is similar to selegiline in most regards. As with selegiline, benefits are modest. The drugs differ primarily in that rasagiline is not converted to amphetamine or methamphetamine.

Pharmacokinetics. Rasagiline is rapidly absorbed, with a bioavailability of 36%. In the liver, the drug undergoes nearly complete metabolism by CYP1A2 (the 1A2 isoenzyme of cytochrome P450). Hepatic impairment and drugs that inhibit CYP1A2 will delay metabolism of rasagiline, causing blood levels of the drug to rise. The drug should be decreased by half in mild hepatic impairment. *Patients with moderate to severe hepatic impairment should not use this drug.*

In contrast to selegiline, rasagiline is not metabolized to amphetamine derivatives. Excretion is primarily via the urine (62%) and feces (7%). The plasma half-life is 3 hours. However, because rasagiline causes irreversible inhibition of MAO-B, clinical effects persist until new MAO-B is synthesized.

Adverse Effects. When used as monotherapy, rasagiline is generally well tolerated. The most common side effects are headache, arthralgia, dyspepsia, depression, and flu-like symptoms. Unlike selegiline, rasagiline does not cause insomnia.

When rasagiline is combined with levodopa, side effects increase. The most common additional reactions are dyskinesias, accidental injury, nausea, orthostatic hypotension, constipation, weight loss, and hallucinations.

Like selegiline, rasagiline may pose a risk for hypertensive crisis (owing to inhibition of MAO-A, especially at higher doses), and hence patients should be instructed to avoid tyramine-containing foods and certain drugs, including sympathomimetic agents.

Rasagiline may increase the risk for malignant melanoma, a potentially deadly cancer of the skin. Periodic monitoring of the skin is recommended.

Drug and Food Interactions. Rasagiline has the potential to interact adversely with multiple drugs. Drugs that should be used with *caution* include:

- Levodopa. Like selegiline, rasagiline can intensify adverse responses to levodopa-derived dopamine. If the patient develops dopaminergic side effects, including dyskinesias or hallucinations, reducing the dosage of levodopa, not rasagiline, should be considered.
- CYP1A2 inhibitors. Blood levels of rasagiline can be raised by ciprofloxacin and other drugs that inhibit CYP1A2, the hepatic enzyme that inactivates rasagiline. For patients taking these drugs, the daily dosage should be reduced.

Drugs and foods that are *contraindicated* include:

- MAO inhibitors. Combining rasagiline with another MAO inhibitor increases the risk of hypertensive crisis. At least 2 weeks should separate the use of these drugs.
- Sympathomimetics. These drugs (e.g., amphetamines, ephedrine, phenylephrine, pseudoephedrine) increase the risk of hypertensive crisis and must be avoided.
- Tyramine-containing foods. These foods increase the risk for hypertensive crisis and must be avoided.
- Antidepressants. Combining rasagiline with mirtazapine, SSRIs, serotonin/norepinephrine reuptake inhibitors, and tricyclic antidepressants may pose a risk for hyperpyrexia and death. These drugs should be discontinued at least 2 weeks before starting rasagiline. Fluoxetine (an SSRI) should be discontinued at least 5 weeks before starting rasagiline.
- Analgesics. Combining rasagiline with meperidine, methadone, or tramadol may pose a risk for serious reactions, including coma, respiratory depression, convulsions, hypertension, hypotension, and even death. At least 2 weeks should separate the use of these drugs.
- Dextromethorphan. Combining rasagiline with dextromethorphan may pose a risk for brief episodes of psychosis and bizarre behavior.
- Cyclobenzaprine. This drug is structurally related to the tricyclic antidepressants, so it should be avoided.

Amantadine

Actions and Uses

Amantadine (generic), formerly available as *Symmetrel,* was developed as an antiviral agent (see Chapter 93), and was later found effective in PD. Possible mechanisms include inhibition of dopamine uptake, stimulation of dopamine release, blockade of cholinergic receptors, antagonism of *N*-methyl-D-aspartate (NMDA) receptors, and blockade of glutamate receptors. Responses develop rapidly—often within 2 to 3 days—but are much less profound than with levodopa or the dopamine agonists. Furthermore, responses may begin to diminish within 3 to 6 months. Accordingly, amantadine is not considered a first-line agent. However, the drug may be helpful for managing dyskinesias caused by levodopa.

Adverse Effects

Amantadine can cause adverse CNS effects (confusion, light-headedness, anxiety) and peripheral effects that are thought to result from muscarinic blockade (blurred vision, urinary retention, dry mouth, constipation). All of these are generally mild when amantadine is used alone. However, if amantadine is combined with an anticholinergic agent, both the CNS and peripheral responses will be intensified.

Patients taking amantadine for 1 month or longer often develop *livedo reticularis,* a condition characterized by mottled discoloration of the skin. Livedo reticularis is benign and gradually subsides after amantadine withdrawal.

Preparations, Dosage, and Administration

Amantadine is supplied in 100-mg tablets and capsules and in a syrup (10 mg/mL). The usual dosage is 100 mg twice daily, which may be increased to 400 mg/day in divided doses. If the patient is taking high doses of other drugs for PD, the recommended starting dose of amantadine is 100 mg/day with subsequent increases up to 200 mg in divided doses. Because amantadine is eliminated primarily by the kidneys, dosage must be reduced in patients with renal impairment.

Amantadine often loses effectiveness after several months. If effects diminish, they can be restored by increasing the dosage or by interrupting treatment for several weeks.

Centrally Acting Anticholinergic Drugs

Anticholinergic drugs have been used in PD since 1867, making them the oldest medicines for this disease. These drugs alleviate symptoms by blocking muscarinic receptors in the striatum, thereby improving the balance between dopamine and acetylcholine. Anticholinergic drugs can reduce tremor and possibly rigidity, but not bradykinesia. These drugs are less effective than levodopa or the dopamine agonists but are better tolerated. Today, anticholinergics are used as second-line therapy for tremor. They are most appropriate for younger patients with mild symptoms. Anticholinergics are generally avoided in older patients, who are intolerant of CNS side effects (sedation, confusion, delusions, and hallucinations).

Safety Alert

BEERS CRITERIA

Anticholinergic drugs have been designated as potentially inappropriate for use in geriatric patients. The anticholinergics most commonly prescribed for management of Parkinson disease are benztropine [Cogentin] and trihexyphenidyl.

Although the anticholinergic drugs used today are somewhat selective for cholinergic receptors in the CNS, they can also block cholinergic receptors in the periphery. As a result, they can cause dry mouth, blurred vision, photophobia, urinary retention, constipation, and tachycardia. These effects are usually dose limiting. Blockade of cholinergic receptors in the eye may precipitate or aggravate glaucoma. Accordingly, intraocular pressure should be measured periodically. Peripheral anticholinergic effects are discussed in Chapter 14.

The anticholinergic agents used most often are *benztropine* [Cogentin] and *trihexyphenidyl,* formerly available as *Artane.* Doses are low initially and then gradually increased, until the desired response is achieved or until side effects become intolerable. For trihexyphenidyl, the initial dosage is 1 mg once a day. This may be increased by 2 mg every 3 to 5 days up to a maximum of 15 mg/day. For benztropine, the initial dosage is 0.5 to 1 mg at bedtime. This may be increased by 0.5 mg every 5 to 6 days up to a maximum dose of 6 mg/day. If anticholinergic drugs are discontinued abruptly, symptoms of parkinsonism may be intensified.

NONMOTOR SYMPTOMS AND THEIR MANAGEMENT

In addition to experiencing characteristic motor symptoms, about 90% of patients with PD develop nonmotor symptoms, notably autonomic disturbances, sleep disturbances, depression, dementia, and psychosis. Management is addressed in two evidence-based AAN guidelines: *Practice Parameter: Evaluation and Treatment of Depression, Psychosis, and Dementia in Parkinson Disease* and *Practice Parameter: Treatment of Nonmotor Symptoms of Parkinson Disease*.

Autonomic Symptoms

Disruption of autonomic function can produce a variety of symptoms, including constipation, urinary incontinence, drooling, orthostatic hypotension, cold intolerance, and erectile dysfunction. The intensity of these symptoms increases in parallel with the intensity of motor symptoms. Erectile function can be managed with sildenafil [Viagra] and other inhibitors of type 5 phosphodiesterase (see Chapter 66). Orthostatic hypotension can be improved by increasing intake of salt and fluid, and possibly by taking fludrocortisone, a mineralocorticoid (see Chapter 60). Urinary incontinence may improve with oxybutynin and other peripherally acting anticholinergic drugs (see Chapter 14). Constipation can be managed by getting regular exercise and maintaining adequate intake of fluid and fiber. Polyethylene glycol (an osmotic laxative) or a stool softener (e.g., docusate) may also be tried (see Chapter 79).

Sleep Disturbances

PD is associated with *excessive daytime sleepiness* (EDS), *periodic limb movements of sleep* (PLMS), and *insomnia* (difficulty falling asleep and staying asleep). EDS may respond to modafinil [Provigil, Alertec 🍁], a nonamphetamine CNS stimulant (see Chapter 36). For PLMS, levodopa/carbidopa should be considered; the nonergot dopamine agonists—pramipexole and ropinirole—may also help. Insomnia may be improved by levodopa/carbidopa and melatonin (see Chapter 34). Levodopa/carbidopa helps by reducing motor symptoms that can impair sleep. Melatonin helps by making people feel they are sleeping better, even though objective measures of sleep quality may not improve.

Depression

About 50% of PD patients develop depression, partly in reaction to having a debilitating disease and partly due to the disease process itself. According to the AAN guidelines, only one drug—*amitriptyline*—has been proved effective in these patients. Unfortunately, amitriptyline, a tricyclic antidepressant, has anticholinergic effects that can exacerbate dementia, and antiadrenergic effects that can exacerbate orthostatic hypotension. Data for other antidepressants, including SSRIs and bupropion, are insufficient to prove or disprove efficacy in PD.

Dementia

Dementia occurs in 40% of PD patients. The AAN guidelines recommend considering treatment with two drugs: *donepezil* and *rivastigmine*. Both drugs are cholinesterase inhibitors developed for Alzheimer's disease (see Chapter 22). In patients with PD, these drugs can produce a modest improvement in cognitive function, without causing significant worsening of motor symptoms, even though these drugs increase availability of acetylcholine at central synapses.

Psychosis

In patients with PD, psychosis is usually caused by the drugs taken to control motor symptoms. Most of these drugs—levodopa, dopamine agonists, amantadine, and anticholinergic drugs—can cause hallucinations. Therefore, if psychosis develops, dopamine agonists, amantadine, and anticholinergic drugs should be withdrawn, and the dosage of levodopa should be reduced to the lowest effective amount. If antipsychotic medication is needed, *first-generation* antipsychotics should be *avoided* because all of these drugs block receptors for dopamine, and hence can intensify motor symptoms. Accordingly, the AAN guidelines recommend considering two second-generation antipsychotics: *clozapine* and *quetiapine*. Because clozapine can cause agranulocytosis, many clinicians prefer quetiapine. The guidelines recommend against routine use of olanzapine, another second-generation agent. The antipsychotic drugs are discussed in Chapter 31.

KEY POINTS

- PD is a neurodegenerative disorder that produces characteristic motor symptoms: tremor at rest, rigidity, postural instability, and bradykinesia.
- In addition to motor symptoms, PD can cause nonmotor symptoms, including autonomic dysfunction, sleep disturbances, depression, psychosis, and dementia.
- The primary pathology in PD is degeneration of neurons in the substantia nigra that supply dopamine to the striatum. The result is an imbalance between dopamine and acetylcholine.
- Motor symptoms are treated primarily with drugs that directly or indirectly activate dopamine receptors. Drugs that block cholinergic receptors can also be used.
- Levodopa (combined with carbidopa) is the most effective treatment for motor symptoms.
- Levodopa relieves motor symptoms by undergoing conversion to dopamine in surviving nerve terminals in the striatum.
- The enzyme that converts levodopa to dopamine is called a decarboxylase.
- Acute loss of response to levodopa occurs in two patterns: gradual wearing off, which develops at the end of the dosing interval, and abrupt loss of effect ("on-off" phenomenon), which can occur at any time during the dosing interval.
- The principal adverse effects of levodopa are nausea, dyskinesias, hypotension, and psychosis.
- First-generation antipsychotic drugs block dopamine receptors in the striatum, and can thereby negate the effects of levodopa. Two second-generation antipsychotics—clozapine and quetiapine—do not block dopamine receptors in the striatum, and hence can be used safely to treat levodopa-induced psychosis.
- Combining levodopa with a nonselective MAO inhibitor can result in hypertensive crisis.
- Because amino acids compete with levodopa for absorption from the intestine and for transport across the blood-brain barrier, high-protein meals can reduce therapeutic effects.
- Carbidopa enhances the effects of levodopa by preventing decarboxylation of levodopa in the intestine and peripheral tissues. Because carbidopa cannot cross the blood-brain barrier, it does not prevent conversion of levodopa to dopamine in the brain.
- Pramipexole, an oral nonergot dopamine agonist, is a first-line drug for motor symptoms. It can be used alone in early PD and combined with levodopa in advanced PD.

- Pramipexole and other dopamine agonists relieve motor symptoms by causing direct activation of dopamine receptors in the striatum.
- The major adverse effects of pramipexole—nausea, dyskinesia, postural hypotension, and hallucinations—result from excessive activation of dopamine receptors.
- Entacapone, a COMT inhibitor, is combined with levodopa to enhance levodopa's effects. The drug inhibits metabolism of levodopa by COMT in the intestine and peripheral tissues, thereby making more levodopa available to the brain.
- Selegiline and rasagiline enhance responses to levodopa by inhibiting MAO-B, the brain enzyme that inactivates dopamine.
- Anticholinergic drugs relieve symptoms of PD by blocking cholinergic receptors in the striatum.

Please visit **http://evolve.elsevier.com/Lehne** for chapter-specific NCLEX® examination review questions.

Summary of Major Nursing Implications[a]

LEVODOPA/CARBIDOPA [RYTARY, SINEMET, DUOPA]

Preadministration Assessment

Therapeutic Goal

The goal of treatment is to improve the patient's ability to carry out activities of daily living. Levodopa does not cure PD or delay its progression.

Baseline Data

Assess motor symptoms—bradykinesia, akinesia, postural instability, tremor, rigidity—and the extent to which they interfere with activities of daily living (e.g., ability to work, dress, bathe, walk).

Identifying High-Risk Patients

Because some studies suggest that levodopa and MAO inhibitors can activate malignant melanoma, for patients taking these drugs it is important to perform a careful skin assessment and to monitor the skin for changes.

Exercise *caution* in patients with cardiac disease and psychiatric disorders and in patients taking selective MAO-B inhibitors.

Implementation: Administration

Route

Oral.

Administration

Motor symptoms may make self-medication challenging. Assist the patient with dosing when needed. Patients may require assistive devices for opening medication containers at home. Ask the pharmacist to avoid using childproof containers that can be challenging to open. If appropriate, involve family members in medicating outpatients. **Inform patients that levodopa may be taken with food to reduce nausea and vomiting. However, high-protein meals should be avoided.**

So that expectations may be realistic, **inform patients that benefits of levodopa may be delayed for weeks to months.** This knowledge will facilitate adherence.

Ongoing Evaluation and Interventions

Evaluating Therapeutic Effects

Evaluate for improvements in activities of daily living and for reductions in bradykinesia, postural instability, tremor, and rigidity.

Managing Acute Loss of Effect

Off times can be reduced by combining levodopa/carbidopa with a dopamine agonist (e.g., pramipexole), a COMT inhibitor (e.g., entacapone), or an MAO-B inhibitor (e.g., rasagiline). **Forewarn patients about possible abrupt loss of therapeutic effects, and instruct them to notify the prescriber if this occurs. Avoiding high-protein meals may help.**

Minimizing Adverse Effects

Nausea and Vomiting. **Inform patients that nausea and vomiting can be reduced by taking levodopa with food. Instruct patients to notify the prescriber if nausea and vomiting persist or become severe.**

Dyskinesias. **Inform patients about possible levodopa-induced movement disorders (tremor, dystonic movements, twitching) and instruct them to notify the prescriber if these develop.** Giving amantadine may help.

If the hospitalized patient develops dyskinesias, withhold levodopa and consult the prescriber about a possible reduction in dosage.

Dysrhythmias. **Inform patients about signs of excessive cardiac stimulation (palpitations, tachycardia, irregular heartbeat) and instruct them to notify the prescriber if these occur.**

Orthostatic Hypotension. **Inform patients about symptoms of hypotension (dizziness, light-headedness) and advise them to sit or lie down if these occur. Advise patients to move slowly when sitting up or standing up.**

Psychosis. **Inform patients about possible levodopa-induced psychosis (visual hallucinations, vivid dreams, paranoia), and instruct them to notify the prescriber if these develop. Treatment with clozapine or quetiapine can help.**

Minimizing Adverse Interactions

First-Generation Antipsychotic Drugs. These can block responses to levodopa and should be avoided. Two

Continued

Summary of Major Nursing Implications[a]—cont'd

second-generation antipsychotics—clozapine and quetiapine—can be used safely.

MAO Inhibitors. Concurrent use of levodopa and a nonselective MAO inhibitor can produce severe hypertension. Withdraw nonselective MAO inhibitors at least 2 weeks before initiating levodopa.

Anticholinergic Drugs. These can enhance therapeutic responses to levodopa, but they also increase the risk of adverse psychiatric effects.

High-Protein Meals. Amino acids compete with levodopa for absorption from the intestine and for transport across the blood-brain barrier. **Instruct patients not to take levodopa/carbidopa with a high-protein meal.**

DOPAMINE AGONISTS

Apomorphine
Bromocriptine
Cabergoline
Pramipexole
Ropinirole
Rotigotine

Preadministration Assessment

Therapeutic Goal

The goal of treatment is to improve the patient's ability to carry out activities of daily living. Dopamine agonists do not cure PD or delay its progression.

Apomorphine is reserved for rescue treatment of hypomobility during off episodes in patients with advanced PD.

Baseline Data

Assess motor symptoms—bradykinesia, akinesia, postural instability, tremor, rigidity—and the extent to which these interfere with activities of daily living (e.g., ability to work, dress, bathe, walk).

Identifying High-Risk Patients

Use *all dopamine agonists* with *caution* in older adult patients and in those with psychiatric disorders. Use *pramipexole* with *caution* in patients with kidney dysfunction. Avoid *ropinirole* during pregnancy. Use *pramipexole* and *ropinirole* with *caution* in patients prone to compulsive behavior.

Implementation: Administration

Route

Oral. Cabergoline, bromocriptine, pramipexole, ropinirole.

Subcutaneous. Apomorphine.

Transdermal. Rotigotine.

Administration

Parkinsonism may make self-medication impossible. Assist the patient with dosing when needed. Assistive devices may be needed for home use. If appropriate, involve family members in medicating outpatients.

Inform patients that oral dopamine agonists may be taken with food to reduce nausea and vomiting.

To minimize adverse effects, dosage should be low initially and then gradually increased.

Reduce dosage of pramipexole in patients with significant renal dysfunction.

Ongoing Evaluation and Interventions

Evaluating Therapeutic Effects

Evaluate for improvements in activities of daily living and for reductions in bradykinesia, postural instability, tremor, and rigidity.

Minimizing Adverse Effects

Nausea and Vomiting. **Inform patients that nausea and vomiting can be reduced by taking oral dopamine agonists with food. Instruct patients to notify the prescriber if nausea and vomiting persist or become severe. Instruct patients taking apomorphine to pretreat with trimethobenzamide [Tigan], an antiemetic.**

Orthostatic Hypotension. **Inform patients about symptoms of orthostatic hypotension (dizziness, light-headedness on standing) and advise them to sit or lie down if these occur. Advise patients to move slowly when sitting up or standing up.**

Dyskinesias. **Inform patients about possible movement disorders (tremor, dystonic movements, twitching), and instruct them to notify the prescriber if these develop.**

Hallucinations. **Forewarn patients that dopamine agonists can cause hallucinations, especially in older adults, and instruct them to notify the prescriber if these develop.**

Sleep Attacks. **Warn patients that pramipexole, ropinirole, rotigotine, and apomorphine may cause sleep attacks. Instruct patients that if a sleep attack occurs, they should inform the prescriber and avoid potentially hazardous activities (e.g., driving).**

Fetal Injury. **Inform patients of childbearing age that ropinirole may harm the developing fetus, and advise them to use effective birth control.** If pregnancy occurs and will be continued, switching to a different dopamine agonist is advised.

Impulse Control Disorders. *Pramipexole* and *ropinirole* may induce *compulsive, self-rewarding behaviors,* including compulsive gambling, eating, shopping, and hypersexuality. Risk factors include relative youth, a family or personal history of alcohol abuse, and a novelty-seeking personality. Before prescribing these drugs, clinicians should screen patient for compulsive behaviors.

[a]Patient education information is highlighted as **blue text.**

CHAPTER

22 Drugs for Alzheimer's Disease

Alzheimer's disease (AD) is a devastating illness characterized by progressive memory loss, impaired thinking, neuropsychiatric symptoms (e.g., hallucinations, delusions), and inability to perform routine tasks of daily living. More than 5 million older Americans have AD. It is the sixth leading cause of death, with an annual cost of about $226 billion. Major pathologic findings are cerebral atrophy, degeneration of cholinergic neurons, and the presence of neuritic plaques and neurofibrillary tangles—all of which begin to develop years before clinical symptoms appear. This neuronal damage is irreversible, so AD cannot be cured. Drugs in current use do little to relieve symptoms or prevent neuronal loss. Furthermore, for many patients there is no significant delay in the progression of AD or cognitive decline.

PATHOPHYSIOLOGY

The underlying cause of AD is unknown. Scientists have discovered important pieces of the AD puzzle, but still don't know how they fit together. It may well be that AD results from a combination of factors, rather than from a single cause.

Degeneration of Neurons

Neuronal degeneration occurs in the hippocampus early in AD, followed later by degeneration of neurons in the cerebral cortex and subsequent decline in cerebral volume. The hippocampus serves an important role in memory. The cerebral cortex is central to speech, perception, reasoning, and other higher functions. As hippocampal neurons degenerate, short-term memory begins to fail. As cortical neurons degenerate, patients begin having difficulty with language. With advancing cortical degeneration, more severe symptoms appear. These include complete loss of speech, loss of bladder and bowel control, and complete inability for self-care. AD eventually destroys enough brain function to cause death.

Reduced Cholinergic Transmission

In patients with advanced AD, levels of acetylcholine are 90% below normal. Loss of acetylcholine is significant for two reasons. First, acetylcholine is an important transmitter in the hippocampus and cerebral cortex, regions where neuronal degeneration occurs. Second, acetylcholine is critical to forming memories, and its decline has been linked to memory loss. However, cholinergic transmission is essentially normal in patients with mild AD. Hence, loss of cholinergic function cannot explain the cognitive deficits that occur early in the disease process.

Beta-Amyloid and Neuritic Plaques

Neuritic plaques, which form outside neurons, are a hallmark of AD. These spherical bodies are composed of a central core of *beta-amyloid* (a protein fragment) surrounded by neuron remnants. Neuritic plaques are seen mainly in the hippocampus and cerebral cortex.

In patients with AD, beta-amyloid is present in high levels and may contribute to neuronal injury. Accumulation of beta-amyloid begins early in the disease process, perhaps 10 to 20 years before the first symptoms of AD appear. Because of the central role that beta-amyloid appears to play in AD, treatments directed against beta-amyloid are in development.

Neurofibrillary Tangles and Tau

Like neuritic plaques, neurofibrillary tangles are a prominent feature of AD. These tangles, which form inside neurons, result when the orderly arrangement of microtubules becomes disrupted (Fig. 22.1). The underlying cause is production of an abnormal form of tau, a protein that, in healthy neurons, forms cross-bridges between microtubules and thereby keeps their configuration stable. In patients with AD, tau twists into paired helical filaments that form tangles.

Apolipoprotein E4

Apolipoprotein E (apoE), long known for its role in cholesterol transport, may also contribute to AD. ApoE has three forms, named apoE2, apoE3, and apoE4. Only one form—apoE4—is associated with AD. Genetic research has shown that individuals

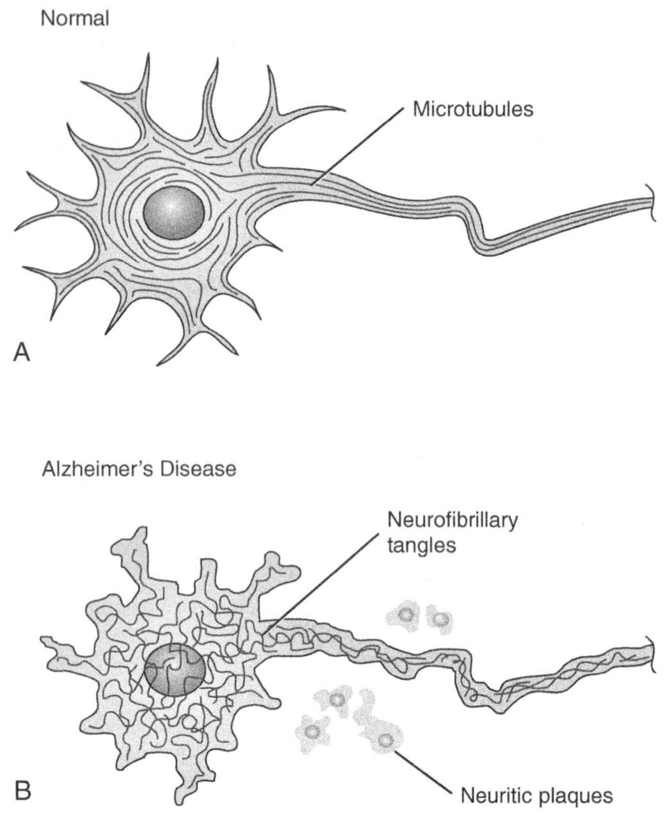

Fig. 22.1 ▪ Histologic changes in Alzheimer's disease. **A,** Healthy neuron. **B,** Neuron affected by Alzheimer's disease, showing characteristic intracellular neurofibrillary tangles. Note also extracellular neuritic plaques.

with one or two copies of the gene that codes for apoE4 are at increased risk for AD; however, many people with AD do not have the gene for apoE4.

Endoplasmic Reticulum–Associated Binding Protein

The discovery of endoplasmic reticulum–associated binding protein (ERAB) adds another piece to the AD puzzle. ERAB is present in high concentration in the brains of patients with AD. These high concentrations of ERAB enhance the neurotoxic effects of beta-amyloid.

Homocysteine

Elevated plasma levels of homocysteine are associated with an increased risk for AD. Fortunately, the risk can be easily reduced: Levels of homocysteine can be lowered by eating foods rich in folic acid and vitamins B_6 and B_{12}, or by taking dietary supplements that contain these compounds.

RISK FACTORS AND SYMPTOMS

Risk Factors

The major known risk factor for AD is advancing age. In 90% of patients, the age of onset is 65 years or older. After age 65 years, the risk for acquiring AD increases exponentially, doubling every 10 years until age 85 to 90 years, after which the risk for getting AD levels off or declines. The only other known risk factor is a family history of AD. Being female *may* be a risk factor. However, the higher incidence of AD in women may occur simply because women generally live longer than men. Other possible risk factors include head injury, low educational level, production of apoE4, high levels of homocysteine, low levels of folic acid, estrogen/progestin therapy, sedentary lifestyle, and nicotine in cigarette smoke.

TABLE 22.1 ▪ Symptoms of Alzheimer's Disease

MILD SYMPTOMS
Confusion and memory loss
Disorientation; getting lost in familiar surroundings
Problems with routine tasks
Changes in personality and judgment
MODERATE SYMPTOMS
Difficulty with activities of daily living, such as feeding and bathing
Anxiety, suspiciousness, agitation
Sleep disturbances
Wandering, pacing
Difficulty in recognizing family and friends
SEVERE SYMPTOMS
Loss of speech
Loss of appetite; weight loss
Loss of bladder and bowel control
Total dependence on caregiver

Symptoms

The symptoms of Alzheimer's disease progress relentlessly from mild to moderate to severe (Table 22.1). Symptoms typically begin after age 65 years, but may appear in people as young as 40 years. Early in the disease, patients begin to experience memory loss and confusion. They may be disoriented and get lost in familiar surroundings. Judgment becomes impaired and personality may change. As the disease progresses, patients have increasing difficulty with self-care. From 70% to 90% eventually develop behavioral problems (wandering, pacing, agitation, screaming). Symptoms may intensify in the evening, a phenomenon known as "sundowning." In the final stages of AD, the patient is unable to recognize close family members or communicate in any way. All sense of identity is lost, and the individual is completely dependent on others for survival. The time from onset of symptoms to death may be 20 years or longer, but it is usually 4 to 8 years. Although there is no clearly effective therapy for *core symptoms,* other symptoms (e.g., incontinence, depression) can be treated.

Prototype Drugs

ALZHEIMER'S DISEASE

Cholinesterase Inhibitors

Donepezil [Aricept]

***N*-Methyl-D-Aspartate (NMDA) Receptor Antagonists**

Memantine [Namenda, Namenda XR]

DRUGS FOR COGNITIVE IMPAIRMENT

Ideally, the goal of AD treatment is to improve symptoms and reverse cognitive decline. Unfortunately, available drugs can't do this. At best, drugs currently in use may slow loss of memory and cognition, and prolong independent function. However, for many patients, even these modest goals are elusive.

Four drugs are approved for treating AD dementia. Three of the drugs—donepezil, galantamine, and rivastigmine—are cholinesterase inhibitors. The fourth drug—memantine—blocks neuronal receptors for *N*-methyl-D-aspartate (NMDA). Treatment of dementia with these drugs can yield improvement that is statistically significant but clinically marginal. As one expert put it, benefits of these drugs are equivalent to losing half a pound after taking a weight-loss drug for 6 months: The loss may be statistically significant, but it has little clinical significance. Given the modest benefits of these drugs, evidence-based clinical guidelines do not recommend that all patients receive drug therapy; this decision is left to the patient, family, and prescriber. No single drug is more effective than the others, so selection should be based on tolerability, ease of use, and cost. Research has not established an optimal treatment duration. Severity indications for drug choice are shown in Table 22.2.

Cholinesterase Inhibitors

The cholinesterase inhibitors were the first drugs approved by the U.S. Food and Drug Administration (FDA) to treat AD. In clinical trials, these drugs produced modest improvements in cognition, behavior, and function, and slightly delayed disease progression. Three cholinesterase inhibitors are available.

Group Properties

Mechanism of Action. Cholinesterase inhibitors prevent the breakdown of acetylcholine by acetylcholinesterase (AChE) and thereby increase the availability of acetylcholine at cholinergic synapses. In patients with AD, the result is enhanced transmission by central cholinergic neurons that have not yet been destroyed. Cholinesterase inhibitors do not cure AD, nor do they stop disease progression—although they may slow progression by a few months.

Therapeutic Effect. All cholinesterase inhibitors are approved for patients with *mild to moderate* symptoms, and one agent—donepezil—is also approved for those with *severe* symptoms. Unfortunately, treatment benefits only 1 in 12 patients. Among those who do benefit, improvements are seen in quality of life and cognitive functions (e.g., memory, thought, reasoning). However, these improvements are modest and last a short time. There is no convincing evidence of marked improvement or significant delay of disease progression. Nonetheless, although improvements are neither universal, dramatic, nor long-lasting and although side effects are common, the benefits may still be worth the risks for some patients.

TABLE 22.2 ▪ Drugs for Alzheimer's Disease: Severity Indications

Drug	Indication (AD Severity)
CHOLINESTERASE INHIBITORS	
Donepezil [Aricept]	Mild to severe
Rivastigmine [Exelon]	Mild to moderate
Galantamine [Razadyne, Razadyne ER, Reminyl ER 🍁]	Mild to moderate
NMDA ANTAGONIST	
Memantine [Namenda, Namenda XR]	Moderate to severe

AD, Alzheimer's disease; *NMDA, N*-methyl-D-aspartate.

Adverse Effects. By elevating acetylcholine in the periphery, all cholinesterase inhibitors can cause typical cholinergic side effects. Gastrointestinal effects—*nausea, vomiting, dyspepsia, diarrhea*—occur often. *Dizziness* and *headache* are also common. Elevation of acetylcholine at synapses in the lungs can cause *bronchoconstriction.* Accordingly, cholinesterase inhibitors should be used with caution in patients with asthma or chronic obstructive pulmonary disease (COPD).

Cardiovascular effects, although uncommon, are a serious concern. Increased activation of cholinergic receptors in the heart can cause symptomatic bradycardia, leading to fainting, falls, fall-related fractures, and pacemaker placement. If a patient is experiencing bradycardia, fainting, or falls, drug withdrawal may be indicated, especially if cognitive benefits are lacking.

Drug Interactions. Drugs that block cholinergic receptors (e.g., anticholinergic agents, first-generation antihistamines, tricyclic antidepressants, conventional antipsychotics) can reduce therapeutic effects and should be avoided.

Dosage and Duration of Treatment. Dosage should be carefully titrated, and treatment should continue as long as clinically indicated. The highest doses produce the greatest benefits—but also the most intense side effects. Accordingly, dosage should be low initially and then gradually increased to the highest tolerable amount. Treatment can continue indefinitely or until side effects become intolerable or benefits are lost.

Properties of Individual Cholinesterase Inhibitors

These drugs have not been directly compared with one another for efficacy. However, they appear to offer equivalent benefits. Accordingly, selection among them is based on side effects, ease of dosing, and cost.

Donepezil. Donepezil [Aricept] is indicated for mild, moderate, or severe AD. The drug causes reversible inhibition of AChE—but is more selective for the form of AChE found in the brain than that found in the periphery. Like other cholinesterase inhibitors, donepezil does not affect the underlying disease process.

Donepezil is well absorbed after oral administration and undergoes metabolism by hepatic CYP2D6 and CYP3A4 isoenzymes. Elimination is mainly in the urine and partly in the bile. Donepezil is highly protein bound and has a prolonged plasma half-life of 70 hours. According to FDA labeling, it takes about 15 days for donepezil to achieve steady state.

Although donepezil is somewhat selective for brain cholinesterase, it can still cause peripheral cholinergic effects; nausea and diarrhea are most common. Like other drugs in this class, donepezil can cause bradycardia, fainting, falls, and fall-related fractures. To minimize side effects, patients are stabilized on the initial dosage for 1 to 3 months before an increase in dosage.

Donepezil is available in three oral formulations: standard tablets (5, 10, and 23 mg), orally disintegrating tablets (5 and 10 mg), and oral solution (1 mg/mL). With all formulations, dosing is done once daily late in the evening, with or without food. To minimize side effects, dosage should be slowly titrated. The initial dosage is 5 mg once daily. After 4 to 6 weeks, dosage may be increased to 10 mg once daily. For patients with moderate or severe AD who have taken 10 mg daily for at least 3 months, dosage may be increased to 23 mg once daily. However, at this dosage, the likelihood of side effects is greatly increased.

Rivastigmine. Rivastigmine [Exelon] is approved for AD and for dementia of Parkinson disease. Unlike donepezil, which causes reversible inhibition of

TABLE 22.3 ▪ Drugs for Alzheimer's Disease: Pharmacokinetic Properties

Drug	Route	Peak	Half-Life	Metabolism	Excretion
Donepezil [Aricept]	PO	3 hr (8 hr for 23-mg tablet)	70 hr	Hepatic (CYP2D6, CYP3A4 and glucuronidation)	Urine (primary), bile
Rivastigmine [Exelon]	PO, transdermal	PO: 1 hr Transdermal: >8 hr	1.5 hr	AChE in the brain	Urine (primary), feces
Galantamine [Razadyne, Razadyne ER Reminyl ER 🍁]	PO	IR tablet without food: 1 hr IR tablet with food: 2.5 hr ER tablet: 5 hr	7 hr	Hepatic (predominantly CYP2D6 and CYP3A4)	Urine
Memantine [Namenda, Namenda XR]	PO	3–7 hr	60–80 hr	Hepatic (primarily non-CYP450)	Urine

AChE, Acetylcholinesterases; *ER,* extended release; *Hr,* hour(s); *IR,* immediate release.

AChE, rivastigmine causes *irreversible* inhibition. As with other cholinesterase inhibitors, benefits in AD are modest.

Like other cholinesterase inhibitors, rivastigmine can cause peripheral cholinergic side effects. These occur with more frequency compared to the other two drugs. With oral dosing, the most common cholinergic effects are nausea, vomiting, diarrhea, abdominal pain, and anorexia. Weight loss (7% of initial weight) occurs in 18% to 26% of patients. By enhancing cholinergic transmission, rivastigmine can intensify symptoms in patients with peptic ulcer disease, bradycardia, sick sinus syndrome, urinary obstruction, and lung disease; caution is advised. Like other drugs in this class, rivastigmine can cause bradycardia, fainting, falls, and fall-related fractures. Blood levels are lower with transdermal dosing than with oral dosing, and hence the intensity of side effects is lower as well. Rivastigmine has no significant drug interactions, probably because it does not interact with hepatic drug-metabolizing enzymes.

Pharmacokinetics of rivastigmine and other drugs in this chapter are provided in Table 22.3. Preparation, dosage, and administration are provided in Table 22.4.

Galantamine. Galantamine [Razadyne, Razadyne ER, Reminyl ER 🍁] is a reversible cholinesterase inhibitor indicated for mild to moderate AD. The drug is prepared by extraction from daffodil bulbs. In clinical trials, galantamine improved cognitive function, behavioral symptoms, quality of life, and the ability to perform activities of daily living. However, as with other cholinesterase inhibitors, benefits were modest and short lasting.

The most common adverse effects are nausea, vomiting, diarrhea, anorexia, and weight loss. Nausea and other GI complaints are greater than with donepezil, but less than with oral rivastigmine. By increasing cholinergic stimulation in the heart, galantamine can cause bradycardia, fainting, falls, and fall-related fractures. Like other cholinesterase inhibitors, galantamine can cause bronchoconstriction, and hence must be used with caution in patients with asthma or COPD. Drugs that block cholinergic receptors (e.g., anticholinergic agents, first-generation antihistamines, tricyclic antidepressants, conventional antipsychotics) can reduce therapeutic effects, and should be avoided.

Memantine

Memantine [Namenda, Namenda XR] is a first-in-class NMDA receptor antagonist. Unlike the cholinesterase inhibitors, which can be used for mild AD, memantine is indicated only for *moderate or severe* AD. We don't yet know if memantine is more effective than the cholinesterase inhibitors, but we do know it's better tolerated. Although memantine helps treat symptoms of AD, there is no evidence that it modifies the underlying disease process.

Therapeutic Effects

In patients with moderate to severe AD, memantine appears to confer modest benefits. For many patients, the drug can slow the decline in function, and, in some cases, it may actually cause symptoms to improve. In one study, patients taking memantine for 28 weeks scored higher on tests of cognitive function and day-to-day function than did those taking placebo, suggesting that memantine slowed functional decline. In another study, treatment with memantine plus donepezil (a cholinesterase inhibitor) was compared with donepezil alone. The result? After 24 weeks, those taking the combination showed less decline in cognitive and day-to-day function than those taking donepezil alone, suggesting that either (1) the two agents confer independent benefits or (2) they act synergistically to enhance each other's effects. Of note, although memantine can benefit patients with moderate to severe AD, it does not benefit patients with mild AD.

Mechanism of Action

Memantine modulates the effects of glutamate (the major excitatory transmitter in the central nervous system) at NMDA receptors, which are believed to play a critical role in learning and memory. The NMDA receptor—a transmembrane protein with a central channel—regulates calcium entry into neurons. Binding of glutamate to the receptor promotes calcium influx.

Under healthy conditions, an action potential releases a burst of glutamate into the synaptic space. Glutamate then binds with the NMDA receptor and displaces magnesium from the receptor channel, permitting calcium entry (Fig. 22.2A). Glutamate then quickly dissociates from the receptor, permitting magnesium to reblock the channel, and thereby prevents further calcium influx. The brief period of calcium entry constitutes a "signal" in the learning and memory process.

Under pathologic conditions, there is slow but steady leakage of glutamate from the presynaptic neuron and surrounding glia. As a result, the channel in the NMDA receptor is kept open, thereby allowing excessive influx of calcium (Fig. 22.2B). High intracellular calcium has two effects: (1) impaired learning and memory (because the "noise" created by excessive calcium overpowers the signal created when calcium enters in response to glutamate released by a nerve impulse); and (2) neurodegeneration (because too much intracellular calcium is toxic).

How does memantine help? It blocks calcium influx when extracellular glutamate is low, but permits calcium influx when extracellular glutamate is high. As shown in Fig. 22.2C, when the glutamate level is low, memantine is able to occupy the NMDA receptor channel, and thereby block the steady entry of calcium. As a result, the level of intracellular calcium is able to normalize. Then, when a burst of glutamate is released in response to an action potential, the resulting high level of

TABLE 22.4 ■ Drugs for Alzheimer's Disease: Preparations, Dosage, and Administration

Drug	Preparations	Dosing Schedule	Administration
Donepezil [Aricept]	Tablet: 5, 10, 23 mg ODT tablet: 5, 10 mg Oral solution: 1 mg/mL	*Mild to moderate AD:* 5 mg/day. After 4–6 weeks, may increase to 10 mg/day *Severe AD:* 10 mg/day. After 3 months, may increase to 23 mg/day	Administer at bedtime. Administer with or without food. The 23-mg tablets must be swallowed whole. Dissolve ODT tablets on the tongue followed by water.
Rivastigmine [Exelon]	Capsule: 1.5, 3, 4.5, 6 mg Oral solution: 2 mg/mL 24-hr transdermal patch: 4.6, 9.5, 13.3 mg	*Mild to moderate AD:* Oral: 1.5 mg twice daily. May increase weekly by 3 mg/day to a maximum of 6 mg twice daily Patch: 4.6-mg patch daily. May increase to a higher dose, if needed *Severe AD:* Initially 4.6-mg patch titrated up to a maximum of 13.3 mg/day	Oral drug: Administer with morning and evening meal. Patch: A single patch is applied once daily to the chest, upper arm, upper back, or lower back after removing the previous patch. The site should be changed daily, and not repeated for at least 14 days. Bathing should not affect treatment.
Galantamine [Razadyne, Razadyne ER, Reminyl ER ♣]	IR tablet: 4, 8, 12 mg Oral solution: 4 mg/mL ER tablet: 8, 16, 24 mg	IR tablets and oral solution: 4 mg twice daily for 4 weeks; may increase dosage by 4 mg twice daily every 4 weeks. Maintenance: 8 to 12 mg twice daily Extended-release capsules: 8 mg once daily for 4 weeks; may increase to 16 mg once daily for 4 weeks and then to 24 mg once daily. Maintenance: 16 to 24 mg/day For patients with moderate hepatic or renal impairment, maximal dose is 16 mg/day. Avoid in patients with severe impairment.	IR: Administer with morning and evening meal. ER: Drug should be swallowed whole.
Memantine [Namenda, Namenda XR]	IR tablet: 5, 10 mg Oral solution: 2 mg/mL, 10 mg/5 mL ER capsules: 7, 14, 21, 28 mg	IR tablets and oral solution: • 5 mg/day (5 mg once daily) for 1 week or more • 10 mg/day (5 mg twice daily) for 1 week or more • 15 mg/day (5 mg and 10 mg in separate doses) for 1 week or more • 20 mg/day (10 mg twice daily) for maintenance ER capsules: • 7 mg once daily for 1 week or more • 14 mg once daily for 1 week or more • 21 mg once daily for 1 week or more • 21 mg once daily for maintenance Dosage should be reduced in patients with moderate renal impairment and discontinued in patients with severe renal impairment.	IR: Administer with or without food. ER tablets: May be swallowed whole *or* the contents may be emptied into a soft food such as applesauce. Contents must not be crushed or chewed. Oral solution: Administer using the provided device. Do not mix with other solutions for administration.

AD, Alzheimer's disease; *ER,* extended release; *IR,* immediate release; *NMDA, N*-methyl-D-aspartate; *ODT,* orally disintegrating tablets.

extracellular glutamate is able to displace memantine, causing a brief period of calcium entry. Because intracellular calcium is now low, normal signaling can occur. When glutamate diffuses away from the receptor, memantine reblocks the channel and thereby stops further calcium entry, despite continuing low levels of glutamate in the synapse.

Pharmacokinetics

Memantine is well absorbed after oral dosing, both in the presence and absence of food. Plasma levels peak in 3 to 7 hours. The drug undergoes little metabolism and is excreted largely unchanged in the urine. The half-life is long—60 to 80 hours. Clearance is reduced in patients with renal impairment.

Adverse Effects

Memantine is well tolerated. The most common side effects are *dizziness, headache, confusion,* and *constipation.* In clinical trials, the incidence of these effects was about the same as in patients taking placebo.

Drug Interactions

In theory, combining memantine with another NMDA antagonist, such as amantadine [Symmetrel] or ketamine [Ketalar], could have an undesirable additive effect. Accordingly, such combinations should be used with caution.

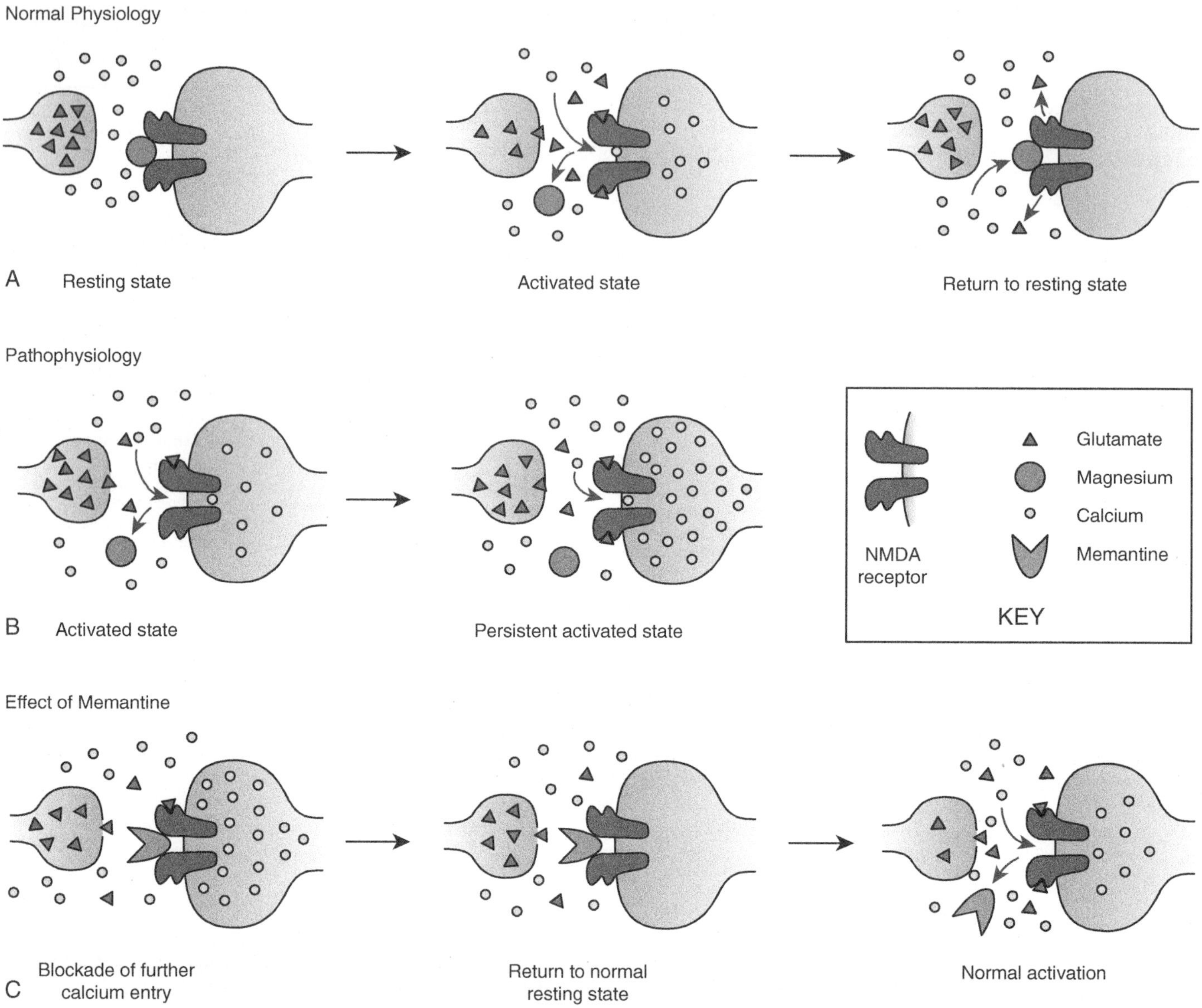

Fig. 22.2 ▪ Memantine mechanism of action.

A, *Normal physiology.* In the resting postsynaptic neuron, magnesium occupies the *N*-methyl-D-aspartate (NMDA) receptor channel, blocking calcium entry. Binding of glutamate to the receptor displaces magnesium, which allows calcium to enter. When glutamate dissociates from the receptor, magnesium returns to the channel and blocks further calcium inflow. The brief period of calcium entry constitutes a "signal" in the learning and memory process. **B,** *Pathophysiology.* Slow but steady leakage of glutamate from the presynaptic neuron keeps the NMDA receptor in a constantly activated state. This allows excessive calcium influx, which can impair memory and learning and can eventually cause neuronal death. **C,** *Effect of memantine.* Memantine blocks calcium entry when extracellular glutamate is low, and thereby stops further calcium entry, which allows intracellular calcium levels to normalize. When a burst of glutamate is released in response to an action potential, the resulting high level of glutamate is able to displace memantine, causing a brief period of calcium entry. Not shown: When glutamate diffuses away, memantine reblocks the channel, and thereby stops further calcium entry, despite continuing low levels of glutamate in the synapse.

Sodium bicarbonate and other drugs that alkalinize the urine can greatly decrease the renal excretion of memantine. Accumulation of the drug to toxic levels might result.

Preparations, Dosage, and Administration

Memantine is available in three oral formulations: IR tablets (5 and 10 mg), sold as *Namenda*; ER capsules (7, 14, 21, and 28 mg), sold as *Namenda XR*; and a solution (2 mg/mL), sold as *Namenda*. With all three, dosing may be done with or without food. Dosage must be titrated as described in Table 22.4. In patients with severe renal impairment, a dosage reduction may be needed, regardless of the formulation used.

DRUGS FOR NEUROPSYCHIATRIC SYMPTOMS

Neuropsychiatric symptoms (e.g., agitation, aggression, delusions, hallucinations) occur in more than 80% of people with AD. Although multiple drug classes—antipsychotics, cholinesterase inhibitors, mood stabilizers, antidepressants, anxiolytics, NMDA receptor antagonists—have been tried as treatment, very few are effective, and even then benefits are limited. There *is* convincing evidence that neuropsychiatric symptoms can be reduced with two atypical antipsychotics: *risperidone* [Risperdal] and *olanzapine* [Zyprexa]. However, benefits are modest, and these drugs slightly *increase* mortality, mainly from cardiovascular events and infection. Cholinesterase inhibitors may offer modest help. There is little or no evidence for a benefit from conventional antipsychotics (e.g., haloperidol, chlorpromazine), mood stabilizers (valproate, carbamazepine, lithium), antidepressants, or memantine.

CAN WE PREVENT ALZHEIMER'S DISEASE OR DELAY COGNITIVE DECLINE?

Despite extensive research to find ways to prevent Alzheimer's disease or to delay the cognitive decline associated with this condition, at this time we have very little good evidence supporting the association of any *modifiable* factor—diet, exercise, social interaction, economic status, nutritional supplements, medications, environmental toxins—with reduced risk for AD. Previously, it was thought that vitamin E was an exception to the rule; however, an updated 2016 Cochrane review found no evidence that vitamin E prevented progression or improved cognitive function. In the meantime, research continues with the hope of a breakthrough.

KEY POINTS

- AD is a relentless illness characterized by progressive memory loss, impaired thinking, neuropsychiatric symptoms, and inability to perform routine tasks of daily living.
- The histopathology of AD is characterized by neuritic plaques, neurofibrillary tangles, and degeneration of cholinergic neurons in the hippocampus and cerebral cortex.
- Neuritic plaques are spherical, extracellular bodies that consist of a beta-amyloid core surrounded by remnants of axons and dendrites.
- In patients with AD, beta-amyloid is present in high levels and may contribute to neuronal injury.
- Neurofibrillary tangles result from production of a faulty form of tau, a protein that in healthy neurons serves to maintain the orderly arrangement of neurotubules.
- The major known risk factor for AD is advancing age.
- AD dementia can be treated with cholinesterase inhibitors or memantine. Although these drugs produced statistically significant symptomatic improvement in clinical trials, benefits in most patients are marginal.
- Cholinesterase inhibitors (e.g., donepezil) increase the availability of acetylcholine at cholinergic synapses, and thereby enhance transmission by cholinergic neurons that have not yet been destroyed by AD.
- Cholinesterase inhibitors produce modest improvements in cognition, behavior, and function in 1 out of 12 AD patients.
- Cholinesterase inhibitors do not cure AD, and they do not stop disease progression.
- The efficacy of all cholinesterase inhibitors appears equal.
- By elevating acetylcholine in the periphery, all cholinesterase inhibitors can cause typical cholinergic side effects. Gastrointestinal effects—nausea, vomiting, dyspepsia, diarrhea—are most common. Of greater concern, by increasing acetylcholine in the heart, these drugs can cause bradycardia, leading to fainting, falls, fall-related fractures, and pacemaker placement.
- Drugs that block cholinergic receptors (e.g., first-generation antihistamines, tricyclic antidepressants, conventional antipsychotics) can reduce responses to cholinesterase inhibitors.
- Memantine is the first representative of a new class of drugs for AD, the NMDA receptor antagonists. Benefits derive from modulating the effects of glutamate at NMDA receptors.
- Unlike cholinesterase inhibitors, all of which can be used for mild AD, memantine is approved only for moderate to severe AD.
- Like the cholinesterase inhibitors, memantine has only modest beneficial effects.
- Memantine appears devoid of significant adverse effects.
- There is no solid evidence that drugs, nutrients, supplements, exercise, cognitive training, or any other intervention can prevent AD or delay cognitive decline.

Please visit **http://evolve.elsevier.com/Lehne** for chapter-specific NCLEX® examination review questions.

CHAPTER

23 Drugs for Multiple Sclerosis

Multiple sclerosis (MS) is a chronic inflammatory autoimmune disorder that damages the myelin sheath of neurons in the central nervous system (CNS), causing a wide variety of sensory, motor, and cognitive deficits. Initially, most patients experience periods of acute clinical exacerbations (relapses) alternating with periods of complete or partial recovery (remissions). Over time, symptoms usually grow progressively worse—although the course of the disease is unpredictable and highly variable. Among young adults, MS causes more disability than any other neurologic disease. Nonetheless, most patients manage to lead fairly normal lives, and life expectancy is only slightly reduced.

Drug therapy of MS changed dramatically in 1993, the year the first disease-modifying agent was approved. Before this time, treatment was purely symptomatic. We had no drugs that could alter the disease process. By using disease-modifying drugs, we can now slow the progression of MS, decrease the frequency and intensity of relapses, and delay permanent neurologic loss. As a result, we can significantly improve prognosis, especially if treatment is started early.

OVERVIEW OF MS AND ITS TREATMENT

Pathophysiology

What's the Primary Pathology of MS?

The pathologic hallmark of MS is the presence of multifocal regions of inflammation and myelin destruction in the CNS (brain, spinal cord, and optic nerve). Because of demyelination, axonal conduction is slowed or blocked, giving rise to a host of neurologic signs and symptoms. As inflammation subsides, damaged tissue is replaced by astrocyte-derived filaments, forming scars known as *scleroses,* hence the disease name. It is important to note that, in addition to stripping off myelin, inflammation may injure the underlying axon and may also damage oligodendrocytes, the cells that produce CNS myelin. Axon injury can also occur in the *absence* of inflammation and can be seen early in the course of the disease.

How Does Inflammation Occur?

The mechanism appears to be autoimmune: Cells of the immune system mistakenly identify components of myelin as being foreign, and hence mount an attack against them. For the attack to occur, circulating lymphocytes (T cells) and monocytes (macrophages) must adhere to the endothelium of CNS blood vessels, migrate across the vessel wall, and then initiate the inflammatory process. The end result is an inflammatory cascade that destroys myelin and may also injure the axonal membrane and nearby oligodendrocytes.

What Initiates the Autoimmune Process?

No one knows. The most likely candidates are genetics, environmental factors, and microbial pathogens. We suspect a *genetic link* for two reasons. First, the risk of MS for first-degree relatives of someone with the disease is 10 to 20 times higher than the risk for people in the general population. Second, the risk of MS differs for members of different races. For example, the incidence is highest among Caucasians (especially those of northern European descent), much lower among Asians, and nearly zero among Inuits (the indigenous people of the Arctic). We suspect *environmental factors* because the risk is not the same in all places: In the United States, MS is more common in northern states than in southern states; around the globe, MS is most common in countries that have a moderately cool climate, whether in the northern or southern hemisphere; and, as we move from the equator toward the poles, the incidence of MS increases. *Microbial pathogens* suspected of initiating autoimmunity include Epstein-Barr virus, human herpesvirus 6, and *Chlamydia pneumoniae.* The bottom line? MS appears to be a disease that develops in genetically vulnerable people following exposure to an environmental or microbial factor that initiates autoimmune activity.

What Happens When an Acute Attack Is Over?

When inflammation subsides, some degree of recovery occurs, at least in the early stages of the disease. Three mechanisms are involved: (1) partial remyelination, (2) functional axonal compensation (axons redistribute their sodium channels from the nodes of Ranvier to the entire region of demyelination), and (3) development of alternative neuronal circuits that bypass the damaged region. Unfortunately, with recurrent episodes of demyelination, recovery becomes less and less complete. Possible reasons include mounting astrocytic scarring, irreversible axonal injury, and the death of neurons and oligodendrocytes.

Does MS Injure the Myelin Sheath of Peripheral Neurons?

No. Myelin in the periphery is made by Schwann cells, whereas myelin in the CNS is made by oligodendrocytes. Although myelin produced by these two cell types is very similar, it is not identical. Because peripheral myelin differs somewhat from CNS myelin, the immune system does not identify peripheral myelin as foreign, and hence this myelin is spared.

Signs and Symptoms

People with MS can experience a wide variety of signs and symptoms. Depending on where CNS demyelination occurs, a patient may experience paresthesias (numbness, tingling, "pins and needles" sensation), muscle or motor problems (weakness, clumsiness, ataxia, spasms, spasticity, tremors, cramps), visual impairment (blurred vision, double vision, blindness), bladder and bowel symptoms (incontinence, urinary urgency, urinary hesitancy, constipation), sexual dysfunction, disabling fatigue, emotional lability, depression, cognitive impairment, slurred speech, dysphagia, dizziness, vertigo, neuropathic pain, and more. The intensity of these symptoms is determined by the size of the region of demyelination. To quantify the impact of MS symptoms, most clinicians employ the Kurtzke Expanded Disability Status Scale (EDSS), an instrument that measures the impact of MS on nine different functional systems (e.g., visual, sensory, cerebellar). The results are tabulated and reported on a scale from 0 to 10, with 0 representing no disability and 10 representing death. An EDSS of 4 or greater indicates difficulties with ambulation. The EDSS form is available online at https://www.nationalmssociety.org/NationalMSSociety/media/MSNationalFiles/Brochures/10-2-3-29-EDSS_Form.pdf. Symptoms of MS are discussed further under *Drugs Used to Manage MS Symptoms.*

MS Subtypes

There are four subtypes of MS—relapsing-remitting, secondary progressive, primary progressive, and progressive-relapsing—defined by the clinical course the disease follows. Symptom patterns that characterize the MS subtypes are shown in Fig. 23.1.

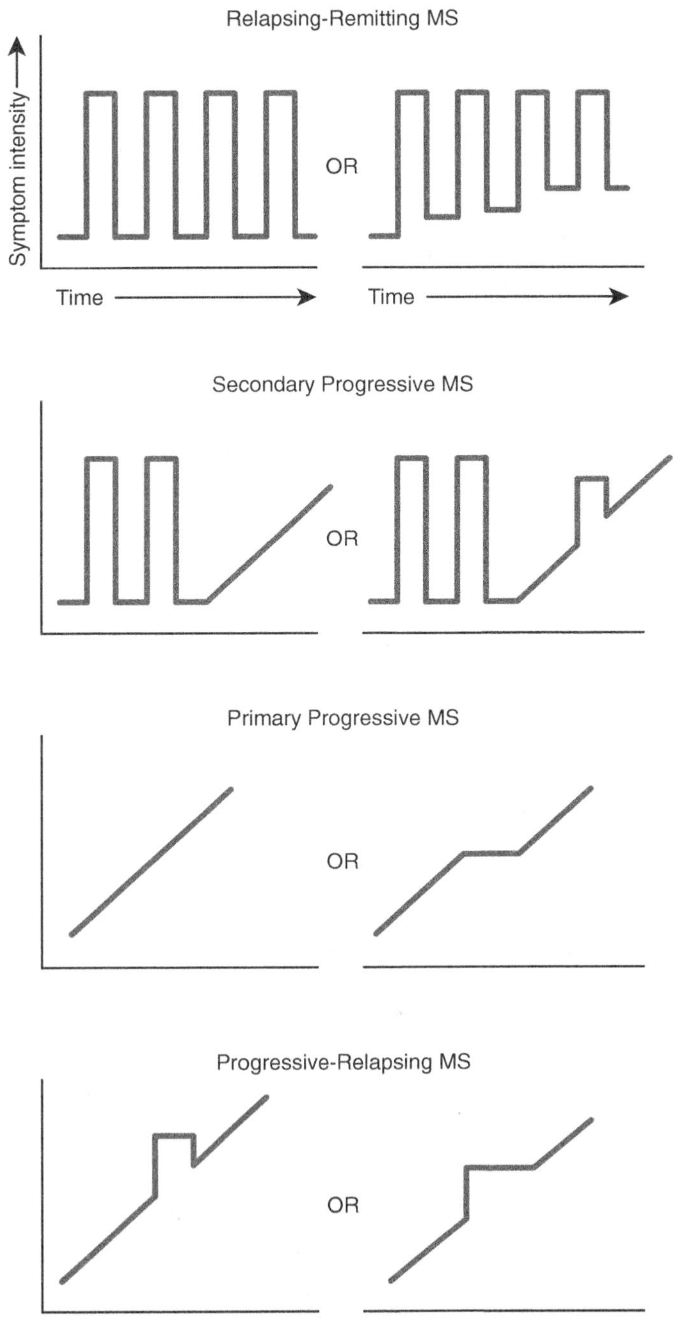

Fig. 23.1 ■ Symptom patterns that define the four subtypes of MS.

Relapsing-Remitting MS

This subtype is characterized by recurrent, clearly defined episodes of neurologic dysfunction (relapses) separated by periods of partial or full recovery (remissions). Between 85% and 90% of patients have this form initially. Symptoms develop over several days and then typically resolve within weeks. The average patient has two relapses every 3 years. Specific signs and symptoms during an attack depend on the size and location of CNS lesions and hence vary from one attack to the next and from one patient to another. The disease usually begins in the second or third decade of life and affects twice as many women as men.

Secondary Progressive MS

This subtype occurs when a patient with relapsing-remitting MS develops steadily worsening dysfunction—with or without occasional plateaus, acute exacerbations, or minor remissions. Within 10 to 20 years of symptom onset, about 50% of patients with relapsing-remitting MS develop secondary progressive MS.

Primary Progressive MS

In this subtype, symptoms grow progressively more intense from the outset, although some patients may experience occasional plateaus or even temporary improvement. Clear remissions, however, do not occur. Only 10% of patients have this form of MS.

Progressive-Relapsing MS

This subtype, which is rare, looks like primary progressive MS, but with acute exacerbations superimposed on the steady intensification of symptoms.

Drug Therapy Overview

In patients with MS, drugs are employed to (1) modify the disease process, (2) treat an acute relapse, and (3) manage symptoms. We have no drugs that can cure MS.

Disease-Modifying Therapy

Disease-modifying drugs can decrease the frequency and severity of relapses, reduce development of brain lesions, decrease future disability, and help maintain quality of life. In addition, they may prevent permanent damage to axons. However, it is important to note that, although these drugs can slow disease progression, they do not work for all patients. Those with relapsing-remitting MS benefit most.

There are two main groups of disease-modifying drugs: *immunomodulators* and *immunosuppressants*. The immunomodulators—dimethyl fumarate, fingolimod, glatiramer acetate, natalizumab, teriflunomide, and interferon beta—are safer than mitoxantrone (the major immunosuppressant in use), and hence are generally preferred. Other immunosuppressants (e.g., azathioprine, methotrexate, cyclophosphamide) are sometimes prescribed for the management of MS, but they have not received approval from the U.S. Food and Drug Administration (FDA) for this use.

Relapsing-Remitting MS. All patients with relapsing-remitting MS—regardless of age, frequency of attacks, or level of disability—should receive one of the immunomodulators:

- Interferon beta-1a [Avonex], for IM use
- Interferon beta-1a [Rebif], for subQ use
- Interferon beta-1b [Betaseron, Extavia], for subQ use
- Dimethyl fumarate [Tecfidera], for PO use
- Glatiramer acetate [Copaxone], for subQ use
- Natalizumab [Tysabri], for IV use
- Fingolimod [Gilenya], for PO use
- Teriflunomide [Aubagio], for PO use

Treatment should begin *as soon as possible* after relapsing-remitting MS has been diagnosed. Early treatment can help prevent axonal injury and may thereby prevent permanent neurologic deficits.

Treatment should continue indefinitely. The principal reasons for stopping would be toxicity or a clear lack of effect. Unfortunately, if disease-modifying therapy is stopped, disease progression may return to the pretreatment rate.

If treatment with an immunomodulator fails to prevent severe relapses or disease progression, treatment with mitoxantrone (an immunosuppressant) should be considered. However, keep in mind that mitoxantrone can cause serious toxicity (e.g., myelosuppression, heart damage), and hence should be reserved for patients who truly need it.

Secondary Progressive MS. *Interferon beta* can benefit certain patients with secondary progressive MS, specifically, those who still experience acute relapses. For these people, interferon beta can reduce the severity and frequency of attacks, and can reduce development of magnetic resonance imaging (MRI)–detectable brain lesions. Whether other disease-modifying drugs can help is unclear.

Mitoxantrone can decrease clinical attack rate, reduce development of new brain lesions, and slow progression of disability. However, although the drug is effective, cardiotoxicity precludes long-term use.

Progressive-Relapsing MS. Mitoxantrone is the only disease-modifying drug approved for this disorder. Unfortunately, benefits are generally modest.

Primary Progressive MS. No disease-modifying therapy has been shown effective against this form of MS. However, ongoing studies with immunosuppressants (e.g., methotrexate, azathioprine, cyclophosphamide) are encouraging.

Treating an Acute Episode (Relapse)

A short course of a *high-dose IV glucocorticoid* (e.g., 500 mg to 1 gm of methylprednisolone daily for 3 to 5 days) is the preferred treatment for an acute relapse. Glucocorticoids suppress inflammation and can thereby reduce the severity and duration of a clinical attack. As discussed in Chapter 72, these drugs are very safe when used short term, elevation of blood glucose being the principal concern. By contrast, long-term exposure can cause osteoporosis and other serious adverse effects. Accordingly, frequent use (more than 3 times a year) or prolonged use (longer than 3 weeks at a time) should be avoided.

Acute relapse may also be treated with *IV gamma globulin.* This option can be especially helpful in patients intolerant of or unresponsive to glucocorticoids. Results have been good.

Drug Therapy of Symptoms

All four subtypes of MS share the same symptoms (e.g., fatigue, spasticity, pain, bladder dysfunction, bowel dysfunction, sexual dysfunction). Accordingly, the drugs used for symptom management are the same for all patients, regardless of MS subtype. Specific treatments are discussed under *Drugs Used to Manage MS Symptoms.*

DISEASE-MODIFYING DRUGS I: IMMUNOMODULATORS

Six immunomodulators are available: dimethyl fumarate [Tecfidera], glatiramer acetate [Copaxone], natalizumab [Tysabri], fingolimod [Gilenya], teriflunomide [Aubagio], and interferon beta [Avonex, Rebif, Betaseron, Extavia]. Unfortunately, some of the drugs that are most effective in decreasing the relapse rate may cause more adverse effects. For example, natalizumab may decrease the relapse rate by 68%, but it is potentially more dangerous than other drugs. Therefore, selection among these drugs is based primarily on drug risks versus benefits and patient tolerability. If a particular drug is intolerable or ineffective, a different one should be tried.

PATIENT-CENTERED CARE ACROSS THE LIFE SPAN

Drugs for Multiple Sclerosis

Life Stage	Patient Care Concerns
Children	These drugs are not indicated as treatment for children with the exception of mitoxantrone, which is also used to treat leukemia in children.
Pregnant women	Teriflunomide is Pregnancy Risk Category X.[a] It can cause major birth defects. Mitoxantrone is Pregnancy Risk Category D. The mechanism by which the drug causes teratogenesis in animals occurs in humans; therefore, there is a high likelihood of human fetal risk. Glatiramer acetate is Pregnancy Risk Category B because there is no evidence of harm in animal research on rats and rabbits. Because this may not be an adequate predictor of human response, the FDA recommends avoidance of pregnancy while taking this drug. The remaining drugs are Pregnancy Risk Category C. For these, human information is insufficient but fetal abnormalities have occurred in animal research. As with other drugs for MS, pregnancy should be avoided.
Breast-feeding women	Excretion of all these drugs in breast milk has not been determined, with the exception of mitoxantrone, for which drug concentrations remain significant up to 3 to 4 weeks following the last dose. Because these drugs can cause significant adverse reactions, breast-feeding is not recommended.
Older adults	There are no contraindications for use in older adults; however, the health status of the patient, along with comorbidities and their treatment, needs to be considered in planning to ensure optimal outcomes.

[a]As of 2020, the FDA will no longer use Pregnancy Risk Categories. Please refer to Chapter 9 for more information.

Interferon Beta Preparations

Description and Mechanism

Interferon beta is a naturally occurring glycoprotein with antiviral, antiproliferative, and immunomodulatory actions. Natural interferon beta is produced in response to viral invasion and other biologic inducers. In patients with MS, it is believed to help in two ways. First, it inhibits the migration of proinflammatory leukocytes across the blood-brain barrier, preventing these cells from reaching neurons of the CNS. Second, it suppresses T-helper cell activity.

Prototype Drugs

DRUGS FOR MULTIPLE SCLEROSIS

Immunomodulators

Interferon beta

Immunosuppressants

Mitoxantrone

Two forms of interferon beta are used clinically: *interferon beta-1a* [Avonex, Rebif] and *interferon beta-1b* [Betaseron, Extavia]. Both forms are manufactured using recombinant DNA technology. Interferon beta-1a contains 166 amino acids plus glycoproteins and is identical to natural human interferon beta with respect to amino acid content. Interferon beta-1b contains 165 amino acids and has no glycoproteins and hence differs somewhat from the natural compound. The two preparations of interferon beta-1a are administered by different routes: Avonex (IM) and Rebif (subQ). The two preparations of interferon beta-1b—Betaseron and Extavia—are identical.

Therapeutic Use

All four interferon beta products are approved for relapsing forms of MS. These drugs can decrease the frequency and severity of attacks, reduce the number and size of MRI-detectable lesions, and delay the progression of disability. Benefits with Rebif, Betaseron, and Extavia may be somewhat greater than with Avonex, perhaps because Avonex is given less frequently and in lower dosage.

In addition to its use in relapsing MS, interferon beta-1b [Betaseron] is approved for patients with secondary progressive MS.

Adverse Effects and Drug Interactions

Interferon beta is generally well tolerated, although side effects are common.

Flu-like Reactions. Flu-like reactions occur often. Symptoms include headache, fever, chills, malaise, muscle aches, and stiffness. Fortunately, these diminish over time, despite continued interferon beta use. Symptoms can be minimized by (1) starting with a low dose and then slowing titrating up to the full dose, and (2) giving an analgesic-antipyretic medication (i.e., acetaminophen; ibuprofen or another nonsteroidal anti-inflammatory drug).

Hepatotoxicity. Interferon beta can injure the liver, typically causing an asymptomatic increase in circulating liver enzymes. Very rarely, patients develop hepatitis or even liver failure. To monitor for hepatotoxicity, liver function tests (LFTs) should be performed at baseline, 1 month later, then every 3 months for 1 year, and every 6 months thereafter. If LFTs indicate significant liver injury, a temporary reduction in dosage or interruption of treatment is indicated. When liver function returns to normal, treatment can resume, but careful monitoring is required. Interferon beta should be used with caution in patients who abuse alcohol, use hepatotoxic medications, or have active liver disease or a history of liver disease.

Myelosuppression. Interferon beta can suppress bone marrow function, thereby decreasing production of all blood cell types. To monitor for myelosuppression, complete blood counts (CBCs) should be obtained at baseline, every 3 months for 1 year, and every 6 months thereafter.

Injection-Site Reactions. Subcutaneous injection (of Rebif or Betaseron) can cause pain, erythema (redness), maculopapular or vesicular rash, and itching. Physical measures to reduce discomfort include rotating the injection site, applying ice (briefly) before and after the injection, and applying a warm, moist compress after the injection. Oral diphenhydramine [Benadryl] or topical hydrocortisone can reduce persistent itching and erythema. However, *continuous* use of topical hydrocortisone should be avoided, owing to a risk of skin damage. Very rarely, subQ injections (of Betaseron, Extavia, or Rebif) have caused local necrosis. Intramuscular injection (of Avonex) can cause discomfort and bruising.

Depression. Interferon beta may promote or exacerbate depression. Some patients may experience suicidal ideation and even attempt suicide.

Neutralizing Antibodies. Like all other foreign proteins, interferon beta is immunogenic, and hence can stimulate production of antibodies against itself. If present in sufficiently high titers, these neutralizing antibodies can decrease clinical benefits.

Drug Interactions. Exercise caution when combining interferon beta with other drugs that can suppress the bone marrow or cause liver injury.

Preparations, Dosage, and Administration

Avonex (Interferon Beta-1a for IM Use). Avonex is available in pre-filled, single-use syringes (30 mcg/0.5 mL) and as a powder (30 mcg/0.5 mL when reconstituted with sterile water). The dosage is 30 mcg IM once a week. Store both Avonex powder and pre-filled syringes at 36°F to 46°F (2°C to 8°C). If refrigeration is unavailable, the drug may be stored at or below 77°F (25°C) for up to 30 days. Injections are made late in the day so that flu-like symptoms occur during sleep.

Rebif (Interferon Beta-1a for SubQ Use). Rebif is available in pre-filled, single-use syringes containing either 8.8 mcg/0.2 mL, 22 mcg/0.5 mL, or 44 mcg/0.5 mL. Injections are made subQ 3 times a week, preferably in late afternoon or evening, at least 48 hours apart, and on the same days each week (e.g., Monday, Wednesday, Friday). Dosage is titrated to achieve a target dose of either 22 mcg or 44 mcg 3 times a week. If the target is 22 mcg 3 times a week, administration is begun at 4.4 mcg 3 times a week for 2 weeks, then increased to 11 mcg 3 times a week for 2 weeks, and then increased to 22 mcg 3 times a week. If the target is 44 mcg 3 times a week, administration is begun at 8.8 mcg 3 times a week for the first 2 weeks, then increased to 22 mcg 3 times a week for 2 weeks, and then increased to 44 mcg 3 times a week thereafter. Ideally, Rebif should be refrigerated at 36°F to 46°F (2°C to 8°C); however, if refrigeration is unavailable, it may be stored at or below 77°F (25°C) for up to 30 days.

Betaseron and Extavia (Interferon Beta-1b for SubQ Use). Betaseron and Extavia are supplied as a powder (300 mcg) in single-use vials. Just before use, the drug is reconstituted to form a 250-mcg/mL solution. Doses are given subQ every other day. Dosage is titrated as follows: 62.5 mcg/dose for weeks 1 and 2; 125 mcg/dose for weeks 3 and 4; 187.5 mcg/dose for weeks 4 and 5; and 250 mcg/dose thereafter. Store the powder at room temperature. Following reconstitution, the drug solution may be stored up to 3 hours refrigerated.

Dimethyl Fumarate

Therapeutic Use

Dimethyl fumarate (DMF) [Tecfidera] is approved for management of relapsing MS. It reduces relapse rates and slows disease progression. In some countries it has been used in the management of psoriasis; however, it has not received approval for this use in the United States or Canada.

Description and Mechanism

DMF is an immunomodulator that promotes apoptosis (self-destruction) of activated T lymphocytes and inhibits migration of lymphocytes into the CNS. Its exact mechanism of action is unknown; however, its effects are widely believed to be the result of activation of the Nrf2 antioxidant response pathway. This pathway protects cells from oxidative stress and provides anti-inflammatory effects.

Pharmacokinetics

Before systemic absorption, DMF undergoes rapid hydrolysis to its active metabolite, monomethyl fumarate (MMF). DMF has a half-life of approximately 1 hour. Peak activity of its active metabolite occurs in 2 to 2.5 hours. Approximately 60% is eliminated through the respiratory system. The remainder is primarily eliminated through the urine with a small amount excreted in feces.

Adverse Effects

The most common side effect is flushing. The most serious adverse effect is lymphopenia with a resulting increased risk of infections. Other common adverse effects are discussed in this section.

Flushing. Many patients experience a vascular flush that is manifested by a warmth and redness of the skin that may be accompanied by sensations of mild burning or itching. The effect decreases over time; however, initially it may be helpful to administer a non–enteric-coated aspirin 30 minutes before administration. Flushing may also be decreased by taking the drug with food.

Gastrointestinal Discomfort. Gastrointestinal disturbances may take a variety of forms. These include abdominal pain, diarrhea, and nausea and vomiting. These symptoms tend to decrease considerably over time. The Canadian label suggests temporarily decreasing the dosage from 240 mg to 120 mg if the symptoms worsen.

Infections. A decrease in lymphocytes may occur. This increases the risk of infections and may be serious. It is important to obtain a baseline CBC; thereafter, a CBC should be obtained at least annually to monitor for lymphopenia and sooner if the patient develops signs or symptoms of infection.

Rash. An erythematous rash may occur. This may be accompanied by pruritus.

Alterations in Laboratory Analyses. Patients taking DMF have developed elevations in hepatic enzymes and proteinuria. The significance of these findings is unknown. Rarely is the drug discontinued for these reasons; however, Canadian labeling recommends baseline and yearly evaluations of hepatic transaminases and a urinalysis as a cautionary measure.

Drug Interactions

DMF can decrease the body's response to vaccines. Patients should not receive live virus vaccines when taking this drug as this could allow vaccine-related infection to occur. It is also advisable to avoid other immunosuppressants when taking this drug to avoid additive immunosuppressive effects.

Preparations, Dosage, and Administration

See Table 23.1 for preparation, dosage, and administration of DMF and other drugs in this chapter.

Glatiramer Acetate

Therapeutic Use

Glatiramer acetate [Copaxone], also known as *copolymer-1,* is used for long-term therapy of relapsing-remitting MS. Like interferon beta, glatiramer can reduce the frequency and severity of relapses, decrease MRI-detectable lesions, and delay the progression of disability. Glatiramer requires more frequent injections than interferon beta, and is less well tolerated.

Description and Mechanism

Glatiramer is a polypeptide composed of four amino acids: L-alanine, L-glutamate, L-lysine, and L-tyrosine. The drug is similar in structure to myelin basic protein, a component of the axonal myelin sheath. In patients with MS, the drug promotes a "T-cell shift." That is, it decreases production of

TABLE 23.1 ▪ Disease-Modifying Drugs for MS

Drug	Preparation	Route	Maintenance Dose	Administration and Storage	Adverse Effects
Interferon beta-1a [Avonex]	Pre-filled syringe: 30 mcg/0.5 mL Powder: 30 mcg, reconstitute with 0.5 mL sterile water	IM	30 mcg once a week	Rotate injection sites. Administer late in the day so that flu-like symptoms occur during sleep. Store both powder and pre-filled syringes at 36°F to 46°F (2°C to 8°C). If refrigeration is unavailable, store at or below 77°F (25°C) for up to 30 days.	Flu-like symptoms Liver injury Myelosuppression Injection-site reactions
Interferon beta-1a [Rebif]	Pre-filled syringe: 8.8 mcg/0.2 mL, 22 mcg/0.5 mL, or 44 mcg/0.5 mL	subQ	44 mcg 3 times a week at least 48 hours apart	Refrigerate at 36°F to 46°F (2°C to 8°C). If refrigeration is unavailable, store at or below 77°F (25°C) for up to 30 days.	
Interferon beta-1b [Betaseron, Extavia]	Powder: 300 mcg, reconstitute to 250-mcg/mL solution	subQ	250 mcg every other day	Rotate injection sites. Store powder at room temperature. May be refrigerated up to 3 hours following reconstitution.	
Dimethyl fumarate [Tecfidera]	ER capsule: 120, 240 mg	PO	120 mg or 240 mg twice daily	Administer with or without food.	Flushing GI discomfort Infections Rash
Glatiramer acetate [Copaxone]	Pre-filled syringe: 20 mg/mL glatiramer plus 40 mg of mannitol	subQ	20 mg once daily	Let syringe warm at room temperature for 20 minutes before administration. Refrigerate at 36°F to 46°F (2°C to 8°C).	Injection-site reactions Postinjection reaction
Natalizumab [Tysabri]	Concentrate: 300 mg/15 mL for dilution to 100 mL	IV	300 mg every 4 weeks	Infuse over 1 hour. Observe during administration and for 1 hour afterward. Stop infusion immediately if signs or symptoms of hypersensitivity develop.	Progressive multifocal leukoencephalopathy Liver injury Allergic reactions
Fingolimod [Gilenya]	Capsules: 0.5 mg	PO	0.5 mg once daily	Administer with or without food	Bradycardia Infections Liver injury Macular edema Fetal harm
Teriflunomide [Aubagio]	Tablets: 7, 14 mg	PO	7 mg or 14 mg once daily	Administer with or without food	Neutropenia Alopecia Infections Liver injury Fetal harm
Mitoxantrone [Novantrone]	Solution: 2 mg/mL in 10-, 12.5-, and 15-mL vials	IV	12 mg/m^2[a] every 3 months	Dilute with at least 50 mL NS or D_5W. Infuse over 15–30 minutes into a free-flowing IV line. Do not mix with other drugs.	Myelosuppression Cardiotoxicity Fetal harm

[a]Maximum lifetime dose is 140 mg/m^2 (because of cardiotoxicity).
D_5W, 5% dextrose in water; *ER,* extended release; *NS,* normal saline.

proinflammatory TH1 cells and increases production of anti-inflammatory TH2 cells. The anti-inflammatory cells migrate across the blood-brain barrier at sites of inflammation, and then suppress the inflammatory attack on myelin.

Adverse Effects and Drug Interactions

Glatiramer is generally well tolerated. Injection-site reactions—pain, erythema, pruritus (itching), induration (pitting)—are most common. About 10% of patients experience a self-limited postinjection reaction—characterized by flushing, palpitations, severe chest pain, anxiety, laryngeal constriction, and urticaria—that typically lasts 15 to 20 minutes. No specific treatment is indicated. Unlike interferon beta, glatiramer does *not* cause flu-like symptoms, myelosuppression, or liver toxicity. No significant interactions with other MS drugs have been observed.

Natalizumab

Natalizumab [Tysabri], a recombinant monoclonal antibody, was introduced in 2004 and then withdrawn a few months later in response to three reports of progressive multifocal leukoencephalopathy (PML), a severe infection of the brain. The drug was reintroduced in 2006, but with protective restrictions on who can prescribe, dispense, administer, and receive it. Before natalizumab can be administered, everyone involved with the drug—patients, physicians, pharmacists, infusion nurses, and infusion centers—must be registered with the TOUCH Prescribing Program.

Therapeutic Uses

Natalizumab is approved for two autoimmune diseases: MS and Crohn's disease (an inflammatory disorder of the bowel). Its use in the management of Crohn's disease is discussed in Chapter 80.

Natalizumab is approved only for *monotherapy* of *relapsing forms of MS.* In the AFFIRM trial, which compared natalizumab with placebo, natalizumab reduced the annualized rate of relapse by 68% and reduced the number of new or enlarging brain lesions by 83%. These benefits are superior to other immunomodulators. However, owing to the risk of PML, natalizumab should not be combined with other disease-modifying drugs.

Mechanism of Action

In patients with MS, natalizumab prevents circulating leukocytes (T cells and monocytes) from leaving the vasculature and thereby prevents these cells from migrating to sites where they can do harm. To exit the vasculature, activated leukocytes must first adhere to the vascular endothelium, a process that requires the interaction of two types of molecules: (1) *integrins* (adhesion molecules) expressed on the surface of leukocytes and (2) *integrin receptors* expressed on cells of the vascular epithelium. Natalizumab binds with integrin molecules on leukocytes, and thereby renders these cells unable to bind with integrin receptors on the capillary wall. As a result, the leukocytes cannot cross the capillary wall, and hence are unable to exit the vasculature to reach their sites of inflammatory action. In patients with MS, natalizumab prevents activated leukocytes from crossing the blood-brain barrier.

Adverse Effects

Natalizumab is generally well tolerated. The most common reactions are headache and fatigue. Other common reactions include abdominal discomfort, arthralgia, depression, diarrhea, gastroenteritis, urinary tract infections, and lower respiratory tract infections. The most serious effects are PML, liver injury, and hypersensitivity reactions.

Progressive Multifocal Leukoencephalopathy. Shortly after natalizumab was released, there were reports of PML, a serious, often fatal infection of the CNS caused by reactivation of the JC virus, an opportunistic pathogen resistant to all available drugs. Of the patients who survive PML, 80% to 90% are left highly disabled. As of May 2011, there had been 124 reported cases of PML among 83,300 natalizumab recipients worldwide, making the incidence 1.4 cases per 1000 patients. Risk for PML increases over time: The longer natalizumab is used, the higher the risk. Why does natalizumab promote PML? Because it suppresses immune function. Risk is increased by other immunosuppressant drugs and by HIV/AIDS and other conditions that compromise cell-mediated immunity.

To reduce the risk of PML, natalizumab is available only through the *TOUCH Prescribing Program.* Patients, prescribers, infusion nurses, infusion centers, and pharmacies associated with infusion centers must all register with the program. In addition, prescribers and patients must understand the risks of natalizumab, including PML and other opportunistic infections—and patients must be screened for PML before each infusion. Also, patients should be informed about symptoms of PML—progressive weakness on one side of the body; clumsiness of the limbs; disturbed vision; changes in thinking, memory, or orientation—and instructed to report them immediately.

Hepatotoxicity. Like interferon beta, natalizumab can injure the liver. Patients should be informed about signs of liver injury—jaundice, nausea, vomiting, fatigue, anorexia, stomach pain, darkening of the urine—and instructed to report these immediately. If significant liver injury is diagnosed, natalizumab should be discontinued.

Hypersensitivity Reactions. Natalizumab can cause a variety of allergic reactions, manifesting as hives, itching, chest pain, dizziness, chills, rash, flushing, and hypotension. Severe reactions (e.g., anaphylaxis) usually develop within 2 hours of infusion onset, but can also develop later. The risk of a severe reaction is increased by the presence of neutralizing antibodies. If a severe reaction develops, natalizumab should be discontinued and never used again.

Neutralizing Antibodies. Antibodies against natalizumab develop in about 6% of patients. These antibodies greatly decrease the efficacy of natalizumab and increase the risk of hypersensitivity and infusion reactions.

Drug Interactions

Immunosuppressants (e.g., mitoxantrone, azathioprine, methotrexate, cyclophosphamide) increase the risk of PML and other opportunistic infections. Accordingly, these drugs should be discontinued at least 3 months before natalizumab is started.

Fingolimod

Fingolimod [Gilenya] is a first-in-class *sphingosine 1-phosphate receptor modulator.* The drug was approved in 2010 for reducing the frequency of MS exacerbations and delaying disability in patients with relapsing forms of the disease. In clinical trials, fingolimod was somewhat more effective than interferon beta. Unfortunately, although effective, fingolimod can cause significant adverse effects. Accordingly, it is commonly reserved for patients who cannot tolerate injections or who have not responded well to other immunomodulators.

Pharmacokinetics

Fingolimod is administered PO, and absorption is nearly complete (93%) both in the presence and absence of food. Plasma levels peak 12 to 16 hours after dosing. Protein binding in blood is high (99.7%). In the liver, some of the drug is converted to its active form—*fingolimod phosphate*—and some is converted to inactive metabolites through the actions of several isoenzymes of cytochrome P450 (CYP). Most (81%) of the drug is eliminated in the urine in the form of inactive metabolites, and much less (2.5%) is eliminated in the feces as fingolimod itself or fingolimod phosphate. The drug has a long half-life (6 to 9 days), and hence it takes a long time (1 to 2 months) for plasma levels to reach plateau. Likewise, it takes a long time for blood levels to decline when treatment stops.

Mechanism of Action

Fingolimod, in the form of fingolimod phosphate, binds with high affinity to a class of molecules known as *sphingosine 1-phosphate (S1P) receptors,* which help regulate multiple processes. How does fingolimod help in MS? It binds with S1P receptors on lymphocytes, causing their sequestration in lymph nodes. As a result, there are fewer lymphocytes in peripheral blood, and hence fewer lymphocytes enter the brain. This reduction in lymphocytes reduces the inflammation that underlies neuronal injury.

Adverse Effects

Fingolimod can cause multiple adverse effects. The most common are headache, diarrhea, cough, back pain, influenza, and elevation of liver enzymes. The most serious are bradycardia, macular edema, infection, fetal harm, and liver injury. Because S1P receptors help regulate multiple processes—including heart rate, vascular tone, airway resistance, neuronal excitability, neurogenesis, angiogenesis, and auditory and vestibular function—this variety of adverse effects should be no surprise.

Bradycardia. Fingolimod reduces heart rate. This effect is maximal within 6 hours after the first daily dose, and then diminishes following each subsequent dose over the next month. For most patients, bradycardia is asymptomatic, although some experience dizziness, fatigue, palpitations, or chest pain, all of which resolve within 24 hours. Owing to the risk of bradycardia, patients should be observed for 6 hours after their first dose, whether initiating therapy or reinstituting therapy following an interruption in treatment of 2 weeks or longer. If symptomatic bradycardia occurs, heart rate can be increased with atropine (a muscarinic antagonist) or with isoproterenol (a beta-adrenergic agonist).

Patients at risk for bradycardia include those with heart failure, ischemic heart disease, or pre-existing bradycardia, and those taking certain antidysrhythmic drugs, especially beta blockers and two of the calcium channel blockers: verapamil and diltiazem. An electrocardiogram (ECG) should be obtained for these patients (if a recent ECG is not available).

Macular Edema. Fingolimod can cause macular edema (swelling of the macula of the eye) owing to leakage and accumulation of fluid. In clinical trials, the incidence was 0.4%. Risk is increased by diabetes and uveitis. To monitor for macular edema, patients should undergo an ophthalmologic examination at baseline, 3 to 4 months after starting treatment, and whenever their vision changes. Patients should be instructed to inform the prescriber if they experience vision problems (blurriness, shadows, sensitivity to light, altered color vision, blind spot in the center of the visual field). Fortunately, macular edema generally resolves with or without stopping fingolimod, although some patients have visual deficits even after the edema is gone.

Liver Injury. Fingolimod can cause liver injury, manifesting as elevations in circulating liver transaminases. LFTs should be performed at baseline and whenever signs of liver injury appear. Patients should be informed about signs of liver injury (nausea, vomiting, anorexia, stomach pain, fatigue, dark urine, jaundice) and instructed to inform the prescriber if these develop. If LFTs confirm significant liver damage, fingolimod should be discontinued.

Infection. Fingolimod causes a 20% to 30% decrease in circulating lymphocytes, and thereby increases the risk of infection. Risk is increased during treatment and for 2 months after stopping. Live virus vaccines should not be used during this time. Patients with an active infection should not use the drug. Inform patients about signs of infection (fever, fatigue, chills, body aches) and instruct them to contact the prescriber if these develop. If a serious infection is diagnosed, interruption of treatment should be considered.

Patients who have not had chickenpox (varicella-zoster virus [VZV] infection) and have not received VZV vaccine should be tested for VZV antibodies before starting fingolimod. Antibody-negative patients should be given VZV vaccine, and fingolimod started 1 month later.

Safety Alert

PREGNANCY RISKS

The onset of MS typically occurs between the ages of 20 and 40 years. Because this is during the period when women are in their peak childbearing years, it is essential to consider safety issues related to pregnancy. With the exception of glatiramer acetate, all of the drugs used to treat MS are potentially teratogenic or lethal to embryos. Women of childbearing age should be informed about the risk of fetal harm and be advised to use two effective forms of contraception, both during treatment and for 2 months after stopping.

Reduced Lung Function. Fingolimod can cause a dose-dependent decrease in lung function. Patients should be advised to inform the prescriber if they experience new or worsening dyspnea (shortness of breath).

Hazardous Agents Requiring Special Handling. Fingolimod may present a hazard for nurses, especially pregnant nurses who administer this drug. Special handling is required for administration. See Chapter 3, Table 3.1, for administration and handling guidelines established by the National Institute for Occupational Safety and Health (NIOSH).

Drug Interactions

Ketoconazole. Ketoconazole, an antifungal drug, inhibits some CYP isoenzymes and can thereby increase fingolimod levels (by as much as 70%). Patients should be monitored for fingolimod toxicity.

Cardiac Drugs. Drugs that slow heart rate (e.g., beta blockers, verapamil, diltiazem) can intensify fingolimod-induced bradycardia. Owing to its effects on heart function, fingolimod may increase the risk of torsades de pointes (a potentially fatal dysrhythmia) if combined with a class IA antidysrhythmic drug (e.g., quinidine, procainamide, disopyramide) or a class III antidysrhythmic drug (amiodarone, sotalol). Patients using any of these combinations should be monitored.

Vaccines. Because fingolimod suppresses immune function, it can reduce the immune response to all vaccines and can increase the risk of infection from live virus vaccines. Accordingly, vaccinations should not be attempted while using fingolimod or for 2 months after stopping it.

Drugs That Suppress Immune Function. Combining fingolimod with an immunosuppressant, certain anticancer drugs, or another immunomodulator will cause more immunosuppression than when fingolimod is used alone, thereby increasing the risk of infection.

Teriflunomide

Therapeutic Use

Teriflunomide [Aubagio] is an immunomodulatory drug that is approved for management of relapsing forms of MS. It reduces relapse rates and disability progression when used alone, and augments clinical benefits when combined with interferon beta or glatiramer.

Mechanism of Action

Teriflunomide is a pyrimidine synthesis inhibitor. (Pyrimidine is one of the building blocks of DNA.) In inhibiting pyrimidine synthesis, this drug decreases T-cell and B-cell proliferation and activation. It also has anti-inflammatory effects. It is important to note that teriflunomide is a metabolite of leflunomide [Arava], a drug used to treat rheumatoid arthritis.

Pharmacokinetics

Greater than 99% of the drug is protein bound. Peak levels occur 1 to 4 hours following administration. It undergoes enterohepatic recycling, which is believed to contribute to its long half-life of approximately 2.5 to 3 weeks. Excretion occurs primarily via feces and urine.

Adverse Effects

Over 10% of patients taking teriflunomide will develop headaches, nausea, diarrhea, neutropenia, and alopecia. They may also develop low phosphate levels, high liver enzyme levels (especially alanine aminotransferase), and an increase in infections such as influenza. Less common, but potentially high-risk adverse effects include severe hyperkalemia, hypertension, peripheral neuropathy, and an increase in malignancies. Renal failure may also occur, but this is a short-term effect.

Fetal and Infant Harm. Teriflunomide can cause serious birth defects. Not only may this occur if it is taken by pregnant women, but also birth defects may occur if a woman is impregnated by a man who is taking teriflunomide. For these reasons, it is essential to rule out pregnancy before initiating therapy and to use a highly reliable form of birth control during and following treatment until serum drug levels indicate that it is safe to become pregnant. It is essential that patients understand the need to check drug levels as teriflunomide may be detectable for 2 years after cessation of therapy.

Contraindications

Teriflunomide is contraindicated in patients who have severe hepatic impairment. It also should not be administered to women who are pregnant or who are at an increased risk of becoming pregnant due to poor adherence to reliable contraception methods.

Drug Interactions

Numerous drug interactions occur with teriflunomide, so it is always essential to check for interactions before administration. Here we discuss some of the most common or significant interactions.

Leflunomide. While all immunomodulators and immunosuppressants present additive risks when given with teriflunomide, leflunomide is particularly risky. Recall that teriflunomide is a metabolite of leflunomide, so taking both drugs can logically increase teriflunomide serum concentrations to toxic levels. Further, when taken together, these drugs have been associated with hepatic failure, interstitial lung disease, bone marrow suppression, severe dermatologic conditions such as Stevens-Johnson syndrome and toxic epidermal necrolysis, and a marked increase in sepsis. Deaths related to these conditions have occurred.

Live Virus Vaccines. When live virus vaccines are given to patients taking teriflunomide, the immunosuppressant effects of teriflunomide may allow development of the infection that the vaccine is given to prevent. For this reason, live virus vaccines should not be given until at least 3 months following teriflunomide therapy.

Bile Acid Sequestrants and Activated Charcoal. Both bile acid sequestrants (administered to decrease cholesterol levels) and activated charcoal (given to manage poisonings) decrease serum levels of teriflunomide. This interaction can be advantageous when used to enhance teriflunomide elimination in the event of hepatotoxicity, dangerous adverse effects, or pregnancy. Without this action to promote drug elimination, drug levels may remain detectable for up to 2 years.

Monitoring

Before initiating therapy, laboratory studies—including CBC, electrolytes, hepatic enzymes, serum creatinine, and bilirubin—should be performed to establish baseline values. These levels should be reassessed twice yearly to monitor for complications. Additionally, signs and symptoms should be assessed through a targeted history and physical examination.

Hazardous Agents Requiring Special Handling

Because exposure to teriflunomide may cause developmental abnormalities, the NIOSH identifies teriflunomide as a hazardous drug requiring special handling. See Chapter 3, Table 3.1, for administration and handling guidelines.

DISEASE-MODIFYING DRUGS II: IMMUNOSUPPRESSANTS

At this time, only one immunosuppressant—mitoxantrone—is approved by the FDA for treating MS. Mitoxantrone, originally used for cancer, produces greater immunosuppression than the immunomodulators, but is also more toxic. In addition to mitoxantrone, several other anticancer/immunosuppressant drugs are employed in MS, although they are not FDA approved for this use.

Mitoxantrone

Mitoxantrone [Novantrone] was developed to treat cancer (see Chapter 102), and then later approved for MS. The drug poses a significant risk of toxicity, and hence is generally reserved for patients who cannot be treated with safer agents.

Therapeutic Use

Mitoxantrone is approved for decreasing neurologic disability and clinical relapses in patients with

- Worsening relapsing-remitting MS
- Secondary progressive MS
- Progressive-relapsing MS

For these patients, the drug may delay the time to relapse and the time to disability progression. In addition, it may decrease the number of new MRI-detectable lesions. Mitoxantrone is *not* effective against primary progressive MS.

Mechanism of Action

Mitoxantrone is a cytotoxic drug that binds with DNA and inhibits topoisomerase II. These actions inhibit DNA and RNA synthesis, and promote cross-linking and breakage of DNA strands. In cell culture, mitoxantrone is toxic to all cells, whether dividing or not. However, in clinical practice, the drug appears especially toxic to tissues with a high percentage of actively dividing cells (bone marrow, hair follicles, GI mucosa). In patients with MS, mitoxantrone suppresses production of immune system cells (B lymphocytes, T lymphocytes, and macrophages), and thereby decreases autoimmune destruction of myelin. Additional protection may derive from reducing antigen presentation and reducing production of cytokines (e.g., interleukin-2, tumor necrosis factor [TNF]–alpha, interferon gamma) that participate in the immune response.

Pharmacokinetics

Following IV infusion, mitoxantrone undergoes rapid, widespread distribution. Elimination occurs slowly, primarily by hepatic metabolism and biliary excretion. In patients with liver dysfunction, clearance of the drug is delayed, thereby increasing the risk of toxicity. Accordingly, mitoxantrone should not be given to patients with liver disease. To assess liver status, LFTs should be performed at baseline and before each infusion. If LFTs are abnormal, the drug should be withheld.

Adverse Effects

Mitoxantrone can cause a variety of adverse effects. Myelosuppression, cardiotoxicity, and fetal injury are the greatest concerns.

Myelosuppression. Toxicity to the bone marrow cells (myelosuppression) can decrease production of platelets and all blood cells. Loss of neutrophils, which is maximal 10 to 14 days after dosing, increases the risk of *severe infection.* Patients should be advised to avoid contact with people who have infections and to report signs of infection (fever, chills, cough, hoarseness) immediately. Also, patients should not be immunized with a live virus vaccine (because the vaccine itself could cause infection). To guide mitoxantrone use, CBCs should be obtained at baseline, before each infusion, 10 to 14 days after each infusion, and whenever signs of infection develop. The drug should be held and the prescriber notified if the neutrophil count falls below 1500 cells/mm^3.

Cardiotoxicity. Mitoxantrone can cause irreversible injury to the heart, manifesting as a reduced left ventricular ejection fraction (LVEF) or outright heart failure. Injury may become apparent during treatment or months to years after drug use has ceased. Cardiotoxicity is directly related to the cumulative lifetime dose. Risk increases significantly if the cumulative dose exceeds 140 mg/m^2, and hence the total should not exceed this amount. Mitoxantrone should not be given to patients with cardiac impairment. Accordingly, LVEF should be determined before the first dose; if the LVEF is less than 50%, mitoxantrone should be withheld. During treatment, LVEF should be measured before every dose and whenever signs of heart failure develop (e.g., peripheral edema, fatigue, shortness of breath).

Fetal Harm. Mitoxantrone has the potential for fetal harm. In animal studies, extremely low doses were associated with growth delay and premature delivery. To date, teratogenicity of mitoxantrone has not been proved. However, because mitoxantrone has the same mechanism as known teratogens, its teratogenicity can be inferred. Women of childbearing age should avoid becoming pregnant, and pregnancy should be ruled out before each dose. Additionally, mitoxantrone is excreted in breast milk. In fact, the drug has been detected in breast milk as long as 28 days after the last dose. Because it can cause serious adverse effects in infants, breast-feeding should be discontinued if this drug is prescribed.

Other Adverse Effects. Because mitoxantrone is especially toxic to tissues with a high percentage of dividing cells, it can cause reversible hair loss and injury to the GI mucosa, resulting in stomatitis and GI distress. The drug can also cause nausea, vomiting, menstrual irregularities (e.g., amenorrhea), and symptoms of allergy (itching, rash, hypotension, shortness of breath). In addition, mitoxantrone can impart a harmless, blue-green tint to the skin, sclera, and urine; patients should be forewarned. Very rarely, patients taking mitoxantrone for MS have developed acute myelogenous leukemia, although a causal relationship has not been established.

Monitoring

To minimize risk, we need to

- Perform CBCs at baseline, before each dose, and 10 to 14 days after each dose.
- Perform LFTs at baseline and before each dose.
- Perform a pregnancy test before each dose.
- Determine LVEF before each dose and whenever signs of heart failure develop.

Hazardous Agents Requiring Special Handling

Mitoxantrone is classified by the NIOSH as a hazardous drug that requires special handling by nurses and other healthcare workers. See Chapter 3, Table 3.1, for administration and handling guidelines.

Preparations, Dosage, and Administration

Mitoxantrone [Novantrone] is available in solution (2 mg/mL) in 10-, 12.5-, and 15-mL multiuse vials. For patients with MS, the dosage is 12 mg/m^2 every 3 months, infused IV over 5 to 30 minutes. The maximum lifetime cumulative dose is 140 mg/m^2. Before infusing, dilute each dose with at least 50 mL of normal saline or 5% dextrose in water; then administer into a free-flowing IV line. Extravasation can cause severe local injury. Accordingly, if extravasation occurs, discontinue the infusion immediately and restart in a different vein. Don't mix mitoxantrone with other drugs.

DRUGS USED TO MANAGE MS SYMPTOMS

MS is associated with an array of potentially debilitating symptoms. Accordingly, effective management is essential for maintaining productivity and quality of life. However, despite the importance of symptom management, the discussion that follows is brief because all of the drugs employed are discussed in other chapters. For more details on symptom management, the web site of the

National Multiple Sclerosis Society—www.nationalmssociety.org—is a good resource.

Bladder Dysfunction

Bladder dysfunction is very common, occurring in up to 90% of patients. The underlying cause is disruption of nerve traffic in areas of the CNS that control the bladder detrusor muscle and bladder sphincter. (Recall that coordinated contraction of the detrusor and relaxation of the sphincter are required for normal voiding.) Three types of bladder dysfunction may be seen: detrusor hyperreflexia, detrusor-sphincter dyssynergia, and flaccid bladder. All three can be successfully managed.

Detrusor hyperreflexia results from decreased inhibition of the bladder reflex and manifests as urinary frequency, urinary urgency, nocturia, and incontinence. Relief is accomplished with anticholinergic drugs, which relax the detrusor and thereby permit a normal volume of urine to accumulate before bladder emptying. Options include *tolterodine* [Detrol], *oxybutynin* [Ditropan, Oxytrol], *darifenacin* [Enablex], and *solifenacin* [VESIcare].

Detrusor-sphincter dyssynergia is characterized by a lack of synchronization between detrusor contraction and sphincter relaxation. The result is difficulty in initiating or stopping urination, and incomplete bladder emptying. Some patients respond to *alpha-adrenergic blocking agents,* such as phenoxybenzamine [Dibenzyline], tamsulosin [Flomax], or terazosin [Hytrin], all of which promote sphincter relaxation. However, most patients require intermittent or continuous catheterization.

In patients with *flaccid bladder,* there is a loss of reflex detrusor contraction, resulting in impaired bladder emptying. In some cases, the condition responds to *bethanechol* [Urecholine], a muscarinic agonist that directly stimulates the detrusor. However, as with detrusor-sphincter dyssynergia, many patients require intermittent or continuous catheterization.

Bowel Dysfunction

Constipation is relatively common, whereas fecal incontinence is relatively rare. Constipation can be managed by increasing dietary fiber and fluids, taking fiber supplements, performing regular exercise, and, if needed, using a bulk-forming laxative such as *psyllium* [Metamucil] and stool softeners such as docusate sodium [Colace]. Fecal incontinence can be managed by establishing a regular bowel routine and, if needed, using a bulk-forming laxative (to improve stool consistency) and/or using an anticholinergic agent (e.g., hyoscyamine) to reduce bowel motility. Be aware, however, that excessive slowing of bowel motility can produce constipation.

Fatigue

Fatigue develops in up to 90% of patients. The underlying cause is unknown. Regular exercise can help. The most common drug therapies are *amantadine* [Symmetrel] and *modafinil* [Provigil, Alertec 🍁]. Both are generally well tolerated. *Methylphenidate* [Ritalin] and *amphetamine mixture* [Adderall] are the next options. *Selective serotonin reuptake inhibitors* (SSRIs) can reduce fatigue, and hence are a good choice for patients who are also depressed.

Depression

Depression is seen in about 70% of MS patients. In these people, depression may be reactive—that is, it may be an emotional response to having a chronic, progressive, disabling disease—or it may be the result of MS-induced injury to neurons that help regulate mood. Depression can be treated with antidepressant drugs and with counseling. For drug therapy, the *SSRIs,* such as fluoxetine [Prozac] and sertraline [Zoloft], can elevate mood but often seem to increase fatigue. In contrast, *bupropion* [Wellbutrin], which has stimulant properties, can relieve depression and may help fight fatigue. The *tricyclic antidepressants,* such as amitriptyline and nortriptyline [Pamelor], can treat pain, sleep disturbances, and incontinence (owing to detrusor hyperreflexia) in addition to improving mood.

Cognitive Dysfunction

About 50% of people with MS experience cognitive dysfunction at some time in the course of the disease. Fortunately, only 5% to 10% experience dysfunction severe enough to significantly interfere with daily living. Memory impairment is the most common problem. Other problems include impaired concentration, reasoning, and problem solving. Cognitive impairment is caused in part by demyelination of CNS neurons and in part by depression, anxiety, stress, and fatigue. By protecting against demyelination, disease-modifying drugs can decrease the degree of cognitive loss. *Donepezil* [Aricept], a cholinesterase inhibitor developed for Alzheimer's disease, may offer modest benefits, as may *memantine* [Namenda], an *N*-methyl-D-aspartate receptor blocker developed for Alzheimer's disease (see Chapter 22).

Sexual Dysfunction

Among MS patients, sexual dysfunction may affect as many as 91% of men and 72% of women. Among men, erectile dysfunction is the most common complaint. Among women, complaints include vaginal dryness, reduced libido, and decreased vaginal and clitoral sensation. Possible causes of sexual dysfunction include depression, side effects of drugs, and injury to neurons of the lower spinal cord. Erectile dysfunction can be treated with *sildenafil* [Viagra], *vardenafil* [Levitra], and other inhibitors of phosphodiesterase type 5 (see Chapter 66). Vaginal dryness can be managed with a water-soluble personal lubricant (e.g., K-Y Jelly).

Neuropathic Pain

Neuropathic pain results from injury to neurons (in contrast to nociceptive pain, which results from injury to peripheral tissues). Neuropathic pain responds poorly to traditional analgesics, but often does respond to certain antiepileptic drugs and antidepressants. The antiepileptic drugs employed include *carbamazepine* [Tegretol], *gabapentin* [Neurontin], and *oxcarbazepine* [Trileptal]. The antidepressants employed, all from the tricyclic family, include *nortriptyline* [Pamelor], *imipramine* [Tofranil], and *amitriptyline.* Please note that pain relief with antidepressants occurs even in patients who are *not* depressed, and hence is not simply the result of elevating mood.

Ataxia and Tremor

Ataxia (loss of coordination) and tremor are relatively common and are often disabling. Unfortunately, they are also largely unresponsive to treatment. Drugs that may offer some relief include *clonazepam* [Klonopin], *primidone* [Mysoline], and *propranolol* [Inderal]. A physical therapist can provide gait training, and an occupational therapist can provide equipment to help maintain independence.

Spasticity

Spasticity can range in severity from mild muscle tightness to painful muscle spasms, usually in the legs. Clinically significant spasticity occurs in more than 40% of patients. Interestingly, spasticity can be beneficial for some patients: By making the legs more rigid, spasticity can facilitate standing and walking.

Spasticity can be managed with drug therapy and with nondrug measures (physical therapy, stretching, regular exercise). The drugs used most are *baclofen* [Lioresal] and *tizanidine* [Zanaflex]. However, dosage must be carefully controlled because high doses of either agent can exacerbate MS-related muscle weakness. Tizanidine causes less weakness than baclofen but poses a risk of liver injury, sedation, and dry mouth. Alternatives to baclofen and tizanidine include *diazepam* [Valium] and *botulinum toxin* [Botox]. Intrathecal infusion of baclofen is a very effective option but is also invasive. In 2014 the American Academy of Neurology published *Complementary and Alternative Medicine in Multiple Sclerosis.* In this evidence-based report, oral cannabis extract received a high (Level A) recommendation for the management of spasticity and non-neuropathic pain.

Dizziness and Vertigo

Dizziness and vertigo result from lesions in the CNS pathways that normally provide a sense of equilibrium. Both symptoms are relatively common and can be reduced with several drugs. Among these are *meclizine* [Antivert] (a drug for motion sickness) and *ondansetron* [Zofran] (a powerful antiemetic).

Dalfampridine to Improve Walking

Actions and Uses

In 2010, the FDA approved oral dalfampridine [Ampyra] to improve walking in patients with MS, making dalfampridine the first and only drug approved specifically to manage an MS symptom. All other drugs approved for MS are used to decrease relapse rates or to prevent accumulation of disability. In clinical trials, improvements in walking speed were modest: Only one-third of patients were able to walk faster, and the increase in speed was only 20%. Nonetheless, because impaired walking is one of the most common and debilitating sequelae of MS, any hope for improvement is welcome. How does dalfampridine work? The drug blocks potassium channels. Although the precise mechanism underlying clinical improvement is unclear, a good guess is that blockade of neuronal potassium channels reduces leakage of current from demyelinated axons, and thereby improves conduction.

Pharmacokinetics

Dalfampridine is absorbed rapidly and completely after oral dosing. With the extended-release formulation, plasma levels peak in 3 to 4 hours. Most of each dose is eliminated intact in the urine. Very little metabolism occurs. In patients with normal kidney function, or with mild renal impairment, the half-life is 6 hours. By contrast, in patients with severe renal impairment, the half-life increases to 19 hours.

Adverse Effects

The most common adverse effect is urinary tract infection. Between 5% and 10% of those taking dalfampridine experience insomnia, headache, dizziness, weakness, nausea, balance disorder, and back pain. Much more troubling, high doses (20 mg twice daily) pose a risk of *seizures*. Accordingly, dosage must not exceed 20 mg/day. Renal impairment can raise blood levels of dalfampridine and can thereby increase the risk of seizures.

Preparations, Dosage, and Administration

Dalfampridine [Ampyra] is supplied in 10-mg extended-release tablets for oral dosing, with or without food. Tablets must be swallowed intact, without dividing, crushing, or chewing. For patients with normal kidney function or with mild renal impairment, the recommended dosage is 10 mg every 12 hours. Patients with moderate or severe renal impairment should not use this drug.

KEY POINTS

- MS is a chronic inflammatory autoimmune disorder that damages the myelin sheath of neurons in the CNS. Because of demyelination, axonal conduction is slowed or blocked, giving rise to a host of sensory, motor, and cognitive deficits. When inflammation subsides, some degree of recovery occurs, at least in the early stage of the disease.
- In addition to stripping off myelin, inflammation may injure the underlying axon and may also injure nearby oligodendrocytes, the cells that make CNS myelin.
- What causes MS? There is general agreement that MS develops in genetically vulnerable people following exposure to an environmental or microbial factor that initiates autoimmune activity.
- There are four subtypes of MS: relapsing-remitting (the most common form), secondary progressive, primary progressive, and progressive-relapsing.
- In patients with MS, drugs are employed to (1) modify the disease process, (2) treat acute relapses, and (3) manage symptoms. We have no drugs to cure MS.
- Disease-modifying drugs can decrease the frequency and severity of relapses, reduce development of brain lesions, decrease future disability, and help maintain quality of life. In addition, they may prevent permanent damage to axons.
- There are two main groups of disease-modifying drugs: immunomodulators and immunosuppressants.
- The immunomodulators—interferon beta, dimethyl fumarate, glatiramer acetate, natalizumab, fingolimod, and teriflunomide—are safer than mitoxantrone (the only FDA-approved immunosuppressant for MS), and hence are generally preferred.
- All patients with relapsing-remitting MS should receive an immunomodulator—interferon beta, dimethyl fumarate, glatiramer acetate, natalizumab, fingolimod, or teriflunomide—beginning as soon as possible after diagnosis and continuing indefinitely.
- Interferon beta and glatiramer are administered by self-injection (IM or subQ) and dimethyl fumarate, fingolimod, and teriflunomide are administered PO. Natalizumab is administered by IV infusion in a specialized center.
- Interferon beta is generally well tolerated, although side effects—flu-like reactions, liver injury, myelosuppression, injection-site reactions—are relatively common.
- The most common side effect of dimethyl fumarate is flushing; the most serious adverse effect is lymphopenia, with a resulting increase in the risk of infections.
- Dimethyl fumarate can decrease the body's response to live virus vaccines; patients should not receive live virus vaccines when taking this drug.
- Glatiramer is less well tolerated than interferon beta, and requires more frequent injections.
- The most common side effects of glatiramer are injection-site reactions (pain, erythema, pruritus, induration), and the most disturbing side effect is brief but severe chest pain after the injection. Unlike interferon beta, glatiramer does not cause flu-like symptoms or myelosuppression.
- Fingolimod (as fingolimod phosphate) binds with sphingosine 1-phosphate receptors on lymphocytes, and thereby keeps them sequestered in lymph nodes. As a result, fewer lymphocytes enter the brain, and hence axonal damage from inflammation is reduced.
- Although effective, fingolimod can cause a host of adverse effects (e.g., bradycardia, infection, macular edema, liver injury, fetal harm).
- Natalizumab can cause progressive multifocal leukoencephalopathy (PML), a severe CNS infection caused by reactivation of the JC virus. To reduce the risk of PML, natalizumab must not be combined with other immunosuppressant drugs, must not be given to patients with HIV/AIDS and other conditions that compromise cell-mediated immunity, and must be used in accord with the TOUCH Prescribing Program.
- Teriflunomide has a very long half-life of approximately 2.5 to 3 weeks and may be detectable in the serum as long as 2 years after cessation of therapy.
- Teriflunomide can cause serious birth defects if taken by pregnant women, and birth defects may occur if a woman is impregnated by a man who is taking teriflunomide.
- Patients taking teriflunomide should not take leflunomide as this combination has resulted in conditions that have been fatal.
- Patients taking teriflunomide should avoid live virus vaccines.
- Mitoxantrone is the only immunosuppressant currently approved for MS.

Continued

- Mitoxantrone suppresses immune function more strongly than the immunomodulators, but is also more toxic. Accordingly, the drug is generally reserved for patients who are unresponsive to, or intolerant of, an immunomodulator.
- In patients with MS, mitoxantrone suppresses production of immune system cells and thereby decreases autoimmune destruction of myelin.
- The major side effects of mitoxantrone are myelosuppression, cardiotoxicity, and fetal injury.
- The risk of cardiotoxicity from mitoxantrone increases significantly if the lifetime cumulative dose exceeds 140 mg/m^2, and hence the total dose should not exceed this amount.
- A short course of high-dose IV glucocorticoids (e.g., methylprednisolone) is the preferred treatment for an acute MS relapse. Intravenous gamma globulin is an option.

Please visit **http://evolve.elsevier.com/Lehne** for chapter-specific NCLEX® examination review questions.

Summary of Major Nursing Implications[a]

INTERFERON BETA

Interferon beta-1a [Avonex, Rebif]
Interferon beta-1b [Betaseron, Extavia]

Preadministration Assessment

Therapeutic Goal

All preparations of beta interferon are used to decrease the frequency and severity of relapses and slow disease progression in patients with relapsing forms of MS. In addition, *interferon beta-1b* [Betaseron, Extavia] is used to treat secondary progressive MS.

Baseline Data

Obtain baseline LFTs and CBC.

Identifying High-Risk Patients

Exercise caution in patients who abuse alcohol, in those with active liver disease or a history of liver disease, and in those taking drugs that can cause liver injury or suppress the bone marrow.

Implementation: Administration

Routes

Intramuscular. Avonex (interferon beta-1a).

Subcutaneous. Rebif (interferon beta-1a); Betaseron and Extavia (interferon beta-1b).

Administration

For all four formulations of interferon beta, instruct patients to store the drug under refrigeration, teach them how to self-inject, and advise them to rotate the injection site.

Avonex. **Instruct patients to inject Avonex IM once a week.**

Rebif. **Instruct patients to inject Rebif subQ 3 times a week, preferably in the late afternoon or evening, at least 48 hours apart, and on the same days each week (e.g., Monday, Wednesday, Friday).**

Betaseron and Extavia. **Instruct patients to reconstitute powdered Betaseron and Extavia just before use and to inject them subQ every other day.**

Ongoing Evaluation and Interventions

Evaluating Therapeutic Effects

Indices of success include a reduction in the frequency and intensity of relapses, a reduction in new MRI-detectable lesions, and improvement in the EDSS score.

Minimizing Adverse Effects

Flu-like Reactions. Flu-like reactions—headache, fever, chills, malaise, muscle aches, stiffness—are common early in therapy, but later diminish. To minimize symptoms, begin therapy with low doses, and then slowly titrate to full doses. **Inform patients that symptoms can be reduced by taking an analgesic-antipyretic medication (i.e., acetaminophen, ibuprofen, or another nonsteroidal anti-inflammatory drug).**

Hepatotoxicity. Interferon beta can cause liver injury. To monitor for hepatotoxicity, obtain LFTs at baseline, 1 month later, then every 3 months for 1 year, and every 6 months thereafter. If LFTs indicate significant injury, interferon should be given in reduced dosage or discontinued. When liver function returns to normal, treatment can resume with careful monitoring.

Myelosuppression. Interferon beta can decrease production of all blood cell types. To monitor for myelosuppression, obtain CBCs at baseline, every 3 months for 1 year, and every 6 months thereafter.

Injection-Site Reactions. Subcutaneous injection (of Rebif, Betaseron, or Extavia) can cause pain, erythema, maculopapular or vesicular rash, and itching. **Inform patients that they can reduce discomfort by physical measures—rotating the injection site, applying ice (briefly) before and after the injection, and applying a warm, moist compress—and that they can reduce persistent itching and erythema with oral diphenhydramine [Benadryl] or topical hydrocortisone. Instruct patients to avoid continuous exposure to topical hydrocortisone, owing to a risk of skin damage.**

Forewarn patients that IM injection (of Avonex) can cause discomfort and bruising.

Minimizing Adverse Interactions

Hepatotoxic and Myelosuppressant Drugs. Exercise caution when combining interferon beta with other drugs that can suppress the bone marrow or cause liver injury.

Summary of Major Nursing Implications[a]—cont'd

DIMETHYL FUMARATE

Preadministration Assessment

Therapeutic Goal

The goal is to decrease the frequency and severity of relapses and to slow disease progression in patients with relapsing forms of MS.

Baseline Data

Obtain LFTs, a CBC, and urinalysis.

Identifying High-Risk Patients

DMF should be avoided in patients with active infection. Use DMF with caution in patients taking immunosuppressants and other immunomodulators. Animal studies have demonstrated risks in the development and behavior of offspring; therefore, it is important to weigh risks and benefits carefully before prescribing this drug to a pregnant woman.

Implementation: Administration

Route

Oral.

Administration

Instruct patients that DMF can be taken with or without food but that it must be swallowed intact.

Ongoing Evaluation and Interventions

Evaluating Therapeutic Effects

Indices of success include a reduction in the frequency and intensity of relapses, a reduction in new MRI-detectable lesions, and improvement in the EDSS score.

Monitoring

Obtain a CBC if signs or symptoms of infection occur; otherwise, monitor for lymphopenia and other hematologic changes with an annual CBC. Obtain LFTs whenever signs or symptoms of liver injury appear. Conduct a urinalysis yearly to monitor for proteinuria.

Minimizing Adverse Effects

Flushing. Discomfort related to flushing may be helped by administering a non–enteric-coated aspirin 30 minutes before administration. Flushing may also be decreased by taking the drug with food. In some cases, the prescriber may elect to decrease the dosage temporarily.

Liver Injury. DMF has the potential to injure the liver. **Inform patients about signs of liver injury (nausea, vomiting, anorexia, stomach pain, fatigue, dark urine, jaundice), and instruct them to tell the prescriber if these develop.**

Infection. DMF increases the risk of infection. Do not start DMF in patients with an active infection. **Inform patients about signs of infection (fever, fatigue, chills, body aches), and instruct them to contact the prescriber if these develop.** If a serious infection is diagnosed, interruption of treatment should be considered.

Drugs That Suppress Immune Function. Combining DMF with an immunosuppressant, another immunomodulator, or other drugs that depress immune responses will cause more immunosuppression than when DMF is used alone. **Inform patients about the increased risk of infection.**

Vaccines. DMF can increase the risk of infection from live virus vaccines. **Instruct patients to avoid live virus vaccines while taking DMF.**

GLATIRAMER ACETATE

Preadministration Assessment

Therapeutic Goal

The goal is to decrease the frequency and severity of relapses and to slow disease progression in patients with relapsing-remitting MS.

Implementation: Administration

Route

Subcutaneous.

Administration

Teach patients how to self-inject the drug (subQ) into the arm, abdomen, hip, or thigh. Advise patients to store glatiramer under refrigeration at 36°F to 46°F (2°C to 8°C).

Ongoing Evaluation and Interventions

Evaluating Therapeutic Effects

Indices of success include a reduction in the frequency and intensity of relapses, a reduction in new MRI-detectable lesions, and improvement in the EDSS score.

Minimizing Adverse Effects

Injection-Site Reactions. **Forewarn patients that glatiramer may cause pain, erythema, pruritus, and induration at the injection site.**

Immediate Postinjection Reaction. **Forewarn patients that glatiramer may cause an uncomfortable and disturbing set of systemic symptoms—flushing, palpitations, chest pain, anxiety, laryngeal constriction, urticaria—that may persist for 15 to 20 minutes after the injection. No specific intervention is needed.**

NATALIZUMAB

Preadministration Assessment

Therapeutic Goal

Natalizumab is used to either (1) decrease the frequency and severity of relapses and slow disease progression in patients with relapsing forms of MS who have failed to respond to at least one other immunomodulating drug or (2) treat patients with moderate to severe Crohn's disease who have been unresponsive to or intolerant of other therapies, including inhibitors of TNF-alpha.

Baseline Data

Obtain an MRI scan of the brain at baseline and every 6 months thereafter. Obtain a baseline evaluation for PML.

Continued

Summary of Major Nursing Implications[a]—cont'd

Identifying High-Risk Patients

Natalizumab is *contraindicated* for patients with PML, for patients taking immunosuppressive drugs, and for patients with HIV/AIDS and other conditions that compromise cell-mediated immunity.

Implementation: Administration

Route

Intravenous.

Administration

Dilute concentrated natalizumab in 100 mL of 0.9% sodium chloride injection and infuse over a 1-hour span. If any signs of hypersensitivity develop, stop the infusion immediately.

Ongoing Evaluation and Interventions

Evaluating Therapeutic Effects

Indices of success include a reduction in the frequency and intensity of relapses, a reduction in new MRI-detectable lesions, and improvement in the EDSS score.

Minimizing Adverse Effects

Progressive Multifocal Leukoencephalopathy. Natalizumab increases the risk of PML, a severe infection of the CNS with no effective treatment. To reduce the risk of PML, do not give natalizumab to patients taking immunosuppressants or to patients with HIV/AIDS and other conditions that compromise cell-mediated immunity. Screen for PML before each infusion. **Inform patients about symptoms of PML (e.g., progressive weakness on one side of the body; clumsiness of the limbs; disturbed vision; changes in thinking, memory, and orientation), and instruct them to report these immediately.** All patients, prescribers, infusion nurses, infusion centers, and pharmacies associated with infusion centers must register with the *TOUCH Prescribing Program* and must comply with its provisions.

Hepatotoxicity. Natalizumab can injure the liver. **Inform patients about signs of liver injury—jaundice, nausea, vomiting, fatigue, darkening of the urine—and instruct them to report these immediately.** Discontinue natalizumab if significant liver injury is diagnosed.

Hypersensitivity Reactions. Natalizumab can cause severe hypersensitivity reactions (e.g., anaphylaxis), usually within 2 hours of starting the infusion. Monitor patients for a reaction during the infusion and for 1 hour after. If a severe reaction develops, discontinue natalizumab and never use it again.

Drug Interactions

Immunosuppressants (e.g., mitoxantrone, azathioprine, methotrexate, cyclophosphamide) increase the risk of PML and other opportunistic infections, and hence should be discontinued at least 3 months before starting natalizumab.

FINGOLIMOD

Preadministration Assessment

Therapeutic Goal

The goal is to decrease the frequency and severity of relapses and to slow disease progression in patients with relapsing forms of MS.

Baseline Data

Obtain a pregnancy test, LFTs, CBC, ophthalmologic examination, and a test for VZV antibodies. Obtain an ECG for patients with cardiac risk factors.

Identifying High-Risk Patients

Fingolimod is *contraindicated* during pregnancy and in patients with active infection. Use fingolimod with *caution* in patients with diabetes, uveitis, heart failure, ischemic heart diseases, or bradycardia, and in those taking ketoconazole, immunosuppressants, immunomodulators, anticancer drugs, beta blockers, verapamil, diltiazem, class IA antidysrhythmics, and class III antidysrhythmics.

Implementation: Administration

Route

Oral.

Administration

Instruct patients to take fingolimod once daily, with or without food.

Ongoing Evaluation and Interventions

Evaluating Therapeutic Effects

Indices of success include a reduction in the frequency and intensity of relapses, a reduction in new MRI-detectable lesions, and improvement in the EDSS score.

Monitoring

Obtain an ophthalmologic examination at baseline, 3 to 4 months after starting treatment, and whenever there is a change in vision.

Obtain LFTs at baseline and whenever signs of liver injury appear.

Minimizing Adverse Effects

Bradycardia. Fingolimod reduces heart rate, especially after the first dose. Symptoms include dizziness, fatigue, palpitations, and chest pain, all of which resolve within 24 hours. **Inform patients that, after receiving the first dose, they must be observed in the provider's office for 6 hours.** For patients who develop symptoms, heart rate can be increased with atropine or isoproterenol. **Inform patients that the risk of bradycardia will return if treatment is interrupted for 2 weeks or longer, and hence observation for 6 hours will be needed when they first resume treatment.**

Summary of Major Nursing Implications[a]—cont'd

Patients at risk for bradycardia include those with heart failure, ischemic heart disease, or pre-existing bradycardia, and those taking certain antidysrhythmic drugs, especially beta blockers and two of the calcium channel blockers: verapamil and diltiazem. Obtain an ECG for these people if a recent ECG is unavailable.

Macular Edema. Fingolimod can cause macular edema. Risk is increased by diabetes and uveitis. To monitor for macular edema, patients should undergo an ophthalmologic examination at baseline, 3 to 4 months after starting treatment, and whenever their vision changes. **Instruct patients to inform the prescriber if they experience vision problems (blurriness, shadows, sensitivity to light, altered color vision, blind spot in the center of the visual field).**

Liver Injury. Fingolimod can injure the liver. LFTs should be performed at baseline and whenever signs of liver injury appear. **Inform patients about signs of liver injury (nausea, vomiting, anorexia, stomach pain, fatigue, dark urine, jaundice), and instruct them to tell the prescriber if these develop.** If LFTs confirm significant liver damage, fingolimod should be discontinued.

Infection. Fingolimod increases the risk of infection during treatment and for 2 months after stopping. **Instruct patients to avoid live virus vaccines during this time.** Do not start fingolimod in patients with an active infection. **Inform patients about signs of infection (fever, fatigue, chills, body aches), and instruct them to contact the prescriber if these develop.** If a serious infection is diagnosed, interruption of treatment should be considered.

Patients who have not had chickenpox (VZV infection) and have not received VZV vaccine should be tested for VZV antibodies before starting treatment. Give antibody-negative patients VZV vaccine, and start fingolimod 1 month later.

Fetal Harm. Fingolimod is teratogenic and lethal to embryos. **Inform women of childbearing age about the risk of fetal harm, and instruct them to use two effective forms of contraception, both during treatment and for 2 months after stopping.**

Use During Breast-feeding. Fingolimod is excreted in the milk of rats and probably in the milk of humans. **Inform patients about the potential risks to the infant, and advise them to avoid breast-feeding while using fingolimod and for some time after stopping.**

Reduced Lung Function. Fingolimod can cause a dose-dependent decrease in lung function. **Advise patients to inform the prescriber if they experience new or worsening dyspnea.**

Minimizing Adverse Interactions

Ketoconazole. Ketoconazole inhibits some CYP isoenzymes, and can thereby greatly increase fingolimod levels. Monitor patients closely for fingolimod toxicity.

Cardiac Drugs. Drugs that slow heart rate (e.g., beta blockers, verapamil, diltiazem) can intensify fingolimod-induced bradycardia. Monitor these patients closely.

Combining fingolimod with a class IA antidysrhythmic drug (e.g., quinidine, procainamide, disopyramide) or a class III antidysrhythmic drug (amiodarone, sotalol) may increase the risk of torsades de pointes, a potentially fatal dysrhythmia. Monitor these patients closely.

Drugs That Suppress Immune Function. Combining fingolimod with an immunosuppressant, certain anticancer drugs, or another immunomodulator will cause more immunosuppression than when fingolimod is used alone. **Inform patients about the increased risk of infection.**

Vaccines. Fingolimod can reduce the immune response to all vaccines and can increase the risk of infection from live virus vaccines. **Advise patients to avoid vaccines while using fingolimod or for 2 months after stopping.**

TERIFLUNOMIDE

Preadministration Assessment

Therapeutic Goal

The goal is to decrease the frequency and severity of relapses and to slow disease progression in patients with relapsing forms of MS.

Baseline Data

Obtain a CBC and electrolyte, hepatic enzyme, serum creatinine, and bilirubin levels.

Identifying High-Risk Patients

Teriflunomide should be avoided in patients with active infection. Use cautiously in patients taking immunosuppressants and other immunomodulators. It is *contraindicated* in patients who have severe hepatic impairment. It should not be administered to women who are pregnant or who are at an increased risk of becoming pregnant due to poor adherence to reliable contraception methods. Women who have taken this drug should not become pregnant within 2 years of stopping the drug. Because it is stored in sperm, it should not be administered to men who are not willing to take responsibility to prevent pregnancy in female partners.

Implementation: Administration

Route

Oral.

Administration

Instruct patients that teriflunomide should be taken every day. It may be taken with or without food.

Ongoing Evaluation and Interventions

Evaluating Therapeutic Effects

Indices of success include a reduction in the frequency and intensity of relapses, a reduction in new MRI-detectable lesions, and improvement in the EDSS score.

Monitoring

A baseline CBC and electrolyte, hepatic enzyme, serum creatinine, and bilirubin levels should be established before initiation of therapy; then values should be checked twice a year.

Continued

Summary of Major Nursing Implications[a]—cont'd

Minimizing Adverse Effects

Liver Injury. Teriflunomide has the potential to injure the liver. **Inform patients about signs of liver injury (nausea, vomiting, anorexia, stomach pain, fatigue, dark urine, jaundice), and instruct them to tell the prescriber if these develop.**

Infection. Teriflunomide increases the risk of infection. It should not be started if the patient has an active infection. **Inform patients to avoid contact with people with infections and take care when in places where people who are ill are likely to congregate, such as medical clinics or emergency departments. Inform patients about signs of infection (fever, fatigue, chills, body aches), and instruct them to contact the prescriber if these develop.** If a serious infection is diagnosed, interruption of treatment should be considered.

Drugs That Suppress Immune Function. Combining teriflunomide with an immunosuppressant, another immunomodulator, or other drugs that depress immune responses will cause more immunosuppression than when it is used alone. **Inform patients about the increased risk of infection.**

Vaccines. Teriflunomide can increase the risk of infection from live virus vaccines. **Instruct patients to avoid live virus vaccines while taking this drug.**

Fetal Harm. Teriflunomide can cause birth defects. **It is essential to advise men and women who want to have children to stop taking the drug and continue to use birth control until serum drug levels are low enough to be safe.** Because it may take up to 2 years to reach desired levels, bile acid sequestrants and activated charcoal may be administered to decrease serum levels of teriflunomide.

MITOXANTRONE

Preadministration Assessment

Therapeutic Goal

The goal is to decrease the frequency and severity of relapses and to slow disease progression in patients with secondary progressive MS, progressive-relapsing MS, and worsening relapsing-remitting MS.

Baseline Data

Obtain a pregnancy test, LFTs, CBC, and LVEF determination.

Identifying High-Risk Patients

Mitoxantrone is *contraindicated* during pregnancy and for patients with abnormal LFTs or an LVEF below 50%.

Implementation: Administration

Route

Intravenous.

Administration

Infuse over 5 to 30 minutes through a free-flowing IV line. If extravasation occurs, discontinue the infusion immediately and restart in a different vein. Don't mix mitoxantrone with other drugs.

Ongoing Evaluation and Interventions

Evaluating Therapeutic Effects

Indices of success include a reduction in the frequency and intensity of relapses, a reduction in new MRI-detectable lesions, and improvement in the EDSS score.

Monitoring

Perform CBCs before each dose, 10 to 14 days after each dose, and whenever signs of infection develop.

Perform LFTs before each dose.

Perform a pregnancy test before each dose.

Determine LVEF before each dose and whenever signs of heart failure develop.

Minimizing Adverse Effects

Myelosuppression. Mitoxantrone can decrease production of platelets and all blood cells. Neutrophil loss increases the risk of severe infection, and hence the drug should be withheld if the neutrophil count drops below 1500 cells/mm^3. **Advise patients to avoid contact with people who have infections, and instruct them to report signs of infection (fever, chills, cough, hoarseness) immediately.** Do not give patients a live virus vaccine.

Cardiotoxicity. Mitoxantrone can cause irreversible injury to the heart, manifesting as a reduced LVEF or outright heart failure. Cardiotoxicity is directly related to the cumulative lifetime dose, which must not exceed 140 mg/m^2. Withhold mitoxantrone if the LVEF drops below 50%. **Inform patients about symptoms of heart failure (e.g., shortness of breath, fatigue, peripheral edema), and instruct them to report these immediately.**

Fetal Harm. Mitoxantrone must not be used during pregnancy. Rule out pregnancy before each infusion. Warn women of childbearing age to avoid pregnancy. If pregnancy occurs, offer counseling about possible pregnancy termination.

Urine and Tissue Discoloration. **Warn patients that mitoxantrone can impart a harmless, blue-green tint to the urine, skin, and sclera.**

[a]Patient education information is highlighted as **blue text.**

CHAPTER

24 Drugs for Seizure Disorders

The term *epilepsy* refers to a group of chronic neurologic disorders characterized by recurrent seizures, brought on by excessive excitability of neurons in the brain. Symptoms can range from brief periods of unconsciousness to violent convulsions. Patients may also experience problems with learning, memory, and mood, which can be just as troubling as their seizures.

In the United States, about 2.9 million people have epilepsy, according to the Centers for Disease Control and Prevention. Every year, about 150,000 new cases are diagnosed. The incidence is highest in the very young and in older adults. Between 60% and 70% of patients can be rendered seizure-free with drugs. Unfortunately, this means that 30% to 40% cannot. The total direct and indirect costs of epilepsy are estimated at $15.5 billion a year.

The terms *seizure* and *convulsion* are not synonymous. *Seizure* is a general term that applies to all types of epileptic events. In contrast, *convulsion* has a more limited meaning, applying only to abnormal motor phenomena, for example, the jerking movements that occur during a tonic-clonic attack. Accordingly, although all convulsions may be called seizures, it is not correct to call all seizures convulsions. Absence seizures, for example, manifest as brief periods of unconsciousness, which may or may not be accompanied by involuntary movements. Because not all epileptic seizures involve convulsions, we will refer to the agents used to treat epilepsy as *antiepileptic drugs* (AEDs), rather than anticonvulsants.

SEIZURE GENERATION

Seizures are initiated by synchronous, high-frequency discharge from a group of hyperexcitable neurons, called a *focus*. A focus may result from several causes, including congenital defects, hypoxia at birth, head trauma, brain infection, stroke, cancer, and genetic disorders. Seizures occur when discharge from a focus spreads to other brain areas, thereby recruiting normal neurons to discharge abnormally. The overt manifestations of any particular seizure disorder depend on the location of the seizure focus and the neuronal connections to that focus. The connections to the focus determine the brain areas to which seizure activity can spread.

TYPES OF SEIZURES

Seizure can be divided into two broad categories: *partial (focal) seizures* and *generalized seizures.* In partial seizures, seizure activity undergoes a very limited spread to adjacent cortical areas beyond the focus. In generalized seizures, focal seizure activity is conducted widely throughout both hemispheres. As a rule, partial seizures and generalized seizures are treated with different drugs; however, there are some exceptions. (Table 24.1).

Partial Seizures

Partial seizures fall into three groups: simple partial seizures, complex partial seizures, and partial seizures that evolve into secondarily generalized seizures.

Simple Partial Seizures

These seizures manifest with discrete symptoms that are determined by the brain region involved. Hence, the patient may experience discrete motor symptoms (e.g., twitching thumb), sensory symptoms (e.g., local numbness; auditory, visual, or olfactory hallucinations), autonomic symptoms (e.g., nausea, flushing, salivation, urinary incontinence), or psychoillusory symptoms (e.g., feelings of unreality, fear, or depression). Simple partial seizures are distinguished from complex partial seizures in that there is *no loss of consciousness.* These seizures persist for 20 to 60 seconds.

Complex Partial Seizures

These seizures are characterized by *impaired consciousness* and lack of responsiveness. At seizure onset, the patient becomes motionless and stares with a fixed gaze. This state is followed by a period of *automatism,* in which the patient performs repetitive, purposeless movements, such as lip smacking or hand wringing. Seizures last 45 to 90 seconds.

Secondarily Generalized Seizures

These seizures begin as simple or complex partial seizures, and then evolve into generalized tonic-clonic seizures. Consciousness is lost. These seizures last 1 to 2 minutes.

TABLE 24.1 ■ Drugs for Specific Types of Seizures

Seizure Type	Drugs Used for Treatment: Traditional AEDs	Drugs Used for Treatment: Newer AEDs
PARTIAL		
Simple partial, complex partial, and secondarily generalized	Carbamazepine Fosphenytoin Phenobarbital Phenytoin Primidone Valproic acid	Eslicarbazepine Ezogabine Felbamate Gabapentin Lacosamide Lamotrigine Levetiracetam Oxcarbazepine Perampanel Pregabalin Tiagabine Topiramate Vigabatrin Zonisamide
PRIMARY GENERALIZED		
Tonic-clonic	Carbamazepine Fosphenytoin Phenobarbital Phenytoin Primidone Valproic acid	Lamotrigine Levetiracetam Perampanel Topiramate
Absence	Ethosuximide Valproic acid	Lamotrigine
Myoclonic	Valproic acid	Lamotrigine Levetiracetam Topiramate

AEDs, Antiepileptic drugs.

Generalized Seizures

Generalized seizures may be convulsive or nonconvulsive. As a rule, they produce immediate loss of consciousness. The major generalized seizures are discussed briefly in the sections that follow.

Tonic-Clonic Seizures

In tonic-clonic seizures (formerly known as grand mal seizures), neuronal discharge spreads throughout both hemispheres of the cerebral cortex. These seizures manifest as major convulsions, characterized by a period of muscle rigidity (tonic phase) followed by synchronous muscle jerks (clonic phase). Tonic-clonic seizures often cause urination, but not defecation. Convulsions may be preceded by a loud cry, caused by forceful expiration of air across the vocal cords. Tonic-clonic seizures are accompanied by marked impairment of consciousness and are followed by a period of central nervous system (CNS) depression, referred to as the *postictal state.* The seizure itself typically lasts 90 seconds or less.

Absence Seizures (Petit Mal)

Absence seizures are characterized by loss of consciousness for a brief time (10 to 30 seconds). Seizures usually involve mild, symmetric motor activity (e.g., eye blinking) but may occur with no motor activity at all. The patient may experience hundreds of absence attacks a day. Absence seizures occur primarily in children and usually cease during the early teen years.

Atonic Seizures

These seizures are characterized by sudden loss of muscle tone. If seizure activity is limited to the muscles of the neck, "head drop" occurs. However, if the muscles of the limbs and trunk are involved, a "drop attack" can occur, causing the patient to suddenly collapse. Atonic seizures occur mainly in children.

Myoclonic Seizures

These seizures consist of sudden muscle contraction that lasts for just 1 second. Seizure activity may be limited to one limb (focal myoclonus), or it may involve the entire body (massive myoclonus).

Status Epilepticus

Status epilepticus (SE) is defined as a seizure that persists for 15 to 30 minutes or longer or a series of recurrent seizures during which the patient does not regain consciousness. There are several types of SE, including generalized convulsive SE, absence SE, and myoclonic SE. Generalized convulsive SE, which can be life threatening, is discussed later in this chapter.

Febrile Seizures

Fever-associated seizures are common among children ages 6 months to 5 years. Febrile seizures typically manifest as generalized tonic-clonic convulsions of short duration. Children who experience these seizures are *not* at high risk of developing epilepsy later in life.

Mixed Seizures: Lennox-Gastaut Syndrome

Lennox-Gastaut syndrome is a severe form of epilepsy that usually develops during the preschool years. The syndrome is characterized by developmental delay and a mixture of partial and generalized seizures. Seizure types include partial, atonic, tonic, generalized tonic-clonic, and atypical absence. In children with Lennox-Gastaut syndrome, seizures can be very difficult to manage.

HOW ANTIEPILEPTIC DRUGS WORK

We have long known that AEDs can (1) suppress discharge of neurons within a seizure focus and (2) suppress propagation of seizure activity from the focus to other areas of the brain. However, until recently we didn't know how these effects were achieved. It now appears that nearly all AEDs act through five basic mechanisms: suppression of sodium influx, suppression of calcium influx, promotion of potassium efflux, blockade of receptors for glutamate, and potentiation or increase of gamma-aminobutyric acid (GABA). Categorization of AEDs by mechanism of action, where known, is displayed in Table 24.1.

Suppression of Sodium Influx

Before discussing AED actions, we need to review sodium channel physiology. Neuronal action potentials are propagated by influx of sodium through sodium channels, which are gated pores in the cell membrane that control sodium entry. For sodium influx to occur, the channel must be in an *activated state.* Immediately following sodium entry, the channel goes into an *inactivated state,* during which further sodium entry is prevented. Under normal circumstances, the inactive channel very quickly returns to the activated state, thereby permitting more sodium entry and propagation of another action potential.

Several AEDs, including phenytoin, carbamazepine, and lamotrigine, reversibly bind to sodium channels while they are in the inactivated state, and thereby prolong channel inactivation. By delaying return to the active state, these drugs decrease the ability of neurons to fire at high frequency. As a result, seizures that depend on high-frequency discharge are suppressed.

Suppression of Calcium Influx

In axon terminals, influx of calcium through voltage-gated calcium channels promotes transmitter release. Hence, drugs that block these calcium channels can suppress transmission. Ethosuximide acts by this mechanism.

Promotion of Potassium Efflux

During an action potential, influx of sodium causes neurons to depolarize, and then efflux of potassium causes neurons to repolarize. One AED—ezogabine—acts on voltage-gated potassium channels to facilitate potassium efflux. This action is believed to underlie the drug's ability to slow repetitive neuronal firing and thereby provide seizure control.

Antagonism of Glutamate

Glutamic acid (glutamate) is the primary excitatory transmitter in the CNS. The compound works through two receptors, known as (1) NMDA receptors (*N*-methyl-D-aspartate receptors) and (2) AMPA receptors (alpha-amino-3-hydroxy-5-methyl-4-isoxazole propionic acid receptors). Perampanel is an AMPA glutamate receptor antagonist. Two other drugs—felbamate and topiramate—block the actions of glutamate at NMDA receptors, and thereby suppress neuronal excitation.

Potentiation of GABA

Several AEDs potentiate the actions of GABA, an inhibitory neurotransmitter that is widely distributed throughout the brain. By augmenting the inhibitory influence of GABA, these drugs decrease neuronal excitability and thereby suppress seizure activity. Drugs increase the influence of GABA by several mechanisms. Benzodiazepines and barbiturates enhance the effects of GABA by mechanisms that involve direct binding to GABA receptors. Gabapentin promotes GABA release. Tiagabine inhibits GABA reuptake, and vigabatrin inhibits the enzyme that degrades GABA, and thereby increases GABA availability.

BASIC THERAPEUTIC CONSIDERATIONS

Therapeutic Goal and Treatment Options

The goal in treating epilepsy is to reduce seizures to an extent that enables the patient to live a normal or near-normal life. Ideally, treatment should eliminate seizures entirely. However, this may not be possible without causing intolerable side effects. Therefore, we must balance the desire for complete seizure control against the acceptability of side effects.

Epilepsy may be treated with drugs or with nondrug therapies. As noted, drugs can benefit from 60% to 70% of patients. This means that, of the 2.9 million Americans with epilepsy, between 870,000 and 1.16 million *cannot* be treated successfully with drugs. For these people, nondrug therapy may well help. Three options exist: neurosurgery, vagus nerve stimulation, and the ketogenic diet. Of the three, neurosurgery has the best success rate, but vagus nerve stimulation is used most widely.

Diagnosis and Drug Selection

Control of seizures requires proper drug selection. As indicated in Table 24.1, many AEDs are selective for specific seizure disorders. Phenytoin, for example, is useful for treating tonic-clonic and partial seizures but not absence seizures. Conversely, ethosuximide is active against absence seizures but not against tonic-clonic or partial seizures. Only one drug—valproic acid—appears effective against practically all forms of epilepsy. Because most AEDs are selective for certain seizure disorders, effective treatment requires a proper match between the drug and the seizure. To make this match, the seizure type must be accurately diagnosed.

Making a diagnosis requires physical, neurologic, and laboratory evaluations along with a thorough history. The history should determine the age at which seizures began, the frequency and duration of seizure events, precipitating factors, and times when seizures occur. Physical and neurologic evaluations may reveal signs of head injury or other disorders that could underlie seizure activity, although in many patients the physical and neurologic evaluations may be normal. An electroencephalogram is essential for diagnosis. Other diagnostic tests that may be employed include computed tomography, positron emission tomography, and magnetic resonance imaging.

Pharmacologic management with AEDs is highly individualized. Very often, patients must try several AEDs before a regimen that is both effective and well tolerated can be established. Initial treatment should be done with just one AED. If this drug fails, it should be discontinued and a different AED should be tried. If this second drug fails, two options are open: (1) treatment with a third AED alone, or (2) treatment with a combination of AEDs.

Drug Evaluation

Once an AED has been selected, a trial period is needed to determine its effectiveness. During this time there is no guarantee that seizures will be controlled. Until seizure control is certain, the patient should be warned not to participate in driving and other activities that could be hazardous should a seizure occur.

During the process of drug evaluation, adjustments in dosage are often needed. No drug should be considered ineffective until it has been tested in sufficiently high dosages and for a reasonable time. Knowledge of plasma drug levels can be a valuable tool for establishing dosage and evaluating the effectiveness of a specific drug.

Maintenance of a seizure frequency chart is important. The chart should be kept by the patient or a family member and should contain a complete record of all seizure events. This record will enable the prescriber to determine whether treatment has been effective. The nurse should teach the patient how to create and use a seizure frequency chart.

Monitoring Plasma Drug Levels

Monitoring plasma levels of AEDs is common. Safe and effective levels have been firmly established for most AEDs (Table 24.2). Monitoring these levels can help guide dosage adjustments.

Monitoring plasma drug levels is especially helpful when treating major convulsive disorders (e.g., tonic-clonic seizures). Because these seizures can be dangerous and because delay of therapy may allow the condition to worsen, rapid control of seizures is desirable. However, because these seizures occur infrequently, a long time may be needed to establish control if clinical outcome is relied on as the only means of determining an effective dosage. By adjusting initial doses on the basis of plasma drug levels (rather than on the basis of seizure control), we can readily achieve drug levels that are likely to be effective, thereby increasing our chances of establishing control quickly.

Measurements of plasma drug levels are less important for determining effective dosages for absence seizures. Because absence seizures occur very frequently (up to several hundred a day), observation of the patient is the best means for establishing an effective dosage: if seizures stop, dosage is sufficient; if seizures continue, more drug is needed.

In addition to serving as a guide for dosage adjustment, knowledge of plasma drug levels can serve as an aid to (1) monitoring patient adherence, (2) determining the cause of lost seizure control, and (3) identifying causes of toxicity, especially in patients taking more than one drug.

Promoting Patient Adherence

Epilepsy is a chronic condition that requires regular and continuous therapy. As a result, seizure control is highly dependent on patient adherence. In fact, it is estimated that nonadherence accounts for about 50% of all treatment failures. Accordingly, promoting adherence should be a priority for all members of the healthcare team. Measures that can help include:

- Educating patients and families about the chronic nature of epilepsy and the importance of adhering to the prescribed regimen.
- Monitoring plasma drug levels to encourage and evaluate adherence.
- Deepening patient and family involvement by having them maintain a seizure frequency chart.

Withdrawing Antiepileptic Drugs

Some forms of epilepsy undergo spontaneous remission, and hence discontinuing treatment may eventually be appropriate. Unfortunately, there are no firm guidelines to indicate the most appropriate time to withdraw AEDs. However, once the decision to discontinue treatment has been made, agreement does exist on how drug withdrawal should be accomplished. The most important rule is that *AEDs be withdrawn slowly* (over a period of 6 weeks to several months). Failure to gradually reduce dosage is a frequent cause of SE. If the patient is taking two drugs to control seizures, they should be withdrawn sequentially, not simultaneously.

Suicide Risk With Antiepileptic Drugs

In 2008, the U.S. Food and Drug Administration (FDA) warned that all AEDs can increase suicidal thoughts and behavior. However, data gathered since 2008 suggest that the risk may be lower than previously believed and may apply only to certain AEDs.

The FDA based its warning on data from 199 placebo-controlled studies involving 11 different AEDs taken by 43,892 patients being treated for epilepsy, psychiatric disorders, and various pain disorders. After analyzing these data, the FDA concluded that when compared with patients taking a placebo, patients taking AEDs had twice the risk of suicidal thoughts and behaviors. Of note, risk was higher among patients taking AEDs for epilepsy than among patients taking these drugs for other conditions, such as migraine, neuropathic pain, or psychiatric illness. Although the analysis was limited to 11 drugs,

TABLE 24.2 ▪ Preparations, Dosage, and Administration of Antiepileptic Drugs (AEDs)

Drug	Preparations	Daily Maintenance Dosage[a] Adults (mg)	Daily Maintenance Dosage[a] Children[b] (mg/kg)	Target Serum Level[b] (mcg/mL)	Administration
TRADITIONAL AEDS					
Carbamazepine [Tegretol, Tegretol-XR, Carbatrol, Equetro, Epitol, Carnexiv]	IR tablets: 200 mg Chewable tablets: 100 mg ER tablets: 100, 200, 400 mg ER capsules: 100, 200, 300 mg Oral suspension: 20 mg/mL IV: 200 mg/20 mL (10 mg/mL)	800–1200	10–35	4–12	Administer IR and chewable tablets with food. ER capsules may be opened and sprinkled on soft food, but contents should not be crushed or chewed. ER tablets should be administered whole, with food. Suspensions should be shaken well before administering. Do not administer this with other liquid medications. IV solutions should be administered over 30 minutes.
Ethosuximide [Zarontin]	Capsules: 250 mg Syrup: 250 mg/5 mL	750	20	40–100[b]	Administer with or without food.
Fosphenytoin [Cerebyx]	Solution for injection: 100 mg PE/2 mL, 500 mg PE/10 mL	4–6 mg PE/kg/day	ND	10–20 as phenytoin	IV administration should not exceed 150 mg PE/min in adults or 1–3 PE/kg/min in children. May be administered IM. Is compatible with other IV solutions.
Phenobarbital [Phenobarb 🍁]	Tablets: 15, 16.2, 30, 32.4, 60, 64.8, 97.2, 100 mg Elixir: 20 mg/5 mL Oral solution: 20 mg/5 mL Solution for injection: 65, 130 mg/mL	50–120	3–8	15–45	Administer oral preparations with or without food. IV administration should not exceed 60 mg/min for adults or 30 mg/min for children. IM administration should not exceed 5 mL per site and should be injected deep into the muscle.
Phenytoin [Dilantin-125, Dilantin Infatab, Phenytek (ER capsules), Dilantin (ER capsules)]	Chewable tablets: 50 mg Capsules: 30, 100, 200, 300 mg Oral suspension: 125 mg/5 mL Solution for injection: 50 mg/mL	300–600	4–8	10–20	Food can affect absorption. Administer with or without food, but if administered with food, the food type and amount should be standardized to prevent fluctuations in drug levels. IM and subQ administration can cause tissue damage. Dosage may need to be divided among several injection sites. Is not compatible with most IV solutions, especially those containing dextrose. IV administration should not exceed 50 mg/min in adults or 1 to 3 mg/kg/min in children. Monitor IV site for infiltration as this can cause tissue necrosis.
Primidone [Mysoline]	Tablets: 50, 250 mg	500–750	10–25	5–12[c]	Administer with or without food.

Continued

TABLE 24.2 ▪ Preparations, Dosage, and Administration of Antiepileptic Drugs (AEDs)—cont'd

Drug	Preparations	Daily Maintenance Dosage[a] Adults (mg)	Children[b] (mg/kg)	Target Serum Level[b] (mcg/mL)	Administration
Valproic acid [Depakene, Depakote, Depakote Sprinkles, Epival 🍁, Depakote ER]	See Table 24.5	500–3000	15–60	50–100	Administer with or without food. Administering with food will decrease nausea. ER tablets should be administered whole. Sprinkle capsules may be opened and sprinkled on soft food, but contents should not be crushed or chewed. Product labeling advises limiting IV administration to no faster than 20 mg/min.
NEWER AEDS					
Eslicarbazepine [Aptiom]	Tablets: 400, 600, 800 mg	800–1600	NA	ND	Administer with or without food.
Ezogabine [Potiga]	Tablets: 50, 200, 300, 400 mg	600–1200	ND	ND	Administer with or without food. Tablets should be swallowed whole
Felbamate [Felbatol]	Tablets: 400, 600 mg Oral suspension: 600 mg/5 mL	1200–3600	15–45	ND	Administer with or without food. Shake suspension prior to administration.
Gabapentin [Neurontin]	Tablets: 600, 800 mg Capsule: 100, 300, 400, 600, 800 mg Oral solution: 250 mg/5 mL	1200–3600	25–50	12–20	Administer with or without food. Administering first dose at bedtime is preferred because it may cause excessive sleepiness.
Lacosamide [Vimpat]	Tablets: 50, 100, 150, 200 mg Oral solution: 10 mg/mL IV solution: 200 mg/20 mL	200–400	ND	ND	Administer oral forms with or without food. U.S. labeling recommends administering IV solutions over 15–60 minutes. Canadian labeling recommends administration over 30–60 minutes.
Lamotrigine [Lamictal, Lamictal ODT, Lamictal XR]	Tablets: 25, 100, 150, 200 mg Chewable tablets: 5, 25 mg ODT: 25, 50, 100, 200 mg ER tablets: 25, 50, 100, 200, 250, 300 mg	400–600[c,d]	5[c,d]	3–14	Administer with or without food. Place ODT tablets on tongue to dissolve. Chewable tablets should be chewed or dissolved in small amounts of juice or water. ER tables should be swallowed whole.
Levetiracetam [Keppra, Keppra XR]	IR tablets: 250, 500, 750, 1000 mg ER tablets: 500, 750 mg ODT: 250, 500, 750, 1000 mg Oral solution: 100 mg/mL IV solution: 500 mg/5 mL, 500 mg/100 mL, 1 gm/100 mL, 1.5 gm/100 mL	2000–3000	40–100	10–40	Administer with or without meals. Both IR and ER tablets should be swallowed whole. Infuse IV over 15 minutes.
Oxcarbazepine [Trileptal Oxtellar XR]	IR tablets: 150, 300, 600 mg ER tablets: 150, 300, 600 mg Oral suspension: 300 mg/5 mL	900–2400 1200–2400	30–46 20–29 kg: 900 mg/day; 29.1–39 kg: 1200 mg/day; >39 kg: 1800 mg/day	3–40	IR and suspension: Administer with or without food. ER: Administer on empty stomach. Tablets should be swallowed whole

TABLE 24.2 ■ Preparations, Dosage, and Administration of Antiepileptic Drugs (AEDs)—cont'd

Drug	Preparations	Daily Maintenance Dosage[a] Adults (mg)	Children[b] (mg/kg)	Target Serum Level[b] (mcg/mL)	Administration
Perampanel [Fycompa]	Tablets: 2, 4, 6, 8, 10, 12 mg	8–12	NA	ND	Administer at bedtime with or without food.
Pregabalin [Lyrica]	Capsules: 25, 50, 75, 100, 150, 200, 225, 300 mg Oral solution: 20 mg/mL	150–600	ND	ND	Administer with or without food.
Rufinamide [Banzel]	Tablets: 200, 400 mg Oral suspension: 40 mg/mL	3200	45	ND	Administer with food. Tablets may be crushed. Shake suspension well before administering.
Tiagabine [Gabitril]	Tablets: 2, 4, 12, 16 mg	16–32	0.4[d]	ND	Administer with food.
Topiramate [Topamax, Trokendi XR, Qudexy XR]	Tablets: 25, 50, 100, 200 mg Sprinkle capsules: 15, 25 mg ER sprinkle capsules: 25, 50, 100, 150, 200 mg ER capsules: 25, 50, 100, 200 mg	100–400	3–9	5–25	Administer with or without food. IR tablets are very bitter if crushed. Sprinkle capsules may be opened and sprinkled on soft food, but contents should not be crushed or chewed. Solid ER capsules should be swallowed whole.
Vigabatrin [Sabril]	Tablets: 500 mg Solution: 500 mg	3000–6000	50–150	ND	Administer with or without food.
Zonisamide [Zonegran]	Capsules: 25, 50, 100 mg	200–400	4–12	10–40	Administer with or without food. Capsules should be swallowed whole.

[a]Dosing for AEDs is highly individualized. These represent averages, which may be subtherapeutic for some patients while toxic for others.
[b]Monitoring the clinical response rather than plasma drug levels is the preferred method for dosage determination.
[c]Dosage must be decreased in patients taking valproic acid.
[d]Dosage must be increased in patients taking drugs that induce hepatic drug-metabolizing enzymes.
EC, Enteric coated; *ER,* extended release; *NA,* not applicable; *ND,* not determined; *ODT,* orally disintegrating tablet; *PE,* phenytoin equivalent; *XR,* extended-release.

the FDA applied its warning to *all* AEDs. However, in the FDA's own analysis, the association between suicide and AED use had statistical significance with just two drugs: topiramate and lamotrigine. Furthermore, with two other drugs—valproic acid and carbamazepine—their analysis showed some *protection* against suicidality.

Since the FDA issued its warning, other large studies have been conducted to clarify the relationship between AEDs and suicidality. Unfortunately, these studies have yielded conflicting results. Nonetheless, they do suggest three things. First, only some AEDs—especially topiramate and lamotrigine—are likely to increase suicidality, not all AEDs as warned by the FDA. Second, the risk of suicidal behavior may be related more to the illness than the medication: By analyzing data on 5,130,795 patients, researchers in the United Kingdom found that AEDs produced a small increase in suicidal behavior in patients with *depression,* but did *not* increase suicidal behavior in patients with *epilepsy* or *bipolar disorder.* And third, even if AEDs do promote suicidality, AED-related suicide attempts and completed suicides are very rare.

Given the uncertainty regarding AEDs and suicidality, what should the clinician do? Because epilepsy itself carries a risk for suicide and because patients with epilepsy often have depression and/or anxiety (which increase the risk of suicide), prudence dictates the screening of all patients for suicide risk, whether or not AEDs increase that risk. In addition, once treatment begins, all patients should be monitored for increased anxiety, agitation, mania, and hostility—signs that may indicate the emergence or worsening of depression, and an increased risk of suicidal thoughts or behavior. Patients, families, and caregivers should be alerted to these signs and advised to report them immediately. Finally, two AEDs—topiramate and lamotrigine—should be used with special caution, given their significant association with suicidality.

Safety Alert

ANTIEPILEPTIC DRUGS AND ORAL CONTRACEPTIVES

Eight AEDs—carbamazepine, eslicarbazepine, lamotrigine, oxcarbazepine, phenytoin, phenobarbital, rufinamide, and topiramate—decrease the effectiveness of oral contraceptives. Four of these—carbamazepine, phenytoin, phenobarbital, and topiramate—are associated with harm to the human fetus. If it is necessary to prescribe any of these drugs, it is important to advise the patient of the risks and the need for additional contraceptives if pregnancy is not desired.

TABLE 24.3 ■ Comparison of Traditional and Newer Antiepileptic Drugs

	AED Group	
Area of Comparison	Traditional AEDs[a]	Newer AEDs[b]
Efficacy	Well established	Equally good (probably), but less well established
Clinical experience	Extensive	Less extensive
Therapeutic niche	Well established	Evolving
Tolerability	Less well tolerated	Better tolerated (usually)
Pharmacokinetics	Often complex	Less complex
Drug interactions	Extensive, owing to induction of drug-metabolizing enzymes	Limited, owing to little or no induction of drug-metabolizing enzymes
Safety in pregnancy	Less safe	Safer
Cost	Less expensive	More expensive

[a]Carbamazepine, ethosuximide, fosphenytoin, phenobarbital, phenytoin, primidone, and valproic acid.
[b]Ezogabine, felbamate, gabapentin, lacosamide, lamotrigine, levetiracetam, oxcarbazepine, pregabalin, rufinamide, tiagabine, topiramate, vigabatrin, and zonisamide.

CLASSIFICATION OF ANTIEPILEPTIC DRUGS

The AEDs can be grouped into two major categories: *traditional AEDs* and *newer AEDs.* The traditional group has seven major members. The group of newer AEDs has 15 members. As shown in Table 24.3, both groups have their advantages and disadvantages. For example, clinical experience with the older AEDs is more extensive than with the newer ones, and the older drugs cost less. Both facts make the older drugs attractive. However, the older AEDs also have drawbacks, including troublesome side effects and complex drug interactions. Of importance, drugs in both groups appear equally effective—although few direct comparisons have been made. The bottom line? Neither group is clearly superior. Hence, when selecting an AED, drugs in both groups should be considered.

TRADITIONAL ANTIEPILEPTIC DRUGS

The traditional AEDs have been in use for decades. Because of this extensive clinical experience, the efficacy and therapeutic niche of the traditional AEDs are well established. As a result, these drugs are prescribed more widely than the newer AEDs.

Although familiarity makes the traditional AEDs appealing, these drugs do have drawbacks. In general, they are less well tolerated than the newer AEDs, and they pose a greater risk to the developing fetus. Furthermore, owing to effects on drug-metabolizing enzymes (either induction or inhibition), they have complex interactions with other drugs, including other AEDs.

In the discussion that follows, we focus on the major traditional AEDs. They are phenytoin, fosphenytoin, carbamazepine, valproic acid, ethosuximide, phenobarbital, and primidone.

Prototype Drugs

DRUGS FOR EPILEPSY

Traditional Agents
Phenytoin

Newer Agents
Oxcarbazepine

Phenytoin

Phenytoin [Dilantin, Phenytek] serves as our prototype for the traditional antiepileptic drugs. It is one of our most widely used traditional AEDs, despite having tricky kinetics and troublesome side effects. The drug is active against partial seizures as well as primary generalized tonic-clonic seizures. Phenytoin is of historic importance in that it was the first drug to suppress seizures without depressing the entire CNS. Consequently, phenytoin heralded the development of selective medications that could treat epilepsy while leaving most CNS functions undiminished.

Mechanism of Action

At the concentrations achieved clinically, phenytoin causes selective inhibition of sodium channels. Specifically, the drug slows recovery of sodium channels from the inactive state back to the active state. As a result, entry of sodium into neurons is inhibited, and hence action potentials are suppressed. Blockade of sodium entry is limited to neurons that are hyperactive. As a result, the drug suppresses activity of seizure-generating neurons while leaving healthy neurons unaffected.

Pharmacokinetics

Phenytoin has unusual pharmacokinetics that must be accounted for in therapy. Absorption varies substantially among patients.

In addition, because of saturation kinetics, small changes in dosage can produce disproportionately large changes in serum drug levels. As a result, a dosage that is both effective and safe is difficult to establish.

Absorption. Absorption varies between the different oral formulations of phenytoin. With the oral suspension and chewable tablets absorption is relatively fast, whereas with the extended-release capsules absorption is delayed and prolonged.

In the past, there was concern that absorption also varied between preparations of phenytoin made by different manufacturers. However, it is now clear that all FDA-approved equivalent products have equivalent bioavailability. As a result, switching from one brand of phenytoin to another produces no more variability than switching between different lots of phenytoin produced by the same manufacturer.

Metabolism. The capacity of the liver to metabolize phenytoin is very limited. Doses of phenytoin needed to produce therapeutic effects are only slightly smaller than the doses needed to saturate the hepatic enzymes that metabolize phenytoin. Consequently, if phenytoin is administered in doses only slightly greater than those needed for therapeutic effects, the liver's capacity to metabolize the drug will be overwhelmed, causing plasma levels of phenytoin to rise dramatically. This unusual relationship between dosage and plasma levels is illustrated in Fig. 24.1A. As you can see, once plasma levels have reached the therapeutic range, small changes in dosage produce large changes in plasma levels. As a result, small increases in dosage can cause toxicity, and small decreases can cause therapeutic failure. This relationship makes it difficult to establish and maintain a dosage that is both safe and effective.

Fig. 24.1B indicates the relationship between dosage and plasma levels that exists for most drugs. As indicated, this relationship is *linear,* in contrast to the nonlinear relationship that exists for phenytoin. Accordingly, for most drugs, if the patient is taking doses that produce plasma levels that are within the therapeutic range, small deviations from that dosage produce only small deviations in plasma drug levels. Because of this relationship, with most drugs it is relatively easy to maintain plasma levels that are safe and effective.

Because of saturation kinetics, the half-life of phenytoin varies with dosage. At low doses, the half-life is relatively short—about 8 hours. However, at higher doses, the half-life becomes prolonged—in some cases up to 60 hours. At higher doses, there is more drug present than the liver can process. As a result, metabolism is delayed, causing the half-life to increase.

Therapeutic Uses

Epilepsy. Phenytoin can be used to treat all major forms of epilepsy except absence seizures. The drug is especially effective against tonic-clonic seizures, and is a drug of choice for treating these seizures in adults and older children. (Carbamazepine is preferred to phenytoin for treating tonic-clonic seizures in young children.) Although phenytoin can be used to treat simple and complex partial seizures, the drug is less effective against these seizures than against tonic-clonic seizures. Phenytoin can be administered IV to treat generalized convulsive SE, but other drugs are preferred.

Cardiac Dysrhythmias. Phenytoin is active against certain types of dysrhythmias. Antidysrhythmic applications are discussed in Chapter 49.

Adverse Effects

Effects on the CNS. Although phenytoin acts on the CNS in a relatively selective fashion to suppress seizures, the drug can still cause CNS side effects—especially when dosage is excessive. At therapeutic levels (10 to 20 mcg/mL), sedation and other CNS effects are mild. At plasma levels above 20 mcg/mL, toxicity can occur. Nystagmus (continuous back-and-forth movements of the eyes) is relatively common. Other manifestations of excessive dosage include sedation, ataxia (staggering gait), diplopia (double vision), and cognitive impairment.

Gingival Hyperplasia. Gingival hyperplasia (excessive growth of gum tissue) is characterized by swelling, tenderness, and bleeding of the gums. In extreme cases, patients require gingivectomy (surgical removal of excess gum tissue). Gingival hyperplasia is seen in about 20% of patients who take phenytoin. Can risk be reduced? Yes. Evidence indicates that supplemental folic acid (0.5 mg/day) may prevent gum overgrowth. In

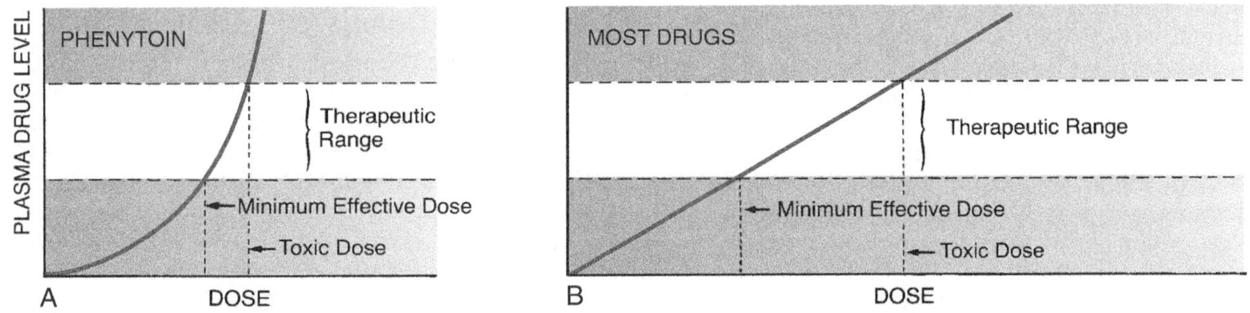

Fig. 24.1 ■ Relationship between dose and plasma level for phenytoin compared with most other drugs.

A, Within the therapeutic range, small increments in phenytoin dosage produce sharp increases in plasma drug levels. This relationship makes it difficult to maintain plasma phenytoin levels within the therapeutic range. **B,** Within the therapeutic range, small increments in dosage of most drugs produce small increases in drug levels. With this relationship, moderate fluctuations in dosage are unlikely to result in either toxicity or therapeutic failure.

addition, risk can be minimized by good oral hygiene, including dental flossing and gum massage. Patients should be taught these techniques and encouraged to practice them.

Dermatologic Effects. Between 2% and 5% of patients develop a morbilliform (measles-like) rash. Rarely, morbilliform rash progresses to much more severe reactions: *Stevens-Johnson syndrome* (SJS) or *toxic epidermal necrolysis* (TEN). Product labeling warns that the risk of developing SJS/TEN is strongly associated with a genetic mutation known as *human leukocyte antigen (HLA)-B*1502,* which occurs almost exclusively in people of Asian descent. For this reason, phenytoin should not be prescribed for patients known to have this mutation.

Effects in Pregnancy. Phenytoin is a teratogen. It can cause cleft palate, heart malformations, and *fetal hydantoin syndrome,* characterized by growth deficiency, motor or mental deficiency, microcephaly, craniofacial distortion, positional deformities of the limbs, hypoplasia of the nails and fingers, and impaired neurodevelopment. Phenytoin should be used during pregnancy only if safer alternatives are not effective and if the benefits of seizure control are deemed to outweigh the risk to the fetus.

Phenytoin can decrease synthesis of vitamin K–dependent clotting factors and can thereby cause *bleeding tendencies in newborns.* The risk of neonatal bleeding can be decreased by giving prophylactic vitamin K to the mother for 1 month before and during delivery, and to the infant immediately after delivery.

Cardiovascular Effects. When phenytoin is administered by IV injection (to treat SE), cardiac dysrhythmias and hypotension may result. These dangerous responses can be minimized by injecting phenytoin slowly and in dilute saline solution (see the Safety Alert for IV Administration of Phenytoin).

Safety Alert

IV ADMINISTRATION OF PHENYTOIN

The chemical and pharmacodynamic properties of phenytoin present unique challenges for intravenous administration. These can be managed through safe administration.

1. To prevent development of significant hypotension and cardiac dysrhythmias during IV administration of phenytoin, administration should not exceed 50 mg/min in adults or either 1–3 mg/kg/min or 50 mg/min (whichever is slower) in children. Cardiac rhythm should be monitored during administration.
2. Phenytoin should never be mixed with or piggybacked onto dextrose solutions. Instead, it should be given directly into a large vein. Product labeling recommends flushing with saline both before and following intravenous administration.
3. Phenytoin can cause severe tissue damage if the solution infiltrates the area surrounding the IV site. This risk can be decreased by initiating infusion in a large peripheral or central vein. Close monitoring for extravasation is essential.

Purple Glove Syndrome. Very rarely, IV phenytoin has been associated with purple glove syndrome, a painful condition characterized by swelling and discoloration of the hands and arms. In some cases, this has led to ischemia and necrosis. This potential effect is yet another reason supporting administration into a large vein rather than the smaller veins in the lower arm or hand.

Other Adverse Effects. Hirsutism (overgrowth of hair in unusual places) can be a disturbing response, especially in young women. Interference with vitamin D metabolism may cause *rickets* and *osteomalacia* (softening of the bones). Interference with vitamin K metabolism can lower prothrombin levels, thereby causing *bleeding tendencies in newborns.* Very rarely, *liver damage* may occur, probably because of drug allergy.

Drug Interactions

Phenytoin interacts with a large number of drugs. The more important interactions are discussed in the following section.

Interactions Resulting From Induction of Hepatic Drug-Metabolizing Enzymes. Phenytoin stimulates synthesis of hepatic drug-metabolizing enzymes CYP2C8, CYP2C9, CYP3A4 and, to a lesser degree, CYP2B6. As a result, phenytoin can decrease the effects of other drugs, including *oral contraceptives, warfarin* (an anticoagulant), and *glucocorticoids* (anti-inflammatory/immunosuppressive drugs). Because avoiding pregnancy is desirable while taking antiseizure medications and because phenytoin can decrease the effectiveness of oral contraceptives, the provider may need to increase the contraceptive dosage or switch to an alternative form of contraception.

Drugs That Increase Plasma Levels of Phenytoin. Because the therapeutic range of phenytoin is narrow, slight increases in phenytoin levels can cause toxicity. Consequently, caution must be exercised when phenytoin is used with drugs that can increase its level. Drugs known to elevate phenytoin levels include *diazepam* (an antianxiety agent and AED), *isoniazid* (a drug for tuberculosis), *cimetidine* (a drug for gastric ulcers), and *alcohol* (when taken acutely). These agents increase phenytoin levels by reducing the rate at which phenytoin is metabolized. *Valproic acid* (an AED) elevates levels of free phenytoin by displacing phenytoin from binding sites on plasma proteins.

Drugs That Decrease Plasma Levels of Phenytoin. *Carbamazepine, phenobarbital,* and *alcohol* (when used chronically) can accelerate the metabolism of phenytoin, thereby decreasing its level. Breakthrough seizures can result.

CNS Depressants. The depressant effects of *alcohol, barbiturates,* and *other CNS depressants* will add to those of phenytoin. Advise patients to avoid alcohol and all other drugs with CNS-depressant actions.

Preparations, Dosage, and Administration

Preparations. Phenytoin [Dilantin, Phenytek] is available in solution for injection and in three oral formulations: (1) chewable tablets (50 mg), marketed as *Dilantin Infatab;* (2) an oral suspension (125 mg/5 mL), marketed as *Dilantin-125;* and (3) extended-release (ER) capsules (30, 100, 200, and 300 mg), marketed as *Dilantin* and *Phenytek.* Phenytoin products made by different manufacturers have equivalent bioavailability. Therefore, although switching between products from different manufacturers was a concern in the past, it is not a concern today.

Dosage. *Dosing is highly individualized.* Initial doses are usually given 3 times a day. Once a maintenance dosage has been established, once-a-day dosing is often possible (using ER capsules). For *adults,* a typical initial dosage is 100 to 125 mg 3 times a day; maintenance dosages usually range between 300 and 600 mg/day. For *children,* a typical initial dosage is 2.5 mg/kg twice a day; maintenance dosages usually range between 4 and 8 mg/kg/day.

Plasma drug levels are often monitored as an aid to establishing dosage. *The dosing objective is to produce levels between 10 and 20 mcg/mL.* Levels below 10 mcg/mL are too low to control seizures; levels above 20 mcg/mL produce toxicity. Because phenytoin has a relatively narrow therapeutic range (between 10 and 20 mcg/mL) and because of the nonlinear relationship between phenytoin dosage and phenytoin plasma levels, once a safe and effective dosage has been established, the patient should adhere to it rigidly.

When treatment is discontinued, dosage should be reduced gradually. Abrupt withdrawal may precipitate seizures.

Administration. *Oral* preparations may cause gastric discomfort. Patients should be informed that gastric upset can be reduced by administering phenytoin with or immediately after a meal. Patients using the oral suspension should shake it well before dispensing, as failure to do so can result in uneven dosing.

Intravenous administration is used to treat generalized convulsive SE. It is imperative that infusions be performed slowly (no faster than 50 mg/min) because rapid administration can cause cardiovascular collapse. Phenytoin should not be added to an existing IV infusion, because mixing phenytoin with other solutions is likely to produce a precipitate. Solutions of phenytoin are highly alkaline and can cause local venous irritation. Irritation can be reduced by flushing the IV needle or catheter with sterile saline immediately after completing the infusion.

Fosphenytoin

Mechanism of Action

Fosphenytoin [Cerebyx] is a prodrug that is converted to phenytoin when metabolized. It is recommended as a substitute for oral phenytoin when the oral route is contraindicated.

Therapeutic Uses

Because fosphenytoin is converted to phenytoin, therapeutic uses are the same as those of phenytoin. It is active against both generalized tonic-clonic seizures and partial seizures.

Pharmacokinetics

The pharmacokinetic properties of fosphenytoin and other drugs are provided separately (Table 24.4).

Adverse Effects

Adverse effects of fosphenytoin are the same as those of phenytoin with one notable exception. During IV infusion, temporary paresthesias and itching, especially in the groin area, may occur. This infusion-related reaction will resolve when the infusion rate is decreased or within 10 minutes following completion of the infusion.

Unique Dosing

Fosphenytoin has a unique dosing system. Although 150 mg of fosphenytoin will hydrolyze to 100 mg of phenytoin, rather than use standard milligram dosing, fosphenytoin is dosed in phenytoin equivalents (PE). Using this alternative, fosphenytoin 1 mg PE equals phenytoin 1 mg.

Specific preparations, dosage, and administration of fosphenytoin and other drugs in this chapter are available in Table 24.2.

Safety Alert

INTRAVENOUS ADMINISTRATION OF FOSPHENYTOIN

If the rate of fosphenytoin administration exceeds 150 mg phenytoin equivalents (PE) per minute, severe hypotension and cardiac arrhythmias may occur. Cardiac monitoring is needed when administering this drug.

Carbamazepine

Carbamazepine [Tegretol, Tegretol-XR, Carbatrol, Epitol, Equetro, Carnexiv] is commonly used for epilepsy therapy. The drug is active against partial seizures and tonic-clonic seizures but not absence seizures.

PATIENT-CENTERED CARE ACROSS THE LIFE SPAN

Antiepileptic Drugs

Life Stage	Patient Care Concerns
Children	Currently approved antiepileptic drugs are approved for children with the exception of eslicarbazepine. Though approved for pediatric use, prescription labeling for many AEDs mentions inadequate studies in younger children.
Pregnant women	Valproate is Pregnancy Risk Category X.[a] It should not be prescribed for pregnant women. Carbamazepine, phenytoin, phenobarbital, and topiramate are Pregnancy Risk Category D. Fetal harm has been documented in humans for these drugs, so it is essential to weigh benefits versus risks. The remaining drugs are Pregnancy Risk Category C. Fetal harm has been documented in animal studies but not in humans. The lack of documented harm in humans often reflects a lack of studies rather than positive outcomes. Canadian labeling prohibits the prescribing of vigabatrin to pregnant women. In order to increase data on pregnancy outcomes, pregnant women taking AEDs are encouraged to enroll in the North American AED Pregnancy Registry at www.aedpregnancyregistry.org.
Breast-feeding women	Manufacturers advise carefully weighing the benefits of breast-feeding over the risks of adverse effects in the infant. Of note, for women taking vigabatrin, Canadian labeling contraindicates breast-feeding.
Older adults	Beers Criteria lists carbamazepine, oxcarbazepine, and phenobarbital among the drugs deemed possibly inappropriate for adults age 65 and older. Because elderly patients are at increased risk of adverse events (e.g., falls secondary to sedation), cautious prescribing of all AEDs, often at lower initial doses, is advisable.

[a]As of 2020, the FDA will no longer use Pregnancy Risk Categories. Please refer to Chapter 9 for more information.

TABLE 24.4 ▪ Pharmacokinetics of Antiepileptic Drugs (AEDs)[a]

Drug	Route	Peak	Half-Life[b]	Metabolism	Induces Hepatic Drug Metabolism	Excretion
Carbamazepine	PO, IV	Suspension: 1.5 hr IR: 4–5 hr ER: 3–26 hr	Variable due to auto-induction. Initially 25–65 hr; after stabilization, 8–14 hr (children) to 12–17 hr (adults)	CYP3A4 (induces its own metabolism)	Yes	Urine (primary), feces
Ethosuximide	PO	1–7 hr	Children: 30 hr Adults: 50–60 hr	CYP3A4, CYP2E1	No	Urine
Phenobarbital	PO, IM, IV	PO: 1.4 hr IV: 15 min	Children: 110 hr (range 60–180 hr) Adults: 79 hr (range 53–118 hr)	CYP2C9 (primary), CYP2C19, CYP2E1	Yes	Urine (primary), feces
Phenytoin	PO, IV	IR: 1.5–3 hr ER: 4–12 hr	7–42 hr	CYP2C9, CYP2C19	Yes	Urine
Fosphenytoin	IM, IV	IV: 15 min IM: 30 min	Conversion to phenytoin: 15 min	Initial conversion to phenytoin: probably phosphatases	Yes	Following conversion to phenytoin: Urine
Primidone	PO	0.5–9 hr	5–16 hr	Hepatic via oxidation	Yes	Urine
Valproic acid	PO, IV	IR: 4 hr ER: 4–17 hr	9–19 hr	Hepatic via glucuronide conjugation and mitochondrial beta-oxidation	No	Urine
Eslicarbazepine	PO	1–4 hr	13–20 hr	Hydrolysis	Yes	Urine
Ezogabine	PO	0.5–2 hr	7–11 hr	Glucuronidation, acetylation	No	Urine (primary), feces
Felbamate	PO	2–6 hr	20–23 hr	CYP3A4	Yes	Urine
Gabapentin	PO	2–4 hr	Children: 4.7 hr Adults: 5–7 hr	Not metabolized	No	Urine
Lacosamide	PO, IV	1–4 hr	13 hr	CYP3A4, CYP2C9, CYP2C19	No	Urine
Lamotrigine	PO	IR: 1–4 hr ER: 4–11 hr	25–33 hr as monotherapy	Hepatic via glucuronidation (primary), renal	No	Urine
Levetiracetam	PO, IV	Solution: 1 hr IR: 1 hr ER: 4 hr	Children: 7.2–9.3 hr (MHD) Adults: 9–11 hr (MHD)	Hydrolysis by enzymes in the blood	No	Urine
Oxcarbazepine	PO	IR: 3–4 hr (MHD) ER: 7 hr	Children: 4.8–9 hr Adults: 9–11 hr	Hepatic cytosolic enzymes MHD, then glucuronide conjugation	Yes[c]	Urine
Perampanel	PO	2–2.5 hr Food delays by 1–2 hr	105 hr	CYP3A4/5, (primary), CYP1A2, CYP2B6	Yes (weak)	Feces (primary), urine
Pregabalin	PO	1.5 hr Food delays by 1.5 hr	6.3 hr	Negligible	No	Urine
Rufinamide	PO	4–6 hr	6–10 hr	Carboxylesterase-mediated hydrolysis		Urine
Tiagabine	PO	45 min	Children: 2–10 hr Adults: 7–9 hr	CYP3A4 (major)	No	Feces (primary), urine

TABLE 24.4 ■ Pharmacokinetics of Antiepileptic Drugs (AEDs)[a]—cont'd

Drug	Route	Peak	Half-Life[b]	Metabolism	Induces Hepatic Drug Metabolism	Excretion
Topiramate	PO	IR: 1–4.3 hr ER: 20–24 hr	Children: 12–13 hr Adults: 19–23 hr	Minimal via hydroxylation, hydrolysis, glucuronidation	No	Urine
Vigabatrin	PO	1 hr Food delays by 1 hr	Children: 5.5–9.5 hr Adults: 10.5 hr	Negligible	Yes	Urine
Zonisamide	PO	2–6 hr	63 hr (range 50–68 hr)	CYP3A4	No	Urine

[a]Peaks and half-lives are often highly variable and dependent on multiple individual factors.
[b]Half-lives are based on monotherapy. Administration of other drugs can significantly alter timing. Those with prolonged half-lives may take many days or even weeks to reach a steady state.
[c]Oxcarbazepine does not induce enzymes that metabolize AEDs, but does induce enzymes that metabolize other drugs.
ER, Extended release; *hr,* hour(s); *IR,* immediate release; *MHD,* 10-monohydroxy metabolite (the active metabolite); *min,* minute(s); *PE,* phenytoin equivalent; *PO,* by mouth.

Mechanism of Action

Carbamazepine suppresses high-frequency neuronal discharge in and around seizure foci. The mechanism appears to be the same as that of phenytoin: delayed recovery of sodium channels from their inactivated state.

Therapeutic Uses

Epilepsy. Carbamazepine is effective against tonic-clonic, simple partial, and complex partial seizures. Because the drug causes fewer adverse effects than phenytoin and phenobarbital, it is often preferred to these agents. Many prescribers consider carbamazepine the drug of first choice for partial seizures. Carbamazepine is not effective against absence, myoclonic, or atonic seizures.

Bipolar Disorder. Carbamazepine can provide symptomatic control in patients with bipolar disorder (manic-depressive illness), and is often effective in patients who are refractory to lithium. The role of carbamazepine in bipolar disorder is discussed in Chapter 33.

Trigeminal and Glossopharyngeal Neuralgias. A neuralgia is a severe, stabbing pain that occurs along the course of a nerve. Carbamazepine can reduce neuralgia associated with the trigeminal and glossopharyngeal nerves. The mechanism is unknown. It should be noted that although carbamazepine can reduce pain in these specific neuralgias, it is not generally effective as an analgesic, and it is not indicated for other kinds of pain.

Adverse Effects

CNS Effects. In contrast to phenytoin and phenobarbital, carbamazepine has minimal effects on cognitive function. This is a primary reason for selecting carbamazepine over other antiseizure drugs.

Carbamazepine can cause a variety of *neurologic effects,* including visual disturbances (nystagmus, blurred vision, diplopia), ataxia, vertigo, unsteadiness, and headache. These reactions are common during the first weeks of treatment, affecting 35% to 50% of patients. Fortunately, tolerance usually develops with continued use. These effects can be minimized by initiating therapy at low doses and giving the largest portion of the daily dose at bedtime.

Hematologic Effects. Carbamazepine-induced bone marrow suppression can cause *leukopenia, anemia,* and *thrombocytopenia.* However, serious reactions are rare. Thrombocytopenia and anemia, which have an incidence of 5%, respond to drug discontinuation. Leukopenia, which has an incidence of 10%, is usually transient and subsides even with continued drug use. Accordingly, carbamazepine should not be withdrawn unless the white blood cell count drops below 3000/mm^3.

Fatal *aplastic anemia* has occurred during carbamazepine therapy. This reaction is extremely rare, having an incidence of 1 in 200,000.

To reduce the risk of serious hematologic effects, complete blood counts should be performed before treatment and periodically thereafter. Patients with pre-existing hematologic abnormalities should not use this drug. Patients should be informed about manifestations of hematologic abnormalities (fever, sore throat, pallor, weakness, infection, easy bruising, petechiae) and instructed to notify the prescriber if these occur.

Birth Defects. Carbamazepine is teratogenic. In humans, the drug is associated with a 2.6-fold increase in the risk of spina bifida, a neural tube defect. Because it can harm the fetus, carbamazepine should be used only if the benefits of seizure control are deemed to outweigh risks to the fetus.

Hypo-osmolarity and Hyponatremia. Carbamazepine can inhibit renal excretion of water, apparently by promoting secretion of antidiuretic hormone. Water retention can reduce the osmolarity of blood and other body fluids, thereby posing a threat to patients with heart failure. Hyponatremia is a particular concern and appears to be dose-dependent. Periodic monitoring of serum sodium levels is recommended.

Dermatologic Effects. Carbamazepine has been associated with several dermatologic effects, including morbilliform rash (10% incidence), photosensitivity reactions, SJS, and TEN. Mild reactions can often be treated with prednisone (an anti-inflammatory agent) or an antihistamine. Severe reactions—SJS and TEN—necessitate drug withdrawal.

TABLE 24.5 ■ Oral Preparations of Valproic Acid and Its Derivatives

Chemical Form	Brand Name	Product Description	Comments
Valproic acid	Depakene	Capsules (250 mg)	Immediate release; GI upset is common.
Valproate	Depakene	Syrup (250 mg/5 mL)	Immediate release; GI upset is common.
Divalproex sodium	Depakote, Epival ♣	Tablets, delayed-release, enteric-coated (125, 250, 500 mg)	Released over 8–12 hr, so *not* for once-daily administration. *Not interchangeable with Depakote ER* (extended-release tablets) because rate of drug release is different. Less GI upset than Depakene.
	Depakote ER	Tablets, extended-release, enteric-coated (250, 500 mg)	Released over 18–24 hr, so *can* be administered once daily. *Not interchangeable with regular Depakote* (delayed-release tablets) because rate of drug release is different. Less GI upset than Depakene.
	Depakote	"Sprinkle" capsules containing enteric-coated granules (125 mg)	Immediate release. Less GI upset than Depakene. May swallow capsule whole or open and sprinkle granules on a small amount (1 tsp) of soft food.

A major risk factor for SJS/TEN is HLA-B*1502, a genetic variation seen primarily in people of Asian descent. Among people with the variant gene, about 5% develop SJS/TEN with carbamazepine. Accordingly, to reduce the risk of severe reactions, the FDA recommends that before receiving carbamazepine, patients of Asian descent be tested for HLA-B*1502. Of note, this was the first time that the FDA recommended genetic screening for a major drug. As discussed previously, the presence of HLA-B*1502 *may* also increase the risk of SJS/TEN in patients taking phenytoin. Accordingly, phenytoin should not be used as an alternative to carbamazepine in patients with the mutation.

Drug-Drug and Drug-Food Interactions

Induction of Drug-Metabolizing Enzymes. Carbamazepine induces hepatic drug-metabolizing enzymes, and hence can increase the rate at which it and other drugs are inactivated. Accelerated inactivation of *oral contraceptives* and *warfarin* is of particular concern.

Phenytoin and Phenobarbital. Both phenytoin and phenobarbital induce hepatic drug metabolism. Thus, if either drug is taken with carbamazepine, induction of metabolism is likely to be greater than with carbamazepine alone. Accordingly, phenytoin and phenobarbital can further accelerate the metabolism of carbamazepine, thereby decreasing its effects.

Grapefruit Juice. As discussed in Chapter 6, grapefruit juice can inhibit the metabolism of many drugs, thereby causing their plasma levels to rise. Grapefruit juice can increase peak and trough levels of carbamazepine by 40%. Advise patients to avoid grapefruit juice.

Valproic Acid

Valproic acid [Depakene, Depakote, Depakote ER, Depakote Sprinkles, Depacon, Epival ♣] is an important AED used widely to treat all major seizure types. In addition to its use in epilepsy, valproic acid is used for bipolar disorder and migraine headache.

Nomenclature

Valproic acid is available in three closely related chemical forms (Table 24.5): (1) valproic acid, (2) the sodium salt of valproic acid, known as *valproate,* and (3) *divalproex sodium,* a combination of valproic acid plus its sodium salt. All three forms have identical antiseizure actions. In this chapter, the term *valproic acid* is used in reference to all three.

Mechanism of Action

Valproic acid appears to act by three mechanisms. First, it shares the same mechanism as phenytoin and carbamazepine: suppression of high-frequency neuronal firing through blockade of sodium channels. Second, it suppresses calcium influx through T-type calcium channels. Third, it may augment the inhibitory influence of GABA.

Therapeutic Uses

Valproic acid is considered a first-line drug for all partial and generalized seizures. As mentioned previously, this drug also is indicated for management of bipolar disorder (see Chapter 33) and migraine headache prophylaxis (see Chapter 30).

Adverse Effects

Valproic acid is generally well tolerated and causes minimal sedation and cognitive impairment. Gastrointestinal effects are most common. Hepatotoxicity and pancreatitis are rare but serious. Owing to teratogenic effects, valproic acid should be avoided during pregnancy.

Gastrointestinal Effects. Nausea, vomiting, and indigestion are common but transient. These effects are most intense with formulations that are not enteric coated. Gastrointestinal reactions can be minimized by administering valproic acid with food and by using an enteric-coated product (see Table 24.5).

Hepatotoxicity. Rarely, valproic acid has been associated with fatal liver failure. Most deaths have occurred within the first few months of therapy. The overall incidence of fatal hepatotoxicity is about 1 in 40,000. However, in high-risk patients—children younger than 2 years receiving multidrug therapy—the incidence is much higher: 1 in 500. To minimize the risk of fatal liver injury, the following guidelines have been established:

- Don't use valproic acid in conjunction with other drugs in children younger than 2 years.
- Don't use valproic acid in patients with pre-existing liver dysfunction.
- Evaluate liver function at baseline and periodically thereafter. (Unfortunately, monitoring liver function may fail to provide advance warning of severe hepatotoxicity. Fatal liver failure can develop so rapidly that it is not preceded by an abnormal test result.)
- Inform patients about signs and symptoms of liver injury (reduced appetite, malaise, nausea, abdominal pain, jaundice), and instruct them to notify the prescriber if these develop.
- Use valproic acid in the lowest effective dosage.

Pancreatitis. Life-threatening pancreatitis may develop in children and adults. Some cases have been hemorrhagic, progressing rapidly from initial symptoms to death. Pancreatitis can develop soon after starting therapy or after years of drug use. Patients should be informed about signs of pancreatitis (abdominal pain, nausea, vomiting, anorexia) and instructed to obtain immediate evaluation if these develop. If pancreatitis is diagnosed, valproic acid should be withdrawn, and alternative medication should be substituted as indicated.

Pregnancy-Related Harm. Valproic acid is *highly teratogenic,* especially when taken during the first trimester. The risk of a major congenital malformation is 4 times higher than with other AEDs. Neural tube defects (e.g., spina bifida) are the greatest concern. The risk is 1 in 20 among women taking valproic acid versus 1 in 1000 among women in the general population. In addition to neural tube defects, valproic acid can cause five other major congenital malformations: atrial septal defect, cleft palate, hypospadias, polydactyly, and craniosynostosis.

Exposure to valproic acid *in utero* can also *impair cognitive function.* Research also indicates an increased risk of autism.

Obviously, valproic acid should be avoided by women of childbearing potential unless it is the only AED that will work. Women who *must* use the drug should use an effective form of contraception and should take folic acid supplements, which can help protect against neural tube damage in case pregnancy occurs.

Hyperammonemia. Combining valproic acid with topiramate poses a risk of hyperammonemia (excessive ammonia in the blood), which may occur with or without encephalopathy. Symptoms include vomiting, lethargy, altered level of consciousness, and altered cognitive function. If these symptoms develop, hyperammonemic encephalopathy should be suspected, and blood ammonia should be measured. As a rule, symptoms abate following removal of either drug.

Other Adverse Effects. Valproic acid may cause *rash, weight gain, hair loss, tremor,* and *blood dyscrasias* (leukopenia, thrombocytopenia, red blood cell aplasia). Significant CNS effects are uncommon.

Drug Interactions

Phenobarbital. Valproic acid decreases the rate at which phenobarbital is metabolized. Blood levels of phenobarbital may rise by 40%, resulting in significant CNS depression. When the combination is used, levels of phenobarbital should be monitored, and if they rise too high, phenobarbital dosage should be reduced.

Phenytoin. Valproic acid can displace phenytoin from binding sites on plasma proteins. The resultant increase in free phenytoin may lead to phenytoin toxicity. Phenytoin levels and clinical status should be monitored.

Topiramate. See previous discussion of *Hyperammonemia.*

Carbapenem Antibiotics. Two carbapenem antibiotics—meropenem and imipenem/cilastatin—can reduce plasma levels of valproic acid. Breakthrough seizures have occurred. Of note, increasing the dosage of valproic acid may be insufficient to overcome this effect. Accordingly, meropenem and imipenem/cilastatin should be avoided in patients taking valproic acid.

Ethosuximide

Mechanism of Action

Ethosuximide [Zarontin] suppresses neurons in the thalamus that are responsible for generating absence seizures. The specific mechanism is inhibition of low-threshold calcium currents, known as T currents. Ethosuximide does not block sodium channels and does not enhance GABA-mediated neuronal inhibition.

Therapeutic Use

Ethosuximide is the drug of choice for absence seizures, the only indication it has. Absence seizures are eliminated in 60% of patients, and in newly diagnosed patients practical control is achieved in 80% to 90% of cases.

Adverse Effects

Ethosuximide is generally devoid of significant adverse effects and interactions. During initial treatment, it may cause *drowsiness, dizziness,* and *lethargy.* These diminish with continued use. *Nausea* and *vomiting* may occur and can be reduced by administering the drug with food. Rare but serious reactions include *systemic lupus erythematosus, leukopenia, aplastic anemia,* and *Stevens-Johnson syndrome.*

Phenobarbital

Phenobarbital, one of our oldest AEDs, is effective and inexpensive, and it can be administered just once a day. Unfortunately, certain side effects—lethargy, depression, learning impairment—can be significant. Hence, although phenobarbital was used widely in the past, it has largely been replaced by newer drugs that are equally effective but better tolerated.

Phenobarbital belongs to the barbiturate family. However, in contrast to most barbiturates, which produce generalized depression of the CNS, phenobarbital is able to suppress seizures at doses that produce only moderate disruption of CNS function. Because it can reduce seizures without causing sedation, phenobarbital is classified as an *anticonvulsant barbiturate* (to distinguish it from most other barbiturates, which are employed as sedatives or "sleeping pills").

The basic pharmacology of the barbiturates is discussed in Chapter 34. Discussion here is limited to the use of phenobarbital for seizures.

Mechanism of Action

Phenobarbital suppresses seizures by potentiating the effects of GABA. Specifically, the drug binds to GABA receptors, causing the receptors to respond more intensely to GABA itself.

Therapeutic Uses

Epilepsy. Phenobarbital is effective against partial seizures and generalized tonic-clonic seizures but not absence seizures. Intravenous phenobarbital can be used for generalized convulsive SE, but other antiseizure drugs are preferred. This drug has a long half-life of 4 days; it takes 2 to 3 weeks for plasma levels to reach plateau (steady state). To address this concern, loading doses are often given to increase serum levels. Loading doses are higher than typical doses. For example, doses that are twice normal can be given for the first 4 days.

Sedation and Induction of Sleep. Like other barbiturates, phenobarbital can be used for sedation and to promote sleep at night. These applications are discussed in Chapter 34.

Adverse Effects

Neuropsychologic Effects. Drowsiness is the most common CNS effect. During the initial phase of therapy, sedation develops in practically all patients. With continued treatment, tolerance to sedation develops. Some children experience paradoxical responses: Instead of becoming sedated, they may become irritable and hyperactive. Depression may occur in adults. Older adult patients may experience agitation and confusion.

Physical Dependence. Like all other barbiturates, phenobarbital can cause physical dependence. However, at the doses employed to treat epilepsy, significant dependence is unlikely.

Exacerbation of Intermittent Porphyria. Phenobarbital and other barbiturates can increase the risk of acute intermittent porphyria. Accordingly, barbiturates are absolutely contraindicated for patients with a history of this disorder. The relationship of barbiturates to intermittent porphyria is discussed in Chapter 34.

Use in Pregnancy. Use of phenobarbital during pregnancy poses a significant risk of major fetal malformations. Women who take phenobarbital during pregnancy or become pregnant while taking the drug should be informed of the potential risk to the fetus.

Like phenytoin, phenobarbital can decrease synthesis of vitamin K–dependent clotting factors and can thereby cause *bleeding tendencies in newborns.* The risk of neonatal bleeding can be decreased by administering vitamin K to the mother for 1 month before delivery and during delivery, and to the infant immediately after delivery.

Other Adverse Effects. Like phenytoin, phenobarbital can interfere with the metabolism of vitamins D and K. Disruption of vitamin D metabolism can cause *rickets* and *osteomalacia.*

Toxicity

When taken in moderately excessive doses, phenobarbital causes nystagmus and ataxia. Severe overdose produces generalized CNS depression; death results from depression of respiration. Barbiturate toxicity and its treatment are discussed in Chapter 34.

Drug Interactions

Induction of Drug-Metabolizing Enzymes. Phenobarbital induces the hepatic drug-metabolizing enzymes CYP1A2, CYP2A6, CYP2C8, CYP2C9, CYP3A4 and, to a lesser degree CYP2B6. As a result, it can accelerate the metabolism of drugs that are substrates for these enzymes, causing a loss of therapeutic effects. This is of particular concern with oral contraceptives and warfarin.

CNS Depressants. Being a CNS depressant itself, phenobarbital can intensify CNS depression caused by other drugs (e.g., alcohol, benzodiazepines, opioids). Severe respiratory depression and coma can result. Patients should be warned against combining phenobarbital with other drugs that have CNS-depressant actions.

Valproic Acid. Valproic acid is an AED that has been used in combination with phenobarbital. By competing with phenobarbital for drug-metabolizing enzymes, valproic acid can increase plasma levels of phenobarbital by approximately 40%. Hence, when this combination is used, the dosage of phenobarbital must be reduced.

Drug Withdrawal

When phenobarbital is withdrawn, dosage should be reduced gradually, because abrupt withdrawal can precipitate SE. Patients should be warned of this danger and instructed not to discontinue phenobarbital too quickly.

Primidone

Mechanism of Action

Primidone [Mysoline] is nearly identical in structure to phenobarbital. As a result, the pharmacology of both agents is very similar.

Therapeutic Uses

Primidone is effective against tonic-clonic, simple partial, and complex partial seizures. The drug is not active against absence seizures.

As a rule, primidone is employed in combination with another AED, usually phenytoin or carbamazepine. Primidone is never taken together with phenobarbital because phenobarbital is an active metabolite of primidone, so concurrent use would be irrational.

Adverse Effects

Sedation, ataxia, and dizziness are common during initial treatment but diminish with continued drug use. Like phenobarbital, primidone can cause confusion in older adults and paradoxical hyperexcitability in children. A sense of acute intoxication can occur shortly after dosing. As with phenobarbital, primidone is absolutely contraindicated for patients with acute intermittent porphyria. Serious adverse reactions (acute psychosis, leukopenia, thrombocytopenia, systemic lupus erythematosus) can occur but are rare.

Drug Interactions

Drug interactions for primidone are similar to those for phenobarbital. Primidone can induce hepatic drug-metabolizing enzymes and can thereby reduce the effects of oral contraceptives, warfarin, and other drugs. In addition, primidone can intensify responses to other CNS depressants.

NEWER ANTIEPILEPTIC DRUGS

The group of newer AEDs has 15 members. Because clinical experience with the newer drugs is less than that of traditional AEDs, they are prescribed less often. Oxcarbazepine and lamotrigine are the primary exceptions to this rule.

Do the newer AEDs have properties that make them appealing? Certainly. As a group, they are better tolerated than the traditional AEDs and may pose a smaller risk to the developing fetus. Furthermore, only one—oxcarbazepine—induces drug-metabolizing enzymes to a significant degree, and hence interactions with other drugs, including other AEDs, are relatively minor.

The subject of approved indications for the newer AEDs requires comment. When these drugs were introduced, FDA-approved indications were limited to *adjunctive* therapy of certain seizure disorders. None of these drugs was approved for *monotherapy* because clinical trials were limited to patients who were refractory to traditional AEDs. When the trials were conducted, rather than switching patients from a traditional AED to the experimental AED, the experimental AED was *added* to the existing regimen. Hence, when the trials were completed, all we knew for sure was that the new AED was effective when used together with an older AED. We had no data on use of the newer AED alone. As a result, the FDA had no option but to approve the new drug for adjunctive therapy. Since being released, seven of the newer AEDs have received FDA approval for monotherapy. These are eslicarbazepine, felbamate, lacosamide, lamotrigine, oxcarbazepine, topiramate, and vigabatrin.

To help prescribers be more comfortable with the newer AEDs, two organizations—the American Academy of Neurology (AAN) and American Epilepsy Society (AES)—convened a panel to evaluate the efficacy and tolerability of these drugs. For some of the newer AEDs, the AAN/AES panel recommended uses not yet approved by the FDA. These recommendations, along with FDA-approved indications, are discussed in the sections that follow.

Oxcarbazepine

Oxcarbazepine [Oxtellar XR, Trileptal] will serve as our prototype for the newer AEDs. It is a derivative of carbamazepine; therefore, they share some of the same features.

Mechanism of Action

Antiseizure effects result from blockade of voltage-sensitive sodium channels in neuronal membranes, an action that stabilizes hyperexcitable neurons and thereby suppresses seizure spread. The drug does not affect neuronal GABA receptors.

Therapeutic Uses

Oxcarbazepine is indicated for both monotherapy and adjunctive therapy for management of partial seizures. It is approved for use in both adults and children. As monotherapy, it is approved for children 4 years of age and older; as adjunctive therapy, it may be prescribed for children as young as 2 years. Of note, in Canada, this drug is approved only for children age 6 years and older.

Adverse Effects

CNS Effects. The most common adverse effects are dizziness, drowsiness, double vision, nystagmus, headache, and ataxia. Patients should avoid driving and other hazardous activities, unless the degree of drowsiness is low.

Hyponatremia. Clinically significant *hyponatremia* (sodium concentration below 125 mmol/L) develops in 2.5% of patients. Signs include nausea, drowsiness, headache, and confusion. If oxcarbazepine is combined with other drugs that can decrease sodium levels (especially diuretics), monitoring of sodium levels may be needed.

Hypothyroidism. Hypothyroidism occurs more commonly in pediatric patients but may also occur in adults. Clinical manifestations of hypothyroidism include lethargy, cold intolerance, dry skin with brittle hair, and constipation. Additional manifestations in children include growth delay and decreased activity. For most children, there will be a tendency for school performance to decline; however, if the child was previously hyperactive, the hypoactivity that often accompanies hypothyroidism may improve school performance. Laboratory studies to assess thyroid function (e.g., thyroid-stimulating hormone [TSH] and free T_4) are necessary if there is suspicion of hypothyroidism. If hypothyroidism is confirmed, the drug should be discontinued. A euthyroid state resumes after therapy is discontinued.

Hematologic Abnormalities. Oxcarbazepine does not usually cause the severe hematologic abnormalities seen with carbamazepine; however, they have occurred rarely. Accordingly, routine monitoring of blood counts is not usually required unless the patient is at risk; however, some experts suggest periodic monitoring is appropriate. In either case, patients should be assessed for evidence of blood dyscrasias (e.g., pallor, fatigue, weakness, exercise intolerance, fever, infection, easy bleeding or bruising, petechiae), and a complete blood count (CBC) should be ordered for confirmation as needed.

Skin Reactions. Like carbamazepine, oxcarbazepine can cause *serious skin reactions,* including SJS and TEN. There is 30% cross-sensitivity among patients with hypersensitivity to carbamazepine. Accordingly, patients with a history of severe reactions to either drug should probably not use the other.

Hypersensitivity Reactions. Oxcarbazepine has been associated with serious *multiorgan hypersensitivity reactions.* Although manifestations vary, patients typically present with fever and rash, associated with one or more of the following: lymphadenopathy, hematologic abnormalities, pruritus, hepatitis, nephritis, hepatorenal syndrome, oliguria, arthralgia, or asthenia. If this reaction is suspected, oxcarbazepine should be discontinued.

Use in Pregnancy and Breast-Feeding

Oxcarbazepine may pose a risk of birth defects. Accordingly, women of childbearing age should use effective contraception. The drug should be avoided if possible by women who are already pregnant. In addition, because both oxcarbazepine and its metabolite are excreted in breast milk, the drug should be avoided by women who are breast-feeding.

Drug Interactions

Phenytoin. Oxcarbazepine's interaction with phenytoin has multiple implications. Oxcarbazepine inhibits the enzymes that metabolize phenytoin, thus raising phenytoin levels. Conversely, phenytoin may decrease serum concentrations of oxcarbazepine. When this combination is used, phenytoin toxicity and subtherapeutic levels of oxcarbazepine can result. Phenytoin and oxcarbazepine levels should be monitored and dosages adjusted accordingly.

Perampanel, Phenobarbital, and Valproic Acid. Perampanel can increase serum levels of oxcarbazepine. Valproic acid can decrease levels of oxcarbazepine. Phenobarbital can decrease serum levels of oxcarbazepine's active metabolite. If these drugs are given together, oxcarbazepine levels will need to be monitored and dosages adjusted accordingly.

Eslicarbazepine. Oxcarbazepine can increase serum levels of eslicarbazepine. This combination is not recommended.

Oral Contraceptives. Oxcarbazepine induces enzymes that metabolize both estrogens and progestins, which are ingredients in *oral contraceptives*. Accordingly, women who are at risk of becoming pregnant should employ an alternative birth control method.

Sodium-Depleting Drugs. Sodium-depleting drugs can increase the risk of hyponatremia. Oxcarbazepine should be used with caution in patients taking *diuretics* and other drugs that can lower sodium levels.

Alcohol. Alcohol can intensify CNS depression caused by oxcarbazepine. It should be avoided.

Lamotrigine

Mechanism of Action

Lamotrigine [Lamictal] has a broad spectrum of antiseizure activity. Benefits derive mainly from blocking sodium channels and partly from blocking calcium channels. Both actions decrease release of glutamate, an excitatory neurotransmitter.

Therapeutic Uses

Lamotrigine is FDA approved for (1) adjunctive therapy of partial seizures in adults and children over 2 years old, (2) adjunctive therapy of generalized seizures associated with Lennox-Gastaut syndrome in adults and children older than 2 years, (3) adjunctive therapy of primary generalized tonic-clonic seizures in adults and children older than 2 years, and (4) monotherapy of partial seizures in patients at least 16 years old who are converting from another AED. In addition, the AAN/AES guidelines recommend using lamotrigine for absence seizures. Lamotrigine is also FDA approved for long-term maintenance therapy of bipolar disorder (see Chapter 33). Investigational uses include myoclonic, absence, and temporal lobe seizures.

Drug Interactions

The half-life is dramatically affected by drugs that induce or inhibit hepatic drug-metabolizing enzymes. Enzyme inducers (e.g., carbamazepine, phenytoin, phenobarbital) decrease the half-life of lamotrigine to 10 hours, whereas valproate (an enzyme inhibitor) increases the half-life to about 60 hours. Lamotrigine itself is not an inducer or inhibitor of drug metabolism.

Estrogens can lower lamotrigine levels while lamotrigine may lower progestin levels. This can create unique concerns for the provider caring for a woman of childbearing age who wants to take oral contraceptives.

Adverse Effects

Common side effects include *dizziness, diplopia (double vision), blurred vision, nausea, vomiting,* and *headache.* Of much greater concern, patients may develop *life-threatening rashes,* including SJS and TEN. Deaths have occurred. The incidence of severe rash is about 0.8% in patients younger than 16 years and 0.3% in adults. Concurrent use of valproic acid increases this risk. If a rash develops, lamotrigine should be withdrawn immediately.

Very rarely, patients experience *aseptic meningitis* (inflammation of the meninges in the absence of bacterial infection). Patients who develop symptoms of meningitis—headache, fever, stiff neck, nausea, vomiting, rash, sensitivity to light—should undergo immediate evaluation to determine the cause. Treatable causes should be managed as indicated. If no clear cause other than lamotrigine is identified, discontinuation of lamotrigine should be considered.

Risk for *suicide* may be greater than with most other AEDs. Screen patients for suicidality before starting treatment, and monitor for suicidality during the treatment course.

When used during pregnancy, lamotrigine may pose a small risk of *cleft lip* and *cleft palate*. Whether the drug poses other risks in pregnancy or in breast-feeding has not been determined.

Gabapentin

Mechanism of Action

Gabapentin [Neurontin] is an analog of GABA but does not directly affect GABA receptors. Its precise mechanism of action is unknown, but it may enhance GABA release, thereby increasing GABA-mediated inhibition of neuronal firing.

Therapeutic Uses

Gabapentin has a broad spectrum of antiseizure activity. However, its only FDA-approved use in epilepsy is adjunctive therapy of partial seizures (with or without secondary generalization). The AAN/AES guidelines also recommend the drug for monotherapy of partial seizures. Gabapentin also has approval for treating postherpetic neuralgia. Interestingly, more than 80% of prescriptions are written for off-label uses, including relief of neuropathic pain (other than postherpetic neuralgia), prophylaxis of migraine, treatment of fibromyalgia, and relief of postmenopausal hot flashes. However, benefits in these disorders are modest, at best. Gabapentin does not appear effective in bipolar disorder.

Drug Interactions

Unlike most AEDs, gabapentin is devoid of significant interactions. It doesn't induce or inhibit drug-metabolizing enzymes, and doesn't affect the metabolism of other drugs. As a result, gabapentin is well suited for combined use with other AEDs.

Adverse Reactions

Gabapentin is very well tolerated. The most common side effects are somnolence, dizziness, ataxia, fatigue, nystagmus, and peripheral edema. These are usually mild to moderate and often diminish with continued drug use. Patients should avoid driving and other hazardous activities until they are confident they are not impaired. Safety in pregnancy and breast-feeding has not been established. Until further data are available, manufacturers recommend that gabapentin should be used by nursing women only if the benefits of breast-feeding outweigh the risks to the infant.

Safety Alert

MULTIPLE FORMULATIONS OF GABAPENTIN

Two forms of gabapentin are *not currently indicated* for management of epilepsy and, therefore, should not be confused with the form of gabapentin known as Neurontin.

- Gabapentin ER [Gralise] is approved for management of postherpetic neuralgia.
- Gabapentin enacarbil [Horizant], a prodrug form of gabapentin, is approved for treatment of moderate to severe restless legs syndrome.

Owing to differences in pharmacokinetics, these forms of gabapentin are *not interchangeable with each other or with Neurontin.*

Pregabalin

Mechanism of Action

Pregabalin [Lyrica], an analog of GABA, is much like gabapentin. Although pregabalin is an analog of GABA, the drug does not bind with GABA receptors or with benzodiazepine receptors, and hence does not work by mimicking or enhancing the inhibitory actions of GABA. Although the precise mechanism of action has not been established, we do know that pregabalin can bind with calcium channels on nerve terminals, and can thereby inhibit calcium influx, which in turn can inhibit release of several neurotransmitters, including glutamate, norepinephrine, and substance P. Reduced transmitter release may underlie seizure control and relief of neuropathic pain.

Therapeutic Uses

Like gabapentin, pregabalin is used for seizures and neuropathic pain. Pregabalin has four approved indications: neuropathic pain associated with diabetic neuropathy, postherpetic neuralgia, adjunctive therapy of partial seizures, and fibromyalgia. Fibromyalgia is discussed in Chapter 107.

Adverse Effects

Pregabalin can cause a variety of adverse effects. The most common are *dizziness* and *somnolence,* which often persist as long as the drug is being taken. *Blurred vision* may develop during early therapy, but resolves with continued drug use. About 8% of patients experience significant *weight gain* (7% or more of body weight in just a few months). Other adverse effects include *difficulty thinking, headache, peripheral edema,* and *dry mouth.*

Postmarketing reports indicate a risk of *hypersensitivity reactions,* including life-threatening *angioedema,* characterized by swelling of the face, tongue, lip, gums, throat, and larynx. Patients should discontinue pregabalin immediately at the first sign of angioedema or any other hypersensitivity reaction (blisters, hives, rash, dyspnea, wheezing).

According to product labeling, three out of over 10,000 patients developed *rhabdomyolysis* (muscle breakdown) during premarketing development. However, it is not clear that pregabalin was the cause. Nonetheless, patients should be instructed to report signs of muscle injury (pain, tenderness, weakness). If rhabdomyolysis is diagnosed, or even suspected, pregabalin should be withdrawn.

Abuse Potential and Physical Dependence

In contrast to most other antiseizure agents, pregabalin is regulated under the Controlled Substances Act. In clinical trials, 4% to 12% of patients reported euphoria as a side effect. When given to recreational users of sedative-hypnotic drugs, pregabalin produced subjective effects perceived as similar to those of diazepam [Valium]. On the basis of these data, the Drug Enforcement Agency has classified pregabalin under Schedule V of the Controlled Substances Act.

Abrupt discontinuation can cause insomnia, nausea, headache, diarrhea, and other symptoms that suggest physical dependence. To avoid withdrawal symptoms, pregabalin should be discontinued slowly, over 1 week or more.

Reproductive Toxicity

Pregabalin has demonstrated adverse effects on reproduction in both male and female animals. Data on human reproduction are lacking

When given to pregnant female rats and rabbits, pregabalin caused fetal growth delay, fetal death, structural abnormalities (e.g., skeletal and visceral malformation), and impaired function of the nervous system and reproductive system. Given this outcome, choice of a different AED is recommended for pregnant women.

When given to male rats before and during mating with untreated females, pregabalin decreased sperm counts and motility, decreased fertility, reduced fetal weight, and caused fetal abnormalities. Men using the drug should be informed about the possibility of decreased fertility and male-mediated teratogenicity. Men taking pregabalin should wear a condom when having sex with a woman of childbearing age.

Use in Breast-Feeding

We do not know with certainty whether pregabalin is excreted in breast milk. Until additional data are available, it is best for the patient to either stop nursing or stop taking pregabalin unless it is determined that the benefits of breast-feeding outweigh the risks of pregabalin exposure to the infant.

Drug Interactions

Alcohol, opioids, benzodiazepines, and other CNS depressants may intensify the depressant effects of pregabalin. Accordingly, such combinations should be avoided.

Extensive studies have failed to show pharmacokinetic interactions with any other drugs. Pregabalin does not inhibit cytochrome P450 isoenzymes.

Whether it can induce these isoenzymes is unknown. Pregabalin does not interact with oral contraceptives and does not alter the kinetics of any antiseizure drugs studied (carbamazepine, lamotrigine, phenobarbital, phenytoin, topiramate, valproic acid, and tiagabine).

Levetiracetam

Mechanism of Action

Levetiracetam [Keppra] is a unique agent that is chemically and pharmacologically different from all other AEDs. How levetiracetam acts is unknown; however, we know that it does not bind to receptors for GABA or any other known neurotransmitter.

Therapeutic Uses

In the United States, the drug is approved for adjunctive therapy of (1) myoclonic seizures in adults and adolescents age 12 years and older, (2) partial-onset seizures in adults and children age 4 years and older, and (3) primary generalized tonic-clonic seizures in adults and children age 6 years and older. Unlabeled uses include migraine, bipolar disorder, and new-onset pediatric epilepsy. In Europe, the drug is approved for monotherapy of partial seizures, for which it is highly effective.

Adverse Effects

In 2017, Health Canada reported a possible link between levetiracetam and renal injury. Other than this potential exception, adverse effects are generally mild to moderate. The most common are drowsiness and asthenia (lack of strength, weakness). Neuropsychiatric symptoms (agitation, anxiety, depression, psychosis, hallucinations, depersonalization) occur in less than 1% of patients. In contrast to other AEDs, levetiracetam does not impair speech, concentration, or other cognitive functions.

Safety for use during pregnancy or breast-feeding has not been determined. However, because it can be detected in breast milk, breast-feeding is not recommended by the manufacturer.

Drug Interactions

Unlike most other AEDs, levetiracetam does not interact with other drugs. It does not alter plasma concentrations of oral contraceptives, warfarin, digoxin, or other AEDs. These benefits are primarily attributable to the fact that levetiracetam is not metabolized by P450 isoenzymes.

Topiramate

Mechanism of Action

Topiramate [Topamax] is another broad-spectrum antiseizure agent. Seizure reduction occurs by four mechanisms: (1) potentiation of GABA-mediated inhibition, (2) blockade of voltage-dependent sodium channels, (3) blockade of calcium channels, and (4) blockade of receptors for glutamate, an excitatory neurotransmitter.

Therapeutic Uses

The drug is FDA approved for (1) *adjunctive* treatment of adults and children 2 years and older with partial seizures, primary generalized tonic-clonic seizures, and seizures associated with Lennox-Gastaut syndrome; (2) *monotherapy* of adults and children 2 years and older with partial seizures or primary generalized tonic-clonic seizures; and (3) prophylaxis of migraine in adults (see Chapter 30). Unlabeled uses include bipolar disorder, cluster headaches, neuropathic pain (including the pain of diabetic neuropathy), infantile spasms, essential tremor, binge-eating disorder, bulimia nervosa, and weight loss. Studies also show promise for the management of alcohol and cocaine dependence.

Adverse Effects

Although topiramate is generally well tolerated, it can cause multiple adverse effects. Common effects include somnolence, dizziness, ataxia, nervousness, diplopia, nausea, anorexia, and weight loss. Cognitive effects (confusion, memory difficulties, altered thinking, reduced concentration, difficulty finding words) can occur, but the incidence is low at recommended dosages. Kidney stones and paresthesias occur rarely.

Topiramate can cause *metabolic acidosis*. The drug inhibits carbonic anhydrase and thereby increases renal excretion of bicarbonate, which causes plasma pH to fall. Hyperventilation is the most characteristic symptom. Mild to moderate metabolic acidosis develops in 30% of adult patients, but severe acidosis is rare. Risk factors include renal disease, severe respiratory disorders, diarrhea, and a ketogenic diet. Prolonged metabolic acidosis can lead to kidney stones, fractures, and growth delay. Serum bicarbonate should be measured at baseline and periodically thereafter. Advise patients to inform the prescriber if they experience hyperventilation and other symptoms (fatigue, anorexia). If metabolic acidosis is diagnosed, topiramate should be given in reduced dosage or discontinued.

Topiramate can cause *hypohidrosis* (reduced sweating), thereby posing a risk of hyperthermia. Significant hyperthermia is usually associated with vigorous activity and an elevated environmental temperature.

There have been case reports of *angle-closure glaucoma*. Left untreated, this rapidly leads to blindness. Patients should be informed about symptoms of glaucoma (ocular pain, unusual redness, sudden worsening or blurring of vision) and instructed to seek immediate attention if these develop. Fortunately, topiramate-induced glaucoma is rare.

When taken during the first trimester of pregnancy, topiramate increases the risk of *cleft lip* and *cleft palate*. Although the *relative* risk seems high (a 20-fold increase), the *absolute* risk is still low (between 0.07% and 1.4%). Topiramate should be used only if the benefits of maternal seizure control are deemed to outweigh the risk to the fetus. Women using topiramate should use an effective form of birth control or should switch to a safer antiseizure drug if pregnancy is intended.

Risk for *suicide* may be greater than with most other AEDs. Screen patients for suicidality before starting treatment, and monitor for suicidality during the treatment course.

Drug Interactions

Phenytoin and carbamazepine can decrease levels of topiramate by about 45%. Topiramate may increase levels of phenytoin.

Tiagabine

Mechanism of Action

Tiagabine [Gabitril] blocks reuptake of GABA by neurons and glia. As a result, the inhibitory influence of GABA is intensified, and seizures are suppressed.

Therapeutic Uses

Tiagabine is FDA approved only for adjunctive therapy of partial seizures in patients at least 12 years old. Off-label uses include management of generalized anxiety disorder, multiple sclerosis, neuropathic pain, post-traumatic stress disorder, psychosis, and spasticity. Recent studies show promise for use of tiagabine in migraine prophylaxis as well as management of bipolar disorder and insomnia. However, owing to a risk of seizures (see *Adverse Effects*), such off-label use is discouraged.

Adverse Effects

Tiagabine is generally well tolerated. Common adverse effects are dizziness, somnolence, asthenia, nausea, nervousness, and tremor. Like most other AEDs, tiagabine can cause dose-related cognitive effects (e.g., confusion, abnormal thinking, trouble in concentrating).

Tiagabine has *caused* seizures in some patients—but only in those using the drug off-label (i.e., those using the drug for a condition other than epilepsy). A few patients have developed SE, which can be life threatening. In most cases, seizures occurred soon after starting tiagabine or after increasing the dosage. Because of seizure risk, off-label use of tiagabine usually should be avoided. Why are people without epilepsy at risk? Possibly because they are not taking AEDs. Remember, tiagabine is approved only for adjunctive use with other AEDs. It may be that these drugs protect against tiagabine-induced seizures. Because patients without epilepsy take tiagabine by itself, they are not protected from seizure development.

Drug Interactions

Tiagabine does not alter the metabolism or serum concentrations of other AEDs. However, levels of tiagabine can be decreased by phenytoin, phenobarbital, and carbamazepine—all of which induce drug-metabolizing enzymes.

Zonisamide

Mechanism of Action

Zonisamide [Zonegran] belongs to the same chemical family as the sulfonamide antibiotics, but lacks antimicrobial activity. In animal models, zonisamide suppresses focal seizure activity and spread. The underlying mechanism appears to be a blockade of neuronal sodium channels and calcium channels.

Therapeutic Uses

Zonisamide is approved only for adjunctive therapy of partial seizures in adults. This drug is sometimes used off-label for the management of bipolar disorder, migraine prophylaxis, and Parkinson disease.

Adverse Effects

The most common adverse effects are drowsiness, dizziness, anorexia, headache, and nausea. Metabolic acidosis is also common. Like most other AEDs, zonisamide can impair speech, concentration, and other cognitive processes. Because the drug can reduce alertness and impair cognition, patients should avoid driving and other hazardous activities until they know how the drug affects them.

Zonisamide can have severe *psychiatric effects*. During clinical trials, 2.2% of patients either discontinued treatment or were hospitalized because of severe depression; 1.1% attempted suicide.

Like all other sulfonamides, zonisamide can trigger *hypersensitivity reactions*, including some that are potentially fatal (e.g., SJS, TEN, fulminant hepatic necrosis). Accordingly, zonisamide is contraindicated for patients with a history of sulfonamide hypersensitivity. Patients who develop a rash should be followed closely, because rash can evolve into a more serious event. If severe hypersensitivity develops, zonisamide should be withdrawn immediately. Fortunately, serious reactions and fatalities are rare.

Zonisamide has adverse effects on the kidneys. In clinical trials, about 4% of patients developed *nephrolithiasis* (kidney stones). The risk can be reduced by drinking 6 to 8 glasses of water a day (to maintain hydration and urine flow). Patients should be informed about signs of kidney stones (sudden back pain, abdominal pain, painful urination, bloody or dark urine) and instructed to report them immediately. In addition to nephrolithiasis, zonisamide can *impair glomerular filtration*. Because of its effects on the kidney, zonisamide should be used with caution in patients with kidney disease.

Like topiramate, zonisamide inhibits carbonic anhydrase and can thereby cause *metabolic acidosis*. The condition develops in up to 90% of children and 43% of adults, usually early in treatment. Risk is increased by renal disease, respiratory disease, diarrhea, and following a ketogenic diet. Metabolic acidosis can delay growth in children and, over time, can lead to kidney stones and fractures in all patients. Advise patients to report hyperventilation and other signs of metabolic acidosis (e.g., fatigue, anorexia). Determine plasma bicarbonate at baseline and periodically thereafter. If metabolic acidosis is diagnosed, zonisamide should be discontinued or given in reduced dosage.

Rarely, zonisamide causes *hypohidrosis* (decreased sweating) and *hyperthermia* (elevation of body temperature). Pediatric patients may be at special risk. In warm weather, hypohidrosis may lead to heat stroke and subsequent hospitalization. Patients should be monitored closely for reduced sweating and increased body temperature.

Use in Pregnancy and Breast-Feeding

Zonisamide is teratogenic and lethal to embryos in laboratory animals. Cardiovascular abnormalities are common. Women of childbearing age should use effective contraception. Zonisamide should be avoided during pregnancy unless the benefits to the mother are deemed to outweigh the potential risks to the fetus. Zonisamide is readily excreted in breast milk. To avoid the potential for serious adverse effects in infants, patients taking zonisamide should not breast-feed.

Drug and Food Interactions

Levels of zonisamide can be affected by agents that induce or inhibit CYP3A4. Inducers of CYP3A4—including St. John's wort (an herbal supplement used for depression) and several AEDs (e.g., phenytoin, phenobarbital, carbamazepine)—can accelerate the metabolism of zonisamide and can thereby reduce the drug's half-life (to as little as 27 hours). Conversely, inhibitors of CYP3A4—including grapefruit juice, azole antifungal agents (e.g., ketoconazole), and several protease inhibitors (e.g., ritonavir)—can slow the metabolism of zonisamide and thereby prolong and intensify its effects.

Felbamate

Mechanism of Action

Felbamate [Felbatol] increases seizure threshold and suppresses seizure spread. The underlying mechanism is unknown. Unlike some AEDs, such as phenobarbital and benzodiazepines, felbamate does not interact with GABA receptors and does not enhance the inhibitory actions of GABA.

Therapeutic Uses

Felbamate is an effective AED with a broad spectrum of antiseizure activity. It is approved for (1) adjunctive or monotherapy in adults with partial seizures (with or without generalization), and (2) adjunctive therapy in children with Lennox-Gastaut syndrome. Because adverse effects can be severe, use of the drug is very limited.

Adverse Effects

Felbamate can cause *aplastic anemia*. Fatality rates varying from 20% to 30% to as high as 70% have been attributed to this drug. Because of this danger, felbamate has a black box warning for this concern.

Felbamate can also cause *liver damage*. Because of the risk of liver failure, felbamate should not be used by patients with pre-existing liver dysfunction. In addition, patients taking the drug should be monitored for indications of liver injury.

The most common adverse effects are GI disturbances (anorexia, nausea, vomiting) and CNS effects (insomnia, somnolence, dizziness, headache, diplopia). These occur more frequently when felbamate is combined with other drugs.

Drug Interactions

Felbamate can alter plasma levels of other AEDs and vice versa. Felbamate increases levels of phenytoin and valproic acid. Levels of felbamate are increased by valproic acid and reduced by phenytoin and carbamazepine. Increased levels of phenytoin and valproic acid (and possibly felbamate) could lead to toxicity; reduced levels of felbamate could lead to therapeutic failure. Therefore, to keep levels of these drugs within the therapeutic range, their levels should be monitored and dosages adjusted accordingly.

Lacosamide

Mechanism of Action

Benefits of lacosamide [Vimpat] appear to derive from slow inactivation of sodium channels. This results in stabilization of hyperexcitable neuronal membranes and subsequent inhibition of repetitive firing.

Therapeutic Uses

Lacosamide is indicated for add-on therapy of partial-onset seizures in patients age 17 years and older. In patients with refractory partial-onset seizures, adding lacosamide to the regimen reduced seizure frequency by 50% or more in roughly 40% of those treated. Monotherapy was added as an indication in 2015 labeling updates. Compared with other drugs for partial-onset seizures, lacosamide has two advantages. First, it has few drug interactions. Second, it can be administered IV as well as orally.

Adverse Effects

Lacosamide is generally well tolerated. The most common adverse effects are dizziness, headache, diplopia, and nasopharyngitis. Other effects include vomiting, fatigue, incoordination, blurred vision, tremor, somnolence, and cognitive changes (e.g., impaired memory, confusion, attention disruption). Lacosamide can prolong the PR interval, so it should be used with caution in patients with cardiac conduction problems and in those taking other drugs that prolong the PR interval. About 1% of patients experience euphoria. As a result, lacosamide is classified as a Schedule V drug under the Controlled Substances Act. Like other AEDs, lacosamide carries a small risk of suicidal thoughts or behavior.

Drug Interactions

Lacosamide has few drug interactions. In clinical trials, it had little effect on plasma levels of other AEDs; however, carbamazepine, fosphenytoin, phenytoin, and phenobarbital may decrease the serum concentration of lacosamide. As noted, lacosamide should be used with caution in patients taking other drugs that can prolong the PR interval (e.g., beta blockers, calcium channel blockers).

Rufinamide

Mechanism of Action

Rufinamide [Banzel] has actions similar to some other AEDs (e.g., phenytoin, carbamazepine) in that rufinamide appears to suppress seizure activity by prolonging the inactive state of neuronal sodium channels.

Therapeutic Uses

Rufinamide is approved as add-on therapy for seizures associated with Lennox-Gastaut syndrome, a severe form of childhood epilepsy. In clinical trials, the drug reduced seizure frequency and severity.

Adverse Effects

Adverse effects differ somewhat between children and adults. In children, the most common adverse effects are somnolence, vomiting, and headache. In adults, the most common effects are dizziness, fatigue, nausea, and somnolence. Rufinamide can reduce the QT interval on the electrocardiogram, so it should not be used by patients with familial short QT syndrome. Like all other AEDs, rufinamide may increase suicidal thoughts and behavior.

Drug Interactions

Four AEDs—carbamazepine, phenobarbital, phenytoin, and primidone—can significantly *reduce* levels of rufinamide. Because rufinamide is not metabolized by P450 isoenzymes, induction of cytochrome P450 cannot be the mechanism. One AED—valproic acid—can *increase* rufinamide levels by up to 70%. Rufinamide causes mild induction of CYP3A4 and can thereby reduce levels of ethinyl estradiol and norethindrone, common components of oral contraceptives. An alternative form of contraception may be needed. Because rufinamide shortens the QT interval, other drugs that shorten the interval (e.g., digoxin) should be used with caution.

Vigabatrin

Mechanism of Action

Benefits of Vigabatrin [Sabril] derive from inhibiting GABA transaminase, the enzyme that inactivates GABA in the CNS. By preventing GABA inactivation, vigabatrin increases GABA availability and thereby enhances GABA-mediated inhibition of neuronal activity. Unfortunately, although vigabatrin is effective, it is also dangerous: The drug can cause *permanent* loss of vision.

Therapeutic Uses

Vigabatrin has two indications: (1) add-on therapy of complex partial seizures in adults who are refractory to other drugs and (2) monotherapy of infantile spasms in children ages 6 months to 2 years. Vigabatrin is the first drug approved in the United States for infantile spasms, a severe seizure disorder that occurs in children during the first year of life.

Adverse Effect: Vision Loss

Vigabatrin can cause *irreversible* loss of peripheral vision. Some degree of visual field reduction occurs in 30% or more of patients. Additionally, damage to the central part of the retina can reduce visual acuity. Some patients experience retinal damage within days to weeks of treatment onset, while others may use the drug for months to years before damage occurs.

To reduce the extent of damage, vision should be tested at baseline and every 3 months thereafter. If vision loss is detected, vigabatrin should be discontinued. Stopping will not reverse damage that has already occurred, but may limit development of further damage. Unfortunately, even with periodic testing, some patients will develop severe vision loss.

Owing to the risk of vision loss, vigabatrin is available only through a restricted use program, known as SHARE (Support, Help, and Resources for Epilepsy). The goal is to monitor for vision damage and discontinue the drug as soon as possible when damage is detected. SHARE requires registration by prescribers, pharmacists, adult patients, and parents/guardians of young patients. In addition, the program requires that adult and pediatric patients undergo regular vision testing.

Other Adverse Effects

In clinical trials, the most common adverse effects in *adults* (who received vigabatrin plus other AEDs) were headache, somnolence, fatigue, dizziness, convulsions, increased weight, visual field defects, and depression. Like other AEDs, vigabatrin can promote suicidal thoughts and behavior. Among *children*, the most common adverse effects were somnolence, bronchitis, and otitis media.

Drug Interactions

The risk of retinal damage is increased by combining vigabatrin with other drugs that can directly damage the retina (e.g., hydroxychloroquine) or with drugs that can promote glaucoma (e.g., glucocorticoids, tricyclic antidepressants). Vigabatrin can reduce levels of phenytoin (by inducing CYP2C9, the 2C9 isoenzyme of cytochrome P450) and can increase levels of clonazepam (by a mechanism that is unknown).

Ezogabine

Mechanism of Action

Ezogabine [Potiga] is a first-in-class potassium channel opener. Ezogabine activates voltage-gated potassium channels in the neuronal membrane and thereby facilitates potassium efflux. As a result, repetitive neuronal firing and related seizure activity are reduced.

Therapeutic Uses

Ezogabine is approved for adjunctive treatment of partial-onset seizures.

Adverse Effect: Vision Loss

Previously, adverse effects due to ezogabine were thought to be minimal. Fortunately, subjects enrolled in clinical trials continued in extension trials postmarketing. As a result of the postmarketing trials, researchers discovered that prolonged use of ezogabine can lead to retinal abnormalities. Moreover, of those taking the drug for 4 years, approximately a third of patients demonstrated retinal changes on eye examinations, and some of those had associated vision loss. As a result of this finding, ezogabine is recommended for use only for those in whom other antiepileptic drugs do not work and in whom benefits exceed the risk of vision loss.

Other Adverse Effects

Approximately 2% of patients taking ezogabine experience urinary retention. As previously mentioned, ezogabine activates voltage-gated potassium channels in the neuronal membrane and thereby facilitates potassium efflux. Unfortunately, ezogabine also activates potassium channels in the bladder epithelium and thereby promotes urinary retention, a unique side effect among the AEDs. Because of its effects on the bladder, ezogabine should be used with caution (if at all) in patients with pre-existing voiding difficulty.

Long-term use of ezogabine can also cause blue, gray-blue, and brown skin discoloration. This occurs most commonly in the nailbed and perioral area; however, it may become generalized. The drug can impart a red-orange color to urine. This effect is dose related and doesn't occur in most patients. When it does, it is harmless and unrelated to urinary retention.

The most common adverse reactions are somnolence, dizziness, fatigue, confusion, vertigo, tremor, incoordination, double vision, memory impairment, and reduced strength. In addition, ezogabine can cause hallucinations and other symptoms of psychosis.

Ezogabine has the potential for abuse and is under review for possible regulation as a controlled substance. Like all other AEDs, ezogabine may increase the risk of suicidal thinking or behavior.

Drug Interactions

In contrast to many AEDs, ezogabine has few interactions with other drugs. Both carbamazepine and phenytoin can decrease plasma concentrations of the drug, so higher doses of ezogabine may be needed when adding either drug to the medication regimen.

Eslicarbazepine

Mechanism of Action

The mechanism of action of eslicarbazepine [Aptiom] appears to be related to blockade of sodium channels. It is a prodrug that is metabolized to its active eslicarbazepine metabolite on first-pass metabolism.

Therapeutic Uses

Eslicarbazepine is approved for the management of partial seizures. It may be used as either monotherapy or as an adjunct to ongoing therapy.

Adverse Effects

The majority of eslicarbazepine's adverse effects are related to actions on the CNS. These include dizziness and sedation. More than 10% of patients have developed headache and diplopia.

Drug Interactions

Eslicarbazepine is a CYP2C19 inhibitor and a CYP3A4 inducer. This is the mechanism behind many of the interactions with this drug.

When prescribed with phenytoin, eslicarbazepine can increase phenytoin levels and phenytoin can decrease eslicarbazepine levels. Carbamazepine and phenobarbital can also decrease levels of eslicarbazepine.

Other significant interactions may occur with statins, hormonal contraceptives, and warfarin. Eslicarbazepine can lower levels of all these drugs. Dosage adjustments may be required, and alternate forms of birth control may need to be considered.

Perampanel

Mechanism of Action

Its antiepileptic effects are the result of AMPA glutamate antagonism. It blocks AMPA glutamate receptors on post-synaptic neurons.

Therapeutic Uses

Perampanel is approved for adjunctive therapy for treatment of both tonic-clonic seizures and partial seizures. It is not approved for use in children under 12 years of age.

Adverse Effects

Perampanel has been associated with serious psychiatric reactions. These include anger, aggression, hostility, violence, and even homicidal ideation. This atypical anger and aggression may occur in as many as 20% of patients taking the drug.

Other than hostility, the most common adverse effects are dizziness, drowsiness, fatigue, and headache. Nausea, vomiting, abdominal discomfort, and weight gain may also occur.

Drug Interactions

Perampanel can decrease the effectiveness of hormonal contraceptives, particularly progestins. It can enhance the effect of CNS depressants, thus increasing risks related to sedation and, if significant, respiratory drive.

Phenytoin, carbamazepine, and oxcarbazepine can decrease perampanel levels by 50% or more through hepatic enzyme induction. Care must be undertaken to adjust for this when making adjustments in therapy.

Safety Alert

MANAGEMENT OF EPILEPSY DURING PREGNANCY

The risk to a fetus from uncontrolled seizures is greater than the risk from AEDs. Therefore, patients with major seizure disorders should continue to take AEDs throughout pregnancy. To minimize fetal risk, the lowest effective dosage should be determined and maintained, and just one drug should be used whenever possible.

To reduce the risk of neural tube defects that can occur with AEDs, pregnant patients should take supplemental folic acid before conception and throughout pregnancy. A dose of 2 mg/day has been recommended.

Maternal and fetal/infant bleeding risks are also a concern. *Phenobarbital, phenytoin, carbamazepine,* and *primidone* reduce levels of vitamin K–dependent clotting factors by inducing hepatic enzymes, increasing the risk of bleeding. To reduce the risk, pregnant patients should be given 10 mg of vitamin K daily during the last few weeks of pregnancy, and the fetus should be given a 1-mg IM injection of vitamin K at birth.

MANAGEMENT OF GENERALIZED CONVULSIVE STATUS EPILEPTICUS

Convulsive SE is defined as a continuous series of tonic-clonic seizures that lasts for at least 20 to 30 minutes. Consciousness is lost during the entire attack. Tachycardia, elevation of blood pressure, and hyperthermia are typical. Metabolic sequelae include hypoglycemia and acidosis. If SE persists for more than 20 minutes, it can cause permanent neurologic injury (cognitive impairment, memory loss, worsening of the underlying seizure disorder) and even death.

Generalized convulsive SE is a medical emergency that requires immediate treatment. Ideally, treatment should commence within 5 minutes of seizure onset. Speed is important because as time passes SE becomes more and more resistant to therapy.

The goal of treatment is to maintain ventilation, correct hypoglycemia, and terminate the seizure. An IV line is established to draw blood for analysis of glucose levels, electrolyte levels, and drug levels. The line is also used to administer glucose and AEDs. The benzodiazepine *lorazepam* is recommended for first-line management of status epilepticus. *Diazepam,* also a benzodiazepine, may be used if lorazepam is not readily available. Both drugs can terminate seizures quickly. Diazepam has a short duration of action, and hence must be administered repeatedly. In contrast, effects of lorazepam last up to 72 hours. Because of its prolonged effects, lorazepam is generally preferred. The usual dosage for lorazepam is 4 mg IV administered at a maximum rate of 2 mg/min. The initial dose for diazepam is 5 to 10 mg IV every 5 to 10 minutes administered at a maximum rate of 5 mg/min. The total dose of diazepam should not exceed 30 mg. If SE occurs outside the hospital setting, diazepam rectal gel 10 mg can be inserted and repeated once, if needed.

Once seizures are controlled, either *phenytoin* [Dilantin] or *fosphenytoin* [Cerebyx] may be given for long-term suppression. For patients who cannot take hydantoin AEDs, *valproic acid* or *levetiracetam* may be used. Because the effects of diazepam are short lived, follow-up treatment with a long-acting drug is essential when diazepam is used for initial control. However, when lorazepam is used for initial control, follow-up therapy may be unnecessary.

KEY POINTS

- Seizures are initiated by discharge from a group of hyperexcitable neurons, called a focus.
- In partial seizures, excitation undergoes limited spread from the focus to adjacent cortical areas.
- In generalized seizures, excitation spreads widely throughout both hemispheres of the brain.
- AEDs act through four basic mechanisms: blockade of sodium channels, blockade of calcium channels, blockade of receptors for glutamate (an excitatory neurotransmitter), and potentiation of GABA (an inhibitory neurotransmitter).
- The goal in treating epilepsy is to reduce seizures to an extent that enables the patient to live a normal or near-normal life. Complete elimination of seizures may not be possible without causing intolerable side effects.
- AEDs can be divided into two main groups: traditional AEDs and newer AEDs.
- Many AEDs are selective for particular seizure types; therefore, successful treatment depends on choosing the correct drug.
- Monitoring plasma drug levels can be valuable for adjusting dosage, monitoring adherence, determining the cause of lost seizure control, and identifying the cause of toxicity, especially in patients taking more than one drug.
- Nonadherence accounts for nearly half of all treatment failures. Promoting adherence is a priority.

- Withdrawal of AEDs must be done gradually, because abrupt withdrawal can trigger SE.
- Some AEDs may pose a risk of suicidal thoughts and behavior.
- Most AEDs cause CNS depression, which can be deepened by concurrent use of other CNS depressants (e.g., alcohol, antihistamines, opioids, other AEDs).
- Phenytoin is active against partial seizures and tonic-clonic seizures but not absence seizures.
- The capacity of the liver to metabolize phenytoin is limited. As a result, doses only slightly greater than those needed for therapeutic effects can push phenytoin levels into the toxic range.
- The therapeutic range for phenytoin is 10 to 20 mcg/mL.
- When phenytoin levels rise above 20 mcg/mL, CNS toxicity develops. Signs include nystagmus, sedation, ataxia, diplopia, and cognitive impairment.
- Phenytoin causes gingival hyperplasia in 20% of patients.
- Rarely, phenytoin causes severe skin reactions: Stevens-Johnson syndrome (SJS) or toxic epidermal necrolysis (TEN). Risk *may* be increased by the HLA-B*1502 gene variation, seen almost exclusively in patients of Asian descent.
- Like phenytoin, carbamazepine is active against partial seizures and tonic-clonic seizures.
- Because carbamazepine is better tolerated than phenytoin, it is often preferred.
- Carbamazepine can cause leukopenia, anemia, and thrombocytopenia—and, very rarely, fatal aplastic anemia. To reduce the risk of serious hematologic toxicity, complete blood counts should be obtained at baseline and periodically thereafter.
- Like phenytoin, carbamazepine can cause SJS/TEN. Risk is *clearly* increased by the HLA-B*1502 gene variation. Accordingly, the FDA recommends that Asian patients should be screened for this variant before using the drug.
- Valproic acid is a broad-spectrum AED, having activity against partial seizures and most generalized seizures, including tonic-clonic, absence, atonic, and myoclonic seizures.
- Valproic acid can cause potentially fatal liver injury, especially in children under 2 years old who are taking other AEDs.
- Valproic acid can cause potentially fatal pancreatitis.
- Valproic acid is highly teratogenic, and can reduce the IQ of children exposed to it *in utero.* Accordingly, valproic acid should not be used during pregnancy, unless it is the only AED that works.
- In contrast to other barbiturates, phenobarbital is able to suppress seizures without causing generalized CNS depression.
- Phenytoin, carbamazepine, and phenobarbital induce the synthesis of hepatic drug-metabolizing enzymes, and can thereby accelerate inactivation of other drugs. Inactivation of oral contraceptives and warfarin is of particular concern.
- AEDs can interact with one another in complex ways, causing their blood levels to change. Dosages must be adjusted to compensate for these interactions.
- All traditional AEDs (and some newer AEDs) can harm the developing fetus, especially during the first trimester. However, the fetus and mother are at greater risk from uncontrolled seizures than from AEDs. Accordingly, women with major seizure disorders should continue taking AEDs throughout pregnancy.
- Fetal risk can be minimized by avoiding valproic acid and by using just one AED (if possible) in the lowest effective dosage.
- Initial control of generalized convulsive SE is accomplished with an IV benzodiazepine—either diazepam or lorazepam. When diazepam is used, follow-up treatment with phenytoin or fosphenytoin is essential for prolonged seizure suppression.

Please visit **http://evolve.elsevier.com/Lehne** for chapter-specific NCLEX® examination review questions.

Summary of Major Nursing Implications[a]

NURSING IMPLICATIONS THAT APPLY TO ALL ANTIEPILEPTIC DRUGS

Preadministration Assessment

Therapeutic Goal

The goal of treatment is to minimize or eliminate seizure events, thereby allowing the patient to live a normal or near-normal life.

Baseline Data

Before initiating treatment, it is essential to know the type of seizure involved (e.g., absence, generalized tonic-clonic) and how often seizure events occur.

Implementation: Administration

Dosage Determination

Dosages are often highly individualized and difficult to establish. Clinical evaluation of therapeutic and adverse effects is essential to establish a dosage that is both safe and effective. For several AEDs (especially those used to treat tonic-clonic seizures), knowledge of plasma AED levels can facilitate dosage adjustment.

Promoting Adherence

Seizure control requires rigid adherence to the prescribed regimen; nonadherence is a major cause of therapeutic failure. **To promote adherence, educate patients about the importance**

Continued

Summary of Major Nursing Implications[a]—cont'd

of taking AEDs exactly as prescribed. Monitoring plasma AED levels can motivate adherence and facilitate assessment of nonadherence.

Ongoing Evaluation and Interventions

Evaluating Therapeutic Effects

Teach the patient (or a family member) to maintain a seizure frequency chart, indicating the date, time, and nature of all seizure events. The prescriber can use this record to evaluate treatment, make dosage adjustments, and alter drug selections.

Minimizing Danger From Uncontrolled Seizures

Advise patients to avoid potentially hazardous activities (e.g., driving, operating dangerous machinery) until seizure control is achieved. Also, because seizures may recur after they are largely under control, advise patients to carry some form of identification (e.g., Medic Alert bracelet) to aid in diagnosis and treatment if a seizure occurs.

Minimizing Adverse Effects

CNS Depression. Most AEDs depress the CNS. Signs of CNS depression (sedation, drowsiness, lethargy) are most prominent during the initial phase of treatment and decline with continued drug use. **Forewarn patients about CNS depression, and advise them to avoid driving and other hazardous activities if CNS depression is significant.**

Withdrawal Seizures. Abrupt discontinuation of AEDs can lead to status epilepticus (SE). Consequently, medication should be withdrawn slowly (over 6 weeks to several months). **Inform patients about the dangers of abrupt drug withdrawal, and instruct them never to discontinue drug use without consulting the prescriber. Advise patients who are planning a trip to carry extra medication to ensure an uninterrupted supply in the event they become stranded where medication is unavailable.**

Usage in Pregnancy. In most cases, the risk from uncontrolled seizures exceeds the risk from medication; hence, women with major seizure disorders should continue to take AEDs during pregnancy. However, the lowest effective dosage should be employed and, if possible, only one drug should be used. One AED—valproic acid—should be avoided: The drug is highly teratogenic and can decrease the IQ of children exposed to it *in utero.* To reduce the risk of neural tube defects, **advise women to take folic acid supplements before and throughout pregnancy.**

Suicidal Thoughts and Behavior. The AEDs pose a small risk of suicidal thoughts and behavior. Screen for suicidality before starting treatment. **Educate patients, families, and caregivers about signs that may precede suicidal behavior (e.g., increased anxiety, agitation, mania, or hostility), and advise them to report these immediately.**

Minimizing Adverse Interactions

CNS Depressants. Drugs with CNS-depressant actions (e.g., alcohol, antihistamines, barbiturates, opioids) will intensify the depressant effects of AEDs, thereby posing a serious risk. **Warn patients against using alcohol and other CNS depressants.**

PHENYTOIN

Nursing implications for phenytoin include those presented below as well as those presented under *Nursing Implications That Apply to All Antiepileptic Drugs.*

Preadministration Assessment

Therapeutic Goal

Oral phenytoin is used to treat partial seizures (simple and complex) and tonic-clonic seizures. Intravenous phenytoin is used to treat convulsive SE.

Identifying High-Risk Patients

Intravenous phenytoin is *contraindicated* for patients with sinus bradycardia, sinoatrial block, second- or third-degree atrioventricular block, or Stokes-Adams syndrome.

Implementation: Administration

Routes

Oral, IV, and (rarely) IM.

Administration

Oral. **Instruct patients to take phenytoin exactly as prescribed. Inform them that once a safe and effective dosage has been established, small deviations in dosage can lead to toxicity or to loss of seizure control.**

Advise patients to take phenytoin with meals to reduce gastric discomfort.

Instruct patients to shake the phenytoin oral suspension before dispensing to provide consistent dosing.

Intravenous. To minimize the risk of severe reactions (e.g., cardiovascular collapse), infuse phenytoin slowly (no faster than 50 mg/min).

Do not mix phenytoin solutions with other drugs.

To minimize venous inflammation at the injection site, flush the needle or catheter with saline immediately after completing the phenytoin infusion.

Ongoing Evaluation and Interventions

Minimizing Adverse Effects

CNS Effects. **Inform patients that excessive doses can produce sedation, ataxia, diplopia, and interference with cognitive function. Instruct them to notify the prescriber if these occur.**

Gingival Hyperplasia. **Inform patients that phenytoin often promotes overgrowth of gum tissue. To minimize harm and discomfort, teach them proper techniques of brushing, flossing, and gum massage—and suggest taking 0.5 mg of folic acid every day.**

Use in Pregnancy. Phenytoin can cause fetal hydantoin syndrome and bleeding tendencies in the neonate. Decrease bleeding risk by giving the mother vitamin K for 1 month before delivery and during delivery and to the infant immediately after delivery. Decrease the risk of fetal hydantoin syndrome by using the lowest effective phenytoin dosage.

Dermatologic Reactions. **Inform patients that phenytoin can cause a morbilliform (measles-like) rash that may progress to much more serious conditions: Stevens-Johnson syndrome**

Summary of Major Nursing Implications[a]—cont'd

(SJS) or toxic epidermal necrolysis (TEN). Instruct patients to notify the prescriber immediately if a rash develops. Use of phenytoin should stop. As with carbamazepine (see later in this summary), the risk of SJS/TEN may be increased by a genetic variation known as HLA-B*1502, seen primarily in patients of Asian descent.

Withdrawal Seizures. Abrupt discontinuation of phenytoin can trigger convulsive SE. **Warn patients against abrupt cessation of treatment.**

Minimizing Adverse Interactions

Phenytoin is subject to a large number of significant interactions with other drugs; a few are noted below. **Warn patients against use of any drugs not specifically approved by the prescriber.**

CNS Depressants. **Warn patients against the use of alcohol and all other drugs with CNS-depressant properties, including opioids, barbiturates, and antihistamines.**

Warfarin and Oral Contraceptives. Phenytoin can decrease the effects of these agents (as well as other drugs) by inducing hepatic drug-metabolizing enzymes. Dosages of warfarin and oral contraceptives may need to be increased.

CARBAMAZEPINE

Nursing implications for carbamazepine include those presented below as well as those presented under *Nursing Implications That Apply to All Antiepileptic Drugs.*

Preadministration Assessment

Therapeutic Goal

Carbamazepine is used to treat partial seizures (simple and complex) and tonic-clonic seizures.

Baseline Data

Obtain complete blood counts before treatment.

Identifying High-Risk Patients

Carbamazepine is *contraindicated* for patients with a history of bone marrow depression or adverse hematologic reactions to other drugs. Screen Asian patients for the HLA-B*1502 gene variation, which increases the risk of SJS/TEN.

Implementation: Administration

Route

Oral.

Administration

Advise patients to administer carbamazepine with meals to decrease gastric upset.

To minimize adverse CNS effects, use low initial doses and give the largest portion of the daily dose at bedtime.

Ongoing Evaluation and Interventions

Minimizing Adverse Effects

CNS Effects. Carbamazepine can cause headache, visual disturbances (nystagmus, blurred vision, diplopia), ataxia, vertigo, and unsteadiness. To minimize these effects, initiate therapy with low doses and have the patient take the largest part of the daily dose at bedtime.

Hematologic Effects. Carbamazepine can cause leukopenia, anemia, thrombocytopenia, and, very rarely, fatal aplastic anemia. To reduce the risk of serious hematologic effects, (1) obtain complete blood counts at baseline and periodically thereafter, (2) avoid carbamazepine in patients with pre-existing hematologic abnormalities, and (3) **inform patients about manifestations of hematologic abnormalities (fever, sore throat, pallor, weakness, infection, easy bruising, petechiae), and instruct them to notify the prescriber if these occur.**

Birth Defects. Carbamazepine can cause neural tube defects. Use in pregnancy only if the benefits of seizure suppression outweigh the risks to the fetus.

Severe Skin Reactions. Carbamazepine can cause SJS/TEN, especially among patients with HLA-B*1502, a genetic variation seen almost exclusively in patients of Asian descent. To reduce risk, the FDA recommends that patients of Asian descent be tested for HLA-B*1502. If SJS/TEN develops, carbamazepine should be discontinued. Because HLA-B*1502 may also increase the risk of SJS/TEN in response to phenytoin, phenytoin should not be used as an alternative to carbamazepine in patients with the mutation.

Minimizing Adverse Interactions

Interactions Due to Induction of Drug Metabolism. Carbamazepine can decrease responses to other drugs by inducing hepatic drug-metabolizing enzymes. Effects on oral contraceptives and warfarin are of particular concern. Patients using these drugs will require increased dosages to maintain therapeutic responses.

Phenytoin and Phenobarbital. These drugs can decrease responses to carbamazepine by inducing drug-metabolizing enzymes (beyond the degree of induction caused by carbamazepine itself). Dosage of carbamazepine may need to be increased.

Grapefruit Juice. Grapefruit juice can increase levels of carbamazepine. **Instruct patients not to drink grapefruit juice.**

VALPROIC ACID

Nursing implications for valproic acid include those presented here as well as those presented earlier in this summary under *Nursing Implications That Apply to All Antiepileptic Drugs.*

Preadministration Assessment

Therapeutic Goal

Valproic acid is used to treat all major seizure disorders: tonic-clonic, absence, myoclonic, atonic, and partial (simple, complex, and secondarily generalized).

Baseline Data

Obtain baseline tests of liver function.

Identifying High-Risk Patients

Valproic acid is *contraindicated* for patients with significant hepatic dysfunction and for children younger than 3 years

Continued

Summary of Major Nursing Implications[a]—cont'd

who are taking other AEDs. Avoid valproic acid during pregnancy.

Implementation: Administration

Routes

Oral, IV.

Administration

Advise patients to take valproic acid with meals, and instruct them to ingest tablets and capsules intact, without crushing or chewing.

Ongoing Evaluation and Interventions

Minimizing Adverse Effects

Gastrointestinal Effects. Nausea, vomiting, and indigestion are common. These can be reduced by using an enteric-coated formulation (see Table 24.5) and by taking valproic acid with meals.

Hepatotoxicity. Rarely, valproic acid has caused fatal liver injury. To minimize risk, (1) don't use valproic acid in conjunction with other drugs in children younger than 3 years; (2) don't use valproic acid in patients with pre-existing liver dysfunction; (3) evaluate liver function at baseline and periodically thereafter; (4) **inform patients about signs and symptoms of liver injury (reduced appetite, malaise, nausea, abdominal pain, jaundice), and instruct them to notify the prescriber if these develop;** and (5) use valproic acid in the lowest effective dosage.

Pancreatitis. Valproic acid can cause life-threatening pancreatitis. **Inform patients about signs of pancreatitis (abdominal pain, nausea, vomiting, anorexia) and instruct them to get an immediate evaluation if these develop.** If pancreatitis is diagnosed, valproic acid should be withdrawn.

Pregnancy-Related Harm. Valproic acid may cause neural tube defects and other congenital malformations, especially when taken during the first trimester. In addition, the drug can reduce the IQ of children exposed to it *in utero.* Valproic acid should be avoided by women of childbearing potential—unless it is the only AED that will work. **Advise women who must use valproic acid to use an effective form of birth control and to take 5 mg of folic acid daily (to reduce the risk of neural tube defects if pregnancy should occur).**

Hyperammonemia. Combining valproic acid with topiramate poses a risk of hyperammonemia. If symptoms develop (vomiting, lethargy, altered level of consciousness and/or cognitive function), blood ammonia should be measured. If the level is excessive, either valproic acid or topiramate should be withdrawn.

Minimizing Adverse Interactions

Antiepileptic Drugs. Valproic acid can elevate plasma levels of phenytoin and phenobarbital. Levels of phenobarbital and phenytoin should be monitored and their dosages adjusted accordingly.

Topiramate. See *Hyperammonemia* above.

Carbapenem Antibiotics. Meropenem and imipenem/cilastatin can reduce plasma levels of valproic acid. Breakthrough seizures have occurred. These antibiotics should be avoided in patients taking valproic acid.

PHENOBARBITAL

Nursing implications that apply to the antiseizure applications of phenobarbital include those presented below and those presented under *Nursing Implications That Apply to All Antiepileptic Drugs.* Nursing implications that apply to the barbiturates as a group are summarized in Chapter 34.

Preadministration Assessment

Therapeutic Goal

Oral phenobarbital is used for partial seizures (simple and complex) and tonic-clonic seizures. Intravenous therapy is used for convulsive SE.

Identifying High-Risk Patients

Phenobarbital is *contraindicated* for patients with a history of acute intermittent porphyria.

Use with *caution* during pregnancy.

Implementation: Administration

Routes

Oral and IV.

Administration

Oral. A loading schedule may be employed to initiate treatment. Monitor for excessive CNS depression when these large doses are used.

Intravenous. Rapid IV infusion can cause severe adverse effects. Perform infusions slowly.

Ongoing Evaluation and Interventions

Minimizing Adverse Effects

Neuropsychologic Effects. **Warn patients that sedation may occur during the initial phase of treatment. Advise them to avoid hazardous activities if sedation is significant.**

Inform parents that children may become irritable and hyperactive, and instruct them to notify the prescriber if these behaviors occur.

Exacerbation of Intermittent Porphyria. Phenobarbital can exacerbate acute intermittent porphyria, so it is absolutely contraindicated for patients with a history of this disorder.

Use in Pregnancy. **Warn patients of childbearing age that barbiturates may cause birth defects.**

Withdrawal Seizures. Abrupt withdrawal of phenobarbital can trigger seizures. **Warn patients against abrupt cessation of treatment.**

Minimizing Adverse Interactions

Interactions Caused by Induction of Drug Metabolism. Phenobarbital induces hepatic drug-metabolizing enzymes, and can thereby decrease responses to other drugs. Effects on *oral contraceptives* and *warfarin* are a particular concern; their dosages should be increased.

Summary of Major Nursing Implications[a]—cont'd

CNS Depressants. **Warn patients against use of alcohol and all other drugs with CNS-depressant properties (e.g., opioids, benzodiazepines).**

Valproic Acid. Valproic acid increases blood levels of phenobarbital. To avoid toxicity, reduce phenobarbital dosage.

OXCARBAZEPINE

Nursing implications for carbamazepine include those presented below as well as those presented under *Nursing Implications That Apply to All Antiepileptic Drugs.*

Preadministration Assessment

Therapeutic Goal

Oxcarbazepine is used as adjunctive therapy to treat partial seizures.

Baseline Data

Obtain complete blood counts before treatment.

Identifying High-Risk Patients

Oxcarbazepine is *contraindicated* for patients with a history of hypersensitivity to carbamazepine.

Implementation: Administration

Route

Oral.

Administration. **Advise patients that oxcarbazepine may be taken with or without food. Extended release formulations should be swallowed whole.**

Ongoing Evaluation and Interventions

Minimizing Adverse Effects

CNS Effects. Oxcarbazepine can cause dizziness and drowsiness. **Advise patients to avoid driving and other hazardous activities as long as drowsiness is a problem.**

Hyponatremia. Clinically significant hyponatremia is a risk for patients taking oxcarbazepine. **Advise patients to report symptoms of nausea, drowsiness, headache, and confusion.** If hyponatremia is suspected, a serum sodium level is needed to determine if this has occurred. Because the symptoms of hyponatremia are similar to the side effects of the drug, periodic monitoring of sodium levels may be indicated.

Hypothyroidism. Oxcarbazepine can cause hypothyroidism. Periodic evaluations of TSH and free T_4 are advised. **Counsel patients to report symptoms of lethargy, cold intolerance, dry skin with brittle hair, and constipation. Advise parents to report growth delays, decreased energy, and alterations in school performance for children taking this drug.**

Birth Defects. Oxcarbazepine can cause birth defects. Use in pregnancy only if the benefits of seizure suppression outweigh the risks to the fetus. **Notify women of childbearing age that oxcarbazepine decreases the effectiveness of oral contraceptives. An alternate form of birth control is needed.**

Severe Skin Reactions. Oxcarbazepine can cause serious skin reactions, including SJS/TEN. There is 30% cross-sensitivity among patients with hypersensitivity to carbamazepine. Accordingly, patients with a history of severe reactions to either drug should probably not use the other. **Instruct patients to notify the prescriber if skin changes occur while taking this drug.**

Multiorgan Hypersensitivity. If patient taking oxcarbazepine presents with fever and rash associated with one or more of the following: lymphadenopathy, hematologic abnormalities, pruritus, hepatitis, nephritis, hepatorenal syndrome, oliguria, arthralgia, or asthenia, hypersensitivity should be suspected. Oxcarbazepine should be discontinued.

Hematologic Effects. Oxcarbazepine can rarely cause blood dyscrasias (leukopenia, anemia, and thrombocytopenia). To reduce the risk of serious hematologic effects, (1) monitor patients for evidence of anemia (e.g., pallor, fatigue, weakness, exercise intolerance), leukopenia (fever, infection), and thrombocytopenia (easy bleeding or bruising, petechiae) and obtain complete blood counts if these occur, (2) avoid oxcarbazepine in patients with pre-existing hematologic abnormalities, and (3) **inform patients about manifestations of hematologic abnormalities and instruct them to notify the prescriber if these occur.**

Minimizing Adverse Interactions

Interactions Due to Induction of Drug Metabolism. Oxcarbazepine can decrease responses to other drugs by inducing hepatic drug-metabolizing enzymes. Patients using these drugs may require medication adjustments to maintain therapeutic responses.

Oral Contraceptives. As mentioned previously, oxcarbazepine reduces the effectiveness of oral contraceptives. **Advise women at risk of becoming pregnant that alternative birth control is required.**

Phenytoin. Oxcarbazepine inhibits the enzymes that metabolize phenytoin while phenytoin may decrease serum concentrations of oxcarbazepine. This can result in phenytoin toxicity and subtherapeutic oxcarbazepine levels. Phenytoin and oxcarbazepine levels should be monitored and dosages adjusted accordingly.

Perampanel, Phenobarbital, and Valproic Acid. Perampanel can increase serum levels of oxcarbazepine. Valproic acid can decrease levels of oxcarbazepine. Phenobarbital can decrease serum levels of oxcarbazepine's active metabolite. If these drugs are given together oxcarbazepine levels will need to be monitored and dosages adjusted accordingly.

Eslicarbazepine. Oxcarbazepine can increase serum levels of eslicarbazepine. This combination is not recommended.

Sodium-Depleting Drugs. Sodium-depleting drugs such as diuretics can increase the risk of hyponatremia. **Instruct patients on the symptoms of hyponatremia (nausea, drowsiness, headache, and confusion) and encourage them to notify the prescriber if these occur.**

Alcohol. Alcohol can increase the CNS effects caused by oxcarbazepine. **Instruct patients not to drink alcohol while taking this drug.**

[a]Patient education information is highlighted as **blue text.**

CHAPTER

25 Drugs for Muscle Spasm and Spasticity

Prototype Drugs

MUSCLE SPASM

Centrally Acting Muscle Relaxer for Spasticity
Baclofen [Lioresal, Gablofen]

Centrally Acting Muscle Relaxer for Localized Muscle Spasm
Cyclobenzaprine [Fexmid, formerly Flexeril]

Direct-Acting Muscle Relaxer
Dantrolene [Dantrium]

In this chapter we consider two groups of drugs that cause skeletal muscle relaxation. One group is used for localized muscle spasm. The other is used for spasticity. As a rule, the drugs used to treat spasticity do not relieve acute muscle spasm and vice versa. Hence, the two groups are not interchangeable. Ten muscle relaxants are currently approved for these purposes (Table 25.1).With the exception of one direct-acting muscle relaxer, these drugs produce their effects through actions in the central nervous system (CNS).

DRUGS FOR SPASTICITY

The term *spasticity* refers to a group of movement disorders of CNS origin. These disorders are characterized by heightened muscle tone, spasm, and loss of dexterity. The most common causes are multiple sclerosis and cerebral palsy. Other causes include traumatic spinal cord lesions and stroke. Spasticity is managed with a combination of drugs and physical therapy.

Four drugs—baclofen, diazepam, dantrolene, and tizanidine—can relieve spasticity. Baclofen, diazepam, and tizanidine act in the CNS; dantrolene acts directly on skeletal muscle. Diazepam [Valium] is a member of the benzodiazepine family. Although diazepam is the only benzodiazepine labeled for treating spasticity, other benzodiazepines have been used off-label for this purpose. The basic pharmacology of the benzodiazepines is discussed in Chapter 34.

Baclofen

Baclofen [Lioresal, Gablofen] will serve as our prototype for centrally acting drugs that relieve spasticity. Baclofen is helpful in relieving spasm related to multiple sclerosis and some spinal cord injuries. It is not approved for management of spasticity related to cerebral palsy, stroke, Parkinson disease, or Huntington's chorea.

Mechanism of Action

Baclofen acts within the spinal cord to suppress hyperactive reflexes involved in the regulation of muscle movement. The precise mechanism of reflex attenuation is unknown. Because baclofen is a structural analog of the inhibitory neurotransmitter GABA, it may act by mimicking the actions of GABA on spinal neurons. Baclofen has no direct effects on skeletal muscle.

Therapeutic Use

As mentioned earlier, baclofen can reduce spasticity associated with multiple sclerosis and spinal cord injury. The drug decreases flexor and extensor spasms and suppresses resistance to passive movement. These actions reduce the discomfort of spasticity and allow increased performance. Because baclofen has no direct muscle-relaxant action, it does not decrease muscle strength. For this reason, baclofen is preferred to dantrolene, a direct-acting muscle relaxer, when spasticity is associated with significant muscle weakness.

TABLE 25.1 ■ Muscle Relaxants

Drug	Preparation	Indication	Usual Adult Oral Maintenance Dosage	Administration	Common Adverse Effects	Notes
CENTRALLY ACTING MUSCLE RELAXANTS						
Baclofen [Lioresal, Gablofen]	Tablets: 10, 20 mg Suspension: 1, 5 mg/mL Cream: 1%, 2% Intrathecal solution[a]: 50 mcg/mL (0.05 mg/mL), 10 mg/5 mL, 10,000 mcg/20 mL (10 mg/20 mL), 20,000 mcg/20 mL, 40,000 mcg/20 mL (40 mg/20 mL)	Spasticity due to spinal cord injury or CNS condition	15–20 mg 3 or 4 times/day	Administer with or without food. Intrathecal use requires an FDA-approved implantable pump.	CNS depression, dizziness, headache, nausea, vomiting, constipation, urinary retention	Abrupt withdrawal can cause seizures and hallucinations. Taper slowly over at least 1–2 weeks.
Carisoprodol [Soma]	Tablets: 250, 350 mg	Musculoskeletal pain and muscle spasms	250–350 mg 3 or 4 times/day	Administer with or without food.	CNS depression, dizziness, headaches, euphoria	Controlled substance (Schedule IV) Avoid in patients with porphyria.
Chlorzoxazone [Lorzone, Parafon Forte DSC]	Tablets: 375, 500, 750 mg	Musculoskeletal pain and muscle spasms	500–750 mg 3 or 4 times/day	Administer with or without food.	CNS depression, dizziness	Paradoxical CNS stimulation may occur. May color urine orange to purple-red. Rare hepatotoxicity can be fatal.
Cyclobenzaprine [Fexmid, Amrix]	IR tablets: 5, 7.5, 10 mg ER capsules: 15, 30 mg Suspension: 1 mg/mL Cream: 5%, 20 mg/gm	Musculoskeletal pain and muscle spasms	IR (tablets or solution): 10 mg 3 times/day ER: 15 or 30 mg once daily	Administer with or without food. Capsules should be swallowed whole or may be opened and sprinkled on soft food, but contents should not be crushed or chewed.	CNS depression, dizziness, anticholinergic effects (dry mouth, blurred vision, photophobia, urinary retention, constipation)	Administration with food increases bioavailability.[b] Contraindicated for patients taking MAO inhibitors. May cause serotonin syndrome in patients taking SSRIs and related antidepressants
Diazepam [Valium]	Tablets: 2, 5, 10 mg Oral solution: 1 mg/mL Oral concentrate: 5 mg/mL Rectal gel: 2.5, 10, 20 mg Injection solution: 5 mg/mL Auto-injector: 10 mg/2 mL	Spasticity due to spinal cord injury or CNS condition Muscle spasms associated with localized musculoskeletal pain, inflammation, or trauma	2–10 mg 3 or 4 times/day	Administer with food or nonalcoholic drink. Dilute oral concentrate before administration. IV push administration should not exceed 1–2 mg/min. Rectal administration requires that the ready band is visible.	CNS depression, hypotension	Controlled substance (C-IV) May cause paradoxical CNS stimulation and/or antegrade amnesia.

Continued

TABLE 25.1 ▪ Muscle Relaxants—cont'd

Drug	Preparation	Indication	Usual Adult Oral Maintenance Dosage	Administration	Common Adverse Effects	Notes
Metaxalone [Skelaxin]	Tablets: 400, 800 mg	Musculoskeletal pain and muscle spasms	800 mg 3 or 4 times/day	Administer with or without food.	CNS depression, dizziness, headache	Administration with food increases bioavailability.[b] May cause liver damage. May cause serotonin syndrome in patients taking serotonergic drugs (e.g., SSRIs and related antidepressants).
Methocarbamol [Robaxin]	Tablets: 500, 750 mg Injection solution: 1000 mg/10 mL	Musculoskeletal pain and muscle spasms	1000 mg 4 times/day	Administer with or without food. May be crushed. IV push administration should not exceed a rate of 3 mL/min. Limit IM injection to 5 mL per site.	CNS depression, amnesia, headache, hypotension, bradycardia, nausea	Have patient stay in a lying position for 10–15 min after IV administration. Less sedation than most. May color urine green to brown-black.
Orphenadrine [Norflex]	ER tablets: 100 mg Injection solution: 30 mg/mL	Musculoskeletal pain and muscle spasms	100 mg twice daily	Have patient swallow the tablet whole.	CNS depression, headache, euphoria, palpitations, tachycardia, anticholinergic effects (dry mouth, blurred vision, photophobia, urinary retention, constipation)	May worsen cardiac conditions such as heart failure.
Tizanidine [Zanaflex]	Tablets: 2, 4 mg Capsules: 2, 4, 6 mg	Spasticity due to spinal cord injury or CNS condition	8 mg every 6–8 hr	Administer with or without food. Capsule contents may be sprinkled on soft food.	CNS depression, dizziness, hypotension, weakness, bradycardia, dry mouth	Administration with food increases bioavailability.[b] May cause liver damage. More sedation than most. Hallucinations and psychosis may occur.
DIRECT-ACTING MUSCLE RELAXANTS						
Dantrolene [Dantrium, Revonto, Ryanodex]	Capsules: 25, 50, 100 mg IV solution: 20, 250 mg	Spasticity due to spinal cord injury or CNS condition	100 mg 3 times/day	Administer with or without food. Capsule contents may be sprinkled on soft food.	Muscle weakness, drowsiness, dysphagia, hoarseness, nausea, erectile dysfunction, diarrhea. Flushing with IV administration.	IV formulation is used for malignant hypothermia. Hepatic toxicity can be life-threatening.

[a]Gablofen is dosed in micrograms; Lioresal is dosed in milligrams.
[b]Increases in bioavailability can increase adverse effects. To stabilize dosing, administer consistently either with or without food.
ER, Extended release; *IR*, immediate release.

Pharmacokinetics

Baclofen peaks about 1 hour after oral administration. Half-life is approximately 4 to 4.5 hours. Following hepatic metabolism of a portion of the drug, excretion occurs primarily in the urine with greater than 70% of the drug unchanged.

Adverse Effects

The most common side effects involve the CNS and GI tract. Serious adverse effects are rare.

CNS Effects. Baclofen is a CNS depressant and hence frequently causes *drowsiness, dizziness, weakness,* and *fatigue.* These responses are most intense during the early phase of therapy and diminish with continued drug use. CNS depression can be minimized with doses that are small initially and then gradually increased. Patients should be cautioned to avoid alcohol and other CNS depressants, because baclofen will potentiate the depressant actions of these drugs.

Overdose can produce *coma* and *respiratory depression.* Because there is no antidote to baclofen overdose, treatment for overdose is supportive.

Withdrawal. Although baclofen does not appear to cause physical dependence, abrupt discontinuation has been associated with adverse reactions. Abrupt withdrawal of *oral* baclofen can cause visual hallucinations, paranoid ideation, and seizures. Accordingly, withdrawal should be done slowly (over 1 to 2 weeks). Abrupt withdrawal of *intrathecal* baclofen can be more dangerous. Potential reactions include high fever, altered mental status, exaggerated rebound spasticity, and muscle rigidity that, in rare cases, has advanced to rhabdomyolysis (muscle breakdown), multiple organ system failure, and death. To avoid these serious consequences, the infusion system must be programmed properly and carefully monitored.

Other Adverse Effects. Baclofen causes *nausea, vomiting, constipation,* and *urinary retention* in about 8% to 10% of patients. Patients should be warned about these possible reactions.

Preparations, Dosage, and Administration

Oral. Baclofen [Lioresal, Gablofen] is available in 10- and 20-mg tablets for oral use. The recommended initial starting dose is 5 mg 3 times a day and then gradually increased by 5 mg every 3 days up to a maximum dose of 80 mg/day. Maintenance dosages range from 15 to 20 mg administered 3 to 4 times a day. Because 5-mg tablets are not available, the patient will need to be taught how to accurately halve a tablet if 5- or 15-mg doses are prescribed.

Intrathecal. Baclofen can be administered by intrathecal infusion using an implantable pump. The typical maintenance dosage is 300 to 800 mcg/day for spinal cord spasticity and 90 to 703 mcg/day for spasticity of cerebral origin. Intrathecal administration is reserved for patients who are unresponsive to or intolerant of oral baclofen.

Contraindications and Interactions

Alcohol and Other CNS Depressants. Baclofen can cause additive CNS depression when given with CNS depressant agents such as alcohol, opioids, or benzodiazepines. Any centrally acting muscle relaxant in combination with a CNS depressant can cause severe respiratory depression. Patients must be advised to avoid these combinations.

Urinary Retention. Baclofen can cause acute urinary retention. Patients with a history of benign prostatic hypertrophy and those taking drugs that can cause urinary retention (e.g., anticholinergics) should be monitored closely for this complication.

Psychiatric Conditions. Baclofen may exacerbate psychotic conditions and confusion. Patients with a history of schizophrenia or other psychiatric illnesses may require close observation to determine progression of symptoms.

Dantrolene

Dantrolene [Dantrium] will serve as our prototype for direct-acting drugs that relieve spasticity.

Mechanism of Action

Unlike baclofen, which acts within the CNS, dantrolene acts directly on skeletal muscle. The drug relieves spasm by suppressing release of calcium from the sarcoplasmic reticulum (SR), and hence the muscle is less able to contract. Fortunately, therapeutic doses have only minimal effects on contraction of smooth muscle and cardiac muscle.

Therapeutic Uses

Spasticity. Dantrolene can relieve spasticity associated with multiple sclerosis, cerebral palsy, and spinal cord injury. Unfortunately, because dantrolene suppresses spasticity by causing a generalized reduction in the ability of skeletal muscle to contract, treatment may be associated with a significant reduction in strength. As a result, overall function may be reduced rather than improved. Accordingly, care must be taken to ensure that the benefits of therapy (reduced spasticity) outweigh the harm (reduced strength).

Malignant Hyperthermia. Malignant hyperthermia is a rare, life-threatening syndrome that can be triggered by any general anesthetic (except nitrous oxide) and by succinylcholine, a neuromuscular blocking agent. Prominent symptoms are muscle rigidity and profound elevation of temperature. The heat of malignant hyperthermia is generated by muscle contraction occurring secondary to massive release of calcium from the SR. Dantrolene relieves symptoms by acting on the SR to block calcium release. Malignant hyperthermia is discussed in Chapter 16.

Pharmacokinetics

The half-life of dantrolene ranges from 4 to 11 hours. It undergoes hepatic metabolism to its active metabolites. Excretion is primarily via feces with lesser excretion in urine.

Adverse Effects

Hepatic Toxicity. Dose-related liver damage is the most serious adverse effect. The incidence is 1 in 1000. Deaths have occurred. Hepatotoxicity is most common in women over age 35 years. By contrast, liver injury is rare in children under 10 years. To reduce the risk of liver damage, liver function tests (LFTs) should be performed at baseline and periodically thereafter. If LFTs indicate liver injury, dantrolene should be withdrawn. Because of the potential for liver damage, dantrolene should be administered in the lowest effective dosage and for the shortest time necessary.

Other Adverse Effects. *Muscle weakness, drowsiness,* and *diarrhea* are the most common side effects. Muscle weakness is a direct extension of dantrolene's pharmacologic action. Other disturbing reactions include *dysphagia and hoarseness, nausea and vomiting,* and *erectile dysfunction.* Almost a third of patients receiving IV dantrolene will experience flushing.

Preparations, Dosage, and Administration

Preparations. Dantrolene sodium [Dantrium] is available in 25-, 50-, and 100-mg capsules for oral use for management of spasticity. For management of malignant hyperthermia, it is available as a powder to be reconstituted for IV injection.

Use in Spasticity. For treatment of spasticity, dosing is oral. The initial adult dosage is 25 mg once daily. The usual maintenance dosage is 100 mg 3 to 4 times a day. If beneficial effects do not develop within 45 days, dantrolene should be stopped.

Use in Malignant Hyperthermia

Preoperative Prophylaxis. Patients with a history of malignant hyperthermia can be given dantrolene for prophylaxis before elective surgery. The dosage is 4 to 8 mg/kg/day in four divided doses for 1 to 2 days preceding surgery.

Treatment of an Ongoing Crisis. For treatment of malignant hyperthermia, dantrolene is administered by IV push. The initial dose is 2 to 5 mg/kg. Administration is repeated until symptoms are controlled or until a total dose of 10 mg/kg has been given. Other management measures are discussed in Chapter 16.

DRUGS FOR LOCALIZED MUSCLE SPASM

Muscle spasm is defined as involuntary contraction of a muscle or muscle group. Muscle spasm is often painful and reduces the ability to function. Spasm can result from a variety of causes, including epilepsy, hypocalcemia, acute and chronic pain syndromes, and trauma (localized muscle injury). Discussion here is limited to spasm resulting from acute musculoskeletal injury.

Treatment of acute muscle spasm involves physical measures as well as drug therapy. Examples of these measures include physical therapy, specific exercises, whirlpool baths, and heat application. Although application of cold compresses is commonly used initially following a musculoskeletal injury, its purpose is to relieve pain and reduce swelling, not to relieve muscle spasm. Current evidence does not support cold treatments for management of muscle spasm.

For drug therapy, two groups of medicines are used: (1) analgesics such as acetaminophen or nonsteroidal anti-inflammatory drugs (NSAIDs), and (2) centrally acting muscle relaxants. These analgesics are discussed in Chapter 71. The centrally acting muscle relaxants used to relieve muscle spasm are carisoprodol, chlorzoxazone, cyclobenzaprine, diazepam, metaxalone, methocarbamol, and orphenadrine. Cyclobenzaprine [Fexmid, formerly Flexeril] will serve as our prototype for drugs used to treat local muscle spasm.

Cyclobenzaprine

Mechanism of Action

Cyclobenzaprine is a centrally acting skeletal muscle relaxant. Its activity takes place primarily in the brainstem and results in a reduction of tonic motor activity.

Therapeutic Use

Cyclobenzaprine is a centrally acting skeletal muscle relaxant used for the relief of muscle spasm and associated pain. It is considered the most efficacious of the drugs used for this purpose; therefore, it is typically the drug of first choice for acute muscle spasm. It is ineffective as a treatment for spasticity.

Pharmacokinetics

Immediate-release cyclobenzaprine peaks at approximately 4 hours. The peak time for the extended-release formulation is around 7 to 8 hours. Half-life ranges from 8 to 37 hours in patients with normal liver function and may extend to as long as 188 hours with hepatic impairment. The drug may undergo significant enterohepatic recirculation. Metabolism occurs via CYP3A4, CYP1A2, and CYP2D6 isoenzymes.

Of note, plasma concentrations tend to be higher in older adults and in those with liver impairment. These patients should receive lower doses and should be monitored closely for evidence of overdose.

Adverse Effects

CNS Effects. Cyclobenzaprine is a CNS depressant. Common CNS depressant effects include *drowsiness, dizziness,* and *fatigue.* As with baclofen, these responses are most intense during the early phase of therapy and diminish with continued drug use.

Anticholinergic Effects. Cyclobenzaprine is structurally similar to tricyclic antidepressants (see Chapter 32). This similarity explains the presence of anticholinergic effects. Common anticholinergic adverse effects include dry mouth, blurred vision, photophobia, urinary retention, constipation.

Cardiac Rhythm Disturbances. Cyclobenzaprine can cause cardiac rhythm disturbances similar to those of tricyclic antidepressants. These include a wide variety of dysrhythmias, including sinus tachycardia and significant conduction delays.

Preparations, Dosage, and Administration. Cyclobenzaprine is available as immediate-release tablets (5 mg, 7.5 mg, 10 mg), extended-release capsules (15 mg, 30 mg), an oral suspension (1 mg/mL), and a topical cream (5%, 20 mg/gm). It is usually begun at 5 mg three times daily; however, it may be increased to 7.5 or 10 mg three times a day if needed. It is recommended for short-term use, not to exceed 2 to 3 weeks.

Contraindications and Interactions

Antidepressants. Cyclobenzaprine use is contraindicated for patients taking monoamine oxidase (MAO) inhibitors. For patients previously undergoing therapy with MAO inhibitors, at least 2 weeks must have passed after discontinuing the drug before starting cyclobenzaprine. Failure to do so has led to potentially fatal serotonin syndrome manifested by high fever, seizures, and rhabdomyolysis.

Serotonin syndrome may also occur if cyclobenzaprine is given with SSRIs, SNRIs, and tricyclic antidepressants. Symptoms may range from mild agitation and tremor to the high fevers and seizures that can occur with MAO inhibitors.

Safety Alert

MANIFESTATIONS OF SEROTONIN SYNDROME

System	Manifestation
Central nervous system	Agitation, restlessness, confusion, hallucinations, headache, unconsciousness
Autonomic nervous system	Hyperthermia, diaphoresis, blood pressure elevation, tachycardia, pupil dilation
Neuromuscular system	Tremor, hyperreflexia, ataxia, muscle twitching, muscle rigidity, seizures
Gastrointestinal system	Nausea, vomiting, diarrhea

PATIENT-CENTERED CARE ACROSS THE LIFE SPAN

Centrally Acting Muscle Relaxants

Life Stage	Patient Care Concerns
Children	Chlorzoxazone, orphenadrine and tizanidine are not approved for use in children.
Pregnant women	Cyclobenzaprine is Pregnancy Risk Category B.[a] Diazepam is Pregnancy Risk Category D. The remaining drugs are Pregnancy Risk Category C except for metaxalone, for which a designation was not determined. Diazepam is associated with low birth weights, prematurity, hypoglycemia, and respiratory depression. Neonatal withdrawal syndrome has been observed with benzodiazepines (e.g., alprazolam, diazepam, lorazepam) and baclofen. Animal studies have yielded adverse events for baclofen, carisoprodol, tizanidine, and dantrolene. There are no (or insufficient) animal studies conducted for chlorzoxazone, methocarbamol, and orphenadrine. Animal studies did not identify any adverse events for metaxalone.
Breast-feeding women	These drugs can cause adverse effects in infants. Breast-feeding is not recommended.
Older adults	At the dosage required to have adequate effect, these drugs may cause sedation and cognitive impairment, thus creating a fall risk. Carisoprodol, chlorzoxazone, cyclobenzaprine, metaxalone, methocarbamol, and orphenadrine are listed in Beers Criteria as potentially inappropriate for older adults. Cyclobenzaprine and orphenadrine have more anticholinergic effects (e.g., blurred vision, constipation, urinary retention, elevated heart rate), which may create additional problems for older adult patients. Long-acting benzodiazepines such as diazepam are particularly troublesome because older adult patients tend to have a slower metabolism. Elimination may be delayed, and active drug may accumulate.

[a]As of 2020, the FDA will no longer use Pregnancy Risk Categories. Please refer to Chapter 9 for more information.

Alcohol and Other CNS Depressants. Cyclobenzaprine will cause additive CNS depression when given with other CNS depressants such as alcohol. Patients must be advised to avoid these combinations.

OTHER CENTRALLY ACTING MUSCLE RELAXANTS

We have discussed our prototype drugs—baclofen, dantrolene, and cyclobenzaprine—in detail. All centrally acting muscle relaxants have similar pharmacologic properties, so we will consider the remaining (nonprototype) agents as a group.

Mechanism of Action

For most centrally acting muscle relaxants, the mechanism of spasm relief is unclear. In laboratory animals, high doses can depress spinal motor reflexes. However, these doses are much higher than those used in humans. Hence, many investigators believe that relaxation of spasm results primarily from the *sedative properties* of these drugs and not from specific actions exerted on CNS pathways that control muscle tone.

The drugs for spasticity—diazepam and tizanidine—are thought to relieve spasm by enhancing presynaptic inhibition of motor neurons in the CNS. Diazepam promotes presynaptic inhibition by enhancing the effects of gamma-aminobutyric acid (GABA), an inhibitory neurotransmitter. Tizanidine promotes inhibition by acting as an agonist at presynaptic $alpha_2$ receptors.

Therapeutic Use

Tizanidine is indicated for treating spasticity and has been used off-label to treat acute back pain. Carisoprodol, chlorzoxazone, metaxalone, methocarbamol, and orphenadrine are used to relieve localized muscle spasm. Diazepam is approved for treatment of both spasticity and muscle spasm.

Adverse Effects

CNS Depression. All of the centrally acting muscle relaxants can produce generalized depression of the CNS. *Drowsiness, dizziness,* and *light-headedness* are common. Patients should be warned not to participate in hazardous activities (e.g., driving) if CNS depression is significant. In addition, they should be advised to avoid alcohol and all other CNS depressants.

Hepatic Toxicity. *Tizanidine* [Zanaflex] and *metaxalone* [Skelaxin] can cause liver damage. Liver function should be assessed before starting treatment and periodically thereafter. If liver injury develops, these drugs should be discontinued. If the patient has pre-existing liver disease, these drugs should be avoided.

Chlorzoxazone [Lorzone, Parafon Forte DSC] can cause hepatitis and potentially fatal hepatic necrosis. Because of this potential for harm, and because other drugs are more effective, the risk of harm generally exceeds the drug's benefits.

Safety Alert

CENTRALLY ACTING MUSCLE RELAXANTS

The CNS depressant effect of centrally acting muscle relaxants may cause severe drowsiness initially. Patients should be advised not to drive or engage in activities that may be hazardous as long as these effects persist.

Physical Dependence. Chronic, high-dose therapy can cause physical dependence, manifesting as a potentially life-threatening abstinence syndrome, if these drugs are abruptly withdrawn. Accordingly, withdrawal should be done slowly. Two of the muscle relaxants, diazepam and carisoprodol, are Schedule IV controlled drugs.

Other Adverse Effects. *Cyclobenzaprine* and *orphenadrine* have significant anticholinergic (atropine-like) properties, and hence may cause dry mouth, blurred vision, photophobia, urinary retention, and constipation.

Methocarbamol may turn urine brown, black, or dark green. *Chlorzoxazone* may color urine orange to purple-red. This appears to be dose-related. The effect is harmless.

Tizanidine can cause dry mouth, hypotension, hallucinations, and psychotic symptoms. Tizanidine is similar to clonidine and can cause hypotension. When discontinuing this drug, it may be necessary to taper dosage to avoid rebound hypertension.

Carisoprodol can be hazardous to patients predisposed to intermittent porphyria. It is contraindicated for patients with this condition.

Dosage and Administration

All centrally acting skeletal muscle relaxants can be administered orally (see Table 25.1). In addition, methocarbamol, orphenadrine, and diazepam can be administered by IM and IV injection, baclofen and cyclobenzaprine can be administered topically, and baclofen can be administered intrathecally.

KEY POINTS

- Localized muscle spasm is treated with centrally acting muscle relaxants and over-the-counter analgesics such as acetaminophen or NSAIDs.
- Spasticity is treated with four drugs: baclofen, diazepam, dantrolene, and tizanidine.
- All centrally acting muscle relaxants produce generalized CNS depression.
- Chlorzoxazone, a central muscle relaxant, is less effective than other available drugs and can cause fatal hepatic necrosis. Accordingly, the risk for harm usually exceeds benefits.
- Baclofen relieves spasticity by mimicking the inhibitory actions of GABA in the CNS.
- In contrast to all other drugs discussed in this chapter, dantrolene acts directly on muscle to promote relaxation.
- Abrupt discontinuation of intrathecal baclofen can lead to rhabdomyolysis, multiple organ system failure, and death.
- With prolonged use, dantrolene can cause potentially fatal liver damage. Monitor liver function and minimize dosage and duration of treatment.
- In addition to relief of spasticity, dantrolene is used to treat malignant hyperthermia, a potentially fatal condition caused by succinylcholine and general anesthetics.

Please visit http://evolve.elsevier.com/Lehne for chapter-specific NCLEX® examination review questions.

Summary of Major Nursing Implications[a]

DRUGS USED TO TREAT MUSCLE SPASM: CENTRALLY ACTING SKELETAL MUSCLE RELAXANTS

Except where noted, the nursing implications summarized below apply to all centrally acting muscle relaxants (see Table 25.1) used to treat muscle spasm.

Preadministration Assessment

Therapeutic Goal

Relief of signs and symptoms of muscle spasm.

Baseline Data

For patients taking metaxalone and tizanidine, obtain baseline LFTs.

Identifying High-Risk Patients

Avoid *chlorzoxazone, metaxalone,* and *tizanidine* in patients with liver disease.

Implementation: Administration

Routes

Oral. All central skeletal muscle relaxants.

Parenteral. *Methocarbamol* and *diazepam* may be given IM and IV as well as PO.

Dosage

See Table 25.1 for adult PO maintenance dosages.

Implementation: Measures to Enhance Therapeutic Effects

The treatment plan should include appropriate physical measures (e.g., immobilization of the affected muscle, application of cold compresses, whirlpool baths, and physical therapy).

Ongoing Evaluation and Interventions

Minimizing Adverse Effects

CNS Depression. All central muscle relaxants cause CNS depression. **Inform patients about possible depressant effects (drowsiness, dizziness, light-headedness, fatigue) and advise them to avoid driving and other hazardous activities if significant impairment occurs.**

Hepatic Toxicity. *Metaxalone* and *tizanidine* can cause liver damage. Obtain LFTs before treatment and periodically thereafter. If liver damage develops, discontinue treatment. Avoid these drugs in patients with pre-existing liver disease.

Chlorzoxazone can cause hepatitis and potentially fatal hepatic necrosis. Drug risks tend to exceed drug benefits. **Advise patients on signs and symptoms of liver injury (malaise, nausea, jaundice), and advise them to report these symptoms to their provider.**

Minimizing Adverse Interactions

CNS Depressants. **Caution patients to avoid CNS depressants (e.g., alcohol, benzodiazepines, opioids, antihistamines)**

Summary of Major Nursing Implications[a]—cont'd

because these drugs will intensify the depressant effects of muscle relaxants.

Avoiding Withdrawal Reactions

Central muscle relaxants can cause physical dependence. To avoid an abstinence syndrome, withdraw gradually. **Warn patients against abrupt discontinuation of treatment.**

BACLOFEN

Preadministration Assessment

Therapeutic Goal

Relief of signs and symptoms of spasticity.

Baseline Data

Assess for spasm, rigidity, pain, range of motion, and dexterity. Obtain baseline LFTs.

Implementation: Administration

Routes

Oral, intrathecal.

Administration

Patients with muscle spasm may be unable to self-medicate. Provide assistance if needed.

Ongoing Evaluation and Interventions

Evaluating Therapeutic Effects

Monitor for reductions in rigidity, muscle spasm, and pain and for improvements in dexterity and range of motion.

Minimizing Adverse Effects

CNS Depression. Baclofen is a CNS depressant. **Inform patients about possible depressant effects (drowsiness, dizziness, light-headedness, fatigue) and advise them to avoid driving and other hazardous activities if significant impairment occurs.**

Minimizing Adverse Interactions

CNS Depressants. **Caution patients to avoid CNS depressants (e.g., alcohol, benzodiazepines, opioids, antihistamines) because these drugs will intensify the depressant effects of baclofen.**

Avoiding Withdrawal Reactions

Oral Baclofen. Abrupt withdrawal can cause visual hallucinations, paranoid ideation, and seizures. **Caution patients against abrupt discontinuation of treatment.**

Intrathecal Baclofen. Abrupt discontinuation can cause multiple adverse effects, including rhabdomyolysis, multiple organ system failure, and death. Make sure the infusion system is programmed properly and monitored with care.

DANTROLENE

The nursing implications summarized here apply only to the use of dantrolene for spasticity.

Preadministration Assessment

Therapeutic Goal

Relief of signs and symptoms of spasticity.

Baseline Data

Assess for spasm, rigidity, pain, range of motion, and dexterity. Obtain baseline LFTs.

Identifying High-Risk Patients

Dantrolene is *contraindicated* for patients with active liver disease (e.g., cirrhosis, hepatitis).

Implementation: Administration

Route

Oral.

Administration

Patients with muscle spasm may be unable to self-medicate. Provide assistance if needed.

Ongoing Evaluation and Interventions

Monitoring

Therapeutic Effects. Monitor for reductions in rigidity, spasm, and pain and for improvements in dexterity and range of motion.

Adverse Effects. Monitor LFTs and assess for reduced muscle strength.

Minimizing Adverse Effects

CNS Depression. Dantrolene is a CNS depressant. **Inform patients about possible depressant effects (drowsiness, dizziness, light-headedness, fatigue) and advise them to avoid driving and other hazardous activities if significant impairment occurs.**

Hepatic Toxicity. Dantrolene is hepatotoxic. Assess liver function at baseline and periodically thereafter. If signs of liver dysfunction develop, withdraw dantrolene. **Inform patients about signs of liver dysfunction (e.g., jaundice, abdominal pain, malaise) and instruct them to seek medical attention if these develop.**

Muscle Weakness. Dantrolene can decrease muscle strength. Evaluate muscle function to ensure that benefits of therapy (decreased spasticity) are not outweighed by reductions in strength.

Minimizing Adverse Interactions

CNS Depressants. **Warn patients to avoid CNS depressants (e.g., alcohol, benzodiazepines, opioids, antihistamines), because these drugs will intensify depressant effects of dantrolene.**

CYCLOBENZAPRINE

Preadministration Assessment

Therapeutic Goal

Relief of localized pain and muscle spasm.

Continued

Summary of Major Nursing Implications[a]—cont'd

Baseline Data

Assess for spasm, rigidity, pain, range of motion, and dexterity.

Implementation: Administration

Routes

Oral, topical.

Administration

Administer with or without food. (Administration with food increases bioavailability.) Capsules may be either swallowed whole or opened to sprinkle the contents on soft food. If sprinkled on food, the content should not be chewed or crushed.

Ongoing Evaluation and Interventions

Evaluating Therapeutic Effects

Monitor for decreased pain and muscle spasm and for improvement in movement if this was a limitation.

Minimizing Adverse Effects

CNS Depression. Cyclobenzaprine is a CNS depressant. **Inform patients about possible depressant effects (drowsiness, dizziness, light-headedness, fatigue) and advise them to avoid driving and other hazardous activities if significant impairment occurs.**

Minimizing Adverse Interactions

CNS Depressants. **Caution patients to avoid CNS depressants (e.g., alcohol, benzodiazepines, opioids, antihistamines) because these drugs will intensify the depressant effects of baclofen.**

Anticholinergic Effects. Cyclobenzaprine can cause dry mouth, blurred vision, photophobia, urinary retention, and constipation. **Advise patients to chew sugar-free gum to relieve dry mouth. Wearing sunglasses can help manage photophobia related to dilated pupils. Increases in fiber and fluid intake, with or without a stool softener, can help with constipation. Advise patients to report any incidence of urinary retention to their healthcare provider.**

DIAZEPAM

Nursing implications for diazepam and the other benzodiazepines are summarized in Chapter 34.

[a]Patient education information is highlighted as **blue text.**

CHAPTER

26 Local Anesthetics

Local anesthetics are drugs that suppress pain by blocking impulse conduction along axons. Conduction is blocked only in neurons located near the site of administration. The great advantage of local anesthesia, compared with inhalation anesthesia, is that pain can be suppressed without causing generalized depression of the entire nervous system. Local anesthetics carry much less risk than do general anesthetics.

We begin the chapter by considering the pharmacology of the local anesthetics as a group. After that, we discuss three prototypic agents: procaine, lidocaine, and cocaine. We conclude by discussing specific routes of anesthetic administration.

BASIC PHARMACOLOGY OF LOCAL ANESTHETICS

Classification

There are two major groups of local anesthetics: *esters* and *amides*. The ester-type anesthetics, represented by *procaine* [Novocain], contain an ester linkage in their structure. In contrast, the amide-type agents, represented by *lidocaine* [Xylocaine], contain an amide linkage. The ester-type agents and amide-type agents differ in two important ways: (1) method of inactivation and (2) promotion of allergic responses. Contrasts between the esters and amides are shown in Table 26.1.

Mechanism of Action

Local anesthetics stop axonal conduction by *blocking sodium channels* in the axonal membrane. Recall that propagation of an action potential requires movement of sodium ions from outside the axon to the inside. This influx takes place through specialized sodium channels. By blocking axonal sodium channels, local anesthetics prevent sodium entry, and thereby block conduction.

Selectivity of Anesthetic Effects

Local anesthetics are nonselective modifiers of neuronal function. That is, they will block action potentials in all neurons to which they have access. The only way to achieve selectivity is by delivering the anesthetic to a limited area.

Although local anesthetics can block traffic in all neurons, blockade develops more rapidly in some neurons than in others. Specifically, small, nonmyelinated neurons are blocked more rapidly than large, myelinated neurons. Because of this differential sensitivity, some sensations are blocked sooner than others. Specifically, perception of pain is lost first, followed in order by perception of cold, warmth, touch, and deep pressure.

The effects of local anesthetics are not limited to sensory neurons: These drugs also block conduction in motor neurons, which is why your face looks funny when you leave the dentist.

Time Course of Local Anesthesia

Ideally, local anesthesia would begin promptly and would persist no longer (or shorter) than needed. Unfortunately, although onset of anesthesia is usually rapid (Tables 26.2 and 26.3), duration of anesthesia is often less than ideal. In some cases, anesthesia persists longer than needed. In others, repeated administration is required to maintain anesthesia of sufficient duration.

Onset of local anesthesia is determined largely by the molecular properties of the anesthetic. Before anesthesia can occur, the anesthetic must diffuse from its site of administration to its sites of action within the axon membrane. Anesthesia is delayed until this movement has occurred. The ability of an anesthetic to penetrate the axon membrane is determined by three properties: *molecular size, lipid solubility,* and *degree of ionization at tissue pH.* Anesthetics of small size, high lipid solubility, and low ionization cross the axon membrane rapidly. In contrast, anesthetics of large size, low lipid solubility, and high ionization cross slowly. Obviously, anesthetics that penetrate the axon most rapidly have the fastest onset.

Termination of local anesthesia occurs as molecules of anesthetic diffuse out of neurons and are carried away in the blood. The same factors that determine onset of anesthesia (molecular size, lipid solubility, degree of ionization) also help determine duration. In addition, *regional blood flow* is an important determinant of how long anesthesia will last. In areas where blood flow is high, anesthetic is carried away quickly, and effects terminate with relative haste. In regions where blood flow is low, anesthesia is more prolonged.

Use With Vasoconstrictors

Local anesthetics are frequently administered in combination with a vasoconstrictor, usually *epinephrine.* The vasoconstrictor decreases local blood flow and thereby delays systemic absorption of the anesthetic. Delaying absorption has two benefits: It *prolongs anesthesia* and *reduces the risk of toxicity.* First, because absorption is slowed, less anesthetic is used. Second, by slowing absorption, a more favorable balance is established between the rate of entry of anesthetic into circulation and the rate of its conversion into inactive metabolites.

It should be noted that absorption of the vasoconstrictor itself can result in systemic toxicity (e.g., palpitations, tachycardia, nervousness, hypertension). If adrenergic stimulation from absorption of epinephrine is excessive, symptoms can be controlled with alpha- and beta-adrenergic antagonists.

TABLE 26.1 ▪ Contrasts Between Ester and Amide Local Anesthetics

Property	Ester-type Anesthetics	Amide-type Anesthetics
Characteristic chemistry	Ester bond	Amide bond
Representative agent	Procaine	Lidocaine
Incidence of allergic reactions	Low	Very low
Method of metabolism	Plasma esterases	Hepatic enzymes

Pharmacokinetics

Absorption and Distribution

Although administered for local effects, local anesthetics do get absorbed into the blood and become distributed to all parts of the body. The rate of absorption is determined largely by blood flow to the site of administration.

Metabolism

The process by which a local anesthetic is metabolized depends on the class—ester or amide—to which it belongs. *Ester-type* local anesthetics are metabolized in the blood by enzymes known as *esterases.* In contrast, *amide-type* anesthetics are metabolized by enzymes in the *liver.* For both types of anesthetic, metabolism results in inactivation.

The balance between rate of absorption and rate of metabolism is clinically significant. If a local anesthetic is absorbed

TABLE 26.2 ▪ Topical Local Anesthetics: Brand Names, Indications, and Time Course of Action

Chemical Class	Generic Name	Brand Name	Indications: Skin	Indications: Mucous Membranes	Time Course of Action[a]: Peak Effect (min)	Time Course of Action[a]: Duration (min)
Amides	Dibucaine	Nupercainal	✓		Less than 5	15–45
	Lidocaine[b]	Xylocaine, Lidoderm, others	✓	✓	2–5	15–45
Esters	Benzocaine	Many names	✓	✓	Less than 5	15–45
	Cocaine	Generic only	✓	✓	1–5	30–60
	Tetracaine[b]	Numfast	✓	✓	3–8	30–60
Others	Dyclonine	Sucrets (spray)		✓	Less than 10	Less than 60
	Pramoxine	Tronothane, others	✓		3–5	—

[a]Based primarily on application to mucous membranes.
[b]Also administered by injection.

TABLE 26.3 ▪ Injectable Local Anesthetics: Brand Names and Time Course of Action

Chemical Class	Generic Name	Brand Name	Time Course of Action[a]: Onset (min)	Time Course of Action[a]: Duration (hr)
Amides	Lidocaine[b]	Xylocaine	Less than 2	0.5–1
	Bupivacaine	Marcaine, Sensorcaine	5	2–4
	Mepivacaine	Carbocaine, Polocaine	3–5	0.75–1.5
	Prilocaine	Citanest	Less than 2	1 or more
	Ropivacaine	Naropin	10–30[c]	0.5–6[c]
Esters[d]	Procaine	Novocain	2–5	0.25–1
	Chloroprocaine	Nesacaine	6–12	0.5
	Tetracaine[b]	None	15 or less	2–3

[a]Values are for *infiltration* anesthesia in the absence of epinephrine (epinephrine prolongs duration two- to threefold).
[b]Also administered topically.
[c]Values are for epidural administration (without epinephrine).
[d]Because of the risk of allergic reactions, the ester anesthetics are rarely administered by injection.

more slowly than it is metabolized, its level in blood will remain low, and systemic reactions will be minimal. Conversely, if absorption outpaces metabolism, plasma drug levels will rise, and the risk of systemic toxicity will increase.

Adverse Effects

Adverse effects can occur locally or distant from the site of administration. Local effects are less common.

Central Nervous System

When absorbed in sufficient amounts, local anesthetics cause central nervous system (CNS) excitation followed by depression. During the excitation phase, *seizures* may occur. If needed, excessive excitation can be managed with an IV benzodiazepine (diazepam or midazolam). Depressant effects range from *drowsiness* to *unconsciousness* to *coma*. Death can occur secondary to *depression of respiration*. If respiratory depression is prominent, mechanical ventilation with oxygen is indicated.

Cardiovascular System

When absorbed in sufficient amounts, local anesthetics can affect the heart and blood vessels. In the heart, these drugs suppress excitability in the myocardium and conducting system, and thereby can cause *bradycardia, heart block, reduced contractile force,* and even *cardiac arrest*. In blood vessels, anesthetics relax vascular smooth muscle; the resultant vasodilation can cause *hypotension*. As discussed in Chapter 49, the cardiosuppressant actions of one local anesthetic—lidocaine—are used to treat dysrhythmias.

Allergic Reactions

An array of hypersensitivity reactions, ranging from *allergic dermatitis* to *anaphylaxis,* can be triggered by local anesthetics. These reactions, which are relatively uncommon, are much more likely with the *ester-type* anesthetics (e.g., procaine) than with the amides. Patients allergic to one ester-type anesthetic are likely to be allergic to all other ester-type agents. Fortunately, cross-hypersensitivity between the esters and amides has not been observed. Therefore, the amides can be used when allergies contraindicate use of ester-type anesthetics. Because they are unlikely to cause hypersensitivity reactions, the amide-type anesthetics have largely replaced the ester-type agents when administration by injection is required.

Use in Labor and Delivery

Local anesthetics can depress uterine contractility and maternal effort. Both actions can *prolong labor.* Also, local anesthetics can cross the placenta, causing *bradycardia and CNS depression in the neonate.*

Methemoglobinemia

Topical *benzocaine* can cause methemoglobinemia, a blood disorder in which hemoglobin is modified such that it cannot release oxygen to tissues. If enough hemoglobin is converted to methemoglobin, death can result. Methemoglobinemia has been associated with benzocaine liquids, sprays, and gels. Most cases were in children under 2 years of age treated with benzocaine gel for teething pain. Because of this risk, topical benzocaine should not be used in children younger than 2 years of age without the advice of a healthcare professional, and should be used with caution in older children and adults when applied to mucous membranes of the mouth.

PROPERTIES OF INDIVIDUAL LOCAL ANESTHETICS

Procaine

Procaine [Novocain] is the prototype of the ester-type local anesthetics. The drug is not effective topically, and must be given by injection. Administration in combination with epinephrine delays absorption. Although procaine is readily absorbed, systemic toxicity is rare because plasma esterases rapidly convert the drug to inactive, nontoxic products. Being an ester-type anesthetic, procaine poses a greater risk of allergic reactions than do the amide-type anesthetics. Individuals allergic to procaine should be considered allergic to all other ester-type anesthetics, but not to the amides.

Prototype Drugs

LOCAL ANESTHETICS

Ester-Type Local Anesthetics
Procaine

Amide-Type Local Anesthetics
Lidocaine

For many years, procaine was the preferred injectable local anesthetic. However, with the development of newer agents, use of procaine has sharply declined. Once popular in dentistry, procaine is rarely employed in that setting today.

Preparations

Procaine hydrochloride [Novocain] is available in solution for administration by injection. Epinephrine (at a final concentration of 1 : 100,000 or 1 : 200,000) may be combined with procaine to delay absorption.

Lidocaine

Lidocaine, introduced in 1948, is the prototype of the amide-type agents. One of today's most widely used local anesthetics, lidocaine can be administered topically and by injection. Anesthesia with lidocaine is more rapid, more intense, and more prolonged than an equal dose of procaine. Effects can be extended by coadministration of epinephrine. Allergic reactions are rare, and individuals allergic to ester-type anesthetics are not cross-allergic to lidocaine. If plasma levels of lidocaine climb too high, CNS and cardiovascular toxicity can result. Inactivation is by hepatic metabolism.

In addition to its use in local anesthesia, lidocaine is employed to treat dysrhythmias (see Chapter 49). Control of dysrhythmias results from suppression of cardiac excitability secondary to blockade of cardiac sodium channels.

Preparations

Lidocaine hydrochloride [Xylocaine, others] is available in several formulations (cream, ointment, jelly, solution, aerosol, patch) for topical administration. Lidocaine for injection is available in concentrations ranging from 0.5% to 5%. Some injectable preparations contain epinephrine (1 : 50,000, 1 : 100,000, or 1 : 200,000).

Cocaine

Cocaine was our first local anesthetic. It is an ester-type anesthetic. In addition to causing local anesthesia, cocaine has pronounced effects on the sympathetic and central nervous systems. These sympathetic and CNS effects are due largely to blocking the reuptake of norepinephrine by adrenergic neurons.

Anesthetic Use

Cocaine is an excellent local anesthetic. Administered topically, the drug is employed for anesthesia of the ear, nose, and throat. Anesthesia develops rapidly and persists for about an hour. Unlike other local anesthetics, cocaine causes intense vasoconstriction (by blocking norepinephrine uptake at sympathetic nerve terminals on blood vessels). Accordingly, the drug should not be given in combination with epinephrine or any other vasoconstrictor. Despite its ability to constrict blood vessels, cocaine is readily absorbed following application to mucous membranes. Significant effects on the brain and heart can result. The drug is inactivated by plasma esterases and liver enzymes.

CNS Effects

Cocaine produces generalized CNS stimulation. Moderate doses cause euphoria, talkativeness, reduced fatigue, and increased sociability and alertness. Excessive doses can cause seizures. Excitation is followed by CNS depression. Respiratory arrest and death can result.

Although cocaine does not seem to cause substantial physical dependence, psychologic dependence can be profound. The drug is subject to widespread abuse and is classified under Schedule II of the Controlled Substances Act. Cocaine abuse is discussed in Chapter 40.

Cardiovascular Effects

Cocaine stimulates the heart and causes vasoconstriction. These effects result from (1) central stimulation of the sympathetic nervous system and (2) blockade of norepinephrine uptake in the periphery. Stimulation of the heart can produce *tachycardia* and potentially fatal *dysrhythmias*. Vasoconstriction can cause *hypertension*. Cocaine presents an especially serious risk to individuals with cardiovascular disease (e.g., hypertension, dysrhythmias, angina pectoris).

Preparations and Administration

Cocaine hydrochloride is available as a topical solution (4% and 10%). For application to the ear, nose, or throat, a 4% solution is usually employed. The drug must be dispensed in accord with the Controlled Substances Act.

Other Local Anesthetics

In addition to the drugs discussed previously, several other local anesthetics are available. These agents differ with respect to indications, route of administration, mode of elimination, duration of action, and toxicity.

The local anesthetics can be grouped according to route of administration: topical versus injection. (Very few agents are administered by both routes, primarily because the drugs that are suitable for topical application are usually too toxic for parenteral use.) Table 26.2 lists the topically administered local anesthetics along with brand names and time course of action. Table 26.3 presents equivalent information for the injectable agents.

CLINICAL USE OF LOCAL ANESTHETICS

Local anesthetics may be administered *topically* (for surface anesthesia) and *by injection* (for infiltration anesthesia, nerve block anesthesia, intravenous regional anesthesia, epidural anesthesia, and spinal anesthesia). The uses and hazards of these anesthesia techniques are discussed in the sections that follow.

Topical Administration

Surface anesthesia is accomplished by applying the anesthetic directly to the skin or a mucous membrane. The agents employed most commonly are *lidocaine, tetracaine,* and *cocaine.*

Therapeutic Uses

Local anesthetics are applied to the *skin* to relieve pain, itching, and soreness of various causes, including infection, thermal burns, sunburn, diaper rash, wounds, bruises, abrasions, plant poisoning, and insect bites. Application may also be made to *mucous membranes* of the nose, mouth, pharynx, larynx, trachea, bronchi, vagina, and urethra. In addition, local anesthetics may be used to relieve discomfort associated with hemorrhoids, anal fissures, and pruritus ani.

Systemic Toxicity

Topical anesthetics applied to the skin can be absorbed in amounts sufficient to produce serious or even life-threatening effects. Cardiac toxicity can result in bradycardia, heart block, or cardiac arrest. CNS toxicity can result in seizures, respiratory depression, and coma. Obviously, the risk of toxicity increases with the amount absorbed, which is determined primarily by (1) the amount applied, (2) skin condition, and (3) skin temperature. Accordingly, to minimize the amount absorbed, and thereby minimize risk, patients should:

- Apply the smallest amount needed.
- Avoid application to large areas.
- Avoid application to broken or irritated skin.
- Avoid strenuous exercise, wrapping the site, and heating the site, all of which can accelerate absorption by increasing skin temperature.

Administration by Injection

Injection of local anesthetics carries significant risk and requires special skills. Injections are usually performed by an anesthesiologist. Because severe systemic reactions may occur, equipment for resuscitation should be immediately available. Also, an IV line should be in place to permit rapid treatment of toxicity. Inadvertent injection into an artery or vein can cause severe toxicity. To ensure the needle is not in a blood vessel, it should be aspirated before injection. Following administration, the patient should be monitored for cardiovascular status, respiratory function, and state of consciousness. To reduce the risk of toxicity, local anesthetics should be administered in the lowest effective dose.

Infiltration Anesthesia

Infiltration anesthesia is achieved by injecting a local anesthetic directly into the immediate area of surgery or manipulation. Anesthesia can be prolonged by combining the anesthetic with epinephrine. The agents employed most frequently for infiltration anesthesia are *lidocaine* and *bupivacaine*.

Nerve Block Anesthesia

Nerve block anesthesia is achieved by injecting a local anesthetic into or near nerves that supply the surgical field, but at a site distant from the field itself. This technique has the advantage of producing anesthesia with doses that are smaller than those needed for infiltration anesthesia. Drug selection is based on required duration of anesthesia. For shorter procedures, *lidocaine* or *mepivacaine* might be used. For longer procedures, *bupivacaine* would be appropriate.

Intravenous Regional Anesthesia

Intravenous regional anesthesia is employed to anesthetize the extremities—hands, feet, arms, and lower legs, but not the entire leg (because too much anesthetic would be needed). Anesthesia is produced by injection into a distal vein of an arm or leg. Before giving the anesthetic, blood is removed from the limb (by gravity or by application of an Esmarch bandage), and a tourniquet is applied to the limb (proximal to the site of anesthetic injection) to prevent anesthetic from entering the systemic circulation. To ensure complete blockade of arterial flow throughout the procedure, a double tourniquet is used. Following injection, the anesthetic diffuses out of the vasculature and becomes evenly distributed to all areas of the occluded limb. When the tourniquet is loosened at the end of surgery, about 15% to 30% of administered anesthetic is released into the systemic circulation. *Lidocaine—without epinephrine*—is the preferred agent for this type of anesthesia.

Epidural Anesthesia

Epidural anesthesia is achieved by injecting a local anesthetic into the epidural space (i.e., within the spinal column but outside the dura mater). A catheter placed in the epidural space allows administration by bolus or by continuous infusion. Following administration, diffusion of anesthetic across the dura into the subarachnoid space blocks conduction in nerve roots and in the spinal cord itself. Diffusion through intervertebral foramina blocks nerves located in the paravertebral region. With epidural administration, anesthetic can reach the systemic circulation in significant amounts. As a result, when the technique is used during delivery, neonatal depression may result. *Lidocaine* and *bupivacaine* are popular drugs for epidural anesthesia. Because of the risk of death from cardiac arrest, the concentrated (0.75%) solution of bupivacaine must not be used in obstetric patients.

Spinal (Subarachnoid) Anesthesia

Technique. Spinal anesthesia is produced by injecting local anesthetic into the subarachnoid space. Injection is made in the lumbar region below the termination of the cord. Spread of anesthetic within the subarachnoid space determines the level of anesthesia achieved. Movement of anesthetic within the subarachnoid space is determined by two factors: (1) the density of the anesthetic solution and (2) the position of the patient. Anesthetics employed most commonly are *bupivacaine, lidocaine,* and *tetracaine.* All must be free of preservatives.

Adverse Effects. The most significant adverse effect of spinal anesthesia is hypotension. Blood pressure is reduced by venous dilation secondary to blockade of sympathetic nerves. (Loss of venous tone decreases the return of blood to the heart, causing a reduction in cardiac output and a corresponding fall in blood pressure.) Loss of venous tone can be compensated for by placing the patient in a 10- to 15-degree head-down position, which promotes venous return to the heart. If blood pressure cannot be restored through head-down positioning, drugs may be indicated; ephedrine and phenylephrine have been employed to promote vasoconstriction and enhance cardiac performance.

Autonomic blockade may disrupt function of the intestinal and urinary tracts, causing fecal incontinence and either urinary incontinence or urinary retention. The prescriber should be notified if the patient fails to void within 8 hours of the end of surgery.

Spinal anesthesia frequently causes headache. These "spinal" headaches are posture dependent and can be relieved by having the patient assume a supine position.

KEY POINTS

- Local anesthetics stop nerve conduction by blocking sodium channels in the axon membrane.
- Small, nonmyelinated neurons are blocked more rapidly than large, myelinated neurons.
- There are two classes of local anesthetics: ester-type anesthetics and amide-type anesthetics.
- Ester-type anesthetics (e.g., procaine) occasionally cause allergic reactions and are inactivated by esterases in the blood.
- Amide-type anesthetics (e.g., lidocaine) rarely cause allergic reactions and are inactivated by enzymes in the liver.
- Onset of anesthesia occurs most rapidly with anesthetics that are small, lipid soluble, and nonionized at physiologic pH.
- Termination of local anesthesia is determined in large part by regional blood flow. Coadministration of epinephrine, a vasoconstrictor, will prolong anesthesia.
- Local anesthetics can be absorbed in amounts sufficient to cause systemic toxicity. Principal concerns are cardiac dysrhythmias and CNS effects (seizures, unconsciousness, coma). Death can occur.
- The risk of systemic toxicity from topical anesthetics applied to the *skin* can be reduced by (1) using the smallest amount needed, (2) avoiding application to large areas, (3) avoiding application to broken or irritated skin, and (4) avoiding strenuous exercise and use of dressings or heating pads (which can increase absorption by increasing skin temperature).

Please visit **http://evolve.elsevier.com/Lehne** for chapter-specific NCLEX® examination review questions.

Summary of Major Nursing Implications[a]

TOPICAL LOCAL ANESTHETICS

Benzocaine
Cocaine
Dibucaine
Dyclonine
Lidocaine
Pramoxine
Prilocaine
Tetracaine

Preadministration Assessment

Therapeutic Goal

Reduction of discomfort associated with local disorders of the skin and mucous membranes.

Continued

Summary of Major Nursing Implications[a]—cont'd

Identifying High-Risk Patients

Ester-type local anesthetics are *contraindicated* for patients with a history of serious allergic reactions to these drugs. Avoid topical *benzocaine* in children under the age of 2 years.

Implementation: Administration

Routes

Topical application to skin and mucous membranes.

Administration

Apply in the lowest effective dosage to the smallest area required. If possible, avoid application to skin that is abraded or otherwise injured. Wear gloves when applying the anesthetic.

Ongoing Evaluation and Interventions

Minimizing Adverse Effects

Systemic Toxicity. Absorption into the general circulation can cause systemic toxicity. Effects on the heart (bradycardia, atrioventricular [AV] heart block, cardiac arrest) and CNS (excitation, possibly including seizures, followed by depression) are of greatest concern. Monitor blood pressure, pulse rate, respiratory rate, and state of consciousness. Have facilities for cardiopulmonary resuscitation available.

The risk of systemic toxicity is determined by the extent of absorption. To minimize absorption, apply topical anesthetics to the smallest surface area needed and, when possible, avoid application to injured skin.

Topical benzocaine can cause methemoglobinemia. Death can result. **Warn parents to avoid the use of topical benzocaine in children younger than 2 years unless approved by a healthcare professional.** For older children and adults, exercise caution when topical benzocaine is applied to mucous membranes of the mouth.

Allergic Reactions. Severe allergic reactions are rare but can occur. Allergic reactions are most likely with ester-type anesthetics. Avoid ester-type agents in patients with a history of allergy to these drugs.

INJECTED LOCAL ANESTHETICS

Bupivacaine
Chloroprocaine
Lidocaine
Mepivacaine
Prilocaine
Procaine
Ropivacaine
Tetracaine

Preadministration Assessment

Therapeutic Goal

Production of local anesthesia for surgical, dental, and obstetric procedures.

Identifying High-Risk Patients

Ester-type local anesthetics are *contraindicated* for patients with a history of serious allergic reactions to these drugs.

Implementation: Administration

Preparation of the Patient

The nurse may be responsible for preparing the patient to receive an injectable local anesthetic. Preparation includes cleansing the injection site, shaving the site when indicated, and placing the patient in a position appropriate to receive the injection. Children, older adults, and uncooperative patients may require restraint before injection by some routes.

Administration

Injection of local anesthetics is performed by clinicians with special training in their use (e.g., physicians, dentists, nurse practitioners, nurse anesthetists).

Ongoing Evaluation and Interventions

Minimizing Adverse Effects

Systemic Reactions. Absorption into the general circulation can cause systemic toxicity. Effects on the CNS and heart are of greatest concern. CNS toxicity manifests as a brief period of excitement, possibly including seizures, followed by CNS depression, which can result in respiratory depression. Cardiotoxicity can manifest as bradycardia, AV heart block, and cardiac arrest. Monitor blood pressure, pulse rate, respiratory rate, and state of consciousness. Have facilities for cardiopulmonary resuscitation available. Manage CNS excitation with IV benzodiazepines, infusion of 20% lipid emulsion, or small doses of IV propofol.

Allergic Reactions. Severe allergic reactions are rare but can occur. These are most likely with ester-type anesthetics. Avoid ester-type agents in patients with a history of allergy to these drugs.

Labor and Delivery. Use of local anesthetics during delivery can cause bradycardia and CNS depression in the newborn. Monitor cardiac status. Avoid concentrated (0.75%) bupivacaine.

Self-Inflicted Injury. Because anesthetics eliminate pain and because pain can be a warning sign of complications, patients recovering from anesthesia must be protected from inadvertent harm until the anesthetic wears off. **Caution the patient against activities that might result in unintentional harm.**

Spinal Headache and Urinary Retention. Patients recovering from spinal anesthesia may experience headache and urinary retention. Headache is posture dependent and can be minimized by having the patient remain supine for about 12 hours. Notify the prescriber if the patient fails to void within 8 hours.

[a]Patient education information is highlighted as **blue text.**

CHAPTER

27 General Anesthetics

General anesthetics are drugs that produce unconsciousness and a lack of responsiveness to all painful stimuli. In contrast, *local anesthetics* do not reduce consciousness, and they blunt sensation only in a limited area (see Chapter 26).

General anesthetics can be divided into two groups: (1) inhalation anesthetics and (2) intravenous anesthetics. The inhalation anesthetics are the main focus of this chapter.

When considering the anesthetics, we need to distinguish between the terms *analgesia* and *anesthesia.* Analgesia refers specifically to loss of sensibility to pain. In contrast, anesthesia refers not only to loss of pain but to loss of all other sensations (e.g., touch, temperature, taste) and to loss of consciousness as well. Hence, while analgesics (e.g., aspirin, morphine) can selectively reduce pain without affecting other sensory modalities and without reducing consciousness, the general anesthetics have no such selectivity: During general anesthesia, all sensation is lost, and consciousness is lost too.

The development of general anesthetics has had an incalculable impact on the surgeon's art. The first general anesthetic—ether—was introduced by William T. Morton in 1846. Before this, surgery was a brutal and exquisitely painful ordeal, undertaken only in the most desperate circumstances. Immobilization of the surgical field was accomplished with the aid of strong men and straps. Survival of the patient was determined by the surgeon's speed rather than finesse. With the advent of general anesthesia, all of this changed. General anesthesia produced a patient who slept through surgery and experienced no pain. These changes allowed surgeons to develop the lengthy and intricate procedures that are routine today. Such procedures were unthinkable before general anesthetics became available.

General anesthetics are also used to facilitate other procedures, including endoscopy, urologic procedures, radiation therapy, electroconvulsive therapy, transbronchial biopsy, and various cardiologic procedures.

INHALATION ANESTHETICS

BASIC PHARMACOLOGY OF INHALATION ANESTHETICS

In this section, we consider the inhalation anesthetics as a group. Our focus is on properties of an ideal anesthetic, pharmacokinetics of inhalation anesthetics, adverse effects of the inhalation anesthetics, and drugs employed as adjuncts to anesthesia.

Properties of an Ideal Inhalation Anesthetic

An ideal inhalation anesthetic would produce unconsciousness, analgesia, muscle relaxation, and amnesia. Furthermore, induction of anesthesia would be brief and pleasant, as would the process of emergence. Depth of anesthesia could be raised or lowered with ease. Adverse effects would be minimal, and the margin of safety would be large. As you might guess, the ideal inhalation anesthetic does not exist: No single agent has all of these qualities.

Balanced Anesthesia

The term *balanced anesthesia* refers to the use of a combination of drugs to accomplish what we cannot achieve with an inhalation anesthetic alone. Put another way, balanced anesthesia is a technique employed to compensate for the lack of an ideal anesthetic. Drugs are combined in balanced anesthesia to ensure that induction is smooth and rapid and that analgesia and muscle relaxation are adequate. The agents used most commonly to achieve these goals are (1) propofol and short-acting barbiturates (for induction of anesthesia), (2) neuromuscular blocking agents (for muscle relaxation), and (3) opioids and nitrous oxide (for analgesia). The primary benefit of combining drugs to achieve surgical anesthesia is that doing so permits full general anesthesia at doses of the inhalation anesthetic that are lower (safer) than those that would be required if surgical anesthesia were attempted using an inhalation anesthetic alone.

Molecular Mechanism of Action

Our understanding of how inhalation anesthetics act has changed dramatically. In the past, we believed that anesthetics worked through nonspecific effects on neuronal membranes. Today, we believe they work through selective alteration of synaptic transmission. However, despite recent advances, we still don't know with certainty just how these drugs work.

More than 100 years ago, scientists postulated that inhalation anesthetics produced their effects through nonspecific interactions with lipid components of the neuronal cell membrane. This long-standing theory was based on the observation that there was a direct correlation between the potency of an anesthetic and its lipid solubility. That is, the more readily an anesthetic could dissolve in the lipid matrix of the neuronal membrane, the more readily that agent could produce anesthesia, hence the theory that anesthetics dissolve into neuronal membranes, disrupt their structure, and thereby suppress axonal conduction and possibly synaptic transmission. However, this theory was called into question by an important observation: Enantiomers of the same anesthetic have different actions. Recall that enantiomers are simply mirror-image molecules that have identical atomic components and hence have identical physical properties, including lipid solubility. Therefore, because enantiomers have the same ability to penetrate the axonal membrane but do not have the same ability to produce anesthesia, a property other than lipid solubility must underlie anesthetic actions.

Inhalation anesthetics work by *enhancing transmission at inhibitory synapses* and by *depressing transmission at excitatory synapses.* Except for nitrous oxide, all of the agents used today enhance activation of receptors for gamma-aminobutyric acid (GABA), the principal inhibitory transmitter in the central nervous system (CNS). As a result, these drugs promote generalized inhibition of CNS function. It should be noted that anesthetics do not activate GABA receptors directly. Rather, by binding with the GABA receptor, they increase receptor sensitivity to activation by GABA itself. How does nitrous oxide work? Probably by blocking the actions of *N*-methyl-D-aspartate (NMDA), an excitatory neurotransmitter. Nitrous oxide appears to bind with the NMDA receptor and thereby prevent receptor activation by NMDA itself.

Minimum Alveolar Concentration

The minimum alveolar concentration (MAC), also known as the median alveolar concentration, is an index of inhalation anesthetic potency. The MAC is defined as *the minimum concentration of drug in the alveolar air that will produce immobility in 50% of patients exposed to a painful stimulus.* Note that, by this definition, a *low* MAC indicates *high* anesthetic potency.

From a clinical perspective, knowledge of the MAC of an anesthetic is of great practical value: The MAC tells us approximately how much anesthetic the inspired air must contain to produce anesthesia. A low MAC indicates that the inspired air needs to contain only low concentrations of the anesthetic to produce surgical anesthesia. The opposite is true for drugs with a high MAC. Fortunately, most inhalation anesthetics have low MACs (Table 27.1). However, one important agent—nitrous oxide—has a very high MAC. The MAC is so high, in fact, that surgical anesthesia cannot be achieved using nitrous oxide alone.

Please note that to produce general anesthesia in *all* patients the inspired anesthetic concentration should be 1.2 to 1.5 times the MAC. If the concentration were simply equal to the MAC, 50% of patients would receive less than they need.

Pharmacokinetics

Uptake and Distribution

To produce therapeutic effects, an inhalation anesthetic must reach a CNS concentration sufficient to suppress neuronal excitability. The principal determinants of anesthetic concentration are (1) uptake from the lungs and (2) distribution to the CNS and other tissues. The kinetics of anesthetic uptake and distribution are complex, and we will not cover them in depth.

Uptake. A major determinant of anesthetic uptake is the concentration of anesthetic in the inspired air: The greater the anesthetic concentration, the more rapid uptake will be. Other factors that influence uptake are pulmonary ventilation, solubility of the anesthetic in blood, and blood flow through the lungs. An increase in any of these will increase the speed of uptake.

Distribution. Distribution to specific tissues is determined largely by regional blood flow. Anesthetic levels rise rapidly in the brain, kidney, heart, and liver—tissues that receive the largest fraction of the cardiac output. Anesthetic levels in these

TABLE 27.1 ▪ Properties of the Major Inhalation Anesthetics

Drug	MAC (%)	Analgesic Effect	Effect on Blood Pressure	Effect on Respiration	Muscle Relaxant Effect	Extent of Metabolism
Nitrous oxide	105	++++	→	→	0	0
Desflurane	4.58	++	↓	↓↓	++	0.02%
Enflurane	1.68	++	↓	↓↓	++	2.4%
Isoflurane	1.15	++	↓	↓↓	++	0.2%
Sevoflurane	1.71	++	↓	↓↓	++	3%

MAC, Minimum alveolar concentration.

tissues equilibrate with those in blood 5 to 15 minutes after inhalation starts. In skin and skeletal muscle—tissues with an intermediate blood flow—equilibration occurs more slowly. The most poorly perfused tissues—fat, bone, ligaments, and cartilage—are the last to equilibrate with anesthetic levels in the blood.

Elimination

Export in the Expired Breath. Inhalation anesthetics are eliminated almost entirely via the lungs; hepatic metabolism is minimal. The same factors that determine anesthetic uptake (pulmonary ventilation, blood flow to the lungs, anesthetic solubility in blood and tissues) also determine the rate of elimination. Because blood flow to the brain is high, anesthetic levels in the brain drop rapidly when administration is stopped. Anesthetic levels in tissues that have a lower blood flow decline more slowly. Because anesthetic levels in the CNS decline more rapidly than levels in other tissues, patients can awaken from anesthesia long before all anesthetic has left the body.

Metabolism. Most inhalation anesthetics undergo very little metabolism. Hence, metabolism does not influence the time course of anesthesia. However, because some metabolites can be toxic, metabolism is nonetheless clinically relevant.

Adverse Effects

The adverse effects discussed here apply to the inhalation anesthetics as a group. Not all of these effects are seen with every anesthetic.

Respiratory and Cardiac Depression

Depression of respiratory and cardiac function is a concern with virtually all inhalation anesthetics. Doses only 2 to 4 times greater than those needed for surgical anesthesia are sufficient to cause potentially lethal depression of pulmonary and cardiac function. To compensate for respiratory depression and to maintain a steady rate of administration, almost all patients require mechanical support of ventilation.

Sensitization of the Heart to Catecholamines

Some anesthetics—most notably *enflurane*—may increase the sensitivity of the heart to stimulation by catecholamines (e.g., norepinephrine, epinephrine). While in this sensitized state, the heart may develop dysrhythmias in response to catecholamines. Exposure to catecholamines may result from two causes: (1) release of endogenous catecholamines (in response to pain or other stimuli of the sympathetic nervous system) and (2) topical application of catecholamines to control bleeding in the surgical field.

Malignant Hyperthermia

Malignant hyperthermia is a rare but potentially fatal reaction that can be triggered by all inhalation anesthetics (except nitrous oxide). Predisposition to the reaction is genetic. Malignant hyperthermia is characterized by muscle rigidity and a profound elevation of temperature—sometimes to as high as 43°C (109°F). Left untreated, the reaction can rapidly prove fatal. The risk of malignant hyperthermia is greatest when an inhalation anesthetic is combined with *succinylcholine,* a neuromuscular blocker that also can trigger the reaction. Diagnosis and management of malignant hyperthermia are discussed in Chapter 16.

Safety Alert

MALIGNANT HYPERTHERMIA

Malignant hyperthermia, while rare, can be fatal. Administration of inhaled anesthetics with the neuromuscular blocker succinylcholine can increase this risk in genetically predisposed individuals. If malignant hyperthermia is present in a patient's family medical history, it is imperative to relay this information to the anesthetist or the team performing surgery.

Aspiration of Gastric Contents

During the state of anesthesia, reflexes that normally prevent aspiration of gastric contents into the lungs are absent. Aspiration of gastric fluids can cause bronchospasm and pneumonia. Use of an endotracheal tube isolates the trachea and can thereby help prevent these complications.

Hepatotoxicity

Rarely, patients receiving inhalation anesthesia develop serious liver dysfunction. The risk is about equal with all anesthetics.

Toxicity to Operating Room Personnel

Chronic exposure to low levels of anesthetics may harm operating room personnel. Suspected reactions include headache, reduced alertness, and spontaneous abortion. Risk can be reduced by venting anesthetic gases from the operating room.

Drug Interactions

Several classes of drugs—analgesics, CNS depressants, CNS stimulants—can influence the amount of anesthetic required to produce anesthesia. Opioid analgesics allow a reduction in anesthetic dosage. When opioids are present, analgesia needn't be produced by the anesthetic alone. Similarly, because CNS depressants (barbiturates, benzodiazepines, alcohol) add to the depressant effects of anesthetics, concurrent use of CNS depressants lowers the required dose of anesthetic. Conversely, concurrent use of CNS stimulants (amphetamines, cocaine) increases the required dose of anesthetic.

Adjuncts to Inhalation Anesthesia

Adjunctive drugs are employed to complement the beneficial effects of inhalation anesthetics and to counteract their adverse effects. Some adjunctive agents are administered before surgery, some during, and some after.

Preanesthetic Medications

Preanesthetic medications are administered for three main purposes: (1) reducing anxiety, (2) producing perioperative amnesia, and (3) relieving preoperative and postoperative pain. In addition, preanesthetic medications may be used to suppress certain adverse responses: excessive salivation, excessive bronchial secretion, coughing, bradycardia, nausea, and vomiting.

Benzodiazepines. Benzodiazepines are given preoperatively to reduce anxiety and promote amnesia. When administered properly, these drugs produce sedation with little or no respiratory depression. Intravenous midazolam [Versed] is used most often.

Opioids. Opioids (e.g., morphine, fentanyl) are administered to relieve preoperative and postoperative pain. These drugs may also help by suppressing cough.

Opioids can have adverse effects. Because they depress the CNS, opioids can delay awakening after surgery. Effects on the bowel and urinary tract may result in postoperative constipation and urinary retention. Stimulation of the chemoreceptor trigger zone promotes vomiting. Opioid-induced respiratory depression combined with anesthetic-induced respiratory depression increases the risk of postoperative respiratory distress.

Alpha$_2$-Adrenergic Agonists. Two alpha$_2$ agonists—clonidine and dexmedetomidine—are employed as adjuncts to anesthesia. Both produce their effects through actions in the CNS.

Clonidine is used to treat hypertension and pain. When administered before surgery, the drug reduces anxiety and causes sedation. In addition, it permits a reduction in anesthetic and analgesic dosages. Analgesic properties of clonidine are discussed further in Chapter 28; antihypertensive properties are discussed in Chapters 19 and 47. The formulation used for analgesia is marketed under the brand name *Duraclon;* the formulation for hypertension is marketed as *Catapres.*

Dexmedetomidine [Precedex] is a highly selective alpha$_2$-adrenergic agonist currently approved only for short-term sedation in critically ill patients. However, the drug is also used for other purposes, including enhancement of sedation and analgesia in patients undergoing anesthesia. The pharmacology of dexmedetomidine is discussed further in Chapter 28.

Anticholinergic Drugs. Anticholinergic drugs (e.g., atropine) may be given to decrease the risk of bradycardia during surgery. Surgical manipulations can trigger parasympathetic reflexes, which in turn can produce profound vagal slowing of the heart. Pretreatment with a cholinergic antagonist prevents bradycardia from this cause.

At one time, anticholinergic drugs were needed to prevent excessive bronchial secretions associated with anesthesia. Older anesthetic agents (e.g., ether) irritate the respiratory tract and thereby cause profuse bronchial secretions. Cholinergic blockers were given to suppress this response. Because the inhalation anesthetics used today are much less irritating, bronchial secretions are minimal. Consequently, although anticholinergic agents are still employed as adjuncts to anesthesia, their purpose is no longer to suppress bronchial secretions (although they may still help by suppressing salivation).

Neuromuscular Blocking Agents. Most surgical procedures require skeletal muscle relaxation, a state achieved with neuromuscular blockers (e.g., succinylcholine, pancuronium). By using these drugs, we can reduce the dose of general anesthetic because we don't need the very high doses of anesthetic that would be required if we tried to produce muscle relaxation with the anesthetic alone.

Muscle relaxants can have adverse effects. Neuromuscular blocking agents prevent contraction of all skeletal muscles, including the diaphragm and other muscles of respiration. Accordingly, patients require mechanical support of ventilation during surgery. Patients recovering from anesthesia may have reduced respiratory capacity owing to residual neuromuscular blockade. Accordingly, respiration must be monitored until recovery is complete.

It is important to appreciate that neuromuscular blockers produce a state of total flaccid paralysis. In this condition, a patient could be fully awake while seeming asleep. Incidents in which paralyzed patients have been awake during surgery but unable to communicate their agony are all too common: Every year in the United States, of the 21 million people who undergo anesthesia, an estimated 1 in every 2000 patients wakes up during the procedure. Because neuromuscular blockade can obscure depth of anesthesia and because failure to maintain adequate anesthesia can result in true horror, the clinician administering anesthesia must be especially watchful to ensure that the anesthetic dosage is adequate.

Postanesthetic Medications

Analgesics. Analgesics are needed to control postoperative pain. If pain is severe, opioids are indicated. For mild pain, acetaminophen-containing drugs may suffice.

Antiemetics. Patients recovering from anesthesia often experience nausea and vomiting. This can be suppressed with antiemetics. Among the most effective is *ondansetron* [Zofran], a drug developed to suppress nausea and vomiting in patients undergoing cancer chemotherapy. Other commonly used antiemetics are *promethazine* and *droperidol.*

Muscarinic Agonists. Abdominal distention (from atony of the bowel) and urinary retention are potential postoperative complications. Both conditions can be relieved through activation of muscarinic receptors. The muscarinic agonist employed most often is *bethanechol.*

Dosage and Administration

Administration of inhalation anesthetics is performed only by anesthesiologists (physicians) and anesthetists (nurses). Clinicians who lack the training of these specialists have no authority to administer anesthesia. Because knowledge of anesthetic dosage and administration is the responsibility of specialists and because this text is designed for beginning students, details on dosage and administration are not presented. If you need this information, consult a textbook of anesthesiology.

Classification of Inhalation Anesthetics

Inhalation anesthetics fall into two basic categories: *gases* and *volatile liquids.* The gases, as their name implies, exist in a gaseous state at atmospheric pressure. The volatile liquids exist in a liquid state at atmospheric pressure but can be easily volatilized (converted to a vapor) for administration by inhalation. The inhalation anesthetics in current use are listed in Table 27.2. The volatile liquids—enflurane, isoflurane, desflurane,

TABLE 27.2 ■ Classification of the Inhalation Anesthetics

	Anesthetic	
Class	Generic Name	Brand Name
Volatile Liquids	Enflurane	Ethrane
	Isoflurane	Forane
	Desflurane	Suprane
	Sevoflurane	Ultane, Sevorane 🍁
Gases	Nitrous oxide	None

and sevoflurane—are similar to one another in structure and function. The only gas in current use is nitrous oxide.

PROPERTIES OF INDIVIDUAL INHALATION ANESTHETICS

Isoflurane

Isoflurane [Forane] is the prototype of the volatile inhalation anesthetics. This drug was introduced in 1983 and is widely used in the United States. Before the advent of this drug, the most common drug employed for anesthesia was halothane, which was discontinued owing to its hepatotoxicity and the availability of newer agents.

Prototype Drugs

GENERAL ANESTHETICS

Inhalation Anesthetics

Isoflurane
Nitrous oxide

Intravenous Anesthetics

Propofol
Ketamine

Anesthetic Properties

Potency. Isoflurane is a high-potency anesthetic, and hence has a low MAC (1.15%), indicating that unconsciousness can be produced when the drug's concentration in alveolar air is only 1.15%.

Time Course. Induction of anesthesia is smooth and relatively rapid. Depth of anesthesia can be adjusted with speed and ease, and patients emerge from anesthesia rapidly. Although isoflurane can act quickly, in actual practice induction is usually produced with propofol, a rapid-acting anesthetic, as isoflurane is a respiratory irritant with an unpleasant odor and can cause coughing or breath-holding. Once the patient is unconscious, depth of anesthesia can be raised or lowered with ease. Patients awaken about 20 minutes after ceasing isoflurane inhalation.

Analgesia. Isoflurane is a weak analgesic. Consequently, when the drug is used for surgical anesthesia, coadministration of a strong analgesic is usually required. The analgesics most commonly employed are opioids (e.g., morphine) and nitrous oxide.

Muscle Relaxation. Although isoflurane has muscle-relaxant actions, the degree of relaxation is generally inadequate for surgery. Accordingly, concurrent use of a neuromuscular blocking agent (e.g., pancuronium) is usually required. Although relaxation of skeletal muscle is only moderate, isoflurane does promote relaxation of uterine smooth muscle. Consequently, when used in obstetrics, isoflurane may inhibit uterine contractions, delaying delivery and possibly increasing postpartum bleeding.

Adverse Effects

Hypotension. Isoflurane causes a dose-dependent reduction in blood pressure through peripheral vasodilation primarily in skin and muscle.

Respiratory Depression. Like other volatile liquids, isoflurane produces depression of respiration. To ensure adequate oxygenation, two measures are implemented: (1) mechanical or manual ventilatory support and (2) enrichment of the inspired gas mixture with oxygen.

Other Adverse Effects

Postoperative nausea and vomiting may occur, but these reactions are less common with isoflurane than with older anesthetics (e.g., ether). By decreasing blood flow to the kidney, isoflurane and other inhaled anesthetics can cause a substantial decrease in urine output.

Elimination

Isoflurane is eliminated almost entirely in the expired breath; only 0.2% undergoes metabolism. As you can see in Table 27.1, the percentage metabolized is much less than that of almost any other inhalational agent.

Enflurane

Enflurane [Ethrane] has pharmacologic properties very similar to those of isoflurane. Enflurane was introduced in 1973 and became quite popular. However, with the introduction of newer agents with preferable kinetics and fewer risks, use of enflurane has declined.

Comparison of enflurane with isoflurane reveals important similarities and a few significant differences. Both anesthetics are very potent: the MAC of enflurane is 1.68%, compared with 1.15% for isoflurane. As with isoflurane, induction of anesthesia is smooth and rapid, and depth of anesthesia can be changed quickly and easily. Like isoflurane, enflurane produces substantial depression of respiration. Accordingly, patients are likely to need ventilatory support; the concentration of inspired oxygen should be at least 35%. Muscle relaxation induced by enflurane is equal to that of isoflurane. However, despite this action, a neuromuscular blocker is usually employed (to permit a reduction of enflurane dosage). Like isoflurane, enflurane can suppress uterine contractions, impeding labor. Enflurane can also sensitize the myocardium to catecholamines, although this effect is much less than with older anesthetic agents. Because this effect is minimal, enflurane remains safe in combination with exogenous administration of epinephrine during procedures. High doses of enflurane can induce seizures, a response not seen with isoflurane; therefore, enflurane should be avoided in patients with a history of seizure disorders. Like isoflurane, enflurane is eliminated primarily in the exhaled breath as the intact parent compound. About 2% is eliminated by hepatic metabolism.

Desflurane

Desflurane [Suprane] is nearly identical in structure to isoflurane. Induction occurs more rapidly than with any other volatile anesthetic, depth of anesthesia can be changed quickly, and recovery occurs only minutes after ceasing administration. Desflurane is indicated for maintenance of anesthesia in adults and children and for induction of anesthesia in adults. The drug is not approved for induction in children and infants owing to a high incidence of respiratory difficulties (laryngospasm, apnea, increased secretions), which are caused by the drug's pungency. Like isoflurane, desflurane can cause respiratory depression and hypotension secondary to vasodilation. During induction, or in response to an abrupt increase in desflurane blood levels, heart rate and blood pressure may increase, causing tachycardia and hypertension. Postoperative nausea and vomiting are possible. Malignant hypertension has occurred in experimental animals. Desflurane undergoes even less metabolism than isoflurane. Hence, the risk of postoperative organ injury is probably low.

Sevoflurane

Sevoflurane [Ultane, Sevorane 🍁] is similar to desflurane. The drug is approved for induction and maintenance of anesthesia in adults and children. As with desflurane, induction is rapid, depth of anesthesia can be adjusted easily, and recovery occurs minutes after ceasing inhalation. Because onset and recovery occur quickly, sevoflurane is widely used for outpatient procedures. In contrast to desflurane, sevoflurane has a pleasant odor and is not a respiratory irritant. Accordingly, the drug is suitable for mask induction in children. Sevoflurane has a MAC of 1.71% and is eliminated primarily in the exhaled breath; about 3% gets metabolized. Adverse effects are minimal. The most common problem is postoperative nausea and vomiting. In contrast to desflurane, sevoflurane does not cause tachycardia or hypertension. Occasionally, sevoflurane produces extreme heat and even fire in the administration apparatus, usually when the CO_2 adsorbent in the apparatus has become desiccated.

Nitrous Oxide

Nitrous oxide (aka "laughing gas") differs from the volatile liquid anesthetics with respect to pharmacologic properties and uses. Pharmacologically, nitrous oxide is unique in two ways: (1) it has very low *anesthetic* potency, whereas the anesthetic potency of the other inhalational agents is high, and (2) it has very high *analgesic* potency, whereas the analgesic potency of other inhalational agents is low. Because of these properties, nitrous oxide has a unique pattern of use: owing to its low anesthetic potency, nitrous oxide is never employed as a primary anesthetic. However, owing to its high analgesic potency, nitrous oxide is frequently combined with other inhalational agents to enhance analgesia.

Because nitrous oxide has such low anesthetic potency, *it is virtually impossible to produce surgical anesthesia employing nitrous oxide alone.* The MAC of nitrous oxide is very high—greater than 100%. This tells us that even if it were possible to administer 100% nitrous oxide (i.e., inspired gas that contains only nitrous oxide and no oxygen), this would still be insufficient to produce surgical anesthesia. Because practical considerations (i.e., the need to administer at least 30% oxygen) limit the maximum usable concentration of nitrous oxide to 70% and because much higher concentrations are needed to produce surgical anesthesia, it is clear that full anesthesia cannot be achieved with nitrous oxide alone.

Despite its low anesthetic potency, nitrous oxide is one of our most widely used inhalational agents: *Many patients undergoing general anesthesia receive nitrous oxide to supplement the analgesic effects of the primary anesthetic.* As indicated in Table 27.1, the analgesic effects of nitrous oxide are substantially greater than those of the other inhalational agents. In fact, nitrous oxide is such a potent analgesic that inhaling 20% nitrous oxide can produce pain relief equivalent to that of morphine. The advantage of providing analgesia with nitrous oxide, rather than relying entirely on the primary anesthetic, is that the dosage of the primary anesthetic can be significantly decreased—usually by 50% or more. As a result, respiratory depression and cardiac depression are reduced, and emergence from anesthesia is accelerated. When employed in combination with other inhalation anesthetics, nitrous oxide is administered at a concentration of 70%.

At therapeutic concentrations, nitrous oxide has no serious adverse effects. The drug is not toxic to the CNS and does not cause cardiovascular or respiratory depression. Furthermore, the drug is not likely to precipitate malignant hyperthermia. The major concern with nitrous oxide is postoperative *nausea* and *vomiting,* which occur more often with this agent than with any other inhalation anesthetic.

In certain settings, nitrous oxide can be used alone—but only for *analgesia,* not anesthesia. Nitrous oxide alone is used for analgesia in dentistry and during delivery.

INTRAVENOUS ANESTHETICS

Intravenous anesthetics may be used alone or to supplement the effects of inhalational agents. When combined with an inhalation anesthetic, IV agents offer two potential benefits: (1) they permit dosage of the inhalational agent to be reduced, and (2) they produce effects that cannot be achieved with an inhalational agent alone. Three of the drug families discussed in this section—opioids, barbiturates, and benzodiazepines—are considered in other chapters. Accordingly, discussion here is limited to their use in anesthesia.

SHORT-ACTING BARBITURATES (OXYBARBITURATES)

Short-acting barbiturates, administered intravenously, are employed for *induction of anesthesia.* One agent is available: *methohexital sodium* [Brevital].

Methohexital

Methohexital [Brevital] is an ultrashort-acting barbiturate, similar to thiopental. Although thiopental was extremely effective for induction of anesthesia, production of the drug ceased in 2011 because of its use in human executions. Methohexital, like thiopental, acts rapidly to produce unconsciousness. Analgesic and muscle-relaxant effects are weak.

Methohexital and other barbiturates were once mainstays of anesthesia induction, but use has decreased secondary to the availability of propofol, a general anesthetic agent. Methohexital has a rapid onset and short duration. Unconsciousness occurs 10 to 20 seconds after IV injection. If methohexital is not followed by inhalation anesthesia, the patient will wake up in about 10 minutes.

The time course of anesthesia is determined by methohexital's pattern of distribution. Methohexital is lipid soluble, and therefore enters the brain rapidly to begin its effects. Anesthesia is terminated as methohexital undergoes redistribution from the brain and blood to other tissues. Practically no metabolism of the drug takes place between giving the injection and the time of waking.

Like most of the inhalation anesthetics, methohexital causes cardiovascular and respiratory depression. If administered too rapidly, the drug may cause apnea. Increase in heart rate may be seen owing to baroreceptor reflex–mediated sympathetic nervous system stimulation.

BENZODIAZEPINES

When administered in large doses, benzodiazepines produce unconsciousness and amnesia. Because of this ability, IV benzodiazepines are occasionally given to induce anesthesia. However, short-acting barbiturates are generally preferred. Three benzodiazepines—*diazepam, lorazepam,* and *midazolam*—are administered IV for induction. Diazepam is the prototype for the group. The basic pharmacology of the benzodiazepines is discussed in Chapter 34.

Diazepam

Induction with IV diazepam [Valium] occurs more slowly than with barbiturates. Unconsciousness develops in about 1 minute. Diazepam causes very little muscle relaxation and no analgesia. Cardiovascular depression and respiratory depression are usually only moderate. However, on occasion respiratory depression is severe. Therefore, whenever diazepam is administered IV, facilities for respiratory support must be immediately available.

Midazolam

Intravenous midazolam [Versed] may be used for *induction of anesthesia* and to produce *conscious sedation.* When used for induction, midazolam is usually combined with a short-acting barbiturate. Unconsciousness develops in 80 seconds.

Conscious sedation can be produced by combining midazolam with an opioid analgesic (e.g., morphine, fentanyl). The state is characterized by sedation, analgesia, amnesia, and lack of anxiety. The patient is unperturbed and passive, but responsive to commands, such as "open your eyes." Conscious sedation persists for an hour or so and is suitable for minor surgeries and endoscopic procedures.

Midazolam can cause dangerous cardiorespiratory effects, including respiratory depression and respiratory and cardiac arrest. Accordingly, the drug should be used only in a setting that permits constant monitoring of cardiac and respiratory status. Facilities for resuscitation must be immediately available. The risk of adverse effects can be minimized by injecting midazolam slowly (over 2 or more minutes) and by waiting another 2 or more minutes for full effects to develop before dosing again.

OTHER INTRAVENOUS ANESTHETICS

Propofol

Actions and Uses

Propofol [Diprivan] is our most widely used IV anesthetic. About 90% of patients who undergo anesthesia receive the drug. Propofol is indicated for induction and maintenance of general anesthesia as part of a balanced anesthesia technique. In addition, the drug can be used to sedate patients undergoing mechanical ventilation, radiation therapy, and diagnostic procedures (e.g., endoscopy, magnetic resonance imaging). Propofol works by promoting release of GABA, the major inhibitory neurotransmitter in the brain. The result is generalized CNS depression. Propofol has no analgesic actions. Propofol has a rapid onset and ultrashort duration. Unconsciousness develops in less than 60 seconds after IV injection, but lasts only 3 to 5 minutes. Redistribution from the brain to other tissues explains the rapid awakening. For extended sedation, a continuous low-dose infusion is used, not to exceed 4 mg/kg/hr.

Adverse Effects

Propofol can cause profound *respiratory depression* (including apnea) and *hypotension.* The drug has a relatively narrow therapeutic range and can cause death from respiratory arrest. To reduce risk, propofol should be used with caution in older adults, hypovolemic patients, and patients with compromised cardiac function. With all patients, facilities for respiratory support should be immediately available.

Propofol poses a high risk of *bacterial infection.* Propofol is not water soluble and hence must be formulated in a lipid-based medium, which is ideal for bacterial growth. In surgical patients, the use of preparations that have become contaminated after opening has caused sepsis and death. To minimize the risk of infection, propofol solutions and opened vials should be discarded within 6 hours. Unopened vials should be stored at 22°C (72°F).

Propofol can cause transient pain at the site of IV injection. This can be minimized by using a large vein and by injecting IV lidocaine (a local anesthetic) at the site just before injecting propofol.

Rarely, prolonged high-dose infusion leads to *propofol infusion syndrome,* characterized by metabolic acidosis, cardiac failure, renal failure, and rhabdomyolysis. Deaths have occurred. Traumatic brain injury and young age are major risk factors. Risk can be minimized by using a low-dose infusion (no more than 4 mg/kg/hr) and by daily monitoring of plasma creatine phosphokinase (CPK), a marker for skeletal and cardiac muscle injury. If CPK rises above 5000 units/L, the propofol infusion should stop immediately.

Abuse

Although not regulated as a controlled substance, propofol is subject to abuse, primarily by anesthesiologists, nurse anesthetists, and other medical professionals, all of whom have easy access to the drug. Why is access easy? First, propofol is widely available in operating rooms, endoscopy suites, and physicians' offices. Second, because propofol is not a controlled substance, supplies are not closely monitored.

The appeal of propofol is unique. As a rule, clinicians don't use the drug to produce a "high." Rather, they use it to produce instantaneous (but brief) sleep, after which they wake up feeling refreshed. When patients awake after getting propofol, they are often talkative and report feeling elated and even euphoric. Animal studies show a profound effect on the brain's reward center.

Unfortunately, although propofol can make us feel good, it can also kill: Because propofol has a low therapeutic index, death from overdose is not uncommon. In 2009, propofol made the headlines as the cause of death for singer Michael Jackson.

Despite its clear potential for abuse and despite a recommendation from the American Society of Anesthesiologists propofol remains unregulated under the Controlled Substances Act. The principal reason, apparently, is that propofol is not readily available to the public, and hence regulation is seen as unnecessary.

Etomidate

Etomidate [Amidate] is a potent hypnotic agent used for induction of surgical anesthesia. Unconsciousness develops rapidly and lasts about 5 minutes. The drug has no analgesic actions. Adverse effects associated with single injections include transient apnea, venous pain at the injection site, and suppression of plasma cortisol levels for 6 to 8 hours. Repeated administration can cause hypotension, oliguria, electrolyte disturbances, and a high incidence (50%) of postoperative nausea and vomiting. Cardiovascular effects are less than with barbiturates, and hence the drug is preferred for patients with cardiovascular disorders.

Ketamine

Anesthetic Effects

Ketamine [Ketalar] produces a state known as *dissociative anesthesia* in which the patient feels dissociated from his or her environment. In addition, the drug causes sedation, immobility, analgesia, and amnesia; responsiveness to pain is lost. Induction is rapid and emergence begins within 10 to 15 minutes. Full recovery, however, may take several hours.

Adverse Psychologic Reactions

During recovery from ketamine, about 12% of patients experience unpleasant psychologic reactions, including hallucinations, disturbing dreams, and delirium. These emergence reactions usually fade in a few hours, although they sometimes last up to 24 hours. To minimize these reactions, the patient should be kept in a soothing, stimulus-free environment until recovery is complete. Premedication with diazepam or midazolam reduces the risk of an adverse reaction. Emergence reactions are least likely in children younger than 15 years and in adults older than 65 years. Despite its potential for unpleasant psychologic effects, ketamine has become a popular drug of abuse (see Chapter 40).

Therapeutic Uses

Ketamine is especially valuable for anesthesia in patients undergoing minor surgical and diagnostic procedures. The drug is frequently used to facilitate the changing of burn dressings. Because of its potential for adverse psychologic effects, ketamine should generally be avoided in patients with a history of psychiatric illness, although the drug has produced rapid relief in patients with intractable depression (see Chapter 32). Owing to its potential for abuse, ketamine is regulated as a Schedule III drug.

Neuroleptic-Opioid Combination: Droperidol Plus Fentanyl

A unique state, known as *neuroleptanalgesia,* can be produced with a combination of fentanyl, a potent opioid, plus droperidol, a neuroleptic (antipsychotic) agent.

Neuroleptanalgesia is characterized by quiescence, indifference to surroundings, and insensitivity to pain. The patient appears to be asleep but is not (i.e., complete loss of consciousness does not occur). In large part, neuroleptanalgesia is similar to the dissociative anesthesia produced by ketamine. Neuroleptanalgesia is employed for diagnostic and minor surgical procedures (e.g., bronchoscopy, repeated changing of burn dressings).

Droperidol prolongs the QT interval on the electrocardiogram, indicating that it can cause potentially fatal dysrhythmias. Accordingly, droperidol should be used only when safer drugs are ineffective or intolerable. Droperidol is contraindicated for patients with existing QT prolongation, and should be used with great caution in those at risk of developing QT prolongation. The issue of drug-induced QT prolongation is discussed in Chapter 7.

Other adverse effects include hypotension and respiratory depression. Respiratory depression can be severe and may persist for hours. Respiratory assistance is usually required. Like other neuroleptics, droperidol blocks receptors for dopamine, and should not be given to patients with Parkinson disease.

For some procedures, the combination of fentanyl plus droperidol is supplemented with nitrous oxide. The state produced by this three-drug regimen is called *neuroleptanesthesia*. Neuroleptanesthesia produces more analgesia and a greater reduction of consciousness than does neuroleptanalgesia. Neuroleptanesthesia can be used for major surgical procedures, but with the advent of newer inhaled anesthetics, it is not commonly used.

KEY POINTS

- General anesthetics produce unconsciousness and insensitivity to painful stimuli. In contrast, analgesics reduce sensitivity to pain but do not reduce consciousness.
- The term *balanced anesthesia* refers to the use of several drugs to ensure that induction of anesthesia is smooth and rapid and that analgesia and muscle relaxation are adequate.
- The minimum alveolar concentration (MAC) of an inhalation anesthetic is defined as the minimum concentration of drug in alveolar air that will produce immobility in 50% of patients exposed to a painful stimulus. A *low* MAC indicates *high* anesthetic potency!
- Inhalational agents work by enhancing transmission at inhibitory synapses and by inhibiting transmission at excitatory synapses.
- Inhalation anesthetics are eliminated almost entirely in the expired air. As a rule, they undergo minimal hepatic metabolism.
- The principal adverse effects of general anesthetics are depression of respiration and cardiac performance.
- Malignant hyperthermia is a rare genetically determined, life-threatening reaction to general anesthetics. Coadministration of succinylcholine, a neuromuscular blocker, increases the risk of the reaction.
- By enhancing analgesia, opioids reduce the required dosage of general anesthetic.
- By enhancing muscle relaxation, neuromuscular blockers reduce the required dosage of general anesthetic.
- Nitrous oxide differs from other general anesthetics in two important ways: (1) it has a very high MAC and therefore cannot be used alone to produce general anesthesia, and (2) it has high analgesic potency and therefore is frequently combined with other general anesthetics to supplement their analgesic effects.
- Propofol, a rapid-acting agent with an ultrashort duration, is widely used alone (for diagnostic procedures) and combined with an inhalation anesthetic (as a component of balanced anesthesia).
- Ketamine is an IV anesthetic that produces a state known as dissociative anesthesia. Patients recovering from ketamine may experience adverse psychologic reactions.

Please visit **http://evolve.elsevier.com/Lehne** for chapter-specific NCLEX® examination review questions.

Summary of Major Nursing Implications

ALL INHALATION ANESTHETICS

Desflurane
Enflurane
Isoflurane
Nitrous oxide
Sevoflurane

Nursing management of the patient receiving general anesthesia is almost exclusively preoperative and postoperative; intraoperative management is the responsibility of anesthesiologists and anesthetists. Accordingly, our summary of anesthesia-related nursing implications is divided into two sections: (1) implications that pertain to the preoperative patient and (2) implications that pertain to the postoperative patient. Intraoperative implications are not considered.

The nursing implications here are limited to ones that are directly related to anesthesia. Nursing implications regarding the overall management of the surgical patient (i.e., implications unrelated to anesthesia) are not presented. (Overall nursing management of the surgical patient is discussed fully in your medical-surgical text.)

Nursing implications for drugs employed as adjuncts to anesthesia (barbiturates, benzodiazepines, anticholinergic agents, opioids, neuromuscular blocking agents) are discussed

Summary of Major Nursing Implications—cont'd

in other chapters. Only those implications that apply specifically to their adjunctive use are addressed here.

Preoperative Patients: Counseling, Assessment, and Medication

Counseling

Anxiety is common among patients anticipating surgery: the patient may fear the surgery itself or may be concerned about the possibility of waking up or experiencing pain during the procedure. Because excessive anxiety can disrupt the smoothness of the surgical course (in addition to being distressing to the patient), you should attempt to dispel preoperative fears. To some extent, fear can be allayed by reassuring the patient that anesthesia will keep him or her asleep for the entire procedure, will prevent pain, and will create amnesia about the experience.

Assessment

Medication History. The patient may be taking drugs that can affect responses to anesthetics. Drugs that act on the respiratory and cardiovascular systems are of particular concern. To decrease the risk of adverse interactions, obtain a thorough history of drug use. *All* drugs—prescription medications, over-the-counter preparations, and illicit agents—should be considered. With illicit drugs (e.g., heroin, barbiturates) and with alcohol, it is important to determine both the duration of use and the amount used per day.

Respiratory and Cardiovascular Function. Most general anesthetics produce cardiovascular and respiratory depression. To evaluate the effects of anesthesia, baseline values for blood pressure, heart rate, and respiration are required. Also, any disease of the cardiovascular and respiratory systems should be noted.

Preoperative Medication

Preoperative medications (e.g., benzodiazepines, opioids, anticholinergic agents) are employed to (1) calm the patient, (2) provide analgesia, and (3) counteract adverse effects of general anesthetics. Because preoperative medication can have a significant impact on the overall response to anesthesia, it is important that these drugs be given at an appropriate time—typically 30 to 60 minutes before surgery. Because preoperative medication may produce drowsiness or hypotension, the patient should remain in bed. A calm environment will complement the effect of sedatives.

Postoperative Patients: Ongoing Evaluation and Interventions

When receiving a patient for postoperative care, you should know all of the drugs the patient has received in the hospital (anesthetics and adjunctive medications). In addition, you should know what medications the patient was taking at home, especially drugs for hypertension. With this information, you will be able to anticipate the time course of emergence from anesthesia as well as potential drug-related postoperative complications.

Evaluations and Interventions That Pertain to Specific Organ Systems

Cardiovascular and Respiratory Systems. Anesthetics depress cardiovascular and respiratory function. Monitor vital signs until they return to baseline. Determine blood pressure, pulse rate, and respiration immediately upon receipt of the patient, and repeat monitoring at brief intervals until recovery is complete. During the recovery period, observe the patient for respiratory and cardiovascular distress. Be alert for (1) reductions in blood pressure; (2) altered cardiac rhythm; and (3) shallow, slow, or noisy breathing. Ensure that the airway remains patent. Have facilities for respiratory support available.

Central Nervous System. Return of CNS function is gradual, and precautions are needed until recovery is complete. When appropriate, employ side rails or straps to avoid accidental falls. Assist ambulation until the patient is able to stand steadily. During the early stage of emergence, the patient may be able to hear, even though he or she may appear unconscious. Accordingly, exercise discretion in what you say.

Gastrointestinal Tract. Bowel function may be compromised by the surgery itself or by the drugs employed as adjuncts to anesthesia (e.g., opioids, anticholinergics). Constipation or atony of the bowel may occur. Monitor bowel function. A bowel regimen with sennosides, docusate, or metoclopramide should be initiated after surgery. (These drugs are discussed in Chapter 79.) Determine bowel sounds before giving oral medications.

Nausea and vomiting are potential postanesthetic reactions. To reduce the risk of aspiration, position the patient with his or her head to the side. Have equipment for suctioning available. Antiemetic medication may be needed.

Urinary Tract. Anesthetics and their adjuncts can disrupt urinary tract function. Anesthetics can decrease urine production by reducing renal blood flow. Opioids and anticholinergic drugs can cause urinary retention. Monitor urine output. If the patient fails to void, follow hospital protocol. Catheterization may be needed.

Management of Postoperative Pain

As anesthesia wears off, the patient may experience postoperative pain. An opioid may be required. Because respiratory depression from opioids will add to residual respiratory depression from anesthesia, use opioids with caution; balance the need to relieve pain against the need to maintain ventilation.

CHAPTER

28 Opioid Analgesics, Opioid Antagonists, and Nonopioid Centrally Acting Analgesics

Analgesics are drugs that relieve pain without causing loss of consciousness. In this chapter, we focus mainly on the opioid analgesics, the most effective pain relievers available. The opioid family, whose name derives from *opium,* includes such widely used agents as morphine, fentanyl, codeine, and oxycodone [OxyContin].

OPIOID ANALGESICS

INTRODUCTION TO THE OPIOIDS

Terminology

An *opioid* (previously known as a narcotic) is any drug, natural or synthetic, that has actions similar to those of morphine. The term *opiate* is more specific and applies only to compounds present in opium (e.g., morphine, codeine).

Endogenous Opioid Peptides

The body has three families of peptides—*enkephalins, endorphins,* and *dynorphins*—that have opioid-like properties. Although we know that endogenous opioid peptides serve as neurotransmitters, neurohormones, and neuromodulators, their precise physiologic role is not fully understood. Endogenous opioid peptides are found in the central nervous system (CNS) and in peripheral tissues.

Opioid Receptors

There are three main classes of opioid receptors, designated *mu, kappa,* and *delta.* From a pharmacologic perspective, mu receptors are the most important because opioid analgesics act primarily by activating mu receptors, although they also produce weak activation of kappa receptors. As a rule, opioid analgesics do not interact with delta receptors. In contrast to opioid analgesics, endogenous opioid peptides act through all three opioid receptors, including delta receptors. Important responses to activation of mu and kappa receptors are shown in Table 28.1.

Mu Receptors

Responses to activation of mu receptors include analgesia, respiratory depression, euphoria, and sedation. In addition, mu activation is related to physical dependence.

A study in genetically engineered mice underscores the importance of mu receptors in drug action. In this study, researchers studied mice that lacked the gene for mu receptors. When these mice were given morphine, the drug had no effect. It did not produce analgesia or physical dependence, and it did not reinforce social behaviors that are thought to indicate subjective effects. Hence, at least in mice, mu receptors appear both necessary and sufficient to mediate the major actions of opioid drugs.

TABLE 28.1 ■ Important Responses to Activation of Mu and Kappa Receptors

	Receptor Type	
Response	**Mu**	**Kappa**
Analgesia	✓	✓
Respiratory depression	✓	
Sedation	✓	✓
Euphoria	✓	
Physical dependence	✓	
Decreased GI motility	✓	✓

TABLE 28.2 ■ Drug Actions at Mu and Kappa Receptors

	Receptor Type	
Drugs	**Mu**	**Kappa**
PURE OPIOID AGONISTS		
Morphine, codeine, meperidine, and other morphine-like drugs	Agonist	Agonist
AGONIST-ANTAGONIST OPIOIDS		
Pentazocine, nalbuphine, butorphanol	Antagonist	Agonist
Buprenorphine	Partial agonist	Antagonist
PURE OPIOID ANTAGONISTS		
Naloxone, naltrexone, others	Antagonist	Antagonist

TABLE 28.3 ■ Opioid Analgesics: Abuse Liability and Maximal Pain Relief

Drug and Category	CSA[a] Schedule	Abuse Liability	Maximal Pain Relief
STRONG OPIOID AGONISTS			
Alfentanil	II	High	High
Fentanyl	II	High	High
Hydromorphone	II	High	High
Levorphanol	II	High	High
Meperidine	II	High	High
Methadone	II	High	High
Morphine	II	High	High
Oxymorphone	II	High	High
Remifentanil	II	—	High
Sufentanil	II	High	High
MODERATE TO STRONG OPIOID AGONISTS			
Codeine	II	Moderate	Low
Hydrocodone	II	Moderate	Moderate
Oxycodone	II	Moderate	Moderate to high
Tapentadol	II	Moderate	Moderate to high
AGONIST-ANTAGONIST OPIOIDS			
Buprenorphine	III	Low	Moderate to high
Butorphanol	IV	Low	Moderate to high
Nalbuphine	NR[b]	Low	Moderate to high
Pentazocine	IV	Low	Moderate

[a]*CSA,* Controlled Substances Act.
[b]*NR,* Not regulated under the Controlled Substances Act.

Kappa Receptors

As with mu receptors, activation of kappa receptors can produce analgesia and sedation. In addition, kappa activation may underlie psychotomimetic effects seen with certain opioids.

Classification of Drugs That Act at Opioid Receptors

Drugs that act at opioid receptors are classified on the basis of how they affect receptor function. At each type of receptor, a drug can act in one of three ways: as an *agonist, partial agonist,* or *antagonist.* (Recall from Chapter 5 that a partial agonist is a drug that produces low to moderate receptor activation when administered alone, but will block the actions of a full agonist if the two are given together.) Based on these actions, drugs that bind opioid receptors fall into three major groups: (1) pure opioid agonists, (2) agonist-antagonist opioids, and (3) pure opioid antagonists. The actions of drugs in these groups at mu and kappa receptors are shown in Table 28.2.

Pure Opioid Agonists

The pure opioid agonists activate mu receptors and kappa receptors. By doing so, the pure agonists can produce analgesia, euphoria, sedation, respiratory depression, physical dependence, constipation, and other effects. As indicated in Table 28.3, the pure agonists can be subdivided into two groups: *strong opioid agonists* and *moderate to strong opioid agonists.* Morphine is the prototype of the strong agonists. Codeine is the prototype of the moderate to strong agonists.

Agonist-Antagonist Opioids

Four agonist-antagonist opioids are available: pentazocine, nalbuphine, butorphanol, and buprenorphine. The actions of these drugs at mu and kappa receptors are shown in Table 28.2. When administered alone, the agonist-antagonist opioids produce analgesia. However, if given to a patient who is taking a pure opioid agonist, these drugs can *antagonize* analgesia caused by the pure agonist. Pentazocine [Talwin] is the prototype of the agonist-antagonists.

Pure Opioid Antagonists

The pure opioid antagonists act as antagonists at mu and kappa receptors. These drugs do not produce analgesia or any of the other effects caused by opioid agonists. Their principal use is reversal of respiratory and CNS depression caused by overdose with opioid agonists. In addition, one of these drugs—methylnaltrexone—is used to treat opioid-induced constipation. Naloxone [Narcan] is the prototype of the pure opioid antagonists.

Prototype Drugs

OPIOID ANALGESICS AND ANTAGONISTS

Pure Opioid Agonists
Morphine

Agonist-Antagonist Opioids
Pentazocine

Pure Opioid Antagonists
Naloxone

BASIC PHARMACOLOGY OF THE OPIOIDS

Morphine

Morphine is the prototype of the strong opioid analgesics and remains the standard by which newer opioids are measured. Morphine has multiple pharmacologic effects, including analgesia, sedation, euphoria, respiratory depression, cough suppression, and suppression of bowel motility.

Source

Morphine is found in the seedpod of the poppy plant *Papaver somniferum*. The drug is prepared by extraction from opium (the dried juice of the poppy seedpod). In addition to morphine, opium contains two other medicinal compounds: codeine (an analgesic) and papaverine (a smooth muscle relaxant).

Overview of Pharmacologic Actions

Morphine has multiple pharmacologic actions. In addition to relieving pain, the drug causes drowsiness and mental clouding, reduces anxiety, and creates a sense of well-being. Through actions in the CNS and periphery, morphine can cause respiratory depression, constipation, urinary retention, orthostatic hypotension, emesis, miosis, cough suppression, and biliary colic. With prolonged use, the drug produces tolerance and physical dependence.

Individual effects of morphine may be beneficial, detrimental, or both. For example, analgesia is clearly beneficial, whereas respiratory depression and urinary retention are clearly detrimental. Certain other effects, such as sedation and reduced bowel motility, may be beneficial or detrimental, depending on the circumstances of drug use.

Therapeutic Use: Relief of Pain

The principal indication for morphine is relief of moderate to severe pain. The drug can relieve postoperative pain, pain of labor and delivery, and chronic pain caused by cancer and other conditions. In addition, morphine can be used to relieve pain of myocardial infarction and dyspnea associated with left ventricular failure and pulmonary edema—although it is no longer the drug of choice for these disorders. Morphine may also be administered preoperatively for sedation and reduction of anxiety.

Morphine relieves pain without affecting other senses (e.g., sight, touch, smell, hearing) and without causing loss of consciousness. The drug is more effective against dull, constant pain than against sharp, intermittent pain. However, even sharp pain can be relieved by large doses. The ability of morphine to cause mental clouding, sedation, euphoria, and anxiety reduction can contribute to relief of pain.

The use of morphine and other opioids to relieve pain is discussed further in this chapter and in Chapter 29.

Mechanism of Analgesic Action. Morphine and other opioid agonists appear to relieve pain by mimicking the actions of endogenous opioid peptides, primarily at mu receptors. This hypothesis is based on the following observations:

- Opioid peptides and morphine-like drugs both produce analgesia when administered to experimental subjects.
- Opioid peptides and morphine-like drugs share structural similarities.
- Opioid peptides and morphine-like drugs bind to the same receptors in the CNS.
- The receptors to which opioid peptides and morphine-like drugs bind are located in regions of the brain and spinal cord associated with perception of pain.
- Subjects rendered tolerant to analgesia from morphine-like drugs show cross-tolerance to analgesia from opioid peptides.
- The analgesic effects of opioid peptides and morphine-like drugs can both be blocked by the same antagonist: naloxone.

From these data we can postulate that (1) opioid peptides serve a physiologic role as modulators of pain perception and (2) morphine-like drugs produce analgesia by mimicking the actions of endogenous opioid peptides.

Adverse Effects

Respiratory Depression. Respiratory depression is the most serious adverse effect. At equianalgesic doses, all of the pure opioid agonists depress respiration to the same extent. Death following overdose is almost always from respiratory arrest. Opioids depress respiration primarily through activation of mu receptors, although activation of kappa receptors also contributes.

The time course of respiratory depression varies with route of administration. Depressant effects begin about 7 minutes after IV injection, 30 minutes after IM injection, and up to 90 minutes after subQ injection. With all three routes, significant depression may persist for 4 to 5 hours. When morphine is administered by spinal injection, onset of respiratory depression may be delayed for hours; be alert to this possibility.

With prolonged use of opioids, tolerance develops to respiratory depression. Huge doses that would be lethal to a nontolerant individual have been taken by opioid addicts without noticeable effect. Similarly, tolerance to respiratory depression develops during long-term clinical use of opioids (e.g., in patients with cancer).

When administered at usual therapeutic doses, opioids rarely cause significant respiratory depression. However, although uncommon, substantial respiratory depression can nonetheless occur. Accordingly, respiratory rate should be determined before opioid administration. If the rate is less than 12 breaths per minute, the opioid should be withheld and the prescriber notified. Certain patients, including the very young, older adults, and those with respiratory disease (e.g., asthma, emphysema), are especially sensitive to respiratory depression, and hence must be monitored closely. Outpatients should be informed about the risk of respiratory depression and instructed to notify the prescriber if respiratory distress occurs.

Respiratory depression is increased by concurrent use of other drugs with CNS-depressant actions (e.g., alcohol, barbiturates, benzodiazepines). Accordingly, these drugs should be avoided. Outpatients should be warned against the use of alcohol and all other CNS depressants.

Pronounced respiratory depression can be reversed with naloxone [Narcan], an opioid antagonist. However, dosing must be carefully titrated, because excessive doses will completely block the analgesic effects of morphine, causing pain to return.

Safety Alert

RESPIRATORY ARREST

Opioid medications can cause respiratory arrest in both opioid-naïve and opioid-tolerant patients. Monitor level of consciousness, respiratory rate, and oxygen saturation in patients receiving opioid medications. When administering opioids, assess initial vital signs and withhold medication and notify the provider if the patient has a decreased level of consciousness or respiratory rate less than 12 breaths per minute.

Constipation. Opioids promote constipation through actions in the CNS and gastrointestinal (GI) tract. Specifically, by activating mu receptors in the gut, these drugs can suppress propulsive intestinal contractions, intensify nonpropulsive contractions, increase the tone of the anal sphincter, and inhibit secretion of fluids into the intestinal lumen. As a result, constipation can develop after a few days of opioid use. Potential complications of constipation include fecal impaction, bowel perforation, rectal tearing, and hemorrhoids.

Opioid-induced constipation can be managed with a combination of pharmacologic and nonpharmacologic measures. The goal is to produce a soft, formed stool every 1 to 2 days. Principal nondrug measures are physical activity and increased intake of fiber and fluids (for prevention) and enemas (for treatment). Most patients also require *prophylactic drugs:* A stimulant laxative, such as senna, is given to counteract reduced bowel motility; a stool softener, such as docusate [Colace], plus polyethylene glycol (an osmotic laxative) can provide additional benefit. If these prophylactic drugs prove inadequate, the patient may need *rescue therapy* with a strong osmotic laxative, such as lactulose or sodium phosphate. As a last resort, patients may be given *methylnaltrexone* [Relistor], an oral drug that blocks mu receptors in the intestine. As discussed later in the chapter, methylnaltrexone can't cross the blood-brain barrier, and hence does not reverse opioid-induced analgesia.

Because of their effects on the intestine, opioids are highly effective for treating diarrhea. In fact, antidiarrheal use of these drugs preceded analgesic use by centuries. The impact of opioids on intestinal function is an interesting example of how an effect can be detrimental (constipation) or beneficial (relief of diarrhea), depending on who is taking the medication. Opioids employed specifically to treat diarrhea are discussed in Chapter 80.

Orthostatic Hypotension. Morphine-like drugs lower blood pressure by blunting the baroreceptor reflex and by dilating peripheral arterioles and veins. Peripheral vasodilation results primarily from morphine-induced release of histamine. Hypotension is mild in the recumbent patient but can be significant when the patient stands up. Patients should be informed about symptoms of hypotension (light-headedness, dizziness) and instructed to sit or lie down if they occur. Also, patients should be informed that hypotension can be minimized by moving slowly when changing from a supine or seated position to an upright position. Patients should be warned against walking if hypotension is substantial. Hospitalized patients may require ambulatory assistance. Hypotensive drugs can exacerbate opioid-induced hypotension.

Urinary Retention. Morphine can cause urinary hesitancy and urinary retention. Three mechanisms are involved. First, morphine increases tone in the bladder sphincter. Second, morphine increases tone in the detrusor muscle, thereby elevating pressure within the bladder, causing a sense of urinary urgency. Third, in addition to its direct effects on the urinary tract, morphine may interfere with voiding by suppressing awareness of bladder stimuli. To reduce discomfort, patients should be encouraged to void every 4 hours. Urinary hesitancy or retention is especially likely in patients with benign prostatic hypertrophy. Drugs with anticholinergic properties (e.g., tricyclic antidepressants, antihistamines) can exacerbate the problem.

Urinary retention should be assessed by monitoring intake and output and by palpating the lower abdomen every 4 to 6 hours for bladder distention. If a change in intake/output ratio develops or if bladder distention is detected or if the patient reports difficulty voiding, the prescriber should be notified. Catheterization may be required.

In addition to causing urinary retention, morphine may decrease urine production largely by decreasing renal blood flow and partly by promoting release of antidiuretic hormone.

Cough Suppression. Morphine-like drugs act at opioid receptors in the medulla to suppress cough. Suppression of spontaneous cough may lead to accumulation of secretions in the airway. Accordingly, patients should be instructed to actively cough at regular intervals. Lung status should be assessed by auscultation for crackles. The ability of opioids to suppress cough is put to clinical use in the form of codeine- and hydrocodone-based cough remedies.

Biliary Colic. Opioids can induce spasm of the common bile duct, causing pressure within the biliary tract to rise dramatically. Symptoms range from epigastric distress to biliary colic. In patients with pre-existing biliary colic, opioids, especially morphine, may intensify pain rather than relieve pain. Nevertheless, it is important to treat pain and not withhold opioids for treatment of severe pain. Certain opioids (e.g., meperidine) cause less smooth muscle spasm than morphine, and hence are less likely to exacerbate biliary colic.

Emesis. Morphine promotes nausea and vomiting through direct stimulation of the chemoreceptor trigger zone of the medulla. Emetic reactions are greatest with the initial dose and then diminish with subsequent doses. Nausea and vomiting are uncommon in recumbent patients, but occur in 15% to 40% of ambulatory patients, suggesting a vestibular component. Nausea and vomiting can be reduced by pretreatment with an antiemetic (e.g., prochlorperazine) and by having the patient remain still.

Elevation of Intracranial Pressure. Morphine can elevate intracranial pressure (ICP). The mechanism is indirect: By suppressing respiration, morphine increases the CO_2 content of blood, which dilates the cerebral vasculature, causing ICP to rise. Accordingly, if respiration is maintained at a normal rate, ICP will remain normal too.

Euphoria/Dysphoria. *Euphoria* is defined as an exaggerated sense of well-being. Morphine often produces euphoria when given to patients in pain. Although euphoria can enhance pain relief, it also contributes to the drug's potential for abuse. Euphoria is caused by activation of mu receptors.

In some individuals, morphine causes *dysphoria* (a sense of anxiety and unease). Dysphoria is uncommon among patients in pain, but may occur when morphine is taken in the absence of pain.

Sedation. When administered to relieve pain, morphine is likely to cause drowsiness and some mental clouding. Although these effects can complement analgesic actions, they can also be detrimental. Outpatients should be warned about CNS depression and advised to avoid hazardous activities (e.g., driving) if sedation is significant. Sedation can be minimized by (1) taking smaller doses more often, (2) using opioids that have short half-lives, and (3) giving small doses of a CNS stimulant (methylphenidate or dextroamphetamine) in the morning and early afternoon. A nonamphetamine stimulant—modafinil [Provigil, Alertec 🍁] or armodafinil [Nuvigil]—may also be tried.

Miosis. Morphine and other opioids cause pupillary constriction (miosis). In response to toxic doses, the pupils may constrict to "pinpoint" size. Because miosis can impair vision in dim light, room light should be kept bright during waking hours.

Birth Defects. Morphine and other opioids increase the risk of serious birth defects by two- to threefold, although the absolute risk remains low. The Centers for Disease Control and Prevention (CDC) released preliminary data showing that when opioids are taken just before conception or during early pregnancy, they increase the risk of congenital heart defects, including atrioventricular septal defects, hypoplastic left heart syndrome, and conoventricular septal defects. In addition, opioids increase the risk of spina bifida and gastroschisis (protrusion of the intestine through the abdominal wall near the umbilicus). Clearly, opioids should be avoided before and during pregnancy.

Neurotoxicity. Opioid-induced neurotoxicity can cause delirium, agitation, myoclonus, hyperalgesia, and other symptoms. Primary risk factors are renal impairment, pre-existing cognitive impairment, and prolonged high-dose opioid use. Management consists of hydration and dose reduction. For patients who must take opioids long term, opioid rotation (periodically switching from one opioid to another) may reduce neurotoxicity development.

Adverse Effects From Prolonged Use. Clinical and preclinical studies indicate that prolonged use of opioids can cause hormonal changes and can alter immune function. Hormonal changes include a progressive decline in cortisol levels, an increase in prolactin levels, and a decrease in levels of luteinizing hormone, follicle-stimulating hormone, testosterone, and estrogen. With prolonged opioid exposure, immune function is suppressed. Are these changes clinically relevant? Because there is lack of adequately designed controlled clinical trials, we don't really know.

Pharmacokinetics

To relieve pain, morphine must cross the blood-brain barrier and enter the CNS. Because the drug has poor lipid solubility, it does not cross the barrier easily. Consequently, only a small fraction of each dose reaches sites of analgesic action. Because the blood-brain barrier is not well developed in infants, these patients generally require lower doses than do older children and adults.

Morphine is inactivated by hepatic metabolism. When taken by mouth, the drug must pass through the liver on its way to the systemic circulation. Much of an oral dose is inactivated during this first pass through the liver. Consequently, oral doses need to be substantially larger than parenteral doses to achieve equivalent analgesic effects. In patients with liver disease, analgesia and other effects may be intensified and prolonged. Accordingly, it may be necessary to reduce the dosage or lengthen the dosing interval.

Tolerance and Physical Dependence

With continuous use, morphine can cause tolerance and physical dependence. These phenomena, which are generally inseparable, reflect cellular adaptations that occur in response to prolonged opioid exposure.

Tolerance. Tolerance can be defined as a state in which a larger dose is required to produce the same response that could formerly be produced with a smaller dose. Alternatively, tolerance can be defined as a condition in which a particular dose now produces a smaller response than it did when treatment began. Because of tolerance, dosage must be increased to maintain analgesic effects.

Tolerance develops to many—but not all—of morphine's actions. With prolonged treatment, tolerance develops to *analgesia, euphoria,* and *sedation.* As a result, with long-term therapy, an increase in dosage may be required to maintain these desirable effects. Fortunately, as tolerance develops to these therapeutic effects, tolerance also develops to *respiratory depression.* As a result, the high doses needed to control pain in the tolerant individual are not associated with increased respiratory depression.

Very little tolerance develops to *constipation* and *miosis.* Even in highly tolerant users, constipation remains a chronic problem, and constricted pupils are characteristic.

Cross-tolerance exists among the opioid agonists (e.g., oxycodone, methadone, fentanyl, codeine, heroin). Accordingly, individuals tolerant to one of these agents will be tolerant to all the others. No cross-tolerance exists between opioids and general CNS depressants (e.g., barbiturates, ethanol, benzodiazepines, general anesthetics).

Physical Dependence. Physical dependence is defined as a state in which an abstinence syndrome will occur if drug use is abruptly stopped. Opioid dependence results from adaptive cellular changes that occur in response to the continuous presence of these drugs. Although the exact nature of these changes is unknown, it is clear that once these compensatory changes have taken place, the body requires the continued presence of opioids to function normally. If opioids are withdrawn, an abstinence syndrome usually will follow.

The intensity and duration of the opioid abstinence syndrome depends on two factors: the half-life of the drug being used and the degree of physical dependence. With opioids that have relatively short half-lives (e.g., morphine), symptoms of abstinence are intense but brief. In contrast, with opioids that have long half-lives (e.g., methadone), symptoms are less intense but more prolonged. With any opioid, the intensity of withdrawal symptoms parallels the degree of physical dependence.

For individuals who are highly dependent, the abstinence syndrome can be extremely unpleasant. Initial reactions include yawning, rhinorrhea, and sweating. Onset occurs about 10 hours after the final dose. These early responses are followed by anorexia, irritability, tremor, and "gooseflesh"—hence the term *cold turkey.* At its peak, the syndrome manifests as violent sneezing, weakness, nausea, vomiting, diarrhea, abdominal cramps, bone and muscle pain, muscle spasm, and kicking movements—hence, "kicking the habit." Giving an opioid at any time during withdrawal rapidly reverses all signs and symptoms. Left untreated, the morphine withdrawal syndrome runs its course in 7 to 10 days. It should be emphasized that, although withdrawal from opioids is unpleasant, the syndrome is rarely dangerous. In contrast, withdrawal from general CNS depressants (e.g., barbiturates, alcohol) can be lethal (see Chapter 34).

To minimize the abstinence syndrome, opioids should be withdrawn gradually. When the degree of dependence is moderate, symptoms can be avoided by administering progressively smaller doses over 3 days. When the patient is highly dependent, dosage should be tapered more slowly—over 7 to 10 days. With a proper withdrawal schedule, withdrawal symptoms will resemble those of a mild case of flu—even when the degree of dependence is high.

It is important to note that physical dependence is rarely a complication when opioids are taken *acutely* to treat pain. Hospitalized patients receiving morphine 2 to 3 times a day for up to 2 weeks show no significant signs of dependence. If morphine is withheld from these patients, no significant signs of withdrawal can be detected. The issue of physical dependence as a clinical concern is discussed further later in the chapter.

Infants exposed to opioids *in utero* may be born drug dependent. If the infant is not provided with opioids, an abstinence syndrome will ensue. Signs of withdrawal include excessive crying, sneezing, tremor, hyperreflexia, fever, and diarrhea. The infant can be treated for opioid dependence by administering opiates in progressively smaller doses.

Cross-dependence exists among pure opioid agonists. As a result, any pure agonist will prevent withdrawal in a patient who is physically dependent on any other pure agonist.

Abuse Liability

Morphine and the other opioids are subject to abuse, largely because of their ability to cause pleasurable experiences (e.g., euphoria, sedation, a sensation in the lower abdomen resembling orgasm). Physical dependence contributes to abuse: Once dependence exists, the ability of opioids to ward off withdrawal serves to reinforce their desirability in the mind of the abuser.

The abuse liability of the opioids is reflected in their classification under the Controlled Substances Act. (The provisions of this act are discussed in Chapter 37.) As shown in Table 28.3, morphine and all other strong opioid agonists are classified under Schedule II. This classification reflects a moderate to high abuse liability. The agonist-antagonist opioids have a lower abuse liability and hence are classified under Schedule IV (butorphanol, pentazocine) or Schedule III (buprenorphine), or have no classification at all (nalbuphine). Healthcare personnel who prescribe, dispense, and administer opioids must adhere to the procedures set forth in the Controlled Substances Act.

Fortunately, abuse is rare when opioids are employed to treat pain. The issue of abuse as a clinical concern is addressed in depth later in the chapter.

Precautions

Some patients are more likely than others to experience adverse effects. Common sense dictates that opioids be used with special caution in these people. Conditions that can predispose patients to adverse reactions are discussed in the sections that follow.

Decreased Respiratory Reserve. Because morphine depresses respiration, it can further compromise respiration in patients with impaired pulmonary function. Accordingly, the drug should be used with caution in patients with asthma, emphysema, kyphoscoliosis, chronic cor pulmonale, and extreme obesity. Caution is also needed in patients taking other drugs that can depress respiration (e.g., barbiturates, benzodiazepines, general anesthetics).

Labor and Delivery. Use of morphine during delivery can suppress uterine contractions and cause respiratory depression in the neonate. Following delivery, respiration in the neonate should be monitored closely. Respiratory depression can be reversed with naloxone. The use of opioids in obstetrics is discussed in depth later in the chapter.

Head Injury. Morphine and other opioids must be used with caution in patients with head injury. Head injury can cause respiratory depression accompanied by elevation of ICP. Morphine can exacerbate these symptoms. In addition, because miosis, mental clouding, and vomiting can be valuable diagnostic signs following head injury and because morphine can cause these same effects, the use of opioids can confound diagnosis.

Other Precautions. *Infants* and *older adult patients* are especially sensitive to morphine-induced respiratory depression. In patients with *inflammatory bowel disease,* morphine may cause toxic megacolon or paralytic ileus. Because morphine and all other opioids are inactivated by liver enzymes, effects may be intensified and prolonged in patients with *liver impairment.* Doses should also be monitored closely and decreased in patients with renal impairment, as morphine metabolites are largely excreted by the kidneys. Severe hypotension may occur in patients with pre-existing *hypotension* or *reduced blood volume.* In patients with *benign prostatic hypertrophy,* opioids may cause acute urinary retention; repeated catheterization may be required.

Drug Interactions

The major interactions between morphine and other drugs are shown in Table 28.4. Some interactions are adverse, and some are beneficial.

CNS Depressants. All drugs with CNS-depressant actions (e.g., barbiturates, benzodiazepines, alcohol) can intensify sedation and respiratory depression caused by morphine and other opioids. Outpatients should be warned against the use of alcohol and all other CNS depressants.

Anticholinergic Drugs. These agents (e.g., antihistamines, tricyclic antidepressants, atropine-like drugs) can exacerbate morphine-induced constipation and urinary retention.

Hypotensive Drugs. Antihypertensive drugs and other drugs that lower blood pressure can exacerbate morphine-induced hypotension.

Monoamine Oxidase Inhibitors. The combination of meperidine (a morphine-like drug) with a monoamine oxidase inhibitor (MAOI) has produced a syndrome characterized by excitation, delirium, hyperpyrexia, convulsions, and severe respiratory depression. Deaths have occurred. Although this

TABLE 28.4 ■ Interactions of Morphine-Like Drugs With Other Drugs

Interacting Drugs	Outcome of the Interaction
ADVERSE INTERACTIONS	
CNS depressants Barbiturates Benzodiazepines Alcohol General anesthetics Antihistamines Phenothiazines	Increased respiratory depression and sedation
Agonist-antagonist opioids	Precipitation of a withdrawal reaction
Anticholinergic drugs Atropine-like drugs Antihistamines Phenothiazines Tricyclic antidepressants	Increased constipation and urinary retention
Hypotensive agents	Increased hypotension
Monoamine oxidase inhibitors	Hyperpyrexic coma
BENEFICIAL INTERACTIONS	
Amphetamines	Increased analgesia and decreased sedation
Antiemetics	Suppression of nausea and vomiting
Naloxone	Suppression of symptoms of opioid overdose
Dextromethorphan	Increased analgesia; possible reduction in tolerance

reaction has not been reported with combined use of an MAOI and morphine, prudence suggests that practitioners employ caution when combining the two.

Agonist-Antagonist Opioids. Agonist-antagonist opioids (e.g., pentazocine, buprenorphine) can precipitate a withdrawal syndrome if given to an individual physically dependent on a pure opioid agonist. The basis of this reaction is considered later in the chapter. Patients taking pure opioid agonists should be weaned from these drugs before beginning treatment with an agonist-antagonist.

Opioid Antagonists. Opioid antagonists (e.g., naloxone) can counteract most actions of morphine and other pure opioid agonists. Opioid antagonists are employed primarily to treat opioid overdose. The actions and uses of the opioid antagonists are discussed in detail later in the chapter.

Other Interactions. *Antiemetics* of the phenothiazine type (e.g., promethazine [Phenergan]) may be combined with opioids to reduce nausea and vomiting. *Amphetamines, clonidine,* and *dextromethorphan* can enhance opioid-induced analgesia. *Amphetamines* can also offset sedation.

Toxicity

Clinical Manifestations. Opioid overdose produces a classic triad of signs: *coma, respiratory depression,* and *pinpoint pupils.* Coma is profound, and the patient cannot be aroused. Respiratory rate may be as low as 2 to 4 breaths per minute. Although the pupils are constricted initially, they may dilate as hypoxia sets in (secondary to respiratory depression). Hypoxia may cause blood pressure to fall. Prolonged hypoxia may result in shock. When death occurs, respiratory arrest is almost always the immediate cause.

Treatment. Treatment consists primarily of *ventilatory support* and giving an *opioid antagonist.* Naloxone [Narcan] is the traditional antagonist of choice. The pharmacology of the opioid antagonists is discussed later.

Preparations

Morphine Alone. Morphine sulfate, by itself, is available in 9 formulations:

- IR tablets (15 and 30 mg)
- ER tablets (15, 20, 30, 50, 60, 80, 100, and 200 mg) sold as *MS Contin*
- ER capsules (10, 20, 30, 40, 45, 50, 60, 70, 75, 80, 90, 100, 120, 130, 150, and 200 mg) sold as *Kadian, Avinza,* and *M-Eslon* 🍁
- Standard oral solution (10 and 20 mg/5 mL)
- Concentrated oral solution (100 mg/5 mL)
- Rectal suppositories (5, 20, and 30 mg)
- Intramuscular solution for auto-injection (10 mg/0.7 mL)
- Standard solution for injection (0.5, 1, 2, 4, 5, 8, 10, 15, 25, and 50 mg/mL) sold as *Astramorph PF, Duramorph,* and *Infumorph*
- ER liposomal solution for injection (10 mg/mL) sold as *DepoDur*

Morphine/Naltrexone [Embeda]. Embeda contains a fixed-dose combination of morphine and naltrexone, an opioid antagonist. The product is designed to discourage morphine abuse. Embeda capsules are filled with tiny pellets that have an outer layer of ER morphine and an inner core of naltrexone. When the capsules are swallowed intact, only the morphine is absorbed. However, if the pellets are crushed, the naltrexone will be absorbed too, thereby blunting the effects of the morphine. As a result, potential abusers cannot get a quick high by crushing the pellets to release all of the morphine at once. However, abusers can still get high by simply taking a large dose. Embeda capsules are more expensive than other ER morphine products and should be prescribed only when abuse appears likely.

Alcohol can accelerate the release of morphine from Embeda pellets. As a result, the entire dose can be absorbed quickly—rather than over 24 hours—thereby causing a potentially fatal spike in morphine blood levels. Accordingly, patients should be warned against alcohol consumption.

Embeda capsules are available in six morphine/naltrexone strengths: 20 mg/0.8 mg, 30 mg/1.2 mg, 50 mg/2 mg, 60 mg/2.4 mg, 80 mg/3.2 mg, and 100 mg/4 mg. Dosing is done once or twice daily. Patients can swallow Embeda capsules whole, or they can open the capsules and sprinkle the pellets on applesauce, which must be ingested without chewing.

Dosage and Administration

General Guidelines. Dosage must be individualized. High doses are required for patients with a low tolerance to pain or with extremely painful disorders. Patients with sharp, stabbing pain need higher doses than patients with dull pain. Older adults generally require lower doses than younger adults. Neonates require relatively low doses because their blood-brain barrier is not fully developed. For all patients, dosage should be reduced as pain subsides. Outpatients should be warned not to increase dosage without consulting the prescriber.

Before an opioid is administered, respiratory rate, blood pressure, and pulse rate should be determined. The drug should be withheld and the prescriber notified if respiratory rate is below 12 breaths per minute, if blood pressure is significantly below the pretreatment value, or if pulse rate is significantly above or below the pretreatment value.

Routes and Dosages

Oral. Oral dosing is generally reserved for patients with chronic severe pain, such as that associated with cancer. Because oral morphine undergoes extensive metabolism on its first pass through the liver, oral doses are usually higher than parenteral doses. A typical dosage is 10 to 30 mg repeated every 4 hours as needed. However, oral dosing is highly individualized, and some patients may require 75 mg or more. Controlled-release formulations may be administered every 8 to 12 hours, and the ER formulation [Avinza] is given every 24 hours. Patients should be instructed to swallow these products intact, without crushing or chewing. Also, *warn patients using Avinza or Embeda capsules not to drink alcohol,* which can accelerate the release of morphine from these products.

Intramuscular and Subcutaneous. Both routes are painful and unreliable and should generally be avoided. For adults, dosing is initiated at 5 to 10 mg every 4 hours and then adjusted up or down as needed. The usual dosage for children is 0.1 to 0.2 mg/kg repeated every 4 hours as needed.

Intravenous. Intravenous morphine should be injected slowly (over 4 to 5 minutes). Rapid IV injection can cause severe adverse effects (profound hypotension, cardiac arrest, respiratory arrest) and should be avoided. When IV injections are made, an opioid antagonist (e.g., naloxone) and facilities for respiratory support should be available. Injections should be given with the patient lying down to minimize hypotension. The usual dose for adults is 4 to 10 mg (diluted in 4 to 5 mL of sterile water for injection). The usual pediatric dose is 0.05 to 0.1 mg/kg.

Epidural and Intrathecal. When morphine is employed for spinal analgesia, epidural injection is preferred to intrathecal. With either route, onset of analgesia is rapid and the duration prolonged (up to 24 hours). The most troubling side effects are delayed respiratory depression and delayed cardiac depression. Be alert for possible late reactions. The usual adult epidural dose is 5 mg. Intrathecal doses are much smaller—about one-tenth the epidural dose.

The *extended-release liposomal formulation* [DepoDur], used only for postsurgical pain, is intended for *epidural use only.* Inadvertent intrathecal and subarachnoid administration has been associated with profound and prolonged respiratory depression, which can be managed with a naloxone infusion. Dosing is highly individualized and must account for age, body mass, physical status, history of opioid use, risk factors for respiratory depression, and medications to be coadministered before and during surgery.

Other Strong Opioid Agonists

In an effort to produce a strong analgesic with a low potential for respiratory depression and abuse, pharmaceutical scientists have created many new opioid analgesics. However, none of the newer pure opioid agonists can be considered truly superior to morphine: These drugs are essentially equal to morphine with respect to analgesic action, abuse liability, and the ability to cause respiratory depression. Also, to varying degrees, they all cause sedation, euphoria, constipation, urinary retention, cough suppression, hypotension, and miosis. However, despite their similarities to morphine, the newer drugs do have unique qualities. Hence one agent may be more desirable than another in a particular clinical setting. With all of the newer pure opioid agonists, toxicity can be reversed with an opioid antagonist (e.g., naloxone). Important differences between morphine and the newer strong opioid analgesics are discussed in the following sections. Table 28.5 shows dosages, routes, and time courses for morphine and the newer agents.

Fentanyl

Fentanyl [Duragesic, Abstral, Actiq, Fentora, Ionsys, Lazanda, Subsys] is a strong opioid analgesic with a high milligram potency (about 100 times that of morphine). Seven formulations are available, for administration by four different routes: parenteral, transdermal, transmucosal, and intranasal. Depending on the route, fentanyl may be used for surgical analgesia, chronic pain control, and control of breakthrough pain in patients taking other opioids. All preparations are regulated under Schedule II of the Controlled Substances Act.

Fentanyl, regardless of route, has the same adverse effects as other opioids: respiratory depression, sedation, constipation, urinary retention, and nausea. Of these, respiratory depression is the greatest concern. Signs of toxicity can be reversed with an opioid antagonist (e.g., naloxone).

Fentanyl is metabolized by CYP3A4 (the 3A4 isoenzyme of cytochrome P450), and hence fentanyl levels can be increased by CYP3A4 inhibitors (e.g., ritonavir, ketoconazole). Patients taking these inhibitors should be closely monitored for severe respiratory depression and other signs of toxicity.

Parenteral. Parenteral fentanyl [generic], administered IM or IV, is employed primarily for induction and maintenance of surgical anesthesia. The drug is well suited for these applications owing to its rapid onset and short duration. Most effects are like those of morphine. In addition, fentanyl can cause muscle rigidity, which can interfere with induction of anesthesia. As discussed in Chapter 27, the combination of fentanyl plus droperidol is used to produce a state known as "neuroleptanalgesia."

Transdermal System. The fentanyl transdermal system [Duragesic] consists of a fentanyl-containing patch that is applied to the skin of the upper torso. The drug is slowly released from the patch and absorbed through the skin, reaching effective levels in 24 hours. Levels remain steady for another 48 hours, after which the patch should be replaced. If a new patch is not applied, effects will nonetheless persist for several hours, owing to continued absorption of residual fentanyl remaining in the skin.

Transdermal fentanyl is indicated only for persistent severe pain in patients who are already opioid tolerant. Use in nontolerant patients can cause fatal respiratory depression. The patch should not be used in children younger than 2 years or in anyone younger than 18 years who weighs less than 110 pounds. Also, the patch should not be used for postoperative pain, intermittent pain, or pain that responds to a less powerful analgesic.

Like other strong opioids, fentanyl overdose poses a risk of fatal respiratory depression. If respiratory depression develops, it may persist for hours following patch removal, owing to continued absorption of fentanyl from the skin.

Fentanyl patches are available in five strengths, which deliver fentanyl to the systemic circulation at rates of 12.5, 25, 50, 75, and 100 mcg/hr. The smallest effective patch should be used. If a dosage greater than 100 mcg/hr is required, a combination of patches can be applied. Once the patch is in place, it must not be exposed to direct heat (e.g., heating pads, hot baths, electric blankets), because doing so can accelerate fentanyl release, as can fever, sunbathing, and strenuous exercise. Because full analgesic effects can take up to 24 hours to develop, PRN therapy with a short-acting opioid may be required until the patch takes effect. As with other long-acting opioids, if breakthrough pain occurs, supplemental dosing with a short-acting opioid is indicated. For the majority of patients, patches can be replaced every 72 hours, although some may require a new patch in 48 hours. Used or damaged patches should be folded in half with the medication side touching and flushed down the toilet. Unused patches should be stored out of reach of children.

Transdermal Iontophoretic System. The transdermal iontophoretic system [Ionsys]—a self-contained credit card–sized device—is the first needle-free patient-activated system for on-demand delivery of analgesia. The device, which is applied to the skin, delivers fentanyl by iontophoresis, a process in which a low-intensity electrical field (generally imperceptible to the patient) drives the drug across the skin and into the systemic circulation. Ionsys is approved only for acute management of postoperative pain in hospitalized adult patients and should be removed before discharge. Pain control is equivalent to that achieved with an IV patient-controlled analgesia pump.

TABLE 28.5 ▪ Clinical Pharmacology and Pharmacokinetics of Pure Opioid Agonists

Drug and Route[a]	Equianalgesic Dose (mg)[b]	Time Course of Analgesic Effects			Metabolism	Excretion
		Onset (min)	Peak (min)	Duration (hr)		
Codeine					Hepatic CYP450[c]: 2D6	Renal
PO	200	30–45	60–120	4–6		
Fentanyl					Hepatic CYP450[c]: 3A4	Renal
IM	0.1	7–8	—	1–2		
IV	0.1	—	—	0.5–1		
Transdermal	—	Delayed	24–72	72		
Transmucosal[d]	—	10–15	20	1–2		
Nasal spray	—	10–15	15–20	1–2		
Hydrocodone					Hepatic CYP450[c]: 3A4, 2B6, 2D6	Renal
PO (IR)	30	10–30	30–60	4–6		
PO (ER)	30	—	360–600	14–16		
Hydromorphone					Hepatic	Renal, gastrointestinal (bile)
PO (IR)	7.5	30	90–120	4		
PO (ER)	7.5	—	360–480	18–24		
IM	1.5	15	30–60	4–5		
IV	1.5	10–15	15–30	2–3		
subQ	1.5	15	30–90	4		
Levorphanol					Hepatic	Renal
PO	4	10–60	90–120	6–8		
IM	2	—	60	6–8		
IV	2	—	Within 20	6–8		
subQ	2	—	60–90	6–8		
Meperidine					Hepatic: CYP450[c]: 2B6	Renal
PO	300	15	60–90	2–4		
IM	75	10–15	30–50	2–4		
IV	75	1	5–7	2–4		
subQ	75	10–15	30–50	2–4		
Methadone					Hepatic CYP450[c]: 2B6, 3A4	Gastrointestinal (feces), renal
PO	20	30–60	90–120	4–6[e]		
IM	10	10–20	60–120	4–5[e]		
IV	10	—	15–30	3–4[e]		
Morphine					Hepatic, gastrointestinal	Gastrointestinal (feces), renal
PO (IR)	30	—	60–120	4–5		
PO (ER)	30	—	420	8–12		
IM	10	10–30	30–60	4–5		
IV	10	—	20	4–5		
subQ	10	10–30	50–90	4–5		
Epidural	—	15–60	—	Up to 24		
Intrathecal	—	15–60	—	Up to 24		
Oxycodone					Hepatic CYP450[c]: 3A4, 2D6	Renal
PO (IR)	20	15–30	60	3–4		
PO (ER)	20	—	120–180	Up to 12		
Oxymorphone					Hepatic	Gastrointestinal (feces), renal
PO (IR)	10	—	—	4–6		
PO (ER)	10	—	—	Up to 12		
IM	1	10–15	30–90	3–6		
IV	1	5–10	15–30	3–4		
subQ	1	10–20	—	3–6		
Rectal	10	15–30	120	3–6		
Tapentadol					Hepatic CYP450[c]: 2C9/19	Renal
PO	100	45–60	90–120	4–8		

[a]IM administration should be avoided whenever possible.
[b]Dose in milligrams that produces a degree of analgesia equivalent to that produced by a 10-mg IM dose of morphine.
[c]CYP450: Cytochrome P450–enzyme specific.
[d]Data are for the Actiq lozenge on a stick.
[e]With repeated doses, methadone's duration of action may increase up to 48 hours.
ER, Extended release; *IR,* immediate release.

Ionsys consists of a plastic case that houses a 3-volt battery, electronic control, and a reservoir containing 10.8 mg of fentanyl hydrochloride. The upper surface of the device has a recessed dosing button and a light; the lower surface has adhesive to hold the device to the skin. When pain relief is needed, the patient presses the dosing button twice within 3 seconds, causing delivery of a 40-mcg dose over a 10-minute interval. A green light blinks continuously while delivery takes place. One Ionsys device can be used for 24 hours or delivery of 80 doses, whichever comes first. Ionsys should be applied to intact nonirritated, nonirradiated skin of the chest or outer upper arm. Excessive hair should be removed by clipping, not shaving. All patients should be titrated to comfort with an appropriate analgesic before Ionsys is employed.

Transmucosal. Fentanyl for transmucosal administration is available in four formulations: lozenges on a stick [Actiq], buccal tablets [Fentora], sublingual spray [Subsys], and sublingual tablets [Abstral]. All five products are approved only for *breakthrough cancer pain in patients at least 18 years old who are already taking opioids around-the-clock and have developed some degree of tolerance,* defined as needing, for 1 week or longer, at least: 60 mg of oral morphine a day, or 30 mg of oral oxycodone a day, or 25 mg of oral oxymorphone a day, or 8 mg of oral hydromorphone a day, or 25 mcg of fentanyl per hour, or an equianalgesic dose of another opioid. Transmucosal fentanyl must not be used for acute pain, postoperative pain, headache, or athletic injuries. Furthermore, it is essential to appreciate that the dose of fentanyl in these formulations is sufficient to kill nontolerant individuals, especially children. Accordingly, these products must be stored in a secure, child-resistant location.

All fentanyl transmucosal formulations are regulated as Schedule II products. Owing to risks of misuse, abuse, and overdose, all transmucosal fentanyl products are available only through a restricted distribution program, called the TIRF REMS (Transmucosal Immediate Release Fentanyl Risk Evaluation and Mitigation Strategy) Access program. The patient must enroll in this program to receive these products, and they are available only through pharmacies enrolled in the TIRF REMS program.

Adverse effects of transmucosal fentanyl are like those of other opioid preparations. The most common are dizziness, anxiety, confusion, nausea, vomiting, constipation, dyspnea, weakness, and headache. The biggest concerns are respiratory depression and shock.

Because of differences in bioavailability, *transmucosal fentanyl products are not interchangeable on a microgram-for-microgram basis.* For example, a 100-mcg buccal tablet produces about the same fentanyl blood level as does a 200-mcg lozenge. Accordingly, if a patient switches from one transmucosal product to another, dosage of the new product must be titrated to determine a strength that is safe and effective.

Lozenge on a Stick. The fentanyl lozenge on a stick [Actiq]—also known as oral transmucosal fentanyl citrate (OTFC)—consists of a raspberry-flavored lozenge on a plastic handle and looks much like a lollipop. Six strengths are available: 200, 400, 600, 800, 1200, and 1600 mcg.

To administer the unit, patients place it between the cheek and the lower gum and actively suck it. Periodically, the unit should be moved from one side of the mouth to the other. Consumption of the entire lozenge should take 15 minutes. As the patient sucks, some of the drug is absorbed directly and rapidly through the oral mucosa, and some is swallowed and absorbed slowly from the GI tract. Analgesia begins in 10 to 15 minutes, peaks in 20 minutes, and persists 1 to 2 hours.

Dosing should begin with a 200-mcg unit. If breakthrough pain persists, the patient can take another 200-mcg unit 15 minutes after finishing the first one (i.e., 30 minutes after starting the first). Unit size should be gradually increased until an effective dose is determined. If the patient needs more than 4 units/day, it may be time to give a higher dose of his or her long-acting opioid.

To promote safe and effective use of the Actiq system, the manufacturer provides an Actiq Welcome Kit as well as a Child Safety Kit with the initial drug supply. The kit contains educational materials and safe storage containers for unused, partially used, and completely used units.

Buccal Tablets. Fentanyl buccal tablets [Fentora] are available in five strengths: 100, 200, 400, 600, and 800 mcg. Patients should place the tablet above a rear molar between the cheek and the gum and let it dissolve in place, usually in 15 to 30 minutes. Remaining fragments should be swallowed with a glass of water. Patients should not split, chew, suck, or swallow the tablets. The initial dose is 100 mcg. If 100 mcg is inadequate, another 100 mcg can be taken in 30 minutes. During each subsequent episode, dosage may be gradually increased, if needed, until an effective dose is established.

Sublingual Spray. Fentanyl sublingual spray [Subsys] is available in doses of 100, 200, 400, 600, 800, 1200, and 1600 mcg/spray. Individual doses of Subsys are supplied in single-use spray units. Once the medication is dispensed under the tongue, the spray unit must be disposed of in a disposal bag provided by the manufacturer. The initial dosage should be 100 mcg. If pain is not relieved by 30 minutes after the first dose, one additional dose may be administered. Use should be limited to four doses per day.

Sublingual Tablets. Fentanyl sublingual tablets [Abstral] are available in six strengths: 100, 200, 300, 400, 600, and 800 mcg. Each strength is a different color and shape. Patients should place the tablet on the floor of the mouth directly under the tongue, and allow it to dissolve completely. If the mouth is dry, it should be moistened with water before dosing. Tablets must not be chewed, sucked, or swallowed. Patients should not eat or drink until the tablet is gone.

The initial dosage is 100 mcg. If 100 mcg is inadequate, another 100 mcg can be taken in 30 minutes. No more than two doses should be used for any pain episode, and patients should wait at least 2 hours before dosing again. With each subsequent episode, the dose should be titrated until a safe and effective dose is identified.

Intranasal. Fentanyl nasal spray [Lazanda] is much like transmucosal fentanyl. Like transmucosal fentanyl, Lazanda is indicated only for *breakthrough cancer pain in patients at least 18 years old who are already taking opioids around-the-clock and have developed some degree of tolerance.* The spray must not be used for acute pain, postoperative pain, headache, or athletic injuries. Because of differences in bioavailability, Lazanda is not interchangeable with other fentanyl products on a microgram-for-microgram basis. Adverse effects are like those of other opioid preparations. The biggest concerns are respiratory depression and shock. As with the transmucosal products, the dose of fentanyl in Lazanda can be fatal to nontolerant individuals, so the spray must be stored in a secure, child-resistant location.

Intranasal fentanyl is supplied in 5-mL bottles that have a metered-dose nasal spray pump. Each bottle contains enough solution for 8 sprays. Three strengths are available: 100, 300, or 400 mcg/spray. Dosing starts with 100 mcg. If needed, dosage can be titrated upward at subsequent pain episodes as follows: 200 mcg (100 mcg in each nostril), 400 mcg (400 mcg in 1 nostril), and then 800 mcg (400 mcg in 2 nostrils). Patients should allow at least 2 hours between doses. If more than 5 days elapse since the last dose, the bottle should be discarded and replaced with a new one.

Alfentanil and Sufentanil

Alfentanil [Alfenta] and sufentanil [Sufenta] are intravenous opioids related to fentanyl. Both drugs are used for induction of anesthesia, for maintenance of anesthesia (in combination with other agents), and as sole anesthetic agents. Pharmacologic effects are like those of morphine. Sufentanil has an especially high milligram potency (about 1000 times that of morphine). Alfentanil is about 10 times more potent than morphine. Both drugs have a rapid onset, and both are Schedule II agents.

Remifentanil

Remifentanil [Ultiva] is an intravenous opioid with a rapid onset and brief duration. The brief duration results from rapid metabolism by plasma and tissue esterases and not from hepatic metabolism or renal excretion. Like fentanyl, remifentanil is about 100 times more potent than morphine. Remifentanil is approved for analgesia during surgery and during the immediate postoperative period. Administration is by continuous IV infusion. Effects begin in minutes, and terminate 5 to 10 minutes after the infusion is stopped. For surgical analgesia, the infusion rate is 0.05 to 2 mcg/kg/min. For postoperative analgesia, the infusion rate is 0.025 to 0.2 mcg/kg/min. Adverse effects during the infusion include respiratory depression, hypotension, bradycardia, and muscle rigidity sufficient to compromise breathing. Postinfusion effects include nausea, vomiting, and headache. Remifentanil is regulated as a Schedule II substance.

Meperidine

Meperidine [Demerol] shares the major pharmacologic properties of morphine. With parenteral and oral administration, analgesia is strong. Meperidine was once considered a first-line drug for relief of moderate to severe pain. Now, use of meperidine is in decline for several reasons. First, the drug has a short half-life, so dosing must be repeated at short intervals. Second, meperidine interacts adversely with a number of drugs. Third, with continuous use, there is a risk of harm owing to accumulation of a toxic metabolite. Accordingly, routine use of the drug should be avoided. However, meperidine may still be appropriate for patients who can't take other opioids and for patients with drug-induced rigors or postanesthesia shivering.

Meperidine can interact with MAOIs to cause excitation, delirium, hyperpyrexia, and convulsions. Coma and death can follow. The underlying mechanism appears to be excessive activation of serotonin receptors owing to meperidine-induced blockade of serotonin reuptake. Clearly, the combination of meperidine with an MAOI should be avoided. Other drugs that increase serotonin availability (e.g., tricyclic antidepressants, selective serotonin reuptake inhibitors [SSRIs]) may also pose a risk.

Repeated dosing results in accumulation of normeperidine, a toxic metabolite that can cause dysphoria, irritability, tremors, and seizures. To avoid toxicity, *treatment should not exceed 48 hours, and the dosage should not exceed 600 mg/24 hr.*

Meperidine is available in tablets (50 and 100 mg) and a syrup (10 mg/mL) for oral use, and in solution (10, 25, 50, 75, and 100 mg/mL) for injection (IV, IM, or subQ). The usual adult dosage is 50 to 150 mg (IM, subQ, or PO) repeated every 3 to 4 hours as needed—up to a maximum of 600 mg/day. The usual dosage for children is 1 to 1.8 mg/kg (IM, subQ, or PO) repeated every 3 to 4 hours as needed. As noted, prolonged use must be avoided.

Methadone

Methadone [Diskets, Dolophine, Methadose] has pharmacologic properties very similar to those of morphine. The drug is effective orally and has a long duration of action. Repeated dosing can result in accumulation. Methadone is used to relieve pain and to treat opioid addiction. Use of methadone for pain control has declined at an average of 3.2% per year between 2006 and 2013. This is likely due to the increases in overdose and death from using this drug. The use of methadone in drug-abuse treatment programs is discussed in Chapter 40.

Methadone prolongs the QT interval, and hence may pose a risk of potentially fatal dysrhythmias. Torsades de pointes has developed in patients taking 65 to 400 mg/day. To reduce risk, methadone should be used with great caution—if at all—in patients with existing QT prolongation or a family history of long QT syndrome, and in those taking other QT-prolonging drugs (e.g., amiodarone, quinidine, erythromycin, tricyclic antidepressants). In addition, all patients should receive an electrocardiogram (ECG) before treatment, 30 days later, and annually thereafter. If the QT interval exceeds 500 msec, stopping methadone or reducing the dosage should be considered.

There have been increasing reports of deaths and life-threatening side effects (especially dysrhythmias and respiratory depression) among patients taking methadone to relieve pain. Although this number is declining, methadone was still involved in 3400 deaths in 2014. It accounted for 39.8% of single-drug deaths. The overdose death rate for methadone is significantly greater than that for other opioid pain relievers for multidrug and single-drug deaths. The presumed cause of toxicity is high drug levels, owing largely to excessive dosage. To reduce risk, patients should be warned against taking more methadone than was prescribed and should be cautioned to avoid other CNS depressants, such as benzodiazepines, alcohol, and other opioids. Drugs that inhibit CYP3A4 (the enzyme that metabolizes methadone) can raise methadone levels, and hence should be used with care. Among these inhibitors are clarithromycin, azole antifungal drugs, and HIV protease inhibitors.

Methadone is supplied in IR tablets (5, 10, and 40 mg) and in solution (1, 2, and 10 mg/mL) for oral use, and in solution (10 mg/mL) for IM and subQ injection. In addition, the drug is available in dispersible 40-mg tablets for detoxification and maintenance of opioid addicts. Usual oral analgesic doses for adults range from 2.5 to 20 mg repeated every 3 to 4 hours as needed.

Hydromorphone, Oxymorphone, and Levorphanol

Basic Pharmacology. All three drugs are strong opioid agonists with pharmacologic actions like those of morphine, and all three are indicated for moderate to severe pain. Dosages and time courses are shown in Table 28.5. Adverse effects include respiratory depression, sedation, cough suppression, constipation, urinary retention, nausea, and vomiting. Of note, hydromorphone may cause less nausea than morphine. Toxicity can be reversed with an opioid antagonist (e.g., naloxone). All three drugs are Schedule II agents.

Preparations, Dosage, and Administration

Hydromorphone. Hydromorphone [Dilaudid, Exalgo, Jurnista 🍁] is available in six formulations:

- IR tablets (2, 4, and 8 mg) sold as *Dilaudid*
- ER tablets (8, 12, 16, and 32 mg) sold as *Exalgo* and *Jurnista* 🍁
- Oral liquid (1 mg/mL) sold as *Dilaudid*
- Rectal suppositories (3 mg) sold as *Dilaudid*
- Solutions (1, 2, 4, and 10 mg/mL), sold as *Dilaudid,* for IM and subQ injection
- Powder (250 mg), sold as *Dilaudid-HP,* to be reconstituted to a 10-mg/mL solution for IM and subQ injection

With the IR tablets, the usual adult dosage is 2 mg every 4 to 6 hours. With the ER tablets, dosage is based on how much opioid was being used before switching to the ER tablets. With the oral liquid, the usual adult dosage is 2.5 to 10 mg every 3 to 6 hours. With the rectal suppositories, the usual dosage is 3 mg every 6 to 8 hours. With subQ and IM injection, dosages range from 1 to 4 mg every 4 to 6 hours.

Oxymorphone. Oxymorphone [Opana] is available in three formulations:

- IR tablets (5 and 10 mg) sold as *Opana*
- ER tablets (5, 7.5, 10, 15, 20, 30, and 40 mg) sold as *Opana ER*
- Solution (1 mg/mL), sold as *Opana,* for IM, IV, or subQ injection

All oxymorphone tablets should be taken on an empty stomach, because dosing with food can produce excessive peak levels. Also, alcohol should be avoided, as it can increase blood levels of oral oxymorphone. For oral therapy in opioid-naïve patients, the usual initial dosage is 10 to 20 mg every 4 to 6 hours (using IR tablets) or 5 mg every 12 hours (using ER tablets). For IV therapy, the initial dose is 0.5 mg. Usual subQ and IM dosages are 1 to 1.5 mg every 4 to 6 hours as needed.

Levorphanol. Levorphanol is available in 2-mg oral tablets. The usual adult oral dosage is 2 mg, repeated in 6 to 8 hours as needed.

Moderate to Strong Opioid Agonists

The moderate to strong opioid agonists are similar to morphine in most respects. Like morphine, these drugs produce analgesia, sedation, and euphoria. In addition, they can cause respiratory depression, constipation, urinary retention, cough suppression, and miosis. Differences between the moderate to strong opioids and morphine are primarily quantitative: The moderate to strong opioids produce less analgesia and respiratory depression than morphine and have a somewhat lower potential for abuse. As with morphine, toxicity from the moderate to strong agonists can be reversed with naloxone.

Codeine

Codeine is indicated for relief of mild to moderate pain. The drug is usually administered by mouth. Side effects are dose limiting. As a result, although taking codeine can produce significant pain relief, the degree of pain relief that can be achieved *safely* is quite low—much lower than with morphine. When taken in its usual analgesic dose (30 mg), codeine produces about as much pain relief as 325 mg of aspirin or 325 mg of acetaminophen.

In the liver, about 10% of each dose of codeine undergoes conversion to *morphine,* the active form of codeine. The enzyme responsible is CYP2D6 (the 2D6 isoenzyme of cytochrome P450). Among people who lack an effective gene for CYP2D6, codeine cannot be converted to morphine, and hence codeine cannot produce analgesia. Conversely, among ultrarapid metabolizers, who carry multiple copies of the CYP2D6 gene, codeine is unusually effective. Ultrarapid metabolism occurs in 7% of whites, 3% of blacks, and 1% of Hispanics and Asians.

Very rarely, severe toxicity develops in breast-fed infants whose mothers are taking codeine. The cause is high levels of morphine in breast milk, owing to ultrarapid codeine metabolism. Nursing mothers who are taking codeine should be alert for signs of infant intoxication—excessive sleepiness, breathing difficulties, lethargy, poor feeding—and should seek medical attention if these develop.

For analgesic use, codeine is formulated alone and in combination with nonopioid analgesics (either aspirin or acetaminophen). Because codeine and nonopioid analgesics relieve pain by different mechanisms, the combinations can produce greater pain relief than either agent alone. Codeine alone is classified under Schedule II of the Controlled Substances Act. The combination preparations are classified under Schedule III. Although codeine is classified along with morphine in Schedule II, the abuse liability of codeine appears to be significantly lower.

Codeine is an extremely effective cough suppressant and is widely used for this action. The antitussive dose (10 mg) is lower than analgesic doses. Codeine is formulated in combination with various agents to suppress cough. These mixtures are classified under Schedule V.

Preparations, Dosage, and Administration. Codeine is administered orally. The drug is available in tablets (15, 30, and 60 mg) and in solution (30 mg/5 mL).

The usual analgesic dosage for adults is 15 to 60 mg PO every 3 to 6 hours (up to a maximum of 120 mg/24 hr). The usual analgesic dosage for children 1 year and older is 0.5 mg/kg PO every 4 to 6 hours (up to a maximum of 60 mg/24 hr).

Oxycodone

Oxycodone [OxyContin, Roxicodone, OxyIR ♣] has analgesic actions equivalent to those of codeine. Administration is oral. Oxycodone is available by itself in IR tablets (5, 10, 15, 20, and 30 mg), IR capsules (5 mg), extended-release tablets (10, 15, 20, 30, 40, 60, and 80 mg), and oral solutions (1 and 20 mg/mL). In addition, the drug is available in combination with aspirin (as Percodan), acetaminophen (as Percocet, Roxicet, others), and ibuprofen (as Combunox). All formulations are classified under Schedule II.

Extended-release oxycodone [OxyContin] is a long-acting analgesic designed to relieve moderate to severe pain around-the-clock for an extended time. Dosing is done every 12 hours—not PRN. If breakthrough pain occurs, supplemental dosing with a short-acting analgesic is indicated.

Owing to increasing reports of OxyContin abuse, safety warnings have been strengthened, and in 2010 the product was reformulated. The new formulation bears the imprint *OP*; the old formulation bears the imprint *OC*. Why the reformulation? Because abusers could crush the OxyContin OC tablets and then "snort" the resulting powder, or dissolve the powder in water and inject it IV. Both practices allowed *immediate* absorption of the entire dose, and thereby produced blood levels that were much higher than those produced when the tablets were ingested whole and absorbed gradually. The result was an intense "high" coupled with a risk of fatal respiratory depression. Compared with the old tablets, OxyContin OP tablets are much harder to crush into a powder. And if exposed to water or alcohol, the tablets form a gummy blob, rather than a solution that can be drawn into a syringe and injected.

To minimize risk, patients should swallow OxyContin tablets whole, without breaking, crushing, or chewing. Furthermore, the 80-mg formulation must be reserved for patients who are already opioid tolerant. As with all other opioids, concerns about abuse and addiction should not interfere with using OxyContin to manage pain. Rather, the drug must simply be prescribed appropriately and then used as prescribed.

Like OxyContin OP, one *immediate-release* formulation [Oxecta] and one extended-release capsule [Xtampza ER] are designed to discourage abuse. If Oxecta tablets are crushed and snorted, they will burn the nasal passages. The Xtampza ER capsules are composed of microspheres formulated with inactive ingredients that are less susceptible to crushing, grinding, or snorting. If the tablets or microspheres are exposed to a solvent (e.g., water, alcohol), they will form a gel that can't be drawn into a syringe. However, the formulations do nothing to deter oral abuse.

Hydrocodone

Hydrocodone has analgesic actions equivalent to those of codeine. The drug is taken orally to relieve pain and to suppress cough. The usual dosage is 5 mg. For analgesic use, hydrocodone is available alone or in combination with acetaminophen or ibuprofen. For cough suppression, the drug is combined with antihistamines and nasal decongestants. Brand names for combination products containing hydrocodone include *Vicodin, Vicoprofen,* and *Lortab.*

Two extended-release formulas [Zohydro ER, Hysingla ER] are also available. All of these combination products are currently classified under Schedule II.

Tapentadol

Actions and Uses. Tapentadol [Nucynta] is indicated for oral therapy of moderate to severe pain—acute or chronic—in patients age 18 years and older. Analgesic effects are equivalent to those of oxycodone. Like other opioids, tapentadol can cause CNS depression and respiratory depression, and has a significant potential for abuse. However, the drug differs from other opioids in two important ways. First, in addition to activating mu opioid receptors, tapentadol *blocks reuptake of norepinephrine,* similar to tramadol, discussed later in this chapter. Second, tapentadol causes less constipation than traditional opioids. Because tapentadol is relatively new, and hence experience with the drug is limited, it would seem prudent to reserve tapentadol for patients who need a strong opioid but cannot tolerate the GI side effects of traditional agents.

Adverse Effects. The most common adverse effects are nausea, vomiting, headache, dizziness, and drowsiness. Like other opioids, tapentadol can cause respiratory depression, and hence should be avoided in patients with pre-existing respiratory depression and in those with acute or severe asthma. As noted, the drug causes less constipation than other opioids. Nonetheless, tapentadol is contraindicated in patients with paralytic ileus. As discussed later in this chapter, tramadol, a drug similar to tapentadol, poses a risk of seizures. To date, seizures have not been reported with tapentadol. Nonetheless, caution should be exercised in patients with a history of seizure disorders. Owing to its abuse potential, tapentadol is classified as a Schedule II substance. Patients should be monitored for abuse and addiction. Tapentadol is classified in FDA Pregnancy Risk Category C,[a] indicating that no adequate studies in pregnant patients have been performed.

Drug Interactions. The depressant effects of tapentadol can add with those of other agents (e.g., alcohol, opioids, barbiturates, benzodiazepines) and can thereby increase the risk of respiratory depression, sedation, and even coma. Because tapentadol can increase serum levels of norepinephrine (by blocking norepinephrine uptake), combined use with an MAOI might result in hypertensive crisis (see Chapter 32). Accordingly, tapentadol should not be used within 14 days of taking an MAOI. Package labeling says that a life-threatening serotonin syndrome could result from combining tapentadol

[a]As of 2020, the FDA will no longer use Pregnancy Risk Categories. Please refer to Chapter 9 for more information.

with an SSRI (e.g., fluoxetine), a serotonin/norepinephrine reuptake inhibitor (e.g., venlafaxine), a tricyclic antidepressant (e.g., amitriptyline), or a serotonin agonist (e.g., eletriptan). However, in clinical trials, combined use with an SSRI had no ill effects. Tapentadol neither inhibits nor induces P450 enzymes, and hence clinically relevant interactions involving the cytochrome P450 system seem unlikely.

Preparations, Dosage, and Administration. Tapentadol is available in two formulations: IR tablets (50, 75, and 100 mg), sold as *Nucynta,* and ER tablets (50, 100, 150, 200, and 250 mg), sold as *Nucynta ER.* The IR tablets are indicated only for moderate to severe *acute* pain. The ER tablets are indicated only for moderate to severe *chronic* pain, and then only in patients who require continuous, around-the-clock treatment with an opioid analgesic. Dosages are as follows:

- *IR tablets:* The recommended dosage is 50, 75, or 100 mg every 4 to 6 hours. When initiating treatment, a second dose can be given 1 hour after the first. The maximum dosage on the first day is 700 mg. The maximum dosage on all subsequent days is 600 mg. In patients with moderate hepatic impairment, the dosage should be no more than 50 mg every 8 hours. In patients with severe hepatic or renal impairment, tapentadol should not be used.
- *ER tablets:* The initial dosage is 50 mg twice a day, and the maximum dosage is 250 mg twice a day. For patients with moderate hepatic impairment, the initial dosage is 50 mg once a day, and the maximum dosage is 100 mg once a day. As with the IR tablets, the ER tablets should not be used in patients with severe hepatic or renal impairment.

Agonist-Antagonist Opioids

Four agonist-antagonist opioids are available: pentazocine, nalbuphine, butorphanol, and buprenorphine. With the exception of buprenorphine, these drugs act as antagonists at mu receptors and agonists at kappa receptors (see Table 28.2). Compared with pure opioid agonists, the agonist-antagonists have a low potential for abuse, produce less respiratory depression, and generally have less powerful analgesic effects. If given to a patient who is physically dependent on a pure opioid agonist, these drugs can precipitate withdrawal. The clinical pharmacology of the agonist-antagonists is shown in Table 28.6.

Pentazocine

Actions and Uses. Pentazocine [Talwin] was the first agonist-antagonist opioid available and can be considered the prototype for the group. The drug is indicated for mild to moderate pain. Pentazocine is much less effective than morphine against severe pain.

Pentazocine acts as an *agonist* at kappa receptors and as an *antagonist* at mu receptors. By activating kappa receptors, the drug produces analgesia, sedation, and respiratory depression. However, unlike the respiratory depression caused by morphine, *respiratory depression caused by pentazocine is limited:* Beyond a certain dose, no further depression occurs. Because it lacks agonist actions at mu receptors, pentazocine produces little or no euphoria. In fact, at supratherapeutic doses, pentazocine produces unpleasant reactions (anxiety, strange thoughts, nightmares, hallucinations). These psychotomimetic effects may result from activation of kappa receptors. Because of its subjective effects, pentazocine has a low potential for abuse and is classified under Schedule IV.

Adverse effects are generally like those of morphine. However, in contrast to the pure opioid agonists, pentazocine increases cardiac work. Accordingly, a pure agonist (e.g., morphine) is preferred to pentazocine for relieving pain in patients with myocardial infarction.

If administered to a patient who is physically dependent on a pure opioid agonist, pentazocine can precipitate withdrawal. Recall that mu receptors mediate physical dependence on pure opioid agonists and that pentazocine acts as an antagonist at these receptors. By blocking access of the pure agonist to mu receptors, pentazocine will prevent receptor activation, thereby triggering withdrawal. Accordingly, *pentazocine and other drugs that block mu receptors should never be administered to a person who is physically dependent on a pure opioid agonist.* If a pentazocine-like agent is to be used, the pure opioid agonist must be withdrawn first.

TABLE 28.6 ▪ Clinical Pharmacology of Opioid Agonist-Antagonists

		Time Course of Analgesic Effects		
Drug and Route[a]	Equianalgesic Dose (mg)[b]	Onset (min)	Peak (min)	Duration (hr)
Buprenorphine				
IM	0.3	15	60	Up to 6
IV	0.3	Under 15	Under 60	Up to 6
Butorphanol				
IM	2–3	10	30–60	3–4
IV	2–3	2–3	30–60	3–4
Intranasal	2–3	Within 15	60–120	4–5
Nalbuphine				
IM	10	Within 15	60	3–6
IV	10	2–3	30	3–6
SubQ	10	Within 15	60	3–6
Pentazocine				
PO	—	15–30	60–90	3[c]
IM	30	15–20	30–60	4–6[c]
IV	30	2–3	15–30	4–6[c]
SubQ	30	15–20	30–60	4–6[c]

[a]IM administration should be avoided whenever possible.
[b]Dose in milligrams that produces a degree of analgesia equivalent to that produced by a 10-mg IM dose of morphine.
[c]Duration may increase greatly in patients with liver disease.

Physical dependence can occur with pentazocine, but symptoms of withdrawal are generally mild (e.g., cramps, fever, anxiety, restlessness). Treatment is rarely required. As with pure opioid agonists, toxicity from pentazocine can be reversed with naloxone.

Preparations, Dosage, and Administration. Pentazocine is available alone for parenteral therapy and in combination with naloxone for oral therapy.

Parenteral. For parenteral therapy, pentazocine is available in solution (30 mg/mL) sold as *Talwin.* Administration may be subQ, IM, or IV. The usual dosage is 30 mg every 3 to 4 hours, but no more than 360 mg/day.

Oral. For oral therapy, pentazocine is available in combination with naloxone (50 mg/0.5 mg) and is sold as *Talwin NX.* The usual dosage is 1 tablet every 3 to 4 hours, but may be increased to 2 tablets every 3 to 4 hours if needed, for a daily maximum of 12 tablets (600 mg pentazocine).

Nalbuphine

Nalbuphine has pharmacologic actions similar to those of pentazocine. The drug is an agonist at kappa receptors and an antagonist at mu receptors. At low doses, nalbuphine has analgesic actions equal to those of morphine. However, as dosage increases, a ceiling to analgesia is reached. As a result, the maximal pain relief that can be produced with nalbuphine is much lower than with morphine. As with pain relief, there is also a ceiling to respiratory depression. Like pentazocine, nalbuphine can cause psychotomimetic reactions. With prolonged treatment, physical dependence can develop. Symptoms of abstinence are less intense than with morphine but more intense than with pentazocine. When used during labor and delivery, nalbuphine has caused serious adverse effects, including bradycardia in the fetus and apnea, cyanosis, and hypotonia in the neonate. Accordingly, use during labor and delivery should be avoided. Nalbuphine has a low abuse potential and is not regulated under the Controlled Substances Act. As with the pure opioid agonists, toxicity can be reversed with naloxone. Like pentazocine, nalbuphine will precipitate a withdrawal reaction if administered to an individual physically dependent on a pure opioid agonist. Nalbuphine is supplied in solution (10 and 20 mg/mL) for IV, IM, and subQ injection. The usual adult dosage is 10 mg repeated every 3 to 6 hours as needed.

Butorphanol

Butorphanol has actions similar to those of pentazocine. The drug is an agonist at kappa receptors and an antagonist at mu receptors. Analgesic effects are less than those of morphine. As with pentazocine, there is a "ceiling" to respiratory depression. The drug can cause psychotomimetic reactions, but these are rare. Butorphanol increases cardiac work and should not be given to patients with myocardial infarction. Physical dependence can occur, but symptoms of withdrawal are relatively mild. The drug may induce a withdrawal reaction in patients physically dependent on a pure opioid agonist. Butorphanol has a low potential for abuse and is regulated as a Schedule IV substance. Toxicity can be reversed with naloxone.

Butorphanol is administered parenterally (IM and IV) and by nasal spray (primarily to treat migraine). The usual adult IV dosage is 1 mg every 3 to 4 hours as needed. The usual IM dosage is 2 mg every 3 to 4 hours as needed. The usual intranasal dosage is 1 mg (1 spray from the metered-dose spray device) repeated in 60 to 90 minutes if needed. The two-dose sequence may then be repeated every 3 to 4 hours as needed.

Buprenorphine

Basic Pharmacology. Buprenorphine [Buprenex, Butrans, Belbuca, Suboxone] differs significantly from other opioid agonist-antagonists. The drug is a partial agonist at mu receptors and an antagonist at kappa receptors. Analgesic effects are like those of morphine, but significant tolerance has not been observed. Although buprenorphine can depress respiration, severe respiratory depression has not been reported. Like pentazocine, buprenorphine can precipitate a withdrawal reaction in persons physically dependent on a pure opioid agonist. Physical dependence on buprenorphine develops, but symptoms of abstinence are delayed: Peak responses may not occur until 2 weeks after the final dose was taken. Although pretreatment with naloxone can prevent toxicity from buprenorphine, naloxone cannot readily reverse toxicity that has already developed. (Buprenorphine binds very tightly to its receptors, and hence cannot be readily displaced by naloxone.) Buprenorphine is classified as a Schedule III substance. In addition to its use for analgesia, buprenorphine is used to treat opioid addiction (see Chapter 40).

Buprenorphine prolongs the QT interval, posing a risk of potentially fatal dysrhythmias. Accordingly, the drug should not be used by patients with long QT syndrome or a family history of long QT syndrome, or by patients using QT-prolonging drugs (e.g., quinidine, amiodarone).

The risk of adverse effects may be increased by coexisting conditions, including psychosis, alcoholism, adrenocortical insufficiency, and severe liver or renal impairment. In addition, buprenorphine can cause spasm of the sphincter of Oddi (where the bile duct and pancreatic duct enter the duodenum) and can thereby pose a risk to patients with pancreatitis or biliary disease.

Preparations. Buprenorphine is available in six formulations: transdermal patch, solution for injection, sublingual tablets, buccal strips, an intradermal implant, and a sublingual film. The patch and solution are approved for pain management. The sublingual products are approved only for opioid addiction—but are used off-label for pain management.

Transdermal Patch. The buprenorphine patch, sold as *Butrans,* is indicated for moderate to severe chronic pain in patients who need continuous analgesia for an extended time. The patch is applied once every 7 days. Five strengths are available, delivering 5, 7.5, 10, 15, or 20 mcg/hr. The lowest strength is used for opioid-naïve patients or for those using an opioid in low dosage (e.g., oral morphine, 30 mg/day). Dosage may be titrated to the next higher strength after a minimum of 72 hours. Breakthrough pain can be managed with acetaminophen, a nonsteroidal anti-inflammatory drug, or a short-acting opioid.

Patches are applied to eight sites: upper outer arm, upper front of chest, upper side of chest, and upper back—on the right and left sides of the body. The site should be rotated when a new patch is applied, and no site should be reused within 21 days. The site should be hairless, or nearly so. If needed, hair can be removed by clipping, not by shaving. The site may be cleaned, but only with water, not with soaps, alcohol, or abrasives. No lotion or oil should be applied. Patches should not be cut or exposed to heat, including heating pads, heated waterbeds, hot baths, saunas, heat lamps, or extended sunshine. If a patch falls off during the 7-day dosing interval, a new patch should be applied, but at a different site. If patch use is stopped, opioids should not be given for 24 hours.

Solution for Injection. Buprenorphine solution (0.3 mg/mL), sold as *Buprenex,* is indicated only for parenteral management of pain. Dosing is by IM or slow IV injection. The usual dosage for patients ages 13 years and older is 0.3 mg repeated every 6 hours as needed.

Sublingual Tablets and Sublingual Film. Buprenorphine is available in two sublingual formulation, tablets and films. *Suboxone* tablets and films contain a mixture of buprenorphine/naloxone (2 mg/0.5 mg, 4 mg/1 mg, 8 mg/2 mg, or 12 mg/3 mg). *Zubsolv* tablets are available in additional strengths (0.7 mg/0.18 mg, 1.4 mg/0.36 mg, 2.9 mg/0.71 mg, 5.7 mg/1.4 mg, 8.6 mg/2.1 mg, and 11.4 mg/2.9 mg). Both sublingual formulations are approved only for managing opioid addiction. However, they are also used off-label for analgesia. For opioid addiction, dosing is done once a day. For pain management, dosing is done 3 or 4 times a day. The use of these sublingual products is restricted in the United States. To prescribe Suboxone or Zubsolv, a provider must undergo training and register for appropriate access. Use of these products for opioid addiction is discussed further in Chapter 40.

Soluble Buccal Film. Buprenorphine buccal film [Belbuca] is made using a drug-delivery technology known as BioErodible MucoAdhesive. Seven film strengths are available: 75 mcg, 150 mcg, 300 mcg, 450 mcg, 600 mcg, 750 mcg, and 900 mcg. A single dose of the film is about 1- to 2-cm square and very thin, with a yellow side (that delivers the buprenorphine) and a white side (that indicates the strength). Patients should press the yellow side against the inside of the cheek for 5 seconds and then leave it there. If the site is dry, it should be moistened first with saliva or water. Patients can drink after 5 minutes but should avoid eating until the film has dissolved (in 15 to 30 minutes). A new film is applied every 12 to 24 hours initially. Dosing is begun at 75 mcg and can be titrated up no sooner than every 4 days. Patients should not tear, chew, or swallow the film.

Intradermal Implant. In 2016, the FDA approved Probuphine, the first implant used to treat opioid-dependent patients. Probuphine contains 74.2 mg of buprenorphine within 4 flexible 1-inch rods. These rods are inserted on the inside of the upper arm and deliver a continuous dose of buprenorphine over 6 months. As with other implants, complications can occur, including nerve or blood vessel injury, and migration, protrusion, or expulsion of the implant.

CLINICAL USE OF OPIOIDS

Dosing Guidelines

Pain Assessment

Assessment is an essential component of pain management. Pain status should be evaluated before opioid administration and about 1 hour after. Unfortunately, because pain is a subjective experience, affected by multiple factors (e.g., cultural influences, patient expectations, associated disease), there is no reliable objective method for determining just how much discomfort the patient is feeling. That is, we cannot measure pain with instruments equivalent to those employed to monitor blood pressure, bone loss, and other physiologic parameters. As a result, assessment must ultimately be based on the patient's description of his or her experience. Accordingly, you should ask the patient where the pain is located, what type of pain is present (e.g., dull, sharp, stabbing), how the pain changes with time, what makes the pain better, what makes it worse, and how much does it impair his or her ability to function. In addition, you should assess for psychologic factors that can reduce pain threshold (anxiety, depression, fear, anger).

When attempting to assess pain, keep in mind that, on occasion, what the patient says may not accurately reflect his or her experience. For example, a few patients who are pain free may claim to feel pain so as to receive medication for its euphoriant effects. Conversely, some patients may claim to feel fine even though they have considerable discomfort. Reasons for underreporting pain include fear of addiction, fear of needles, and a need to be stoic and bear the pain. Patients suspected of underreporting pain must be listened to with care if their true pain status is to be evaluated.

Pain assessment is further discussed in Chapter 29.

Dosage Determination

Dosage of opioid analgesics must be adjusted to accommodate individual variation. "Standard" doses cannot be relied upon as appropriate for all patients. For example, if a "standard" 10-mg dose of morphine were employed for all adults, only 70% would receive adequate relief; the other 30% would be undertreated. Not all patients have the same tolerance for pain, and hence some need larger doses than others for the same disorder. Some conditions hurt more than others. For example, patients recovering from open chest surgery are likely to experience greater pain and need larger doses than patients recovering from an appendectomy. Older adult patients metabolize opioids slowly and therefore require lower doses than younger adults. Because the blood-brain barrier of newborns is poorly developed, these patients are especially sensitive to opioids; therefore, they generally require smaller doses (on a milligram-per-kilogram basis) than do older infants and young children.

Dosing Schedule

Opioids should be administered on a fixed schedule (e.g., every 4 hours) rather than PRN for the first 24 hours of treatment in a postoperative setting. With a fixed schedule, each dose is given before pain returns, thereby sparing the patient needless discomfort. In contrast, when PRN dosing is employed, there can be a long delay between onset of pain and production of relief: Each time pain returns, the patient must call the nurse, wait for the nurse to respond, wait for the nurse to evaluate the pain, wait for the nurse to sign out medication, wait for the nurse to prepare and administer the injection, and then wait for the drug to undergo absorption and finally produce analgesia. This delay causes unnecessary discomfort and creates anxiety about pain recurrence. Use of a fixed dosing schedule reduces these problems. As discussed in this chapter, allowing the patient to self-administer opioids with a patient-controlled analgesia (PCA) device can provide even greater protection against pain recurrence than can be achieved by having the nurse administer opioids on a fixed schedule. The differences between PRN dosing, fixed-schedule dosing, and the use of a PCA device are shown in Fig. 28.1.

Avoiding a Withdrawal Reaction

When opioids are administered in high doses for 20 days or more, clinically significant physical dependence may develop. Under these conditions, abrupt withdrawal will precipitate an abstinence syndrome. To minimize symptoms of abstinence, opioids should be withdrawn slowly, tapering the dosage over 3 days. If the degree of dependence is especially high, as can occur in opioid addicts, dosage should be tapered over 7 to 10 days.

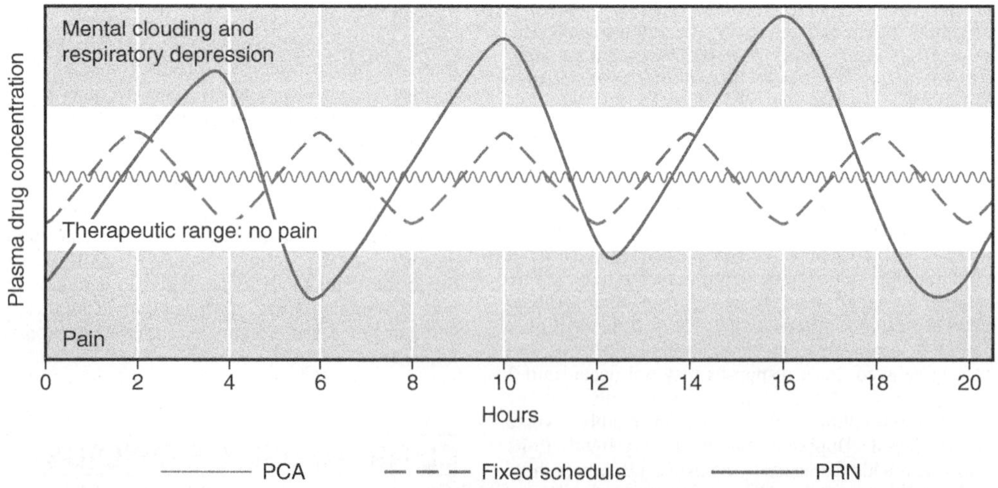

Fig. 28.1 ▪ Fluctuation in opioid blood levels seen with three dosing procedures. Note that, with PRN dosing, opioid levels can fluctuate widely, going from subtherapeutic to excessive and back again. In contrast, when opioids are administered with a PCA device or on a fixed schedule, levels stay within the therapeutic range, allowing continuous pain relief with minimal adverse effects.

Physical Dependence, Abuse, and Addiction as Clinical Concerns

Some health professionals may harbor strong fears about the ability of opioids to cause addiction. Because of these fears, providers may prescribe less pain medication than patients need, and nurses may administer less than was prescribed. The result, according to one estimate, is that only 25% of patients receive doses of opioids that are sufficient to relieve suffering. One pain specialist described this situation as follows: "The excessive and unrealistic concern about the dangers of addiction in the hospitalized medical patient is a significant and potent force for the undertreatment with narcotics [opioids]."

When treating a patient for pain, you may have to decide how much opioid to give and when to give it. If you are excessively concerned about the ability of opioids to cause physical dependence and addiction, you will be unable to make a rational choice. Furthermore, in your role as patient advocate, it is your responsibility to intervene and request an increase in dosage if the prescribed dosage has proved inadequate. If you fear that dosage escalation may cause addiction, you are less likely to make the request.

The objective of the following discussion is to dispel concerns about dependence, abuse, and addiction in the medical patient so that these concerns do not result in undermedication and needless suffering.

Definitions

Before we can discuss the clinical implications of physical dependence, abuse, and addiction, we need to define these terms.

Physical Dependence. As noted, physical dependence is a state in which an abstinence syndrome will occur if the dependence-producing drug is abruptly withdrawn. *Physical dependence is NOT the same as addiction.*

Abuse. Abuse can be broadly defined as *drug use that is inconsistent with medical or social norms.* By this definition, abuse is determined primarily by the reason for drug use and by the setting in which that use occurs—and not by the pharmacologic properties of the drug itself. For example, whereas it is *not* considered abuse to administer 20 mg of morphine in a hospital to relieve pain, it *is* considered abuse to administer the same dose of the same drug on the street to produce euphoria. The concept of abuse is discussed at length in Chapter 37.

Addiction. Addiction is defined by the American Society of Addiction Medicine as *primary, chronic disease characterized by an individual pathologically pursuing rewards and/or relief by substance use and other behaviors.* Note that nowhere in this definition is addiction equated with physical dependence. In fact, physical dependence is not even part of the definition. The concept of addiction is discussed further in Chapter 37.

Although physical dependence is not required for addiction to occur, physical dependence *can* contribute to addictive behavior. If an individual has already established a pattern of compulsive drug use, physical dependence can reinforce that pattern. For the individual with a marginal resolve to discontinue opioid use, the desire to avoid symptoms of withdrawal may be sufficient to promote continued drug use. However, in the presence of a strong desire to become drug free, physical dependence, by itself, is insufficient to motivate continued addictive behavior.

Minimizing Fears About Physical Dependence

For two important reasons, there is little to fear regarding physical dependence on opioids in the hospitalized patient:

- Development of significant physical dependence is extremely rare when opioids are used short term to relieve pain. For most patients, the doses employed and the duration of treatment are insufficient to cause significant dependence.
- Even when physical dependence *does* occur, patients rarely develop addictive behavior and continue opioid administration after their pain has subsided. The vast majority of patients who become physically dependent in a clinical setting simply go through gradual withdrawal and never take opioids again. This observation emphasizes the point that physical dependence per se is insufficient to cause addiction.

We can conclude, therefore, that there is no justification for withholding opioids from patients in pain on the basis of concerns about physical dependence.

Minimizing Fears About Addiction

The principal reason for abandoning fears about opioid addiction in patients is simple: *Development of addiction to opioids as a result of clinical exposure to these drugs is extremely rare.* Results of the Boston Collaborative Drug Study showed that of 12,000 hospitalized patients taking opioids, only 4 became drug abusers. Furthermore, if abuse or addiction *does* occur, it is probable that these behaviors reflect tendencies that existed before the patient entered the hospital, and hence are not the result of inappropriate medical use of opioids during the hospital stay.

For the purpose of this discussion, the population can be divided into two groups: individuals who are prone to drug abuse and individuals who are not. One source estimates that about 8% of the population is prone to drug abuse, whereas the other 92% is not. Individuals who are prone to drug abuse have a tendency to abuse drugs inside the hospital and out. Nonabusers, on the other hand, will not abuse drugs in a clinical setting or anywhere else. Withholding analgesics from abuse-prone individuals is not going to reverse their tendency to abuse drugs. Conversely, administering opioids to non–abuse-prone persons will not convert them into abusers.

If a patient who did not formerly abuse opioids does abuse these drugs following therapeutic exposure, you should not feel responsible for having created an addict. That is, if a patient tries to continue opioid use after leaving the hospital, it is probable that the patient was abuse prone before you met him or her. Therefore, the pattern of abuse that emerged during clinical exposure to opioids was the result of factors that existed before the patient entered the hospital—and not the consequence of therapy. The only action that might have prevented opioid abuse by such a patient would have been to withhold opioids entirely—an action that would not have been acceptable.

Balancing the Need to Provide Pain Relief With the Desire to Minimize Abuse

Although concerns about opioid abuse in the clinical setting are small, they cannot be dismissed entirely. You are still obligated to administer opioids with discretion in an effort to minimize abuse. The first step is to identify patients at risk for abuse by using a screening tool, such as *NIDA-Modified ASSIST,* available at www.drugabuse.gov/nidamed/screening/nmassist.pdf. When nonabusers say they need more pain relief, believe them and provide it. In contrast, when a likely abuser requests more analgesic, some healthy skepticism is in order. When there is doubt as to whether a patient is abuse prone or not, logic dictates giving the patient the benefit of the doubt and providing the medication. If the patient is an abuser, little harm will result from giving unneeded medication. However, if the patient is a nonabuser, failure to provide medication would intensify suffering for no justifiable reason.

To minimize physical dependence and abuse, opioid analgesics should be administered in the lowest effective dosages for the shortest time needed. Be aware, however, that larger doses are needed for patients who have more intense pain and for those who have developed tolerance. As pain diminishes, opioid dosage should be reduced. As soon as possible, the patient should be switched to a nonopioid analgesic, such as aspirin or acetaminophen.

When working with opioids, as with any other drugs, you must balance the risks of therapy against the benefits. The risk of addiction from therapeutic use of opioids is real but very small. Consequently, concerns about addiction should play a real but secondary role in making decisions about giving these drugs. Dosages should be sufficient to relieve pain. Suffering because of insufficient dosage is unacceptable. However, it is also unacceptable to promote possible abuse through failure to exercise good judgment.

Patient-Controlled Analgesia

PCA is a method of drug delivery that permits the patient to self-administer parenteral (transdermal, IV, subQ, epidural) opioids on an "as-needed" basis. PCA has been employed primarily for relief of pain in postoperative patients. Other candidates include patients experiencing pain caused by cancer, trauma, myocardial infarction, vaso-occlusive sickle cell crisis, and labor. As discussed in the sections that follow, PCA offers several advantages over opioids administered by the nurse.

PCA Devices

PCA was made possible by the development of reliable PCA devices. At this time, only one kind of PCA device is available: an electronically controlled infusion pump that can be activated by the patient to deliver a preset bolus dose of an opioid, which is delivered through an indwelling catheter. In addition to providing bolus doses on demand, some PCA pumps can deliver a basal infusion of opioid.

An essential feature of all PCA pumps is a timing control. This control limits the total dose that can be administered each hour, thereby minimizing the risk of overdose. In addition, the timing control regulates the minimum interval (e.g., 10 minutes) between doses. This interval, referred to as the "lock-out" or "delay" interval, prevents the patient from administering a second dose before the first has had time to produce its full effect.

Drug Selection and Dosage Regulation

The opioid used most extensively for PCA is morphine. Other pure opioid agonists (e.g., methadone, hydromorphone, fentanyl) have also been employed, as have agonist-antagonist opioids (e.g., nalbuphine, buprenorphine).

Before starting PCA, the postoperative patient should be given an opioid loading dose (e.g., 2 to 10 mg of morphine). Once effective opioid levels have been established with the loading dose, PCA can be initiated, provided the patient has recovered sufficiently from anesthesia. For PCA with morphine, initial bolus doses of 1 mg are typical. The size of the bolus should be increased if analgesia is inadequate and decreased if excessive sedation occurs.

Comparison of PCA With Traditional IM Therapy

The objective of therapy with analgesics is to provide comfort while minimizing sedation and other side effects, especially respiratory depression. This objective is best achieved by maintaining plasma levels of opioids that have minimal fluctuations. In this manner, side effects from excessively high levels can be avoided, as can the return of severe pain when levels dip too low.

In the traditional management of postoperative pain, patients are given an IM injection of an opioid every 3 to 4 hours. With this dosing schedule, plasma drug levels can vary widely. Shortly after the injection, plasma levels may rise very high, causing excessive sedation and possibly respiratory depression. Late in the dosing interval, pain may return as plasma levels drop to their lowest point. In addition, multiple IM injections can be painful to the patient and cause negative side effects, including bruising and hematoma formation.

In contrast to traditional therapy, PCA is ideally suited to maintain steady levels of opioids because it relies on small doses given frequently (e.g., 1 mg of morphine every 10 minutes) rather than on large doses given infrequently (e.g., 20 mg of morphine every 3 hours). Maintenance of steady drug levels can be facilitated further if the PCA device is capable of delivering a basal infusion. Because plasma drug levels remain relatively steady, PCA can provide continuous pain control while avoiding the adverse effects associated with excessive drug levels.

An additional advantage of PCA is rapid relief. Because the patient can self-administer a parenteral dose of opioid as soon as pain begins to return, there is minimal delay between detection of pain and restoration of an adequate drug level. With traditional therapy, the patient must wait for the nurse to respond to a request for more drug; this delay allows pain to grow more intense.

Studies indicate that PCA is associated with accelerated recovery. When compared with patients receiving traditional IM analgesia, postoperative patients receiving PCA show improved early mobilization, greater cooperation during physical therapy, and a shorter hospital stay.

Patient and Family Education

Patient education is important for successful PCA. Surgical patients should be educated preoperatively. Education should include an explanation of what PCA is, along with instruction on how to activate the PCA device.

Patients should be told not to fear overdose; the PCA device will not permit self-administration of excessive doses. Families should be informed that activating the device for the patient while he or she is sleeping can lead to drug overdose. Patients should be informed that there is a time lag (about 10 minutes) between activation of the device and production of maximal analgesia. To reduce discomfort associated with physical therapy, changing of dressings, ambulation, and other potentially painful activities, patients should be taught to activate the pump prophylactically (e.g., 10 minutes before the anticipated activity).

Using Opioids for Specific Types of Pain

Postoperative Pain

Opioid analgesics offer several benefits to the postoperative patient. The most obvious is increased comfort through reduction of pain. In addition, by reducing painful sensation, opioids can facilitate early movement and intentional cough. In patients who have undergone thoracic surgery, opioids permit chest movement that would otherwise be too uncomfortable for adequate ventilation. By promoting ventilation, opioids can reduce the risk of hypoxia and pneumonitis.

Opioids are not without drawbacks for the postoperative patient. These agents can cause constipation and urinary retention. Suppression of reflex cough can result in respiratory tract complications. In addition, analgesia may delay diagnosis of postoperative complications—because pain will not be present to signal them.

Obstetric Analgesia

When administered to relieve pain during delivery, opioids such as morphine or meperidine may depress fetal respiration and uterine contractions when administered parenterally. Although these drugs are still used for relief of labor pain, regional and epidural modes of analgesia are often favored for pain relief in childbirth. For patients who are hesitant to use these more invasive methods, providers are employing newer opioid medications. Fentanyl, sufentanil, alfentanil, and remifentanil have a short duration of action and should not produce significant neonatal depression. The mixed opioid agonist-antagonists—nalbuphine, butorphanol, pentazocine, and buprenorphine—offer increased pain relief without causing further respiratory depression in higher doses. Even if these newer medications are used, however, respiration in the neonate should be monitored closely after delivery. Naloxone can reverse respiratory depression and should be on hand.

Myocardial Infarction

Morphine is the opioid of choice for decreasing pain of myocardial infarction. With careful control of dosage, morphine can reduce discomfort without causing excessive respiratory depression and adverse cardiovascular effects. In addition, by lowering blood pressure, morphine can decrease cardiac work. If excessive hypotension or respiratory depression occurs, it can be reversed with naloxone. Because *pentazocine* and *butorphanol* increase cardiac work and oxygen demand, these agonist-antagonist opioids should generally be avoided.

Head Injury

Opioids must be employed with caution in patients with head injury. Head injury can cause respiratory depression accompanied by elevation of ICP; opioids can exacerbate these symptoms. In addition, because miosis, mental clouding, and vomiting can be valuable diagnostic signs following head injury and because opioids can cause these same effects, the use of opioids can complicate diagnosis.

Cancer-Related Pain

Treating chronic pain of cancer differs substantially from treating acute pain of other disorders. When treating cancer pain, the objective is to maximize comfort. Psychologic and physical dependence are minimal concerns. Patients should be given as much medication as needed to relieve pain. In the words of one pain specialist, "No patient should wish for death because of the physician's reluctance to use adequate amounts of opioids." With proper therapy, cancer pain can be effectively managed in about 90% of patients. Cancer pain is discussed fully in Chapter 29.

Chronic Noncancer Pain

In patients with chronic pain of nonmalignant origin, opioids can reduce discomfort, improve mood, and enhance function. Accordingly, pain experts now recommend that opioids not be withheld from these people after other therapies have failed. Nonetheless, because of concerns about addiction, tolerance, adverse effects, diversion to street use, and regulatory action, physicians and nurse practitioners are often reluctant to prescribe these drugs. To some degree, all of these concerns are legitimate. However, patients still have a right to effective treatment. Hence there is a need to balance patients' rights with prescribers' concerns. To help achieve that balance, the American Academy of Pain Medicine and the American Pain Society issued guidelines for the use of opioids in patients with chronic noncancer pain. Provisions include:

- Using opioids only after nonopioid analgesics or more conservative methods have failed
- Discussing the benefits and risks of long-term opioids with the patient
- When possible, using only one prescriber and one pharmacy
- Ensuring comprehensive follow-up to assess efficacy and side effects of treatment, and to monitor for signs of opioid abuse
- Stopping opioids after an attempt at opioid rotation has produced inadequate benefit
- Fully documenting the entire process

REMS to Reduce Opioid-Related Morbidity, Mortality, and Abuse

The FDA introduced a Risk Evaluation and Mitigation Strategy (REMS) for prescription opioids to reduce injuries and death from prescription opioids and to reduce abuse. Why is this REMS needed? Because efforts to improve pain management have led to a 10-fold increase in opioid prescriptions, accompanied by a substantial increase in abuse, serious injuries, and deaths. In 2015, accidental overdose with prescription opioids resulted in 20,101 fatalities, more than from heroin and cocaine combined.

What does the REMS consist of? The central component is education for prescribers (e.g., physicians, nurse practitioners, physician assistants) and patients. Training for prescribers will focus on patient selection, balancing the risks and benefits of opioids, monitoring treatment, and recognizing opioid misuse, abuse, and addiction. In addition, prescribers will be taught how to counsel patients on the safe use of opioids and will be given written instructions for their patients. When patients have a prescription filled, the pharmacy will provide a medication guide. The companies that market opioids develop and pay for all training, but the content is reviewed by the FDA.

Do the new REMS have limitations? Yes. First, prescriber participation is *voluntary,* not mandatory. Prescribers who choose not to accept training may do so. Second, the REMS does not apply to all opioids. With the exception of transmucosal fentanyl and sublingual buprenorphine, IR products are largely exempt because they are considered safer than long-acting and ER products. Yes, IR products can cause death. However, the risk is much higher with long-acting and ER products, because the dose of opioid is much greater than it is in IR products. Products currently covered by the REMS include the following:

- Buprenorphine, transdermal [Butrans], buccal film [Belbuca], and sublingual [Suboxone]
- Fentanyl, transdermal [Duragesic] and transmucosal [Abstral, Actiq, Fentora, Subsys]
- Hydrocodone [Hysingla ER and Zohydro ER]
- Hydromorphone [Exalgo]
- Methadone [Dolophine and Methadose]
- Morphine [Avinza, Kadian, MS Contin]
- Morphine/naltrexone [Embeda]
- Oxycodone [OxyContin and Xtampza ER]
- Oxymorphone [Opana ER]
- Tapentadol [Nucynta ER]

PATIENT-CENTERED CARE ACROSS THE LIFE SPAN

Opioid Analgesics

Life Stage	Patient Care Concerns
Infants	Regular use of opioids during pregnancy can cause physical dependence in the fetus, resulting in withdrawal after delivery.
Children	Adequately assess pain with a standardized pain scale. Aspirin, as an adjuvant to opioids, should be avoided due to risk of Reye's syndrome. There remains a lack of research regarding best practice in the treatment of chronic noncancer pain in children.
Pregnant women	Taking opioids in early pregnancy can increase the risk of congenital heart defects, spina bifida, and gastroschisis.
Breast-feeding women	Limited data suggest small amounts of opioids are excreted in breast milk. This can result in infant drowsiness.
Older adults	Persistent pain is often undertreated in the frail older adult population. The American Geriatrics Association recommends that providers consider treating moderate to severe uncontrolled pain with opiates after a trial of acetaminophen.

OPIOID ANTAGONISTS

Opioid antagonists are drugs that block the effects of opioid agonists. Principal uses are treatment of opioid overdose, relief of opioid-induced constipation, reversal of postoperative opioid effects (e.g., respiratory depression, ileus), and management of opioid addiction. Four pure antagonists are available: naloxone [Narcan], methylnaltrexone [Relistor], naloxegol [Movantik], alvimopan [Entereg], and naltrexone [ReVia, Vivitrol].

Naloxone

Mechanism of Action

Naloxone [Narcan] is a structural analog of morphine that acts as a competitive antagonist at opioid receptors, thereby blocking opioid actions. Naloxone can reverse most effects of the opioid agonists, including respiratory depression, coma, and analgesia.

Pharmacologic Effects

When administered in the absence of opioids, naloxone has no significant effects. If administered before giving an opioid, naloxone will block opioid actions. If administered to a patient who is already receiving opioids, naloxone will reverse analgesia, sedation, euphoria, and respiratory depression. If administered to an individual who is physically dependent on opioids, naloxone will precipitate an immediate withdrawal reaction.

Pharmacokinetics

Naloxone may be administered IV, IM, or subQ. After IV injection, effects begin almost immediately and persist about 1 hour. Following IM or subQ injection, effects begin within 2 to 5 minutes and persist several hours. Elimination is by hepatic metabolism. The half-life is approximately 2 hours. Naloxone cannot be used orally because of rapid first-pass inactivation.

Therapeutic Uses

Reversal of Opioid Overdose. Naloxone is the drug of choice for treating overdose with a pure opioid agonist. The drug reverses respiratory depression, coma, and other signs of opioid toxicity. Naloxone can also reverse toxicity from agonist-antagonist opioids (e.g., pentazocine, nalbuphine). However, the doses required may be higher than those needed to reverse poisoning by pure agonists.

Dosage must be carefully titrated when treating toxicity in opioid addicts because the degree of physical dependence in these individuals is usually high, and hence an excessive dose of naloxone can transport the patient from a state of poisoning to one of acute withdrawal. Accordingly, treatment should be initiated with a series of small doses rather than one large dose. Because the half-life of naloxone is shorter than that of most opioids, repeated dosing is required until the crisis has passed.

In some cases of accidental poisoning, there may be uncertainty as to whether unconsciousness is due to opioid overdose or to overdose with a general CNS depressant (e.g., barbiturate, alcohol, benzodiazepine). When uncertainty exists, naloxone is nonetheless indicated. If the cause of poisoning is a barbiturate or another general CNS depressant, naloxone will be of no benefit—but neither will it cause any harm. If a cumulative dose of 10 mg fails to elicit a response, it is unlikely that opioids are involved, and hence other intoxicants should be suspected.

In 2016, the FDA approved the use of naloxone by caregivers of patients using opioids. This decision was secondary to the increase in deaths from opioid overdose. Two formulations are available for outpatient use; nasal spray [Narcan Nasal

Spray] and auto-injector [Evzio]. Both of these drugs are administered by caregivers for the emergency treatment of known or suspected opioid overdose in settings outside of the hospital. After administration, emergency medical care is indicated immediately for continued treatment.

Reversal of Postoperative Opioid Effects. Following surgery, naloxone may be employed to reverse excessive respiratory and CNS depression caused by opioids given preoperatively or intraoperatively. Dosage should be titrated with care; the objective is to achieve adequate ventilation and alertness without reversing opioid actions to the point of unmasking pain.

Reversal of Neonatal Respiratory Depression. When opioids are given for analgesia during labor and delivery, respiratory depression may occur in the neonate. If respiratory depression is substantial, naloxone should be administered to restore ventilation.

Preparations, Dosage, and Administration

Preparations and Routes. Naloxone [Narcan, Evzio] is available in solution (0.4 and 1 mg/mL) for IV, IM, and subQ injection, an auto-injector (2 mg/0.4 mL) sold as *Evzio,* and in a nasal spray (0.4 mg/1 mL and 2 mg/1 mL) sold as *Narcan Nasal Spray.*

Opioid Overdose. If the patient is in a setting outside the hospital, two options are available for caregivers: nasal spray or auto-injector. When using Narcan Nasal Spray, one spray is administered to one nostril, delivering 4 mg of naloxone. If there is no response, additional doses may be given every 2 to 3 minutes until emergency medical services arrive. The auto-injector [Evzio] is a cartridge containing one dose of naloxone that is delivered to the muscle or skin of the outer thigh. The cartridge uses an electronic voice instruction system and blinking lights to help guide the caregiver through proper administration. As with the nasal spray, additional doses may be administered every 2 to 3 minutes until additional medical support arrives.

If the patient is hospitalized, the initial dose is 0.4 mg for adults and 10 mcg/kg for children. The preferred route is IV. However, if IV administration is not possible, then IM or subQ injection may be employed. Dosing is repeated at 2- to 3-minute intervals until a satisfactory response has been achieved. Additional doses may be needed at 1- to 2-hour intervals for up to 72 hours, depending on the duration of the offending opioid.

Postoperative Opioid Effects. Initial therapy for adults consists of 0.1 to 0.2 mg IV repeated every 2 to 3 minutes until an adequate response has been achieved. Additional doses may be required at 1- to 2-hour intervals.

Neonatal Respiratory Depression. The initial dose is 10 mcg/kg (IV, IM, or subQ). This dose is repeated every 2 to 3 minutes until respiration is satisfactory.

Other Opioid Antagonists

Methylnaltrexone

Actions and Therapeutic Use. Methylnaltrexone [Relistor] and naloxegol [Movantik] are selective mu opioid antagonists indicated for opioid-induced constipation in patients with chronic pain who are taking opioids continuously to relieve pain and who have not responded to standard laxative therapy. Benefits derive from blocking mu opioid receptors in the GI tract. Both drugs work in the periphery, and hence do not block opioid receptors in the CNS. Accordingly, the drug does not decrease analgesia and cannot precipitate opioid withdrawal.

Pharmacokinetics. Methylnaltrexone is rapidly absorbed following subQ injection, reaching peak plasma levels within 30 minutes. Naloxegol can be taken orally on a daily basis and has a slightly longer half-life (6 to 11 hours) than methylnaltrexone. Methylnaltrexone undergoes minimal metabolism and is excreted in the urine (50%) and feces (50%), primarily as unchanged drug. The terminal half-life is 8 hours. Naloxegol is metabolized in the liver and largely excreted in the feces (68%).

Adverse Effects, Precautions, and Drug Interactions. Methylnaltrexone and naloxegol are generally well tolerated. The most common adverse effects are *abdominal pain, flatulence, nausea, dizziness,* and *diarrhea.* In the event of severe or persistent diarrhea, the drug should be discontinued. In patients with known or suspected mechanical GI obstruction, methylnaltrexone and naloxegol should be avoided. No significant drug interactions have been reported with methylnaltrexone. Naloxegol should be used with caution in patients taking 3A4 inhibitors.

Preparations, Dosage, and Administration. Methylnaltrexone [Relistor] is available in solution (12 mg/0.6 mL) for subQ injection into the upper arm, abdomen, or thigh. Because defecation can occur rapidly, a bathroom should be immediately available. Dosing is usually done once every 48 hours and should not exceed once every 24 hours. Dosage is based on weight as follows: 8 mg for patients from 38 kg to under 62 kg (84 lb to under 136 lb); 12 mg for patients 62 to 114 kg (136 to 251 lb); and 0.15 mg/kg for patients under 38 kg or over 114 kg. In patients with severe renal impairment, defined as creatinine clearance below 30 mL/min, dosage should be reduced by 50%. Methylnaltrexone should be stored at room temperature and protected from light.

Naloxegol [Movantik] is available in 12.5- and 25-mg tablets for oral administration. Usual dosing is 25 mg daily taken 1 hour before the first meal or 2 hours after the meal. The dose may be decreased by half if the patient does not tolerate initial therapy.

Alvimopan

Like methylnaltrexone, alvimopan [Entereg] is a selective, peripherally acting mu opioid antagonist developed to counteract the adverse effects of opioids on bowel function. At therapeutic doses, alvimopan does not reduce opioid-mediated analgesia, in part because of limited ability to cross the blood-brain barrier. In contrast to methylnaltrexone, which is approved for long-term therapy of constipation in patients taking opioids for chronic pain, alvimopan is approved only for short-term therapy of opioid-induced ileus following partial small or large bowel resection with primary anastomosis. The goal is to accelerate time to recovery of upper and lower bowel function, which can be impaired by opioids used for analgesia during and after surgery.

When used short term in postoperative patients, alvimopan is very well tolerated. However, when used long term in patients taking opioids for chronic pain, the drug has been associated with an increased incidence of myocardial infarction, although a causal relationship has not been established. Because myocardial infarction may be a risk with prolonged dosing, the drug is approved only for short-term (7-day) use and only for hospitalized patients. Furthermore, hospitals that dispense the drug must enroll in the Entereg Access Support and Education program, designed to minimize risk of myocardial infarction.

Alvimopan is available in 12-mg capsules for oral dosing. The regimen consists of 12 mg given 0.5 to 5 hours before surgery, followed by 12 mg twice daily (beginning the day after surgery) for a total of 15 doses or less.

Naltrexone

Naltrexone [ReVia, Vivitrol], given PO or IM, is a pure opioid antagonist used for opioid and alcohol abuse. In opioid abuse, the goal is to prevent euphoria if the abuser should take an opioid. Because naltrexone can precipitate a withdrawal reaction in persons who are physically dependent on opioids, candidates for treatment must be rendered opioid free before naltrexone is started. Although naltrexone can block opioid-induced euphoria, the drug does not prevent craving for opioids. As a result, many addicts fail to comply with treatment. Therapy with naltrexone has been considerably less successful than with methadone, a drug that eliminates craving for opioids while blocking euphoria. Use of naltrexone for alcohol dependence and opioid addiction is discussed in Chapter 38.

When dosage is excessive, naltrexone can cause hepatocellular injury. Accordingly, the drug is contraindicated for patients with acute hepatitis or liver failure. Warn patients about the possibility of liver injury, and advise them to discontinue the drug if signs of hepatitis develop.

Intramuscular administration can cause injection-site reactions, which are sometimes severe. Moderate reactions include pain, tenderness, induration, swelling, erythema, bruising, and pruritus. Severe reactions—cellulitis, hematoma, abscess, necrosis—can cause significant scarring and may require surgical intervention.

TABLE 28.7 ■ Clinical Pharmacology and Pharmacokinetics of Nonopioid Analgesics

Drug and Route	Time Course of Analgesic Effects: Onset (min)	Peak (min)	Half-Life (hr)	Metabolism	Excretion
Clonidine				Hepatic CYP450[a]	Renal, gastrointestinal (bile and feces)
PO	30–45	60–120	4–6		
Dexmedatomidine				Hepatic CYP450[a]: 2A6	Renal, gastrointestinal (feces)
IV	—	6	2		
Tramadol				Hepatic CYP450[a]: 3A4, 2B6, 2D6	Renal
PO (IR)	60	120	6–7		
PO (ER)	—	720	8		
Ziconotide				Renal, hepatic, pulmonary	Renal minimally
IT	—	—	4–5		

[a]CYP450: Cytochrome P450–enzyme specific.
IT, Intrathecally.

Naltrexone is available in two formulations: (1) 50-mg tablets, marketed as *ReVia,* for oral dosing; and (2) an ER suspension (380 mg/vial), marketed as *Vivitrol,* for IM dosing. For oral therapy, a typical dosing schedule consists of 100 mg on Monday and Wednesday and 150 mg on Friday. Alternatively, the drug can be administered daily in 50-mg doses. For IM dosing, the usual regimen is 380 mg once a month.

NONOPIOID CENTRALLY ACTING ANALGESICS

Four centrally acting analgesics—tramadol [Ultram], clonidine [Catapres, Duraclon], ziconotide [Prialt], and dexmedetomidine [Precedex]—relieve pain by mechanisms largely or completely unrelated to opioid receptors (Table 28.7). These drugs cause little or no respiratory depression, physical dependence, or abuse, and, with the exception of tramadol (Schedule IV), are not regulated under the Controlled Substances Act.

Tramadol

Tramadol [Ultram, Ultram ER, Ryzolt, Rybix ODT] is a moderately strong analgesic with a low potential for dependence, abuse, or respiratory depression. The drug relieves pain through a combination of opioid and nonopioid mechanisms.

Mechanism of Action

Tramadol is an analog of codeine that relieves pain in part through weak agonist activity at mu opioid receptors. However, it seems to work primarily by blocking uptake of norepinephrine and serotonin, thereby activating monoaminergic spinal inhibition of pain. Naloxone, an opioid antagonist, only partially blocks tramadol's effects.

Therapeutic Use

Tramadol is approved for moderate to moderately severe pain. The drug is less effective than morphine and no more effective than codeine combined with aspirin or acetaminophen. Analgesia begins 1 hour after oral dosing, is maximal at 2 hours, and continues for 6 hours.

Adverse Effects

Tramadol has been used by millions of patients, and serious adverse effects have been rare. Respiratory depression is minimal at recommended doses. The most common side effects are *sedation, dizziness, headache, dry mouth,* and *constipation. Seizures* have been reported in over 280 patients, and hence the drug should be avoided in patients with epilepsy and other neurologic disorders. Severe allergic reactions occur rarely. Although generally very safe, tramadol can be fatal in overdose, especially when combined with another CNS depressant.

Drug Interactions

Tramadol can intensify responses to *CNS depressants* (e.g., alcohol, benzodiazepines), and therefore should not be combined with these drugs.

By inhibiting uptake of norepinephrine, tramadol can precipitate a hypertensive crisis if combined with a *monoamine oxidase inhibitor.* Accordingly, the combination is absolutely contraindicated.

By inhibiting uptake of serotonin, tramadol can cause *serotonin syndrome* in patients taking *drugs that enhance serotonergic transmission.* Among these are SSRIs, serotonin/norepinephrine reuptake inhibitors, tricyclic antidepressants, MAOIs, and triptans. If these drugs must be combined with tramadol, the patient should be monitored carefully, especially during initial therapy and times of dosage escalation.

Abuse Liability

Abuse liability is low, and hence tramadol is listed as Schedule IV under the Controlled Substances Act. Nonetheless, there have been reports of abuse, dependence, withdrawal, and intentional overdose, presumably for subjective effects. Consequently, tramadol should not be given to patients with a history of drug abuse, and the recommended dosage should not be exceeded.

Warning: Suicide

Tramadol can be a vehicle for suicide. When taken alone, and especially when combined with another CNS depressant, tramadol can cause severe respiratory and CNS depression. Deaths have occurred, primarily in patients with a history of emotional disturbance, suicidal ideation or behavior, or misuse of alcohol and/or other CNS depressants. To reduce risk, tramadol should not be prescribed for patients who are suicidal or addiction prone, and should be used with caution in patients who are depressed, taking sedatives or antidepressants, or prone to excessive alcohol use.

Preparations, Dosage, and Administration

Tramadol is available alone and in combination with acetaminophen. Tramadol alone is available in three formulations: (1) 50-mg IR tablets, sold as *Ultram;* (2) 50-mg orally disintegrating tablets (ODTs), sold as *Rybix ODT;* and (3) ER tablets (100, 200, and 300 mg), sold as *Ultram ER, ConZip,* and *Ryzolt.* Dosages are as follows:

- *IR tablets* [Ultram] and *ODTs* [Rybix ODT]—The recommended adult dosage is 50 to 100 mg every 4 to 6 hours as needed, up to a maximum of 400 mg/day. In patients with significant renal or hepatic impairment, the dosing interval should be increased to 12 hours, and the total daily dose should not exceed 200 mg (with renal impairment) or 100 mg (with hepatic impairment). Inform patients that the ODTs should be placed on the tongue until dissolved (about 1 minute) and then swallowed, with or without water.
- *ER tablets* [Ultram ER, ConZip, Ryzolt]—For patients who are not currently taking IR tramadol, the dosage is 100 mg once a day initially, and then titrated every 5 days in 100-mg increments to a maximum of 300 mg once a day. For patients currently taking IR tramadol, the initial once-daily dosage should equal the total daily dosage of IR tramadol (rounded *down* to the nearest 100 mg). Dosage can then be titrated up or down as needed. ER tramadol should not be used by patients with severe hepatic or renal impairment.

Tramadol *combined with acetaminophen* [Ultracet] is indicated for short-term therapy of acute pain. Each tablet contains 37.5 mg tramadol and 325 mg acetaminophen. The recommended dosage is 2 tablets every 4 to 6 hours (but should not exceed 8 tablets/day). Treatment should not exceed 5 days.

Clonidine

Clonidine [Catapres, Duraclon] has two approved applications: treatment of hypertension and relief of severe pain. To relieve pain, clonidine is administered by continuous epidural infusion. To treat hypertension, the drug is given by mouth or as a transdermal patch. Because the antihypertensive pharmacology of clonidine differs dramatically from its analgesic pharmacology, antihypertensive pharmacology is discussed separately (in Chapters 19 and 47). To avoid errors, you should know that the brand name employed for clonidine depends on the application: When used for pain relief, clonidine is marketed as *Duraclon;* when used for hypertension, the drug is marketed as *Catapres.* Clonidine has no abuse potential and is not regulated under the Controlled Substances Act.

Mechanism of Pain Relief

As discussed in Chapter 19, clonidine is an alpha$_2$-adrenergic agonist. The drug appears to relieve pain by binding with presynaptic and postsynaptic alpha$_2$ receptors in the spinal cord. The result is blockade of nerve traffic in pathways that transmit pain signals from the periphery to the brain. Pain relief is not blocked by opioid antagonists.

Analgesic Use

Clonidine, in combination with an opioid analgesic, is approved for treating severe cancer pain that cannot be relieved by an opioid alone. Administration is by continuous infusion through an implanted epidural catheter. The drug is more effective against neuropathic pain (electrical, burning, or shooting in nature) than diffuse (unlocalized) visceral pain. Pain relief occurs only in regions innervated by sensory nerves that come from the part of the spinal cord where clonidine is present in high concentration.

Adverse Effects

Hypotension. The greatest concern is severe hypotension secondary to extensive vasodilation. The cause of vasodilation is activation of alpha$_2$ receptors in the CNS. Hypotension is most likely during the first 4 days of treatment—and is most intense following infusion into the upper thoracic region of the spinal cord. Because of the risk of hypotension, vital signs should be monitored closely, especially during the first few days. Hypotension can be managed by infusing IV fluids. If necessary, IV ephedrine can be used to promote vasoconstriction.

Bradycardia. Clonidine can slow heart rate. The underlying mechanism is activation of alpha$_2$ receptors in the CNS. Severe bradycardia can be managed with atropine.

Rebound Hypertension. As discussed in Chapter 19, abrupt discontinuation of clonidine can cause rebound hypertension. Accordingly, when the drug is withdrawn, dosage should be tapered over 2 to 4 days. Rebound hypertension can be managed with IV clonidine or labetalol.

Catheter-Related Infection. Infection is common with implanted epidural catheters. If the patient develops a fever of unknown origin, infection should be suspected.

Other Adverse Effects. As with oral clonidine, epidural clonidine can cause *dry mouth, dizziness, sedation, anxiety,* and *depression.*

Contraindications

Because of the risk of severe hypotension and bradycardia, epidural clonidine is contraindicated for patients who are hemodynamically unstable and for obstetric, postpartum, or surgical patients. Additional contraindications are infection at the site of infusion, administration above the C4 dermatome, and use by patients receiving anticoagulants.

Preparations, Dosage, and Administration

Clonidine for analgesia [Duraclon] is available in 10-mL vials containing 100 or 500 mcg/mL. The drug is administered through an implanted epidural catheter using a continuous infusion device. The initial infusion rate is 30 mcg/hr.

Ziconotide

Ziconotide [Prialt] is a centrally acting analgesic with a novel structure and mechanism. Administration is intrathecal (IT). The drug is indicated only for severe chronic pain in patients for whom IT therapy is warranted and who are intolerant of or refractory to other treatments, including systemic and IT morphine. In clinical trials, analgesic responses were modest (at least in opioid-resistant patients), and adverse effects (e.g., hallucinations, confusion, muscle injury) were common. Accordingly, ziconotide cannot be considered a first-choice drug.

Mechanism of Action

Ziconotide is a small synthetic peptide equivalent to a peptide found naturally in *Conus magus,* a marine snail. The drug is a selective antagonist at N-type voltage-sensitive calcium channels on neurons. Benefits derive from blocking calcium channels on primary nociceptive afferent neurons in the dorsal horn of the spinal cord, an action that prevents transmission of pain signals from the periphery to the brain. To maximize analgesia and minimize effects on peripheral nerves, ziconotide must be administered by IT infusion. The drug does not interact with opioid receptors and does not cause tolerance, physical dependence, or respiratory depression. Abrupt discontinuation does not cause a withdrawal syndrome.

Clinical Trials

Ziconotide was evaluated in three randomized, placebo-controlled trials involving patients with severe intractable pain. In all three trials, pain relief was modest. In one trial, for example, patients had severe pain that was unresponsive to IT morphine, IT clonidine, and/or IT bupivacaine. At baseline, mean pain scores were 81 mm, as measured with a Visual Analog Scale of Pain Intensity (where 100 mm equals the worst pain possible and 0 mm equals no pain). Patients were randomized to receive IT ziconotide or IT placebo. The result? At the end of 3 weeks, the mean improvement in pain scores was only 12% in the ziconotide group, compared with 5% in the placebo group. Only 16% of ziconotide recipients improved by 30% or more, and nearly 50% did not respond at all. Keep in mind, however, that none of these patients responded to IT morphine either. Hence, before concluding that ziconotide is not very effective, it would be nice to see whether the drug works well in patients who do respond to morphine.

Adverse Effects

Adverse CNS effects—mainly cognitive impairment and psychiatric symptoms—are common. In clinical trials, patients reported the following cognitive effects: *confusion, memory impairment, speech impairment, aphasia,* and *abnormal thinking.* As a rule, these resolved within 2 weeks after stopping treatment. The most common psychiatric effect—*hallucinations*—developed in 12% of patients. Ziconotide can also cause *paranoid reactions* and *depression.* Use of ziconotide is contraindicated in patients with a pre-existing history of psychosis.

Ziconotide can cause *muscle injury.* In clinical trials, 40% of patients had abnormally high serum levels of creatine kinase (CK), a marker for muscle breakdown. However, serious muscle pain, soreness, or weakness was uncommon. Because of the risk of muscle injury, serum CK should be monitored. In patients with high CK levels combined with symptoms of muscle injury, the prescriber should consider reducing ziconotide dosage or discontinuing treatment.

Drug Interactions

Formal studies on drug interactions have not been conducted. However, given that ziconotide is a peptide that is not metabolized by CYP450 isoenzymes, the drug is unlikely to affect the disposition of most other drugs, which *are* metabolized by CYP450 isoenzymes. Combined use with CNS depressants may increase the risk of adverse CNS events, such as dizziness and confusion. Combined use with *systemic* opioids appears safe, but combined use with *intrathecal* opioids is not recommended.

Preparations, Dosage, and Administration

Ziconotide [Prialt] is available in single-use vials (25 and 100 mcg/mL) for IT infusion using a programmable microinfusion device, either external or implanted. The initial infusion rate is 0.1 mcg/hr (2.4 mcg/day). The rate may be gradually increased in steps of 0.1 mcg/hr every 2 to 3 days, up to a maximum of 0.8 mcg/hr (19.2 mcg/day) at the end of 3 weeks. Dosage adjustments are based on pain relief and tolerability of side effects.

Dexmedetomidine

Actions and Therapeutic Use

Dexmedetomidine [Precedex], like clonidine, is a selective alpha$_2$-adrenergic agonist. The drug acts in the CNS to cause sedation and analgesia. The drug has two approved indications: (1) short-term sedation in critically ill patients who are initially intubated and undergoing mechanical ventilation and (2) sedation for nonintubated patients before and/or during surgical and other procedures. However, in addition to these approved uses, dexmedetomidine has a variety of off-label uses, including sedation during awake craniotomy, prevention and treatment of postanesthetic shivering, and enhancement of sedation and analgesia in patients undergoing general anesthesia. In contrast to clonidine, which is administered by epidural infusion, dexmedetomidine is administered by IV infusion.

Adverse Effects

The most common adverse effects are *hypotension* and *bradycardia.* The mechanism is activation of alpha$_2$-adrenergic receptors in the CNS and periphery, which results in decreased release of norepinephrine from sympathetic neurons innervating the heart and blood vessels. If these cardiovascular effects are too intense, they can be managed in several ways, including (1) decreasing or stopping the infusion, (2) infusing fluid, and (3) elevating the lower extremities. Giving a muscarinic antagonist (e.g., atropine) can increase heart rate.

Additional adverse effects include *nausea, dry mouth,* and *transient hypertension.* Importantly, dexmedetomidine does *not* cause respiratory depression.

Drug Interactions

Dexmedetomidine can enhance the actions of anesthetics, sedatives, hypnotics, and opioids. Excessive CNS depression can be managed by reducing the dosage of dexmedetomidine or the other agents.

Preparations, Dosage, and Administration

Dexmedetomidine [Precedex] is supplied in solution (100 mcg/mL), which must be diluted to 4 mcg/mL before use. Administration is by IV infusion. For *intensive care sedation,* treatment consists of a loading dose (1 mcg/kg infused over 10 minutes) followed by a maintenance infusion of 0.2 to 0.7 mcg/kg/hr for no more than 24 hours. For *procedural sedation,* treatment typically consists of a loading dose (1 mcg/kg infused over 10 minutes) followed by a maintenance infusion of 0.2 to 1 mcg/kg/hr.

KEY POINTS

- Analgesics are drugs that relieve pain without causing loss of consciousness.
- Opioids are the most effective analgesics available.
- There are three major classes of opioid receptors, designated mu, kappa, and delta.
- Morphine and other pure opioid agonists relieve pain by mimicking the actions of endogenous opioid peptides—primarily at mu receptors, and partly at kappa receptors.
- Opioid-induced sedation and euphoria can complement pain relief.
- Because opioids produce euphoria and other desirable subjective effects, they have a high liability for abuse.
- Respiratory depression is the most serious adverse effect of the opioids.
- Other important adverse effects are constipation, urinary retention, orthostatic hypotension, emesis, miosis, birth defects, and elevation of ICP.
- Because of first-pass metabolism, oral doses of morphine must be larger than parenteral doses to produce equivalent analgesic effects.
- Because the blood-brain barrier is poorly developed in infants, these patients need smaller doses of opioids (adjusted for body weight) than do older children and adults.
- With prolonged opioid use, tolerance develops to analgesia, euphoria, sedation, and respiratory depression, but not to constipation and miosis.
- Cross-tolerance exists among the various opioid agonists, but not between opioid agonists and general CNS depressants.
- With prolonged opioid use, physical dependence develops. An abstinence syndrome will occur if the opioid is abruptly withdrawn.
- In contrast to the withdrawal syndrome associated with general CNS depressants, the withdrawal syndrome associated with opioids, although unpleasant, is not dangerous.
- To minimize symptoms of abstinence, opioids should be withdrawn gradually.
- Precautions to opioid use include pregnancy, labor and delivery, head injury, and decreased respiratory reserve.
- Patients taking opioids should avoid alcohol and other CNS depressants because these drugs can intensify opioid-induced sedation and respiratory depression.
- Patients taking opioids should avoid anticholinergic drugs (e.g., antihistamines, tricyclic antidepressants, atropine-like drugs) because these drugs can exacerbate opioid-induced constipation and urinary retention.
- Opioid overdose produces a classic triad of signs: coma, respiratory depression, and pinpoint pupils.
- All strong opioid agonists are essentially equal to morphine with regard to analgesia, abuse liability, and respiratory depression.
- Use of meperidine should be avoided so as to prevent accumulation of normeperidine, a toxic metabolite.
- Like morphine, codeine and other moderate to strong opioid agonists produce analgesia, sedation, euphoria, respiratory depression, constipation, urinary retention, cough suppression, and miosis. These drugs differ from morphine in that they produce less analgesia and respiratory depression and have a lower potential for abuse.
- The combination of codeine with a nonopioid analgesic (e.g., aspirin, acetaminophen) produces greater pain relief than can be achieved with either agent alone.
- Most agonist-antagonist opioids act as agonists at kappa receptors and antagonists at mu receptors.
- Pentazocine and other agonist-antagonist opioids produce less analgesia than morphine and have a lower potential for abuse.
- With agonist-antagonist opioids, there is a ceiling to respiratory depression.
- If given to a patient who is physically dependent on pure opioid agonists, an agonist-antagonist will precipitate withdrawal.
- Pure opioid antagonists act as antagonists at mu receptors and kappa receptors.
- Naloxone and other pure opioid antagonists can reverse respiratory depression, coma, analgesia, and most other effects of pure opioid agonists. The only exception is methylnaltrexone, which doesn't cross the blood-brain barrier.
- Pure opioid antagonists are used primarily to treat opioid overdose. Two agents—methylnaltrexone and naloxegol—are used for opioid-induced constipation, and another—alvimopan—for opioid-induced ileus.
- If administered in excessive dosage to an individual who is physically dependent on opioid agonists, naloxone will precipitate an immediate withdrawal reaction.
- Opioid dosage must be individualized. Patients with a low tolerance to pain or with extremely painful conditions need high doses. Patients with sharp, stabbing pain need higher doses than patients with dull pain. Older adults generally require lower doses than younger adults. Neonates require relatively low doses.

- As a rule, opioids should be administered on a fixed schedule for the first 24 hours postoperatively (with supplemental doses for breakthrough pain) rather than PRN.
- Most PCA devices are electronically controlled pumps that can be activated by the patient to deliver a preset dose of opioid through an indwelling catheter. Some PCA devices also deliver a basal opioid infusion.
- PCA devices provide steady plasma drug levels, thereby maintaining continuous pain control while avoiding unnecessary sedation and respiratory depression.
- Use of parenteral opioids during delivery can suppress uterine contractions and cause respiratory depression in the neonate.
- Addiction is a primary chronic disease characterized by an individual pathologically pursuing rewards and/or relief by substance use and other behaviors. Physical dependence and addiction are not the same.
- Abuse is defined as drug use that is inconsistent with medical or social norms.
- Because of excessive and inappropriate fears about addiction and abuse, providers frequently prescribe less pain medication than patients need, and nurses frequently administer less medication than was prescribed.
- Dispel your concerns about abuse and addiction, and give your patients the medication they need to relieve suffering. That's what opioids are for, after all.

Please visit http://evolve.elsevier.com/Lehne for chapter-specific NCLEX® examination review questions.

Summary of Major Nursing Implications[a]

PURE OPIOID AGONISTS

Alfentanil
Codeine
Fentanyl
Hydrocodone
Hydromorphone
Levorphanol
Meperidine
Methadone
Morphine
Oxycodone
Oxymorphone
Remifentanil
Sufentanil
Tapentadol

Preadministration Assessment

Therapeutic Goal

Relief or prevention of moderate to severe pain while causing minimal respiratory depression, constipation, urinary retention, and other adverse effects.

Baseline Data

Pain Assessment. Assess pain before administration and 1 hour later. Determine the location, time of onset, and quality of pain (e.g., sharp, stabbing, dull). Also, assess for psychologic factors that can lower pain threshold (anxiety, depression, fear, anger). Because pain is subjective and determined by multiple factors (e.g., cultural influences, patient expectations, associated disease), there is no reliable objective method for determining how much discomfort the patient is experiencing. Ultimately, you must rely on your ability to interpret what patients have to say about their pain. When listening to patients, be aware that a few may claim discomfort when their pain is under control, and others may claim to feel fine when they actually hurt.

Vital Signs. Before administration, determine respiratory rate, blood pressure, and pulse rate.

Identifying High-Risk Patients

All opioids are *contraindicated* for premature infants (both during and after delivery). *Morphine* is *contraindicated* following biliary tract surgery. *Meperidine* is *contraindicated* for patients taking MAOIs.

Use opioids with *caution* in patients with head injury, profound CNS depression, coma, respiratory depression, pulmonary disease (e.g., emphysema, asthma), cardiovascular disease, hypotension, reduced blood volume, benign prostatic hypertrophy, urethral stricture, and liver impairment. *Caution* is also required when treating infants, older adult or debilitated patients, and patients receiving MAOIs, CNS depressants, anticholinergic drugs, and hypotensive agents. In addition, use opioids with *caution* in patients deemed at high risk of opioid abuse.

Implementation: Administration

Routes

Oral, IM, IV, subQ, rectal, epidural, intrathecal, transdermal (fentanyl), and transmucosal (fentanyl). Routes for specific opioids are shown in Tables 28.5 and 28.6.

Dosage

General Guidelines. Adjust dosage to meet individual needs. Higher doses are required for patients with low pain tolerance or with especially painful conditions. Patients with sharp, stabbing pain need higher doses than patients with dull, constant pain. Older adult patients generally require lower doses than younger adults. Neonates require relatively low doses because the blood-brain barrier is poorly developed. For all patients, dosage should be reduced as pain subsides.

Oral doses are larger than parenteral doses. Check to ensure that the dose is appropriate for the intended route.

Tolerance may develop with prolonged treatment, necessitating dosage escalation.

Warn outpatients not to increase dosage without consulting the prescriber.

Dosage in Patients With Cancer. Treatment of cancer pain is done long term. The objective is to maximize comfort.

Continued

Physical dependence is a minor concern. Cancer patients should receive opioids on a fixed schedule around-the-clock—not PRN. If breakthrough pain occurs, fixed dosing should be supplemented PRN with a short-acting opioid. Because of tolerance to opioids or intensification of pain, dosage escalation may be required. Hence, patients should be re-evaluated on a regular basis to determine if pain control is adequate.

Discontinuing Opioids. Although significant dependence in hospitalized patients is rare, it can occur. To minimize symptoms of abstinence, withdraw opioids slowly, tapering the dosage over 3 days. **Warn outpatients against abrupt discontinuation of treatment.**

Administration

Before administration, determine respiratory rate, blood pressure, and pulse rate. Withhold medication and notify the prescriber if respiratory rate is at or below 12 breaths per minute, if blood pressure is significantly below the pretreatment value, or if pulse rate is significantly above or below the pretreatment value.

As a rule, opioids should be administered on a fixed schedule during the first 24 hours postoperatively, with supplemental doses as needed.

Perform IV injections slowly (over 4 to 5 minutes). Rapid injection may produce severe adverse effects (profound hypotension, respiratory arrest, cardiac arrest) and should be avoided. When making an IV injection, have an opioid antagonist (e.g., naloxone) and facilities for respiratory support available.

Perform injections (especially IV) with the patient lying down to minimize hypotension.

Warn patients using fentanyl patches to avoid exposing the patch to direct heat (e.g., heating pad, hot tub) because doing so can accelerate fentanyl release.

Warn patients not to crush or chew controlled-release oxycodone [OxyContin] tablets.

Warn patients using morphine/naltrexone [Embeda] not to crush or chew the capsules or to drink alcohol, because these actions can accelerate absorption of morphine from the product.

Instruct patients using tramadol ODTs [Rybix ODT] to place the tablet on the tongue until it dissolves (about 1 minute) and then to swallow with or without water.

Opioid agonists are regulated under the Controlled Substances Act and must be dispensed accordingly. All pure agonists are Schedule II substances.

Concern for Opioid Abuse as a Factor in Dosage and Administration. Although opioids have a high potential for abuse, abuse is rare in the clinical setting. Consequently, when balancing the risk of abuse against the need to relieve pain, do not give excessive weight to concerns about abuse. The patient must not be allowed to suffer because of your unwarranted fears about abuse and dependence.

Although abuse is rare in the clinical setting, it can occur. To keep abuse to a minimum: (1) screen patients for abuse risk, (2) exercise clinical judgment when interpreting requests for opioid doses that seem excessive, (3) use opioids in the lowest effective doses for the shortest time required, (4) reserve opioid analgesics for patients with moderate to severe pain, and (5) switch to a nonopioid analgesic when the intensity of pain no longer justifies an opioid.

Responses to analgesics can be reinforced by nondrug measures, such as positioning the patient comfortably, showing concern and interest, and reassuring the patient that the medication will provide relief. Rest, mood elevation, and diversion can raise pain threshold and should be promoted. Conversely, anxiety, depression, fatigue, fear, and anger can lower pain threshold and should be minimized.

Ongoing Evaluation and Interventions

Evaluating Therapeutic Effects

Evaluate for pain control 1 hour after opioid administration. If analgesia is insufficient, consult the prescriber about an increase in dosage. Patients taking opioids chronically for suppression of cancer pain should be re-evaluated on a regular basis to determine whether dosage is adequate.

Minimizing Adverse Effects

Respiratory Depression. Monitor respiration in all patients. If respiratory rate is 12 breaths per minute or less, withhold medication and notify the prescriber. **Warn outpatients about respiratory depression, and instruct them to notify the prescriber if respiratory distress occurs.**

Certain patients, including the very young, older adults, and those with respiratory disease (e.g., asthma, emphysema), are especially sensitive to respiratory depression and must be monitored closely.

Delayed respiratory depression may develop following spinal administration of morphine. Be alert to this possibility.

When employed during labor and delivery, opioids may cause respiratory depression in the neonate. Monitor the infant closely. Have naloxone available to reverse opioid toxicity.

Sedation. **Inform patients that opioids may cause drowsiness. Warn them against doing hazardous activities (e.g., driving) if sedation is significant.** Sedation can be minimized by (1) using smaller doses given more frequently, (2) using opioids with short half-lives, and (3) giving small doses of a CNS stimulant (methylphenidate, dextroamphetamine) in the morning and early afternoon. Modafinil, a nonamphetamine stimulant, may also be tried.

Orthostatic Hypotension. Monitor blood pressure and pulse rate. **Inform patients about symptoms of hypotension (dizziness, light-headedness), and advise them to sit or lie down if these occur. Inform patients that hypotension can be minimized by moving slowly when standing. Warn patients against walking if hypotension is significant.** If indicated, assist hospitalized patients with ambulation.

Constipation. The risk of constipation can be reduced by maintaining physical activity, increasing intake of fiber and fluids, and prophylactic treatment with a stimulant laxative (e.g., senna, bisacodyl) plus a stool softener (e.g., docusate) and perhaps polyethylene glycol (an osmotic laxative). A strong osmotic laxative (e.g., lactulose, sodium phosphate) may be used for rescue therapy. If these measures fail, methylnaltrexone or naloxegol (opioid antagonists) may help.

Urinary Retention. To evaluate urinary retention, monitor intake and output, and palpate the lower abdomen for bladder distention every 4 to 6 hours. If there is a change in intake/output ratio, if bladder distention is detected, or if the patient reports difficulty voiding, notify the prescriber. Catheterization may be required. Difficulty with voiding is especially likely in men with benign prostatic hypertrophy. **Because opioids may suppress awareness of bladder stimuli, encourage patients to void every 4 hours.**

Biliary Colic. By constricting the common bile duct, morphine can increase pressure within the biliary tract, thereby causing severe pain. Biliary colic may be less pronounced with meperidine.

Emesis. Initial doses of opioids may cause nausea and vomiting. These reactions can be minimized by pretreatment with an antiemetic (e.g., promethazine) and by having the patient remain still. Tolerance to emesis develops quickly.

Cough Suppression. Cough suppression may result in accumulation of secretions in the airway. **Instruct patients to cough at regular intervals.** Auscultate the lungs for crackles.

Miosis. Miosis can impair vision in dim light. Keep hospital room lighting bright during waking hours.

Neurotoxicity. Neurotoxicity—delirium, agitation, myoclonus, hyperalgesia—can develop with prolonged high-dose therapy. Symptoms can be reduced with hydration, dose reduction, and opioid rotation.

Birth Defects. When taken just before conception or during early pregnancy, opioids increase the risk of spina bifida, gastroschisis, and congenital heart defects (e.g., atrioventricular septal defects, hypoplastic left heart syndrome, conoventricular septal defects). Use of opioids before and during pregnancy should be discouraged.

Opioid Dependence in the Neonate. The infant whose mother abused opioids during pregnancy may be born drug dependent. Observe the infant for signs of withdrawal (e.g., excessive crying, sneezing, tremor, hyperreflexia, fever, diarrhea), which usually develop within a few days after birth. The infant can be weaned from drug dependence by administering dilute paregoric in progressively smaller doses.

Dysrhythmias. Methadone prolongs the QT interval, and hence can pose a risk of fatal dysrhythmias. Use methadone with great caution in patients with existing QT prolongation or a family history of long QT syndrome, and in those taking other QT-prolonging drugs (e.g., amiodarone, quinidine, erythromycin, tricyclic antidepressants). All patients should receive an ECG before treatment, 30 days later, and annually thereafter. If the QT interval exceeds 500 msec, stopping methadone or reducing the dosage should be considered.

Minimizing Adverse Interactions

CNS Depressants. Opioids can intensify responses to other CNS depressants (e.g., barbiturates, benzodiazepines, alcohol, antihistamines), thereby presenting a risk of profound sedation and respiratory depression. **Warn patients against the use of alcohol and other depressants.**

Anticholinergic Drugs. These agents (e.g., atropine-like drugs, tricyclic antidepressants, phenothiazines, antihistamines) can exacerbate opioid-induced constipation and urinary retention.

Hypotensive Drugs. Antihypertensive agents and other drugs that lower blood pressure can exacerbate opioid-induced orthostatic hypotension.

Opioid Antagonists. Opioid antagonists (e.g., naloxone) can precipitate an abstinence syndrome if administered in excessive dosage to a patient who is physically dependent on opioids. To avoid this problem, carefully titrate the dosage of the antagonist.

Agonist-Antagonist Opioids. These drugs (e.g., pentazocine, nalbuphine) can precipitate an abstinence syndrome if administered to a patient who is physically dependent on a pure opioid agonist. Before administering an agonist-antagonist, make certain the patient has been withdrawn from opioid agonists.

MAOIs. Combining *meperidine* or *tapentadol* with an MAOI can cause delirium, hyperthermia, rigidity, convulsion, coma, and death. Obviously, these combinations must be avoided.

CYP3A4 Inhibitors. Inhibitors of CYP3A4 (e.g., ritonavir, ketoconazole) can increase levels of *fentanyl,* thereby posing a risk of fatal respiratory depression. Monitor patients using this combination with care.

AGONIST-ANTAGONIST OPIOIDS

Buprenorphine
Butorphanol
Nalbuphine
Pentazocine

Except for the differences presented in the following sections, the nursing implications for these drugs are much like those for the pure opioid agonists.

Therapeutic Goal

Relief of moderate to severe pain.

Routes

Oral, IV, IM, and subQ. Routes for individual agents are shown in Table 28.6.

Differences From Pure Opioid Agonists

Maximal pain relief with the agonist-antagonists is generally lower than with pure opioid agonists.

Most agonist-antagonists have a ceiling to respiratory depression, thereby minimizing concerns about insufficient oxygenation.

Agonist-antagonists cause little euphoria. Hence, abuse liability is low.

Agonist-antagonists increase cardiac work and should not be given to patients with acute myocardial infarction.

Because of their antagonist properties, agonist-antagonists can precipitate an abstinence syndrome in patients physically dependent on opioid agonists. Accordingly, patients must be withdrawn from pure opioid agonists before receiving an agonist-antagonist.

NALOXONE

Therapeutic Goal

Reversal of postoperative opioid effects, opioid-induced neonatal respiratory depression, and overdose with pure opioid agonists.

Routes

Intravenous, IM, and subQ. For initial treatment, administer IV. Once opioid-induced CNS depression and respiratory depression have been reversed, IM or subQ administration may be employed.

Dosage

Titrate dosage carefully. In opioid addicts, excessive doses can precipitate withdrawal. In postoperative patients, excessive doses can unmask pain by reversing opioid-mediated analgesia.

[a]Patient education information is highlighted as **blue text.**

CHAPTER

29 Pain Management in Patients With Cancer

Our topic—management of cancer pain—is of note both for its good news and its bad news. The good news is that cancer pain can be relieved with simple interventions in 90% of patients. The bad news is that, despite the availability of effective treatments, pain goes unrelieved far too often. Multiple factors contribute to undertreatment (Table 29.1). Important among these are inadequate prescriber training in pain management, unfounded fears of addiction (shared by prescribers, patients, and families), and a healthcare system that focuses more on treating disease than relieving suffering.

Pain has a profound impact on both the patient and family. Pain undermines quality of life for the patient and puts a heavy burden on the family. Unrelieved pain compromises the patient's ability to work, enjoy leisure activities, and fulfill his or her role in the family and in society at large. Furthermore, pain can impede recovery, hasten death from cancer, and possibly even create a risk of suicide.

Every patient has the right to expect that pain management will be an integral part of treatment throughout the course of his or her disease. The goal is to minimize pain and thereby maintain a reasonable quality of life, including the ability to function at work and at play, and within the family and society. In addition, if the cancer is incurable, treatment should permit the patient a relatively painless death when that time comes.

PATHOPHYSIOLOGY OF PAIN

What Is Pain?

The International Association for the Study of Pain defines pain as "an unpleasant sensory and emotional experience associated with actual or potential tissue damage, or described in terms of such damage." Note that, by this definition, pain is not simply a sensory experience resulting from activation of pain receptors. Rather, it also includes the patient's emotional and cognitive responses to both the sensation of pain and the underlying cause (e.g., tissue damage caused by cancer). Most importantly, we must appreciate that pain is inherently *personal and subjective*. Hence, when assessing pain, the most reliable method is to have the patient describe his or her experience.

Neurophysiologic Basis of Painful Sensations

The following discussion is a simplified version of how we perceive pain. Nonetheless, it should be adequate as a basis for understanding the interventions used for pain relief.

Sensation of pain is the net result of activity in two opposing neuronal pathways. The first pathway carries pain impulses from their site of origin to the brain and thereby generates pain sensation. The second pathway, which originates in the brain, suppresses impulse conduction along the first pathway and thereby diminishes pain sensation.

Pain impulses are initiated by activation of pain receptors, which are simply free nerve endings. These receptors can be activated by three types of stimuli: mechanical (e.g., pressure), thermal, and chemical (e.g., bradykinin, serotonin, histamine). In addition, *prostaglandins* and *substance P* can enhance the sensitivity of pain receptors to activation, although these compounds do not activate pain receptors directly.

Conduction of pain impulses from the periphery to the brain occurs by way of a multineuron pathway. The first neuron carries impulses from the periphery to a synapse in the spinal cord, where it releases either *glutamate* or *substance P* as a transmitter. The next neuron carries the impulse up the cord

TABLE 29.1 ■ Barriers to Cancer Pain Management

BARRIERS RELATED TO HEALTHCARE PROFESSIONALS
Inadequate knowledge of pain management
Poor assessment of pain
Concerns stemming from regulations on controlled substances
Fear of patient addiction
Concern about side effects of analgesics
Concern about tolerance to analgesics
BARRIERS RELATED TO PATIENTS
Reluctance to report pain
Fear of distracting physicians from treating the cancer
Fear that pain means the cancer is worse
Concern about not being a "good" patient
Reluctance to take pain medication
Fear of addiction or being thought of as an addict
Worries about unmanageable side effects
Concern about becoming tolerant to pain medications
Inability to pay for treatment
BARRIERS RELATED TO THE HEALTHCARE SYSTEM
Low priority given to cancer pain management
Inadequate reimbursement: The most appropriate treatment may not be reimbursed
Restrictive regulation of controlled substances
Treatment is unavailable or access is limited

Adapted from Jacox A, Carr DB, Payne R, et al: Management of Cancer Pain (Clinical Practice Guideline No. 9; AHCPR Publication No. 94-0592). Rockville, MD: Agency for Health Care Policy and Research, 1994.

to a synapse in the thalamus. And the next neuron carries impulses from the thalamus to the cerebral cortex.

The brain is able to suppress pain conduction using endogenous opioid compounds, especially *enkephalins* and *beta-endorphin.* These compounds are released at synapses in the brain and spinal cord. Release within the spinal cord is controlled by a descending neuronal pathway that originates in the brain. The opioids that we give as drugs (e.g., morphine) produce analgesia by activating the same receptors that are activated by this endogenous pain-suppressing system.

Nociceptive Pain Versus Neuropathic Pain

In patients with cancer, pain has two major forms, referred to as *nociceptive* and *neuropathic.* Nociceptive pain results from injury to *tissues,* whereas neuropathic pain results from injury to *peripheral nerves.* These two forms of pain respond differently to analgesic drugs. Accordingly, it is important to differentiate between them. Among cancer patients, nociceptive pain is more common than neuropathic pain.

Nociceptive pain has two forms, known as *somatic* and *visceral.* Somatic pain results from injury to somatic tissues (e.g., bones, joints, muscles), whereas visceral pain results from injury to visceral organs (e.g., small intestine). Patients generally describe somatic pain as localized and sharp. In contrast, they describe visceral pain as vaguely localized with a diffuse, aching quality. Both forms of nociceptive pain respond well to *opioid analgesics* (e.g., morphine). In addition, they may respond to *nonopioids* (e.g., ibuprofen).

Neuropathic pain produces different sensations than does nociceptive pain and responds to a different group of drugs. Patients describe neuropathic pain with such words as "burning," "shooting," "jabbing," "tearing," "numb," "dead," and "cold." Unlike nociceptive pain, neuropathic pain responds poorly to opioid analgesics. However, it does respond to drugs known collectively as *adjuvant analgesics.* Among these are certain antidepressants (e.g., duloxetine), anticonvulsants (e.g., carbamazepine, gabapentin), and local anesthetics/antidysrhythmics (e.g., lidocaine).

Pain in Cancer Patients

Among patients with cancer, pain can be caused by the cancer itself and by therapeutic interventions. Cancer can cause pain through direct invasion of surrounding tissues (e.g., nerves, muscles, visceral organs) and through metastatic invasion at distant sites. Metastases to bone are very common, causing pain in up to 50% of patients. Cancer can cause neuropathic pain through infiltration of nerves, and visceral pain through infiltration, obstruction, and compression of visceral structures.

The incidence and intensity of cancer-induced pain is a function of cancer type and the stage of disease progression. Among patients with advanced disease, about 75% experience significant pain. Of these, 40% to 50% report moderate to severe pain, and 25% to 30% report very severe pain.

Therapeutic interventions—especially chemotherapy, radiation, and surgery—cause significant pain in at least 25% of patients, and probably more. Chemotherapy can cause painful mucositis, diffuse neuropathies, and aseptic necrosis of joints. Radiation can cause osteonecrosis, chronic visceral pain, and peripheral neuropathy (secondary to causing fibrosis of nerves). Surgery can cause a variety of pain syndromes, including phantom limb syndrome and postmastectomy syndrome.

MANAGEMENT STRATEGY

Management of cancer pain is an ongoing process that involves repeating cycles of assessment, intervention, and reassessment. The goal is to create and implement a flexible treatment plan that can meet the changing needs of the individual patient. Fig. 29.1 shows the steps involved. Management begins with a comprehensive assessment. Once the nature of the pain has been determined, a treatment modality is selected. Analgesic drugs are preferred, and hence are usually tried first. If drugs are ineffective, other modalities can be implemented. Among these are radiation, surgery, and nerve blocks. After each intervention, pain is reassessed. Once relief has been achieved, the effective intervention is continued, accompanied by frequent reassessments. If severe pain returns or new pain develops, a new comprehensive assessment should be performed—followed by appropriate interventions and reassessment. Throughout this process, the healthcare team should make every effort to ensure active involvement of the patient and his or her family. Without their involvement, maximal benefits cannot be achieved.

ASSESSMENT AND ONGOING EVALUATION

Assessment is the foundation of treatment. In the absence of thorough assessment, effective pain management is impossible. Assessment begins with a comprehensive evaluation and then

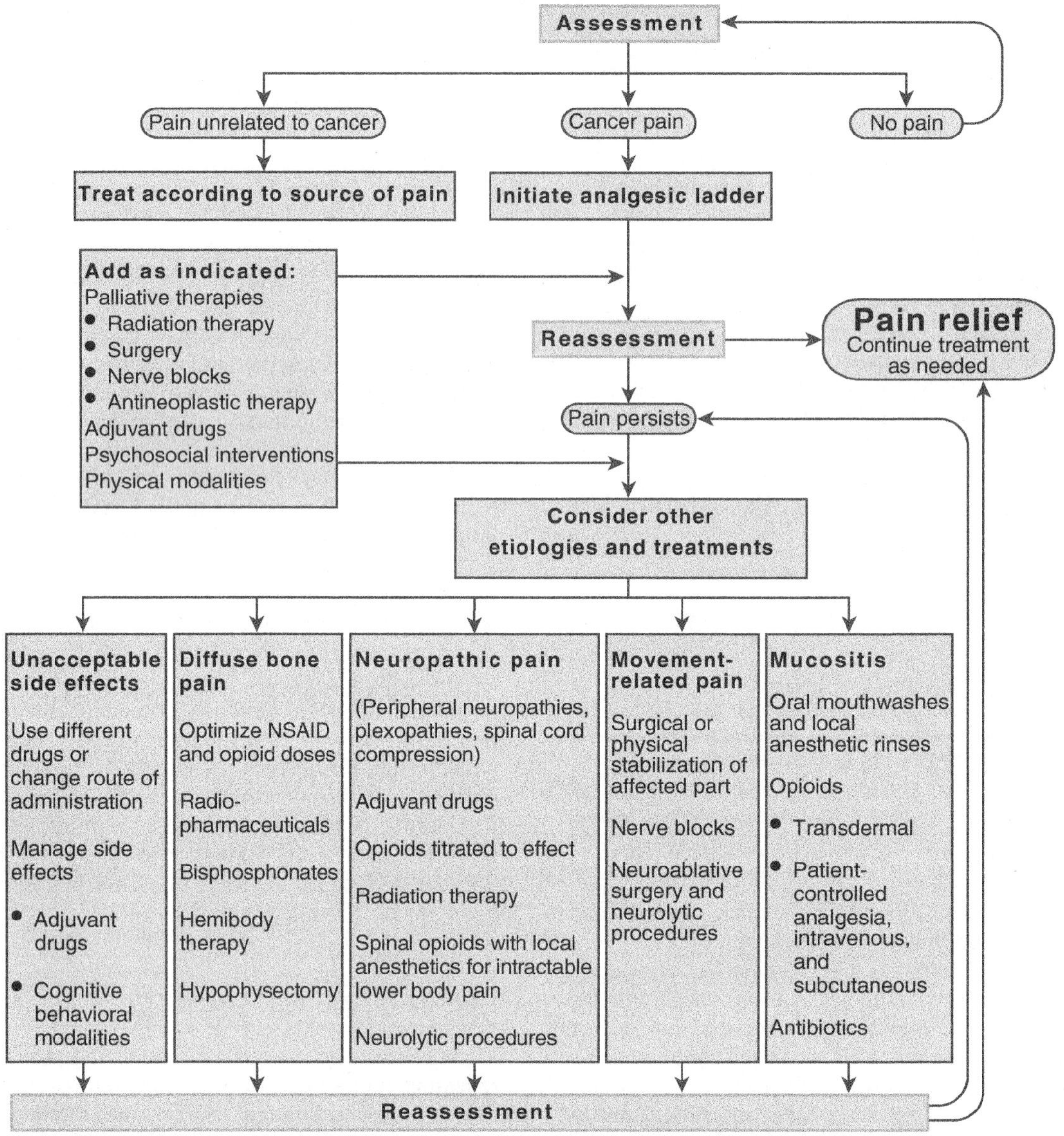

Fig. 29.1 ■ Flow chart for pain management in patients with cancer.
NSAID, Nonsteroidal anti-inflammatory drug. (Adapted from Jacox A, Carr DB, Payne R, et al: Management of Cancer Pain [Clinical Practice Guideline No. 9; AHCPR Publication No. 94-0592]. Rockville, MD: Agency for Health Care Policy and Research, 1994.)

continues with regular follow-up evaluations. The initial assessment provides the basis for designing the treatment program. Follow-ups let us know how well treatment is working.

Comprehensive Initial Assessment

The initial assessment employs an extensive array of tests. The primary objective is to characterize the pain and identify its cause. This information provides the basis for designing a pain management plan. In addition, by documenting the patient's baseline pain status, the initial assessment provides a basis for evaluating the efficacy of treatment.

Assessment of Pain Intensity and Character: The Patient Self-Report

The patient's description of his or her pain is the cornerstone of pain assessment. No other component of assessment is more important! Remember, pain is a personal experience. Accordingly, if we want to assess pain, we must rely on the patient to tell us about it. Furthermore, we must act on what the patient says—even if we personally believe the patient may not be telling the truth.

The best way to ensure an accurate report is to ask the right questions and listen carefully to the answers. We cannot elicit comprehensive information by asking, "How do you feel?" Rather, we must ask a series of specific questions. The answers should be recorded on a pain inventory form. The following information should be obtained:

Onset and temporal pattern: When did your pain begin? How often does it occur? Has the intensity increased, decreased, or remained constant? Does the intensity vary throughout the day?

Location: Where is your pain? Do you feel pain in more than one place? Ask patients to point to the exact location of the pain, either on themselves, on you, or on a full-body drawing.

Quality: What does your pain feel like? Is it sharp or dull? Does it ache? Is it shooting or stabbing? Burning or tingling? These questions can help distinguish neuropathic pain from nociceptive pain.

Intensity: On a scale of 0 to 10, with 0 being no pain and 10 the most intense pain you can imagine, how would you rank your pain now? How would you rank your pain at its worst? And at its best? A pain intensity scale (see *Pain Intensity Scales* later in this section) can be very helpful for this assessment.

Modulating factors: What makes your pain worse? What makes it better?

Previous treatment: What treatments have you tried to relieve your pain (e.g., analgesics, acupuncture, relaxation techniques)? Are they effective now? If not, were they ever effective in the past?

Impact: How does the pain affect your ability to function, both physically and socially? For example, does the pain interfere with your general mobility, work, eating, sleeping, socializing, or sex life?

Physical and Neurologic Examinations

The physical and neurologic examinations help to further characterize the pain, identify its source, and identify any complications related to the underlying pathology. The clinician should examine the site of pain and determine if palpation or manipulation makes it worse. Nonverbal cues (e.g., protecting the painful area, limited movement in an arm or leg) that may indicate pain should be noted. Common patterns of referred pain should be assessed. For example, if the patient has hip pain, the assessment should determine whether the pain actually originates in the hip or is referred pain caused by pathology in the lumbar spine. Potential neurologic complications should be considered. For example, patients with back pain should be evaluated for impaired motor and sensory function in the limbs, and for impaired rectal and urinary sphincter function, which may indicate spinal cord involvement.

Diagnostic Tests

Diagnostic tests are performed to identify the underlying cause of pain (e.g., progression of cancer, tissue injury caused by cancer treatments). The battery of diagnostic tests includes imaging studies (e.g., computed tomography scan, magnetic resonance imaging), neurophysiologic tests, and tests for tumor markers in blood. To ensure that abnormalities identified in the diagnostic tests really do explain the patient's pain, these findings should be correlated with findings from the physical and neurologic examinations.

Psychosocial Assessment

Psychosocial assessment is directed at both the patient and his or her family. The information is used in making pain management decisions. Some important issues to address include:

- The impact of significant pain on the patient in the past
- The patient's usual coping responses to pain and stress
- The patient's preferences regarding pain management methods
- The patient's concerns about using opioids and other controlled substances (anxiolytics, stimulants)
- Changes in the patient's mood (anxiety, depression) brought on by cancer and pain
- The impact of cancer and its treatment on the family
- The level of care the family can provide and the potential need for outside help (e.g., palliative care or hospice)

Pain Intensity Scales

Pain intensity scales are useful tools for assessing pain intensity. Representative scales are shown in Figs. 29.2 and 29.3. The *descriptive scale* and *numeric scale* (see Fig. 29.2) are used for adults and older children. The *pain affect FACES scale* (see Fig. 29.3) is used for young children and for patients with cognitive impairment, who may have difficulty understanding the descriptive and numeric scales.

Pain intensity scales are valuable not only for assessing pain intensity, but also for *setting pain relief goals and evaluating treatment.* When setting goals, the patient and prescriber should agree on a target pain intensity rating that will permit the patient to participate in recovery activities, perform activities of daily living, and enjoy activities that contribute to quality of life. The objective of treatment is to reduce pain to the agreed-upon level—and lower, if possible.

Ongoing Evaluation

Once a treatment plan has been implemented, pain should be reassessed frequently. The objective is to determine the efficacy of treatment and to allow early diagnosis and treatment of new pain. Each time an analgesic drug is administered, pain should be evaluated after sufficient time has elapsed for the drug to take effect. Because most patients are treated at home, patients and caregivers should be taught to conduct and document pain evaluations. The prescriber will use the documented record to make adjustments to the pain management plan.

Prescribers, patients, and caregivers should be alert for new pain. In the majority of cases, new pain results from a new cause (e.g., metastasis, infection, fracture). Accordingly, whenever new pain occurs, a rigorous diagnostic work-up is indicated.

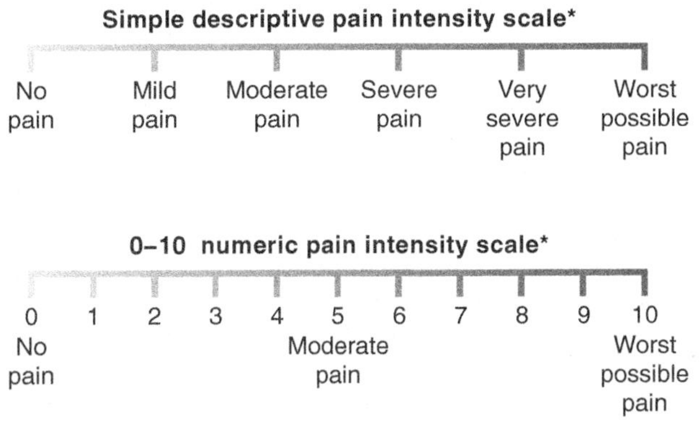

Fig. 29.2 ■ Linear pain intensity scales.
*If used as a graphic rating scale, a 10-cm baseline is recommended. (From Acute Pain Management Guideline Panel: Acute Pain Management: Operative or Medical Procedures and Trauma [Clinical Practice Guideline No. 1; AHCPR Publication No. 92-0032]. Rockville, MD: Agency for Health Care Policy and Research, 1992.)

Fig. 29.3 ■ Wong-Baker FACES pain rating scale.
Explain to the patient that the first face represents a person who feels happy because he or she has no pain and that the other faces represent people who feel sad because they have pain, ranging from a little to a lot. Explain that face 10 represents a person who hurts as much as you can imagine but that you don't have to be crying to feel this bad. Ask the patient to choose the face that best reflects how he or she is feeling. The numbers below the faces correspond to the values in the numeric pain scale shown in Fig. 29.2. (From Hockenberry MJ, Wilson D: Wong's Essentials of Pediatric Nursing, 8th ed. St. Louis: Elsevier, 2009.)

Barriers to Assessment

Pain assessment relies heavily on a report from the patient. Unfortunately, the report is not always accurate: Some patients report more pain than they have, some report less, and some are unable to report at all. With other patients, cultural and language differences impede assessment. In all cases, reliance on behavioral cues and facial expression is a poor substitute for an accurate report by the patient.

Many patients underreport pain, frequently because of misconceptions. Some fear addiction to opioids, and hence want to minimize opioid use. Some believe they are expected to be stoic and "tough it out." Some deny their pain because they fear pain signifies disease progression. When underreporting of pain is suspected, the patient should be interviewed in an effort to discover the reason. If a misconception is responsible for underreporting, educating the patient can help fix the problem.

Some patients fear they may be denied sufficient pain medication, and hence, to ensure adequate dosing, report more pain than they actually have. When exaggeration is suspected, the patient should be reassured that adequate pain relief will be provided and should be taught that inaccurate reporting serves only to make appropriate treatment more difficult.

Language barriers and cultural barriers can impede pain assessment. For patients who do not speak English, a translator should be provided. Obtaining a pain rating scale in the patient's own language would assist in accurate assessment. *A pain affect FACES scale* can be useful, as facial expressions reflecting discomfort are the same in all cultures. Cultural beliefs may cause some patients to hide overt expression of pain and report less pain than is present. The interviewer should be alert to this possibility.

When assessing pain, we must keep in mind that behavior and facial expression may be poor indicators of pain status. For example, in patients approaching the end of life, behavioral cues of pain (e.g., vocalizing, grimacing) are often absent. Other patients may simply have good coping skills, and hence may smile and move around in apparent comfort, even though they are in considerable pain. Because appearances can be deceiving, we must not rely on them to assess pain.

Assessment in young children and other nonverbal patients is a special challenge. By definition, nonverbal patients are unable to self-report pain. Accordingly, we must use less reliable methods of assessment, including observing the patient for cues. Assessment in children is discussed further under *Pain Management in Special Populations.*

DRUG THERAPY

Analgesic drugs are the most powerful weapons we have for overcoming cancer pain. With proper use, these agents can relieve pain in 90% of patients. Because analgesics are so effective, drug therapy is the principal modality for pain treatment. Three types of analgesics are employed:

- Nonopioid analgesics (nonsteroidal anti-inflammatory drugs [NSAIDs] and acetaminophen)
- Opioid analgesics (e.g., oxycodone, fentanyl, morphine)
- Adjuvant analgesics (e.g., amitriptyline, carbamazepine, dextroamphetamine)

These classes differ in their abilities to relieve pain. With the nonopioid and adjuvant analgesics, there is a ceiling to how much relief we can achieve. In contrast, there is no ceiling to relief with the opioids.

Selection among the analgesics is based on pain intensity and pain type. To help guide drug selection, the World Health Organization (WHO) devised a drug selection ladder (Fig. 29.4). The first step of the ladder—for mild to moderate pain—consists of nonopioid analgesics: NSAIDs and acetaminophen. The second step—for more severe pain—*adds* opioid analgesics of moderate strength (e.g., oxycodone, hydrocodone). The top step—for severe pain—substitutes powerful opioids (e.g., morphine, fentanyl) for the weaker ones. Adjuvant analgesics, which are especially effective against neuropathic pain, can be used on any step of the ladder. Specific drugs to *avoid* are listed in Table 29.2.

Traditionally, patients have been given opioid analgesics only after a trial with nonopioids has failed. Guidelines from the National Comprehensive Cancer Network (NCCN) recommend a different approach, in which initial drug selection is based on pain intensity. Specifically, if the patient reports pain in the 4 to 10 range (as measured on a numeric rating scale), then treatment should start directly with an opioid; an initial trial with a nonopioid is considered unnecessary. If the patient reports pain in the 1 to 3 range, then treatment usually begins with a nonopioid, although starting with an opioid remains an alternative.

It is common practice to combine an opioid with a nonopioid because the combination can be more effective than either drug alone. When pain is only moderate, opioids and nonopioids can be given in a fixed-dose combination formulation, thereby simplifying dosing. However, when pain is severe, these drugs must be given separately because, with a fixed-dose combination, side effects of the nonopioid would become intolerable as the dosage grew large, and hence would limit how much opioid could be given.

Drug therapy of cancer pain should adhere to the following principles:

- Perform a comprehensive pretreatment assessment to identify pain intensity and the underlying cause.
- Individualize the treatment plan.
- Use the WHO analgesic ladder and NCCN guidelines to guide drug selection.
- Use oral therapy whenever possible.
- Avoid IM injections whenever possible.
- For persistent pain, administer analgesics on a fixed schedule around-the-clock (ATC), and provide additional rescue doses of a short-acting agent if breakthrough pain occurs.
- Evaluate the patient frequently for pain relief and drug side effects.

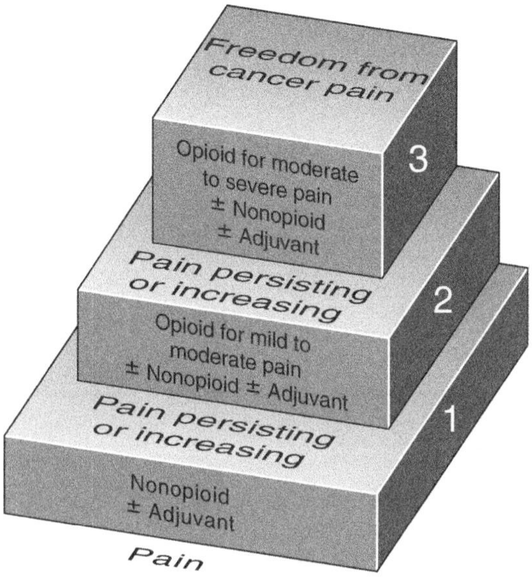

Fig. 29.4 ▪ The WHO analgesic ladder for cancer pain management.
Note that steps represent pain intensity. Accordingly, if a patient has intense pain at the outset, then treatment can be initiated with an opioid (step 2), rather than trying a nonopioid first (step 1). (Adapted from Cancer Pain Relief, 2nd ed. Geneva: World Health Organization, 1996.)

Nonopioid Analgesics

The nonopioid analgesics—NSAIDs and acetaminophen—constitute the first rung of the WHO analgesic ladder. These agents are the initial drugs of choice for patients with mild pain. There is a ceiling to how much pain relief nonopioid drugs can provide, so there is no benefit to exceeding recommended dosages (Table 29.3). Acetaminophen is about equal to the NSAIDs in *analgesic* efficacy but lacks *anti-inflammatory* actions. Because of this difference and others, acetaminophen is considered separately later in the chapter. The NSAIDs and acetaminophen are discussed in Chapter 71.

Nonsteroidal Anti-Inflammatory Drugs

NSAIDs (e.g., aspirin, ibuprofen) can produce a variety of effects. Primary beneficial effects are pain relief, suppression of inflammation, and reduction of fever. Primary adverse effects are gastric ulceration, acute renal failure, and bleeding. In addition, all NSAIDs *except aspirin* increase the risk of thrombotic events (e.g., myocardial infarction, stroke). In contrast to opioids, NSAIDs do not cause tolerance, physical dependence, or psychologic dependence.

NSAIDs are effective analgesics that can relieve mild to moderate pain. All of the NSAIDs have essentially equal analgesic efficacy, although individual patients may respond better to one NSAID than to another. NSAIDs relieve pain by a mechanism different from that of the opioids. As a result, combined use of an NSAID with an opioid can produce greater pain relief than either agent alone.

TABLE 29.2 ▪ Drugs That Are Not Recommended for Treating Cancer Pain

Drug Class	Drug	Why the Drug Is Not Recommended
OPIOIDS		
Pure agonists	Meperidine	A toxic metabolite accumulates with prolonged use
	Codeine	Maximal pain relief is limited owing to dose-limiting side effects
Agonist-antagonists	Buprenorphine Butorphanol Nalbuphine Pentazocine	Ceiling to analgesic effects; can precipitate withdrawal in opioid-dependent patients; cause psychotomimetic reactions
OPIOID ANTAGONISTS	Naloxone Naltrexone	Can precipitate withdrawal in opioid-dependent patients; limit use to the reversal of life-threatening respiratory depression caused by opioid overdose
BENZODIAZEPINES	Diazepam Lorazepam others	Sedation from benzodiazepines limits opioid dosage; no demonstrated analgesic action
BARBITURATES	Secobarbital others	Sedation from barbiturates limits opioid dosage; no demonstrated analgesic action
MISCELLANEOUS	Marijuana	Side effects (dysphoria, drowsiness, hypotension, bradycardia) preclude routine use as an analgesic

TABLE 29.3 ■ Dosages for Nonopioid Analgesics: Acetaminophen and Selected NSAIDs

Drug	Usual Adult Dosage[a]	
	Body Weight 50 kg or More	**Body Weight Less Than 50 kg**
Acetaminophen	650 mg every 4 hr *or* 975 mg every 6 hr	10–15 mg/kg every 4 hr *or* 15–20 mg/kg every 4 hr (rectal)
NSAIDs: SALICYLATES		
Aspirin	650 mg every 4 hr *or* 975 mg every 6 hr	10–15 mg/kg every 4 hr *or* 15–20 mg/kg every 4 hr (rectal)
Magnesium salicylate [Doan's][b]	650 mg every 4 hr	—
NSAIDs: PROPIONIC ACID DERIVATIVES		
Fenoprofen	300–600 mg every 6 hr	—
Ibuprofen [Motrin, Advil, others]	400–800 mg every 6 hr	10 mg/kg every 6–8 hr
Ketoprofen	25–60 mg every 6–8 hr	—
Naproxen [Naprosyn]	250–275 mg every 6–8 hr	5 mg/kg every 8 hr
Naproxen sodium [Anaprox, Aleve, Naprelan, others]	275 mg every 6–8 hr	—
NSAIDs: SELECTIVE COX-2 INHIBITORS		
Celecoxib [Celebrex]	200 mg every 12 hr	—
NSAIDs: MISCELLANEOUS		
Diflunisal	500 mg every 12 hr	—
Etodolac	200–400 mg every 6–8 hr	—
Meclofenamate sodium	50–100 mg every 6 hr	—
Mefenamic acid [Ponstel, Ponstan 🍁]	250 mg every 6 hr	—

[a]All dosages are oral except where indicated.

[b]Magnesium salicylate is nonacetylated, and hence, unlike aspirin, is safe for patients with thrombocytopenia.

NSAIDs produce their effects—both good and bad—by inhibiting cyclooxygenase (COX), an enzyme that has two forms, known as COX-1 and COX-2. Most NSAIDs inhibit both COX-1 and COX-2, although a few are selective for COX-2. The selective COX-2 inhibitors (e.g., celecoxib [Celebrex]) cause less GI damage than the nonselective inhibitors. Unfortunately, the selective inhibitors pose a greater risk of thrombotic events, and hence long-term use of these drugs is not recommended.

For patients undergoing chemotherapy, inhibition of platelet aggregation by NSAIDs is a serious concern. Many anticancer drugs suppress bone marrow function and thereby decrease platelet production. The resultant thrombocytopenia puts patients at risk of bruising and bleeding. Obviously, this risk will be increased by drugs that inhibit platelet function. Among the conventional NSAIDs, only one subclass—the nonacetylated salicylates (e.g., magnesium salicylate)—does not inhibit platelet aggregation, and hence is safe for patients with thrombocytopenia. All other conventional NSAIDs should be avoided. *Aspirin* should be avoided because it causes *irreversible* inhibition of platelet aggregation. Hence, its effects persist for the life of the platelet (about 8 days). Because COX-2 inhibitors do not affect platelets, these drugs are safe for patients with thrombocytopenia.

Acetaminophen

Acetaminophen [Tylenol, others] is similar to the NSAIDs in some respects and different in others. Like the NSAIDs, acetaminophen is an effective analgesic, and hence can relieve mild to moderate pain. Benefits derive from inhibiting COX in the central nervous system (CNS), but not in the periphery. Combining acetaminophen with an opioid can produce greater analgesia than either drug alone (because acetaminophen and opioids relieve pain by different mechanisms).

Acetaminophen differs from the NSAIDs in several important ways. Because it does not inhibit COX in the periphery, acetaminophen lacks anti-inflammatory actions, does not inhibit platelet aggregation, and does not promote gastric ulceration, renal failure, or thrombotic events. Because acetaminophen does not affect platelets, the drug is safe for patients with thrombocytopenia.

Acetaminophen has important interactions with two other drugs: alcohol and warfarin (an anticoagulant). Combining acetaminophen with alcohol, even in moderate amounts, can result in potentially fatal liver damage. Accordingly, patients taking acetaminophen should minimize alcohol consumption. Acetaminophen also can increase the risk of bleeding in patients taking warfarin. The mechanism appears to be inhibition of warfarin metabolism, which causes warfarin to accumulate to toxic levels.

Opioid Analgesics

Opioids are the most effective analgesics available, and hence are the primary drugs for treating moderate to severe cancer pain. With proper dosing, opioids can safely relieve pain in about 90% of cancer patients. Unfortunately, many patients are denied adequate doses, owing largely to unfounded fears of addiction.

Opioids produce a variety of pharmacologic effects. In addition to analgesia, they can cause sedation, euphoria, constipation, respiratory depression, urinary retention, and miosis. With continuous use, tolerance develops to most of these effects, with the notable exceptions of constipation and miosis. Continuous use also results in physical dependence, which must not be equated with addiction.

The opioids are discussed in Chapter 28. Discussion here focuses on their use in patients with cancer.

Mechanism of Action and Classification

Opioid analgesics relieve pain by mimicking the actions of endogenous opioid peptides (enkephalins, dynorphins, endorphins), primarily at mu receptors and partly at kappa receptors.

Based on their actions at mu and kappa receptors, the opioids fall into two major groups: (1) *pure (full) agonists* (e.g., morphine) and (2) *agonist-antagonists* (e.g., butorphanol). The pure agonists can be subdivided into (1) agents for mild to moderate pain and (2) agents for moderate to severe pain. The pure agonists act as agonists at mu receptors *and* at kappa receptors. In contrast, the agonist-antagonists act as agonists only at kappa receptors; at mu receptors, these drugs act as *antagonists.* Because their agonist actions are limited to kappa receptors, the agonist-antagonists have a ceiling to their analgesic effects. Furthermore, because of their antagonist actions, the agonist-antagonists can block access of the pure agonists to mu receptors and can thereby prevent the pure agonists from relieving pain. Accordingly, agonist-antagonists are not recommended for managing cancer pain.

Tolerance and Physical Dependence

Over time, opioids cause tolerance and physical dependence. These phenomena, which are generally inseparable, reflect neuronal adaptations to prolonged opioid exposure. Some degree of tolerance and physical dependence develops after 1 to 2 weeks of opioid use.

Tolerance. Tolerance can be defined as a state in which a specific dose (e.g., 10 mg of morphine) produces a smaller effect than it could when treatment began. Put another way, tolerance is a state in which dosage must be increased to maintain the desired response. In patients with cancer, however, a need for larger doses isn't always a sign of tolerance. In fact, it's usually a sign that pain is getting worse (owing to disease progression).

Tolerance develops to some opioid effects but not to others. Tolerance develops to analgesia, euphoria, respiratory depression, and sedation. In contrast, little or no tolerance develops to constipation or miosis.

There is cross-tolerance among opioids. Accordingly, significant tolerance to one opioid confers a similar degree of tolerance to all others.

Physical Dependence. Physical dependence is a state in which an abstinence syndrome will occur if a drug is abruptly withdrawn. With opioids, the abstinence syndrome can be very unpleasant—but not dangerous. The intensity and duration of the abstinence syndrome are determined in part by the duration of drug use and in part by the half-life of the drug taken. Because drugs with a short half-life leave the body rapidly, the abstinence syndrome is brief but intense. Conversely, for drugs with long half-lives, the syndrome is prolonged but relatively mild. The abstinence syndrome can be minimized by withdrawing opioids slowly (i.e., by giving progressively smaller doses over several days). Please note that *physical dependence is not the same as addiction!*

Addiction

Opioid addiction is an important issue in pain management—not because addiction occurs (it rarely does), but because *inappropriate fears of addiction* are a major cause for undertreatment.

The American Society of Addiction Medicine defines addiction as *a primary, chronic disease characterized by an individual pathologically pursuing rewards and/or relief by substance use and other behaviors.* According to this definition, addiction is primarily a *behavior pattern*—and is *not* equated with physical dependence. Although it is true that physical dependence can contribute to addictive behavior, other factors—especially *psychologic dependence*—are the primary underlying cause. All cancer patients who take opioids chronically develop substantial physical dependence, but only a few (<1%) develop addictive behavior. Most patients, if their cancer were cured, would simply go through gradual withdrawal and never think about or use opioids again. Clearly, these patients cannot be considered addicted, despite their physical dependence.

Because of misconceptions about opioid addiction, prescribers often order lower doses than patients need, nurses administer lower doses than were ordered, patients report less pain than they actually have, and family members discourage opioid use. The end result? The majority of cancer patients receive lower doses of opioids than they need. To improve this unacceptable situation we must educate physicians, nurses, patients, and family members. Specifically, we must teach them about the nature of addiction and inform them that development of addiction in the therapeutic setting is very rare. Hopefully, this information will dispel unfounded fears of addiction and will thereby help ensure delivery of opioids in doses that are sufficient to relieve suffering.

Drug Selection

Preferred Opioids. For all cancer patients, *pure opioid agonists* are preferred to the agonist-antagonists. If pain is not too intense, a moderately strong opioid (e.g., oxycodone) is appropriate. If pain is moderate to severe, a strong opioid (e.g., morphine) should be used. Because morphine is inexpensive, available in multiple dosage forms, and clinically well understood, this opioid is used more than any other.

Opioid Rotation. Opioid rotation—switching from one opioid to another—is now an accepted practice. Because opioids have different side effect profiles, rotation can help minimize adverse effects while maintaining good analgesia. To make the switch, the current opioid is stopped abruptly and immediately replaced with an equianalgesic dose of an alternative opioid.

Opioids to Use With Special Caution. *Methadone* [Dolophine, Methadose] must be used with caution. Methadone has a prolonged half-life, which makes dosage titration difficult. If dosing is not done skillfully, this drug can accumulate to dangerous levels, causing excessive sedation and respiratory depression.

Codeine deserves special comment. Although codeine is capable of producing significant analgesia, side effects limit the dose that can be given. As a result, the degree of pain relief that can be achieved safely is quite low.

Opioids to Avoid. *Meperidine* [Demerol], a pure opioid agonist, may be used for a few days, but no longer. When the drug is taken chronically, a toxic metabolite—normeperidine—can accumulate, thereby posing a risk of adverse CNS effects (dysphoria, agitation, seizures).

The *agonist-antagonists*—buprenorphine, butorphanol, nalbuphine, and pentazocine—should be avoided for several reasons. First, they are less effective than pure opioid agonists, and hence, there is little reason to choose them. Second, if given to a patient who is physically dependent on a pure opioid agonist, these drugs can prevent the pure agonist from working and can thereby block analgesia and precipitate withdrawal. Third, the agonist-antagonists can cause adverse psychologic reactions (nightmares, hallucinations, dysphoria).

Dosage

Dosage must be individualized. The objective is to find a dosage that can relieve pain without causing intolerable side effects. For patients with moderate pain and low opioid tolerance, very low doses (e.g., 2 mg of parenteral morphine every 4 hours) can be sufficient. In contrast, when pain is severe or tolerance is high, much larger doses (e.g., 600 mg of parenteral morphine every few hours) may be required. The upper limit to dosage is determined only by the intensity of side effects. Accordingly, as pain and/or tolerance increase, dosage should be increased until pain is relieved—unless intolerable side effects (e.g., excessive respiratory depression) occur first.

The dosing schedule is determined by the temporal pattern of the pain. If pain is intermittent and infrequent, PRN dosing can suffice. However, because most patients have persistent pain, PRN dosing is inappropriate. Instead, dosing should be done *on a fixed schedule* ATC. A fixed schedule can prevent opioid levels from becoming subtherapeutic and can thereby prevent pain recurrence. As a result, the patient is spared needless suffering, both from the pain itself and from anxiety about its return.

What dose should be used when switching from one opioid to another or from one route of administration to another? To help make this decision, an equianalgesic table should be consulted. Equianalgesic tables indicate equivalent analgesic doses for different opioids and for the same opioid administered by different routes.

Routes of Administration

Because most patients with cancer pain must take analgesics continuously, the route should be as convenient, affordable, and noninvasive as possible. Oral administration meets these criteria best, and hence is preferred for most patients. If oral medication cannot be used, the preferred alternative routes are rectal and transdermal: Both are relatively convenient, affordable, and noninvasive. If these routes are ineffective or inappropriate, then parenteral administration (IV or subQ) is indicated (IM injections should be avoided). For patients who cannot be managed with IV or subQ therapy, more invasive routes—intraspinal or intraventricular—can be tried.

Oral. Oral administration is the preferred route for chronic therapy because oral dosing is cheap, convenient, and noninvasive. Accordingly, in the absence of contraindications (e.g., vomiting, inability to swallow), oral therapy should be considered for all patients. Opioids are available in several formulations (e.g., tablets, capsules, solution) for oral use. To reduce the number of daily doses, a long-acting formulation (e.g., controlled-release morphine) can be used. Because oral opioids undergo substantial first-pass metabolism, oral doses must be larger than parenteral doses to achieve equivalent analgesic effects.

Rectal. Rectal administration is an alternative for patients who cannot take drugs by mouth. Two opioids—morphine and hydromorphone—are available in rectal formulations (suppositories). When switching from oral to rectal administration, dosing is begun with the same dose that was used orally, and then adjusted as needed. Rectal administration is inappropriate for patients with diarrhea or lesions of the rectum or anus. Also, children frequently object to this route.

Transdermal. Transdermal administration is a preferred alternative to oral therapy. Only one pure opioid agonist—fentanyl [Duragesic]—is available for chronic transdermal use. Fentanyl patches provide steady analgesia for 72 hours, and hence are appropriate for patients with pain that is continuous and does not fluctuate much in intensity. Absorption from the patch is very slow. As a result, when the first patch is applied, effective analgesia may take 12 to 24 hours to develop. During this time, PRN therapy with a short-acting opioid may be required. Fentanyl patches are available in five strengths, allowing dosage to be matched with pain intensity. As with other long-acting opioids, rescue doses with a short-acting opioid are needed when breakthrough pain occurs.

Intravenous and Subcutaneous. Intravenous and subQ administration are acceptable alternatives when less invasive routes (oral, transdermal, rectal) cannot be used. The IV and subQ routes have two advantages: (1) onset of analgesia is quick and (2) these routes permit rapid escalation of dosage. Obvious disadvantages are inconvenience and increased cost. In addition, frequent subQ dosing is uncomfortable. Conditions that might justify IV or subQ administration include:

- Persistent nausea and vomiting (which preclude oral dosing)
- Inability to swallow (which precludes oral dosing)
- Delirium or stupor (which precludes oral dosing)
- Pain that requires a large number of pills (which makes oral dosing inconvenient)
- Unstable pain that requires rapid dosage escalation (which precludes oral, rectal, and transdermal administration)

Dosages for IV and subQ administration are the same.

Intramuscular. Intramuscular administration should be avoided. IM injections are painful, and hence unacceptable for repeated dosing. In addition, absorption from IM sites is inconsistent, hence pain relief is unpredictable.

Intraspinal. Intraspinal administration is reserved for patients with intractable pain that cannot be controlled with less invasive routes (e.g., IV, subQ). In this technique, opioids are delivered to the epidural or subarachnoid space via a percutaneous catheter connected to an infusion pump or injection port. By using this route, we can achieve high opioid concentrations at receptors on pain pathways in the spinal cord. It is important to note, however, that effects will not be limited to the spinal cord: Intraspinal opioids undergo absorption into the blood in amounts sufficient to cause systemic effects. In fact, blood levels may be equivalent to those achieved with conventional routes (e.g., subQ). Intraspinal administration is especially useful for patients with severe pain in the lower body: Pain is relieved in up to 90% of appropriate candidates. Patients who are tolerant to opioids delivered by other routes will also be tolerant to opioids given intraspinally, and hence dosage should be adjusted accordingly. Patients should have access to rescue medication in case breakthrough pain occurs, owing either to delivery system malfunction or inadequate dosing. Side effects with intraspinal administration are the same as with other routes. In addition, there is a risk of *delayed* respiratory depression as well as infection associated with the catheter.

Intraventricular. Like intraspinal administration, intraventricular administration is reserved for patients whose pain cannot be controlled with less invasive routes. In this procedure, morphine is delivered to the cerebral ventricles via a catheter connected to an external infusion pump (for continuous administration) or a subcutaneous reservoir (for intermittent administration). Because morphine is delivered directly to the brain, bypassing the blood-brain barrier, analgesia can be achieved with extremely low doses (e.g., 5 mg daily). Pain is relieved in 90% of patients. Intraventricular administration is especially helpful for patients with intractable pain caused by head and neck malignancies or tumors that affect the brachial plexus.

Patient-Controlled Analgesia. Patient-controlled analgesia (PCA) is a method of drug delivery that permits patients to control the amount of opioid they receive. PCA is accomplished using a PCA device to deliver opioids through an indwelling IV or subQ catheter. The PCA device is an electronically controlled infusion pump that (1) delivers a continuous basal infusion of opioid and (2) can be activated manually by the patient to deliver additional bolus doses for breakthrough pain. To prevent an overdose, the device (1) limits the total dose of opioid that can be delivered per hour and (2) sets a minimum interval (e.g., 10 minutes) between bolus doses, thereby preventing the patient from giving a second dose before the first one can take full effect. PCA devices are safe for use in the hospital and at home, but should not be used by patients who are sedated or confused. PCA administration is discussed in Chapter 28.

Managing Breakthrough Pain

Many patients whose pain is well controlled most of the day experience transient episodes of moderate to severe pain, known as breakthrough pain. Breakthrough pain develops quickly, reaches peak intensity in minutes, and may persist from minutes to hours (the median duration is 30 minutes). At least 50% of cancer patients experience these episodes, typically 1 to 4 times a day. Breakthrough pain may occur spontaneously, or it may be precipitated by coughing or other movements. In contrast to end-of-dose pain, which occurs because analgesic levels are lowest at that time, breakthrough pain can occur at any time during the dosing interval.

All patients receiving ATC opioids for persistent pain should have access to a rescue medication to manage breakthrough pain. Because breakthrough pain is both severe and self-limited, the best medication is a strong opioid with a rapid onset and short duration. The rapid onset permits speedy relief, and the short duration facilitates dosage titration. For ease of administration, oral, transmucosal, and intranasal formulations are preferred; examples include immediate-release oral morphine, transmucosal fentanyl [Abstral, Actiq, Fentora, Onsolis, Subsys], and fentanyl nasal spray [Lazanda].

Managing Side Effects

Side effects of the opioids include respiratory depression, constipation, sedation, orthostatic hypotension, miosis, nausea, and vomiting. All can be effectively managed. In many patients, side effects can be reduced simply by decreasing the dosage (typically by 25%). If dosage reduction causes pain to return, adding a nonopioid analgesic may take care of the problem. Over time, tolerance develops to sedation, respiratory depression, nausea, and vomiting—but not to constipation or miosis.

Respiratory Depression. Respiratory depression is the most serious side effect of the opioids; death can result. Fortunately, when dosage and monitoring are appropriate, significant respiratory depression is rare. Pain counteracts the depressant actions of opioids. Hence, as pain decreases, respiratory depression may deepen.

Respiratory depression is greatest at the outset of treatment and then decreases as tolerance develops. As a result, small initial doses of opioids (e.g., 5 mg of IV morphine every hour) can pose a greater risk than much larger doses (e.g., 1000 mg of IV morphine every hour) later on.

Significant respiratory depression is most likely when dosage is being titrated up. The best way to assess the risk of impending respiratory depression is to monitor opioid-induced sedation. An increase in sedation generally precedes an increase in respiratory depression, so if excessive sedation is observed, further dosing should be delayed.

Respiratory depression is increased by other drugs with CNS-depressant actions (e.g., alcohol, barbiturates, benzodiazepines). Accordingly, these agents should be avoided.

Severe respiratory depression can be reversed with *naloxone* [Narcan], a pure opioid antagonist. However, caution is required: Excessive dosing will reverse analgesia, thereby putting the patient in great pain. Accordingly, naloxone dosage must be titrated carefully.

When death is near, should opioids be withheld out of fear that respiratory depression may bring death sooner? For several reasons, the answer is no. First, significant respiratory depression is rare in the tolerant patient. Hence, concerns about hastening death are largely unfounded. Second, unrelieved pain can itself hasten death. Third, when death is imminent, it is more important to provide comfort than to prolong life. Accordingly, adequate opioids should be provided, even if doing so means life ends a bit sooner.

Constipation. Constipation occurs in most patients. Opioids promote constipation by decreasing propulsive intestinal contractions, increasing nonpropulsive contractions, increasing the tone of the anal sphincter, and reducing fluid secretion into the intestinal lumen. No tolerance to these effects develops. To reduce constipation, all patients should increase dietary fiber and fluid. However, most patients also need pharmacologic help. Options include stool softeners (e.g., docusate), stimulant laxatives (e.g., senna), osmotic laxatives (e.g., sodium phosphate), and methylnaltrexone [Relistor], which blocks opioid receptors in the intestine. For prophylaxis of constipation, current guidelines recommend daily therapy with a combination product, such as Senokot-S, which contains both senna and docusate. Strong osmotic laxatives are reserved for severe constipation. Methylnaltrexone [Relistor] is indicated only for constipation in patients when other measures are unsuccessful. Drugs with anticholinergic properties (e.g., tricyclic antidepressants, antihistamines) can exacerbate opioid-induced constipation (by further depressing bowel function), and hence should be avoided.

Sedation. Sedation is common early in therapy, but tolerance develops quickly. If sedation persists, it can be reduced by giving smaller doses of the opioid more frequently, while keeping the total daily dose the same. This dosing schedule decreases peak opioid levels and reduces excessive CNS depression. If necessary, sedation can be opposed with a CNS stimulant (e.g., caffeine, methylphenidate, dextroamphetamine, modafinil).

Nausea and Vomiting. Initial doses of opioids may cause nausea and vomiting. Fortunately, tolerance develops rapidly. Nausea and vomiting can be minimized by pretreatment with an antiemetic (e.g., prochlorperazine, metoclopramide). A serotonin antagonist (e.g., granisetron, ondansetron) may also be tried, but these drugs may increase constipation.

Other Side Effects. Opioids promote histamine release, and can thereby cause *itching,* which can be relieved with an antihistamine (e.g., diphenhydramine).

Opioids increase the tone in the urinary bladder sphincter, and can thereby cause *urinary retention.* Benign prostatic hypertrophy and use of anticholinergic drugs will exacerbate the problem. Patients should be monitored for urinary retention and encouraged to void every 4 hours.

Opioids can cause *orthostatic hypotension.* Patients should be informed about symptoms of hypotension (light-headedness, dizziness) and instructed to sit or lie down if they occur. Orthostatic hypotension can be minimized by moving slowly when changing from a supine or seated position to an upright posture.

Opioid-induced *neurotoxicity* is a recently recognized syndrome. Symptoms include delirium, agitation, myoclonus, and hyperalgesia. Primary risk factors are renal impairment, pre-existing cognitive impairment, and prolonged high-dose opioid use. Management consists of hydration, dose reduction, and opioid rotation.

Adjuvant Analgesics

Adjuvant analgesics are used to *complement* the effects of opioids. Accordingly, these drugs are employed in *combination* with opioids—not as substitutes. Adjuvant analgesics can (1) enhance analgesia from opioids, (2) help manage concurrent symptoms that exacerbate pain, and (3) treat side effects caused by opioids. Several of the adjuvants are especially useful for *neuropathic pain.* The adjuvant analgesics differ from opioids in that pain relief is limited and less predictable, and often develops slowly.

Adjuvant agents may be employed at any step on the analgesic ladder. The adjuvants are interesting in that, although they can relieve pain, all of them were developed to treat other conditions (e.g., depression, seizures, dysrhythmias). Accordingly, it is important to reassure patients that the adjuvant is being used to alleviate pain and not for its original purpose. Dosages for the adjuvant analgesics are shown in Table 29.4.

Antidepressants

Tricyclic Antidepressants. *Amitriptyline* [Elavil] and other tricyclic antidepressants (TCAs) can reduce pain of *neuropathic* origin. TCAs have analgesic effects of their own and they enhance the effects of opioids, and may thereby allow a reduction in opioid dosage. As a side benefit, TCAs can elevate mood. Important adverse effects are orthostatic hypotension, sedation, anticholinergic effects (dry mouth, urinary retention, constipation), and weight gain (secondary to improved appetite). Dosing at bedtime takes advantage of sedative effects and minimizes hypotension during the day. Effects begin in 1 to 2 weeks and reach their maximum in 4 to 6 weeks. The TCAs are discussed in Chapter 32.

Other Antidepressants. In addition to the tricyclic agents, certain other antidepressants (e.g., bupropion, duloxetine, venlafaxine) can help with neuropathic pain.

Antiseizure Drugs

Certain antiseizure drugs can help relieve *neuropathic pain.* Acute pain (sharp, darting pain) is especially responsive, although other forms of neuropathic pain (cramping pain, aching pain, burning pain) also respond. Analgesia is thought to result from suppressing spontaneous neuronal firing. Of the available antiseizure drugs, gabapentin [Neurontin] and pregabalin [Lyrica] are used most widely. Carbamazepine [Tegretol] is an additional option, but carbamazepine is myelosuppressive and must be used with caution in patients receiving anticancer drugs that suppress bone marrow function. As discussed in Chapter 24, caution is also needed in patients of Asian descent, owing to an increased risk of severe dermatologic reactions. Another drug—*gabapentin* [Neurontin]—is also very effective and causes fewer side effects than carbamazepine. Dosage should be low initially (100 mg once a day) and then gradually increased; dosages as high as 1200 mg 3 times a day have been employed. Antiseizure drugs are discussed in Chapter 24.

Topical Anesthetics

Lidocaine [Lidoderm] is considered a second-line agent for *neuropathic pain.* It is supplied in a topical 5% patch that may be applied to the area of pain for up to 12 hours. Lidocaine is discussed in Chapter 26 and 49.

CNS Stimulants

The CNS stimulants, such as *dextroamphetamine* [Dexedrine] and *methylphenidate* [Ritalin], have two beneficial effects: They can enhance opioid-induced analgesia, and they can counteract opioid-induced sedation. In addition, they can be used for rapid elevation of mood. Principal adverse effects are weight loss (from appetite suppression) and insomnia (from CNS stimulation). To minimize interference with sleep, dosing late in the day should be avoided. The CNS stimulants are discussed in Chapter 36.

Glucocorticoids

Although glucocorticoids lack direct analgesic actions, they can help manage painful cancer-related conditions. Because glucocorticoids can reduce cerebral and spinal edema, they are essential for the emergency management of elevated intracranial pressure and epidural spinal cord compression. Similarly, glucocorticoids are part of the standard therapy for tumor-induced spinal cord compression. In addition to these benefits, glucocorticoids can improve appetite and impart a general sense of well-being; both actions help in managing anorexia (loss of appetite) and cachexia (weakness and emaciation) associated with terminal illness.

Glucocorticoids are very safe when used short term (even in high doses) and very dangerous when used long term (even in low doses). In particular, long-term therapy can cause adrenal insufficiency, osteoporosis, glucose intolerance (hyperglycemia),

TABLE 29.4 ■ Adjuvant Drugs for Cancer Pain

Drug	Usual Adult Dosage	Beneficial Actions
TRICYCLIC ANTIDEPRESSANTS		
Amitriptyline [Elavil]	25–150 mg/day PO	Reduce neuropathic pain
Desipramine [Norpramin][a]	10–150 mg/day PO	
Doxepin [Sinequan 🍁][a]	25–150 mg/day PO	
Imipramine [Tofranil]	20–100 mg/day PO	
Nortriptyline [Aventyl 🍁, Pamelor][a]	10–150 mg/day PO	
OTHER ANTIDEPRESSANTS		
Duloxetine [Cymbalta]	30–60 mg/day PO	Reduce neuropathic pain
Venlafaxine [Effexor][a]	37.5–225 mg/day PO	
ANTISEIZURE DRUGS		
Carbamazepine [Tegretol]	200–1600 mg/day PO	Reduce neuropathic pain
Gabapentin [Neurontin]	300–3600 mg/day PO	
Lamotrigine [Lamictal][a]	25–400 mg/day PO	
Phenytoin [Dilantin][a]	300–500 mg/day PO	
Pregabalin [Lyrica]	100–600 mg/day PO	
TOPICAL ANESTHETICS		
Lidocaine [Lidoderm]	Apply 5% topical patch for up to 12 hours daily	Reduce neuropathic pain
CNS STIMULANTS		
Dextroamphetamine [Dexedrine]	5–10 mg/day PO	Enhance analgesia and reduce sedation from opioids
Methylphenidate [Ritalin]	10–15 mg/day PO	
GLUCOCORTICOIDS		
Dexamethasone [Decadron, others]	16–96 mg/day PO or IV	Reduce pain associated with brain metastases and epidural spinal cord compression
Prednisone	40–100 mg/day PO	
BISPHOSPHONATES		
Pamidronate	60–90 mg IV once	Reduce hypercalcemia and possibly bone pain
Zoledronic acid	4 mg IV once	

[a]Off-label use.

increased vulnerability to infection, thinning of the skin, and, possibly, peptic ulcer disease. The risk of osteoporosis can be reduced by giving calcium supplements and vitamin D along with calcitonin or a bisphosphonate (e.g., etidronate). The glucocorticoids are discussed in Chapter 72.

Bisphosphonates

Bisphosphonates, such as *zoledronic acid* and *pamidronate* [Aredia], can reduce cancer-related *bone pain* in some patients. Bone pain is common when cancers metastasize to bone. The cause of pain may be tumor-induced bone resorption, which can also cause hypercalcemia, osteoporosis, and related fractures. Bisphosphonates inhibit bone resorption and are approved for treating hypercalcemia of malignancy and bone metastases in breast cancer—but not bone pain itself. However, when these drugs are given to treat hypercalcemia, many patients report a reduction in bone pain, although others do not. Hence, although these drugs appear promising, their use for management of bone pain is still considered investigational. The bisphosphonates are discussed in Chapter 75.

NONDRUG THERAPY

Invasive Procedures

Invasive therapies are the last resort for relieving intractable pain. Hence, for most patients, all other options should be exhausted first.

Neurolytic Nerve Block

The goal of this procedure is to destroy neurons that transmit pain from a limited area, thereby providing permanent pain relief. Nerve destruction is accomplished through local injection of a neurolytic (neurotoxic) substance, typically alcohol or phenol. To ensure that the correct nerves are destroyed, reversible nerve block is done first, using a local anesthetic. If the local anesthetic relieves the pain, a neurolytic agent is then applied to the same site. Neurolytic nerve block can eliminate pain in up to 80% of patients. However, even if pain relief is only partial, the procedure can still permit some reduction in opioid dosage and can thereby decrease side effects, such as sedation and constipation. When nerve block is successful and opioids are discontinued, opioid dosage should be tapered gradually to avoid withdrawal. Nerve block is not without risk. Potential complications include hypotension, paresis (slight paralysis), paralysis, and disruption of bowel and bladder function (e.g., diarrhea, incontinence). The incidence of complications ranges from 0.5% to 2%.

Neurosurgery

Neurosurgeons can relieve cancer pain in several ways. They can destroy neurons that transmit pain signals; they can implant opioid infusion systems; and, in a procedure known as neuroaugmentation, they can implant electrodes to stimulate neurons that release endogenous opioid peptides (e.g., endorphins). Nerve damage incurred during these surgeries can result in neurologic deficits and new pain. Less than 10% of cancer patients undergo neurosurgery for pain relief.

Tumor Surgery

When curative excision of a tumor is not feasible, it may still be appropriate to surgically debulk the tumor with the goal of relieving pain. Unfortunately, palliative debulking provides only temporary relief: Growth of residual cancer cells eventually causes pain to return. Radiation therapy after the surgery may extend pain relief.

Radiation Therapy

Radiation therapy relieves pain by causing tumor regression. Palliative treatment can be directed at primary tumors and at metastases anywhere in the body.

Radiation can be delivered in four forms: *brachytherapy* (implanted radioactive pellets), *teletherapy* (external beam radiation), *radiofrequency ablation,* and *intravenous radiopharmaceuticals.* With brachytherapy, cell kill is limited to the immediate area of the implanted pellets; hence, the technique is suited only for localized tumors. With teletherapy, cell kill can be localized or widespread, depending on the size of the beam employed; hence, the technique can be used for both localized tumors and metastases. Radiofrequency ablation uses a thin, needle-like probe inserted into a tumor through an incision in the skin. The probe extends electrodes that emit high-frequency electrical current, producing heat to destroy cancer cells; hence, the technique is best suited for localized tumors. Intravenous radiopharmaceuticals travel throughout the body, and hence are best suited for widespread metastases.

With radiation therapy, as with chemotherapy, damage to normal tissue is dose limiting. Therefore, the challenge is to deliver a dose of radiation that is large enough to kill cancer cells, but not so large that it causes intolerable damage to healthy tissue.

Some side effects of radiation occur early and some are late. Early effects develop during or immediately after radiation exposure. Late reactions develop months or years later. The most common early effects are skin inflammation and lesions of the GI mucosa. Fortunately, in the regimens employed for palliation, these acute effects are generally mild. The most common late reaction is fibrosis, which occurs mainly in tissues that have a limited ability to regenerate (e.g., brain, peripheral neurons, lung). Late reactions are of limited concern, however, because most patients die from their cancer before late reactions can develop.

Physical and Psychosocial Interventions

Physical and psychosocial interventions can help reduce pain, but the degree of relief is limited. Accordingly, these interventions should be used only in conjunction with drug therapy—not as substitutes.

Physical Interventions

Physical interventions (e.g., heat, massage, vibration) can help relieve aches and pains associated with cancer.

Heat. Application of heat can benefit the patient in at least two ways: (1) heat promotes vasodilation and can thereby increase delivery of oxygen and nutrients to damaged tissue, and (2) heat increases elasticity in muscle and can thereby reduce stiffness. Heat may be applied in several ways, including the use of hot compresses, hot water bottles, and electric heating pads. Heat may be harmful to tissues exposed to radiation, and hence these tissues should be avoided. There is some concern that heat may actually stimulate tumor growth and metastatic spread, although convincing data are lacking.

Cold. Application of cold can reduce inflammation and muscle spasm. Cold can be applied using ice packs, chemical gel packs, and towels soaked in ice water. Application should last no longer than 15 minutes. Cold should not be applied to areas damaged by radiation. In addition, because cold promotes vasoconstriction, it should be avoided in patients with peripheral vascular disease, Raynaud's phenomenon, and all other disorders that can be exacerbated by vasoconstriction.

Massage. Massage is primarily a comfort measure that provides relief through distraction and relaxation. In addition, massage may help ease discomfort at specific sites by increasing local circulation.

Exercise. Exercise can reduce subacute and chronic pain by increasing muscle strength and joint mobility. Additional benefits include improved cardiovascular conditioning and restoration of coordination and balance. Range-of-motion exercises can preserve strength and joint function. When patients cannot perform these exercises on their own, family members should be taught to assist. Although weight-bearing exercise is desirable, it should be avoided in patients who are at risk of fractures because of tumor invasion or osteoporosis.

Acupuncture and Transcutaneous Electrical Nerve Stimulation. In theory, these techniques reduce pain by stimulating peripheral nerves, which in turn activate central pain-modulating pathways. Acupuncture is performed by inserting solid needles through the skin into the underlying muscle. Studies regarding acupuncture for the treatment of cancer pain are few and are not well designed. At this time, there is insufficient evidence to determine whether acupuncture is effective in treating cancer pain. Transcutaneous electrical nerve stimulation (TENS) is performed using low-voltage cutaneous electrodes. Three small randomized controlled trials (RCTs) regarding TENS revealed conflicting results. Until larger RCTs are completed, the efficacy of TENS for the treatment of cancer pain is uncertain. Because the efficacy of these techniques is questionable, pain status must be closely monitored if they are used.

Psychosocial Interventions

Psychosocial interventions can help patients cope by (1) increasing the sense of control over pain, (2) reversing negative thoughts and feelings, and (3) offering social support. Interventions that require learning and practice should be introduced early so that they can be perfected while the patient still has sufficient energy and strength to learn them.

Relaxation and Imagery. The aim of these techniques is to reduce pain by inducing both mental relaxation (alleviation of anxiety) and physical relaxation (release of tension in skeletal muscles). These techniques are easy to learn and require little or no special equipment. Examples include (1) meditation, (2) slow, rhythmic breathing, (3) imagining a peaceful scene (e.g., gentle waves breaking on a secluded, sunny beach), and (4) active listening to recorded music (e.g., tapping a finger in time to an enjoyable tune).

Cognitive Distraction. The goal of cognitive distraction is to divert attention away from pain and associated negative emotions. Distractions may be internal or external. Examples of internal distractions include praying, counting or singing in one's head, and repeating positive thoughts. External distractions include watching TV, listening to music, and talking with friends.

Peer Support Groups. Support groups composed of other cancer patients can help members cope with pain and all other sequelae of their disease. These groups can provide emotional support, cancer-related information, and a sense of social belonging. Talking with other cancer survivors can be especially helpful for the newly diagnosed. Some support groups welcome patients who have any form of cancer; others are dedicated to just one form of the disease (e.g., breast cancer). Resources for locating a support group in your community include the National Cancer Institute's Information Service (1-800-4-CANCER) and your local chapter of the American Cancer Society, whose phone number can be found through an Internet search.

PAIN MANAGEMENT IN SPECIAL POPULATIONS

Older Adults

In older adult patients, two issues are of special concern: (1) undertreatment of pain and (2) increased risk of adverse effects. Paradoxically, a third issue—heightened drug sensitivity—contributes to both problems.

Heightened Drug Sensitivity

Older adults are more sensitive to drugs than are younger adults, owing largely to a decline in organ function. In particular, rates of hepatic metabolism and renal excretion decline with age. As a result, drugs tend to accumulate in the body, causing responses to be more intense and prolonged.

Undertreatment of Pain

Undertreatment is common in older adults. In addition to the usual reasons (fears about tolerance, addiction, adverse effects, and regulatory actions), older adults are denied adequate medication for two more reasons: difficulties with assessment and erroneous ideas about "old age."

Assessment is made difficult by cognitive impairment (e.g., delirium, dementia) and by impairment of vision and hearing. As a result, self-reporting of pain may be inaccurate or even impossible. Because of these obstacles, special effort must be made to help ensure that assessment is accurate. However, because accuracy cannot be guaranteed, frequent reassessment is recommended.

Misconceptions about older adults contribute to undertreatment. Specifically, providers may believe (incorrectly) that dosage should be low because (1) older adults are relatively insensitive to pain; (2) if pain occurs, older adults can tolerate it well; and (3) older adults are highly sensitive to opioid side effects. The first two concepts have no basis in fact and therefore must not be allowed to influence treatment. Although there is some truth to the third concept, concern about side effects is no excuse for inadequate dosing.

Increased Risk of Side Effects and Adverse Interactions

For several reasons, older adult patients may experience more side effects than younger adults. As noted, drug elimination in older adults is impaired, posing a risk that drug levels may rise dangerously high. However, with careful dosing, drug levels can be kept within a range that is both safe and effective. Drugs with prolonged half-lives (e.g., methadone) pose an increased risk of excessive accumulation, and should be avoided.

The risk of gastric ulceration and renal toxicity from NSAIDs is increased in older patients. Gastric erosion can be reduced by concurrent therapy with misoprostol or a proton pump inhibitor (e.g., esomeprazole). There is no specific way to prevent renal toxicity. The best we can do is to monitor closely for evolving kidney damage.

Older adult patients are at increased risk of adverse drug-drug interactions. In addition to the disorder that's causing pain, older adults are likely to have other disorders and to require more drugs than younger adults. The risk of serious injury from drug interactions can be reduced by careful drug selection and by monitoring for potential reactions.

Young Children

Management of cancer pain in children is much like management in adults. The principal difference is that assessment in children is more difficult. In addition, children frequently experience more pain from chemotherapy and other interventions than from the cancer itself.

Assessment

Assessment must be tailored to the child's developmental level and personality. Selecting an appropriate assessment method is especially important for children with developmental delays, learning disabilities, and emotional disturbances. Assessment can be greatly facilitated by open communication about pain between the child, family, and healthcare team.

Assessment methods include self-reporting, behavioral observation, and measurement of physiologic parameters (e.g., heart rate, blood pressure, respiratory rate, sweating). As stressed earlier, self-reporting is preferred and should be employed whenever appropriate. Behavioral observation is a distant second choice. Because many factors other than pain can alter physiologic parameters, measuring these is the least reliable way to assess pain.

Verbal Children. For children who can verbalize and are older than 4 years, self-reporting is the most reliable way to assess pain. Because children rarely claim to have pain that isn't there, there is little risk of error from overreporting.

However, there *is* a significant risk of error from underreporting. Children may report less pain than they have for several reasons. These include (1) fear that revealing their pain will lead to additional injections and other painful procedures, (2) lack of awareness that healthcare workers can help their pain go away, (3) a desire to protect their parents from the knowledge that their cancer is getting worse, and (4) a desire to please. Because the self-report may conceal pain, it can be helpful to supplement the self-report with behavioral observation (see later in this section).

Preverbal and Nonverbal Children. Because preverbal and nonverbal children cannot self-report pain, a less reliable method must be used for assessment. The principal alternative is *behavioral observation.* Behavioral cues suggesting pain include vocalization (crying, whining, groaning), facial expression (grimacing, frowning, reduced affect), muscle tension, inability to be consoled, protection of body areas, and reduced activity. The biggest drawback to behavioral observation is the risk of a false-negative conclusion. That is, a child may be in pain although his or her behavior may lead the observer to conclude otherwise. For example, sleeping, watching TV, or laughing may suggest that a child is comfortable. However, these behaviors can actually represent an attempt to control pain. Similarly, although sitting quietly might indicate comfort, it could also mean that moving and talking are painful. When behavioral observation leaves doubt about whether the child is in pain, a trial with an analgesic can help confirm the assessment.

Treatment

Therapy of cancer pain in children is essentially the same as in adults. As in adults, drugs are the cornerstone of treatment; nondrug therapies are used only as supplements. Drug selection is guided by the WHO analgesic ladder. Because of the risk of Reye's syndrome, children with influenza or chickenpox should not receive NSAIDs, including aspirin. Acetaminophen is a safe alternative. As in adults, oral dosing is preferred. More invasive routes should be reserved for patients who cannot take drugs by mouth. Children generally object to rectal administration and may refuse treatment by this route. Administration with a PCA device is an option for children older than 7 years.

Neonates and infants are highly sensitive to drugs, and hence must be treated with special caution. Drug sensitivity occurs for two reasons: (1) the blood-brain barrier is incompletely formed, giving drugs ready access to the CNS, and (2) the kidneys and liver are poorly developed, causing drug elimination to be slow. Because of heightened drug sensitivity, neonates and infants are at increased risk of respiratory depression from opioids. Accordingly, when opioids are given to nonventilated infants, the initial dosage should be very low (about one-third the dosage employed for older children). Furthermore, use of opioids should be accompanied by intensive monitoring of respiration.

Opioid Use Disorder

When treating cancer pain in patients with opioid use disorder, we have two primary obligations: we must try to (1) relieve the pain and (2) avoid giving opioids simply because the patient wants to get high. Both obligations are difficult to meet. Because of the challenge, treatment should be directed by a clinician trained in substance abuse as well as pain management.

Concerns about abuse can result in undertreatment of pain. This must be avoided. Remember, patients who abuse opioids feel pain like everyone else and therefore need opioids like everyone else. Clinicians must take special care not to withhold opioids because they have confused relief-seeking behavior with drug-seeking behavior. In the end, we have little choice but to base treatment on the patient's self-report of pain. Hence, if the patient tells us that pain is persisting, adequate doses of opioids should be provided.

Because of opioid tolerance, initial doses in patients with opioid use disorder must be higher than in patients who do not abuse opioids. To estimate how high the initial dosage should be, we must try to estimate the existing degree of tolerance by interviewing the patient about the extent of opioid use.

As with other adults, drug selection can be guided by the WHO analgesic ladder and the NCCN guidelines. If pain is sufficient to justify opioids, then opioids should be used; nonopioids (NSAIDs and acetaminophen) should not be substituted for opioids out of concern for addiction. If the patient is on methadone maintenance, methadone can be used for the pain. However, because regulations limit the dosage of methadone that drug-abuse clinics can dispense, the increased dosage required to manage pain will have to come from another source. One group of opioids—the agonist-antagonists—will precipitate withdrawal in opioid abusers, and hence must never be prescribed for these patients.

Drug delivery with a PCA device can be helpful. By using a PCA device, we can avoid potential conflicts between the patient and the clinician, who would otherwise have to administer each dose. Excessive dosing can be prevented by setting the PCA device to limit how much opioid the patient can self-administer.

PATIENT EDUCATION

Patient education is an integral part of cancer pain management. When education is successful, it can help reduce anxiety, dispel hopelessness, facilitate assessment, enhance compliance, decrease complications, provide a sense of control, and enable patients to take an active role in their care. All of these will promote pain relief.

General Issues

Common sense tells us that patient education should be accurate, comprehensive, and understandable. To reinforce communication, information should be presented at least twice and in more than one way. Major topics to discuss are (1) the nature and causes of pain, (2) assessment and the importance of honest self-reporting, and (3) plans for drug and nondrug therapy. Patients should be encouraged to express their fears and concerns about cancer, cancer pain, and pain treatment—and they should be reassured that pain can be effectively controlled in most cases. All patients should receive a written pain management plan. To facilitate ongoing education, patients should be invited to contact care providers whenever they feel the need—be it to discuss specific concerns with treatment or simply to acquire new information. Finally, patients should know when and how to contact the prescriber to report treatment failure, serious side effects, or new pain.

Drug Therapy

The goal in teaching patients about analgesic drugs is to maximize pain relief and minimize harm. To help achieve this goal, patients should know the following about each drug they take:

- Drug name and therapeutic category
- Dosage size and dosing schedule
- Route and technique of administration
- Expected therapeutic response and when it should develop
- Duration of treatment
- Method of drug storage and disposal
- Symptoms of major adverse effects and measures to minimize discomfort and harm
- Major adverse drug-drug and drug-food interactions
- Whom to contact in the event of therapeutic failure, severe adverse effects, or severe adverse interactions

The dosing schedule should be discussed. Patients should understand that PRN dosing is appropriate only if pain is intermittent. When pain is persistent, as it is for most patients, the objective is to *prevent* pain from returning. Hence, dosing should be done on a fixed schedule ATC, not PRN. However, even with ATC dosing, breakthrough pain can occur. Hence, patients should be taught what drug and dosage to use for rescue treatment.

Fears based on misconceptions about opioids can impair compliance and can thereby impair pain control. The misconceptions that influence compliance the most relate to tolerance, physical dependence, addiction, and side effects. To correct these misconceptions, and thereby dispel fears and improve compliance, the following topics should be discussed:

- *Tolerance*—Some patients fear that, because of tolerance, taking opioids now will decrease their effectiveness later. Hence, to help ensure pain relief in the future, they limit opioid use now and thus suffer needless pain. These patients should be reassured that if tolerance does develop, efficacy can be restored by increasing the dosage; tolerance does not mean that efficacy is lost.
- *Physical Dependence and Addiction*—Many patients fear opioid addiction, and hence are reluctant to take these drugs. This fear is based largely on the misconception that physical dependence (which eventually develops in all patients) equals addiction. Patients should be taught that physical dependence is not the same as addiction and that physical dependence itself is nothing to fear. In addition, they should be taught that the behavior pattern that constitutes addiction rarely develops in people who take opioids in a therapeutic setting.
- *Fear of Severe Side Effects*—Some patients fear that opioids cannot relieve pain without causing severe side effects. These patients should be reassured that when used correctly, opioids are both safe and effective. The most dangerous side effect—respiratory depression—is uncommon.

The rationale for using an adjuvant analgesic should be discussed. With all of the adjuvants, the objective is to *complement* the effects of opioid and nonopioid analgesics. Adjuvants are not intended to substitute for these drugs. Furthermore, because the drugs we use as adjuvants were originally developed to treat disorders other than pain, the rationale for prescribing specific adjuvants should be explained. For example, when duloxetine is prescribed, the patient should understand that the objective is to relieve neuropathic pain and not depression, the disorder for which this drug was originally developed.

Basic issues related to patient education in drug therapy are discussed in Chapter 2.

Nondrug Therapy

Education regarding nondrug therapy focuses on psychosocial interventions. Patients should understand that these interventions are intended as complements to analgesics—not as alternatives. Techniques for imagery, relaxation, and distraction should be introduced early in treatment. Family caregivers should be taught how to apply heat and cold and how to give a therapeutic massage. Patients should be informed about the benefits of peer support groups and given assistance in locating one.

THE JOINT COMMISSION PAIN MANAGEMENT STANDARDS

Thanks to *The Joint Commission* (TJC), undertreatment of pain will no longer be tolerated. TJC is the authority that accredits hospitals and other healthcare institutions in the United States. TJC established a set of standards designed to make assessment and management of pain a priority in the nation's healthcare system. Under the standards, *accountability for pain management is shifted from individual practitioners to the institution as a whole.* Compliance is mandatory: Healthcare organizations that fail to meet the standards will lose accreditation. Loss of accreditation would mean loss of insurance reimbursement and would disqualify teaching hospitals from offering training programs. Hence, thanks to the enforcement power wielded by TJC, healthcare institutions in the United States now have a very real incentive to correct the persistent problem of pain undertreatment. It should be noted that the standards are *not* a guideline on how to treat specific kinds of pain. Rather, they focus on (1) the rights of patients to receive appropriate assessment and management of pain, and (2) ways for institutions to establish a formalized, systematic approach to pain management that involves interdisciplinary teams whose members have clearly identified responsibilities. Specific provisions include the following:

- Institutions must recognize assessment and management of pain as a right of all patients.
- Institutions must assess patients for pain and if pain is present, identify its nature and intensity.
- Institutions must educate patients and their families about pain management and must provide ready access to educational materials.
- Institutions must educate clinical staff about assessment and management of pain and must document the education provided.

- Institutions must establish a system to monitor pain management, including a system of checks and balances in which individuals who assess and manage pain are monitored for compliance with standards set by the institution.
- Institutions must monitor patient satisfaction with pain management.
- Discharge planning must provide for continuing reassessment and management of pain.

A statement from TJC regarding its pain standards can be found on its web site at https://jointcommission.org/topics/pain_management.aspx.

KEY POINTS

- Cancer pain can be relieved in 90% of patients.
- Despite the availability of effective treatments, cancer pain goes unrelieved in a large number of patients.
- Barriers to pain relief include inadequate prescriber training, fears of addiction, and a healthcare system that until recently has put a low priority on pain management.
- Pain is a personal, subjective experience that encompasses not only the sensory perception of pain but also the patient's emotional and cognitive responses to both the painful sensation and the underlying disease.
- Pain has two major forms: nociceptive pain, which results from injury to tissues, and neuropathic pain, which results from injury to peripheral nerves.
- Management of cancer pain is an ongoing process that involves repeated cycles of assessment, intervention, and reassessment. The goal is to create an individualized treatment plan that can meet the changing needs of the patient.
- The patient self-report is the cornerstone of assessment.
- Behavioral observation is a poor substitute for the patient self-report as a method of assessment.
- Analgesic drugs are the principal modality for treating cancer pain.
- Three groups of analgesics are employed: nonopioid analgesics (NSAIDs and acetaminophen), opioid analgesics, and adjuvant analgesics.
- Drug selection is guided by the WHO analgesic ladder: As pain intensity increases, treatment progresses from nonopioid analgesics to opioids of moderate strength (e.g., oxycodone) and then to powerful opioids (e.g., morphine). Adjuvant analgesics can be used at any time. If pain is already intense, treatment can start with an opioid, rather than trying a nonopioid first.
- Because nonopioids and opioids relieve pain by different mechanisms, combining an opioid with a nonopioid can be more effective than either drug alone.
- NSAIDs produce their effects by inhibiting cyclooxygenase (COX), an enzyme with two basic forms: COX-1 and COX-2.
- Most NSAIDs inhibit both COX-1 and COX-2. A few NSAIDs are COX-2 selective.
- Principal adverse effects of the NSAIDs are GI injury, acute renal failure, and bleeding. In addition, all NSAIDs except aspirin pose a risk of thrombotic events.
- The COX-2 inhibitors cause less GI injury than the nonselective NSAIDs, but they pose a greater risk of thrombotic events. Accordingly, long-term use of COX-2 inhibitors is not recommended.
- By inhibiting platelet aggregation, NSAIDs increase the risk of bruising and bleeding in patients with thrombocytopenia, a common side effect of cancer chemotherapy.
- In contrast to opioids, NSAIDs do not cause tolerance, physical dependence, or psychologic dependence.
- Acetaminophen relieves pain but, unlike the NSAIDs, does not suppress inflammation, inhibit platelet aggregation, or promote gastric ulceration or renal failure.
- Because acetaminophen does not affect platelets, the drug is safe for patients with thrombocytopenia.
- Combining acetaminophen with alcohol, even in moderate amounts, can result in potentially fatal liver damage.
- Opioids are the most effective analgesics available, and hence are the primary drugs for treating moderate to severe cancer pain.
- Opioids are especially effective against nociceptive pain; efficacy against neuropathic pain is limited.
- Opioid analgesics relieve pain by mimicking the actions of endogenous opioid peptides (enkephalins, dynorphins, endorphins), primarily at mu receptors in the CNS.
- The opioids fall into two major groups: pure (full) agonists (e.g., morphine) and agonist-antagonists (e.g., butorphanol).
- There is a ceiling to pain relief with the agonist-antagonists, but not with the pure agonists. Hence, for patients with cancer, pure agonists are generally preferred.
- For most patients, opioids should be given on a fixed schedule ATC, with additional doses provided for breakthrough pain. PRN dosing should be limited to patients with intermittent pain.
- Oral administration is preferred for most patients; transdermal administration is a good alternative.
- Intramuscular opioids are painful and should be avoided.
- PCA is a desirable method of opioid delivery because it gives patients more control over their treatment.
- An equianalgesia table can facilitate dosage selection when switching from one opioid to another or from one route to another.
- Over time, opioids cause tolerance, a state in which a specific dose produces a smaller effect than it could when treatment began.
- Tolerance develops to analgesia, euphoria, respiratory depression, and sedation, but not to constipation or miosis.
- Over time, opioids produce physical dependence, a state in which an abstinence syndrome will occur if the drug is abruptly withdrawn. *Note:* Physical dependence is NOT the same as addiction!
- Addiction is a behavior pattern characterized by continued use of a psychoactive substance despite physical,

psychologic, or social harm. *Note:* Addiction is NOT the same as physical dependence!

- Addiction to opioids is very rare in people taking these drugs to relieve pain.
- Misconceptions about opioid addiction are a major cause for undertreatment of cancer pain. Accordingly, we must correct these misconceptions by teaching physicians, nurses, patients, and family members that (1) addiction is not the same as physical dependence, and (2) addiction is very rare in therapeutic settings.
- Respiratory depression is the most dangerous side effect of the opioids. Fortunately, significant respiratory depression is rare.
- Respiratory depression is increased by other drugs with CNS-depressant actions (e.g., alcohol, barbiturates, benzodiazepines). Accordingly, combining these agents with opioids should be avoided.
- Severe respiratory depression can be reversed with naloxone [Narcan], an opioid antagonist. However, because excessive naloxone will reverse opioid analgesia and precipitate withdrawal, dosage must be titrated carefully.
- Opioids cause constipation in most patients. No tolerance develops. Constipation can be minimized by increasing dietary fiber and fluids, and by taking one or more appropriate drugs (stool softener, stimulant laxative, osmotic laxative, peripherally acting opioid antagonist).
- Use of meperidine (a pure opioid agonist) should be avoided because a toxic metabolite can accumulate.
- Agonist-antagonist opioids must not be given to patients taking pure opioid agonists because doing so could reduce analgesia and precipitate withdrawal.
- Adjuvant analgesics can enhance analgesia from opioids, help manage concurrent symptoms that exacerbate pain, and treat side effects caused by opioids. In addition, several adjuvants are effective against neuropathic pain.
- Adjuvant analgesics are given to complement the effects of opioids. Accordingly, these drugs are employed in combination with opioids—not as substitutes.
- Invasive therapies (nerve blocks, neurosurgical procedures) are the last resort for relieving intractable pain. All other options should be exhausted before these are tried.
- Physical interventions (e.g., heat, cold, massage, acupuncture, TENS) and psychosocial interventions (e.g., relaxation, imagery, cognitive distraction, peer support groups) can help reduce pain, but the degree of relief is limited. Accordingly, these interventions should be used only in conjunction with drug therapy—not as substitutes.
- Older adults are more sensitive to drugs than are younger adults. The principal reason is drug accumulation secondary to a decline in hepatic metabolism and renal excretion.
- Undertreatment of pain is especially common in older adults. Undertreatment is inexcusable and must not be allowed.
- Older adults are at risk of increased side effects and adverse drug interactions. Careful drug selection and monitoring can minimize risk.
- Management of cancer pain in children is much like management in adults, except that assessment is more difficult.
- For children who can verbalize and are older than 4 years, self-reporting is the most reliable way to assess pain. The self-report can be supplemented with behavioral observation to enhance accuracy.
- Preverbal and nonverbal children cannot self-report pain, and a less reliable assessment method must be used. The principal option is behavioral observation, a method that carries a significant risk of underassessment.
- When opioid abusers get cancer, they feel pain and need relief like anyone else. If their pain is sufficient to justify opioids, then opioids should be used—nonopioids should not be substituted for opioids out of concern for addiction.
- Pain management standards from TJC are designed to make pain relief an institutional priority, and hence should greatly reduce the incidence of pain undertreatment.

Please visit **http://evolve.elsevier.com/Lehne** for chapter-specific NCLEX® examination review questions.

CHAPTER

30 Drugs for Headache

Headache is a common symptom that can be triggered by a variety of stimuli, including stress, fatigue, acute illness, and sensitivity to alcohol. Many people experience mild, episodic headaches that can be relieved with over-the-counter medications, such as aspirin, acetaminophen [Tylenol, others], and ibuprofen [Motrin, Advil, others]. For these individuals, medical intervention is unnecessary. In contrast, some people experience severe recurrent, debilitating headaches that are frequently unresponsive to aspirin-like drugs. For these individuals, medical attention is merited. In this chapter, we focus on severe forms of headache—specifically, migraine, cluster, and tension-type headaches.

When attempting to treat headache, we must differentiate between headaches that have an identifiable underlying cause (e.g., severe hypertension; hyperthyroidism; tumors; infection; disorders of the eyes, ears, nose, sinuses, and throat) and headaches that have no identifiable cause (e.g., migraine and cluster headaches). If there is a clear cause, it should be treated directly.

As we consider drugs for headache, keep three basic principles in mind. First, antiheadache drugs may be used in two ways: to abort an ongoing attack or to prevent an attack from occurring. Second, not all patients with a particular type of headache respond to the same drugs. Hence, therapy must be individualized. Third, several of the drugs employed to treat severe headaches (e.g., ergotamine, opioids) can cause physical dependence. Accordingly, every effort should be made to keep dependence from developing. If dependence does develop, a withdrawal procedure is needed.

MIGRAINE HEADACHE

CHARACTERISTICS, PATHOPHYSIOLOGY, AND OVERVIEW OF TREATMENT

Characteristics

Migraine headache is characterized by throbbing head pain of moderate to severe intensity that may be unilateral (60%) or bilateral (40%). Most patients also experience nausea and vomiting, along with neck pain and sensitivity to light and sound. Physical activity intensifies the pain. During a prolonged attack, patients develop *hyperalgesia* (augmented responses to painful stimuli) and *allodynia* (painful responses to normally innocuous stimuli). Migraines usually develop in the morning after arising. Pain increases gradually and lasts 4 to 72 hours (median duration 24 hours). On average, attacks occur 1.5 times a month. Precipitating factors include anxiety, fatigue, stress, menstruation, alcohol, weather changes, and tyramine-containing foods.

Migraine has two primary forms: migraine *with aura* and migraine *without aura.* In migraine with aura, the headache is preceded by visual symptoms (flashes of light, a blank area in the field of vision, zigzag patterns). Of the two forms, migraine without aura is more common, affecting about 70% of migraineurs.

Migraine afflicts 37 million people in the United States and over 1 billion worldwide. The headaches are more common and more severe in females, with a lifetime incidence of 43%, compared with 18% in males. About 65% of migraineurs are women in their late teens, 20s, or 30s. With some women, migraine attacks are worse during menstruation but subside during pregnancy and cease after menopause, indicating a hormonal component to the attacks. A family history of the disease is typical.

Migraine is highly debilitating. An attack can prevent participation in social and leisure activities, and can result in lost productivity at home, school, and work. According to the World Health Organization, disability caused by a severe migraine attack equals that caused by quadriplegia, psychosis, or dementia.

Pathophysiology

Migraine headache is a *neurovascular* disorder that involves *dilation* and *inflammation* of intracranial blood vessels. Headache generation begins with neural events that trigger vasodilation. Vasodilation then leads to pain, which leads to further neural activation, thereby amplifying pain-generating signals. Neurons of the trigeminal vascular system, which innervate intracranial blood vessels, are key components.

The exact cause of migraine pain is not completely understood although vasodilation and inflammation are clearly involved. Available data suggest that two compounds—*calcitonin gene–related peptide* (CGRP) and *serotonin* (5-hydroxytryptamine [5-HT])—play important roles. The role of CGRP is to *promote migraine,* and the role of 5-HT is to *suppress* migraine. Data that implicate CGRP as a cause of migraine include the following:

- Plasma levels of CGRP rise during a migraine attack.
- Stimulation of neurons of the trigeminal vascular system promotes release of CGRP, which in turn promotes vasodilation and release of inflammatory neuropeptides.
- Dosing with sumatriptan, a drug that relieves migraine, lowers elevated levels of CGRP.
- Sumatriptan can suppress release of CGRP from cultured trigeminal neurons.

Data that support a protective role for 5-HT include the following:

- Plasma levels of 5-HT drop by 50% during a migraine attack.
- Depletion of 5-HT with reserpine can precipitate an attack in migraine-prone individuals.
- Administration of 5-HT or sumatriptan, both of which activate 5-HT receptors, can abort an ongoing attack.

Overview of Treatment

Drugs for migraine are employed in two ways: to abort an ongoing attack and to prevent attacks from occurring. Drugs used to abort an attack fall into two groups: nonspecific analgesics (aspirin-like drugs and opioid analgesics) and migraine-specific drugs (serotonin$_{1B/1D}$ receptor agonists [triptans] and ergot alkaloids). Drugs employed for prophylaxis include beta blockers (e.g., propranolol), tricyclic antidepressants (e.g., amitriptyline), and antiepileptic drugs (e.g., divalproex).

Nondrug measures can help. Patients should try to control or eliminate triggers and should maintain a regular pattern of eating, sleeping, and exercise. Why? Because in people with migraine the brain seems to have a low tolerance for the ups and downs of life. Once an attack has begun, the migraineur should retire to a dark, quiet room. Placing an ice pack on the neck and scalp can help.

TABLE 30.1 ▪ Migraine Headache: Drugs for Abortive Therapy

NONSPECIFIC ANALGESICS
Aspirin-like Drugs
Acetaminophen + aspirin + caffeine [Excedrin Migraine]
Nonsteroidal anti-inflammatory drugs (e.g., aspirin, naproxen, diclofenac)
Opioid Analgesics
Butorphanol
Meperidine [Demerol]
MIGRAINE-SPECIFIC DRUGS
Selective Serotonin$_{1B/1D}$ Receptor Agonists (Triptans)
Almotriptan [Axert]
Eletriptan [Relpax]
Frovatriptan [Frova]
Naratriptan [Amerge]
Rizatriptan [Maxalt]
Sumatriptan [Imitrex, Sumavel DosePro]
Zolmitriptan [Zomig]
Ergot Alkaloids
Dihydroergotamine [D.H.E. 45, Migranal]
Ergotamine [Ergomar]
Ergotamine + caffeine [Cafergot, Migergot]

ABORTIVE THERAPY

The objective of abortive therapy is to eliminate headache pain and suppress associated nausea and vomiting. Treatment should commence at the earliest sign of an attack. Because migraine causes GI disturbances (nausea, vomiting, and gastric stasis), oral therapy may be ineffective once an attack has begun. Hence, for treatment of an established attack, a drug that can be administered by injection, nasal spray, or rectal suppository may be best. As noted, two types of drugs are used: nonspecific analgesics and migraine-specific agents. Representative drugs are listed in Table 30.1.

Drug selection depends on the intensity of the attack. For mild to moderate symptoms, an *aspirin-like drug* (e.g., aspirin, naproxen) may be sufficient. For moderate to severe symptoms, patients should take a *migraine-specific drug,* such as a serotonin$_{1B/1D}$ agonist, or—less frequently used—an ergot alkaloid (ergotamine or dihydroergotamine). If these agents fail to relieve pain, an *opioid analgesic* (e.g., butorphanol, meperidine) may be needed. Note that opioids should be reserved for treatment in patients with migraines resistant to all other treatments.

Use of abortive medications (both nonspecific and migraine-specific) should be limited to 1 or 2 days a week. More frequent use can lead to *medication overuse headache* (MOH), also known as drug-induced headache or drug-rebound headache (Box 30.1).

Antiemetics are important adjuncts to migraine therapy. By reducing nausea and vomiting, these drugs can (1) make the patient more comfortable and (2) permit therapy with oral antimigraine drugs. Two antiemetics—*metoclopramide* [Reglan] and *prochlorperazine*—are used most often. Of the two, metoclopramide is preferred. In addition to suppressing nausea and vomiting, metoclopramide can reverse gastric stasis caused by the attack and can thereby facilitate absorption of oral antimigraine drugs. Like metoclopramide, prochlorperazine suppresses nausea and vomiting. However, because of its anticholinergic actions, prochlorperazine can make gastric stasis even worse.

si

BOX 30.1 ▪ SPECIAL INTEREST TOPIC

MEDICATION OVERUSE HEADACHE: TOO MUCH OF A GOOD THING

People who take headache medicine every day often develop medication overuse headaches (MOHs). An MOH is a chronic headache that develops in response to frequent use of headache medicines and that resolves days to weeks after the overused drug is withdrawn. The stage for MOH is set when headache drugs are taken too often, especially if the dosage is high. Discontinuing the medication brings on the MOH, which causes the patient to resume taking medicine—setting up a repeating cycle of MOH, followed by medication use and discontinuation, followed by another MOH, and so on. One reason the cycle gets established is that patients don't realize that the drugs they're taking to *treat* headache can, if taken too often, become the *cause* of headache. Failing to recognize MOH for what it is, patients take more and more medicine to make their headaches go away, but only succeed in making MOH worse.

Almost all of the medicines used for abortive headache therapy can cause MOH: analgesics (aspirin-like drugs, opioids), triptans, ergotamine (but not dihydroergotamine), and caffeine.

How can MOH be treated? The only hope is to stop taking all headache medicines. Unfortunately, when medication is withdrawn, headaches increase for a while. Their duration and intensity depend on the drug that was overused. With triptans, withdrawal headaches are relatively mild and often resolve in a few days. In contrast, with analgesics or ergots, withdrawal headaches are more intense and may persist for 2 weeks or more.

Small studies have demonstrated the positive effects of high-dose glucocorticoids as treatment for medication withdrawal. In these studies, duration of withdrawal headaches was shorter in those taking high-dose glucocorticoids than in the nontreatment group. Unfortunately, there are no other controlled studies regarding glucocorticoids or any other medications at this time, so it is not currently recommended to treat withdrawal headaches with headache medication or other analgesics.

Several measures can *decrease the risk* of developing MOH. The most important is to limit the use of abortive medicines. If possible, patients should take these drugs no more than 2 or 3 times a week—and doses should be no higher than actually needed. Alternating headache medicines may help too, because this would limit exposure to any one drug. If headaches begin to occur more than 2 or 3 times a month, prophylactic therapy should be tried. Implementing nondrug measures—stress reduction, avoidance of triggers, getting sufficient sleep, relaxation techniques, and biofeedback—can reduce the need for headache medicines and decrease exposure to drugs that cause MOH.

Analgesics

Aspirin-like Drugs

Aspirin, acetaminophen, naproxen, diclofenac, and other aspirin-like analgesics can provide adequate relief of mild to moderate migraine attacks. In fact, when combined with metoclopramide (to enhance absorption), aspirin may work as well as sumatriptan, a highly effective antimigraine drug. Moreover, the combination of aspirin plus metoclopramide costs less than sumatriptan and causes fewer adverse effects.

Acetaminophen can be used alone if the episode is non-incapacitating, otherwise it should be used only in combination with other drugs. One effective combination, marketed as *Excedrin Migraine,* consists of acetaminophen, aspirin, and caffeine.

Opioid Analgesics

Opioid analgesics are reserved for severe migraine that has not responded to first-line medications. The agents used most often are *meperidine* [Demerol] and *butorphanol nasal spray* [Stadol NS]. Of the two, butorphanol is preferred. Why? Because meperidine can cause all of the adverse effects associated with other pure opioid agonists (e.g., respiratory depression, sedation, constipation) and also has significant abuse potential. These drawbacks are less pronounced with butorphanol.

Serotonin$_{1B/1D}$ Receptor Agonists (Triptans)

The serotonin$_{1B/1D}$ receptor agonists, also known as *triptans,* are first-line drugs for terminating a migraine attack. These agents relieve pain by constricting intracranial blood vessels and suppressing release of inflammatory neuropeptides. All are well tolerated. Rarely, they cause symptomatic coronary vasospasm.

Sumatriptan

Sumatriptan [Imitrex, Sumavel DosePro] was the first triptan available and will serve as our prototype for the group. The drug can be administered by mouth, nasal inhalation, or subQ injection.

Mechanism of Action. Sumatriptan, an analog of 5-HT, causes selective activation of 5-HT$_{1B}$ and 5-HT$_{1D}$ receptors (5-HT$_{1B/1D}$ receptors). The drug has no affinity for 5-HT$_2$ or 5-HT$_3$ receptors, nor does it bind to adrenergic, dopaminergic, muscarinic, or histaminergic receptors. Binding to 5-HT$_{1B/1D}$ receptors on intracranial blood vessels causes vasoconstriction. Binding to 5-HT$_{1B/1D}$ receptors on sensory nerves of the trigeminal vascular system suppresses release of CGRT, a compound that promotes release of inflammatory neuropeptides. As a result, sumatriptan reduces release of inflammatory neuropeptides and thereby diminishes perivascular inflammation. Both actions—vasoconstriction and decreased perivascular inflammation—help relieve migraine pain.

Therapeutic Use. Sumatriptan is taken to abort an ongoing migraine attack. The drug relieves headache and associated symptoms (nausea, neck pain, photophobia, phonophobia). In clinical trials, sumatriptan gave complete relief to the majority of patients. Beneficial effects begin about 15 minutes after subQ or intranasal dosing and 30 to 60 minutes after oral dosing. Complete relief occurs in 40% to 60% of patients 2 hours after subQ dosing, in 30% to 60% of patients 2 hours after intranasal dosing, in 18% of patients 2 hours after transdermal dosing, and in 50% to 60% of patients 4 hours after oral dosing. Unfortunately, headache returns in about 40% of patients within 24 hours. In comparison, the 24-hour recurrence rate with dihydroergotamine is only 14%. In patients who respond to subQ sumatriptan, subsequent administration of oral sumatriptan can delay recurrence but does not prevent it. In addition to migraine, sumatriptan is approved for cluster headaches.

Pharmacokinetics. With oral or intranasal dosing, bioavailability is low (about 15%). The transdermal system has even lower bioavailability (about 6%), whereas with subQ dosing, bioavailability is high (97%). As a result, oral and intranasal doses are considerably higher than subQ and transdermal doses. Sumatriptan undergoes extensive hepatic metabolism, primarily by monoamine oxidase (MAO), followed by excretion in the urine. The half-life is short—about 2.5 hours.

Adverse Effects. Sumatriptan is generally well tolerated. Most side effects are transient and mild. Coronary vasospasm is the biggest concern.

Chest Symptoms. About 50% of patients experience unpleasant chest symptoms, usually described as "heavy arms" or "chest pressure" rather than pain. These symptoms are transient and *not* related to ischemic heart disease. Possible causes are pulmonary vasoconstriction, esophageal spasm, intercostal muscle spasm, and bronchoconstriction. Patients should be forewarned of these symptoms and reassured that they are not dangerous.

Coronary Vasospasm. Very rarely, sumatriptan and other triptans can cause angina secondary to coronary vasospasm. Electrocardiographic changes have been observed in patients with coronary artery disease (CAD) or Prinzmetal's (vasospastic) angina. To reduce the risk of angina, avoid sumatriptan in patients with risk factors for CAD until CAD has been ruled out. These patients include postmenopausal women, men older than 40 years, smokers, and patients with hypertension, hypercholesterolemia, diabetes, or a family history of CAD. Owing to the risk of coronary vasospasm, sumatriptan is contraindicated for patients with a history of ischemic heart disease, myocardial infarction (MI), uncontrolled hypertension, or other heart disease.

Teratogenesis. Sumatriptan should be avoided during pregnancy. When given daily to pregnant rabbits, the drug was embryolethal at blood levels only 3 times higher than those achieved with a 6-mg subQ injection in humans (a typical dose). Accordingly, unless the prescriber directs otherwise, women should be instructed to avoid the drug if they are pregnant or think they might be, if they are trying to become pregnant, or if they are not using an adequate form of contraception. Sumatriptan is classified in U.S. Food and Drug Administration (FDA) Pregnancy Risk Category C.[a]

Other Adverse Effects. Mild reactions include *vertigo, malaise, fatigue,* and *tingling sensations.* Transient pain and redness may occur at sites of subQ injection. The intranasal formulation tastes bad and may irritate the nose and throat.

[a]As of 2020, the FDA will no longer use Pregnancy Risk Categories. Please refer to Chapter 9 for more information.

Safety Alert

SEROTONIN RECEPTOR AGONISTS

Serotonin receptor agonists can cause vasoconstriction and coronary vasospasm. These drugs should not be administered to patients with coronary artery disease, current symptoms of angina, or uncontrolled hypertension.

Drug Interactions

Ergot Alkaloids and Other Triptans. Sumatriptan, other triptans, and ergot alkaloids (e.g., ergotamine, dihydroergotamine) all cause vasoconstriction. Accordingly, if one triptan is combined with another or with an ergot alkaloid, excessive and prolonged vasospasm could result. Accordingly, sumatriptan should not be used within 24 hours of an ergot derivative or another triptan.

Monoamine Oxidase Inhibitors. Monoamine oxidase inhibitors (MAOIs) can suppress hepatic degradation of sumatriptan, causing its plasma level to rise. Toxicity can result. Accordingly, sumatriptan should not be combined with an MAOI and should not be used within 2 weeks of stopping an MAOI.

Selective Serotonin Reuptake Inhibitors (SSRIs) and Serotonin/Norepinephrine Reuptake Inhibitors (SNRIs). As discussed in Chapter 32, the SSRIs (e.g., fluoxetine [Prozac]) and SNRIs (e.g., duloxetine [Cymbalta]) indirectly activate serotonin receptors in the brain (by increasing the availability of serotonin at brain synapses). If receptor activation is excessive, serotonin syndrome can occur. Signs and symptoms include altered mental status (agitation, confusion, disorientation, anxiety, hallucinations, poor concentration) as well as incoordination, myoclonus, hyperreflexia, excessive sweating, tremor, and fever. Deaths have occurred. Because the triptans *directly* activate serotonin receptors and the SSRIs and SNRIs *indirectly* activate serotonin receptors, you can see how combining these drugs could lead to excessive receptor activation. Accordingly, these combinations should not be used.

Preparations, Dosage, and Administration

Subcutaneous, Using a Needle. Sumatriptan succinate [Imitrex] for subQ injection is available in two strengths: 4 mg and 6 mg. Both strengths are supplied in a STATdose Pen for self-injection. The maximum single dose is 6 mg. The maximum that may be given in 24 hours is two 6-mg doses, separated by at least 1 hour.

Subcutaneous, Using a Needle-Free Device. The sumatriptan needle-free device [Sumavel DosePro] uses pressurized nitrogen to push a sumatriptan solution (6 mg) through the skin into the subcutaneous tissue. Injections are made into the thigh or abdomen. Bioavailability and dosage are the same as when using a needle. Injection pain is the same too.

Oral. Sumatriptan [Imitrex], by itself, is available in 25-, 50-, and 100-mg tablets. The usual dose is 25 mg, but doses as high as 100 mg may be tried. If, after 2 hours, the response to the first dose is unsatisfactory, a second dose may be given.

Oral sumatriptan is also available with naproxen in fixed-dose combination tablets marketed as *Treximet* (see *Other Abortive Agents* later in this chapter).

Nasal Spray. Sumatriptan [Imitrex] is available in 5- and 20-mg unit-dose spray devices. The initial dose is 5, 10, or 20 mg, which can be repeated in 2 hours if needed. The maximum 24-hour dose is 40 mg.

Nasal Powder. Capsules containing 11 mg of sumatriptan are available for nasal inhalation and sold as *Onzetra Xsail.* The initial dose is one capsule inhaled through each nostril. This dose may be repeated in 2 hours. The maximum 24-hour dose is 44 mg.

Other Serotonin$_{1B/1D}$ Receptor Agonists

In addition to sumatriptan, the triptan family includes six other drugs: naratriptan [Amerge], rizatriptan [Maxalt], zolmitriptan [Zomig], almotriptan [Axert], frovatriptan [Frova], and eletriptan [Relpax]. All six are administered orally, and one—zolmitriptan—is also given by nasal spray. All six are essentially equal to sumatriptan with respect to efficacy and safety, and all have the same mechanism of action: activation of 5-$HT_{1B/1D}$ receptors with subsequent intracranial vasoconstriction and decreased perivascular inflammation. All are in FDA Pregnancy Risk Category C.[b] Because the triptans are very similar, selection among them is based on differences in kinetics, side effects, and drug interactions. Dosage and time course are shown in Table 30.2.

Zolmitriptan. Zolmitriptan [Zomig, Zomig ZMT] is indicated for terminating an ongoing migraine attack. The drug is similar to sumatriptan with regard to mechanism, efficacy, time course, side effects, and interactions. Zolmitriptan is formulated for oral and intranasal use. Two oral preparations are available: tablets (2.5 and 5 mg), sold as *Zomig,* and melt-in-the-mouth wafers (2.5 and 5 mg), sold as *Zomig ZMT.* Zomig ZMT dissolves in saliva on the tongue. Because no water is needed, the drug can be taken conveniently as soon as an aura is perceived. Be aware, however, that onset of effects is no faster than with standard Zomig tablets. With either formulation, a 2.5-mg dose produces the most favorable response/tolerability ratio. Intranasal zolmitriptan, sold as *Zomig,* is available in a 2.5- and 5-mg single-dose spray device. Effects begin in 15 minutes, compared with 45 minutes for the oral products. However, although the nasal spray is faster, it does have one drawback: It tastes bad (albeit not as bad as sumatriptan nasal spray). Regardless of the formulation, about 65% of patients respond within 2 hours. If headache persists, dosing can be repeated 2 hours after the initial dose. The maximum dose per 24 hours is 10 mg. Headache recurs in 8% to 32% of patients. Adverse effects are generally mild and transient. Like sumatriptan, zolmitriptan causes harmless, transient chest discomfort. Of much greater concern, the drug can cause coronary vasospasm, and hence is contraindicated for patients with ischemic heart disease, prior MI, or uncontrolled hypertension. Like sumatriptan, zolmitriptan should not be administered within 24 hours of an ergot alkaloid or another triptan, or within 2 weeks of stopping an MAOI. To avoid serotonin syndrome, zolmitriptan should not be combined with an SSRI or SNRI.

Naratriptan. Naratriptan [Amerge] is indicated for oral therapy of an ongoing migraine attack. Compared with most other triptans, naratriptan has a slower onset and longer duration. Because effects persist, the 24-hour migraine recurrence rate may be reduced. Naratriptan is available in 1- and 2.5-mg tablets. The 2.5-mg strength is more effective but causes more side effects. The initial dose is 1 or 2.5 mg. Dosing may be repeated in 4 hours if needed. The maximum daily dose is 5 mg. Like other triptans, naratriptan causes transient chest discomfort. Also like other triptans, the drug can cause coronary vasospasm, and hence it is contraindicated for patients with ischemic heart disease, prior MI, or uncontrolled hypertension. To avoid excessive vasospasm, naratriptan should not be administered within 24 hours of an ergot alkaloid or another triptan. Like other triptans, naratriptan should not be combined with an SSRI or SNRI, owing to the risk of serotonin syndrome. In contrast to some triptans, naratriptan can be used safely with an MAOI.

Rizatriptan. Rizatriptan [Maxalt, Maxalt MLT] may be the most consistently effective triptan for terminating an ongoing migraine attack. The drug is similar to sumatriptan with regard to mechanism, efficacy, time course, side effects, and interactions. Rizatriptan is available in two oral formulations: standard tablets [Maxalt] and melt-in-the-mouth wafers [Maxalt MLT] that can be taken without water. Both formulations come in 5- and 10-mg strengths. The initial dose is 5 or 10 mg. Dosing may be repeated in 2 hours if needed. No more than 30 mg should be taken per day. Adverse effects are generally mild and transient. Like other triptans, rizatriptan causes harmless, transient chest discomfort. Also like other triptans, the drug can cause coronary vasospasm, and hence is contraindicated for patients with ischemic heart disease, prior MI, or uncontrolled hypertension. To avoid excessive vasospasm, rizatriptan should not be administered within 24 hours of an ergot alkaloid or another triptan, or within 2 weeks of stopping an MAOI. Like other triptans, rizatriptan should not be combined with an SSRI or SNRI, owing to the risk of serotonin syndrome. Propranolol can raise levels of rizatriptan, and hence a dosage reduction may be needed. Rizatriptan may harm the developing fetus: In rats, the drug increased perinatal mortality, reduced learning capacity, and decreased pre- and post-weaning weight. However, postmarketing studies suggest that, in humans, rizatriptan may not increase the risk of congenital anomalies or spontaneous abortion. As these studies were done on small populations, the drug should be used with caution in pregnant patients until further research is completed.

Almotriptan. Almotriptan [Axert] is indicated for oral therapy of an ongoing migraine attack. The drug is similar to sumatriptan with regard to mechanism, efficacy, and time course—and is better tolerated. Almotriptan is available in 6.25- and 12.5-mg tablets. The initial dose is 6.25 or 12.5 mg. Dosing can be repeated in 2 hours if headache persists. The maximum dose per 24 hours is 25 mg. Adverse effects are minimal. Like other triptans, almotriptan can cause harmless, transient chest discomfort—but the incidence is very low (only 0.3%). Also like other triptans, the drug can cause coronary vasospasm, and hence is contraindicated for patients with ischemic heart disease, prior MI, or uncontrolled hypertension. Almotriptan is metabolized by CYP3A4 (the 3A4 isoenzyme of cytochrome P450), and hence a dosage reduction is recommended if the drug is combined with a potent CYP3A4 inhibitor (e.g., ketoconazole, itraconazole, clarithromycin, ritonavir). To avoid excessive vasospasm, almotriptan should not be administered within 24 hours of an ergot alkaloid or another triptan. Like other triptans, almotriptan should not be combined with an SSRI or SNRI, owing to a risk of serotonin syndrome. In contrast to some triptans, almotriptan can be combined safely with an MAOI.

Frovatriptan. Frovatriptan [Frova] is indicated for oral therapy of an ongoing migraine attack. The drug is similar to other triptans with regard to mechanism and side effects—but is less effective and has very different kinetics. Effects begin slowly, but are sustained—thanks to the drug's long half-life (26 hours). Although the number of patients responding at 2 hours is low (37% to 46%), rates of headache recurrence are low too (7% to 23%)—lower than with any other triptan. Frovatriptan is available in 2.5-mg tablets. The initial dose is 2.5 mg. If headache recurs after initial relief, dosing can be repeated—but no sooner than 2 hours after the first dose. If there was no response to the first dose, repeat dosing is unlikely to help. The maximum dose per 24 hours is 7.5 mg. Adverse effects are mild and transient. Like sumatriptan, frovatriptan can cause harmless, transient chest discomfort. In addition, the drug can cause coronary vasospasm, and hence is contraindicated for patients with ischemic heart disease, prior MI, or uncontrolled hypertension. To avoid excessive vasospasm, frovatriptan should not be administered within 24 hours of an ergot alkaloid or another triptan. However, it can be used concurrently with an MAOI. Like other triptans, frovatriptan should not be combined with an SSRI or SNRI, owing to the risk of serotonin syndrome.

Eletriptan. Eletriptan [Relpax] is indicated for oral therapy of an ongoing migraine attack. The drug is at least as effective as oral sumatriptan and may have a faster onset. Eletriptan is available in 20- and 40-mg tablets. The initial dose is 20 or 40 mg, which can be repeated in 2 hours if needed. The total dose in 24 hours should not exceed 80 mg. Like other triptans, eletriptan can cause transient chest discomfort. Also like other triptans, it can cause coronary vasospasm, and hence is contraindicated for patients with ischemic heart disease, prior MI, or uncontrolled hypertension. To avoid excessive vasospasm, eletriptan should not be administered within 24 hours of an ergot alkaloid or another triptan. However, the drug may be used concurrently with an MAOI, as eletriptan is not broken down by MAO. Eletriptan is metabolized in the liver by CYP3A4, and hence strong inhibitors of CYP3A4 (e.g., ketoconazole, itraconazole, clarithromycin, ritonavir) may cause toxicity by raising eletriptan levels. Accordingly, eletriptan should not be used within 72 hours of these drugs. Eletriptan levels may also be raised by verapamil, a moderate CYP3A4 inhibitor used for migraine prophylaxis; caution is advised. Like other triptans, eletriptan should not be combined with an SSRI or SNRI, owing to the risk of serotonin syndrome.

Prototype Drugs

DRUGS FOR MIGRAINE HEADACHE

Nonsteroidal Anti-Inflammatory Drugs
Aspirin

Selective Serotonin Receptor Agonists
Sumatriptan

Ergot Alkaloids
Ergotamine

Ergot Alkaloids

Ergotamine

Mechanism of Antimigraine Action. Ergotamine has complex actions, and the precise mechanism by which it aborts

[b]As of 2020, the FDA will no longer use Pregnancy Risk Categories. Please refer to Chapter 9 for more information.

TABLE 30.2 ■ Clinical Pharmacology of the Triptans

Generic Name [Brand Name]	Route	Onset (min)	Duration	Half-Life (hr)	Dosage	Contraindicated Drugs: SSRIs, SNRIs, Triptans, Ergots	Contraindicated Drugs: MAOIs	Contraindicated Drugs: CYP3A4 Inhibitors	Comments
Sumatriptan									
[Imitrex]	Oral	30–60	Short	2.5	25, 50, or 100 mg; may repeat in 2 hr (max. 200 mg/24 hr)	✓	✓		First triptan available and best understood. Available in three fast-acting formulations: nasal spray, an auto-injector for subQ dosing (using a needle), and a needle-free device for subQ dosing [Sumavel DosePro].
[Imitrex]	Nasal spray	15–20			5 or 20 mg; may repeat in 2 hr (max. 40 mg/24 hr)				
[Onzetra Xsail]	Nasal capsule	10–120			11 mg (1 capsule) per nostril; may repeat in 2 hr (max. 44 mg/24 hr)				
[Imitrex]	SubQ, with needle	10–15			6 mg; may repeat in 1 hr (max. 12 mg/24 hr)				
[Sumavel DosePro]	SubQ, needle-free	10			6 mg; may repeat in 1 hr (max. 12 mg/24 hr)				
Almotriptan [Axert]	Oral	30–120	Short	3–4	6.25 or 12.5 mg; may repeat in 2 hr (max. 25 mg/24 hr)	✓			Incidence of chest discomfort (pain, tightness, pressure) is lower than with other triptans. Decrease dosage if combined with a CYP3A4 inhibitor.
Eletriptan [Relpax]	Oral	60	Short	4	20 or 40 mg; may repeat in 2 hr (max. 40 mg/24 hr)	✓		✓	Bioavailability increased by high-fat meal. Good balance between fast onset and long duration.
Frovatriptan [Frova]	Oral	120–180	Long	26	2.5 mg; may repeat in 2 hr	✓			Slowest onset, longest half-life, and lowest rate of headache recurrence. Decrease dose if combined with propranolol.
Naratriptan [Amerge]	Oral	60–180	Intermediate	6	1 or 2.5 mg; may repeat in 4 hr (max. 5 mg/24 hr)	✓			Slower onset and longer duration than most triptans.
Rizatriptan [Maxalt, Maxalt MLT]	Oral	30–120	Short	2–3	5 or 10 mg; may repeat in 2 hr (max. 30 mg/24 hr)	✓	✓		May be the most consistently effective triptan. Decrease dose if combined with propranolol. Available in melt-in-the-mouth wafers [Maxalt MLT] that can be taken without water.
Zolmitriptan									
[Zomig, Zomig ZMT]	Oral	45	Short	3	2.5 or 5 mg; may repeat in 2 hr (max. 10 mg/24 hr)	✓	✓		Available in a fast-acting nasal spray and in melt-in-the-mouth wafers [Zomig ZMT] that can be taken without water.
[Zomig]	Nasal spray	15			2.5 or 5 mg; may repeat in 2 hr (max. 10 mg/24 hr)				

CYP3A4, 3A4 isoenzyme of cytochrome P450; *MAOIs,* monoamine oxidase inhibitors; *SNRIs,* serotonin/norepinephrine reuptake inhibitors; *SSRIs,* selective serotonin reuptake inhibitors.

migraine is unknown. Ergotamine can alter transmission at serotonergic, dopaminergic, and alpha-adrenergic junctions. Current evidence suggests that antimigraine effects are related to agonist activity at subtypes of serotonin receptors, specifically 5-HT_{1B} and 5-HT_{1D} receptors. Additional evidence indicates that ergotamine can block inflammation associated with the trigeminal vascular system, perhaps by suppressing release of CGRP. Relief may also be related to vascular effects. In cranial arteries, ergotamine acts directly to promote constriction and reduce the amplitude of pulsations. In addition, the drug can affect blood flow by depressing the vasomotor center.

Therapeutic Uses. Ergotamine is used as a second-line drug for stopping an ongoing migraine attack in patients who have not responded to a triptan. Owing to the risk of dependence (see *Physical Dependence* later in this chapter), ergotamine should not be taken daily on a long-term basis.

Pharmacokinetics. Administration may be oral, sublingual, or rectal. Bioavailability with oral and sublingual administration is low. Bioavailability with rectal administration is higher. Although the half-life of ergotamine is only 2 hours, pharmacologic effects can still be observed 24 hours after dosing. Ergotamine undergoes metabolism by CYP3A4 followed by excretion in the bile.

Adverse Effects. Ergotamine is well tolerated at usual therapeutic doses. The drug can stimulate the chemoreceptor trigger zone, causing *nausea and vomiting* in about 10% of patients, thereby augmenting nausea and vomiting caused by the migraine itself. Concurrent treatment with metoclopramide or a phenothiazine antiemetic (e.g., prochlorperazine) can help reduce these responses. Other common side effects include *weakness in the legs, myalgia, numbness and tingling in the fingers and toes, angina-like pain,* and *tachycardia or bradycardia.*

Overdose. Acute or chronic overdose can cause serious toxicity referred to as *ergotism.* In addition to the adverse effects seen at therapeutic doses, overdose can cause ischemia secondary to constriction of peripheral arteries and arterioles: the extremities become cold, pale, and numb; muscle pain develops; and gangrene may eventually result. Patients should be informed about these responses and instructed to seek immediate medical attention if they develop. The risk of ergotism is highest in patients with sepsis, peripheral vascular disease, and renal or hepatic impairment. Management consists of discontinuing ergotamine, followed by measures to maintain circulation (treatment with anticoagulants and with IV nitroprusside, phentolamine, or nitroglycerin as appropriate).

Drug Interactions

Triptans. Ergotamine should not be combined with triptans (e.g., sumatriptan, zolmitriptan) because a prolonged vasospastic reaction could occur. To avoid this problem, dosing with ergotamine and serotonin agonists should be separated by at least 24 hours.

CYP3A4 Inhibitors. Potent inhibitors of CYP3A4 can raise ergotamine to dangerous levels, posing a risk of intense vasospasm. Cerebral and/or peripheral ischemia can result. Accordingly, concurrent use with CYP3A4 inhibitors is contraindicated. Drugs to avoid include certain HIV protease inhibitors (e.g., ritonavir, nelfinavir), azole antifungal drugs (e.g., ketoconazole, itraconazole), and macrolide antibiotics (e.g., erythromycin, clarithromycin). Less potent inhibitors (e.g., saquinavir, nefazodone, fluconazole, grapefruit juice) should be used with caution.

Physical Dependence. Regular daily use of ergotamine, even in moderate doses, can cause physical dependence. The withdrawal syndrome is characterized by headache, nausea, vomiting, and restlessness. That is, withdrawal resembles a migraine attack. Patients who experience these symptoms are likely to resume taking the drug, thereby perpetuating the cycle of dependence. Hospitalization may be required to break the cycle. To avoid dependence, dosage and duration of treatment must be restricted (see dosing guidelines later in this section).

Contraindications. Ergotamine is contraindicated for patients with hepatic or renal impairment, sepsis (gangrene has resulted), CAD, peripheral vascular disease, and uncontrolled hypertension and for those taking potent inhibitors of CYP3A4. In addition, the drug should not be taken during pregnancy. Why? Ergotamine can promote uterine contractions, and hence might cause fetal harm or abortion. In fact, because of its effects on the uterus, ergotamine is classified in FDA Pregnancy Risk Category X[c]: The risk of use by pregnant patients clearly outweighs any possible benefits. Warn women of childbearing age to avoid pregnancy while using this drug.

Preparations, Dosage, and Administration. Ergotamine by itself is available in tablets for sublingual use. In addition, ergotamine is available in combination with caffeine for oral and rectal dosing.

Sublingual. Ergotamine tartrate [Ergomar] is supplied in 2-mg tablets for sublingual use. One tablet should be placed under the tongue immediately after onset of aura or headache. If needed, additional tablets can be administered at 30-minute intervals—up to a maximum of 3 tablets/24 hr or 5 tablets/wk.

Oral. Tablets for oral dosing, sold as *Cafergot,* contain 1 mg ergotamine tartrate and 100 mg caffeine. Two tablets are taken immediately after onset of aura or headache. One additional tablet can be administered every 30 minutes—up to a maximum of 6 per attack or 10 per week.

Rectal. Suppositories for rectal dosing, sold as *Migergot,* contain 2 mg ergotamine tartrate and 100 mg caffeine. No more than 5 suppositories should be administered per week.

Dihydroergotamine

Therapeutic Uses. Parenteral dihydroergotamine [D.H.E. 45, Migranal]—given IM, IV, or subQ—is a second-line drug for terminating a migraine attack. The drug also may be given by intranasal spray. A formulation for oral inhalation is undergoing review by the FDA. Intranasal dihydroergotamine is less effective than intranasal sumatriptan but is associated with a lower rate of migraine recurrence.

Pharmacologic Effects. The actions of dihydroergotamine are similar to those of ergotamine. Like ergotamine, dihydroergotamine alters transmission at serotonergic, dopaminergic, and alpha-adrenergic junctions. In contrast to ergotamine, dihydroergotamine causes little nausea and vomiting, no physical dependence, and minimal peripheral vasoconstriction (when used alone). Diarrhea, however, is prominent.

Pharmacokinetics. Dihydroergotamine may be administered parenterally or by nasal spray—but not by mouth (owing to extensive first-pass metabolism). In the liver, the drug is metabolized by CYP3A4. An active metabolite (8′-hydroxydihydroergotamine) contributes to therapeutic effects. The half-life of dihydroergotamine plus the active metabolite is about 21 hours.

Drug Interactions. As with ergotamine, dihydroergotamine should not be combined with potent inhibitors of CYP3A4,

[c]As of 2020, the FDA will no longer use Pregnancy Risk Categories. Please refer to Chapter 9 for more information.

and should not be administered within 24 hours of a serotonin agonist (e.g., sumatriptan).

Contraindications. Like ergotamine, dihydroergotamine is contraindicated for patients with CAD, peripheral vascular disease, sepsis, pregnancy, and hepatic or renal impairment, and for patients taking triptans or potent inhibitors of CYP3A4.

Parenteral Administration. Dihydroergotamine mesylate [D.H.E. 45] is available in solution (1 mg/mL) for IM, IV, and subQ administration.

Intramuscular and Subcutaneous. The initial dose is 1 mg immediately after symptom onset. Additional 1-mg doses may be given hourly—but the total dose should not exceed 3 mg/24 hr for IM or subQ administration. With either route, the total dose should not exceed 6 mg/wk.

Intravenous. One milligram is given initially, followed by 1 mg an hour later if needed. Dosage should not exceed 2 mg/24 hr or 6 mg/wk.

Intranasal Administration. The nasal spray device [Migranal] delivers 0.5 mg of dihydroergotamine per actuation. The dosage is 1 spray in each nostril, repeated in 15 minutes, for a total of 2 mg. Pain is relieved in up to 64% of patients within 2 hours. The 24-hour recurrence rate is 14%.

Other Abortive Agents

Sumatriptan/Naproxen

Sumatriptan and naproxen (a nonsteroidal anti-inflammatory drug) are available in a fixed-dose combination under the brand name *Treximet.* Each tablet contains 85 mg sumatriptan and 500 mg naproxen. In clinical trials, the combination was better than either agent alone at relieving the pain of a migraine attack. In addition, the combination effectively reduced nausea and sensitivity to both light and sound. Presumably, the superior benefits of the combination derive from attacking migraine by multiple mechanisms: naproxen reduces pain and inflammation, while sumatriptan causes vasoconstriction and inhibits release of inflammatory neuropeptides.

PREVENTIVE THERAPY

Prophylactic therapy can reduce the frequency, intensity, and duration of migraine attacks, and can improve responses to abortive drugs. Preventive treatment is indicated for patients who have frequent attacks (three or more a month), attacks that are especially severe, or attacks that do not respond adequately to abortive agents. Preferred drugs for prophylaxis include propranolol, divalproex, and amitriptyline. All three are effective and well tolerated, and with all three, benefits take 4 to 6 weeks to develop. Major preventive agents are listed in Table 30.3.

Beta Blockers

Beta blockers are first-line drugs for migraine prevention. Of the available beta blockers, *propranolol* is used most often. Treatment can reduce the number and intensity of attacks in 70% of patients. Benefits take a few weeks to develop. The most common side effects are extreme tiredness and fatigue, which occur in about 10% of patients. In addition, the drug can exacerbate symptoms of asthma and may promote depression. If rizatriptan is used for abortive therapy, its dosage must be reduced. The usual maintenance dosage for propranolol is 80 to 240 mg/day, taken either as a single dose (using a long-acting formulation) or in two divided doses (using a short-acting formulation). In addition to propranolol, four other beta blockers—*timolol, atenolol, metoprolol,* and *nadolol*—can help prevent migraine attacks. In contrast, beta blockers that possess intrinsic sympathomimetic activity (e.g., acebutolol, pindolol) are *not* effective. The basic pharmacology of the beta blockers is discussed in Chapter 18.

TABLE 30.3 ▪ Migraine Headache: Drugs for Preventive Therapy

BETA-ADRENERGIC BLOCKING AGENTS
Metoprolol [Lopressor]
Propranolol [Inderal]
ANTIEPILEPTIC DRUGS
Divalproex [Depakote ER]
Topiramate [Topamax]
TRICYCLIC ANTIDEPRESSANTS
Amitriptyline [Elavil]
ESTROGENS (FOR MENSTRUALLY ASSOCIATED MIGRAINE)
Estrogen gel
Estrogen patch [Alora, Climara, Vivelle-Dot]

Antiepileptic Drugs

Several drugs that were developed for epilepsy can reduce migraine attacks. Proof of efficacy is strongest for divalproex [Depakote ER] and topiramate [Topamax]. Gabapentin [Neurontin] and tiagabine [Gabitril] appear promising, although extensive proof of efficacy is lacking.

Divalproex

Divalproex [Depakote ER], employed first for epilepsy and later for bipolar disorder (manic-depressive illness), is now approved for prophylaxis of migraine too. The drug is a form of valproic acid (see Chapter 24). Divalproex reduces the incidence of attacks by 50% or more in 30% to 50% of patients. However, when attacks do occur, their intensity and duration are not diminished. In migraineurs, the most common side effect is nausea. Other side effects include fatigue, weight gain, tremor, bone loss, and reversible hair loss. Potentially fatal pancreatitis and hepatitis occur rarely. Divalproex can cause neural tube defects in the developing fetus, and hence is contraindicated during pregnancy. The drug is available in delayed-release and extended-release tablets. The dosage range is 500 to 1000 mg/day.

Topiramate

Topiramate [Topamax], originally developed for epilepsy, was approved for migraine prophylaxis in 2004. Benefits take several weeks to develop and appear equal to those of beta blockers, tricyclic antidepressants, or divalproex. However, topiramate costs much more than these drugs. In clinical trials, topiramate reduced migraine frequency by at least 50% in 83% of adolescents and about 50% of adults. The drug also reduced the need for rescue medication. Unfortunately, side effects are common, especially paresthesias, fatigue, and cognitive dysfunction (psychomotor slowing, word-finding difficulty, impairment of concentration and memory). Other side effects include metabolic acidosis and moderate weight loss (owing to anorexia, nausea, and diarrhea). To minimize side effects, dosage should be low initially and then gradually increased. The recommended titration schedule is 25 mg in the evening the first week, 25 mg in the morning and evening the second week, 25 mg in the morning and 50 mg in the evening the third week, and 50 mg in the morning and evening thereafter. The basic pharmacology of topiramate is discussed in Chapter 24.

Tricyclic Antidepressants

Tricyclic antidepressants can prevent migraine and tension-type headaches in some patients. The underlying mechanism has not been established, but may involve inhibiting reuptake of serotonin, making more of the transmitter available for action. The tricyclic agent used most often is *amitriptyline* [Elavil]. Benefits equal those of propranolol. The dosage range is 25 to 150 mg once daily at bedtime. Because amitriptyline is effective in patients who are not depressed, it would seem that benefits do not depend on elevation of mood. Like other tricyclic antidepressants, amitriptyline can cause hypotension and anticholinergic effects (dry mouth, constipation, urinary retention, blurred vision, tachycardia). Excessive doses can cause dysrhythmias. The basic pharmacology of amitriptyline is discussed in Chapter 32.

Estrogens and Triptans for Menstrually Associated Migraine

Menstrually associated migraine is defined as migraine that routinely occurs within 2 days of the onset of menses. An important trigger is the decline in estrogen levels that precedes menstruation. For many women, menstrually associated migraine can be prevented by taking estrogen supplements, which compensate for the premenstrual estrogen drop. Topical preparations—estrogen gel and estrogen patches [e.g., Climara]—work well. Effective dosages are 1.5 mg/day for the gel and 100 mcg/day for the patches. Dosing is done for 7 days each month, beginning 2 days before the expected attack.

Perimenstrual triptans can also help. For example, frovatriptan, naratriptan, and zolmitriptan can reduce the frequency, intensity, and duration of menstrually associated migraine. Dosing is done for 6 days each month, beginning 2 days before the expected onset of menses.

In addition, naproxen sodium at a dosage of 550 mg twice daily, given 6 days before to 7 days after menses, has demonstrated effectiveness in the prevention of migraine.

Other Drugs for Prophylaxis

Calcium Channel Blockers

Of the calcium channel blockers (CCBs) evaluated for migraine prevention, two originally appeared useful: *verapamil* and *nimodipine*. It has since been determined that the studies completed on verapamil and nimodipine demonstrated low levels of evidence to support their use in migraine prophylaxis. Currently, the role of CCBs in migraine prophylaxis remains unclear; until more evidence is obtained, their use cannot be supported. The basic pharmacology of CCBs is discussed in Chapter 45.

Botulinum Toxin

In 2010, the FDA approved injections of botulinum toxin A [Botox] for prevention of headaches in adults with *chronic* migraine (defined as having 15 or more headache days per month), but not for patients with less frequent headaches. Treatment consists of 31 injections, made into muscles of the scalp, neck, and upper back. Treatment is expensive and benefits are modest: On average, patients experience about 2 fewer headache days a month.

Angiotensin-Converting Enzyme Inhibitors (ACEIs) and Angiotensin II Receptor Blockers (ARBs)

For prophylaxis of migraine, ACEIs and ARBs are considered third-line drugs. Benefits are limited to a 25% reduction in migraine days. Side effects include hyperkalemia, hypotension, volume depletion, and angioedema. When used during pregnancy, these drugs can injure the developing fetus. How ACEIs and ARBs reduce migraine attacks is unknown, although it is thought that they may stabilize blood vessels and alter sympathetic activity. The basic pharmacology of these drugs is discussed in Chapter 44.

Supplements

Riboflavin. Riboflavin (vitamin B_2) can reduce the number and severity of migraine attacks, but benefits are modest and develop slowly. In one study, migraineurs with frequent attacks took 400 mg of riboflavin a day. After 3 months, the number of attacks was decreased by 37%. In addition, the average duration of each attack also declined. Side effects were minimal.

Coenzyme Q-10. In two studies, daily therapy with coenzyme Q-10 (CoQ-10) produced a significant reduction in the occurrence of migraine attacks when compared with placebo. Subjects took 150 mg of CoQ-10 each morning or 100 mg 3 times daily. After 3 months, the number of days on which headaches occurred declined by at least 50% in 61% and 47% of study participants, respectively. However, although headache frequency declined, headache intensity was not affected. CoQ-10 was well tolerated.

Butterbur. Extracts made from the root of *Petasites hybridus*, a plant whose common name is butterbur, can reduce the frequency of migraine attacks. In a double-blind, placebo-controlled trial, about 1 in 5 patients taking 75 mg of extract twice daily experienced a 50% or greater reduction in migraine frequency. The only side effects were mild GI symptoms (e.g., nausea, burping, stomach pain). However, butterbur root contains pyrrolizidine alkaloids, which, if not removed during processing, can cause liver damage and cancer. In the study noted, the preparation employed, sold as *Petadolex*, was pyrrolizidine free.

CLUSTER HEADACHES

CHARACTERISTICS

Cluster headaches occur in a series or "cluster" of attacks. Each attack lasts 15 minutes to 2 hours and is characterized by severe, throbbing unilateral pain in the orbital-temporal area (i.e., near the eye). A typical cluster consists of one or two such attacks every day for 2 to 3 months. An attack-free interval of months to years separates each cluster. Along with headache, patients usually experience lacrimation, conjunctival redness, nasal congestion, rhinorrhea, ptosis (drooping eyelid), and miosis (constriction of the pupil)—all on the same side as the headache. Although related to migraine, cluster headaches differ in several ways: (1) they are not preceded by an aura, (2) they do not cause nausea and vomiting, (3) they can be more debilitating, (4) they are less common and occur mostly in males (5 : 1), (5) they are not associated with a family history of attacks, and (6) management is different.

DRUG THERAPY

Prophylaxis

Primary therapy is directed at prophylaxis. Effective agents include *systemic corticosteroids (betamethasone), verapamil,* and *lithium*. A small study revealed relief of attacks in 85% of patients receiving a suboccipital injection of betamethasone dipropionate and betamethasone disodium phosphate. Verapamil may also be considered for preventing chronic cluster headache. This drug is effective, easy to use, and safe. Lithium is considered a second-line drug for prophylaxis. The drug is effective, but it can cause multiple adverse effects, and dosing is difficult. To ensure therapeutic effects and minimize toxicity, blood levels of lithium must be monitored; the target range is 0.4 to 1 mEq/L. With all of these drugs, prophylactic therapy should be limited to the cluster cycle and then discontinued when the current cycle is over. Drugs for prophylaxis are listed in Table 30.4.

Treatment

If an attack occurs despite preventive therapy, it can be aborted with *sumatriptan* or *oxygen*. Sumatriptan (6 mg subQ) is the treatment of choice for cluster headaches. Inhaling 100% oxygen (6 to 12 L/min for 15 to 20 minutes) is also highly effective and has virtually no adverse effects. In the past, *ergot preparations* (e.g., intravenous dihydroergotamine, sublingual ergotamine) were commonly used. However, their use today is limited, as modern trials are small in population and lack evidence that these drugs work any better at relieving cluster headaches than placebo.

TENSION-TYPE HEADACHE

CHARACTERISTICS

Tension-type headaches (formerly called muscle-contraction headaches) are the most common headache type. These headaches are characterized by

TABLE 30.4 ▪ Drugs Used for Prophylaxis of Cluster Headache

Drug[a]	Usual Daily Dosage (mg)
CALCIUM CHANNEL BLOCKERS	
Verapamil [Calan, others]	240–420
NEUROSTABILIZERS	
Divalproex [Depakote]	500–1500
Lithium [Lithobid]	600–1200[b]
Topiramate [Topamax]	50–200
NONSTEROIDAL ANTI-INFLAMMATORY DRUGS	
Indomethacin	100–150
Naproxen	1000–1500
SYSTEMIC CORTICOSTEROID	
Betamethasone dipropionate/ betamethasone disodium phosphate	12.46/5.26 suboccipital injection once
Prednisone	40–80
ERGOT ALKALOIDS	
Ergotamine	1.2

[a]None of the drugs listed is approved by the FDA for cluster headache prophylaxis.
[b]Dosage is adjusted on the basis of serum lithium levels.

moderate, nonthrobbing pain, usually located in a "headband" distribution. Headache is often associated with scalp tingling and a sense of tightness or pressure in the head and neck. Precipitating factors include eye strain, aggravation, frustration, and life's daily stresses. Depressive symptoms (sleep disturbances, including early and frequent awakening) are often present. Tension headaches may be episodic or chronic. By definition, chronic tension-type headaches occur 15 or more days per month for at least 6 months.

TREATMENT

An acute attack of mild to moderate intensity can be relieved with a nonopioid analgesic: acetaminophen or a nonsteroidal anti-inflammatory drug (e.g., aspirin, ibuprofen, naproxen). An analgesic-sedative combination (e.g., aspirin-butalbital) may also be used. However, because of their potential for dependence and abuse, these combinations should be reserved for acute therapy of episodic attacks; they are inappropriate for patients with chronic daily headaches.

For prophylaxis, *amitriptyline* [Elavil], a tricyclic antidepressant, is the drug of choice. Dosing at bedtime will help relieve any depression-related sleep disturbances in addition to protecting against headache. Amitriptyline can cause anticholinergic side effects (e.g., dry mouth, constipation) and poses a risk of cardiotoxicity at high doses (see Chapter 32).

In addition to receiving drugs, patients should be taught how to manage stress. Instruction should include cognitive coping skills and information on relaxation techniques (e.g., massage, hot baths, biofeedback, deep muscle relaxation).

KEY POINTS

- Migraine is a neurovascular disorder involving dilation and inflammation of intracranial arteries.
- Antimigraine drugs are used in two ways: abortive and prophylactic.
- The goal of abortive therapy is to eliminate headache pain and associated nausea and vomiting.
- The goal of prophylactic therapy is to reduce the incidence and intensity of migraine attacks.
- There are two kinds of drugs for abortive therapy: nonspecific analgesics (aspirin-like drugs and opioids) and migraine-specific drugs (triptans and ergot alkaloids).
- Aspirin-like analgesics (e.g., acetaminophen, aspirin, naproxen) are effective for abortive therapy of mild to moderate migraine.
- Opioid analgesics (e.g., butorphanol, meperidine) are reserved for severe migraine that has not responded to other drugs.
- Triptans (e.g., sumatriptan) are first-line drugs for abortive therapy of moderate to severe migraine.
- Triptans activate $5\text{-HT}_{1B/1D}$ receptors and thereby constrict intracranial blood vessels and suppress release of inflammatory neuropeptides.
- All triptans are available in oral formulations, which have a relatively slow onset. Two triptans—sumatriptan and zolmitriptan—are available in fast-acting formulations (either nasal spray, subQ injection, or both).
- Triptans can cause coronary vasospasm, and hence are contraindicated for patients with ischemic heart disease, prior MI, or uncontrolled hypertension.
- Triptans should not be combined with one another or with ergot derivatives because excessive vasoconstriction could occur.
- Triptans should not be combined with SSRIs or SNRIs because serotonin syndrome could occur.
- Ergotamine is a second-line drug for abortive therapy of severe migraine.
- Overdose with ergotamine can cause ergotism, a serious condition characterized by severe tissue ischemia secondary to generalized constriction of peripheral arteries.
- Ergotamine must not be taken routinely because physical dependence will occur.
- Ergotamine can cause uterine contractions and must not be taken during pregnancy.
- Ergotamine must not be combined with potent inhibitors of CYP3A4, owing to a risk of intense vasoconstriction and associated ischemia.
- Prophylactic therapy is indicated for migraineurs who have frequent attacks (two or more a month), especially severe attacks, or attacks that do not respond adequately to abortive agents.
- Propranolol, divalproex, and amitriptyline are preferred drugs for migraine prophylaxis.
- Estrogen supplements can help prevent menstrual-associated migraine.

Please visit **http://evolve.elsevier.com/Lehne** for chapter-specific NCLEX® examination review questions.

Summary of Major Nursing Implications[a]

SEROTONIN$_{1B/1D}$ RECEPTOR AGONISTS (TRIPTANS)

Almotriptan
Eletriptan
Frovatriptan
Naratriptan
Rizatriptan
Sumatriptan
Zolmitriptan

Preadministration Assessment

Therapeutic Goal

Termination of migraine headache.

Baseline Data

Determine the age at onset, frequency, location, intensity, and quality (throbbing or nonthrobbing) of headaches as well as the presence or absence of a prodromal aura. Assess for trigger factors (e.g., stress, anxiety, fatigue) and for a family history of severe headache.

Assess for possible underlying causes of headache (e.g., severe hypertension; hyperthyroidism; infection; tumors; disorders of the eyes, ears, nose, sinuses, or throat), which should be treated if present.

Identifying High-Risk Patients

All triptans are *contraindicated* for patients with ischemic heart disease, prior MI, or uncontrolled hypertension, and for patients taking ergot alkaloids, other triptans, SSRIs, or SNRIs. *Sumatriptan, rizatriptan,* and *zolmitriptan* are *contraindicated* for patients taking MAOIs. *Eletriptan* is contraindicated for patients taking strong inhibitors of CYP3A4.

Implementation: Administration

Routes

Oral. All triptans.
Subcutaneous. Sumatriptan.
Intranasal. Sumatriptan and zolmitriptan.
Transdermal. Sumatriptan.

Dosage and Administration

Instruct patients to administer triptans immediately after onset of symptoms.

Teach patients how to use the sumatriptan auto-injector, the iontophoretic transdermal system, and the needle-free injection device.

Implementation: Measures to Enhance Therapeutic Effects

Educate patients in ways to control, avoid, or eliminate trigger factors (e.g., stress, fatigue, anxiety, alcohol, tyramine-containing foods).

Teach patients biofeedback or another relaxation technique. Advise patients to rest in a quiet, dark room for 2 to 3 hours after drug administration and to apply an ice pack to the neck and scalp.

Ongoing Evaluation and Interventions

Evaluating Therapeutic Effects

Determine the size and frequency of doses used and the extent to which therapy has reduced the intensity and duration of attacks.

Minimizing Adverse Effects

Coronary Vasospasm. All triptans can cause coronary vasospasm with resultant anginal pain. Avoid these drugs in patients with ischemic heart disease, prior MI, or uncontrolled hypertension. In patients with risk factors for CAD, rule out CAD before giving triptans.

Teratogenesis. *Sumatriptan* can cause birth defects in laboratory animals, and hence must not be used during pregnancy. *Rizatriptan* may also pose fetal risk.

Minimizing Adverse Interactions

Ergot Alkaloids and Other Triptans. Combining a triptan with an ergot alkaloid (e.g., ergotamine, dihydroergotamine) or another triptan can cause prolonged vasospasm. Do not administer a triptan within 24 hours of an ergot alkaloid or another triptan.

SSRIs and SNRIs. These drugs should not be combined with a triptan, owing to the risk of serotonin syndrome.

MAOIs. MAOIs can intensify the effects of *sumatriptan, rizatriptan,* and *zolmitriptan.* Patients should not combine these drugs with an MAOI or use them within 2 weeks of stopping an MAOI.

CYP3A4 Inhibitors. Ketoconazole, ritonavir, and other strong inhibitors of CYP3A4 can raise levels of *eletriptan* and *almotriptan.* Toxicity can result. Eletriptan must not be combined with these inhibitors. Almotriptan can be combined with a CYP3A4 inhibitor, but almotriptan dosage must be reduced.

Propranolol. Propranolol can raise levels of *rizatriptan.* Dosage of the triptan should be reduced.

ERGOTAMINE AND DIHYDROERGOTAMINE

Preadministration Assessment

Therapeutic Goal

Termination of migraine or cluster headache.

Baseline Data

See *Serotonin$_{1B/1D}$ Receptor Agonists (Triptans).*

Identifying High-Risk Patients

Ergot alkaloids are *contraindicated* in patients with hepatic or renal impairment, sepsis, CAD, or peripheral vascular disease, and for patients who are pregnant, taking triptans, or taking potent inhibitors of CYP3A4.

Implementation: Administration

Routes

Ergotamine Alone. Sublingual.
Ergotamine Plus Caffeine. Oral, rectal.
Dihydroergotamine. Nasal spray, IM, IV, and subQ.

Summary of Major Nursing Implications[a]—cont'd

Dosage and Administration

Instruct patients to begin dosing immediately upon onset of symptoms.

Nausea and vomiting from the headache and from ergotamine itself may prevent complete absorption of oral ergotamine. Concurrent treatment with metoclopramide or another antiemetic can minimize these effects. (Nausea and vomiting are minimal with dihydroergotamine.)

Ergotamine (but not dihydroergotamine) can cause physical dependence and serious toxicity if dosage is excessive. **Inform patients about the risks of dependence and toxicity and the importance of not exceeding the prescribed dosage.**

Implementation: Measures to Enhance Therapeutic Effects

Educate patients in ways to control, avoid, or eliminate trigger factors (e.g., stress, fatigue, anxiety, alcohol, tyramine-containing foods).

Teach patients about relaxation techniques (e.g., biofeedback, deep muscle relaxation). Advise patients to rest in a quiet, dark room for 2 to 3 hours after drug administration and to apply an ice pack to the neck and scalp.

Ongoing Evaluation and Interventions

Evaluating Therapeutic Effects

Determine the size and frequency of doses used and the extent to which therapy has reduced the intensity and duration of attacks.

Minimizing Adverse Effects

Nausea and Vomiting. *Ergotamine* promotes nausea and vomiting. Minimize these by concurrent therapy with metoclopramide or a phenothiazine-type antiemetic.

Ergotism. Toxicity (ergotism) can result from acute or chronic overdose. **Teach patients the early manifestations of ergotism (muscle pain; paresthesias in fingers and toes; extremities become cold, pale, and numb) and instruct them to seek immediate medical attention if they develop.** Treat by withdrawing ergotamine and administering drugs (anticoagulants, phentolamine, IV nitroprusside, IV nitroglycerin) as appropriate to maintain circulation.

Physical Dependence. *Ergotamine* can cause physical dependence. **Warn patients not to overuse the drug because physical dependence can result. Teach patients the signs and symptoms of withdrawal (headache, nausea, vomiting, restlessness), and instruct them to inform the prescriber if these develop during a drug-free interval.** Patients who become dependent may require hospitalization to bring about withdrawal.

Abortion. Ergot alkaloids are uterine stimulants that can cause abortion in high doses. **Warn women of childbearing age to avoid pregnancy while using these drugs.**

Minimizing Adverse Interactions

Inhibitors of CYP3A4. *Ergotamine* and *dihydroergotamine* must not be combined with potent inhibitors of CYP3A4, which can raise these drugs to toxic levels, thereby posing a risk of intense vasoconstriction and associated ischemia. Drugs to avoid include certain HIV protease inhibitors (e.g., ritonavir, nelfinavir), azole antifungal drugs (e.g., ketoconazole, itraconazole), and macrolide antibiotics (e.g., erythromycin, clarithromycin).

[a]Patient education information is highlighted as **blue text.**

CHAPTER

31 Antipsychotic Agents and Their Use in Schizophrenia

The antipsychotic agents are a chemically diverse group of compounds used for a broad spectrum of psychotic disorders. Specific indications include schizophrenia, delusional disorders, bipolar disorder, depressive psychoses, and drug-induced psychoses. In addition to their psychiatric applications, the antipsychotics are used to suppress emesis and to treat Tourette's syndrome and Huntington's chorea. As a rule, antipsychotics should not be used to treat dementia-related psychosis in older adults, owing to a risk of increased mortality.

Since their introduction in the early 1950s, the antipsychotic agents have catalyzed revolutionary change in the management of psychotic illnesses. Before these drugs were available, psychoses were largely untreatable and patients were fated to a life of institutionalization. With the advent of antipsychotic medications, many patients with schizophrenia and other severe psychotic disorders have been able to leave psychiatric hospitals and return to the community. Others have been spared hospitalization entirely. For those who must be institutionalized, antipsychotic drugs have at least reduced suffering.

The antipsychotic drugs fall into two major groups: (1) *first-generation antipsychotics* (FGAs), also known as *conventional antipsychotics,* and (2) *second-generation antipsychotics* (SGAs), also known as *atypical antipsychotics.* Both groups are equally effective. All of the FGAs produce strong blockade of dopamine in the central nervous system (CNS). As a result, they all can cause serious movement disorders, known as *extrapyramidal symptoms* (EPS). The SGAs produce moderate blockade of receptors for dopamine and much stronger blockade of receptors for serotonin. Because dopamine receptor blockade is only moderate, the risk of EPS is lower than with the FGAs. However, although the SGAs carry a reduced risk of EPS, they carry a significant risk of *metabolic effects*—weight gain, diabetes, and dyslipidemia—that can cause cardiovascular events and early death.

SGAs outsell the FGAs by a factor of 10. Given that the SGAs are no more effective than the FGAs and carry significant risks that the FGAs don't have, why are SGAs so widely prescribed? The main reason is inappropriate off-label use, such as controlling agitation in nursing home residents. In addition, aggressive marketing has created the *perception* of clinical superiority, even though the FGAs are just as good.

SCHIZOPHRENIA: CLINICAL PRESENTATION AND ETIOLOGY

Clinical Presentation

Schizophrenia is a chronic psychotic illness characterized by disordered thinking and a reduced ability to comprehend reality. Symptoms usually emerge during adolescence or early adulthood. In the United States, about 3.2 million people are affected.

Prototype Drugs

ANTIPSYCHOTIC AGENTS

Traditional Antipsychotics
Chlorpromazine (a low-potency agent)
Haloperidol (a high-potency agent)

Atypical Antipsychotics
Clozapine

Three Types of Symptoms

Symptoms of schizophrenia can be divided into three groups: positive symptoms, negative symptoms, and cognitive symptoms. Positive and negative symptoms are shown in Table 31.1.

Positive Symptoms and Negative Symptoms. Positive symptoms can be viewed as an exaggeration or distortion of normal function, whereas negative symptoms can be viewed as a loss or diminution of normal function. Positive symptoms include hallucinations, delusions, agitation, tension, and paranoia. Negative symptoms include lack of motivation, poverty of speech, blunted affect, poor self-care, and social withdrawal. Positive and negative symptoms respond equally to FGAs and SGAs.

TABLE 31.1 ■ Positive and Negative Symptoms of Schizophrenia

Positive Symptoms	Negative Symptoms
Hallucinations	Social withdrawal
Delusions	Emotional withdrawal
Disordered thinking	Lack of motivation
Disorganized speech	Poverty of speech
Combativeness	Blunted affect
Agitation	Poor insight
Paranoia	Poor judgment
	Poor self-care

Cognitive Symptoms. Cognitive symptoms include disordered thinking, reduced ability to focus attention, and prominent learning and memory difficulties. Subtle changes may appear years before symptoms become florid, when thinking and speech may be completely incomprehensible to others. Cognitive symptoms may respond equally to FGAs and SGAs.

Acute Episodes

During an acute schizophrenic episode, delusions (fixed false beliefs) and hallucinations are frequently prominent. Delusions are typically religious, grandiose, or persecutory. Auditory hallucinations, which are more common than visual hallucinations, may consist of voices arguing or commenting on one's behavior. The patient may feel controlled by external influences. Disordered thinking and loose association may render rational conversation impossible. Affect may be blunted or labile. Misperception of reality may result in hostility and lack of cooperation. Impaired self-care skills may leave the patient disheveled and dirty. Patterns of sleeping and eating are usually disrupted.

Residual Symptoms

After florid symptoms (e.g., hallucinations, delusions) of an acute episode remit, less vivid symptoms may remain. These include suspiciousness, poor anxiety management, and diminished judgment, insight, motivation, and capacity for self-care. As a result, patients frequently find it difficult to establish close relationships, maintain employment, and function independently in society. Suspiciousness and poor anxiety management contribute to social withdrawal. Inability to appreciate the need for continued drug therapy may cause nonadherence, resulting in relapse and perhaps hospital readmission.

Long-Term Course

The long-term course of schizophrenia is characterized by episodic acute exacerbations separated by intervals of partial remission. As the years pass, some patients experience progressive decline in mental status and social functioning. However, many others stabilize, or even improve. Maintenance therapy with antipsychotic drugs reduces the risk of acute relapse, but may fail to prevent long-term deterioration.

Etiology

Although there is strong evidence that schizophrenia has a biologic basis, the exact etiology is unknown. Genetic, perinatal, neurodevelopmental, and neuroanatomic factors may all be involved. Possible primary defects include excessive activation of CNS receptors for dopamine, and insufficient activation of CNS receptors for glutamate. Although psychosocial stressors can precipitate acute exacerbations in susceptible patients, they are not considered causative.

FIRST-GENERATION (CONVENTIONAL) ANTIPSYCHOTICS

The FGAs have been in use for decades, and their pharmacology is well understood. Accordingly, it seems appropriate to begin with these drugs, even though their use has greatly declined. Besides, because the pharmacology of the FGAs and SGAs is very similar, once you understand the FGAs, you will know a great deal about the SGAs as well.

Group Properties

In this section we discuss pharmacologic properties shared by all FGAs. Much of our attention focuses on adverse effects. Of these, extrapyramidal side effects are of particular concern. Because of these neurologic side effects, the FGAs are also known as *neuroleptics.*

Classification

The FGAs can be classified by potency or chemical structure. From a clinical viewpoint, classification by potency is more helpful.

Classification by Potency. First-generation antipsychotics can be classified as *low potency, medium potency,* or *high potency* (Table 31.2). The low-potency drugs, represented by chlorpromazine, and the high-potency drugs, represented by haloperidol, are of particular interest.

It is important to note that, although the FGAs differ from one another in potency, they all have the same ability to relieve symptoms of psychosis. Recall that the term *potency* refers only to the size of the dose needed to elicit a given response; potency implies nothing about the maximal effect a drug can produce. Hence, when we say that haloperidol is more potent than chlorpromazine, we only mean that the dose of haloperidol required to relieve psychotic symptoms is smaller than the required dose of chlorpromazine. We do not mean that haloperidol can produce greater effects. When administered in therapeutically equivalent doses, both drugs elicit an equivalent antipsychotic response.

If low-potency and high-potency neuroleptics are equally effective, why distinguish between them? The answer is that, although these agents produce identical *antipsychotic* effects, they differ significantly in *side effects.* Hence, by knowing the potency category to which a particular neuroleptic belongs, we can better predict its undesired responses. This knowledge is useful in drug selection and in providing patient care and education.

Chemical Classification. The FGAs fall into four major chemical categories (Table 31.3). One of these categories, the phenothiazines, has three subgroups. Drugs in all groups are equivalent with respect to antipsychotic actions, and hence chemical classification is not emphasized in this chapter.

Two chemical categories—*phenothiazines* and *butyrophenones*—deserve attention. The phenothiazines were the first modern antipsychotic agents. Chlorpromazine, our prototype of

TABLE 31.2 ▪ Antipsychotic Drugs: Relative Potency and Incidence of Selected Side Effects

			Incidence of Side Effects							
Drug	Brand Name	Equivalent Oral Dose (mg)[a]	Extrapyramidal Effects[b]	Sedation	Orthostatic Hypotension	Anticholinergic Effects	Metabolic Effects: Weight Gain, Diabetes Risk, Dyslipidemia	Significant QT Prolongation	Prolactin Elevation	Metabolized by CYP3A4
FIRST-GENERATION (CONVENTIONAL) ANTIPSYCHOTICS										
Low Potency										
Chlorpromazine	Generic only	100	Moderate	High	High	Moderate	Moderate	Yes	Low	—
Molindone	Generic only	10	Moderate	High	Low	Moderate	None	No	Low	—
Thioridazine	Generic only	100	Low	High	High	High	Moderate	Yes	Low	—
Medium Potency										
Loxapine	Loxitane	13	Moderate	Moderate	Low	Low	Low	No	Moderate	—
Perphenazine	Generic only	8	Moderate	Moderate	Low	Low	—	No	Low	—
Thiothixene	Generic only	2	High	Low	Moderate	Low	Moderate	No	Moderate	—
High Potency										
Fluphenazine	Generic only	1	Very high	Low	Low	Low	—	No	Moderate	—
Haloperidol	Generic only	2	Very high	Low	Low	Low	Moderate	Yes	Moderate	—
Pimozide	Orap	1	High	Moderate	Low	Moderate	—	Yes	Moderate	—
Trifluoperazine	Generic only	1	High	Low	Low	Low	—	No	Moderate	—
SECOND-GENERATION (ATYPICAL) ANTIPSYCHOTICS										
Aripiprazole	Abilify	2	Very low	Low	Low	None	None/low	Yes	Low	Yes
Asenapine	Saphris	4	Moderate	Moderate	Moderate	Low	Low	Yes	Low	Slightly
Brexpiprazole	Rexulti	2	Very low	Very low	Low	None	Low	No	Low	Yes
Cariprazine	Vraylar	1.5	Very low	Moderate	Low	Low	Moderate	No	No	Yes
Clozapine	Clozaril, FazaClo, Versacloz	75	Very low	High	Moderate	High	High	Yes	Low	Yes
Iloperidone	Fanapt	4	Very low	Moderate	Moderate	Moderate	Moderate	Yes	Low	Yes
Lurasidone	Latuda	10	Moderate	Moderate	Low	None	None/low	No	Low	Yes
Olanzapine	Zyprexa	3	Low	Moderate	Moderate	Moderate	High	No	Low	No
Paliperidone	Invega	2	Moderate	Low	Low	None	Moderate	Yes	High	Slightly
Quetiapine	Seroquel	95	Very low	Moderate	Moderate	None	Moderate/high	Yes	Low	Yes
Risperidone	Risperdal	1	Moderate	Low	Low	None	Moderate	Yes	High	No
Ziprasidone	Geodon, Zeldox 🍁	20	Low	Moderate	Moderate	None	None/low	Yes	Low	Yes

[a]Doses listed are the therapeutic equivalent of 100 mg of oral chlorpromazine.
[b]Incidence here refers to *early* extrapyramidal reactions (acute dystonia, parkinsonism, akathisia). The incidence of *late* reactions (tardive dyskinesia) is the same for all traditional antipsychotics.

TABLE 31.3 ▪ Antipsychotic Drugs: Routes and Dosages

Chemical Group and Generic Name	Brand Name	Route	Usual Total Daily Dose for Schizophrenia (mg)[a]
FIRST-GENERATION (CONVENTIONAL) ANTIPSYCHOTICS			
Phenothiazine: Aliphatic			
Chlorpromazine	Generic only	PO, IM, IV	300–1000
Phenothiazine: Piperidine			
Thioridazine	Generic only	PO	300–800
Phenothiazine: Piperazine			
Fluphenazine	Generic only	PO, IM	5–20
Perphenazine	Generic only	PO	12–64
Trifluoperazine	Generic only	PO	15–50
Thioxanthene			
Thiothixene	Generic only	PO	15–50
Butyrophenone			
Haloperidol	Generic only	PO, IM	6–40
Dihydroindolone			
Molindone	Generic only	PO	50–75
Dibenzoxazepine			
Loxapine	Loxitane	PO	30–100
SECOND-GENERATION (ATYPICAL) ANTIPSYCHOTICS			
Aripiprazole	Abilify	PO	10–30
Asenapine	Saphris	Sublingual	10–20
Brexpiprazole	Rexulti	PO	2–4
Cariprazine	Vraylar	PO	1.5–6
Clozapine	Clozaril, FazaClo, Versacloz	PO	150–600
Iloperidone	Fanapt	PO	12–24
Lurasidone	Latuda	PO	40–160
Olanzapine	Zyprexa	PO, IM	5–30
Paliperidone	Invega	PO	3–12
Quetiapine	Seroquel	PO	300–750
Risperidone	Risperdal	PO, IM	2–8
Ziprasidone	Geodon, Zeldox 🍁	PO, IM	8–160

[a]Higher doses may be given for acute symptom management or in patients with refractory symptoms.

the low-potency neuroleptics, belongs to this family. The butyrophenones stand out because they are the family to which haloperidol belongs. Haloperidol is the prototype of the high-potency FGAs.

Mechanism of Action

The FGAs block a variety of receptors within and outside the CNS. To varying degrees, they block receptors for dopamine, acetylcholine, histamine, and norepinephrine. There is little question that blockade at these receptors is responsible for the major *adverse effects* of the antipsychotics. However, because the etiology of psychotic illness is unclear, the relationship of receptor blockade to *therapeutic effects* can only be guessed. The current dominant theory suggests that FGA drugs suppress symptoms of psychosis by blocking dopamine$_2$ (D_2) receptors in the mesolimbic area of the brain. In support of this theory is the observation that all of the FGAs produce D_2 receptor blockade. Furthermore, there is a close correlation between the clinical potency of these drugs and their potency as D_2 receptor antagonists.

Therapeutic Use: Schizophrenia

Schizophrenia is the primary indication for antipsychotic drugs. These agents effectively suppress symptoms during acute psychotic episodes and, when taken chronically, can greatly reduce the risk of relapse. Initial effects may be seen in 1 to 2 days, but substantial improvement usually takes 2 to 4 weeks, and full effects may not develop for several months. Positive symptoms (e.g., delusions, hallucinations) may respond somewhat better than negative symptoms (e.g., social and emotional withdrawal, blunted affect, poverty of speech) or cognitive dysfunction (e.g., disordered thinking, learning and memory difficulties). All of the FGA agents are equally effective, although individual patients may respond better to one FGA than to another. Consequently, selection among these drugs is based primarily on their side effect profiles, rather than on therapeutic effects. It must be noted that antipsychotic drugs do not alter the underlying pathology of schizophrenia. Hence, treatment is not curative—it offers only symptomatic relief. Management of schizophrenia is discussed later in the chapter.

Neuroleptics may be employed acutely to help manage patients with bipolar disorder going through a severe manic phase. Neuroleptic medications are also used to treat Tourette's syndrome, a rare inherited disorder characterized by severe motor tics, barking cries, grunts, and outbursts of obscene language. Additional applications include suppression of emesis through dopamine receptor blockade, relief of symptoms caused by Huntington's chorea, and treatment of organic mental syndromes.

Adverse Effects

The antipsychotic drugs block several kinds of receptors and produce an array of side effects, including a variety of undesired effects. However, these drugs are generally very safe; death from overdose is practically unheard of. Among the many side effects FGAs can produce, the most troubling are the extrapyramidal reactions—especially tardive dyskinesia (TD).

Extrapyramidal Symptoms (EPS). EPS are movement disorders resulting from effects of antipsychotic drugs on the extrapyramidal motor system. The extrapyramidal system is the same neuronal network whose malfunction is responsible for the movement disorders of Parkinson disease (PD). Although the exact cause of EPS is unclear, blockade of D_2 receptors is strongly suspected.

Four types of EPS occur. They differ with respect to time of onset and management. Three of these reactions—acute dystonia, parkinsonism, and akathisia—occur early in therapy and can be managed with a variety of drugs. The fourth reaction—tardive dyskinesia—occurs late in therapy and has no satisfactory treatment. Characteristics of EPS are shown in Table 31.4.

The *early* reactions occur *less frequently* with *low-potency* agents (e.g., chlorpromazine) than with high-potency agents (e.g., haloperidol). In contrast, the risk of TD is equal with all FGAs.

Safety Alert

EXTRAPYRAMIDAL SYMPTOMS

For many patients, EPS are uncomfortable, disturbing, and sometimes, dangerous. Some manifestations of EPS, such as tardive dyskinesia, are irreversible. It is crucial for the RN to monitor patients treated with antipsychotic medications for evidence of EPS, and to report this immediately if present.

Acute Dystonia. Acute dystonia can be both disturbing and dangerous. The reaction develops within the first few days of therapy and frequently within hours of the first dose. Typically, the patient develops severe spasm of the muscles of the tongue, face, neck, or back. Oculogyric crisis (involuntary upward deviation of the eyes) and opisthotonus (tetanic spasm of the back muscles causing the trunk to arch forward, while the head and lower limbs are thrust backward) may also occur. Severe cramping can cause joint dislocation. Laryngeal dystonia can impair respiration.

Intense dystonia is a crisis that requires rapid intervention. Initial treatment consists of an anticholinergic medication (e.g., benztropine, diphenhydramine) administered IM or IV. As a rule, symptoms resolve within 5 minutes of IV dosing and within 15 to 20 minutes of IM dosing.

It is important to differentiate between acute dystonia and psychotic hysteria. Misdiagnosis of acute dystonia as hysteria could result in giving bigger antipsychotic doses, thereby causing the acute dystonia to become even worse.

Parkinsonism. Antipsychotic-induced parkinsonism is characterized by bradykinesia, mask-like facies, drooling, tremor, rigidity, shuffling gait, cogwheeling, and stooped posture. Symptoms develop within the first month of therapy and are indistinguishable from those of idiopathic PD.

Neuroleptics cause parkinsonism by blocking dopamine receptors in the striatum. Because idiopathic PD is also due to reduced activation of striatal dopamine receptors (see Chapter

TABLE 31.4 ▪ Extrapyramidal Side Effects of Antipsychotic Drugs

Type of Reaction	Time of Onset	Features	Management
EARLY REACTIONS			
Acute dystonia	A few hours to 5 days	Spasm of muscles of tongue, face, neck, and back; opisthotonus	Anticholinergic drugs (e.g., benztropine) IM or IV.
Parkinsonism	5–30 days	Bradykinesia, mask-like facies, tremor, rigidity, shuffling gait, drooling, cogwheeling, stooped posture	Anticholinergics (e.g., benztropine, diphenhydramine), amantadine, or both. For severe symptoms, switch to a second-generation antipsychotic.
Akathisia	5–60 days	Compulsive, restless movement; symptoms of anxiety, agitation	Reduce dosage or switch to a low-potency antipsychotic. Treat with a benzodiazepine, beta blocker, or anticholinergic drug.
LATE REACTION			
Tardive dyskinesia	Months to years	Oral-facial dyskinesias, choreoathetoid movements	Best approach is prevention; no reliable treatment. Discontinue all anticholinergic drugs. Give benzodiazepines. Reduce antipsychotic dosage. For severe TD, switch to a second-generation antipsychotic.

21), it is no wonder that PD and neuroleptic-induced parkinsonism share the same symptoms.

Neuroleptic-induced parkinsonism is treated with some of the drugs used for idiopathic PD. Specifically, centrally acting *anticholinergic drugs* (e.g., benztropine, diphenhydramine) and *amantadine* may be employed. Levodopa and direct dopamine agonists (e.g., bromocriptine) should be avoided because these drugs activate dopamine receptors and might thereby counteract the beneficial effects of antipsychotic treatment.

Use of antiparkinsonism drugs should not continue indefinitely. Antipsychotic-induced parkinsonism tends to resolve spontaneously, usually within months of its onset. Accordingly, antiparkinsonism drugs should be withdrawn after a few months to determine whether they are still needed.

If parkinsonism is severe, switching to an SGA is likely to help. As discussed later, the risk of parkinsonism with the SGAs is much lower than with FGAs.

Akathisia. Akathisia is characterized by pacing and squirming brought on by an uncontrollable need to be in motion. This profound sense of restlessness can be very disturbing. The syndrome usually develops within the first 2 months of treatment. Like other early EPS, akathisia occurs most frequently with high-potency FGAs.

Three types of drugs have been used to suppress symptoms: *beta blockers, benzodiazepines,* and *anticholinergic drugs.* Although these drugs can help, reducing antipsychotic dosage or switching to a low-potency FGA may be more effective.

It is important to differentiate between akathisia and exacerbation of psychosis. If akathisia were to be confused with anxiety or psychotic agitation, it is likely that antipsychotic dosage would be increased, thereby making akathisia more intense.

Tardive Dyskinesia. TD, the most troubling EPS, develops in 15% to 20% of patients during long-term therapy with FGAs. The risk is related to duration of treatment and dosage size. For many patients, symptoms are irreversible.

TD is characterized by involuntary choreoathetoid (twisting, writhing, worm-like) movements of the tongue and face. Patients may also present with lip-smacking movements, and their tongues may flick out in a "fly-catching" motion. One of the earliest manifestations of TD is slow, worm-like movement of the tongue. Involuntary movements that involve the tongue and mouth can interfere with chewing, swallowing, and speaking. Eating difficulties can result in malnutrition and weight loss. Over time, TD produces involuntary movements of the limbs, toes, fingers, and trunk. For some patients, symptoms decline following a dosage reduction or drug withdrawal. For others, TD is irreversible.

The cause of TD is complex and incompletely understood. One theory suggests that symptoms result from excessive *activation* of dopamine receptors. It is postulated that, in response to chronic receptor blockade, dopamine receptors of the extrapyramidal system undergo a functional change such that their sensitivity to activation is increased. Stimulation of these "supersensitive" receptors produces an imbalance in favor of dopamine and thereby produces abnormal movement. In support of this theory is the observation that symptoms of TD can be reduced (temporarily) by *increasing* antipsychotic dosage, which increases dopamine receptor blockade. (Because symptoms eventually return even though antipsychotic dosage is kept high, dosage elevation cannot be used to treat TD.)

There is no reliable management for TD. Measures that may be tried include gradually withdrawing anticholinergic drugs, giving benzodiazepines, and reducing the dosage of the offending FGA. For patients with severe TD, switching to an SGA agent may help because SGAs are less likely to promote TD.

Because TD has no reliable means of treatment, prevention is the best approach. Antipsychotic drugs should be used in the lowest effective dosage for the shortest time required. After 12 months, the need for continued therapy should be assessed. If drug use must continue, a neurologic evaluation should be done at least every 3 months to detect early signs of TD. For patients with chronic schizophrenia, dosage should be tapered periodically (at least annually) to determine the need for continued treatment.

Other Adverse Effects

Neuroleptic Malignant Syndrome. Neuroleptic malignant syndrome (NMS) is a rare but serious reaction that carries a 5% to 20% risk of mortality. Primary symptoms are "lead pipe" rigidity, sudden high fever (temperature may exceed 41°C), sweating, and autonomic instability, manifested as dysrhythmias and fluctuations in blood pressure. Level of consciousness may rise and fall, the patient may appear confused or mute, and seizures or coma may develop. Death can result from respiratory failure, cardiovascular collapse, dysrhythmias, and other causes. NMS is more likely with high-potency FGAs than with low-potency FGAs.

Safety Alert

NEUROLEPTIC MALIGNANT SYNDROME

Neuroleptic malignant syndrome can be fatal if not treated promptly. The RN must recognize the signs and symptoms of NMS and report them immediately. Treatment with dantrolene and bromocriptine may be ordered by the provider.

Treatment consists of supportive measures, drug therapy, and immediate withdrawal of antipsychotic medication. Hyperthermia should be controlled with cooling blankets and antipyretics (e.g., aspirin, acetaminophen). Hydration should be maintained with fluids. Benzodiazepines may relieve anxiety and help reduce blood pressure and tachycardia. Two drugs—*dantrolene* and *bromocriptine*—may be especially helpful. Dantrolene is a direct-acting muscle relaxant (see Chapter 25). In patients with NMS, this drug reduces rigidity and hyperthermia. Bromocriptine is a dopamine receptor agonist (see Chapter 21) that may relieve CNS toxicity.

Resumption of antipsychotic therapy carries a small risk of NMS recurrence. The risk can be minimized by (1) waiting at least 2 weeks before resuming antipsychotic treatment, (2) using the lowest effective dosage, and (3) avoiding high-potency agents. If a second episode occurs, switching to an SGA may help.

Anticholinergic Effects. First-generation agents produce varying degrees of muscarinic cholinergic blockade (see Table 31.2) and can elicit the full spectrum of anticholinergic responses (dry mouth, blurred vision, photophobia, urinary hesitancy, constipation, tachycardia). Patients should be informed about these responses and taught how to minimize danger and discomfort. As indicated in Table 31.2, anticholinergic effects are more likely with low-potency FGAs than with high-potency FGAs. Anticholinergic effects and their management are discussed in detail in Chapter 14.

Orthostatic Hypotension. Antipsychotic drugs promote orthostatic hypotension by blocking $alpha_1$-adrenergic receptors on blood vessels. Alpha-adrenergic blockade prevents compensatory vasoconstriction when the patient stands, thereby causing blood pressure to fall. Patients should be informed about signs of hypotension (light-headedness, dizziness) and advised to sit or lie down if these occur. In addition, patients should be informed that hypotension can be minimized by moving slowly when assuming an erect posture. With hospitalized patients, blood pressure and pulses should be checked before dosing and 1 hour after. Measurements should be made while the patient is lying down and again after the patient has been sitting or standing for 1 to 2 minutes. If blood pressure is low or if pulse rate is high, the dose should be withheld and the prescriber consulted. Hypotension is more likely with low-potency FGAs than with the high-potency FGAs (see Table 31.2). Tolerance to hypotension develops in 2 to 3 months.

Sedation. Sedation is common during the early days of treatment but subsides within a week or so. Neuroleptic-induced sedation is thought to result from blockade of $histamine_1$ receptors in the CNS. Daytime sedation can be minimized by giving the entire daily dose at bedtime. Patients should be warned against participating in hazardous activities (e.g., driving) until sedative effects diminish.

Neuroendocrine Effects. Antipsychotics increase levels of circulating *prolactin* by blocking the inhibitory action of dopamine on prolactin release. Elevation of prolactin levels promotes *gynecomastia* (breast growth) and *galactorrhea* in up to 57% of women. Up to 97% of women experience menstrual irregularities. Gynecomastia and galactorrhea can also occur in males. Because prolactin can promote growth of prolactin-dependent carcinoma of the breast, neuroleptics should be avoided in patients with this form of cancer. (It should be noted that although FGAs can promote the growth of cancers that already exist, there is no evidence that FGAs actually *cause* cancer.)

Seizures. First-generation agents can reduce seizure threshold, thereby increasing the risk of seizure activity. The risk of seizures is greatest in patients with seizure disorders. These patients should be monitored, and if loss of seizure control occurs, the dosage of their antiseizure medication must be increased.

Sexual Dysfunction. First-generation agents can cause sexual dysfunction in women and men. In women, these drugs can suppress libido and impair the ability to achieve orgasm. In men, FGAs can suppress libido and cause erectile and ejaculatory dysfunction; the incidence is 25% to 60%. Drug-induced sexual dysfunction can make treatment unacceptable to sexually active patients, thereby leading to poor compliance. A reduction in dosage or switching to a high-potency FGA may reduce adverse sexual effects. Patients should be counseled about possible sexual dysfunction and encouraged to report any problems.

Agranulocytosis. Agranulocytosis is a rare but serious reaction. Among the FGAs, the risk is highest with chlorpromazine and certain other phenothiazines. Because agranulocytosis severely compromises the ability to fight infection, a white blood cell (WBC) count should be done whenever signs of infection (e.g., fever, sore throat) appear. If agranulocytosis is diagnosed, the neuroleptic should be withdrawn. Agranulocytosis will then reverse.

Severe Dysrhythmias. Four FGAs—*chlorpromazine, haloperidol, thioridazine,* and *pimozide*—pose a risk of fatal cardiac dysrhythmias. The mechanism is prolongation of the QT interval, an index of cardiac function that can be measured with an electrocardiogram (ECG). As discussed in Chapter 7, drugs that prolong the QT interval increase the risk of torsades de pointes, a dysrhythmia that can progress to fatal ventricular fibrillation. To reduce the risk of dysrhythmias, patients should undergo an ECG and serum potassium determination before treatment and periodically thereafter. In addition, they should avoid other drugs that cause QT prolongation (see Chapter 7), as well as drugs that can increase levels of these four FGAs.

Effects in Older Adult Patients With Dementia. When used off-label to treat older adult patients with dementia-related psychosis, all antipsychotics (FGAs and SGAs) about double the rate of mortality. Most deaths result from heart-related events (e.g., heart failure, sudden death) or from infection (mainly pneumonia). Because antipsychotics are not approved for treating dementia-related psychosis and because doing so increases the risk of death, such use is not recommended.

Signs of Withdrawal and EPS in Neonates. Neonates exposed to antipsychotic drugs (first or second generation) during the third trimester of pregnancy may experience EPS and/or signs of withdrawal. Symptoms include tremor, agitation, sleepiness, difficulty feeding, severe breathing difficulty, and altered muscle tone (increased or decreased). Fortunately, the risk appears low. Neonates who present with EPS or signs of withdrawal should be monitored. Some will recover within hours or days, but others may require prolonged hospitalization. Despite the risk to the infant, women who become pregnant should not discontinue their medication without consulting the prescriber.

Dermatologic Effects. Drugs in the *phenothiazine* class can sensitize the skin to ultraviolet light, thereby increasing the risk of severe sunburn. Patients should be warned against excessive exposure to sunlight and advised to apply a sunscreen and wear protective clothing. Phenothiazines can also produce pigmentary deposits in the skin as well as in the cornea and lens of the eye.

Handling antipsychotics can cause contact dermatitis in patients and healthcare workers. Dermatitis can be prevented by avoiding direct contact with these drugs.

Physical and Psychologic Dependence

Development of physical and psychologic dependence is rare. Patients should be reassured that addiction and dependence are not likely.

Although physical dependence is minimal, abrupt withdrawal of FGAs *can* precipitate a mild abstinence syndrome. Symptoms, which are related to chronic cholinergic blockade, include restlessness, insomnia, headache, gastric distress, and sweating. The syndrome can be avoided by withdrawing FGAs gradually.

Drug Interactions

Anticholinergic Drugs. Drugs with anticholinergic properties will intensify anticholinergic responses to neuroleptics. Patients should be advised to avoid all drugs with anticholinergic actions, including antihistamines and certain over-the-counter sleep aids.

CNS Depressants. Neuroleptics can intensify CNS depression caused by other drugs. Patients should be warned against using alcohol and all other drugs with CNS-depressant actions (e.g., antihistamines, benzodiazepines, barbiturates).

Levodopa and Direct Dopamine Receptor Agonists. Levodopa (a drug for PD) may counteract the antipsychotic effects of neuroleptics. Conversely, neuroleptics may counteract the therapeutic effects of levodopa. These interactions occur because levodopa and neuroleptics have opposing effects on receptors for dopamine: Levodopa activates dopamine receptors, whereas neuroleptics cause receptor blockade. Like levodopa, the direct dopamine receptor agonists (e.g., bromocriptine) activate dopamine receptors, and hence have interactions with neuroleptics identical to those of levodopa.

Toxicity

First-generation antipsychotics are very safe; death by overdose is extremely rare. With chlorpromazine, for example, the therapeutic index is about 200. That is, the lethal dose is 200 times the therapeutic dose.

Overdose produces hypotension, CNS depression, and extrapyramidal reactions. Extrapyramidal reactions can be treated with antiparkinsonism drugs. Hypotension can be treated with IV fluids plus an alpha-adrenergic agonist (e.g., phenylephrine). There is no specific antidote to CNS depression. Excess drug can be removed from the stomach by gastric lavage. Emetics cannot be used because their effects would be blocked by the antiemetic action of the neuroleptic.

Properties of Individual Agents

All of the FGAs are equally effective at alleviating symptoms of schizophrenia, although individual patients may respond better to one FGA than to another. Differences among these agents relate primarily to side effects (see Table 31.2). Because the high-potency agents produce fewer side effects than the low-potency agents, high-potency agents are used more often.

High-Potency Agents

Compared with the low-potency FGAs, the high-potency FGAs cause more early EPS, but cause less sedation, orthostatic hypotension, and anticholinergic effects. Because they cause fewer side effects, high-potency agents are generally preferred for initial therapy.

Haloperidol

Actions and Uses. Haloperidol, a member of the *butyrophenone* family, is the prototype of the high-potency FGAs. Principal indications are schizophrenia and acute psychosis. In addition, haloperidol is a preferred agent for Tourette's syndrome. The drug can also be used to control severe behavioral problems in children (e.g., combative, explosive hyperexcitability unrelated to any immediate provocation), but only as a last resort. Haloperidol is used more than other FGAs. The pharmacokinetics of haloperidol and other drugs can be found in Table 31.5.

Adverse Effects. As indicated in Table 31.2, early extrapyramidal reactions (acute dystonia, parkinsonism, akathisia) occur frequently, whereas sedation, hypotension, and anticholinergic effects are uncommon. Note that the incidence of these reactions is opposite to that seen with the low-potency agents. However, the incidence of TD is the same as with all other FGAs. Neuroendocrine effects—galactorrhea, gynecomastia, menstrual irregularities—are seen occasionally. NMS, photosensitivity, convulsions, and impotence are rare.

Haloperidol can prolong the QT interval, and hence may pose a risk of *serious dysrhythmias,* especially when given IV and/or in high doses. The drug should be used with caution in patients with dysrhythmia risk factors, including long QT syndrome, hypokalemia or hyperkalemia, or a history of dysrhythmias, heart attack, or severe heart failure. Combined use

TABLE 31.5 ▪ Pharmacokinetic Properties of Antipsychotic Medications

Drug	Route	Peak (hr)[a]	Half-Life (hr)[a]	Metabolism	Excretion
FIRST-GENERATION ANTIPSYCHOTICS					
Chlorpromazine [generic only]	PO/IM/IV	1–4	23–37	Hepatic	Renal
Haloperidol [generic only]	PO/IM	2–6	23–37	Hepatic	Renal
SECOND-GENERATION ANTIPSYCHOTICS					
Aripiprazole [Abilify]	PO/IM	3–5	75	Hepatic	Gastrointestinal,[b] renal
Asenapine [Saphris]	PO	1	24	Hepatic	Renal
Brexpiprazole [Rexulti]	PO	4	91	Hepatic	Gastrointestinal,[b] renal
Cariprazine [Vraylar]	PO	3–6	24–48	Hepatic	Renal
Clozapine [Clozaril]	PO	3	12	Hepatic	Renal, gastrointestinal[b]
Iloperidone [Fanapt]	PO	2–4	18–37	Hepatic	Renal, gastrointestinal[b]
Lurasadone [Latuda]	PO	1–3	18	Hepatic	Gastrointestinal,[b] urine
Olanzapine [Zyprexa]	PO/IM	6	30	Hepatic	Renal
Quetiapine [Seroquel]	PO	1.5	6	Hepatic	Gastrointestinal,[b] renal
Risperidone [Risperdal]	PO/IM	1	24	Hepatic	Renal
Ziprasidone [Geodon]	PO/IM	6–8	7	Hepatic	Gastrointestinal[b]

[a]Oral administration.
[b]Feces.

with other QT-prolonging drugs (e.g., amiodarone, erythromycin, quinidine) should be avoided.

Preparations. Haloperidol for oral use is available in tablets (0.5, 1, 2, 5, 10, and 20 mg) and a liquid concentrate (2 mg/mL), both sold generically. *Haloperidol lactate* is available for IV and IM administration for acute therapy in a 5-mg/mL solution [Haldol], although IV administration is not FDA approved. *Haloperidol decanoate* is available as a 50-mg/mL and 100-mg/mL oily suspension [Haldol Decanoate] only for IM dosing as a depot preparation used for long-term therapy.

Dosage and Administration

ORAL. The initial dosage for adults is 0.5 to 2 mg taken 2 or 3 times a day. For severe illness, daily doses up to 100 mg have been employed. Once symptoms have been controlled, the dosage should be reduced to the lowest effective amount.

INTRAVENOUS OR INTRAMUSCULAR. For *acute therapy* of severe psychosis, haloperidol lactate is administered IV or IM in doses of 2 to 5 mg. Dosing may be repeated as often as every 60 minutes, although intervals of 4 to 8 hours may be satisfactory. Once symptoms are under control, the patient should be switched to oral therapy.

For *long-term therapy,* haloperidol decanoate is given once every 4 weeks by deep IM injection—but only to patients already stabilized on oral haloperidol. The initial dose is 10 to 20 times the current oral dose—but no greater than 100 mg. Maintenance doses are 10 to 15 times the previous oral dose.

Other High-Potency Agents

Fluphenazine. Fluphenazine is a high-potency agent indicated for schizophrenia and other psychotic disorders. The drug belongs to the piperazine subclass of phenothiazines. As with other high-potency agents, the most common adverse effects are early EPS: acute dystonia, parkinsonism, and akathisia. The risk of TD equals that of other FGAs. Effects seen occasionally include sedation, orthostatic hypotension, anticholinergic effects, gynecomastia, galactorrhea, and menstrual irregularities. NMS, convulsions, and agranulocytosis are rare.

Fluphenazine may be given PO or IM. For oral use, the drug is available in tablets (1, 2.5, 5, and 10 mg), an elixir (2.5 mg/5 mL), and an oral concentrate (5 mg/1 mL). The initial *oral* dosage is 2.5 to 10 mg/day, given in divided doses every 6 to 8 hours. Daily dosages greater than 3 mg are rarely needed, although some patients may require as much as 30 mg. Once symptoms have been controlled, the dosage should be reduced to the lowest effective amount, typically 1 to 5 mg/day taken as a single dose.

Two injectable preparations are available: *fluphenazine hydrochloride* (2.5 mg/mL) and *fluphenazine decanoate* (25 mg/mL). Both are given IM. Fluphenazine hydrochloride is a fast-acting preparation used for acute therapy. The usual dosage is 2.5 to 10 mg/day, given in divided doses every 6 to 8 hours. Fluphenazine decanoate is a depot preparation used for long-term therapy—but only in patients already stabilized on oral fluphenazine (or another phenothiazine antipsychotic). Intramuscular doses are based on the oral dosage. A reasonable conversion ratio is 12.5 mg of IM fluphenazine every 3 weeks for each 10 mg of oral fluphenazine taken daily.

Trifluoperazine. Trifluoperazine is a high-potency agent used for schizophrenia and other psychotic disorders. The drug belongs to the piperazine subclass of phenothiazines. The most common adverse effects are early extrapyramidal reactions (acute dystonia, parkinsonism, akathisia). Effects seen occasionally include sedation, orthostatic hypotension, anticholinergic effects, gynecomastia, galactorrhea, menstrual irregularities, and TD. NMS, convulsions, and agranulocytosis are rare. Trifluoperazine is available in tablets (1, 2, 5, and 10 mg) for oral use. Dosing is begun at 2 to 5 mg twice daily in hospitalized or highly supervised patients. Outpatients may begin at 1 to 2 mg twice daily. In both patient groups, doses are then increased until an optimal response has been produced, usually with 15 to 20 mg/day.

Pimozide. Pimozide [Orap] is a high-potency FGA approved only for treating *Tourette's syndrome,* a rare disorder characterized by severe motor tics and uncontrollable grunts, barking cries, and outbursts of obscene language. Like other neuroleptics, pimozide can cause sedation, postural hypotension, and extrapyramidal reactions (acute dystonia, parkinsonism, akathisia, TD).

Pimozide can prolong the QT interval, and hence poses a risk of fatal cardiac dysrhythmias. Sertraline [Zoloft] increases this risk by raising pimozide levels, and hence the two drugs should not be combined. Similarly, combining citalopram [Celexa] or escitalopram [Lexapro, Cipralex 🍁] with pimozide can prolong the QT interval (by an unknown mechanism), and hence these combinations should be avoided.

Pimozide is available in tablets (1 and 2 mg) for oral therapy. The initial dosage is 1 to 2 mg/day in divided doses. Dosage should be slowly increased to a maintenance level of 10 mg/day or 0.2 mg/kg/day (whichever is less).

Medium-Potency Agents

Loxapine. Loxapine [Loxitane, Adasuve] is a medium-potency agent indicated only for schizophrenia. The side effect profile is similar to that of fluphenazine. The drug is available in capsules (5, 10, 25, and 50 mg) sold as *Loxitane* for oral use. The initial dosage is 10 mg twice a day. Dosage is increased until symptoms are controlled, typically with 60 to 100 mg/day in divided doses. The dosage should be reduced for maintenance therapy; the usual range is 20 to 60 mg/day. *Adasuve* is used for acute treatment of agitation associated with schizophrenia. Adasuve is available as a 10-mg inhaled powder. Only one inhalation is recommended in a 24-hour period.

Perphenazine. Perphenazine is a medium-potency agent used for schizophrenia and other psychotic disorders. Its side effect profile is like that of fluphenazine. The drug is available alone in tablets (2, 4, 8, and 16 mg) or in combination with amitriptyline (2/10, 2/25, 4/10, 4/25, and 4/50 mg) for oral use. The initial dosage in outpatients is 4 to 8 mg 3 times daily. Hospitalized patients may receive 8 to 16 mg 2 to 4 times daily. Once symptoms have been controlled, the dosage should be reduced to the lowest effective amount.

Thiothixene. Thiothixene [Navane] is a medium-potency agent approved only for schizophrenia. The most common adverse effects are early extrapyramidal reactions (acute dystonia, parkinsonism, akathisia) and anticholinergic effects. Side effects seen occasionally include galactorrhea, gynecomastia, menstrual irregularities, sedation, orthostatic hypotension, and TD. Agranulocytosis, NMS, and convulsions are rare. Thiothixene is available in capsules (1, 2, 5, and 10 mg) for oral use. The initial dosage is 2 mg 3 times daily. Dosage is increased until an optimal response has been achieved, usually with 20 to 30 mg/day.

Low-Potency Agents

Chlorpromazine. Chlorpromazine was the first modern antipsychotic medication. None of the newer FGAs is superior at relieving symptoms of psychotic illnesses. Chlorpromazine is a low-potency FGA and belongs to the phenothiazine family.

Therapeutic Uses. Principal indications are schizophrenia and other psychotic disorders. Additional psychiatric indications are schizoaffective disorder and the manic phase of bipolar disorder. Other uses include suppression of emesis, relief of intractable hiccups, and control of severe behavioral problems in children.

Adverse Effects. The most common adverse effects are sedation, orthostatic hypotension, and anticholinergic effects (dry mouth, blurred vision, urinary retention, photophobia, constipation, tachycardia). Neuroendocrine effects (galactorrhea, gynecomastia, menstrual irregularities) are seen on occasion. Photosensitivity reactions are possible, and patients should be advised to minimize unprotected exposure to sunlight. Because chlorpromazine is a low-potency neuroleptic, the risk of early extrapyramidal reactions (dystonia, akathisia, parkinsonism) is relatively low. However, the risk of TD is the same as with all other FGAs. Chlorpromazine lowers seizure threshold. Accordingly, patients with seizure disorders should be especially diligent about taking antiseizure medication. Like haloperidol, chlorpromazine can prolong the QT interval, and hence may pose a risk of fatal dysrhythmias, especially in patients with dysrhythmia risk factors (e.g., long QT syndrome, hypokalemia, hyperkalemia, history of cardiac dysrhythmias). Agranulocytosis and NMS occur rarely.

Drug Interactions. Chlorpromazine can intensify responses to CNS depressants (e.g., antihistamines, benzodiazepines, barbiturates) and anticholinergic drugs (e.g., antihistamines, tricyclic antidepressants, atropine-like drugs).

PREPARATIONS, DOSAGE, AND ADMINISTRATION. Chlorpromazine is available in two formulations: *tablets* (10, 25, 50, 100, and 200 mg) and *solution for injection* (25 mg/mL).

ORAL THERAPY. The initial dosage for adults is 25 mg 3 times a day. Dosage should be gradually increased until symptoms are controlled. The usual maintenance dosage is 400 mg/day. Older adult patients require less drug than younger patients.

PARENTERAL THERAPY. Parenteral therapy is indicated for acutely psychotic, hospitalized patients. Intramuscular administration is preferred to IV administration. (Intravenous chlorpromazine is highly irritating and generally avoided.) The initial dose is 25 to 50 mg. Dosage may be increased gradually to a maximum of 400 mg every 4 to 6 hours. Once symptoms are controlled, oral therapy should be substituted for parenteral therapy.

Thioridazine. Thioridazine is a low-potency FGA that prolongs the QT interval, and hence can cause fatal cardiac dysrhythmias. Because of this danger, the drug should be reserved for treating schizophrenia in patients who have not responded to safer agents. The most common adverse effects are sedation, orthostatic hypotension, anticholinergic effects, weight gain, and inhibition of ejaculation. Effects seen occasionally include extrapyramidal reactions (dystonia, parkinsonism, akathisia, TD), neuroendocrine effects (galactorrhea, gynecomastia, menstrual irregularities), and photosensitivity reactions. NMS, convulsions, agranulocytosis, and pigmentary retinopathy occur rarely. Principal interactions are with anticholinergic drugs and CNS depressants. Thioridazine is available in tablets (10, 15, 25, 50, 100, 150, and 200 mg) for oral dosing. The initial dosage is 50 to 100 mg 3 times a day. Dosage may be gradually increased until symptoms are controlled, but should not exceed 800 mg/day. The usual maintenance dosage is 200 to 800 mg/day in two to four divided doses.

Molindone. Molindone is a low-potency FGA approved only for the treatment of schizophrenia. The most common adverse effects are sedation, orthostatic hypotension, anticholinergic effects, weight gain, and inhibition of ejaculation. Molindone has the potential to cause agranulocytosis. Therefore, CBC should be monitored frequently during the first few months of treatment and molindone should be discontinued in patients with an absolute neutrophil count (ANC) less than 1000/mm^3. Molindone is available in 5, 10, and 25 mg tablets. Usual initial dosing is 50 to 75 mg daily in 3 or 4 divided doses.

SECOND-GENERATION (ATYPICAL) ANTIPSYCHOTICS

The SGAs, also known as *atypical antipsychotics,* were introduced in the 1990s and quickly took over 90% of the market, owing to the perception of superior efficacy and greater safety. However, neither initial perception has held up. Thanks to two large government-sponsored studies, one in the United States and the other in Great Britain, we now know that in most cases SGAs and FGAs are equally effective. As for major side effects, the SGAs *are* less likely to cause EPS, including TD. However, the SGAs carry an even greater risk of their own, namely, serious metabolic effects—weight gain, diabetes, and dyslipidemia—that can lead to cardiovascular events and premature death. Furthermore, like the FGAs, the SGAs can cause sedation and orthostatic hypotension, and can increase the risk of death when used to treat dementia-related psychosis in older adults. Finally, even though SGAs have no clear clinical advantage over FGAs, the SGAs cost 10 to 20 times as much.

In addition to their use in schizophrenia, all of the SGAs are approved for bipolar disorder (see Chapter 33).

Clozapine

Clozapine [Clozaril, FazaClo, Versacloz] was the first SGA and will serve as our prototype for the group—even though other SGAs are now used more widely. This drug is our most effective agent for schizophrenia, the only indication it has. However, because clozapine can cause agranulocytosis, it should be reserved for patients who have not responded to safer alternatives.

Mechanism of Action

Antipsychotic effects result from blockade of receptors for dopamine and serotonin (5-hydroxytryptamine [5-HT]). Like the FGAs, clozapine blocks D_2 dopamine receptors, but its affinity for these receptors is relatively low. In contrast, the drug produces strong blockade of 5-HT_2 serotonin receptors. Combined blockade of D_2 receptors and 5-HT_2 receptors is thought to underlie therapeutic effects. Low affinity for D_2 receptors may explain why SGAs cause fewer EPS than do the FGAs. In addition to blocking receptors for dopamine and serotonin, clozapine blocks receptors for norepinephrine (alpha$_1$), histamine, and acetylcholine.

Therapeutic Use

Schizophrenia. Clozapine is approved for relieving general symptoms of schizophrenia and for reducing suicidal behavior in patients with schizophrenia or schizoaffective disorder who are at chronic suicide risk. The drug is highly effective and often works when all other antipsychotics have failed. Unfortunately, clozapine can cause fatal agranulocytosis (discussed later in this chapter), and hence should be reserved for patients with severe disease who have not responded to safer alternatives. Like the FGAs, clozapine improves positive, negative, and cognitive symptoms of schizophrenia. Because the incidence of EPS with clozapine is low, the drug is well suited for patients who have experienced severe EPS with an FGA.

Levodopa-Induced Psychosis. Psychosis is a common side effect of levodopa, a drug used for PD. Clozapine is preferred to FGAs for treatment. As discussed in Chapter 21, the movement disorders of PD result from insufficient dopamine in the striatum, a component of the extrapyramidal system. Levodopa reduces symptoms of PD by increasing dopamine availability. Because FGAs cause profound blockade of dopamine receptors in the striatum, they will intensify symptoms of PD. In contrast, clozapine causes little or no blockade of striatal dopamine receptors, and hence can alleviate levodopa-induced psychosis without making symptoms of PD worse. The average dosage of clozapine required is only 25 mg a day—about 20 times less than the dosage for schizophrenia.

Adverse Effects and Interactions

Common adverse effects include sedation and weight gain (from blocking histamine$_1$ [H_1] receptors); orthostatic hypotension (from blocking alpha-adrenergic receptors); and dry mouth, blurred vision, urinary retention, constipation, and tachycardia (from blocking muscarinic cholinergic receptors). Neuroendocrine effects (galactorrhea, gynecomastia, amenorrhea) and interference with sexual function are minimal. Compared with the FGAs, clozapine carries a low risk of extrapyramidal effects, including TD.

Agranulocytosis. Clozapine produces agranulocytosis in 1% to 2% of patients. The overall risk of death is about 1 in 5000. The usual cause is gram-negative sepsis. Agranulocytosis typically occurs during the first 6 months of treatment, and the onset is usually gradual. Why agranulocytosis occurs is unknown.

Because of the risk of fatal agranulocytosis, providers must enroll in the Risk Evaluation and Mitigation Strategies (REMS) program to be able to prescribe clozapine. This ensures that providers receive education regarding mandatory monitoring of the WBC count *and* ANC. Before starting clozapine, both the total WBC count and ANC must be in the normal range (i.e., WBC count of 3500/mm^3 or greater and ANC of 2000/mm^3 or greater). During treatment, the WBC count and ANC must be monitored weekly for the first 6 months, then every 2 weeks for the following 6 months. After 1 year of treatment, WBC and ANC monitoring is decreased to monthly. Additional testing may be completed when considering the possibility of neutropenia, when adding other antipsychotics, or when clinically indicated. If the total WBC count falls below 3000/mm^3 or if the ANC falls below 1500/mm^3, treatment should be interrupted. When subsequent *daily* monitoring indicates that counts have risen above these values, clozapine can be resumed. If the total WBC count falls below 2000/mm^3 or if the ANC falls below 1000/mm^3, clozapine should be permanently discontinued. Blood counts should be monitored for 4 weeks after drug withdrawal.

Patients should be informed about the risk of agranulocytosis and told that clozapine will not be dispensed if the blood tests have not been done. Also, patients should be informed about early signs of infection (fever, sore throat, fatigue, mucous membrane ulceration) and instructed to report these immediately.

Metabolic Effects: Weight Gain, Diabetes, and Dyslipidemia. Clozapine and the other SGAs can cause a group of closely linked metabolic effects—obesity, diabetes, and dyslipidemia—all of which increase the risk of cardiovascular events. As indicated in Table 31.2, risk is highest with clozapine and olanzapine, and lowest with aripiprazole, lurasidone, and ziprasidone.

Weight gain is the metabolic effect of greatest concern because it seems to underlie development of diabetes and dyslipidemia. Among patients taking clozapine, weight gain can be significant. Patients should be informed about the possibility. Body mass index should be measured at baseline, at every visit for 6 months, and every 3 months thereafter. In addition, waist circumference should be measured at baseline and annually thereafter. If significant weight gain occurs, it can be managed with a combination of lifestyle measures and *metformin,* an oral drug used for diabetes. In one study, metformin was more effective than lifestyle measures and the combination of metformin plus lifestyle measures was more effective than either intervention alone. Antipsychotic drugs promote weight gain through blockade of H_1 receptors in the brain; they also cause a decrease in body temperature, which decreases energy expenditure.

Clozapine and all other SGAs can cause *new-onset diabetes.* Patients taking these drugs have developed typical diabetes symptoms, including hyperglycemia, polyuria, polydipsia, polyphagia, and dehydration. In extreme cases, hyperglycemia has led to ketoacidosis, hyperosmolar coma, and even death. Because of diabetes risk, fasting blood sugar should be measured before starting clozapine, 12 weeks later, and annually thereafter. Patients with documented diabetes at treatment onset should be monitored for worsening of glucose control. All patients should be informed about symptoms of diabetes and instructed to report them. If diabetes develops, it can be managed with insulin or an oral antidiabetic drug, such as metformin. Discontinuing clozapine is also an option. However, if the drug has produced control of psychotic symptoms, continuing clozapine and treating the diabetes would seem preferable.

Dyslipidemia associated with clozapine and other SGAs can manifest as increased total cholesterol, LDL cholesterol, and triglycerides, along with decreased HDL cholesterol. This lipid profile increases the risk of atherosclerosis and coronary heart disease. To monitor effects on lipids, a fasting lipid profile should be obtained at baseline and every 6 months thereafter. A fasting lipid profile should be obtained more frequently for patients on high-risk medications, including clozapine and olanzapine.

Seizures. Generalized tonic-clonic convulsions occur in 3% of patients. The risk of seizures is dose related. Patients should be warned not to drive or to participate in other potentially hazardous activities if a seizure has occurred. Patients with a history of seizure disorders should use the drug with great caution.

Extrapyramidal Symptoms. Although the risk of EPS with SGAs is relatively low, it is not zero. Hence, like the FGAs, clozapine and other SGAs can cause parkinsonism, acute dystonia, akathisia, and TD.

Myocarditis. Very rarely, clozapine has been associated with myocarditis (inflammation of the heart muscle), which can be fatal. If a patient develops signs and symptoms (e.g., unexplained fatigue, dyspnea, tachypnea, chest pain, palpitations), clozapine should be withheld until myocarditis has been ruled out. If myocarditis is diagnosed, clozapine should not be used again.

Orthostatic Hypotension. Clozapine can cause orthostatic hypotension, sometimes with fainting. Rarely, collapse is severe, and accompanied by respiratory and/or cardiac arrest. Hypotension is most likely during initial dosage titration, especially if dosage escalation is rapid.

Effects in Older Adult Patients With Dementia. Like the FGAs, the SGAs about double the rate of mortality when used off-label to treat dementia-related psychosis in older adults. Accordingly, because SGAs are not approved for this use and because they pose a risk to these patients, it is clear that SGAs should not be prescribed for this condition.

Drug Interactions. Because it can cause agranulocytosis, clozapine is contraindicated for patients taking other drugs that can suppress bone marrow function, including many anticancer drugs.

Drugs that induce cytochrome P450 isoenzymes (e.g., phenytoin, rifampin) can lower clozapine levels, and drugs that inhibit P450 isoenzymes (e.g., ketoconazole, erythromycin) can raise clozapine levels. These inducers and inhibitors should be used with caution.

Preparations, Dosage, and Administration

Clozapine is available in standard tablets (12.5, 25, 50, 100, and 200 mg) sold as *Clozaril,* in a 50-mg/mL suspension sold as *Versacloz,* and in orally disintegrating tablets (12.5, 25, 100, 150, and 200 mg) sold as *FazaClo.* To minimize side effects, treatment should begin with a 12.5-mg dose, followed by 25 mg once or twice daily. Dosage is then increased by 25 mg/day until it reaches 300 to 450 mg/day. Further increases can be made once or twice weekly in increments no larger than 100 mg. The usual maintenance dosage is 300 to 600 mg/day in three divided doses. The maximum dosage is 900 mg/day. If therapy is interrupted for greater than 48 hours, it should resume with a 12.5-mg dose and then follow the original titration guidelines. Because of the risk of agranulocytosis, dispensing is normally limited to a 1-week supply.

Other Second-Generation Antipsychotics

Risperidone

Risperidone [Risperdal, Risperdal Consta] is a rapid-acting drug originally approved for schizophrenia and then later approved for acute bipolar mania. Most recently, the drug was approved for children with autism spectrum disorder, with the goal of reducing irritability-associated symptoms such as tantrums, aggression, mood swings, and self-injury. In patients with schizophrenia, risperidone improves positive symptoms, negative symptoms, and cognitive function. Like other SGAs, it causes fewer EPS than FGAs. Risperidone is structurally unrelated to clozapine.

Mechanism of Action. We know that risperidone binds to multiple receptors, but we don't know with certainty how clinical benefits are produced. Risperidone is a powerful antagonist at 5-HT_2 receptors and a less powerful antagonist at D_2 receptors. Antagonism at both sites probably underlies therapeutic effects. Risperidone does not block cholinergic receptors but does block H_1 receptors as well as alpha-adrenergic receptors.

Therapeutic Effects. Risperidone relieves positive and negative symptoms of schizophrenia and improves cognitive function. Significant improvement may be seen in 1 week. In patients with severe TD, risperidone may have an antidyskinetic effect.

Adverse Effects. Side effects are generally infrequent and mild, and only rarely require discontinuation of treatment. The incidence of EPS is very low at the recommended dosage. However, at dosages above 10 mg/day, there is a dose-related increase in EPS. With the long-acting IM formulation, the incidence of EPS is substantial (about 25%). Risperidone increases prolactin levels, but symptoms (gynecomastia, galactorrhea) are uncommon. Like most other SGAs, risperidone can cause metabolic effects: weight gain, diabetes, and dyslipidemia. Adverse effects that have led to drug discontinuation include agitation, dizziness, somnolence, and fatigue. Excessive doses have caused sedation, difficulty in concentrating, and disruption of sleep. When used off-label to treat older adult patients with dementia-related psychosis, risperidone doubles or triples the risk of stroke and nearly doubles the risk of death (usually from cardiac events or pneumonia).

Preparations, Dosage, and Administration

Schizophrenia, Oral Therapy. For oral therapy, risperidone is available in film-coated tablets (0.25, 0.5, 1, 2, 3, and 4 mg) and solution (1 mg/mL), both sold as *Risperdal,* and in orally disintegrating tablets (0.5, 1, 2, 3, and 4 mg) sold as *Risperdal M-TAB.* The recommended dosage is 1 mg twice daily the first day, 2 mg twice daily the second day, and 3 mg twice daily thereafter. Dosages above 2 or 3 mg twice daily do not increase therapeutic effects, but do increase the risk of EPS and other side effects. Dosage should be reduced in patients with renal or hepatic impairment.

Schizophrenia, Intramuscular Therapy. Intramuscular risperidone [Risperdal Consta] is a depot preparation used only for *long-term* therapy. In this formulation, risperidone is bound to a matrix that has been encapsulated within microspheres. Following IM injection, the matrix gradually breaks down to release free drug. Importantly, significant release doesn't begin until 2 to 3 weeks after the injection, producing therapeutic levels 4 to 6 weeks after the injection. Because effects are delayed, patients should take an oral antipsychotic during the first 3 weeks of Risperdal Consta use. The IM dosage range is 25 to 50 mg every 2 weeks. Risperdal Consta is supplied in a kit that contains 2 mL of diluent plus risperidone in microspheres (12.5, 25, 37.5, or 50 mg).

Bipolar Disorder. Dosage for bipolar disorder is presented in Chapter 33.

Irritability Associated With Autism Spectrum Disorder. The initial dosage is 0.25 mg/day (for children under 20 kg) and 0.5 mg/day (for children 20 kg and over). After a minimum of 4 days, dosage may be increased to the recommended maintenance level of 0.5 mg/day (for children under 20 kg) or 1 mg/day (for children 20 kg and over). If needed, dosage may be slowly titrated higher. For all children, the total daily dose can be administered as a single dose or as two divided doses of equal size.

Safe Handling and Administration. In 2016, the National Institute for Occupations Safety and Health (NIOSH), a division of the Centers for Disease Control and Prevention, published a list of drugs considered to be potentially hazardous in healthcare settings. Risperidone was included in this list secondary to its potential to cause fetal harm. Exposure to these drugs can pose a reproductive risk to healthcare workers who administer these drugs. To promote safe administration, NIOSH suggests donning a protective gown and two sets of gloves when cutting or crushing tablets and administering liquid formulations or injections. For further information on this report, visit https://www.cdc.gov/niosh/topics/antineoplastic/pdf/hazardous-drugs-list_2016-161.pdf.

Paliperidone

Paliperidone [Invega, Invega Sustenna, Invega Trinza] is approved for acute therapy of schizoaffective disorder and for acute and maintenance therapy of schizophrenia. The drug is the active metabolite of risperidone (9-hydroxyrisperidone), and hence has the same adverse and therapeutic effects as risperidone itself. The two drugs differ primarily in that paliperidone is not extensively metabolized, and has no significant kinetic interactions with other drugs. Also, in contrast to risperidone, paliperidone is dosed just once a day, and doesn't require initial dosage titration. Paliperidone can prolong the QT interval, and hence should not be combined with other QT-prolonging drugs.

Paliperidone for *oral therapy* [Invega] is available in extended-release tablets (1.5, 3, 6, and 9 mg) that employ the so-called osmotic-release oral system (OROS) for delivery. Dosing is done once daily in the morning, with or without food. Patients should be instructed to swallow the tablets whole, without crushing, chewing, or dividing. Also, they should be informed that Invega tablets have a nonabsorbable shell that passes intact into the stool. For patients with normal renal function, the usual dosage is 6 mg/day. For patients with moderate renal impairment (creatinine clearance 50 to 80 mL/min), dosage must not exceed 6 mg/day. For patients with severe renal impairment (creatinine clearance 10 to 50 mL/min), dosage should not exceed 3 mg/day.

Paliperidone for *parenteral therapy* is available in two extended-release suspensions. Invega Sustenna is available as an extended-release suspension (39, 79, 117, 156, and 234 mg) in pre-filled syringes. The usual dosing schedule for this depot preparation is 234 mg on day 1 and 156 mg on day 8, both injected into the deltoid muscle, followed by monthly maintenance doses (117 mg) injected into either the deltoid or gluteal muscle. The maintenance range is 79 to 234 mg once a month. As Invega Trinza is administered only every 3 months, it is indicated only in patients who have received Invega Sustenna and have remained stable for at least 4 months. The IM injection dose ranges from 273 mg to 819 mg, depending on the last dose of Invega Sustenna.

Safe Handling and Administration. As paliperidone is a metabolite of risperidone, NIOSH recommends the same procedures for administration as previously outlined. For further information on this report, visit https://www.cdc.gov/niosh/topics/antineoplastic/pdf/hazardous-drugs-list_2016-161.pdf.

Olanzapine

Olanzapine [Zyprexa] is an SGA approved for (1) schizophrenia, (2) maintenance therapy of bipolar disorder, (3) acute agitation associated with schizophrenia and bipolar mania, and (4) treatment-resistant major depression (in combination with fluoxetine). In addition, olanzapine is used off-label to suppress nausea and vomiting in cancer patients. The drug is similar to clozapine in structure and actions, but carries little or no risk of agranulocytosis (although it can cause leukopenia/neutropenia). The risk of metabolic effects is higher than with most other SGAs.

Mechanism of Action. Olanzapine blocks receptors for serotonin, dopamine, histamine, acetylcholine, and norepinephrine. Therapeutic effects are believed to result from blocking $5\text{-}HT_2$ and D_2 receptors. Adverse effects result in part from blocking receptors for histamine, acetylcholine, and norepinephrine.

Therapeutic Uses

Schizophrenia. In patients with schizophrenia, olanzapine is at least as effective as haloperidol or risperidone and produces fewer EPS than either drug. Comparative trials with clozapine reveal that olanzapine is not inferior to clozapine in patients previously refractory to treatment. Interestingly, olanzapine can relieve psychosis induced by drugs taken for PD, without reversing antiparkinsonism effects.

Bipolar Disorder. Olanzapine is approved for monotherapy of acute mania in patients with bipolar disorder. Benefits appear equal to those of lithium, a drug of choice for this condition (see Chapter 33).

Adverse Effects With Oral Olanzapine. Regarding *serious* adverse effects, olanzapine is a mixed blessing: The drug carries a low risk of EPS but carries a high risk of metabolic effects. Acute EPS are minimal when olanzapine is used at the recommended dosage. Among the SGAs, olanzapine (along with clozapine) poses the highest risk of serious metabolic effects: weight gain, diabetes, and dyslipidemia—all of which can lead to adverse cardiovascular events and premature death. Like all other antipsychotic drugs, olanzapine can increase mortality in older adult patients with dementia-related psychosis.

Olanzapine can cause *leukopenia/neutropenia* and can thereby increase the risk of infection. Accordingly, for patients at high risk—including those with pre-existing low WBC counts and those with a history of drug-induced leukopenia/neutropenia—complete blood counts should be conducted often during the first few months of treatment. If the ANC falls below $1000/mm^3$, olanzapine should be discontinued, and the patient should be monitored for fever and other signs of infection. Neutrophil counts should be monitored until they return to normal.

Mild effects are relatively common. Olanzapine causes somnolence in 26% of patients, presumably by blocking H_1 receptors. Blockade of muscarinic receptors causes constipation and other anticholinergic effects. $Alpha_1$-adrenergic blockade causes orthostatic hypotension. Following an overdose, the signs and symptoms may include slurred speech, ataxia, nystagmus, hypotension, respiratory depression, and drowsiness.

In 2016, the FDA posted a new alert associating the use of olanzapine with a rare skin condition known as *drug reaction with eosinophilia and systemic symptoms* (DRESS). Over 23 cases of DRESS have been reported, including one death. DRESS can cause injury to multiple organ systems and carries a mortality rate of up to 10%. Patients that develop fever, swollen glands, and rash while taking olanzapine should seek medical attention immediately.

Adverse Effects With Long-Acting IM Olanzapine. Overdose with the long-acting IM depot preparation of olanzapine [Zyprexa Relprevv] is dangerous. Principal concerns are CNS depression (ranging from mild sedation to coma) and/or delirium (confusion, disorientation, agitation, anxiety). Patients may also experience EPS, joint pain, ataxia, aggression, dizziness, weakness, hypertension, and convulsions. Symptoms typically develop within 1 to 3 hours of dosing, but may also develop later. After the injection, patients should be observed by a healthcare provider for at least 3 hours, and should be warned against driving and other hazardous activities for the remainder of the day.

Preparations. For oral therapy, olanzapine is available in standard tablets (2.5, 5, 7.5, 10, 15, and 20 mg) sold as *Zyprexa,* in orally disintegrating tablets (5, 10, 15, and 20 mg) sold as *Zyprexa Zydis,* and in capsules combined with fluoxetine (3 mg olanzapine/25 mg fluoxetine, 6 mg/25 mg, 6 mg/50 mg, 12 mg/25 mg, and 12 mg/50 mg), sold as *Symbyax,* used for acute treatment of depressive episodes in bipolar disorder as well as treatment-resistant major depression.

For IM therapy, olanzapine is available in two formulations: short acting and long acting. The *short-acting* formulation, sold as *Zyprexa IntraMuscular,* is supplied as a powder (10 mg olanzapine) to be reconstituted with 2.1 mL of sterile water. The *long-acting* depot formulation, sold as *Zyprexa Relprevv,* is supplied as a powder (210, 300, and 405 mg olanzapine pamoate in single-use vials) to be reconstituted with the diluent supplied. The volume of diluent depends on the intended dose and the vial used.

Dosage and Administration

Schizophrenia. The recommended *oral* dosage is 5 to 10 mg once a day for the first few days, and 10 mg once a day thereafter. Dosages greater than 10 mg/day are not more effective, but do increase the risk of side effects. *Intramuscular* doses depend on the formulation. With the *short-acting* formulation, the usual dosage is 2.5 to 10 mg. With the *long-acting* formulation, the usual dosage is 150 to 300 mg every 2 weeks, or 405 mg every 4 weeks. After the injection, patients should be watched for at least 3 hours for signs of overdose (see previous section).

Bipolar Disorder. For bipolar disorder, we can use olanzapine alone [Zyprexa, Zyprexa Zydis] or olanzapine/fluoxetine [Symbyax]. The dosage for olanzapine alone is presented in Chapter 33. The dosage range for olanzapine/fluoxetine is 6 to 12 mg/day of olanzapine plus 25 or 50 mg/day of fluoxetine.

Treatment-Resistant Major Depression. Major depression is treated with olanzapine/fluoxetine [Symbyax], not with olanzapine alone. The initial dosage is olanzapine 6 mg/fluoxetine 25 mg given once daily in the evening. Daily dosages for maintenance range from 6 to 18 mg olanzapine plus 25 or 50 mg fluoxetine.

Ziprasidone

Ziprasidone [Geodon, Zeldox 🍁] is an SGA indicated for schizophrenia and acute bipolar mania. In patients with schizophrenia, ziprasidone can improve positive symptoms, negative symptoms, and cognitive function, while causing fewer EPS than FGAs. Like some other SGAs, ziprasidone can cause significant prolongation of the QT interval and can thereby cause potentially fatal dysrhythmias.

Mechanism of Action. Ziprasidone blocks multiple receptor types, including D_2, 5-HT_2, H_1, and alpha-adrenergic receptors. In addition, it blocks reuptake of two transmitters: serotonin and norepinephrine. As with other SGAs, therapeutic effects are believed to result from blockade of D_2 and 5-HT_2 receptors. Blockade of serotonin and norepinephrine uptake may provide antidepressant effects.

Adverse Effects. Ziprasidone is generally well tolerated. The most common side effects are somnolence (perhaps from H_1 blockade), orthostatic hypotension (perhaps from alpha-adrenergic blockade), and rash (the side effect most responsible for discontinuing the drug). EPS are seen in about 5% of patients. Like other SGAs, ziprasidone can promote weight gain, diabetes, and dyslipidemia. However, the risk is low. Like other antipsychotic drugs, ziprasidone may increase mortality in older adult patients with dementia-related psychosis.

Like olanzapine, ziprasidone can cause *leukopenia/neutropenia* and can thereby increase the risk of infection. For patients at high risk (e.g., those with pre-existing low WBC counts, those with a history of drug-induced leukopenia/neutropenia), complete blood counts should be conducted often during the first few months of treatment. If the ANC falls below 1000/mm^3, ziprasidone should be discontinued and the patient should be monitored for fever and other signs of infection. Neutrophil counts should be monitored until they return to normal.

Ziprasidone *prolongs the QT interval* and thereby poses a risk of torsades de pointes, a dysrhythmia that can progress to fatal ventricular fibrillation. QT prolongation is greater than with haloperidol but less than with thioridazine. Because of QT prolongation, ziprasidone should not be given to patients with risk factors for torsades de pointes, the most important being hypokalemia, hypomagnesemia, bradycardia, congenital QT prolongation, or a history of dysrhythmias, myocardial infarction, or severe heart failure.

Drug Interactions. Ziprasidone should not be combined with other drugs that prolong the QT interval. Among these are tricyclic antidepressants, thioridazine, several antidysrhythmic drugs (e.g., amiodarone, dofetilide, quinidine), and certain antibiotics (e.g., clarithromycin, erythromycin, moxifloxacin).

Drugs that induce CYP3A4 (e.g., rifampin, phenytoin) can accelerate the metabolism of ziprasidone, and may thereby decrease its levels. Conversely, drugs that inhibit CYP3A4 (e.g., ketoconazole) may increase ziprasidone levels.

Preparations. Ziprasidone [Geodon, Zeldox 🍁] is available in capsules (20, 40, 60, and 80 mg) for oral dosing and 20-mg single-use vials for IM injection.

Dosage and Administration

Schizophrenia, Oral. The initial dosage is 20 mg twice daily taken with food. The maximum is 80 mg twice daily.

Schizophrenia, Intramuscular. Two dosing schedules may be employed: (1) 10-mg doses given at least 2 hours apart up to a maximum of 40 mg/day or (2) 20-mg doses administered at least 4 hours apart up to a maximum of 40 mg/day. Intramuscular therapy for more than 3 days has not been studied. If long-term treatment is indicated, switch to oral ziprasidone.

Bipolar Disorder. Dosage for bipolar disorder is presented in Chapter 33.

Safe Handling and Administration. Ziprasidone, like risperidone and paliperidone, has the potential to cause reproductive harm in healthcare workers exposed during administration. NIOSH recommends the same procedures for administration as outlined previously. For further information, visit https://www.cdc.gov/niosh/topics/antineoplastic/pdf/hazardous-drugs-list_2016-161.pdf.

Quetiapine

Actions and Uses. Quetiapine [Seroquel] is an SGA indicated for schizophrenia, major depression, and acute episodes of mania and depression in patients with bipolar disorder. In patients with schizophrenia, the drug can improve positive symptoms, negative symptoms, and cognitive function. Like other SGAs, quetiapine produces strong blockade of 5-HT_2 receptors and weaker blockade of D_2 receptors. Blockade of both receptor types is believed responsible for beneficial effects. In addition to blocking receptors for serotonin and dopamine, quetiapine blocks H_1 receptors and alpha-adrenergic receptors, but does not block receptors for acetylcholine.

Adverse Effects. Quetiapine carries a moderate risk of serious metabolic effects (i.e., weight gain, diabetes, and dyslipidemia). As with other SGAs, the risk of EPS is low at therapeutic doses. Despite structural similarity to clozapine, quetiapine does not pose a risk of agranulocytosis. Common side effects include sedation (from H_1 blockade) and orthostatic hypotension (from alpha blockade). Like other antipsychotics, quetiapine increases the risk of death in older adult patients with dementia-related psychosis.

Cataracts are a concern. Cataracts developed in dogs fed 4 times the maximum human dose for 6 or 12 months. Lens changes have also developed in patients; quetiapine may have been the cause. Because quetiapine may pose a risk of cataracts, the manufacturer recommends examining the lenses for cataracts at baseline and every 6 months thereafter.

Like ziprasidone, quetiapine can *prolong the QT interval,* thereby posing a risk of torsades de pointes. Accordingly, quetiapine should not be given to patients with risk factors for torsades de pointes (e.g., hypokalemia; hypomagnesemia; bradycardia; congenital QT prolongation; a history of dysrhythmias, myocardial infarction, or severe heart failure) or to patients taking drugs that prolong the QT interval.

Drug Interactions. Metabolism of quetiapine is accelerated by drugs that induce CYP3A4 (e.g., phenytoin, rifampin). As a result, a larger dose of quetiapine may be needed to maintain antipsychotic effects. Conversely, drugs that inhibit CYP3A4 (e.g., ketoconazole, itraconazole, fluconazole, erythromycin) may increase levels of quetiapine and may thereby cause toxicity. Caution is advised.

As noted, quetiapine should not be combined with other drugs that prolong the QT interval. Agents to avoid include tricyclic antidepressants, thioridazine, certain antidysrhythmic drugs (e.g., amiodarone, dofetilide, quinidine), and certain antibiotics (e.g., clarithromycin, erythromycin, moxifloxacin).

Preparations. Quetiapine is available in immediate-release tablets (25, 50, 100, 200, 300, and 400 mg) marketed as *Seroquel* and in extended-release tablets (50, 150, 200, 300, and 400 mg) marketed as *Seroquel XR.*

Dosage and Administration

Schizophrenia. With the *immediate-release* tablets, the initial dosage is low—25 mg twice a day—to minimize orthostatic hypotension. Dosage is gradually increased over the next 3 days to a maintenance level of 400 to 800 mg/day, given in two or three divided doses. For patients who may be especially sensitive to quetiapine (e.g., older adults, those with hepatic impairment, those predisposed to hypotension), a slower titration rate and lower maintenance dosage may be advisable.

With the *extended-release* tablets, dosing begins at 300 mg once daily and is later increased to a maintenance level of 400 to 800 mg once daily. Patients currently using immediate-release quetiapine may be switched to extended-release quetiapine at the equivalent total daily dosage.

Major Depression. The recommended dosage is 150 to 300 mg once daily, using the extended-release formulation.

Bipolar Disorder. Dosage for bipolar disorder is presented in Chapter 33.

Aripiprazole

Contrasts With Other SGAs. Aripiprazole [Abilify, Abilify Maintena] is the first representative of a unique class of antipsychotic drugs, referred to by some as *dopamine system stabilizers* (DSSs). Approved indications are schizophrenia, acute bipolar mania, major depressive disorder, agitation associated with schizophrenia or bipolar mania, and irritability associated with autism spectrum disorder. Aripiprazole has a more favorable safety profile than any other SGA, but may be less effective than some. In patients with schizophrenia, aripiprazole is like other SGAs: it improves cognitive function, positive symptoms, and negative symptoms, while posing a low risk of EPS and TD. In contrast to other SGAs, aripiprazole is unlikely to cause significant metabolic effects, hypotension, or prolactin release, and poses no risk of anticholinergic effects or dysrhythmias. However, like all other antipsychotics, the drug may increase mortality in older adults with dementia-related psychosis.

Mechanism of Action. Like other antipsychotic drugs, aripiprazole can affect multiple receptor types. It blocks H_1, 5-HT_2, and $alpha_1$ receptors, and has mixed effects on 5-HT_1 and D_2 receptors. The drug does not block cholinergic receptors.

As with other SGAs, therapeutic effects are believed to result from interaction with dopamine and serotonin receptors. However, the nature of the interaction differs: Whereas other SGAs act as *pure antagonists* at dopamine and serotonin receptors, aripiprazole acts as a *partial agonist* at 5-HT_1 and D_2 receptors, and as a pure antagonist only at 5-HT_2 receptors. Because aripiprazole is a partial agonist at 5-HT_1 and D_2 receptors, net effects on receptor activity will depend on how much transmitter (dopamine or serotonin) is present. Specifically, at synapses where transmitter concentrations are *low,* aripiprazole will bind to receptors and thereby cause *moderate activation.* Conversely, at synapses where transmitter concentrations are *high,* aripiprazole will compete with the transmitter for receptor binding, and hence will *reduce receptor activation.* Because of this ability to modulate the activity of dopamine receptors—rather than simply cause receptor activation or blockade—aripiprazole has been dubbed a DSS. Researchers suggest that dopamine system stabilization explains why aripiprazole can improve positive and negative symptoms of schizophrenia while having little or no effect on the extrapyramidal system or prolactin release.

Adverse Effects. Aripiprazole is generally well tolerated. The most common side effects are headache, agitation, nervousness, anxiety, insomnia, nausea, vomiting, dizziness, and somnolence. The incidence of EPS is very low. Only a few cases of NMS have been reported. Among the SGAs, aripiprazole (along with ziprasidone) poses the lowest risk of weight gain, diabetes, and dyslipidemia. Although aripiprazole can block $alpha_1$-adrenergic receptors, the incidence of orthostatic hypotension is low (1.9% vs. 1% in patients on placebo). Aripiprazole does not prolong the QT interval, and hence does not pose a risk of dysrhythmias. Also, the drug has little or no effect on prolactin levels, and hence does not cause gynecomastia or galactorrhea. Like other antipsychotic drugs, aripiprazole may increase mortality in older adult patients with dementia-related psychosis.

Drug Interactions. Drugs that induce CYP3A4 (e.g., barbiturates, carbamazepine, phenytoin, rifampin) can accelerate metabolism of aripiprazole and can thereby reduce its blood level. Conversely, drugs that inhibit CYP3A4 (e.g., ketoconazole, itraconazole, fluconazole, erythromycin) can increase aripiprazole levels, as can drugs that inhibit CYP2D6 (e.g., quinidine, fluoxetine, paroxetine).

Preparations. Aripiprazole for *oral therapy* is available in standard tablets (2, 5, 10, 15, 20, and 30 mg) and solution (1 mg/mL), both sold as *Abilify,* and in orally disintegrating tablets (10 and 15 mg). Aripiprazole for IM therapy is available in single-use vials (7.5 mg/mL) sold as *Abilify* and extended-release injections sold as *Abilify Maintena.*

Dosage and Administration

Schizophrenia. The recommended oral dosage—both initial and maintenance—is 10 or 15 mg once a day, administered with or without food. Dosages above 15 mg/day do not increase therapeutic effects, but can intensify side effects. Dosage should be doubled for patients taking inducers of CYP3A4 and cut in half for patients taking inhibitors of CYP3A4 or CYP2D6. The extended-release depot preparation [Abilify Maintena] is available in 300-mg and 400-mg doses to be given once monthly.

Major Depressive Disorder. The recommended initial dosage is 2 to 5 mg PO a day. Dosage may be increased by up to 5 mg/day, but at intervals of no less than 1 week. Dosages above 15 mg/day have not been studied. As with oral therapy of schizophrenia, dosage should be doubled for patients taking inducers of CYP3A4 and cut in half for patients taking inhibitors of CYP3A4 or CYP2D6.

Bipolar Disorder. Dosage for bipolar disorder is presented in Chapter 33.

Irritability Associated With Autism Spectrum Disorder. The initial dosage is 2 mg/day, and the usual maintenance dosage is 5 to 15 mg/day.

Agitation Associated With Schizophrenia or Bipolar Mania. The recommended dosage is 9.75 mg IM once. As with oral therapy, dosage should be doubled for patients taking inducers of CYP3A4 and cut in half for patients taking inhibitors of CYP3A4 or CYP2D6.

Cariprazine

Cariprazine [Vraylar] is an antipsychotic medication whose exact mechanism is unknown. It is thought to act much like aripiprazole, through partial agonist activity at 5-HT_1 and D_2 receptors, and as a pure antagonist only at 5-HT_2 receptors. Approved indications are schizophrenia, acute bipolar mania, or treatment of mixed episodes associated with bipolar I disorder. Further information regarding cariprazine is located in Table 31.3 and Table 31.5.

Brexpiprazole

Brexpiprazole [Rexulti], an additional SGA, was approved in 2015 for the treatment of schizophrenia and as an adjunct drug to antidepressants for the treatment of major depressive disorder (MDD). Like aripiprazole and cariprazine, brexpiprazole is thought to work on both serotonin and dopamine receptors. Further information regarding brexpiprazole is located in Table 31.3 and Table 31.5.

Asenapine

Therapeutic Use. Asenapine [Saphris] is an SGA indicated for (1) acute and maintenance therapy of schizophrenia in adults and (2) acute monotherapy or acute adjunctive therapy (with lithium or valproate) of manic or mixed manic episodes associated with bipolar disorder. In clinical trials, benefits appeared modest. Asenapine is formulated as a sublingual tablet to allow absorption directly across the oral mucosa. The drug carries a low risk of weight gain, diabetes, or dyslipidemia and has few interactions with other agents. Because of its unique properties, asenapine is well suited for patients who (1) have difficulty swallowing or (2) cannot tolerate the metabolic side effects of some other SGAs.

Mechanism of Action. Asenapine can block D_2, 5-HT_2, H_1, and alpha-adrenergic receptors, but has little effect on muscarinic receptors. As with other SGAs, clinical benefits appear to result from blockade of D_2 and 5-HT_2 receptors. Blockade of H_1 and alpha-adrenergic receptors contributes to side effects.

Adverse Effects. Asenapine is generally well tolerated. The risk of anticholinergic effects, prolactin elevation, and metabolic effects (weight gain, diabetes, dyslipidemia) is low. Blockade of H_1 receptors can promote drowsiness, and blockade of alpha-adrenergic receptors can promote hypotension. In clinical trials, higher doses were associated with EPS. Asenapine can prolong the QT interval, and hence should be avoided by patients with risk factors for QT prolongation, including use of other drugs that can prolong the QT interval. Asenapine has local anesthetic properties, and hence can numb the mouth when the sublingual tablets dissolve. Like other antipsychotic drugs, asenapine may increase mortality in older adult patients with dementia-related psychosis. Rarely, patients have experienced severe allergic reactions, including angioedema and life-threatening anaphylaxis.

Drug Interactions. Asenapine is largely devoid of significant drug interactions. In theory, drugs such as fluvoxamine (Luvox), which strongly inhibit CYP1A2, can increase serum levels of asenapine.

Preparations, Dosage, and Administration. Asenapine [Saphris] is formulated in 2.5-, 5- and 10-mg sublingual tablets. Instruct patients to place the tablet under the tongue, where it will dissolve in a few seconds. This dosing method has two benefits. First, it greatly increases absorption (by avoiding first-pass metabolism). Second, patients can't "cheek" the drug to avoid being medicated because, if asenapine is cheeked, it will simply dissolve and be absorbed across the oral mucosa. Warn patients not to swallow the tablets, and instruct them to avoid eating and drinking for 10 minutes after dosing. Also, tell them not to be alarmed if their mouth gets numb when the tablet dissolves (asenapine can act like a local anesthetic). The usual dosage is 5 mg twice daily for patients with schizophrenia and 10 mg twice daily for patients with bipolar disorder. Increasing the dosage above 10 mg twice daily offers no clinical benefit, but *will* increase the risk of certain side effects. No dosage adjustment is needed in patients with renal impairment or in patients with mild or moderate hepatic impairment. However, in patients with severe hepatic impairment, asenapine should be avoided.

Iloperidone

Actions and Therapeutic Use. Iloperidone [Fanapt] is a chemical relative of risperidone. As with other SGAs, benefits derive from blocking D_2 and 5-HT_2 receptors. In clinical trials, efficacy equaled that of risperidone and haloperidol. Iloperidone is better tolerated than some other SGAs, but still carries a significant risk of weight gain, hypotension, and QT effects.

Adverse Effects. The most common adverse effects are dry mouth, somnolence, fatigue, nasal congestion, and orthostatic hypotension, which can be severe during initial therapy. The incidence of EPS is very low. Iloperidone carries a low risk of diabetes and dyslipidemia, but can cause significant weight gain. The drug prolongs the QT interval and hence poses a risk of serious dysrhythmias. Like other antipsychotic drugs, iloperidone may increase mortality in older adult patients with dementia-related psychosis.

Drug Interactions. Strong inhibitors of CYP2D6 (e.g., paroxetine) or CYP3A4 (e.g., ketoconazole) can increase levels of iloperidone and can thereby increase QT prolongation. Accordingly, in patients taking such inhibitors, dosage of iloperidone should be reduced. Iloperidone should not be combined with other drugs that prolong the QT interval (e.g., amiodarone, quinidine).

Preparations, Dosage, and Administration. Iloperidone [Fanapt] is supplied in tablets (1, 2, 4, 6, 8, 10, and 12 mg) for oral dosing. A 4-day titration pack (2 tablets each of 1, 2, 4, and 6 mg) is available to start treatment. The usual maintenance dosage is 6 to 12 mg twice daily. To minimize hypotension during initial therapy, dosage should be titrated as follows: on days 1, 2, 3, 4, 5, 6, and 7, give twice-daily doses of 1, 2, 4, 6, 8, 10, and 12 mg, respectively. Dosage should be reduced by 50% in patients taking strong inhibitors of CYP2D6 or CYP3A4. Patients with significant hepatic impairment should avoid this drug.

Lurasidone

Actions and Therapeutic Use. Lurasidone [Latuda] is indicated for schizophrenia and acute depressive bipolar disorder. In clinical trials, dosages of 20, 40, 80, and 120 mg/day were clearly superior to placebo. As with other SGAs, benefits derive from blocking D_2 and 5-HT_2 receptors.

Adverse Effects. In clinical trials, the most common adverse events were somnolence, akathisia, parkinsonism, nausea, agitation, and anxiety. Lurasidone does not cause anticholinergic effects or orthostatic hypotension, or prolong the QT interval, and the risk of metabolic effects (diabetes, weight gain, dyslipidemia) is low. Like other antipsychotic drugs, lurasidone may increase mortality in older adult patients with dementia-related psychosis.

Drug Interactions. Because lurasidone is metabolized by CYP3A4, its levels can be increased by CYP3A4 inhibitors and reduced by CYP3A4 inducers. Accordingly, use of the drug with strong inhibitors (e.g., ketoconazole) or strong inducers (e.g., rifampin) of CYP3A4 is *contraindicated.*

Preparations, Dosage, and Administration. Lurasidone [Latuda] is supplied in tablets (20, 40, 60, 80, and 120 mg) for dosing with food (at least 350 calories). The usual initial dosage is 40 mg once daily for schizophrenia and 20 mg daily for acute depressive bipolar disorder. The maximum dosage is 160 mg once daily. Increasing the daily dose to 120 mg does not increase benefits, but does increase the risk of dystonia and other side effects. Dosage should not exceed 40 mg once daily in patients with moderate to severe liver impairment or moderate to severe renal impairment, or in patients taking a moderate inhibitor of CYP3A4. Patients taking a strong inhibitor of CYP3A4 should not use the drug.

DEPOT ANTIPSYCHOTIC PREPARATIONS

Depot antipsychotics are long-acting, injectable formulations used for long-term maintenance therapy of schizophrenia. The objective is to prevent relapse and maintain the highest possible level of functioning. As a rule, the rate of relapse is lower with depot therapy than with oral therapy. Depot preparations are valuable for all patients who need long-term treatment—not just for patients who have difficulty with adherence. There is no evidence that depot preparations pose an increased risk of side effects, including NMS and TD. In fact, because depot therapy permits a reduction in the total drug burden (the dose per unit time is lower than with oral therapy), the risk of TD is actually reduced.

Seven depot preparations are currently available: *haloperidol decanoate* [Haldol Decanoate], *fluphenazine decanoate* (generic only), *risperidone microspheres* [Risperdal Consta], *paliperidone palmitate* [Invega Sustenna], *paliperidone palmitate* [Invega Trinza], *aripiprazole* [Abilify Maintena], and *olanzapine pamoate* [Zyprexa Relprevv]. Following the injection, active drug is slowly absorbed into the blood. Because of this slow, steady absorption, plasma levels remain relatively constant between doses. The dosing interval is 2 to 4 weeks. Typical maintenance dosages are shown in Table 31.6.

TABLE 31.6 ▪ Depot Antipsychotic Preparations

Drug	Route	Typical Maintenance Dosage
Haloperidol decanoate [Haldol Decanoate]	IM	50–200 mg every 4 weeks
Fluphenazine decanoate (generic only)	IM, subQ	12.5–50 mg every 2 weeks
Risperidone microspheres [Risperdal Consta]	IM	25–50 mg every 2 weeks
Paliperidone palmitate [Invega Sustenna]	IM	117 mg every 4 weeks
Paliperidone palmitate [Invega Trinza]	IM	273–819 mg every 12 weeks
Olanzapine pamoate [Zyprexa Relprevv]	IM	150–300 mg every 2 weeks *or* 405 mg every 4 weeks
Aripiprazole [Abilify Maintena]	IM	400 mg every 4 weeks

MANAGEMENT OF SCHIZOPHRENIA

Drug Therapy

Drug therapy of schizophrenia has three major objectives: (1) suppression of acute episodes, (2) prevention of acute exacerbations, and (3) maintenance of the highest possible level of functioning.

Drug Selection

Like all other drugs, antipsychotics should be selected on the basis of effectiveness, tolerability, and cost. Currently, SGAs are prescribed 10 times more often than FGAs, but that may change. When the SGAs were introduced, available data suggested they were more effective than FGAs and also safer. However, we now know otherwise. A comparative effectiveness review, published in 2012, compared FGAs with SGAs in the treatment of schizophrenia in adults. In 113 studies, clozapine was more effective than chlorpromazine in treating the core illness of schizophrenia. Yet when looking at functional outcomes, quality of life, and adverse events, there was no difference between the FGAs and SGAs. Regarding serious side effects, SGAs were initially thought to be safer than FGAs because SGAs pose a lower risk of EPS. However, over time, it became clear that SGAs posed a serious risk of their own: potentially fatal metabolic effects. Hence, rather than being *free* of serious side effects, the SGAs simply substituted a new serious effect for the old one. As for cost, FGAs are much cheaper. For example, haloperidol costs only $50 a year, risperidone costs about $600 a year, and olanzapine costs about $1120 a year. In summary, here's what we know:

- Most FGAs and SGAs are equally effective, except for clozapine, which is more effective than the rest.
- Whereas FGAs pose a greater risk of EPS, SGAs pose a significant risk of metabolic effects, which may be more detrimental than EPS.
- FGAs cost much less than SGAs.

Given this information, which drug should we choose? That's still hard to answer. With regard to efficacy and safety, no single agent is clearly superior to the others. So we're back to our initial selection criteria: efficacy, safety, and cost. For a patient who is treatment resistant, a trial with clozapine might be reasonable. For a patient with a history of diabetes or dyslipidemia, an FGA might be a good choice, as might aripiprazole or ziprasidone, two SGAs with a low risk of metabolic effects. If there's no clinical reason to select an SGA over an FGA, cost considerations would suggest choosing an FGA.

Dosing

Dosing with antipsychotics is highly individualized. Older adult patients require relatively small doses—typically 30% to 50% of those for younger patients. Poorly responsive patients may need larger doses. However, very large doses should generally be avoided because huge doses are probably no more effective than moderate doses and will increase the risk of side effects.

Dosage size and timing are likely to change over the course of therapy. During the initial phase, antipsychotics should be administered in divided daily doses. Once an effective dosage has been determined, the entire daily dose can often be given at bedtime. Because antipsychotics cause sedation, bedtime dosing helps promote sleep while decreasing daytime drowsiness. Doses used early in therapy to gain rapid control of behavior are often very high. For long-term therapy, the dosage should be reduced to the lowest effective amount.

Routes

Oral. Oral dosing is preferred for most patients. Antipsychotics are available in tablets, capsules, and liquids for oral use.

The liquid formulations require special handling. These preparations are concentrated and must be diluted before use. Dilution may be performed with a variety of fluids, including milk, fruit juices, and carbonated beverages. Some oral liquids are light sensitive and must be stored in amber or opaque containers. Liquid formulations of *phenothiazines* can cause contact dermatitis; nurses and patients should take care to avoid skin contact with these preparations.

Sublingual. One SGA—*asenapine* [Saphris]—is administered as a sublingual tablet designed to be absorbed through the oral mucosa (to avoid first-pass hepatic metabolism). This route has the additional advantage of preventing "cheeking," as doing so will simply cause the drug to be absorbed as intended.

Intramuscular. Intramuscular injection is generally reserved for patients with severe acute schizophrenia and for long-term maintenance. Depot preparations are given every 2 to 4 weeks (see Table 31.6).

Inhaled. Loxapine [Adasuve] is a formula used for acute treatment of agitation associated with schizophrenia. Adasuve is available as a 10-mg inhaled powder. Only one inhalation is recommended in a 24-hour period.

Initial Therapy

With adequate dosing, symptoms begin to resolve within 1 to 2 days. However, significant improvement takes 1 to 2 weeks, and a full response may not be seen for several months.

Some symptoms resolve sooner than others. During the first week, the goal is to reduce agitation, hostility, anxiety, and tension and to normalize patterns of sleeping and eating. Over the next 6 to 8 weeks, symptoms should continue to steadily improve. The goals over this interval are increased socialization and improved self-care, mood, and formal thought processes. Of the patients who have not responded within 6 weeks, 50% are likely to respond by the end of 12 weeks.

Maintenance Therapy

Schizophrenia is a chronic disorder that usually requires prolonged treatment. The purpose of long-term therapy is to reduce the recurrence of acute florid episodes and to maintain the highest possible level of functioning. Unfortunately, although long-term treatment can be very effective, it also carries a risk of adverse effects, especially TD.

Following control of an acute episode, antipsychotic therapy should continue for at least 12 months. Withdrawal of medication before this time is associated with a 55% incidence of relapse, compared with only 20% in patients who continue drug use. Accordingly, patients must be convinced to continue therapy for the entire 12-month course, even though they may be symptom free and consider themselves "cured."

After 12 months, an attempt may be made to discontinue drug use, provided symptoms have been absent for this period of time. Drug continuation past 12 months may be needed to maintain patient stability. About 25% of patients do not need drugs beyond this time. To avoid a withdrawal reaction, dosage should be tapered gradually. It is important that medication not be withdrawn at a time of stress (e.g., when the patient is being discharged following hospitalization). If relapse occurs following withdrawal, treatment should be reinstituted. For many patients, resumption of therapy controls symptoms and prevents further deterioration.

When long-term therapy is conducted, dosage should be adjusted with care. To reduce the risk of TD and other adverse effects, a minimum effective dosage should be established. Annual attempts should be made to lower the dosage or to discontinue treatment entirely.

Long-acting (depot) antipsychotics are especially well suited for prolonged treatment. Depot therapy has three major advantages over oral therapy: (1) the relapse rate may be lower, (2) drug levels are more stable between doses, and (3) the total dose per unit time is lower, thereby reducing the risk of adverse effects, including TD. In the United States, only a small number of patients receive depot therapy. The low rate is based in large part on the widely held (but unfounded) perception that depot therapy is for patients who suffer recurrent relapse because of persistent nonadherence with oral therapy.

Adjunctive Drugs

Benzodiazepines (e.g., lorazepam, alprazolam) can suppress anxiety and promote sleep. Whether they also improve core symptoms of schizophrenia is uncertain. In patients experiencing an acute psychotic episode, benzodiazepines can help suppress anxiety, irritability, and agitation. In addition, benzodiazepines may allow the dosage of antipsychotic medication to be reduced.

Antidepressants are appropriate when schizophrenia is associated with depressive symptoms. Only one study has examined continued adjunctive use of an antidepressant with an antipsychotic medication. This tricyclic antidepressant, imipramine, was shown to be helpful in the treatment of depression. Although imipramine was successful in preventing relapse, many providers are choosing newer forms of antidepressants (serotonin/norepinephrine reuptake inhibitors, selective serotonin reuptake inhibitors), as they are thought to have fewer anticholinergic side effects. Antidepressant dosage is the same as for major depression. The ideal duration is unknown.

Promoting Adherence

Poor adherence is a common cause of therapeutic failure and underlies a significant proportion of hospital readmissions. Adherence can be difficult to achieve because treatment is prolonged and because patients may fail to appreciate the need for therapy, or they may be unwilling or unable to take medicine as prescribed. In addition, side effects can discourage adherence. Adherence can be enhanced by

- Ensuring that the medication given to hospitalized patients is actually swallowed and not "cheeked."
- Encouraging family members to oversee medication for outpatients.
- Providing patients with written and verbal instructions on dosage size and timing, and encouraging them to take their medicine exactly as prescribed.
- Informing patients and their families that antipsychotics must be taken on a regular schedule to be effective, and hence should not be used PRN.
- Informing patients about side effects of treatment and teaching them how to minimize undesired responses.
- Assuring patients that antipsychotic drugs do not cause addiction.
- Establishing a good therapeutic relationship with the patient and family.
- Using an IM depot preparation (e.g., fluphenazine decanoate, haloperidol decanoate) for long-term therapy.

Nondrug Therapy

Although drugs can be of great benefit in schizophrenia, medication alone does not constitute optimal treatment. The acutely ill patient needs care, support, and protection; a period of hospitalization may be essential. Counseling can offer the patient and family insight into the nature of schizophrenia and can facilitate adjustment and rehabilitation. Although conventional psychotherapy is of little value in reducing symptoms of schizophrenia, establishing a good therapeutic relationship can help promote adherence and can help the prescriber evaluate the patient, which in turn can facilitate dosage adjustment and drug selection. Behavioral therapy can help reduce stress. Vocational training in a sheltered environment offers the hope of productivity and some measure of independence. Ideally, the patient will be provided with a comprehensive therapeutic program to complement the benefits of medication. Unfortunately, ideal situations don't always exist, leaving many patients to rely on drugs as their sole treatment modality.

KEY POINTS

- Schizophrenia is the principal indication for antipsychotic drugs, although many are also used for bipolar disorder.
- Schizophrenia is a chronic illness characterized by disordered thinking and reduced comprehension of reality. Positive symptoms include hallucinations, delusions, and agitation. Negative symptoms include blunted affect, poverty of speech, and social withdrawal. Cognitive dysfunction manifests as disordered thinking, reduced ability to focus attention, plus learning and memory difficulties.
- Antipsychotic drugs fall into two major groups: first-generation antipsychotics (FGAs) and second-generation antipsychotics (SGAs).
- The drugs in both groups are equally effective at treating schizophrenia.
- Despite initial impressions, the SGAs are no safer than FGAs—they simply produce different adverse reactions. Whereas FGAs carry a high risk of extrapyramidal symptoms (EPS), the SGAs carry a high risk of metabolic effects.
- Drugs in both generations increase the risk of mortality in older adult patients with dementia-related psychosis.
- Therapeutic responses to antipsychotic drugs develop slowly, often taking several months to exert maximal effects.
- First-generation antipsychotics are thought to relieve symptoms of schizophrenia by causing strong blockade of D_2 receptors.
- Second-generation antipsychotics are thought to relieve symptoms of schizophrenia by causing moderate blockade of D_2 receptors and strong blockade of 5-HT_2 receptors.
- The major concern with FGAs is production of EPS, which can occur early in treatment (acute dystonia, parkinsonism, and akathisia) or late in treatment (tardive dyskinesia).
- Acute dystonia and parkinsonism respond to anticholinergic drugs (e.g., benztropine). Akathisia is harder to treat but may respond to anticholinergic drugs, benzodiazepines, or beta blockers.
- Tardive dyskinesia (TD) has no reliable treatment. For patients with severe TD, switching to an SGA may help.
- The risk of early EPS is much greater with high-potency FGAs than with low-potency FGAs, whereas the risk of TD is equal with both groups.
- The risk of sedation, orthostatic hypotension, and anticholinergic effects is greater with the low-potency FGAs than with the high-potency FGAs.

- FGAs can cause neuroleptic malignant syndrome, characterized by muscular rigidity, high fever, and autonomic instability. Deaths have occurred. Dantrolene and bromocriptine are used for treatment.
- Antipsychotic drugs can increase levels of circulating prolactin by blocking the inhibitory action of dopamine on prolactin release.
- Levodopa can counteract the beneficial effects of FGA drugs, and vice versa, because levodopa activates dopamine receptors, whereas FGAs block dopamine receptors.
- Haloperidol [Haldol] is the prototype of the high-potency FGAs.
- Second-generation antipsychotics differ from FGAs in three important ways: (1) they block receptors for serotonin in addition to receptors for dopamine; (2) they carry a lower risk of EPS, including TD; and (3) they carry a higher risk of serious metabolic effects—weight gain, diabetes, and dyslipidemia—that can lead to adverse cardiovascular events and premature death.
- Among the SGAs, the risk of metabolic effects is greatest with clozapine and olanzapine.
- Clozapine, the first SGA, is the most effective antipsychotic drug available.
- Clozapine can cause potentially fatal agranulocytosis. Hence, regular blood tests are mandatory and the drug should be reserved for patients who have not responded to other antipsychotics.
- Antipsychotic depot preparations (e.g., haloperidol decanoate, fluphenazine decanoate) are used for long-term maintenance therapy of schizophrenia.

Please visit **http://evolve.elsevier.com/Lehne** for chapter-specific NCLEX® examination review questions.

Summary of Major Nursing Implications[a]

FIRST-GENERATION (CONVENTIONAL) ANTIPSYCHOTICS

Chlorpromazine
Fluphenazine
Haloperidol
Loxapine
Molindone
Perphenazine
Pimozide
Thioridazine
Thiothixene
Trifluoperazine

Except where indicated, the nursing implications that follow apply to all FGAs.

Preadministration Assessment

Therapeutic Goal

Treatment of schizophrenia has three goals: suppression of acute episodes, prevention of acute exacerbations, and maintenance of the highest possible level of functioning.

Baseline Data

Patients should receive a thorough mental status examination and a physical examination.

Observe and record such factors as overt behavior (e.g., gait, pacing, restlessness, volatile outbursts), emotional state (e.g., depression, agitation, mania), intellectual function (e.g., stream of thought, coherence, hallucinations, delusions), and responsiveness to the environment.

Obtain a complete family and social history.

Determine vital signs and obtain complete blood counts, electrolytes, and evaluations of hepatic, renal, and cardiovascular function.

Identifying High-Risk Patients

First-generation antipsychotics are *contraindicated* for patients who are comatose or severely depressed and for patients with Parkinson disease, prolactin-dependent carcinoma of the breast, bone marrow depression, and severe hypotension or hypertension. Use with *caution* in patients with glaucoma, adynamic ileus, prostatic hypertrophy, cardiovascular disease, hepatic or renal dysfunction, and seizure disorders.

Avoid *chlorpromazine, thioridazine, haloperidol,* and *pimozide* in patients with risk factors for torsades de pointes (e.g., hypokalemia, hypomagnesemia, bradycardia, congenital QT prolongation, or a history of dysrhythmias, myocardial infarction, or severe heart failure) and for those taking drugs that prolong the QT interval.

Generally *avoid all FGAs* in older adults with dementia-related psychosis.

Implementation: Administration

Routes

Oral, inhalation, IM, IV, and subQ. Routes for individual agents are shown in Tables 31.3 and 31.6.

Administration

Dosing. Divided daily doses are employed initially. Once an effective dosage has been determined, the entire daily dose is usually administered at bedtime, thereby promoting sleep and minimizing daytime sedation. For long-term therapy, the smallest effective dosage should be employed.

Oral Liquids. Oral liquid formulations must be protected from light. Concentrated formulations should be diluted just before use. Dilution in fruit juice improves palatability.

Oral liquids can cause contact dermatitis. **Warn patients against making skin contact with these drugs, and instruct them to flush the affected area with water if a spill occurs.**

Continued

Summary of Major Nursing Implications[a]—cont'd

Take care to avoid skin contact with these preparations yourself.

Intramuscular. Make injections into the deltoid or gluteal muscle. Rotate the injection site. Depot preparations are administered every 2 to 4 weeks.

Implementation: Measures to Enhance Therapeutic Effects

Promoting Adherence

Poor adherence is a common cause of therapeutic failure and rehospitalization. To improve adherence:

- Ensure that medication is actually swallowed and not "cheeked."
- **Encourage family members to oversee medication for outpatients.**
- **Provide patients with written and verbal instructions on dosage size and timing, and encourage them to take their medicine as prescribed.**
- **Inform patients and their families that antipsychotic drugs must be taken on a regular schedule.**
- **Inform patients about side effects and teach them how to minimize undesired responses.**
- **Assure patients that antipsychotic drugs do not cause addiction.**
- Establish a good therapeutic relationship with the patient and family.
- Use a depot preparation (e.g., paliperidone palmitate) for long-term therapy.

Nondrug Therapy

Acutely ill patients need care, support, and protection; hospitalization may be essential. **Educate the patient and family about the nature of schizophrenia to facilitate adjustment and rehabilitation.** Behavioral therapy can help reduce stress. Vocational training in a sheltered environment offers the hope of productivity and some measure of independence.

Ongoing Evaluation and Interventions

Evaluating Therapeutic Effects

Success is indicated by improvement in psychotic symptoms. Evaluate for suppression of hallucinations, delusions, agitation, tension, and hostility, and for improvement in judgment, insight, motivation, affect, self-care, social skills, anxiety management, and patterns of sleeping and eating.

Minimizing Adverse Effects

Early EPS: Acute Dystonia, Parkinsonism, and Akathisia. These reactions develop within hours to months after starting treatment. The risk is greatest with high-potency FGAs. Take care to differentiate these reactions from worsening of psychotic symptoms. **Inform patients and their families about symptoms (e.g., muscle spasm of tongue, face, neck, or back; tremor; rigidity; restless movement), and instruct them to notify the prescriber if these appear.** Acute dystonia and parkinsonism respond to anticholinergic drugs (e.g., benztropine). Akathisia may respond to anticholinergic drugs, beta blockers, or benzodiazepines. For severe parkinsonism, switch to an SGA.

Late EPS: Tardive Dyskinesia. TD develops after months or years of continuous therapy. The risk is equal with all FGAs. **Inform patients and their families about early signs (e.g., fine, worm-like movements of the tongue), and instruct them to notify the prescriber if these develop.** Although there is no reliable treatment, the following measures are recommended: discontinue all anticholinergic drugs; give a benzodiazepine; and discontinue the antipsychotic, or at least reduce the dosage. For severe TD, switch to an SGA.

Neuroleptic Malignant Syndrome. NMS is a rare reaction that carries a 5% to 20% risk of death. Symptoms include rigidity, fever, sweating, dysrhythmias, and fluctuations in blood pressure. NMS is most likely with high-potency FGAs.

Treatment consists of supportive measures (use of cooling blankets, rehydration), drug therapy (dantrolene, bromocriptine), and immediate withdrawal of the neuroleptic. If neuroleptic therapy is resumed after symptoms subside, the lowest effective dosage of a low-potency drug should be employed. If a second episode occurs, switching to an SGA may help.

Anticholinergic Effects. **Inform patients about possible anticholinergic effects (dry mouth, blurred vision, photophobia, urinary hesitancy, constipation, tachycardia, suppression of sweating), and teach them how to minimize discomfort.** A summary of nursing implications for anticholinergic effects is given in Chapter 14. Anticholinergic effects are most likely with low-potency FGAs.

Orthostatic Hypotension. **Inform patients about signs of hypotension (light-headedness, dizziness) and advise them to sit or lie down if these occur. Inform patients that hypotension can be minimized by moving slowly when standing up.** Orthostatic hypotension is most likely with low-potency FGAs.

In hospitalized patients, measure blood pressure and pulses before dosing and 1 hour after. Make these measurements while the patient is lying down and again after he or she has been sitting or standing for 1 to 2 minutes. If blood pressure is low, withhold medication and consult the prescriber.

Sedation. Sedation is most intense during the first weeks of therapy and declines with continued drug use. **Warn patients about sedative effects, and advise them to avoid hazardous activity until sedation subsides.** Sedation is most likely with low-potency FGAs.

Seizures. Neuroleptics reduce seizure threshold, thereby increasing the risk of seizures, especially in patients with epilepsy and other seizure disorders. For patients with seizure disorders, adequate doses of antiseizure medication must be employed. Monitor the patient for seizure activity; if loss of seizure control occurs, dosage of antiseizure medication must be increased.

Sexual Dysfunction. In women, FGAs can suppress libido and impair the ability to achieve orgasm. In men, FGAs can suppress libido and cause erectile and ejaculatory dysfunction. **Counsel patients about possible sexual dysfunction and encourage them to report problems.** Dosage reduction or switching to a high-potency FGA may help.

Summary of Major Nursing Implications[a]—cont'd

Dermatologic Effects. **Inform patients that phenothiazines can sensitize the skin to ultraviolet light, thereby increasing the risk of sunburn. Advise them to avoid excessive exposure to sunlight, apply a sunscreen, and wear protective clothing.**

Oral liquid formulations can cause contact dermatitis. **Warn patients to avoid skin contact with these drugs.**

Neuroendocrine Effects. **Inform patients that FGAs can cause galactorrhea, gynecomastia, and menstrual irregularities.**

Antipsychotics can promote growth of prolactin-dependent carcinoma of the breast and must not be used by patients with this cancer.

Agranulocytosis. Agranulocytosis greatly diminishes the ability to fight infection. **Inform patients about early signs of infection (fever, sore throat), and instruct them to notify the prescriber if these develop.** If blood tests indicate agranulocytosis, the antipsychotic should be withdrawn.

Severe Dysrhythmias. *Chlorpromazine, haloperidol, thioridazine,* and *pimozide* prolong the QT interval and can thereby induce torsades de pointes, a dysrhythmia that can progress to fatal ventricular fibrillation. To reduce risk, (1) ensure that potassium and magnesium levels are normal, (2) avoid other drugs that cause QT prolongation, and (3) avoid drugs that can increase levels of the antipsychotic drug being used.

Signs of Withdrawal and EPS in Neonates. Neonates exposed to antipsychotic drugs during the third trimester may experience EPS and/or signs of withdrawal. Symptoms include tremor, agitation, sleepiness, difficulty feeding, severe breathing difficulty, and altered muscle tone (increased or decreased). Neonates who develop EPS or signs of withdrawal should be monitored. Hospitalization may be required. **Advise patients who become pregnant not to discontinue their medication without consulting the prescriber.**

Death in Older Adult Dementia Patients. All FGAs increase the risk of mortality when used to treat dementia-related psychosis in older adult patients, an application use for which these drugs are not approved. Avoid FGAs in these patients.

Minimizing Adverse Interactions

Anticholinergics. Drugs with anticholinergic properties will intensify anticholinergic responses to FGAs. **Instruct patients to avoid all drugs with anticholinergic properties, including the antihistamines and certain over-the-counter sleep aids.**

CNS Depressants. First-generation agents will intensify CNS depression caused by other drugs. **Warn patients against use of alcohol and all other drugs with CNS-depressant properties (e.g., barbiturates, opioids, antihistamines, benzodiazepines).**

Levodopa and Direct Dopamine Receptor Agonists. Levodopa and the dopamine receptor agonists (e.g., bromocriptine) promote activation of dopamine receptors and may thereby diminish the therapeutic effects of FGAs. Accordingly, patients taking FGAs should not use these drugs.

QT-Prolonging Drugs. Drugs that prolong the QT interval increase the risk of dysrhythmias in patients taking *thioridazine, haloperidol,* and *pimozide,* and hence must be avoided. Agents to avoid include tricyclic antidepressants, thioridazine, several antidysrhythmic drugs (e.g., amiodarone, dofetilide, quinidine), and certain antibiotics (e.g., clarithromycin, erythromycin, moxifloxacin).

SECOND-GENERATION (ATYPICAL) ANTIPSYCHOTICS

Aripiprazole
Asenapine
Brexpiprazole
Cariprazine
Clozapine
Iloperidone
Lurasidone
Olanzapine
Paliperidone
Quetiapine
Risperidone
Ziprasidone

Except where indicated, the nursing implications that follow apply to all SGAs.

Preadministration Assessment

Therapeutic Goal

See *First-Generation (Conventional) Antipsychotics.*

Baseline Data

See *First-Generation (Conventional) Antipsychotics.* Also, obtain baseline measurements of weight, waist circumference, fasting blood glucose, and fasting lipid levels. For patients taking *quetiapine,* examine the lenses for cataracts. For patients taking *clozapine,* obtain baseline values for total WBC count and ANC.

Identifying High-Risk Patients

Use all SGAs, especially *clozapine* and *olanzapine,* with *caution* in patients with diabetes.

Clozapine is *contraindicated* for patients with a history of bone marrow depression or clozapine-induced agranulocytosis, and for those taking myelosuppressive drugs (e.g., many anticancer drugs).

Use *clozapine* with *caution* in patients with seizure disorders.

Ziprasidone is *contraindicated* for patients with risk factors for torsades de pointes (e.g., hypokalemia, hypomagnesemia, bradycardia, congenital QT prolongation, or a history of dysrhythmias, myocardial infarction, or severe heart failure) and for those taking drugs that prolong the QT interval. Use *aripiprazole, asenapine, clozapine, iloperidone, quetiapine, risperidone,* and *paliperidone* with caution in these patients.

Generally *avoid all SGAs* in older adults with dementia-related psychosis.

Continued

Summary of Major Nursing Implications[a]—cont'd

Implementation: Administration

Routes

Oral, IM, and sublingual. Routes for individual agents are shown in Tables 31.3 and 31.5. Risperidone, paliperidone, and ziprasidone have the potential to cause reproductive harm to healthcare workers exposed during administration. NIOSH suggests donning a protective gown and two sets of gloves when crushing or splitting tablets or during handling or administration of oral or injectable liquids.

Dosing

To minimize side effects, dosage should be low initially and increased gradually.

Implementation: Measures to Enhance Therapeutic Effects

Promoting Adherence

See *First-Generation (Conventional) Antipsychotics.*

Ongoing Evaluation and Interventions

Evaluating Therapeutic Effects

See *First-Generation (Conventional) Antipsychotics.*

Minimizing Adverse Effects

Compared with the FGAs, the SGAs carry a low risk of sexual dysfunction, neuroendocrine effects, and extrapyramidal reactions, including TD—but they carry a high risk of metabolic effects.

Orthostatic Hypotension and Anticholinergic Effects. See *First-Generation (Conventional) Antipsychotics.*

Agranulocytosis. *Clozapine* produces agranulocytosis in 1% to 2% of patients, typically during the first 6 months of treatment. Deaths from gram-negative septicemia have occurred.

Regular hematologic monitoring is mandatory: WBC count and ANC must be determined weekly for the first 6 months, biweekly from months 6 to 12, then monthly thereafter. Additional testing may be completed when considering the possibility of neutropenia, when adding other antipsychotics, or when clinically indicated. If the total WBC count falls below 3000/mm^3 or if the ANC falls below 1500/mm^3, treatment should be interrupted. When subsequent *daily* monitoring indicates that cell counts have risen above these values, clozapine can be resumed. If the total WBC count falls below 2000/mm^3 or if the ANC falls below 1000/mm^3, clozapine should be permanently discontinued. Continue monitoring blood counts for 4 weeks.

Warn patients about the risk of agranulocytosis, and inform them that clozapine will not be dispensed without repeated proof of blood counts. Inform patients about early signs of infection (fever, sore throat, fatigue, mucous membrane ulceration), and instruct them to report these immediately.

Leukopenia/Neutropenia. *Olanzapine* and *ziprasidone* can cause *leukopenia/neutropenia* and can thereby increase the risk of infection. For patients at high risk (e.g., those with a pre-existing low WBC count, those with a history of drug-induced leukopenia/neutropenia), conduct complete blood counts frequently during the first few months of treatment. If the ANC falls below 1000/mm^3, these drugs should be discontinued and the patient monitored for fever and other signs of infection. Neutrophil counts should be monitored until they return to normal.

Metabolic Effects: Weight Gain, Diabetes, and Dyslipidemia. All SGAs—especially *clozapine* and *olanzapine*—can promote weight gain, which can lead to diabetes and dyslipidemia. To monitor weight gain, determine weight at baseline and every 3 months thereafter. Also, determine waist circumference at baseline and annually thereafter. **Inform patients about the risk of weight gain and encourage them to control caloric intake and get regular exercise.** If significant weight gain occurs, it can be managed with a combination of diet, exercise, and metformin.

To monitor for diabetes, measure fasting blood glucose at baseline, 12 weeks later, and annually thereafter. In patients with documented diabetes at baseline, monitor for worsening of glucose control. **Inform all patients about symptoms of diabetes—hyperglycemia, polyuria, polydipsia, polyphagia, dehydration—and instruct them to tell the prescriber if they occur.** If diabetes develops, it can be managed with insulin or an oral antidiabetic drug (e.g., metformin).

To monitor for *dyslipidemia,* obtain a fasting lipid profile at baseline, 12 weeks, and at least every 5 years thereafter.

Seizures. *Clozapine* causes generalized tonic-clonic seizures in 3% of patients. **Warn patients against driving and other hazardous activities if seizures have occurred.**

Sedation. All SGAs—especially *clozapine* and *olanzapine*—can cause sedation. **Warn patients against driving and participating in other hazardous activities if impairment is significant.**

Extrapyramidal Symptoms. Like the FGAs, the SGAs can cause acute dystonia, parkinsonism, akathisia, and tardive dyskinesia—although the risk is lower than with the FGAs. For nursing implications, see *First-Generation (Conventional) Antipsychotics.*

Myocarditis. Very rarely, *clozapine* causes myocarditis. **Inform patients about signs and symptoms (e.g., unexplained fatigue, dyspnea, tachypnea, chest pain, palpitations), and advise them to seek immediate medical attention if these develop.** Withhold clozapine until myocarditis has been ruled out. If myocarditis is diagnosed, the drug should never be used again.

Dysrhythmias. Eight SGAs—*aripiprazole, asenapine, clozapine, iloperidone, paliperidone, quetiapine, risperidone,* and *ziprasidone*—may prolong the QT interval, posing a risk of torsades de pointes, a potentially fatal dysrhythmia. To reduce the risk of dysrhythmias (1) ensure that potassium and magnesium levels are normal, (2) avoid other drugs that cause QT prolongation, and (3) avoid drugs that can increase levels of ziprasidone.

Signs of Withdrawal and EPS in Neonates. Neonates exposed to antipsychotic drugs during the third trimester may experience EPS and/or signs of withdrawal. Symptoms include tremor, agitation, sleepiness, difficulty feeding, severe breathing difficulty, and altered muscle tone (increased or decreased). Neonates who present with EPS or signs of withdrawal should

Summary of Major Nursing Implications[a]—cont'd

be monitored. Hospitalization may be required. **Advise women who become pregnant not to discontinue their medication without consulting the prescriber.**

Death in Older Adult Dementia Patients. All SGAs increase the risk of mortality when used to treat dementia-related psychosis in older adults, an application for which these drugs are not approved. Avoid SGAs in these patients.

Cataracts. *Quetiapine* may pose a risk of cataracts. Examine the lenses for cataracts at baseline and every 6 months thereafter.

Minimizing Adverse Interactions

CNS Depressants. Second-generation antipsychotics may intensify CNS depression caused by other drugs. **Warn patients against the use of alcohol and all other drugs with CNS-depressant properties (e.g., barbiturates, opioids, antihistamines, benzodiazepines).**

Levodopa and Direct Dopamine Receptor Agonists. Levodopa and the dopamine receptor agonists (e.g., bromocriptine) promote activation of dopamine receptors and may thereby diminish therapeutic effects of the SGAs. Patients taking antipsychotics should not use these drugs.

Myelosuppressive Drugs. *Clozapine* must not be given to patients taking other drugs that can suppress bone marrow function (e.g., many anticancer agents).

QT-Prolonging Drugs. Drugs that prolong the QT interval increase the risk of dysrhythmias in patients taking *aripiprazole, asenapine, clozapine, iloperidone, paliperidone, quetiapine, risperidone*, and *ziprasidone,* and hence must be avoided. Agents to avoid include tricyclic antidepressants, thioridazine, several antidysrhythmic drugs (e.g., amiodarone, dofetilide, quinidine), and certain antibiotics (e.g., clarithromycin, erythromycin, moxifloxacin).

Inducers and Inhibitors of CYP3A4. Drugs that induce CYP3A4 (e.g., barbiturates, carbamazepine, phenytoin, rifampin) can reduce levels of *aripiprazole, iloperidone, lurasidone, quetiapine,* and *ziprasidone,* and may thereby cause therapeutic failure. Conversely, drugs that inhibit CYP3A4 (e.g., ketoconazole, itraconazole, fluconazole, erythromycin) can increase levels of these five drugs and may thereby increase toxicity. Use *caution* if these combinations are employed. Use of *lurasidone* with strong CYP3A4 inhibitors or inducers is *contraindicated.*

[a]Patient education information is highlighted as **blue text**.

CHAPTER

32 Antidepressants

Our principal focus in this chapter is drugs used to treat major depression. In addition, we consider four somatic (nondrug) therapies. We begin by discussing depression itself and the basic approach to treatment. After that, we discuss the antidepressant drugs and the somatic therapies.

MAJOR DEPRESSION: CLINICAL FEATURES, PATHOGENESIS, AND TREATMENT OVERVIEW

Depression is the most common psychiatric disorder. In the United States, about 15 million adults are affected per year. The incidence in women is twice that in men. The risk of suicide among depressed people is high. Unfortunately, depression is underdiagnosed and undertreated: Only 35% of depressed individuals had seen a mental health provider. This is especially sad in that treatment can help many people: About 30% of those given antidepressants achieve full remission; an additional 20% to 30% achieve at least a 50% reduction in symptom severity.

CLINICAL FEATURES

The principal symptoms of major depression are *depressed mood* and *loss of pleasure or interest in all or nearly all of one's usual activities and pastimes.* Associated symptoms include insomnia (or sometimes hypersomnia); anorexia and weight loss (or sometimes hyperphagia and weight gain); mental slowing and loss of concentration; feelings of guilt, worthlessness, and helplessness; thoughts of death and suicide; and overt suicidal behavior. For a diagnosis to be made, symptoms must be present most of the day nearly every day for at least 2 weeks.

It is important to distinguish between major depression and normal grief or sadness. Whereas major depression is an illness, grief or sadness is not. Rather, grief and sadness are appropriate reactions to a major life stressor (e.g., death of a loved one, loss of a job). In most cases, grief and sadness resolve spontaneously over several weeks and do not require medical intervention. However, if symptoms are unusually intense and if they fail to resolve within an appropriate time, a major depressive episode may have been superimposed. If this occurs, treatment is indicated.

PATHOGENESIS

The etiology of major depression is complex and incompletely understood. For some individuals, depression seems to descend "out of the blue"; otherwise healthy people—unexpectedly and without apparent cause—find themselves feeling profoundly depressed. For many others, depressive episodes are brought on by stressful life events, such as bereavement, loss of a job, or childbirth (Box 32.1). Since depression does not occur in everyone, it would appear that some people are more vulnerable than others. Factors that may contribute to vulnerability include genetic heritage, a difficult childhood, and chronic low self-esteem.

Clinical observations made in the 1960s led to formulation of the *monoamine-deficiency hypothesis of depression,* which asserts that depression is caused by a functional deficiency of monoamine neurotransmitters (norepinephrine, serotonin, or both). Findings that support the hypothesis include (1) induction of depression with reserpine, a drug that depletes monoamines from the brain; (2) induction of depression with inhibitors of tyrosine hydroxylase, an enzyme needed for monoamine transmitter synthesis; and (3) relief of depression with drugs that intensify monoamine-mediated neurotransmission. Although these observations lend support to the monoamine-deficiency hypothesis, it is clear that the hypothesis is too simplistic. However, despite its shortcomings, the monoamine-deficiency hypothesis does provide a useful conceptual framework for understanding antidepressant drugs.

TREATMENT OVERVIEW

Depression can be treated with three major modalities: (1) pharmacotherapy, (2) depression-specific psychotherapy (e.g., cognitive behavioral therapy or interpersonal psychotherapy), and (3) somatic therapies, such as electroconvulsive therapy and transcranial magnetic stimulation. For patients with mild to moderate depression, drug therapy and psychotherapy can be equally effective. For those with more severe depression,

si BOX 32.1 ▪ SPECIAL INTEREST TOPIC

PERIPARTUM DEPRESSION

The vast majority of women (about 80%) experience depressive symptoms after giving birth. For most, the symptoms are mild and transient, reflecting a condition sometimes called the "baby blues." For others, symptoms are severe and persistent, reflecting true postpartum depression, a condition that merits rapid medical attention.

An estimated 60% to 70% of women experience depression postpartum, and in 50% of these depression begins *before* delivery—hence the term *peripartum depression.* Symptoms include tearfulness, sadness, nervousness, irritability, and anxiety, along with difficulty eating and sleeping. The new mother may feel overwhelmed, vulnerable, weak, and alone. She may cry for no clear reason. Her self-esteem and self-confidence may decline, and she may feel unqualified to care for her baby. Fortunately, all of these symptoms pass quickly: They develop a few days after delivery and are gone by day 10. Because these symptoms are so common, they're considered a normal postpartum event. Treatment is neither necessary nor recommended.

True peripartum depression is different. The condition is much less common than the "baby blues" but much more serious. Left untreated, peripartum depression lasts for months and is likely to become worse as time passes. The condition is detrimental to the mother, and it can adversely affect the child, preventing secure attachment and impairing cognitive, emotional, and behavioral development. Immediate intervention is indicated.

What is true peripartum depression? It's an episode of major depression that starts in the weeks before or just after giving birth. Otherwise, the diagnostic criteria are the same as for all other episodes of major depression. According to the *Diagnostic and Statistical Manual of Mental Disorders, Fifth Edition* (DSM-5), for a depressive episode to qualify as having peripartum onset, symptoms must begin within *4 weeks* of delivery. However, most clinicians who study the disorder use a different criterion: To them, depression is considered postpartum if it begins within *3 months* of delivery—not just within 4 weeks.

Who is likely to suffer peripartum depression? Sometimes the condition occurs in first-time mothers, and sometimes it doesn't strike until a second, third, or fourth child is born. Among first-time mothers, the incidence is between 8% and 15% (about 1 in 8). For women with a history of the disorder, the risk increases to 33% (1 in 3). In addition to a prior history of the disorder, risk factors include a history of depression unrelated to childbirth, history of premenstrual dysphoric disorder (i.e., severe premenstrual syndrome), and major stress related to family, work, or residence (e.g., death of a loved one, loss of a job, moving away from a familiar town or city).

The underlying cause of peripartum depression is unknown, but several factors are thought to contribute. Heading the list is the sharp drop in estrogen and progesterone levels that occurs after delivery. (Levels of these hormones increase 10-fold during pregnancy and return to baseline after the placenta is expelled.) However, since hormone levels fall in all women but only some get peripartum depression, other factors—physical, emotional, and social—must be involved. The birthing process may leave women feeling weak and fatigued. Caring for a baby, who needs round-the-clock attention and feeding, exacerbates tiredness and exhaustion. Emotional and social factors may also play a role. Feelings of loss are common: Women experience loss of freedom, loss of control, and even loss of identity. Stress increases substantially, owing to increased workload and responsibilities, coupled with feelings of self-doubt and inadequacy, and compounded by a self-imposed (albeit highly unrealistic) expectation to be a "perfect" parent. Stress can be made even worse by financial insecurity and inadequate support from one's partner, family, and friends. Thyroid insufficiency may also contribute: Levels of thyroid hormone often decline after delivery, causing symptoms that can mimic depression. Accordingly, thyroid levels should be checked and, if indicated, replacement therapy should be implemented.

Screening for peripartum depression should be contemplated in all women, although evidence is lacking regarding universal screening. Women with multiple risk factors should be strongly considered. Screening can be accomplished with a quick test: the Edinburgh Postnatal Depression Scale.

Treatment of peripartum depression is much like treatment of major depression unrelated to pregnancy. The goal is to

Continued

si

PERIPARTUM DEPRESSION—cont'd

normalize mood and to optimize maternal and social functioning. The principal treatment modalities are psychotherapy and antidepressant drugs, both of which can be effective. In addition, the woman should be encouraged to nurture herself. She should

- Reduce isolation (by going out for at least a short time each day).
- Ensure adequate rest (by doing only what's really needed and letting the rest go).
- Spend time alone with her partner.

Other beneficial measures include joining a support group for new mothers and recruiting family members and friends to assist with household and baby-related chores.

Although antidepressants are clearly appropriate, there are few published data to guide selection. In one study of women with postpartum depression, fluoxetine [Prozac], a selective serotonin reuptake inhibitor (SSRI), was compared with psychotherapy. Both treatments were equally effective, and both were superior to placebo. Efficacy has also been demonstrated for sertraline [Zoloft], venlafaxine [Effexor], and certain tricyclic antidepressants (TCAs). For initial therapy, an SSRI is an attractive choice because these drugs are effective and well tolerated and present little risk of toxicity if taken in overdose. However, if a woman has responded to an antidepressant from a different class in the past, that drug should be tried first. To minimize side effects, dosage should be low initially (50% of the usual starting dosage) and then gradually increased. To reduce the risk of relapse, treatment should continue for at least 6 months after symptoms have resolved. Unfortunately, even then the relapse rate is high: Between 50% and 85% of patients experience at least one more depressive episode. With each succeeding episode, the risk of another recurrence increases. Accordingly, long-term prophylactic therapy should be considered.

Which antidepressants can be taken safely while breast-feeding? All of these drugs can be detected in breast milk—but levels of some are lower (safer) than levels of others. Sertraline, for example, appears safe. Studies show that drug activity in breast-fed infants is extremely low, and no adverse reactions have been observed. The TCAs (e.g., nortriptyline, desipramine) also appear safe: Levels are too low for detection in breast-fed infants, and follow-up studies have found no developmental deficits. In contrast to sertraline and the TCAs, fluoxetine appears unsafe: The drug and its metabolites reach therapeutic levels in breast-fed infants; potential consequences include colic and impaired weight gain. Infants of breast-feeding mothers on antidepressants should be monitored closely for these side effects.

a combination of drug therapy and psychotherapy is better than either intervention alone. Electroconvulsive therapy can be used when a rapid response is needed or when drugs and psychotherapy have not worked. For all patients, aerobic exercise and resistance training can improve mood.

Prototype Drugs

ANTIDEPRESSANTS

Selective Serotonin Reuptake Inhibitors
Fluoxetine

Serotonin/Norepinephrine Reuptake Inhibitors
Venlafaxine

Tricyclic Antidepressants
Imipramine

Monoamine Oxidase Inhibitors
Phenelzine

Atypical Antidepressants
Bupropion

DRUGS USED FOR DEPRESSION

Drugs are the primary therapy for major depression. However, benefits are limited mainly to patients with *severe* depression. In patients with *mild to moderate* depression, antidepressants have little or no beneficial effect.

Available antidepressants are listed in Table 32.1. As indicated, these drugs fall into five major classes: selective serotonin reuptake inhibitors (SSRIs), serotonin/norepinephrine reuptake inhibitors (SNRIs), tricyclic antidepressants (TCAs), monoamine oxidase inhibitors (MAOIs), and atypical antidepressants. All of these classes are equally effective, as are the individual drugs within each class. Hence, differences among these drugs relate mainly to side effects and drug interactions.

BASIC CONSIDERATIONS

In this section we consider basic issues that apply to all antidepressant drugs. The information on suicide risk is especially important.

Time Course of Response

With all antidepressants, symptoms resolve slowly. Initial responses develop in 1 to 3 weeks. Maximal responses may not be seen until 12 weeks. Because therapeutic effects are delayed, antidepressants cannot be used PRN. Furthermore, a therapeutic trial should not be considered a failure until a drug has been taken for at least 1 month without success.

Drug Selection

Because all antidepressants have nearly equal efficacy, selection among them is based largely on tolerability and safety. Additional considerations are drug interactions, patient preference, and cost. The usual drugs of first choice are the SSRIs, SNRIs,

TABLE 32.1 ▪ Antidepressant Classes and Adult Dosages

Generic Name	Brand Name	Initial Dose[a,b] (mg/day)	Maintenance Dose[a] (mg/day)
SELECTIVE SEROTONIN REUPTAKE INHIBITORS (SSRIs)			
Citalopram	Celexa	20	20–40
Escitalopram	Lexapro, Cipralex 🍁	10	10–20
Fluoxetine	Prozac, Serafem	20	20–80
Fluvoxamine[c]	Generic	50	100–300
Paroxetine	Paxil, Pexeva	20	20–50
Sertraline	Zoloft	50	50–200
SEROTONIN/NOREPINEPHRINE REUPTAKE INHIBITORS (SNRIs)			
Desvenlafaxine	Pristiq	50	50–100
Duloxetine	Cymbalta	30	60–120
Levomilnacipran	Fetzima	20	40–120
Venlafaxine	Effexor XR	37.5–75	75–375
TRICYCLIC ANTIDEPRESSANTS (TCAs)			
Amitriptyline	Generic only	25–50	100–300
Clomipramine[c]	Anafranil	25	100–250
Desipramine	Norpramin	25–50	100–300
Doxepin	Generic only[d]	25–50	75–300
Imipramine	Tofranil	25–50	100–300
Maprotiline	Generic only	75	100–150
Nortriptyline	Pamelor	25–50	50–150
Protriptyline	Vivactil	15–30	20–60
Trimipramine	Surmontil	75–100	75–300
MONOAMINE OXIDASE INHIBITORS (MAOIs)			
Isocarboxazid	Marplan	10–20	30–60
Phenelzine	Nardil	45	60–90
Selegiline (transdermal)	Emsam	6	6–12
Tranylcypromine	Parnate	10–30	30–60
ATYPICAL ANTIDEPRESSANTS			
Amoxapine	Generic only	100	200–400
Bupropion	Wellbutrin, others	200	300–450
Mirtazapine	Remeron	15	15–45
Nefazodone	Generic only	200	300–600
Trazodone	Generic only	150	150–600
Trazodone ER	Oleptro	150	150–375
Vilazodone	Viibryd	10	40

[a]Doses listed are *total daily doses.* Depending on the drug and the patient, the total dose may be given in a single dose or in divided doses.
[b]Initial doses are employed for 4 to 8 weeks, the time required for most symptoms to respond. Dosage is gradually increased as required.
[c]Fluvoxamine and clomipramine are not approved for major depression.
[d]Doxepin is also available in a low-dose formulation, sold as *Silenor,* for treating insomnia.

bupropion, and mirtazapine. Older antidepressants—TCAs and MAOIs—have more adverse effects and are less well tolerated than the first-line agents, and hence are generally reserved for patients who have not responded to the first-line drugs.

In some cases, the side effects of a drug, when matched to the right patient, can actually be beneficial. Here are some examples:

- For a patient with fatigue, choose a drug that causes central nervous system (CNS) stimulation (e.g., fluoxetine, bupropion).
- For a patient with insomnia, choose a drug that causes substantial sedation (e.g., mirtazapine).
- For a patient with sexual dysfunction, choose bupropion, a drug that enhances libido.

- For a patient with chronic pain, choose duloxetine or a TCA, drugs that can relieve chronic pain.

Managing Treatment

Once a drug has been selected for initial treatment, it should be used for 4 to 8 weeks to assess efficacy. As a rule, dosage should be low initially (to reduce side effects), and then gradually increased (see Table 32.1). If the initial drug is not effective, prescribers have four major options:

- Increase the dosage.
- Switch to another drug in the same class.
- Switch to another drug in a different class.
- Add a second drug, such as lithium or an atypical antidepressant.

After symptoms are in remission, treatment should continue for at least 4 to 9 months to prevent relapse. To this end, patients should be encouraged to take their drugs even if they are symptom free and hence feel that continued dosing is unnecessary. When antidepressant therapy is discontinued, dosage should be gradually tapered over several weeks because abrupt withdrawal can trigger withdrawal symptoms.

Suicide Risk With Antidepressant Drugs

Patients with depression often think about or attempt suicide. During treatment with antidepressants, especially early on, the risk of suicide may actually *increase.* Which antidepressants increase the risk of suicide? All of them do. According to two recent reports, risk appears equal for all antidepressant groups and for all individual drugs within those groups. In recognition of this risk, all antidepressants now carry a black box warning about a possible increase in suicidal thoughts or behavior. Concerns about antidepressant-induced suicide apply mainly to children, adolescents, and adults younger than 25 years.

To reduce the risk of suicide, patients taking antidepressant drugs should be observed closely for suicidality, worsening mood, and unusual changes in behavior. Close observation is especially important during the first few months of therapy and whenever antidepressant dosage is changed (either increased or decreased). Ideally, the patient or caregiver should meet with the prescriber at least weekly during the first 4 weeks of treatment, then biweekly for the next 4 weeks, then once 1 month later, and periodically thereafter. Phone contact may be appropriate between visits. In addition, family members or caregivers should monitor the patient *daily,* being alert for symptoms of decline (e.g., anxiety, agitation, panic attacks, insomnia, irritability, hostility, impulsivity, hypomania, and, of course, emergence of suicidality). If these symptoms are severe or develop abruptly, the patient should see his or her prescriber immediately.

Because antidepressant drugs can be used to *commit* suicide, two precautions should be observed. First, prescriptions should be written for the smallest number of doses consistent with good patient management. Second, dosing of inpatients should be directly observed to ensure that each dose is swallowed and not "cheeked," thereby preventing the patient from accumulating multiple doses that might be taken with suicidal intent.

What should be done if suicidal thoughts emerge during drug therapy or if depression is persistently worse while taking drugs? One option is to switch to another antidepressant. However, as noted, the risk of suicidality appears equal with all antidepressants. Another option is to stop antidepressants entirely. However, this option is probably unwise, because the long-term risk of suicide from untreated depression is much greater than the long-term risk associated with antidepressant drugs. If the risk of suicide appears high, temporary hospitalization may be the best protection.

SELECTIVE SEROTONIN REUPTAKE INHIBITORS

The SSRIs were introduced in 1987 and have since become our most commonly prescribed antidepressants. These drugs are indicated for major depression as well as several other psychologic disorders (Table 32.2). Characteristic side effects are nausea, agitation/insomnia, and sexual dysfunction (especially anorgasmia). The SSRIs can interact adversely with MAOIs and other serotonergic drugs, and hence these combinations must be avoided. In addition, when used late in pregnancy, SSRIs can lead to a withdrawal syndrome and persistent pulmonary hypertension in the infant. Like all other antidepressants, SSRIs may increase the risk of suicide. Compared with the TCAs and MAOIs, SSRIs are equally effective, better tolerated, and much safer. Death by overdose is extremely rare.

Fluoxetine

Fluoxetine [Prozac, Prozac Weekly, Sarafem], the first SSRI available, will serve as our prototype for the group. At one time, this drug was the most widely prescribed antidepressant in the world.

Mechanism of Action

The mechanism of action of fluoxetine and the other SSRIs is depicted in Fig. 32.1. As shown, SSRIs selectively block neuronal reuptake of serotonin (5-hydroxytryptamine [5-HT]), a monoamine neurotransmitter. As a result of reuptake blockade,

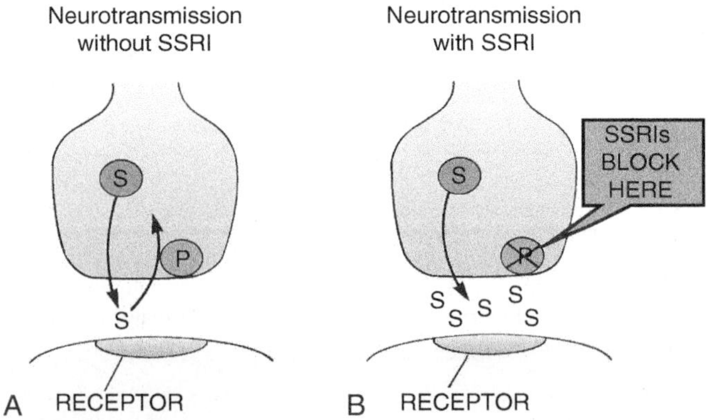

Fig. 32.1 ■ Mechanism of action of selective serotonin reuptake inhibitors.
A, Under drug-free conditions, the actions of serotonin are terminated by active uptake of the transmitter back into the nerve terminals from which it was released. **B,** By inhibiting the reuptake pump for serotonin, the SSRIs cause the transmitter to accumulate in the synaptic space, thereby intensifying transmission. (P, reuptake pump; S, serotonin; SSRI, selective serotonin reuptake inhibitor.)

TABLE 32.2 ■ Therapeutic Uses of Selective Serotonin Reuptake Inhibitors and Serotonin/Norepinephrine Reuptake Inhibitors

	Therapeutic Use[a]								
Drug	Major Depression	OCD	Panic Disorder	Social Phobia	Gad	Ptsd	PMDD	Bulimia Nervosa	Chronic Pain Disorders[b]
Citalopram [Celexa]	A	U	U	U	U	U	U		
Escitalopram [Lexapro]	A	U	U		A	U			
Fluoxetine [Prozac]	A	A	A	U	U	U	A	A	
Fluvoxamine	U	A	U	A	U	U	U	U	
Paroxetine [Paxil]	A	A	A	A	A	A	A		
Sertraline [Zoloft]	A	A	A	A	U	A	A		
Desvenlafaxine [Pristiq]	A		U	U	U				U
Duloxetine [Cymbalta]	A				A				A
Levomilnacipran [Fetzima]	A				U				U
Venlafaxine [Effexor]	A		A	A	A				U

[a]A, approved use; U, unlabeled use.
[b]Chronic musculoskeletal pain, neuropathic pain, or fibromyalgia.
GAD, Generalized anxiety disorder; *OCD,* obsessive-compulsive disorder; *PMDD,* premenstrual dysphoric disorder; *PTSD,* post-traumatic stress disorder.

TABLE 32.3 ■ Pharmacokinetic Properties of Antidepressants

Drug	Route	Half-Life (hr)	Metabolism	Excretion
SELECTIVE SEROTONIN REUPTAKE INHIBITORS (SSRIs)				
Fluoxetine [Prozac]	PO	48[a]	Hepatic; CYP2D6	Renal
Sertraline [Zoloft]	PO	24	Hepatic	Renal, gastrointestinal (feces)
Fluvoxamine	PO	15	Hepatic	Renal
Paroxetine [Paxil]	PO	20	Hepatic	Renal
Citalopram	PO	35	Hepatic	Renal, gastrointestinal (feces)
SEROTONIN/NOREPINEPHRINE REUPTAKE INHIBITORS (SNRIs)				
Venlafaxine [Effexor XR][b]	PO	5	Hepatic	
Desvenlafaxine [Pristiq]	PO	11	Hepatic	Renal
Duloxetine [Cymbalta]	PO	12	Hepatic; CYP2D6	Urine, gastrointestinal (feces)

[a]The half-life of fluoxetine's major metabolite, norfluoxetine, is 168 hours.
[b]Venlafaxine is metabolized into desvenlafaxine.

the concentration of 5-HT in the synapse increases, causing increased activation of postsynaptic 5-HT receptors. This mechanism is consistent with the theory that depression stems from a *deficiency* in monoamine-mediated transmission—and hence should be relieved by drugs that can intensify monoamine effects.

It is important to appreciate that blockade of 5-HT reuptake, by itself, cannot fully account for therapeutic effects. Clinical responses to SSRIs (relief of depressive symptoms) and the biochemical effect of the SSRIs (blockade of 5-HT reuptake) do not occur in the same time frame. That is, whereas SSRIs block 5-HT reuptake within hours of dosing, relief of depression takes several weeks to fully develop. This delay suggests that therapeutic effects are the result of adaptive cellular changes that take place in response to prolonged reuptake blockade. Fluoxetine and the other SSRIs do not block reuptake of dopamine or norepinephrine (NE). In contrast to the TCAs (see later in chapter), fluoxetine does not block cholinergic, histaminergic, or alpha$_1$-adrenergic receptors. Furthermore, fluoxetine produces CNS excitation rather than sedation.

Therapeutic Uses

Fluoxetine is used primarily for major depression. In addition, the drug is approved for bipolar disorder (see Chapter 33), obsessive-compulsive disorder (see Chapter 35), panic disorder (see Chapter 35), bulimia nervosa, and premenstrual dysphoric disorder (see Chapter 61). Unlabeled uses include post-traumatic stress disorder, social phobia, alcoholism, attention-deficit/hyperactivity disorder, migraine, and Tourette's syndrome. The pharmacokinetic properties of fluoxetine and other SSRIs are located in Table 32.3.

Adverse Effects

Fluoxetine is safer and better tolerated than TCAs and MAOIs. Death from overdose with fluoxetine alone has not been reported. In contrast to TCAs, fluoxetine does not block receptors for histamine, NE, or acetylcholine, and hence does not cause sedation, orthostatic hypotension, anticholinergic effects, or cardiotoxicity. The most common side effects are sexual dysfunction, nausea, headache, and manifestations of CNS stimulation, including nervousness, insomnia, and anxiety. Weight gain can also occur.

Sexual Dysfunction. Fluoxetine causes sexual problems (impotence, delayed or absent orgasm, delayed or absent ejaculation, decreased sexual interest) in nearly 70% of men and women. The underlying mechanism is unknown.

Sexual dysfunction can be managed in several ways. In some cases, reducing the dosage or taking "drug holidays" (e.g., discontinuing medication on Fridays and Saturdays) can help. Another solution is to add a drug that can overcome the problem. Among these are yohimbine, buspirone [BuSpar], and two typical antidepressants: bupropion [Wellbutrin, others] and nefazodone. Drugs such as sildenafil [Viagra] can also help: In *men,* these drugs improve erectile dysfunction, as well as arousal, ejaculation, orgasm, and overall satisfaction; in *women,* they can improve delayed orgasm. If all of these measures fail, the patient can try a different antidepressant. Agents that cause the least sexual dysfunction are the same two atypical antidepressants just mentioned.

Sexual problems often go unreported, either because patients are uncomfortable in discussing them or because patients don't realize their medicine is the cause. Accordingly, patients should be informed about the high probability of sexual dysfunction and told to report any problems so that they can be addressed.

Weight Gain. Like many other antidepressants, fluoxetine and other SSRIs cause weight gain. When these drugs were first introduced, researchers thought they caused weight *loss.* During the first few weeks of therapy patients lose weight, perhaps because of drug-induced nausea and vomiting. However, with long-term treatment, the lost weight is regained. Furthermore, about one-third of patients continue to gain weight. Although the reason is unknown, a good possibility is decreased sensitivity of 5-HT receptors that regulate appetite.

Serotonin Syndrome. By increasing serotonergic transmission in the brainstem and spinal cord, fluoxetine and other SSRIs can cause serotonin syndrome. This syndrome usually begins 2 to 72 hours after treatment onset. Signs and symptoms include altered mental status (agitation, confusion, disorientation, anxiety, hallucinations, poor concentration) as well as incoordination, myoclonus, hyperreflexia, excessive sweating, tremor, and fever. Deaths have occurred. The syndrome resolves spontaneously after discontinuing the drug. The risk of serotonin syndrome is increased by concurrent use of MAOIs and other drugs (see *Drug Interactions,* later in this chapter).

Withdrawal Syndrome. Abrupt discontinuation of SSRIs can cause a withdrawal syndrome. Symptoms include dizziness, headache, nausea, sensory disturbances, tremor, anxiety, and dysphoria. These begin within days to weeks of the last dose, and then persist for 1 to 3 weeks. Resumption of drug use will make symptoms subside. The withdrawal syndrome can be minimized by tapering the dosage slowly. Of the SSRIs in use today, fluoxetine is least likely to cause a withdrawal reaction. Because fluoxetine has a prolonged half-life, plasma levels decline slowly when dosing is stopped. When SSRIs are discontinued, it is important to distinguish between symptoms of withdrawal and return of depression.

Neonatal Effects From Use in Pregnancy. Use of fluoxetine and other SSRIs late in pregnancy poses a small risk of two adverse effects in the newborn: (1) *neonatal abstinence syndrome* (NAS) and (2) *persistent pulmonary hypertension of the newborn* (PPHN). NAS is characterized by irritability, abnormal crying, tremor, respiratory distress, and possibly seizures. The syndrome can be managed with supportive care and generally abates within a few days. PPHN, which compromises tissue oxygenation, carries a significant risk of death and, among survivors, a risk of cognitive delay, hearing loss, and neurologic abnormalities. Treatment measures include providing ventilatory support, giving oxygen and nitric oxide (to dilate pulmonary blood vessels), and giving IV sodium bicarbonate (to maintain alkalosis) and dopamine or dobutamine (to increase cardiac output and thereby maintain pulmonary perfusion). Infants exposed to SSRIs late in gestation should be monitored closely for NAS and PPHN.

Teratogenesis. Do fluoxetine and other SSRIs cause birth defects? Probably not. And if they do, the risk appears to be very low. Two SSRIs—*paroxetine* and *fluoxetine*—may cause septal heart defects. But even with these agents, the absolute risk is very low.

Safety Alert

SUICIDE RISK

Antidepressants may increase the risk of suicide in depressed patients, especially during the early phase of treatment. The risk of antidepressant-induced suicide is greatest among children, adolescents, and young adults. Patients starting treatment or changing doses must be monitored closely for suicidal behavior.

Extrapyramidal Side Effects. SSRIs cause extrapyramidal symptoms (EPS) in about 0.1% of patients. This is much less frequent than among patients taking antipsychotic medications (see Chapter 31). Among patients taking SSRIs, the most common EPS is akathisia, characterized by restlessness and agitation. However, parkinsonism, dystonic reactions, and tardive dyskinesia can also occur. EPS typically develop during the first month of treatment. The risk is increased by concurrent use of an antipsychotic drug. The underlying cause of SSRI-induced EPS may be alteration of serotonergic transmission within the extrapyramidal system. For a detailed discussion of EPS, refer to Chapter 31.

Bruxism. SSRIs may cause bruxism (clenching and grinding of teeth). However, since bruxism usually occurs during sleep, the condition often goes unrecognized. Sequelae of bruxism include headache, jaw pain, and dental problems (e.g., cracked fillings).

How do SSRIs cause bruxism? One theory is that they inhibit release of dopamine, a neurotransmitter that suppresses activity in certain muscles, including those of the jaw. By decreasing dopamine availability, SSRIs could release these muscles from inhibition, and excessive activity could result. This same mechanism may be responsible for SSRI-induced EPS.

One option to decrease bruxism is to reduce the SSRI dosage. However, this may cause depression to return. Other options include switching to a different class of antidepressant, use of a mouth guard, and treatment with low-dose buspirone (5 to 10 mg 1 to 3 times a day).

Bleeding Disorders. Fluoxetine and other SSRIs can increase the risk of bleeding in the GI tract and at other sites by impeding platelet aggregation. Platelets require 5-HT for aggregation, but can't make it themselves, and hence must take 5-HT up from the blood; by blocking 5-HT uptake, SSRIs suppress aggregation. The SSRIs cause a threefold increase in the risk of GI bleeding. However, the absolute risk is still low (about 1%). Caution is advised in patients with ulcers or a history of GI bleeding, in patients older than 60 years, and in patients taking nonsteroidal anti-inflammatory drugs (NSAIDs) or anticoagulants.

Fluoxetine and other SSRIs have been associated with an increased risk of hemorrhagic stroke. However, a causal relationship has not been established.

Hyponatremia. Fluoxetine can cause hyponatremia (serum sodium below 135 mEq/L), probably by increasing secretion of antidiuretic hormone. Most cases involve older adult patients taking thiazide diuretics. Accordingly, when fluoxetine is used in older adult patients, sodium should be measured at baseline and periodically thereafter.

Other Adverse Effects. Fluoxetine may cause *dizziness* and *fatigue;* patients who experience intense dizziness and fatigue should be warned against driving and other hazardous activities. *Skin rash,* which can be severe, has occurred in 4% of patients; in most cases, rashes readily respond to drug therapy (antihistamines, glucocorticoids) or to withdrawal of fluoxetine. Other common reactions include *diarrhea* and *excessive sweating.*

Drug Interactions

MAOIs and Other Drugs That Increase the Risk of Serotonin Syndrome. MAOIs increase 5-HT availability, and hence greatly increase the risk of serotonin syndrome. Accordingly, the use of MAOIs with SSRIs is *contraindicated.* Because MAOIs cause *irreversible* inhibition of monoamine oxidase (MAO; see further discussion later in this chapter), their effects persist long after dosing stops. Therefore, MAOIs should be withdrawn at least 14 days before starting an SSRI. Because fluoxetine and its active metabolite have long half-lives, at least 5 weeks should elapse between stopping fluoxetine and starting an MAOI. For other SSRIs, at least 2 weeks should elapse between treatment cessation and starting an MAOI.

Other drugs that increase the risk of serotonin syndrome include the serotonergic drugs listed in Table 32.4, drugs that inhibit CYP2D6 (and thereby raise fluoxetine levels), tramadol (an analgesic), and linezolid (an antibiotic that inhibits MAO).

Tricyclic Antidepressants and Lithium. Fluoxetine can elevate plasma levels of TCAs and lithium. Exercise caution if fluoxetine is combined with these agents.

Antiplatelet Drugs and Anticoagulants. Antiplatelet drugs (e.g., aspirin, NSAIDs) and anticoagulants (e.g., warfarin) increase the risk of GI bleeding. Exercise caution if fluoxetine is combined with these drugs.

The risk of bleeding with *warfarin* is compounded by a pharmacokinetic interaction. Because fluoxetine is highly bound to plasma proteins, it can displace other highly bound drugs. Displacement of warfarin is of particular concern. Monitor responses to warfarin closely.

Drugs That Are Substrates for or Inhibitors of CYP2D6. Fluoxetine and most other SSRIs are inactivated by CYP2D6. Accordingly, drugs that inhibit this enzyme can raise SSRI levels, thereby posing a risk of toxicity.

In addition to being a substrate for CYP2D6, fluoxetine itself can *inhibit* CYP2D6. As a result, fluoxetine can raise levels of other drugs that are CYP2D6 substrates. Among these are TCAs, several antipsychotics, and two antidysrhythmics: propafenone and flecainide. Combined use of fluoxetine with these drugs should be done with caution.

Preparations, Dosage, and Administration

Preparations. Fluoxetine is available in several oral formulations and is sold under three brand names: Prozac, Prozac Weekly, and Sarafem. Products available under each brand name are as follows:

- *Prozac*: oral solution (20 mg/5 mL)
- *Prozac:* tablets (10, 20, and 40 mg)
- *Prozac Weekly:* delayed-release, enteric-coated capsules (90 mg)
- *Sarafem:* tablets (10 and 20 mg)

In addition to these single-ingredient products, fluoxetine is available in a fixed-dose combination with olanzapine (an antipsychotic), sold as *Symbyax,* for treating bipolar disorder (see Chapter 33) and treatment-resistant major depression (see Chapter 32).

TABLE 32.4 ▪ Drugs That Promote Activation of Serotonin Receptors

Drug	Mechanism
SELECTIVE SEROTONIN REUPTAKE INHIBITORS (SSRIs)	
Citalopram [Celexa] Escitalopram [Lexapro, Cipralex 🍁] Fluoxetine [Prozac] Fluvoxamine Paroxetine [Paxil] Sertraline [Zoloft]	Block 5-HT reuptake and thereby increase 5-HT in the synapse
SEROTONIN/NOREPINEPHRINE REUPTAKE INHIBITORS (SNRIs)	
Desvenlafaxine [Pristiq] Duloxetine [Cymbalta] Levomilnacipran [Fetzima] Venlafaxine [Effexor XR]	Same as SSRIs
TRICYCLIC ANTIDEPRESSANTS (TCAs)	
Amitriptyline Clomipramine [Anafranil] Desipramine [Norpramin] Doxepin Imipramine [Tofranil] Trimipramine [Surmontil]	Same as SSRIs
MONOAMINE OXIDASE INHIBITORS (MAOIs)	
Isocarboxazid [Marplan] Phenelzine [Nardil] Selegiline [Emsam]	Inhibit neuronal breakdown of 5-HT by MAO, and thereby increase stores of 5-HT available for release
ATYPICAL ANTIDEPRESSANTS	
Mirtazapine [Remeron]	Promotes release of 5-HT
Nefazodone	Same as SSRIs
Trazodone [Oleptro]	Same as SSRIs
ANALGESICS	
Meperidine [Demerol]	Same as SSRIs *and* MAOIs
Methadone [Dolophine]	Same as SSRIs *and* MAOIs
Tramadol [Ultram]	Same as SSRIs
TRIPTAN ANTIMIGRAINE DRUGS	
Almotriptan [Axert] Eletriptan [Relpax] Frovatriptan [Frova] Rizatriptan [Maxalt] Sumatriptan [Imitrex] Zolmitriptan [Zomig]	Cause direct activation of serotonin receptors
OTHERS	
St. John's wort	Same as SSRIs *and* MAOIs
Linezolid [Zyvox]	Same as MAOIs

5-HT, 5-Hydroxytryptamine (serotonin); *MAO,* monoamine oxidase.

Dosage for Depression

Daily Dosing. The recommended initial dosage is 20 mg/day, taken with or without food. If needed, dosage may be increased gradually to a maximum of 80 mg/day. However, doses greater than 20 mg/day may increase adverse effects without increasing benefits. For older adult patients and patients with impaired liver function, the dosage should be low initially and then cautiously increased if needed. Since fluoxetine often impairs sleep, evening dosing should generally be avoided.

Weekly Dosing. Patients who have been treated successfully with 20 mg of fluoxetine daily for at least 13 weeks can be switched to once-weekly dosing (using 90-mg delayed-release capsules) for maintenance. Weekly dosing is initiated 7 days after the last 20-mg dose of daily fluoxetine.

Withdrawal. When discontinuing the drug, dosage should be reduced gradually.

Other SSRIs

In addition to fluoxetine, five other SSRIs are available: citalopram [Celexa], escitalopram [Lexapro, Cipralex 🍁], fluvoxamine [generic], paroxetine [Paxil, Pexeva], and sertraline [Zoloft]. All five are similar to fluoxetine. Antidepressant effects equal those of TCAs. Characteristic side effects are nausea, insomnia, headache, nervousness, weight gain, sexual dysfunction, hyponatremia, GI bleeding, and NAS and PPHN (in infants who were exposed to these drugs late in gestation). Serotonin syndrome is a potential complication with all SSRIs, especially if these agents are combined with MAOIs or other serotonergic drugs. The principal differences among the SSRIs relate to duration of action. Patients who experience intolerable adverse effects with one SSRI may find a different SSRI more acceptable. As with fluoxetine, withdrawal should be done slowly. In contrast to the TCAs, the SSRIs do not cause hypotension or anticholinergic effects, and with the exception of fluvoxamine they do not cause sedation. When taken in overdose, these drugs do not cause cardiotoxicity. Therapeutic uses for individual SSRIs are shown in Table 32.2.

Sertraline

Sertraline [Zoloft] is much like fluoxetine: both drugs block reuptake of 5-HT, both relieve symptoms of major depression, both cause CNS stimulation rather than sedation, and both have minimal effects on seizure threshold and the electrocardiogram (ECG). Sertraline is indicated for major depression, panic disorder, obsessive-compulsive disorder, post-traumatic stress disorder, premenstrual dysphoric disorder, and social anxiety disorder (social phobia). The drug is used off-label to treat generalized anxiety disorder, impulse control disorders, mild dementia-associated agitation in nonpsychotic patients, eating disorders, and paraphilia.

Common side effects include headache, tremor, insomnia, agitation, nervousness, nausea, diarrhea, weight gain, and sexual dysfunction. Treatment may also increase the risk of suicide. Because of the risk of serotonin syndrome, sertraline must not be combined with MAOIs and other serotonergic drugs (see Table 32.4). MAOIs should be withdrawn at least 14 days before starting sertraline, and sertraline should be withdrawn at least 14 days before starting an MAOI. Because of a risk of pimozide-induced dysrhythmias, sertraline (which raises pimozide levels) and pimozide should not be combined. Like fluoxetine and other SSRIs, sertraline poses a risk of hyponatremia, GI bleeding, and NAS and PPHN when used late in pregnancy.

Sertraline is available in tablets (25, 50, and 100 mg) and a concentrated oral solution (20 mg/mL). For treatment of depression, the initial adult daily dosage is 50 mg, administered in the morning or evening. After 4 to 8 weeks, the dosage may be increased by 50-mg increments to a maximum of 200 mg/day. When discontinuing the drug, dosage should be reduced gradually.

Fluvoxamine

Like other SSRIs, fluvoxamine produces powerful and selective inhibition of 5-HT reuptake. The drug is approved for obsessive-compulsive disorder and social anxiety disorder. Unlabeled uses include major depression, panic disorder, generalized anxiety disorder, post-traumatic stress disorder, premenstrual dysphoric disorder, and bulimia nervosa.

Common side effects include nausea, vomiting, dry mouth, headache, constipation, weight gain, and sexual dysfunction. In contrast to other SSRIs, fluvoxamine has moderate sedative effects, although it nonetheless can cause insomnia. Some patients have developed abnormal liver function tests. Accordingly, liver function should be assessed before treatment and weekly during the first month of therapy. Like other SSRIs, fluvoxamine interacts adversely with MAOIs and other serotonergic drugs, and hence these combinations must be avoided. As with other SSRIs, fluvoxamine poses a risk of hyponatremia, GI bleeding, and NAS and PPHN in infants exposed to the drug *in utero*.

Fluvoxamine is available in immediate-release (IR) tablets (25, 50, and 100 mg) and extended-release (ER) capsules (100 and 150 mg). With the IR formulation, dosing begins at 50 mg once a day at bedtime, and can be gradually increased to a maximum of 300 mg/day, given in two divided doses when the daily total exceeds 100 mg. With the CR capsules, dosing begins at 100 mg once daily, and can be gradually increased to 300 mg once daily. With either formulation, drug withdrawal should be done gradually.

Paroxetine

Like other SSRIs, paroxetine [Paxil, Paxil CR, Pexeva] produces powerful and selective inhibition of 5-HT reuptake. The drug is indicated for major depression, obsessive-compulsive disorder, social anxiety disorder, panic disorder, generalized anxiety disorder, post-traumatic stress disorder, and premenstrual dysphoric disorder. Paroxetine is used off-label to treat bipolar disorder, eating disorders, impulse control disorders, obsessive-compulsive disorder in children, mild dementia-associated agitation in nonpsychotic patients, and paraphilia.

Side effects are dose-dependent and generally mild. Early reactions include nausea, somnolence, sweating, tremor, and fatigue. These tend to diminish over time. After 5 to 6 weeks, the major complaints are headache, weight gain, and sexual dysfunction. Like fluoxetine, paroxetine causes signs of CNS stimulation (increased awakenings, reduced time in rapid-eye-movement sleep, insomnia). In contrast to TCAs, paroxetine has no effect on heart rate, blood pressure, or the ECG, but it does have some antimuscarinic effects. Like other SSRIs, paroxetine interacts adversely with MAOIs and other serotonergic drugs, and hence these combinations must be avoided. Also, like other SSRIs, paroxetine can increase the risk of GI bleeding and can cause hyponatremia (especially in older adult patients taking thiazide diuretics). As with other SSRIs, use late in pregnancy can result in NAS and PPHN. In addition, paroxetine, but not other SSRIs (except possibly fluoxetine), poses a small risk of cardiovascular birth defects, primarily ventricular septal defects. Because of this risk, the drug is classified in the U.S. Food and Drug Administration's Pregnancy Risk Category D.[a] Like all other antidepressants, paroxetine may increase the risk of suicide, especially in children and young adults.

Paroxetine is available as two salts: paroxetine *hydrochloride* and paroxetine *mesylate*. Although the two preparations have not been compared directly, effects are likely to be identical. The hydrochloride salt is available in IR tablets (10, 20, 30, and 40 mg) sold as *Paxil* and in ER tablets (12.5, 25, and 37.5 mg) sold as *Paxil CR*. Please note that the ER tablets are *not* longer-acting than the IR tablets. Rather, the ER tablets are designed to dissolve in the lower intestine, and hence may cause less GI disturbance than the IR tablets. The mesylate salt [Pexeva] is available in tablets (10, 20, 30, and 40 mg).

The initial dosage for depression is 20 mg/day (25 mg/day for Paxil CR). The entire daily dose is administered in the morning (to minimize sleep disturbance) and with food (to minimize GI upset). Dosage may be increased gradually (at intervals of at least 1 week) to a maximum of 50 mg/day (65 mg/day for Paxil CR). When discontinuing the drug, dosage should be reduced gradually.

Citalopram

Citalopram [Celexa] is very similar to fluoxetine and the other SSRIs. Benefits derive from selective blockade of 5-HT reuptake. The drug does not block receptors for acetylcholine, NE, or histamine. Its only approved indication is major depression. Unlabeled uses include panic disorder, social anxiety disorder, generalized anxiety disorder, obsessive-compulsive disorder, post-traumatic stress disorder, and premenstrual dysphoric disorder.

The most common adverse effects are nausea, somnolence, dry mouth, and sexual dysfunction. Additional side effects include weight gain, tachycardia, postural hypotension, headache, paresthesias, hyponatremia, and increased risk of GI bleeding. Large doses are teratogenic in animals. Citalopram enters breast milk in amounts sufficient to cause somnolence, reduced feeding, and weight loss in the infant. Use late in pregnancy can result in NAS and PPHN in the infant. Like all other antidepressants, citalopram may increase the risk of suicide, especially in children and young adults.

Citalopram prolongs the QT interval, and hence may pose a risk of fatal dysrhythmias, especially when the dosage exceeds 40 mg/day. Risk is increased in patients with heart disease, long QT syndrome, and low blood levels of potassium and magnesium. Because of the risk of serotonin syndrome, citalopram should not be combined with MAOIs or other serotonergic drugs. Allow at least 14 days to pass between stopping an MAOI and starting citalopram, or vice versa.

Citalopram [Celexa] is available in tablets (10, 20, and 40 mg) and an oral solution (10 mg/5 mL). The drug may be taken in the morning or evening, with or without food. The initial dosage for depression is 20 mg

[a]As of 2020, the FDA will no longer use Pregnancy Risk Categories. Please refer to Chapter 9 for more information.

once a day. Dosage may be increased slowly to a maximum of 40 mg/day in patients younger than 60 years. Doses above 40 mg/day offer no increase in benefits, but do increase the risk of dysrhythmias and other adverse effects. Dosage should remain low in older adult patients and in those with liver impairment. When discontinuing citalopram, dosage should be reduced gradually.

Escitalopram

Escitalopram [Lexapro, Cipralex 🍁] is the *S*-isomer of citalopram [Celexa], which is a 50 : 50 mixture of *S*- and *R*-isomers. The *S*-isomer (escitalopram) is responsible for antidepressant effects. The *R*-isomer has no antidepressant actions, but does contribute to side effects. Accordingly, escitalopram retains the therapeutic benefits of citalopram, but may be better tolerated. Otherwise, the pharmacology of the two drugs is largely the same. Escitalopram is approved for major depression and generalized anxiety disorder. Escitalopram has been used off-label for panic disorder. The drug can also reduce hot flashes in some menopausal women.

Like citalopram and other SSRIs, escitalopram is generally well tolerated. In clinical trials, the most common side effects were nausea, insomnia, somnolence, sweating, and fatigue. In addition, 9% of males reported ejaculatory disorders. However, the true incidence of sexual dysfunction may be higher because the incidence of sexual problems reported during clinical trials is usually considerably lower than the incidence seen in actual practice. As with other SSRIs, combined use with MAOIs and other serotonergic drugs increases the risk of serotonin syndrome. At least 14 days should separate the use of MAOIs and escitalopram. Like citalopram and other SSRIs, escitalopram increases the risk of hyponatremia and GI bleeding, and, when used late in pregnancy, may cause NAS or PPHN in the newborn. Like all other antidepressants, this drug can increase the risk of suicide, especially in children and young adults.

Escitalopram [Lexapro, Cipralex 🍁] is available in tablets (5, 10, and 20 mg) and an oral solution (5 mg/5 mL). The recommended initial dosage is 10 mg/day, taken in the morning or evening, with or without food. In clinical trials, dosages above 10 mg/day did not increase antidepressant effects, but did intensify side effects. There is no need to reduce the dosage in older adult patients or in patients with either hepatic impairment or mild to moderate renal impairment. However, in patients with severe renal impairment, a dosage reduction may be required. When discontinuing the drug, dosage should be reduced gradually.

PATIENT-CENTERED CARE ACROSS THE LIFE SPAN

Antidepressants

Life Stage	Patient Care Concerns
Infants	Use of SSRIs in late pregnancy poses a small risk of neonatal abstinence syndrome (NAS), characterized by abnormal crying, irritability, tremor, and possible seizures.
Children/adolescents	Antidepressants may increase the risk of suicide, especially during the early phase of treatment.
Pregnant women	Use of SSRIs late in pregnancy may promote persistent pulmonary hypertension of the newborn (PPHN).
Breast-feeding women	Antidepressants are generally safe in breast-feeding women. Sertraline has been shown to be especially safe.
Older adults	Treatment with SSRIs or SNRIs is generally safe, providing less medication interaction and smaller side effect profiles.

SEROTONIN/NOREPINEPHRINE REUPTAKE INHIBITORS

Four drugs—venlafaxine, desvenlafaxine, duloxetine, and levomilnacipran—block neuronal reuptake of serotonin *and* NE, with minimal effects on other transmitters or receptors. Pharmacologic effects are similar to those of the SSRIs, although the SSRIs may be better tolerated. The SNRIs are indicated for major depression as well as other disorders (see Table 32.2).

Venlafaxine

Venlafaxine [Effexor XR], the first SNRI available, is approved for major depression, generalized anxiety disorder, social anxiety disorder (social phobia), and panic disorder. The drug produces powerful blockade of NE and 5-HT reuptake and weak blockade of dopamine reuptake. The relationship of these actions to therapeutic effects is uncertain. Venlafaxine does not block cholinergic, histaminergic, or alpha$_1$-adrenergic receptors. Despite impressions that venlafaxine may be superior to SSRIs, when compared directly in clinical trials, the drugs were about equally effective—and SSRIs are probably safer.

Venlafaxine can cause a variety of adverse effects. The most common is nausea (37% to 58%), followed by headache, anorexia, nervousness, sweating, somnolence, and insomnia. Dose-dependent weight loss may occur secondary to anorexia. Venlafaxine can also cause dose-related sustained diastolic hypertension; blood pressure should be monitored. Sexual dysfunction (e.g., impotence, anorgasmia) may occur too. Some patients experience sustained mydriasis (dilation of the pupil), which can increase the risk of eye injury in those with elevated intraocular pressure or glaucoma. Like the SSRIs, venlafaxine can cause hyponatremia, especially in older adult patients taking diuretics. Like all other antidepressants, venlafaxine may increase the risk of suicide, especially in children and young adults.

Combined use of venlafaxine with MAOIs and other serotonergic drugs (see Table 32.4) increases the risk of serotonin syndrome, a potentially fatal reaction. If the clinical situation demands, venlafaxine may be cautiously combined with an SSRI or another SNRI. However, combined use with an MAOI is *contraindicated.* Accordingly, MAOIs should be withdrawn at least 14 days before starting venlafaxine. When switching from venlafaxine to an MAOI, venlafaxine should be discontinued 7 days before starting the MAOI.

As with the SSRIs, use of venlafaxine late in pregnancy can result in a neonatal withdrawal syndrome, characterized by irritability, abnormal crying, tremor, respiratory distress, and possibly seizures. Symptoms, which can be managed with supportive care, generally abate within a few days.

Abrupt discontinuation can cause an intense withdrawal syndrome. Symptoms include anxiety, agitation, tremors, headache, vertigo, nausea, tachycardia, and tinnitus. Worsening of pretreatment symptoms may also occur. Withdrawal symptoms can be minimized by tapering the dosage over 2 to 4 weeks. Warn patients not to stop venlafaxine abruptly.

Venlafaxine is available in three formulations: IR tablets (25, 37.5, 50, 75, and 100 mg) sold generically, extended-release (ER) tablets (37.5, 75, 150, and 225 mg) sold generically, and ER capsules (37.5, 75, and 150 mg) sold as *Effexor XR.* The ER capsules and ER tablets are bioequivalent. All doses should be taken with food. Inform patients that the ER tablets should be swallowed intact, but the ER capsules can be opened and sprinkled on applesauce. For treatment of depression, the recommended initial dosage is 75 mg/day (taken in two or three divided doses using IR tablets, or in a single dose using ER tablets or ER capsules). If needed, the dosage may be gradually increased. The usual maximum dosage is 375 mg/day (225 mg/day for Effexor XR). However, dosages as large as 375 mg/day have been used for severely depressed patients. Dosage should be reduced in patients with liver disease and possibly in those with kidney disease. As with all other antidepressants, dosage should be tapered slowly when treatment is stopped.

Desvenlafaxine

Desvenlafaxine [Pristiq] is the major active metabolite of venlafaxine. Accordingly, the actions and adverse effects of both drugs are similar. Like venlafaxine, desvenlafaxine is a strong inhibitor of 5-HT and NE reuptake and does not block cholinergic, histaminergic, or alpha$_1$-adrenergic receptors. At this time, desvenlafaxine is approved only for major depression, in contrast to venlafaxine, which is approved for major depression, generalized anxiety disorder, panic disorder, and social phobia.

Adverse effects are like those of venlafaxine. The most common are nausea, headache, dizziness, insomnia, diarrhea, dry mouth, sweating, and constipation. Sexual effects include erectile dysfunction and decreased libido. Like all other antidepressants, desvenlafaxine may increase the risk of suicide in children and young adults. Some neonates exposed to the drug *in utero* have required prolonged hospitalization, respiratory support, and tube feeding. Additional concerns include hyponatremia, sustained hypertension, serotonin syndrome, bleeding, seizures, and withdrawal symptoms if the drug is discontinued abruptly.

As with venlafaxine, combining desvenlafaxine with another serotonergic drug increases the risk of serotonin syndrome. Combined use with an SSRI or another SNRI may be done cautiously. In contrast, combined use with an MAOI is *contraindicated.* Accordingly, MAOIs should be withdrawn at least 14 days before starting desvenlafaxine, and desvenlafaxine should be withdrawn at least 7 days before starting an MAOI.

Desvenlafaxine [Pristiq] is available in 25-, 50- and 100-mg ER tablets, which should be swallowed whole with fluid, and not crushed, chewed, or dissolved. The recommended dosage is 50 mg once daily, taken with or without food, about the same time each day. Increasing the dose above 50 mg/day offers no therapeutic benefit, but does increase the risk of side effects. In patients with severe renal impairment (creatinine clearance less than 30 mL/min), the dosage should be reduced to 50 mg every other day. There is no need to reduce the dosage in patients with moderate renal impairment or in those with liver impairment of any degree. To minimize withdrawal reactions, the drug should be discontinued slowly (by gradually increasing the dosing interval).

Duloxetine

Mechanism of Action and Therapeutic Uses

Duloxetine [Cymbalta] was the second SNRI approved for major depression. The drug is a powerful inhibitor of 5-HT and NE reuptake, and a much weaker inhibitor of dopamine reuptake. Duloxetine does not bind with receptors for NE, serotonin, dopamine, acetylcholine, or histamine, and does not inhibit MAO.

Data on the antidepressant effects of duloxetine are limited. Clinical trials have shown that duloxetine is clearly superior to *placebo:* Treatment reduces depressive symptoms and may also reduce physical pain associated with depression (e.g., backache). Furthermore, benefits may develop quickly, in some cases within 2 weeks of starting treatment. Limited studies have compared duloxetine to SSRIs (fluoxetine and escitalopram), as well as to venlafaxine and desvenlafaxine. There does not appear to be any difference in efficacy when treating depression with duloxetine. In addition, duloxetine seems less well tolerated than the other medications commonly used to treat depression. As a result, there is no basis for choosing duloxetine over other antidepressants.

In addition to its use in depression, duloxetine is approved for fibromyalgia, generalized anxiety disorder, pain of diabetic peripheral neuropathy, and chronic musculoskeletal pain, including low back pain and pain from osteoarthritis. The drug is used off-label for *stress* urinary incontinence (in contrast to *urge* urinary incontinence).

Adverse Effects

Duloxetine is generally well tolerated. In clinical trials, the most common adverse effects were nausea, dry mouth, insomnia, somnolence, constipation, reduced appetite, fatigue, increased sweating, and blurred vision. Duloxetine can cause a small increase in blood pressure, and hence blood pressure should be measured at baseline and periodically thereafter. Duloxetine promotes mydriasis, and hence should not be used by patients with uncontrolled narrow-angle glaucoma.

Liver toxicity is a concern. Elevation of serum transaminases, indicating liver damage, occurs in about 1% of patients. There have been reports of hepatitis, hepatomegaly, cholestatic jaundice, and elevation of transaminases to more than 20 times the upper limit of normal. To reduce risk, duloxetine should not be given to patients with pre-existing liver disease or to those who drink alcohol heavily.

As with venlafaxine, abrupt cessation of treatment can cause a withdrawal syndrome. Symptoms include nausea, vomiting, dizziness, headache, nightmares, and paresthesias. To minimize risk, duloxetine should be withdrawn slowly. Like all other antidepressants, duloxetine may increase the risk of suicide, especially in children and young adults.

Effects in Pregnancy and Lactation

Animal studies indicate that duloxetine interferes with fetal and postnatal development, causing reduced fetal weight, decreased postnatal survival, and neurologic disturbances. Use of duloxetine late in pregnancy can also lead to withdrawal syndrome in the infant. The drug is excreted in the milk of lactating rats. Two studies completed in pregnant women indicated that the occurrence of fetal malformation was no greater in the group receiving duloxetine than in the general population. One completed study found duloxetine in the breast milk of six lactating women who received 40 mg twice daily for 3.5 days; the daily infant dose was minimal. However, these studies were small, and until the larger studies are completed, use of duloxetine during pregnancy and lactation is not recommended.

Drug Interactions

The combination of duloxetine with heavy alcohol consumption greatly increases the risk of liver damage. Accordingly, duloxetine should not be prescribed to patients with substantial alcohol intake.

Like venlafaxine and other drugs that block 5-HT reuptake, duloxetine can cause serotonin syndrome if combined with an MAOI or any other serotonergic drug. MAOIs should be withdrawn at least 14 days before starting duloxetine, and duloxetine should be withdrawn at least 5 days before starting an MAOI.

Drugs that inhibit CYP1A2 or CYP2D6 can increase duloxetine levels, and may thereby cause toxicity. Inhibitors of CYP1A2 include cimetidine [Tagamet], fluvoxamine, and ciprofloxacin [Cipro]. Inhibitors of CYP2D6 include fluoxetine [Prozac], paroxetine [Paxil], and quinidine.

Duloxetine is a moderate inhibitor of CYP2D6, and hence may raise levels of drugs that are extensively metabolized by this enzyme. Among these are certain TCAs (e.g., amitriptyline, nortriptyline), type IC antidysrhythmics (propafenone [Rythmol] and flecainide [Tambocor]), and phenothiazines, including thioridazine. Interaction with thioridazine is of special concern owing to a risk of serious ventricular dysrhythmias. Accordingly, the two drugs should not be combined.

Preparations, Dosage, and Administration

Duloxetine [Cymbalta] is available in delayed-release capsules (20, 30, and 60 mg) that should be swallowed whole, with or without food. The usual dosage for depression is 40 to 60 mg/day initially, followed by 60 to 120 mg/day for maintenance. For all other indications—depression, generalized anxiety disorder, pain of diabetic neuropathy, and chronic musculoskeletal pain—the dosage is 30 mg once daily for 1 week, followed by 60 mg once daily for maintenance. When treatment is discontinued, dosage should be tapered slowly.

Levomilnacipran

Levomilnacipran [Fetzima] is an SNRI approved for major depressive disorder in 2013. In clinical studies, patients taking levomilnacipran showed significant clinical improvement in depressive symptoms. Side effects were similar to those of the other SNRIs, including erectile dysfunction, constipation, and nausea. Levomilnacipran is available in 20-, 40-, 80-, and 120-mg capsules and is taken once daily. Usual dosing is 40 to 120 mg daily.

TRICYCLIC ANTIDEPRESSANTS

The first TCA—imipramine—was introduced to psychiatry in the late 1950s. Since then, the ability of TCAs to relieve depressive symptoms has been firmly established. For decades, TCAs were drugs of first choice for depression. However, owing to the development of safer alternatives, especially the SSRIs, the use of TCAs has greatly declined. The most common adverse effects are sedation, orthostatic hypotension, and anticholinergic effects. The most dangerous effect is cardiac toxicity. When taken in overdose, TCAs can readily prove lethal. Like all other antidepressants, TCAs may increase the risk of suicide. Because all of the TCAs have similar properties, we will discuss these drugs as a group, rather than focusing on a representative prototype.

Chemistry

The structure of imipramine, a representative TCA, is very similar to the structure of the phenothiazine antipsychotics. Because of this similarity, TCAs and phenothiazines have several actions in common. Specifically, both groups produce varying degrees of *sedation, orthostatic hypotension,* and *anticholinergic effects.*

Mechanism of Action

The TCAs block neuronal reuptake of two monoamine transmitters: NE and 5-HT. As a result, TCAs increase the concentration of these transmitters at CNS synapses, and thereby intensify their effects. As indicated in Table 32.5, some TCAs block reuptake of NE *and* 5-HT, whereas others block reuptake of only NE. As with the SSRIs, biochemical effects (blockade of transmitter reuptake) occur within hours, whereas therapeutic effects (relief of depression) develop over several weeks. This delay suggests that antidepressant effects are due to adaptive changes brought on by prolonged reuptake blockade, and not to reuptake blockade directly.

Pharmacokinetics

The half-lives of TCAs are long and variable. Because their half-lives are long, TCAs can usually be administered in a single daily dose. Because their half-lives are variable, TCAs require individualization of dosage.

Therapeutic Uses

Depression. TCAs are effective agents for major depression. These drugs can elevate mood, increase activity and alertness, decrease morbid preoccupation, improve appetite, and normalize sleep patterns. Despite their efficacy, TCAs are generally considered second-line drugs, owing to the development of safer and better tolerated alternatives.

Bipolar Disorder. Bipolar disorder (manic-depressive illness) is characterized by alternating episodes of mania and depression (see Chapter 33). TCAs can help during depressive episodes.

Fibromyalgia Syndrome. Fibromyalgia syndrome is a chronic disorder characterized by diffuse musculoskeletal pain, profound fatigue, disturbed sleep, and cognitive dysfunction. As discussed in Chapter 107, TCAs are the most effective drugs we have for reducing symptoms.

Other Uses. TCAs can benefit patients with neuropathic pain (see Chapter 29), chronic insomnia (see Chapter 34), attention-deficit/hyperactivity disorder (see Chapter 36), and panic disorder or obsessive-compulsive disorder (see Chapter 35).

Adverse Effects

The most common adverse effects are orthostatic hypotension, sedation, and anticholinergic effects. The most serious adverse effect is cardiotoxicity. These effects occur because, in addition to blocking reuptake of NE and 5-HT, TCAs cause direct blockade of receptors for histamine and acetylcholine. Adverse effects of individual agents are shown in Table 32.5.

Orthostatic Hypotension. Orthostatic hypotension is the most serious of the common adverse responses to TCAs. Hypotension is due in large part to blockade of $alpha_1$-adrenergic receptors on blood vessels. Patients should be informed that they can minimize orthostatic hypotension by moving slowly when assuming an upright posture. In addition, patients should be instructed to sit or lie down if symptoms (dizziness, lightheadedness) occur. For hospitalized patients, blood pressure and pulse rate should be monitored on a regular schedule (e.g., 4 times a day). These measurements should be taken while the patient is lying down and again after the patient has been sitting or standing for 1 to 2 minutes. If blood pressure is low or pulse rate is high, medication should be withheld and the prescriber notified.

Anticholinergic Effects. The TCAs block muscarinic cholinergic receptors and can thereby cause an array of anticholinergic effects (dry mouth, blurred vision, photophobia, constipation, urinary hesitancy, and tachycardia). Patients should be informed about possible anticholinergic responses and instructed in ways to minimize discomfort. A detailed discussion of anticholinergic effects and their management is presented in Chapter 14.

Diaphoresis. Despite their anticholinergic properties, TCAs often cause diaphoresis (sweating). The mechanism of this paradoxical effect is unknown.

Sedation. Sedation is a common response to TCAs. The cause is blockade of histamine receptors in the CNS. Patients should be advised to avoid hazardous activities if sedation is prominent.

Cardiac Toxicity. Tricyclics can adversely affect cardiac function. However, in the absence of an overdose or pre-existing cardiac impairment, serious effects are rare. The TCAs affect the heart by (1) decreasing vagal influence on the heart (secondary to muscarinic blockade) and (2) acting directly on the bundle of His to slow conduction. Both effects increase the risk of dysrhythmias. To minimize risk, all patients should undergo ECG evaluation before treatment and periodically thereafter. Risk of cardiac toxicity may be higher with desipramine than with other TCAs.

Seizures. TCAs lower seizure threshold and thereby increase seizure risk. Exercise caution in patients with seizure disorders.

Hypomania. On occasion, TCAs produce too much of a good thing, elevating mood from depression all the way to hypomania (mild mania). If hypomania develops, the patient should be evaluated to determine whether elation is drug induced or the result of bipolar disorder.

Suicide Risk. As discussed earlier in this chapter, TCAs and all other antidepressants may increase the risk of suicide in depressed patients, especially during the early phase of treatment. The risk of antidepressant-induced suicide is greatest among children, adolescents, and young adults.

Drug Interactions

Monoamine Oxidase Inhibitors. The combination of a TCA with an MAOI can lead to *severe hypertension,* owing to excessive adrenergic stimulation of the heart and blood vessels. Excessive adrenergic stimulation occurs because (1) inhibition of MAO causes accumulation of NE in adrenergic neurons and (2) blockade of NE reuptake by the tricyclics decreases NE inactivation. Because of the potential for hypertensive crisis, combined therapy with TCAs and MAOIs is generally avoided.

Direct-Acting Sympathomimetic Drugs. Tricyclics *potentiate* responses to direct-acting sympathomimetics (i.e., drugs such as epinephrine and dopamine that produce their effects by direct interaction with adrenergic receptors). Because TCAs block uptake of these agents into adrenergic nerve terminals, they prolong the presence of these agents in the synaptic space.

Indirect-Acting Sympathomimetic Drugs. TCAs *decrease* responses to indirect-acting sympathomimetics (i.e., drugs such as ephedrine and amphetamine that promote release of transmitter from adrenergic nerves). TCAs block uptake of these agents into adrenergic nerves, thereby preventing them from reaching their site of action within the nerve terminal.

TABLE 32.5 ▪ Antidepressants: Adverse Effects and Impact on Neurotransmitters

Drug	Transmitters Affected[a]	Agitation/ Insomnia	Anticholinergic Activity	Sedation	Hypotension	Seizure Risk	Cardiac Toxicity	Weight Gain	Sexual Dysfunction	Other Side Effects
SELECTIVE SEROTONIN REUPTAKE INHIBITORS (SSRIs)										
Citalopram	5-HT	++	0/+		0	0/+	0	+	+++	GI bleeding, hyponatremia, NAS and PPHN in newborns. Citalopram may cause dysrhythmias.[c]
Escitalopram	5-HT	++	0/+	0/+	0	0/+	0	+	+++	
Fluoxetine	5-HT	++	0	[b]	0	0/+	0/+	+	+++	
Fluvoxamine	5-HT	++	0/+	0/+	0	0/+		+	+++	
Paroxetine	5-HT	++	0/+	[b]	0	0/+	0	+	+++	
Sertraline	5-HT	++	0	[b]	0	0/+	0	+	+++	
SEROTONIN/NOREPINEPHRINE REUPTAKE INHIBITORS (SNRIs)										
Desvenlafaxine	NE, 5-HT	++	0	0	0	0/+	0/+	0	++	
Duloxetine	NE, 5-HT	++	0	0	0/+	0/+	0/+	0/+	+	Hepatotoxicity
Venlafaxine	NE, 5-HT	++	0	0	0	0/+	0/+	0	+++	
Levomilnacipran	NE, 5-HT	++	0	0	0	[d]	0/+	0	++	Hyponatremia
TRICYCLIC ANTIDEPRESSANTS (TCAs)										
Amitriptyline	NE, 5-HT	0/+	++++	+++	++	++	+++	+++	++	
Clomipramine	NE, 5-HT	+	++	++	++	+++	+++	++	++	
Doxepin	NE, 5-HT	0/+	++	+++	++	++	+++	+++	++	
Imipramine	NE, 5-HT	+	++	++	++	++	+++	++	++	
Trimipramine	NE, 5-HT	0/+	+++	+++	++	++	+++	++	++	
Desipramine	NE	+	+	[b]	+	+++	+++	+	++	
Maprotiline	NE	+	++	++	+	+++	++	+	++	
Nortriptyline	NE	+	+	+	+	+	++	++	++	
Protriptyline	NE	++	++	[b]	+	++	+++	+	++	
MONOAMINE OXIDASE INHIBITORS (MAOIs)										
Isocarboxazid	NE, 5-HT, DA	++	0	+	+	0	0	+	++	Hypertensive crisis from tyramine in food[e]
Phenelzine	NE, 5-HT, DA	++	0	+	+	0	0	+	++	
Selegiline	NE, 5-HT, DA	++	0	0	0	0	0	0	+	
Tranylcypromine	NE, 5-HT, DA	++	0	[b]	+	0	0	+	++	
ATYPICAL ANTIDEPRESSANTS										
Amoxapine	NE, ↓DA[f]	0/+	+	+	+	++	++	+	++	Parkinsonism
Bupropion	DA	++	0/+	[b]	0	+++	0	0	[g]	Seizures
Mirtazapine	NE, 5-HT	0/+	0/+	++++	0/+	0	0	++++	0	
Nefazodone	5-HT	0/+	0/+	++	0	0	0/+	0/+	0/+	
Trazodone	5-HT	0/+	0/+	++++	+	0	0/+	+	+[h]	Priapism
Vilazodone	5-HT	++	0	++	0	0	0	0	++	Bleeding, hyponatremia

[a]All of the antidepressants *increase* synaptic activity of the transmitters indicated—with the exception of amoxapine, which increases activity of NE, but *blocks* receptors for DA. The TCAs, SSRIs, SNRIs, amoxapine, bupropion, nefazodone, and trazodone decrease transmitter reuptake; vilazodone blocks transmitter reuptake and directly activates 5-HT receptors; MAOIs block transmitter breakdown; and mirtazapine promotes transmitter release.
[b]Produces moderate *stimulation,* not sedation.
[c]NAS, neonatal abstinence syndrome; PPHN, persistent pulmonary hypertension of the newborn.
[d]Levomilnacipran was not tested in patients with seizure disorders.
[e]Hypertensive crisis is not a risk with low-dose (6 mg/day) transdermal selegiline, and possibly not with higher doses.
[f]Amoxapine blocks *reuptake* of NE and blocks *receptors* for DA.
[g]Bupropion may increase sexual desire.
[h]Trazodone can cause priapism (persistent painful erection).
DA, Dopamine; *5-HT,* 5-hydroxytryptamine (serotonin); *NE,* norepinephrine.

electroshock, patients are treated with two drugs: a *short-acting neuromuscular blocker* (succinylcholine) and a *short-acting intravenous anesthetic* (e.g., propofol, etomidate, methohexital). The neuromuscular blocker prevents shock-induced seizure movements, which are both hazardous and unnecessary for a therapeutic response. The IV anesthetic prevents conscious awareness of the ECT procedure (without interfering with beneficial actions). Patients may also receive an anticholinergic drug (e.g., glycopyrrolate) to minimize bradycardia and salivation.

ECT can terminate an ongoing depression episode, but a single series of treatments cannot prevent recurrence. Accordingly, some patients are now given "maintenance" treatments, at weekly or monthly intervals. In one study, the relapse rate at 6 months in the absence of maintenance was 73%, compared with only 8% when maintenance ECT was used. Maintenance with antidepressant drugs (e.g., lithium plus amitriptyline) is another option, but appears significantly less effective than maintenance with ECT.

ECT is very safe. There are no absolute contraindications to its use. The principal adverse effect is amnesia, primarily for events immediately surrounding treatment. However, patients may also experience some loss of older memories, but these usually return within 6 months. There is also transient impairment of cognitive function. Minor adverse effects, which occur immediately after treatment, include nausea, headache, confusion, and muscle discomfort.

TRANSCRANIAL MAGNETIC STIMULATION

Like ECT, transcranial magnetic stimulation (TMS) is reserved for patients with major depression that has not responded to antidepressant drugs. Magnetic stimulation is accomplished using the *NeuroStar TMS System,* a device that employs an insulated magnetic coil, placed against the scalp, to deliver pulsed magnetic fields to the left dorsolateral prefrontal cortex. The magnetic fields induce electrical currents in the brain, which in turn cause neuronal depolarization and other changes in brain activity. A full course of treatment consists of daily 40-minute sessions for 6 weeks or so. How effective is TMS? Trial results have been inconsistent. In some trials, TMS was just as effective as ECT, but in other trials, TMS was less effective. How safe is TMS? The procedure is generally well tolerated. Principal adverse effects are transient headaches and scalp discomfort. Patients may also experience eye pain, toothache, muscle twitching, and seizures. Cognitive changes have not been reported.

VAGUS NERVE STIMULATION

The Vagus Nerve Stimulation (VNS) Therapy System is approved for adjunctive long-term therapy of patients with "treatment-resistant depression" (TRD), which the manufacturer defines as major depression that has not responded to at least four different antidepressant drugs. The VNS Therapy System—an implanted device that delivers electrical pulses to the vagus nerve—was first developed to treat drug-resistant seizure disorders. In the course of that research, mood elevation was observed in some patients. A trial was then conducted in patients with TRD. However, the results were equivocal. Newer small studies show possible promise in patients with severe refractory depression. The mechanism by which VNS alleviates depression (if it really does) is unknown. The principal side effects of VNS are hoarseness, voice alteration, cough, and dyspnea, all of which tend to diminish over time. The cost of the VNS system, along with surgical implantation and calibration, is about $25,000.

LIGHT THERAPY

Exposure to bright light is an effective treatment of SAD and of nonseasonal major depression. The more intense the light, the greater the response. Light can be beneficial alone, and can enhance the response to antidepressant drugs. How does light relieve depression? Possibly by enhancing serotonergic neurotransmission. Light therapy is attractive, owing to low cost and low risk.

KEY POINTS

- The principal symptoms of major depression are depressed mood and loss of pleasure or interest in one's usual activities and pastimes.
- Patients with mild depression can be treated equally well with antidepressant drugs or psychotherapy. Patients with severe depression respond better to a combination of drugs plus psychotherapy than to either intervention alone.
- Patients with depression often think about or attempt suicide. During treatment with antidepressants, especially initially, the risk of suicide may *increase.* To reduce the risk of suicide, patients should be followed closely by family members, caregivers, and the prescriber. Suicide risk is greatest in children and young adults.
- All antidepressants appear equally effective. Differences relate primarily to side effects, drug interactions, and cost.
- Therapeutic responses to antidepressants develop slowly. Initial responses develop in 1 to 3 weeks. Maximal responses may not be seen until 12 weeks.
- Antidepressant therapy should continue for 4 to 9 months after symptoms resolve.
- SSRIs block reuptake of serotonin, and thereby intensify transmission at serotonergic synapses. Over time, this induces adaptive cellular responses that are ultimately responsible for relieving depression.
- SSRIs have two major advantages over TCAs: they cause fewer side effects and are safer when taken in overdose.
- Most SSRIs have stimulant properties, and hence can cause insomnia and agitation. This contrasts with TCAs, which cause sedation.
- Like most other antidepressants, SSRIs can cause weight gain.
- Sexual dysfunction (e.g., impotence, anorgasmia) is more common with SSRIs than with most other antidepressants.
- SSRIs can cause serotonin syndrome, especially when combined with MAOIs. Symptoms include agitation, confusion, hallucinations, hyperreflexia, tremor, and fever.

Continued

Combined use of SSRIs and MAOIs is contraindicated, and combined use with other serotonergic drugs (see Table 32.4) should be done with extreme caution, if at all.

- SNRIs block reuptake of serotonin and norepinephrine. Effects are similar to those of the SSRIs.
- The most common side effects of SNRIs include nausea, insomnia, and hypertension. SNRIs can also contribute to sexual dysfunction.
- SNRIs, like SSRIs, can cause serotonin syndrome.
- TCAs block reuptake of NE and 5-HT and thereby intensify transmission at noradrenergic and serotonergic synapses. Over time, this induces adaptive cellular responses that are ultimately responsible for relieving depression.
- The most common adverse effects of TCAs are sedation, orthostatic hypotension, and anticholinergic effects (e.g., dry mouth, constipation).
- The most serious adverse effect of TCAs is cardiotoxicity, which can be lethal if an overdose is taken.
- TCAs can cause a hypertensive crisis if combined with an MAOI. Accordingly, the combination is generally avoided.
- TCAs intensify responses to direct-acting sympathomimetics (e.g., epinephrine) and diminish responses to indirect-acting sympathomimetics (e.g., amphetamine).
- MAOIs increase neuronal stores of NE and 5-HT, and thereby intensify transmission at noradrenergic and serotonergic synapses. Over time, this induces adaptive cellular responses that are ultimately responsible for relieving depression.
- MAOIs are as effective as SSRIs and TCAs, but are potentially more hazardous.
- MAOIs are first-choice drugs only for patients with atypical depression.
- Like SSRIs and SNRIs (and unlike TCAs), MAOIs cause direct CNS stimulation.
- Like TCAs (and unlike SSRIs or SNRIs), MAOIs cause orthostatic hypotension.
- Patients taking MAOIs must not eat tyramine-rich foods because hypertensive crisis can result. Hypertensive crisis can be treated with an IV vasodilator (e.g., sodium nitroprusside, labetalol, phentolamine).
- MAOIs must not be combined with indirect-acting sympathomimetics (e.g., amphetamine, cocaine) because hypertensive crisis can result.
- MAOIs must not be combined with SSRIs, SNRIs, or other serotonergic drugs because serotonin syndrome could result.
- ECT relieves depression faster than antidepressant drugs, and often helps when antidepressants have failed.
- ECT as practiced today is safer and less traumatic than in the past, owing to adjunctive use of (1) a short-acting IV anesthetic (e.g., propofol, etomidate) to produce unconsciousness and (2) a short-acting muscle relaxant (succinylcholine) to prevent convulsions.

Please visit **http://evolve.elsevier.com/Lehne** for chapter-specific NCLEX® examination review questions.

Summary of Major Nursing Implications[a]

IMPLICATIONS THAT APPLY TO ALL ANTIDEPRESSANTS

Psychologic Assessment

Observe and record the patient's behavior. Factors to assess include affect, thought content, interest in the environment, appetite, sleep patterns, and appearance.

Reducing the Risk of Suicide

Depression carries a risk of suicide, which may increase during the initial phase of antidepressant therapy or when antidepressant dosage is changed. The risk is greatest among children and young adults. **Advise family members and caregivers to monitor for symptoms of clinical decline (e.g., anxiety, agitation, panic attacks, insomnia, irritability, hostility, impulsivity, hypomania, and emergence of suicidal thoughts) and to immediately report symptoms that are severe or develop abruptly.** Arrange for the patient or caregiver to meet with the prescriber at least weekly during the first 4 weeks of treatment, then biweekly for the next 4 weeks, then once 1 month later, and periodically thereafter.

Patients who are so depressed that they are a risk to themselves and others should be hospitalized until symptoms are under control. Suicide potential should be evaluated carefully. To prevent patients from accumulating a potentially lethal supply of medication, ensure that each dose is swallowed and not "cheeked." Provide outpatients with no more than a 1-week supply of medication at a time. For patients considered at high risk of suicide, TCAs and MAOIs should be avoided; SSRIs are much safer.

Promoting Adherence

Inform the patient that antidepressant effects usually develop slowly, over 1 to 3 weeks. This knowledge will make expectations more realistic, which should help promote adherence.

Premature discontinuation of therapy can result in relapse. **Educate patients about the importance of taking their medication as prescribed, even though they may be symptom free and therefore feel "cured."** In general, treatment should continue for 4 to 9 months after symptoms resolve.

Nondrug Therapy

For patients with severe depression, treatment with drugs alone is not optimal. Emotional support and psychotherapy can complement and reinforce responses to antidepressants. ECT may be indicated for suicidal patients and for patients who fail to respond to antidepressant drugs and psychotherapy. Other options include low-dose IV ketamine, transcranial magnetic stimulation, and vagus nerve stimulation.

Evaluating Therapeutic Effects

Assess patients for improvement in symptoms, especially depressed mood and loss of interest or pleasure in usual activities.

Summary of Major Nursing Implications[a]—cont'd

SELECTIVE SEROTONIN REUPTAKE INHIBITORS

Citalopram
Escitalopram
Fluoxetine
Fluvoxamine
Paroxetine
Sertraline

SEROTONIN/NOREPINEPHRINE REUPTAKE INHIBITORS

Desvenlafaxine
Duloxetine
Levomilnacipran
Venlafaxine

In addition to the implications summarized later, see the previous discussion on *Implications That Apply to All Antidepressants*.

Preadministration Assessment

Therapeutic Goal

Alleviation of Symptoms of Major Depression. All SSRIs except fluvoxamine and all SNRIs are approved for treating depression.

Other Goals. SSRIs and SNRIs are used to relieve the symptoms of many psychologic disorders, including obsessive-compulsive disorder, panic disorder, social phobia, generalized anxiety disorder, post-traumatic stress disorder, premenstrual dysphoric disorder, chronic pain, and bulimia nervosa (see Table 32.2).

Identifying High-Risk Patients

SSRIs and SNRIs are *contraindicated* for patients taking MAOIs, and should be used with *caution* in patients taking other serotonergic drugs. Use with *caution* in patients with liver disease, in older adults, and in patients who are pregnant or breast-feeding.

Implementation: Administration

Route

Oral.

Administration

All SSRIs and SNRIs may be administered with food. Dosing in the morning minimizes sleep disruption.

Warn patients not to discontinue treatment once mood has improved, since doing so could lead to relapse.

Ongoing Evaluation and Interventions

Minimizing Adverse Effects

Suicide Risk. See *Implications That Apply to All Antidepressants.*

CNS Stimulation. *Citalopram, escitalopram, fluoxetine, paroxetine,* and *sertraline* as well as all the SNRIs can cause nervousness, insomnia, and anxiety. These reactions may respond to a decrease in dosage. (Fluvoxamine causes mild sedation.)

Serotonin Syndrome. Symptoms of this potentially fatal syndrome include agitation, confusion, disorientation, anxiety, hallucinations, poor concentration, incoordination, myoclonus, hyperreflexia, excessive sweating, tremor, and fever. The risk is reduced by avoiding concurrent use of MAOIs and certain other drugs (see later in summary under *Minimizing Adverse Interactions*). Serotonin syndrome resolves spontaneously after discontinuing the SSRI.

Sexual Dysfunction. **Inform patients about possible sexual dysfunction (anorgasmia, impotence, decreased libido), and encourage them to report problems.** Management strategies include dosage reduction, drug holidays, adding a drug to counteract sexual dysfunction (e.g., sildenafil, buspirone), and switching to an antidepressant that causes less sexual dysfunction (e.g., bupropion, nefazodone, mirtazapine).

Dizziness and Fatigue. **Inform patients about possible dizziness and fatigue when using SSRIs, and advise them to exercise caution while performing hazardous tasks (e.g., driving).**

Rash. *Fluoxetine* may cause rash. **Inform patients about the risk of rash, and instruct them to notify the prescriber if one develops.** Treatment consists of drug therapy (antihistamines, glucocorticoids) or withdrawal of fluoxetine.

Neonatal Abstinence Syndrome (NAH) and Persistent Pulmonary Hypertension of the Newborn (PPHN). Use of SSRIs late in pregnancy poses a small risk of NAS and PPHN. Newborns exposed to SSRIs *in utero* should be monitored for both disorders. If NAS occurs, it can be managed with supportive care, and generally abates within a few days. Treatment measures for PPHN include providing mechanical ventilatory support, giving inhaled nitric oxide and oxygen, and giving IV sodium acetate and dopamine.

Teratogenesis. Two SSRIs—*fluoxetine* and *paroxetine*—pose a small risk of birth defects, especially ventricular septal defects and other cardiovascular anomalies. Other SSRIs are preferred during pregnancy.

Dysrhythmias. *Citalopram* may cause severe dysrhythmias, especially when doses are too high. **Warn patients not to exceed 40 mg/day.** Use with caution in patients with dysrhythmia risk factors, including heart disease, long QT syndrome, and low blood levels of potassium or magnesium. SNRIs are noted to cause tachycardia in many patients.

GI Bleeding. SSRIs and SNRIs impair platelet aggregation and can thereby increase the risk of GI bleeding. Exercise caution in older adult patients, patients with ulcers or a history of GI bleeding, and patients taking antiplatelet drugs or anticoagulants.

Hyponatremia. SSRIs and SNRIs can cause hyponatremia, primarily in older adult patients taking diuretics. When SSRIs and diuretics are used in older adult patients, serum sodium should be measured at baseline and periodically thereafter.

Bruxism. SSRIs and SNRIs can cause bruxism (clenching and grinding of teeth), usually during sleep. **Alert patients to the sequelae of bruxism (headache, jaw pain, and dental problems, such as cracked fillings).** If these develop, investigate whether an SSRI is the cause. Bruxism can be managed by

Continued

(1) reducing the SSRI dosage (but then depression may return), (2) switching to a different class of antidepressants, (3) using a mouth guard, and (4) treating with low-dose buspirone.

Minimizing Adverse Interactions

MAOIs and Other Drugs That Increase the Risk of Serotonin Syndrome. MAOIs greatly increase the risk of serotonin syndrome, and hence should be withdrawn at least 14 days before starting an SSRI. The risk of serotonin syndrome can also be increased by other serotonergic drugs (see Table 32.4) and by tramadol (an analgesic) and linezolid (an antibiotic that inhibits MAO). Withdraw fluoxetine at least 5 weeks before starting an MAOI, and withdraw other SSRIs at least 2 weeks before starting an MAOI.

TCAs and Lithium. Fluoxetine can increase levels of these drugs. Exercise caution.

Antiplatelet Drugs and Anticoagulants. Antiplatelet drugs (e.g., aspirin, NSAIDs) and anticoagulants (e.g., warfarin) increase the risk of GI bleeding. Exercise caution.

The risk of bleeding with *warfarin* is compounded by a pharmacokinetic interaction with *fluoxetine,* which can displace warfarin from binding sites on plasma proteins, causing levels of free warfarin to rise. Monitor responses to warfarin closely.

Drugs That Are Substrates for or Inhibitors of CYP2D6. Drugs that inhibit CYP2D6 can raise levels of SSRIs and SNRIs, and can thereby pose a risk of toxicity. In addition to being substrates for CYP2D6, two SSRIs—*fluoxetine* and *paroxetine*—can *inhibit* CYP2D6 and can thereby raise levels of other drugs that are CYP2D6 substrates, including TCAs, some antipsychotics, and two antidysrhythmic drugs: propafenone and flecainide. Exercise caution.

TRICYCLIC ANTIDEPRESSANTS

Amitriptyline
Clomipramine
Desipramine
Doxepin
Imipramine
Maprotiline
Nortriptyline
Protriptyline
Trimipramine

In addition to the implications summarized later, see the previous discussion on *Implications That Apply to All Antidepressants*.

Preadministration Assessment

Therapeutic Goal

Alleviation of symptoms of major depression.

Baseline Data

Assess psychologic status. Arrange for an ECG, especially for patients with cardiac disease and those older than 40 years.

Identifying High-Risk Patients

TCAs are generally *contraindicated* for patients taking MAOIs.

Use TCAs with *caution* in patients with cardiac disorders (e.g., coronary heart disease, progressive heart failure, paroxysmal tachycardia), elevated intraocular pressure, urinary retention, hyperthyroidism, seizure disorders, and liver or kidney dysfunction.

Doxepin is *contraindicated* for patients with glaucoma or a tendency to urinary retention.

Maprotiline is *contraindicated* for patients with seizure disorders.

Implementation: Administration

Route

Oral.

Administration

Instruct patients to take medication daily as prescribed and not PRN. Warn patients not to discontinue treatment once mood has improved, since doing so may result in relapse. Once an effective dosage has been established, the entire daily dose can usually be taken at bedtime.

Ongoing Evaluation and Interventions

Minimizing Adverse Effects

Suicide Risk. See *Implications That Apply to All Antidepressants.*

Orthostatic Hypotension. **Inform patients about symptoms of hypotension (dizziness, light-headedness), and advise them to sit or lie down if these occur. Inform patients that hypotension can be minimized by moving slowly when assuming an erect posture.** For hospitalized patients, monitor blood pressure and pulse rate on a regular schedule; take measurements while the patient is lying down and again after the patient has been sitting or standing for 1 to 2 minutes. If blood pressure is low or pulse rate is high, withhold medication and inform the prescriber.

Anticholinergic Effects. **Inform patients about possible anticholinergic effects (dry mouth, blurred vision, photophobia, urinary hesitancy, constipation, tachycardia), and advise them to notify the prescriber if these are troublesome.** A detailed summary of nursing implications for anticholinergic drugs is presented in Chapter 14.

Diaphoresis. TCAs promote sweating (despite their anticholinergic properties). Excessive sweating may necessitate frequent changes of bedding and clothing.

Sedation. Sedation is most intense during the first weeks of therapy and declines with continued drug use. **Advise patients to avoid hazardous activities (e.g., driving, operating dangerous machinery) if sedation is significant.** Giving TCAs at bedtime minimizes daytime sedation and promotes sleep.

Cardiotoxicity. TCAs can disrupt cardiac function, but usually only when taken in excessive doses or by patients with heart disease. All patients should receive an ECG before treatment and periodically thereafter. Risk of cardiac toxicity may be higher with *desipramine* than with other TCAs.

Seizures. TCAs decrease seizure threshold. Exercise caution in patients with seizure disorders.

Hypomania. TCAs may shift mood from depression up to hypomania. If hypomania develops, the patient must be evaluated to determine whether elation is drug induced or indicates bipolar disorder.

Minimizing Adverse Interactions

MAO Inhibitors. Rarely, the combination of a TCA and an MAOI has produced hypertensive episodes and hypertensive crisis. Exercise caution if this combination is employed.

Sympathomimetic Agents. TCAs decrease the effects of indirect-acting sympathomimetics (e.g., ephedrine, amphetamine), but potentiate the actions of direct-acting sympathomimetics (e.g., epinephrine, dopamine). If sympathomimetics are to be used, these effects must be accounted for.

Anticholinergic Agents. Drugs capable of blocking muscarinic receptors will enhance the anticholinergic effects of TCAs. **Warn patients against concurrent use of other anticholinergic drugs (e.g., scopolamine, antihistamines, phenothiazines).**

CNS Depressants. These will enhance the depressant effects of TCAs. **Warn patients against using alcohol and all other drugs with CNS-depressant properties (e.g., opioids, antihistamines, barbiturates, benzodiazepines).**

MONOAMINE OXIDASE INHIBITORS

Isocarboxazid
Phenelzine
Selegiline
Tranylcypromine

In addition to the implications summarized later, see the previous discussion on *Implications That Apply to All Antidepressants*.

Preadministration Assessment

Therapeutic Goal

Alleviation of symptoms of major depression, especially atypical depression.

Identifying High-Risk Patients

MAOIs are *contraindicated* for patients taking SSRIs; for patients with pheochromocytoma, heart failure, liver disease, severe renal impairment, cerebrovascular defect (known or suspected), cardiovascular disease, and hypertension; and for patients older than 60 years (because of possible cerebral sclerosis associated with vessel damage).

Use with *caution* in patients taking serotonergic drugs.

Implementation: Administration

Routes

Oral. Isocarboxazid, phenelzine, tranylcypromine.

Transdermal. Selegiline.

Administration

All MAOIs. **Instruct patients to take MAOIs every day as prescribed—not PRN. Warn patients not to discontinue treatment once mood has improved, since doing so may result in relapse.**

Transdermal Selegiline. **Instruct patients to apply the Emsam patch to dry intact skin of the upper torso, upper thigh, or outer surface of the upper arm once every 24 hours.**

Ongoing Evaluation and Interventions

Minimizing Adverse Effects

Suicide Risk. See *Implications That Apply to All Antidepressants.*

Hypertensive Crisis. Dietary tyramine, certain other dietary constituents (see Table 32.6), and indirect-acting sympathomimetics (e.g., amphetamine, methylphenidate, ephedrine, cocaine) can precipitate a hypertensive crisis in patients taking MAOIs.

Inform patients about symptoms of hypertensive crisis—severe headache, tachycardia, hypertension, nausea, vomiting, confusion, and profuse sweating—and instruct them to seek immediate medical attention if these develop.

To reduce the risk of hypertensive crisis, the following precautions must be observed:

- Do not give MAOIs to patients who are suicidal or who are considered incapable of rigid adherence to dietary constraints.
- **Forewarn patients about the hazard of hypertensive crisis and the need to avoid tyramine-rich foods and sympathomimetic drugs.** (Patients on low-dose transdermal selegiline needn't avoid tyramine-containing foods, but do need to avoid sympathomimetic drugs.)
- **Provide patients with a list of specific foods to avoid (see Table 32.6).**
- **Instruct patients to avoid all drugs not approved by the prescriber.**

If hypertensive crisis develops, blood pressure can be lowered with an IV vasodilator, such as sodium nitroprusside, labetalol, or phentolamine.

Orthostatic Hypotension. **Inform patients about signs of hypotension (dizziness, light-headedness), and advise them to sit or lie down if these occur. Inform patients that hypotension can be minimized by moving slowly when standing up.** For the hospitalized patient, monitor blood pressure and pulse rate on a regular schedule. Take these measurements while the patient is lying down and again after the patient has been sitting or standing for 1 to 2 minutes. If blood pressure is low, withhold medication and inform the prescriber.

Skin Rash. Application-site rash is common with transdermal selegiline, and can be managed with a topical glucocorticoid.

Minimizing Adverse Interactions

All Drugs. MAOIs can interact adversely with many other drugs. **Instruct the patient to avoid all medications—prescription and nonprescription—that have not been specifically approved by the prescriber.**

Indirect-Acting Sympathomimetics. Concurrent use with MAOIs can precipitate a hypertensive crisis. **Warn patients against use of any indirect-acting sympathomimetics (e.g., ephedrine, methylphenidate, amphetamines, cocaine).**

Tricyclic Antidepressants. Concurrent use with MAOIs can produce hypertensive episodes and hypertensive crisis. Use this combination with caution.

Serotonergic Drugs. Combining MAOIs with other serotonergic drugs (see Table 32.4) poses a risk of serotonin syndrome. Accordingly, these combinations should generally be avoided.

Antihypertensive Drugs. These drugs will potentiate the hypotensive effects of MAOIs. If these agents are combined, monitor blood pressure periodically.

Meperidine. Meperidine can produce hyperthermia in patients taking MAOIs and hence should be avoided.

[a]Patient education information is highlighted as **blue text.**

CHAPTER

33 Drugs for Bipolar Disorder

Our topic for this chapter is *bipolar disorder* (BPD). The disease afflicts an estimated 4.4% of the adult population—more than 6.7 million Americans. The mainstays of long-term therapy are lithium and divalproex sodium (valproate), drugs that can stabilize mood. Many patients also receive an antipsychotic agent, and some may require an antidepressant. BPD is a chronic condition that requires lifelong treatment.

CHARACTERISTICS OF BIPOLAR DISORDER

BPD is a severe biologic illness characterized by recurrent fluctuations in mood. Typically, patients experience alternating episodes in which mood is abnormally elevated or abnormally depressed—separated by periods in which mood is relatively normal. Symptoms usually begin in adolescence or early adulthood, but can occur before adolescence or as late as the fifth decade of life. In the absence of treatment, episodes of mania or depression generally persist for several months. As time passes, manic and depressive episodes tend to recur more frequently. Although the precise etiology of BPD is unknown, it is clear that symptoms are caused by altered brain physiology—not by a character flaw or an unstable personality.

Types of Mood Episodes Seen in Bipolar Disorder

Patients with BPD may experience four types of mood episodes: pure manic, hypomanic, major depressive, and mixed.

Pure Manic Episode (Euphoric Mania)

Manic episodes are characterized by persistently heightened, expansive, or irritable mood—typically associated with hyperactivity, excessive enthusiasm, and flight of ideas. Manic individuals display overactivity at work and at play and have a reduced need for sleep. Mania produces excessive sociability and talkativeness. Extreme self-confidence, grandiose ideas, and delusions of self-importance are common. Manic individuals often indulge in high-risk activities (e.g., questionable business deals, reckless driving, gambling, sexual indiscretions), giving no forethought to the consequences. In severe cases, symptoms may resemble those of paranoid schizophrenia (hallucinations, delusions, bizarre behavior).

Hypomanic Episode (Hypomania)

Hypomania can be viewed as a mild form of mania. As in mania, mood is persistently elevated, expansive, or irritable. However, symptoms are not severe enough to cause marked impairment in social or occupational functioning, or to require hospitalization. Psychotic symptoms are absent.

Major Depressive Episode (Depression)

A major depressive episode is characterized by depressed mood and loss of pleasure or interest in all or nearly all of one's usual activities and pastimes. Associated symptoms include disruption of sleeping and eating patterns; difficulty in concentrating; feelings of guilt, worthlessness, and helplessness; and thoughts of death and suicide. The characteristics of major depression are discussed further in Chapter 32.

Mixed Episode

In a true mixed episode, patients experience symptoms of mania and depression simultaneously. Patients may be agitated and irritable (as in mania), but may also feel worthless and depressed. The combination of high energy and depression puts them at significant risk of suicide.

Patterns of Mood Episodes

Among people with BPD, mood episodes can occur in a variety of patterns. Contrary to popular belief, not all patients alternate repeatedly between mania and depression. Some experience repeated episodes of mania, and some experience repeated episodes of depression (with an occasional episode of mania). Mood may be normal between episodes of mania and depression, or it may be slightly elevated (hypomania) or slightly depressed (dysphoria).

Mood episodes can vary greatly with respect to how often they occur and how long they last. A single episode may last for days, weeks, months, or more than a year. In the absence of treatment, episodes of mania or hypomania typically last a few months, whereas episodes of major depression typically last at least 6 months. On average, people with BPD experience only four episodes during the first 10 years of their illness. However, some people cycle much more rapidly, experiencing many episodes every year.

On the basis of mood episode type and frequency, BPD can be subdivided into two major categories:

- *Bipolar I Disorder*—Patients experience manic or mixed episodes and usually depressive episodes too.
- *Bipolar II Disorder*—Patients experience hypomanic or depressive episodes, but not manic or mixed episodes.

Etiology

Theories regarding the etiology of BPD continue to evolve. In the past, there was general agreement that BPD was due primarily to an imbalance in neurotransmitters. Today, researchers suspect the real cause may be disruption of neuronal growth and survival. First, neuroimaging studies have shown an association between prolonged mood disorders and atrophy of specific brain regions—especially the subgenual prefrontal cortex, an area involved in emotionality. Second, mood-stabilizing drugs can prevent or reverse neuronal atrophy in patients with BPD, apparently by influencing signaling pathways that regulate neuronal growth and survival.

Prototype Drugs

MOOD-STABILIZING DRUGS FOR BIPOLAR DISORDER

Lithium
Valproic acid
Carbamazepine

TREATMENT OF BIPOLAR DISORDER

Drug Therapy

Types of Drugs Employed

BPD is treated with three major groups of drugs: mood stabilizers, antipsychotics, and antidepressants. In addition, benzodiazepines are frequently used for sedation.

Mood Stabilizers. Mood stabilizers are drugs that (1) relieve symptoms during manic and depressive episodes, (2) prevent recurrence of manic and depressive episodes, and (3) do not worsen symptoms of mania or depression or accelerate the rate of cycling. The principal mood stabilizers are *lithium* and two drugs originally developed for epilepsy: *divalproex sodium* (valproate) and *carbamazepine.* These drugs are the mainstays of treatment. The pharmacology of lithium and the antiepileptic drugs is discussed later in the chapter.

Antipsychotics. In patients with BPD, antipsychotic drugs are given to help control symptoms during severe manic episodes, even if psychotic symptoms are absent. Although antipsychotics can be used alone, they are usually employed in combination with a mood stabilizer. For reasons discussed later in this chapter, the second-generation antipsychotics (e.g., olanzapine, risperidone) are generally preferred to the first-generation agents (e.g., haloperidol).

Antidepressants. Antidepressants may be needed during a depressive episode. However, in patients with BPD, antidepressants are almost always combined with a mood stabilizer because of the long-held belief that when used alone, antidepressants may elevate mood so much that a hypomanic or manic episode will result. However, data indicate that the risk of inducing mania may be much lower than previously thought. Nonetheless, until the issue is fully resolved, it would seem prudent to continue the traditional practice of using an antidepressant only if a mood stabilizer is being used as well.

Although antidepressants have been studied extensively in patients with major depression, very little research has been done in patients with BPD. As a result, we lack reliable information on which to base drug selection. Even so, experts do have their preferences. Among clinicians with extensive experience in BPD, the following are considered antidepressants of choice: *bupropion* [Wellbutrin], *venlafaxine* [Effexor XR], and the *selective serotonin reuptake inhibitors* (SSRIs), such as fluoxetine [Prozac] and sertraline [Zoloft]. The pharmacology of these drugs is discussed in Chapter 32.

Drug Selection

Acute Therapy: Manic Episodes. Two mood stabilizers—lithium and valproate—are preferred drugs for acute management of manic episodes in combination with a second-generation (atypical) antipsychotic medication. Lithium is the drug of choice. If the patient does not respond adequately to lithium or valproate alone, the drugs may be used together. Responses to mood stabilizers develop slowly, taking 2 or more weeks to become maximal.

Seven second-generation antipsychotic medications are approved for the management of acute manic or mixed episodes occurring in bipolar depression. These medications are often used for short-term management of severe mania as adjunctive therapy to the mood stabilizers. Table 33.1 lists common dosages for treatment.

If needed for episodes of severe mania, a benzodiazepine (e.g., lorazepam [Ativan]) may be added to the regimen for acute management of symptoms (insomnia, anxiety, agitation). For patients with hypoactive mania an antipsychotic may be employed as monotherapy; olanzapine or risperidone would be a good choice.

Acute Therapy: Depressive Episodes. Depressive episodes may be treated with a mood stabilizer, an atypical antipsychotic, or with a mood stabilizer or antipsychotic *plus* an antidepressant—but rarely with an antidepressant alone (because hypomania or mania might result). If depression is mild, monotherapy with a mood stabilizer (lithium or valproate) may be sufficient. If the mood stabilizer is inadequate, an antidepressant or antipsychotic can be added. Benefits may be limited with the addition of an antidepressant. Preferred antidepressants are bupropion, venlafaxine, or an SSRI (fluoxetine). There is even a combination drug that consists of an atypical antipsychotic and an SSRI specifically designed for this purpose (see Table 33.1).

Long-Term Preventive Treatment. The purpose of long-term therapy is to prevent recurrence of both mania and depression. As a rule, one or more mood stabilizers are employed. Drug selection is based on what worked acutely. For example, if the patient responded to acute therapy with lithium alone, then lithium alone should be tried long term. Other long-term options include valproate alone, and valproate plus lithium. More recently, antipsychotic agents have been employed for long-term maintenance, either as monotherapy or in combination with a mood stabilizer.

TABLE 33.1 ▪ Adult Oral Dosages for Atypical Antipsychotics Used in Bipolar Disorder

Drug	Dosage
Aripiprazole [Abilify]	*Acute Mania:* Start with 15 mg once daily and increase to 30 mg once daily if needed. Do not exceed 30 mg daily.
Asenapine [Saphris]	*Acute Mania/Mixed Episode:* Start with 10 mg daily and increase to 20 mg once daily if needed.
Cariprazine [Vraylar]	*Acute Mania/Mixed Episode:* Start with 1.5 mg on day 1. Increase to 3 mg daily on day 2. May adjust in 1.5–3 mg increments, as indicated. Do not exceed 6 mg daily.
Lurasidone [Latuda]	*Depressive Episodes:* Start with 20 mg daily. May increase as indicated to a maximum of 120 mg daily. Doses of >80 mg daily may not show additional benefit when compared to side effects.
Olanzapine [Zyprexa]	*Acute Mania:* Start with 10–15 mg once daily. Increase in 5-mg/day increments, as indicated. The effective range is 5–20 mg once daily. *Maintenance Therapy:* The effective range is 5–20 mg once daily.
Olanzapine/fluoxetine [Symbyax]	*Depressive Episodes:* Start with 6 mg olanzapine/25 mg fluoxetine once daily in the evening. The effective range for antidepressant effects is olanzapine 6–12 mg and fluoxetine 25–50 mg.
Quetiapine [Seroquel]	*Acute Mania (with normal liver function):* Give in two divided doses as follows: 100 mg on day 1, 200 mg on day 2, 300 mg on day 3, and 400 mg on day 4. If needed, increase to 600 mg on day 5 and 800 mg on day 6. *Acute Mania (with liver impairment):* Give 25 mg on day 1, then increase by 25–50 mg/day until symptoms are controlled or side effects are intolerable, whichever comes first. *Depressive Episodes:* Give once-daily doses at bedtime as follows: 50 mg on day 1, 100 mg on day 2, 200 mg on day 3, and 300 mg on day 4; if needed, increase to 400 mg on day 5, and 600 mg on day 8.
Risperidone, short-acting [Risperdal]	*Acute Mania:* Start with 2–3 mg once daily; increase to a maximum of 6 mg once daily, if needed.
Risperidone, long-acting [Risperdal Consta]	*Maintenance Therapy:* Start with 25 mg IM every 2 weeks. After at least 4 weeks, dosage may be increased to 37.5 mg IM every 2 weeks, and after at least 4 more weeks, increased again to 50 mg IM every 2 weeks.
Ziprasidone [Geodon]	*Acute Mania:* On day 1, give 80 mg (in two divided doses with food). On day 2, increase to 60 or 80 mg twice daily. Based on tolerability and efficacy, adjust dosage within the range of 40–80 mg twice daily. *Maintenance Therapy:* The effective range is 15–30 mg daily.

Promoting Adherence

Poor patient adherence can frustrate attempts to treat a manic episode. Patients may resist treatment because they fail to see anything wrong with their thinking or behavior. Furthermore, the experience is not necessarily unpleasant. In fact, individuals going through a manic episode may well enjoy it. As a result, to ensure adherence, short-term hospitalization may be required. To achieve this, collaboration with the patient's family may be needed. Since hospitalization per se won't guarantee success, lithium administration should be directly observed to ensure that each dose is actually taken.

After an acute manic episode has been controlled, long-term prophylactic therapy is indicated, making adherence an ongoing issue. To promote adherence, the patient and family should be educated about the nature of BPD and the importance of taking medication as prescribed. Family members can help ensure adherence by overseeing medication use and by urging the patient to visit his or her prescriber or a psychiatric clinic if a pattern of nonadherence develops.

Nondrug Therapy

Education and Psychotherapy

Ideally, BPD should be treated with a combination of drugs and adjunctive psychotherapy (individual, group, or family); drug therapy alone is not optimal. BPD is a chronic illness that requires supportive therapy and education for the patient and family. Counseling can help patients cope with the sequelae of manic episodes, such as strained relationships, reduced self-confidence, and a sense of shame regarding uncontrolled behavior. Certain life stresses (e.g., moving, job loss, bereavement, childbirth) can precipitate a mood change. Therapy can help reduce the destabilizing impact of these events. Patients should be taught to recognize early symptoms of mood change and encouraged to contact their primary clinician immediately if these develop. Additional measures by which patients can help themselves include the following:

- Maintaining a stable sleep pattern.
- Maintaining a regular pattern of activity.
- Avoiding alcohol and psychoactive street drugs.
- Enlisting the support of family and friends.
- Taking steps to reduce stress at work.
- Keeping a mood chart to monitor progress.

Electroconvulsive Therapy

Electroconvulsive therapy (ECT) is an effective intervention that can be lifesaving in patients with severe mania or severe depression. However, ECT is not a treatment of first choice. It should be reserved for patients who have not responded adequately to drugs. Candidates for ECT include patients with psychotic depression, severe nonpsychotic depression, severe mania, and rapid-cycling BPD. Details of ECT are discussed in Chapter 32.

MOOD-STABILIZING DRUGS

As noted, mood stabilizers are drugs that can relieve an acute manic or depressive episode and can prevent symptoms from recurring—all without aggravating mania or depression, and without accelerating cycling. The agents used most often are lithium, valproate, and carbamazepine.

Lithium

Lithium [Lithobid, Carbolith ♣] can stabilize mood in patients with BPD. Beneficial effects were first described in 1949 by psychiatrist John Cade of Australia. Because of concerns about toxicity, lithium was not approved for use in the United States until 1970. Lithium has a low therapeutic index. As a result, toxicity can occur at blood levels only slightly greater than therapeutic levels. Accordingly, monitoring lithium levels is mandatory.

Chemistry

Lithium is a simple inorganic ion that carries a single positive charge. In the periodic table of elements, lithium is in the same group as potassium and sodium. Not surprisingly, lithium has properties in common with both elements. Lithium is found naturally in animal tissues but has no known physiologic function.

Therapeutic Uses

Lithium is a drug of choice for controlling acute manic episodes in patients with BPD and for long-term prophylaxis against recurrence of mania or depression. In manic patients, lithium reduces euphoria, hyperactivity, and other symptoms but does not cause sedation. Antimanic effects begin 5 to 7 days after treatment onset, but full benefits may not develop for 2 to 3 weeks. Lithium is considered the drug of choice for all patients experiencing an acute manic episode, regardless of clinical presentation.

Mechanism of Action

Although lithium has been studied extensively, the precise mechanism by which it stabilizes mood is unknown. In the past, research focused on three aspects of brain neurochemistry: (1) altered distribution of certain ions (calcium, sodium, magnesium) that are critical to neuronal function; (2) altered synthesis and release of norepinephrine, serotonin, and dopamine; and (3) effects on second messengers (e.g., cyclic AMP, phosphatidylinositol), which mediate intracellular responses to neurotransmitters. Unfortunately, this research has failed to provide a definitive explanation of how lithium works. Current neurochemical research suggests that lithium may work by (1) altering glutamate uptake and release, (2) blocking the binding of serotonin to its receptors, and/or (3) inhibiting glycogen synthase kinase-3 beta.

There has been growing interest in the neurotrophic and neuroprotective actions of lithium. As noted previously, there is evidence that symptoms of BPD may result from neuronal atrophy in certain brain areas. In animal studies, "therapeutic" doses of lithium doubled the level of neurotrophic Bcl-2 proteins. In addition, lithium has been shown to facilitate the regeneration of damaged optic nerves. In patients with BPD taking lithium long term, the volume of the subgenual prefrontal cortex is greater than in untreated patients. Furthermore, lithium can increase total gray matter in regions known to atrophy in BPD, including the prefrontal cortex, hippocampus, and caudate nucleus. All of these studies suggest that the benefits of lithium may result at least in part from an ability to protect against neuronal atrophy and/or promote neuronal growth.

Pharmacokinetics

Absorption and Distribution. Lithium is well absorbed following oral administration. The drug distributes evenly to all tissues and body fluids.

Excretion. Lithium has a short half-life owing to rapid renal excretion. Because of its short half-life (and high toxicity), the drug must be administered in divided daily doses. Large single daily doses cannot be used, even when a slow-release preparation is prescribed. Because lithium is excreted by the kidneys, it must be employed with great care in patients with renal impairment.

Renal excretion of lithium is affected by blood levels of sodium. Specifically, lithium excretion is *reduced* when levels of sodium are *low* because the kidney processes lithium and sodium in the same way. Hence, when the kidney senses that sodium levels are inadequate, it retains lithium in an attempt to compensate. Because of this relationship, in the presence of low sodium, lithium can accumulate to toxic levels. Accordingly, it is important that sodium levels remain normal. Patients should be instructed to maintain normal sodium intake. Obviously, a sodium-free diet cannot be used. Because diuretics promote sodium loss, these agents must be employed with caution. Also, sodium loss secondary to diarrhea can be sufficient to cause lithium accumulation. The patient should be told about this possibility.

Dehydration will cause lithium retention by the kidneys, posing the risk of accumulation to dangerous levels. Potential causes of dehydration include hot weather and diarrhea. Counsel patients to maintain adequate hydration.

Monitoring Plasma Lithium Levels. Measurement of plasma lithium levels is an essential component of treatment. *Lithium levels must be kept below 1.5 mEq/L; levels greater than this can produce significant toxicity.* Lithium levels should range from 0.4 to 1 mEq/L. Generally, levels are desired between 0.6 and 0.8 mEq/L. Levels of 0.8 to 1 mEq/L may be more effective, but carry greater risk of adverse effects. Blood for lithium determinations should be drawn in the morning, 12 hours after the evening dose. During maintenance therapy, lithium levels should be measured every 3 to 6 months.

Adverse Effects

The adverse effects of lithium can be divided into two categories: (1) effects that occur at excessive lithium levels and (2) effects that occur at therapeutic lithium levels. In the discussion that follows, adverse effects produced at excessive lithium levels are considered as a group. Effects produced at therapeutic levels are considered individually.

Adverse Effects That Occur When Lithium Levels Are Excessive. Certain toxicities are closely correlated with the concentration of lithium in blood. As indicated in Table 33.2, mild responses (e.g., fine hand tremor, GI upset, thirst, muscle weakness) can develop at lithium levels that are still within the therapeutic range (i.e., below 1.5 mEq/L). When plasma levels exceed 1.5 mEq/L, more serious toxicities appear. At drug levels above 2.5 mEq/L, death can occur. Patients should

TABLE 33.2 ▪ Toxicities Associated With Excessive Plasma Level of Lithium

Plasma Lithium Level (mEq/L)	Signs of Toxicity
Below 1.5	Nausea, vomiting, diarrhea, thirst, polyuria, lethargy, slurred speech, muscle weakness, fine hand tremor
1.5–2	Persistent GI upset, coarse hand tremor, confusion, hyperirritability of muscles, ECG changes, sedation, incoordination
2–2.5	Ataxia, giddiness, high output of dilute urine, serious ECG changes, fasciculations, tinnitus, blurred vision, clonic movements, seizures, stupor, severe hypotension, coma, death (usually secondary to pulmonary complications)
Above 2.5	Symptoms may progress rapidly to generalized convulsions, oliguria, and death

ECG, Electrocardiogram; *GI,* gastrointestinal.

be informed about early signs of toxicity and instructed to interrupt lithium dosing if these appear. In adherent patients, the most common cause of lithium accumulation is sodium depletion.

To keep lithium levels within the therapeutic range, plasma drug levels should be monitored routinely. Levels should be measured every 2 to 3 days at the beginning of treatment and every 3 to 6 months during maintenance therapy.

Treatment of acute overdose is primarily supportive; there is no specific antidote. The severely intoxicated patient should be hospitalized. Hemodialysis is an effective means of lithium removal and should be considered whenever drug levels exceed 2.5 mEq/L.

Adverse Effects That Occur at Therapeutic Levels of Lithium

Early Adverse Effects. Several responses occur early in treatment and then usually subside. *Gastrointestinal effects* (e.g., nausea, diarrhea, abdominal bloating, anorexia) are common but transient. About 30% of patients experience *transient fatigue, muscle weakness, headache, confusion,* and *memory impairment. Polyuria* and *thirst* occur in 30% to 50% of patients and may persist.

Tremor. Patients may develop a fine hand tremor, especially in the fingers, that can interfere with writing and other motor skills. Lithium-induced tremor can be augmented by stress, fatigue, and certain drugs (antidepressants, antipsychotics, caffeine). Tremor can be reduced with a beta blocker (e.g., propranolol) and by measures that reduce peak levels of lithium (i.e., dosage reduction, the use of divided doses, or the use of a sustained-release formulation).

Polyuria. Polyuria occurs in 50% to 70% of patients taking lithium chronically. In some patients, daily urine output may exceed 3 L. Lithium promotes polyuria by antagonizing the effects of antidiuretic hormone. To maintain adequate hydration, patients should be instructed to drink 8 to 12 glasses of fluids daily. Polyuria, nocturia, and excessive thirst can discourage patients from adhering to the regimen.

Lithium-induced polyuria can be reduced with *amiloride* [Midamor], a potassium-sparing diuretic. Amiloride appears to help by reducing the entry of lithium into epithelial cells of the renal tubule. Polyuria can also be reduced with a thiazide diuretic. However, because thiazides can lower levels of sodium (see Chapter 41), and would thereby increase lithium retention, amiloride is preferred.

Renal Toxicity. Chronic lithium use has been associated with degenerative changes in the kidney. The risk of renal injury can be reduced by keeping the dosage low and, when possible, avoiding long-term lithium therapy. Kidney function should be assessed before treatment and once a year thereafter.

Goiter and Hypothyroidism. Lithium can reduce incorporation of iodine into thyroid hormone and can inhibit thyroid hormone secretion. With long-term use, the drug can cause *goiter* (enlargement of the thyroid gland). Although usually benign, lithium-induced goiter is sometimes associated with *hypothyroidism.* Treatment with thyroid hormone (levothyroxine) or withdrawal of lithium will reverse both goiter and hypothyroidism. Levels of thyroid hormones—triiodothyronine (T_3) and thyroxine (T_4)—and levels of thyroid-stimulating hormone (TSH) should be measured before giving lithium and annually thereafter.

Teratogenesis. Lithium may—or may not—be a teratogen. In older studies, lithium appeared to have significant teratogenic effects: Drug use during the first trimester of pregnancy was associated with an 11% incidence of birth defects (usually malformations of the heart). However, in more recent studies, lithium showed little or no teratogenic potential. Nonetheless, lithium is still classified in U.S. Food and Drug Administration Pregnancy Risk Category D.[a] To minimize any potential fetal risk, *lithium should be avoided during the first trimester of pregnancy,* and unless the benefits of therapy clearly outweigh the risks, it should be avoided during the remainder of pregnancy as well. Women of childbearing age should be counseled to avoid pregnancy while taking lithium. Also, pregnancy should be ruled out before initiating lithium therapy.

Use in Lactation. Lithium readily enters breast milk and can achieve concentrations that might harm the nursing infant. Consequently, breast-feeding during lithium therapy should be discouraged.

Other Side Effects. Lithium can cause mild, reversible *leukocytosis* (10,000 to 18,000 white blood cells/mm^3); complete blood counts with a differential should be obtained before treatment and annually thereafter. Possible *dermatologic reactions* include psoriasis, acne, folliculitis, and alopecia.

Drug Interactions

Diuretics. Diuretics promote sodium loss and can thereby increase the risk of lithium toxicity. Toxicity can occur because in the presence of low sodium renal excretion of lithium is reduced, causing lithium levels to rise.

Nonsteroidal Anti-Inflammatory Drugs (NSAIDs). NSAIDs can increase lithium levels by as much as 60%. By suppressing prostaglandin synthesis in the kidney, NSAIDs can increase renal reabsorption of lithium (and also sodium), causing lithium levels to rise. NSAIDs known to increase lithium levels include ibuprofen [Motrin, others], naproxen [Naprosyn],

[a]As of 2020, the FDA will no longer use Pregnancy Risk Categories. Please refer to Chapter 9 for more information.

TABLE 33.3 ▪ Lithium Preparations

Formulation	Lithium Content[a]	Brand Name
Capsules	4.06 mEq lithium (150 mg Li_2CO_3)	Generic only
	8.12 mEq lithium (300 mg Li_2CO_3)	Carbolith ♣
	16.24 mEq lithium (600 mg Li_2CO_3)	Generic only
Oral solution	Lithium citrate 8 mEq/5 mL (300 mg Li_2CO_3)	Generic only
Tablets: immediate-release	8.12 mEq lithium (300 and 450 mg Li_2CO_3)	Generic only
Tablets: slow-release	8.12 mEq lithium (300 and 450 mg Li_2CO_3)	Lithobid

[a]Lithium content is expressed in two ways: milliequivalents (mEq) of lithium ion and milligrams (mg) of lithium carbonate.

piroxicam [Feldene], indomethacin [Indocin], and celecoxib [Celebrex]. Interestingly, aspirin (the prototype NSAID) and sulindac [Clinoril] do *not* increase lithium levels. Accordingly, if a mild analgesic is needed, aspirin or sulindac would be a good choice.

Anticholinergic Drugs. Anticholinergics can cause urinary hesitancy. Coupled with lithium-induced polyuria, this can result in considerable discomfort. Accordingly, patients should avoid drugs with prominent anticholinergic actions (e.g., antihistamines, phenothiazine antipsychotics, tricyclic antidepressants).

Preparations, Dosage, and Administration

Preparations and Administration. *Lithium carbonate* is supplied in capsules, standard tablets, and slow-release tablets (Table 33.3). *Lithium citrate* syrup is also available in a solution of 8 mEq/5 mL. Gastric upset can be reduced by administering lithium with meals or milk.

Dosing. Lithium dosing is highly individualized. Dosage adjustments are based on plasma drug levels and clinical response.

Plasma levels should be kept within the therapeutic range. Lithium levels should range from 0.4 to 1 mEq/L. (Levels of 0.6 to 0.8 mEq/L are effective for most patients.) To avoid serious toxicity, *lithium levels should not exceed 1.5 mEq/L.*

Knowledge of plasma drug levels is not the only guide to lithium dosing; the clinical response is at least as important. Accordingly, when evaluating lithium dosage, we must not forget to look at the patient. Laboratory tests are all well and good, but they are not a substitute for clinical assessment. For example, if blood levels of lithium appear proper but clinical evaluation indicates toxicity, there is no question as to what should be done: Reduce the dosage—despite the apparent acceptability of the dosage as reflected by plasma lithium levels.

Because of its short half-life and low therapeutic index, *lithium cannot be administered in a single daily dose.* With once-a-day dosing, peak levels would be excessive. Hence, a typical dosage is 300 mg taken 3 or 4 times a day. A dosage of 600 mg twice a day is acceptable, provided a slow-release formulation is employed. However, even these preparations cannot be given once daily.

Antiepileptic Drugs

Three antiepileptic drugs—divalproex sodium, carbamazepine, and lamotrigine—can suppress mania and/or depression and stabilize mood in patients with BPD. The efficacy of these agents is firmly established. In fact, one drug—divalproex sodium—is so effective that it has replaced lithium as the drug of choice for many patients. The basic pharmacology of the antiepileptic drugs and their use in seizure disorders are discussed in Chapter 24. Discussion here focuses on their use in BPD.

Divalproex Sodium (Valproate)

Divalproex sodium[b] [Depakote, Epival ♣], or simply valproate, was the first antiseizure agent approved for BPD. Valproate can control symptoms in acute manic episodes and can help prevent relapse into mania. However, the drug is less effective at treatment and prevention of depressive episodes. As with lithium, benefits appear to result at least in part from neurotrophic and neuroprotective effects. In patients with BPD, valproate compares favorably with lithium: both drugs are highly effective, and valproate works faster and has a higher therapeutic index and a more desirable side effect profile. However, lithium *is* superior in two important respects. First, lithium is better at reducing the risk of suicide. Second, lithium is more effective at preventing relapses. Nonetheless, because of its rapid onset, safety, and overall efficacy, valproate has become a first-line treatment for BPD. The starting dosage for acute mania in adults is 250 mg 3 times a day or 500 mg once daily at bedtime. Typical maintenance dosages range from 1000 to 2500 mg/day. The target trough plasma level is 50 to 120 mcg/mL.

Although valproate has a higher therapeutic index than lithium and is generally better tolerated, it *can* cause serious toxicity. Of greatest concern are rare cases of thrombocytopenia, pancreatitis, and liver failure—all of which require immediate drug withdrawal. In addition, valproate is a teratogen, and hence should not be used during pregnancy. Gastrointestinal disturbances (nausea, vomiting, diarrhea, dyspepsia, indigestion) are common. Despite causing GI distress, valproate frequently causes weight gain, a serious and chronic complication of treatment.

Carbamazepine

Carbamazepine [Tegretol, Equetro] is approved for treatment and prevention of manic episodes in patients with BPD. Like valproate, carbamazepine appears less effective at treatment and prevention of depression. For treatment of acute manic episodes, the dosage should be low initially (200 mg twice daily) and then gradually increased. The maximum dosage is 1600 mg/day. The target trough plasma level is 4 to 12 mcg/mL. Neurologic side effects (visual disturbances, ataxia, vertigo, unsteadiness, headache) are common early in treatment, but generally resolve despite continued drug use. Hematologic effects (leukopenia, anemia, thrombocytopenia, aplastic anemia) are relatively uncommon, but can be severe. Accordingly, complete blood counts, including platelets, should be obtained at baseline and periodically thereafter. Carbamazepine induces

[b]As discussed in Chapter 24, divalproex sodium [Depakote] is a mixture of valproic acid [Depakene, Depacon] and its sodium salt (sodium valproate). Only divalproex sodium is approved for BPD, although all three preparations have identical actions.

cytochrome P450 isoenzymes and can thereby accelerate its own metabolism and the metabolism of other drugs (e.g., oral contraceptives, warfarin, valproate, tricyclic antidepressants). To maintain efficacy, dosages of carbamazepine and these other drugs should be increased as needed.

Drug products containing carbamazepine are available under four brand names: *Carbatrol, Equetro, Epitol,* and *Tegretol.* Carbamazepine formulations with any of these names can be used for BPD. However, only one product—Equetro—is actually *approved* for BPD.

Lamotrigine

Lamotrigine [Lamictal] is indicated for long-term maintenance therapy of BPD. The goal is to prevent affective relapses into mania or depression. Lamotrigine may be used alone or in combination with other mood-stabilizing agents. Side effects include headache, dizziness, double vision, and, rarely, life-threatening rashes (Stevens-Johnson syndrome, toxic epidermal necrolysis). To minimize the risk of serious rash, dosage should be low initially (25 to 50 mg/day) and then gradually increased. The target maintenance dosage is 200 mg/day (if used alone), 100 mg/day (if combined with valproate), or 400 mg/day (if combined with carbamazepine or some other inducer of cytochrome P450).

ANTIPSYCHOTIC DRUGS

In patients with BPD, antipsychotic drugs are used *acutely* to control symptoms during manic episodes, and *long term* to help stabilize mood. These drugs benefit patients with or without psychotic symptoms. Although antipsychotics can be used alone, they are usually employed in combination with a mood stabilizer, typically lithium or valproate.

As discussed in Chapter 31, the antipsychotic drugs fall into two major groups: first-generation antipsychotics (conventional antipsychotics) and second-generation antipsychotics (atypical antipsychotics). Compared with the conventional agents, the atypical agents carry a lower risk of extrapyramidal side effects, including tardive dyskinesia. Accordingly, the atypical agents are preferred for BPD.

Eight atypical antipsychotics—*olanzapine* [Zyprexa], *quetiapine* [Seroquel], *risperidone* [Risperdal], *aripiprazole* [Abilify], *lurasidone* [Latuda], *cariprazine* [Vraylar], *asenapine* [Saphris], and *ziprasidone* [Geodon]—are approved for BPD. (Another one—*clozapine* [Clozaril]—although highly effective in BPD, is not used owing to a risk of agranulocytosis.) All of these drugs are effective against acute mania, when used alone or combined with lithium or valproate. Currently, only three atypical agents—aripiprazole, olanzapine, and ziprasidone—are approved for long-term use to prevent recurrence of mood episodes. Dosages for patients with BPD are shown in Table 33.1.

Pharmacology of the antipsychotics is presented in Chapter 31.

KEY POINTS

- BPD is treated with three kinds of drugs: mood stabilizers, antipsychotic drugs, and antidepressants.
- Mood stabilizers are drugs that (1) relieve symptoms during manic and depressive episodes; (2) prevent recurrence of manic and depressive episodes; and (3) do not worsen symptoms of mania or depression and do not accelerate the rate of cycling.
- Antipsychotic drugs are used acutely to treat manic episodes, and long term to help stabilize mood. Benefits occur in patients with and without psychotic symptoms.
- In patients with bipolar depression, using an antidepressant alone may induce mania—although the risk appears lower than previously believed. Nonetheless, to minimize risk of mania, antidepressants should not be routinely used alone; rather, they should be combined with a mood-stabilizing drug.
- Lithium and valproate are the preferred mood stabilizers for BPD.
- To minimize the risk of toxicity, lithium levels must be monitored. The trough level, measured 12 hours after the evening dose, should be less than 1.5 mEq/L.
- Common side effects that occur at therapeutic lithium levels include tremor, goiter, and polyuria.
- Lithium may be teratogenic, and hence should be avoided during the first trimester of pregnancy. Also, unless the benefits outweigh the risks, lithium should be avoided during the second and third trimesters too.
- A reduction in sodium levels will reduce lithium excretion, causing lithium to accumulate—possibly to toxic levels. Patients must maintain normal sodium intake and levels.
- Lithium levels can be increased by diuretics (especially thiazides) and by several nonsteroidal anti-inflammatory drugs.

Please visit **http://evolve.elsevier.com/Lehne** for chapter-specific NCLEX® examination review questions.

Summary of Major Nursing Implications[a]

LITHIUM

Preadministration Assessment

Therapeutic Goal

Control of acute manic episodes in patients with BPD, and prophylaxis against recurrent mania and depression in patients with BPD.

Baseline Data

Make baseline determinations of cardiac status (electrocardiogram, blood pressure, pulse), hematologic status (complete blood counts with differential), serum electrolytes, renal function (serum creatinine, creatinine clearance, urinalysis), and thyroid function (T_3, T_4, and TSH).

Summary of Major Nursing Implications[a]—cont'd

Identifying High-Risk Patients

Lithium should be *avoided* during the first trimester of pregnancy and used with *caution* during the remainder of pregnancy and in the presence of renal disease, cardiovascular disease, dehydration, sodium depletion, and concurrent therapy with diuretics.

Implementation: Administration

Route

Oral.

Administration

Advise patients to administer lithium with meals or milk to decrease gastric upset. Instruct patients to swallow slow-release tablets intact, without crushing or chewing.

Promoting Adherence

Rigid adherence to the prescribed regimen is important. Deviations in dosage size and timing can cause toxicity. Inadequate dosing may cause relapse.

To promote adherence, educate patients and families about the nature of BPD and the importance of taking lithium as prescribed. Encourage family members to oversee lithium use, and advise them to urge the patient to visit the prescriber or a psychiatric clinic if a pattern of nonadherence develops.

When medicating inpatients, observe the patient to make certain that each lithium dose is ingested.

Ongoing Evaluation and Interventions

Monitoring Summary

Lithium Levels. Monitor lithium levels to ensure that they remain within the therapeutic range (0.4 to 1 mEq/L). Levels should be measured every 2 to 3 days during initial therapy, and every 3 to 6 months during maintenance. Blood for lithium determination should be drawn in the morning, 12 hours after the evening dose.

Other Parameters to Monitor. Evaluate the patient at least once a year for hematologic status (complete blood count with differential), serum electrolytes, renal function (serum creatinine, creatinine clearance, urinalysis), and thyroid function (T_3, T_4, and TSH).

Evaluating Therapeutic Effects

Evaluate the patient for abatement of manic symptoms (e.g., flight of ideas, pressured speech, hyperactivity) and for mood stabilization.

Minimizing Adverse Effects

Effects Caused by Excessive Drug Levels. Excessive lithium levels can result in serious adverse effects (see Table 33.2). Lithium levels must be monitored (see *Monitoring Summary* earlier in chapter) and dosage adjusted accordingly.

Teach patients the signs of toxicity, and instruct them to withhold medication and notify the prescriber if they develop.

Renal impairment can cause lithium accumulation. Kidney function should be assessed before treatment and once yearly thereafter.

Sodium deficiency can cause lithium to accumulate. **Instruct patients to maintain normal sodium intake. Inform patients that diarrhea can cause significant sodium loss.** Diuretics promote sodium excretion and must be used with caution.

In the event of severe toxicity, hospitalization may be required. If lithium levels exceed 2.5 mEq/L, hemodialysis should be considered.

Tremor. Lithium can cause fine hand tremor that can interfere with motor skills. Tremor can be reduced with a beta blocker (e.g., propranolol) and by measures that reduce peak lithium levels (dosage reduction; use of divided doses or a sustained-release formulation).

Hypothyroidism and Goiter. Lithium can promote goiter (thyroid enlargement) and frank hypothyroidism. Plasma levels of T_3, T_4, and TSH should be measured before treatment and yearly thereafter. Treat hypothyroidism with levothyroxine.

Renal Toxicity. Lithium can cause renal damage. Kidney function should be assessed before treatment and yearly thereafter. If renal impairment develops, lithium dosage must be reduced.

Polyuria. Lithium increases urine output. Polyuria can be suppressed with amiloride (a potassium-sparing diuretic). **Instruct patients to drink 8 to 12 glasses of fluid daily to maintain hydration.**

Use in Pregnancy and Lactation. Lithium may cause birth defects. The drug should be avoided during pregnancy, especially in the first trimester. **Counsel women of childbearing age about the importance of avoiding pregnancy.** Rule out pregnancy before initiating therapy.

Lithium enters breast milk. **Advise patients to avoid breast-feeding.**

Minimizing Adverse Interactions

Diuretics. By promoting sodium loss, diuretics can reduce lithium excretion, thereby causing lithium levels to rise. Monitor closely for signs of toxicity.

Anticholinergic Drugs. By causing urinary hesitancy, drugs with anticholinergic actions (e.g., antihistamines, phenothiazine antipsychotics, tricyclic antidepressants) can intensify discomfort associated with lithium-induced diuresis.

Nonsteroidal Anti-Inflammatory Drugs. Several NSAIDs (e.g., ibuprofen, naproxen, celecoxib), but *not* aspirin or sulindac, can increase renal reabsorption of lithium, thereby causing lithium levels to rise. If a mild analgesic is needed, aspirin or sulindac would be a good choice.

[a]Patient education information is highlighted as **blue text.**

CHAPTER

34 Sedative-Hypnotic Drugs

The sedative-hypnotics are drugs that depress central nervous system (CNS) function. With some of these drugs, CNS depression is more generalized than with others. The sedative-hypnotics are used primarily for two common disorders: anxiety and insomnia. Agents given to relieve anxiety are known as *antianxiety agents* or *anxiolytics*. Agents given to promote sleep are known as *hypnotics*. The distinction between antianxiety effects and hypnotic effects is often a matter of dosage: typically, sedative-hypnotics relieve anxiety in low doses and induce sleep in higher doses. Hence, a single drug may be considered both an antianxiety agent and a hypnotic agent, depending upon the reason for its use and the dosage employed.

There are three major groups of sedative-hypnotics: barbiturates (e.g., secobarbital), benzodiazepines (e.g., diazepam), and benzodiazepine-like drugs (e.g., zolpidem). The barbiturates were introduced in the early 1900s, the benzodiazepines in the 1950s, and the benzodiazepine-like drugs in the 1990s. Although barbiturates were widely used as sedative-hypnotics in the past, they are rarely used for this purpose today, having been replaced by the newer drugs.

Before the benzodiazepines became available, anxiety and insomnia were treated with barbiturates and other *general CNS depressants*—drugs with multiple undesirable qualities. First, these drugs are powerful respiratory depressants that can readily prove fatal in overdose. Second, because they produce subjective effects that many individuals find desirable, most general CNS depressants have a high potential for abuse. Third, with prolonged use, most of these drugs produce significant tolerance and physical dependence. And fourth, barbiturates and some other CNS depressants induce synthesis of hepatic drug-metabolizing enzymes and can thereby decrease responses to other drugs. Because the benzodiazepines are just as effective as the general CNS depressants but do not share their undesirable properties, the benzodiazepines are preferred to the general CNS depressants for treating anxiety and insomnia.

We begin by discussing the basic pharmacology of the sedative-hypnotics and end by discussing their use in insomnia. Use of these drugs for anxiety disorders is addressed in Chapter 35.

BENZODIAZEPINES

Benzodiazepines, along with the newer benzodiazepine receptor agonists, are drugs of first choice for anxiety and insomnia. In addition, these drugs are used to induce general anesthesia and to manage seizure disorders, muscle spasm, and withdrawal from alcohol.

Benzodiazepines were introduced in the late 1950s and remain important today. Perhaps the most familiar member of the family is diazepam [Valium]. The most frequently prescribed members are lorazepam [Ativan] and alprazolam [Xanax, Xanax XR, Niravam].

The popularity of the benzodiazepines as sedatives and hypnotics stems from their superiority over the alternatives: barbiturates and other general CNS depressants. The benzodiazepines are safer than the general CNS depressants and have a lower potential for abuse. In addition, benzodiazepines produce less tolerance and physical dependence and are subject to fewer drug interactions. Contrasts between benzodiazepines and barbiturates are shown in Table 34.1.

Because all of the benzodiazepines produce nearly identical effects, we will consider the family as a group, rather than selecting a representative member as a prototype.

Overview of Pharmacologic Effects

Practically all responses to benzodiazepines result from actions in the CNS. Benzodiazepines have few direct actions outside the CNS. All of the benzodiazepines produce a similar spectrum of responses. However, because of pharmacokinetic differences, individual benzodiazepines may differ in clinical applications.

Central Nervous System. All beneficial effects of benzodiazepines, and most adverse effects, result from depressant actions in the CNS. With increasing dosage, effects progress from sedation to hypnosis to stupor.

Benzodiazepines depress neuronal function at multiple sites in the CNS. They *reduce anxiety* through effects on the limbic system, a neuronal network associated with emotionality. They *promote sleep* through effects on cortical areas and on the sleep-wakefulness "clock." They *induce muscle relaxation* through effects on supraspinal motor areas, including

TABLE 34.1 ■ Contrasts Between Benzodiazepines and Barbiturates

Area of Comparison	Benzodiazepines	Barbiturates
Relative safety	High	Low
Maximal ability to depress CNS function	Low	High
Respiratory depressant ability	Low	High
Suicide potential	Low	High
Ability to cause physical dependence	Low[a]	High
Potential to develop tolerance	Low	High
Abuse potential	Low	High
Ability to induce hepatic drug metabolism	Low	High

[a]Although dependence is low in most patients, significant dependence *can* develop with long-term, high-dose use.

the cerebellum. Two important side effects—*confusion* and *anterograde amnesia*—result from effects on the hippocampus and cerebral cortex.

Cardiovascular System. When taken *orally,* benzodiazepines have almost no effect on the heart and blood vessels. In contrast, when administered *intravenously,* even in therapeutic doses, benzodiazepines can produce profound hypotension and cardiac arrest.

Respiratory System. In contrast to the barbiturates, the benzodiazepines are weak respiratory depressants. When taken alone in therapeutic doses, benzodiazepines produce little or no depression of respiration—and with toxic doses, respiratory depression is moderate at most. With oral therapy, clinically significant respiratory depression occurs only when benzodiazepines are combined with other CNS depressants (e.g., opioids, barbiturates, alcohol).

Although benzodiazepines generally have minimal effects on respiration, they can be a problem for patients with respiratory disorders. In patients with chronic obstructive pulmonary disease, benzodiazepines may worsen hypoventilation and hypoxemia. In patients with obstructive sleep apnea (OSA), benzodiazepines may exacerbate apneic episodes. In patients who snore, benzodiazepines may convert partial airway obstruction into OSA.

Molecular Mechanism of Action

Benzodiazepines *potentiate the actions of gamma-amino-butyric acid* (GABA), an inhibitory neurotransmitter found throughout the CNS. These drugs enhance the actions of GABA by binding to specific receptors in a supramolecular structure known as the GABA receptor–chloride channel complex (Fig. 34.1). Note that benzodiazepines do not act as direct GABA agonists—they simply intensify the effects of GABA.

Because benzodiazepines act by amplifying the actions of endogenous GABA, rather than by directly mimicking GABA, there is a limit to how much CNS depression benzodiazepines can produce. This explains why benzodiazepines are so much

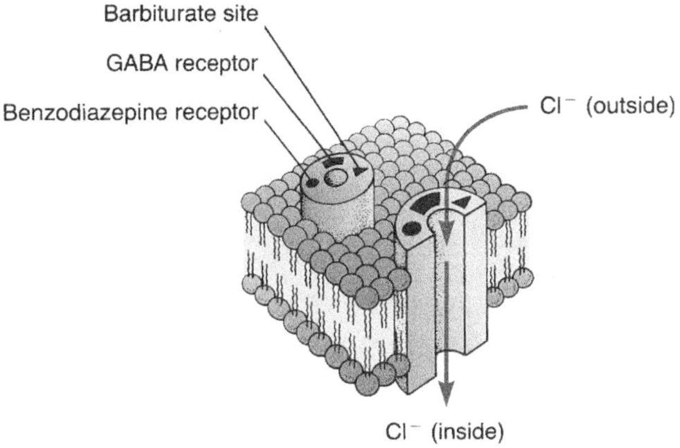

Fig. 34.1 ■ Schematic model of the GABA receptor–chloride channel complex showing binding sites for benzodiazepines and barbiturates.
The GABA receptor–chloride channel complex, which spans the neuronal cell membrane, can exist in an open or closed configuration. Binding of GABA to its receptor on the complex causes the chloride channel to *open.* The resulting inward flow of chloride ions hyperpolarizes the neuron (makes the cell highly negative inside) and thereby decreases its ability to fire. Hence GABA is an *inhibitory* neurotransmitter. Binding of a *benzodiazepine* to its receptor on the complex increases the frequency of channel opening, thereby increasing chloride influx. Hence, benzodiazepines enhance the inhibitory effects of GABA. Effects of *barbiturates* on the chloride channel are dose dependent: at low doses, barbiturates enhance the actions of GABA (by prolonging the duration of channel opening); at high doses, barbiturates directly mimic the actions of GABA.

safer than the barbiturates—drugs that can directly mimic GABA. Since benzodiazepines simply potentiate the inhibitory effects of endogenous GABA and since the amount of GABA in the CNS is finite, there is a built-in limit to the depth of CNS depression the benzodiazepines can produce. In contrast, because the barbiturates are direct-acting CNS depressants, maximal effects are limited only by the amount of barbiturate administered.

Pharmacokinetics

Absorption and Distribution. Most benzodiazepines are well absorbed following oral administration. Because of their high lipid solubility, benzodiazepines readily cross the blood-brain barrier to reach sites in the CNS.

Metabolism. Most benzodiazepines undergo extensive metabolic alterations. With few exceptions, the *metabolites are pharmacologically active.* As a result, responses produced by administering a particular benzodiazepine often persist long after the parent drug has disappeared. Hence, there may be a poor correlation between the plasma half-life of the parent drug and the duration of pharmacologic effects. Flurazepam, for example, whose plasma half-life is only 2 to 3 hours, is converted into an active metabolite with a half-life of 50 hours. Hence, giving flurazepam produces long-lasting effects, even though flurazepam itself is gone from the plasma in 8 to 12 hours (about four half-lives).

In patients with liver disease, metabolism of benzodiazepines may be reduced, thereby prolonging excretion and intensifying responses. Because certain benzodiazepines (oxazepam, temazepam, and lorazepam) undergo very little metabolic

TABLE 34.2 ▪ Applications of the Benzodiazepines

	Approved Applications						
Drug	Anxiety	Insomnia	Seizures	Muscle Spasm, Spasticity	Alcohol Withdrawal	Anesthesia Induction or Preanesthesia	Panic Disorder
Alprazolam [Xanax, Xanax XR, Niravam]	✓						✓
Chlordiazepoxide [Librium]	✓				✓		✓
Clonazepam [Klonopin, Rivotril 🍁]			✓				✓
Clorazepate [Tranxene-T]	✓		✓		✓		
Diazepam [Valium, Diastat AcuDial]	✓		✓	✓	✓	✓	
Estazolam (generic only)		✓					
Flurazepam (generic only)		✓					
Lorazepam [Ativan]	✓	✓	✓				
Midazolam [Versed]						✓[a]	
Oxazepam (generic only)	✓				✓		
Quazepam [Doral]		✓					
Temazepam [Restoril]		✓					
Triazolam [Halcion]		✓					

[a]Midazolam, in conjunction with an opioid analgesic, is also used to produce *conscious sedation,* a semiconscious state suitable for minor surgeries and endoscopic procedures.

alteration, they may be preferred for patients with hepatic impairment.

Time Course of Action. Benzodiazepines differ significantly from one another with respect to time course. Specifically, they differ in onset and duration of action, and tendency to accumulate with repeated dosing.

Because all benzodiazepines have essentially equivalent pharmacologic actions, selection among them is based largely on differences in time course. For example, if a patient needs medication to accelerate falling asleep, a benzodiazepine with a rapid onset (e.g., triazolam) would be indicated. However, if medication is needed to prevent waking later in the night, a benzodiazepine with a slower onset (e.g., estazolam) would be preferred. For treatment of anxiety, a drug with an intermediate duration is desirable. For treatment of any benzodiazepine-responsive condition in older adults, a drug such as lorazepam, which is not likely to accumulate with repeated dosing, is generally preferred.

Therapeutic Uses

The benzodiazepines have three principal indications: (1) anxiety, (2) insomnia, and (3) seizure disorders. In addition, they are used as preoperative medications and to treat muscle spasm and withdrawal from alcohol. Although all benzodiazepines share the same pharmacologic properties, and therefore might be equally effective for all applications, not every benzodiazepine is actually employed for all potential uses. The principal factors that determine the actual applications of a particular benzodiazepine are (1) the pharmacokinetic properties of the drug itself and (2) research and marketing decisions of pharmaceutical companies. Specific applications of individual benzodiazepines are shown in Table 34.2.

Anxiety. Benzodiazepines are drugs of first choice for acute anxiety. Although all benzodiazepines have anxiolytic actions, only six are marketed for this indication (see Table 34.2). Anxiolytic effects result from depressing neurotransmission in the limbic system and cortical areas. Use of benzodiazepines to treat anxiety disorders is discussed in Chapter 35.

Insomnia. Benzodiazepines are preferred drugs for insomnia. These drugs decrease latency time to falling asleep, reduce awakenings, and increase total sleeping time. The role of benzodiazepines in managing insomnia is discussed in depth later.

Seizure Disorders. Four benzodiazepines—diazepam, clonazepam, lorazepam, and clorazepate—are employed for seizure disorders. Antiseizure applications are discussed in Chapter 24.

Muscle Spasm. One benzodiazepine—diazepam—is used to relieve muscle spasm and spasticity (see Chapter 25). Effects on muscle tone are secondary to actions in the CNS. Diazepam cannot relieve spasm without causing sedation.

Alcohol Withdrawal. Diazepam and other benzodiazepines may be administered to ease withdrawal from alcohol (see Chapter 38). Benefits derive from cross-dependence with alcohol, which enables benzodiazepines to suppress symptoms brought on by alcohol abstinence.

Perioperative Applications. Two benzodiazepines—diazepam [Valium] and midazolam [Versed]—are approved and given IV for *induction of anesthesia.* In addition, midazolam (in combination with an opioid analgesic) can be used to produce *conscious sedation,* a semiconscious state suitable for endoscopic procedures and minor surgeries. Benzodiazepines are also used for *preoperative sedation.* All of these applications are discussed in Chapter 27.

Adverse Effects

Benzodiazepines are generally well tolerated, and serious adverse reactions are rare. In contrast to barbiturates and other general CNS depressants, benzodiazepines are remarkably safe.

CNS Depression. When taken to promote sleep, benzodiazepines cause drowsiness, light-headedness, incoordination, and difficulty in concentrating. When these effects occur at bedtime, they are generally inconsequential. However, if sedation and other manifestations of CNS depression persist beyond waking, interference with daytime activities can result.

Anterograde Amnesia. Benzodiazepines can cause anterograde amnesia (impaired recall of events that take place after dosing). Anterograde amnesia has been especially troublesome with *triazolam* [Halcion]. If patients complain of forgetfulness, the possibility of drug-induced amnesia should be evaluated.

Sleep Driving and Other Complex Sleep-Related Behaviors. Patients taking benzodiazepines in sleep-inducing doses may carry out complex behaviors and then have no memory of their actions. Reported behaviors include sleep driving, preparing and eating meals, and making phone calls. Although these events can occur with normal doses, they are more likely when doses are excessive and when benzodiazepines are combined with alcohol and other CNS depressants. Because of the potential for harm, benzodiazepines should be withdrawn if sleep driving is reported. To minimize withdrawal symptoms, dosing should be tapered slowly, rather than discontinued abruptly.

Paradoxical Effects. When employed to treat anxiety, benzodiazepines sometimes cause paradoxical responses, including insomnia, excitation, euphoria, heightened anxiety, and rage. If these occur, the benzodiazepine should be withdrawn.

Respiratory Depression. Benzodiazepines are weak respiratory depressants. The risk of death from overdose with oral benzodiazepines alone is low. Hence, in contrast to the barbiturates, benzodiazepines present little risk as vehicles for suicide. It must be emphasized, however, that although respiratory depression with *oral* therapy is rare, benzodiazepines can cause severe respiratory depression when administered *intravenously.* In addition, substantial respiratory depression can result from combining oral benzodiazepines with other CNS depressants (e.g., alcohol, barbiturates, opioids).

Abuse. Benzodiazepines have a lower abuse potential than barbiturates and most other general CNS depressants. The behavior pattern that constitutes "addiction" is uncommon among people who take benzodiazepines for therapeutic purposes. When asked about their drug use, individuals who regularly abuse drugs rarely express a preference for benzodiazepines over barbiturates. Because their potential for abuse is low, the benzodiazepines are classified under Schedule IV of the Controlled Substances Act. This contrasts with the barbiturates, most of which are classified under Schedule III.

Use in Pregnancy and Lactation. Benzodiazepines are highly lipid soluble and can readily cross the placental barrier. Use of benzodiazepines during the first trimester of pregnancy is associated with an increased risk of congenital malformations, such as cleft lip, inguinal hernia, and cardiac anomalies. Use near term can cause CNS depression in the neonate. Because they may represent a risk to the fetus, most benzodiazepines are classified in U.S. Food and Drug Administration (FDA) Pregnancy Risk Category D.[a] Five of these drugs—estazolam, flurazepam, quazepam, temazepam, and triazolam—are in Category X.[b] Women of childbearing age should be warned about the potential for fetal harm and instructed to discontinue benzodiazepines if pregnancy occurs.

Benzodiazepines enter breast milk with ease and may accumulate to toxic levels in the breast-fed infant. Accordingly, these drugs should be avoided by nursing mothers.

Other Adverse Effects. Occasional reactions include weakness, headache, blurred vision, vertigo, nausea, vomiting, epigastric distress, and diarrhea. Neutropenia and jaundice occur rarely. Rarely, benzodiazepines may cause severe allergic reactions, including angioedema and anaphylaxis.

Drug Interactions

Benzodiazepines undergo very few important interactions with other drugs. Unlike barbiturates, benzodiazepines do not induce hepatic drug-metabolizing enzymes. Hence, benzodiazepines do not accelerate the metabolism of other drugs.

CNS Depressants. The CNS-depressant actions of benzodiazepines add to those of other CNS depressants (e.g., alcohol, barbiturates, opioids). Hence, although benzodiazepines are very safe when used alone, they can be extremely hazardous in combination with other depressants. Combined overdose with a benzodiazepine plus another CNS depressant can cause profound respiratory depression, coma, and death. Patients should be warned against the use of alcohol and all other CNS depressants.

Tolerance and Physical Dependence

Tolerance. With prolonged use of benzodiazepines, tolerance develops to some effects but not to others. No tolerance develops to anxiolytic effects, and tolerance to hypnotic effects is generally low. In contrast, significant tolerance develops to antiseizure effects. Patients tolerant to barbiturates, alcohol, and other general CNS depressants show some cross-tolerance to benzodiazepines.

Physical Dependence. Benzodiazepines can cause physical dependence—but the incidence of *substantial* dependence is low. When benzodiazepines are discontinued following short-term use at therapeutic doses, the resulting withdrawal syndrome is generally mild and often goes unrecognized. Symptoms include anxiety, insomnia, sweating, tremors, and dizziness. Withdrawal from long-term, high-dose therapy can cause more serious reactions, such as panic, paranoia, delirium, hypertension, muscle twitches, and outright convulsions. Symptoms of withdrawal are usually more intense with benzodiazepines that have a short duration of action. With one agent—*alprazolam* [Xanax, Xanax XR, Niravam]—dependence may be a greater problem than with other benzodiazepines. Because the benzodiazepine withdrawal syndrome can resemble an anxiety disorder, it is important to differentiate withdrawal symptoms from the return of the original symptoms of anxiety.

The intensity of withdrawal symptoms can be minimized by discontinuing treatment gradually. Doses should be slowly tapered over several weeks or months. Substituting a benzodiazepine with a long half-life for one with a short half-life is also helpful. Patients should be warned against abrupt cessation of treatment. Following discontinuation of treatment, patients should be monitored for 3 weeks for indications of withdrawal or recurrence of original symptoms.

Acute Toxicity

Oral Overdose. When administered in excessive dosage by mouth, benzodiazepines rarely cause serious toxicity.

[a,b]As of 2020, the FDA will no longer use Pregnancy Risk Categories. Please refer to Chapter 9 for more information.

Symptoms include drowsiness, lethargy, and confusion. Significant cardiovascular and respiratory effects are uncommon. If an individual known to have taken an overdose of benzodiazepines does exhibit signs of serious toxicity, it is probable that another drug was taken too.

Intravenous Toxicity. When injected IV, even in therapeutic doses, benzodiazepines can cause severe adverse effects. Life-threatening reactions (e.g., profound hypotension, respiratory arrest, cardiac arrest) occur in about 2% of patients.

General Treatment Measures. Benzodiazepine-induced toxicity is managed with supportive care. Currently, the use of activated charcoal is not recommended, as the risks outweigh the benefits. Respiration should be monitored and the airway kept patent. Support of blood pressure with IV fluids may be required.

Treatment With Flumazenil. Flumazenil [Romazicon] is a competitive benzodiazepine receptor antagonist. The drug can reverse the sedative effects of benzodiazepines but may not reverse respiratory depression. Flumazenil is approved for benzodiazepine overdose and for reversing the effects of benzodiazepines following general anesthesia. The principal adverse effect is precipitation of seizures. This is most likely in patients taking benzodiazepines to treat epilepsy and in patients who are physically dependent on benzodiazepines. Flumazenil is administered IV. Doses are injected over 15 seconds and may be repeated every minute as needed up to a dose of 3 mg. The first dose is 0.2 mg, the second is 0.3 mg, and all subsequent doses are 0.5 mg. Effects of flumazenil fade in about 1 hour, hence repeated doses may be required.

Preparations, Dosage, and Administration

Preparations and Dosage. Preparations and dosages for *insomnia* are presented later in the chapter. Preparations and dosages of benzodiazepines used for other disorders are presented in Chapter 24, Chapter 25, Chapter 27, and Chapter 35.

Routes. All benzodiazepines can be administered orally. In addition, two agents—diazepam and lorazepam—may be administered parenterally (IM and IV). When used for sedation or induction of sleep, benzodiazepines are almost always administered by mouth. Parenteral administration is reserved for emergencies, including acute alcohol withdrawal, severe anxiety, and status epilepticus.

Oral. Patients should be advised to take oral benzodiazepines with food if gastric upset occurs. Also, they should be instructed to swallow sustained-release formulations intact, without crushing or chewing. Patients should be warned not to increase the dosage or discontinue therapy without consulting the prescriber.

For treatment of insomnia, benzodiazepines should be given on an intermittent schedule (e.g., 3 or 4 days a week) in the lowest effective dosage for the shortest duration required. This will minimize physical dependence and associated drug-dependency insomnia.

Intravenous. Intravenous administration is hazardous and must be performed with care. Life-threatening reactions (severe hypotension, respiratory arrest, cardiac arrest) have occurred. In addition, IV administration carries a risk of venous thrombosis, phlebitis, and vascular impairment.

To reduce complications, the following precautions should be taken: (1) inject the drug slowly; (2) take care to avoid intra-arterial injection and extravasation; (3) if direct venous injection is impossible, make the injection into infusion tubing as close to the vein as possible; (4) follow the manufacturer's instructions regarding suitable diluents for preparing solutions; and (5) have facilities for resuscitation available.

Intramuscular. If IM administration is needed, *lorazepam* is the preferred benzodiazepine to use, owing to consistent absorption from IM sites. Absorption of IM diazepam is erratic and may be delayed. Accordingly, IM diazepam should be avoided.

Prototype Drugs

SEDATIVE-HYPNOTIC DRUGS

Benzodiazepines
Triazolam

Benzodiazepine-like Drugs
Zaleplon
Zolpidem

Barbiturates
Secobarbital

Melatonin Receptor Agonists
Ramelteon

Orexin Receptor Antagonists
Suvorexant

BENZODIAZEPINE-LIKE DRUGS

Three benzodiazepine-like drugs are available: zolpidem, zaleplon, and eszopiclone. All three are preferred agents for insomnia. They are not indicated for anxiety. These drugs are structurally different from benzodiazepines, but nonetheless share the same mechanism of action: They all act as *agonists at the benzodiazepine receptor site* on the GABA receptor–chloride channel complex. Like the benzodiazepines, these drugs have a low potential for tolerance, dependence, and abuse, and are classified as Schedule IV substances.

Zolpidem

Zolpidem [Ambien, Ambien CR, Edluar, Intermezzo, Zolpimist], our most widely used hypnotic, is approved only for short-term management of insomnia. However, although approval is limited to short-term use, many patients have taken the drug long term with no apparent tolerance or increase in adverse effects. All zolpidem formulations have a rapid onset, and hence can help people who have difficulty falling asleep. In addition, the extended-release formulation—Ambien CR—can help people who have difficulty maintaining sleep.

Although structurally unrelated to the benzodiazepines, zolpidem binds to the benzodiazepine receptor site on the GABA receptor–chloride channel complex and shares some properties of the benzodiazepines. Like the benzodiazepines, zolpidem can reduce sleep latency and awakenings and can prolong sleep duration. The drug does not significantly reduce time in rapid-eye-movement (REM) sleep and causes little or no rebound insomnia when therapy is discontinued. In contrast to the benzodiazepines, zolpidem lacks anxiolytic, muscle relaxant, and anticonvulsant actions because zolpidem doesn't bind with all benzodiazepine receptors. Rather, binding is limited to the $benzodiazepine_1$ subtype of benzodiazepine receptors. The pharmacokinetics of zolpidem is displayed in Table 34.3.

Zolpidem has a side effect profile like that of the benzodiazepines. *Daytime drowsiness* and *dizziness* are most

TABLE 34.3 ■ Pharmacokinetic Properties of Sedative-Hypnotic Drugs

Drug	Route	Peak[a] (hr)	Half-Life[a] (hr)	Metabolism	Excretion
BENZODIAZEPINE-LIKE DRUGS					
Eszopiclone [Lunesta]	PO	1–2	6	Hepatic	Renal
Zaleplon [Sonata]	PO	1	1	Hepatic	Renal
Zolpidem [Ambien]	PO, SL	2	2.5	Hepatic	Gastrointestinal (bile, feces), renal
MELATONIN RECEPTOR AGONIST					
Ramelteon [Rozarem]	PO	1	2–5	Hepatic	Renal
OREXIN RECEPTOR ANTAGONIST					
Suvorexant [Belsomra]	PO	2	12	Hepatic	Gastrointestinal (feces), renal

[a]With oral administration.

common, and these occur in only 1% to 2% of patients. Like the benzodiazepines, zolpidem has been associated with *sleep driving* and other *sleep-related complex behaviors.* At therapeutic doses, zolpidem causes little or no respiratory depression. Safety in pregnancy has not been established. According to the FDA, zolpidem may pose a small risk of anaphylaxis and angioedema.

Short-term treatment is not associated with significant tolerance or physical dependence. Withdrawal symptoms are minimal or absent. Similarly, the abuse liability of zolpidem is low. Accordingly, the drug is classified under Schedule IV of the Controlled Substances Act.

Like other sedative-hypnotics, zolpidem can intensify the effects of other CNS depressants. Accordingly, patients should be warned against combining zolpidem with alcohol and all other drugs that depress CNS function.

Zolpidem is available in four formulations: (1) immediate-release tablets (5 and 10 mg) sold as *Ambien,* (2) extended-release tablets (6.25 and 12.5 mg) sold as *Ambien CR,* (3) an oral spray (5 mg) sold as *Zolpimist,* and (4) sublingual tablets sold as *Edluar* (5 and 10 mg) or *Intermezzo* (1.75 and 3.5 mg). With the immediate-release tablets, sublingual tablets, and oral spray, the usual dose is 10 mg. The initial dose should be reduced to 5 mg for older adult and debilitated patients and for those with hepatic insufficiency. With the extended-release tablets, the usual dose is 12.5 mg (or 6.25 mg for older adult or debilitated patients). All formulations have a rapid onset, and hence should be taken just before bedtime. This timing will promote sleep while minimizing daytime sedation.

Zaleplon

Zaleplon [Sonata] is the first representative of a new class of hypnotics, the pyrazolopyrimidines. The drug is approved only for short-term management of insomnia, but prolonged use does not appear to cause tolerance. Like zolpidem, zaleplon binds to the benzodiazepine$_1$ receptor site on the GABA receptor–chloride channel complex, enhancing the depressant actions of endogenous GABA. In contrast to zolpidem, zaleplon has a very rapid onset and short duration of action, and hence is good for helping patients fall asleep, but not for maintaining sleep.

Zaleplon is well tolerated. The most common side effects are headache, nausea, drowsiness, dizziness, myalgia, and abdominal pain. Like the benzodiazepines, zaleplon has been associated with rare cases of sleep driving and other complex sleep-related behaviors. Respiratory depression has not been observed. Physical dependence is minimal, the only sign being mild rebound insomnia the first night after drug withdrawal. Next-day sedation and hangover have not been reported. Like the benzodiazepines, zaleplon has a low potential for abuse, and hence is classified as a Schedule IV drug.

Cimetidine (a drug for peptic ulcer disease) inhibits hepatic aldehyde oxidase and can thereby greatly increase levels of zaleplon. Accordingly, dosage of zaleplon must be reduced if these drugs are used concurrently.

Zaleplon [Sonata] is available in 5- and 10-mg capsules. The usual dose is 10 mg. The dose should be reduced to 5 mg for (1) older adults, (2) small individuals, (3) patients with liver impairment, and (4) patients taking cimetidine. The maximum dose is 20 mg. Dosing is usually done just before retiring. However, dosing may also be done after going to bed on nights when sleep fails to come.

Eszopiclone

Eszopiclone [Lunesta], like zaleplon and zolpidem, binds selectively with the benzodiazepine$_1$ receptor on the GABA receptor–chloride channel complex and thereby enhances the depressant actions of endogenous GABA.

Eszopiclone is approved for treating insomnia, with no limitation on how long it can be used. This contrasts with zaleplon and zolpidem, which are approved for short-term use only. Does this mean that eszopiclone is safer than the other two drugs or less likely to promote tolerance? Not necessarily. It only means that the manufacturer of eszopiclone conducted a prolonged (6-month) study, whereas the manufacturers of the other two drugs did not. In that prolonged study, eszopiclone reduced sleep latency and nighttime awakening, increased total sleep time and sleep quality, had no significant effect on sleep architecture, and showed no indication of tolerance.

Eszopiclone is generally well tolerated. The most common adverse effect is a bitter aftertaste, reported by 17% of patients dosed with 2 mg and 34% of those dosed with 3 mg. Other common effects are headache, somnolence, dizziness, and dry mouth. Rebound insomnia may occur on the first night after discontinuing the drug. Like the benzodiazepines and the other benzodiazepine-like drugs, eszopiclone has been associated with cases of sleep driving and other sleep-related complex behaviors. Rarely, eszopiclone may cause anaphylaxis or angioedema. Eszopiclone has a low potential for abuse and hence is classified as a Schedule IV drug.

Eszopiclone [Lunesta] is available in 1-, 2-, and 3-mg tablets. For adults, the recommended starting dose is 1 mg, taken just before bedtime. The dose can be raised to 3 mg if needed. For patients with severe hepatic impairment, older adult patients, and for those taking inhibitors of CYP3A4 (e.g., ketoconazole), the maximum dose is 2 mg.

RAMELTEON: A MELATONIN AGONIST

Ramelteon [Rozerem] is a hypnotic with a unique mechanism of action: activation of receptors for melatonin. The drug is approved for treating chronic insomnia characterized by difficulty with sleep onset, but not with sleep maintenance. Long-term use is permitted. Of the major drugs for insomnia, ramelteon is the only one not regulated as a controlled substance.

Therapeutic Use

Ramelteon has a rapid onset (about 30 minutes) and short duration, and hence is good for inducing sleep but not maintaining sleep. There are no significant residual effects on the day after dosing. Nor is there any rebound insomnia when treatment is stopped after 35 consecutive nights of use. When approving the drug, the FDA put no limit on how long it may be used.

Mechanism of Action

Ramelteon activates receptors for melatonin—specifically the MT_1 and MT_2 subtypes, which are key mediators of the normal sleep-wakefulness cycle. Sleep promotion derives primarily from activating MT_1 receptors. (Under physiologic conditions, activation of MT_1 receptors by endogenous melatonin induces sleepiness.) Ramelteon does not activate MT_3 receptors, which help regulate numerous systems unrelated to sleep. Selectivity for MT_1 and MT_2 receptors explains why ramelteon is superior to melatonin itself for treating insomnia (Box 34.1). Ramelteon does not bind with the GABA receptor–chloride channel complex, or with receptors for neuropeptides, benzodiazepines, dopamine, serotonin, norepinephrine, acetylcholine, or opioids.

Adverse Effects

Ramelteon is very well tolerated. In clinical trials, the incidence of adverse effects was nearly identical to that of placebo. The most common side effects are somnolence, dizziness, and fatigue. According to the FDA, ramelteon may share the ability of benzodiazepines to cause sleep driving and other sleep-related complex behaviors. Very rarely, patients have reported hallucinations, agitation, and mania.

Ramelteon can increase levels of prolactin and reduce levels of testosterone. As a result, the drug has the potential to cause

si BOX 34.1 ■ SPECIAL INTEREST TOPIC

MELATONIN, KEEPER OF THE CIRCADIAN CLOCK

Melatonin is a hormone that helps regulate our circadian clock, the time-keeping mechanism that controls our sleep-wakefulness cycle. Principal uses for melatonin are insomnia and jet lag. Of note, melatonin is the only hormone that can be purchased without a prescription. The compound is available in health-food stores, vitamin shops, and even airport newsstands.

Melatonin is produced by the pineal gland, a structure located at the base of the brain. Secretion is suppressed by environmental light and stimulated by darkness. Normally, secretion is low during the day, begins to rise around 9:00 PM, reaches a peak between 2:00 AM and 4:00 AM, and returns to baseline by morning. Signals that control secretion travel along a multineuron pathway that connects the retina to the pineal gland. Nocturnal secretion peaks early in life and then remains steady from adolescence through old age. In blind people, melatonin secretion has no predictable pattern. In insomniacs, melatonin levels are low.

When taken to promote sleep, melatonin has two beneficial actions. First, low doses can reset the circadian clock. Second, higher doses exert direct hypnotic effects. Melatonin receptors on the suprachiasmatic nucleus (the anatomic site of the circadian clock) probably mediate clock resetting by exogenous melatonin. Whether these receptors also mediate direct hypnotic effects is unknown.

What's the effect of melatonin on insomnia? Several trials indicate that it promotes sleep. For example, doses of 0.3 to 1 mg taken 1 to 2 hours before bedtime can hasten sleep onset and the time to rapid-eye-movement (REM) sleep without reducing total time in REM sleep. During a 6-month study, patients taking *Circadin*[a]—a 2-mg sustained-release formulation—experienced consistent improvements in sleep latency, sleep quality, and morning alertness, with no withdrawal symptoms or rebound insomnia when dosing was stopped. In blind insomniacs, taking melatonin for 3 weeks normalized the melatonin production cycle and relieved insomnia.

Can melatonin ease symptoms of jet lag? Probably. Of all treatments for jet lag, melatonin is the most widely studied. To date, there have been 11 double-blind, placebo-controlled trials. In eight of these trials, melatonin produced significant benefit. Of the three negative studies, two were too small to permit firm conclusions, and one involved subjects whose baseline circadian rhythm may have been inappropriate for evaluation. How does melatonin help ease jet lag? It resets the circadian clock to the new time zone.

What side effects does melatonin have? When used short term in low doses (e.g., under 2 mg), melatonin has no observable adverse effects. However, short-term use of large doses can cause hangover, headache, nightmares, hypothermia, and transient depression. In one case, reversible psychosis occurred with a huge daytime dose. Possible adverse effects of long-term use are unknown.

Two melatonin formulations are available: immediate release (IR) and sustained release (SR). The IR products are best for people with trouble falling asleep, and the SR products are best for people with trouble staying asleep. For both types of product, strengths typically range from 0.3 to 3 mg. Today, most commercial melatonin is synthesized in the laboratory. Melatonin from animal sources should be avoided, owing to a risk of contamination.

Although melatonin is a hormone, it is marketed as a dietary supplement—not as a drug. As a result, melatonin is not regulated by the FDA and has not been reviewed for safety and efficacy. Because melatonin is not regulated, commercial preparations may have impurities and may not contain the exact amount of melatonin advertised on the label.

[a]Not available in the United States.

amenorrhea, galactorrhea, reduced libido, and fertility problems. If these occur, the prescriber should be consulted.

Postmarketing reports indicate a small risk of severe allergic reactions. Rarely, patients have experienced angioedema of the tongue, glottis, or larynx. Some patients also experienced dyspnea and throat constriction, suggestive of anaphylaxis. Patients who experience these symptoms should discontinue ramelteon and never use it again.

Physical Dependence and Abuse

There is no evidence that taking ramelteon leads to physical dependence or abuse. As a result, ramelteon is the first FDA-approved sleep remedy that is not regulated under the Controlled Substances Act.

Drug Interactions

Fluvoxamine [Luvox], a strong inhibitor of CYP1A2, can increase levels of ramelteon more than 50-fold. Accordingly, the combination should be avoided. Weaker inhibitors of CYP1A2 should be used with caution. Alcohol can intensify sedation, and hence should be avoided.

Precautions

Ramelteon should be used with caution by patients with moderate hepatic impairment and should be avoided by those with severe hepatic impairment. Because ramelteon promotes sedation, patients should be advised to avoid dangerous activities, such as driving or operating heavy machinery.

Use in Pregnancy and Breast-Feeding

Very high doses (197 times the human dose) are teratogenic in rats. Effects during human pregnancy have not been studied. Until more is known, prudence dictates avoiding the drug during pregnancy (or at least using it with caution). Ramelteon is not recommended for use by nursing mothers.

Preparations, Dosage, and Administration

Ramelteon [Rozerem] is available in 8-mg tablets. The usual dosage is 8 mg taken 30 minutes before bedtime. Because food reduces absorption, ramelteon should not be taken with or immediately after a high-fat meal.

SUVOREXANT: AN OREXIN ANTAGONIST

Suvorexant [Belsomra] is a sedative that selectively blocks receptors for orexin, a neurotransmitter in the brain that promotes wakefulness. The drug is approved for treating chronic insomnia characterized by difficulty with sleep onset and/or sleep maintenance. Similar to the benzodiazepine-like drugs, suvorexant is regulated as a Schedule IV substance.

Adverse Effects

The most common side effects are somnolence, headache, dizziness, diarrhea, dry mouth, and cough. Hallucinations, sleep paralysis (an inability to speak or move for up to several minutes during sleep-wake transitions), and vivid, disturbing perceptions have been reported by some patients.

Physical Dependence and Abuse

Suvorexant is classified by the U.S. Drug Enforcement Administration (DEA) as a Schedule IV medication. An abuse study conducted with suvorexant revealed that patients had similar subjective ratings of "drug liking" as that of zolpidem, also a Schedule IV drug. Patients with a history of drug abuse or addiction may be at an increased risk for abuse of suvorexant.

Drug Interactions

Use with strong inhibitors of CYP3A (ketoconazole, clarithromycin, others) can increase the effects of suvorexant; therefore, such use is not recommended. Suvorexant can also increase digoxin levels; therefore, close monitoring is indicated.

Precautions

Suvorexant should be used with caution by patients with compromised respiratory function, such as severe chronic obstructive pulmonary disease (COPD) or obstructive sleep apnea (OSA). Because suvorexant promotes sedation, its use is contraindicated in patients with narcolepsy.

Use in Pregnancy and Breast-Feeding

Adequate human studies on the effects of suvorexant in pregnant women are lacking. Administration to pregnant rats resulted in decreased fetal body weight with increased doses. It remains unknown if suvorexant is expressed in breast milk. When using this medication during pregnancy, benefits should clearly outweigh the risks

Preparations, Dosage, and Administration

Suvorexant [Belsomra] is available in 5-, 10-, 15-, and 20-mg tablets. The usual dosage is 10 mg taken 30 minutes before bedtime.

BARBITURATES

The barbiturates have been available for more than 100 years. These drugs cause relatively nonselective depression of CNS function and are the prototypes of the general CNS depressants. Because they depress multiple aspects of CNS function, barbiturates can be used for daytime sedation, induction of sleep, suppression of seizures, and general anesthesia. Barbiturates cause tolerance and dependence, have a high abuse potential, and are subject to multiple drug interactions. Moreover, barbiturates are powerful respiratory depressants that can be fatal in overdose. Because of these undesirable properties, barbiturates are used much less than in the past, having been replaced by newer and safer drugs—primarily the benzodiazepines and benzodiazepine-like drugs (e.g., zolpidem). However, although their use has declined greatly, barbiturates still have important applications in seizure control and anesthesia. Moreover, barbiturates are valuable from an instructional point of view: By understanding these prototypic agents, we gain an understanding of the general CNS depressants as a group, along with an appreciation of why barbiturates are no longer used for anxiety and insomnia.

Safety Alert

BARBITURATES

Barbiturates are powerful respiratory depressants that can be fatal in overdose. Respiratory depression does not decrease with drug tolerance.

TABLE 34.4 ■ Characteristics of Barbiturate Subgroups

			Time Course		
Barbiturate Subgroup	Representative Drug	Lipid Solubility	Onset (min)	Duration (hr)	Applications
Ultrashort-acting	Methohexital	High	0.5	0.2	Induction of anesthesia; treatment of seizures
Short- to intermediate-acting	Secobarbital	Moderate	10–15	3–4	Treatment of insomnia
Long-acting	Phenobarbital	Low	60 or less	10–12	Treatment of seizures

Classification

The barbiturates fall into three groups—ultrashort-acting, short- to intermediate-acting, and long-acting—based on duration of action. As indicated in Table 34.4, their duration of action is inversely related to their lipid solubility. Barbiturates with the highest lipid solubility have the shortest duration of action. Conversely, barbiturates with the lowest lipid solubility have the longest duration.

Duration of action influences the clinical applications of barbiturates. The ultrashort-acting agents (e.g., methohexital) are used for induction of anesthesia. The short- to intermediate-acting agents (e.g., secobarbital) are used as sedatives and hypnotics. The long-acting agents (e.g., phenobarbital) are used primarily as antiseizure drugs.

Mechanism of Action

Like benzodiazepines, barbiturates bind to the GABA receptor–chloride channel complex (see Fig. 34.1). By doing so, these drugs can (1) enhance the inhibitory actions of GABA and (2) directly mimic the actions of GABA.

Because barbiturates can directly mimic GABA, there is no ceiling to the degree of CNS depression they can produce. Hence, in contrast to the benzodiazepines, these drugs can readily cause death by overdose. Although barbiturates can cause general depression of the CNS, they show some selectivity for depressing the *reticular activating system* (RAS), a neuronal network that helps regulate the sleep-wakefulness cycle. By depressing the RAS, barbiturates produce sedation and sleep.

Pharmacologic Effects

CNS Depression. Most effects of barbiturates—both therapeutic and adverse—result from generalized depression of CNS function. With increasing dosage, responses progress from sedation to sleep to general anesthesia.

Most barbiturates can be considered nonselective CNS depressants. The main exception is phenobarbital, a drug used to control seizures. Seizure control is achieved at doses that have minimal effects on other aspects of CNS function.

Cardiovascular Effects. At hypnotic doses, barbiturates produce modest reductions in blood pressure and heart rate. In contrast, toxic doses can cause profound hypotension and shock. At high doses, barbiturates depress the myocardium and vascular smooth muscle, along with all other electrically excitable tissues.

Induction of Hepatic Drug-Metabolizing Enzymes. Barbiturates stimulate synthesis of hepatic microsomal enzymes, the principal drug-metabolizing enzymes of the liver. As a result, barbiturates can accelerate their own metabolism and the metabolism of many other drugs.

Barbiturates stimulate drug metabolism by promoting synthesis of porphyrin. Porphyrin is then converted into heme, which in turn is incorporated into cytochrome P450, a key component of the hepatic drug-metabolizing system.

Tolerance and Physical Dependence

Tolerance. Tolerance is defined as reduced drug responsiveness that develops over the course of repeated drug use. When barbiturates are taken regularly, tolerance develops to many—but not all—of their CNS effects. Specifically, tolerance develops to sedative and hypnotic effects and to other effects that underlie barbiturate abuse. However, even with chronic use, *very little tolerance develops to toxic effects.*

In the tolerant user, doses must be increased to produce the same intensity of response that could formerly be achieved with smaller doses. Hence, individuals who take barbiturates for prolonged periods—be it for therapy or recreation—require steadily increasing doses to achieve the effects they desire.

It is important to note that *very little tolerance develops to respiratory depression.* Because tolerance to respiratory depression is minimal and because tolerance does develop to therapeutic effects with continued treatment, the lethal (respiratory-depressant) dose remains relatively constant while the therapeutic dose climbs higher and higher (Fig. 34.2). As tolerance to therapeutic effects increases, the therapeutic dose grows steadily closer to the lethal dose—a situation that is clearly hazardous.

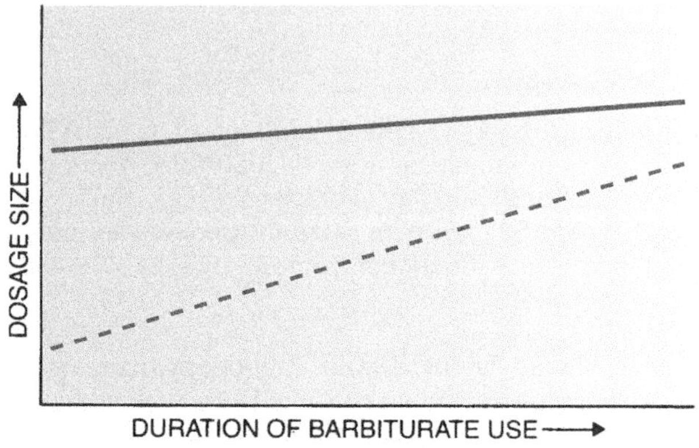

Fig. 34.2 ■ Development of tolerance to the toxic and subjective effects of barbiturates.
With prolonged barbiturate use, tolerance develops. However, less tolerance develops to toxic effects than to desired effects. Consequently, as duration of use increases, the difference between the dose producing desirable effects and the dose producing toxicity becomes progressively smaller, thereby increasing the risk of serious harm.

As a rule, tolerance to one general CNS depressant bestows tolerance to all other general CNS depressants. Hence, there is cross-tolerance among barbiturates, alcohol, benzodiazepines, general anesthetics, and certain other agents. Tolerance to barbiturates and the other general CNS depressants does *not* produce significant cross-tolerance with opioids (e.g., morphine).

Physical Dependence. Prolonged use of barbiturates results in physical dependence, a state in which continued use is required to avoid an abstinence syndrome. Physical dependence results from adaptive neurochemical changes that occur in response to chronic drug exposure.

Individuals who are physically dependent on barbiturates exhibit cross-dependence with other general CNS depressants. Because of cross-dependence, a person physically dependent on barbiturates can prevent withdrawal symptoms by taking any other general CNS depressant (e.g., alcohol, benzodiazepines). As a rule, cross-dependence exists among all of the general CNS depressants. However, there is no significant cross-dependence with opioids.

The general CNS-depressant abstinence syndrome can be severe. Abrupt withdrawal from general CNS depressants is more dangerous than withdrawal from opioids. Although withdrawal from opioids is certainly unpleasant, the risk of serious injury is low. In contrast, the abstinence syndrome associated with general CNS depressants can be fatal.

The following description illustrates how dangerous withdrawal from general CNS depressants can be. Early reactions include weakness, restlessness, insomnia, hyperthermia, orthostatic hypotension, confusion, and disorientation. By the third day, major convulsive episodes may develop. Approximately 75% of patients experience psychotic delirium (a state similar to alcoholic delirium tremens). In extreme cases, these symptoms may be followed by exhaustion, cardiovascular collapse, and death. The entire abstinence syndrome evolves over approximately 8 days. Symptom intensity can be greatly reduced by withdrawing barbiturates and other general CNS depressants slowly.

A long-acting barbiturate (e.g., phenobarbital) may be administered to facilitate the withdrawal process. Because of cross-dependence, phenobarbital can substitute for other CNS depressants and can thereby suppress symptoms of withdrawal. Because phenobarbital is eliminated from the body slowly, treatment permits a gradual transition from a drug-dependent state to a drug-free state. When phenobarbital is given to aid withdrawal, its dosage should be reduced gradually over 10 days to 3 weeks.

It is important to note that physical dependence should not be equated with addiction. Addiction is defined as a primary chronic disease characterized by an individual pathologically pursuing rewards and/or relief by substance use and other behaviors. Although physical dependence can contribute to this behavior pattern, physical dependence by itself will neither cause nor sustain addictive behavior. The distinction between addiction and physical dependence is discussed further in Chapter 37.

Therapeutic Uses

Seizure Disorders. Phenobarbital is used for seizure disorders (see Chapter 24). This drug suppresses seizures at doses that are essentially nonsedative.

Induction of Anesthesia. One highly lipid-soluble barbiturate—methohexital sodium [Brevital]—is used to induce general anesthesia (see Chapter 27). Unconsciousness develops within seconds of IV injection.

Insomnia. By depressing the CNS, barbiturates can promote sleep. However, because they can cause multiple undesired effects, barbiturates have been replaced by benzodiazepines and related drugs as treatments of choice for insomnia.

Other Uses. Barbiturates have been used to treat acute manic states and delirium. In children, they can decrease restlessness secondary to colic, pylorospasm, and whooping cough. In addition, they can help reduce anxiety in children before minor dental and medical procedures. Excessive excitation from overdose with CNS stimulants (e.g., amphetamine, theophylline, ephedrine) can be decreased with barbiturates. They can also be employed for emergency treatment of convulsions caused by tetanus, eclampsia, and epilepsy. When administered in anesthetic doses, barbiturates can help reduce mortality from head injury; deep anesthesia reduces the brain's requirements for oxygen and glucose and thereby helps preserve CNS function. However, until anesthetic levels are achieved, barbiturates *increase* sensitivity to pain, and hence should not be used until pain is under control.

Adverse Effects

Respiratory Depression. Barbiturates reduce ventilation by two mechanisms: (1) depression of brainstem neurogenic respiratory drive and (2) depression of chemoreceptive mechanisms that control respiratory drive. Doses only 3 times greater than those needed to induce sleep can cause complete suppression of the neurogenic respiratory drive. With severe overdose, barbiturates can cause apnea and death.

For most patients, the degree of respiratory depression produced at therapeutic doses is not significant. However, in older adult patients and in those with respiratory disease, therapeutic doses can compromise respiration substantially. Combining a barbiturate with another CNS depressant intensifies respiratory depression.

Suicide. Barbiturates have a low therapeutic index. Accordingly, overdose can readily cause death. Because of their toxicity, the barbiturates are employed as vehicles for suicide, and hence should not be dispensed to patients with suicidal tendencies.

Abuse. Barbiturates produce subjective effects that many individuals find desirable. As a result, they are popular drugs of abuse. The barbiturates that are most prone to abuse are those in the short- to intermediate-acting group (e.g., secobarbital). Individual barbiturates within the group are classified under Schedule III of the Controlled Substances Act, reflecting their high potential for abuse. Although barbiturates are frequently abused in nonmedical settings, they are rarely abused during medical use.

Acute Toxicity

Acute intoxication with barbiturates is a medical emergency: Left untreated, overdose can be fatal. Poisoning is often the result of attempted suicide, although it can also occur by accident (usually in children and drug abusers). Since acute toxicity from barbiturates and other general CNS depressants is very similar, the discussion that follows applies to all of these drugs.

Symptoms. Acute overdose produces a classic triad of symptoms: *respiratory depression, coma,* and *pinpoint pupils.* (Pupils may later dilate as hypoxia caused by respiratory depression sets in.) The three classic symptoms are frequently accompanied by *hypotension* and *hypothermia.* Death is likely to result from pulmonary complications and renal failure.

Treatment. Proper management requires an intensive care unit. With vigorous treatment, most patients recover fully.

Treatment has two main objectives: (1) removal of barbiturate from the body and (2) maintenance of an adequate oxygen supply to the brain. Oxygenation can be maintained by keeping the airway patent and giving oxygen.

Several measures can promote barbiturate removal. Unabsorbed drug can be adsorbed when in the stomach through the use of activated charcoal. For phenobarbital and other barbiturates that are excreted intact in the urine, forced diuresis and alkalinization of the urine may facilitate their renal excretion.

Steps should be taken to prevent hypotension and loss of body heat. Blood pressure can be supported with fluid replacement and norepinephrine. Body heat can be maintained with blankets and warming devices.

Barbiturate poisoning has no specific antidote. CNS stimulants should definitely *not* be employed. Not only are stimulants ineffective, they are also dangerous: Their use in barbiturate poisoning has been associated with a significant increase in mortality. Naloxone, a drug that can reverse poisoning by opioids, is *not* effective against poisoning by barbiturates.

Administration

Oral. Oral administration is employed for daytime sedation and to treat insomnia. Patients should be warned not to increase their dosage or to discontinue treatment without consulting the prescriber. Dosages should be reduced for older adult patients. When terminating therapy, the dosage should be gradually tapered.

Intravenous. Intravenous administration is reserved for general anesthesia and emergency treatment of convulsions. Injections should be made slowly to minimize respiratory depression and hypotension. Blood pressure, pulses, and respiration should be monitored, and facilities for resuscitation should be available. The patient should be under continuous observation. Extravasation may result in local necrosis, hence care must be taken to ensure that extravasation does not occur. Solutions that are cloudy or contain a precipitate should not be used. Intra-arterial injection should be avoided, owing to a risk of gangrene secondary to prolonged arteriospasm.

Intramuscular. Barbiturate solutions are highly alkaline and can cause pain and necrosis when injected IM. Consequently, IM injection is generally avoided. Injection in the vicinity of peripheral nerves can cause irreversible neurologic injury.

MANAGEMENT OF INSOMNIA

Insomnia can be defined as an inability to sleep well. Some people have difficulty falling asleep, some have difficulty maintaining sleep, some are troubled by early morning awakening, and some have sleep that is not refreshing. Insomnia is transient for some people and chronic for others. In any given year, about 30% of Americans experience intermittent insomnia, and about 10% experience chronic insomnia.

As a result of sleep loss, insomniacs experience daytime drowsiness along with impairment of mood, memory, coordination, and the ability to concentrate and make decisions. Chronic insomnia is a major risk factor for automotive and industrial accidents, marital and social problems, major depression, coronary heart disease, and metabolic and endocrine dysregulation.

Loss of sleep is often the result of a medical condition. Psychiatric disorders often disturb sleep, and pain can keep anyone awake. Sleep is frequently lost owing to concern regarding impending surgery and other procedures.

At one time or another, nearly everyone suffers from situational insomnia. Worry about exams may keep students awake. Job-related pressures may deprive workers of sleep. Unfamiliar surroundings may keep travelers awake. Major life stressors (bereavement, divorce, loss of job) frequently disrupt sleep. Other factors, such as uncomfortable bedding, excessive noise, and bright light, can rob us of sound sleep.

Sleep Phases

The sleeping state has two primary phases: *rapid-eye-movement* (REM) sleep and *non–rapid-eye-movement* (NREM) sleep. NREM sleep is further divided into four stages, labeled I, II, III, and IV. Sleep is relatively light in stages I and II, and deep in stages III and IV. REM sleep is the phase when most recallable dreams occur. In a typical night, we go through four to six REM periods. The percentage of time spent in each sleep phase is as follows:

- Stage I: 5%
- Stage II: 50% to 60%
- Stages III and IV: 10% to 20%
- REM: 20% to 25%

Basic Principles of Management

Cause-Specific Therapy

Treatment is highly dependent on the cause of insomnia. Accordingly, if therapy is to succeed, the underlying reason for sleep loss must be determined. To make this assessment, a thorough history is required.

When the cause of insomnia is a known medical disorder, primary therapy should be directed at the underlying illness; hypnotics should be employed only as adjuncts. For example, if pain is the reason for lost sleep, analgesics should be prescribed. If insomnia is secondary to major depression, antidepressants are the appropriate treatment. If anxiety is the cause of insomnia, the patient should receive an anxiolytic.

Nondrug Therapy

For many insomniacs, nondrug measures may be all that is needed to promote sleep. For some individuals, avoidance of naps and adherence to a regular sleep schedule are sufficient. For others, decreased consumption of caffeine-containing beverages (e.g., coffee, tea, cola drinks) may fix the problem. Still others may benefit from restful activity as bedtime nears. If environmental factors are responsible for lack of sleep, the patient should be taught how to correct them or compensate for them. All patients should be counseled about sleep fitness (also known as sleep hygiene). Rules for sleep fitness are shown in Table 34.5.

TABLE 34.5 ■ Rules for Sleep Fitness

- Establish a regular time to go to bed and a regular time to rise—even on weekends. This will help reset your biologic clock.
- Sleep only as long as needed to feel refreshed. Too much time in bed causes fragmented and shallow sleep. In contrast, restricting time in bed helps consolidate and deepen sleep.
- Insulate your bedroom against light and sounds that disturb your sleep (e.g., install carpeting and insulated curtains).
- Keep your bedroom temperature moderate. High temperature may disturb sleep.
- Exercise daily, but not later than 7:00 PM. Regular exercise helps deepen sleep.
- Schedule outdoor time at the same time each day.
- Avoid daytime naps. Staying awake during the day helps you sleep at night.
- Avoid caffeine, especially in the evening.
- Avoid consuming too much fluid in the evening so as to minimize nighttime trips to the bathroom.
- Avoid alcohol in the evening. Although alcohol can help you fall asleep, it causes sleep to be fragmented.
- Avoid tobacco; it disturbs sleep (and shortens your life, too).
- Try having a light snack near bedtime, as hunger can disturb sleep. But don't eat heavily.
- Relax before bedtime with soft music, mild stretching, yoga, or pleasurable reading.
- Avoid bright light—including television, computers, and video games—before going to bed.
- Leave your problems outside the bedroom. Reserve time earlier in the evening to work on problems and to plan tomorrow's activities.
- Reserve your bedroom for sleeping and sex. This will help condition your brain to see the bedroom as a place where sleep happens. Don't eat, read, or watch TV in bed.
- If you don't fall asleep within 20 minutes or so, get up and do something relaxing (e.g., read, listen to music, watch TV), and then return to bed when you feel drowsy. Repeat as often as required.
- Don't look at the clock if you wake up during the night. If necessary, turn its face away from the bed.

Research has shown that *cognitive behavioral therapy* is *superior* to drug therapy for both short-term and long-term management of chronic insomnia in older adults. Cognitive and behavioral interventions include sleep restriction, control of the bedroom environment, progressive relaxation, and education about sleep hygiene. The American Academy of Sleep Medicine considers these interventions both effective and reliable, and hence recommends them as first-line therapy for chronic insomnia, even if drug therapy is also employed.

Therapy With Hypnotic Drugs

Hypnotics should be used only when insomnia cannot be managed by other means. Hence, before resorting to drugs, we should implement nondrug measures, and we should treat any pathology that may underlie inadequate sleep.

Drug therapy of transient insomnia should be short term (just 2 to 3 weeks). The patient should be reassessed on a regular basis to determine whether drug therapy is still needed.

Escalation of dosage should be avoided. A need for increased dosage suggests development of tolerance. If hypnotic effects are lost in the course of treatment, it is preferable to interrupt therapy rather than to elevate dosage. Interruption will allow tolerance to decline, thereby restoring responsiveness to treatment.

In certain patients, hypnotics must be employed with special caution. Patients who snore heavily and those with respiratory disorders have reduced respiratory reserve, which can be further compromised by the respiratory-depressant actions of hypnotics. Hypnotic agents are generally contraindicated for use during pregnancy; these drugs have the potential to cause fetal harm, and their use is rarely an absolute necessity.

Patients taking hypnotics should be forewarned that residual CNS depression may persist the next day. Although CNS depression may not be pronounced, it may still compromise intellectual or physical performance.

When hypnotics are employed, care must be taken to prevent *drug-dependency insomnia,* a condition that can lead to inappropriate prolongation of therapy. Drug-dependency insomnia

TABLE 34.6 ▪ Major Drugs for Insomnia

Drug	Time Course		Use in Insomnia		Bedtime Dosage (mg)	
	Onset (min)	Duration	DFA	DMS	Younger Adult	Older Adult
BENZODIAZEPINES						
Triazolam [Halcion]	15–30	Short	✓		0.125–0.25	0.125
Flurazepam[a] (generic only)	30–60	Long	✓	✓	15–30	15
Quazepam[a] [Doral]	20–45	Long	✓	✓	15	7.5
Estazolam (generic only)	15–60	Intermediate		✓	1–2	0.5–1
Temazepam [Restoril]	45–60	Intermediate		✓	15–30	7.5–15
BENZODIAZEPINE-LIKE DRUGS						
Eszopiclone [Lunesta]	30	Intermediate	✓	✓	2–3	1–2
Zolpidem						
Extended-release tablets [Ambien CR]	30	Intermediate	✓	✓	12.5	6.25
Immediate-release tablets [Ambien]	30	Short	✓		10	5
Sublingual [Intermezzo]	30	Short	✓	✓	1.75 for females and 3.5 for males	1.75
Sublingual [Edluar]	30	Short	✓		10	5
Oral spray [Zolpimist]	30	Short	✓		5–10	5
Zaleplon [Sonata]	15–30	Ultrashort	✓		5–10	5
MELATONIN RECEPTOR AGONIST						
Ramelteon [Rozerem]	30	Short	✓		8	8
OREXIN RECEPTOR ANTAGONIST						
Suvorexant [Belsomra]	30	Intermediate	✓	✓	10	10

[a]Because of its long duration, this drug is not generally recommended.
DFA, Difficulty falling asleep; *DMS,* difficulty maintaining sleep.

is a particular problem with older hypnotics (e.g., barbiturates); it develops as follows:

1. Insomnia motivates treatment with hypnotics.
2. With continuous drug use, low-level physical dependence develops.
3. Upon cessation of treatment, a mild withdrawal syndrome occurs and disrupts sleep.
4. Failing to recognize that the inability to sleep is a manifestation of drug withdrawal, the patient becomes convinced that insomnia has returned and resumes drug use.
5. Continued drug use leads to heightened physical dependence, making it even more difficult to withdraw medication without producing another episode of drug-dependency insomnia.

To minimize drug-dependency insomnia, hypnotics should be employed judiciously. That is, they should be used in the lowest effective dosage for the shortest time required.

Major Hypnotics Used for Treatment

Insomnia can be treated with prescription drugs, nonprescription drugs, and alternative medicines. Among the prescription drugs, benzodiazepines and the benzodiazepine-like drugs (zolpidem, zaleplon, and eszopiclone) are drugs of choice. Older sedative-hypnotics, such as barbiturates, are rarely used. Nonprescription drugs and alternative medicines are much less effective than the first-choice drugs, and hence should be reserved for people whose insomnia is mild.

As shown in Table 34.6, hypnotic drugs differ with respect to onset and duration of action, and hence differ in their applications. Drugs with a rapid onset (e.g., zolpidem) are good for patients who have difficulty falling asleep, whereas drugs with a long duration (e.g., estazolam) are good for patients who have difficulty maintaining sleep. Drugs such as flurazepam, which have both a rapid onset and long duration, are good for patients with both types of sleep problems.

Benzodiazepines

Benzodiazepines are drugs of first choice for short-term treatment of insomnia. These agents are safe and effective and lack the undesirable properties that typify barbiturates and other older hypnotics. Benzodiazepines have a low abuse potential, cause minimal tolerance and physical dependence, present a minimal risk of suicide, and undergo few interactions with other drugs. Only five benzodiazepines are marketed specifically for use as hypnotics (see Table 34.6). However, any benzodiazepine with a short to intermediate onset could be employed.

Benzodiazepines have multiple desirable effects on sleep: they decrease the interval to sleep onset, decrease the number of awakenings, and increase total sleeping time. In addition, they impart a sense of deep and refreshing sleep. With most benzodiazepines, tolerance to hypnotic actions develops slowly, allowing them to be used nightly for several weeks without a noticeable loss in hypnotic effects. Furthermore, with most benzodiazepines, treatment does not significantly reduce the amount of time spent in REM sleep, and withdrawal is not associated with significant rebound insomnia.

Two agents—*triazolam* [Halcion] and *flurazepam*—can be considered prototypes of the benzodiazepines used to promote sleep. Triazolam has a rapid onset and short duration, making it a good choice for patients who have difficulty in falling asleep (as compared with difficulty in maintaining sleep). Flurazepam has a delayed onset and more prolonged duration, making it an effective agent for patients who have difficulty in maintaining sleep. However, because flurazepam has a relatively long half-life, the drug is likely to cause daytime drowsiness, and hence is not used widely today. Triazolam has a much shorter half-life than flurazepam, which is both good news and bad news. The good news is that because it leaves the body rapidly, triazolam does not cause daytime sedation. The bad news is that because triazolam is rapidly cleared, treatment is associated with two problems: (1) tolerance to hypnotic effects can develop quickly—in 11 to 18 days, which is much faster than with other benzodiazepines, and (2) triazolam causes more rebound insomnia than other benzodiazepines.

The pharmacology of the benzodiazepines is discussed earlier.

Benzodiazepine-like Drugs: Zolpidem, Zaleplon, and Eszopiclone

Zolpidem [Ambien, Ambien CR, Edluar, Intermezzo, Zolpimist], zaleplon [Sonata], and eszopiclone [Lunesta] are drugs of first choice for insomnia. In fact, one of these drugs—zolpidem—is prescribed more often than any other hypnotic. All three drugs have the same mechanism as the benzodiazepines—and all three are as effective as the benzodiazepines, and may be safer for long-term use. Furthermore, whereas benzodiazepines are contraindicated during pregnancy, the benzodiazepine-like drugs are not (although use during pregnancy should be discouraged). All three drugs have a rapid onset, and hence can help people with difficulty in *falling* asleep. Also, with zolpidem and eszopiclone, effects persist long enough to help people who have difficulty in *staying* asleep. In contrast, effects of zaleplon fade too rapidly to help people with trouble in staying asleep. However, zaleplon is great for people who wake up in the middle of the night. Owing to its ultrashort duration, zaleplon can be taken a few hours before rising and still not cause drowsiness during the day. Of the three drugs, only eszopiclone has been proved effective for long-term use. However, even though long-term studies for zaleplon and zolpidem are lacking, it seems likely that they too would retain efficacy when taken long term. The pharmacology of the benzodiazepine-like drugs is discussed previously in this chapter.

Ramelteon

Ramelteon [Rozerem] is a melatonin agonist approved for long-term therapy of insomnia. The drug has a rapid onset and short duration, and hence is good for inducing sleep, but not for maintaining sleep. Ramelteon does not cause tolerance or dependence, and is not regulated as a controlled substance. The pharmacology of ramelteon is discussed earlier in this chapter.

Suvorexant

Suvorexant [Belsomra] is an orexin receptor antagonist approved for both onset and maintenance of sleep. As there is a risk for dependence, it is a Schedule IV drug, similar to the benzodiazepine-like drug zolpidem.

Other Hypnotics

Antidepressants

Trazodone. Trazodone [Oleptro] is an atypical antidepressant with strong sedative actions. The drug can decrease sleep latency and prolong sleep duration, and does not cause tolerance or physical dependence. Trazodone is especially useful in the treatment of insomnia resulting from the use of antidepressants that cause significant CNS stimulation (e.g., fluoxetine [Prozac], bupropion [Wellbutrin]). Principal adverse effects are daytime grogginess and postural hypotension. (Hypotension results from alpha-adrenergic blockade.) The basic pharmacology of trazodone is presented in Chapter 32.

Doxepin. Doxepin is an old tricyclic antidepressant (TCA) with strong sedative actions. The formulation (3- and 6-mg tablets) is sold as *Silenor*. In clinical trials of adults with chronic insomnia, Silenor increased total sleep time and maintained the effect for over 12 weeks. These benefits probably derive from blocking receptors for histamine. The initial dosage for patients age 65 and older is 3 mg, taken within 30 minutes of bedtime. The initial dosage for patients under age 65 is 6 mg. Both dosages are much lower than the dosages used for depression (75 to 150 mg/day).

In the low doses used for sleep maintenance, doxepin is well tolerated. The most common adverse effects are sedation, nausea, and upper respiratory infection. In the high doses used for depression, doxepin can cause hypotension, dysrhythmias, and anticholinergic effects (e.g., dry mouth, constipation, urinary retention, blurred vision). Owing to the risk of anticholinergic effects, Silenor is contraindicated for patients with untreated narrow-angle glaucoma or severe urinary retention. In addition, Silenor is contraindicated for patients who have taken a monoamine oxidase inhibitor within the past 2 weeks. Unlike the benzodiazepines and benzodiazepine-like drugs, Silenor has little or no potential for abuse, and hence is not regulated under the Controlled Substances Act. Accordingly, the drug may be especially appropriate when drug abuse is a concern.

The basic pharmacology of doxepin and other TCAs is presented in Chapter 32.

Antihistamines

Two antihistamines—diphenhydramine [Nytol, Sominex, others] and doxylamine [Unisom]—are FDA approved for use as "sleep aids" and can be purchased without a prescription. These drugs are less effective than benzodiazepines and benzodiazepine-like drugs, and tolerance develops quickly (in 1 to 2 weeks). Daytime drowsiness and anticholinergic effects (e.g., dry mouth, blurred vision, urinary hesitancy, constipation) are common.

Alternative Medicines

Of the alternative medicines employed to promote sleep, only one—melatonin—appears moderately effective (see Box 34.1). Several others—valerian root, chamomile, passionflower, lemon balm, and lavender—have very mild sedative effects, but proof of benefits in insomnia is lacking.

KEY POINTS

- Drugs used to treat anxiety disorders are called antianxiety agents, anxiolytics, or tranquilizers.
- Drugs that promote sleep are called hypnotics.
- Barbiturates and other general CNS depressants are undesirable in that they can cause fatal respiratory depression, have a high potential for abuse, cause significant tolerance and physical dependence, and often induce hepatic drug-metabolizing enzymes.
- Benzodiazepines are preferred to barbiturates and other general CNS depressants because they are much safer, have a low abuse potential, cause less tolerance and dependence, and don't induce drug-metabolizing enzymes.
- Although benzodiazepines can cause physical dependence, the withdrawal syndrome is usually mild (except in patients who have undergone prolonged high-dose therapy).
- To minimize withdrawal symptoms, benzodiazepines should be discontinued gradually, over several weeks or even months.
- Benzodiazepines cause minimal respiratory depression when used alone, but can cause profound respiratory depression when combined with other CNS depressants (e.g., opioids, alcohol).
- Benzodiazepines produce their effects by enhancing the actions of GABA, the principal inhibitory neurotransmitter in the CNS.
- Although benzodiazepines undergo extensive metabolism, in most cases the metabolites are pharmacologically active. As a result, responses produced by administering a particular benzodiazepine often persist long after the parent drug has disappeared from the blood.
- All of the benzodiazepines have essentially equivalent pharmacologic actions; hence, selection among them is based in large part on differences in time course.
- The principal indications for benzodiazepines are anxiety, insomnia, and seizure disorders.
- The principal adverse effects of benzodiazepines are daytime sedation and anterograde amnesia.
- Rarely, patients taking benzodiazepines to promote sleep carry out sleep driving and other complex behaviors, and then have no memory of their actions.
- Flumazenil, a benzodiazepine receptor antagonist, can be used to treat benzodiazepine overdose.
- Like the benzodiazepines, the benzodiazepine-like drugs—zaleplon [Sonata], eszopiclone [Lunesta], and zolpidem [Ambien, others]—produce their effects by enhancing the actions of GABA.
- When insomnia has a treatable cause (e.g., pain, depression, schizophrenia), primary therapy should be directed at the underlying illness; hypnotics should be used only as adjuncts.
- Cognitive behavioral therapy is highly effective for insomnia, and hence is considered first-line treatment, even if drugs are also employed.
- Benzodiazepines and the benzodiazepine-like drugs (zolpidem, zaleplon, eszopiclone) are drugs of choice for insomnia.
- When benzodiazepines are used for transient insomnia, treatment should last only 2 to 3 weeks.

Please visit **http://evolve.elsevier.com/Lehne** for chapter-specific NCLEX® examination review questions.

Summary of Major Nursing Implications[a]

BENZODIAZEPINES

Alprazolam
Chlordiazepoxide
Clonazepam
Clorazepate
Diazepam
Estazolam
Flurazepam
Lorazepam
Midazolam
Oxazepam
Quazepam
Temazepam
Triazolam

The nursing implications summarized here apply to the sedative-hypnotic benzodiazepines and their use in insomnia.

Preadministration Assessment

Therapeutic Goal

Benzodiazepines are used to promote sleep, relieve symptoms of anxiety (see Chapter 35), suppress seizure disorders (see Chapter 24), relax muscle spasm (see Chapter 25), and ease withdrawal from alcohol (see Chapter 38). They are also used for preanesthetic medication and to induce general anesthesia (see Chapter 27).

Baseline Data

Determine the nature of the sleep disturbance (prolonged latency, frequent awakenings, early morning awakening) and how long it has lasted. Assess for a possible underlying cause (e.g., medical illness, psychiatric illness, use of caffeine and other stimulants, poor sleep hygiene, major life stressor).

Continued

Summary of Major Nursing Implications[a]—cont'd

Identifying High-Risk Patients

Benzodiazepines are *contraindicated* during pregnancy and for patients who experience sleep apnea. Use with *caution* in patients with suicidal tendencies or a history of substance abuse.

Implementation: Administration

Routes

Oral. All benzodiazepines.

IM and IV. Diazepam and lorazepam.

Rectal. Diazepam.

Administration

Oral. **Advise patients to administer benzodiazepines with food if gastric upset occurs. Instruct patients to swallow sustained-release formulations intact, without crushing or chewing.**

Warn patients not to increase the dosage or discontinue treatment without consulting the prescriber.

To minimize physical dependence when treating insomnia, use intermittent dosing (3 or 4 nights a week) and the lowest effective dosage for the shortest duration required.

To minimize abstinence symptoms, taper the dosage gradually (over several weeks or even months).

Intravenous. Perform IV injections with care. Life-threatening reactions (severe hypotension, respiratory arrest, cardiac arrest) have occurred, along with less serious reactions (venous thrombosis, phlebitis, vascular impairment). To reduce complications, follow these guidelines: (1) make injections slowly; (2) take care to avoid intra-arterial injection and extravasation; (3) if direct venous injection is impossible, inject into infusion tubing as close to the vein as possible; (4) follow the manufacturer's instructions regarding suitable diluents for preparing solutions; and (5) have facilities for resuscitation available.

Implementation: Measures to Enhance Therapeutic Effects

Educate patients about sleep fitness (see Table 34.5). Reassure patients with situational insomnia that sleep patterns will normalize once the precipitating stressor has been eliminated. Ensure that correctable underlying causes of insomnia (psychiatric or medical illness, use of stimulant drugs) are being managed.

Ongoing Evaluation and Interventions

Evaluating Therapeutic Effects

Insomnia is usually self-limiting. Consequently, drug therapy is usually short term. Benzodiazepines should be discontinued periodically to determine whether they are still required. If insomnia is long term, make a special effort to identify possible underlying causes (e.g., psychiatric illness, medical illness, use of caffeine and other stimulants).

Minimizing Adverse Effects

CNS Depression. Drowsiness may be present the next day when benzodiazepines are used for insomnia. **Warn patients about possible residual CNS depression and advise them to avoid hazardous activities (e.g., driving) if daytime sedation is significant.**

Sleep Driving and Other Complex Sleep-Related Behaviors. Rarely, patients taking benzodiazepines to promote sleep may carry out complex behaviors (e.g., sleep driving, eating, making phone calls), and then have no memory of the event. To reduce the risk of these events, dosage should be as low as possible, and alcohol and other CNS depressants should be avoided. **Inform patients about the possibility of complex sleep-related behaviors and instruct them to notify the prescriber if they occur.** If the patient reports driving while asleep, the benzodiazepine should be withdrawn (albeit slowly).

Paradoxical Effects. **Inform patients about possible paradoxical reactions (rage, excitement, heightened anxiety), and instruct them to notify the prescriber if these occur.** If the reaction is verified, benzodiazepines should be withdrawn.

Physical Dependence. With most benzodiazepines, significant physical dependence is rare. However, with one agent—alprazolam [Xanax, Xanax XR, Niravam]—substantial dependence has been reported. With all benzodiazepines, development of dependence can be minimized by using the lowest effective dosage for the shortest time necessary and by using intermittent dosing when treating insomnia.

When dependence is mild, withdrawal can elicit insomnia and other symptoms that resemble anxiety. These must be distinguished from a return of the patient's original sleep disorder. **Warn patients about possible drug-dependency insomnia during or after benzodiazepine withdrawal.**

When dependence is severe, withdrawal reactions may be serious (panic, paranoia, delirium, hypertension, convulsions). To minimize symptoms, withdraw benzodiazepines slowly (over several weeks or months). **Warn patients against abrupt discontinuation of treatment.** After drug cessation, patients should be monitored for 3 weeks for signs of withdrawal or recurrence of original symptoms.

Abuse. The abuse potential of the benzodiazepines is low. However, some individuals do abuse them. Be alert to requests for increased dosage, since this may reflect an attempt at abuse. Benzodiazepines are classified under Schedule IV of the Controlled Substances Act and must be dispensed accordingly.

Use in Pregnancy and Lactation. Benzodiazepines may injure the developing fetus, especially during the first trimester. **Inform women of childbearing age about the potential for fetal harm and warn them against becoming pregnant.** If pregnancy occurs, benzodiazepines should be withdrawn.

Benzodiazepines readily enter breast milk and may accumulate to toxic levels in the infant. **Warn mothers against breast-feeding.**

Minimizing Adverse Interactions

CNS Depressants. Combined overdose with a benzodiazepine plus another CNS depressant can cause profound respiratory depression, coma, and death. **Warn patients against the use of alcohol and all other CNS depressants (e.g., opioids, barbiturates, antihistamines).**

[a]Patient education information is highlighted as **blue text.**

CHAPTER

35 Management of Anxiety Disorders

Anxiety is an uncomfortable state that has both psychologic and physical components. The psychologic component can be characterized with terms such as *fear, apprehension, dread,* and *uneasiness.* The physical component manifests as tachycardia, palpitations, trembling, dry mouth, sweating, weakness, fatigue, and shortness of breath.

Anxiety is a nearly universal experience that often serves an adaptive function. When anxiety is moderate and situationally appropriate, therapy may not be needed or even desirable. In contrast, when anxiety is persistent and disabling, intervention is clearly indicated.

Anxiety disorders are among the most common psychiatric illnesses. In the United States, about 25% of people develop pathologic anxiety at some time in their lives. As a rule, the incidence is higher in women than in men.

In this chapter, we focus on five of the more common anxiety disorders: generalized anxiety disorder, panic disorder, obsessive-compulsive disorder, social anxiety disorder, and post-traumatic stress disorder. Although each type is distinct, they all have one element in common: an unhealthy level of anxiety. In addition, with all anxiety disorders, depression is frequently comorbid.

Fortunately, anxiety disorders often respond well to treatment—either psychotherapy or drug therapy, or both. For most patients, a combination of psychotherapy and drug therapy is more effective than either modality alone.

As indicated in Table 35.1, two classes of drugs are used most: *serotoninergic reuptake inhibitors* (SRIs) and *benzodiazepines*. Benzodiazepines are used primarily for two conditions: generalized anxiety disorder (GAD) and panic disorder (PD). In contrast, the SRIs are now used for *all* anxiety disorders. It should be noted that although SRIs were developed as antidepressants, they can be very effective against anxiety—whether or not depression is present.

GENERALIZED ANXIETY DISORDER

Characteristics

GAD is a chronic condition characterized by uncontrollable worrying. Of all anxiety disorders, GAD is the least likely to remit. Most patients with GAD also have another psychiatric disorder, usually depression. GAD should not be confused with *situational anxiety,* which is a normal response to a stressful situation (e.g., family problems, exams, financial difficulties); symptoms may be intense, but they are temporary.

The hallmark of GAD is unrealistic or excessive anxiety about several events or activities (e.g., work or school performance) that lasts 6 months or longer. Other psychologic manifestations include vigilance, tension, apprehension, poor concentration, and difficulty falling or staying asleep. Somatic manifestations include trembling, muscle tension, restlessness, and signs of autonomic hyperactivity, such as palpitations, tachycardia, sweating, and cold, clammy hands.

Prototype Drugs

DRUGS FOR ANXIETY DISORDERS

Serotonergic Reuptake Inhibitors (SRIs)

Paroxetine (selective serotonin reuptake inhibitor [SSRI])
Venlafaxine (serotonin-norepinephrine reuptake inhibitor [SNRI])

Nonbenzodiazepine-Nonbarbiturates

Buspirone

Benzodiazepines

Diazepam

Treatment

GAD can be managed with nondrug therapy and with drugs. Nondrug approaches include supportive therapy, cognitive behavioral therapy (CBT), biofeedback, and relaxation training. These can help relieve symptoms and improve coping skills in anxiety-provoking situations. When symptoms are mild, nondrug therapy may be all that is needed. However, if symptoms are intensely uncomfortable or disabling, drugs are indicated. Current U.S. Food and Drug Administration (FDA)–approved first-line choices are SRIs (including both SSRIs and SNRIs) and buspirone. Second-line choices include the benzodiazepines. With the benzodiazepines, onset of relief

TABLE 35.1 ■ Drugs for Anxiety Disorders

Anxiety Disorder	Benzodiazepines	SSRIs	Others
Generalized anxiety disorder	Alprazolam Chlordiazepoxide Clorazepate Diazepam Lorazepam Oxazepam	Escitalopram Paroxetine	Buspirone Duloxetine Venlafaxine
Panic disorder	Alprazolam Clonazepam	Fluoxetine Paroxetine Sertraline	Venlafaxine
Obsessive-compulsive disorder		Citalopram Escitalopram Fluoxetine Fluvoxamine Paroxetine Sertraline	
Social anxiety disorder		Fluvoxamine Paroxetine Sertraline	Venlafaxine
Post-traumatic stress disorder		Fluoxetine Paroxetine Sertraline	Venlafaxine

SSRIs, Selective serotonin reuptake inhibitors.

is rapid. In contrast, with buspirone and the antidepressants, onset is delayed. Accordingly, benzodiazepines can be utilized for immediate stabilization, especially when anxiety is severe. However, for long-term management, buspirone and the antidepressants are preferred. Because GAD is a chronic disorder, initial drug therapy should be prolonged, lasting at least 12 months and possibly longer. Unfortunately, even after extended treatment, drug withdrawal frequently results in relapse. Hence, for many patients, drug therapy must continue indefinitely. Although other drugs are recommended for the treatment of GAD, they are currently used off-label.

Serotonergic Reuptake Inhibitors

Both SSRIs and SNRIs are considered first-line treatment for generalized anxiety disorder. At this time, only four antidepressants—venlafaxine [Effexor XR], duloxetine [Cymbalta], paroxetine [Paxil], and escitalopram [Lexapro, Cipralex ♣]—are approved for GAD. Venlafaxine and duloxetine are SNRIs; paroxetine and escitalopram are SSRIs. All four drugs are especially well suited for patients who have depression in addition to GAD. However, they are also effective even when depression is absent. Anxiolytic effects develop slowly: Initial responses can be seen in a week, but optimal responses require several more weeks to develop. Because relief is delayed, the antidepressants cannot be used PRN. Compared with benzodiazepines, the antidepressants do a better job of decreasing cognitive and psychic symptoms of anxiety, but are not as good at decreasing somatic symptoms. In contrast to the benzodiazepines, antidepressants have no potential for abuse. However, abrupt discontinuation *can* produce withdrawal symptoms.

Venlafaxine, an SNRI, was the first antidepressant approved for GAD. The drug has proven effective for both short-term and long-term use. The most common side effect is nausea, which develops in 37% of patients. Fortunately, nausea subsides despite continued treatment. Other common reactions include headache, anorexia, nervousness, sweating, daytime somnolence, and insomnia. In addition, venlafaxine can cause hypertension, although this is unlikely at the doses used in GAD. Combining venlafaxine with a monoamine oxidase inhibitor can result in serious toxicity, and hence must be avoided. Venlafaxine is available in two formulations: standard tablets (generic only) and extended-release capsules [Effexor XR]. Only the extended-release formulation is approved for GAD. The initial dosage is 37.5 mg once a day, and the maintenance range is 75 to 225 mg once a day.

Duloxetine, like venlafaxine, is an SNRI. The usual dosage, both initial and maintenance, is 30 to 60 mg once a day.

Paroxetine and *escitalopram* are the only SSRIs approved for GAD. These drugs are as effective as the benzodiazepines, but less well tolerated. For paroxetine, the initial dosage is 20 mg once a day in the morning. Dosage can be gradually increased to a maintenance range of 20 to 50 mg/day. For escitalopram, dosing begins at 10 mg once daily and can be increased to 20 mg once daily after a week. Treatment beyond 8 weeks has not been studied.

The basic pharmacology of venlafaxine, paroxetine, escitalopram, and duloxetine is discussed in Chapter 32.

Buspirone

Actions and Therapeutic Use. Buspirone [BuSpar] is an anxiolytic drug that differs significantly from the benzodiazepines. Most notably, buspirone is *not* a central nervous system (CNS) depressant. For treatment of anxiety, buspirone is as effective as the benzodiazepines and has two distinct advantages: It has no abuse potential and does not intensify the effects of CNS depressants (benzodiazepines, alcohol, barbiturates, and related drugs). Its major disadvantage is that anxiolytic effects develop *slowly:* Initial responses take a week to appear, and several more weeks must pass before responses peak. Because therapeutic effects are delayed, buspirone is not suitable for PRN use or for patients who need immediate relief. Because buspirone has no abuse potential, it may be especially appropriate for patients known to abuse alcohol and other drugs.

Because it lacks depressant properties, buspirone is an attractive alternative to benzodiazepines in patients who require long-term therapy but cannot tolerate benzodiazepine-induced sedation and psychomotor slowing. Buspirone is labeled only for *short-term* treatment of anxiety. However, the drug has been taken for as long as a year with no reduction in benefit. Buspirone does not display cross-dependence with benzodiazepines. Hence, when patients are switched from a benzodiazepine to buspirone, the benzodiazepine must be tapered slowly. Furthermore, since the effects of buspirone are delayed, buspirone should be initiated 2 to 4 weeks before beginning benzodiazepine withdrawal. In contrast to benzodiazepines, buspirone lacks sedative, muscle relaxant, and anticonvulsant actions—and hence cannot be used for insomnia, muscle spasm, or epilepsy.

The mechanism by which buspirone relieves anxiety has not been established. The drug binds with high affinity to receptors for serotonin and with lower affinity to receptors for dopamine. Buspirone does not bind to receptors for gamma-aminobutyric acid (GABA) or benzodiazepines.

Pharmacokinetics. Buspirone is well absorbed following oral administration, but undergoes extensive metabolism on its first pass through the liver. Administration with food delays absorption but enhances bioavailability (by reducing first-pass metabolism). The drug is excreted in part by the kidneys, primarily as metabolites.

Adverse Effects. Buspirone is generally well tolerated. The most common reactions are *dizziness, nausea, headache, nervousness, sedation, light-headedness,* and *excitement.* Furthermore, it poses little or no risk of suicide; huge doses (375 mg/day) have been given to healthy volunteers with only moderate adverse effects (nausea, vomiting, dizziness, drowsiness, miosis).

Drug and Food Interactions. Levels of buspirone can be greatly increased (5- to 13-fold) by *erythromycin* and *ketoconazole.* Levels can also be increased by *grapefruit juice.* Elevated levels may cause drowsiness and subjective effects (dysphoria, feeling "spacey"). Buspirone does not enhance the depressant effects of alcohol, barbiturates, and other general CNS depressants.

Tolerance, Dependence, and Abuse. Buspirone has been used for up to a year without evidence of tolerance, physical dependence, or psychologic dependence. No withdrawal symptoms have been observed upon termination. There is no cross-tolerance or cross-dependence between buspirone and the sedative-hypnotics (e.g., benzodiazepines, barbiturates). Buspirone appears to have no potential for abuse, and hence is not regulated under the Controlled Substances Act.

Preparations, Dosage, and Administration. Buspirone tablets [BuSpar] are available in four strengths: 5, 10, 15, and 30 mg. The initial dosage is 7.5 mg 2 times a day. Dosage may be increased to a maximum of 60 mg/day.

Benzodiazepines

Benzodiazepines are second-choice drugs for anxiety. As discussed in Chapter 34, benefits derive from enhancing responses to GABA, an inhibitory neurotransmitter. Onset of benefits is immediate, and the margin of safety is high. Although this class of drugs is particularly helpful in the treatment of acute anxiety, the potential for dependence and abuse with benzodiazepines has led to a decline in their use. Principal side effects are sedation and psychomotor slowing. Patients should be warned about these effects and informed that they will subside in 7 to 10 days. Because of their abuse potential, benzodiazepines should be used with caution in patients known to abuse alcohol or other psychoactive substances.

Long-term use of benzodiazepines carries a risk of physical dependence. Withdrawal symptoms include panic, paranoia, and delirium. These can be especially troubling for patients with GAD. Furthermore, they can be confused with a return of pretreatment symptoms. Accordingly, clinicians must differentiate between a withdrawal reaction and relapse. To minimize withdrawal symptoms, benzodiazepines should be tapered gradually—over a period of several months. If relapse occurs, treatment should resume.

Of the 13 benzodiazepines available, 6 are approved for anxiety. The agents prescribed most often are alprazolam [Xanax, Xanax XR, Niravam] and lorazepam [Ativan]. However, there is no proof that any one benzodiazepine is clearly superior to the others. Hence, selection among them is largely a matter of prescriber preference. Dosages for anxiety are shown in Table 35.2.

PANIC DISORDER

Characteristics

Panic disorder is characterized by recurrent, intensely uncomfortable episodes known as *panic attacks.* A panic attack is an abrupt surge of intense fear or intense discomfort during which four or more of the following are present:

- Palpitations, pounding heart, racing heartbeat
- Sweating
- Trembling or shaking
- Sensation of shortness of breath or smothering
- Feeling of choking
- Chest pain or discomfort
- Nausea or abdominal distress
- Feeling dizzy, unsteady, light-headed, or faint
- Chills or heat sensations
- Paresthesias (numbness or tingling sensations)
- Derealization (feelings of unreality) or depersonalization (feeling detached from oneself)
- Fear of losing control or going crazy
- Fear of dying

Panic symptoms reach a peak in a few minutes, and then dissipate within 30 minutes. Many patients go to an emergency department because they think they are having a heart attack. Some patients experience panic attacks daily; others have only one or two a month. Panic disorder is a common condition

TABLE 35.2 ▪ Dosages of Benzodiazepines Approved for Anxiety

		Dosage	
Generic Name	Brand Name	Initial	Usual Range (mg/day)
Alprazolam	Xanax, Niravam Xanax XR	0.25–0.5 mg 3 times/day 0.5–1 mg once/day	0.5–4 0.5–4
Chlordiazepoxide	Librium	—	15–100
Clorazepate	Tranxene-T	—	15–60
Diazepam	Valium	—	4–40
Lorazepam	Ativan	0.5–1 mg 3 times/day	2–6
Oxazepam	Generic only	—	30–120

that affects 1.6% of Americans at some time in their lives. The incidence in women is two to three times the incidence in men. Onset of panic disorder usually occurs in the late teens or early 20s.

Perhaps 50% of patients who get panic disorder also experience *agoraphobia,* a condition characterized by anxiety about being in places or situations from which escape might be difficult or embarrassing, or in which help might be unavailable in the event that a panic attack should occur. Agoraphobia leads to avoidance of certain places (e.g., elevators, bridges, tunnels, movie theaters) and situations (e.g., being outside the home alone; being in a crowd; standing in line; driving in traffic; traveling by bus, train, or plane). In extreme cases, agoraphobics may never set foot outside the home. Because of avoidance behavior, agoraphobia can severely limit occupational and social options.

Malfunction of the brain's "alarm system" is the suspected etiology of panic attacks. This malfunction may result from abnormalities in noradrenergic systems, serotonergic systems, and/or benzodiazepine receptors. Genetic vulnerability also may play a role.

Treatment

Between 70% and 90% of patients with panic disorder respond well to treatment. Two modalities may be employed: drug therapy and CBT. Combining drug therapy with CBT is more effective than either modality alone. As a rule, patients experience rapid and significant improvement. Drug therapy helps suppress panic attacks, while CBT helps patients become more comfortable with situations and places they've been avoiding. Additional benefit can be derived from avoiding caffeine and sympathomimetics (which can trigger panic attacks), avoiding sleep deprivation (which can predispose to panic attacks), and doing regular aerobic exercise (which can reduce anxiety).

Drug therapy should continue for at least 6 to 9 months. Stopping sooner is associated with a high rate of relapse.

Antidepressants

Panic disorder responds well to all four classes of antidepressants: SSRIs, SNRIs, tricyclic antidepressants (TCAs), and monoamine oxidase inhibitors (MAOIs). With all four, full benefits take 6 to 12 weeks to develop. Owing to better tolerability, SSRIs are generally preferred. The basic pharmacology of the antidepressants is discussed in Chapter 32.

Selective Serotonin Reuptake Inhibitors. The SSRIs are first-line drugs for panic disorder. At this time, only three SSRIs—fluoxetine [Prozac], paroxetine [Paxil], and sertraline [Zoloft]—are approved for this condition. However, the other SSRIs appear just as effective. The SSRIs decrease anticipatory anxiety, avoidance behavior, and the frequency and intensity of attacks. Furthermore, SSRIs decrease panic attacks regardless of whether the patient is actually depressed. However, if the patient does have coexisting depression, antidepressants will benefit the depression and panic disorder simultaneously. Common side effects include nausea, headache, insomnia, weight gain, and sexual dysfunction. In addition, SSRIs can *increase* anxiety early in treatment. To minimize exacerbation of anxiety, dosage should be low initially and then gradually increased as follows

- *Paroxetine*—initial, 10 mg/day; target range, 20 to 40 mg/day
- *Fluoxetine*—initial, 10 mg/day; maintenance, 20 mg/day
- *Sertraline*—initial, 25 mg/day; target range, 50 to 200 mg/day

Venlafaxine. In patients with panic disorder, extended-release venlafaxine [Effexor XR], an SNRI, can induce remission, prevent relapse, and improve quality of life. In clinical trials, efficacy was equal to that of paroxetine, an SSRI. The initial dosage is 37.5 mg/day for 7 days. Daily maintenance doses range between 75 mg and 225 mg. The pharmacology of venlafaxine is discussed in Chapter 32.

Tricyclic Antidepressants. The TCAs (e.g., imipramine [Tofranil], clomipramine [Anafranil]) are second-line drugs for panic disorder. They should be used only after a trial with at least one SSRI has failed. Although TCAs are as effective as SSRIs, they are less well tolerated. The most common side effects are sedation, orthostatic hypotension, and anticholinergic effects: dry mouth, blurred vision, urinary retention, constipation, and tachycardia. Of greater concern, TCAs can cause fatal dysrhythmias if taken in overdose. As with the SSRIs, dosage should be low initially and then gradually increased. For clomipramine, the initial dosage is 25 mg/day, and the target range is 50 to 200 mg/day. For imipramine, the initial dosage is 10 mg/day, and the target range is 100 to 300 mg/day.

Monoamine Oxidase Inhibitors. Although MAOIs (e.g., phenelzine) are very effective in panic disorder, they are difficult to use. MAOIs can cause significant side effects, including orthostatic hypotension, weight gain, and sexual dysfunction. In addition, they can cause hypertensive crisis if the patient takes certain drugs or consumes foods rich in tyramine. Because of these drawbacks, MAOIs are considered last-line drugs for panic disorder.

Benzodiazepines. Although benzodiazepines are effective in panic disorder, as in GAD, they are now considered second-line drugs because, unlike the SSRIs, benzodiazepines pose a risk of abuse, dependence, and rapid re-emergence of symptoms after discontinuation. Of the available benzodiazepines, the agents used most often are alprazolam [Xanax, Niravam], clonazepam [Klonopin, Rivotril 🍁], and lorazepam [Ativan]. All three provide rapid and effective protection against panic attacks. These drugs also reduce anticipatory anxiety and phobic avoidance.

Safety Alert

BENZODIAZEPINES

Benzodiazepines can cause physical dependence, which can make withdrawal extremely hard for some patients. The difficulty is that withdrawal produces intense anxiety, which people with panic disorder may find intolerable. To minimize withdrawal symptoms, benzodiazepines should be withdrawn very slowly—over a period of several months.

OBSESSIVE-COMPULSIVE DISORDER

Characteristics

Obsessive-compulsive disorder (OCD) is a potentially disabling condition characterized by persistent obsessions and compulsions that cause marked distress, consume at least 1 hour a day, and significantly interfere with daily living. An *obsession* is defined as a recurrent, persistent thought, impulse, or mental image that is unwanted and distressing, and comes involuntarily to mind despite attempts to ignore or suppress it. Common obsessions include fear of contamination (e.g., acquiring a disease by touching another person), aggressive impulses (e.g., harming a family member), a need for orderliness or symmetry (e.g., personal bathroom items must be arranged in a precise way), and repeated doubts (e.g., did I unplug the iron?). A *compulsion* is a repetitive behavior or mental act that the patient is driven to perform in response to his or her obsessions. In the patient's mind, carrying out the compulsion is essential to prevent some horrible event from occurring (e.g., death of a loved one). If performing the compulsion is suppressed or postponed, the patient experiences increased anxiety. Common compulsions include hand washing, mental counting, arranging objects symmetrically, and hoarding. Patients usually understand that their compulsive behavior is excessive and senseless, but nonetheless are unable to stop.

Treatment

Patients with OCD respond to drugs and to behavioral therapy. Optimal treatment consists of both. As a last resort, patients with severe, resistant OCD can be treated with deep brain stimulation.

Behavioral therapy is probably more important in OCD than in any other psychiatric disorder. In the technique employed, patients are exposed to sources of their fears, while being encouraged to refrain from acting out their compulsive rituals. When no dire consequences come to pass, despite the absence of "protective" rituals, patients are able to gradually give up their compulsive behavior. Although this form of therapy causes great anxiety, the success rate is high.

Five drugs are approved for OCD: four SSRIs and one TCA (clomipramine). All five enhance serotonergic transmission. The SSRIs are better tolerated than clomipramine, and hence are preferred.

Selective Serotonin Reuptake Inhibitors

The SSRIs are first-line drugs for OCD. Only four SSRIs—fluoxetine [Prozac], fluvoxamine [Luvox], sertraline [Zoloft], and paroxetine [Paxil]—are approved for OCD. However, the remaining two—citalopram [Celexa] and escitalopram [Lexapro, Cipralex ♣]—are also effective. All six reduce symptoms by enhancing serotonergic transmission. They all are equally effective, although individual patients may respond better to one than to another. With all six, beneficial effects develop slowly, taking several months to become maximal. Common side effects include nausea, headache, insomnia, and sexual dysfunction. Weight gain can also occur. Despite this array of side effects, SSRIs are safer than clomipramine and better tolerated. Dosages are as follows:

- *Citalopram*—20 mg once daily initially, increased to a maximum of 40 mg/day
- *Escitalopram*—10 mg once daily initially, increased to a maximum of 20 mg/day
- *Fluoxetine*—20 mg in the morning initially, increased to a maximum of 80 mg/day
- *Fluvoxamine*—50 mg at bedtime initially, increased to a maximum of 300 mg/day
- *Paroxetine*—20 mg in the morning initially, increased to a maximum of 60 mg/day
- *Sertraline*—50 mg once daily initially, increased to a maximum of 200 mg/day

Therapy of an initial episode should continue for at least 1 year, after which discontinuation can be tried. Withdrawal should be done slowly, reducing the dosage by 25% every 1 to 2 months. Unfortunately, relapse is common; estimates range from 23% to as high as 90%. If relapse continues to occur after three or four attempts at withdrawal, lifelong treatment may be indicated.

Deep Brain Stimulation

An implantable neurostimulator from Medtronics is approved for treating severe treatment-resistant OCD. The neurostimulator is a small battery-powered device with wires connected to electrodes. The device itself is surgically implanted in the abdomen or near the collarbone, and the electrodes are placed deep in the brain. When activated, the device delivers intermittent electrical stimulation that blocks nerve traffic. After 12 months of treatment, symptom reduction, on average, was 40%. Candidates for deep brain stimulation must first fail treatment with psychotherapy and with three or more drugs.

SOCIAL ANXIETY DISORDER (SOCIAL PHOBIA)

Characteristics

Social anxiety disorder, formerly known as social phobia, is characterized by an intense, irrational fear of situations in which one might be scrutinized by others, or might do something that is embarrassing or humiliating. Exposure to the feared situation almost always elicits anxiety. As a result, the person avoids the situation or, if it can't be avoided, endures it with intense anxiety (manifestations include blushing, stuttering, sweating, palpitations, dry throat, and muscle tension and twitches).

Social anxiety disorder has two principal forms: generalized and performance only. In the generalized form, the person fears nearly all social and performance situations. In the performance-only form, fear is limited to speaking or performing in public.

Social anxiety disorder can be very debilitating. In younger people, it can delay social development, inhibit participation in social activities, impair acquisition of friends, and make dating difficult or even impossible. It can also preclude the pursuit of higher education. In older people, it can severely limit social and occupational options.

Social anxiety disorder is one of the most common psychiatric disorders, and *the* most common anxiety disorder. In the United States, 13% to 14% of the population is affected at some time in their lives. The disorder typically begins during the teenage years; left untreated, it is likely to continue lifelong.

Treatment

Social anxiety disorder can be treated with psychotherapy, drug therapy, or both. Studies indicate that psychotherapy—both cognitive and behavioral—can be as effective as drugs. However, a combination of psychotherapy *plus* drugs is likely to be more effective than either modality alone.

The SSRIs are considered first-line drugs for most patients. These drugs are especially well suited for patients who fear multiple situations and are obliged to face those situations on a regular basis. Only two SSRIs—paroxetine [Paxil] and sertraline [Zoloft]—are approved for social anxiety disorder, but available data indicate that the other SSRIs are effective too. Initial effects take about 4 weeks to develop; optimal effects are seen in 8 to 12 weeks. Patients should be informed that benefits will be delayed. For paroxetine, the initial dosage is 20 mg once a day in the morning. The usual maintenance range is 20 to 40 mg/day. Treatment should continue for at least 1 year, after which gradual withdrawal can be tried. Unfortunately, withdrawal frequently results in relapse.

Benzodiazepines (e.g., clonazepam [Klonopin, Rivotril ♣], alprazolam [Xanax]) are an option for some patients. These drugs are well tolerated and their benefits are immediate, unlike those of the SSRIs. As a result, benzodiazepines can provide rapid relief and can be used PRN. Accordingly, these drugs are well suited for people whose fear is limited to performance situations and who must face those situations only occasionally. The usual dosage is 1 to 3 mg/day for clonazepam, and 1 to 6 mg/day for alprazolam.

Propranolol [Inderal] and other beta blockers can benefit patients with performance anxiety. When taken 1 to 2 hours before a scheduled performance, beta blockers can reduce symptoms caused by autonomic hyperactivity (e.g., tremors, sweating, tachycardia, palpitations). Doses are relatively small—only 10 to 80 mg for propranolol.

POST-TRAUMATIC STRESS DISORDER

Characteristics

Post-traumatic stress disorder (PTSD) develops following a *traumatic event* that elicited an immediate reaction of *fear, helplessness,* or *horror.* PTSD has three core symptoms: *re-experiencing* the event, *avoiding reminders* of the event (coupled with generalized emotional numbing), and a persistent state of *hyperarousal.* A traumatic event is one that involves a threat of injury or death, or a threat to one's physical integrity. Many events meet this criterion. Among these are physical or sexual assault, rape, torture, combat, industrial explosions, serious accidents, natural disasters, being taken hostage, displacement as a refugee, and terrorist attacks. It should be noted that PTSD can affect persons who were only *witnesses* to a traumatic event—not just those who were directly involved.

The epidemiology of PTSD is revealing. In the United States, more than 8 million Americans have PTSD in any given year, making PTSD the fourth most common psychiatric disorder. PTSD develops in 4% of men at some time in their lives and in 10% to 14% of women. Traumatic events that involve interpersonal violence (e.g., assault, rape, torture) are more likely to cause PTSD than are traumatic events that do not (e.g., car accidents, natural disasters). For example, among rape victims, the incidence of PTSD is 45.9% for women and 65% for men. In contrast, among natural disaster survivors, the incidence is 5.4% for women and 3.7% for men. Combat carries a high risk of PTSD; the disorder develops in up to 40% of soldiers who go to war.

Treatment

PTSD can be treated with psychotherapy and with drugs, as described in an evidence-based guideline—*VA/DoD Clinical Practice Guideline for the Management of Post-Traumatic Stress*—released by the Department of Veterans Affairs and Department of Defense in 2010. Two basic types of psychotherapy are recommended: *trauma-focused therapy* and *stress inoculation training*. Trauma-focused therapy uses a variety of cognitive behavioral techniques, including a very effective one known as *exposure therapy,* in which patients repeatedly reimagine traumatic events as a way to make those events lose their power. Stress inoculation training helps patients identify cues that can trigger fear and anxiety, and then teaches them techniques to cope with those disturbing reactions.

Regarding drugs, evidence of efficacy is strongest for three SSRIs (fluoxetine, paroxetine, and sertraline) and one SNRI (venlafaxine). Of these four drugs, only two—paroxetine [Paxil] and sertraline [Zoloft]—are FDA approved for PTSD. If none of the first-line drugs is effective, the guidelines suggest several alternatives: mirtazapine, a TCA (amitriptyline or imipramine), or an MAOI (phenelzine). Current evidence does *not* support the use of monotherapy with bupropion, buspirone, trazodone, or a benzodiazepine.

KEY POINTS

- Anxiety is an uncomfortable state that has psychologic manifestations (fear, apprehension, dread, uneasiness) and physical manifestations (tachycardia, palpitations, trembling, dry mouth, sweating, weakness, fatigue, shortness of breath).
- When anxiety is persistent and disabling, intervention is indicated.
- As a rule, optimal therapy of anxiety disorders consists of psychotherapy combined with drug therapy.
- The drugs used most often for anxiety disorders are serotonergic reuptake inhibitors and benzodiazepines.
- Benzodiazepines are used primarily for panic disorder (PD) and generalized anxiety disorder (GAD), whereas SRIs are used for *all* anxiety disorders.
- GAD is a chronic condition characterized by uncontrollable worrying.
- First-line drugs for GAD are SRIs, buspirone, and benzodiazepines.
- SRIs (venlafaxine, paroxetine, escitalopram, and duloxetine) are especially well suited for treating patients who have depression in addition to GAD. However, they are also effective even when depression is absent.
- With buspirone, venlafaxine, paroxetine, escitalopram, and duloxetine, anxiolytic effects are delayed. Accordingly, these drugs are best suited for long-term management—not rapid relief.
- Buspirone has three advantages over benzodiazepines: It does not cause CNS depression, has no abuse potential, and does not intensify the effects of CNS depressants.
- Buspirone levels can be increased by erythromycin, ketoconazole, and grapefruit juice.
- Benzodiazepines suppress symptoms of GAD immediately. Accordingly, these drugs are preferred agents for rapid stabilization, especially when anxiety is severe.
- Benzodiazepines are CNS depressants and hence can cause sedation and psychomotor slowing. In addition, they can intensify CNS depression caused by other drugs.
- Benzodiazepines have some potential for abuse, and hence should be used with caution in patients known to abuse alcohol or other psychoactive drugs.
- When taken long term, benzodiazepines can cause physical dependence. To minimize withdrawal symptoms, dosage

should be tapered gradually—over a period of several months.

- Patients with panic disorder experience recurrent panic attacks, characterized by palpitations, pounding heart, chest pain, derealization or depersonalization, and fear of dying or going crazy.
- Many patients with panic disorder also experience agoraphobia, a condition characterized by anxiety about being in places or situations from which escape might be difficult or embarrassing, or in which help might be unavailable if a panic attack should occur.
- SSRIs are first-line drugs for panic disorder.
- SSRIs decrease the frequency and intensity of panic attacks, anticipatory anxiety, and avoidance behavior, and they work regardless of whether the patient has depression.
- Obsessive-compulsive disorder (OCD) is characterized by persistent obsessions and compulsions that cause marked distress, consume at least 1 hour a day, and significantly interfere with daily living.
- SSRIs are first-line drugs for OCD.
- Social anxiety disorder, formerly known as social phobia, is characterized by an intense, irrational fear of being scrutinized by others or of doing something that could be embarrassing or humiliating.
- The SSRIs are first-line drugs for most patients with social anxiety disorder.
- When social anxiety disorder is limited to fear of speaking or performing in public and when these situations arise infrequently, PRN treatment with a benzodiazepine may be preferred to long-term treatment with an SSRI.
- Post-traumatic stress disorder (PTSD) develops following a traumatic event that elicited an immediate reaction of fear, helplessness, or horror.
- PTSD has three core symptoms: re-experiencing, avoidance/emotional numbing, and hyperarousal.
- Events that can lead to PTSD include physical or sexual assault, rape, torture, combat, industrial explosions, serious accidents, natural disasters, being taken hostage, displacement as a refugee, and terrorist attacks.
- According to a VA/DoD guideline, PTSD can be treated with psychotherapy and with drugs.
- Two SSRIs—paroxetine and sertraline—are approved by the FDA for first-line drug treatment of PTSD. Additional drugs used for treatment of PTSD include venlafaxine (an SNRI), TCAs, and MAOIs.

Please visit **http://evolve.elsevier.com/Lehne** for chapter-specific NCLEX® examination review questions.

CHAPTER

36 Central Nervous System Stimulants and Attention-Deficit/Hyperactivity Disorder

CENTRAL NERVOUS SYSTEM STIMULANTS

Central nervous system (CNS) stimulants increase the activity of CNS neurons. Most stimulants act by enhancing neuronal excitation. A few act by suppressing neuronal inhibition. In sufficient doses, all stimulants can cause convulsions.

Clinical applications of the CNS stimulants are limited. Currently these drugs have two principal indications: attention-deficit/hyperactivity disorder (ADHD) and narcolepsy.

Please note that CNS stimulants are not the same as antidepressants. The antidepressants act selectively to elevate mood, and hence can relieve depression without affecting other CNS functions. In contrast, CNS stimulants cannot elevate mood without producing generalized excitation. Accordingly, the role of stimulants in treating depression is minor.

Our principal focus is on *amphetamines, methylphenidate* [Ritalin, others], and *methylxanthines* (e.g., caffeine). These are by far the most widely used stimulant drugs.

AMPHETAMINES

The amphetamine family consists of amphetamine, dextroamphetamine, methamphetamine, and lisdexamfetamine. All are powerful CNS stimulants. In addition to their CNS actions, amphetamines have significant peripheral actions—actions that can cause cardiac stimulation and vasoconstriction. The amphetamines have a high potential for abuse.

Chemistry

Dextroamphetamine and Levamphetamine. Amphetamines are molecules with an asymmetric carbon atom. As a result, amphetamines can exist as mirror images of each other. Such compounds are termed *optical isomers* or *enantiomers*. Dextroamphetamine and levamphetamine both contain the same atomic components, but those components are arranged differently around the asymmetric carbon. Because of this structural difference, these compounds have somewhat different properties. For example, dextroamphetamine is more selective than levamphetamine for causing stimulation of the CNS, and hence produces fewer peripheral side effects.

Prototype Drugs

Central Nervous System Stimulants

Amphetamines
Amphetamine sulfate

Amphetamine-like Drugs
Methylphenidate

Methylxanthines
Caffeine

Drugs for Attention-Deficit/Hyperactivity Disorder

CNS Stimulants
Methylphenidate

Nonstimulants
Atomoxetine

Amphetamine. The term *amphetamine* refers not to a single compound but rather to a 50:50 mixture of dextroamphetamine and levamphetamine. (In chemistry, we refer to such equimolar mixtures of enantiomers as racemic.)

Lisdexamfetamine. Lisdexamfetamine [Vyvanse] is a prodrug composed of dextroamphetamine covalently linked to L-lysine. Following oral dosing, the drug undergoes rapid hydrolysis by enzymes in the intestine and liver to yield lysine and free dextroamphetamine, the active form of the drug. If lisdexamfetamine is inhaled or injected, hydrolysis will not take place, and hence the drug is not effective by these routes. Accordingly, it may have a lower abuse potential than other forms of amphetamine.

Methamphetamine. Methamphetamine is simply dextroamphetamine with an additional methyl group.

Mechanism of Action

The amphetamines act primarily by causing release of norepinephrine (NE) and dopamine (DA), and partly by inhibiting reuptake of both transmitters. These actions take place in the CNS and in peripheral nerves. Most pharmacologic effects result from release of NE.

Pharmacologic Effects

Central Nervous System. The amphetamines have prominent effects on mood and arousal. At usual doses, they increase wakefulness and alertness, reduce fatigue, elevate mood, and augment self-confidence and initiative. Euphoria, talkativeness, and increased motor activity are likely. Task performance that had been reduced by fatigue or boredom improves.

Amphetamines can stimulate respiration and suppress appetite and the perception of pain. Stimulation of the medullary respiratory center increases respiration. Effects on the hypothalamic feeding center depress appetite. By a mechanism that is not understood, amphetamines can enhance the analgesic effects of morphine and other opioids.

Cardiovascular System. Cardiovascular effects occur secondary to release of NE from sympathetic neurons. Norepinephrine acts in the heart to increase heart rate, atrioventricular conduction, and force of contraction. Excessive cardiac stimulation can cause dysrhythmias. In blood vessels, NE promotes constriction. Excessive vasoconstriction can cause hypertension.

Tolerance

With regular amphetamine use, tolerance develops to elevation of mood, suppression of appetite, and stimulation of the heart and blood vessels. In highly tolerant users, doses up to 1000 mg (IV) every few *hours* may be required to maintain *euphoric* effects. This compares with *daily* doses of 5 to 30 mg for nontolerant individuals.

Physical Dependence

Chronic amphetamine use produces physical dependence. If amphetamines are abruptly withdrawn from a dependent person, an abstinence syndrome will ensue. Symptoms include exhaustion, depression, prolonged sleep, excessive eating, and a craving for more amphetamine. Sleep patterns may take months to normalize.

Abuse

Because amphetamines can produce euphoria (extreme mood elevation), they have a high potential for abuse. Psychologic dependence can occur. (Users familiar with CNS stimulants find the psychologic effects of amphetamines nearly identical to those of cocaine.) Because of their abuse potential, all amphetamines, including lisdexamfetamine, are classified under Schedule II of the Controlled Substances Act and must be dispensed accordingly. Whenever amphetamines are used therapeutically, their potential for abuse must be weighed against their potential benefits.

Adverse Effects

CNS Stimulation. Stimulation of the CNS can cause insomnia, restlessness, and extreme loquaciousness. These effects can occur at therapeutic doses.

Weight Loss. By suppressing appetite, amphetamines can cause weight loss.

Cardiovascular Effects. At recommended doses, stimulants produce a small increase in heart rate and blood pressure. For most patients, these increases lack clinical significance. However, for patients with pre-existing cardiovascular disease, stimulants may cause dysrhythmias, anginal pain, or hypertension. Accordingly, amphetamines must be employed with extreme caution in these people. Any patient who develops cardiovascular symptoms (e.g., chest pain, shortness of breath, fainting) while using a stimulant should be evaluated immediately.

Do amphetamines increase the risk of *sudden death*? Probably not. Sudden death in children on these medications is very rare, and evidence is conflicting regarding the risk of sudden death. Should children *routinely* receive an electrocardiogram (ECG) before using these drugs? Probably not—despite a 2008 statement from the American Heart Association (AHA) saying it would be reasonable to consider obtaining an ECG in children being evaluated for stimulant therapy of ADHD. Why is the AHA concerned? Because 14 children, 5 with heart defects, died suddenly while using Adderall, a mixture of amphetamine and dextroamphetamine. However, given that millions of children have used the drug, the death rate is no greater than would be expected for a group this size, whether or not Adderall was being used. The bottom line? First, there are conflicting data showing that stimulants increase the risk of sudden death, even in children with heart disease. Second, there are no data showing that limiting the use of stimulants in children with heart defects will protect them from sudden death. And third, there are no data showing that screening for heart disease with an ECG before starting stimulants will be of benefit. Therefore, it would seem that *routine* ECGs are unnecessary before starting a child on stimulant therapy, especially if there is no evidence of heart disease. However, if there *is* evidence of heart disease, or evidence of hereditary cardiovascular defects, an ECG might be appropriate.

Psychosis. Excessive amphetamine use produces a state of paranoid psychosis, characterized by hallucinations and paranoid delusions (suspiciousness, feelings of being watched). Amphetamine-induced psychosis looks very much like schizophrenia. Symptoms are thought to result from the release of DA. Consistent with this hypothesis is the observation that symptoms can be alleviated with a DA receptor blocking agent (e.g., haloperidol). Following amphetamine withdrawal, psychosis usually resolves spontaneously within a week.

In some individuals, amphetamines can unmask latent schizophrenia. For these people, symptoms of psychosis do not clear spontaneously, and hence psychiatric care is indicated.

Acute Toxicity

Symptoms. Overdose produces dizziness, confusion, hallucinations, paranoid delusions, palpitations, dysrhythmias, and hypertension. Death is rare. Fatal overdose is associated with convulsions, coma, and cerebral hemorrhage.

Treatment. Hallucinations can be controlled with atypical antipsychotic drugs (e.g., olanzapine). An alpha-adrenergic blocker (e.g., phentolamine) can reduce hypertension (by promoting vasodilation). Owing to its ability to block alpha receptors, chlorpromazine helps lower blood pressure. Seizures can be managed with diazepam.

Therapeutic Uses

Attention-Deficit/Hyperactivity Disorder. The role of amphetamines in ADHD is discussed later in this chapter.

Narcolepsy. Narcolepsy is a disorder characterized by daytime somnolence and uncontrollable attacks of sleep. By stimulating the CNS, amphetamines can promote arousal and thereby alleviate symptoms.

Safety Alert

AMPHETAMINES

Amphetamines have a high potential for abuse and dependence. In patients who use amphetamines chronically, withdrawal may occur if use of these medications is suddenly stopped.

Preparations, Dosage, and Administration

Four members of the amphetamine family are used clinically: dextroamphetamine sulfate, an amphetamine/dextroamphetamine mixture, lisdexamfetamine, and methamphetamine. In clinical practice, amphetamines are given *orally.* (These drugs are not approved for IV administration. Amphetamines for IV use are available only through illegal sources.) All amphetamines are regulated under Schedule II of the Controlled Substances Act and must be dispensed accordingly.

Dextroamphetamine Sulfate. Dextroamphetamine is available in immediate-release (IR) and extended-release (ER) formulations. Both are indicated for ADHD.

Immediate Release. IR dextroamphetamine is available in 2.5-, 5-, 7.5-, 10-, 15-, 20-, and 30-mg tablets sold as *Zenzedi* and as a 5-mg/mL solution sold as *Procentra.* Effects begin rapidly and last 4 to 6 hours. The usual maintenance dosage for ADHD is 5 to 10 mg once or twice daily, up to 40 mg/day.

Extended Release. ER dextroamphetamine [Dexedrine] is available in 5-, 10-, and 15-mg capsules. Effects begin rapidly and last 6 to 10 hours. The usual maintenance dosage for ADHD is 5 mg once or twice daily.

Amphetamine/Dextroamphetamine Mixture. Amphetamine/dextroamphetamine mixture is available in IR [Adderall] and ER [Adderall XR] formulations. Both are used for ADHD.

Immediate Release. Adderall is available in IR tablets (5, 7.5, 10, 12.5, 15, 20, and 30 mg). Effects begin rapidly and last 4 to 6 hours. The usual maintenance dosage for ADHD is 5 mg twice daily, taken in the morning and 4 to 6 hours later.

Extended Release. Adderall XR is available in 5-, 10-, 15-, 20-, 25-, and 30-mg ER capsules. Half the dose is released immediately, and the remainder is released 4 hours later. As a result, effects begin rapidly and last 10 to 12 hours. The usual maintenance dosage for ADHD is 20 mg once daily in the morning. This is equivalent to taking 10 mg of IR Adderall at 8:00 AM and again around noon.

Lisdexamfetamine. Lisdexamfetamine [Vyvanse] is available in capsules (10, 20, 30, 40, 50, 60, and 70 mg) and chewable tablets (10, 20, 30, 40, 50, and 60 mg). Effects begin rapidly and persist about 13 hours. Dosing is done once daily in the morning without regard to meals. The capsules may be swallowed intact, or their contents may be dissolved in water and swallowed immediately. The usual daily maintenance dosage for ADHD is 30 mg.

Methamphetamine. Methamphetamine [Desoxyn] is indicated for ADHD, although it is not a preferred treatment for this condition. The drug is available in 5-mg IR tablets. The usual regimen for ADHD is 20 to 25 mg/day, administered in two divided doses.

METHYLPHENIDATE AND DEXMETHYLPHENIDATE

Methylphenidate and dexmethylphenidate are nearly identical in structure and pharmacologic actions. Furthermore, the pharmacology of both drugs is nearly identical to that of the amphetamines.

Methylphenidate

Although methylphenidate [Ritalin, Metadate, Methylin, Concerta, Daytrana, Biphentin 🍁] is structurally dissimilar from the amphetamines, the pharmacologic actions of these drugs are essentially the same. Consequently, methylphenidate can be considered an amphetamine in all but structure and name. Methylphenidate and amphetamine share the same mechanism of action (promotion of NE and DA release, and inhibition of NE and DA reuptake), adverse effects (insomnia, reduced appetite, emotional lability), and abuse liability (Schedule II). Like amphetamine, methylphenidate is not a single compound, but rather a 50:50 mixture of dextro and levo isomers. The dextro isomer is highly active; the levo isomer is not. Methylphenidate has two indications: ADHD and narcolepsy.

Preparations, Dosage, and Administration

Methylphenidate is available in three types of formulations: IR, sustained-release (SR), and once-daily doses. All three are indicated for ADHD. As a rule, the SR and IR formulations must be taken 2 or 3 times a day.

Immediate Release. Ritalin and Methylin are available in standard tablets (5, 10, and 20 mg), chewable tablets (2.5, 5, and 10 mg), and an oral solution (5 and 10 mg/5 mL). Effects begin rapidly and last 3 to 5 hours. Because effects are brief, dosing must be done 2 or 3 times a day. The usual maintenance dosage for ADHD is 5 mg twice daily, with a maximum dose of 60 mg daily in two or three divided doses.

Sustained Release. Ritalin-SR and Metadate ER are available in 20-mg tablets, and Quillivant XR is available in a 25-mg/5 mL oral suspension or as Quillichew ER in 20-, 30-, and 40-mg chewable tablets. Effects are delayed and last 6 to 8 hours. Dosing is done once or twice daily. For children with ADHD, the usual maintenance dosage is 20 to 40 mg in the morning, supplemented with 20 mg in the early afternoon if needed.

Once-Daily Dosing. Five products are available. Their brand names are Concerta, Metadate CD, Aptensio XR, Ritalin LA, and Daytrana. With all five, dosing is done once daily in the morning; no afternoon dose is needed.

Concerta. Concerta tablets—formulated as an osmotic-release oral system (OROS)—consist of an outer coating of IR methylphenidate and a special inner core that releases the remainder of each dose gradually. As a result, effects begin rapidly and last 10 to 12 hours. Because of their special architecture, Concerta tablets must be swallowed whole, not crushed or chewed. The tablet shell may not dissolve fully in the GI tract. Accordingly, patients should be informed that they may see tablet "ghosts" in the stool. Concerta tablets are available in four strengths: 18, 27, 36, and 54 mg.

Dosage depends on whether the patient is already taking methylphenidate (IR or SR). For children *not* already taking methylphenidate, the initial dosage is 18 mg once daily in the morning. Dosage can be increased to a maximum of 72 mg once daily. For children who *are* taking methylphenidate (IR or SR), the initial dosage of Concerta is as follows:

- For those taking 5 mg (2 or 3 times a day) of IR methylphenidate or 20 mg once daily of SR methylphenidate, start with 18 mg of Concerta.
- For those taking 10 mg (2 or 3 times a day) of IR or 40 mg once daily of SR, start with 36 mg of Concerta.
- For those taking 15 mg (2 or 3 times a day) of IR or 60 mg once daily of SR, start with 54 mg of Concerta.

Metadate CD. Metadate CD is available in 10-, 20-, 30-, 40-, 50-, and 60-mg capsules that contain IR and delayed-release beads. The beads release

30% of the dose rapidly and the remaining 70% 4 hours later. As a result, plasma levels peak twice—at 1.5 and 4.5 hours. This is the same pattern produced by taking IR methylphenidate twice daily. For ADHD patients *not* already taking methylphenidate, the initial dosage is 20 mg once daily in the morning. This can be gradually increased to a maximum of 60 mg once daily. For patients who *are* already taking methylphenidate, start with 20 mg of Metadate CD once daily (for those taking 10 mg of IR methylphenidate twice daily) or with 40 mg of Metadate CD once daily (for those taking 20 mg of IR methylphenidate twice daily). If needed, Metadate CD capsules can be opened and sprinkled on a small amount of soft food (e.g., applesauce) right before ingestion.

Aptensio XR. Aptensio XR is formulated in capsules (10, 15, 20, 30, 40, 50, and 60 mg) that contain delayed-release beads. Therapeutic effects begin rapidly and persist for 12 hours. The capsules may be swallowed intact or opened to permit sprinkling the beads onto applesauce or some other soft food. Aptensio XR capsules are approved for treating ADHD in children, adolescents, and adults.

Ritalin LA. Ritalin LA is formulated as ER capsules (10, 20, 30, 40, and 60 mg). The product is much like Metadate CD in that some of the dose is released immediately and the rest 4 hours later. Dosing is done *once daily in the morning.* As with Metadate CD and Concerta, dosage depends on whether the patient is already taking methylphenidate (IR or SR). For children *not* already taking methylphenidate, the initial dosage is 20 mg. Dosage can be gradually increased to a maximum of 60 mg. For children who *are* taking methylphenidate (IR or SR), the initial dosage is as follows:

- For those taking 10 mg twice daily of IR methylphenidate or 20 mg once daily of SR methylphenidate, start with 20 mg of Ritalin LA.
- For those taking 15 mg twice daily of IR, start with 30 mg of Ritalin LA.
- For those taking 20 mg twice daily of IR or 40 mg once daily of SR, start with 40 mg of Ritalin LA.
- For those taking 30 mg twice daily of IR or 60 mg once daily of SR, start with 60 mg of Ritalin LA.

Daytrana. Daytrana—a *transdermal methylphenidate patch*—is the first nonoral treatment for ADHD. Following patch application, blood levels of methylphenidate rise slowly and peak in about 9 hours, after which the patch should be removed. Because of the slow rise, effects are delayed about 2 hours. Furthermore, effects will persist for about 3 hours after patch removal. Daytrana patches are available in four sizes—12.5, 18.75, 25, and 37.5 cm^2—that deliver 10, 15, 20, and 30 mg/9 hr, respectively. Treatment should begin with the smallest patch, even in patients already taking methylphenidate PO. If needed, larger patches can be tried at weekly intervals. Patients should apply the patch to the hip in the morning—alternating hips each day—and remove it no more than 9 hours later. (They can remove it sooner to terminate effects early.) Application to inflamed skin or application of heat will accelerate drug absorption, and hence should be avoided. Patients should be informed that bathing, showering, and swimming will not dislodge the patch.

Side effects of the patch are like those of oral methylphenidate, with two exceptions. First, users may experience erythema and pruritus at the application site. Second, exposing the skin to methylphenidate can cause a *hypersensitivity reaction.* If hypersensitivity develops, the patient may be unable to use *any* methylphenidate formulation—transdermal or oral—ever again.

Dexmethylphenidate

Dexmethylphenidate [Focalin, Focalin XR], a drug for ADHD, is simply the dextro isomer of methylphenidate. As noted, the dextro isomer accounts for most of the pharmacologic activity of methylphenidate, a 50:50 mixture of dextro and levo isomers. Accordingly, the pharmacology of dexmethylphenidate is nearly identical to that of methylphenidate. The only difference is that the dosage of dexmethylphenidate is one-half the dosage of methylphenidate. Dexmethylphenidate is available in IR tablets (2.5, 5, and 10 mg) marketed as *Focalin,* and in ER capsules (5, 10, 15, 20, 25, 30, 35, and 40 mg) marketed as *Focalin XR.* Both formulations may be administered with or without food. For children currently treated with methylphenidate, the initial dosage of dexmethylphenidate is one-half the methylphenidate dosage. For children who are *not* currently being treated, the initial dosage is 2.5 mg twice daily using Focalin or 10 mg once daily using Focalin XR. The maximum dosage is 10 mg twice daily for Focalin and 40 mg once daily for Focalin XR. Dexmethylphenidate is a Schedule II drug and must be dispensed accordingly.

METHYLXANTHINES

The methylxanthines are methylated derivatives of xanthine, hence the family name. These compounds consist of a xanthine nucleus with one or more methyl groups attached. Caffeine, the most familiar member of the family, will serve as our prototype.

PATIENT-CENTERED CARE ACROSS THE LIFE SPAN

Stimulants

Life Stage	Patient Care Concerns
Infants	Caffeine citrate [Cafcit] is used for neonatal apnea. Other CNS stimulants should be avoided in this population.
Children	The stimulant class of drugs for treatment of ADHD has been proven safe and effective for this population. Atomoxetine, a nonstimulant for ADHD, may cause suicidal thinking in children and adolescents.
Pregnant women	Caffeine may pose a small risk of birth defects, although human data are lacking. Methylphenidate and atomoxetine are classified as FDA Pregnancy Risk Category C,[a] as adverse fetal effects have been demonstrated in animal studies.
Breast-feeding women	Stimulants, such as methylphenidate, do not have any reported side effects in the breast-feeding infant. There are limited to no data on nonstimulants and the effects on breast-feeding infants.
Older adults	Most studies focus on patients older than 65 years, since stimulants are often used for the treatment of apathy, depression, and fatigue in the older adult population. Stimulants should be avoided in patients with cardiac disease or glaucoma. Consider a lower starting dose, and monitor heart rate, blood pressure, and weight.

[a]As of 2020, the FDA will no longer use Pregnancy Risk Categories. Please refer to Chapter 9 for more information.

Caffeine

Caffeine is consumed worldwide for its stimulant effects. In the United States, per capita consumption is about 200 mg/day, mostly in the form of coffee. Although clinical applications of caffeine are few, caffeine remains of interest because of its widespread ingestion for nonmedical purposes.

Dietary Sources

Caffeine can be found in chocolates, desserts, soft drinks, and beverages prepared from various natural products. Common dietary sources are coffee, tea, and cola drinks. The caffeine in cola drinks derives partly from the cola nut and partly from caffeine added by the manufacturer. Caffeine is also present in many noncola soft drinks. The caffeine content of some common foods and beverages is shown in Table 36.1.

TABLE 36.1 ■ Dietary Caffeine

Product	Amount	Caffeine (mg)
COFFEE		
Brewed (typical)	8 oz	60–180
Instant	8 oz	30–120
Espresso	1.5 oz	77
Decaffeinated	8 oz	1–5
TEA		
Brewed	8 oz	35–40
Herbal tea	8 oz	0
Iced tea mix, decaffeinated	8 oz	<5
SODA AND ENERGY DRINKS		
Energy drink	12 oz	71
Diet cola	12 oz	47
Cola	12 oz	45
Orange soda	12 oz	40
Concentrated energy drink	2 oz	200
Caffeinated water	16 oz	100
ICE CREAM AND YOGURT		
Coffee ice cream	½ cup	20–30
Coffee yogurt	4 oz	22
MISCELLANEOUS		
Cocoa	8 oz	2–50
Chocolate milk	1.5 oz	3–11
Milk chocolate bar	1.5 oz	10
Dark chocolate bar	1.5 oz	31

Mechanism of Action

Several mechanisms of action have been proposed. These include (1) reversible blockade of adenosine receptors, (2) enhancement of calcium permeability in the sarcoplasmic reticulum, and (3) inhibition of cyclic nucleotide phosphodiesterase, resulting in accumulation of cyclic adenosine monophosphate (cyclic AMP). Blockade of adenosine receptors appears responsible for most effects.

Pharmacologic Effects

Central Nervous System. In low doses, caffeine decreases drowsiness and fatigue and increases the capacity for prolonged intellectual exertion. With increasing dosage, caffeine produces nervousness, insomnia, and tremors. When administered in very large doses, caffeine can cause convulsions. Despite popular belief, there is little evidence that caffeine can restore mental function during intoxication with alcohol, although it might delay passing out.

Heart. High doses of caffeine stimulate the heart. When caffeinated beverages are consumed in excessive amounts, dysrhythmias may result.

Blood Vessels. Caffeine affects blood vessels in the periphery differently from those in the CNS. In the periphery, caffeine promotes *vasodilation,* whereas in the CNS, caffeine promotes *vasoconstriction.* Constriction of cerebral blood vessels is thought to underlie the drug's ability to relieve headache.

Bronchi. Caffeine and other methylxanthines cause relaxation of bronchial smooth muscle and thereby promote bronchodilation. Theophylline is an especially effective bronchodilator, and hence can be used to treat asthma (see Chapter 76).

Kidney. Caffeine is a diuretic. The mechanism underlying increased urine formation is likely related to suppression of antidiuretic hormone in the posterior pituitary.

Reproduction. Caffeine readily crosses the placenta and may pose a risk of birth defects, although that risk appears low. When applied to cells in culture, caffeine can cause chromosomal damage and mutations. However, the concentrations required are much greater than can be achieved by drinking caffeinated beverages. Also, although there is clear proof that caffeine can cause birth defects in animals, studies have failed to document birth defects in humans. Although caffeine-induced birth defects seem unlikely, caffeine *has* been associated with low birth weight.

According to a meta-analysis reported in 2010, consuming less than 300 mg of caffeine daily does *not* increase the risk of preterm birth. An additional review in 2013 revealed that restricting caffeine consumption during the second and third trimesters of pregnancy did not affect birth weight or length of gestation. Whether higher doses might increase risk is unclear.

Pharmacokinetics

Caffeine is readily absorbed from the GI tract and achieves peak plasma levels within 1 hour. Plasma half-life ranges from 3 to 7 hours. Elimination is by hepatic metabolism.

Therapeutic Uses

Neonatal Apnea. Premature infants may experience prolonged apnea (lasting 15 seconds or more) along with bradycardia. Hypoxemia and neurologic damage may result. Caffeine and other methylxanthines can reduce the number and duration of apnea episodes and can promote a more regular pattern of breathing.

Promoting Wakefulness. Caffeine is used commonly to aid in staying awake. The drug is marketed in various over-the-counter preparations [Maximum Strength NoDoz, Vivarin, others] for this purpose. Of course, individuals desiring increased alertness can get just as much caffeine by drinking coffee or some other caffeine-containing beverage.

Other Applications. Intravenous caffeine can help relieve headache induced by spinal puncture. The drug is used orally to enhance analgesia induced by opioids and by nonopioid analgesics (e.g., aspirin).

Acute Toxicity

Caffeine toxicity is characterized by intensification of the responses seen at low doses. Stimulation of the CNS results in excitement, restlessness, and insomnia; if the dosage is very high, convulsions may occur. Tachycardia and respiratory stimulation are likely. Sensory phenomena (ringing in the ears, flashing lights) are common. Death from caffeine overdose is rare. When fatalities have occurred, between 5 and 10 gm have been ingested.

Preparations, Dosage, and Administration

For Promoting Wakefulness. Caffeine is available in three formulations for promoting wakefulness: 200-mg tablets, 200-mg capsules, and 75-mg lozenges. The usual dosage is 100 to 200 mg every 3 to 4 hours as needed.

For Neonatal Apnea. Caffeine citrate [Cafcit] is used for neonatal apnea. The drug is available in oral and IV solutions. Both have the same concentration: 20 mg/mL. Treatment consists of an IV loading dose (20 mg/

kg) followed every 24 hours by an oral or IV maintenance dose (5 mg/kg). *Note:* The amount of caffeine *base* in a 20-mg dose of caffeine citrate is only 10 mg (i.e., one-half of the total dose on a milligram basis).

MISCELLANEOUS CNS STIMULANTS

Modafinil

Therapeutic Use

Modafinil [Provigil, Alertec ♣], a unique nonamphetamine stimulant, is approved for promoting wakefulness in patients with excessive sleepiness associated with three disorders: narcolepsy, shift-work sleep disorder (SWSD), and obstructive sleep apnea/hypopnea syndrome (OSAHS). However, although the drug has only three *approved* uses, most prescriptions (95%) are written for off-label uses, including fatigue, depression, ADHD, jet lag, and sleepiness caused by medications. Investigational uses include ADHD and fatigue associated with multiple sclerosis. The military studied the drug for use in sustaining alertness in helicopter pilots and found it superior to placebo.

In clinical trials, modafinil has been moderately effective. In patients with narcolepsy, modafinil increased wakefulness, but only to about 50% of the level seen in normal people. In contrast, methylphenidate and dextroamphetamine increase wakefulness to about 70% of normal. In patients with SWSD and OSAHS, benefits are about the same as those seen in narcolepsy.

Mechanism of Action

How modafinil works remains unclear. The drug does seem to influence hypothalamic areas involved in maintaining the normal sleep-wakefulness cycle. Also, there is evidence that modafinil inhibits the activity of sleep-promoting neurons (in the ventrolateral preoptic nucleus) by blocking reuptake of norepinephrine.

Pharmacokinetics

Modafinil is rapidly absorbed from the GI tract. Plasma levels peak in 2 to 4 hours. Food decreases the rate of absorption but not the extent. Elimination is by hepatic metabolism followed by renal excretion. The half-life is about 15 hours.

Adverse Effects

Modafinil is generally well tolerated. The most common adverse effects are headache, nausea, nervousness, diarrhea, and rhinitis. Modafinil does not disrupt nighttime sleep. In clinical trials, only 5% of patients dropped out because of undesired effects. Initially, the drug was believed devoid of cardiovascular effects. However, we now know it can increase heart rate and blood pressure, apparently by altering autonomic function. Subjective effects—euphoria; altered perception, thinking, and feeling—are like those of other CNS stimulants. However, modafinil has less abuse potential, and hence is regulated as a Schedule IV substance. Physical dependence and withdrawal have not been reported. Modafinil is embryotoxic in laboratory animals, and hence should be avoided during pregnancy.

Postmarketing reports link modafinil to rare cases of serious skin reactions, including Stevens-Johnson syndrome, erythema multiforme, and toxic epidermal necrolysis. Patients should be informed about signs of these reactions—swelling or rash, especially in the presence of fever or changes in the oral mucosa—and instructed to discontinue the drug if they develop.

Drug Interactions

Modafinil inhibits some forms of cytochrome P450 (CYP) and induces others. Induction of CYP3A4 (the 3A4 isoenzyme of P450) may accelerate the metabolism of oral contraceptives, cyclosporine, and certain other drugs, thereby causing their levels to decline. Caution is advised.

Preparations, Dosage, and Administration

Modafinil is available in 100- and 200-mg tablets. For patients with narcolepsy or OSAHS, the usual dosage is 200 mg/day, taken as a single dose in the morning. For patients with SWSD, the usual dosage is 200 mg/day, taken as a single dose 1 hour before the shift starts. For patients with severe hepatic impairment, doses should be decreased by 50%. Dosage reduction may also be needed in older adults.

Armodafinil

Armodafinil [Nuvigil] is simply the *R*-enantiomer of modafinil, a mixture of *R*- and *S*-enantiomers. Armodafinil differs from modafinil in that the *R*-enantiomer (armodafinil) has a somewhat longer half-life than the *S*-enantiomer component of modafinil. Otherwise, the two drugs are essentially identical, although armodafinil costs more. Armodafinil has the same indications as modafinil—improving wakefulness in people with narcolepsy, SWSD, and OSAHS—and has similar adverse effects, including the potential for rare but severe skin reactions. Like modafinil, armodafinil is classified as a Schedule IV substance. Armodafinil is available in 50-, 150-, and 250-mg tablets. The recommended dosage for narcolepsy and OSAHS is 150 or 250 mg, taken in the morning. The recommended dosage for SWSD is 150 mg, taken 1 hour before the work shift.

Doxapram

Doxapram [Dopram] stimulates the CNS at all levels. The drug is employed clinically to stimulate respiration. However, since the doses required are close to those that can produce generalized CNS stimulation and convulsions, doxapram must be used with great care. Furthermore, although doxapram is labeled for the treatment of general CNS depressant overdose, its use for this purpose should be discontinued: Experience has shown that respiratory depression from CNS depressant overdose can be managed more safely and effectively with mechanical support of ventilation than with pharmacologic stimulation of respiration.

ATTENTION-DEFICIT/HYPERACTIVITY DISORDER

Our discussion of ADHD has two parts. We begin by addressing basic concepts in ADHD—specifically, signs and symptoms, etiology, and treatment strategy. After that, we discuss the pharmacology of the drugs used for treatment.

BASIC CONSIDERATIONS

ADHD in Children

ADHD is the most common neuropsychiatric disorder of childhood, affecting 5% to 11% of school-age children. The incidence in boys is two to three times the incidence in girls. Symptoms begin between ages 3 and 7, usually persist into the teens, and often persist into adulthood. The majority (60% to 70%) of children respond well to stimulant drugs. Methylphenidate [Ritalin, Concerta, others] is the agent employed most.

Signs and Symptoms

ADHD is characterized by *inattention, hyperactivity,* and *impulsivity.* Affected children are fidgety, unable to concentrate on schoolwork, and unable to wait their turn; switch excessively from one activity to another; call out excessively in class; and never complete tasks. To make a diagnosis, symptoms must appear before age 12 years and be present for at least 6 months. Since other disorders—especially anxiety and depression—may cause similar symptoms, diagnosis must be done carefully.

ADHD can be subclassified as predominantly inattentive type, predominantly hyperactive-impulsive type, or combined type, depending on the symptom profile. Former names for ADHD—*hyperkinetic syndrome* and *minimal brain dysfunction*—are misleading and have been abandoned.

Etiology

Although various theories have been proposed, the underlying pathophysiology of ADHD is only partly understood. Neuroimaging studies indicate structural and functional abnormalities in multiple brain areas, including the frontal cortex, basal ganglia, brainstem, and cerebellum—regions involved with regulating attention, impulsive behavior, and motor activity. Several theories implicate dysregulation in neuronal pathways that employ NE, DA, and serotonin as transmitters. These theories would be consistent with the effects of atomoxetine (which blocks NE reuptake), imipramine (which blocks NE and serotonin uptake), and stimulant drugs (which promote the release of NE and DA and to some degree block their uptake). Genetic factors play a significant role.

Management Overview

Multiple strategies may be employed to manage ADHD. In addition to drugs, which are considered first-line treatment, the management program can include family therapy, parent training, and cognitive therapy for the child. Guidelines issued by the American Academy of Pediatrics emphasize the importance of a comprehensive treatment program involving collaboration among clinicians, families, and educators. For long-term gains, a combination of cognitive therapy and stimulant drugs appears most effective. Of the drugs employed for ADHD, stimulants are most effective, and so are considered agents of choice. The nonstimulants (e.g., atomoxetine, guanfacine, clonidine) are less effective than stimulants, and hence are considered second-choice drugs.

ADHD in Adults

In about 30% to 60% of cases, childhood ADHD persists into adulthood. In the United States, about 8 million adults are afflicted, although an estimated 90% are undiagnosed and untreated. Symptoms include poor concentration, stress intolerance, antisocial behavior, outbursts of anger, and inability to maintain a routine. Also, adults with ADHD experience more job loss, divorce, and driving accidents. As in childhood ADHD, therapy with a stimulant drug is the foundation of treatment. Methylphenidate is prescribed most often. About 33% of adults fail to respond to stimulants or cannot tolerate their side effects. For these patients, a trial with a nonstimulant may help. Combining behavioral therapy with drug therapy may be more effective than drug therapy alone.

DRUGS USED FOR ADHD

CNS Stimulants

Stimulant drugs are the mainstay of ADHD therapy. Drugs with proven efficacy include *methylphenidate* [Ritalin, Concerta, others], *dexmethylphenidate* [Focalin], *dextroamphetamine/amphetamine mixture* [Adderall], and *lisdexamfetamine* [Vyvanse]. There are no data to support the use of one stimulant over another. If one stimulant is ineffective, another should be tried before considering a second-line agent.

The response to stimulants can be dramatic. These drugs can increase attention span and goal-oriented behavior while decreasing impulsiveness, distractibility, hyperactivity, and restlessness. Tests of cognitive function (memory, reading, arithmetic) often improve significantly. Unfortunately, although benefits can be dramatic initially, in children they diminish after 2 to 3 years. This finding was initially reported in a 2009 paper: *MTA at 8 Years: Prospective Follow-up of Children Treated for Combined-Type ADHD in a Multisite Study.* The findings were corroborated in a systematic review of long-term outcomes in ADHD in 2012. Nonetheless, stimulant therapy can still buy time to teach children behavioral strategies to help them combat inattention and hyperactivity over the long term.

Although reduction of impulsiveness and hyperactivity with a stimulant may seem paradoxical, it isn't. Stimulants don't suppress rowdy behavior directly. Rather, they improve attention and focus. Impulsiveness and hyperactivity decline because the child is now able to concentrate on the task at hand. It should be noted that stimulants do not create *positive* behavior; they only reduce *negative* behavior. Accordingly, stimulants cannot give a child good study skills and other appropriate behaviors. Rather, these must be learned once the disruptive behavior is no longer an impediment.

The dosing schedule employed is important and is determined by the time course of the formulation selected. As discussed previously and shown in Table 36.2, CNS stimulants are available in IR, SR, and 24-hour formulations. With the IR and SR formulations, the child usually takes two or three doses a day. In contrast, the 24-hour formulations are taken just once a day (in the morning). Not only is once-daily dosing more convenient, it spares the child any embarrassment or stigma associated with taking medicine at school. Accordingly, 24-hour formulations (e.g., Adderall XR, Concerta, Daytrana) are generally preferred. With all formulations, dosage should be low initially and then gradually increased. Maintenance dosage is determined by monitoring for improvement in symptoms and the appearance of side effects.

Principal adverse effects of the stimulants are *insomnia* and *growth suppression.* Insomnia results from CNS stimulation and can be minimized by reducing the size of the afternoon dose and taking it no later than 4:00 PM. Growth suppression occurs secondary to appetite suppression. Growth reduction can be minimized by administering stimulants during or after meals (which reduces the impact of appetite suppression). In addition, some clinicians recommend taking "drug holidays" on weekends and in the summer (which creates an opportunity for growth to catch up). However, other clinicians argue against this strategy because depriving children of medication during these unstructured times can be hard on them. When stimulants are discontinued, a rebound increase in growth will take place; as a result, adult height may not be affected. Other adverse effects include *headache* and *abdominal pain,* which have an incidence of 10%, and *lethargy* and *listlessness,* which can occur when dosage is excessive.

Nonstimulants

Several nonstimulants are used for ADHD, although only three of them—atomoxetine, guanfacine, and clonidine—are approved by the U.S. Food and Drug Administration (FDA) for this use. The nonstimulants are less effective than the stimulants, and hence are considered second-choice drugs. For treatment of ADHD, the nonstimulants may be employed as monotherapy or as add-on therapy with a stimulant. Unlike the stimulants, the nonstimulants are not regulated as controlled substances.

Atomoxetine, a Norepinephrine Uptake Inhibitor

Description and Therapeutic Effects. Atomoxetine [Strattera] is a unique drug approved for ADHD in children and adults. It was the first *nonstimulant* approved for ADHD,[a] and one of only three drugs approved for ADHD in adults (the

[a]Some older nonstimulants, such as imipramine and bupropion, although *used* for ADHD, are not actually *approved* for ADHD.

TABLE 36.2 ■ Major Drugs for Attention-Deficit/Hyperactivity Disorder

Drug	Brand Name	Duration (hr)	Dosing Schedule	Usual Pediatric Maintenance Dosage
STIMULANTS				
Methylphenidate				
Immediate Release	Ritalin, Methylin	3–5	2 or 3 times daily	10 mg at 8:00 AM and noon, and 5 mg at 4:00 PM
Sustained Release	Ritalin-SR, Metadate ER, Quillivant XR, Quillichew ER	6–8	Once or twice daily	20 or 40 mg in AM plus 20 mg in the early PM if needed
24-Hour	Concerta	10–12	Once daily	36 mg in the AM
	Aptensio XR	12	Once daily	10 mg in the AM
	Metadate CD	8–12	Once daily	30 mg in the AM
	Ritalin LA	8–12	Once daily	30 mg in the AM
	Daytrana	10–12	Once daily	One 15- or 20-mg patch, applied in the AM and removed 9 hr later
Dexmethylphenidate				
Immediate Release	Focalin	4–5	Twice daily	10 mg in the AM plus 10 mg in the early PM
Sustained Release	Focalin XR	12	Once daily	10 mg in the AM
Dextroamphetamine				
Immediate Release	Zenzedi, Procentra	4–6	Once or twice daily	5 mg in the AM
Sustained Release	Dexedrine	6–10	Once or twice daily	10 mg at 8:00 AM
Amphetamine Mixture				
Immediate Release	Adderall	4–6	Twice daily	5 mg in the AM and 4–6 hr later
Sustained Release	Adderall XR	10–12	Once daily	20 mg in the AM
Lisdexamfetamine				
Sustained Release	Vyvanse	13	Once daily	30 mg in the AM
NONSTIMULANTS				
Atomoxetine	Strattera	24	Once or twice daily	80 mg in the AM *or* 40 mg in the AM and early PM
Guanfacine	Intuniv	24	Once daily	1–4 mg in the AM
Clonidine	Kapvay	24	Twice daily	0.1–0.2 mg in the AM and PM

others are amphetamine/dextroamphetamine mixture [Adderall XR] and lisdexamfetamine [Vyvanse]). In contrast to the CNS stimulants, atomoxetine has no potential for abuse, and hence is not regulated as a controlled substance. As a result, prescriptions can be refilled over the phone, making atomoxetine more convenient than the stimulants. Like the long-acting stimulants, atomoxetine can be administered just once a day.

In clinical trials comparing atomoxetine with placebo in children or adults with ADHD, atomoxetine was clearly superior at reducing symptoms. Benefits were similar whether the drug was given once a day or in two divided doses. It should be noted that responses develop slowly: The initial response takes a few days to develop, and the maximal response is seen in 1 to 3 weeks. This contrasts with the CNS stimulants, whose effects are near maximal with the first dose.

How does atomoxetine compare with stimulants for treating children with ADHD? In two older 3-week randomized trials, comparing atomoxetine with either methylphenidate [Concerta] or an amphetamine [Adderall XR], the stimulants were superior: More children responded to the stimulants, symptom reduction was greater, and benefits developed more quickly. These results were reinforced in a large 6-week placebo-controlled trial, in which a stimulant—methylphenidate [Concerta]—was again clearly superior to atomoxetine.

Mechanism of Action. Atomoxetine is a *selective inhibitor of NE reuptake,* and hence causes NE to accumulate at synapses. Although the precise relationship between this neurochemical action and symptom relief is unknown, it would appear that *adaptive changes* that occur following uptake blockade underlie benefits. Uptake blockade occurs immediately, whereas full therapeutic effects are not seen for at least a week—suggesting that, after uptake blockade occurs, additional processes must take place before benefits can be seen.

Pharmacokinetics. Atomoxetine is rapidly and completely absorbed following oral administration. Plasma levels peak in 1 to 3 hours, depending on whether the drug was taken without or with food. Atomoxetine is metabolized in the liver, primarily by CYP2D6 (the 2D6 isoenzyme of cytochrome P450). For most patients, the half-life is 5 hours. However, for 5% to 10% of patients, the half-life is much longer: 24 hours. These patients have an atypical form of CYP2D6, which metabolizes atomoxetine slowly. Dosage should be reduced in these people.

Adverse Effects. Like the CNS stimulants, atomoxetine is generally well tolerated. In clinical trials, the most common effects were GI reactions (dyspepsia, nausea, and vomiting), reduced appetite, dizziness, somnolence, mood swings, and trouble sleeping. Sexual dysfunction and urinary retention were seen in adults. Severe allergic reactions, including angioneurotic edema, occurred rarely. If allergy develops, patients should discontinue the drug and contact their prescriber immediately.

Atomoxetine may cause *suicidal thinking* in children and adolescents, but not in adults. Fortunately, the incidence is relatively low: about 4 cases per 1000 patients. Risk is greatest during the first few months of treatment. Young patients should be monitored closely for suicidal thinking and behavior, and for signs of clinical worsening (e.g., agitation, irritability).

Appetite suppression may result in *weight loss and growth delay.* Among children who took atomoxetine for 18 months or longer, mean height and weight percentiles declined. Because experience with the drug is limited, we don't know whether expected adult height will be affected, nor do we know whether "drug holidays" would have an impact on growth.

Atomoxetine poses a small risk of *severe liver injury* that may progress to outright liver failure, resulting in death or the need for a liver transplant. Patients should be informed about signs of liver injury—jaundice, dark urine, abdominal tenderness, unexplained flu-like symptoms—and instructed to report these immediately. In the event of jaundice or laboratory evidence of liver injury, atomoxetine should be discontinued.

Atomoxetine *may raise or lower blood pressure.* During clinical trials, some patients experienced a small increase in blood pressure and heart rate. Accordingly, atomoxetine should be used with caution by patients with hypertension or tachycardia. During postmarketing surveillance, some patients experienced *hypotension and syncope* (fainting). Patients should be informed of this possibility and advised to sit or lie down if they feel faint.

Drug Interactions. Combining atomoxetine with a *monoamine oxidase inhibitor* (e.g., isocarboxazid [Marplan], phenelzine [Nardil]) can cause hypertensive crisis, owing to accumulation of NE at synapses in the periphery. Accordingly, these drugs must not be used together or within 3 weeks of each other.

Inhibitors of CYP2D6 can increase levels of atomoxetine, and hence must be used with caution. Common examples include paroxetine [Paxil], fluoxetine [Prozac], and quinidine.

Role in ADHD Therapy. Atomoxetine is recommended for treatment of ADHD in cases in which there may be concern for stimulant abuse or there exists a strong aversion to treatment with stimulant medications. Because CNS stimulants are more effective and have a long record of safety and efficacy, it would seem prudent to reserve atomoxetine for patients who are unresponsive to or intolerant of the stimulants. In the absence of a compelling reason, patients doing well on the stimulants shouldn't switch.

Preparations, Dosage, and Administration. Atomoxetine [Strattera] is available in capsules (10, 18, 25, 40, 60, 80, and 100 mg) that should be swallowed whole, with or without food. Dosage is based on body weight as follows:

- Children who weigh *less than 70 kg*—Start with 0.5 mg/kg/day and then, after at least 3 days, increase to the recommended target of 1.2 mg/kg/day. The maximum dosage is 1.4 mg/kg/day or 100 mg, whichever is smaller.
- Children who weigh *more than 70 kg and all adults*—Start with 40 mg/day and then, after at least 3 days, increase to the recommended target of 80 mg/day. Do not exceed 100 mg/day.

Two dosing schedules may be used: Patients may either (1) take the total daily dose all at once in the morning or (2) divide the dosage up, taking half in the morning and half in the late afternoon or early evening. Note that, with either schedule, dosing during school hours is unnecessary.

Dosage should be reduced in patients who are slow metabolizers, either because of hepatic insufficiency or atypical CYP2D6.

Alpha$_2$-Adrenergic Agonists

Two alpha$_2$-adrenergic agonists—guanfacine and clonidine—are approved for ADHD. Both drugs appear less effective than CNS stimulants. Principal side effects are sedation, hypotension, and fatigue. Unlike the CNS stimulants, guanfacine and clonidine are not controlled substances and do not cause anorexia or insomnia. The basic pharmacology of these drugs is discussed in Chapter 19.

Guanfacine. Available in an ER formulation, sold as *Intuniv,* guanfacine is used for treating children and adolescents with ADHD. In clinical trials, ER guanfacine improved hyperactivity and inattention. Benefits were greater than with placebo, but less than reported with stimulants. The exact mechanism behind guanfacine is unknown. We do know that guanfacine activates presynaptic alpha$_2$-adrenergic receptors in the brain. However, we don't know how this action relates to clinical benefits. Principal side effects are somnolence, fatigue, and reduced blood pressure. Effects on blood pressure are most pronounced during initial therapy and whenever dosage is increased. Abrupt discontinuation can cause rebound hypertension. In contrast to the stimulants, guanfacine causes weight gain rather than weight loss, causes somnolence rather than insomnia, and is not regulated under the Controlled Substances Act. Who should receive guanfacine? Because the drug does not cause anorexia or insomnia, it might be especially good for children who cannot tolerate these effects of stimulants. Guanfacine can also be combined with a stimulant to treat severe ADHD.

For treatment of ADHD, guanfacine [Intuniv] is available in ER tablets (1, 2, 3, and 4 mg), which should be swallowed intact, without chewing, cutting, or crushing. Dosing with a high-fat meal increases absorption and should be avoided. Dosage starts at 1 mg/day for at least 1 week, and can be increased at intervals of 1 week (or longer) by 1 mg/day. Children switching from IR guanfacine should use the same titration schedule, regardless of the dosage they had been taking. For all children, the maximum dosage is 4 mg/day. When guanfacine is discontinued, dosage should be tapered by 1 mg/day every 3 to 7 days. Abrupt discontinuation should be avoided, owing to a risk of rebound hypertension. The IR formulation used for hypertension, sold as *Tenex,* is discussed in Chapter 19.

Clonidine. ER clonidine [Kapvay] is much like ER guanfacine [Intuniv]. Both drugs are alpha$_2$ agonists, both were developed for hypertension, and both had been used off-label in ADHD for years. In clinical trials of ADHD, ER clonidine was superior to placebo when used alone and provided additional symptom relief when combined with a stimulant. As with guanfacine, principal side effects are somnolence, fatigue, and hypotension. Somnolence can be made worse by alcohol and other CNS depressants. Hypotension can be made worse by antihypertensive agents. Because clonidine can lower blood pressure (and slow heart rate too), blood pressure and heart rate should be measured at baseline, following each dose increase, and periodically thereafter. Like guanfacine, clonidine does not cause anorexia or insomnia and is not a controlled substance. For treatment of ADHD, clonidine [Kapvay] is supplied in 0.1- and 0.2-mg ER tablets, which should be swallowed whole without crushing, cutting, or chewing. Dosing may be done with or without food. The initial dosage is 0.1 mg in the evening, and the maximum dosage is 0.2 mg twice a day. Dosage is titrated, at intervals of 1 week or longer, as follows:

- 0.1 mg in PM
- 0.1 mg in AM and 0.1 mg in PM

- 0.1 mg in AM and 0.2 mg in PM
- 0.2 mg in AM and 0.2 mg in PM

When treatment stops, dosage should be reduced by 0.1 mg every 3 to 7 days to avoid rebound hypertension. Clonidine formulations used for hypertension, marketed as *Catapres* and *Catapres-TTS,* are discussed in Chapter 19.

Antidepressants

Three antidepressants—desipramine, imipramine, and bupropion—can reduce behavioral symptoms in children with ADHD. However, these antidepressants are less effective than CNS stimulants and are not approved for ADHD. Accordingly, they are generally reserved for children who have not responded to trials with at least two different stimulants.

Tricyclic Antidepressants. Desipramine [Norpramin] and imipramine [Tofranil] can reduce symptoms in children with ADHD. These drugs decrease hyperactivity but have little effect on impulsivity and inattention. Responses develop slowly. Beneficial effects begin in 2 to 3 weeks and reach a maximum at around 6 weeks. Tolerance frequently develops within a few months. In contrast to the stimulants, which can be discontinued on weekends, antidepressants must be taken continuously. Adverse effects include sedation and anticholinergic effects (e.g., dry mouth, blurred vision, urinary retention, constipation). More importantly, sudden death (from cardiotoxicity) has occurred in at least three children. Compared with stimulants, antidepressants have their benefits (no insomnia, abuse potential, or suppression of appetite and growth) as well as their drawbacks (anticholinergic effects, delayed onset, tolerance, less efficacy, risk of sudden death). Because these antidepressants are less effective and more dangerous than the stimulants, they are considered second-line drugs. Dosages for ADHD range from 2 to 5 mg/kg/day, administered in two or three divided doses. The basic pharmacology of the antidepressants is presented in Chapter 32.

Bupropion. Bupropion [Wellbutrin] can reduce behavioral symptoms of ADHD, but is less effective than stimulants. The drug lacks the adverse effects associated with tricyclic antidepressants (e.g., cardiotoxicity, anticholinergic effects) but does pose a risk of seizures. Like the tricyclic antidepressants, bupropion is considered a second-line drug for ADHD. Dosage is 100 to 150 mg twice a day. The basic pharmacology of bupropion is presented in Chapter 32.

KEY POINTS

- The amphetamine family consists of dextroamphetamine, amphetamine (a racemic mixture of dextroamphetamine and levamphetamine), methamphetamine, and lisdexamfetamine.
- The amphetamines work primarily by promoting neuronal release of NE and DA, and partly by blocking NE and DA reuptake.
- Through actions in the CNS, the amphetamines can increase wakefulness and alertness, reduce fatigue, elevate mood, stimulate respiration, and suppress appetite.
- By promoting release of NE from peripheral neurons, amphetamines can cause vasoconstriction and cardiac effects (increased heart rate, increased atrioventricular conduction, and increased force of contraction).
- The most common adverse effects of amphetamines are insomnia and weight loss. Amphetamines may also cause psychosis and cardiovascular effects (dysrhythmias, angina, hypertension).
- Amphetamines have a high abuse potential (owing to their ability to elevate mood), and hence are classified as Schedule II drugs.
- The principal indication for amphetamines is ADHD.
- The pharmacology of methylphenidate is nearly identical to that of the amphetamines.
- Methylphenidate and other CNS stimulants are the most effective drugs for ADHD, and hence are considered agents of first choice.
- Methylphenidate and other CNS stimulants reduce symptoms of ADHD by enhancing the patient's ability to focus.
- Only three nonstimulants—atomoxetine, guanfacine, and clonidine—are approved for ADHD.
- In treatment of ADHD, the nonstimulants may be used alone or as add-on therapy with a stimulant.
- Compared with the CNS stimulants, the nonstimulants are less effective in ADHD, but also are safer and have a lower potential for abuse.
- Caffeine and other methylxanthines act primarily by blocking adenosine receptors.
- Responses to caffeine are dose dependent: low doses decrease drowsiness and fatigue; higher doses cause nervousness, insomnia, and tremors; and huge doses cause convulsions.
- Caffeine has two principal uses: treatment of apnea in premature infants and reversal of drowsiness.

Please visit **http://evolve.elsevier.com/Lehne** for chapter-specific NCLEX® examination review questions.

Summary of Major Nursing Implications[a]

AMPHETAMINES, METHYLPHENIDATE, AND DEXMETHYLPHENIDATE

Preadministration Assessment

Therapeutic Goal

Reduction of symptoms in children and adults with ADHD. Reduction of sleep attacks in patients with narcolepsy.

Baseline Data

Children With ADHD. Document the degree of inattention, impulsivity, hyperactivity, and other symptoms of ADHD. Symptoms must be present for at least 6 months to allow a diagnosis of ADHD. Obtain baseline values of height and weight.

Narcolepsy. Document the degree of daytime sleepiness and the frequency and circumstances of sleep attacks.

Identifying High-Risk Patients

All amphetamines are *contraindicated* for patients with symptomatic cardiovascular disease, advanced atherosclerosis, hypertension, hyperthyroidism, agitated states, and a history of drug abuse, and in those who have taken monoamine

Continued

Summary of Major Nursing Implications[a]—cont'd

oxidase inhibitors within the previous 2 weeks. *Amphetamine/dextroamphetamine mixture* [Adderall XR] is *generally contraindicated* for patients with structural cardiac defects.

Implementation: Administration

Routes

Oral. Amphetamines, methylphenidate, and dexmethylphenidate.

Transdermal. Methylphenidate only.

Administration

Oral. **Instruct patients to swallow long-acting formulations intact, without crushing or chewing.**

Advise parents that children with ADHD should take the morning dose after breakfast and the last daily dose by 4:00 PM.

Transdermal. **Instruct patients using transdermal methylphenidate [Daytrana] to apply one patch to alternating hips each morning and to remove each patch not more than 9 hours after applying it. Instruct patients to avoid application to skin that is inflamed.**

Ongoing Evaluation and Interventions

Evaluating Therapeutic Effects

Children With ADHD. Monitor for reductions in symptoms (impulsiveness, hyperactivity, inattention) and for improvement in cognitive function.

Minimizing Adverse Effects

Excessive CNS Stimulation. CNS stimulants can cause restlessness and insomnia. **Advise patients to use the smallest dose required and to avoid dosing late in the day. Advise patients to minimize or eliminate dietary caffeine (e.g., coffee, tea, caffeinated soft drinks).**

Weight Loss. Appetite suppression can cause weight loss. **Advise patients to take the morning dose after breakfast and the last daily dose early in the afternoon to minimize interference with eating.**

Cardiovascular Effects. **Warn patients about cardiovascular responses (palpitations, hypertension, angina, dysrhythmias), and instruct them to notify the prescriber if these develop.**

Very rarely, children using stimulants for ADHD have experienced sudden cardiac death. In response, the AHA says it is reasonable to consider giving a child an ECG before starting stimulant therapy. However, there is conflicting evidence that stimulants actually cause sudden death, or that withholding stimulants will protect from sudden death, or that screening for cardiac defects with an ECG will be of any benefit. Therefore, it would seem that routine ECG screening is unnecessary, especially in children with no signs or symptoms of heart defects. However, if there *is* evidence of existing heart disease, or evidence of hereditary cardiovascular defects, an ECG might be appropriate.

Psychosis. If amphetamine-induced psychosis develops, therapy should be discontinued. For most individuals, symptoms resolve within a week. For some patients, drug-induced psychosis may represent unmasking of latent schizophrenia, indicating a need for psychiatric care.

Withdrawal Reactions. Abrupt discontinuation can produce extreme fatigue and depression. Minimize by withdrawing amphetamines and methylphenidate gradually.

Hypersensitivity Reactions. *Transdermal methylphenidate* [Daytrana] can cause hypersensitivity reactions, which may necessitate discontinuing *all* methylphenidate products, oral as well as transdermal. **Inform patients about signs of hypersensitivity—erythema, edema, papules, vesicles—and instruct them to inform the prescriber if these develop.**

Minimizing Abuse

If the medical history reveals that the patient is prone to drug abuse, monitor use of these drugs closely.

CAFFEINE

General Considerations

Caffeine is usually administered to promote wakefulness. **Warn patients against habitual caffeine use to compensate for chronic lack of sleep. Advise patients to consult the prescriber if fatigue is persistent or recurrent.**

Minimizing Adverse Effects

Cardiovascular Effects

Inform patients about cardiovascular responses to caffeine (palpitations, rapid pulse, dizziness), and instruct them to discontinue caffeine if these occur.

Excessive CNS Stimulation

Warn patients that overdose can cause convulsions. Advise them to ingest no more caffeine than needed.

[a]Patient education information is highlighted as **blue text**.

CHAPTER

37 Substance Use Disorders I: Basic Considerations

Mind-altering drugs have intrigued human beings since the dawn of civilization. Throughout history, people have taken drugs to elevate mood, release inhibitions, distort perceptions, induce hallucinations, and modify thinking. Many of those who take mind-altering drugs restrict usage to socially approved patterns. However, many others self-administer drugs to excess. Excessive drug use is our focus in this chapter and the three that follow.

Drug abuse extracts a huge toll on the individual and on society. Tobacco alone kills about 480,000 Americans each year. Alcohol and illicit drugs kill an additional 100,000. In addition to putting people at risk of death, drug abuse puts them at risk of long-term illness and impairs their ability to fulfill role obligations at home, school, and work. The economic burden of drug abuse is staggering: The combined direct and indirect costs from abusing nicotine, alcohol, and illicit substances are estimated at over $700 *billion* each year.

Drug abuse confronts clinicians in a variety of ways, making knowledge of abuse a necessity. Important areas in which expertise on drug abuse may be applied include (1) diagnosis and treatment of acute toxicity, (2) diagnosis and treatment of secondary medical complications of drug abuse, (3) the facilitation of drug withdrawal, and (4) education and counseling to maintain long-term abstinence.

Our discussion of drug abuse occurs in two stages. In this chapter, we discuss basic concepts in drug abuse. In Chapters 38, 39, and 40, we focus on the pharmacology of specific abused agents and methods of treatment.

DEFINITIONS

Drug Abuse

Drug abuse can be defined as *using a drug in a fashion inconsistent with medical or social norms.* Traditionally, the term also implies drug usage that is harmful to the individual or society. As we shall see, although we can give abuse a general definition, deciding whether a particular instance of drug use constitutes "abuse" is often difficult.

Whether drug use is considered abuse depends, in part, on the purpose for which a drug is taken. Not everyone who takes large doses of psychoactive agents has a disorder. For example, we do not consider it abuse to take large doses of opioids long term to relieve pain caused by cancer. However, we do consider it abusive for an otherwise healthy individual to take those same opioids in the same doses to produce euphoria.

Abuse can have different degrees of severity. Some people, for example, use heroin only occasionally, whereas others use it habitually and compulsively. Although both patterns of drug use are socially condemned, and therefore constitute abuse, there is an obvious quantitative difference between taking heroin once or twice and taking it routinely and compulsively.

Note that, by the definition earlier in this section, drug abuse is culturally defined. Because abuse is culturally defined and because societies differ from one another and are changeable, there can be wide variations in what is labeled abuse. What is defined as abuse can vary from one culture to another. For example, in the United States, moderate consumption of alcohol is not usually considered abuse. In contrast, any ingestion of alcohol may be considered abuse in some Muslim societies. Furthermore, what is defined as abuse can vary from one time to another within the same culture. For example, when a few Americans first experimented with lysergic acid diethylamide (LSD) and other psychedelic drugs, these agents were legal and their use was not generally disapproved. However, when use of psychedelics became widespread, our societal posture changed and legislation was passed to make the manufacture, sale, and use of these drugs illegal.

Within the United States, there is divergence of opinion about what constitutes drug abuse. For example, some people would consider any use of marijuana to be abuse, whereas others would call smoking marijuana abusive only if it were done *habitually*. Similarly, although many Americans do not consider cigarette smoking abuse (even though the practice is compulsive and clearly harmful to the individual and society), others believe very firmly that cigarette smoking is a blatant form of abuse.

As we can see, distinguishing between culturally acceptable drug use and drug use that is to be called abuse is more in the realm of social science than pharmacology. Accordingly, since this is a pharmacology text and not a sociology text, we will not attempt to define just what patterns of drug use do or do not constitute abuse. Instead, we will focus on the pharmacologic properties of abused drugs—leaving distinctions about what is and is not abuse to sociologists and legislators. Fortunately, we can identify the drugs that tend to be abused and discuss their pharmacology without having to resolve all arguments about what patterns of use should or should not be considered abusive.

Substance Use Disorder

According to the American Psychiatric Association (APA), substance use disorder (SUD) is defined as *a cluster of cognitive, behavioral, and physiological symptoms indicating that the individual continues using the substance despite significant substance-related problems*. Please note that nowhere in this definition is SUD equated with physical dependence. As discussed elsewhere in this chapter, although physical dependence can contribute to addictive behavior, it is neither necessary nor sufficient for addiction to occur.

Other Definitions

Tolerance results from regular drug use and can be defined as a state in which a particular dose elicits a smaller response than it did with initial use. As tolerance increases, higher and higher doses are needed to elicit desired effects.

Cross-tolerance is a state in which tolerance to one drug confers tolerance to another. Cross-tolerance generally develops among drugs within a particular class, and not between drugs in different classes. For example, tolerance to one opioid (e.g., heroin) confers cross-tolerance to other opioids (e.g., morphine), but not to central nervous system (CNS) depressants, psychostimulants, psychedelics, or nicotine.

Psychologic dependence can be defined as an intense subjective need for a particular psychoactive drug.

Physical dependence can be defined as a state in which an abstinence syndrome will occur if drug use is discontinued. Physical dependence is the result of neuroadaptive processes that take place in response to prolonged drug exposure.

Cross-dependence refers to the ability of one drug to support physical dependence on another drug. When cross-dependence exists between drug A and drug B, taking drug A will prevent withdrawal in a patient physically dependent on drug B, and vice versa. As with cross-tolerance, cross-dependence generally exists among drugs in the same pharmacologic family, but not between drugs in different families.

A *withdrawal syndrome* is a constellation of signs and symptoms that occurs in physically dependent individuals when they discontinue drug use. Quite often, the symptoms seen during withdrawal are opposite to effects the drug produced before it was withdrawn. For example, discontinuation of a CNS depressant can cause CNS excitation.

DIAGNOSTIC CRITERIA REGARDING SUBSTANCE USE DISORDER

Substance use disorder is best defined as continued use of a substance despite significant substance-related problems. There exists a change in brain circuitry that persists despite detoxification. Diagnosis of substance abuse disorder is based on behaviors related to continued use of a substance.

Tolerance and withdrawal are among the criteria established by the APA for having a substance use disorder. Please note, however, that tolerance and withdrawal, by themselves, are neither necessary nor sufficient for a substance use disorder to exist. Put another way, the pattern of drug use that constitutes a substance use disorder can exist in persons who are not physically dependent on drugs and who have not developed tolerance. Because this distinction is extremely important, we will express it another way: *Being physically dependent on a drug is not the same as having a disorder!* Many people are physically dependent but do not meet the criteria for a substance use disorder. These people are not considered to have SUD because they do not demonstrate the behavior pattern that constitutes substance dependence. Patients with terminal cancer, for example, are often physically dependent on opioids. However, since their lives are not disrupted by their medication (quite the contrary), their drug use does not meet the criteria for a substance use disorder. Similarly, some degree of physical dependence occurs in all patients who take phenobarbital to control seizure disorders. However, despite their physical dependence, patients with seizure do not carry out stereotypic addictive behavior and therefore do not have a substance use disorder.

Having stressed that physical dependence and SUD are different from each other, we must note that the two states are not entirely unrelated. As discussed in the sections that follow, although physical dependence is not the same as SUD, physical dependence often contributes to addictive behavior.

FACTORS THAT CONTRIBUTE TO SUBSTANCE USE DISORDER

Substance use disorder is the end result of a progressive involvement with drugs. Taking psychoactive drugs is usually initiated out of curiosity. From this initial involvement, the user can progress to occasional use. Occasional use can then evolve into compulsive use. Factors that play a role in the progression from experimental use to compulsive use are discussed in the sections that follow.

Reinforcing Properties of Drugs

Although there are several reasons for initiating drug use (e.g., curiosity, peer pressure), individuals would not continue drug use unless drugs produced desirable feelings or experiences. By making people feel "good," drugs reinforce the reasons for their use. Conversely, if drugs did not give people experiences that they found desirable, the reasons for initiating drug use would not be reinforced, and drug use would stop.

Reinforcement by drugs can occur in two ways. First, drugs can give the individual an experience that is pleasurable. Cocaine, for example, produces a state of euphoria. Second, drugs can reduce the intensity of unpleasant experiences. For example, drugs can reduce anxiety and stress.

The reinforcing properties of drugs can be clearly demonstrated in experiments with animals. In the laboratory, animals will self-administer most of the drugs that are abused by humans (e.g., opioids, barbiturates, alcohol, cocaine, amphetamines, phencyclidine, nicotine, caffeine). When these drugs are made freely available, animals develop patterns of drug use that are similar to those of humans. Animals will self-administer these drugs (except for nicotine and caffeine) in preference to eating, drinking, and sex. When permitted, they often die from lack of food and fluid. These observations strongly suggest that pre-existing psychopathology is not necessary for drug abuse to develop. Rather, these studies suggest that drug abuse results, in large part, from the reinforcing properties of drugs themselves.

Physical Dependence

As defined earlier in this chapter, physical dependence is a state in which an abstinence syndrome will occur if drug use is discontinued. The degree of physical dependence is determined largely by dosage and duration of drug use. Physical dependence is greatest in people who take large doses for a long time. The more physically dependent a person is, the more intense the withdrawal syndrome. Substantial physical dependence develops to the opioids (e.g., morphine, heroin) and CNS depressants (e.g., barbiturates, alcohol). Physical dependence tends to be less prominent with other abused drugs (e.g., psychostimulants, psychedelics, marijuana).

Physical dependence can contribute to compulsive drug use. Once dependence has developed, the desire to avoid withdrawal becomes a motivator for continued dosing. Furthermore, if the drug is administered after the onset of withdrawal, its ability to alleviate the discomfort of withdrawal can reinforce its desirability. Please note, however, that although physical dependence plays a role in the abuse of drugs, physical dependence should not be viewed as the primary cause of addictive behavior. Rather, physical dependence is just one of several factors that can contribute to the development and continuation of compulsive use.

Psychologic Dependence

Psychologic dependence is defined as *an intense subjective need for a drug.* Individuals who are psychologically dependent feel very strongly that their sense of well-being is dependent upon continued drug use; a sense of "craving" is felt when the drug is unavailable. There is no question that psychologic dependence can be a major factor in addictive behavior. For example, it is psychologic dependence—and not physical dependence—that plays the principal role in causing renewed use of opioids by addicts who had previously gone through withdrawal.

Social Factors

Social factors can play an important role in the development of SUD. The desire for social status and approval is a common reason for initiating drug use. Also, since initial drug experiences are frequently unpleasant, the desire for social approval can be one of the most compelling reasons for repeating drug use after the initial exposure. For example, most people do not especially enjoy their first cigarette; were it not for peer pressure, many would quit before they smoked enough for it to become pleasurable. Similarly, initial use of heroin, with its associated nausea and vomiting, is often deemed unpleasant; peer pressure is a common reason for continuing heroin use long enough to develop tolerance to these undesirable effects.

Drug Availability

Drug availability is clearly a factor in the development and maintenance of abuse. Abuse can flourish only in environments where drugs can be readily obtained. In contrast, where procurement is difficult, abuse is minimal. The ready availability of drugs in hospitals and clinics is a major reason for the unusually high rate of addiction among pharmacists, nurses, and physicians.

Vulnerability of the Individual

Some individuals are more prone to becoming drug abusers than others. By way of illustration, let's consider three individuals from the same social setting who have equal access to the same psychoactive drug. The first person experiments with the drug briefly and never uses it again. The second person progresses from experimentation to occasional use. The third goes on to take the drug compulsively. Since social factors, drug availability, and the properties of the drug itself are the same for all three people, these factors cannot explain the three different patterns of drug use. We must conclude, therefore, that the differences must lie in the people: one individual was not prone to drug abuse, one had only moderate tendencies toward abuse, and the third was highly vulnerable to becoming an abuser.

Several psychologic factors have been associated with tendencies toward drug abuse. Drug abusers are frequently individuals who are impulsive, have a low tolerance for frustration, and are rebellious against social norms. Other psychologic factors that seem to predispose individuals to abusing drugs include depressive disorders, anxiety disorders, and antisocial personality. It is also clear that individuals who abuse one type of drug are likely to abuse other drugs.

There is speculation that some instances of drug abuse may actually represent self-medication to relieve emotional discomfort. For example, some people may use alcohol and other depressants to control severe anxiety. Although their drug use may appear excessive, it may be no more than they need to neutralize intolerable feelings.

Genetics also contributes to drug abuse. Vulnerability to alcoholism, for example, may result from an inherited predisposition.

NEUROBIOLOGY OF SUBSTANCE USE DISORDER

Repeated use of a drug contributes to the transition from voluntary drug use to compulsive use by causing molecular changes in the brain. Each time the drug is taken, it causes changes that promote further drug use. With repeated drug exposure, these changes are reinforced, making drug use increasingly more difficult to control.

Molecular changes occur in the so-called *reward circuit*—a system that normally serves to reinforce behaviors essential for survival, such as eating and reproductive activities. Neurons of the reward circuit originate in the ventral tegmental area of the midbrain and project to the nucleus accumbens. Their major transmitter is *dopamine.* Under normal circumstances, biologically critical behavior, such as sexual intercourse, activates the circuit. The resultant release of dopamine rewards and reinforces the behavior. Like natural positive stimuli, addictive drugs can also activate the circuit and thereby cause dopamine release. In fact, drugs are so effective at activating the circuit that the amount of dopamine released may be 2 to 10 times the amount released by natural stimuli. Ultimately, whether the system is activated by use of drugs or by behavior essential for survival, the outcome is the same: a tendency to repeat the behavior that turned the system on. With repeated activation over time, the system undergoes synaptic remodeling, thereby consolidating changes in brain function. This neural remodeling persists after drug use has ceased.

An important aspect of drug-induced remodeling is a phenomenon known as *down-regulation,* which serves to *reduce* the response to drugs. Because drugs release abnormally large amounts of dopamine, the reward circuit is put in a state of excessive activation. In response, the brain (1) produces less dopamine and (2) reduces the number of dopamine receptors. As a result, responses to drugs are reduced. Unfortunately, the ability of natural stimuli to activate the circuit is reduced as well. In the absence of pleasurable feelings from natural stimuli, the abuser is left feeling flat, lifeless, and depressed. The good news is that, when drug use stops, neural remodeling tends to gradually reverse.

PRINCIPLES OF SUBSTANCE USE DISORDER TREATMENT

Substance use disorder is a treatable disease of the brain. With therapy, between 40% and 60% of addicts can reduce drug use. The first science-based guide on addiction therapy—*Principles of Drug Addiction Treatment*—was published by the National Institute on Drug Abuse in 1999, and later revised in 2009 and 2012. The guide centers on 13 principles of effective treatment, shown in Table 37.1.

TABLE 37.1 ▪ Principles of Substance Use Treatment

1. **Substance use disorder is a complex but treatable disease that affects brain function and behavior.** Drugs of abuse alter brain structure and function, resulting in changes that persist long after drug use has stopped. These persistent changes may explain why former abusers are at the risk of relapse after prolonged abstinence.
2. **No single treatment is appropriate for everyone.** It is critical to match treatment settings, interventions, and services to each patient's problems and needs.
3. **Treatment must be readily available.** Treatment applicants can be lost if treatment is not immediately available or readily accessible. As with other chronic diseases, the earlier treatment is offered in the disease process, the greater the likelihood of positive outcomes.
4. **Effective treatment must attend to multiple needs of the individual, not solely drug use.** In addition to addressing drug use, treatment must address the individual's medical, psychologic, social, vocational, and legal problems.
5. **Remaining in treatment for an adequate time is critical.** Treatment duration is based on individual need. Most patients require at least 3 months of treatment to significantly reduce or stop drug use. Additional treatment can produce further progress. As with other chronic illnesses, relapses can occur, signaling a need for treatment to be reinstated or adjusted. Programs should include strategies to prevent patients from leaving prematurely.
6. **Individual and/or group counseling and other behavioral therapies are the most common forms of drug abuse treatment.** In therapy, patients address motivation, build skills to resist drug use, replace drug-using activities with constructive and rewarding activities, and improve problem-solving abilities. Behavioral therapy also addresses incentives for abstinence and facilitates interpersonal relationships. Ongoing group therapy and other peer support programs can help maintain abstinence.
7. **Medication can be an important element of treatment, especially when combined with counseling and other behavioral therapies.** Methadone, buprenorphine, and naltrexone can help persons addicted to opioids. Nicotine replacement therapy (e.g., patches, gum), bupropion, and varenicline can help persons addicted to nicotine. Disulfiram, naltrexone, topiramate, and acamprosate can help persons addicted to alcohol.
8. **Because needs of the individual can change, the plan for treatment and services must be reassessed continually and modified as indicated.** At different times during treatment, a patient may develop a need for medications, medical services, family therapy, parenting instruction, vocational rehabilitation, and social and legal services.
9. **Many individuals with substance use disorder also have other mental disorders, which must be addressed.** Because drug addiction often co-occurs with other mental illnesses, patients presenting with one condition should be assessed for other conditions and treated as indicated.
10. **Medically assisted detoxification is only the first stage of treatment and, by itself, does little to change long-term drug use.** Medical detoxification manages the acute physical symptoms of withdrawal—and can serve as a precursor to effective long-term treatment.
11. **Treatment needn't be voluntary to be effective.** Sanctions or enticements coming from the family, employer, or criminal justice system can significantly increase treatment entry, retention, and success.
12. **Drug use during treatment must be monitored continuously, as relapses during treatment do occur.** Knowing that drug use is being monitored (e.g., through urinalysis) can help the patient withstand urges to use drugs. Monitoring also can provide early evidence of drug use, thereby allowing timely adjustment of the treatment program.
13. **Treatment programs should provide assessment for HIV/AIDS, hepatitis B and C, tuberculosis, and other infectious diseases, along with counseling, to help patients modify behaviors that place them or others at risk.**

HIV/AIDS, Human immunodeficiency virus/acquired immunodeficiency syndrome.
Adapted from National Institute on Drug Abuse: Principles of Drug Addiction Treatment: A Research-Based Guide, 3rd ed. (Publication No. 12-4180). Bethesda, MD: National Institutes of Health, 2012.

Ideally, the goal of treatment is *complete cessation* of drug use. However, total abstinence is not the only outcome that can be considered successful. Treatment that changes drug use from compulsive to moderate will permit increased productivity, better health, and a decrease in socially unacceptable behavior. Clearly, this outcome is beneficial both to the individual and to society—even though some degree of drug use continues. It must be noted, however, that in the treatment of some forms of abuse, nothing short of total abstinence can be considered a true success. Experience has shown that abusers of *cigarettes, alcohol,* and *opioids* are rarely capable of sustained moderation. Hence, for many of these individuals, abstinence must be complete if there is to be any hope of avoiding a return to compulsive use.

Recovery from addiction is a prolonged process that typically requires multiple treatment episodes because addiction is a *chronic, relapsing* illness. As such, periods of treatment-induced abstinence will very likely be followed by relapse. This does not mean that treatment has failed. Rather, it simply means that at least one more treatment episode is needed. Eventually, many patients achieve stable, long-term abstinence, along with a more productive and rewarding life.

Because addiction is a complex illness that affects all aspects of life, the treatment program must be comprehensive and multifaceted. In addition to addressing drug use itself, the program should address any related medical, psychologic, social, vocational, and legal problems. Obviously, treatment must be tailored to the individual; no single approach works for all people. Multiple techniques are employed. Techniques with proven success include (1) group and individual therapy directed at resolving emotional problems that underlie drug use, (2) substituting alternative rewards for the rewards of drug use, (3) threats and external pressure to discourage drug use, and (4) the use of pharmacologic agents to modify the effects of abused drugs. The most effective treatment programs incorporate two or more of these methods.

THE CONTROLLED SUBSTANCES ACT

The *Comprehensive Drug Abuse Prevention and Control Act* of 1970, known informally as the *Controlled Substances Act* (CSA), is the principal federal legislation addressing drug abuse. One objective of the CSA is to reduce the chances that drugs originating from legitimate sources will be diverted to abusers. To accomplish this goal, the CSA sets forth regulations for the handling of controlled substances by manufacturers, distributors, pharmacists, nurses, and physicians. Enforcement of the CSA is the responsibility of the *Drug Enforcement Agency* (DEA), an arm of the U.S. Department of Justice.

Record Keeping

To keep track of controlled substances that originate from legitimate sources, a written record must be made of all transactions involving these agents. Every time a controlled substance is purchased or dispensed, the transfer must be recorded. Physicians, pharmacists, and hospitals must keep an inventory of all controlled substances in stock. This inventory must be reported to the DEA every 2 years. Although not specifically obliged to do so by the CSA, many hospitals use medication dispensing machines that count the controlled substances dispensed during each shift.

DEA Schedules

Each drug preparation regulated under the CSA has been assigned to one of five categories: Schedule I, II, III, IV, or V. Drugs in Schedule I have a high potential for abuse and no approved medical use in the United States. In contrast, drugs in Schedules II through V all have approved applications. Assignment to Schedules II through V is based on abuse potential and potential for causing physical or psychologic dependence. Of the drugs that have medical applications, those in Schedule II have the highest potential for abuse and dependence. Drugs in the remaining schedules have decreasing abuse and dependence liabilities. Table 37.2 lists the primary drugs that come under the five DEA Schedules.

Scheduling of drugs under the CSA undergoes periodic re-evaluation. With increased understanding of the abuse and dependence liabilities of a drug, the DEA may choose to reassign it to a different Schedule. For example, hydrocodone (a commonly used opioid) was switched from Schedule III to Schedule II.

Prescriptions

The CSA places restrictions on prescribing drugs in Schedules II through V. (Drugs in Schedule I have no approved uses, and hence are not prescribed.) Only prescribers registered with the DEA are authorized to prescribe controlled drugs. Regulations on prescribing controlled substances are summarized in the sections that follow.

Schedule II

All prescriptions for Schedule II drugs must be typed or filled out in ink or indelible pencil and signed by the prescriber. Alternatively, prescribers may submit prescriptions using an electronic prescribing procedure. Oral prescriptions may be called in, but only in emergencies, and a written prescription must follow within 72 hours. Prescriptions for Schedule II drugs cannot be refilled. However, a DEA rule allows a prescriber to write multiple prescriptions on the same day—for the same patient and same drug—to be filled sequentially for up to a 90-day supply.

Schedules III and IV

Prescriptions for drugs in Schedules III and IV may be oral, written, or electronic. If authorized by the prescriber, these prescriptions may be refilled up to 5 times. Refills must be made within 6 months of the original order. If additional medication is needed beyond the amount provided for in the original prescription, a new prescription must be written.

Schedule V

The same regulations for prescribing drugs in Schedules III and IV apply to drugs in Schedule V. In addition, Schedule V drugs may be dispensed without a prescription provided the following conditions are met: (1) the drug is dispensed by a pharmacist; (2) the amount dispensed is very limited; (3) the recipient is at least 18 years old and can prove it; (4) the pharmacist writes and initials a record indicating the date, the name and amount of the drug, and the name and address

TABLE 37.2 ▪ Drug Enforcement Agency Classification of Controlled Substances

Schedule I Drugs	Schedule II Drugs	Schedule III Drugs	Schedule IV Drugs	Schedule V Drugs
Opioids	**Opioids**	**Opioids**	**Opioids**	**Opioids**
Acetylmethadol	Alfentanil	Buprenorphine	Butorphanol	Diphenoxylate plus
Heroin	Codeine	Paregoric	Pentazocine	atropine
Normethadone	Fentanyl	**Cannabinoids**	**Stimulants**	**Miscellaneous**
Many others	Hydrocodone	Dronabinol (THC)	Diethylpropion	Pregabalin
Psychedelics	Hydromorphone	**Stimulants**	Fenfluramine	
Bufotenin	Levorphanol	Benzphetamine	Mazindol	
Diethyltryptamine	Meperidine	Phendimetrazine	Pemoline	
Dimethyltryptamine	Methadone	**Barbiturates**	Phentermine	
Ibogaine	Morphine	Aprobarbital	**Barbiturates**	
d-Lysergic acid diethylamide	Opium tincture	Butabarbital	Methohexital	
(LSD)	Oxycodone	Talbutal	Phenobarbital	
Mescaline	Oxymorphone	Thiamylal	**Benzodiazepines**	
3,4-Methylenedioxy-	Remifentanil	Thiopental	Alprazolam	
methamphetamine	Sufentanil	**Miscellaneous**	Chlordiazepoxide	
(MDMA)	**Psychostimulants**	**Depressants**	Clonazepam	
Psilocin	Amphetamine	Methyprylon	Clorazepate	
Psilocybin	Cocaine	**Anabolic Steroids**	Diazepam	
Cannabis Derivatives	Dextroamphetamine	Fluoxymesterone	Estazolam	
Marijuana	Methamphetamine	Methyltestosterone	Flurazepam	
Others	Methylphenidate	Nandrolone	Lorazepam	
Gamma-hydroxybutyrate	Phenmetrazine	Oxandrolone	Midazolam	
Methaqualone	**Barbiturates**	Stanozolol	Oxazepam	
	Amobarbital	Testosterone	Prazepam	
	Pentobarbital	Many others	Quazepam	
	Secobarbital	**Others**	Temazepam	
	Miscellaneous	Ketamine	Triazolam	
	Depressants		**Benzodiazepine-like Drugs**	
	Glutethimide		Zaleplon	
			Zolpidem	
			Miscellaneous Depressants	
			Chloral hydrate	
			Dichloralphenazone	
			Ethchlorvynol	
			Ethinamate	
			Meprobamate	
			Paraldehyde	
			Tramadol	

of the recipient; and (5) state and local laws do not prohibit dispensing Schedule V drugs without a prescription.

Labeling

When drugs in Schedules II, III, and IV are dispensed, their containers must bear this label: *Caution—Federal law prohibits the transfer of this drug to any person other than the patient for whom it was prescribed.* The label must also indicate whether the drug belongs to Schedule II, III, or IV. The symbols C-II, C-III, and C-IV are used to indicate the Schedule.

State Laws

All states have their own laws regulating drugs of abuse. In many cases, state laws are more stringent than federal laws. As a rule, whenever there is a difference between state and federal laws, the more restrictive of the two takes precedence.

KEY POINTS

- Drug abuse can be defined as drug use that is inconsistent with medical or social norms.
- Drug abuse is a culturally defined term. What is considered abuse can vary from one culture to another and from one time to another within the same culture.
- Substance use disorder can be defined as a chronic, relapsing brain disease characterized by compulsive drug seeking and use, despite harmful consequences. Note that physical dependence is not required for SUD to exist.
- Tolerance is a state in which a particular drug dose elicits a smaller response than it formerly did.
- Cross-tolerance is a state in which tolerance to one drug confers tolerance to another drug.
- Psychologic dependence is defined as an intense subjective need for a particular psychoactive drug.
- Physical dependence is a state in which an abstinence syndrome will occur if drug use is discontinued. Physical dependence is *not* the same as addiction.
- Cross-dependence refers to the ability of one drug to support physical dependence on another drug.
- A withdrawal syndrome is a group of signs and symptoms that occur in physically dependent individuals when they discontinue drug use.
- Although tolerance and withdrawal are among the diagnostic criteria for substance dependence, they are neither necessary nor sufficient for a diagnosis.
- Although physical dependence is not the same as SUD, physical dependence can certainly contribute to addictive behavior.
- Drugs can reinforce their own use by providing pleasurable experiences, reducing the intensity of unpleasant experiences, and warding off a withdrawal syndrome.
- All addictive drugs activate the brain's dopamine reward circuit. Over time, they cause adaptive changes in the circuit that make it more and more difficult to control use.
- Some individuals, because of psychologic or genetic factors, are more prone to SUD than others.
- Because SUD is a chronic, relapsing illness, recovery is a prolonged process that typically requires multiple episodes of treatment.
- The ideal goal of treatment is complete abstinence. However, treatment that substantially reduces drug use can still be considered a success.
- Under the Controlled Substances Act, drugs in Schedule I have a high potential for abuse and no medically approved use in the United States. Drugs in Schedules II through V have progressively less abuse potential and are all medically approved.

Please visit **http://evolve.elsevier.com/Lehne** for chapter-specific NCLEX® examination review questions.

CHAPTER

38 Substance Use Disorders II: Alcohol

Alcohol (ethyl alcohol, ethanol) is the most commonly used and abused psychoactive agent in the United States. Although alcohol does have some therapeutic applications, the drug is of interest primarily for its nonmedical use. When consumed in moderation, alcohol prolongs life and reduces the risk of dementia and cardiovascular disorders. Conversely, when consumed in excess, alcohol does nothing but diminish life in both quality and quantity.

In approaching our study of alcohol, we begin by discussing the basic pharmacology of alcohol, and then we discuss alcohol use disorder and the drugs employed for treatment.

BASIC PHARMACOLOGY OF ALCOHOL

Central Nervous System Effects

Acute Effects

Alcohol has two acute effects on the brain: (1) general depression of central nervous system (CNS) function and (2) activation of the reward circuit.

For many years, we believed that alcohol simply dissolved into the neuronal membrane, thereby disrupting the ordered arrangement of membrane phospholipids. However, we now know that alcohol interacts with specific proteins—certain receptors, ion channels, and enzymes—that regulate neuronal excitability. Three target proteins are of particular importance, namely (1) receptors for gamma-aminobutyric acid (GABA), (2) receptors for glutamate, and (3) the 5-HT_3 subset of receptors for serotonin (5-hydroxytryptamine [5-HT]). The *depressant* effects of alcohol result from binding with receptors for GABA (the principal inhibitory transmitter in the CNS) and receptors for glutamate (a major excitatory transmitter in the CNS). When alcohol binds with GABA receptors, it enhances GABA-mediated inhibition, causing widespread depression of CNS activity. When alcohol binds with glutamate receptors, it blocks glutamate-mediated excitation and thereby reduces overall CNS activity. The *rewarding* effects of alcohol result from binding with 5-HT_3 receptors in the brain's reward circuit. When these receptors are activated (by serotonin), they promote release of dopamine, the major transmitter of the reward system. When alcohol binds with these receptors, it enhances serotonin-mediated release of dopamine and intensifies the reward process.

The depressant effects of alcohol are dose dependent. When dosage is low, higher brain centers (cortical areas) are primarily affected. As dosage increases, more primitive brain areas (e.g., medulla) become depressed. With depression of cortical function, thought processes and learned behaviors are altered, inhibitions are released, and self-restraint is replaced by increased sociability and expansiveness. Cortical depression also impairs motor function. As CNS depression deepens, reflexes diminish greatly and consciousness becomes impaired. At very high doses, alcohol produces a state of general anesthesia. (Alcohol can't be used for anesthesia because the doses required are close to lethal.) Table 38.1 shows the effects of alcohol as a function of blood alcohol level and indicates the brain areas involved.

Chronic Effects

When consumed chronically and in excess, alcohol can produce severe neurologic and psychiatric disorders. Injury to the CNS is caused by the direct actions of alcohol and by the nutritional deficiencies often seen in chronic heavy drinkers.

Two neuropsychiatric syndromes are common in patients with AUD: *Wernicke's encephalopathy* and *Korsakoff's psychosis*. Both disorders are caused by thiamine deficiency, which results from poor diet and alcohol-induced suppression of thiamine absorption. Wernicke's encephalopathy is characterized by confusion, nystagmus, and abnormal ocular movements. This syndrome is readily reversible with thiamine. Korsakoff's psychosis is characterized by polyneuropathy, inability to convert short-term memory into long-term memory, and confabulation (unconscious filling of gaps in memory with fabricated facts and experiences). Korsakoff's psychosis is not reversible.

Perhaps the most dramatic effect of long-term excessive alcohol consumption is enlargement of the cerebral ventricles, presumably in response to atrophy of the cerebrum itself. These gross anatomic changes are associated with impairment of memory and intellectual function. With cessation of drinking, ventricular enlargement and cognitive deficits partially reverse, but only in some individuals.

TABLE 38.1 ▪ Central Nervous System Responses at Various Blood Alcohol Levels[a]

Blood Alcohol Level (%)	Pharmacologic Response	Brain Area Affected
0.50	Peripheral collapse	Medulla
0.45	Respiratory depression	
0.40	Stupor, coma	Diencephalon
0.35	Apathy, inertia	
0.30	Altered equilibrium	Cerebellum
	Double vision	Occipital lobe
0.25	Altered perception	
0.20	Reduced motor skills	Parietal lobe
	Slurred speech	
0.15	Tremors	
	Ataxia	
	Reduced attention	Frontal lobe
0.10	Loquaciousness	
	Altered judgment	
0.05	Increased confidence	
	Euphoria, decreased inhibitions	

[a]According to the National Institute on Alcohol Abuse and Alcoholism.

Impact on Cognitive Function

Low to moderate drinking helps preserve cognitive function in older people and may protect against development of dementia.

Effect on Sleep

Although alcohol is commonly used as a sleep aid, it actually disrupts sleep. Drinking can alter sleep cycles, decrease total sleeping time, and reduce the quality of sleep. In addition, alcohol can intensify snoring and exacerbate obstructive sleep apnea. Having a drink with dinner won't affect sleep, but drinking late in the evening will.

Other Pharmacologic Effects

Cardiovascular System

When alcohol is consumed acutely and in moderate doses, cardiovascular effects are minor. The most prominent effect is *dilation of cutaneous blood vessels,* causing increased blood flow to the skin. By doing so, alcohol imparts a sensation of warmth—but at the same time promotes loss of heat.

Although the cardiovascular effects of moderate alcohol consumption are unremarkable, chronic and excessive consumption is clearly harmful. Abuse of alcohol results in *direct damage to the myocardium,* thereby increasing the risk of heart failure. Some investigators believe that alcohol may be the major cause of cardiomyopathy in the Western world.

In addition to damaging the heart, alcohol produces a dose-dependent *elevation of blood pressure.* The cause is vasoconstriction in vascular beds of skeletal muscle brought on by increased activity of the sympathetic nervous system. Estimates suggest that heavy drinking may be responsible for 10% of all cases of hypertension.

Not all of the cardiovascular effects of alcohol are deleterious: There is clear evidence that people who drink *moderately* (2 drinks a day or less for men, 1 drink a day or less for women) experience less ischemic stroke, coronary artery disease (CAD), myocardial infarction (MI), and heart failure than do abstainers. It is important to note, however, that *heavy* drinking (5 or more drinks/day) *increases* the risk of heart disease and stroke. Moderate drinking protects against heart disease primarily by raising levels of high-density lipoprotein (HDL) cholesterol. As discussed in Chapter 50, HDL cholesterol protects against CAD, whereas low-density lipoprotein (LDL) cholesterol promotes CAD. Of all the agents that can raise HDL cholesterol, alcohol is one of the most effective known. In addition to raising HDL cholesterol, alcohol may confer protection through four other mechanisms: decreasing platelet aggregation, decreasing levels of fibrinogen (the precursor of fibrin, which reinforces clots), increasing levels of tissue plasminogen activator (a clot-dissolving enzyme), and suppressing the inflammatory component of atherosclerosis. The degree of cardiovascular protection is nearly equal for beer, wine, and distilled spirits. That is, protection is determined primarily by the *amount* of alcohol consumed—not by the particular beverage the alcohol is in. Also, the *pattern* of drinking matters: protection is greater for people who drink moderately 3 or 4 days a week than for people who drink just 1 or 2 days a week. Finally, cardioprotection is greatest for those with an *un*healthy lifestyle: Among people who exercise, eat fruits and vegetables, and do not smoke, alcohol has little or no effect on the incidence of coronary events; conversely, among people who lack these behaviors, moderate alcohol intake is associated with a 50% reduction in coronary risk.

Glucose Metabolism

Alcohol has several effects on glucose metabolism that may decrease the risk for type 2 diabetes. For example, alcohol raises levels of adiponectin, a compound that enhances insulin sensitivity. In addition, alcohol suppresses gluconeogenesis, blunts the postprandial rise in blood glucose, and lowers fasting levels of both glucose and insulin.

Bone Health

Alcohol increases bone mineral density, probably by increasing levels of sex hormones.

Respiration

Like all other CNS depressants, alcohol depresses respiration. Respiratory depression from moderate drinking is negligible. However, when consumed in excess, alcohol can cause death by respiratory arrest. The respiratory depressant effects of alcohol are potentiated by other CNS depressants (e.g., benzodiazepines, opioids, barbiturates).

Liver

Alcohol-induced liver damage can progress from fatty liver to hepatitis to cirrhosis, depending on the amount consumed. Acute drinking causes reversible accumulation of fat and protein in the liver. With more chronic drinking, nonviral *hepatitis* develops in about 90% of heavy users. In 8% to 20% of patients with chronic alcohol use disorder (AUD), hepatitis evolves into cirrhosis—a condition characterized by proliferation of fibrous tissue and destruction of liver parenchymal cells. Although various factors other than alcohol can cause cirrhosis, alcohol abuse is unquestionably the major cause of *fatal* cirrhosis.

Stomach

Excessive use of alcohol can cause *erosive gastritis.* About one-third of patients with AUD have this disorder. Two mechanisms are involved. First, alcohol stimulates secretion of gastric acid. Second, when present in high concentrations, alcohol can injure the gastric mucosa directly.

Kidney

Alcohol is a diuretic. It promotes urine formation by inhibiting the release of antidiuretic hormone (ADH) from the pituitary. Because ADH acts on the kidney to promote water reabsorption, thereby decreasing urine formation, a reduction in circulating ADH will increase urine production.

Pancreas

Approximately 35% of cases of acute pancreatitis can be attributed to alcohol, making alcohol the second most common cause of the disorder. Flare-ups typically occur after a bout of heavy drinking. Only 10% of patients with AUD develop pancreatitis, and then only after years of overindulgence.

Sexual Function

Alcohol has both psychologic and physiologic effects related to human sexual behavior. Although alcohol is not exactly an aphrodisiac, its ability to release inhibitions has been known to motivate sexual activity. Ironically, the physiologic effects of alcohol may frustrate attempts at consummating the activity that alcohol inspired: Objective measurements in males and females show that alcohol significantly decreases our physiologic capacity for sexual responsiveness. In males, long-term use of alcohol may induce *feminization.* Symptoms include testicular atrophy, impotence, sterility, and breast enlargement.

Cancer

Alcohol—even in moderate amounts—is associated with an increased risk of several common cancers. Among these are cancers of the breast, liver, rectum, and aerodigestive tract, which includes the lips, tongue, mouth, nose, throat, vocal cords, and portions of the esophagus and trachea. According to a 2016 study, alcohol consumption is linked to seven cancers. The fraction attributable to alcohol is highest for aerodigestive tract cancers. People who drink more than 50 gm of alcohol daily (12 oz beer, 5 oz wine, or 1.25 oz of hard alcohol are all about 14 gm) are at 4 to 7 times increased risk of developing these types of cancers. The risk is somewhat lower for liver, breast, and colorectal cancer (1.5 times increased risk). The bottom line? Data suggest that, regarding cancer risk, no amount of alcohol can be considered safe—although risk is lowest with moderate drinking (2 drinks or less a day for men and 1 drink or less a day for women).

Pregnancy

Effects of alcohol on the developing fetus are dose-dependent. The risk of fetal injury is greatest with heavy drinking and much lower with light drinking. Is there some low level of drinking that is *completely* safe? We don't know.

Fetal alcohol exposure can cause structural and functional abnormalities, ranging from mild neurobehavioral deficits to facial malformation and developmental delay. The term *fetal alcohol spectrum disorder* (FASD) is used in reference to the *full range* of outcomes—from mild to severe—that drinking during pregnancy can cause. In contrast, the term *fetal alcohol syndrome* (FAS) is reserved for the most severe cases of FASD, characterized by craniofacial malformations, growth restriction (including microcephaly), and neurodevelopmental abnormalities, manifesting during childhood as cognitive and social dysfunction. In addition to causing FASD and FAS, heavy drinking during pregnancy can result in stillbirth, spontaneous abortion, and giving birth to an alcohol-dependent infant.

Is *light* drinking safe during pregnancy? The data are unclear. Two studies published in 2010 suggest that light drinking may carry little risk. One study, conducted in the United Kingdom, found no clinically relevant behavioral or cognitive problems in 5-year-olds whose mothers consumed 1 to 2 drinks a week during pregnancy. The other study, conducted in Australia, found no link between *low to moderate* alcohol consumption during pregnancy and alcohol-related birth defects (ARBDs), although the same study did show that *heavy* drinking was associated with a fourfold increased risk of an ARBD. These results are consistent with other recent studies, which have failed to show a relationship between occasional or light drinking during pregnancy and abnormalities in newborns or older children. However, since all of these studies were observational, rather than randomized controlled trials, the negative results might be explained by confounding factors, especially educational level, income, or access to prenatal care. Furthermore, since the follow-up time for these studies was relatively short (only 5 years), the long-term effects of light drinking remain unknown. What's the bottom line? If there *is* some amount of alcohol that is safe during pregnancy, that amount is very low. Accordingly, despite the studies noted, the American College of Obstetricians and Gynecologists (ACOG) continues to maintain its long-held position that no amount of alcohol can be considered safe during pregnancy. Therefore, in the interests of fetal health, all women should be advised to avoid alcohol *entirely* while pregnant or trying to conceive. Having said that, it is important to appreciate that a few drinks early in pregnancy are not likely to harm the fetus. Consequently, if a woman consumed a little alcohol before realizing she was pregnant, she should be reassured that the risk to the fetus—if any—is extremely low.

Lactation

The concentration of alcohol in breast milk parallels the concentration in blood. Recent data indicate that drinking while breast-feeding can adversely affect the infant's feeding and behavior.

Impact on Longevity

The effects of alcohol on life span depend on the amount consumed. *Heavy* drinkers have a higher mortality rate than the population at large. Causes of death include cirrhosis, respiratory disease, cancer, and fatal accidents. The risk of mortality associated with alcohol abuse increases markedly in individuals who consume 6 or more drinks a day.

Interestingly, people who consume *moderate* amounts of alcohol live *longer* than those who abstain—and combining regular exercise with moderate drinking prolongs life even more. Compared with nondrinkers, moderate drinkers have a 30% lower mortality rate, a 50% lower incidence of MI, and a 59% lower incidence of heart failure. According to a study by the American Medical Association, if all Americans were to give up drinking, deaths from heart disease would *increase* by 81,000 a year. Hence, for people who already *are* moderate drinkers, continued moderate drinking would seem beneficial. Conversely, despite the apparent benefits of drinking—and the apparent health disadvantage of abstinence—no one is recommending that abstainers take up drinking. Furthermore, when the risks of alcohol outweigh any possible benefits—such as in pregnancy—then alcohol consumption should be avoided entirely.

How does alcohol prolong life? In large part by reducing cardiovascular disease. For people who drink red wine, a small benefit may come from *resveratrol,* although the amount present appears too small to have a significant effect (see Chapter 108).

Pharmacokinetics

Absorption

Alcohol is absorbed from the stomach and small intestine. About 20% of ingested alcohol is absorbed from the stomach. Gastric absorption is relatively slow and is delayed even further by the presence of food. Milk is especially effective at delaying absorption. Absorption from the small intestine is rapid and largely independent of food; about 80% of ingested alcohol is absorbed from this site. Because most alcohol is absorbed from the small intestine, gastric emptying time is a major determinant of individual variation in alcohol absorption.

Distribution

Because alcohol is both nonionic and water soluble, it distributes well to all tissues and body fluids. The drug crosses the blood-brain barrier with ease, allowing alcohol in the brain to equilibrate rapidly with alcohol in the blood. Alcohol also crosses the placenta and hence can affect the developing fetus.

Distribution in body water partly explains why women are more sensitive to alcohol than men. As a rule, women have a lower percentage of body water than men. Hence, when a woman drinks, the alcohol is diluted in a smaller volume of water, causing the concentration of alcohol in tissues and fluids to be relatively high, which causes the effects of alcohol to be more intense.

Metabolism

Alcohol is metabolized in both the liver and stomach. The liver is the primary site. The process begins with conversion of alcohol to acetaldehyde, a reaction catalyzed by *alcohol dehydrogenase.* This reaction is slow and puts a limit on the rate at which alcohol can be inactivated. Once formed, acetaldehyde undergoes *rapid* conversion by aldehyde dehydrogenase to acetic acid. Through a series of reactions, acetic acid is then used to synthesize cholesterol, fatty acids, and other compounds.

The kinetics of alcohol metabolism differ from those of most other drugs. With most drugs, as plasma drug levels rise, the amount of drug metabolized per unit of time increases too. This is not true for alcohol: As the alcohol content of blood increases, there is almost no change in the speed of alcohol breakdown. That is, alcohol is metabolized at a relatively *constant rate*—regardless of how much alcohol is present. The average rate at which individuals can metabolize alcohol is about *15 mL (0.5 oz) per hour.*

TABLE 38.2 ▪ Alcohol Content of Beer, Wine, and Whiskey

	Wine	Beer	Whiskey
Usual serving	1 glass	1 can or bottle	1 shot
Serving size	150 mL (5 oz)	360 mL (12 oz)	45 mL (1.5 oz)
Alcohol concentration	12%[a]	5%[b]	40%[c]
Alcohol per serving	18 mL[d] (0.6 oz)	18 mL[e] (0.6 oz)	18 mL[f] (0.6 oz)

[a]The alcohol content of wine varies from 8% to 20%; typical table wines contain 12%.
[b]The alcohol content of beer varies: 5% alcohol is typical of American premium beers; cheaper American beers and light beers have less alcohol (2.4% to 5%); and imported or craft beers may have more alcohol (6% to 10%). Beer sold in Europe may have 7% to 8% alcohol.
[c]Whiskeys and other distilled spirits (e.g., rum, vodka, gin) are usually 80 proof (40% alcohol) but may also be 100 proof (50% alcohol).
[d]The alcohol in a 5-ounce glass of wine varies from 12 to 30 mL, depending on the alcohol concentration in the wine. Wine with 12% alcohol has 18 mL of alcohol per 5-ounce glass.
[e]The alcohol in a 12-ounce can of beer varies from 9 to 29 mL, depending on the alcohol concentration in the beer. Beer with 5% alcohol has 18 mL per 12-ounce can.
[f]The alcohol in a 1.5-ounce shot of whiskey can be either 18 or 22.5 mL, depending on the proof of the whiskey. Eighty-proof whiskey has 18 mL of alcohol per 1.5-ounce serving.

Because alcohol is metabolized at a slow and constant rate, there is a limit to how much alcohol one can consume without having the drug accumulate. For practical purposes, that limit is about *1 drink per hour.* Consumption of more than 1 drink per hour—be that drink beer, wine, straight whiskey, or a cocktail—will result in alcohol accumulation.

The information in Table 38.2 helps explain why we can't metabolize more than 1 drink's worth of alcohol per hour. Beer, wine, and whiskey differ from one another with respect to alcohol concentration and usual serving size. However, despite these differences, it turns out that the average can of beer, the average glass of wine, and the average shot of whiskey all contain the same amount of alcohol—namely, 18 mL (0.6 oz). Since the liver can metabolize about 15 mL of alcohol per hour and since the average alcoholic drink contains 18 mL of alcohol, 1 drink contains just about the amount of alcohol that the liver can comfortably process each hour. Consumption of more than 1 drink per hour will overwhelm the capacity of the liver for alcohol metabolism, and therefore alcohol will accumulate.

When used on a regular basis, alcohol induces hepatic drug-metabolizing enzymes, thereby increasing the rate of its own metabolism and that of other drugs. As a result, individuals who consume alcohol routinely in high amounts can metabolize the drug faster than people who drink occasionally and moderately.

Males and females differ with respect to activity of alcohol dehydrogenase in the stomach. Specifically, women have lower activity than men. As a result, gastric metabolism of alcohol is significantly less in women. This difference partly explains why women achieve higher blood alcohol levels than men after consuming the same number of drinks.

Blood Levels of Alcohol

Since alcohol in the brain rapidly equilibrates with alcohol in the blood, blood levels of alcohol are predictive of CNS effects. The behavioral effects associated with specific blood levels are shown in Table 38.1. The earliest effects (euphoria, reduced inhibitions, increased confidence) are seen when blood alcohol content is about 0.05%. As blood alcohol rises, intoxication becomes more intense. When blood alcohol exceeds 0.4%, there is a substantial risk of respiratory depression, peripheral collapse, and death. In the United States, a level of 0.08% defines intoxication.

Tolerance

Chronic consumption of alcohol produces tolerance. As a result, to alter consciousness, people who drink on a regular basis require larger amounts of alcohol than people who drink occasionally. Tolerance to alcohol confers cross-tolerance to general anesthetics, barbiturates, and other general CNS depressants. However, no cross-tolerance develops to opioids. Tolerance subsides within a few weeks following drinking cessation.

Although tolerance develops to many of the effects of alcohol, *very little tolerance develops to respiratory depression.* Consequently, the lethal dose of alcohol for chronic heavy drinkers is not much bigger than the lethal dose for nondrinkers. Individuals with AUD may tolerate blood alcohol levels as high as 0.4% (5 times the amount defined by law as intoxicating) with no marked reduction in consciousness. However, if blood levels rise only slightly above this level, death may ensue.

Physical Dependence

Chronic use of alcohol produces physical dependence. If alcohol is withdrawn abruptly, an abstinence syndrome will result. The intensity of the abstinence syndrome is proportional to the degree of physical dependence. Individuals who are physically dependent on alcohol show cross-dependence with other general CNS depressants (e.g., barbiturates, chloral hydrate, benzodiazepines) but not with opioids. The alcohol withdrawal syndrome and its management are discussed in detail later in this chapter.

Drug Interactions

CNS Depressants

The CNS effects of alcohol are additive with those of other CNS depressants (e.g., barbiturates, benzodiazepines, opioids). Consumption of alcohol with other CNS depressants intensifies the psychologic and physiologic manifestations of CNS depression and greatly increases the risk of death from respiratory depression.

Nonsteroidal Anti-Inflammatory Drugs

Like alcohol, aspirin, ibuprofen, and other nonsteroidal anti-inflammatory drugs (NSAIDs) can injure the GI mucosa. The combined effects of alcohol and NSAIDs can result in significant gastric bleeding.

Acetaminophen

The combination of acetaminophen [Tylenol, others] with alcohol poses a risk of potentially fatal liver injury. The interaction between alcohol and acetaminophen is discussed further in Chapter 71.

Safety Alert

ACETAMINOPHEN AND ALCOHOL

There is evidence that relatively modest alcohol consumption (2 to 4 drinks a day) can cause fatal liver damage when combined with acetaminophen taken in normal therapeutic doses. Accordingly, some authorities recommend that people who drink take no more than 2 gm of acetaminophen a day (i.e., half the normal dosage).

Disulfiram

The combination of alcohol with disulfiram [Antabuse] can cause a variety of adverse effects, some of which are dangerous. These effects, and the use of disulfiram to maintain abstinence, are discussed later.

Antihypertensive Drugs

Since alcohol raises blood pressure, it tends to counteract the effects of antihypertensive medications. However, elevation of blood pressure is significant only when alcohol dosage is high. Conversely, when the dosage is low, alcohol may actually help: Among hypertensive men, light to moderate alcohol consumption is associated with a reduced risk for both cardiovascular mortality and all-cause mortality.

Acute Overdose

Acute overdose produces vomiting, coma, pronounced hypotension, and respiratory depression. The combination of vomiting and unconsciousness can result in aspiration, which in turn can result in pulmonary obstruction and pneumonia. Alcohol-induced hypotension results from a direct effect on peripheral blood vessels and cannot be corrected with vasoconstrictors (e.g., epinephrine). Hypotension can lead to renal failure (secondary to compromised renal blood flow) and cardiovascular shock, a common cause of alcohol-related death. Although death can also result from respiratory depression, this is not the usual cause.

Because symptoms of acute alcohol poisoning can mimic symptoms of other pathologies (e.g., diabetic coma, skull fracture), a definitive diagnosis may not be possible without measuring alcohol in the blood, urine, or expired air. The smell of "alcohol" on the breath is not a reliable means of diagnosis, since the breath odors we associate with alcohol are due to impurities in alcoholic beverages—and not to alcohol itself. Hence, these odors may or may not be present.

Alcohol poisoning is treated like poisoning with all other general CNS depressants. Details of management are discussed in Chapter 34. Alcohol can be removed from the body by gastric lavage and dialysis. Stimulants (e.g., caffeine) should not be given.

Precautions and Contraindications

Alcohol can injure the GI mucosa and should not be consumed by persons with *peptic ulcer disease.* Alcohol is harmful to the liver and should not be used by individuals with *liver disease.* Alcohol should be avoided during *pregnancy,* owing to the risk of FASD (including FAS), stillbirth, spontaneous abortion, and neurodevelopmental abnormalities.

Alcohol must be used with caution by patients with *epilepsy.* During alcohol use, the CNS is depressed. When alcohol consumption ceases, the CNS undergoes rebound excitation; seizures can result.

Alcohol causes a dose-related increase in the risk of *breast cancer.* All women—and especially those at high risk—should minimize alcohol consumption. Alcohol also increases the risk of cancer of the liver, rectum, and aerodigestive tract.

Alcohol can cause serious adverse effects if combined with *CNS depressants, NSAIDs, acetaminophen, vasodilators,* and *disulfiram.* These combinations should be avoided.

Therapeutic Uses

Although our emphasis has been on the nonmedical use of alcohol, it should be remembered that alcohol does have therapeutic applications.

Topical

Topical alcohol can be an effective skin disinfectant.

Oral

Oral alcohol is frequently used as self-medication for insomnia—although it can actually disrupt sleep.

Local Injection

Injection of alcohol in the vicinity of nerves produces nerve block. This technique can relieve pain from trigeminal neuralgia, inoperable carcinoma, and other causes.

PATIENT-CENTERED CARE ACROSS THE LIFE SPAN

Alcohol

Life Stage	Patient Care Concerns
Infants	See "Breast-feeding women," below.
Children/ adolescents	Adolescents are more sensitive to alcohol-induced memory impairment than adults, but less sensitive to the motor effects of alcohol. Alcohol exposure during adolescence affects brain functioning during adulthood.
Pregnant women	The use of alcohol while pregnant can cause structural and functional abnormalities in the fetus. These abnormalities are termed fetal alcohol spectrum disorder (FASD). It is recommended that pregnant women abstain from alcohol.
Breast-feeding women	The concentration of alcohol in breast milk parallels the concentration in blood. Breast-feeding while consuming alcohol can affect infant behavior.
Older adults	Aging lowers the body's tolerance for alcohol. Many older adults may not metabolize alcohol as efficiently as younger adults. Many older adults take medications that interact with alcohol.

ALCOHOL USE DISORDER (AUD)

Alcohol use disorder is a chronic, relapsing disorder characterized by impaired control over drinking, preoccupation with alcohol consumption, use of alcohol despite awareness of adverse consequences, and distortions in thinking, especially as evidenced by denial of a drinking problem. The development and manifestations of AUD are influenced by genetic, psychosocial, and environmental factors. The disease is progressive and often fatal. In the United States, about 6% of the adult population are diagnosed with AUD.

Alcohol use disorder is defined as a problematic pattern of alcohol use leading to clinically significant impairment or distress occurring within a 12-month period. Manifestations of alcohol use disorder can include recurrent alcohol use in situations in which it is physically hazardous; recurrent use resulting in a failure to fulfill major role obligations at work, school, or home; and spending a great deal of time in activities necessary to obtain alcohol, use alcohol, or recover from alcohol.

In the United States, misuse of alcohol is responsible for 6 million nonfatal injuries and 85,000 deaths each year. Causes of death range from liver disease to automobile wrecks. Fully 50% of all fatal highway crashes are alcohol related. Among teens, alcohol-related crashes are the leading cause of death. Alcohol also causes industrial accidents and is responsible for 40% of industrial fatalities.

Alcohol abuse is a major public health problem, and its consequences are numerous. AUD produces psychologic derangements, including anxiety, depression, and suicidal ideation. Malnutrition, secondary to inadequate diet and malabsorption, is common. Poor work performance and disruption of family life reflect the social deterioration suffered by individuals with AUD. Alcohol abuse during pregnancy can result in FASD (including FAS), stillbirth, and spontaneous abortion. Lastly, chronic alcohol abuse is harmful to the body; consequences include liver disease, cardiomyopathy, and brain damage—not to mention injury and death from accidents.

Chronic alcohol consumption produces substantial tolerance. Tolerance is both pharmacokinetic (accelerated alcohol metabolism) and pharmacodynamic. Pharmacodynamic tolerance is evidenced by an increase in the blood alcohol level required to produce intoxication. Individuals with AUD may tolerate blood alcohol levels of 200 to 400 mg/dL—2.5 to 5 times the level that defines legal intoxication—with no marked reduction in consciousness. It should be noted, however, that very little tolerance develops to respiratory depression. Hence, as the person with AUD consumes increasing amounts in an effort to feel good, the risk of death from respiratory arrest gets increasingly high. Cross-tolerance exists with general anesthetics and other CNS depressants, but not with opioids.

Chronic use of alcohol produces physical dependence, and abrupt withdrawal produces an abstinence syndrome. When the degree of physical dependence is low, withdrawal symptoms are mild (disturbed sleep, weakness, nausea, anxiety, mild tremors) and last less than a day. In contrast, when the degree of dependence is high, withdrawal symptoms can be severe. Initial symptoms appear 12 to 72 hours after the last drink and continue 5 to 7 days. Early manifestations include cramps, vomiting, hallucinations, and intense tremors; heart rate, blood pressure, and temperature may rise, and tonic-clonic seizures may develop. As the syndrome progresses, disorientation and loss of insight occur. A few individuals with AUD (fewer than 5%) experience *delirium tremens* (severe persecutory hallucinations). Hallucinations can be so vivid and lifelike that people often can't distinguish them from reality. In extreme cases,

TABLE 38.3 ▪ Screening Instrument: The Alcohol Use Disorders Identification Test (AUDIT)

	0	1	2	3	4	Score
1. How often do you have a drink containing alcohol?	Never	Monthly or less	2 to 4 times a month	2 to 3 times a week	4 or more times a week	
2. How many drinks containing alcohol do you have on a typical day when you are drinking?	1 or 2	3 or 4	5 or 6	7 to 9	10 or more	
3. How often do you have 5 or more drinks on one occasion?	Never	Less than monthly	Monthly	Weekly	Daily or almost daily	
4. How often during the last year have you found that you were not able to stop drinking once you had started?	Never	Less than monthly	Monthly	Weekly	Daily or almost daily	
5. How often during the last year have you failed to do what was normally expected of you because of drinking?	Never	Less than monthly	Monthly	Weekly	Daily or almost daily	
6. How often during the last year have you needed a first drink in the morning to get yourself going after a heavy drinking session?	Never	Less than monthly	Monthly	Weekly	Daily or almost daily	
7. How often during the last year have you had a feeling of guilt or remorse after drinking?	Never	Less than monthly	Monthly	Weekly	Daily or almost daily	
8. How often during the last year have you been unable to remember what happened the night before because of your drinking?	Never	Less than monthly	Monthly	Weekly	Daily or almost daily	
9. Have you or someone else been injured because of your drinking?	No		Yes, but not in the last year		Yes, during the last year	
10. Has a relative, friend, doctor, or other healthcare worker been concerned about your drinking or suggested you cut down?	No		Yes, but not in the last year		Yes, during the last year	
Total Score						

Instructions to patient: Circle the option that best describes your answer to each question.
Scoring: Record the score (0, 1, 2, 3, or 4) for each response in the blank box at the end of each line, and then add up the total score. The maximum possible is 40. A total score of 8 or more for men up to age 60 (or 4 or more for women, adolescents, and men over 60) is considered a positive screen. For patients with totals near the cut-points, clinicians may wish to examine individual responses to questions and clarify them during the clinical examination.
Reprinted with permission from the World Health Organization. To reflect standard drink sizes in the United States, the number of drinks in question 3 was changed from 6 to 5.

alcohol withdrawal can result in cardiovascular collapse and death. Drugs used to ease withdrawal are discussed later in this chapter.

In 2008, the National Institute on Alcohol Abuse and Alcoholism (NIAAA) updated its document titled *Helping Patients Who Drink Too Much: A Clinician's Guide,* which contains clear, concise information on screening, counseling, and treatment of alcohol use disorders. By following this guide, clinicians can help reduce morbidity and mortality among people who drink more than is safe, defined as more than 4 drinks in a day (or 14/week) for men, or more than 3 drinks in a day (or 7/week) for women. Helping patients involves four simple steps:

- Ask about alcohol use.
- Assess for alcohol use disorders using the Alcohol Use Disorders Identification Test (AUDIT).
- Advise and assist (brief intervention).
- At follow-up: continue support.

This process is founded in part on two lines of evidence. First, we can identify people who misuse alcohol with an easily administered questionnaire, such as the AUDIT (Table 38.3).[a] Second, for many people, alcohol consumption can be reduced through brief interventions, such as offering feedback and advice about drinking and about setting goals. Long-term follow-up studies have shown that these simple interventions can decrease hospitalization and lower mortality rates. The guide is available at www.niaaa.nih.gov/guide.

[a]Rapid *screening* can be accomplished with a single question: How many times in the past year have you had *x* or more drinks in a day? ($x = 5$ for men and 4 for women). A positive response is defined as 1 or more. If this simple screen is positive, a more detailed diagnostic interview is indicated.

To help individuals who drink too much, the NIAAA created an interactive web site, located at rethinkingdrinking.niaaa.nih.gov. Content includes tools to identify and manage problem drinking, plus a calculator for determining the alcohol content of various beverages.

DRUGS FOR ALCOHOL USE DISORDER

In the United States, about 1 million people with AUD seek treatment every year. Although the success rate is discouraging—nearly 50% relapse during the first few months—treatment should nonetheless be tried. The objective is to modify drinking patterns (i.e., to reduce or completely eliminate alcohol consumption). Drugs can help in two ways. First, they can facilitate withdrawal. Second, they can help maintain abstinence once withdrawal has been accomplished.

Drugs Used to Facilitate Withdrawal

Management of withdrawal depends on the degree of dependence. When dependence is mild, withdrawal can be accomplished on an outpatient basis without drugs. However, when dependence is great, withdrawal carries a risk of death. Accordingly, hospitalization and drug therapy are indicated. The goals of management are to minimize symptoms of withdrawal, prevent seizures and delirium tremens, and facilitate transition to a program for maintaining abstinence. In theory, any drug that has cross-dependence with alcohol (i.e., any of the general CNS depressants) should be effective. However, in actual practice, benzodiazepines are the drugs of choice. The benefits of benzodiazepines and other drugs used during withdrawal are shown in Table 38.4.

Benzodiazepines

Of the drugs used to facilitate alcohol withdrawal, benzodiazepines are the most effective. Furthermore, they are safe. In patients with severe alcohol dependence, benzodiazepines can stabilize vital signs, reduce symptom intensity, and decrease the risk of seizures and delirium tremens. Although all benzodiazepines are effective, agents with longer half-lives are generally preferred because they provide the greatest protection against seizures and breakthrough symptoms. The benzodiazepines employed most often are chlordiazepoxide [Librium, others], clorazepate [Tranxene], oxazepam (generic only), and lorazepam [Ativan]. Traditionally, benzodiazepines have been administered around-the-clock on a fixed schedule. However, PRN administration (in response to symptoms) is just as effective and permits speedier withdrawal.

TABLE 38.4 ■ Drugs Used to Facilitate Alcohol Withdrawal

Drug	Benefit During Withdrawal
BENZODIAZEPINES	
Chlordiazepoxide Clorazepate Diazepam Lorazepam Oxazepam	Decrease withdrawal symptoms; stabilize vital signs; prevent seizures and delirium tremens
BETA-ADRENERGIC BLOCKERS	
Atenolol Propranolol	Improve vital signs; decrease craving; decrease autonomic component of withdrawal symptoms
CENTRAL ALPHA$_2$-ADRENERGIC AGONIST	
Clonidine	Decreases autonomic component of withdrawal symptoms
ANTIEPILEPTIC DRUG	
Carbamazepine	Decreases withdrawal symptoms; prevents seizures

Adjuncts to Benzodiazepines

Combining a benzodiazepine with another drug may improve withdrawal outcome. Agents that have been tried include carbamazepine (an antiepileptic drug), clonidine (an alpha$_2$-adrenergic agonist), and atenolol and propranolol (beta-adrenergic blockers). Carbamazepine may reduce withdrawal symptoms and the risk of seizures. Clonidine and the beta blockers reduce the autonomic component of withdrawal symptoms. In addition, the beta blockers may improve vital signs and decrease craving. It should be stressed, however, that these drugs are not very effective as monotherapy. Hence, they should be viewed only as adjuncts to benzodiazepines—not as substitutes.

Drugs Used to Maintain Abstinence

Once detoxification has been accomplished, the goal is to prevent—or at least minimize—future drinking. The ideal goal is complete abstinence. However, if drinking must resume, keeping it to a minimum is still beneficial, since doing so will reduce alcohol-related morbidity.

In trials of drugs used to maintain abstinence, several parameters are used to measure efficacy. These include:

- Proportion of patients who maintain complete abstinence
- Days to relapse
- Number of drinking days
- Number of drinks per drinking day

In the United States, only three drugs—disulfiram, naltrexone, and acamprosate—are approved for maintaining abstinence. Disulfiram works by causing an unpleasant reaction if alcohol is consumed. Naltrexone blocks the pleasurable effects of alcohol and decreases craving. Acamprosate reduces some of the unpleasant feelings (e.g., tension, dysphoria, anxiety) brought on by alcohol abstinence. Of the three drugs, naltrexone appears most effective. However, even with this agent, benefits are modest.

Owing to the risk of relapse, prolonged treatment is needed. The minimum duration is 3 months. However, continuing for a year or more is not unreasonable. If the first drug fails, clinicians often try a different one.

Disulfiram Aversion Therapy

Therapeutic Effects. Disulfiram [Antabuse] helps individuals with AUD avoid drinking by causing unpleasant effects if alcohol is ingested. Disulfiram has no applications outside the treatment of AUD.

Although disulfiram has been employed for decades, its efficacy is only moderate. In clinical trials, there is emerging evidence that the drug may be only slightly better than placebo at maintaining long-term abstinence; however, long-term studies have not been completed. Disulfiram does decrease the frequency of drinking after relapse has occurred—presumably because of the unpleasant reaction that the patient is now familiar with. Supervised administration of disulfiram may be more effective than when patients self-administer the drug.

Mechanism of Action. Disulfiram disrupts alcohol metabolism by causing *irreversible inhibition of aldehyde dehydrogenase,* the enzyme that converts acetaldehyde to acetic acid. As a result, if alcohol is ingested, *acetaldehyde* will accumulate to toxic levels, producing unpleasant and potentially harmful effects.

Pharmacologic Effects. The constellation of effects caused by alcohol plus disulfiram is referred to as *acetaldehyde syndrome,* a potentially dangerous event. In its "mild" form, the syndrome manifests as nausea, copious vomiting, flushing, palpitations, headache, sweating, thirst, chest pain, weakness, blurred vision, and hypotension; blood pressure may ultimately decline to shock levels. This reaction, which may last from 30 minutes to several hours, can be brought on by consuming as little as 7 mL of alcohol.

In its most severe manifestation, the acetaldehyde syndrome is life threatening. Possible reactions include marked respiratory depression, cardiovascular collapse, cardiac dysrhythmias, MI, acute congestive heart failure, convulsions, and death. Clearly, the acetaldehyde syndrome is not simply unpleasant; this syndrome can be extremely hazardous and must be avoided.

In the absence of alcohol, disulfiram rarely causes significant effects. Drowsiness and skin eruptions may occur during initial use, but they diminish with time.

Patient Selection. Owing to the severity of the acetaldehyde syndrome, candidates must be carefully chosen. People with AUD who lack the determination to stop drinking should not receive disulfiram. In other words, disulfiram must not be administered to individuals who are likely to attempt drinking while undergoing treatment.

Patient Education. Patient education is an extremely important component of therapy. Patients must be thoroughly informed about the potential hazards of treatment. Patients should be made aware that the effects of disulfiram will persist about 2 weeks after the last dose, and hence continued abstinence is necessary. Individuals using disulfiram should be encouraged to carry identification indicating their status.

Safety Alert

DISULFIRAM

Patients must be made aware that consuming any alcohol while taking disulfiram may produce a severe, potentially fatal, reaction. Patients must be warned to avoid all forms of alcohol, including alcohol found in sauces and cough syrups, and alcohol applied to the skin in aftershave lotions, colognes, and liniments.

Preparations, Dosage, and Administration. Disulfiram [Antabuse] is supplied in 250- and 500-mg tablets. At least 12 hours must elapse between the patient's last drink and starting treatment. The initial dosage is 500 mg once daily for 1 to 2 weeks. Maintenance dosages range from 125 to 500 mg/day, usually taken as a single dose in the morning. Therapy may last months or even years.

Naltrexone

Naltrexone [ReVia, Vivitrol] is a pure opioid antagonist that decreases craving for alcohol and blocks alcohol's reinforcing (pleasurable) effects. Patients with AUD report that naltrexone decreases their "high." Although the mechanism underlying these effects is uncertain, one possibility is blockade of dopamine release secondary to blockade of opioid receptors. Naltrexone is generally well tolerated. Nausea is the most common adverse effect, followed by headache, anxiety, and sedation. Because naltrexone is an opioid antagonist, the drug will precipitate withdrawal if given to a patient who is opioid dependent. Conversely, if a patient taking naltrexone needs emergency treatment with an opioid analgesic, high doses of the opioid will be required.

Naltrexone was approved for AUD on the basis of randomized clinical trials that combined extensive counseling along with the drug. In these trials, naltrexone cut the relapse rate by 50%. Compared with patients taking placebo, those taking naltrexone reported less craving for alcohol, fewer days drinking, fewer drinks per occasion, and reduced severity of alcohol-related problems. In contrast to the original trials, a more recent trial, conducted by the U.S. Department of Veterans Affairs, failed to show any benefit of naltrexone in maintaining abstinence. Why did naltrexone work in the original trials but not in the more recent one? The most likely reason is that the subjects in the two trials were very different: The veterans with AUD suffered from chronic AUD, had little or no social support, and received minimal counseling during the trial, whereas subjects in the earlier studies were younger, had good support systems, and received extensive counseling along with naltrexone. Hence, the new study does not prove that naltrexone doesn't work. Rather, it proves only that naltrexone doesn't work for all individuals and that it doesn't work in the absence of adequate counseling.

Naltrexone is available in two formulations: 50-mg tablets [ReVia] for oral use and a 380-mg depot formulation [Vivitrol] for IM injection. The oral dosage is 50 mg once a day. The IM dosage is 380 mg once a month. Depot naltrexone is especially good when patient adherence is a concern. As with disulfiram, patients must stop drinking before starting naltrexone.

The basic pharmacology of naltrexone is discussed in Chapter 28.

Acamprosate

Therapeutic Use. Acamprosate is approved for maintaining abstinence in patients with alcohol dependence following detoxification. Benefits derive from reducing unpleasant feelings (e.g., tension, dysphoria, anxiety) brought on by abstinence. This effect contrasts with the effects of disulfiram (which makes drinking unpleasant) and naltrexone (which blocks the pleasant feelings that alcohol can cause). Acamprosate should be used only as part of a comprehensive management program that includes psychosocial support.

In clinical trials, acamprosate was moderately effective. Compared with patients taking placebo, those taking acamprosate abstained from their first drink longer, had greater rates of complete abstinence, and were abstinent for more total days. Benefits may be related to the degree of alcohol dependence: The greater the dependence, the more likely that acamprosate will help. Among patients who lack psychosocial support, little or no benefit is seen.

Mechanism of Action. Just how acamprosate works is unknown. One theory suggests that acamprosate enhances inhibitory neurotransmission (mediated by GABA) and suppresses excitatory neurotransmission (mediated by glutamate), and thereby restores a balance between these transmitter systems. When given to alcohol-dependent animals, the drug reduces voluntary alcohol intake. Acamprosate is devoid of direct anxiolytic, anticonvulsant, and antidepressant activity, and does not cause alcohol aversion.

Pharmacokinetics. Acamprosate is administered orally, and bioavailability is low (11%). Food reduces absorption even further. The drug has a long half-life (20 to 33 hours), and hence about 5 days are required for plasma levels to reach a plateau. Acamprosate does not undergo metabolism, and is excreted unchanged in the urine.

Adverse Effects and Drug Interactions. Acamprosate is generally well tolerated. With most adverse effects, the incidence is no greater than with placebo. The principal exception is diarrhea, which occurs in 17% of acamprosate users compared with 10% of those taking placebo. Reports of suicide-related events (suicidal ideation, suicide attempts, completed suicide) are rare, but more common than with placebo. Acamprosate can cause fetal malformations in animals (at doses close to those used by humans). Accordingly, it would seem prudent to avoid this drug during pregnancy, especially since alternatives are available. Acamprosate has no potential for dependence or abuse, and appears devoid of significant drug interactions.

Preparations, Dosage, and Administration. Acamprosate is available in 333-mg delayed-release tablets. The recommended dosage is 2 tablets (666 mg) 3 times a day, taken with meals. (The reason for administration with meals is to promote compliance—not to influence absorption or GI effects.) Dosing should start immediately after detoxification is over and should continue even if relapse occurs. For patients with *mild* renal impairment, the recommended initial dosage is 333 mg 3 times a day. If the patient has *severe* renal impairment, acamprosate should not be used.

Nutritional Support, Fluid Replacement, and Antibiotics

Malnutrition is a common problem in the patient with chronic AUD. The underlying causes are poor diet and malabsorption of nutrients and vitamins. Malabsorption results from alcohol-induced damage to the GI mucosa. Poor diet occurs in part because individuals with AUD meet up to 50% of their caloric needs with alcohol and therefore consume suboptimal amounts of foods with high nutritional value. Because of their poor nutritional state, these patients are in need of fat, protein, and vitamins. The B vitamins (thiamine, folic acid, cyanocobalamin) are especially needed. To correct nutritional deficiencies, a program of dietary modification and vitamin supplements should be implemented.

Individuals with AUD frequently require fluid replacement therapy. Fluids are needed to replace fluids lost because of gastritis or because of vomiting associated with withdrawal.

KEY POINTS

- Alcohol is generally beneficial when consumed in moderation and always detrimental when consumed in excess.
- Alcohol causes CNS depression by enhancing the depressant effects of GABA and reducing the excitatory effects of glutamate.
- As blood levels of alcohol rise, CNS depression progresses from cortical areas to more primitive brain areas (e.g., medulla).
- Long-term, excessive drinking reduces the size of the cerebrum.
- Alcohol produces a dose-dependent increase in blood pressure.
- Moderate drinking is defined as 2 drinks per day or less for men and 1 drink per day or less for women.
- Moderate drinking significantly reduces the risk of CAD, MI, ischemic stroke, and heart failure—primarily by raising HDL cholesterol and partly by suppressing platelet aggregation, reducing fibrin formation, enhancing fibrinolysis, and suppressing the inflammatory component of atherosclerosis.
- Excessive drinking causes direct damage to the myocardium.
- Like all other CNS depressants, alcohol depresses respiration.
- Chronic, heavy drinking can cause hepatitis and cirrhosis. People with liver disease should avoid alcohol.
- Heavy drinking can cause erosive gastritis.
- Alcohol is a diuretic.
- Alcohol, even in low doses, increases the risk of breast cancer, as well as cancers of the liver, rectum, and aerodigestive tract.
- Excessive drinkers die younger than the population at large.
- Because of the cardioprotective effects of alcohol, moderate drinkers live longer than those who abstain.
- Alcohol dehydrogenase is the rate-limiting enzyme in alcohol metabolism.
- Alcohol is metabolized at a constant rate, regardless of how high blood levels rise. In contrast, the rate of metabolism of most drugs increases as their blood levels rise.
- Most people can metabolize about 1 drink per hour—be it beer, wine, straight whiskey, or a cocktail. Consuming more than 1 drink per hour causes alcohol to accumulate.
- Chronic drinking produces tolerance to many of alcohol's effects—but not to respiratory depression.
- Tolerance to alcohol confers cross-tolerance to general anesthetics, barbiturates, and other general CNS depressants—but not to opioids.
- The CNS-depressant effects of alcohol are additive with those of other CNS depressants.
- The combined effects of alcohol and NSAIDs can cause significant gastric bleeding. People with peptic ulcer disease should avoid alcohol.
- The combination of alcohol and acetaminophen can cause fatal hepatic failure.
- Alcohol use during pregnancy can result in FASD (including FAS), stillbirth, and spontaneous abortion. Women who are pregnant or trying to conceive should not drink.
- Benzodiazepines (e.g., chlordiazepoxide, diazepam, lorazepam) are drugs of choice for facilitating withdrawal in alcohol-dependent individuals. Benzodiazepines suppress symptoms because of cross-dependence with alcohol.

Continued

- Three drugs are approved for maintaining alcohol abstinence: disulfiram, naltrexone, and acamprosate.
- Disulfiram blocks aldehyde dehydrogenase. As a result, if alcohol is consumed, acetaldehyde will accumulate, thereby causing a host of unpleasant and potentially dangerous symptoms.
- Naltrexone blocks opioid receptors and thereby decreases craving for alcohol and blocks alcohol's reinforcing effects.
- Acamprosate decreases tension, anxiety, and other unpleasant feelings caused by the absence of alcohol. The underlying mechanism is unclear.

Please visit **http://evolve.elsevier.com/Lehne** for chapter-specific NCLEX® examination review questions.

Summary of Major Nursing Implications[a]

DISULFIRAM

Preadministration Assessment

Therapeutic Goal

Maintaining alcohol abstinence.

Patient Selection

Candidates for therapy must be chosen carefully. Disulfiram must not be given to patients who are likely to attempt drinking while taking this drug.

Identifying High-Risk Patients

Disulfiram is *contraindicated* for patients suspected of being incapable of abstinence from alcohol; for patients with myocardial disease, coronary occlusion, or psychosis; and for patients who have recently received alcohol, metronidazole, or alcohol-containing medications (e.g., cough syrups, tonics).

Implementation: Administration

Route

Oral.

Administration

Instruct the patient not to administer the first dose until at least 12 hours after his or her last drink.

Dosing is done once daily and may continue for months or even years.

Inform patients that tablets may be crushed or mixed with liquid.

Implementation: Measures to Enhance Therapeutic Effects

Patient education is essential for safety. **Inform patients about the potential hazards of treatment, and warn them to avoid all forms of alcohol, including alcohol in vinegar, sauces, and cough syrups, and alcohol applied to the skin in aftershave lotions, colognes, and liniments. Inform patients that the effects of disulfiram will persist about 2 weeks after the last dose and that alcohol must not be consumed during this time. Encourage patients to carry identification to alert emergency healthcare personnel to their condition.**

[a]Patient education information is highlighted as **blue text.**

CHAPTER

39 Substance Use Disorders III: Nicotine and Smoking

Cigarette smoking remains the greatest single cause of preventable illness and premature death. In the United States, smoking kills more than 480,000 adults each year—about 1 of every 5 deaths. Around the world, tobacco kills more than 6 million people each year. On average, male smokers die 13.2 years prematurely, and female smokers die 14.5 years prematurely. According to the Centers for Disease Control and Prevention, most deaths result from lung cancer (127,700), coronary heart disease (99,300), and chronic airway obstruction (100,600). Not only do cigarettes kill people who smoke, but every year, through secondhand smoke, cigarettes kill about 41,000 nonsmoking Americans, and about 600,000 nonsmokers worldwide. The direct medical costs of smoking exceed $170 billion a year. Indirect costs, including lost time from work and disability, add up to an additional $156 billion. In the United States, the prevalence of smoking among adults fell steadily from 1965 (42%) through the 1980s and 1990s, but decreased only slightly between 2004 (20.9%) and 2015 (15.1%).

Although tobacco smoke contains many dangerous compounds, nicotine is of greatest concern. Other hazardous components in tobacco smoke include carbon monoxide, hydrogen cyanide, ammonia, nitrosamines, and tar. Tar is composed of various polycyclic hydrocarbons, some of which are proven carcinogens.

What is the regulatory status of cigarettes? Good question, given that cigarettes are the single most dangerous product available to U.S. consumers. Until recently, cigarettes had avoided virtually all federal regulation. However, strong regulations are now in place. Under the *Family Smoking Prevention and Tobacco Control Act*, the U.S. Food and Drug Administration (FDA) now has the authority to:

- Strengthen advertising restrictions, including the prohibition on marketing to youth.
- Require revised and more prominent warning labels.
- Require disclosure of all ingredients in tobacco products and restrict harmful additives.
- Monitor nicotine yields, and mandate gradual nicotine reduction to nonaddictive levels.

BASIC PHARMACOLOGY OF NICOTINE

Mechanism of Action

The effects of nicotine result from actions at nicotinic receptors. Whether these receptors are activated or inhibited depends on nicotine dosage. *Low* doses *activate* nicotinic receptors; *high* doses *block* them. The amount of nicotine received from cigarettes is relatively low. Accordingly, cigarette smoking causes receptor *activation.*

Nicotine can activate nicotinic receptors at several locations. Most effects result from activating nicotinic receptors in autonomic ganglia and the adrenal medulla. In addition, nicotine can activate nicotinic receptors in the carotid body, aortic arch, and central nervous system (CNS). As discussed later, actions in the CNS mimic those of cocaine and other highly addictive substances. When present at the levels produced by smoking, nicotine has no significant effect on nicotinic receptors of the neuromuscular junction.

Pharmacokinetics

Absorption of nicotine depends on whether the delivery system is a cigarette or e-cigarette, a cigar, or smokeless tobacco. Nicotine in cigarette smoke is absorbed primarily from the lungs. When cigarette smoke is inhaled, between 90% and 98% of nicotine in the lungs enters the blood. Unlike nicotine in cigarette smoke, nicotine in cigar smoke is absorbed primarily from the mouth, as is nicotine in smokeless tobacco.

Nicotine can cross membranes easily and is widely distributed throughout the body. The drug readily enters breast milk, reaching levels that can be toxic to the nursing infant. Nicotine also crosses the placental barrier and can cause fetal harm. When inhaled in cigarette smoke, nicotine reaches the brain in just 10 seconds.

Nicotine is rapidly metabolized to inactive products. Nicotine and its metabolites are excreted by the kidney. The drug's half-life is 1 to 2 hours.

Pharmacologic Effects

The pharmacologic effects discussed in this section are associated with *low* doses of nicotine. These are the effects caused by smoking cigarettes. Responses to *high* doses are discussed under *Acute Poisoning*.

Cardiovascular Effects

The cardiovascular effects of nicotine result primarily from activating nicotinic receptors in *sympathetic ganglia* and the *adrenal medulla*. Activation of these receptors promotes the release of norepinephrine from sympathetic nerves and the release of epinephrine (and some norepinephrine) from the adrenals. Norepinephrine and epinephrine act on the cardiovascular system to constrict blood vessels, accelerate the heart, and increase the force of ventricular contraction. The net result is elevation of blood pressure and increased cardiac work. These effects underlie cardiovascular deaths.

GI Effects

Nicotine influences GI function primarily by activating nicotinic receptors in *parasympathetic* ganglia, thereby increasing secretion of gastric acid and augmenting tone and motility of GI smooth muscle. In addition, nicotine can promote vomiting. Nicotine-induced vomiting results from a complex process that involves nicotinic receptors in the aortic arch, carotid sinus, and CNS.

CNS Effects

Nicotine is a CNS stimulant. The drug stimulates respiration and produces an arousal pattern on an electroencephalograph. Moderate doses can cause tremors, and high doses can cause convulsions.

Nicotine has multiple psychologic effects. The drug increases alertness, facilitates memory, improves cognition, reduces aggression, and suppresses appetite. In addition, by promoting the release of dopamine, nicotine activates the brain's "pleasure system" located in the mesolimbic area. The effects of nicotine on the pleasure system are identical to those of other highly addictive drugs, including cocaine, amphetamines, and opioids.

Effects During Pregnancy and Lactation

Nicotine exposure during gestation can harm the fetus, and nicotine in breast milk can harm the nursing infant. Nonetheless, as discussed in Box 39.1, since pharmaceutical nicotine is safer than tobacco smoke, it is reasonable to consider using nicotine therapy during pregnancy to help a patient quit smoking.

Tolerance and Dependence

Tolerance

Tolerance develops to some effects of nicotine but not to others. Tolerance does develop to nausea and dizziness, which are common in the unseasoned smoker. In contrast, *very little tolerance develops to the cardiovascular effects:* Veteran smokers continue to experience increased blood pressure and increased cardiac work whenever they smoke.

Dependence

Chronic cigarette smoking results in dependence. By definition, this means that individuals who discontinue smoking will experience an abstinence syndrome. Prominent symptoms are craving, nervousness, restlessness, irritability, impatience, increased hostility, insomnia, impaired concentration, increased appetite, and weight gain. Symptoms begin about 24 hours after smoking has ceased and can last for weeks to months. Women report more discomfort than men. Experience has shown that abrupt discontinuation may be preferable to gradual reduction. (All that gradual reduction seems to do is prolong the suffering.)

Acute Poisoning

Nicotine is highly toxic. Doses as low as 40 mg can be fatal. Toxicity is underscored by the use of nicotine as an insecticide. Common causes of nicotine poisoning include ingestion of tobacco by children and exposure to nicotine-containing insecticides.

Symptoms

The most prominent symptoms involve the cardiovascular, GI, and central nervous systems. Specific symptoms include nausea, salivation, vomiting, diarrhea, cold sweats, disturbed hearing and vision, confusion, and faintness; pulses may be rapid, weak, and irregular. Death results from respiratory paralysis, which is caused by direct effects of nicotine on the muscles of respiration, as well as by effects in the CNS.

Treatment

Management centers on reducing nicotine absorption and supporting respiration; there is no specific antidote to nicotine poisoning. Absorption of ingested nicotine can be reduced by giving activated charcoal. If respiration is depressed, ventilatory assistance is indicated. Since nicotine undergoes rapid metabolic inactivation, recovery from the acute phase of poisoning can occur within hours.

Chronic Toxicity From Smoking

According to a 2004 report from the U.S. Surgeon General, the adverse consequences of smoking are more extensive than previously understood. It is now clear that chronic smoking can injure nearly every organ of the body. We already knew that smoking could cause cardiovascular disease, chronic lung disease, and cancers of the larynx, lung, esophagus, oral cavity, and bladder. New additions to the list include leukemia, cataracts, pneumonia, periodontal disease, type 2 diabetes, abdominal aortic aneurysm, and cancers of the cervix, kidney, pancreas, and stomach. Smoking during pregnancy increases the risk of low birth weight, preterm labor, stillbirth, miscarriage, spontaneous abortion, perinatal mortality, and sudden infant death. The leading causes of smoking-related death are lung cancer, ischemic heart disease, and chronic airway obstruction.

Prototype Drugs

DRUGS TO AID SMOKING CESSATION

Nicotine-Based Products

Nicotine patch [Nicoderm CQ]
Nicotine gum [Nicorette]
Nicotine lozenge [Nicorette Lozenge]
Nicotine nasal spray [Nicotrol NS]
Nicotine inhaler [Nicotrol Inhaler]

Nicotine-Free Products

Varenicline
Bupropion

BOX 39.1 ■ SPECIAL INTEREST TOPIC

SMOKING CESSATION DURING PREGNANCY

Smoking is the largest modifiable risk factor for pregnancy-related morbidity and mortality. Smoking increases the risk of ectopic pregnancy, placenta previa, placental abruption, chorioamnionitis, stillbirth, preterm birth, and spontaneous abortion. In addition, fetal exposure increases the risk of low birth weight, perinatal mortality, sudden infant death syndrome (SIDS), and cognitive, behavioral, and emotional deficits in childhood.

Of the many harmful chemicals in tobacco smoke, reproductive toxicity is due in large part to just three: *nicotine, carbon monoxide,* and *oxidizing agents.* Nicotine reduces placental blood flow (by promoting vasoconstriction), delays or impairs fetal brain development (by direct neurotoxic effects), inhibits maturation of fetal pulmonary cells, and increases the risk of SIDS. Carbon monoxide reduces the oxygen-carrying capacity of blood and, in high levels, is neuroteratogenic. Oxidizing agents increase the risk of thrombotic events, and by decreasing the availability of nitrous oxide (a smooth muscle relaxant), they contribute to placental vasoconstriction and preterm labor.

Clearly, smoking during pregnancy is dangerous. Ideally, female smokers should quit before conception or early in pregnancy. However, quitting later is still beneficial. To aid in smoking cessation, the authors of *Treating Tobacco Use and Dependence: 2008 Update* recommend that clinicians offer effective interventions at the first prenatal visit and throughout the course of pregnancy as needed. Intensive person-to-person psychosocial intervention should be offered to all pregnant smokers. Pharmacologic intervention—mainly *nicotine replacement therapy* (NRT)—may also be offered, but only if psychosocial intervention alone has failed. Of note, quit rates with a combination of psychosocial intervention plus NRT are higher than with psychosocial intervention alone.

What do we know about NRT during pregnancy? Not as much as we would like. Studies on the efficacy of NRT in pregnant smokers have been inconclusive—probably because the nicotine dosage was too low. (During the later stages of pregnancy, nicotine is metabolized at a high rate. Hence, if conventional NRT doses are used, nicotine blood levels may be too low to be effective.) Nonetheless, even if we are uncertain about NRT *efficacy,* it seems likely that NRT is much *safer* than smoking. After all, cigarette smoke contains thousands of harmful chemicals (in addition to nicotine), whereas NRT contains nicotine only. In fact, among pregnant patients who switched from smoking to NRT, there was no evidence of serious adverse effects, and there was an important benefit: birth weight was increased.

Who should use NRT? According to a 2009 review,[a] the use of NRT should be based on the number of cigarettes smoked. Pregnant patients who smoke no more than five cigarettes a day should be offered psychosocial support, but not NRT. Conversely, pregnant patients who smoke more should be offered NRT along with psychosocial support.

What about bupropion and varenicline? Compared with NRT, bupropion lacks the potential adverse effects of nicotine; however, its side effect of appetite suppression is not desirable for the pregnant patient and developing fetus. One prominent voice—the American College of Obstetricians and Gynecologists (ACOG)—says that bupropion may be considered when behavioral interventions have failed. However, another prominent voice—the Motherisk Program—says that bupropion should be avoided until we know more about its safety and efficacy. As for varenicline, we have no human data on safety in pregnancy, but we do have animal data showing fetal harm. Accordingly, varenicline should not be used.

[a]Osadchy A, Kazmin A, Koren G: Nicotine replacement therapy during pregnancy: recommended or not recommended? J Obstet Gynaecol Can 31:744–747, 2009.

PHARMACOLOGIC AIDS TO SMOKING CESSATION

Cigarettes are highly addictive, which makes giving them up very hard. Nonetheless, abstinence *can* be achieved. Every year, about 41% of Americans who smoke make one or more attempts to quit. Of those who try to quit without formal help, only 4% to 7% achieve long-term success. In contrast, when a combination of counseling and drugs is employed, the 6-month abstinence rate approaches 25%. However, even with the aid of counseling and drugs, the first attempt usually fails. In fact, most people try to quit 5 to 7 times before they ultimately succeed. As time without a cigarette increases, the chances of relapse get progressively smaller: Of those who quit for a year, only 15% smoke again; and of those who quit for 5 years, only 3% smoke again.

Long-term smokers should be assured that quitting offers important health benefits. Regardless of how long you have smoked, quitting can reduce the risk of developing a tobacco-related disease, slow the progression of an established tobacco-related disease, and increase life expectancy. These benefits apply not only to people who quit while they are young and healthy, but also to people who quit after age 65 years and to those with established tobacco-related disease. Data from the Nurses' Health Study indicate that former smokers eventually achieve the same disease-risk status as never smokers, even with respect to lung cancer. The risk of chronic obstructive pulmonary disease or death from a heart attack declines to that of never smokers in 20 years, and the risk of lung cancer reaches that of never smokers in 30 years.

Seven drug products have been shown to aid smoking cessation (Table 39.1). Of these seven products, five contain nicotine and two don't. The nicotine-based products—nicotine gum, nicotine lozenge, nicotine patch, nicotine inhaler, and nicotine nasal spray—are employed as nicotine replacement therapy (NRT). The nicotine-free products—sustained-release bupropion (bupropion SR) [Zyban, Buproban] and varenicline [Chantix, Champix ♣]—are taken to decrease nicotine craving and to suppress symptoms of withdrawal. The most effective drug therapies for smoking cessation are varenicline alone and the nicotine patch combined with a short-acting nicotine product (i.e., nasal spray or gum). At this time, we cannot predict who

TABLE 39.1 ■ Pharmacologic Aids for Smoking Cessation

Product	Common Side Effects	Advantages	Disadvantages
NICOTINE-BASED PRODUCTS			
Nicotine patch [Nicorette Invisipatch ♣, NicoDerm CQ]	Transient itching, burning, and redness under the patch; insomnia	Nonprescription; provides a steady level of nicotine; easy to use; unobtrusive	User cannot adjust dose if craving occurs; nicotine released more slowly than in other products
Nicotine gum [Nicorette, others]	Mouth and throat irritation, aching jaw muscles, dyspepsia	Nonprescription; user controls dose	Unpleasant taste; requires proper chewing technique; cannot eat or drink while chewing the gum; can damage dental work and is difficult for denture wearers to use
Nicotine lozenge [Nicorette Lozenge]	Hiccups, dyspepsia, mouth irritation, nausea	Nonprescription; user controls dose; easier to use than nicotine gum	Cannot eat or drink while the lozenge is in the mouth
Nicotine nasal spray [Nicotrol NS]	During first week: mouth and throat irritation, rhinitis, sneezing, coughing, teary eyes	User controls dose; fastest nicotine delivery and highest nicotine levels of all nicotine-based products	Prescription required; most irritating nicotine-based product; device visible when used
Nicotine inhaler [Nicotrol Inhaler]	Mouth and throat irritation, cough	User controls dose; mimics hand-to-mouth motion of smoking	Prescription required; slow onset and low nicotine levels; frequent puffing needed; device visible when used
NICOTINE-FREE PRODUCTS			
Varenicline [Chantix, Champix ♣]	Nausea, sleep disturbances, headaches, abnormal dreams	Easy to use (pill); no nicotine; most effective pharmacologic aid to smoking cessation	Prescription required; may cause neuropsychiatric disturbances, including suicidal thoughts and actions
Bupropion [Zyban, Buproban]	Insomnia, dry mouth, agitation	Easy to use (pill); no nicotine; promotes weight loss, which may limit cessation-related weight gain; first-choice drug for smokers with depression	Prescription required; carries a small risk of seizures

will respond best to a particular product. Accordingly, selection should be based on patient preference, success with a particular product in the past, and side effects.

Interventions for smoking cessation can be found in *Treating Tobacco Use and Dependence: 2008 Update,* a clinical practice guideline issued by the U.S. Public Health Service. As stated in the guideline, tobacco dependence is a chronic condition that warrants repeated intervention until long-term abstinence is achieved. This is the same philosophy that guides the treatment of dependence on other highly addictive substances, including cocaine and heroin. Tobacco dependence can be treated with two methods: drugs and counseling. Both methods are effective, but a combination of both is more effective than either one alone. Accordingly, the guidelines recommend that all patients who want to quit be offered (1) at least one smoking cessation drug (bupropion, varenicline, or a nicotine-based product) along with (2) counseling, be it one-on-one, in a group, or over the phone (dial 1-800-QUITNOW in the United States or 1-877-513-5333 in Canada). The overall intervention strategy is summarized in the "5 A's" model for treating tobacco use and dependence:

Ask (screen all patients for tobacco use).
Advise tobacco users to quit.
Assess willingness to make a quit attempt.
Assist with quitting (offer medication and provide or refer to counseling).
Arrange follow-up contacts, beginning within the first week after the quit date.

TABLE 39.2 ■ Internet-Based Resources for Smoking Cessation

UNITED STATES

- U.S. Department of Health and Human Services: https://www.surgeongeneral.gov/library/reports/index.html
- Centers for Disease Control and Prevention: http://www.cdc.gov/tobacco/quit_smoking/
- American Lung Association: http://www.lungusa.org/stop-smoking/

CANADA

- Health Canada: https://www.canada.ca/en/health-canada/services/health-concerns/tobacco.html
- The Lung Association: https://www.lung.ca/lung-health/smoking-and-tobacco/how-quit-smoking

For additional information on smoking cessation, visit the Internet sites for Canada and the United States listed in Table 39.2.

Nicotine Replacement Therapy

NRT allows smokers to substitute a pharmaceutical source of nicotine for the nicotine in cigarettes—and then gradually to withdraw the replacement nicotine. This is analogous to using methadone to wean addicts from heroin.

Five FDA-approved formulations are available: chewing gum, lozenges, transdermal patches, a nasal spray, and an

TABLE 39.3 ■ Nicotine Transdermal Systems (Patches)

Brand Name	Surface Area (cm^2)	Hours/Day in Place	Dose Absorbed	Duration of Use: Per Patch Size	Duration of Use: Total
Nicoderm CQ Step 1	30	24	21 mg over 24 hr	First 4–6 wk	8–10 wk
Nicoderm CQ Step 2	20	24	14 mg over 24 hr	Next 2 wk	
Nicoderm CQ Step 3	10	24	7 mg over 24 hr	Next 2 wk	
Nicorette Invisipatch Step 1 🍁	22.5	16	25 mg over 16 hr	First 8 wk	12 wk
Nicorette Invisipatch Step 2 🍁	13.5	16	15 mg over 16 hr	Next 2 wk	
Nicorette Invisipatch Step 3 🍁	9	16	10 mg over 16 hr	Next 2 wk	

inhaler (see Table 39.1). With the gum, lozenges, patches, and inhaler, blood levels of nicotine rise slowly and remain relatively steady. Because nicotine levels rise slowly, these delivery systems produce less pleasure than cigarettes, but nonetheless do relieve symptoms of withdrawal. With the nasal spray, blood levels of nicotine rise rapidly, much as they do with smoking. Hence the nasal spray provides some of the subjective pleasure that smoking does.

Long-term quit rates are significantly greater with NRT than with placebo—although absolute success rates remain low. For example, the 1-year success with nicotine patches is about 25%, compared with 9% for placebo. Success rates are highest when replacement therapy is combined with counseling.

Nicotine products are classified in FDA Pregnancy Risk Category C[a] (chewing gum, lozenge) or Category D (patch, inhaler, nasal spray). Accordingly, they should generally be avoided during pregnancy. However, since smoking is probably more harmful than NRT, use of NRT during pregnancy is worth consideration (see Box 39.1).

Nicotine Chewing Gum (Nicotine Polacrilex)

Nicotine chewing gum [Nicorette, others] is composed of a gum base plus nicotine polacrilex, an ion exchange resin to which nicotine is bound. The gum must be chewed to release the nicotine. Following release, nicotine is absorbed across the oral mucosa into the systemic circulation. Like other forms of NRT, nicotine gum doubles the cessation success rate.

The most common adverse effects are mouth and throat soreness, jaw muscle ache, eructation (belching), and hiccups. Using optimal chewing technique minimizes these problems.

Patients should be advised to chew the gum slowly and intermittently for about 30 minutes. Rapid chewing can release too much nicotine at one time, resulting in effects similar to those of excessive smoking (e.g., nausea, throat irritation, hiccups). Because foods and beverages can reduce nicotine absorption, patients should not eat or drink while chewing or for 15 minutes before chewing.

Nicotine gum is available in two strengths: 2 mg/piece and 4 mg/piece. Dosing is individualized and based on the degree of nicotine dependence. For initial therapy, patients with low to moderate nicotine dependence (those who smoke their first cigarette after 30 minutes of waking) should use the 2-mg strength; highly dependent patients (those who smoke their first cigarette within 30 minutes of waking) should use the 4-mg strength. The average adult dosage is 9 to 12 pieces a day. The maximum daily dosage is 24 pieces. Experience indicates that dosing on a fixed schedule (one piece every 2 to 3 hours) is more effective than PRN dosing for achieving abstinence.

After 3 months without cigarettes, patients should discontinue nicotine use. Withdrawal should be done gradually. Use of nicotine gum beyond 6 months is not recommended.

Nicotine Lozenges (Nicotine Polacrilex)

The pharmacology of nicotine lozenges [Nicorette Lozenge] is very similar to that of nicotine gum. Both products contain nicotine bound to polacrilex. Sucking on the lozenge releases nicotine, which is then absorbed across the oral mucosa into the systemic circulation. Like nicotine gum and other forms of NRT, nicotine lozenges double the cessation success rate.

The most common adverse effects are mouth irritation, dyspepsia, nausea, and hiccups—all of which can be made worse by taking two lozenges at once or by taking several lozenges in immediate succession.

Administration consists of placing the lozenge in the mouth and allowing it to dissolve, which takes 20 to 30 minutes. Users should not eat or drink for 15 minutes before dosing and while the lozenge is in the mouth. Also, they should not chew or swallow the lozenge.

Like nicotine gum, nicotine lozenges are available in two strengths: 2 mg and 4 mg. Dosing with the lozenges is the same as with the gum. Users should consume no more than 5 lozenges every 6 hours and no more than 20 lozenges per day. The recommended dosing schedule is 1 lozenge every 1 to 2 hours for the first 6 weeks; 1 every 2 to 4 hours for the next 3 weeks; and 1 every 4 to 8 hours for the next 3 weeks, after which dosing should stop.

Nicotine Transdermal Systems (Patches)

Nicotine transdermal systems are nicotine-containing adhesive patches that, after application to the skin, slowly release their nicotine content. The nicotine is absorbed into the skin and then into the blood, producing steady blood levels. Use of the patch about doubles the cessation success rate.

Two systems are available: NicoDerm CQ and Nicorette Invisipatch 🍁. Both can be purchased without a prescription. As indicated in Table 39.3, the patches come in different sizes. The larger patches release more nicotine.

Nicotine patches are applied once a day to clean, dry, nonhairy skin of the upper body or upper arm. The site should be changed daily and not reused for at least 1 week. NicoDerm

[a]As of 2020, the FDA will no longer use Pregnancy Risk Categories. Please refer to Chapter 9 for more information.

CQ patches are left in place for 24 hours and then immediately replaced with a fresh one. In contrast, Nicorette patches are applied in the morning and removed 16 hours later at bedtime. This pattern is intended to simulate nicotine dosing produced by smoking.

Most patients begin with a large patch and then use progressively smaller patches over several weeks. Certain patients (those with cardiovascular disease, those who weigh less than 100 pounds, or those who smoke less than one-half pack of cigarettes a day) should begin with a smaller patch.

Adverse effects are generally mild. Short-lived erythema, itching, and burning occur under the patch in 35% to 50% of users. In 14% to 17% of users, persistent erythema occurs, lasting up to 24 hours after patch removal. Patients who experience severe, persistent local reactions (e.g., severe erythema, itching, edema) should discontinue the patch and contact a physician or nurse practitioner.

Nicotine Inhaler

The nicotine inhaler [Nicotrol Inhaler] differs from other NRT products in that it looks much like a cigarette. Puffing on it delivers the nicotine. Because of this delivery method, using the inhaler can substitute for the hand-to-mouth behavior of smoking. In addition to nicotine, the inhaler contains menthol, which is intended to create a sensation in the back of the throat reminiscent of that caused by smoke. Like other forms of NRT, the inhaler doubles cessation success rates.

The nicotine inhaler consists of a mouthpiece and a sealed tubular cartridge. Inside the cartridge is a porous plug containing 10 mg of nicotine. Inserting the cartridge into the mouthpiece breaks the seal. Puffing on the mouthpiece draws air over the plug and thereby draws nicotine vapor into the mouth. Most of the nicotine is absorbed through the *oral mucosa*—not in the lungs. As a result, blood levels rise slowly and peak 10 to 15 minutes after puffing stops. Blood levels are less than half those achieved with cigarettes. Each cartridge can deliver 300 to 400 puffs. Benefits are greatest with frequent puffing over 20 minutes, after which the cartridge is discarded. Patients generally use 6 to 16 cartridges a day for 3 months, and then taper off over 2 to 3 months.

Adverse effects are mild. The most frequent are dyspepsia, coughing, throat irritation, oral burning, and rhinitis. The inhaler should not be used by patients with asthma. Because the cartridges contain dangerous amounts of nicotine, they should be kept away from children and pets.

Nicotine Nasal Spray

Nicotine nasal spray [Nicotrol NS] differs from other NRT formulations in that blood levels of nicotine rise *rapidly* after each administration, thereby closely simulating smoking. Because nicotine levels rise rapidly, the spray provides some of the subjective pleasure associated with cigarettes. As with other forms of NRT, the spray doubles smoking cessation rates.

The spray device delivers 0.5 mg of nicotine per activation. Two sprays (one in each nostril) constitute one dose and are equivalent to the amount of nicotine absorbed from one cigarette. Treatment should be started with 1 or 2 doses per hour—and never more than 5 doses per hour, or 40 doses a day. After 4 to 6 weeks, dosing should be gradually reduced and then stopped.

Quitting success with the spray has been good news and bad news. The good news, as reported in one study, is that 27% of users avoided smoking for 1 year—about twice the abstinence rate achieved with placebo. The bad news is that many patients continued to use the spray, being unwilling or unable to give it up. Nonetheless, since the spray delivers nicotine without the additional hazards in cigarettes, using the spray is clearly preferable to smoking.

Adverse effects are mild and temporary. At first, most users experience rhinitis, sneezing, coughing, watering eyes, and nasal and throat irritation. Fortunately, these effects abate in a few days. Nicotine nasal spray should be avoided by patients with sinus problems, allergies, or asthma.

Bupropion SR

Bupropion SR [Zyban, Buproban], an atypical antidepressant, was the first non-nicotine drug approved as an aid to smoking cessation. The drug is structurally similar to amphetamine and, like amphetamine, causes CNS stimulation and suppresses appetite. In people trying to quit cigarettes, bupropion reduces the urge to smoke and reduces some symptoms of nicotine withdrawal (e.g., irritability, anxiety). The drug is effective in the presence and absence of depression. Although the mechanism of action is uncertain, benefits may derive from blocking uptake of norepinephrine and dopamine. For use in depression, bupropion is sold under the brand name Wellbutrin.

Like the NRT products, bupropion SR doubles the cessation success rate. In one trial, patients were given bupropion SR (100, 150, or 300 mg/day) or placebo. At 7 weeks, abstinence rates were 19% with placebo, and 29%, 39%, and 44% with increasing dosages of bupropion SR. At 12 weeks, abstinence rates were lower: 12% with placebo and 20%, 23%, and 23% with increasing dosages of bupropion SR. Combining a nicotine patch with bupropion SR is somewhat more effective than either treatment alone.

Adverse effects are generally mild. The most common are dry mouth and insomnia. High doses (above 450 mg/day) are associated with a 0.4% risk of seizures. However, at the doses employed for smoking cessation (300 mg/day), seizures have not been reported. Nonetheless, bupropion SR should be avoided in patients with seizure risk factors, such as head trauma, history of seizures, anorexia nervosa, cocaine use, and alcohol withdrawal. Because it suppresses appetite, bupropion SR can cause weight loss. Bupropion SR should not be combined with a monoamine oxidase inhibitor. Nor should it be given to patients taking Wellbutrin, which is just another name for bupropion itself.

The usual regimen is 150 mg in the morning for 3 days, followed by 150 mg twice a day for 7 to 12 weeks. To minimize interference with sleep, the second dose should be taken as early in the day as possible—but at least 8 hours after the morning dose. Because onset of effects is delayed, dosing should begin 1 to 2 weeks before attempting to give up cigarettes.

The basic pharmacology of bupropion is discussed in Chapter 32.

Varenicline

Varenicline [Chantix, Champix 🍁], a partial agonist at nicotinic receptors, is our most effective aid to smoking cessation. In clinical trials, more patients achieved abstinence with varenicline than with bupropion SR or the nicotine patch. Estimated abstinence rates after 6 months were 33.2% with varenicline,

24.2% with bupropion SR, and 23.4% with a nicotine patch. The most common side effect is nausea. The most troubling side effects are psychologic changes. Unlike bupropion SR and NRT, varenicline does *not* cause weight loss.

Mechanism of Action

Varenicline acts as a *partial agonist* at a subset of nicotinic receptors—known as alpha$_4$beta$_2$ nicotinic receptors—whose activation promotes release of dopamine, the compound that mediates the pleasurable effects of nicotine. Compared with nicotine, varenicline binds alpha$_4$beta$_2$ receptors with greater affinity. Hence, when varenicline is present, access of nicotine to these receptors is blocked. Because varenicline is a partial agonist, receptor binding results in mild activation, which promotes some dopamine release and thereby helps reduce both nicotine craving and the intensity of withdrawal symptoms. At the same time, the presence of varenicline prevents intense receptor activation by nicotine itself and thereby blocks the reward that nicotine can provide.

Pharmacokinetics

Varenicline is readily absorbed from the GI tract, both in the presence and absence of food. Plasma levels peak about 4 hours after dosing. Binding to plasma proteins is low (20%). Metabolism is minimal, and hence most of each dose (92%) is excreted unchanged in the urine. The plasma half-life is 17 to 24 hours. Moderate to severe renal impairment delays excretion and increases varenicline blood levels.

Adverse Effects

In clinical trials, dose-dependent *nausea* was the most common adverse effect, occurring in 30% to 40% of users. Nausea is mild to moderate initially and becomes less severe over time. Other common reactions include sleep disturbances, headaches, abnormal dreams, constipation, dry mouth, flatulence, vomiting, and altered sense of taste. Mild physical dependence develops, but there have been no reports of abuse or addictive behavior. Rarely, varenicline has been associated with seizures, diabetes, dizziness, disturbed vision, and moderate and severe skin reactions, although a causal relationship has not been established.

Early postmarketing reports indicated that varenicline can cause serious *neuropsychiatric effects,* including mood changes, erratic behavior, and suicidality. At that time, the FDA placed a black box warning on varenicline for this reason. In 2016, the FDA removed the warning, as these cases were deemed more rare than initially expected. Nevertheless, all patients should be advised to contact their prescriber if they experience a significant change in behavior or mental status. Varenicline should be used with caution in patients with a history of psychiatric disease.

In 2011, the FDA warned that varenicline can increase the risk of cardiovascular events (e.g., angina pectoris, peripheral edema, hypertension, nonfatal myocardial infarction) in patients with stable cardiovascular disease. After that, a Canadian study revealed a similar risk in patients *without* cardiovascular disease. Fortunately, cardiovascular risk appears to be small—much smaller than the risk posed by smoking. Nonetheless, patients should be warned about cardiovascular risk and instructed to notify the prescriber if they experience new or worsening cardiovascular symptoms and to seek immediate medical attention if symptoms of myocardial infarction appear.

Owing to concerns about unpredictable physical and psychiatric adverse effects, authorities in the United States have banned the use of varenicline by truck drivers, bus drivers, airplane pilots, and air traffic controllers.

Drug Interactions

Varenicline does not affect the major components of the cytochrome P450 system. Studies with bupropion, transdermal nicotine, digoxin, warfarin, cimetidine, and metformin have shown no significant interactions. To date, no clinically significant interactions with other drugs have been reported.

Preparations, Dosage, and Administration

Varenicline is formulated in 0.5- and 1-mg tablets. To reduce nausea, each dose should be taken after eating and with a full glass of water. Dosing should begin 8 to 35 days before smoking is stopped. Titrate dosage as follows: on days 1 through 3, take 0.5 mg once daily; on days 4 through 7, take 0.5 mg twice daily; then take 1 mg twice daily for 12 weeks. If abstinence has been achieved, an additional 12 weeks of treatment is recommended. Patients who fail to stop smoking after the initial 12 weeks or who relapse after a full course of treatment should be encouraged to try again when conditions are deemed favorable. Patients with severe renal impairment should begin therapy at 0.5 mg once daily and increase to 0.5 mg twice daily if tolerated. Patients with end-stage renal disease undergoing dialysis should take a maximum of 0.5 mg once daily. Dosage adjustment is unnecessary in patients with mild to moderate renal impairment.

Products That Are Not Recommended

According to *Treating Tobacco Use and Dependence: 2008 Update,* there is insufficient proof to recommend the following drugs as aids to smoking cessation: naltrexone, silver acetate, beta blockers, benzodiazepines, and antidepressants other than bupropion SR, including the selective serotonin reuptake inhibitors.

Although not mentioned in the 2008 Update, *electronic cigarettes,* or *e-cigarettes,* should be avoided. E-cigarettes are battery-powered, cigarette-shaped devices that release a puff of vaporized nicotine, sometimes together with flavoring and other chemicals. According to analyses conducted by the FDA, the amount of nicotine per puff can vary widely, and the vapor may contain trace amounts of diethylene glycol and/or other contaminants. E-cigarettes are promoted on the Internet as aids to quit smoking, but are not FDA-approved for this use (or any other use, for that matter). At this writing, the FDA is attempting to regulate e-cigarettes as drug-delivery devices (which seems reasonable), but is meeting resistance from the courts. The bottom line: Because the dose of nicotine with e-cigarettes is unpredictable and because data on safety and efficacy are lacking, the use of e-cigarettes should be discouraged—especially since products of known safety and efficacy are available.

KEY POINTS

- Cigarette smoking kills about 480,000 American adults each year, making smoking the largest preventable cause of premature death.
- The principal cause of death among smokers is lung cancer, followed closely by heart disease.
- Nicotine in cigarette smoke is absorbed from the lungs, whereas nicotine in cigar smoke and smokeless tobacco is absorbed from the mouth.
- By activating nicotinic receptors in sympathetic ganglia and the adrenal medulla, nicotine causes vasoconstriction, increases heart rate, and increases force of ventricular contraction, thereby elevating blood pressure and increasing cardiac work. These effects underlie cardiovascular deaths.
- Through actions in the CNS, nicotine increases alertness, facilitates memory, improves cognitive function, reduces aggression, and suppresses appetite. In addition, by promoting the release of dopamine, nicotine activates the same pleasure circuit involved in addiction to cocaine, amphetamines, and opioids.
- Although tolerance develops to some effects of nicotine, very little tolerance develops to cardiovascular effects: Veteran smokers continue to experience an increase in blood pressure and cardiac work whenever they smoke.
- Nicotine causes physical dependence. Withdrawal is characterized by craving, nervousness, restlessness, irritability, impatience, increased hostility, insomnia, impaired concentration, increased appetite, and weight gain.
- Nicotine for replacement therapy is available in five FDA-approved delivery systems: chewing gum, lozenges, transdermal patches, nasal spray, and an inhaler.
- Although nicotine is harmful during pregnancy, NRT is probably safer than smoking, and hence use of NRT during pregnancy is worth consideration.
- Bupropion SR [Zyban, Buproban], which blocks reuptake of norepinephrine and dopamine, helps smokers quit by reducing nicotine craving and withdrawal symptoms.
- Varenicline [Chantix, Champix ♣] acts as a partial agonist at a specific subset of nicotinic receptors and thereby reduces nicotine craving and withdrawal symptoms. In addition, the drug blocks access of nicotine itself to those receptors and thereby prevents nicotine from producing pleasurable effects.
- The most effective drug/therapies for smoking cessation are varenicline alone and the nicotine patch combined with PRN nicotine nasal spray or nicotine gum.
- With the aid of counseling and pharmacotherapy, about 30% of smokers who attempt to quit can expect to achieve long-term abstinence.

Please visit **http://evolve.elsevier.com/Lehne** for chapter-specific NCLEX® examination review questions.

CHAPTER

40 Substance Use Disorders IV: Major Drugs of Abuse Other Than Alcohol and Nicotine

In this chapter, we discuss all of the major drugs of abuse except alcohol (see Chapter 38) and nicotine (see Chapter 39). As indicated in Table 40.1, abused drugs fall into seven major categories: (1) opioids, (2) psychostimulants, (3) depressants, (4) psychedelics, (5) dissociative drugs, (6) anabolic steroids, and (7) miscellaneous drugs of abuse. The basic pharmacology of many of these drugs is presented in previous chapters, so their discussion here is brief. Agents that have not been addressed previously (e.g., marijuana, *d*-lysergic acid diethylamide [LSD]) are discussed in depth.

HEROIN, OXYCODONE, AND OTHER OPIOIDS

The opioids (e.g., heroin, oxycodone, meperidine) are major drugs of abuse. As a result, most opioids are classified as Schedule II substances. The basic pharmacology of the opioids is discussed in Chapter 28.

Patterns of Use

Opioid use disorder (OUD) is encountered in all segments of society. Formerly, OUD was limited almost exclusively to lower socioeconomic groups residing in cities. Today, however, opioid abuse is more widespread, occurring in small towns as well as big cities, and among the rich and middle class as well as the poor.

For most people with OUD, initial exposure to opioids occurs either recreationally (i.e., illicitly) or in the context of pain management in a medical setting. The overwhelming majority of individuals who go on to abuse opioids begin their drug use illicitly. Only an exceedingly small percentage of those exposed to opioids therapeutically develop a pattern of compulsive drug use.

TABLE 40.1 ▪ Pharmacologic Categorization of Abused Drugs

Category	Examples
OPIOIDS	Heroin Hydromorphone Meperidine Morphine Oxycodone
PSYCHOSTIMULANTS	Cocaine Dextroamphetamine Methamphetamine Methylphenidate
DEPRESSANTS	
Barbiturates	Amobarbital Pentobarbital Phenobarbital Secobarbital
Benzodiazepines	Diazepam Lorazepam
Miscellaneous	Alcohol Gamma-hydroxybutyrate Meprobamate Methaqualone
PSYCHEDELICS	Dimethyltryptamine LSD Mescaline Psilocybin
DISSOCIATIVE DRUGS	Ketamine Phencyclidine
ANABOLIC STEROIDS	Nandrolone Oxandrolone Testosterone
MISCELLANEOUS	Amyl nitrite Dextromethorphan Marijuana Nicotine Nitrous oxide

Opioid abuse by healthcare providers deserves special consideration. It is well established that physicians, nurses, and pharmacists, as a group, abuse opioids to a greater extent than all other groups with similar educational backgrounds. The vulnerability of healthcare professionals to opioid abuse is due primarily to drug access.

Subjective and Behavioral Effects

Moments after IV injection, heroin produces sensations of pleasure, relaxation, warmth, and thirst. This initial reaction, known as a "rush" or "kick," persists for about 45 seconds. After this, the user experiences a prolonged sense of euphoria (well-being); there is a feeling that "all is well with the world." These extended effects, rather than the initial rush, are the primary reason for opioid abuse.

Interestingly, when individuals first use opioids, nausea and vomiting are prominent, and an overall sense of *dysphoria* may be felt. In many cases, were it not for peer pressure, individuals would not continue opioid use long enough to allow these unpleasant reactions to be replaced by a more agreeable experience.

Preferred Drugs and Routes of Administration

Which opioids do people abuse? Practically all of them. In the past, heroin was the most commonly abused opioid drug, but no longer, although its use is increasing. Prescription opioid analgesics were abused much more commonly than heroin, but with the opioid epidemic and increases in deaths from overdose, heroin is becoming more available and is cheaper than opioids. In 2015, more than 3.4 million Americans reported past-month abuse of opioids and 325,000 people reported that they had used heroin within the past month (www.samhsa.gov/data/sites/default/files/NSDUH).

Heroin

Among street users, heroin is the traditional opioid of choice. Because of its high lipid solubility, heroin crosses the blood-brain barrier with ease, causing effects that are both immediate and intense. This combination of speed and intensity sets heroin apart from other opioids.

Heroin can be administered in several ways. The order of preference is IV injection, smoking, and nasal inhalation (known as sniffing or snorting). Intravenous injection produces effects with the greatest intensity and fastest onset (7 to 8 seconds). When heroin is smoked or snorted, effects develop more slowly, peaking in 10 to 15 minutes. Among users who seek treatment, injection is the predominant method of administration. However, because sniffing and smoking are safer and easier than injection, these routes have become increasingly popular.

It should be noted that, when heroin is administered orally or subcutaneously, as opposed to intravenously, its effects cannot be distinguished from those of morphine and other opioids. This observation is not surprising given that, once in the brain, heroin is rapidly converted into morphine, its active form.

Oxycodone

In many parts of the United States, people are abusing the *controlled-release* formulation of oxycodone [OxyContin], an opioid similar to morphine. The controlled-release tablets were designed to provide steady levels of oxycodone over an extended time, and are safe and effective when swallowed intact. However, abusers do not ingest the tablets whole. Rather, they crush the tablets; then they either snort the powder or dissolve it in water and then inject it intravenously. As a result, the entire dose is absorbed *immediately,* producing blood levels that are dangerously high. Thousands of deaths have been reported. The risk of respiratory depression and death is greatest in people who have not developed tolerance to opioids.

In an effort to reduce OxyContin abuse, the controlled-release tablets were reformulated in 2010. The new formulation bears the imprint OP, rather than OC, which appeared on the old formulation. Compared with the old tablets, OxyContin OP tablets are much harder to crush into a powder. And if exposed to water or alcohol, the tablets just form a gel, rather than a solution that can be drawn into a syringe and injected. However, there is no evidence that OxyContin OP tablets are less subject to abuse, diversion, overdose, or development of OUD than the old tablets.

Meperidine

Nurses and physicians who abuse opioids may select meperidine [Demerol], a drug with distinct advantages for these users.

First, unlike heroin, meperidine is highly effective when administered orally, and hence abuse need not be associated with telltale signs of repeated injections. Second, meperidine produces less pupillary constriction than other opioids, thereby minimizing awkward questions about miosis. Lastly, meperidine has minimal effects on smooth muscle function, making constipation and urinary retention less problematic than with other opioids.

Tolerance and Physical Dependence

Tolerance

With prolonged opioid use, tolerance develops to some pharmacologic effects, but not others. Effects to which tolerance does develop include euphoria, respiratory depression, and nausea. In contrast, little or no tolerance develops to constipation and miosis. Because tolerance to respiratory depression develops in parallel with tolerance to euphoria, respiratory depression does not increase as higher doses are taken to produce desired subjective effects. Persons tolerant to one opioid are cross-tolerant to other opioids. However, there is no cross-tolerance between opioids and general central nervous system (CNS) depressants (e.g., barbiturates, benzodiazepines, alcohol).

Physical Dependence

Long-term use produces substantial physical dependence. The abstinence syndrome resulting from opioid withdrawal is described in Chapter 28. It is important to note that, although the opioid withdrawal syndrome can be extremely unpleasant, it is rarely dangerous.

Following the acute abstinence syndrome, which fades in 10 days, patients with opioid use disorder may experience a milder but protracted phase of withdrawal. This second phase, which may persist for months, is characterized by insomnia, irritability, and fatigue. Gastrointestinal hyperactivity and premature ejaculation may also occur.

Treatment of Acute Toxicity

Treatment of acute opioid toxicity is discussed in Chapter 28 and summarized here. Overdose produces a classic triad of symptoms: *respiratory depression, coma,* and *pinpoint pupils. Naloxone* [Narcan], an opioid antagonist, is the treatment of choice. This agent rapidly reverses all signs of opioid poisoning. However, dosage must be titrated carefully because if too much is given, the patient will swing from a state of intoxication to one of withdrawal. Owing to its short half-life, naloxone must be readministered every few hours until opioid concentrations have dropped to nontoxic levels, which may take days. Failure to repeat naloxone dosing may result in the death of patients who had earlier been rendered symptom free.

Detoxification

Persons who are physically dependent on opioids experience unpleasant symptoms if drug use is abruptly discontinued. Techniques for minimizing discomfort are presented later in this chapter.

Methadone Substitution

Methadone, a long-acting oral opioid, is the agent most commonly employed for easing withdrawal. The first step in methadone-aided withdrawal is to substitute methadone for the opioid upon which the individual is dependent. Because opioids display cross-dependence with one another, methadone will prevent an abstinence syndrome. Once the subject has been stabilized on methadone, withdrawal is accomplished by administering methadone in gradually smaller doses. The resultant abstinence syndrome is mild, with symptoms resembling those of moderate influenza. The entire process of methadone substitution and withdrawal takes about 10 days.

When substituting methadone for another opioid, suppression of the abstinence syndrome requires that methadone dosage be closely matched to the existing degree of physical dependence. Hence, to ensure that methadone dosing is adequate, the extent of physical dependence must be assessed. This can be accomplished by taking a history on the extent of drug use and by observing the patient for symptoms of withdrawal. Of the two approaches, observation is the more reliable. Estimates of drug use based on patient histories may be unreliable because (1) street users don't know the purity of the drugs they have taken, (2) claims of drug use may be inflated in hopes of receiving larger doses of methadone, and (3) healthcare professionals with OUD may report minimal consumption to downplay the extent of use. Because information from patients with OUD is not likely to permit accurate assessment of dependence, it is essential to observe the patient to make certain methadone dosage is sufficient to suppress withdrawal.

The use of methadone for *maintenance therapy* and *suppressive therapy* is discussed later in this chapter.

Buprenorphine

Buprenorphine is an agonist-antagonist opioid. Like methadone, buprenorphine can be substituted for the opioid on which an individual with OUD is physically dependent and can thereby prevent symptoms of withdrawal. After the individual is stabilized on buprenorphine, the dosage is gradually reduced, thereby keeping symptoms of withdrawal to a minimum. Use of buprenorphine for *maintenance therapy* is discussed later.

Clonidine-Assisted Withdrawal

Clonidine is a centrally acting alpha$_2$-adrenergic agonist. When administered to an individual physically dependent on opioids, clonidine can suppress some symptoms of abstinence. Clonidine is most effective against symptoms related to autonomic hyperactivity (nausea, vomiting, diarrhea). Modest relief is provided from muscle aches, restlessness, anxiety, and insomnia. Opioid craving is not diminished. The basic pharmacology of clonidine is discussed in Chapter 19.

Rapid and Ultrarapid Withdrawal

In both procedures, the patient is given an opioid *antagonist* (naloxone or naltrexone) to precipitate immediate withdrawal and thereby accelerate the withdrawal process. The ultrarapid procedure is carried out under general anesthesia or heavy sedation with IV midazolam [Versed]. In both procedures, clonidine may be added to ease symptoms. These procedures permit a rapid switch to maintenance therapy with an opioid antagonist. However, they are no more effective than standard withdrawal techniques, and they are considerably more expensive.

Drugs for Long-Term Management of Opioid Use Disorder

Three kinds of drugs are employed for long-term management: *opioid agonists, opioid agonist-antagonists,* and *opioid antagonists.* Opioid agonists (methadone) and agonist-antagonists (buprenorphine) substitute for the abused opioid and are given to patients who are not yet ready for detoxification. In contrast, opioid antagonists (naltrexone) are used to discourage renewed opioid use after detoxification has been accomplished. Drugs

TABLE 40.2 ■ Drugs for Long-Term Management of Opioid Use Disorder

Drug	Brand Name	Formulation	Dosing Schedule	CSA Schedule	Comments
OPIOID AGONIST					
Methadone	Methadose	Concentrated oral liquid	Once daily	II	Methadone maintenance may be provided only by Opioid Treatment Programs certified by the federal Substance Abuse and Mental Health Services Administration and approved by the designated state authority.
OPIOID AGONIST-ANTAGONIST					
Buprenorphine	Suboxone[a] Suboxone[a]	Sublingual tablet Sublingual film	Once daily Once daily	III	Suboxone may be prescribed in a primary care setting by any physician or nurse practitioner who has received authorized training and has registered with the Substance Abuse and Mental Health Services Administration.
OPIOID ANTAGONIST					
Naltrexone	ReVia Vivitrol	Oral tablet Extended-release suspension for IM injection	Once daily Once a month	NR	Naltrexone is not a controlled substance, and hence prescribers do not require special training or certification. Intramuscular naltrexone [Vivitrol] is the only drug approved for opioid use disorder that is given monthly, rather than daily. Before receiving naltrexone, patients must undergo opioid detoxification.

[a]In addition to buprenorphine, Suboxone contains naloxone, an opioid antagonist, to discourage IV dosing.
CSA, Controlled Substances Act; *NR,* not regulated under the CSA.

used for long-term management of opioid use disorder are shown in Table 40.2.

Methadone

In addition to its role in facilitating opioid withdrawal, methadone [Methadose] can be used for *maintenance therapy* and *suppressive therapy.* These strategies are employed to modify drug-using behavior in patients who are not ready to try withdrawal.

Methadone maintenance consists of transferring the patient from the abused opioid to oral methadone. By taking methadone, the individual avoids both withdrawal and the need to procure illegal drugs. Maintenance dosing is done once a day. Maintenance is most effective when done in conjunction with nondrug measures directed at altering patterns of drug use.

Suppressive therapy is done to prevent the reinforcing effects of opioid-induced euphoria. Suppression is achieved by giving the patient progressively larger doses of methadone until a very high dose (120 mg/day) is reached. Building up to this dose creates a high degree of tolerance, and hence no subjective effects are experienced from the methadone itself. Because cross-tolerance exists among opioids, once the patient is tolerant to methadone, taking street drugs, even in high doses, cannot produce significant desirable effects. As a result, individuals made tolerant with methadone will be less likely to seek out illicit opioids.

The use of methadone to treat opioid use disorder is restricted to Opioid Treatment Programs approved by the designated state authority and certified by the federal Substance Abuse and Mental Health Services Administration. These restrictions on the nonanalgesic use of methadone are needed to control abuse of methadone, a Schedule II drug with the same abuse liability as morphine and other strong opioids.

The basic pharmacology of methadone is presented in Chapter 28.

Buprenorphine

Buprenorphine [Suboxone] is an agonist-antagonist opioid. The drug is a partial agonist at mu receptors and a full antagonist at kappa receptors. Buprenorphine can be used for maintenance therapy and to facilitate detoxification (see earlier section in this chapter). When used for maintenance, buprenorphine alleviates craving, reduces the use of illicit opioids, and increases retention in therapeutic programs.

Unlike methadone, which is available only through certified Opioid Treatment Programs, buprenorphine can be prescribed and dispensed in general medical settings, such as primary care offices. Prescribers must receive at least 8 hours of authorized training and must register with the Substance Abuse and Mental Health Services Administration.

Buprenorphine has several properties that make it attractive for treating OUD. Because it is a partial agonist at mu receptors, it has a low potential for abuse—but can still suppress craving for opioids. If the dosage is sufficiently high, buprenorphine can completely block access of strong opioids to mu receptors and can thereby prevent opioid-induced euphoria. With buprenorphine, there is a ceiling to respiratory depression, which makes it safer than methadone. Development of physical dependence is low, and hence withdrawal is relatively mild.

Buprenorphine is currently available in three formulations that are dosed once a day. One formulation—sublingual tablets—contains buprenorphine *alone.* The other two formulations—sublingual tablets and sublingual films, both marketed as *Suboxone*—contain buprenorphine *combined with naloxone.* Generic buprenorphine is used for the first few days of treatment, and then Suboxone is used for long-term maintenance. The naloxone in Suboxone is there to discourage IV abuse. If taken intravaneously, the naloxone in Suboxone will precipitate withdrawal. However, with sublingual administration, very little naloxone is absorbed, and hence, when the drug is administered as intended, the risk of withdrawal is low. Nonetheless, because there *is* a small risk with sublingual Suboxone, treatment is initiated with generic buprenorphine, thereby allowing substitution of buprenorphine for the abused opioid. Thereafter, Suboxone is taken for maintenance.

The basic pharmacology of buprenorphine is presented in Chapter 28.

Naltrexone

After a patient has undergone opioid detoxification, naltrexone [ReVia, Vivitrol], a pure opioid antagonist, can be used to discourage renewed opioid abuse. Benefits derive from blocking euphoria and all other opioid-induced effects. By preventing pleasurable effects, naltrexone eliminates the reinforcing properties of opioid use. When the recovering patient learns that taking an opioid cannot produce the desired response, drug-using behavior will cease. Naltrexone is not a controlled substance, and hence prescribers require no special training or certification.

Naltrexone is available in oral and IM formulations. The oral formulation, sold as ReVia, is dosed once a day. The IM formulation, sold as Vivitrol, is dosed once a month. At this time, Vivitrol is the only long-acting drug for managing opioid use disorder. All other drugs must be taken every day.

The basic pharmacology of naltrexone is presented in Chapter 28.

Sequelae of Compulsive Opioid Use

Surprisingly, chronic opioid use has very few *direct* detrimental effects. Patients in treatment programs have been maintained on high doses of methadone for a decade with no significant impairment of health. Furthermore, individuals on methadone maintenance can be successful socially and at work. It appears, then, that opioid use is not necessarily associated with poor health, lack of productivity, or inadequate social interaction.

Although opioids have few direct ill effects, there are many *indirect* hazards. These risks stem largely from the lifestyle of the opioid user and from impurities common to street drugs. Infections secondary to sharing nonsterile needles occur frequently. The infections that opioid abusers acquire include septicemia, cellulitis, abscesses, endocarditis, tuberculosis, hepatitis C, and HIV. Foreign-body emboli have resulted from impurities in opioid preparations. Opioid users suffer an unusually high death rate. Some deaths reflect the violent nature of the subculture in which opioid use often takes place. Many others result from accidental overdose.

GENERAL CNS DEPRESSANTS

The family of CNS depressants consists of barbiturates, benzodiazepines, alcohol, and other agents. With the exception of the benzodiazepines, all of these drugs are more alike than different. The benzodiazepines have properties that set them apart. The basic pharmacology of the benzodiazepines, barbiturates, and most other CNS depressants is presented in Chapter 34; the pharmacology of alcohol is presented in Chapter 38. Discussion here is limited to abuse of these drugs.

Barbiturates

The barbiturates embody all of the properties that typify general CNS depressants, and hence can be considered prototypes of the group. Depressant effects are dose dependent and range from mild sedation to sleep to coma to death. With prolonged use, barbiturates produce tolerance and physical dependence.

The abuse liability of the barbiturates stems from their ability to produce subjective effects similar to those of alcohol. The barbiturates with the highest potential for abuse have a short to intermediate duration of action. These agents—amobarbital, pentobarbital, and secobarbital—are classified under Schedule II of the Controlled Substances Act. Other barbiturates appear under Schedules III and IV. Despite legal restrictions, barbiturates are available cheaply and in abundance.

Tolerance

Regular use of barbiturates produces tolerance to some effects, but not to others. Tolerance to subjective effects is significant. As a result, progressively larger doses are needed to produce desired psychologic responses. Unfortunately, very little tolerance develops to respiratory depression. Consequently, as barbiturate use continues, the dose needed to produce subjective effects moves closer and closer to the dose that can cause respiratory arrest. (Note that this differs from the pattern seen with opioids, in which tolerance to subjective effects and to respiratory depression develop in parallel.) Individuals tolerant to barbiturates show cross-tolerance with other CNS depressants (e.g., alcohol, benzodiazepines, general anesthetics). However, little or no cross-tolerance develops to opioids.

Physical Dependence and Withdrawal Techniques

Chronic barbiturate use can produce substantial physical dependence. Cross-dependence exists between barbiturates and other CNS depressants, but not with opioids. When physical dependence is great, the associated abstinence syndrome can be severe—sometimes fatal. In contrast, the opioid abstinence syndrome, although unpleasant, is rarely life threatening.

One technique for easing barbiturate withdrawal employs phenobarbital, a barbiturate with a long half-life. Because of cross-dependence, substitution of phenobarbital for the abused barbiturate suppresses symptoms of abstinence. Once the patient has been stabilized, the dosage of phenobarbital is gradually tapered off, thereby minimizing symptoms of abstinence.

Acute Toxicity

Overdose with barbiturates produces a triad of symptoms: *respiratory depression, coma,* and *pinpoint pupils*—the same symptoms that accompany opioid poisoning. Treatment is directed at maintaining respiration and removing the drug; endotracheal intubation and ventilatory assistance may be required. Details of management are presented in Chapter 34. Barbiturate overdose has no specific antidote. Naloxone, which reverses poisoning by opioids, is not effective against poisoning by barbiturates.

Benzodiazepines

Benzodiazepines differ significantly from barbiturates. Benzodiazepines are much safer than the barbiturates, and overdose with *oral* benzodiazepines *alone* is rarely lethal. However, the risk of death is greatly increased when oral benzodiazepines are combined with other CNS depressants (e.g., alcohol, barbiturates) or when benzodiazepines are administered IV. If severe overdose occurs, signs and symptoms can be reversed with *flumazenil* [Romazicon, Anexate ♣], a benzodiazepine antagonist. As a rule, tolerance and physical dependence are only moderate when benzodiazepines are taken for legitimate indications, but can be substantial when these drugs are abused. In patients who develop physical dependence, the abstinence syndrome can be minimized by withdrawing benzodiazepines very slowly—over a period of months. The abuse liability of the benzodiazepines is much lower than that of the barbiturates. As a result, all benzodiazepines are classified under Schedule IV of the Controlled Substances Act. Benzodiazepines are discussed in Chapter 34.

PSYCHOSTIMULANTS

Discussion here focuses on two CNS stimulants that have a high potential for abuse: cocaine and methamphetamine. Because of their considerable abuse liability, these drugs are classified as Schedule II agents. (If they lacked approved medical uses, they would be classified in Schedule I.) In addition to stimulating the CNS, methamphetamine and cocaine can stimulate the heart, blood vessels, and other structures under sympathetic control. Because of these peripheral actions, these stimulants are also referred to as *sympathomimetics.*

Stimulants with little or no abuse potential are not addressed in this chapter. Included in this group are Schedule III stimulants (e.g., benzphetamine), Schedule IV stimulants (e.g., diethylpropion), and stimulants that are not regulated at all (e.g., caffeine, ephedrine).

Cocaine

Cocaine is a stimulant extracted from the leaves of the coca plant. The drug has CNS effects similar to those of the amphetamines. In addition, cocaine can produce local anesthesia as well as vasoconstriction and cardiac stimulation. Among abusers, a form of cocaine known as "crack" is used widely. Crack is extremely addictive, and the risk of lethal overdose is high.

According to the National Survey on Drug Use and Health, cocaine use has declined. In 2015, 2.4 million Americans age 18 and older reported using cocaine in any form, compared with 5.5 million in 2005.

Forms

Cocaine is available in two forms: *cocaine hydrochloride* and *cocaine base* (alkaloidal cocaine, freebase cocaine, "crack"). Cocaine base is heat stabile, whereas cocaine hydrochloride is not. Cocaine hydrochloride is available as a white powder that is frequently diluted ("cut") before sale. Cocaine base is sold in the form of crystals ("rocks") that consist of nearly pure cocaine. Cocaine base is widely known by the street name "crack," a term inspired by the sound the crystals make when heated.

Routes of Administration

Cocaine *hydrochloride* is usually administered *intranasally.* The drug is "snorted" and absorbed across the nasal mucosa into the bloodstream. A few users (about 5%) administer cocaine hydrochloride IV. Cocaine hydrochloride cannot be smoked because it is unstable at high temperature.

Cocaine *base* is administered by *smoking,* a process referred to as "freebasing." Smoking delivers large amounts of cocaine to the lungs, where absorption is very rapid. Subjective and physiologic effects are equivalent to those elicited by IV injection.

Subjective Effects and Cocaine Use Disorder

At usual doses, cocaine produces euphoria similar to that produced by amphetamines. In a laboratory setting, individuals familiar with the effects of cocaine are unable to distinguish between cocaine and amphetamine. Cocaine causes euphoria through inhibition of neuronal reuptake of dopamine and thereby increases activation of dopamine receptors in the brain's reward circuit.

As with many other psychoactive drugs, the intensity of subjective responses depends on the rate at which plasma drug levels rise. Because cocaine levels rise relatively slowly with intranasal administration and almost instantaneously with IV injection or smoking, responses produced by intranasal cocaine are much less intense than those produced by the other two routes.

When crack cocaine is smoked, desirable subjective effects begin to fade within minutes and are often replaced by dysphoria. In an attempt to avoid dysphoria and regain euphoria, the user may administer repeated doses at short intervals. This usage pattern—termed *bingeing*—can rapidly lead to cocaine use disorder.

Acute Toxicity: Symptoms and Treatment

Overdose is frequent, and deaths have occurred. Mild overdose produces agitation, dizziness, tremor, and blurred vision. Severe overdose can produce hyperpyrexia, convulsions, ventricular dysrhythmias, and hemorrhagic stroke. Angina pectoris and myocardial infarction may develop secondary to coronary artery spasm. Psychologic manifestations of overdose include severe anxiety, paranoid ideation, and hallucinations (visual, auditory, and/or tactile). Because cocaine has a short half-life, symptoms subside in 1 to 2 hours.

Although there is no specific antidote to cocaine toxicity, most symptoms can be controlled with drugs. Intravenous *diazepam* or *lorazepam* can reduce anxiety and suppress seizures. *Diazepam* may also alleviate hypertension and dysrhythmias, since these result from increased central sympathetic activity. If hypertension is severe, it can be corrected with IV *nitroprusside.* Dysrhythmias associated with prolonging the QT interval may respond to *hypertonic sodium bicarbonate.* Although beta blockers can suppress dysrhythmias, they might further compromise coronary perfusion (by preventing $beta_2$-mediated coronary vasodilation). Reduction of thrombus formation with aspirin can lower the risk of myocardial ischemia. Hyperthermia should be reduced with external cooling.

Chronic Toxicity

When administered intranasally on a long-term basis, cocaine can cause atrophy of the nasal mucosa and loss of sense of smell. In extreme cases, necrosis and perforation of the nasal septum occur. Nasal pathology results from local ischemia secondary to chronic vasoconstriction. Injury to the lungs can occur from smoking cocaine base.

Use During Pregnancy

Cocaine is highly lipid soluble and readily crosses the placenta, allowing it to accumulate in the fetal circulation. Data from 2013 revealed that babies born to mothers who used cocaine during pregnancy were more likely to be born early, to have smaller heads and decreased length, and to have lower birth weights than babies born to mothers who did not use cocaine. In addition, the effects on babies born to prenatal users of cocaine can last well into childhood, causing deficits in attention, memory, and language development.

Tolerance, Dependence, and Withdrawal

In animal models, regular administration of cocaine results in *increased* sensitivity to the drug, not tolerance. Whether this holds true for humans is not clear.

The degree of physical dependence produced by cocaine is in dispute. Some observers report little or no evidence of withdrawal following cocaine discontinuation. In contrast, others report symptoms similar to those associated with amphetamine withdrawal: dysphoria, craving, fatigue, depression, and prolonged sleep.

Treatment of Cocaine Use Disorder

Although achieving complete abstinence from cocaine is extremely difficult, treatment *can* greatly reduce cocaine use. For the individual with cocaine use disorder, psychosocial therapy is the cornerstone of treatment. This therapy is directed at motivating users to commit to a drug-free life, and then helping them work toward that goal. A combination of individual therapy and group drug counseling is most effective, producing a 70% reduction in cocaine use at 12-month follow-up.

Can medication help with cocaine use disorder? To date, no drug has been proved broadly effective in treating cocaine abuse. However, ongoing work with two agents is encouraging:

- *Anticocaine vaccine*—Subjects receiving the vaccine develop antibodies that bind with cocaine and thereby render the cocaine inactive. The higher the antibody titer, the greater the reduction in cocaine use. Phase I human testing recruitment began in 2016.
- *Disulfiram* [Antabuse]—Subjects receiving a combination of disulfiram plus cognitive behavioral therapy reduced their cocaine use from 2 or 3 times daily to 0.5 times daily. Disulfiram is the same drug we discussed in Chapter 38 for treating alcohol abuse.

Methamphetamine

The basic pharmacology of the amphetamine family is discussed in Chapter 36. Discussion here is limited to abuse of methamphetamine.

Description and Routes

Methamphetamine is a white crystalline powder that readily dissolves in water or alcohol. The drug may be swallowed, "snorted," smoked, or injected IV. Owing to its potential for abuse, methamphetamine is classified as a Schedule II drug.

Patterns of Use

Use of methamphetamine declined between the years of 2006 and 2012. Yet, we are now seeing an increase in use. According to the 2015 National Survey on Drug Use and Health, use of methamphetamine within the past month by Americans age 12 years and older increased from 569,000 in 2014 to 898,000 in 2015.

Subjective and Behavioral Effects

As discussed in Chapter 36, amphetamines act primarily by increasing the release of norepinephrine and dopamine, and partly by reducing the reuptake of both transmitters. By doing so, methamphetamine produces arousal and elevation of mood. Euphoria is likely and talkativeness is prominent. A sense of increased physical strength and mental capacity occurs. Self-confidence rises. Users feel little or no need for food and sleep.

Adverse Psychologic Effects

All amphetamines can produce a psychotic state characterized by delusions, paranoia, and auditory and visual hallucinations, making patients look as if they suffer from schizophrenia. Although psychosis can be triggered by a single dose, it occurs more commonly with long-term abuse. Methamphetamine-induced psychosis usually resolves spontaneously following drug withdrawal. If needed, an antipsychotic agent (e.g., olanzapine) can be given to suppress symptoms.

Adverse Cardiovascular Effects

Because of its sympathomimetic actions, methamphetamine can cause vasoconstriction and excessive stimulation of the heart, leading to hypertension, angina pectoris, and dysrhythmias. Overdose may also cause cerebral and systemic vasculitis and renal failure. Changes in cerebral blood vessels can lead to stroke. Vasoconstriction can be relieved with an alpha-adrenergic blocker (e.g., phentolamine). Cardiac stimulation can be reduced with a mixed alpha and beta blocker (e.g., labetalol).

Other Adverse Effects

By suppressing appetite, methamphetamine can cause significant weight loss. Use during pregnancy increases the risk of preterm birth, hypertension, placental abruption, intrauterine growth restriction, and neonatal death. Heavy use can promote severe tooth decay, known informally as "meth mouth." Causes include reduced salivation, grinding and clenching of the teeth, increased consumption of sugary drinks, and neglect of oral hygiene. Lastly, methamphetamine can cause direct injury to dopaminergic nerve terminals in the brain, leading to prolonged deficits in cognition and memory.

Tolerance, Dependence, and Withdrawal

Long-term use results in tolerance to mood elevation, appetite suppression, and cardiovascular effects. Although physical dependence is only moderate, psychologic dependence can be intense. Methamphetamine withdrawal can produce dysphoria and a strong sense of craving. Other symptoms include fatigue, prolonged sleep, excessive eating, and depression. Depression can persist for months and is a common reason for resuming drug use.

Treatment

Amphetamine-type substance use disorder responds well to cognitive behavioral therapy. One such approach, known as the Matrix Model, combines group therapy, individual therapy, family education, drug testing, and encouragement to participate in non–drug-related activities. At this time, no medications are approved for treatment. However, encouraging results have been achieved with two drugs: *bupropion* [Wellbutrin, Zyban], currently approved for major depression and smoking cessation, and *modafinil* [Provigil, Alertec 🍁], a nonamphetamine stimulant currently approved for narcolepsy, shift-work sleep disorder, and obstructive sleep apnea/hypopnea syndrome. An additional drug, ibudilast, is in clinical trials. Preliminary results indicate that ibudilast may dampen cravings for methamphetamine and improve cognitive functioning.

Synthetic Cathinones

Synthetic cathinones are drugs better known by their street name, "bath salts." These drugs are closely related to the naturally occurring khat plant, found in East Africa and southern Arabia. Bath salts have appeared on the market within the past few years, and are touted as substitutes to other psychostimulants, such as cocaine or methamphetamine.

Bath salts are consumed by injecting, swallowing, snorting, or smoking. Often, bath salts are sold in packets of white power or tablets labeled "not for human consumption" or as plant food or cleaning substances. They are structurally related to amphetamines and are thought to increase dopamine, serotonin, and norepinephrine levels. This leads to feelings of euphoria and alertness. Onset of duration is fairly quick with overall duration of 2 to 4 hours.

Multiple negative psychologic effects have been noted with the use of bath salts, including paranoia, aggression, hallucinations, panic attacks, agitation, and delirium. Physical effects range from nose bleeds and sweating to renal failure and death. Bath salts were formerly available over the counter in gas stations and convenience stores, but due to their negative effects and many emergency room visits, bath salts are banned for sale and use in all 50 states.

MARIJUANA AND RELATED PREPARATIONS

Marijuana is the most commonly used illicit drug in the United States. Over 128 million Americans have tried it at least once. In 2015, over 22 million Americans age 12 and older used marijuana. Among youth, rates of daily marijuana use are the highest since the 1970s. Results of the 2016 *Monitoring the Future* survey show that 5.4% of 8th-graders and 14% of 10th-graders reported using marijuana in the past month. Monthly marijuana use among 12th-graders has risen to 22.5%.

Cannabis sativa: The Source of Marijuana

Marijuana is prepared from *Cannabis sativa,* the Indian hemp plant—an unusual plant in that it has separate male and female forms. Psychoactive compounds are present in all parts of the male and female plants. However, the greatest concentration of psychoactive substances is found in the flowering tops of the female plants.

The two most common *Cannabis* derivatives are *marijuana* and *hashish.* Marijuana is a preparation consisting of leaves and flowers of male and female plants. Alternative names for marijuana include *grass, weed, pot,* and *dope.* The terms *joint* and *reefer* refer to marijuana cigarettes. Hashish is a dried preparation of the resinous exudate from female flowers. Hashish is considerably more potent than marijuana.

Psychoactive Component

The major psychoactive substance in *Cannabis sativa* is delta-9-tetrahydrocannabinol (THC), an oily chemical with high lipid solubility.

The THC content of *Cannabis* preparations is variable. The highest concentrations are found in the flowers of the female plant. The lowest concentrations are in the seeds. Depending on growing conditions and the strain of the plant, THC in marijuana preparations may range from 1% to 11%.

Mechanism of Action

Psychologic effects of THC result from activating specific cannabinoid receptors in the brain. The endogenous ligand for these receptors appears to be *anandamide,* a derivative of arachidonic acid unique to the brain. The concentration of cannabinoid receptors is highest in brain regions associated with pleasure, memory, thinking, concentration, appetite, sensory perception, time perception, and coordination of movement.

There is evidence that marijuana may act in part through the same reward system as do opioids and cocaine. Both heroin and cocaine produce pleasurable sensations by promoting a release of dopamine in the brain's reward circuit. In rats, intravenous THC also causes dopamine release. Interestingly, the release of dopamine by THC is blocked by naloxone, a drug that blocks the effects of opioids. This suggests that THC causes the release of dopamine by first causing a release of endogenous opioids.

Pharmacokinetics

Administration by Smoking

When marijuana or hashish is smoked, about 60% of the THC content is absorbed. Absorption from the lungs is rapid. Subjective effects begin in minutes and peak 10 to 20 minutes later. Effects from a single marijuana cigarette may persist for 2 to 3 hours. Termination results from metabolism of THC to inactive products.

Oral Administration

When marijuana or hashish is ingested, practically all of the THC undergoes absorption. However, the majority is inactivated on its first pass through the liver. Hence, only 6% to 20% of absorbed drug actually reaches the systemic circulation. Because of this extensive first-pass metabolism, oral doses must be 3 to 10 times greater than smoked doses to produce equivalent effects. With oral dosing, effects are delayed and prolonged: Responses begin in 30 to 50 minutes and persist up to 12 hours.

Behavioral and Subjective Effects

Marijuana produces three principal subjective effects: *euphoria, sedation,* and *hallucinations.* This set of responses is unique to marijuana; no other psychoactive drug causes all three. Because of this singular pattern of effects, marijuana is in a class by itself.

Effects of Low to Moderate Doses

Responses to low doses of THC are variable and depend on several factors, including dosage size and route, setting of drug use, and expectations and previous experience of the user. The following effects are common: euphoria and relaxation; gaiety and a heightened sense of the humorous; increased sensitivity to visual and auditory stimuli; enhanced sense of touch, taste, and smell; increased appetite and ability to appreciate the flavor of food; and distortion of time perception such that short spans seem much longer than they really are. In addition to these effects, which might be considered pleasurable (or at least innocuous), moderate doses can produce undesirable responses. Among these are impairment of short-term memory; decreased capacity to perform multistep tasks; slowed reaction time and impairment of motor coordination (which can make driving dangerous); altered judgment and decision making (which can lead to high-risk sexual behavior); temporal disintegration (inability to distinguish between past, present, and future); depersonalization (a sense of strangeness about the self); decreased ability to perceive the emotions of others; and reduced interpersonal interaction.

High-Dose Effects

In high doses, marijuana can have serious adverse psychologic effects. The user may experience hallucinations, delusions, and paranoia. Euphoria may be displaced by intense anxiety, and a dissociative state may occur in which the user feels "outside of himself or herself." In extremely high doses, marijuana can produce a state resembling toxic psychosis, which may persist for weeks. Because of the widespread use of marijuana, psychiatric emergencies caused by the drug are relatively common.

Not all users are equally vulnerable to the adverse psychologic effects of marijuana. Some individuals experience ill effects only at extremely high doses. In contrast, others routinely experience adverse effects at moderate doses.

Effects of Chronic Use

Chronic, excessive use of marijuana is associated with a behavioral phenomenon known as an *amotivational syndrome,* characterized by apathy, dullness, poor grooming, reduced interest in achievement, and disinterest in the pursuit of conventional goals. The precise relationship between marijuana and development of the syndrome is not known, nor is it certain what other factors may contribute. Available data do not suggest that the amotivational syndrome is due to organic brain damage.

Role in Schizophrenia

Marijuana use is associated with an increased risk of schizophrenia. In young people with no history of psychotic symptoms, marijuana increases the risk of symptom occurrence. In people who already have symptoms, marijuana may prolong symptom persistence. In the stabilized schizophrenic, marijuana may precipitate an acute psychotic episode.

Physiologic Effects

Cardiovascular Effects

Marijuana produces a dose-related increase in heart rate. Increases of 20 to 50 beats/min are typical. However, rates up to 140 beats/min are not uncommon. Pretreatment with propranolol prevents marijuana-induced tachycardia but does not block the drug's subjective effects. Marijuana causes orthostatic hypotension and pronounced reddening of the conjunctivae. These responses apparently result from vasodilation.

Respiratory Effects

When used *acutely,* marijuana produces *bronchodilation.* However, when smoked chronically, the drug causes airway constriction. In addition, chronic use is closely associated with the development of bronchitis, sinusitis, and asthma. Lung cancer is another possible outcome. Animal studies have shown that tar from marijuana smoke is a more potent carcinogen than tar from cigarette smoke.

Effects on Reproduction

Research in animals has shown multiple effects on reproduction. In males, marijuana decreases spermatogenesis and testosterone levels. In females, the drug reduces levels of follicle-stimulating hormone, luteinizing hormone, and prolactin.

Multiple effects may be seen in babies and children who were exposed to marijuana *in utero.* Some babies present with trembling, altered responses to visual stimuli, and a high-pitched cry. Preschoolers may have a decreased ability to perform tasks that involve memory and sustained attention. Schoolchildren may exhibit deficits in memory, attentiveness, and problem solving.

Altered Brain Structure

Long-term marijuana use is associated with structural changes in the brain. Specifically, the volume of the hippocampus and amygdala is reduced, by an average of 12% and 7.1%, respectively. We don't know whether volume reduction is due to reduced cell size, reduced synaptic density, or loss of glial cells and/or neurons. Interestingly, hippocampal volume loss occurs primarily in the left hemisphere.

Tolerance and Dependence

When taken in extremely high doses, marijuana can produce tolerance and physical dependence. Neither effect, however, is remarkable. Some tolerance develops to the cardiovascular, perceptual, and motor effects of marijuana. Little or no tolerance develops to subjective effects.

To demonstrate physical dependence on marijuana, the drug must be given in very high doses—and even then the degree of dependence is only moderate. Symptoms brought on by abrupt discontinuation of high-dose marijuana include irritability, restlessness, nervousness, insomnia, reduced appetite, and weight loss. Tremor, hyperthermia, and chills may occur too. Symptoms subside in 3 to 5 days. With moderate marijuana use, no withdrawal symptoms occur.

Therapeutic Use

In the United States, there are no approved medical uses for marijuana itself. However, there *are* U.S. Food and Drug Administration (FDA)–approved uses for two *purified* cannabinoids: THC and dronabinol, an analog of THC. A third cannabinoid preparation—nabiximols—is approved in Canada.

Approved Uses for Cannabinoids

Suppression of Emesis. Intense nausea and vomiting are common side effects of cancer chemotherapy. In certain patients, these responses can be suppressed more effectively with cannabinoids than with traditional antiemetics (e.g., prochlorperazine, metoclopramide). At this time, two cannabinoids—*dronabinol* [Marinol] and *nabilone* [Cesamet]—are available for antiemetic use. Dronabinol, a synthetic form of THC, is a Schedule III drug. Nabilone, a THC derivative, is a Schedule II drug. Dosage forms and dosages are presented in Chapter 80.

Appetite Stimulation. Dronabinol is FDA approved for stimulating appetite in patients with AIDS. By relieving anorexia, treatment may prevent or reverse loss of weight.

Relief of Neuropathic Pain. In 2005, Canadian regulators approved *nabiximols* [Sativex 🍁], administered by oral spray, for treating neuropathic pain caused by multiple sclerosis (MS). Nabiximols is a mixture of two cannabinoids: THC and cannabidiol. Because the cannabinoids in Sativex are absorbed through the oral mucosa, the product has a rapid onset (like smoked marijuana), while being devoid of the dangerous tars in marijuana smoke. In the United States, nabiximols is under study for treating intractable cancer pain. However, the drug is not yet approved in the United States, and cannot be legally imported, owing to its current classification as a Schedule I substance.

Unapproved Uses for Cannabinoids

Glaucoma. In patients with glaucoma, smoking marijuana may reduce intraocular pressure. Unfortunately, marijuana may also reduce blood flow to the optic nerve. We don't know whether the drug improves vision.

Multiple Sclerosis. Whether smoked or ingested, marijuana appears to reduce spasticity and tremor of MS. Oral cannabinoids may also reduce urge incontinence. As previously mentioned, cannabinoids can reduce neuropathic pain of MS.

Medical Research on Marijuana

Proponents of making marijuana available by prescription argue that smoked marijuana can reduce chronic pain, suppress nausea caused by chemotherapy, improve appetite in patients with AIDS, lower intraocular pressure in patients with glaucoma, and suppress spasticity associated with MS and spinal cord injury. However, the evidence supporting most of these claims is weak—largely because federal regulations had effectively barred marijuana research.

In 1999, two developments opened the doors to marijuana research. First, an expert panel, convened by the National Academy of Sciences' Institute of Medicine, recommended that clinical trials on marijuana proceed. Because smoking marijuana poses a risk of lung cancer and other respiratory disorders, the panel also recommended development of a rapid-onset nonsmoked delivery system. In response to this report and to pressure from scientists and voters, the government created new guidelines that loosened restraints on marijuana research. Under the guidelines, researchers will be allowed to purchase marijuana directly from the federal government. (On behalf of the government, the University of Mississippi maintains a plot of marijuana on 1.8 closely guarded acres.) The only catch is that all proposed research must be approved by the FDA, the National Institute on Drug Abuse, and the Drug Enforcement Agency (DEA). Due to the increase in the legalization of marijuana, medical studies have increased. In 2016 multiple studies were conducted regarding marijuana's role in the treatment of epilepsy and migraine headaches, as well as its effects on the general health of frequent users.

Legal Status of Medical Marijuana

United States. Twenty-eight states[a] and the District of Columbia have enacted laws that eliminate criminal penalties for medical use of marijuana, and more states are considering doing the same. Because of the new state laws, patients can now possess and use small amounts of marijuana for medical purposes. In most of these states, qualified patients must have a debilitating medical condition plus documentation from their physicians that medical use of marijuana "may be of benefit."

What about federal marijuana regulations? Because marijuana is classified by the DEA as a Schedule I substance, physicians still cannot *prescribe* the drug—all they can do is *suggest* it may be of benefit. Furthermore, in 2005, the U.S. Supreme Court ruled that DEA legislation trumps the new state laws, and hence people who use or provide medical marijuana can still be prosecuted under federal law, even in states where medical marijuana has been legalized. In a (delayed) response to this ruling, the Department of Justice, in 2009, instructed U.S. attorneys not to use federal resources to prosecute people whose actions comply with state laws that allow medical marijuana use. Hence, although patients may be breaking federal law, the Department of Justice will not prosecute them.

Canada. Medical use of marijuana has been legal in Canada since 2001, when the Marijuana Medical Access Regulations took effect. Patients with documentation from a physician can get their marijuana through Health Canada, or they can get a license to grow their own. Marijuana supplies for Health Canada are grown and distributed by Prairie Plant Systems.

Comparison of Marijuana With Alcohol

In several important ways, responses to marijuana and alcohol are quite different. Whereas increased hostility and aggression are common sequelae of alcohol consumption, aggressive behavior is rare among marijuana users. Although loss of judgment and control can occur with either drug, these losses are greater with alcohol. For the marijuana user, increased appetite and food intake are typical. In contrast, heavy drinkers often suffer nutritional deficiencies. Lastly, whereas marijuana can cause toxic psychosis, dissociative phenomena, and paranoia, these severe acute psychologic reactions rarely occur with alcohol.

Synthetic Marijuana

Synthetic cannabis blends showed up on the market in the early 2000s. They became popular because of their availability and their lack of traces in drug tests. They were initially legal, as they were thought to contain blends of natural herbs sprayed

---

[a]Alaska, Arizona, Arkansas, California, Colorado, Connecticut, Delaware, Florida, Hawaii, Illinois, Louisiana, Maine, Maryland, Michigan, Minnesota, Montana, Nevada, New Hampshire, New Jersey, New Mexico, New York, North Dakota, Ohio, Oregon, Pennsylvania, Rhode Island, Vermont, and Washington.

with chemicals that mimic the effects of THC. These chemicals come in two classes: THC analogs and other compounds.

Although synthetic marijuana was once thought harmless, the American Association of Poison Control Centers reported more than 7000 calls regarding synthetic marijuana in a 2-year period. In addition, several deaths and many episodes of florid psychosis and toxicity are possibly related to synthetic marijuana use. Side effects include hypertension, nausea, vomiting, anxiety, agitation, paranoid behavior, hallucinations, and catatonic state. By 2011, the FDA had placed many of these chemicals on the controlled substances list as Schedule I drugs, making them illegal to possess. However, more than 500 compounds exist; therefore, synthetic marijuana is still available. Many organizations, including the U.S. military, have banned all similar compounds.

PSYCHEDELICS

The psychedelics are a fascinating drug family for which LSD can be considered the prototype. Other family members include mescaline, dimethyltryptamine (DMT), psilocin, and salvia. The psychedelics are so named because of their ability to produce what has been termed a *psychedelic state.* Individuals in this state show an increased awareness of sensory stimuli and are likely to perceive the world around them as beautiful and harmonious; the normally insignificant may assume exceptional meaning, the "self" may seem split into an "observer" and a "doer," and boundaries between "self" and "nonself" may fade, producing a sense of unity with the cosmos.

Psychedelic drugs are often referred to as *hallucinogens* or *psychotomimetics.* These names reflect their ability to produce hallucinations as well as mental states that resemble psychoses.

Although psychedelics can cause hallucinations and psychotic-like states, these are not their most characteristic effects. The characteristic that truly distinguishes the psychedelics from other agents is their *ability to bring on the same types of alterations in thought, perception, and feeling that otherwise occur only in dreams.* In essence, the psychedelics seem able to activate mechanisms for dreaming without causing unconsciousness.

d-Lysergic Acid Diethylamide (LSD)

History

The first person to experience LSD was a Swiss chemist named Albert Hofmann. In 1943, 5 years after LSD was first synthesized, Hofmann accidentally ingested a minute amount of the drug. The result was a dream-like state accompanied by perceptual distortions and vivid hallucinations. The high potency and unusual actions of LSD led to speculation that it might provide a model for studying psychosis. Unfortunately, that speculation did not prove correct: Extensive research has shown that the effects of LSD cannot be equated with idiopathic psychosis. With the realization that LSD did not produce a "model psychosis," medical interest in the drug declined. Not everyone, however, lost interest; during the 1960s, nonmedical experimentation flourished. This widespread use caused substantial societal concern, and by 1970 LSD had been classified as a Schedule I substance. Nonetheless, street use of LSD continues.

Mechanism of Action

LSD acts at multiple sites in the brain and spinal cord. However, effects are most prominent in the cerebral cortex and the locus ceruleus. Effects are thought to result from activation of serotonin$_2$ receptors. This concept has been reinforced by the observation that *ritanserin,* a selective blocker of serotonin$_2$ receptors, can prevent the effects of LSD in animals.

Time Course

LSD is usually administered orally but can also be injected or smoked. With oral dosing, initial effects can be felt in minutes. Over the next few hours, responses become progressively more intense, and then subside 8 to 12 hours later.

Subjective and Behavioral Effects

Responses to LSD can be diverse, complex, and changeable. The drug can alter thinking, feeling, perception, sense of self, and sense of relationship with the environment and other people. LSD-induced experiences may be sublime or terrifying. Just what will be experienced during any particular "trip" cannot be predicted.

Perceptual alterations can be dramatic. Colors may appear iridescent or glowing, kaleidoscopic images may appear, and vivid hallucinations may occur. Sensory experiences may merge so that colors seem to be heard and sounds seem to be visible. Afterimages may occur, causing current perceptions to overlap with preceding perceptions. The LSD user may feel a sense of wonderment and awe at the beauty of commonplace things.

LSD can have a profound impact on affect. Emotions may range from elation, good humor, and euphoria to sadness, dysphoria, and fear. The intensity of emotion may be overwhelming.

Thoughts may turn inward. Attitudes may be re-evaluated, and old values assigned new priorities. A sense of new and important insight may be felt. However, despite the intensity of these experiences, enduring changes in beliefs, behavior, and personality are rare.

Physiologic Effects

LSD has few physiologic effects. Activation of the sympathetic nervous system can produce tachycardia, elevation of blood pressure, mydriasis, piloerection, and hyperthermia. Neuromuscular effects (tremor, incoordination, hyperreflexia, and muscular weakness) may also occur.

Tolerance and Dependence

Tolerance to LSD develops rapidly. Substantial tolerance can be seen after just three or four daily doses. Tolerance to subjective and behavioral effects develops to a greater extent than to cardiovascular effects. Cross-tolerance exists with mescaline and psilocybin, but not with DMT. Since DMT is similar to LSD, the absence of cross-tolerance is surprising. There is no cross-tolerance with amphetamines or THC. Upon cessation of LSD use, tolerance rapidly fades. Abrupt withdrawal of LSD is not associated with an abstinence syndrome. Hence there is no evidence for physical dependence.

Toxicity

Toxic reactions are primarily psychologic. LSD has never been a direct cause of death, although fatalities have occurred from accidents and suicides.

Acute panic reactions are relatively common and may be associated with a fear of disintegration of the self. Such "bad trips" can usually be managed by a process of "talking down" (providing emotional support and reassurance in a nonthreatening environment). Panic episodes can also be managed with an antianxiety agent, such as diazepam. Neuroleptics (e.g., haloperidol, chlorpromazine) may actually intensify the experience, and hence their use is questionable.

A small percentage of former LSD users experience episodic visual disturbances, referred to as *flashbacks* by users and *hallucinogen persisting perception disorder* (HPPD) by clinicians. These disturbances may manifest as geometric pseudohallucinations, flashes of color, or positive afterimages. Visual disturbances may be precipitated by several factors, including marijuana use, fatigue, stress, and anxiety. Phenothiazines exacerbate these experiences rather than providing relief. HPPD appears to be caused by permanent changes in the visual system.

In addition to panic reactions and visual disturbances, LSD can cause other adverse psychologic effects. Depressive episodes, dissociative reactions, and distortions of body image may occur. When an LSD experience has been intensely terrifying, the user may be left with persistent residual fear. The drug may also cause prolonged psychotic reactions. In contrast to acute effects, which differ substantially from symptoms of schizophrenia, prolonged psychotic reactions mimic schizophrenia faithfully.

Potential Therapeutic Uses

LSD has no recognized therapeutic applications. The drug has been evaluated in subjects with alcohol use disorder, opioid use disorder, and psychiatric disorders, including depression, anxiety, and obsessive-compulsive disorder. In addition, LSD has been studied as a possible means of promoting psychologic well-being in patients with terminal cancer. With the possible exception of some psychiatric disorders (e.g., depression, anxiety), LSD has proved either ineffective or impractical.

Salvia

Salvia divinorum is a hallucinogenic herb native to southern Mexico and to Central and South America. Its primary psychoactive component is *salvinorin A,* a potent activator of kappa opioid receptors. The genus *Salvia,* a part of the mint family, is commonly known as sage—hence the colorful street names for *S. divinorum:* Magic Mint, Diviner's Sage, and Sage of the Seers. Salvia is legal in some states, illegal in others, and not yet regulated under the Controlled Substances Act.

Salvia is used extensively in the United States, primarily by teens and young adults. In 2015, 1.8% of high school seniors reported using the drug in the past year. About 15% of Americans older than 12 years report having used a hallucinogen such as salvia at least once in their lives (https://www.drugabuse.gov/drugs-abuse/hallucinogens).

How is salvia administered? Among Mexican Indians, the traditional method is to chew the leaves or drink a liquid extract. In contrast, recreational users usually smoke the dried leaves, either in a pipe or rolled in a joint. When the smoke is inhaled, salvinorin A undergoes rapid absorption from the lungs. As a result, psychologic effects begin quickly (in less than 1 minute) and then quickly fade (typically in 5 to 10 minutes).

Like other psychedelic drugs, salvia induces a dream-like state of unreality. Users may lose awareness of their own bodies and of the room they are in. They may feel they are floating, traveling through time and space, or merging with or transforming into objects. Some feel they are being twisted or pulled. There may be a sense of overlapping realities and of being in several places at once. Speech may become slurred, and sentences may lack fluent structure. Uncontrollable laughter may break out. Possible physical effects include chills, dizziness, nausea, incoordination, and bradycardia. Whether saliva poses long-term health risks has not been studied. However, we do know that Mexican Indians have used the drug for generations, with no apparent ill effects.

Mescaline, Psilocin, Psilocybin, and Dimethyltryptamine

In addition to LSD and salvia, the family of psychedelic drugs includes mescaline, psilocin, psilocybin, DMT, and several related compounds. Some psychedelics are synthetic, and some occur naturally. DMT and LSD represent the synthetic compounds. Mescaline, a constituent of the peyote cactus, and psilocin and psilocybin, constituents of "magic mushrooms," represent compounds found in nature.

The subjective and behavioral effects of the miscellaneous psychedelic drugs are similar to those of LSD. Like LSD, these drugs can elicit modes of thought, perception, and feeling that are normally restricted to dreams. In addition, they can cause hallucinations and induce mental states that resemble psychosis.

The miscellaneous psychedelics differ from LSD with respect to potency and time course. LSD is the most potent of the psychedelics, producing its full spectrum of effects at doses as low as 0.5 mcg/kg. Psilocin and psilocybin are 100 times less potent than LSD, and mescaline is 4000 times less potent than LSD. Whereas the effects of LSD are prolonged (responses may last 12 or more hours), the effects of mescaline and DMT are shorter: Responses to mescaline usually fade within 8 to 12 hours, and responses to DMT fade within 1 to 2 hours.

None of these psychedelics is approved for medical use. The use of psilocybin in patients with terminal cancer and obsessive-compulsive disorder is under investigation.

DISSOCIATIVE DRUGS

The dissociative drugs—phencyclidine and ketamine—were originally developed as surgical anesthetics. When taken recreationally, these drugs distort perception of sight and sound, and produce feelings of dissociation (detachment) from the environment. High doses can produce sedation, immobility, analgesia, and amnesia.

Phencyclidine

Phencyclidine ("PCP," "angel dust," "peace pill") was originally developed as an anesthetic for animals. The drug was tried briefly as a general anesthetic for humans, but was withdrawn, owing to severe emergence delirium. Although rejected for therapeutic use, phencyclidine has become widely used as a drug of abuse, largely because it can be synthesized easily by amateur chemists, making it cheap and abundant. The popularity of phencyclidine is disturbing in that a high incidence of adverse effects makes phencyclidine one of the most dangerous drugs of abuse.

Chemistry and Pharmacokinetics

Chemistry. Phencyclidine is a weak organic base with high lipid solubility. The drug is chemically related to ketamine, an unusual general anesthetic (see Chapter 27 and later in this chapter).

Pharmacokinetics. Phencyclidine can be administered orally, intranasally, intravenously, and by smoking. For administration by smoking, the drug is usually sprinkled on plant matter (e.g., oregano, parsley, tobacco, marijuana). Because of its high lipid solubility, phencyclidine is readily absorbed from all sites.

Once absorbed, phencyclidine undergoes substantial gastroenteric recirculation. Because it is a base, phencyclidine in the blood can be drawn into the acidic environment of the stomach (by the pH partitioning effect); from the stomach, the drug reenters the intestine, from which it is reabsorbed into the blood. This cycling from blood to GI tract and back prolongs the drug's sojourn in the body. Elimination occurs eventually through a combination of hepatic metabolism and renal excretion.

Mechanism of Action

Phencyclidine acts in the cerebral cortex and limbic system, where it blocks a subset of receptors for glutamate, known as *N*-methyl-D-aspartate (NMDA) receptor complexes. These glutamate receptors are involved in multiple processes, including learning, memory, emotionality, and perception of pain.

Subjective and Behavioral Effects

Phencyclidine produces a unique set of effects. Hallucinations are prominent. In addition, the drug can produce CNS depression, CNS excitation, and analgesia.

Effects of Low to Moderate Doses. At low doses, phencyclidine produces effects like those of alcohol. Low-dose intoxication is characterized by euphoria, release of inhibitions, and emotional lability. Nystagmus, slurred speech, and motor incoordination may occur too.

As dosage increases, the clinical picture becomes more variable and complex. Symptoms include excitation, disorientation, anxiety, disorganized thoughts, altered body image, and reduced perception of tactile and painful stimuli. Mood may be volatile and hostile. Bizarre behavior may develop. Heart rate and blood pressure are elevated.

High-Dose (Toxic) Effects. High doses can cause severe adverse physiologic and psychologic effects. Death may result from several causes.

Psychologic effects include hallucinations, confusional states, combativeness, and psychosis. The psychosis closely resembles schizophrenia and may persist for weeks. Individuals with pre-existing psychoses are especially vulnerable to psychotogenic effects and may attempt suicide.

Physiologic effects of high-dose phencyclidine are varied. Extreme overdose can produce hypertension, coma, seizures, and muscular rigidity associated with severe hyperthermia and rhabdomyolysis (disintegration of muscle tissue).

Managing Toxicity. Treatment is primarily supportive. Psychotic reactions are best managed by isolation from external stimuli. "Talking down" is not effective, and the benefits of antipsychotic drugs, such as haloperidol, are limited. Physical restraint may be needed to prevent self-inflicted harm and to protect others from assault. If respiration is depressed, mechanical support of ventilation may be needed. Severe hypertension can be managed with nitroprusside, a vasodilator. Seizures can be controlled with IV diazepam. If fever is high, external cooling can lower temperature. By promoting muscle relaxation, dantrolene [Dantrium] can reduce heat generation and the risk of rhabdomyolysis.

Elimination of phencyclidine can be accelerated by continuous gastric lavage and by acidification of the urine with ammonium chloride. Continuous lavage is effective because gastroenteric recirculation keeps delivering drug to the stomach. Acidification of urine may promote phencyclidine excretion by reducing tubular reabsorption of this weak base.

Ketamine

Ketamine is a dissociative anesthetic used in animals and humans (see Chapter 27). The drug can also produce rapid relief of depression. Medicinal ketamine is formulated as an injectable liquid. For recreational use, the liquid is evaporated off, leaving a powder that can be snorted or ingested. Doses typically range from 50 to 200 mg. Much of the ketamine sold on the street was diverted from veterinary offices. Ketamine is regulated as a Schedule III substance.

Ketamine is similar to phencyclidine in structure, mechanism, and effects, although its duration of action is shorter. When the drug is snorted, effects begin in 5 to 15 minutes and persist about an hour. Moderate doses produce effects ranging from a dream-like state to a pleasant sensation of floating to a sense of being separated from one's body. Some users experience a state known as the *K-hole,* likened to a near-death experience in which there is a sense of rising above one's body. For some, the K-hole experience is accompanied by a sense of inner peace and radiant light. For others, the K-hole experience is characterized by a terrifying sense of nearly complete sensory detachment. At high doses, ketamine can cause hallucinations, delirium, amnesia, elevation of blood pressure, and potentially fatal disruption of respiration. Even higher doses can produce unconsciousness and fatal cardiovascular collapse.

Because of its depressant and amnesic effects, ketamine has been used to facilitate sexual assault. The drug is colorless, tasteless, and odorless, and hence can be added to a beverage without detection.

DEXTROMETHORPHAN

Dextromethorphan (DXM) is a cough suppressant widely available in over-the-counter cough and cold remedies (see Chapter 77). At the low doses needed for cough suppression, DXM is devoid of psychologic effects. However, at doses 5 to 10 times higher, DXM can cause euphoria, disorientation, paranoia, and altered sense of time, as well as visual, auditory, and tactile hallucinations. These effects are produced by dextrorphan, a metabolite of DXM that blocks receptors for NMDA. Note that this is the same mechanism used by phencyclidine and ketamine. Many of the products that contain DXM also contain other drugs, including acetaminophen, antihistamines, phenylephrine, and pseudoephedrine. Therefore, when excessive doses are taken, users are subject to toxicity from these compounds as well as from DXM itself. The principal users of DXM are adolescents and teenagers. Between 1999 and 2004, reports of DXM abuse in these groups rose 10-fold. Many products contain DXM, including Coricidin HBP Cough & Cold, Robitussin DM, and Vicks NyQuil Cough Syrup.

3,4-METHYLENEDIOXYMETHAMPHETAMINE (MDMA, ECSTASY)

MDMA, also known as "ecstasy," is a complex drug with stimulant and psychedelic properties. The drug is structurally related to methamphetamine (a stimulant) and mescaline (a hallucinogen). Low doses produce mild LSD-like psychedelic effects; higher doses produce amphetamine-like stimulant effects. These effects result from (1) blocking reuptake of serotonin and (2) promoting the release of serotonin, dopamine, and norepinephrine. Although MDMA can produce effects that are clearly pleasurable, it can also be dangerous; the biggest concerns are neurotoxicity, seizures, excessive cardiovascular stimulation, and hyperthermia and its sequelae. MDMA is classified as a Schedule I drug.

Time Course and Dosage

MDMA is usually dosed orally, but may also be snorted, injected, or inserted as a rectal suppository. With oral administration, effects begin in 20 minutes, peak in 2 to 3 hours, and persist 4 to 5 hours. The usual dose is 100 mg or less.

Who Uses MDMA and Why?

MDMA is used primarily by adolescents and young adults in cities, in the suburbs, and in rural areas. According to a survey conducted in 2015, the use of ecstasy in school-age children has continued to steadily decline.

Why do people take MDMA? Because it makes them feel very good. The drug can elevate mood, increase sensory awareness, and heighten sensitivity to music. It can also facilitate interpersonal relationships: Users report a sense of closeness with others, a lowering of defenses, reduced anxiety, enhanced communication, and increased sociability.

Adverse Effects

MDMA is not free of risks. The drug can injure serotonergic neurons, stimulate the heart, and raise body temperature to a dangerous level. In addition, it can cause neurologic effects (e.g., seizures, spasmodic jerking, jaw clenching, teeth grinding) and a host of adverse psychologic effects (e.g., confusion, anxiety, paranoia, panic attacks, visual hallucinations, and suicidal thoughts and behavior). Every year, MDMA is associated with several thousand admissions to emergency departments, mainly because of seizures.

MDMA can damage serotonergic neurons, perhaps irreversibly. When administered to rats and primates in doses only 2 to 4 times greater than those that produce hallucinations in humans, MDMA causes *irreversible destruction of serotonergic neurons,* resulting in passivity and insomnia. At least three lines of evidence suggest that MDMA is also neurotoxic in humans. First, MDMA causes dose-related impairment of memory, a brain function mediated in part by serotonin. Memory impairment persists long after MDMA was last taken. Second, the cerebrospinal fluid of long-term MDMA users contains abnormally low concentrations of serotonin metabolites, suggesting a loss of serotonergic neurons. And third, using positron emission tomography to study former MDMA users, researchers demonstrated decreased binding of a ligand selective for the serotonin transporter, indicating damage to serotonergic neurons. In this study, reductions in ligand binding correlated with the extent of MDMA use and not with the duration of abstinence.

MDMA can cause hyperthermia in association with dehydration, hyponatremia, and rhabdomyolysis. Treatment consists of rapid cooling, rehydration, and the administration of dantrolene [Dantrium], a drug that relaxes skeletal muscle, thereby reducing heat generation and the risk of rhabdomyolysis. The risk of hyperthermia and dehydration could be greatly reduced by providing ample fluids at dance parties known as "raves" and other events where MDMA is likely to be used.

Because of its amphetamine-like actions, MDMA can increase heart rate, blood pressure, and myocardial oxygen consumption. Remarkably, the increases in heart rate and blood pressure equal those produced by maximal doses of dobutamine, a powerful adrenergic agonist (see Chapter 17). Cardiovascular stimulation poses a special risk to users with heart disease.

Potential Medical Use

Despite its potential for adverse effects, MDMA also has the potential for therapeutic good, owing largely to its ability to decrease feelings of fear and defensiveness and promote feelings of love, trust, and compassion. Small clinical trials of MDMA for the treatment of post-traumatic stress disorder and in patients with severe anxiety related to terminal cancer were promising, revealing reduced fear of death and decreased anxiety in patients taking MDMA.

INHALANTS

The inhalants are a diverse group of drugs that have one characteristic in common: administration by inhalation. These drugs can be divided into three classes: anesthetics, volatile nitrites, and organic solvents.

Anesthetics

Provided that dosage is modest, anesthetics produce subjective effects similar to those of alcohol (euphoria, exhilaration, loss of inhibitions). The anesthetics that have been abused most are *nitrous oxide* ("laughing gas") and *ether.* One reason for the popularity of these drugs is ease of administration: Both agents can be used without exotic equipment. For nitrous oxide, ready availability also promotes use: Small cylinders of the drug, marketed for aerating whipping cream, can be purchased without restriction.

Volatile Nitrites

Four volatile nitrites—*amyl nitrite, butyl nitrite, isobutyl nitrite,* and *cyclohexyl nitrite*—are subject to abuse. These drugs are abused by homosexual males because of an ability to relax the anal sphincter, and by males in general because of a reputed ability to prolong and intensify sexual orgasm.

The most pronounced pharmacologic effect of volatile nitrites is *venodilation,* which causes a pooling of blood in veins, which in turn causes a profound drop in systolic blood pressure. The result is dizziness, light-headedness, palpitations, and possibly pulsatile headache. Effects begin seconds after inhalation and fade rapidly. The primary toxicity is methemoglobinemia, which can be treated with methylene blue and supplemental oxygen.

Nitrites are available from medical and nonmedical sources. Amyl nitrite is used for angina pectoris. Cyclohexyl nitrite is present in room odorizers. Butyl nitrite and isobutyl nitrite are present in products made solely for recreational use. On the street, preparations of amyl nitrite are known as "poppers" or "snappers." These terms reflect the popping sound made by amyl nitrite ampules when snapped open to allow inhalation.

Organic Solvents

A wide assortment of solvents have been inhaled to induce intoxication. These compounds include *toluene, gasoline, lighter fluid, paint thinner, nail-polish remover, benzene, acetone, chloroform,* and *model-airplane glue.* These agents are used primarily by children and the very poor—people who, because of age or insufficient funds, lack access to more conventional drugs of abuse. In recent years, the use of inhalants by young children and teens has been rising.

Administration

Solvents are administered by three processes, referred to as "bagging," "huffing," and "sniffing." Bagging is performed by pouring solvent in a bag and inhaling the vapor. Huffing is performed by pouring the solvent on a rag and inhaling the vapor. Sniffing is performed by inhaling the solvent directly from its container.

Acute Pharmacologic Effects

The acute effects of organic solvents are somewhat like those of alcohol (euphoria, impaired judgment, slurred speech, flushing, CNS depression). In addition, these compounds can cause visual hallucinations and disorientation with respect to time and place. High doses can result in sudden death. Possible causes include anoxia, respiratory depression, vagal stimulation (which slows heart rate), and dysrhythmias.

Chronic Toxicity

Prolonged use is associated with multiple toxicities. For example, chloroform is toxic to the heart, liver, and kidneys, and toluene can cause severe brain damage and bone marrow depression. Many solvents can damage the heart; fatal dysrhythmias have occurred secondary to drug-induced heart block.

Management

Management of acute toxicity is strictly supportive. The objective is to stabilize vital signs. We have no antidotes for volatile solvents.

ANABOLIC STEROIDS

Many athletes take anabolic steroids (androgens) to enhance athletic performance. The principal benefit is increased muscle mass and strength. Because of the massive doses that are employed, the risk of adverse effects is substantial. With long-term steroid use, a disorder develops. Because of their abuse potential, most androgens are now classified as Schedule III drugs. The basic pharmacology of androgens and their abuse by athletes are discussed in Chapter 65.

KEY POINTS

- Abuse of OxyContin and other opioid analgesics remains more common than abuse of heroin, although the use of heroin is increasing.
- Because heroin is very lipid soluble, initial effects are more intense and occur faster than with other opioids.
- With opioids, tolerance to respiratory depression develops in parallel with tolerance to euphoria. As a result, respiratory depression does not increase as higher doses are taken to produce desired subjective effects.
- Persons tolerant to one opioid are cross-tolerant to all other opioids.
- Although the opioid withdrawal syndrome can be extremely unpleasant, it is rarely dangerous.
- Opioid overdose produces a classic triad of symptoms: respiratory depression, coma, and pinpoint pupils. Death can result.
- Naloxone, an opioid antagonist, is the treatment of choice for opioid overdose.
- Naloxone dosage must be titrated carefully because too much naloxone will transport the patient from a state of intoxication to one of withdrawal. Also, since the half-life of naloxone is shorter than the half-lives of the opioids, naloxone must be administered repeatedly until the crisis is over.
- Because of cross-dependence, methadone can ease withdrawal symptoms in opioid-dependent individuals. To ease withdrawal, methadone is substituted for the abused opioid and then gradually tapered.
- For patients with opioid use disorder who are not ready for withdrawal, methadone can be used for maintenance therapy or for suppressive therapy. In maintenance therapy, the methadone dosage is equivalent to the dosage of the abused opioid, thereby preventing withdrawal. In suppressive therapy, the abuser is rendered opioid tolerant with very high doses of methadone; as a result, the use of street opioids can no longer produce subjective effects.

Continued

- Buprenorphine is an alternative to methadone for detoxification and maintenance of patients with opioid use disorder.
- In contrast to methadone, which is available only through approved Opioid Treatment Programs, buprenorphine can be prescribed in a primary care setting by any physician or nurse practitioner who has (1) received at least 8 hours of approved training and (2) registered with the Substance Abuse and Mental Health Services Administration.
- After a patient has undergone opioid detoxification, naltrexone, an opioid antagonist, can be used to discourage renewed opioid abuse.
- A sustained-release IM formulation of naltrexone can be dosed just once a month, unlike all other drugs for managing opioid use disorder, which must be dosed once a day.
- With barbiturates, tolerance develops to subjective effects but not to respiratory depression. As a result, as increasingly large doses are taken to produce subjective effects, the risk of serious respiratory depression increases. (Note that this differs from the situation with opioids.)
- Individuals who are tolerant to barbiturates show cross-tolerance with other CNS depressants (e.g., alcohol, benzodiazepines, general anesthetics) but not with opioids.
- Individuals who are physically dependent on barbiturates show cross-dependence with other CNS depressants, but not with opioids.
- When physical dependence on barbiturates (and other CNS depressants) is great, the associated abstinence syndrome can be severe—sometimes fatal. (Note that this differs from the situation with opioids.)
- Overdose with barbiturates produces the same triad of symptoms seen with opioids: respiratory depression, coma, and pinpoint pupils. Death can result.
- In contrast to opioid overdose, barbiturate overdose has no antidote, and hence treatment is only supportive.
- In contrast to overdose with opioids or barbiturates, overdose with benzodiazepines alone is rarely fatal.
- If necessary, benzodiazepine overdose can be treated with flumazenil, a benzodiazepine antagonist.
- The psychologic effects of cocaine result from activation of dopamine receptors secondary to cocaine-induced blockade of dopamine reuptake.
- Severe overdose with cocaine can produce hyperpyrexia, convulsions, ventricular dysrhythmias, and hemorrhagic stroke; death has occurred. Psychologic effects of overdose include severe anxiety, paranoid ideation, and hallucinations.
- There is no specific antidote to cocaine overdose. Intravenous diazepam can suppress anxiety, seizures, hypertension, and dysrhythmias. Intravenous nitroprusside or phentolamine can treat severe hypertension.
- In animals, regular use of cocaine produces sensitization—not tolerance. Whether this is true for humans is unclear.
- Whether cocaine causes significant physical dependence is in dispute.
- Psychosocial therapy is considered the cornerstone of treatment for cocaine use disorder. Adding disulfiram may also help.
- In addition to CNS stimulation, methamphetamine causes vasoconstriction and stimulates the heart. Cardiovascular stimulation may result in hypertension, angina, dysrhythmias, and stroke.
- Regular use of methamphetamine can produce a state that closely resembles paranoid schizophrenia.
- Although physical dependence on methamphetamine is only moderate, psychologic dependence can be intense. Withdrawal can produce dysphoria and a strong sense of craving.
- The major psychoactive substance in marijuana is delta-9-tetrahydrocannabinol (THC).
- THC produces its psychologic effects by activating cannabinoid receptors in the brain.
- Marijuana has three principal subjective effects: euphoria, sedation, and hallucinations.
- Physiologic effects of marijuana, as well as tolerance and physical dependence, are minimal.
- Marijuana has no approved medical uses, although THC and other purified cannabinoids do.
- Psychedelic drugs produce alterations in thought, perception, and feeling that otherwise occur only in dreams.
- Psychedelic drugs are also known as hallucinogens or psychotomimetics—names that reflect their ability to produce hallucinations and mental states that resemble psychosis.
- Lysergic acid diethylamide (LSD) can be considered the prototype of the psychedelic drugs.
- LSD produces its effects by activating serotonin$_2$ receptors in the brain.
- Although tolerance develops to LSD, physiologic effects and physical dependence are minimal.
- Acute panic reactions to LSD can be managed by "talking down" and by treatment with benzodiazepines. Neuroleptic drugs (e.g., haloperidol) may intensify the reaction.
- LSD users may experience episodic visual disturbances after discontinuing the drug. In many cases, the underlying cause is a permanent change in the visual system.
- Some LSD users experience prolonged psychotic reactions that closely resemble schizophrenia.
- Phencyclidine (PCP) is a dissociative anesthetic that produces alcohol-like effects at low doses and hallucinations and psychotic reactions at high doses.
- Extreme overdose with phencyclidine can produce hypertension, coma, and seizures, as well as muscular rigidity associated with severe hyperthermia and rhabdomyolysis.
- There is no specific antidote to phencyclidine overdose. "Talking down" is not effective, and antipsychotic drugs are of limited help.
- Ecstasy (MDMA) produces psychedelic effects at low doses and amphetamine-like stimulation at higher doses.
- Ecstasy can cause irreversible destruction of serotonergic neurons.

Please visit **http://evolve.elsevier.com/Lehne** for chapter-specific NCLEX® examination review questions.

UNIT VI

DRUGS THAT AFFECT FLUID AND ELECTROLYTE BALANCE

CHAPTER

41 Diuretics

Diuretics are drugs that increase the output of urine. These agents have two major applications: (1) treatment of hypertension and (2) mobilization of edematous fluid associated with heart failure, cirrhosis, or kidney disease. In addition, because of their ability to maintain urine flow, diuretics are used to prevent renal failure.

REVIEW OF RENAL ANATOMY AND PHYSIOLOGY

Understanding the diuretic drugs requires a basic knowledge of the anatomy and physiology of the kidney. Therefore, let's review these topics before discussing the diuretics themselves.

Anatomy

The basic functional unit of the kidney is the *nephron.* As indicated in Fig. 41.1, the nephron has four functionally distinct regions: (1) the *glomerulus,* (2) the *proximal convoluted tubule,* (3) the *loop of Henle,* and (4a, 4b) the *distal convoluted tubule.* All nephrons are oriented within the kidney such that the upper portion of Henle's loop is located in the renal cortex and the lower end of the loop descends toward the renal *medulla.* Without this orientation, the kidney could not produce concentrated urine.

In addition to the nephrons, the *collecting ducts* (the tubules into which the nephrons pour their contents) play a critical role in kidney function. The final segment of the distal convoluted tubule (4b) plus the collecting duct into which it empties (5) can be considered a single functional unit: the *distal nephron.*

Physiology

Overview of Kidney Functions

The kidney serves three basic functions: (1) cleansing of extracellular fluid (ECF) and maintenance of ECF volume and composition; (2) maintenance of acid-base balance; and (3) excretion of metabolic wastes and foreign substances (e.g., drugs, toxins). Of the three, maintenance of ECF volume and composition is the one that diuretics affect most.

The Three Basic Renal Processes

Effects of the kidney on ECF are the net result of three basic processes: (1) *filtration,* (2) *reabsorption,* and (3) *active secretion.* To cleanse the entire ECF, a huge volume of plasma must be filtered. Furthermore, to maintain homeostasis, practically everything that has been filtered must be reabsorbed—leaving behind only a small volume of urine for excretion.

Filtration. Filtration occurs at the *glomerulus* and is the first step in urine formation. Virtually all small molecules (electrolytes, amino acids, glucose, drugs, metabolic wastes) that are present in plasma undergo filtration. In contrast, cells and large molecules (lipids, proteins) remain behind in the blood. The most prevalent constituents of the filtrate are sodium ions and chloride ions. Bicarbonate ions and potassium ions are also present, but in smaller amounts.

The filtration capacity of the kidney is very large. Each minute the kidney produces 125 mL of filtrate, which adds up to 180 L/day. Since the total volume of ECF is only 12.5 L, the kidneys can process the equivalent of all the ECF in the body every 100 minutes. Hence, the ECF undergoes complete cleansing about 14 times each day.

Be aware that filtration is a *nonselective process* and therefore cannot regulate the composition of urine. Reabsorption and secretion—processes that display a significant degree of selectivity—are the primary determinants of what the urine ultimately contains. Of the two, reabsorption is by far the more important.

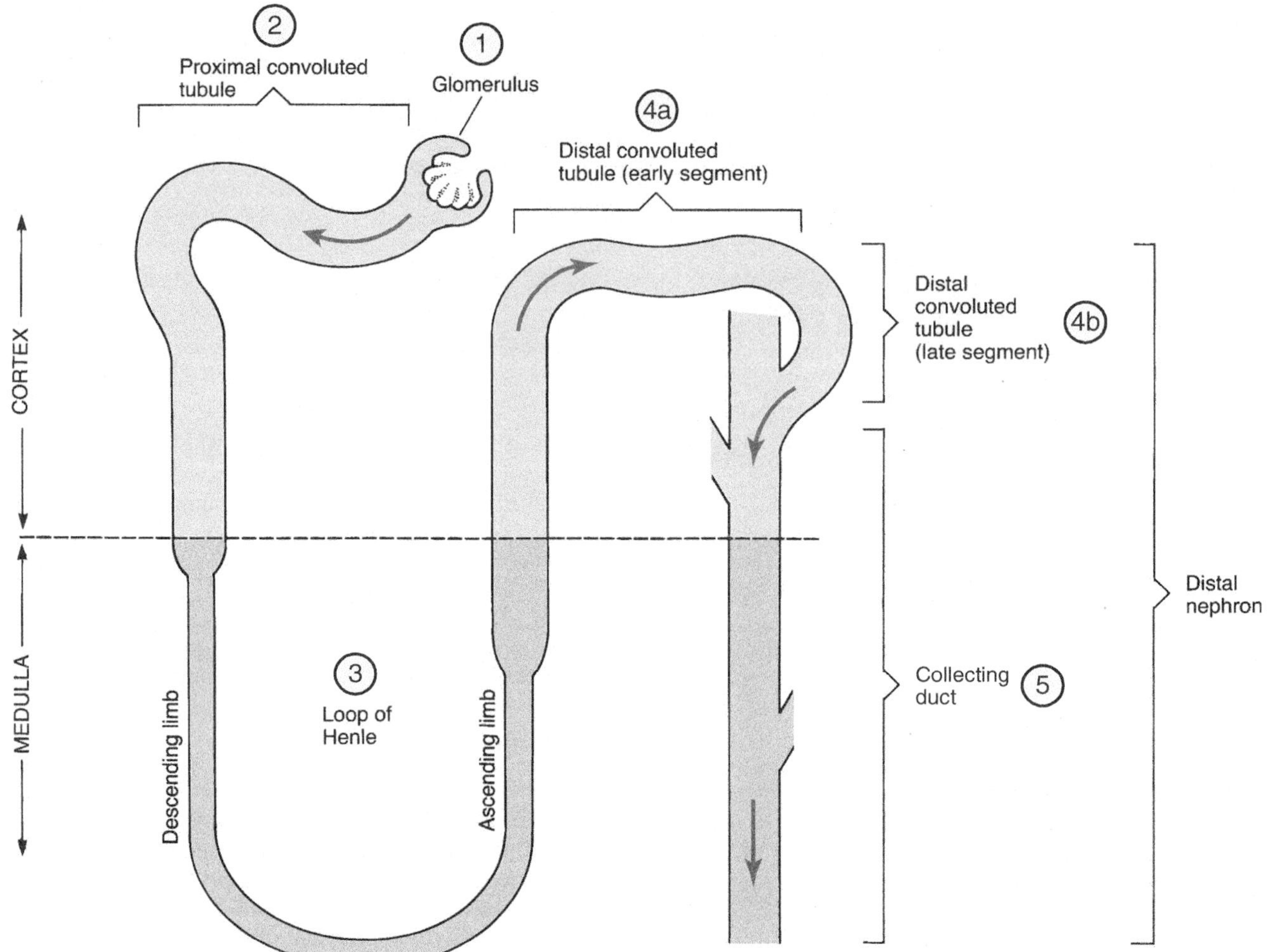

Fig. 41.1 ■ Schematic representation of a nephron and collecting duct.

Reabsorption. More than 99% of the water, electrolytes, and nutrients that are filtered at the glomerulus undergo reabsorption. This conserves valuable constituents of the filtrate while allowing wastes to undergo excretion. Reabsorption of solutes (e.g., electrolytes, amino acids, glucose) takes place by way of *active transport.* Water then follows passively along the osmotic gradient created by solute reuptake. Specific sites along the nephron at which reabsorption takes place are discussed later in this chapter. Diuretics work primarily by interfering with reabsorption.

Active Tubular Secretion. The kidney has two major kinds of "pumps" for active secretion. These pumps transport compounds from the plasma into the lumen of the nephron. One pump transports *organic acids* and the other transports *organic bases.* Together, these pumps can promote the excretion of a wide assortment of molecules, including metabolic wastes, drugs, and toxins. The pumps for active secretion are located in the *proximal convoluted tubule.*

Processes of Reabsorption That Occur at Specific Sites Along the Nephron

Because most diuretics act by disrupting solute reabsorption, to understand the diuretics, we must first understand the major processes by which nephrons reabsorb filtered solutes. Because sodium and chloride ions are the predominant solutes in the filtrate, reabsorption of these ions is of greatest interest. As we discuss reabsorption, numeric values are given for the percentage of solute reabsorbed at specific sites along the nephron. Bear in mind that these values are only approximate. Fig. 41.2 depicts the sites of sodium and chloride reabsorption, indicating the amount of reabsorption that occurs at each site.

Proximal Convoluted Tubule. The proximal convoluted tubule (PCT) has a high reabsorptive capacity. *A large fraction (about 65%) of filtered sodium and chloride is reabsorbed at the PCT.* In addition, essentially all of the bicarbonate and potassium in the filtrate is reabsorbed here. As sodium, chloride, and other solutes are actively reabsorbed, water follows passively. Since solutes and water are reabsorbed to an equal extent, the tubular urine remains isotonic (300 mOsm/L). By the time the filtrate leaves the PCT, sodium and chloride are the only solutes that remain in significant amounts.

Loop of Henle. The *descending limb* of the loop of Henle is freely permeable to water. Hence, as tubular urine moves down the loop and passes through the hypertonic environment of the renal medulla, water is drawn from the loop into the interstitial space. This process decreases the volume of the tubular urine and causes the urine to become concentrated (tonicity increases to about 1200 mOsm/L).

Within the thick segment of the *ascending limb* of the loop of Henle, about *20% of filtered sodium and chloride is*

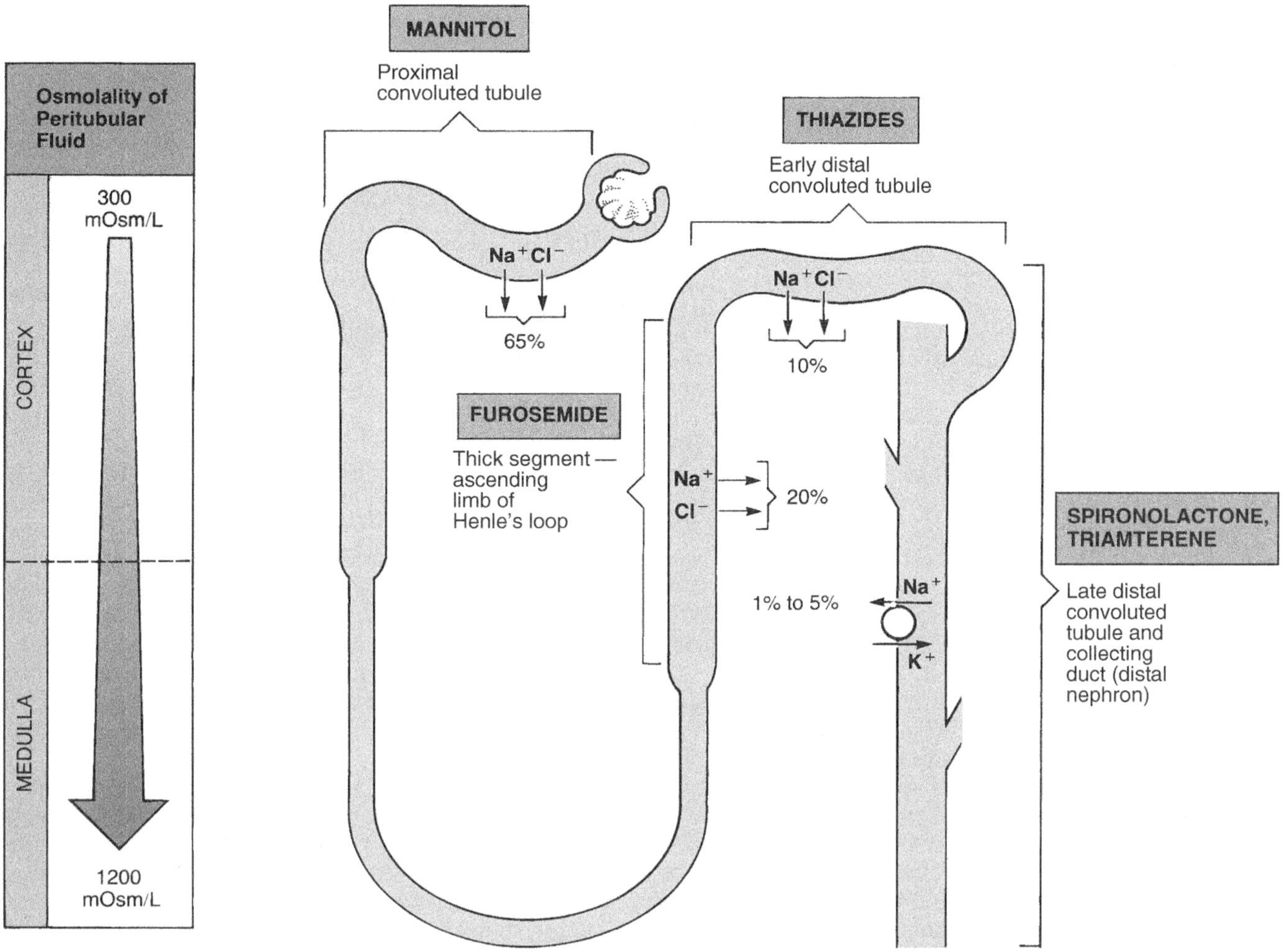

Fig. 41.2 ■ Schematic diagram of a nephron showing sites of sodium absorption and diuretic action.
The percentages indicate how much of the filtered sodium and chloride are reabsorbed at each site.

reabsorbed (see Fig. 41.2). Since, unlike the descending limb, the ascending limb is not permeable to water, water must remain in the loop as reabsorption of sodium and chloride takes place. This process causes the tonicity of the tubular urine to return to that of the original filtrate (300 mOsm/L).

Distal Convoluted Tubule (Early Segment). About 10% of filtered sodium and chloride is reabsorbed in the early segment of the distal convoluted tubule. Water follows passively.

Distal Nephron: Late Distal Convoluted Tubule and Collecting Duct. The distal nephron is the site of two important processes. The first involves exchange of sodium for potassium and is under the influence of aldosterone. The second determines the final concentration of the urine and is regulated by antidiuretic hormone (ADH). Although sodium-potassium exchange is discussed in more detail, we will not continue discussion of ADH, as it has little to do with the actions of diuretics.

Sodium-Potassium Exchange. Aldosterone, the principal mineralocorticoid of the adrenal cortex, stimulates reabsorption of sodium from the distal nephron. At the same time, aldosterone causes potassium to be secreted. Although not directly coupled, these two processes—sodium retention and potassium excretion—can be viewed as an exchange mechanism. This exchange is shown in Fig. 41.2. Aldosterone promotes sodium-potassium exchange by stimulating cells of the distal nephron to synthesize more of the pumps responsible for sodium and potassium transport.

Prototype Drugs

DIURETICS

Loop Diuretics
Furosemide

Thiazide Diuretics
Hydrochlorothiazide

Potassium-Sparing Diuretics
Spironolactone
Triamterene

INTRODUCTION TO DIURETICS

How Diuretics Work

Most diuretics share the same basic mechanism of action: blockade of sodium and chloride reabsorption. By blocking the reabsorption of these prominent solutes, diuretics create osmotic pressure within the nephron that prevents the passive reabsorption of water. Hence, diuretics cause water and solutes to be retained within the nephron and thereby promote the excretion of both.

The increase in urine flow that a diuretic produces is directly related to the amount of sodium and chloride reabsorption that it blocks. Accordingly, drugs that block solute reabsorption to the greatest degree produce the most profound diuresis. Since the amount of solute in the nephron becomes progressively smaller as filtrate flows from the proximal tubule to the collecting duct, *drugs that act early in the nephron have the opportunity to block the greatest amount of solute reabsorption. As a result, these agents produce the greatest diuresis.* Conversely, since most of the filtered solute has already been reabsorbed by the time the filtrate reaches the distal parts of the nephron, diuretics that act at distal sites have very little reabsorption available to block. Consequently, such agents produce relatively scant diuresis.

It is instructive to look at the quantitative relationship between blockade of solute reabsorption and production of diuresis. Recall that the kidneys produce 180 L of filtrate a day, practically all of which is normally reabsorbed. With filtrate production at this volume, a diuretic will increase daily urine output by 1.8 L for each 1% of solute reabsorption that is blocked. A 3% blockade of solute reabsorption will produce 5.4 L of urine a day—a rate of fluid loss that would reduce body weight by 12 pounds in 24 hours. Clearly, with only a small blockade of reabsorption, diuretics can produce a profound effect on the fluid and electrolyte composition of the body.

Adverse Impact on Extracellular Fluid

To promote excretion of water, diuretics must interfere with the normal operation of the kidney. By doing so, diuretics can cause *hypovolemia* (from excessive fluid loss), *acid-base imbalance,* and *altered electrolyte levels.* These adverse effects can be minimized by using short-acting diuretics and by timing drug administration such that the kidney is allowed to operate in a drug-free manner between periods of diuresis. Both measures will give the kidney periodic opportunities to readjust the ECF so as to compensate for any undesired alterations produced under the influence of diuretics.

Classification of Diuretics

There are four major categories of diuretic drugs: (1) *loop diuretics* (e.g., furosemide); (2) *thiazide diuretics* (e.g., hydrochlorothiazide); (3) *osmotic diuretics* (e.g., mannitol); and (4) *potassium-sparing diuretics.* The last group, the potassium-sparing agents, can be subdivided into *aldosterone antagonists* (e.g., spironolactone) and *nonaldosterone antagonists* (e.g., triamterene).

In addition to the four major categories of diuretics, there is a fifth group: the *carbonic anhydrase inhibitors.* Although the carbonic anhydrase inhibitors are classified as diuretics, these drugs are employed primarily to lower intraocular pressure (IOP) and not to increase urine production. Consequently, the carbonic anhydrase inhibitors are discussed in Chapter 104.

LOOP DIURETICS

The loop agents are the most effective diuretics available. These drugs produce more loss of fluid and electrolytes than any other diuretics. They are known as *loop diuretics* because their site of action is in the loop of Henle.

Furosemide

Furosemide [Lasix] is the most frequently prescribed loop diuretic and will serve as our prototype for the group.

Mechanism of Action

Furosemide acts in the thick segment of the ascending limb of Henle's loop to block reabsorption of sodium and chloride (see Fig. 41.2). By blocking solute reabsorption, furosemide prevents passive reabsorption of water. Since a substantial amount (20%) of filtered NaCl is normally reabsorbed in the loop of Henle, interference with reabsorption here can produce profound diuresis.

Pharmacokinetics

Furosemide can be administered orally, IV, and IM. With oral administration, diuresis begins in 60 minutes and persists for 8 hours. Oral therapy is used when rapid onset is not required. Effects of IV furosemide begin within 5 minutes and last for 2 hours. Intravenous therapy is used in critical situations (e.g., pulmonary edema) that demand immediate mobilization of fluid. Furosemide undergoes hepatic metabolism followed by renal excretion.

Therapeutic Uses

Furosemide is a powerful drug that is generally reserved for situations that require rapid or massive mobilization of fluid. This drug should be avoided when less efficacious diuretics (thiazides) will suffice. Conditions that justify use of furosemide include (1) pulmonary edema associated with congestive heart failure (CHF); (2) edema of hepatic, cardiac, or renal origin that has been unresponsive to less efficacious diuretics; and (3) hypertension that cannot be controlled with other diuretics. Furosemide is especially useful in patients with severe renal impairment, since, unlike the thiazides (see later in the chapter), the drug can promote diuresis even when renal blood flow and glomerular filtration rate (GFR) are low. If treatment with furosemide alone is insufficient, a thiazide diuretic may be added to the regimen. There is no benefit to combining furosemide with another loop diuretic.

Adverse Effects

Hyponatremia, Hypochloremia, and Dehydration. Furosemide can produce excessive loss of sodium, chloride, and water. Severe dehydration can result. Signs of evolving dehydration include dry mouth, unusual thirst, and oliguria (scanty urine output). Impending dehydration can also be anticipated from excessive loss of weight. If dehydration occurs, furosemide should be withheld.

Dehydration can promote thrombosis and embolism. Symptoms include headache and pain in the chest, calves, or pelvis. The prescriber should be notified if these develop.

The risk of dehydration and its sequelae can be minimized by initiating therapy with low doses, adjusting the dosage carefully, monitoring weight loss every day, and administering furosemide on an intermittent schedule.

Safety Alert

FUROSEMIDE

Use of furosemide can produce excessive loss of sodium, chloride, and water. Severe dehydration can result. Dehydration can promote hypotension, thrombosis, and embolism.

Hypotension. Furosemide can cause a substantial drop in blood pressure. At least two mechanisms are involved: (1) loss of volume and (2) relaxation of venous smooth muscle, which reduces venous return to the heart. Signs of hypotension include dizziness, light-headedness, and fainting. If blood pressure falls precipitously, furosemide should be discontinued. Because of the risk of hypotension, blood pressure should be monitored routinely.

Outpatients should be taught to monitor their blood pressure and instructed to notify the prescriber if it drops substantially. Also, patients should be informed about symptoms of postural hypotension (dizziness, light-headedness) and advised to sit or lie down if these occur. Patients should be taught that postural hypotension can be minimized by rising slowly.

Hypokalemia. Potassium is lost through increased secretion in the distal nephron. If serum potassium falls below 3.5 mEq/L, fatal dysrhythmias may result. As discussed later under *Drug Interactions,* loss of potassium is of special concern for patients taking digoxin, a drug for heart failure. Hypokalemia can be minimized by consuming potassium-rich foods (e.g., dried fruits, nuts, spinach, potatoes, bananas), taking potassium supplements, or using a potassium-sparing diuretic.

Ototoxicity. Rarely, loop diuretics cause hearing impairment. With furosemide, deafness is transient. With ethacrynic acid (another loop diuretic), irreversible hearing loss may occur. The ability to impair hearing is unique to the loop diuretics. Diuretics in other classes are not ototoxic. Because of the risk of hearing loss, caution is needed when loop diuretics are used in combination with other ototoxic drugs (e.g., aminoglycoside antibiotics).

Hyperglycemia. Elevation of plasma glucose is a potential, albeit uncommon, complication of furosemide therapy. Hyperglycemia appears to result from inhibition of insulin release. Increased glycogenolysis and decreased glycogen synthesis may also contribute. When furosemide is taken by a diabetic patient, he or she should be especially diligent about monitoring blood glucose content.

Hyperuricemia. Elevation of plasma uric acid is a frequent side effect of treatment. For most patients, furosemide-induced hyperuricemia is asymptomatic. However, for patients predisposed to gout, elevation of uric acid may precipitate a gouty attack. Patients should be informed about symptoms of gout (tenderness or swelling in joints) and instructed to notify the prescriber if these develop.

Use in Pregnancy. When administered to pregnant laboratory animals, loop diuretics have caused maternal death, abortion, fetal resorption, and other adverse effects. There are no definitive studies on loop diuretics during human pregnancy. However, given the toxicity displayed in animals, prudence dictates that pregnant patients use these drugs only if absolutely required.

Impact on Lipids, Magnesium, and Calcium. Furosemide reduces high-density lipoprotein (HDL) cholesterol and raises low-density lipoprotein (LDL) cholesterol and triglycerides. Although these undesirable effects by themselves can increase the risk of coronary heart disease, they are more than balanced by the beneficial effects of the diuretic therapy on the heart. That is, despite adverse effects on lipids, loop diuretics reduce the risk of coronary mortality by 25%.

Furosemide increases urinary excretion of magnesium, posing a risk of magnesium deficiency. Symptoms include muscle weakness, tremor, twitching, and dysrhythmias.

Furosemide increases urinary excretion of calcium. This action has been exploited to treat hypercalcemia.

PATIENT-CENTERED CARE ACROSS THE LIFE SPAN

Diuretics

Life Stage	Patient Care Concerns
Infants	See "Breast-feeding women," below.
Children/adolescents	Diuretics can be used safely in children, just in smaller doses. Side effect profiles are similar to those for adults.
Pregnant women	Animal studies revealed that furosemide can cause maternal death, abortion, and fetal resorption. Risks and benefits must be considered for administration during pregnancy.
Breast-feeding women	Furosemide may decrease breast milk production through excessive diuresis. Data are lacking regarding transmission of drug from mother to infant via breast milk.
Older adults	Diuretics are the most common cause of adverse medication reactions and interactions in older adults. Monitor closely for dehydration and cardiac dysrhythmias.

Drug Interactions

Digoxin. Digoxin is used for heart failure (see Chapter 48) and cardiac dysrhythmias (see Chapter 49). In the presence of low potassium, the risk of serious digoxin-induced toxicity (ventricular dysrhythmias) is greatly increased. Because loop diuretics promote potassium loss, the use of these drugs in combination with digoxin can increase the risk of dysrhythmia. This interaction is unfortunate in that most patients who take digoxin for heart failure must also take a diuretic as well. To reduce the risk of toxicity, potassium levels should be monitored routinely; when indicated, potassium supplements or a potassium-sparing diuretic should be given.

Ototoxic Drugs. The risk of furosemide-induced hearing loss is increased by concurrent use of other ototoxic drugs—especially aminoglycoside antibiotics (e.g., gentamicin). Accordingly, combined use of these drugs should be avoided.

Potassium-Sparing Diuretics. The potassium-sparing diuretics (e.g., spironolactone, triamterene) can help counterbalance the potassium-wasting effects of furosemide, thereby reducing the risk of hypokalemia.

Lithium. Lithium is used to treat bipolar disorder (see Chapter 33). In patients with low sodium, excretion of lithium is reduced. Hence, by lowering sodium levels, furosemide can cause lithium to accumulate to toxic levels. Accordingly, lithium levels should be monitored; if they climb too high, lithium dosage should be reduced.

Antihypertensive Agents. The hypotensive effects of furosemide add to those of other hypotensive drugs. To avoid excessive reduction of blood pressure, patients may need to reduce or eliminate the use of other hypotensive medications.

Nonsteroidal Anti-Inflammatory Drugs (NSAIDs). Aspirin and other NSAIDs can attenuate the diuretic effects of furosemide. The mechanism appears to be inhibition of prostaglandin synthesis in the kidney. Part of the diuretic effect of furosemide results from increasing renal blood flow, which is thought to occur through a prostaglandin-mediated process. By inhibiting prostaglandin synthesis, NSAIDs prevent the increase in renal blood flow and thereby partially blunt diuretic effects.

Preparations, Dosage, and Administration

Oral. Furosemide [Lasix] is available in tablets (20, 40, and 80 mg) and in solution (10 mg/mL, 40 mg/5 mL) for oral use. The initial dosage for adults is 20 to 80 mg/day as a single dose. The maximum daily dosage is 600 mg. Twice-daily dosing (8:00 AM and 2:00 PM) is common. Dosing late in the day produces nocturia and should be avoided.

Parenteral. Furosemide is available in solution (10 mg/mL) for IV and IM administration. The usual dosage for adults is 20 to 40 mg, repeated in 1 or 2 hours if needed. Intravenous administration should be done slowly (over 1 to 2 minutes). For high-dose therapy, furosemide can be administered by continuous infusion at a rate of 4 mg/min or slower.

Other Loop Diuretics

In addition to furosemide, three other loop diuretics are available: *ethacrynic acid* [Edecrin], *torsemide* [Demadex], and *bumetanide* [Burinex 🍁, generic only in United States]. All three are much like furosemide. They all promote diuresis by inhibiting sodium and chloride reabsorption in the thick ascending limb of the loop of Henle. All are approved for edema caused by heart failure, chronic renal disease, and cirrhosis, but only torsemide, like furosemide, is also approved for hypertension. All can cause ototoxicity, hypovolemia, hypotension, hypokalemia, hyperuricemia, hyperglycemia, and disruption of lipid metabolism, specifically, reduction of HDL cholesterol and elevation of LDL cholesterol and triglycerides. Lastly, they all share the same drug interactions: Their effects can be blunted by NSAIDs, they can intensify ototoxicity caused by aminoglycosides, they can increase cardiotoxicity caused by digoxin, and they can cause lithium to accumulate to toxic levels. Routes, dosages, and time courses are shown in Table 41.1.

THIAZIDES AND RELATED DIURETICS

The thiazide diuretics (also known as benzothiadiazides) have effects similar to those of the loop diuretics. Like the loop diuretics, thiazides increase renal excretion of sodium, chloride, potassium, and water. In addition, thiazides elevate plasma levels of uric acid and glucose. The principal difference between the thiazides and loop diuretics is that the maximum diuresis produced by the thiazides is considerably lower than the maximum diuresis produced by the loop diuretics. In addition, whereas loop diuretics can be effective even when urine flow is decreased, thiazides cannot.

Hydrochlorothiazide

Hydrochlorothiazide is the most widely used thiazide diuretic and will serve as our prototype for the group. Because of its use in hypertension, a very common disorder, hydrochlorothiazide is one of our most widely used drugs.

Mechanism of Action

Hydrochlorothiazide promotes urine production by blocking the reabsorption of sodium and chloride in the *early segment of the distal convoluted tubule* (see Fig. 41.2). Retention of sodium and chloride in the nephron causes water to be retained as well, thereby producing an increased flow of urine. Because only 10% of filtered sodium and chloride is normally reabsorbed at the site where thiazides act, the maximum urine flow these drugs can produce is lower than with the loop diuretics.

The ability of thiazides to promote diuresis is dependent on adequate kidney function. These drugs are ineffective when GFR is low (less than 15 to 20 mL/min). Hence, in contrast to the loop diuretics, thiazides cannot be used to promote fluid loss in patients with severe renal impairment.

Pharmacokinetics

Diuresis begins about 2 hours after oral administration. Effects peak within 4 to 6 hours and may persist up to 12 hours. Most of the drug is excreted unchanged in the urine.

Therapeutic Uses

Essential Hypertension. The primary indication for hydrochlorothiazide is hypertension, a condition for which thiazides are often drugs of first choice. For many hypertensive patients, blood pressure can be controlled with a thiazide alone, although many other patients require multiple-drug therapy. The role of thiazides in hypertension is discussed in Chapter 47.

Edema. Thiazides are preferred drugs for mobilizing edema associated with mild to moderate heart failure. They are also given to mobilize edema associated with hepatic or renal disease.

Diabetes Insipidus. Diabetes insipidus is a rare condition characterized by excessive production of urine. In patients with this disorder, thiazides reduce urine production by 30% to 50%. The mechanism of this paradoxical effect is unclear.

Protection Against Postmenopausal Osteoporosis. Thiazides promote tubular reabsorption of calcium and may thereby decrease the risk of osteoporosis in postmenopausal women. Here's how. Before menopause, estrogen from the ovaries acts on renal tubules to promote calcium reabsorption. When menopause occurs, estrogen levels drop, allowing renal excretion of calcium to increase. The resultant decrease in circulating calcium promotes mobilization of calcium from bone and thereby increases the risk of osteoporosis. Because thiazides promote renal calcium retention, they may counteract the calcium loss associated with menopause and may thereby help preserve bone integrity.

TABLE 41.1 ■ Loop Diuretics: Routes, Time Course, and Dosage

		Time Course			
Drug	**Route**	**Onset (min)**	**Duration (hr)**	**Dosage (mg)**	**Doses/Day**
Furosemide [Lasix]	Oral	Within 60	6–8	20–80	1–2
	IV or IM	Within 5	2	20–40	1–2
Ethacrynic acid [Edecrin]	Oral	Within 30	6–8	50–100	1–2
	IV	Within 5	2	50	1–2
Bumetanide [Burinex 🍁, generic only in United States]	Oral	30–60	4–6	0.5–2	1
	IV	Within a few	0.5–1	0.5–1	1–3
Torsemide [Demadex]	Oral	Within 60	6–8	5–20	1
	IV	Within 10	6–8	5–20	1

TABLE 41.2 ▪ Thiazides and Related Diuretics: Dosages and Time Course of Effects

Generic Name	Brand Name	Time Course: Onset (hr)	Time Course: Duration (hr)	Optimal Oral Adult Dosage (mg/day)
THIAZIDES				
Chlorothiazide	Diuril	1–2	6–12	500–1000
Hydrochlorothiazide	Microzide	2	6–12	12.5–25
Methyclothiazide	Enduron	2	24	2.5–5
RELATED DRUGS				
Chlorthalidone	Thalitone	2	24–72	50–100
Indapamide	Lozide 🍁, generic only in the United States	1–2	Up to 36	2.5–5
Metolazone	Generic only	1	12–24	2.5–20

Adverse Effects

The adverse effects of thiazide diuretics are similar to those of the loop diuretics. In fact, with the exception that thiazides are not ototoxic, the adverse effects of the thiazides and loop diuretics are nearly identical.

Hyponatremia, Hypochloremia, and Dehydration. Loss of sodium, chloride, and water can lead to hyponatremia, hypochloremia, and dehydration. However, since the diuresis produced by thiazides is moderate, these drugs have a smaller impact on sodium, chloride, and water than do the loop diuretics. To evaluate fluid and electrolyte status, electrolyte levels should be determined periodically, and the patient should be weighed on a regular basis.

Hypokalemia. Like the loop diuretics, the thiazides can cause hypokalemia from excessive potassium excretion. As noted, potassium loss is of particular concern for patients taking digoxin. Potassium levels should be measured periodically; if serum potassium falls below 3.5 mEq/L, treatment with potassium supplements or a potassium-sparing diuretic should be instituted. Hypokalemia can be minimized by eating potassium-rich foods.

Hyperglycemia. Like the loop diuretics, the thiazides can elevate plasma levels of glucose. Significant hyperglycemia develops only in diabetic patients, who should be especially diligent about monitoring blood glucose. To maintain normal glucose levels, the diabetic patient may require larger doses of insulin or an oral hypoglycemic drug.

Hyperuricemia. The thiazides, like the loop diuretics, can cause retention of uric acid, thereby elevating plasma uric acid. Although hyperuricemia is usually asymptomatic, it may precipitate gouty arthritis in patients with a history of the disorder. Plasma levels of uric acid should be measured periodically.

Impact on Lipids and Magnesium. Thiazides can increase levels of LDL cholesterol, total cholesterol, and triglycerides. Thiazides increase excretion of magnesium, sometimes causing magnesium deficiency. Symptoms include muscle weakness, tremor, twitching, and dysrhythmias.

Drug Interactions

The important drug interactions of the thiazides are nearly identical to those of the loop diuretics. By promoting potassium loss, thiazides can increase the risk of toxicity from *digoxin.* By lowering blood pressure, thiazides can augment the effects of other *antihypertensive drugs.* By promoting sodium loss, thiazides can reduce renal excretion of *lithium,* thereby causing the drug to accumulate, possibly to toxic levels. *NSAIDs* may blunt the diuretic effects of thiazides. By counterbalancing the potassium-wasting effects of the thiazides, the *potassium-sparing diuretics* can help prevent excessive potassium loss. In contrast to the loop diuretics, the thiazides can be combined with *ototoxic agents* without an increased risk of hearing loss.

Preparations, Dosage, and Administration

Hydrochlorothiazide is supplied in capsules (12.5 mg) and tablets (12.5, 25, and 50 mg). Like most other thiazides, hydrochlorothiazide is administered only by mouth. The usual adult dosage is 25 to 50 mg once or twice daily. To minimize nocturia, the drug should not be administered late in the day. To minimize electrolyte imbalance, the drug should be administered on an intermittent basis (e.g., every other day). In addition to being marketed alone, hydrochlorothiazide is available in fixed-dose combinations with potassium-sparing diuretics and a long list of other drugs: beta blockers, angiotensin-converting enzyme inhibitors, angiotensin receptor blockers, calcium channel blockers, hydralazine, clonidine, and methyldopa (see Chapter 47).

Other Thiazide-Type Diuretics

In addition to hydrochlorothiazide, five other thiazides (and related drugs) are approved for use in the United States (Table 41.2). All have pharmacologic properties similar to those of hydrochlorothiazide. With the exception of chlorothiazide, these drugs are administered only by mouth. Chlorothiazide can be administered IV as well as PO. Although the thiazides differ from one another in milligram potency (see Table 41.2), at therapeutically equivalent doses, all elicit the same degree of diuresis. Although most have the same onset time (1 to 2 hours), these drugs differ significantly with respect to duration of action. As with hydrochlorothiazide, disturbance of electrolyte balance can be minimized through alternate-day dosing. Nocturia can be minimized by avoiding dosing in the late afternoon. Table 41.2 lists three drugs—chlorthalidone, indapamide, and metolazone—that are not true thiazides. However, these agents are very similar to thiazides both in structure and function, and hence are included in the group.

POTASSIUM-SPARING DIURETICS

The potassium-sparing diuretics can elicit two potentially useful responses. First, they produce a modest increase in urine production. Second, they produce a substantial *decrease in potassium excretion.* Because their diuretic effects are limited, the potassium-sparing drugs are rarely employed alone to promote diuresis. However, because of their marked ability to decrease potassium excretion, these drugs are often used to counteract potassium loss caused by thiazide and loop diuretics.

There are two subcategories of potassium-sparing diuretics: *aldosterone antagonists* and *nonaldosterone antagonists.* In the United States, only one aldosterone antagonist—spironolactone—is used for diuresis.[a] Two nonaldosterone

[a]Another aldosterone antagonist—*eplerenone* [Inspra]—is available, but the drug is not considered a diuretic. The basic pharmacology of eplerenone and its main use, heart failure, are discussed in Chapters 44 and 47, respectively.

TABLE 41.3 ■ Potassium-Sparing Diuretics: Names, Dosages, and Time Course of Effects

Generic Name	Brand Name	Time Course: Onset (hr)	Time Course: Duration (hr)	Usual Adult Dosage (mg/day)
Spironolactone	Aldactone	24–48	48–72	25–200
Triamterene	Dyrenium	2–4	12–16	50–300
Amiloride	Midamor	2	24	5–20

antagonists—triamterene and amiloride—are currently employed.

Spironolactone

Mechanism of Action

Spironolactone [Aldactone] blocks the actions of aldosterone in the distal nephron. Since aldosterone acts to promote sodium uptake in exchange for potassium secretion (see Fig. 41.2), inhibition of aldosterone has the opposite effect: *retention of potassium and increased excretion of sodium.* The diuresis caused by spironolactone is scanty because most of the filtered sodium load has already been reabsorbed by the time the filtrate reaches the distal nephron. (Recall that the degree of diuresis a drug produces is directly proportional to the amount of sodium reuptake that it blocks.)

The effects of spironolactone are delayed, taking up to 48 hours to develop (Table 41.3). Recall that aldosterone acts by stimulating cells of the distal nephron to synthesize the proteins required for sodium and potassium transport. By preventing aldosterone's action, spironolactone blocks the synthesis of *new* proteins, but does not stop existing transport proteins from doing their job. Therefore, effects are not visible until the existing proteins complete their normal life cycle—a process that takes 1 or 2 days.

Therapeutic Uses

Hypertension and Edema. Spironolactone is used primarily for hypertension and edema. Although it can be employed alone, the drug is used most commonly in combination with a thiazide or loop diuretic. The purpose of spironolactone in these combinations is to counteract the potassium-wasting effects of the more powerful diuretics. Spironolactone also makes a small contribution to diuresis.

Heart Failure. In patients with severe heart failure, spironolactone reduces mortality and hospital admissions. Benefits derive from protective effects of aldosterone blockade in the heart and blood vessels (see Chapter 48).

Other Uses. In addition to the applications already discussed, spironolactone can be used for primary hyperaldosteronism (see Chapter 60), premenstrual syndrome (see Chapter 61), polycystic ovary syndrome (see Chapter 63), and acne in young women (see Chapter 105).

Adverse Effects

Hyperkalemia. The potassium-sparing effects of spironolactone can result in hyperkalemia, a condition that can produce fatal dysrhythmias. Although hyperkalemia is most likely when spironolactone is used alone, it can also develop when spironolactone is used in conjunction with potassium-wasting agents (thiazides and loop diuretics). If serum potassium rises above 5 mEq/L or if signs of hyperkalemia develop (e.g., abnormal heart rhythm), spironolactone should be discontinued and potassium intake restricted. Injection of insulin can help lower potassium levels by promoting potassium uptake into cells.

Endocrine Effects. Spironolactone is a steroid derivative with a structure similar to that of steroid hormones (e.g., progesterone, estradiol, testosterone). As a result, spironolactone can cause a variety of endocrine effects, including *gynecomastia, menstrual irregularities, impotence, hirsutism,* and *deepening of the voice.*

Benign and Malignant Tumors. When given long term to rats in doses 25 to 250 times those used in humans, spironolactone has caused benign adenomas of the thyroid and testes, malignant mammary tumors, and proliferative changes in the liver. The risk of tumors in humans from use of normal doses is unknown.

Drug Interactions

Thiazide and Loop Diuretics. Spironolactone is frequently combined with thiazide and loop diuretics. The goal is to counteract the potassium-wasting effects of the more powerful diuretic.

Agents That Raise Potassium Levels. Because of the risk of hyperkalemia, caution must be employed when combining spironolactone with potassium supplements, salt substitutes (which contain potassium chloride), or another potassium-sparing diuretic. In addition, three groups of drugs—angiotensin-converting enzyme (ACE) inhibitors, angiotensin receptor blockers, and direct renin inhibitors—can elevate potassium levels (by suppressing aldosterone secretion), and hence should be combined with spironolactone only when clearly necessary.

Preparations, Dosage, and Administration

Spironolactone [Aldactone] is dispensed in tablets (25, 50, and 100 mg) for oral dosing. The usual adult dosage is 25 to 100 mg/day. Spironolactone is also marketed in a fixed-dose combination with hydrochlorothiazide under the brand name *Aldactazide*.

Safe Handling and Administration. In 2016, the National Institute for Occupational Safety and Health (NIOSH), a division of the Centers for Disease Control and Prevention, published a list of drugs considered to be potentially hazardous in healthcare settings. Spironolactone was included in this list secondary to its potential to cause fetal harm. Exposure to these drugs can pose a reproductive risk to healthcare workers who administer these drugs. To promote safe administration, NIOSH suggests donning a protective gown and two sets of gloves when cutting or crushing tablets. For further information on this report, visit https://www.cdc.gov/niosh/topics/antineoplastic/pdf/hazardous-drugs-list_2016-161.pdf.

Triamterene

Mechanism of Action

Like spironolactone, triamterene [Dyrenium] disrupts sodium-potassium exchange in the distal nephron. However, in contrast to spironolactone, which reduces ion transport *indirectly* through blockade of aldosterone, triamterene is a *direct inhibitor of the exchange mechanism itself.* The net effect of inhibition is a decrease in sodium reabsorption and a reduction in potassium secretion. Hence, sodium excretion is increased, while potassium is conserved. Because it inhibits ion transport directly, triamterene acts much more quickly than spironolactone. Initial responses develop in hours, compared with days for spironolactone. As with spironolactone, diuresis with triamterene is minimal.

Therapeutic Uses

Triamterene can be used alone or in combination with other diuretics to treat *hypertension* and *edema.* When used alone, triamterene produces mild diuresis. When combined with other diuretics (e.g., furosemide, hydrochlorothiazide), triamterene augments diuresis and helps counteract the potassium-wasting effects of the more powerful diuretic. It is the latter effect for which triamterene is principally employed.

Adverse Effects

Hyperkalemia. Excessive potassium accumulation is the most significant adverse effect. Hyperkalemia is most likely when triamterene is used alone, but can also occur when the drug is combined with thiazides or loop diuretics. Caution should be employed when triamterene is used in conjunction with another potassium-sparing diuretic or with potassium supplements or salt substitutes. In addition, caution is needed if the drug is combined with an ACE inhibitor, angiotensin receptor blocker, or direct renin inhibitor.

Other Adverse Effects. Relatively common side effects include *nausea, vomiting, leg cramps,* and *dizziness.* Blood dyscrasias occur rarely.

Preparations, Dosage, and Administration

Triamterene [Dyrenium] is available in 50- and 100-mg capsules for oral use. The usual initial dosage is 100 mg twice a day. The maximum dosage is 300 mg/day. Triamterene is also marketed in fixed-dose combinations with hydrochlorothiazide under the brand names *Dyazide* and *Maxzide.*

Amiloride

Pharmacologic Properties

Amiloride has actions similar to those of triamterene. Both drugs inhibit potassium loss by direct blockade of sodium-potassium exchange in the distal nephron. Also, both drugs produce only modest diuresis. Although it can be employed alone as a diuretic, amiloride is used primarily to counteract potassium loss caused by more powerful diuretics (thiazides, loop diuretics). The major adverse effect is hyperkalemia. Accordingly, concurrent use of other potassium-sparing diuretics or potassium supplements must be monitored closely. Caution is needed if the drug is combined with an ACE inhibitor, angiotensin receptor blocker, or direct renin inhibitor.

Preparations, Dosage, and Administration

Amiloride is supplied in 5-mg tablets for oral use. Dosing is begun at 5 mg/day and may be increased to a maximum of 20 mg/day. Amiloride is available in a fixed-dose combination with hydrochlorothiazide.

MANNITOL: AN OSMOTIC DIURETIC

Osmotic diuretics differ from other diuretics with regard to mechanism and uses. At this time, mannitol is the only osmotic diuretic available in the United States. Three related drugs—urea, glycerin, and isosorbide—have been withdrawn.

Mechanism of Diuretic Action

Mannitol [Osmitrol] is a simple six-carbon sugar that embodies the four properties of an ideal osmotic diuretic. Specifically, the drug:

- Is freely filtered at the glomerulus.
- Undergoes minimal tubular reabsorption.
- Undergoes minimal metabolism.
- Is pharmacologically inert (i.e., it has no direct effects on the biochemistry or physiology of cells).

Following IV administration, mannitol is filtered by the glomerulus. However, unlike other solutes, the drug undergoes minimal reabsorption. As a result, most of the filtered drug remains in the nephron, creating an osmotic force that inhibits passive reabsorption of water. Hence, urine flow increases. The degree of diuresis produced is directly related to the concentration of mannitol in the filtrate: The more mannitol present, the greater the diuresis. Mannitol has no significant effect on the excretion of potassium and other electrolytes.

Pharmacokinetics

Mannitol does not diffuse across the GI epithelium and cannot be transported by the uptake systems that absorb dietary sugars. Accordingly, to reach the circulation, the drug must be given parenterally. Following IV injection, mannitol distributes freely to extracellular water. Diuresis begins in 30 to 60 minutes and persists 6 to 8 hours. Most of the drug is excreted intact in the urine.

Therapeutic Uses

Prophylaxis of Renal Failure. Under certain conditions (e.g., dehydration, severe hypotension, hypovolemic shock), blood flow to the kidney is decreased, causing a great reduction in filtrate volume. When the volume of filtrate is this low, transport mechanisms of the nephron are able to reabsorb virtually all of the sodium and chloride present, causing complete reabsorption of water as well. As a result, urine production ceases, and kidney failure ensues. The risk of renal failure can be reduced with mannitol. Here's how. Because filtered mannitol is not reabsorbed—even when filtrate volume is small—filtered mannitol will remain in the nephron, drawing water with it. Hence, mannitol can preserve urine flow and may thereby prevent renal failure. Thiazides and loop diuretics are not as effective for this application because, under conditions of low filtrate production, there is such an excess of reabsorptive capacity (relative to the amount of filtrate) that these drugs are unable to produce sufficient blockade of reabsorption to promote diuresis.

Reduction of Intracranial Pressure. Intracranial pressure (ICP) that has been elevated by cerebral edema can be reduced with mannitol. The drug lowers ICP because its presence in the blood vessels of the brain creates an osmotic force that draws edematous fluid from the brain into the blood. There is no risk of increasing cerebral edema because mannitol cannot exit the capillary beds of the brain.

Reduction of Intraocular Pressure. Mannitol and other osmotic agents can lower IOP by rendering the plasma hyperosmotic with respect to intraocular fluids. The hyperosmotic plasma creates an osmotic force that draws ocular fluid into the blood. Use of mannitol to lower IOP is reserved for patients who have not responded to more conventional treatment.

Adverse Effects

Edema. Mannitol can leave the vascular system at all capillary beds except those of the brain. When the drug exits capillaries, it draws water along, causing edema. Mannitol must be used with extreme caution in patients with heart disease, since it may precipitate CHF and pulmonary edema. If signs of pulmonary congestion or CHF develop, use of the drug must cease immediately. Mannitol must also be discontinued if patients with heart failure or pulmonary edema develop renal failure, because the resultant accumulation of mannitol would increase the risk of cardiac or pulmonary injury.

Other Adverse Effects. Common responses include headache, nausea, and vomiting. Fluid and electrolyte imbalance may also occur.

Preparations, Dosage, and Administration

Mannitol [Osmitrol] is administered by IV infusion. Solutions for IV use range in concentration from 5% to 25%. Dosing is complex and varies with the objective of therapy (prevention of renal failure, lowering of ICP, lowering of IOP). The usual adult dosage for preventing renal failure is 50 to 100 gm over 24 hours. The infusion rate should be set to elicit a urine flow of at least 30 to 50 mL/hr. It should be noted that mannitol may crystallize out of solution if exposed to low temperature. Accordingly, preparations should be observed for crystals before use. Preparations that contain crystals should be warmed (to redissolve the mannitol) and then cooled to body temperature for administration. A filter needle is employed to withdraw mannitol from the vial, and an in-line filter is used to prevent crystals from entering the circulation. If urine flow declines to a very low rate or ceases entirely, the infusion should be stopped.

KEY POINTS

- More than 99% of the water, electrolytes, and nutrients that are filtered at the glomerulus undergo reabsorption.
- Most diuretics block active reabsorption of sodium and chloride, and thereby prevent passive reabsorption of water.
- The amount of diuresis produced is directly related to the amount of sodium and chloride reabsorption blocked.
- Drugs that act early in the nephron are in a position to block the greatest amount of solute reabsorption, and hence produce the greatest diuresis.
- Loop diuretics block sodium and chloride reabsorption in the loop of Henle.
- Loop diuretics produce the greatest diuresis.
- In contrast to thiazide diuretics, loop diuretics are effective even when the glomerular filtration rate is low.
- Loop diuretics can cause dehydration through excessive fluid loss.
- Loop diuretics can cause hypotension by decreasing blood volume and relaxing venous smooth muscle.
- Loop diuretics can cause hearing loss which, fortunately, is usually reversible.
- Hypokalemia caused by loop diuretics is a special problem for patients taking digoxin.
- Thiazide diuretics block sodium and water reabsorption in the early distal convoluted tubule.
- Thiazide diuretics produce less diuresis than loop diuretics.
- Thiazide diuretics are ineffective when glomerular filtration rate is low.
- Like the loop diuretics, thiazide diuretics can cause dehydration and hypokalemia. However, thiazides do not cause hearing loss.
- Thiazide-induced hypokalemia is a special problem for patients taking digoxin.
- Potassium-sparing diuretics act by directly or indirectly blocking sodium-potassium "exchange" in the distal convoluted tubule.
- Potassium-sparing diuretics cause only modest diuresis.
- Potassium-sparing diuretics are used primarily to counteract potassium loss in patients taking loop diuretics or thiazides.
- The principal adverse effect of potassium-sparing diuretics is hyperkalemia.
- Because of the risk of hyperkalemia, use caution when combining potassium-sparing diuretics with one another or with potassium supplements, and in patients taking ACE inhibitors, angiotensin receptor blockers, or direct renin inhibitors.
- Loop diuretics and thiazides are used to treat hypertension and edema associated with heart failure, cirrhosis, and kidney disease.

Please visit **http://evolve.elsevier.com/Lehne** for chapter-specific NCLEX® examination review questions.

Summary of Major Nursing Implications[a]

LOOP DIURETICS

Bumetanide
Ethacrynic acid
Furosemide
Torsemide

Preadministration Assessment

Therapeutic Goal

Loop diuretics are indicated for patients with (1) pulmonary edema associated with congestive heart failure; (2) edema of hepatic, cardiac, or renal origin that has been unresponsive to less effective diuretics; (3) hypertension that cannot be controlled with thiazide and potassium-sparing diuretics; and (4) all patients who need diuretic therapy but have low renal blood flow.

Baseline Data

For all patients, obtain baseline values for weight, blood pressure (sitting and supine), pulse, respiration, and electrolytes (sodium, potassium, chloride). For patients with edema, record sites and extent of edema. For patients with ascites, measure abdominal girth. For acutely ill patients (e.g., severe CHF), assess lung sounds.

Identifying High-Risk Patients

Use with *caution* in patients with cardiovascular disease, renal impairment, diabetes mellitus, or a history of gout, and in patients who are pregnant or taking digoxin, lithium, ototoxic drugs, NSAIDs, or antihypertensive drugs.

Implementation: Administration

Routes

Furosemide and Bumetanide. Oral, IV, IM.
Ethacrynic Acid and Torsemide. Oral, IV.

Administration

Oral. Dosing may be done once daily, twice daily, or on alternate days. **Instruct patients who are using once-a-day or alternate-day dosing to take their medication in the morning. Instruct patients using twice-a-day dosing to take their medication at 8:00 AM and 2:00 PM (to minimize nocturia).**

Advise patients to administer furosemide with food if GI upset occurs.

Parenteral. Administer IV injections slowly (over 1 to 2 minutes). For high-dose therapy, administer by continuous infusion. Discard discolored solutions.

Summary of Major Nursing Implications[a]—cont'd

Promoting Adherence

Increased frequency of urination is inconvenient and can discourage adherence. **To promote adherence, inform patients that treatment will increase urine volume and frequency of voiding, and that these effects will subside 6 to 8 hours after dosing. Inform patients that nighttime diuresis can be minimized by avoiding dosing late in the day.**

Ongoing Evaluation and Interventions

Evaluating Therapeutic Effects

Monitor blood pressure and pulse rate, weigh the patient daily, and evaluate for decreased edema.

Monitor intake and output. Notify the prescriber if oliguria (urine output less than 25 mL/hr) or anuria (no urine output) develops.

Instruct outpatients to weigh themselves daily (using the same scale), preferably in the morning before eating. Also, instruct them to maintain a weight record and to report excessive weight gain or loss.

In acute conditions requiring rapid diuresis and careful monitoring, a Foley catheter may be used. The catheter should be emptied before drug injection, and output should be monitored hourly and recorded.

Minimizing Adverse Effects

Hyponatremia, Hypochloremia, and Dehydration. Loss of sodium, chloride, and water can cause hyponatremia, hypochloremia, and severe dehydration. Signs of dehydration include dry mouth, unusual thirst, and oliguria. Withhold the drug if these appear.

Dehydration can promote thromboembolism. Monitor the patient for symptoms (headache; pain in the chest, calves, or pelvis), and notify the prescriber if these develop.

The risk of dehydration and its sequelae can be minimized by (1) initiating therapy with low doses, (2) adjusting the dosage carefully, (3) monitoring weight loss daily, and (4) using an intermittent dosing schedule.

Hypotension. Monitor blood pressure. If it falls precipitously, withhold medication and notify the prescriber.

Teach patients to monitor their blood pressure, and instruct them to notify the prescriber if it drops substantially.

Inform patients about signs of postural hypotension (dizziness, light-headedness), and advise them to sit or lie down if these occur. Inform patients that postural hypotension can be minimized by rising slowly and by dangling legs off the bed before standing.

Hypokalemia. If serum potassium falls below 3.5 mEq/L, fatal dysrhythmias may result. Hypokalemia can be minimized by consuming potassium-rich foods (e.g., nuts, dried fruits, spinach, citrus fruits, potatoes, bananas), taking potassium supplements, or using a potassium-sparing diuretic. **Teach patients the signs and symptoms of hypokalemia (e.g., irregular heartbeat, muscle weakness, cramping, flaccid paralysis, leg discomfort, extreme thirst, confusion), and stress the importance of showing up for regular blood tests.**

Ototoxicity. **Inform patients about possible hearing loss and instruct them to notify the prescriber if a hearing deficit develops.** Exercise caution when loop diuretics are used concurrently with other ototoxic drugs, especially aminoglycosides.

Hyperglycemia. Loop diuretics may elevate blood glucose levels in diabetic patients. **Advise these patients to be especially diligent about monitoring blood glucose.**

Hyperuricemia. Loop diuretics frequently cause *asymptomatic* hyperuricemia, although gout-prone patients may experience a gouty attack. **Inform patients about signs of gout (tenderness or swelling in joints), and instruct them to notify the prescriber if these occur.**

Minimizing Adverse Interactions

Digoxin. By lowering potassium levels, loop diuretics increase the risk of fatal dysrhythmias from digoxin. Serum potassium levels must be monitored and maintained above 3.5 mEq/L.

Lithium. Loop diuretics can suppress lithium excretion, thereby causing the drug to accumulate, possibly to toxic levels. Plasma lithium should be monitored routinely. If drug levels become elevated, lithium dosage should be reduced.

Ototoxic Drugs. The risk of hearing loss from loop diuretics is increased in the presence of other ototoxic drugs, especially aminoglycosides. Exercise caution when such combinations are employed.

THIAZIDES AND RELATED DIURETICS

Chlorothiazide
Chlorthalidone
Hydrochlorothiazide
Indapamide
Methyclothiazide
Metolazone

Thiazide diuretics have actions much like those of the loop diuretics. Hence, nursing implications for the thiazides are nearly identical to those of the loop diuretics.

Preadministration Assessment

Therapeutic Goal

Thiazide diuretics are indicated for hypertension and edema.

Baseline Data

For all patients, obtain baseline values for weight, blood pressure (sitting and supine), pulse, respiration, and electrolytes (sodium, chloride, potassium). For patients with edema, record sites and extent of edema.

Identifying High-Risk Patients

Use with *caution* in patients with cardiovascular disease, renal impairment, diabetes mellitus, or a history of gout and in patients taking digoxin, lithium, or antihypertensive drugs.

Implementation: Administration

Routes

Oral. All thiazide-type diuretics.

Intravenous. Chlorothiazide.

Continued

Summary of Major Nursing Implications[a]—cont'd

Administration

Dosing may be done once daily, twice daily, or on alternate days. **When once-a-day dosing is employed, instruct patients to take their medicine early in the day to minimize nocturia. When twice-a-day dosing is employed, instruct patients to take their medicine at 8:00 AM and 2:00 PM.**

Advise patients to administer thiazides with or after meals if GI upset occurs.

Promoting Adherence

See nursing implications for *Loop Diuretics.*

Ongoing Evaluation and Interventions

Evaluating Therapeutic Effects

See nursing implications for *Loop Diuretics.*

Minimizing Adverse Effects

Like the loop diuretics, thiazides can cause *hyponatremia, hypochloremia, dehydration, hypokalemia, hypotension, hyperglycemia,* and *hyperuricemia.* For implications regarding these effects, see nursing implications for *Loop Diuretics.*

Minimizing Adverse Interactions

Like loop diuretics, thiazides can interact adversely with *digoxin* and *lithium.* For implications regarding these interactions, see nursing implications for *Loop Diuretics.*

POTASSIUM-SPARING DIURETICS

Amiloride
Spironolactone
Triamterene

Preadministration Assessment

Therapeutic Goal

Potassium-sparing diuretics are given primarily to counterbalance the potassium-losing effects of thiazide diuretics and loop diuretics.

Baseline Data

Obtain baseline values for serum potassium, along with baseline values for weight, blood pressure (sitting and supine), pulse, respiration, sodium, and chloride. For patients with edema, record sites and extent of edema.

Identifying High-Risk Patients

Potassium-sparing diuretics are *contraindicated* for patients with hyperkalemia and should be used with *caution* in patients taking potassium supplements or another potassium-sparing diuretic. Use with *caution* in patients taking ACE inhibitors, angiotensin receptor blockers, and direct renin inhibitors.

Implementation: Administration

Route

Oral. Spironolactone has the potential to cause reproductive harm to healthcare workers exposed during administration. NIOSH suggests donning a protective gown and two sets of gloves when crushing or splitting tablets.

Administration

Advise patients to take these drugs with or after meals if GI upset occurs.

Ongoing Evaluation and Interventions

Evaluating Therapeutic Effects

Monitor serum potassium levels on a regular basis. The objective is to maintain serum potassium levels between 3.5 and 5 mEq/L.

Minimizing Adverse Effects

Hyperkalemia. Hyperkalemia is the principal adverse effect. **Instruct patients to restrict intake of potassium-rich foods.** If serum potassium levels rise above 5 mEq/L, or if signs of hyperkalemia develop (e.g., abnormal cardiac rhythm), withhold medication and notify the prescriber. Insulin can be given to (temporarily) decrease potassium levels.

Endocrine Effects. *Spironolactone* may cause *menstrual irregularities* and *impotence.* **Inform patients about these effects, and instruct them to notify the prescriber if they occur.**

Minimizing Adverse Interactions

Drugs That Raise Potassium Levels. Owing to a risk of hyperkalemia, use caution when combining a potassium-sparing diuretic with potassium supplements, salt substitutes, or with another potassium-sparing diuretic. Generally avoid combined use with ACE inhibitors, angiotensin receptor blockers, and direct renin inhibitors.

[a]Patient education information is highlighted as **blue text.**

CHAPTER

42 Agents Affecting the Volume and Ion Content of Body Fluids

The drugs discussed in this chapter are used to correct disturbances in the volume and ionic composition of body fluids. Three groups of agents are considered: (1) drugs used to correct disorders of fluid volume and osmolality, (2) drugs used to correct disturbances of hydrogen ion concentration (acid-base status), and (3) drugs used to correct electrolyte imbalances.

DISORDERS OF FLUID VOLUME AND OSMOLALITY

Good health requires that both the volume and osmolality of extracellular and intracellular fluids remain within a normal range. If a substantial alteration in either the volume or osmolality of these fluids develops, significant harm can result.

Maintenance of fluid volume and osmolality is primarily the job of the kidneys, and, even under adverse conditions, renal mechanisms usually succeed in keeping the volume and composition of body fluids within acceptable limits. However, circumstances can arise in which the regulatory capacity of the kidneys is exceeded. When this occurs, disruption of fluid volume, osmolality, or both can result.

Abnormal states of hydration can be divided into two major categories: volume contraction and volume expansion. *Volume contraction* is defined as a *decrease* in total body water; conversely, *volume expansion* is defined as an *increase* in total body water. States of volume contraction and volume expansion have three subclassifications based on alterations in extracellular osmolality. For volume contraction, the subcategories are *isotonic contraction, hypertonic contraction,* and *hypotonic contraction.* Volume expansion may also be subclassified as *isotonic, hypertonic,* or *hypotonic.* Descriptions and causes of these abnormal states are discussed in the sections that follow.

In the clinical setting, changes in osmolality are described in terms of the sodium content of plasma. Sodium is used as the reference for classification because this ion is the principal extracellular solute. (Recall that plasma sodium content ranges from 135 to 145 mEq/L.) In most cases, the total osmolality of plasma is about 2 times the osmolality of sodium. That is, total plasma osmolality usually ranges from 280 to 300 mOsm/kg water.

Volume Contraction

Isotonic Contraction

Definition and Causes. Isotonic contraction is defined as volume contraction in which *sodium and water are lost in isotonic proportions.* Hence, although there is a decrease in the total volume of extracellular fluid, there is no change in osmolality. Causes of isotonic contraction include vomiting, diarrhea, kidney disease, and misuse of diuretics. Isotonic contraction is characteristic of cholera, an infection that produces vomiting and severe diarrhea.

Treatment. Lost volume should be replaced with fluids that are isotonic to plasma. This can be accomplished by infusing isotonic (0.9%) sodium chloride in sterile water, a solution in which both sodium and chloride are present at a concentration of 145 mEq/L. Volume should be replenished slowly to avoid pulmonary edema.

Hypertonic Contraction

Definition and Causes. Hypertonic contraction is defined as volume contraction in which *loss of water exceeds loss of sodium.* Hence, there is a reduction in extracellular fluid volume coupled with an increase in osmolality. Because of extracellular hypertonicity, water is drawn out of cells, thereby producing intracellular dehydration and partial compensation for lost extracellular volume.

Causes of hypertonic contraction include excessive sweating, osmotic diuresis, and feeding excessively concentrated foods to infants. Hypertonic contraction may also develop secondary to extensive burns or disorders of the central nervous system (CNS) that render the patient unable to experience or report thirst.

Treatment. Volume replacement in hypertonic contraction should be accomplished with hypotonic fluids (e.g., 0.45% sodium chloride) or with fluids that contain no solutes at all. Initial therapy may consist simply of drinking water.

Alternatively, 5% dextrose can be infused intravenously. (Since dextrose is rapidly metabolized to carbon dioxide and water, dextrose solutions can be viewed as the osmotic equivalent of water alone.) Volume replenishment should be done in stages. About 50% of the estimated loss should be replaced during the first few hours of treatment. The remainder should be replenished over 1 to 2 days.

Hypotonic Contraction

Definition and Causes. Hypotonic contraction is defined as volume contraction in which *loss of sodium exceeds loss of water.* Hence, both the volume and osmolality of extracellular fluid are reduced. Because intracellular osmolality now exceeds extracellular osmolality, extracellular volume becomes diminished further by movement of water into cells.

The principal cause of hypotonic contraction is excessive loss of sodium through the kidneys. This may occur because of diuretic therapy, chronic renal insufficiency, or lack of aldosterone (the adrenocortical hormone that promotes renal retention of sodium).

Treatment. If hyponatremia is mild, and if renal function is adequate, hypotonic contraction can be corrected by infusing *isotonic* sodium chloride solution for injection. When this is done, plasma tonicity will be adjusted by the kidneys. However, if the sodium loss is severe, a *hypertonic* (e.g., 3%) solution of sodium chloride should be infused. Administration should continue until plasma sodium concentration has been raised to about 130 mEq/L. Patients should be monitored for signs of fluid overload (distention of neck veins, peripheral or pulmonary edema). When hypotonic contraction is due to aldosterone insufficiency, patients should receive hormone replacement therapy along with intravenous infusion of isotonic sodium chloride.

Volume Expansion

Volume expansion is defined as an *increase in the total volume of body fluid.* As with volume contraction, volume expansion may be *isotonic, hypertonic,* or *hypotonic.* Volume expansion may result from an overdose with therapeutic fluids (e.g., sodium chloride infusion) or may be associated with disease states, such as heart failure, nephrotic syndrome, or cirrhosis of the liver with ascites. The principal drugs employed to correct volume expansion are *diuretics* and the *agents used for heart failure.* These drugs are discussed in Chapters 41 and 48, respectively. A specific form of volume expansion known as hypervolemic hyponatremia can be treated with a vasopressin antagonist, such as conivaptan or tolvaptan (see Chapter 59).

ACID-BASE DISTURBANCES

Maintenance of acid-base balance is a complex process, the full discussion of which is beyond the scope of this text. Hence, discussion here is condensed.

Acid-base status is regulated by multiple systems. The most important are (1) the bicarbonate–carbonic acid buffer system, (2) the respiratory system, and (3) the kidneys. The respiratory system influences pH through control of CO_2 exhalation. Because CO_2 represents volatile carbonic acid, exhalation of CO_2 tends to elevate pH (reduce acidity), whereas retention of CO_2 (secondary to respiratory slowing) tends to lower pH. The kidneys influence pH by regulating bicarbonate excretion. By *retaining* bicarbonate, the kidneys can raise pH. Conversely, by increasing bicarbonate *excretion,* the kidneys can lower pH and thereby compensate for alkalosis.

There are four principal types of acid-base imbalance: (1) respiratory alkalosis, (2) respiratory acidosis, (3) metabolic alkalosis, and (4) metabolic acidosis. Causes and treatments are discussed in the sections that follow.

Respiratory Alkalosis

Causes

Respiratory alkalosis is produced by hyperventilation. Deep and rapid breathing increases CO_2 loss, which in turn lowers the pCO_2 (partial pressure of carbon dioxide) of blood and increases pH. Mild hyperventilation may result from a number of causes, including hypoxia, pulmonary disease, and drugs (especially aspirin and other salicylates). Severe hyperventilation can be caused by CNS injury and hysteria.

Treatment

Management of respiratory alkalosis is dictated by the severity of pH elevation. When alkalosis is mild, no specific treatment is indicated. Severe respiratory alkalosis resulting from hysteria can be controlled by having the patient rebreathe his or her CO_2-laden expired breath. This can be accomplished by holding a paper bag over the nose and mouth. A sedative (e.g., diazepam [Valium]) can help suppress the hysteria.

Respiratory Acidosis

Causes

Respiratory acidosis results from retention of CO_2 secondary to hypoventilation. Reduced CO_2 exhalation raises plasma pCO_2, which in turn causes plasma pH to fall. Primary causes of impaired ventilation are (1) depression of the medullary respiratory center and (2) pathologic changes in the lungs (e.g., status asthmaticus, airway obstruction). Over time, the kidneys compensate for respiratory acidosis by excreting less bicarbonate.

Treatment

Primary treatment of respiratory acidosis is directed at correcting respiratory impairment. The patient may also need oxygen and ventilatory assistance. Infusion of sodium bicarbonate may be indicated if acidosis is severe.

Metabolic Alkalosis

Causes

Metabolic alkalosis is characterized by increases in both the pH and bicarbonate content of plasma. Causes include excessive loss of gastric acid (through vomiting or suctioning) and administration of alkalinizing salts (e.g., sodium bicarbonate). The body compensates for metabolic alkalosis by (1) hypoventilation (which causes retention of CO_2), (2) increased renal excretion of bicarbonate, and (3) accumulation of organic acids.

Treatment

In most cases, metabolic alkalosis can be corrected by infusing a solution of *sodium chloride plus potassium chloride.* This facilitates renal excretion of bicarbonate and thereby promotes normalization of plasma pH. When alkalosis is severe, direct correction of pH is indicated. This can be accomplished by infusing dilute (0.1 N) *hydrochloric acid* through a central venous catheter or by administering an acid-forming salt, such as *ammonium chloride*. However, ammonium chloride must not be given to patients with liver failure because the drug is likely to cause hepatic encephalopathy.

Metabolic Acidosis

Causes

Principal causes of metabolic acidosis are chronic renal failure, loss of bicarbonate during severe diarrhea, and metabolic disorders that result in overproduction of lactic acid (lactic acidosis) or ketoacids (ketoacidosis). Metabolic acidosis may also result from poisoning by methanol and certain medications (e.g., aspirin and other salicylates).

Treatment

Treatment consists of correcting the underlying cause of acidosis and administering an alkalinizing salt (e.g., sodium bicarbonate, sodium carbonate) if the acidosis is severe.

When an alkalinizing salt is indicated, *sodium bicarbonate* is generally preferred. Administration may be oral or intravenous. If acidosis is mild, oral administration is preferred. Intravenous infusion is usually reserved for severe reductions of pH. When sodium bicarbonate is given IV to treat acute severe acidosis, caution must be exercised to avoid excessive elevation of plasma pH because rapid conversion from acidosis to alkalosis can be hazardous. Also, because of the sodium content of sodium bicarbonate, care should be taken to avoid hypernatremia.

POTASSIUM IMBALANCES

Potassium is the most abundant *intracellular* cation, having a concentration within cells of about 150 mEq/L. In contrast, *extracellular* concentrations are low (4 to 5 mEq/L). Potassium plays a major role in conducting nerve impulses and maintaining the electrical excitability of muscle. Potassium also helps regulate acid-base balance.

Regulation of Potassium Levels

Serum levels of potassium are regulated primarily by the kidneys. Under steady-state conditions, urinary output of potassium equals intake. Renal excretion of potassium is increased by aldosterone, an adrenal steroid that promotes conservation of sodium while increasing potassium loss. Potassium excretion is also increased by most diuretics. Potassium-sparing diuretics (e.g., spironolactone) are the exception.

Potassium levels are influenced by extracellular pH. In the presence of extracellular *alkalosis,* potassium uptake by cells is *enhanced,* causing a *reduction* in extracellular potassium levels. Conversely, extracellular *acidosis* promotes the exit of potassium from cells, thereby causing extracellular *hyperkalemia.*

Insulin has a profound effect on potassium: In high doses, insulin stimulates potassium uptake by cells. This ability has been used to treat hyperkalemia.

Hypokalemia

Causes and Consequences

Hypokalemia is defined as a deficiency of potassium in the blood. By definition, hypokalemia exists when serum potassium levels fall below 3.5 mEq/L. The most common cause is treatment with a thiazide or loop diuretic (see Chapter 41). Other causes include insufficient potassium intake; alkalosis and excessive insulin (both of which decrease extracellular potassium levels by driving potassium into cells); increased renal excretion of potassium (e.g., as caused by aldosterone); and potassium loss associated with vomiting, diarrhea, and abuse of laxatives. Hypokalemia may also occur because of excessive potassium loss in sweat. As a rule, potassium depletion is accompanied by loss of chloride. Insufficiency of both ions produces *hypokalemic alkalosis.*

Hypokalemia has adverse effects on skeletal muscle, smooth muscle, blood pressure, and the heart. Symptoms include weakness or paralysis of skeletal muscle, a risk of fatal dysrhythmias, and intestinal dilation and ileus. In patients taking digoxin (a cardiac drug), hypokalemia is the principal cause of digoxin toxicity. For all people, hypokalemia increases the risk of hypertension and stroke.

Prevention and Treatment

Potassium depletion can be treated with three potassium salts: potassium chloride, potassium phosphate, and potassium bicarbonate. These may also be used for prophylaxis against potassium insufficiency. For either treatment or prophylaxis, the preferred salt is *potassium chloride* because chloride deficiency frequently coexists with potassium deficiency.

Potassium chloride may be administered PO or IV. Oral therapy is preferred for prophylaxis and for treating mild deficiency. Intravenous therapy is reserved for severe deficiency and for patients who cannot take potassium by mouth.

Oral Potassium Chloride

Uses, Dosage, and Preparations. Oral potassium chloride may be used for both prevention and treatment of potassium deficiency. Dosages for prevention range from 16 to 24 mEq/day. Dosages for deficiency range from 40 to 100 mEq/day.

Oral potassium chloride is available in solution and in solid formulations: immediate-release tablets, sustained-release tablets, effervescent tablets, and powders. *The sustained-release tablets (e.g., Klor-Con, Micro-K) are preferred* because they are more convenient and better tolerated than the other formulations, and hence offer the best chance of patient adherence.

Adverse Effects. Potassium chloride irritates the GI tract, frequently causing abdominal discomfort, nausea, vomiting, and diarrhea. With the exception of the sustained-release tablets, solid formulations can produce high local concentrations of potassium, resulting in severe intestinal injury (ulcerative lesions, bleeding, perforation); death has occurred. To minimize GI effects, oral potassium chloride should be taken with meals or a full glass of water. If symptoms of irritation occur, dosing should be discontinued. Rarely, oral potassium chloride produces hyperkalemia. This dangerous development is much more likely with IV therapy.

Intravenous Potassium Chloride. Intravenous potassium chloride is indicated for prevention and treatment of hypokalemia. Intravenous solutions must be diluted (preferably to 40 mEq/L or less) as they are extremely irritating to the veins.

> **Safety Alert**
>
> **POTASSIUM**
>
> Intravenous potassium must be infused slowly (generally no faster than 10 mEq/hr in adults). Potassium chloride must never be administered by IV push. In fact, potassium chloride is one of the agents used in lethal injections, as rapid infusion results in cardiac arrest.

The principal complication is *hyper*kalemia, which can prove fatal. To reduce the risk of hyperkalemia, serum potassium levels should be measured before the infusion and periodically throughout the treatment interval. Also, renal function should be assessed before and during treatment to ensure adequate output of urine. If renal failure develops, the infusion should be stopped immediately. Changes in the electrocardiogram (ECG) can be an early indication that potassium toxicity is developing.

Contraindications to Potassium Use. Potassium should be avoided under conditions that predispose to hyperkalemia (e.g., severe renal impairment, use of potassium-sparing diuretics, hypoaldosteronism). Potassium must also be avoided when hyperkalemia already exists.

Hyperkalemia

Causes

Hyperkalemia (excessive elevation of serum potassium) can result from a number of causes. These include severe tissue trauma, untreated Addison's disease, acute acidosis (which draws potassium out of cells), acute renal failure, misuse of potassium-sparing diuretics, and overdose with IV potassium.

Consequences

The most serious consequence of hyperkalemia is disruption of the electrical activity of the heart. Because hyperkalemia alters the generation and conduction of cardiac impulses, alterations in the ECG and cardiac rhythm are usually the earliest signs that potassium levels are growing dangerously high. With mild elevation of serum potassium (5 to 7 mEq/L), the T wave heightens and the PR interval becomes prolonged. When serum potassium reaches 8 to 9 mEq/L, cardiac arrest can occur, possibly preceded by ventricular tachycardia or fibrillation.

Effects of hyperkalemia are not limited to the heart. Noncardiac effects include confusion, anxiety, dyspnea, weakness or heaviness of the legs, and numbness or tingling of the hands, feet, and lips.

Treatment

Treatment is begun by withholding any foods that contain potassium and any medicines that promote potassium accumulation (e.g., potassium-sparing diuretics, potassium supplements). After this, management consists of measures that (1) counteract potassium-induced cardiotoxicity and (2) lower extracellular levels of potassium. Specific steps include (1) infusion of a *calcium salt* (e.g., calcium gluconate) to offset effects of hyperkalemia on the heart; (2) infusion of *glucose* and *insulin* to promote uptake of potassium by cells and thereby decrease extracellular potassium levels; and (3) if acidosis is present (which is likely), infusion of *sodium bicarbonate* to move pH toward alkalinity and thereby increase cellular uptake of potassium. If these measures prove inadequate, steps can be taken to remove potassium. These include (1) oral or rectal administration of *sodium polystyrene sulfonate* [Kayexalate, Kionex], an exchange resin that absorbs potassium; and (2) peritoneal or extracorporeal dialysis.

MAGNESIUM IMBALANCES

Magnesium is required for the activity of many enzymes and for binding of messenger RNA to ribosomes. In addition, magnesium helps regulate neurochemical transmission and the excitability of muscle. The concentration of magnesium within cells is about 40 mEq/L, much higher than its concentration outside cells (about 2 mEq/L).

Hypomagnesemia

Causes and Consequences

Low levels of magnesium may result from a variety of causes, including diarrhea, hemodialysis, kidney disease, and prolonged IV feeding with magnesium-free solutions. Hypomagnesemia may also be seen in chronic alcoholics and in people with diabetes or pancreatitis. Frequently, patients with magnesium deficiency also present with hypocalcemia and hypokalemia.

Prominent symptoms of hypomagnesemia involve cardiac and skeletal muscle. In the presence of low levels of magnesium, release of acetylcholine at the neuromuscular junction is enhanced. This can increase muscle excitability to the point of tetany. Hypomagnesemia also increases excitability of neurons in the CNS, causing disorientation, psychoses, and seizures.

In the kidneys, hypomagnesemia may lead to nephrocalcinosis (formation of minuscule calcium stones within nephrons). Renal injury occurs when the stones become large enough to block the flow of tubular urine.

Prevention and Treatment

Frank hypomagnesemia is treated with parenteral magnesium sulfate. For prophylaxis against magnesium deficiency, an oral preparation (magnesium oxide) may be used.

Magnesium Oxide. Tablets of magnesium oxide may be taken as supplements to dietary magnesium to help prevent hypomagnesemia. With any oral magnesium preparation, excessive doses may cause diarrhea. The adult dosage for preventing deficiency is 400 to 800 mg daily.

Magnesium Sulfate

Uses, Administration, and Dosage. Magnesium sulfate (IM or IV) is the preferred treatment for severe hypomagnesemia. The IM dosage is 0.5 to 1 gm 4 times a day. For IV therapy, a 10% solution can be used, infused at a rate of 1.5 mL/min or less.

Adverse Effects. Excessive levels of magnesium cause *neuromuscular blockade.* Paralysis of the respiratory muscles is of particular concern. By suppressing neuromuscular transmission, magnesium excess can intensify the effects of neuromuscular blocking agents (e.g., succinylcholine, atracurium). Hence, caution must be exercised in patients receiving these drugs. The neuromuscular blocking actions of magnesium can be counteracted with calcium. Accordingly, when parenteral magnesium is being employed, an injectable form of calcium (e.g., calcium gluconate) should be immediately available.

In the heart, excessive magnesium can suppress impulse conduction through the atrioventricular (AV) node. Accordingly, magnesium sulfate is contraindicated for patients with AV heart block.

To minimize the risk of toxicity, serum magnesium levels should be monitored. Respiratory paralysis occurs at 12 to 15 mEq/L. When magnesium levels exceed 25 mEq/L, cardiac arrest may set in.

Hypermagnesemia

Toxic elevation of magnesium levels is most common in patients with renal insufficiency, especially when magnesium-containing antacids or cathartics are being used. Symptoms of mild intoxication include muscle weakness (resulting from inhibition of acetylcholine release), hypotension, sedation, and ECG changes. As noted, respiratory paralysis is likely when plasma levels reach 12 to 15 mEq/L. At higher magnesium concentrations, there is a risk of cardiac arrest. Muscle weakness and paralysis can be counteracted with IV calcium.

KEY POINTS

- Treat isotonic volume contraction with isotonic (0.9%) sodium chloride.
- Treat hypertonic volume contraction with hypotonic (e.g., 0.45%) sodium chloride.
- Treat hypotonic volume contraction with hypertonic (e.g., 3%) sodium chloride.
- Treat volume expansion with diuretics.
- Treat respiratory or metabolic acidosis with sodium bicarbonate.
- Treat respiratory alkalosis by having patients inhale 5% CO_2 or rebreathe their expired air.
- Treat metabolic alkalosis with an infusion of sodium chloride plus potassium chloride. For severe cases, infuse 0.1% hydrochloric acid or ammonium chloride.
- Treat moderate hypokalemia with potassium chloride in sustained-release tablets.
- Treat severe hypokalemia with IV potassium chloride.
- To treat hyperkalemia, begin by withdrawing potassium-containing foods and drugs that promote potassium accumulation (e.g., potassium supplements, potassium-sparing diuretics). Subsequent measures include (1) infusing a calcium salt to offset the cardiac effects of potassium, (2) infusing glucose and insulin to promote potassium uptake by cells, and (3) infusing sodium bicarbonate if acidosis is present.
- Treat hypomagnesemia with IM or IV magnesium sulfate. For prophylaxis, give oral magnesium (e.g., magnesium oxide).

Please visit **http://evolve.elsevier.com/Lehne** for chapter-specific NCLEX® examination review questions.

UNIT VII

DRUGS THAT AFFECT THE HEART, BLOOD VESSELS, AND BLOOD

CHAPTER 43

Review of Hemodynamics

Hemodynamics is the study of the movement of blood throughout the circulatory system, along with the regulatory mechanisms and driving forces involved. Concepts introduced here reappear throughout the chapters on cardiovascular drugs, so we urge you to review these now. Because this is a pharmacology text and not a physiology text, discussion is limited to hemodynamic factors that have particular relevance to the actions of drugs.

OVERVIEW OF THE CIRCULATORY SYSTEM

The circulatory system has two primary functions: (1) delivery of oxygen, nutrients, hormones, electrolytes, and other essentials to cells and (2) removal of carbon dioxide and metabolic wastes from cells. In addition, the system helps fight infection.

The circulatory system has two major divisions: the *pulmonary circulation* and the *systemic circulation.* The pulmonary circulation delivers blood to the lungs. The systemic circulation delivers blood to all other organs and tissues. The systemic circulation is also known as the *greater circulation* or *peripheral circulation.*

Components of the Circulatory System

The circulatory system is composed of the *heart* and *blood vessels.* The heart is the pump that moves blood through the arterial tree. The blood vessels have several functions:

- *Arteries* transport blood under high pressure to tissues.
- *Arterioles* are control valves that regulate local blood flow.
- *Capillaries* are the sites for exchange of fluid, oxygen, carbon dioxide, nutrients, hormones, and wastes.
- *Venules* collect blood from the capillaries.
- *Veins* transport blood back to the heart. In addition, veins serve as a major reservoir for blood.

Arteries and veins differ with respect to distensibility (elasticity). Arteries are very muscular, and hence do not readily stretch. As a result, large increases in arterial pressure (AP) cause only small increases in arterial diameter. Veins are much less muscular, and hence are 6 to 10 times more distensible. As a result, small increases in venous pressure cause large increases in vessel diameter; this produces a large increase in venous volume.

Distribution of Blood

The adult circulatory system contains about 5 L of blood, which is distributed throughout the system. As indicated in Fig. 43.1, 9% is in the pulmonary circulation, 7% is in the heart, and 84% is in the systemic circulation. Within the systemic circulation, however, distribution is uneven: most (64%) of the blood is in veins, venules, and venous sinuses; the remaining 20% is in arteries (13%) and arterioles or capillaries (7%). The large volume of blood in the venous system serves as a reservoir.

What Makes Blood Flow?

Blood moves within vessels because the force that drives flow is greater than the resistance to flow. As shown in Fig. 43.2, the force that drives blood flow is the pressure gradient between two points in a vessel. Blood will flow from the point where pressure is higher toward the point where pressure is lower. Resistance to flow is determined by the

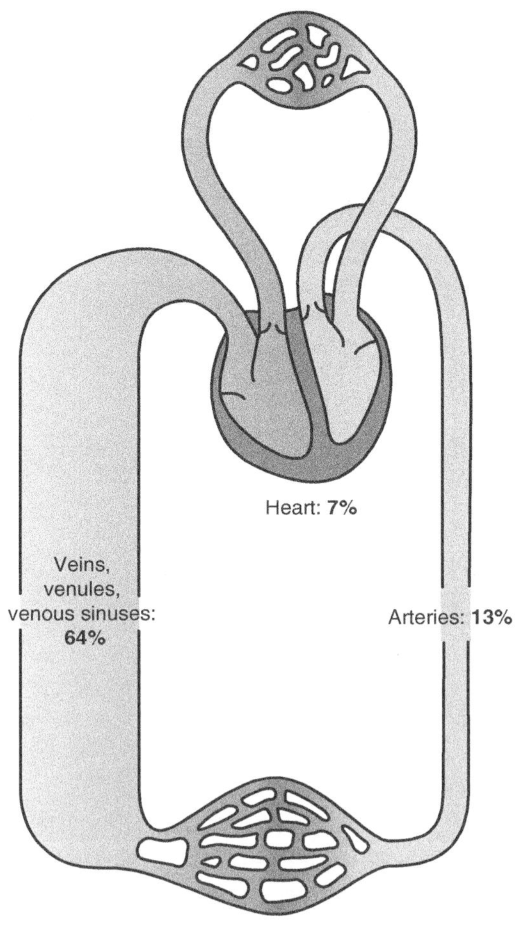

Fig. 43.1 ■ Distribution of blood in the circulatory system. A large percentage of the blood resides in the venous system.

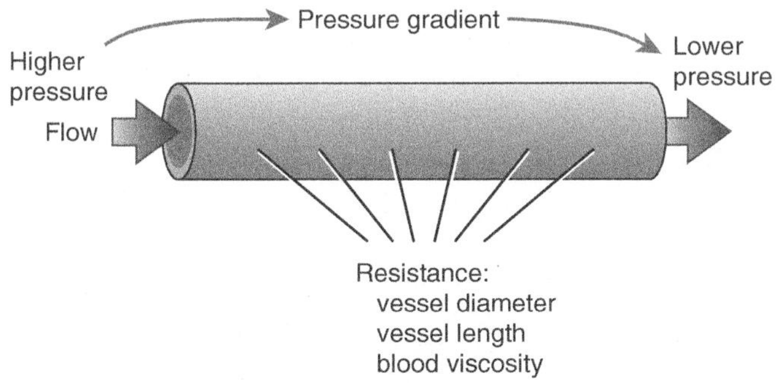

Fig. 43.2 ■ Forces that promote and impede flow of blood. Blood flows from the point of higher pressure toward the point of lower pressure. Resistance to flow is determined by vessel diameter, vessel length, and blood viscosity.

diameter and length of the vessel and by blood viscosity. From a pharmacologic viewpoint, the most important determinant of resistance is vessel diameter: The larger the vessel, the smaller the resistance. Accordingly, when vessels dilate, resistance declines, causing blood flow to increase. When vessels constrict, resistance rises, causing blood flow to decline. To maintain adequate flow when resistance rises, blood pressure must rise as well.

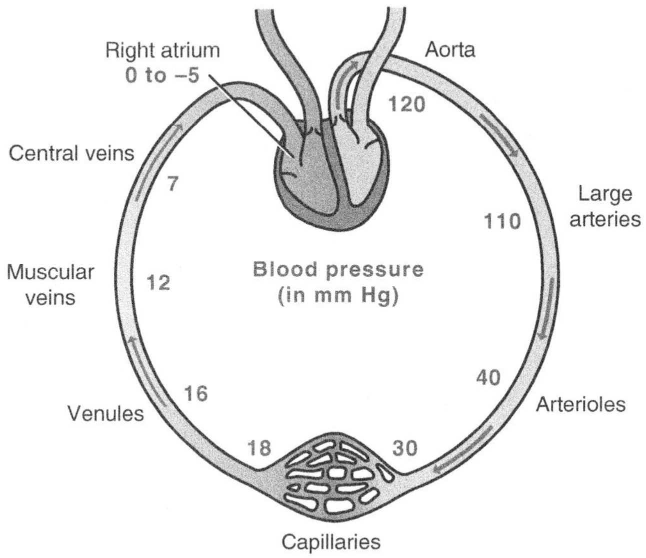

Fig. 43.3 ■ Distribution of pressure within the systemic circulation.
Pressure is highest when blood leaves the left ventricle, falls to only 18 mm Hg as blood exits capillaries, and reaches negative values within the right atrium.

How Does Blood Get Back to the Heart?

As indicated in Fig. 43.3, pressure falls progressively as blood moves through the systemic circulation. Pressure is 120 mm Hg when blood enters the aorta, 30 mm Hg when blood enters capillaries, and only 18 mm Hg when blood leaves capillaries; pressure then drops to negative values (0 to −5 mm Hg) in the right atrium. (Negative atrial pressure is generated by expansion of the chest during inspiration.)

Given that pressure is only 18 mm Hg when blood leaves capillaries, we must ask, "How does blood get back to the heart?" In addition to the small pressure head in venules, three mechanisms help ensure venous return. First, negative pressure in the right atrium helps "suck" blood toward the heart. Second, constriction of smooth muscle in the venous wall increases venous pressure, which helps drive blood toward the heart. Third, and most important, the combination of venous valves and skeletal muscle contraction constitutes an auxiliary "venous pump." As shown in Fig. 43.4A, the veins are equipped with a system of one-way valves. When skeletal muscles contract (Fig. 43.4B), venous blood is squeezed toward the heart—the only direction the valves will permit.

REGULATION OF CARDIAC OUTPUT

In the average adult, cardiac output is about 5 L/min. Hence, every minute the heart pumps the equivalent of all the blood in the body. In this section, we consider the major factors that determine how much blood the heart pumps.

Determinants of Cardiac Output

The basic equation for cardiac output is:

$$CO = HR \times SV$$

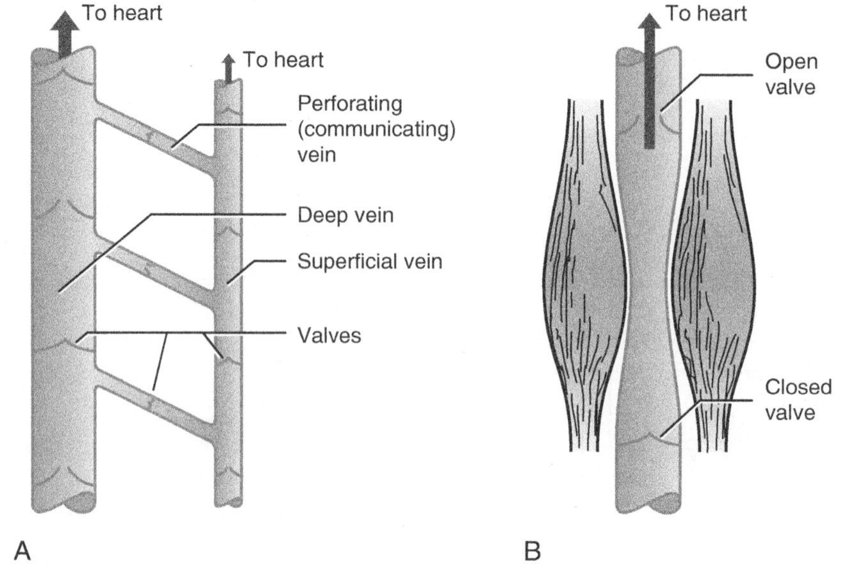

Fig. 43.4 ■ Venous valves and the auxiliary venous "pump."
A, Veins and their one-way valves in the leg. The configuration of these valves ensures that blood will move toward the heart. **B,** Contraction of skeletal muscle pumps venous blood toward the heart.

where CO is cardiac output, HR is heart rate, and SV is stroke volume. According to the equation, an increase in HR or SV will increase CO, whereas a decrease in HR or SV will decrease CO. For the average person, heart rate is about 70 beats/min and stroke volume is about 70 mL. Multiplying these, we get 4.9 L/min—the average value for CO.

Heart Rate

Heart rate is controlled primarily by the autonomic nervous system (ANS). Rate is increased by the sympathetic branch acting through $beta_1$-adrenergic receptors in the sinoatrial (SA) node. Rate is decreased by the parasympathetic branch acting through muscarinic receptors in the SA node. Parasympathetic impulses reach the heart via the vagus nerve.

Stroke Volume

Stroke volume is determined largely by three factors: (1) myocardial contractility, (2) cardiac afterload, and (3) cardiac preload. *Myocardial contractility* is defined as the force with which the ventricles contract. Contractility is determined primarily by the degree of cardiac dilation, which in turn is determined by the amount of venous return. The importance of venous return in regulating contractility and SV is discussed separately later in this chapter. In addition to regulation by venous return, contractility can be increased by the sympathetic nervous system, acting through $beta_1$-adrenergic receptors in the myocardium.

Preload

Preload is formally defined as the amount of tension (stretch) applied to a muscle before contraction. In the heart, stretch is determined by ventricular filling pressure, that is, the *force of venous return:* The greater filling pressure is, the more the ventricles will stretch. Cardiac preload can be expressed as either *end-diastolic volume* or *end-diastolic pressure.* As discussed later in this chapter, an increase in preload will increase SV, whereas a decrease in preload will reduce SV. Frequently, the terms *preload* and *force of venous return* are used interchangeably—although they are not truly equivalent.

Afterload

Afterload is formally defined as the load against which a muscle exerts its force (i.e., the load a muscle must overcome in order to contract). For the heart, afterload is the *arterial pressure* that the left ventricle must overcome to eject blood. Common sense tells us that if afterload increases, SV will decrease. Conversely, if afterload falls, SV will rise. Cardiac afterload is determined primarily by the degree of peripheral resistance, which in turn is determined by constriction and dilation of arterioles. That is, when arterioles constrict, peripheral resistance rises, causing AP (afterload) to rise as well. Conversely, when arterioles dilate, peripheral resistance falls, causing AP to decline.

Starling's Law of the Heart

Starling's law states that the force of ventricular contraction is proportional to muscle fiber length (up to a point). Accordingly, as fiber length (ventricular diameter) increases, there is a corresponding increase in contractile force (Fig. 43.5). Because of this built-in mechanism, when more blood enters the heart, more is pumped out. As a result, the healthy heart is able to precisely match its output with the volume of blood delivered by veins. That is, when venous return increases, CO increases correspondingly. Conversely, when venous return declines, CO declines to precisely the same extent. Hence, under normal, nonstressed conditions, SV is determined by factors that regulate venous return.

Why does contractile force change as a function of fiber length (ventricular diameter)? Recall that muscle contraction results from the interaction of two proteins: actin and myosin. As the heart stretches in response to increased ventricular filling, actin and myosin are brought into a more optimal alignment with each other, which allows them to interact with greater force.

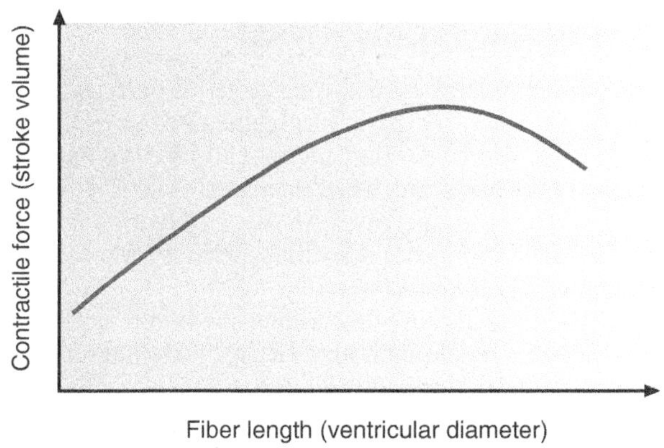

Fig. 43.5 ■ The Starling relationship between myocardial fiber length and contractile force.
An increase in fiber length produces a corresponding increase in contractile force. Fiber length increases as the ventricles enlarge during filling. Increased contractile force is reflected by increased stroke volume.

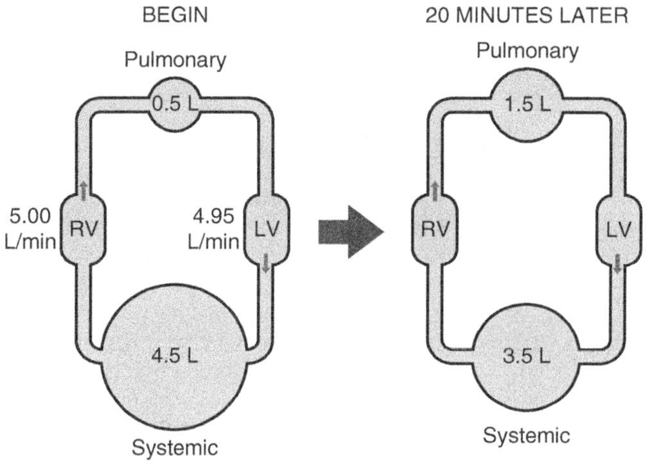

Fig. 43.6 ■ Systemic-pulmonary imbalance that develops when the output of the left and right ventricles is not identical.
In this example, the output of the left ventricle (LV) is 1% less than the output of the right ventricle (RV). Hence, while the right ventricle pumps 5000 mL/min, the left pumps only 4950 mL/min—50 mL/min less than the right side. This causes blood to back up in the pulmonary circulation. After 20 minutes, 1000 mL of blood has shifted from the systemic circulation to the pulmonary circulation. Death would ensue in less than 40 minutes. Numbers in the pulmonary and systemic circulations indicate volume of blood in liters.

Factors That Determine Venous Return

Having established that venous return is the primary determinant of SV (and hence CO), we need to understand the factors that determine venous return. With regard to pharmacology, the most important factor is *systemic filling pressure* (i.e., the force that returns blood to the heart). The normal value for filling pressure is 7 mm Hg. This value can be raised to 17 mm Hg by constriction of veins. Filling pressure can also be raised by an increase in blood volume. Conversely, filling pressure, and hence venous return, can be lowered by venodilation or by reducing blood volume. Blood volume and venous tone can both be altered with drugs.

In addition to systemic filling pressure, three other factors influence venous return: (1) the auxiliary muscle pumps discussed earlier, (2) resistance to flow between peripheral vessels and the right atrium, and (3) right atrial pressure, elevation of which will impede venous return. None of these factors can be directly influenced with drugs.

Starling's Law and Maintenance of Systemic-Pulmonary Balance

Because the myocardium operates in accord with Starling's law, the right and left ventricles always pump exactly the same amount of blood. When venous return increases, SV of the right ventricle increases, thereby increasing delivery of blood to the pulmonary circulation, which in turn delivers more blood to the left ventricle; this increases filling of the left ventricle, which causes *its* SV to increase. Because an increase in venous return causes the output of *both* ventricles to increase, blood flow through the systemic and pulmonary circulations is always in balance, as long as the heart is healthy.

In the failing heart, Starling's law breaks down. That is, force of contraction no longer increases in proportion to increased ventricular filling. As a result, blood backs up behind the failing ventricle (Fig. 43.6). In this example, output of the left ventricle is 1% less than the output of the right ventricle, which causes blood to back up in the pulmonary circulation. In only 20 minutes, this small imbalance between left and right ventricular output shifts a liter of blood from the systemic circulation to the pulmonary circulation. In less than 40 minutes, death from pulmonary congestion would ensue. This example underscores the importance of systemic-pulmonary balance and the critical role of Starling's mechanism in maintaining it.

REGULATION OF ARTERIAL PRESSURE

Arterial pressure is the driving force that moves blood through the arterial side of the systemic circulation. The general formula for AP is:

$$AP = PR \times CO$$

where AP is arterial pressure, PR is peripheral resistance, and CO is cardiac output. Accordingly, an increase in PR or CO will increase AP, whereas a decrease in PR or CO will decrease AP. Peripheral resistance is regulated primarily through constriction and dilation of arterioles. Cardiac output is regulated by the mechanisms discussed previously. Regulation of AP through processes that alter PR and CO is discussed in the sections that follow.

Overview of Control Systems

Under normal circumstances, AP is regulated primarily by three systems: the ANS, the renin-angiotensin-aldosterone system (RAAS), and the kidneys. These systems differ greatly with regard to time frame of response. The ANS acts in two ways: (1) it responds rapidly (in seconds or minutes) to acute changes in blood pressure and (2) it provides steady-state control. The RAAS responds more slowly, taking hours or days to influence AP. The kidneys are responsible for long-term control, and hence may take days or weeks to adjust AP.

Arterial pressure is also regulated by a fourth system: a family of natriuretic peptides. These peptides come into play primarily under conditions of volume overload.

Steady-State Control by the ANS

The ANS regulates AP by adjusting CO and PR. Sympathetic tone to the heart increases HR and contractility, thereby increasing CO. In contrast, parasympathetic tone slows the heart and thereby reduces CO. As discussed in Chapter 13, constriction of blood vessels is regulated exclusively by the sympathetic branch of the ANS; blood vessels have no parasympathetic innervation. Steady-state sympathetic tone provides a moderate level of vasoconstriction. The resultant resistance to blood flow maintains AP. Complete elimination of sympathetic tone would cause AP to fall by 50%.

Rapid Control by the ANS: The Baroreceptor Reflex

The baroreceptor reflex serves to maintain AP at a predetermined level. When AP changes, the reflex immediately attempts to restore AP to the preset value.

The reflex works as follows. Baroreceptors (pressure sensors) in the aortic arch and carotid sinus sense AP and relay this information to the vasoconstrictor center of the medulla. When AP changes, the vasoconstrictor center compensates by sending appropriate instructions to arterioles, veins, and the heart. For example, when AP drops, the vasoconstrictor center causes (1) constriction of nearly all arterioles, thereby increasing PR; (2) constriction of veins, thereby increasing venous return; and (3) acceleration of HR (by increasing sympathetic impulses to the heart and decreasing parasympathetic impulses). The combined effect of these responses is to restore AP to the preset level. When AP rises too high, opposite responses occur: The reflex dilates arterioles and veins and slows the heart.

The baroreceptor reflex is poised for rapid action—but not for sustained action. When AP falls or rises, the reflex acts within seconds to restore the preset pressure. However, when AP *remains* elevated or lowered, the system resets to the new pressure within 1 to 2 days. After this, the system perceives the new (elevated or reduced) pressure as "normal" and ceases to respond.

Drugs that lower AP will trigger the baroreceptor reflex. For example, if we administer a drug that dilates arterioles, the resultant drop in PR will reduce AP, causing the baroreceptor reflex to activate. The most noticeable response is *reflex tachycardia.* The baroreceptor reflex can temporarily negate efforts to lower AP with drugs.

The Renin-Angiotensin-Aldosterone System

The RAAS supports AP by causing (1) constriction of arterioles and veins and (2) retention of water by the kidneys. Vasoconstriction is mediated by a hormone named *angiotensin II.* Water retention is mediated in part by *aldosterone* through retention of sodium. Responses develop in hours (vasoconstriction) to days (water retention). The RAAS and its role in controlling blood pressure are discussed in Chapter 44.

Renal Retention of Water

When AP remains low for a long time, the kidneys respond by retaining water, which in turn causes AP to rise. Pressure rises because fluid retention increases blood volume, which increases venous pressure, which increases venous return, which increases CO, which increases AP. Water retention is a mechanism for maintaining AP over long periods (weeks, months, years).

Reduction in AP causes the kidneys to retain water because low AP reduces renal blood flow (RBF), which in turn reduces glomerular filtration rate (GFR). Because less fluid is filtered, less urine is produced, and therefore more water is retained. Low AP activates the RAAS, causing levels of angiotensin II and aldosterone to rise. Angiotensin II causes constriction of renal blood vessels and thereby further decreases RBF and GFR. Aldosterone promotes renal retention of sodium, which causes water to be retained along with it.

Postural Hypotension

Postural hypotension, also known as *orthostatic hypotension,* is a reduction in AP that can occur when we move from a supine or seated position to an upright position. The cause of hypotension is pooling of blood in veins, which decreases venous return, which in turn decreases CO. Between 300 and 800 mL of blood can pool in veins when we stand, causing CO to drop by as much as 2 L/min. Blood collects in veins when we stand, as gravity increases the pressure that blood exerts on veins. Because veins are not very muscular, they are unable to retain their shape when pressure increases, and hence they stretch. The resultant increase in venous volume allows blood to pool.

Two mechanisms help overcome postural hypotension. One is the system of auxiliary venous pumps, which promote venous return. In fact, in healthy individuals, these auxiliary pumps usually prevent postural hypotension from occurring in the first place. When postural hypotension does occur, the baroreceptor reflex can restore AP by (1) constricting veins and arterioles and (2) increasing HR.

In patients taking drugs that interfere with venoconstriction, postural hypotension is more intense and more prolonged. Hypotension is more intense because venous pooling is greater. Hypotension is more prolonged because there is no venoconstriction to help reverse venous pooling. As with drugs that reduce AP by dilating arterioles, drugs that reduce AP by relaxing veins can trigger the baroreceptor reflex and can thereby cause reflex tachycardia.

Natriuretic Peptides

Natriuretic peptides serve to protect the cardiovascular system in the event of volume overload, a condition that increases preload and thereby increases CO and AP. Volume overload is caused by excessive retention of sodium and water. Natriuretic peptides work primarily by (1) reducing blood volume and (2) promoting dilation of arterioles and veins. Both actions lower AP.

The family of natriuretic peptides has three principal members: *atrial natriuretic peptide* (ANP), *B-* or *brain natriuretic peptide* (BNP), and *C-natriuretic peptide* (CNP). ANP is produced by myocytes of the atria; BNP is produced by myocytes of the ventricles (and to a lesser extent by cells in the brain, where BNP was discovered); and CNP is produced by cells of the vascular endothelium. When blood volume is excessive, all three peptides are released. (Release of ANP and BNP is triggered by stretching of the atria and ventricles, which occurs because of increased preload.)

ANP and BNP have similar actions. Both peptides reduce blood volume and increase venous capacitance, and thereby reduce cardiac preload. Three processes are involved. First, ANP and BNP shift fluid from the vascular system to the extravascular compartment; the underlying mechanism is increased vascular permeability. Second, these peptides act on the kidney to cause diuresis (loss of water) and natriuresis (loss of sodium). Third, they promote dilation of arterioles and veins, in part by suppressing sympathetic outflow from the central nervous system. In addition to these actions, ANP and BNP help protect the heart during the early phase of heart failure by suppressing both the RAAS and sympathetic outflow, and by inhibiting proliferation of myocytes. Although CNP shares some actions of ANP and BNP, its primary action is to promote vasodilation.

KEY POINTS

- Arterioles serve as control valves to regulate local blood flow.
- Veins are a reservoir for blood.
- Arteries are not very distensible. As a result, large increases in arterial pressure (AP) cause only small increases in arterial diameter.
- Veins are highly distensible. As a result, small increases in venous pressure cause large increases in venous diameter.
- The adult circulatory system contains 5 L of blood, 64% of which is in systemic veins.
- Vasodilation reduces resistance to blood flow, whereas vasoconstriction increases resistance to flow.
- In addition to the small pressure head in venules, three mechanisms help ensure venous return to the heart: (1) negative pressure in the right atrium sucks blood toward the heart; (2) constriction of veins increases venous pressure and thereby drives blood toward the heart; and (3) contraction of skeletal muscles, in conjunction with one-way venous valves, pumps blood toward the heart.
- Heart rate is increased by sympathetic nerve impulses and decreased by parasympathetic impulses.
- Stroke volume is determined by myocardial contractility, cardiac preload, and cardiac afterload.
- Preload is defined as the amount of tension (stretch) applied to a muscle before contraction. In the heart, preload is determined by the force of venous return.
- Afterload is defined as the load against which a muscle exerts its force. For the heart, afterload is the AP that the left ventricle must overcome to eject blood.
- Cardiac afterload is determined primarily by peripheral resistance, which in turn is determined by the degree of constriction in arterioles.
- Starling's law states that the force of ventricular contraction is proportional to myocardial fiber length. Because of this relationship, when more blood enters the heart, more is pumped out. As a result, the healthy heart is able to precisely match output with venous return.
- The most important determinant of venous return is systemic filling pressure, which can be raised by constricting veins and increasing blood volume.
- Because cardiac muscle operates under Starling's law, the right and left ventricles always pump exactly the same amount of blood (assuming the heart is healthy). Hence, balance between the pulmonary and systemic circulations is maintained.
- Arterial pressure is regulated by the ANS, the RAAS, the kidneys, and natriuretic peptides.
- The ANS regulates AP (1) through tonic control of heart rate and peripheral resistance and (2) through the baroreceptor reflex.
- The baroreceptor reflex is useful only for short-term control of AP. When pressure remains elevated or lowered, the system resets to the new pressure within 1 to 2 days, and hence ceases to respond.
- Drugs that lower AP trigger the baroreceptor reflex and thereby cause reflex tachycardia. Hence, the baroreceptor reflex can temporarily negate efforts to lower AP with drugs.
- The RAAS supports AP by causing (1) constriction of arterioles and veins and (2) retention of water by the kidneys. Vasoconstriction is mediated by angiotensin II; water retention is mediated in part by aldosterone.
- The kidneys provide long-term control of blood pressure by regulating blood volume.
- Postural (orthostatic) hypotension is caused by decreased venous return secondary to pooling of blood in veins, which can occur when we assume an erect posture.
- Drugs that dilate veins intensify and prolong postural hypotension. As with other drugs that reduce AP, venodilators can trigger the baroreceptor reflex and can thereby cause reflex tachycardia.
- Natriuretic peptides defend the cardiovascular system from volume overload—primarily by reducing blood volume and promoting vasodilation.

Please visit **http://evolve.elsevier.com/Lehne** for chapter-specific NCLEX® examination review questions.

CHAPTER

44 Drugs Acting on the Renin-Angiotensin-Aldosterone System

In this chapter we consider four families of drugs: angiotensin-converting enzyme (ACE) inhibitors, angiotensin II receptor blockers (ARBs), direct renin inhibitors (DRIs), and aldosterone antagonists. With all four groups, effects result from interfering with the renin-angiotensin-aldosterone system (RAAS). The ACE inhibitors, available for more than three decades, have established roles in the treatment of hypertension, heart failure, and diabetic nephropathy; in addition, these drugs are indicated for myocardial infarction (MI) and prevention of cardiovascular events in patients at risk. Indications for ARBs are limited to hypertension, heart failure, diabetic nephropathy, and prevention of cardiovascular events in patients at risk. The aldosterone antagonist eplerenone has only two indications: hypertension and heart failure; spironolactone is also used to prevent diuretic-induced hypokalemia and to treat hyperaldosteronism. Current indications for DRIs are limited to hypertension. We begin by reviewing the physiology of the RAAS, and then we discuss the drugs that affect it.

PHYSIOLOGY OF THE RENIN-ANGIOTENSIN-ALDOSTERONE SYSTEM

The RAAS plays an important role in regulating blood pressure, blood volume, and fluid and electrolyte balance. In addition, the system appears to mediate certain pathophysiologic changes associated with hypertension, heart failure, and MI. The RAAS exerts its effects through angiotensin II and aldosterone.

Types of Angiotensin

Before considering the physiology of the RAAS, we need to introduce the angiotensin family, which consists of angiotensin I, angiotensin II, and angiotensin III. All three compounds are small polypeptides. Angiotensin I is the precursor of angiotensin II (Fig. 44.1) and has only weak biologic activity. In contrast, angiotensin II has strong biologic activity. Angiotensin III, which is formed by degradation of angiotensin II, has moderate biologic activity.

Actions of Angiotensin II

Angiotensin II participates in all processes regulated by the RAAS. The most prominent actions of angiotensin II are vasoconstriction and stimulation of aldosterone release. Both actions raise blood pressure. In addition, angiotensin II (as well as aldosterone) can act on the heart and blood vessels to cause pathologic changes in their structure and function.

Vasoconstriction

Angiotensin II is a powerful vasoconstrictor. The compound acts directly on vascular smooth muscle (VSM) to cause contraction. Vasoconstriction is prominent in arterioles and less so in veins. As a result of angiotensin-induced vasoconstriction, blood pressure rises. In addition to its direct action on blood vessels, angiotensin II can cause vasoconstriction indirectly by acting on (1) sympathetic neurons to promote norepinephrine release, (2) the adrenal medulla to promote epinephrine release, and (3) the central nervous system to increase sympathetic outflow to blood vessels.

Release of Aldosterone

Angiotensin II acts on the adrenal cortex to promote synthesis and secretion of aldosterone, whose actions are discussed in an upcoming section. The adrenal cortex is highly sensitive to angiotensin II, and hence angiotensin II can stimulate aldosterone release even when angiotensin II levels are too low to induce vasoconstriction. Aldosterone secretion is enhanced when sodium levels are low and when potassium levels are high.

Alteration of Cardiac and Vascular Structure

Angiotensin II may cause pathologic structural changes in the heart and blood vessels. In the heart, it may cause *hypertrophy* (increased cardiac mass) and *remodeling* (redistribution of mass within the heart). In hypertension, angiotensin II may be responsible for increasing the thickness of blood vessel walls. In atherosclerosis, it may be responsible for thickening the

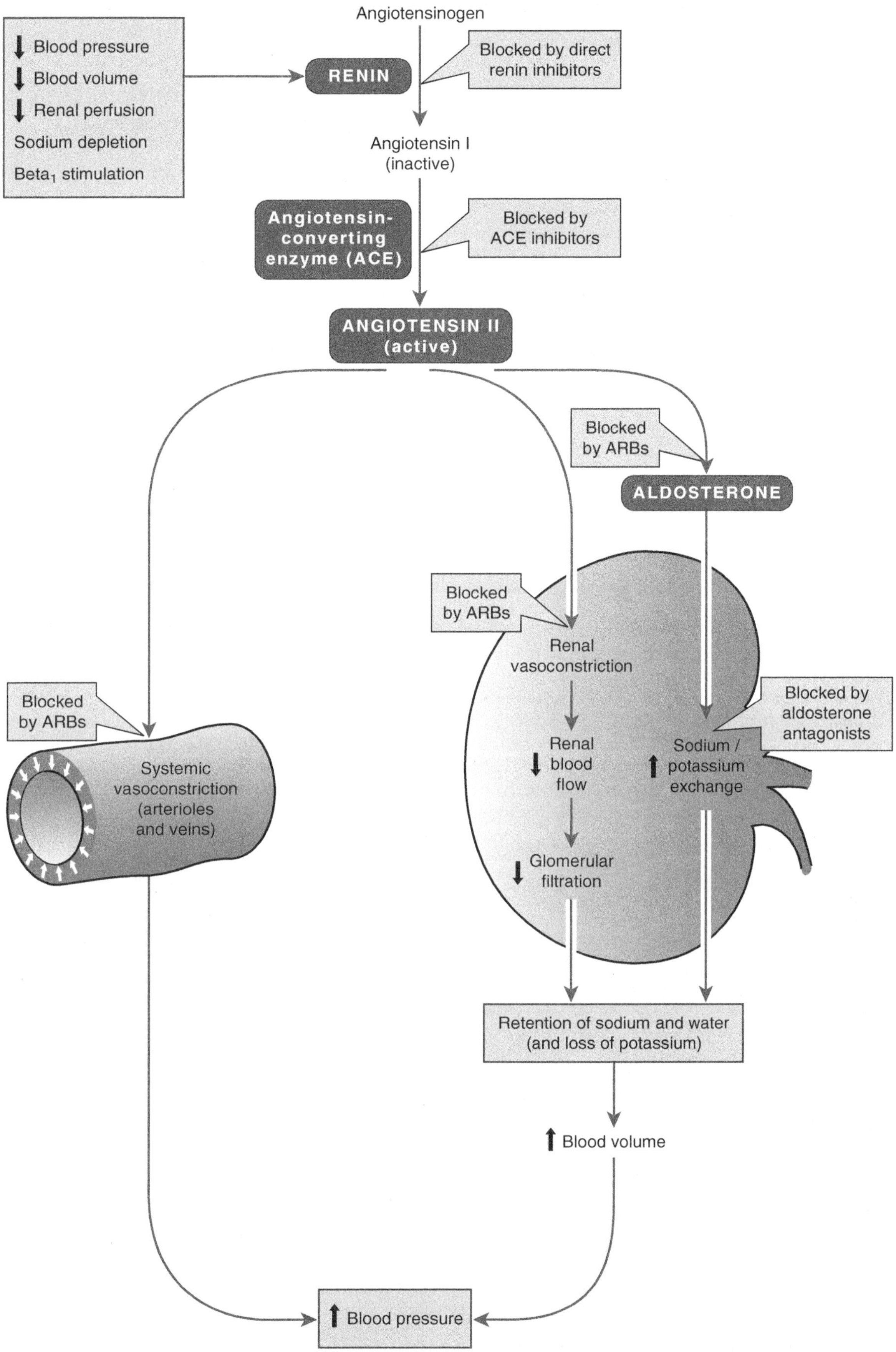

Fig. 44.1 ■ Regulation of blood pressure by the renin-angiotensin-aldosterone system. In addition to the mechanisms depicted, angiotensin II can raise blood pressure by (1) acting on the distal nephron to promote reabsorption of sodium and (2) increasing vasoconstriction by three mechanisms: promoting release of norepinephrine from sympathetic nerves; promoting release of epinephrine from the adrenal medulla; and acting in the central nervous system to increase sympathetic outflow to blood vessels. (*ARBs,* Angiotensin receptor blockers.)

intimal surface of blood vessels. And in heart failure and MI, it may be responsible for causing cardiac hypertrophy and fibrosis. Known effects of angiotensin II that could underlie these pathologic changes include:

- Increased migration, proliferation, and hypertrophy of VSM cells
- Increased production of extracellular matrix by VSM cells
- Hypertrophy of cardiac myocytes
- Increased production of extracellular matrix by cardiac fibroblasts

Actions of Aldosterone

Regulation of Blood Volume and Blood Pressure

After being released from the adrenal cortex, aldosterone acts on distal tubules of the kidney to cause retention of sodium and excretion of potassium and hydrogen. Because retention of sodium causes water to be retained as well, aldosterone increases blood volume, which causes blood pressure to rise.

Pathologic Cardiovascular Effects

Until recently, knowledge of aldosterone's actions was limited to effects on the kidney. Now, however, we know that aldosterone can cause more harmful effects. Like angiotensin II, aldosterone can promote cardiac remodeling and fibrosis. In addition, aldosterone can activate the sympathetic nervous system and suppress uptake of norepinephrine in the heart, thereby predisposing the heart to dysrhythmias. Also, aldosterone can promote vascular fibrosis (which decreases arterial compliance), and it can disrupt the baroreceptor reflex. These adverse effects appear to be limited to states such as heart failure, in which levels of aldosterone can be extremely high.

PATIENT-CENTERED CARE ACROSS THE LIFE SPAN

RAAS Inhibitors

Life Stage	Patient Care Concerns
Infants	Captopril and enalapril have been used in infants safely for management of hypertension (HTN).
Children/ adolescents	Some ACE inhibitors and ARBs are approved for use in children over the age of 6 for treatment of HTN.
Pregnant women	Animal studies revealed that drugs that block the RAAS should be avoided in pregnancy, especially in the second and third trimesters. ACE inhibitors, ARBs, and DRIs are classified in FDA Pregnancy Risk Category D.[a]
Breast-feeding women	Data are lacking regarding effects on the infant when breast-feeding. Caution is advised.
Older adults	The SCOPE and LIFE trials revealed a 25% decrease in stroke in patients ages 55–80 years using losartan when compared with atenolol. A 20% decreased risk of new-onset diabetes was seen with candesartan when compared with placebo.

[a]As of 2020, the FDA will no longer use Pregnancy Risk Categories. Please refer to Chapter 9 for more information.

Formation of Angiotensin II by Renin and Angiotensin-Converting Enzyme

Angiotensin II is formed through two sequential reactions. The first is catalyzed by renin, the second by ACE.

Renin

Renin catalyzes the formation of *angiotensin I* from *angiotensinogen.* This reaction is the rate-limiting step in angiotensin II formation. Renin is produced by juxtaglomerular cells of the kidney and undergoes controlled release into the bloodstream, where it cleaves angiotensinogen into angiotensin I.

Regulation of Renin Release. Since renin catalyzes the rate-limiting step in angiotensin II formation and since renin must be released into the blood in order to act, the factors that regulate renin release regulate the rate of angiotensin II formation.

Release of renin can be triggered by multiple factors (see Fig. 44.1). Release *increases* in response to a *decline* in blood pressure, blood volume, plasma sodium content, or renal perfusion pressure. Reduced renal perfusion pressure is an especially important stimulus for renin release and can occur in response to (1) stenosis of the renal arteries, (2) reduced systemic blood pressure, and (3) reduced plasma volume (brought on by dehydration, hemorrhage, or chronic sodium depletion). For the most part, these factors increase renin release through effects exerted locally in the kidney. However, some of these factors may also promote renin release through activation of the sympathetic nervous system. (Sympathetic nerves increase secretion of renin by causing stimulation of $beta_1$-adrenergic receptors on juxtaglomerular cells.)

Release of renin is *suppressed* by factors opposite to those that cause release. That is, renin secretion is inhibited by elevation of blood pressure, blood volume, and plasma sodium content. Hence, as blood pressure, blood volume, and plasma sodium content increase in response to renin release, further release of renin is suppressed. In this regard, we can view release of renin as being regulated by a classic negative feedback loop.

Angiotensin-Converting Enzyme (Kinase II)

ACE catalyzes the conversion of angiotensin I (inactive) into angiotensin II (highly active). ACE is located on the luminal surface of all blood vessels. The vasculature of the lungs is especially rich in the enzyme. Because ACE is abundant, conversion of angiotensin I into angiotensin II occurs almost instantaneously after angiotensin I has been formed. ACE is a relatively nonspecific enzyme that can act on a variety of substrates in addition to angiotensin I.

Nomenclature regarding ACE can be confusing and requires comment. As just noted, ACE can act on several substrates. When the substrate is angiotensin I, we refer to the enzyme as ACE. However, when the enzyme is acting on other substrates, we refer to it by different names. Of importance to us, when the substrate is a hormone known as *bradykinin,* we refer to the enzyme as *kinase II.* So, please remember, whether we call it ACE or kinase II, we're talking about the same enzyme.

Regulation of Blood Pressure by the Renin-Angiotensin-Aldosterone System

The RAAS is poised to help regulate blood pressure. Factors that lower blood pressure turn the RAAS on; factors that raise blood pressure turn it off. However, although the RAAS does indeed contribute to blood pressure control, its role in *normovolemic, sodium-replete* individuals is only modest. In contrast, the system can be a major factor in maintaining blood pressure in the presence of *hemorrhage, dehydration,* or *sodium depletion.*

The RAAS, acting through angiotensin II, raises blood pressure through two basic processes: vasoconstriction and renal retention of water and sodium. Vasoconstriction raises blood pressure by increasing total peripheral resistance; retention of water and sodium raises blood pressure by increasing blood volume. Vasoconstriction occurs within minutes to hours of activating the system, and hence can raise blood pressure quickly. In contrast, days, weeks, or even months are required for the kidney to raise blood pressure by increasing blood volume.

Angiotensin II acts in two ways to promote renal retention of water. First, by constricting renal blood vessels, angiotensin II reduces renal blood flow and thereby reduces glomerular filtration. Second, angiotensin II stimulates release of aldosterone from the adrenal cortex. Aldosterone then acts on renal tubules to promote retention of sodium and water and excretion of potassium.

Tissue (Local) Angiotensin II Production

In addition to the traditional RAAS that we've been discussing, in which angiotensin II is produced in the blood and then carried to target tissues, angiotensin II is produced in individual tissues. This permits discrete, local effects of angiotensin II independent of the main system. Interference with local production of angiotensin II may underlie some effects of the ACE inhibitors.

It is important to note that some angiotensin II is produced by pathways that *do not involve* ACE. As a result, drugs that inhibit ACE cannot completely block angiotensin II production.

Prototype Drugs

DRUGS ACTING ON THE RAAS SYSTEM

Angiotensin-Converting Enzyme (ACE) Inhibitor
Captopril

Angiotensin II Receptor Blocker
Losartan

Direct Renin Inhibitor
Aliskiren

Aldosterone Antagonist
Eplerenone

ANGIOTENSIN-CONVERTING ENZYME INHIBITORS

The ACE inhibitors are important drugs for *treating* hypertension, heart failure, diabetic nephropathy, and MI. In addition, they are used to *prevent* adverse cardiovascular events in patients at risk. Their most prominent adverse effects are cough, angioedema, first-dose hypotension, and hyperkalemia. For all of these agents, beneficial effects result largely from suppressing formation of angiotensin II. Because the similarities among ACE inhibitors are much more striking than their differences, we will discuss these drugs as a group, rather than selecting a prototype to represent them.

Mechanism of Action and Overview of Pharmacologic Effects

As shown in Fig. 44.2, ACE inhibitors produce their beneficial effects and adverse effects by (1) reducing levels of angiotensin II (through inhibition of ACE) and (2) increasing levels of bradykinin (through inhibition of kinase II). By reducing levels of angiotensin II, ACE inhibitors can dilate blood vessels (primarily arterioles and to a lesser extent veins), reduce blood volume (through effects on the kidney), and, importantly, prevent or reverse pathologic changes in the heart and blood vessels mediated by angiotensin II and aldosterone. Inhibition of ACE can also cause hyperkalemia and fetal injury. Elevation of

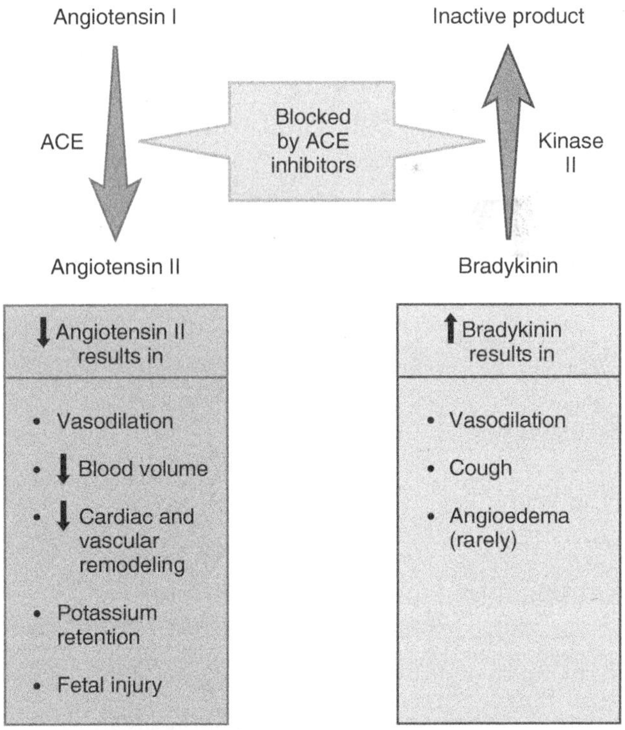

Fig. 44.2 ■ Overview of ACE inhibitor actions and pharmacologic effects.
Angiotensin-converting enzyme (ACE) and *kinase II* are two names for the same enzyme. When angiotensin II is the substrate, we call the enzyme ACE; when bradykinin is the substrate, we call it kinase II. Inhibition of this enzyme decreases *production* of angiotensin II (thereby *reducing* angiotensin II levels) and decreases *breakdown* of bradykinin (thereby *increasing* bradykinin levels).

bradykinin causes vasodilation (secondary to increased production of prostaglandins and nitric oxide) and can also promote cough and angioedema.

Pharmacokinetics

Regarding pharmacokinetics, the following generalizations apply:

- Nearly all ACE inhibitors are administered *orally.* The only exception is enalaprilat (the active form of enalapril), which is given IV.
- Except for captopril and moexipril, all oral ACE inhibitors can be administered with food.
- With the exception of captopril, all ACE inhibitors have prolonged half-lives, and hence can be administered just once or twice a day. Captopril is administered 2 or 3 times a day.
- With the exception of lisinopril, all ACE inhibitors are *prodrugs* that must undergo conversion to their active form in the small intestine and liver. Lisinopril is active as given.
- All ACE inhibitors are *excreted by the kidneys.* As a result, nearly all can accumulate to dangerous levels in patients with kidney disease, and hence *dosages must be reduced in these patients.* Only one agent—fosinopril—does not require a dosage reduction.

Therapeutic Uses

When the ACE inhibitors were introduced, their only indication was hypertension. Today, they are also used for heart failure, acute MI, left ventricular (LV) dysfunction, and diabetic and nondiabetic nephropathy. In addition, they can help prevent MI, stroke, and death in patients at high risk for cardiovascular events. It should be noted that no single ACE inhibitor is approved for all of these conditions (Table 44.1). However, given that all ACE inhibitors are very similar, it seems likely that all may produce similar benefits.

Hypertension. All ACE inhibitors are approved for hypertension. These drugs are especially effective against malignant hypertension and hypertension secondary to renal arterial stenosis. They are also useful against essential hypertension of mild to moderate intensity—although maximal benefits may take several weeks to develop.

In patients with essential hypertension, the mechanism underlying blood pressure reduction is not fully understood. *Initial* responses are proportional to circulating angiotensin II levels and are clearly related to reduced formation of that compound. (By lowering angiotensin II levels, ACE inhibitors dilate blood vessels and reduce blood volume; both actions help lower blood pressure.) However, with *prolonged* therapy, blood pressure often undergoes additional decline. During this phase, there is no relationship between reductions in blood

TABLE 44.1 ▪ ACE Inhibitors: Approved Indications and Adult Dosages

Generic Name	Brand Name	Approved Indications	Starting Dosage[a]	Usual Maintenance Dosage[a]
Benazepril	Lotensin	Hypertension	10 mg once/day	20–80 mg/day in 1 or 2 doses
Captopril	Capoten	Hypertension Heart failure LVD after MI Diabetic nephropathy	25 mg 2 or 3 times/day 6.25–12.5 mg 3 times/day 12.5 mg 3 times/day 25 mg 3 times/day	25–50 mg 2 or 3 times/day 50 mg 3 times/day 50 mg 3 times/day 25 mg 3 times/day
Enalapril	Vasotec, Epaned	Hypertension Heart failure Asymptomatic LVD	2.5–5 mg once/day 2.5 mg twice/day 2.5 mg twice/day	10–40 mg/day in 1 or 2 doses 10–20 mg twice/day 10 mg twice/day
Enalaprilat	Generic only	Hypertension	1.25 mg every 6 hr	Not used for maintenance
Fosinopril	Generic only	Hypertension Heart failure	10 mg once/day 5–10 mg once/day	20–40 mg/day in 1 or 2 doses 20–40 mg once/day
Lisinopril	Prinivil, Zestril, Qbrelis	Hypertension Heart failure Acute MI	10 mg once/day 2.5–5 mg once/day 5 mg once/day	10–40 mg once/day 20–40 mg once/day 10 mg once/day
Moexipril	Generic only	Hypertension	7.5 mg once/day	7.5–30 mg/day in 1 or 2 doses
Perindopril	Aceon, Coversyl 🍁	Hypertension Stable CAD	4 mg once/day 4 mg once/day	4–8 mg/day in 1 or 2 doses 8 mg once/day
Quinapril	Accupril	Hypertension Heart failure	1020 mg/day 5 mg twice/day	20–80 mg/day in 1 or 2 doses 20–40 mg twice/day
Ramipril	Altace	Hypertension Heart failure after MI Prevention of MI, stroke, and death in people at high risk for CVD	2.5 mg once/day 1.25–2.5 mg twice/day 2.5 mg/day for 1 wk	2.5–20 mg/day in 1 or 2 doses 5 mg twice/day 10 mg once/day
Trandolapril	Mavik	Hypertension Heart failure after MI LVD after MI	1 mg once/day 1 mg once/day 1 mg once/day	2–4 mg once/day 4 mg once/day 4 mg once/day

[a]For all ACE inhibitors except fosinopril, dosage must be reduced in patients with significant renal impairment.
CAD, Coronary artery disease; *CVD,* cardiovascular disease; *LVD,* left ventricular dysfunction; *MI,* myocardial infarction.

pressure and reductions in *circulating* angiotensin II. It may be that the delayed response is due to reductions in *local* angiotensin II levels—reductions that would not be revealed by measuring angiotensin II in the blood.

ACE inhibitors offer several advantages over most other antihypertensive drugs. In contrast to the sympatholytic agents, ACE inhibitors do not interfere with cardiovascular reflexes. Hence, exercise capacity is not impaired and orthostatic hypotension is minimal. In addition, these drugs can be used safely in patients with bronchial asthma, a condition that precludes the use of beta$_2$-adrenergic antagonists. ACE inhibitors do not promote hypokalemia, hyperuricemia, or hyperglycemia—side effects seen with thiazide diuretics. Furthermore, they do not induce lethargy, weakness, or sexual dysfunction—responses that are common with other antihypertensive agents. Most importantly, *ACE inhibitors reduce the risk of cardiovascular mortality caused by hypertension.* The only other drugs proved to reduce hypertension-associated mortality are beta blockers and diuretics (see Chapter 47).

Heart Failure. ACE inhibitors produce multiple benefits in heart failure. By lowering arteriolar tone, these drugs improve regional blood flow, and, by reducing cardiac afterload, they increase cardiac output. By causing venous dilation, they reduce pulmonary congestion and peripheral edema. By dilating blood vessels in the kidney, they increase renal blood flow and thereby promote excretion of sodium and water. This loss of fluid has two beneficial effects: (1) it helps reduce edema, and (2) by lowering blood volume, it decreases venous return to the heart and thereby reduces right-heart workload. Lastly, by suppressing aldosterone and reducing local production of angiotensin II in the heart, ACE inhibitors may prevent or reverse pathologic changes in cardiac structure. Although only seven ACE inhibitors are approved for heart failure (see Table 44.1), both the American Heart Association and the American College of Cardiology have concluded that the ability to improve symptoms and prolong survival is a class effect. The use of ACE inhibitors in heart failure is discussed further in Chapter 48.

Myocardial Infarction. ACE inhibitors can reduce mortality following acute MI (heart attack). In addition, they decrease the chance of developing overt heart failure. Treatment should begin as soon as possible after infarction and should continue for at least 6 weeks. In patients who develop overt heart failure, treatment should continue long term. As for patients who do not develop heart failure, there are no data to indicate whether or not continued treatment would be beneficial. At this time, only three ACE inhibitors—captopril, lisinopril, and trandolapril—are approved for patients with MI.

Diabetic and Nondiabetic Nephropathy. ACE inhibitors can benefit patients with diabetic nephropathy, the leading cause of end-stage renal disease in the United States. In patients with overt nephropathy, as indicated by proteinuria of more than 500 mg/day, ACE inhibitors can slow progression of renal disease. In patients with less advanced nephropathy (30 to 300 mg proteinuria/day), ACE inhibitors can delay onset of overt nephropathy. These benefits were first demonstrated in patients with type 1 diabetes (insulin-dependent diabetes mellitus) and were later demonstrated in patients with type 2 diabetes (non–insulin-dependent diabetes mellitus). More recently, ACE inhibitors have been shown to provide similar benefits in patients with nephropathy unrelated to diabetes.

The principal protective mechanism appears to be reduction of glomerular filtration pressure. ACE inhibitors lower filtration pressure by reducing levels of angiotensin II, a compound that can raise filtration pressure by two mechanisms. First, angiotensin II raises systemic blood pressure, which raises pressure in the afferent arteriole of the glomerulus (Fig. 44.3). Second, it constricts the efferent arteriole, thereby generating back-pressure in the glomerulus. The resultant increase in filtration pressure promotes injury. By reducing levels of angiotensin II, ACE inhibitors lower glomerular filtration pressure and thereby slow development of renal injury.

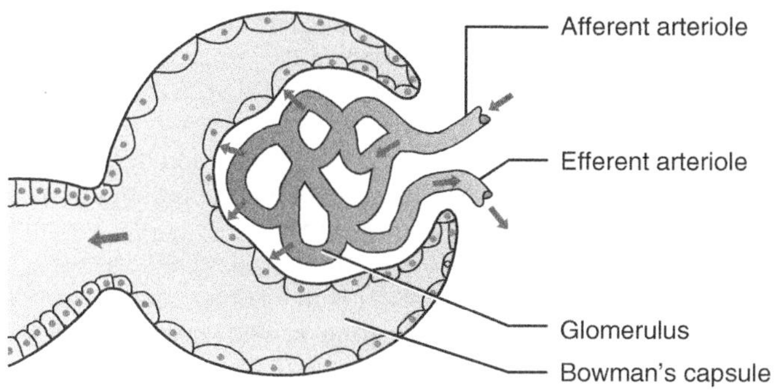

Fig. 44.3 ▪ Elevation of glomerular filtration pressure by angiotensin II.
Angiotensin II increases filtration pressure by (1) increasing pressure in the afferent arteriole (secondary to increasing systemic arterial pressure) and (2) constricting the efferent arteriole, thereby generating back-pressure in the glomerulus.

At this time, the only ACE inhibitor approved for nephropathy is captopril. However, the American Diabetes Association considers benefits in diabetic nephropathy to be a class effect, and hence recommends choosing an ACE inhibitor based on its cost and likelihood of patient adherence.

Can ACE inhibitors be used for *primary prevention* of diabetic nephropathy? No. Although use of these agents can slow progression of kidney disease, they ultimately do not prevent it. This conclusion is based on multiple small studies, as well as the *Renin-Angiotensin System Study* (RASS), which evaluated the effects of an ACE inhibitor (*enalapril* [Vasotec]) and an ARB (*losartan* [Cozaar]) in patients with type 1 diabetes who did not have hypertension or any signs of early kidney disease. Both drugs failed to protect the kidney: Compared with patients receiving placebo, those receiving enalapril or losartan developed the same degree of microalbuminuria (an early sign of kidney damage), the same decline in kidney function, and the same changes in glomerular structure (as shown by microscopic analysis of kidney biopsy samples). Hence, although ACE inhibitors may slow progression of established nephropathy, they do not protect against kidney damage.

Prevention of MI, Stroke, and Death in Patients at High Cardiovascular Risk. One ACE inhibitor (*ramipril* [Altace]) is approved for reducing the risk of MI, stroke, and death from cardiovascular causes in patients at *high* risk for a major cardiovascular event—high risk being defined by (1) a history of stroke, coronary artery disease, peripheral vascular disease, or diabetes, combined with (2) at least one other risk factor, such as hypertension, high LDL cholesterol, low HDL cholesterol, or cigarette smoking. Ramipril was approved for this use based on results of the *Heart Outcomes Prevention Evaluation* (HOPE) trial, a large study in which patients at high cardiovascular risk took either ramipril (10 mg/day) or placebo. Follow-up time was 5 years. The combined endpoint of MI, stroke, or death from cardiovascular causes was significantly lower in the ramipril group (14% vs. 18%)—a 22% reduction in risk. Possible mechanisms underlying benefits include reduced vascular resistance and protection of the heart, blood vessels, and kidneys from the damage that angiotensin II and aldosterone can cause over time.

Like ramipril, *perindopril* [Aceon, Coversyl ♣] can reduce morbidity and mortality in patients at risk for major cardiovascular events. However, the drug is not yet approved for this use. Benefits were demonstrated in the *EURopean trial On reduction of cardiac events with Perindopril in stable coronary Artery disease* (EUROPA). Patients in EUROPA were at lower risk than those in HOPE.

Can ACE inhibitors other than ramipril and perindopril also reduce cardiovascular risk? Possibly. However, at this time there is insufficient evidence to say for sure.

Diabetic Retinopathy. The RASS trial showed that at least one ACE inhibitor—*enalapril*—can reduce the risk of diabetic retinopathy in *some* patients. Specifically, in patients with *type 1 diabetes* who do not have hypertension, nephropathy, or established retinopathy, enalapril prevented or slowed development of retinal change. However, in patients with type 1 diabetes and *established* retinopathy, enalapril had no benefit. In patients with *type 2 diabetes,* enalapril had no benefit, regardless of retinopathy status.

Adverse Effects

ACE inhibitors are generally well tolerated. Some adverse effects (e.g., first-dose hypotension, hyperkalemia) are due to a reduction in angiotensin II, whereas others (cough, angioedema) are due to elevation of bradykinin.

First-Dose Hypotension. A precipitous drop in blood pressure may occur following the first dose of an ACE inhibitor. This reaction is caused by widespread vasodilation secondary to abrupt lowering of angiotensin II levels. First-dose hypotension is most likely in patients with severe hypertension, in patients taking diuretics, and in patients who are sodium depleted or volume depleted. To minimize the first-dose effect, initial doses should be low. Also, diuretics should be temporarily discontinued, starting 2 to 3 days before beginning an ACE inhibitor. Blood pressure should be monitored for several hours following the first dose of an ACE inhibitor. If hypotension develops, the patient should assume a supine position. If necessary, blood pressure can be raised with an infusion of normal saline.

Cough. All ACE inhibitors can cause persistent dry, irritating, nonproductive cough. Severity can range from a scratchy throat to severe hacking cough. The underlying cause is accumulation of bradykinin secondary to inhibition of kinase II (another name for ACE). Cough occurs in about 10% of patients and is the most common reason for discontinuing therapy. Factors that increase the risk of cough include advanced age, female sex, and Asian ancestry. Cough begins to subside 3 days after discontinuing an ACE inhibitor and is gone within 10 days.

Hyperkalemia. Inhibition of aldosterone release (secondary to inhibition of angiotensin II production) can cause potassium retention by the kidney. As a rule, significant potassium accumulation is limited to patients taking potassium supplements, salt substitutes (which contain potassium), or a potassium-sparing diuretic. For most other patients, hyperkalemia is rare. Patients should be instructed to avoid potassium supplements and potassium-containing salt substitutes unless they are prescribed.

Renal Failure. ACE inhibitors can cause severe renal insufficiency in patients with *bilateral renal artery stenosis or stenosis in the artery to a single remaining kidney.* In patients with renal artery stenosis, the kidneys release large amounts of renin. The resulting high levels of angiotensin II serve to maintain glomerular filtration by two mechanisms: elevation of blood pressure and constriction of efferent glomerular arterioles (see Fig. 44.3). When ACE is inhibited, causing angiotensin II levels to fall, the mechanisms that had been supporting glomerular filtration fail, causing urine production to drop precipitously. Not surprisingly, *ACE inhibitors are contraindicated for patients with bilateral renal artery stenosis (or stenosis in the artery to a single remaining kidney).*

Fetal Injury. For a long time, we have known that use of ACE inhibitors during the *second* and *third* trimesters of pregnancy can injure the developing fetus. Specific effects include hypotension, hyperkalemia, skull hypoplasia, pulmonary hypoplasia, anuria, renal failure (reversible and irreversible), and death. Women who become pregnant while using ACE inhibitors should discontinue treatment as soon as possible. Infants who have been exposed to ACE inhibitors during the second or third trimester should be closely monitored for hypotension, oliguria, and hyperkalemia.

Are ACE inhibitors safe *early* in pregnancy? Possibly. Even though an article in the *New England Journal of Medicine* reported that among 209 children exposed to ACE inhibitors during the first trimester, 18 (8.7%) had major congenital malformations, compared with 3.2% of controls, these data contrast with animal studies, which suggest that such malformations are not likely. Furthermore, no mechanism by which ACE inhibitors might disrupt early embryogenesis is known. It is now thought that the malformations attributed to ACE inhibitors are more related to hypertension in pregnancy, not the drug itself. As there is lack of complete data, however, the U.S. Food and Drug Administration (FDA) still classifies ACE inhibitors in Pregnancy Risk Category D,[a] which indicates they should be avoided in pregnancy.

Angioedema. Angioedema is a potentially fatal reaction that develops in up to 1% of patients. Symptoms, which result from increased capillary permeability, include giant wheals and edema of the tongue, glottis, lips, eyes, and pharynx. Severe reactions should be treated with subcutaneous epinephrine. If angioedema develops, ACE inhibitors should be discontinued and never used again. Angioedema is caused by accumulation of bradykinin secondary to inhibition of kinase II.

Safety Alert

ACE INHIBITORS

ACE inhibitors can cause angioedema, a potentially life-threatening reaction. If patients report edema of the tongue, lips, or eyes, emergency care should be sought immediately, and the patient must never take ACE inhibitors again.

[a]As of 2020, the FDA will no longer use Pregnancy Risk Categories. Please refer to Chapter 9 for more information.

Neutropenia. Neutropenia, with its associated risk of infection, is a rare but serious complication. Neutropenia is most likely in patients with renal impairment and in those with collagen vascular diseases (e.g., systemic lupus erythematosus, scleroderma). These patients should be followed closely. Fortunately, neutropenia is reversible when detected early. If neutropenia develops, ACE inhibitors should be withdrawn immediately. Neutrophil counts should normalize in approximately 2 weeks. In the absence of early detection, neutropenia may progress to fatal agranulocytosis. Patients should be informed about early signs of infection (e.g., fever, sore throat) and instructed to report them immediately. Neutropenia is more common with captopril than with other ACE inhibitors.

Drug Interactions

Diuretics. Diuretics may intensify first-dose hypotension. To prevent this interaction, diuretics should be withdrawn 2 to 3 days before giving an ACE inhibitor. Diuretic therapy can be resumed later if needed.

Antihypertensive Agents. The hypotensive effects of ACE inhibitors are often additive with those of other antihypertensive drugs (e.g., diuretics, sympatholytics, vasodilators, calcium channel blockers). When an ACE inhibitor is added to an antihypertensive regimen, dosages of other drugs may require reduction.

Drugs That Raise Potassium Levels. ACE inhibitors increase the risk of hyperkalemia caused by *potassium supplements and potassium-sparing diuretics.* The risk of hyperkalemia is increased because, by suppressing aldosterone secretion, ACE inhibitors can reduce excretion of potassium. To minimize the risk of hyperkalemia, potassium supplements and potassium-sparing diuretics should be employed only when clearly indicated.

Lithium. ACE inhibitors can cause lithium to accumulate to toxic levels. Lithium levels should be monitored frequently.

Nonsteroidal Anti-Inflammatory Drugs (NSAIDs). Aspirin, ibuprofen, and other NSAIDs may reduce the antihypertensive effects of ACE inhibitors.

Preparations, Dosage, and Administration

Except for enalaprilat, all ACE inhibitors are administered orally. Of the oral products, all are available in single-drug formulations. Most are also available in fixed-dose combinations with hydrochlorothiazide, a thiazide diuretic, and one agent—perindopril—is available combined with indapamide. Three ACE inhibitors—benazepril, perindopril, and trandolapril—are available combined with calcium channel blockers. Except for captopril and moexipril, all oral formulations may be administered without regard to meals; captopril and moexipril should be administered 1 hour before meals. Dosages for all ACE inhibitors (except fosinopril) should be reduced in patients with renal impairment. Dosages for specific indications are shown in Table 44.1. Formulations are described in the list that follows:

- Benazepril is available alone (5-, 10-, 20-, and 40-mg tablets) as *Lotensin,* combined with hydrochlorothiazide as *Lotensin HCT,* and combined with amlodipine as *Lotrel.*
- Captopril is available alone (12.5-, 25-, 50-, and 100-mg tablets) as *Capoten,* and combined with hydrochlorothiazide.
- Enalapril is available alone (2.5-, 5-, 10-, and 20-mg tablets) as *Vasotec,* as a 1 mg/mL oral solution sold as *Epaned,* and combined with hydrochlorothiazide as *Vaseretic.*
- Enalaprilat, the active form of enalapril, is available in solution (1.25 mg/mL) for IV therapy of severe hypertension. Enalaprilat is the only ACE inhibitor that is given IV.
- Fosinopril is available alone (10-, 20-, and 40-mg tablets) as *Monopril,* and combined with hydrochlorothiazide.
- Lisinopril is available alone (2.5-, 5-, 10-, 20-, 30-, and 40-mg tablets) as *Prinivil* and *Zestril,* as a 1 mg/mL oral solution sold as *Qbrelis,* and combined with hydrochlorothiazide.
- Moexipril is available alone (7.5- and 15-mg tablets) and combined with hydrochlorothiazide.
- Perindopril is available alone (2-, 4-, and 8-mg tablets) as *Aceon* and *Coversyl* ♣, in combination with amlodipine (3.5/2.5-, 7/5-, and 14/10-mg tablets) sold as *Prestalia,* and combined with indapamide (2/0.625, 4/1.25, and 8/2.5 mg) as *Coversyl Plus* ♣.
- Quinapril is available alone (5-, 10-, 20-, and 40-mg tablets) as *Accupril,* and combined with hydrochlorothiazide as *Accuretic.*
- Ramipril is available alone (1.25-, 2.5-, 5-, and 10-mg capsules) as *Altace,* and combined with hydrochlorothiazide (2.5/12.5, 5/12.5, 10/12.5, 5/25, 10/25 mg) as *Altace HCT* ♣.
- Trandolapril is available alone (1-, 2-, and 4-mg tablets) as *Mavik,* and combined with verapamil as *Tarka.* The drug is not available in combination with hydrochlorothiazide.

ANGIOTENSIN II RECEPTOR BLOCKERS

The ARBs are relatively new, and their indications are evolving. Initially, ARBs were approved only for hypertension. Today, they also are approved for treating heart failure, diabetic nephropathy, and MI, and for prevention of MI, stroke, and death in people at high risk for cardiovascular events.

Like the ACE inhibitors, ARBs decrease the influence of angiotensin II. However, the mechanisms involved differ: Whereas ACE inhibitors block *production* of angiotensin II, ARBs block the *actions* of angiotensin II. Because both groups interfere with angiotensin II, they both have similar effects. They differ primarily in that ARBs pose a much lower risk of cough or hyperkalemia.

Given that ACE inhibitors and ARBs have very similar effects, are these drugs clinically interchangeable? No. We have clear and extensive evidence that ACE inhibitors decrease cardiovascular morbidity and mortality. The evidence for ARBs is less convincing. Accordingly, until more is known, ACE inhibitors are preferred. For patients who cannot tolerate ACE inhibitors, ARBs are an appropriate second choice.

Eight ARBs are available. All eight are very similar; hence, we will discuss them as a group, rather than choosing one as a prototype.

Mechanism of Action and Overview of Pharmacologic Effects

ARBs block access of angiotensin II to its receptors in blood vessels, the adrenals, and all other tissues. As a result, ARBs have effects much like those of the ACE inhibitors. By blocking angiotensin II receptors on blood vessels, ARBs cause dilation of arterioles and veins. By blocking angiotensin II receptors in the heart, ARBs can prevent angiotensin II from inducing pathologic changes in cardiac structure. By blocking angiotensin II receptors in the adrenals, ARBs decrease release of aldosterone and can thereby increase renal excretion of sodium and water. Sodium and water excretion is further increased through dilation of renal blood vessels.

In contrast to the ACE inhibitors, ARBs do *not* inhibit kinase II, and hence do not increase levels of bradykinin in the lung. As a result, ARBs have a lower risk of cough, the most common reason for stopping ACE inhibitors.

Therapeutic Uses

Hypertension. All ARBs are approved for hypertension. Reductions in blood pressure equal those seen with ACE inhibitors. Whether ARBs share the ability of ACE inhibitors to reduce mortality has not been established.

Heart Failure. Currently, only two ARBs—*valsartan* [Diovan] and *candesartan* [Atacand]—are approved for heart failure. In clinical trials, these drugs reduced symptoms, decreased hospitalizations, improved functional capacity, and increased LV ejection fraction. More importantly, they prolonged survival. Because experience with these drugs is limited, they should be reserved for patients who cannot tolerate ACE inhibitors (because of cough). Although the other ARBs are not yet approved for heart failure, most authorities believe they are effective.

Diabetic Nephropathy. Two ARBs—*irbesartan* [Avapro] and *losartan* [Cozaar]—are approved for managing nephropathy in hypertensive patients with type 2 diabetes. In clinical trials, these drugs delayed development of overt nephropathy and slowed progression of established nephropathy. Benefits are due in part to reductions in blood pressure and in part to mechanisms that have not been determined. How do ARBs compare with ACE inhibitors? Although both groups of drugs can delay progression of nephropathy, only the ACE inhibitors have been shown to reduce mortality. As noted previously, neither ARBs nor ACE inhibitors are effective for primary prevention of diabetic nephropathy.

Myocardial Infarction. One ARB—*valsartan* [Diovan]—is approved for reducing cardiovascular mortality in post-MI patients with heart failure or LV dysfunction. Approval was based on the results of a major trial—the *Valsartan in Acute Myocardial Infarction Trial* (VALIANT)—that showed that valsartan was as effective as captopril at reducing short-term and long-term mortality in these patients.

Stroke Prevention. One ARB—*losartan* [Cozaar]—is approved for reducing the risk of stroke in patients with hypertension and LV hypertrophy. In clinical studies, stroke prevention with losartan was better than with atenolol (a beta blocker), even though both drugs produced an equivalent decrease in blood pressure. This observation indicates that the benefits of losartan cannot be explained on the basis of reduced blood pressure alone.

Prevention of MI, Stroke, and Death in Patients at High Cardiovascular Risk. One ARB—*telmisartan* [Micardis]—is approved for reducing the risk of MI, stroke, and death from cardiovascular causes in patients age 55 years and older, but only if they are intolerant of ACE inhibitors. (Recall that ramipril, an ACE inhibitor, is also approved for preventing MI, stroke, and death in high-risk patients.) Approval of telmisartan was based on the ONTARGET study, which showed that telmisartan was similar to ramipril with regard to reducing cardiovascular morbidity and mortality. Of note, combining telmisartan with ramipril was no more effective than either agent alone, but did increase the risk of adverse events. Can other ARBs reduce cardiovascular risk? Possibly, but proof is lacking.

Diabetic Retinopathy. In the RASS study mentioned earlier, benefits of the ARB *losartan* [Cozaar] were like those of enalapril: In patients with type 1 diabetes without established retinopathy, losartan slowed the development and progression of retinopathy, but it had no benefit in patients with established retinopathy. In patients with type 2 diabetes, the drug offered no benefit at all, regardless of retinopathy status.

Adverse Effects

All of the ARBs are well tolerated. In contrast to ACE inhibitors, ARBs do not cause clinically significant hyperkalemia. Furthermore, because ARBs do not promote accumulation of bradykinin in the lung, they have a lower incidence of cough.

Angioedema. Like the ACE inhibitors, ARBs can cause angioedema, although the incidence may be lower with ARBs. If angioedema occurs, ARBs should be withdrawn immediately and never used again. Severe reactions are treated with subcutaneous epinephrine.

ARBs cause angioedema possibly by increasing bradykinin availability. Unlike ACE inhibitors, ARBs do not inhibit bradykinin breakdown. However, through an indirect mechanism, ARBs may be able to increase local bradykinin synthesis.

Is it reasonable to give an ARB to a patient who developed angioedema with an ACE inhibitor? Sometimes. About 8% of patients who experience angioedema with an ACE inhibitor will also develop angioedema if given an ARB. Nonetheless, switching to an ARB may be worth the risk for specific patients, namely, those with a disorder for which ARBs are known to improve outcomes (i.e., heart failure, diabetes, and MI).

Fetal Harm. Like the ACE inhibitors, ARBs can injure the developing fetus if taken during the second or third trimester of pregnancy, and hence are contraindicated during this period. Also, there is concern that ARBs and ACE inhibitors may harm the fetus earlier in pregnancy, and hence should be discontinued as soon as pregnancy is discovered.

Renal Failure. Like the ACE inhibitors, ARBs can cause renal failure in patients with bilateral renal artery stenosis or stenosis in the artery to a single remaining kidney. Accordingly, ARBs must be used with extreme caution in patients with these conditions.

Drug Interactions

The hypotensive effects of ARBs are additive with those of other antihypertensive drugs. When an ARB is added to an antihypertensive regimen, dosages of the other drugs may require reduction.

Preparations, Dosage, and Administration

All ARBs are administered PO, and all may be taken with or without food. All are available alone, and all but azilsartan are also available in fixed-dose combinations with hydrochlorothiazide, a thiazide diuretic. Dosages for specific indications are shown in Table 44.2. Formulations are described in the list that follows:

- Azilsartan is available alone (40- and 80-mg tablets) as *Edarbi.* Unlike other ARBs, the drug is not available

TABLE 44.2 ■ Angiotensin II Receptor Blockers: Approved Indications and Adult Dosages

Generic Name	Brand Name	Approved Indications	Initial Dosage	Maintenance Dosage
Azilsartan	Edarbi	Hypertension	40–80 mg once/day	80 mg once/day
Candesartan	Atacand	Hypertension Heart failure	16 mg once/day 4 mg once/day	8–32 mg/day in 1 or 2 doses 32 mg once/day
Eprosartan	Teveten	Hypertension	600 mg once/day	400–800 mg/day in 1 or 2 doses
Irbesartan	Avapro	Hypertension Diabetic nephropathy[a]	150 mg once/day 300 mg once/day	150–300 mg once/day 300 mg once/day
Losartan	Cozaar	Hypertension Stroke prevention[b] Diabetic nephropathy[a]	25–50 mg once/day 50 mg once/day 50 mg once/day	25–100 mg/day in 1 or 2 doses 50–100 mg once/day 100 mg once/day
Olmesartan	Benicar, Olmetec ♣	Hypertension	20 mg once/day	20–40 mg once/day
Telmisartan	Micardis	Hypertension Prevention of MI, stroke, and death in people at high risk for CVD but who can't take an ACE inhibitor	40 mg once/day 80 mg once/day	20–80 mg once/day 80 mg once/day
Valsartan	Diovan	Hypertension Heart failure MI	80–160 mg once/day 40 mg twice/day 20 mg twice/day	80–320 mg once/day 40–160 mg twice/day 160 mg twice/day

[a]In patients with type 2 diabetes.
[b]In patients with hypertension and left ventricular hypertrophy.
ACE, Angiotensin-converting enzyme; *CVD,* cardiovascular disease; *MI,* myocardial infarction.

combined with hydrochlorothiazide but is paired with chlorthalidone and marketed as *Edarbyclor.*

- Candesartan is available alone (4-, 8-, 16-, and 32-mg tablets) as *Atacand,* and combined with hydrochlorothiazide as *Atacand HCT.*
- Eprosartan is available alone (400- and 600-mg tablets) as *Teveten,* and combined with hydrochlorothiazide as *Teveten HCT.*
- Irbesartan is available alone (75-, 150-, and 300-mg tablets) as *Avapro,* and combined with hydrochlorothiazide as *Avalide.*
- Losartan is available alone (25-, 50-, and 100-mg tablets) as *Cozaar,* and combined with hydrochlorothiazide as *Hyzaar.*
- Olmesartan is available alone (5-, 20-, and 40-mg tablets) as *Benicar* and *Olmetec* ♣, combined with hydrochlorothiazide as *Benicar HCT* and *Olmetec Plus* ♣, combined with amlodipine as *Azor,* and combined with amlodipine plus hydrochlorothiazide as *Tribenzor.*
- Telmisartan is available alone (20-, 40-, and 80-mg tablets) as *Micardis,* combined with hydrochlorothiazide as *Micardis HCT,* and combined with amlodipine as *Twynsta.*
- Valsartan is available alone (40-, 80-, 160-, and 320-mg tablets) as *Diovan,* combined with hydrochlorothiazide as *Diovan HCT,* combined with amlodipine as *Exforge,* combined with nebivolol as *Byvalson,* and combined with amlodipine plus hydrochlorothiazide as *Exforge HCT.*

A new combination of valsartan and sacubitril, sold as *Entresto*, is approved only for heart failure and is discussed in Chapter 48.

ALISKIREN, A DIRECT RENIN INHIBITOR

DRIs are drugs that act on renin to inhibit the conversion of angiotensinogen into angiotensin I. By decreasing production of angiotensin I, DRIs can suppress the entire RAAS. Currently, only one DRI—*aliskiren* [Tekturna, Rasilez ♣]—is available.

Blood pressure reduction with aliskiren equals that seen with ACE inhibitors. Aliskiren causes less cough and angioedema than the ACE inhibitors, but poses similar risks to the developing fetus.

Mechanism of Action

Aliskiren binds tightly with renin and thereby inhibits the cleavage of angiotensinogen into angiotensin I. Since this reaction is the first and rate-limiting step in the production of angiotensin II and aldosterone, aliskiren can reduce the influence of the entire RAAS. In clinical trials, the drug decreased plasma renin activity by 50% to 80%. Although aliskiren works at an earlier step than either the ACE inhibitors or ARBs, there is no proof that doing so results in superior clinical outcomes.

Therapeutic Use

Aliskiren is approved only for *hypertension.* It may be used alone or in combination with other antihypertensives. In clinical trials, aliskiren reduced blood pressure to the same extent as did ACE inhibitors, ARBs, or calcium channel blockers. Maximal effects developed within 2 weeks. Although aliskiren can reduce blood pressure in hypertensive patients, we don't know whether the drug also reduces negative outcomes (i.e., blindness, stroke, kidney disease, death). In contrast, the ability of ACE inhibitors and ARBs to improve outcomes is well established. Until the long-term benefits and safety of aliskiren are known, older antihypertensives should be considered first. In addition to its use in hypertension, aliskiren was evaluated for treating heart failure and renal failure associated with diabetes. Unfortunately, in the ATMOSPHERE and ALTITUDE trials, aliskiren was no more effective than other current treatments.

Pharmacokinetics

Aliskiren is administered orally, and bioavailability is low (only 2.5%). Dosing with a *high-fat meal* makes availability much lower (about 0.8%). Aliskiren undergoes some metabolism by CYP3A4 (the 3A4 isoenzyme of cytochrome P450), but the extent of metabolism is not known. About 25% of the drug is eliminated unchanged in the urine. The half-life is about 24 hours.

Adverse Effects

Aliskiren is generally well tolerated. At usual doses, the risk of angioedema, cough, or hyperkalemia is low. At high therapeutic doses, some patients experience diarrhea. Like other drugs that affect the RAAS, aliskiren should be avoided during pregnancy.

Angioedema and Cough. With ACE inhibitors, angioedema and cough result from inhibition of kinase II. Because aliskiren does not inhibit kinase II, the risk of these effects is low. In clinical trials, the incidence of cough was 1.1% with aliskiren versus about 10% with an ACE inhibitor. Similarly, the incidence of angioedema was 0.06% with aliskiren versus 1% with an ACE inhibitor. If angioedema does occur, aliskiren should be discontinued immediately.

Gastrointestinal Effects. Aliskiren causes dose-dependent *diarrhea,* seen in 2.3% of patients taking 300 mg/day. Women and older adults are most susceptible. Excessive doses (600 mg/day) are associated with abdominal pain and dyspepsia.

Hyperkalemia. Like the ACE inhibitors, aliskiren rarely causes hyperkalemia when used alone. However, hyperkalemia might be expected if aliskiren were combined with an ACE inhibitor, a potassium-sparing diuretic, or potassium supplements.

Fetal Injury and Death. Although aliskiren has not been studied in pregnant women, the drug is likely to pose a risk of major congenital malformations and fetal death because the risk of these events is well established with other drugs that suppress the RAAS. Therefore, like the ACE inhibitors and ARBs, aliskiren is contraindicated during the second and third trimesters, and should be discontinued as soon as possible when pregnancy occurs.

Drug Interactions

Aliskiren undergoes some metabolism by CYP3A4, but it neither induces nor inhibits the P450 system. In clinical trials, aliskiren had no significant interactions with atenolol, digoxin, amlodipine, or hydrochlorothiazide. However, levels of aliskiren were significantly raised by atorvastatin and ketoconazole (a P450 inhibitor), and significantly lowered by irbesartan. Levels of furosemide were lowered by aliskiren.

Preparations, Dosage, and Administration

Aliskiren is available alone as *Tekturna* and *Rasilez* 🍁, in combination with hydrochlorothiazide as *Tekturna HCT* and *Rasilez HCT* 🍁, and in combination with amlodipine as *Tekamlo.* All formulations are indicated for hypertension.

Aliskiren alone [Tekturna, Rasilez 🍁] is available in 150- and 300-mg tablets. The initial dosage is 150 mg once a day. If control of blood pressure is inadequate, dosage may be increased to 300 mg once a day. Daily doses above 300 mg will not increase benefits, but will increase the risk of diarrhea. Since high-fat meals decrease absorption substantially, each daily dose should be taken at the same time with respect to meals (e.g., 1 hour before dinner), so as to achieve a consistent response.

Aliskiren/hydrochlorothiazide [Tekturna HCT, Rasilez HCT 🍁] tablets are available in four strengths—150 mg/12.5 mg, 150 mg/25 mg, 300 mg/12.5 mg, and 300 mg/25 mg—for once-daily dosing. As with Tekturna, each daily dose should be taken at the same time with respect to meals.

Aliskiren/amlodipine [Tekamlo] tablets are available in four strengths—150 mg/5 mg, 150 mg/10 mg, 300 mg/5 mg, and 300 mg/10 mg—for once-daily dosing. As with Tekturna and Tekturna HCT, each daily dose should be taken at the same time with respect to meals.

ALDOSTERONE ANTAGONISTS

Aldosterone antagonists are drugs that block receptors for aldosterone. Two such agents are available: eplerenone and spironolactone. Both drugs have similar structures and actions, and both are used for the same disorders: hypertension and heart failure. They differ, however, in that spironolactone is less selective than eplerenone. As a result, spironolactone causes more side effects.

Eplerenone

Eplerenone [Inspra] is a first-in-class *selective aldosterone receptor blocker.* The drug is used for hypertension and heart failure and has one significant side effect: hyperkalemia.

Mechanism of Action

Eplerenone produces selective blockade of aldosterone receptors, having little or no effect on receptors for other steroid hormones (e.g., glucocorticoids, progesterone, androgens). In the kidney, activation of aldosterone receptors promotes excretion of potassium and retention of sodium and water. Receptor blockade has the opposite effect: retention of potassium and increased excretion of sodium and water. Loss of sodium and water reduces blood volume, and hence blood pressure. Blockade of aldosterone receptors at nonrenal sites may prevent or reverse pathologic effects of aldosterone on cardiovascular structure and function.

Therapeutic Uses

Hypertension. For treatment of hypertension, eplerenone may be used alone or in combination with other antihypertensive agents. Maximal reductions in blood pressure take about 4 weeks to develop. In clinical trials, reductions in blood pressure were equivalent to those produced by spironolactone and superior to those produced by losartan (an ARB). In patients already using an ACE inhibitor or an ARB, adding eplerenone produced a further reduction in blood pressure.

Although it is clear that eplerenone can lower blood pressure, we have no information on what really matters: the drug's ability to reduce morbidity and mortality in patients with isolated hypertension and lack of LV hypertrophy. Until more is known, eplerenone should be reserved for patients who have not responded to traditional antihypertensive drugs.

Heart Failure. In patients with heart failure, eplerenone can improve symptoms, reduce hospitalizations, and prolong life. Benefits appear to derive from blocking the adverse effects of aldosterone on cardiovascular structure and function. Use of eplerenone in heart failure is discussed in Chapter 48.

Pharmacokinetics

Eplerenone is administered orally, and absorption is not affected by food. Plasma levels peak about 1.5 hours after dosing. Absolute bioavailability is unknown. Eplerenone undergoes metabolism by CYP3A4, followed by excretion in the urine (67%) and feces (32%). The elimination half-life is 4 to 6 hours.

Adverse Effects

Eplerenone is generally well tolerated. The incidence of adverse effects is nearly identical to that of placebo. A few adverse effects—diarrhea, abdominal pain, cough, fatigue, gynecomastia, flu-like syndrome—occur slightly (1% to 2%) more often with eplerenone than with placebo.

Hyperkalemia. The greatest concern is hyperkalemia, which can occur secondary to potassium retention. Because of this risk, combined use with potassium supplements, salt substitutes, or potassium-sparing diuretics (e.g., spironolactone, triamterene) is contraindicated. Combined use with ACE inhibitors or ARBs is permissible, but should be done with caution. Eplerenone is contraindicated for patients with high serum potassium (above 5.5 mEq/L) and for patients with impaired renal function or type 2 diabetes with microalbuminuria, both of which can promote hyperkalemia. Monitoring potassium levels is recommended for patients at risk (e.g., those taking ACE inhibitors or ARBs).

Drug Interactions

Inhibitors of CYP3A4 can increase levels of eplerenone, thereby posing a risk of toxicity. Weak inhibitors (e.g., erythromycin, saquinavir, verapamil, fluconazole) can double eplerenone levels. Strong inhibitors (e.g., ketoconazole, itraconazole) can increase levels fivefold. If eplerenone is combined with a weak inhibitor, eplerenone dosage should be reduced. Eplerenone should not be combined with a strong inhibitor.

Drugs that raise potassium levels can increase the risk of hyperkalemia. Eplerenone should not be combined with potassium supplements, salt substitutes, or potassium-sparing diuretics. Combining eplerenone with ACE inhibitors or ARBs should be done with caution.

Drugs similar to eplerenone (e.g., ACE inhibitors and diuretics) are known to increase levels of *lithium*. Although the combination of eplerenone and lithium has not been studied, caution is nonetheless advised. Lithium levels should be measured frequently.

Preparations, Dosage, and Administration

Eplerenone [Inspra] is available in 25- and 50-mg tablets. The usual starting dosage is 50 mg once a day, taken with or without food. After 4 weeks, dosage can be increased to 50 mg twice daily (if the hypotensive response has been inadequate). Raising the dosage above 100 mg/day is not recommended because doing so is unlikely to increase the therapeutic response, but *will* increase the risk of hyperkalemia. In patients taking weak inhibitors of CYP3A4, the initial dosage should be reduced by 50% (to 25 mg once a day).

Spironolactone

Spironolactone [Aldactone], a much older drug than eplerenone, blocks receptors for aldosterone, but also binds with receptors for other steroid hormones (e.g., glucocorticoids, progesterone, androgens). Blockade of aldosterone receptors underlies beneficial effects in hypertension and heart failure, as well as the drug's major adverse effect: hyperkalemia. Binding with receptors for other steroid hormones underlies additional adverse effects: gynecomastia, menstrual irregularities, impotence, hirsutism, and deepening of the voice. The basic pharmacology of spironolactone and its use in heart failure are discussed in Chapters 41 and 48, respectively.

KEY POINTS

- The RAAS helps regulate blood pressure, blood volume, and fluid and electrolyte balance. The system can promote cardiovascular pathology.
- The RAAS acts through production of angiotensin II and aldosterone.
- Angiotensin II has much greater biologic activity than angiotensin I or angiotensin III.
- Angiotensin II is formed by the actions of two enzymes: renin and ACE.
- Angiotensin II causes vasoconstriction (primarily in arterioles) and release of aldosterone. In addition, angiotensin II can promote pathologic changes in the heart and blood vessels.
- Aldosterone acts on the kidneys to promote retention of sodium and water. In addition, aldosterone can also mediate pathologic changes in cardiovascular function.
- The RAAS raises blood pressure by causing vasoconstriction and by increasing blood volume (secondary to aldosterone-mediated retention of sodium and water).
- In addition to the traditional RAAS, in which angiotensin II is produced in the blood and then carried to target tissues, angiotensin II can be produced locally by individual tissues.
- Beneficial effects of ACE inhibitors result largely from inhibition of ACE and partly from inhibition of kinase II (the name for ACE when the substrate is bradykinin).
- By inhibiting ACE, ACE inhibitors decrease production of angiotensin II. The result is vasodilation, decreased blood volume, and prevention or reversal of pathologic changes in the heart and blood vessels mediated by angiotensin II and aldosterone.
- ACE inhibitors (and ARBs) are used to treat patients with hypertension, heart failure, MI, and established diabetic nephropathy. In addition, they are used to prevent MI, stroke, and death from cardiovascular causes in patients at high risk for a cardiovascular event. Of note, ACE inhibitors (and ARBs) are *not* effective for primary prevention of diabetic nephropathy.
- Preliminary data indicate that ACE inhibitors (and ARBs) can reduce the risk of developing diabetic retinopathy, although they can't slow the progression of established retinopathy.
- ACE inhibitors can produce significant first-dose hypotension by causing a sharp drop in circulating angiotensin II.
- Cough, secondary to accumulation of bradykinin, is the most common reason for discontinuing ACE inhibitors.
- By suppressing aldosterone release, ACE inhibitors can cause hyperkalemia. Exercise caution in patients taking potassium supplements, salt substitutes, or potassium-sparing diuretics.
- ACE inhibitors can cause major fetal malformations and should be avoided during pregnancy. Until recently,

Continued

we thought that risk was limited to exposure during the second and third trimesters. However, new data indicate that exposure during the first trimester may be dangerous as well.

- ACE inhibitors can cause a precipitous drop in blood pressure in patients with bilateral renal artery stenosis (or stenosis in the artery to a single remaining kidney).
- ARBs block the actions of angiotensin II in blood vessels, the adrenals, and all other tissues.
- ARBs are similar to ACE inhibitors in that they cause vasodilation, suppress aldosterone release, promote excretion of sodium and water, reduce blood pressure, and cause birth defects and angioedema.
- ARBs differ from ACE inhibitors in that they have a much lower incidence of hyperkalemia or cough.
- Aliskiren, a DRI, binds tightly with renin and thereby inhibits cleavage of angiotensinogen into angiotensin I. As a result, the drug suppresses the entire RAAS.
- Like the ACE inhibitors and ARBs, aliskiren causes vasodilation, suppresses aldosterone release, promotes excretion of sodium and water, reduces blood pressure, and causes birth defects and angioedema.
- Despite their similarities, aliskiren, ARBs, and ACE inhibitors are not clinically interchangeable.
- Aldosterone antagonists (spironolactone, eplerenone) block receptors for aldosterone.
- By blocking aldosterone receptors, aldosterone antagonists can (1) promote renal excretion of sodium and water (and can thereby reduce blood volume and blood pressure) and (2) prevent or reverse pathologic effects of aldosterone on cardiovascular structure and function.

Please visit **http://evolve.elsevier.com/Lehne** for chapter-specific NCLEX® examination review questions.

Summary of Major Nursing Implications[a]

ANGIOTENSIN-CONVERTING ENZYME INHIBITORS

Benazepril
Captopril
Enalapril
Enalaprilat
Fosinopril
Lisinopril
Moexipril
Perindopril
Quinapril
Ramipril
Trandolapril

Unless indicated otherwise, the implications summarized in the sections that follow pertain to all of the ACE inhibitors.

Preadministration Assessment

Therapeutic Goals

ACE inhibitors are used to:

- Reduce blood pressure in patients with hypertension (*all ACE inhibitors*).
- Improve hemodynamics in patients with heart failure (*captopril, enalapril, fosinopril, lisinopril, quinapril*).
- Slow progression of established diabetic nephropathy (*captopril*).
- Reduce mortality following acute MI (*lisinopril*).
- Treat heart failure after MI (*ramipril, trandolapril*).
- Reduce the risk of MI, stroke, or death from cardiovascular causes in patients at high risk (*ramipril*).
- Reduce cardiovascular mortality or nonfatal MI in patients with stable coronary artery disease (*perindopril*).

Baseline Data

Determine blood pressure, and obtain a white blood cell count and differential.

Identifying High-Risk Patients

ACE inhibitors are *contraindicated* during the second and third trimesters of pregnancy and for patients with (1) bilateral renal artery stenosis (or stenosis in the artery to a single remaining kidney) or (2) a history of hypersensitivity reactions (especially angioedema) to ACE inhibitors.

Exercise *caution* in patients with salt or volume depletion, renal impairment, or collagen vascular disease, and in those taking potassium supplements, salt substitutes, potassium-sparing diuretics, ARBs, aliskiren, or lithium.

Implementation: Administration

Routes

Oral. *All* ACE inhibitors (except enalaprilat).
Intravenous. Enalaprilat.

Dosage and Administration

Dosage is low initially and then gradually increased.

Instruct patients to administer captopril and moexipril at least 1 hour before meals. All other oral ACE inhibitors can be administered with food.

Ongoing Evaluation and Interventions

Monitoring Summary

Monitor blood pressure closely for 2 hours after the first dose and periodically thereafter. Obtain a white blood cell count and differential every 2 weeks for the first 3 months of therapy and periodically thereafter.

Evaluating Therapeutic Effects

Hypertension. Monitor for reduced blood pressure. The usual target pressure is systolic/diastolic of 140/90 mm Hg or 130/80 in patients with diabetes.

Heart Failure. Monitor for a lessening of signs and symptoms (e.g., dyspnea, cyanosis, jugular vein distention, edema).

Summary of Major Nursing Implications[a]—cont'd

Diabetic Nephropathy. Monitor for proteinuria and altered glomerular filtration rate.

Minimizing Adverse Effects

First-Dose Hypotension. Severe hypotension can occur with the first dose. Minimize hypotension by (1) withdrawing diuretics 2 to 3 days before initiating ACE inhibitors and (2) using low initial doses. Monitor blood pressure for 2 hours following the first dose. **Instruct patients to lie down if hypotension develops.** If necessary, infuse normal saline to restore pressure.

Cough. **Warn patients about the possibility of persistent dry, irritating, nonproductive cough. Instruct them to consult the prescriber if cough is bothersome.** Stopping the ACE inhibitor may be indicated.

Hyperkalemia. ACE inhibitors may increase potassium levels. **Instruct patients to avoid potassium supplements and potassium-containing salt substitutes unless they are prescribed by the provider.** Potassium-sparing diuretics must also be avoided.

Fetal Injury. **Warn women of childbearing age that taking ACE inhibitors during the second and third trimesters of pregnancy can cause major fetal injury (hypotension, hyperkalemia, skull hypoplasia, anuria, reversible and irreversible renal failure, death) and that taking these drugs earlier in pregnancy may pose a risk as well.** If the patient becomes pregnant, withdraw ACE inhibitors as soon as possible. Closely monitor infants who have been exposed to ACE inhibitors during the second or third trimester for hypotension, oliguria, and hyperkalemia.

Angioedema. This rare and potentially fatal reaction is characterized by giant wheals and edema of the tongue, glottis, and pharynx. **Instruct patients to seek immediate medical attention if these symptoms develop.** If angioedema is diagnosed, ACE inhibitors should be discontinued and never used again. Treat severe reactions with subcutaneous epinephrine.

Renal Failure. Renal failure is a risk for patients with bilateral renal artery stenosis or stenosis in the artery to a single remaining kidney. ACE inhibitors must be used with extreme caution in these people.

Neutropenia (Mainly With Captopril). Neutropenia poses a high risk of infection. **Inform patients about early signs of infection (fever, sore throat, mouth sores), and instruct them to notify the prescriber if these occur.** If neutropenia develops, withdraw the drug immediately; neutrophil counts should normalize in approximately 2 weeks. Neutropenia is most likely in patients with renal impairment and collagen vascular diseases (e.g., systemic lupus erythematosus, scleroderma); monitor these patients closely.

Minimizing Adverse Interactions

Diuretics. Diuretics may intensify first-dose hypotension. Withdraw diuretics 2 to 3 days before beginning an ACE inhibitor. Diuretics may be resumed later if needed.

Antihypertensive Agents. The antihypertensive effects of ACE inhibitors are additive with those of other antihypertensive drugs (e.g., ARBs, diuretics, sympatholytics, vasodilators, calcium channel blockers). When an ACE inhibitor is added to an antihypertensive regimen, dosages of the other drugs may require reduction.

Drugs That Elevate Potassium Levels. ACE inhibitors increase the risk of hyperkalemia associated with *potassium supplements, potassium-sparing diuretics,* and possibly *aliskiren.* Risk can be minimized by avoiding potassium supplements and potassium-sparing diuretics except when they are clearly indicated.

Lithium. ACE inhibitors can increase serum levels of lithium, causing toxicity. Monitor lithium levels frequently.

Nonsteroidal Anti-Inflammatory Drugs. NSAIDs (e.g., aspirin, ibuprofen) can interfere with the antihypertensive effects of ACE inhibitors. **Advise patients to minimize NSAID use.**

ANGIOTENSIN II RECEPTOR BLOCKERS

Azilsartan
Candesartan
Eprosartan
Irbesartan
Losartan
Olmesartan
Telmisartan
Valsartan

Unless indicated otherwise, the implications summarized here pertain to all of the ARBs.

Preadministration Assessment

Therapeutic Goals

ARBs are used to:

- Reduce blood pressure in patients with hypertension (*all ARBs*).
- Treat heart failure (*candesartan, valsartan*).
- Slow the progression of established diabetic nephropathy (*irbesartan, losartan*).
- Prevent stroke in patients with hypertension and LV hypertrophy (*losartan*).
- Protect against MI, stroke, and death from cardiovascular causes in high-risk patients, but only if they can't tolerate ACE inhibitors (*telmisartan*).
- Treat heart failure after MI (*valsartan*).

Baseline Data

Determine blood pressure.

Identifying High-Risk Patients

ARBs are *contraindicated* during the second and third trimesters of pregnancy and for patients with either (1) bilateral renal artery stenosis (or stenosis in the artery to a single remaining kidney) or (2) a history of hypersensitivity reactions (especially angioedema) to ARBs.

Implementation: Administration

Route

Oral.

Continued

Summary of Major Nursing Implications[a]—cont'd

Dosage and Administration

Inform patients that ARBs may be taken with or without food.

Ongoing Evaluation and Interventions

Evaluating Therapeutic Effects

Hypertension. Monitor for reduced blood pressure. The usual target pressure is systolic/diastolic of 140/90 mm Hg or 130/80 in patients with diabetes.

Heart Failure. Monitor for a lessening of signs and symptoms (e.g., dyspnea, cyanosis, jugular vein distention, edema).

Diabetic Nephropathy. Monitor for proteinuria and altered glomerular filtration rate.

Minimizing Adverse Effects

Angioedema. This rare and potentially fatal reaction is characterized by giant wheals and edema of the tongue, glottis, and pharynx. **Instruct patients to seek immediate medical attention if these symptoms develop.** If angioedema is diagnosed, ARBs should be discontinued and never used again. Treat severe reactions with subcutaneous epinephrine.

Fetal Injury. **Warn women of childbearing age that ARBs can cause fetal injury during the second and third trimesters of pregnancy, and may pose a risk earlier in pregnancy as well.** If the patient becomes pregnant, withdraw ARBs as soon as possible. Closely monitor infants who have been exposed to ARBs during the second or third trimester for hypotension, oliguria, and hyperkalemia.

Renal Failure. Renal failure is a risk for patients with bilateral renal artery stenosis or stenosis in the artery to a single remaining kidney. ARBs are contraindicated for these people.

Minimizing Adverse Interactions

Antihypertensive Agents. The antihypertensive effects of ARBs are additive with those of other antihypertensive drugs (e.g., diuretics, sympatholytics, vasodilators, ACE inhibitors, calcium channel blockers). When an ARB is added to an antihypertensive regimen, dosages of the other drugs may require reduction.

ALISKIREN, A DIRECT RENIN INHIBITOR

Preadministration Assessment

Therapeutic Goal

Reduction of blood pressure in patients with hypertension.

Baseline Data

Determine blood pressure.

Identifying High-Risk Patients

Aliskiren is *contraindicated* during the second and third trimesters of pregnancy.

Exercise *caution* in patients taking potassium supplements, salt substitutes, potassium-sparing diuretics, or ACE inhibitors.

Implementation: Administration

Route

Oral.

Dosage and Administration

Advise patients to take each daily dose at the same time with respect to meals (e.g., 1 hour before dinner). Dosage should be low (150 mg/day) initially, and increased to a maximum of 300 mg/day if needed.

Ongoing Evaluation and Interventions

Minimizing Adverse Effects

Hyperkalemia. Aliskiren may increase potassium levels. **Instruct patients to avoid potassium supplements and potassium-containing salt substitutes unless they are prescribed by the provider.** Potassium-sparing diuretics must also be avoided. Exercise caution in patients taking an ACE inhibitor.

Fetal Injury. **Warn women of childbearing age that aliskiren taken during the second and third trimesters of pregnancy can cause fetal injury (hypotension, hyperkalemia, skull hypoplasia, anuria, reversible and irreversible renal failure, death).** If the patient becomes pregnant, withdraw aliskiren as soon as possible. Closely monitor infants who have been exposed to aliskiren during the second or third trimester for hypotension, oliguria, and hyperkalemia.

Angioedema. This rare and potentially fatal reaction is characterized by giant wheals and edema of the tongue, glottis, and pharynx. **Instruct patients to seek immediate medical attention if these symptoms develop.** If angioedema is diagnosed, aliskiren should be discontinued and never used again. Treat severe reactions with subcutaneous epinephrine.

Minimizing Adverse Interactions

Drugs That Elevate Potassium Levels. Aliskiren increases the risk of hyperkalemia associated with *ACE inhibitors, potassium supplements,* and *potassium-sparing diuretics.* Risk can be minimized by avoiding ACE inhibitors, potassium supplements, and potassium-sparing diuretics except when they are clearly indicated.

Antihypertensive Agents. The antihypertensive effects of aliskiren are additive with those of other antihypertensive drugs (e.g., ACE inhibitors, ARBs, diuretics, sympatholytics, vasodilators, calcium channel blockers). When aliskiren is added to an antihypertensive regimen, dosages of the other drugs may require reduction.

[a]Patient education information is highlighted as **blue text**.

CHAPTER

45 Calcium Channel Blockers

Calcium channel blockers (CCBs) are drugs that prevent calcium ions from entering cells. These agents have their greatest effects on the heart and blood vessels. CCBs are used widely to treat hypertension, angina pectoris, and cardiac dysrhythmias. There remains controversy about the safety of CCBs in patients with heart failure. Alternative names for CCBs are *calcium antagonists* and *slow channel blockers.*

CALCIUM CHANNELS: PHYSIOLOGIC FUNCTIONS AND CONSEQUENCES OF BLOCKADE

Calcium channels are gated pores in the cytoplasmic membrane that regulate entry of calcium ions into cells. Calcium entry plays a critical role in the function of vascular smooth muscle (VSM) and the heart.

Vascular Smooth Muscle

In VSM, calcium channels regulate contraction. When an action potential travels down the surface of a smooth muscle cell, calcium channels open and calcium ions flow inward, thereby initiating the contractile process. If calcium channels are blocked, contraction will be prevented and vasodilation will result.

At therapeutic doses, CCBs act selectively on *peripheral arterioles* and *arteries and arterioles of the heart.* CCBs have no significant effect on veins.

Heart

In the heart, calcium channels help regulate the myocardium, the sinoatrial (SA) node, and the atrioventricular (AV) node. Calcium channels at all three sites are coupled to beta_1-adrenergic receptors.

Myocardium

In cardiac muscle, calcium entry has a positive inotropic effect. That is, calcium increases force of contraction. If calcium channels in atrial and ventricular muscle are blocked, contractile force will diminish.

SA Node

Pacemaker activity of the SA node is regulated by calcium influx. When calcium channels are open, spontaneous discharge of the SA node increases. Conversely, when calcium channels close, pacemaker activity declines. Hence, the effect of calcium channel blockade is to reduce heart rate.

AV Node

Impulses that originate in the SA node must pass through the AV node on their way to the ventricles. Because of this arrangement, regulation of AV conduction plays a critical role in coordinating contraction of the ventricles with contraction of the atria.

The excitability of AV nodal cells is regulated by calcium entry. When calcium channels are open, calcium entry increases and cells of the AV node discharge more readily. Conversely, when calcium channels are closed, discharge of AV nodal cells is suppressed. Hence, the effect of calcium channel blockade is to decrease velocity of conduction through the AV node.

Coupling of Cardiac Calcium Channels to Beta_1-Adrenergic Receptors

In the heart, calcium channels are coupled to beta_1-adrenergic receptors (Fig. 45.1). As a result, when cardiac beta_1 receptors are activated, calcium influx is enhanced. Conversely, when beta_1 receptors are blocked, calcium influx is suppressed. Because of this relationship, CCBs and beta blockers have identical effects on the heart. That is, they both reduce force of contraction, slow heart rate, and suppress conduction through the AV node.

CALCIUM CHANNEL BLOCKERS: CLASSIFICATION AND SITES OF ACTION

Classification

The CCBs used in the United States belong to three chemical families (Table 45.1). The largest family is the *dihydropyridines,* for which *nifedipine* is the prototype. This family name is encountered frequently, and hence the name is worth remembering. The other two families consist of orphans: *verapamil* is the only *phenylalkylamine,* and *diltiazem* is the only *benzothiazepine.* The drug names are important; the family names are not.

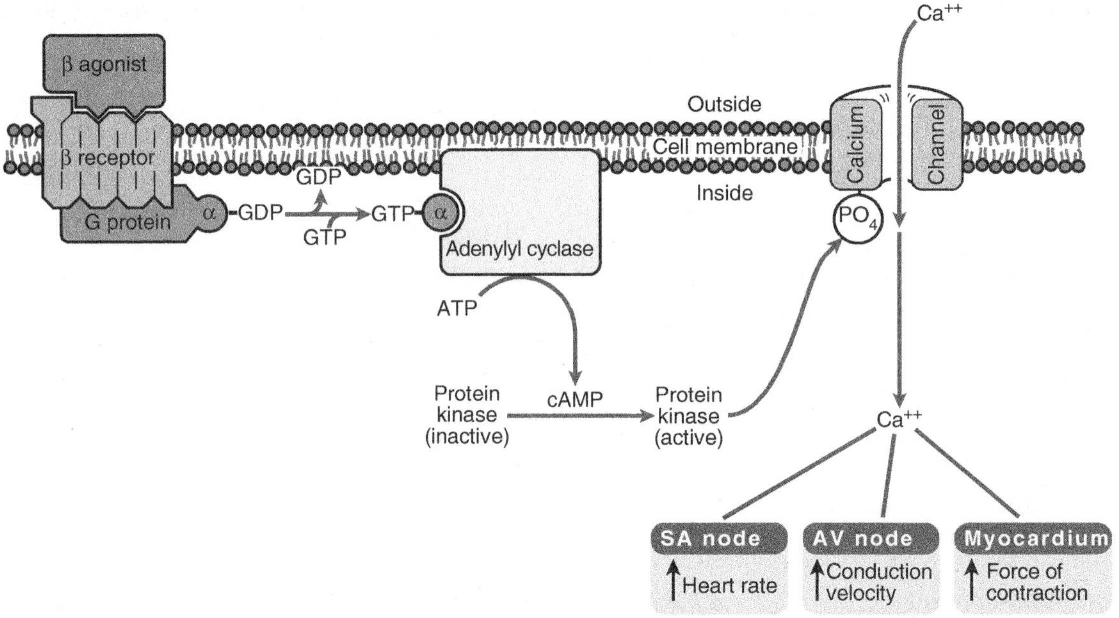

Fig. 45.1 ■ Coupling of cardiac calcium channels with beta$_1$-adrenergic receptors. In the heart, beta$_1$ receptors are coupled to calcium channels. As a result, when cardiac beta$_1$ receptors are activated, calcium influx is enhanced. The process works as follows: Binding of an agonist (e.g., norepinephrine) causes a conformational change in the beta receptor, which in turn causes a change in G protein, converting it from an inactive state (in which GDP is bound to the alpha subunit) to an active state (in which GTP is bound to the alpha subunit). (G protein is so named because it binds guanine nucleotides: GDP and GTP.) Following activation, the alpha subunit dissociates from the rest of G protein and activates adenylyl cyclase, an enzyme that converts ATP to cyclic AMP (cAMP). cAMP then activates protein kinase, an enzyme that phosphorylates proteins—in this case, the calcium channel. Phosphorylation changes the channel such that calcium entry is enhanced when the channel opens. (Opening of the channel is triggered by a change in membrane voltage [i.e., by passage of an action potential].) The effect of calcium entry on cardiac function is determined by the type of cell involved. If the cell is in the SA node, heart rate increases; if the cell is in the AV node, impulse conduction through the node accelerates; and if the cell is part of the myocardium, force of contraction is increased. Because binding of a single agonist molecule to a single beta receptor stimulates the synthesis of many cAMP molecules, with the subsequent activation of many protein kinase molecules, causing the phosphorylation of many calcium channels, this system can greatly amplify the signal initiated by the agonist. (*GDP,* Guanosine diphosphate; *GTP,* guanosine-5′-triphosphate; *cAMP,* cyclic AMP phosphodiesterase; *ATP,* adenosine triphosphate.)

Prototype Drugs

CALCIUM CHANNEL BLOCKERS

Agents That Affect the Heart and Blood Vessels

Verapamil

Dihydropyridines: Agents That Act Mainly on Blood Vessels

Nifedipine

Sites of Action

At therapeutic doses, the dihydropyridines act primarily on arterioles; in contrast, verapamil and diltiazem act on arterioles *and* the heart (see Table 45.1). However, although dihydropyridines don't affect the heart at *therapeutic* doses, *toxic* doses can produce dangerous cardiac suppression (just like verapamil and diltiazem can). The differences in selectivity among CCBs are based on structural differences among the drugs themselves and structural differences among calcium channels.

VERAPAMIL AND DILTIAZEM: AGENTS THAT ACT ON VASCULAR SMOOTH MUSCLE AND THE HEART

Verapamil

Verapamil [Calan, Verelan, Covera-HS ✦] blocks calcium channels in blood vessels and in the heart. Major indications are angina pectoris, essential hypertension, and cardiac dysrhythmias. Verapamil was the first CCB available and will serve as our prototype for the group.

Hemodynamic Effects

The overall hemodynamic response to verapamil is the net result of (1) direct effects on the heart and blood vessels and (2) reflex responses.

TABLE 45.1 ■ Calcium Channel Blockers: Classification, Sites of Action, and Indications

		Indications			
Classification	Sites of Action	Hypertension	Angina	Dysrhythmias	Others
DIHYDROPYRIDINES					
Nifedipine [Adalat CC, Nifediac, Nifedical, Procardia]	Arterioles	✔	✔		a
Amlodipine [Norvasc]	Arterioles	✔	✔		
Clevidipine [Cleviprex]	Arterioles	✔[b]			
Felodipine [Plendil, Renedil 🍁]	Arterioles	✔			
Isradipine [DynaCirc CR]	Arterioles	✔			
Nicardipine [Cardene SR]	Arterioles	✔	✔		
Nimodipine [Nymalize, Nimotop 🍁]	Arterioles				c
Nisoldipine [Sular]	Arterioles	✔			
PHENYLALKYLAMINE					
Verapamil [Calan, Covera-HS 🍁, Verelan]	Arterioles/heart	✔	✔	✔	
BENZOTHIAZEPINE					
Diltiazem [Cardizem, Dilacor XR, Tiazac, others]	Arterioles/heart	✔	✔	✔	

[a]Suppression of preterm labor (off-label use).
[b]Only for IV treatment of *severe* hypertension.
[c]Prophylaxis of neurologic injury after rupture of an intracranial aneurysm.

Direct Effects. By blocking calcium channels in the heart and blood vessels, verapamil has five direct effects:

- Blockade at peripheral arterioles causes dilation, and thereby reduces arterial pressure.
- Blockade at arteries and arterioles of the heart increases coronary perfusion.
- Blockade at the SA node reduces heart rate.
- Blockade at the AV node decreases AV nodal conduction.
- Blockade in the myocardium decreases the force of contraction.

Of the direct effects on the heart, reduced AV conduction is the most important.

Indirect (Reflex) Effects. Verapamil-induced lowering of blood pressure activates the baroreceptor reflex, causing increased firing of sympathetic nerves to the heart. Norepinephrine released from these nerves acts to increase heart rate, AV conduction, and force of contraction. However, since these same three parameters are suppressed by the direct actions of verapamil, the direct and indirect effects tend to neutralize each other.

Net Effect. Because the direct effects of verapamil on the heart are counterbalanced by indirect effects, the drug has little or no net effect on cardiac performance: For most patients, heart rate, AV conduction, and contractility are not noticeably altered. Consequently, the overall cardiovascular effect of verapamil is simply vasodilation accompanied by reduced arterial pressure and increased coronary perfusion.

Pharmacokinetics

Verapamil may be administered orally or IV. The drug is well absorbed following oral administration, but undergoes extensive metabolism on its first pass through the liver. Consequently, only about 20% of an oral dose reaches the systemic circulation. Effects begin 30 minutes after dosing and peak within 5 hours. Elimination is primarily by hepatic metabolism. Because the drug is eliminated by the liver, doses must be reduced substantially in patients with hepatic impairment.

Therapeutic Uses

Angina Pectoris. Verapamil is used widely to treat angina pectoris. The drug is approved for vasospastic angina and angina of effort. Benefits in both disorders derive from vasodilation. The role of verapamil in angina is discussed in Chapter 51.

Essential Hypertension. Verapamil is a second-line agent for chronic hypertension, used after thiazide diuretics. The drug lowers blood pressure by dilating arterioles. The role of verapamil and other CCBs in hypertension is discussed in Chapter 47.

Cardiac Dysrhythmias. Verapamil, administered IV, is used to slow ventricular rate in patients with atrial flutter, atrial fibrillation, and paroxysmal supraventricular tachycardia. Benefits derive from suppressing impulse conduction through the AV node, thereby preventing the atria from driving the ventricles at an excessive rate. Antidysrhythmic applications are discussed in Chapter 49.

Adverse Effects

Common Effects. Verapamil is generally well tolerated. *Constipation* occurs frequently and is the most common complaint. This problem, which can be especially severe in older adults, can be minimized by increasing dietary fluids and fiber. Constipation results from blockade of calcium channels in smooth muscle of the intestine. Other common effects—dizziness, facial flushing, headache, and edema of the ankles and feet—occur secondary to vasodilation.

Cardiac Effects. Blockade of calcium channels in the heart can compromise cardiac function. In the SA node, calcium channel blockade can cause bradycardia; in the AV node, blockade can cause partial or complete AV block; and in the myocardium, blockade can decrease contractility. When the heart is healthy, these effects rarely have clinical significance. However, in patients with certain cardiac diseases, verapamil can seriously exacerbate dysfunction. Accordingly, the drug must be used with special caution in patients with cardiac failure, and it must not be used at all in patients with sick sinus syndrome or second-degree or third-degree AV block.

Other Effects. In older patients, CCBs have been associated with *chronic eczematous eruptions,* typically starting 3 to 6 months after treatment onset. If the reaction is mild, switching to a different CCB may help. If the condition is severe, use of verapamil and other CCBs should stop.

Gingival hyperplasia (overgrowth of gum tissue) has been reported.

Drug and Food Interactions

Digoxin. Like verapamil, digoxin suppresses impulse conduction through the AV node. Accordingly, when these drugs are used concurrently, the risk of AV block is increased. Patients receiving the combination should be monitored closely.

Verapamil increases plasma levels of digoxin by about 60%, thereby increasing the risk of digoxin toxicity. If signs of toxicity appear, digoxin dosage should be reduced.

Beta-Adrenergic Blocking Agents. Beta blockers and verapamil have the same effects on the heart: They decrease heart rate, AV conduction, and contractility. Hence, when a beta blocker and verapamil are used together, there is a risk of excessive cardiosuppression. To minimize risk, beta blockers and IV verapamil should be administered several hours apart.

Grapefruit Juice. Grapefruit juice can inhibit the intestinal and hepatic metabolism of many drugs and thus raise their levels. In a case report on verapamil toxicity, consumption of grapefruit juice and verapamil (360 mg over 24 hours) led to a verapamil blood level of 2772 ng/mL—approximately 8 to 24 times higher than would have been achieved without grapefruit juice.

Toxicity

Clinical Manifestations. Overdose can produce severe hypotension and cardiotoxicity (bradycardia, AV block).

Treatment

General Measures. Verapamil can be removed from the GI tract with gastric lavage followed by activated charcoal. Intravenous calcium gluconate can counteract both vasodilation and negative inotropic effects, but will not reverse AV block.

Hypotension. Hypotension can be treated with IV norepinephrine, which promotes vasoconstriction (by activating $alpha_1$ receptors on blood vessels) and increases cardiac output (by activating $beta_1$ receptors in the heart). Placing the patient in modified Trendelenburg's position (legs elevated) and administering IV fluids may also help.

Bradycardia and AV Block. Bradycardia and AV block can be treated with atropine (an anticholinergic drug that blocks parasympathetic influences on the heart). If pharmacologic measures are inadequate, electronic pacing may be required. Use of glucagon in animal models has improved heart rate through increasing amounts of intracellular cyclic AMP. It has been used successfully in treating human cases of CCB toxicity.

Preparations, Dosage, and Administration

Oral. Verapamil is available in immediate-release (IR) tablets (40, 80, and 120 mg) as *Calan;* extended-release (ER) tablets (120, 180, and 240 mg) as *Calan SR* and *Covera-HS* ♣; and ER capsules (120, 180, 240, and 360 mg) as *Verelan.* In addition, verapamil is available as *Verelan PM* (100-, 200-, and 300-mg capsules), a timed-release formulation that, when administered at bedtime, produces maximum verapamil levels in the morning. The sustained- and timed-release formulations are approved only for hypertension. Instruct patients to swallow these products intact, without crushing or chewing. A fixed-dose combination with trandolapril (an angiotensin-converting enzyme [ACE] inhibitor) is available under the brand name *Tarka.*

The usual initial dosage for *angina pectoris* is 80 to 120 mg 3 times a day. The usual initial dosage for *essential hypertension* is 80 mg 3 times a day (using IR tablets), 180 mg of an ER formulation (administered once a day in the morning with food), or 200 mg of Verelan PM (administered once a day at bedtime). Dosages should be reduced for older adult patients and for patients with advanced renal or liver disease. Dosages for dysrhythmias are presented in Chapter 49.

Intravenous. Intravenous verapamil is used for dysrhythmias. Because IV verapamil can cause severe adverse cardiovascular effects, blood pressure and the electrocardiogram (ECG) should be monitored and equipment for resuscitation should be immediately available. Intravenous dosages for dysrhythmias are presented in Chapter 49.

Diltiazem

Actions and Uses

Like verapamil, diltiazem [Cardizem, Dilacor XR, Tiazac, others] blocks calcium channels in the heart and blood vessels. As a result, the actions and applications of verapamil and diltiazem are very similar. Diltiazem has the same effects on cardiovascular function as verapamil. Both drugs lower blood pressure through arteriolar dilation, and because their direct suppressant actions are balanced by reflex cardiac stimulation, both have little *net* effect on the heart. Like verapamil, diltiazem is used for angina pectoris, essential hypertension, and cardiac dysrhythmias (atrial flutter, atrial fibrillation, and paroxysmal supraventricular tachycardia).

Pharmacokinetics

Oral diltiazem is well absorbed and then extensively metabolized on its first pass through the liver. As a result, bioavailability is only about 50%. Effects begin rapidly (within a few minutes) and peak within half an hour. The drug undergoes nearly complete metabolism before elimination in the urine and feces.

Adverse Effects

Adverse effects are like those of verapamil, except that diltiazem causes less constipation. The most common effects are dizziness, flushing, headache, and edema of the ankles and feet. Like verapamil, diltiazem can exacerbate cardiac dysfunction in patients with bradycardia, sick sinus syndrome, heart failure, or second-degree or third-degree AV block. Like other CCBs, diltiazem may cause chronic eczematous rash in older adults.

Drug and Food Interactions

Like verapamil, diltiazem can exacerbate digoxin-induced suppression of AV conduction and can intensify the cardiosuppressant effects of beta blockers.

PATIENT-CENTERED CARE ACROSS THE LIFE SPAN

Calcium Channel Blockers

Life Stage	Patient Care Concerns
Infants	Verapamil can be used in infants for conversion of certain heart dysrhythmias.
Children/ adolescents	Calcium channel blockers are used in children for hypertension, hypertensive emergencies, and hypertrophic cardiomyopathy.
Pregnant women	Calcium channel blockers are classified in U.S. Food and Drug Administration Pregnancy Risk Category C.[a] There is a risk of fetal death based on animal data, but inadequate human data exist. Therefore, caution is advised during pregnancy.
Breast-feeding women	Certain drugs such as verapamil may pose harm to the infant. For other drugs such as nifedipine, data are lacking regarding transmission of drug from mother to infant via breast milk.
Older adults	In older patients, calcium channel blockers have been associated with chronic eczematous eruptions.

[a]As of 2020, the FDA will no longer use Pregnancy Risk Categories. Please refer to Chapter 9 for more information.

Patients receiving diltiazem concurrently with digoxin or a beta blocker should be monitored closely for cardiac status. As with verapamil, grapefruit juice can significantly increase levels of diltiazem.

Preparations, Dosage, and Administration

Oral diltiazem is available in IR tablets (30, 60, 90, and 120 mg) as *Cardizem,* extended-release (ER) tablets (120, 180, 240, 300, 360, and 420 mg) as *Cardizem LA,* and SR capsules (120, 180, 240, 300, 360, and 420 mg) as *Cardizem CD, Cartia XT, Dilacor XR, Dilt-CD, Dilt-XR, Diltia XT, Taztia XT,* and *Tiazac.* The drug is also available in solution (5 mg/mL) for IV administration. The usual initial dosage for hypertension is 180 mg once a day with Cardizem CD, 60 to 120 mg twice a day with Cardizem, and 180 to 240 mg once a day with Cardizem LA or Dilacor XR. Angina pectoris can be treated with IR tablets (30 mg 4 times a day initially and 60 mg 4 times a day for maintenance). Intravenous diltiazem is reserved for dysrhythmias.

DIHYDROPYRIDINES: AGENTS THAT ACT MAINLY ON VASCULAR SMOOTH MUSCLE

All of the drugs discussed in this section belong to the *dihydropyridine* family. At therapeutic doses, these drugs produce significant blockade of calcium channels in blood vessels and minimal blockade of calcium channels in the heart. The dihydropyridines are similar to verapamil in some respects, but quite different in others.

Nifedipine

Nifedipine [Adalat CC, Nifedical XL, Nifediac CC, Procardia, Procardia XL] was the first dihydropyridine available and will serve as our prototype for the group. Like verapamil, nifedipine blocks calcium channels in VSM and thereby promotes vasodilation. However, in contrast to verapamil, nifedipine produces very little blockade of calcium channels in the heart. As a result, nifedipine cannot be used to treat dysrhythmias, does not cause cardiac suppression, and is less likely than verapamil to exacerbate pre-existing cardiac disorders. Nifedipine also differs from verapamil in that nifedipine is more likely to cause reflex tachycardia. Contrasts between nifedipine and verapamil are shown in Table 45.2.

TABLE 45.2 ■ Comparisons and Contrasts Between Nifedipine and Verapamil

Property	Drug: Nifedipine	Drug: Verapamil
DIRECT EFFECTS ON THE HEART AND ARTERIOLES		
Arteriolar dilation	Yes	Yes
Effects on the heart		
Reduced automaticity	No	Yes
Reduced AV conduction	No	Yes
Reduced contractile force	No	Yes
MAJOR INDICATIONS		
Hypertension	Yes	Yes
Angina pectoris (classic and variant)	Yes	Yes
Dysrhythmias	No	Yes
ADVERSE EFFECTS		
Exacerbation of		
AV block	No	Yes
Sick sinus syndrome	No	Yes
Heart failure	No	Yes
Effects secondary to vasodilation		
Edema (ankles and feet)	Yes	Yes
Flushing	Yes	Yes
Headaches	Yes	Yes
Dizziness	Yes	Yes
Reflex tachycardia	Yes	No
Constipation	No	Yes
DRUG INTERACTIONS		
Intensifies digoxin-induced AV block	No	Yes
Intensifies cardiosuppressant effects of beta blockers	No	Yes
Often combined with a beta blocker to suppress reflex tachycardia	Yes	No

AV, Atrioventricular.

Hemodynamic Effects

Direct Effects. The direct effects of nifedipine on the cardiovascular system are limited to blockade of calcium channels in VSM. Blockade of calcium channels in peripheral arterioles causes vasodilation and thus lowers arterial pressure. Calcium channel blockade in arteries and arterioles of the heart increases coronary perfusion. Because nifedipine does not block cardiac calcium channels at usual therapeutic doses, the drug has no *direct* suppressant effects on automaticity, AV conduction, or contractile force.

Indirect (Reflex) Effects. By lowering blood pressure, nifedipine activates the baroreceptor reflex, thereby causing sympathetic stimulation of the heart. Because nifedipine lacks direct cardiosuppressant actions, cardiac stimulation is unopposed, and hence heart rate and contractile force increase.

It is important to note that reflex effects occur primarily with the *immediate-release* formulation of nifedipine, not with the SR formulation. This is because the baroreceptor reflex is turned on only by a *rapid* fall in blood pressure; a gradual decline will not activate the reflex. With the IR formulation, blood levels of nifedipine rise quickly, and hence blood pressure drops quickly and the reflex is turned on. Conversely, with the SR formulation, blood levels of nifedipine rise slowly, so blood pressure falls slowly and the reflex is blunted.

Net Effect. The overall hemodynamic response to nifedipine is simply the sum of its direct effect (vasodilation) and indirect effect (reflex cardiac stimulation). Accordingly, nifedipine (1) lowers blood pressure, (2) increases heart rate, and (3) increases contractile force. Please note, however, that the reflex increases in heart rate and contractile force are transient and occur primarily with the IR formulation.

Pharmacokinetics

Nifedipine is well absorbed following oral administration, but undergoes extensive first-pass metabolism. As a result, only about 50% of an oral dose reaches the systemic circulation. With the IR formulation, effects begin rapidly and peak in 30 minutes; with the SR formulation, effects begin in 20 minutes and peak in 6 hours. Nifedipine is fully metabolized before excretion in the urine.

Therapeutic Uses

Angina Pectoris. Nifedipine is indicated for vasospastic angina and angina of effort. The drug is usually combined with a beta blocker to prevent reflex stimulation of the heart, which could intensify anginal pain. Long-term use reduces the rates of overt heart failure, coronary angiography, and coronary bypass surgery—but not rates of stroke, myocardial infarction, or death. The role of nifedipine in angina is discussed in Chapter 51.

Hypertension. Nifedipine is used widely to treat *essential hypertension.* Only the ER formulation should be used. In the past, nifedipine was used for *hypertensive emergencies,* but it has largely been replaced by drugs that are safer. The use of CCBs in essential hypertension is discussed in Chapter 47.

Investigational Uses. Nifedipine has been used off-label to *suppress preterm labor* (see Chapter 64).

Adverse Effects

Some adverse effects are like those of verapamil; others are quite different. Like verapamil, nifedipine can cause flushing, dizziness, headache, peripheral edema, and gingival hyperplasia, and may pose a risk of chronic eczematous rash in older patients. In contrast to verapamil, nifedipine causes very little constipation. Also, since nifedipine causes minimal blockade of calcium channels in the heart, the drug is not likely to exacerbate AV block, heart failure, bradycardia, or sick sinus syndrome. Accordingly, nifedipine is preferred to verapamil for patients with these disorders.

A response that occurs with nifedipine that does not occur with verapamil is *reflex tachycardia.* This response is problematic in that it increases cardiac oxygen demand and can thereby increase pain in patients with angina. To prevent reflex tachycardia, nifedipine can be combined with a beta blocker (e.g., metoprolol).

Safety Alert

IMMEDIATE-RELEASE NIFEDIPINE

Immediate-release nifedipine has been associated with increased mortality in patients with myocardial infarction and unstable angina. Other IR CCBs have been associated with an increased risk of myocardial infarction in patients with hypertension. However, in both cases, a causal relationship has not been established. Nonetheless, the National Heart, Lung, and Blood Institute has recommended that *immediate-release* nifedipine, especially in higher doses, be used with great caution, if at all. It is important to note that these adverse effects have not been associated with *sustained-release* nifedipine or with any other long-acting CCB.

Drug Interactions

Beta-Adrenergic Blockers. Beta blockers are combined with nifedipine to prevent reflex tachycardia. It is important to note that, whereas beta blockers can *decrease* the adverse cardiac effects of *nifedipine,* they can *intensify* the adverse cardiac effects of *verapamil* and *diltiazem.*

Toxicity

When taken in excessive dosage, nifedipine loses selectivity. Hence, toxic doses affect the heart in addition to blood vessels. Consequently, the manifestations and treatment of nifedipine overdose are the same as described previously for verapamil.

Preparations, Dosage, and Administration

Nifedipine is available in IR capsules (10 mg) as *Procardia* and in SR tablets (30, 60, and 90 mg) as *Adalat CC, Nifedical XL, Nifediac CC,* and *Procardia XL.* Instruct patients to swallow SR tablets whole, without crushing or chewing.

For treatment of *angina pectoris,* the usual initial dosage is 10 mg 3 times a day. The usual maintenance dosage is 10 to 20 mg 3 times a day. The maximum recommended dosage is 180 mg/day.

For *essential hypertension,* only the SR tablets are approved. The usual initial dosage is 30 mg once a day.

Other Dihydropyridines

In addition to nifedipine, seven other dihydropyridines are available. All are similar to nifedipine. Like nifedipine, these drugs produce greater blockade of calcium channels in VSM than in the heart.

Nicardipine

At therapeutic doses, nicardipine [Cardene, Cardene SR] produces selective blockade of calcium channels in blood vessels and has minimal direct effects on the heart. The drug has two indications: essential hypertension and effort-induced angina pectoris. The most common adverse effects are flushing, headache, asthenia (weakness), dizziness, palpitations, and edema of the ankles and feet. As with other CCBs, eczematous rash may develop in older patients. Gingival hyperplasia (overgrowth of gum tissue) has been reported. Like nifedipine, nicardipine can be combined with a beta blocker to promote therapeutic effects and suppress reflex tachycardia. Nicardipine is available in 20- and 30-mg IR capsules (generic only) and in ER capsules (30, 45, and 60 mg) sold as *Cardene SR.* The usual initial dosage for *angina pectoris* is 20 mg 3 times a day using the IR capsules. The usual initial dosage for *essential hypertension* is 20 mg 3 times a day (using IR capsules) or 30 mg twice a day (using ER capsules).

Amlodipine

At therapeutic doses, amlodipine [Norvasc] produces selective blockade of calcium channels in blood vessels, having minimal direct effects on the heart. Approved indications are essential hypertension and angina pectoris (effort induced and vasospastic). Amlodipine is administered orally and absorbed slowly; peak levels develop in 6 to 12 hours. The drug has a long half-life (30 to 50 hours) and therefore is effective with once-a-day dosing. Principal adverse effects are peripheral and facial edema. Flushing, dizziness, and headache may also occur, as may eczematous rash in older patients. In contrast to other dihydropyridines, amlodipine causes little reflex tachycardia. Amlodipine is available in 2.5-, 5-, and 10-mg tablets. The usual initial dosage for hypertension or angina pectoris is 5 mg once a day. Fixed-dose combinations are also available: amlodipine/benazepril [Lotrel], amlodipine/telmisartan [Twynsta], amlodipine/atorvastatin [Caduet], amlodipine/aliskiren [Tekamlo], amlodipine/olmesartin [Azor], amlodipine/valsartan [Exforge], aliskiren/amlodipine/hydrochlorothiazide [Amturnide], amlodipine/valsartan/hydrochlorothiazide [Exforge HCT], and amlodipine/hydrochlorothiazide/olmesartan [Tribenzor].

Isradipine

Like nifedipine, isradipine (generic only) produces relatively selective blockade of calcium channels in blood vessels. In the United States, the drug is approved only for hypertension. Isradipine is rapidly absorbed following oral administration, but undergoes extensive first-pass metabolism. Parent drug and metabolites are excreted in the urine. The most common side effects are facial flushing, headache, dizziness, and ankle edema. Eczematous rash may develop in older patients. In contrast to nifedipine, isradipine causes minimal reflex tachycardia. The drug is available in capsules (2.5 and 5 mg). The usual antihypertensive dosage is 2.5 to 5 mg twice a day.

Felodipine

Felodipine [Plendil, Renedil 🍁] produces selective blockade of calcium channels in blood vessels. In the United States, the drug is approved only for hypertension. Felodipine is well absorbed following oral administration but undergoes extensive first-pass metabolism. As a result, bioavailability is low—only 20%. Plasma levels peak in 2.5 to 5 hours and then decay with a half-life of 24 hours. Because of its prolonged half-life, felodipine is effective with once-a-day dosing. Characteristic adverse effects are reflex tachycardia, peripheral edema, headache, facial flushing, and dizziness. Eczematous rash may develop in older patients. Gingival hyperplasia has been reported. Felodipine is available in ER tablets (2.5, 5, and 10 mg). The usual dosage for hypertension is 5 to 10 mg once a day.

Nimodipine

Nimodipine [Nymalize, Nimotop 🍁] produces selective blockade of calcium channels in *cerebral blood vessels.* The only approved application is prophylaxis of neurologic injury following rupture of an intracranial aneurysm. Benefits derive from preventing cerebral arterial spasm that follows subarachnoid hemorrhage (SAH) and can result in ischemic neurologic injury. Dosing (60 mg every 4 hours) should begin within 96 hours of SAH and continue for 21 days. Nimotop 🍁 is available in 30-mg liquid-filled capsules for oral administration and as a 60 mg/20 mL oral solution [Nymalize]. *Nimodipine must never be given intravenously,* owing to a risk of potentially fatal cardiovascular events.

Nisoldipine

Like nifedipine, nisoldipine [Sular] produces selective blockade of calcium channels in blood vessels; the drug has minimal direct effects on the heart. The only approved indication is hypertension. Nisoldipine is well absorbed following oral administration, but the first-pass effect limits bioavailability to 5%. Plasma levels peak 6 hours after administration. The most common side effects are dizziness, headache, and peripheral edema. Reflex tachycardia may also occur. As with other CCBs, eczematous rash may develop in older patients. Nisoldipine is available in ER tablets (8.5, 17, 20, 25.5, 30, 34, and 40 mg). The dosage for hypertension is 17 to 60 mg once a day.

Clevidipine

Clevidipine [Cleviprex] is indicated only for *intravenous* therapy of *severe* hypertension, defined as systolic blood pressure above 180 mm Hg or diastolic pressure above 110 mm Hg. The drug has an ultrashort half-life (about 1 minute), owing to rapid inactivation by plasma esterases. Effects are not altered by impairment of liver or kidney function. Because of IV dosing and rapid inactivation, blood pressure falls quickly and then rises quickly when the infusion is slowed or stopped. As a result, responses can be easily titrated. Clevidipine is formulated in a lipid emulsion made from soybean oil and egg yolk phospholipids, and hence is contraindicated for patients allergic to soybeans or eggs. Clevidipine is supplied in single-dose vials (50, 100, or 250 mL) at a concentration of 0.5 mg/mL. For patients with severe hypertension, the infusion rate is 1 to 2 mg/hr initially, and can be doubled every 90 seconds up to a maximum of 32 mg/hr. In clinical trials, the average time to reach the target blood pressure was 10.9 minutes. The most common side effects are headache, nausea, and vomiting. Like other dihydropyridines, clevidipine can cause hypotension and reflex tachycardia.

KEY POINTS

- Calcium channels are gated pores in the cytoplasmic membrane that regulate calcium entry into cells.
- In blood vessels, calcium entry causes vasoconstriction, and hence calcium channel blockade causes vasodilation.
- In the heart, calcium entry increases heart rate, AV conduction, and myocardial contractility, so calcium channel blockade has the opposite effects.
- In the heart, calcium channels are coupled to beta$_1$ receptors, activation of which enhances calcium entry. As a result, calcium channel blockade and beta blockade have identical effects on cardiac function.
- At therapeutic doses, nifedipine and the other dihydropyridines act primarily on VSM; in contrast, verapamil and diltiazem act on VSM *and* on the heart.
- All CCBs promote vasodilation, and hence are useful in hypertension and angina pectoris.
- Because they suppress AV conduction, verapamil and diltiazem are useful for treating cardiac dysrhythmias (in addition to hypertension and angina pectoris).
- Because of their cardiosuppressant effects, verapamil and diltiazem can cause bradycardia, partial or complete AV block, and exacerbation of heart failure.
- Beta blockers intensify cardiosuppression caused by verapamil and diltiazem.
- Nifedipine and other dihydropyridines can cause reflex tachycardia. Tachycardia is most intense with immediate-release formulations, and much less intense with sustained-release formulations.
- Beta blockers can be used to suppress reflex tachycardia caused by nifedipine and other dihydropyridines.
- Because they cause vasodilation, all CCBs can cause dizziness, headache, and peripheral edema.
- In toxic doses, nifedipine and other dihydropyridines can cause cardiosuppression, just like verapamil and diltiazem.
- Immediate-release nifedipine has been associated with increased mortality in patients with myocardial infarction and unstable angina, although a causal relationship has not been established. The National Heart, Lung, and Blood Institute recommends that immediate-release nifedipine, especially in higher doses, be used with great caution, if at all.

Please visit **http://evolve.elsevier.com/Lehne** for chapter-specific NCLEX® examination review questions.

Summary of Major Nursing Implications[a]

VERAPAMIL AND DILTIAZEM

Preadministration Assessment

Therapeutic Goal

Verapamil and diltiazem are indicated for *hypertension, angina pectoris,* and *cardiac dysrhythmias* (atrial fibrillation, atrial flutter, and paroxysmal supraventricular tachycardia).

Baseline Data

For *all patients,* determine blood pressure and pulse rate, and obtain laboratory evaluations of liver and kidney function. For patients with *angina pectoris,* obtain baseline data on the frequency and severity of anginal attacks. For baseline data relevant to *hypertension,* see Chapter 47.

Identifying High-Risk Patients

Verapamil and diltiazem are *contraindicated* for patients with severe hypotension, sick sinus syndrome (in the absence of electronic pacing), and second-degree or third-degree AV block. Use with *caution* in patients with heart failure or liver impairment and in patients taking digoxin or beta blockers.

Implementation: Administration

Routes

Oral, IV.

Administration

Oral. *Verapamil* and *diltiazem* may be used for angina pectoris and essential hypertension. *Verapamil* may be used

Continued

with digoxin to control ventricular rate in patients with atrial fibrillation and atrial flutter.

Extended-release formulations are reserved for essential hypertension. **Instruct patients to swallow extended-release formulations whole, without crushing or chewing.**

Before dosing, measure blood pressure and pulse rate. If hypotension or bradycardia is detected, withhold medication and notify the prescriber.

Intravenous. Intravenous therapy with verapamil or diltiazem is reserved for cardiac dysrhythmias. Perform injections slowly (over 2 to 3 minutes). Monitor the ECG for AV block, sudden reduction in heart rate, and prolongation of the PR or QT interval. Have facilities for cardioversion and cardiac pacing immediately available.

Ongoing Evaluation and Interventions

Evaluating Therapeutic Effects

Angina Pectoris. Keep an ongoing record of anginal attacks, noting the time and intensity of each attack and the likely precipitating event. **Teach outpatients to chart the time, intensity, and circumstances of their attacks, and to notify the prescriber if attacks increase.**

Essential Hypertension. Monitor blood pressure periodically. For most patients, the goal is to reduce systolic/diastolic pressure to a value below 140/90 mm Hg. **Teach patients to self-monitor their blood pressure and to maintain a blood pressure record.**

Minimizing Adverse Effects

Cardiosuppression. Verapamil and diltiazem can cause bradycardia, AV block, and heart failure. **Inform patients about manifestations of cardiac effects (e.g., slow heartbeat, shortness of breath, weight gain) and instruct them to notify the prescriber if these occur.** If cardiac impairment is severe, drug use should stop.

Peripheral Edema. **Inform patients about signs of edema (swelling in ankles or feet), and instruct them to notify the prescriber if these occur.** If necessary, edema can be reduced with a diuretic.

Constipation. Constipation occurs primarily with *verapamil.* **Advise patients that constipation can be minimized by increasing dietary fluid and fiber.**

Minimizing Adverse Interactions

Digoxin. The combination of digoxin with verapamil or diltiazem increases the risk of partial or complete AV block. Monitor for indications of impaired AV conduction (missed beats, slowed ventricular rate).

Verapamil (and possibly diltiazem) can increase plasma levels of digoxin. Digoxin dosage should be reduced.

Beta Blockers. Concurrent use of a beta blocker with verapamil or diltiazem can cause bradycardia, AV block, or heart failure. Monitor closely for cardiac suppression. Administer *intravenous verapamil* and beta blockers several hours apart.

Grapefruit Juice. Grapefruit juice can raise levels of verapamil and diltiazem. Toxicity may result. **Advise patients that it may be prudent to minimize grapefruit juice consumption.**

Managing Acute Toxicity

Remove unabsorbed drug with gastric lavage followed by activated charcoal. Give IV calcium to help counteract excessive vasodilation and reduced myocardial contractility.

To raise blood pressure, give IV norepinephrine. Intravenous fluids and placing the patient in modified Trendelenburg's position can also help.

Bradycardia and AV block can be reversed with atropine and glucagon. If these are inadequate, electronic pacing may be required.

DIHYDROPYRIDINES

Amlodipine
Clevidipine
Felodipine
Isradipine
Nicardipine
Nifedipine
Nimodipine
Nisoldipine

Preadministration Assessment

Therapeutic Goal

Amlodipine, nifedipine, and *nicardipine* are approved for essential hypertension and angina pectoris.

Isradipine, felodipine, and *nisoldipine* are approved for hypertension only.

Nimodipine is used only for subarachnoid hemorrhage.

Clevidipine is used only for IV therapy of *severe* hypertension.

Baseline Data

See nursing implications for *Verapamil and Diltiazem.*

Identifying High-Risk Patients

Use dihydropyridines with *caution* in patients with hypotension, sick sinus syndrome (in the absence of electronic pacing), angina pectoris (because of reflex tachycardia), heart failure, and second-degree or third-degree AV block.

Implementation: Administration

Route

Oral. All dihydropyridines except clevidipine.

Intravenous. Nicardipine, clevidipine.

Administration

Instruct patients to swallow sustained-release formulations whole, without crushing or chewing.

Ongoing Evaluation and Interventions

Evaluating Therapeutic Effects

See nursing implications for *Verapamil and Diltiazem.*

Minimizing Adverse Effects

Reflex Tachycardia. Reflex tachycardia can be suppressed with a beta blocker.

Peripheral Edema. **Inform patients about signs of edema and instruct them to notify the prescriber if these occur.** If necessary, edema can be reduced with a diuretic.

Managing Acute Toxicity

See nursing implications for *Verapamil and Diltiazem.*

[a]Patient education information is highlighted as **blue text**.

CHAPTER

46 Vasodilators

Vasodilation can be produced with a variety of drugs. The major classes of vasodilators, along with representative agents and the chapters in which they are discussed, are shown in Table 46.1. Some of these drugs act primarily on arterioles, some act primarily on veins, and some act on both types of vessels. The vasodilators are widely used, with indications ranging from hypertension to angina pectoris to heart failure. Many of the vasodilators have been discussed in previous chapters. Three agents—hydralazine, minoxidil, and nitroprusside—are introduced here.

In approaching the vasodilators, we begin by considering concepts that apply to the vasodilators as a group. After that we discuss the pharmacology of individual agents.

BASIC CONCEPTS IN VASODILATOR PHARMACOLOGY

Selectivity of Vasodilatory Effects

Vasodilators differ from one another with respect to the types of blood vessels they affect. Some agents (e.g., hydralazine) produce selective dilation of arterioles. Others (e.g., nitroglycerin) produce selective dilation of veins. Still others (e.g., prazosin) dilate arterioles *and* veins. The selectivity of some important vasodilators is shown in Table 46.2.

The selectivity of a vasodilator determines its hemodynamic effects. For example, drugs that dilate *resistance vessels* (arterioles) cause a decrease in cardiac *afterload* (the force the heart works against to pump blood). By decreasing afterload, arteriolar dilators reduce cardiac work while causing cardiac output and tissue perfusion to increase. In contrast, drugs that dilate *capacitance vessels* (veins) reduce the force with which blood is returned to the heart, which reduces ventricular filling. This reduction in filling decreases cardiac *preload* (the degree of stretch of the ventricular muscle before contraction), which in turn decreases the force of ventricular contraction. Hence, by decreasing preload, venous dilators cause a decrease in cardiac work, along with a decrease in cardiac output and tissue perfusion.

Because hemodynamic responses to dilation of arterioles and veins differ, the selectivity of a vasodilator is a major determinant of its effects, both therapeutic and undesired. Undesired effects related to selective dilation of arterioles and veins are discussed later in this chapter. Therapeutic implications of selective dilation are discussed in Chapters 47, 48, 51, 53, and 107.

Overview of Therapeutic Uses

The vasodilators, as a group, have a broad spectrum of uses. Principal indications are essential hypertension, hypertensive crisis, angina pectoris, heart failure, and myocardial infarction. Additional indications include pheochromocytoma, peripheral vascular disease, pulmonary arterial hypertension, and production of controlled hypotension during surgery. The specific applications of any particular agent are determined by its pharmacologic profile. Important facets of that profile are route of administration, site of vasodilation (arterioles, veins, or both), and intensity and duration of effects.

Adverse Effects Related to Vasodilation

Postural Hypotension

Postural (orthostatic) hypotension is defined as a fall in blood pressure brought on by moving from a supine or seated position to an upright position. The underlying cause is relaxation of smooth muscle in *veins*. Because of venous relaxation, gravity causes blood to "pool" in veins, thereby decreasing venous return to the heart. Reduced venous return causes a decrease in cardiac output and a corresponding decrease in blood pressure. Hypotension from venous dilation is minimal in recumbent subjects because when we are lying down, the impact of gravity on venous return is small.

Safety Alert

FALLS

Vasodilators place patients at increased risk of falls. Patients receiving vasodilators should be informed about symptoms of hypotension (light-headedness, dizziness) and advised to sit or lie down if these occur. Failure to follow this advice may result in fainting. Patients should also be taught that they can minimize hypotension by avoiding abrupt transitions from a supine or seated position to an upright position.

Reflex Tachycardia

Reflex tachycardia can be produced by dilation of arterioles *or* veins. The mechanism is this: (1a) *arteriolar* dilation causes a direct decrease in arterial pressure or (1b) *venous* dilation

TABLE 46.1 ■ Types of Vasodilators

Category	Examples	Chapter
DRUGS ACTING ON THE RENIN-ANGIOTENSIN-ALDOSTERONE SYSTEM		
Angiotensin-converting enzyme inhibitors	Captopril Enalapril	44
Angiotensin II receptor blockers	Losartan Valsartan	44
Direct renin inhibitors	Aliskiren	44
Organic nitrates	Isosorbide dinitrate Nitroglycerin	51
Calcium channel blockers	Diltiazem Nifedipine Verapamil	45
SYMPATHOLYTIC DRUGS		
Alpha-adrenergic blockers	Phenoxybenzamine Phentolamine Prazosin Terazosin	18
Adrenergic neuron blockers	Reserpine	19
Centrally acting agents	Clonidine Methyldopa	19
Drugs for pulmonary arterial hypertension	Bosentan Epoprostenol	107
Other important vasodilators	Hydralazine Minoxidil Nitroprusside	46

TABLE 46.2 ■ Vasodilator Selectivity

	Site of Vasodilation	
Vasodilator	Arterioles	Veins
Hydralazine	+	
Minoxidil	+	
Diltiazem	+	
Nifedipine	+	
Verapamil	+	
Prazosin	+	+
Terazosin	+	+
Phentolamine	+	+
Nitroprusside	+	+
Captopril	+	+
Enalapril	+	+
Losartan	+	+
Aliskiren	+	+
Nitroglycerin		+
Isosorbide dinitrate		+

reduces cardiac output, which in turn reduces arterial pressure; (2) baroreceptors in the aortic arch and carotid sinus sense the drop in pressure and relay this information to the vasomotor center of the medulla; and (3) in an attempt to bring blood pressure back up, the medulla sends impulses along sympathetic nerves instructing the heart to beat faster.

Reflex tachycardia is undesirable for two reasons. First, tachycardia can put an unacceptable burden on the heart. Second, if the vasodilator was given to reduce blood pressure, tachycardia would raise pressure and thereby negate the desired effect.

To help prevent vasodilator-induced reflex tachycardia, patients can be pretreated with a beta blocker (e.g., metoprolol), which will block sympathetic stimulation of the heart.

Expansion of Blood Volume

Prolonged use of *arteriolar* or *venous* dilators can cause an increase in blood volume (secondary to prolonged reduction of blood pressure). The increase in volume represents an attempt by the body to restore blood pressure to pretreatment levels.

First, reduced blood pressure triggers secretion of aldosterone by the adrenal glands. Aldosterone then acts on the kidney to promote retention of sodium and water, thereby increasing blood volume. Second, by reducing arterial pressure, vasodilators decrease both renal blood flow and glomerular filtration rate; because filtrate volume is decreased, the kidney is able to reabsorb an increased fraction of filtered sodium and water, which causes blood volume to expand.

Increased blood volume can negate the beneficial effects of the vasodilator. For example, if volume increases during the treatment of hypertension, blood pressure will rise and the benefits of therapy will be canceled. To prevent the kidney from neutralizing the beneficial effects of vasodilation, patients often receive concurrent therapy with a diuretic, which prevents fluid retention and volume expansion.

PHARMACOLOGY OF INDIVIDUAL VASODILATORS

In this section we focus on three drugs: hydralazine, minoxidil, and sodium nitroprusside. All of the other vasodilators are discussed in other chapters (see Table 46.1).

Hydralazine

Cardiovascular Effects

Hydralazine causes selective dilation of arterioles. The drug has little or no effect on veins. Arteriolar dilation results from a direct action on vascular smooth muscle (VSM). The exact mechanism is unknown. In response to arteriolar dilation, peripheral resistance and arterial blood pressure fall. In addition, heart rate and myocardial contractility increase, largely by reflex mechanisms. Because hydralazine acts selectively on arterioles, postural hypotension is minimal.

Pharmacokinetics

Absorption and Time Course of Action. Hydralazine is readily absorbed following oral administration. Effects begin within 45 minutes and persist for 6 hours or longer. With parenteral administration, effects begin faster (within 10 minutes) and last 2 to 4 hours.

Metabolism. Hydralazine is inactivated by a metabolic process known as *acetylation.* The ability to acetylate drugs is genetically determined. Some people are rapid acetylators; some are slow acetylators. The distinction between rapid and slow acetylators can be clinically significant because individuals who acetylate hydralazine slowly are likely to have higher blood levels of the drug, which can result in excessive vasodilation and other undesired effects. To avoid hydralazine accumulation, dosage should be reduced in slow acetylators.

Therapeutic Uses

Essential Hypertension. Oral hydralazine can be used to lower blood pressure in patients with essential hypertension. The regimen almost always includes a beta blocker, and may include a diuretic as well. Although commonly employed in the past, hydralazine has been largely replaced by newer antihypertensive agents (see Chapter 47).

Hypertensive Crisis. Parenteral hydralazine is used to lower blood pressure rapidly in severe hypertensive episodes. The drug should be administered in small incremental doses. If dosage is excessive, severe hypotension may replace the hypertension.

Heart Failure. As discussed in Chapter 48, hydralazine (usually in combination with isosorbide dinitrate) can be used short term to reduce afterload in patients with heart failure. With prolonged therapy, tolerance to hydralazine develops.

Adverse Effects

Reflex Tachycardia. By lowering arterial blood pressure, hydralazine can trigger reflex stimulation of the heart, thereby causing cardiac work and myocardial oxygen demand to increase. Because hydralazine-induced reflex tachycardia is frequently severe, the drug is usually combined with a beta blocker.

Increased Blood Volume. Hydralazine-induced hypotension can cause sodium and water retention and a corresponding increase in blood volume. A diuretic can prevent volume expansion.

Systemic Lupus Erythematosus–like Syndrome. Hydralazine can cause an acute rheumatoid syndrome that closely resembles systemic lupus erythematosus (SLE). Symptoms include muscle pain, joint pain, fever, nephritis, pericarditis, and the presence of antinuclear antibodies. The syndrome occurs most frequently in slow acetylators and is rare when dosage is kept below 200 mg/day. If an SLE-like reaction occurs, hydralazine should be discontinued. Symptoms are usually reversible but may take 6 or more months to resolve. In some cases, rheumatoid symptoms persist for years.

Other Adverse Effects. Common responses include *headache, dizziness, weakness,* and *fatigue.* These reactions are related to hydralazine-induced hypotension.

Drug Interactions

Hydralazine can be combined with a *beta blocker* to protect against reflex tachycardia and with a *diuretic* to prevent sodium and water retention and expansion of blood volume. Drugs that lower blood pressure will intensify hypotensive responses to hydralazine. Accordingly, if hydralazine is used with other *antihypertensive agents,* care is needed to avoid excessive hypotension. In the treatment of heart failure, hydralazine is usually combined with *isosorbide dinitrate,* a drug that dilates veins.

Preparations, Dosage, and Administration

Preparations. Hydralazine is available in tablets (10, 25, 50, and 100 mg) for oral use and in solution (20 mg/mL in 1-mL ampules) for parenteral administration. Hydralazine is also available in a fixed-dose combination with isosorbide dinitrate (a vasodilator), sold as *BiDil.* As discussed in Chapters 8 and 48, BiDil is the first drug product approved for treating a specific ethnic group—namely, African Americans.

Oral Therapy. Dosage should be low initially (10 mg 4 times a day) and then gradually increased. Rapid increases may produce excessive hypotension. Usual maintenance dosages for adults range from 25 to 100 mg twice a day. Daily doses greater than 200 mg are associated with an increased incidence of adverse effects and should be avoided.

Parenteral Therapy. Parenteral administration (IV and IM) is reserved for hypertensive crises. The usual dose is 20 to 40 mg, repeated as needed. Blood pressure should be monitored frequently to minimize excessive hypotension. In most cases, patients can be switched from parenteral hydralazine to oral therapy within 48 hours.

Minoxidil

Minoxidil produces more intense vasodilation than hydralazine but also causes more severe adverse reactions. Because it is both very effective and very dangerous, minoxidil is reserved for patients with severe hypertension unresponsive to safer drugs.

Cardiovascular Effects

Like hydralazine, minoxidil produces selective dilation of *arterioles.* Little or no venous dilation occurs. Arteriolar dilation decreases peripheral resistance and arterial blood pressure. In response, reflex mechanisms increase heart rate and myocardial contractility. Both responses can increase cardiac oxygen demand and can thereby exacerbate angina pectoris.

Vasodilation results from a direct action on VSM. To relax VSM, minoxidil must first be metabolized to minoxidil sulfate. This metabolite then causes potassium channels in VSM to open. The resultant efflux of potassium hyperpolarizes VSM cells, thereby reducing their ability to contract.

Pharmacokinetics

Minoxidil is rapidly and completely absorbed following oral administration. Vasodilation is maximal within 2 to 3 hours and then gradually declines. Residual effects may persist for 2 days or more. Minoxidil is extensively metabolized. Metabolites and parent drug are eliminated in the urine. The drug's half-life is 4.2 hours.

Therapeutic Uses

The only cardiovascular indication for minoxidil is *severe hypertension.* Because of its serious adverse effects, minoxidil is reserved for patients who have not responded to safer drugs. To minimize adverse responses (reflex tachycardia, expansion of blood volume, pericardial effusion), minoxidil should be used with a beta blocker plus intensive diuretic therapy.

Topical minoxidil [Rogaine, others] is used to promote hair growth in balding men and women (see Chapter 105).

Adverse Effects

Reflex Tachycardia. Blood pressure reduction triggers reflex tachycardia, a serious effect that can be minimized by co-treatment with a beta blocker.

Sodium and Water Retention. Fluid retention is both common and serious. Volume expansion may be so severe as to cause cardiac decompensation. Management of fluid retention requires a loop diuretic (e.g., furosemide) used alone or in combination with a thiazide diuretic. If diuretics are inadequate, dialysis must be employed or minoxidil must be withdrawn.

Hypertrichosis. About 80% of patients taking minoxidil for 4 weeks or more develop hypertrichosis (excessive growth of hair). Hair growth begins on the face and later develops on the arms, legs, and back. Hypertrichosis appears to result from proliferation of epithelial cells at the base of the hair follicle; vasodilation may also be involved. Hairiness is a cosmetic problem that can be controlled by shaving or using a depilatory. However, many patients find hypertrichosis both unmanageable and intolerable and refuse to continue treatment.

Pericardial Effusion. Rarely, minoxidil-induced fluid retention results in pericardial effusion (fluid accumulation beneath the pericardium). In most cases, pericardial effusion is asymptomatic. However, in some cases, fluid accumulation becomes so great as to cause cardiac tamponade (compression of the heart with a resultant decrease in cardiac performance). If tamponade occurs, it must be treated by pericardiocentesis or surgical drainage.

Other Adverse Effects. Minoxidil may cause *nausea, headache, fatigue, breast tenderness, glucose intolerance, thrombocytopenia,* and *skin reactions* (rashes, Stevens-Johnson syndrome). In addition, the drug has caused *hemorrhagic cardiac lesions* in experimental animals.

Preparations, Dosage, and Administration

Minoxidil is supplied in 2.5- and 10-mg tablets. The initial dosage is 5 mg once a day. The maximum dosage is 100 mg/day. The usual adult dosage is 10 to 40 mg/day administered in single or divided doses. When a rapid response is needed, a loading dose of 5 to 20 mg is given, followed by doses of 2.5 to 10 mg every 4 hours.

PATIENT-CENTERED CARE ACROSS THE LIFE SPAN

Vasodilators

Life Stage	Patient Care Concerns
Infants	Hydralazine is used in infants as young as 1 month for management of hypertensive crisis and chronic hypertension. Sodium nitroprusside is used in heart failure and for management of hypertensive emergency.
Children/adolescents	Hydralazine and sodium nitroprusside can be used safely in children, just in smaller doses. Side effect profiles are similar to those of adults.
Pregnant women	Hydralazine, sodium nitroprusside, and minoxidil are classified in U.S. Food and Drug Administration Pregnancy Risk Category C.[a] Benefits should outweigh the risks.
Breast-feeding women	Data are lacking regarding transmission of drug from mother to infant via breast milk. Sodium nitroprusside causes potential adverse effects in the infant.
Older adults	Monitor for falls, as there is increased risk with polypharmacy and associated orthostatic hypotension.

[a]As of 2020, the FDA will no longer use Pregnancy Risk Categories. Please refer to Chapter 9 for more information.

Sodium Nitroprusside

Sodium nitroprusside [Nitropress, Nipride ♣] is potent and efficacious and acts faster than any other vasodilator available. Because of these qualities, nitroprusside is a drug of choice for hypertensive emergencies.

Cardiovascular Effects

In contrast to hydralazine and minoxidil, nitroprusside causes *venous* dilation in addition to *arteriolar* dilation. Curiously, although nitroprusside is an effective arteriolar dilator, reflex tachycardia is minimal. Administration is by IV infusion, and effects begin at once. By adjusting the infusion rate, blood pressure can be decreased to almost any level desired. When the infusion is stopped, blood pressure returns to pretreatment levels in minutes. Nitroprusside can trigger retention of sodium and water; furosemide can help counteract this effect.

Mechanism of Action

Once in the body, nitroprusside breaks down to release *nitric oxide,* which then activates *guanylate cyclase,* an enzyme present in VSM. Guanylate cyclase catalyzes the production of *cyclic GMP,* which, through a series of reactions, causes vasodilation. This mechanism is similar to that of nitroglycerin.

Metabolism

Nitroprusside contains five *cyanide groups,* which are split free in the first step of nitroprusside metabolism. *Nitric oxide,* the active component, is released next. Both reactions take place in smooth muscle. Once freed, the cyanide groups are converted to *thiocyanate* by the liver, using *thiosulfate* as a cofactor. Thiocyanate is eliminated by the kidneys over several days.

Therapeutic Uses

Hypertensive Emergencies. Nitroprusside is used to lower blood pressure rapidly in hypertensive emergencies. Oral antihypertensive medication should be initiated simultaneously. During nitroprusside treatment, furosemide may be needed to prevent excessive retention of fluid.

Other Uses. Nitroprusside is approved for producing controlled hypotension during surgery (to reduce bleeding in the surgical field) and for acute decompensated heart failure. In addition, the drug has been employed investigationally to treat myocardial infarction.

Adverse Effects

Excessive Hypotension. If administered too rapidly, nitroprusside can cause a precipitous drop in blood pressure, resulting in headache, palpitations, nausea, vomiting, and sweating. Blood pressure should be monitored continuously.

Cyanide Poisoning. Rarely, lethal amounts of cyanide have accumulated. Cyanide buildup is most likely in patients with liver disease and in those with low stores of thiosulfate, the cofactor needed for cyanide detoxification. The chances of cyanide poisoning can be minimized by avoiding rapid infusion (faster than 5 mcg/kg/min) and by coadministering thiosulfate. If cyanide toxicity occurs, nitroprusside should be withdrawn.

Thiocyanate Toxicity. When nitroprusside is given for several days, thiocyanate may accumulate. Although much less hazardous than cyanide, thiocyanate can also cause adverse effects. These effects, which involve the central nervous system, include disorientation, psychotic behavior, and delirium. To minimize toxicity, patients receiving nitroprusside for more than 3 days should undergo monitoring of plasma thiocyanate, which must be kept below 0.1 mg/mL.

Preparations, Dosage, and Administration

Sodium nitroprusside [Nitropress] is available in powdered form (50 mg) to be dissolved and then diluted for IV infusion. Fresh solutions may have a faint brown color. Solutions that are deeply colored (blue, green, dark red) should be discarded. Nitroprusside in solution can be degraded by light, and hence should be protected with an opaque material.

Blood pressure can be adjusted to practically any level by increasing or decreasing the rate of infusion. The initial infusion rate is 0.3 mcg/kg/min. The maximal rate is 10 mcg/kg/min. If infusion at the maximal rate for 10 minutes fails to produce an adequate drop in blood pressure, administration should stop. During the infusion, blood pressure should be monitored continuously, with either an arterial line or an electronic monitoring device. No other drugs should be mixed with the nitroprusside solution.

KEY POINTS

- Some vasodilators are selective for arterioles, some are selective for veins, and some dilate both types of vessel.
- Drugs that dilate arterioles reduce cardiac afterload and can thereby reduce cardiac work while increasing cardiac output and tissue perfusion.
- Drugs that dilate veins reduce cardiac preload and can thereby reduce cardiac work, cardiac output, and tissue perfusion.
- Principal indications for vasodilators are essential hypertension, hypertensive crisis, angina pectoris, heart failure, and myocardial infarction.
- Drugs that dilate veins can cause orthostatic hypotension.
- Drugs that dilate arterioles or veins can cause reflex tachycardia, which increases cardiac work and elevates blood pressure. Reflex tachycardia can be blunted with a beta blocker.
- Drugs that dilate arterioles or veins can cause fluid retention, which can be blunted with a diuretic.
- Hydralazine causes selective dilation of arterioles.
- Hydralazine can cause a syndrome that resembles SLE.
- Minoxidil causes selective and profound dilation of arterioles.
- Minoxidil can cause hypertrichosis.
- Sodium nitroprusside dilates arterioles and veins.
- Prolonged infusion of nitroprusside can result in toxic accumulation of cyanide and thiocyanate.

Please visit **http://evolve.elsevier.com/Lehne** for chapter-specific NCLEX® examination review questions.

CHAPTER

47 Drugs for Hypertension

Hypertension (elevated blood pressure [BP]) is a common chronic disorder that affects about 2 million American children, 85 million American adults, and over 1 billion people worldwide. According to the World Health Organization, hypertension is the leading global risk for mortality, and has increased nearly 20% from 25.1 million in 1990 to 30.8 million in 2013. Left untreated, hypertension can lead to heart disease, kidney disease, and stroke. Conversely, a treatment program of lifestyle modifications and drug therapy can reduce BP and the risk of long-term complications. However, although we can reduce symptoms and long-term consequences, we can't cure hypertension. As a result, treatment must continue lifelong, making nonadherence a significant problem. Despite advances in management, hypertension remains undertreated: Among Americans with the disease, only 74% undergo treatment, and only 48% take sufficient medicine to bring their BP under control.

We can treat hypertension with 14 classes of drugs. Fortunately, all 14 were introduced in previous chapters. In this chapter, rather than struggling with a huge array of new drugs, all you have to do is learn the antihypertensive applications of drugs you already know about.

In 2017 the American College of Cardiology, the American Heart Association, and The Task Force on Clinical Practice Guidelines issued a new guideline for hypertension entitled *2017 ACC/AHA/AAPA/ABC/ACPM/AGS/APhA/ASH/ASPC/NMA/PCNA Guideline for the Prevention, Detection, Evaluation and Management of High Blood Pressure in Adults.* Clinical practice recommendations throughout this chapter reflect those in the 2017 hypertension guidelines except where noted otherwise.[a]

BASIC CONSIDERATIONS IN HYPERTENSION

In this section, we consider three issues: (1) classification of BP based on values for systolic and diastolic pressure, (2) types of hypertension, and (3) the damaging effects of chronic hypertension.

CLASSIFICATION OF BLOOD PRESSURE

The 2017 hypertension guidelines define four BP categories: normal, elevated, stage 1 hypertension, and stage 2 hypertension.

[a]Although the 2017 hypertension guideline is the most influential guideline in the United States, it is not the only authoritative guideline available. Treatment guidelines have been released by several organizations, including the American Society of Hypertension, the Canadian Hypertension Education Program, the European Society of Hypertension in conjunction with the European Society of Cardiology, and the World Health Organization in conjunction with the International Society of Hypertension.

These categories are defined solely by systolic and diastolic blood pressures. These new guidelines do not differentiate between patient age or comorbidities.

TYPES OF HYPERTENSION

There are two broad categories of hypertension: *primary hypertension* and *secondary hypertension.* Primary hypertension is by far the most common form of hypertensive disease. Less than 10% of people with hypertension have a secondary form.

Primary (Essential) Hypertension

Primary hypertension is defined as hypertension that has no identifiable cause. A diagnosis of primary hypertension is made by ruling out probable specific causes of BP elevation. Primary hypertension is a chronic, progressive disorder. In the absence of treatment, patients will experience a continuous, gradual rise in BP over the rest of their lives.

In the United States, primary hypertension affects about 30% of adults. However, not all groups are at equal risk: Older people are at higher risk than younger people; African Americans are at higher risk than Caucasian Americans; and postmenopausal women are at higher risk than premenopausal women.

Although the cause of primary hypertension is unknown, the condition *can* be successfully treated. Please understand, however, that treatment is not curative: Drugs can lower BP, but they can't eliminate the underlying pathology. Consequently, treatment must continue lifelong.

Primary hypertension is also referred to as *essential hypertension.* This alternative name preceded the term *primary hypertension* and reflects our ignorance about the cause of the problem. Historically, it had been noted that as people grew older, their BP rose. Why older people had elevated BP was (and remains) unknown. One hypothesis noted that as people aged, their vascular systems offered greater resistance to blood flow. To move blood against this increased resistance, a compensatory increase in BP was required. Therefore, the hypertension that occurred with age was seen as being "essential" for providing adequate tissue perfusion—hence, the term *essential hypertension.* Over time, the term came to be applied to all cases of hypertension for which an underlying cause could not be found.

Secondary Hypertension

Secondary hypertension is defined as an elevation of BP brought on by an identifiable primary cause. Because secondary hypertension results from an identifiable cause, it may be possible to treat that cause directly, rather than relying on antihypertensive drugs for symptomatic relief. As a result, some individuals can actually be cured. For example, if hypertension occurs secondary to pheochromocytoma (a catecholamine-secreting tumor), surgical removal of the tumor may produce permanent cure. When cure is not possible, secondary hypertension can be managed with the same drugs used for primary hypertension.

CONSEQUENCES OF HYPERTENSION

Chronic hypertension is associated with increased morbidity and mortality. Left untreated, prolonged elevation of BP can lead to heart disease (myocardial infarction [MI], heart failure, angina pectoris), kidney disease, and stroke. The degree of injury is directly related to the degree of pressure elevation: The higher the pressure, the greater the risk. Among people 40 to 70 years old, the risk of cardiovascular disease is doubled for each 20 mm Hg increase in SBP or each 10 mm Hg increase in DBP—beginning at 115/75 mm Hg and continuing through 185/155 mm Hg. For people older than 50 years, elevated *systolic* BP poses a greater risk than elevated *diastolic* BP. For patients of all ages, hypertension-related deaths result largely from cerebral hemorrhage, renal failure, heart failure, and MI.

Unfortunately, despite its potential for serious harm, hypertension usually remains asymptomatic until long after injury has begun to develop. As a result, the disease can exist for years before overt pathology is evident. Because injury develops slowly and progressively, and because hypertension rarely causes discomfort, many people who have the disease don't know it. Furthermore, many who do know it forgo treatment anyway, largely because hypertension doesn't make them feel bad—that is, until it's too late.

MANAGEMENT OF CHRONIC HYPERTENSION

In this section we consider treatments for chronic hypertension. We begin by addressing patient evaluation and other basic issues, after which we discuss the two modes of management: lifestyle modifications and drug therapy.

BASIC CONSIDERATIONS

Diagnosis

Diagnosis should be based on several BP readings, not just one. If an initial screen shows that BP is elevated (but does not represent an immediate danger), measurement should be repeated on two subsequent office visits. At each visit, two measurements should be made, at least 5 minutes apart. The patient should be seated in a chair—not on an examination table—with his or her feet on the floor. High readings should be confirmed in the contralateral arm. If the mean of all readings shows that SBP is indeed greater than 130 mm Hg or that DBP is greater than 80 mm Hg, a diagnosis of hypertension can be made.

Ideally, diagnosis would be based on *ambulatory blood pressure monitoring* (ABPM) because office-based measurements are often abnormally high, causing individuals to be diagnosed with hypertension when they don't really have it. By contrast, when BP is measured with ABPM, false-positive diagnoses can be avoided. Accordingly, some experts recommend that office-based measurements be used only for *screening* and that treatment be postponed until the diagnosis is confirmed using ABPM. In this way, the risks and expense of unnecessary treatment will be avoided.

Benefits of Lowering Blood Pressure

Multiple clinical trials have demonstrated unequivocally that when the BP of hypertensive individuals is lowered, morbidity is decreased and life is prolonged. Treatment reduces the incidence of stroke by 35% to 40%, MI by 20% to 25%, and heart failure by more than 50%. Although reductions in mortality are less dramatic, they are nonetheless significant: Among patients with stage 1 hypertension plus additional cardiovascular risk factors, one death would be prevented for every 11 patients who reduced SBP by 12 mm Hg for a period of 10 years. Among those with hypertension plus cardiovascular disease or target-organ damage, one death would be prevented for every 9 patients who achieved a sustained 12 mm Hg reduction in pressure.

Patient Evaluation

Evaluation of patients with hypertension has two major objectives. Specifically, we must assess for (1) identifiable causes of hypertension and (2) factors that increase cardiovascular risk. To aid evaluation, diagnostic tests are required.

Hypertension With a Treatable Cause

As discussed earlier, some forms of hypertension result from a treatable cause, such as Cushing's syndrome, pheochromocytoma, and the use of oral contraceptives. Patients should be evaluated for these causes and managed appropriately. In many cases, direct treatment of the underlying cause can control BP, eliminating the need for further antihypertensive therapy.

Factors That Increase Cardiovascular Risk

Two types of factors—existing target-organ damage and major cardiovascular risk factors—increase the risk of cardiovascular events in people with hypertension. When these factors are present, aggressive therapy is indicated. Accordingly, to select appropriate interventions, we must identify patients with the following types of *target-organ damage:*

- Heart disease:
  - Left ventricular hypertrophy
  - Angina pectoris
  - Prior MI
  - Prior coronary revascularization
  - Heart failure
- Stroke or transient ischemic attack
- Chronic kidney disease
- Peripheral arterial disease
- Retinopathy

We must also identify patients with the following *major cardiovascular risk factors* (other than hypertension):

- Cigarette smoking
- Physical inactivity
- Dyslipidemia
- Diabetes
- Microalbuminuria
- Advancing age (older than 55 years for men, older than 65 years for women)
- Family history of premature cardiovascular disease

Diagnostic Tests

The following tests should be done in all patients: electrocardiogram; complete urinalysis; hemoglobin and hematocrit; and blood levels of sodium, potassium, calcium, creatinine, glucose, uric acid, triglycerides, and cholesterol (total, LDL, and HDL cholesterol).

Treatment Goals

The ultimate goal in treating hypertension is to reduce cardiovascular and renal morbidity and mortality. Hopefully this can be accomplished without decreasing quality of life with the drugs used. For all patients regardless of age, the goal is to maintain SBP below 130 mm Hg and DBP below 80 mm Hg. These numbers have decreased from the prior guidelines.

Therapeutic Interventions

We can reduce BP in two ways: We can implement healthy lifestyle changes, and we can treat with antihypertensive drugs. For all patients, a combination of lifestyle changes and drugs is indicated. Lifestyle changes and drug therapy are discussed in detail in the sections that follow.

LIFESTYLE MODIFICATIONS

Lifestyle changes offer multiple cardiovascular benefits with little cost and minimal risk. When implemented before hypertension develops, they may actually prevent hypertension. When implemented after hypertension has developed, they can lower BP, possibly decreasing or eliminating the need for drugs. Lastly, lifestyle modifications can decrease other cardiovascular risk factors. Accordingly, all patients should be strongly encouraged to adopt a healthy lifestyle. Key components are discussed in the sections that follow.

Sodium Restriction

Reducing sodium chloride (salt) intake can lower BP in people with hypertension and can help prevent overt hypertension in those with prehypertension. In addition, salt restriction can enhance the hypotensive effects of drugs. However, the benefits of sodium restriction are both small and short lasting: Over time, BP returns to its original level, despite continued salt restriction. Nonetheless, the Department of Health and Human Services *Dietary Guidelines for Americans 2015-2020* recommends that people consume no more than 2300 mg of sodium a day. In patients at higher risk for cardiovascular disease (African Americans, patients older than 51 years, and those who have hypertension, diabetes, or chronic kidney disease), the recommendation is even lower, at 1500 mg of sodium daily. This recommendation is undergoing evaluation, because this decrease has not yet shown any benefit in patient outcomes. To facilitate salt restriction, patients should be given information on the salt content of foods.

Experts disagree about the relationship between salt intake and BP in *normotensive* patients. In particular, they disagree as to whether a high-salt diet *causes* hypertension. For people with normal BP, a low-salt diet may be considered healthy or unnecessary, depending on the expert you consult.

The DASH Eating Plan

Two studies have shown that we can reduce BP by adopting a healthy diet, known as the Dietary Approaches to Stop Hypertension (DASH) eating plan. This diet is rich in fruits, vegetables, and low-fat dairy products, and low in total fat, saturated fats, and cholesterol. In addition, the plan encourages intake of whole-grain products, fish, poultry, and nuts, and recommends minimal intake of red meat and sweets. Details are available online at https://www.nhlbi.nih.gov/health/health-topics/topics/dash/.

Alcohol Restriction

Excessive alcohol consumption can raise BP and create resistance to antihypertensive drugs. Accordingly, patients should limit alcohol intake: Most men should consume no more than 1 ounce/day; women and lighter weight men should consume no more than 0.5 ounce/day. (One ounce of ethanol is equivalent to about two mixed drinks, two glasses of wine, or two cans of beer.)

Aerobic Exercise

Regular aerobic exercise (e.g., walking, swimming, bicycling) can reduce BP by about 10 mm Hg. In addition, exercise reduces the risk of cardiovascular disease and reduces all-cause mortality. In normotensive people, exercise decreases the risk of developing hypertension. Accordingly, patients should be encouraged to develop an exercise program if they have not already done so. An activity as simple as brisk walking 30 to 45 minutes most days of the week is beneficial.

Smoking Cessation

Smoking is a major risk factor for cardiovascular disease. Each time a cigarette is smoked, BP rises. In patients with hypertension, smoking can reduce the effects of antihypertensive drugs. Clearly, all patients who smoke should be strongly encouraged to quit. (Pharmacologic aids to smoking cessation are discussed in Chapter 39.) As a rule, the use of nicotine replacement products (e.g., nicotine gum, nicotine patch) does not elevate BP. The cardiovascular benefits of quitting become evident within 1 year.

Weight Loss

Weight loss can reduce BP in 60% to 80% of overweight hypertensive individuals and can enhance responses to antihypertensive drugs. Consequently, a program of weight management and exercise is recommended for patients who are overweight.

Maintenance of Potassium and Calcium Intake

Potassium has a beneficial effect on BP. In patients with hypertension, potassium can lower BP. In normotensive people, high potassium intake helps protect against hypertension, whereas low intake elevates BP. For optimal cardiovascular effects, all people should take in 4700 mg of potassium a day. Preferred sources are fresh fruits and vegetables. If hypokalemia develops secondary to diuretic therapy, dietary intake may be insufficient to correct the problem. In this case, the patient may need to use a potassium supplement, a potassium-sparing diuretic, or a potassium-containing salt substitute.

Although adequate calcium is needed for overall good health, the impact of calcium on BP is only modest. In epidemiologic studies, high calcium intake is associated with a reduced incidence of hypertension. Among patients with hypertension, a few may be helped by increasing calcium intake. To maintain good health, calcium intake should be 1000 mg/day for men ages 25 to 65 years and women ages 19 to 50 years, and 1500 mg/day for men and women older than 65.

DRUG THERAPY

Drug therapy, together with lifestyle modifications, can control BP in all patients with chronic hypertension. The decision to use drugs should be the result of collaboration between prescriber and patient. We have a wide assortment of antihypertensive drugs. Consequently, for the majority of patients, it should be possible to establish a program that is effective and yet devoid of objectionable side effects.

Prototype Drugs

DRUGS FOR HYPERTENSION

Diuretics
Hydrochlorothiazide
Spironolactone

Beta-Adrenergic Blockers
Propranolol
Metoprolol

Inhibitors of the Renin-Angiotensin-Aldosterone System
Captopril (ACE inhibitor)
Losartan (angiotensin II receptor blocker)
Aliskiren (direct renin inhibitor)
Eplerenone (aldosterone antagonist)

Calcium Channel Blockers
Verapamil
Nifedipine

Review of Blood Pressure Control

Before discussing the antihypertensive drugs, we need to review the major mechanisms by which BP is controlled. This information will help you understand the mechanisms by which drugs lower BP.

Principal Determinants of Blood Pressure

The principal determinants of BP are shown in Fig. 47.1. As indicated, arterial pressure is the product of cardiac output and peripheral resistance. An increase in either will increase BP.

Cardiac Output. Cardiac output is influenced by four factors: (1) heart rate, (2) myocardial contractility (force of contraction), (3) blood volume, and (4) venous return of blood to the heart. An increase in any of these will increase cardiac output, thereby causing BP to rise. Conversely, a decrease in

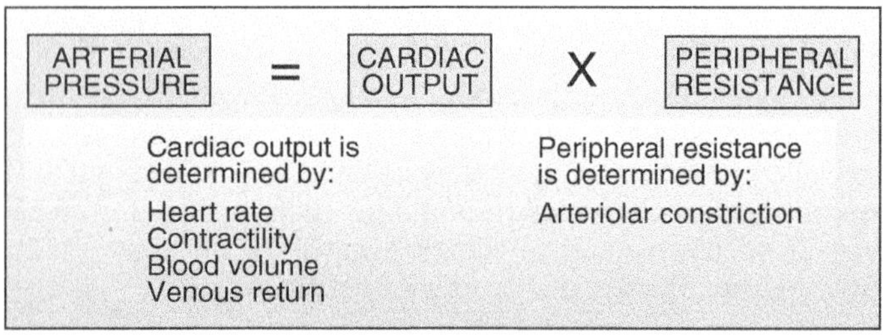

Fig. 47.1 ■ Primary determinants of arterial blood pressure.

these factors will make BP fall. Hence, to reduce BP, we might give a beta blocker to reduce cardiac output, or a diuretic to reduce blood volume, or a venodilator to reduce venous return.

Peripheral Vascular Resistance. Vascular resistance is increased by arteriolar constriction. Accordingly, we can reduce BP with drugs that promote arteriolar dilation.

Systems That Help Regulate Blood Pressure

Having established that BP is determined by heart rate, myocardial contractility, blood volume, venous return, and arteriolar constriction, we can now examine how these factors are regulated. Three regulatory systems are of particular significance: (1) the sympathetic nervous system, (2) the renin-angiotensin-aldosterone system (RAAS), and (3) the kidney.

Sympathetic Baroreceptor Reflex. The sympathetic nervous system employs a reflex circuit—the baroreceptor reflex—to keep BP at a preset level. This circuit operates as follows:

1. Baroreceptors in the aortic arch and carotid sinus sense BP and relay this information to the brainstem.
2. When BP is perceived as too low, the brainstem sends impulses along sympathetic nerves to stimulate the heart and blood vessels.
3. BP is then elevated by (a) activation of $beta_1$ receptors in the heart, resulting in increased cardiac output; and (b) activation of vascular $alpha_1$ receptors, resulting in vasoconstriction.
4. When BP has been restored to an acceptable level, sympathetic stimulation of the heart and vascular smooth muscle subsides.

The baroreceptor reflex frequently opposes our attempts to reduce BP with drugs. Opposition occurs because the "set point" of the baroreceptors is high in people with hypertension. That is, the baroreceptors are set to perceive excessively high BP as "normal" (i.e., appropriate). As a result, the system operates to maintain BP at pathologic levels. Consequently, when we attempt to lower BP using drugs, the reduced (healthier) pressure is interpreted by the baroreceptors as below what it should be, and, in response, signals are sent along sympathetic nerves to "correct" the reduction. These signals produce reflex tachycardia and vasoconstriction—responses that can counteract the hypotensive effects of drugs. Clearly, if treatment is to succeed, the regimen must compensate for the resistance offered by this reflex. Taking a *beta blocker,* which will block reflex tachycardia, can be an effective method of compensation. Fortunately, when BP has been suppressed with drugs for an extended time, the baroreceptors become reset at a lower level. Consequently, as therapy proceeds, sympathetic reflexes offer progressively less resistance to the hypotensive effects of medication.

Renin-Angiotensin-Aldosterone System. The RAAS can elevate BP, negating the hypotensive effects of drugs. The RAAS is discussed in Chapter 44 and reviewed briefly here.

The RAAS elevates BP beginning with the release of renin from juxtaglomerular cells of the kidney. These cells release renin in response to reduced renal blood flow, reduced blood volume, reduced BP, and activation of $beta_1$-adrenergic receptors on the cell surface. Following its release, *renin* catalyzes the conversion of angiotensinogen into angiotensin I, a weak vasoconstrictor. After this, *angiotensin-converting enzyme* (ACE) acts on angiotensin I to form *angiotensin II,* a compound that constricts systemic and renal blood vessels. Constriction of systemic blood vessels elevates BP by increasing peripheral resistance. Constriction of renal blood vessels elevates BP by reducing glomerular filtration, which causes retention of salt and water, which in turn increases blood volume and BP. In addition to causing vasoconstriction, angiotensin II causes release of *aldosterone* from the adrenal cortex. Aldosterone acts on the kidney to further increase retention of sodium and water.

Because drug-induced reductions in BP can activate the RAAS, this system can counteract the effect we are trying to achieve. We have five ways to cope with this problem. First, we can suppress renin release with *beta blockers.* Second, we can prevent conversion of angiotensinogen to angiotensin I with a *direct renin inhibitor.* Third, we can prevent the conversion of angiotensin I into angiotensin II with an *ACE inhibitor.* Fourth, we can block receptors for angiotensin II with an *angiotensin II receptor blocker.* And fifth, we can block receptors for aldosterone with an *aldosterone antagonist.*

Renal Regulation of Blood Pressure. As discussed in Chapter 43, the kidney plays a central role in long-term regulation of BP. When BP falls, glomerular filtration rate (GFR) falls too, thereby promoting retention of sodium, chloride, and water. The resultant increase in blood volume increases venous return to the heart, causing an increase in cardiac output, which in turn increases arterial pressure. We can neutralize renal effects on BP with *diuretics.*

Antihypertensive Mechanisms: Sites of Drug Action and Effects Produced

As discussed earlier, drugs can lower BP by reducing heart rate, myocardial contractility, blood volume, venous return, and the tone of arteriolar smooth muscle. In this section we survey the principal mechanisms by which drugs produce these effects.

The major mechanisms for lowering BP are shown in Fig. 47.2 and Table 47.1. The figure depicts the principal sites at which antihypertensive drugs act. The table shows the effects elicited when drugs act at these sites. The numbering system used in the sections that follow corresponds with the system used in Fig. 47.2 and Table 47.1.

1—Brainstem

Antihypertensive drugs acting in the brainstem suppress sympathetic outflow to the heart and blood vessels, resulting in decreased heart rate, decreased myocardial contractility, and vasodilation. Vasodilation contributes the most to reducing

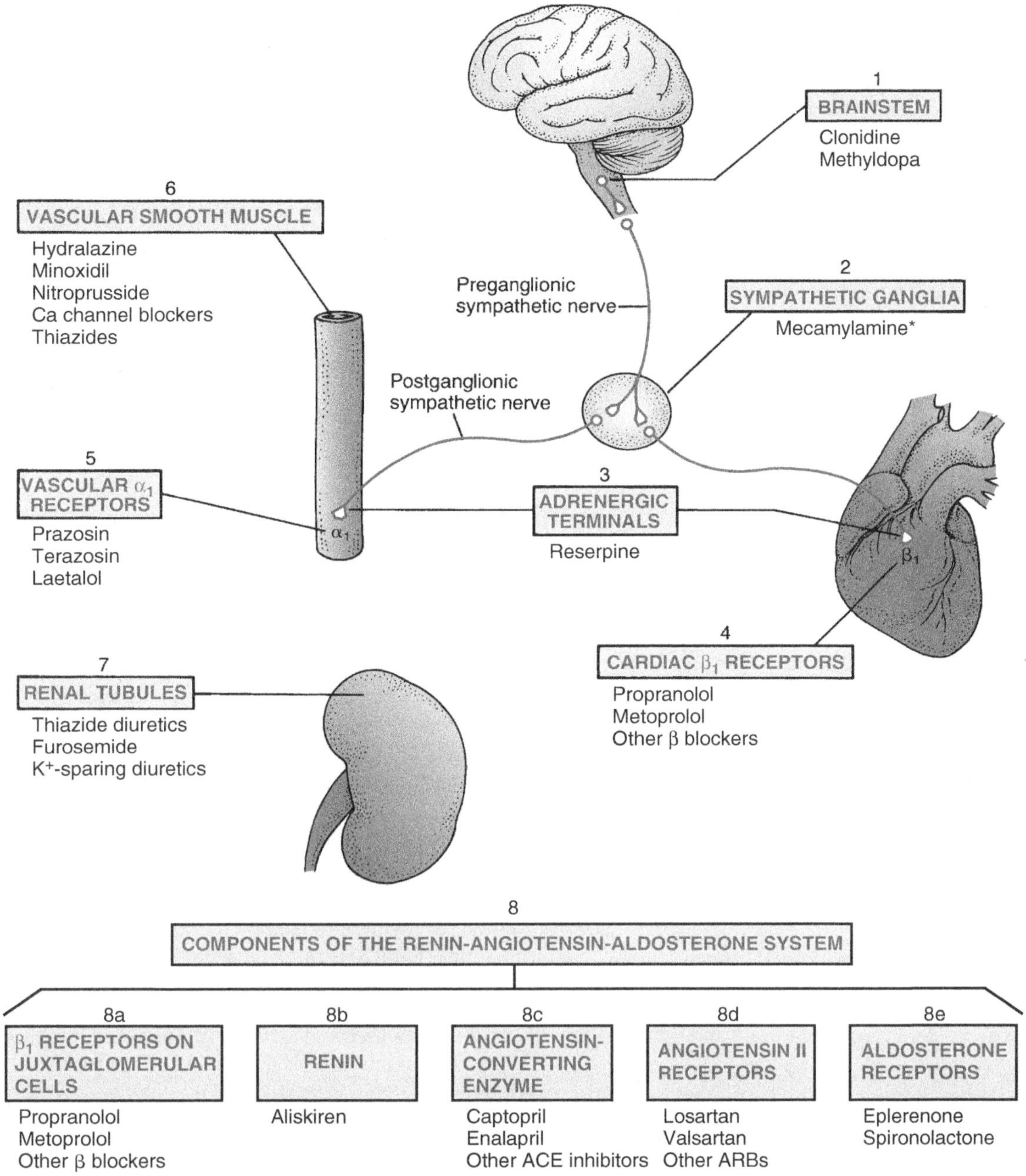

Fig. 47.2 ■ Sites of action of antihypertensive drugs.
Note that some antihypertensive agents act at more than one site: beta (β) blockers act at sites 4 and 8a, and thiazides act at sites 6 and 7. The hemodynamic consequences of drug actions at the sites depicted are shown in Table 47–1. (*ACE,* Angiotensin-converting enzyme; *ARB,* angiotensin II receptor blocker.)
*No longer available in the United States.

BP. Dilation of arterioles reduces BP by decreasing vascular resistance. Dilation of veins reduces BP by decreasing venous return to the heart.

2—Sympathetic Ganglia

Ganglionic blockade reduces sympathetic stimulation of the heart and blood vessels. Antihypertensive effects result primarily from dilation of arterioles and veins. Ganglionic blocking agents produce such a profound reduction in BP that they are used rarely, and then only for hypertensive emergencies. Because use is so limited, the last one available—mecamylamine—was voluntarily withdrawn from the U.S. market.

3—Terminals of Adrenergic Nerves

Antihypertensive agents that act at adrenergic nerve terminals decrease the release of norepinephrine, resulting in decreased sympathetic stimulation of the heart and blood vessels. These drugs, known as adrenergic neuron blocking agents, are used

TABLE 47.1 ■ Antihypertensive Effects Elicited by Drug Actions at Specific Sites

Site of Drug Action[a]	Representative Drug	Drug Effects
1. Brainstem	Clonidine	Suppression of sympathetic outflow decreases sympathetic stimulation of the heart and blood vessels.
2. Sympathetic ganglia	Mecamylamine[b]	Ganglionic blockade reduces sympathetic stimulation of the heart and blood vessels.
3. Adrenergic nerve terminals	Reserpine	Reduced norepinephrine release decreases sympathetic stimulation of the heart and blood vessels.
4. Cardiac beta$_1$ receptors	Metoprolol	Beta$_1$ blockade decreases heart rate and myocardial contractility.
5. Vascular alpha$_1$ receptors	Prazosin	Alpha$_1$ blockade causes vasodilation.
6. Vascular smooth muscle	Hydralazine	Relaxation of vascular smooth muscle causes vasodilation.
7. Renal tubules	Hydrochlorothiazide	Promotion of diuresis decreases blood volume.
Components of the renin-angiotensin-aldosterone system (8a to 8e)		
8a. Beta$_1$ receptors on juxtaglomerular cells	Metoprolol	Beta$_1$ blockade suppresses renin release, resulting in (1) vasodilation secondary to reduced production of angiotensin II and (2) prevention of aldosterone-mediated volume expansion.
8b. Renin	Aliskiren	Inhibition of renin suppresses formation of angiotensin I, which in turn decreases formation of angiotensin II and thereby reduces (1) vasoconstriction and (2) aldosterone-mediated volume expansion.
8c. Angiotensin-converting enzyme (ACE)	Captopril	Inhibition of ACE decreases formation of angiotensin II and thereby prevents (1) vasoconstriction and (2) aldosterone-mediated volume expansion.
8d. Angiotensin II receptors	Losartan	Blockade of angiotensin II receptors prevents angiotensin-mediated vasoconstriction and aldosterone-mediated volume expansion.
8e. Aldosterone receptors	Eplerenone	Blockade of aldosterone receptors in the kidney promotes excretion of sodium and water and thereby reduces blood volume.

[a]Site numbers in this table correspond with site numbers in Fig. 47.2.
[b]No longer available in the United States.

only rarely. In the United States, reserpine is the only drug in this class still on the market.

4—Beta$_1$-Adrenergic Receptors on the Heart

Blockade of cardiac beta$_1$ receptors prevents sympathetic stimulation of the heart. As a result, heart rate and myocardial contractility decline.

5—Alpha$_1$-Adrenergic Receptors on Blood Vessels

Blockade of vascular alpha$_1$ receptors promotes dilation of arterioles and veins. Arteriolar dilation reduces peripheral resistance. Venous dilation reduces venous return to the heart.

6—Vascular Smooth Muscle

Several antihypertensive drugs (see Fig. 47.2) act directly on vascular smooth muscle to cause relaxation. One of these agents—sodium nitroprusside—is used only for hypertensive emergencies. The rest are used for chronic hypertension.

7—Renal Tubules

Diuretics act on renal tubules to promote salt and water excretion. As a result, blood volume declines, causing BP to fall.

8—Components of the RAAS (8a to 8e)

8a—Beta$_1$ Receptors on Juxtaglomerular Cells. Blockade of beta$_1$ receptors on juxtaglomerular cells suppresses release of renin. The resultant decrease in angiotensin II levels has three effects: peripheral vasodilation, renal vasodilation, and suppression of aldosterone-mediated volume expansion.

8b—Renin. Inhibition of renin decreases conversion of angiotensinogen into angiotensin I and thereby suppresses the entire RAAS. The result is peripheral vasodilation, renal vasodilation, and suppression of aldosterone-mediated volume expansion.

8c—Angiotensin-Converting Enzyme. Inhibitors of ACE suppress formation of angiotensin II. The result is peripheral vasodilation, renal vasodilation, and suppression of aldosterone-mediated volume expansion.

8d—Angiotensin II Receptors. Blockade of angiotensin II receptors prevents the actions of angiotensin II. Hence blockade results in peripheral vasodilation, renal vasodilation, and suppression of aldosterone-mediated volume expansion.

8e—Aldosterone Receptors. Blockade of aldosterone receptors in the kidney promotes excretion of sodium and water, and thereby reduces blood volume.

Classes of Antihypertensive Drugs

In this section we consider the principal drugs employed to treat *chronic* hypertension. Drugs for hypertensive emergencies and hypertensive disorders of pregnancy are considered separately.

Individual antihypertensive drugs and their classes are shown in Table 47.2. Combination products are shown in Table 47.3.

Diuretics

Diuretics are a mainstay of antihypertensive therapy. These drugs reduce BP when used alone, and they can enhance the

TABLE 47.2 ▪ Drugs for Chronic Hypertension

Diuretics	Sympatholytics	RAAS Suppressants	Others
Thiazides and Related Diuretics Chlorothiazide Chlorthalidone Hydrochlorothiazide Indapamide Methyclothiazide Metolazone **Loop Diuretics** Bumetanide Ethacrynic acid Furosemide Torsemide **Potassium-Sparing Diuretics** Amiloride Spironolactone Triamterene	**Beta Blockers** Acebutolol (has ISA) Atenolol Betaxolol Bisoprolol Metoprolol Nadolol Nebivolol Penbutolol (has ISA) Pindolol (has ISA) Propranolol Timolol **Alpha$_1$ Blockers** Doxazosin Prazosin Terazosin **Alpha/Beta Blockers** Carvedilol Labetalol **Centrally Acting Alpha$_2$ Agonists** Clonidine Guanabenz Guanfacine Methyldopa **Adrenergic Neuron Blockers** Reserpine	**ACE Inhibitors** Benazepril Captopril Enalapril Fosinopril Lisinopril Moexipril Perindopril Quinapril Ramipril Trandolapril **Angiotensin II Receptor Blockers** Azilsartan Candesartan Eprosartan Irbesartan Losartan Olmesartan Telmisartan Valsartan **Direct Renin Inhibitor** Aliskiren **Aldosterone Antagonists** Eplerenone Spironolactone	**Direct-Acting Vasodilators** Hydralazine Minoxidil **Calcium Channel Blockers** Amlodipine Diltiazem (non-DHP) Felodipine Isradipine Nicardipine Nifedipine Nimodipine Nisoldipine Verapamil (non-DHP)

DHP, Dihydropyridine; *ISA,* intrinsic sympathomimetic activity; *RAAS,* renin-angiotensin-aldosterone system.

effects of other hypotensive drugs. The basic pharmacology of the diuretics is discussed in Chapter 41.

Thiazide Diuretics. Thiazide diuretics (e.g., hydrochlorothiazide, chlorthalidone) are first-line drugs for hypertension. They reduce BP by two mechanisms: reduction of blood volume and reduction of arterial resistance. Reduced blood volume is responsible for initial antihypertensive effects. Reduced vascular resistance develops over time and is responsible for long-term antihypertensive effects. The mechanism by which thiazides reduce vascular resistance has not been determined.

Of the thiazides available, hydrochlorothiazide is used most widely. In fact, hydrochlorothiazide is used more widely than any other antihypertensive drug. Nonetheless, other thiazides, especially chlorthalidone, may be more effective.

The principal adverse effect of thiazides is *hypokalemia.* This can be minimized by consuming potassium-rich foods (e.g., bananas, citrus fruits) and using potassium supplements or a potassium-sparing diuretic. Other side effects include *dehydration, hyperglycemia,* and *hyperuricemia.*

Thiazides are superior to calcium channel blockers and ACE inhibitors as monotherapy, and therefore are preferred.

Loop Diuretics. Loop diuretics (e.g., furosemide) produce much greater diuresis than the thiazides. For most individuals with chronic hypertension, the amount of fluid loss that loop diuretics can produce is greater than needed or desirable. Consequently, loop diuretics are not used routinely for hypertension. Rather, they are reserved for (1) patients who need greater diuresis than can be achieved with thiazides and (2) patients with a low GFR (because thiazides won't work when GFR is low). Like the thiazides, the loop diuretics lower BP by reducing blood volume and promoting vasodilation.

Most adverse effects are like those of the thiazides: *hypokalemia, dehydration, hyperglycemia,* and *hyperuricemia.* In addition, loop diuretics can cause *hearing loss.*

Potassium-Sparing Diuretics. The degree of diuresis induced by the potassium-sparing agents (e.g., spironolactone) is small. Consequently, these drugs have only modest hypotensive effects. However, because of their ability to conserve potassium, these drugs can play an important role in an antihypertensive regimen. Specifically, they can balance potassium loss caused by thiazides or loop diuretics. The most significant adverse effect of the potassium-sparing agents is *hyperkalemia.* Because of the risk of hyperkalemia, potassium-sparing diuretics must not be used in combination with one another or with potassium supplements. Also, they should not be used routinely with ACE inhibitors, angiotensin II receptor blockers, or aldosterone antagonists, all of which promote significant hyperkalemia.

Sympatholytics (Antiadrenergic Drugs)

Sympatholytic drugs suppress the influence of the sympathetic nervous system on the heart, blood vessels, and other structures. These drugs are used widely for hypertension.

TABLE 47.3 ▪ Combination Products for Chronic Hypertension

Generic Name	Brand Name
TWO-DRUG COMBINATIONS	
Thiazide Plus a Beta Blocker	
Hydrochlorothiazide + metoprolol	Lopressor HCT
Hydrochlorothiazide + bisoprolol	Ziac
Hydrochlorothiazide + pindolol	Viskazide 🍁
Bendroflumethiazide + nadolol	Corzide
Chlorthalidone + atenolol	Tenoretic
Thiazide Plus an ACE Inhibitor	
Hydrochlorothiazide + captopril	Generic only
Hydrochlorothiazide + benazepril	Lotensin HCT
Hydrochlorothiazide + enalapril	Vaseretic
Hydrochlorothiazide + fosinopril	Generic only
Hydrochlorothiazide + lisinopril	Zestoretic
Hydrochlorothiazide + moexipril	Generic only
Hydrochlorothiazide + quinapril	Accuretic
Indapamide + perindopril	Coversyl Plus 🍁
Thiazide Plus an ARB	
Hydrochlorothiazide + losartan	Hyzaar
Hydrochlorothiazide + valsartan	Diovan HCT
Hydrochlorothiazide + candesartan	Atacand HCT
Hydrochlorothiazide + eprosartan	Teveten HCT
Hydrochlorothiazide + irbesartan	Avalide
Hydrochlorothiazide + telmisartan	Micardis HCT
Hydrochlorothiazide + olmesartan	Benicar HCT, Olmetec Plus 🍁
Thiazide Plus a Potassium-Sparing Diuretic	
Hydrochlorothiazide + spironolactone	Aldactazide
Hydrochlorothiazide + triamterene	Dyazide, Maxzide
Hydrochlorothiazide + amiloride	Moduretic
Thiazide Plus an Alpha$_2$ Agonist	
Chlorthalidone + clonidine	Clorpres
Hydrochlorothiazide + methyldopa	Generic only
Thiazide Plus a Direct-Acting Vasodilator	
Hydrochlorothiazide + hydralazine	Generic only
CCB Plus an ACE Inhibitor	
Amlodipine + benazepril	Lotrel
Felodipine + enalapril	Generic only
Verapamil + trandolapril	Tarka
CCB Plus an ARB	
Amlodipine + olmesartan	Azor
Amlodipine + valsartan	Exforge
Amlodipine + telmisartan	Twynsta
Aliskiren (a DRI) Plus Another Drug	
Aliskiren + amlodipine	Tekamlo
Aliskiren + hydrochlorothiazide	Tekturna HCT, Rasilez HCT 🍁
THREE-DRUG COMBINATIONS	
Hydrochlorothiazide + amlodipine + valsartan	Exforge HCT
Hydrochlorothiazide + amlodipine + olmesartan	Tribenzor
Hydrochlorothiazide + amlodipine + aliskiren	Amturnide

ACE, Angiotensin-converting enzyme; *ARB*, angiotensin II receptor blocker; *CCB*, calcium channel blocker; *DRI*, direct renin inhibitor.

As indicated in Table 47.2, there are five subcategories of sympatholytic drugs: (1) beta blockers, (2) alpha$_1$ blockers, (3) alpha/beta blockers, (4) centrally acting alpha$_2$ agonists, and (5) adrenergic neuron blockers.

Beta-Adrenergic Blockers. Like the thiazides, beta blockers (e.g., propranolol, metoprolol) are widely used antihypertensive drugs. However, despite their efficacy and frequent use, the exact mechanism by which they reduce BP is somewhat uncertain. Beta blockers are less effective in African Americans than in whites.

The beta blockers have at least four useful actions in hypertension. First, blockade of cardiac beta$_1$ receptors decreases heart rate and contractility, thereby causing cardiac output to decline. Second, beta blockers can suppress reflex tachycardia caused by vasodilators. Third, blockade of beta$_1$ receptors on juxtaglomerular cells of the kidney reduces release of renin and thereby reduces angiotensin II–mediated vasoconstriction and aldosterone-mediated volume expansion. Fourth, long-term use of beta blockers reduces peripheral vascular resistance by a mechanism that is unknown. This action could readily account for most of their antihypertensive effects.

Three beta blockers have *intrinsic sympathomimetic activity* (see Table 47.2). That is, they can produce mild activation of beta receptors while blocking receptor activation by strong agonists (e.g., norepinephrine). As a result, heart rate at rest is slowed less than with other beta blockers. Accordingly, if a patient develops symptomatic bradycardia with another beta blocker, switching to one of these may help.

Beta blockers can produce several adverse effects. Blockade of cardiac beta$_1$ receptors can produce *bradycardia, decreased atrioventricular (AV) conduction,* and *reduced contractility.* Consequently, beta blockers should not be used by patients with sick sinus syndrome or second- or third-degree AV block, and they must be used with care in patients with heart failure. Blockade of beta$_2$ receptors in the lung can promote *bronchoconstriction.* Accordingly, beta blockers should be avoided by patients with asthma. If an asthmatic individual absolutely must use a beta blocker, a beta$_1$-selective agent (e.g., metoprolol) should be employed. Beta blockers can mask signs of hypoglycemia; therefore, they must be used with caution in patients with diabetes. Potential side effects of beta blockers include depression, insomnia, bizarre dreams, and sexual dysfunction; however, a review of older clinical trials has shown that the risk is small or nonexistent.

The basic pharmacology of the beta blockers is discussed in Chapter 18.

Alpha$_1$ Blockers. The alpha$_1$ blockers (e.g., doxazosin, terazosin) prevent stimulation of alpha$_1$ receptors on arterioles and veins, thereby preventing sympathetically mediated vasoconstriction. The resultant vasodilation reduces both peripheral resistance and venous return to the heart.

The most disturbing side effect of alpha blockers is *orthostatic hypotension.* Hypotension can be especially severe with the initial dose. Significant hypotension continues with subsequent doses but is less profound.

The American College of Cardiology recommends that alpha blockers *not* be used as first-line therapy for hypertension. In a huge clinical trial known as the Antihypertensive and Lipid-Lowering Treatment to Prevent Heart Attack Trial (ALLHAT), in which doxazosin was compared with chlorthalidone (a thiazide diuretic), patients taking doxazosin experienced 25% more cardiovascular events and were twice as likely to be hospitalized for heart failure. It is not clear whether doxazosin *increased* cardiovascular risk or chlorthalidone *decreased* risk. Either way, the diuretic is clearly preferred to the alpha blocker.

The basic pharmacology of the alpha blockers is discussed in Chapter 18.

Alpha/Beta Blockers: Carvedilol and Labetalol. Carvedilol and labetalol are unusual in that they can block alpha$_1$ receptors as well as beta receptors. Blood pressure reduction results from a combination of actions: (1) alpha$_1$ blockade promotes dilation of arterioles and veins, (2) blockade of cardiac beta$_1$ receptors reduces heart rate and contractility, and (3) blockade of beta$_1$ receptors on juxtaglomerular cells suppresses release of renin. Presumably, these drugs also share the ability of other beta blockers to reduce peripheral vascular resistance. Like other nonselective beta blockers, labetalol and carvedilol can exacerbate bradycardia, AV heart block, and asthma. Blockade of venous alpha$_1$ receptors can produce postural hypotension.

Centrally Acting Alpha$_2$ Agonists. As discussed in Chapter 19, these drugs (e.g., clonidine, methyldopa) act within the brainstem to suppress sympathetic outflow to the heart and blood vessels. The result is vasodilation and reduced cardiac output, both of which help lower BP. All central alpha$_2$ agonists can cause *dry mouth* and *sedation.* In addition, clonidine can cause severe *rebound hypertension* if treatment is abruptly discontinued. Additional adverse effects of methyldopa are *hemolytic anemia* (accompanied by a positive direct Coombs' test) and *liver disorders.*

Adrenergic Neuron Blockers. Reserpine—the only adrenergic neuron blocker still available—depletes norepinephrine from postganglionic sympathetic nerve terminals, reducing sympathetic stimulation of the heart and blood vessels. The result is a drop in cardiac output and blood pressure. In addition to its peripheral effects, reserpine depletes serotonin and catecholamines from neurons in the central nervous system, causing deep emotional depression. Accordingly, reserpine is absolutely contraindicated for patients with a history of depressive illness. Because reserpine can cause depression and because more desirable antihypertensive drugs are available, reserpine is not a preferred agent for treating hypertension. The basic pharmacology of reserpine is discussed in Chapter 19.

Direct-Acting Vasodilators: Hydralazine and Minoxidil

Hydralazine and minoxidil reduce BP by promoting dilation of *arterioles.* Neither drug causes significant dilation of veins. Because venous dilation is minimal, the risk of orthostatic hypotension is low. With both drugs, the lowering of BP may be followed by reflex tachycardia, renin release, and fluid retention. Reflex tachycardia and release of renin can be prevented with a beta blocker. Fluid retention can be prevented with a diuretic.

The most disturbing adverse effect of *hydralazine* is a syndrome resembling *systemic lupus erythematosus* (SLE). Fortunately, this reaction is rare at recommended doses. If an SLE-like reaction occurs, hydralazine should be withdrawn. Hydralazine is considered a third-line drug for chronic hypertension.

Minoxidil is potentially more harmful than hydralazine. By causing fluid retention, minoxidil can promote *pericardial effusion* (accumulation of fluid beneath the myocardium) that in some cases progresses to *cardiac tamponade* (compression of the heart). A less serious effect is *hypertrichosis* (excessive hair growth). Because of its capacity for significant side effects, minoxidil is not used routinely for chronic hypertension. Instead, the drug is reserved for patients with severe hypertension that has not responded to safer drugs.

The basic pharmacology of hydralazine and minoxidil is discussed in Chapter 46.

Calcium Channel Blockers

The calcium channel blockers (CCBs) fall into two groups: dihydropyridines (e.g., nifedipine) and nondihydropyridines (e.g., verapamil and diltiazem). Drugs in both groups promote dilation of arterioles. In addition, verapamil and diltiazem have direct suppressant effects on the heart.

Like other vasodilators, CCBs can cause *reflex tachycardia.* This reaction is greatest with the dihydropyridines and minimal with verapamil and diltiazem. Reflex tachycardia is low with verapamil and diltiazem because of cardiosuppression. Since dihydropyridines do not block cardiac calcium channels, reflex tachycardia with these drugs can be substantial.

Because of their ability to compromise cardiac performance, verapamil and diltiazem must be used cautiously in patients with bradycardia, heart failure, or AV heart block. These precautions do not apply to dihydropyridines.

The immediate-release formulation of *nifedipine* has been associated with increased mortality in patients with MI and unstable angina. Thus the National Heart, Lung, and Blood Institute has recommended that the use of immediate-release nifedipine be discontinued for treatment of hypertensive emergency.

The basic pharmacology of the CCBs is discussed in Chapter 45.

Drugs That Suppress the RAAS

Because the RAAS plays an important role in controlling BP, drugs that suppress the system—especially the ACE inhibitors—have a significant role in controlling hypertension. The basic pharmacology of these drugs is discussed in Chapter 44.

ACE Inhibitors. The ACE inhibitors (e.g., captopril, enalapril) lower BP by preventing the formation of angiotensin II and thereby preventing angiotensin II–mediated vasoconstriction and aldosterone-mediated volume expansion. In hypertensive diabetic patients with renal damage, these actions slow the progression of kidney injury. Like the beta blockers, ACE inhibitors are less effective in African Americans than in whites. Principal adverse effects are *persistent cough, first-dose hypotension, angioedema,* and *hyperkalemia* (secondary to suppression of aldosterone release). Because of the risk of hyperkalemia, combined use with potassium supplements or potassium-sparing diuretics is generally avoided. ACE inhibitors can cause serious *fetal harm,* especially during the second and third trimesters of pregnancy, and hence must not be given to pregnant women. ACE inhibitors—along with angiotensin receptor blockers (ARBs) and direct renin inhibitors (DRIs)—are the only antihypertensive drugs specifically contraindicated during pregnancy.

Angiotensin II Receptor Blockers. ARBs lower BP in much the same way as do ACE inhibitors. Like the ACE inhibitors, ARBs prevent angiotensin II–mediated vasoconstriction and release of aldosterone. The only difference is that ARBs do so by blocking the *actions* of angiotensin II, whereas ACE inhibitors block the *formation* of angiotensin II. Both groups lower BP to the same extent. Like the ACE inhibitors, ARBs can cause *fetal harm* and must not be used during pregnancy. In contrast to ACE inhibitors, ARBs have a low incidence of inducing cough or significant hyperkalemia, but they do cause angioedema.

Direct Renin Inhibitors. DRIs act directly on renin to inhibit conversion of angiotensinogen into angiotensin I. As a result, DRIs can suppress the entire RAAS. At this time, only one DRI—*aliskiren* [Tekturna, Rasilez ♣]—is available. Antihypertensive effects equal those of ACE inhibitors, ARBs, and CCBs. Compared with ACE inhibitors, aliskiren causes less hyperkalemia, cough, or angioedema—but poses a similar risk of *fetal harm.* In addition, aliskiren causes *diarrhea* in 2.3% of patients. Also, in patients with type 2 diabetes mellitus, the use of aliskiren has demonstrated an increased incidence of renal impairment, hypotension, and hyperkalemia. Because of these findings, the use of aliskiren is contraindicated in patients with diabetes mellitus who are also taking an ACE inhibitor or ARB. Although we know that aliskiren can lower BP, we don't yet know if it reduces adverse outcomes (e.g., stroke, kidney failure, MI). Accordingly, until experience with the drug is more extensive, other antihypertensives should be considered first.

Aldosterone Antagonists. Aldosterone antagonists lower BP by promoting renal excretion of sodium and water. Only two agents are available: *eplerenone* and *spironolactone.* (In case you're confused about spironolactone, yes, it's the same drug we discussed earlier under *potassium-sparing diuretics.* We're discussing it here because it produces diuresis through aldosterone receptor blockade.) Both spironolactone and eplerenone promote renal retention of potassium, and hence pose a risk of *hyperkalemia.* Accordingly, they should not be given to patients with existing hyperkalemia and should not be combined with potassium-sparing diuretics or potassium supplements. Combined use with ACE inhibitors, ARBs, and DRIs is permissible, but must be done with caution. Spironolactone is discussed in Chapter 41, and eplerenone is discussed in Chapter 44.

Fundamentals of Hypertension Drug Therapy

Treatment Algorithm

The basic approach to treating hypertension was published with the 2017 guidelines in the *Journal of the American College of Cardiology* and can be found online at http://www.onlinejacc.org/content/early/2017/11/04/j.jacc.2017.11.006?_ga=2.176790566.2093167245.1516654950-136371117.1515608281. As shown in the algorithm at this link, lifestyle changes should be instituted first. If these fail to lower BP enough, drug therapy should be started, and the lifestyle changes should continue. Treatment often begins with a single drug. If needed, another drug may be *added* (if the initial drug was well tolerated but inadequate) or *substituted* (if the initial drug was poorly tolerated). However, before another drug is considered, possible reasons for failure of the initial drug should be assessed. Among these are insufficient dosage, poor adherence, excessive salt intake, and the presence of secondary hypertension. If treatment with two drugs is unsuccessful, a third and even fourth may be added.

Initial Drug Selection

Initial drug selection is determined by the presence or absence of a *compelling indication,* defined as a comorbid condition for which a specific class of antihypertensive drugs has been shown to improve outcomes. Initial drugs for patients with and without compelling indications are discussed in the sections that follow.

Patients Without Compelling Indications. For initial therapy in the absence of a compelling indication, a *thiazide diuretic* is currently recommended for most patients. This preference is based on long-term controlled trials showing conclusively that thiazides can reduce morbidity and mortality in hypertensive patients, and are well tolerated and inexpensive too. Other options for initial therapy—*ACE inhibitors, ARBs,* and *CCBs*—equal diuretics in their ability to lower BP. However, they may not be as effective at reducing morbidity and mortality. Accordingly, these drugs should be reserved for special indications and for patients who have not responded to thiazides. Certain other alternatives—*centrally acting sympatholytics, adrenergic neuron blockers,* and *direct-acting vasodilators*—are associated with a high incidence of adverse effects, and hence are not well suited for initial monotherapy. One last alternative—*alpha$_1$ blockers*—is no longer recommended as first-line therapy. As noted, when the alpha blocker doxazosin was compared with the diuretic chlorthalidone, doxazosin was associated with a much higher incidence of adverse cardiovascular events.

Patients With Compelling Indications. For patients with hypertension plus certain comorbid conditions (e.g., heart failure, diabetes), there is strong evidence that specific antihypertensive drugs can reduce morbidity and mortality. Drugs shown to improve outcomes for six comorbid conditions are indicated in Table 47.4. Clearly, these drugs should be used for initial therapy. If needed, other antihypertensive agents can be added to the regimen. Management of hypertension in patients with diabetes and renal disease—two specific comorbid conditions—is discussed further under *Individualizing Therapy.*

Adding Drugs to the Regimen

Rationale for Drug Selection. When using two or more drugs to treat hypertension, each drug should come from a different class. That is, each drug should have a different mechanism of action. In accord with this guideline, it would be appropriate to combine a beta blocker, a diuretic, and a vasodilator, since each lowers BP by a different mechanism. In contrast, it would be inappropriate to combine two thiazide diuretics or two beta blockers or two vasodilators.

TABLE 47.4 ■ Classes of Antihypertensive Drugs Recommended for Initial Therapy of Hypertension in Patients With Certain High-Risk Comorbid Conditions

	Heart Failure	Recurrent Stroke Prevention	High Risk of CAD	Post–Myocardial Infarction	Diabetes	Chronic Kidney Disease
Recommended Drug Classes for Treatment of HTN	• ACE inhibitor • Aldosterone antagonist • ARB • Beta blocker • CCB • Diuretic	• ACE inhibitor • Diuretic	• ACE inhibitor • Beta blocker • CCB • Diuretic	• ACE inhibitor • Aldosterone antagonist • Beta blocker	• ACE inhibitor • ARB • Beta blocker • CCB • Diuretic	• ACE inhibitor • ARB

ACE, Angiotensin-converting enzyme; *ARB,* angiotensin II receptor blocker; *CAD,* coronary artery disease; *CCB,* calcium channel blocker.
Data from The Seventh Report of the Joint National Committee on Prevention, Detection, Evaluation, and Treatment of High Blood Pressure. *JAMA* 289:2560–2572, 2003.

Benefits of Multidrug Therapy. Treatment with multiple drugs offers significant benefits. First, by employing drugs that have different mechanisms, we can increase the chance of success: Targeting BP control at several sites is likely to be more effective than targeting at one site. Second, when drugs are used in combination, each can be administered in a lower dosage than would be possible if it were used alone. As a result, both the frequency and the intensity of side effects are reduced. Third, when proper combinations are selected, one agent can offset the adverse effects of another. For example, if a vasodilator is used alone, reflex tachycardia is likely. However, if a vasodilator is combined with a beta blocker, reflex tachycardia will be minimal.

Dosing

For each drug in the regimen, *dosage should be low initially and then gradually increased.* For most people with chronic hypertension, the disease poses no immediate threat. Hence, there is no need to lower BP rapidly using large doses. Also, when BP is reduced slowly, baroreceptors gradually reset to the new lower pressure. As a result, sympathetic reflexes offer less resistance to the hypotensive effects of therapy. Finally, since there is no need to drop BP rapidly and since higher doses carry a higher risk of adverse effects, the use of high initial doses would needlessly increase the risk of adverse effects.

Step-Down Therapy

After BP has been controlled for at least 1 year, an attempt should be made to reduce dosages and the number of drugs in the regimen. Of course, lifestyle modifications should continue. When reductions are made slowly and progressively, many patients are able to maintain BP control with less medication—and some can be maintained with no medication at all. If drugs are discontinued, regular follow-up is essential, because BP usually returns to hypertensive levels—although it may take years to do so.

Individualizing Therapy

Patients With Comorbid Conditions

Comorbid conditions complicate treatment. Two conditions that are especially problematic—renal disease and diabetes—are discussed here. Preferred drugs for patients with these and other comorbid conditions are shown in Table 47.4. Drugs to avoid in patients with specific comorbid conditions are summarized in Table 47.5.

Renal Disease. Nephrosclerosis (hardening of the kidney) secondary to hypertension is among the most common causes of progressive renal disease. Pathophysiologic changes include degeneration of renal tubules and fibrotic thickening of the glomeruli, both of which contribute to renal insufficiency. Nephrosclerosis sets the stage for a downward spiral: Renal insufficiency causes water retention, which in turn causes BP to rise higher, which in turn promotes even more renal injury, and so forth. Accordingly, early detection and treatment are essential. To slow progression of renal damage, the most important action is to lower BP. The target BP in all patients is now below 120/80 mm Hg. Although all classes of antihypertensive agents are effective in nephrosclerosis, ACE inhibitors and ARBs work best. Hence, in the absence of contraindications, all patients should get one of these drugs. In most cases, a diuretic is used too. In patients with advanced renal insufficiency, thiazide diuretics are ineffective, hence a loop diuretic should be employed. Potassium-sparing diuretics should be avoided.

Diabetes. In patients with diabetes, the target BP is the same as with all other populations. Preferred antihypertensive drugs are ACE inhibitors, ARBs, CCBs, and diuretics (in low doses). In patients with diabetic nephropathy, ACE inhibitors and ARBs can slow the progression of renal damage and reduce albuminuria. In diabetic patients, as in nondiabetics, beta blockers and diuretics can decrease morbidity and mortality. Keep in mind, however, that beta blockers can suppress glycogenolysis and mask early signs of hypoglycemia; therefore, they must be used with caution. Thiazides and loop diuretics promote hyperglycemia, and hence should be used with care.

How do ACE inhibitors compare with CCBs in patients with hypertension and diabetes? In one large study, patients taking nisoldipine (a CCB) had a higher incidence of MI than did patients taking enalapril (an ACE inhibitor). Because the study was not placebo controlled, it was impossible to distinguish between two possible interpretations: (1) the CCB increased the risk of MI or (2) the ACE inhibitor protected against MI.

TABLE 47.5 ▪ Comorbid Conditions That Require Cautious Use or Complete Avoidance of Certain Antihypertensive Drugs

Comorbid Condition	Drugs to Be Avoided or Used With Caution	Reason for Concern
CARDIOVASCULAR DISORDERS		
Heart failure	Verapamil Diltiazem	These drugs act on the heart to decrease myocardial contractility and can thereby further reduce cardiac output.
AV heart block	Beta blockers Labetalol Verapamil Diltiazem	These drugs act on the heart to suppress AV conduction and can thereby intensify AV block.
Coronary artery disease	Hydralazine	Reflex tachycardia induced by hydralazine can precipitate an anginal attack.
Post–myocardial infarction	Hydralazine	Reflex tachycardia induced by hydralazine can increase cardiac work and oxygen demand.
OTHER DISORDERS		
Dyslipidemia	Beta blockers Diuretics	These drugs may exacerbate dyslipidemia.
Renal insufficiency	K^+-sparing diuretics K^+ supplements	Use of these agents can lead to dangerous accumulations of potassium.
Asthma	Beta blockers Labetalol	$Beta_2$ blockade promotes bronchoconstriction.
Depression	Reserpine	Reserpine can cause depression.
Diabetes mellitus	Thiazides Furosemide Beta blockers	Thiazides and furosemide promote hyperglycemia, and beta blockers suppress glycogenolysis and can mask signs of hypoglycemia.
Gout	Thiazides Furosemide	These diuretics promote hyperuricemia.
Hyperkalemia	K^+-sparing diuretics ACE inhibitors Direct renin inhibitors Aldosterone antagonists	These drugs cause potassium accumulation.
Hypokalemia	Thiazides Furosemide	These drugs cause potassium loss.
Collagen diseases	Hydralazine	Hydralazine can precipitate a lupus erythematosus–like syndrome.
Liver disease	Methyldopa	Methyldopa is hepatotoxic.
Preeclampsia	ACE inhibitors ARBs Direct renin inhibitors	These drugs can injure the fetus.

ACE, Angiotensin-converting enzyme; *ARBs,* angiotensin II receptor blockers; *AV,* atrioventricular.

Either way, it seems clear that ACE inhibitors are better than CCBs for patients with hypertension and diabetes.

Patients in Special Populations

African Americans. Hypertension is a major health problem for African American adults. Hypertension develops earlier, has a much higher incidence, and is likely to be more severe. As a result, African Americans face a greater risk of heart disease, end-stage renal disease, and stroke. Compared with the general population, African Americans experience a 50% higher rate of death from heart disease, are twice as likely to die from stroke, and are six times more likely to experience hypertension-related end-stage renal disease.

With timely treatment, this disparity can be greatly reduced, if not eliminated. We know that blacks and whites respond equally to treatment (although not always to the same drugs). The primary problem is that hypertension often goes untreated among African Americans until after significant organ damage has developed. If hypertension were diagnosed and treated earlier, the prognosis would be greatly improved. Accordingly, it is important that African Americans undergo routine monitoring of BP. If hypertension is diagnosed, treatment should begin at once. Because African Americans have a high incidence of salt sensitivity and cigarette use, lifestyle modifications are an important component of treatment.

African Americans respond better to some antihypertensive drugs than to others. Controlled trials have shown that *diuretics* can decrease morbidity and mortality in blacks. Accordingly, diuretics are drugs of first choice. *CCBs* and alpha/beta blockers are also effective. In contrast, monotherapy with *beta blockers* or *ACE inhibitors* is less effective in blacks than in whites. Nonetheless, beta blockers and ACE inhibitors should be used if they are strongly indicated for a comorbid condition. For example, ACE inhibitors should be used in black patients who have type 1 diabetes with proteinuria. Also, ACE inhibitors should be used in patients with hypertensive nephrosclerosis, a condition for which ACE inhibitors are superior to CCBs. When BP cannot be adequately controlled with a single drug, several two-drug combinations are recommended: an ACE inhibitor plus a thiazide diuretic, an ACE inhibitor plus a CCB, and a beta blocker plus a thiazide.

In 2010, the International Society on Hypertension in Blacks (ISHIB) issued updated guidelines on managing hypertension in African Americans. Because hypertension takes a high toll on the black community, these guidelines call for strict new BP goals: under 135/85 mm Hg for most patients, and under 130/80 mm Hg for those at high risk of a cardiovascular event. Some experts, however, have criticized these goals, arguing there is insufficient evidence to support them.

Children and Adolescents. The incidence of secondary hypertension in children is much higher than in adults. Accordingly, efforts to diagnose and treat an underlying cause should be especially diligent. For children with primary hypertension, treatment is the same as for adults—although doses are lower and should be adjusted with care. Because ACE inhibitors and ARBs can cause fetal harm, they should be avoided in girls who are sexually active or pregnant.

Older Adults. By age 65 years, most Americans have hypertension. Furthermore, high BP in this group almost always presents as *isolated systolic hypertension;* DBP is usually normal or low. The good news, as shown in the Hypertension in the Very Elderly Trial (HYVET), is that treatment can reduce the incidence of heart failure, fatal stroke, and all-cause mortality. The bad news is that most older people are not treated.

Because cardiovascular reflexes are blunted in older adults, treatment carries a significant risk of orthostatic hypotension. Accordingly, initial doses should be low—about one-half those used for younger adults—and dosage escalation should be done slowly. Drugs that are especially likely to cause orthostatic hypotension (e.g., reserpine, $alpha_1$ blockers, alpha/beta blockers) should be used with caution.

Minimizing Adverse Effects

Antihypertensive drugs can produce many unwanted effects, including hypotension, sedation, and sexual dysfunction. (Although not stressed previously, practically all antihypertensive drugs can interfere with sexual function.)

The fundamental strategy for decreasing side effects is to tailor the regimen to the sensitivities of the patient. Simply put, if one drug causes effects that are objectionable, a more acceptable drug should be substituted. The best way to identify unacceptable responses is to encourage patients to report them.

Adverse effects caused by the exacerbation of comorbid diseases are both predictable and avoidable. We know, for example, that beta blockers can intensify AV block, and hence should not be taken by people with these disorders. Other conditions that can be aggravated by antihypertensive drugs are listed in Table 47.5. To help avoid drug-disease mismatches, the medical history should identify all comorbid conditions. With this information, the prescriber can choose drugs that are least likely to make the comorbid condition worse.

PATIENT-CENTERED CARE ACROSS THE LIFE SPAN

Hypertension

Life Stage	Patient Care Concerns
Infants	See "Breast-feeding women," below.
Children/adolescents	No data are available on the long-term effects of antihypertensive drugs on growth and development of children. Drugs recommended for treatment of hypertension in children 1 to 18 years old include ACE inhibitors, diuretics, beta blockers, and calcium channel blockers.
Pregnant women	Drugs of choice in treating pregnant women with mild preeclampsia include labetalol and methyldopa. Magnesium sulfate is used in the prevention of seizures in severe preeclampsia or for the treatment of seizures in eclampsia.
Breast-feeding women	Effects of RAAS-blocking drugs have not been studied in breast-feeding. Beta blockers, such as metoprolol, appear safe for the breast-feeding infant. Diuretics appear safe, but may suppress lactation.
Older adults	Older adults benefit from SBPs <145 mm Hg. Treatment with ACE inhibitors, diuretics, and/or beta blockers is reasonable. Caution must be taken to avoid overdiuresis when using diuretics in the older adult population.

High initial doses and rapid dosage escalation can increase the incidence and severity of adverse effects. Accordingly, doses should be low at first and then gradually increased. Remember, there is usually no need to reduce BP rapidly. Hence, large initial doses that can produce a rapid fall in BP but also produce adverse effects should be avoided.

Promoting Adherence

The major cause of treatment failure in patients with chronic hypertension is lack of adherence to the prescribed regimen. In this section we consider the causes of nonadherence and discuss some solutions.

Why Adherence Is Often Hard to Achieve

Much of the difficulty in promoting adherence stems from the nature of hypertension itself. Hypertension is a chronic, slowly progressing disease that is devoid of overt symptoms through much of its course. Because symptoms are absent, it can be difficult to convince patients that they are ill and need treatment. In addition, since there are no symptoms to relieve, drugs cannot produce an obvious therapeutic response. In the absence of such a response, it can be difficult for patients to believe that their medication is doing anything useful.

Because hypertension progresses very slowly, the disease tends to encourage procrastination. For most people, the adverse effects of hypertension will not become manifest for many years. Realizing this, patients may reason (incorrectly) that they can postpone therapy without significantly increasing risk.

The negative aspects of treatment also contribute to nonadherence. Antihypertensive regimens can be complex and expensive. In addition, treatment must continue lifelong. Lastly, antihypertensive drugs can cause a number of adverse effects, ranging from sedation to hypotension to impaired sexual function. It is difficult to convince people who are feeling good to take drugs that may make them feel worse. Some people may decide that exposing themselves to the negative effects of therapy today is paying too high a price to avoid the adverse consequences of hypertension at some indefinite time in the future.

Ways to Promote Adherence

Patient Education. Adherence requires motivation, and patient education can help provide it. Patients should be taught about the consequences of hypertension and the benefits of treatment. Because hypertension does not cause discomfort, it may not be clear to patients that their condition is indeed serious. Patients must be helped to understand that, left untreated, hypertension can cause heart disease, kidney disease, and stroke. In addition, patients should appreciate that, with proper therapy, the risks of these long-term complications can be minimized, resulting in a longer and healthier life. Lastly, patients must understand that drugs do not cure hypertension—they only control symptoms. Hence, for treatment to be effective, medication must be taken lifelong.

Teach Self-Monitoring. Patients should be taught the goal of treatment (usually maintenance of BP below 120/80 mm Hg), and they should be taught to monitor and record their BP daily. This increases patient involvement and provides positive feedback that can help promote adherence.

Minimize Side Effects. If we expect patients to comply with long-term treatment, we must keep adverse effects to a minimum. As discussed previously, adverse effects can be minimized by (1) encouraging patients to report side effects, (2) discontinuing objectionable drugs and substituting more acceptable ones, (3) avoiding drugs that can exacerbate comorbid conditions, and (4) using doses that are initially low and gradually increased.

Establish a Collaborative Relationship. The patient who feels like a collaborative partner in the treatment program is more likely to comply than is the patient who feels that treatment is being imposed. Collaboration allows the patient to help set treatment goals, create the treatment program, and evaluate progress. In addition, a collaborative relationship facilitates communication about side effects.

Simplify the Regimen. Antihypertensive regimens may consist of several drugs taken multiple times a day. Such complex regimens deter adherence. To promote adherence, the dosing schedule should be as simple as possible. Once an effective regimen has been established, dosing just once or twice daily should be tried. If an appropriate combination product is available (e.g., a fixed-dose combination of a thiazide diuretic plus an ACE inhibitor), the combination product may be substituted for its components.

Other Measures. Adherence can be promoted by giving positive reinforcement when therapeutic goals are achieved. Involvement of family members can be helpful. Also, adherence can be promoted by scheduling office visits at convenient times and by following up when appointments are missed. For many patients, antihypertensive therapy represents a significant economic burden; devising a regimen that is effective but inexpensive will help.

DRUGS FOR HYPERTENSIVE EMERGENCIES

A hypertensive emergency exists when *diastolic* BP exceeds 120 mm Hg. The severity of the emergency is determined by the likelihood of organ damage. When excessive BP is associated with papilledema (edema of the retina), intracranial hemorrhage, MI, or acute congestive heart failure, a severe emergency exists—and BP must be lowered rapidly (within 1 hour). If severe hypertension is present but does not yet pose an immediate threat of organ damage, reducing BP more slowly (over 24 to 48 hours) is preferable. Because rapid reductions can cause cerebral ischemia, MI, and renal failure, pressure should be reduced gradually whenever possible.

The major drugs used for hypertensive emergencies are discussed here. All reduce BP by causing vasodilation, and all are given IV.

Sodium Nitroprusside

When acute severe hypertension demands a rapid but controlled reduction in BP, IV nitroprusside [Nitropress] is usually the drug of first choice. Nitroprusside is a direct-acting vasodilator that relaxes smooth muscle of arterioles and veins. Effects begin in seconds and then fade rapidly when administration ceases. Nitroprusside is administered by continuous IV infusion using an infusion pump to control the rate. The usual rate is 0.3 to 3 mcg/kg/min. To avoid hypotension, continuous BP monitoring is required. Because nitroprusside has an extremely short duration, hypotension can be corrected quickly by reducing the rate of infusion. Prolonged infusion (longer than 72 hours) can produce toxic accumulation of thiocyanate and should be avoided. The basic pharmacology of nitroprusside is discussed in Chapter 46.

Fenoldopam

Fenoldopam [Corlopam] is an IV drug indicated for short-term management of hypertensive emergencies. Benefits equal those of nitroprusside. Fenoldopam lowers BP by activating $dopamine_1$ receptors on arterioles to cause vasodilation. In animal models, the drug dilates renal, coronary, mesenteric, and peripheral vessels.

Fenoldopam differs from other antihypertensives in that it helps maintain (or even improve) renal function. Two mechanisms are involved. First, the drug dilates renal blood vessels, increasing renal blood flow (despite reducing arterial pressure). Second, fenoldopam promotes sodium and water excretion through direct effects on renal tubules.

Fenoldopam has a rapid onset and short duration. Effects begin in less than 5 minutes. The drug undergoes rapid hepatic metabolism followed by renal excretion. Its plasma half-life is only 5 minutes.

Fenoldopam is generally well tolerated. The most common side effects are hypotension, headache, flushing, dizziness, and reflex tachycardia—all of which occur secondary to vasodilation. Tachycardia may cause ischemia in patients with angina. Combined use with a beta blocker can minimize tachycardia, but may also result in excessive lowering of BP. Fenoldopam can elevate intraocular pressure, and hence should be used with caution in patients with glaucoma.

Fenoldopam is administered by continuous IV infusion. To minimize tachycardia, the initial dosage should be low. The typical infusion rate is 0.25

to 0.5 mcg/kg/min. With continuous 24-hour infusion, no tolerance develops to antihypertensive effects, and there is no rebound increase in BP when the infusion is stopped. With a 48-hour infusion, some tolerance may develop. Oral antihypertensive therapy can be added as soon as BP has stabilized.

Labetalol

Labetalol blocks alpha- and beta-adrenergic receptors. Blood pressure is reduced by arteriolar dilation secondary to alpha blockade. Beta blockade prevents reflex tachycardia in response to reduced arterial pressure, and hence the drug is probably safe for patients with angina or MI. Beta blockade can aggravate bronchial asthma, heart failure, AV block, cardiogenic shock, and bradycardia. Accordingly, labetalol should not be given to patients with these disorders. Administration is by slow IV injection.

Clevidipine

Clevidipine [Cleviprex] is a dihydropyridine CCB with an ultrashort half-life (about 1 minute). Administration is by IV infusion. As with nitroprusside, effects begin rapidly and then fade rapidly when the infusion is slowed or stopped. As a result, BP can be easily titrated. For patients with severe hypertension, the infusion rate is 1 to 2 mg/hr initially, and can be doubled every 3 minutes up to a maximum of 32 mg/hr. In clinical trials, the average time to reach the target BP was 10.9 minutes. The most common side effects are headache, nausea, and vomiting. The basic pharmacology of clevidipine is discussed in Chapter 45.

DRUGS FOR HYPERTENSIVE DISORDERS OF PREGNANCY

Hypertension is the most common complication of pregnancy, with an incidence of about 10%. When hypertension develops, it is essential to distinguish between chronic hypertension and preeclampsia. Chronic hypertension is relatively benign, whereas preeclampsia can lead to life-threatening complications for the patient and the fetus.

CHRONIC HYPERTENSION

Chronic hypertension, seen in 5% of pregnancies, is defined as hypertension that was present before pregnancy or that developed before the 20th week of gestation. Persistent *severe* hypertension carries a risk to both the patient and the fetus. Potential adverse outcomes include placental abruption, maternal cardiac decompensation, premature birth, fetal growth delay, central nervous system hemorrhage, and renal failure. The goal of treatment is to minimize the risk of hypertension to the patient and fetus while avoiding drug-induced harm to the fetus. With the exception of ACE inhibitors, ARBs, and DRIs, antihypertensive drugs that were being taken before pregnancy can be continued. *ACE inhibitors, ARBs, and DRIs are contraindicated owing to their potential for harm* (fetal growth delay, congenital malformations, neonatal renal failure, neonatal death). When drug therapy is initiated *during* pregnancy, *methyldopa* or *labetalol* are the traditional agents of choice. These drugs have limited effects on uteroplacental and fetal hemodynamics, and do not adversely affect the fetus or neonate. Regardless of the drug selected, treatment should not be too aggressive because an excessive drop in BP could compromise uteroplacental blood flow.

According to guidelines issued by the American College of Obstetricians and Gynecologists (ACOG), "severe" hypertension requires treatment, whereas "mild" hypertension generally does not. (The ACOG defines severe hypertension as SBP above 160 mm Hg or DBP above 110 mm Hg, and mild hypertension as SBP 140 to 159 mm Hg or DBP 90 to 109 mm Hg.) There is good evidence that treating severe hypertension reduces risk. In contrast, there is little evidence that treating mild hypertension offers significant benefit.

Patients who have chronic hypertension during pregnancy are at increased risk of developing preeclampsia (see next section). Unfortunately, reducing BP does *not* lower this risk.

PREECLAMPSIA AND ECLAMPSIA

Preeclampsia is a multisystem disorder characterized by the combination of elevated BP (above 130/90 mm Hg) and proteinuria (300 mg or more in 24 hours) that develops after the 20th week of gestation. The disorder occurs in about 5% of pregnancies. Rarely, women with preeclampsia develop seizures. If seizures do develop, the condition is then termed *eclampsia.* Risk factors for preeclampsia include black race, chronic hypertension, diabetes, collagen vascular disorders, and previous preeclampsia. The etiology of preeclampsia is complex and incompletely understood.

Preeclampsia poses serious risks for the fetus and mother. Risks for the fetus include intrauterine growth restriction, premature birth, and even death. The mother is at risk for seizures (eclampsia), renal failure, pulmonary edema, stroke, and death.

Management of preeclampsia is based on the severity of the disease, the status of mother and fetus, and the length of gestation. The objective is to preserve the health of the mother and deliver an infant who will not require intensive and prolonged neonatal care. Success requires close maternal and fetal monitoring. Although drugs can help reduce BP, delivery is the only cure.

Management of *mild* preeclampsia is controversial and depends on the duration of gestation. If preeclampsia develops near term, and if fetal maturity is certain, induction of labor is advised. However, if mild preeclampsia develops earlier in gestation, experts disagree about what to do. Suggested measures include bed rest, prolonged hospitalization, treatment with antihypertensive drugs, and prophylaxis with an anticonvulsant. Studies to evaluate these strategies have generally failed to demonstrate benefits from any of them, including treatment with antihypertensive drugs.

The definitive intervention for *severe* preeclampsia is delivery. However, making the choice to induce labor presents a dilemma. Since preeclampsia can deteriorate rapidly, with grave consequences for the patient and fetus, immediate delivery is recommended. However, if the fetus is not sufficiently mature, immediate delivery could threaten its life. Do we deliver the fetus immediately, which would eliminate risk for the patient but present a serious risk for the fetus—or do we postpone delivery, which would reduce risk for the fetus but greatly increase risk for the patient? If the patient elects to postpone delivery, then BP can be lowered with drugs. Because severe preeclampsia can be life threatening, treatment must be done in a tertiary care center to permit close monitoring. The major objective is to prevent maternal cerebral complications (e.g., hemorrhage, encephalopathy). The drug of choice for lowering

BP is *labetalol* (20 mg by IV bolus over 2 minutes); dosing may be repeated at 10-minute intervals up to a total of 300 mg.

Because severe preeclampsia can evolve into eclampsia, an antiseizure drug may be given for prophylaxis. *Magnesium sulfate* is the drug of choice. In one study, prophylaxis with magnesium sulfate reduced the risk of eclampsia by 58% and the risk of death by 45%. Dosing is the same as for treating eclampsia.

If eclampsia develops, magnesium sulfate is the preferred drug for seizure control. Initial dosing consists of a 4- to 6-gm IV loading dose followed by 5 gm IM injected into each buttock. Maintenance consists of continuous IV infusion of 1 to 2 gm/hr or 5 gm IM injected into alternating buttocks every 4 hours. To ensure therapeutic effects and prevent toxicity, blood levels of magnesium, as well as presence of patellar reflex, should be monitored. The target range for serum magnesium is 4 to 7 mEq/L (the normal range for magnesium is 1.5 to 2 mEq/L).

Can drugs help prevent preeclampsia in those at risk? Yes. When started before 16 weeks of gestation, low-dose *aspirin* reduces risk by about 50%. Similarly, *L-arginine* (combined with antioxidant vitamins) can also help. By contrast, several other preparations—magnesium, zinc, vitamin C, vitamin E, fish oil, and diuretics—appear to offer no protection at all.

KEY POINTS

- Hypertension is defined as SBP greater than 130 mm Hg or DBP greater than 80 mm Hg.
- Primary hypertension (essential hypertension), defined as hypertension with no identifiable cause, is the most common form of hypertension.
- Untreated hypertension can lead to heart disease, kidney disease, and stroke.
- In patients older than 50, elevated *systolic* BP represents a greater cardiovascular risk than elevated *diastolic* BP.
- The goal of antihypertensive therapy is to decrease morbidity and mortality without decreasing quality of life. For most patients, this goal is achieved by maintaining BP between 120/80 and 130/80 mm Hg.
- To reduce BP, two types of treatment may be used: drug therapy and lifestyle modification (smoking cessation, reduction of salt and alcohol intake, following the DASH diet, and increasing aerobic exercise).
- The baroreceptor reflex, the kidneys, and the RAAS can oppose our attempts to lower BP with drugs. We can counteract the baroreceptor reflex with a beta blocker, the kidneys with a diuretic, and the RAAS with an ACE inhibitor, ARB, DRI, or aldosterone antagonist.
- Thiazide diuretics (e.g., hydrochlorothiazide, chlorthalidone) and loop diuretics (e.g., furosemide) reduce BP in two ways: they reduce blood volume (by promoting diuresis) and they reduce arterial resistance (by an unknown mechanism).
- Loop diuretics should be reserved for (1) patients who need greater diuresis than can be achieved with thiazides and (2) patients with a low GFR (because thiazides don't work when GFR is low).
- Beta blockers (e.g., metoprolol) appear to lower BP primarily by reducing peripheral vascular resistance; the mechanism is unknown. They may also lower BP by decreasing myocardial contractility and suppressing reflex tachycardia (through $beta_1$ blockade in the heart), and by decreasing renin release (through $beta_1$ blockade in the kidney).
- Calcium channel blockers (e.g., diltiazem, nifedipine) reduce BP by promoting dilation of arterioles.
- ACE inhibitors, ARBs, and DRIs lower BP by preventing angiotensin II–mediated vasoconstriction and aldosterone-mediated volume expansion. ACE inhibitors work by blocking the formation of angiotensin II, whereas ARBs block the actions of angiotensin II. DRIs prevent formation of angiotensin I and thereby shut down the entire RAAS.
- Aldosterone antagonists lower BP by preventing aldosterone-mediated retention of sodium and water in the kidney.
- Thiazide diuretics are preferred drugs for initial therapy of uncomplicated hypertension.
- When a combination of drugs is used for hypertension, each drug should have a different mechanism of action.
- Dosages of antihypertensive drugs should be low initially and increased gradually. This approach minimizes adverse effects and permits baroreceptors to reset to a lower pressure.
- Lack of patient adherence is the major cause of treatment failure in antihypertensive therapy.
- Adherence is difficult to achieve because (1) hypertension has no symptoms (so drug benefits aren't obvious); (2) hypertension progresses slowly (so patients think they can postpone treatment); and (3) treatment is complex and expensive, continues lifelong, and can cause adverse effects.
- A severe hypertensive emergency exists when *diastolic* BP exceeds 120 mm Hg and there is ongoing end-organ damage.
- Nitroprusside (IV) is a drug of choice for hypertensive emergencies.
- Hypertension is the most common complication of pregnancy.
- Methyldopa and labetalol are drugs of choice for treating chronic hypertension of pregnancy.

Please visit **http://evolve.elsevier.com/Lehne** for chapter-specific NCLEX® examination review questions.

Summary of Major Nursing Implications[a]

ANTIHYPERTENSIVE DRUGS

Preadministration Assessment

Therapeutic Goal

The goal of antihypertensive therapy is to prevent the long-term sequelae of hypertension (heart disease, kidney disease, stroke) while minimizing drug effects that can reduce quality of life. For most patients, BP should be reduced to less than 130/80 mm Hg.

Baseline Data

The following tests should be done in all patients: BP; electrocardiogram; complete urinalysis; hemoglobin and hematocrit; and blood levels of sodium, potassium, calcium, creatinine, glucose, uric acid, triglycerides, and cholesterol (total, LDL, and HDL cholesterol).

Identifying High-Risk Patients

When taking the patient's drug history, attempt to identify drugs that can raise BP or that can interfere with the effects of antihypertensive drugs. Some drugs of concern are listed later under *Minimizing Adverse Interactions.*

The patient history should identify comorbid conditions that either contraindicate the use of specific agents (e.g., AV block contraindicates use of beta blockers) or require that drugs be used with special caution (e.g., thiazide diuretics must be used with caution in patients with gout or diabetes). For risk factors that pertain to specific antihypertensive drugs, see the chapters in which those drugs are discussed.

Implementation: Administration

Routes

All drugs for chronic hypertension are administered orally.

Dosage

To minimize adverse effects, dosages should be low initially and increased gradually. It is counterproductive to employ high initial dosages that produce a rapid fall in pressure while also producing intense adverse effects that can discourage adherence. After 12 months of successful treatment, dosage reductions should be tried.

Implementation: Measures to Enhance Therapeutic Effects

Lifestyle Modifications

In hypertensive patients, lifestyle changes can reduce BP and increase responsiveness to antihypertensive drugs. These changes should be tried for 6 to 12 months before implementing drug therapy and should continue even if drugs are required.

Weight Reduction. **Help patients develop an exercise and weight management program if needed.**

Sodium Restriction. **Encourage patients to consume no more than 2300 mg of salt daily and provide them with information on the salt content of foods.**

DASH Diet. **Encourage patients to adopt a diet rich in fruits, vegetables, and low-fat dairy products, and low in total fat, unsaturated fat, and cholesterol.**

Alcohol Restriction. **Encourage patients to limit alcohol consumption to 1 ounce/day (for most men) and 0.5 ounce/day (for women and lighter weight men).** One ounce of ethanol is equivalent to about two mixed drinks, two glasses of wine, or two cans of beer.

Exercise. **Encourage patients with a sedentary lifestyle to perform 30 to 45 minutes of aerobic exercise (e.g., walking, swimming, bicycling) most days of the week.**

Smoking Cessation. **Strongly encourage patients to quit smoking. Teach patients about aids for smoking cessation (e.g., nicotine patch, bupropion, varenicline).**

Promoting Adherence

Nonadherence is the major cause of treatment failure. Achieving adherence is difficult for several reasons: hypertension is devoid of overt symptoms; drugs don't make people feel better (but can make them feel worse); regimens can be complex and expensive; complications of hypertension take years to develop, thereby providing a misguided rationale for postponing treatment; and treatment usually lasts lifelong.

Provide Patient Education. **Educate patients about the long-term consequences of hypertension and the ability of lifestyle changes and drug therapy to decrease morbidity and prolong life. Inform patients that drugs do not cure hypertension; therefore, the medication prescribed must usually be taken lifelong.**

Encourage Self-Monitoring. **Make certain that patients know the treatment goal (usually reduction of BP to less than 130/80 mm Hg), and teach them to monitor and chart their own BP.** This will increase their involvement and help them see the benefits of treatment.

Minimize Adverse Effects. Adverse drug effects are an obvious deterrent to adherence. Measures to reduce undesired effects are discussed under *Minimizing Adverse Effects.*

Establish a Collaborative Relationship. **Encourage patients to be active partners in setting treatment goals, creating a treatment program, and evaluating progress.**

Simplify the Regimen. An antihypertensive regimen can consist of several drugs taken multiple times a day. Once an effective regimen has been established, attempt to switch to once-a-day or twice-a-day dosing. If an appropriate combination product is available (e.g., a fixed-dose combination of a thiazide diuretic plus an ACE inhibitor), substitute the combination product for its components.

Other Measures. Additional measures to promote adherence include providing positive reinforcement when treatment goals are achieved, involving family members in the treatment program, scheduling office visits at convenient times, following up on patients who miss an appointment, and devising a program that is effective but keeps costs low.

Continued

Summary of Major Nursing Implications[a]—cont'd

Ongoing Evaluation and Interventions

Evaluating Treatment

Monitor BP periodically. The usual goal is to reduce it to less than 130/80 mm Hg. **Teach patients to self-monitor their BP and to maintain a BP record.**

Minimizing Adverse Effects

General Considerations. The fundamental strategy for decreasing adverse effects is to tailor the regimen to the sensitivities of the patient. If a drug causes objectionable effects, a more acceptable drug should be substituted.

Inform patients about the potential side effects of treatment, and encourage them to report objectionable responses.

Avoid drugs that can exacerbate comorbid conditions. For example, don't give beta blockers to patients who have bradycardia, AV block, or asthma. Table 47.5 lists drugs to avoid in patients with specific disorders.

Initiate therapy with low doses and increase them gradually.

Adverse Effects of Specific Drugs. For measures to minimize adverse effects of specific antihypertensive drugs (e.g., beta blockers, diuretics, ACE inhibitors), see the chapters in which those drugs are discussed.

Minimizing Adverse Interactions

When taking the patient history, identify drugs that can raise BP or interfere with the effects of antihypertensive drugs. Drugs of concern include oral contraceptives, nonsteroidal anti-inflammatory drugs, glucocorticoids, appetite suppressants, tricyclic antidepressants, monoamine oxidase inhibitors, cyclosporine, erythropoietin, alcohol (in large quantities), and nasal decongestants and other cold remedies.

Antihypertensive regimens frequently contain two or more drugs, posing a potential risk of adverse interactions (e.g., ACE inhibitors can increase the risk of hyperkalemia caused by potassium-sparing diuretics). For interactions that pertain to specific antihypertensive drugs, see the chapters in which those drugs are discussed.

[a]Patient education information is highlighted as **blue text.**

CHAPTER

48 Drugs for Heart Failure

Heart failure is a disease with two major forms: (1) heart failure with left ventricular (LV) systolic dysfunction, also known as heart failure with reduced LV ejection fraction (HFrEF) and (2) diastolic heart failure, also known as heart failure with preserved LV ejection fraction (HFpEF). In this chapter, discussion is limited to the first form. Accordingly, for the rest of this chapter, the term *heart failure* (HF) will be used to denote the first form only.

Heart failure is a progressive, often fatal disorder characterized by ventricular dysfunction, reduced cardiac output, insufficient tissue perfusion, and signs of fluid retention (e.g., peripheral edema, shortness of breath). The disease affects nearly 6 million Americans and is responsible for about 285,000 deaths every year. Of those who have HF, 20% are likely to die within 1 year, and 50% within 5 years. Heart failure is primarily a disease of older adults, affecting 4% to 8% of those at age 65 years and more than 9% to 12% of those older than 80 years. Direct and indirect healthcare costs of HF are estimated at more than $30 billion yearly. With improved evaluation and care, many hospitalizations could be prevented, quality of life could be improved, and life expectancy could be extended.

In the past, HF was commonly referred to as *congestive heart failure.* This term was used because HF frequently causes fluid accumulation (congestion) in the lungs and peripheral tissues. However, because many patients do not have signs of pulmonary or systemic congestion, the term *heart failure* is now preferred.

Drugs recommended for treatment include diuretics, inhibitors of the renin-angiotensin-aldosterone system (RAAS), beta blockers, and digoxin. In this chapter, only digoxin is discussed at length. The other drugs are presented at length in previous chapters, so discussion here is limited to their use in heart failure.

To understand HF and its treatment, you need a basic understanding of hemodynamics. In particular, you need to understand the role of venous pressure, afterload, and Starling's mechanism in determining cardiac output. You also need to understand the roles of the baroreceptor reflex, the RAAS, and the kidneys in regulating arterial pressure. You can refresh your memory of these concepts by reading Chapter 43.

PATHOPHYSIOLOGY OF HEART FAILURE

Heart failure is a syndrome in which the heart is unable to pump sufficient blood to meet the metabolic needs of tissues. The syndrome is characterized by signs of *inadequate tissue perfusion* (fatigue, shortness of breath, exercise intolerance) and/or signs of *volume overload* (venous distention, peripheral and pulmonary edema). The major underlying causes of HF are chronic hypertension and myocardial infarction. Other causes include valvular heart disease, coronary artery disease, congenital heart disease, dysrhythmias, and aging of the myocardium. In its earliest stage, HF is asymptomatic. As failure progresses, fatigue and shortness of breath develop. As cardiac performance declines further, blood backs up behind the failing ventricles, causing venous distention, peripheral edema, and pulmonary edema. Heart failure is a chronic disorder that requires continuous treatment with drugs.

Cardiac Remodeling

In the initial phase of failure, the heart undergoes remodeling, a process in which the ventricles dilate (grow larger), hypertrophy (increase in wall thickness), and become more spherical (less cylindrical). These alterations in cardiac geometry increase wall stress and reduce LV ejection fraction. Remodeling occurs in response to cardiac injury brought on by infarction and other causes. The remodeling process is driven primarily by neurohormonal systems, including the sympathetic nervous system (SNS) and the RAAS. In addition to promoting remodeling, neurohormonal factors promote cardiac fibrosis and myocyte death. The net result of these pathologic changes—remodeling, fibrosis, and cell death—is progressive decline in cardiac output. As a rule, cardiac remodeling precedes development of symptoms and continues after they appear. As a result, cardiac performance continues to decline.

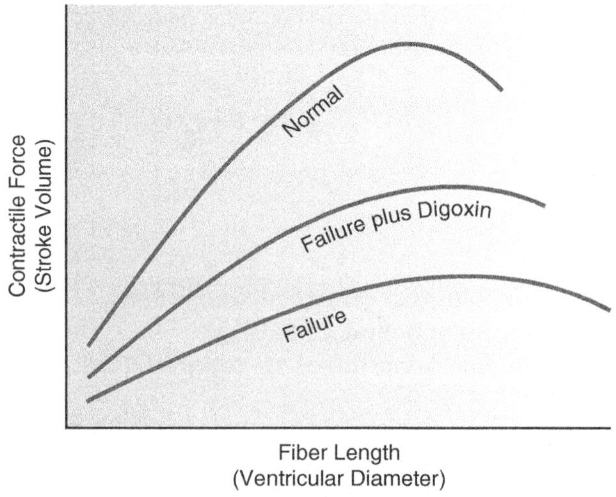

Fig. 48.1 ■ Relationship of ventricular diameter to contractile force.
In the normal heart and the failing heart, increased fiber length produces increased contractile force. However, for any given fiber length, contractile force in the failing heart is much less than in the healthy heart. By increasing cardiac contractility, digoxin shifts the relationship between fiber length and stroke volume in the failing heart toward that in the normal heart.

Physiologic Adaptations to Reduced Cardiac Output

In response to reductions in cardiac pumping ability, the body undergoes several adaptive changes. Some of these help improve tissue perfusion; others compound existing problems.

Cardiac Dilation

Dilation of the heart is characteristic of HF. Cardiac dilation results from a combination of increased venous pressure (see the following text) and reduced contractile force. Reduced contractility lowers the amount of blood ejected during systole, causing end-systolic volume to rise. The increase in venous pressure increases diastolic filling, which causes the heart to expand even further.

Because of Starling's mechanism, the increase in heart size that occurs in HF helps improve cardiac output. That is, as the heart fails and its volume expands, contractile force increases, causing a corresponding increase in stroke volume. However, please note that the maximal contractile force that can be developed by the failing heart is considerably lower than the maximal force of the healthy heart. This limitation is reflected in the curve for the failing heart shown in Fig. 48.1.

If cardiac dilation is insufficient to maintain cardiac output, other factors come into play. As discussed further in the text, these are not always beneficial.

Increased Sympathetic Tone

Heart failure causes arterial pressure to fall. In response, the baroreceptor reflex increases sympathetic output to the heart, veins, and arterioles. At the same time, parasympathetic effects on the heart are reduced. The consequences of increased sympathetic tone are summarized as follows:

- *Increased heart rate.* Acceleration of heart rate increases cardiac output, thereby helping improve tissue perfusion. However, if heart rate increases too much, there will be insufficient time for complete ventricular filling, and cardiac output will fall.
- *Increased contractility.* Increased myocardial contractility has the obvious benefit of increasing cardiac output. The only detriment is an increase in cardiac oxygen demand.
- *Increased venous tone.* Elevation of venous tone increases venous pressure and thereby increases ventricular filling. Because of Starling's mechanism, increased filling increases stroke volume. Unfortunately, if venous pressure is excessive, blood will back up behind the failing ventricles, thereby aggravating pulmonary and peripheral edema. Furthermore, excessive filling pressure can dilate the heart so much that stroke volume will begin to decline.
- *Increased arteriolar tone.* Elevation of arteriolar tone increases arterial pressure, thereby increasing perfusion of vital organs. Unfortunately, increased arterial pressure also means the heart must pump against greater resistance. Since cardiac reserve is minimal in HF, the heart may be unable to meet this challenge, and output may fall.

Water Retention and Increased Blood Volume

Mechanisms. Water retention results from two mechanisms. First, reduced cardiac output causes a reduction in renal blood flow, which in turn decreases glomerular filtration rate (GFR). As a result, urine production is decreased and water is retained. Retention of water increases blood volume.

Second, HF activates the RAAS. Activation occurs in response to reduced blood pressure and reduced renal blood flow. Once activated, the RAAS promotes water retention by increasing circulating levels of *aldosterone* and *angiotensin II.* Aldosterone acts directly on the kidneys to promote retention of sodium and water. Angiotensin II causes constriction of renal blood vessels, which decreases renal blood flow and thereby further decreases urine production. In addition, angiotensin II causes constriction of systemic arterioles and veins, and thereby increases venous and arterial pressure.

Consequences. As with other adaptive responses to HF, increased blood volume can be beneficial or harmful. Increased blood volume increases venous pressure and thereby increases venous return. As a result, ventricular filling and stroke volume are increased. The resultant increase in cardiac output can improve tissue perfusion. However, as noted, if venous pressure is too high, edema of the lungs and periphery may result. More importantly, *if the increase in cardiac output is insufficient to maintain adequate kidney function, renal retention of water will progress unabated. The resultant accumulation of fluid will cause severe cardiac, pulmonary, and peripheral edema—and, ultimately, death.*

Natriuretic Peptides

In response to stretching of the atria and dilation of the ventricles, the heart releases two natriuretic peptides: atrial natriuretic peptide (ANP) and B-natriuretic peptide (BNP). As discussed in Chapter 43, these hormones promote dilation of arterioles and veins, and also promote a loss of sodium and water through the kidneys. Hence, they tend to counterbalance vasoconstriction caused by the SNS and angiotensin II, as well as retention of sodium and water caused by the RAAS. However, as HF progresses, the effects of ANP and BNP eventually become overwhelmed by the effects of the SNS and RAAS.

Levels of circulating BNP are an important index of cardiac status in HF patients and so can be a predictor of long-term survival. High levels of BNP indicate poor cardiac health and can predict a lower chance of survival. Conversely, low levels of BNP indicate better cardiac health and can predict a higher chance of survival. This information can be helpful when assessing the hospitalized patient at discharge: The lower the BNP level, the greater the chances of long-term survival.

The Vicious Cycle of "Compensatory" Physiologic Responses

As discussed earlier, reduced cardiac output leads to compensatory responses: (1) cardiac dilation, (2) activation of the SNS, (3) activation of the RAAS, and (4) retention of water and expansion of blood volume. Although these responses represent the body's attempt to compensate for reduced cardiac output, they can actually make matters worse: Excessive heart rate can reduce ventricular filling; excessive arterial pressure can lower cardiac output; and excessive venous pressure can cause pulmonary and peripheral edema. Thus, as depicted in Fig. 48.2, the "compensatory" responses can create a self-sustaining cycle of maladaptation that further impairs cardiac output and tissue perfusion. If cardiac output becomes too low to maintain sufficient production of urine, the resultant accumulation of water will eventually be fatal. The actual cause of death is complete cardiac failure secondary to excessive cardiac dilation and cardiac edema.

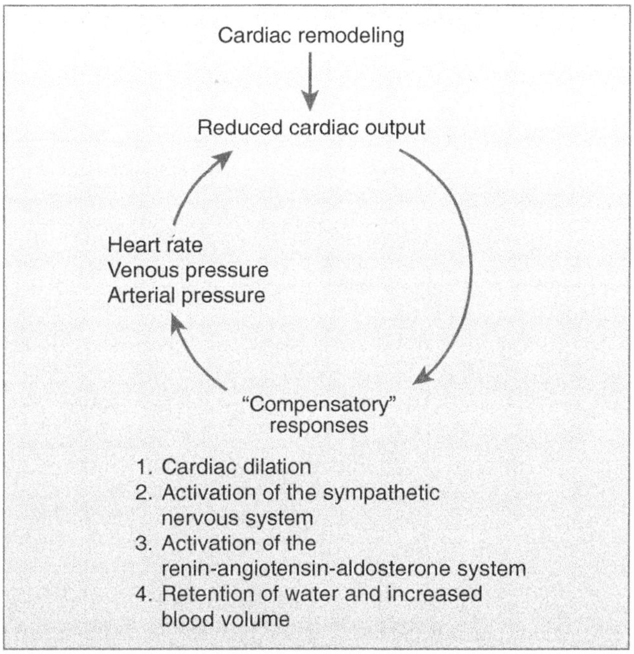

Fig. 48.2 ▪ The vicious cycle of maladaptive compensatory responses to a failing heart.

Signs and Symptoms of Heart Failure

The prominent signs and symptoms of HF are a direct consequence of the pathophysiology just described. Decreased tissue perfusion results in reduced exercise tolerance, fatigue, and shortness of breath; shortness of breath may also reflect pulmonary edema. Increased sympathetic tone produces tachycardia. Increased ventricular filling, reduced systolic ejection, and myocardial hypertrophy result in cardiomegaly (increased heart size). The combination of increased venous tone plus increased blood volume helps cause pulmonary edema, peripheral edema, hepatomegaly (increased liver size), and distention of the jugular veins. Weight gain results from fluid retention.

Classification of Heart Failure Severity

There are two major schemes for classifying HF severity. One scheme, established by the New York Heart Association (NYHA), classifies HF based on the functional limitations it causes. A newer scheme, proposed jointly by the American College of Cardiology (ACC) and the American Heart Association (AHA), is based on the observation that HF is a progressive disease that moves through stages of increasing severity.

The NYHA scheme, which has four classes, can be summarized as follows:

- Class I—No limitation of ordinary physical activity
- Class II—Slight limitation of physical activity: normal activity produces fatigue, dyspnea, palpitations, or angina
- Class III—Marked limitation of physical activity: even mild activity produces symptoms
- Class IV—Symptoms occur at rest

The ACC/AHA scheme, which also has four stages, can be summarized as follows:

- Stage A—At high risk for HF but without structural heart disease or symptoms of HF
- Stage B—Structural heart disease but without symptoms of HF
- Stage C—Structural heart disease with prior or current symptoms of HF
- Stage D—Advanced structural heart disease with marked symptoms of HF at rest, and requiring specialized

ACC/AHA Stage	NYHA Functional Classification
A At high risk for HF but without structural heart disease or symptoms of HF	
B Structural heart disease but without symptoms of HF	I Asymptomatic
C Structural heart disease with prior or current symptoms of HF	II Symptomatic with moderate exertion
	III Symptomatic with minimal exertion
D Advanced structural heart disease with marked symptoms of HF at rest despite maximal medical therapy. Specialized interventions (e.g., heart transplant, mechanical assist device) required	IV Symptomatic at rest

Fig. 48.3 ■ American College of Cardiology/American Heart Association (ACC/AHA) stages and New York Heart Association (NYHA) functional classification of heart failure.

interventions (e.g., heart transplant, mechanical assist device)

Please note that the ACC/AHA scheme is intended to complement the NYHA scheme, not replace it. The relationship between the two is shown in Fig. 48.3.

OVERVIEW OF DRUGS USED TO TREAT HEART FAILURE

For routine therapy, heart failure is treated with three types of drugs: (1) diuretics, (2) agents that inhibit the RAAS, and (3) beta blockers. Other agents (e.g., digoxin, dopamine, hydralazine) may be used as well.

Diuretics

Diuretics are first-line drugs for all patients with signs of volume overload or with a history of volume overload. By reducing blood volume, these drugs can decrease venous pressure, arterial pressure (afterload), pulmonary edema, peripheral edema, and cardiac dilation. However, excessive diuresis must be avoided: If blood volume drops too low, cardiac output and blood pressure may fall precipitously, thereby further compromising tissue perfusion. For the most part, the benefits of diuretics are limited to symptom reduction. As a rule, these drugs do not prolong survival. The basic pharmacology of the diuretics is discussed in Chapter 41.

Thiazide Diuretics

The thiazide diuretics (e.g., hydrochlorothiazide) produce moderate diuresis. These oral agents are used for long-term therapy of HF when edema is not too great. Since thiazides are ineffective when GFR is low, these drugs cannot be used if cardiac output is greatly reduced. The principal adverse effect of the thiazides is *hypokalemia,* which increases the risk of *digoxin-induced dysrhythmias* (see later in this chapter).

Loop Diuretics

The loop diuretics (e.g., furosemide) produce profound diuresis. In contrast to the thiazides, these drugs can promote fluid loss even when GFR is low. Therefore, loop diuretics are preferred to thiazides when cardiac output is greatly reduced. Administration may be oral or IV. Because they can mobilize large volumes of water and because they work when GFR is low, loop diuretics are drugs of choice for patients with severe HF. Like the thiazides, these drugs can cause *hypokalemia,* thereby increasing the risk of *digoxin toxicity.* In addition, loop diuretics can cause severe *hypotension* secondary to excessive volume reduction.

Potassium-Sparing Diuretics

In contrast to the thiazides and loop diuretics, the potassium-sparing diuretics (e.g., spironolactone, triamterene) promote only scant diuresis. In patients with HF, these drugs are employed to counteract potassium loss caused by thiazide and loop diuretics, thereby lowering the risk of digoxin-induced dysrhythmias. Not surprisingly, the principal adverse effect of the potassium-sparing drugs is *hyperkalemia.* Because *angiotensin-converting enzyme (ACE) inhibitors* and *angiotensin II receptor blockers (ARBs)* also carry a risk of hyperkalemia, caution is needed if these drugs are combined with a potassium-sparing diuretic. Accordingly, when therapy with an ACE inhibitor or ARB is initiated, the potassium-sparing diuretic should be discontinued. It can be resumed later if needed.

One potassium-sparing diuretic—spironolactone—prolongs survival in patients with HF primarily by blocking receptors for aldosterone, not by causing diuresis. This drug and a related agent—eplerenone—are discussed later under *Aldosterone Antagonists.*

Drugs That Inhibit the RAAS

The RAAS plays an important role both in cardiac remodeling and in the hemodynamic changes that occur in response to reduced cardiac output. Accordingly, agents that inhibit the

RAAS can be highly beneficial. Five groups of drugs are available: ACE inhibitors, ARBs, angiotensin receptor neprilysin inhibitors (ARNIs), direct renin inhibitors (DRIs), and aldosterone antagonists. Of the five, the ACE inhibitors have been studied most thoroughly in HF. The basic pharmacology of the RAAS inhibitors is presented in Chapter 44.

Prototype Drugs

DRUGS FOR HEART FAILURE

Diuretics

Hydrochlorothiazide
Furosemide

Inhibitors of the Renin-Angiotensin-Aldosterone System

Captopril (ACE inhibitor)
Losartan (angiotensin II receptor blocker)
Entresto (angiotensin receptor neprilysin inhibitor)
Eplerenone (aldosterone antagonist)

Beta Blockers

Metoprolol

Inotropic Agents

Digoxin (a cardiac glycoside)
Dopamine (a sympathomimetic)

Vasodilators

Isosorbide dinitrate plus hydralazine

ACE Inhibitors

ACE inhibitors (e.g., captopril, enalapril) are a cornerstone of HF therapy. These drugs can improve functional status and prolong life. In one trial, the 2-year mortality rate for patients taking enalapril was 47% lower than the rate for patients taking placebo. Other large, controlled trials have shown similar benefits. Accordingly, in the absence of specific contraindications, all patients with HF should receive one of these drugs. Although ACE inhibitors can be used alone, they are usually combined with a beta blocker and a diuretic.

ACE inhibitors help by blocking the production of angiotensin II, decreasing the release of aldosterone, and suppressing the degradation of kinins. As a result, they improve hemodynamics and favorably alter cardiac remodeling.

Hemodynamic Benefits. By suppressing production of angiotensin II, ACE inhibitors cause dilation of arterioles and veins, and they decrease release of aldosterone. Resulting benefits in HF are as follows:

- *Arteriolar dilation* improves regional blood flow in the kidneys and other tissues. By reducing afterload, it increases stroke volume and cardiac output. Increased renal blood flow promotes excretion of sodium and water.
- *Venous dilation* reduces venous pressure and thereby reduces pulmonary congestion, peripheral edema, preload, and cardiac dilation.
- *Suppression of aldosterone release* enhances excretion of sodium and water, while causing retention of potassium.

Interestingly, suppression of angiotension II production diminishes over time, suggesting that long-term benefits are the result of some other action.

Impact on Cardiac Remodeling. With continued use, ACE inhibitors have a favorable impact on cardiac remodeling. Elevation of kinins is largely responsible. This statement is based in part on the observation that, in experimental models, giving a kinin receptor blocker decreases beneficial effects on remodeling. Also, we know that suppression of angiotensin II production diminishes over time, and so reduced angiotensin II cannot fully explain long-term benefits.

Adverse Effects. The principal adverse effects of the ACE inhibitors are *hypotension* (secondary to arteriolar dilation), *hyperkalemia* (secondary to decreased aldosterone release), *intractable cough,* and *angioedema.* In addition, these drugs can cause *renal failure in patients with bilateral renal artery stenosis.* If taken during pregnancy—especially the second and third trimesters—ACE inhibitors can cause *fetal injury.* Accordingly, if pregnancy occurs, these drugs should be discontinued. Because of their ability to elevate potassium levels, ACE inhibitors should be used with caution in patients taking potassium supplements or a potassium-sparing diuretic (e.g., spironolactone, triamterene).

Dosage. Adequate dosage is still debated in the literature: Higher dosages may be associated with increased survival, but conflicting evidence remains. Results of the Assessment of Treatment with Lisinopril and Survival (ATLAS) trial indicate that the doses needed to increase survival are higher than those needed to produce hemodynamic changes. In contrast to the ATLAS trial, the NETWORK trial and the High Dose Enalapril Study Group did not find a difference in mortality between patients on low-dose or high-dose ACE inhibitors. Treatment with ACE inhibitors should be initiated at low doses and slowly titrated upward if the patient tolerates treatment. Target dosages associated with disease modification are shown in Table 48.1. These dosages should be used unless side effects make them intolerable.

Angiotensin II Receptor Blockers

In patients with HF, the effects of ARBs are similar—but not identical—to those of ACE inhibitors. Hemodynamic effects of both groups are much the same. Clinical trials have shown that ARBs improve LV ejection fraction, reduce HF symptoms, increase exercise tolerance, decrease hospitalization, enhance quality of life, and, most importantly, reduce mortality. However, because ARBs do not increase levels of kinins, their effects on cardiac remodeling are less favorable than those of ACE inhibitors. For this reason, and because clinical experience with ACE inhibitors is much greater than with ARBs, ACE inhibitors are generally preferred. For now, ARBs should be reserved for HF patients who cannot tolerate ACE inhibitors, usually owing to intractable cough. (Because ARBs do not increase bradykinin levels, they do not cause cough.)

Angiotensin Receptor Neprilysin Inhibitor

Sacubitril/Valsartan [Entresto]. Sacubitril/valsartan [Entresto] is a newly approved drug that functions in two different manners. Sacubitril is a new class of drug, called an ARNI (angiotensin receptor neprilysin inhibitor). In simple terms, Entresto increases natriuretic peptides while suppressing the negative effects of the RAAS. As discussed earlier in the chapter, ANP and BNP are important indices of cardiac status in HF

TABLE 48.1 ▪ Inhibitors of the Renin-Angiotensin-Aldosterone System Used in Heart Failure

Drug	Initial Daily Dose	Maximum Daily Dose
ACE INHIBITORS		
Captopril [Capoten]	6.25 mg 3 times	150 mg 3 times
Enalapril [Vasotec]	2.5 mg twice	10–20 mg twice
Fosinopril [generic only]	10 mg once	80 mg once
Lisinopril [Zestril, Prinivil]	2.5–5 mg once	20–40 mg once
Quinapril [Accupril]	5 mg once	20 mg twice
Ramipril [Altace]	2.5 mg twice	5 mg twice
Trandolapril [Mavik]	1 mg once	4 mg once
ANGIOTENSIN II RECEPTOR BLOCKERS		
Candesartan [Atacand]	4 mg once	32 mg once
Losartan [Cozaar]	25–50 mg once	50–100 mg once
Valsartan [Diovan]	40 mg twice	160 mg twice
ANGIOTENSIN RECEPTOR NEPRILYSIN INHIBITOR		
Sacubitril/Valsartan [Entresto]	24/26 mg twice	97/103 mg twice
ALDOSTERONE ANTAGONISTS		
Eplerenone [Inspra]	25 mg once	50 mg once
Spironolactone [Aldactone]	25 mg once	25 mg once or twice

patients. Entresto is approved for patients with Class II–IV HF to be used in place of an ACE inhibitor or ARB.

In the PARADIGM-HF study, Entresto was superior to enalapril alone when looking at the overall endpoints of reduction in hospitalizations, risk of all-cause mortality, and risk of death from cardiovascular causes. In fact, the study was terminated early secondary to the overwhelmingly positive results.

As Entresto contains an ARB, the contraindications and side effects are similar. Entresto can cause angioedema, hyperkalemia, and hypotension. Administration should be avoided in pregnancy, as its use can cause fetal harm.

Aldosterone Antagonists

In patients with HF, aldosterone antagonists—*spironolactone* [Aldactone] and *eplerenone* [Inspra]—can reduce symptoms, decrease hospitalizations, and prolong life. These benefits were first demonstrated with spironolactone in the Randomized Aldactone Evaluation Study (RALES). Similar results were later obtained with eplerenone. Current guidelines recommend adding an aldosterone antagonist to standard HF therapy, but only in patients with persistent symptoms despite adequate treatment with an ACE inhibitor and a beta blocker.

Aldosterone antagonists work primarily by blocking aldosterone receptors in the heart and blood vessels. To understand these effects, we need to review the role of aldosterone in HF. In the past, researchers believed that aldosterone's only action was to promote renal retention of sodium (and water) in exchange for excretion of potassium. However, we now know that aldosterone has additional—and more harmful—effects. Among these are:

- Promotion of myocardial remodeling (which impairs pumping)
- Promotion of myocardial fibrosis (which increases the risk of dysrhythmias)
- Activation of the SNS and suppression of norepinephrine uptake in the heart (both of which can promote dysrhythmias and ischemia)
- Promotion of vascular fibrosis (which decreases arterial compliance)
- Promotion of baroreceptor dysfunction

During HF, activation of the RAAS causes levels of aldosterone to rise. In some patients, levels reach 20 times normal. As aldosterone levels grow higher, harmful effects increase, and prognosis becomes progressively worse.

Drugs can reduce the impact of aldosterone by either decreasing aldosterone production or blocking aldosterone receptors. ACE inhibitors, ARBs, and DRIs decrease aldosterone production; spironolactone and eplerenone block aldosterone receptors. Although ACE inhibitors and ARBs can reduce aldosterone production, they do not block it entirely. Furthermore, production is suppressed for only a relatively short time. Hence, when ACE inhibitors or ARBs are used alone, detrimental effects of aldosterone can persist. However, when an aldosterone antagonist is added to the regimen, any residual effects are eliminated. As a result, symptoms of HF are improved and life is prolonged.

Aldosterone antagonists have one major adverse effect: *hyperkalemia.* The underlying cause is renal retention of potassium. Risk is increased by renal impairment and by using an ACE inhibitor or ARB. To minimize risk, potassium levels and renal function should be measured at baseline and periodically thereafter. Potassium supplements should be discontinued.

Spironolactone—but not eplerenone—poses a significant risk of *gynecomastia* (breast enlargement) in men, a condition that can be both cosmetically troublesome and painful. In the RALES trial, 10% of males experienced painful breast enlargement.

Direct Renin Inhibitors

As discussed in Chapter 44, DRIs can shut down the entire RAAS. In theory, their benefits in HF should equal those of the ACE inhibitors and ARBs. At this time, only one DRI—*aliskiren* [Tekturna]—is available. In recent trials, aliskiren did not improve outcomes in hospitalized patients with heart failure. Because of these findings, aliskiren is approved for hypertension, but is not approved for HF.

Beta Blockers

The role of beta blockers in HF continues to evolve. Previously, HF was considered an absolute contraindication to these drugs. After all, blockade of cardiac $beta_1$-adrenergic receptors *reduces* contractility—an effect that is clearly detrimental, given that contractility is already compromised in the failing heart. However, it is now clear that with careful control of dosage, beta blockers can improve patient status. Controlled trials have shown that three beta blockers—*carvedilol* [Coreg], *bisoprolol* [Zebeta], and *sustained-release metoprolol* [Toprol XL]—when added to conventional therapy, can improve LV ejection fraction, increase exercise tolerance, slow progression of HF, reduce the need for hospitalization, and, most importantly, prolong survival. Accordingly, beta blockers are now recommended as first-line therapy for most patients. These drugs can even be used in patients with severe disease (NYHA Class IV), provided the patient is euvolemic and hemodynamically stable. Although the mechanism underlying benefits is uncertain, likely possibilities include protecting the heart from excessive sympathetic stimulation and protecting against dysrhythmias. Because excessive beta blockade can reduce contractility, doses must be very low initially and then gradually increased. Full benefits may not be seen for 1 to 3 months. Among patients with HF, the principal adverse effects are (1) fluid retention and worsening of HF, (2) fatigue, (3) hypotension, and (4) bradycardia or heart block. The basic pharmacology of the beta blockers is discussed in Chapter 18.

Ivabradine (Corlanor)

In 2015, the FDA approved ivabradine [*Corlanor*] for use in patients with stable, symptomatic heart failure and LVEF <35% in sinus rhythm with heart rates >70 BPM on maximally tolerated doses of beta blockers. It may also be used in patients who have a contraindication to beta blocker use.

Ivabradine causes a dose-dependent reduction in heart rate by blocking channels responsible for cardiac pacemaker current. Although the drug slows heart rate, it does not possess negative inotropic effects or cause QTc prolongation. When used in recommended doses, heart rate reduction is approximately 10 beats/min.

The SHIFT (Systolic Heart failure treatment with the I_f inhibitor ivabradine Trial) study was a randomized, double-blind trial comparing ivabradine to placebo in 6558 adults. End results revealed that the use of ivabradine reduced the risk of hospitalization for worsening heart failure or cardiovascular death. Given these findings, ivabradine may be a useful alternative for patients with heart failure who need additional beta blockade above what is currently available.

Inotropic Agents

Digoxin

Digoxin belongs to a class of drugs known as *cardiac glycosides,* agents best known for their *positive inotropic actions,* that is, their ability to increase myocardial contractile force. By increasing contractile force, digoxin can increase cardiac output. In addition, it can alter the electrical activity of the heart, and it can favorably affect neurohormonal systems. Unfortunately, although digoxin can reduce symptoms of HF, it does not prolong life. Used widely in the past, *digoxin is considered a second-line agent today.* The pharmacology of digoxin is discussed later.

Inotropic Agents (Other Than Digoxin)

In addition to digoxin, we have two other types of inotropic drugs: sympathomimetics and phosphodiesterase (PDE) inhibitors. Unlike digoxin, which can be taken orally, these other inotropics must be given by IV infusion. Accordingly, their use is restricted to acute care of hospitalized patients. Because digoxin can be given PO, it is the only inotropic agent suited for long-term therapy.

Sympathomimetic Drugs: Dopamine and Dobutamine. The basic pharmacology of dopamine and dobutamine is presented in Chapter 17. Discussion here is limited to their use in HF. Both drugs are administered by IV infusion.

Dopamine. Dopamine is a catecholamine that can activate (1) $beta_1$-adrenergic receptors in the heart, (2) dopamine receptors in the kidney, and (3) at high doses, $alpha_1$-adrenergic receptors in blood vessels. Activation of $beta_1$ receptors increases myocardial contractility, thereby improving cardiac performance. $Beta_1$ activation also increases heart rate, creating a risk of tachycardia. Activation of dopamine receptors dilates renal blood vessels, thereby increasing renal blood flow and urine output. Activation of $alpha_1$ receptors increases vascular resistance (afterload) and can thereby reduce cardiac output. Dopamine is administered by continuous infusion. Constant monitoring of blood pressure, the electrocardiogram (ECG), and urine output is required. Dopamine is employed as a short-term rescue measure for patients with severe acute cardiac failure.

Dobutamine. Dobutamine is a synthetic catecholamine that causes selective activation of $beta_1$-adrenergic receptors. By doing so, the drug can increase myocardial contractility and can thereby improve cardiac performance. Like dopamine, dobutamine can cause tachycardia and induce myocardial ischemia. In contrast to dopamine, dobutamine does not activate $alpha_1$ receptors and therefore does not increase vascular resistance. As a result, the drug is generally preferred to dopamine for short-term treatment of acute HF. Administration is by continuous infusion.

Phosphodiesterase Inhibitors

Milrinone. Milrinone has been called an inodilator because it increases myocardial contractility *and* promotes vasodilation. Increased contractility results from accumulation of cyclic AMP (cAMP) secondary to inhibition of phosphodiesterase type 3 (PDE3), an enzyme that degrades cAMP. Milrinone is administered by IV infusion and is indicated only for short-term therapy of severe HF. The initial dose is 25 to 75 mcg/kg over 10 to 20 minutes. The maintenance infusion is 0.375 to 0.75 mcg/kg/min. Use should be reserved for patients with severe reduction in cardiac output resulting in decreased organ perfusion, as inotropes can induce dysrhythmias and cause myocardial ischemia from increased metabolic demand.

Vasodilators (Other Than ACE Inhibitors and ARBs)

Isosorbide Dinitrate Plus Hydralazine

For treatment of HF, isosorbide dinitrate (ISDN) and hydralazine are usually combined. The combination represents an alternative to ACE inhibitors or ARBs. However, ACE inhibitors and ARBs are generally preferred.

Isosorbide dinitrate [Isordil Titradose] belongs to the same family as nitroglycerin. Like nitroglycerin, ISDN causes selective dilation of *veins.* In patients with severe refractory HF, the drug can reduce congestive symptoms and improve exercise capacity. In addition to its hemodynamic actions, ISDN may inhibit abnormal myocyte growth and thus may delay cardiac remodeling. Principal adverse effects are *orthostatic hypotension* and *reflex tachycardia.* The basic pharmacology of ISDN and other organic nitrates is discussed in Chapter 51.

Hydralazine causes selective dilation of *arterioles.* By doing so, the drug can improve cardiac output and renal blood flow. For treatment of HF, hydralazine is always used in combination with ISDN, since hydralazine by itself is not very effective. Principal adverse effects are *hypotension, tachycardia,* and a syndrome that resembles *systemic lupus erythematosus.* The basic pharmacology of hydralazine is discussed in Chapter 46.

BiDil, a fixed-dose combination of hydralazine and isosorbide dinitrate, is indicated for treating HF—but only in African Americans, making *BiDil* the first medication approved for a specific ethnic group. Can *BiDil* help people in other ethnic groups? Probably, but data are lacking: The manufacturer tested the product only in African Americans. As discussed in Chapter 8, testing was limited primarily because of regulatory and market incentives, not because there were data suggesting it wouldn't work for others. Of course, now that *BiDil* is approved, clinicians may prescribe it for anyone they see fit. Each *BiDil* tablet contains 37.5 mg hydralazine and 20 mg isosorbide dinitrate. The recommended dosage is 1 or 2 tablets 3 times a day.

Intravenous Vasodilators for Acute Care

Nitroglycerin. Intravenous nitroglycerin is a powerful *venodilator* that produces a dramatic reduction in venous pressure. Effects have been described as being equivalent to "pharmacologic phlebotomy." In HF, nitroglycerin is used to relieve acute severe pulmonary edema. Principal adverse effects are *hypotension* and resultant *reflex tachycardia.* The basic pharmacology of nitroglycerin is discussed in Chapter 51.

Sodium Nitroprusside. Sodium nitroprusside [Nitropress] acts rapidly to dilate *arterioles* and *veins*. Arteriolar dilation reduces afterload and thereby increases cardiac output. Venodilation reduces venous pressure and thereby decreases pulmonary and peripheral congestion. The drug is indicated for short-term therapy of severe refractory HF. The principal adverse effect is *profound hypotension*. Blood pressure must be monitored continuously. The basic pharmacology of nitroprusside is discussed in Chapter 46.

Nesiritide. Nesiritide [Natrecor] is a synthetic form of human BNP indicated only for short-term IV therapy of hospitalized patients with acutely decompensated HF, characterized by increased pulmonary capillary wedge pressure (PCWP) and dyspnea at rest. Nesiritide is produced by recombinant DNA technology and has the same amino acid sequence as naturally occurring BNP. The drug was approved after a relatively small trial—Vasodilation in the Management of Acute Congestive Heart Failure (VMAC)—and showed a modest decrease in dyspnea and PCWP. However, a much larger trial—Acute Study of Clinical Effectiveness of Nesiritide in Decompensated Heart Failure (ASCEND-HF)—failed to show *any* benefit: The incidence of dyspnea, rehospitalization, and 30-day mortality was the same for patients receiving nesiritide as it was for patients receiving placebo. Worse yet, although nesiritide offered no benefit, it nearly doubled the incidence of hypotension. These results led the authors to conclude that "Nesiritide cannot be recommended for routine use in the broad population of patients with heart failure."

Mechanism of Action. Nesiritide affects hemodynamics by three mechanisms: suppression of the RAAS, suppression of sympathetic outflow from the central nervous system (CNS), and direct dilation of arterioles and veins. In patients with HF, benefits derive primarily from direct vasodilation. To promote vasodilation, nesiritide binds with receptors on vascular smooth muscle (VSM), and thereby stimulates production of cyclic GMP (cGMP), a second messenger that causes VSM to relax. This mechanism is similar to that of nitroglycerin, which also stimulates cGMP production. However, whereas nitroglycerin acts primarily on veins, nesiritide dilates arterioles as well. By dilating arterioles and veins, nesiritide reduces both preload and afterload. The net result is a decrease in PCWP and increased cardiac output. Also, by dilating afferent renal arterioles, nesiritide increases GFR, and thereby increases excretion of sodium and water. The result is a reduction in blood volume, which further reduces cardiac preload.

Pharmacokinetics. With continuous infusion, nesiritide achieves steady-state levels that are 3 to 6 times greater than the level of endogenous BNP present at baseline. Nesiritide is eliminated by three mechanisms: (1) proteolytic cleavage by endopeptidases present on the luminal surface of blood vessels; (2) binding to clearance receptors on the surface of cells, followed by cellular uptake and proteolytic cleavage; and (3) renal filtration. The drug's half-life is short, about 18 minutes.

Adverse Effects. The principal adverse effect is symptomatic *hypotension*. In the ASCEND-HF trial, hypotension developed in 26.6% of patients receiving nesiritide, compared with 15.3% of those receiving placebo. The risk of hypotension is increased by high doses of nesiritide and by concurrent use of ACE inhibitors and other vasodilators. In addition to causing hypotension, nesiritide can cause ventricular tachycardia, headache, back pain, dizziness, and nausea. An analysis of several clinical trials suggested that nesiritide may cause renal damage. However, ASCEND-HF revealed no evidence of renal harm.

Preparations, Dosage, and Administration. Nesiritide [Natrecor] is available in 1.5-mg, single-use vials. The powder must be dissolved and then diluted to a final concentration of 6 mcg/mL. Dosing consists of an initial IV bolus (2 mcg/kg) followed by continuous infusion (0.01 mcg/kg/min), typically lasting 48 hours or less. If symptomatic hypotension develops, the infusion should be slowed or stopped.

DIGOXIN, A CARDIAC GLYCOSIDE

Digoxin [Lanoxin] belongs to a family of drugs known as *cardiac glycosides*. These drugs are prepared by extraction from *Digitalis purpurea* (purple foxglove) and *Digitalis lanata* (Grecian foxglove), and so are also known as *digitalis glycosides*. In the United States, digoxin is the only cardiac glycoside available.

Digoxin has profound effects on the mechanical and electrical properties of the heart. In addition, it has important neurohormonal effects. In patients with HF, benefits derive from increased myocardial contractility and from effects on neurohormonal systems as well.

Digitalis is a dangerous drug because it can cause severe dysrhythmias at doses close to the therapeutic range. Owing to its prodysrhythmic actions, digoxin must be used with respect, caution, and skill.

Digoxin is indicated for HF and for control of dysrhythmias (see Chapter 49). When used for HF, digoxin can reduce symptoms, increase exercise tolerance, and decrease hospitalizations. However, the drug does *not* prolong life. Furthermore, when used by women, it may actually *shorten* life (Box 48.1). Because benefits are limited to symptomatic relief and because the risk of toxicity is substantial, *digoxin is now considered a second-line drug for treating HF.*

Chemistry

Digoxin consists of three components: a steroid nucleus, a lactone ring, and three molecules of digitoxose (a sugar). It is because of the sugars that digoxin is known as a glycoside. The region of the molecule composed of the steroid nucleus plus the lactone ring (i.e., the region without the sugar molecules) is responsible for the pharmacologic effects of digoxin. The sugars only increase solubility.

Mechanical Effects on the Heart

Digoxin exerts a *positive inotropic action* on the heart. That is, the drug *increases the force of ventricular contraction* and can thereby increase cardiac output.

Mechanism of Inotropic Action

Digoxin increases myocardial contractility by inhibiting an enzyme known as *sodium, potassium-ATPase* (Na^+/K^+-ATPase). By way of an indirect process described in the paragraphs that follow, inhibition of Na^+/K^+-ATPase promotes calcium accumulation within myocytes. The calcium then augments contractile force by facilitating the interaction of myocardial contractile proteins: actin and myosin.

To understand how inhibition of Na^+/K^+-ATPase causes intracellular calcium to rise, we must first understand the normal role of Na^+/K^+-ATPase in myocytes. That role is shown in Fig. 48.4. As indicated, when an action potential passes along the myocyte membrane (sarcolemma), Na^+ ions and Ca^{++} ions enter the cell, and K^+ ions exit. Once the action potential has passed, these ion fluxes must be reversed so that the original ionic balance of the cell can be restored. Na^+/K^+-ATPase is critical to this process. Na^+/K^+-ATPase acts as a "pump" to draw extracellular K^+ ions into the cell, while simultaneously extruding intracellular Na^+. The energy required for pumping Na^+ and K^+ is provided by the breakdown of ATP—hence the name Na^+/K^+-ATPase. To complete the normalization of cellular ionic composition, Ca^{++} ions must leave the cell. Extrusion of Ca^{++} is accomplished through an exchange process in which extracellular Na^+ ions are taken into the cell while Ca^{++} ions exit. This exchange of Na^+ for Ca^{++} is a passive (energy-independent) process.

We can now answer the question, how does inhibition of Na^+/K^+-ATPase increase intracellular Ca^{++}? By inhibiting Na^+/K^+-ATPase, digoxin prevents the myocyte from restoring its proper ionic composition following the passage of an action potential. Inhibition of Na^+/K^+-ATPase blocks uptake of K^+ and extrusion of Na^+. Therefore, with each successive action potential, intracellular K^+ levels decline and intracellular Na^+ levels rise. It is this rise in Na^+ that leads to the rise in intracellular Ca^{++}. In the presence of excess intracellular Na^+, further Na^+ entry is suppressed. Since Na^+ entry is suppressed, the passive exchange of Ca^{++} for Na^+ cannot take place, and so Ca^{++} accumulates within the cell.

Relationship of Potassium to Inotropic Action

Potassium ions compete with digoxin for binding to Na^+/K^+-ATPase. This competition is of great clinical significance. Because potassium competes with digoxin, when potassium levels are low, binding of digoxin to Na^+/K^+-ATPase increases. This increase can produce excessive inhibition of Na^+/K^+-ATPase

si

BOX 48.1 ▪ SPECIAL INTEREST TOPIC

ATTENTION: DIGOXIN MAY BE HAZARDOUS TO WOMEN'S HEALTH

Researchers who conducted a reanalysis of older data discovered that for women with heart failure digoxin may do more harm than good. The Digitalis Investigation Group[a] (DIG) reported the results of a large randomized, placebo-controlled trial designed to assess the impact of digoxin on morbidity and mortality in patients with heart failure. The study enrolled 6801 patients (men and women) with heart failure and followed them for an average of 37 months. They all took an ACE inhibitor and a diuretic; half also received digoxin, and the other half received a placebo. The result? Digoxin improved symptoms and decreased hospitalizations, but did not reduce mortality. The overall death rate was 35%, regardless of whether patients took digoxin or placebo. However, the data were not analyzed for possible gender-related effects. Accordingly, Rathore et al.[b] performed a retrospective analysis of the DIG data to determine whether digoxin had different effects in men and women. Among men, digoxin had no significant impact on mortality, mirroring the overall mortality seen previously. However, among *women*, digoxin produced a small but significant *increase* in mortality: After 37 months, the death rate was 28.9% for women taking placebo compared with 33.1% for those taking digoxin—an increase of 4.2%.

Although the Rathore et al. study suggests that for female patients the benefits of digoxin therapy (primarily a small [4%] decrease in the risk of hospitalization) may not justify the risk of possible drug-induced death, a further study including over 35,000 patients demonstrated no difference in mortality between men and women taking digoxin for the treatment of heart failure.[c]

Why did digoxin possibly increase the mortality rate in women in the Rathore et al. study? We don't know. Possibilities include sex-based differences in autonomic function, muscle metabolism, signal transduction, or myocardial cell growth and function. However, there may be a simpler answer: Among the women who died, digoxin plasma levels may have been excessive. It is well established that digoxin can be lethal at high levels. In the DIG trial, digoxin levels were measured only in randomly selected patients, and so Rathore et al. lacked the data needed to determine whether deaths were related to high drug levels. If high digoxin levels were indeed responsible for the observed mortality increase, then the take-home message is obvious: We must keep digoxin doses low.

As a rule, the drug should be reserved for patients who have not responded adequately to first-line medicines: ACE inhibitors or ARBs, diuretics, and beta blockers. Furthermore, digoxin levels should be kept as low as possible (0.5 to 0.8 ng/mL is a reasonable initial target).

[a]The Digitalis Investigation Group: The effect of digoxin on mortality and morbidity in patients with heart failure. N Engl J Med 336:525–533, 1997.
[b]Rathore SS, Wang Y, Krumholz H: Sex-based differences in the effect of digoxin for the treatment of heart failure. N Engl J Med 347:1403–1411, 2002.
[c]Flory JH, Ky B, Haynes K, et al: Observational cohort study of the safety of digoxin use in women with heart failure. BMJ Open 2:e000888:1–7, 2012.

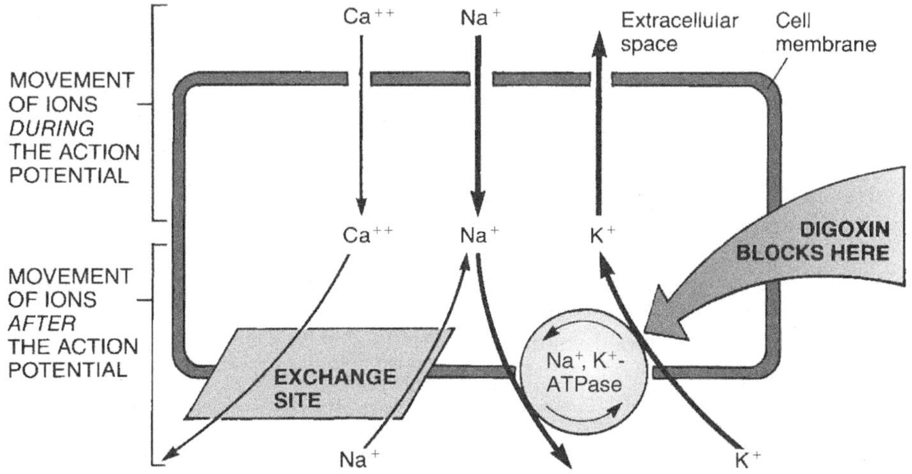

Fig. 48.4 ▪ Ion fluxes across the cardiac cell membrane.
During the action potential, Na^+ and Ca^{++} enter the cardiac cell and K^+ exits. Following the action potential, Na^+/K^+-ATPase pumps Na^+ out of the cell and takes up K^+. Ca^{++} leaves the cell in exchange for the uptake of Na^+. By inhibiting Na^+/K^+-ATPase, digoxin prevents the extrusion of Na^+, causing Na^+ to accumulate inside the cell. The resulting buildup of intracellular Na^+ suppresses the Na^+-Ca^{++} exchange process, thereby causing intracellular levels of Ca^{++} to rise.

with resultant toxicity. Conversely, when levels of potassium are high, inhibition of Na^+/K^+-ATPase by digoxin is reduced, causing a reduction in the therapeutic response. Because an increase in potassium can impair therapeutic responses, whereas a decrease in potassium can cause toxicity, it is imperative that potassium levels be kept within the normal physiologic range: 3.5 to 5 mEq/L.

Hemodynamic Benefits in Heart Failure

Increased Cardiac Output

In patients with HF, increased myocardial contractility increases cardiac output. By increasing contractility, digoxin shifts the relationship of fiber length to stroke volume in the failing heart toward that in the healthy heart. Consequently, at any given heart size, the stroke volume of the failing heart increases, causing cardiac output to rise.

Consequences of Increased Cardiac Output

As a result of increased cardiac output, three major secondary responses occur: (1) sympathetic tone declines, (2) urine production increases, and (3) renin release declines. These responses can reverse virtually all signs and symptoms of HF. However, they do not correct the underlying problem of cardiac remodeling.

Decreased Sympathetic Tone. By increasing contractile force and cardiac output, digoxin increases arterial pressure. In response, sympathetic nerve traffic to the heart and blood vessels is reduced via the baroreceptor reflex. (Recall that a compensatory *increase* in sympathetic tone had taken place because of HF.)

The decrease in sympathetic tone has several beneficial effects. First, heart rate is reduced, thereby allowing more complete ventricular filling. Second, afterload is reduced (because of reduced arteriolar constriction), thereby allowing more complete ventricular emptying. Third, venous pressure is reduced (because of reduced venous constriction), thereby reducing cardiac distention, pulmonary congestion, and peripheral edema.

Increased Urine Production. The increase in cardiac output increases renal blood flow and thereby increases production of urine. The resultant loss of water reduces blood volume, which in turn reduces cardiac distention, pulmonary congestion, and peripheral edema.

Decreased Renin Release. In response to increased arterial pressure, renin release declines, causing levels of aldosterone and angiotensin II to decline as well. The decrease in angiotensin II decreases vasoconstriction, thereby further reducing afterload and venous pressure. The decrease in aldosterone reduces retention of sodium and water, which reduces blood volume, which in turn further reduces venous pressure.

Summary of Hemodynamic Effects

We can see that, through direct and indirect mechanisms, digoxin has the potential to reverse all of the overt manifestations of HF: cardiac output improves, heart rate decreases, heart size declines, constriction of arterioles and veins decreases, water retention reverses, blood volume declines, peripheral and pulmonary edema decrease, and water weight is lost. In addition, exercise tolerance improves and fatigue is reduced. There is, however, one important caveat: Although digoxin can produce substantial improvement in HF symptoms, it does not prolong life.

Neurohormonal Benefits in Heart Failure

At dosages below those needed for positive inotropic effects, digoxin can modulate the activity of neurohormonal systems. The underlying mechanism is inhibition of Na^+/K^+-ATPase.

In the kidney, digoxin can suppress renin release. By inhibiting Na^+/K^+-ATPase in renal tubules, digoxin decreases tubular absorption of sodium. As a result, less sodium is presented to the distal tubule, and so renin release is suppressed.

Through effects on the vagus nerve, digoxin can decrease sympathetic outflow from the CNS. Specifically, by inhibiting Na^+/K^+-ATPase in vagal afferent fibers, digoxin increases the sensitivity of cardiac baroreceptors. As a result, these receptors discharge more readily, thereby signaling the CNS to reduce sympathetic traffic to the periphery.

How important are these effects on renin and sympathetic tone? No one knows for sure. However, they are probably just as important as inotropic effects, and perhaps even more important.

Electrical Effects on the Heart

The effects of digoxin on the electrical activity of the heart are of therapeutic and toxicologic importance. It is because of its electrical effects that digoxin is useful for treating dysrhythmias (see Chapter 49). Ironically, these same electrical effects are responsible for *causing* dysrhythmias, the most serious adverse effect of digoxin.

The electrical effects of digoxin can be bewildering in their complexity. Through a combination of actions, digoxin can alter the electrical activity in noncontractile tissue (sinoatrial [SA] node, atrioventricular [AV] node, Purkinje fibers) as well as in ventricular muscle. In these various regions, digoxin can alter automaticity, refractoriness, and impulse conduction. Whether these parameters are increased or decreased depends on cardiac status, digoxin dosage, and the region involved.

Although the electrical effects of digoxin are many and varied, only a few are clinically significant. These are discussed in the sections that follow.

Mechanisms for Altering Electrical Activity of the Heart

Digoxin alters the electrical properties of the heart by *inhibiting Na^+/K^+-ATPase* and by *enhancing vagal influences on the heart*. By inhibiting Na^+/K^+-ATPase, digoxin alters the distribution of ions (Na^+, K^+, Ca^{++}) across the cardiac cell membrane. This change in ion distribution can alter the electrical responsiveness of the cells involved. Since hypokalemia intensifies inhibition of Na^+/K^+-ATPase, hypokalemia intensifies alterations in cardiac electrical properties.

Digoxin acts in two ways to enhance vagal effects on the heart. First, the drug acts in the CNS to increase the firing rate of vagal fibers that innervate the heart. Second, digoxin increases the responsiveness of the SA node to acetylcholine (the neurotransmitter released by the vagus). The net result of these vagotonic effects is (1) decreased automaticity of the SA node and (2) decreased conduction through the AV node.

Effects on Specific Regions of the Heart

In the SA node, digoxin decreases automaticity (by the vagotonic mechanisms just mentioned). In the AV node, digoxin decreases conduction velocity and prolongs the effective refractory period. These effects, which can promote varying degrees of AV block, result primarily from the drug's vagotonic actions. In Purkinje fibers, digoxin-induced inhibition of Na^+/K^+-ATPase results in increased automaticity; this increase can generate ectopic foci that, in turn, can cause ventricular dysrhythmias. In the ventricular myocardium, digoxin acts to shorten the effective refractory period and (possibly) increase automaticity.

Adverse Effects I: Cardiac Dysrhythmias

Dysrhythmias are the most serious adverse effect of digoxin. They result from altering the electrical properties of the heart. Fortunately, when used in the dosages recommended today, dysrhythmias are uncommon.

What kinds of dysrhythmias can occur? Digoxin can mimic practically all types of dysrhythmias. Atrioventricular block with escape beats is among the most common. Ventricular flutter and ventricular fibrillation are the most dangerous.

Because serious dysrhythmias are a potential consequence of therapy, all patients should be evaluated frequently for changes in heart rate and rhythm. If significant changes occur, digoxin should be withheld and the prescriber consulted. Outpatients should be taught to monitor their pulses and instructed to report any significant changes in rate or regularity.

Mechanism of Ventricular Dysrhythmia Generation

Digoxin-induced ventricular dysrhythmias result from a combination of four factors:

- Decreased automaticity of the SA node
- Decreased impulse conduction through the AV node
- Spontaneous discharge of Purkinje fibers (caused in part by increased automaticity)
- Shortening of the effective refractory period in ventricular muscle

Increased Purkinje fiber discharge and shortening of the ventricular effective refractory period predispose the ventricles to developing ectopic beats. Potential ectopic beats become manifest because the effects of digoxin on the SA and AV nodes decrease the ability of the normal pacemaker to drive the ventricles, allowing ventricular ectopic beats to take over.

Predisposing Factors

Hypokalemia. *The most common cause of dysrhythmias in patients receiving digoxin is hypokalemia secondary to the use of diuretics.* Less common causes include vomiting and diarrhea. Hypokalemia promotes dysrhythmias by increasing digoxin-induced inhibition of Na^+/K^+-ATPase, which in turn leads to increased automaticity of Purkinje fibers. Because low potassium can precipitate dysrhythmias, *it is imperative that serum potassium levels be kept within the normal range.* If diuretic therapy causes potassium levels to fall, a potassium-sparing diuretic (e.g., spironolactone) can be prescribed to correct the problem. Potassium supplements may be used too. Patients should be taught to recognize symptoms of hypokalemia (e.g., muscle weakness) and instructed to notify the prescriber if these develop.

Elevated Digoxin Levels. *Digoxin has a narrow therapeutic range: Drug levels only slightly higher than the therapeutic range greatly increase the risk of toxicity.* Possible causes of excessive digoxin levels include (1) intentional or accidental overdose, (2) increased digoxin absorption, and (3) decreased digoxin elimination.

If digoxin levels are kept within the optimal therapeutic range—now considered to be 0.5 to 0.8 ng/mL—the chances of a dysrhythmia will be reduced. However, it is important to note that careful control over drug levels does not eliminate the risk. As already discussed, there is only a loose relationship between digoxin levels and clinical effects. As a result, some patients may experience dysrhythmias even when drug levels are within what is normally considered a safe range.

Heart Disease. The ability of digoxin to cause dysrhythmias is greatly increased by the presence of heart disease. Doses of digoxin that have no adverse effects on healthy volunteers can precipitate serious dysrhythmias in patients with HF. The probability and severity of a dysrhythmia are directly related to the severity of the underlying disease. Since heart disease is the reason for taking digoxin, it should be no surprise that people taking the drug are at risk of dysrhythmias.

Diagnosing Digoxin-Induced Dysrhythmias

Diagnosis is not easy, largely because the failing heart is prone to spontaneous dysrhythmias. Hence, when a dysrhythmia occurs, we cannot simply assume that digoxin is the cause: The possibility that the dysrhythmia is the direct result of heart disease must be considered. Compounding diagnostic difficulties is the poor correlation between plasma digoxin levels and dysrhythmia onset. Because of this loose association, the presence of an apparently excessive digoxin level does not necessarily indicate that digoxin is responsible for the problem. Laboratory data required for diagnosis include digoxin level, serum electrolytes, and an ECG. Ultimately, diagnosis is based on experience and clinical judgment. Resolution of the dysrhythmia following digoxin withdrawal confirms the diagnosis.

Managing Digoxin-Induced Dysrhythmias

With proper treatment, digoxin-induced dysrhythmias can almost always be controlled. Basic management measures are as follows:

- *Withdraw digoxin and potassium-wasting diuretics.* For many patients, no additional treatment is needed. To help ensure that medication is stopped, a written order to withhold digoxin should be made.
- *Monitor serum potassium.* If the potassium level is low or nearly normal, potassium (IV or PO) should be administered. Potassium displaces digoxin from Na^+/K^+-ATPase and thereby helps reverse toxicity. However, if potassium levels are high or if AV block is present, no more potassium should be given. Under these conditions, more potassium may cause complete AV block.
- Some patients may require an antidysrhythmic drug. *Phenytoin* and *lidocaine* are most effective. Quinidine, another antidysrhythmic drug, can cause plasma levels of digoxin to rise, and so should not be used.
- Patients who develop bradycardia or AV block can be treated with atropine. (Atropine blocks the vagal influences that underlie bradycardia and AV block.) Alternatively, electronic pacing may be employed.
- When overdose is especially severe, digoxin levels can be lowered using *Fab antibody fragments* [Digifab]. Following IV administration, these fragments bind digoxin and thereby prevent it from acting. Treatment is expensive: A full neutralizing dose costs $3000 to $4000. *Cholestyramine* and *activated charcoal,* agents that also bind digoxin, can be administered orally to suppress absorption of digoxin from the GI tract.

Adverse Effects II: Noncardiac Adverse Effects

The principal noncardiac toxicities of digoxin concern the GI system and the CNS. Since adverse effects on these systems frequently precede development of dysrhythmias, symptoms involving the GI tract and CNS can provide advance warning of more serious toxicity. Accordingly, patients should be taught to recognize these effects and instructed to notify the prescriber if they occur.

Anorexia, nausea, and *vomiting* are the most common GI side effects. These responses result primarily from stimulation of the chemoreceptor trigger zone of the medulla. Digoxin rarely causes diarrhea.

Fatigue is the most frequent CNS effect. *Visual disturbances* (e.g., blurred vision, yellow tinge to vision, appearance of halos around dark objects) are also relatively common.

Adverse Effects III: Measures to Reduce Adverse Effects

Patient education can help reduce the incidence of toxicity. Patients should be warned about digoxin-induced dysrhythmias and instructed to take their medication exactly as prescribed. In addition, they should be informed about symptoms of developing toxicity (altered heart rate or rhythm, visual or GI disturbances) and instructed to notify the prescriber if these develop. If a potassium supplement or potassium-sparing diuretic is part of the regimen, it should be taken exactly as ordered.

Drug Interactions

Digoxin is subject to a large number of significant drug interactions. Some are pharmacodynamic and some are pharmacokinetic. Several important interactions are discussed in the sections that follow. Interactions are shown in Table 48.2.

Diuretics

Thiazide diuretics and *loop diuretics* promote loss of potassium and thereby increase the risk of digoxin-induced dysrhythmias. Accordingly, when digoxin and these diuretics are used concurrently, serum potassium levels must be monitored and maintained within the normal range (3.5 to 5 mEq/L). If hypokalemia develops, potassium levels can be restored with potassium supplements, a potassium-sparing diuretic, or both.

ACE Inhibitors and ARBs

These drugs can increase potassium levels and can thereby decrease therapeutic responses to digoxin. Exercise caution if an ACE inhibitor or ARB is combined with potassium supplements or a potassium-sparing diuretic.

Sympathomimetics

Sympathomimetic drugs (e.g., dopamine, dobutamine) act on the heart to increase the rate and force of contraction. The increase in contractile force can add to the positive inotropic effects of digoxin. These complementary actions can be beneficial. In contrast, the ability of sympathomimetics to increase heart rate may be detrimental in that the risk of a tachydysrhythmia is increased.

Quinidine

Quinidine is an antidysrhythmic drug that can cause plasma levels of digoxin to rise. Quinidine increases digoxin levels by (1) displacing digoxin from tissue binding sites and (2) reducing renal excretion of digoxin. By elevating levels of free digoxin, quinidine can promote digoxin toxicity. Accordingly, concurrent use of quinidine and digoxin should be avoided.

TABLE 48.2 ■ Drug Interactions With Digoxin

Drug	Effect
PHARMACODYNAMIC INTERACTIONS	
Thiazide diuretics Loop diuretics Succinylcholine	Promote potassium loss and thereby increase the risk of digoxin-induced dysrhythmias
Beta blockers Verapamil Diltiazem	Decrease contractility and heart rate
Sympathomimetics	Increase contractility and heart rate
PHARMACOKINETIC INTERACTIONS	
Cholestyramine Kaolin-pectin Metoclopramide Neomycin Sulfasalazine	Decrease digoxin levels by decreasing digoxin absorption or bioavailability
Aminoglycosides Antacids Colestipol Azithromycin Clarithromycin Erythromycin Omeprazole Tetracycline	Increase digoxin levels by increasing digoxin absorption or bioavailability
Alprazolam Amiodarone Atorvastatin Captopril Diltiazem Nifedipine Nitrendipine Propafenone Quinidine Verapamil	Increase digoxin levels by decreasing excretion of digoxin, altering distribution of digoxin, or both

Verapamil

Verapamil, a calcium channel blocker, can significantly increase plasma levels of digoxin. If the combination is employed, digoxin dosage must be reduced. In addition, verapamil can suppress myocardial contractility and can thereby counteract the benefits of digoxin.

Pharmacokinetics

Absorption

Absorption with digoxin tablets is variable, ranging between 60% and 80%, and can be decreased by certain foods and drugs. Meals high in bran can decrease absorption significantly, as can cholestyramine, kaolin-pectin, and certain other drugs (see Table 48.2). Of note, taking digoxin with meals decreases the rate of absorption but not the extent.

In the past, there was considerable variability in the absorption of digoxin from tablets prepared by different manufacturers. This variability resulted from differences in the rate and extent of tablet dissolution. Because of this variable bioavailability, it had been recommended that patients not switch between different digoxin brands. Today, bioavailability of digoxin in tablets produced by different companies is fairly uniform, making brands of digoxin more interchangeable than in the past. However, given the narrow therapeutic range of digoxin, some authorities still recommend that patients not switch between brands of digoxin tablets—even when prescriptions are written generically—except with the approval and supervision of the prescriber.

Distribution

Digoxin is distributed widely and crosses the placenta. High levels are achieved in cardiac and skeletal muscle, owing largely to binding to Na^+/K^+-ATPase. About 23% of digoxin in plasma is bound to proteins, mainly albumin.

Elimination

Digoxin is eliminated primarily by *renal excretion.* Hepatic metabolism is minimal. Because digoxin is eliminated by the kidneys, renal impairment can lead to toxic accumulation. Accordingly, dosage must be reduced if kidney function declines. Because digoxin is not metabolized to a significant extent, changes in liver function do not affect digoxin levels.

Half-Life and Time to Plateau

The half-life of digoxin is about 1.5 days. Therefore, in the absence of a loading dose, about 6 days (four half-lives) are required to reach plateau. When use of the drug is discontinued, another 6 days are required for digoxin stores to be eliminated.

Single-Dose Time Course

Effects of a single oral dose begin 30 minutes to 2 hours after administration and peak within 4 to 6 hours. Effects of IV digoxin begin rapidly (within 5 to 30 minutes) and peak in 1 to 4 hours.

A Note on Plasma Digoxin Levels

Most hospitals are equipped to measure plasma levels of digoxin. The optimal range is 0.5 to 0.8 ng/mL. Levels above 1 ng/mL offer no additional benefits but do increase the risk of toxicity. Knowledge of plasma levels can be useful for

- Establishing dosage
- Monitoring compliance
- Diagnosing toxicity
- Determining the cause of therapeutic failure

Once a stable blood level has been achieved, routine measurement of digoxin levels can be replaced with an annual measurement. Additional measurements may be useful when

- Digoxin dosage is changed
- Symptoms of HF intensify
- Kidney function deteriorates
- Signs of toxicity appear
- Drugs that can affect digoxin levels are added to or deleted from the regimen

Although knowledge of digoxin plasma levels can aid the clinician, it must be understood that the extent of this aid is limited. The correlation between plasma levels of digoxin and clinical effects—both therapeutic and adverse—is not very tight: Drug levels that are safe and effective for patient A may be subtherapeutic for patient B and toxic for patient C. Because of interpatient variability, knowledge of digoxin levels does not permit precise predictions of therapeutic effects or toxicity. Hence, information regarding drug levels must not be relied on too heavily. Rather, this information should be seen as but one factor among several to be considered when evaluating clinical responses.

Preparations, Dosage, and Administration

Preparations

Digoxin is available in three formulations:

- Tablets—0.125 and 0.25 mg
- Pediatric elixir—0.05 mg/mL
- Solution for injection—0.1 and 0.25 mg/mL

Administration

Digoxin can be administered *orally* and *intravenously. Intramuscular* administration should be avoided, owing to a risk of tissue damage and severe pain. Before dosing, the rate and regularity of the heartbeat should be determined. If heart rate is less than 60 beats/min or if a change in rhythm is detected, digoxin should be withheld and the prescriber notified. When digoxin is given IV, cardiac status should be monitored continuously for 1 to 2 hours.

Dosage in Heart Failure

Most patients can be treated with initial and maintenance dosages of 0.125 mg/day. Doses above 0.25 mg/day are rarely used or needed. The target plasma drug level is 0.5 to 0.8 ng/mL.

Digitalization

The term *digitalization* refers to the use of a loading dose to achieve high plasma levels of digoxin quickly. (As noted, 6 days are needed for drug levels to reach plateau if no loading dose is employed.) Although digitalization was common in the past, the practice is now considered both unnecessary and inappropriate in the treatment of chronic heart failure.

MANAGEMENT OF HEART FAILURE

Our discussion of HF management is based on recommendations in the practice guideline: *2013 ACCF/AHA Guideline for the Management of Heart Failure,* and on an update—*2016 ACC/AHA/HFSA Focused Update on New Pharmacological Therapy for Heart Failure.* These guidelines approach HF as a progressive disease that advances through four stages of increasing severity. Management for each stage is discussed next.

Stage A

By definition, patients in ACC/AHA Stage A have no symptoms of HF and no structural or functional cardiac abnormalities—but they do have behaviors or conditions strongly associated with developing HF. Important among these are hypertension, coronary artery disease, diabetes, family history of cardiomyopathy, and a personal history of alcohol abuse, rheumatic fever, or treatment with a cardiotoxic drug (e.g., doxorubicin, trastuzumab).

Management is directed at reducing risk. Hypertension, hyperlipidemia, and diabetes should be controlled, as should ventricular rate in patients with supraventricular tachycardias. An ACE inhibitor or ARB can be useful for patients with diabetes, atherosclerosis, or hypertension. Patients should cease behaviors that increase HF risk, especially smoking and alcohol abuse. (Excessive, chronic consumption of alcohol is a leading cause of cardiomyopathy. In patients with HF, acute alcohol consumption can suppress contractility.) There is no evidence that getting regular exercise can prevent development of HF, although exercise does have other health benefits. Routine use of dietary supplements to prevent structural heart disease is not recommended.

Stage B

Like patients in Stage A, those in Stage B have no signs or symptoms of HF, but they do have structural heart disease that is strongly associated with the development of HF. Among these structural changes are LV hypertrophy or fibrosis, LV dilation or hypocontractility, valvular heart disease, and previous myocardial infarction.

The goal of management is to prevent development of symptomatic HF. The approach is to implement measures that can prevent further cardiac injury, delaying the progression of remodeling and LV dysfunction. Specific measures include all those discussed for Stage A. In addition, treatment with an ACE inhibitor plus a beta blocker is recommended for all patients with a reduced ejection fraction, history of myocardial infarction, or both. For patients who cannot tolerate ACE inhibitors, an ARB may be used instead. As in Stage A, there is no evidence that using dietary supplements or getting regular exercise can help prevent progression to symptomatic HF.

Stage C

Patients in Stage C have symptoms of HF and also have structural heart disease. As discussed earlier, symptoms include dyspnea, fatigue, peripheral edema, and distention of the jugular veins. Treatment has four major goals: (1) relief of pulmonary and peripheral congestive symptoms, (2) improvement of functional capacity and quality of life, (3) slowing of cardiac remodeling and progression of LV dysfunction, and (4) prolongation of life. Treatment measures include those recommended for Stages A and B, plus those discussed in the sections that follow.

Drug Therapy

Drug therapy for HF has changed dramatically over the past 15 to 20 years. Formerly, digoxin was a mainstay of treatment. Today, its role is secondary. First-line therapy now consists of three drugs: a diuretic, an ACE inhibitor or ARB, and a beta blocker. As a rule, digoxin is added only when symptoms cannot be managed with the preferred agents.

Diuretics. All patients with evidence of fluid retention should restrict salt intake and use a diuretic. Diuretics are the only reliable means of correcting fluid overload. Furthermore, these drugs produce symptomatic improvement faster than any other drugs. If renal function is good, a thiazide diuretic will work. However, if renal function is significantly impaired, as it is in most patients, a loop diuretic will be needed. Efficacy of diuresis is best assessed by daily measurement of body weight. Once fluid overload has been corrected, diuretic therapy should continue to prevent recurrence. Diuretics should not be used alone. Rather, for most patients, they should be combined with an ACE inhibitor (or ARB) plus a beta blocker. Since aspirin and other nonsteroidal anti-inflammatory drugs (NSAIDs) can decrease the effects of diuretics and increase the incidence of acute kidney injury when used in combination with an ACE inhibitor and a diuretic, these agents should be avoided. As noted, although diuretics reduce symptoms, they do not prolong survival.

ACE Inhibitors and ARBs. In the absence of specific contraindications (e.g., pregnancy), all patients with Stage C HF should receive an ACE inhibitor. If fluid retention is evident, a diuretic should be used as well. Symptomatic improvement may take weeks or even months to develop. However, even in the absence of symptomatic improvement, ACE inhibitors may prolong life. Dosage should be sufficient to reduce mortality (see Table 48.1). For patients who cannot tolerate ACE inhibitors (owing to intractable cough or angioedema), ARBs remain the recommended alternative.

Beta Blockers. In the absence of specific contraindications, all patients with Stage C HF should receive an approved beta blocker (e.g., carvedilol). As with ACE inhibitors, symptomatic improvement may not be evident for months. Nonetheless, life may be prolonged even in the absence of clinical improvement.

Aldosterone Antagonists. Adding an aldosterone antagonist (spironolactone or eplerenone) to standard therapy (i.e., diuretic, ACE inhibitor or ARB, and a beta blocker) is reasonable in patients with moderately severe or severe symptoms of HF following a heart attack. However, aldosterone antagonists must not be used if kidney function is impaired or serum potassium is elevated. Monitoring renal function and potassium levels is imperative.

Digoxin. Digoxin may be used in combination with ACE inhibitors (or ARBs), diuretics, and beta blockers to improve clinical status. However, although digoxin can reduce symptoms, it does not prolong life. The usual dosage is 0.125 mg/day. Adjustments are based on clinical response. Digoxin may be started early to help improve symptoms, or it may be reserved for patients who have not responded adequately to a diuretic, ACE inhibitor or ARB, and beta blocker.

Isosorbide Dinitrate/Hydralazine. Adding ISDN/hydralazine is *recommended* to improve outcomes in self-described African Americans who have moderate to severe symptoms despite optimal therapy with ACE inhibitors, beta blockers, and diuretics. For all other patients who continue to have symptoms despite treatment with standard therapy, adding ISDN/hydralazine to the regimen is considered *reasonable.* For patients who cannot tolerate ACE inhibitors or ARBs, *substitution* of ISDN/hydralazine is considered reasonable.

Drugs to Avoid

Patients in Stage C should avoid three classes of drugs: antidysrhythmics, calcium channel blockers (CCBs), and NSAIDs (e.g., aspirin). Reasons for not using these drugs are as follows:

- *Antidysrhythmic agents*—These drugs have cardiosuppressant and prodysrhythmic actions that can make HF worse. Only two agents—amiodarone [Cordarone] and dofetilide [Tikosyn]—have been proven not to reduce survival.
- *Calcium channel blockers*—These drugs can make HF worse and may increase the risk of adverse cardiovascular events. Only the long-acting dihydropyridine CCBs, such as amlodipine [Norvasc], have been shown not to reduce survival.
- *NSAIDs*—These drugs promote sodium retention and peripheral vasoconstriction. Both actions can make HF worse. In addition, NSAIDs can reduce the efficacy and intensify the toxicity of diuretics and ACE inhibitors. Hence, even though aspirin has beneficial effects on coagulation, it should still be avoided unless clinically indicated for conditions such as myocardial infarction.

Device Therapy

Implanted Cardioverter-Defibrillators. Cardiac arrest and fatal ventricular dysrhythmias are relatively common complications of HF. Accordingly, implantable cardioverter-defibrillators are now recommended for primary or secondary prevention to reduce mortality in selected patients.

Cardiac Resynchronization. When the left and right ventricles fail to contract at the same time, cardiac output is further compromised. Synchronized contractions can be restored with a biventricular pacemaker. In clinical trials, cardiac resynchronization improved exercise tolerance and quality of life and reduced all-cause mortality.

Exercise Training

In the past, bed rest was recommended owing to concern that physical activity might accelerate progression of LV dysfunction. However, we now know that inactivity is actually detrimental: It reduces conditioning, worsens exercise intolerance, and contributes to HF symptoms. Conversely, studies have shown that exercise training can improve clinical status, increase exercise capacity, and improve quality of life. Accordingly, exercise training should be considered for all stable patients.

Evaluating Treatment

Evaluation is based on symptoms and physical findings. Reductions in dyspnea on exertion, paroxysmal nocturnal dyspnea, and orthopnea (difficulty breathing, except in the upright position) indicate success. The physical examination should assess for reductions in jugular distention, edema, and crackles. Success is also indicated by increased capacity for physical activity. Accordingly, patients should be interviewed to determine improvements in the maximal activity they can perform without symptoms, the type of activity that regularly produces symptoms, and the maximal activity they can tolerate. (Activity is defined as walking, stair climbing, activities of daily living, or any other activity that is appropriate.) Successful treatment should also improve health-related quality of life in general. Thus the interview should look for improvements in sleep, sexual function, outlook on life, cognitive function (alertness, memory, concentration), and ability to participate in usual social, recreational, and work activities.

Routine measurement of ejection fraction or maximal exercise capacity is not recommended. Although the degree of reduction in ejection fraction measured at the beginning of therapy is predictive of outcome, improvement in the ejection fraction does not necessarily indicate the prognosis has changed.

As noted earlier, a reduction in circulating BNP indicates improvement. The lower BNP is, the better the odds of long-term survival.

Stage D

Patients in Stage D have advanced structural heart disease and marked symptoms of HF at rest, despite treatment with maximal dosages of medications used in Stage C. Repeated and prolonged hospitalization is common. For eligible candidates, the best long-term solution is a heart transplant. An implantable LV mechanical assist device can be used as a "bridge" in patients awaiting a transplant and to prolong life in those who are not transplant eligible.

Management focuses largely on the control of fluid retention, which underlies most signs and symptoms. Intake and output should be monitored closely, and the patient should be weighed daily. Fluid retention can usually be treated with a loop diuretic, perhaps combined with a thiazide. If volume overload becomes severe, the patient should be hospitalized and given an IV diuretic. If needed, IV dopamine or IV dobutamine can be added to increase renal blood flow, thereby enhancing diuresis. Patients should not be discharged until a stable and effective oral diuretic regimen has been established.

What about beta blockers and ACE inhibitors? These agents may be tried, but doses should be low and responses monitored with care. In Stage D, beta blockers pose a significant risk of making HF worse, and ACE inhibitors may induce profound hypotension or renal failure.

When severe symptoms persist despite application of all recommended therapies, options for end-of-life care should be discussed with the patient and family.

KEY POINTS

- Heart failure with LV systolic dysfunction, referred to simply as *heart failure* (HF) in this chapter, is characterized by ventricular dysfunction, reduced cardiac output, signs of inadequate tissue perfusion (fatigue, shortness of breath, exercise intolerance), and signs of fluid overload (venous distention, peripheral edema, pulmonary edema).
- The initial phase of HF consists of cardiac remodeling—a process in which the ventricles dilate (grow larger), hypertrophy (increase in wall thickness), and become more spherical—coupled with cardiac fibrosis and myocyte death. As a result of these changes, cardiac output is reduced.
- Reduced cardiac output leads to compensatory responses: (1) activation of the SNS, (2) activation of the RAAS, and (3) retention of water and expansion of blood volume. As a result of volume expansion, cardiac dilation increases.
- If the compensatory responses are not sufficient to maintain adequate production of urine, body water will continue to accumulate, eventually causing death (from complete cardiac failure secondary to excessive cardiac dilation and cardiac edema).
- There are three major groups of drugs for heart failure: diuretics, ACE inhibitors or ARBs, and beta blockers. Digoxin, which had been used widely in the past, may be added as indicated.
- Diuretics are first-line drugs for all patients with fluid overload. By reducing blood volume, these drugs can decrease venous pressure, arterial pressure, pulmonary edema, peripheral edema, and cardiac dilation.
- Although diuretics can reduce symptoms of HF, they do not prolong survival.

Continued

- Thiazide diuretics are ineffective when GFR is low, and cannot be used if cardiac output is greatly reduced.
- Loop diuretics are effective even when GFR is low, and are preferred to thiazides for most patients.
- Thiazide diuretics and loop diuretics can cause hypokalemia and can increase the risk of digoxin-induced dysrhythmias.
- Potassium-sparing diuretics are used to counteract potassium loss caused by thiazide diuretics and loop diuretics.
- Potassium-sparing diuretics can cause hyperkalemia. By doing so, they can increase the risk of hyperkalemia in patients taking ACE inhibitors or ARBs.
- In patients with HF, ACE inhibitors improve functional status and reduce mortality. In the absence of specific contraindications, all patients should be prescribed one.
- ACE inhibitors block formation of angiotensin II, promote accumulation of kinins, and reduce aldosterone release. As a result, these drugs cause dilation of veins and arterioles, promote renal excretion of water, and favorably alter cardiac remodeling.
- By dilating arterioles, ACE inhibitors (1) improve regional blood flow in the kidneys and other tissues and (2) reduce cardiac afterload, which causes stroke volume and cardiac output to rise.
- By dilating veins, ACE inhibitors reduce venous pressure, which in turn reduces pulmonary congestion, peripheral edema, preload, and cardiac dilation.
- By suppressing aldosterone release, ACE inhibitors increase excretion of sodium and water, and decrease excretion of potassium.
- By increasing levels of kinins (and partly by decreasing levels of angiotensin II), ACE inhibitors can favorably alter cardiac remodeling.
- Major side effects of ACE inhibitors are hypotension, hyperkalemia, cough, angioedema, and birth defects.
- ARBs share the beneficial hemodynamic effects of ACE inhibitors, but not the beneficial effects on cardiac remodeling.
- In patients with HF, ARBs should be reserved for patients intolerant of ACE inhibitors (usually owing to cough).
- In patients with HF, aldosterone antagonists (e.g., spironolactone, eplerenone) reduce symptoms and prolong life. Benefits derive from blocking aldosterone receptors in the heart and blood vessels.
- Beta blockers can prolong survival in patients with HF, and are considered first-line therapy.
- To avoid excessive cardiosuppression, beta-blocker dosage must be very low initially and then gradually increased.
- Isosorbide dinitrate (which dilates veins) plus hydralazine (which dilates arterioles) can be used in place of an ACE inhibitor (or ARB) if an ACE inhibitor (or ARB) cannot be used.
- BiDil, a fixed-dose combination of hydralazine and isosorbide dinitrate, is approved specifically for treating HF in African Americans.
- Digoxin and other inotropic agents increase the force of myocardial contraction and thereby increase cardiac output.
- Of the available inotropic agents, digoxin is the only one that is both effective and safe when used *orally* and the only one suitable for long-term use.
- Digoxin increases contractility by inhibiting myocardial Na^+/K^+-ATPase, thereby (indirectly) increasing intracellular calcium, which in turn facilitates the interaction of actin and myosin.
- Potassium competes with digoxin for binding to Na^+/K^+-ATPase. Therefore, if potassium levels are low, excessive inhibition of Na^+/K^+-ATPase can occur, resulting in toxicity. Conversely, if potassium levels are high, insufficient inhibition can occur, resulting in therapeutic failure. Accordingly, it is imperative to keep potassium levels in the normal physiologic range: 3.5 to 5 mEq/L.
- By increasing cardiac output, digoxin can reverse all of the overt manifestations of HF: cardiac output improves, heart rate decreases, heart size declines, constriction of arterioles and veins decreases, water retention reverses, blood volume declines, peripheral and pulmonary edema decrease, water weight is lost, and exercise tolerance improves. Unfortunately, although digoxin can improve symptoms, it does not prolong life.
- In patients with HF, benefits of digoxin are not due solely to improved cardiac output; neurohormonal effects are important too.
- Digoxin causes dysrhythmias by altering the electrical properties of the heart (secondary to inhibition of Na^+/K^+-ATPase).
- The most common reason for digoxin-related dysrhythmias is diuretic-induced hypokalemia.
- If a severe digoxin overdose is responsible for dysrhythmias, digoxin levels can be lowered using Fab antibody fragments [Digifab].
- In addition to dysrhythmias, digoxin can cause GI effects (anorexia, nausea, vomiting) and CNS effects (fatigue, visual disturbances). Gastrointestinal and CNS effects often precede dysrhythmias and therefore can provide advance warning of serious toxicity.
- Digoxin has a narrow therapeutic range.
- Digoxin is eliminated by renal excretion.
- Although routine monitoring of digoxin levels is generally unnecessary, monitoring can be helpful when dosage is changed, symptoms of HF intensify, kidney function declines, signs of toxicity appear, or drugs that affect digoxin levels are added to or deleted from the regimen.
- Maintenance doses of digoxin are based primarily on observation of the patient: Doses should be large enough to minimize symptoms of HF but not so large as to cause adverse effects.
- Maintenance doses of digoxin must be reduced if renal function declines.
- Therapy of Stage C HF has four major goals: (1) relief of pulmonary and peripheral congestion, (2) improvement of functional status and quality of life, (3) delay of progression of cardiac remodeling and LV dysfunction, and (4) prolongation of life.
- For routine therapy, Stage C HF is treated with a diuretic, an ACE inhibitor or an ARB, and a beta blocker.

Please visit **http://evolve.elsevier.com/Lehne** for chapter-specific NCLEX® examination review questions.

Summary of Major Nursing Implications[a]

DIGOXIN

Preadministration Assessment

Therapeutic Goal

Digoxin is used to treat HF and dysrhythmias. Be sure to confirm which disorder the drug has been ordered for.

Baseline Data

Assess for signs and symptoms of HF, including fatigue, weakness, cough, breathing difficulty (orthopnea, dyspnea on exertion, paroxysmal nocturnal dyspnea), jugular distention, and edema.

Determine baseline values for maximal activity without symptoms, activity that regularly causes symptoms, and maximal tolerated activity.

Laboratory tests should include an ECG, serum electrolytes, measurement of ejection fraction, and evaluation of kidney function.

Identifying High-Risk Patients

Digoxin is *contraindicated* for patients experiencing ventricular fibrillation, ventricular tachycardia, or digoxin toxicity.

Exercise *caution* in the presence of conditions that can predispose the patient to serious adverse responses to digoxin, such as hypokalemia, partial AV block, advanced HF, or renal impairment.

Implementation: Administration

Routes

Oral, slow IV injection.

Administration

Oral. Determine heart rate and rhythm before administration. If heart rate is less than 60 beats/min or if a change in rhythm is detected, withhold digoxin and notify the prescriber.

Warn patients not to "double up" on doses in attempts to compensate for missed doses.

Intravenous. Monitor cardiac status closely for 1 to 2 hours following IV injection.

Promoting Adherence

Because digoxin has a narrow therapeutic range, rigid adherence to the prescribed dosage is essential. **Inform patients that failure to take digoxin exactly as prescribed may lead to toxicity or therapeutic failure.** If poor adherence is suspected, serum drug levels may help in assessing the extent of nonadherence.

Implementation: Measures to Enhance Therapeutic Effects

Advise patients to limit salt intake to 1500 mg/day and to avoid excessive fluids. Advise patients who drink alcohol to consume no more than one drink each day. Help patients establish an appropriate program of regular mild exercise (e.g., walking, cycling). Precipitating factors for HF (e.g., hypertension, valvular heart disease) should be corrected.

Ongoing Evaluation and Interventions

Evaluating Therapeutic Effects

Evaluation is based on symptoms and physical findings. Assess for reductions in orthopnea, dyspnea on exertion, paroxysmal nocturnal dyspnea, neck vein distention, edema, and crackles, and for increased capacity for physical activity. In addition, assess for improvements in sleep, sexual function, outlook on life, cognitive function, and ability to participate in social, recreational, and work activities.

Plasma BNP levels reflect cardiac status: The lower the level, the better the odds for long-term survival.

Measurement of plasma drug levels can help determine the cause of therapeutic failure. The optimal range for digoxin is 0.5 to 0.8 ng/mL.

Minimizing Adverse Effects

Cardiotoxicity. Dysrhythmias are the most serious adverse effect of digoxin. Monitor hospitalized patients for alterations in heart rate or rhythm, and withhold digoxin if significant changes develop.

Inform outpatients about the danger of dysrhythmias. Teach them to monitor their pulses for rate and rhythm, and instruct them to notify the prescriber if significant changes occur. Provide the patient with an ECG rhythm strip; this can be used by providers unfamiliar with the patient (e.g., when the patient is traveling) to verify suspected changes in rhythm.

Hypokalemia, usually diuretic induced, is the most frequent underlying cause of dysrhythmias. Monitor serum potassium concentrations. If hypokalemia develops, potassium levels can be raised with potassium supplements, a potassium-sparing diuretic, or both. **Teach patients to recognize early signs of hypokalemia (e.g., muscle weakness), and instruct them to notify the prescriber if these develop.** Severe vomiting and diarrhea can increase potassium loss; exercise caution if these events occur.

To treat digoxin-induced dysrhythmias: (1) withdraw digoxin and diuretics (make sure that a written order for digoxin withdrawal is made); (2) administer potassium (unless potassium levels are above normal or AV block is present); (3) administer an antidysrhythmic drug (phenytoin or lidocaine, but not quinidine) if indicated; (4) manage bradycardia with atropine or electrical pacing; and (5) treat with Fab fragments if toxicity is life threatening.

Noncardiac Effects. *Nausea, vomiting, anorexia, fatigue,* and *visual disturbances* (blurred or yellow vision) frequently foreshadow more serious toxicity (dysrhythmias) and should be reported immediately. **Inform patients about these early indications of toxicity, and instruct them to notify the prescriber if they develop.**

Minimizing Adverse Interactions

Diuretics. *Thiazide diuretics* and *loop diuretics* increase the risk of dysrhythmias by promoting potassium loss. Monitor potassium levels. If hypokalemia develops, it should be corrected with potassium supplements, a potassium-sparing diuretic, or both.

ACE Inhibitors and ARBs. These drugs can elevate potassium levels and decrease therapeutic responses to digoxin. Exercise caution if an ACE inhibitor or ARB is combined with potassium supplements or a potassium-sparing diuretic.

Sympathomimetic Agents. Sympathomimetic drugs (e.g., dopamine, dobutamine) stimulate the heart, thereby increasing the risk of tachydysrhythmias and ectopic pacemaker activity. When sympathomimetics are combined with digoxin, monitor closely for dysrhythmias.

Quinidine. Quinidine can elevate plasma levels of digoxin. If quinidine is employed concurrently with digoxin, digoxin dosage must be reduced. Do not use quinidine to treat digoxin-induced dysrhythmias.

[a]Patient education information is highlighted as **blue text**.

CHAPTER

49 Antidysrhythmic Drugs

A dysrhythmia is defined as *an abnormality in the rhythm of the heartbeat.* In their mildest forms, dysrhythmias have only modest effects on cardiac output. However, in their most severe forms, dysrhythmias can so disable the heart that no blood is pumped at all. Because of their ability to compromise cardiac function, dysrhythmias are associated with a high degree of morbidity and mortality.

There are two basic types of dysrhythmias: *tachydysrhythmias* (dysrhythmias in which heart rate is increased) and *bradydysrhythmias* (dysrhythmias in which heart rate is slowed). In this chapter, we consider only the tachydysrhythmias. This is by far the largest group of dysrhythmias and the group that responds best to drugs. We do not discuss the bradydysrhythmias because they are few in number and are commonly treated with electronic pacing. When drugs are indicated, atropine is usually the agent of choice.

It is important to appreciate that virtually all of the drugs used to treat dysrhythmias can also *cause* dysrhythmias. These drugs can create new dysrhythmias and worsen existing ones. Because of these prodysrhythmic actions, antidysrhythmic drugs should be employed only when the benefits of treatment clearly outweigh the risks.

For two reasons, the use of antidysrhythmic drugs is declining. First, research has shown that some of these agents actually *increase* the risk of death. Second, nonpharmacologic therapies—especially implantable defibrillators and radiofrequency ablation—have begun to replace drugs as the preferred treatment for many dysrhythmia types.

A note on terminology: Dysrhythmias are also known as *arrhythmias.* Since the term *arrhythmia* denotes an *absence* of cardiac rhythm, whereas *dysrhythmia* denotes an *abnormal* rhythm, dysrhythmia would seem the more appropriate term.

CARDIAC ELECTROPHYSIOLOGY, DYSRHYTHMIAS, AND THE ANTIDYSRHYTHMIC DRUGS

In this section we discuss background information that will help you understand the actions and uses of antidysrhythmic drugs. We begin by reviewing the electrical properties of the heart and the electrocardiogram (ECG). Next, we discuss how dysrhythmias are generated. After that, we discuss classification of the antidysrhythmic drugs, as well as the ability of these drugs to *cause* dysrhythmias. We conclude by discussing the major dysrhythmias and the basic principles that guide antidysrhythmic therapy.

ELECTRICAL PROPERTIES OF THE HEART

Dysrhythmias result from alteration of the electrical impulses that regulate cardiac rhythm—and antidysrhythmic drugs control rhythm by correcting or compensating for these alterations. Accordingly, to understand both the generation and treatment of dysrhythmias, we must first understand the electrical properties of the heart. Therefore, we begin by reviewing (1) pathways and timing of impulse conduction, (2) cardiac action potentials, and (3) basic elements of the ECG.

Impulse Conduction: Pathways and Timing

For the heart to pump effectively, contraction of the atria and ventricles must be coordinated. Coordination is achieved through precise timing and routing of impulse conduction. In the healthy heart, impulses originate in the sinoatrial (SA) node, spread rapidly through the atria, pass slowly through the atrioventricular (AV) node, and then spread rapidly through the ventricles via the His-Purkinje system (Fig. 49.1).

SA Node

Under normal circumstances, the SA node serves as the pacemaker for the heart. Pacemaker activity results from spontaneous phase 4 depolarization (discussed later in this chapter). Because cells of the sinus node usually discharge faster than other cells that display automaticity, the SA node normally dominates all other potential pacemakers.

After the SA node discharges, impulses spread rapidly through the atria along the *internodal pathways.* This rapid conduction allows the atria to contract in unison.

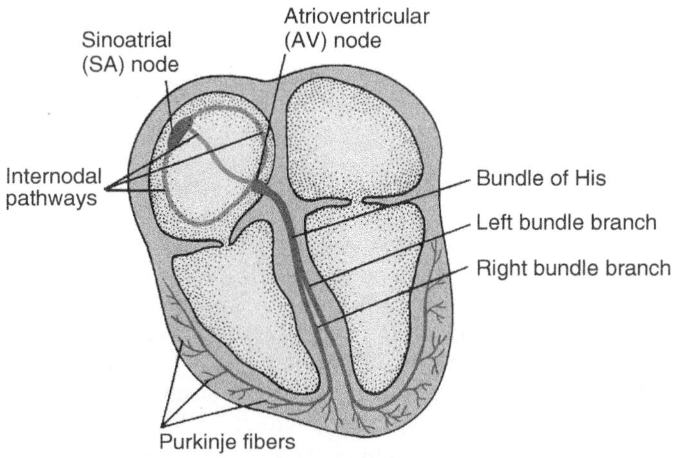

Fig. 49.1 ■ Cardiac conduction pathways.

AV Node

Impulses originating in the atria must travel through the AV node to reach the ventricles. In the healthy heart, impulses arriving at the AV node are delayed before going on to excite the ventricles. This delay provides time for blood to fill the ventricles before ventricular contraction.

His-Purkinje System

The fibers of the His-Purkinje system consist of specialized conducting tissue. The function of these fibers is to conduct electrical excitation very rapidly to all parts of the ventricles. Stimulation of the His-Purkinje system is caused by impulses leaving the AV node. These impulses are conducted rapidly down the bundle of His, enter the right and left bundle branches, and then distribute to the many fine branches of the Purkinje fibers (see Fig. 49.1). Because impulses travel quickly through this system, all regions of the ventricles are stimulated almost simultaneously, producing synchronized ventricular contraction with resultant forceful ejection of blood.

Cardiac Action Potentials

Cardiac cells can initiate and conduct action potentials, consisting of self-propagating waves of depolarization followed by repolarization. As in neurons, cardiac action potentials are generated by the movement of ions into and out of cells. These ion fluxes take place by way of specific channels in the cell membrane. In the resting cardiac cell, negatively charged ions cover the inner surface of the cell membrane while positively charged ions cover the external surface. Because of this separation of charge, the cell membrane is said to be *polarized.* Under proper conditions, channels in the cell membrane open, allowing positively charged ions to rush in. This influx eliminates the charge difference across the cell membrane, and so the cell is said to depolarize. Following depolarization, positively charged ions are extruded from the cell, causing the cell to return to its original polarized state.

In the heart, two kinds of action potentials occur: *fast potentials* and *slow potentials.* These potentials differ with respect to the mechanisms by which they are generated, the kinds of cells in which they occur, and the drugs to which they respond.

Profiles of fast and slow potentials are depicted in Fig. 49.2. Please note that action potentials in this figure represent the electrical activity of *single cardiac cells.* Such single-cell recordings, which are made using experimental preparations, should not be confused with the ECG, which is made using surface electrodes, and thus reflects the electrical activity of the entire heart.

Fast Potentials

Fast potentials occur in fibers of the *His-Purkinje system* and in *atrial and ventricular muscle.* These responses serve to conduct electrical impulses rapidly throughout the heart.

As shown in Fig. 49.2A, fast potentials have five distinct phases, labeled 0, 1, 2, 3, and 4. As we discuss each phase, we focus on its ionic basis and its relationship to the actions of antidysrhythmic drugs.

Phase 0. In phase 0, the cell undergoes *rapid depolarization* in response to *influx of sodium ions.* Phase 0 is important in that the speed of phase 0 depolarization determines the velocity

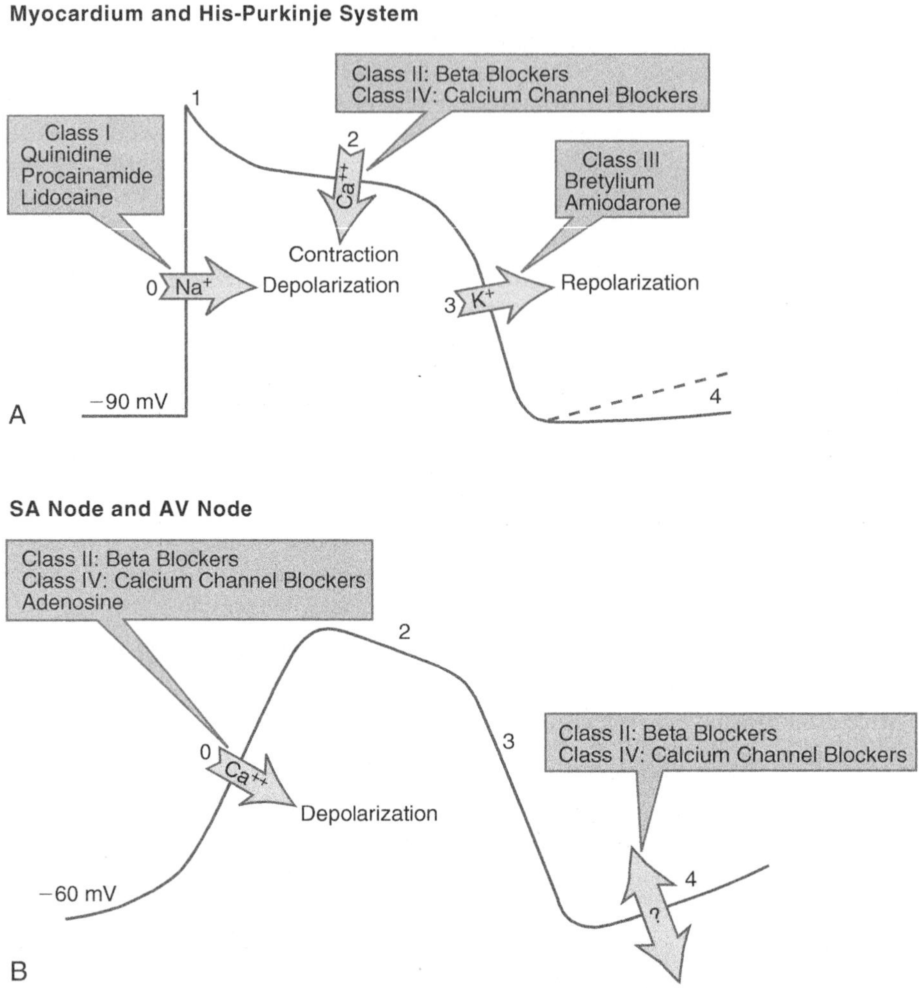

Fig. 49.2 ■ Ion fluxes during cardiac action potentials and effects of antidysrhythmic drugs.

A, Fast potential of the His-Purkinje system and atrial and ventricular myocardium. Blockade of sodium influx by class I drugs slows conduction in the His-Purkinje system. Blockade of calcium influx by beta blockers and calcium channel blockers decreases contractility. Blockade of potassium efflux by class III drugs delays repolarization and thereby prolongs the effective refractory period. **B,** Slow potential of the sinoatrial (SA) node and atrioventricular (AV) node. Blockade of calcium influx by beta blockers, calcium channel blockers, and adenosine slows AV conduction. Beta blockers and calcium channel blockers decrease SA nodal automaticity (phase 4 depolarization); the ionic basis of this effect is not understood.

of impulse conduction. Drugs that decrease the rate of phase 0 depolarization (by blocking sodium channels) slow impulse conduction through the His-Purkinje system and myocardium.

Phase 1. During phase 1, rapid (but partial) repolarization takes place. Phase 1 has no relevance to antidysrhythmic drugs.

Phase 2. Phase 2 consists of a prolonged plateau in which the membrane potential remains relatively stable. During this phase, *calcium* enters the cell and promotes contraction of atrial and ventricular muscle. Drugs that reduce calcium entry during phase 2 do *not* influence *cardiac rhythm.* However, since calcium influx is required for contraction, these drugs *can* reduce myocardial contractility.

Phase 3. In phase 3, rapid repolarization takes place. This repolarization is caused by *extrusion of potassium* from the cell. Phase 3 is relevant in that delay of repolarization prolongs the action potential duration and thereby prolongs the effective refractory period (ERP). (The ERP is the time during which a cell is unable to respond to excitation and initiate a new action potential. Therefore, extending the ERP prolongs the minimum interval between two propagating responses.) Phase 3 repolarization can be delayed by drugs that block potassium channels.

Phase 4. During phase 4, two types of electrical activity are possible: (1) the membrane potential may remain *stable* (solid line in Fig. 49.2A) or (2) the membrane may undergo *spontaneous depolarization* (dashed line in Fig. 49.2A). In cells undergoing spontaneous depolarization, the membrane potential gradually rises until a threshold potential is reached. At this point, rapid phase 0 depolarization takes place, setting off a new action potential. Hence, it is phase 4 depolarization that gives cardiac cells *automaticity* (i.e., the ability to initiate an action potential through self-excitation). The capacity for self-excitation makes potential pacemakers of all cells that have it.

Under normal conditions, His-Purkinje cells undergo very slow spontaneous depolarization, and myocardial cells do not undergo any. However, under pathologic conditions, significant phase 4 depolarization may occur in all of these cells, especially in Purkinje fibers. When this happens, a dysrhythmia can result.

Slow Potentials

Slow potentials occur in cells of the *SA node* and *AV node.* The profile of a slow potential is depicted in Fig. 49.2B. Like fast potentials, slow potentials are generated by ion fluxes. However, the specific ions involved are not the same for every phase.

From a physiologic and pharmacologic perspective, slow potentials have three features of special significance: (1) phase 0 depolarization is slow and mediated by calcium influx, (2) these potentials conduct slowly, and (3) spontaneous phase 4 depolarization in the SA node normally determines heart rate.

Phase 0. Phase 0 (depolarization phase) of slow potentials differs significantly from phase 0 of fast potentials. As we can see from Fig. 49.2, whereas phase 0 of fast potentials is caused by a *rapid influx of sodium,* phase 0 of slow potentials is caused by *slow influx of calcium.* Because calcium influx is slow, the rate of depolarization is slow; and because depolarization is slow, these potentials conduct slowly. This explains why impulse conduction through the AV node is delayed. Phase 0 of the slow potential is of therapeutic significance in that drugs that suppress calcium influx during phase 0 can slow (or stop) AV conduction.

Phases 2 and 3. Slow potentials lack a phase 1 (see Fig. 49.2B). Phases 2 and 3 of the slow potential are not significant with respect to the actions of antidysrhythmic drugs.

Phase 4. Cells of the SA node and AV node undergo spontaneous phase 4 depolarization. The ionic basis of this phenomenon is complex and incompletely understood.

Under normal conditions, the rate of phase 4 depolarization in cells of the SA node is faster than in all other cells of the heart. As a result, the SA node discharges first and determines heart rate. Hence, the SA node is referred to as the cardiac *pacemaker.*

As shown in Fig. 49.2B, two classes of drugs (beta blockers and calcium channel blockers) can suppress phase 4 depolarization. By doing so, these agents can decrease automaticity in the SA node.

The Electrocardiogram

The ECG provides a graphic representation of cardiac electrical activity. The ECG can be used to identify dysrhythmias and monitor responses to therapy. (*Note:* In referring to the electrocardiogram, two abbreviations may be used: EKG and ECG.)

The major components of an ECG are shown in Fig. 49.3. As we can see, three features are especially prominent: the P wave, the QRS complex, and the T wave. The P wave is caused by *depolarization in the atria.* Therefore, the P wave corresponds to atrial contraction. The QRS complex is caused by *depolarization of the ventricles,* so the QRS complex corresponds to ventricular contraction. If conduction through the ventricles is slowed, the QRS complex will widen. The T wave is caused by *repolarization of the ventricles,* so this wave is not associated with overt physical activity of the heart.

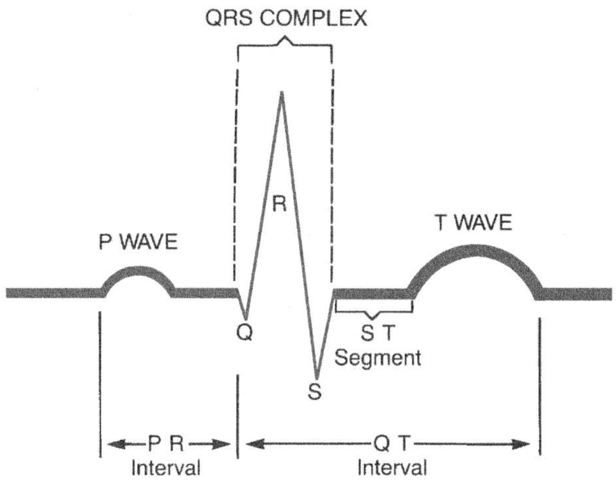

Fig. 49.3 ■ The electrocardiogram.

In addition to the features just described, the ECG has three other components of interest: the PR interval, the QT interval, and the ST segment. The PR interval is defined as the time between the onset of the P wave and the onset of the QRS complex. Lengthening of this interval indicates a delay in conduction through the AV node. Several drugs increase the PR interval. The QT interval is defined as the time between the onset of the QRS complex and completion of the T wave. This interval is prolonged by drugs that delay ventricular repolarization. The ST segment is the portion of the ECG that lies between the end of the QRS complex and the beginning of the T wave. Digoxin depresses the ST segment.

GENERATION OF DYSRHYTHMIAS

Dysrhythmias arise from two fundamental causes: *disturbances of impulse formation* (automaticity) and *disturbances of impulse conduction.* One or both of these disturbances underlie all dysrhythmias. Factors that may alter automaticity or conduction include hypoxia, electrolyte imbalance, cardiac surgery, reduced coronary blood flow, myocardial infarction, and antidysrhythmic drugs.

Disturbances of Automaticity

Disturbances of automaticity can occur in any part of the heart. Cells normally capable of automaticity (cells of the SA node, AV node, and His-Purkinje system) can produce dysrhythmias if their normal rate of discharge changes. In addition, dysrhythmias may be produced if tissues that do not normally express automaticity (atrial and ventricular muscle) develop spontaneous phase 4 depolarization.

Altered automaticity in the SA node can produce tachycardia or bradycardia. Excessive discharge of sympathetic neurons that innervate the SA node can augment automaticity to such a degree that sinus tachycardia results. Excessive vagal (parasympathetic) discharge can suppress automaticity to such a degree that sinus bradycardia results.

Increased automaticity of Purkinje fibers is a common cause of dysrhythmias. The increase can be brought on by injury and by excessive stimulation of Purkinje fibers by the sympathetic nervous system. If Purkinje fibers begin to discharge faster than the SA node, they will escape control by the SA node; potentially serious dysrhythmias can result.

Under special conditions, automaticity may develop in cells of atrial and ventricular muscle. If these cells fire faster than the SA node, dysrhythmias will result.

PATIENT-CENTERED CARE ACROSS THE LIFE SPAN

Antidysrhythmic Drugs

Life Stage	Patient Care Concerns
Infants	See "Breast-feeding women," below.
Children/adolescents	Some antidysrhythmic drugs can be used safely in children, just in smaller doses. These include disopyramide, flecainide, and sotalol. Side effect profiles are similar to those of adults.
Pregnant women	Many of the drugs discussed in this chapter are classified in FDA Pregnancy Risk Category C or D.[a] Animal studies show adverse fetal effects, and in Category D,[a] there is evidence of human fetal risk. Benefits should outweigh the risks. Dronedarone is classified in Pregnancy Risk Category X.[a]
Breast-feeding women	For most of the drugs discussed in this chapter, data are lacking regarding transmission of drug from mother to infant via breast milk. Breast-feeding is contraindicated in women taking dronedarone.
Older adults	Aging alters the absorption, distribution, metabolism, and elimination of antidysrhythmic drugs. Liver and kidney function must be monitored, and antiarrhythmic dosing may need to be adjusted for age. Older adult patients are also more susceptible to the side effects of many antidysrhythmics, including bradycardia, orthostatic hypotension, urinary retention, and falls.

[a]As of 2020, the FDA will no longer use Pregnancy Risk Categories. Please refer to Chapter 9 for more information.

Disturbances of Conduction

Atrioventricular Block

Impaired conduction through the AV node produces varying degrees of AV block. If impulse conduction is delayed (but not prevented entirely), the block is termed *first degree.* If some impulses pass through the node but others do not, the block is termed *second degree.* If all traffic through the AV node stops, the block is termed *third degree.*

Reentry (Recirculating Activation)

Reentry, also referred to as recirculating activation, is a generalized mechanism by which dysrhythmias can be produced. Reentry causes dysrhythmias by establishing a localized, self-sustaining circuit capable of repetitive cardiac stimulation. Reentry results from a unique form of conduction disturbance. The mechanism of reentrant activation and the effects of drugs on this process are described here.

In normal impulse conduction, electrical impulses travel down both branches of the Purkinje fiber to cause excitation of the muscle at two locations (Fig. 49.4A). Impulses created within the muscle travel in both directions (to the right and to the left) away from their sites of origin. Those impulses that are moving toward each other meet midway between the two branches of the Purkinje fiber. Since in the wake of both impulses the muscle is in a refractory state, neither impulse can proceed further, so both impulses stop.

In a reentrant circuit (Fig. 49.4B), there is a region of one-way conduction block of one branch of the Purkinje fiber. This region prevents conduction of impulses downward (toward the muscle) but does not prevent impulses from traveling upward. (Impulses can travel back up the block because impulses in muscle are very strong, and hence are able to pass the block, whereas impulses in the Purkinje fiber are weaker, and so are unable to pass.) A region of one-way block is essential for reentrant activation.

How does one-way block lead to reentrant activation? As an impulse travels down the Purkinje fiber, it is blocked in one branch but continues unimpeded in the other branch. Upon reaching the tip of the second (unblocked) branch, the impulse stimulates the muscle. As previously described, the impulse in the muscle travels to the right and to the left away from its site of origin. However, in this new situation, as the impulse travels toward the impaired branch of the Purkinje fiber, it meets no impulse coming from the other direction and continues on, resulting in stimulation of the terminal end of the first (blocked) branch. This stimulation causes an impulse to travel backward up the blocked branch of the Purkinje fiber. Since blockade of conduction in that branch is one way (downward only), the impulse can pass upward through the region of block and then back down into the unblocked branch, causing reentrant activation of this branch. Under proper conditions, the impulse will continue to cycle indefinitely, resulting in repetitive ectopic beats.

There are two mechanisms by which drugs can abolish a reentrant dysrhythmia. First, drugs can improve conduction in the sick branch of the Purkinje fiber and can thereby eliminate the one-way block (Fig. 49.4C). Alternatively, drugs can suppress conduction in the sick branch, thereby converting one-way block into two-way block (Fig. 49.4D).

CLASSIFICATION OF ANTIDYSRHYTHMIC DRUGS

According to the Vaughan Williams classification scheme, the antidysrhythmic drugs fall into five groups (Table 49.1). There are four major classes of antidysrhythmic drugs (classes I, II, III, and IV) and a fifth group that includes adenosine and digoxin. Membership in classes I through IV is determined by the effects on ion movements during slow and fast potentials (see Fig. 49.2).

Class I: Sodium Channel Blockers

Class I drugs block cardiac sodium channels (see Fig. 49.2A). By doing so, these drugs slow impulse conduction in the atria, ventricles, and His-Purkinje system. Class I constitutes the largest group of antidysrhythmic drugs.

Class II: Beta Blockers

Class II consists of beta-adrenergic blocking agents. As suggested by Fig. 49.2, these drugs reduce calcium entry (during fast and slow potentials), and they depress phase 4 depolarization (in slow potentials only). Beta blockers have three prominent effects on the heart:

- In the SA node, they reduce automaticity.
- In the AV node, they slow conduction velocity.
- In the atria and ventricles, they reduce contractility.

Cardiac effects of the beta blockers are nearly identical to those of the calcium channel blockers.

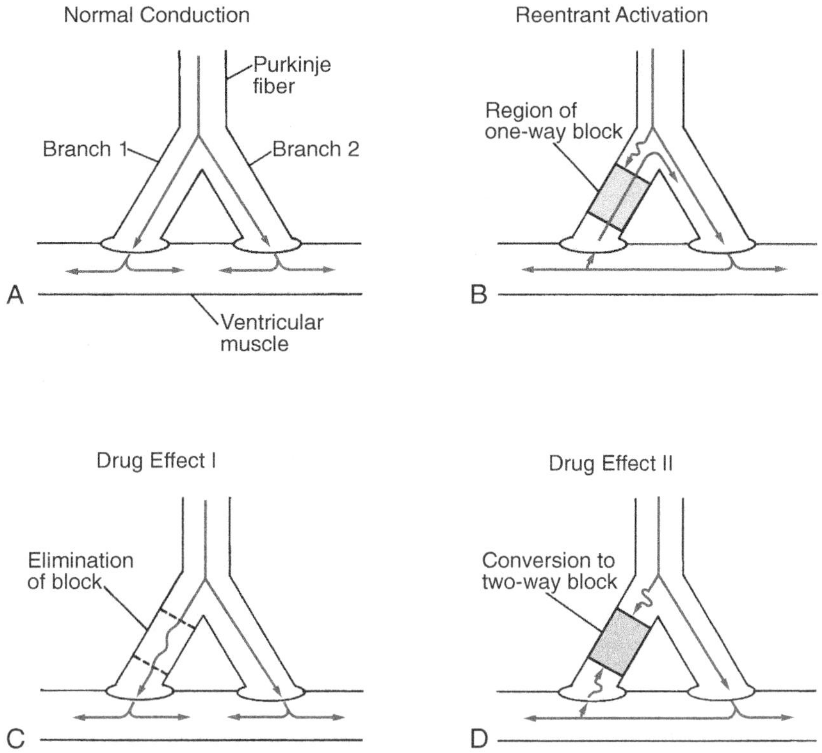

Fig. 49.4 ■ Reentrant activation: mechanism and drug effects.
A, In normal conduction, impulses from the branched Purkinje fiber stimulate the strip of ventricular muscle in two places. Within the muscle, waves of excitation spread from both points of excitation, meet between the Purkinje fibers, and cease further travel. **B,** In the presence of one-way block, the strip of muscle is excited at only one location. Impulses spreading from this area meet no impulses coming from the left and, therefore, can travel far enough to stimulate branch 1 of the Purkinje fiber. This stimulation passes back up the fiber, past the region of one-way block, and then stimulates branch 2, causing reentrant activation. **C,** Elimination of reentry by a drug that improves conduction in the sick branch of the Purkinje fiber. **D,** Elimination of reentry by a drug that further suppresses conduction in the sick branch, thereby converting one-way block into two-way block.

Class III: Potassium Channel Blockers (Drugs That Delay Repolarization)

Class III drugs block potassium channels (see Fig. 49.2A) and thereby delay repolarization of fast potentials. By delaying repolarization, these drugs prolong both the action potential duration and the effective refractory period.

Class IV: Calcium Channel Blockers

Only two calcium channel blockers—verapamil and diltiazem—are employed as antidysrhythmics. As indicated in Fig. 49.2, calcium channel blockade has the same impact on cardiac action potentials as does beta blockade. Accordingly, verapamil, diltiazem, and beta blockers have nearly identical effects on cardiac function—namely, reduction of automaticity in the SA node, delay of conduction through the AV node, and reduction of myocardial contractility. Antidysrhythmic benefits derive from suppressing AV nodal conduction.

Other Antidysrhythmic Drugs

Adenosine and digoxin do not fit into the four major classes of antidysrhythmic drugs. Both drugs suppress dysrhythmias by decreasing conduction through the AV node and reducing automaticity in the SA node.

PRODYSRHYTHMIC EFFECTS OF ANTIDYSRHYTHMIC DRUGS

Virtually all of the drugs used to treat dysrhythmias have prodysrhythmic (proarrhythmic) effects. That is, *all of these drugs can worsen existing dysrhythmias and generate new ones.* This ability was documented dramatically in the Cardiac Arrhythmia Suppression Trial (CAST), in which use of class IC drugs (encainide and flecainide) to prevent dysrhythmias after myocardial infarction actually *doubled the rate of mortality.* Because of their prodysrhythmic actions, antidysrhythmic drugs should be used only when dysrhythmias are symptomatically significant and only when the potential benefits clearly outweigh the risks. Applying this guideline, it would be inappropriate to give antidysrhythmic drugs to a patient with nonsustained ventricular tachycardia, since this dysrhythmia does not significantly reduce cardiac output. Conversely, when a patient is facing death from ventricular fibrillation, any therapy that might work must be tried. In this case, the risk of prodysrhythmic

TABLE 49.1 ■ Vaughan Williams Classification of Antidysrhythmic Drugs

CLASS I: SODIUM CHANNEL BLOCKERS
Class IA
Quinidine
Procainamide [Procan ♣, generic in United States]
Disopyramide [Norpace, Norpace CR]
Class IB
Lidocaine [Xylocaine]
Phenytoin [Dilantin]
Mexiletine
Class IC
Flecainide
Propafenone [Rythmol, Rythmol SR]
CLASS II: BETA BLOCKERS
Propranolol [Inderal LA]
Acebutolol [Sectral]
Esmolol [Brevibloc]
CLASS III: POTASSIUM CHANNEL BLOCKERS (DRUGS THAT DELAY REPOLARIZATION)
Amiodarone [Cordarone, Pacerone]
Dronedarone [Multaq]
Sotalol [Betapace, Betapace AF]
Dofetilide [Tikosyn]
Ibutilide [Corvert]
CLASS IV: CALCIUM CHANNEL BLOCKERS
Verapamil [Calan, Covera-HS, Verelan]
Diltiazem [Cardizem, Dilacor-XR, Tiazac, others]
OTHER ANTIDYSRHYTHMIC DRUGS
Adenosine [Adenocard]
Digoxin [Lanoxin]

Safety Alert

ANTIDYSRHYTHMIC DRUGS

All of these drugs can worsen existing dysrhythmias and generate new ones. Regardless of the particular circumstances of drug use, all patients must be followed closely.

Of the mechanisms by which drugs can cause dysrhythmias, one deserves special mention: prolongation of the QT interval. As discussed in Chapter 7, drugs that prolong the QT interval increase the risk of *torsades de pointes,* a dysrhythmia that can progress to fatal ventricular fibrillation. All class IA and class III agents cause QT prolongation, and so must be used with special caution.

effects is clearly outweighed by the potential benefits of stopping the fibrillation.

OVERVIEW OF COMMON DYSRHYTHMIAS AND THEIR TREATMENT

The common dysrhythmias can be divided into two major groups: *supraventricular dysrhythmias* and *ventricular dysrhythmias.* In general, ventricular dysrhythmias are more dangerous than supraventricular dysrhythmias. With either type, intervention is required only if the dysrhythmia interferes with effective ventricular pumping. Treatment often proceeds in two phases: (1) *termination* of the dysrhythmia (with electrical countershock, drugs, or both), followed by (2) *long-term suppression* with drugs. Dysrhythmias can also be treated with an implantable cardioverter-defibrillator (ICD) or by destroying small areas of cardiac tissue using radiofrequency (RF) catheter ablation.

It is important to appreciate that drug therapy of dysrhythmias is highly empiric (i.e., based largely on the response of the patient and not on scientific principles). In practice, this means that even after a dysrhythmia has been identified, we cannot predict with certainty just which drugs will be effective. Frequently, trials with several drugs are required before the control of rhythm is achieved. In the discussion that follows, only first-choice drugs are considered.

Supraventricular Dysrhythmias

Supraventricular dysrhythmias are dysrhythmias that arise in areas of the heart above the ventricles (atria, SA node, AV node). Supraventricular dysrhythmias per se are not especially harmful because dysrhythmic activity within the atria does not significantly reduce cardiac output (except in patients with valvular disorders and heart failure [HF]). Supraventricular tachydysrhythmias *can* be dangerous, however, in that atrial impulses are likely to traverse the AV node, resulting in excitation of the ventricles. If the atria drive the ventricles at an excessive rate, diastolic filling will be incomplete and cardiac output will decline. Hence, when treating supraventricular tachydysrhythmias, the objective is frequently the slowing of ventricular rate (by blocking impulse conduction through the AV node) and not elimination of the dysrhythmia itself. Of course, if treatment did abolish the dysrhythmia, this outcome would not be unwelcome. Acute treatment of supraventricular dysrhythmias is accomplished with vagotonic maneuvers, direct-current (DC) cardioversion, and certain drugs: class II agents, class IV agents, adenosine, and digoxin.

Atrial Fibrillation

Atrial fibrillation is the most common sustained dysrhythmia, affecting about 4 million people in the United States. The disorder is caused by multiple atrial ectopic foci firing randomly; each focus stimulates a small area of atrial muscle. This chaotic excitation produces a highly irregular atrial rhythm. Depending upon the extent of impulse transmission through the AV node, ventricular rate may be very rapid or nearly normal.

In addition to compromising cardiac performance, atrial fibrillation carries a high risk of stroke because, in patients with atrial fibrillation, some blood can become trapped in the atria (rather than flowing straight through to the ventricles), thereby permitting formation of a clot. When normal sinus rhythm is restored, the clot may become dislodged; then it may travel to the brain to cause stroke.

Treatment of atrial fibrillation has two goals: improvement of ventricular pumping and prevention of stroke. Pumping can be improved by either (1) restoring normal sinus rhythm or (2) slowing ventricular rate. The preferred method is to slow ventricular rate by *long-term* therapy with a beta blocker (atenolol or metoprolol) or a cardioselective calcium channel blocker (diltiazem or verapamil), both of which impede conduction through the AV node. For patients who elect to restore normal rhythm, options are DC cardioversion, short-term treatment with drugs (e.g., amiodarone, sotalol), or RF ablation of the dysrhythmia source.

To prevent stroke, patients are treated with warfarin or newer anticoagulants. For those undergoing treatment to restore normal sinus rhythm, warfarin should be taken for 3 weeks before the procedure and for 4 weeks after. For those taking an antidysrhythmic drug long term to control ventricular rate, warfarin must be taken long term too. Alternatives to warfarin include four oral anticoagulants (apixaban [Eliquis], dabigatran [Pradaxa], edoxaban [Savaysa], and rivaroxaban [Xarelto]) and antiplatelet drugs (aspirin alone or aspirin plus clopidogrel).

Atrial Flutter

Atrial flutter is caused by an ectopic atrial focus discharging at a rate of 250 to 350 times a minute. Ventricular rate is considerably slower, however, because the AV node is unable to transmit impulses at this high rate. Typically, one atrial impulse out of two reaches the ventricles. The treatment of choice is DC cardioversion, which almost always converts atrial flutter to normal sinus rhythm. Cardioversion may also be achieved with IV ibutilide. To prevent the dysrhythmia from recurring, patients may need long-term therapy with drugs—either a class IC agent (flecainide or propafenone) or a class III agent (amiodarone, dronedarone, sotalol, dofetilide).

There are two alternatives to cardioversion: (1) RF ablation of the dysrhythmia focus and (2) control of ventricular rate with drugs. As with atrial fibrillation, ventricular rate is controlled with drugs that suppress AV conduction: verapamil, diltiazem, or a beta blocker.

Like atrial fibrillation, atrial flutter poses a risk of stroke, which can be reduced by treatment with anticoagulants.

Sustained Supraventricular Tachycardia (SVT)

Sustained SVT is usually caused by an AV nodal reentrant circuit. Heart rate is increased to 150 to 250 beats/min. SVT often responds to interventions that increase vagal tone, such as carotid sinus massage or the Valsalva maneuver. If these are ineffective, an IV beta blocker or calcium channel blocker can be tried. With these drugs, ventricular rate will be slowed even if the dysrhythmia persists. Once the dysrhythmia has been controlled, beta blockers and/or calcium channel blockers can be taken orally to prevent recurrence. As a last resort, amiodarone can be used for prevention.

Ventricular Dysrhythmias

In contrast to atrial dysrhythmias, which are generally benign, ventricular dysrhythmias can cause significant disruption of cardiac pumping. Accordingly, the usual objective is to abolish the dysrhythmia. Cardioversion is often the treatment of choice. When antidysrhythmic drugs are indicated, agents in class I or class III are usually employed.

Sustained Ventricular Tachycardia

Ventricular tachycardia arises from a single, rapidly firing ventricular ectopic focus, typically located at the border of an old infarction. The focus drives the ventricles at a rate of 150 to 250 beats/min. Because the ventricles cannot pump effectively at these rates, immediate intervention is required. Cardioversion is the treatment of choice. If cardioversion fails to normalize rhythm, IV procainamide should be administered; lidocaine and amiodarone are alternatives. For long-term management, drugs (e.g., sotalol, amiodarone) or an ICD may be employed.

Ventricular Fibrillation

Ventricular fibrillation is a life-threatening emergency that requires immediate treatment. This dysrhythmia results from the asynchronous discharge of multiple ventricular ectopic foci. Because many different foci are firing and because each focus initiates contraction in its immediate vicinity, localized twitching takes place all over the ventricles, making coordinated ventricular contraction impossible. As a result, the pumping action of the heart stops. In the absence of blood flow, the patient becomes unconscious and cyanotic. If heartbeat is not restored rapidly, death soon follows. Electrical countershock (defibrillation) is applied to eliminate fibrillation and restore cardiac function. Amiodarone can be used for acute and long-term suppression.

Premature Ventricular Complexes (PVCs)

PVCs are beats that occur before they should in the cardiac cycle. These beats are caused by ectopic ventricular foci. PVCs may arise from a single ectopic focus or from several foci. In the absence of additional signs of heart disease, PVCs are benign and not usually treated. However, in the presence of acute myocardial infarction, PVCs may predispose the patient to ventricular fibrillation. In this case, therapy is required. A beta blocker is the agent of choice.

Digoxin-Induced Ventricular Dysrhythmias

Digoxin toxicity can mimic practically all types of dysrhythmias. Varying degrees of AV block are among the most common. Ventricular flutter and ventricular fibrillation are the most dangerous. Digoxin causes dysrhythmias by increasing automaticity in the atria, ventricles, and His-Purkinje system, and by decreasing conduction through the AV node.

With proper treatment, digoxin-induced dysrhythmias can almost always be controlled. Treatment is discussed in Chapter 48. If antidysrhythmic drugs are required, lidocaine and phenytoin are the agents of choice. In patients with digoxin toxicity, DC cardioversion may bring on ventricular fibrillation. Accordingly, this procedure should be used only when absolutely required.

Torsades de Pointes

Torsades de pointes is an atypical, rapid, undulating ventricular tachydysrhythmia that can evolve into potentially fatal ventricular fibrillation. The main factor associated with development of torsades de pointes is prolongation of the QT interval, which can be caused by a variety of drugs, including class IA and class III antidysrhythmic agents. Acute management consists of IV magnesium plus cardioversion for sustained ventricular tachycardia.

PRINCIPLES OF ANTIDYSRHYTHMIC DRUG THERAPY

Balancing Risks and Benefits

Therapy with antidysrhythmic drugs is based on a simple but important concept: Treat only if there is a clear benefit—and then only if the benefit outweighs the risks. As a rule, this means that intervention is needed only when the dysrhythmia interferes with ventricular pumping.

Treatment offers two potential benefits: reduction of symptoms and reduction of mortality. Symptoms that can be reduced include palpitations, angina, dyspnea, and faintness. For most antidysrhythmic drugs, there is little or no evidence of reduced mortality. In fact, mortality may actually increase.

Antidysrhythmic therapy carries considerable risk. Because of their *prodysrhythmic actions,* antidysrhythmic drugs can exacerbate existing dysrhythmias and generate new ones. Examples abound: Toxic doses of digoxin can generate a wide variety of dysrhythmias; drugs that prolong the QT interval can cause torsades de pointes; many drugs can cause ventricular ectopic beats; several drugs (quinidine, flecainide, propafenone) can cause atrial flutter; and one drug—flecainide—can produce incessant ventricular tachycardia. Because of their prodysrhythmic actions, antidysrhythmic drugs can *increase mortality.* Other adverse effects include HF and third-degree AV block (caused by calcium channel blockers and beta blockers), as well as many noncardiac effects, including severe diarrhea (quinidine), a lupus-like syndrome (procainamide), and pulmonary toxicity (amiodarone).

Properties of the Dysrhythmia to Be Considered

Sustained Versus Nonsustained Dysrhythmias

As a rule, nonsustained dysrhythmias require intervention only when they are symptomatic; in the absence of symptoms, treatment is usually unnecessary. In contrast, sustained dysrhythmias can be dangerous; therefore, the benefits of treatment generally outweigh the risks.

Asymptomatic Versus Symptomatic Dysrhythmias

No study has demonstrated a benefit to treating dysrhythmias that are asymptomatic or minimally symptomatic. In contrast, therapy may be beneficial for dysrhythmias that produce symptoms (palpitations, angina, dyspnea, faintness).

Supraventricular Versus Ventricular Dysrhythmias

Supraventricular dysrhythmias are generally benign. The primary harm comes from driving the ventricles too rapidly to allow adequate filling. The goal of treatment is to either (1) terminate the dysrhythmia or (2) prevent excessive atrial beats from reaching the ventricles (using a beta blocker, calcium channel blocker, or digoxin). In contrast to supraventricular dysrhythmias, ventricular dysrhythmias frequently interfere with pumping. Accordingly, the goal of treatment is to terminate the dysrhythmia and prevent its recurrence.

Phases of Treatment

Treatment has two phases: acute and long term. The goal of acute treatment is to terminate the dysrhythmia. For many dysrhythmias, termination is accomplished with DC cardioversion (electrical countershock) or vagotonic maneuvers (e.g., carotid sinus massage) rather than drugs. The goal of long-term therapy is to prevent dysrhythmias from recurring. Quite often, the risks of long-term prophylactic therapy outweigh the benefits.

Long-Term Treatment: Drug Selection and Evaluation

Selecting a drug for long-term therapy is largely empiric. There are many drugs that might be employed, and we usually can't predict which one is going to work. Therefore, finding an effective drug is done by trial and error.

Drug selection can be aided with electrophysiologic testing. In these tests, a dysrhythmia is generated artificially by programmed electrical stimulation of the heart. If a candidate drug is able to suppress the electrophysiologically induced dysrhythmia, it may also work against the real thing.

Holter monitoring can be used to evaluate treatment. A Holter monitor is a portable ECG device that is worn by the patient around-the-clock. If Holter monitoring indicates that dysrhythmias are still occurring with the present drug, a different drug should be tried.

Minimizing Risks

Several measures can help minimize risk. These include:

- Starting with low doses and increasing them gradually.
- Using a Holter monitor during initial therapy to detect danger signs—especially QT prolongation, which can precede torsades de pointes.
- Monitoring plasma drug levels. Unfortunately, although drug levels can be good predictors of noncardiac toxicity (e.g., quinidine-induced nausea), they are less helpful for predicting adverse cardiac effects.

PHARMACOLOGY OF THE ANTIDYSRHYTHMIC DRUGS

As discussed earlier in this chapter, the antidysrhythmic drugs fall into four main groups—classes I, II, III, and IV—plus a fifth group that includes adenosine and digoxin. The pharmacology of these drugs is presented here and in Table 49.2.

CLASS I: SODIUM CHANNEL BLOCKERS

Class I antidysrhythmic drugs block cardiac sodium channels. By doing so, they decrease conduction velocity in the atria, ventricles, and His-Purkinje system.

There are three subgroups of class I agents. Drugs in all three groups block sodium channels. In addition, class IA agents delay repolarization, whereas class IB agents accelerate repolarization. Class IC agents have pronounced prodysrhythmic actions.

The class I drugs are similar in action and structure to the local anesthetics. In fact, one of these drugs—lidocaine—has both local anesthetic and antidysrhythmic applications.

Class IA Agents

Quinidine

Quinidine is the oldest, best studied, and most widely used class IA drug. Accordingly, quinidine will serve as our prototype for the group. Like other antidysrhythmic agents, quinidine has prodysrhythmic actions.

TABLE 49.2 ▪ Properties of Antidysrhythmic Drugs

Drug	Usual Route	Effects on the ECG	Major Antidysrhythmic Applications
CLASS IA			
Quinidine	PO	Widens QRS, prolongs QT	Broad spectrum: used for long-term suppression of ventricular and supraventricular dysrhythmias
Procainamide	PO	Widens QRS, prolongs QT	Broad spectrum: similar to quinidine, but toxicity makes it less desirable for long-term use
Disopyramide	PO	Widens QRS, prolongs QT	Ventricular dysrhythmias
CLASS IB			
Lidocaine	IV	No significant change	Ventricular dysrhythmias
Phenytoin	PO	No significant change	Digoxin-induced ventricular dysrhythmias
Mexiletine	PO	No significant change	Ventricular dysrhythmias
CLASS IC			
Flecainide	PO	Widens QRS, prolongs PR	Maintenance therapy of supraventricular dysrhythmias
Propafenone	PO	Widens QRS, prolongs PR	Maintenance therapy of supraventricular dysrhythmias
CLASS II			
Propranolol	PO	Prolongs PR, bradycardia	Dysrhythmias caused by excessive sympathetic activity; control of ventricular rate in patients with supraventricular tachydysrhythmias
Acebutolol	PO	Prolongs PR, bradycardia	Premature ventricular beats
Esmolol	IV	Prolongs PR, bradycardia	Control of ventricular rate in patients with supraventricular tachydysrhythmias
CLASS III			
Amiodarone	PO, IV	Prolongs QT and PR, widens QRS	Life-threatening ventricular dysrhythmias, atrial fibrillation[a]
Dronedarone	PO	Prolongs QT and PR, widens QRS	Atrial flutter, atrial fibrillation
Sotalol	PO, IV	Prolongs QT and PR, bradycardia	Life-threatening ventricular dysrhythmias, atrial fibrillation/flutter
Dofetilide	PO	Prolongs QT	Highly symptomatic atrial dysrhythmias
Ibutilide	IV	Prolongs QT	Atrial flutter, atrial fibrillation
CLASS IV			
Verapamil	PO	Prolongs PR, bradycardia	Control of ventricular rate in patients with supraventricular tachydysrhythmias
Diltiazem	IV	Prolongs PR, bradycardia	Same as verapamil
OTHERS			
Adenosine	IV	Prolongs PR	Termination of paroxysmal supraventricular tachycardia
Digoxin	PO, IV	Prolongs PR, depresses ST	Control of ventricular rate in patients with supraventricular tachydysrhythmias

[a]Amiodarone is widely used for atrial fibrillation, but it is not approved for this use.

Prototype Drugs

ANTIDYSRHYTHMIC DRUGS

Class I: Sodium Channel Blockers

Quinidine (class IA)
Lidocaine (class IB)

Class II: Beta Blockers

Propranolol

Class III: Drugs That Delay Repolarization

Amiodarone

Class IV: Calcium Channel Blockers

Verapamil

Others

Adenosine
Digoxin

Chemistry and Source. Quinidine is similar to quinine in structure and actions. The natural source of both drugs is the bark of the South American cinchona tree. Accordingly, these agents are referred to as *cinchona alkaloids.* Like quinine, quinidine has antimalarial and antipyretic properties.

Effects on the Heart. By blocking sodium channels, quinidine *slows impulse conduction* in the atria, ventricles, and His-Purkinje system. In addition, the drug *delays repolarization* at these sites, apparently by blocking potassium channels. Both actions contribute to suppression of dysrhythmias.

Quinidine is strongly *anticholinergic* (atropine-like) and blocks vagal input to the heart. The resultant *increase* in SA nodal automaticity and AV conduction can drive the ventricles at an excessive rate. To prevent excessive ventricular stimulation, patients are usually pretreated with digoxin, verapamil, or a beta blocker, all of which suppress AV conduction.

TABLE 49.3 ▪ Pharmacokinetic Properties of Antidysrhythmic Drugs

Drug	Usual Route	Peak (hr)	Half-Life (hr)	Metabolism	Excretion
Quinidine	PO	0.5–1.5	6–8	Hepatic	Renal
Procainamide [Procan 🍁]	IV	—	3–4	Hepatic	Renal
Lidocaine [Xylocaine]	IV	—	1.5–2	Hepatic	Renal
Amiodarone	PO	—	600–2640	Hepatic	Gastrointestinal (bile)
Dronedarone [Multaq]	PO	3–6	13–19	Hepatic	Gastrointestinal (feces)
Dofetilide [Tikosyn]	PO	2–3	10	Hepatic (minor)	Renal

Effects on the ECG. Quinidine has two pronounced effects on the ECG. The drug *widens the QRS complex* (by slowing depolarization of the ventricles) and *prolongs the QT interval* (by delaying ventricular repolarization).

Therapeutic Uses. Quinidine is a broad-spectrum agent active against *supraventricular* and *ventricular dysrhythmias.* The drug's principal indication is long-term suppression of dysrhythmias, including SVT, atrial flutter, atrial fibrillation, and sustained ventricular tachycardia. An analysis of older studies indicates that quinidine may actually *increase* mortality in patients with *atrial flutter* and *atrial fibrillation.*

In addition to its antidysrhythmic applications, quinidine is a drug of choice for severe *malaria* (see Chapter 98). The pharmacokinetics of quinidine and other antidysrhythmics can be found in Table 49.3.

Adverse Effects

Diarrhea. Diarrhea and other GI symptoms develop in about 33% of patients. These reactions can be immediate and intense, frequently forcing discontinuation of treatment. Gastric upset can be reduced by administering quinidine with food.

Cinchonism. Cinchonism is characterized by tinnitus (ringing in the ears), headache, nausea, vertigo, and disturbed vision. These can develop with just one dose.

Cardiotoxicity. At high concentrations, quinidine can cause severe cardiotoxicity (sinus arrest, AV block, ventricular tachydysrhythmias, asystole). These reactions occur secondary to increased automaticity of Purkinje fibers and reduced conduction throughout all regions of the heart.

As cardiotoxicity develops, the ECG changes. Important danger signals are *widening of the QRS complex* (by 50% or more) and *excessive prolongation of the QT interval.* Notify the prescriber immediately if these changes occur.

Arterial Embolism. Embolism is a potential complication of treating atrial *fibrillation.* During atrial fibrillation, thrombi may form in the atria. When sinus rhythm is restored, these thrombi may be dislodged and cause embolism. To reduce the risk of embolism, anticoagulant therapy is given for 3 to 4 weeks before quinidine and is maintained for an additional 4 weeks. Signs of embolism (e.g., sudden chest pain, dyspnea) should be reported immediately.

Other Adverse Effects. Quinidine can cause alpha-adrenergic blockade, resulting in vasodilation and subsequent *hypotension.* This reaction is much more serious with IV therapy than with oral therapy. Rarely, quinidine has caused *hypersensitivity reactions,* including fever, anaphylactic reactions, and thrombocytopenia.

Drug Interactions

Digoxin. Quinidine can double digoxin levels. The increase is caused by displacing digoxin from plasma albumin and by decreasing digoxin elimination. When these drugs are used concurrently, digoxin dosage must be reduced. Also, patients should be monitored closely for digoxin toxicity (dysrhythmias). Because of its interaction with digoxin, quinidine is a last-choice drug for treating digoxin-induced dysrhythmias.

Other Interactions. Because of its anticholinergic actions, quinidine can intensify the effects of other atropine-like drugs; one possible result is excessive tachycardia. Phenobarbital, phenytoin, and other drugs that induce hepatic drug metabolism can shorten the half-life of quinidine by as much as 50%. Quinidine can intensify the effects of warfarin by an unknown mechanism.

Preparations, Dosage, and Administration

Preparations. Quinidine is available as two salts: *quinidine sulfate* and *quinidine gluconate.* Because these salts have different molecular weights, equal doses (on a milligram basis) do not provide equal amounts of quinidine. A 200-mg dose of quinidine sulfate is equivalent to 275 mg of quinidine gluconate. Quinidine sulfate is available in immediate-release tablets (200 and 300 mg) and extended-release tablets (300 mg). Quinidine gluconate is available in sustained-release tablets (324 mg) and in solution (80 mg/mL) for parenteral use.

Dosage. The usual dosage of quinidine sulfate is 200 to 400 mg every 6 hours. The usual dosage of quinidine gluconate is 324 to 648 mg every 8 to 12 hours. Dosage is adjusted to produce plasma quinidine levels between 2 and 5 mcg/mL.

Administration. Quinidine is almost always administered by mouth. Intramuscular administration is painful and produces erratic absorption. Intravenous injection carries a high risk of adverse cardiovascular reactions; therefore, continuous cardiovascular monitoring is required.

Procainamide

Procainamide [Procan 🍁] is similar to quinidine in actions and uses. Like quinidine, procainamide is active against a broad spectrum of dysrhythmias. Unfortunately, serious side effects frequently limit its use.

Effects on the Heart and ECG. Like quinidine, procainamide blocks cardiac sodium channels, thereby decreasing conduction velocity in the atria, ventricles, and His-Purkinje system. Also, the drug delays repolarization. In contrast to quinidine, procainamide is only weakly anticholinergic, and hence is not likely to increase ventricular rate. Effects on the ECG are the same as with quinidine: widening of the QRS complex and prolongation of the QT interval.

Therapeutic Uses. Procainamide is effective against a broad spectrum of atrial and ventricular dysrhythmias. Like quinidine, the drug can be used for long-term suppression. However, since prolonged therapy is often associated with serious adverse effects, procainamide is less desirable than quinidine for long-term use. In contrast to quinidine, procainamide can be used to terminate ventricular tachycardia and ventricular fibrillation.

Adverse Effects

Systemic Lupus Erythematosus–Like Syndrome. Prolonged treatment with procainamide is associated with severe immunologic reactions. Within a year, about 70% of patients develop antinuclear antibodies (ANAs)—antibodies directed against the patient's own nucleic acids. If procainamide is continued, between 20% and 30% of patients with ANAs go on to develop symptoms resembling those of systemic lupus erythematosus (SLE). These symptoms include pain and inflammation of the joints, pericarditis, fever, and hepatomegaly. When procainamide is withdrawn, symptoms usually slowly subside. If the patient has a life-threatening dysrhythmia for which no alternative drug is available, procainamide can be continued and the symptoms of SLE controlled with a nonsteroidal anti-inflammatory drug (e.g., aspirin) or a glucocorticoid. All patients taking procainamide chronically should be tested for ANAs. If the ANA titer rises, discontinuation of treatment should be considered.

Blood Dyscrasias. About 0.5% of patients develop blood dyscrasias, including neutropenia, thrombocytopenia, and agranulocytosis. Fatalities have occurred. These reactions usually develop during the first 12 weeks of treatment. Complete blood counts should be obtained weekly during this time and periodically thereafter. Also, complete blood counts should be obtained promptly at the first sign of infection, bruising, or bleeding. If blood counts indicate bone marrow suppression, procainamide should be withdrawn. Hematologic status usually returns to baseline within 1 month.

Cardiotoxicity. Procainamide has cardiotoxic actions like those of quinidine. Warning signs are QRS widening (more than 50%) and excessive QT prolongation. If these develop, the drug should be withheld and the prescriber informed.

Other Adverse Effects. Like quinidine, procainamide can cause *GI symptoms* and *hypotension.* However, these are much less prominent than with quinidine. Procainamide is a derivative of procaine (a local anesthetic); therefore, its use is contraindicated in patients with a history of procaine allergy. As with quinidine, *arterial embolism* may occur during treatment of atrial fibrillation.

Preparations, Dosage, and Administration

Oral. Procainamide is available in capsules (250, 375, and 500 mg) and sustained-release tablets (250, 500, and 750 mg) in Canada. The usual maintenance dosage is 50 mg/kg/day in divided doses. The capsules are administered every 3 to 4 hours and the sustained-release tablets every 6 hours. Dosage is adjusted to maintain plasma drug levels between 4 and 8 mcg/mL.

Parenteral. Procainamide is available in solution (100 and 500 mg/mL) for IM and IV administration. Intramuscular injection is made deep into the gluteal muscle; dosage is 0.5 to 1 gm repeated every 4 to 8 hours.

Intravenous infusion may be performed at an initial rate of 20 to 50 mg/min (maximal loading dose is 1500 mg). After the loading period, an infusion rate of 2 to 6 mg/min should be employed. Once the dysrhythmia has been controlled, the patient should be switched to oral procainamide. Three hours should elapse between terminating the infusion and the first oral dose.

Disopyramide

Disopyramide [Norpace, Norpace CR] is a class I drug with actions like those of quinidine. However, because of prominent side effects, indications for disopyramide are limited.

Effects on the Heart and ECG. Cardiac effects are similar to those of quinidine. By blocking sodium channels, disopyramide decreases conduction velocity in the atria, ventricles, and His-Purkinje system. In addition, the drug delays repolarization. Anticholinergic actions are greater than those of quinidine. In contrast to quinidine, disopyramide causes a pronounced reduction in contractility. Like quinidine, disopyramide widens the QRS complex and prolongs the QT interval.

Adverse Effects. *Anticholinergic responses* are most common. These include dry mouth, blurred vision, constipation, and urinary hesitancy or retention. Urinary retention frequently requires discontinuation of treatment.

Because of its negative inotropic effects, disopyramide can cause *severe hypotension* (secondary to reduced cardiac output) and can *exacerbate heart failure.* The drug should not be administered to patients with HF or to patients taking a beta blocker. Whenever disopyramide is used, pressor drugs should be immediately available.

Therapeutic Uses. Disopyramide is indicated only for ventricular dysrhythmias (PVCs, ventricular tachycardia, ventricular fibrillation). The drug is reserved for patients who cannot tolerate safer medications (e.g., quinidine, procainamide).

Preparations, Dosage, and Administration. Disopyramide [Norpace, Norpace CR] is available in immediate- and extended-release capsules (100 and 150 mg). An initial loading dose (200 to 300 mg) is followed by maintenance doses (100 to 200 mg) every 6 hours.

Class IB Agents

As a group, class IB agents differ from quinidine and the other class IA agents in two respects: (1) whereas class IA agents *delay* repolarization, class IB agents *accelerate* repolarization; and (2) class IB agents have little or no effect on the ECG.

Lidocaine

Lidocaine [Xylocaine], an intravenous agent, is used only for ventricular dysrhythmias. In addition to its antidysrhythmic applications, lidocaine is employed as a local anesthetic (see Chapter 26).

Effects on the Heart and ECG. Lidocaine has three significant effects on the heart: (1) like other class I drugs, lidocaine blocks cardiac sodium channels and thereby *slows conduction* in the atria, ventricles, and His-Purkinje system; (2) the drug *reduces automaticity* in the ventricles and His-Purkinje system by a mechanism that is poorly understood; and (3) lidocaine *accelerates repolarization* (shortens the action potential duration and ERP). In contrast to quinidine and procainamide, lidocaine is devoid of anticholinergic properties. Also, lidocaine has no significant impact on the ECG: A small reduction in the QT interval may occur, but there is no QRS widening.

Antidysrhythmic Use. Antidysrhythmic use of lidocaine is limited to short-term therapy of *ventricular dysrhythmias.* Lidocaine is not active against supraventricular dysrhythmias.

Adverse Effects. Lidocaine is generally well tolerated. However, adverse central nervous system (CNS) effects can occur. High therapeutic doses can cause *drowsiness, confusion,* and *paresthesias.* Toxic doses may produce *seizures* and *respiratory arrest.* Consequently, whenever lidocaine is used, equipment for resuscitation must be available. Seizures can be managed with diazepam.

Preparations, Dosage, and Administration. Administration is parenteral only. The usual route is IV. Intramuscular injection can be used in emergencies. Blood pressure and the ECG should be monitored for signs of toxicity.

Intravenous. Lidocaine [Xylocaine] preparations intended for IV administration are clearly labeled as such. They contain no preservatives or catecholamines. (Lidocaine used for local anesthesia frequently contains epinephrine.) Preparations that contain epinephrine or another catecholamine must never be administered IV, since doing so can cause severe hypertension and life-threatening dysrhythmias.

Intravenous therapy is initiated with a loading dose followed by continuous infusion for maintenance. The usual loading dose is 50 to 100 mg (1 mg/kg) administered at a rate of 25 to 50 mg/min. An infusion rate of 1 to 4 mg/min is used for maintenance; the rate is adjusted on the basis of cardiac response. Intravenous lidocaine should be discontinued as soon as possible, usually within 24 hours. Lidocaine for IV administration is supplied in concentrated and dilute formulations. The concentrated formulations must be diluted with 5% dextrose in water.

To avoid toxicity, dosage should be reduced in patients with impaired hepatic function or impaired hepatic blood flow (e.g., older adult patients; patients with cirrhosis, shock, or HF).

Phenytoin

Phenytoin is an antiseizure drug that is also used to treat digoxin-induced dysrhythmias. The basic pharmacology of phenytoin is shown in Chapter 24. Discussion here is limited to antidysrhythmic applications.

Effects on the Heart and ECG. Like lidocaine, phenytoin reduces automaticity (especially in the ventricles) and has little or no effect on the ECG. In contrast to lidocaine (and practically all other antidysrhythmic agents), phenytoin increases AV nodal conduction.

Pharmacokinetics. Phenytoin has two unfortunate kinetics properties. First, metabolism of the drug is subject to wide interpatient variation. Second, doses only slightly greater than therapeutic are likely to cause toxicity. Because of these characteristics, maintenance of therapeutic plasma levels (5 to 20 mcg/mL) is difficult.

Adverse Effects and Interactions. The most common adverse reactions are sedation, ataxia, and nystagmus. With too-rapid IV administration, phenytoin can cause hypotension, dysrhythmias, and cardiac arrest. Gingival hyperplasia is a frequent complication of long-term treatment. Phenytoin is subject to multiple undesirable drug interactions (see Chapter 24).

Antidysrhythmic Applications. Phenytoin has been used for digoxin-induced dysrhythmias and for acute and chronic suppression of ventricular dysrhythmias. The ability of phenytoin to increase AV nodal conduction can help counteract the reduction in AV conduction caused by digoxin intoxication. Phenytoin should not be used to treat atrial fibrillation or atrial flutter because enhanced AV conduction could increase the number of atrial impulses reaching the ventricles, thereby driving the ventricles at an excessive rate.

Dosage and Administration. Phenytoin can be given PO or IV. For PO therapy, a loading dose (14 mg/kg) is followed by daily maintenance doses (200 to 400 mg).

Intravenous dosing is reserved for severe acute dysrhythmias. Blood pressure and the ECG must be monitored continuously. Phenytoin is not soluble in water and must be diluted in the medium supplied by the manufacturer. This medium is highly alkaline (pH 12) and will cause phlebitis if given by continuous infusion. Consequently, dosing is by intermittent injections. Intravenous injections must be performed slowly (50 mg/min or less), because rapid injection can cause cardiovascular collapse. Treatment is begun with a series of loading doses (100 mg every 5 minutes until the dysrhythmia has been controlled or until a maximum dose of 20 mg/kg is reached). Maintenance dosages range from 200 to 400 mg/day.

Mexiletine

Mexiletine is an oral analog of lidocaine used for symptomatic ventricular dysrhythmias. Principal indications are PVCs and sustained ventricular tachycardia. Like lidocaine, mexiletine does not alter the ECG. The drug is eliminated by hepatic metabolism, so effects may be prolonged in patients with liver disease or reduced hepatic blood flow. The most common adverse effects are GI (nausea, vomiting, diarrhea, constipation) and neurologic (tremor, dizziness, sleep disturbances, psychosis, convulsions). About 40% of patients find these intolerable. Like other class I agents, mexiletine has prodysrhythmic properties. The initial dosage is 200 mg every 8 hours. The maintenance dosage is 200 to 300 mg every 8 hours. All doses should be taken with food.

Mexiletine is also used to alleviate persistent pain of diabetic neuropathy. Benefits derive from lidocaine-like anesthetic actions. Because mexiletine can *cause* dysrhythmias, it should not be used by diabetic patients with heart disease.

Class IC Agents

Class IC antidysrhythmics block cardiac sodium channels and thereby reduce conduction velocity in the atria, ventricles, and His-Purkinje system. In addition, these drugs delay ventricular repolarization, causing a small increase in the effective refractory period. All class IC agents can exacerbate existing dysrhythmias and create new ones. Currently, only two class IC agents are available: flecainide and propafenone.

Flecainide

Flecainide is active against a variety of ventricular and supraventricular dysrhythmias. However, use is restricted largely to maintenance therapy of supraventricular dysrhythmias. Like other class IC agents, flecainide decreases cardiac conduction and increases the effective refractory period. Prominent effects on the ECG are prolongation of the PR interval and widening of the QRS complex. Excessive QRS widening indicates a need for dosage reduction. Flecainide has prodysrhythmic effects. As a result, the drug can intensify existing dysrhythmias and provoke new ones. In patients with asymptomatic ventricular tachycardia associated with acute myocardial infarction, flecainide has caused a twofold increase in mortality. Flecainide decreases myocardial contractility and can thereby exacerbate or precipitate HF. Accordingly, the drug should not be combined with other agents that can decrease contractile force (e.g., beta blockers, verapamil, diltiazem). Elimination is by hepatic metabolism and renal excretion. Flecainide is available in tablets (50, 100, and 150 mg) for oral dosing. Dosage is low initially (50 to 100 mg every 12 hours) and then gradually increased to a maximum of 400 mg/day. Because of its potential for serious side effects, flecainide should be reserved for severe ventricular dysrhythmias that have not responded to safer drugs. Patients should be monitored closely.

Propafenone

Propafenone [Rythmol, Rythmol SR] is similar to flecainide in actions and uses. By blocking cardiac sodium channels, the drug decreases conduction velocity in the atria, ventricles, and His-Purkinje system. In addition, it causes a small increase in the ventricular ERP. Prominent effects on the ECG are QRS widening and PR prolongation. Like flecainide, propafenone has prodysrhythmic actions that can exacerbate existing dysrhythmias and create new ones. It is not known if propafenone, like flecainide, increases mortality in patients with asymptomatic ventricular dysrhythmias after myocardial infarction. Propafenone has beta-adrenergic blocking properties and can thereby decrease myocardial contractility and promote bronchospasm. Accordingly, the drug should be used with caution in patients with HF, AV block, or asthma. Noncardiac adverse effects are generally mild and include dizziness, altered taste, blurred vision, and GI symptoms (abdominal discomfort, anorexia, nausea, vomiting). Because of its prodysrhythmic actions, propafenone should be reserved for patients who have not responded to safer drugs. Propafenone is available in immediate-release tablets (150 and 225 mg) and extended-release capsules (225, 325, and 425 mg). For the immediate-release tablets, the dosage is 150 mg every 8 hours initially, and can be gradually increased to 300 mg every 8 hours. For the extended-release capsules, the dosage is 225 mg every 12 hours initially; it can be gradually increased to 425 mg every 12 hours.

CLASS II: BETA BLOCKERS

Class II consists of beta-adrenergic blocking agents. At this time only four beta blockers—propranolol, acebutolol, esmolol, and sotalol—are approved for treating dysrhythmias. One of these drugs—sotalol—also blocks potassium channels; it is discussed under class III. The basic pharmacology of the beta blockers is presented in Chapter 18. Discussion here is limited to their antidysrhythmic use.

Propranolol

Propranolol [Inderal LA] is considered a nonselective beta-adrenergic antagonist, in that it blocks both $beta_1$- and $beta_2$-adrenergic receptors. $Beta_1$ blockade affects the heart, and $beta_2$ blockade affects the bronchi.

Effects on the Heart and ECG

Blockade of cardiac $beta_1$ receptors attenuates sympathetic stimulation of the heart. The result is (1) decreased automaticity of the SA node, (2) decreased velocity of conduction through the AV node, and (3) decreased myocardial contractility. The reduction in AV conduction velocity translates to a prolonged PR interval on the ECG.

It is worth noting that cardiac $beta_1$ receptors are functionally coupled to calcium channels and that $beta_1$ blockade causes these channels to close. Therefore, the effects of beta blockers on heart rate, AV conduction, and contractility all result from decreased calcium influx. Because beta blockers and calcium channel blockers both decrease calcium entry, the cardiac effects of these drugs are very similar.

Therapeutic Use

Propranolol is especially useful for treating dysrhythmias caused by excessive sympathetic stimulation of the heart. Among these are sinus tachycardia, severe recurrent ventricular tachycardia, exercise-induced tachydysrhythmias, and paroxysmal atrial tachycardia evoked by emotion or exercise. In patients with supraventricular tachydysrhythmias, propranolol has two beneficial effects: (1) suppression of excessive discharge of the SA node and (2) slowing of ventricular rate by decreasing transmission of atrial impulses through the AV node.

Adverse Effects

Beta blockers are generally well tolerated. Principal adverse effects concern the heart and bronchi. By blocking cardiac $beta_1$ receptors, propranolol can cause *heart failure, AV block,* and *sinus arrest. Hypotension* can occur secondary to reduced cardiac output. In patients with asthma, blocking $beta_2$ receptors in the lung can cause *bronchospasm.* Because of its cardiac and pulmonary effects, propranolol should be used cautiously in patients with asthma, and it is contraindicated in patients with sinus bradycardia, high-degree heart block, and HF.

Dosage and Administration

Propranolol can be administered orally and, in life-threatening emergencies, by IV injection. Dosages with either route show wide individual variation. Oral dosages range from 10 to 30 mg every 6 to 8 hours. The usual IV dose is 1 to 3 mg injected at a rate of 1 mg/min.

Acebutolol

Acebutolol [Sectral] is a cardioselective beta blocker approved for oral therapy of PVCs. Adverse effects are like those of propranolol: bradycardia, HF, AV block, and—despite cardioselectivity—bronchospasm. Accordingly, acebutolol should be used cautiously in patients with asthma, and is contraindicated in patients with HF, severe bradycardia, and AV block. Acebutolol can also cause adverse immunologic reactions; titers of ANAs may rise, resulting in myalgia, arthralgia, and arthritis. For suppression of PVCs, the initial dosage is 200 mg twice daily. Usual maintenance dosages range from 600 to 1200 mg/day.

Esmolol

Esmolol [Brevibloc] is a cardioselective beta blocker with a very short half-life (9 minutes). Administration is by IV infusion. The drug is employed for immediate control of ventricular rate in patients with SVT, atrial flutter, and atrial fibrillation. Use is short term only (e.g., in patients with dysrhythmias associated with surgery). The most common adverse reaction is hypotension. However, like other beta blockers, esmolol can also cause bradycardia, heart block, HF, and bronchospasm (at higher doses). In addition, pain can occur at the infusion site. Esmolol is available in two concentrations: 10 and 20 mg/mL. Treatment begins with a loading dose (500 mcg/kg) infused over 1 minute. The usual maintenance infusion rate is 100 mcg/kg/min.

CLASS III: POTASSIUM CHANNEL BLOCKERS (DRUGS THAT DELAY REPOLARIZATION)

Five class III antidysrhythmics are available: *amiodarone, dronedarone, dofetilide, ibutilide,* and *sotalol* (which is also a beta blocker). All five delay repolarization of fast potentials. Hence, all five prolong the action potential duration and ERP. By doing so, they prolong the QT interval. In addition, each drug can affect the heart in other ways, so they are not interchangeable.

Amiodarone

Amiodarone [Cordarone, Pacerone] is a class III antidysrhythmic agent that has complex effects on the heart. The drug is highly effective against both atrial and ventricular dysrhythmias. Unfortunately, serious toxicities (e.g., lung damage, visual impairment) are common and may persist for months after treatment has stopped. Because of toxicity, amiodarone is *approved* only for life-threatening ventricular dysrhythmias that have been refractory to safer agents. Nonetheless, because of its efficacy, amiodarone is one of our most frequently prescribed antidysrhythmic drugs, used for atrial and ventricular dysrhythmias alike.

Amiodarone is available for oral and IV use. Indications, electrophysiologic effects, time course of action, and adverse effects differ for each route. Accordingly, oral and IV therapy are discussed separately.

Oral Therapy

Therapeutic Use. Although amiodarone is very effective, concerns about toxicity limit its indications. In the United States, oral amiodarone is *approved* only for long-term therapy of two life-threatening ventricular dysrhythmias: *recurrent ventricular fibrillation* and *recurrent hemodynamically unstable ventricular tachycardia.* Treatment should be reserved for patients who have not responded to safer drugs.

Amiodarone is our most effective drug for *atrial fibrillation* and is prescribed widely to treat this dysrhythmia—even though it is not approved for this use. The drug is given to convert atrial fibrillation to normal sinus rhythm and to maintain normal sinus rhythm following conversion.

Effects on the Heart and ECG. Amiodarone has complex effects on the heart. Like all other drugs in this class, amiodarone delays repolarization, and thereby prolongs the action potential duration and ERP. The underlying cause of these effects may be blockade of potassium channels. Additional cardiac effects include reduced automaticity in the SA node, reduced contractility, and reduced conduction velocity in the AV node, ventricles, and His-Purkinje system. These occur secondary to blockade of sodium channels, calcium channels, and beta receptors. Prominent effects on the ECG are QRS widening and prolongation of the PR and QT intervals. Amiodarone also acts on coronary and peripheral blood vessels to promote dilation.

Adverse Effects. Amiodarone produces many serious adverse effects. Furthermore, because the drug's half-life is protracted, toxicity can continue for weeks or months after drug withdrawal. To reduce adverse events, the U.S. Food and Drug Administration (FDA) requires that all patients using amiodarone be given a Medication Guide describing potential toxicities.

Pulmonary Toxicity. Lung damage—hypersensitivity pneumonitis, interstitial/alveolar pneumonitis, pulmonary fibrosis—is the greatest concern. Symptoms (dyspnea, cough, chest pain) resemble those of HF and pneumonia. Pulmonary toxicity develops in 2% to 17% of patients and carries a 10% risk of mortality. Patients at highest risk are those receiving long-term, high-dose therapy. A baseline chest x-ray and pulmonary function test are recommended. Pulmonary function should be monitored throughout treatment. If lung injury develops, amiodarone should be withdrawn.

Cardiotoxicity. Amiodarone may cause a paradoxical increase in dysrhythmic activity. In addition, by suppressing the SA and AV nodes, the drug can cause sinus bradycardia and AV block. By reducing contractility, amiodarone can precipitate HF.

Thyroid Toxicity. Amiodarone may cause hypothyroidism or hyperthyroidism. Accordingly, thyroid function should be assessed at baseline and periodically during treatment. Hypothyroidism can be treated with thyroid hormone supplements. Hyperthyroidism can be treated with an antithyroid drug (e.g., methimazole) or thyroidectomy. Discontinuing amiodarone should be considered.

Liver Toxicity. Amiodarone can injure the liver. Accordingly, tests of liver function should be obtained at baseline and periodically throughout treatment. If circulating liver enzymes exceed 3 times the normal level, amiodarone should be discontinued. Signs and symptoms of liver injury, which are seen only rarely, include anorexia, nausea, vomiting, malaise, fatigue, itching, jaundice, and dark urine.

Ophthalmic Effects. Rarely, amiodarone has been associated with optic neuropathy and optic neuritis, sometimes progressing to blindness. However, the absolute risk is small. Patients who develop changes in visual acuity or peripheral vision should undergo ophthalmologic evaluation. If optic neuropathy or neuritis is diagnosed, discontinuation of amiodarone should be considered.

Virtually all patients taking amiodarone develop corneal microdeposits. Fortunately, these deposits have little or no effect on vision, and so rarely necessitate the cessation of amiodarone.

Toxicity in Pregnancy and Breast-Feeding. Amiodarone crosses the placental barrier and enters breast milk, and can thereby harm the developing fetus and breast-feeding infant. Accordingly, pregnancy and breast-feeding should be avoided while using the drug and for several months after stopping it.

Dermatologic Toxicity. Patients frequently experience *photosensitivity reactions* (skin reactions triggered by exposure to ultraviolet radiation). To reduce risk, patients should avoid sunlamps, and should wear sunblock and protective clothing when outdoors. With frequent and prolonged sun exposure, exposed skin may turn *bluish-gray*. Fortunately, this discoloration resolves within months after amiodarone is discontinued.

Other Adverse Effects. Possible *CNS reactions* include ataxia, dizziness, tremor, mood alteration, and hallucinations. *Gastrointestinal reactions* (anorexia, nausea, vomiting) are common.

Drug Interactions. Amiodarone is subject to significant interactions with many drugs. The result can be toxicity or reduced therapeutic effects. Accordingly, combined use with these drugs should be avoided. When it cannot, the patient should be monitored closely. Interactions of concern include the following:

- Amiodarone can *increase* levels of several drugs, including quinidine, procainamide, phenytoin, digoxin, diltiazem, warfarin, cyclosporine, and three statins: lovastatin, simvastatin, and atorvastatin. Dosages of these agents often require reduction.
- Amiodarone levels can be *increased* by grapefruit juice and by inhibitors of CYP3A4. Toxicity can result.
- Amiodarone levels can be *reduced* by cholestyramine (which decreases amiodarone absorption) and by agents that induce CYP3A4 (e.g., St. John's wort, rifampin).
- The risk of severe dysrhythmias is increased by diuretics (because they can reduce levels of potassium and magnesium) and by drugs that prolong the QT interval, of which there are many.
- Combining amiodarone with a beta blocker, verapamil, or diltiazem can lead to excessive slowing of heart rate.

Dosage. Oral amiodarone [Cordarone, Pacerone] is available in tablets (100, 200, and 400 mg). Treatment should be initiated in a hospital. The following schedule is used for loading: 800 to 1600 mg daily for 1 to 3 weeks, followed by 600 to 800 mg daily for 4 weeks. The daily maintenance dosage is 400 mg.

Intravenous Therapy

Therapeutic Use. Intravenous amiodarone is approved only for initial treatment and prophylaxis of recurrent ventricular fibrillation and hemodynamically unstable ventricular tachycardia in patients refractory to safer drugs. For these indications, amiodarone may be lifesaving.

In addition to its approved uses, IV amiodarone has been used with success against other dysrhythmias, including atrial fibrillation, AV nodal reentrant tachycardia, and shock-resistant ventricular fibrillation.

Effects on the Heart and ECG. In contrast to oral amiodarone, which affects multiple aspects of cardiac function, IV amiodarone affects primarily the AV node. Specifically, the drug slows AV conduction and prolongs AV refractoriness. Both effects probably result from antiadrenergic actions. The mechanism underlying antidysrhythmic effects is unknown.

Adverse Effects. The most common adverse effects are hypotension and bradydysrhythmias. Hypotension develops in 15% to 20% of patients, and may require discontinuation of treatment. Bradycardia or AV block occurs in 5% of patients; discontinuation of treatment or insertion of a pacemaker may be needed. Infusions containing more than 2 mg/mL (in 5% dextrose in water) produce a high incidence of phlebitis, and hence they should be administered through a central venous line. Torsades de pointes in association with QT prolongation occurs rarely.

Dosage. Dosing is complex. During the first 24 hours, a total dose of 1050 mg is infused. After that, a maintenance infusion (0.5 mg/min) is given around-the-clock. The usual duration of treatment is 2 to 4 days. However, maintenance infusions may be continued for up to 3 weeks before switching to oral amiodarone.

Dronedarone

Dronedarone [Multaq], a derivative of amiodarone, is indicated for oral therapy of *atrial flutter* and *paroxysmal or persistent atrial fibrillation,* but *not* permanent atrial fibrillation. The manufacturer hoped to create a drug with the high efficacy of amiodarone, but with less toxicity. Unfortunately, although dronedarone is somewhat less toxic than amiodarone, it is also less effective. Furthermore, in patients with HF or permanent atrial fibrillation, dronedarone doubles the risk of death. Dronedarone has a much shorter half-life than amiodarone, so adverse effects resolve more quickly.

Effects on the Heart and ECG

Like other class III agents, dronedarone blocks cardiac potassium channels and thereby delays repolarization. In addition, dronedarone can block sodium channels (like class I agents), beta-adrenergic receptors (like class II agents), and calcium channels (like class IV agents). Just how these actions contribute to antidysrhythmic benefits is unclear. Prominent effects on the ECG are PR and QT prolongation and widening of the QRS complex.

Adverse Effects

The most common side effects are diarrhea, weakness, nausea, and skin reactions. In contrast to amiodarone, dronedarone does *not* cause significant thyroid toxicity, pulmonary toxicity (e.g., pulmonary fibrosis, pneumonitis), or ocular toxicity (e.g., corneal microdeposits, optic neuropathy)—although it can cause liver toxicity. Dronedarone can increase skin sensitivity to sunlight, but it does not cause the bluish-gray skin discoloration seen with amiodarone. Furthermore, because dronedarone has a much shorter half-life than amiodarone, adverse effects that *do* occur have a much shorter duration.

Cardiac Effects. In patients with *severe heart failure,* dronedarone doubles the risk of death, as shown in the ANDROMIDA trial. Accordingly, dronedarone is contraindicated in patients with New York Heart Association (NYHA)

Class IV HF and in patients with NYHA Class II or III HF with recent decompensation that required hospitalization.

In patients with *permanent atrial fibrillation* (as opposed to paroxysmal or persistent atrial fibrillation), dronedarone doubles the risk of death, as shown in the PALLAS trial. Accordingly, dronedarone should not be used in these patients.

Dronedarone reduces SA nodal automaticity and AV nodal conduction, posing a risk of bradycardia and heart block. Accordingly, the drug is contraindicated in patients with sick sinus syndrome or second- or third-degree AV block (unless a pacemaker is in use), and in patients with bradycardia below 50 beats/min.

Dronedarone prolongs the QT interval (by about 10 msec). Accordingly, the drug should not be used in patients with a QT interval greater than 500 msec or in patients taking drugs or supplements that cause QT prolongation.

Liver Toxicity. Dronedarone has been associated with rare cases of severe liver injury, including two that required a liver transplant. Accordingly, patients should be warned about signs and symptoms of liver injury (e.g., anorexia, nausea, vomiting, malaise, fatigue, itching, jaundice, dark urine), and instructed to contact their provider immediately if these develop. Providers should consider monitoring for liver enzymes in blood, especially during the first 6 months of treatment.

Toxicity in Pregnancy and Breast-Feeding. Dronedarone is a proven teratogen and must not be used during pregnancy. In animal studies, doses at or below the mean recommended human dose have produced visceral, skeletal, and external malformations. Accordingly, dronedarone is classified in FDA Pregnancy Risk Category X[a]: risks to the developing fetus clearly outweigh any possible benefit. Women of childbearing age should be counseled about using effective contraception.

We know that dronedarone is excreted in the milk of rats, but information in lactating women is lacking. Nonetheless, owing to the potential risk to nursing infants, dronedarone is contraindicated for use by breast-feeding mothers.

Drug Interactions

Dronedarone is subject to multiple drug interactions, many involving CYP3A4.

- *Strong inhibitors of hepatic CYP3A4* (e.g., ketoconazole, clarithromycin, ritonavir) can make dronedarone accumulate to dangerous levels. Accordingly, concurrent use of these inhibitors is contraindicated. Grapefruit juice, which strongly inhibits *intestinal* CYP3A4, can raise dronedarone levels threefold and so should also be avoided. Moderate inhibitors of hepatic CYP3A4 (e.g., verapamil, diltiazem) should be used with caution.
- *Strong inducers of CYP3A4* (e.g., rifampin, carbamazepine, St. John's wort) can reduce dronedarone levels by as much as 80% and can thereby greatly reduce dysrhythmia control.
- In addition to being a substrate for CYP3A4, dronedarone can inhibit this enzyme. Accordingly, dronedarone can raise levels of other drugs that are *CYP3A4 substrates*. Substrates with a narrow therapeutic range (e.g., tacrolimus, sirolimus, warfarin) should be used with caution.
- Dronedarone can inhibit CYP2D6 and can thereby increase levels of *CYP2D6 substrates* (e.g., beta blockers, tricyclic antidepressants). Concurrent use of these agents should be done with caution.
- *Beta blockers*, which suppress the SA node and AV conduction, can intensify dronedarone-induced bradycardia and can also increase the risk of AV block.
- Like the beta blockers, two *calcium channel blockers—verapamil* and *diltiazem*—also suppress the SA node and AV conduction and pose the same risk as the beta blockers do. In addition, verapamil and diltiazem can inhibit CYP3A4 and can thereby raise dronedarone levels, making the risk of cardiosuppression even greater.
- *Drugs and supplements that prolong the QT interval* (e.g., phenothiazines, tricyclic antidepressants, class I and class III antidysrhythmics) can intensify dronedarone-induced QT prolongation, and can thereby increase the risk of torsades de pointes. Accordingly, these drugs are contraindicated for use with dronedarone.

Contraindications

Dronedarone has the following contraindications:

- NYHA Class IV HF *or* NYHA Class II or III HF with recent decompensation requiring hospitalization
- Liver or lung toxicity related to previous amiodarone use
- Permanent atrial fibrillation
- Second- or third-degree AV block or sick sinus syndrome (except in patients using a pacemaker)
- Bradycardia below 50 beats/min
- PR interval greater than 280 msec
- QT interval greater than 500 msec
- Use of drugs or supplements that prolong the QT interval
- Use of strong inhibitors of CYP3A4
- Pregnancy
- Breast-feeding
- Severe liver impairment

Preparations, Dosage, and Administration

Dronedarone [Multaq] is supplied in 400-mg tablets for oral dosing. The recommended dosage is 400 mg twice daily, taken with the morning and evening meals. Note that, unlike amiodarone, dronedarone does not require a loading dose.

Sotalol

Actions and Uses

Sotalol [Betapace, Betapace AF] is a beta blocker that also delays repolarization. Hence, the drug has combined class II and class III antidysrhythmic properties. Prodysrhythmic properties are pronounced. Sotalol was initially approved only for ventricular dysrhythmias, such as sustained ventricular tachycardia, that are considered life threatening. Later, it was approved for prophylaxis and treatment of atrial flutter and fibrillation, but only if symptoms are severe. The drug is not approved for hypertension or angina pectoris (the primary indications for other beta blockers).

Pharmacokinetics

Sotalol is administered orally and undergoes nearly complete absorption. The drug is excreted unchanged in the urine. Its half-life is 12 hours.

Adverse Effects

The major adverse effect is torsades de pointes, a serious dysrhythmia that develops in about 5% of patients. Risk is increased by hypokalemia and by other drugs that prolong the QT interval.

[a]As of 2020, the FDA will no longer use Pregnancy Risk Categories. Please refer to Chapter 9 for more information.

At therapeutic doses, sotalol produces substantial beta blockade. It can cause bradycardia, AV block, HF, and bronchospasm. Accordingly, the usual contraindications to beta blockers apply.

Preparations, Dosage, and Administration

Sotalol is available under two brand names: *Betapace* and *Betapace AF.* Betapace (80-, 120-, 160-, and 240-mg tablets) is intended for treating ventricular dysrhythmias. Betapace AF (80-, 120-, and 160-mg tablets) is intended for treating atrial fibrillation and atrial flutter. Although tablets are the same under both brand names, packaging differs: Packaging for Betapace provides information specific for treating ventricular dysrhythmias, whereas packaging for Betapace AF provides information specific for treating atrial dysrhythmias. For both types of dysrhythmias, treatment should start in a hospital. Dosing for both is the same: The initial dosage is 160 mg/day (in two divided doses), and the usual maintenance dosage is 160 to 320 mg/day in two or three divided doses. The dosing interval should be increased in patients with renal impairment.

Dofetilide

Therapeutic Use

Dofetilide [Tikosyn] is an oral class III antidysrhythmic indicated for restoring and maintaining normal sinus rhythm in patients with atrial flutter or atrial fibrillation. The drug causes dose-related QT prolongation and thereby poses a serious risk of torsades de pointes. Accordingly, it should be reserved for patients with highly symptomatic atrial dysrhythmias. Initial treatment requires continuous ECG monitoring in a hospital. Dosage must be carefully titrated on the basis of renal function tests. Dofetilide is available only through authorized hospitals and prescribers.

Effects on the Heart and ECG

Like other class III agents, dofetilide blocks cardiac potassium channels and delays repolarization, prolonging the QT interval. Dofetilide does not affect the PR interval or widen the QRS complex, and it has no effect on cardiac beta receptors or sodium channels.

Adverse Effects

By increasing the QT interval, dofetilide predisposes to *torsades de pointes,* which can progress to fatal ventricular fibrillation. The risk is directly related to dofetilide blood levels and is increased by hypokalemia and by other drugs that cause QT prolongation. To assess risk, an ECG should be obtained at baseline, and ECG monitoring should be continuous during initial treatment. Dofetilide is contraindicated for patients with a baseline QT interval greater than 440 msec (or greater than 500 msec in patients with ventricular conduction abnormalities). Other side effects include headache, chest pain, and dizziness.

Drug Interactions

Drugs that are excreted by renal cation pumps can interfere with the excretion of dofetilide, thereby causing its levels to rise. Accordingly, concurrent use of these drugs (e.g., cimetidine, trimethoprim, ketoconazole, prochlorperazine, megestrol) is contraindicated.

Drugs that prolong the QT interval may increase the risk of dysrhythmias and so should be avoided. Among these are class I and class III antidysrhythmics, phenothiazines, tricyclic antidepressants, and some macrolide antibiotics.

Combining verapamil with dofetilide increases the risk of torsades de pointes and should be avoided.

Preparations, Dosage, and Administration

Dofetilide [Tikosyn] is available in capsules (125, 250, and 500 mcg) for oral dosing. Because of the risk of dysrhythmias, treatment must be initiated in a hospital with *continuous ECG monitoring for at least 3 days.* Because dysrhythmia risk is directly related to plasma drug levels, which in turn are directly related to creatinine clearance (a measure of renal function), *creatinine clearance must be monitored.* Dosage should be reduced with decreasing creatinine clearance as follows: For patients with normal renal function (creatinine clearance greater than 60 mL/min), give 500 mcg twice a day; for creatinine clearance 40 to 60 mL/min, give 250 mcg twice a day; for creatinine clearance 20 to 39 mL/min, give 125 mcg twice a day; and for creatinine clearance below 20 mL/min, withhold dofetilide. If the QT interval becomes excessively prolonged (greater than 500 msec, or greater than 550 msec in patients with ventricular conduction abnormalities), dosage should be reduced.

Ibutilide

Ibutilide [Corvert] is an IV agent used to terminate atrial flutter and atrial fibrillation of recent onset (i.e., that has been present no longer than 90 days). Conversion to sinus rhythm occurs during the infusion or within 90 minutes of its termination. Ibutilide is more effective against atrial flutter (49% to 70% success) than atrial fibrillation (22% to 43% success). Like other class III agents, ibutilide blocks potassium channels and thereby prolongs the action potential duration and QT interval. Up to 8% of patients develop torsades de pointes, frequently in association with QT prolongation. Oral doses are teratogenic and embryocidal in rats. For patients who weigh over 60 kg, the dosage is 1 mg infused over 10 minutes. If the dysrhythmia does not convert within 10 minutes of terminating the infusion, a second 1-mg infusion may be tried.

CLASS IV: CALCIUM CHANNEL BLOCKERS

Only two calcium channel blockers—*verapamil* [Calan, Verelan] and *diltiazem* [Cardizem, Dilacor-XR, Tiazac, others]—are able to block calcium channels in the heart. Accordingly, they are the only calcium channel blockers used to treat dysrhythmias. Their basic pharmacology is discussed in Chapter 45. Consideration here is limited to their use against dysrhythmias.

Effects on the Heart and ECG

Blockade of cardiac calcium channels has three effects:

- Slowing of SA nodal automaticity
- Delay of AV nodal conduction
- Reduction of myocardial contractility

Note that these are identical to the effects of beta blockers, which makes sense in that beta blockers promote calcium channel closure in the heart. The principal effect on the ECG is prolongation of the PR interval, reflecting delayed AV conduction.

Therapeutic Uses

Verapamil and diltiazem have two antidysrhythmic uses. First, they can slow ventricular rate in patients with atrial fibrillation or atrial flutter. Second, they can terminate SVT caused by an AV nodal reentrant circuit. In both cases, benefits derive from suppressing AV nodal conduction. With IV administration, effects can be seen in 2 to 3 minutes. Verapamil and diltiazem are not active against ventricular dysrhythmias.

Adverse Effects

Although generally safe, these drugs *can* cause undesired effects. Blockade of cardiac calcium channels can cause *bradycardia, AV block,* and *heart failure.* Blockade of calcium channels in vascular smooth muscle can cause vasodilation, resulting in *hypotension* and *peripheral edema.* Blockade of calcium channels in intestinal smooth muscle can produce *constipation.*

Drug Interactions

Both verapamil and diltiazem can elevate levels of *digoxin,* thereby increasing the risk of digoxin toxicity. Also, since digoxin shares with verapamil and diltiazem the ability to decrease AV conduction, combining digoxin with either drug increases the risk of AV block.

Because verapamil, diltiazem, and *beta blockers* have nearly identical suppressant effects on the heart, combining verapamil or diltiazem with a beta blocker increases the risk of bradycardia, AV block, and HF.

Preparations, Dosage, and Administration

Verapamil. Dosing may be IV or oral. Intravenous therapy is preferred for initial treatment. Oral therapy is used for maintenance.

Verapamil for intravenous use is supplied in solution (5 mg/2 mL). The initial dose is 5 to 10 mg injected slowly (over 2 to 3 minutes). If the dysrhythmia persists, an additional 10 mg may be administered in 30 minutes. An IV infusion (0.375 mg/min) can be used for maintenance. Intravenous verapamil can cause serious cardiovascular effects. Accordingly, blood pressure and the ECG should be monitored, and equipment for resuscitation should be immediately available.

Verapamil for oral use is available in immediate- and sustained-release tablets. The maintenance dosage is 40 to 120 mg 3 or 4 times a day.

Diltiazem. Like verapamil, diltiazem may be given IV or PO. Intravenous therapy is preferred for initial treatment, and oral therapy is used for maintenance.

Intravenous therapy is initiated with an IV bolus (0.25 mg/kg). If the response is inadequate, a second bolus (0.35 mg/kg) may be administered in 15 minutes. If appropriate, initial therapy may be followed with a continuous IV infusion (up to 24 hours' duration) at a rate of 5 to 15 mg/hr.

Diltiazem for oral use is available in immediate-release and extended-release tablets. Maintenance dosing is 360 to 480 mg daily taken in four divided doses.

OTHER ANTIDYSRHYTHMIC DRUGS

Adenosine

Adenosine [Adenocard], a naturally occurring nucleotide, is a drug of choice for terminating paroxysmal SVT. Adenosine has an extremely short half-life and thus must be administered IV. Adverse effects are minimal because adenosine is rapidly cleared from the blood.

Effects on the Heart and ECG

Adenosine decreases automaticity in the SA node and greatly slows conduction through the AV node. The most prominent ECG change is prolongation of the PR interval, brought on by delayed AV conduction. Adenosine works in part by inhibiting cyclic AMP–induced calcium influx, thereby suppressing calcium-dependent action potentials in the SA and AV nodes.

Therapeutic Use

Adenosine is approved only for termination of paroxysmal SVT, including Wolff-Parkinson-White syndrome. The drug is not active against atrial fibrillation, atrial flutter, or ventricular dysrhythmias.

Pharmacokinetics

Adenosine has an extremely short half-life (estimated at 1.5 to 10 seconds), owing primarily to rapid uptake by cells and partly to deactivation by circulating adenosine deaminase. Because of its rapid clearance, adenosine must be administered by IV bolus, as close to the heart as possible.

Adverse Effects

Adverse effects are short lived, lasting less than 1 minute. The most common are sinus bradycardia, dyspnea (from bronchoconstriction), hypotension and facial flushing (from vasodilation), and chest discomfort (perhaps from stimulation of pain receptors in the heart).

Drug Interactions

Methylxanthines (aminophylline, theophylline, caffeine) block receptors for adenosine. Hence, asthma patients taking aminophylline or theophylline need larger doses of adenosine, and even then adenosine may not work.

Dipyridamole, an antiplatelet drug, blocks cellular uptake of adenosine and can thereby intensify its effects.

Preparations, Dosage, and Administration

Adenosine [Adenocard] is supplied in solution (3 mg/mL) for bolus IV administration. The injection should be made as close to the heart as possible and should be followed by a saline flush. The initial dose is 6 mg. If there is no response in 1 or 2 minutes, 12 mg may be tried and repeated once. If a response is going to occur, it should happen as soon as the drug reaches the AV node.

Digoxin

Although its primary indication is HF, digoxin [Lanoxin] is also used to treat supraventricular dysrhythmias. The basic pharmacology of digoxin is discussed in Chapter 48. Consideration here is limited to treatment of dysrhythmias.

Effects on the Heart

Digoxin suppresses dysrhythmias by decreasing conduction through the AV node and by decreasing automaticity in the SA node. The drug decreases AV conduction by (1) a direct depressant effect on the AV node and by (2) acting in the CNS to increase vagal (parasympathetic) impulses to the AV node. Digoxin decreases automaticity of the SA node by increasing vagal traffic to the node and by decreasing sympathetic traffic. It should be noted that, although digoxin decreases automaticity in the SA node, it can *increase* automaticity in *Purkinje fibers.* The latter effect contributes to dysrhythmias *caused* by digoxin.

Effects on the ECG

By slowing AV conduction, digoxin prolongs the PR interval. The QT interval may be shortened, reflecting accelerated repolarization of the ventricles. Depression of the ST segment is common. The T wave may be depressed or even inverted. There is little or no change in the QRS complex.

Adverse Effects and Interactions

The major adverse effect is *cardiotoxicity* (dysrhythmias). Risk is increased by hypokalemia, which can result from concurrent therapy with diuretics (thiazides and loop diuretics). Accordingly, it is essential that potassium levels be kept within the normal range (3.5 to 5 mEq/L). The most common adverse effects are GI disturbances (anorexia, nausea, vomiting, abdominal discomfort). CNS responses (fatigue, visual disturbances) are also relatively common.

Antidysrhythmic Uses

Digoxin is used only for supraventricular dysrhythmias. The drug is inactive against ventricular dysrhythmias.

Atrial Fibrillation and Atrial Flutter. Digoxin can be used to slow ventricular rate in patients with atrial fibrillation and atrial flutter. Ventricular rate is decreased by reducing the number of atrial impulses that pass through the AV node.

Supraventricular Tachycardia. Digoxin may be employed acutely and chronically to treat SVT. Acute therapy is used to abolish the dysrhythmia. Chronic therapy is used to prevent its return. Digoxin suppresses SVT by increasing cardiac vagal tone and by decreasing sympathetic tone.

Dosage and Administration

Oral therapy is generally preferred. The initial dosage is 1 to 1.5 mg administered in three or four doses over 24 hours. The maintenance dosage is 0.125 to 0.5 mg/day. This dose should be decreased in patients with renal impairment.

KEY POINTS

- Dysrhythmias result from alteration of the electrical impulses that regulate cardiac rhythm. Antidysrhythmic drugs control rhythm by correcting or compensating for these alterations.
- In the healthy heart, the SA node is the pacemaker.
- Impulses originating in the SA node must travel through the AV node to reach the ventricles. Impulses arriving at the AV node are delayed before going on to excite the ventricles.
- The His-Purkinje system conducts impulses rapidly throughout the ventricles, thereby causing all parts of the ventricles to contract in near synchrony.
- The heart employs two kinds of action potentials: fast potentials and slow potentials.
- Fast potentials occur in the His-Purkinje system, atrial muscle, and ventricular muscle.
- Slow potentials occur in the SA node and AV node.
- Phase 0 of fast potentials (depolarization) is generated by rapid influx of sodium. Because depolarization is fast, these potentials conduct rapidly.
- During phase 2 of fast potentials, calcium enters myocardial cells, thereby promoting contraction.
- Phase 3 of fast potentials (repolarization) is generated by rapid extrusion of potassium.
- Phase 0 of slow potentials (depolarization) is caused by slow influx of calcium. Because depolarization is slow, these potentials conduct slowly.
- Spontaneous phase 4 depolarization—of fast or slow potentials—gives cells automaticity.
- Spontaneous phase 4 depolarization of cells in the SA node normally determines heart rate.
- The P wave of an ECG is caused by depolarization of the atria.
- The QRS complex is caused by depolarization of the ventricles. Widening of the QRS complex indicates slowed conduction through the ventricles.
- The T wave is caused by repolarization of the ventricles.
- The PR interval represents the time between onset of the P wave and onset of the QRS complex. PR prolongation indicates delayed AV conduction.
- The QT interval represents the time between onset of the QRS complex and completion of the T wave. QT prolongation indicates delayed ventricular repolarization.
- Dysrhythmias arise from disturbances of impulse formation (automaticity) or impulse conduction.
- Reentrant dysrhythmias result from a localized, self-sustaining circuit capable of repetitive cardiac stimulation.
- Tachydysrhythmias can be divided into two major groups: supraventricular tachydysrhythmias and ventricular tachydysrhythmias. In general, ventricular tachydysrhythmias disrupt cardiac pumping more than do supraventricular tachydysrhythmias.
- Treatment of supraventricular tachydysrhythmias is often directed at blocking impulse conduction through the AV node, rather than at eliminating the dysrhythmia.
- Treatment of ventricular dysrhythmias is usually directed at eliminating the dysrhythmia.
- All antidysrhythmic drugs are also prodysrhythmic (proarrhythmic). That is, they all can worsen existing dysrhythmias and generate new ones.
- Class I antidysrhythmic drugs block cardiac sodium channels and thereby slow impulse conduction through the atria, ventricles, and His-Purkinje system.
- Slowing ventricular conduction widens the QRS complex.
- Quinidine (a class IA drug) blocks sodium channels and delays ventricular repolarization. Delaying ventricular repolarization prolongs the QT interval.
- Quinidine causes diarrhea and other GI symptoms in 33% of patients. These effects frequently force drug withdrawal.
- Quinidine can cause dysrhythmias. Widening of the QRS complex (by 50% or more) and excessive prolongation of the QT interval are warning signs.
- Quinidine can raise digoxin levels. If the drugs are used together, digoxin dosage must be reduced.
- Class IB agents differ from class IA agents in two ways: they accelerate repolarization and have little or no effect on the ECG.
- Lidocaine (a class IB agent) is used only for ventricular dysrhythmias. The drug is not active against supraventricular dysrhythmias.
- Lidocaine undergoes rapid inactivation by the liver. As a result, it must be administered by continuous IV infusion.
- Propranolol and other class II drugs block cardiac $beta_1$ receptors.
- By blocking cardiac $beta_1$ receptors, propranolol attenuates sympathetic stimulation of the heart and thereby decreases SA nodal automaticity, AV conduction velocity, and myocardial contractility.
- By decreasing AV conduction velocity, propranolol prolongs the PR interval.
- The effects of propranolol on the heart result (ultimately) from suppressing calcium entry. Therefore, the cardiac effects of propranolol and the effects of calcium channel blockers are nearly identical.
- Propranolol is especially useful for treating dysrhythmias caused by excessive sympathetic stimulation of the heart.
- In patients with supraventricular tachydysrhythmias, propranolol helps by (1) slowing discharge of the SA node and (2) decreasing impulse conduction through the AV node, which prevents the atria from driving the ventricles at an excessive rate.
- Class III antidysrhythmics block potassium channels and thereby delay repolarization of fast potentials. As a result, they prolong the action potential duration and the effective refractory period. By delaying ventricular repolarization, they prolong the QT interval.
- Amiodarone (a class III agent) is highly effective against atrial and ventricular dysrhythmias, but can cause multiple serious adverse effects, including damage to the lungs, eyes, liver, and thyroid.
- Dronedarone, a derivative of amiodarone, is somewhat less toxic than amiodarone, but also less effective. In patients with heart failure or permanent atrial fibrillation, dronedarone doubles the risk of death.

- Verapamil and diltiazem (class IV antidysrhythmics) block cardiac calcium channels and thereby reduce automaticity of the SA node, slow conduction through the AV node, and decrease myocardial contractility. These effects are identical to those of the beta blockers.
- By suppressing AV conduction, verapamil and diltiazem prolong the PR interval.
- Verapamil and diltiazem are used to slow ventricular rate in patients with atrial fibrillation or atrial flutter and to terminate SVT caused by an AV nodal reentrant circuit. In both cases, benefits derive from suppressing AV nodal conduction.
- Adenosine is a drug of choice for terminating paroxysmal SVT.
- Adenosine has a very short half-life (less than 10 seconds) and must be given by IV bolus.

Please visit **http://evolve.elsevier.com/Lehne** for chapter-specific NCLEX® examination review questions.

Summary of Major Nursing Implications[a]

Summaries are limited to the major antidysrhythmic drugs. Summaries for beta blockers (propranolol, acebutolol, and esmolol), phenytoin, calcium channel blockers (verapamil and diltiazem), and digoxin appear in Chapters 18, 24, 45, and 48, respectively.

QUINIDINE

Preadministration Assessment

Therapeutic Goal

The usual goal is long-term suppression of atrial and ventricular dysrhythmias.

Baseline Data

Obtain a baseline ECG and laboratory evaluation of liver function. Determine blood pressure.

Identifying High-Risk Patients

Quinidine is *contraindicated* for patients with a history of hypersensitivity to quinidine or other cinchona alkaloids and for patients with complete heart block, digoxin toxicity, or conduction disturbances associated with marked QRS widening and QT prolongation.

Exercise *caution* in patients with partial AV block, HF, hypotensive states, and hepatic dysfunction.

Implementation: Administration

Routes

Usual Route. Oral.

Rare Routes. IM and IV.

Administration

Advise patients to take quinidine with meals. Warn them not to crush or chew sustained-release formulations.

Dosage size depends on the particular quinidine salt being used: 200 mg of quinidine sulfate is equivalent to 275 mg of quinidine gluconate.

Ongoing Evaluation and Interventions

Evaluating Therapeutic Effects

Monitor for beneficial changes in the ECG. Plasma drug levels should be kept between 2 and 5 mcg/mL.

Minimizing Adverse Effects

Diarrhea. Diarrhea and other GI disturbances occur in one-third of patients and frequently force drug withdrawal. **Inform patients that they can reduce GI effects by taking quinidine with meals.**

Cinchonism. **Inform patients about symptoms of cinchonism (tinnitus, headache, nausea, vertigo, disturbed vision), and instruct them to notify the prescriber if these develop.**

Cardiotoxicity. Monitor the ECG for signs of cardiotoxicity, especially widening of the QRS complex (by 50% or more) and excessive prolongation of the QT interval. Monitor pulses for significant changes in rate or regularity. If signs of cardiotoxicity develop, withhold quinidine and notify the prescriber.

Arterial Embolism. Embolism may occur during therapy of atrial fibrillation. Risk is reduced by treatment with an anticoagulant (e.g., warfarin, dabigatran). Observe for signs of thromboembolism (e.g., sudden chest pain, dyspnea), and report these immediately.

Minimizing Adverse Interactions

Digoxin. Quinidine can double digoxin levels. When these drugs are combined, digoxin dosage should be reduced. Monitor patients for digoxin toxicity (dysrhythmias).

PROCAINAMIDE

Preadministration Assessment

Therapeutic Goal

Procainamide is indicated for acute and long-term management of ventricular and supraventricular dysrhythmias. Because procainamide can be toxic with long-term use, quinidine is preferred to procainamide for chronic suppression.

Baseline Data

Obtain a baseline ECG, complete blood count, and laboratory evaluations of liver and kidney function. Determine blood pressure.

Identifying High-Risk Patients

Procainamide is *contraindicated* for patients with systemic lupus erythematosus (SLE), complete AV block, and second-

Continued

Summary of Major Nursing Implications[a]—cont'd

degree or third-degree AV block in the absence of an electronic pacemaker, and patients with a history of procaine allergy.

Exercise *caution* in patients with hepatic or renal dysfunction.

Implementation: Administration

Routes

Oral, IM, IV.

Administration

Instruct patients to administer procainamide at evenly spaced intervals around-the-clock. Warn patients not to crush or chew sustained-release formulations.

When switching from IV procainamide to oral procainamide, allow 3 hours to elapse between stopping the infusion and giving the first oral dose.

Give IM injections deep into the gluteal muscle.

Ongoing Evaluation and Interventions

Evaluating Therapeutic Effects

Monitor the ECG for beneficial changes. Plasma drug levels should be kept between 3 and 10 mcg/mL.

Minimizing Adverse Effects

SLE-like Syndrome. Prolonged therapy can produce a syndrome resembling SLE. **Inform patients about manifestations of SLE (joint pain and inflammation; hepatomegaly; unexplained fever; soreness of the mouth, throat, or gums), and instruct them to notify the prescriber if these develop.** If SLE is diagnosed, procainamide should be discontinued. If discontinuation is impossible, signs and symptoms can be controlled with a nonsteroidal anti-inflammatory drug (e.g., aspirin) or a glucocorticoid. The ANA titer should be measured periodically, and if it rises, procainamide withdrawal should be considered.

Blood Dyscrasias. Procainamide can cause agranulocytosis, thrombocytopenia, and neutropenia. Deaths have occurred. Obtain complete blood counts weekly during the first 3 months of treatment and periodically thereafter. **Instruct patients to inform the prescriber at the first sign of infection (fever, chills, sore throat), bruising, or bleeding.** If subsequent blood counts indicate hematologic disturbance, discontinue procainamide immediately.

Cardiotoxicity. Procainamide can cause dysrhythmias. Monitor pulses for changes in rate or regularity. Monitor the ECG for excessive QRS widening (greater than 50%) and for PR prolongation. If these occur, withhold procainamide and notify the prescriber.

Arterial Embolism. Embolism may occur during therapy of atrial fibrillation. Risk is reduced by treatment with an anticoagulant (e.g., warfarin, dabigatran). Observe for signs of thromboembolism (e.g., sudden chest pain, dyspnea), and report these immediately.

LIDOCAINE

Preadministration Assessment

Therapeutic Goal

Acute management of ventricular dysrhythmias.

Baseline Data

Obtain a baseline ECG and determine blood pressure.

Identifying High-Risk Patients

Lidocaine is *contraindicated* for patients with Stokes-Adams syndrome, Wolff-Parkinson-White syndrome, and severe degrees of SA, AV, or intraventricular block in the absence of electronic pacing.

Exercise *caution* in patients with hepatic dysfunction or impaired hepatic blood flow.

Implementation: Administration

Routes

Usual. IV.

Emergencies. IM.

Administration

Intravenous. Make certain the lidocaine preparation is labeled for IV use (i.e., is devoid of preservatives and catecholamines). Dilute concentrated preparations with 5% dextrose in water.

The initial dose is 50 to 100 mg (1 mg/kg) infused at a rate of 25 to 50 mg/min. For maintenance, monitor the ECG and adjust the infusion rate on the basis of cardiac response. The usual rate is 1 to 4 mg/min.

Intramuscular. Reserve for emergencies. The usual dose is 300 mg injected into the deltoid muscle. Switch to IV lidocaine as soon as possible.

Ongoing Evaluation and Interventions

Evaluating Therapeutic Effects

Continuous ECG monitoring is required. Plasma drug levels should be kept between 1.5 and 5 mcg/mL.

Minimizing Adverse Effects

Excessive doses can cause convulsions and respiratory arrest. Equipment for resuscitation should be available. Seizures can be managed with diazepam.

AMIODARONE

Preadministration Assessment

Therapeutic Goal

Oral Therapy. Long-term treatment of (1) atrial fibrillation and (2) life-threatening recurrent ventricular fibrillation or recurrent hemodynamically unstable ventricular tachycardia in patients who have not responded to safer drugs.

Intravenous Therapy. Initial treatment of recurrent ventricular fibrillation, shock-resistant ventricular fibrillation,

Summary of Major Nursing Implications[a]—cont'd

recurrent hemodynamically unstable ventricular tachycardia, atrial fibrillation, and AV nodal reentrant tachycardia.

Baseline Data

Obtain a baseline ECG, eye examination, and chest x-ray, along with potassium and magnesium levels, and tests for thyroid, pulmonary, and liver function.

Identifying High-Risk Patients

Amiodarone is *contraindicated* for patients with severe sinus node dysfunction or second- or third-degree AV block, and for women who are pregnant or breast-feeding.

Exercise *caution* in patients with thyroid disorders, hypokalemia, or hypomagnesemia.

Implementation: Administration

Routes

Oral. Used for maintenance therapy of atrial and ventricular dysrhythmias.

Intravenous. Used for acute therapy of atrial and ventricular dysrhythmias.

Administration and Dosage

Oral. Initiate treatment in a hospital. High doses are used initially (800 to 1600 mg/day for 1 to 3 weeks). The usual maintenance dosage is 400 mg/day.

Intravenous. Administer by continuous IV infusion, starting with a rapid infusion rate and later reducing the rate for maintenance. Intravenous treatment may last from 2 days to 3 weeks.

Ongoing Evaluation and Interventions

Evaluating Therapeutic Effects

Monitor for beneficial changes in the ECG.

Minimizing Adverse Effects

Pulmonary Toxicity. Amiodarone can cause potentially fatal lung damage (hypersensitivity pneumonitis, interstitial/alveolar pneumonitis, and pulmonary fibrosis). Obtain a baseline chest x-ray and pulmonary function test, and monitor pulmonary function throughout treatment. **Inform patients about signs of lung injury (dyspnea, cough, chest pain), and instruct them to report these immediately.** Treatment consists of withdrawing amiodarone and providing supportive care, sometimes including glucocorticoids.

Cardiotoxicity. Amiodarone can cause HF and atrial and ventricular dysrhythmias. *Patients with pre-existing heart failure must not use the drug.* **Warn patients about signs of HF (e.g., shortness of breath, reduced exercise tolerance, fatigue, tachycardia, weight gain), and instruct them to report these immediately.**

Liver Toxicity. Amiodarone can injure the liver. Obtain tests of liver function at baseline and periodically during treatment. If circulating liver enzymes exceed 3 times the normal level, amiodarone should be withdrawn. **Inform patients about signs and symptoms of liver injury (e.g., anorexia, nausea, vomiting, malaise, fatigue, itching, jaundice, dark urine), and instruct them to report them immediately.**

Thyroid Toxicity. Amiodarone can cause hypothyroidism and hyperthyroidism. Obtain tests of thyroid function at baseline and periodically during treatment. Treat hypothyroidism with thyroid hormone supplements. Treat hyperthyroidism with an antithyroid drug (e.g., methimazole) or thyroidectomy. Stopping amiodarone should be considered.

Toxicity in Pregnancy and Breast-Feeding. Amiodarone can harm the developing fetus and breast-feeding infant. **Warn patients to avoid pregnancy and breast-feeding while using amiodarone and for several months after stopping.**

Ophthalmic Effects. Amiodarone has been associated with optic neuropathy and optic neuritis, sometimes progressing to blindness. Obtain ophthalmic tests, including funduscopy and a slit-lamp examination, at baseline and periodically during treatment. **Advise patients to report reductions in visual acuity or peripheral vision.** If optic neuropathy or neuritis is diagnosed, discontinuing amiodarone should be considered.

Virtually all patients develop corneal microdeposits. In most cases, the deposits have no effect on vision and thus only rarely lead to the discontinuation of amiodarone.

Dermatologic Effects. Photosensitivity reactions are common. **Advise patients to avoid sunlamps and to wear sunscreen and protective clothing when outdoors.** With prolonged sun exposure, skin may develop a bluish-gray discoloration, which typically resolves a few months after amiodarone is stopped.

Minimizing Adverse Interactions

Amiodarone is subject to significant interactions with many drugs. Interactions of special concern are presented here.

Drugs Whose Levels Can Be Increased by Amiodarone. Amiodarone can increase levels of several drugs, including quinidine, procainamide, phenytoin, digoxin, diltiazem, warfarin, cyclosporine, and three statins: lovastatin, simvastatin, and atorvastatin. Dosages of these agents often require reduction.

Drugs That Can Reduce Amiodarone Levels. Amiodarone levels can be reduced by cholestyramine (which decreases amiodarone absorption) and by agents that induce CYP3A4 (e.g., St. John's wort, rifampin). Monitor to ensure that amiodarone is still effective.

Drugs That Can Increase the Risk of Dysrhythmias. The risk of severe dysrhythmias is increased by diuretics (because they can reduce levels of potassium and magnesium) and by drugs that prolong the QT interval.

Drugs That Can Cause Bradycardia. Combining amiodarone with a beta blocker, verapamil, or diltiazem can lead to excessive slowing of heart rate.

Grapefruit Juice. Grapefruit juice inhibits CYP3A4 and can raise levels of amiodarone. Toxicity can result. **Advise patients to avoid grapefruit juice.**

[a]Patient education information is highlighted as **blue text.**

CHAPTER

50 Prophylaxis of Atherosclerotic Cardiovascular Disease: Drugs That Help Normalize Cholesterol and Triglyceride Levels

Our main topic for the chapter is drugs used to lower cholesterol. Drugs used to lower triglycerides (TGs) are considered as well. Cholesterol has a large impact on *atherosclerosis* (thickening of the coronary arteries), also known as atherosclerotic cardiovascular disease (ASCVD). ASCVD includes the vessels of the heart as well as the brain. Damage to these vessels can result in myocardial infarction (MI) or stroke. Moderate cardiac ASCVD usually manifests first as anginal pain. Severe cardiac ASCVD sets the stage for acute coronary syndrome (ACS) and MI. In the United States, cardiac ASCVD is the leading killer of men and women, causing 801,000 deaths in 2013. According to the American Heart Association, about 92 million Americans have heart disease or a history of stroke. More than half of these people are women.

How does ASCVD develop? Very briefly, it begins as a fatty streak in the arterial wall. This is followed by deposition of fibrous plaque. As atherosclerotic plaque grows, it impedes coronary blood flow, causing anginal pain. Worse yet, atherosclerosis encourages formation of thrombi, which can block flow to the brain and heart entirely, thereby causing MI and stroke.

It is important to appreciate that atherosclerosis is not limited to arteries of the heart or brain: Atherosclerotic plaque can develop in any artery and can thereby compromise circulation to any tissue. Furthermore, adverse effects can occur at sites distant from the original lesion: A ruptured lesion can produce a thrombus, which can travel downstream to block a new vessel. Blockage in the lungs is of particular concern.

The risk of developing ASCVD is directly related to increased levels of blood cholesterol in the form of low-density lipoproteins (LDLs). By reducing levels of LDL cholesterol, we can slow progression of atherosclerosis, reduce the risk of serious ASCVD and its potential consequences, and prolong life. The preferred method for lowering LDL cholesterol is modification of diet combined with exercise. Drugs are employed only when diet modification and exercise are insufficient.

We approach our primary topic—cholesterol and its impact on ASCVD—in three stages. First, we discuss cholesterol itself, plasma lipoproteins (structures that transport cholesterol in blood), and the process of atherogenesis. Second, we discuss guidelines for cholesterol screening and the management of high cholesterol. Third, we discuss the pharmacology of the cholesterol-lowering drugs, as well as drugs used to lower TGs.

CHOLESTEROL

Cholesterol has several physiologic roles. Of greatest importance, cholesterol is a component of all cell membranes and membranes of intracellular organelles. In addition, cholesterol is required for synthesis of certain hormones (e.g., estrogen, progesterone, testosterone) and for synthesis of bile salts, which are needed to absorb and digest dietary fats. Also, cholesterol is deposited in the stratum corneum of the skin, where it reduces evaporation of water and blocks transdermal absorption of water-soluble compounds.

Some of our cholesterol comes from dietary sources (exogenous cholesterol), and some is manufactured by cells (endogenous cholesterol), primarily in the liver. More cholesterol comes from endogenous production than from the diet. A critical step in hepatic cholesterol synthesis is catalyzed by an enzyme named *3-hydroxy-3-methylglutaryl coenzyme A reductase,* or simply *HMG-CoA reductase.* As discussed later in the chapter, drugs that inhibit this enzyme—the statins—are our most effective and widely used cholesterol-lowering agents.

An increase in dietary cholesterol produces only a small increase in cholesterol in the blood, primarily because a rise in cholesterol intake inhibits endogenous cholesterol synthesis. Interestingly, an increase in dietary saturated fats produces a substantial (15% to 25%) increase in circulating cholesterol because the liver uses saturated fats to make cholesterol. Accordingly, when we want to reduce cholesterol levels, it is more important to reduce intake of saturated fats than to reduce intake of cholesterol itself, although cholesterol intake should definitely be lowered.

PLASMA LIPOPROTEINS

Structure and Function of Lipoproteins

Function

Lipoproteins serve as carriers for transporting lipids—cholesterol and TGs—in blood. Like all other nutrients and metabolites, lipids use the bloodstream to move throughout the body. However, being lipids, cholesterol and TGs are not water soluble, and hence cannot dissolve directly in plasma. Lipoproteins provide a means of solubilizing these lipids, thereby permitting transport.

Basic Structure

The basic structure of lipoproteins is depicted in Fig. 50.1. As indicated, lipoproteins are tiny spherical structures that consist of a *hydrophobic core,* composed of cholesterol and TGs, surrounded by a *hydrophilic shell,* composed primarily of phospholipids. Because the hydrophilic shell completely covers the lipid core, the entire structure is soluble in the aqueous environment of the plasma.

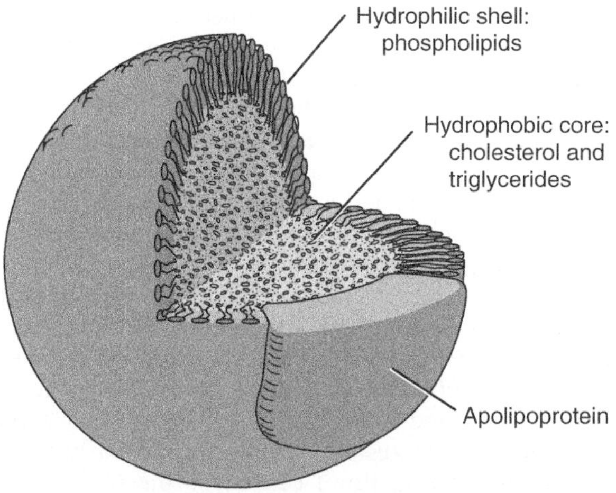

Fig. 50.1 ■ Basic structure of plasma lipoproteins.

Apolipoproteins

All lipoproteins have one or more *apolipoprotein* molecules embedded in their shell (see Fig. 50.1). Apolipoproteins, which constitute the protein component of lipoproteins, have three functions:

- They serve as recognition sites for cell-surface receptors and thereby allow cells to bind with and ingest lipoproteins.
- They activate enzymes that metabolize lipoproteins.
- They increase the structural stability of lipoproteins.

The apolipoproteins of greatest clinical interest are labeled A-I, A-II, and B-100. All lipoproteins that deliver cholesterol and TGs to nonhepatic tissues contain *apolipoprotein B-100.* Conversely, all lipoproteins that transport lipids from nonhepatic tissues back to the liver (i.e., that remove lipids from tissues) contain *apolipoprotein A-I.*

Classes of Lipoproteins

There are six major classes of plasma lipoproteins. Distinctions among classes are based on size, density, apolipoprotein content, transport function, and primary core lipids (cholesterol or TG). From a pharmacologic perspective, the features of greatest interest are *lipid content, apolipoprotein content,* and *transport function.*

For two reasons, the topic of lipoprotein *density* deserves comment. First, naming of lipoprotein types is based on their density. Second, differences in density provide the basis for the physical isolation and subsequent measurement of plasma lipoproteins, as is done in research and clinical laboratories. The various classes of lipoproteins differ in density because they differ in their percentage of composition of lipid and protein. Because protein is denser than lipid, lipoproteins that have a high percentage of protein (and a low percentage of lipid) have a relatively high density. Conversely, lipoproteins with a lower percentage of protein have a lower density.

Of the six major classes of lipoproteins, three are especially important in coronary atherosclerosis. These classes are named (1) very-low-density lipoproteins (VLDLs), (2) low-density lipoproteins (LDLs), and (3) high-density lipoproteins (HDLs). Properties of these classes are shown in Table 50.1.

Very-Low-Density Lipoproteins

VLDLs contain mainly *triglycerides* (and some cholesterol), and they account for nearly all of the TGs in blood. The main physiologic role of VLDLs is to *deliver triglycerides* from the liver to adipose tissue and muscle, which can use the TGs as fuel. Each VLDL particle contains one molecule of *apolipoprotein B-100,* which allows VLDLs to bind with cell-surface receptors and thereby transfer their lipid content to cells.

The role of VLDLs in atherosclerosis is unclear. Although several studies suggest a link between elevated levels of VLDLs and development of atherosclerosis, this link has not been firmly established. However, we do know that elevation of TG levels (above 500 mg/dL) increases the risk of *pancreatitis.*

Low-Density Lipoproteins

LDLs contain *cholesterol* as their primary core lipid, and they account for the majority (60% to 70%) of all cholesterol in blood. The physiologic role of LDLs is *delivery of cholesterol*

TABLE 50.1 ▪ Properties of the Plasma Lipoproteins That Affect Atherosclerosis

Lipoprotein Class	Major Core Lipids	Apolipoproteins	Transport Function	Influence on Atherosclerosis
VLDL	Triglycerides	B-100, E, others	Delivery of triglycerides to nonhepatic tissues	*Probably contribute* to atherosclerosis
LDL	Cholesterol	B-100	Delivery of cholesterol to nonhepatic tissues	*Definitely contribute* to atherosclerosis
HDL	Cholesterol	A-I, A-II, A-IV	Transport of cholesterol from nonhepatic tissues back to the liver	*Protect* against atherosclerosis

HDL, High-density lipoprotein; *LDL,* low-density lipoprotein; *VLDL,* very-low-density lipoprotein.

to nonhepatic tissues. Each LDL particle contains one molecule of *apolipoprotein B-100,* which is needed for the binding of LDL particles to LDL receptors on cells. LDLs can be viewed as by-products of VLDL metabolism, in that the lipids and apolipoproteins that compose LDLs are remnants of VLDL degradation.

Cells that require cholesterol meet their needs through endocytosis (engulfment) of LDLs from the blood. The process begins with the binding of LDL particles to LDL receptors on the cell surface. When cellular demand for cholesterol increases, cells synthesize more LDL receptors and thereby increase their capacity for LDL uptake. Accordingly, cells that are unable to make more LDL receptors cannot increase cholesterol absorption. Increasing the number of LDL receptors on cells is an important mechanism by which certain drugs increase LDL uptake and thereby reduce LDL levels in blood.

Of all lipoproteins, LDLs make the greatest contribution to coronary atherosclerosis. The probability of developing ASCVD is directly related to the level of LDLs in blood. Conversely, by reducing LDL levels, we decrease the risk of ASCVD. Accordingly, *when cholesterol-lowering drugs are used, the main goal is to reduce elevated LDL levels.* Multiple studies have shown that by reducing LDL levels we can arrest or perhaps even reverse atherosclerosis and can thereby reduce mortality from ASCVD. In fact, for each 1% reduction in the LDL level, there is about a 1% reduction in the risk of a major cardiovascular (CV) event.

High-Density Lipoproteins

Like LDLs, HDLs contain *cholesterol* as their primary core lipid and account for 20% to 30% of all cholesterol in the blood. In contrast to LDLs, whose function is the delivery of cholesterol to peripheral tissues, HDLs carry cholesterol from peripheral tissues back to the liver. That is, *HDLs promote cholesterol removal.*

The influence of HDLs on ASCVD is dramatically different from that of LDLs. Whereas elevation of LDLs *increases* the risk of ASCVD, elevation of HDLs *reduces* the risk of ASCVD. That is, high HDL levels actively protect against ASCVD.

LDL Cholesterol Versus HDL Cholesterol

The previous discussion shows that not all cholesterol in plasma has the same impact on ASCVD. As stated, a rise in cholesterol associated with LDLs increases the risk of ASCVD. In contrast, a rise in cholesterol associated with HDLs lowers the risk. Consequently, when speaking of plasma cholesterol levels, we need to distinguish between cholesterol that is associated with HDLs and cholesterol that is associated with LDLs. To make this distinction, we use the terms *HDL cholesterol* and *LDL cholesterol.* Because LDL cholesterol promotes atherosclerosis, it has been dubbed *bad cholesterol.* Conversely, because HDL seems to protect against atherosclerosis, it is often called *good cholesterol* or *healthy cholesterol.*

ROLE OF LDL CHOLESTEROL IN ATHEROSCLEROSIS

LDLs initiate and fuel development of atherosclerosis. The process begins with the transport of LDLs from the arterial lumen into endothelial cells that line the lumens of blood vessels. From there, they move into the space that underlies the arterial epithelium. Once in the subendothelial space, components of LDLs undergo *oxidation.* This step is critical in that oxidized LDLs:

- Attract monocytes from the circulation into the subendothelial space, after which the monocytes are converted to macrophages (which are critical to atherogenesis)
- Inhibit macrophage mobility, thereby keeping macrophages at the site of atherogenesis
- Undergo uptake by macrophages (macrophages do not take up LDLs that have not been oxidized)
- Are cytotoxic, and hence can damage the vascular endothelium directly

As macrophages engulf more and more cholesterol, they become large and develop large vacuoles. When macrophages assume this form, they are referred to as *foam cells.* Foam cell accumulation beneath the arterial epithelium produces a *fatty streak,* which makes the surface of the arterial wall lumpy, causing blood flow to become turbulent. Continued accumulation of foam cells can eventually cause rupture of the endothelium, thereby exposing the underlying tissue to the blood. This results in platelet adhesion and formation of microthrombi. As the process continues, smooth muscle cells migrate to the site, synthesis of collagen increases, and there can be repeated rupturing and healing of the endothelium. The end result is a mature atherosclerotic lesion, characterized by a large lipid core and a tough *fibrous cap.* In less mature lesions, the fibrous cap is not strong, and hence the lesions are unstable and more likely to rupture. As a result, arterial pressure and shear forces (from turbulent blood flow) can cause the cap to rupture. Accumulation of platelets at the site of rupture can rapidly cause thrombosis and can thereby cause infarction. Infarction is less likely at sites of mature atherosclerotic lesions. The atherosclerotic process is depicted in Fig. 50.2.

It is important to appreciate that atherogenesis involves more than just deposition of lipids. In fact, atherogenesis is now considered primarily a chronic *inflammatory process*. When LDLs penetrate the arterial wall, they cause mild injury. The injury, in turn, triggers an inflammatory response that includes infiltration of macrophages, T lymphocytes, and other potentially noxious chemicals (e.g., C-reactive protein [CRP]). In the late stage of the disease process, inflammation can weaken atherosclerotic plaque, leading to plaque rupture and subsequent thrombosis.

2013 ACC/AHA GUIDELINES ON THE TREATMENT OF BLOOD CHOLESTEROL TO REDUCE ATHEROSCLEROTIC CARDIOVASCULAR RISK

It is well established that high levels of cholesterol (primarily LDL cholesterol) cause substantial morbidity and mortality, and that aggressive treatment can save lives. Accordingly, periodic cholesterol screening and risk assessment are recommended. If the assessment indicates ASCVD risk, lifestyle changes—especially diet and exercise—should be implemented. If ASCVD risk is high, LDL-lowering drugs should be added to the regimen.

In 1988, the National Cholesterol Education Program (NCEP) began issuing guidelines on cholesterol detection and management. The most recent update was issued in 2001 and amended in 2004, and new guidelines were developed in 2013 in partnership with the American College of Cardiology (ACC) and the American Heart Association (AHA). A summary of the 2013 guidelines—*2013 ACC/AHA Guideline on the Treatment of Blood Cholesterol to Reduce Atherosclerotic Cardiovascular Risk in Adults: A Report of the American College of Cardiology/American Heart Association Task Force on Practice Guidelines*—was published in *Circulation* and is available at http://circ.ahajournals.org/content/early/2013/11/11/01.cir.0000437738.63853.7a.

Like earlier NCEP guidelines, the 2013 ACC/AHA cholesterol guideline focuses on the role of high cholesterol in ASCVD and stresses the importance of treatment. However, the new guideline focuses specifically on identifying patients who are most likely to benefit from cholesterol-lowering therapy instead of targeting specific cholesterol goals.

Cholesterol Screening

Adults

Management of high LDL cholesterol begins with screening, generally done every 5 years for adults older than 20 years. The ATP III guidelines recommended a more thorough screen than before, consisting of total cholesterol, LDL cholesterol, HDL cholesterol, and TGs. Blood for these tests should be drawn after fasting. Previous to the new guidelines, total cholesterol and LDL cholesterol levels were placed into classifications. With the introduction of the new guidelines, patients should be considered for statin treatment if they fall into one of four different risk categories (Table 50.2).

TABLE 50.2 ■ Statin Benefit Groups as Defined by the 2013 ACC/AHA Blood Cholesterol Guidelines

Individuals with clinical atherosclerotic cardiovascular disease (ASCVD)
Individuals with primary elevations of LDL cholesterol (LDL-C) ≥190 mg/dL
Individuals 40 to 75 years of age with diabetes with LDL-C 70 to 189 mg/dL
Individuals without clinical ASCVD or diabetes who are 40 to 75 years of age with LDL-C 70 to 189 mg/dL and an estimated 10-year ASCVD risk of 7.5% or higher

TABLE 50.3 ■ NCEP Classification of Cholesterol Levels for Children and Adolescents[a]

Category	Total Cholesterol (mg/dL)	LDL Cholesterol (mg/dL)
Acceptable	<170	<110
Borderline	170–199	110–129
Elevated	≥200	≥130

[a]HDL levels should be greater than or equal to 35 mg/dL and triglycerides should be less than or equal to 150 mg/dL.
Data from National Cholesterol Education Program: Report of the Expert Panel on Blood Cholesterol Levels in Children and Adolescents. Pediatrics 89(3 Pt 2):525–584, 1992.

Children and Adolescents

Elevated cholesterol in pediatric patients is a growing concern and is not addressed in the 2013 ACC/AHA blood cholesterol guidelines. However, it is addressed in other guidelines, including one created in 2011 by an expert panel appointed by the National Heart, Lung, and Blood Institute, and endorsed by the American Academy of Pediatrics. This report—*Expert Panel on Integrated Guidelines for Cardiovascular Health and Risk Reduction in Children and Adolescents*—is available at www.nhlbi.nih.gov/guidelines/cvd_ped/summary.htm#chap9.

The guideline recommends lipid screening for *all* children between ages 9 and 11 years, followed by another screen between ages 18 and 21 years. For children with a family history of high cholesterol or heart disease, screening should start sooner: between ages 2 and 8 years. Cholesterol classification for children and adolescents is presented in Table 50.3.

If LDL cholesterol is high, all patients and their families should receive nutritional counseling. In addition, patients should focus on weight control and increased activity, as indicated. Should children use cholesterol-lowering drugs? For two reasons, the answer is "Probably not." First, these children are in no immediate danger: Their risk of developing clinically significant ASCVD in the next 20 years is close to zero. And second, the only data from randomized, controlled trials were for children with familial hypercholesterolemia. No data exist to show that these drugs will improve outcomes when given to children with secondary lipid disorders.

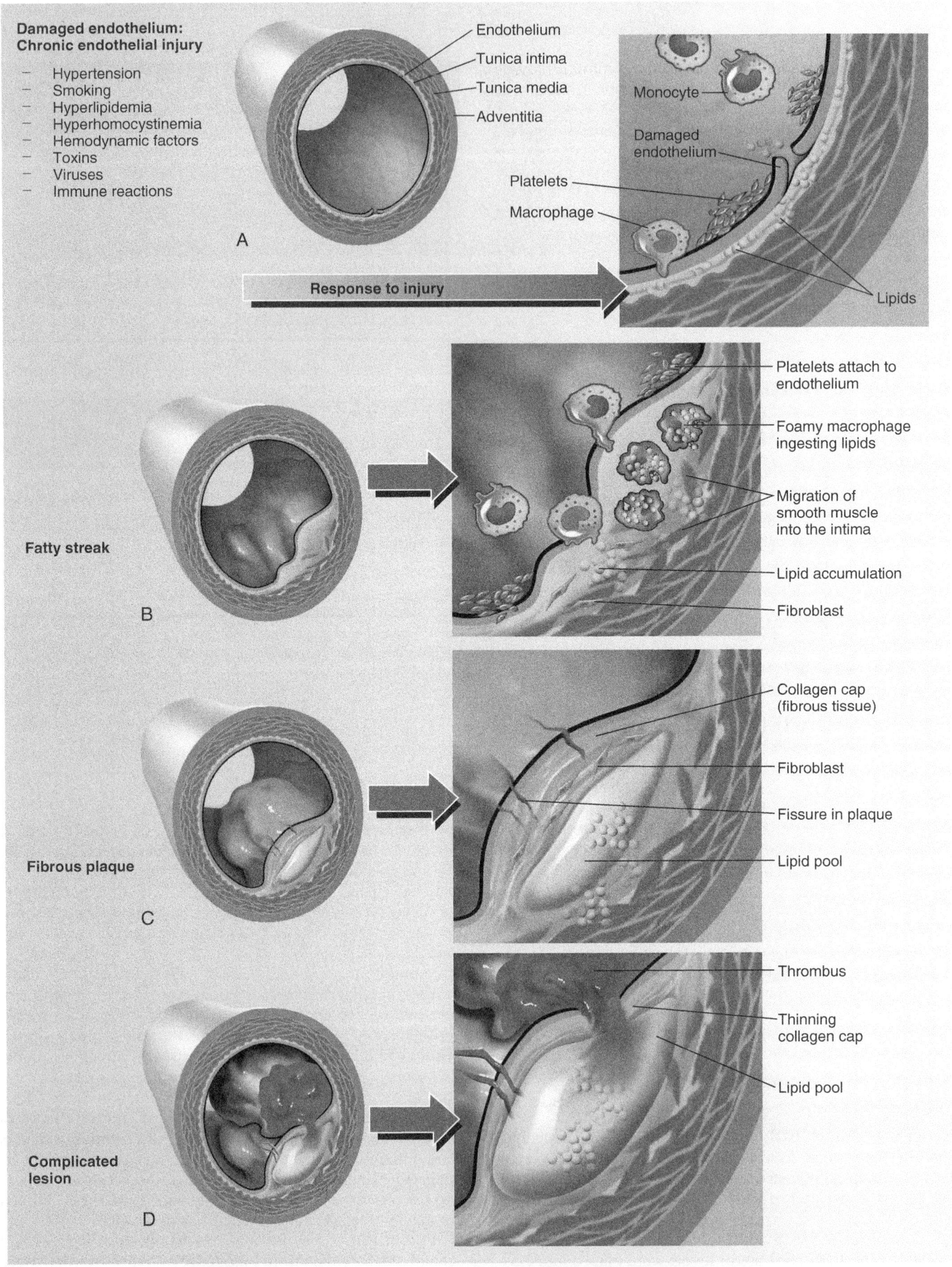

Fig. 50.2 ▪ **Progression of atherosclerosis.**

A, Damaged endothelium. **B,** Diagram of fatty streak and lipid core formation. **C,** Diagram of fibrous plaque. Raised plaques are visible: some are yellow and some are white. **D,** Diagram of a complicated lesion, showing a thrombus (in red) and collagen (in blue). (From McCance KL, Huether SE: Pathophysiology: The Biologic Basis for Disease in Adults and Children, 7th ed. St. Louis: Elsevier, 2014.)

PATIENT-CENTERED CARE ACROSS THE LIFE SPAN

Treating Dyslipidemia

Life Stage	Patient Care Concerns
Infants	See "Breast-feeding women," below.
Children/ adolescents	Lovastatin, simvastatin, pravastatin, and atorvastatin are approved for use in children. It is recommended to avoid statin use in children younger than 10 years.
Pregnant women	Statins are classified in FDA Pregnancy Risk Category X.[a] They are contraindicated in pregnancy. Ezetimibe and fibrates are classified in Pregnancy Risk Category C,[a] hence benefit should outweigh risk.
Breast-feeding women	Effects of statins, ezetimibe, and fibrates have not been studied in breast-feeding. Given the possibility of harm, benefit should outweigh risk.
Older adults	In patients age 65 years and older, statins, compared to placebo, significantly reduced the risk of MI, as well as the risk of stroke, by 23.8%. However, the cost-benefit evaluation of treatment in older adults should be considered.

[a]As of 2020, the FDA will no longer use Pregnancy Risk Categories. Please refer to Chapter 9 for more information.

ASCVD Risk Assessment

Under the 2013 ACC/AHA guidelines, ASCVD risk assessment is directed at determining the patient's *absolute risk of developing clinical coronary disease over the next 10 years.* The mode of intervention is then determined by the individual's degree of risk.

Factors in Risk Assessment

To assess the ASCVD risk for an individual, we need three kinds of information. Specifically, we need to (1) identify ASCVD risk factors, (2) calculate 10-year ASCVD risk, and (3) identify ASCVD risk equivalents.

Identifying ASCVD Risk Factors. Major risk factors that modify LDL treatment goals include positive risk factors (advancing age, African American race, hypertension, cigarette smoking, and low HDL cholesterol) and one negative risk factor (high HDL cholesterol). (LDL itself is not listed because the reason for counting these risk factors is to modify treatment of high LDL.)

We know that diabetes is a very strong predictor of developing ASCVD. Accordingly, we no longer consider diabetes to be a risk *factor.* Instead, for the purpose of risk assessment, diabetes is now considered an ASCVD risk *equivalent.* That is, having diabetes is considered equivalent to having ASCVD as a predictor of a major coronary event.

Calculating 10-Year ASCVD Risk. The 2013 ACC/AHA cholesterol guideline defines high ASCVD risk as 7.5% or greater. Some people are automatically in this risk group—specifically, those with existing ASCVD and those with diabetes. For all other people, 10-year risk must be calculated. The instrument employed most often is the Framingham Risk Prediction Score, which takes five factors into account: age, total cholesterol, HDL cholesterol, smoking status, and systolic blood pressure. These are similar to risk factors noted earlier. Framingham scores can be determined using either (1) the tables for men and women shown in Fig. 50.3 or (2) a web-based risk calculator, such as the one provided by the ACC/AHA at http://tools.acc.org/ASCVD-Risk-Estimator-Plus/#!/calculate/estimate/.

Identifying ASCVD Risk Equivalents. An ASCVD risk equivalent is a condition that poses the same risk of a major coronary event as does established ASCVD (i.e., more than 20% risk of a major event within 10 years). There are two basic ASCVD risk equivalents:

- Diabetes
- The presence of multiple risk factors that confer an ASCVD 10-year risk score 7.5% or more

Identifying an Individual's ASCVD Risk Category

Under the 2013 ACC/AHA cholesterol guideline, there are four categories of patients who would benefit from statin treatment of cholesterol (see Table 50.2). Category assignment is based on (1) the presence or absence of ASCVD (or an ASCVD risk equivalent, such as diabetes), (2) the number of risk factors the individual has (other than high LDL cholesterol), and (3) the individual's 10-year ASCVD score. Although this assessment sounds complicated, it's not. Let's consider the hypothetical case of Ralph J. and follow along by looking at Fig. 50.3. Mr. J. is 62 years old, hypertensive, and he smokes—but, remarkably, his HDL cholesterol is high (above 60 mg/dL). He has no family history of premature ASCVD, does not have ASCVD himself, and does not have diabetes. His 10-year Framingham Risk Prediction Score is 11%. Because his estimated 10-year ASCVD score is greater than 7.5%, Mr. J. should be considered for moderate- to high-intensity drug therapy (Fig. 50.4). This is even easier if you use an online risk assessment tool, such as the ones available at https://www.cvdriskchecksecure.com/framinghamriskscore.aspx.

Final Note: Each Type of Dyslipidemia a Patient Has Contributes Independently to ASCVD Risk

Patients are likely to have more than one type of dyslipidemia—for example, high LDL cholesterol combined with low HDL cholesterol and high TGs—and each of these disorders contributes *independently* to CV risk. This means that fixing just one of these problems will not eliminate the risk posed by the others. Accordingly, to get maximal risk reduction, we must correct all lipid abnormalities that are present.

Treatment of High LDL Cholesterol

Treatment of high LDL cholesterol is based on the individual's ASCVD risk category or the presence of other comorbidities such as diabetes. Treatment may be started with a high-intensity statin or a moderate-intensity statin depending on the patient's risk factors (see Fig. 50.4 and Table 50.4). To reduce LDL levels, the 2013 ACC/AHA guideline recommends two forms of intervention: (1) therapeutic lifestyle changes (TLCs) and (2) drug therapy. For some people, cholesterol can be reduced adequately with TLCs alone. Others require TLCs *plus* cholesterol-lowering drugs. Please note: Drugs should be used only as an *adjunct* to TLCs—not as a *substitute.*

Estimate of 10-year risk for MEN

Age	Points
20–34	−9
35–39	−4
40–44	0
45–49	3
50–54	6
55–59	8
60–64	10
65–69	11
70–74	12
75–79	13

Total Cholesterol	Points Age 20–39	Age 40–49	Age 50–59	Age 60–69	Age 70–79
<160	0	0	0	0	0
160–199	4	3	2	1	0
200–239	7	5	3	1	0
240–279	9	6	4	2	1
≥280	11	8	5	3	1

	Points Age 20–39	Age 40–49	Age 50–59	Age 60–69	Age 70–79
Nonsmoker	0	0	0	0	0
Smoker	8	5	3	1	1

HDL (mg/dL)	Points
≥60	−1
50–59	0
40–49	1
<40	2

Systolic BP (mm Hg)	If Untreated	If Treated
<120	0	0
120–129	0	1
130–139	1	2
140–159	1	2
≥160	2	3

Point Total	10-Year Risk %
<0	<1
0	1
1	1
2	1
3	1
4	1
5	2
6	2
7	3
8	4
9	5
10	6
11	8
12	10
13	12
14	16
15	20
16	25
≥17	≥30

10-Year Risk ______%

Estimate of 10-year risk for WOMEN

Age	Points
20–34	−7
35–39	−3
40–44	0
45–49	3
50–54	6
55–59	8
60–64	10
65–69	12
70–74	14
75–79	16

Total Cholesterol	Points Age 20–39	Age 40–49	Age 50–59	Age 60–69	Age 70–79
<160	0	0	0	0	0
160–199	4	3	2	1	1
200–239	8	6	4	2	1
240–279	11	8	5	3	2
≥280	13	10	7	4	2

	Points Age 20–39	Age 40–49	Age 50–59	Age 60–69	Age 70–79
Nonsmoker	0	0	0	0	0
Smoker	9	7	4	2	1

HDL (mg/dL)	Points
≥60	−1
50–59	0
40–49	1
<40	2

Systolic BP (mm Hg)	If Untreated	If Treated
<120	0	0
120–129	1	3
130–139	2	4
140–159	3	5
≥160	4	6

Point Total	10-Year Risk %
<9	<1
9	1
10	1
11	1
12	1
13	2
14	2
15	3
16	4
17	5
18	6
19	8
20	11
21	14
22	17
23	22
24	27
≥25	≥30

10-Year Risk ______%

Fig. 50.3 ■ Tables for calculating Framingham Risk Prediction Scores.
To determine an individual's 10-year risk of developing clinical coronary disease, simply circle the appropriate points for each of the five risk factors considered (age, total cholesterol, smoking status, HDL cholesterol, and systolic blood pressure) and then add up the points. The point total indicates the 10-year risk. For example, a total of 13 points indicates a 10-year risk of 12% for men. (Framingham scores can also be determined using a web-based calculator, such as the one at https://www.cvdriskchecksecure.com/framinghamriskscore.aspx.)

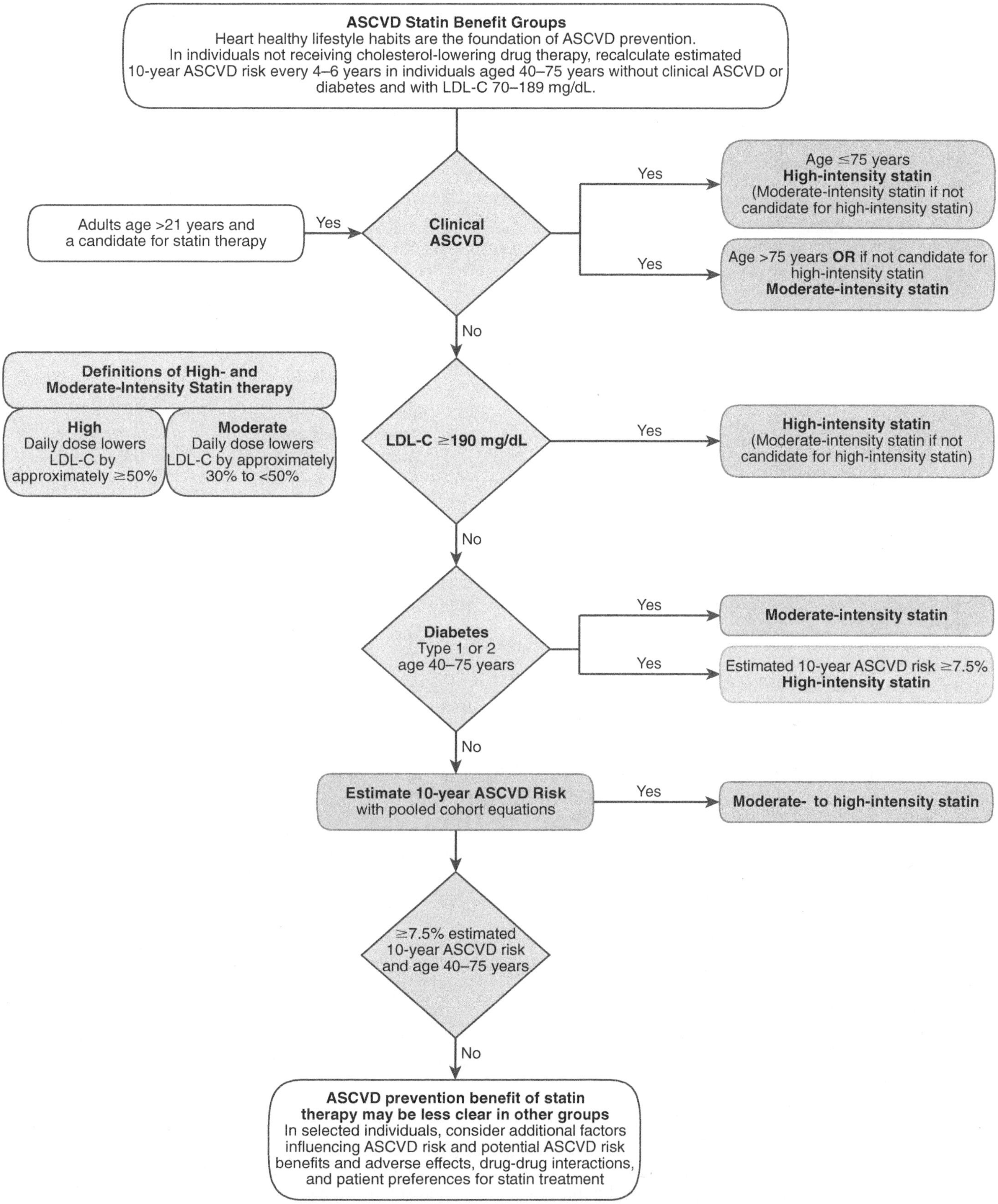

Fig. 50.4 ■ **Recommendations for statin therapy for ASCVD prevention.**

TABLE 50.4 ▪ High-, Moderate-, and Low-Intensity Statin Therapy

High-Intensity Therapy	Moderate-Intensity Therapy	Low-Intensity Therapy
Daily dose lowers LCL-C on average by ≥ 50%	Daily dose lowers LDL-C on average by ~30% to <50%	Daily dose lowers LDL-C on average by <30%
Atorvastatin: 40–80 mg Rosuvastatin: 20 mg	Atorvastatin: 10 mg Rosuvastatin: 10 mg Simvastatin: 20–40 mg Pravastatin: 40 mg Lovastatin: 40 mg	Simvastatin: 10 mg Pravastatin: 10–20 mg Lovastatin: 20 mg

Adapted from 2013 ACC/AHA Guideline on the Treatment of Blood Cholesterol to Reduce Atherosclerotic Cardiovascular Risk in Adults: *A Report of the American College of Cardiology/American Heart Association Task Force on Practice Guidelines.* Available at http://circ.ahajournals.org/content/early/2013/11/11/01.cir.0000437738.63853.7a.

Therapeutic Lifestyle Changes

Therapeutic lifestyle changes are nondrug measures used to lower LDL cholesterol. TLCs focus on four main issues: diet, exercise, weight control, and smoking cessation. These measures are first-line treatment for LDL reduction and should be implemented before drug therapy. However, TLCs can be a challenge because some people do not eat healthier diets or exercise. Physical conditions such as arthritis can limit attempts at exercise, and economic and time limitations can be a barrier to healthier eating.

The TLC Diet. This diet has two objectives: (1) reducing LDL cholesterol and (2) establishing and maintaining a healthy weight. The central feature of the diet is reduced intake of cholesterol and saturated fats: Individuals should limit intake of cholesterol to 200 mg/day or less and intake of saturated fat to 7% or less of total calories. Intake of *trans fats*—found primarily in snack crackers, commercial baked goods, and fried foods—should be minimized. (Many food manufacturers are adding "no trans fat" labels to their product labels, making shopping somewhat easier.)

If the basic TLC diet fails to lower LDL cholesterol adequately, ATP III recommends two additional measures: increased intake of soluble fiber (10 to 25 gm/day; oatmeal is a good source) and increased intake of plant stanols and sterols (2 gm/day). Plant stanols and sterols are cholesterol-lowering chemicals found (albeit in very small amounts) in certain vegetable oils (e.g., canola), nuts (walnuts are a good source), certain fruits, and most beans and many other vegetables. They are also found in some of the cholesterol-lowering margarines, commonly advertised as "buttery spreads" (see later in this chapter under *Plant Stanol and Sterol Esters*).

Exercise. An inactive lifestyle carries an increased risk of ASCVD. Conversely, participating in regular exercise lowers ASCVD risk. Running and swimming, for example, can decrease LDL cholesterol and elevate HDL cholesterol, thereby reducing risk. In addition, exercise can reduce blood pressure, improve overall CV performance, and decrease insulin resistance (important because many people with high cholesterol also have diabetes). Accordingly, ATP III encourages regular physical activity (defined as 30 to 60 minutes of activity on most days). Improvements in the plasma lipid profile depend more on the total time spent exercising than on the intensity of exercise or improvements in fitness.

Smoking Cessation. Smoking cigarettes raises LDL cholesterol and lowers HDL cholesterol, thereby increasing the risk of ASCVD. Smokers should be strongly encouraged to quit—and nonsmokers should be urged not to start. Drugs to aid smoking cessation are discussed in Chapter 39.

Weight Control. Weight loss can reduce both LDL cholesterol and ASCVD risk. This is especially important for people with metabolic syndrome (discussed in an upcoming section).

Drug Therapy

Drugs are not the first-line therapy for lowering LDL cholesterol. Rather, drugs should be employed only if TLCs fail to reduce LDL cholesterol to an acceptable level—and then only if the combination of elevated LDL cholesterol and the patient's ASCVD risk category justify drug use. When drugs are used, it is essential that lifestyle modification continues because the beneficial effects of diet and drugs are additive; drugs alone may be unable to achieve the LDL goal. It is important to note that the principal benefit of drug therapy is *primary prevention:* Drugs are much better at preventing or slowing ASCVD than at promoting regression of established coronary atherosclerosis. Furthermore, because LDL cholesterol levels will return to pretreatment values if drugs are withdrawn, *treatment must continue lifelong.* Patients should be made aware of this requirement.

Table 50.5 shows properties of the drug families used to lower LDL cholesterol. The most effective agents are the *HMG-CoA reductase inhibitors* (e.g., atorvastatin [Lipitor]), usually referred to simply as *statins.* Lesser used alternatives are *bile-acid sequestrants* (e.g., cholestyramine) and *niacin* (nicotinic acid). Although *fibrates* are listed in Table 50.5, these drugs are used primarily to reduce levels of TGs—not LDLs. Treatment is initiated with a single drug, almost always a statin. If the statin is ineffective, a bile-acid sequestrant can be added to the regimen.

In addition to lowering LDL cholesterol, drugs may be used to raise HDL cholesterol. The most effective agents are niacin and the fibrates. However, virtually all of the drugs that we use to lower LDL cholesterol have the added benefit of

TABLE 50.5 ▪ Drugs Used to Improve Plasma Levels of LDLs, HDLs, and Triglycerides

	HMG-CoA Reductase Inhibitors (Statins)[a]	Bile Acid Sequestrants	Fibrates	Ezetimibe	Monoclonal Antibody (PCSK9) Inhibitors
Results of Treatment					
Effect on LDL	↓ 21%–63%	↓ 15%–30%	↓ 6%-10%, but may increase if TGs are high	↓ 19%	↓ 63%–71%
Effect on HDL	↑ 5%–22%	↑ 3%–5%	↑ 10%–20%	↑ 1%–4%	↑ 6%
Effect on TG	↓ 6%–43%	↓ or no change	↓ 20%–50%	↓ 5%–10%	↓ 11%–16%
Clinical Trial Results	Reduced major coronary events, stroke, ASCVD deaths, and total mortality	Reduced major coronary events and ASCVD deaths	Reduced major coronary events	Impact on coronary events and mortality has not been established	Reduced major coronary events and stroke

[a]Use caution in patients taking fibrates and agents that inhibit CYP3A4 (the 3A4 isoenzyme of P450), including cyclosporine, macrolide antibiotics (e.g., erythromycin), azole antifungal drugs (e.g., ketoconazole), and HIV protease inhibitors (e.g., ritonavir).
ASCVD, Atherosclerotic cardiovascular disease; *HDL,* high-density lipoprotein; *LDL,* low-density lipoprotein; *TG,* triglyceride.
Data from the Executive Summary of the Third Report of the National Cholesterol Education Program (NCEP) Expert Panel on Detection, Evaluation, and Treatment of High Blood Cholesterol in Adults (Adult Treatment Panel III). *JAMA* 285:2486–2497, 2001. Data on ezetimibe are from other sources.

increasing HDL cholesterol, at least to some degree. This rise of HDL, therefore, can be considered a beneficial "side effect."

Secondary Treatment Targets

Metabolic Syndrome

The term *metabolic syndrome (also known as syndrome X)* refers to a group of metabolic abnormalities associated with an increased risk of ASCVD and type 2 diabetes. The metabolic abnormalities involved are high blood glucose, high TGs, high apolipoprotein B, low HDL, small LDL particles, a prothrombotic state, and a proinflammatory state. Hypertension is both common and important.

How is metabolic syndrome diagnosed? According to a joint scientific statement—issued by the International Diabetes Federation Task Force on Epidemiology and Prevention; the National Heart, Lung, and Blood Institute; the American Heart Association; the World Heart Federation; the International Atherosclerosis Society; and the International Association for the Study of Obesity—metabolic syndrome is diagnosed when three or more of the following are present:

- *High TG levels*—150 mg/dL or higher (or undergoing drug therapy for high TGs)
- *Low HDL cholesterol*—below 40 mg/dL for men or below 50 mg/dL for women (or undergoing drug therapy for reduced HDL)
- *Hyperglycemia*—fasting blood glucose 100 mg/dL or higher (or undergoing drug therapy for hyperglycemia/diabetes mellitus)
- *High blood pressure*—systolic 130 mm Hg or higher and/or diastolic 85 mm Hg or higher (or undergoing drug therapy for hypertension)
- *Waist circumference 40 inches or more for most men or 35 inches or more for most women* (these limits can vary depending on ethnicity, country, or geographic region within a country)

Treatment has two primary goals: reducing the risk of atherosclerotic disease and reducing the risk of type 2 diabetes. According to ATP III, basic therapy consists of weight control and increased physical activity, which, together, can reduce all symptoms of the metabolic syndrome. In addition, specific treatment should be directed at lowering blood pressure and TG levels. Patients should take low-dose aspirin to reduce the risk of thrombosis, unless they are at high risk of intracranial bleeds (hemorrhagic stroke).

Although the term *metabolic syndrome* is widely used, there is debate about its clinical relevance. In the CV community, most clinicians believe the term has great utility. By contrast, in the diabetes community, many clinicians feel the term is misleading, in that it implies the existence of a specific disease entity, even though it is defined only by a cluster of risk factors that may or may not have a common underlying cause. Furthermore, they point out that the risk associated with a diagnosis of metabolic syndrome is no greater than the sum of the risks of its components. Accordingly, until there is more proof that the metabolic syndrome actually exists, they believe the term serves no clinical purpose and hence should be avoided. This position was voiced in a joint statement from the American Diabetes Association and the European Association for the Study of Diabetes. The American Heart Association and the National Heart, Lung, and Blood Institute countered with a joint statement of their own, reasserting their belief that the metabolic syndrome is an important clinical entity. Although the two camps disagree about whether the metabolic syndrome is an actual disease, both sides strongly agree that the risk factors that define the syndrome should be identified and treated.

One final point: Whether or not you think *metabolic syndrome* is a useful term, you will still see lots of patients who meet the criteria. The fact is, patients with several of these risk factors are much more common than patients with just one.

High Triglycerides

High TG levels (above 200 mg/dL) may be an independent risk factor for ASCVD. In clinical practice, high TGs are seen most often in patients with metabolic syndrome. However, high levels may also be associated with inactive lifestyle, cigarette smoking, excessive alcohol intake, type 2 diabetes, certain genetic disorders, and high carbohydrate intake (when carbohydrates account for more than 60% of total caloric intake). In most patients with high TG levels, the first treatment goal is to achieve the original LDL goal. Dietary modification is always recommended. Statins being taken to lower cholesterol may help lower TGs as well, perhaps to a satisfactory level. However, if TG levels remain unacceptably high, medications specific to TGs—and fibrates—may be needed. Unfortunately, when these drugs are combined with cholesterol-lowering drugs (as they often are), the adverse effects of cholesterol-lowering agents may be intensified.

DRUGS AND OTHER PRODUCTS USED TO IMPROVE PLASMA LIPID LEVELS

As discussed earlier in this chapter, the lipid abnormality that contributes most to CV disease is high LDL cholesterol. Accordingly, we will focus primarily on drugs for this disorder. Nonetheless, we also need to consider other lipid abnormalities, especially (1) high total cholesterol,[a] (2) low HDL cholesterol, and (3) high TGs.

Some drugs for dyslipidemias are more selective than others. That is, whereas some drugs may improve just one dyslipidemia (e.g., high TGs), others may improve two or more dyslipidemias. The highly selective agents can be useful as add-ons, to "target" a particular lipid abnormality when other medications prove inadequate.

Drugs that lower *LDL cholesterol* levels include HMG-CoA reductase inhibitors (statins), bile-acid sequestrants, and ezetimibe. All are effective to varying degrees. The HMG-CoA reductase inhibitors—the statins—are more effective than the others, cause fewer adverse effects, are better tolerated, and are more likely to improve clinical outcomes.

As we consider the drugs for lipid disorders, you should be aware of the following: Although all of these drugs can improve lipid profiles, not all of them improve clinical outcomes (reduced morbidity and mortality). This leads us to question whether some of the lipid abnormalities are a true cause of pathophysiology and ultimate death, or whether they are simply "associated markers" of some other pathophysiology that we don't yet understand.

[a]Note that total cholesterol is slightly different from the simple sum of LDL cholesterol (LDL-C) plus HDL cholesterol (HDL-C); triglycerides (TG) also contribute to the value, as in the following equation: total cholesterol = HDL-C + LDL-C + (TG/5) (provided TG levels are below 400 mg/dL).

Prototype Drugs

LDL CHOLESTEROL- AND TRIGLYCERIDE-LOWERING DRUGS

HMG-CoA Reductase Inhibitors (Statins)
Lovastatin

Bile-Acid Sequestrants
Colesevelam

Others
Ezetimibe

HMG-CoA Reductase Inhibitors (Statins)

HMG-CoA reductase inhibitors, commonly called *statins* (because their generic names all end in *statin*), are the most effective drugs for lowering LDL and total cholesterol. In addition, they can raise HDL cholesterol and lower TGs in some patients. Most important, these drugs have been shown to improve clinical outcomes, including a lowering of the risk of heart failure, MI, and sudden death. Because of these benefits, and because so many people have ASCVD risks associated with dyslipidemias, statins are among our most widely prescribed drugs—and have earned tens of billions for their makers.

Beneficial Actions

The statins have several actions that can benefit patients with (or at risk of) atherosclerosis. The most obvious and important are reductions of LDL cholesterol.

Reduction of LDL Cholesterol. Statins have a profound effect on LDL cholesterol. Low doses decrease LDL cholesterol by about 25%, and larger doses decrease levels by as much as 63% (Table 50.6). Reductions are significant within 2 weeks and maximal within 4 to 6 weeks. Because cholesterol synthesis normally increases during the night, statins are most effective when given in the evening. If statin therapy is stopped, serum cholesterol will return to pretreatment levels within weeks to months. Therefore, treatment should continue lifelong, unless serious adverse effects or specific contraindications (especially pregnancy or muscle damage) arise. The mechanism by which statins reduce cholesterol levels is discussed under *Mechanism of Cholesterol Reduction.*

Elevation of HDL Cholesterol. Statins can increase levels of HDL cholesterol. Recall that low levels of HDL cholesterol (below 40 mg/dL) are an independent risk factor for ASCVD. Hence, by raising HDL cholesterol, statins may help reduce the risk of CV events in yet another way. The objective is to raise levels to 50 mg/dL or more.

Reduction of Triglyceride Levels. Although statins mainly affect cholesterol synthesis and thereby lower LDL cholesterol levels, these drugs may also lower TGs. Just why these "anti-cholesterol" drugs lower TGs is unknown, but the response has been amply documented. Please note that although statins may reduce TG levels, they are not actually prescribed for this action. Hence TG reduction is usually a beneficial side effect in patients taking statins to lower their LDL cholesterol. Of note, the ability to lower TGs seems to be short lived, and hence a drug designed to lower TGs eventually may need to be added.

TABLE 50.6 ▪ HMG-CoA Reductase Inhibitors: Selected Aspects of Clinical Pharmacology

Drug	% Change in Serum Lipids[a]			Effect of CYP3A4 Inhibitors on Statin Levels[b]	Effect of Renal or Hepatic Impairment on Statin Levels
	LDL-C	HDL-C	TGs		
Atorvastatin [Lipitor]	↓ 25–60	↑ 5–15	↓ 15–50	Moderate ↑	No change with renal disease; significant ↑ with hepatic impairment
Fluvastatin [Lescol, Lescol XL]	↓ 20–40	↑ 2–11	↓ 10–25	None	No change with renal disease; possible ↑ with hepatic impairment
Lovastatin [Altoprev, Mevacor]	↓ 20–40	↑ 5–10	↓ 5–25	Significant ↑	↑ with significant renal impairment; no change with hepatic impairment
Pitavastatin [Livalo]	↓ 40–45	↑ 6–8	↓ 15–30	Little or none	↑ with significant renal impairment; little or no change with hepatic impairment
Pravastatin [Pravachol]	↓ 20–40	↑ 1–15	↓ 10–25	None	Potential ↑ with either renal or hepatic impairment
Rosuvastatin [Crestor]	↓ 30–60	↑ 3–20	↓ 10–40	None	↑ levels with severe renal impairment or hepatic dysfunction
Simvastatin [Zocor]	↓ 25–50	↑ 7–15	↓ 8–40	Significant ↑	Potential ↑ with severe renal or hepatic impairment

[a]The values were obtained from a variety of studies and do not reflect dose dependency of drug responses.
[b]Inhibitors of CYP3A4 (the 3A4 isoenzyme of P450) include itraconazole, ketoconazole, erythromycin, clarithromycin, HIV protease inhibitors, cyclosporine, nefazodone, and substances in grapefruit juice.
↑, Increase; ↓, decrease.
HDL-C, High-density lipoprotein cholesterol; *LDL-C,* low-density lipoprotein cholesterol; *TGs,* triglycerides.

Nonlipid Beneficial CV Actions. There is increasing evidence that statins do more than just alter lipid levels. Specifically, they can promote atherosclerotic plaque stability (by decreasing plaque cholesterol content), reduce inflammation at the plaque site, slow progression of coronary artery calcification, improve abnormal endothelial function, enhance the ability of blood vessels to dilate, reduce the risk of atrial fibrillation, and reduce the risk of thrombosis by (1) inhibiting platelet deposition and aggregation and (2) suppressing production of thrombin, a key factor in clot formation. All of these actions help reduce the risk of CV events.

Increased Bone Formation. There is evidence that statins may promote bone formation and may thereby reduce the risk of osteoporosis and related fractures. This has been shown in several case-control studies in humans. However, other case-control studies have failed to demonstrate a protective effect. In addition, six randomized controlled trials of statins in 3022 postmenopausal women failed to show a difference in bone density. Until randomized controlled trials are completed in other populations, osteoporosis should be managed with bisphosphonates and/or other drugs with proven efficacy (see Chapter 75).

Mechanism of Cholesterol Reduction

The mechanism by which statins decrease LDL cholesterol levels is complex and depends ultimately on *increasing the number of LDL receptors on hepatocytes* (liver cells). The process begins with inhibition of hepatic HMG-CoA reductase, the rate-limiting enzyme in cholesterol biosynthesis. In response to decreased cholesterol production, hepatocytes synthesize more HMG-CoA reductase. As a result, cholesterol synthesis is largely restored to pretreatment levels. However—and for reasons that are not fully understood—inhibition of cholesterol synthesis causes hepatocytes to synthesize more LDL receptors. As a result, hepatocytes are better able to remove more LDLs from the blood. In patients who are genetically unable to synthesize LDL receptors, statins fail to reduce LDL levels, indicating that (1) inhibition of cholesterol synthesis, by itself, is not sufficient to explain cholesterol-lowering effects; and (2) for statins to be effective, synthesis of LDL receptors must increase.

In addition to inhibiting HMG-CoA reductase, statins decrease production of apolipoprotein B-100. As a result, hepatocytes decrease production of VLDLs. This lowers VLDL levels and TG levels too since they're the main lipid in VLDLs. Also, statins raise HDL levels by 5% to 22%.

Clinical Trials

Statins slow the progression of ASCVD and decrease the risk of stroke, hospitalization, cardiac events, peripheral vascular disease, and death. Benefits are seen in men and women, and in apparently healthy people, as well as in those with a history of CV events. Hence, the statins are useful for both primary and secondary prevention. Furthermore, these drugs can help people with even *normal* LDL levels, in addition to those whose LDL level is high. Statins may also have some added protective effects in people with diabetes.

Secondary Prevention Studies. In patients with evidence of existing ASCVD (angina pectoris or previous MI), statins reduce the risk of death from cardiac causes. This was first demonstrated conclusively in the landmark *Scandinavian Simvastatin Survival Study* (4S). After 4.9 to 6.3 years of follow-up, the death rate was 12% among patients taking placebo and 8% among those taking simvastatin—a 30% decrease in overall mortality. Benefits were due to a decrease in cardiac-related mortality; deaths from noncardiac causes were the same in both groups.

The *Cholesterol and Recurrent Events* (CARE) trial demonstrated the ability of statins to reduce the risk of stroke in addition to coronary events. In this study, 4159 people with a history of MI were given pravastatin (40 mg daily) or placebo. After 5 years, the incidence of MI (fatal or nonfatal) was 13.2% in those taking placebo and 10.2% in those taking the drug. Pravastatin also produced a 26% decrease in the risk of stroke.

The *Pravastatin or Atorvastatin Evaluation and Infection Therapy* (PROVE-IT) trial was the first to show that *intensive* reductions in LDL with statin therapy provide more CV protection than moderate reductions. In PROVE-IT, 4162 patients with ACS were randomized to either a moderate statin regimen (pravastatin, 40 mg daily) or an intensive statin regimen (atorvastatin, 80 mg daily). The result? LDL levels in the moderate group dropped to 95 mg/dL, compared with 62 mg/dL in the intensive group. Furthermore, not only did intensive therapy produce a greater decrease in LDL cholesterol, it also produced a greater reduction in adverse outcomes: After 24 months, the incidence of CV events (death, MI, unstable angina, or revascularization) was only 22.4% in the intensive group compared with 26.3% in the moderate group. These results led the ATP III panel to recommend lower target LDL levels in patients at very high CV risk.

Primary Prevention Studies. Two major studies have demonstrated the ability of statins to reduce mortality in people with no previous history of coronary events. In the first trial—the *West of Scotland Coronary Prevention Study* (WOSCOPS)—6595 men with high cholesterol were given either pravastatin (40 mg/day) or placebo. During an average follow-up of 4.9 years, 4.1% of those taking placebo died, compared with only 3.2% of those taking the statin. The second trial—the *Air Force/Texas Coronary Atherosclerosis Prevention Study* (AFCAPS/TexCAPS)—enrolled 6605 low-risk patients: men and women with average cholesterol levels (221 mg/dL) and no history of CV events. The subjects were randomly assigned to receive lovastatin (20 to 40 mg/day) or placebo. After an average follow-up of 5.5 years, the incidence of first major coronary events was 5.5% for those taking placebo and 3.5% for those taking the drug—representing a 36% decrease in risk.

Primary Prevention in Patients With Normal Cholesterol Levels. The landmark *Heart Protection Study,* published in 2002, was the first major trial to demonstrate that statins can reduce the risk of major coronary events in people who have normal levels of cholesterol. This double-blind, placebo-controlled trial enrolled 20,536 high-risk British patients: men and women with diabetes, prior MI, stroke, or prior angioplasty. Some had high levels of LDL and total cholesterol; others had normal levels. Subjects were randomly assigned to receive either simvastatin (40 mg/day) or placebo. After 5 years, the incidence of death was 12.9% in the treatment group, compared with 14.7% in the placebo group. Death from ASCVD was reduced by 18%. In addition, simvastatin reduced the risk of nonfatal MI by 38% and of stroke by 25%, and reduced the need for coronary revascularization (e.g., angioplasty) by 30%. Most strikingly, benefits were seen in patients whose LDL cholesterol was *normal* or *low,* as well as in those whose levels were high. These data suggest a radical shift in practice. Specifically, they suggest we should treat people at high ASCVD risk—not just those with high cholesterol levels. Obviously, doing so would greatly expand the number of patients receiving statin therapy.

A more recent trial—*Justification for the Use of Statins in Prevention: an Intervention Trial Evaluating Rosuvastatin* (JUPITER)—reinforced the results of the Heart Protection Study. The study demonstrated that rosuvastatin can reduce the risk of coronary events in people with normal LDL levels, but with high levels of CRP and other risk factors for ASCVD.

Prevention in Patients With Diabetes. Results of the *Collaborative Atorvastatin Diabetes Study* (CARDS) indicate that statin therapy can reduce the risk of CV events in diabetes patients, even if LDL levels are normal. This randomized trial, conducted in Britain and Ireland, enrolled 2838 patients with type 2 diabetes who had no history of CV disease. Half received 10 mg of atorvastatin [Lipitor] daily, and half received a placebo. After a mean of 4 years, the combined incidence of acute coronary events, coronary revascularization, and stroke was only 5.8% in the atorvastatin group, compared with 9% in the placebo group, representing a 36% reduction in risk. These results suggest that statin therapy could benefit most patients with diabetes, regardless of their LDL level.

Therapeutic Uses

When the statins were introduced, they were approved only for hypercholesterolemia (elevated LDL cholesterol levels) in adults. As understanding of their benefits grew, so has the list of indications. Today the statins have nearly a dozen U.S. Food and Drug Administration (FDA)–approved indications, and these drugs can be prescribed for young patients, as well as for adults. Indications for individual statins are shown in Table 50.7. Major indications are discussed in the sections that follow.

Hypercholesterolemia. Statins are the most effective drugs we have for lowering LDL cholesterol. In sufficient dosage, statins can decrease LDL cholesterol by more than 60%. For many patients, the treatment goal is to drop LDL cholesterol to below 100 mg/dL. For patients at very high CV risk, a target of 70 mg/dL may be appropriate.

Primary and Secondary Prevention of CV Events. As discussed, statins can reduce the risk of CV events (e.g., MI,

TABLE 50.7 ▪ HMG-CoA Reductase Inhibitors: FDA-Approved Indications

Indication	Atorvastatin [Lipitor]	Fluvastatin [Lescol, Lescol XL]	Lovastatin [Altoprev, Mevacor]	Pitavastatin [Livalo]	Pravastatin [Pravachol]	Rosuvastatin [Crestor]	Simvastatin [Zocor]
Primary hypercholesterolemia	✓	✓	✓	✓	✓	✓	✓
Homozygous familial hyperlipidemia	✓					✓	✓
Heterozygous familial hypercholesterolemia in adolescents	✓		✓		✓	✓	✓
Mixed dyslipidemia	✓	✓	✓	✓	✓	✓	✓
Primary dysbetalipoproteinemia	✓				✓	✓	✓
Primary prevention of coronary events	✓		✓		✓	✓[a]	✓
Secondary prevention of CV events	✓	✓	✓		✓		✓
Increasing HDL cholesterol in primary hypercholesterolemia	✓		✓	✓		✓	✓
Slowing progression of coronary atherosclerosis		✓	✓		✓	✓	

[a]Rosuvastatin is approved for primary prevention in patients who have *normal* LDL cholesterol and no clinical evidence of ASCVD, but who do have high levels of C-reactive protein combined with other risk factors for CV disease.

angina, stroke) in patients who have never had one (primary prevention), and they can reduce the risk of a subsequent event after one has occurred (secondary prevention). Risk reduction is related to the reduction in LDL: the greater the LDL reduction, the greater the reduction in risk.

Primary Prevention in People With Normal LDL Levels. One agent—*rosuvastatin* [Crestor]—is now approved for reducing the risk of CV events in people with *normal* levels of LDL and no clinically evident ASCVD, but who do have an increased risk based on advancing age, high levels of *high-sensitivity C-reactive protein,* and at least one other risk factor for CV disease (e.g., hypertension, low HDL, smoking). Approval for this use was based in large part on results of the JUPITER trial.

Post-MI Therapy. Patients who have survived an MI and who were not on statin therapy at the time of the event are routinely started on a statin, the rationale being "better late than never." The current trend is to begin statins as soon as the patient is stabilized and able to take oral drugs. Other drugs for MI are discussed in Chapter 53.

Diabetes. Cardiovascular disease is the primary cause of death in people with diabetes. Hence, to reduce mortality, controlling CV risk factors—especially hypertension and high cholesterol—is as important as controlling high blood glucose. The American Diabetes Association recommends a statin for all patients older than 40 years whose LDL cholesterol is greater than 100 mg/dL. The American College of Physicians recommends a statin for (1) all patients with type 2 diabetes plus diagnosed ASCVD—*even if they don't have high cholesterol;* and (2) all adults with type 2 diabetes plus one additional risk factor (e.g., hypertension, smoking, age older than 55 years)—*even if they don't have high cholesterol.* Taken together, these guidelines suggest that most patients with diabetes should receive a statin.

Potential Uses. Potential uses of statins extend well beyond diabetes and CV disorders. Judging from preliminary evidence, these drugs may eventually be used to prevent and/or treat a variety of conditions, including Alzheimer's disease, kidney disease, multiple sclerosis, macular degeneration, glaucoma, rheumatoid arthritis, weak or brittle bones, and even certain cancers.

Influenza is associated with an increase in the risk for ACS, stroke, and venous thromboembolism. This is related to the increase in proinflammatory cytokines released during influenza. It is thought that statins can decrease this cytokine release and improve influenza-associated morbidity and mortality. A 10-year retrospective cohort study of older adults revealed that statins can protect against influenza morbidity in people taking statins as an outpatient. It also noted that there was an increase in the mortality of hospitalized patients admitted with influenza when their statin was stopped. Although this information is promising, more research is needed.

Pharmacokinetics

Statins are administered orally. The amount absorbed ranges between 30% and 90%, depending on the drug. Regardless of how much is absorbed, most of an absorbed dose is extracted from the blood on its first pass through the liver, the principal site at which statins act. Only a small fraction of each dose reaches the systemic circulation. Statins undergo rapid hepatic metabolism followed by excretion primarily in the bile. Only four agents—*lovastatin, pitavastatin, pravastatin,* and *simvastatin*—undergo clinically significant (10% to 20%) excretion in the urine.

Three statins—*atorvastatin, lovastatin,* and *simvastatin*—are metabolized by CYP3A4 (the 3A4 isoenzyme of cytochrome P450). As a result, levels of these drugs can be lowered by agents that induce CYP3A4 synthesis and speed up the metabolic inactivation of the statin. More importantly, statin levels can be increased—sometimes dramatically—by agents that inhibit CYP3A4 (see *With Drugs That Inhibit CYP3A4* later in this chapter).

One agent—*rosuvastatin*—reaches abnormally high levels in people of Asian heritage. At usual therapeutic doses, rosuvastatin levels in these patients are about twice those in Caucasians. Accordingly, if rosuvastatin is used by Asians, dosage should be reduced.

Adverse Effects

Statins are generally well tolerated. Side effects are uncommon. Some patients develop headache, rash, memory loss, or GI disturbances (dyspepsia, cramps, flatulence, constipation, abdominal pain). However, these effects are usually mild and transient. Serious adverse effects—hepatotoxicity and myopathy—are relatively rare. Some statins pose a greater risk than others, as noted here.

Myopathy/Rhabdomyolysis. Statins can injure muscle tissue. *Mild injury* occurs in 5% to 10% of patients. Characteristic symptoms are muscles aches, tenderness, or weakness that may be diffuse or localized to certain muscle groups. Rarely, mild injury progresses to *myositis,* defined as muscle inflammation associated with moderate elevation of creatine kinase (CK), an enzyme released from injured muscle. Release of potassium from muscle may cause blood potassium concentrations to rise. Rarely, myositis progresses to potentially fatal *rhabdomyolysis,* defined as muscle disintegration or dissolution. Release of muscle components leads to marked elevations of blood CK (greater than 10 times the upper limit of normal [ULN]) and elevations of free myoglobin. High levels of CK, in turn, may cause *renal impairment,* as excess CK can plug up the glomeruli, thereby preventing normal filtration.

Fortunately, fatal rhabdomyolysis is extremely rare: The overall incidence is less than 0.15 case per 1 million prescriptions. Nonetheless, patients should be informed about the risk of myopathy and instructed to notify the prescriber if unexplained muscle pain or tenderness occurs. How statins cause myopathy is unknown.

Several factors increase the risk of myopathy. Among these are advanced age, small body frame, frailty, multisystem disease (e.g., chronic renal insufficiency, especially associated with diabetes), use of statins in high doses, low vitamin D and coenzyme Q levels, concurrent use of fibrates (which can cause myopathy too), and the use of drugs that can raise statin levels (see the following paragraphs). In addition, hypothyroidism increases risk. Accordingly, if muscle pain develops, thyroid function should be assessed. Measurement of CK levels can facilitate diagnosis. Levels should be determined at baseline and again if symptoms of myopathy appear. If the CK level is more than 10 times the ULN, the statin should be discontinued. If the level is less than 10 times the ULN, the statin can be continued, provided myopathy symptoms and the CK level are followed weekly. However, given that weekly blood tests are expensive and inconvenient, it may be best to stop the statin and re-evaluate therapy, even when CK levels *are* less than 10 times the ULN. Routine monitoring of CK in asymptomatic patients is unnecessary.

What is the rhabdomyolysis risk with individual statins? Of the seven statins in current use, *rosuvastatin* [Crestor] poses the highest risk of rhabdomyolysis. But even with this drug, the absolute number of cases is extremely low. With the other statins, the risk is even lower.

Should concerns about myopathy discourage statin use? Definitely not! Remember: The risk of serious myopathy is extremely low, whereas the risk of untreated LDL cholesterol is very high. Accordingly, when statins are used to lower cholesterol, the benefits of therapy (reduction of CV events) far outweigh the small risk of myopathy. Additional strategies for the management of myalgia include replacement of vitamin D and coenzyme Q and switching statins. Studies reveal that replacement of vitamin D and coenzyme Q can reduce myalgias in patients with low levels. Switching statins can be effective, as patients may not have myalgias when taking a different drug, even if it is within the same class.

Hepatotoxicity. Liver injury, as evidenced by elevations in serum transaminase levels, develops in 0.5% to 2% of patients treated 1 year or longer. However, jaundice and other clinical signs are rare. Progression to outright liver failure occurs very rarely. Because of the risk of liver injury, product labeling recommends that liver function tests (LFTs) be done before treatment and then if clinically indicated after starting the drug. If serum transaminase levels rise to 3 times the ULN and remain there, statins should be discontinued. Transaminase levels decline to pretreatment levels following drug withdrawal.

Should statins be used by patients with active liver disease? The answer depends on the disease. In patients with viral or alcoholic hepatitis, statins should be avoided. However, in patients with the most common cause of hepatitis—nonalcoholic fatty liver disease—statins are acceptable therapy. In fact, in these patients, not only can statins reduce cholesterol levels, they may also decrease liver inflammation, improve LFTs, and reduce steatosis (fatty infiltration in the liver). Should LFTs be monitored? Yes—at baseline and as clinically indicated thereafter. If LFTs climb to 3 times the ULN, statin use should stop.

New-Onset Diabetes. The risk of developing new-onset diabetes while taking a statin is 1 in 500 patients prescribed a statin. Yet many of the patients in these studies had prediabetes before taking a statin. It is unclear whether taking a statin accelerates the advancement from prediabetes to diabetes. Despite the possibility, the CV benefits of taking a statin far outweigh the risk, and management should not change.

Memory Loss. Some patients have reported reversible memory loss or confusion that improves after stopping statin therapy. Although memory loss may occur, there is an overall lack of evidence surrounding these reports. A large review of 41 different studies completed in 2013 found no connection between memory loss and statin use. What the evidence does reveal is a possible increase in memory loss in patients taking any type of cholesterol-reducing medication, not just statins. As this issue remains unclear, patients should still report confusion or memory loss to their provider.

Cataracts. An analysis of military healthcare records between 2003 and 2010 revealed a 27% increase of cataracts in patients who had taken a statin for at least 90 days when compared with patients not taking statins. More recently, two larger studies were completed in the older adult population, and similar results were found. The reason for this association is unknown. The greatest risk appears to be in patients taking simvastatin, lovastatin, and atorvastatin. Overall, the risk remains small, and statin therapy should be continued in patients when indicated.

Drug Interactions

With Other Lipid-Lowering Drugs. Combining a statin with most other lipid-lowering drugs (except probably the bile-acid sequestrants) can increase the incidence and severity of the most serious statin-related adverse events: muscle injury, liver injury, and kidney damage. The increase in risk occurs primarily with fibrates (gemfibrozil, fenofibrate), which are commonly combined with statins. The bottom line: When statins are combined with other lipid-lowering agents, use extra caution and monitor for adverse effects more frequently.

With Drugs That Inhibit CYP3A4. Drugs that inhibit CYP3A4 can raise levels of *lovastatin* and *simvastatin* substantially, and can raise levels of *atorvastatin* moderately, by slowing their inactivation. Important inhibitors of CYP3A4 include macrolide antibiotics (e.g., erythromycin), azole antifungal drugs (e.g., ketoconazole, itraconazole), HIV protease inhibitors (e.g., ritonavir), amiodarone (an antidysrhythmic drug), and cyclosporine (an immunosuppressant). If these drugs are combined with a statin, increased caution is advised. Some authorities recommend an automatic reduction in statin dosage if these inhibitors are used.

As discussed in Chapter 6, chemicals in grapefruit and grapefruit juice can inhibit CYP3A4. Furthermore, the inhibition may persist for 3 days or more after eating the fruit or drinking its juice. Accordingly, statin users should avoid grapefruits and their juice.

Use in Pregnancy

Statins are classified in FDA Pregnancy Risk Category X[b]: The risks to the fetus outweigh any potential benefits of treatment. Some statins have caused fetal malformation in animal models—but only at doses far higher than those used in humans. To date, teratogenic effects in humans have not been reported. Nonetheless, because statins inhibit synthesis of cholesterol and because cholesterol is required for the synthesis of cell membranes as well as several fetal hormones, concern regarding human fetal injury remains. Moreover, there is no compelling reason to continue lipid-lowering drugs during pregnancy: Stopping the statin for 9 months is not going to cause a sudden, dangerous rise in cholesterol levels or risk of ASCVD. Women of childbearing age should be informed about the potential for fetal harm and warned against becoming pregnant. If pregnancy occurs and the patient plans to continue the pregnancy, statins should be discontinued.

Preparations, Dosage, and Administration

Statins are available alone and in fixed-dose combinations. The single-ingredient products are discussed here. The combination products are discussed later in the chapter under the heading *Drug Combinations*.

Seven statins are available for use alone: atorvastatin, fluvastatin, lovastatin, pitavastatin, pravastatin, rosuvastatin,

[b]As of 2020, the FDA will no longer use Pregnancy Risk Categories. Please refer to Chapter 9 for more information.

TABLE 50.8 ■ HMG-CoA Reductase Inhibitors: Preparations, Dosage, and Administration

Drug	Dosage	Administration With Regard to Meals	Dosage Changes in Special Populations	Preparations
Atorvastatin [Lipitor]	*Initial:* 10 mg at bedtime *Maximum:* 80 mg at bedtime	Take without regard to meals	No changes needed	*Lipitor (tablets):* 10, 20, 40, 80 mg
Fluvastatin [Lescol, Lescol XL]	*Initial:* 20–40 mg at bedtime *Maximum, Lescol:* 40 mg twice a day *Maximum, Lescol XL:* 80 mg at bedtime	Take without regard to meals	Reduce dosage for severe renal impairment	*Lescol (capsules):* 20, 40 mg *Lescol XL (extended-release tablets):* 80 mg
Lovastatin [Altoprev, Mevacor; generics]	*Initial:* 20 mg *Maximum:* 40 mg twice daily or 80 mg at bedtime	Take immediate-release tablets with evening meal to increase absorption. Take extended-release tablets at bedtime.	Reduce dosage for severe renal impairment	*Altoprev (extended-release tablets):* 20, 40, 60 mg *Mevacor and generics (tablets):* 10, 20, 40 mg
Pitavastatin [Livalo]	*Initial:* 2 mg once daily at any time of day *Maximum:* 4 mg once daily	Take without regard to meals	Reduce dosage for moderate to severe renal impairment	*Livalo (tablets):* 1, 2, 4 mg
Pravastatin [Pravachol; generics]	*Initial:* 40 mg at bedtime *Maximum:* 80 mg at bedtime	Take without regard to meals	Reduce dosage for moderate to severe renal impairment	*Pravachol and generics (tablets):* 10, 20, 40, 80 mg
Rosuvastatin [Crestor]	*Initial:* 5–20 mg at bedtime *Maximum:* 40 mg at bedtime	Take without regard to meals	Reduce dosage for severe renal impairment Reduce dosage in Asian patients	*Crestor (tablets):* 5, 10, 20, 40 mg
Simvastatin [Zocor; generics]	*Initial:* 10–20 mg at bedtime *Maximum:* 40 mg/day	Take without regard to meals	Reduce dosage for severe renal impairment	*Zocor and generics (tablets):* 5, 10, 20, 40, 80 mg

and simvastatin. Information on preparations, dosage, and administration is shown in Table 50.8.

Dosing is done once daily, preferably in the *evening* either with the evening meal or at bedtime. Because endogenous cholesterol synthesis increases during the night, statins have the greatest impact when given in the evening.

Drug Selection

Several factors bear on statin selection, including the LDL goal, drug interactions, kidney function, safety in Asian patients, and price.

LDL Goal. If a 30% to 40% reduction in LDL is deemed sufficient, any statin will do. However, if LDL must be lowered by more than 40%, then atorvastatin or simvastatin may be preferred. Furthermore, not only are these two drugs highly effective, clinical experience with them is extensive.

Drug Interactions. Drugs that inhibit CYP3A4 can raise levels of atorvastatin, lovastatin, and simvastatin, thereby increasing the risk of toxicity, especially myopathy and liver injury. Accordingly, in patients taking a CYP3A4 inhibitor, other statins may be preferred.

Kidney Function. For patients with normal renal function, any statin is acceptable. However, for patients with significant renal impairment, atorvastatin and fluvastatin are preferred (because no dosage adjustment is needed).

Safety in Asians. The same dose of *rosuvastatin,* when given to Asian and Caucasian subjects, may produce twofold higher blood levels in the Asians. Accordingly, when rosuvastatin is used in Asians, start with the lowest available dosage and monitor diligently.

Price. Six statins—lovastatin, pravastatin, atorvastatin, fluvastatin, rosuvastatin, and simvastatin—are now available as generic products, and hence are cheaper than all other statins.

A Word Regarding Niacin (Nicotinic Acid)

Niacin was once thought to be beneficial in the reduction of LDL and TG levels. However, despite these previously demonstrated favorable effects on lipid levels, niacin does little to improve outcomes and carries much potential harm. Therefore, in 2016, a panel of experts recommended that niacin be removed from the guidelines for use in hypertriglyceridemia and in lowering LDL cholesterol.

Bile-Acid Sequestrants

Bile-acid sequestrants reduce LDL cholesterol levels. In the past, these drugs were a mainstay of lipid-lowering therapy. Today, they are used primarily as adjuncts to statins. Three agents are available: colesevelam, cholestyramine, and colestipol. Colesevelam is newer than the other two and is better tolerated.

Colesevelam

Colesevelam [Welchol] is the drug of choice when a bile-acid sequestrant is indicated. Like the older sequestrants, colesevelam is a nonabsorbable resin that binds (sequesters) bile acids and other substances in the GI tract and thereby prevents their absorption and promotes their excretion. Colesevelam is preferred to the older sequestrants for three reasons: (1) the drug is better tolerated (less constipation, flatulence, bloating, and cramping); (2) it does not reduce absorption of fat-soluble vitamins (A, D, E, and K); and (3) it does not significantly reduce the absorption of statins, digoxin, warfarin, and most other drugs studied.

In addition to its beneficial effects on plasma lipids, colesevelam is approved for adjunctive therapy of hyperglycemia in patients with type 2 diabetes. Diabetes and its management are the subject of Chapter 57.

Effect on Plasma Lipoproteins. The main response to bile-acid sequestrants is a reduction in LDL cholesterol. LDL decline begins during the first week of therapy and becomes maximal (about a 20% drop) within about a month. When these drugs are discontinued, LDL cholesterol returns to pretreatment levels in 3 to 4 weeks.

Bile-acid sequestrants may increase VLDL levels in some patients. In most cases, the elevation is transient and mild. However, if VLDL levels are elevated before treatment, the increase induced by the bile-acid sequestrants may be sustained and substantial. Accordingly, bile-acid sequestrants are not drugs of choice for lowering LDL cholesterol in patients with high VLDL levels.

Pharmacokinetics. Bile-acid sequestrants are biologically inert. Also, they are insoluble in water, cannot be absorbed from the GI tract, and are not attacked by digestive enzymes. Following oral administration, they simply pass through the intestine and are excreted in the feces.

Mechanism of Action. The bile-acid sequestrants lower LDL cholesterol through a mechanism that ultimately depends on increasing LDL receptors on hepatocytes. As background, you need to know that bile acids secreted into the intestine are normally reabsorbed and reused. Bile-acid sequestrants prevent this reabsorption. Following oral dosing, these drugs form an insoluble complex with bile acids in the intestine; this complex prevents the reabsorption of bile acids and thereby accelerates their excretion. Because bile acids are normally reabsorbed, the increase in excretion creates a demand for increased synthesis, which takes place in the liver. Since bile acids are made from cholesterol, liver cells require an increased cholesterol supply to increase bile acid production. The required cholesterol is provided by LDL. To avail themselves of more LDL cholesterol, liver cells increase their number of LDL receptors, thereby increasing their capacity for LDL uptake. The result is an increase in LDL uptake from plasma, which decreases circulating LDL levels. Individuals who are genetically incapable of increasing LDL receptor synthesis are unable to benefit from these drugs.

Therapeutic Use. Colesevelam is indicated as adjunctive therapy to diet and exercise for reducing LDL cholesterol in patients with primary hypercholesterolemia. The drug may be used alone, but usually is combined with a statin. On average, colesevelam alone can lower LDL cholesterol by about 20% (the typical range is between 15% and 30%). In contrast, combined therapy with a statin can reduce LDL cholesterol by up to 50%.

Adverse Effects. The bile-acid sequestrants are not absorbed from the GI tract, and hence are devoid of systemic effects. Accordingly, they are safer than all other lipid-lowering drugs.

Adverse effects are limited to the GI tract. *Constipation* is the main complaint. This can be minimized by increasing dietary fiber and fluids. If necessary, a mild laxative may be used. Other GI effects include *bloating, indigestion,* and *nausea.* The older agents—cholestyramine and colestipol—can decrease fat absorption and may thereby *decrease uptake of fat-soluble vitamins.* However, this does not seem to be a problem with colesevelam.

Drug Interactions. The bile-acid sequestrants can form insoluble complexes with other drugs. Medications that undergo binding cannot be absorbed, and hence are not available for systemic effects. Drugs known to form complexes with the sequestrants include thiazide diuretics, digoxin, warfarin, and some antibiotics. To reduce formation of sequestrant-drug complexes, oral medications that are known to interact should be administered either 1 hour before the sequestrant or 4 hours after.

Preparations, Dosage, and Administration. Colesevelam [Welchol] is supplied in tablets (625 mg) and as a powder (1.875 and 3.75 gm) for making an oral suspension. With the tablets, the initial adult dosage is 3 tablets (1.9 gm) twice daily or 6 tablets (3.8 gm) once daily. With the oral suspension, the initial adult dosage is 1.875 gm twice daily or 3.75 gm once daily. All doses are taken with food and water. Of note, the dosage for colesevelam is much smaller than that of cholestyramine (4 to 24 gm/day) or colestipol (5 to 30 gm/day).

Older Agents: Cholestyramine and Colestipol

Cholestyramine and colestipol have been available for decades, but have been largely replaced by colesevelam because colesevelam is better tolerated, does not impede absorption of fat-soluble vitamins, and has minimal effects on other drugs. Although cholestyramine and colestipol are very safe, they frequently cause constipation, abdominal discomfort, and bloating.

Cholestyramine [Questran, Questran Light, Prevalite] is supplied in powdered form. Instruct patients to mix the powder with fluid, because swallowing it dry can cause esophageal irritation and impaction. Appropriate liquids for mixing include water, fruit juices, and soups. Pulpy fruits with a high fluid content (e.g., applesauce, crushed pineapple) may also be used. The dosage range is 4 to 24 gm/day.

Colestipol hydrochloride [Colestid] is supplied in granular form (5 gm) and in 1-gm tablets. The dosage for the *granules* is 5 to 30 gm/day administered in one or more doses. Instruct patients to mix the granules with fluids or pulpy fruits before ingestion. The dosage for the *tablets* is 2 to 16 gm/day administered in one or more doses. Tablets should be swallowed whole and taken with fluid.

Ezetimibe

Ezetimibe [Zetia, Ezetrol 🍁] is a unique drug for reducing plasma cholesterol. Benefits derive from blocking cholesterol absorption.

Mechanism of Action and Effect on Plasma Lipoproteins

Ezetimibe acts on cells of the brush border of the small intestine to inhibit dietary cholesterol absorption. The drug also inhibits reabsorption of cholesterol secreted in the bile. Treatment reduces plasma levels of total cholesterol, LDL cholesterol, TGs, and apolipoprotein B. In addition, ezetimibe can produce a small *increase* in HDL cholesterol.

Therapeutic Use

Ezetimibe is indicated as an adjunct to diet modification for reducing total cholesterol, LDL cholesterol, and apolipoprotein B in patients with primary hypercholesteremia. The drug is approved for monotherapy and for combined use with a statin. In clinical trials, ezetimibe alone reduced LDL cholesterol by about 19%, increased HDL cholesterol by 1% to 4%, and decreased TGs by 5% to 10%. When ezetimibe was combined with a statin, the reduction in LDL cholesterol was about 25% greater than with the statin alone. Despite these desirable effects on blood lipids, there is no evidence that ezetimibe reduces atherosclerosis or improves clinical outcomes.

Pharmacokinetics

Ezetimibe is administered orally, and absorption is not affected by food. In the intestinal wall and liver, ezetimibe undergoes extensive conversion to ezetimibe glucuronide, an active metabolite. Both compounds—ezetimibe itself and its main metabolite—are eliminated primarily in the bile. The elimination half-life is about 22 hours.

Adverse Effects

Ezetimibe is generally well tolerated. During clinical trials, the incidence of significant side effects was nearly identical to that seen with placebo. However, during postmarketing surveillance, there have been reports of myopathy, rhabdomyolysis, hepatitis, pancreatitis, and thrombocytopenia. In contrast to the bile-acid sequestrants, ezetimibe does not cause constipation and other adverse GI effects.

Drug Interactions

Statins. In patients taking a statin, adding ezetimibe slightly increases the risk of liver damage (as indicated by elevated transaminase levels). If the drugs are combined, transaminase levels should be monitored before starting therapy, as well as whenever clinically indicated thereafter. Combining ezetimibe with a statin may also increase the risk of myopathy.

Fibrates. Both ezetimibe and fibrates (gemfibrozil and fenofibrate) can increase the cholesterol content of bile and can thereby increase the risk of gallstones. Both also increase the risk of myopathy. Accordingly, combined use is not recommended.

Bile-Acid Sequestrants. Cholestyramine (and possibly colestipol) can significantly decrease the absorption of ezetimibe. To minimize effects on absorption, ezetimibe should be administered at least 2 hours before a sequestrant or more than 4 hours after.

Cyclosporine. Cyclosporine may greatly increase levels of ezetimibe. If the drugs are combined, careful monitoring is needed.

Caution

In patients with hepatic impairment, bioavailability of ezetimibe is significantly increased. At this time, we do not know if increased availability is harmful. Until more is known, patients with moderate or severe hepatic insufficiency should not be given the drug.

Preparations, Dosage, and Administration

Ezetimibe [Zetia, Ezetrol 🍁] is available in 10-mg tablets. The recommended dosage is 10 mg once a day, taken with or without food. If ezetimibe is combined with a statin, both drugs can be taken at the same time. If ezetimibe is combined with a bile-acid sequestrant, ezetimibe should be taken 2 hours before the sequestrant or 4 hours after.

Fibric Acid Derivatives (Fibrates)

The fibric acid derivatives, also known as fibrates, are the most effective drugs we have for lowering TG levels. In addition, these drugs can raise HDL cholesterol, but have little or no effect on LDL cholesterol. Furthermore, there is no proof that fibrates reduce mortality from ASCVD. Fibrates can increase the risk of bleeding in patients taking warfarin (an anticoagulant) and the risk of rhabdomyolysis in patients taking statins. Because of these and other undesired effects, and because mortality is not reduced, fibrates are considered third-line drugs for managing lipid disorders. In the United States, three preparations are available: gemfibrozil [Lopid], fenofibrate [Tricor, others], and fenofibric acid [TriLipix, Fibricor], a delayed-release preparation.

Gemfibrozil

Gemfibrozil [Lopid] decreases TG (VLDL) levels and raises HDL cholesterol levels. The drug does not reduce LDL cholesterol to a significant degree. Its principal indication is hypertriglyceridemia.

Effect on Plasma Lipoproteins. Gemfibrozil decreases plasma TG content by lowering VLDL levels. Maximum reductions in VLDLs range from 40% to 55%, and are achieved within 3 to 4 weeks of treatment. Gemfibrozil can raise HDL cholesterol by 6% to 10%. In patients with normal TG levels, the drug can produce a small reduction in LDL levels. However, if TG levels are high, gemfibrozil may actually increase LDL levels.

Mechanism of Action. Gemfibrozil and other fibrates appear to work by interacting with a specific receptor subtype—known as peroxisome proliferator-activated receptor alpha (PPAR alpha)—present in the liver and brown adipose tissue. Activation of PPAR alpha leads to (1) increased synthesis of lipoprotein lipase (LPL) and (2) reduced production of apolipoprotein C-III (an inhibitor of LPL). Both actions accelerate the clearance of VLDLs and thereby reduce levels of TGs. How do fibrates elevate HDL levels? By activating PPAR alpha, fibrates increase production of apolipoproteins A-I and A-II, which in turn facilitates HDL formation.

Therapeutic Use. Gemfibrozil is used primarily to *reduce high levels of plasma triglycerides* (VLDLs). Treatment is limited to patients who have not responded adequately to weight control and diet modification. Gemfibrozil can also reduce LDL cholesterol slightly. However, other drugs (statins, cholestyramine, colestipol) are much more effective.

Gemfibrozil can be used to *raise HDL cholesterol,* although it is not approved for this application. When tested in patients with normal LDL cholesterol and low HDL cholesterol, gemfibrozil reduced the risk of major CV events—but did not reduce *mortality* from ASCVD. Because LDL cholesterol was normal, it appears that benefits were due primarily to elevation of HDL cholesterol, along with reduction of plasma TGs.

Adverse Effects. Gemfibrozil is generally well tolerated. The most common reactions are rash and GI disturbances (nausea, abdominal pain, diarrhea).

Gallstones. Gemfibrozil increases biliary cholesterol saturation, thereby increasing the risk of gallstones. Patients should be informed about manifestations of gallbladder disease (e.g., upper abdominal discomfort, intolerance of fried foods, bloating) and instructed to notify the prescriber at once if these develop. Patients with pre-existing gallbladder disease should not take the drug.

Myopathy. Like the statins, gemfibrozil and other fibrates can cause myopathy. Warn patients to report any signs of muscle injury, such as tenderness, weakness, or unusual muscle pain.

Liver Injury. Gemfibrozil is hepatotoxic. The drug can disrupt liver function and may also pose a risk of liver cancer. Periodic tests of liver function are recommended.

Drug Interactions. *Gemfibrozil displaces warfarin from plasma albumin,* thereby increasing anticoagulant effects. Prothrombin time (international normalized ratio) should be measured frequently to assess coagulation status. Warfarin dosage may need to be reduced.

As noted, gemfibrozil increases the risk of *statin-induced myopathy.* Accordingly, the combination of a statin with gemfibrozil should be used with great caution, if at all.

Preparations, Dosage, and Administration. Gemfibrozil [Lopid] is available in 600-mg tablets. The adult dosage is 600 mg twice a day. Dosing is done 30 minutes before the morning and evening meals.

Fenofibrate

Actions and Uses. Fenofibrate [Tricor, Antara, Lofibra, Triglide, Lipofen, Lipidil 🍁] is indicated for hypertriglyceridemia in patients who have not responded to dietary measures. The drug lowers TGs by decreasing levels of VLDLs.

Pharmacokinetics. Fenofibrate is well absorbed from the GI tract, especially in the presence of food. Once absorbed, the drug is rapidly converted to fenofibric acid, its active form. In the blood, the drug is 98% protein bound. Elimination is the result of hepatic metabolism followed by renal excretion. The plasma half-life is about 20 hours.

Adverse Effects and Drug Interactions. The most common adverse effects are rash and GI disturbances. Like gemfibrozil, fenofibrate can cause gallstones and liver injury. In animal models, doses 1 to 6 times the maximum human dose caused cancers of the pancreas and liver. Like gemfibrozil, fenofibrate can increase the risk of bleeding with warfarin and the risk of myopathy with statins.

Preparations, Dosage, and Administration. Fenofibrate is available in several formulations that differ with respect to dosage and the impact of food on absorption. Four products are discussed here.

Tricor tablets (48 and 145 mg) are made using NanoCrystal technology to enhance absorption. As a result, dosing can be done with or without food. The dosage range is 48 to 145 mg/day.

Triglide tablets (160 mg), like Tricor tablets, may be administered with or without food. The dosage is 160 mg/day.

Antara capsules (30 and 90 mg), which contain micronized particles, must be administered with food to maximize absorption. The dosage range is 30 to 90 mg/day.

Lofibra capsules (67, 134, and 200 mg) contain micronized particles. Like Antara, Lofibra must be administered with food to maximize absorption. The dosage range is 67 to 200 mg/day.

Fenofibric Acid

Fenofibric acid [TriLipix, Fibricor] is the active metabolite of fenofibrate. Accordingly, the pharmacology of the drug is much like that of the parent compound. Fenofibric acid stands out from other fibrates for being the only group member *approved* for use with a statin. However, there is no proof that combining the drug with a statin reduces the risk of a major CV event. Furthermore, just like other fibrates, fenofibric acid can cause myopathy, and hence combined use with a statin still poses significant myopathy risk. Therefore, the combination must be employed with great care. Fenofibric acid is available in delayed-release capsules (45 and 135 mg, sold as *TriLipix;* 35 and 105 mg, sold as *Fibricor*). Daily dosages for hypertriglyceridemia range from 35 to 135 mg. In patients with mild to moderate renal impairment, a low dosage (45 mg/day) should be used. When combined with a statin for patients with mixed dyslipidemias, fenofibric acid should be dosed at 135 mg/day.

Monoclonal Antibodies (Proprotein Convertase Subtilisin/Kexin Type 9 [PCSK9] Inhibitors)

Alirocumab [Praluent] and evolocumab [Repatha] compose a new type of drug class used for patients with high LDL levels, specifically in patients with heterozygous familial hypercholesterolemia or with atherosclerotic heart problems who need additional lowering of LDL cholesterol. The PCSK9 inhibitors are indicated as an adjunct to diet modification and maximally tolerated statin therapy for reducing total LDL cholesterol.

Mechanism of Action and Effect on Plasma Lipoproteins

Proprotein convertase subtilisin kexin type 9 (PCSK9) is a protein that binds to low-density lipoprotein receptors (LDLR) within the liver. LDLR is the primary receptor that clears circulating LDL. When PCSK9 binds to LDLR, there is an increase in LDL cholesterol, because LDLR cannot clear LDL. By inhibiting PCSK9, we can free up LDLR and decrease circulating levels of LDL in the blood.

Pharmacokinetics

PCSK9 inhibitors are administered subcutaneously. Because monoclonal antibodies are composed of protein, no specific metabolism studies were conducted. It is thought that the proteins degrade to small peptides and amino acids within the body. Both drugs have a long half-life of 11 to 20 days.

Adverse Effects

Hypersensitivity. Hypersensitivity reactions, including vasculitis, rash, and urticaria requiring hospitalization, have been noted with use of PCSK9 inhibitors.

Immunogenicity. As this class of drug is composed of protein, there is a risk for developing antibodies; 4.8% of patients treated with alirocumab and 0.1% treated with evolocumab developed antibodies to the drug after initiating treatment. These patients also had a higher incidence of injection site reactions compared with patients who did not develop antibodies.

Drug Interactions

Neither drug is noted to have any significant drug interactions.

Preparations, Dosage, and Administration

Alirocumab [Praluent] is available in 75 and 150 mg/mL single-dose pre-filled pens and syringes. The recommended dosage is 75 mg subcutaneously every 2 weeks. If the LDL cholesterol response is inadequate, the dose may be increased to 150 mg every 2 weeks. Injection may be administered into the thigh, abdomen, or upper arm.

Evolocumab [Repatha], like alirocumab, is administered subcutaneously every 2 weeks. The recommended dose is 140 mg. Repatha is available in 140 mg/mL single-use pre-filled syringes or in a 140 mg/mL single-use SureClick auto-injector. Alternate dosing of 420 mg can also be administered every 4 weeks.

Drug Combinations

Simvastatin/Ezetimibe [Vytorin]

Actions and Uses. Simvastatin and ezetimibe are available in fixed-dose combination tablets sold as *Vytorin.* Vytorin has only one indication: hypercholesterolemia. Because ezetimibe has a different mechanism of action than simvastatin, the combination can lower cholesterol more effectively than simvastatin alone.

With this combination, the dose of simvastatin required to effectively lower cholesterol may be lower than the dose required when simvastatin is used alone. As a result, the risk of statin-related adverse effects can be reduced. Additional benefits of the combination are convenience (take just one pill instead of two) and reduced cost (the combination costs less than both drugs purchased separately).

Despite the advantages of Vytorin, some authorities are concerned that the combination may be less beneficial than simvastatin alone. This concern is based on four facts:

- We have proof that simvastatin *alone* can decrease adverse outcomes (i.e., MI and other CV events).
- We have no proof that the combination can decrease adverse outcomes of elevated cholesterol (even though it *can* reduce levels of cholesterol).
- In addition to lowering cholesterol, statins have other beneficial actions (e.g., they often lower elevated TGs).
- When ezetimibe and simvastatin are combined, cholesterol goals can be met using simvastatin in reduced dosage (which is a problem for reasons discussed in the paragraph that follows).

Because the combination permits a reduction in simvastatin dosage, there is concern that although the target cholesterol goal may be reached, the reduction in adverse outcomes may be smaller than when cholesterol is lowered using simvastatin alone. Despite concerns, the FDA reviewed the evidence and determined that, although there was no significant change in carotid artery thickness after taking Vytorin, there was a significant decrease in LDL cholesterol in people taking Vytorin, which may decrease CV risk. For this reason, the FDA recommends that patients continue treatment on Vytorin.

Adverse Effects and Drug Interactions. Vytorin is generally well tolerated. However, myopathy is a concern (because both drugs can cause muscle injury). Concurrent use of a fibrate, which can also cause myopathy, increases risk. The risk of myopathy and other adverse effects is also increased by inhibitors of CYP3A4, the enzyme that inactivates simvastatin. Because Vytorin contains a statin, the product is contraindicated for women who are pregnant and for patients with liver disease.

Preparations, Dosage, and Administration. Vytorin tablets contain 10 mg of ezetimibe plus either 10, 20, 40, or 80 mg of simvastatin. The usual starting dosage is 10 mg ezetimibe/20 mg simvastatin each day. Dosing is done once daily, preferably in the evening. The simvastatin dosage can be increased as needed and tolerated.

Atorvastatin/Amlodipine [Caduet]

Atorvastatin and amlodipine (a calcium channel blocker) are available in fixed-dose combination tablets under the brand name *Caduet.* This is the first single product indicated for dyslipidemia combined with hypertension and/or angina. The combination has one advantage over taking each drug separately: fewer pills to swallow. Eleven amlodipine/atorvastatin combinations are available: 2.5 mg amlodipine with either 10, 20, or 40 mg atorvastatin; 5 mg amlodipine with either 10, 20, 40, or 80 mg atorvastatin; and 10 mg amlodipine with either 10, 20, 40, or 80 mg atorvastatin. Dosage is individualized on the basis of therapeutic response and tolerance of adverse effects. The pharmacology of amlodipine and other calcium channel blockers is discussed in Chapter 45.

Fish Oil

Consuming fatty fish or fish-oil supplements was once associated with a decreased risk of ASCVD and ASCVD-related death. Unfortunately, recent studies have revealed that consuming fish oil provides no advantage in the prevention of heart disease in high-risk populations. Yet, it is still believed that taking fish oil can reduce the incidence of heart dysrhythmias after MI or heart failure.

Fish oil may be beneficial in the prevention of heart dysrhythmias because it contains two "heart healthy" compounds: *eicosapentaenoic acid* (EPA) and *docosahexaenoic acid* (DHA). Both compounds are long-chain, omega-3 polyunsaturated fatty acids, with a methyl group at one end and a carboxyl group at the other. They are called *omega-3 fatty acids* because they have a double bond located three carbons in from the methyl terminus.

How do omega-3 fatty acids help us? The answer is unclear. Benefits of lower doses (850 mg to 1 gm) may result from reducing platelet aggregation; reducing thrombosis (by effects on platelets and the vascular endothelium); reducing inflammation (which may help stabilize atherosclerotic plaques); and reducing blood pressure and cardiac dysrhythmias.

As the evidence is so new regarding lack of benefit in the primary prevention of heart disease, the American Heart Association still recommends eating at least two servings of fish a week. Fish with high concentrations of EPA and DHA are preferred. Among these are mackerel, halibut, herring, salmon, albacore tuna, and trout. The goal is to take in, on average, about 1 gm of fish oil a day.

Because fish concentrate certain environmental contaminants—especially methylmercury, dioxins, and polychlorinated biphenyls (PCBs)—eating fish carries some risk. Methylmercury can cause heart disease as well as neurologic damage, manifesting as tremor, numbness, tingling, altered vision, and impaired concentration. Exposure *in utero* or during early childhood can lead to developmental delay, blindness, and seizures. With dioxin and PCBs, carcinogenesis is the major concern. Does this mean we should avoid eating fish? No. For postmenopausal women and for men who are middle-aged or older, the benefits of fish outweigh the risks. For women who are pregnant or breast-feeding, fish consumption should be limited to 12 ounces a week, and certain species—swordfish, king mackerel, shark, and golden snapper, all of which may have high levels of methylmercury—should be avoided entirely. Young children should limit fish consumption too. For people who like salmon, dioxin exposure can be reduced by eating wild salmon, which contains much less dioxin than farm-raised salmon. Exposure to all contaminants can be reduced by using fish-oil supplements, which have much less contamination than fish themselves.

Lovaza

Lovaza is the brand name for the first preparation of omega-3-acid ethyl esters approved by the FDA. The product, available only by prescription, contains a combination of EPA and DHA. Lovaza is approved as an adjunct to dietary measures to reduce very high levels of TGs (500 mg/dL or greater). When used alone, Lovaza can reduce TG levels by 20% to 50%. Combining it with simvastatin produces a further decrease. Because large doses of omega-3 fatty acids can impair platelet function, leading to prolonged bleeding time, the product should be used with care in patients taking anticoagulants or antiplatelet drugs, including aspirin. Lovaza is supplied in 1-gm, liquid-filled, soft-gelatin capsules that contain approximately 465 mg of EPA and approximately 375 mg of DHA. The recommended dosage is 4 gm/day, taken either all at once (4 capsules) or in two doses (2 capsules twice a day).

Plant Stanol and Sterol Esters

Stanol esters and sterol esters, which are analogs of cholesterol, can reduce intestinal absorption of cholesterol (by 10%) and can thereby reduce levels of LDL cholesterol (by 14%). These compounds do not affect HDL levels or TG levels. ATP III recommends adding plant stanols or sterols to the diet if the basic TLC diet fails to reduce LDL cholesterol to the target level. Where can you get plant stanols and sterols? Two good sources are the *Benecol* brand of margarine and soft spreads sold under the brand name *Promise.*

Cholestin

Cholestin is the brand name for a dietary supplement that can lower cholesterol levels. The product is made from rice fermented with red yeast. Its principal active ingredient—*lovastatin*—is identical to the active ingredient in Mevacor, a brand-name, cholesterol-lowering drug. In addition to lovastatin, Cholestin contains at least seven other HMG-CoA reductase inhibitors (statins).

Several clinical trials have demonstrated that Cholestin can lower cholesterol levels, although none has studied its effects on CV events. In a trial conducted at Tufts University School of Medicine, Cholestin reduced total cholesterol by 11.4% and LDL cholesterol by 21%, and increased HDL cholesterol by 14.6%. Similarly, in a study conducted at the University of California at Los Angeles Medical School, Cholestin reduced total cholesterol by 16% and LDL cholesterol by 22%. Whether Cholestin also reduces the incidence of ASCVD is unknown.

Information on Cholestin is lacking in four important areas: clinical benefits, adverse effects, drug interactions, and precise mechanism of action. As noted, there are no data on the ability of Cholestin to reduce the risk of MI, stroke, or any other CV event. In contrast, the clinical benefits of prescription statins (lovastatin and all the others) are fully documented. There is little or no information on the adverse effects or drug interactions of Cholestin. In contrast, the safety (and hazards) of prescription statins, as well as their drug interactions, have been studied extensively.

The mechanism by which Cholestin lowers cholesterol levels is only partly understood. The recommended daily dose of Cholestin contains only 5 mg of lovastatin and varying doses of other HMG-CoA reductase inhibitors, compared with 10 mg for the lowest recommended dose of Mevacor. Hence, it seems unlikely that the statins in Cholestin can fully account for the supplement's ability to reduce cholesterol levels. This implies that Cholestin has one or more active ingredients that have not yet been identified. What they are and how they may work is a mystery.

What's the bottom line? Until more is known about Cholestin, stick with statins—medications of proven safety and efficacy. Furthermore, for people with health insurance, using statins is cheaper: Most insurers will cover the cost of statins, but will not pay for Cholestin.

KEY POINTS

- Lipoproteins are structures that transport lipids (cholesterol and triglycerides [TGs]) in blood.
- Lipoproteins consist of a hydrophobic core, a hydrophilic shell, plus at least one apolipoprotein, which serves as a recognition site for receptors on cells.
- Lipoproteins that contain apolipoprotein B-100 transport cholesterol and/or TGs from the liver to peripheral tissues.
- Lipoproteins that contain apolipoproteins A-I or A-II transport cholesterol from peripheral tissues back to the liver.
- There are three major types of lipoproteins: VLDLs (very-low-density lipoproteins), LDLs (low-density lipoproteins), and HDLs (high-density lipoproteins).
- VLDLs transport TGs to peripheral tissues.
- The contribution of VLDLs to ASCVD is unclear.
- LDLs transport cholesterol to peripheral tissues.
- Elevation of LDL cholesterol greatly increases the risk of ASCVD.
- By reducing LDL cholesterol levels, we can arrest or reverse atherosclerosis, and can thereby reduce morbidity and mortality from ASCVD.
- HDLs transport cholesterol back to the liver.
- HDLs protect against ASCVD.
- Atherogenesis is a chronic inflammatory process that begins with accumulation of LDLs beneath the arterial endothelium, followed by oxidation of LDLs.
- All adults older than 20 years should be screened every 5 years for total cholesterol, LDL cholesterol, HDL cholesterol, and TGs.
- Treatment of high LDL cholesterol is based on the individual's 10-year risk of having a major coronary event.
- Individuals with established ASCVD or an ASCVD risk equivalent (e.g., diabetes) are in the highest 10-year risk group.
- Diet modification along with exercise is the primary method for reducing LDL cholesterol. Drugs are employed only if diet modification and exercise fail to reduce LDL cholesterol to the target level.
- Therapy with cholesterol-lowering drugs must continue lifelong. If these drugs are withdrawn, cholesterol levels will return to pretreatment values.
- Statins (HMG-CoA reductase inhibitors) are the most effective drugs for lowering LDL cholesterol, and they cause few adverse effects.
- Statins can slow progression of ASCVD, decrease the number of adverse cardiac events, and reduce mortality.
- Statins reduce LDL cholesterol levels by increasing the number of LDL receptors on hepatocytes, thereby enabling hepatocytes to remove more LDLs from the blood. The process by which LDL receptor number is increased begins with inhibition of HMG-CoA reductase, the rate-limiting enzyme in cholesterol synthesis.
- Four statins—atorvastatin, fluvastatin, lovastatin, and simvastatin—are metabolized by CYP3A4, and hence their levels can be increased by CYP3A4 inhibitors (e.g., cyclosporine, erythromycin, ketoconazole, ritonavir).
- Statins can cause liver damage. Tests of liver function should be done at baseline and as clinically indicated thereafter.
- Statins can cause myopathy. Patients who experience unusual muscle pain, soreness, tenderness, and/or weakness should inform their provider. A marker for muscle injury—creatine kinase (CK)—should be measured at baseline, before starting the drug, and whenever signs or symptoms that could be due to myositis or myopathy develop.
- Statins should not be used during pregnancy.
- Bile-acid sequestrants (e.g., colesevelam) reduce LDL cholesterol levels by increasing the number of LDL receptors on hepatocytes. The mechanism is complex and begins with preventing reabsorption of bile acids in the intestine.
- Bile-acid sequestrants are not absorbed from the GI tract, and hence do not cause systemic adverse effects. However, they can cause constipation and other GI effects. (GI effects with one agent—colesevelam—are minimal.)
- Older bile-acid sequestrants form complexes with other drugs and thereby prevent their absorption. Accordingly, oral medications should be administered 1 hour before the sequestrant or 4 hours after. With a newer sequestrant—colesevelam—these interactions are minimal.
- Ezetimibe lowers LDL cholesterol by reducing cholesterol absorption in the small intestine.
- Like the statins, ezetimibe can cause muscle injury.
- Gemfibrozil and other fibrates are the most effective drugs for lowering TG levels.
- Like the statins, the fibrates can cause muscle injury.

Please visit **http://evolve.elsevier.com/Lehne** for chapter-specific NCLEX® examination review questions.

Summary of Major Nursing Implications[a]

IMPLICATIONS THAT APPLY TO ALL DRUGS THAT LOWER LDL CHOLESTEROL

Preadministration Assessment

Baseline Data

Obtain laboratory values for total cholesterol, LDL cholesterol, HDL cholesterol, and TGs (VLDLs).

Identifying ASCVD Risk Factors

The patient history and physical examination should identify ASCVD risk factors. These include smoking, advancing age, a personal history of ASCVD, reduced levels of HDL cholesterol (below 40 mg/dL), and hypertension.

In the past, diabetes was considered an ASCVD risk factor. However, because the association between diabetes and

Summary of Major Nursing Implications[a]—cont'd

ASCVD is so strong, diabetes is now considered an ASCVD risk *equivalent* (i.e., it poses the same 10-year risk of a major coronary event as ASCVD itself).

Measures to Enhance Therapeutic Effects

Diet Modification

Diet modification should precede and accompany drug therapy for elevated LDL cholesterol. **Inform patients about the importance of diet in controlling cholesterol levels, and arrange for dietary counseling. Advise patients to limit consumption of cholesterol (to below 200 mg/day) and saturated fat (to below 7% of caloric intake). If these measures fail to reduce LDL cholesterol to the target level, advise patients to add soluble fiber and plant stanols or sterols to the regimen.**

Exercise

Regular exercise can reduce LDL cholesterol and elevate HDL cholesterol, reducing the risk of ASCVD. **Help the patient establish an appropriate exercise program.**

Reduction of ASCVD Risk Factors

Correctable ASCVD risk factors should be addressed. **Encourage smokers to quit.** Disease states that promote ASCVD—diabetes mellitus and hypertension—must be treated.

Promoting Compliance

Drug therapy for elevated LDL cholesterol must continue lifelong; if drugs are withdrawn, cholesterol levels will return to pretreatment values. **Inform patients about the need for continuous therapy, and encourage them to adhere to the prescribed regimen.**

HMG-COA REDUCTASE INHIBITORS (STATINS)

Atorvastatin
Fluvastatin
Lovastatin
Pitavastatin
Pravastatin
Rosuvastatin
Simvastatin

In addition to the implications discussed below, *see earlier in this summary* for implications that apply to all drugs that lower LDL cholesterol.

Preadministration Assessment

Therapeutic Goal

Statins, in combination with diet modification and exercise, are used primarily to lower levels of LDL cholesterol. Additional indications are shown in Table 50.7.

Baseline Data

Obtain a baseline lipid profile, consisting of total cholesterol, LDL cholesterol, HDL cholesterol, and TGs (VLDLs). Also, obtain baseline LFTs and a CK level.

Identifying High-Risk Patients

Statins are *contraindicated* for patients with viral or alcoholic hepatitis and for women who are pregnant.

Exercise *caution* in patients with nonalcoholic fatty liver disease, in those who consume alcohol to excess, and in those taking fibrates or ezetimibe or agents that inhibit CYP3A4 (e.g., cyclosporine, erythromycin, ketoconazole, ritonavir). Use *rosuvastatin* with *caution* in Asian patients.

Implementation: Administration

Route

Oral.

Administration

Instruct patients to take lovastatin with the evening meal; all other statins can be administered without regard to meals. Advise patients that dosing in the evening is preferred for all statins.

Ongoing Evaluation and Interventions

Evaluating Therapeutic Effects

Cholesterol levels should be monitored monthly early in treatment and at longer intervals thereafter.

Minimizing Adverse Effects

Statins are very well tolerated. Side effects are uncommon, and serious adverse effects—hepatotoxicity and myopathy—are relatively rare.

Hepatotoxicity. Statins can injure the liver, but jaundice and other clinical signs are rare. Liver function should be assessed before treatment and as clinically indicated thereafter. If serum transaminase becomes persistently excessive (more than 3 times the ULN), statins should be discontinued. Statins should be avoided in patients with alcoholic or viral hepatitis, but may be used in patients with nonalcoholic fatty liver disease.

Myopathy. Statins can cause muscle injury. If statins are not withdrawn, injury may progress to severe myositis or potentially fatal rhabdomyolysis. **Inform patients about the risk of myopathy, and instruct them to notify the prescriber if unexplained muscle pain or tenderness develops.** If muscle pain does develop, the CK level should be measured, and if it is more than 10 times the ULN, the statin should be withdrawn or changed.

Minimizing Adverse Interactions

The risk of myopathy is increased by (1) gemfibrozil, fenofibrate, and ezetimibe, which promote myopathy themselves; and by (2) inhibitors of CYP3A4—such as cyclosporine, macrolide antibiotics (e.g., erythromycin), azole antifungal drugs (e.g., ketoconazole), and HIV protease inhibitors (e.g., ritonavir)—which can cause statin levels to rise. The combination of a statin with any of these drugs should be used with caution.

Use in Pregnancy

Statins are contraindicated during pregnancy. **Inform women of childbearing age about the potential for fetal harm and warn them against becoming pregnant.** If pregnancy occurs and the patient intends to continue the pregnancy, statins should be withdrawn.

Continued

Summary of Major Nursing Implications[a]—cont'd

BILE-ACID SEQUESTRANTS

Cholestyramine
Colesevelam
Colestipol

In addition to the implications discussed here, *see earlier in this summary* for implications that apply to all drugs that lower LDL cholesterol.

Preadministration Assessment

Therapeutic Goal

Bile-acid sequestrants, in conjunction with diet modification and exercise (and a statin if necessary), are used to reduce elevated levels of LDL cholesterol.

Baseline Data

Obtain laboratory values for total cholesterol, LDL cholesterol, HDL cholesterol, and TGs (VLDLs).

Implementation: Administration

Route

Oral.

Administration

Instruct patients to mix cholestyramine powder and colestipol granules with water, fruit juice, soup, or pulpy fruit (e.g., applesauce, crushed pineapple) to reduce the risk of esophageal irritation and impaction. Inform patients that the sequestrants are not water soluble, so the mixtures will be cloudy suspensions, not clear solutions.

Ongoing Evaluation and Interventions

Evaluating Therapeutic Effects

Cholesterol levels should be monitored monthly early in treatment and at longer intervals thereafter.

Minimizing Adverse Effects

Constipation. *Cholestyramine* and *colestipol*—but not colesevelam—can cause constipation. **Inform patients that constipation can be minimized by increasing dietary fiber and fluids. A mild laxative may be used if needed. Instruct patients taking cholestyramine or colestipol to notify the prescriber if constipation becomes bothersome, in which case a switch to colesevelam should be considered.**

Vitamin Deficiency. *Cholestyramine* and *colestipol*—but not colesevelam—can impair absorption of fat-soluble vitamins (A, D, E, and K). Vitamin supplements may be required. Colesevelam does not reduce vitamin absorption.

Minimizing Adverse Interactions

Cholestyramine and *colestipol*—but not colesevelam—can bind with other drugs and prevent their absorption. **Advise patients to administer other medications 1 hour before these sequestrants or 4 hours after.**

GEMFIBROZIL

Preadministration Assessment

Therapeutic Goal

Gemfibrozil, in conjunction with diet modification, is used to reduce elevated levels of TGs (VLDLs). The drug is not very effective at lowering LDL cholesterol. It may also be used to raise low levels of HDL cholesterol.

Baseline Data

Obtain laboratory values for total cholesterol, LDL cholesterol, HDL cholesterol, and TGs (VLDLs).

Identifying High-Risk Patients

Gemfibrozil is *contraindicated* for patients with liver disease, severe renal dysfunction, and gallbladder disease.

Use with *caution* in patients taking statins or warfarin.

Implementation: Administration

Route

Oral.

Administration

Instruct patients to administer gemfibrozil 30 minutes before the morning and evening meals.

Ongoing Evaluation and Interventions

Evaluating Therapeutic Effects

Obtain periodic tests of blood lipids.

Minimizing Adverse Effects

Gallstones. Gemfibrozil increases gallstone development. **Inform patients about symptoms of gallbladder disease (e.g., upper abdominal discomfort, intolerance of fried foods, bloating), and instruct them to notify the prescriber if these develop.**

Myopathy. Gemfibrozil can cause muscle damage. **Warn patients to report any signs of muscle injury, such as tenderness, weakness, or unusual muscle pain.**

Liver Disease. Gemfibrozil may disrupt liver function. Cancer of the liver may also be a risk. Obtain periodic tests of liver function.

Minimizing Adverse Interactions

Warfarin. Gemfibrozil enhances the effects of warfarin, thereby increasing the risk of bleeding. Obtain more frequent measurements of prothrombin time and assess the patient for signs of bleeding. Reduction of warfarin dosage may be required, and reassessment and readjustment of the warfarin dosage may be needed if the fibrate is stopped.

Statins. Gemfibrozil and statins both cause muscle injury. Risks rise when both are used. Use the combination with caution.

[a]Patient education information is highlighted as **blue text.**

CHAPTER

51 Drugs for Angina Pectoris

Angina pectoris is defined as sudden pain beneath the sternum, often radiating to the left shoulder, left arm, and jaw. Anginal pain is precipitated when the oxygen supply to the heart is insufficient to meet oxygen demand. Most often, angina occurs secondary to atherosclerosis of the coronary arteries, so angina should be seen as a symptom of a disease and not as a disease in its own right. In the United States, more than 10 million people have chronic stable angina; about 500,000 new cases develop annually.

Drug therapy of angina has two goals: (1) prevention of myocardial infarction (MI) and death and (2) prevention of myocardial ischemia and anginal pain. Two types of drugs are employed to decrease the risk of MI and death: cholesterol-lowering drugs and antiplatelet drugs. These agents are discussed in Chapters 50 and 52, respectively.

In this chapter, we focus on antianginal drugs (i.e., drugs that prevent myocardial ischemia and anginal pain). There are three main families of antianginal agents: *organic nitrates* (e.g., nitroglycerin), *beta blockers* (e.g., metoprolol), and *calcium channel blockers* (e.g., verapamil). In addition, a fourth agent—*ranolazine*—can be combined with these drugs to supplement their effects. Most of the chapter focuses on the organic nitrates. Beta blockers and calcium channel blockers are discussed at length in previous chapters; consideration of these drugs here is limited to their use in angina.

DETERMINANTS OF CARDIAC OXYGEN DEMAND AND OXYGEN SUPPLY

Before discussing angina pectoris, we need to review the major factors that determine cardiac oxygen demand and supply.

Oxygen Demand

The principal determinants of cardiac oxygen demand are heart rate, myocardial contractility, and, most importantly, intramyocardial wall tension. Wall tension is determined by two factors: cardiac preload and cardiac afterload. (Preload and afterload are defined in Chapter 43.) In summary, cardiac oxygen demand is determined by (1) heart rate, (2) contractility, (3) preload, and (4) afterload. Drugs that reduce these factors reduce oxygen demand.

Oxygen Supply

Cardiac oxygen supply is determined by myocardial blood flow. Under resting conditions, the heart extracts nearly all of the oxygen delivered to it by the coronary vessels. Therefore, the only way to accommodate an increase in oxygen demand is to increase blood flow. When oxygen demand increases, coronary arterioles dilate; the resultant decrease in vascular resistance allows blood flow to increase. During exertion, coronary blood flow increases four- to fivefold. It is important to note that myocardial perfusion takes place only during diastole (i.e., when the heart relaxes). Perfusion does not take place during systole because the vessels that supply the myocardium are squeezed shut when the myocardium contracts.

ANGINA PECTORIS: PATHOPHYSIOLOGY AND TREATMENT STRATEGY

Angina pectoris has three forms: (1) *chronic stable angina* (exertional angina), (2) *variant angina* (Prinzmetal's or vasospastic angina), and (3) *unstable angina*. Our focus is on stable angina and variant angina. Consideration of unstable angina is brief.

Chronic Stable Angina (Exertional Angina)

Pathophysiology

Stable angina is triggered most often by an increase in physical activity. Emotional excitement, large meals, and cold exposure may also precipitate an attack. Because stable angina usually occurs in response to strain, this condition is also known as *exertional angina* or *angina of effort.*

The underlying cause of exertional angina is coronary artery disease (CAD), a condition characterized by deposition of fatty plaque in the arterial wall. If an artery is only partially blocked by plaque, blood flow will be reduced and angina pectoris will result. However, if complete vessel blockage occurs, blood flow will stop and MI (heart attack) will result.

The impact of CAD on the balance between myocardial oxygen demand and oxygen supply is shown in Fig. 51.1. In both the healthy heart and the heart with CAD, oxygen supply and oxygen demand are in balance during rest. In the presence of CAD, resting oxygen demand is met through dilation of arterioles distal to the partial occlusion. This dilation reduces resistance to blood flow, compensating for the increase in resistance created by plaque.

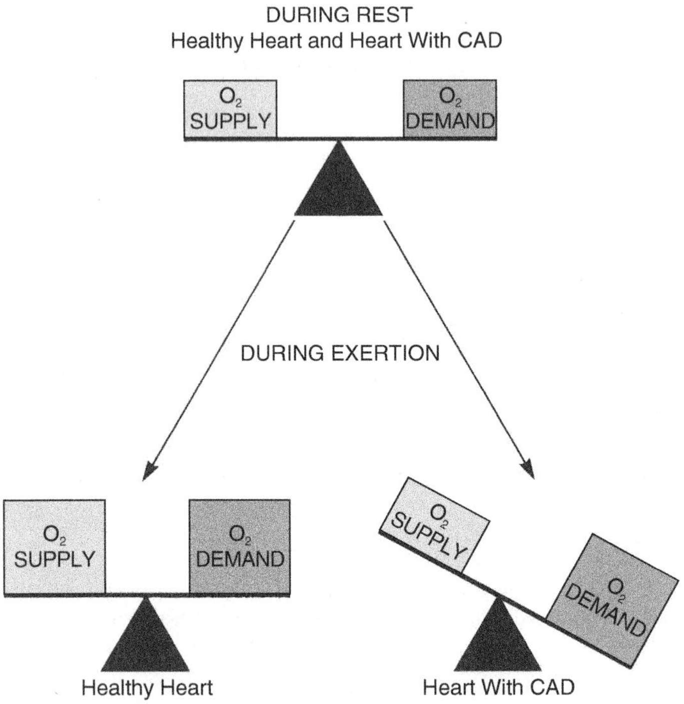

Fig. 51.1 ▪ Effect of exertion on the balance between oxygen supply and oxygen demand in the healthy heart and the heart with CAD.
In the healthy heart, O_2 supply and O_2 demand are always in balance; during exertion, coronary arteries dilate, producing an increase in blood flow to meet the increase in O_2 demand. In the heart with CAD, O_2 supply and O_2 demand are in balance only during rest. During exertion, dilation of coronary arteries cannot compensate for the increase in O_2 demand, and an imbalance results.

The picture is very different during exertion. In the healthy heart, as cardiac oxygen demand rises, coronary arterioles dilate, causing blood flow to increase. The increase keeps oxygen supply in balance with oxygen demand. By contrast, in people with CAD, arterioles in the affected region are already fully dilated during rest. Thus, when exertion occurs, there is no way to increase blood flow to compensate for the increase in oxygen demand. The resultant imbalance between oxygen supply and oxygen demand causes anginal pain.

Treatment Strategy

The goal of antianginal therapy is to reduce the intensity and frequency of anginal attacks. Because anginal pain results from an imbalance between oxygen supply and oxygen demand, logic dictates two possible remedies: (1) increase cardiac oxygen supply or (2) decrease oxygen demand. Since the underlying cause of stable angina is occlusion of the coronary arteries, there is little we can do to increase cardiac oxygen supply. Therefore, the first remedy is not a real option. Consequently, all we really can do is *decrease cardiac oxygen demand.* As discussed earlier, oxygen demand can be reduced with drugs that decrease heart rate, contractility, afterload, and preload.

Overview of Therapeutic Agents

Stable angina can be treated with three main types of drugs: *organic nitrates, beta blockers,* and *calcium channel blockers.* As previously noted, *ranolazine* can be combined with these drugs for additional benefit. All four groups relieve the pain of stable angina primarily by decreasing cardiac oxygen demand (Table 51.1). Please note that drugs provide only symptomatic relief; they do not affect the underlying pathology. To reduce the risk of MI, all patients should receive an antiplatelet drug (e.g., aspirin) unless it is contraindicated. Other measures to reduce the risk of infarction are discussed later under *Drugs Used to Prevent Myocardial Infarction and Death.*

Nondrug Therapy

Patients should attempt to avoid factors that can precipitate angina. These include overexertion, heavy meals, emotional stress, and exposure to cold.

TABLE 51.1 ▪ Mechanisms of Antianginal Action

	Mechanism of Pain Relief	
Drug Class	Stable Angina	Variant Angina
Nitrates	*Decrease oxygen demand* by dilating veins, which decreases preload	*Increase oxygen supply* by relaxing coronary vasospasm
Beta Blockers	*Decrease oxygen demand* by decreasing heart rate and contractility	Not used
Calcium Channel Blockers	*Decrease oxygen demand* by dilating arterioles, which decreases afterload (all calcium blockers), and by decreasing heart rate and contractility (verapamil and diltiazem)	*Increase oxygen supply* by relaxing coronary vasospasm
Ranolazine	*Appears to decrease oxygen demand,* possibly by helping the myocardium generate energy more efficiently	Not used

Risk factors for stable angina should be corrected. Important among these are smoking, hypertension, hyperlipidemia, and a sedentary lifestyle. Patients should be strongly encouraged to quit smoking. Patients with a sedentary lifestyle should be encouraged to establish a regular program of aerobic exercise (e.g., walking, jogging, swimming, biking). Hypertension and hyperlipidemia are major risk factors and should be treated. These disorders are discussed in Chapters 47 and 50, respectively.

Variant Angina (Prinzmetal's Angina, Vasospastic Angina)

Pathophysiology

Variant angina is caused by *coronary artery spasm,* which restricts blood flow to the myocardium. Hence, as in stable angina, pain is secondary to insufficient oxygenation of the heart. In contrast to stable angina, whose symptoms occur primarily at times of exertion, variant angina can produce pain at any time, even during rest and sleep. Frequently, variant angina occurs in conjunction with stable angina. Alternative names for variant angina are *vasospastic angina* and *Prinzmetal's angina.*

Treatment Strategy

The goal is to reduce the incidence and severity of attacks. In contrast to stable angina, which is treated primarily by reducing oxygen demand, variant angina is treated by *increasing cardiac oxygen supply.* This makes sense in that the pain is caused by a reduction in oxygen supply, rather than by an increase in demand. Oxygen supply is increased with vasodilators, which prevent or relieve coronary artery spasm.

Overview of Therapeutic Agents

Vasospastic angina is treated with two groups of drugs: *calcium channel blockers* and *organic nitrates.* Both relax coronary artery spasm. Beta blockers and ranolazine, which are effective in stable angina, are not effective in variant angina. As with stable angina, therapy is symptomatic only; drugs do not alter the underlying pathology.

Unstable Angina

Pathophysiology

Unstable angina is a medical emergency. Symptoms result from severe CAD complicated by vasospasm, platelet aggregation, and transient coronary thrombi or emboli. The patient may present with either symptoms of angina at rest, new-onset exertional angina, or intensification of existing angina. Unstable angina poses a much greater risk of death than stable angina, but a smaller risk of death than MI. The risk of dying is greatest initially and then declines to baseline in about 2 months.

Treatment

In March 2012, the American College of Cardiology (ACC) and the American Heart Association (AHA) issued updated guidelines for the diagnosis and management of unstable angina. The document—*2012 ACCF/AHA Focused Update Incorporated Into the ACC/AHA 2007 Guidelines for the Management of Patients with Unstable Angina and Non–ST-Segment Elevation Myocardial Infarction*—is available free at www.acc.org and www.americanheart.org. According to the guideline, the treatment strategy is to *maintain oxygen supply* and *decrease oxygen demand.* The goal is to reduce pain and prevent progression to MI or death. All patients should be hospitalized. Acute management consists of anti-ischemic therapy combined with antiplatelet and anticoagulation therapy.

Anti-ischemic therapy consists of:

- Nitroglycerin—give three doses sublingually every 5 minutes (tablet or spray) and follow with IV therapy in the event of persistent ischemia or hypertension.
- A beta blocker—give the first dose IV if chest pain is ongoing. If beta blockers are contraindicated, substitute a nondihydropyridine calcium channel blocker (verapamil or diltiazem).
- Supplemental oxygen—for patients with cyanosis or respiratory distress.
- Intravenous morphine sulfate—if pain is not relieved immediately by nitroglycerin, or if pulmonary congestion or severe agitation is present.
- An angiotensin-converting enzyme inhibitor—for patients with left ventricular dysfunction or congestive heart failure. Angiotensin receptor blockers are a reasonable alternative in patients who have intolerance to angiotensin-converting enzyme inhibitors.

Antiplatelet therapy, which should be started promptly, consists of:

- Aspirin—continue indefinitely.
- Clopidogrel [Plavix], prasugrel [Effient], or ticagrelor [Brilinta]—continue for up to 2 months.
- Abciximab [ReoPro], a glycoprotein IIb/IIIa inhibitor—but only if angioplasty is planned.
- Eptifibatide [Integrilin] or tirofiban [Aggrastat] (both are glycoprotein IIb/IIIa inhibitors)—but only in high-risk patients with continuing ischemia, and only if angioplasty is *not* planned.

Anticoagulant therapy consists of subcutaneous low-molecular-weight heparin (e.g., enoxaparin [Lovenox]), direct thrombin inhibitors (bivalirudin [Angiomax]), factor Xa inhibitors (fondaparinux [Arixtra]), or IV unfractionated heparin.

ORGANIC NITRATES

The organic nitrates are the oldest and most frequently used antianginal drugs. These agents relieve angina by causing vasodilation. Nitroglycerin, the most familiar organic nitrate, will serve as our prototype.

Prototype Drugs

DRUGS FOR ANGINA PECTORIS

Organic Nitrates
Nitroglycerin

Beta Blockers
Metoprolol
Propranolol

Calcium Channel Blockers
Nifedipine
Verapamil

Drug That Increases Myocardial Efficiency
Ranolazine

Nitroglycerin

Nitroglycerin has been used to treat angina since 1879. The drug is effective, fast acting, and inexpensive. Despite availability of newer antianginal agents, nitroglycerin remains the drug of choice for relieving an acute anginal attack.

Vasodilator Actions

Nitroglycerin acts directly on vascular smooth muscle (VSM) to promote vasodilation. At usual therapeutic doses, the drug acts primarily on *veins.* Dilation of arterioles is only modest.

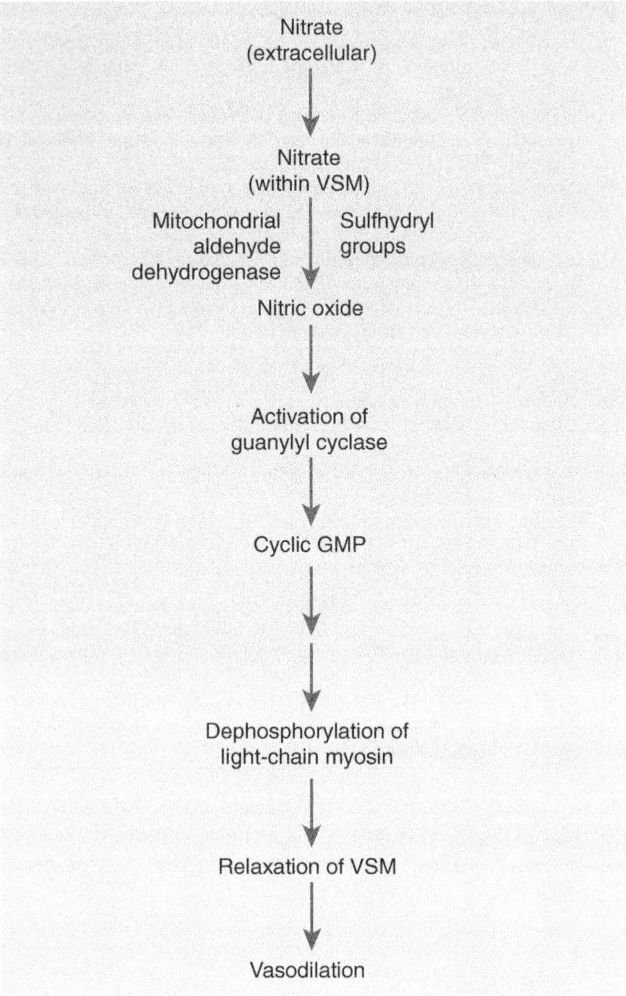

Fig. 51.2 ■ Biochemistry of nitrate-induced vasodilation. Note that sulfhydryl groups are needed to catalyze the conversion of nitrate to its active form, nitric oxide. If sulfhydryl groups are depleted from VSM, tolerance to nitrates will occur.

The biochemical events that lead to vasodilation are outlined in Fig. 51.2. The process begins with uptake of nitrate by VSM, followed by conversion of nitrate to its active form: *nitric oxide.* As indicated, conversion requires the presence of *sulfhydryl groups.* Nitric oxide then activates guanylyl cyclase, an enzyme that catalyzes the formation of cyclic GMP (cGMP). Through a series of reactions, elevation of cGMP leads to dephosphorylation of light-chain myosin in VSM. (Recall that, in all muscles, phosphorylated myosin interacts with actin to produce contraction.) As a result of dephosphorylation, myosin is unable to interact with actin, and so VSM relaxes, causing vasodilation. For our purposes, the most important aspect of this sequence is the conversion of nitrate to its active form—nitric oxide—in the presence of a sulfhydryl source.

Mechanism of Antianginal Effects

Stable Angina. Nitroglycerin decreases the pain of exertional angina primarily by *decreasing cardiac oxygen demand.* Oxygen demand is decreased as follows: By dilating veins, nitroglycerin decreases venous return to the heart, and thereby decreases ventricular filling; the resultant decrease in wall tension (preload) decreases oxygen demand.

In patients with stable angina, nitroglycerin does not appear to increase blood flow to ischemic areas of the heart. This statement is based on two observations. First, nitroglycerin does not dilate atherosclerotic coronary arteries. Second, when nitroglycerin is injected directly into coronary arteries during an anginal attack, it does not relieve pain. Both observations suggest that pain relief results from effects of nitroglycerin on peripheral blood vessels—not from effects on coronary blood flow.

Variant Angina. In patients with variant angina, nitroglycerin acts by relaxing or preventing spasm in coronary arteries. Hence, the drug *increases oxygen supply.* It does not reduce oxygen demand.

Pharmacokinetics

Absorption. Nitroglycerin is *highly lipid soluble* and crosses membranes with ease. Because of this property, nitroglycerin can be administered by uncommon routes (sublingual, buccal, transdermal), as well as by more conventional routes (oral, intravenous).

Metabolism. Nitroglycerin undergoes *rapid inactivation* by hepatic enzymes (organic nitrate reductases). As a result, the drug has a plasma half-life of only 5 to 7 minutes. When nitroglycerin is administered orally, most of each dose is destroyed on its first pass through the liver.

Adverse Effects

Nitroglycerin is generally well tolerated. Principal adverse effects—headache, hypotension, and tachycardia—occur secondary to vasodilation.

Headache. Initial therapy can produce severe headache. This response diminishes over the first few weeks of treatment. In the meantime, headache can be reduced with aspirin, acetaminophen, or some other mild analgesic.

Orthostatic Hypotension. Relaxation of VSM causes blood to pool in veins when the patient assumes an erect posture. Pooling decreases venous return to the heart, which reduces cardiac output, causing blood pressure to fall. Symptoms of orthostatic hypotension include light-headedness and dizziness. Patients should be instructed to sit or lie down if these occur. Lying with the feet elevated promotes venous return and can help restore blood pressure.

Reflex Tachycardia. Nitroglycerin lowers blood pressure—primarily by decreasing venous return and partly by dilating arterioles. By lowering blood pressure, the drug can activate the baroreceptor reflex, causing sympathetic stimulation of the heart. The resultant increase in both heart rate and contractile force increases cardiac oxygen demand, which negates the benefits of therapy. Pretreatment with a beta blocker or verapamil (a calcium channel blocker that directly suppresses the heart) can prevent sympathetic cardiac stimulation.

Drug Interactions

Hypotensive Drugs. Nitroglycerin can intensify the effects of other hypotensive agents. Consequently, care should be exercised when nitroglycerin is used concurrently with beta blockers, calcium channel blockers, diuretics, and all other drugs that can lower blood pressure, including inhibitors of phosphodiesterase type 5 (PDE5). Also, patients should be advised to avoid alcohol.

Nitroglycerin and the PDE5 inhibitors both increase cGMP (nitrates increase cGMP formation, and PDE5 inhibitors decrease

Safety Alert

PHOSPHODIESTERASE TYPE 5 INHIBITORS

As discussed in Chapter 66, PDE5 inhibitors—sildenafil [Viagra], tadalafil [Cialis], avanafil [Stendra], and vardenafil [Levitra]—are used for erectile dysfunction. All of these drugs can greatly intensify nitroglycerin-induced vasodilation. Life-threatening hypotension can result. Accordingly, concurrent use of PDE5 inhibitors with nitroglycerin is *absolutely contraindicated.*

cGMP breakdown). Therefore, if these drugs are combined, levels of cGMP can rise dangerously high, causing excessive vasodilation and a precipitous drop in blood pressure.

Beta Blockers, Verapamil, and Diltiazem. These drugs can suppress nitroglycerin-induced tachycardia. Beta blockers do so by preventing sympathetic activation of $beta_1$-adrenergic receptors on the heart. Verapamil and diltiazem prevent tachycardia through direct suppression of pacemaker activity in the sinoatrial node.

Tolerance

Tolerance to nitroglycerin-induced vasodilation can develop rapidly (over the course of a single day). One possible mechanism is depletion of sulfhydryl groups in VSM: In the absence of sulfhydryl groups, nitroglycerin cannot be converted to nitric oxide, its active form. Another possible mechanism is reversible oxidative injury to mitochondrial aldehyde dehydrogenase, an enzyme needed to convert nitroglycerin into nitric oxide. Patients who develop tolerance to nitroglycerin display cross-tolerance to all other nitrates and vice versa. Development of tolerance is most likely with high-dose therapy and uninterrupted therapy. To prevent tolerance, nitroglycerin and other nitrates should be used in the lowest effective dosages; long-acting formulations (e.g., patches, sustained-release preparations) should be used on an intermittent schedule that allows at least 8 drug-free hours every day, usually during the night. If pain occurs during the nitrate-free interval, it can be managed with sparing use of a short-acting nitrate (e.g., sublingual nitroglycerin) or by adding a beta blocker or calcium channel blocker to the regimen. Tolerance can be reversed by withholding nitrates for a short time.

Preparations and Routes of Administration

Nitroglycerin is available in several formulations for administration by several routes. This proliferation of dosage forms reflects efforts to delay hepatic metabolism and prolong therapeutic effects.

All nitroglycerin preparations produce qualitatively similar responses; differences relate only to onset and duration of action (Table 51.2). With two preparations, effects begin rapidly (in 1 to 5 minutes) and then diminish in less than 1 hour. With three others, effects begin slowly but last several hours. Only one preparation—sublingual isosorbide dinitrate tablets—has both a rapid onset and a long duration.

Applications of specific preparations are based on their time course. Preparations with a *rapid onset* are employed to *terminate an ongoing anginal attack.* When used for this purpose, rapid-acting preparations are administered as soon as pain begins. Rapid-acting preparations can also be used for *acute prophylaxis of angina.* For this purpose, they are taken just before anticipated exertion. *Long-acting preparations* are used to provide *sustained protection* against anginal attacks. To provide protection, they are administered on a fixed schedule (but one that permits at least 8 drug-free hours each day).

TABLE 51.2 ▪ Organic Nitrates: Time Course of Action

Drug and Dosage Form	Onset[a]	Duration[b]
NITROGLYCERIN		
Sublingual tablets	Rapid (1–3 min)	Brief (30–60 min)
Sublingual powder	Rapid (1–3 min)	Brief (30–60 min)
Translingual spray	Rapid (2–3 min)	Brief (30–60 min)
Oral capsules, SR	Slow (20–45 min)	Long (3–8 hr)
Transdermal patches	Slow (30–60 min)	Long (24 hr)[c]
Topical ointment	Slow (20–60 min)	Long (2–12 hr)
ISOSORBIDE MONONITRATE		
Oral tablets, IR	Slow (30–60 min)	Long (6–10 hr)
Oral tablets, SR	Slow (30–60 min)	Long (7–12 hr)
ISOSORBIDE DINITRATE		
Sublingual tablets	Rapid (2–5 min)	Long (1–3 hr)
Oral tablets, IR	Slow (20–40 min)	Long (4–6 hr)
Oral tablets, SR	Slow (30 min)	Long (6–8 hr)
Oral capsules, SR	Slow (30 min)	Long (6–8 hr)

[a]Nitrates with a *rapid* onset have two uses: (1) termination of an ongoing anginal attack and (2) short-term prophylaxis before anticipated exertion. Of the rapid-acting nitrates, nitroglycerin (sublingual tablet, sublingual powder, or translingual spray) is preferred to the others for terminating an ongoing attack.
[b]*Long-acting* nitrates are used for sustained prophylaxis (prevention) of anginal attacks. All cause tolerance if used without interruption.
[c]Although patches can release nitroglycerin for up to 24 hours, they should be removed after 12 to 14 hours to avoid tolerance.
IR, Immediate release; *SR,* sustained release.

Brand names and dosages for nitroglycerin preparations are shown in Table 51.3.

Sublingual Tablets and Powder. When administered sublingually (beneath the tongue), nitroglycerin is absorbed directly through the oral mucosa into the bloodstream. Hence, unlike orally administered drugs, which must pass through the liver on their way to the systemic circulation, sublingual nitroglycerin bypasses the liver and thereby temporarily avoids inactivation. Because the liver is bypassed, sublingual doses can be low (between 0.3 and 0.6 mg). These doses are about 10 times lower than those required when nitroglycerin is dosed orally.

Effects of sublingual nitroglycerin begin rapidly—in 1 to 3 minutes—and persist up to 1 hour. Because sublingual administration works fast, this route is ideal for (1) terminating an ongoing attack and (2) short-term prophylaxis when exertion is anticipated.

To terminate an acute anginal attack, sublingual nitroglycerin should be administered as soon as pain begins. Administration should not be delayed until the pain has become severe. According to current guidelines, if pain is not relieved in 5 minutes, the

TABLE 51.3 ■ Organic Nitrates: Brand Names and Dosages

Drug and Formulation	Brand Name	Usual Dosage
NITROGLYCERIN		
Sublingual tablets	Nitrostat	0.3–0.6 mg as needed every 5 min for maximum of three doses
Sublingual powder	GONITRO	1–2 packets (400 mcg/packet, up to three packets in a 15-min period)
Translingual spray	Nitrolingual Pumpspray, NitroMist	1–2 sprays (up to 3 sprays in a 15-min period)
Oral capsules, SR	Nitro-Time	2.5–6.5 mg 3 or 4 times daily; to avoid tolerance, administer only once or twice daily; do not crush or chew
Transdermal patches	Nitro-Dur	1 patch a day; to avoid tolerance, remove after 12–14 hr, allowing 10–12 patch-free hours each day. Patches come in sizes that release 0.1–0.8 mg/hr.
Topical ointment	Nitro-Bid	1–2 inches (7.5–40 mg) every 4–6 hr
Intravenous	Generic only	5 mcg/min initially, then increased gradually as needed (max 200 mcg/min); tolerance develops with prolonged continuous infusion
ISOSORBIDE MONONITRATE		
Oral tablets, IR	Generic only	20 mg twice daily; to avoid tolerance, take the first dose upon awakening and the second dose 7 hr later
Oral tablets, SR	Imdur	60–240 mg once daily; do not crush or chew
ISOSORBIDE DINITRATE		
Sublingual tablets	Generic only	2.5–5 mg before activities that may cause angina. For acute angina, 2.5–5 mg every 5 min for maximum of three doses. Do not crush or chew
Oral tablets, IR	Isordil Oral Titradose	10–40 mg 2 or 3 times daily; to avoid tolerance, take the last dose no later than 7:00 PM
Oral tablets, SR	Generic only	40 mg every 6–12 hr; to avoid tolerance, take only once or twice daily (at 8:00 AM and 2:00 PM)
Oral capsules, SR	Dilatrate-SR	40 mg every 6–12 hr; to avoid tolerance, take only once or twice daily (at 8:00 AM and 2:00 PM)

IR, Immediate release; *SR,* sustained release.

patient should call 911 or report to an emergency department, since anginal pain that does not respond to nitroglycerin may indicate MI. While awaiting emergency care, the patient can take 1 more tablet, and then a third tablet 5 minutes later.

Sublingual administration is unfamiliar to most patients. Accordingly, education is needed. The patient should be instructed to place the tablet or empty the powder packet under the tongue and leave it there while it dissolves. Nitroglycerin tablets and powder formulated for sublingual use are ineffective if swallowed.

Nitroglycerin tablets available today have good chemical stability. When stored properly, they should remain effective until the expiration date on the container. To ensure good stability, the tablets should be stored moisture free at room temperature in their original container, which should be closed tightly after each use.

Sustained-Release Oral Capsules. Sustained-release oral capsules are intended for long-term prophylaxis only; these formulations cannot act fast enough to terminate an ongoing anginal attack. Sustained-release capsules contain a large dose of nitroglycerin that is slowly absorbed across the GI wall. In theory, doses are large enough so that amounts of nitroglycerin sufficient to produce a therapeutic response will survive passage through the liver. Because they produce sustained blood levels of nitroglycerin, these formulations can cause tolerance. To reduce the risk of tolerance, these products should be taken only once or twice daily. Patients should be instructed to swallow sustained-release capsules intact.

Transdermal Delivery Systems. Nitroglycerin patches contain a reservoir from which nitroglycerin is slowly released. Following release, the drug is absorbed through the skin and then into the blood. The rate of release is constant and, depending on the patch used, can range from 0.1 to 0.8 mg/hr. Effects begin within 30 to 60 minutes and persist as long as the patch remains in place (up to 14 hours). Patches are applied once daily to a hairless area of skin. The site should be rotated to avoid local irritation.

Tolerance develops if patches are used continuously (24 hours a day every day). Accordingly, a daily "patch-free" interval of 10 to 12 hours is recommended. This can be accomplished by applying a new patch each morning, leaving it in place for 12 to 14 hours, and then removing it in the evening.

Because of their long duration, patches are well suited for sustained prophylaxis. Since patches have a delayed onset, they cannot be used to abort an ongoing attack.

Translingual Spray. Nitroglycerin can be delivered to the oral mucosa using a metered-dose spray device. Each activation delivers a 0.4-mg dose. Indications for nitroglycerin spray are the same as for sublingual tablets: suppression of an acute anginal attack and prophylaxis of angina when exertion is anticipated. As with sublingual tablets, no more than three doses should be administered within a 15-minute interval. *Instruct patients not to inhale the spray.*

Topical Ointment. Topical nitroglycerin ointment is used for sustained protection against anginal attacks. The ointment is applied to the skin of the chest, back, abdomen, or anterior thigh. (Since nitroglycerin acts primarily by dilating peripheral veins, there is no mechanistic advantage to applying topical nitroglycerin directly over the heart.) Following topical application, nitroglycerin is absorbed through the skin and then into the blood. Effects begin in 20 to 60 minutes and may persist up to 12 hours.

Nitroglycerin ointment (2%) is dispensed from a tube, and the length of the ribbon squeezed from the tube determines dosage. (One inch contains about 15 mg of nitroglycerin.) The usual adult dosage is 1 to 2 inches applied every 4 to 6 hours. The ointment should be spread over an area at least 2.5 inches by 3.5 inches and then covered with plastic wrap. Sites of application should be rotated to minimize skin irritation. As with other long-acting formulations, uninterrupted use can cause tolerance.

Intravenous Infusion. Intravenous nitroglycerin is employed only rarely to treat angina pectoris. When used for angina, IV nitroglycerin is limited to patients who have failed to respond to other medications. Additional uses of IV nitroglycerin include treatment of heart failure associated with acute MI, treatment of perioperative hypertension, and production of controlled hypotension for surgery.

Intravenous nitroglycerin has a very short duration, so continuous infusion is required. The infusion rate is 5 mcg/min initially; it is then increased gradually until an adequate response has been achieved. Heart rate and blood pressure must be monitored continuously.

Stock solutions of nitroglycerin must be diluted for IV use. Because ampules of nitroglycerin prepared by different manufacturers can differ in both volume and nitroglycerin concentration, the label must be read carefully when dilutions are made.

Administer using a glass IV bottle and the administration set provided by the manufacturer. Nitroglycerin absorbs into standard polyvinyl chloride tubing, so this tubing should be avoided.

Discontinuing Nitroglycerin

Long-acting preparations (transdermal patches, topical ointment, sustained-release oral tablets or capsules) should be discontinued slowly. If they are withdrawn abruptly, vasospasm may result.

Summary of Therapeutic Uses

Acute Therapy of Angina. For acute treatment of angina pectoris, nitroglycerin is administered in sublingual tablets and a translingual spray. Both formulations can be used to abort an ongoing anginal attack and to provide prophylaxis in anticipation of exertion.

Sustained Therapy of Angina. For sustained prophylaxis against angina, nitroglycerin is administered in the following formulations: transdermal patches, topical ointment, and sustained-release oral capsules.

Intravenous Therapy. Intravenous nitroglycerin is indicated for perioperative control of blood pressure, production of controlled hypotension during surgery, and treatment of heart failure associated with acute MI. In addition, IV nitroglycerin is used to treat unstable angina and chronic angina when symptoms cannot be controlled with preferred medications.

Isosorbide Mononitrate and Isosorbide Dinitrate

Both of these drugs have pharmacologic actions identical to those of nitroglycerin. Both drugs are used for angina, both are taken orally, and both produce headache, hypotension, and reflex tachycardia. Differences between them relate only to route of administration and time course of action. Time course determines whether a particular drug or dosage form will be used for acute therapy, sustained prophylaxis, or both. As with nitroglycerin, tolerance can develop to long-acting preparations. To avoid tolerance, the dosing schedule for long-acting preparations should allow at least 12 drug-free hours a day. Time courses are shown in Table 51.2. Brand names and dosages are shown in Table 51.3. A fixed-dose combination of isosorbide dinitrate plus hydralazine is discussed in Chapter 48.

BETA BLOCKERS

Beta blockers (e.g., propranolol, metoprolol) are first-line drugs for *angina of effort,* but are *not* effective against vasospastic angina. When administered on a fixed schedule, beta blockers can provide sustained protection against effort-induced anginal pain. Exercise tolerance is increased, and the frequency and intensity of anginal attacks are lowered. All of the beta blockers appear equally effective. In addition to reducing anginal pain, beta blockers decrease the risk of death, especially in patients with a prior MI.

Beta blockers reduce anginal pain primarily by *decreasing cardiac oxygen demand,* principally through blockade of $beta_1$ receptors in the heart, which decreases heart rate and contractility. Beta blockers reduce oxygen demand further by causing a modest reduction in arterial pressure (afterload). In addition to decreasing oxygen demand, beta blockers help increase oxygen supply. By slowing heart rate, they increase time in diastole and thereby increase the time during which blood flows through myocardial vessels. (Recall that blood does not flow in these vessels during systole.) In patients taking vasodilators (e.g., nitroglycerin), beta blockers provide the additional benefit of blunting reflex tachycardia.

For treatment of stable angina, dosage should be low initially and then gradually increased. The dosing goal is to reduce resting heart rate to 50 to 60 beats/min and to limit exertional heart rate to about 100 beats/min. Beta blockers should not be withdrawn abruptly, since doing so can increase the incidence and intensity of anginal attacks, and may even precipitate MI.

Beta blockers can produce a variety of adverse effects. Blockade of cardiac $beta_1$ receptors can produce *bradycardia, decreased atrioventricular (AV) conduction,* and *reduction of contractility.* Consequently, beta blockers should not be used by patients with sick sinus syndrome, heart failure, or second-degree or third-degree AV block. Blockade of $beta_2$ receptors in the lung can promote bronchoconstriction. Accordingly, beta blockers should be used with caution by patients with asthma. If an asthmatic individual absolutely must use a beta blocker, a $beta_1$-selective agent (e.g., metoprolol) should be chosen. Beta blockers can mask signs of hypoglycemia and therefore must be used with caution in patients with diabetes. Rarely, these drugs cause adverse central nervous system effects, including *insomnia, depression,* and *bizarre dreams.*

The basic pharmacology of the beta blockers is discussed in Chapter 18.

CALCIUM CHANNEL BLOCKERS

The calcium channel blockers (CCBs) used most frequently are *verapamil, diltiazem,* and *nifedipine* (a dihydropyridine-type calcium channel blocker). Accordingly, our discussion focuses on these three drugs. *All three* can block calcium channels in VSM, primarily in arterioles. The result is arteriolar dilation and reduction of peripheral resistance (afterload). In addition, all three can relax coronary vasospasm. *Verapamil* and *diltiazem* also block calcium channels in the heart and can thereby decrease heart rate, AV conduction, and contractility.

Calcium channel blockers are used to treat both stable and variant angina. In *variant angina,* these drugs promote relaxation of coronary artery spasm, *increasing cardiac oxygen supply.* In *stable angina,* they promote relaxation of peripheral arterioles; the resultant decrease in afterload *reduces cardiac oxygen demand.* Verapamil and diltiazem can produce modest additional reductions in oxygen demand by suppressing heart rate and contractility.

The major adverse effects of the CCBs are cardiovascular. Dilation of peripheral arterioles lowers blood pressure and can thereby induce *reflex tachycardia.* This reaction is greatest with nifedipine and minimal with verapamil and diltiazem. Because of their suppressant effects on the heart, verapamil and diltiazem must be used cautiously in patients taking beta blockers and in patients with bradycardia, heart failure, or AV block. These precautions do not apply to nifedipine or other dihydropyridines.

The basic pharmacology of the CCBs is discussed in Chapter 45.

RANOLAZINE

Actions and Therapeutic Use

Ranolazine [Ranexa] represented the first new class of antianginal agents to be approved in more than 25 years. In clinical trials, the drug reduced the number of angina episodes per week and increased exercise tolerance. However, these benefits were modest, and were smaller in women than in men. Unlike most other antianginal drugs, ranolazine does not reduce heart rate, blood pressure, or vascular resistance. However, it *can* prolong the QT interval, and is subject to multiple drug interactions. Ranolazine works by reducing accumulation of sodium and calcium in myocardial cells, which might help the myocardium use energy more efficiently. However, the exact mechanism of action is unknown. Despite limited efficacy, many drug interactions, and a risk of dysrhythmias (see text that follows), ranolazine is now approved as a first-line drug for angina. It may be combined with nitrates, beta blockers, amlodipine (a CCB), and other drugs used for angina treatment.

Pharmacokinetics

Absorption from the GI tract is highly variable, but not affected by food. Plasma levels peak 2 to 5 hours after dosing. In the liver, ranolazine undergoes rapid and extensive metabolism, mainly by CYP3A4 (the 3A4 isoenzyme of cytochrome P450). The drug has a plasma half-life of 7 hours and is excreted in the urine (75%) and feces (25%), almost entirely as metabolites.

Adverse Effects

QT Prolongation. Ranolazine can cause a dose-related increase in the QT interval and may thereby increase the risk of torsades de pointes, a serious ventricular dysrhythmia. Accordingly, the drug is contraindicated for patients with pre-existing QT prolongation and for those taking other drugs that can increase the QT interval. In addition, ranolazine is contraindicated for patients at risk of developing high levels of the drug—namely, patients with hepatic impairment or those taking drugs that inhibit CYP3A4. The issue of drug-induced QT prolongation is discussed in Chapter 7.

Elevation of Blood Pressure. In patients with severe renal impairment, ranolazine can raise blood pressure by about 15 mm Hg. Accordingly, blood pressure should be monitored often in these people.

Other Adverse Effects. The most common adverse effects are constipation, dizziness, nausea, and headache.

Drug Interactions

CYP3A4 Inhibitors. Agents that inhibit CYP3A4 can increase levels of ranolazine and can thereby increase the risk of torsades de pointes. Accordingly, moderate or strong CYP3A4 inhibitors should be avoided. Among these agents are grapefruit juice, HIV protease inhibitors (e.g., ritonavir), macrolide antibiotics (e.g., erythromycin), azole antifungal drugs (e.g., itraconazole), and some calcium channel blockers.

QT Drugs. Drugs that prolong the QT interval (e.g., quinidine, sotalol) can increase the risk of torsades de pointes in patients taking ranolazine, and hence should be avoided. Chapter 7 presents a comprehensive list of QT drugs.

Calcium Channel Blockers. Most CCBs—but not amlodipine—can inhibit CYP3A4 and thus increase levels of ranolazine. Accordingly, when the use of ranolazine plus a CCB is indicated, amlodipine is the only CCB that should be used.

Preparations, Dosage, and Administration

Ranolazine [Ranexa] is formulated in extended-release tablets (500 and 1000 mg) that should be swallowed intact, with or without food. Dosing begins at 500 mg twice daily, and it may be increased to a maximum of 1000 mg twice daily. Ranolazine may be used in combination with a nitrate, beta blocker, or amlodipine (a CCB), and other drugs for angina.

TREATMENT MEASURES

Guidelines for Management of Chronic Stable Angina

In 1999, three organizations—the American Heart Association, the American College of Cardiology, and the American College of Physicians–American Society of Internal Medicine—joined forces to produce the first national guidelines on the management of chronic stable angina. The 1999 guidelines were updated in 2002 and again in 2007. Both updates—*ACC/AHA 2002 Guideline Update for the Management of Patients with Chronic Stable Angina,* and *2007 Chronic Angina Focused Update of the ACC/AHA 2002 Guidelines for the Management of Patients with Chronic Stable Angina*—are available free online at circ.ahajournals.org. The discussion that follows reflects recommendations in these guidelines.

Treatment of stable angina has two objectives: (1) prevention of MI and death, and (2) reduction of cardiac ischemia and associated anginal pain. Although both goals are desirable, prevention of MI and death is clearly more important. If two treatments are equally effective at decreasing anginal pain but one also decreases the risk of death, then the latter is preferred.

Drugs Used to Prevent Myocardial Infarction and Death

We now have medical treatments that can decrease the risk of MI and death in patients with chronic stable angina. Therapy directed at preventing MI and death is a new paradigm in the management of stable angina, and all practitioners should become familiar with it.

Antiplatelet Drugs. These agents decrease platelet aggregation and thereby decrease the risk of thrombus formation in coronary arteries. The most effective agents are *aspirin* and *clopidogrel.* In patients with stable angina, low-dose aspirin produces a 33% decrease in the risk of adverse cardiovascular events. Benefits of clopidogrel seem equal to those of aspirin, although they are not as well documented. The guidelines recommend that all patients with stable angina take 75 to 162 mg of aspirin daily, unless there is a specific reason not to. Aspirin, clopidogrel, and other antiplatelet drugs are discussed in Chapter 52.

Cholesterol-Lowering Drugs. Elevated cholesterol is a major risk factor for coronary atherosclerosis. Drugs that lower cholesterol can slow the progression of CAD, stabilize atherosclerotic plaques, and even cause plaque regression. Therapies that reduce cholesterol are associated with decreased mortality from coronary heart disease. For example, in patients with established CAD, taking simvastatin can decrease the risk of mortality by 35%. Because of the well-established benefits of cholesterol-lowering therapy, the guidelines recommend that all patients with stable angina receive a cholesterol-lowering drug. The pharmacology of the cholesterol-lowering drugs is discussed in Chapter 50.

Angiotensin-Converting Enzyme (ACE) Inhibitors. There is strong evidence that, in patients with CAD, ACE inhibitors greatly reduce the incidence of adverse outcomes. In the Heart Outcomes Prevention Evaluation (HOPE) trial, for example, ramipril reduced the incidence of stroke, MI, and cardiovascular death. Among one subset of patients—those with diabetes—benefits were particularly striking. Ramipril decreased the risk of stroke by 33%, MI by 22%, and cardiovascular death by 37%. In addition, ramipril reduced the risk of nephropathy, retinopathy, and other microvascular complications of diabetes. Because of these well-documented benefits, the guidelines recommend ACE inhibitors for most patients with established CAD, and especially for those with diabetes. The pharmacology of the ACE inhibitors is discussed in Chapter 44.

Antianginal Agents: Drugs Used to Reduce Anginal Pain

The goal of antianginal therapy is to achieve complete (or nearly complete) elimination of anginal pain, along with a return to normal activities. This should be accomplished with a minimum of adverse drug effects.

The basic strategy of antianginal therapy is to provide baseline protection using one or more long-acting drugs (beta blocker, CCB, long-acting nitrate) supplemented with sublingual nitroglycerin when breakthrough pain occurs. A flow plan for drug selection is shown in Fig. 51.3. As indicated, treatment is approached sequentially. Progression from one step to the next is based on patient response. Some patients can be treated with a single long-acting drug, some require two or three, and some require revascularization.

Initial treatment consists of sublingual nitroglycerin plus a long-acting antianginal drug. Beta blockers are the preferred agents for baseline therapy because they can decrease mortality, especially in patients with a prior MI. In addition to providing prophylaxis, beta blockers suppress nitrate-induced reflex tachycardia.

If a beta blocker is inadequate, or if there are contraindications to beta blockade, a long-acting CCB should be added or substituted. Dihydropyridine-type CCBs (e.g., nifedipine) lack cardiosuppressant actions and are safer than beta blockers for patients with bradycardia, AV block, or heart failure. When a CCB is to be *combined* with a beta blocker, a dihydropyridine is preferred to verapamil or diltiazem because verapamil and diltiazem will intensify the cardiosuppressant actions of the beta blocker, whereas a dihydropyridine CCB will not.

If a CCB is inadequate, or if there are contraindications to calcium channel blockade, a long-acting nitrate (e.g., transdermal nitroglycerin) should be added or substituted. However, because tolerance can develop quickly, these nitrate preparations are less well suited than beta blockers or CCBs for continuous protection.

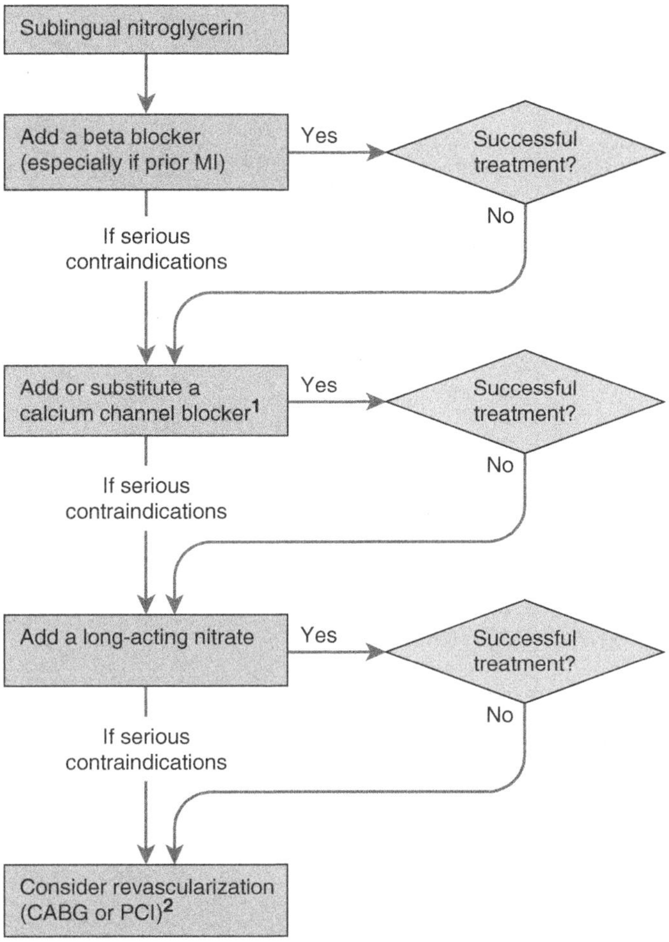

Fig. 51.3 ■ Flow plan for antianginal drug selection in patients with chronic stable angina.
[1]Avoid short-acting dihydropyridines.
[2]At any point in this process, based on coronary anatomy, severity of angina symptoms, and patient preference, it is reasonable to consider evaluation for coronary revascularization (PCI or CABG). Unless a patient is documented to have left main, three-vessel, or two-vessel CAD with significant stenosis of the proximal left anterior descending coronary artery, there is no demonstrated survival advantage associated with CABG or PCI in low-risk patients with chronic stable angina. Accordingly, medical therapy should be attempted in most patients before considering PCI or CABG. (Adapted from Gibbons RJ, Chatterjee K, Daley J, et al: ACC/AHA 2002 Guideline Update for the Management of Patients with Chronic Stable Angina: *A report of the American College of Cardiology/American Heart Association Task Force on Practice Guidelines [Committee to Update the 1999 Guidelines for the Management of Patients with Chronic Stable Angina].* 2002. Available online at circ.ahajournals.org.)

Note that, as we proceed along the drug-selection flow plan, drugs are *added* to the regimen, resulting in treatment with two or more agents. Combination therapy increases our chances of success because oxygen demand is decreased by multiple mechanisms: Beta blockers reduce heart rate and contractility; CCBs reduce afterload (by dilating arterioles); and nitrates reduce preload (by dilating veins).

If combined treatment with a beta blocker, CCB, and long-acting nitrate fails to provide relief, coronary artery bypass graft (CABG) surgery or percutaneous coronary intervention (PCI) may be indicated. Note that these invasive procedures should be considered only after more conservative treatment has been tried.

How should we treat angina in patients who have a coexisting condition? The antianginal drugs employed—nitrates, beta blockers, and CCBs—are the same ones used in patients who have angina alone. However, when selecting among these drugs, we must consider the coexisting disorder as well as the angina. For example, as noted earlier, in patients with asthma, CCBs are preferred to beta blockers (because beta blockers promote bronchoconstriction, whereas CCBs do not). Table 51.4 shows more than 20 coexisting conditions and indicates which antianginal agents to use, as well as which ones to avoid.

Reduction of Risk Factors

The treatment program should reduce anginal risk factors: Smokers should quit; sedentary patients should get aerobic exercise; and patients with diabetes, hypertension, or high cholesterol should receive appropriate therapy.

Smoking. Smoking increases the risk of cardiovascular mortality by 50%. Fortunately, smoking cessation greatly decreases cardiovascular risk. Accordingly, all patients who smoke should be strongly encouraged to quit. Smoking cessation is discussed in Chapter 39.

High Cholesterol. As noted, high cholesterol levels increase the risk of adverse cardiovascular events, and therapies that

TABLE 51.4 ▪ Choosing Between Beta Blockers and Calcium Channel Blockers for Treating Angina in Patients Who Have a Coexisting Condition

Coexisting Condition	Recommended Treatment (Alternative Treatment)	Drugs to Avoid
MEDICAL CONDITIONS		
Systemic hypertension	Beta blockers (long-acting, slow-release CCBs)	
Migraine or vascular headache	Beta blockers (verapamil or diltiazem)	
Asthma or COPD with bronchospasm	Verapamil or diltiazem	Beta blockers
Hyperthyroidism	Beta blockers	
Raynaud's disease	Long-acting, slow-release CCBs	Beta blockers
Type 1 diabetes	Beta blockers, particularly if prior MI, or long-acting, slow-release CCBs	
Type 2 diabetes	Beta blockers or long-acting, slow-release CCBs	
Depression	Long-acting, slow-release CCBs	Beta blockers
Mild peripheral vascular disease	Beta blockers or long-acting, slow-release CCBs	
Severe peripheral vascular disease with ischemia at rest	Long-acting, slow-release CCBs	Beta blockers
CARDIAC DYSRHYTHMIAS AND CONDUCTION ABNORMALITIES		
Sinus bradycardia	Long-acting, slow-release CCBs that do not decrease heart rate	Beta blockers, diltiazem, verapamil
Sinus tachycardia (not due to heart failure)	Beta blockers	
Supraventricular tachycardia	Verapamil, diltiazem, or beta blockers	
AV block	Long-acting, slow-release CCBs that do not slow AV conduction	Beta blockers, diltiazem, verapamil
Rapid atrial fibrillation (with digoxin)	Verapamil, diltiazem, or beta blockers	
Ventricular dysrhythmias	Beta blockers	
LEFT VENTRICULAR DYSFUNCTION		
Congestive heart failure		
Mild (LVEF ≥40%)	Beta blockers	
Moderate to severe (LVEF <40%)	Amlodipine or felodipine (nitrates)	Diltiazem, verapamil
Left-sided valvular heart disease		
Mild aortic stenosis	Beta blockers	
Aortic insufficiency	Long-acting, slow-release dihydropyridine CCBs	
Mitral regurgitation	Long-acting, slow-release dihydropyridine CCBs	
Mitral stenosis	Beta blockers	
Hypertropic cardiomyopathy	Beta blockers, verapamil, diltiazem	Dihydropyridine CCBs, nitrates

AV, Atrioventricular; *CCB,* calcium channel blocker; *COPD,* chronic obstructive pulmonary disease; *LVEF,* left ventricular ejection fraction; *MI,* myocardial infarction.

Adapted from Gibbons RJ, Chatterjee K, Daley J, et al: ACC/AHA 2002 Guideline Update for the Management of Patients with Chronic Stable Angina: *A report of the American College of Cardiology/American Heart Association Task Force on Practice Guidelines (Committee to Update the 1999 Guidelines for the Management of Patients with Chronic Stable Angina).* 2002. Available online at circ.ahajournals.org/.

reduce cholesterol reduce that risk. Accordingly, all patients with high cholesterol levels should receive cholesterol-lowering therapy.

Hypertension. High blood pressure increases the risk of cardiovascular mortality, and lowering blood pressure reduces the risk. Accordingly, all patients with hypertension should receive treatment. Blood pressure should be reduced to 140/90 mm Hg or less. In patients with additional risk factors (e.g., diabetes, heart failure, retinopathy), the target blood pressure is 130/80 mm Hg or less. Management of hypertension is discussed in Chapter 47.

Diabetes. Both type 1 (insulin-dependent) and type 2 (non–insulin-dependent) diabetes increase the risk of cardiovascular mortality. Type 1 increases the risk 3- to 10-fold; type 2 increases the risk 2- to 4-fold. Although there is good evidence that tight glycemic control decreases the risk of microvascular complications of diabetes, there is little evidence to show that tight glycemic control decreases the risk of cardiovascular complications. Nonetheless, it is prudent to strive for optimal glycemic control.

Physical Inactivity. Increased physical activity has multiple benefits. In patients with chronic stable angina, exercise increases exercise tolerance and the sense of well-being, and decreases anginal symptoms, cholesterol levels, and objective measures of ischemia. Accordingly, the guidelines recommend that patients perform 30 to 60 minutes of a moderate-intensity activity 3 to 4 times a week. Such activities include walking, jogging, cycling, and other aerobic exercises. Exercise by moderate- to high-risk patients should be medically supervised.

Management of Variant Angina

Treatment of vasospastic angina can proceed in three steps. For initial therapy, either a calcium channel blocker or a long-acting nitrate is selected. If either drug alone is inadequate, then combined therapy with a calcium channel blocker *plus* a nitrate should be tried. If the combination fails to control symptoms, CABG surgery may be indicated. Beta blockers are not effective in vasospastic angina.

KEY POINTS

- Anginal pain occurs when cardiac oxygen supply is insufficient to meet cardiac oxygen demand.
- Cardiac oxygen demand is determined by heart rate, contractility, preload, and afterload. Drugs that reduce these factors can help relieve anginal pain.
- Cardiac oxygen supply is determined by myocardial blood flow. Drugs that increase oxygen supply will reduce anginal pain.
- Angina pectoris has three forms: chronic stable angina, variant (vasospastic) angina, and unstable angina.
- The underlying cause of stable angina is coronary artery atherosclerosis.
- The underlying cause of variant angina is coronary artery spasm.
- Drugs relieve pain of stable angina by decreasing cardiac oxygen demand. They do not increase oxygen supply.
- Drugs relieve pain of variant angina by increasing cardiac oxygen supply. They do not decrease oxygen demand.
- Nitroglycerin and other organic nitrates are vasodilators.
- To cause vasodilation, nitroglycerin must first be converted to nitric oxide, its active form. This reaction requires a sulfhydryl source.
- Nitroglycerin relieves pain of stable angina by dilating veins, which decreases venous return, which decreases preload, which decreases oxygen demand.
- Nitroglycerin relieves pain of variant angina by relaxing coronary vasospasm, which increases oxygen supply.
- Nitroglycerin is highly lipid soluble, and therefore is readily absorbed through the skin and oral mucosa.
- Nitroglycerin undergoes very rapid inactivation in the liver. Hence, when the drug is administered orally, most of each dose is destroyed before reaching the systemic circulation.
- When nitroglycerin is administered sublingually, it is absorbed directly into the systemic circulation and therefore temporarily bypasses the liver. Hence, to produce equivalent effects, sublingual doses can be much smaller than oral doses.
- Nitroglycerin causes three characteristic side effects: headache, orthostatic hypotension, and reflex tachycardia. All three occur secondary to vasodilation.
- Reflex tachycardia from nitroglycerin can be prevented with a beta blocker, verapamil, or diltiazem.
- Continuous use of nitroglycerin can produce tolerance within 24 hours. The mechanism may be depletion of sulfhydryl groups.
- To prevent tolerance, nitroglycerin should be used in the lowest effective dosage, and long-acting formulations should be used on an intermittent schedule that allows at least 8 drug-free hours every day, usually during the night.
- Nitroglycerin preparations that have a rapid onset (e.g., sublingual nitroglycerin) are used to abort an ongoing anginal attack and to provide acute prophylaxis when exertion is expected. Administration is PRN.
- Nitroglycerin preparations that have a long duration (e.g., patches, sustained-release oral capsules) are used for extended protection against anginal attacks. Administration is on a fixed schedule (but one that allows at least 8 drug-free hours a day).
- Nitroglycerin should be used cautiously with most vasodilators and must not be used at all with sildenafil [Viagra] and other PDE5 inhibitors.
- Beta blockers prevent pain of stable angina primarily by decreasing heart rate and contractility, which reduces cardiac oxygen demand.
- Beta blockers are administered on a fixed schedule, not PRN.
- Beta blockers are not used for variant angina.
- CCBs relieve the pain of stable angina by reducing cardiac oxygen demand. Two mechanisms are involved. First, all

Continued

CCBs relax peripheral arterioles and decrease afterload. Second, verapamil and diltiazem reduce heart rate and contractility (in addition to decreasing afterload).

- CCBs relieve pain of variant angina by increasing cardiac oxygen supply. The mechanism is relaxation of coronary artery spasm.
- When a CCB is combined with a beta blocker, a dihydropyridine (e.g., nifedipine) is preferred to verapamil or diltiazem. Verapamil and diltiazem will intensify cardiosuppression caused by the beta blocker, whereas a dihydropyridine will not.
- Ranolazine appears to reduce anginal pain by helping the heart generate energy more efficiently.
- Ranolazine should not be used alone. Rather, it should be combined with a nitrate, a beta blocker, or the CCB amlodipine.
- Ranolazine increases the QT interval and may pose a risk of torsades de pointes, a serious ventricular dysrhythmia.
- In patients with chronic stable angina, treatment has two objectives: (1) prevention of MI and death and (2) prevention of anginal pain.
- The risk of MI and death can be decreased with two types of drugs: (1) antiplatelet agents (e.g., aspirin, clopidogrel) and (2) cholesterol-lowering drugs.
- Anginal pain is prevented with one or more long-acting antianginal drugs (beta blocker, CCB, long-acting nitrate) supplemented with sublingual nitroglycerin when breakthrough pain occurs.
- As a rule, revascularization with CABG surgery or PCI is indicated only after treatment with two or three antianginal drugs has failed.

Please visit http://evolve.elsevier.com/Lehne for chapter-specific NCLEX® examination review questions.

Summary of Major Nursing Implications[a]

NITROGLYCERIN

Preadministration Assessment

Therapeutic Goal

Reduction of the frequency and intensity of anginal attacks.

Baseline Data

Obtain baseline data on the frequency and intensity of anginal attacks, the location of anginal pain, and the factors that precipitate attacks.

The patient interview and physical examination should identify risk factors for angina pectoris, including treatable contributing pathophysiologic conditions (e.g., hypertension, hyperlipidemia).

Identifying High-Risk Patients

Use with *caution* in hypotensive patients and in patients taking drugs that can lower blood pressure, including alcohol and antihypertensive medications. Use with sildenafil [Viagra] and other PDE5 inhibitors is *contraindicated.*

Implementation: Administration

Routes and Administration

Sublingual Tablets or Powder

Use. Prophylaxis or termination of an acute anginal attack.

Technique of Administration. **Instruct patients to place the tablet or empty the powder under the tongue and leave it there until fully dissolved; these medications should not be swallowed.**

Instruct patients to call 911 or go to an emergency department if pain is not relieved in 5 minutes. While awaiting emergency care, they can take 1 more dose, and then a third 5 minutes later.

Instruct patients to store tablets in a dry place at room temperature in their original container, which should be closed tightly after each use. Under these conditions, the tablets should remain effective until the expiration date on the container.

Sustained-Release Oral Capsules

Use. Sustained protection against anginal attacks. To avoid tolerance, administer only once or twice daily.

Technique of Administration. **Instruct patients to swallow these preparations intact, without chewing or crushing.**

Transdermal Delivery Systems

Use. Sustained protection against anginal attacks.

Technique of Administration. **Instruct patients to apply transdermal patches to a hairless area of skin, using a new patch and a different site each day.**

Instruct patients to remove the patch after 12 to 14 hours, allowing 10 to 12 "patch-free" hours each day. This will prevent tolerance.

Translingual Spray

Use. Prophylaxis or termination of an acute anginal attack.

Technique of Administration. **Instruct patients to direct the spray against the oral mucosa. Warn patients not to inhale the spray.**

Topical Ointment

Use. Sustained protection against anginal attacks. **Instruct patients to remove any remaining ointment before applying a new dose.**

Technique of Administration. (1) Squeeze a ribbon of ointment of prescribed length onto the applicator paper provided; (2) using the applicator paper, spread the ointment over an area at least 2.5 inches by 3.5 inches (application may be made to the chest, back, abdomen, upper arm, or anterior thigh); and (3) cover the ointment with plastic wrap. Avoid touching the ointment.

Instruct patients to rotate the application site to minimize local irritation.

Summary of Major Nursing Implications[a]—cont'd

Intravenous

Uses. (1) Angina pectoris refractory to more conventional therapy, (2) perioperative control of blood pressure, (3) production of controlled hypotension during surgery, and (4) heart failure associated with acute MI.

Technique of Administration. Infuse IV using a glass IV bottle and the administration set provided by the manufacturer; avoid standard IV tubing. Check the stock solution label to verify volume and concentration, which can differ among manufacturers. Dilute stock solutions before use.

Administer by continuous infusion. The rate is slow initially (5 mcg/min) and then gradually increased until an adequate response is achieved.

Monitor cardiovascular status constantly.

Terminating Therapy

Warn patients against abrupt withdrawal of long-acting preparations (transdermal systems, topical ointment, sustained-release tablets and capsules).

Implementation: Measures to Enhance Therapeutic Effects

Reducing Risk Factors

Precipitating Factors. **Advise patients to avoid activities that are likely to elicit an anginal attack (e.g., overexertion, heavy meals, emotional stress, cold exposure).**

Exercise. Encourage patients who have a sedentary lifestyle to establish a regular program of aerobic exercise (e.g., walking, jogging, swimming, biking).

Smoking Cessation. Strongly encourage patients to quit smoking.

Contributing Disease States. Ensure that patients with contributing pathology (especially hypertension or hypercholesterolemia) are receiving appropriate treatment.

Ongoing Evaluation and Interventions

Evaluating Therapeutic Effects

Instruct patients to keep a record of the frequency and intensity of anginal attacks, the location of anginal pain, and the factors that precipitate attacks.

Minimizing Adverse Effects

Headache. **Inform patients that headache will diminish with continued drug use. Advise patients that headache can be relieved with aspirin, acetaminophen, or some other mild analgesic.**

Orthostatic Hypotension. **Inform patients about symptoms of hypotension (e.g., dizziness, light-headedness), and advise them to sit or lie down if these occur. Inform patients that hypotension can be minimized by moving slowly when changing from a sitting or supine position to an upright posture.**

Reflex Tachycardia. This reaction can be suppressed by concurrent treatment with a beta blocker, verapamil, or diltiazem.

Minimizing Adverse Interactions

Hypotensive Agents, Including PDE5 Inhibitors. Nitroglycerin can interact with other hypotensive drugs to produce excessive lowering of blood pressure. **Advise patients to avoid alcohol.** Exercise caution when nitroglycerin is used in combination with beta blockers, calcium channel blockers, diuretics, and all other drugs that can lower blood pressure.

Warn patients not to combine nitroglycerin with a PDE5 inhibitor (e.g., sildenafil [Viagra]), because life-threatening hypotension can result.

ISOSORBIDE MONONITRATE AND ISOSORBIDE DINITRATE

Both drugs have pharmacologic actions identical to those of nitroglycerin. Differences relate only to dosage forms, routes of administration, and time course of action. Therefore, the implications presented for nitroglycerin apply to these drugs as well.

[a]Patient education information is highlighted as **blue text**.

CHAPTER

52 Anticoagulant, Antiplatelet, and Thrombolytic Drugs

The drugs discussed here are used to prevent formation of thrombi (intravascular blood clots) and to dissolve thrombi that have already formed. These drugs act in several ways: some suppress coagulation, some inhibit platelet aggregation, and some promote clot degradation. They all interfere with normal hemostasis. As a result, they all carry a significant risk of bleeding.

COAGULATION: PHYSIOLOGY AND PATHOPHYSIOLOGY

HEMOSTASIS

Hemostasis is the physiologic process by which bleeding is stopped. Hemostasis occurs in two stages: (1) formation of a platelet plug, followed by (2) reinforcement of the platelet plug with fibrin. Both processes are set in motion by blood vessel injury.

Stage One: Formation of a Platelet Plug

Platelet aggregation is initiated when platelets come in contact with collagen on the exposed surface of a damaged blood vessel. In response to contact with collagen, platelets adhere to the site of vessel injury. Adhesion initiates platelet *activation,* which in turn leads to massive platelet *aggregation.*

Platelet aggregation is a complex process that ends with formation of *fibrinogen bridges* between *glycoprotein IIb/IIIa (GP IIb/IIIa) receptors* on adjacent platelets (Fig. 52.1). For these bridges to form, GP IIb/IIIa receptors must first undergo activation—that is, they must undergo a configurational change that allows them to bind with fibrinogen. As indicated in Fig. 52.1A, activation of GP IIb/IIIa can be stimulated by multiple factors, including thromboxane A_2 (TXA_2), thrombin, collagen, platelet activation factor, and ADP. Under the influence of these factors, GP IIb/IIIa changes its shape, binds with fibrinogen, and thereby causes aggregation (Fig. 52.1B). The aggregated platelets constitute a plug that stops bleeding. This plug is unstable, however, and must be reinforced with *fibrin* if protection is to last.

Stage Two: Coagulation

Coagulation is defined as production of *fibrin,* a thread-like protein that reinforces the platelet plug. Fibrin is produced by two convergent pathways (Fig. 52.2), referred to as the *contact activation pathway* (also known as the *intrinsic pathway*) and the *tissue factor pathway* (also known as the *extrinsic pathway*). The two pathways converge at factor Xa, after which they employ the same final series of reactions. In both pathways, each reaction in the sequence amplifies the reaction that follows. Hence, once this sequence is initiated, it becomes self-sustaining and self-reinforcing.

The *tissue factor pathway* is turned on by trauma to the vascular wall, which triggers release of tissue factor,[a] also

[a]FYI: The term *tissue factor* refers not to a single compound but rather to a complex of several compounds, including a proteolytic enzyme and phospholipids released from tissue membranes.

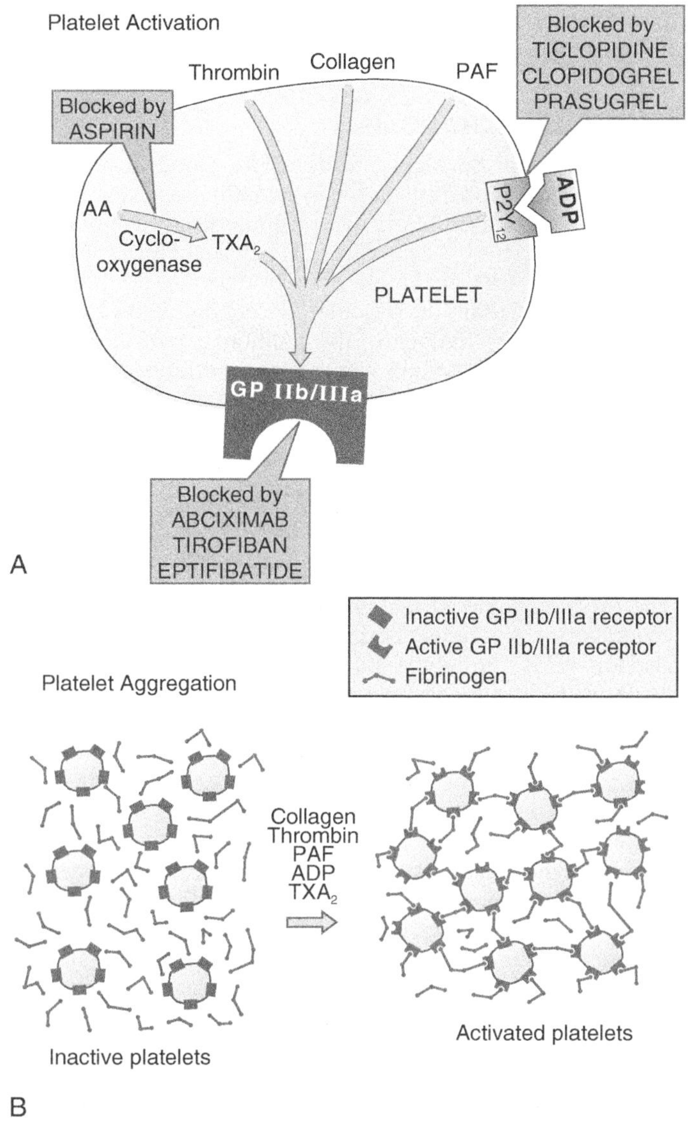

Fig. 52.1 ▪ **Mechanism of platelet aggregation and actions of antiplatelet drugs.**

A, Multiple factors—TXA_2, thrombin, collagen, PAF, and ADP—promote activation of the GP IIb/IIIa receptor. Each platelet has 50,000 to 80,000 GP IIb/IIIa receptors, although only one is shown. **B,** Activation of the GP IIb/IIIa receptor permits binding of fibrinogen, which causes aggregation by forming cross-links between platelets. After aggregation occurs, the platelet plug is reinforced with fibrin (not shown). (*AA,* Arachidonic acid; *ADP,* adenosine diphosphate; *GP IIb/IIIa,* glycoprotein IIb/IIIa receptor; *PAF,* platelet activation factor; *$P2Y_{12}$,* $P2Y_{12}$ ADP receptor; *TXA_2,* thromboxane A_2.)

known as *tissue thromboplastin.* Tissue factor then combines with and thereby activates factor VII, which in turn activates factor X, which then catalyzes the conversion of *prothrombin* (factor II) into *thrombin* (factor IIa). Thrombin then does three things. First, it catalyzes the conversion of fibrinogen into fibrin. Second, it catalyzes the conversion of factor V into *its* active form (Va), a compound that greatly increases the activity of factor Xa, even though it has no direct catalytic activity of its own. Third, thrombin catalyzes the conversion of factor VIII into *its* active form (VIIIa), a compound that greatly increases the activity of factor IXa in the contact activation pathway.

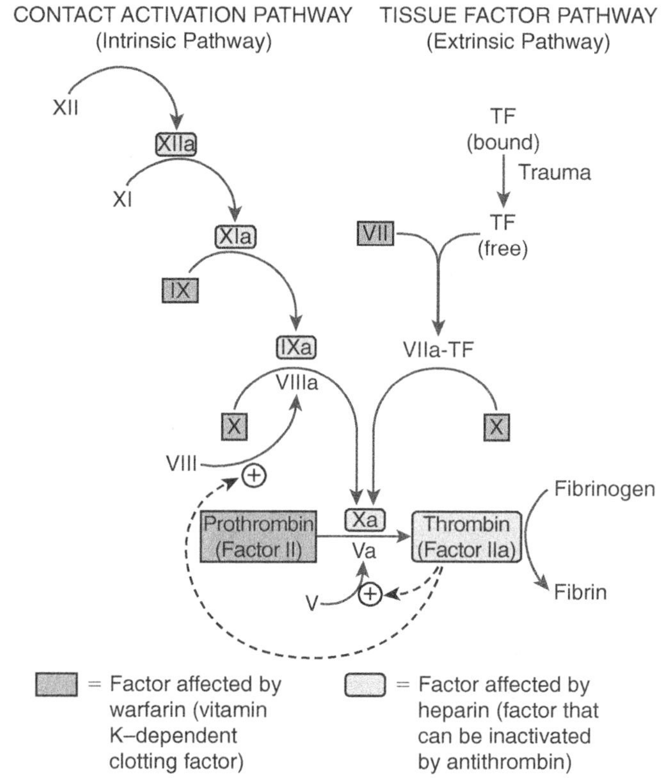

Fig. 52.2 ▪ **Outline of coagulation pathways showing factors affected by warfarin and heparin.**

TF, tissue factor. Common names for factors shown in roman numerals: V, proaccelerin; VII, proconvertin; VIII, antihemophilic factor; IX, Christmas factor; X, Stuart factor; XI, plasma thromboplastin antecedent; and XII, Hageman factor. The letter "a" after a factor's name (e.g., factor VIIIa) indicates the active form of the factor.

The *contact activation pathway* is turned on when blood makes contact with collagen that has been exposed as a result of trauma to a blood vessel wall. Collagen contact stimulates conversion of factor XII into its active form, XIIa (see Fig. 52.2). Factor XIIa then activates factor XI, which activates factor IX, which activates factor X. After this, the contact activation pathway is the same as the tissue factor pathway. As noted, factor VIIIa, which is produced under the influence of thrombin, greatly increases the activity of factor IXa, even though it has no direct catalytic activity of its own.

Important to our understanding of anticoagulant drugs is the fact that *four coagulation factors—factors VII, IX, X, and II (prothrombin)—require vitamin K for their synthesis.* These factors appear in green boxes in Fig. 52.2. The significance of the vitamin K–dependent factors will become apparent when we discuss warfarin, an oral anticoagulant.

Keeping Hemostasis Under Control

To protect against widespread coagulation, the body must inactivate any clotting factors that stray from the site of vessel injury. Inactivation is accomplished with *antithrombin,* a protein that forms a complex with clotting factors and thereby inhibits their activity. The clotting factors that can be neutralized by antithrombin appear in yellow in Fig. 52.2. As we shall see,

Prototype Drugs

ANTICOAGULANT, ANTIPLATELET, AND THROMBOLYTIC DRUGS

Anticoagulants

Drugs That Activate Antithrombin

Heparin (unfractionated)
Enoxaparin (low-molecular-weight heparin)

Vitamin K Antagonist

Warfarin

Direct Thrombin Inhibitors

Dabigatran

Direct Factor Xa Inhibitors

Rivaroxaban
Apixaban

Antiplatelet and Thrombolytic Drugs

Antiplatelet Drugs

Aspirin (cyclooxygenase [COX] inhibitor)
Clopidogrel ($P2Y_{12}$ ADP receptor antagonist)
Abciximab (glycoprotein IIb/IIIa receptor antagonist)

Thrombolytic Drugs

Streptokinase
Alteplase (tissue-type plasminogen activator)

antithrombin is intimately involved in the action of *heparin,* an injectable anticoagulant drug.

Physiologic Removal of Clots

As healing of an injured vessel proceeds, removal of the clot is eventually necessary. The body accomplishes this with *plasmin,* an enzyme that degrades the fibrin meshwork of the clot. Plasmin is produced through the activation of its precursor, *plasminogen.* The *fibrinolytic drugs* (e.g., alteplase) act by promoting conversion of plasminogen into plasmin.

THROMBOSIS

A thrombus is a blood clot formed within a blood vessel or within the heart. Thrombosis (thrombus formation) reflects pathologic functioning of hemostatic mechanisms.

Arterial Thrombosis

Formation of an arterial thrombus begins with adhesion of platelets to the arterial wall. (Adhesion is stimulated by damage to the wall or rupture of an atherosclerotic plaque.) Following adhesion, platelets release ADP and TXA_2, and thereby attract additional platelets to the evolving thrombus. With continued platelet aggregation, occlusion of the artery takes place. As blood flow comes to a stop, the coagulation cascade is initiated, causing the original plug to undergo reinforcement with fibrin. The consequence of an arterial thrombus is localized tissue injury owing to lack of perfusion.

Venous Thrombosis

Venous thrombi develop at sites where blood flow is slow. Stagnation of blood initiates the coagulation cascade, resulting in the production of fibrin, which enmeshes red blood cells and platelets to form the thrombus. The typical venous thrombus has a long tail that can break off to produce an *embolus.* Such emboli travel within the vascular system and become lodged at faraway sites, frequently the pulmonary arteries. Hence, unlike an arterial thrombus, whose harmful effects are localized, injury from a venous thrombus occurs secondary to embolization at a site distant from the original thrombus.

OVERVIEW OF DRUGS FOR THROMBOEMBOLIC DISORDERS

The drugs considered fall into three major groups: (1) anticoagulants, (2) antiplatelet drugs, and (3) thrombolytic drugs, also known as fibrinolytic drugs. *Anticoagulants* (e.g., heparin, warfarin, dabigatran) disrupt the coagulation cascade and thereby suppress production of fibrin. *Antiplatelet drugs* (e.g., aspirin, clopidogrel) inhibit platelet aggregation. *Thrombolytic drugs* (e.g., alteplase) promote lysis of fibrin, causing dissolution of thrombi. Drugs that belong to these groups are shown in Table 52.1.

Although the anticoagulants and the antiplatelet drugs both suppress thrombosis, they do so by different mechanisms. As a result, they differ in their effects and applications. The *antiplatelet drugs* are most effective at preventing *arterial* thrombosis, whereas *anticoagulants* are most effective against *venous* thrombosis.

ANTICOAGULANTS

By definition, anticoagulants are drugs that *reduce formation of fibrin.* Two basic mechanisms are involved. One anticoagulant—warfarin—inhibits the *synthesis* of clotting factors, including factor X and thrombin. All other anticoagulants inhibit the *activity* of clotting factors: either factor Xa or thrombin, or both.

Traditionally, anticoagulants have been grouped into two major classes: *oral anticoagulants* and *parenteral anticoagulants.* This scheme was reasonable because, until recently, all oral anticoagulants belonged to just one pharmacologic class: the vitamin K antagonists, of which warfarin is the principal member. Today, however, anticoagulants in two other pharmacologic classes—direct factor Xa inhibitors and direct thrombin inhibitors—can also be administered by mouth (see Table 52.1). Hence, grouping the anticoagulants by route of administration makes less sense than in the past. Accordingly, these drugs are grouped only by pharmacologic class and not by whether they are given orally or by injection.

Heparin and Its Derivatives: Drugs That Activate Antithrombin

All drugs in this group share the same mechanism of action. Specifically, they greatly enhance the activity of *antithrombin,*

TABLE 52.1 ■ Overview of Drugs for Thromboembolic Disorders

Generic Name	Brand Name	Route	Action	Therapeutic Use
ANTICOAGULANTS			Anticoagulants decrease formation of fibrin	Used primarily to prevent thrombosis in *veins* and the *atria of the heart*
Vitamin K Antagonist				
Warfarin	Coumadin	PO		
Heparin and Its Derivatives: Drugs That Activate Antithrombin				
Heparin (unfractionated)		SubQ, IV		
LMW heparins				
Dalteparin	Fragmin	SubQ		
Enoxaparin	Lovenox	SubQ		
Fondaparinux	Arixtra	SubQ		
Direct Thrombin Inhibitors				
Hirudin Analogs				
Bivalirudin	Angiomax	IV		
Desirudin	Iprivask	SubQ		
Other Direct Thrombin Inhibitors				
Argatroban	Acova	IV		
Dabigatran	Pradaxa, Pradax 🍁	PO		
Direct Factor Xa Inhibitors				
Rivaroxaban	Xarelto	PO		
Apixaban	Eliquis	PO		
Edoxaban	Savaysa	PO		
Antithrombin (AT)				
Recombinant human AT	ATryn	IV		
Plasma-derived AT	Thrombate III	IV		
ANTIPLATELET DRUGS			Antiplatelet drugs suppress platelet aggregation	Used primarily to prevent thrombosis in *arteries*
Cyclooxygenase Inhibitor				
Aspirin		PO		
$P2Y_{12}$ Adenosine Diphosphate Receptor Antagonists				
Clopidogrel	Plavix	PO		
Prasugrel	Effient	PO		
Ticagrelor	Brilinta	PO		
Protease-Activated Receptor-1 (PAR-1) Antagonists				
Vorapaxar	Zontivity	PO		
Glycoprotein IIb/IIIa Receptor Antagonists				
Abciximab	ReoPro	IV		
Eptifibatide	Integrilin	IV		
Tirofiban	Aggrastat	IV		
Other Antiplatelet Drugs				
Dipyridamole	Persantine	PO		
Cilostazol	Pletal	PO		
THROMBOLYTIC (FIBRINOLYTIC) DRUGS			Thrombolytic drugs promote breakdown of fibrin in thrombi	Used to dissolve newly formed thrombi
Alteplase	Activase	IV		
Reteplase	Retavase	IV		
Tenecteplase	TNKase	IV		

LMW, Low molecular weight.

a protein that inactivates two major clotting factors: *thrombin* and *factor Xa.* In the absence of thrombin and factor Xa, production of fibrin is reduced, and hence clotting is suppressed.

Our discussion focuses on three preparations: *unfractionated heparin,* the *low-molecular-weight (LMW) heparins,* and *fondaparinux.* Although all three activate antithrombin, they do not have equal effects on thrombin and factor Xa. Specifically, heparin reduces the activity of thrombin and factor Xa more or less equally; the LMW heparins reduce the activity of factor Xa more than they reduce the activity of thrombin; and fondaparinux causes selective inhibition of factor Xa, having no effect on thrombin. Properties of the three preparations are shown in Table 52.2.

Heparin (Unfractionated)

Heparin is a rapid-acting anticoagulant administered only by injection. Heparin differs from warfarin (an oral anticoagulant)

TABLE 52.2 ▪ Comparison of Drugs That Activate Antithrombin

Property	Unfractionated Heparin	Low-Molecular-Weight Heparins	Fondaparinux
Molecular weight range	3000–30,000	1000–9000	1728
Mean molecular weight	12,000–15,000	4000–5000	1728
Mechanism of action	Activation of antithrombin, resulting in the inactivation of factor Xa and thrombin	Activation of antithrombin, resulting in preferential inactivation of factor Xa, plus some inactivation of thrombin	Activation of antithrombin, resulting in selective inactivation of factor Xa
Routes	IV, subQ	SubQ only	SubQ only
Nonspecific binding	Widespread	Minimal	Minimal
Laboratory monitoring	aPTT monitoring is essential	No aPTT monitoring required	No aPTT monitoring required
Dosage	Dosage must be adjusted on the basis of aPTT	Dosage is fixed	Dosage is fixed
Setting for use	Hospital	Hospital or home	Hospital or home

aPTT, Activated partial thromboplastin time; *LMW,* low molecular weight.

in several respects, including mechanism, time course, indications, and management of overdose.

Chemistry. Heparin is not a single molecule, but rather a mixture of long polysaccharide chains, with molecular weights that range from 3000 to 30,000. The active region is a unique pentasaccharide (five-sugar) sequence found randomly along the chain. An important feature of heparin's structure is the presence of many negatively charged groups. Because of these negative charges, heparin is highly polar, and hence cannot readily cross membranes.

Mechanism of Anticoagulant Action. Heparin suppresses coagulation by helping antithrombin inactivate clotting factors, primarily thrombin and factor Xa. As shown in Fig. 52.3, binding of heparin to antithrombin produces a conformational change in antithrombin that greatly enhances its ability to inactivate both thrombin and factor Xa. However, the process of inactivating these two clotting factors is distinct. To inactivate thrombin, heparin must simultaneously bind with both thrombin and antithrombin, thereby forming a ternary complex. In contrast, to inactivate factor Xa, heparin binds only with antithrombin; heparin itself does not bind with factor Xa.

By activating antithrombin, and thereby promoting the inactivation of thrombin and factor Xa, heparin ultimately suppresses the formation of fibrin. Since fibrin forms the framework of thrombi in *veins,* heparin is especially useful for prophylaxis of *venous thrombosis.* Because thrombin and factor Xa are inhibited as soon as they bind with the heparin-antithrombin complex, the anticoagulant effects of heparin develop *quickly* (within minutes of IV administration). This contrasts with warfarin, whose full effects are not seen for *days.*

Pharmacokinetics

Absorption and Distribution. Because of its polarity and large size, heparin is unable to cross membranes, including those of the GI tract. Consequently, heparin cannot be absorbed if given orally and therefore must be given by injection (IV or subQ). Since it cannot cross membranes, heparin does not traverse the placenta and does not enter breast milk.

Protein and Tissue Binding. Heparin binds nonspecifically to plasma proteins, mononuclear cells, and endothelial cells. As a result, plasma levels of free heparin can be highly variable. Because of this variability, intensive monitoring is required (see later in this section).

Metabolism and Excretion. Heparin undergoes hepatic metabolism followed by renal excretion. Under normal conditions, the half-life is short (about 1.5 hours). However, in patients with hepatic or renal impairment, the half-life is increased.

Time Course. Therapy is sometimes initiated with a bolus IV injection, and effects begin immediately. Duration of action is brief (hours) and varies with dosage. Effects are prolonged in patients with hepatic or renal impairment.

Therapeutic Uses. Heparin is a preferred anticoagulant for use during *pregnancy* (because it doesn't cross the placenta) and in situations that require rapid onset of anticoagulant effects, including *pulmonary embolism* (PE) and *massive deep vein thrombosis* (DVT). In addition, heparin is used for patients undergoing *open heart surgery* and *renal dialysis;* during these procedures, heparin serves to prevent coagulation in devices of extracorporeal circulation (heart-lung machines, dialyzers). Low-dose therapy is used to *prevent postoperative venous thrombosis.* Heparin may also be useful for treating *disseminated intravascular coagulation,* a complex disorder in which fibrin clots form throughout the vascular system and in which bleeding tendencies may be present; bleeding can occur because massive fibrin production consumes available supplies of clotting factors. Heparin is also used as an adjunct to thrombolytic therapy of *acute myocardial infarction* (MI).

Adverse Effects

Hemorrhage. Bleeding develops in about 10% of patients and is the principal complication of treatment. Hemorrhage can occur at any site and may be fatal. Patients should be monitored closely for signs of blood loss. These include reduced blood pressure, increased heart rate, bruises, petechiae, hematomas, red or black stools, cloudy or discolored urine, pelvic pain (suggesting ovarian hemorrhage), headache or faintness (suggesting cerebral hemorrhage), and lumbar pain (suggesting adrenal hemorrhage). If bleeding develops, heparin should be withdrawn. Severe overdose can be treated with *protamine sulfate* (see *Protamine Sulfate for Heparin Overdose*).

The risk of hemorrhage can be decreased in several ways. First, dosage should be carefully controlled so that the activated partial thromboplastin time or anti-factor Xa levels (see later in this chapter) do not exceed the recommended safe limits. In addition, candidates for heparin therapy should be screened

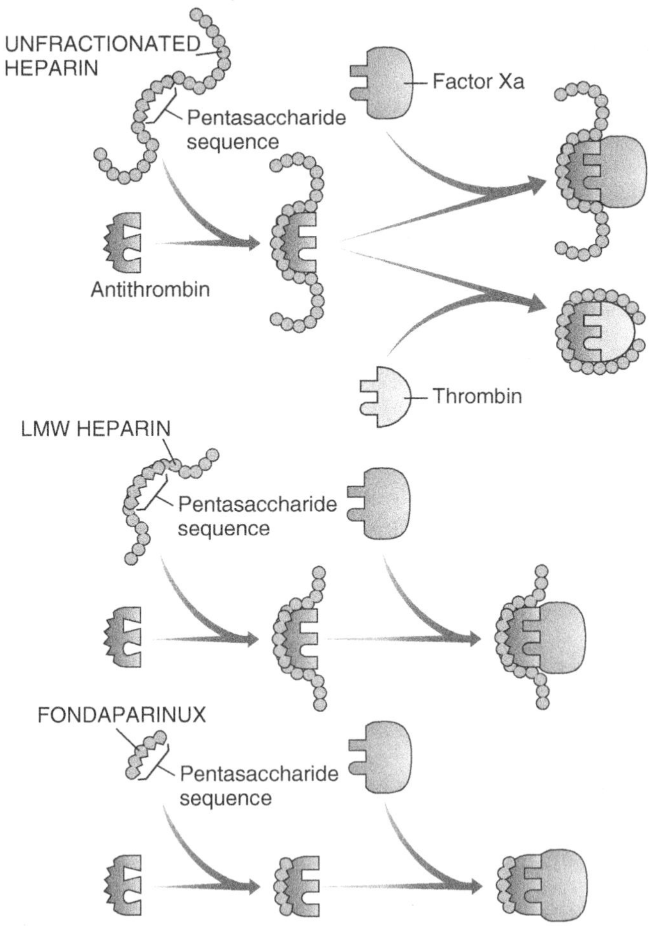

Fig. 52.3 ▪ Mechanism of action of heparin, LMW heparins, and fondaparinux.
All three drugs share a pentasaccharide sequence that allows them to bind with—and activate—antithrombin, a protein that inactivates two major clotting factors: thrombin and factor Xa. All three drugs enable antithrombin to inactivate factor Xa, but only heparin also facilitates inactivation of thrombin. *Upper Panel:* Unfractionated heparin binds with antithrombin, causing a conformational change in antithrombin that greatly increases its ability to interact with factor Xa and thrombin. When the heparin-antithrombin complex binds with thrombin, heparin changes its conformation so that both heparin and antithrombin come in contact with thrombin. Formation of this ternary complex is necessary for thrombin inactivation. Inactivation of factor Xa is different: It requires contact only between activated antithrombin and factor Xa; contact between heparin and factor Xa is unnecessary. *Middle Panel:* Low-molecular-weight (LMW) heparins have the same pentasaccharide sequence as unfractionated heparin and can bind with and activate antithrombin. However, in contrast to unfractionated heparin, most molecules of LMW heparin can inactivate only factor Xa. They are unable to inactivate thrombin because most molecules of LMW heparin are too small to form a ternary complex with thrombin and antithrombin. *Lower Panel:* Fondaparinux is a synthetic pentasaccharide identical in structure to the antithrombin binding sequence found in unfractionated heparin and LMW heparins. Being even smaller than LMW heparins, fondaparinux is too small to form a ternary complex with thrombin and can only inactivate factor Xa.

for risk factors (see *Warnings and Contraindications*). Finally, antiplatelet drugs (e.g., aspirin, clopidogrel) should be avoided.

Spinal/Epidural Hematoma. Heparin and all other anticoagulants pose a risk of spinal or epidural hematoma in patients undergoing spinal puncture or spinal/epidural anesthesia. Pressure on the spinal cord caused by the bleed can result in prolonged or permanent paralysis. Risk of hematoma is increased by:

- Use of an indwelling epidural catheter
- Use of other anticoagulants (e.g., warfarin, dabigatran)
- Use of antiplatelet drugs (e.g., aspirin, clopidogrel)
- History of traumatic or repeated epidural or spinal puncture
- History of spinal deformity, spinal injury, or spinal surgery

Patients should be monitored for signs and symptoms of neurologic impairment. If impairment develops, immediate intervention is needed.

Heparin-Induced Thrombocytopenia. Heparin-induced thrombocytopenia (HIT) is a potentially fatal immune-mediated disorder characterized by reduced platelet counts (thrombocytopenia) and a seemingly paradoxical *increase* in thrombotic events. The underlying cause is development of antibodies against heparin–platelet protein complexes. These antibodies activate platelets and damage the vascular endothelium, thereby promoting both thrombosis and a rapid loss of circulating platelets. Thrombus formation poses a risk of DVT, PE, cerebral thrombosis, and MI. Ischemic injury secondary to thrombosis in the limbs may require amputation of an arm or leg. Coronary thrombosis can be fatal. The primary treatment for HIT is discontinuation of heparin and, if anticoagulation is still needed, substitution of a nonheparin anticoagulant (e.g., argatroban). The incidence of HIT is between 0.2% and 5% among patients who receive heparin for more than 4 days.

HIT should be suspected whenever platelet counts fall significantly or when thrombosis develops despite adequate anticoagulation. Accordingly, to reduce the risk of HIT, patients should be monitored for signs of thrombosis and for reductions in platelets. Platelet counts should be determined frequently (2 to 3 times a week) during the first 3 weeks of heparin use, and monthly thereafter. If severe thrombocytopenia develops (platelet count below 100,000/mm^3), heparin should be discontinued.

Hypersensitivity Reactions. Because commercial heparin is extracted from animal tissues, these preparations may be contaminated with antigens that can promote allergy. Possible allergic responses include chills, fever, and urticaria. Anaphylactic reactions are rare.

Other Adverse Effects. Subcutaneous dosing may produce local irritation and hematoma. Vasospastic reactions that persist for several hours may develop after 1 or more weeks of treatment. Long-term, high-dose therapy may cause osteoporosis.

Safety Alert

ANTICOAGULANT, ANTIPLATELET, AND THROMBOLYTIC DRUGS

All the drugs discussed in this chapter increase the risk of patient bleeding. Careful assessment of mental status, blood pressure, heart rate, and mucous membranes should be completed to assess for internal bleeding.

Warnings and Contraindications

Warnings. Heparin must be used with extreme caution in all patients who have a high likelihood of bleeding. Among these are individuals with hemophilia, increased capillary permeability, dissecting aneurysm, peptic ulcer disease, severe hypertension, or threatened abortion. Heparin must also be used cautiously in patients with severe disease of the liver or kidneys.

Contraindications. Heparin is contraindicated for patients with thrombocytopenia and uncontrollable bleeding. In addition, heparin should be avoided both during and immediately after surgery of the eye, brain, or spinal cord. Lumbar puncture and regional anesthesia are additional contraindications.

Drug Interactions. In heparin-treated patients, platelet aggregation is the major remaining defense against hemorrhage. Aspirin and other drugs that depress platelet function or affect coagulation will weaken this defense, and hence must be employed with caution.

Protamine Sulfate for Heparin Overdose. Protamine sulfate is an antidote to severe heparin overdose. Protamine is a small protein that has multiple positively charged groups. These groups bond ionically with the negative groups on heparin, thereby forming a heparin-protamine complex that is devoid of anticoagulant activity. Neutralization of heparin occurs immediately and lasts for 2 hours, after which additional protamine may be needed. Protamine is administered by slow IV injection (no faster than 20 mg/min or 50 mg in 10 minutes). Dosage is based on the fact that 1 mg of protamine will inactivate 100 units of heparin. Hence, for each 100 units of heparin in the body, 1 mg of protamine should be injected.

Laboratory Monitoring. The objective of anticoagulant therapy is to reduce blood coagulability to a level that is low enough to prevent thrombosis but not so low as to promote spontaneous bleeding. Because heparin levels can be highly variable, achieving this goal is difficult and requires careful control of dosage based on frequent tests of coagulation. There are two tests used to monitor the effects of heparin.

Activated Partial Thromboplastin Time. The laboratory test employed most commonly is the *activated partial thromboplastin time* (aPTT). The normal value for the aPTT is 40 seconds. At therapeutic levels, heparin *increases* the aPTT by a factor of 1.5 to 2, making the aPTT 60 to 80 seconds. Since heparin has a rapid onset and brief duration, if an aPTT value should fall outside the therapeutic range, coagulability can be quickly corrected through an adjustment in dosage: if the aPTT is too long (more than 80 seconds), the dosage should be lowered; conversely, if the aPTT is too short (less than 60 seconds), the dosage should be increased. Measurements of aPTTs should be made frequently (every 4 to 6 hours) during the initial phase of therapy. Once an effective dosage has been established, measuring aPTT once a day will suffice.

Anti-Factor Xa Heparin Assay. A newer way to monitor heparin levels is being used in many facilities. Unlike aPTT, the anti-Xa assay directly measures heparin and its activity. In addition, aPTT levels can be affected by other physiologic variables, such as high levels of factor VIII. Anti-Xa levels are not altered by these variables, making the test potentially more accurate. Antithrombin binding to Xa is increased in patients receiving heparin. The anti-Xa assay measures the amount of Xa activity and is, therefore, directly inversely proportional to heparin activity in the bloodstream. Much like aPTT, anti-factor Xa levels guide titration of IV heparin. Levels of 0.3 to 0.7 IU/mL are considered within therapeutic range for anticoagulation with unfractionated heparin. One drawback of measuring anti-Xa levels is an increase in cost compared with monitoring aPTT.

Prescription and Preparations

Prescription. Heparin is prescribed in units, not in milligrams. The heparin unit is an index of anticoagulant activity. Heparin dosage is titrated on the basis of laboratory monitoring, and hence dosage can be adjusted as needed based on test results.

Preparations. Heparin sodium is supplied in single-dose vials; multidose vials; and unit-dose, preloaded syringes that have their own needles. Concentrations range from 1000 to 20,000 units/mL. Heparin sodium for use in heparin locks is supplied in *dilute* solutions (10 and 100 units/mL) that are too weak to produce systemic anticoagulant effects.

Dosage and Administration

General Considerations. Heparin is administered by injection only. Two routes are employed: *intravenous* (either intermittent or continuous) and *subcutaneous.* Intramuscular injection causes hematoma and must not be done. Heparin is not administered orally because heparin is too large and too polar to permit intestinal absorption.

Dosage varies by indication. Postoperative prophylaxis of thrombosis, for example, requires relatively small doses. In other situations, such as open heart surgery, much larger doses are needed. The dosages given here are for "general anticoagulant therapy." Because heparin is formulated in widely varying concentrations, you must read the label carefully to ensure that dosing is correct.

Continuous IV Infusion. Intravenous infusion provides steady levels of heparin. Dosing may consist of an initial weight-based bolus followed by a weight-based infusion titrated to laboratory results. Whether a bolus is indicated depends on the indication for treatment and the facility policy. During the initial phase of treatment, the aPTT or anti-Xa level should be measured once every 6 hours and the infusion rate adjusted accordingly. Heparin should be infused using an infusion pump, and the rate should be checked every 30 to 60 minutes.

Low-Dose Therapy. Heparin in low doses is given for prophylaxis against thromboembolism in hospitalized patients. Doses of 5000 units are given every 8 to 12 hours for the duration of hospitalization. Low-dose heparin is also employed as adjunctive therapy for patients with MI. During low-dose therapy, monitoring of the aPTT is not usually required.

Low-Molecular-Weight Heparins

Group Properties. LMW heparins are simply heparin preparations composed of molecules that are shorter than those found in unfractionated heparin. LMW heparins are as effective as unfractionated heparin and are easier to use because they can be given using a fixed dosage and don't require aPTT monitoring. As a result, LMW heparins can be used at home, whereas unfractionated heparin must be given in a hospital when administering intravenously. Because of these advantages, LMW heparins are now considered first-line therapy for prevention and treatment of DVT. In the United States, two LMW heparins are available: enoxaparin [Lovenox] and dalteparin [Fragmin]. Differences between LMW heparins and unfractionated heparin are shown in Table 52.2.

Production. LMW heparins are made by depolymerizing unfractionated heparin (i.e., breaking unfractionated heparin into smaller pieces). Molecular weights in LMW preparations range between 1000 and 9000, with a mean of 4000 to 5000. In comparison, molecular weights in unfractionated heparin range between 3000 and 30,000, with a mean of 12,000 to 15,000.

Mechanism of Action. Anticoagulant activity of LMW heparin is mediated by the same active pentasaccharide sequence

PATIENT-CENTERED CARE ACROSS THE LIFE SPAN

Anticoagulants

Life Stage	Patient Care Concerns
Infants	Heparin is commonly used in infants needing anticoagulation. Argatroban has been used successfully in infants with HIT. Warfarin is also administered to infants.
Children/adolescents	Many anticoagulants can be used safely in children, just in smaller doses. Side effect profiles are similar to that of adults.
Pregnant women	Warfarin is classified in FDA Pregnancy Risk Category X[a] and is contraindicated in pregnancy. LMW heparins and unfractionated heparin are commonly used in pregnancy. In pregnant women with HIT, argatroban is a safe alternative.
Breast-feeding women	Data are lacking regarding safety of these medications in breast-feeding. Warfarin and heparin are both safe to use.
Older adults	Atrial fibrillation becomes more common with age. In older adults, benefit must outweigh risk of bleeding secondary to falls, decreased renal function, or polypharmacy.

[a]As of 2020, the FDA will no longer use Pregnancy Risk Categories. Please refer to Chapter 9 for more information.

that mediates anticoagulant action of unfractionated heparin. However, because LMW heparin molecules are short, they do not have quite the same effect as unfractionated heparin. Specifically, whereas unfractionated heparin is equally good at inactivating factor Xa *and* thrombin, *LMW heparins preferentially inactivate factor Xa,* being much less able to inactivate thrombin. Why the difference? To inactivate thrombin, a heparin chain must not only contain the pentasaccharide sequence that activates antithrombin, it must also be long enough to provide a binding site for thrombin. This binding site is necessary because inactivation of thrombin requires simultaneous binding of thrombin with heparin and antithrombin (see Fig. 52.3). In contrast to unfractionated heparin chains, most (but not all) LMW heparin chains are too short to allow thrombin binding, and hence LMW heparins are less able to inactivate thrombin.

Therapeutic Use. LMW heparins are *approved* for (1) prevention of DVT following abdominal surgery, hip replacement surgery, or knee replacement surgery; (2) treatment of established DVT, with or without PE; and (3) prevention of ischemic complications in patients with unstable angina, non–Q-wave MI, and ST-elevation MI (STEMI). In addition, these drugs have been used extensively *off label* to prevent DVT after general surgery and in patients with multiple trauma and acute spinal injury. When used for prophylaxis or treatment of DVT, LMW heparins are at least as effective as unfractionated heparin, and possibly more effective.

Pharmacokinetics. Compared with unfractionated heparin, LMW heparins have higher bioavailability and longer half-lives. Bioavailability is higher because LMW heparins do not undergo nonspecific binding to proteins and tissues, and hence are more available for anticoagulant effects. Half-lives are prolonged (up to 6 times longer than that of unfractionated heparin) because LMW heparins undergo less binding to macrophages, and hence undergo slower clearance by the liver. Because of increased bioavailability, plasma levels of LMW heparin are highly predictable. As a result, these drugs can be given using a fixed dosage, with no need for routine monitoring of coagulation. Because of their long half-lives, LMW heparins can be given just once or twice a day.

Administration, Dosing, and Monitoring. All LMW heparins are administered subQ. Dosage is sometimes based on body weight, depending on indication. Because plasma levels of LMW heparins are predictable for any given dose, these drugs can be employed using a fixed dosage without laboratory monitoring. This contrasts with unfractionated heparin, which requires dosage adjustments on the basis of aPTT measurements. Because LMW heparins have an extended half-life, dosing can be done once or twice daily. For prophylaxis of DVT, dosing is begun in the perioperative period and continued 5 to 10 days.

Adverse Effects and Interactions. Bleeding is the major adverse effect. However, the incidence of bleeding complications is less than with unfractionated heparin. Despite the potential for bleeding, LMW heparins are considered safe for outpatient use. Like unfractionated heparin, LMW heparins can cause immune-mediated *thrombocytopenia.* As with unfractionated heparin, overdose with LMW heparins can be treated with protamine sulfate.

Like unfractionated heparin, LMW heparins can cause *severe neurologic injury,* including permanent paralysis, when given to patients undergoing *spinal puncture* or *spinal or epidural anesthesia.* The risk of serious harm is increased by concurrent use of antiplatelet drugs (e.g., aspirin, clopidogrel) or anticoagulants (e.g., warfarin, dabigatran). Patients should be monitored closely for signs of neurologic impairment.

Individual Preparations. In the United States, two LMW heparins are available: enoxaparin and dalteparin. Additional LMW heparins are available in other countries. Each preparation is unique, so clinical experience with one may not apply fully to the other.

Enoxaparin. Enoxaparin [Lovenox] was the first LMW heparin available in the United States. The drug is prepared by depolymerization of unfractionated porcine heparin. Molecular weights range between 2000 and 8000.

Enoxaparin is approved for prevention of DVT following hip and knee replacement surgery or abdominal surgery in patients considered at high risk of thromboembolic complications (e.g., obese patients, those over age 40, and those with malignancy or a history of DVT or pulmonary embolism [PE]). The drug is also approved for treatment of DVT or PE, and for preventing ischemic complications in patients with unstable angina, non–Q-wave MI, or STEMI.

In the event of overdose, hemorrhage can be controlled with protamine sulfate. The dosage is 1 mg of protamine sulfate for each milligram of enoxaparin administered.

ADMINISTRATION AND DOSAGE. Enoxaparin is administered by deep subQ injection. For patients with normal renal function (or moderate renal impairment), dosages are as follows:

- *Prevention of DVT after hip or knee replacement surgery*—30 mg every 12 hours, starting 12 to 24 hours after surgery and continuing 7 to 10 days.
- *Prevention of DVT after abdominal surgery*—40 mg once daily, beginning 2 hours before surgery and continuing 7 to 10 days.

- *Treatment of established DVT*—1 mg/kg every 12 hours for 7 days.
- *Patients with unstable angina or non–Q-wave MI*—1 mg/kg every 12 hours (in conjunction with oral aspirin, 100 to 325 mg once daily) for 2 to 8 days.
- *Patients with acute STEMI*—30 mg/kg by IV bolus plus 1 mg/kg subQ, followed by 1 mg/kg subQ every 12 hours for up to 8 days.

For patients with severe renal impairment, dosage should be reduced.

Dalteparin. Dalteparin [Fragmin] was the second LMW heparin approved in the United States. The drug is prepared by depolymerization of porcine heparin. Molecular weights range between 2000 and 9000, the mean being 5000. Approved indications are prevention of DVT following hip replacement surgery or abdominal surgery in patients considered at high risk of thromboembolic complications, prevention of ischemic complications in patients with unstable angina or non–Q-wave MI, and management of symptomatic venous thromboembolism (VTE). Administration is by deep subQ injection. Dosages are as follows:

- *Prevention of DVT after hip replacement surgery*—2500 units 1 or 2 hours before surgery, 2500 units that evening (at least 6 hours after the first dose), and then 5000 units once daily for 5 to 10 days.
- *Prevention of DVT after abdominal surgery*—2500 units once daily for 5 to 10 days, starting 1 to 2 hours before surgery. In high-risk patients, this dose is increased to 5000 units once daily, starting the night before surgery.
- *Patients with unstable angina or non–Q-wave MI*—120 units/kg (but not more than 10,000 units total) every 12 hours for 5 to 8 days. Concurrent therapy with aspirin (75 to 165 mg/day) is required.
- *Patients with symptomatic VTE*—200 units/kg (but not more than 18,000 units total) once daily for 1 month, then 150 units/kg (but not more than 18,000 IU total) once daily for months 2 through 6.

Overdose is treated with 1 mg of protamine sulfate for every 100 units of dalteparin administered.

Fondaparinux

Actions. Fondaparinux [Arixtra] is a synthetic subQ anticoagulant that enhances the activity of antithrombin *to cause selective inhibition of factor Xa.* The result is reduced production of thrombin, and hence reduced coagulation. Note that fondaparinux differs from the heparin preparations, which cause inactivation of thrombin as well as factor Xa.

Fondaparinux is closely related in structure and function to heparin and the LMW heparins. Structurally, fondaparinux is a pentasaccharide identical to the antithrombin-binding region of the heparins. Hence, like the heparins, fondaparinux is able to induce a conformational change in antithrombin, thereby increasing the activity of antithrombin—but only against factor Xa, not against thrombin. Why is fondaparinux selective for factor Xa? Because the drug is quite small—even smaller than the LMW heparins. As a result, it is too small to form a complex with both antithrombin and thrombin, and hence cannot reduce thrombin activity (see Fig. 52.3).

Fondaparinux has no effect on prothrombin time, aPTT, bleeding time, or platelet aggregation.

Therapeutic Use. Fondaparinux is approved for (1) preventing DVT following hip fracture surgery, hip replacement surgery, knee replacement surgery, or abdominal surgery; (2) treating acute PE (in conjunction with warfarin); and (3) treating acute DVT (in conjunction with warfarin). The drug is somewhat more effective than enoxaparin (an LMW heparin) at preventing DVT, but may cause slightly more bleeding. Anticoagulation may persist for 2 to 4 days after the last dose. Fondaparinux is administered using a fixed dosage, and does not require routine laboratory monitoring.

Pharmacokinetics. Fondaparinux is administered subQ. Bioavailability is 100%. Plasma levels peak 2 hours after dosing. The drug is eliminated by the kidneys with a half-life of 17 to 21 hours. The half-life is increased in patients with renal impairment.

Adverse Effects. As with other anticoagulants, *bleeding* is the biggest concern. The risk is increased by advancing age and renal impairment. Fondaparinux should be used with caution in patients with moderate renal impairment, defined as creatinine clearance (CrCl) of 30 to 50 mL/min, and avoided in patients with severe renal impairment, defined as CrCl below 30 mL/min. The drug should also be avoided for prophylactic use in patients weighing less than 50 kg because low body weight increases bleeding risk. Following surgery, at least 6 hours should elapse before starting fondaparinux. Aspirin and other drugs that interfere with hemostasis should be used with caution. In contrast to overdose with heparin or LMW heparins, overdose with fondaparinux cannot be treated with protamine sulfate.

Fondaparinux does not promote immune-mediated HIT, although it still can lower platelet counts. During clinical trials, *thrombocytopenia* developed in 3% of patients. Platelet counts should be monitored, and if they fall below 100,000/mm^3, fondaparinux should be discontinued.

In patients undergoing anesthesia using an epidural or spinal catheter, fondaparinux (as well as other anticoagulants) can cause *spinal or epidural hematoma,* which can result in permanent paralysis. However, in clinical trials, when fondaparinux was administered no sooner than 2 hours after catheter removal, no hematomas were reported.

Preparations, Dosage, and Administration. Fondaparinux [Arixtra] is available in single-dose, pre-filled syringes (2.5, 5, 7.5, and 10 mg). Dosing is done once a day by subQ injection.

For *prevention of DVT,* the recommended dosage is 2.5 mg once a day, starting 6 to 8 hours after surgery. The usual duration is 5 to 9 days.

For *treatment of acute DVT or acute PE,* dosage is based on body weight as follows: for patients under 50 kg, 5 mg once daily; for patients 50 to 100 kg, 7.5 mg once daily, and for patients over 100 kg, 10 mg once daily. The usual duration is 5 to 9 days.

Warfarin, a Vitamin K Antagonist

Warfarin [Coumadin, Jantoven], a vitamin K antagonist, is our oldest *oral* anticoagulant. The drug is similar to heparin in some respects and quite different in others. Like heparin, warfarin is used to prevent thrombosis. In contrast to heparin, warfarin has a delayed onset, which makes it inappropriate for emergencies. However, because it doesn't require injection, warfarin is well suited for long-term prophylaxis. Like heparin, warfarin carries a significant risk of hemorrhage, which is amplified by the many drug interactions to which warfarin is subject.

History

The history of warfarin underscores its potential for harm. Warfarin was discovered after a farmer noticed that his cattle bled after eating spoiled clover silage. The causative agent was identified as bishydroxycoumarin (dicumarol). Research into derivatives of dicumarol led to the synthesis of warfarin. When warfarin was first developed, clinical use was ruled out, owing to concerns about hemorrhage. So, instead of becoming a medicine, warfarin was used to kill rats. The drug proved especially effective in this application and remains one of our most widely used rodenticides. Clinical interest in warfarin was renewed following the report of a failed suicide attempt using huge doses of a warfarin-based rat poison. The clinical trials triggered by that event soon demonstrated that warfarin could be employed safely to treat humans.

Mechanism of Action

Warfarin suppresses coagulation by decreasing production of four clotting factors, namely, factors VII, IX, X, and prothrombin. These factors are known as *vitamin K–dependent clotting factors,* because an active form of vitamin K is needed to make them. Warfarin works by inhibiting *vitamin K epoxide reductase complex 1* (VKORC1), the enzyme needed to convert vitamin K to the required active form. Because of its mechanism, warfarin is referred to as a *vitamin K antagonist,* a term that is somewhat misleading because it implies antagonism of vitamin K *actions,* not antagonism of vitamin K *activation.* In therapeutic doses, warfarin reduces production of vitamin K–dependent clotting factors by 30% to 50%.

Pharmacokinetics

Absorption, Distribution, and Elimination. Warfarin is readily absorbed after oral dosing. Once in the blood, about 99% of warfarin binds to albumin. Warfarin molecules that remain free (unbound) can readily cross membranes, including those of the placenta and milk-producing glands. Warfarin is inactivated in the liver, mainly by CYP2C9, the 2C9 isoenzyme of cytochrome P450. Metabolites are excreted in the urine and feces.

Time Course. Although warfarin acts quickly to inhibit clotting factor *synthesis,* noticeable *anticoagulant effects* are delayed because warfarin has no effect on clotting factors already in circulation. Hence, until these clotting factors decay, coagulation remains unaffected. Since decay of clotting factors occurs with a half-life of 6 hours to 2.5 days (depending on the clotting factor under consideration), initial responses may not be evident until 8 to 12 hours after the first dose. Peak effects take several days to develop.

After warfarin is discontinued, coagulation remains inhibited for 2 to 5 days because warfarin has a long half-life (1.5 to 2 days). Hence, synthesis of new clotting factors remains suppressed, despite stopping dosing.

Therapeutic Uses

Overview of Uses. Warfarin is employed most frequently for long-term prophylaxis of thrombosis. Specific indications are (1) prevention of venous thrombosis and associated PE, (2) prevention of thromboembolism in patients with prosthetic heart valves, and (3) prevention of thrombosis in patients with atrial fibrillation. The drug has also been used to reduce the risk of recurrent transient ischemic attacks (TIAs) and recurrent MI. Because onset of effects is delayed, warfarin is not useful in emergencies. When rapid action is needed, anticoagulant therapy can be initiated with heparin.

Atrial Fibrillation. As discussed in Chapter 49, atrial fibrillation carries a high risk of stroke secondary to clot formation in the atrium. (If the clot becomes dislodged, it can travel to the brain and block an artery, thereby causing ischemic stroke.) So, when people have atrial fibrillation, anticoagulant therapy is given long term to prevent clot formation. Until recently, warfarin was the only oral anticoagulant available, and hence has been the reference standard for stroke prevention. However, four novel oral anticoagulants (NOACs)—dabigatran [Pradaxa, Pradax ♣], apixaban [Eliquis], edoxaban [Savaysa], and rivaroxaban [Xarelto]—which are much easier to use than warfarin, are likely to replace warfarin as the treatment of choice for many patients.

Monitoring Treatment

The anticoagulant effects of warfarin are evaluated by monitoring *prothrombin time* (PT)—a coagulation test that is especially sensitive to alterations in vitamin K–dependent factors. The average pretreatment value for PT is 12 seconds. Treatment with warfarin prolongs PT.

Traditionally, PT test results had been reported as a *PT ratio,* which is simply the ratio of the patient's PT to a control PT. However, there is a serious problem with this form of reporting: Test results can vary widely among laboratories. The underlying cause of variability is thromboplastin, a critical reagent employed in the PT test. To ensure that test results from different laboratories are comparable, results are now reported in terms of an *international normalized ratio* (INR). The INR is determined by multiplying the observed PT ratio by a correction factor specific to the particular thromboplastin preparation employed for the test.

The objective of treatment is to raise the INR to an appropriate value. Recommended INR ranges are shown in Table 52.3. As indicated, an INR of 2 to 3 is appropriate for most

TABLE 52.3 ▪ Monitoring Warfarin Therapy: Recommended Ranges of Prothrombin Time–Derived Values

	Recommended Ranges	
Condition Being Treated	**Observed PT Ratio[a]**	**INR[b]**
Acute myocardial infarction[c]	1.3–1.5	2–3
Atrial fibrillation[c]	1.3–1.5	2–3
Valvular heart disease[c]	1.3–1.5	2–3
Pulmonary embolism	1.3–1.5	2–3
Venous thrombosis[d]	1.3–1.5	2–3
Tissue heart valves[c]	1.3–1.5	2–3
Mechanical heart valves	1.5–2	3–4.5
Systemic embolism		
Prevention	1.3–1.5	2–3
Recurrent	1.5–2	2–3

[a]Observed PT ratio is the ratio of patient's PT to a control PT value. In this table, the reagent used to determine the control PT value is one of the preparations of rabbit brain thromboplastin employed in the United States. Had a different preparation of thromboplastin been used, the observed PT ratio could be very different.
[b]INR (international normalized ratio) is calculated from the observed PT ratio. The INR is equivalent to the PT ratio that would have been obtained if the patient's PT has been compared to a PT value obtained using the International Reference Preparation, a standardized human brain thromboplastin prepared by the World Health Organization. In contrast to PT ratios, INR values are comparable from one laboratory to the next throughout the United States and the rest of the world.
[c]For prevention of ischemic stroke and systemic embolism.
[d]Prophylaxis in high-risk surgery; treatment.

patients—although for some patients the target INR is 2.5 to 3.5. If the INR is below the recommended range, warfarin dosage should be increased. Conversely, if the INR is above the recommended range, dosage should be reduced. Unfortunately, since warfarin has a delayed onset and prolonged duration of action, the INR cannot be altered quickly: Once the dosage has been changed, it may take a week or more to reach the desired INR.

INR must be determined frequently during warfarin therapy. PT should be measured daily during the first 5 days of treatment, twice a week for the next 1 to 2 weeks, once a week for the next 1 to 2 months, and every 2 to 4 weeks thereafter. In addition, PT should be determined whenever a drug that interacts with warfarin is added to or deleted from the regimen.

INR can now be monitored at home. Several devices are available, including *CoaguChek* and the *ProTime Microcoagulation System.* These small, hand-held machines are easy to use, provide reliable results, and determine PT and INR values. In addition, the ProTime meter can be programmed by the prescriber with upper and lower INR values appropriate for the individual patient. When this is done, the meter will display either *In Range, INR High,* or *INR Low,* depending on the degree of anticoagulation. Home monitoring is more convenient than laboratory monitoring and gives patients a sense of empowerment. In addition, it improves anticoagulation control. In theory, home monitoring should help reduce bleeding (from excessive anticoagulation) and thrombosis (from insufficient anticoagulation). The CoaguChek meter costs about $1300 and the ProTime meter costs about $2700 to $3500. Each test costs about $10.

Adverse Effects

Hemorrhage. Bleeding is the major complication of warfarin therapy. Hemorrhage can occur at any site. Patients should be monitored closely for signs of bleeding (reduced blood pressure, increased heart rate, bruises, petechiae, hematomas, red or black stools, cloudy or discolored urine, pelvic pain, headache, and lumbar pain). If bleeding develops, warfarin should be discontinued. Severe overdose can be treated with *vitamin K* (discussed later). Patients should be encouraged to carry identification (e.g., Medic Alert bracelet) to inform emergency personnel of warfarin use. Of note, compared with warfarin, the newer oral anticoagulants—apixaban, rivaroxaban, edoxaban, and dabigatran—pose a significantly lower risk of serious bleeds.

Several measures can reduce the risk of bleeding. Candidates for treatment must be carefully screened for risk factors (see *Warnings and Contraindications*). INR must be measured frequently. A variety of drugs can potentiate warfarin's effects (see *Drug Interactions* later in this section), and hence must be used with care. Patients should be given detailed verbal and written instructions regarding signs of bleeding, dosage size and timing, and scheduling of INR tests. When a patient is incapable of accurate self-medication, a responsible individual must supervise treatment. Patients should be advised to make a record of each dose, rather than relying on memory. A soft toothbrush can reduce gingival bleeding. An electric razor can reduce cuts from shaving.

Warfarin intensifies bleeding during surgery. Accordingly, surgeons must be informed of warfarin use. Patients anticipating elective procedures should discontinue warfarin several days before the appointment. If an emergency procedure must be performed, injection of vitamin K can help suppress bleeding.

Does warfarin increase bleeding during dental surgery? Yes, but not that much. Accordingly, most patients needn't interrupt warfarin for dental procedures, including dental surgery. However, it is important that the INR be in the target range.

Fetal Hemorrhage and Teratogenesis From Use During Pregnancy. Warfarin can cross the placenta and affect the developing fetus. Fetal hemorrhage and death have occurred. In addition, warfarin can cause gross malformations, central nervous system (CNS) defects, and optic atrophy. Accordingly, *warfarin is classified in U.S. Food and Drug Administration (FDA) Pregnancy Risk Category X*[b]*: The risks to the developing fetus outweigh any possible benefits of treatment.* Women of childbearing age should be informed about the potential for teratogenesis and advised to postpone pregnancy. If pregnancy occurs, the possibility of termination should be discussed. If an anticoagulant is needed during pregnancy, heparin or LMW heparin, which does not cross the placenta, should be employed.

Use During Lactation. Warfarin enters breast milk. Women should be advised against breast-feeding.

Other Adverse Effects. Adverse effects other than hemorrhage are uncommon. Possible undesired responses include skin necrosis, alopecia, urticaria, dermatitis, fever, GI disturbances, and red-orange discoloration of urine, which must not be confused with hematuria. Long-term warfarin use (more than 12 months) may weaken bones and thereby increase the risk of fractures.

Drug Interactions

General Considerations. Warfarin is subject to a large number of clinically significant adverse interactions—perhaps more than any other drug. As a result of interactions, anticoagulant effects may be reduced to the point of permitting thrombosis, or they may be increased to the point of causing hemorrhage. Patients must be informed about the potential for hazardous interactions and instructed to avoid *all* drugs not specifically approved by the prescriber. This prohibition includes prescription drugs and over-the-counter products.

Interactions between warfarin and other drugs are shown in Table 52.4. As indicated, the interactants fall into three major categories: (1) *drugs that increase anticoagulant effects,* (2) *drugs that promote bleeding,* and (3) *drugs that decrease anticoagulant effects.* The major mechanisms by which anticoagulant effects can be *increased* are (1) displacement of warfarin from plasma albumin, (2) inhibition of the hepatic enzymes that degrade warfarin, and (3) decreased synthesis of clotting factors. The major mechanisms for *decreasing* anticoagulant effects are (1) acceleration of warfarin degradation through induction of hepatic drug-metabolizing enzymes, (2) increased synthesis of clotting factors, and (3) inhibition of warfarin absorption. Mechanisms by which drugs can *promote bleeding,* and thereby complicate anticoagulant therapy, include (1) inhibition of platelet aggregation, (2) inhibition of clotting factors, and (3) generation of GI ulcers.

The existence of an interaction between warfarin and another drug does not absolutely preclude using the combination. The interaction does mean, however, that the combination must be used with due caution. The potential for harm is greatest when an interacting drug is being added to or withdrawn from the regimen. At these times, PT must be monitored, and the dosage of warfarin adjusted to compensate for the impact of removing or adding an interacting drug.

Specific Interacting Drugs. Of the many drugs listed in Table 52.4, a few are especially likely to produce interactions of clinical significance. Four are discussed here.

Heparin. The interaction of heparin with warfarin is obvious: Being an anticoagulant itself, heparin directly increases the bleeding tendencies brought on by warfarin. Yet because onset of a therapeutic INR when starting warfarin therapy may take a few days, heparin is often administered alongside warfarin during this time. Combined therapy with heparin plus warfarin must be performed with care.

Aspirin. Aspirin inhibits platelet aggregation. By blocking aggregation, aspirin can suppress formation of the platelet plug that initiates hemostasis. To make matters worse, aspirin can act directly on the GI tract to cause ulcers, thereby initiating bleeding. Therefore, when the antifibrin effects of warfarin are coupled with the antiplatelet and ulcerogenic effects of aspirin, the potential for hemorrhage is significant. Accordingly, patients should be warned specifically against using any product that contains aspirin, unless the provider has prescribed aspirin therapy. Drugs similar to aspirin (e.g., indomethacin, ibuprofen) should be avoided as well.

Nonaspirin Antiplatelet Drugs. Like aspirin, other antiplatelet drugs can increase the risk of bleeding with warfarin.

[b]As of 2020, the FDA will no longer use Pregnancy Risk Categories. Please refer to Chapter 9 for more information.

TABLE 52.4 ■ Interactions Between Warfarin and Other Drugs

Drug Category	Mechanism of Interaction	Representative Interacting Drugs
Drugs that *increase* the effects of warfarin	Displacement of warfarin from albumin	Aspirin and other salicylates Sulfonamides
	Inhibition of warfarin degradation	Acetaminophen Amiodarone Azole antifungal agents Cimetidine Disulfiram Leflunomide Trimethoprim-sulfamethoxazole
	Decreased synthesis of clotting factors	Certain parenteral cephalosporins, including cefoperazone and cefamandole
Drugs that *promote bleeding*	Inhibition of platelet aggregation	Abciximab Aspirin and other salicylates Cilostazol Clopidogrel Dipyridamole Eptifibatide Prasugrel Ticagrelor Ticlopidine Tirofiban
	Inhibition of clotting factors and/or thrombin	Antimetabolites Apixaban Argatroban Bivalirudin Dabigatran Desirudin Fondaparinux Heparins Rivaroxaban
	Promotion of ulcer formation	Aspirin Glucocorticoids Indomethacin Phenylbutazone
Drugs that *decrease* the effects of warfarin	Induction of drug-metabolizing enzymes	Carbamazepine Phenobarbital Phenytoin Rifampin
	Promotion of clotting factor synthesis	Oral contraceptives Vitamin K_1
	Reduction of warfarin absorption	Cholestyramine Colestipol

Accordingly, these drugs (e.g., clopidogrel, dipyridamole, ticlopidine, abciximab) should be used with caution.

Acetaminophen. In the past, acetaminophen was considered safe for patients on warfarin. In fact, acetaminophen was routinely recommended as an aspirin substitute for patients who needed a mild analgesic. Now, however, it appears that acetaminophen can increase the risk of bleeding: Compared with nonusers of acetaminophen, those who take just 4 regular-strength tablets a day for a week are 10 times more likely to have a dangerously high INR. Unlike aspirin, which promotes bleeding by inhibiting platelet aggregation, acetaminophen is believed to inhibit warfarin degradation, thereby raising warfarin levels. At this time, the interaction between acetaminophen and warfarin has not been proven. Nonetheless, when the drugs are combined, the INR should be monitored closely.

Other Notable Interactions. Several drugs, including *phenobarbital, carbamazepine,* and *rifampin,* are powerful inducers of hepatic drug-metabolizing enzymes. As a result, these drugs can accelerate warfarin degradation, thereby decreasing anticoagulant effects. Accordingly, if one of these drugs is added to the regimen, warfarin dosage must be increased. Of equal importance, when an inducer is withdrawn, causing rates of drug metabolism to decline, a compensatory decrease in warfarin dosage must be made.

Intravaginal miconazole can intensify the anticoagulant effects of warfarin. (Miconazole is the antifungal agent found in Monistat brand vaginal suppositories and cream, used for vaginal candidiasis [yeast infection].) One woman using the combination reported bruising, bleeding gums, and a nosebleed. We have long known that *systemic* miconazole (as well as other azole antifungal agents) can inhibit the metabolism of warfarin and can thereby cause warfarin levels to rise. Apparently, intravaginal miconazole can be absorbed in amounts sufficient to do the same. Because of this interaction, women taking warfarin should not use intravaginal miconazole. If the drugs must be used concurrently, anticoagulation should be monitored closely and warfarin dosage reduced as indicated.

Like the azole antifungal agents, *cimetidine* (a drug for ulcers) and *disulfiram* (a drug for alcoholism) can inhibit warfarin metabolism and can thereby increase anticoagulant effects.

Vitamin K increases clotting factor synthesis and can thereby decrease anticoagulant effects.

Sulfonamide antibacterial drugs can displace warfarin from albumin and thereby increase anticoagulant effects.

Leflunomide [Arava], a drug for arthritis, can significantly increase the INR in just a few days, probably by inhibiting warfarin degradation. Case reports suggest that two other antiarthritic agents—*glucosamine* and *chondroitin*—may also potentiate warfarin action.

Warnings and Contraindications

Like heparin, warfarin is contraindicated for patients with severe thrombocytopenia or uncontrollable bleeding and for patients undergoing lumbar puncture, regional anesthesia, or surgery of the eye, brain, or spinal cord. Also like heparin, warfarin must be used with extreme caution in patients at high risk of bleeding, including those with hemophilia, increased capillary permeability, dissecting aneurysm, GI ulcers, and severe hypertension, and in women anticipating abortion. In addition, warfarin is contraindicated in the presence of vitamin K deficiency, liver disease, and alcoholism—conditions that can disrupt hepatic synthesis of clotting factors. Warfarin is also contraindicated during pregnancy and lactation.

Vitamin K_1 for Warfarin Overdose

The effects of warfarin overdose can be overcome with vitamin K_1 (phytonadione). Vitamin K_1 antagonizes warfarin's actions and can thereby reverse warfarin-induced inhibition of clotting factor synthesis. (Vitamin K_3—menadione—has no effect on warfarin action.)

Vitamin K may be given orally or IV; subQ administration is less effective and should be avoided. Intravenous vitamin K acts faster than oral vitamin K, but can cause severe anaphylactoid reactions, characterized by flushing, hypotension, and cardiovascular collapse. To reduce this risk, vitamin K should be diluted and infused slowly.

As a rule, small doses—2.5 mg PO or 0.5 to 1 mg IV—are preferred. Large doses (e.g., 10 mg PO) can cause prolonged resistance to warfarin, thereby hampering restoration of anticoagulation once bleeding is under control.

If vitamin K fails to control bleeding, levels of clotting factors can be raised quickly by infusing fresh whole blood, fresh-frozen plasma, or plasma concentrates of vitamin K–dependent clotting factors.

What About Dietary Vitamin K?

Like medicinal vitamin K, dietary vitamin K can reduce the anticoagulant effects of warfarin. Dietary sources include mayonnaise, canola oil, soybean oil, and green leafy vegetables. Must patients avoid these foods? No. But they should keep intake of vitamin K constant. If vitamin K intake does increase, then warfarin dosage should be increased as well. Conversely, if vitamin K intake decreases, the warfarin dosage should decrease too.

Contrasts Between Warfarin and Heparin

Although heparin and warfarin are both anticoagulants, they differ in important ways (Table 52.5). Whereas warfarin is given orally, heparin is given by injection. Although both drugs decrease fibrin formation, they do so by different mechanisms: heparin inactivates thrombin and factor Xa, whereas warfarin inhibits synthesis of clotting factors. Heparin and warfarin differ with respect to time course of action: effects of heparin begin and fade rapidly, whereas effects of warfarin begin slowly but persist several days. Different tests are used to monitor therapy. Changes in aPTT are used to monitor heparin treatment; changes in PT are used to monitor warfarin. Finally, these drugs differ with respect to management of overdose. Protamine is given to counteract heparin; vitamin K_1 is given to counteract warfarin.

Dosage

Basic Considerations. Dosage requirements for warfarin vary widely among individuals, and hence dosage must be tailored to each patient. Traditionally, dosage adjustments have been done empirically (i.e., by trial and error). Dosing is usually begun at 2 to 5 mg/day. Maintenance dosages, which typically range from 2 to 10 mg/day, are determined by the target INR value. For most patients, dosage should be adjusted to produce an INR between 2 and 3.

Genetics and Dosage Adjustment. Patients with variant genes that code for VKORC1 and CYP2C9 are at increased risk of warfarin-induced bleeding, and hence require reduced doses. As noted previously, VKORC1 is the target enzyme that warfarin inhibits, and CYP2C9 is the enzyme that metabolizes warfarin. Variations in VKORC1 increase the enzyme's sensitivity to inhibition by warfarin, and variations in CYP2C9 delay warfarin breakdown. With either variation, effects of warfarin are increased. To reduce the risk of bleeding, the FDA now recommends—but does not require—that patients undergo genetic testing for these variants. Dosage reductions based on this information can be determined using the calculator at www.warfarindosing.org.

TABLE 52.5 ■ Contrasts Between Heparin and Warfarin

	Heparin	Warfarin
Mechanism of action	Activates antithrombin, which then inactivates thrombin and factor Xa	Inhibits synthesis of vitamin K–dependent clotting factors, including prothrombin and factor X
Route	IV or subQ	PO
Onset	Rapid (minutes)	Slow (hours)
Duration	Brief (hours)	Prolonged (days)
Monitoring	aPTT or anti-Xa heparin assay	PT (INR)[a]
Antidote for overdose	Protamine	Vitamin K_1

aPTT, Activated partial thromboplastin time; *PT,* prothrombin time.
[a]Test results are reported as an INR (international normalized ratio).

Preparations

Warfarin sodium [Coumadin, Jantoven] is available in tablets (1, 2, 2.5, 3, 4, 5, 6, 7.5, and 10 mg) for oral use. In addition, warfarin is available in a formulation for parenteral dosing, which is not commonly done.

Direct Thrombin Inhibitors

The anticoagulants discussed in this section work by direct inhibition of thrombin. Hence, they differ from the heparin-like anticoagulants, which inhibit thrombin indirectly (by enhancing the activity of antithrombin). One of the direct thrombin inhibitors—dabigatran—is administered PO; another—desirudin—is administered subQ; and two others—bivalirudin and argatroban—are administered by continuous IV infusion. Only the subQ and PO drugs are suitable for outpatient use.

Dabigatran Etexilate

Dabigatran etexilate [Pradaxa, Pradax ♣] is an *oral* prodrug that undergoes rapid conversion to *dabigatran*, a reversible, direct thrombin inhibitor. Compared with warfarin—our oldest oral anticoagulant—dabigatran has five major advantages: rapid onset; no need to monitor anticoagulation; few drug-food interactions; lower risk of major bleeding; and, since responses are predictable, the same dose can be used for all patients, regardless of age or weight. Contrasts between dabigatran and warfarin are shown in Table 52.6.

Mechanism of Action. Dabigatran is a direct, reversible inhibitor of thrombin. The drug binds with and inhibits thrombin that is free in the blood, as well as thrombin that is bound to clots. In contrast, heparin inhibits only free thrombin. By inhibiting thrombin, dabigatran (1) prevents the conversion of fibrinogen into fibrin and (2) prevents the activation of factor XIII, and thereby prevents the conversion of soluble fibrin into insoluble fibrin.

Therapeutic Use

Atrial Fibrillation. In the United States, dabigatran is approved for the treatment of DVT and PE, as well as for prevention of stroke and systemic embolism in patients with nonvalvular atrial fibrillation. Approval was based on the RE-LY trial, in which over 18,000 patients were randomized to receive either dabigatran (110 or 150 mg twice daily) or warfarin (dosage adjusted to produce an INR of 2 to 3). At the lower dabigatran dose (110 mg twice daily), the incidence of bleeding with dabigatran was less than with warfarin, but protection against stroke was less too. By contrast, at the higher dose (150 mg twice daily), the incidence of bleeding with dabigatran

TABLE 52.6 ▪ Properties of Oral Anticoagulants

	Warfarin [Coumadin]	Rivaroxaban [Xarelto]	Apixaban [Eliquis]	Edoxaban [Savaysa]	Dabigatran Etexilate [Pradaxa, Pradax ♣]
Mechanism	Decreased synthesis of vitamin K–dependent clotting factors	Inhibition of factor Xa	Inhibition of factor Xa	Inhibition of factor Xa	Direct inhibition of thrombin
Indications					
Atrial fibrillation	Yes	Yes	Yes	Yes	Yes
Heart valve replacement	Yes	No	No	No	No
Knee or hip replacement	Yes	Yes	No	No	Yes
Onset	Delayed (days)	Rapid (hours)	Rapid (hours)	Rapid (hours)	Rapid (hours)
Duration	Prolonged	Short	Short	Short	Short
Antidote available	Yes (oral/parenteral vitamin K)	No	No	No	No
Drug-food interactions	Many	Few	Few	Few	Few
INR testing needed	Yes	No	No	No	No
Dosage	Adjusted based on INR	Fixed	Fixed	Fixed	Fixed
Doses/day	One	One	Two	One	Two
Clinical experience	Extensive	Limited	Limited	Limited	Limited
Advantages, summary	Decades of clinical experience Precise dosage timing not critical, owing to long duration Antidote available for overdose	Rapid onset Fixed dosage No blood tests needed Less bleeding and hemorrhagic stroke Few drug-food interactions	Same as rivaroxaban	Same as rivaroxaban	Same as rivaroxaban
Disadvantages, summary	Delayed onset Blood tests required No fixed dosage Many drug-food interactions	Dosing on time is important, owing to short duration No antidote to overdose Limited clinical experience	Same as rivaroxaban	Same as rivaroxaban	Same as rivaroxaban *plus* GI disturbances are common

equaled that with warfarin, but the incidence of stroke or embolism was significantly lower. On the basis of these results, the FDA concluded that, for patients with atrial fibrillation, the benefit/risk profile of dabigatran was better at 150 mg twice daily than at 110 mg twice daily, and hence they approved the higher dose for these patients.

Knee or Hip Replacement. Dabigatran is approved for prevention of VTE following knee or hip replacement surgery. The dosage is 220 mg once daily, following an initial dose of 110 mg.

DVT/PE Treatment. In 2014, the FDA approved dabigatran for the treatment of DVT and PE in patients who have been treated with a parenteral anticoagulant for 5 to 10 days, and to reduce the risk of recurrent DVT and PE in patients who have been previously treated. The dose for treatment is 150 mg twice daily.

Pharmacokinetics. Dabigatran etexilate is well absorbed from the GI tract, both in the presence and absence of food. (Food delays absorption but does not reduce the extent of absorption.) Plasma levels peak about 1 hour after dosing in the absence of food, and 3 hours after dosing in the presence of food. In the blood, plasma esterases rapidly convert dabigatran etexilate to dabigatran, the drug's active form. Protein binding in blood is low (about 35%). Dabigatran is not metabolized by hepatic enzymes. Elimination is primarily renal. The half-life is 13 hours in patients with normal renal function (CrCl 50 mL/min or higher), and it increases to 18 hours in patients with moderate renal impairment (CrCl 30 to 50 mL/min).

Adverse Effects

Bleeding. Like all other anticoagulants, dabigatran can cause bleeding. In the RE-LY trial, about 17% of patients taking 150 mg of dabigatran twice daily experienced bleeding of any intensity, and 3% experienced major bleeding. Patients who develop pathologic bleeding should stop taking the drug. Compared with warfarin, dabigatran is safer, posing a much lower risk of hemorrhagic stroke and other major bleeds.

Because dabigatran is not highly protein bound, dialysis can remove much of the drug (about 60% over 2 to 3 hours).

Because dabigatran is eliminated primarily in the urine, maintaining adequate diuresis is important.

Owing to bleeding risk, dabigatran should be stopped before elective surgery. For patients with normal renal function (CrCl 50 mL/min or higher), dosing should stop 1 or 2 days before surgery. For patients with renal impairment (CrCl below 50 mL/min), dosing should stop 3 to 5 days before surgery.

Gastrointestinal Disturbances. About 35% of patients experience *dyspepsia* (abdominal pain, bloating, nausea, vomiting) and/or *gastritis-like symptoms* (esophagitis, gastroesophageal reflux disease, gastric hemorrhage, erosive gastritis, hemorrhagic gastritis, GI ulcer). Symptoms of *dyspepsia* can be reduced by taking dabigatran with food and by using an acid-suppressing drug (proton pump inhibitor or histamine$_2$ receptor blocker). If these measures don't help, patients may try a switch to warfarin, which carries a much lower risk of adverse GI effects.

Drug Interactions. Dabigatran is not metabolized by hepatic P450 enzymes, nor is it an inhibitor or inducer of these enzymes. Accordingly, dabigatran does not have metabolic interactions with other drugs.

Dabigatran etexilate is a substrate for intestinal *P-glycoprotein,* the transporter protein that can pump dabigatran and other drugs back into the intestine. Drugs that inhibit P-glycoprotein can increase dabigatran absorption and blood levels, and drugs that induce P-glycoprotein can decrease dabigatran absorption and blood levels. Combined use with a P-glycoprotein *inhibitor* (e.g., ketoconazole, amiodarone, verapamil, quinidine) could cause bleeding from excessive dabigatran levels, and hence these combinations should be avoided. Combined use with a P-glycoprotein *inducer* appears to be safe, even though it might reduce beneficial effects somewhat.

Bleeding risk is increased by other drugs that impair hemostasis.

Preparations, Dosage, Administration, and Storage

Preparations. Dabigatran etexilate [Pradaxa] is available in three strengths: 75-, 110-, and 150-mg capsules.

Administration. Dosing may be done with or without food. Patients should swallow the capsules intact. If the capsules are crushed, chewed, or opened, absorption will be increased by 75%, thereby posing a risk of bleeding.

Dosage for Atrial Fibrillation. The usual dosage is 150 mg twice daily. If a dose is missed, it should be taken as soon as possible on the same day. However, if the missed dose cannot be taken at least 6 hours before the next scheduled dose, the missed dose should be skipped.

In patients with significant renal impairment (CrCl 15 to 30 mL/min), the dosage is 75 mg twice a day. For patients with greater renal impairment (CrCl below 15 mL/min), no dosing recommendation can be made.

Switching From Warfarin to Dabigatran. Discontinue warfarin, wait until the INR falls below 2, and then start dabigatran.

Switching From Dabigatran to Warfarin. Because onset of warfarin's effects is delayed, warfarin should be started before stopping dabigatran, based on CrCl as follows:

- CrCl above 50 mL/min—start warfarin 3 days before stopping dabigatran.
- CrCl 31 to 50 mL—start warfarin 2 days before stopping dabigatran.
- CrCl 15 to 30 mL—start warfarin 1 day before stopping dabigatran.
- CrCl below 15 mL/min—no recommendation can be made.

Storage. Dabigatran is unstable, especially when exposed to moisture. To maintain efficacy, the drug must be stored in the manufacturer-supplied bottle, which has a desiccant cap. Patients should open just one bottle at a time and should not distribute dabigatran to any other container, such as a weekly pill organizer. Current labeling says that once the bottle is opened, dabigatran should be used within 30 days. However, recent evidence indicates that dabigatran capsules maintain efficacy for 4 months, provided they are stored in the original container—away from excessive moisture, heat, and cold—with the cap tightly closed after each use.

Hirudin Analogs

Bivalirudin

Actions and Use. Bivalirudin [Angiomax], an IV direct thrombin inhibitor, has actions like those of dabigatran. The drug is a synthetic 20–amino acid peptide that is chemically related to *hirudin,* an anticoagulant isolated from the saliva of leeches.

Bivalirudin is given in combination with aspirin, clopidogrel, or prasugrel to prevent clot formation in patients undergoing coronary angioplasty. At this time, the standard therapy for these patients is aspirin combined with a platelet GP IIb/IIIa inhibitor combined with low-dose, unfractionated heparin. Bivalirudin, an alternative to heparin in this regimen, has been studied in combination with aspirin, as well as GP IIb/IIIa inhibitors. In one trial—the Hirulog Angioplasty Study—bivalirudin plus aspirin was compared with heparin plus aspirin. Bivalirudin was at least as effective as heparin at preventing ischemic complications (MI, abrupt vessel closure, death), and caused fewer bleeding complications. In a subgroup of patients—those with postinfarction angina—bivalirudin was significantly *more* effective than heparin.

Adverse Effects. The most common side effects are back pain, nausea, hypotension, and headache. Other relatively common effects (incidence greater than 5%) include vomiting, abdominal pain, pelvic pain, anxiety, nervousness, insomnia, bradycardia, and fever.

Bleeding is the effect of greatest concern. However, compared with heparin, bivalirudin causes fewer incidents of major bleeding (3.7% vs. 9.3%), and fewer patients require transfusions (2% vs. 5.7%). Coadministration of bivalirudin with heparin, warfarin, or thrombolytic drugs increases the risk of bleeding.

Pharmacokinetics. With IV dosing, anticoagulation begins immediately. Drug levels are maintained by continuous infusion. Bivalirudin is eliminated primarily by renal excretion and partly by proteolytic cleavage. The half-life is short (25 minutes) in patients with normal renal function, but may be longer in patients with renal impairment. Coagulation returns to baseline about 1 hour after stopping the infusion. Anticoagulation can be monitored by measuring activated clotting time.

Comparison With Heparin. Bivalirudin is just as effective as heparin and has several advantages: It works independently of antithrombin, inhibits clot-bound thrombin as well as free thrombin, and causes less bleeding and fewer ischemic events. However, the drug has one disadvantage: Bivalirudin is more expensive than heparin. One single-use vial, good for a full course of treatment, costs about $1000, compared with $10 for an equivalent course of heparin. However, the manufacturer estimates that reductions in bleeding and ischemic complications would save, on average, $1000 per patient, which would offset the greater cost of bivalirudin. The bottom line? Bivalirudin works as well as heparin, is safer, and may be equally cost effective—and hence is considered an attractive alternative to heparin for use during angioplasty.

Preparations, Dosage, and Administration. Bivalirudin [Angiomax] is supplied as a lyophilized powder (250 mg) for reconstitution in sterile water. Dosing consists of an initial IV bolus (0.75 mg/kg) followed by continuous infusion (1.75 mg/kg/hr) for the duration of the procedure, and up to 4 hours after. If necessary, bivalirudin may be infused for up to 20 additional hours at a rate of 0.2 mg/kg/hr. Treatment should begin just before angioplasty. Dosage should be reduced in patients with severe renal impairment. All patients should take aspirin (300 to 325 mg).

Desirudin. Desirudin [Iprivask] is a direct thrombin inhibitor similar to bivalirudin. However, unlike bivalirudin, which is given by IV infusion, desirudin is given by subQ injection. Desirudin is indicated for prevention of DVT in patients undergoing elective hip replacement surgery. In clinical trials, patients experienced fewer thromboembolic events than those given unfractionated heparin or enoxaparin, an LMW heparin.

Desirudin is completely absorbed following subQ injection, achieving peak plasma levels in 1 to 3 hours. Elimination is primarily by renal excretion and partly by proteolytic cleavage. In patients with normal renal function, the elimination half-life is 2 to 3 hours. By contrast, in those with severe renal impairment, the half-life is greatly prolonged (up to 12 hours).

As with other anticoagulants, hemorrhage is the adverse effect of greatest concern. In clinical trials, the incidence of hemorrhage was 30% in the desirudin group, compared with 33% in the enoxaparin group and 20% in the heparin group. Less serious effects include wound secretion, injection-site mass, anemia, nausea, and deep thrombophlebitis.

In patients undergoing spinal or epidural anesthesia, desirudin may cause spinal or epidural hematoma, which can result in long-term or even permanent paralysis. Hematoma risk is increased by the use of other drugs that impair hemostasis (e.g., nonsteroidal anti-inflammatory drugs [NSAIDs], antiplatelet drugs, warfarin, heparin). Patients should be monitored for signs of neurologic impairment and given immediate treatment if they develop.

Desirudin [Iprivask] is supplied as a lyophilized powder (15 mg) in single-use vials. Immediately after reconstitution (with 0.5 mL of 3% mannitol in sterile water), the drug is administered by deep subQ injection into the thigh or abdominal wall. For patients with normal renal function, the dosage is 15 mg every 12 hours, beginning 5 to 15 minutes before hip surgery (but after induction of regional block anesthesia, if used). For patients with *moderate* renal impairment (CrCl 30 to 50 mL/min), dosage is reduced to 5 mg every 12 hours. For those with *severe* renal impairment (CrCl below 30 mL/min), dosage is reduced to 1.7 mg every 12 hours. For all patients, the usual duration of treatment is 9 to 12 days.

Argatroban. Like bivalirudin, argatroban is an IV anticoagulant that works by direct inhibition of thrombin. The drug is indicated for prophylaxis and treatment of thrombosis in patients with HIT. In clinical trials, argatroban reduced development of new thrombosis and permitted restoration of platelet counts. Like other anticoagulants, argatroban poses a risk of hemorrhage. About 12% of patients experience hematuria. Allergic reactions (dyspnea, cough, rash), which develop in 10% of patients, occur almost exclusively in those receiving either thrombolytic drugs (e.g., alteplase) or contrast media for coronary angioplasty. Argatroban has a short half-life (about 45 minutes), owing to rapid metabolism by the liver. Treatment is monitored by measuring the aPTT. When infusion of argatroban is discontinued, the aPTT returns to baseline in 2 to 4 hours.

Argatroban is supplied in 2.5-mL single-dose vials (100 mg/mL) intended for dilution followed by continuous IV infusion. Dosage depends on the setting as follows:

- *For prophylaxis and treatment of thrombosis in patients with HIT and normal liver function* (but who are *not* undergoing percutaneous coronary intervention [PCI])—The initial infusion rate is 2 mcg/kg/min. In patients with liver dysfunction, the initial rate is only 0.5 mcg/kg/min. Dosage is adjusted to maintain the aPTT at 1.5 to 3 times the baseline value.
- *For prevention of thrombosis in patients with or at risk of HIT who are undergoing PCI*—Give an IV bolus (350 mcg/kg) followed by continuous IV infusion (25 mcg/kg/min). Adjust the infusion rate (and perhaps give a second IV bolus) to achieve the desired activated clotting time.

Direct Factor Xa Inhibitors

Rivaroxaban

Actions and Uses. Rivaroxaban [Xarelto] is an *oral* anticoagulant that causes selective inhibition of factor Xa (activated factor X). Unlike fondaparinux (previously discussed), which acts indirectly, rivaroxaban binds directly with the active center of factor Xa and thereby inhibits production of thrombin. Compared with warfarin, our oldest oral anticoagulant, rivaroxaban has several advantages: rapid onset, fixed dosage, lower bleeding risk, few drug interactions, and no need for INR monitoring. Rivaroxaban has three approved uses: (1) prevention of DVT and PE following total hip or knee replacement surgery, (2) prevention of stroke in patients with atrial fibrillation, and (3) treatment of DVT and PE unrelated to orthopedic surgery. Contrasts with warfarin are shown in Table 52.6.

Clinical Trials

Knee and Hip Replacement Patients. In a series of trials known as RECORD (Regulation of Coagulation in Orthopedic Surgery to Prevent Deep Vein Thrombosis and Pulmonary Embolism), rivaroxaban was compared with enoxaparin (an LMW heparin) in patients who had undergone hip or knee replacement surgery. Patients who received rivaroxaban (10 mg once daily) were much less likely to experience DVT, VTE, PE, or death, compared with patients who received enoxaparin (40 mg once daily or 30 mg twice daily). With both drugs, the incidence of major bleeding episodes was low (0.2%).

Nonvalvular Atrial Fibrillation Patients. In a trial known as ROCKET AF, rivaroxaban was compared with warfarin for preventing stroke in patients with nonvalvular atrial fibrillation (i.e., patients with atrial fibrillation who do not have a prosthetic heart valve or hemodynamically significant valve disease). Rivaroxaban was at least as effective as warfarin and carried the same risk of major hemorrhagic events of all kinds—but had a lower risk for intracranial bleeds and fatal bleeds.

Pharmacokinetics. Rivaroxaban is administered orally, and bioavailability is high (80% to 90%). Plasma levels peak 2 to 4 hours after dosing. Protein binding in blood is substantial (92% to 95%). Rivaroxaban undergoes partial metabolism by CYP3A4 (the 3A4 isoenzyme of cytochrome P450) and is a substrate for P-glycoprotein, an efflux transporter that helps remove rivaroxaban from the body. Rivaroxaban is eliminated in the urine (36% as unchanged drug) and feces (7% as unchanged drug), with a half-life of 5 to 9 hours. In patients with renal impairment or hepatic impairment, rivaroxaban levels may accumulate.

Adverse Effects

Bleeding. Bleeding is the most common adverse effect and can occur at any site. Patients have experienced epidural hematoma, as well as major intracranial, retinal, adrenal, and GI bleeds. Some people have died. Bleeding risk is increased by other drugs that impede hemostasis. How does rivaroxaban compare with warfarin? The risk of hemorrhagic stroke and other major bleeds is significantly lower with rivaroxaban.

In the event of overdose, we have no specific antidote to reverse this drug's anticoagulant effects. However we *can* prevent further absorption of ingested rivaroxaban with activated charcoal (see Chapter 109). Treatment with several agents—recombinant factor VIIa, prothrombin complex concentrate (PCC), or activated PCC—can be considered. Preliminary studies of PCC have been promising, but more testing must be completed. Because rivaroxaban is highly protein bound, dialysis is unlikely to remove it from the blood.

Spinal/Epidural Hematoma. Like all other anticoagulants, rivaroxaban poses a risk of spinal or epidural hematoma in patients undergoing spinal puncture or epidural anesthesia. Prolonged or permanent paralysis can result. Rivaroxaban should be discontinued at least 18 hours before removing an epidural catheter; once the catheter is out, another 6 hours should elapse before rivaroxaban is restarted. If a traumatic puncture occurs, rivaroxaban should be delayed for at least 24 hours. Anticoagulant-related spinal/epidural hematoma is discussed further earlier in this chapter (see *Adverse Effects* under Heparin).

Drug Interactions. Levels of rivaroxaban can be altered by drugs that inhibit or induce CYP3A4 and P-glycoprotein. Specifically, in patients with *normal renal function,* drugs that inhibit CYP3A4 strongly *and also* inhibit P-glycoprotein (e.g., ketoconazole, itraconazole, ritonavir) can raise rivaroxaban levels enough to increase the risk of bleeding. Similarly, in patients with *renal impairment,* drugs that inhibit CYP3A4 moderately *and also* inhibit P-glycoprotein (e.g., amiodarone, dronedarone, quinidine, diltiazem, verapamil, ranolazine, macrolide antibiotics) can raise rivaroxaban levels enough to increase the risk of bleeding. Conversely, drugs that induce CYP3A4 strongly *and also* induce P-glycoprotein (e.g., carbamazepine, phenytoin, rifampin, St. John's wort) may reduce rivaroxaban levels enough to increase the risk of thrombotic events. Of note, rivaroxaban itself does not inhibit or induce cytochrome P450 enzymes or P-glycoprotein, and hence is unlikely to alter the effects of other drugs.

Owing to the risk of bleeding, rivaroxaban should not be combined with other anticoagulants. Concurrent use with antiplatelet drugs and fibrinolytics should be done with caution.

Precautions

Renal Impairment. Renal impairment can delay excretion of rivaroxaban and can thereby increase the risk of bleeding. Accordingly, rivaroxaban should be avoided in patients with *severe* renal impairment, indicated by a CrCl below 30 mL/min. In patients with moderate renal impairment (CrCl 30 to 50 mL/min), rivaroxaban should be used with caution. If renal failure develops during treatment, rivaroxaban should be discontinued.

Hepatic Impairment. In clinical trials, rivaroxaban levels and anticoagulation were excessive in patients with moderate hepatic impairment. Accordingly, in patients with moderate or severe hepatic impairment, rivaroxaban should not be used.

Pregnancy. Rivaroxaban appears unsafe in pregnancy. The drug increases the risk of pregnancy-related hemorrhage and may have detrimental effects on the fetus. When pregnant rabbits were given high doses (10 mg/kg or more) during organogenesis, rivaroxaban increased fetal resorption, decreased fetal weight, and decreased the number of live fetuses. However, dosing of rats and rabbits early in pregnancy was not associated with gross fetal malformations. Rivaroxaban is classified in FDA Pregnancy Risk Category C[c], and should be used only if the benefits are deemed to outweigh the risks to the mother and fetus.

Preparations, Dosage, and Administration. Rivaroxaban [Xarelto] is supplied in tablets (10, 15, and 20 mg). Whether dosing is done with food depends on the setting, as discussed later.

Prevention of DVT. The recommended dosage is 10 mg once a day, *with or without food,* starting 6 to 10 hours after knee or hip replacement surgery. If a dose is missed, it should be taken as soon as possible, and the next dose should be taken as originally scheduled. Treatment duration is 12 days following knee replacement and 35 days following hip replacement.

Nonvalvular Atrial Fibrillation. Dosing is done once a day *with the evening meal.* For patients with normal renal function, the dosage is 20 mg once daily, and for patients with moderate renal impairment, the dosage is 15 mg once daily. Patients with severe renal impairment should not use this drug.

Treatment of DVT/PE. Dosing is started at 15 mg twice daily for the first 21 days, and then increased to 20 mg daily. Doses should be taken at approximately the same time each day.

Apixaban

Actions and Uses. Apixaban [Eliquis] is an additional *oral* anticoagulant that causes selective inhibition of factor Xa. Apixaban inhibits free and clot-bound factor Xa, as well as prothrombinase activity. Apixaban has three approved uses: (1) prevention of stroke and systemic embolism in patients with nonvalvular atrial fibrillation, (2) treatment of DVT/PE, and (3) prophylaxis of DVT in patients undergoing hip or knee replacement.

Pharmacokinetics. Apixaban is administered orally, and bioavailability is moderate (~50%). Plasma levels peak 2 to 4 hours after dosing. Protein binding in blood is substantial (87%). Apixaban undergoes partial metabolism by CYP3A4. Apixaban is eliminated in the urine and feces, with a half-life of 12 hours after repeated dosing. In patients with renal impairment, apixaban levels may accumulate.

Adverse Effects

Bleeding. As with rivaroxaban, bleeding is the most common adverse effect and can occur at any site. Bleeding risk is increased by other drugs that impede hemostasis. How does apixaban compare with warfarin? The risk of hemorrhagic stroke and other major bleeds is significantly lower with apixaban.

In the event of overdose, we have no specific antidote to reverse this drug's anticoagulant effects. Treatment with several agents—recombinant factor VIIa, PCC, or activated PCC—can be considered, but testing has not been completed. Like rivaroxaban, apixaban is highly protein bound. Dialysis is unlikely to remove it from the blood.

Drug Interactions. Levels of rivaroxaban can be altered by drugs that inhibit or induce CYP3A4 and P-glycoprotein. Specifically, in patients with *normal renal function,* drugs that inhibit CYP3A4 strongly *and also* inhibit P-glycoprotein (e.g., ketoconazole, itraconazole, ritonavir) can raise apixaban levels enough to increase the risk of bleeding. Conversely, drugs that induce CYP3A4 strongly *and also* induce P-glycoprotein (e.g., carbamazepine, phenytoin, rifampin, St. John's wort) may reduce apixaban levels enough to increase the risk of thrombotic events.

Precautions

Renal Impairment. Renal impairment can delay excretion of apixaban, increasing the risk of bleeding. In patients with renal impairment, defined as a serum creatinine level greater than or equal to 1.5 mg/dL, apixaban dosing is decreased.

Pregnancy. Studies of apixaban in pregnant patients are lacking. The drug may increase the risk of hemorrhage during pregnancy and delivery. Apixaban is classified in FDA Pregnancy Risk Category B.[d]

Preparations, Dosage, and Administration. Apixaban [Eliquis] is supplied in tablets (2.5 and 5 mg). The recommended dose for most patients with atrial fibrillation is 5 mg taken orally twice daily. In patients with renal impairment, dosing is decreased to 2.5 mg twice daily.

For the treatment of DVT, the dose is doubled to 10 mg twice daily. For prophylaxis after orthopedic surgery, the dose is only 2.5 mg twice daily.

Edoxaban

Edoxaban [Savaysa] is a newer *oral* anticoagulant that also causes selective inhibition of factor Xa. Edoxaban has two approved uses: (1) prevention of stroke and systemic embolism in patients with nonvalvular atrial fibrillation and (2) treatment of DVT/PE. Because it is a novel oral anticoagulant, like apixaban and rivaroxaban, edoxaban causes adverse effects and has drug interactions similar to these drugs.

Preparations, Dosage, and Administration. Edoxaban is available in 15-, 30-, and 60-mg tablets. The suggested dose for patients with atrial fibrillation is 60 mg orally daily. Treatment for DVT and PE is weight based. For patients who weigh less than 60 kg, the dose is 30 mg daily. For patients who weigh more than 60 kg, this dose is doubled to 60 mg daily. As with the other NOACs, doses should be decreased in patients with renal impairment.

Antithrombin

As discussed earlier, antithrombin (AT) is an endogenous compound that suppresses coagulation, primarily by inhibiting thrombin and factor Xa. Clinically, AT is used to prevent thrombosis in patients with inherited AT deficiency. Currently, we have two AT preparations, marketed as *ATryn* and *Thrombate III. ATryn* is made by recombinant DNA technology; Thrombate III is made by extraction from human plasma. Nonetheless, the actions of both products are the same: suppression of coagulation mediated by thrombin and factor Xa.

Recombinant Human Antithrombin

Production. Recombinant human AT (rhAT), sold as *ATryn,* is produced in goats that have been given the DNA sequence for human AT, along with genetic instructions that cause the AT to be expressed into their milk. The

[c]As of 2020, the FDA will no longer use Pregnancy Risk Categories. Please refer to Chapter 9 for more information.

[d]As of 2020, the FDA will no longer use Pregnancy Risk Categories. Please refer to Chapter 9 for more information.

rhAT produced in goats is nearly identical to endogenous AT: Both compounds have the same sequence of amino acids, but they have different patterns of glycosylation. (Glycosylation refers to sugar derivatives attached to the amino acid backbone of rhAT.) rhAT is the first drug produced in transgenic animals to be approved for use in the United States.

Therapeutic Use. rhAT is approved for prevention of perioperative or peripartum thromboembolic events in patients with inherited AT deficiency, a disorder that puts these people at high risk of VTE. In fact, to protect against thromboembolism, these people typically require lifelong therapy with an anticoagulant, usually warfarin. During surgery or childbirth, the risk of thrombosis increases. However, there is also an obvious increase in the risk of serious bleeding. Accordingly, when patients with hereditary AT deficiency are facing childbirth or surgery, anticoagulant therapy is usually discontinued—reducing the risk of bleeding, but *increasing* the risk of thrombosis. To reduce that risk of thrombosis, rhAT is given until anticoagulant therapy can be safely resumed. In clinical trials, rhAT prevented thromboembolism associated with childbirth or surgery in 30 of 31 patients with inherited AT deficiency.

Adverse Effects. The principal concern is hemorrhage. To minimize risk, AT activity should be monitored, and if it rises too high, the rhAT dosage should be reduced. In addition to causing outright hemorrhage, rhAT may cause hematoma, hematuria, and hemarthrosis. Infusion-site reactions are common.

Because rhAt is derived from goats' milk, there is a risk of hypersensitivity reactions. Accordingly, patients should be closely observed during the infusion period. If signs of a hypersensitivity reaction develop (e.g., hives, generalized urticaria, wheezing, hypotension), rhAT should be discontinued immediately.

Interaction With Heparin. As discussed earlier, heparin produces its anticoagulant effects by enhancing the actions of AT. Accordingly, if rhAT is given to a patient taking heparin, anticoagulation will be greatly increased, thereby posing a risk of bleeding. Accordingly, if heparin is used with rhAT, tests for anticoagulation should be performed often, especially during the first hours following the initiation or termination of rhAT use.

Comparison With Plasma-Derived AT. rhAT has two advantages over plasma-derived AT. First, supplies of rhAT are more abundant because supplies are not limited by the availability of human volunteers. Second, rhAT is safer because plasma-derived AT carries a risk of infection, especially hepatitis C, whereas rhAT carries no such risk.

Preparations, Dosage, and Administration. rhAT [ATryn] is supplied as a powder (1750 units) in single-use vials for reconstitution with 10 mL of sterile water, followed by further dilution before IV infusion. Treatment consists of a 15-minute loading infusion followed immediately by a continuous maintenance infusion. The loading infusion should begin before delivery or 24 hours before surgery, and should continue until normal maintenance coagulation can be re-established. Dosage size is based on the patient's AT activity and body weight. The goal is to maintain AT activity between 80% and 120% of normal. During the maintenance infusion, AT activity should be monitored periodically, and the dosage adjusted accordingly.

Plasma-Derived Antithrombin

Plasma-derived AT [Thrombate III] is made by extraction from the plasma of human volunteers. Thrombate III is like rhAT in most regards: Both drugs share the same indication (prevention of thromboembolic events associated with surgery or childbirth in patients with inherited AT deficiency), both pose a risk of hemorrhage, both increase the anticoagulant effects of heparin, and both are given by IV infusion. The drugs differ primarily in that plasma-derived AT carries a risk of hepatitis C and other infections, whereas rhAT does not. Thrombate III is supplied as a powder (500 and 1000 units) in single-use vials and must be reconstituted with sterile water before use. As with rhAT, dosage is based on AT activity and body weight.

ANTIPLATELET DRUGS

Antiplatelet drugs suppress platelet aggregation. Since a platelet core constitutes the bulk of an *arterial thrombus,* the principal indication for the antiplatelet drugs is prevention of thrombosis in *arteries.* In contrast, the principal indication for anticoagulants (e.g., heparin, warfarin) is prevention of thrombosis in veins.

There are three major groups of antiplatelet drugs: aspirin (a "group" with one member), $P2Y_{12}$ ADP receptor antagonists, and GP IIb/IIIa receptor antagonists. As indicated in Fig. 52.1, aspirin and the $P2Y_{12}$ ADP receptor antagonists affect only one pathway in platelet activation, and hence their antiplatelet effects are limited. In contrast, the GP IIb/IIIa antagonists block the final common step in platelet activation, and hence have powerful antiplatelet effects. Properties of the major classes of antiplatelet drugs are shown in Table 52.7.

Aspirin

The basic pharmacology of aspirin is discussed in Chapter 71. Consideration here is limited to aspirin's role in preventing arterial thrombosis.

Mechanism of Antiplatelet Action

Aspirin suppresses platelet aggregation by causing *irreversible inhibition of cyclooxygenase,* an enzyme required by platelets to synthesize TXA_2. As noted, TXA_2 is one of the factors that can promote platelet activation. In addition to activating platelets, TXA_2 acts on vascular smooth muscle to promote vasoconstriction. Both actions promote hemostasis. By inhibiting cyclooxygenase, aspirin suppresses both TXA_2-mediated

TABLE 52.7 ■ Properties of the Major Classes of Antiplatelet Drugs

	Aspirin, a Cyclooxygenase Inhibitor	$P2Y_{12}$ Adenosine Diphosphate (ADP) Receptor Blockers	Protease-Activated Receptor-1 (PAR-1) Antagonists	Glycoprotein (GP) IIb/IIIa Receptor Blockers
Representative drug	Aspirin	Clopidogrel [Plavix]	Vorapaxar [Zontivity]	Tirofiban [Aggrastat]
Mechanism of antiplatelet action	Irreversibly inhibits cyclooxygenase, and thereby blocks synthesis of TXA_2	Irreversibly blocks receptors for ADP[a]	Reversibly blocks the protease-activated receptor-1 (PAR-1) expressed on platelets	Reversibly blocks receptors for GP IIb/IIIa
Route	PO	PO	PO	IV infusion
Duration of effects	Effects persist 7–10 days after the last dose	Effects persist 7–10 days after the last dose[a]	Effects persist 7–10 days after the last dose	Effects stop within 4 hr of stopping the infusion
Cost	$3/month	$87/month	$320/month	$1000/course

[a]The ADP receptor blocker ticagrelor [Brilinta] causes reversible ADP receptor blockade, so effects wear off faster than with clopidogrel.
TXA_2, Thromboxane A_2.

vasoconstriction and platelet aggregation, thereby reducing the risk of arterial thrombosis. Because inhibition of cyclooxygenase by aspirin is irreversible and because platelets lack the machinery to synthesize new cyclooxygenase, the effects of a single dose of aspirin persist for the life of the platelet (7 to 10 days).

In addition to inhibiting the synthesis of TXA_2, aspirin can inhibit synthesis of *prostacyclin* by the blood vessel wall. Since prostacyclin has effects that are exactly opposite to those of TXA_2—namely, suppression of platelet aggregation and promotion of vasodilation—suppression of prostacyclin synthesis can partially offset the beneficial effects of aspirin therapy. Fortunately, aspirin is able to inhibit synthesis of TXA_2 at doses that are lower than those needed to inhibit synthesis of prostacyclin. Accordingly, if we keep the dosage of aspirin *low* (325 mg/day or less), we can minimize inhibition of prostacyclin production while maintaining inhibition of TXA_2 production.

Indications for Antiplatelet Therapy

Antiplatelet therapy with aspirin has multiple indications of proven efficacy:

- *Ischemic stroke* (to reduce the risk of death and nonfatal stroke)
- *TIAs* (to reduce the risk of death and nonfatal stroke)
- *Chronic stable angina* (to reduce the risk of MI and sudden death)
- *Unstable angina* (to reduce the combined risk of death and nonfatal MI)
- *Coronary stenting* (to prevent reocclusion)
- *Acute MI* (to reduce the risk of vascular mortality)
- *Previous MI* (to reduce the combined risk of death and nonfatal MI)
- *Primary prevention of MI* (to prevent a first MI in men and in women age 65 and older)

In all of these situations, prophylactic therapy with aspirin can reduce morbidity, and possibly mortality. Primary prevention of MI is discussed next.

Primary Prevention of MI. In 2009, the U.S. Preventive Services Task Force (USPSTF) issued updated guidelines on the use of aspirin for primary prevention of MI. The USPSTF recommends the use of aspirin for men ages 45 to 79 years and women ages 55 to 79 years when the potential benefit of a reduction in MI outweighs the potential harm of an increase in GI hemorrhage. Cardiovascular risk is based on five factors—age, gender, cholesterol levels, blood pressure, and smoking status—and can be calculated using an online risk assessment tool, such as those at www.med-decisions.com. Although the optimal aspirin dosage for primary prevention is unknown, low doses (e.g., 81 mg/day) appear as effective as higher ones.

Adverse Effects

Even in low doses, aspirin increases the risk of GI bleeding and hemorrhagic stroke. Among middle-aged people taking aspirin for 5 years, the estimated rate of major GI bleeding episodes is 2 to 4 per 1000 patients, and the rate of hemorrhagic stroke is 0 to 2 episodes per 1000 patients. Use of enteric-coated or buffered aspirin may *not* reduce the risk of GI bleeding. Benefits of treatment must be weighed against bleeding risks. If GI bleeding occurs, adding a proton pump inhibitor (e.g., omeprazole [Prilosec]) to reduce gastric acidity can help.

Dosing

Dosage for preventing cardiovascular events should be low. Maximal inhibition of platelet cyclooxygenase, and hence maximal effects on platelet function, can be produced in a few days by taking 81 mg/day. Dosages above 81 mg/day offer no increase in benefits, but do increase the risk of GI bleeding and stroke. Accordingly, for *chronic therapy,* a dosage of 81 mg/day is probably adequate. A higher dosage (e.g., 325 mg/day) is indicated for *initial* treatment of an acute event, such as MI, to establish full antiplatelet effects rapidly—after which 81 mg/day can be taken for maintenance.

$P2Y_{12}$ Adenosine Diphosphate Receptor Antagonists

Drugs in this class block $P2Y_{12}$ ADP receptors on the platelet surface, preventing ADP-stimulated aggregation (see Fig. 52.1). Three $P2Y_{12}$ ADP receptor antagonists are available. Two of them—clopidogrel and prasugrel—cause *irreversible* receptor blockade, and the third—ticagrelor—causes *reversible* receptor blockade. Clopidogrel, prasugrel, and ticagrelor are used for secondary prevention of atherothrombotic events in patients with acute coronary syndromes (ACS), defined as unstable angina or MI. All three drugs are taken orally and can cause serious bleeding.

Clopidogrel

Clopidogrel [Plavix] is an oral antiplatelet drug with effects much like those of aspirin. The drug is taken to prevent stenosis of coronary stents and for secondary prevention of MI, ischemic stroke, and other vascular events.

Antiplatelet Actions. Clopidogrel blocks $P2Y_{12}$ ADP receptors on platelets and thereby prevents ADP-stimulated platelet aggregation. As with aspirin, antiplatelet effects are irreversible, and hence persist for the life of the platelet. Effects begin 2 hours after the first dose and plateau after 3 to 7 days of treatment. At the recommended dosage, platelet aggregation is inhibited by 40% to 60%. Platelet function and bleeding time return to baseline 7 to 10 days after the last dose.

Pharmacokinetics. Clopidogrel is rapidly absorbed from the GI tract, both in the presence and absence of food. Bioavailability is about 50%. Clopidogrel is a *prodrug* that undergoes metabolism to its active form, primarily by hepatic CYP2C19 (the 2C19 isoenzyme of cytochrome P450). People with variant forms of the CYP2C19 gene are *poor metabolizers* of clopidogrel, and hence may not benefit adequately from the drug.

Therapeutic Use. Clopidogrel is used widely to prevent blockage of coronary artery stents and to reduce thrombotic events—MI, ischemic stroke, and vascular death—in patients with ACS and in those with atherosclerosis documented by recent MI, recent stroke, or established peripheral arterial disease. In patients with ACS, clopidogrel should always be combined with aspirin (75 to 325 mg once daily).

Clopidogrel should not be used in poor metabolizers. As noted, people with variant forms of the CYP2C19 gene cannot reliably convert clopidogrel to its active form. When treated with standard dosages of clopidogrel, these poor metabolizers exhibit a higher rate of cardiovascular events compared with normal metabolizers. Poor metabolizers can be identified by testing a blood or saliva sample for CYP2C19 variants, or by simply measuring the platelet response to treatment. Unfortunately, even with this information, the course of action is not clear. Yes, we could give poor metabolizers higher doses—but doses that might be safe and effective have not been established. As an alternative, poor metabolizers could be treated with either prasugrel [Effient] or ticagrelor [Brilinta], two other $P2Y_{12}$ ADP receptor antagonists discussed later.

Adverse Effects. Clopidogrel is generally well tolerated. Adverse effects are about the same as with aspirin. The most common complaints are abdominal pain, dyspepsia, diarrhea, and rash.

Bleeding. Like all other antiplatelet drugs, clopidogrel poses a risk of serious bleeding. However, compared with aspirin, clopidogrel causes less GI bleeding (2% vs. 2.7%) and less intracranial hemorrhage (ICH) (0.4% vs. 0.5%). Owing to bleeding risk, clopidogrel should be discontinued 5 days before elective surgery. If possible, major bleeding should be managed without discontinuing clopidogrel, since discontinuation would increase the risk of a thrombotic event.

Patients should be told about the risk of bleeding and warned that they may bruise or bleed more easily, and that bleeding will take longer than usual to stop. Also, patients should be informed about signs of bleeding (e.g., blood in the urine, black tarry stools, vomitus that looks like coffee grounds) and instructed to contact the prescriber if these develop. Finally, patients who develop these symptoms should be warned not to stop clopidogrel until the prescriber says they should.

Thrombotic Thrombocytopenic Purpura (TTP). Rarely, patients develop TTP, a potentially fatal condition characterized by thrombocytopenia, hemolytic anemia, neurologic symptoms, renal dysfunction, and fever. Most cases occur during the first 2 weeks of treatment. TTP is a serious disorder that requires urgent treatment, including plasmapheresis.

Drug Interactions

Drugs That Promote Bleeding. Clopidogrel should be used with caution in patients taking other drugs that promote bleeding (e.g., heparin, warfarin, aspirin, and NSAIDs).

Proton Pump Inhibitors (PPIs). Omeprazole [Prilosec, Losec 🍁] and other PPIs suppress secretion of gastric acid (see Chapter 78), and hence are often combined with clopidogrel to protect against GI bleeding. Unfortunately, PPIs may also reduce the antiplatelet effects of clopidogrel. PPIs inhibit CYP2C19, the enzyme that converts clopidogrel to its active form. Hence the dilemma: If clopidogrel is used alone, there is a significant risk of GI bleeding; however, if clopidogrel is combined with a PPI to reduce the risk of GI bleeding, antiplatelet effects may be reduced as well. After considering the available evidence, three organizations—the American College of Cardiology, the American Heart Association, and the American College of Gastroenterology—issued a consensus document on the problem. This document concludes that although PPIs may reduce the antiplatelet effects of clopidogrel somewhat, there is no evidence that the reduction is large enough to be clinically relevant. Accordingly, for patients who have risk factors for GI bleeding (e.g., advanced age, use of NSAIDs or anticoagulants), the benefits of combining a PPI with clopidogrel probably outweigh any risk from reduced antiplatelet effects—and hence combining a PPI with clopidogrel is probably acceptable for these people. Conversely, for patients who lack risk factors for GI bleeding, combined use of clopidogrel with a PPI may reduce the benefits of clopidogrel without offering any meaningful GI protection; hence, combining a PPI with clopidogrel in these patients should probably be avoided. When a PPI *is* used with clopidogrel, pantoprazole [Protonix] would be a good choice because when compared with other PPIs, pantoprazole causes less inhibition of CYP2C19.

CYP2C19 Inhibitors (Other Than PPIs). Like the PPIs, several other drugs can inhibit CYP2C19. Among these are cimetidine, fluoxetine, fluvoxamine, fluconazole, ketoconazole, voriconazole, etravirine, felbamate, and ticlopidine. Since these drugs may reduce the antiplatelet effects of clopidogrel (by reducing its activation), use of alternative drugs is preferred.

Preparations, Dosage, and Administration. Clopidogrel [Plavix] is available in 75-mg tablets. The usual maintenance dosage is 75 mg once a day, taken with or without food. A 300-mg loading dose may be used for some patients. The optimal duration of treatment is unknown. Dosage needn't be changed for older adult patients or those with renal impairment. Patients being treated for ACS should take daily aspirin (75 to 325 mg). Clopidogrel should be withdrawn 5 days before elective surgery and resumed as soon as possible.

Prasugrel

Actions and Uses. Prasugrel [Effient], a close relative of clopidogrel, is an oral antiplatelet drug approved for prevention of thrombotic events in patients with ACS. Like clopidogrel, prasugrel is a prodrug that undergoes conversion to an active metabolite, which then blocks $P2Y_{12}$ ADP receptors on platelets, causing irreversible inhibition of platelet aggregation. Prasugrel is more effective than clopidogrel and has fewer drug interactions, but causes more major bleeding.

Clinical Trial. In a trial known as TRITON-TIMI, prasugrel was compared directly with clopidogrel. The trial enrolled over 13,000 patients with ACS who were scheduled for coronary angioplasty, also known as *percutaneous coronary intervention.* The goal with both drugs was to prevent thrombotic complications, including stent restenosis. Patients taking prasugrel experienced fewer thrombotic events, but more major bleeding.

Pharmacokinetics. Prasugrel is rapidly absorbed after oral dosing, both in the presence and absence of food. Activation takes place in two steps. The process begins with hydrolysis by esterases in the intestine, and ends with conversion to the active metabolite in the liver, primarily by CYP3A4 and CYP2B6, two isoenzymes of cytochrome P450. (Note that activation of prasugrel differs from activation of clopidogrel, which is mediated by CYP2C19.) The entire activation process is fast: Plasma levels of the active metabolite peak about 30 minutes after dosing. Elimination of the active form is primarily by hepatic metabolism, followed by excretion in the urine and feces. The active metabolite has a half-life of 7 hours. In patients who weigh less than 60 kg, total exposure to the active metabolite is 30% to 40% higher than in heavier patients. Accordingly, these lighter patients may need a dosage reduction.

Adverse Effects. The principal adverse effect is *bleeding,* which occurs more often with prasugrel than with clopidogrel. According to results of TRITON-TIMI, among patients not undergoing coronary artery bypass surgery (CABG), the incidence of major bleeding was 2.4% with prasugrel versus 1.8% with clopidogrel, and the incidence of life-threatening bleeding was 0.4% versus 0.1%. Among patients who required CABG surgery, the incidence of major bleeding was greatly increased: 18.8% with prasugrel versus 2.7% with clopidogrel. Accordingly, if CABG surgery is anticipated, prasugrel should not be started. Prasugrel should be avoided by patients at increased risk of bleeding, including patients with active pathologic bleeding, patients over the age of 75, and patients with a history of TIAs or stroke. If possible, major bleeding should be managed without discontinuing prasugrel, since discontinuation would increase the risk of a thrombotic event.

Rarely, patients experience *hypersensitivity reactions,* including potentially life-threatening angioedema. Onset may occur within hours of the first dose, or after 5 to 10 days of treatment.

Data from TRITON-TIMI suggest that prasugrel may increase the risk of *cancer.* Among patients using the drug, there was a 62% increase in the rate of new and worsening solid tumors. However, we don't know of any plausible mechanism of tumor promotion. The FDA is monitoring for more cancer cases.

Drug Interactions. Other drugs that promote bleeding (e.g., warfarin, heparin, fibrinolytic drugs, chronic NSAIDs) will increase the risk of a serious bleed, and hence should be used with great caution. PPIs, which may slow the activation of clopidogrel (by inhibiting CYP2C19), do *not* prevent the activation of prasugrel. Also, according to the prasugrel package insert, drugs that induce or inhibit CYP3A4 do *not* have a significant impact on prasugrel activity.

Preparations, Dosage, and Administration. Prasugrel [Effient] is supplied in 5- and 10-mg tablets for oral dosing, with or without food. Treatment consists of a 60-mg loading dose, followed by once-daily 10-mg maintenance doses. For patients who weigh less than 60 kg, maintenance doses may be reduced to 5 mg. All patients should take aspirin daily (80 to 325 mg).

Ticagrelor

Actions and Uses. Ticagrelor [Brilinta] is a $P2Y_{12}$ ADP receptor antagonist indicated for prevention of thrombotic events in patients with ACS and to prevent further CV events in patients with a history of MI. The drug inhibits platelet aggregation by blocking $P2Y_{12}$ ADP receptors on the platelet surface. In contrast to clopidogrel and prasugrel, which cause *irreversible* receptor blockade, ticagrelor causes *reversible* blockade, and hence the effects of ticagrelor wear off faster.

Clinical Trial. In a trial known as PLATO, ticagrelor was compared directly with clopidogrel in patients with recent-onset ACS (within the previous 24 hours). The trial randomized over 18,000 patients to receive either ticagrelor (180 mg once followed by 90 mg twice daily) or clopidogrel (300 mg once followed by 75 mg once daily). All patients also took a daily aspirin. Compared with clopidogrel, ticagrelor produced a greater reduction in MI, stroke, stent restenosis, and cardiovascular death. Unfortunately, these advantages were offset by a greater risk of hemorrhagic events, including fatal intracranial bleeding.

Pharmacokinetics. Ticagrelor is administered by mouth, and food has little effect on absorption. Plasma levels peak 1.5 hours after dosing. Bioavailability is 36%. Unlike clopidogrel and prasugrel, which are prodrugs, ticagrelor is active as administered. In the liver, CYP3A4 converts much of each dose to an active metabolite. Later, the parent drug and active metabolite undergo inactivation by CYP3A4, followed by excretion in the feces (58%) and urine (26%). The elimination half-life is 7 hours for ticagrelor itself and 9 hours for the active metabolite.

Adverse Effects. The most common adverse effects are bleeding and dyspnea. Other adverse effects include headache, cough, dizziness, nausea, noncardiac chest pain, diarrhea, and bradycardia, including ventricular pauses.

Bleeding. Like all other antiplatelet drugs, ticagrelor poses a risk of serious bleeding. In the PLATO study, serious non-CABG bleeding developed in 4.5% of patients taking ticagrelor, compared with 3.8% of patients taking clopidogrel. However, the incidence of CABG-related bleeding was the same with both drugs. Because of bleeding risk, ticagrelor should be discontinued 5 days before elective surgery, and then resumed as soon as possible after the surgery is done.

Dyspnea. In the PLATO study, dyspnea developed in 13.8% of patients taking ticagrelor, compared with 7.8% of patients taking clopidogrel. Dyspnea was usually mild to moderate and often resolved despite continued drug use. Ticagrelor-related dyspnea does not require any specific intervention.

Ventricular Pauses. Ticagrelor can cause ventricular pauses. In the PLATO trial, ventricular pauses were relatively common early in treatment (6% with ticagrelor vs. 3.5% with clopidogrel), but were much less common after 1 month (2.2% with ticagrelor vs. 1.6% with clopidogrel).

Drug Interactions

Aspirin. Aspirin in *low* doses—75 to 100 mg/day—enhances the effects of ticagrelor. However, *higher* doses—more than 100 mg/day—actually *reduce* the benefits of ticagrelor. Accordingly, patients should be warned against taking more than 100 mg of aspirin a day.

Drugs That Promote Bleeding. Anticoagulants (e.g., warfarin, heparin, dabigatran), fibrinolytics (e.g., alteplase, reteplase), and antiplatelet drugs (e.g., aspirin, abciximab) will increase the risk of a serious bleed, and hence should be used with great caution.

Inhibitors and Inducers of CYP3A4. Because ticagrelor and its active metabolite are eliminated by CYP3A4, drugs that induce CYP3A4 (e.g., rifampin, phenytoin, phenobarbital, carbamazepine) can reduce the therapeutic effects of both compounds, and drugs that inhibit CYP3A4 (e.g., ketoconazole, itraconazole, clarithromycin, telithromycin, ritonavir, saquinavir) can increase the risk of toxicity (by allowing both compounds to accumulate to dangerous levels).

Statins. Ticagrelor inhibits CYP3A4 and can thereby increase levels of *simvastatin* and *lovastatin*. To avoid toxicity, dosages of these statins should not exceed 40 mg/day.

Digoxin. Ticagrelor and its active metabolite can inhibit P-glycoprotein, a transport molecule that promotes renal, hepatic, and intestinal elimination of drugs (see Chapter 4). P-glycoprotein inhibition is of particular concern with digoxin, a heart drug with a low margin of safety. To avoid toxicity, digoxin levels should be checked during initial ticagrelor use, and whenever ticagrelor dosage is changed.

Contraindications and Precautions. Ticagrelor is contraindicated for patients with active pathologic bleeding, a history of ICH, or severe hepatic impairment. In patients with moderate hepatic impairment, ticagrelor should be used with caution (because levels of ticagrelor itself and its active metabolite could become excessive, thereby increasing the risk of bleeding).

Preparations, Dosage, and Administration. Ticagrelor [Brilinta] is supplied in 90-mg tablets for dosing with or without food. Following an initial loading dose (180 mg) combined with 325 mg of aspirin, patients take 90 mg twice daily. Daily aspirin (75 to 100 mg) should be continued as well.

Protease-Activated Receptor-1 (PAR-1) Antagonists

Vorapaxar

Uses. Vorapaxar [Zontivity] is approved for use in conjunction with aspirin and/or clopidogrel in the reduction of thrombotic CV events in patients with a history of MI or PAD. When used with other antiplatelet agents, vorapaxar reduces the rate of cardiovascular death, MI, stroke, and urgent coronary revascularization.

Mechanism of Action. Protease-activated receptor-1 (PAR-1) antagonists mediate the effects of thrombin, and these receptors are located on the surface of platelets. By reversibly antagonizing these receptors, vorapaxar inhibits thrombin-induced and thrombin receptor agonist peptide (TRAP)-induced platelet aggregation. Vorapaxar does not work on ADP receptors.

Pharmacokinetics. Vorapaxar is well absorbed following oral administration. Antiplatelet effects begin within 1 hour. The drug undergoes extensive hepatic metabolism followed by excretion in the feces. Vorapaxar has a long half-life (8 days). Effects persist for 7 to 10 days after drug withdrawal (i.e., until new platelets have been synthesized).

Adverse Effects

Bleeding. Like all other antiplatelet drugs, vorapaxar poses a risk of serious bleeding. In the GUSTO study, serious non-CABG bleeding developed in 3% of patients taking vorapaxar. This is similar to the rates seen with ticagrelor in the PLATO trial.

Preparations, Dosage, and Administration. Vorapaxar is available in 2.08-mg tablets. The recommended dosage is one tablet daily with or without food. Vorapaxar should be administered with clopidogrel and/or aspirin, as it has not been studied alone in the prevention of thrombotic CV events.

Glycoprotein IIb/IIIa Receptor Antagonists

Group Properties

The GP IIb/IIIa receptor antagonists, sometimes called "super aspirins," are the most effective antiplatelet drugs on the market. Three agents are available: abciximab, tirofiban, and eptifibatide. All three are administered IV, usually in combination with aspirin and low-dose heparin. Dosages are shown in Table 52.8.

Actions. The GP IIb/IIIa antagonists cause *reversible* blockade of platelet GP IIb/IIIa receptors and thereby inhibit the final step in aggregation (see Fig. 52.1). As a result, these drugs can prevent aggregation stimulated by all factors, including collagen, TXA_2, ADP, thrombin, and platelet activation factor.

Therapeutic Use. The GP IIb/IIIa antagonists are used short term to prevent ischemic events in patients with ACS and those undergoing PCI.

Acute Coronary Syndromes. ACS have two major manifestations: unstable angina and non-STEMI. In both cases, symptoms result from thrombosis triggered by disruption of atherosclerotic plaque. When added to traditional drugs for ACS (heparin and aspirin), GP IIb/IIIa antagonists reduce the risk of ischemic complications.

TABLE 52.8 ■ Dosages for Glycoprotein IIb/IIIa Receptor Antagonists

Application	Tirofiban [Aggrastat]	Eptifibatide [Integrilin]	Abciximab [ReoPro]
Acute coronary syndromes (ACS)	0.4 mcg/kg/min for 30 min, then 0.1 mcg/kg/min for 48–108 hr	180-mcg/kg bolus, then 2 mcg/kg/min for up to 72 hr	0.25-mg/kg bolus, then 10 mcg/kg/min for 18–24 hr
Percutaneous coronary intervention[a] (PCI) following treatment for ACS	Continue 0.1 mcg/kg/min for the procedure and 12–24 hr after	Consider decreasing the infusion rate to 0.5 mcg/kg/min for the procedure and 20–24 hr after	Continue 10 mcg/kg/min for the procedure and 1 hr after
PCI without prior treatment for ACS	Not FDA approved for this application	135-mcg/kg bolus before procedure, then 0.5 mcg/kg/min for 20–24 hr	0.25-mg/kg bolus 10–60 min before procedure, then 0.125 mcg/kg/min (max. 10 mcg/min) for 12 hr

[a]Balloon or laser angioplasty, or atherectomy.
FDA, U.S. Food and Drug Administration.

Percutaneous Coronary Intervention. GP IIb/IIIa antagonists reduce the risk of rapid reocclusion following coronary artery revascularization with PCI (balloon or laser angioplasty, or atherectomy using an intra-arterial rotating blade). Reocclusion is common because PCI damages the arterial wall, encouraging platelet aggregation.

Properties of Individual GP IIb/IIIa Antagonists

Abciximab

Description and Use. Abciximab [ReoPro] is a purified Fab fragment of a monoclonal antibody. The drug binds to platelets in the vicinity of GP IIb/IIIa receptors and thereby prevents the receptors from binding fibrinogen. Abciximab, in conjunction with aspirin and heparin, is approved for IV therapy of ACS and for patients undergoing PCI. In addition, studies indicate it can accelerate revascularization in patients undergoing thrombolytic therapy for acute MI. Antiplatelet effects persist for 24 to 48 hours after stopping the infusion.

Adverse Effects and Interactions. Abciximab doubles the risk of major bleeding, especially at the PCI access site in the femoral artery. The drug may also cause GI, urogenital, and retroperitoneal bleeds. However, it does not increase the risk of fatal hemorrhage or hemorrhagic stroke. In the event of severe bleeding, infusion of abciximab and heparin should be discontinued. Other drugs that impede hemostasis will increase bleeding risk.

Eptifibatide. Eptifibatide [Integrilin] is a small peptide that causes reversible and highly selective inhibition of GP IIb/IIIa receptors. The drug is approved for patients with ACS and those undergoing PCI. Antiplatelet effects reverse within 4 hours of stopping the infusion. The most important adverse effect is bleeding, which occurs most often at the site of PCI catheter insertion, and in the GI and urinary tracts. As with other GP IIb/IIIa inhibitors, the risk of bleeding is increased by concurrent use of other drugs that impede hemostasis.

Tirofiban. Tirofiban [Aggrastat] causes selective and reversible inhibition of GP IIb/IIIa receptors. The drug—neither an antibody nor a peptide—was modeled after a platelet inhibitor isolated from the venom of the saw-scaled viper, a snake indigenous to Africa. Like other GP IIb/IIIa inhibitors, tirofiban is used to reduce ischemic events associated with ACS and PCI. Platelet function returns to baseline within 4 hours of stopping the infusion. Bleeding is the primary adverse effect. The risk of bleeding can be increased by other drugs that suppress hemostasis.

Other Antiplatelet Drugs

Dipyridamole

Dipyridamole [Persantine] suppresses platelet aggregation, perhaps by increasing plasma levels of adenosine. The drug is approved only for prevention of thromboembolism following heart valve replacement. For this application, dipyridamole is always combined with warfarin. The recommended dosage is 75 to 100 mg 4 times a day. A fixed-dose combination of dipyridamole and aspirin (discussed next) is indicated for recurrent stroke.

Dipyridamole Plus Aspirin

Actions and Use. Dipyridamole combined with aspirin is available in a fixed-dose formulation sold as *Aggrenox.* The product is used to prevent recurrent ischemic stroke in patients who have had a previous stroke or TIA. Both drugs—aspirin and dipyridamole—suppress platelet aggregation. However, since they do so by different mechanisms, the combination is more effective than either drug alone.

Clinical Trial. The benefit of combining aspirin and dipyridamole was demonstrated in the second *European Stroke Prevention Study* (ESPS-2), a randomized controlled trial that enrolled over 6000 patients who had suffered a prior ischemic stroke or TIA. Some patients took aspirin alone (25 mg twice daily), some took dipyridamole alone (200 mg twice daily), some took both drugs, and some took placebo. After 24 months, the incidence of fatal or nonfatal ischemic stroke was reduced by 16% with dipyridamole alone, 18% with aspirin alone, and 37% with the combination. Unfortunately, ESPS-2 was tainted by scientific scandal (one investigator, who later resigned, was charged with creating and falsifying data). Although all fraudulent data were discarded before publication, some authorities remain skeptical of the results.

Adverse Effects. The most common adverse effects of the combination are headache, dizziness, and GI disturbances (nausea, vomiting, diarrhea, abdominal pain, dyspepsia). Of course, bleeding is a concern: The product can cause hemorrhage (3.2% vs. 1.5% with placebo), nosebleed (2.4% vs. 1.5%), and purpura (1.4% vs. 0.4%). The aspirin in Aggrenox poses a risk of GI bleeding from peptic ulcers.

Preparations, Dosage, and Administration. Aggrenox capsules contain 25 mg of aspirin and 200 mg of extended-release dipyridamole. The recommended dosage is 2 capsules a day—one in the morning and one at night. It is important to note that the daily dose of aspirin (50 mg) is lower than the dose recommended to prevent MI (at least 80 mg/day). Accordingly, supplemental aspirin may be needed.

Cilostazol

Actions and Therapeutic Use. Cilostazol [Pletal], a platelet inhibitor and vasodilator, is indicated for *intermittent claudication.* (Intermittent claudication is a syndrome characterized by pain, cramping, and weakness of the calf muscles brought on by walking and relieved by resting a few minutes. The underlying cause is atherosclerosis in the legs.) Cilostazol suppresses platelet aggregation by inhibiting type 3 phosphodiesterase (PDE3) in platelets, and promotes vasodilation by inhibiting PDE3 in blood vessels (primarily in the legs). Inhibition of platelet aggregation is greater than with aspirin, ticlopidine, or dipyridamole. Full effects take up to 12 weeks to develop, but reverse quickly (within 48 hours) following drug withdrawal.

Adverse Effects. Cilostazol causes a variety of untoward effects. The most common is headache (34%). Others include diarrhea, abnormal stools, palpitations, dizziness, and peripheral edema.

Other drugs that inhibit PDE3 have increased mortality in patients with heart failure. Whether cilostazol represents a risk is unknown. Nonetheless, heart failure is a contraindication to cilostazol use.

Drug and Food Interactions. Cilostazol is metabolized by hepatic CYP3A4, so cilostazol levels can be increased by CYP3A4 inhibitors (e.g., ketoconazole, itraconazole, erythromycin, fluoxetine, fluvoxamine, nefazodone, sertraline, and grapefruit juice). Metabolism of cilostazol can also be inhibited by omeprazole.

Preparations, Dosage, and Administration. Cilostazol [Pletal] is available in 50- and 100-mg tablets. The usual dosage is 100 mg twice daily, taken 30 minutes before or 2 hours after breakfast and the evening meal. Dosage should be reduced to 50 mg twice daily in patients taking omeprazole and drugs or foods that inhibit CYP3A4.

THROMBOLYTIC (FIBRINOLYTIC) DRUGS

As their name implies, thrombolytic drugs are given to remove thrombi that have already formed. This contrasts with the anticoagulants, which are given to prevent thrombus formation. In the United States, three thrombolytic drugs are available: alteplase, reteplase, and tenecteplase. These drugs are employed acutely and only for severe thrombotic disease: acute MI, PE, and ischemic stroke. Principal differences among the drugs concern specific uses, duration of action, and ease of dosing. All thrombolytics pose a risk of serious bleeding, and hence should be administered only by clinicians skilled in their use. Because of their mechanism, thrombolytic drugs are also known as *fibrinolytics* (and informally as *clot busters*). Properties of individual agents are shown in Table 52.9.

Alteplase (tPA)

Description and Mechanism

Alteplase [Activase, Cathflo Activase]—also known as *tissue plasminogen activator*—is identical to naturally occurring human tPA. The drug is manufactured using recombinant DNA technology.

The drug first binds with *plasminogen* to form an active complex. The alteplase-plasminogen complex then catalyzes the conversion of other plasminogen molecules into *plasmin,* an enzyme that digests the fibrin meshwork of clots. In addition to digesting fibrin, plasmin degrades fibrinogen and other clotting factors. These actions don't contribute to lysis of thrombi, but they do increase the risk of hemorrhage.

Therapeutic Uses

Alteplase has three major indications: (1) acute MI, (2) acute ischemic stroke, and (3) acute massive PE. In all three settings, timely intervention is essential: The sooner alteplase is administered, the better the outcome.

The importance of early intervention was first demonstrated in GUSTO-I (Global Utilization of Streptokinase and tPA for Occluded Coronary Arteries), a huge trial that evaluated the benefits of two thrombolytic drugs—alteplase (tPA) and streptokinase—in patients with acute MI. Results for alteplase were as follows: Among patients treated within 2 hours of symptom onset, the death rate was only 5.4%; among those treated 2 to 4 hours after symptom onset, the rate increased to 6.6%; and among those treated 4 to 6 hours after symptom onset, the rate jumped to 9.4%. Clearly, outcomes are best when thrombolytic therapy is started quickly, preferably within 2 to 4 hours of symptom onset, and even earlier if possible. Thrombolytic therapy of acute MI is discussed further in Chapter 53.

In addition to its use for acute thrombotic disease, alteplase can be used to restore patency in a clogged central venous catheter.

Pharmacokinetics

Alteplase is a large molecule that must be administered parenterally, almost always by IV infusion. The drug has a very short

TABLE 52.9 ■ Properties of Thrombolytic (Fibrinolytic) Drugs

	Alteplase (tPA)	Tenecteplase	Reteplase
Brand name	Activase, Cathflo Activase	TNKase	Retavase
Description	A compound identical to human tPA	Modified form of tPA with a prolonged half-life	A compound that contains the active sequence of amino acids present in tPA
Source	All three drugs are made using recombinant DNA technology		
Mechanism	All three drugs promote conversion of plasminogen to plasmin, an enzyme that degrades the fibrin matrix of thrombi		
Indications			
Acute MI	Yes	Yes	Yes
Acute ischemic stroke	Yes	No	No
Acute pulmonary embolism	Yes	No	No
Clearing a blocked central venous catheter	Yes	No	No
Adverse effect: Bleeding	With all three drugs, bleeding is the primary adverse effect		
Half-life (min)	5	20–24	13–16
Dosage and administration for acute MI	*Intravenous:* 15-mg bolus, then 50 mg infused over 30 min, then 35 mg infused over 60 min[a]	*Intravenous:* Single bolus based on body weight (see text)	*Intravenous:* 10-unit bolus 2 times, separated by 30 min

[a]Dosage for patients who weigh more than 67 kg.

MI, Myocardial infarction; *tPA,* tissue plasminogen activator.

half-life (5 minutes), owing to rapid hepatic inactivation. Within 5 minutes of stopping an infusion, 50% of the drug is cleared from the blood. About 80% is cleared within 10 minutes.

Adverse Effect: Bleeding

Bleeding is the major complication of treatment. ICH is by far the most serious concern. Bleeding occurs for two reasons: (1) plasmin can destroy pre-existing clots and can thereby promote recurrence of bleeding at sites of recently healed injury, and (2) by degrading clotting factors, plasmin can disrupt coagulation and can thereby interfere with new clot formation in response to vascular injury. Likely sites of bleeding include recent wounds, sites of needle puncture, and sites at which an invasive procedure has been performed. Anticoagulants and antiplatelet drugs further increase hemorrhage risk. Accordingly, high-dose therapy with these drugs must be avoided until thrombolytic effects of alteplase have abated.

Management of bleeding depends on severity. Oozing at sites of cutaneous puncture can be controlled with a pressure dressing. If severe bleeding occurs, alteplase should be discontinued. Patients who require blood replacement can be given whole blood or blood products (packed red blood cells, fresh-frozen plasma). As a rule, blood replacement restores hemostasis. However, if this approach fails, excessive fibrinolysis can be reversed with IV *aminocaproic acid* [Amicar], a compound that prevents activation of plasminogen and directly inhibits plasmin.

The risk of bleeding can be lowered by:

- Minimizing physical manipulation of the patient
- Avoiding subQ and IM injections
- Minimizing invasive procedures
- Minimizing concurrent use of anticoagulants (e.g., heparin, warfarin, dabigatran)
- Minimizing concurrent use of antiplatelet drugs (e.g., aspirin, clopidogrel)

Owing to the risk of hemorrhage, alteplase and other thrombolytic drugs must be avoided in patients at high risk for bleeding complications and must be used with great caution in patients at lower risk of bleeding. Absolute and relative contraindications to thrombolytic therapy are shown in Table 52.10.

Preparations

Alteplase is available under two brand names: *Activase* (50 and 100 mg/vial) and *Cathflo Activase* (2 mg/vial). Activase is used to treat thrombotic disorders. Cathflo Activase is used to clear clogged central venous catheters. Both products are supplied as a powder to be reconstituted with sterile water. After reconstitution, the solution should stand a few minutes to allow dissipation of any large bubbles.

Dosage and Administration

Acute Myocardial Infarction (Activase Only). Alteplase is usually given by an "accelerated" or "front-loaded" schedule, in which the infusion time is only 90 minutes, compared with 3 hours as routinely done in the past. Dosage is based on patient weight, but should not exceed 100 mg because doses in excess of 100 mg are associated with an increased risk of intracranial bleeding.

For patients who weigh *over 67 kg,* the *total* dose is 100 mg, administered in three phases: a 15-mg IV bolus, followed by 50 mg infused over 30 minutes, followed in turn by 35 mg infused over 60 minutes.

For patients who weigh *under 67 kg,* the *maximum* dose is 100 mg, administered in three phases: a 15-mg IV bolus, followed by 0.75 mg/kg (max. 50 mg) infused over 30 minutes, followed in turn by 0.5 mg/kg (max. 35 mg) infused over 60 minutes.

Acute Ischemic Stroke (Activase Only). The recommended dosage is 0.9 mg/kg (max. 90 mg) infused IV over 60 minutes, with 10% of the dose given as an initial IV bolus over 1 minute.

TABLE 52.10 ▪ Contraindications and Cautions Regarding Thrombolytic Use for Myocardial Infarction

ABSOLUTE CONTRAINDICATIONS
• Any prior intracranial hemorrhage
• Known structural cerebral vascular lesion
• Ischemic stroke within past 3 months *except* ischemic stroke within 4.5 hr
• Known intracranial neoplasm
• Active internal bleeding (other than menses)
• Suspected aortic dissection
RELATIVE CONTRAINDICATIONS/CAUTIONS
• Severe, uncontrolled hypertension on presentation (blood pressure above 180/110 mm Hg)
• History of chronic, severe, poorly controlled hypertension
• History of prior ischemic stroke, dementia, or known intracerebral pathology not covered in absolute contraindications
• Current use of anticoagulants in therapeutic doses (INR 2–3 or greater); known bleeding diathesis
• Traumatic or prolonged (more than 10 min) CPR or major surgery (less than 3 wk ago)
• Recent internal bleeding (within 2–4 wk)
• Noncompressible vascular punctures
• Pregnancy
• Active peptic ulcer

CPR, Cardiopulmonary resuscitation; *INR,* international normalized ratio.

Pulmonary Embolism (Activase Only). The recommended dosage is 100 mg infused IV over 2 hours.

Clearing a Central Venous Catheter (Cathflo Activase Only). Use a dilute solution (1 mg/mL). Dosage is based on patient weight. For patients who weigh *30 kg or more,* instill 2 mg in 2 mL of solution. For patients who weigh *10 kg to 29 kg,* instill a volume equal to 110% of the internal volume of the catheter, but no more than 2 mL (2 mg of alteplase).

Tenecteplase

Tenecteplase [TNKase], a variant of human tPA (alteplase), is approved only for acute MI. Except for the substitution of three amino acids, the drug is structurally identical to tPA. However, because of this small structural change, the pharmacokinetics of tenecteplase is much different. Specifically, tenecteplase is 80 times more resistant than tPA to circulating inhibitors and has a much longer half-life (20 to 24 minutes vs. 5 minutes for tPA). Like tPA, tenecteplase acts by converting plasminogen into plasmin, an enzyme that digests fibrin clots. Tenecteplase is just as safe and effective as tPA, but much easier to use: Whereas tPA must be infused over 90 minutes, tenecteplase is given as a single IV bolus. As a result, thrombolysis develops faster, and emergency personnel are spared the trouble of monitoring a prolonged infusion. Because tenecteplase is so easy to administer, it has the potential to allow dosing before the patient reaches a hospital.

Tenecteplase was compared with tPA in the second Assessment of the Safety and Efficacy of a New Thrombolytic (ASSENT-2) study, which enrolled 16,949 patients. Tenecteplase was given as a 5-second IV bolus; tPA was infused over 90 minutes. The median time between symptom onset and starting treatment was 2.7 hours for tenecteplase and 2.8 hours for tPA. Thirty days after treatment, outcomes were equivalent with respect to mortality (6.2% with each drug), ICH (0.93% with tenecteplase vs. 0.94% with tPA), and total stroke (1.78% vs. 1.66% with tPA). Of significance, the incidence of major hemorrhage (other than intracranial) was *lower* with tenecteplase (4.7% vs. 5.9%).

Tenecteplase dosage is based on body weight as follows:

- Below 60 kg: dose 30 mg
- 60 to 69.9 kg: dose 35 mg
- 70 to 79.9 kg: dose 40 mg
- 80 to 89.9 kg: dose 45 mg
- Above 90 kg: dose 50 mg

Reteplase

Reteplase [Retavase] is a derivative of tPA produced by recombinant DNA technology. In contrast to tPA itself, which contains 527 amino acids, reteplase is composed of only 355 amino acids. Like tPA, reteplase converts plasminogen to plasmin, which in turn digests the fibrin matrix of the thrombus. Reteplase has a short half-life (13 to 16 minutes), owing to rapid clearance by the liver and kidneys. As with other thrombolytic drugs, bleeding is the major adverse effect. The risk of bleeding is increased by concurrent use of heparin, aspirin, and other drugs that impair hemostasis.

Reteplase is approved only for acute MI. Treatment consists of two 10-unit doses separated by 30 minutes. Each dose is given by IV bolus injected over a 2-minute interval. Reteplase should not be administered through a line that contains heparin. If a heparin-containing line must be used, it should be flushed before giving reteplase.

KEY POINTS

- Hemostasis occurs in two stages: formation of a platelet plug, followed by coagulation (i.e., production of fibrin, a protein that reinforces the platelet plug).
- Platelet aggregation depends on activation of platelet glycoprotein (GP) IIb/IIIa receptors, which bind fibrinogen to form cross-links between platelets.
- Fibrin is produced by two pathways—the contact activation pathway (aka intrinsic pathway) and the tissue factor pathway (aka extrinsic pathway)—that converge at clotting factor Xa, which catalyzes formation of thrombin, which in turn catalyzes formation of fibrin.
- Four factors in the coagulation pathways require an activated form of vitamin K for their synthesis.
- Plasmin, the active form of plasminogen, serves to degrade the fibrin meshwork of clots.
- A thrombus is a blood clot formed within a blood vessel or the atria of the heart.
- Arterial thrombi begin with formation of a platelet plug, which is then reinforced with fibrin.
- Venous thrombi begin with formation of fibrin, which then enmeshes red blood cells and platelets.
- Arterial thrombi are best prevented with antiplatelet drugs (e.g., aspirin, clopidogrel), whereas venous thrombi are best prevented with anticoagulants (e.g., heparin, warfarin, dabigatran).
- Heparin is a large polymer (molecular weight range, 3000 to 30,000) that carries many negative charges.
- Heparin suppresses coagulation by helping antithrombin inactivate thrombin and factor Xa.
- Heparin is administered IV or subQ. Because of its large size and negative charges, heparin is unable to cross membranes, and hence cannot be administered PO.
- Anticoagulant effects of heparin develop within minutes of IV administration.
- The major adverse effect of heparin is bleeding.
- Severe heparin-induced bleeding can be treated with protamine sulfate, a drug that binds heparin and thereby stops it from working.
- Heparin-induced thrombocytopenia is a potentially fatal condition caused by development of antibodies against heparin–platelet protein complexes.
- Heparin is contraindicated for patients with thrombocytopenia or uncontrollable bleeding, and must be used with extreme caution in all patients for whom there is a high likelihood of bleeding.
- Heparin therapy is monitored by measuring the activated partial thromboplastin time (aPTT) or anti-Xa heparin assay. The target aPTT is 60 to 80 seconds (i.e., 1.5 to 2 times the normal value of 40 seconds). The target anti-Xa level is 0.3 to 0.7 IU/mL.
- Low-molecular-weight (LMW) heparins are produced by breaking molecules of unfractionated heparin into smaller pieces.
- In contrast to unfractionated heparin, which inactivates factor Xa and thrombin equally, LMW heparins preferentially inactivate factor Xa.
- In contrast to unfractionated heparin, LMW heparins do not bind nonspecifically to plasma proteins and tissues. As a result, their bioavailability is high, making their plasma levels predictable.
- Because plasma levels of LMW heparins are predictable, these drugs can be administered using a fixed dosage, with no need for routine laboratory monitoring. As a result, LMW heparins can be used at home.
- Warfarin is our oldest *oral* anticoagulant.
- Warfarin prevents the activation of vitamin K and thereby blocks the biosynthesis of vitamin K–dependent clotting factors.
- Anticoagulant responses to warfarin develop slowly and persist for several days after warfarin is discontinued.
- Warfarin is used to prevent venous thromboembolism (VTE) and to prevent stroke and systemic embolism in patients with atrial fibrillation.
- Warfarin therapy is monitored by measuring prothrombin time (PT). Results are expressed as an international normalized ratio (INR). An INR of 2 to 3 is the target for most patients.
- Bleeding is the major complication of warfarin therapy.
- Genetic testing for variant genes that code for VKORC1 and CYP2C9 can identify people with increased sensitivity to warfarin, and who therefore may need a dosage reduction.
- Moderate warfarin overdose is treated with vitamin K.
- Warfarin must not be used during pregnancy. The drug can cause fetal malformation, CNS defects, and optic atrophy.
- Warfarin is subject to a large number of clinically significant drug interactions. Drugs can increase anticoagulant effects

by displacing warfarin from plasma albumin, by inhibiting hepatic enzymes that degrade warfarin, and by decreasing synthesis of clotting factors. Drugs can decrease anticoagulant effects by inducing hepatic drug-metabolizing enzymes, increasing synthesis of clotting factors, and inhibiting warfarin absorption. Drugs that promote bleeding, such as heparin and aspirin, will obviously increase the risk of bleeding in patients taking warfarin. Instruct patients to avoid all drugs—prescription and nonprescription—that have not been specifically approved by the prescriber.

- Dabigatran is an oral anticoagulant that works by direct inhibition of thrombin.
- Dabigatran is an alternative to warfarin for chronic anticoagulation in patients with atrial fibrillation.
- Compared with warfarin, dabigatran has five *advantages:* rapid onset, fixed dosage, no need for coagulation testing, few drug-food interactions, and a lower risk of hemorrhagic stroke and other major bleeds.
- Compared with warfarin, dabigatran has three *disadvantages:* no antidote, limited clinical experience, and more GI disturbances (dyspepsia, ulceration, gastritis, etc.).
- Rivaroxaban, edoxaban, and apixaban are oral anticoagulants that work by direct inhibition of factor Xa.
- Like dabigatran, rivaroxaban, edoxaban, and apixaban are safer than warfarin and easier to use.
- Aspirin and other antiplatelet drugs suppress thrombus formation in arteries.
- Aspirin inhibits platelet aggregation by causing irreversible inhibition of cyclooxygenase. Since platelets are unable to synthesize new cyclooxygenase, inhibition persists for the life of the platelet (7 to 10 days).
- In its role as an antiplatelet drug, aspirin is given for multiple purposes, including primary prevention of myocardial infarction (MI), acute management of MI, and reduction of cardiovascular events in patients with unstable angina, chronic stable angina, ischemic stroke, or a history of transient ischemic attacks (TIAs).
- When used to suppress platelet aggregation, aspirin is administered in low doses—typically 80 to 325 mg/day.
- Clopidogrel suppresses platelet aggregation by causing irreversible blockade of $P2Y_{12}$ ADP receptors on the platelet surface.
- Clopidogrel is a prodrug that undergoes conversion to its active form by hepatic CYP2C19.
- Patients with an inherited deficiency in CYP2C19 may have an unreliable response to clopidogrel.
- The major adverse effect of clopidogrel is bleeding.
- The GP IIb/IIIa receptor blockers (e.g., abciximab) inhibit the final common step in platelet aggregation, and hence are the most effective antiplatelet drugs available.
- Alteplase (tPA) and other thrombolytic drugs (aka fibrinolytic drugs) are used to dissolve existing thrombi (rather than prevent thrombi from forming).
- Thrombolytic drugs work by converting plasminogen to plasmin, an enzyme that degrades the fibrin matrix of thrombi.
- Thrombolytic therapy is most effective when started early (e.g., for acute MI, within 4 to 6 hours of symptom onset, and preferably sooner).
- Thrombolytic drugs carry a significant risk of bleeding. Intracranial hemorrhage is the greatest concern.

Please visit **http://evolve.elsevier.com/Lehne** for chapter-specific NCLEX® examination review questions.

Summary of Major Nursing Implications[a]

HEPARIN

Preadministration Assessment

Therapeutic Goal

The objective is to prevent thrombosis without inducing spontaneous bleeding.

Heparin is the preferred anticoagulant for use during pregnancy and in situations that require rapid onset of effects, including PE, evolving stroke, and massive DVT. Other indications include open heart surgery, renal dialysis, and disseminated intravascular coagulation. Low doses are used to prevent postoperative venous thrombosis and to enhance thrombolytic therapy of MI.

Baseline Data

Obtain baseline values for blood pressure, heart rate, complete blood cell counts, platelet counts, hematocrit, and aPTT.

Identifying High-Risk Patients

Heparin is *contraindicated* for patients with severe thrombocytopenia or uncontrollable bleeding and for patients undergoing lumbar puncture, regional anesthesia, or surgery of the eye, brain, or spinal cord.

Use with *extreme caution* in patients at high risk of bleeding, including those with hemophilia, increased capillary permeability, dissecting aneurysm, GI ulcers, or severe hypertension. Caution is also needed in patients with severe hepatic or renal impairment.

Implementation: Administration

Routes

Intravenous (continuous infusion or intermittent) and subQ. Avoid IM injections!

Administration

General Considerations. Dosage is prescribed in units, not milligrams. Heparin preparations vary widely in concentration; read the label carefully to ensure correct dosing.

Continuous IV Infusion. Administer with a continuous infusion pump or some other approved volume-control unit. Policy may require that dosage be double-checked by a second person. Check the infusion rate every 30 to 60 minutes. During

Continued

Summary of Major Nursing Implications[a]—cont'd

the early phase of treatment, the aPTT or anti-Xa level should be determined every 6 hours. Check the site of needle insertion periodically for extravasation.

Ongoing Evaluation and Interventions

Evaluating Treatment

We evaluate treatment by measuring the aPTT or the anti-Xa level. Heparin should increase the aPTT by 1.5- to 2-fold above baseline. Therapeutic range for anti-Xa level is 0.3 to 0.7 IU/mL.

Minimizing Adverse Effects

Hemorrhage. Heparin overdose may cause hemorrhage. Monitor closely for signs of bleeding. These include reduced blood pressure, elevated heart rate, discolored urine or stool, bruises, petechiae, hematomas, persistent headache or faintness (suggestive of cerebral hemorrhage), pelvic pain (suggestive of ovarian hemorrhage), and lumbar pain (suggestive of adrenal hemorrhage). Laboratory data suggesting hemorrhage include reductions in the hematocrit and blood cell counts. If bleeding occurs, heparin should be discontinued. Severe overdose can be treated with *protamine sulfate* administered by slow IV injection. The risk of bleeding can be reduced by ensuring that the aPTT or the anti-Xa levels are not above recommended range according to facility protocol.

Heparin-Induced Thrombocytopenia. HIT, characterized by reduced platelet counts and increased thrombotic events, poses a risk of DVT, PE, cerebral thrombosis, MI, and ischemic injury to the arms and legs. To reduce risk, monitor platelet counts 2 to 3 times a week during the first 3 weeks of heparin use, and monthly thereafter. If severe thrombocytopenia develops (platelet count below 100,000/mm^3), discontinue heparin and, if anticoagulation is still needed, substitute another anticoagulant, such as argatroban.

Spinal/Epidural Hematoma. Heparin and all other anticoagulants pose a risk of spinal or epidural hematoma in patients undergoing spinal puncture or spinal/epidural anesthesia. Prolonged or permanent paralysis can result. Risk of hematoma is increased by several factors, including use of an indwelling epidural catheter, use of other anticoagulants (e.g., warfarin, dabigatran), and use of antiplatelet drugs (e.g., aspirin, clopidogrel). Monitor for signs and symptoms of neurologic impairment. If impairment develops, immediate intervention is needed.

Hypersensitivity Reactions. Allergy may develop to antigens in heparin preparations. To minimize the risk of severe reactions, administer a small test dose before the full therapeutic dose.

Minimizing Adverse Interactions

Antiplatelet Drugs. Concurrent use of aspirin, clopidogrel, and other antiplatelet drugs increases the risk of bleeding. Use these agents with caution.

WARFARIN, A VITAMIN K ANTAGONIST

Preadministration Assessment

Therapeutic Goal

The goal is to prevent thrombosis without inducing spontaneous bleeding. Specific indications include prevention of venous thrombosis and associated PE, prevention of thromboembolism in patients with prosthetic heart valves, and prevention of stroke and systemic embolism in patients with atrial fibrillation.

Baseline Data

Obtain a thorough medical history. Be sure to identify use of any medications that might interact adversely with warfarin. Obtain baseline values of vital signs and PT. Genetic testing for variants of CYP2C9 and VKORC1 may be done to identify patients who may require a reduction in warfarin dosage.

Identifying High-Risk Patients

Warfarin is *contraindicated* in the presence of vitamin K deficiency, liver disease, alcoholism, thrombocytopenia, uncontrollable bleeding, pregnancy, and lactation, and for patients undergoing lumbar puncture, regional anesthesia, or surgery of the eye, brain, or spinal cord.

Use with *extreme caution* in patients at high risk of bleeding, including those with hemophilia, increased capillary permeability, dissecting aneurysm, GI ulcers, and severe hypertension.

Use with *caution* in patients with variant forms of CYP2C9 or VKORC1.

Implementation: Administration

Route

Oral.

Administration

For most patients, dosage is adjusted to maintain an INR value of 2 to 3. Maintain a flow chart for hospitalized patients indicating INR values, dose, and administration time.

Implementation: Measures to Enhance Therapeutic Effects

Promoting Adherence

Safe and effective therapy requires rigid adherence to the dosing schedule. Achieving adherence requires active and informed participation by the patient. **Provide the patient with detailed written and verbal instructions regarding the purpose of treatment, dosage size and timing, and the importance of careful adherence to the dosing schedule. Also, provide the patient with a chart on which to keep an ongoing record of warfarin use.** If the patient is incompetent (e.g., mentally ill, alcoholic, senile), ensure that a responsible individual supervises treatment.

Summary of Major Nursing Implications[a]—cont'd

Nondrug Measures

Advise the patient to (1) avoid prolonged immobility, (2) elevate the legs when sitting, (3) avoid garments that can restrict blood flow in the legs, (4) participate in exercise activities, and (5) wear support hose. These measures will reduce venous stasis and will thereby reduce the risk of thrombosis.

Ongoing Evaluation and Interventions

Monitoring Treatment

Evaluate therapy by monitoring PT. Test results are reported as an *international normalized ratio* (INR). For most patients, the target INR is 2 to 3. If the INR is below this range, dosage should be increased. Conversely, if the INR is above this range, dosage should be reduced.

The INR should be determined frequently: daily during the first 5 days, twice a week for the next 1 to 2 weeks, once a week for the next 1 to 2 months, and every 2 to 4 weeks thereafter. In addition, the INR should be determined whenever a drug that interacts with warfarin is added to or withdrawn from the regimen.

When appropriate, teach patients how to monitor their PT and INR at home.

Minimizing Adverse Effects

Hemorrhage. Hemorrhage is the major complication of warfarin therapy. **Warn patients about the danger of hemorrhage, and inform them about signs of bleeding. These include reduced blood pressure, elevated heart rate, discolored urine or stools, bruises, petechiae, hematomas, persistent headache or faintness (suggestive of cerebral hemorrhage), pelvic pain (suggestive of ovarian hemorrhage), and lumbar pain (suggestive of adrenal hemorrhage).** Laboratory data suggesting hemorrhage include reductions in the hematocrit and blood cell counts.

Instruct the patient to withhold warfarin and notify the prescriber if signs of bleeding are noted. Advise the patient to wear some form of identification (e.g., Medic Alert bracelet) to alert emergency personnel to warfarin use.

To reduce the incidence of bleeding, **advise the patient to avoid excessive consumption of alcohol. Suggest use of a soft toothbrush to prevent bleeding from the gums. Advise patients to shave with an electric razor.**

Warfarin intensifies bleeding during surgical procedures. **Instruct the patient to make certain the surgeon is aware of warfarin use.** Warfarin should be discontinued several days before elective procedures. If emergency surgery must be performed, vitamin K_1 can help reduce bleeding.

Warfarin-induced bleeding can be controlled with vitamin K_1. For most patients, oral vitamin K will suffice. For patients with severe bleeding or a very high INR, vitamin K is given by injection (usually IV).

Use in Pregnancy and Lactation. Warfarin can cross the placenta, causing fetal hemorrhage and malformation. **Inform those of childbearing age about potential risks to the fetus, and warn them against becoming pregnant.** If pregnancy develops, termination should be considered.

Warfarin enters breast milk and may harm the nursing infant. **Warn patients against breast-feeding.**

Minimizing Adverse Interactions

Inform patients that warfarin is subject to a large number of potentially dangerous drug interactions. Instruct them to avoid all drugs—prescription and nonprescription—that have not been specifically approved by the prescriber. Before treatment, take a complete medication history to identify any drugs that might interact adversely with warfarin.

CLOPIDOGREL, A $P2Y_{12}$ ADENOSINE DIPHOSPHATE RECEPTOR ANTAGONIST

Preadministration Assessment

Therapeutic Goal

Clopidogrel is used to prevent blockage of coronary artery stents and to reduce thrombotic events—MI, ischemic stroke, and vascular death—in patients with ACS and in those with atherosclerosis documented by recent MI, recent stroke, or established peripheral arterial disease.

Baseline Data

Consider testing for variants of the CYP2C19 gene to determine whether the patient is a poor metabolizer of clopidogrel.

Identifying High-Risk Patients

Clopidogrel is *contraindicated* in patients with active pathologic bleeding, including ICH and bleeding ulcers. Use with *caution* in patients taking other drugs that promote bleeding. *Generally avoid* clopidogrel in poor metabolizers of the drug.

Implementation: Administration

Route

Oral.

Administration

Instruct patients to take clopidogrel once a day, with or without food.

Ongoing Evaluation and Interventions

Promoting Beneficial Effects

Instruct patients being treated for ACS to take aspirin (75 to 325 mg) once daily.

Minimizing Adverse Effects

Bleeding. Clopidogrel poses a risk of serious bleeding. Avoid clopidogrel in patients with active pathologic bleeding, and use with caution in patients taking other drugs that promote bleeding. If possible, manage major bleeding without stopping clopidogrel, since discontinuation would increase the risk of a thrombotic event.

Inform patients about the risk of bleeding, and warn them that:

- **You may bruise more easily.**
- **You may bleed more easily.**

Continued

Summary of Major Nursing Implications[a]—cont'd

- You are more likely to get nosebleeds.
- Bleeding will take longer than usual to stop.

Instruct patients to contact the prescriber if they experience any of these symptoms of bleeding:

- Unexpected bleeding
- Bleeding that lasts a long time
- Blood in the urine, indicated by discoloration (pink, red, brown)
- Blood in stools (indicated by red, black, tarry stools)
- Bruising with no obvious cause
- Vomiting blood, which may look like coffee grounds

Instruct patients that, even if these symptoms occur, they should continue taking clopidogrel until the prescriber says they should stop.

Instruct patients to discontinue clopidogrel 5 days before elective surgery.

Thrombotic Thrombocytopenic Purpura (TTP). Rarely, patients develop TTP, a potentially fatal condition characterized by thrombocytopenia, hemolytic anemia, neurologic symptoms, renal dysfunction, and fever. If TTP is diagnosed, urgent treatment—including plasmapheresis—is required.

Minimizing Adverse Interactions

Drugs That Promote Bleeding. Use with caution in patients taking other drugs that promote bleeding (e.g., heparin, warfarin, dabigatran, aspirin, and nonaspirin NSAIDs).

Proton Pump Inhibitors (PPIs). The PPIs can help prevent clopidogrel-related GI bleeding—but may reduce the benefits of clopidogrel by inhibiting CYP2C19, the hepatic enzyme that converts clopidogrel to its active form. In patients with risk factors for GI bleeding (e.g., advanced age, use of NSAIDs or anticoagulants), the benefits of combining a PPI with clopidogrel probably outweigh any risk from reduced antiplatelet effects. Conversely, in patients who lack risk factors for GI bleeding, combined use of clopidogrel with a PPI may reduce the benefits of clopidogrel without offering any meaningful GI protection—and hence combining a PPI with clopidogrel in these patients should probably be avoided. When a PPI *is* used with clopidogrel, pantoprazole is a good choice because, compared with other PPIs, pantoprazole causes less inhibition of CYP2C19.

CYP2C19 Inhibitors (Other Than PPIs). Like the PPIs, several other drugs can inhibit CYP2C19. Among these are cimetidine, fluoxetine, fluvoxamine, fluconazole, ketoconazole, voriconazole, etravirine, felbamate, and ticlopidine. Since these drugs may reduce the antiplatelet effects of clopidogrel, using an alternative to these drugs is preferred.

THROMBOLYTIC (FIBRINOLYTIC) DRUGS

Alteplase (tPA)
Reteplase
Tenecteplase

Preadministration Assessment

Therapeutic Goal

All three thrombolytic drugs are used for acute MI, and one drug—alteplase—is also used for ischemic stroke and PE, and, in low dosage, for clearing blocked central venous catheters.

Baseline Data

Obtain baseline values for blood pressure, heart rate, platelet counts, hematocrit, aPTT, PT, and fibrinogen level.

Identifying High-Risk Patients

Thrombolytic drugs are *contraindicated* for patients with active bleeding, aortic dissection, acute pericarditis, cerebral neoplasm, cerebrovascular disease, or a history of intracranial bleeding.

Use with *great caution* in patients with relative contraindications, including pregnancy, severe hypertension, ischemic stroke within the prior 6 months, and major surgery within the prior 2 to 4 weeks. See Table 52.10 for other absolute and relative contraindications.

Implementation: Administration

Route

Intravenous.

Administration (for Acute MI)

Alteplase. Administer as an initial IV bolus followed by a 90-minute IV infusion.

Tenecteplase. Administer as a single IV bolus.

Reteplase. Administer as two IV boluses, separated by 30 minutes.

Ongoing Evaluation and Interventions

Minimizing Adverse Effects

Hemorrhage. Thrombolytics may cause bleeding; ICH is the greatest concern. To reduce the risk of major bleeding, minimize manipulation of the patient, avoid subQ and IM injections, minimize invasive procedures, and minimize concurrent use of anticoagulants and antiplatelet drugs. Manage oozing at cutaneous puncture sites with a pressure dressing.

Minimizing Adverse Interactions

Anticoagulants and Antiplatelet Drugs. Anticoagulants (e.g., heparin, warfarin, dabigatran) and antiplatelet drugs (e.g., aspirin, clopidogrel) increase the risk of bleeding from antithrombotics. Avoid high-dose therapy with these drugs until thrombolytic effects have subsided.

[a]Patient education information is highlighted as **blue text**.

CHAPTER

53 Management of ST-Elevation Myocardial Infarction

Myocardial infarction (MI), also known as heart attack, is defined as necrosis of the myocardium (heart muscle) resulting from local ischemia (deficient blood flow). The underlying cause is partial or complete blockage of a coronary artery. When blockage is complete, the area of infarction is much larger than when the blockage is partial. In this chapter, discussion is limited to acute MI caused by *complete* interruption of regional myocardial blood flow. This class of MI is called *ST-elevation MI* (STEMI), because it causes elevation of the ST segment on the electrocardiogram (ECG). Management of STEMI differs from management of non–ST-elevation MI, which occurs when blockage of blood flow is only partial.

In the United States, STEMI strikes about 258,000 people each year and is the most common cause of death. Between 20% and 30% of STEMI victims die before reaching the hospital, another 5% to 6% die in the hospital, and 7% to 18% die within a year of hospital discharge. Risk factors for STEMI include advanced age, a family history of MI, sedentary lifestyle, high serum cholesterol, hypertension, smoking, and diabetes. The objectives of this chapter are to describe the pathophysiology of STEMI and to discuss interventions that can help reduce morbidity and mortality.

PATHOPHYSIOLOGY OF STEMI

Acute MI occurs when blood flow to a region of the myocardium is stopped owing to platelet plugging and thrombus formation in a coronary artery—almost always at the site of a fissured or ruptured atherosclerotic plaque. Myocardial injury is ultimately the result of an imbalance between oxygen demand and oxygen supply.

In response to local ischemia, a dramatic redistribution of ions takes place. Hydrogen ions accumulate in the myocardium, and calcium ions become sequestered in mitochondria. The resultant acidosis and functional calcium deficiency alter the distensibility of cardiac muscle. Sodium ions accumulate in myocardial cells and promote edema. Potassium ions are lost from myocardial cells, setting the stage for dysrhythmias.

Local metabolic changes begin rapidly following coronary arterial occlusion. Within seconds, metabolism shifts from aerobic to anaerobic. High-energy stores of ATP and creatine phosphate become depleted. As a result, contraction ceases in the affected region.

If blood flow is not restored, cell death begins within 20 minutes. Clear indices of cell death—myocyte disruption, coagulative necrosis, elevation of cardiac proteins in serum—are present by 24 hours. By 4 days, monocyte infiltration and removal of dead myocytes weaken the infarcted area, making it vulnerable to expansion and rupture. Structural integrity is partially restored with the deposition of collagen, which begins in 10 to 12 days and ends with dense scar formation by 4 to 6 weeks.

Myocardial injury also triggers ventricular remodeling, a process in which ventricular mass increases and the chambers change in volume and shape. Remodeling is driven in part by local production of angiotensin II. Ventricular remodeling increases the risk of heart failure and death.

The degree of residual cardiac impairment depends on how much of the myocardium was damaged. With infarction of 10% of left ventricular (LV) mass, the ejection fraction is reduced. With 25% LV infarction, cardiac dilation and heart failure occur. With 40% LV infarction, cardiogenic shock and death are likely.

DIAGNOSIS OF STEMI

Acute STEMI is diagnosed by the presence of chest pain, characteristic ECG changes, and elevated serum levels of myocardial cellular components (troponin, creatine kinase). Other symptoms include sweating, weakness, and a sense of impending doom. Of note, about 20% of people with STEMI experience no symptoms.

Chest Pain

Patients undergoing STEMI typically experience severe substernal pressure that they characterize as unbearable crushing or constricting pain. The pain often radiates down the arms and up to the jaw. STEMI can be differentiated from angina

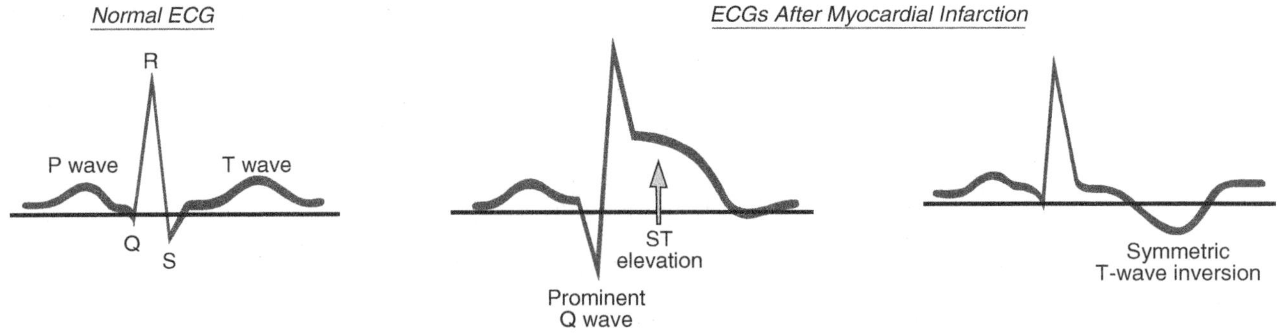

Fig. 53.1 ■ **ECG changes associated with ST-elevation myocardial infarction.**

pectoris in that pain caused by STEMI lasts longer (20 to 30 minutes) and is not relieved by nitroglycerin. Some patients confuse the pain of STEMI with indigestion.

ECG Changes

Acute STEMI produces changes in the ECG because conduction of electrical impulses through the heart becomes altered in the region of injury. Elevation of the ST segment, which defines STEMI, occurs almost immediately in response to acute ischemia (Fig. 53.1). Following a period of ST-segment elevation, a prominent Q wave (more than 40 milliseconds in duration) develops in the majority of patients. (Q waves are small or absent in the normal ECG.) Over time, the ST segment returns to baseline, after which a symmetric inverted T wave appears. This T-wave inversion may resolve within weeks to months. Q waves may resolve over a period of years.

Biochemical Markers for MI

When myocardial cells undergo necrosis, they release intracellular proteins (e.g., cardiac troponins, creatine kinase). Hence, elevations in these proteins in blood can be diagnostic of STEMI.

Today, cardiac-derived troponins—*cardiac troponin I* and *cardiac troponin T*—are considered the best serum markers for STEMI. These proteins are components of the sarcomere, and are distinct from their counterparts in skeletal muscle. Under normal conditions, troponin I and troponin T are undetectable in blood. However, when STEMI occurs, their levels rise dramatically, often to 100-fold or more above the lower limits of detection. Cardiac troponins become detectable 2 to 4 hours after symptom onset, peak in 10 to 24 hours, and return to undetectable in 5 to 14 days. Measurements of troponin I and troponin T are more sensitive than measurements of other biochemical markers for STEMI and produce fewer false-positive or false-negative results.

Before cardiac troponins became the preferred biomarkers for STEMI, clinicians relied on measurement of the MB isoenzyme of creatine kinase (CK-MB). Since CK-MB is found primarily in cardiac muscle rather than skeletal muscle, an increase in serum CK-MB is highly suggestive of cardiac injury. Following MI, serum levels of CK-MB begin to rise in 4 to 8 hours, peak in 24 hours, and return to baseline in 36 to 72 hours. In some patients, the increase in CK-MB may be too small to allow a definitive diagnosis, even though significant myocardial injury has occurred.

MANAGEMENT OF STEMI

The acute phase of management refers to the interval between the onset of symptoms and discharge from the hospital (usually 6 to 10 days). The goal is to bring cardiac oxygen supply back into balance with oxygen demand. This can be accomplished by reperfusion therapy, which restores blood flow to the myocardium, and by reducing myocardial oxygen demand. The first few hours of treatment are most critical. The major threats to life during acute STEMI are ventricular dysrhythmias, cardiogenic shock, and heart failure.

To aid clinicians in the management of STEMI, the American College of Cardiology Foundation (ACCF), the American Heart Association (AHA), and the Society for Cardiovascular Angiography and Interventions (SCAI) have updated a series of evidence-based guidelines, including the following:

- 2013 ACCF/AHA Guideline for the Management of ST-Elevation Myocardial Infarction: A Report of the American College of Cardiology Foundation/American Heart Association Task Force on Practice Guidelines
- 2015 ACC/AHA/SCAI Focused Update on Primary Percutaneous Coronary Intervention for Patients with ST-Elevation Myocardial Infarction: An Update of the 2011 ACCF/AHA/SCAI Guideline for Percutaneous Coronary Intervention and the 2013 ACCF/AHA Guideline for the Management of ST-Elevation Myocardial Infarction.

These guidelines are available at http://professional.heart.org/professional/GuidelinesStatements/searchresults.jsp?q=&y=&t=1001. The discussion that follows reflects recommendations in these documents.

Routine Drug Therapy

When a patient presents with suspected STEMI, several interventions should begin immediately. The objective is to minimize possible myocardial necrosis while waiting for a clear diagnosis. Once STEMI has been diagnosed, more definitive therapy—reperfusion—can be implemented (see *Reperfusion Therapy*).

Oxygen

Supplemental oxygen, administered by nasal cannula, can increase arterial oxygen saturation and can thereby increase oxygen delivery to the ischemic myocardium. Accordingly, current guidelines recommend giving oxygen to all patients with reduced arterial oxygen saturation (below 90%). However, although oxygen is recommended and using it seems to make sense, the practice is not evidence based. That is, we have no hard evidence to show that oxygen is beneficial. In fact, there is some evidence that oxygen may actually be harmful, causing mortality to increase rather than decline.

Aspirin

Aspirin suppresses platelet aggregation, producing an immediate antithrombotic effect. In the Second International Study of Infarct Survival (ISIS-2), aspirin caused a substantial reduction in mortality. Moreover, benefits were synergistic with fibrinolytic drugs: mortality was 13.2% with fibrinolytics alone, and it dropped to 8% with the addition of aspirin. Because of these benefits, virtually all patients with evolving STEMI should get aspirin. Therapy should begin immediately after onset of symptoms and should continue indefinitely. The first dose (162 to 325 mg) should be chewed to allow rapid absorption across the buccal mucosa. Prolonged therapy (with 81 to 162 mg/day) reduces the risk of reinfarction, stroke, and death.

Nonaspirin Nonsteroidal Anti-Inflammatory Drugs

According to the 2013 guideline, routine use of nonsteroidal anti-inflammatory drugs (NSAIDs) other than aspirin should be *discontinued.* Unlike aspirin, these agents increase the risk of mortality, reinfarction, hypertension, heart failure, and myocardial rupture.

Morphine

Intravenous morphine is the treatment of choice for STEMI-associated pain. In addition to relieving pain, morphine can improve hemodynamics. By promoting venodilation, the drug reduces cardiac preload. By promoting modest arterial dilation, morphine may cause some reduction in afterload. The combined reductions in preload and afterload lower cardiac oxygen demand, helping preserve the ischemic myocardium.

Beta Blockers

When given to patients undergoing acute STEMI, beta blockers (e.g., atenolol, metoprolol) reduce cardiac pain, infarct size, and short-term mortality. Recurrent ischemia and reinfarction are also decreased. Reduction in myocardial wall tension may decrease the risk of myocardial rupture. Continued use of an oral beta blocker increases long-term survival. Unfortunately, although nearly all patients can benefit from beta blockers, many don't get them. Furthermore, among patients who *do* get a beta blocker, the dosage is often too low.

Benefits result from several mechanisms. As STEMI evolves, traffic along sympathetic nerves to the heart increases greatly, as does the number of beta receptors in the heart. As a result, heart rate and force of contraction rise substantially, increasing cardiac oxygen demand. By preventing beta-receptor activation, beta blockers reduce heart rate and contractility, and thereby reduce oxygen demand. They reduce oxygen demand even more by lowering blood pressure. By prolonging diastolic filling time, beta blockers increase coronary blood flow and myocardial oxygen supply. Additional benefits derive from antidysrhythmic actions.

Beta blockers should be used routinely in the absence of specific contraindications (e.g., bradycardia, significant LV dysfunction). The initial dose may be oral or IV; oral dosing is used thereafter. Treatment with an oral beta blocker should begin within 24 hours. Beta blockers are especially good for patients with reflex tachycardia, systolic hypertension, atrial fibrillation, and atrioventricular conduction abnormalities. Contraindications include overt severe heart failure, pronounced bradycardia, persistent hypotension, advanced heart block, and cardiogenic shock. The basic pharmacology of the beta blockers is presented in Chapter 18.

Nitroglycerin

In patients with STEMI, nitroglycerin has several beneficial effects: It can (1) reduce preload and thereby reduce oxygen demand; (2) increase collateral blood flow in the ischemic region of the heart; (3) control hypertension caused by STEMI-associated anxiety; and (4) limit infarct size and improve LV function. However, despite these useful effects, nitroglycerin does not reduce mortality. Nonetheless, since the drug is easily administered, offers hemodynamic benefits, and helps relieve ischemic chest pain, it continues to be used. According to the current guidelines, patients with ongoing ischemic discomfort should be given sublingual nitroglycerin (0.4 mg) every 5 minutes for a total of three doses, and then be assessed to determine whether IV nitroglycerin should be given. Indications for IV therapy include persisting ischemic discomfort, hypertension, and pulmonary congestion. Nitroglycerin should be avoided in patients with hypotension (systolic pressure below 90 mm Hg), severe bradycardia (heart rate below 50 beats/min), marked tachycardia (heart rate above 100 beats/min), or suspected right ventricular infarction. In addition, nitroglycerin should be avoided in patients who have taken sildenafil, avanafil, or vardenafil for erectile dysfunction or pulmonary hypertension within the past 24 hours, or tadalafil within the past 48 hours.

Reperfusion Therapy

The goal of reperfusion therapy is to restore blood flow through the blocked coronary artery. Reperfusion is the most effective way to preserve myocardial function and limit infarct size. How do we accomplish reperfusion? Either with fibrinolytic drugs (also known as thrombolytic drugs) or with percutaneous coronary intervention (PCI), usually balloon angioplasty coupled with the placement of a stent. Both options are very effective. However, PCI is generally preferred. The relative advantages of fibrinolytic therapy and primary PCI are shown in Table 53.1. With either intervention, rapid implementation is essential.

Primary Percutaneous Coronary Intervention

The term *primary PCI* refers to the use of angioplasty, rather than fibrinolytic therapy, to recanalize an occluded coronary artery. In almost all cases, PCI consists of balloon angioplasty coupled with placement of a drug-eluting stent. Under current guidelines, the institutional goal is to implement PCI within 90 minutes of initial patient contact. As discussed later in the chapter, all patients undergoing PCI should receive an anticoagulant (IV heparin, bivalirudin) combined with antiplatelet drugs: aspirin plus either clopidogrel, ticagrelor, or prasugrel, and perhaps a glycoprotein (GP) IIb/IIIa inhibitor.

The success rate with primary PCI is somewhat higher than with fibrinolytic therapy. Moreover, studies indicate that the benefits of PCI last longer. After 30 days, the rate of death, reinfarction, or disabling stroke following PCI is 8% versus

TABLE 53.1 ▪ Comparison of Fibrinolytic Therapy With Primary PCI

ADVANTAGES OF FIBRINOLYTIC THERAPY
• More universal access
• Shorter time to treatment
• Results less dependent on physician experience
• Lower system cost
ADVANTAGES OF PRIMARY PCI
• Higher initial reperfusion rates
• Less residual stenosis
• Lower recurrence rates of ischemia/infarction
• Does not promote intracranial bleeding
• Defines coronary anatomy and LV function
• Can be used when fibrinolytic therapy is contraindicated

LV, Left ventricular; *PCI,* percutaneous coronary intervention.

13.7% following fibrinolytic therapy using tissue plasminogen activator (tPA). After 7.8 years, the rate of all-cause mortality following PCI is 34.88% versus 41.3% with streptokinase—the difference being due entirely to lower cardiovascular mortality in PCI-treated patients. Benefits of primary PCI over fibrinolytic therapy are greatest in high-risk patients.

Fibrinolytic Therapy

Fibrinolytic drugs dissolve clots by converting plasminogen into plasmin, a proteolytic enzyme that digests the fibrin meshwork that holds clots together. In the United States, three fibrinolytic drugs are available for treatment of myocardial infarction: *alteplase (tPA), reteplase,* and *tenecteplase.* The basic pharmacology of these drugs is discussed in Chapter 52. Discussion here is limited to their use in STEMI.

Fibrinolytic therapy is most effective when presentation is early. When thrombolytics are given soon enough, the occluded artery can be opened in 80% of patients. Current guidelines suggest a target of 30 minutes or less for the time between entering the emergency department and starting fibrinolysis. Clinical trials have shown that timely therapy improves ventricular function, limits infarct size, and reduces mortality. Restoration of blood flow reduces or eliminates chest pain and often reduces ST elevation. Current guidelines restrict fibrinolytic therapy to patients with ischemic pain that has been present no more than 12 to 24 hours. Patients for whom fibrinolytic therapy is contraindicated are listed in Table 53.2.

Under *typical* conditions, all fibrinolytics are equally beneficial. However, under *ideal* conditions (i.e., treatment within 4 to 6 hours of pain onset), alteplase is most effective, especially in patients younger than 75 years, as shown in a trial known as GUSTO-I. Unfortunately, alteplase is very expensive.

The major complication of fibrinolytic therapy is bleeding, which occurs in 1% to 5% of patients. Intracranial hemorrhage (ICH) is the greatest concern. ICH has an incidence of 0.5% to 1%, and is most likely in older adults. Nonetheless, the benefits of fibrinolysis generally outweigh the risks.

As discussed in the following sections, all patients undergoing fibrinolytic therapy should receive an anticoagulant (IV heparin, bivalirudin, enoxaparin, fondaparinux) plus antiplatelet drugs (aspirin plus clopidogrel—but not a GP IIb/IIIa inhibitor, such as abciximab).

TABLE 53.2 ▪ Contraindications and Cautions Regarding Fibrinolytic Use for Myocardial Infarction

ABSOLUTE CONTRAINDICATIONS
• Any prior intracranial hemorrhage
• Known structural cerebrovascular lesion
• Ischemic stroke within past 3 months *except* ischemic stroke within 4.5 hr
• Known intracranial neoplasm
• Active internal bleeding (other than menses)
• Severe uncontrolled hypertension (unresponsive to emergency therapy)
• Suspected aortic dissection
• For streptokinase, prior treatment within the previous 6 months
• Intracranial or intraspinal surgery within 2 months
• Significant closed head or facial trauma within 3 months
RELATIVE CONTRAINDICATIONS/CAUTIONS
• Severe, uncontrolled hypertension on presentation (blood pressure above 180/110 mm Hg)
• History of chronic, severe, poorly controlled hypertension
• History of prior ischemic stroke (>3 months ago), dementia, or known intracerebral pathology not covered in contraindications
• Current use of anticoagulants in therapeutic doses (INR 2–3 or greater); known bleeding diathesis
• Traumatic or prolonged (>10 min) CPR or major surgery (<3 wk ago)
• Recent internal bleeding (within 2–4 wk)
• Noncompressible vascular punctures
• Pregnancy
• Active peptic ulcer
• Oral anticoagulant therapy

CPR, Cardiopulmonary resuscitation; *INR,* international normalized ratio.

Adapted from O'Gara PT, Kushner FG, Ascheim DD, et al: 2013 ACCF/AHA Guideline for the Management of ST-Elevation Myocardial Infarction: A report of the American College of Cardiology Foundation/American Heart Association Task Force on Practice Guidelines. *J Am Coll Cardiol* 61(4):e78–e140.

Adjuncts to Reperfusion Therapy

Anticoagulants

Heparin. Heparin is a parenteral anticoagulant that was used widely to treat MI before fibrinolytics and primary PCI became available. The drug was shown to decrease mortality, reinfarction, stroke, pulmonary embolism, and deep vein thrombosis. Today, heparin is used in conjunction with fibrinolytics and PCI to reduce the risk of thrombosis. The main complication of heparin is bleeding.

Heparin is recommended for all STEMI patients undergoing fibrinolytic therapy or PCI. For those receiving fibrinolytic drugs, treatment should begin before giving the fibrinolytic and should continue for at least 48 to 72 hours after. For patients undergoing PCI, heparin is given once, immediately before the procedure.

Heparin is available as the intact (unfractionated) drug and in low-molecular-weight (LMW) forms. When heparin is used as an adjunct to fibrinolytic therapy, selection of a heparin product depends on duration of use. For treatment lasting less than 48 hours, *unfractionated* heparin can be employed. However, for treatment lasting more than 48 hours, enoxaparin

[Lovenox], an *LMW* heparin, should be chosen because prolonged use of unfractionated heparin poses a risk of heparin-induced thrombocytopenia. Enoxaparin is given in a 30-mg IV bolus in patients younger than 75 years, followed by administration of subcutaneous enoxaparin 1 mg/kg every 12 hours. Patients 75 years and older should not receive an IV bolus. When using enoxaparin, dosing should be adjusted for creatinine clearance less than 30 mL/min. Enoxaparin should be continued throughout the hospitalization, for up to a period of 8 days, or until revascularization.

Fondaparinux. Fondaparinux [Arixtra] is a selective factor Xa inhibitor. It is recommended as an alternative therapy to heparin for adjunctive use in patients undergoing reperfusion therapy with fibrinolytics. Due to its association with catheter thrombosis, fondaparinux is not recommended for use as the sole anticoagulant in patients undergoing PCI.

Initial dosing is 2.5 mg IV, then 2.5 mg subcutaneously starting the following day. Like enoxaparin, fondaparinux should be continued for the length of the hospitalization, for up to a period of 8 days, or until revascularization. Fondaparinux is contraindicated in patients with a creatinine clearance of less than 30 mL/min.

Bivalirudin. Bivalirudin [Angiomax], a direct thrombin inhibitor, is the preferred agent of use over unfractionated heparin with GP IIb/IIIa inhibitor (abciximab) in patients undergoing PCI who are at high risk of bleeding. In addition, bivalirudin is used as an alternative to heparin in patients with known heparin-induced thrombosis who are undergoing fibrinolytic therapy.

Bivalirudin is given IV. Initial dosing for patients undergoing PCI is a 0.75-mg/kg bolus, and then continued infusion at 1.75 mg/kg/hr. Doses should be reduced for patients with a creatinine clearance of less than 30 mL/min.

Antiplatelet Drugs

Thienopyridines: Clopidogrel, Ticagrelor, and Prasugrel. Clopidogrel [Plavix], ticagrelor [Brilinta], and prasugrel [Effient] suppress platelet aggregation by blocking receptors for adenosine diphosphate. These drugs are recommended for all MI patients undergoing PCI. In all cases, clopidogrel, ticagrelor, or prasugrel should be *combined* with aspirin. In patients undergoing PCI with stenting, duration of treatment should be at least 12 months, unless the risk of bleeding outweighs the benefits of continued drug use. In patients undergoing fibrinolytic therapy, clopidogrel is the only recommended antiplatelet drug. Dosing should continue for at least 14 days up to a period of 1 year.

Glycoprotein IIb/IIIa Inhibitors. The GP IIb/IIIa inhibitors (e.g., abciximab [ReoPro]) are powerful intravenous antiplatelet drugs that inhibit the final step in platelet aggregation. These drugs are recommended for patients undergoing PCI, but not for those undergoing fibrinolytic therapy. Of the three GP IIb/IIIa inhibitors available, abciximab is preferred. Treatment should begin as soon as possible before PCI and should continue for 12 hours after.

Aspirin. As discussed earlier, *low-dose* aspirin (81 to 162 mg/day) should be taken indefinitely by all people who have had an MI. This should be combined with antiplatelet drugs (clopidogrel, ticagrelor, prasugrel) for a period of 1 year. The duration of therapy does not change with the placement of a drug-eluting stent or bare metal stent.

Safety Alert

INCREASED RISK FOR BLEEDING

All of the anticoagulant and antiplatelet drugs mentioned increase the risk for bleeding. The nurse must be diligent in assessing for and reporting any signs and symptoms of bleeding, including decreased level of consciousness, painful or swollen joints, oozing gums, hematuria, or decrease in platelet or hemoglobin values.

Angiotensin-Converting Enzyme Inhibitors and Angiotensin II Receptor Blockers

When used following acute STEMI, angiotensin-converting enzyme (ACE) inhibitors (e.g., captopril, lisinopril) decrease short-term mortality in all patients and long-term mortality in patients with reduced LV function. Benefits derive from reducing preload and afterload, promoting water loss, and favorably altering ventricular remodeling. Because of their benefits, ACE inhibitors are recommended for all STEMI patients in the absence of specific contraindications. Treatment should start within 24 hours of symptom onset. The possibility that long-term therapy may also benefit patients who do not have LV dysfunction is being evaluated in large-scale trials. The major adverse effects of ACE inhibitors are hypotension and cough. Contraindications to ACE inhibitors are hypotension, bilateral renal artery stenosis, renal failure, and a history of ACE inhibitor–induced cough or angioedema. The basic pharmacology of the ACE inhibitors is described in Chapter 44.

Therapy with angiotensin II receptor blockers (ARBs) in STEMI patients has not been studied as extensively as has therapy with ACE inhibitors. However, one major trial—Valsartan in Acute Myocardial Infarction Trial (VALIANT)—demonstrated that, in patients with post-MI heart failure or LV dysfunction, valsartan (an ARB) was as effective as captopril (an ACE inhibitor) at reducing short-term and long-term mortality. In the current guidelines, ARBs are recommended for STEMI patients who are intolerant of ACE inhibitors and have heart failure or reduced LV function.

Calcium Channel Blockers

Because of their antianginal, vasodilatory, and antihypertensive actions, calcium channel blockers (CCBs) were presumed beneficial for patients with acute STEMI and were once used widely. However, in large-scale controlled trials, CCBs failed to decrease mortality during or after acute STEMI. Accordingly, CCBs are not recommended for routine use. However, since the effects of CCBs on the heart are nearly identical to those of beta blockers, current guidelines state that it is reasonable to use one of two CCBs—verapamil or diltiazem—when beta blockers are either ineffective or contraindicated to relieve ongoing ischemia or control a rapid ventricular rate caused by atrial fibrillation or atrial flutter. CCBs should not be used if the patient has heart failure, LV dysfunction, or atrioventricular block.

COMPLICATIONS OF STEMI

MI predisposes the heart and vascular system to serious complications. Among the most severe are ventricular dysrhythmias, cardiogenic shock, and heart failure.

Ventricular Dysrhythmias

These dysrhythmias develop frequently and are the major cause of death following MI. Sudden death from dysrhythmias occurs in 15% of patients during the first hour. Ultimately, ventricular dysrhythmias cause 60% of infarction-related deaths. Acute management of ventricular fibrillation consists of defibrillation followed by IV amiodarone for 24 to 48 hours. Programmed ventricular stimulation with guided antidysrhythmic therapy may be lifesaving for some patients.

Attempts to prevent dysrhythmias by giving antidysrhythmic drugs *prophylactically* have failed to reduce mortality. Worse yet, attempted prophylaxis of ventricular dysrhythmias with two drugs—encainide and flecainide—actually *increased* mortality. Similarly, when quinidine was employed to prevent supraventricular dysrhythmias, it too increased mortality. Therefore, since prophylaxis with antidysrhythmic drugs does not reduce mortality—and may in fact increase mortality—antidysrhythmic drugs should be withheld until a dysrhythmia actually occurs.

Cardiogenic Shock

Shock results from greatly reduced tissue perfusion secondary to impaired cardiac function. Shock develops in 7% to 10% of patients in the first few days after MI and has a mortality rate of up to 50% in hospitalized patients. Patients at highest risk are those with large infarcts, a previous infarct, a low ejection fraction (less than 35%), diabetes, and advanced age. Drug therapy includes inotropic agents (e.g., dopamine, dobutamine) to increase cardiac output and vasodilators (nitroglycerin, nitroprusside) to improve tissue perfusion and to reduce cardiac work and oxygen demand. Unfortunately, although these drugs can improve hemodynamic status, they do not seem to reduce mortality. Restoration of cardiac perfusion with PCI or coronary artery bypass grafting may be of value.

Heart Failure

Heart failure secondary to acute MI can be treated with a combination of drugs. A diuretic (e.g., furosemide) is given to decrease preload and pulmonary congestion. Inotropic agents (e.g., digoxin) increase cardiac output by enhancing contractility. Vasodilators (e.g., nitroglycerin, nitroprusside) improve hemodynamic status by reducing preload, afterload, or both. ACE inhibitors (or ARBs), which reduce both preload and afterload, can be especially helpful. Beta blockers may also improve outcome. Drug therapy of heart failure is discussed in Chapter 48.

Cardiac Rupture

Weakening of the myocardium predisposes the heart wall to rupture. Following rupture, shock and circulatory collapse develop rapidly. Death is often immediate. Fortunately, cardiac rupture is relatively rare (less than 2% incidence). Patients at highest risk are those with a large anterior infarction. Cardiac rupture is most likely within the first days after MI. Early treatment with vasodilators and beta blockers may reduce the risk of wall rupture.

SECONDARY PREVENTION OF STEMI

As a rule, patients who survive the acute phase of STEMI can be discharged from the hospital as early as 72 hours after admission if they remain free of complications. However, they are still at risk of reinfarction (5% to 15% incidence within the first year) and other complications (e.g., dysrhythmias, heart failure). Outcome can be improved with risk factor reduction, exercise, and long-term therapy with drugs.

Reduction of risk factors for MI can increase long-term survival. Patients who smoke must be encouraged to quit; the goal is total cessation. Patients with high serum cholesterol should be given an appropriate dietary plan and, if necessary, treated with a high-dose statin. Hypertension and diabetes increase the risk of mortality and must be controlled. For patients with hypertension, blood pressure should be decreased to below 140/90 mm Hg. For patients with diabetes, the goal is a level of hemoglobin A1C below 7%.

Exercise training can be valuable for two reasons: it reduces complications associated with prolonged bed rest and it accelerates return to an optimal level of functioning. The goal is 30 minutes of exercise at least 3 to 4 days a week. Although exercise is safe for most patients, there is concern about cardiac risk and impairment of infarct healing in patients whose infarct is large.

All post-MI patients should take four drugs: (1) a beta blocker; (2) an ACE inhibitor or an ARB; either (3a) an antiplatelet drug (aspirin or clopidogrel, ticagrelor, or prasugrel) or (3b) an anticoagulant (warfarin); and (4) a statin. All four should be taken indefinitely.

Estrogen therapy for postmenopausal women is not effective as secondary prevention and should not be initiated.

KEY POINTS

- MI is necrosis of the myocardium secondary to acute occlusion of a coronary artery. The usual cause is platelet plugging and thrombus formation at the site of a ruptured atherosclerotic plaque.
- STEMI is diagnosed by the presence of chest pain, characteristic ECG changes, and elevated serum levels of cardiac troponins.
- Aspirin suppresses platelet aggregation, decreasing mortality, reinfarction, and stroke. All patients should chew a 162- to 325-mg dose on hospital admission and should take 81 to 162 mg/day indefinitely after discharge. In patients undergoing acute STEMI, beta blockers reduce cardiac pain, infarct size, short-term mortality, recurrent ischemia, and reinfarction. Continued use increases

long-term survival. All patients should receive a beta blocker in the absence of specific contraindications.

- Oxygen, morphine, and nitroglycerin are considered routine therapy for suspected STEMI. They should be started, as appropriate, soon after symptom onset.
- Reperfusion therapy, which restores blood flow through blocked coronary arteries, is the most beneficial treatment for STEMI.
- Reperfusion can be accomplished with PCI or with fibrinolytic drugs. Both approaches are highly effective, but PCI is now generally preferred.
- PCI usually consists of balloon angioplasty coupled with placement of a drug-eluting stent.
- Fibrinolytic drugs dissolve clots by converting plasminogen into plasmin, an enzyme that digests the fibrin meshwork that holds clots together.
- Typically, all fibrinolytic drugs are equally effective. However, when treatment is initiated within 4 to 6 hours of pain onset, alteplase is most effective.
- The major complication of fibrinolytic therapy is bleeding. Intracranial hemorrhage is the greatest concern.
- Heparin is recommended for all patients undergoing fibrinolytic therapy or PCI.
- Aspirin (an antiplatelet drug) combined with clopidogrel is recommended for all patients undergoing reperfusion therapy with a fibrinolytic drug.
- Glycoprotein IIb/IIIa inhibitors (e.g., abciximab) are powerful IV antiplatelet drugs that can enhance the benefits of primary PCI.
- In patients with acute MI, ACE inhibitors decrease mortality, severe heart failure, and recurrent MI. All patients should receive an ACE inhibitor in the absence of specific contraindications. For patients who cannot tolerate ACE inhibitors, an ARB may be used instead.
- To lower the risk of a second MI, all patients should decrease cardiovascular risk factors (e.g., smoking, hypercholesterolemia, hypertension, diabetes), exercise for 30 minutes at least 3 or 4 days a week, and undergo long-term therapy with four drugs: a beta blocker, an ACE inhibitor or an ARB, an antiplatelet drug or warfarin, and a statin.

Please visit **http://evolve.elsevier.com/Lehne** for chapter-specific NCLEX® examination review questions.

CHAPTER

54 Drugs for Hemophilia

Hemophilia is a rare genetic bleeding disorder seen almost exclusively in males. About 70% of cases result from inheriting a defective gene from the mother. The other 30% result from a spontaneous gene mutation.

Hemophilia has two forms: hemophilia A and hemophilia B. In hemophilia A, there is a deficiency of clotting factor VIII (aka antihemophilic factor). In hemophilia B, there is a deficiency of clotting factor IX (aka Christmas factor, named for Stephen Christmas, the first boy diagnosed with the disease). Hemophilia A is about 6 times more prevalent than hemophilia B, occurring in 1 of every 5000 males, compared with 1 of every 30,000 males for hemophilia B.

When hemophilia is managed well, the prognosis is good. Patients starting treatment today can live healthy, near-normal lives. The foundation of treatment is clotting factor replacement, which may be given on a regular schedule (to prevent bleeds from occurring) or "on demand" (to stop an ongoing bleed). Unfortunately, although treatment is highly effective, it is also very expensive: For patients undergoing prophylactic treatment, the cost for clotting factors alone ranges between $60,000 and $150,000 a year.

BASIC CONSIDERATIONS

Pathophysiology

In people with hemophilia, there is a failure of hemostasis, the process by which bleeding is stopped. As discussed in Chapter 52, hemostasis occurs in two stages: (1) formation of a platelet plug followed by (2) production of fibrin, a protein that reinforces the platelet plug. In patients with hemophilia, platelet aggregation proceeds normally, but fibrin production does not. The underlying problem is a deficiency of clotting factors—specifically, factor VIII (in hemophilia A) and factor IX (in hemophilia B). As shown in Fig. 54.1, both factors are part of the contact activation (intrinsic) coagulation pathway, and both—in their activated forms—are needed to catalyze the conversion of factor X to *its* active form (factor Xa), which in turn catalyzes the conversion of prothrombin to thrombin, which catalyzes the formation of fibrin. If either factor VIII or factor IX is deficient, the contact activation pathway will not work properly, causing clot formation to be delayed. As a result, bleeding will continue longer than in the population at large.

It should be noted that the degree of factor deficiency—and thus the likelihood of serious bleeding—depends on the nature of the underlying gene mutation. In some patients, the mutation produces a severe deficiency, resulting in a high probability of prolonged bleeding. In others, the mutation causes mild deficiency, so the tendency to bleed is low.

Inheritance Pattern

The genes for factors VIII and IX are *recessive,* and both are carried on the X chromosome. Because males have only one X chromosome, a male with a defective gene will have hemophilia. In contrast, a female with a defective gene on one X chromosome will usually be an asymptomatic carrier, since she still has a functioning gene on her other X chromosome. Be aware, however, that although females are usually asymptomatic carriers, there are two situations in which females *can* have hemophilia: (1) a female could be born with defective genes on *both* X chromosomes, which is rare; and (2) a female who was born with one defective gene could experience *inactivation* of the good gene. Boys whose mothers are carriers have a 1 in 2 chance of inheriting the disease. Girls whose mothers are carriers have a 1 in 2 chance of being carriers themselves. Males with hemophilia cannot pass the disease on to their sons, but all of their daughters will be carriers. The risk of acquiring hemophilia is shared by all races and ethnic groups.

Clinical Features

Hemophilia may be severe, moderate, or mild, depending on the degree of clotting factor deficiency. Patients with severe hemophilia may experience life-threatening hemorrhage in response to minor trauma, whereas those with mild hemophilia may experience little or no excessive bleeding. Table 54.1 presents the defining characteristics of severe, moderate, and mild hemophilia.

Severe Hemophilia

In patients with severe hemophilia, the concentration of clotting factor VIII or IX is very low—less than 1% of normal. As a result, these patients experience frequent bleeds within joints and soft tissues, especially muscle. Trauma or surgery can cause profuse hemorrhage. Joint bleeding occurs most often in the knee, followed in turn by the elbow, ankle, shoulder, and hip. Bleeding in these joints causes swelling and intense

TABLE 54.1 ▪ Clinical Classification of Hemophilia Severity

Disease Parameter	Disease Severity: Severe	Moderate	Mild
Clotting factor level (VIII or IX)	Less than 1% of normal	Between 1% and 5% of normal	Between 6% and 49% of normal
Bleeding tendency	Can bleed with very mild injury	Can bleed with moderate injury	Can bleed with severe injury, surgery, or invasive procedures
Bleeding frequency	May bleed once or twice a week	May bleed once a month	May never have a bleeding episode
Occurrence of joint bleeding	Frequent	Less frequent	Infrequent, but can occur in response to severe injury

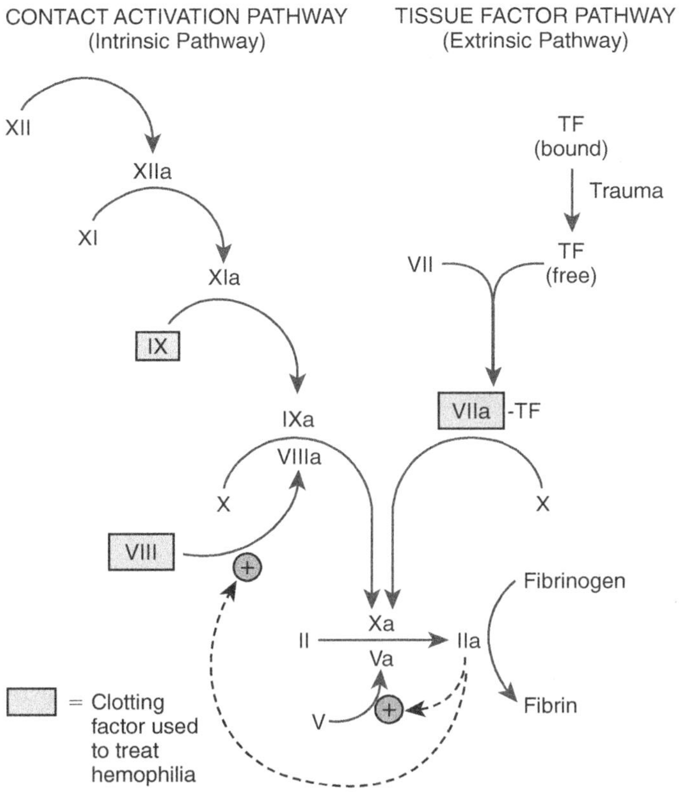

Fig. 54.1 ▪ The coagulation cascade showing clotting factors used to treat hemophilia.

TF, tissue factor. Common names for factors shown in roman numerals: II, prothrombin; IIa, thrombin; VII, proconvertin; VIII, antihemophilic factor; IX, Christmas factor; X, Stuart factor; XI, plasma thromboplastin antecedent; and XII, Hageman factor. The letter "a" after a factor's name (e.g., factor VIIIa) indicates the active form of the factor. Note that factors VIII and IX, which are deficient in hemophilia A and B, respectively, are part of the contact activation (intrinsic) coagulation pathway. The symbol [⊕] indicates acceleration of the reaction.

pain. With recurrent episodes, permanent injury to the joint develops. In addition to occurring in joints, bleeding may occur in muscles, mucous membranes (e.g., nosebleeds), the GI and urinary tracts, near the pharynx (which can cause life-threatening restriction of airflow), and within the skull (which carries a 30% risk of death). Among patients with hemophilia A, about 60% have severe disease. In contrast, among patients with hemophilia B, only 20% to 45% have severe disease. Although severe hemophilia can be devastating, most patients can live normal and productive lives, thanks to the availability of safe factor concentrates for replacement therapy.

PATIENT-CENTERED CARE ACROSS THE LIFE SPAN

Drugs for Hemophilia

Life Stage	Patient Care Concerns
Infants	See "Breast-feeding women," below.
Children/adolescents	Factor replacement and desmopressin can be used safely in children, just in smaller doses. Side effect profiles are similar to those of adults.
Pregnant women	Factor VIII and factor IX concentrates are classified in U.S. Food and Drug Administration Pregnancy Risk Category C.[a] There have been no controlled human studies. Weigh risk versus benefit.
Breast-feeding women	Caution is advised when breast-feeding. There is a lack of data regarding antihemophilic factors in human milk.
Older adults	Patients with hemophilia are now living longer secondary to treatment. Individualized doses are suggested for many of the drugs in this chapter. Cumulative inhibitor risk increases with age.

[a]As of 2020, the FDA will no longer use Pregnancy Risk Categories. Please refer to Chapter 9 for more information.

Moderate Hemophilia

In patients with moderate hemophilia, the concentration of factor VIII or factor IX is between 1% and 5% of normal. Excessive bleeding in response to minor trauma is unlikely. However, serious bleeding *can* be induced by significant trauma, tooth extractions, and surgery. Joint bleeding may occur, but the frequency is much lower than with severe hemophilia.

Mild Hemophilia

In patients with mild hemophilia, the concentration of clotting factors is between 6% and 49% of normal. Joint bleeding is uncommon, but can be induced by severe injury or surgery.

Overview of Therapy

Whenever possible, treatment should be guided by a team of specialists at a hemophilia treatment center. Typically, the team consists of a hematologist, orthopedist, dietitian, psychologist, physical therapist, occupational therapist, genetics counselor, infectious disease specialist, social worker, and nurse coordinator.

The cornerstone of treatment is *replacement therapy* with factor VIII (hemophilia A) or factor IX (hemophilia B). In the past, factor replacement was performed only to terminate a bleeding episode. Today, however, there is increasing emphasis on primary prophylaxis, especially for young children. By minimizing bleeding episodes, prophylaxis can minimize long-term damage to joints.

For some patients with mild *hemophilia A,* bleeding can be stopped with *desmopressin,* a drug that promotes release of factor VIII from the vascular endothelium. Desmopressin has the advantage of being much cheaper than factor VIII, and can be administered by nasal spray as well as by IV infusion. Keep in mind, however, that repeated use of desmopressin can deplete stored factor VIII, making the drug ineffective until more factor VIII is made.

Antifibrinolytic drugs (i.e., drugs that prevent the breakdown of fibrin) can be used as adjuncts to factors VIII and IX in special situations, such as tooth extractions. Two antifibrinolytic drugs are available: aminocaproic acid and tranexamic acid.

In some patients receiving factor VIII or factor IX, antibodies against the factor develop. These antibodies, referred to as *inhibitors,* prevent the factor from working. When inhibitors are present, bleeding can be stopped by infusing *activated factor VII recombinant.* Other treatments are also available, as discussed under *Managing Patients Who Develop Inhibitors.*

Pain Management

How should we manage bleeding-related pain? For mild pain, *acetaminophen* [Tylenol, others] is the drug of choice. For severe pain, an *opioid analgesic* may be needed. Regardless of pain severity, *aspirin should be avoided* because aspirin causes irreversible inhibition of platelet aggregation and can thus increase bleeding risk. Aspirin can also induce GI ulceration and bleeding, an obvious problem.

Can we use nonsteroidal anti-inflammatory drugs (NSAIDs) other than aspirin? As a rule, these agents should also be avoided. Like aspirin, most NSAIDs inhibit platelet aggregation (although the inhibition is reversible rather than irreversible). Also, like aspirin, most NSAIDs can promote GI ulceration and bleeding (although the risk is somewhat lower than with aspirin).

What about the second-generation NSAIDs, known as cyclooxygenase-2 (COX-2) inhibitors? As discussed in Chapter 71, the COX-2 inhibitors (e.g., celecoxib) do not suppress platelet aggregation, and they cause less GI ulceration and bleeding than traditional NSAIDs. Accordingly, these agents are clearly preferred to traditional NSAIDs, although their safety in hemophilia has not been proved.

Immunization

Children with hemophilia should undergo the normal immunization schedule (see Chapter 68). Some clinicians inject vaccines subQ, rather than IM, to avoid muscle hemorrhage. However, since the efficacy of subQ vaccination is not certain, and since most patients tolerate IM injections without bleeding, IM vaccination is generally preferred. The risk of bleeding after IM injection can be reduced by prolonged application of pressure.

To minimize the risk of hepatitis, all patients with newly diagnosed hemophilia should be vaccinated for hepatitis A and hepatitis B, as should all other patients with hemophilia who are not seropositive for hepatitis A or B. Family members who administer clotting factors at home should also be immunized, provided they test negative for hepatitis.

PREPARATIONS USED TO TREAT HEMOPHILIA

Factor VIII Concentrates

Factor VIII concentrates are the mainstay of hemophilia A treatment. A concentrate is a powdered formulation in which the amount of factor VIII is very high. When treatment is needed, the powder is dissolved in a sterile solution and administered IV.

All factor VIII concentrates available today are very safe. They carry essentially no risk of HIV/AIDS, and little or no risk of hepatitis.

Prototype Drugs

DRUGS FOR HEMOPHILIA

Factor VIII concentrates
Factor IX concentrates
Desmopressin

Production Methods and Product Safety

Factor VIII concentrates are made in two basic ways: (1) purification from human plasma and (2) production in cell culture using recombinant DNA technology. Recombinant factor VIII is somewhat safer than plasma-derived factor VIII, but is also more expensive. All factor VIII products, whether recombinant or plasma derived, are equally effective. Available products are shown in Table 54.2.

Plasma-Derived Factor VIII. Before 1985, factor VIII produced from donor plasma often contained viral contaminants. As a result, nearly all people with hemophilia developed hepatitis and/or HIV/AIDS. Today, however, the risk of viral contamination is exceedingly low. Donated plasma is now screened for viral pathogens—specifically, human immunodeficiency virus (HIV), hepatitis A virus (HAV), hepatitis B virus (HBV), hepatitis C virus (HCV), and parvovirus B19. Techniques for inactivating *lipid-coated* viruses (HIV, HBV, and HCV) are also employed. Unfortunately, viruses that lack a lipid coat, such as HAV and parvovirus B19, are not eliminated.

There is one additional concern: *prions.* These strange proteins, which are responsible for Creutzfeldt-Jakob disease (CJD, the human form of "mad cow disease"), are not susceptible

TABLE 54.2 ▪ Some Factor VIII and Factor IX Concentrates

Type of Preparation	Factor VIII	Factor IX
RECOMBINANT		
Third generation	Advate Xyntha	BeneFix
Second generation	Helixate FS Kogenate FS	
First generation	Recombinate	
PLASMA-DERIVED		
Ultrapure	Hemofil-M Monoclate-P Wilate[a,b]	AlphaNine SD Bebulin[c] Mononine Profilnine SD[c]
Intermediate and high purity	Alphanate[a] Koate-DVI[a] Humate-P[a]	

[a]Contains von Willebrand factor in addition to factor VIII.
[b]Approved only for von Willebrand's disease.
[c]Contains factors II, VII, and X, in addition to factor IX.

to any known inactivation technique, so the possibility of transmitting CJD remains.

Plasma-derived factor VIII is available in varying degrees of purity. The ultrapure products (e.g., Hemofil-M) are prepared using monoclonal antibodies.

Recombinant Factor VIII. Recombinant factor VIII has traditionally been produced in culture, using hamster cells that have been genetically transformed. We now have a product called hrFVIII that was developed in a human host cell. All recombinant factor VIII products are very safe and are considered the agents of choice for treating hemophilia A.

During the manufacturing process, most recombinant factor VIII products are exposed to bovine serum albumin (BSA), human serum albumin (HSA), or both. Because BSA or HSA could, in theory, be a source of viruses or prions, manufacturing processes that reduce the use of BSA and HSA have been developed. As a result, we now have three "generations" of recombinant products:

- *First-generation product*—Recombinate—is made using BSA in the cell culture, and contains HSA as a stabilizer in the vial.
- *Second-generation products*—Helixate FS and Kogenate FS—are made using HSA in the cell culture, but they contain neither BSA nor HSA in the vial.
- *Third-generation products*—Advate and Xyntha—are not exposed to BSA or HSA during cell culture, and they contain neither BSA nor HSA in the vial.

Theoretically, the third-generation products—Advate and Xyntha—which are never exposed to any proteins of animal or human origin, are safer than the first- or second-generation products. However, there are no published data showing this is the case. With all three generations, the risk of human viral contamination is essentially zero. Transmission of HIV, HBV, or HCV has not been reported.

Safety Alert

FACTOR VIII CONCENTRATES

Factor VIII concentrates can cause allergic reactions, which can range from mild to severe. Symptoms of a mild reaction include hives, rash, urticaria, stuffy nose, and fever. These can be managed with an antihistamine (e.g., diphenhydramine [Benadryl]). Rarely, anaphylaxis may develop. Symptoms of this potentially fatal reaction include wheezing, tightness in the throat, shortness of breath, and swelling in the face. The treatment of choice is epinephrine, injected subQ.

Dosage and Administration

On-Demand Therapy. On-demand therapy is indicated for patients who are bleeding or about to undergo surgery. As a rule, administration is by slow IV push done over 5 to 10 minutes. Continuous infusion may also be done, but only by a clinician with special training.

Dosage depends primarily on the site and severity of the bleed. Table 54.3 shows approximate dosages for a variety of bleeding situations. The dosing target is expressed as a percentage of normal factor VIII activity. For example, when treating a joint bleed, the dosing target is 40% of the normal activity level.

How can we calculate dosage? By knowing that *for each unit of factor VIII we give per kilogram of body weight, we will raise factor VIII activity in plasma by 2%.* Therefore, to calculate dosage, we simply multiply the patient's weight by the target activity level for factor VIII and then divide by 2. To help guide dosing, we can measure factor VIII activity in plasma before and after treatment. However, although knowledge of factor VIII activity is helpful, dosage is ultimately determined by the clinical response.

Prophylactic Therapy. For prophylaxis, factor VIII is administered on a regular schedule. The goal is to *prevent* bleeding and thereby prevent life-threatening hemorrhage and long-term injury to joints. Children with severe hemophilia are the primary candidates for prophylaxis. Treatment is often done at home. The goal is to maintain factor VIII activity above 1% of normal. As a rule, this can be achieved by infusing factor VIII concentrate every other day or 3 times a week. Recombinant factor VIII products are generally preferred, although plasma-derived products, which are just as effective and much less expensive, may also be used.

To facilitate frequent IV administration, a central venous access device can be installed. Options include an external catheter (e.g., Hickman catheter) or an implanted venous port (e.g., Port-A-Cath). Both types of device are intended for long-term use and can remain in place for several years. It should be noted, however, that although these devices make prophylaxis much easier, they do carry risks, especially infection and thrombosis.

Factor IX Concentrates

Therapeutic Use, Production, and Safety

Factor IX concentrates are the mainstay of treatment for hemophilia B. The pharmacology of these concentrates is nearly identical to that of the factor VIII concentrates. Like the factor

TABLE 54.3 ■ Estimated Dosages for Factor VIII and Factor IX

Type of Hemorrhage	Target Activity Level[a] Factor VIII (Hemophilia A)	Factor IX (Hemophilia B)
Joint	40%–60%	40%–60%
Muscle (except the iliopsoas muscle)	40%–60%	40%–60%
Iliopsoas muscle[b]		
Initial	80%–100%	60%–80%
Maintenance	30%–60%	30%–60%
CNS/Head		
Initial	80%–100%	60%–80%
Maintenance	50%	30%
Throat and neck		
Initial	80%–100%	60%–80%
Maintenance	50%	30%
Gastrointestinal		
Initial	80%–100%	60%–80%
Maintenance	50%	30%
Renal	50%	40%
Deep laceration	50%	40%
Surgical		
Initial	80%–100%	60%–80%
Maintenance	50%	50%

[a]Target activity levels are expressed as a percentage of normal activity level.
[b]The iliopsoas is a compound muscle consisting of the iliacus and psoas major muscles, located in the groin region.
CNS, Central nervous system.
Data from World Federation of Hemophilia: Guidelines for the Management of Hemophilia. 2012. (Available as of February 6, 2014, at www.wfh.org/en/resources/wfh-treatment-guidelines.)

VIII concentrates, the factor IX concentrates are made either by extraction from donor plasma or by recombinant DNA technology. None of the products in current use poses a risk of HIV/AIDS. However, the plasma-derived products may carry a very small risk of hepatitis A, parvovirus B19, or CJD. Because recombinant factor IX [BeneFix] is, in theory, safer than plasma-derived factor IX [Bebulin, Mononine, Profilnine SD, others], recombinant factor IX is considered the preparation of choice. Like factor VIII, factor IX can cause allergic reactions.

Dosage and Administration

On-Demand Therapy. On-demand therapy, administered by IV push, should be initiated at the earliest sign of bleeding. As with factor VIII, dosage is determined primarily by the site and severity of bleeding. However, factors VIII and IX differ in that, on a unit-per-kilogram (unit/kg) basis, we need twice as much factor IX to achieve an equivalent increase in plasma factor level. Hence, with factor IX, *for each unit we give per kilogram of body weight, we will raise the plasma activity level by 1%* (compared with 2% for each unit/kg of factor VIII). To calculate dosage, we simply multiply the patient's weight by the target factor IX activity level (expressed as a percentage of normal factor IX activity level), as in this example:

$$50\,(\text{kg body weight}) \times 40\,(\text{target }\%) = 2000\,(\text{units of factor IX})$$

As with factor VIII therapy, we can measure plasma levels of factor IX activity to guide treatment—although the dose depends ultimately on the clinical response.

Prophylactic Therapy. As with factor VIII, prophylaxis is done to prevent bleeding and thus prevent injury to joints. The dosing goal is to maintain factor IX levels above 1% of normal. Because factor IX has a longer half-life than factor VIII (18 to 24 hours vs. 8 to 12 hours), prophylaxis can be done less often (twice a week rather than 3 times a week). The usual dose is 20 to 40 units/kg.

Desmopressin

Therapeutic Use

Desmopressin [DDAVP, Stimate], an analog of antidiuretic hormone, can stop or prevent bleeding in patients with *mild* hemophilia A. The drug works by releasing stored factor VIII from the vascular endothelium. Levels of factor VIII begin to rise within 30 minutes of dosing and to peak within 90 to 120 minutes. Desmopressin can be used to stop episodes of trauma-induced bleeding and can be given preoperatively to maintain hemostasis during surgery. Desmopressin does not release factor IX and so cannot be used to treat hemophilia B. Principal adverse effects are fluid retention and hyponatremia. The basic pharmacology of desmopressin, along with its use in hypothalamic diabetes insipidus, is discussed in Chapter 59.

Preparations, Dosage, and Administration

For treatment of hemophilia A, desmopressin may be administered IV or by intranasal spray. An oral formulation is available, but is not indicated for hemophilia.

For *intravenous therapy,* desmopressin [DDAVP] is formulated in a concentrated solution (4 mcg/mL) that must be diluted in 0.9% saline. The usual dosage is 0.3 mcg/kg infused over 15 to 30 minutes.

For *intranasal therapy,* desmopressin is available under two brand names: *DDAVP,* which delivers 10 mcg/spray, and *Stimate,* which delivers 150 mcg/spray. Only Stimate is used for hemophilia. For patients who weigh 50 kg or more, the dosage is 150 mcg/nostril, for a total of 300 mcg. For patients who weigh less than 50 kg, the dosage is one spray (150 mcg) in just one nostril.

Antifibrinolytic Agents

Antifibrinolytic agents inhibit the normal process of fibrin breakdown. When a clot is no longer needed, an enzyme called *plasmin* dissolves the fibrin meshwork that holds the clot together and thereby promotes clot removal. Unfortunately, in people with hemophilia, fibrin breakdown can lead to a resumption of bleeding. Accordingly, by preserving fibrin with an antifibrinolytic drug, we can help keep bleeding under control. Because of their mechanism, antifibrinolytic drugs are most useful for *preventing recurrent* bleeding and less useful for stopping an ongoing bleed.

Two antifibrinolytic drugs are currently available: *aminocaproic acid* and *tranexamic acid.* Both agents act primarily by preventing the formation of plasmin from its precursor (plasminogen). These drugs are most useful for controlling bleeding in mucous membranes (of the nose, mouth, and throat), as well as bleeding caused by dental extractions—presumably because fibrinolytic activity at all of these sites is especially high.

Aminocaproic Acid

Aminocaproic acid is available in solution (250 mg/mL) for IV use, and in tablets (500 and 1000 mg) and solution (250 mg/mL) for oral use. Dosages to prevent or treat serious bleeding are as follows:

- *Oral therapy, adults*—give 5 gm for the first hour, then 1 or 1.25 gm every hour

- *IV therapy, adults*—infuse 4 to 5 gm over the first hour, then infuse at a rate of 1 gm/hr
- *Oral therapy, children*—give 100 mg/kg for the first hour, then 33.3 mg/kg every hour
- *IV therapy, children*—infuse 100 mg/kg over the first hour, then infuse at a rate of 33.3 mg/kg/hr

In all cases, continue dosing for 8 hours or until bleeding stops.

Tranexamic Acid

For treatment of hemophilia, tranexamic acid [Cyklokapron] is available in solution (100 mg/mL) for IV dosing. To control bleeding associated with dental extractions, the recommended dosage is 10 mg/kg immediately before the extraction, followed by doses of 10 mg/kg 3 to 4 times a day for 2 to 8 days. Dosage should be decreased in patients with renal impairment.

As discussed in Chapter 64, an oral formulation of tranexamic acid, marketed as *Lysteda,* is used to treat heavy cyclic menstrual bleeding.

Managing Patients Who Develop Inhibitors

Patients receiving factor VIII or factor IX can develop antibodies against the factor. These antibodies, referred to as inhibitors, neutralize the clotting factor and thereby render factor replacement ineffective. In most cases, the antibodies develop early, typically after only 9 to 12 courses of treatment.

Some patients are more likely to develop inhibitors than others. Among patients with *severe* hemophilia A, between 20% and 30% develop antibodies to factor VIII, compared with 3% to 13% of those with *mild* hemophilia A. Among patients with severe hemophilia B, between 2% and 12% develop antibodies to factor IX. The risk of inhibitor development among African American and Hispanic patients is unusually high (up to 50%).

The titer of inhibitors to factor VIII is measured using the Bethesda assay. In this procedure, serial dilutions of patient plasma are mixed with an equal volume of normal plasma, after which factor VIII activity in the mixture is measured. The dilution that inhibits 50% of factor VIII activity defines the inhibitor titer. For example, if the 1:40 dilution inhibits 50% of the factor VIII activity, the patient is said to have a titer of 40 *Bethesda units* (BU) of factor VIII inhibitor.

For some patients, *immune tolerance therapy* (ITT) can eliminate inhibitor production. The procedure involves repeated administration of factor replacement products over an extended time. The success rate is high (63% to 83%) for patients with hemophilia A and very low for those with hemophilia B. A low antibody titer (less than 5 BU) increases the chances of success. If ITT fails to stop antibody production, then hemostasis must be achieved with drugs, as discussed in the sections that follow.

Drugs for Patients With Factor VIII Inhibitors

To control bleeding in patients with inhibitors to factor VIII, the preferred treatments are (1) activated factor VII and (2) anti-inhibitor coagulant complex. Neither option is clearly superior to the other. Accordingly, selection between them is based on previous response and prescriber preference.

Activated Factor VII (Factor VIIa). Factor VIIa [NovoSeven RT], manufactured by recombinant DNA technology, can control bleeding in patients with inhibitors to factor VIII or factor IX. Factor VIIa has the same action as factors VIII and IX. That is, it catalyzes the conversion of factor X to its active form. Therefore, by giving factor VIIa, we can bypass neutralization of factors VIII and IX and allow clotting to proceed normally.

Factor VIIa is generally well tolerated. No human proteins are used in making this agent, so there is no risk of transmitting a human virus. Rarely, thrombotic events have occurred—arterial thrombosis, cerebral sinus thrombosis, and myocardial infarction (MI). In most cases, these events were seen when NovoSeven RT was used off-label to stop bleeding in nonhemophiliacs, including patients with acute intracerebral hemorrhage.

Factor VIIa is supplied as a powder in single-use vials (1, 2, 5, and 8 mg) and must be reconstituted with a prepackaged diluent before use. Administration is by IV bolus. The usual dosage is 90 mcg/kg, repeated every 2 hours until bleeding stops. However, some patients require much higher doses (e.g., 300 mcg/kg). Treatment is very expensive: A single 90-mcg/kg dose for a 70-kg patient costs about $13,000. The drug should be stored under refrigeration.

Anti-Inhibitor Coagulant Complex (AICC). AICC [Feiba[a]], made from pooled human plasma, contains variable amounts of clotting factors II, VII, IX, and X—in both their activated and nonactivated forms. AICC is indicated for patients with inhibitors to factor VIII or factor IX who are bleeding or about to undergo surgery. Benefits are believed to derive from factors VIIa and Xa, which bypass factors VIII and IX in the coagulation cascade.

Because AICC is made from human plasma, there is a theoretical risk of transmitting viral or prion disease. AICC also contains multiple coagulation factors, so it poses a risk of thrombotic complications, specifically MI and disseminated intravascular coagulation (DIC). Fortunately, these events are very rare. The risk of MI or DIC is increased with repeated dosing and by liver disease.

Preparations of Feiba are standardized in *units.* The usual dosage is 50 to 100 units/kg, infused IV at a rate no faster than 2 units/kg/min. Dosing can be repeated every 6 hours, but the total daily dose must not exceed 200 units/kg.

Factor VIII Concentrate. If the inhibitor titer is very low (< 5 BU), we may be able to overcome inhibition with high doses of factor VIII itself. However, if the inhibitor titer is high, then factor VIII will not work, and the agents previously discussed must be employed.

Porcine Factor VIII. Porcine factor VIII (factor VIII from pigs) can establish hemostasis in patients with hemophilia A who have developed antibodies to human factor VIII. Porcine factor VIII may be produced in two ways: by extraction from pig blood and by recombinant DNA technology. Recombinant porcine factor VIII is now in clinical trials.

Antibodies to human factor VIII can cross-react with porcine factor VIII. However, the degree of cross-reactivity is low. Accordingly, if the antibody titer is not too high (≤ 50 BU/mL), porcine factor VIII is likely to work. If the titer exceeds 50 BU/mL, significant neutralization of the porcine factor can occur.

Drugs for Patients With Factor IX Inhibitors

Treatment options for patients with factor IX inhibitors are limited. In contrast to factor VIII inhibitors, which may be overcome with large doses of human factor VIII or porcine factor VIII, factor IX inhibitors are difficult to overcome with any preparation of factor IX available. Furthermore, elimination of factor IX inhibitors with ITT often fails. Currently, factor VIIa and AICC are the treatments of choice. Both options are effective because they bypass the blockade caused by the inhibitor.

[a]Feiba stands for factor VIII inhibitor bypassing activity.

KEY POINTS

- Hemophilia is a bleeding disorder seen almost exclusively in males. The underlying cause is a genetically based deficiency of clotting factors.
- Hemophilia has two forms: hemophilia A (factor VIII deficiency) and hemophilia B (factor IX deficiency).
- Hemophilia may be severe, moderate, or mild, depending on the degree of clotting factor deficiency.
- Patients with severe hemophilia may experience life-threatening hemorrhage in response to minor trauma, whereas those with mild hemophilia may experience little or no excessive bleeding.
- Repeated bleeding in the knee and other joints can cause permanent joint damage.
- The cornerstone of hemophilia treatment is replacement therapy with factor VIII (hemophilia A) or factor IX (hemophilia B).
- Replacement therapy may be done prophylactically (to prevent bleeding and thus prevent joint injury) or on demand (to stop an ongoing bleed or to prevent excessive bleeding during surgery).
- Clotting factor products are made in two basic ways: extraction from donor plasma and production in cell culture using recombinant DNA technology.
- All clotting factor concentrates, whether plasma derived or recombinant, are equally effective.
- All clotting factor concentrates in use today are very safe: They carry no risk of transmitting HIV/AIDS and little or no risk of transmitting hepatis or CJD. However, because recombinant factors are, in theory, slightly safer than plasma-derived factors, recombinant factors are considered the treatment of choice.
- As a rule, clotting factors are given by slow IV push. Continuous infusion may also be done, but only by a clinician with special training.
- Clotting factor dosage depends primarily on the site and severity of the bleed.
- A dose of 1 unit of factor VIII/kg will raise the plasma level of factor VIII activity by 2%, whereas 1 unit of factor IX/kg will raise the plasma level of factor IX activity by only 1%.
- Although we can monitor the activity of clotting factors in blood to help guide treatment, dosage is ultimately determined by the clinical response.
- For prophylaxis, clotting factor concentrates are administered on a regular schedule, usually every other day to 3 times a week for factor VIII and twice a week for factor IX. With both factors, the goal is to maintain plasma factor levels above 1% of normal.
- To facilitate frequent IV administration during prophylaxis, a central venous access device can be installed.
- Clotting factor concentrates can cause allergic reactions. Mild reactions can be managed with an antihistamine (e.g., diphenhydramine [Benadryl]). The most severe reaction—anaphylaxis—is treated with subQ epinephrine.
- For some patients with mild hemophilia A, bleeding can be stopped with desmopressin, a drug that promotes the release of stored factor VIII. Desmopressin does not release factor IX, and so cannot treat hemophilia B.
- Two drugs—aminocaproic acid and tranexamic acid—can suppress fibrinolysis and can promote hemostasis in hemophilia A and hemophilia B. These antifibrinolytic agents are more effective for preventing recurrent bleeding than for stopping an ongoing bleed.
- Development of inhibitors (antibodies that neutralize factor VIII or factor IX) is a serious complication of hemophilia therapy.
- Activated factor VII (factor VIIa) and AICC are preferred agents for controlling bleeding when inhibitors of factor VIII or factor IX are present.
- People with hemophilia should avoid aspirin and other traditional NSAIDs because these agents suppress platelet aggregation and promote GI ulceration and bleeding. Second-generation NSAIDs (COX-2 inhibitors) are *probably* safe.

Please visit **http://evolve.elsevier.com/Lehne** for chapter-specific NCLEX® examination review questions.

Summary of Major Nursing Implications[a]

FACTOR VIII AND FACTOR IX CONCENTRATES

Preadministration Assessment

Therapeutic Goal

Factor VIII is indicated for replacement therapy in patients with hemophilia A, and factor IX is indicated for replacement therapy in patients with hemophilia B.

Both factors may be given prophylactically (to prevent bleeding and subsequent joint injury) or "on demand" (to stop ongoing bleeding or prevent excessive bleeding during anticipated surgery).

Baseline Data

Obtain a baseline level for activity of factor VIII or factor IX.

Identifying High-Risk Patients

Use with *caution* in patients with a history of allergic reactions to the factor concentrate.

Summary of Major Nursing Implications[a]—cont'd

Implementation: Administration

Route

Intravenous.

Administration

Administer by slow IV push or continuous infusion.

Record the following each time you give a factor concentrate:

- Time and date
- Infusion site and rate
- Total dose
- Manufacturer, brand name, lot number, and expiration date of the factor concentrate

Teach home caregivers about:

- **The importance of having an assistant, who can give aid or call for help if complications arise**
- **The importance and proper method of hand washing**
- **Making dosage calculations**
- **Reconstituting the powdered factor concentrate**
- **Infusion technique**
- **Cleanup and waste disposal**
- **Recording the time, date, and other information listed in this section**

Ongoing Evaluation and Interventions

Evaluating Therapeutic Effects

Success is indicated by preventing bleeding (during prophylactic therapy) or controlling bleeding (during on-demand therapy). With both forms of therapy, monitoring activity levels of factor VIII or factor IX can help guide treatment.

Minimizing Adverse Effects

Allergic Reactions. Clotting factor concentrates can cause allergic reactions, ranging from mild to severe. **Inform patients about symptoms of mild reactions (e.g., hives, rash, urticaria, stuffy nose, fever), and advise them to take an antihistamine (e.g., diphenhydramine) if these occur. Inform patients about symptoms of anaphylaxis (wheezing, tightness in the throat, shortness of breath, swelling in the face), and instruct them to seek immediate emergency care if these develop.** The treatment of choice is epinephrine, injected subQ.

Minimizing Adverse Interactions

Aspirin. **Warn patients not to use aspirin, a drug that inhibits platelet aggregation and can cause GI ulceration and bleeding.**

NSAIDs Other Than Aspirin. **Advise patients that first-generation NSAIDs (e.g., ibuprofen, naproxen) have actions similar to those of aspirin, and hence should be avoided.**

Advise patients that second-generation NSAIDs (e.g., celecoxib), which do not inhibit platelets and cause minimal GI effects, are *probably* safe.

[a]Patient education information is highlighted as **blue text**.

CHAPTER

55 Drugs for Deficiency Anemias

Anemia is defined as a decrease in the number, size, or hemoglobin content of erythrocytes (red blood cells [RBCs]). Causes include blood loss, hemolysis, bone marrow dysfunction, and deficiencies of substances essential for RBC formation and maturation. Most deficiency anemias result from deficiency of iron, vitamin B_{12}, or folic acid. Accordingly, this chapter focuses on anemias caused by these deficiencies. To facilitate discussion, we begin by reviewing RBC development.

RED BLOOD CELL DEVELOPMENT

RBCs begin their development in the bone marrow and then mature in the blood. As developing RBCs grow and divide, they evolve through four stages (Fig. 55.1). In their earliest stage, RBCs lack hemoglobin and are known as *proerythroblasts.* In the next stage, they gain hemoglobin and are called *erythroblasts.* Both the erythroblasts and the proerythroblasts reside in bone marrow. After the erythroblast stage, RBCs evolve into *reticulocytes* (immature erythrocytes) and enter the systemic circulation. Following the reticulocyte stage, circulating RBCs reach full maturity and are referred to as *erythrocytes.*

Development of RBCs requires the cooperative interaction of several factors: bone marrow must be healthy; erythropoietin (a stimulant of RBC maturation) must be present; iron must be available for hemoglobin synthesis; and other factors, including vitamin B_{12} and folic acid, must be available to

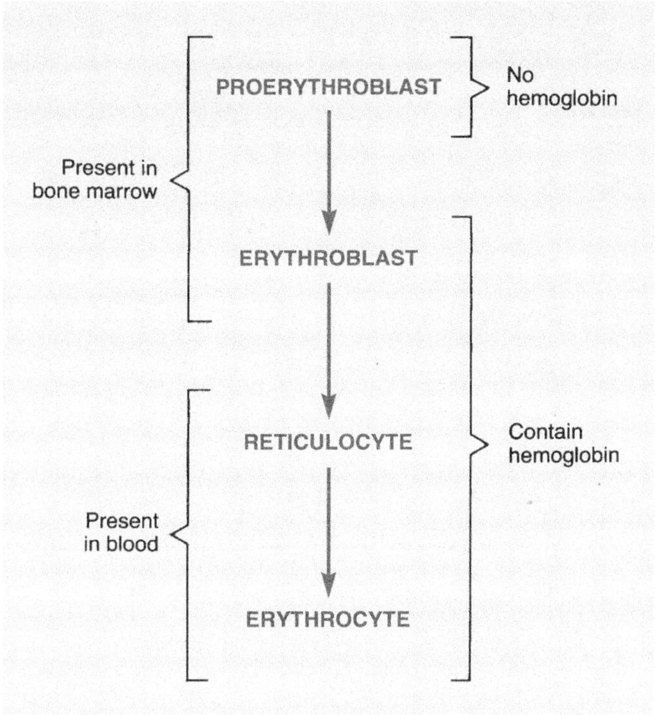

Fig. 55.1 ■ Stages of red blood cell development.

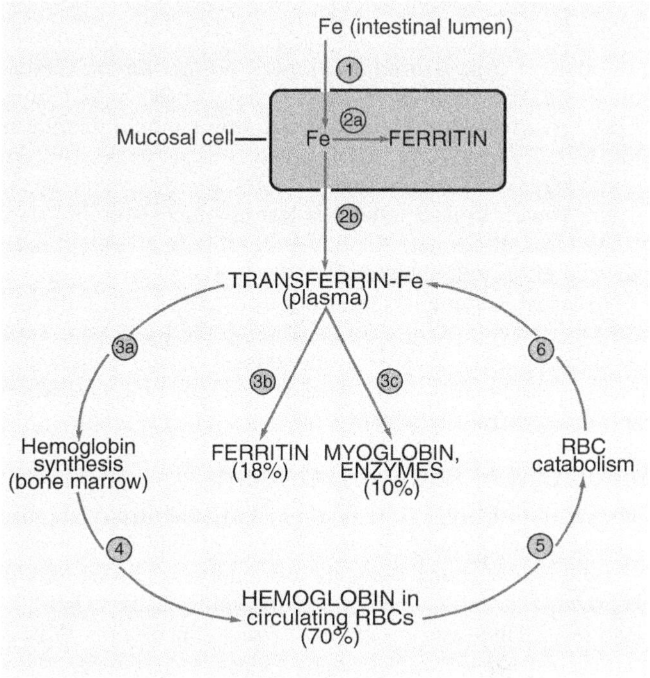

Fig. 55.2 ■ Fate of iron in the body.
Pathways labeled with circled numbers are explained in the text. Values in parentheses indicate percentage of total body stores. Elimination of iron is not shown, because most iron is rigidly conserved. (*Fe,* Iron; *RBC,* red blood cell.)

support synthesis of DNA. If any of these is absent or amiss, anemia will result.

IRON DEFICIENCY

Iron deficiency is the most common nutritional deficiency and the most common cause of nutrition-related anemia. Worldwide, people with iron deficiency number in the hundreds of millions. In the United States, about 5% of the population is iron deficient.

BIOCHEMISTRY AND PHYSIOLOGY OF IRON

To understand the consequences of iron deficiency, as well as the rationale behind iron therapy, we must first understand the biochemistry and physiology of iron. This information is reviewed here.

Metabolic Functions

Iron is essential to the function of hemoglobin, myoglobin (the oxygen-storing molecule of muscle), and a variety of iron-containing enzymes. Most (70% to 80%) of the body's iron is present in hemoglobin. A much smaller amount (10%) is present in myoglobin and iron-containing enzymes.

Fate in the Body

The major pathways for iron movement and utilization are shown in Fig. 55.2. In the discussion that follows, the numbers in parentheses refer to the circled numbers in the figure.

Uptake and Distribution

The life cycle of iron begins with (1) uptake of iron into mucosal cells of the small intestine. These cells absorb 5% to 20% of dietary iron. Their maximum absorptive capacity is 3 to 4 mg/day. Iron in the ferrous form (Fe^{++}) is absorbed more readily than iron in the ferric form (Fe^{+++}). Vitamin C enhances absorption, and food reduces absorption.

Following uptake, iron can either (2a) undergo storage within mucosal cells in the form of *ferritin* (a complex consisting of iron plus a protein used to store iron) or (2b) undergo binding to *transferrin* (the iron transport protein) for distribution throughout the body.

Utilization and Storage

Iron that is bound to transferrin can undergo one of three fates. The majority of transferrin-bound iron (3a) is taken up by cells of the bone marrow for incorporation into hemoglobin. Small amounts (3b) are taken up by the liver and other tissues for storage as ferritin. Lastly (3c), some of the iron in plasma is taken up by muscle (for production of myoglobin), and some is taken up by all other tissues (for production of iron-containing enzymes).

Recycling

As Fig. 55.2 depicts, iron associated with hemoglobin undergoes continuous recycling. After hemoglobin is made in bone marrow, iron re-enters the circulation (4) as a component of hemoglobin in erythrocytes. (The iron in circulating erythrocytes accounts for about 70% of total body iron.) After 120 days of useful life, RBCs are catabolized (5). Iron released by this process re-enters the plasma bound to transferrin (6), and then the cycle begins anew.

Elimination

Excretion of iron is minimal. Under normal circumstances, only 1 mg of iron is excreted each day. At this rate, if none of the lost iron were replaced, body stores would decline by only 10% a year.

Iron leaves the body by several routes. Most excretion occurs via the bowel. Iron in ferritin is lost as mucosal cells slough off, and iron also enters the bowel in bile. Small amounts are excreted in urine and sweat.

Note that, although very little iron leaves the body as a result of excretion (i.e., normal physiologic loss), substantial amounts can leave because of blood loss. Hence, menorrhagia (excessive menstrual flow), hemorrhage, and blood donations can all cause iron deficiency.

Regulation of Body Iron Content

The amount of iron in the body is regulated through control of intestinal absorption. As noted, most of the iron that enters the body stays in the body. If all dietary iron were readily absorbed, body iron content would rapidly accumulate to a toxic level. However, *excessive buildup is prevented through control of iron uptake: As body stores rise, uptake of iron declines; conversely, as body stores become depleted, uptake increases.* For example, when body stores of iron are high, only 2% to 3% of dietary iron is absorbed. In contrast, when body stores are depleted, as much as 20% may be absorbed.

Daily Requirements

Requirements for iron are determined largely by the rate of erythrocyte production. When RBC production is low, iron needs are low too. Conversely, when RBC production is high, iron needs rise. Accordingly, among infants and children—individuals whose rapid growth rate requires massive RBC synthesis—iron requirements are high (relative to body weight). In contrast, the daily iron needs of adults are relatively low. Adult men need only 8 mg of dietary iron each day. Adult women need considerably more (15 to 18 mg/day), to replace iron lost through menstruation.

During pregnancy, requirements for iron increase dramatically, owing to (1) expansion of maternal blood volume and (2) production of RBCs by the fetus. In most cases, the iron needs of pregnant women are too great to be met by diet alone. Consequently, iron supplements (about 27 mg/day) are recommended during pregnancy and for 2 to 3 months after delivery.

Table 55.1 shows the recommended dietary allowances (RDAs) of iron as a function of age. The RDA values in the table are about 10 times greater than actual physiologic need because, on average, only 10% of dietary iron is absorbed. Therefore, if physiologic requirements are to be met, the diet must contain 10 times more iron than we need.

Dietary Sources

Iron is available in foods of plant and animal origin. Foods especially rich in iron include egg yolk, brewer's yeast, and wheat germ. Other foods with high iron content include muscle meats, fish, fowl, cereal grains, beans, and green leafy vegetables. Foods that do not provide much iron include milk and most nongreen vegetables. Because iron can be extracted from cooking utensils, using iron pots and pans can augment dietary iron. Except for individuals who have very high iron requirements (infants, pregnant patients, those undergoing chronic blood loss), the average diet is sufficient to meet iron needs.

TABLE 55.1 ▪ Recommended Dietary Allowances (RDAs) for Iron

Life Stage	Age	RDA for Iron (mg/day)
Infants	7–12 mo	11
Children	1–3 yr	7
	4–8 yr	10
Males	9–13 yr	8
	14–18 yr	11
	≥ 19 yr	8
Females: nonpregnant, nonlactating	9–13 yr	8
	14–18 yr	15
	19–50 yr	18
	≥ 51 yr	8
Females: pregnant	14–50 yr	27[a]
Females: lactating	14–18 yr	10
	19–50 yr	9

[a]Iron requirements during pregnancy cannot be met through dietary sources alone, so supplements are recommended.

IRON DEFICIENCY: CAUSES, CONSEQUENCES, AND DIAGNOSIS

Causes

Iron deficiency results when there is an imbalance between iron uptake and iron demand. As a rule, the imbalance results from increased demand—not from reduced uptake. The most common causes of increased iron demand (and resulting iron deficiency) are (1) blood volume expansion during pregnancy coupled with RBC synthesis by the growing fetus; (2) blood volume expansion during infancy and early childhood; and (3) chronic blood loss, usually of GI or uterine origin. Rarely, iron deficiency results from reduced iron uptake; potential causes include gastrectomy and sprue.

Consequences

Iron deficiency has multiple effects, the most conspicuous being *iron deficiency anemia.* In the absence of iron for hemoglobin synthesis, red blood cells become *microcytic* (small) and *hypochromic* (pale). The reduced oxygen-carrying capacity of blood results in listlessness, fatigue, and pallor of the skin and mucous membranes. If tissue oxygenation is severely compromised, tachycardia, dyspnea, and angina may result. In addition to causing anemia, iron deficiency impairs myoglobin production and synthesis of iron-containing enzymes. In young children, iron deficiency can cause developmental problems, and in school-age children, iron deficiency may impair cognition.

Diagnosis

The hallmarks of iron deficiency anemia are (1) the presence of microcytic, hypochromic erythrocytes and (2) the absence

TABLE 55.2 ■ Iron Preparations Available for Oral Therapy

Iron Preparation	Brand Names	Description
Ferrous iron salts:		
Ferrous sulfate	Feosol, FeroSul, Slow FE, others	All four compounds are salts of the ferrous form of iron
Ferrous gluconate	Fergon, Floradix, others	
Ferrous fumarate	Ferro-Sequels, Hemocyte, Palafer ♣, others	
Ferrous aspartate	FE Aspartate	
Ferrous bisglycinate	Ferrochel, others	An iron–amino acid chelate
Ferric ammonium citrate	Iron Citrate	A ferric iron salt
Carbonyl iron	Feosol, Ircon, Icar, others	Microparticles of elemental iron
Heme-iron polypeptide	Proferrin	Hemoglobin extracted from porcine RBCs
Polysaccharide iron complex	Niferex-150 Forte, Ferrex 150, Triferexx 150 ♣, others	Ferric iron complexed to hydrolyzed starch

of hemosiderin (aggregated ferritin) in bone marrow. Additional laboratory data that can help confirm a diagnosis include reduced RBC count, reduced reticulocyte hemoglobin content, reduced hemoglobin and hematocrit values, reduced serum iron content, and increased serum iron-binding capacity (IBC).[a]

When a diagnosis of iron deficiency anemia is made, it is imperative that the underlying cause be determined. This is especially true when the suspected cause is GI-related blood loss, because GI blood loss may be indicative of peptic ulcer disease or GI cancer, conditions that demand immediate treatment.

ORAL IRON PREPARATIONS

As shown in Table 55.2, iron for oral therapy is available in multiple forms. Of these, the ferrous salts (especially ferrous sulfate) and carbonyl iron are used most often. Accordingly, the discussion here is limited to these iron preparations.

Ferrous Iron Salts

We have two basic types of iron salts: ferrous salts and ferric salts. This discussion is limited to the ferrous iron salts because they are absorbed 3 times more readily than the ferric salts, and so are more widely used. Four ferrous iron salts are available: ferrous sulfate, ferrous gluconate, ferrous fumarate, and ferrous aspartate. All four are equally effective, and with all four, GI disturbances are the major adverse effects.

Ferrous Sulfate

Indications. Ferrous sulfate is the treatment of choice for iron deficiency anemia. It is also the preferred drug for *preventing* deficiency when iron needs cannot be met by diet alone (e.g., during pregnancy or chronic blood loss). Ferrous sulfate costs less than ferrous gluconate or ferrous fumarate, but has equal efficacy and tolerability.

Adverse Effects

GI Disturbances. The most significant adverse effects involve the GI tract. These effects, which are dose dependent, include nausea, pyrosis (heartburn), bloating, constipation, and diarrhea. Gastrointestinal reactions are most intense during initial therapy and become less disturbing with continued drug use. Because of their GI effects, oral iron preparations can aggravate peptic ulcers, regional enteritis, and ulcerative colitis. Accordingly, patients with these disorders should not take iron by mouth. In addition to its other GI effects, oral iron may impart a dark green or black color to stools. This effect is harmless and should not be interpreted as a sign of GI bleeding.

Staining of Teeth. Liquid iron preparations can stain the teeth. This can be prevented by (1) diluting liquid preparations with juice or water, (2) administering the iron through a straw or with a dropper, and (3) rinsing the mouth after administration.

Toxicity. Iron in large amounts is toxic. Poisoning is almost always the result of accidental or intentional overdose, not from therapeutic doses. Death from iron ingestion is rare in adults. By contrast, *in young children, iron-containing products are the leading cause of poisoning fatalities.* For children, the lethal dose of elemental iron is 2 to 10 gm. To reduce the risk of pediatric poisoning, iron should be stored in childproof containers and kept out of reach.

Symptoms. The effects of iron poisoning are complex. Early reactions include nausea, vomiting, diarrhea, and shock. These are followed by acidosis, gastric necrosis, hepatic failure, pulmonary edema, and vasomotor collapse.

Diagnosis and Treatment. With rapid diagnosis and treatment, mortality from iron poisoning is low (about 1%). Serum iron should be measured and the intestine x-rayed to determine if unabsorbed tablets are present. Whole bowel irrigation with a polyethylene glycol electrolyte solution (GoLYTELY) may speed the passage of tablets through the GI tract, but there is lack of evidence regarding improvement in outcomes with this technique.

If the plasma level of iron is high (above 500 mcg/dL), it should be lowered with parenteral *deferoxamine* [Desferal]. Another oral drug—*deferasirox* [Exjade]—is indicated for patients with chronic iron overload caused by blood transfusions. Both agents—deferoxamine and deferasirox—adsorb iron and thereby prevent toxic effects. The pharmacology of these drugs is discussed in Chapter 109.

Drug Interactions. Interaction of iron with other drugs can alter the absorption of iron, the other drug, or both. *Antacids* reduce the absorption of iron. Coadministration of iron with tetracyclines decreases absorption of both. *Ascorbic acid* (vitamin C) promotes iron absorption but also increases its adverse effects. Accordingly, attempts to enhance iron uptake by combining iron with ascorbic acid offer no advantage over a simple increase in iron dosage.

Preparations. Ferrous sulfate is available in standard tablets, and in enteric-coated and sustained-release formulations. The enteric-coated and sustained-release products are designed to reduce gastric disturbances. Unfortunately, although side effects may be lowered, these special formulations have disadvantages. First, iron may be released at variable rates, causing

[a]Serum IBC measures iron binding by transferrin. An *increase* in IBC indicates an increase in the amount of transferrin that is *not* carrying any iron, and so signals reduced iron availability.

TABLE 55.3 ■ Commonly Used Oral Iron Preparations

Iron Preparation	% Elemental Iron (by weight)	Dose Providing 100 mg Elemental Iron
FERROUS IRON SALTS		
Ferrous sulfate	20	500 mg
Ferrous sulfate (dried)	30	330 mg
Ferrous fumarate	33	300 mg
Ferrous gluconate	11.6	860 mg
Ferrous aspartate	16	625 mg
ELEMENTAL IRON		
Carbonyl iron	100	100 mg

variable and unpredictable absorption. Second, these preparations are expensive. Standard tablets do not share these drawbacks.

Some iron products are formulated with vitamin C. The goal is to improve absorption. Unfortunately, the amount in most products is too low to help: More than 200 mg of vitamin C is needed to enhance the absorption of 30 mg of elemental iron.

Brand names for ferrous sulfate products include *Feosol, FeroSul, Slow FE,* and *Ferodan* 🍁.

Dosage and Administration

General Considerations. Dosing with oral iron can be complicated in that oral iron salts differ with regard to percentage of elemental iron (Table 55.3). Ferrous sulfate, for example, contains 20% iron by weight. In contrast, ferrous gluconate contains only 11.6% iron by weight. Consequently, to provide equivalent amounts of elemental iron, we must use different doses of these iron salts. For example, if we want to provide 100 mg of elemental iron using ferrous sulfate, we need to administer a 500-mg dose. To provide this same amount of elemental iron using ferrous fumarate, the dose would be only 300 mg. In the following discussion, dosage values refer to milligrams of elemental iron and not to milligrams of any particular iron compound needed to provide that amount of elemental iron.

Food affects therapy in two ways. First, food helps protect against iron-induced GI distress. Second, food decreases iron absorption by 50% to 70%. Therefore, we have a dilemma: *Absorption is best* when iron is taken *between* meals, but *GI distress is lowest* when iron is taken *with* meals. As a rule, iron should be administered between meals, maximizing absorption. If necessary, the dosage can be lowered to render GI effects more acceptable.

For two reasons, it may be desirable to take iron *with* food during *initial* therapy. First, since the GI effects of iron are most intense when treatment commences, the salving effects of food can be especially beneficial early on. Second, by reducing GI discomfort during the early phase of therapy, dosing with food can help promote adherence.

Use in Iron Deficiency Anemia. Dosing with oral iron represents a compromise between a desire to replenish lost iron rapidly and a desire to keep GI effects to a minimum. For most adults, this compromise can best be achieved by giving 65 mg 3 times a day, yielding a total daily dose of about 200 mg. Since there is a ceiling to intestinal absorption of iron, doses above this amount provide only a modest increase in therapeutic effect. On the other hand, at dosages greater than 200 mg/day, GI disturbances become disproportionately high. Hence, elevation of the daily dose above 200 mg would enhance adverse effects without offering a significant increase in benefits. When treating iron deficiency in infants and children, a typical dosage is 5 mg/kg/day administered in three or four divided doses.

Timing of administration is important: Doses should be spaced evenly throughout the day. This schedule gives the bone marrow a continuous iron supply and thereby maximizes RBC production.

Duration of therapy is determined by the therapeutic objective. If correction of anemia is the sole objective, a few months of therapy is sufficient. However, if the objective also includes replenishing ferritin, treatment must continue another 4 to 6 months. It should be noted, however, that drugs are usually unnecessary for ferritin replenishment: In most cases, diet alone can do the job. Accordingly, once anemia has been corrected, pharmaceutical iron can usually be stopped.

Prophylactic Use. Pregnant women are the principal candidates for prophylactic therapy. A total daily dose of 27 mg, taken between meals, is recommended. Other candidates include infants, children, and women experiencing menorrhagia.

Ferrous Gluconate, Ferrous Fumarate, and Ferrous Aspartate

In addition to ferrous sulfate, three other oral ferrous salts are available: ferrous gluconate [Fergon, Floradix], ferrous fumarate [Ferro-Sequels, Hemocyte, Palafer 🍁, others], and ferrous aspartate [FE Aspartate]. Except for differences in percentage of iron content (see Table 55.3), all of these preparations are equivalent. Therefore, when dosage is adjusted to provide equal amounts of elemental iron, ferrous gluconate, ferrous fumarate, and ferrous aspartate produce pharmacologic effects identical to those of ferrous sulfate. All four agents produce equivalent therapeutic responses, and all four cause the same degree of GI distress. Patients who fail to respond to one will not respond to the others. Patients who cannot tolerate the GI effects of one will find the others intolerable too.

Carbonyl Iron

Carbonyl iron is pure elemental iron in the form of microparticles, which confer good bioavailability. Therapeutic efficacy equals that of the ferrous salts. Because of the microparticles, iron is absorbed slowly, so the risk of toxicity is reduced. Compared with ferrous sulfate, carbonyl iron requires a much higher dosage to cause serious harm. Because of this increased margin of safety, carbonyl iron should pose a reduced risk to children in the event of accidental ingestion.

Carbonyl iron is available in several formulations, including (1) 45-mg tablets, marketed as *Feosol;* (2) 65-mg tablets, marketed as *Ircon;* (3) 90-mg film-coated tablets marketed as *Ferralet 90;* (4) 15-mg chewable tablets, marketed as *Icar;* and (5) a suspension (15 mg/1.25 mL), also marketed as *Icar.* Because these products contain 100% iron, rather than an iron salt, there should be no confusion about dosage: 100 mg of any formulation provides 100 mg of elemental iron. The usual dosage is 50 mg, 3 times a day.

PARENTERAL IRON PREPARATIONS

Iron is available in four forms for parenteral therapy. However, only one of these forms—iron dextran—is approved for iron deficiency of all causes. Approval of the other three forms—iron sucrose, sodium–ferric gluconate complex, and ferumoxytol—is limited to treating iron deficiency anemia in patients with chronic kidney disease.

Iron Dextran

Iron dextran [INFeD, Dexferrum, Dexiron ♣] is the most frequently used parenteral iron preparation. The drug is a complex consisting of ferric hydroxide and dextrans (polymers of glucose). The rate of response to parenteral iron is equal to that of oral iron.

> **Safety Alert**
>
> **IRON DEXTRAN**
>
> Iron dextran is not without risk—fatal anaphylactic reactions have occurred. This preparation should be used for the treatment of iron deficiency only in patients in whom oral administration is infeasible or ineffective. A test dose is required before administration.

Indications

Iron dextran is reserved for patients with a clear diagnosis of iron deficiency and for whom oral iron is either ineffective or intolerable. Primary candidates for parenteral iron are patients who, because of intestinal disease, are unable to absorb iron taken orally. Iron dextran is also indicated when blood loss is so great (500 to 1000 mL/wk) that oral iron cannot be absorbed fast enough to meet hematopoietic needs. Parenteral iron may also be employed when there is concern that oral iron might exacerbate pre-existing disease of the stomach or bowel. Lastly, parenteral iron can be given to the rare patient for whom the GI effects of oral iron are intolerable.

Adverse Effects

Anaphylactic Reactions. Potentially fatal anaphylaxis is the most serious adverse effect. These reactions are triggered by dextran in the product, not by the iron. Although anaphylactic reactions are rare, their possibility demands that iron dextran be used only when clearly required. Furthermore, whenever iron dextran is administered, injectable epinephrine and facilities for resuscitation should be at hand. To reduce risk, each full dose must be preceded by a small test dose. However, be aware that even the test dose can trigger anaphylactic and other hypersensitivity reactions. In addition, even when the test dose is uneventful, patients can still experience anaphylaxis.

Other Adverse Effects. Hypotension is common in patients receiving parenteral iron. In addition, iron dextran can cause headache, fever, urticaria, and arthralgia. More serious reactions—circulatory failure and cardiac arrest—may also occur. When administered IM, iron dextran can cause persistent pain and prolonged, localized discoloration. Very rarely, tumors develop at sites of IM injection. Intravenous administration may result in lymphadenopathy and phlebitis.

Preparations, Dosage, and Administration

Preparations. Iron dextran [INFeD, Dexferrum, Dexiron ♣] is available in single-dose vials (1 and 2 mL) that contain 50 mg/mL of elemental iron.

Dosage. Dosage determination is complex. Dosage depends on the degree of anemia, the weight of the patient, and the presence of persistent bleeding. For patients with iron deficiency anemia who are not losing blood, the equation in Fig. 55.3 provides a guideline for estimating total iron dosage.

Administration. Iron dextran may be administered IM or IV. Intravenous administration is preferred. This route is just as effective as IM administration but causes fewer anaphylactic reactions and other adverse effects.

Intravenous. To minimize anaphylactic reactions, IV iron dextran should be administered by the following protocol: (1) administer a small test dose (25 mg over 5 minutes) and observe the patient for at least 15 minutes; (2) if the test dose appears safe, slowly administer a larger dose (100 mg over a 10- to 15-minute interval); and (3) if the 100-mg dose is uneventful, additional doses may be given as needed on a daily basis.

Intramuscular. Intramuscular iron dextran has significant drawbacks and should be avoided. Disadvantages include persistent pain and discoloration at the injection site, possible development of tumors, and a greater risk of anaphylaxis. When IM administration must be performed, iron dextran should be injected deep into each buttock using the Z-track technique. (Z-track injection keeps the iron dextran deep in the muscle, minimizing leakage and surface discoloration.) As with IV iron dextran, a small test dose should precede the full therapeutic dose.

Sodium–Ferric Gluconate Complex, Iron Sucrose, and Ferumoxytol

Sodium–ferric gluconate complex (SFGC), iron sucrose, and ferumoxytol represent alternatives to iron dextran for parenteral iron therapy. With all three drugs, the risk of anaphylaxis is very low, and so there is little or no need for giving test doses. As a result, these drugs are more convenient than iron dextran. Unfortunately, indications for these drugs are limited to treatment of iron deficiency anemia in patients with chronic kidney disease (CKD). They are not approved for iron deficiency from other causes.

Sodium–Ferric Gluconate Complex

SFGC, sold under the brand name *Ferrlecit*, is a parenteral iron product indicated for iron deficiency anemia in patients with CKD who are undergoing chronic hemodialysis. The drug is always used in conjunction with erythropoietin, an agent that stimulates RBC production (see Chapter 56). SFGC can cause transient flushing and hypotension, associated with lightheadedness, malaise, fatigue, weakness, and severe pain in the chest, back, flanks, or groin. This reaction can be minimized by infusing the drug slowly. In contrast to iron dextran, SFGC poses little risk of anaphylaxis. SFGC is supplied in 5-mL ampules that contain 62.5 mg of elemental iron. Dilution is not required (but may be done) before the infusion. For most patients, a single dose consists of 125 mg (the contents of 2 ampules) infused slowly (over 10 minutes or more). The typical patient requires a cumulative dose of 1 gm (eight 125-mg infusions on separate days). Every time the drug is administered, facilities for cardiopulmonary resuscitation should be immediately available.

Iron Sucrose

Like SFGC, iron sucrose [Venofer] is a parenteral form of iron indicated for iron deficiency anemia in patients with CKD. However, in contrast to SFGC, whose indications are limited to CKD patients undergoing hemodialysis in conjunction with erythropoietin therapy, iron sucrose is indicated for a broader range of CKD patients, specifically

- Non–dialysis-dependent (NDD) patients receiving erythropoietin
- NDD patients *not* receiving erythropoietin
- Hemodialysis-dependent (HDD) patients receiving erythropoietin
- Peritoneal dialysis–dependent (PDD) patients receiving erythropoietin

The most common adverse effects of iron sucrose are hypotension and cramps. The drug has also been associated with heart failure, sepsis, and taste perversion. Life-threatening hypersensitivity reactions are very rare: No cases were observed during clinical trials, and only 27 cases (out of 450,000 patients) were reported

$$\text{mg iron} = 0.66 \times \text{kg body weight} \times \left(100 - \frac{\text{Hemoglobin value in g/dL}}{14.8}\right)$$

Fig. 55.3 ■ Formula for estimating total dosage of parenteral iron dextran.

during postmarketing surveillance. Nonetheless, facilities for cardiopulmonary resuscitation should be available during administration. However, in contrast to iron dextran, no test dose is needed.

Iron sucrose is supplied in 2.5, 5, and 10-mL single-dose vials. Administration is IV, either by (1) slow injection (1 mL/min) or (2) infusion (dilute iron sucrose in up to 100 mL of 0.9% saline and infuse over 15 minutes or longer). Iron sucrose should not be mixed with other drugs or with parenteral nutrition solutions. All patients should receive a *total* dose of 1000 mg, but the dosing schedule and administration technique depend on the patient as follows:

- HDD patients—Give ten 100-mg doses during each of 10 consecutive dialysis sessions. Administer by slow IV injection or IV infusion.
- NDD patients—Give five 200-mg doses on separate occasions over a 14-day span. Administer by slow IV injection.
- PDD patients—Give two 300-mg doses 14 days apart, then one 400-mg dose 14 days later. Administer by slow IV infusion.

Ferumoxytol

Ferumoxytol [Feraheme] is a parenteral form of iron indicated for iron deficiency anemia in all patients with CKD, whether or not they are on dialysis or using erythropoietin. Compared with SFGC and iron sucrose, ferumoxytol is much more convenient because it requires only 2 doses (given over 3 to 8 days), whereas SFGC and iron sucrose require 3 to 10 doses (given over several weeks).

Ferumoxytol is generally well tolerated. The most common adverse effects are nausea, dizziness, hypotension, headache, vomiting, and edema. In clinical trials, about 0.2% of patients experienced serious hypersensitivity reactions. Accordingly, facilities for cardiopulmonary resuscitation should be immediately available. However, in contrast to iron dextran, no test dose is needed.

Because of its unique composition (ferumoxytol is a superparamagnetic form of iron oxide), the drug can interfere with magnetic resonance imaging studies. This interference is most profound 1 to 2 days after dosing, but can persist for up to 3 months. Fortunately, ferumoxytol does not interfere with other forms of diagnostic imaging, including x-rays, computed tomography, positron emission tomography, ultrasound, or nuclear medicine imaging.

Ferumoxytol [Feraheme] is supplied in 17-mL single-dose vials (30 mg elemental iron/mL). Administration is by slow IV injection, defined here as 1 mL/sec (30 mg/sec). The usual dosage is 510 mg on day 1, followed by another 510 mg 3 to 8 days later. Additional doses may be given as needed. Following each injection, patients should be monitored for at least 30 minutes for hypotension and hypersensitivity reactions. For patients on dialysis, dosing should be done at least 1 hour after starting dialysis, and only after blood pressure has stabilized.

GUIDELINES FOR TREATING IRON DEFICIENCY

Assessment

Before starting therapy, the cause of iron deficiency must be determined. Without this information, appropriate treatment is impossible. Potential causes of deficiency include pregnancy, bleeding, inadequate diet, and, rarely, impaired intestinal absorption.

The objective is to increase production of hemoglobin and erythrocytes. When therapy is successful, reticulocytes will increase within 4 to 7 days; within 1 week, increases in hemoglobin and the hematocrit will be apparent; and within 1 month, hemoglobin levels will rise by at least 2 gm/dL. If these responses fail to occur, the patient should be evaluated for (1) compliance, (2) continued bleeding, (3) inflammatory disease (which can interfere with hemoglobin production), and (4) malabsorption of oral iron.

Routes of Administration

Iron preparations are available for oral, IV, and IM administration. Oral iron is preferred because it is safer than parenteral iron and just as effective. Parenteral iron should be used only when oral iron is ineffective or intolerable. Of the two parenteral routes, IV is safer and preferred.

Duration of Therapy

Therapy with oral iron should be continued until hemoglobin levels become normal (about 15 gm/dL). This phase of treatment may require 1 to 2 months. After this, continued treatment can help replenish stores of ferritin. However, for most patients, dietary iron alone is sufficient.

Therapeutic Combinations

As a rule, combinations of antianemic agents should be avoided. Combining oral iron with parenteral iron can lead to iron toxicity. Accordingly, the use of oral iron should cease before giving iron injections. Combinations of iron with vitamin B_{12} or folic acid should be avoided; as discussed in the following sections, using these combinations can confuse interpretation of hematologic responses.

VITAMIN B_{12} DEFICIENCY

The term *vitamin B_{12}* refers to a group of compounds with similar structures. These compounds are large molecules that contain an atom of cobalt. Because of the cobalt atom, members of the vitamin B_{12} family are known as *cobalamins.*

The most prominent consequences of vitamin B_{12} deficiency are *anemia* and *injury to the nervous system.* Anemia reverses rapidly following vitamin B_{12} administration. Neurologic damage takes longer to repair and, in some cases, may never fully resolve. Additional effects of B_{12} deficiency include GI disturbances and impaired production of white blood cells and platelets.

BIOCHEMISTRY AND PHYSIOLOGY OF VITAMIN B_{12}

To understand the consequences of vitamin B_{12} deficiency and the rationale behind therapy, we must first understand the normal biochemistry and physiology of B_{12}. This information is reviewed here.

Metabolic Function

Vitamin B_{12} is essential for the synthesis of DNA, and so is required for the growth and division of virtually all cells. The mechanism by which the vitamin influences DNA synthesis is depicted in Fig. 55.4. As indicated, vitamin B_{12} helps catalyze the conversion of folic acid to its active form. Active folic acid then participates in several reactions essential for DNA synthesis. Hence, *it is by permitting utilization of folic acid that vitamin B_{12} influences cell growth and division*—and it is the absence of usable folic acid that underlies the blood cell abnormalities seen during B_{12} deficiency.

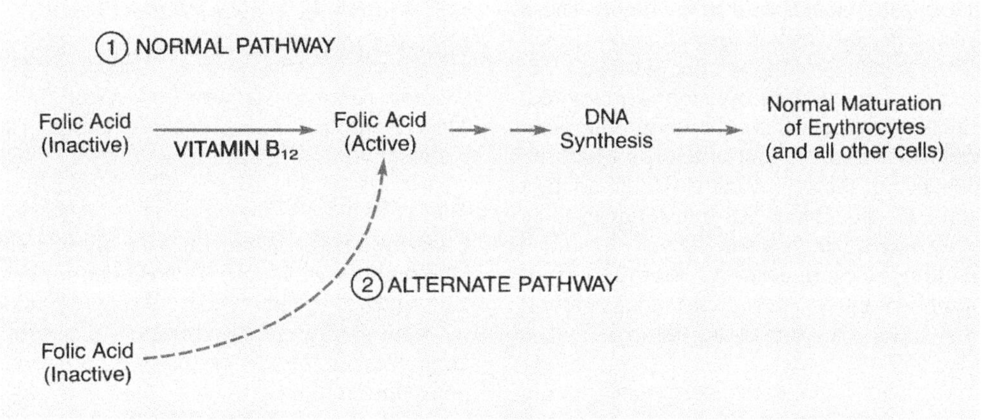

Fig. 55.4 ▪ Relationship of folic acid and vitamin B_{12} to DNA synthesis and cell maturation. Folic acid requires activation to be of use. Normally, activation occurs via a vitamin B_{12}-dependent pathway. However, when folic acid is present in large amounts, activation can occur via an alternate pathway, bypassing the need for B_{12}.

Fate in the Body

Absorption

Efficient absorption of B_{12} requires *intrinsic factor,* a compound secreted by parietal cells of the stomach. Following ingestion, vitamin B_{12} forms a complex with intrinsic factor. Upon reaching the ileum, the B_{12}–intrinsic factor complex interacts with specific receptors on the intestinal wall, causing the complex to be absorbed. In the absence of intrinsic factor, absorption of vitamin B_{12} is greatly reduced. However, about 1% of the amount present can still be absorbed by passive diffusion; no intrinsic factor is needed.

Distribution and Storage

Following absorption, the vitamin B_{12}–intrinsic factor complex dissociates. Free B_{12} then binds to *transcobalamin II* for transport to tissues. Most vitamin B_{12} goes to the liver and is stored. Total body stores of B_{12} are tiny, ranging from 2 to 3 mg by most estimates.

Elimination

Excretion of vitamin B_{12} takes place very slowly: Each day, about 0.1% of the total body store is lost. Because B_{12} is excreted so slowly, years are required for B_{12} deficiency to develop—even when none of the lost B_{12} is replaced.

Daily Requirements

Because very little vitamin B_{12} is excreted and because body stores are small to begin with, daily requirements for this vitamin are minuscule. The average adult needs about 2.4 mcg of B_{12} per day. Children need even less.

Dietary Sources

The ability to biosynthesize vitamin B_{12} is limited to microorganisms; higher plants and animals can't make it. The microorganisms that make B_{12} reside in the soil, sewage, and the intestines of humans and other animals. Unfortunately, vitamin B_{12} produced in the human GI tract is unavailable for absorption. Consequently, humans must obtain the majority of their B_{12} by consuming animal products. Liver and dairy products are especially good sources. Between 10% and 30% of adults older than 50 years are unable to absorb vitamin B_{12} found naturally in foods. Accordingly, these people should meet their requirements by consuming B_{12}-fortified foods or a B_{12}-containing vitamin supplement.

VITAMIN B_{12} DEFICIENCY: CAUSES, CONSEQUENCES, AND DIAGNOSIS

Causes

In the majority of cases, vitamin B_{12} deficiency is the result of *impaired absorption.* Only rarely is insufficient B_{12} in the diet the cause. Potential causes of poor absorption include (1) regional enteritis, (2) celiac disease (a malabsorption syndrome involving abnormalities in the intestinal villi), and (3) development of antibodies directed against the vitamin B_{12}–intrinsic factor complex. In addition, because stomach acid is required to release vitamin B_{12} from foods, the vitamin cannot be absorbed if acid secretion is significantly reduced, as often happens in older adults and in those taking acid-suppressing drugs.

Most frequently, impaired absorption of vitamin B_{12} occurs secondary to a lack of intrinsic factor. The usual causes are atrophy of gastric parietal cells and surgery of the stomach (total gastric resection).

When vitamin B_{12} deficiency is caused by an absence of intrinsic factor, the resulting syndrome is called *pernicious anemia*—a term suggesting a highly destructive or fatal condition. Pernicious anemia is an old term that dates back to a time when, for most patients, vitamin B_{12} deficiency had no effective therapy and the condition was uniformly fatal. Today, vitamin B_{12} deficiency secondary to lack of intrinsic factor can be managed successfully, so the label *pernicious* no longer has its original, ominous connotation.

Consequences

Many of the consequences of B_{12} deficiency result from disruption of DNA synthesis. The tissues affected most are those with a high proportion of cells undergoing growth and division. Accordingly, B_{12} deficiency has profound effects on the bone marrow (the site where blood cells are produced) and the epithelial cells lining the mouth and GI tract.

Megaloblastic Anemia

The most conspicuous consequence of B_{12} deficiency is an anemia in which large numbers of *megaloblasts* (oversized erythroblasts) appear in the bone marrow and in which *macrocytes* (oversized erythrocytes) appear in the blood. These strange cells are produced because of impaired DNA synthesis: Lacking sufficient DNA, growing cells are unable to divide; hence, as erythroblasts mature and their division is prevented, oversized cells result. Most megaloblasts die within the bone marrow; only a few evolve into the macrocytes that can be seen in the blood. Because of these unusual cells, the anemia associated with vitamin B_{12} deficiency is often referred to as either *megaloblastic* or *macrocytic* anemia.

Severe anemia is the principal cause of mortality from B_{12} deficiency. Anemia produces peripheral and cerebral hypoxia. Heart failure and dysrhythmias are the usual cause of death.

It is important to note that the hematologic effects of vitamin B_{12} deficiency can be reversed with large doses of *folic acid.* As indicated in Fig. 55.4, when folic acid is present in large amounts, some of it can be activated by an alternate pathway that is independent of vitamin B_{12}. This pathway bypasses the metabolic block caused by B_{12} deficiency, permitting DNA synthesis to proceed.

Neurologic Damage

Deficiency of vitamin B_{12} causes demyelination of neurons, primarily in the spinal cord and brain. A variety of signs and symptoms can result. Early manifestations include paresthesias (tingling, numbness) of the hands and feet and a reduction in deep tendon reflexes. Late-developing responses include loss of memory, mood changes, hallucinations, and psychosis. If vitamin B_{12} deficiency is prolonged, neurologic damage can become permanent.

The precise mechanism by which B_{12} deficiency results in neuronal damage is unknown. We do know, however, that *neuronal damage is not related to effects on folic acid or DNA.* That is, the mechanism that underlies neuronal damage is different from the mechanism that underlies disruption of hematopoiesis. Consequently, although administering large doses of folic acid can correct the hematologic consequences of B_{12} deficiency, folic acid will not improve the neurologic picture.

Other Effects

As noted, vitamin B_{12} deficiency can adversely affect virtually all tissues in which a high proportion of cells are undergoing growth and division. Therefore, in addition to disrupting the production of erythrocytes, lack of B_{12} also prevents the bone marrow from making leukocytes (white blood cells) and thrombocytes (platelets). Loss of these blood elements can lead to infection and spontaneous bleeding. Disruption of DNA synthesis can also suppress division of the cells that form the epithelial lining of the mouth, stomach, and intestine, causing oral ulceration and a variety of GI disturbances.

Diagnosis

When megaloblastic anemia occurs, it may be due to vitamin B_{12} deficiency or other causes, especially a lack of folic acid. Hence, if therapy is to be appropriate, a definitive diagnosis must be made. Two tests are particularly helpful. The first is obvious: measurement of plasma B_{12}. The second procedure, known as the Schilling test, measures vitamin B_{12} absorption. The combination of megaloblastic anemia plus low plasma vitamin B_{12} plus evidence of B_{12} malabsorption permits a clear diagnosis of vitamin B_{12} deficiency.

VITAMIN B_{12} PREPARATIONS: CYANOCOBALAMIN

Cyanocobalamin is a purified, crystalline form of vitamin B_{12}. This compound is the drug of choice for all forms of B_{12} deficiency.

Adverse Effects

Cyanocobalamin is generally devoid of serious adverse effects. One potential response, *hypokalemia,* may occur as a natural consequence of increased erythrocyte production. Erythrocytes incorporate significant amounts of potassium. Therefore, as large numbers of new erythrocytes are produced, levels of free potassium may fall.

Preparations, Dosage, and Administration

Cyanocobalamin can be given orally, intranasally, and by IM or subQ injection. Most pharmacology texts, including prior editions of this one, will tell you that oral therapy is appropriate only for people who absorb B_{12} well; all other patients (i.e., those with impaired absorption) should use intranasal or parenteral therapy. However, this statement is not correct. Although it *is* true that various conditions—including lack of intrinsic factor, low gastric acidity, and regional enteritis—severely impair B_{12} absorption, these conditions do not prevent absorption entirely. Hence, even people with impaired absorption can still be treated orally; the only catch is that doses must be very high. Is there any advantage to oral therapy compared with parenteral therapy? Yes. First, oral therapy is more comfortable (injections sometimes hurt). Second, oral therapy is more convenient (because it avoids regular trips to the physician for injections).

Oral. Oral cyanocobalamin is appropriate for most people with mild to moderate B_{12} deficiency, regardless of the cause. (The principal exception is patients with severe neurologic involvement.) If the B_{12} deficiency is due to malabsorption, dosages must be high—typically 1000 to 10,000 mcg/day. To ensure that absorption has been adequate, B_{12} levels should be measured periodically.

In addition to treating patients with B_{12} deficiency, oral cyanocobalamin can be used as a dietary supplement. The usual dosage is 1000–2000 mcg/day.

Seven oral formulations are available: standard tablets (50, 100, 250, 500, 1000, 2000, and 2500 mcg), extended-release tablets (1000, 1500, and 5000 mcg), capsules (1000, 3000, and 5000 mcg), sublingual tablets (500, 1000, 2500, 3000, 5000, and 6000 mcg), oral dissolving tablets (1500 mcg), chewable tablets (250, 500, and 750 mcg), and a solution for sublingual use (5000 mcg/mL).

Parenteral. Parenteral cyanocobalamin (generic only) can be administered by *IM or deep subQ injection. Cyanocobalamin must NOT be given IV.* Intramuscular and subQ injections are generally well tolerated, although they occasionally cause pain and other local reactions.

Parenteral administration is indicated for patients with impaired B_{12} absorption—although most of these people can be treated with oral cyanocobalamin instead. If the cause of malabsorption is irreversible (e.g., parietal cell atrophy, total gastrectomy), therapy must continue lifelong. A typical dosing schedule for megaloblastic anemia is 100 mcg IM or deep subQ daily for 7 days. If there is a positive response after this time, continue to administer 100 mcg every other day for 7 doses, then decrease to every 3 to 4 days for another 2 to 3 weeks. After anemia has been corrected, doses of 100 mcg are administered monthly for life.

Intranasal. Intranasal cyanocobalamin [Nascobal] represents a convenient alternative to IM or subQ injection for people who cannot take cyanocobalamin by mouth. Efficacy of intranasal cyanocobalamin has not been determined for patients with nasal congestion, allergic rhinitis, or upper respiratory infections. Accordingly, until more is known, patients with these disorders should not use this formulation until symptoms subside. Hot foods or liquids can increase nasal secretions, which might flush cyanocobalamin gel from the nose. Accordingly, hot foods should not be eaten within 1 hour before or 1 hour after administering the drug.

Intranasal cyanocobalamin is available in a metered-dose formulation called *Nascobal,* which delivers 500 mcg/actuation. The dosing schedule is 500 mcg in one nostril once a week.

GUIDELINES FOR TREATING VITAMIN B_{12} DEFICIENCY

Route of B_{12} Administration

As discussed previously, oral therapy can be used for most patients, including those with conditions that impair B_{12} absorption. The major exception is patients with severe neurologic deficits caused by B_{12} deficiency. For these people, parenteral cyanocobalamin is indicated.

Treatment of Moderate B_{12} Deficiency

The primary manifestations of moderate B_{12} deficiency are megaloblasts in the bone marrow and macrocytes in peripheral blood. Moderate deficiency does not cause leukopenia, thrombocytopenia, or neurologic complications. Moderate deficiency can be managed with vitamin B_{12} alone; no other measures are required.

Treatment of Severe B_{12} Deficiency

Severe deficiency produces multiple effects, all of which must be attended to. Unlike mild deficiency, in which erythrocytes are the only blood cells affected, severe deficiency disrupts production of all blood cells. Loss of erythrocytes leads to hypoxia, cerebrovascular insufficiency, and heart failure. Loss of leukocytes encourages infection, and loss of thrombocytes promotes bleeding. In addition to causing serious hematologic deficits, severe B_{12} deficiency has adverse effects on the nervous system and GI tract.

Following treatment with vitamin B_{12} plus folic acid, recovery from anemia occurs quickly. Within 1 to 2 days, megaloblasts disappear from the bone marrow; within 3 to 5 days, reticulocyte counts become elevated; by day 10, the hematocrit begins to rise; and within 14 to 21 days, the hematocrit becomes normal.

Recovery from neurologic damage is slow and depends on how long the damage had been present. When deficits have been present for only 2 to 3 months, recovery is relatively fast. When deficits have been present for many months or for years, recovery is slow: Months may pass before any improvement is apparent, and complete recovery may never occur.

Long-Term Treatment

For patients who lack intrinsic factor or who suffer from some other permanent cause of vitamin B_{12} malabsorption, lifelong treatment is required. Traditional therapy consists of monthly IM or subQ injections of cyanocobalamin. However, *large* daily oral doses can be just as effective, as can weekly intranasal doses. During prolonged therapy, treatment should be periodically assessed: plasma levels of vitamin B_{12} should be measured every 3 to 6 months, blood samples should be examined for the return of macrocytes, and blood counts should be performed.

Potential Hazard of Folic Acid

Treatment with folic acid can exacerbate the neurologic consequences of B_{12} deficiency. Recall that folic acid, by itself, can reverse the *hematologic* effects of B_{12} deficiency—but will not alleviate *neurologic* deficits. So, by correcting the most obvious manifestation of B_{12} deficiency (anemia), folic acid can mask the fact that deficiency of B_{12} still exists. As a result, *the use of folic acid can lead to undertreatment with B_{12} itself* and can thereby permit neurologic damage to progress. Clearly, folic acid is not a substitute for vitamin B_{12}, and vitamin B_{12} deficiency should never be treated with folic acid alone. Whenever folic acid is employed during the treatment of vitamin B_{12} deficiency, extra care must be taken to ensure that B_{12} dosage is adequate.

FOLIC ACID DEFICIENCY

In one respect, folic acid deficiency is identical to vitamin B_{12} deficiency: In both states, *megaloblastic anemia* is the most conspicuous pathology. However, in other important ways, folic acid deficiency and vitamin B_{12} deficiency are dissimilar (Table 55.4). Consequently, when a patient presents with megaloblastic anemia, it is essential to determine whether the cause is deficiency of folic acid, vitamin B_{12}, or both.

PHYSIOLOGY AND BIOCHEMISTRY OF FOLIC ACID

Metabolic Function

As noted when we discussed vitamin B_{12}, folic acid (also known as *folate*) is an essential factor for DNA synthesis. Without folic acid, DNA replication and cell division cannot proceed.

To be usable, dietary folic acid must first be converted to an active form. Under normal conditions, activation occurs through a pathway that employs vitamin B_{12} (see Fig. 55.4). However, when large amounts of folate are ingested, some can be activated through an alternate pathway—one that does not employ vitamin B_{12}. Hence, even in the absence of vitamin B_{12}, if sufficient amounts of folic acid are consumed, active folate will be available for DNA synthesis.

Fate in the Body

Folic acid is absorbed in the early segment of the small intestine, and then transported to the liver and other tissues, where it is either used or stored.

TABLE 55.4 ▪ Vitamin B_{12} Deficiency Versus Folic Acid Deficiency

	Vitamin B_{12} Deficiency	Folic Acid Deficiency
Usual cause	Vitamin B_{12} malabsorption from lack of intrinsic factor	Low dietary folic acid
Primary hematologic effect	Megaloblastic anemia	Megaloblastic anemia
Neurologic effect	Damage to brain and spinal cord	None[a]
Diagnosis	Low plasma vitamin B_{12}; low B_{12} absorption (Schilling test)	Low plasma folic acid
Treatment (usual route)	Cyanocobalamin (PO or IM)	Folic acid (PO)
Usual duration of therapy	Lifelong	Short term

[a]Folic acid deficiency early in pregnancy can cause neural tube defects in the fetus.

Folic acid in the liver undergoes extensive enterohepatic recirculation. That is, folate from the liver is excreted into the intestine, after which it is reabsorbed and then returned to the liver through the hepatic-portal circulation. This enterohepatic recirculation helps salvage up to 200 mcg of folate per day. Accordingly, the process is an important way to maintain folate stores.

In contrast to vitamin B_{12}, folic acid is not conserved rigidly: every day, significant amounts are excreted. As a result, if intake of folic acid were to cease, signs of deficiency would develop rapidly (within weeks if body stores were already low).

Daily Requirements

The RDA of folic acid, as set by the Food and Nutrition Board of the Institute of Medicine, is 400 mcg for adult males and for adult females who are neither pregnant nor lactating. RDAs during pregnancy and lactation increase to 600 mcg and 500 mcg, respectively. Although the RDA for adult females is set at 400 mcg, women of childbearing age should consume even more: 400 to 800 mcg of *supplemental* folate, in addition to the folate in food (see *Dietary Sources*). Individuals with malabsorption syndromes (e.g., tropical sprue) may require as much as 2000 mcg (2 mg) per day; at these high doses, folate will be taken up in sufficient quantity despite impaired absorption.

Dietary Sources

Folic acid is present in all foods. Good sources include peas, lentils, oranges, whole-wheat products, asparagus, beets, broccoli, and spinach. Also, many grain products (e.g., cereals, bread, pasta, rice, flour) are now fortified with folic acid.

FOLIC ACID DEFICIENCY: CAUSES, CONSEQUENCES, AND DIAGNOSIS

Causes

Folic acid deficiency has two principal causes: (1) poor diet (especially in patients with alcohol use disorder), and (2) malabsorption secondary to intestinal disease. Rarely, certain drugs may cause folate deficiency.

Alcohol Use Disorder

Alcohol use disorder, either acute or chronic, may be the most common cause of folate deficiency. Deficiency results for two reasons: (1) insufficient folic acid in the diet and (2) derangement of enterohepatic recirculation secondary to alcohol-induced injury to the liver. Fortunately, with improved diet and reduced alcohol consumption, alcohol-related folate deficiency will often reverse.

Sprue

Sprue is an intestinal malabsorption syndrome that decreases folic acid uptake. Since sprue does not block folate absorption entirely, deficiency can be corrected by giving large doses of folic acid orally.

Consequences

With the important exception that folic acid deficiency does not injure the nervous system, the effects of folate deficiency are identical to those of vitamin B_{12} deficiency. As with B_{12} deficiency, the most prominent consequence of folate deficiency is *megaloblastic anemia.* In addition, like B_{12} deficiency, lack of folic acid may result in leukopenia, thrombocytopenia, and injury to the oral and GI mucosa. Since we already noted that many of the consequences of vitamin B_{12} deficiency result from depriving cells of active folic acid, the similarities between folate deficiency and vitamin B_{12} deficiency should be no surprise.

The Developing Fetus

Folic acid deficiency *very early* in pregnancy can cause neural tube defects (e.g., spina bifida, anencephaly). Accordingly, it is imperative that all women of reproductive age ensure adequate folate levels *before* pregnancy occurs. To accomplish this, the U.S. Preventive Services Task Force now recommends that *all women who may become pregnant consume 400 to 800 mcg of supplemental folic acid each day—in addition to the folate they get from food.*

Other Consequences

As discussed in Chapter 81, folic acid deficiency may increase the risk of colorectal cancer and atherosclerosis.

Diagnosis

When patients present with megaloblastic anemia, it is essential to distinguish between folic acid deficiency and vitamin B_{12} deficiency as the cause by comparing plasma levels of folate and vitamin B_{12}. If folic acid levels are low and vitamin B_{12} levels are normal, a diagnosis of folic acid deficiency is suggested. Conversely, if folate levels are normal and B_{12} is low, B_{12} deficiency would be the likely diagnosis. A decision against folic acid deficiency would be strengthened if neurologic deficits were observed.

FOLIC ACID PREPARATIONS

Nomenclature

Two forms of folic acid are available. One form is inactive as administered (but undergoes activation after being absorbed).

The second form is active to start with. Both forms have several generic names: the *inactive* form is referred to as *folacin, folate, pteroylglutamic acid,* or *folic acid;* the *active* form is referred to as *leucovorin calcium, folinic acid,* or *citrovorum factor.* The inactive form is by far the most commonly used.

Folic Acid (Pteroylglutamic Acid)

Chemistry

Folic acid is inactive as administered and cannot support DNA synthesis. Activation takes place rapidly following absorption.

Indications

Folic acid has three uses: (1) treatment of megaloblastic anemia resulting from folic acid deficiency; (2) prophylaxis of folate deficiency, especially during pregnancy and lactation; and (3) initial treatment of severe megaloblastic anemia resulting from vitamin B_{12} deficiency.

Adverse Effects

Oral folic acid is nontoxic when used *short term.* Massive dosages (e.g., as much as 15 mg) have been taken with no ill effects. However, as noted in Chapter 81, even moderately large doses (1000 mcg/day), when taken *long term,* may pose a nonsignificant increase in the risk of some cancers, including colorectal cancer and cancer of the prostate.

Safety Alert

FOLIC ACID

If taken in large-enough doses, folic acid can correct the hematologic consequences of vitamin B_{12} deficiency, masking the fact that a vitamin B_{12} deficiency still exists. Since folic acid will not prevent the neurologic consequences of B_{12} deficiency, this masking effect may allow the development of irreversible damage to the nervous system. Therefore, folate should not be used indiscriminately. Unless specifically indicated, consumption of folic acid should not exceed 1000 mcg/day, and whenever folic acid is given to patients known to have a deficiency in vitamin B_{12}, care must be taken to ensure that the vitamin B_{12} dosage is adequate.

Formulations and Routes of Administration

Folic acid is available in tablets (0.4, 0.8, and 1 mg) for oral use and in a 5-mg/mL solution for IM, IV, or subQ injection. As a rule, injections are reserved for patients with severely impaired GI absorption.

Dosage

For treatment of folate-deficient megaloblastic anemia in adults, the usual oral dosage is 1000 to 2000 mcg/day. Once symptoms have resolved, the maintenance dosage is 400 mcg/day. For prophylaxis during pregnancy and lactation, doses up to 1000 mcg/day may be used.

Leucovorin Calcium (Folinic Acid)

Leucovorin calcium is an active form of folic acid used primarily as an adjunct to cancer chemotherapy (see Chapter 102). Leucovorin is not used routinely to correct folic acid deficiency because folic acid is just as effective and cheaper.

GUIDELINES FOR TREATING FOLIC ACID DEFICIENCY

Choice of Treatment Modality

The modality for treating folic acid deficiency should be matched with the cause. If the deficiency is due to poor diet, it should be corrected by dietary measures—not with supplements (except for women who may become pregnant). Ingestion of one serving of a fresh vegetable or one glass of fruit juice a day will often suffice. In contrast, when folate deficiency is the result of malabsorption, diet alone cannot correct the deficiency, and supplemental folate will be needed.

Route of Administration

Oral administration is preferred for most patients. Unlike vitamin B_{12}, folic acid is rarely administered by injection. Even in the presence of intestinal disease, oral folic acid can be effective, provided the dosage is high enough.

Prophylactic Use of Folic Acid

Folic acid should be taken prophylactically only when clearly appropriate. The principal candidates for prophylactic folate are women who might become pregnant and women who are pregnant or lactating. Because folic acid may mask vitamin B_{12} deficiency, indiscriminate use of folate should be avoided.

Treatment of Severe Deficiency

Folic acid deficiency can produce severe megaloblastic anemia. To ensure a rapid response, therapy should be initiated with an IM injection of folic acid and vitamin B_{12}. (Because of the metabolic interrelationship between folic acid and vitamin B_{12}, combining these agents accelerates recovery.) After the initial injection, treatment should be continued with folic acid alone. Folic acid should be given orally in a dosage of 1000 to 2000 mcg/day for 1 to 2 weeks. After this, maintenance doses of 400 mcg/day may be required.

Therapy is evaluated by monitoring the hematologic picture. When treatment has been effective, megaloblasts will disappear from the bone marrow within 48 hours; the reticulocyte count will increase measurably within 2 to 3 days; and the hematocrit will begin to rise in the second week.

KEY POINTS

- The principal cause of iron deficiency is increased iron demand secondary to (1) maternal and fetal blood volume expansion during pregnancy; (2) blood volume expansion during infancy and early childhood; or (3) chronic blood loss, usually of GI or uterine origin.
- The major consequence of iron deficiency is microcytic, hypochromic anemia.
- Ferrous sulfate, given PO, is the drug of choice for iron deficiency.
- Iron-deficient patients who cannot tolerate or absorb oral ferrous salts are treated with parenteral iron—usually iron dextran administered IV.
- The major adverse effects of ferrous sulfate are GI disturbances. These are best managed by reducing the dosage (rather than by administering the drug with food, which would greatly reduce absorption).
- Parenteral iron dextran carries a significant risk of fatal anaphylactic reactions. The risk is much lower with other parenteral iron products (e.g., iron sucrose).
- When iron dextran is used, a small test dose is required before each full dose. Be aware, however, that patients can experience anaphylaxis and other hypersensitivity reactions from the test dose, and patients who did not react to the test dose may still have these reactions with the full dose.
- The principal cause of vitamin B_{12} deficiency is impaired absorption secondary to lack of intrinsic factor.
- The principal consequences of B_{12} deficiency are megaloblastic (macrocytic) anemia and neurologic injury.
- Vitamin B_{12} deficiency caused by malabsorption is treated lifelong with cyanocobalamin. Traditional treatment consists of IM injections administered monthly. However, large oral doses administered daily are also effective, as are intranasal doses (administered weekly with Nascobal).
- For initial therapy of severe vitamin B_{12} deficiency, parenteral folic acid is given along with cyanocobalamin.
- When folic acid is combined with vitamin B_{12} to treat B_{12} deficiency, it is essential that the dosage of B_{12} be adequate because folic acid can mask continued B_{12} deficiency (by improving the hematologic picture), while allowing the neurologic consequences of B_{12} deficiency to progress.
- The principal causes of folic acid deficiency are poor diet (usually in patients with alcohol use disorder) and malabsorption secondary to intestinal disease.
- The principal consequences of folic acid deficiency are megaloblastic anemia and neural tube defects in the developing fetus.
- To prevent neural tube defects, all women who may become pregnant should ingest 400 to 800 mcg of supplemental folate daily, in addition to the folate they get in food.

Please visit **http://evolve.elsevier.com/Lehne** for chapter-specific NCLEX® examination review questions.

Summary of Major Nursing Implications[a]

IRON PREPARATIONS

Carbonyl iron
Ferric ammonium citrate
Ferrous aspartate
Ferrous bisglycinate
Ferrous fumarate
Ferrous gluconate
Ferrous sulfate
Ferumoxytol
Heme-iron polypeptide
Iron dextran
Iron sucrose
Polysaccharide iron complex
Sodium–ferric gluconate complex (SFGC)

Except where indicated, the implications summarized here apply to all iron preparations.

Preadministration Assessment

Therapeutic Goal

Prevention or treatment of iron deficiency anemias.

Baseline Data

Before treatment, assess the degree of anemia. Fatigue, listlessness, and pallor indicate mild anemia; dyspnea, tachycardia, and angina suggest severe anemia. Laboratory findings indicative of anemia are subnormal hemoglobin levels, subnormal hematocrit, subnormal hemosiderin in bone marrow, and the presence of microcytic, hypochromic erythrocytes.

The cause of iron deficiency (e.g., pregnancy, occult bleeding, menorrhagia, inadequate diet, malabsorption) must be determined.

Identifying High-Risk Patients

All iron preparations are *contraindicated* for patients with anemias other than iron deficiency anemia.

Parenteral preparations are *contraindicated* for patients who have had a severe allergic reaction to them in the past.

Use *oral* preparations with *caution* in patients with peptic ulcer disease, regional enteritis, and ulcerative colitis.

Implementation: Administration

Routes

Oral. Ferrous sulfate, ferrous fumarate, ferrous gluconate, ferrous aspartate, ferrous bisglycinate, ferric ammonium citrate, carbonyl iron, heme-iron polypeptide, polysaccharide iron complex, SFGC.

Parenteral. Iron dextran, SFGC, iron sucrose, ferumoxytol.

Oral Administration

Food reduces GI distress from oral iron but also greatly reduces absorption. **Instruct patients to administer oral iron between**

Summary of Major Nursing Implications[a]—cont'd

meals to maximize uptake. If GI distress is intolerable, the dosage may be reduced. If absolutely necessary, oral iron may be administered with meals.

Liquid preparations can stain the teeth. **Instruct patients to dilute liquid preparations with juice or water, administer them through a straw, and rinse the mouth after.**

Warn patients not to crush or chew sustained-release preparations.

Warn patients against ingesting iron salts together with antacids or tetracyclines.

Inform patients that oral iron preparations differ and warn them against switching from one to another.

Parenteral Administration: Iron Dextran

Iron dextran may be given IV or IM. Intravenous administration is safer and preferred.

Intravenous. To minimize anaphylactic reactions, follow this protocol: (1) Infuse 25 mg as a test dose and observe the patient for at least 15 minutes. (2) If the test dose appears safe, infuse 100 mg over 10 to 15 minutes. (3) If the 100-mg dose proves uneventful, give additional doses as needed every 24 hours.

Intramuscular. Intramuscular injection can cause significant adverse reactions (anaphylaxis, persistent pain, localized discoloration, promotion of tumors) and is generally avoided. Make injections deep into each buttock using the Z-track technique. Give a 25-mg test dose and wait 1 hour before giving the full therapeutic dose.

Parenteral Administration: SFGC

To minimize adverse reactions, precede the first full dose with a test dose (25 mg infused IV over 60 minutes). Administer therapeutic doses by slow IV infusion (no faster than 12.5 mg/min).

Parenteral Administration: Iron Sucrose

Hemodialysis-Dependent Patients. Administer iron sucrose directly into the dialysis line. Do not mix with other drugs or with parenteral nutrition solutions. Administer by either (1) slow injection (1 mL/min) or (2) infusion (dilute iron sucrose in up to 100 mL of 0.9% saline and infuse over 15 minutes or longer).

Peritoneal Dialysis–Dependent Patients. Administer by slow infusion.

Non–Dialysis-Dependent Patients. Administer by slow injection.

Parenteral Administration: Ferumoxytol

Give 510 mg by slow IV injection, defined here as 1 mL/sec (30 mg/sec), taking about 17 seconds for the total 510-mg dose. Repeat 3 to 8 days later.

Implementation: Measures to Enhance Therapeutic Effects

If the diet is low in iron, advise the patient to increase consumption of iron-rich foods (e.g., egg yolks, brewer's yeast, wheat germ, muscle meats, fish, fowl).

Ongoing Evaluation and Interventions

Evaluating Therapeutic Responses

Evaluate treatment by monitoring hematologic status. Reticulocyte counts should increase within 4 to 7 days, hemoglobin content and the hematocrit should begin to rise within 1 week, and hemoglobin levels should rise by at least 2 gm/dL within 1 month. If these responses do not occur, evaluate the patient for adherence, persistent bleeding, inflammatory disease, and malabsorption.

Minimizing Adverse Effects

GI Disturbances. **Forewarn patients about possible GI reactions (nausea, vomiting, constipation, diarrhea) and inform them these will diminish over time.** If GI distress is severe, the dosage may be reduced, or if absolutely necessary, iron may be administered with food.

Inform patients that iron will impart a harmless dark green or black color to stools.

Anaphylactic Reactions. Parenteral iron dextran (and, rarely, SFGC, iron sucrose, and ferumoxytol) can cause potentially fatal anaphylaxis. Before giving parenteral iron, ensure that injectable epinephrine and facilities for resuscitation are immediately available. After administration, observe the patient for 60 minutes. Give test doses as described earlier. Precede all doses of iron dextran with a test dose; test doses are unnecessary with iron sucrose and ferumoxytol.

Managing Acute Toxicity. Iron poisoning can be fatal to young children. **Instruct parents to store iron out of reach and in childproof containers.** If poisoning occurs, rapid treatment is imperative. Use gastric lavage to remove iron from the stomach. Administer deferoxamine if plasma levels of iron exceed 500 mcg/mL. Manage acidosis and shock as required.

CYANOCOBALAMIN (VITAMIN B_{12})

Preadministration Assessment

Therapeutic Goal

Correction of megaloblastic anemia and other sequelae of vitamin B_{12} deficiency.

Baseline Data

Assess the extent of vitamin B_{12} deficiency. Record signs and symptoms of anemia (e.g., pallor, dyspnea, palpitations, fatigue). Determine the extent of neurologic damage. Assess GI involvement.

Baseline laboratory data include plasma vitamin B_{12} levels, erythrocyte and reticulocyte counts, and hemoglobin and hematocrit values. Bone marrow may be examined for megaloblasts. A Schilling test may be ordered to assess vitamin B_{12} absorption.

Identifying High-Risk Patients

Use with *caution* in patients receiving folic acid.

Implementation: Administration

Routes and Administration

Administration may be IM, subQ, oral, or intranasal. For most patients, lifelong treatment is required. Traditional therapy

Continued

Summary of Major Nursing Implications[a]—cont'd

consists of IM or subQ injections administered monthly. However, treatment can be just as effective with large daily oral doses or with intranasal doses (administered weekly with Nascobal). **Inform patients that intranasal doses should not be administered within 1 hour before or 1 hour after consuming hot foods or hot liquids.**

Implementation: Measures to Enhance Therapeutic Effects

Promoting Adherence

Patients with permanent impairment of B_{12} absorption require lifelong B_{12} therapy. To promote adherence, **educate patients about the nature of their condition, and impress upon them the need for monthly injections, daily oral therapy, or weekly intranasal therapy.** Schedule appointments for injections at convenient times.

Improving Nutrition

When B_{12} deficiency is not due to impaired absorption, a change in diet may accelerate recovery. **Advise the patient to increase consumption of B_{12}-rich foods (e.g., muscle meats, dairy products).**

Ongoing Evaluation and Interventions

Evaluating Therapeutic Effects

Assess for improvements in hematologic and neurologic status. Over a period of 2 to 3 weeks, megaloblasts should disappear, reticulocyte counts should rise, and the hematocrit should normalize. Neurologic damage may take months to improve; in some cases, full recovery may never occur.

For patients receiving long-term therapy, vitamin B_{12} levels should be measured every 3 to 6 months, and blood counts should be performed.

Minimizing Adverse Effects

Hypokalemia may develop during the first days of therapy. Monitor serum potassium levels and observe the patient for signs of potassium insufficiency. **Teach patients the signs and symptoms of hypokalemia (e.g., muscle weakness, irregular heartbeat), and instruct them to report these immediately.**

Minimizing Adverse Interactions

Folic acid can correct hematologic effects of vitamin B_{12} deficiency, but not the neurologic effects. By improving the hematologic picture, folic acid can mask ongoing B_{12} deficiency, resulting in undertreatment and progression of neurologic injury. Accordingly, when folic acid and cyanocobalamin are used concurrently, special care must be taken to ensure that the cyanocobalamin dosage is adequate.

FOLIC ACID (FOLACIN, FOLATE, PTEROYLGLUTAMIC ACID)

Preadministration Assessment

Therapeutic Goal

Folic acid is used for (1) treatment of megaloblastic anemia resulting from folic acid deficiency; (2) initial treatment of severe megaloblastic anemia resulting from vitamin B_{12} deficiency; and (3) prevention of folic acid deficiency, especially in women who might become pregnant and in women who are pregnant or lactating.

Baseline Data

Assess the extent of folate deficiency. Record signs and symptoms of anemia (e.g., pallor, dyspnea, palpitations, fatigue). Determine the extent of GI damage.

Baseline laboratory data include serum folate levels, erythrocyte and reticulocyte counts, and hemoglobin and hematocrit values. In addition, bone marrow may be evaluated for megaloblasts. To rule out vitamin B_{12} deficiency, vitamin B_{12} determinations and a Schilling test may be ordered.

Identifying High-Risk Patients

Folic acid is *contraindicated* for patients with pernicious anemia (except during the acute phase of treatment). Inappropriate use of folic acid by these patients can mask signs of vitamin B_{12} deficiency, allowing further neurologic deterioration.

Implementation: Dosage and Administration

Routes

Oral, subQ, IV, and IM. Oral administration is most common and preferred. Injections are employed only when intestinal absorption is severely impaired.

Dosage

Prevention of Neural Tube Defects. To reduce the risk of neural tube defects, women who might become pregnant should consume 400 to 800 mcg of supplemental folate daily—in addition to the folate they get from food.

Treatment of Folate-Deficient Megaloblastic Anemia. The initial oral dosage is 1000 to 2000 mcg/day. Once symptoms have resolved, the maintenance dosage is 400 mcg/day.

Implementation: Measures to Enhance Therapeutic Effects

Improving Nutrition

If the diet is deficient in folic acid, advise the patient to increase consumption of folate-rich foods (e.g., green vegetables, liver). If alcoholism underlies dietary deficiency, offer counseling for alcoholism, as well as dietary advice.

Ongoing Evaluation and Interventions

Evaluating Therapeutic Effects

Monitor hematologic status. Within 2 weeks, megaloblasts should disappear, reticulocyte counts should increase, and the hematocrit should begin to rise.

[a]Patient education information is highlighted as **blue text.**

CHAPTER

56 Hematopoietic Agents

HEMATOPOIETIC GROWTH FACTORS

Hematopoiesis is the process by which our bodies make red blood cells, white blood cells, and platelets. The process is regulated in part by hematopoietic growth factors—naturally occurring hormones that stimulate the proliferation and differentiation of hematopoietic stem cells, and enhance function in the mature forms of those cells. In a laboratory setting, hematopoietic growth factors can cause stem cells to form colonies of mature blood cells. Because of this action, some hematopoietic growth factors are also known as *colony-stimulating factors.* Therapeutic applications of hematopoietic growth factors include (1) acceleration of neutrophil and platelet repopulation after cancer chemotherapy, (2) acceleration of bone marrow recovery after an autologous bone marrow transplantation (BMT), and (3) stimulation of erythrocyte production in patients with chronic renal failure (CRF).

The names used for the hematopoietic growth factors are a potential source of confusion. Each product has a biologic name, a generic name, and one or more proprietary (brand) names. The biologic, generic, and proprietary names for available products are shown in Table 56.1.

ERYTHROPOIETIC GROWTH FACTORS

Erythropoietic growth factors—also known as *erythropoiesis stimulating agents* (ESAs)—stimulate production of erythrocytes (red blood cells [RBCs]). Because they increase RBC production, ESAs represent an alternative to infusions for patients with low RBC counts, including patients with CRF and cancer patients undergoing myelosuppressive chemotherapy. Unfortunately, although these drugs can be beneficial, postmarketing surveillance has shown clear evidence of harm. In all patients, ESAs may increase the risk of stroke, heart failure, blood clots, myocardial infarction (MI), and death. In patients with cancer, ESAs may shorten time to tumor progression and reduce overall survival. Because of this potential for harm, use of ESAs has dropped sharply, especially among patients with cancer.

In the United States, two ESAs are available: epoetin alfa (erythropoietin) and darbepoetin alfa (a long-acting form of erythropoietin). A third ESA—methoxy polyethylene glycol–epoetin beta (a very-long-acting form of erythropoietin), sold as *Mircera*—was formerly available only in other countries, but is now available for hemodialysis patients in authorized clinics within the United States.

Prototype Drugs

HEMATOPOIETIC AGENTS

Erythropoietic Growth Factors
Epoetin alfa (erythropoietin)

Leukopoietic Growth Factors
Filgrastim (granulocyte colony-stimulating factor)

Thrombopoietic Growth Factors
Oprelvekin

Epoetin Alfa (Erythropoietin)

Epoetin alfa [Epogen, Procrit, Eprex ♣] is a growth factor produced by recombinant DNA technology. Chemically, the compound is a glycoprotein containing 165 amino acids. The protein portion of epoetin alfa is identical to that of human erythropoietin, a naturally occurring hormone. Epoetin alfa is used to maintain erythrocyte counts in (1) patients with CRF, (2) patients with nonmyeloid malignancies who have anemia secondary to chemotherapy, and (3) HIV-infected patients taking zidovudine. In addition, the drug can be used to elevate erythrocyte counts in anemic patients before elective surgery.

TABLE 56.1 ■ Nomenclature for Hematopoietic Growth Factors

	Pharmacologic Names	
Biologic Name	**Generic Name**	**Brand Name**
ERYTHROPOIETIC GROWTH FACTORS		
Erythropoietin	Darbepoetin alfa Epoetin alfa	Aranesp Epogen, Procrit, Eprex ♣
LEUKOPOIETIC GROWTH FACTORS		
Granulocyte colony-stimulating factor (G-CSF)	Filgrastim Pegfilgrastim	Neupogen Neulasta
Granulocyte-macrophage colony-stimulating factor (GM-CSF)	Sargramostim	Leukine
THROMBOPOIETIC GROWTH FACTOR		
Interleukin-11	Oprelvekin	Generic only

Physiology

Erythropoietin is a glycoprotein hormone that stimulates production of RBCs in the bone marrow. The hormone is produced by peritubular cells in the proximal tubules of the kidney. In response to anemia or hypoxia, circulating levels of erythropoietin rise dramatically, triggering an increase in erythrocyte synthesis. However, because production of erythrocytes requires iron, folic acid, and vitamin B_{12}, the response to erythropoietin is minimal if any of these is deficient.

Erythropoietin has significant physiologic effects outside the hematopoietic system. Animal studies indicate that erythropoietin is secreted by cells of many organs, including the brain, bone marrow, liver, heart, kidney, uterus, testes, and blood vessels—and that receptors for erythropoietin are present at most of these sites. Actions of the hormone include modulation of angiogenesis (blood vessel formation) and maintenance of cellular integrity (by inhibiting apoptotic mechanisms of cell injury). In the future, these actions may be exploited to treat a variety of disorders, including stroke, diabetic nephropathy, multiple sclerosis, MI, and heart failure (HF).

Therapeutic Uses

Anemia of Chronic Renal Failure. Epoetin alfa can partially reverse anemia associated with CRF, reducing—but not eliminating—the need for transfusions. Benefits accrue to patients on dialysis as well as those who do not yet require dialysis. Initial effects can be seen within 1 to 2 weeks. Hemoglobin reaches maximal acceptable levels (10 to 11 gm/dL) in 2 to 3 months. Unfortunately, although treatment reduces the need for transfusions, it does *not* improve quality of life, decrease fatigue, or prevent progressive renal deterioration.

For therapy to be effective, iron stores must be adequate. Transferrin saturation should be at least 20%, and ferritin concentration should be at least 100 ng/mL. If pretreatment assessment indicates these values are low, they must be restored with iron supplements.

Chemotherapy-Induced Anemia. Epoetin alfa is used to treat chemotherapy-induced anemia in patients with *nonmyeloid malignancies,* reducing the need for periodic transfusions. Since transfusions require hospitalization, whereas epoetin can be self-administered at home, epoetin therapy can spare patients considerable inconvenience. Because epoetin works slowly (the hematocrit may take 2 to 4 weeks to recover), transfusions are still indicated when rapid replenishment of RBCs is required. Please note that epoetin is not approved for patients with *leukemias* and *other myeloid malignancies* because the drug may stimulate proliferation of these cancers. Furthermore, since ESAs can shorten survival time in *all* cancer patients, epoetin is indicated only when the goal of cancer therapy is *palliation.* When the goal is *cure,* ESAs should not be used. (It makes no sense to give a potentially lethal drug to a patient who might be cured.) A new clinical guideline—*American Society of Hematology/American Society of Clinical Oncology Clinical Practice Guideline Update on the Use of Epoetin and Darbepoetin in Adult Patients with Cancer*—provides detailed information on using ESAs in patients with cancer.

HIV-Infected Patients Taking Zidovudine. Epoetin alfa is approved for treating anemia caused by therapy with zidovudine (AZT) in patients with AIDS. For these patients, treatment can maintain or elevate erythrocyte counts and reduce the need for transfusions. However, if endogenous levels of erythropoietin are at or above 500 milliunits/mL, raising them further with epoetin is unlikely to help.

Anemia in Patients Facing Surgery. Epoetin may be given to increase erythrocyte levels in anemic patients scheduled for elective surgery. The drug should be used only when significant blood loss is anticipated—but should not be used before cardiac or vascular surgery. For surgical patients, epoetin offers two benefits: (1) it decreases the need for transfusions, and (2) by increasing erythrocyte synthesis, it allows patients to predeposit more blood in anticipation of transfusion needs.

Pharmacokinetics

Epoetin alfa is administered parenterally (IV or subQ). The drug cannot be given orally because, being a glycoprotein, it would be degraded in the GI tract. The plasma half-life is highly variable and unchanged by dialysis.

Adverse Effects and Interactions

Epoetin alfa is generally well tolerated. Although the drug is a protein, no serious allergic reactions have been reported. The most significant adverse effect is hypertension. There are no significant drug interactions. As discussed later under *Warnings,* improper use of epoetin alfa has been associated with serious cardiovascular events, tumor progression, and deaths.

Hypertension. In patients with CRF, epoetin is frequently associated with an increase in blood pressure. The extent of hypertension is directly related to the rate of rise in the hematocrit. To minimize risk, blood pressure should be monitored and, if necessary, controlled with antihypertensive drugs. If hypertension cannot be controlled, epoetin dosage should be reduced. In patients with pre-existing hypertension (a common complication of CRF), it is imperative that blood pressure be under control before epoetin use. About 30% of dialysis patients receiving epoetin require an adjustment in their antihypertensive therapy once the hematocrit has been normalized.

Cardiovascular Events. Epoetin has been associated with an increase in serious cardiovascular events. Among these are cardiac arrest, hypertension, HF, and thrombotic events, including stroke and MI. Risk is greatest when (1) the hemoglobin level exceeds 11 gm/dL or (2) the rate of rise in hemoglobin exceeds 1 gm/dL in any 2-week interval. Accordingly, dosage should be reduced when hemoglobin approaches 11 gm/dL or when the rate of rise exceeds 1 gm/dL in 2 weeks—and, in most patients, dosing should be temporarily stopped if hemoglobin rises to 11 gm/dL or more. To prevent clotting in the dialysis machine, CRF patients on dialysis may need increased anticoagulation with heparin.

Autoimmune Pure Red-Cell Aplasia. Very, very rarely, treatment with epoetin leads to pure red-cell aplasia (PRCA), a condition characterized by severe anemia and a complete absence of erythrocyte precursor cells in bone marrow. The cause is production of neutralizing antibodies directed against epoetin itself, as well as any native erythropoietin the body is still able to produce. In the absence of epoetin and erythropoietin, production of RBCs ceases. Because patients can no longer make erythrocytes, transfusions are required for survival. If evidence of PRCA develops, epoetin should be discontinued and blood should be assessed for neutralizing antibodies.

Safety Alert

DOSAGES

To minimize the risk of serious adverse events, the dosage of epoetin alfa and all other ESAs should be the lowest needed to gradually raise hemoglobin content to the lowest level sufficient to reduce the need for RBC transfusions. In most cases, hemoglobin level should not exceed 11 gm/dL. When ESAs are administered in doses sufficient to raise hemoglobin above this level, risk of serious cardiovascular events and death is increased.

Warnings

Cancer Patients. Postmarketing reports indicate that ESAs can accelerate tumor progression and shorten life in certain cancer patients—especially when hemoglobin has been driven above 12 gm/dL. In patients with advanced head and neck cancer who are undergoing radiation therapy, ESAs have shortened the time to tumor progression. In patients with metastatic breast cancer who are receiving chemotherapy, ESAs have shortened overall survival and increased deaths from tumor progression. Also, ESAs have increased the risk of death in patients with active malignant disease who are not receiving either radiation or chemotherapy, so ESAs are contraindicated for this group.

Renal Failure Patients. In patients with anemia of chronic renal failure, ESAs can increase the risk of serious cardiovascular events and death if hemoglobin levels are driven too high. Accordingly, dosage should be individualized to produce hemoglobin levels no higher than 10 to 11 gm/dL.

Preoperative Patients. When given to preoperative patients to reduce the need for RBC transfusion, ESAs have increased the risk of deep vein thrombosis—but only in patients who were not given an anticoagulant. Accordingly, anticoagulant therapy should be considered for all preoperative patients receiving an ESA.

Risk Evaluation and Mitigation Strategy

All Patients. Because ESAs can cause serious adverse effects, these drugs must be prescribed and used under a Risk Evaluation and Mitigation Strategy (REMS), mandated by the U.S. Food and Drug Administration (FDA). Under the REMS, all patients must receive a Medication Guide that explains the risks and benefits of ESAs. The goal is to help patients make an informed decision when use of an ESA is under consideration. The guide also informs patients about what they can do to minimize risk.

Cancer Patients. The *ESA APPRISE Oncology Program*[a] sets additional requirements for using ESAs in cancer patients. Prescribers must enroll in ESA APPRISE, complete a brief training module, discuss the risks and benefits of ESAs with the patient, and sign a form acknowledging that the discussion took place. Hospitals that dispense ESAs must be enrolled in ESA APPRISE and must ensure that all ESA prescribers are enrolled as well. Prescribers who use ESAs for patients who do not have cancer are not required to enroll in ESA APPRISE.

PATIENT-CENTERED CARE ACROSS THE LIFE SPAN

Hematopoietic Agents

Life Stage	Patient Care Concerns
Infants	See "Breast-feeding women," below.
Children/ adolescents	Many hematopoietics can be used safely in children, just in smaller doses. Side effect profiles are similar to those of adults.
Pregnant women	Animal studies indicate that hematopoietics can cause fetal harm, and they are classified in FDA Pregnancy Risk Category C.[a] Risks and benefits must be considered for administration during pregnancy.
Breast-feeding women	Colony-stimulating factors are normal components of human breast milk. Infant harm has not been demonstrated. No special precautions are required during breast-feeding.
Older adults	Hematopoietic agents do not lower mortality or cardiovascular risk in older adults. However, recent studies have shown improved quality of life in older adults with more physiologically normal hemoglobin. Hematopoietic agents can help achieve this.

[a]As of 2020, the FDA will no longer use Pregnancy Risk Categories. Please refer to Chapter 9 for more information.

Monitoring

Hemoglobin level should be measured at baseline and twice weekly thereafter until the target level has been reached and a maintenance dose established. Complete blood counts with a differential should be done routinely. Blood chemistry—blood urea nitrogen (BUN), uric acid, creatinine, phosphorus, and potassium—should be monitored. Iron should be measured periodically and maintained at an adequate level.

Preparations, Dosage, and Administration

Preparations. Epoetin alfa [Epogen, Procrit, Eprex 🍁] is supplied in 1-mL single-dose vials (2000, 3000, 4000, 10,000, and 40,000 units) and in 1- and 2-mL multidose vials (10,000 and 20,000 units). Vials should not be shaken (because epoetin is a protein that can be denatured by agitation). Don't mix epoetin with other drugs. Store at 2°C to 8°C (36°F to 46°F); don't freeze.

General Dosing Guidelines. *Use the lowest dosage needed to gradually increase the hemoglobin concentration to the lowest level sufficient to reduce the need for RBC transfusion.* For most patients, the target

[a]ESA (erythropoiesis stimulating agent) APPRISE (Assisting Providers and Cancer Patients with Risk Information for the Safe Use of ESAs) Oncology Program.

hemoglobin level is 10 to 11 gm/dL. *Regimens that raise hemoglobin above 11 gm/dL are associated with an increased risk of serious cardiovascular events and death.* Accordingly, dosage should be reduced when hemoglobin approaches 11 gm/dL or when hemoglobin increases by more than 1 gm/dL in any 2-week interval. For most patients, if hemoglobin rises above 11 gm/dL, withhold treatment until hemoglobin drops below 11 gm/dL. When treatment resumes, decrease the dose by 25%, and then titrate upward as needed.

Dosing in Patients With Chronic Renal Failure

Route. Administration may be IV or subQ. When epoetin alfa first came into use, IV administration was preferred, in part because subQ administration was reputedly painful and in part because bioavailability following subQ injection is reduced—although the half-life is prolonged. A study comparing IV therapy with subQ therapy indicated that both methods produce equivalent effects. Furthermore, with subQ administration, 30% less epoetin is required, and reported discomfort at the injection site is minimal. However, IV is currently the preferred route for administration.

Dosage. The initial dosage is 50 to 100 units/kg 3 times a week. Administration is by IV bolus for dialysis patients and by IV bolus or subQ injection for nondialysis patients. Once hemoglobin has risen high enough to avoid transfusions, an individualized maintenance dosage should be established: For dialysis patients, the median maintenance dosage is 75 units/kg 3 times a week; for nondialysis patients, the median maintenance dosage is 75 to 100 units/kg once a week. If hemoglobin rises above 11 gm/dL (for patients on dialysis) or 10 gm/dL (for patients not on dialysis), epoetin should be temporarily withheld.

Dosing in Patients Receiving Cancer Chemotherapy. Two dosing schedules may be used: once weekly or thrice weekly.

Once-Weekly Dosing. The initial dosage is 40,000 units subQ each week. If, after 4 weeks of therapy, hemoglobin has not increased by at least 1 gm/dL, the dosage should be increased to 60,000 units once weekly. If hemoglobin has not increased by 1 gm/dL after 4 weeks, treatment should stop, since further increases are not likely to succeed. When treatment *does* work, dosing should cease when chemotherapy stops.

Thrice-Weekly Dosing. The initial dosage is 150 units/kg subQ 3 times a week. If the response is inadequate by 8 weeks, the dosage may be increased to 300 units/kg 3 times a week. Dosing should cease when chemotherapy stops.

Dosing in HIV-Infected Patients Taking Zidovudine. Before treatment, measure the endogenous erythropoietin level. If this level is already at or above 500 milliunits/mL, epoetin alfa is unlikely to help.

The initial dosage is 100 units/kg (IV or subQ injection) 3 times a week for 8 weeks. If the response is insufficient, the dosage may be increased by increments of 50 to 100 units/kg until a maximum of 300 units/kg 3 times a week has been reached. If hemoglobin rises above 12 gm/dL, epoetin should be temporarily withheld.

Dosing in Anemic Patients Scheduled for Surgery. The recommended dosage is 300 units/kg/day subQ for 15 days starting 10 days before surgery.

Darbepoetin Alfa (Erythropoietin, Long Acting)

Actions and Therapeutic Use

Darbepoetin alfa [Aranesp] is a long-acting analog of epoetin alfa. Both drugs act on erythroid progenitor cells to stimulate production of erythrocytes. Darbepoetin differs structurally from epoetin in that it has two additional carbohydrate chains. Because of these chains, darbepoetin is cleared more slowly than epoetin, and thus has a longer half-life (49 hours vs. 18 to 24 hours). As a result, darbepoetin can be administered less frequently.

Darbepoetin is indicated for (1) anemia associated with CRF and (2) anemia associated with cancer chemotherapy. In patients with CRF, darbepoetin can reduce the need for erythrocyte infusions—but it does not reduce the incidence of renal events, cardiovascular events, or death, nor does it decrease fatigue or improve quality of life. In patients with cancer, treatment is limited to those with nonmyeloid malignancies whose anemia is caused by chemotherapy, and not by the cancer itself. Furthermore, since darbepoetin may increase the risk of cancer-related death, it should be used only when the objective of cancer therapy is palliation, not when the objective is cure.

Adverse Effects and Warnings

Darbepoetin is generally well tolerated. As with epoetin, the most common problem is hypertension. The risk can be minimized by ensuring that the rate of rise in hemoglobin does not exceed 1 gm/dL every 2 weeks. If hypertension develops, it should be controlled with antihypertensive drugs. Patients already taking antihypertensive drugs may need to increase their dosage.

Like epoetin alfa, darbepoetin increases the risk of PRCA, MI, HF, stroke, cardiac arrest, and other cardiovascular events, especially when the hemoglobin level exceeds 11 gm/dL or when the rate of rise in hemoglobin exceeds 1 gm/dL in 2 weeks.

Like epoetin alfa, darbepoetin can promote tumor progression and shorten survival in some cancer patients, and thus should not be used when the objective of chemotherapy is cure.

Monitoring

When initiating darbepoetin or changing dosage, the hemoglobin level should be measured weekly until it stabilizes. Thereafter, hemoglobin should be measured at least once a month.

Preparations, Dosage, and Administration

Preparations and Storage. Darbepoetin alfa [Aranesp] is available in 1-mL single-dose vials (25, 40, 60, 100, 200, and 300 mcg/mL and 150 mcg/0.75 mL) and pre-filled single-dose syringes and auto-injectors (10 mcg/0.4 mL, 25 mcg/0.42 mL to 500 mcg/mL). Administration is by subQ and IV injection. Don't dilute darbepoetin or mix it with other drugs. Because darbepoetin is a protein that can be denatured by agitation, do not shake the drug. Discard preparations that are discolored or contain particles. Store at 2°C to 8°C (36°F to 46°F); don't freeze.

General Dosing Guidelines. The treatment goal is to reduce the need for transfusions. Dosage should be reduced when hemoglobin approaches 11 gm/dL or when hemoglobin increases by more than 1 gm/dL in any 2-week interval. If hemoglobin rises to 11 gm/dL or higher, withhold treatment until hemoglobin drops below 11 gm/dL. When treatment resumes, decrease the dose by 25%, and then titrate upward as needed.

Dosing in Patients With Chronic Renal Failure. The initial dosage is 0.45 mcg/kg, given either IV or subQ once a week. If hemoglobin rises above 11 gm/dL (for patients on dialysis) or 10 gm/dL (for patents not on dialysis), treatment should be temporarily withheld. Because responses develop gradually, dosage should be adjusted no more than once every 4 weeks. Quite often, the maintenance dosage is less than the initial dosage.

When switching from epoetin to darbepoetin, the new dosage and dosing frequency are based on the existing epoetin usage. For example, patients receiving 5000 to 11,000 units of epoetin each week should receive 25 mcg of darbepoetin each week. If the epoetin dosing frequency was 2 to 3 times a week, darbepoetin should be given once a week; if epoetin was given once a week, darbepoetin should be given once every 2 weeks.

Dosing in Patients Undergoing Cancer Chemotherapy. The initial dosage is 2.25 mcg/kg subQ once a week or 500 mcg subQ every 3 weeks. If the increase in hemoglobin is less than 1 gm/dL after 6 weeks, dosage should be increased to 4.5 mcg once a week. If the increase in hemoglobin exceeds 1 gm/dL in 2 weeks, or if hemoglobin rises high enough to avoid transfusions, dosage should be reduced by 40%. Dosing should cease when chemotherapy stops.

LEUKOPOIETIC GROWTH FACTORS

The leukopoietic growth factors stimulate production of leukocytes (white blood cells). Three preparations are available: filgrastim, pegfilgrastim, and sargramostim.

Filgrastim (Granulocyte Colony-Stimulating Factor)

Filgrastim [Neupogen] is a leukopoietic growth factor produced by recombinant DNA technology. The drug is essentially identical in structure and actions to human granulocyte colony-stimulating factor (G-CSF), a naturally occurring hormone. Filgrastim has three principal uses: elevation of neutrophil counts in cancer patients, mobilization of hematopoietic progenitor cells into peripheral blood for apheresis collection, and treatment of severe chronic neutropenia.

Physiology

G-CSF acts on cells in bone marrow to increase production of neutrophils (granulocytes). In addition, it enhances phagocytic and cytotoxic actions of mature neutrophils. The hormone is produced by monocytes, fibroblasts, and endothelial cells in response to inflammation and allergic challenge, suggesting that its natural role is to help fight infection and cancer.

Therapeutic Uses

Patients Undergoing Myelosuppressive Chemotherapy. Filgrastim is given to reduce the risk of infection in patients undergoing cancer chemotherapy. Many anticancer drugs act on the bone marrow to suppress production of neutrophils, greatly increasing the risk of infection. By stimulating neutrophil production, filgrastim can decrease infection risk. Clinical trials have shown that treatment (1) reduces the incidence of severe neutropenia, (2) produces a dose-dependent increase in circulating neutrophils, (3) reduces the incidence of infection, (4) reduces the need for hospitalization, and (5) reduces the need for IV antibiotics. Because filgrastim stimulates proliferation of bone marrow cells, it should be used with great caution in patients with cancers that originated in the marrow.

Patients Undergoing Bone Marrow Transplantation. Filgrastim is given to shorten the duration of neutropenia in patients who have undergone high-dose chemotherapy followed by BMT. As noted, the drug is not used when the cancer is of myeloid origin.

Harvesting of Hematopoietic Stem Cells. Hematopoietic stem cells (HSCs) are harvested before bone marrow ablation with high-dose chemotherapy. Following chemotherapy, the HSCs are infused back into the patient to accelerate repopulation of the bone marrow. Treatment with filgrastim before harvesting increases the number of circulating HSCs and therefore facilitates collection. If treatment with filgrastim alone is inadequate, a drug called plerixafor (discussed later) can be added to increase the HSC yield.

Severe Chronic Neutropenia. Filgrastim provides effective treatment for *congenital neutropenia* (Kostmann's syndrome), a condition characterized by pronounced neutropenia and frequent, severe infections. Therapy helps resolve existing infections and decreases the incidence of subsequent infections. Because treatment is chronic, the cost is very high. In addition to congenital neutropenia, filgrastim is used in patients with *idiopathic neutropenia* and *cyclic neutropenia.*

Investigational Uses. Filgrastim can reverse *zidovudine-induced neutropenia* in HIV-infected patients. However, the drug does not reduce the incidence of opportunistic infections. In patients with *acute myelogenous leukemia,* filgrastim has been given to stimulate division of cancer cells, making them more sensitive to chemotherapeutic agents. Filgrastim has also been employed in patients with *aplastic anemia* and *myelodysplasia.*

Pharmacokinetics

Administration is parenteral (IV or subQ). Filgrastim cannot be used orally because, being a protein, it would be destroyed in the GI tract. The drug is eliminated by renal excretion. Its serum half-life is about 3.5 hours.

Adverse Effects and Interactions

When used short term, filgrastim is generally devoid of serious adverse effects. There are no drug interactions of note.

Bone Pain. Filgrastim causes bone pain in about 25% of patients. Pain is dose related and usually mild to moderate. In most cases, relief can be achieved with a nonopioid analgesic (e.g., acetaminophen). If not, an opioid may be tried.

Leukocytosis. When administered in doses greater than 5 mcg/kg/day, filgrastim has caused white blood cell counts to rise above 100,000/mm^3 in 2% of patients. Although no adverse effects were associated with this degree of leukocytosis, avoiding leukocytosis would nonetheless be prudent. Excessive white cell counts can be avoided by obtaining complete blood counts twice weekly during treatment and by reducing filgrastim dosage if leukocytosis develops.

Other Adverse Effects. Treatment frequently causes elevation of plasma uric acid, lactate dehydrogenase, and alkaline phosphatase. Increases are usually moderate and reverse spontaneously. Long-term therapy has caused splenomegaly.

Preparations, Dosage, and Administration

Preparations and Storage. Filgrastim [Neupogen] solution for injection is supplied in two concentrations: (1) 300 mcg in 1-mL and 480 mcg in 1.6-mL single-dose vials, and (2) 300 mcg/0.5 mL and 480 mcg/0.8 mL pre-filled syringes. The drug is stored at 2°C to 8°C (36°F to 46°F)—not frozen.

Dosage and Administration

General Considerations. Before administration, filgrastim can be kept at room temperature for up to 24 hours. Each vial or syringe should be used only once, and should not be agitated.

Cancer Chemotherapy. The usual dosage is 5 mcg/kg once daily, given IV or subQ. Therapy should start no sooner than 24 hours after termination of chemotherapy and should continue up to 2 weeks after the expected chemotherapy-induced nadir, or until the absolute neutrophil count has reached 10,000/mm^3. Administer by subQ bolus, short IV infusion, or continuous IV or subQ infusion. A complete blood count and platelet count should be obtained before treatment and twice weekly during treatment.

Bone Marrow Transplantation. The initial dosage is 10 mcg/kg/day, administered by slow IV or subQ infusion. During the period of neutrophil recovery, dosage is titrated against the neutrophil count.

Harvesting of Hematopoietic Stem Cells. The usual dosage is 10 mcg/kg/day IV (by bolus or infusion), starting at least 4 days before the first leukapheresis procedure, and continuing until the last leukapheresis.

Severe Chronic Neutropenia. For congenital neutropenia, the initial dosage is 6 mcg/kg subQ twice a day. The maintenance dosage is 6 mcg/kg/day.

Tbo-filgrastim (Granulocyte Colony-Stimulating Factor). Tbo-filgrastim [Granix], like filgrastim, also acts by stimulating the production of neutrophils. It is indicated for the treatment of neutropenia in patients with non-myeloid malignancy who are undergoing chemotherapy. When compared to filgrastim in trials, tbo-filgrastim provided similar results, but at a decreased cost. Tbo-filgrastim is supplied in pre-filled syringes (300 mcg/0.5 mL, 480 mcg/0.8 mL). The usual dose is 5 mcg/kg subQ daily, starting 24 hours after chemotherapy.

Pegfilgrastim (Granulocyte Colony-Stimulating Factor, Long Acting)

Pegfilgrastim [Neulasta] is a long-acting derivative of filgrastim [Neupogen]. Both drugs stimulate myeloid cells to increase production of neutrophils. Pegfilgrastim is made by conjugating filgrastim with polyethylene glycol (PEG), in a process known as pegylation. Pegylation increases the size of filgrastim and thereby delays its excretion by the kidneys. As a result, the drug's half-life is greatly increased—from 3.5 hours (for native filgrastim) up to about 17 hours. Because pegfilgrastim has a longer half-life than filgrastim, the drug is easier to use: A course of treatment consists of just one dose, rather than one dose every day for 2 weeks. At this time, pegfilgrastim has only one approved application: to decrease the incidence of infection, as indicated by febrile neutropenia, in patients undergoing chemotherapy of nonmyeloid malignancies. As discussed previously, filgrastim has additional uses.

Adverse effects are much like those of filgrastim. Bone pain is the most common, occurring in 26% of patients. About 6% require an opioid analgesic for relief. Other side effects include reversible elevations of lactate dehydrogenase, alkaline phosphatase, and uric acid.

Preparations, Dosage, and Administration

Pegfilgrastim [Neulasta] is available in solution (6 mg/0.6 mL) in pre-filled, single-dose syringes. For all patients, treatment consists of one 6-mg subQ dose, injected 24 hours after each round of chemotherapy. Because stimulated myeloid cells are highly vulnerable to anticancer drugs and because pegfilgrastim has a prolonged duration of action, at least 14 days must elapse between injecting pegfilgrastim and the next round of chemotherapy. Accordingly, if the scheduled interval between rounds of chemotherapy is less than 15 days (24 hours plus 14 days), pegfilgrastim cannot be used. Instead, filgrastim, with its shorter duration of action, should be employed. Pegfilgrastim has not been evaluated in infants, children, or adolescents who weigh less than 45 kg. Accordingly, the drug should not be used in these patients.

Sargramostim (Granulocyte-Macrophage Colony-Stimulating Factor)

Sargramostim [Leukine] is a hematopoietic growth factor produced by recombinant DNA technology. The drug is nearly identical in structure and actions to human granulocyte-macrophage colony-stimulating factor (GM-CSF), a naturally occurring hormone. Sargramostim is given to accelerate bone marrow recovery following BMT.

Physiology

GM-CSF acts on cells in bone marrow to increase production of neutrophils, monocytes, macrophages, and eosinophils. In addition, the hormone acts on the mature forms of these cells to enhance their function. For example, GM-CSF acts on neutrophils and macrophages to increase their chemotactic, antifungal, and antiparasitic actions. Also, the hormone acts on monocytes and polymorphonuclear leukocytes to enhance their actions against cancer cells. GM-CSF is synthesized by T lymphocytes, monocytes, fibroblasts, and endothelial cells. Like G-CSF, GM-CSF is produced in response to inflammation and allergic challenge, suggesting that its natural role is to help fight infection and cancer.

Therapeutic Uses

Adjunct to Autologous Bone Marrow Transplantation. Sargramostim can accelerate myeloid recovery in cancer patients who have undergone autologous BMT following high-dose chemotherapy (with or without concurrent irradiation). The drug is approved for promoting myeloid recovery following BMT in patients with acute lymphoblastic leukemia, non-Hodgkin's lymphoma, and Hodgkin's disease. In these patients, sargramostim can (1) accelerate neutrophil engraftment, (2) reduce the duration of antibiotic use, (3) reduce the duration of infectious episodes, and (4) reduce the duration of hospitalization.

Treatment of Failed Bone Marrow Transplants. Sargramostim is approved for patients in whom an autologous or allogenic bone marrow transplant has failed to take. For these patients, the drug can produce a significant increase in survival time.

Patients With Acute Myelogenous Leukemia (AML). Sargramostim is given following induction chemotherapy in older patients with AML. The goal is to accelerate neutrophil recovery and reduce the incidence of life-threatening infections.

Investigational Uses. In *HIV-infected patients,* sargramostim can reverse neutropenia caused by zidovudine (a drug that inhibits HIV replication) and by ganciclovir (a drug for cytomegalovirus retinitis).

In patients with *aplastic anemia* (a syndrome characterized by pancytopenia and high mortality from infection and bleeding), sargramostim can increase neutrophil counts and reduce the incidence and severity of infections.

Sargramostim is beneficial for patients with *myelodysplastic syndrome* (MDS), a chronic disorder characterized by greatly reduced hematopoiesis. Patients with MDS are neutropenic, thrombocytopenic, and anemic, putting them at high risk for serious infections and bleeding. The syndrome has a mortality rate of 66%—and those who survive often develop leukemia. Treatment with sargramostim can increase counts of neutrophils, eosinophils, and monocytes. However, the premalignant clone still exists and may eventually cause leukemia.

Pharmacokinetics

Sargramostim is administered by IV infusion. Since the drug is a protein and thus would be degraded in the digestive tract, it cannot be administered by mouth. Other aspects of its kinetics are unremarkable.

Adverse Effects and Interactions

Sargramostim is generally well tolerated. A variety of acute reactions have been observed, including diarrhea, weakness, rash, malaise, and bone pain that can be managed with nonopioid analgesics (e.g., acetaminophen). Pleural and pericardial effusions have occurred, but only when sargramostim dosage was massive (16 times the recommended dosage). There are no drug interactions of note.

Leukocytosis and Thrombocytosis. Stimulation of the bone marrow can cause excessive production of white blood cells and platelets. Complete blood counts should be done twice weekly during therapy. If the white cell count rises above 50,000/mm^3, if the absolute neutrophil count rises above 20,000/mm^3, or if the platelet count rises above 500,000/mm^3, sargramostim should be interrupted or the dosage reduced.

Preparations, Dosage, and Administration

Preparations. Sargramostim [Leukine] is available in concentrated solution (500 mcg/mL) and as a powder (250 mcg) to be reconstituted for IV infusion. To reconstitute the powder, add 1 mL of sterile water and gently swirl; don't shake.

Dilution. To prepare the final infusion solution, dilute the concentrated solution in either (1) 0.9% sodium chloride (if the final concentration of sargramostim is to be 10 mcg/mL or more) or (2) 0.9% sodium chloride plus 0.1% albumin (if the final concentration is to be less than 10 mcg/mL). Since the solution contains no antibacterial preservatives, it should be used as soon as possible—and no later than 6 hours after preparation.

Storage. All sargramostim preparations should be stored at 2°C to 8°C (36°F to 46°F)—never frozen.

Dosage and Administration. To accelerate myeloid recovery after autologous BMT, the recommended dosage is 250 mcg/m^2 (as a 2-hour IV infusion) administered once daily for 21 days beginning 2 to 4 hours after the bone marrow infusion.

For patients in whom an autologous or allogenic bone marrow transplant has failed or in whom engraftment has been delayed, the recommended dosage is 250 mcg/m^2 (as a 2-hour IV infusion) administered once daily for 14 days. After a 7-day hiatus, the 14-day series of infusions can be repeated, if needed.

After another 7-day hiatus, the 14-day series can be repeated once more, if needed. If the graft still has not taken, further treatment is unlikely to help.

To accelerate neutrophil recovery following chemotherapy for AML, the recommended dosage is 250 mcg/m²/day (as a 4-hour IV infusion), starting on day 11 (or 4 days after completing the course of chemotherapy). Continue daily infusions for 42 days, or until the absolute neutrophil count exceeds 1500 cells/mm³ on 3 consecutive days, whichever is less.

THROMBOPOIETIC GROWTH FACTOR

Thrombopoietic growth factors are endogenous compounds that stimulate production of thrombocytes (platelets). At this time, oprelvekin is the only thrombopoietic growth factor available. Two drugs with similar actions—romiplostim and eltrombopag—are discussed in the section that follows.

Oprelvekin (Interleukin-11)

Oprelvekin is a thrombopoietic growth factor produced by recombinant DNA technology. The drug is a protein nearly identical in structure and actions to human *interleukin-11,* a cytokine produced in bone marrow. Oprelvekin is given to stimulate platelet production in patients undergoing myelosuppressive chemotherapy for nonmyeloid cancers.

Actions

Oprelvekin acts on platelet progenitor cells to increase platelet production. Specifically, it stimulates proliferation of hematopoietic stem cells and megakaryocyte progenitor cells, and thereby increases synthesis of megakaryocytes, the cells that fragment into large numbers of platelets. In addition to promoting megakaryocyte *synthesis,* oprelvekin induces megakaryocyte *maturation.* The net result is increased platelet production. In patients treated with oprelvekin daily for 14 days, platelet counts begin to increase 5 to 9 days after the first injection, peak about 7 days after the last injection, and return to baseline 14 days after that.

Therapeutic Use

Oprelvekin is administered to patients undergoing myelosuppressive chemotherapy to minimize thrombocytopenia (platelet deficiency) and to decrease the need for platelet transfusions. Because it stimulates the bone marrow, oprelvekin should *not* be given to patients with cancers of myeloid origin.

In clinical trials, oprelvekin was effective for some patients but not for others. To assess its benefits, oprelvekin was given to patients who had required platelet transfusions following earlier rounds of chemotherapy. Some patients were on moderately myelosuppressive regimens and some were on highly suppressive regimens. Among those on moderately suppressive regimens, 30% were spared the need for platelet transfusions by combining oprelvekin with chemotherapy. Among those on highly suppressive regimens, only 13% were spared the need for platelet transfusions. Hence, although oprelvekin can increase platelet counts and decrease the need for platelet transfusions, not all patients benefit equally. As these data indicate, the more myelosuppressive the regimen, the less helpful oprelvekin is likely to be.

Pharmacokinetics

Oprelvekin is administered by subQ injection. (The drug is a protein and so cannot be administered by mouth.) Serum levels peak about 3 hours after administration. Elimination is by hepatic and renal tubular metabolism, followed by excretion of the metabolites in urine.

Adverse Effects

Fluid Retention. Oprelvekin causes retention of sodium and water by the kidney. The result is *peripheral edema* and a 10% to 15% *expansion of plasma volume.* Expansion of plasma volume decreases both the hematocrit and hemoglobin concentration, causing anemia. As a result, about 48% of patients experience dyspnea (shortness of breath on exertion). Because of fluid retention, oprelvekin should be used with caution in patients with a history of HF or pleural effusion. Fluid balance should be monitored throughout treatment. Following oprelvekin withdrawal, fluid balance normalizes within days.

Cardiac Dysrhythmias. Tachycardia, atrial fibrillation, and atrial flutter are common. The cause of cardiac effects is unclear, although expansion of plasma volume is suspected. Oprelvekin does not affect the heart directly.

Severe Allergic Reactions. Oprelvekin has been associated with severe allergic reactions, including anaphylaxis. Signs of oprelvekin-induced allergy include rash, urticaria, flushing, fever, hypotension, joint pain, chest pain, wheezing, shortness of breath, and edema of the face, tongue, and larynx. Patients and healthcare providers should be alert for these reactions; if allergy is diagnosed, oprelvekin should be withdrawn and never used again.

Effects on the Eye. Conjunctival injection (red eye) is common. The incidence is 19% in adults. Other ophthalmic effects are transient visual blurring and papilledema (edema of the optic disk).

Preparations, Dosage, and Administration

Preparation. Oprelvekin is supplied as a powder in 5-mg single-dose vials. To reconstitute, add 1 mL of Sterile Water for Injection (supplied with the drug) and gently swirl; don't shake. Neither the powder nor the diluent contains preservatives, so the solution must be used within 3 hours to avoid infection. Oprelvekin and its diluent should be refrigerated at 2°C to 8°C (36°F to 46°F).

Dosage and Administration. Oprelvekin is administered by subQ injection into the abdomen, thigh, hip, or upper arm. The recommended adult dosage is 50 mcg/kg once daily. Dosing should begin 4 to 6 hours after chemotherapy and should continue until the platelet count rises above 50,000/mm³—but should not continue beyond 21 days. Treatment should cease 2 days before the next round of chemotherapy.

DRUGS THAT MIMIC HEMATOPOIETIC GROWTH FACTORS OR ENHANCE THEIR ACTIONS

In this section we consider three drugs—romiplostim, eltrombopag, and plerixafor—that are not structurally related to any endogenous hematopoietic growth factor. Nonetheless, two of these drugs—romiplostim and eltrombopag—have effects similar to those of an endogenous growth factor. And the third drug—plerixafor—is used to enhance the effects of an endogenous growth factor.

THROMBOPOIETIN RECEPTOR AGONISTS

Like oprelvekin, the thrombopoietin receptor agonists (TRAs) stimulate production of platelets. However, TRAs and oprelvekin do so by different mechanisms. Currently, two TRAs are available: romiplostim and eltrombopag. Both are used to increase platelet production in patients with *idiopathic thrombocytopenic purpura* (ITP), also known as *immune thrombocytopenic purpura.* In contrast, oprelvekin is used to increase platelet production in patients undergoing cancer chemotherapy.

Romiplostim

Therapeutic Use: Idiopathic Thrombocytopenic Purpura

Romiplostim [Nplate] is indicated for subQ treatment of ITP, a disorder characterized by *low platelet counts* secondary to (1) immune-mediated platelet destruction and (2) impaired platelet production. Symptoms include easy bruising, superficial bleeding, prolonged bleeding from cuts, spontaneous bleeding from the gums or nose, blood in the urine or stools, heavy menstrual bleeding, and profuse bleeding during surgery. Traditional treatments—glucocorticoids, IV immunoglobulins, and splenectomy—are designed to *reduce platelet destruction* through inhibiting production of antiplatelet antibodies. Removal of the spleen removes the main source of antibody production. Romiplostim is indicated only after one or more of these traditional measures have failed. In patients who have not already undergone splenectomy, treatment with romiplostim may render splenectomy unnecessary.

Mechanism of Action

In contrast to traditional treatments, which reduce platelet destruction, romiplostim *increases platelet production.* Romiplostim is a unique kind of molecule known as a *peptibody* (a combination of a peptide and an antibody). Benefits derive from mimicking the actions of *thrombopoietin,* an endogenous compound that stimulates the proliferation and differentiation of megakaryocytes, the cells that fragment into platelets. Romiplostim stimulates megakaryocytes by binding to the same receptor used by thrombopoietin. Platelet counts begin rising 4 to 9 days after a single subQ dose, peak between days 12 and 16, and then decline to pretreatment levels by day 28.

Pharmacokinetics

The pharmacokinetics of romiplostim is highly variable. Plasma levels peak between 7 and 50 hours after subQ dosing. Serum concentrations vary between patients and do not correlate well with dosage. The half-life ranges from 1 to 34 days.

Adverse Effects

The most common adverse effects are arthralgia, dizziness, insomnia, pain in the extremities, abdominal pain, myalgia, shoulder pain, dyspepsia, and paresthesias. When romiplostim is discontinued, platelet counts may drop below pretreatment levels, increasing the risk of bleeding. Uncommon but serious effects are *bone marrow fibrosis* (replacement of blood-forming cells with fibrotic tissue), *hematologic malignancy* (from stimulation of bone marrow cells), and *thrombotic/thromboembolic complications* (from excessive production of platelets).

Preparations, Dosage, and Administration

Romiplostim [Nplate] is supplied as a powder (250 and 500 mcg in single-use vials) for reconstitution in sterile water to a final concentration of 500 mcg/mL. Treatment consists of a weekly subQ injection. The initial dose is 1 mcg/kg, and the maximum dose is 10 mcg/kg. After the initial dose, dosage is increased or decreased by 1 mcg/kg/wk to achieve and maintain platelet counts equal to or above 50×10^9/L. If platelet counts rise above 400×10^9/L, romiplostim should be discontinued.

Eltrombopag

Actions and Therapeutic Use

Eltrombopag [Promacta] is indicated for oral therapy of ITP in patients who have not responded adequately to at least one traditional intervention (i.e., glucocorticoids, IV immunoglobulins, or splenectomy), as well as for treatment of thrombocytopenia in patients with chronic hepatitis C to allow and maintain interferon-based therapy. Like romiplostim, eltrombopag increases platelet production by activating the thrombopoietin receptor on megakaryocytes, causing these cells to proliferate and differentiate.

Pharmacokinetics

Eltrombopag is administered by mouth. Food reduces absorption by 60%, and polycations (e.g., calcium, aluminum, magnesium) reduce absorption by 70%. The drug undergoes extensive hepatic metabolism, followed by excretion in the feces (59%) and urine (31%). In patients with hepatic impairment, drug exposure is increased by 41% (with mild impairment) and by 80% to 93% (with moderate to severe impairment). Drug exposure is also affected by race: Among patients of black ancestry, total exposure is increased by 40%, and among patients of East Asian ancestry, total exposure is increased by 70%.

Adverse Effects

Eltrombopag is generally well tolerated, but nonetheless can cause serious adverse effects. Like romiplostim, eltrombopag may cause *bone marrow fibrosis, hematologic malignancy,* and *thrombotic/thromboembolic events,* and may pose a risk of *bleeding* from a rapid drop in platelet counts when treatment is stopped. In addition, the drug may cause *liver injury.* Accordingly, liver function tests—alanine aminotransferase (ALT), aspartate aminotransferase, and bilirubin—should be performed at baseline, every 2 weeks during the dosage adjustment phase, and every month thereafter. Eltrombopag should be discontinued if ALT levels exceed 3 times the upper limit of normal, or if there are clinical symptoms of liver injury.

Drug Interactions

Absorption of eltrombopag can be greatly reduced by polycations (i.e., calcium, magnesium, aluminum, selenium, zinc). Accordingly, at least 4 hours should separate administration of eltrombopag and drugs (e.g., antacids) or supplements that contain these elements.

Preparations, Dosage, and Administration

Eltrombopag [Promacta] is supplied in 12.5-, 25-, 50-, 75-, and 100-mg tablets for once-daily oral dosing on an empty stomach (i.e., at least 1 hour before a meal or 2 hours after). Do not administer within 4 hours of drugs and supplements that contain calcium, magnesium, or other polycations. The usual initial dosage is 50 mg once daily for patients with ITP. The maximum dosage is 75 mg once daily. After the initial dose, dosage is increased or decreased by 25 mg/day to achieve and maintain platelet counts equal to or above 50×10^9/L. If platelet counts rise above 400×10^9/L, eltrombopag should be discontinued. The initial dosage should be reduced to 25 mg/day in patients with liver impairment and in those of East Asian ancestry (i.e., Chinese, Japanese, Korean, Taiwanese).

PLERIXAFOR

Plerixafor [Mozobil] is a CXCR4 antagonist used in conjunction with G-CSF to increase the harvest of HSCs before bone marrow ablation with high-dose chemotherapy in patients with multiple myeloma or non-Hodgkin's lymphoma. Once chemotherapy is completed, the harvested HSCs are infused back into the patient to accelerate repopulation of the bone marrow. In many patients, treatment with G-CSF alone can mobilize sufficient HSCs for bone marrow rescue. When G-CSF alone is inadequate, plerixafor is added to increase the yield. Plerixafor works by blocking a receptor known as CXCR4, which plays an important role in holding HSCs in bone marrow. By blocking CXCR4, plerixafor promotes the release of HSCs from the bone marrow to peripheral blood, where these cells can be harvested for subsequent bone marrow rescue.

Plerixafor is administered by subQ injection, and plasma levels peak 30 to 60 minutes after dosing. The drug is eliminated intact in the urine. In patients with normal renal function, the half-life is 3 to 5 hours. In patients with significant renal impairment, the half-life is prolonged.

Plerixafor is generally well tolerated. The incidence of most side effects is the same as with placebo. Side effects that do occur more often with plerixafor include injection-site reactions, diarrhea, nausea, and dizziness.

Plerixafor is supplied in 20 mg/mL vials for subQ dosing. Treatment is done in conjunction with G-CSF as follows: (1) patients receive once-daily doses of G-CSF, starting at least 4 days before the first HSC collection and continuing until the last HSC collection, and (2) after at least 4 days of pretreatment with G-CSF, patients receive up to 4 once-daily doses of plerixafor, each dose beginning 11 hours before an HSC collection. For patients with normal renal function, a single dose of plerixafor is 0.24 mg/kg (but no more than 40 mg total). For patients with reduced renal function (creatinine clearance below 50 mL/min), the dosage is 0.16 mg/kg (but no more than 27 mg total).

KEY POINTS

- Epoetin is given to increase red blood cell counts and thereby decrease the need for transfusions. Specific indications include anemia associated with (1) chronic renal failure, (2) myelosuppressive cancer chemotherapy, and (3) zidovudine therapy in patients with HIV/AIDS.
- By increasing the hematocrit, epoetin can cause or exacerbate hypertension.
- Epoetin increases the risk of cardiovascular events (e.g., cardiac arrest, stroke, HF, MI), especially when the hemoglobin level exceeds 11 gm/dL or the rate of rise in hemoglobin exceeds 1 gm/dL in 2 weeks.
- In some cancer patients, epoetin can accelerate tumor progression and shorten life.
- Owing to the risk of serious toxicity, epoetin must be prescribed and used under a new Risk Evaluation and Mitigation Strategy (REMS).
- Filgrastim is given to elevate neutrophil counts and thereby reduce the risk of infection. Specific indications are chronic severe neutropenia and neutropenia associated with cancer chemotherapy or BMT.
- The principal adverse effects of filgrastim are bone pain and leukocytosis.
- Sargramostim is used to accelerate recovery from BMT, treat patients in whom a bone marrow transplant has failed, and accelerate neutrophil recovery in patients undergoing chemotherapy for AML.
- The principal adverse effect of sargramostim is leukocytosis.
- Oprelvekin is given to stimulate platelet production in patients undergoing myelosuppressive chemotherapy for nonmyeloid cancers. The goal is to minimize thrombocytopenia and platelet transfusions.
- The principal adverse effects of oprelvekin are fluid retention (which causes edema and anemia), cardiac dysrhythmias (tachycardia, atrial fibrillation, and atrial flutter), and severe allergic reactions, including anaphylaxis.
- TRAs are used to increase platelet production in patients with ITP after traditional methods of treatment have failed.
- Uncommon but serious effects of TRAs include bone marrow fibrosis, hematologic malignancy, and thrombotic/thromboembolic complications.
- Since epoetin alfa, filgrastim, sargramostim, and oprelvekin stimulate proliferation of bone marrow cells, these drugs should be used with great caution, if at all, in patients with cancers of bone marrow origin.

Please visit **http://evolve.elsevier.com/Lehne** for chapter-specific NCLEX® examination review questions.

Summary of Major Nursing Implications[a]

EPOETIN ALFA (ERYTHROPOIETIN)

Preadministration Assessment

Therapeutic Goal

Epoetin is used to restore and maintain erythrocyte counts, and thereby decrease the need for transfusions, in patients with CRF, HIV-infected patients receiving zidovudine, anemic patients facing elective surgery, and cancer patients receiving myelosuppressive chemotherapy, but only if the goal of chemotherapy is palliation, not cure. For most patients, the hemoglobin level should not exceed 10 or 11 mg/dL.

Baseline Data

All Patients. Obtain blood pressure; blood chemistry (BUN, uric acid, creatinine, phosphorus, potassium); complete blood counts with differential and platelet count; hemoglobin level; degree of transferrin saturation (should be at least 20%); and ferritin concentration (should be at least 100 ng/mL).

HIV-Infected Patients. Obtain an erythropoietin level. If the level is above 500 milliunits/mL, epoetin is unlikely to help.

Identifying High-Risk Patients

Avoid epoetin alfa in patients with uncontrolled hypertension, hypersensitivity to mammalian cell–derived products or albumin, or cancer of myeloid origin.

Implementation: Administration

Routes

IV and subQ.

Handling and Storage

Epoetin alfa is supplied in single-use and multiuse vials; don't re-enter the single-use vials. Don't agitate. Don't mix with other drugs. Discard the unused portion of the vial. Store at 2°C to 8°C (36°F to 46°F); don't freeze.

Administration

Chronic Renal Failure. Administer by IV bolus or subQ injection.

Chemotherapy-Induced Anemia. Administer by subQ injection.

Zidovudine-Induced Anemia. Administer by IV or subQ injection.

Surgery Patients. Administer by subQ injection.

Ongoing Evaluation and Interventions

Monitoring Summary

Measure hemoglobin level twice weekly until the maximum acceptable level has been achieved (10 or 11 mg/dL for most patients) and a maintenance dosage established. Measure hemoglobin periodically thereafter. Obtain complete blood counts with a differential and platelet counts routinely. Monitor

Continued

blood chemistry, including BUN, uric acid, creatinine, phosphorus, and potassium. Monitor iron stores and maintain at an adequate level. Monitor blood pressure.

Minimizing Adverse Effects

Hypertension. Monitor blood pressure and, if necessary, control with antihypertensive drugs. If hypertension cannot be controlled, reduce epoetin dosage. In patients with preexisting hypertension (a common complication of CRF), make certain that blood pressure is controlled before epoetin use.

Cardiovascular Events. Epoetin has been associated with an increase in cardiovascular events (e.g., cardiac arrest, stroke, HF, and MI). Risk is greatest when the hemoglobin level exceeds 11 gm/dL or the rate of rise in hemoglobin exceeds 1 gm/dL in 2 weeks. To minimize risk, reduce dosage when hemoglobin approaches 11 gm/dL or when the rate of rise exceeds 1 gm/dL in 2 weeks, and temporarily stop dosing if hemoglobin rises to 11 gm/dL or more. CRF patients on dialysis may need a higher dosage of heparin to prevent clotting in the dialysis machine.

For patients taking the drug before elective surgery, anticoagulant treatment can reduce the risk of deep vein thrombosis.

Cancer Patients: Tumor Progression and Shortened Survival. Epoetin can accelerate tumor progression and shorten survival in some cancer patients. To reduce risk, dosage should be no higher than needed to bring hemoglobin gradually up to 12 gm/dL. Also, epoetin should be used only in cancer patients who are undergoing chemotherapy or radiation therapy. Those who are not receiving chemotherapy or radiation therapy should not take this drug.

Autoimmune Pure Red-Cell Aplasia. Epoetin use may lead to pure red-cell aplasia (PRCA), owing to production of neutralizing antibodies directed against epoetin and native erythropoietin. If evidence of PRCA develops, epoetin should be discontinued and blood assessed for neutralizing antibodies. If PRCA is diagnosed, transfusions will be needed for life.

Patient Education. **Give all patients a Medication Guide that explains the risks and benefits of epoetin so that they can make an informed decision on whether to use this drug.**

FILGRASTIM (GRANULOCYTE COLONY-STIMULATING FACTOR)

Preadministration Assessment

Therapeutic Goal

Filgrastim is given to promote neutrophil recovery in cancer patients following myelosuppressive chemotherapy or BMT. The drug is also used to treat severe chronic neutropenia.

Baseline Data

Obtain complete blood counts and platelet counts.

Identifying High-Risk Patients

Filgrastim is *contraindicated* for patients with hypersensitivity to *Escherichia coli*–derived proteins.

Use with *caution* in patients with cancers of bone marrow origin.

Implementation: Administration

Routes

IV, subQ.

Handling and Storage

Filgrastim is supplied in single-use vials. Don't re-enter the vial; discard the unused portion. Don't agitate. Store at 2°C to 8°C (36°F to 46°F); don't freeze. Before administration, filgrastim may be kept at room temperature for up to 24 hours.

Administration

Cancer Chemotherapy. Administer by subQ bolus, short IV infusion, or continuous IV or subQ infusion.

Bone Marrow Transplantation. Administer by slow IV or subQ infusion.

Chronic Severe Neutropenia. Inject subQ daily.

Ongoing Evaluation and Interventions

Evaluating Therapeutic Effects.

Obtain complete blood counts twice weekly. Discontinue treatment when the absolute neutrophil count reaches 10,000/mm^3.

Minimizing Adverse Effects

Bone Pain. Evaluate for bone pain and treat with a nonopioid analgesic (e.g., acetaminophen). Consider an opioid analgesic if the nonopioid is insufficient.

Leukocytosis. Massive doses can cause leukocytosis (white blood cell counts above 100,000/mm^3). If leukocytosis develops, reduce filgrastim dosage.

SARGRAMOSTIM (GRANULOCYTE-MACROPHAGE COLONY-STIMULATING FACTOR)

Preadministration Assessment

Therapeutic Goal

Sargramostim is used to accelerate myeloid recovery in cancer patients who have undergone autologous BMT following high-dose chemotherapy (with or without concurrent irradiation). In addition, the drug is approved for treatment of patients for whom an autologous or allogenic bone marrow transplant has failed to take. Sargramostim is also used to accelerate neutrophil recovery in older patients receiving induction chemotherapy for AML.

Baseline Data

Obtain complete blood counts with differential and platelet count.

Identifying High-Risk Patients

Sargramostim is *contraindicated* in the presence of hypersensitivity to yeast-derived products and excessive leukemic myeloid blasts in bone marrow or peripheral blood.

Exercise *caution* in patients with cardiac disease, hypoxia, peripheral edema, pleural or pericardial effusion, or cancers of bone marrow origin.

Implementation: Administration

Route

IV (by infusion).

Handling and Storage

Sargramostim is supplied in concentrated solution and as a powder, which must be reconstituted for IV infusion. To

Summary of Major Nursing Implications[a]—cont'd

reconstitute the powder, add 1 mL of sterile water and gently swirl. Before infusing, dilute the concentrated solution or reconstituted powder. Administer as soon as possible after diluting—and no later than 6 hours after reconstitution. Store sargramostim (powder, reconstituted powder, final IV solution) at 2°C to 8°C (36°F to 46°F) until used.

Administration

Administer by 2-hour or 4-hour IV infusion.

Ongoing Evaluation and Interventions

Minimizing Adverse Effects

Leukocytosis and Thrombocytosis. Obtain complete blood counts with differential and platelet counts twice weekly. If the white blood cell count rises above 50,000/mm^3, if the absolute neutrophil count rises above 20,000/mm^3, or if the platelet count rises above 500,000/mm^3, temporarily interrupt sargramostim or reduce the dosage.

OPRELVEKIN (INTERLEUKIN-11)

Preadministration Assessment

Therapeutic Goal

Oprelvekin is given to minimize thrombocytopenia and the need for platelet transfusions in patients undergoing myelosuppressive therapy for nonmyeloid cancers.

Baseline Data

Determine baseline blood cell counts and platelet count, hematocrit, and fluid and electrolyte status.

Identifying High-Risk Patients

Use with *caution* in patients with cancers of myeloid origin; in patients taking diuretics or ifosfamide; and in patients with a history of atrial dysrhythmias, HF, pleural effusion, or papilledema.

Implementation: Administration

Route

SubQ.

Handling and Storage

Oprelvekin is supplied in single-use vials; don't re-enter the vial. Don't agitate. Don't mix with other drugs. Discard the unused portion of the vial. Store at 2°C to 8°C (36°F to 46°F); don't freeze.

Administration

Administer once daily beginning 4 to 6 hours after chemotherapy. Continue for 21 days or until platelet counts exceed 50,000/mm^3—whichever comes first.

Ongoing Evaluation and Interventions

Monitoring Summary

Monitor platelet counts from the time of the expected nadir until the count exceeds 50,000/mm^3. Monitor blood cell counts, fluid status, and electrolyte status.

Minimizing Adverse Effects

Fluid Retention. Fluid retention can result in edema, expanded plasma volume, anemia, and dyspnea. **Instruct patients with a history of congestive heart failure or pleural effusion to contact the prescriber if dyspnea worsens.**

Cardiac Dysrhythmias. Oprelvekin can cause tachycardia, atrial flutter, and atrial fibrillation. Use caution in patients with a history of these disorders.

ROMIPLOSTIM

Preadministration Assessment

Therapeutic Goal

Romiplostim is given to increase platelet production in patients with ITP that has not responded to other conventional treatments.

Baseline Data

Determine baseline blood cell counts and platelet count.

Identifying High-Risk Patients

Use with *caution* in patients with cancers of myeloid origin, patients with hematologic malignancies, and patients with hepatic or renal impairment.

Implementation: Administration

Route

SubQ.

Handling and Storage

Romiplostim is supplied in single-use vials; don't re-enter the vial. Don't agitate. Protect the reconstituted medication from light. Don't mix with other drugs. Discard the unused portion of the vial. Store at 2°C to 8°C (36°F to 46°F); don't freeze.

Administration

Administer 1 mcg/kg once weekly and adjust dose based on platelet response. Use lowest effective dose to maintain platelets above 50,000/mm^3.

Ongoing Evaluation and Interventions

Monitoring Summary

Monitor platelet counts from the time of the expected nadir until the count exceeds 50,000/mm^3. Monitor blood cell counts weekly until platelet counts are stable for 4 weeks. Then monitor platelets and blood count every 2 months thereafter.

Minimizing Adverse Effects

Thrombosis/Thromboembolism. Romiplostim should not be used to normalize platelet counts. Depending on current platelet count, doses should be adjusted per package recommendations. In patients with chronic liver disease, portal vein thrombosis has been reported with romiplostim use. Use cautiously in this population of patients.

[a]Patient education information is highlighted as **blue text**.

UNIT VIII DRUGS FOR ENDOCRINE DISORDERS

CHAPTER 57

Drugs for Diabetes Mellitus

JOSHUA J. NEUMILLER

DIABETES MELLITUS

BASIC CONSIDERATIONS

The term *diabetes mellitus* is derived from the Greek word for *fountain* and the Latin word for *honey.* The term describes one of the prominent symptoms of untreated diabetes: production of large volumes of glucose-rich urine. Indeed, long ago, the disease we now call diabetes was "diagnosed" by the sweet smell of urine—and, yes, by its sweet taste, too. In this chapter we use the terms *diabetes mellitus* and *diabetes* interchangeably.

Diabetes is primarily a disorder of carbohydrate metabolism. Symptoms mainly result from a deficiency of insulin, from cellular resistance to insulin's actions, or both. The principal sign of diabetes is *sustained hyperglycemia,* which results from impaired glucose uptake by cells and from increased glucose production. When hyperglycemia develops, it can quickly lead to polyuria, polydipsia, ketonuria, and weight loss. Over time, hyperglycemia can lead to heart disease, renal failure, blindness, neuropathy, amputations, impotence, and stroke. There is an often-overlooked point about diabetes: In addition to affecting carbohydrate metabolism, insulin deficiency disrupts metabolism of proteins and lipids as well. We refer to regulation of blood glucose levels as *glycemic control.*

In the United States, diabetes is the most common endocrine disorder and was the seventh leading cause of death by disease in 2010. According to the 2014 National Diabetes Fact Sheet, compiled by the Centers for Disease Control and Prevention, about 29 million Americans have diabetes, and over one-quarter of them have not yet been diagnosed. Another 86 million or so Americans are estimated to have prediabetes and are at increased risk of developing diabetes in the future.

We need to do a better job of diagnosing diabetes and treating it—and we need to do what we can to reduce the risk of developing the disease in the first place. Unfortunately, a major risk factor for developing diabetes is genetics, a factor that can't be modified. Nonetheless, we can still reduce risk significantly by adopting a healthy lifestyle, centered on engaging in physical activity and establishing a healthy diet.

Types of Diabetes Mellitus

There are two main forms of diabetes mellitus: type 1 diabetes mellitus (often abbreviated as T1DM) and type 2 diabetes mellitus (often abbreviated as T2DM). Both forms have similar signs and symptoms. Major differences concern etiology, prevalence, treatments, and outcomes (illness severity and deaths). The distinguishing characteristics of type 1 and type 2 diabetes are shown in Table 57.1 and discussed here. Another important form—gestational diabetes—is discussed later under *Diabetes and Pregnancy.* While there are additional forms of diabetes, they are relatively rare and will not be discussed specifically here.

Type 1 Diabetes

Type 1 diabetes accounts for about 5% of all diabetes cases. According to the American Diabetes Association (ADA), approximately 1.25 million American children and adults have type 1 diabetes. In the past, type 1 diabetes was called *juvenile-onset diabetes mellitus* or *insulin-dependent diabetes mellitus (IDDM).* These terms have fallen out of favor, however, because type 2 diabetes is becoming more common in children, and many people with type 2 diabetes use insulin to manage their diabetes. Accordingly, the terms *juvenile-onset diabetes mellitus* and *IDDM* are no longer clinically useful. Generally, type 1 diabetes develops during childhood or adolescence, and symptom onset is relatively abrupt. That being said, type 1 diabetes can develop at any age, including during adulthood.

The primary defect in type 1 diabetes is destruction of pancreatic beta cells—the cells responsible for insulin synthesis

TABLE 57.1 ▪ Characteristics of Type 1 and Type 2 Diabetes Mellitus

	Type of Diabetes Mellitus	
Characteristics	**Type 1**	**Type 2**
Age of onset	Usually childhood or adolescence	Usually older than 40 years
Speed of onset	Abrupt	Gradual
Family history	Frequently negative	Frequently positive
Prevalence	Approximately 5% of people with diabetes have type 1 diabetes	90%–95% of people with diabetes have type 2 diabetes
Etiology	Autoimmune process	Unknown—but there is a strong familial association, suggesting heredity is a risk factor
Primary defect	Loss of pancreatic beta cells	Insulin resistance and inappropriate insulin secretion
Insulin levels	Reduced early in the disease and completely absent later	Levels may be low (indicating deficiency), normal, or high (indicating resistance)
Treatment	Insulin replacement is mandatory, along with strict dietary control	Treat with an oral antidiabetic or non-insulin injectable agent and/or insulin, but always in combination with a reduced-calorie diet and appropriate exercise
Blood glucose	Levels fluctuate widely in response to infection, exercise, and changes in caloric intake and insulin dose	Levels are generally more stable than in type 1 diabetes
Symptoms	Polyuria, polydipsia, polyphagia, weight loss	May be asymptomatic initially
Body composition	Usually thin and undernourished at diagnosis	Frequently obese
Ketosis	Common, especially if insulin dosage is insufficient	Uncommon

and release into the bloodstream. Insulin levels are reduced early in the disease and usually fall to zero later. Beta cell destruction is the result of an autoimmune process (i.e., the patient's immune system inappropriately wages war against its own beta cells). The trigger for this immune response is not entirely known, but genetic, environmental, and infectious factors likely play a role.

Type 2 Diabetes

Type 2 diabetes is the most prevalent form of diabetes, accounting for 90% to 95% of all diagnosed cases. In the past, type 2 diabetes was called *non–insulin-dependent diabetes mellitus (NIDDM)* or *adult-onset diabetes mellitus.* As just discussed for type 1 diabetes, these terms are no longer clinically useful since insulin is commonly used by people with type 2 diabetes, and type 2 diabetes can occur in all age groups. The disease most commonly begins in middle age and progresses gradually. In contrast to type 1 diabetes, type 2 diabetes carries little risk of ketoacidosis. However, type 2 diabetes does carry the same long-term risks as type 1 diabetes (see *Long-Term Complications of Diabetes*).

Symptoms of type 2 diabetes usually result from a combination of *insulin resistance* and *impaired insulin secretion.* In contrast to patients with type 1 diabetes, many people with type 2 diabetes are capable of insulin synthesis. In fact, early in the disease, insulin levels tend to be normal or slightly elevated, a state known as *hyperinsulinemia.* However, although insulin is still produced, its secretion is no longer tightly coupled to plasma glucose content: release of insulin is delayed and peak output is subnormal. More importantly, the target tissues of insulin (liver, muscle, adipose tissue) exhibit insulin resistance: For a given blood insulin level, cells in these tissues are less able to take up and metabolize the glucose available to them. Insulin resistance appears to result from three causes: reduced binding of insulin to its receptors, reduced receptor numbers, and reduced receptor responsiveness. Over time, hyperglycemia leads to diminished pancreatic beta cell function, and hence insulin production and secretion eventually decline as the beta cells work harder to overcome insulin resistance within the tissues.

Although the underlying causes of type 2 diabetes are not entirely known, there is a strong familial association, suggesting that genetics plays a role. This possibility was reinforced by a study that implicated the gene for *insulin receptor substrate-2 (IRS-2),* a compound that helps mediate intracellular responses to insulin. Type 2 diabetes is likewise tightly linked to weight gain and obesity.

Short-Term Complications of Diabetes

The principal short-term complications of diabetes are hyperglycemia and hypoglycemia. *Hyperglycemia,* or high blood glucose, can result from a variety of factors, such as when drug doses are insufficient. Conversely, *hypoglycemia* is a term used to describe a blood sugar that is too low. A variety of factors can likewise contribute to the development of hypoglycemia, such as when the insulin dosage is excessive compared with the body's metabolic needs. *Ketoacidosis,* a potentially fatal acute complication, develops when hyperglycemia becomes severe and is allowed to persist. As already noted, ketoacidosis is rare with type 2 diabetes, and relatively common in patients with type 1 diabetes. All three complications are discussed later.

Long-Term Complications of Diabetes

The long-term consequences of type 1 and type 2 diabetes usually take years to develop. The overwhelming majority of deaths in people with diabetes result from long-term complications, not from acute episodes of hyperglycemia, hypoglycemia, or ketoacidosis. Ironically, among patients with type 1 diabetes, insulin therapy can be viewed as having made long-term complications possible: Before the discovery of insulin, people with type 1 diabetes usually died long before chronic complications could arise.

Most long-term complications occur secondary to disruption of blood flow, owing to either macrovascular or microvascular damage. There is strong evidence that optimal control of blood glucose can reduce *microvascular* injury. Good glycemic control may also reduce *macrovascular* injury, although other measures (e.g., exercise, healthy diet, control of blood pressure and blood lipids) are probably just as, if not more, important.

Macrovascular Damage

Cardiovascular disease (CVD) is the leading cause of death among people with diabetes. Diabetes carries an increased risk of heart disease, hypertension, and stroke. Much of this pathology is due to atherosclerosis, which develops earlier in people with diabetes than in those without diabetes and progresses faster too. Macrovascular complications result from a combination of hyperglycemia and altered lipid metabolism.

Microvascular Damage

Damage to small blood vessels and capillaries (the microvasculature) is common in diabetes. The basement membrane of capillaries thickens, causing blood flow in these narrow vessels to fall. Pathology in small blood vessels contributes to kidney damage (nephropathy), blindness (retinopathy), and various neuropathies. Microvascular injury is directly related to the degree and duration of hyperglycemia.

Retinopathy. Diabetes is the major cause of blindness among American adults. Visual losses result most commonly from damage to retinal capillaries. Microaneurysms may occur, followed by scarring and proliferation of new vessels; the overgrowth of new retinal capillaries reduces visual acuity. Capillary damage may also impair vision by causing local ischemia (reductions of local blood flow), which can kill retinal cells. Retinopathy is accelerated by hyperglycemia, hypertension, and smoking. Accordingly, these risk factors should be controlled or eliminated. All patients with diabetes, whether type 1 or type 2, should have a comprehensive eye examination every 1 to 2 years.

Nephropathy. Diabetic damage to the kidneys—diabetic nephropathy—is characterized by albuminuria (the spilling of protein into the urine), reduced glomerular filtration, and increased blood pressure. Diabetic nephropathy is the most common cause of end-stage renal disease, a condition that requires dialysis or a kidney transplant for survival, with diabetes listed as the primary cause of kidney failure in 44% of all cases in 2011. In the same year, nearly 50,000 people with diabetes began treatment for kidney failure due to diabetes.

We can screen for kidney damage by testing for *microalbuminuria* (the presence of small amounts of albumin in the urine). Recall that albumin is the blood's major protein. When the kidney is healthy, the urine contains no albumin because albumin is so large that it cannot be filtered by the healthy glomerulus. However, when the glomerulus is damaged, even slightly, some albumin gets filtered and enters the urine. If renal function undergoes further decline, larger amounts of albumin will enter the urine, causing *macroalbuminuria* and, eventually, renal failure.

Treatment of diabetes can delay the onset of nephropathy and reduce its severity. The Diabetes Control and Complications Trial (DCCT) revealed that "tight" glucose control decreases the risk of nephropathy by 35% to 57% in people with type 1 diabetes. As discussed in Chapter 44, treatment with an *angiotensin-converting enzyme* (ACE) *inhibitor* or an *angiotensin II receptor blocker* (ARB) can slow progression of mild to moderate nephropathy that is already present. However, these drugs are not effective for primary prevention. Of note, ACE inhibitors and ARBs have an additional benefit: They can help control hypertension, a common complication of diabetes.

Sensory and Motor Neuropathy. Nerve degeneration often begins early in the course of diabetes, but symptoms are usually absent for years. Sensory and motor nerves may be affected. Symptoms of diabetic neuropathy—which are usually bilateral and symmetric—include tingling sensations in the fingers and toes (paresthesias), increased pain or decreased ability to feel pain, suppression of reflexes, and loss of other sensations (especially vibratory sensation). These changes are one of the reasons why a complete foot examination for people with diabetes includes not only an examination for sores and possible infections, but also for sensory responses. The clinician will use a small filament or other stiff or sharp object to prod the bottoms of the feet, without the patient looking. Failure to detect the stimuli gives a good indication that neuropathies are developing.

Nerve damage is directly related to sustained hyperglycemia, which may cause metabolic disturbances in nerves or may injure the capillaries that supply nutrients to the nerves. In the DCCT, "tight" glycemic control reduced the incidence of peripheral neuropathy by 60%.

Autonomic Neuropathy: Gastroparesis. Diabetic gastroparesis (delayed stomach emptying) affects 20% to 30% of patients with long-standing diabetes. Manifestations include nausea, vomiting, delayed gastric emptying, and gastric or intestinal distention. Injury to the autonomic nerves that control GI motility seems to be the underlying cause. Symptoms can be reduced with *metoclopramide* [Reglan], a dopamine antagonist that promotes gastric emptying (see Chapter 80). In addition to affecting autonomic nerves that innervate the GI tract, diabetes can affect autonomic nerves that innervate other structures. Autonomic neuropathies can be particularly problematic when they blunt an individual's ability to sense the symptoms of hypoglycemia.

Amputations Secondary to Infection. Diabetes is responsible for an estimated 60% of all lower limb amputations in the United States. The underlying cause is typically a severe infection, which can develop following local trauma, be it major or minor. There are three reasons why serious infection can occur. First, hyperglycemia provides a glucose-rich environment for bacteria to grow. Second, diabetes can suppress immune function and thereby compromise host defenses against infection. And third, diabetic neuropathy can prevent the patient from feeling discomfort and other sensations that would signal that a serious infection is developing. Because of these factors, an infection that would be inconsequential and self-limiting in those without diabetes can become very serious in a person with diabetes. If the infection spreads and becomes gangrenous, the only realistic and effective solution is amputation. Because of these possibilities, regular *foot examinations* and *foot care* are an important part of diabetes management.

Erectile Dysfunction. The combination of blood vessel injury and neuropathy can cause erectile dysfunction (ED). Among men with diabetes, the estimated incidence of ED is 35% to 75%. Treatment with sildenafil [Viagra] and related drugs can often help.

Diabetes and Pregnancy

Before the discovery of insulin, virtually all babies born to mothers with severe diabetes died during infancy. Although insulin therapy has greatly improved outcomes, successful management of the diabetic pregnancy remains a challenge. Three factors contribute to the problem. First, the placenta produces hormones that antagonize insulin's actions. Second, production of cortisol, a hormone that promotes hyperglycemia, increases threefold during pregnancy. Both factors increase the body's need for insulin. And third, because glucose can pass freely from the maternal circulation to the fetal circulation, hyperglycemia in the mother will stimulate excessive secretion of insulin in the fetus. The resultant hyperinsulinism can have multiple adverse effects on the fetus.

Successful management of diabetes during pregnancy demands that proper glucose levels be maintained in both the mother and fetus. Achieving glucose control requires diligence on the part of the mother and her prescriber. Some experts on diabetes in pregnancy advise that blood glucose levels must be monitored 6 to 7 times a day. Insulin dosage and food intake must be adjusted accordingly.

Gestational diabetes is defined as diabetes that appears in the pregnant patient during pregnancy and then subsides after delivery. Gestational diabetes is managed in much the same manner as any other diabetic pregnancy: Blood glucose should be monitored and then controlled with diet and medication. In most cases, the diabetic state disappears almost immediately after delivery, permitting discontinuation of medication. However, if the diabetic state persists beyond parturition, it is no longer considered gestational and should be diagnosed and treated accordingly.

Insulin is considered the preferred agent for managing both pre-existing type 1 and type 2 diabetes during pregnancy. While metformin is sometime used during pregnancy in the setting of type 2 diabetes, long-term studies on fetal outcomes are lacking. Women with type 2 diabetes who discontinue oral medications can resume oral therapy after delivery.

Diagnosis

Diagnosis of diabetes was once made solely by measuring blood levels of glucose. However, in 2010, the ADA added the hemoglobin A1C—a test that provides an estimate of glycemic control over the previous 2 to 3 months—as an acceptable method of diagnosing diabetes. For all of these tests, diagnostic values of diabetes are shown in Table 57.2.

Tests Based on Blood Levels of Glucose

Excessive plasma glucose is diagnostic of diabetes. Several tests may be employed: a fasting plasma glucose (FPG) test,

TABLE 57.2 ▪ Criteria for the Diagnosis of Diabetes Mellitus

Fasting plasma glucose ≥ 126 mg/dL[a]
Or
Casual plasma glucose ≥ 200 mg/dL *plus* symptoms of diabetes[b]
Or
Oral glucose tolerance test (OGTT): 2-hr plasma glucose ≥ 200 mg/dL[c]
Or
Hemoglobin A1C 6.5% or higher

[a]*Fasting* is defined as no caloric intake for at least 8 hours.
[b]*Casual* is defined as any time of day without regard to meals. Classic symptoms of diabetes include polyuria, polydipsia, and unexplained weight loss.
[c]In this OGTT, plasma glucose content is measured 2 hours after ingesting the equivalent of 75 gm of anhydrous glucose dissolved in water. The OGTT is not recommended or needed for routine clinical use.
Data from Standards of Medical Care in Diabetes—2017. Diabetes Care 40(Suppl 1):S11–S25, 2017.

an oral glucose tolerance test (OGTT), or a random plasma glucose test in patients exhibiting classic symptoms of hyperglycemia or hyperglycemic crisis. Unless there is a clear clinical diagnosis (such as patients in hyperglycemic crises or with classic symptoms of hyperglycemia), a second test is required for diagnostic confirmation. The ADA recommends that the same test be repeated without delay using a new blood sample, although using an alternative diagnostic measure is also an appropriate option.

Fasting Plasma Glucose Test. To determine FPG levels, blood is drawn at least 8 hours after the last meal. In normoglycemic individuals, FPG levels are less than 100 mg/dL. If FPG glucose levels are 126 mg/dL or higher, diabetes is indicated. For those individuals falling between 100 and 125 mg/dL, they are considered to be at increased risk for diabetes (often referred to as prediabetes as discussed in more detail in the *Increased Risk for Diabetes (Prediabetes)* section later).

Oral Glucose Tolerance Test (OGTT). This test is often used when diabetes is suspected but could not be definitively diagnosed by measuring fasting glucose levels or by measuring hemoglobin A1C. The OGTT is performed by giving an oral glucose load (equivalent to 75 gm of anhydrous glucose dissolved in water) and measuring plasma glucose levels 2 hours later. In individuals who do not have diabetes, 2-hour glucose levels will be below 140 mg/dL. Diabetes is suggested if 2-hour plasma glucose levels are 200 mg/dL or higher. The OGTT test is more expensive and time consuming than the alternatives and is not used routinely. Similar to the earlier discussion for FPG, patients falling between 140 and 199 mg/dL during an OGTT are considered to have prediabetes.

Random Plasma Glucose Test. For this test, blood can be drawn at any time, without regard to meals. Fasting is not required. Of note, the test can be performed in the office, using a finger-stick blood sample and the same type of test device employed by patients at home. A plasma glucose level that is 200 mg/dL or higher suggests diabetes. However, to make a definitive diagnosis, the patient must also display classic signs of diabetes: polyuria, polydipsia, and rapid weight loss. Ketonuria may also be present, but only if blood glucose is extremely high.

Hemoglobin A1C

As described later under *Monitoring Treatment,* levels of hemoglobin A1C, or simply A1C, reflect average blood glucose levels over the previous 2 to 3 months. Accordingly, if a patient's A1C is high, we know that his or her glucose levels have been high for a relatively long time. In other words, we know that he or she has diabetes. An A1C value of 6.5% or higher is considered diagnostic.

It is important to note that the A1C test is not necessarily accurate in all patients because some people have conditions that can affect hemoglobin levels or the lifespan of erythrocytes (red blood cells), thus skewing the results of this test. Among these are pregnancy, chronic kidney or liver disease, recent severe bleeding or blood transfusion, and certain blood disorders, including thalassemia, iron deficiency anemia, and anemia related to vitamin B_{12} deficiency.

Increased Risk for Diabetes (Prediabetes)

As briefly noted earlier, increased risk for diabetes (sometimes referred to as prediabetes) is a state defined by *impaired fasting plasma glucose* (FPG between 100 and 125 mg/dL), *impaired glucose tolerance* (2-hour OGTT result of 140 to 199 mg/dL), or an A1C of 5.7% to 6.4%. These values are below those that define diabetes, but are too high to be considered normal. People with "prediabetes" are at increased risk of developing type 2 diabetes and CVD—but not the microvascular complications associated with diabetes (i.e., retinopathy, nephropathy, neuropathy). The risk of CVD can be reduced by dietary modifications, increased physical activity, and, if indicated, use of appropriate drugs to control blood lipids and blood pressure. The risk of progression to diabetes may be reduced by diet and exercise, and possibly by certain oral antidiabetic drugs (such as metformin).

It is important to note that many people who meet the criteria for "prediabetes" never go on to develop diabetes—even if they *don't* modify their lifestyle and even if they *don't* take antidiabetic drugs. Hence, although "prediabetes" indicates an increased *risk* of diabetes, it by no means guarantees that diabetes will occur.

Overview of Treatment

The primary goals of treating type 1 or type 2 diabetes are to: (1) prevent long-term complications, especially CVD, retinopathy, kidney disease, and amputations; and (2) manage the symptoms of hyperglycemia. To minimize these complications, treatment must keep glucose levels as close to "normal" as safely possible. In addition, treatment must keep blood pressure and blood lipids within an acceptable range. In both type 1 and type 2 diabetes, proper diet and adequate physical activity are central components of management.

Type 1 Diabetes

Preventing complications of diabetes requires a comprehensive plan directed at glycemic control and reduction of cardiovascular risk factors. Glycemic control in the setting of type 1 diabetes is accomplished with an integrated program of diet, self-monitoring of blood glucose (SMBG), physical activity, and insulin replacement. Of importance, glycemic control must be achieved *safely,* that is, adequately controlling glycemia while minimizing the risk of hypoglycemia. An essential component of treatment—education of the patient and his or her caregivers about diet, physical activity, and drugs—is usually left to the nurse and a dietitian or nutritionist.

Dietary Measures. *Proper diet, balanced by insulin replacement, is the cornerstone of treatment.* Because patients with type 1 diabetes are often thin, the dietary goal is to maintain weight—not lose it. The ADA recommends that all people with type 1 diabetes be offered intensive insulin therapy education on the need to couple insulin administration with carbohydrate intake. While it is widely accepted that such educational interventions are useful for people with type 1 diabetes, studies examining the ideal amount of carbohydrate are largely inconclusive. So how should people with diabetes be advised to eat? Evidence suggests that there is no ideal percentage of calories that should be ingested from carbohydrate, fat, or protein. Accordingly, macronutrient distribution for any given individual should be based on his or her current eating patterns, preferences, and goals. Ultimately, there is no "one-size-fits-all" eating pattern for individuals with diabetes.

Physical Activity. Unless specifically contraindicated, regular physical activity should be part of the management program. Physical activity increases cellular responsiveness to insulin and may also increase glucose tolerance. Accordingly, the ADA recommends that patients perform at least 150 minutes per week of physical activity of moderate to vigorous intensity, spread over at least 3 days per week. Implementation of resistance exercise programs and flexibility and balance training are also recommended (especially for older adults with diabetes). Because strenuous exercise can produce hypoglycemia, patient and provider must work to establish a safe balance between activity level, caloric intake, and insulin dosage. Unfortunately, although the benefits of physical activity are well established, long-term adherence to a program is often difficult to maintain.

Insulin Replacement. *Among patients with type 1 diabetes, survival requires daily dosing with insulin.* Before insulin replacement became available, people with type 1 diabetes invariably died within a few years after disease onset. The cause of death was usually ketoacidosis. It is essential to coordinate insulin dosage with carbohydrate intake. If carbohydrate intake is too great or too small with respect to insulin dosage, hyperglycemia or hypoglycemia will result.

While insulin is the cornerstone of management in type 1 diabetes, the use of other medications as add-on therapy to insulin may be encountered in clinical practice.

Managing Hypertension and Dyslipidemia. As noted earlier, an ACE inhibitor (e.g., lisinopril) or an ARB (e.g., losartan) can reduce the risk of diabetic nephropathy progression, a long-term consequence of poor glycemic control, in patients with signs of albuminuria. Because of this, ACE inhibitors and ARBs are preferred agents for managing hypertension in patients with albuminuria. For patients with diabetes who do not have albuminuria, antihypertensive medications that have been demonstrated to reduce cardiovascular events in patients with diabetes can be used, including: ACE inhibitors, ARBs, thiazide-like diuretics (e.g., hydrochlorothiazide), or dihydropyridine calcium channel blockers (e.g., amlodipine). The current goal, as set by the ADA, is to keep blood pressure at or below 140/90 mm Hg, with blood pressure targets such as 130/80 mm Hg appropriate for some individuals.

To reduce high levels of LDL cholesterol, statins (e.g., atorvastatin) are preferred drugs. Not only do statins reduce cardiovascular events in patients with high cholesterol, they reduce cardiovascular events in patients with normal or low cholesterol. Another cholesterol-lowering drug—colesevelam—is discussed separately later because of its recognized role in managing diabetes. See Chapter 50 for a discussion of lipid-lowering therapies.

Type 2 Diabetes

As with type 1 diabetes, preventing long-term complications requires a comprehensive treatment plan. Lifestyle measures (diet and physical activity) and drug therapy are the foundation of glycemic control. Physical activity provides the additional benefit of promoting glucose uptake by muscle, even when insulin levels are low. In addition to glycemic control, the plan should address other factors that can increase morbidity and mortality. Accordingly, all patients should be screened and treated for hypertension, nephropathy, retinopathy, and neuropathy. In addition, dyslipidemias (high LDL cholesterol, low HDL cholesterol, and high triglycerides) should be corrected.

Recommendations for glycemic control have changed. Until recently, treatment was started with lifestyle measures *alone;* drugs were added only if these measures failed. Today, treatment is started with lifestyle measures *plus* drug therapy. We no longer wait to use drugs. As a result, glycemic control is established sooner, and the risk of long-term complications is lowered.

Type 2 diabetes can be treated with a variety of oral and injectable drugs. Among the oral drugs, metformin is used most widely. Among the injectable drugs, insulin is used most widely. Although wide use of insulin may surprise you, it shouldn't. Remember, as type 2 diabetes progresses, less and less insulin is produced. As a result, it is common for people with type 2 diabetes to eventually require insulin therapy, although insulin (particularly basal, or long-acting, insulins) can also be used early in the course of type 2 diabetes as well.

Given the many drugs available for type 2 diabetes, how does one decide which drugs to use for a given patient? As recommended in the 2017 ADA Standards of Medical Care in Diabetes, there are a number of patient-specific considerations that come into play when deciding on a course of treatment. To treat type 2 diabetes, the Standards of Care recommends a four-step approach:

Step 1. At diagnosis, initiate lifestyle changes *plus* metformin.

Step 2. Continue lifestyle changes plus metformin, and *add* a second drug, either a sulfonylurea, a thiazolidinedione, a dipeptidyl peptidase-4 (DPP-4) inhibitor, a sodium-glucose cotransporter 2 (SGLT-2) inhibitor, a glucagon-like peptide-1 (GLP-1) receptor agonist, or basal insulin. The choice of agent is made in light of relative efficacy, hypoglycemia risk, weight-related considerations, side effect profile, and cost.

Step 3. Progress from step 2 to a three-drug combination (inclusive of metformin). Again, the choice of regimen used is determined based on drug- and patient-specific considerations.

Step 4. If three-drug combination therapy that includes basal insulin fails to achieve treatment goals after approximately 3 months, it is recommended to proceed to a combination injectable regimen inclusive of insulin and possibly a GLP-1 receptor agonist.

Treatment should start at step 1, and then progress to steps 2, 3, and 4 if needed. The exception to this stepwise approach is in patients who have an A1C of 7.5% at the time of diagnosis, in which case it is recommended to start dual therapy (that is, start at step 2). Additionally, patients who have an A1C of 10% or greater or who are markedly symptomatic may be started on combination injectable therapy immediately.

Determining Appropriate Glycemic Goals

In both type 1 and type 2 diabetes, it is important to determine appropriate glycemic goals for the individual based on his or her lifestyle and other patient-specific considerations. The process of maintaining glucose levels within a normal range around-the-clock is often referred to as "tight glycemic control." Maintaining tight glycemic control is difficult but can be worth the trouble, especially for young patients with type 1 diabetes. However, for many patients with type 2 diabetes, the risks of tight control may be greater than the benefits. Table 57.3 shows current recommendations regarding glycemic goals.

Type 1 Diabetes

Benefits. The benefits of tight glycemic control in type 1 diabetes were demonstrated conclusively in the Diabetes Control and Complications Trial (DCCT), in which patients received either *conventional insulin therapy* (1 or 2 injections a day) or *intensive insulin therapy* (4 injections a day). After 6.5 years, the patients who received intensive therapy experienced a 50% decrease in clinically significant kidney disease, a 35% to 57% decrease in neuropathy, and a 76% decrease in serious ophthalmic complications. Moreover, the onset of ophthalmic problems was delayed and the progression of existing problems was slowed. In addition to reducing these *microvascular* complications, "tight control" decreased *macrovascular* complications: 17-year follow-up data from the DCCT showed a significant reduction in myocardial infarction, coronary revascularization, and angina. Hence, with rigorous control of blood glucose, the high degree of morbidity and mortality traditionally associated with type 1 diabetes can be markedly reduced.

TABLE 57.3 ▪ General Glycemic Treatment Targets for Nonpregnant Adults With Diabetes

A1C	<7.0%[a]
Premeal plasma glucose	80–130 mg/dL[a]
Peak postmeal plasma glucose	<180 mg/dL[a]

[a]Goals should be individualized based on:
- Duration of diabetes
- Age/life expectancy
- Comorbid conditions
- Known cardiovascular disease or advanced microvascular complications
- Hypoglycemia unawareness
- Other individualized considerations

Data from Standards of Medical Care in Diabetes—2017. Diabetes Care 40(Suppl 1):S11–S25, 2017.

Drawbacks. The greatest concern of intensive therapy and strict glycemic goals is *hypoglycemia.* Because glucose levels are kept relatively low, even a modest overdose with insulin can cause blood glucose to fall too low, so the possibility of hypoglycemia increases. Also, a meal that is skipped or exercise that is too strenuous can do the same. Results of the DCCT showed that compared with patients using conventional therapy, those using intensive insulin therapy experienced 3 times as many hypoglycemic events requiring the assistance of another person and 3 times as many episodes of hypoglycemia-induced coma or seizures. In addition, patients on intensive insulin therapy experienced greater *weight gain* (about 10 pounds, on average). Other disadvantages are greater inconvenience, increased complexity, increased cost of therapy, and a need for greater patient motivation.

Type 2 Diabetes

In patients with type 2 diabetes, benefits of tight glycemic control are limited mainly to *microvascular* complications; tight control probably does little to reduce *macrovascular* complications, as evidenced by studies performed to date. Furthermore, benefits accrue more to younger adults with *recent-onset* disease than to older adults with *well-established* disease. As in type 1 diabetes, tight glycemic control poses a significant risk of *hypoglycemia* and *weight gain.* In addition, tight control may increase the risk of *death.*

The effects of tight glycemic control in type 2 diabetes were demonstrated in four landmark trials:

- United Kingdom Prospective Diabetes Study (UKPDS)
- Action to Control Cardiovascular Risk in Diabetes (ACCORD)
- Action in Diabetes and Vascular Disease: Preterax and Diamicron Modified Release Controlled Evaluation (ADVANCE)
- Veterans Affairs Diabetes Trial (VADT)

These large randomized trials differed in patient populations: Whereas the UKPDS trial enrolled younger adults with recent-onset diabetes and no prior cardiovascular events, the ACCORD, ADVANCE, and VADT trials enrolled older adults with long-standing diabetes, as well as established CVD or cardiovascular risk factors.

Results of the UKPDS trial, released in 1998, showed a significant reduction in *micro*vascular complications—but little or no reduction in *macro*vascular complications or death. In one branch of the study, nonobese patients were given either intensive therapy or conventional therapy. Mean values for A1C were 7% in the intensive group and 7.9% in the conventional group. Compared with patients in the conventional group, patients in the intensive group had a 12% reduction in total diabetes-related endpoints (cardiovascular, retinal, and renal damage). However, a reduction in microvascular complications (especially retinal damage) accounted for most of the benefit.

Results of ACCORD, ADVANCE, and VADT were released in 2008. As in the UKPDS trial, tight glycemic control failed to reduce stroke, amputations, all-cause mortality, or mortality from cardiovascular causes. In fact, in the ACCORD trial, intensive therapy was associated with an *increased* risk of death. Tight control also increased the risk of severe hypoglycemia and weight gain. The ADVANCE trial did show a reduction in microvascular outcomes, but the ACCORD trial did not.

Taken together, these four studies suggest that tight glycemic control is most appropriate for younger adults who have recent-onset type 2 diabetes and no cardiovascular complications. Because even short periods of hyperglycemia may increase the risk of complications, optimal therapy should be started as soon as diabetes is diagnosed.

Who should *not* receive intensive therapy? Intensive glycemic control may be inappropriate for patients with

- Long-standing type 2 diabetes
- Advanced microvascular or macrovascular complications
- Extensive comorbid conditions
- A history of severe hypoglycemia
- Limited life expectancy
- Limited resources and a limited support system

For these patients, an A1C goal above 7% may be more appropriate than a goal below 7% (see Table 57.3).

Monitoring Treatment

We need monitoring to (1) determine whether glucose levels are being maintained in a safe range, both short term and long term, and (2) guide changes in treatment when the range is not satisfactory or safe. SMBG levels are the standard method for day-to-day monitoring. As mentioned previously, A1C is measured to assess long-term glycemic control.

Self-Monitoring of Blood Glucose

SMBG is recommended for all patients who use insulin. That is, SMBG is recommended for all patients with type 1 diabetes and for all patients with type 2 diabetes receiving insulin. It is additionally used by most patients with type 2 diabetes using other therapies as well. Many devices for measuring blood glucose (generally called glucometers) are available. With most of them, the patient places a small drop of capillary blood (e.g., from a finger stick) on a chemically treated strip, which is then analyzed by the machine. The test is rapid and can be performed in almost any setting. Information on blood glucose concentration provides a guide for "fine tuning" dosages of insulin and other antidiabetic drugs. The frequency of SMBG for any given patient can vary widely based on the therapies the patient uses and how active he or she is. A patient on metformin monotherapy may need to check his or her blood sugar only once a week, as an example, while a patient with type 1 diabetes on an intensive insulin regimen may check up to 8 times a day or more. Frequently used target values for blood glucose are 80 to 130 mg/dL before meals and less than 180 mg/dL 1 to 2 hours after meals.

Newly diagnosed patients tend to be diligent about testing their blood. This is good because it provides essential information for adjusting treatment on a day-to-day basis. Unfortunately, just as many patients start out by getting proper exercise and eating right, and then go back to their old habits; they often follow the same pattern regarding SMBG.

A final note on SMBG: Glucometers are both amazing and sophisticated—and often not used to their full potential. By pushing a few buttons, you can get the current blood glucose measurement and can then label the reading as to when it was taken (e.g., after exercise, before a meal). Many meters can calculate the average glucose level at a given time of day, track trends in glucose levels over a variety of time ranges, or give just about any other information you might want or need. Some meters even come equipped with a USB that can be plugged directly into the patient's computer to analyze the data. However, there's a problem: To use a glucometer properly, and take full advantage of the information it can provide, you need to be able to read, understand, and follow the directions—directions that can be both complicated and lengthy.

Continuous Glucose Monitoring (CGM)

Using CGM is another tool for monitoring glucose. CGM measures interstitial glucose (which correlates well with plasma glucose). CGM devices are worn for a period of time—often for 6 or 7 days—and read the interstitial glucose level every 5 minutes or so, depending on the specific device. CGMs are programmed to include sophisticated alarms for hypoglycemic and hyperglycemic excursions and can interface with insulin pumps and even smartphones. In September 2016 the U.S. Food and Drug Administration (FDA) approved the first "hybrid closed-loop system," which integrates CGM technology with insulin pump technology. Essentially the system will adjust insulin delivery automatically based on what is happening with the patient's glucose levels.

Monitoring of Hemoglobin A1C

Measurement of hemoglobin A1C—also called *glycosylated hemoglobin* or *glycated hemoglobin*—provides an index of *average glucose levels* over the prior 2 to 3 months. Glucose interacts spontaneously with hemoglobin in red blood cells to form glycosylated derivatives, the most prevalent being A1C. With prolonged hyperglycemia, levels of A1C gradually increase. Since red blood cells have a long life span (120 days), levels of A1C reflect average glucose levels over an extended time. Hence, by measuring A1C every 3 to 6 months, we can get a picture of long-term glycemic control. Please note, however, that measuring A1C tells us nothing about acute, hour-to-hour swings in blood glucose. Accordingly, although measuring A1C is an important part of diabetes management, it is clearly no substitute for SMBG.

How is testing done? Current tests use a tiny capillary blood sample from a finger stick and yield results in minutes, while the patient is still in the office. A1C values can also be obtained as part of a routine blood panel.

How are test results expressed? Results are usually reported as a *percentage of total hemoglobin in blood* (e.g., 7%). In addition, they may be reported as a value for *estimated Average Glucose* (eAG), expressed as mg of glucose/dL of blood (i.e., the same units patients see every day when doing SMBG). Selected A1C values and their eAG equivalents are shown in Table 57.4.

What's the A1C target level? The general goal is to keep the A1C below 7%. Although an A1C goal of below 7% is good for most patients, a less stringent goal (e.g., below 8%) may be appropriate for some patients, such as those with a history of severe hypoglycemia, limited life expectancy, or advanced microvascular or macrovascular complications.

INSULIN

Insulin is used to treat all patients with type 1 diabetes and many patients with type 2 diabetes. Our discussion of insulin is divided into three sections: physiology, preparations and administration, and therapeutic use.

PHYSIOLOGY

Structure

The structure of insulin is shown in Fig. 57.1. As indicated, insulin consists of two amino acid chains: the "A" (acidic)

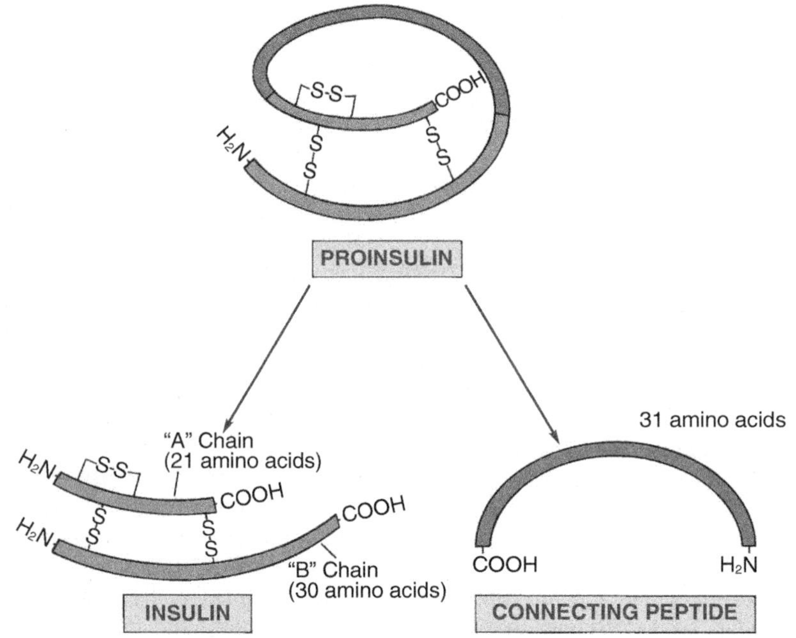

Fig. 57.1 ▪ Conversion of proinsulin to insulin.
Proinsulin is the immediate precursor of the insulin secreted by our pancreas. Enzymes clip off connecting peptide (C-peptide) to release active insulin, composed of two peptide chains (A and B) connected by two disulfide (S–S) bonds. Since C-peptide arises only from endogenous insulin, its presence in blood indicates that at least some pancreatic insulin is being made.

TABLE 57.4 ▪ Hemoglobin A1C Levels and Their Corresponding eAG Levels[a]

A1C Level (% of Total Hb)	Corresponding Mean Plasma Glucose (eAG) Level: mg/dL	mmol/L
6	126	7.0
7[b]	**154**	**8.6**
8	183	10.2
9	212	11.8
10	240	13.4
11	269	14.9
12	298	16.5

[a]The formula to convert from A1C (%) to average glucose concentration equivalents (expressed in mg/dL) is: eAG = (A1C × 28.7) – 46.7.
[b]An A1C level of 7 and below is the desired goal.
eAG, Estimated average glucose in blood; *Hb,* hemoglobin.
Data from Standards of Medical Care in Diabetes—2017. Diabetes Care 40(Suppl 1):S11–S25, 2017.

Prototype Drugs

DRUGS FOR DIABETES MELLITUS

Insulin Preparations
Insulin lispro (short duration, rapid acting)
Regular insulin (short duration, short acting)
NPH insulin (intermediate duration)
Insulin glargine (long duration)
Insulin degludec (ultra-long duration)

Biguanides
Metformin

Sulfonylureas
Glyburide

Meglitinides (Glinides)
Repaglinide

Thiazolidinediones (Glitazones)
Pioglitazone

Alpha-Glucosidase Inhibitors
Acarbose

Gliptins (DPP-4 Inhibitors)
Sitagliptin

SGLT-2 Inhibitors
Empagliflozin

GLP-1 Receptor Agonists
Exenatide

chain and the "B" (basic) chain. The A and B chains are linked to each other by two disulfide bridges.

Biosynthesis

Insulin is synthesized in the pancreas by beta cells within the islets of Langerhans. The immediate precursor of insulin is called proinsulin.

Proinsulin consists of insulin itself plus a peptide loop that runs from the A chain to the B chain. This loop is named *connecting peptide* or *C-peptide.* In the final step of insulin synthesis, C-peptide is enzymatically clipped from the proinsulin molecule.

Measurement of plasma C-peptide levels offers a way to assess residual capacity for insulin synthesis. Since commercial insulin preparations lack C-peptide and since endogenous C-peptide is present only as a by-product of insulin biosynthesis, the presence of C-peptide in the blood indicates the pancreas is still producing some insulin of its own.

Secretion

The principal stimulus for insulin release is a rise in blood glucose, and the most common cause of glucose elevation is eating a meal, especially one rich in carbohydrates. Under normal conditions, there is tight coupling between rising levels of blood glucose and increased secretion of insulin. Insulin release may also be triggered by amino acids, fatty acids, ketone bodies, and gut hormones such as GLP-1 (more on this later).

The sympathetic nervous system provides additional control of release. Activation of $beta_2$-adrenergic receptors in the pancreas *promotes* secretion of insulin. Conversely, activation of alpha-adrenergic receptors in the pancreas *inhibits* insulin release. Of the two modes of regulation, activation of beta receptors is more important.

Metabolic Actions

The metabolic actions of insulin are primarily *anabolic* (i.e., conservative, constructive). Insulin promotes the conservation of energy and the buildup of energy stores, such as glycogen. The hormone also promotes cell growth and division.

Insulin acts in two ways to promote anabolic effects. First, it stimulates cellular transport (uptake) of glucose, amino acids, nucleotides, and potassium. Second, insulin promotes synthesis of complex organic molecules. Under the influence of insulin and other factors, glucose is converted into glycogen (the liver's way to store glucose for later use), amino acids are assembled into proteins, and fatty acids are incorporated into triglycerides. The principal metabolic actions of insulin are shown in Table 57.5.

TABLE 57.5 ▪ Metabolic Actions of Insulin

Substance Affected	Insulin Action	Site of Action
CARBOHYDRATES	↑ Glucose uptake	Muscle, adipose tissue
	↑ Glucose oxidation	Muscle
	↑ Glucose storage ↑ Glycogen synthesis ↓ Glycogenolysis	Muscle, liver
	Gluconeogenesis[a]	Liver
AMINO ACIDS AND PROTEINS	↑ Amino acid uptake	Muscle
	↓ Amino acid release	Muscle
	↑ Protein synthesis	Muscle
LIPIDS	↑ Triglyceride synthesis	Adipose tissue
	↓ Release of FFA and glycerol	Adipose tissue
	↓ Oxidation of FFA to ketoacids[b]	Liver

[a]Because of decreased delivery of substrate (fatty acids and amino acids) to the liver.
[b]Because of decreased delivery of FFA to the liver.
FFA, Free fatty acids.

Metabolic Consequences of Insulin Deficiency

Insulin deficiency puts the body into a *catabolic* mode (i.e., a metabolic state that favors the breakdown of complex molecules into their simpler constituents). Hence, in the absence of insulin, glycogen is converted into glucose, proteins are degraded into amino acids, and fats are converted to glycerol (glycerin) and free fatty acids. These catabolic effects contribute to the signs and symptoms of diabetes. Note that the catabolic effects resulting from insulin deficiency are opposite to the anabolic effects when insulin levels are normal.

Insulin deficiency promotes *hyperglycemia* by three mechanisms: (1) increased glycogenolysis, (2) increased gluconeogenesis, and (3) reduced glucose utilization. *Glycogenolysis,* by definition, generates free glucose by breaking down glycogen. The raw materials that allow increased *gluconeogenesis* are the amino acids and fatty acids produced by metabolic breakdown of proteins and fats. *Reduced glucose utilization* occurs because insulin deficiency decreases cellular uptake of glucose and decreases conversion of glucose to glycogen.

PREPARATIONS AND ADMINISTRATION

There are many insulin preparations or formulations. Major differences concern time course, appearance (clear or cloudy), concentration, and route of administration. Because of these differences, insulin preparations cannot be used interchangeably. In fact, if a patient is given the wrong preparation, the consequences can be dire. Unfortunately, medication errors with insulins remain all too common, which explains why insulin appears on all lists of "high-alert" agents.

Sources of Insulin

All forms of insulin currently manufactured in the United States are produced using recombinant DNA technology. Some products, referred to as *human insulin,* are identical to insulin produced by the human pancreas. Other products, referred to as *human insulin analogs,* are modified forms of human insulin. The analogs have the same pharmacologic actions as human insulin, but have different time courses.

Types of Insulin

There are multiple types of insulin: "natural" insulin (also known as regular insulin or native insulin) and a number of modified insulins that have variable time courses of action. Three of the modified insulins—insulin lispro, insulin aspart, and insulin glulisine—act more rapidly than regular insulin but have a shorter duration of action. The exception to this is a formulation of regular insulin that is administered via inhalation, which also acts more rapidly than injectable regular insulin. The other modified insulins act more slowly than regular insulin but have a longer duration of action. Two processes are used to prolong insulin effects: (1) complexing natural insulin with a protein and (2) altering the insulin molecule itself. When the insulin molecule has been altered, we refer to the product as a *human insulin analog.* Specific alterations made to create the insulin analogs are shown in Table 57.6.

TABLE 57.6 ▪ Amino Acids Substitutions in Human Insulin Analogs[a]

Insulin Type	Amino Acids in A-Chain Position			Amino Acids in B-Chain Position					
	A8	A10	A21	B3	B28	B29	B30	B31	B32
HUMAN INSULIN									
Native[b]	Thr	Ilc	Asn	Asn	Pro	Lys	Thr	—	—
HUMAN INSULIN ANALOGS									
Glargine	Thr	Ilc	Gly	Gly	Pro	Lys	Thr	Arg	Arg
Aspart	Thr	Ilc	Asn	Asn	Asp	Lys	Thr	—	—
Lispro	Thr	Ilc	Asn	Asn	Lys	Pro	Thr	—	—
Glulisine	Thr	Ilc	Asn	Lys	Pro	Glu	Thr	—	—
Detemir	Thr	Ilc	Asn	Asn	Pro	Lys[c]	[d]	—	—

[a]The human insulin analogs have the same physiologic effects as native human insulin—they just have different pharmacokinetics, such as onset and duration of action.
[b]Human insulin (i.e., the form of insulin made by the human pancreas) is also known as *native insulin.*
[c]A fatty-acid chain has been added to the lysine in position B29.
[d]The amino acid normally in position B30 has been deleted.
Arg, Arginine; *Asn,* asparagine; *Asp,* aspartic acid; *Glu,* glutamine; *Gly,* glycine; *Ilc,* isoleucine; *Lys,* lysine; *Pro,* proline; *Thr,* threonine.

TABLE 57.7 ▪ Types of Insulin: Time Course of Action After Subcutaneous Injection

Generic Name	Brand Name	Time Course: Onset (min)	Peak (hr)	Duration (hr)
SHORT DURATION: RAPID ACTING				
Insulin lispro	Humalog	15–30	0.5–2.5	3–6
Insulin aspart	NovoLog	10–20	1–3	3–5
Insulin glulisine	Apidra	10–15	1–1.5	3–5
SHORT DURATION: SLOWER ACTING				
Regular insulin	Humulin R, Novolin R	30–60	1–5	6–10
INTERMEDIATE DURATION				
NPH insulin	Humulin N, Novolin N	60–120	6–14	16–24
LONG DURATION				
Insulin glargine (U-100)	Lantus	70	None[a]	18–24
Insulin detemir	Levemir	60–120	None[a]	12–24
ULTRA-LONG DURATION				
Insulin glargine (U-300)	Toujeo	360	None[a]	> 24
Insulin degludec	Tresiba	30–90	None[a]	> 24

[a]Levels are steady with no discernible peak.

When classified according to time course, insulin preparations fall into three major groups: short duration, intermediate duration, and long duration. As shown in Table 57.7, these three main groupings can further be divided based on the properties of the insulins in each group. The short-duration insulins can be subdivided into two groups: rapid acting (insulin lispro, insulin aspart, insulin glulisine, and inhaled human insulin) and slower acting (regular or "natural" insulin). The long-duration insulins can also be subdivided into two groups: long acting (U-100 insulin glargine and insulin detemir) and longer-acting (U-300 insulin glargine and insulin degludec) products that have a duration in excess of 24 hours. Time courses for different insulin types are shown in Fig. 57.2. Selected properties of insulin types are shown in Table 57.8.

Short Duration: Rapid Acting

Short-duration insulins are administered in association with meals to control the postprandial (or after meal) rise in blood glucose. To provide glycemic control between meals and at night, short-acting insulins must be used in conjunction with an intermediate- or long-acting agent in people with type 1 diabetes. *All three of the injectable rapid-acting insulins are formulated as clear solutions,* and all three require a prescription. For routine therapy, all three are given subQ. If needed, all three may also be given IV. These products are rarely used IV, however, because regular insulin is a more cost-effective choice in the inpatient setting.

Insulin Lispro. Insulin lispro [Humalog] is a rapid-acting analog of regular insulin. Effects begin within 15 to 30 minutes

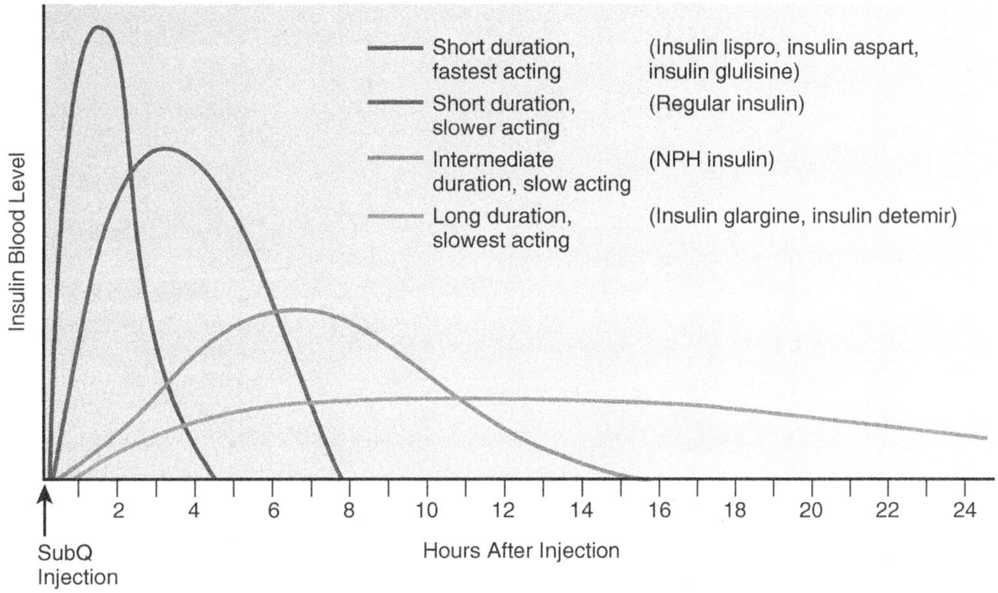

Fig. 57.2 ▪ Time-effect relationship for different types of insulin following subcutaneous injection.

of subQ injection and persist for 3 to 6 hours. Insulin lispro acts faster than regular insulin but has a shorter duration of action. Because of its rapid onset, insulin lispro can be administered immediately before eating, or even after eating in some patients. In contrast, regular insulin is generally administered 30 to 60 minutes before meals. The usual route for insulin lispro is subQ via injection or use in an insulin pump. Insulin lispro (100 units/mL, or U-100) is commercially available in 10-mL vials and as 3-mL pre-filled pens and cartridges. Of note, insulin lispro is also available in a twice-concentrated solution (200 units/mL, or U-200) that is available in pre-filled pen devices. The potential advantage of the concentrated product is to be able to administer larger doses of insulin in a smaller volume for patients requiring large doses at a time.

The structure of insulin lispro is nearly identical to that of natural insulin. The only difference is that the positions of two amino acids have been switched. Because of this switch, molecules of insulin lispro aggregate less than do molecules of regular insulin, which explains why insulin lispro acts more rapidly.

Insulin Aspart. Insulin aspart [NovoLog] is an analog of human insulin with a rapid onset (10 to 20 minutes) and short duration (3 to 5 hours). The drug is structurally identical to human insulin except that one amino acid—proline in position 28 of the B chain—has been changed to aspartic acid. Insulin aspart is very similar to insulin lispro.

Insulin aspart (100 units/mL) is supplied in 10-mL vials and 3-mL pre-filled pens and cartridges. Dosing is almost always done by subQ injection or subQ infusion with an insulin pump. Because insulin aspart acts rapidly, injections should be made 5 to 15 minutes before meals.

Insulin Glulisine. Like insulin lispro and insulin aspart, insulin glulisine [Apidra] is a synthetic analog of natural human insulin with a rapid onset (10 to 15 minutes) and short duration (3 to 5 hours). Owing to its rapid onset, the drug should be administered close to the time of eating. Administration is almost always by subQ injection or continuous subQ infusion. Insulin glulisine (100 units/mL) differs from natural insulin by two amino acids and is available in 10-mL vials and as 3-mL pre-filled insulin pens.

Inhaled Human Insulin. As mentioned briefly before, when regular human insulin is inhaled, the time action profile is altered such that the regular insulin works more quickly and has a shorter duration when compared to regular insulin when injected subQ. Inhaled human insulin [Afrezza] is a mealtime insulin product that can be used in people with type 1 and type 2 diabetes. The insulin product is available commercially in cartridges that contain 4, 8, or 12 units each. The cartridges are inserted into a dry powder inhalation device to administer the insulin by inhalation. The limitation of this particular insulin product is that patients are limited to doses of insulin in increments of 4, 8, or 12 units. For example, if a patient required 24 units of insulin, he or she would need to take 2 inhalations using the 12-unit cartridges (or 3 inhalations with the 8-unit cartridges, and so on).

Short Duration: Slower Acting

Regular Insulin Injection. Regular insulin [Humulin R, Novolin R] is unmodified human insulin. The product can be administered by subQ injection, subQ infusion (although rapid-acting analogs are generally used for this purpose), IM injection (used rarely), and through IV therapy. For IV therapy, only the U-100 formulation should be used.

For routine treatment of diabetes, regular insulin can be (1) injected before meals to control postprandial hyperglycemia and (2) infused subQ to provide basal glycemic control. Following *subQ injection,* molecules of regular insulin form small aggregates (dimers and hexamers) at the injection site. As a result, absorption is slightly delayed. Effects begin in 30 to 60 minutes, peak in 1 to 5 hours, and last up to 10 hours. Onset is slower than with the rapid-acting insulins and faster than with the longer-acting insulins. Because of this delay, most people using insulin pumps use a rapid-acting insulin analog instead of regular insulin.

Regular insulin is supplied as a clear solution. Two concentrations are available: U-100 (100 units/mL) and U-500 (500

TABLE 57.8 ▪ Properties of Insulin Types

Drug	Class	Rx or OTC	Strength[a]	Appearance	Route	Administration Options
SHORT DURATION: RAPID ACTING						
Insulin lispro [Humalog]	HA	Rx	U-100, U-200	Clear	subQ, IV	*subQ inj:* within 15 min before or just after meals *subQ inf:* continuous, with bolus just before meals *IV:* approved route, but rarely used
Insulin aspart [NovoLog]	HA	Rx	U-100	Clear	subQ, IV	*subQ inj:* 5–10 min before meals *subQ inf:* continuous, with bolus 5–10 min before meals *IV:* approved route, but rarely used
Insulin glulisine [Apidra]	HA	Rx	U-100	Clear	subQ, IV	*subQ inj:* within 15 min before meals or within 20 min after *subQ inf:* continuous, with bolus 15–20 min before meals *IV:* approved route, but rarely used
SHORT DURATION: SLOWER ACTING						
Regular insulin [Humulin R, Novolin R]	H	OTC[b]	U-100, U-500	Clear	subQ, IV, IM	*subQ inj:* 30 min before meals *subQ inf:* continuous, with bolus 20–30 min before meals *IV:* for emergencies and glycemic management in the inpatient setting (never use U-500 IV) *IM:* approved route, but rarely used
INTERMEDIATE DURATION						
NPH insulin [Humulin N, Novolin N]	H	OTC	U-100	Cloudy	subQ	*subQ inj:* twice daily at the same times each day; gently agitate before use
LONG DURATION						
U-100 Insulin glargine [Lantus]	HA	Rx	U-100	Clear	subQ	*subQ inj:* once or twice daily at the same time each day
Insulin detemir [Levemir]	HA	Rx	U-100	Clear	subQ	*subQ inj:* once or twice daily at the same time each day
ULTRA-LONG DURATION						
U-300 Insulin glargine [Toujeo]	HA	Rx	U-300	Clear	subQ	*subQ inj:* once daily
Insulin degludec [Tresiba]	HA	Rx	U-100, U-200	Clear	subQ	*subQ inj:* once daily

[a]*U-100,* 100 units/mL; *U-200,* 200 units/mL; *U-300,* 300 units/mL; *U-500,* 500 units/mL.
[b]U-100 formulations are OTC; the U-500 formulation is Rx.
H, Human insulin; *HA,* human insulin analog; *inf,* infusion; *inj,* injection; *OTC,* over the counter (no prescription needed); *Rx,* prescription needed.

units/mL). Regular insulin [Humulin R] is the only type available in a U-500 strength. U-100 preparations are used by most patients. The U-500 concentration is reserved for patients with extreme insulin resistance who take more than 200 units of insulin per day. Because it is so concentrated, U-500 insulin should never be given IV. U-500 insulin is available in 20-mL vials and in pre-filled U-500 insulin pens. When patients are using the vial, it is important to ensure that they are using U-500 insulin syringes; otherwise, they are at serious risk for an overdose of insulin. For this reason, extra caution and education are critical when working with patients using U-500 insulin. Except for the U-500 formulation, all formulations of regular insulin are available without prescription.

Intermediate Duration

Neutral Protamine Hagedorn (NPH) Insulin Suspension. NPH insulin [Humulin N, Novolin N], also known as *isophane insulin,* is prepared by conjugating regular insulin with protamine (a large protein). The presence of protamine decreases the solubility of NPH insulin and thus delays absorption. As a result, onset of action is delayed and duration of action is extended. Because onset is delayed, NPH insulin cannot be administered at mealtime to control postprandial hyperglycemia. Rather, the drug is injected two or three times daily to provide glycemic control between meals and during the night. Of the longer-acting insulins in current use, NPH insulin is the only one suitable for mixing with short-acting insulins. Because protamine is a foreign protein, allergic reactions are possible. NPH insulins are supplied as cloudy suspensions that must be agitated before administration. Administration is by subQ injection only. Like regular insulin, NPH insulins are available without prescription. NPH insulin (100 units/mL) is available in 10-mL vials and in 3-mL pre-filled insulin pens.

Long Duration

Insulin Glargine (U-100). U-100 insulin glargine [Lantus, Basaglar] is a modified human insulin with a prolonged duration of action (up to 24 hours). The drug is indicated for once-daily subQ dosing to treat adults and children with type 1 diabetes and adults with type 2 diabetes. That being said, some patients require twice-daily administration to achieve a full 24 hours of basal coverage. Dosing may be done any time of day (morning, afternoon, or evening), but should be done at the same time every day, if possible.

U-100 insulin glargine differs from natural human insulin by four amino acids. Because of these modifications, insulin glargine has low solubility at physiologic pH. Hence, when injected subQ, it forms microprecipitates that slowly dissolve and thereby release insulin glargine in small amounts over an extended time. In contrast to other long-acting insulins (i.e., NPH insulin, insulin detemir), whose blood levels rise to a peak and then fall to a trough, insulin glargine achieves blood levels that are relatively steady.

U-100 insulin glargine is supplied as a *clear solution* in 10-mL vials containing 100 units/mL, and in pre-filled pens. The drug should not be mixed with other insulins, and it should never be given IV.

Insulin Detemir. Insulin detemir [Levemir] is a human insulin analog with a slow onset. At low doses (0.2 units/kg), effects persist about 12 hours. At higher doses (0.4 units/kg), effects persist for up to 20 to 24 hours. Because of its slow onset and prolonged duration, insulin detemir is used to provide basal glycemic control. It is not given before meals to control postprandial hyperglycemia. Compared with NPH insulin, insulin detemir has a slower onset and longer duration.

Insulin detemir differs from natural insulin in two ways. First, one amino acid has been removed. Second, a 14-carbon fatty-acid chain has been attached to the B chain. Because of these structural changes, molecules of insulin detemir adhere strongly to each other, and hence absorption is delayed. Because of the fatty-acid chain, insulin detemir binds strongly with plasma albumin, and hence distribution to target sites is delayed even further.

Insulin detemir is supplied as a clear, colorless solution (100 units/mL) in 10-mL vials and as a 3-mL *FlexTouch Pen.* Dosing is done once or twice daily by subQ injection. Insulin detemir should not be mixed with other insulins and must not be given IV. The drug is available by prescription only.

Longer Duration (> 24 hours)

Insulin Glargine (U-300). U-300 insulin glargine [Toujeo] is similar to U-100 insulin glargine except that it is three times concentrated, which prolongs its duration of action to be in excess of 24 hours. The drug is indicated for once-daily subQ dosing to treat both type 1 and type 2 diabetes. Because U-300 insulin glargine has a longer duration of action than U-100 insulin glargine, use of this product is an option for those individuals who do not realize a full 24 hours of effect with the U-100 product.

U-300 insulin glargine is supplied as a *clear solution* in pre-filled pens only. The pre-filled pens minimize the risk of insulin overdose. To administer a dose of U-300 insulin, the patient simply dials the desired number of units on the pen, and all volume conversions are made automatically. The pre-filled pens eliminate the risk of overdose with U-100 insulin syringes, for example. The product is dosed once daily.

Insulin Degludec. Insulin degludec [Tresiba] is another longer-acting insulin that can be used in type 1 and type 2 diabetes to provide basal insulin coverage. So how does insulin degludec achieve a longer time action profile? In solution insulin degludec exists as soluble dihexamers. Once injected, however, the degludec dihexamers assemble into multihexamer chains that are quite stable in the subQ tissue. Over time monomers of insulin diffuse from the terminal ends of the long insulin chain, which are then absorbed. The slow dissociation of insulin degludec at the injection site results in a duration of action in excess of 24 hours.

Insulin degludec is available in both U-100 and U-200 concentrations. The more concentrated U-200 product is useful for patients on large doses of insulin. Both concentrations are available in pre-filled insulin pens only. The product is recommended to be dosed once daily for basal insulin needs.

Appearance

In the past, many insulins were formulated as cloudy suspensions, and this was an easy tip-off that the drug must not be injected intravenously. Today, the opposite is true: With the exception of NPH insulins, all insulins made in the United States are formulated as *clear, colorless solutions.* NPH insulin is still a cloudy suspension. Patients should inspect their insulin before using it and should discard the vial if the insulin looks abnormal.

Because most insulin preparations—and not just regular insulin—are now formulated as clear solutions, generalities that applied in the past are no longer true. Accordingly, patients and providers should note the following changes:

In the past: *All insulins available as clear solutions were short acting.* This was true when regular insulin was the only preparation available as a clear solution.

Today: Of the insulins available as clear solutions, four preparations—regular, lispro, aspart, and glulisine insulin—are short acting, and four preparations—detemir, U-100 glargine, U-300 glargine, and degludec insulin—have more prolonged actions.

In the past: *All insulins available as clear solutions could be administered IV.* Again, this was true when regular insulin was the only preparation available as a clear solution.

Today: Of the insulins available as clear solutions, four preparations—regular, aspart, lispro, and glulisine insulin—can be administered IV. The rest—detemir, U-100 glargine, U-300 glargine, and degludec insulin—cannot.

In the past: *All insulins that were clear solutions could be mixed in the same syringe with other insulins.* Again, this was true when regular insulin was the only preparation available as a clear solution.

Today: Of the insulins available as clear solutions, only the short-acting preparations—regular, lispro, aspart, and glulisine insulin—can be mixed with other insulins (usually NPH insulin).

Concentration

In the United States, insulin is available in several concentrations, depending on the product: 100 units/mL (U-100), 200 units/mL (U-200), 300 units/mL (U-300), and 500 units/mL (U-500). U-100 insulins are employed for routine replacement therapy. Most insulin types are available in U-100 formulations. As noted previously, insulin lispro and insulin degludec are available in both U-100 and U-200 concentrations. Insulin glargine is the only insulin product available in a U-300 concentration to be used for basal insulin coverage. Only one product—the *Humulin R* brand of regular insulin—is formulated in the U-500 strength. This product is for patients with severe insulin resistance, generally defined as needing more than 200 units/day.

Mixing Insulins

When the treatment plan calls for using a short-acting insulin in combination with a longer-acting insulin, it is usually desirable to mix the preparations (in a single syringe) rather than inject them separately, so as to eliminate the need for an additional injection. However, although mixing offers convenience, it can alter the time course of the response. Therefore, to ensure a consistent response, mixing should be done only with insulins of proven compatibility. Of the longer-acting insulins in current use, *only NPH insulin is appropriate for mixing with short-acting insulins* (i.e., regular, lispro, aspart, and glulisine insulins). When a mixture is prepared, the short-acting insulin should be drawn into the syringe first to avoid contaminating the stock vial of the short-acting insulin with NPH insulin. As a rule, the mixtures are stable for 28 days. Commercially available premixed combinations are generally preferred due to convenience and accuracy of the mixture. These products are described in Table 57.9.

Administration

Subcutaneous Injection

Insulin is usually given by subQ injection because, owing to its peptide structure, insulin would be inactivated by the digestive system if it were given by mouth. All types of insulins (with the exception of inhaled regular insulin) may be injected subQ.

Preparing for Injection. Initial preparation depends on whether the insulin product is in solution or suspension. With the exception of NPH insulins, all insulins available today are supplied as clear, colorless solutions. These solutions are ready to use—*unless they have become colored or cloudy, or contain a precipitate,* in which case they should be discarded. Because NPH insulins are suspensions, their particles must be evenly dispersed before loading the syringe. Dispersion is accomplished by rolling the vial between the palms of the hands. Mixing must be gentle, because vigorous agitation will cause frothing and render accurate dosing more difficult. If granules or clumps remain after gentle agitation, the vial should be discarded.

Before loading the syringe, the rubber cap should be swabbed with alcohol. Air bubbles should be eliminated from the syringe and needle after loading. The skin should be cleaned with alcohol (or soap and water) before injection.

Injection Sites. The most common sites of subQ injection are the upper arm, thigh, and abdomen (Fig. 57.3). Absorption is fastest and most consistent following abdominal injection, and slowest following injection in the thigh. Because rates of absorption vary among sites, patients should make all injections into the same general area (e.g., thigh or abdomen). To reduce

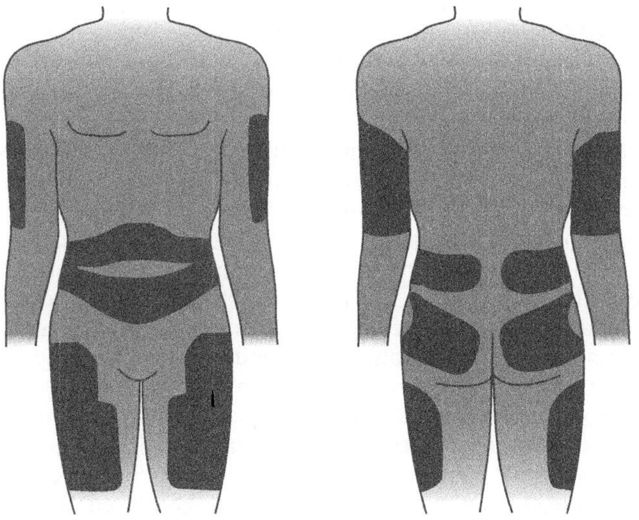

Fig. 57.3 ▪ Possible sites for subcutaneous injection of insulin.

TABLE 57.9 ▪ Premixed Insulin Combinations[a]

Description	Brand Name	Time Course: Onset (min)	Peak (hr)	Duration (hr)
70% NPH insulin/30% regular insulin	Humulin 70/30	30–60	1.5–16	10–16
	Novolin 70/30	30–60	2–12	10–16
70% insulin aspart protamine/30% insulin aspart	NovoLog Mix 70/30	10–20	1–4	15–18
75% insulin lispro protamine/25% insulin lispro	Humalog Mix 75/25	15–30	1–6.5	10–16
50% insulin lispro protamine/50% insulin lispro	Humalog Mix 50/50	15–30	0.8–4.8	10–16

[a]Use only after the dosages and ratios of the components have been established as correct for the patient.

the risk of lipohypertrophy (see the *Other Complications* section), injections within the chosen area should be made in different spots, preferably about 1 inch apart. Ideally, each spot should be used only once a month.

Injection Devices

Syringe and Needle. Syringes and needles for insulin injection are manufactured in several sizes, so they can be matched to individual needs. Three syringe sizes are available: 1 mL, ½ mL, and ⅓ mL, which can deliver up to 100, 50, and 30 units of insulin, respectively. Patients should choose the syringe that best matches their dosage. For example, a patient who injects 25 units of insulin per dose should choose a ⅓-mL syringe, which can deliver up to 30 units of insulin. Patients should use the smallest syringe that will hold the required volume.

Needles for injecting insulin are available in three lengths: 12.7 mm (½ inch), 8 mm (5⁄16 inch), 5 mm (3⁄16 inch), and 4 mm (5⁄32 inch).

As mentioned previously for U-500 insulin, a dedicated insulin syringe is also available for dosing U-500 insulin. The syringe is visibly different from U-100 insulin syringes in that the cap is green and it has "U-500" printed in green just above the plunger of the syringe. The syringe is marked in 5-unit increments and can deliver up to 250 units of U-500 insulin. *U-500 insulin syringes should be used with U-500 insulin only.*

Pen Injectors. These devices are similar to a syringe and needle but are more convenient. Pen injectors look like a fountain pen but have a disposable needle (where the writing tip would be) and a disposable insulin-filled cartridge inside. Administration is accomplished by sticking the needle under the skin and injecting the insulin manually.

Jet Injectors. These devices shoot insulin directly through the skin into subcutaneous tissue. No needle is used. Hence, for patients who dislike needles, a jet injector may be attractive. However, these devices do have a downside. They're expensive and can be difficult to use and are thus very rarely used. Moreover, because insulin is delivered under high pressure, jet injectors can cause stinging, burning, and pain. In addition, bruising can occur in people with reduced subcutaneous fat.

Subcutaneous Infusion

Portable Insulin Pumps. These computerized devices deliver a basal infusion of insulin (usually rapid-acting analogs—lispro, aspart, or glulisine) plus bolus doses before each meal. In other words, the pump uses only one type of insulin for both basal and mealtime coverage. The basal infusion is usually about 1 unit/hr and can be programmed to match the patient's metabolic requirements. Basal rates can even be adjusted to different rates throughout the day, depending on the individualized needs of the patient, and are adjustable in some pumps up to 1/100th of a unit per hour. Mealtime boluses are calculated to match carbohydrate intake and can be adjusted to within 1/10th of a unit. The pumps are about the size of a small cell phone, weigh only 4 ounces, and are worn on the belt or in a pocket. An infusion set delivers insulin from the pump to a subcutaneous catheter, usually located on the abdomen. The infusion set should be replaced about every 3 days, at which time the catheter is moved to a new infusion site (at least 1 inch away from the old one). Because the pump delivers rapid-acting insulin, insulin levels will drop quickly if the pump is removed. Accordingly, the pump should remain in place most of the day. However, it can be removed for an hour or two on special occasions. External insulin pumps generally cost between $3000 and $5000. Infusion sets, insulin, and glucose monitoring materials add another $300 or more per month to the bill.

Implantable Insulin Pumps. These devices are surgically implanted in the abdomen and deliver insulin either intraperitoneally or intravenously. Like external pumps, internal pumps deliver a basal insulin infusion plus bolus doses with meals. Insulin delivery is adjusted by external telemetry. Compared with multiple daily injections, pumps produce superior glycemic control, cause less hypoglycemia and weight gain, and can improve quality of life. As with external pumps, delivery of insulin can be impeded by formation of insulin microprecipitates. Implantable pumps are experimental and not yet available for general use.

Intravenous Infusion

Intravenous infusion is reserved for emergencies that require a rapid reduction in blood glucose and for people being managed in the inpatient setting during hospitalization. Not long ago, regular insulin (U-100 strength) was the only formulation considered safe for IV use. Today, three other short-acting insulins—insulin aspart [Novolog], insulin lispro [Humalog], and insulin glulisine [Apidra]—may also be used. Regular insulin is most commonly used because it is less expensive, and because IV administration does not require absorption from the subQ depot. When used for intravenous infusion, regular human insulin is generally diluted by adding 100 units to 100 mL of 0.9% NaCl or other compatible intravenous fluid. An initial infusion rate of 0.1 unit/kg/hr is often recommended, but infusion rates and insulin doses must be individualized based on individual needs.

Inhalation

Inhaled human insulin [Afrezza] is one mealtime insulin product that provides good glycemic control with a relatively low incidence of hypoglycemia, and it has demonstrated little or no effect on pulmonary function in studies to date. This product is used for mealtime coverage and is inhaled at each meal. While approved for both type 1 and type 2 diabetes, the ability to fine-tune the dose is limited by the availability of 4-, 8-, and 12-unit insulin cartridges.

Storage

Insulin in *unopened vials* should be stored *under refrigeration* until needed. Vials should not be frozen. When stored unopened under refrigeration, insulin can be used up to the expiration date on the vial.

The vial in current use can, in general, be kept at room temperature for up to 1 month without significant loss of activity. The product information for each product should be reviewed for product-specific storage recommendations. Direct sunlight and extreme heat must be avoided. Partially filled vials should be discarded after several weeks if left unused. Injecting insulin stored at room temperature causes less pain than injecting cold insulin and reduces the risk of lipodystrophy.

Mixtures of insulin prepared in *vials* are stable for 1 month at room temperature and for 3 months under refrigeration.

Mixtures of insulin in *pre-filled syringes* (plastic or glass) should be stored in a refrigerator, where they will be stable for at least 1 week and perhaps 2 weeks. The syringe should be stored vertically with the needle pointing up to avoid clogging the needle. Before administration, the syringe should be agitated gently to resuspend the insulin.

THERAPEUTIC USE

Indications

The principal indication for insulin is *diabetes mellitus.* Insulin is required by all patients with type 1 diabetes and by many patients with type 2 diabetes. In fact, most of the insulin sold is used by people with type 2 diabetes—largely due to the fact that type 2 diabetes accounts for 90% to 95% of all cases of diabetes. Intravenous insulin is used to treat *diabetic ketoacidosis.* Because of its ability to promote cellular uptake of potassium and thereby lower plasma potassium levels, insulin infusion is also employed to acutely treat *hyperkalemia.* Lastly, insulin can aid in the *diagnosis of growth hormone (GH) deficiency.*[a] The use of insulin in diabetes is discussed here.

Insulin Therapy of Diabetes

Insulin is given to all patients who have type 1 diabetes and to many who have type 2 diabetes. In addition, insulin is the preferred drug to manage gestational diabetes. In treating these disorders, the objective is to prevent complications by keeping blood glucose within an acceptable range. When therapy is successful, both hyperglycemia and hypoglycemia are minimized, and the long-term complications of diabetes are avoided and/or delayed.

Dosage

To achieve optimal glucose control, insulin dosage must be closely matched with insulin needs. If carbohydrate intake is increased, insulin dosage must be increased too (especially in the case of patients with type 1 diabetes). When a meal is missed or is low in carbohydrates, or when physical activity levels increase, the dosage of insulin must be decreased. Dosing requires additional adjustments to meet specialized needs. For example, insulin needs are *increased* by infection, stress, obesity, the adolescent growth spurt, and in pregnancy after the first trimester. Conversely, insulin needs are *decreased* by exercise and during the first trimester of pregnancy. To ensure that insulin dosage is coordinated with insulin requirements, the patient and the healthcare team must work together to establish an integrated program of nutrition, exercise, insulin replacement therapy, and appropriate blood glucose monitoring.

Total daily dosages may range from 0.1 unit/kg body weight to more than 2.5 units/kg. For patients with type 1 diabetes, initial dosages typically range from 0.5 to 0.6 units/kg/day. For patients with type 2 diabetes, initial dosages typically range from 0.2 to 0.6 units/kg/day. These are generalities, however, and insulin doses are always individualized based on patient-specific needs.

Dosing Schedules

The schedule of insulin administration helps determine the extent to which glucose control can be achieved. Three dosing schedules are compared here. These example regimens include use of (1) a twice-daily premixed insulin regimen, (2) intensive basal/bolus strategy, and (3) continuous subcutaneous insulin infusion (CSII). While three example regimens are discussed, it should be noted that practitioners can use currently available insulin products in a number of ways and combinations to meet patient-specific needs and treatment goals.

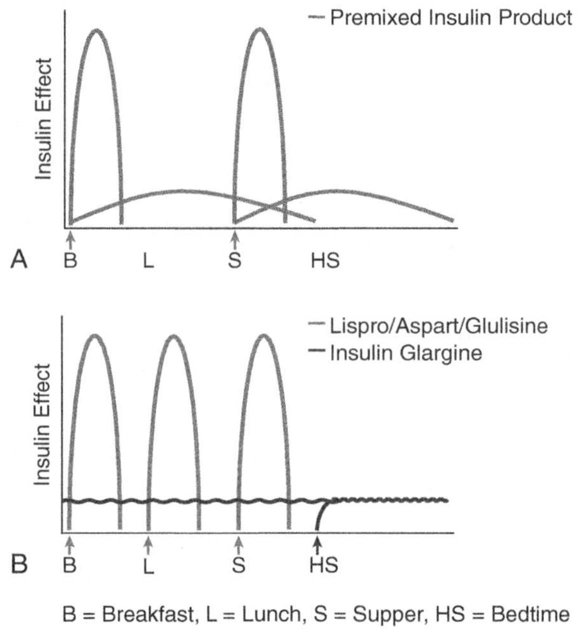

Fig. 57.4 ▪ Examples of insulin dosing schedules.

Twice-Daily Premixed Regimen. There are several premixed insulin products on the market. As shown in Fig. 57.4A, a twice-daily regimen of such a premixed insulin product can be used to provide both basal and prandial insulin coverage. The advantage of this strategy is that patients need only two injections per day. A disadvantage, however, is that if given with breakfast and dinner, there is no mealtime coverage at lunch. Additionally, using a fixed combination does not allow for adjustments of the long-acting or short-acting insulin individually; if the dose is changed, both components are altered.

Intensive Basal/Bolus Strategy. For patients with type 1 diabetes, an intensive basal/bolus strategy is indicated. As shown in Fig. 57.4B, this strategy involves the use of a long-acting insulin (such as insulin glargine [Lantus]) in addition to a short-acting insulin (such as regular insulin, insulin aspart, insulin lispro, or insulin glulisine). This insulin dosing strategy allows for very good basal coverage and the ability to dose a short- or rapid-acting insulin with each meal and as needed to cover snacks or elevated blood glucose levels.

Continuous Subcutaneous Insulin Infusion (CSII). CSII is accomplished using a portable infusion pump connected to an indwelling subcutaneous catheter. Four types of insulin may be used: regular, lispro, aspart, and glulisine. Rapid-acting insulins are most commonly used. To provide a basal level of insulin, the pump is set to infuse insulin continuously at a slow but steady rate. To accommodate insulin needs created by eating, the pump is triggered manually to provide a bolus dose matched in size to the carbohydrate content of each meal. Hence, CSII can adapt to altered insulin needs. While the use of CSII allows for ease of administration, the use of frequent SMBG is essential to achieve optimal glycemic control. Advances in continuous glucose monitoring (CGM) technology have to some degree decreased the need for SMBG in patients using CSII. In 2016

[a]The *insulin hypoglycemia test* can aid in the diagnosis of suspected GH deficiency in preadolescent children who are not growing as fast as their peers. The test is based on the fact that even modest insulin-induced hypoglycemia can trigger GH release, causing blood levels of GH to rise. In children with GH deficiency, the rise in blood GH will be lower than in children with normal pituitary function.

the FDA approved the first "hybrid closed-loop system," which integrates CGM technology with CSII technology. Essentially the system will adjust basal insulin delivery based on what is happening with the patient's glucose levels automatically. This technology certainly doesn't eliminate the need of the patient to be diligent with monitoring and dosing, but it is a step toward a more automated insulin delivery approach. Infusion pumps were further discussed earlier in the section titled *Subcutaneous Infusion* under *Administration.*

Achieving Optimal Glucose Control

As we have seen, the primary requirement for achieving tight glucose control is a method of insulin delivery that permits dosage adjustments that accommodate ongoing variations in insulin needs. Intensive basal/bolus therapy and CSII meet this criterion. In addition to an adaptable method of insulin delivery, achieving tight glucose control requires the following:

- Careful attention to all elements of the treatment program (diet, exercise, insulin replacement therapy)
- Defined glycemic targets
- Self-monitoring of blood glucose in concordance with the patient's individualized management plan
- A high degree of patient motivation
- Extensive patient education

Tight glucose control cannot be achieved without the informed participation of the patient. Accordingly, patients must receive thorough instruction on the following:

- The nature of diabetes
- The importance of optimal glucose control
- The major components of the treatment routine (insulin replacement, SMBG, diet, exercise)
- Procedures for purchasing insulin, syringes, and needles
- The importance of avoiding arbitrary changes between insulins from different manufacturers
- Methods of insulin storage
- Procedures for mixing insulins (if applicable)
- Calculation of dosage adjustments
- Techniques of insulin administration
- Methods for monitoring blood glucose

In the final analysis, responsibility for managing diabetes rests with the patient. The healthcare team can design a treatment program and provide education and guidance. However, optimal glucose control can only be achieved if the patient is actively involved in his or her own therapy.

Complications of Insulin Treatment

Hypoglycemia

Hypoglycemia (generally defined clinically as a blood glucose below 70 mg/dL) occurs when insulin levels exceed insulin needs. A major cause of insulin excess is overdose. Imbalance between insulin levels and insulin needs can also result from reduced intake of food, vomiting and diarrhea (which reduce absorption of nutrients), excessive consumption of alcohol (which promotes hypoglycemia), unusually intense exercise (which promotes cellular glucose uptake and metabolism), and childbirth (which reduces insulin requirements).

Patients with diabetes and their families should be familiar with the signs and symptoms of hypoglycemia. Establishing whether patients are experiencing hypoglycemia and whether they recognize hypoglycemic symptoms is recommended as a critical component of an encounter with a patient with diabetes. Some symptoms result from activation of the sympathetic nervous system; others arise from a lack of glucose within the central nervous system (CNS). When glucose levels fall *rapidly,* activation of the sympathetic nervous system occurs, resulting in tachycardia, palpitations, sweating, and nervousness. However, if glucose declines *gradually,* symptoms may be limited to those of CNS origin. Mild CNS symptoms include headache, confusion, drowsiness, and fatigue. If hypoglycemia is severe, convulsions, coma, and death may follow.

Rapid treatment of hypoglycemia is mandatory: If hypoglycemia is allowed to persist, irreversible brain damage or even death may result. In conscious patients, glucose levels can be restored with a fast-acting oral sugar (e.g., glucose tablets, orange juice, sugar cubes, honey, corn syrup, nondiet soda). However, if the swallowing reflex or the gag reflex is suppressed, nothing should be administered by mouth. In cases of severe hypoglycemia, IV glucose is the preferred treatment. Parenteral *glucagon* is an alternative treatment. (The pharmacology of glucagon is discussed at the end of the chapter.)

In anticipation of hypoglycemic episodes, people with diabetes should always have an oral carbohydrate available (e.g., sugared candy, sugar cubes, glucose tablets). Treatment guidelines from organizations such as the ADA also recommend that patients keep glucagon on hand too—particularly people on insulin therapy or otherwise at increased risk of hypoglycemia. Patients should carry some sort of identification (e.g., Medic Alert bracelet) to inform emergency personnel of their condition.

In some patients, hypoglycemia occurs without producing the symptoms noted here. This is known as *hypoglycemia unawareness*. As a result, the patient remains unaware of hypoglycemia until blood sugar has become dangerously low. Hypoglycemia unawareness is a particular problem among patients practicing tight glucose control. This is because as patients experience more frequent hypoglycemia, they start to have diminished symptoms over time. The risk of dangerous hypoglycemia can be minimized by frequently monitoring blood glucose. Additionally, current recommendations state that treatment goals should be temporarily loosened (such as for several weeks) for people experiencing hypoglycemia unawareness so that they can regain hypoglycemia awareness.

Both severe hypoglycemia and diabetic ketoacidosis (see later section on *Acute Complications of Poor Glycemic Control*) can result in coma. Of the two causes, hypoglycemia is more common. Since treatment of these two conditions is very different (hypoglycemia involves withholding insulin, whereas ketoacidosis requires giving insulin), it is essential that coma from these causes be differentiated. The most definitive diagnosis is made by measuring plasma glucose levels: in hypoglycemic coma, glucose levels are very low; in ketoacidosis, glucose levels are very high.

Other Complications

Hypokalemia. Insulin promotes uptake of potassium by cells. Insulin activates a membrane-bound enzyme—Na^+,K^+-ATPase—that pumps potassium into cells and pumps sodium out. Hence, in addition to lowering blood levels of glucose, insulin can lower blood levels of potassium. When insulin dosage is proper, effects on potassium are unremarkable. However, if insulin dosage is excessive, clinically significant hypokalemia can result. Effects on the heart are of greatest concern: Hypokalemia can reduce contractility and can cause potentially fatal dysrhythmias.

Lipohypertrophy. Lipohypertrophy (accumulation of subcutaneous fat) can occur when insulin is injected too frequently at the same site. Fat accumulates because insulin stimulates fat synthesis. When use of the site is discontinued, excess fat is eventually lost. Lipohypertrophy can be minimized through systematic rotation of injection sites.

Allergic Reactions. Rarely, patients experience systemic allergic responses. These reactions develop rapidly and are characterized by the widespread appearance of red and intensely itchy welts. Breathing difficulty may develop. If severe allergy develops in a patient who nonetheless must continue insulin use, a desensitization procedure can be performed. This process entails giving small initial doses of human insulin, followed by a series of progressively larger doses.

Drug Interactions

Hypoglycemic Agents

Drugs that lower blood glucose levels can intensify hypoglycemia induced by insulin. Among these drugs are *sulfonylureas, glinides,* and *alcohol* (used acutely or long term in excessive doses). When these drugs are combined with insulin, special care must be taken to ensure as best as possible that blood glucose does not fall too low.

Hyperglycemic Agents

Drugs that raise blood glucose (e.g., *glucocorticoids, sympathomimetics*) can counteract the desired effects of insulin. When these agents are combined with insulin, insulin dosage may need to be increased.

Beta-Adrenergic Blocking Agents

Beta blockers can delay awareness of and response to hypoglycemia by masking signs that are associated with stimulation of the sympathetic nervous system (e.g., tachycardia, palpitations) that hypoglycemia normally causes. Furthermore, since beta blockade impairs glycogenolysis, and since glycogenolysis is one means by which the body can respond to and counteract a fall in blood glucose, beta blockers (particularly noncardiac selective beta blockers such as propranolol) can make insulin-induced hypoglycemia even worse by preventing the body's natural counterregulatory response.

NON-INSULIN MEDICATIONS FOR THE TREATMENT OF DIABETES

The non-insulin medications for the treatment of diabetes fall into two major groups: oral drugs and non-insulin injectable drugs. Their actions and major adverse effects are shown in Table 57.10.

ORAL DRUGS

There are seven main families of oral antidiabetic drugs: biguanides, sulfonylureas, meglitinides (glinides), thiazolidinediones (glitazones), alpha-glucosidase inhibitors, DPP-4 inhibitors (gliptins), and sodium-glucose co-transporter 2 (SGLT-2) inhibitors. These agents are approved for use in type 2 diabetes, but agents such as the SGLT-2 inhibitors are used off-label in combination with insulin for the treatment of type 1 diabetes—with clinical studies in progress. In the past, the oral agents were used only after a program of diet modification and exercise had failed to yield sufficient glycemic control. Today, one oral agent—metformin—is usually started immediately after type 2 diabetes has been diagnosed.

The oral agents work in a variety of ways. Some of them—notably the sulfonylureas and glinides (collectively referred to as "insulin secretagogues")—actively drive blood glucose down by increasing insulin release from beta cells of the pancreas. Others—notably metformin (a biguanide), the alpha-glucosidase inhibitors, the DPP-4 inhibitors, and SGLT-2 inhibitors—don't drive blood glucose down; rather, they simply modulate the rise in glucose that happens after a meal. This distinction is not just academic: If taken when blood glucose is normal or low, agents that drive glucose down can cause *hypoglycemia.* Hypoglycemia is not a large risk with the drugs that do not stimulate insulin release from the pancreas.

A note on nomenclature: Traditionally, the oral drugs for diabetes have been referred to as *oral hypoglycemic drugs* or *oral hypoglycemics.* However, this description is inaccurate and is not used in this book. As discussed previously, only some of these drugs drive glucose levels down, and hence only some deserve to be called *hypoglycemics.* A better name for these drugs is *oral antidiabetic agents* or *oral antihyperglycemic agents* because these names apply to all drugs in the group, not just the ones that actively reduce levels of glucose and induce a risk of hypoglycemia.

Biguanides: Metformin

Metformin [Glucophage, Glucophage XR, Fortamet, Glumetza, Riomet], classified chemically as a biguanide, is the drug of choice for initial therapy in most patients with type 2 diabetes. Typically, metformin is started immediately after the diagnosis of type 2 diabetes. The most common side effects are GI disturbances. Lactic acidosis, a potentially fatal complication, is rare.

Mechanism of Action

Metformin lowers blood glucose and improves glucose tolerance in three ways. First, it inhibits glucose production in the liver. Second, it sensitizes insulin receptors in target tissues (fat and skeletal muscle) and thereby increases glucose uptake in response to whatever insulin may be available. And third, it reduces (slightly) glucose absorption in the gut. In contrast to the sulfonylureas (see later), metformin does not stimulate insulin release from the pancreas. As a result, metformin does not actively drive blood glucose levels down, and hence poses little if any added risk of hypoglycemia when used alone.

Pharmacokinetics

Following oral dosing, metformin is slowly absorbed from the small intestine. Of particular interest, metformin is not metabolized. Rather it is excreted unchanged by the kidneys. Hence, in the event of renal impairment, metformin can accumulate to toxic levels.

Therapeutic Uses

Glycemic Control. Metformin is used to lower blood sugar in patients with type 2 diabetes. Metformin may be used alone or in combination with other agents. When used alone, metformin lowers fasting and postprandial blood glucose levels. When metformin is used as a component of combination therapy, the combination lowers blood sugar more effectively than either drug alone—which is to be expected because other available agents act via different mechanisms.

TABLE 57.10 ■ Drugs for Type 2 Diabetes

Class and Specific Agents	Actions	Major Adverse Effects
ORAL DRUGS		
Biguanide		
Metformin [Fortamet, Glucophage, Glumetza, Riomet]	Decreases glucose production by the liver, increases tissue response to insulin	GI symptoms: decreased appetite, nausea, diarrhea Lactic acidosis (rarely)
Second-Generation Sulfonylureas		
Glimepiride [Amaryl] Glipizide [Glucotrol, Glucotrol XL] Glyburide[a] [DiaBeta, Glynase PresTab]	Promote insulin secretion by the pancreas; may also increase tissue response to insulin	Hypoglycemia Weight gain
Meglitinides (Glinides)		
Nateglinide [Starlix] Repaglinide [Prandin, GlucoNorm 🍁]	Promote insulin secretion by the pancreas	Hypoglycemia Weight gain
Thiazolidinediones (Glitazones)		
Pioglitazone [Actos] Rosiglitazone [Avandia]	Decrease insulin resistance and thereby increase glucose uptake by muscle and adipose tissue, and decrease glucose production by the liver	Hypoglycemia, but only in the presence of excessive insulin Heart failure Bladder cancer Fractures (in women) Ovulation, and thus possible unintended pregnancy
Alpha-Glucosidase Inhibitors		
Acarbose [Precose, Glucobay 🍁] Miglitol [Glyset]	Delay carbohydrate digestion and absorption, thereby decreasing the postprandial rise in blood glucose	GI symptoms: flatulence, cramps, abdominal distention, borborygmus
DPP-4 Inhibitors (Gliptins)		
Alogliptin [Nesina] Linagliptin [Tradjenta] Saxagliptin [Onglyza] Sitagliptin [Januvia]	Enhance the activity of incretins (by inhibiting their breakdown by DPP-4), and thereby increase insulin release, reduce glucagon release, and decrease hepatic glucose production	Pancreatitis Hypersensitivity reactions
Sodium-Glucose Co-Transporter 2 (SGLT-2) Inhibitors		
Canagliflozin [Invokana] Dapagliflozin [Farxiga] Empagliflozin [Jardiance]	Increase glucose excretion via the urine by inhibiting SGLT-2 in the kidney tubules, decreasing glucose levels, and inducing weight loss via caloric loss through the urine	Genital mycotic infections Orthostasis
Dopamine Agonist		
Bromocriptine [Cycloset]	Activates dopamine receptors in the CNS; how it improves glycemic control is unknown	Orthostatic hypotension Exacerbation of psychosis
NON-INSULIN INJECTABLE DRUGS		
Incretin Mimetics		
Exenatide [Byetta] Exenatide extended-release [Bydureon] Liraglutide [Victoza] Lixisenatide [Adlyxin] Albiglutide [Tanzeum] Dulaglutide [Trulicity]	Lower blood glucose by slowing gastric emptying, stimulating glucose-dependent insulin release, suppressing postprandial glucagon release, and reducing appetite	Hypoglycemia GI symptoms: nausea, vomiting, diarrhea Pancreatitis Renal insufficiency Thyroid cancer (?) (liraglutide, exenatide extended-release, albiglutide, and dulaglutide)
Amylin Mimetics		
Pramlintide [Symlin]	Delays gastric emptying and suppresses glucagon secretion, decreasing the postprandial rise in glucose	Hypoglycemia Nausea Injection-site reactions

[a]Commonly known as *glibenclamide* outside the United States.

Metformin is well suited for patients who tend to skip meals. When meals are skipped, blood glucose can drop below a level that is healthy. Because metformin does not lower blood glucose any further, it won't make the situation any worse. In contrast, drugs that actively lower blood glucose, such as the sulfonylureas, can drop a normal or slightly low blood glucose into clinically significant hypoglycemia.

Prevention of Type 2 Diabetes. Data from the Diabetes Prevention Program (DPP), a large study sponsored by the National Institutes of Health, indicate that metformin can delay development of type 2 diabetes in high-risk individuals. The DPP enrolled 3234 people ages 25 to 85. All participants had impaired glucose tolerance (as determined by an OGTT), and all were severely overweight. Participants were randomly assigned to one of three protocols: (1) intensive lifestyle changes with the aim of reducing body weight by 7% through moderate exercise (e.g., vigorous walking 30 minutes a day 5 days a week) combined with a low-fat diet, (2) treatment with metformin (850 mg twice daily), or (3) treatment with placebo. The results? Metformin reduced the risk of developing type 2 diabetes by 31%. However, benefits were limited primarily to younger patients and to those who were most overweight; the drug was relatively ineffective in older patients and those less overweight. It must be stressed, however, that metformin is not a substitute for diet and exercise. In fact, the DPP showed that lifestyle changes are even more effective than metformin: The combination of moderate exercise plus weight loss (5% to 7% of initial weight) reduced the average risk of type 2 diabetes by 58%. Benefits were greatest (71%) for people older than 60 years.

Gestational Diabetes. For decades, insulin was considered the preferred, if not the only, antidiabetic drug for managing diabetes during pregnancy, whether the mother had type 1 or type 2 diabetes. Recent clinical studies have compared metformin with insulin in pregnant women with type 2 diabetes. Multiple outcomes were assessed, including glycemic control in the mother and blood glucose and Apgar scores in the neonate. The result? Outcomes with metformin were essentially the same as those with insulin, the traditional agent for managing gestational diabetes—suggesting that metformin may become an acceptable alternative for many women. (Note: The data obtained with metformin do *not* apply to other classes of oral agents, such as the sulfonylureas and glitazones.) That said, the ADA currently states that pregnant women using metformin should be informed that although no adverse effects on the fetus have been thus far demonstrated, long-term studies are currently lacking.

Polycystic Ovary Syndrome (PCOS). PCOS is a combined endocrine/metabolic disorder characterized by androgen excess and insulin resistance. It affects about 5% to 10% of women of reproductive age. Symptoms include irregular periods, anovulation, infertility, acne, and hirsutism. Although not approved for PCOS, metformin can be very helpful. Metformin treatment increases insulin sensitivity and decreases insulin levels, which, through an indirect mechanism, lowers androgen levels. The net result is improved glucose tolerance, improved ovulation, and increased pregnancy rates. PCOS and its management are discussed further in Chapter 63.

Side Effects

The most common side effects are decreased appetite, nausea, and diarrhea. These generally subside over time. However, in 3% to 5% of patients, *GI side effects* lead to discontinuation of treatment. Therefore, the dose of metformin must be titrated up to the target dose to minimize the severity of GI side effects.

Metformin decreases absorption of vitamin B_{12} and folic acid, and can thereby cause deficiencies of both. Deficiency of B_{12}, in turn, can contribute to peripheral neuropathy, a common long-term consequence of diabetes. Based on recent evidence, the ADA states that long-term metformin use may be associated with vitamin B_{12} deficiency and recommends that periodic measurement of B_{12} levels be considered in metformin-treated patients. This is especially true in patients with anemia or symptoms of peripheral neuropathy. As discussed in Chapter 81, deficiency of folic acid during pregnancy can impair development of the CNS, resulting in neural tube defects, which manifest as anencephaly or spina bifida. Nonetheless, current evidence suggests that metformin is safe for use during pregnancy.

In contrast with sulfonylureas (see later), metformin does not cause weight gain. In fact, patients maintain or possibly *lose* weight with metformin therapy. As a result, metformin is considered a "weight-neutral" antidiabetic drug, in contrast with several other antidiabetic drugs that tend to increase weight ("weight-positive"). Appetite suppression and weight loss in response to metformin can occur both in the presence and absence of nausea, indicating that reduced food intake because of metformin-induced nausea is not the only reason for weight loss in those patients who lose weight.

Toxicity: Lactic Acidosis

Metformin inhibits mitochondrial oxidation of lactic acid and can thereby cause lactic acidosis. This condition is a medical emergency and has a mortality rate of about 50%. Fortunately, lactic acidosis is rare (about 3 cases/100,000 patient-years) when metformin is used at recommended doses in patients with good renal function. However, in patients with renal insufficiency, metformin can rapidly accumulate to toxic levels. Accordingly, the drug must never be used by these people. Specifically, metformin is considered contraindicated in patients with an estimated glomerular filtration rate (eGFR) of less than 30 mL/minute/1.73 m^2. Cautious use is additionally recommended in those with an eGFR of less than 45 mL/minute/1.73 m^2. In addition, metformin must be avoided in patients who are prone to increased lactic acid production. Among these are patients with liver disease, severe infection, or a history of lactic acidosis; patients who consume alcohol to excess; and patients with shock and other conditions that can result in hypoxemia.

All patients taking metformin should be informed about early signs of lactic acidosis—hyperventilation, myalgia, malaise, and unusual somnolence—and instructed to report these to the prescriber. Metformin should be withdrawn until lactic acidosis has been ruled out. If lactic acidosis is diagnosed, hemodialysis can correct the condition and remove accumulated metformin.

Because heart failure (HF) can predispose to lactic acidosis, metformin is contraindicated for people with failing hearts. However, in one study, patients with HF who took the drug were *less* likely to die than those who took a sulfonylurea. These data suggest that use of metformin in HF is much safer than previously believed.

Drug Interactions

Alcohol. Like metformin, alcohol can inhibit breakdown of lactic acid and can thereby intensify lactic acidosis caused by metformin. To minimize risk, patients should avoid consuming alcohol in excess, whether acutely or long term. Discontinuing alcohol entirely would be even safer.

Cimetidine. Cimetidine [Tagamet], a histamine$_2$ (H_2) blocker used to reduce gastric acidity, can increase the risk of lactic acidosis. Accordingly, if an H_2 blocker is indicated, another member of this drug family should be used, since cimetidine is the only H_2 blocker that poses this risk.

Iodinated Radiocontrast Media. Intravenous radiocontrast media that contain iodine pose a risk of acute renal failure, which could exacerbate metformin-induced lactic acidosis. To reduce risk, patients should discontinue metformin a day or two before elective radiography. Metformin can then be resumed 48 hours after the procedure, provided lab tests show that renal function is normal.

Preparations, Dosage, and Administration

Metformin is available *alone* in immediate-release (IR) tablets (500, 850, and 1000 mg) as *Glucophage;* in extended-release (ER) tablets (500, 750, and 1000 mg) as *Glucophage XR, Fortamet,* and *Glumetza;* and in an oral solution (500 mg/5 mL) as *Riomet.* In addition, the drug is available in several fixed-dose *combinations* with other drugs for type 2 diabetes mellitus (see later).

With the IR tablets and oral solution, the recommended initial dosage is 500 mg twice daily (taken with the morning and evening meals) or 850 mg once daily, taken with a meal. The usual maintenance dosage is 850 mg twice daily. The maximum dosage is 850 mg 3 times a day (or 2550 mg/day for adults) or 2000 mg/day (for children 10 to 16 years old). There is no evidence that doses above 2000 mg/day are more efficacious.

With the ER tablets, dosing is done once daily with the evening meal. Why the evening meal? Because this timing may enhance absorption, owing to slower GI transit time at night. For previously untreated patients, the initial dosage is 500 mg a day (or 1000 mg once a day using Fortamet). For patients already taking metformin, the total daily dosage remains the same; it's simply taken all at once. The maximum daily dosage is 2000 mg (or 2500 mg using Fortamet).

Sulfonylureas

The sulfonylureas, introduced in the 1950s, were the first oral antihyperglycemic agents available. They work by promoting insulin release and hence are to be used only in type 2 diabetes. The sulfonylureas were a major advance in diabetes therapy: For the first time, some patients could be treated with an oral medication, rather than with daily injections of insulin. The major side effects with these drugs are hypoglycemia and weight gain.

The sulfonylureas fall into two groups: *first-generation (older) agents* and *second-generation (newer) agents.* Both generations reduce glucose levels to the same extent. How do the generations differ? The second-generation agents are *much more potent* than the first-generation agents, and hence dosages are much lower (as much as 1000 times lower in some cases). More importantly, with the second-generation agents *significant drug-drug interactions are less common,* and the outcomes tend to be milder. Because of these differences, the second-generation agents have nearly completely replaced the first-generation agents in clinical practice. Accordingly, our discussion in this chapter is limited to the second-generation agents.

Three second-generation sulfonylureas are currently available (Table 57.11). All have similar actions and side effects, and they all share the same application: treatment of type 2 diabetes.

TABLE 57.11 ▪ Sulfonylureas: Time Course and Dosage

Drug	Duration (hr)	Dosage[a]	Approximate Equivalent Dose (mg/24 hr)[b]
FIRST-GENERATION AGENTS[c]			
Tolbutamide [Orinase]	6–12	*Initial:* 1–2 gm/day in 1–3 doses *Maximum:* 2–3 gm/day in 1–3 doses	1000–1500
Tolazamide (generic only)	12–24	*Initial:* 100–250 mg/day with breakfast *Maximum:* 0.75–1 gm/day in 2 doses	250–375
Chlorpropamide (generic only)	24–60	*Initial:* 250 mg/day with breakfast *Maximum:* 750 mg once a day	250–375
SECOND-GENERATION AGENTS			
Glipizide			
Immediate release [Glucotrol]	10–24	*Initial:* 5 mg/day with breakfast *Maximum:* 40 mg/day in 2 doses	10
Sustained release [Glucotrol XL]	24	*Initial:* 5 mg/day with breakfast *Maximum:* 20 mg/day with breakfast	10
Glyburide			
Nonmicronized [DiaBeta]	16–24	*Initial:* 2.5–5 mg day with breakfast *Maximum:* 20 mg/day in 1 or 2 doses	5
Micronized [Glynase PresTab]	12–24	*Initial:* 1.5–3 mg/day with breakfast *Maximum:* 12 mg/day in 1 or 2 doses	3
Glimepiride [Amaryl]	24	*Initial:* 1–2 mg/day with breakfast *Maximum:* 8 mg/day with breakfast	2

[a]Older adults should use a smaller dose than those noted here.
[b]These values reflect differences in potency and can be used to estimate what dose to use when switching from one sulfonylurea to another.
[c]The first-generation agents are used only rarely.

Mechanism of Action

Sulfonylureas act primarily by stimulating the release of insulin from pancreatic islets. If the pancreas is incapable of insulin synthesis, sulfonylureas will be ineffective—which is why they don't work in patients with type 1 diabetes. With prolonged use, sulfonylureas may increase target cell sensitivity to insulin.

How do sulfonylureas promote insulin release? They bind with and thereby block ATP-sensitive potassium channels in the cell membrane. As a result, the membrane depolarizes, thereby permitting influx of calcium, which in turn causes insulin release.

Therapeutic Use

Sulfonylureas are indicated only for type 2 diabetes. These drugs are of no help to patients with type 1 diabetes. Like all other drugs for type 2 diabetes, the sulfonylureas should be used in conjunction with a lifestyle program inclusive of dietary and physical activity interventions. The sulfonylureas may be used alone or together with other antidiabetic drugs.

Adverse Effects

Hypoglycemia. Sulfonylureas cause a dose-dependent reduction in blood glucose and can thereby cause *hypoglycemia.* Importantly, regardless of what the glucose level is—high, normal, or low—sulfonylureas will make it go lower. If the level is high, reducing it will be therapeutic. However, if the level is normal, reducing it will cause mild hypoglycemia. And if the level is already low, reducing it can cause severe hypoglycemia.

Although sulfonylurea-induced hypoglycemia is usually mild, severe and even fatal cases have occurred. Hypoglycemia is sometimes persistent, requiring the infusion of dextrose for several days. Hypoglycemic reactions are more likely in patients with kidney or liver dysfunction because sulfonylureas are eliminated by hepatic metabolism and renal excretion and hence may accumulate to dangerous levels when liver or kidney function is impaired. If signs of hypoglycemia develop (fatigue, excessive hunger, profuse sweating, palpitations), the patient should treat the hypoglycemia and notify the prescriber.

Drug Interactions

Alcohol. When alcohol is combined with a sulfonylurea (especially a first-generation agent), a disulfiram-like reaction may occur. This syndrome includes flushing, palpitations, and nausea. Disulfiram reactions are discussed in Chapter 38. Also, alcohol can potentiate the hypoglycemic effects of sulfonylureas. Accordingly, patients using the drug must be warned about the risks of alcohol consumption in combination with a sulfonylurea.

Drugs That Can Intensify Hypoglycemia. A variety of drugs, acting by diverse mechanisms, can intensify hypoglycemic responses to most sulfonylureas. Included are *nonsteroidal anti-inflammatory drugs, sulfonamide antibiotics, alcohol* (used acutely in large amounts), and *cimetidine.* Caution must be exercised when a sulfonylurea is used in combination with these drugs.

Beta-Adrenergic Blocking Agents. Beta blockers can diminish the benefits of sulfonylureas by suppressing insulin release. (Recall that activation of beta receptors is one way to promote insulin release.) In addition, because beta blockers can mask sympathetic responses (primarily tachycardia) to declining blood glucose, the use of beta blockers can delay awareness of sulfonylurea-induced hypoglycemia.

Preparations, Dosage, and Administration

This information is shown in Table 57.11.

Meglitinides (Glinides)

Meglitinides—also known as *glinides*—are antidiabetic agents that have the same mechanism as the sulfonylureas: stimulation of pancreatic insulin release. The main difference between the glinides and the sulfonylureas is their pharmacokinetic profile—the glinides are more short acting and are taken with each meal. Only two glinides are available: repaglinide and nateglinide.

Repaglinide

Actions and Uses. Like the sulfonylureas, repaglinide [Prandin, GlucoNorm 🍁] blocks ATP-sensitive potassium channels on pancreatic beta cells and thereby facilitates calcium influx, which leads to increased insulin release. In clinical trials, repaglinide was about as effective as glyburide and glipizide (second-generation sulfonylureas). The drug is approved for type 2 diabetes only. Because repaglinide has the same mechanism as the sulfonylureas, patients who do not respond to sulfonylureas will not respond to this agent either.

Pharmacokinetics. Repaglinide undergoes rapid absorption followed by rapid elimination. Blood levels peak within 1 hour of oral dosing and return to baseline about 4 hours later. Elimination results from hepatic metabolism followed by biliary excretion. The drug's half-life is only 1 hour. Blood levels of insulin rise and fall in parallel with levels of repaglinide—and since levels of repaglinide rise and fall quickly, so do blood levels of insulin.

Adverse Effects. Repaglinide is generally well tolerated. The main significant adverse effect is *hypoglycemia.* In patients with liver dysfunction, metabolism of repaglinide may be slowed, and hence the risk of hypoglycemia may be increased. Because of possible hypoglycemia, it is imperative that patients eat no later than 30 minutes after taking the drug.

Drug Interactions. *Gemfibrozil* [Lopid], a drug used to lower triglyceride levels, can inhibit the metabolism of repaglinide, thereby causing its level to rise. Hypoglycemia can result. If possible, the combination should be avoided.

Preparations, Dosage, and Administration. Repaglinide [Prandin] is available in 0.5-, 1-, and 2-mg tablets. Administration must always be associated with a meal. For patients who have not used another oral antidiabetic drug, the initial dosage is 0.5 mg taken 0 to 30 minutes before each meal. Patients who *have* used another oral antidiabetic drug may take 1 or 2 mg before each meal. The maximum daily dose is 16 mg (4 mg with each meal for up to four meals).

Nateglinide

Basic Pharmacology and Therapeutic Use. The pharmacology of nateglinide [Starlix] is nearly identical to that of repaglinide. Both drugs have the same indication: treatment of type 2 diabetes, either as monotherapy or combined with metformin or a glitazone. They also have the same mechanism of action (promotion of insulin release), the same major adverse effect (hypoglycemia), and perhaps the same major drug interaction (elevation of their blood level by gemfibrozil). The two drugs differ primarily with respect to time course. Specifically, nateglinide has a slightly faster onset (30 minutes vs. 1 hour) and a significantly shorter duration (2 hours vs. 4 hours). Because the glinides and sulfonylureas have the same mechanism of action, nateglinide, like repaglinide, will not work in patients who have not responded to a sulfonylurea. Nateglinide undergoes extensive metabolism by cytochrome P450 enzymes, followed by rapid and complete excretion, primarily in the urine.

Preparations, Dosage, and Administration. Nateglinide [Starlix] is available in 60- and 120-mg tablets. The initial dosage is 120 mg 3 times a day taken 0 to 30 minutes before a meal. For patients with A1C concentrations close to the target value, the initial dosage is lower: 60 mg 3 times a day taken 0 to 30 minutes before a meal. Please note that dosing must always be associated with a meal. Otherwise, nateglinide-induced insulin release could cause hypoglycemia.

Thiazolidinediones (Glitazones)

The thiazolidinediones, also known as *glitazones* or simply *TZDs,* reduce glucose levels primarily by decreasing insulin resistance. These drugs are not related chemically or functionally to sulfonylureas or biguanides. Their only indication is type 2 diabetes, mainly as an add-on to metformin.

The glitazones have a bit of a troubled past. Troglitazone [Rezulin] was the first to receive FDA approval, followed by rosiglitazone [Avandia] and pioglitazone [Actos]. Soon after its approval, troglitazone was withdrawn, owing to a high incidence of severe liver damage that proved fatal in some patients. After that, rosiglitazone came under scrutiny: The drug was at one time thought to be associated with myocardial infarction and sudden cardiac death, and was for a period of time available only under a restricted access program; however, the FDA has since lifted the restrictions for use of rosiglitazone due to more recent evidence that did not show an increased risk for myocardial infarction when compared to other anti-hyperglycemic agents. Due to this previous restriction, however, pioglitazone is the agent most commonly utilized in this class. Accordingly, pioglitazone will be the focus of our discussion about these drugs.

Pioglitazone

Actions and Use. Pioglitazone [Actos] reduces insulin resistance and may also decrease glucose production. The underlying mechanism is activation of a specific receptor type in the cell nucleus, known as the *peroxisome proliferator-activated receptor gamma* (PPAR gamma). By activating PPAR gamma, pioglitazone turns on insulin-responsive genes that help regulate carbohydrate and lipid metabolism. As a result, cellular responses to insulin are increased, thereby promoting (mainly) increased glucose uptake by skeletal muscle and adipose cells, and (partly) decreased glucose production by the liver. Since pioglitazone enhances responses to insulin, insulin must be present for the drug to work.

Pioglitazone is approved as an adjunct to diet and exercise to improve glycemic control in adults with type 2 diabetes. The drug can be used as monotherapy, but is usually combined with metformin, a sulfonylurea, and/or supplemental insulin. Because insulin is required for pioglitazone to work, the drug is not effective in patients with type 1 diabetes.

Pharmacokinetics. Pioglitazone is well absorbed from the GI tract. Blood levels peak about 2 hours after dosing. Food slows absorption (blood levels peak 3 to 4 hours after dosing), but does not reduce the extent of absorption. Pioglitazone undergoes conversion to active and inactive metabolites, mainly by CYP2C8 (the 2C8 isoenzyme of cytochrome P450). Metabolites and parent drug are excreted in the feces (mainly) and urine. The half-lives of pioglitazone and its metabolites are 3 to 7 hours and 16 to 24 hours, respectively.

Adverse Effects. Pioglitazone is generally well tolerated. The most common reactions are upper respiratory tract infection, headache, sinusitis, and myalgia.

The greatest concern is *heart failure* secondary to renal *retention of fluid.* For most patients, fluid retention is not clinically significant. However, for patients with HF, especially severe or uncompensated HF, increased fluid retention can make HF worse. In these individuals, fluid retention is exacerbated when pioglitazone is used in combination with insulin therapy. Accordingly, pioglitazone should be used with caution in patients with *mild* HF and should be avoided by those with *severe* failure. Patients should be informed about signs of HF (dyspnea, edema, fatigue, rapid weight gain) and instructed to consult the prescriber immediately if these develop. If HF is diagnosed, pioglitazone should be discontinued or used in reduced dosage.

While TZDs have a low risk of *hypoglycemia* when used as monotherapy, the risk is increased when pioglitazone is combined with insulin or with drugs that inhibit pioglitazone metabolism. Use these combinations with caution.

Pioglitazone can cause *ovulation* in anovulatory premenopausal women, thereby posing a risk of unintended pregnancy. This effect has not been studied in clinical trials, and hence the incidence is unknown. Women should be informed about the potential for ovulation and educated about contraceptive options.

Postmarketing data indicate an increased risk of *bladder cancer,* associated mainly with long-term, high-dose pioglitazone therapy. Package labeling warns against using pioglitazone in patients with active bladder cancer or with a history of bladder cancer. Patients should be informed about signs of bladder cancer (e.g., blood in the urine, worsening urinary urgency, painful urination) and instructed to contact their prescriber if these develop.

Pioglitazone appears to increase the risk of *fractures* in women, but not in men. Most fractures have occurred in the foot, hand, or upper arm, not the spine. Risk appears greater with long-term, high-dose therapy. Fracture risk can be reduced through measures to maintain bone health. Among these are exercise, ensuring adequate intake of calcium and vitamin D, and, if indicated, the use of drugs for osteoporosis (see Chapter 75).

Pioglitazone is related to troglitazone (a highly hepatotoxic TZD), and hence there is concern that pioglitazone might be *hepatotoxic* too. However, although pioglitazone has been associated with rare cases of hepatic failure, a causal relationship has not been established. Nonetheless, serum alanine aminotransferase (ALT), a marker of liver function, should be measured at baseline and periodically thereafter (e.g., every 3 to 6 months). If ALT levels rise to more than 3 times the upper limit of normal or if jaundice develops, pioglitazone should be withdrawn. Patients should be informed about symptoms of liver injury (nausea, vomiting, abdominal pain, fatigue, anorexia, dark urine, jaundice) and instructed to notify the prescriber if these develop.

Pioglitazone has mixed effects on *plasma lipids.* One effect—elevation of LDL cholesterol—increases cardiovascular risk. Two other effects—elevation of HDL cholesterol and reduction of triglycerides—reduce cardiovascular risk. The net effect appears to be either (1) a reduction in cardiovascular risk or, at worst, (2) no increase in cardiovascular risk. The HF risk mentioned previously must not be overlooked, however.

Drug Interactions. Like pioglitazone, *insulin* promotes fluid retention, and hence the combination poses an increased risk of HF. Accordingly, using pioglitazone and insulin together should be done with caution.

Drugs that induce or inhibit CYP2C8 can alter pioglitazone levels and can thereby alter the glycemic response. Strong inhibitors of CYP2C8—such as gemfibrozil (a cholesterol-lowering agent)—can increase levels of pioglitazone and prolong its half-life, necessitating a reduction in pioglitazone dosage. Conversely, strong inducers of CYP2C8—such as rifampin (a drug for tuberculosis) and cimetidine (a gastric acid suppressant)—can reduce levels of pioglitazone and shorten its half-life, necessitating an increase in pioglitazone dosage.

Preparations, Dosage, and Administration. Pioglitazone [Actos] is available in 15-, 30-, and 45-mg tablets. The initial dosage for monotherapy is 15 or 30 mg once a day, taken with or without food. The maximum dosage is 45 mg once a day for patients not using insulin, but only 30 mg once a day for patients who are using insulin.

Rosiglitazone

Rosiglitazone [Avandia] is used only rarely today even though restrictions on its use have been lifted. Rosiglitazone shares many of the same clinical and safety considerations with pioglitazone.

Alpha-Glucosidase Inhibitors

The alpha-glucosidase inhibitors—acarbose and miglitol—act in the intestine to delay absorption of carbohydrates. These drugs are indicated for type 2 diabetes.

Acarbose

Mechanism of Action. Acarbose [Precose, Glucobay 🍁] delays absorption of dietary carbohydrates and thereby reduces the rise in blood glucose after a meal. To be absorbed, oligosaccharides and complex carbohydrates must be broken down to monosaccharides by alpha-glucosidase, an enzyme located on the brush border of cells that line the intestine. Acarbose inhibits this enzyme and thereby slows digestion of carbohydrates, which reduces the postprandial rise in blood glucose.

Therapeutic Use. Acarbose is indicated for patients with type 2 diabetes. The drug may be used alone or in combination with other antihyperglycemic agents. In clinical trials, 24 weeks of therapy with acarbose alone reduced mean peak postprandial glucose levels by 57 mg/dL, compared with 71 mg/dL for tolbutamide (a sulfonylurea) alone and 85 mg/dL for acarbose plus tolbutamide. In addition to lowering glucose levels after meals, acarbose lowers A1C levels, indicating an overall improvement in glycemic control.

Pharmacokinetics. Acarbose is administered by mouth, and only 2% is absorbed as active drug. As a result, systemic effects are minimal. Because acarbose acts locally in the intestine, lack of absorption is considered beneficial. In the gut, acarbose is converted to inactive products by bacteria and digestive enzymes.

Adverse Effects and Interactions. Acarbose frequently causes *flatulence, cramps, abdominal distention, borborygmus* (rumbling bowel sounds), and *diarrhea.* These responses result from bacterial fermentation of unabsorbed carbohydrates in the colon. Because of the common occurrence of these GI-related side effects, this class of medication is not often used in the United States. In addition to its GI effects, acarbose can decrease absorption of iron, thereby posing a risk of *anemia.*

Hypoglycemia does not occur with acarbose alone, but may develop when acarbose is combined with *insulin* or a *sulfonylurea.* When hypoglycemia develops, sucrose cannot be used for oral therapy because acarbose will impede its hydrolysis and thereby delay absorption. Accordingly, in patients taking acarbose, oral therapy of hypoglycemia must be accomplished with glucose itself.

Long-term, high-dose therapy may cause *liver dysfunction.* Asymptomatic elevation of plasma transaminases (which come from damaged liver cells) occurs in about 15% of patients. However, overt jaundice is rare. Liver function tests should be monitored every 3 months for the first year and periodically thereafter. Liver dysfunction reverses when acarbose is discontinued.

Preparations, Dosage, and Administration. Acarbose [Precose, Glucobay 🍁] is available in tablets (25, 50, and 100 mg) to be taken with the first bite of main meals. The recommended initial dosage is 25 mg 3 times a day. Depending on tolerability and postprandial blood glucose levels, the dosage may be increased at 4- to 8-week intervals. The maximum dosage is 50 mg 3 times a day (for patients under 60 kg) and 100 mg 3 times a day (for patients over 60 kg).

Miglitol

Miglitol [Glyset] is the second alpha-glucosidase inhibitor approved in the United States. Like acarbose, miglitol delays conversion of oligosaccharides and complex carbohydrates to glucose and other monosaccharides, and thereby reduces the postprandial rise in blood glucose. In clinical trials, the drug was especially effective among Latinos and African Americans. Hypoglycemia does not occur with miglitol monotherapy, but may occur if the drug is combined with insulin or a sulfonylurea. Like acarbose, miglitol causes flatulence, abdominal discomfort, and other GI effects. In contrast to acarbose, miglitol has not been associated with liver dysfunction. As with acarbose therapy, oral sucrose cannot be used to treat hypoglycemia. Rather, oral glucose must be given. Miglitol is available in 25-, 50-, and 100-mg tablets. The initial dosage is 25 mg 3 times daily before meals. The maintenance dosage is 50 or 100 mg 3 times a day.

Dipeptidyl Peptidase-4 (DPP-4) Inhibitors (Gliptins)

DPP-4 inhibitors promote glycemic control by enhancing the actions of incretin hormones. Reductions in A1C are modest. Hypoglycemia is uncommon when these drugs are used alone. Pancreatitis and severe hypersensitivity reactions occur rarely.

The ADA considers the DPP-4 inhibitors to be an optional second-line therapy as an add-on to metformin in the treatment of type 2 diabetes. When added to the regimen, the resulting decrease in A1C is about 0.5%. However, for some patients, even this small improvement can be clinically meaningful.

Sitagliptin

Mechanism of Action. Sitagliptin [Januvia] enhances the actions of *incretin hormones,* endogenous compounds that (1) stimulate glucose-dependent release of insulin and (2) suppress postprandial release of glucagon (a hormone that increases glucose production by the liver). Both actions help keep blood glucose from climbing too high. How does sitagliptin boost incretin actions? It inhibits DPP-4, an enzyme that inactivates the incretin hormones. As discussed later in this chapter, another class of drugs—GLP-1 receptor agonists—also boosts incretin actions, but by a different mechanism: Rather than preventing incretin breakdown, they mimic incretin actions.

Therapeutic Use. Sitagliptin is indicated for type 2 diabetes, either as monotherapy or combined with another antidiabetic drug. Like all the other agents for managing diabetes, sitagliptin should be used as an adjunct to diet and exercise.

Pharmacokinetics. Sitagliptin undergoes rapid and nearly complete absorption, both in the presence and absence of food. Blood levels peak about 1 to 4 hours after dosing. Most of the drug is excreted unchanged in the urine. The elimination half-life is about 12 hours.

Adverse Effects and Interactions. Sitagliptin is generally well tolerated. In clinical trials, the most common side effects were upper respiratory tract infection, headache, and inflammation of the nasal passages and throat—at rates similar to those seen with placebo. The incidence of hypoglycemia was about 1.2%, compared with 0.9% with placebo—again a nonsignificant difference.

Rarely, patients have developed *pancreatitis,* including fatal hemorrhagic or necrotizing pancreatitis, according to postmarketing reports. Patients should be informed about signs and symptoms of pancreatitis (e.g., severe and persistent abdominal pain, with or without vomiting) and instructed to stop sitagliptin immediately should they occur. If pancreatitis is confirmed, sitagliptin should not be resumed. We don't know whether patients with a history of pancreatitis are at increased risk, although the FDA recommends cautious use of these agents in such patients.

There have been postmarketing reports of serious *hypersensitivity reactions,* including anaphylaxis, angioedema, and Stevens-Johnson syndrome. However, a causal relationship has not been established. Nonetheless, if a hypersensitivity reaction is suspected, sitagliptin should be discontinued.

Sitagliptin has few drug-drug interactions, which is one benefit of this class of medications.

Preparations, Dosage, and Administration. Sitagliptin [Januvia] is supplied in film-coated tablets (25, 50, and 100 mg). The usual dosage is 100 mg once daily, taken with or without food. Because sitagliptin is eliminated primarily by renal excretion, dosages should be reduced in patients with renal impairment, as indicated by reduced creatinine clearance. Dosage should be reduced to 50 mg once daily (in moderate renal disease) and 25 mg once daily (in severe renal disease).

Saxagliptin

Actions and Therapeutic Use. Like sitagliptin, saxagliptin [Onglyza] is a DPP-4 inhibitor indicated as an adjunct to diet and exercise to improve glycemic control in adults with type 2 diabetes. Saxagliptin may be used as monotherapy or combined with other antidiabetic agents.

Pharmacokinetics. Saxagliptin is well absorbed, both in the presence and absence of food. Plasma levels peak about 2 hours after dosing. Saxagliptin undergoes conversion to an active metabolite by CYP3A4/5 (the 3A4/5 isoenzyme of cytochrome P450). Parent drug and metabolite are excreted in the urine (75%) and feces (22%). To avoid toxicity, dosage must be reduced in patients taking strong CYP3A4/5 inhibitors (e.g., clarithromycin, ketoconazole, nefazodone, nelfinavir, ritonavir) and in those with significant renal impairment.

Adverse Effects. In clinical trials, the most common adverse effects were upper respiratory infection, urinary tract infection, and headache. Saxagliptin can intensify hypoglycemia caused by a sulfonylurea, but causes little or no hypoglycemia when used alone. Like sitagliptin, saxagliptin has been associated with rare cases of pancreatitis and severe hypersensitivity reactions. If symptoms of either develop, saxagliptin should be withdrawn. The prescribing information for saxagliptin also recommends that the agent be used with caution in patients with a history of or increased risk for heart failure. This recommendation is in place because patients taking saxagliptin were found to have a small increase in risk of hospitalization for heart failure in a large cardiovascular outcomes study performed with saxagliptin. The FDA recommends that patients be observed for signs and symptoms of heart failure and that the drug be discontinued should they occur.

Preparations, Dosage, and Administration. Saxagliptin [Onglyza] is supplied in 2.5- and 5-mg tablets for dosing once daily without regard to meals. The usual daily dosage is 5 mg. In patients with mild to moderate renal impairment and in those taking a strong inhibitor of CYP3A4/5, dosage should be reduced to 2.5 mg/day.

Linagliptin

Actions and Therapeutic Use. Linagliptin [Tradjenta] is indicated as an adjunct to diet and exercise to improve glycemic control in adults with type 2 diabetes. As with other gliptins, benefits, which are modest, derive from preserving incretins through inhibition of DPP-4.

Pharmacokinetics. About 30% of each dose is absorbed, both in the presence and absence of food. Plasma levels peak 1.5 hours after dosing. Linagliptin undergoes minimal metabolism. Most of the drug (90%) is excreted unchanged—80% in the feces and 5% in the urine. The effective half-life is 12 hours.

Adverse Effects. Linagliptin is generally well tolerated. The drug has caused hypoglycemia when combined with metformin plus a sulfonylurea, but not when used alone or when combined with just metformin or pioglitazone. Like sitagliptin and saxagliptin, linagliptin has been associated with rare cases of pancreatitis and hypersensitivity reactions. If either of these develop, linagliptin should be withdrawn.

Drug Interactions. Linagliptin is a substrate for P-glycoprotein, a transporter that promotes excretion of linagliptin and other drugs. In theory, drugs that induce P-glycoprotein could reduce levels of linagliptin. Accordingly, the manufacturer recommends that linagliptin not be used with rifampin and other P-glycoprotein inducers.

Preparations, Dosage, and Administration. Linagliptin [Tradjenta] is supplied as 5-mg tablets. The dosage is 5 mg once a day, taken without regard to meals. Unlike dosing with saxagliptin or sitagliptin, dosage needn't be reduced in patients with renal impairment.

Alogliptin

Actions and Therapeutic Use. Alogliptin [Nesina] is another DPP-4 inhibitor indicated to improve glycemic control in adults with type 2 diabetes. As with other DPP-4 inhibitors, alogliptin improves glycemic control by allowing natural incretin hormones to carry out their glucoregulatory functions for a longer period of time.

Pharmacokinetics. The absolute bioavailability of alogliptin is approximately 100% when administered orally. Alogliptin does not undergo extensive metabolism, with the majority of an oral dose excreted unchanged in the urine. Accordingly, this drug is dose-adjusted when used in people with renal impairment. Alogliptin has a terminal half-life of about 20 hours and thus can be administered once daily.

Adverse Effects. As with other DPP-4 inhibitors, alogliptin is generally well tolerated. The most common side effects reported in clinical trials included upper respiratory tract infection and nasopharyngitis. Again, like other agents in this class, hypersensitivity reactions and postmarketing reports of pancreatitis have been noted. Similar to saxagliptin, the label for alogliptin includes a warning related to a potential increased risk of heart failure. Again, similar to saxagliptin, there was a small increase in the number of patients requiring hospitalization for heart failure.

Drug Interactions. Alogliptin is primarily excreted renally, yet no significant drug-drug interactions have been noted with other drugs excreted through the kidneys.

Preparations, Dosage, and Administration. Alogliptin [Nesina] is supplied as 6.25-, 12.5-, and 25-mg tablets. The dosage is 25 mg once daily. Alogliptin is dose-adjusted based on kidney function. Accordingly, the recommended dose is 12.5 mg daily for people with moderate renal impairment and 6.25 mg daily for those with significant renal impairment.

Sodium-Glucose Co-Transporter 2 (SGLT-2) Inhibitors

The kidney plays a major role in glucose homeostasis due to its role in the filtration and reabsorption of glucose in the renal tubules. The transport of glucose from the tubule into the tubular epithelial cells is accomplished by sodium-glucose co-transporters (SGLTs). SGLT-2 is a high-capacity, low-affinity transporter expressed chiefly in the kidney that accounts for approximately 90% of glucose reabsorption in the kidney. SGLT-2 inhibitors have been shown to block the reabsorption of filtered glucose, leading to glucosuria. This mechanism of action has proven clinically useful in patients with type 2 diabetes in terms of improving glycemic control. In addition, the glucosuria associated with SGLT-2 inhibition is associated with caloric loss, thus providing a potential benefit of weight loss. While currently approved agents hold an indication for the management of type 2 diabetes only, these agents are being studied and used off-label in people with type 1 diabetes.

Canagliflozin

Actions and Therapeutic Use. Canagliflozin [Invokana] was the first SGLT-2 inhibitor approved in the United States. By inhibiting SGLT-2 in the kidney, canagliflozin reduces the reabsorption of glucose, thereby increasing urinary glucose excretion. Clinical studies of canagliflozin have shown benefits in terms of improved glycemic control and weight loss. In addition, canagliflozin has been shown to improve cardiovascular and renal outcomes in patients with a history of cardiovascular disease.

Pharmacokinetics. The half-life of canagliflozin is approximately 12 hours when taken orally; thus it can be administered once daily. Peak plasma concentrations are reached within 1 to 2 hours after a given dose.

Adverse Effects. The most common side effects noted with canagliflozin in clinical trials were female genital fungal infections, urinary tract infections, and increased urination. Because SGLT-2 inhibitors increase the amount of sugar present in the urine, the increased risk of such infections is not much of a surprise. In addition, particularly in older adults, use of canagliflozin can lead to postural hypotension and dizziness, particularly if used in combination with diuretics. More serious and rare events have been reported with canagliflozin use, including euglycemic diabetic ketoacidosis (DKA), urosepsis, pyelonephritis, and increased risk of amputation.

Drug Interactions. Coadministration of canagliflozin with UDP-glucuronosyltransferase inducers—such as rifampin, phenytoin, or phenobarbital—can decrease canagliflozin efficacy. Accordingly, if used with such an agent, the 300-mg canagliflozin dose should be considered. Because canagliflozin causes a diuretic effect, the risk of dehydration and hypotension may be increased when used in combination with thiazide and loop diuretics.

Preparations, Dosage, and Administration. Canagliflozin [Invokana] is available as 100- and 300-mg tablets. Canagliflozin is recommended at a starting dose of 100 mg daily taken before the first meal of the day. The dose can be increased to 300 mg once daily, requiring additional glycemic control and an estimated glomerular filtration rate [GFR] of 60 mL/min/1.73 m^2 or greater. The once-daily dose of 100 mg is recommended for individuals with a GFR of less than 60 mL/min/1.73 m^2. Because SGLT-2 inhibitors don't work as well in people with significantly compromised kidney function, canagliflozin is not recommended for people with an estimated GFR below 30 mL/min/1.73 m^2.

Dapagliflozin

Actions and Therapeutic Use. Dapagliflozin [Farxiga] was the second SGLT-2 inhibitor approved in the United States. By inhibiting SGLT-2, dapagliflozin suppresses glucose reuptake from tubular urine and thereby increases urinary glucose excretion. As a result, blood levels of glucose decline and weight loss can be seen.

Pharmacokinetics. The half-life of dapagliflozin following oral administration is approximately 13 hours; thus it can be taken once daily.

Adverse Effects. The most common side effects noted with dapagliflozin in clinical studies were vulvovaginitis and other genital infections, back pain, polyuria, and an increased hematocrit. Orthostasis (particularly if used with diuretics) is possible.

Drug Interactions. Because dapagliflozin induces a diuretic effect in the kidney, the risk of dehydration and hypotension may be increased when used in combination with thiazide and loop diuretics. When used with other antidiabetic agents, patients should also monitor carefully to avoid the possibility of hypoglycemia.

Preparations, Dosage, and Administration. Dapagliflozin [Farxiga] is available as 5- and 10-mg tablets. Dapagliflozin is dosed initially as 5 mg once daily in the morning with or without food. The dose can be subsequently increased to 10 mg once daily, if needed, to achieve desired glycemic control. Because SGLT-2 inhibitors do not work as well in people with diminished kidney function, dapagliflozin is not recommended for use in people with an estimated GFR consistently less than 60 mL/min/1.73 m^2.

Empagliflozin

Actions and Therapeutic Use. Empagliflozin [Jardiance] was the third SGLT-2 inhibitor approved by the FDA. Similar to other medications in this class, empagliflozin increases urinary glucose excretion to decrease glucose levels and weight via caloric loss through the urine. A large cardiovascular outcomes trial performed with empagliflozin showed that this medication can help prevent cardiovascular events in patients with diabetes and established cardiovascular disease.

Pharmacokinetics. The apparent terminal half-life of empagliflozin is approximately 12 hours, allowing for once-daily oral administration.

Adverse Effects. The most common adverse reactions associated with the use of empagliflozin in clinical trials were urinary tract infections and female genital mycotic infections. Similar to other agents in the SGLT-2 inhibitor class, patients taking empagliflozin may be at increased risk for hypotension, more severe urinary tract infections (urosepsis and pyelonephritis), and euglycemic DKA. Patients taking empagliflozin and other agents in this class should be monitored and counseled regarding these potential rare adverse effects.

Drug Interactions. Similar to other SGLT-2 inhibitors, there is an added risk for hypotension and dehydration when used in combination with diuretic medications. When used in combination with insulin and insulin secretagogue medications, there is also an increased risk for hypoglycemic events.

Preparations, Dosage, and Administration. Empagliflozin [Jardiance] is available as 10- and 25-mg tablets. Empagliflozin is dosed initially as 10 mg taken once daily in the morning with or without food. The dose can be increased to 25 mg once daily in patients who require additional glycemic control. Like other medications in this class, empagliflozin is dosed based on renal function. For patients with an eGFR less than 45 mL/min/1.73 m^2, it is recommended that empagliflozin not be initiated. If patients taking empagliflozin experience a drop in their GFR to a level consistently below 45 mL/min/1.73 m^2, it is recommended that the medication be discontinued.

Colesevelam

Colesevelam [Welchol] is best known as a bile-acid sequestrant used to lower plasma cholesterol. However, the drug can also help lower blood glucose. Accordingly, in 2008, the FDA approved colesevelam to treat type 2 diabetes. Since many patients with diabetes also have high cholesterol, a drug with the potential to treat both disorders is welcome. The pharmacology of colesevelam is discussed in Chapter 50.

Bromocriptine

Bromocriptine, marketed as *Cycloset,* is approved as an adjunct to diet and exercise to treat type 2 diabetes. The same drug, marketed as *Parlodel,* has been available for years to treat Parkinson disease (see Chapter 21) and hyperprolactinemia (see Chapter 63). Unfortunately, benefits in diabetes are modest: The typical reduction in A1C is only 0.5%.

How does bromocriptine improve glycemic control? The mechanism is unclear. We do know that bromocriptine is a dopamine agonist that can activate dopamine receptors in the brain. By activating these receptors in the hypothalamus, the drug may reverse an abnormal hypothalamic drive that raises plasma levels of glucose, triglycerides, and free fatty acids in insulin-resistant patients.

We also know that, by activating these receptors, bromocriptine can reset circadian rhythms in people with type 2 diabetes. This action, in turn, may reverse some of the metabolic changes associated with insulin resistance.

Principal adverse effects are nausea, drowsiness, and orthostatic hypotension, which can cause dizziness and fainting. Bromocriptine can also exacerbate psychoses. Of note, the drug appears devoid of cardiovascular toxicity.

For treatment of diabetes, bromocriptine [Cycloset] is available in 0.8-mg tablets, which should be taken with food to decrease GI side effects. Dosing is done once daily, within 2 hours of waking in the morning. The daily dosage is 0.8 mg initially, and then increased by 0.8 mg each week until the maximal dose is reached (4.8 mg) or until side effects become intolerable. While approved, this medication is used very rarely for the treatment of type 2 diabetes.

Oral Combination Products

As noted previously, many patients with type 2 diabetes must take several medications with complementary mechanisms of action to meet glycemic goals. Accordingly, to help minimize the number of pills that patients must take on a daily basis, several oral combination products are commercially available. Since metformin is the recommended first-line agent in combination with lifestyle interventions, most combination products contain metformin with a second antidiabetic agent. Table 57.12 shows combination products available in the United States. Keep in mind, however, that combination products have drawbacks. First, they are often more expensive than taking the components separately. Second, they limit dosing flexibility.

NON-INSULIN INJECTABLE AGENTS

In addition to insulin, we now have two additional classes of injectable agents available for the treatment of diabetes. In the amylin mimetic class, pramlintide—the only amylin mimetic currently on the market—is indicated for type 1 *and* type 2 diabetes patients who are also using mealtime insulin. The other class of drugs—GLP-1 receptor agonists (or incretin mimetics)—is indicated for type 2 diabetes only, yet these drugs are increasingly being used off-label for people with type 1 diabetes. Because all of these agents are injectable, they are often mistaken for insulin products, but they work very differently from insulin.

Glucagon-like Peptide-1 (GLP-1) Receptor Agonists

GLP-1 receptor agonists, often referred to as *incretin mimetics,* work by augmenting the effects of the incretin hormone GLP-1. Under physiologic conditions, GLP-1 and other incretins are released from cells of the GI tract after a meal. Incretin mimetics

TABLE 57.12 ■ Combination Oral Agents for the Treatment of Type 2 Diabetes

Brand Name	Generic Name
Metaglip	Glipizide-metformin
Glucovance	Glyburide-metformin
Jentadueto	Linagliptin-metformin
Kombiglyze XR	Saxagliptin-metformin
Janumet, Janumet XR	Sitagliptin-metformin
Kazano	Alogliptin-metformin
Oseni	Alogliptin-pioglitazone
Duetact	Pioglitazone-glimepiride
ActoPlus Met, ActoPlus Met XR	Pioglitazone-metformin
Avandamet	Rosiglitazone-metformin
Avandaryl	Rosiglitazone-glimepiride
PrandiMet	Repaglinide-metformin
Synjardy, Synjardy XR	Empagliflozin-metformin
Glyxambi	Empagliflozin-linagliptin
Invokamet, Invokamet XR	Canagliflozin-metformin
Xigduo XR	Dapagliflozin-metformin
Qtern	Dapagliflozin-saxagliptin

activate receptors for GLP-1 and thereby cause the same effects as endogenous incretins. That is, they slow gastric emptying, stimulate glucose-dependent release of insulin, inhibit postprandial release of glucagon, and suppress appetite. Due to augmentation of these effects, incretin mimetics are effective in improving glucose control and can induce weight loss. You will recall that DPP-4 inhibitors "boost" the effects of incretin hormones by slowing their degradation by the enzyme DPP-4. GLP-1 receptor agonists, in contrast, are structurally related to the native GLP-1 hormone but are resistant to metabolism by DPP-4. There are currently four GLP-1 receptor agonist products approved in the United States, with multiple other agents currently in development.

Exenatide

Exenatide [Byetta] was the first *incretin mimetic.* The drug is used to improve glucose control in patients with type 2 diabetes. A longer-acting formulation of exenatide known as Exenatide Once Weekly [Bydureon] is also currently available and is dosed once weekly (compared to twice daily with Byetta). Nausea is common, and hypoglycemia can occur, particularly if used in combination with a sulfonylurea.

Description and Actions. Exenatide is a synthetic analog of GLP-1, a peptide hormone in the *incretin* family. Exenatide activates receptors for GLP-1 and thereby causes the same effects as endogenous incretins. That is, it slows gastric emptying, stimulates glucose-dependent release of insulin, inhibits postprandial release of glucagon, and suppresses appetite.

Therapeutic Use. Exenatide is indicated to improve glycemic control in patients with type 2 diabetes. In clinical trials, injecting exenatide [Byetta] 5 or 10 mcg subQ twice daily before the two largest meals of the day produced a modest decrease in fasting blood glucose and a large decrease in postprandial blood glucose. Patients did not gain any weight, and many lost weight. In contrast, injecting exenatide extended-release for injectable suspension [Bydureon] 2 mg subQ once weekly has a greater effect on fasting glucose as opposed to postprandial blood glucose. These differences are related to the varying pharmacokinetic profiles of these two products.

Pharmacokinetics. For exenatide [Byetta], plasma levels peak 2.1 hours after subQ injection and decline with a half-life of 2.4 hours. Exenatide ER suspension [Bydureon], in contrast, is released slowly from microspheres over approximately 10 weeks, with a peak level of drug reached at around 2 weeks after administration. Exenatide is excreted unchanged in the urine. In patients with mild to moderate renal impairment, clearance is reduced only slightly, and hence no dosage reduction is needed. By contrast, in patients with end-stage renal disease, clearance is reduced significantly, and hence the drug should not be used.

Adverse Effects. Dose-related *hypoglycemia* is common when exenatide is combined with a sulfonylurea (but not when combined with metformin). To minimize hypoglycemia, sulfonylurea dosage may need a reduction. *Gastrointestinal effects*—nausea, vomiting, and diarrhea—are common with exenatide [Byetta]. Exenatide ER suspension [Bydureon] is better tolerated in terms of nausea and vomiting, but can result in injection-site irritation and pruritus. In some patients, *anti-exenatide antibodies* develop. These antibodies do not cause adverse effects, but they can reduce exenatide's effects.

Exenatide poses a risk of *pancreatitis.* Severe cases have led to pancreatic necrosis, pancreatic hemorrhage, and even death. Patients should be informed about signs and symptoms of pancreatitis—typically severe and persistent abdominal pain, with or without vomiting—and instructed to stop exenatide immediately if symptoms arise. If pancreatitis is confirmed, exenatide should not be resumed. Patients with a history of pancreatitis should probably not use this drug.

Exenatide can cause *renal impairment,* sometimes requiring hemodialysis or a kidney transplant. Fortunately, the incidence is low—about 1 case for every 13,000 patients. Risk of renal impairment may be increased by nausea, vomiting, or diarrhea, or any other event that can cause dehydration. Exenatide should be avoided in patients with severe renal impairment and should be used with caution in kidney transplant recipients.

In pregnant animals, doses of exenatide only 3 times the human dose caused *fetal harm,* manifesting as reduced growth and skeletal abnormalities. At this time, the drug is classified in FDA Pregnancy Risk Category C,[b] and hence should be used only if the benefits are believed to outweigh the fetal risk. Furthermore, given the established safety and efficacy of insulin in pregnancy, there seems to be little reason to even try exenatide.

There have been postmarketing reports of serious *hypersensitivity reactions,* including anaphylaxis and angioedema. If severe reaction occurs, patients should stop taking exenatide and seek immediate medical attention.

Drug Interactions. Exenatide delays gastric emptying and hence can slow the absorption of oral drugs, thereby decreasing peak plasma levels and prolonging the time to peak serum

[b]As of 2020, the FDA will no longer use Pregnancy Risk Categories. Please refer to Chapter 9 for more information.

levels. Reduced absorption is of particular concern with oral contraceptives and antibiotics, which require high peak concentrations to be maximally effective. To minimize this interaction, give oral drugs at least 1 hour before exenatide.

Preparations, Dosage, and Administration. Exenatide [Byetta] is supplied in pre-filled, 60-dose injector pens that deliver 5 or 10 mcg per dose. Injections are made subQ into the thigh, abdomen, or upper arm. The initial dosage is 5 mcg twice daily, administered 0 to 60 minutes before the morning and evening meals—never after the meal. After 1 month, the dosage may be increased to 10 mcg twice daily. If the patient is taking a sulfonylurea, its dosage may need a reduction (to avoid hypoglycemia). If the patient is taking metformin, no dosage reduction is needed. Because of greatly reduced clearance, exenatide should not be used by patients with severe renal impairment. Exenatide ER suspension [Bydureon] is supplied as 2-mg ER powder in single-dose vials or pens for suspension in diluent for injection. Injections are made subQ in the thigh, abdomen, or upper arm.

Liraglutide

Actions and Uses. Liraglutide [Victoza] is an *incretin mimetic* similar to exenatide. The drug is indicated as an adjunct to diet and exercise to improve glycemic control in adults with type 2 diabetes. Like exenatide, liraglutide is an analog of human GLP-1 that causes direct activation of GLP-1 receptors and thereby slows gastric emptying, stimulates glucose-dependent insulin release, and inhibits postprandial release of glucagon. Liraglutide is more convenient that exenatide (dosing is done just once a day without regard to meals, rather than twice a day before meals).

Liraglutide can be used alone or combined with other antidiabetic drugs. Most often, the drug is combined with metformin, a sulfonylurea, or another agent. Because sulfonylureas actively drive down blood glucose levels, adding liraglutide to a sulfonylurea regimen increases the risk of hypoglycemia. Reducing the sulfonylurea dosage at the start of liraglutide treatment seems to lower the risk.

Liraglutide has been shown to be effective as an add-on to rosiglitazone, a drug that is all but gone from use. Although liraglutide has not been studied as an add-on to pioglitazone (the only other glitazone still on the market), it seems likely that liraglutide would be effective with pioglitazone too.

Pharmacokinetics. Pharmacokinetics of liraglutide are unremarkable. Plasma levels peak 8 to 13 hours after subQ dosing. The drug undergoes metabolic breakdown followed by excretion in the urine and feces. The plasma half-life is 13 hours—long enough to permit once-daily dosing.

Adverse Effects. Dose-related *GI effects* are common, developing in 41% of patients. Specific effects include nausea, diarrhea, and constipation. *Hypoglycemia* can also occur, especially when liraglutide is combined with a sulfonylurea (but not with metformin).

In clinical trials, 8.6% of patients developed *anti-liraglutide antibodies.* This is surprising, given that liraglutide is nearly identical to human GLP-1, and hence should not be antigenic. In theory, these antibodies could neutralize liraglutide. However, to date, there is no evidence this has happened.

Like exenatide, liraglutide has been associated with rare cases of *pancreatitis.* If pancreatitis is suspected, liraglutide should be discontinued immediately. If pancreatitis is confirmed, the drug should never be used again. However, if pancreatitis is ruled out, use of liraglutide can resume.

Like exenatide, liraglutide has been associated with rare cases of *renal impairment,* including new acute renal failure and worsening of chronic renal failure. Most cases occurred in patients who had experienced nausea, vomiting, diarrhea, or any other event that can cause dehydration. Renal impairment may reverse with supportive treatment and discontinuation of liraglutide and any other potentially causative agents.

There is concern that liraglutide may cause thyroid C-cell tumors, including *medullary thyroid carcinoma* (MTC). In tests on rodents, clinically relevant doses have caused C-cell tumors. However, there is no proof that liraglutide has caused these tumors in humans. Nonetheless, the package label bears a black box warning about possible thyroid cancer, including a contraindication against using the drug in patients with a family history of MTC or in those with multiple endocrine neoplasia syndrome type 2.

Drug Interactions. As noted, combined use with a *sulfonylurea* can increase the risk of hypoglycemia. Dosage of the sulfonylurea may need a reduction.

Because liraglutide delays gastric emptying, it might delay the absorption of some oral drugs, thereby reducing their peak serum levels and prolonging the time to peak serum levels.

Preparations, Dosage, and Administration. Liraglutide [Victoza] is supplied in pre-filled multidose injector pens that deliver 0.6, 1.2, or 1.8 mg/dose. Administration is by subQ injection into the abdomen, thigh, or upper arm. Dosing is done once a day, at any time and independent of meals. The initial dosage is low—0.6 mg once a day—to minimize GI side effects. After 1 week, dosage is increased to 1.2 mg once a day. If that dosage proves inadequate, it can be increased to 1.8 mg once a day.

Lixisenatide

Actions and Therapeutic Use. Lixisenatide [Adlyxin] is another short-acting *incretin mimetic* indicated for the treatment of type 2 diabetes mellitus in combination with diet and exercise. Being a shorter-acting agent, lixisenatide is recommended to be administered once daily via subcutaneous injection. The safety and tolerability profile of lixisenatide is very similar to other agents in this therapeutic class.

Preparations, Dosage, and Administration. Lixisenatide [Adlyxin] is commercially available in a pre-filled pen device. The starting dose of lixisenatide is 10 mcg injected once daily within 1 hour before the morning meal. The 10-mcg dose is administered for 14 days. On day 15 of treatment, the dose is recommended to be increased to 20 mcg daily.

Albiglutide

Actions and Therapeutic Use. Albiglutide [Tanzeum] is an *incretin mimetic* indicated as an adjunct to diet and exercise to enhance glycemic control in adults with type 2 diabetes. Like exenatide ER suspension, albiglutide is administered once weekly via subcutaneous injection. The safety and tolerability profile of albiglutide is likewise similar to that of exenatide ER suspension.

Preparations, Dosage, and Administration. Albiglutide [Tanzeum] is supplied as single-dose pens for administration of 30- and 50-mg doses. Albiglutide is recommended to be initiated at 30 mg once weekly. The dose can be increased to 50 mg once weekly in patients requiring additional glycemic control.

Dulaglutide

Actions and Therapeutic Use. Dulaglutide [Trulicity] is a long-acting *incretin mimetic* indicated for the treatment of type 2 diabetes in combination with diet and exercise. It is administered once weekly. As a member of the incretin mimetic class of medications, dulaglutide has an efficacy and safety profile similar to that of other once-weekly products in this drug class.

Preparations, Dosage, and Administration. Dulaglutide [Trulicity] is available in 0.75- and 1.5-mg pre-filled pens for injection. Dulaglutide differs from other once-weekly products, such as exenatide ER and albiglutide, in that it is formulated in solution. This is a potential advantage because the other currently available once-weekly products require reconstitution and preparation before administration. The recommended starting dose of dulaglutide is 0.75 mg subcutaneously once weekly. The dose can be administered at any time of day without regard to meals. Depending on clinical response and if needed for additional glycemic control, the dose may be increased to 1.5 mg weekly.

Amylin Mimetic: Pramlintide

Pramlintide [Symlin] is an *amylin mimetic.* The drug is used to complement the effects of mealtime insulin in patients with type 1 or type 2 diabetes. Severe hypoglycemia is a concern, and nausea is common.

Description and Actions

Pramlintide is a synthetic analog of *amylin,* a peptide hormone made in the pancreas and co-released with insulin. Both amylin and pramlintide, which mimics the effects of amylin, reduce postprandial levels of glucose, mainly by delaying gastric emptying and suppressing glucagon secretion. In addition, both agents act in the brain to increase the sense of satiety, helping to lower caloric intake.

Therapeutic Use

Pramlintide is indicated as a supplement to mealtime insulin in patients with type 1 or type 2 diabetes who have failed to achieve glucose control despite optimal insulin therapy. In clinical trials, adding subQ pramlintide to mealtime insulin decreased postprandial glucose levels, smoothed out glucose fluctuations, and reduced the needed mealtime dose of insulin. Mean reductions in A1C were about 0.39% for those with type 1 diabetes and 0.55% for those with type 2 diabetes.

Pharmacokinetics

Blood levels peak about 20 minutes after subQ injection and decline with a half-life of 49 minutes. Unlike most drugs, pramlintide is metabolized in the kidneys rather than in the liver. One active metabolite has been identified.

Adverse Effects

Hypoglycemia is the biggest concern. Pramlintide does not cause hypoglycemia when used alone, but poses a risk of severe hypoglycemia when combined with insulin, especially in patients with type 1 diabetes. Because pramlintide is specifically indicated for use in combination with mealtime insulin, the risk of hypoglycemia is inherent to its use. As a rule, hypoglycemia develops within 3 hours of dosing. To reduce risk, insulin dosage must be decreased, at least initially. Also, pramlintide should not be given to patients who have hypoglycemia unawareness, a history of poor adherence to their insulin regimen, poor adherence to SMBG, or recurrent hypoglycemia needing assistance.

Nausea occurs early in therapy and is more common in patients with type 1 diabetes (37% to 48%) than type 2 diabetes (28% to 30%). The incidence and severity of nausea can be reduced by gradual titration of dosage.

Injection-site reactions—redness, swelling, or itching—may occur, but generally resolve within a few days to weeks.

Drug Interactions

By delaying gastric emptying, pramlintide can delay the absorption of oral drugs. Accordingly, oral drugs should be taken 1 hour before injecting pramlintide or 2 hours after. Pramlintide should not be combined with other drugs that slow intestinal motility (e.g., antimuscarinic agents, opioid analgesics) or with drugs that slow the absorption of nutrients (e.g., acarbose, miglitol).

Preparations, Dosage, and Administration

Pramlintide [Symlin] is supplied as pre-filled *SymlinPens,* which should be stored under refrigeration, but not frozen. Pens currently in use, which can be kept cool or at room temperature, should be discarded after 28 days.

Dosing is done before major meals that contain at least 250 kcal or 30 gm of carbohydrates. Injections are made subQ into the abdomen or thigh.

In patients with *type 1 diabetes,* the initial dosage is 15 mcg before meals. If there is no serious nausea for 3 days, dosage can be increased in 15-mcg steps to a maximum of 60 mcg. If 30 mcg causes too much nausea, discontinuation should be considered.

In patients with *type 2 diabetes,* the initial dosage is 60 mcg before meals. If there is no serious nausea for 3 to 7 days, dosage may be increased to 120 mcg.

In patients with *type 1* or *type 2 diabetes,* the premeal dose of rapid- or short-acting insulin should be decreased by 50% (to reduce the risk of hypoglycemia). When the maintenance dosage of pramlintide is established, the insulin dosage can be titrated upward as needed to achieve desired glycemic control.

Combination Injectable Agents

In 2017 the first combination injectable agents were made available on the U.S. market. These products contain a fixed-dose combination of a basal insulin with a GLP-1 receptor agonist. The two products currently available include Soliqua 100/33 (insulin glargine, lixisenatide) and Xultophy 100/3.6 (insulin degludec, liraglutide). These products allow patients to receive treatment with both component agents with a single daily injection.

ACUTE COMPLICATIONS OF POOR GLYCEMIC CONTROL

Uncontrolled diabetes will lead to hyperglycemia, which in turn can lead to *diabetic ketoacidosis* (DKA) or *hyperosmolar hyperglycemic state* (HHS). The cardinal feature of both conditions is hyperglycemic crisis and associated loss of fluid and electrolytes. Both conditions can be life threatening, and hence immediate treatment should be implemented. As indicated in Table 57.13, these disorders have two principal differences. First, hyperglycemia is more severe in HHS. Second, whereas ketoacidosis is characteristic of DKA, it is absent in HHS. Treatment of both disorders is similar.

TABLE 57.13 ▪ Contrasts Between Diabetic Ketoacidosis and Hyperosmolar Hyperglycemic State

Characteristic	Diabetic Ketoacidosis (DKA)	Hyperosmolar Hyperglycemic State (HHS)
Patient population	Mainly in type 1 diabetes	More likely in type 2 diabetes
Onset	Rapid	Gradual
Blood glucose (mg/dL)	≥250	≥600
Plasma osmolality (mOsm/L)[a]	<320	>320
pH of arterial blood	≤7.3	≥7.3
Blood ketones	Large increase	Little or no change
Urine ketones	Large increase	Normal or small increase
Urine and breath odor	Urine smells like rotten apples; breath smells sweet or like acetone (nail polish)	Normal

[a]The normal range is 285 to 295 mOsm/L.

DIABETIC KETOACIDOSIS

Diabetic ketoacidosis is a severe manifestation of insulin deficiency. This syndrome is characterized by hyperglycemia, production of ketoacids, hemoconcentration, acidosis, and coma. These symptoms typically evolve quickly, over a period of several hours to a couple of days. Before insulin became available, practically all patients with type 1 diabetes died from ketoacidosis. Today, DKA remains a common complication, especially in pediatric patients. DKA occurs much more often in patients with type 1 diabetes than in those with type 2 diabetes.

Pathogenesis

DKA is brought on by derangements of glucose and fat metabolism. Altered glucose metabolism causes hyperglycemia, water loss, and hemoconcentration. Altered fat metabolism causes production of ketoacids. Fig. 57.5 shows the sequence of metabolic events by which ketoacidosis develops. Note that, in its final stages, the syndrome consists of hemoconcentration and shock in addition to ketoacidosis itself. The alterations in fat and glucose metabolism that lead to ketoacidosis are described in detail next.

Altered Fat Metabolism

Alterations in fat metabolism lead to production of ketoacids. Insulin deficiency promotes lipolysis (breakdown of fats) in adipose tissue. The products of lipolysis are glycerol and free fatty acids (FFA). Both of these metabolites are transported to the liver. In the liver, oxidation of FFA results in the production of two ketoacids (beta-hydroxybutyric acid and acetoacetic acid), also known as ketone bodies. Accumulation of ketoacids puts the body in a state of ketosis. As buildup of ketoacids increases, frank acidosis develops. At this point, the patient's condition changes from ketosis to ketoacidosis. (Ketoacidosis can be distinguished from ketosis by the presence of hyperventilation.) Acidosis contributes to the development of shock.

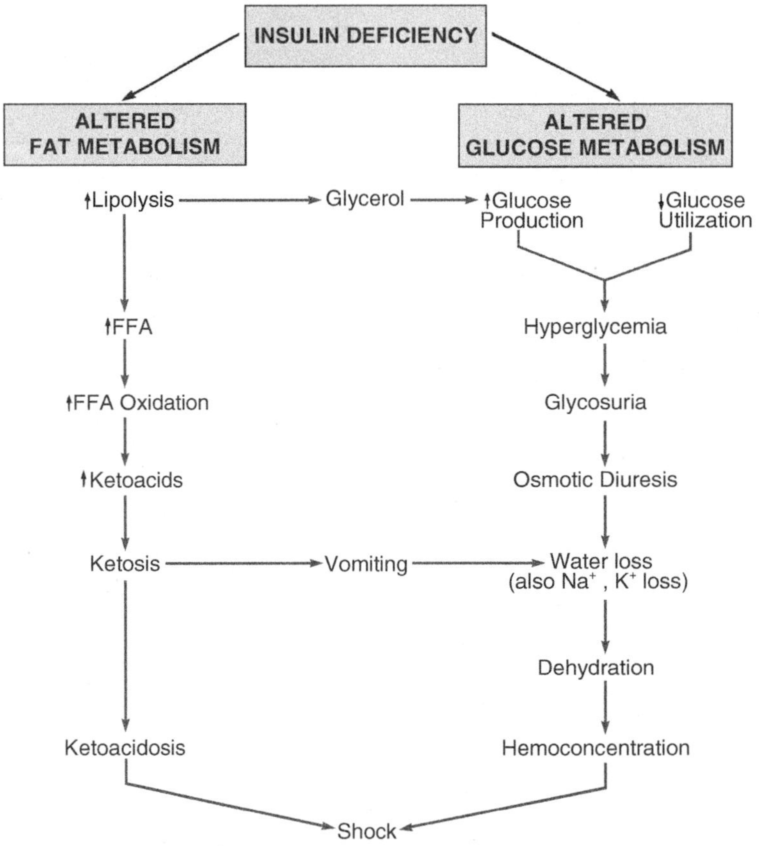

Fig. 57.5 ■ Pathogenesis of diabetic ketoacidosis (DKA).
The syndrome of DKA is caused by severe derangements of glucose metabolism and fat metabolism that occur in response to lack of insulin. (*FFA*, Free fatty acids.)

Ketosis imparts characteristic smells to the urine and breath, which can be useful clues to the patient's condition. Ketones in the urine smell like rotten or decaying apples. Ketones in expired air give off a sweet smell, sometimes called "Juicy Fruit breath," because it smells much like that flavorful chewing gum. Alternatively, the breath may smell like nail polish remover, which contains the ketone acetone. To some degree, the breath of a ketotic person smells like the breath of someone who has been drinking alcohol. Because of this smell—coupled with the neurologic sequelae of ketosis (reduced alertness, impaired gait and balance)—some patients with DKA have been arrested for drunk driving, even though they hadn't been drinking at all.

Altered Glucose Metabolism

Deranged glucose metabolism leads to hyperglycemia, water loss, and hemoconcentration. Insulin deficiency has two direct effects on the metabolism of glucose: (1) an increase in glucose production and (2) a decrease in glucose utilization. (The glycerol released by lipolysis is a substrate for glucose synthesis and therefore helps increase glucose production.) Because more glucose is being made and less is being used, plasma levels of glucose rise, causing hyperglycemia. Glycosuria develops when plasma glucose content becomes so high that the amount of glucose filtered by the glomeruli exceeds the capacity of the renal tubules for glucose reuptake. As the concentration of glucose in the urine increases, osmotic diuresis develops, resulting in the loss of large volumes of water. Vomiting is a direct source of fluid loss and, more importantly, is an impediment to rehydration with oral fluids. (It should be noted that, along with loss of water, sodium and potassium are lost too. These ions are excreted in conjunction with ketone bodies, compounds that carry a negative charge.) As dehydration becomes more severe, hemoconcentration develops. Hemoconcentration causes cerebral dehydration, which, together with acidosis, leads to shock.

Treatment

Diabetic ketoacidosis is a life-threatening emergency. Treatment is directed at correcting hyperglycemia and acidosis, replacing lost water and sodium, and normalizing potassium balance. We begin with IV fluids and electrolytes, followed as soon as possible by IV insulin. Although it might seem reasonable to drive glucose levels down quickly with lots of insulin, doing so is unsafe and should be avoided. Instead, glucose levels should be reduced slowly, by about 50 mg/dL/hr. DKA is managed in the inpatient setting, and institutions have protocols in place to assist with managing patients per the interventions noted above.

HYPEROSMOLAR HYPERGLYCEMIC STATE

HHS, also known as hyperglycemic hyperosmolar nonketotic syndrome (HHNS), is similar to DKA in some respects and different in others. As noted, the central characteristic in both disorders is severe hyperglycemia brought on by insulin deficiency. In HHS, as in DKA, a large amount of glucose is excreted in the urine, carrying a large volume of water with it. The result is dehydration and loss of blood volume, which greatly increases the blood concentrations of electrolytes and nonelectrolytes (particularly glucose)—hence the term hyperosmolar. Loss of blood volume also increases the hematocrit. As a result, the blood "thickens" and blood flow becomes sluggish. How does HHS differ from DKA? As its name indicates, HHS is nonketotic: There is little or no change in ketoacid levels in blood, and hence little or no change in blood pH. In contrast, blood levels of ketoacids rise dramatically in DKA, causing blood pH to fall. Since ketone levels remain close to normal in HHNS, the sweet or acetone-like smell imparted to the urine and breath of the DKA patient is absent. Finally, whereas DKA occurs mainly in patients with type 1 diabetes and develops quickly (usually in association with infection, acute illness, or some other stress), HHS occurs more often in patients with type 2 diabetes and evolves slowly: Metabolic changes typically begin a month or two before signs and symptoms become apparent. If HHS goes untreated, severe dehydration will eventually lead to coma, seizures, and death. As with

DKA, management of HHS is directed at correcting hyperglycemia and dehydration by use of IV insulin, fluids, and electrolytes.

GLUCAGON FOR TREATMENT OF SEVERE HYPOGLYCEMIA

Insulin overdose and the use of insulin secretagogue medications can cause severe hypoglycemia in which the patient is unable to self-treat with oral carbohydrate administration. The preferred treatment is IV glucose. However, if this option is not available, blood glucose can be restored with glucagon.

Glucagon, a polypeptide hormone produced by alpha cells of the pancreas, has effects on carbohydrate metabolism that are opposite to those of insulin. Specifically, glucagon promotes the breakdown of glycogen to glucose, reduces conversion of glucose to glycogen, and stimulates biosynthesis of glucose. Hence, whereas insulin acts to lower plasma glucose, glucagon causes plasma glucose to rise. In addition to these metabolic effects, glucagon acts on GI smooth muscle to promote relaxation.

Glucagon is used to treat severe hypoglycemia in the ambulatory setting. However, in patients with severe hypoglycemia, IV glucose is preferred because it raises blood glucose immediately, whereas responses to glucagon are somewhat delayed. Accordingly, glucagon should be used only if IV glucose is not an option—such as subQ administration in the home setting before emergency services arrive. When glucagon is administered to unconscious patients, the subsequent rise in blood glucose usually restores consciousness in 20 minutes or so. Once consciousness is sufficient for swallowing, oral carbohydrates should be given. These will help prevent recurrence of hypoglycemia and will help replenish hepatic glycogen stores.

Glucagon cannot correct hypoglycemia resulting from starvation. Glucagon acts in large part by promoting glycogen breakdown, and people who are starved have little or no glycogen left.

Glucagon is administered parenterally (IM, subQ, and IV). The drug is supplied in powder form and must be reconstituted to a concentration of 1 mg/mL (or less) using the diluent supplied by the manufacturer. A dose of 0.5 to 1 mg is usually effective.

KEY POINTS

- Diabetes is characterized by sustained hyperglycemia.
- Initial metabolic changes involve glucose and other carbohydrates. If the disease progresses, metabolism of fats and proteins changes as well.
- Diabetes has two major forms: type 1 diabetes and type 2 diabetes.
- Symptoms of type 1 diabetes result from a complete absence of insulin. The underlying cause is autoimmune destruction of pancreatic beta cells.
- Early in the disease process, symptoms of type 2 diabetes result mainly from cellular resistance to insulin's actions, not from insulin deficiency. However, later in the disease process, insulin deficiency develops.
- Type 1 diabetes and type 2 diabetes share the same long-term complications: heart disease, stroke, blindness, renal failure, neuropathy, lower limb amputations, erectile dysfunction, and gastroparesis, among others.
- Diabetes is diagnosed if (1) hemoglobin A1C is 6.5% or higher; (2) fasting plasma glucose is 126 mg/dL or higher; (3) an oral glucose tolerance test (OGTT) results in a blood glucose of 200 mg/dL or higher; or the patient presents with classic symptoms of hyperglycemia and has a random plasma glucose of 200 mg/dL or higher.
- With both type 1 and type 2 diabetes, the goal of treatment is to manage the symptoms of hyperglycemia and reduce long-term complications, including death.
- Type 1 diabetes is treated primarily with insulin replacement.
- Type 2 diabetes is treated with oral antidiabetic drugs or, if needed, with insulin or non-insulin injectable drugs—but always in conjunction with diet modification and exercise.
- In the past, drugs for type 2 diabetes were started only after a program of diet modification and exercise had failed to yield glycemic control. Today, drugs (usually metformin) are started immediately after diagnosis, but always in conjunction with diet modification and exercise.
- In type 1 diabetes, tight glycemic control can markedly reduce long-term complications, as demonstrated in the Diabetes Control and Complications Trial (DCCT).
- In type 2 diabetes, tight glycemic control can decrease microvascular complications, but not necessarily macrovascular complications or mortality, as shown in the ACCORD, ADVANCE, and VADT trials.
- Tight glycemic control increases the risk of severe hypoglycemia and weight gain, and possibly the risk of death.
- For patients with type 1 diabetes and for patients with type 2 diabetes who use insulin, self-monitoring of blood glucose (SMBG) is the standard method for day-to-day monitoring of therapy. The premeal target is 80 to 130 mg/dL, and the peak postmeal target is 180 mg/dL or lower for many patients.
- For patients with type 1 or type 2 diabetes, hemoglobin A1C should be measured every 3 to 6 months to assess long-term glycemic control.
- Insulin is an anabolic hormone. That is, it promotes conservation of energy and buildup of energy stores.
- Insulin has two basic effects: it (1) stimulates cellular uptake of glucose, amino acids, and potassium; and (2) promotes synthesis of complex organic molecules (glycogen, proteins, triglycerides).
- Insulin deficiency puts the body into a catabolic mode. As a result, glycogen is converted to glucose, proteins are degraded to amino acids, and fats are converted to glycerol (glycerin) and free fatty acids.
- Insulin deficiency promotes hyperglycemia by increasing glycogenolysis and gluconeogenesis and by decreasing glucose utilization.
- Multiple insulin products are used in the United States: regular human insulin (injectable and inhaled forms), NPH insulin, and several human insulin analogs: insulin lispro, insulin aspart, insulin glulisine, insulin detemir, insulin glargine, and insulin degludec.
- All insulins used in the United States are produced by recombinant DNA technology.
- Insulin lispro, insulin aspart, insulin glulisine, and regular insulin, when administered via inhalation, have a very rapid onset and short duration.

Continued

- Regular insulin, when used subQ, has a moderately rapid onset and short duration.
- NPH insulin has an intermediate duration of action.
- Insulin glargine (U-100) and insulin detemir have a prolonged duration, with no definite "peak" in either blood levels or hypoglycemic effects. Some patients may still require twice-daily administration with these products.
- Insulin glargine (U-300) and insulin degludec have a very long duration of action, with a duration of effect in excess of 24 hours.
- *All* insulins can be administered subQ, and four preparations—regular, aspart, lispro, and glulisine insulin—can be administered IV as well.
- One insulin preparation—NPH insulin—is a *suspension.* It looks cloudy and should be agitated before being drawn into a syringe. All other insulins are *solutions.* They look clear and do not require agitation.
- Insulin is used to treat all patients with type 1 diabetes and many patients with type 2 diabetes.
- SMBG is an essential component of intensive insulin therapy.
- The most important and common adverse effect of insulin therapy is hypoglycemia (blood glucose below 70 mg/dL), which occurs whenever insulin levels exceed insulin needs. Symptoms include tachycardia, palpitations, sweating, headache, confusion, drowsiness, and fatigue. If hypoglycemia is severe, convulsions, coma, and death may follow.
- Beta blockers can delay awareness of hypoglycemia by masking hypoglycemia-induced signs that are caused by activation of the sympathetic nervous system (e.g., tachycardia, palpitations). In addition, beta blockers inhibit the breakdown of glycogen to glucose and can thereby impede glucose replenishment.
- Insulin-induced hypoglycemia can be treated with a fast-acting oral sugar (e.g., glucose tablets, orange juice, sugar cubes), IV glucose, or parenteral glucagon. (Oral sucrose—aka table sugar—acts slowly and will barely work at all in patients taking acarbose, a drug that prevents intestinal conversion of sucrose into glucose and fructose.)
- Metformin (a biguanide) decreases glucose production by the liver and increases glucose uptake by muscle and adipose tissue.
- The major adverse effects of metformin are GI disturbances: decreased appetite, nausea, and diarrhea. Metformin does *not* cause hypoglycemia when used alone.
- Very rarely, metformin causes lactic acidosis, which can be fatal. The risk of lactic acidosis is increased by renal impairment, which decreases metformin excretion and thereby causes levels to rise rapidly. Metformin is therefore dosed based on renal function.
- Sulfonylureas stimulate release of insulin from the pancreas.
- The major adverse effects of sulfonylureas are hypoglycemia and weight gain.
- Pioglitazone, a thiazolidinedione (glitazone) for type 2 diabetes, increases insulin sensitivity of target cells and thereby increases glucose uptake by muscle and adipose tissue and decreases glucose production by the liver.
- Thiazolidinediones promote water retention and can thereby increase the risk of heart failure. In addition, pioglitazone can cause liver damage, bladder cancer, and fractures, and can cause ovulation in anovulatory premenopausal women, thereby posing a risk of unintended pregnancy.
- Acarbose and miglitol, alpha-glucosidase inhibitors for type 2 diabetes, inhibit digestion and absorption of carbohydrates and thereby reduce the postprandial rise in blood glucose. To be effective, these agents must be taken with every meal.
- The major adverse effects of alpha-glucosidase inhibitors are GI disturbances: flatulence, cramps, and abdominal distention.
- DPP-4 inhibitors are oral medications that, on average, lower A1C by about 0.5%. These agents are generally well tolerated and augment the effects of natural incretin hormones.
- Sodium-glucose co-transporter 2 (SGLT-2) inhibitors lower blood sugar by increasing excretion of glucose via the urine. SGLT-2 inhibitors can increase the risk of genitourinary infections.
- Canagliflozin and empagliflozin, both SGLT-2 inhibitors, have been shown in large cardiovascular outcome trials to prevent cardiovascular events in at-risk patients.
- Incretin mimetics are injectable agents for the treatment of type 2 diabetes. These drugs delay gastric emptying, suppress glucagon release, and stimulate glucose-dependent release of insulin. There are currently six products available within this drug class: exenatide, exenatide ER, liraglutide, lixisenatide, albiglutide, and dulaglutide.
- Incretin mimetics pose a risk of hypoglycemia in patients taking a sulfonylurea, but not in those taking metformin. Nausea is common.
- Pramlintide, an amylin mimetic, is injected subQ before meals to enhance the effects of mealtime insulin in patients with type 1 or type 2 diabetes. The drug delays gastric emptying and suppresses glucagon release and thereby helps reduce postprandial hyperglycemia.
- The combination of pramlintide plus insulin poses a risk of severe hypoglycemia. Nausea is common.
- Fixed-dose injectable combination products containing a basal insulin with a GLP-1 receptor agonist are available. Currently available agents are Soliqua 100/33 (insulin glargine, lixisenatide) and Xultophy 100/3.6 (insulin degludec, liraglutide).

Please visit **http://evolve.elsevier.com/Lehne** for chapter-specific NCLEX® examination review questions.

Summary of Major Nursing Implications[a]

INSULIN

Preadministration Assessment

Therapeutic Goal

Insulin is required by all patients with type 1 diabetes and by some with type 2 diabetes. The goal of insulin therapy is to maintain plasma levels of glucose and A1C within an acceptable range.

Baseline Data

Assess for clinical manifestations of diabetes (e.g., polyuria, polydipsia, polyphagia, weight loss) and for indications of hyperglycemia. Baseline laboratory tests may include casual plasma glucose, FPG, an OGTT, hemoglobin A1C, urinary glucose and ketones, and serum electrolytes.

Assess for baseline knowledge of diabetes and readiness to learn.

Identifying High-Risk Patients

Special care is needed in patients taking drugs that can raise or lower blood glucose levels, including sympathomimetics, glucocorticoids, sulfonylureas, insulin, glinides (e.g., repaglinide), and pramlintide.

Implementation: Administration

Routes

All insulins may be administered subQ, and four preparations—regular, aspart, lispro, and glulisine insulin—may be administered IV too. Regular insulin is also available as a product for inhalation.

Preparing for Subcutaneous Injection

Teach the patient to prepare for subQ injections as follows:

- Before loading the syringe, disperse insulin suspensions (i.e., NPH insulin preparations) by rolling the vial between the palms. Vigorous agitation causes frothing and must be avoided. If granules or clumps remain after mixing, discard the vial.
- Except for NPH insulin, all preparations are formulated as clear, colorless solutions, and hence can be administered without resuspension. If a preparation becomes cloudy or discolored, or if a precipitate develops, discard the vial.
- Before loading the syringe, swab the bottle cap with alcohol.
- Eliminate air bubbles from the syringe and needle after loading.
- Cleanse the skin (with alcohol or soap and water) before injection.

Sites of Injection

Provide the patient with the following instructions regarding sites of subQ injection:

- Usual sites of injection are the abdomen, upper arm, and thigh. To minimize variability in responses, make all injections in just one of these areas. Injections in the abdomen provide the most consistent insulin levels and effects.
- Rotate the injection site within the general area employed (e.g., the abdomen).
- Allow about 1 inch between sites. If possible, use each site just once a month.

Insulin Storage

Teach the patient the following about insulin storage:

- Store unopened vials of insulin in the refrigerator, but do not freeze. When stored under these conditions, insulin can be used up to the expiration date on the vial.
- The vial in current use can typically be stored at room temperature for up to 1 month, but must be kept out of direct sunlight and extreme heat. Discard partially filled vials after several weeks if left unused. Always consult the package insert for specific product storage recommendations.
- Mixtures of insulin prepared in vials may typically be stored for 1 month at room temperature and for 3 months under refrigeration. Always consult the package insert for specific product storage recommendations.
- Mixtures of insulin in pre-filled syringes (plastic or glass) should be stored in a refrigerator, where they will be stable for at least 1 week and perhaps 2 weeks. Store the syringe vertically (needle pointing up) to avoid clogging the needle. Gently agitate the syringe before administration to resuspend the insulin.

Dosage Adjustment

The dosing goal is to maintain blood glucose levels within an acceptable range. Dosage must be adjusted to balance changes in carbohydrate intake and other factors that can decrease insulin needs (strenuous exercise, pregnancy during the first trimester) or increase insulin needs (illness, trauma, stress, adolescent growth spurt, pregnancy after the first trimester).

Patient and Family Education

Patient and family education is an absolute requirement for safe and successful glycemic control. **Ensure that patients and their families receive thorough instruction on the following:**

- The nature of diabetes
- The importance of optimal glucose control
- The major components of the treatment routine—insulin, SMBG, diet, exercise, A1C tests—emphasizing the importance of proper diet and adequate exercise even though insulin is in use
- Procedures for purchasing insulin, syringes, and needles
- Methods of insulin storage
- Procedures for mixing insulins, if appropriate
- Calculation of dosage adjustments
- Techniques of insulin injection
- Rotation of injection sites
- Measurement of blood glucose
- Signs and management of hypoglycemia
- Signs and management of hyperglycemia

Continued

Summary of Major Nursing Implications[a]—cont'd

- **Special problems of diabetic pregnancy**
- **The procedure for obtaining Medic Alert registration**
- **The importance of avoiding arbitrary switches between insulins made by different manufacturers**

Ongoing Evaluation and Interventions

Measures to Evaluate and Enhance Therapeutic Effects

SMBG should be employed to evaluate day-to-day treatment. **Teach patients how to use the glucometer, and encourage them to measure blood glucose before meals and at bedtime.** Hemoglobin A1C should be measured 2 to 4 times a year to assess long-term glycemic control. Measuring urinary glucose is not helpful.

Minimizing Adverse Effects

Hypoglycemia. Hypoglycemia occurs whenever insulin levels exceed insulin needs. **Inform the patient about potential causes of hypoglycemia (e.g., insulin overdose, reduced food intake, vomiting, diarrhea, excessive alcohol intake, unaccustomed exercise, termination of pregnancy), and teach the patient and family members to recognize the early signs and symptoms of hypoglycemia (tachycardia, palpitations, sweating, nervousness, headache, confusion, drowsiness, fatigue).**

Rapid treatment is mandatory. If the patient is conscious, oral carbohydrates are indicated (e.g., glucose tablets, orange juice, sugar cubes). However, if the swallowing or gag reflex is suppressed, nothing should be administered PO. For unconscious patients, IV glucose is the treatment of choice. Parenteral glucagon is an alternative.

Hypoglycemic coma must be differentiated from coma of diabetic ketoacidosis (DKA). The differential diagnosis is made by measuring plasma or urinary glucose: Hypoglycemic coma is associated with very low levels of glucose, whereas high levels signify DKA.

Lipohypertrophy. Accumulation of subcutaneous fat can occur at sites of frequent insulin injection. **Inform the patient that lipohypertrophy can be minimized by systematic rotation of the injection site within the area selected (e.g., abdomen).**

Allergic Reactions. Systemic reactions (widespread urticaria, impairment of breathing) are rare. If systemic allergy develops, it can be reduced through desensitization (i.e., giving small initial doses of human insulin followed by a series of progressively larger doses).

Minimizing Adverse Interactions

Hypoglycemic Agents. Several drugs, including *sulfonylureas, glinides, alcohol* (used acutely), and *beta blockers,* can intensify hypoglycemia induced by insulin. When any of these drugs is combined with insulin, special care must be taken to ensure that blood glucose content does not fall too low.

Hyperglycemic Agents. Several drugs, including thiazide diuretics, glucocorticoids, and sympathomimetics, can raise blood glucose concentration and can thereby counteract the beneficial effects of insulin. When these agents are combined with insulin, increased insulin dosage may be needed.

Beta Blockers. Beta blockade can mask sympathetic responses (e.g., tachycardia, palpitations, tremors) to a steep drop in glucose levels and can thereby delay awareness of insulin-induced hypoglycemia. Also, because beta blockade impairs hepatic conversion of glycogen to glucose (glycogenolysis), beta blockers can make insulin-induced hypoglycemia even worse and can delay recovery from a hypoglycemic event.

METFORMIN

Preadministration Assessment

Therapeutic Goal

Metformin is used in conjunction with good nutrition and exercise to help maintain glycemic control in patients with type 2 diabetes. The drug is also used to prevent type 2 diabetes and to treat women with polycystic ovary syndrome. Metformin is not used for, nor is it effective in, type 1 diabetes.

Identifying High-Risk Patients

Metformin should be used with great caution in patients with or at imminent risk of developing renal insufficiency, liver disease, severe infection, heart failure, a history of lactic acidosis, or shock or other conditions that can cause hypoxemia. It should not be administered to patients who consume excessive amounts of alcohol acutely or long term, until and unless alcohol consumption can be cut back markedly. Likewise, patients for whom the drug is prescribed should be cautioned and encouraged to drink alcohol in moderation.

Implementation: Administration

Route

Oral.

Administration

Advise patients to take immediate-release tablets twice daily, with the morning and evening meals.

Advise patients to take extended-release metformin once daily with the evening meal.

Ongoing Evaluation and Interventions

Minimizing Adverse Effects

Lactic Acidosis. Rarely, metformin causes lactic acidosis, a medical emergency with a 50% mortality rate. Use metformin cautiously in patients with renal insufficiency and other conditions that increase acidosis risk (e.g., liver disease, severe infection, shock) and heart failure. **Inform patients about early signs of lactic acidosis—hyperventilation, myalgia, malaise, and unusual somnolence—and instruct them to seek immediate medical attention if these develop.** Withhold metformin until lactic acidosis has been ruled out. If lactic acidosis is diagnosed, hemodialysis may correct the condition and remove accumulated metformin.

Summary of Major Nursing Implications[a]—cont'd

Gastrointestinal Effects. Metformin can cause nausea, diarrhea, and appetite reduction, which usually subside over time. If these reactions are intolerable and the drug must be stopped, suitable alternative drugs should be started.

Vitamin Deficiency. Metformin can reduce absorption of vitamin B_{12} and folic acid. Monitoring for deficiencies and corrective supplements may be needed.

Minimizing Adverse Interactions

Alcohol. **Inform patients that alcohol increases the risk of lactic acidosis and therefore should be avoided or consumed in moderation.**

SULFONYLUREAS

First-Generation Agents (Rarely Used)

Chlorpropamide
Tolazamide
Tolbutamide

Second-Generation Agents

Glimepiride
Glipizide
Glyburide (glibenclamide)

Preadministration Assessment

Therapeutic Goal

Sulfonylureas are used in conjunction with calorie restriction and exercise to maintain glycemic control in patients with type 2 diabetes. These drugs do not work in patients with type 1 diabetes.

Identifying High-Risk Patients

Sulfonylureas are *contraindicated* during pregnancy and breast-feeding. Sulfonylureas should not be used in conjunction with alcohol.

Use with *caution* in patients with kidney or liver dysfunction.

Implementation: Administration

Route

Oral.

Administration

Advise patients to administer with food if GI upset occurs.

Note that dosages for the second-generation agents, which are preferred, are much lower than dosages for first-generation agents.

Sulfonylureas are intended only as supplemental therapy of type 2 diabetes. Encourage patients to maintain their established program of exercise and caloric restriction.

Ongoing Evaluation and Interventions

Minimizing Adverse Effects

Hypoglycemia. **Inform patients about signs of hypoglycemia (palpitations, tachycardia, sweating, fatigue, excessive hunger), and instruct them to notify the prescriber if these occur.** Treat severe hypoglycemia with IV glucose.

Minimizing Adverse Interactions

Alcohol. Alcohol increases the risk of lactic acidosis. **Instruct patients to avoid alcohol.**

Use in Pregnancy and Lactation

Pregnancy. Discontinue sulfonylureas during pregnancy. If an antidiabetic agent is needed, insulin is the drug of choice.

Lactation. Sulfonylureas are excreted into breast milk, posing a risk of hypoglycemia to the nursing infant. Women who choose to breast-feed should substitute insulin for the sulfonylurea.

GLINIDES (MEGLITINIDES)

Nateglinide
Repaglinide

Preadministration Assessment

Therapeutic Goal

Glinides are used in conjunction with calorie restriction and exercise to maintain glycemic control in patients with type 2 diabetes. Glinides are not used for type 1 diabetes.

Identifying High-Risk Patients

Use with *caution* in patients with liver impairment and those taking gemfibrozil.

Implementation: Administration

Route

Oral.

Administration

Inform patients that dosing must be associated with a meal, and instruct them to take the drug 30 minutes or less before eating.

Ongoing Evaluation and Interventions

Minimizing Adverse Effects

Hypoglycemia. **Inform patients about signs of hypoglycemia (palpitations, tachycardia, sweating, fatigue, excessive hunger), and instruct them to notify the prescriber if these occur.** Treat severe hypoglycemia with IV glucose.

Minimizing Adverse Interactions

Gemfibrozil. Gemfibrozil slows metabolism of glinides and thereby increases their levels and the risk of hypoglycemia. Avoid gemfibrozil if possible.

THIAZOLIDINEDIONES

Pioglitazone
Rosiglitazone

Continued

Summary of Major Nursing Implications[a]—cont'd

Preadministration Assessment

Therapeutic Goal

Thiazolidinediones are used in conjunction with good nutrition and exercise to maintain glycemic control in patients with type 2 diabetes. Pioglitazone is the most frequently used agent in this class, so it will be discussed specifically in this section.

Baseline Data

Obtain a baseline value for serum alanine aminotransferase (ALT).

Identifying High-Risk Patients

Pioglitazone is *contraindicated* for patients with *severe* heart failure, and should be used with *caution* in those with *mild* heart failure or even heart failure risk factors. The drug is also *contraindicated* for patients with active bladder cancer or a history of bladder cancer. Exercise *caution* in patients taking insulin or drugs that inhibit or induce CYP2C8.

Implementation: Administration

Route

Oral.

Administration. **Advise patients to take pioglitazone once daily, with or without food.**

Ongoing Evaluation and Interventions

Minimizing Adverse Effects

Heart Failure. Pioglitazone can cause heart failure secondary to renal retention of fluid. Accordingly, pioglitazone must be used with caution in patients with *mild* heart failure or heart failure risk factors, and must be avoided in those with *severe* failure. **Inform patients about signs of heart failure (dyspnea, edema, weight gain, fatigue), and instruct them to consult the prescriber if these develop.** If heart failure is diagnosed, pioglitazone should be discontinued or used in reduced dosage.

Liver Injury. Pioglitazone may pose a risk of liver injury. Accordingly, ALT should be determined at baseline and periodically thereafter (e.g., every 3 to 6 months). If ALT levels rise to more than 3 times the upper limit of normal or if jaundice develops, pioglitazone should be withdrawn. **Inform patients about symptoms of liver injury (nausea, vomiting, abdominal pain, fatigue, anorexia, dark urine, jaundice), and instruct them to notify the prescriber if these develop.**

Bladder Cancer. Pioglitazone may cause bladder cancer, especially with long-term, high-dose use. Avoid the drug in patients with active bladder cancer or a history of bladder cancer. **Inform patients about signs of bladder cancer (e.g., blood in urine, worsening urinary urgency, painful urination), and instruct them to contact their prescriber if these develop.**

Fractures. Pioglitazone increases the risk of fractures in women (but not in men), especially with long-term, high-dose therapy. **Advise women about measures to maintain bone health, including regular exercise, ensuring adequate intake of calcium and vitamin D, and use of drugs for osteoporosis, if needed.**

Ovulation. Pioglitazone can cause ovulation in premenopausal anovulatory women, thereby posing a risk of unintended pregnancy. **Inform women about this action, and educate them about contraceptive options.**

Minimizing Adverse Interactions

Insulin. Like pioglitazone, insulin increases the risk of fluid retention and the associated risk of heart failure. Use the combination with caution.

Inhibitors and Inducers of CYP2C8. Strong inhibitors of CYP2C8 (e.g., atorvastatin, ketoconazole) can increase pioglitazone levels and prolong its half-life, necessitating a reduction in pioglitazone dosage. Conversely, strong inducers of CYP2C8 (e.g., rifampin, cimetidine) can reduce pioglitazone levels and shorten its half-life, necessitating an increase in pioglitazone dosage. Use caution when pioglitazone is combined with any of these drugs.

[a]Patient education information is highlighted as **blue text**.

CHAPTER

58 Drugs for Thyroid Disorders

Thyroid hormones have profound effects on metabolism, cardiac function, growth, and development. These hormones stimulate the metabolic rate of most cells and increase the force and rate of cardiac contraction. During infancy and childhood, thyroid hormones promote maturation; severe deficiency can produce extreme short stature and permanent mental impairment. Fortunately, most abnormalities of thyroid function can be effectively treated.

We begin our study of thyroid drugs by reviewing thyroid physiology. Next we review the pathophysiology of hypothyroid and hyperthyroid states. Finally, we discuss the agents used for thyroid disorders.

THYROID PHYSIOLOGY

Chemistry and Nomenclature

The thyroid gland produces two active hormones: triiodothyronine (T_3) and thyroxine (T_4, tetraiodothyronine). These hormones have nearly identical structures. The only difference is that T_4 contains four atoms of iodine, whereas T_3 contains three. The biologic effects of T_3 and T_4 are qualitatively similar. However, when compared on a molar basis, T_3 is much more potent.

Preparations of T_3 and T_4 employed clinically, although synthetic, are identical in structure to the naturally occurring hormones. The generic name of synthetic T_3 is *liothyronine,* and the generic name of synthetic T_4 is *levothyroxine.* A fixed-ratio mixture of T_3 plus T_4, known as *liotrix,* is also available.

Synthesis and Fate of Thyroid Hormones

Synthesis

Synthesis of thyroid hormones takes place in four steps (Fig. 58.1). The circled numbers in the figure correspond with the steps that follow.

- *Step 1.* Formation of thyroid hormone begins with the active transport of *iodide* into the thyroid. Under normal conditions, this process produces concentrations of iodide within the thyroid that are 20 to 50 times greater than the concentration of iodide in plasma. When plasma iodide levels are extremely low, intrathyroid iodide content may reach levels that are more than 100 times greater than those in plasma.
- *Step 2.* Following uptake, iodide undergoes oxidation to *iodine,* the active form of iodide. Iodide oxidation is catalyzed by an enzyme called *peroxidase.*
- *Step 3.* In this step, activated iodine becomes incorporated into tyrosine residues that are bound to *thyroglobulin,* a large glycoprotein. One tyrosine molecule may receive either one or two iodine atoms, resulting in the production of monoiodotyrosine (MIT) or diiodotyrosine (DIT), respectively.
- *Step 4.* In this final step, iodinated tyrosine molecules are coupled. Coupling of one DIT with one MIT forms T_3 (step 4A); coupling of one DIT with another DIT forms T_4 (step 4B).

Fate

Thyroid hormones are released from the thyroid gland by a proteolytic process. The amount of T_4 released is substantially greater than the amount of T_3 released. However, much of the T_4 that is released undergoes conversion to T_3 by enzymes in peripheral tissues. In fact, conversion of T_4 to T_3 accounts for the majority (about 80%) of the T_3 found in plasma.

More than 99.5% of the T_3 and T_4 in plasma is bound to plasma proteins. Consequently, only a tiny fraction of circulating thyroid hormone is free to produce biologic effects.

Thyroid hormones are eliminated primarily by hepatic metabolism. Because T_3 and T_4 are extensively bound to plasma proteins, metabolism is slow. As a result, the half-lives of these hormones are prolonged—about 1 day for T_3 and 7 days for T_4.

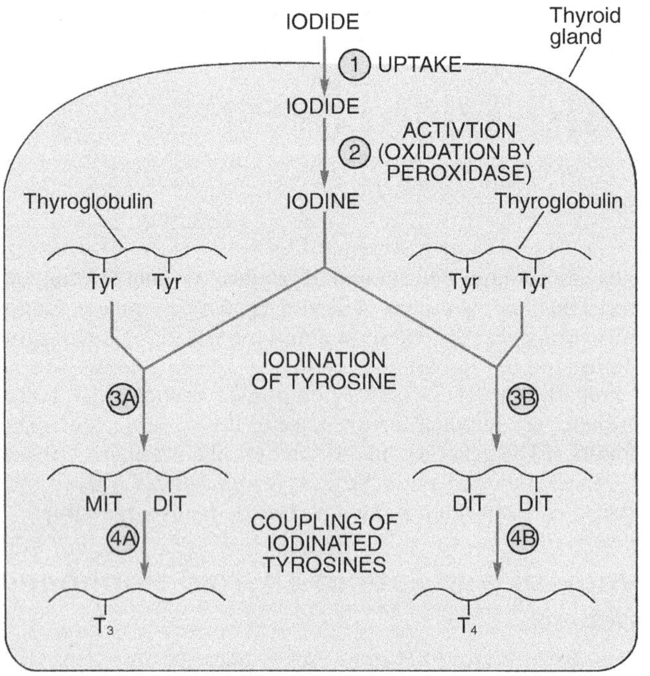

Fig. 58.1 ▪ Steps in thyroid hormone synthesis.
The reactions at each step (circled numbers) are explained in the text. (*DIT*, Diiodotyrosine; *MIT*, monoiodotyrosine; *T_3*, triiodothyronine; *T_4*, thyroxine; *Tyr*, tyrosine.)

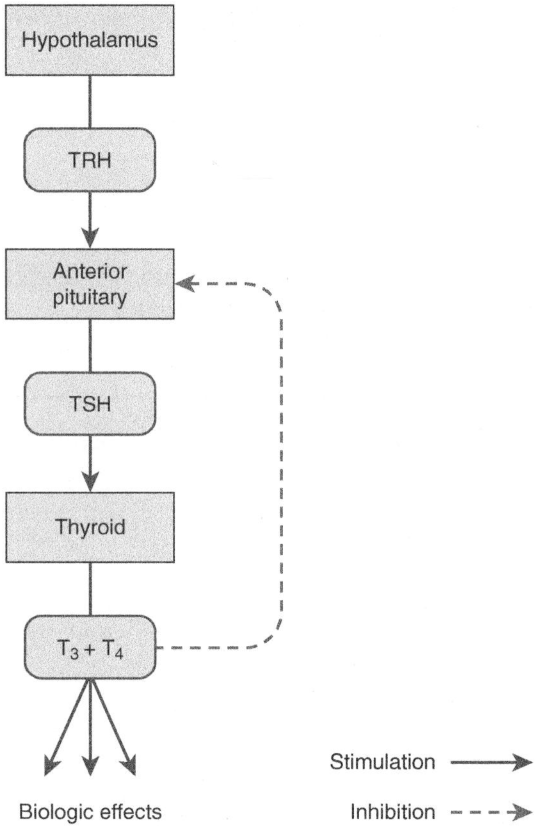

Fig. 58.2 ▪ Regulation of thyroid function.
TRH from the hypothalamus stimulates release of TSH from the pituitary. TSH stimulates all aspects of thyroid function, including release of T_3 and T_4. T_3 and T_4 act on the pituitary to suppress further TSH release. (*T_3*, Triiodothyronine; *T_4*, thyroxine; *TRH*, thyrotropin-releasing hormone; *TSH*, thyrotropin thyroid-stimulating hormone.)

Thyroid Hormone Actions

Thyroid hormones have three principal actions: (1) stimulation of energy use, (2) stimulation of the heart, and (3) promotion of growth and development. Stimulation of energy use elevates the basal metabolic rate, resulting in increased oxygen consumption and increased heat production. Stimulation of the heart increases both the rate and force of contraction, resulting in increased cardiac output and increased oxygen demand. Thyroid effects on growth and development are profound: Thyroid hormones are essential for normal development of the brain and other components of the nervous system, and they have a significant impact on maturation of skeletal muscle.

Thyroid hormones produce their effects by modulating the activity of specific genes. Furthermore, it appears that most, if not all, of the effects of thyroid hormones are mediated by T_3, not by T_4. There is good evidence that T_3 penetrates to the cell nucleus and binds with high affinity to nuclear receptors, which in turn bind to specific DNA sequences. The result is modulation of gene transcription, causing production of proteins that mediate thyroid hormone effects. Although T_4 also binds with nuclear receptors, its affinity is low, and gene transcription is not altered. Hence it would seem that T_4 serves only as a source of T_3, having little or no physiologic effects of its own.

Regulation of Thyroid Function by the Hypothalamus and Anterior Pituitary

The functional relationship between the hypothalamus, anterior pituitary, and thyroid is shown in Fig. 58.2. As indicated, thyrotropin-releasing hormone (TRH), secreted by the hypothalamus, acts on the pituitary to cause secretion of thyrotropin (thyroid-stimulating hormone [TSH]). TSH then acts on the thyroid to stimulate all aspects of thyroid function: Thyroid size is enlarged, iodine uptake is augmented, and synthesis and release of thyroid hormones are increased. In response to rising plasma levels of T_3 and T_4, further release of TSH is suppressed. The stimulatory effect of TSH on the thyroid, followed by the inhibitory effect of thyroid hormones on the pituitary, constitutes a negative feedback loop.

Effect of Iodine Deficiency on Thyroid Function

When iodine availability is diminished, production of thyroid hormones decreases. The ensuing drop in thyroid hormone levels promotes release of TSH, which acts on the thyroid to increase its size (causing goiter) and ability to concentrate iodine. If iodine deficiency is not too severe, the increased capacity for iodine uptake will restore normal production of T_3 and T_4.

THYROID FUNCTION TESTS

Several laboratory tests can be used to evaluate thyroid function. Three are described here. Values indicating euthyroid (normal), hypothyroid, and hyperthyroid states are shown in Table 58.1.

TABLE 58.1 ■ Serum Values for Thyroid Function Tests[a]

	Serum Values		
Thyroid Test	Normal	Hypothyroid	Hyperthyroid
Total T_4 (mcg/dL)	4.5–12.5	Under 4.5	Over 12.5
Free T_4 (ng/dL)	0.9–2	Under 0.9	Over 2
Total T_3 (ng/dL)	80–220	Under 80	Over 220
Free T_3 (pg/dL)	230–620	Under 230	Over 620
TSH (microunits/mL)	0.3–6	Over 6	Under 0.3

[a]Labs have different reference ranges. These are relative ranges and are not absolute.

Serum TSH

Serum TSH determinations are used primarily for screening and diagnosis of hypothyroidism and for monitoring replacement therapy in hypothyroid patients.

Measurement of serum TSH is the most sensitive method for diagnosing hypothyroidism because the anterior pituitary is exquisitely sensitive to changes in thyroid hormone levels. As a result, very small reductions in serum T_3 and T_4 can cause a dramatic rise in serum TSH. Therefore, even when the degree of hypothyroidism is minimal, it will be reflected by an abnormally high level of TSH. When replacement therapy is instituted, the TSH level should return to normal.

Serum TSH determinations can also be used to distinguish primary hypothyroidism from secondary hypothyroidism. In primary (thyroidal) hypothyroidism, TSH levels are *high.* However, in secondary hypothyroidism (hypothyroidism resulting from anterior pituitary dysfunction), TSH levels are low, normal, or even slightly elevated—despite the presence of low levels of T_3 and T_4.

Serum T_4 Test

Testing can measure either *total T_4* (bound plus free) or *free T_4*. Measurement of free T_4 is preferred. The T_4 test can be used to monitor thyroid hormone replacement therapy and to screen for thyroid dysfunction. However, in both cases, measurement of TSH is preferred.

Serum T_3 Test

As with T_4, we can measure either total or free T_3. Measurement of free T_3 is preferred. This test is useful for diagnosing hyperthyroidism. In this disorder, levels of T_3 often rise sooner and to a greater extent than do levels of T_4. T_3 determinations can also be used to monitor thyroid hormone replacement therapy (all thyroid preparations should increase levels of T_3).

THYROID PATHOPHYSIOLOGY

Hypothyroidism

Hypothyroidism can occur at any age. In adults, mild deficiency of thyroid hormone is referred to simply as *hypothyroidism.* Severe deficiency is called *myxedema.* When hypothyroidism occurs in infants, the resulting condition is called *congenital hypothyroidism.*

Hypothyroidism in Adults

Clinical Presentation. Signs and symptoms of hypothyroidism depend on disease severity. With mild hypothyroidism, symptoms are subtle and may go unrecognized for what they are. In contrast, with moderate to severe disease, characteristic signs and symptoms emerge. The face is pale, puffy, and expressionless. The skin is cold and dry. The hair is brittle, and hair loss occurs. Heart rate and temperature are lowered. The patient may complain of lethargy, fatigue, and intolerance to cold. Mentation may be impaired. Thyroid enlargement (goiter) may occur if reduced levels of T_3 and T_4 promote excessive release of TSH.

Causes. Hypothyroidism in the adult is usually due to malfunction of the thyroid itself. In iodine-sufficient countries, the principal cause is *chronic autoimmune thyroiditis* (Hashimoto's thyroiditis). Other causes are insufficient iodine in the diet, surgical removal of the thyroid, and destruction of the thyroid by radioactive iodine. Adult hypothyroidism may also result from insufficient secretion of TSH and TRH.

Therapeutic Strategy. Hypothyroidism in adults requires replacement therapy with thyroid hormones. In almost all cases, treatment must continue lifelong. Today, the standard replacement regimen consists of *levothyroxine* (T_4) alone. Combined therapy with levothyroxine plus liothyronine (T_3) is an option. However, with only three exceptions, all studies to date indicate that combined T_3/T_4 offers no advantage over T_4 alone. (Remember, when we give T_4, much of it is rapidly converted to T_3, the active form of the hormone.) When replacement doses of T_4 are adequate, they can eliminate all signs and symptoms of thyroid deficiency.

Hypothyroidism During Pregnancy

Maternal hypothyroidism can result in permanent neuropsychologic deficits in the child. We have long known that *congenital* hypothyroidism can cause developmental problems (see *Hypothyroidism in Infants*). However, it was not until 1999 that researchers demonstrated that *maternal* hypothyroidism—in the absence of fetal hypothyroidism—can decrease IQ and other aspects of neuropsychologic function in the child. The impact of maternal hypothyroidism is limited largely to the first trimester, a time during which the fetus is unable to produce thyroid hormones of its own. By the second trimester, the fetal thyroid gland is fully functional, and hence the fetus can supply its own hormones from then on. Therefore, to help ensure healthy fetal development, maternal hypothyroidism must be diagnosed and treated very early. Unfortunately, symptoms of hypothyroidism are often nonspecific (irritability, tiredness, poor concentration, etc.) or there may be no symptoms at all. Accordingly, some authorities now recommend routine screening for hypothyroidism as soon as pregnancy is confirmed. If hypothyroidism is diagnosed, replacement therapy should begin immediately.

When women who take thyroid supplements become pregnant, dosage requirements usually increase—often by as much as 50%. The need for increased dosage begins between weeks 4 and 8 of gestation, levels off around week 16, and then remains steady until parturition. To ensure adequate hormone levels, some authorities increase T_4 dosage by 30% as soon as pregnancy is confirmed. Further adjustments are based on serum TSH levels, which should be monitored closely.

Hypothyroidism in Infants

Clinical Presentation. Hypothyroidism in newborns may be permanent or transient. In either case, congenital hypothyroidism can cause delay in mental development and derangement of growth. In the absence of thyroid hormones, the child develops a large and protruding tongue, potbelly, and dwarfish stature. Development of the nervous system, bones, teeth, and muscles is impaired.

Causes. Congenital hypothyroidism usually results from a failure in thyroid development. Other causes include autoimmune disease, severe iodine deficiency, TSH deficiency, and exposure to radioactive iodine *in utero.*

Therapeutic Strategy. Hypothyroidism in newborns requires replacement therapy with thyroid hormones. If treatment is initiated within a few days of birth, physical and mental development will be normal. However, if therapy is delayed beyond 3 to 4 weeks, some permanent disability will be evident, although the physical effects of thyroid deficiency will reverse.

In all children, treatment should continue for 3 years, after which it should be stopped for 4 weeks. The objective is to determine whether thyroid deficiency is permanent or transient. If TSH rises, indicating thyroid hormone production is low, we know the deficiency is permanent, and so replacement therapy should resume. If TSH and T_4 normalize, we know the deficiency was transient, and hence further replacement therapy is unnecessary.

Hyperthyroidism

There are two major forms of hyperthyroidism: *Graves' disease* and *toxic nodular goiter* (also known as *Plummer's disease*). Of the two disorders, Graves' disease is more common. Signs and symptoms of both disorders are similar. The principal difference is that Graves' disease may cause exophthalmos, whereas toxic nodular goiter does not.

Graves' Disease

Graves' disease is the most common cause of excessive thyroid hormone secretion. This disorder occurs most frequently in women ages 20 to 40 years. The incidence in females is 6 times greater than in males.

Clinical Presentation. Most clinical manifestations result from elevated levels of thyroid hormone. Heartbeat is rapid and strong, and dysrhythmias and angina may develop. The central nervous system is stimulated, resulting in nervousness, insomnia, rapid thought flow, and rapid speech. Skeletal muscles may weaken and atrophy. Metabolic rate is raised, resulting in increased heat production, increased body temperature, intolerance to heat, and skin that is warm and moist. Appetite is increased. However, despite increased food consumption, weight loss occurs if caloric intake fails to match the increase in metabolic rate. Collectively, these signs and symptoms are referred to as *thyrotoxicosis.*

In addition to thyrotoxicosis, patients with Graves' disease often present with *exophthalmos* (protrusion of the eyeballs). The underlying cause is an immune-mediated infiltration of the extraocular muscles and orbital fat by lymphocytes, macrophages, plasma cells, mast cells, and mucopolysaccharides.

Cause. Thyroid stimulation in Graves' disease is caused by thyroid-stimulating immunoglobulins (TSIs), which are antibodies produced by an autoimmune process. TSIs increase thyroid activity by stimulating receptors for TSH on the thyroid gland. That is, TSIs mimic the effects of TSH on thyroid function. TSIs are not responsible for exophthalmos.

Treatment. Treatment for Graves' disease is directed at decreasing the production of thyroid hormones. Three modalities are employed: (1) surgical removal of thyroid tissue, (2) destruction of thyroid tissue with radioactive iodine, and (3) suppression of thyroid hormone synthesis with an antithyroid drug (methimazole or propylthiouracil). Radiation is the preferred treatment for adults, whereas antithyroid drugs are preferred for younger patients.

Beta blockers (e.g., propranolol) and nonradioactive iodine may be used as adjunctive therapy. Beta blockers suppress tachycardia by blocking beta receptors on the heart. Nonradioactive iodine inhibits synthesis and release of thyroid hormones.

Since exophthalmos is not the result of hyperthyroidism per se, this condition is not improved by lowering thyroid hormone production. If exophthalmos is severe, it can be treated with surgery or with high doses of oral glucocorticoids.

Toxic Nodular Goiter (Plummer's Disease)

Toxic nodular goiter is the result of a thyroid adenoma. Clinical manifestations are much like those of Graves' disease, except exophthalmos is absent. Toxic nodular goiter is a persistent condition that rarely undergoes spontaneous remission. Treatment modalities are the same as for Graves' disease. However, if an antithyroid drug is used, symptoms return rapidly when the drug is withdrawn. Accordingly, surgery and radiation, which provide long-term control, are often preferred.

Thyrotoxic Crisis (Thyroid Storm)

Thyrotoxic crisis can occur in patients with severe thyrotoxicosis when they undergo major surgery or develop a severe intercurrent illness (e.g., infection, sepsis). The syndrome is characterized by profound hyperthermia (105°F or even higher), severe tachycardia, restlessness, agitation, and tremor. Unconsciousness, coma, hypotension, and heart failure may ensue. These symptoms are produced by excessive levels of thyroid hormones.

Thyrotoxic crisis can be life threatening and requires immediate treatment. High doses of potassium iodide or strong iodine solution are given to suppress thyroid hormone release. Methimazole is given to suppress thyroid hormone synthesis. A beta blocker is given to reduce heart rate. Additional measures include sedation, cooling, and the administration of glucocorticoids and IV fluids.

THYROID HORMONE PREPARATIONS FOR HYPOTHYROIDISM

Thyroid hormones are available as pure synthetic compounds and as extracts of animal thyroid glands. All preparations have qualitatively similar effects. The synthetic preparations are more stable and better standardized than the animal gland extracts. As a result, the synthetics are preferred to the natural products. Properties of thyroid hormone preparations are shown in Table 58.2.

TABLE 58.2 ■ Thyroid Hormone Preparations

Generic Name	Brand Names	Dosage Forms	Approximate Equivalent Dosage[a]	Description
Levothyroxine	Levothroid, Levoxyl, Synthroid	Tablets, injection	50–60 mcg	Synthetic preparation of T_4 identical to the naturally occurring hormone
Liothyronine	Cytomel, Triostat	Tablets, injection	15–37 mcg	Synthetic preparation of T_3 identical to the naturally occurring hormone
Liotrix	Thyrolar	Tablets	60 mcg	Synthetic T_4 plus synthetic T_3 in a 4 : 1 fixed ratio
Thyroid	Armour Thyroid, Nature-Throid, Thyroid USP	Tablets, capsules	60 mg	Desiccated animal thyroid glands (rarely used today)

[a]Approximate dosage needed to produce equivalent effects.

Levothyroxine (T_4)

Levothyroxine [Synthroid, others] is a synthetic preparation of thyroxine, a naturally occurring thyroid hormone. The structure of levothyroxine is identical to that of the natural hormone. Levothyroxine is the drug of choice for most patients who require thyroid hormone replacement. Consequently, levothyroxine will serve as our prototype for the thyroid hormone preparations.

Prototype Drugs

DRUGS FOR THYROID DISORDERS

Drugs for Hypothyroidism

Levothyroxine (T_4)

Drugs for Hyperthyroidism

Methimazole (a thionamide)

Pharmacokinetics

Absorption. Absorption of oral levothyroxine is reduced by food. Accordingly, to minimize variability in blood levels, levothyroxine should be taken on an empty stomach in the morning, at least 30 to 60 minutes before breakfast.

Conversion to T_3. Much of an administered dose of levothyroxine is converted to T_3 in the body. As a result, levothyroxine can produce nearly normal levels of both T_3 and T_4. Hence, for most patients, there is no need to give T_3 along with levothyroxine.

Half-Life and Plasma Levels. Because levothyroxine is highly protein bound (about 99.97%), the hormone has a prolonged half-life (about 7 days). From a clinical perspective, this long half-life is good news and bad news. The good news is that hormone levels remain fairly steady, even with once-a-day dosing, which makes levothyroxine well suited for lifelong therapy. The bad news is that it takes about 1 month (four half-lives) for plasma levels of levothyroxine to reach plateau (steady state). As a result, onset of full effects is delayed.

Therapeutic Uses

Levothyroxine is indicated for all forms of hypothyroidism, regardless of cause. The drug is used for congenital hypothyroidism, myxedema coma, simple goiter, and primary hypothyroidism in adults and children. Levothyroxine is also used to treat hypothyroidism resulting from insufficient TSH (secondary to pituitary malfunction) and from insufficient TRH (secondary to hypothalamic malfunction). In addition, levothyroxine is used to maintain proper levels of thyroid hormones following thyroid surgery, irradiation, and treatment with antithyroid drugs.

Levothyroxine and other thyroid hormones should not be taken to treat obesity. These hormones will accelerate metabolism and promote weight reduction only if the dosage is high enough to establish a pathologic (hyperthyroid) state.

Adverse Effects

When administered in appropriate dosage, levothyroxine rarely causes adverse effects. With an acute overdose, *thyrotoxicosis* may result. Signs and symptoms include tachycardia, angina, tremor, nervousness, insomnia, hyperthermia, heat intolerance, and sweating. The patient should be informed about these signs and instructed to notify the prescriber if they develop. Chronic overdosage is associated with accelerated bone loss and increased risk of atrial fibrillation, especially in older adults. Loss of bone increases the risk of fractures.

Drug Interactions

Drugs That Reduce Levothyroxine Absorption. Absorption of levothyroxine can be reduced by the following drugs:

- Histamine$_2$ (H_2) receptor blockers (e.g., cimetidine [Tagamet])
- Proton pump inhibitors (e.g., lansoprazole [Prevacid]
- Sucralfate [Carafate]
- Cholestyramine [Questran]
- Colestipol [Colestid]
- Aluminum-containing antacids (e.g., Maalox, Mylanta)
- Calcium supplements (e.g., Tums, Os-Cal)
- Iron supplements (e.g., ferrous sulfate)
- Magnesium salts
- Orlistat [Xenical]

To ensure adequate absorption of levothyroxine, patients should separate administration of levothyroxine and these drugs by 4 hours. As noted previously, food also reduces absorption.

Drugs That Accelerate Levothyroxine Metabolism. Several drugs can accelerate the metabolism of levothyroxine. Among these are phenytoin [Dilantin], carbamazepine

[Tegretol, Carbatrol], rifampin [Rifadin], sertraline [Zoloft], and phenobarbital. Accordingly, in order to maintain adequate levothyroxine levels, patients taking these drugs may need to increase their levothyroxine dosage.

Warfarin. Levothyroxine accelerates the degradation of vitamin K–dependent clotting factors. As a result, effects of warfarin (an anticoagulant) are enhanced. If thyroid hormone replacement therapy is started in a patient taking warfarin, the dosage of warfarin may need to be reduced.

Catecholamines. Thyroid hormones increase cardiac responsiveness to catecholamines (epinephrine, dopamine, dobutamine), thereby increasing the risk of catecholamine-induced dysrhythmias. Caution must be exercised when administering catecholamines to patients receiving levothyroxine and other thyroid preparations.

Other Interactions. Levothyroxine can increase requirements for insulin and digoxin. When converting patients from a hypothyroid to a euthyroid state, dosages of insulin and digoxin may need to be increased.

Are Levothyroxine Preparations Interchangeable?

Levothyroxine is available in several brand-name and generic formulations. Whether any of these are interchangeable is in dispute.

Levothyroxine has a narrow therapeutic range, so tight control of plasma drug levels is important. Otherwise, symptoms of hypothyroidism or toxicity will develop. In order to maintain good control, all pills a patient takes must produce the same levothyroxine levels. Accordingly, if a patient switches from one product to another, the new product must be bioequivalent to the old one.

Whether or not any levothyroxine products—brand-name or generic—are truly equivalent is a point of contention. According to the U.S. Food and Drug Administration (FDA), certain formulations of levothyroxine are therapeutically equivalent to others. For example, the FDA maintains that generic levothyroxine made by Mylan is equivalent to two brand-name products: Levoxyl and Synthroid. However, three medical organizations—the American Association of Clinical Endocrinologists (AACE), The Endocrine Society (TES), and the American Thyroid Association (ATA)—*strongly* disagree, as expressed in a 2004 position statement. They believe the FDA's testing procedure was seriously flawed. First, the FDA only measured blood levels of levothyroxine; it did not measure serum TSH, the favored clinical test for assessing thyroid status. Second, and more important, testing was done in *normal* (euthyroid) volunteers. Hence, when blood levels of levothyroxine were measured, the values reflected the sum of endogenous thyroxine plus levothyroxine contributed by the drug—making it impossible to state with precision how much of the total was truly due to the drug. As a result, conclusions regarding the equivalence of levothyroxine products are questionable. Nonetheless, pharmacists may switch patients from one product to another, often without the knowledge of the patient or prescriber—a practice with the potential for causing toxicity or therapeutic failure.

Given the debate about whether certain levothyroxine products are clinically interchangeable, what should the clinician do? In their position statement, the AACE, TES, and ATA recommend the following:

- Maintain patients on the same brand-name levothyroxine product.
- If a switch *is* made (from one branded product to another, from a branded product to a generic product, or from one generic product to another), retest serum TSH in 6 weeks, and adjust the levothyroxine dosage as indicated.
- Advise patients to check with their prescriber before allowing a pharmacist to switch to a different levothyroxine product.

Dosage and Administration I: General Considerations

Routes of Administration. Levothyroxine is almost always administered by mouth. Oral doses should be taken once daily on an empty stomach (to enhance absorption). *Dosing is usually done in the morning, at least 30 to 60 minutes before eating.*

Intravenous administration is used for myxedema coma and for patients who cannot take levothyroxine orally. Intravenous doses are about 50% of the size of oral doses.

Evaluation. The goal of replacement therapy is to provide a dosage that compensates precisely for the existing thyroid deficit. This dosage is determined using a combination of clinical judgment and laboratory tests. When therapy is successful in adults, clinical evaluation should reveal a reversal of the signs and symptoms of thyroid deficiency—and an absence of signs of thyroid excess. Successful therapy of infants is reflected in normalization of intellectual function and normalization of growth and development. Monthly determinations of height provide a good index of success.

Measurement of serum TSH is an important means of evaluation. Successful replacement therapy causes elevated TSH levels to fall. However, TSH will not normalize quickly and often lags behind normalization of serum T_3 and T_4. Hence, evaluation should not be done until 6 to 8 weeks after starting treatment. A TSH target of 0.5 to 2 microunits/mL is appropriate for most patients. Once an adequate replacement dosage is established, TSH levels will remain suppressed for the duration of treatment.

In some cases serum T_4 must be used to evaluate therapy, because TSH secretion remains high in some patients even though levels of thyroid hormones have been restored to normal. When this happens, success is indicated by levels of T_4 in the normal to high-normal range—whether or not TSH values are normal.

Duration of Therapy. For most hypothyroid patients, replacement therapy must be continued for life. Treatment provides symptomatic relief but does not produce cure. Patients must be made fully aware of the chronic nature of their condition. In addition, they should be forewarned that, although therapy will cause symptoms to improve, these improvements do not constitute a reason to interrupt or discontinue drug use.

Dosage and Administration II: Specific Applications

Hypothyroidism in Adults. When calculated on a body weight basis, the average adult dosage is about 1.6 mcg/kg/day. Most patients under the age of 50 can be started on full replacement doses (100 to 125 mcg/day for a 70-kg adult). For older patients, dosage should be low initially and then gradually increased. A typical starting dosage is 25 to 50 mcg/day. For older adults with coronary heart disease, the starting dosage is even lower—between 12.5 and 25 mcg/day.

Myxedema Coma. Myxedema coma is a rare but serious condition that requires rapid treatment. Levothyroxine is administered IV in a dose of 200 to 500 mcg. If required, an additional dose of 100 to 300 mcg can be given 1 day later. Glucocorticoids (e.g., hydrocortisone) are also required.

Congenital Hypothyroidism. In congenital hypothyroidism, thyroid hormone dosage decreases with age. For infants less than 3 months old, the dosage is 10 to 15 mcg/kg/day; for children ages 3 to 6 months, 8 to 10 mcg/kg/day;

for children ages 6 to 12 months, 6 to 8 mcg/kg/day; for children ages 1 to 5 years, 5 to 6 mcg/kg/day; and for children ages 6 to 12 years, 4 to 5 mcg/kg/day. In all cases, dosage is adjusted to normalize TSH and free T_4.

Simple Goiter. In simple goiter, the thyroid is enlarged and levels of thyroid hormones are reduced. Thyroid enlargement is caused by TSH that has been released in response to low levels of thyroid hormones. When treating simple goiter, the goal is to provide full replacement doses of thyroid hormones, so as to suppress further TSH release. For many patients, this can be achieved with 100 to 200 mcg of levothyroxine daily.

Liothyronine (T_3)

Liothyronine [Cytomel, Triostat] is a synthetic preparation of triiodothyronine, a naturally occurring thyroid hormone. The structure of liothyronine is identical to that of thyroid-derived T_3. Since liothyronine is the active form of levothyroxine, the effects of the two drugs are identical.

Contrasts With Levothyroxine

Liothyronine differs from levothyroxine in three important ways: (1) liothyronine has a shorter half-life and shorter duration of action, (2) liothyronine has a more rapid onset, and (3) liothyronine is more expensive. Because of its high price and relatively brief duration of action, liothyronine is less desirable than levothyroxine for long-term use. However, because its effects develop quickly, liothyronine may be superior to levothyroxine in situations that require speedy results, especially myxedema coma.

Evaluation

As with levothyroxine, the dosage of liothyronine is adjusted on the basis of clinical evaluation and laboratory data. Two laboratory tests are useful: free serum T_3 and serum TSH. Since liothyronine is not converted into T_4, plasma levels of T_4 remain low. Hence, T_4 levels cannot be used to assess treatment.

Dosage and Administration

The usual route is oral, using *Cytomel,* although dosing may also be done IV, using *Triostat.* Oral dosage is about 80% of the dosage of levothyroxine. Because of its short half-life, oral liothyronine is taken twice daily, in contrast to levothyroxine, which is taken once daily.

Other Thyroid Preparations

Liotrix

Liotrix [Thyrolar] is a mixture of synthetic T_4 plus synthetic T_3 in a 4:1 fixed ratio. (This ratio is similar to the ratio of these hormones in plasma.) The rationale for using liotrix is that the mixture can produce plasma levels of T_4 and T_3 similar to those that occur naturally. However, since levothyroxine alone produces the same ratio of T_4 to T_3, liotrix offers no advantage over levothyroxine for most indications.

Thyroid (Desiccated)

Thyroid [Armour Thyroid, others] consists of desiccated animal thyroid glands. Standardization is based on content of iodine, levothyroxine, and liothyronine. The ratio of levothyroxine to liothyronine is not less than 5:1. Thyroid is available in tablets (15 to 300 mg). For practical purposes, thyroid is obsolete: Use is limited to patients who have been taking the preparation for years. Thyroid is rarely prescribed for patients starting therapy today.

DRUGS FOR HYPERTHYROIDISM

Antithyroid Drugs: Thionamides

The thionamide drugs—methimazole and propylthiouracil (PTU)—suppress synthesis of thyroid hormones. These agents can be used long term to treat hyperthyroidism, or short term as preparation for subtotal thyroidectomy or therapy with radioactive iodine. Methimazole and PTU are similar in most respects. Primary differences concern pharmacokinetics (Table 58.3) and adverse effects.

Methimazole

Methimazole [Tapazole] is a first-line drug for hyperthyroidism. Benefits derive from inhibiting thyroid hormone synthesis.

TABLE 58.3 ▪ Pharmacokinetics of Methimazole and Propylthiouracil

	Methimazole	Propylthiouracil
Bioavailability	80%–95%	80%–95%
Plasma protein binding	0	75%–80%
Levels in breast milk	Low	Low
Transplacental passage	Higher	Low
Half-life	6–13 hr	1–2 hr
Dosing frequency		
Initial therapy	1–3 times/day	3 or 4 times/day
Maintenance therapy	Once daily	2 or 3 times/day

Methimazole is safer and more convenient than PTU, and hence is preferred for most patients—except women who are pregnant or breast-feeding, and perhaps patients who are in thyrotoxic crisis.

Mechanism of Action. Therapeutic effects result from blocking synthesis of thyroid hormones. Two mechanisms are involved. First, methimazole prevents the oxidation of iodide, thereby inhibiting incorporation of iodine into tyrosine. Second, methimazole prevents iodinated tyrosines from coupling. Both effects result from inhibiting peroxidase, the enzyme that catalyzes both reactions.

Please note that although methimazole prevents thyroid hormone synthesis, it does not destroy existing stores of thyroid hormone. Hence, once therapy has begun, it may take 3 to 12 weeks to produce a euthyroid state.

Pharmacokinetics. Methimazole is well absorbed following oral dosing. Binding to plasma proteins is minimal. The drug readily crosses membranes, including those of the placenta. Levels in breast milk are sufficient to affect the nursing infant. The plasma half-life is 6 to 13 hours—long enough to permit once-a-day dosing.

Therapeutic Uses. Methimazole has four applications in hyperthyroidism:

- It can be used as the sole form of therapy for Graves' disease.
- It can be employed as an adjunct to radiation therapy until the effects of radiation become manifest.
- It can be given to suppress thyroid hormone synthesis in preparation for thyroid gland surgery (subtotal thyroidectomy).
- It can be given to patients experiencing thyrotoxic crisis.

Adverse Effects. Methimazole is generally well tolerated, but should be avoided by women who are pregnant or breast-feeding. In addition, the National Institute for Occupational Safety and Health (NIOSH) has designated methimazole as a hazardous agent; it should be handled with caution by healthcare providers of childbearing age. See Chapter 3, Table 3.1, for administration and handling guidelines.

Agranulocytosis is the most dangerous toxicity. If agranulocytosis occurs, methimazole should be discontinued. Agranulocytosis will then reverse. Treatment with granulocyte colony-stimulating factor (filgrastim [Neupogen]) may accelerate recovery.

> **Safety Alert**
>
> **AGRANULOCYTOSIS**
>
> Agranulocytosis is a serious condition characterized by a dramatic reduction in circulating granulocytes, a type of white blood cell needed to fight infection. The reaction is rare (about 3 cases per 10,000 patients) and usually develops during the first 2 months of therapy. Sore throat and fever may be the earliest indications, and patients should be instructed to report these immediately. Because agranulocytosis often develops rapidly, periodic blood counts cannot guarantee early detection.

Hypothyroidism. When given in high doses, methimazole can convert the patient from a hyperthyroid state to a hypothyroid state. If this occurs, dosage should be reduced. Temporary treatment with thyroid hormone may be required.

Effects in Pregnancy. Methimazole can cause neonatal hypothyroidism, goiter, and even congenital hypothyroidism. Accordingly, the drug should be avoided during the first trimester. Use in the second and third trimesters is considered safe. Compared with methimazole, PTU crosses the placenta poorly, and hence risk to the fetus is low. Accordingly, if a thionamide is needed during the first trimester of pregnancy, PTU is the preferred drug.

Effects in Lactation. Methimazole therapy does not affect thyroid function or intellectual development in breast-fed infants with doses up to 20 mg daily.

Preparations, Dosage, and Administration. Methimazole is supplied in tablets (5 and 10 mg) for oral dosing. For treatment of severe disease, doses are high initially (e.g., 30 to 40 mg once a day) and then decreased for maintenance (5 to 15 mg once a day). As a rule, treatment continues for 1 to 2 years. When methimazole is discontinued, some 30% to 40% of patients remain euthyroid, indicating remission. Others become hyperthyroid in 1 to 4 weeks, indicating relapse. If relapse occurs, another round of methimazole can be tried. Alternatively, the patient can opt for radiation therapy or surgery.

Propylthiouracil

Like methimazole, PTU suppresses synthesis of thyroid hormones and can be used for Graves' disease and other hyperthyroid states. Propylthiouracil, a much older drug than methimazole, is now considered a second-line treatment.

Contrasts With Methimazole. Propylthiouracil is much like methimazole, but with four significant differences:

- First, and most important, PTU can cause severe liver injury, whereas methimazole does not.
- Second, PTU has a shorter half-life than methimazole (90 minutes vs. 6 to 13 hours), and hence requires two or three daily doses rather than one.
- Third, PTU crosses the placenta less readily than does methimazole.
- Fourth, PTU blocks conversion of T_4 to T_3 in the periphery, whereas methimazole does not.

Current Role in Treating Hyperthyroidism. Because PTU is more toxic than methimazole and requires more daily doses, methimazole is preferred for most patients. However, there are three groups for whom PTU is preferred:

- Pregnant women, but only during the first trimester. (Methimazole is preferred during the second and third trimesters.)
- Patients experiencing thyroid storm. (Because PTU can block conversion of T_4 to T_3, it may be more effective than methimazole.)
- Patients who are intolerant of methimazole.

Pharmacokinetics. Propylthiouracil is rapidly absorbed following oral administration. Therapeutic actions begin within 30 minutes. Plasma protein binding is moderate (75% to 80%). The half-life is short (about 90 minutes), and hence PTU must be administered 2 or 3 times a day. Transplacental passage is low, as is entry into breast milk.

Adverse Effects. As with methimazole, adverse effects are relatively rare. Nonetheless, severe adverse effects can occur, especially liver injury and agranulocytosis. The most common undesired effect is rash. PTU may also cause nausea, arthralgia, headache, dizziness, and paresthesias.

Adverse Effects Shared With Methimazole. Like methimazole, PTU has caused rare cases of agranulocytosis and can cause hypothyroidism if the dosage is too high. In addition, PTU can harm the developing fetus and the breast-feeding infant.

Liver Injury. Propylthiouracil has caused rare cases of severe liver injury. Transplants have been required, and deaths have occurred. Children are especially vulnerable. The incidence in children is 1 case in 2000, compared with 1 case in 10,000 for adults. Liver toxicity is unrelated to dosage or duration of treatment. Furthermore, onset is sudden and progression is rapid, and hence performing routine tests of liver function doesn't help. Patients should be forewarned of the potential for liver injury and instructed to promptly report any signs, such as fatigue, weakness, abdominal pain, reduced appetite, dark urine, or yellowing of the eyes or skin. If these signs appear, PTU should be discontinued until hepatotoxicity has been ruled out.

Preparations, Dosage, and Administration. Propylthiouracil is available in 50-mg tablets for oral use. Because of its short half-life, PTU requires multiple daily doses.

Treatment of Graves' Disease. High doses (100 to 300 mg 3 times a day) are used initially. Lower doses (e.g., 50 mg 3 times a day) are used for maintenance. As a rule, treatment continues for 1 to 2 years.

PATIENT-CENTERED CARE ACROSS THE LIFE SPAN

Thyroid Drugs

Life Stage	Patient Care Concerns
Infants	Thyroid hormone preparation is used to treat hypothyroidism in infants. Treatment should continue for 3 years.
Children/ adolescents	Thyroid hormone preparations are used in children and adolescents. Doses are based on clinical response. Antithyroid drugs (methimazole and PTU) are also safe in children. Iodine-131 is not generally used in children.
Pregnant women	Iodine-131 is classified in FDA Pregnancy Risk Category X[a] and is contraindicated in pregnancy. Methimazole should be avoided in the first trimester of pregnancy.
Breast-feeding women	Thyroid hormone preparations and antithyroid medications are generally safe in breast-feeding women.
Older adults	Thyroid gland dysfunction is common in the older adult. This is associated with increased morbidity if not treated. Thyroid hormone preparations and antithyroid medications can be used successfully to treat thyroid dysfunction in the older adult.

[a]As of 2020, the FDA will no longer use Pregnancy Risk Categories. Please refer to Chapter 9 for more information.

Radioactive Iodine (^{131}I)

Physical Properties

Iodine-131 is a radioactive isotope of stable iodine that emits a combination of beta particles and gamma rays. Radioactive decay of ^{131}I takes place rapidly, with a half-life of 8 days.

Hence, after 56 days (seven half-lives), less than 1% of the radioactivity in a dose of ^{131}I remains.

Use in Graves' Disease

Iodine-131 can be used to destroy thyroid tissue in patients with hyperthyroidism. The objective is to produce clinical remission without causing complete destruction of the gland. Unfortunately, delayed hypothyroidism, due to excessive thyroid damage, is a frequent complication.

Effect on the Thyroid. Like stable iodine, ^{131}I is concentrated in the thyroid gland. Destruction of thyroid tissue is produced primarily by emission of beta particles. (The gamma rays from ^{131}I are relatively harmless.) Because beta particles have a very limited ability to penetrate any type of physical barrier, they do not travel outside the thyroid. Hence, damage to surrounding tissue is minimal.

Reduction of thyroid function is gradual. Initial effects become apparent in days or weeks. Full effects develop in 2 to 3 months.

Not all patients respond satisfactorily to a single treatment. About 66% of patients with Graves' disease are cured with a single exposure to ^{131}I. Others require two or more treatments.

Advantages and Disadvantages of ^{131}I Therapy. The advantages of ^{131}I treatment are considerable: (1) low cost; (2) patients are spared the risks, discomfort, and expense of thyroid surgery; (3) death from ^{131}I treatment is extremely rare; and (4) no tissue other than the thyroid is injured (patients should be reassured of this).

Treatment with ^{131}I is not without drawbacks. First, the effect of treatment is delayed, taking several months to become maximal. Second, and more important, treatment is associated with a significant incidence of delayed hypothyroidism. Hypothyroidism results from excessive dosage and occurs in up to 90% of patients within the first year following ^{131}I exposure.

Who Should Be Treated and Who Should Not. Iodine-131 is indicated for adults with hyperthyroidism, as well as in patients who have not responded adequately to antithyroid drugs or to subtotal thyroidectomy.

As a rule, very young children are considered inappropriate candidates. The likelihood of delayed hypothyroidism is higher than in adults. Also, there is concern that administration of ^{131}I to young patients may carry a slight risk of cancer. It should be noted, however, that there is no evidence that the use of ^{131}I in Graves' disease has ever caused cancer of the thyroid or any other tissue. Although ^{131}I is generally avoided in young children, it is commonly used in postpubertal adolescents and young adults.

Iodine-131 is *contraindicated in pregnancy and lactation.* Exposure of the fetus to ^{131}I after the first trimester may damage the immature thyroid, and exposure to radiation at any point in fetal life carries a risk of generalized developmental harm. Accordingly, a negative pregnancy test is required before giving ^{131}I. Because ^{131}I enters breast milk, women receiving this agent should not breast-feed.

Dosage. Dosage of ^{131}I is determined by thyroid size and by the rate of thyroidal iodine uptake. For Graves' disease, the dosage usually ranges between 4 and 10 millicuries (mCi).

Use in Thyroid Cancer

Iodine-131 can be used to destroy malignant thyroid cells. However, since most forms of thyroid cancer do not accumulate iodine, only a small percentage of patients are candidates for ^{131}I therapy.

The doses of ^{131}I used to treat cancer are large, ranging from 50 to 150 mCi. These doses are much higher than those used in Graves' disease. Because high amounts of radioactivity are involved, body wastes must be disposed of properly. In addition, adverse effects from large doses of ^{131}I can be severe: radiation sickness may occur; leukemia may be produced; and bone marrow function may be depressed, resulting in leukopenia, thrombocytopenia, and anemia. Fortunately, these severe effects are rare.

Diagnostic Use

Iodine-131 is employed to diagnose a variety of thyroid disorders, including hyperthyroidism, hypothyroidism, and goiter. Following ^{131}I administration, the thyroid is scanned for uptake of radioactivity; the amount and location of ^{131}I uptake reveal the extent of thyroid activity. Doses for diagnosis are minuscule (less than 1 mCi for children and less than 10 mCi for adults). These tracer doses pose virtually no threat to health. Please note that although ^{131}I can be used for diagnosis, the preferred isotope is ^{123}I.

Preparations

Iodine-131 is supplied in capsules and solution for oral administration. Both preparations are odorless and tasteless. Capsules contain between 0.75 and 100 mCi of ^{131}I. Vials of oral solution contain between 3.5 and 150 mCi of ^{131}I.

Nonradioactive Iodine: Lugol's Solution

Description

Lugol's solution, also known as *strong iodine solution,* is a mixture containing 5% elemental iodine and 10% potassium iodide. The iodine undergoes reduction to iodide within the GI tract before absorption.

Mechanism of Action

When present in high concentrations, iodide has a paradoxical suppressant effect on the thyroid. Three mechanisms are involved. First, high concentrations of iodide decrease iodine uptake by the thyroid. Second, high concentrations of iodide inhibit thyroid hormone synthesis by suppressing both the iodination of tyrosine and the coupling of iodinated tyrosine residues. Third, high concentrations of iodine inhibit release of thyroid hormone into the blood. All three actions combine to decrease circulating levels of T_3 and T_4.

Unfortunately, the effects of iodide on thyroid function cannot be sustained indefinitely. With long-term iodide administration, suppressant effects become weaker. Accordingly, iodide is rarely used alone for thyroid suppression.

Therapeutic Use

Strong iodine solution can be given to hyperthyroid individuals to suppress thyroid function in preparation for thyroidectomy. Initial effects develop within 24 hours. Peak effects develop in 10 to 15 days. In most cases, plasma levels of thyroid hormone are reduced with methimazole before initiating strong iodine solution. Then strong iodine solution (along with more PTU) is administered for the last 10 days before surgery. In addition to its use before thyroidectomy, strong iodine solution is employed in thyrotoxic crisis and as an antiseptic (see Chapter 96).

Adverse Effects

Chronic ingestion of iodine can produce *iodism.* Signs and symptoms include a brassy taste, a burning sensation in the mouth and throat, soreness of the teeth and gums, frontal headache, coryza (nasal inflammation and sneezing), salivation, and various skin eruptions. All of these fade rapidly after iodine use stops.

Overdose

Iodine is corrosive, so overdose will injure the GI tract. Symptoms include abdominal pain, vomiting, and diarrhea. Swelling of the glottis may cause asphyxiation. Treatment consists of gastric lavage (to remove iodine from the stomach) and giving sodium thiosulfate (to reduce iodine to iodide).

Dosage and Administration

When employed to prepare hyperthyroid patients for thyroidectomy, strong iodine solution is administered in a dosage of 5 to 7 drops 3 times daily for 10 days immediately preceding surgery. Iodine solution should be mixed with juice or some other beverage to mask its unpleasant taste. The dosage for thyrotoxic crisis is 10 drops every 8 hours.

Beta Blockers

Propranolol [Inderal LA, InnoPran XL] and other beta blockers can suppress tachycardia and other symptoms of *Graves' disease.* Benefits derive from beta-adrenergic blockade, not from reducing levels of T_3 or T_4. One advantage of beta blockers is that they work quickly, unlike PTU, methimazole, and ^{131}I. Dosages for hyperthyroidism are highly individualized.

Beta blockers are also beneficial in *thyrotoxic crisis.* In the absence of contraindications (e.g., asthma, heart failure), all patients should receive one immediately. Administration may be oral or IV. The dosage for propranolol is 10 to 40 mg PO every 6 to 8 hours, or 0.5 to 1 mg IV repeated every four hours until effects are observed.

The basic pharmacology of beta blockers is discussed in Chapter 18.

KEY POINTS

- The thyroid gland produces two active hormones: triiodothyronine (T_3), which is highly active, and thyroxine (T_4, tetraiodothyronine), which appears inactive.
- Thyroid hormones have three principal actions: stimulation of energy use, stimulation of the heart, and promotion of growth and development.
- Hormonal regulation of thyroid function occurs as follows: TRH from the hypothalamus causes the pituitary to release TSH, which causes the thyroid to make and release T_3 and T_4, which then act on the pituitary to suppress further release of TSH.
- The four steps in thyroid hormone synthesis are (1) uptake of iodide by the thyroid, (2) conversion of iodide to iodine, (3) linking of iodine to tyrosine, and (4) coupling of two iodinated tyrosines to form T_3 or T_4.
- Much of the T_4 released by the thyroid is converted to T_3 in the periphery.
- Low plasma levels of iodine stimulate synthesis of T_3 and T_4.
- In iodine-sufficient countries, the major cause of hypothyroidism is chronic autoimmune thyroiditis (Hashimoto's thyroiditis).
- A goiter is an enlargement of the thyroid.
- Testing serum for elevated levels of TSH is the most sensitive way to diagnose hypothyroidism.
- Most patients with hypothyroidism require lifelong replacement therapy with thyroid hormones.
- Maternal hypothyroidism during the first trimester of pregnancy can result in permanent neuropsychologic deficits in the child.
- Levothyroxine (synthetic T_4) is the drug of choice for most patients who require thyroid hormone replacement.
- There is debate as to whether certain levothyroxine preparations are interchangeable. Until the debate is resolved, it would seem best for patients to use only one product, unless the switch is approved of and monitored by the prescriber.
- Levothyroxine should be taken on an empty stomach in the morning, at least 30 to 60 minutes before eating.
- Chronic overtreatment with levothyroxine can cause atrial fibrillation and bone loss, especially in older adults.
- Many drugs—including cholestyramine [Questran], colestipol [Colestid], sucralfate [Carafate], H_2 receptor blockers, proton pump inhibitors, aluminum-containing antacids, iron supplements, and calcium supplements—can significantly reduce levothyroxine absorption. At least 4 hours should separate administration of levothyroxine and these drugs.
- Levothyroxine can intensify the anticoagulant effects of warfarin.
- Graves' disease is the most common cause of excessive thyroid hormone secretion.
- Graves' disease can be treated by surgical removal of thyroid tissue, destruction of thyroid tissue with radioactive iodine (^{131}I), or treatment with antithyroid drugs (methimazole or propylthiouracil).
- Methimazole, an antithyroid drug, benefits patients with hyperthyroidism by suppressing thyroid hormone synthesis.
- Full benefits of methimazole may take 3 to 12 weeks to develop.
- The most serious adverse effect of methimazole is agranulocytosis.
- Methimazole should be avoided during the first trimester of pregnancy.
- Methimazole is on the NIOSH hazardous drug list and should be handled with caution by healthcare workers of childbearing age
- Full effects of ^{131}I require 2 to 3 months to develop.
- Iodine-131 is contraindicated during pregnancy and lactation.
- Strong iodine solution (Lugol's solution) can be used to suppress thyroid hormone synthesis.

Please visit **http://evolve.elsevier.com/Lehne** for chapter-specific NCLEX® examination review questions.

Summary of Major Nursing Implications[a]

LEVOTHYROXINE (T_4)

Preadministration Assessment

Therapeutic Goal

Resolution of signs and symptoms of hypothyroidism and restoration of normal laboratory values for serum TSH and free T_4.

Baseline Data

Obtain serum levels of TSH and free T_4.

Implementation: Administration

Routes

Oral, IV.

Administration

Oral. **Instruct the patient to take levothyroxine on an empty stomach in the morning, at least 30 to 60 minutes before breakfast.**

Make certain the patient understands that replacement therapy must continue for life. Caution patients against discontinuing treatment without consulting the prescriber.

Intravenous. Intravenous administration is reserved for treating myxedema coma and for patients who cannot take levothyroxine orally.

Ongoing Evaluation and Interventions

Evaluating Therapeutic Effects

Adults. Clinical evaluation should reveal reversal of signs of thyroid deficiency and an absence of signs of thyroid excess (e.g., tachycardia). Laboratory tests should indicate normal plasma levels of TSH and T_4.

Infants. Clinical evaluation should reveal normalization of intellectual function, growth, and development. Monthly measurements of height provide a good index of thyroid sufficiency. Laboratory tests should show normal plasma levels of TSH and T_4. (*Note:* TSH levels may remain high in some children, despite adequate dosing.)

Minimizing Adverse Effects

Thyrotoxicosis. Overdose may cause thyrotoxicosis. **Inform patients about symptoms of thyrotoxicosis (tachycardia, angina, tremor, nervousness, insomnia, hyperthermia, heat intolerance, sweating), and instruct them to notify the prescriber if these develop.**

Atrial Fibrillation and Bone Loss. Chronic overtreatment with levothyroxine can cause atrial fibrillation and fractures (from bone loss), especially in older adults. To prevent overtreatment, measure TSH levels at least once a year.

Minimizing Adverse Interactions

Drugs That Reduce Levothyroxine Absorption. Absorption of levothyroxine can be reduced by multiple drugs, including H_2 receptor blockers, proton pump inhibitors, cholestyramine, colestipol, sucralfate, aluminum-containing antacids, iron supplements, calcium supplements, magnesium salts, and orlistat. **Instruct patients to separate administration of levothyroxine and these drugs by 4 hours.**

Drugs That Accelerate Levothyroxine Metabolism. Several drugs, including carbamazepine, rifampin, phenytoin, phenobarbital, and sertraline, can accelerate metabolism of levothyroxine and can thereby reduce its effects. An increase in levothyroxine dosage may be needed.

Warfarin. Levothyroxine can intensify the effects of warfarin. Warfarin dosage may need to be reduced.

Catecholamines. Thyroid hormones sensitize the heart to catecholamines (epinephrine, dopamine, dobutamine) and may promote dysrhythmias. Exercise caution when catecholamines and levothyroxine are used together.

LIOTHYRONINE (T_3)

With the exceptions noted below, the nursing implications for liothyronine are the same as those for levothyroxine.

Evaluating Therapeutic Effects

Success is indicated by resolution of the signs and symptoms of hypothyroidism and by normalization of plasma T_3 and TSH levels. T_4 levels cannot be used to evaluate therapy.

METHIMAZOLE

Preadministration Assessment

Therapeutic Goals

Methimazole has four indications: (1) reduction of thyroid hormone production in Graves' disease, (2) control of hyperthyroidism until the effects of radiation on the thyroid become manifest, (3) suppression of thyroid hormone production before subtotal thyroidectomy, and (4) treatment of thyrotoxic crisis.

Baseline Data

Obtain serum levels of free T_3 and free T_4.

Identifying High-Risk Patients

Methimazole should be *avoided* during the first trimester of pregnancy.

Implementation: Administration

Route

Oral.

Administration

Instruct the patient to take methimazole once daily, at the same time every day.

Ongoing Evaluation and Interventions

Summary of Monitoring

Evaluate treatment by monitoring for weight gain, decreased heart rate, and other indications that levels of thyroid hormone

Continued

Summary of Major Nursing Implications[a]—cont'd

have declined. Laboratory tests should indicate a decrease in serum free T_3 and free T_4.

Minimizing Adverse Effects

Agranulocytosis. **Inform patients about early signs of agranulocytosis (fever, sore throat), and instruct them to notify the prescriber if these develop.** If follow-up blood tests reveal leukopenia, methimazole should be withdrawn. Giving granulocyte colony-stimulating factor may accelerate recovery.

Hypothyroidism. Methimazole may cause excessive reductions in thyroid hormone synthesis. If signs of hypothyroidism develop or if plasma levels of T_3 and T_4 become subnormal, methimazole dosage should be reduced. Supplemental thyroid hormone may be needed.

Effects in Pregnancy. When used during the first trimester, methimazole can cause neonatal hypothyroidism, goiter, and even congenital hypothyroidism. Use in the second and third trimesters is considered safe. If a thionamide is needed during the first trimester of pregnancy, PTU should be selected.

RADIOACTIVE IODINE (^{131}I)

Use in Graves' Disease

Therapeutic Goal

Suppression of thyroid hormone production.

Identifying High-Risk Patients

Iodine-131 is *contraindicated* during pregnancy and lactation.

Dosage and Administration

Iodine-131 is administered in capsules or an oral liquid. The dosing objective is to reduce thyroid hormone production without causing complete thyroid destruction. The dosage for Graves' disease is 4 to 10 mCi.

Promoting Therapeutic Effects

Responses take 2 to 3 months to develop fully. Methimazole or propylthiouracil may be required during this interval.

Minimizing Adverse Effects

Excessive thyroid destruction can cause hypothyroidism. Patients who develop thyroid insufficiency need thyroid hormone supplements.

Use in Thyroid Cancer

High doses (50 to 150 mCi) are required. These doses can cause radiation sickness, leukemia, and bone marrow depression. Monitor for these effects. Body wastes will be contaminated with radioactivity and must be disposed of appropriately.

Diagnostic Use

Iodine-131 is used to diagnose hyperthyroidism, hypothyroidism, and goiter. Diagnostic doses are so small (less than 10 mCi) as to be virtually harmless.

STRONG IODINE SOLUTION (LUGOL'S SOLUTION)

Preadministration Assessment

Therapeutic Goal

Suppression of thyroid hormone production in preparation for subtotal thyroidectomy. Also used to suppress thyroid hormone release in patients experiencing thyroid storm.

Baseline Data

Obtain tests of thyroid function.

Implementation: Administration

Route

Oral.

Administration

Advise patients to dilute strong iodine solution with fruit juice or another beverage to increase palatability.

Ongoing Evaluation and Interventions

Minimizing Adverse Effects

Mild Toxicity. **Inform patients about symptoms of iodism (brassy taste, burning sensations in the mouth, soreness of gums and teeth), and instruct them to discontinue treatment and notify the prescriber if these occur.** Symptoms fade upon drug withdrawal.

Severe Toxicity. Iodine solution can cause corrosive injury to the GI tract. **Instruct patients to discontinue the drug and notify the prescriber immediately if severe abdominal distress develops.** Treatment includes gastric lavage and giving sodium thiosulfate.

[a]Patient education information is highlighted as **blue text.**

CHAPTER

59 Drugs Related to Hypothalamic and Pituitary Function

The hypothalamus and pituitary are intimately related both anatomically and functionally. Working together, these structures help regulate practically all bodily processes. To achieve their widespread effects, the hypothalamus and pituitary employ at least 15 hormones and releasing factors (Fig. 59.1). As you can imagine, the endocrinology of these structures is exceedingly complex. However, rather than discussing all relevant information in depth, we will focus on just three agents: growth hormone (GH), antidiuretic hormone (ADH), and prolactin. Additional hypothalamic and pituitary hormones of therapeutic interest are considered briefly here and discussed further in other chapters.

OVERVIEW OF HYPOTHALAMIC AND PITUITARY ENDOCRINOLOGY

Anatomic Considerations

The pituitary sits in a depression in the skull located just below the third ventricle of the brain; the hypothalamus is located immediately above (see Fig. 59.1). The pituitary has two divisions: the *anterior pituitary* (or adenohypophysis) and *posterior pituitary* (or neurohypophysis). Both divisions are under hypothalamic control. The hypothalamus communicates with the anterior pituitary by way of release-regulating factors delivered through a system of portal blood vessels. In contrast, communication with the posterior pituitary is neuronal.

Hormones of the Anterior Pituitary

The anterior pituitary produces six major hormones. Production and release of these hormones is controlled largely by the hypothalamus. Functions of the anterior pituitary hormones are as follows:

- *Growth hormone* (GH) stimulates growth in practically all tissues and organs.
- *Corticotropin* (adrenocorticotropic hormone [ACTH]) acts on the adrenal cortex to promote synthesis and release of adrenocortical hormones.
- *Thyrotropin* (thyroid-stimulating hormone [TSH]) acts on the thyroid gland to promote synthesis and release of thyroid hormones.
- *Follicle-stimulating hormone* (FSH) acts on the ovaries to promote follicular growth and development, and acts on the testes to promote spermatogenesis.
- *Luteinizing hormone* (LH) acts on the ovaries to promote ovulation and development of the corpus luteum, and acts on the testes to promote androgen production.
- *Prolactin* stimulates milk production after childbirth.

Hormones of the Posterior Pituitary

The posterior pituitary has only two hormones: *oxytocin* and *antidiuretic hormone.* The principal function of oxytocin is to facilitate uterine contractions at term. ADH promotes renal conservation of water.

Although oxytocin and ADH are considered hormones of the posterior pituitary, these agents are actually synthesized in the hypothalamus. The cells that make oxytocin and ADH are called neurosecretory cells. These cells originate in the hypothalamus and project their axons to the posterior pituitary. Oxytocin and ADH are produced within the bodies of these cells and then undergo transport down axons to the axon

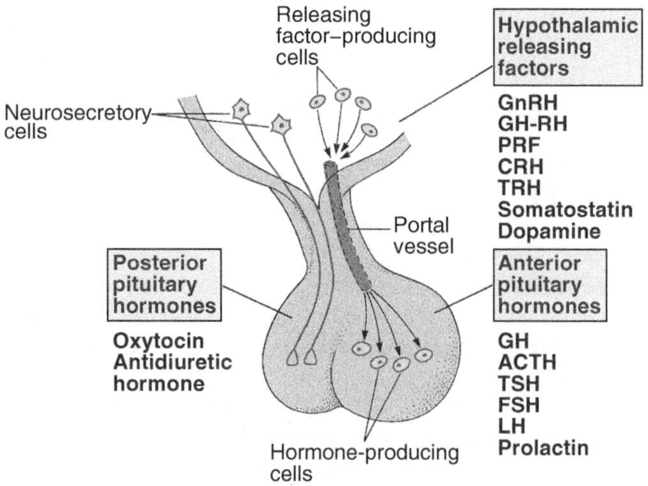

Fig. 59.1 ▪ Hormones and releasing factors of the hypothalamus and pituitary.
Hypothalamic releasing factors: GnRH, gonadotropin-releasing hormone; GH-RH, growth hormone–releasing hormone; PRF, prolactin-releasing factor; CRH, corticotropin-releasing hormone; TRH, thyrotropin-releasing hormone. *Anterior pituitary hormones:* GH, growth hormone; ACTH, adrenocorticotropic hormone (corticotropin); TSH, thyroid-stimulating hormone; FSH, follicle-stimulating hormone; LH, luteinizing hormone.

terminals for storage. When appropriate stimuli impinge upon the bodies of the neurosecretory cells, impulses are sent down the axon, causing hormone release.

Hypothalamic Release-Regulating Factors

The hypothalamus has the primary responsibility for regulating the release of hormones from the *anterior* pituitary. To accomplish this, the hypothalamus employs seven different release-regulating factors. Most of these factors *stimulate* the release of anterior pituitary hormones. However, two of these factors *inhibit* hormone release. The hypothalamic release-regulating factors are delivered to the anterior pituitary via portal blood vessels. Although the hypothalamic releasing factors are of extreme *physiologic* importance, only five of them—growth hormone–releasing hormone, thyrotropin-releasing hormone, gonadotropin-releasing hormone, corticotropin-releasing hormone, and somatostatin—have clinical applications. These are the only hypothalamic release-regulating factors discussed in this chapter.

Feedback Regulation of the Hypothalamus and Anterior Pituitary

With few exceptions, the release of hypothalamic and anterior pituitary hormones is regulated by a *negative feedback loop* (Fig. 59.2). In this example, the loop begins with the secretion of releasing-factor *X* from the hypothalamus. Factor *X* then acts on the anterior pituitary to stimulate release of hormone A. Hormone A then acts on its target gland to promote release of hormone B. Hormone B has two actions: (1) it produces its designated biologic effects and (2) it acts on the hypothalamus and pituitary to inhibit further release of factor *X* and hormone A. This feedback inhibition of the hypothalamus and pituitary suppresses further release of hormone B itself, thereby keeping levels of hormone B within an appropriate range.

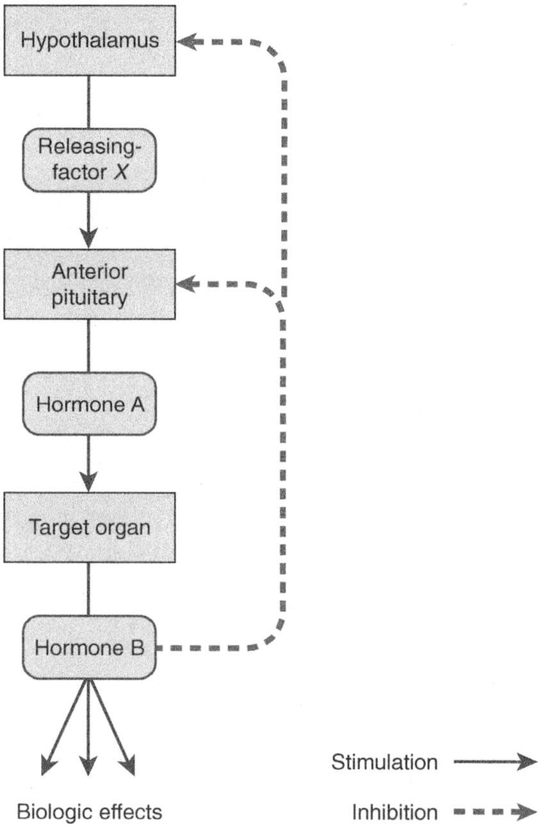

Fig. 59.2 ▪ Negative feedback regulation of the hypothalamus and anterior pituitary.
The feedback loop works as follows: Releasing-factor *X* stimulates the pituitary to release hormone A, which stimulates its target organ, causing release of hormone B. Hormone B then acts on the hypothalamus and pituitary to suppress further release of factor *X* and hormone A, thereby suppressing further release of hormone B itself.

GROWTH HORMONE

Growth hormone is a large polypeptide hormone (191 amino acids) produced by the anterior pituitary. As its name suggests, GH helps regulate growth. Childhood deficiency of GH results in *short stature.* Excessive GH results in *gigantism* (when too much is present before puberty) and *acromegaly* (when too much is present during adulthood).

Physiology

Regulation of Release

Factors that regulate GH release are shown in Fig. 59.3. The hypothalamus first releases growth hormone–releasing hormone (GH-RH), which stimulates release of GH from the pituitary. GH then acts on the liver and other tissues to cause release of *insulin-like growth factor-1* (IGF-1). IGF-1 has two actions: it (1) promotes growth and (2) acts on the hypothalamus and pituitary to suppress release of GH-RH and GH, completing a negative feedback loop.

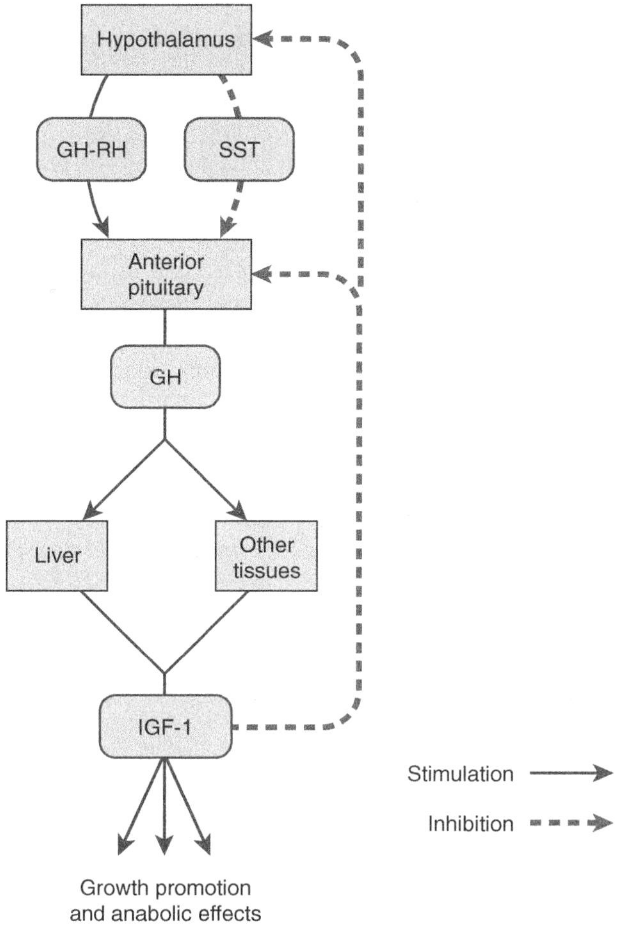

Fig. 59.3 ▪ Regulation of growth hormone release. (*GH,* Growth hormone; *GH-RH,* growth hormone–releasing hormone; *IGF-1,* insulin-like growth factor-1; *SST,* somatostatin.)

One additional hormone, *somatostatin,* helps regulate GH release. Somatostatin is produced in the hypothalamus and acts on the pituitary to *inhibit* GH release.

Biologic Effects

Promotion of Growth. GH, acting through IGF-1, stimulates the growth of practically all organs and tissues. If administered to a GH-deficient child before epiphyseal closure, GH will increase bone length, producing a corresponding increase in height. The size and number of muscle cells are increased, resulting in enlargement of muscle mass, and the internal organs are stimulated to grow in proportion to overall body growth. The only structures that do not respond noticeably are the brain and eyes.

Promotion of Protein Synthesis. For growth to occur, cells must increase production of protein. GH facilitates this process by increasing amino acid uptake and utilization. Since amino acids have substantial nitrogen content, increased protein synthesis results in net nitrogen retention, which is reflected in reduced urinary nitrogen excretion. Increased amino acid utilization also causes blood urea nitrogen to fall.

Effect on Carbohydrate Metabolism. GH reduces glucose utilization, causing a tendency for plasma levels of glucose to rise. When GH is administered to nondiabetics, elevation of blood glucose stimulates release of insulin, thereby maintaining glucose levels within a normal range. In contrast, when GH is administered to patients with type 1 diabetes, insulin cannot be released. As a result, the hyperglycemic action of GH goes unopposed, allowing plasma glucose levels to rise, sometimes dramatically.

Pathophysiology

Growth Hormone Deficiency

Pediatric. GH is essential for normal growth of children, and hence GH deficiency results in *short stature.* Growth is slowed to an equal extent in all parts of the body, and hence the child, although short, has normal proportions. Mental function is not impaired. The only treatment for GH deficiency is replacement therapy with human GH itself (see *Therapeutic Uses* later in this section).

Adult. In adults, GH deficiency causes a syndrome characterized by reduced muscle mass, reduced exercise capacity, increased mortality from cardiovascular causes, and impaired psychosocial function. Onset of GH deficiency may begin in childhood or later in life.

Growth Hormone Excess

Consequences. When GH excess occurs in children, the resulting syndrome is called *gigantism,* and when the excess occurs in adults, the syndrome is called *acromegaly.* The pathophysiology of both syndromes is similar. The principal difference is that GH excess causes children to grow very tall—as much as 7 to 9 feet—owing to stimulation of long bones before epiphyseal closure. In adults, effects on bone growth result in coarse facial features, splayed teeth, and large hands and feet. However, because the epiphyses have already closed, height is not increased. Other manifestations, seen in adults *and* children, include headache, profuse sweating, soft tissue swelling, cardiomegaly, hypertension, arthralgias, and diabetes. Levels of IGF-1 are elevated in all patients. In almost all cases, the cause of GH excess is a pituitary adenoma.

Treatment Overview. Treatment of gigantism requires surgical removal of the pituitary. In contrast, acromegaly may be treated with three modalities: surgery, radiation, or drugs. Surgical excision of the pituitary adenoma is the preferred initial treatment. Radiation therapy may be used as primary treatment or as an adjunct to surgery. When used as primary treatment, radiation takes months to years to produce a full response.

Drugs are generally reserved for patients with large tumors or residual disease despite tumor excision and/or radiation therapy. Four drugs are available: octreotide [Sandostatin, Sandostatin LAR Depot], lanreotide [Somatuline Depot], pasireotide [Signifor LAR], and pegvisomant [Somavert]. The pharmacology of these agents is discussed later under *Drugs for Acromegaly.*

Clinical Pharmacology

Therapeutic Uses

Pediatric Growth Hormone Deficiency. For children with documented GH deficiency, treatment should begin early in life and must stop before epiphyseal closure. To ensure timely termination of treatment, epiphyseal status should be assessed annually. When treatment is started early, adult height may be increased by as much as 6 inches. To monitor treatment, height and weight should be measured monthly. Therapy should continue until a satisfactory adult height has been achieved, until epiphyseal closure occurs, or until a response can no longer be elicited. Efficacy of therapy declines as the patient grows older and is usually lost entirely by age 20 to 24 years. If treatment fails to promote growth, GH should be discontinued and the diagnosis of GH deficiency re-evaluated.

Pediatric Non–Growth-Hormone-Deficient (NGHD) Short Stature. Growth hormone is used for the treatment of children with documented GH deficiency, as well as children with NGHD short stature. These children have normal levels of GH but are nonetheless very short. To qualify for treatment, children must be 2.25 standard deviations below the mean height for their sex and age, which makes them among the shortest 1.2% of their peers. In clinical trials, children who received 6 to 7 injections a week for 4 to 6 years grew an extra 1 to 3 inches, although some did not respond at all. As with treatment of GH-deficient children, the cost is very high.

Pediatric Short Stature Associated With Prader-Willi Syndrome. Prader-Willi syndrome (PWS) is a complex genetic disorder characterized by short stature, mental impairment, incomplete sexual development, behavioral problems, low muscle tone, and the urge to eat constantly. GH is indicated to increase the height of PWS patients, but only if GH deficiency has been documented. However, owing to a risk of sudden death, GH must be avoided in PWS patients who are severely obese, have severe respiratory impairment, or have a history of upper airway obstruction or sleep apnea.

Growth Hormone Deficiency in Adults. In adults with GH deficiency—be it childhood-onset or adult-onset—replacement therapy can increase lean body mass, decrease adipose mass, and increase lumbar spine density. Unfortunately, GH also increases systolic blood pressure and fasting blood glucose. Furthermore, although GH increases muscle mass, it does not increase strength.

Other Uses. In addition to the uses noted previously, GH is approved for pediatric growth failure associated with chronic renal insufficiency, cachexia or wasting in patients with AIDS, short-bowel syndrome, and short stature associated with Turner's syndrome or Noonan's syndrome. Individual GH preparations that are approved for these indications are shown in Table 59.1.

Adverse Effects and Interactions

Hyperglycemia. GH is diabetogenic. When used in patients with pre-existing diabetes, significant hyperglycemia may result. Glucose levels should be monitored, and insulin dosage should be adjusted accordingly.

Neutralizing Antibodies. Over the course of treatment, patients may develop neutralizing antibodies that bind with GH and thereby render the hormone inactive. If these antibodies develop, treatment with mecasermin (recombinant IGF-1, discussed later) may be effective.

Fatality in PWS Patients. Fatalities have occurred in PWS patients treated with GH. Major risk factors are severe obesity, upper airway obstruction, sleep apnea, and respiratory infection. GH is contraindicated in PWS patients who are severely obese or have severe respiratory impairment.

Interaction With Glucocorticoids. Glucocorticoids can oppose the growth-promoting effects of GH. Glucocorticoid replacement doses must be carefully adjusted to avoid growth inhibition.

Preparations, Dosage, and Administration

Preparations: Somatropin. GH for clinical use is available as *somatropin* [Humatrope, Nutropin, others], a molecule produced by recombinant DNA technology. The structure and actions of somatropin are identical to those of GH produced by the human pituitary. At this time, 9 preparations of somatropin are available. They differ with respect to approved indications and dosages (see Table 59.1).

Administration. Administration is parenteral—IM or subQ. Subcutaneous administration is preferred because it is less painful than IM while being just as safe and effective. Subcutaneous administration can be done using either a traditional syringe and needle or a pre-filled injection device. To avoid local tissue atrophy, the injection site should be rotated.

MECASERMIN (INSULIN-LIKE GROWTH FACTOR-1)

Mecasermin [Increlex], produced by recombinant DNA technology, is identical to naturally occurring IGF-1, the compound that mediates the effects of GH. Mecasermin is approved for long-term therapy of growth failure in children with severe primary deficiency of IGF-1, a rare condition seen in about 1:10,000 children worldwide. The drug may also be used in children with GH deficiency who can no longer be treated with GH itself, owing to development of neutralizing antibodies. In children with GH deficiency who are still responsive to GH, treatment with GH is preferred to IGF-1. Mecasermin should not be used after epiphyseal closure or by children with secondary forms of IGF-1 deficiency.

Mecasermin can cause a variety of adverse effects. The most common is hypoglycemia, which develops in nearly 50% of patients, usually during the first weeks of treatment. Hypertrophy of the tonsils develops in 15% of patients, and can be managed by tonsillectomy if needed. Other adverse effects include intracranial hypertension, vomiting, arthralgia, otitis media, elevation of serum aminotransferases and lipids, and overgrowth of fat, facial bones, and the kidneys. Like all other foreign proteins, mecasermin can trigger allergic reactions, both local and systemic.

Mecasermin is supplied in solution (10 mg/mL) in 40-mL multiuse vials. Administration is by subQ injection. The initial dosage is 40 to 80 mcg/kg twice daily. If treatment is well tolerated for at least 1 week, the dosage may be increased by 40 mcg/kg/dose up to a maximum of 120 mcg/kg twice daily. Higher doses, which have not been evaluated, will increase the risk of hypoglycemia. To minimize hypoglycemia, all injections should be made about 20 minutes before or after eating. If hypoglycemia develops despite adequate food intake, the dosage should be reduced. If the patient is unable to eat when a dose is scheduled, that dose should be withheld; subsequent doses should not be increased to make up for the dose that was missed.

PROLACTIN

Prolactin is a polypeptide hormone produced by the anterior pituitary. The principal function of prolactin is stimulation of milk production after parturition. Prolactin deficiency is generally without symptoms, except for disturbance of lactation. In contrast, overproduction of prolactin causes multiple adverse effects.

Regulation of Release

Regulation of prolactin release is predominantly *inhibitory*. Under the influence of dopamine released from the hypothalamus, release of prolactin by the pituitary is *suppressed*. When the release of dopamine declines, release of prolactin is allowed to increase. Another hypothalamic factor, known as prolactin-releasing factor (PRF), *promotes* prolactin release. However, the stimulatory influence of PRF is usually dominated by dopamine-mediated inhibition. The most powerful stimulus

TABLE 59.1 ▪ Somatropin (Human Growth Hormone): Preparations, Indications, and Dosages

Brand Name	Approved Indications	Dosage
Genotropin	GFAW pediatric GH deficiency	0.16–0.24 mg/kg/week subQ, divided into 6 or 7 equal daily doses
	Small for gestational age	Up to 0.48 mg/kg/week subQ, divided into 6 or 7 equal daily doses
	Pediatric NGHD short stature	Up to 0.47 mg/kg/week subQ, divided into 6 or 7 equal daily doses
	GFAW Prader-Willi syndrome	0.24 mg/kg/week subQ, divided into 6 or 7 equal daily doses
	GFAW Turner's syndrome	0.33 mg/kg/week subQ, divided into 6 or 7 equal daily doses
	Adult GH deficiency	0.04–0.08 mg/kg/week subQ, divided into 7 equal daily doses
Humatrope	GFAW pediatric GH deficiency	0.18 mg/kg/week subQ or IM, divided into either (a) 6 equal daily doses or (b) 3 equal doses administered every other day
	Small for gestational age	0.47 mg/kg/week subQ, divided into 6 or 7 daily doses
	Pediatric NGHD short stature	Up to 0.37 mg/kg/week subQ, divided into 6 or 7 equal daily doses
	GFAW Turner's syndrome	0.375 mg/kg/week (max) subQ, divided into either (a) 7 equal daily doses or (b) 3 equal doses administered every other day
	SHOX deficiency	0.35 mg/kg/week subQ, divided in 6 to 7 equal daily doses
	Adult GH deficiency	0.006–0.0125 mg/kg/day subQ
Norditropin	GFAW pediatric GH deficiency	0.024–0.034 mg/kg subQ 6–7 days/week
	Small for gestational age	Up to 0.067 mg/kg/day subQ
	GFAW Turner's syndrome	Up to 0.067 mg/kg/day subQ
	GFAW Noonan's syndrome	Up to 0.066 mg/kg/day subQ
	Adult GH deficiency	0.004–0.016 mg/kg/day subQ
Nutropin, Nutropin AQ	GFAW pediatric GH deficiency	Up to 0.3 mg/kg/week subQ, divided into 7 equal daily doses
	Pediatric NGHD short stature	0.3 mg/kg/week subQ, divided into 7 equal daily doses
	GFAW chronic renal insufficiency	0.35 mg/kg/week subQ, divided into 7 equal daily doses
	GFAW Turner's syndrome	0.375 mg/kg/week subQ, divided into 3–7 equal daily doses
	Adult GH deficiency	0.006 mg/kg/day subQ initially, increased to 0.025 mg/kg/day (max) in patients under 35 yr, or to 0.0125 mg/kg/day (max) in patients over 35 yr
Omnitrope	GFAW pediatric GH deficiency	0.16–0.24 mg/kg/week subQ, divided into 6 or 7 equal daily doses
	GFAW Turner's syndrome	0.33 mg/kg/week subQ, divided into 6 or 7 equal daily doses
	GFAW Prader-Willi syndrome	0.24 mg/kg/week subQ, divided into 6 or 7 equal daily doses
	Small for gestational age	Up to 0.48 mg/kg/week subQ, divided into 6 or 7 equal daily doses
	Pediatric NGHD short stature	0.47 mg/kg/week subQ, divided into 6 or 7 equal daily doses
	Adult GH deficiency	0.04–0.08 mg/kg/week subQ, divided into 7 equal daily doses
Saizen	GFAW pediatric GH deficiency	0.06 mg/kg subQ or IM 3 days/week
	Adult GH deficiency	0.005 mg/kg/day subQ initially, increased to no more than 0.01 mg/kg/day after 4 weeks
Serostim	Cachexia or wasting in AIDS	4–6 mg subQ daily at bedtime (dose depends on patient's weight). For adults under 35 kg, dosage is 0.1 mg/kg subQ once daily at bedtime
Zomacton	GFAW pediatric GH deficiency	0.1 mg/kg subQ 3 times a week

AIDS, Acquired immunodeficiency syndrome; *GFAW,* growth failure associated with; *GH,* growth hormone; *NGHD,* non–growth-hormone-deficient; *SHOX,* short stature homeobox-containing gene.

to prolactin release is suckling, an action that presumably suppresses release of dopamine from the hypothalamus.

Prolactin Hypersecretion

Excessive secretion of prolactin produces adverse effects in males and females. Women may experience amenorrhea, galactorrhea (excessive milk flow), and infertility. In men, libido and potency are reduced; galactorrhea occurs on occasion. Puberty may be delayed in boys and girls. Causes of prolactin hypersecretion include pituitary adenoma, injury to the hypothalamus, and certain drugs (e.g., antipsychotic drugs, estrogens).

Suppressing Prolactin Release With Dopamine Agonists

Excessive secretion of prolactin can be reduced with two dopamine agonists: cabergoline and bromocriptine. These drugs bind with dopamine receptors in the pituitary and thereby exert the same inhibitory influence on prolactin release as does dopamine released from the hypothalamus. Cabergoline is better tolerated than bromocriptine, and dosing is more convenient. As a result, cabergoline is generally preferred. The pharmacology of both drugs and their use in hyperprolactinemia is discussed in Chapter 63. The use of cabergoline and bromocriptine (and other dopamine agonists) in Parkinson disease is discussed in Chapter 21.

ANTIDIURETIC HORMONE (VASOPRESSIN)

Antidiuretic hormone, also known as *vasopressin,* is a nine-peptide hormone that acts on the kidney to cause reabsorption (conservation) of water. Deficiency of ADH produces *hypothalamic diabetes insipidus,* a condition in which large volumes of dilute urine are produced.

Physiology

Actions

ADH promotes *renal conservation of water* through action on the collecting ducts of the kidney to increase their permeability to water. This results in increased water *reabsorption.* Because water is withdrawn from the tubular urine (back into the extracellular space), urine that entered the collecting ducts in a relatively dilute state becomes highly concentrated by the time it leaves.

In addition to its renal actions, ADH can stimulate *contraction of vascular smooth muscle and smooth muscle of the GI tract.* Because of its ability to cause vasoconstriction, ADH is also known as vasopressin. It should be noted that the plasma levels of ADH required to cause smooth muscle contraction are higher than those that occur physiologically.

Production, Storage, and Release

ADH is produced in neurosecretory cells of the hypothalamus, transported down their axons, and then stored in their terminals until released. Release is regulated by the hypothalamus—the brain center responsible for maintaining body fluids at their proper osmolality. When the hypothalamus senses that osmolality has risen too high, it instructs the posterior pituitary to release ADH. The resultant increase in water reabsorption dilutes body fluids, causing osmolality to decline. Release of ADH can also be stimulated by hypotension and by reduced plasma volume.

Pathophysiology: Hypothalamic Diabetes Insipidus

Hypothalamic diabetes insipidus is a syndrome caused by partial or complete deficiency of ADH. The syndrome is characterized by polydipsia (excessive thirst) and excretion of large volumes of dilute urine. Deficiency of ADH may be inherited or may result from head trauma, neurosurgery, cancer, and other causes. The best treatment is replacement therapy with ADH. (In contrast to hypothalamic diabetes insipidus, *nephrogenic diabetes insipidus* results from a failure of the kidney to produce concentrated urine despite adequate levels of ADH.)

Antidiuretic Hormone Preparations

Two preparations with ADH activity are available: *vasopressin* [Vasostrict] and *desmopressin* [DDAVP, Stimate]. Vasopressin is identical in structure to naturally occurring ADH; desmopressin is a structural analog of natural ADH. The preparations differ with respect to route of administration, duration of action, and therapeutic applications (Table 59.2). They also differ in their ability to cause vasoconstriction.

Clinical Pharmacology

Adverse Effects

Water Intoxication. Excessive water retention can cause water intoxication. Early signs include drowsiness, listlessness, and headache. Severe intoxication progresses to convulsions and terminal coma. Patients experiencing early symptoms should notify their prescriber. Treatment includes diuretic therapy and restriction of fluid intake.

A major cause of intoxication is failure to reduce water intake once ADH therapy has begun. Because treatment prevents continued fluid loss, failure to decrease fluid intake will result in water buildup. Hence, at the onset of treatment, patients should be instructed to reduce their accustomed intake of fluid.

The risk of water intoxication is also increased by renal impairment. Accordingly, if creatinine clearance is below 50 mL/min, ADH should not be used.

TABLE 59.2 ■ ADH Preparations

Drug	Routes	Duration of Antidiuretic Action (hr)	Therapeutic Uses	Usual Maintenance Dosage
Desmopressin [DDAVP, Stimate]	Intranasal, subQ, IV, PO	8–20	Diabetes insipidus	*Adults:* 0.1–0.4 mL (10–40 mcg) intranasally 1–3 times/day *or* 0.25–0.5 mL subQ or IV twice daily *or* 0.1–1.2 mg PO daily in 2 or 3 doses *Children:* 0.05–0.3 mL intranasally daily either as a single dose or in 2 doses
			Nocturnal enuresis	0.2–0.6 mg PO at bedtime (intranasal therapy of enuresis is contraindicated)
			Hemophilia	See Chapter 54
Vasopressin [Vasostrict]	IM, subQ[a]	2–8	Diabetes insipidus	*Adults:* 5–10 units IM or subQ 2–3 times/day *Children:* 2.5–10 units IM or subQ 2–3 times/day
			Postoperative abdominal distention	5 units IM initially; then 10 units IM every 3–4 hr
			Abdominal radiography (to dispel gas shadows)	10 units 2 hr before and again 30 min before the procedure
			Cardiac resuscitation	40 units

[a]Sometimes administered intranasally or IV.

Safety Alert

CARDIOVASCULAR EFFECTS OF VASOPRESSIN

Because of its powerful vasoconstrictor actions, *vasopressin* can cause severe adverse cardiovascular effects. (Desmopressin is a weak pressor agent, and hence does not adversely affect hemodynamics.) By constricting arteries of the heart, vasopressin can cause angina pectoris and even myocardial infarction—especially in patients with coronary insufficiency. In addition, vasopressin may cause gangrene by decreasing blood flow in the periphery. Because it can reduce cardiac perfusion, vasopressin must be used with extreme caution in patients with coronary artery disease.

Therapeutic Uses

Diabetes Insipidus. Diabetes insipidus may be treated with either desmopressin or vasopressin. However, *desmopressin* is the agent of choice because it has a long duration of action, is easy to administer (by mouth or intranasal spray), and lacks significant side effects, especially vasoconstriction. The response to treatment is rapid, and urine volume quickly drops to normal. Because desmopressin is expensive and because excessive dosing can result in water intoxication, the smallest effective dosage should be employed.

Cardiac Arrest. For patients in cardiac arrest, vasopressin can be used to enhance cardiopulmonary resuscitation (CPR). Benefits derive from vasopressin-induced vasoconstriction, which, in people receiving CPR, increases blood flow to the heart and brain, improves neurologic outcome, and increases the chances of successful resuscitation.

Other Uses. *Vasopressin* is indicated for postoperative abdominal distention and preparation for abdominal radiography. *Desmopressin* is indicated for nocturnal enuresis (bedwetting), hemophilia A, and von Willebrand's disease. The drug decreases enuresis by reducing urine production, and helps patients with hemophilia A and von Willebrand's disease by promoting the release of clotting factor VIII (see Chapter 54).

ANTIDIURETIC HORMONE (VASOPRESSIN) ANTAGONISTS

Antidiuretic hormone antagonists, also known as vasopressin antagonists, block the effects of ADH (vasopressin) in renal collecting ducts. By doing so, they increase the excretion of free water. Two vasopressin antagonists are available: conivaptan and tolvaptan. These drugs, also known as *vaptans,* have only one indication: treatment of hyponatremia in euvolemic or hypervolemic patients. The principal difference between the two drugs concerns route of administration: conivaptan is administered IV, whereas tolvaptan is administered PO (Table 59.3).

Conivaptan

Conivaptan [Vaprisol] is indicated for short-term *IV* therapy of hyponatremia in euvolemic and hypervolemic hospitalized patients. In patients with euvolemic or hypervolemic hyponatremia, levels of circulating vasopressin are usually high, causing retention of water by the kidney. Conivaptan blocks vasopressin V_2 receptors in renal collecting ducts and thereby promotes "aquaresis" (renal excretion of free water), leaving sodium behind for reabsorption into the blood. As a result, the concentration of sodium in blood rises, thereby correcting the hyponatremia.

The most common adverse effects are infusion-site reactions. Other common reactions include hypokalemia, orthostatic hypotension, headache, fever, constipation, diarrhea, and vomiting. If blood sodium rises too rapidly (more than 12 mEq/L/24 hr), neurons can undergo *osmotic demyelination,* resulting in serious neurologic deficits (e.g., difficulty swallowing, inability to speak, affective changes, seizures, coma, and death). Accordingly, blood sodium should be monitored often and, if the rise is too fast, conivaptan should be interrupted.

Conivaptan is both a substrate for and inhibitor of CYP3A4 (the 3A4 isoenzyme of cytochrome P450). Accordingly, the drug must not be combined with strong inhibitors of CYP3A4 (e.g., itraconazole, clarithromycin, ritonavir), owing to a risk of conivaptan toxicity. Combined use with drugs that are substrates for CYP3A4 should be done with caution.

Conivaptan is supplied in solution (0.2 mg/mL) for IV administration. Dosing consists of an initial loading dose (20 mg over 30 minutes) followed by a continuous infusion (20 mg over 24 hours). A maximum of three additional infusions (20 or 40 mg over 24 hours each) may be done as needed.

DRUGS FOR ACROMEGALY

As discussed earlier, acromegaly results from excessive production of GH by a pituitary tumor, and can be treated with three modalities: surgical excision of the pituitary, irradiation of the pituitary, and drug therapy. As a rule, drugs are reserved for patients who did not respond adequately to surgery and/or radiation, or for whom these modalities are not options. Two types of drugs are available: somatostatin analogs and GH receptor antagonists. Drug therapy is both prolonged and expensive.

Somatostatin Analogs

The somatostatin analogs—octreotide, pasireotide, and lanreotide—are our most effective drugs for suppressing GH release. Benefits derive from mimicking the suppressant actions of somatostatin on the pituitary (see Fig. 59.3). The somatostatin analogs can be used as primary therapy for acromegaly or as an adjunct to surgery and/or radiation. In both cases, the objective is to normalize levels of GH and IGF-1.

Octreotide is available in two formulations: an immediate-release product, sold as *Sandostatin,* and a sustained-release product, sold as *Sandostatin LAR Depot.* Sandostatin is available in solution for IM injection (50, 100, 200, 500, and 1000 mcg/mL) and Sandostatin LAR Depot is available in depot injections (10, 20, and 30 mg). The usual maintenance dosage is 100 mcg subQ 3 times a day (for Sandostatin) or 10 to 30 mg IM once a month (for Sandostatin LAR Depot). Gastrointestinal side effects (nausea, cramps, diarrhea, flatulence) are common initially, but subside in 1 to 2 weeks. Within a year, cholesterol gallstones develop in about 25% of patients, although they are usually asymptomatic.

Pasireotide [Signifor LAR] is supplied in 20-, 40-, and 60-mg vials of powder to be reconstituted for IM injection every 4 weeks. Doses start at 40 mg and can be titrated to effect. The most common side effects are diarrhea and hyperglycemia. Signifor may also cause QT prolongation and bradycardia.

TABLE 59.3 ■ Vasopressin Antagonists

Drug	Indications	Adverse Effects	Availability and Usual Adult Dosage
Conivaptan [Vaprisol]	Euvolemic and hypervolemic hyponatremia	Infusion site reactions, hypokalemia, orthostatic hypotension	IV: 20-mg loading dose followed by a 20-mg infusion over 24 hr. May repeat 24-hr infusion × 3.
Tolvaptan [Samsca]	Euvolemic and hypervolemic hyponatremia	Thirst, dry mouth, polyuria	Tablets: Start 15 mg every 24 hr. May increase to 60 mg every 24 hr if tolerated.

Lanreotide [Somatuline Depot] is supplied in single-use, pre-filled syringes (60, 90, and 120 mg) for deep subQ injection into the buttocks. Dosages range from 60 to 120 mg every 4 weeks. The most common side effect is diarrhea; other common reactions include gallstones, bradycardia, injection-site reactions, and hypo- or hyperglycemia.

Pegvisomant, a Growth Hormone Receptor Antagonist

Pegvisomant [Somavert], a GH receptor antagonist, may be our most effective drug for acromegaly. The goal of therapy is to normalize serum levels of IGF-1. In clinical trials, treatment for 12 months or longer greatly reduced symptoms and normalized IGF-1 levels in nearly all patients (97%). Pegvisomant is generally well tolerated. The most common side effects are injection-site reactions, nausea, diarrhea, chest pain, and flu-like symptoms. In a few patients, serum levels of hepatic transaminases rise, indicating liver injury. Monitoring of hepatic function is recommended. The only known drug interaction is an apparent reduction in pegvisomant effects by opioid analgesics. Why this occurs is a mystery. Pegvisomant is available as a powder (10, 15, and 20 mg) that must be reconstituted with sterile water before use. Administration is by subQ injection. Treatment consists of an initial 40-mg loading dose (given by the prescriber), followed by 10-mg doses injected once daily by the patient. Every 4 to 6 weeks, the level of IGF-1 is measured, and dosage is increased by 5 mg (if the IGF-1 level is still above normal) or decreased by 5 mg (if the IGF-1 level is below normal). Treatment should continue indefinitely.

KEY POINTS

- Release of hormones from the anterior pituitary is stimulated by releasing factors from the hypothalamus and inhibited by negative feedback loops.
- The growth-promoting actions of growth hormone (GH) are mediated by insulin-like growth factor-1 (IGF-1).
- Pediatric GH deficiency causes short stature.
- Adult GH deficiency causes reduced muscle mass, reduced exercise capacity, increased mortality from cardiovascular causes, and impaired psychosocial function.
- Pediatric GH excess causes gigantism.
- Adult GH excess causes acromegaly.
- Among pediatric patients, GH is approved for growth promotion in children who are GH deficient and in children who are very short despite having normal GH levels.
- Exogenous glucocorticoids can inhibit responses to GH.
- GH can elevate glucose levels in patients with diabetes.
- Acromegaly can be treated with three drugs: pegvisomant (a GH receptor antagonist) and two analogs of somatostatin—octreotide and lanreotide—that suppress GH release.
- Prolactin stimulates milk production after delivery.
- Excessive production of prolactin can be suppressed with cabergoline and bromocriptine, drugs that mimic the inhibitory action of hypothalamic dopamine on the pituitary.
- Antidiuretic hormone (ADH) acts on the kidney to cause reabsorption (conservation) of water.
- ADH deficiency results in hypothalamic diabetes insipidus.
- Hypothalamic diabetes insipidus can be treated by replacement therapy with desmopressin, a synthetic form of ADH.
- When initiating ADH replacement therapy, warn the patient to decrease water intake, because failure to do so can cause water intoxication.
- Vasopressin, a drug identical to natural ADH, can cause profound vasoconstriction.
- By promoting vasoconstriction, vasopressin can be lifesaving in patients with cardiac arrest.

Please visit http://evolve.elsevier.com/Lehne for chapter-specific NCLEX® examination review questions.

Summary of Major Nursing Implications[a]

SOMATROPIN (HUMAN GROWTH HORMONE)

The nursing implications here apply only to the use of GH in *pediatric* patients.

Preadministration Assessment

Therapeutic Goal

Normalization of growth and development in children with (1) proven GH deficiency and (2) very short stature despite normal GH levels.

Baseline Data

Assess developmental status (height, weight, etc.) and obtain laboratory data on thyroid function and GH levels.

Identifying High-Risk Patients

GH is *contraindicated* during and after epiphyseal closure, and in children with PWS who are severely obese or have severe respiratory impairment.

Use with *caution* in children with diabetes mellitus and hypothyroidism.

Implementation: Administration

Routes

SubQ (preferred) or IM.

Administration

Provide the following administration instructions:

- **For powdered preparations, reconstitute with the appropriate volume of diluent. *Mix gently; do not shake.***
- **Do not inject if the preparation is cloudy or contains particulate matter.**
- **Rotate the injection site to avoid localized tissue atrophy.**

Ongoing Evaluation and Interventions

Evaluating Treatment

Monitor height and weight monthly. Continue therapy until a satisfactory adult height has been achieved, until epiphyseal closure occurs, or until a response can no longer be elicited (usually by age 20 to 24).

Summary of Major Nursing Implications[a]—cont'd

If no stimulation of growth occurs, discontinue treatment and re-evaluate the diagnosis of GH deficiency.

Minimizing Adverse Effects and Interactions

Hyperglycemia. GH can elevate plasma glucose levels in diabetics. Increase insulin dosage as needed.

Hypothyroidism. GH may suppress thyroid function. Assess thyroid function before treatment and periodically thereafter. If levels of thyroid hormone fall, institute replacement therapy.

Fatality in PWS Patients. Owing to a risk of death, do not give GH to pediatric patients with PWS who are severely obese or who have severe respiratory impairment.

Interaction With Glucocorticoids. Glucocorticoids can oppose the growth-stimulating effects of GH. Carefully adjust glucocorticoid replacement dosage to avoid growth inhibition.

Neutralizing Antibodies. Antibodies that neutralize exogenous GH can develop over the course of treatment. If this happens, mecasermin (recombinant IGF-1) may be an effective alternative to GH.

ANTIDIURETIC HORMONE

Desmopressin
Vasopressin

The nursing implications here apply only to the use of ADH preparations for *hypothalamic diabetes insipidus.*

Preadministration Assessment

Therapeutic Goal

Normalization of urinary water excretion in patients with hypothalamic diabetes insipidus.

Baseline Data

Determine creatinine clearance and fluid and electrolyte status.

Identifying High-Risk Patients

Use *vasopressin* with *caution* in patients with coronary artery disease and other vascular diseases.

Implementation: Administration

Routes

Desmopressin. Intranasal, PO, subQ, IV.

Vasopressin. IM, subQ.

Administration

Teach the patient the technique for intranasal administration. To promote adherence, make certain the patient understands that treatment is lifelong.

Ongoing Evaluation and Interventions

Evaluating Therapeutic Effects

Teach the patient to monitor and record daily intake and output of fluid. If ADH dosage is correct, urine volume should rapidly drop to normal.

Minimizing Adverse Effects

Water Intoxication. Excessive retention of water can produce water intoxication—most often at the beginning of therapy. **Instruct patients to decrease their accustomed fluid intake at the start of treatment. Inform patients about early signs of water intoxication (drowsiness, listlessness, headache), and instruct them to notify the prescriber if these occur.** Treatment includes fluid restriction and diuretic therapy. Avoid ADH in patients with creatinine clearance below 50 mL/min.

Cardiovascular Effects. *Vasopressin*, but not desmopressin, is a powerful vasoconstrictor. Excessive vasoconstriction can produce angina pectoris, myocardial infarction, and gangrene (from extravasation of IV vasopressin). Use vasopressin with caution, especially in patients with coronary insufficiency.

[a]Patient education information is highlighted as **blue text.**

CHAPTER

60 Drugs for Disorders of the Adrenal Cortex

The hormones of the adrenal cortex affect multiple physiologic processes, including maintenance of glucose availability, regulation of water and electrolyte balance, development of sexual characteristics, and life-preserving responses to stress. As you might guess, when production of adrenal hormones goes awry, the consequences can be profound. The two most familiar forms of adrenocortical dysfunction are *Cushing's syndrome,* caused by adrenal hormone excess, and *Addison's disease,* caused by adrenal hormone deficiency.

In approaching the drugs for treating disorders of the adrenal cortex, we begin by reviewing adrenocortical endocrinology. After that, we discuss the disease states associated with adrenal hormone excess and adrenal hormone insufficiency. Having established this background, we discuss the agents used for diagnosis and treatment of adrenocortical disorders.

PHYSIOLOGY OF THE ADRENOCORTICAL HORMONES

The adrenal cortex produces three classes of steroid hormones: *glucocorticoids, mineralocorticoids,* and *androgens.* Glucocorticoids influence carbohydrate metabolism and other processes; mineralocorticoids modulate salt and water balance; and adrenal androgens contribute to expression of sexual characteristics.

Glucocorticoids

Glucocorticoids are so named because they increase the availability of glucose. Of the several glucocorticoids produced by the adrenal cortex, *cortisol* is the most important.

When considering the glucocorticoids, we need to distinguish between *physiologic effects* and *pharmacologic effects. Physiologic effects* occur at *low* levels of glucocorticoids (i.e., the levels produced by release of glucocorticoids from healthy adrenal glands, or by administering glucocorticoids in low doses). *Pharmacologic effects* occur at *high* levels of glucocorticoids. These levels are achieved when glucocorticoids are administered in the large doses required to treat disorders unrelated to adrenocortical function (e.g., allergic reactions, asthma, inflammation, cancer). Pharmacologic levels can also be reached when production of endogenous glucocorticoids is excessive, as occurs in Cushing's disease. Here we focus on the *physiologic* role of glucocorticoids. The use of high-dose glucocorticoids for nonendocrine purposes is discussed in Chapter 72.

Physiologic Effects

Carbohydrate Metabolism. Supplying the brain with glucose is essential for survival. Glucocorticoids help meet this need. Specifically, they promote glucose availability in four ways: (1) stimulation of gluconeogenesis, (2) reduction of peripheral glucose utilization, (3) inhibition of glucose uptake by muscle and adipose tissue, and (4) promotion of glucose storage (in the form of glycogen). All four actions increase glucose availability during fasting and thus help ensure that the brain will not be deprived of its primary source of energy.

The effects of glucocorticoids on carbohydrate metabolism are opposite to those of insulin. That is, whereas insulin lowers plasma levels of glucose, glucocorticoids raise them. When present chronically in high concentrations, glucocorticoids produce symptoms much like those of diabetes.

Protein Metabolism. Glucocorticoids promote protein catabolism (breakdown). This action, which is opposite to that of insulin, provides amino acids for glucose synthesis. If present at high levels for a prolonged time, glucocorticoids will cause muscle wasting, thinning of the skin, and negative nitrogen balance.

Fat Metabolism. Glucocorticoids promote lipolysis (fat breakdown). When present at high levels for an extended time, as occurs in Cushing's syndrome, glucocorticoids cause fat redistribution, giving the patient a "potbelly," "moon face," and "buffalo hump."

Cardiovascular System. Glucocorticoids are required to maintain the functional integrity of the vascular system. When levels of glucocorticoids are depressed, capillary permeability is increased, the ability of vessels to constrict is reduced, and blood pressure falls.

Glucocorticoids have multiple effects on blood cells. These hormones increase red blood cell counts and hemoglobin levels. Of the white blood cells, only counts of polymorphonuclear leukocytes increase. In contrast, counts of lymphocytes, eosinophils, basophils, and monocytes decrease.

Skeletal Muscle. Glucocorticoids support the function of striated muscle, primarily by maintaining circulatory competence. In the absence of sufficient levels of glucocorticoids, muscle perfusion decreases, causing work capacity to decrease as well.

Central Nervous System. Glucocorticoids affect mood, central nervous system (CNS) excitability, and the electroencephalogram. Glucocorticoid insufficiency is associated with depression, lethargy, and irritability. Rarely, outright psychosis occurs. In contrast, when present in excess, glucocorticoids can produce generalized excitation and euphoria.

Stress. In response to stress (e.g., anxiety, exercise, trauma, infection, surgery), the adrenal cortex secretes increased amounts of glucocorticoids, and the adrenal medulla secretes increased amounts of epinephrine. Working together, glucocorticoids and epinephrine serve to maintain blood pressure and blood glucose content. If glucocorticoid levels are inadequate, hypotension and hypoglycemia can occur. If the stress is extreme (e.g., trauma, surgery, severe infection), glucocorticoid deficiency can result in circulatory collapse and death. Accordingly, it is imperative that patients with adrenal insufficiency receive glucocorticoid supplements when severe stress occurs.

Respiratory System in Neonates. During labor and delivery, the adrenals of the full-term fetus release a burst of glucocorticoids. Within hours, these steroids act on the lungs to accelerate their maturation. In the preterm infant, the adrenals produce only small amounts of glucocorticoids. As a result, preterm infants experience a high incidence of respiratory distress syndrome.

PATIENT-CENTERED CARE ACROSS THE LIFE SPAN

Adrenal Cortex Drugs

Life Stage	Patient Care Concerns
Infants	Adrenal replacement medications can be given safely in infants. Indications for treatment include congenital adrenal hyperplasia and adrenal insufficiency.
Children/ adolescents	Long-term use of steroid medications can cause inhibition of bone growth and osteoporosis at any age of life.
Pregnant women	Prednisone is classified in U.S. Food and Drug Administration Pregnancy Risk Category D[a]: There is evidence of human fetal risk. Hydrocortisone is classified in Pregnancy Risk Category C[a]: Risk must be weighed against benefit.
Breast-feeding women	Prednisone is safe to use in lower doses when breast-feeding. As hydrocortisone has not been studied, other glucocorticoids are preferred.
Older adults	Long-term use of glucocorticoids can cause osteoporosis. As some older adults are at increased risk of falls, assessment for safety and fractures should be completed.

[a]As of 2020, the FDA will no longer use Pregnancy Risk Categories. Please refer to Chapter 9 for more information.

Regulation of Synthesis and Secretion

Adrenal storage of glucocorticoids is minimal. Accordingly, the amount of glucocorticoid released from the adrenals closely approximates the amount being made.

Glucocorticoid synthesis and release are regulated by a negative feedback loop (Fig. 60.1). The loop begins with the release of corticotropin-releasing hormone (CRH) from the hypothalamus. CRH acts on the anterior pituitary to promote the release of adrenocorticotropic hormone (ACTH), which stimulates the zona fasciculata of the adrenal cortex, causing synthesis and release of cortisol and other glucocorticoids. Following release, cortisol acts in two ways: (1) it promotes its designated biologic effects and (2) it acts on the hypothalamus and pituitary to suppress further release of CRH and ACTH. Thus, as cortisol levels rise, they act to suppress further stimulation of glucocorticoid production, thereby keeping glucocorticoid levels within an appropriate range.

The hypothalamic-pituitary-adrenal system is activated by signals from the CNS. These signals turn the system on

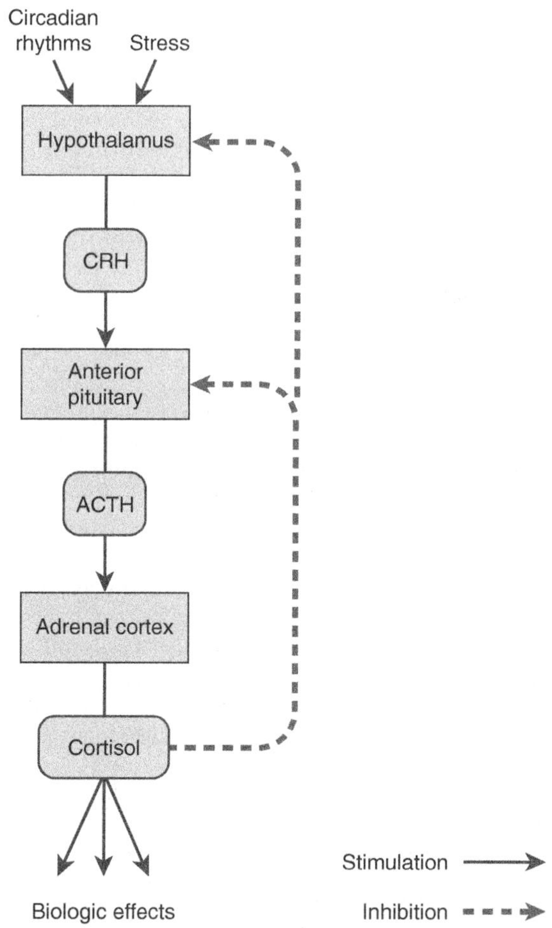

Fig. 60.1 ■ Negative feedback regulation of glucocorticoid synthesis and secretion.
(*ACTH,* Adrenocorticotropic hormone; *CRH,* corticotropin-releasing hormone.)

by causing the hypothalamus to release CRH. Two modes of activation are involved. One provides a basal level of stimulation; the other increases stimulation at times of stress. Basal stimulation follows a circadian rhythm: Cortisol levels are lowest near bedtime, rise during sleep, reach a peak just before waking, and then decline through the day. (Note that this cycle is linked to one's *sleep pattern* and not to the clock. Therefore, for some people, cortisol may peak in the morning, and for others it may peak in the afternoon or evening, depending on when they normally sleep.) When stress occurs, glucocorticoid production goes up. Stressful events that can activate the loop include injury, infection, and surgery. The signals generated by stress produce intense stimulation of the hypothalamus. The resultant release of CRH and ACTH can cause plasma levels of cortisol to increase 10-fold. Because stress is such a powerful stimulus, it overrides feedback inhibition by cortisol.

How much cortisol do the adrenals produce? Basal production ranges between 5 and 10 mg/m^2/day (the equivalent of 20 to 30 mg/day of hydrocortisone or 5 to 7 mg/day of prednisone). When severe stress occurs, production increases 5- to 10-fold—to a maximum of 100 mg/m^2/day.

Mineralocorticoids

The mineralocorticoids influence renal processing of sodium, potassium, and hydrogen. In addition, they have direct effects on the heart and blood vessels. Of the mineralocorticoids made by the adrenal cortex, *aldosterone* is the most important.

Physiologic Effects

Renal Actions. Aldosterone promotes sodium and potassium hemostasis and helps maintain intravascular volume. Specifically, the hormone acts on the collecting ducts of the nephron to promote sodium reabsorption in exchange for secretion of potassium and hydrogen. The total amount of hydrogen and potassium lost equals the amount of sodium reabsorbed. Note that, as sodium is reabsorbed, water is reabsorbed along with it. In the absence of aldosterone, renal excretion of sodium and water is greatly increased, whereas excretion of potassium and hydrogen is reduced. As a result, aldosterone insufficiency causes hyponatremia, hyperkalemia, acidosis, cellular dehydration, and reduction of extracellular fluid volume. Left uncorrected, the condition can lead to renal failure, circulatory collapse, and death.

Cardiovascular Actions. In addition to its effects on the kidneys, aldosterone acts on the heart and blood vessels as well. When aldosterone levels are high, cardiovascular effects are *harmful,* increasing the risk of heart failure and hypertension. Specific cardiovascular effects include (1) promotion of myocardial remodeling (which can impair pumping); (2) promotion of myocardial fibrosis (which increases the risk of dysrhythmias); (3) activation of the sympathetic nervous system and suppression of norepinephrine uptake in the heart (both of which can promote dysrhythmias and ischemia); (4) promotion of vascular fibrosis (which decreases arterial compliance); and (5) disruption of the baroreceptor reflex.

Control of Secretion

Secretion of aldosterone is regulated by the renin-angiotensin-aldosterone system (RAAS), not by ACTH. The mechanisms by which the RAAS regulates aldosterone are discussed in Chapter 44. Note that, because aldosterone is not regulated by ACTH, conditions that alter the secretion of ACTH do not alter the secretion of aldosterone.

Adrenal Androgens

The adrenal cortex produces several steroids that have androgenic properties. *Androstenedione* is representative. Under normal conditions, physiologic effects of adrenal androgens are minimal. In adult males, the influence of adrenal androgens is overshadowed by the effects of testosterone produced by the testes. In adult females, a metabolite of the adrenal androgens—testosterone—contributes to the development of sexual hair and the maintenance of libido. Although adrenal androgens normally have very little effect, when production is excessive, as occurs in congenital adrenal hyperplasia (CAH), virilization can result.

PATHOPHYSIOLOGY OF THE ADRENOCORTICAL HORMONES

Adrenal Hormone Excess

Cushing's Syndrome

Causes. Signs and symptoms of Cushing's syndrome result from excess levels of circulating glucocorticoids. Principal causes are (1) hypersecretion of ACTH by pituitary adenomas (Cushing's disease), (2) hypersecretion of glucocorticoids by adrenal adenomas and carcinomas, and (3) the administration of glucocorticoids in the large doses used to treat arthritis and other nonendocrine disorders.

Clinical Presentation. Cushing's syndrome is characterized by hyperglycemia, glycosuria, hypertension, fluid and electrolyte disturbances, osteoporosis, muscle weakness, myopathy, hirsutism, menstrual irregularities, and decreased resistance to infection. The skin is weakened, resulting in striae (stretch marks) and increased susceptibility to injury. Fat undergoes redistribution to the abdomen, face, and upper back, giving the patient a "potbelly," "moon face," and "buffalo hump." Psychiatric changes are common.

Treatment. Treatment is directed at the cause. The treatment of choice for adrenal adenoma and carcinoma is surgical removal of the diseased adrenal gland. If bilateral adrenalectomy is required, replacement therapy with glucocorticoids and mineralocorticoids will be needed. For patients with inoperable adrenal carcinoma, treatment with *mitotane* may be indicated. Mitotane is an anticancer drug that produces selective destruction of adrenocortical cells. The pharmacology of mitotane is discussed in Chapter 102.

When Cushing's syndrome is caused by pituitary adenoma, surgery is the preferred intervention. Partial removal of the pituitary often lowers ACTH secretion to safe levels, while leaving other pituitary functions intact. If partial adenectomy is unsuccessful, the remainder of the pituitary may be removed. As an alternative, pituitary irradiation may be employed.

The role of drugs in treating Cushing's syndrome is limited. Specifically, drugs are employed only as adjuncts to radiation and surgery—not as the primary intervention. Benefits derive from suppressing glucocorticoid synthesis. The most effective agent is *ketoconazole* [Nizoral], an antifungal drug that also blocks glucocorticoid synthesis. The dosage for suppression of steroid synthesis is initiated at 600 to 800 mg/day—much higher than doses employed for antifungal therapy. At these doses, ketoconazole can cause significant liver dysfunction. The basic pharmacology of ketoconazole is discussed in Chapter 92.

Primary Hyperaldosteronism

Clinical Presentation, Causes, and Diagnosis. Hyperaldosteronism (excessive secretion of aldosterone) causes hypokalemia, metabolic alkalosis, and hypertension and can increase the risk of heart failure. Muscle weakness and changes in the electrocardiogram develop secondary to hypokalemia. Hyperaldosteronism is frequently caused by an aldosterone-producing adrenal adenoma. The condition may also result from bilateral adrenal hyperplasia. Primary hyperaldosteronism can be diagnosed by determining the ratio of plasma aldosterone concentration to plasma renin activity (as discussed in Chapter 44, renin is an enzyme that plays a critical role in the RAAS).

Treatment. Management of hyperaldosteronism depends on the cause. When an adrenal adenoma is responsible, surgical resection of the adrenal gland is usually curative. When bilateral adrenal hyperplasia is the cause, an *aldosterone antagonist* is the preferred treatment. The antagonist employed most frequently is *spironolactone,* a drug we normally think of as a potassium-sparing diuretic. Under the influence of spironolactone, potassium levels may normalize in 2 weeks. To achieve full control of hypertension, an additional diuretic may be required. The basic pharmacology of spironolactone is discussed in Chapter 41, as are alternatives to spironolactone. These include *amiloride* (another potassium-sparing diuretic) and *eplerenone* (a highly selective aldosterone antagonist).

Adrenal Hormone Insufficiency

General Therapeutic Considerations

Chronic adrenal hormone insufficiency can result from multiple causes, including destruction of the adrenals, inborn deficiencies of the enzymes required for glucocorticoid synthesis, and reduced secretion of ACTH and CRH. Regardless of the cause, chronic adrenal insufficiency requires lifelong replacement therapy. All patients require a *glucocorticoid.* Some may require a *mineralocorticoid* as well. Of the glucocorticoids available, *hydrocortisone, prednisone,* and *dexamethasone* are drugs of choice. When a mineralocorticoid is indicated, *fludrocortisone* is the drug of choice.

Replacement therapy should mimic normal patterns of glucocorticoid secretion. Since levels of glucocorticoids normally peak in the morning, the usual practice is to take the entire daily dose immediately after waking up. An alternative is to divide the daily dose, giving two-thirds in the morning and one-third in the afternoon. Mineralocorticoids can be administered once a day. Doses of glucocorticoids and mineralocorticoids should approximate the amounts normally secreted by the adrenals. It is important to note that, when glucocorticoids are employed for replacement therapy, doses are much smaller than the doses employed for nonendocrine disorders.

Safety Alert

STRESS AND GLUCOCORTICOIDS

At times of stress, patients *must* increase their glucocorticoid dosage. Failure to increase the dosage can be fatal.

TABLE 60.1 ■ Guidelines for Giving Supplemental Doses of Glucocorticoids at Times of Stress Related to Medical Conditions and Surgical Procedures

Medical Condition or Surgical Procedure	Supplemental Glucocorticoid Dosage
MINOR	
Inguinal hernia repair Colonoscopy Mild febrile illness Mild to moderate nausea/vomiting Gastroenteritis	Take normal dose of steroids on the day of the procedure.
MODERATE	
Open cholecystectomy Hemicolectomy Significant febrile illness Pneumonia Severe gastroenteritis	50 mg of hydrocortisone IV just before the procedure. Continue with 25 mg hydrocortisone IV every 8 hr for 24 hr, then resume usual replacement dose.
SEVERE	
Major cardiothoracic surgery Whipple procedure Liver resection Pancreatitis	100 mg of hydrocortisone IV just before the procedure. Continue with 50 mg hydrocortisone IV every 8 hr for 24 hr, then resume usual replacement dose.
CRITICALLY ILL	
Sepsis-induced hypotension or shock	50 mg of hydrocortisone IV every 6 hr (or 0.18 mg/kg/hr as continuous infusion) *plus* 50 mg of fludrocortisone until shock resolves, which may take several days to a week or more. Then gradually taper to usual replacement dose, following vital signs and serum sodium.

Recall that healthy adrenals increase their output of glucocorticoids in response to stress. For patients with adrenal insufficiency, the extra glucocorticoids that would normally be supplied by the adrenals must instead be supplied through supplemental dosing. Dosing guidelines related to specific medical conditions and surgical procedures are shown in Table 60.1. For mild or febrile illness, the "3 by 3 rule" applies: Take 3 times the usual dosage for 3 days.

To ensure availability of glucocorticoids in emergencies, patients should carry an adequate supply at all times. This supply should include an injectable preparation plus an oral preparation. Furthermore, the patient should wear some form of identification (e.g., Medic Alert bracelet) to inform emergency personnel about his or her glucocorticoid needs.

Primary Adrenocortical Insufficiency (Addison's Disease)

Causes. Primary adrenocortical insufficiency (PAI), also known as Addison's disease, is a condition in which the adrenal glands are damaged and unable to make glucocorticoids. Most cases (80%) are caused by autoimmune destruction of adrenal tissue. Another 15% are caused by tuberculosis and other infections. Other causes include adrenal hemorrhage, cancers, and certain drugs (e.g., ketoconazole, rifampin).

Clinical Presentation. Symptoms can range from mild (anorexia, nausea, weight loss) to severe (hypotensive crisis). In most patients, PAI follows a chronic course. Patients typically present with nonspecific symptoms: nausea, vomiting, diarrhea, anorexia, weakness, emaciation, and abdominal pain. Hyperkalemia, hyponatremia, and hypotension are present as well. These symptoms result from a deficiency of glucocorticoids and mineralocorticoids that occurs secondary to adrenal atrophy. In addition, patients may develop hyperpigmentation of the skin and mucous membranes. The cause is excessive production of ACTH in attempts to restore depressed levels of glucocorticoids. Severe symptoms of acute adrenal crisis are discussed separately.

Treatment. Replacement therapy with adrenocorticoids is required. *Hydrocortisone,* which has both glucocorticoid and mineralocorticoid activity, is a drug of choice. If additional mineralocorticoid activity is needed, *fludrocortisone,* the only mineralocorticoid available, can be added to the regimen.

Secondary and Tertiary Adrenocortical Insufficiency

Secondary adrenocortical insufficiency results from decreased secretion of ACTH, while tertiary insufficiency results from decreased secretion of CRH. In both cases, adrenal secretion of glucocorticoids is diminished, whereas secretion of mineralocorticoids is usually normal. Glucocorticoid insufficiency produces a characteristic set of symptoms: hypoglycemia, malaise, loss of appetite, and reduced capacity to respond to stress. For secondary and tertiary insufficiency, treatment consists of replacement therapy with a glucocorticoid (e.g., hydrocortisone). Rarely, a mineralocorticoid is needed too.

Acute Adrenal Insufficiency (Adrenal Crisis)

Clinical Presentation. Acute adrenal insufficiency is characterized by hypotension, dehydration, weakness, lethargy, and GI symptoms (e.g., vomiting, diarrhea). Left untreated, the syndrome progresses to shock and then death.

Causes. Adrenal crisis may be brought on by adrenal failure, pituitary failure, or failure to provide patients receiving replacement therapy with adequate doses of glucocorticoids. Adrenal crisis may also be triggered by abrupt withdrawal from chronic high-dose glucocorticoid therapy.

Treatment. Patients require rapid replacement of fluid, salt, and glucocorticoids. They also need glucose for energy. These needs are met by injecting 100 mg of hydrocortisone (as an IV bolus) followed by IV infusion of normal saline with dextrose. Additional hydrocortisone is given by infusion at a rate of 50 mg every 8 hours.

Congenital Adrenal Hyperplasia

Clinical Presentation and Causes. CAH results from an inborn deficiency of enzymes needed for glucocorticoid synthesis, most commonly *21-alpha-hydroxylase.* The ability to make glucocorticoids is reduced, but not eliminated. In an attempt to enhance glucocorticoid synthesis, the pituitary releases large amounts of ACTH, which act on the adrenals to cause growth of adrenal tissue (hyperplasia) and increased synthesis of glucocorticoids and androgens. Synthesis of mineralocorticoids changes very little. Frequently, stimulation of glucocorticoid synthesis may be sufficient to normalize levels of cortisol. Unfortunately, the amounts of ACTH required for normalization are so large that synthesis of adrenal androgens becomes excessive. In girls, increased androgen levels cause masculinization of the external genitalia, but the ovaries, uterus, and fallopian tubes are not affected. Increased androgen levels in boys may cause precocious penile enlargement. In all children, linear growth is accelerated. However, because androgens cause premature closure of the epiphyses, adult height is usually diminished. CAH affects 1 of every 10,000 to 20,000 infants.

Treatment. The objective is to ensure adequate levels of glucocorticoids while preventing excessive production of adrenal androgens. This goal is achieved through lifelong glucocorticoid replacement. *Hydrocortisone, dexamethasone,* and *prednisone* are preferred agents. By supplying glucocorticoids exogenously, we can suppress secretion of ACTH. As a result, the adrenals are no longer stimulated to produce excessive quantities of androgens. As a rule, ACTH suppression can be achieved with daily doses of hydrocortisone equivalent to twice the amount secreted by normal adrenals. To assess treatment, children should be monitored every 3 months for growth rate and signs of virilization.

Screening. The Endocrine Society recommends universal screening of newborns for 21-alpha-hydroxylase deficiency. If the test is positive, follow-up testing should be done to confirm a CAH diagnosis. These recommendations are endorsed by several professional organizations, including the American Academy of Pediatrics, the Pediatric Endocrine Society, the Society for Pediatric Urology, and the CARES Foundation.

AGENTS FOR REPLACEMENT THERAPY IN ADRENOCORTICAL INSUFFICIENCY

Patients with adrenocortical insufficiency require replacement therapy. A glucocorticoid is always required; some patients require a mineralocorticoid too. The principal glucocorticoids employed are *hydrocortisone, dexamethasone,* and *prednisone. Fludrocortisone* is the only mineralocorticoid available.

Note that classification of a drug as a "glucocorticoid" or "mineralocorticoid" may be an oversimplification. A drug that we classify as a glucocorticoid may also exhibit salt-retaining (mineralocorticoid) activity. Conversely, a drug that we classify as a mineralocorticoid may also display typical glucocorticoid activity.

Hydrocortisone

Hydrocortisone is a synthetic steroid with a structure identical to that of cortisol, the principal glucocorticoid produced by the adrenal cortex. Hydrocortisone is a preferred drug for adrenocortical insufficiency and will serve as our prototype of the glucocorticoids employed clinically. Please note that, despite being classified as a glucocorticoid, hydrocortisone also has mineralocorticoid actions.

Prototype Drugs

DRUGS FOR ADRENAL CORTEX DISORDERS

Hydrocortisone (a glucocorticoid)
Fludrocortisone (a mineralocorticoid)

Therapeutic Uses

Replacement Therapy. Hydrocortisone is a preferred drug for all forms of adrenocortical insufficiency. Oral hydrocortisone is ideal for chronic replacement therapy. Parenteral administration is used for acute adrenal insufficiency and to supplement oral doses at times of stress. Because of its mineralocorticoid actions, hydrocortisone may suffice as sole therapy for adrenal insufficiency, even when salt loss is a symptom.

Nonendocrine Applications. Hydrocortisone and other glucocorticoids are used to treat a broad spectrum of nonendocrine disorders, ranging from allergic reactions to inflammation to cancer. The doses required are considerably higher than those employed for replacement therapy. Use of glucocorticoids for nonendocrine diseases is discussed in Chapter 72.

Adverse Effects

When given in the low doses required for replacement therapy, hydrocortisone and other glucocorticoids are devoid of adverse effects. In contrast, when taken chronically in the large doses employed to treat nonendocrine disorders, glucocorticoids are highly toxic. The adverse effects of chronic high-dose therapy include adrenal suppression and promotion of Cushing's syndrome. These adverse effects are discussed in Chapter 72.

Preparations, Dosage, and Administration

Dosages presented here are for oral and parenteral therapy of adrenal insufficiency. Dosages for nonendocrine disorders are found in Chapter 72.

Oral Therapy. *Hydrocortisone base* [Cortef ♣] is available in tablets (5, 10, and 20 mg) for oral therapy of chronic adrenal insufficiency. The total daily dose is 12 to 15 mg/m^2. For adults, this translates to 22 to 25 mg/day. To mimic normal cortisol secretion, patients can take the entire daily dose in the morning, immediately after waking. If this schedule results in afternoon or evening fatigue, patients may split the dosage, taking two-thirds in the morning and one-third around 4:00 PM.

Parenteral Therapy. *Hydrocortisone sodium succinate* [Solu-Cortef] is available in single-use vials (100, 250, 500, and 1000 mg) for IM or IV administration. For emergency treatment, IV doses of 50 to 100 mg are employed (see Table 60.1). When IV injections can't be used, IM doses of 100 to 250 mg may be given instead.

Dexamethasone, Prednisone, and Cortisone

Like hydrocortisone, prednisone and dexamethasone are preferred drugs for oral therapy of chronic adrenal insufficiency. The total initial daily dosage is 0.25 to 0.75 mg for dexamethasone and 5 to 60 mg for prednisone, depending on response. In addition to its use for replacement therapy, dexamethasone is used to diagnose adrenal dysfunction (see later).

Cortisone is a prodrug that undergoes conversion to hydrocortisone (its active form) in the body. The drug has both glucocorticoid and mineralocorticoid activity. For management of chronic adrenal insufficiency, the total daily oral dosage is 12 to 15 mg/m^2.

Fludrocortisone

Fludrocortisone is a potent mineralocorticoid that also possesses significant glucocorticoid activity. Fludrocortisone is the only mineralocorticoid available and is the drug of choice for chronic mineralocorticoid replacement.

Therapeutic Uses

Fludrocortisone is a preferred drug for treating primary adrenal insufficiency, primary hypoaldosteronism, and CAH (when salt wasting is a feature of the syndrome). In most cases, fludrocortisone must be used in combination with a glucocorticoid (e.g., hydrocortisone).

Adverse Effects

Adverse effects are a direct consequence of mineralocorticoid actions. When dosage is too high, salt and water are retained in excess, while excessive amounts of potassium are lost. These effects on salt and water can result in expansion of blood volume, hypertension, edema, cardiac enlargement, and hypokalemia. Patients should be monitored for weight gain, elevation of blood pressure, and hypokalemia. If these changes occur, fludrocortisone should be temporarily withdrawn. Fluid and electrolyte imbalance should resolve spontaneously in a few days.

Preparations, Dosage, and Administration. Fludrocortisone acetate is available in 0.1-mg tablets for oral dosing. The dosage is 0.1 mg/day. If excessive salt retention occurs, the dose should be cut to 0.05 mg/day.

AGENTS FOR DIAGNOSING ADRENOCORTICAL DISORDERS

Cosyntropin

Cosyntropin [Cortrosyn], a synthetic analog of ACTH, acts on the adrenal cortex to stimulate synthesis and secretion of cortisol and other adrenal glucocorticoids. The drug is used to diagnose adrenal insufficiency. In the usual test, patients are given a 250-mcg dose of cosyntropin, injected IM or IV. Plasma cortisol is measured just before the injection and then 30 or 60 minutes later. If cortisol rises to above 20 mcg/dL, the adrenal response is considered normal, and hence primary adrenal insufficiency can be ruled out. If cortisol fails to rise significantly, a diagnosis of primary adrenal insufficiency can be made.

Dexamethasone

Dexamethasone is a synthetic steroid that has pronounced glucocorticoid properties and very little mineralocorticoid activity. The drug is used for replacement therapy, treating nonendocrine disorders, and diagnosing Cushing's syndrome.

KEY POINTS

- The adrenal cortex produces three classes of steroid hormones: glucocorticoids, mineralocorticoids, and androgens.
- Glucocorticoids influence the metabolism of carbohydrates, proteins, and fats. In addition, they affect skeletal muscle, the cardiovascular system, and the CNS. At times of stress, glucocorticoids are essential for survival.
- Synthesis and release of glucocorticoids are regulated by a negative feedback loop involving CRH from the hypothalamus, ACTH from the pituitary, and cortisol from the adrenal cortex.
- Aldosterone, the major mineralocorticoid, acts on the kidney to promote retention of sodium and water and excretion of potassium and hydrogen. Aldosterone also acts directly on the heart and blood vessels, causing harm when its levels are high.
- Glucocorticoid excess causes Cushing's syndrome.
- The principal treatment for Cushing's syndrome is surgical removal of the adrenals (if adrenal adenoma or carcinoma is the cause) or part of the pituitary (if pituitary adenoma is the cause).
- Ketoconazole can be used to suppress synthesis of adrenal steroids in patients with Cushing's syndrome. However, this drug is employed only as an adjunct to surgery or radiation.
- Adrenal insufficiency causes Addison's disease.
- Adrenal insufficiency is treated by replacement therapy with glucocorticoids (e.g., hydrocortisone). Fludrocortisone, a pure mineralocorticoid, may be added if the mineralocorticoid actions of hydrocortisone are inadequate.
- Glucocorticoid replacement therapy may be done by (1) giving the entire daily dose in the morning or by (2) splitting the daily dose, giving two-thirds in the morning and one-third in the afternoon.
- In patients with adrenal insufficiency, it is essential to increase glucocorticoid doses at times of stress (e.g., surgery, infection). Failure to do so may be fatal.
- When used in the low (physiologic) doses needed for replacement therapy, glucocorticoids have no adverse effects. In contrast, when used chronically in the high (pharmacologic) doses needed to treat nonendocrine diseases (e.g., arthritis), glucocorticoids can cause severe adverse effects.
- Cosyntropin, which acts like ACTH, is used only for diagnosis of adrenal insufficiency—not for treatment.

Please visit **http://evolve.elsevier.com/Lehne** for chapter-specific NCLEX® examination review questions.

Summary of Major Nursing Implications[a]

GLUCOCORTICOIDS: HYDROCORTISONE AND CORTISONE

The nursing implications here apply only to the use of glucocorticoids for *replacement therapy.*

Use in Addison's Disease

Administration

Instruct patients to follow the prescribed dosing schedule. Primary options are (1) take the entire daily dose in the morning upon waking or (2) divide the daily dose, taking two-thirds upon waking and one-third in the afternoon.

Make certain the patient understands that replacement therapy must continue lifelong.

Emergency Preparedness

Warn patients that dosage must be increased at times of stress (e.g., infection, surgery, trauma). For mild or febrile illness, the "3 by 3 rule" applies: Take 3 times the usual dosage for 3 days. Advise patients to carry an emergency supply of glucocorticoids—oral and injectable—at all times. Advise patients to wear identification (e.g., Medic Alert bracelet) to inform emergency medical personnel of their glucocorticoid requirements.

Monitoring

Determine electrolyte and glucocorticoid levels at baseline and periodically thereafter.

Use in Congenital Adrenal Hyperplasia

To assess therapy, monitor the child at 3-month intervals for signs of excess androgen production (e.g., excessive growth rate, virilization in girls, precocious penile enlargement in boys). Suppression of these effects indicates success.

Minimizing Adverse Effects

Excessive doses can produce symptoms of Cushing's syndrome. Observe the patient for signs of Cushing's syndrome, and notify the prescriber if these develop.

FLUDROCORTISONE (A MINERALOCORTICOID)

Route

Oral.

Minimizing Adverse Effects

Excessive doses cause retention of sodium and water and excessive excretion of potassium, resulting in expansion of blood volume, hypertension, cardiac enlargement, edema, and hypokalemia. Evaluate patients periodically for clinical status and electrolyte levels. **Inform patients about signs of salt and water retention (e.g., unusual weight gain, swelling of the feet or lower legs) and hypokalemia (e.g., muscle weakness, irregular heartbeat), and instruct them to notify the prescriber if these occur.** Treatment consists of temporary withdrawal of fludrocortisone, after which fluid and electrolyte balance should normalize within days.

[a]Patient education information is highlighted as **blue text.**

UNIT IX WOMEN'S HEALTH

CHAPTER 61

Estrogens and Progestins: Basic Pharmacology and Noncontraceptive Applications

In order to understand pharmacologic properties of manufactured estrogens and progestins, it is important to first understand properties and actions of the endogenous hormones. We begin this chapter with a discussion of how estrogens and progestins regulate physiologic processes.

Estrogens and progestins (also known as progestogens) are hormones with multiple actions. They promote female maturation and help regulate the ongoing activity of female reproductive organs. In addition, they affect bone mineralization and lipid metabolism.

The principal endogenous estrogen is estradiol. The principal endogenous progestational hormone (i.e., progestin) is progesterone. Both hormones are produced by the ovaries. During pregnancy, large amounts are produced by the placenta. In addition, small amounts of estrogens and progestins are produced in peripheral tissues.

Clinical applications of the female sex hormones fall into two major categories: contraceptive and noncontraceptive applications. In this chapter, we focus on noncontraceptive uses. Contraception is discussed in Chapter 62.

THE MENSTRUAL CYCLE

Because much of the clinical pharmacology of the estrogens and progestins is related to their actions during the menstrual cycle, understanding the menstrual cycle is central to understanding these hormones. Accordingly, we begin by reviewing the menstrual cycle. The anatomic and hormonal changes that take place during the cycle are shown in Fig. 61.1. As indicated, the first half of the cycle (days 1 through 14) is called the *follicular phase,* and the second half is called the *luteal phase.* One full cycle typically takes approximately 28 days.

Ovarian and Uterine Events

The menstrual cycle consists of a coordinated series of ovarian and uterine events. In the ovary, the following sequence occurs: (1) Several ovarian follicles ripen; (2) one of the ripe follicles ruptures, causing ovulation; (3) the ruptured follicle evolves into a corpus luteum; and (4) if fertilization does not occur, the corpus luteum atrophies. As these ovarian events are taking place, parallel events take place in the uterus: (1) While ovarian follicles ripen, the endometrium prepares for nidation (implantation of a fertilized ovum) by increasing in thickness and

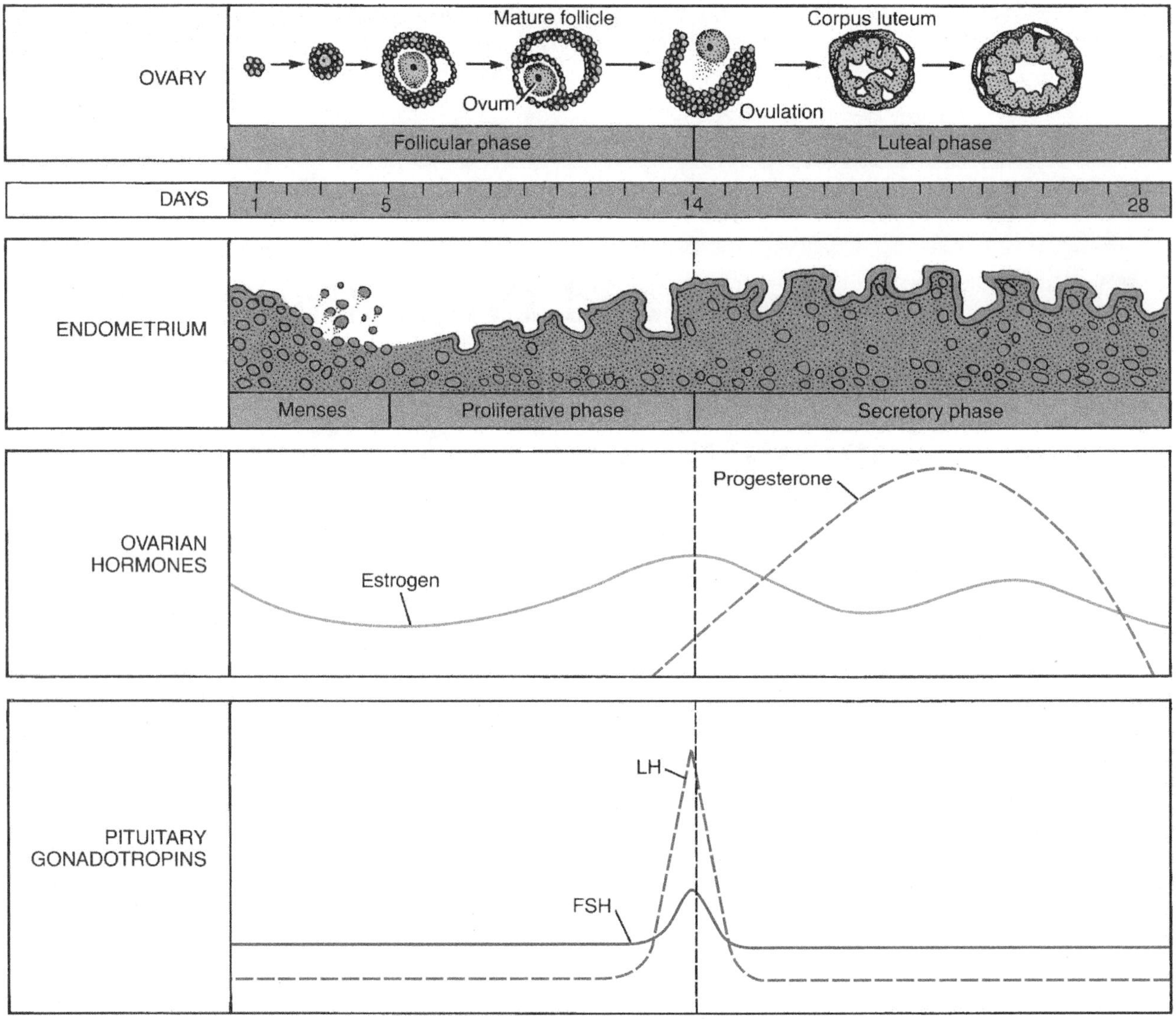

Fig. 61.1 ■ The menstrual cycle: anatomic and hormonal changes. (*FSH*, Follicle-stimulating hormone; *LH*, luteinizing hormone.)

vascularity; (2) following ovulation, the uterus continues its preparation by increasing secretory activity; and (3) if implantation fails to occur, the thickened endometrium breaks down, causing menstruation, and the cycle begins anew.

The Roles of Estrogens and Progesterone

The uterine changes that occur during the cycle are brought about under the influence of estrogens and progesterone produced by the ovaries. During the first half of the cycle, estrogens are secreted by the maturing ovarian follicles. As suggested by Fig. 61.1, these estrogens act on the uterus to cause proliferation of the endometrium. At midcycle, one of the ovarian follicles ruptures and then evolves into a corpus luteum. For most of the second half of the cycle, estrogens and progesterone are produced by the newly formed corpus luteum. These hormones maintain the endometrium in its hypertrophied state. At the end of the cycle, the corpus luteum atrophies, causing production of estrogens and progesterone to decline. In response to the diminished supply of ovarian hormones, the endometrium breaks down.

The Role of Pituitary Hormones

Two anterior pituitary hormones—follicle-stimulating hormone (FSH) and luteinizing hormone (LH)—play central roles in regulating the menstrual cycle. Precisely timed alterations in the secretion of these hormones are responsible for coordinating the structural and secretory changes that occur throughout the menstrual cycle. During the first half of the cycle, FSH acts on the developing ovarian follicles, causing them to mature and secrete estrogens. The resultant rise in estrogen levels exerts a negative feedback influence on the pituitary, thereby suppressing further FSH release. At midcycle, LH levels rise abruptly (see Fig. 61.1). This LH surge causes the dominant follicle to swell rapidly, burst, and release its ovum. Following ovulation, the ruptured follicle becomes a corpus luteum and, under the influence of LH, begins to secrete progesterone.

si

BOX 61.1 ■ SPECIAL INTEREST TOPIC

A NEW DRUG TO INCREASE FEMALE LIBIDO

Research indicates that approximately 10% to 40% of women experience female sexual interest/arousal disorder (FSIAD; formerly called hypoactive sexual desire disorder). The incidence of FSIAD is greatly increased following the hormonal changes associated with menopause.

Over the centuries, treatments to increase a woman's interest in sex have ranged from dangerous (e.g., cantharidin [Spanish fly], the toxic chemical from a beetle that causes irritation and blistering of the mucosa) to ridiculous (e.g., filling the vagina with various horrid substances). More recent management has focused on addressing psychological issues and on the off-label use of drugs such as sildenafil and testosterone (both drugs with varying degrees of success). Some women report that "self-medicating" with recreational drugs such as cocaine and methylphenidate (Ritalin) increase libido, although we would never recommend the use of these substances for that purpose.

In 2015 the U.S. Food and Drug Administration (FDA) approved the first drug to manage FSIAD. Flibanserin (Addyi) is available by prescription for women with low libido not associated with medical or mental health problems, relationship problems, or medication side effects. Unfortunately, it is not indicated for the treatment of women who are postmenopausal.

Unlike drugs for males with sexual dysfunction, which have predictably rapid effects after administration of a single dose, flibanserin requires daily doses for several weeks before benefits are seen. The prescribing information recommends discontinuing the drug if improvement is not seen after 8 weeks.

A number of serious risks are associated with the use of flibanserin. Central nervous system depression and hypotension, with or without syncope, are the most common adverse effects. Flibanserin is a substrate of multiple isoenzymes, most notably CYP3A4, and therefore drug interactions are common. It is also expensive—a month's supply costs approximately $960.

In addition, there exist a couple of restrictions on prescribers and pharmacies. Flibanserin is available only through a Risk Evaluation and Mitigation Strategy (REMS). The Addyi REMS program requires enrollment of and training for any providers wanting to prescribe this drug. In addition, only pharmacies certified with the Addyi REMS program may dispense flibanserin.

Additional information on flibanserin is available at http://www.addyi.com/hcp. Information on the Addyi REMS program is available at https://addyirems.com/AddyiUI/rems/home.action.

ESTROGENS

Biosynthesis and Elimination

Females

In premenopausal women, the ovary is the principal source of estrogen. During the follicular phase of the menstrual cycle, estrogens are synthesized by ovarian follicles; during the luteal phase, estrogens are synthesized by the corpus luteum. The major estrogen produced by the ovaries is *estradiol.* In the periphery, some of the estradiol secreted by the ovaries is converted into *estrone* and *estriol,* hormones that are less potent than estradiol. Estrogens are eliminated by a combination of hepatic metabolism and urinary excretion.

During pregnancy, large quantities of estrogens are produced by the placenta. Excretion of these hormones results in high levels of estrogens in the urine.

Males

Estrogen production is not limited to females. In the human male, small amounts of testosterone are converted into estradiol and estrone by the testes. Enzymatic conversion of testosterone in peripheral tissues (e.g., liver, fat, skeletal muscle) results in additional estrogen production.

Mechanism of Action

Like other steroidal hormones (e.g., testosterone, cortisol), estrogen acts primarily through receptors in the cell nucleus, not on the cell surface. Hence, to produce its effects, estrogen must diffuse into cells, migrate to the nucleus, and then bind with an estrogen receptor (ER). The estrogen-ER complex then binds with an *estrogen response element* on a target gene, altering the rate of gene transcription. It is important to note that not all ERs are found in the nucleus: Some ERs are found on cell membranes. Activating these surface receptors produces a rapid response—more rapid than can be produced by activating nuclear receptors.

There are two forms of ERs, termed *ER alpha* and *ER beta.* ER alpha is highly expressed in the vagina, uterus, ovaries, mammary glands, vascular epithelium, and hypothalamus. ER beta is expressed in the ovary and prostate, and to a lesser extent in the lungs, brain, bones, and blood vessels. Some cells have both types of ERs.

Physiologic and Pharmacologic Effects

Effects on Primary and Secondary Sex Characteristics of Females

Estrogens support the development and maintenance of the female reproductive tract and secondary sex characteristics. These hormones are required for the growth and maturation of the uterus, vagina, fallopian tubes, and breasts. In addition, estrogens direct pigmentation of the nipples and genitalia.

Estrogens have a profound influence on physiologic processes related to reproduction. During the follicular phase of the menstrual cycle, estrogens promote (1) ductal growth in the breast, (2) thickening and cornification of the vaginal epithelium, (3) proliferation of the uterine epithelium, and (4) copious secretion of thickened mucus from endocervical glands. In addition, estrogens increase vaginal acidity (by promoting local deposition of glycogen, which is then acted upon by lactobacilli and corynebacteria to produce lactic acid). At the end of the menstrual cycle, a decline in estrogen levels can bring on menstruation. However, it is the fall in progesterone levels at the end of the cycle that normally causes breakdown of the endometrium and resultant menstrual bleeding. Following menstruation, estrogens promote endometrial restoration.

During pregnancy, the placenta produces estrogen in large amounts. This estrogen stimulates uterine blood flow and growth of uterine muscle. In addition, it acts on the breast to continue ductal proliferation. However, final transformation of the breast for milk production requires the combined influence of estrogen, progesterone, and human placental lactogen.

Metabolic Actions

Endogenous estrogens can affect various nonreproductive tissues. Important among these are bone, cardiovascular, and central nervous systems (CNS). They also have an important roles glucose homeostasis. This is discussed next.

Bone. Estrogens have a positive effect on bone mass. Under normal conditions, bone undergoes continuous remodeling, a process in which bone mineral is resorbed and deposited in equal amounts. The principal effect of estrogens on the process is to block bone resorption (i.e., bone tissue breakdown to release minerals), although estrogens may also promote mineral deposition.

During puberty, the long bones grow rapidly under the combined influence of growth hormone, adrenal androgens, and *low* levels of ovarian estrogens. When estrogen levels grow high enough, they promote epiphyseal closure, and thereby bring linear growth to a stop.

Cardiovascular System. Cardiovascular disease is much less common in premenopausal women. Estrogens have several roles in lowering this risk. For example, estrogen receptors in the vascular smooth muscle respond to activation by decreasing vasoconstriction. Activation of estrogen receptors in vessel endothelium results in the production of nitric oxide, which promotes vasodilation and increased perfusion. Estrogens also decrease atherosclerosis through favorable effects on cholesterol levels: Levels of low-density lipoprotein (LDL) cholesterol are reduced, while levels of high-density lipoprotein (HDL) cholesterol are elevated.

Blood Coagulation. Estrogens both promote and suppress blood coagulation. Estrogens promote coagulation by (1) increasing levels of coagulation factors (e.g., factors II, VII, IX, X, and XII), and by (2) decreasing levels of factors that suppress coagulation (e.g., antithrombin). Estrogens suppress coagulation by increasing the activity of factors that promote breakdown of fibrin, a protein that reinforces blood clots. The net effect—increased or decreased coagulation—may be determined by a hereditary defect in one of these targets.

Central Nervous System. In the CNS, estrogens have a neuroprotective effect by defending neurons from the effects of oxidative stress and injury. They also have a role in neuronal growth and repair via stimulation of nerve growth factors. Estrogen-induced synaptic changes coupled with estrogen-promoted increases in synaptic serotonin, dopamine, and norepinephrine are thought to preserve cognitive function, enhance short-term memory, and regulate mood. Cerebral perfusion is also enhanced via the release of nitric acid and the resulting vasodilation.

Glucose Homeostasis. Estrogen plays an active role in maintaining glucose levels. In conditions that lead to insulin resistance due to impaired transport, estrogen has been shown to increase insulin sensitivity to promote glucose uptake. Estrogens also have a role in insulin secretion and are believed to protect pancreatic islet beta cells from certain types of injury.

Clinical Pharmacology

Now that we have reviewed the effects of endogenous estrogens, let's examine how estrogen preparations are used clinically. We'll begin with a discussion of therapeutic uses.

Therapeutic Uses

Estrogens have contraceptive and noncontraceptive applications. In this chapter, discussion is limited to the noncontraceptive applications. Use of estrogens for contraception is discussed in Chapter 62.

Menopausal Hormone Therapy. Hormone therapy in postmenopausal women is the most common noncontraceptive use of estrogens. When estrogen is used for this purpose, it is usually accompanied by progestins. For this reason, we will cover hormone therapy following the discussion of progestins.

Female Hypogonadism. In the absence of ovarian estrogens, pubertal transformation will not take place. Causes of estrogen deficiency include primary ovarian failure, hypopituitarism, bilateral oophorectomy (removal of both ovaries), and Turner's syndrome (a genetic disorder that impairs gonadal function). In girls with estrogen insufficiency, puberty can be induced by giving exogenous estrogens. This treatment promotes breast development, maturation of the reproductive organs, and development of pubic and axillary hair. To simulate normal patterns of estrogen secretion, the regimen should consist of continuous low-dose therapy (for about a year) followed by cyclic administration of estrogen in higher doses.

Acne. Estrogens, in the form of oral contraceptives, can help control acne. Treatment is limited to those at least 14 or 15 years old who want contraception. The use of estrogen for acne is discussed in Chapter 105.

Cancer Palliation. Estrogens are sometimes used for palliative therapy in the management of advanced prostate cancer in men. It is also used in a select type of metastatic breast cancer in both men and women.

Adverse Effects

The principal concerns with estrogen therapy are the potential for endometrial hyperplasia, endometrial cancer, breast cancer, and cardiovascular thromboembolic events. Of these, the potential for endometrial hyperplasia and endometrial cancer can be resolved by prescribing a progestin, if indicated.

Estrogens have been associated with gallbladder disease, jaundice, and headache. Use during menopause may produce or uncover gallbladder disease. Jaundice may develop in women with pre-existing liver dysfunction, especially those who experienced cholestatic jaundice of pregnancy.

Nausea is the most common undesired response to the estrogens. Fortunately, nausea diminishes with continued use, and is rarely so severe as to necessitate treatment cessation.

Estrogens can increase the risk for headache, especially migraine headache. Fluid retention with edema commonly occurs. Most other adverse effects (e.g., chloasma, a patchy brown facial discoloration) are more of a nuisance than a concern.

Hazardous Drug Status

Estrogen is classified by the National Institute for Occupational Safety and Health (NIOSH) as a hazardous drug because estrogens pose a reproductive risk to healthcare workers who handle them. See Chapter 3, Table 3.1, for administration and handling guidelines.

Safety Alert

ESTROGEN

Endometrial cancer risk is increased in women with a uterus who take unopposed estrogen (i.e., estrogen without a progestin). Estrogen may increase the risk for deep vein thrombosis and stroke.

Estrogen may increase the risk for dementia in women age 65 and older.

Contraindications

Estrogens should not be taken by patients with a history of deep vein thrombosis, pulmonary embolus, or conditions such as stroke or myocardial infarction (MI) that occurred secondary to a thromboembolic event. They should not be prescribed to women who are pregnant or who have vaginal bleeding without a known cause. Patients with a history of liver disease, estrogen-dependent tumors, or breast cancer (except when indicated for management) also should not take estrogens.

Interactions

Estrogens are major substrates of CYP1A2 and CYP3A4. Inducers of these isoenzymes may lower estrogen levels, while drugs that are inhibitors may raise estrogen levels. Additionally, estrogens may decrease the effectiveness of some antidiabetic drugs and thyroid preparations. Estrogens can also interact with anticoagulants and other drugs that affect clotting.

Preparations and Routes of Administration

Estrogen is available in conjugated and esterified forms. Esterified estrogens are plant-based; conjugated estrogens may be either synthetic or natural preparations derived from the urine of pregnant horses.

Oral. Owing to convenience, the oral route is used more than any other. The most active estrogenic compound—estradiol—is available alone and in combination with progestins. Estrogen itself is available in conjugated and esterified forms.

Transdermal. Transdermal estradiol is available in four formulations:

- Emulsion [Estrasorb]
- Spray [Evamist]
- Gels [EstroGel, Elestrin, Divigel]
- Patches [Alora, Climara, Estraderm, Estradot 🍁, Menostar, Vivelle-Dot, Oesclim]

Application is specific to certain body regions. The emulsion is applied once daily to the top of both thighs and the back of both calves. The spray is applied once daily to the forearm. The gel is applied once daily to one arm, from the shoulder to the wrist or to the thigh *(Divigel)*. The patches are applied to the skin of the trunk (but not the breasts). Rates of estrogen absorption with transdermal formulations range from 14 to 60 mcg/24 hr, depending on the product employed.

Compared with oral formulations, the transdermal formulations have four advantages:

- The total dose of estrogen is greatly reduced (because the liver is bypassed).
- There is less nausea and vomiting.
- Blood levels of estrogen fluctuate less.
- There is a lower risk for deep vein thrombosis, pulmonary embolism, and stroke.

Intravaginal. Estrogens for intravaginal administration are available as tablets, creams, and vaginal rings. The tablets [Vagifem], creams [Estrace Vaginal, Premarin Vaginal], and one of the two available vaginal rings [Estring] are used only for local effects, primarily treatment of vulval and vaginal atrophy associated with menopause. The other vaginal ring [Femring] is used for systemic effects (e.g., control of hot flashes and night sweats), as well as local effects (e.g., treatment of vulval and vaginal atrophy).

PATIENT-CENTERED CARE ACROSS THE LIFE SPAN

Estrogens

Life Stage	Patient Care Concerns
Children	Estrogens are not indicated for prepubertal children.
Pregnant women	Estrogens are Pregnancy Risk Category X.[a] They are contraindicated during pregnancy.
Breast-feeding women	Estrogens may affect infant development and may decrease both the quantity and quality of milk produced.
Older adults	Beers Criteria include estrogens among those identified as potentially inappropriate for use in geriatric patients.

[a]As of 2020, the FDA will no longer use Pregnancy Risk Categories. Please refer to Chapter 9 for more information.

Parenteral. Although estrogens are formulated for IV and IM administration, use of these routes is rare. Intravenous administration is generally limited to acute emergency control of heavy uterine bleeding.

SELECTIVE ESTROGEN RECEPTOR MODULATORS (SERMs)

SERMs are drugs that activate estrogen receptors in some tissues and block them in others. These drugs were developed in an effort to provide the benefits of estrogen (e.g., protection against osteoporosis, maintenance of the urogenital tract, reduction of LDL cholesterol) while avoiding its drawbacks (e.g., promotion of breast cancer, uterine cancer, and thromboembolism). Four SERMs are available: tamoxifen [Nolvadex], toremifene [Fareston], raloxifene [Evista], and bazedoxifene [Duavee]. None of these offers all of the benefits of estrogen, and none avoids all of the drawbacks. Three of these—tamoxifen, toremifene, and raloxifene—are classified as hazardous drugs by NIOSH. These require special handling during administration. (See Table 3.1 of Chapter 3 for administration and handling guidelines.)

Tamoxifen was the first SERM to be widely used. By blocking estrogen receptors, tamoxifen (and its active metabolite, endoxifen) can inhibit cell growth in the breast. As a result, the drug is used extensively to prevent and treat breast cancer. Unfortunately, blockade of estrogen receptors also produces hot flashes. By activating estrogen receptors, tamoxifen protects against osteoporosis and has a favorable effect on serum lipids. However, receptor activation also increases the risk for endometrial cancer and thromboembolism. The pharmacology of tamoxifen and toremifene (a close relative of tamoxifen) is discussed in Chapter 103.

Raloxifene is very similar to tamoxifen. The principal difference is that raloxifene does not activate estrogen receptors in the endometrium, and hence does not pose a risk for uterine cancer. Like tamoxifen, raloxifene protects against breast cancer and osteoporosis, increases the risk for thromboembolism, and induces hot flashes. Raloxifene is approved only for the prevention and treatment of osteoporosis and for prevention of breast cancer in high-risk women. Raloxifene is discussed at length in Chapter 75.

In 2013, the FDA approved *Duavee* (conjugated estrogens/bazedoxifene) for the prevention of vasomotor symptoms and osteoporosis in postmenopausal women with a uterus. Duavee is the first drug to combine estrogen with an estrogen agonist/antagonist (bazedoxifene). The bazedoxifene component of Duavee reduces the risk for excessive growth of the lining of the uterus that can occur with the estrogen component. Contraindications to taking Duavee are the same as for other estrogen-containing products.

PROGESTINS

Estrogens and progestins are often prescribed together. Before we discuss these uses, it will be helpful to discuss endogenous progestins. As previously mentioned, progesterone is the principal endogenous progestational hormone. As its name implies, progesterone acts before gestation to prepare the uterus for implantation of a fertilized ovum. In addition, progesterone helps maintain the uterus throughout pregnancy.

Biosynthesis

Progesterone is produced by the ovaries *and* the placenta. Ovarian production occurs during the second half of the menstrual cycle. During this period, progesterone is synthesized by the corpus luteum in response to LH released from the anterior pituitary. If implantation of a fertilized ovum does not occur, progesterone production by the corpus luteum ceases, and menstrual flow begins. However, if implantation *does* take place, the developing trophoblast will produce its own luteotropic hormone—human chorionic gonadotropin (hCG)—that will stimulate the corpus luteum to continue to make progesterone. For the first 7 weeks of gestation, the placenta depends entirely on progesterone from the corpus luteum. However, between weeks 7 and 10, production of progesterone is shared between the corpus luteum and placenta. After 10 weeks of gestation, progesterone made by the placenta is sufficient to support pregnancy, and hence ovarian progesterone production declines. Placental synthesis of progesterone and estrogen continues throughout the pregnancy.

Mechanism of Action

As with estrogen, receptors for progesterone are found in the cell nucleus. Hence, to produce an effect, progesterone must diffuse across the cell membrane, migrate to the nucleus, and then bind with a progesterone receptor (PR). The progesterone-PR complex then binds with a *progesterone regulatory element* on a target gene, thereby rapidly increasing gene transcription. As with estrogen, there are two types of receptors for progesterone, designated PR-A and PR-B. In general, the *stimulatory* actions of progesterone are mediated by PR-B, whereas *inhibitory* actions are mediated by PR-A.

Physiologic Effects

Effects During the Menstrual Cycle

Progesterone is secreted during the second half of the menstrual cycle from a proliferative state into a secretory state. If implantation does not occur, progesterone production by the corpus luteum declines. The resultant fall in progesterone levels is the principal stimulus for the onset of menstruation.

In addition to affecting the endometrium, progesterone affects the endocervical glands, breasts, body temperature, respiration, and mood. Under the influence of progesterone, secretions from endocervical glands become scant and viscous. (In contrast, estrogen makes these secretions profuse and watery.) In addition, progesterone causes the epithelium of the breast to divide and grow. Actions in the CNS may cause depression and sleepiness. By increasing the sensitivity of the respiratory center to CO_2, progesterone causes the partial pressure of carbon dioxide (pCO_2) in blood to fall. At midcycle, when ovulation occurs, progesterone raises body temperature by 0.6°C (1°F).

Effects During Pregnancy

As noted, progesterone levels increase during pregnancy. These high levels suppress contraction of *uterine smooth muscle* and thereby help sustain pregnancy. Unfortunately, progesterone also suppresses contraction of *GI smooth muscle,* which leads to prolonged transit time and constipation. In the *breast,* progesterone promotes growth and proliferation of alveolar tubules (acini), the structures that produce milk. Metabolic effects include suppression of arterial pCO_2, altered serum bicarbonate content, and elevation of serum pH. Finally, progesterone may help suppress the maternal immune system, thereby preventing immune attack on the fetus.

Other Effects

Pharmacologic doses of progesterone can suppress release of pituitary gonadotropins (LH and FSH). This prevents follicular maturation and ovulation. Also, individual progestin preparations display varying degrees of estrogenic, androgenic, and anabolic activity.

Clinical Pharmacology

Therapeutic Uses

Discussion in this chapter is limited to the noncontraceptive uses of progestins. Use for contraception is considered in Chapter 62.

Menopausal Hormone Therapy. The primary noncontraceptive use of progestins is to counteract the adverse effects of estrogen on the endometrium in women undergoing menopausal hormone therapy (HT). This application is discussed later in this chapter.

Dysfunctional Uterine Bleeding. This condition, characterized by heavy irregular bleeding, occurs when progesterone levels are insufficient to balance the stimulatory influence of estrogen on the endometrium. In the absence of sufficient progesterone, estrogen puts the endometrium in a state of continuous proliferation. Since progesterone is unavailable to induce monthly endometrial breakdown, the excessively proliferative endometrium undergoes spontaneous sloughing at irregular intervals. The result is periodic episodes of severe menstrual bleeding. Dysfunctional uterine bleeding is typically associated with anovulatory cycles. The disorder occurs most commonly in adolescents and women approaching menopause. Obese women and those with polycystic ovary syndrome are also susceptible.

Treatment has two objectives: the initial goal is cessation of hemorrhage; the long-term goal is to establish a regular monthly cycle. Excessive bleeding can be stopped by administering a progestin for 10 to 14 days. When dosing is stopped, withdrawal bleeding takes place. Bleeding is likely to be profuse and associated with cramping. Giving an oral contraceptive twice daily for 5 to 7 days can help stabilize the endometrium and thereby reduce bleeding duration.

Cyclic therapy is employed to establish a regular monthly cycle. In one regimen, oral dosing is started 10 to 14 days after the onset of each menstrual period and continued for the next 10 days. Alternatively, a progestin can be given for the first 10 days of each month. Both approaches can promote regular endometrial breakdown and menstruation.

Amenorrhea. Progestins can induce menstrual flow in selected women who are experiencing amenorrhea. If endogenous estrogen levels are adequate, treatment with a progestin for 5 to 10 days will be followed by withdrawal bleeding when the progestin is stopped. If estrogen levels are low, it may be necessary to induce endometrial proliferation with an estrogen before giving the progestin.

Infertility. Progestins are used to support an early pregnancy in women with corpus luteum deficiency syndrome and in women undergoing *in vitro* fertilization (IVF).

Prematurity Prevention. One progestin—*hydroxyprogesterone acetate* [Makena]—is approved for preventing preterm birth in women with a singleton pregnancy and a history of preterm delivery. This use is discussed in Chapter 64.

Endometrial Carcinoma and Hyperplasia. Progestins can provide palliation in women with metastatic endometrial carcinoma, but these drugs do not prolong life. Several months of treatment may be required for a response. The progestins employed are *medroxyprogesterone acetate* and *megestrol acetate*. Medroxyprogesterone acetate is given once weekly by IM injection; megestrol acetate is administered daily by mouth.

Endometrial hyperplasia, a potentially precancerous condition, can be suppressed with progestins. Benefits derive from counteracting the proliferative effects of estrogen. Treatment options include oral therapy with *megestrol acetate* [Megace] or *medroxyprogesterone acetate* [Provera], and local delivery of a *levonorgestrel* using the Mirena IUD.

Safety Alert

ESTROGEN PLUS PROGESTIN

Estrogen plus progestin may increase the risk for thromboembolic events such as deep vein thrombosis, stroke, and pulmonary embolism. It may increase the risk of dementia in women age 65 and older. Estrogen plus progestin also may increase breast cancer risk.

Adverse Effects

Up to 20% of patients may experience breast tenderness, headache, abdominal discomfort, arthralgias, and depression. When used continuously for birth control, progestins greatly decrease production of cervical mucus and cause involution of the endometrial layer. Effects on the endometrium lead to spotting, breakthrough bleeding, and irregular menses. Progestins, in combination with estrogen, increase the risk for breast cancer in postmenopausal women.

PATIENT-CENTERED CARE ACROSS THE LIFE SPAN

Progestins

Life Stage	Patient Care Concerns
Children	Progestins are not indicated for prepubertal children.
Pregnant women	Progestins are Pregnancy Risk Category X.[a] High-dose therapy during the first 4 months of pregnancy has been associated with an increased incidence of birth defects (limb reductions, heart defects, masculinization of the female fetus).
Breast-feeding women	Progestins may contribute to neonatal jaundice.
Older adults	Progestins are indicated only if the patient is taking estrogen and has a uterus.

[a]As of 2020, the FDA will no longer use Pregnancy Risk Categories. Please refer to Chapter 9 for more information.

Hazardous Drug Status

Progestins are classified by the NIOSH as hazardous drugs because they pose a reproductive risk to healthcare workers who handle them. See Chapter 3, Table 3.1, for administration and handling guidelines.

Preparations and Routes of Administration

Progestins are available in oral, IM, subQ, intravaginal, intrauterine, and transdermal formulations. Older oral progestins include *medroxyprogesterone acetate* [Provera], *norethindrone* [Micronor, Nor-QD, others], *norethindrone acetate* [Aygestin], *megestrol acetate* [Megace], *levonorgestrel* [Plan B One-Step, Next Choice], and a micronized formulation of *progesterone* [Prometrium]. Newer oral progestins—*norgestimate* and *drospirenone*—are available in fixed-dose combinations with estradiol sold as Prefest and Angeliq, respectively. Intramuscular progestins are *medroxyprogesterone acetate* [Depo-Provera] and *progesterone* (in oil). *Medroxyprogesterone acetate* is also available in a formulation for subQ injection [Depo-SubQ Provera 104]. *Micronized progesterone* for intravaginal use is available as progesterone gel [Crinone] and a vaginal insert [Endometrin]. Transdermal products are limited to *norethindrone* (formulated with estradiol under the name CombiPatch) and *levonorgestrel* (formulated with estradiol under the name Climara Pro). A second-generation progestin—*etonogestrel*—used for contraception is available by itself as a subQ implant [Nexplanon] and combined with estradiol in a vaginal ring [NuvaRing].

MENOPAUSAL HORMONE THERAPY

Menopausal HT, formerly known as *hormone replacement therapy* (HRT), consists of low doses of estrogen (with or without a progestin) taken to compensate for the loss of estrogen that occurs during menopause. We begin this section with a discussion of menopause.

Physiologic Alterations Accompanying Menopause

Menopause may occur as the result of surgery (i.e., surgical menopause associated with bilateral oophorectomy) or as the result of declining ovarian function associated with aging. Why is estrogen lost with aging? Because ovarian follicles, which are the primary source of estrogen, decline as women grow older. Natural menopause typically begins around age 51 or 52 years, with 95% of women entering menopause between the ages of 45 and 55 years old. During the initial phase, the menstrual cycle becomes irregular, anovulatory cycles may occur, and periods of amenorrhea may alternate with menses. Eventually, ovulation and menstruation cease entirely. Production of ovarian estrogens decreases gradually, coming to a complete stop several years after menstruation has ceased.

Loss of estrogen has multiple effects. Prominent among these are vasomotor symptoms (manifesting as hot flashes, also known as hot flushes and night sweats), sleep disturbances, urogenital atrophy (presenting as vaginal dryness, itching, and burning), bone loss (manifesting as osteoporosis and increased fracture risk), and altered lipid metabolism (presenting as increased levels of LDL cholesterol and reduced levels of HDL cholesterol).

It is typically the vasomotor symptoms that compel most women to seek out HT. Hot flashes and the drenching sweats that accompany them can interfere with daily life and cause sleepless nights. Not only are they uncomfortable, but they may create embarrassing situations, especially for women working with the public where appearances can be important.

Controversy Surrounding Menopausal Hormone Therapy

Given the positive physiologic effects of estrogen and the detrimental physiologic changes that occur with estrogen loss, it might seem logical to prescribe HT for all women experiencing menopause. Indeed, this was once common practice, with therapy that began during perimenopause and continued into later years of life. Then, in the early 2000s, data from two landmark studies, the Women's Health Initiative (WHI) and the Heart and Estrogen/progestin Replacement Study (HERS) and its follow-up (HERS II), demonstrated that, contrary to popular assumptions, the use of HT could increase, rather than prevent, cardiovascular events. Women taking HT in the study also had an increase in thromboembolic events such as deep vein thrombosis and stroke. For women receiving EPT (but not ET), there was a significant increase in the incidence of breast cancer. The reaction in the medical community was strong and swift as many providers stopped prescribing HT altogether and the use of HT declined by 80%.

Over the past decade, increased scrutiny of these early studies yielded concerns that have resulted in a re-examination of these risks. Subjects in those studies tended to be older. For example, *only 3.5% of women in the WHI study were in the age range of 50 to 54 years,* which is the age at which most women currently begin HT. Initial enrollment included women up to 79 years of age. By the time the study was stopped, some of the women were in their 80s! Further, the therapy in those studies was at a higher dose and use was prolonged beyond that of recommended current practice. When WHI data for women ages 50 to 59 taking HT for less than 10 years were examined, it was discovered that the increase in venous thromboembolic episodes was only between 1.1 and 5 out of 1000 women taking ET and 5.1 and 10 out of 1000 women taking EPT. For women taking ET, there was no increase in coronary heart disease (CHD); for women taking EPT, the increase in CHD was 1.1 to 5 out of 1000 women. Moreover, when benefits were examined, *for both ET and EPT, 5.1 to 10 out of 1000 women experienced a reduction in overall mortality compared to women not taking HT.*

Subsequent and ongoing research has provided more insight into the relationships of HT to dosage, time of initiation, length of use, and patient age, which were not adequately accounted for in the original reports from these studies. The more informed view of HT has evolved to a more reasoned approach to HT.

Recognizing that findings based on women older than 60 years of age taking high-dose, long-term HT for over a decade could not be generalized to younger women taking low-dose HT for shorter time intervals, the Endocrine Society undertook an extensive review of published research to determine the benefits and risk for HT in women recently menopausal (i.e., less than 10 years postmenopausal) and aged 50 to 59. Significant findings are summarized in Table 61.1. Not included in the table are the results of benefits related to the vasomotor and urogenital symptoms because the benefit (90% reduction in symptoms) is firmly established. Also not included are many of the previously assumed risks that were not supported in the data.

Based on these findings, especially considering the benefits of overall mortality, it certainly seems unreasonable to refuse HT for women early in menopause once individual risks are ruled out. Unfortunately, this does not address concerns of older women who have indications for therapy. More studies are needed; however, in the meantime, it is important to recognize that risk for complications increases with age.

TABLE 61.1 ■ Benefits and Risks of Menopausal Hormone Therapy

	Number of Fewer Cases Per 1000 Women Age 50–59	
Benefits Over 5 Years	**Estrogen Plus Progestin (EPT)**	**Estrogen Only (ET)**
Coronary heart disease	0.9	3.8
Osteoporotic fractures	4.9	5.9
Breast cancer	—	1.5
Colorectal cancer	1.2	—
Type 2 diabetes mellitus	11	11
Mortality for all causes	5.3 fewer deaths	5 fewer deaths
	Number of Increased Cases Per 1000 Women Age 50–59	
Risk Over 5 Years	**Estrogen Plus Progestin (EPT)**	**Estrogen Only (ET)**
Thromboembolism	5	2
Stroke	1.0	1.2
Breast cancer	6.8	—
Cholecystitis[a]	9.6	14.2

[a]Data specific for cholecystitis are based on a larger demographic because data specific to ages 50–59 were not available.
Data from Postmenopausal Hormone Therapy: An Endocrine Society Scientific Statement. *J Clin Endocrinol Metab,* July 2010, 95(Suppl 1):S1–S66

Benefits and Risks of Hormone Therapy

As with any drug, prescribing decisions require weighing the benefits and risks. It is important to keep in mind that our understanding of the benefits and risks of HT continues to evolve as current research focuses on the new demographic of younger woman taking HT at lower doses over fewer years.

Prototype Drugs

ESTROGENS AND PROGESTINS

Estrogens
Conjugated estrogens [Premarin]
Estradiol

Progestins
Medroxyprogesterone acetate
Norethindrone

General Recommendations

To balance benefits and risks, an individual risk profile should be compiled for every woman considering HT. All candidates for HT should be informed of known risks. Women with multiple risk factors should consider alternative therapies. For most women, the benefits of *long-term* HT for disease prevention do not outweigh the risks, and hence long-term HT should generally be avoided. Conversely, the benefits of short-term therapy (less than 5 years) to treat menopausal symptoms often *do* justify the risks. To keep risk as low as possible, HT should be used in the lowest dosage and for the shortest time needed to accomplish treatment goals.

Regimens for Menopausal Hormone Therapy

There are two basic regimens for HT: estrogen alone (estrogen therapy, or ET) and estrogen plus a progestin (estrogen/progestin therapy, or EPT). The purpose of estrogen in both regimens is to control menopausal symptoms by replacing estrogen that was lost owing to menopause.

The progestin is present for only one reason and that is to counterbalance estrogen-mediated stimulation of the endometrium, which can lead to endometrial hyperplasia and cancer. Progestins should not be prescribed for women who have undergone hysterectomy. Although progestins can protect against estrogen-induced cancer of the *uterus,* progestins appear to *increase* the risk for estrogen-induced cancer of the *breast.* In addition, progestins appear to increase the risk for adverse cardiac events.

Use for Approved Indications

Hormone therapy has only three approved indications:

- Treatment of moderate to severe vasomotor symptoms associated with menopause
- Treatment of moderate to severe symptoms of vulvar and vaginal atrophy associated with menopause
- Prevention of postmenopausal osteoporosis

Hormone therapy should be restricted to achieving one or more of these goals. With the first two indications, duration of treatment is relatively short (typically 3 to 4 years), and hence the risk for harm is relatively low—except for women with established heart disease. In contrast, prevention of osteoporosis requires lifelong HT, and hence the risk for harm is higher.

Treatment of Vasomotor Symptoms. Hormone therapy is the most effective treatment for vasomotor symptoms (hot flashes, night sweats). To increase safety, the lowest effective dosage should be employed. Furthermore, because vasomotor symptoms subside over time, the need for continued HT should be reassessed at regular intervals.

For women with risk factors that contraindicate the use of HT, other options are available, but they are less effective than estrogen. Trials have shown that two antidepressants—*escitalopram* [Lexapro] and *desvenlafaxine* [Pristiq]—can produce a modest but meaningful reduction in both the frequency and severity of hot flashes. Escitalopram is an SSRI; desvenlafaxine is a serotonin/norepinephrine reuptake inhibitor (SNRI). Other SSRIs and SNRIs are likely to be effective as well. *Paroxetine* [Brisdelle], an SSRI, was approved in 2013 for the treatment of vasomotor symptoms in menopause. Paroxetine is used as an antidepressant and is discussed further in Chapter 32.

TABLE 61.2 ▪ Intravaginal Estrogens for Menopausal Hormone Therapy[a]

Generic Name	Brand Name	Usual Maintenance Dosage
VAGINAL CREAMS		
Conjugated estrogens	Premarin	Apply 0.5–2 gm/day (625 mcg conjugated estrogens/gm)[b]
Estradiol	Estrace	Apply 1–2 gm 1–3 times/wk (100 mcg estradiol/gm)
VAGINAL RINGS		
Estradiol	Estring	This 2-mg ring releases 7.5 mcg/day for 90 days
Estradiol acetate	Femring	The 12.4-mg ring releases 50 mcg/day for 90 days[a] The 24.8-mg ring releases 100 mcg/day for 90 days[a]
VAGINAL TABLETS		
Estradiol hemihydrate	Vagifem	Insert 1 tablet (10 mcg) every day for 2 wk, then 1 tablet twice a week thereafter

[a]All intravaginal estrogens are used to treat urogenital atrophy. With one product—Femring—estradiol is absorbed in amounts sufficient to cause systemic effects, both beneficial (e.g., suppression of vasomotor symptoms) and adverse (e.g., increased risk for thrombosis).
[b]Administer cyclically (3 weeks on and 1 week off). For short-term use only.

By contrast, controlled trials have shown that soy isoflavones do *not* reduce hot flashes. In fact, these preparations may make symptoms worse.

Treatment of Symptoms of Vulvar and Vaginal Atrophy. Estrogen is the most effective treatment for reducing symptoms of menopause-related vulvar and vaginal atrophy, characterized by dryness, irritation, itching, and uncomfortable intercourse. Because systemic estrogen carries significant risks, the FDA recommends that if HT is being used solely to manage vulvar and vaginal symptoms, a topical estrogen formulation should be considered. Options include vaginal creams, vaginal tablets, and vaginal rings (Table 61.2). Although long-term data are lacking, it seems likely that topical estrogen is safer than oral estrogen because with nearly all topical formulations blood levels of estrogen remain low. The notable exception is the Femring, which releases enough estrogen to cause significant systemic effects.

Prevention of Osteoporosis. Hormone therapy reduces postmenopausal bone loss, and thereby decreases the risk for osteoporosis and related fractures. Unfortunately, when HT is stopped, bone mass rapidly decreases by about 12%. Hence, to maintain bone health, HT must continue lifelong. As a result, the risk for harm is increased. Accordingly, alternative treatments are preferred. In fact, labeling of HT products now must carry the following advice: *When this product is prescribed solely to prevent postmenopausal osteoporosis, approved nonestrogen treatments should be carefully considered. Furthermore, HT should be considered only for women with significant risk for osteoporosis, and only when that risk outweighs the risks of HT.* As discussed in Chapter 75, effective alternatives to HT include raloxifene [Evista], bisphosphonates (e.g., alendronate

[Fosamax]), calcitonin [Miacalcin], and teriparatide [Forteo]. Of course, all women (not to mention men) should practice primary prevention of bone loss by ensuring adequate intake of calcium and vitamin D, performing regular weight-bearing exercise, and avoiding smoking and excessive alcohol use.

Inappropriate Uses: Attempted Prevention of Heart Disease and Dementia

Heart Disease. HT should *not* be prescribed for the express purpose of preventing CHD. For most women, HT confers no protection, and it may increase the risk for CHD and MI in some women.

To reduce risk for cardiovascular events, postmenopausal women should be counseled about alternative ways to promote cardiovascular health. Among these are avoiding smoking, performing regular aerobic exercise, decreasing intake of saturated fats, and taking prescribed drugs to treat hypertension, diabetes, and high cholesterol.

Alzheimer's Disease. Hormone therapy should not be used to prevent Alzheimer's disease. There is no evidence that either EPT or ET can protect against dementia, whereas there *is* evidence that EPT may *cause* dementia and that ET can increase the combined risk for dementia and mild cognitive impairment.

Safety in Younger Women Who Don't Have a Uterus

For women younger than 60 years who have undergone hysterectomy, HT may be safer than for any other group. There are two reasons why. First, because these women no longer have a uterus, they are treated with estrogen alone, which is somewhat safer than estrogen combined with a progestin. Second, for younger women, the risks of estrogen therapy are lower than for older women. Specifically, compared with older women, younger women are at lower risk for estrogen-induced CHD, MI, and breast cancer. In fact, among younger women, ET appears to protect against CHD and MI, and possibly against breast cancer too.

Discontinuing Hormone Therapy

Unfortunately, discontinuation of HT may cause vasomotor symptoms to return, typically within 4 days of the last HT dose. Women who had severe symptoms before initiating HT are at highest risk for developing intolerable symptoms when they stop.

No firm guidelines exist for stopping hormone therapy. There are two basic methods: immediate cessation and tapering slowly. However, there are no controlled studies to indicate which option might result in fewer symptoms. For women who choose to taper slowly, again there are two basic options, referred to as "dose tapering" and "day tapering." With dose tapering, dosing is done every day, but the size of the daily dose is gradually reduced. If intense symptoms return following a dosage reduction, further reductions should be delayed until symptoms improve. With day tapering, the daily dose remains unchanged, but the number of days between doses is gradually increased—starting with dosing every other day, then every third day, and so on. Regardless of which method is used—dose tapering or day tapering—only the dosage of *estrogen* should be lowered. For women on EPT, the *progestin dosage should remain unchanged* because lowering the progestin dosage might permit estrogen to stimulate endometrial growth, thereby posing a risk for endometrial hyperplasia.

Drug Products for Hormone Therapy

Preparations

Preparations for HT are listed in Tables 61.2, 61.3, and 61.4. Dosing may be oral, transdermal, or intravaginal. The oral estrogens employed most often are conjugated equine estrogens [Premarin] (prepared by extraction from pregnant mares' urine), estradiol [Estrace], and estropipate. For transdermal therapy, estradiol is the only estrogen employed, formulated in patches, gels, a spray, and an emulsion. Oral estrogen/progestin combinations include conjugated equine estrogens/medroxyprogesterone acetate [Prempro, Premphase], estradiol/norethindrone acetate [Activella], and ethinyl estradiol/norethindrone [Femhrt]. Combination estrogen/progestin patches are estradiol/norethindrone [CombiPatch] and estradiol/levonorgestrel [Climara Pro]. Intravaginal products—formulated as tablets, creams, and rings—are used primarily to manage symptoms of urogenital atrophy.

Dosing Schedules

Every woman undergoing systemic HT receives an estrogen, and every woman with a uterus also receives a progestin to

TABLE 61.3 ▪ Oral Drugs for Menopausal Hormone Therapy

Generic Name	Brand Name	Usual Dosage
ESTROGENS		
Conjugated estrogens, equine	Premarin	0.3–1.25 mg/day
Conjugated estrogens A, synthetic	Cenestin	0.3–1.25 mg/day
Conjugated estrogens B, synthetic	Enjuvia	0.3–1.25 mg/day
Esterified estrogens	Menest	0.3–2.5 mg/day
Estradiol, micronized	Estrace	0.5–2 mg/day
Estropipate	Generic only	0.75–6 mg/day
PROGESTINS[a]		
Medroxyprogesterone acetate	Provera	2.5–10 mg
Progesterone (micronized)	Prometrium	200 mg

TABLE 61.3 ▪ Oral Drugs for Menopausal Hormone Therapy—cont'd

Generic Name	Brand Name	Usual Dosage
ESTROGEN/PROGESTIN COMBINATIONS[a]		
Conjugated estrogens/medroxyprogesterone acetate	Prempro	0.3/1.5, 0.45/1.5, 0.625/2.5, or 0.625/5 mg daily
Conjugated estrogens/medroxyprogesterone acetate	Premphase	*Days 1–14:* 0.625 mg estrogen (alone) daily *Days 15–28:* 0.625/5 mg estrogen/progesterone daily
Estradiol/drospirenone	Angeliq	0.5/0.25 or 1/0.5 mg daily
Estradiol/norethindrone acetate	Activella	0.5/0.1 or 1/0.5 mg daily
Estradiol/norgestimate	Prefest	1 mg estradiol every day; 0.09 mg norgestimate in a repeating cycle of 3 days on and 3 days off
Ethinyl estradiol/norethindrone	Femhrt	2.5 mcg/0.5 mg or 5 mcg/1 mg daily
OTHER ESTROGEN COMBINATIONS		
Esterified estrogens/methyltestosterone	Covaryx	1.25 mg/2.5 mg daily
Esterified estrogens/methyltestosterone	Covaryx HS	0.625/1.25 mg daily
Conjugated estrogens/bazedoxifene[b]	Duavee	0.45 mg/20 mg twice daily

[a]Progestins are used to counteract the effects of estrogen on the uterus. The progestins listed can be used when the regimen calls for taking estrogen and progestin separately, rather than using a combination product. In estrogen/progestin regimens, the estrogen is taken daily, and the progestin is taken daily or intermittently (e.g., 14 days on, 14 days off).
[b]Bazedoxifene is an estrogen antagonist/SERM that acts to reduce excessive growth of the uterine lining that can occur with the estrogen component.

TABLE 61.4 ▪ Transdermal Drugs for Menopausal Hormone Therapy

Generic Name	Brand Name	Strength (mcg absorbed/day)	Application
ESTROGENS			
Transdermal Patches			
Estradiol	Menostar	14	Once weekly
	Climara	25, 37.5, 50, 60, 75, 100	Once weekly
	Alora	25, 50, 75, 100	Twice weekly
	Estradot 🍁	25, 37.5, 50, 75, 100	Twice weekly
	Oesclim 🍁	25, 37.5, 50, 75, 100	Twice weekly
	Vivelle-Dot	25, 37.5, 50, 75, 100	Twice weekly
	Estraderm	50, 100	Twice weekly
Topical Emulsion			
Estradiol hemihydrate	Estrasorb	50	Once daily
Transdermal Spray			
Estradiol	Evamist	1.53–4.6 mg is applied[a]	Once daily
Topical Gel			
Estradiol	EstroGel	0.75 mg is applied[a]	Once daily
	Elestrin	0.52 or 1.04 mg is applied[a]	Once daily
	Divigel	0.25, 0.5, or 1 mg is applied[a]	Once daily
ESTROGEN/PROGESTIN COMBINATIONS			
Transdermal Patches			
Estradiol/norethindrone	CombiPatch	50/140, 50/250	Twice weekly
Estradiol/levonorgestrel	Climara Pro	45/15	Once weekly

[a]Application of this dose produces blood levels of estrogen and estrone similar to those seen in the follicular phase of the ovulatory cycle.

counteract the stimulant effects of estrogen on the endometrium. Several dosing schedules may be employed. Estrogen and progestin are commonly administered continuously, thereby eliminating monthly bleeding. An alternative is to give estrogen continuously but give the progestin cyclically (e.g., on calendar days 15 through 28). However, cyclic progestin has the disadvantage of promoting monthly bleeding, which may explain why most women prefer continuous dosing.

Vaginal estrogens can be given continuously for 1 to 2 weeks, followed by dosing 1 to 3 times per week, titrating the dosing schedule based on symptoms. Estring remains in the vagina for 3 months, after which it is removed and replaced with a new ring.

KEY POINTS

- Estradiol is the principal endogenous estrogen.
- Progesterone is the principal endogenous progestational hormone.
- The first half of the 28-day menstrual cycle is called the follicular phase. The second half is called the luteal phase.
- During the follicular phase, estrogens produced by maturing ovarian follicles cause proliferation of the endometrium.
- During the luteal phase, progesterone produced by the corpus luteum causes the endometrium to become more vascular and the endometrial glands to secrete glycogen.
- Toward the end of the menstrual cycle, progesterone levels decline, causing breakdown of the endometrium, which results in menstrual bleeding.
- In addition to their role in the menstrual cycle, estrogens are required for the growth and maturation of the uterus, vagina, fallopian tubes, and breasts. Estrogens also control pigmentation of the nipples and genitalia.
- Estrogens suppress bone mineral resorption, and thereby have a positive effect on bone mass.
- Estrogens raise levels of HDL cholesterol and reduce levels of LDL cholesterol. These actions partially explain the low incidence of coronary heart disease in premenopausal women.
- Nausea is the most common adverse effect of exogenous oral estrogens.
- Prolonged use of estrogens alone is associated with an increased risk for endometrial hyperplasia and endometrial carcinoma. However, when estrogens are used in combination with a progestin, there is little or no risk for this cancer.
- Estrogens are potentially teratogenic. Research has shown that high dose exposure can affect testicular development in the developing male fetus, leading to eventual infertility. Follow-up studies of women who inadvertently took estrogen (as a component in combined oral contraceptives) early during an undiagnosed pregnancy did not identify subsequent abnormalities in their offspring.
- Symptoms of menopause result from a decline in ovarian production of estrogen.
- Menopausal hormone therapy (HT), formerly known as *hormone replacement therapy* (HRT), has three approved indications: suppression of vasomotor symptoms, prevention of urogenital atrophy, and prevention of bone loss and osteoporosis.
- Hormone therapy is not approved for cardiovascular protection, and should not be used for this purpose.
- The Women's Health Initiative (WHI) and the Heart and Estrogen/progestin Replacement Study (HERS)—two large, randomized, placebo-controlled trials—have given us the most statistically valid data to date on the benefits and risks of HT; however, problems related to the advanced age of subjects, high doses of HT, and prolonged regimens resulted in findings that do not reflect optimal recommendations.
- When the Endocrine Society extrapolated findings from research that reflected women younger than 60, HT was found to have far fewer adverse effects and life-promoting benefits.
- We have two basic regimens for HT: estrogen alone (ET) and estrogen combined with a progestin (EPT). The purpose of the estrogen is to manage symptoms caused by estrogen loss. The progestin is present to counteract the adverse effects that unopposed estrogen has on the endometrium. In women who no longer have a uterus, the progestin is omitted.
- The major risks of HT are CHD, MI, DVT, pulmonary embolism, stroke, breast cancer, gallbladder disease, and dementia. Ovarian cancer and lung cancer are also a concern.
- Risk factors associated with HT depend on the regimen and the age of the user. An extrapolation of findings from the WHI by the Endocrine Society found that for women ages 50 to 59, HT resulted in 5 to 5.3 fewer deaths per 1000 women. The risk for adverse events increases with increasing age.
- The benefits of using HT short term to reduce vasomotor symptoms generally outweigh the risks, especially in younger women. To keep risk low, women should use the smallest effective dose for the shortest time needed.
- The benefits of using HT short term to manage urogenital symptoms probably outweigh the risks. If this is the only reason for HT, a topical estrogen should be considered.
- For protection against osteoporosis, HT must be taken long term. When HT is discontinued, 12% of bone mass is lost. Because of the risks associated with prolonged HT, alternative therapies are preferred.
- Premenstrual disorder (PMD) consists of a constellation of psychologic and physical symptoms that develop in the luteal phase of the menstrual cycle and resolve with menses.
- SSRIs are the most effective drugs known for PMD. In addition to relieving psychologic symptoms, they often reduce physical symptoms (e.g., breast tenderness, bloating, headache).

Please visit **http://evolve.elsevier.com/Lehne** for chapter-specific NCLEX® examination review questions.

Summary of Major Nursing Implications[a]

ESTROGENS

Conjugated estrogens
Conjugated estrogens, synthetic
Estradiol
Estradiol acetate
Estropipate
Ethinyl estradiol

Preadministration Assessment

Therapeutic Goal

Estrogens are used primarily for contraception (see Chapter 62) and for menopausal HT, but only to prevent osteoporosis, suppress vasomotor symptoms, and manage symptoms related to vulvar and vaginal atrophy. Indications unrelated to HT are female hypogonadism, prostate cancer, and dysfunctional uterine bleeding.

Baseline Data

Assessment should include a breast examination, pelvic examination, lipid profile, mammography, and blood pressure measurement. If the indication for HT is vasomotor symptoms, menopause should be verified by a serum FSH level.

Identifying High-Risk Patients

Estrogens are *contraindicated* for patients with estrogen-dependent cancers, undiagnosed abnormal vaginal bleeding, active thrombophlebitis or thromboembolic disorders, or a history of estrogen-associated thrombophlebitis, thrombosis, or thromboembolic disorders. In addition, estrogens are *contraindicated* during pregnancy—not because they are especially harmful, but because there is no indication for use in pregnancy.

Implementation: Administration

Routes

Oral, IM, IV, transdermal, and intravaginal.

Administration

Transdermal Patch. **Give the patient the following instructions for using estradiol transdermal patches:**

- **Apply to an area of clean, dry intact skin on the abdomen or some other region of the trunk (but not the breasts or waistline) by pressing the patch firmly in place for 10 seconds.**
- **If the patch falls off, reapply the same patch or, if necessary, apply a new patch.**
- **Remove the old patch and apply a new patch once or twice weekly according to the product specifications.**
- **Rotate the application site such that the same site is not used more than once each week.**

Transdermal Emulsion. **Instruct the patient to apply the emulsion each morning to the top of both thighs and the back of both calves.**

Transdermal Gel. **Instruct the patient to apply the gel once daily after showering to one arm, from the shoulder to the wrist.**

Transdermal Spray. **Instruct the patient to apply 1, 2, or 3 sprays once daily to the inner forearm, and then let it dry at least 2 minutes before dressing and at least 30 minutes before washing.**

Intravaginal Cream. **Instruct the patient to apply estrogen cream high into the vagina, usually at bedtime, using the applicator provided.**

Intravaginal Ring. **Instruct the patient to insert the ring as deeply as possible and to leave it in place for 3 months, after which it should be removed, and then replaced with a new ring if indicated.**

Intravaginal Tablet. **Inform patients that dosing consists of 1 tablet daily for 2 weeks, followed by 1 tablet twice a week thereafter. Instruct patients to insert each tablet as far as comfortably possible using the applicator supplied.**

Dosing Schedules for Hormone Therapy

Women with an intact uterus should receive estrogen plus progestin, whereas women who have had a hysterectomy should use estrogen alone. In both cases, dosing with oral estrogen is done *daily.* With estrogen plus progestin, the progestin component may be given *daily* or cyclically 10 days per month.

Ongoing Evaluation and Interventions

Monitoring Summary

The patient should receive a yearly follow-up breast and pelvic examination.

Minimizing Adverse Effects

Nausea. Nausea is common early in treatment but diminishes with time. **Inform the patient that nausea can be reduced by taking estrogens with food and by dosing at night.**

Endometrial Hyperplasia and Cancer. Menopausal HT with estrogen alone increases the risk for endometrial carcinoma. Adding a progestin lowers this risk to the pretreatment level. **Instruct the patient to notify the prescriber if persistent or recurrent vaginal bleeding develops so that the possibility of endometrial carcinoma can be evaluated.**

Breast Cancer. Estrogen, combined with a progestin, produces a small increase in the risk for breast cancer in postmenopausal women. **To minimize risk, remind patients of the need to receive periodic mammograms.** Estrogen alone *may* increase breast cancer risk, but only when HT is started after menopause onset. Among younger women, estrogen alone may actually *protect* against breast cancer.

Ovarian Cancer. In postmenopausal women, giving ET or EPT may pose a small risk for ovarian cancer. **Advise women using ET or EPT to undergo periodic evaluation for ovarian cancer.**

Lung Cancer. Menopausal EPT, but not ET, may increase the risk for lung cancer. **Advise women using EPT to undergo periodic evaluation for lung cancer.**

Cardiovascular Events. Estrogen plus a progestin increases the risk for CHD, MI, DVT, pulmonary embolism, and stroke. For women over the age of 60, therapy with

Continued

Summary of Major Nursing Implications[a]—cont'd

estrogen alone carries the same risks. For women ages 50 to 59, therapy with estrogen alone increases the risk for DVT, pulmonary embolism, and stroke, but may *protect* against CHD and MI. **To reduce cardiovascular risk, advise women to avoid smoking, perform regular exercise, decrease intake of saturated fats, and take appropriate drugs to treat hypertension, diabetes, and high cholesterol.**

Effects Resembling Those Caused by Oral Contraceptives. Use of estrogens for noncontraceptive purposes can produce adverse effects similar to those caused by oral contraceptives (e.g., abnormal vaginal bleeding, hypertension, benign hepatic adenoma, reduced glucose tolerance). Nursing implications regarding these effects are summarized in Chapter 62.

Minimizing Adverse Interactions. The interactions of estrogens are probably similar to those seen with oral contraceptives. Implications regarding these interactions are summarized in Chapter 62.

PROGESTINS

Drospirenone
Hydroxyprogesterone caproate
Levonorgestrel
Medroxyprogesterone acetate
Megestrol acetate
Norethindrone
Norethindrone acetate
Norgestimate
Norgestrel
Progesterone

Preadministration Assessment

Therapeutic Goal

Progestins are used for contraception (see Chapter 62) and to counteract endometrial hyperplasia that could be caused by unopposed estrogen during HT. Other uses include dysfunctional uterine bleeding, amenorrhea, endometriosis, and support of pregnancy in women with corpus luteum deficiency. Progestins are also used in IVF cycles and to prevent prematurity in women at high risk for preterm birth.

Baseline Data

The physical examination should include breast and pelvic examinations. A pregnancy examination is warranted for premenopausal women.

Identifying High-Risk Patients

Progestins are *contraindicated* in the presence of undiagnosed abnormal vaginal bleeding. *Relative contraindications* include active thrombophlebitis or a history of thromboembolic disorders, active liver disease, and carcinoma of the breast.

Implementation: Administration

Routes

Oral, IM, transdermal, intravaginal.

Administration

Advise patients to take oral progestins with food if GI upset occurs.

Ongoing Evaluation and Interventions

Minimizing Adverse Effects

Gynecologic Effects. Progestins can cause breakthrough bleeding, spotting, and amenorrhea. **Inform patients about potential side effects. Instruct the patient to report any persistent or recurrent vaginal bleeding.**

Teratogenic Effects. High-dose therapy during the first 4 months of pregnancy has been associated with an increased incidence of birth defects (limb reductions, heart defects, masculinization of the female fetus). Accordingly, use of progestins during early pregnancy is not recommended.

[a]Patient education information is highlighted as **blue text.**

CHAPTER

62 Birth Control

Birth control can be accomplished by interfering with the reproductive process at any step from gametogenesis to nidation (implantation of a fertilized ovum). Pharmacologic methods of contraception include oral contraceptives, etonogestrel implants, injectable medroxyprogesterone acetate, intrauterine devices, vaginal rings, and transdermal patches. Nonpharmacologic methods include surgical sterilization (tubal ligation, vasectomy), mechanical devices (condom, diaphragm, cervical cap), and avoiding intercourse during periods of fertility (calendar method, temperature method, cervical mucus method).

Most of this chapter focuses on combination oral contraceptive pills—the most widely used *reversible* form of contraception. Sterilization is used more often, but is not reversible. In preparing to study these agents and other forms of contraception, you should review Chapter 61, paying special attention to information on the menstrual cycle and the physiologic and pharmacologic effects of estrogens and progestins.

EFFECTIVENESS OF BIRTH CONTROL METHODS

The effectiveness of a birth control method can be expressed as the percentage of unplanned pregnancies that occur while using the method. Employing this criterion, Table 62.1 compares the effectiveness of the major birth control methods. As you can see, the most effective methods are Nexplanon, intrauterine devices (IUDs), and sterilization. Oral contraceptives (OCs), Depo-Provera, the contraceptive ring, and the contraceptive patch are close behind. The least reliable methods include barrier methods, periodic abstinence, spermicides, and withdrawal.

Table 62.1 contains two columns of figures, one labeled *theoretical use* and the other *actual use.* The *theoretical use* figures represent pregnancy rates when a method of birth control is employed exactly as it should be (i.e., consistently and with proper technique). The *actual use* figures represent pregnancy rates observed in actual practice. The higher pregnancy rates reported in the *actual use* column are largely an indication that methods of birth control are not always used when and as they should be.

SELECTING A BIRTH CONTROL METHOD

The method of contraception chosen most frequently is sterilization: Female sterilization (tubal ligation) plus male sterilization (vasectomy) are selected by 37% of birth control users. OCs or male condoms are chosen by most of the remaining birth control users. Diaphragms, periodic abstinence, IUDs, and other techniques account for a small fraction of birth control use.

Several factors should be considered when choosing a method of birth control. Chief among these are *effectiveness, safety,* and *personal preference.* As shown in Table 62.1, the most effective methods are etonogestrel subdermal implants [Nexplanon], intramuscular medroxyprogesterone acetate [Depo-Provera], sterilization, and IUDs. Three other methods—OCs, the contraceptive ring [NuvaRing], and the contraceptive patch [Ortho Evra]—are close behind. The remaining methods—condoms, the sponge, diaphragm, cervical cap, spermicides, and periodic abstinence—must be used in a near-perfect fashion to afford any reasonable level of protection.

When factoring safety into the selection equation, several guidelines apply. Combination OCs should be avoided by women with certain cardiovascular disorders (see *Thromboembolic Disorders*), as well as by women older than 35 years who smoke. For women in these categories, an alternative method (e.g., diaphragm, progestin-only pill, or IUD) is preferable. Although OCs are effective and relatively convenient, they can also cause significant side effects. Accordingly, women who consider the benefit/risk ratio unfavorable should be advised about alternative contraceptive techniques. Women who are not in a mutually monogamous relationship, and hence are at risk for a sexually transmitted disease (STD), should not use an IUD.

Personal preference is a major factor in providing the motivation needed for consistent implementation of a birth control method. Because even the best form of contraception

TABLE 62.1 ▪ Effectiveness of Birth Control Methods

Birth Control Method	Failure Rate[a] (%) Actual Use[b]	Theoretical Use[c]
No method	85	85
EXTREMELY EFFECTIVE		
Etonogestrel subdermal implant [Nexplanon]	0.05	0.05
Surgical sterilization		
Female: tubal ligation	0.5	0.5
Male: vasectomy	0.15	0.1
Intrauterine devices		
Copper T 380A [ParaGard]	0.8	0.6
Levonorgestrel T [Mirena]	0.2	0.2
VERY EFFECTIVE		
Oral contraceptives		
Combination pills	8	0.3
Progestin-only pills	8	0.3
Intramuscular medroxyprogesterone acetate [Depo-Provera]	3	0.3
Vaginal contraceptive ring [NuvaRing]	8	0.3
Contraceptive patch [Ortho Evra]	8	0.3
EFFECTIVE		
Condoms		
Male	15	2
Female [FC2 Female Condom]	21	5
Diaphragm with spermicide	16	6
LEAST EFFECTIVE		
Contraceptive sponge [Today Sponge]		
Parous	32	20
Nulliparous	16	9
Spermicide alone	29	18
Periodic abstinence	25	3–5
Withdrawal	27	4

[a]Failure rate: percentage of women who have an unplanned pregnancy during first year of use.
[b]Actual use: failure rate usually observed in actual practice.
[c]Theoretical use: failure rate that would be expected if the birth control method were practiced exactly as it should be.

will be less effective if improperly practiced, the importance of personal preference cannot be overemphasized. Practitioners should take pains to educate patients about the contraceptive methods available so that selection and use can be based on understanding.

Additional factors that bear on selecting a birth control method include family planning goals, age, frequency of sexual intercourse, and the individual's capacity for adherence. If family planning goals have already been met, sterilization of either the male or female partner may be desirable. For women who engage in coitus frequently, OCs or a long-term method (e.g., Nexplanon, Depo-Provera, IUD) are reasonable choices. Conversely, when sexual activity is limited, use of a spermicide, condom, or diaphragm may be more appropriate. Since barrier methods combined with spermicides can offer some protection against STDs (as well as providing contraception), these combinations may be of special benefit to individuals who have multiple partners. If adherence is a problem (as it can be with OCs, condoms, and diaphragms), the use of a long-term method (e.g., vaginal contraceptive ring, IUD, Nexplanon, Depo-Provera) can confer more reliable protection.

To help women select the birth control method that suits them best, Planned Parenthood has created a step-by-step computerized selection tool, accessible online at www.plannedparenthood.org/all-access/my-method-26542.htm. This tool accounts for all of the factors noted earlier.

ORAL CONTRACEPTIVES

There are two main categories of OCs: (1) those that contain an estrogen *plus* a progestin, known as *combination OCs,* and (2) those that contain just a progestin, known as "minipills" or *progestin-only OCs.* Of the two groups, combination OCs are by far the more widely used.

Combination Oral Contraceptives

Since their introduction in the late 1950s, combination OCs have become one of our most widely prescribed families of drugs. These drugs are both safe and effective, although minor side effects are common.

Prototype Drugs

DRUGS FOR BIRTH CONTROL

Combination Oral Contraceptives
Ethinyl estradiol/norethindrone

Progestin-Only Oral Contraceptives
Norethindrone

Long-Acting Contraceptives
Subdermal etonogestrel implant [Implanon]
Depot medroxyprogesterone acetate [Depo-Provera]

Drugs for Emergency Contraception
Levonorgestrel alone [Plan B One-Step]
Ulipristal acetate [Ella]
Ethinyl estradiol/levonorgestrel (the Yuzpe regimen)

Mechanism of Action

Combination OCs reduce fertility primarily by *inhibiting ovulation.* The estrogen in combination OCs suppresses release of follicle-stimulating hormone from the pituitary (and thereby inhibits follicular maturation), and progestin in combination OCs acts in the hypothalamus and pituitary to suppress the midcycle luteinizing hormone surge, which normally triggers ovulation. Secondary mechanisms include thickening of the cervical mucus (creating a barrier to the penetration of sperm) and alteration of the endometrium, making it less hospitable for implantation.

TABLE 62.2 ▪ Progestins Used in Combination Oral Contraceptives

Progestins	Comments
FIRST GENERATION	
Ethynodiol diacetate Norethindrone	Lower risk of thrombosis than with other progestins Mildly androgenic
SECOND GENERATION	
Levonorgestrel Norgestrel	Greater risk of thrombosis than with FGPs More androgenic than FGPs Prolonged half-life
THIRD GENERATION	
Desogestrel Norgestimate	Greater risk of thrombosis than with FGPs (especially desogestrel) Less androgenic than FGPs
FOURTH GENERATION	
Dienogest Drospirenone	For drospirenone *and* dienogest: • Greater risk of thrombosis than with other progestins (especially drospirenone) • Less androgenic than FGPs • Low risk of acne and hirsutism For drospirenone only: • Risk of hyperkalemia

FGPs, First-generation progestins.

Components

Estrogens. Only three estrogens are employed: *ethinyl estradiol, mestranol,* and *estradiol valerate.* Most combination OCs use ethinyl estradiol. A few older products use mestranol, which undergoes conversion to ethinyl estradiol in the body. And one new product—*Natazia*—uses estradiol valerate, which undergoes conversion to estradiol in the body.

Progestins. Combination OCs employ eight different progestins, which can be grouped into four generations (Table 62.2). Progestins in all four generations are equally effective. Differences relate to side effects, especially thrombotic events, androgenic effects (acne, hirsutism, dyslipidemia), and hyperkalemia.

Drospirenone, a fourth-generation progestin, has progestational, antiandrogen, and antialdosterone actions. The drug is a structural analog of spironolactone, a potassium-sparing diuretic that blocks receptors for aldosterone. Drospirenone was developed in an effort to reduce fluid retention caused by the estrogen component in combination OCs. (Estrogens promote fluid retention by activating the renin-angiotensin-aldosterone system. Drospirenone reduces fluid retention by blocking aldosterone receptors, thereby preventing retention of sodium and water. As a result, OCs made with drospirenone may cause less bloating, weight gain, and hypertension than other combination OCs.) The principal concern with drospirenone is *venous thromboembolism,* which occurs more often than with other progestins. Also, drospirenone can cause *hyperkalemia* (secondary to renal retention of potassium).

Effectiveness

As shown in Table 62.1, OCs can be very effective. With perfect use, the failure rate is only 0.3%. However, with typical use, the failure rate is significantly higher: about 8%. Among women of higher weight, efficacy is somewhat reduced. Possible reasons include decreased blood levels of the hormones, sequestration in adipose tissue, and altered metabolism.

TABLE 62.3 ▪ Absolute and Relative Contraindications to the Use of Combination OCs

ABSOLUTE CONTRAINDICATIONS	RELATIVE CONTRAINDICATIONS
Thrombophlebitis, thromboembolic disorders, cerebral vascular disease, coronary occlusion, *or* a past history of these conditions, *or* a condition that predisposes to these disorders	Hypertension
Abnormal liver function	Cardiac disease
Known or suspected breast cancer	Diabetes
Undiagnosed abnormal vaginal bleeding	History of cholestatic jaundice of pregnancy
Known or suspected pregnancy	Gallbladder disease
Smokers over the age of 35	Uterine leiomyoma
	Epilepsy
	Migraine

However, even though efficacy of OCs is slightly reduced in higher-weight women, these drugs are still more reliable than most of the alternatives.

Overall Safety

Determining the relative safety of combination OCs is complex. Part of the difficulty lies with the fact that much of our information on the adverse effects of OCs was gathered when these agents were employed in higher doses than those employed today. Newer data show that today's OCs, as currently prescribed, are considerably safer than indicated by older studies. An additional complication stems from the fact that the risk of mortality associated with OCs is much smaller than the risk associated with pregnancy and delivery. Keeping the above provisos in mind, we can make the following observations on OC safety. Of the contraceptive methods available, OCs produce the broadest spectrum of adverse effects, ranging from nausea to menstrual irregularity to rare thromboembolic disorders. However, despite their wide variety of undesired actions, when used by healthy women, OCs produce no greater mortality than any other form of birth control.

Adverse Effects

Combination OCs can cause a variety of adverse effects. However, although many types of effects may occur, severe effects are rare. Hence, when compared with the serious risks associated with pregnancy and childbirth, the risks of OCs are low. Nonetheless, because OCs are usually taken by women who are healthy and because OCs represent a potential health hazard (albeit small), we must take steps to minimize risk. To this end, a full medical history should be obtained. If the history reveals an *absolute* contraindication to OC use (Table 62.3), OCs should not be prescribed. In women with *relative* contraindications, OCs should be used with caution. Candidates for OCs undergo a physical examination before starting these agents.

Thromboembolic Disorders. Combination OCs have been associated with an increased risk of venous thromboembolism (VTE), arterial thromboembolism, pulmonary embolism, myocardial infarction (MI), and thrombotic stroke. Among OC users, the *relative* risk of a thrombotic event is 2 to 3 times the risk in nonusers. However, the *absolute* risk is still very small: about 8 to 10 events per 10,000 woman-years of OC use. Furthermore, the risk of thrombosis associated with OCs is considerably lower than the risk associated with pregnancy and delivery. OCs promote thrombosis in part by raising levels of clotting factors. Thrombosis is not due to atherosclerosis.

Formerly, we believed that thrombotic events were caused solely by the estrogen in combination OCs. However, it is now clear that the progestin can contribute too. Two newer progestins—*drospirenone* and *desogestrel*—appear to carry the greatest risk.

Fortunately, the risk of thrombotic events with OCs used today is much lower than with the OCs used in the past because the amount of estrogen in OCs has been reduced. When combination OCs first became available, they contained high doses of estrogens (e.g., 100 mcg ethinyl estradiol). Today's OCs contain no more than 50 mcg ethinyl estradiol (and usually less), so the risk of thromboembolism is quite low.

Major factors that increase the risk of thromboembolism are *heavy smoking, a history of thromboembolism,* and *thrombophilias* (genetic disorders that predispose to thrombosis). Additional risk factors include diabetes, hypertension, cerebrovascular disease, coronary artery disease, and surgery in which immobilization increases the risk of postoperative thrombosis.

In the past, OCs were not recommended for women older than 35 years because earlier studies indicated an increase in the risk of MI for this group. However, reanalysis showed that the risk was limited to older women who smoked. With today's low-estrogen OCs, nonsmokers may continue usage until menopause, with no greater risk of MI than among younger women.

Several measures can help minimize thromboembolic phenomena. Specifically:

- The estrogen dose in OCs should be no greater than required for contraceptive efficacy.
- OCs containing drospirenone or desogestrel should generally be avoided as they may pose a higher risk for developing VTE.
- OCs should not be prescribed for heavy smokers, women with a history of thromboembolism, or women with other risk factors for thrombosis.
- OCs should be discontinued at least 4 weeks before surgery in which postoperative thrombosis might be expected.
- Women should be informed about the symptoms of thrombosis and thromboembolism (e.g., leg tenderness or pain, sudden chest pain, shortness of breath, severe headache, sudden visual disturbance) and instructed to consult the prescriber if these occur.

What about the cardiovascular risk for *former* OC users? Data from the Women's Health Initiative suggest that use of OCs in the past may *protect* against cardiovascular disease. Among women with a history of OC use, there was an 8% decrease in the overall incidence of cardiovascular disease, including a reduced risk of angina, MI, peripheral vascular disease, transient ischemic attacks, and elevation of cholesterol.

Can women with a history of thrombosis use drugs for birth control? Yes. Although these women should avoid estrogen/progestin products, they can still use a progestin-only method. Options include the levonorgestrel intrauterine system [Mirena], medroxyprogesterone acetate injection [Depo-Provera], the etonogestrel subdermal implant [Nexplanon], and the "mini-pill"—all of which are discussed later.

Cancer. Oral contraceptives present no known risk of cancer—with the important exception of promoting (not causing) breast cancer growth. The effects of OCs on cancers of the ovaries, endometrium, cervix, and breast have been studied extensively. Effects on three of these cancers are clear: OCs *protect* against ovarian and endometrial cancer, and have *no impact* (positive or negative) on cervical cancer, which is caused by human papillomaviruses.

What about breast cancer? OCs do *not* increase the risk of breast cancer for *most* women. This conclusion is based on data from the Women's Contraceptive and Reproductive Experience (Women's CARE) study. This major study, involving over 9000 women, found no association between present or past use of OCs and the development of breast cancer. This conclusion applied not only to study participants as a whole, but also to women in the following subgroups:

- Those who used OCs with high estrogen content
- Those who used OCs for a prolonged time
- Those who began OC use during adolescence
- Those with a first-degree relative with breast cancer

These results should reassure women who are OC users.

However, although this study shows that OCs do not increase risk for *most* women, the results of another large recent study show that OCs *do* increase risk for *some* women, specifically, women who have the *BRCA1* gene mutation. Even without taking OCs, these women have a very high—50% to 80%—lifetime risk of breast cancer. OCs increase this risk by one-third. The same study found that OCs do *not* increase risk in women with the *BRCA2* mutation.

It is important to note that although OCs do not *cause* breast cancer, estrogens can promote the growth of *existing* breast carcinoma. Accordingly, women with this disease should not take OCs.

Hypertension. Combination OCs can cause hypertension, but the risk with today's low-estrogen preparations is very low. OCs raise blood pressure by increasing blood levels of two compounds: angiotensin (a potent vasoconstrictor) and aldosterone (a hormone that promotes salt and water retention). If hypertension develops, and if OCs are determined to be the cause, two options are open: (1) discontinue the OC or (2) continue the OC and manage the hypertension with drugs.

Abnormal Uterine Bleeding. By altering the endometrium, OCs may decrease or eliminate menstrual flow. In addition, breakthrough bleeding and spotting may occur, especially with the use of extended-cycle OCs (e.g., Seasonique, Seasonale). Spotting and bleeding can also occur with monthly-cycle OCs, most often during the first 3 months when low-estrogen OCs are used. If a period is missed while taking monthly-cycle OCs, the possibility of pregnancy should be assessed. Following discontinuation of OCs, normal menstruation usually resumes, although the first period may be delayed. Women with a pretreatment history of irregular menses will return to their previous pattern when OCs are discontinued.

Use in Pregnancy and Lactation. OCs have no therapeutic role during pregnancy, and hence are *contraindicated for use by pregnant women.* Pregnancy should be ruled out before starting OC use, and if pregnancy should occur despite OC use, use should stop immediately. Woman should be assured,

TABLE 62.4 ■ Side Effects Caused by an Excess of or Deficiency in the Estrogen or Progestin Content of an Oral Contraceptive Regimen

Estrogen		Progestin	
Excess	**Deficiency**	**Excess**	**Deficiency**
Nausea Breast tenderness Edema Bloating Hypertension Migraine Cervical mucorrhea Polyposis	Early or midcycle breakthrough bleeding Increased spotting Hypomenorrhea	Increased appetite Weight gain Depression Tiredness Fatigue Hypomenorrhea Breast regression Monilial vaginitis Acne, oily scalp[a] Hair loss[a] Hirsutism[a]	Late breakthrough bleeding Amenorrhea Hypermenorrhea

[a]Caused by progestins that have strong androgenic activity.

however, that inadvertent use of OCs during early pregnancy poses no risk of fetal harm. Because OCs have no role in pregnancy—and *not* because they are harmful—these drugs are classified in U.S. Food and Drug Administration (FDA) Pregnancy Risk Category X.[a]

Combination OCs enter breast milk and reduce milk production, especially in the early stages of lactation. In contrast, progestin-only OCs have little or no effect on milk production, and hence are preferred for contraception during lactation, at least early on. (Later, when the milk supply is well established, and especially with the addition of solids to the infant's diet, use of combination OCs may resume.)

Nurses of Childbearing Age. In 2016 the National Institute for Occupational Safety and Health (NIOSH) expanded the list of drugs identified as hazardous. (See https://www.cdc.gov/niosh/docs/2016-161/pdfs/2016-161.pdf.) NIOSH requires special handling of drugs identified as hazardous. See Chapter 3, Table 3.1, for administration and handling guidelines. The hazardous drugs mentioned in this chapter are listed in the following box.

Safety Alert

HAZARDOUS DRUGS REQUIRING SPECIAL HANDLING

Dinoprostone	Medroxyprogesterone acetate
Estradiol	Mifepristone
Estrogen/progesterone combinations	Misoprostol
Estrogens, conjugated	Progesterone
Estrogens, esterified	Ulipristal

Stroke in Women With Migraine. When used by women who experience migraine headaches, OCs may increase the risk of thrombotic stroke. However, the absolute increase is low: only 8 cases per 100,000 women at age 20 years, and rising to 80 cases per 100,000 women at age 40 years. Because the risk is low, OCs are generally considered safe for women with migraine, provided they are younger than 35 years, don't smoke, and are healthy, and provided their headaches are not preceded by visual changes known as an aura (migraine with aura has a greater risk of stroke than migraine without aura). Migraine and its management are discussed in Chapter 30.

Benign Hepatic Adenoma. Hepatic adenoma is a rare complication seen in women who use OCs that contain *mestranol.* These highly vascular, nonmalignant tumors are usually picked up as incidental findings on a computed tomography scan or magnetic resonance imaging. If hepatic adenoma is diagnosed, discontinuing OCs usually results in spontaneous tumor regression.

Effects Related to Estrogen or Progestin Imbalance. Many of the mild side effects of combination OCs result from an excess or deficiency of estrogen or progestin. Effects that can result from an excess of estrogen include nausea, breast tenderness, and edema. Progestin excess can increase appetite and cause fatigue and depression. A deficiency in either hormone can cause menstrual irregularities. Side effects related to hormonal imbalance are shown in Table 62.4.

Quite often, these effects can be reduced by adjusting the estrogen/progestin balance of an OC regimen. With most women, therapy is initiated with an OC containing 30 to 35 mcg of ethinyl estradiol. If significant nausea occurs, it can be managed by dosing at bedtime or, if needed, switching to an OC with less estrogen. Using less estrogen can also reduce breast discomfort. During the first 3 months of use, spotting and breakthrough bleeding are common, and usually resolve on their own. If they don't, they can be managed by increasing the estrogen dosage or by using a product that contains a different progestin. For women who experience androgenic effects (e.g., acne, hirsutism), switching to an OC that has drospirenone or dienogest can help. Other side effects can be reduced by making similar adjustments. When substituting one combination OC for another, the change is best made at the beginning of a new cycle.

Hyperkalemia. *Drospirenone,* a fourth-generation progestin, promotes renal retention of potassium and can thereby cause hyperkalemia. Accordingly, the drug is inappropriate for women with conditions that predispose to hyperkalemia (e.g., renal insufficiency, adrenal insufficiency, liver disease).

[a]As of 2020, the FDA will no longer use Pregnancy Risk Categories. Please refer to Chapter 9 for more information.

Furthermore, drospirenone should be used with caution in women taking other drugs that can elevate serum potassium. Important among these are angiotensin-converting enzyme inhibitors, angiotensin II receptor blockers, potassium-sparing diuretics, potassium supplements, and nonsteroidal anti-inflammatory drugs (when taken daily). If women taking these drugs are using a drospirenone-containing OC, potassium levels should be checked during the first cycle of use.

Noncontraceptive Benefits of OCs

OCs decrease the risk of several disorders, including ovarian cancer, endometrial cancer, ovarian cysts, pelvic inflammatory disease (PID), benign breast disease, iron deficiency anemia, and acne. In addition, OCs favorably affect menstrual symptoms: cramps are reduced, menstrual flow is reduced in volume and duration, and menses are more predictable. In women with premenstrual disorder or premenstrual dysphoric disorder, OCs can reduce symptom intensity. In some women with menstrual-associated migraine, OCs can reduce migraine frequency. Surprisingly, OCs may even benefit women with rheumatoid arthritis.

Drug Interactions

Drugs and Herbs That Reduce the Effects of OCs. Products that induce hepatic cytochrome P450 can accelerate OC metabolism and can thereby reduce OC effects. Products that induce P450 include *rifampin* (used for tuberculosis), *ritonavir* (used for HIV infection), several *antiseizure agents* (carbamazepine, phenobarbital, phenytoin, and primidone), and *St. John's wort* (an herb used for depression). Women taking OCs in combination with any of these agents should be alert for indications of reduced OC blood levels, such as breakthrough bleeding or spotting. If these signs appear, it may be necessary to either (1) increase the estrogen dosage of the OC, (2) combine the OC with a second form of birth control (e.g., condom), or (3) switch to an alternative form of birth control.

Drugs Whose Effects Are Reduced by OCs. OCs can decrease the benefits of warfarin and hypoglycemic agents. By increasing levels of clotting factors, OCs can decrease the effectiveness of *warfarin,* an anticoagulant. By increasing levels of glucose, OCs can counteract the benefits of insulin and other hypoglycemic agents used in diabetes. Accordingly, when combined with OCs, warfarin and hypoglycemic agents may require increased dosage.

Drugs Whose Effects Are Increased by OCs. OCs can impair the hepatic metabolism of several agents, including *theophylline, tricyclic antidepressants, diazepam,* and *chlordiazepoxide.* Because of reduced clearance, these drugs may accumulate to toxic levels. If signs of toxicity appear, dosage of these drugs should be reduced.

Preparations

The combination OCs in current use are listed in Tables 62.5 through 62.8. As you can see, nearly all of these products contain the same estrogen: ethinyl estradiol. In contrast, eight different progestins are employed. Products are listed in order of increasing estrogen content. The OCs with low estrogen are safer. As a rule, high-estrogen OCs are reserved for women taking drugs that induce P450. Products with unique properties are discussed next.

Beyaz, Rajani, and Safyral. In addition to an estrogen and a progestin, these combination OCs contain *levomefolate,* a metabolite of folic acid. The purpose is to reduce the risk of fetal neural tube defects—anencephaly and spina bifida—if pregnancy should occur despite contraceptive use. As discussed in Chapter 81, neural tube defects can result if folic acid is low early in pregnancy.

Natazia. Natazia has two unique components: *estradiol valerate* and *dienogest,* a fourth-generation progestin. Estradiol valerate is a prodrug that undergoes rapid conversion to estradiol, the predominant endogenous estrogen. Dienogest, which is much like drospirenone (see discussion of *Components,* earlier), has strong progestational activity and antiandrogenic activity. However, in contrast to drospirenone, dienogest does not cause potassium retention, and hence there is no need to monitor potassium levels. Unlike all other combination OCs, Natazia employs a *four-phase dosing schedule,* in which the amount of estradiol decreases over the monthly cycle and the amount of progestin (dienogest) increases. Because of this schedule, duration of withdrawal bleeding is shorter than with other combination OCs, and the intensity of bleeding is lighter. In women who normally experience heavy or prolonged menstrual bleeding, Natazia can reduce blood loss.

Dosing Schedules

With only one exception, combination OCs are dosed in a *cyclic pattern.* For most products, each cycle is *28 days long* (see Tables 62.5 through 62.7). However, with a few newer products, the cycle is either *extended* (to 91 days) or *continuous* [Amethyst].

28-Day-Cycle Schedules. The 28-day regimens are subdivided into four groups: *monophasic, biphasic, triphasic,* and *quadriphasic (four-phasic).* In a monophasic regimen, the daily doses of estrogen and progestin remain constant throughout the cycle of use. In the other regimens, either the estrogen or the progestin changes (or both change) as the cycle progresses. The biphasic, triphasic, and quadriphasic schedules reflect efforts to more closely simulate ovarian production of estrogens and progestins. However, these preparations appear to offer little or no advantage over monophasic OCs.

Most 28-day cycle products are taken in a repeating sequence consisting of 21 days of an active pill followed by 7 days on which either (1) no pill is taken, (2) an inert pill is taken, or (3) an iron-containing pill is taken. The sequence is begun on either (1) the first day of the menstrual cycle or (2) the first Sunday after the onset of menses. With the first option, protection is conferred immediately, and hence no backup contraception is needed. With a Sunday start, which is done to have menses occur on weekdays rather than the weekend, protection may not be immediate, and hence an alternate form of birth control should be used during the first cycle. With both options, each dose should be taken at the same time every day (e.g., with a meal or at bedtime). Successive dosing cycles should commence every 28 days, even if there is breakthrough bleeding or spotting.

Extended-Cycle and Continuous Schedules. Many healthcare providers recommend taking combination OCs for an extended time, rather than following the traditional 28-day cycle, because doing so decreases episodes of withdrawal bleeding with its associated menstrual pain, premenstrual symptoms, headaches, and other problems. Prolonged use of OCs is possible because these drugs suppress endometrial thickening, and hence monthly bleeding is not required to slough off hypertrophied tissue. At this time, 14 products—*Amethia, Amethia Lo, Ashlyna, Camrese, Camrese Lo, Daysee, Introvale, Jolessa, Quasense, Seasonale, Seasonique, LoSeasonique, Setlakin,* and *Amethyst* —are packaged and marketed for prolonged use. The following regimens are employed:

- *Introvale, Jolessa, Quasense, Seasonale,* and *Setlakin*—active pills for 84 days, then no pills for 7 days

Text continued on p. 762

TABLE 62.5 ▪ Composition of 28-Day Monophasic Combination Oral Contraceptives

Brand Name	mcg	Estrogen	mg	Progestin
Lo Loestrin Fe[a]	10	Ethinyl estradiol	1	Norethindrone
Blisovi 1/20 Blisovi 24 Fe[b] Gildess 1/20 Gildess Fe 1/20 Junel 1/20 Junel Fe 1/20 Junel Fe 24[b] Larin 1/20 Larin Fe 1/20 Larin 24 Fe[b] Loestrin 21 1/20 Loestrin Fe 1/20 Lomedia 24 Fe[b] Mibelas 24 Fe[b] Microgestin 1/20 Microgestin Fe 1/20 Minastrin 24 Fe[b] Tarina Fe 1/20 Taytulla[b]	20	Ethinyl estradiol	1	Norethindrone
Aviane-28 Falmina Lessina Lutera Orsythia Sronyx Vienva	20	Ethinyl estradiol	0.1	Levonorgestrel
Gianvi[c] Loryna Nikki[c] Vestura[c] YAZ[c] Beyaz[c,d] Rajani[d]	20	Ethinyl estradiol	3	Drospirenone
Generess Fe[e] Kaitlib Fe	25	Ethinyl estradiol	0.8	Norethindrone
Kurrelo Levora Marlissa Portia-28	30	Ethinyl estradiol	0.15	Levonorgestrel
Cryselle Elinest Low-Ogestrel Lo/Ovral-28	30	Ethinyl estradiol	0.3	Norgestrel
Blisovi 1.5/30 Gildess 1.5/30 Gildess Fe 1.5/30 Larin 1.5/30 Larin Fe 1.5/30 Junel 1.5/30 Junel Fe 1.5/30 Loestrin 21 1.5/30 Loestrin Fe 1.5/30 Microgestin 1.5/30 Microgestin Fe 1.5/30	30	Ethinyl estradiol	1.5	Norethindrone

Continued

TABLE 62.5 ▪ Composition of 28-Day Monophasic Combination Oral Contraceptives—cont'd

Brand Name	mcg	Estrogen	mg	Progestin
Altavera Apri Desogen Emoquette Enskyce Reclipsen	30	Ethinyl estradiol	0.15	Desogestrel
Ocella Safyral[d] Syeda Yasmin Zarah	30	Ethinyl estradiol	3	Drospirenone
Kelnor 1/35 Zovia 1/35E	35	Ethinyl estradiol	1	Ethynodiol diacetate
Balziva Briellyn Femcon Fe[e] Gildagia Ovcon-35[e] Philith Vyfemla Wymzya Fe[f] Zeosa Zenchent Fe[f]	35	Ethinyl estradiol	0.4	Norethindrone
Brevicon-28 Modicon-28 Necon 0.5/35 Nortrel 0.5/35 Wera	35	Ethinyl estradiol	0.5	Norethindrone
Alyacen 1/35 Cyclafem 1/35 Dasetta 1/35 Necon 1/35 Norinyl 1/35 Nortrel 1/35 Ortho-Novum 1/35 Pirmella 1/35	35	Ethinyl estradiol	1	Norethindrone
Estarylla Mono-Lynah MonoNessa Ortho-Cyclen-28 Previfem Sprintec	35	Ethinyl estradiol	0.25	Norgestimate
Ogestrel	50	Ethinyl estradiol	0.5	Norgestrel
Zovia 1/50	50	Ethinyl estradiol	1	Ethynodiol diacetate
Necon 1/50 Norinyl 1/50	50	Mestranol	1	Norethindrone

[a]The cycle for Lo Loestrin Fe is 24 active tablets followed by 2 0/10 mcg tabs ×2, then 2 ferrous fumarate tablets.
[b]The cycle for Blisovi 24 Fe, Junel Fe 24, Larin 24 Fe, Lomedia 24 Fe, Mibelas 24 Fe, Minastrin 24 Fe, and Taytulla is 24 active tablets followed by 4 ferrous fumarate tablets.
[c]The cycle for Gianvi, YAZ, and Beyaz is 24 active tablets followed by 4 inert tablets.
[d]Each tablet of Beyaz, Rajani, and Safyral contains 0.451 mg levomefolate (a metabolite of folic acid) to help prevent fetal neural tube defects if pregnancy should occur despite contraceptive use.
[e]Generess Fe, Femcon Fe, and Ovcon-35 are the only chewable OCs available (they may also be swallowed whole).
[f]The cycle for Wymzya Fe and Zenchent Fe is 21 active tablets followed by 7 ferrous fumarate tablets.

TABLE 62.6 ▪ Composition of 28-Day Biphasic and Triphasic Combination Oral Contraceptives

Brand Name	mcg	Estrogen	mg	Progestin
BIPHASIC				
Necon 10/11	35 35	Ethinyl estradiol	0.5 1	Norethindrone (phase 1) Norethindrone (phase 2)
Azurette Bekyree Kariva Kimidess Pimtrea Viorele	20 10	Ethinyl estradiol	0.15 0	Desogestrel (phase 1) Desogestrel (phase 2)
TRIPHASIC				
Caziant Cyclessa Velivet	25 25 25	Ethinyl estradiol	0.1 0.125 0.15	Desogestrel (phase 1) Desogestrel (phase 2) Desogestrel (phase 3)
Aranelle Leena Tri-Norinyl	35 35 35	Ethinyl estradiol	0.5 1 0.5	Norethindrone (phase 1) Norethindrone (phase 2) Norethindrone (phase 3)
Ortho-Novum 7/7/7 Pirmella 7/7/7 Dasetta 7/7/7 Cyclafem 7/7/7 Neocon 7/7/7 Nortrel 7/7/7	35 35 35	Ethinyl estradiol	0.5 0.75 1	Norethindrone (phase 1) Norethindrone (phase 2) Norethindrone (phase 3)
Enpresse Levonest Myzilra Trivora	30 40 30	Ethinyl estradiol	0.05 0.075 0.125	Levonorgestrel (phase 1) Levonorgestrel (phase 2) Levonorgestrel (phase 3)
Ortho Tri-Cyclen Lo Tri-Lo-Marzia Tri-Lo-Sprintec	25 25 25	Ethinyl estradiol	0.18 0.215 0.25	Norgestimate (phase 1) Norgestimate (phase 2) Norgestimate (phase 3)
Ortho Tri-Cyclen Tri-Estarylla Tri-Linyah TriNessa Tri-Sprintec Tri-Previfem	35 35 35	Ethinyl estradiol	0.18 0.215 0.25	Norgestimate (phase 1) Norgestimate (phase 2) Norgestimate (phase 3)
Estrostep Fe Tilia Fe Tri-Legest Fe	20 30 35	Ethinyl estradiol	1 1 1	Norethindrone (phase 1) Norethindrone (phase 2) Norethindrone (phase 3)

TABLE 62.7 ▪ Composition of Quadriphasic Combination Oral Contraceptives

Brand Name	mcg	Estrogen	mg	Progestin
Natazia	3 2 2 1	Estradiol valerate	0 2 3 0	Dienogest (phase 1) Dienogest (phase 2) Dienogest (phase 3) Dienogest (phase 4)
Quartette[a] Rivelsa[a]	20 25 30 10	Ethinyl estradiol	0.15 0.15 0.15 0	Levonorgestrel (phase 1) Levonorgestrel (phase 2) Levonorgestrel (phase 3) Levonorgestrel (phase 4)

[a]Quartette and Rivelsa are extended-cycle OCs.

TABLE 62.8 ▪ Extended-Cycle and Continuous OCs

Brand Name	mcg	Estrogen	mg	Progestin
EXTENDED-CYCLE OCS				
Amethia[a] Ashlyna[a] Camrese[a] Daysee[a] Introvale[b] Jolessa[b] Quasense[b] Seasonale[b] Seasonique[a] Setlakin[b]	30	Ethinyl estradiol	0.15	Levonorgestrel
Amethia Lo[a] Camrese Lo[a] LoSeasonique[a]	20	Ethinyl estradiol	0.1	Levonorgestrel
CONTINUOUS OC				
Amethyst[c]	20	Ethinyl estradiol	0.09	Levonorgestrel

[a]The cycle for Amethia, Amethia Lo, Ashlyna, Camrese, Camrese Lo, Daysee, Seasonique, and LoSeasonique is 84 active tablets followed by 7 low-estrogen tablets (10 mcg ethinyl estradiol).
[b]The cycle for Introvale, Jolessa, Quasense, Seasonale, and Setlakin is 84 active tablets followed by 7 inert tablets.
[c]Amethyst is taken continuously, without interruption.

- *Amethia, Amethia Lo, Ashlyna, Camrese, Camrese Lo, Daysee, Seasonique,* and *LoSeasonique*—active pills for 84 days, then low-dose estrogen pills for 7 days
- *Amethyst*—active pills are taken continuously, with no scheduled interruption

Hence, with Introvale, Jolessa, Quasense, Seasonale, Setlakin, Amethia, Amethia Lo, Ashlyna, Camrese, Camrese Lo, Daysee, Seasonique, and LoSeasonique, withdrawal bleeding occurs just 4 times a year, instead of 13 as with conventional cycles. With Amethyst, withdrawal bleeding occurs only when dosing is finally stopped. However, although these regimens decrease episodes of *scheduled* bleeding, *breakthrough bleeding* can be more common.

It is important to note that there is nothing special about the estrogen/progestin combinations used in these extended-cycle products. Put another way, we could get the same results with other combination OCs, provided they are *monophasic.* To achieve an extended schedule, the user would simply purchase four packets of a 28-day product (each of which contains 21 active pills), and then take the active pills for 84 days straight.

What to Do if Doses Are Missed

The chances of ovulation (and hence pregnancy) from missing one OC dose are small. However, the risk of pregnancy becomes progressively larger with each successive omission.

For products that use a *28-day cycle,* the following recommendations apply:

- If *1 or more pills* are missed in the *first week,* take 1 pill as soon as possible and then continue with the pack. Use an additional form of contraception for 7 days.
- If *1 or 2 pills* are missed during the *second or third week,* take 1 pill as soon as possible and then continue with the *active* pills in the pack—but skip the placebo pills and go straight to a new pack once all the active pills have been taken.
- If *3 or more pills* are missed during the *second or third week,* follow the same instructions given for missing 1 or 2 pills, but use an additional form of contraception for 7 days.

Important note: The response to a missed dose of Natazia, as described in the package insert, is more complex than with other combination OCs.

For combination OCs that use an *extended or continuous cycle,* up to 7 days can be missed with little or no increased risk of pregnancy, provided the pills had been taken *continuously for the prior 3 weeks.*

Progestin-Only Oral Contraceptives

Progestin-only OCs, also known as "minipills," contain a progestin but no estrogen. Because they lack estrogen, minipills do not cause thromboembolic disorders, headaches, nausea, or most of the other adverse effects associated with combination OCs. Unfortunately, although slightly safer than combination OCs, the progestin-only preparations are less effective and are more likely to cause irregular bleeding (breakthrough bleeding, spotting, amenorrhea, inconsistent cycle length, variations in the volume and duration of monthly flow). Irregular bleeding is the major drawback of these products and the principal reason that women discontinue them. Nine products are available: *Camila, Errin, Heather, Jolivette, Ortho Micronor, Nor-QD, Heather, Jencycla,* and *Nora-BE.* All contain 0.35 mg *norethindrone.*

Contraceptive effects of the minipill result largely from altering cervical secretions. Under the influence of progestins, cervical glands produce a thick, sticky mucus that acts as a barrier to penetration by sperm. Progestins also modify the endometrium, making it less favorable for implantation. Compared with combination OCs, minipills are weak inhibitors of ovulation, and hence this mechanism contributes little to their effects. Unlike combination OCs, whose administration is cyclic, progestin-only OCs are taken continuously. Use is initiated on day 1 of the menstrual cycle, and 1 pill is taken daily thereafter. A backup contraceptive method should be used for the first 7 days. Dosing should be done at the same time each day.

If one or more doses is missed, the following guidelines apply. If 1 pill is missed, it should be taken as soon as remembered, and backup contraception should be used for at least 2 days. The pills should be resumed as scheduled on the next day. If 2 pills are missed, the regimen should be restarted, and backup contraception should be used for at least 2 days. In addition, if 2 or more pills are missed and no menstrual bleeding occurs, a pregnancy test should be done.

COMBINATION CONTRACEPTIVES WITH NOVEL DELIVERY SYSTEMS

Two combination contraceptives—*a transdermal patch* and a *vaginal ring*—have the same mechanism as combination OCs, but they deliver hormones in novel ways. Like combination OCs, both of these contraceptives contain two hormones—an estrogen and a progestin—that undergo absorption into the systemic circulation, and then prevent pregnancy primarily by suppressing ovulation. What's different is how the hormones are delivered: With the patch, the hormones are absorbed through the skin, and with the vaginal ring, the hormones are absorbed through the vaginal mucosa. Otherwise, the pharmacology of these contraceptives is essentially identical to that of combination OCs.

Transdermal Contraceptive Patch

The *Ortho Evra* and *Xulane* transdermal contraceptive patches have the same mechanism as combination OCs. Furthermore, these products have the same contraceptive efficacy and the same incidence of breakthrough bleeding and spotting. The principal difference between them lies with their dosing schedules: Whereas combination OCs must be taken every day, the patch is applied just once a week. As a result, the patch is more convenient than OCs, and hence adherence is better.

The Ortho Evra patch contains 750 mcg of *ethinyl estradiol* (the estrogen found in most combination OCs) and 6 mg of *norelgestromin* (the active metabolite of norgestimate, a progestin found in some OCs). Each day, the patch releases 20 mcg of ethinyl estradiol and 150 mcg of norelgestromin. Xulane releases 35 mcg of ethinyl estradiol and 150 mcg of norelgestromin. Following release, these hormones penetrate the skin, enter capillaries, and undergo distribution throughout the body. Plasma levels plateau 2 days after the first patch is applied.

Application of the patch is done once a week for 3 weeks, followed by 1 week off (to permit normal menstruation). Patches are applied to the lower abdomen, buttocks, upper outer arm, or upper torso (front or back)—but not to the breasts or to skin that is red, cut, or irritated. To enhance adhesion, the skin should be clean, dry, and free of lotions, creams, or oils. In clinical trials, the pregnancy rate was about 1 for every 100 woman-years of patch use. However, among women who weighed 90 kg (198 lb) or more, the pregnancy rate was significantly higher, suggesting that the patch may be inappropriate for women in this weight group.

When should patch use begin? For women not currently using OCs, the first patch should be applied during the first 24 hours of the menstrual period. For women switching from OCs, the first patch should be applied on the first day of withdrawal bleeding.

In clinical trials, 4.6% of patches became partially or completely detached. When this occurs, the patch should be reattached or replaced. If the patch has been off less than 24 hours, backup contraception is unnecessary. However, if the patch has been off more than 24 hours, a new cycle should be started, accompanied by backup contraception during the first 7 days.

The most common adverse effects are breast discomfort, headache, local irritation, nausea, and menstrual cramps. Compared with Triphasil (a combination OC), the patch produces a higher incidence of breast discomfort and dysmenorrhea. Contraindications and drug interactions are the same as for combination OCs.

Does the patch cause more VTE than do OCs? Possibly. Three epidemiologic studies have examined the question. In two of the studies, the risk of VTE in women using the patch was double the risk in women using combination OCs. However, in the third study, there was no difference in risk. Of note, women who use the patch are exposed to 60% more estrogen than women who use an OC containing 35 mcg of estrogen. The higher estrogen exposure could increase the risk of VTE.

Vaginal Contraceptive Ring

NuvaRing is a hormonal contraceptive device designed for vaginal insertion. Like combination OCs, the ring contains an estrogen/progestin combination that prevents pregnancy largely by suppressing ovulation. Adverse effects, drug interactions, warnings, and contraindications for the ring are the same as for combination OCs. The ring is made of transparent, flexible material and looks like a very skinny doughnut, with an overall diameter of 2.1 inches and a cross-sectional diameter of one-eighth inch. Insertion is done by the user.

The NuvaRing contains 2.7 mg of *ethinyl estradiol* and 11.7 mg of *etonogestrel* (the active metabolite of desogestrel, a progestin found in some OCs). Each day, the ring releases 15 mcg of ethinyl estradiol and 120 mcg of etonogestrel. Following release, the hormones penetrate the vaginal mucosa, undergo absorption into the blood, and then distribute throughout the body. Contraception results from systemic effects—not from local effects in the vagina.

One ring is inserted once each month, left in place for 3 weeks, and then removed; a new ring is inserted 1 week later. During the ring-free week, withdrawal bleeding occurs. The new ring should be inserted on schedule, even if bleeding is still ongoing. If a ring is expelled before 3 weeks have passed, it can be washed off in warm water (not hot water) and reinserted. If the expelled ring cannot be reused, a new one should be inserted. If more than 3 hours elapse between ring expulsion and reinsertion, contraceptive effects may be diminished, and hence backup contraception should be used for 7 days.

For women not currently using contraception, ring use should start anytime during days 1 through 5 of the menstrual cycle, even if bleeding is ongoing; backup contraception should be used during the first 7 days.

The most common adverse effects are vaginitis, headaches, upper respiratory infection, leukorrhea, sinusitis, weight gain, and nausea. Common reasons for discontinuing the ring include foreign body sensations, coital problems, ring expulsion, vaginal symptoms, headache, and emotional lability. The risk of serious adverse effects—thrombosis, embolism, and hypertension—is the same as with combination OCs.

LONG-ACTING CONTRACEPTIVES

Subdermal Etonogestrel Implants

A subdermal system [Nexplanon] for delivery of etonogestrel is available for long-term, reversible contraception. As shown in Table 62.1, Nexplanon is among the most effective contraceptives available.

Description

Nexplanon consists of a single 4-cm rod that contains 68 mg of etonogestrel, a synthetic progestin. The rod is implanted subdermally in the groove between the biceps and triceps in the nondominant arm. Etonogestrel then diffuses slowly and continuously, providing blood levels sufficient for contraception for 3 years, after which the rod is removed. If continued contraception is desired, a new rod is implanted.

Mechanism of Action

Etonogestrel suppresses ovulation and thickens cervical mucus. In addition, it causes the endometrium to become involuted and hence hostile to implantation.

Pharmacokinetics

Daily release of etonogestrel is 60 to 70 mcg initially and gradually declines to 25 to 30 mcg over 3 years. Absorbed drug is slowly metabolized by the liver. When the rod is removed, etonogestrel becomes undetectable within 5 to 7 days.

Drug Interactions

Agents that induce hepatic enzymes—such as barbiturates, phenytoin, rifampin, carbamazepine, topiramate, HIV protease inhibitors, and St. John's wort—may reduce the efficacy of Nexplanon. Accordingly, Nexplanon should not be used by women taking these drugs.

Adverse Effect: Irregular Bleeding

In women using Nexplanon, bleeding episodes are irregular and unpredictable. In clinical trials, amenorrhea occurred in 22% of women; infrequent bleeding (less than 3 bleeding or spotting episodes in 90 days) occurred in 34% of women; frequent bleeding (more than 5 bleeding or spotting episodes in 90 days) occurred in 7% of women, and prolonged bleeding (more than 14 days of bleeding in 90 days) occurred in 18%

of women. Despite effects on bleeding, levels of hemoglobin were unaffected over 3 years. The general pattern of irregular and unpredictable bleeding does not change while using Nexplanon. Bleeding irregularities are the leading reason for discontinuing the device.

Use During Breast-Feeding

Nexplanon is safe to use during breast-feeding after the 21st postpartum day. Very little etonogestrel is excreted in breast milk. In a controlled clinical trial, there were no significant effects on the physical or psychomotor development of infants. Also, Nexplanon had no effect on the production or quality of milk, even when implanted just a few days postpartum.

Depot Medroxyprogesterone Acetate

Depot medroxyprogesterone acetate (DMPA), injected IM or subQ, protects against pregnancy for 3 months or longer by inhibiting secretion of gonadotropins. The drug thereby (1) inhibits follicular maturation and ovulation, (2) thickens the cervical mucus, and (3) causes thinning of the endometrium, making implantation unlikely. When injections are discontinued, return of fertility is delayed (by an average of 9 months).

DMPA is available in two formulations for contraception. One is injected IM [Depo-Provera] and the other is injected subQ [Depo-SubQ Provera 104]. Dosages are 150 mg and 104 mg, respectively, injected once every 3 months. To ensure that the recipient is not pregnant, the first dose should be given either (1) during the first 5 days of a normal menstrual period, (2) within the first 5 days postpartum (if not breast-feeding), or (3) at the sixth week postpartum (if exclusively breast-feeding).

Most adverse effects are like those seen with other progestin-only contraceptives. Menstrual disturbances are common; menstruation may be irregular at first and then, after 6 to 12 months, may cease entirely. Mild weight gain (about 3.5 lb) is likely during the first year. Women may also experience abdominal bloating, headache, depression, and decreased libido. However, it is unclear whether DMPA is the cause. Although DMPA has produced uterine and mammary cancers in animals, a large-scale study has shown no increase in the risk of cervical, ovarian, or breast cancer in women—and the risk of endometrial cancer is actually reduced.

DMPA poses a risk of reversible bone loss, but this risk does not outweigh the benefits of treatment. During the first 1 to 2 years of DMPA use, bone mineral density (BMD) declines rapidly, at a rate of 1% to 2% per year. However, after this time, the rate of bone loss slows down. Importantly, when DMPA is discontinued, BMD returns to pretreatment levels, typically within 30 months. Whether DMPA-induced bone loss increases the risk of fractures is unclear. While this story was still evolving, the FDA revised the label for DMPA to include a black box warning that recommends against using the drug for more than 2 years. However, in the light of data gathered, this warning appears unwarranted. Accordingly an American College of Obstetricians and Gynecologists committee counseled that practitioners should not let concerns about bone loss deter them from prescribing DMPA or cause them to limit prescriptions to 2 years. In addition, the committee recommended against routine testing of BMD in women on DMPA. When counseling patients about this issue, practitioners should point out that any risk of fracture with DMPA is theoretical, whereas the risks associated with pregnancy are very real.

Intrauterine Devices

IUDs are among the most reliable forms of reversible birth control (see Table 62.1). In addition, the IUDs available today are very safe when used by appropriate patients. Worldwide, more than 85 million women use these devices. However, IUDs are not popular in the United States: Among women who use birth control, only 5.5% choose an IUD. Nonuse of IUDs is largely the legacy of the Dalkon Shield, a poorly designed IUD associated with a high rate of pelvic infection.

Two forms of IUDs are available: (1) the *copper T 380A* [ParaGard] and (2) those containing *levonorgestrel* [Kyleena, Liletta, Mirena, and Skyla]. Both forms are extremely effective. IUDs are placed within 7 days of the onset of menses, and a replacement can be inserted during any phase of the menstrual cycle. ParaGard can remain in place for 10 years, Mirena and Kyleena for 5 years, and Liletta and Skyla for 3 years. These devices prevent conception by producing a harmless local inflammatory response that is spermicidal. ParaGard, whose active ingredient is copper, may also inhibit implantation. Levonorgestrel also causes endometrial involution and thickening of the cervical mucus. Neither form prevents ovulation.

With proper counseling and patient selection, both IUDs are very safe. The principal risk is PID secondary to an STD. Accordingly, IUDs should be used only by women with a low risk for STDs—that is, by women who are monogamous and are confident that their partners are too. The risk for PID is highest during the first 20 days after insertion, with a rate of 9.7 cases per 1000 woman-years of use. One month after insertion, the risk declines to only 1.4 cases per 1000 woman-years of use.

IUDs can cause cramping and alteration of menses. Cramping is most intense upon IUD insertion and can be minimized by applying a topical anesthetic (2% lidocaine intracervical gel) or by premedicating with ibuprofen. With ParaGard, monthly bleeding is increased. With levonorgestrel, light spotting and amenorrhea are common.

In addition to providing long-term contraception, Mirena and ParaGard have other uses. Owing to its ability to greatly reduce menstrual bleeding, Mirena is approved for treating *menorrhagia* (heavy menstrual bleeding) in women who want to use an IUD for contraception. As discussed in Box 62.1, ParaGard can be used for *emergency contraception.* In one study, the pregnancy rate with postcoital placement was reduced to 0.2%.

SPERMICIDES

Spermicides are chemical surfactants that kill sperm by destroying their cell membrane. These drugs are available in the form of a foam, gel, jelly, suppository, vaginal film, and contraceptive sponge. All formulations can be purchased without a prescription. When used alone, spermicides are only moderately effective (see Table 62.1). Combined use with a diaphragm or condom increases efficacy. As shown in Table 62.9, spermicidal preparations contain *nonoxynol 9.*

Spermicides are generally devoid of serious side effects. Studies show no relationship between spermicides and birth defects. However, there is some evidence that nonoxynol 9 may *increase* the risk of HIV transmission. The apparent mechanism is promotion of vaginal, cervical, anal, and rectal lesions that facilitate HIV penetration to cells. Allergic reactions (to the drug or vehicle) occur in some women.

Correct use is required for contraceptive efficacy. The spermicide must be applied before intercourse, but no more than 1 hour in advance (when used alone). Containers for foam preparations must be shaken thoroughly before each use to ensure dispersal of the spermicide. Suppositories should be inserted at least 10 to 15 minutes before intercourse to allow time for dissolution. Spermicides should be reapplied each time intercourse is anticipated. Douching should be postponed for at least 6 hours following coitus.

The contraceptive sponge [Today Sponge] is a soft, porous, polyurethane disk impregnated with 1000 mg of nonoxynol 9. When inserted to cover the cervix, it protects against conception by (1) releasing spermicide, (2) absorbing seminal fluid, and (3) blocking penetration of sperm. Unlike other spermicide products, which must be reapplied before each act of intercourse, a single sponge is effective for 24 hours, regardless of how often coitus takes place. After 24 hours, the sponge should be removed. The rate of unintended pregnancy with the sponge is high: 16% among typical *nulliparous* users, and 32% among *parous* users. The most common adverse effects are vaginal irritation and dryness.

si

BOX 62.1 ■ SPECIAL INTEREST TOPIC

EMERGENCY CONTRACEPTION

Emergency contraception (EC) is defined as contraception that is implemented *after* intercourse. Women can use EC to prevent pregnancy following unprotected intercourse, which can result from sexual assault, contraceptive failure (e.g., broken condom), or other reasons. Safe and effective methods of EC have been available for decades. However, products marketed specifically for EC are relatively new.

In the United States, nearly 50% of women ages 15 to 44 years report having had at least one unintended pregnancy. Among teenagers, 88% of pregnancies are unintended. Of the 6 million pregnancies that occur each year, about 3.5 million are accidental. Every year, unintended pregnancies lead to 1.4 million abortions and 1.1 million births that women did not want—at least not yet. Clearly, if EC were used widely, most abortions and unwanted births could be avoided.

EC can be accomplished in two basic ways: Taking an *emergency contraceptive pill* (ECP), also known as a *morning-after pill,* or inserting a copper-T intrauterine device (IUD). Taking an ECP is most common. Furthermore, of the three basic types of ECPs—progestin-only pills, ulipristal-containing pills, and estrogen/progestin pills—the progestin-only pills are used most widely.

Progestin-Only ECPs

Three progestin-only products are available: Plan B One-Step, Next Choice One Dose, and Next Choice. All three contain *levonorgestrel.* These products are packaged and marketed specifically for emergency contraception. This contrasts with the estrogen/progestin products, which are marketed as oral contraceptives (OCs), but can be used off-label for EC.

Plan B One-Step and Next Choice One Dose

Plan B One-Step and Next Choice One Dose consist of a single high-dose (1.5-mg) tablet of levonorgestrel, a progestin found in many combination OCs. The package insert calls for taking the tablet within 72 hours of unprotected intercourse. However, although early implementation is best, Plan B One-Step, Next Choice One Dose, and other ECPs can still be effective when started up to 5 days after intercourse. Success is indicated by onset of menstrual bleeding in about 21 days.

Plan B One-Step reduces the odds of pregnancy by 89% and Next Choice One Dose prevented 84% of expected pregnancies, which is better than it may seem. In the absence of these two medications, the pregnancy rate from a single act of unprotected intercourse is about 8% (i.e., 8 women in 100 would become pregnant). However, among women using Plan B One-Step or Next Choice One Dose, only 1 and 1.3 in 100 is likely to become pregnant—a reduction of 89% and 84%, respectively.

Plan B One-Step and Next Choice One Dose work primarily by delaying or stopping ovulation. Inhibition of fertilization may also contribute. Of note, levonorgestrel is *not* effective after fertilization has occurred.

The major side effects of Plan B One-Step are heavier menstrual bleeding, nausea, abdominal pain, headache, and dizziness. Nausea can be reduced by taking an antiemetic (e.g., prochlorperazine) 1 hour before dosing. Importantly, if pregnancy does occur, having used levonorgestrel will not increase the risk of major congenital malformations, pregnancy complications, or any other adverse pregnancy outcomes.

These drugs will not terminate an existing pregnancy and will not harm a fetus if present. Recall that pregnancy is defined as implantation of a fertilized egg. Since Plan B One-Step and Next Choice One Dose act before fertilization and implantation, they cannot be considered abortifacients.

Plan B One-Step and Next Choice One Dose are now available over the counter. No prescription is required.

Next Choice

Next Choice consists of two 0.75-mg tablets of levonorgestrel (one-half the amount in a single Plan B One-Step or Next Choice One Dose tablet). According to the package insert, women should take 1 tablet within 72 hours of intercourse, and a second tablet 12 hours later. However, taking both tablets at the same time is just as effective. (This is equivalent to taking 1 tablet of Plan B One-Step or Next Choice One Step.) As with Plan B One-Step and Next Choice One Dose, these ECPs can still be effective when started up to 5 days after intercourse, but are most effective when taken earlier. Adverse effects are similar to those of Plan B One-Step and Next Choice One Dose. If vomiting occurs within 2 hours of dosing, a repeat dose may be required. Like Plan B One-Step, Next Choice can be obtained without a prescription.

Ulipristal Acetate ECP

Ulipristal acetate [Ella] is a drug that acts as an agonist/antagonist at receptors for progestin. Like levonorgestrel, ulipristal acetate prevents conception primarily by suppressing ovulation. Despite this similarity, ulipristal acetate and levonorgestrel differ in two important ways. First, ulipristal acetate remains highly effective when taken up to *5* days (120 hours) after intercourse, whereas levonorgestrel is most effective when taken within *3* days (72 hours) of intercourse. Second, whereas levonorgestrel [Plan B One-Step, Next Choice, Next Choice One Dose] is available without a prescription, ulipristal acetate [Ella] requires a prescription for all women, regardless of age. The dosage for ulipristal acetate is 1 tablet (30 mg), taken up to 5 days after unprotected intercourse. Principal adverse effects are headache, nausea, dysmenorrhea, and abdominal pain. If vomiting occurs within 3 hours of dosing, an additional dose may be required.

Estrogen/Progestin ECPs (Yuzpe Regimen)

The *Yuzpe regimen,* first described in 1974 by Professor A. Alfred Yuzpe, consists of two doses of an OC that contains an estrogen (ethinyl estradiol) plus a progestin (levonorgestrel or norgestrel). The first dose should be taken within 72 hours of unprotected intercourse, and the second dose 12 hours later. Pregnancy is prevented by interfering with ovulation, fertilization, and implantation. Like other ECPs, this regimen will not cause abortion. Compared with Plan B One-Step, this regimen is less effective (75% vs. 89%) and causes more nausea (50% vs. 13.3%)

Continued

EMERGENCY CONTRACEPTION—cont'd

and vomiting (19% vs. 6%). However, because other ECPs are more effective, better tolerated, and more readily available, these alternatives are used infrequently.

Mifepristone as an ECP

One drug—*mifepristone (RU 486)*—can prevent pregnancy *or* cause abortion, depending on when it is taken. If mifepristone is taken within 5 days of unprotected intercourse, it will prevent pregnancy from occurring, and thus can be considered an ECP. However, if mifepristone is taken after this time, it may terminate pregnancy that has already begun, and thus can be considered an abortifacient. When used as an ECP, mifepristone is 100% effective. The drug is available in the United States but is not approved for EC.

The Copper IUD

Insertion of a *copper IUD* (*ParaGard*) within 5 days of unprotected intercourse can prevent pregnancy in most women. The method is more than 99.9% effective, allowing less than 1 pregnancy for every 1000 IUD recipients. IUD insertion has the additional benefit of providing ongoing contraception for up to 10 years. Although using an IUD for EC is highly effective, the technique does have drawbacks: the IUD is expensive, not all women are candidates, and obtaining one quickly may be difficult.

TABLE 62.9 ■ Spermicides

Formulation	Active Ingredient	Brand Name
Foam	Nonoxynol 9 (12.5%)	Delfen Contraceptive
Jelly	Nonoxynol 9 (3%)	Gynol II Extra Strength Contraceptive[a]
Gel	Nonoxynol 9 (4%)	Conceptrol Disposable Contraceptive
	Nonoxynol 9 (3.5%)	Advantage 24[a]
	Nonoxynol 9 (2.2%)	K-Y Plus[a]
	Nonoxynol 9 (2%)	Shur Seal[a]
Suppository	Nonoxynol 9 (2.27%)	Encare
	Nonoxynol 9 (100 mg)	Semicid
Sponge	Nonoxynol 9 (1000 mg)	Today Sponge
Vaginal film	Nonoxynol 9 (28%)	VCF

[a]Intended for use only in combination with a vaginal diaphragm.

BARRIER DEVICES

Barrier devices—male condoms, female condoms, diaphragms, and the cervical cap—are *nonpharmacologic* options for birth control. Of the barrier devices available, condoms for men are by far the most commonly employed.

DRUGS FOR MEDICAL ABORTION

Mifepristone (RU 486) With Misoprostol

Mifepristone (RU 486) [Mifeprex] is a synthetic steroid that blocks receptors for progesterone and glucocorticoids. In the United States, the drug has one approved indication: termination of early intrauterine pregnancy; co-treatment with misoprostol is usually required. In addition, mifepristone is the most effective drug known for emergency contraception, although it is not used routinely for this purpose (see Box 62.1).

Mifepristone, followed by misoprostol, is a safe and effective alternative to surgery for termination of early pregnancy. Together, these drugs terminate pregnancy in about 95% of women. Principal adverse effects are abdominal pain and vaginal bleeding, which are unavoidable aspects of abortion. There is also a small risk of infection. In contrast to surgical abortion, which is generally unavailable before 8 weeks of gestation, abortion with mifepristone is performed early—within 7 weeks of conception.

Mechanism of Action

Mifepristone acts through blockade of progesterone receptors. Although mifepristone also blocks receptors for glucocorticoids, this action does not contribute to abortion. In the pregnant uterus, the drug has three effects. First, blockade of progesterone receptors leads to decidual breakdown and detachment of the conceptus. Second, mifepristone promotes cervical softening and dilation. Third, mifepristone increases uterine production of prostaglandins and renders the myometrium more responsive to the contractile effects of these prostaglandins. All three effects lead to expulsion of the conceptus. If mifepristone alone fails to induce abortion, the patient is given 400 mcg of oral misoprostol, a synthetic prostaglandin that reinforces uterine contractions induced by mifepristone. The pharmacology of misoprostol is discussed separately under *Prostaglandins*.

Adverse Effects

The most common side effects are bleeding, cramping, nausea, vomiting, diarrhea, and headache. The most serious adverse effects are severe bleeding and sepsis.

Successful abortion necessarily causes abdominal pain (cramping) and bleeding. Nearly all women experience these events. About 80% of patients experience transient cramping, beginning 1 hour after taking misoprostol; most women require an opioid analgesic for relief. Bleeding and spotting typically last 9 to 16 days. However, in some women, bleeding persists for 30 days or more. About 1% of women experience severe bleeding; treatment measures include curettage, uterotonic drugs (e.g., methylergonovine, ergonovine), and infusion of fluids, blood, or both.

Mifepristone/misoprostol has been associated with a few cases of serious bacterial infection, including very rare cases of fatal septic shock. Accordingly, patients and providers should be alert for typical signs of sepsis (sustained fever of 100.4°F or higher, severe abdominal pain, pelvic tenderness). However, in two confirmed cases of sepsis caused by *Clostridium sordellii*, these signs were absent. Instead, the patients presented with nausea, vomiting, and diarrhea, without fever or abdominal pain. In patients with typical or atypical presentation, the possibility of infection should be evaluated immediately.

The bleeding caused by mifepristone/misoprostol could mask bleeding due to a ruptured ectopic pregnancy. Accordingly, before mifepristone/misoprostol is used, ectopic pregnancy must be ruled out. This is best done by a routine ultrasound examination.

Misoprostol (but not mifepristone), a proven teratogen, can cause Möbius' syndrome, a rare fetal anomaly. Hence if the mifepristone/misoprostol fails to induce abortion, performing surgical abortion should be considered.

Contraindications

Major contraindications to mifepristone/misoprostol are ectopic pregnancy, hemorrhagic disorders, or use of anticoagulant drugs. Because mifepristone blocks receptors for glucocorticoids, it should not be used in women with adrenal insufficiency or in those on long-term glucocorticoid therapy.

Preparations, Dosage, and Administration

Mifepristone [Mifeprex] is supplied in single-dose packets containing three 200-mg tablets. The dosage is 600 mg taken all at once—followed in 2 days by 400 mcg of misoprostol (if mifepristone did not induce complete abortion by itself). Mifepristone is available only through qualified physicians; it is not sold in pharmacies.

FDA-Approved Protocol for Abortion

Under the FDA-approved protocol, induction of abortion with mifepristone/misoprostol requires *two visits to a qualified physician*. To dispense mifepristone, a physician must be qualified to determine pregnancy duration and to diagnose ectopic pregnancy. In addition, the physician must either (1) be able to perform surgical abortion (in the event mifepristone/misoprostol fails) as well as curettage (in the event of severe bleeding) or (2) have a commitment from a colleague to perform these procedures.

Prostaglandins: Misoprostol, Carboprost, and Dinoprostone

Prostaglandins are synthesized in all tissues of the body, where they act as local hormones. Unlike true hormones, which travel to distant sites to produce their effects, prostaglandins act on the very tissues in which they are made; degradation of prostaglandins is so rapid that they rarely escape their tissue of origin intact. Although the prostaglandins produce a broad spectrum of physiologic effects, their clinical use is limited. In obstetrics, prostaglandins are indicated for induction of abortion, cervical ripening before labor induction, and control of postpartum hemorrhage. The use of prostaglandins for abortion is discussed here. Their use for cervical ripening and control of postpartum hemorrhage is discussed in Chapter 64.

Nomenclature

Nomenclature regarding the prostaglandins can be confusing and hence deserves clarification. Each prostaglandin has three names: a traditional name, an official generic name, and a brand name. Misoprostol, carboprost, and dinoprostone are *generic names*. For carboprost, the traditional name is *15-methyl-prostaglandin F_2 alpha* and the brand name is *Hemabate*. For dinoprostone, the traditional name is *prostaglandin E_2*; brand names are *Cervidil, Prepidil,* and *Prostin E2* 🍁. For misoprostol, a synthetic *analog of prostaglandin E_1*, the brand name is *Cytotec*.

Physiologic and Pharmacologic Effects

Uterine Stimulation. Prostaglandins increase the force, frequency, and duration of uterine contractions. In the early months of pregnancy, the uterus is more responsive to prostaglandins than to oxytocin. During the second and third trimesters, prostaglandins can induce contractions of sufficient strength to cause complete evacuation of the uterus.

Like oxytocin, prostaglandins appear to have a physiologic role as promoters of uterine contraction, spontaneous labor, and delivery. Observations supporting this statement include: (1) Exogenous prostaglandins can induce uterine contractions that are very similar in frequency and duration to contractions that occur spontaneously; (2) the ability of the uterus to synthesize prostaglandins increases at term; (3) the prostaglandin content of amniotic fluid, umbilical blood, and maternal blood increases at term and during labor; and (4) labor is delayed and prolonged by agents that inhibit prostaglandin synthesis.

Cervical Softening. Local application of prostaglandins produces cervical softening. This softening results from breakdown of collagen and hence mimics the process by which natural cervical ripening occurs. Softening of the cervix does not depend on uterine stimulation.

Therapeutic Uses

Abortion. All three prostaglandins—misoprostol, carboprost, and dinoprostone—can be used to induce abortion. Misoprostol (in combination with methotrexate or mifepristone [RU 486]) is used *early* in pregnancy, as well as in the *second trimester*. Carboprost and dinoprostone are used in the *second trimester only*. With all three drugs, uterine contractions develop slowly. As a result, about 18 hours must pass between dosing and expulsion of the fetus. Unlike other abortifacients, prostaglandins are not feticidal, and hence the aborted fetus may show transient signs of life. Following passage of the fetus and placenta, the patient should be examined for possible cervical or uterine laceration.

Control of Postpartum Hemorrhage. *Carboprost* is indicated for control of postpartum hemorrhage. The drug is reserved for bleeding that has been refractory to more conventional agents (oxytocin, ergot alkaloids). In these situations, carboprost may be lifesaving. Use of carboprost to control postpartum hemorrhage is discussed in Chapter 64.

Induction of Labor. *Misoprostol* has been used to induce labor. The regimen recommended by the American College of Obstetricians and Gynecologists consists of 25 mcg vaginally repeated every 3 to 6 hours as needed.

Cervical Ripening. *Dinoprostone* and *misoprostol* can be used to initiate ripening of the cervix before induction of labor. This application is discussed in Chapter 64.

Adverse Effects

Gastrointestinal reactions are extremely common with dinoprostone and result from the ability of prostaglandins to stimulate smooth muscle of the alimentary canal. Vomiting and diarrhea occur in up to 62% of those treated. Nausea also occurs often. These responses can be reduced by pretreatment with antiemetic and antidiarrheal medications.

Intense uterine contractions can result in *cervical or uterine laceration*. The patient should be examined thoroughly for trauma following expulsion of the fetus and placenta.

Fever is seen with dinoprostone. When hyperthermia develops, it is important to distinguish between drug-induced fever and pyrexia resulting from endometritis. With dinoprostone, there is a 10% incidence of headache, shivering, and chills.

Precautions and Contraindications

Prostaglandins are *contraindicated* for women with active disease of the heart, lungs, kidneys, or liver. Carboprost should be avoided in women with a history of asthma or hypertension.

Preparations, Dosage, and Administration

Dinoprostone. Dinoprostone [Prepidil, Cervidil, Prostin E2 🍁] is available in three formulations: (1) 20-mg vaginal suppositories, (2) 10-mg vaginal inserts, and (3) a 0.5-mg gel. Dinoprostone suppositories [Prostin E2 🍁] are used for abortion. The gel [Prepidil] and vaginal inserts [Cervidil] are used for cervical ripening.

For *induction of abortion* (weeks 12 to 20), one 20-mg vaginal suppository is inserted initially, followed by one suppository every 3 to 5 hours as needed.

Carboprost Tromethamine. Carboprost tromethamine [Hemabate] is available in solution (250 mcg/mL) for IM administration. For *induction of abortion* (weeks 13 to 20), the dosage is 250 mcg initially followed by 250 mcg every 1.5 to 3.5 hours as needed. For *control of postpartum bleeding*, a single 250-mcg dose is injected.

Misoprostol. Misoprostol [Cytotec] is available in 100- and 200-mcg tablets. For induction of abortion in the *first trimester*, misoprostol is used in combination with mifepristone; dosing options for misoprostol include 400 mcg PO and 800 mcg vaginally. For induction of abortion in the *second trimester*, the dosage is 200 mcg administered vaginally every 6 to 12 hours until abortion occurs.

KEY POINTS

- The most effective methods of birth control are etonogestrel subdermal implants [Nexplanon], intramuscular medroxyprogesterone acetate [Depo-Provera], IUDs, and sterilization. OCs and transdermal patches are a close second.
- Sterilization is the most common form of birth control. OCs and male condoms come next.
- A long-term method of birth control (e.g., Nexplanon, Depo-Provera, IUD) is a good choice when adherence is a problem.

Continued

- There are two main categories of OCs: (1) combination OCs, which contain an estrogen plus a progestin, and (2) progestin-only OCs (aka minipills).
- Almost all combination OCs use the same estrogen: ethinyl estradiol. In contrast, eight different progestins are employed.
- Combination OCs act primarily by inhibiting ovulation.
- Although combination OCs can cause a variety of adverse effects, serious events are rare.
- Thrombotic events with combination OCs are caused by the progestin as well as the estrogen.
- The risk of thrombotic events is lowest with combination OCs that (1) have a low dose of estrogen and (2) contain a first-generation progestin. Conversely, risk is high with OCs that contain drospirenone or desogestrel.
- The risk of thrombotic events is increased in women who smoke and in those with thrombophilias.
- When used by nonsmoking women with normal cardiovascular function, OCs produce no greater mortality than other active forms of birth control.
- Combination OCs *protect* against ovarian and endometrial cancer and do *not* increase the risk of breast cancer.
- OCs are contraindicated during pregnancy, not because they are dangerous, but because they have no legitimate use during pregnancy. If accidental pregnancy occurs, OCs should be discontinued.
- The efficacy of OCs can be reduced by agents that induce hepatic drug-metabolizing enzymes (e.g., rifampin, phenobarbital, St. John's wort).
- Because they lack estrogen, progestin-only OCs are safer than combination OCs—but are less effective and cause more menstrual irregularity.
- Progestin-only OCs prevent pregnancy by causing production of thick, sticky mucus (which creates a barrier to migration of sperm) and by suppressing endometrial growth (which discourages nidation).
- Subdermal etonogestrel implants [Nexplanon] are active for 3 years and are among the most effective contraceptives available.
- Nexplanon has the same mechanism as progestin-only pills: production of thick, sticky mucus and involution of the endometrium.
- Injectable medroxyprogesterone acetate [Depo-Provera] is active for 3 months and is one of the most effective contraceptives available.
- Depo-Provera prevents pregnancy mainly by suppressing ovulation. In addition, it thickens cervical mucus and alters the endometrium such that nidation is discouraged.

Please visit **http://evolve.elsevier.com/Lehne** for chapter-specific NCLEX® examination review questions.

Summary of Major Nursing Implications[a]

COMBINATION ORAL CONTRACEPTIVES

Preadministration Assessment

Therapeutic Goal

Prevention of unwanted pregnancy.

Baseline Data

Assess for a history of hypertension, diabetes, thrombophlebitis, thromboembolic disorders, cerebrovascular disease, coronary artery disease, breast carcinoma, estrogen-dependent neoplasm, and benign or malignant liver tumors.

Identifying High-Risk Patients

Absolute contraindications to OC use are thromboembolic disorders, cerebrovascular disease, coronary occlusion, abnormal liver function, known or suspected breast carcinoma, undiagnosed abnormal genital bleeding, known or suspected pregnancy, and smokers older than 35. *Relative contraindications* are diabetes, hypertension, cardiac disease, history of cholestatic jaundice of pregnancy, gallbladder disease, uterine leiomyoma, epilepsy, and migraine.

Women anticipating elective surgery in which postoperative immobilization increases the risk of thrombosis should stop OCs before surgery.

Implementation: Administration

Dosing Schedule

Provide the patient with the following dosing instructions:

- Initiate dosing on the first day of menses, or the first Sunday after the onset of menses.
- For most combination OCs, the approved dosing schedule consists of 21 days of active drug followed by 7 days off (for the 7 "off" days, the manufacturer may provide inert tablets, iron-containing tablets, or no tablets).
- For all OCs, take pills at the same time each day (e.g., with a meal, at bedtime).

Responding to Missed Doses

For women using a 28-day-cycle combination OC—except *Natazia*—provide the following instructions regarding missed doses:

- If *1 or more pills* are missed in the *first week*, take 1 pill as soon as possible and then continue with the pack. Use an additional form of contraception for 7 days.
- If *1 or 2 pills* are missed during the *second* or *third week*, take 1 pill as soon as possible and then continue with the active pills in the pack—but skip the placebo pills and go straight to a new pack once all the active pills have been taken.
- If *3 or more pills* are missed during the *second* or *third week*, follow the same instructions given for missing 1 or 2 pills, but use an additional form of contraception for 7 days.

Note: The response to a missed dose of Natazia is more complex than with other combination OCs. Consult the package insert for details.

Inform women using an *extended-cycle* or *continuous* OC that once the pills have been taken daily for at least 3 weeks, up to 7 days can be missed with little or no increased risk of pregnancy.

Postpartum Use

Inform the patient that OCs can be initiated 2 weeks after delivery if breast-feeding is not intended. (For breast-feeding

Summary of Major Nursing Implications[a]—cont'd

patients, the progestin-only minipill can be started immediately postpartum.)

Promoting Adherence

Counsel the patient about the importance of taking OCs as prescribed. Encourage the patient to read the package insert provided with combination OCs.

Ongoing Evaluation and Interventions

Minimizing Adverse Effects

Thrombotic Disorders. Combination OCs slightly increase the risk of thrombosis and thromboembolism. To minimize the risk of a thrombotic event, (1) use OCs of low estrogen content, (2) avoid OCs that contain drospirenone or desogestrel, (3) avoid OCs in women with known risk factors for thrombotic disorders, and (4) discontinue OCs at least 4 weeks before elective surgery in which postoperative thrombosis might be expected. Inform the patient about symptoms of thrombosis and thromboembolism (e.g., leg tenderness or pain, sudden chest pain, shortness of breath, severe headache, sudden visual disturbance), and instruct her to notify the prescriber if these develop.

Hypertension. Perform periodic determinations of blood pressure. If hypertension is detected, discontinue OCs. Blood pressure usually normalizes. However, for women with chronic hypertension, OCs can be used as long as the blood pressure is normal.

Abnormal Uterine Bleeding. During initial use, combination OCs may cause breakthrough bleeding or spotting. This usually resolves with continued use. Bleeding is less likely with low-estrogen OCs.

Instruct the patient to notify the prescriber if two consecutive periods are missed; the possibility of pregnancy must be evaluated.

Instruct the patient to notify the prescriber if bleeding irregularities persist; an alternative OC may be tried.

Inform the patient that once OCs are discontinued, menses quickly return to normal.

Use in Pregnancy and Lactation. OCs are contraindicated during pregnancy, not because they are dangerous, but because they have no therapeutic role. Pregnancy should be ruled out before OC use. Instruct the patient to discontinue OC use if accidental pregnancy should occur.

Inform the patient that OCs can reduce milk production early in lactation. Once the milk supply is established, OC use can be resumed.

Stroke in Women With Migraine. When used by women with migraine, OCs may increase the risk of thrombotic stroke. To minimize risk, OCs should be reserved for migraineurs who are under age 35, don't smoke, are generally healthy, and have migraine without aura.

Hyperkalemia. Combination OCs that contain *drospirenone* (e.g., YAZ) pose a risk of hyperkalemia and hence should not be used by (1) women with conditions that predispose to hyperkalemia (e.g., renal insufficiency, adrenal insufficiency, liver disease) or by (2) women taking drugs that can increase potassium levels (see *Drugs That Elevate Potassium,* later).

Minimizing Adverse Interactions

Agents That Reduce OC Levels. Levels of OCs can be reduced by agents that induce hepatic drug-metabolizing enzymes (e.g., phenobarbital, phenytoin, troglitazone, rifampin, ritonavir, St. John's wort). Advise women who are taking these agents to be alert for indications of reduced OC levels (e.g., breakthrough bleeding, spotting) and to notify the prescriber if these occur. An increase in OC dosage or the use of an alternative method of birth control may be required.

Drugs Whose Effects Are Reduced by OCs. OCs can reduce the effects of some drugs, including *warfarin, insulin,* and some *oral hypoglycemics.* When combined with OCs, these drugs may require a greater-than-normal dosage.

Drugs Whose Effects Are Increased by OCs. OCs can increase blood levels of several drugs, including *theophylline* and *imipramine.* Women using these drugs in combination with OCs should be alert for signs of toxicity; dosage reduction for theophylline or imipramine may be required.

Drugs That Elevate Potassium. Drugs that elevate serum potassium (e.g., potassium supplements, potassium-sparing diuretics, angiotensin-converting enzyme inhibitors, and angiotensin receptor blockers) should be avoided by women using OCs that contain *drospirenone,* which promotes potassium retention.

PROGESTIN-ONLY ORAL CONTRACEPTIVES

Preadministration Assessment

Therapeutic Goal

Prevention of unwanted pregnancy.

Implementation: Administration

Dosing Schedule

Instruct the patient to initiate the minipill on day 1 of the menstrual cycle and to take 1 pill every day thereafter. Pills should be taken at the same time each day (e.g., with a meal, at bedtime).

Responding to Missed Doses

Provide the patient with the following instructions regarding missed doses:

- If 1 pill is missed, take it as soon as the omission is remembered. Use a backup form of contraception for 2 days.
- If 2 pills are missed, take 2 pills as soon as the omission is remembered, and use a backup form of contraception for 2 days.
- If 3 pills are missed, the minipill should be stopped. Do not resume use until menstruation occurs or until pregnancy has been ruled out.

Ongoing Evaluation and Interventions

Minimizing Adverse Effects

Menstrual Irregularities. Breakthrough bleeding, spotting, amenorrhea, inconsistent cycle length, and variations in the amount and duration of monthly flow are common and unavoidable. Forewarn the patient of these effects.

[a]Patient education information is highlighted as **blue text.**

CHAPTER

63 Drug Therapy for Infertility

Infertility (subfertility) is defined as a decrease in the ability to reproduce. This contrasts with sterility, which is the complete absence of reproductive ability. About 10% of couples attempting to have children experience infertility. Failure to conceive may be due to reproductive dysfunction of the male partner, the female partner, or both. When medical treatment is implemented, approximately one-half of infertile couples achieve pregnancy. So far, drug therapy of female infertility has been considerably more successful than drug therapy of male infertility.

In treating infertility, the chances of success are greatly enhanced by accurate diagnosis. A thorough history of both partners is essential, including information on frequency and timing of coitus and the use of drugs that might lower fertility. Routine evaluation should include a semen analysis, determination of fallopian tube patency, and assessment of ovulation. If the patient reports regular menstrual cycles, ovulation is presumed, and hence there is no need to determine estrogen and progesterone levels.

In this chapter, we discuss infertility in two stages. First, we discuss the underlying causes of reproductive dysfunction. Second, we discuss the fertility-promoting drugs. As preparation to study these agents, you should review Chapter 61 for information on the menstrual cycle and information on the biosynthesis and physiologic and pharmacologic effects of estrogens and progestins. Pay special attention to the roles of gonadotropin-releasing hormone (GnRH), luteinizing hormone (LH), and follicle-stimulating hormone (FSH).

INFERTILITY: CAUSES AND TREATMENT STRATEGIES

Female Infertility

Female infertility can result from dysfunction in all phases of the reproductive process. The most critical phases are follicular maturation, ovulation, transport of the ovum through the fallopian tubes, fertilization of the ovum, nidation (implantation), and growth and development of the conceptus. These events can take place only if the ovaries, uterus, hypothalamus, and pituitary are functioning properly. If the activity of any of these structures is disturbed, fertility can be impaired.

Anovulation and Failure of Follicular Maturation

In the absence of adequate hormonal stimulation, ovarian follicles will not ripen and ovulation will not take place. Frequently, these causes of infertility can be corrected with drugs. The agents used to promote follicular maturation and/or ovulation are *clomiphene, menotropins, follitropins* (e.g., urofollitropin), and *human chorionic gonadotropin* (hCG). Clomiphene induces follicular maturation and ovulation by promoting release of FSH and LH from the pituitary gland; in some cases, induction of ovulation requires co-treatment with hCG. Menotropins and follitropins are used in conjunction with hCG: Menotropins and follitropins act directly on the ovary to promote follicular development; after follicles have matured, hCG is given to induce ovulation. Because hCG acts on mature follicles to cause ovulation, the drug is used only after follicular maturation has been induced with another agent (menotropins, a follitropin, or clomiphene). The pharmacology of clomiphene, menotropins, follitropins, and hCG is discussed later in this chapter.

Unfavorable Cervical Mucus

In the periovulatory period, the cervical glands normally secrete large volumes of thin, watery mucus. These secretions, which are produced under the influence of estrogen, facilitate passage of sperm through the cervical canal. If the cervical mucus is scant or of inappropriate consistency (thick, sticky), sperm will be unable to pass through to the uterus. Production of unfavorable mucus may occur spontaneously or as a side effect of clomiphene.

Cervical mucus can be restored to its proper volume and consistency by administering estrogen. Two regimens have been employed. In one, ethinyl estradiol is given beginning early in the menstrual cycle (on day 6, 7, or 8) and continued through day 12 or 13; dosages range from 20 to 80 mcg/day. In the other regimen, conjugated estrogens are administered from day 5 through day 15 of the cycle; dosages range from 2.5 to 5 mg/day. When used to counteract the effects of clomiphene on the cervical mucus, estrogens are administered for 10 days beginning 1 day after the last clomiphene dose.

Hyperprolactinemia

Elevation of prolactin levels may be caused by a pituitary adenoma or by disturbed regulation of the healthy pituitary gland. Amenorrhea, galactorrhea, and infertility may all occur in association with excessive prolactin. The mechanism by which hyperprolactinemia impairs fertility is unknown. Hyperprolactinemia can be treated with *cabergoline, bromocriptine,* and other dopamine agonists.

Endometriosis

Endometriosis is a condition in which endometrial tissue has become implanted outside the uterus, usually on the ovaries, pelvic peritoneum, or rectovaginal septum. These endometrial implants respond to hormonal stimulation in much the same way as the normally situated endometrium. Endometriosis is a common cause of infertility. When pregnancies do occur, the rate of spontaneous abortion is high (about 50%).

The mechanism by which endometriosis reduces fertility is not always clear. In some cases, infertility results from ovarian or tubal adhesions that impede transport of the ovum. However, when endometriosis is mild, a visible cause of infertility may be absent.

Endometriosis can be treated with surgery, drugs, or both. Surgery reduces symptoms of endometriosis *and* increases fertility. In contrast, although drugs can reduce discomfort, they do *not* enhance fertility. First-line agents for pain relief are *nonsteroidal anti-inflammatory drugs* (NSAIDs) and *combination oral contraceptives. Gonadotropin-releasing hormone agonists*—goserelin, leuprolide, and nafarelin—are also effective, but can't be used long term, owing to side effects, especially osteoporosis and hot flashes.

Polycystic Ovary Syndrome

Polycystic ovary syndrome (PCOS) is a combined endocrine-metabolic disorder characterized by androgen excess and insulin resistance. Symptoms include irregular periods, anovulation, infertility, acne, and hirsutism. About 50% of patients are obese. PCOS increases the risk for diabetes, hyperlipidemia, hypertension, and cancer of the ovaries and endometrium. The syndrome was first described in a woman whose ovaries were enlarged and covered with multiple fluid-filled cysts—thus the name of the condition. However, the presence of cysts is not required for a positive diagnosis. PCOS is the most common endocrine disorder in young women, affecting 5% to 7% of women of reproductive age.

PCOS can be treated with lifestyle changes and drugs. The goal is to restore regular menstruation and ovulation, to reverse hyperandrogenism (eliminating acne and hirsutism), and to decrease the long-term risk for diabetes, cancer, and heart disease. Treatment options include the following:

- *Weight loss* can reduce insulin and androgen levels, improve insulin sensitivity, restore menstruation and ovulation, and increase pregnancy rates.
- *Clomiphene* [Clomid, Serophene] is considered a first-line drug for inducing ovulation. It may be used alone or in combination with metformin.
- *Metformin* [Glucophage, others], a drug for type 2 diabetes, increases insulin sensitivity and decreases insulin levels, which, through an indirect mechanism, lowers androgen levels. The net result is improved glucose tolerance, improved ovulation, and increased pregnancy rates.
- *Pioglitazone* [Actos], another drug for type 2 diabetes, acts like metformin, causing an increase in insulin sensitivity and a decrease in insulin levels and androgen levels. However, pioglitazone can harm the fetus, and hence should not be used by women trying to become pregnant.
- *Oral contraceptives* can restore regular periods and reduce acne and hirsutism, but obviously won't improve fertility.
- *Spironolactone* has antiandrogenic actions and can thereby decrease hirsutism and acne. The drug can harm the fetus and therefore must not be used during pregnancy.

Male Infertility

For about 50% of infertile couples, failure to conceive is due to reproductive dysfunction in the male. The most common cause is decreased density or motility of sperm, or semen of abnormal volume or quality. Erectile dysfunction (ED) is another contributing factor. In most cases, infertility in males is not associated with an identifiable endocrine disorder. Unfortunately, with the exception of ED, male infertility is generally unresponsive to drugs.

Hypogonadotropic Hypogonadism

A few males may be incapable of spermatogenesis owing to insufficient gonadotropin secretion. In these rare cases, drugs may help. If the gonadotropin deficiency is only partial, sperm counts can be increased using hCG (alone or in combination with menotropins). If the deficiency is severe, treatment with androgens is required (see Chapter 65). If therapy with hCG and menotropins is intended, the patient should be informed that treatment will be both prolonged (3 to 4 years) and expensive.

Erectile Dysfunction

Inability to achieve erection can cause male infertility. Sildenafil [Viagra] and other drugs for ED are discussed in Chapter 66.

Idiopathic Male Infertility

Idiopathic infertility is defined as infertility for which no cause can be identified. About 25% to 40% of male infertility is idiopathic. Since the cause is unknown, targeted drug therapy is impossible. Accordingly, treatment is empiric (trial and error). Several drugs, including androgens and hCG, have been administered in the hope of improving idiopathic infertility in males. However, success is rare.

DRUGS USED TO TREAT FEMALE INFERTILITY

Drugs for Controlled Ovarian Stimulation

The term *controlled ovarian stimulation* refers to the use of drugs to facilitate follicular maturation and ovulation. Following ovulation, fertilization can be accomplished either naturally (through sexual intercourse) or through assisted reproductive technology (e.g., *in vitro* fertilization). Of the drugs used for ovarian stimulation, six are used to promote follicular maturation, two are used to stimulate ovulation, and two are used to prevent premature stimulation of ovulation by endogenous hormones (Table 63.1).

Clomiphene

Therapeutic Use. Clomiphene [Clomid, Serophene] is used to promote follicular maturation and ovulation in selected infertile women.

Mechanism of Fertility Promotion. Clomiphene blocks receptors for estrogen. Receptor blockade in the hypothalamus and pituitary makes it appear to these structures that estrogen

TABLE 63.1 ■ Drugs for Controlled Ovarian Stimulation

Generic Name	Brand Name	Mechanism of Action
DRUGS THAT PROMOTE FOLLICULAR MATURATION		
Clomiphene	Clomid, Serophene	Clomiphene blocks estrogen receptors in the hypothalamus and pituitary, and thereby causes a compensatory increase in the release of LH and FSH, which then act on the ovary to promote follicular maturation (and possibly ovulation).
Menotropins	Repronex ♣, Menopur	Menotropins is a 50:50 mixture of FSH and LH that acts on the ovary to promote follicular maturation. Treatment is followed by hCG to induce ovulation.
Follitropins		Follitropins are preparations of FSH that act on the ovary to promote follicular maturation. Treatment is followed by hCG to induce ovulation.
Follitropin alfa	Gonal-f, Gonal-f RFF	
Follitropin beta	Follistim AQ, Puregon ♣	
Urofollitropin	Bravelle	
Lutropin alfa	Generic only	Lutropin alfa is a recombinant form of LH used in combination with follitropin alfa [Gonal-f, Gonal-f RFF] to promote follicular maturation. Treatment is followed by hCG to induce ovulation.
DRUGS THAT STIMULATE OVULATION		
Human chorionic gonadotropin (hCG)	Novarel, Pregnyl	hCG is similar in structure and identical in action to LH. The drug acts on the ovary to induce ovulation.
Choriogonadotropin alfa	Ovidrel	Choriogonadotropin is a recombinant form of hCG that acts on the ovary to induce ovulation.
DRUGS THAT PREVENT PREMATURE OVULATION		
Ganirelix Cetrorelix	Generic only Cetrotide	These drugs are GnRH antagonists that block endogenous release of LH and thereby prevent possible premature ovulation in women receiving drugs to promote follicular maturation.

levels are low. In response, the pituitary increases secretion of gonadotropins (LH and FSH), and these hormones then stimulate the ovary, promoting follicular maturation and ovulation. In properly selected patients, the ovulation rate is about 90%. Because of its mechanism of action, clomiphene can induce ovulation only if the pituitary is capable of producing LH and FSH, and only if the ovaries are capable of responding. Success is impossible in women with primary pituitary or ovarian failure. Accordingly, pituitary and ovarian function should be verified before clomiphene therapy. If treatment produces follicular maturation but ovulation fails to occur, it may be possible to induce ovulation by adding hCG to the regimen.

Monitoring. Effects on the ovary can be monitored with serial ultrasound examinations. When treatment is successful, the scans will show progressive follicular enlargement, followed by conversion of the follicle to a corpus luteum after ovulation occurs.

Adverse Effects. Common side effects include hot flashes (similar to the vasomotor responses of menopause), nausea, abdominal discomfort, bloating, and breast engorgement. Some patients experience visual disturbances (blurred vision, visual flashes), which usually reverse following drug withdrawal. Multiple births (usually twins) occur in 8% to 10% of clomiphene-facilitated pregnancies. Patients should be told of this possibility.

Very rarely, clomiphene can cause ovarian hyperstimulation. Symptoms include low abdominal pain, pressure, weight gain, and swelling. Hyperstimulation can be minimized by avoiding unnecessarily large doses. If undue ovarian enlargement occurs, clomiphene use should cease. The ovaries will then regress to normal size.

Some actions of clomiphene may *interfere* with conception. Luteal-phase defect may be induced, but can be corrected by giving progesterone. Because it has antiestrogenic actions, clomiphene may force the production of scant and viscous cervical mucus; estrogen therapy can render cervical secretions more hospitable to sperm.

Preparations, Dosage, and Administration. Clomiphene [Clomid, Serophene] is supplied in 50-mg oral tablets. The initial course of treatment consists of 50 mg once daily for 5 days. If cyclic menstrual bleeding has been occurring, therapy should begin on the fifth day after the onset of menses. If menstruation has been absent, dosing can start any time (assuming pregnancy has been ruled out). If the first course of treatment fails to induce ovulation, a second 5-day course (using 100 mg/day) may be tried. The second course may begin as early as 30 days after the previous one. Doses may be increased in subsequent courses. However, doses above 100 mg/day are rarely needed. Once a dose that induces ovulation has been established, that dose should be used for a maximum of three cycles. If pregnancy has not occurred, further treatment is unlikely to succeed. When ovulation does occur, it is usually within 5 to 10 days after the last clomiphene dose; patients should be instructed to have coitus at least every other day during this interval.

Hazardous Drugs and Special Administration Requirements. In 2016 the National Institute for Occupational Safety and Health (NIOSH) expanded the list of drugs identified as hazardous. (See https://www.cdc.gov/niosh/docs/2016-161/pdfs/2016-161.pdf.) Clomiphene is included on that list. NIOSH requires special handling of drugs identified as hazardous. The Safety Alert box that follows lists all the hazardous drugs in this chapter. See Chapter 3, Table 3.1, for administration and handling guidelines.

Safety Alert

HAZARDOUS DRUGS REQUIRING SPECIAL HANDLING

Cabergoline	Human chorionic gonadotropin
Cetrorelix	Menotropins
Clomiphene	
Ganirelix	

PATIENT-CENTERED CARE ACROSS THE LIFE SPAN

Infertility Drugs

Life Stage	Patient Care Concerns
Children	Drugs for infertility are inappropriate for prepubertal children. In males, hCG may be prescribed for prepubertal cryptorchidism; however, this may cause precocious puberty.
Pregnant women	Infertility drugs are not indicated for women who are already pregnant. Clomiphene, cetrorelix, ganirelix, follitropins, human chorionic gonadotropin, choriogonadotropin alfa, and menotropins are Pregnancy Risk Category X.[a] Animal and/or human developmental abnormalities and abortions have occurred. Bromocriptine and cabergoline are Pregnancy Risk Category B.[a]
Breast-feeding women	Bromocriptine, cabergoline, and clomiphene may decrease milk production. Breast-feeding is contraindicated when taking lutropin alfa, follitropins, and cetrorelix. Manufacturers recommend caution when taking clomiphene and hCG. While FDA labeling does not contraindicate breast-feeding by women taking menotropins and ganirelix, the manufacturer does not recommend it. As with all drugs, benefits should be weighed against risks.
Older adults	Infertility drugs are not typically recommended for older patients; however, there are no age-related contraindications.

[a]As of 2020, the FDA will no longer use Pregnancy Risk Categories. Please refer to Chapter 9 for more information.

Menotropins

Menotropins [Repronex ♣, Menopur]—also known as human menopausal gonadotropin, or hMG—consists of equal amounts of LH and FSH activity. Commercial menotropins is prepared by extraction from the urine of postmenopausal women.

Therapeutic Actions and Uses

Anovulatory Women. Menotropins, in conjunction with hCG, is used to promote follicular maturation and ovulation in anovulatory patients. Menotropins acts directly on the ovaries to cause maturation of follicles. Once follicles have ripened, hCG is given to induce ovulation.

Menotropins is employed when gonadotropin secretion by the pituitary is insufficient to provide adequate ovarian stimulation. Candidates must have ovaries capable of responding to FSH and LH; menotropins is of no help in women with primary ovarian failure. Among properly selected patients, the rate of ovulation approaches 100%. It should be noted that menotropins is very expensive.

Ovulatory Women. Menotropins can be used to induce the development of multiple follicles in ovulatory women participating in an *in vitro* fertilization program.

Men. Menotropins has been used off-label to promote spermatogenesis in males with primary or secondary hypogonadotropic hypogonadism.

Adverse Effects. The most serious adverse response is *ovarian hyperstimulation syndrome,* a condition characterized by sudden enlargement of the ovaries. Mild to moderate ovarian enlargement is common, occurring in about 20% of patients. This condition is benign and resolves spontaneously after discontinuing drug use. Of greater concern is ovarian enlargement that occurs rapidly and that may be accompanied by ascites, pleural effusion, and considerable pain. If this manifestation of ovarian stimulation occurs, menotropins should be withdrawn and the patient hospitalized. Treatment is usually supportive (bed rest, analgesics, fluid and electrolyte replacement). Paracentesis can be used to remove some excess ascitic fluid. If rupture of ovarian cysts occurs, surgery may be required to stop bleeding. Enlargement of the ovaries is most likely during the first 2 weeks of treatment. To ensure early detection, the patient should be examined at least every other day while taking menotropins and for 2 weeks after stopping. Ovarian stimulation can be minimized by keeping the dosage as low as possible.

Pregnancies facilitated by menotropins often result in *multiple births:* 15% of pregnancies result in twins, and 5% of pregnancies result in three or more babies.

Monitoring Therapy. Ovarian responses to menotropins must be monitored to determine timing of hCG administration and to minimize the risk for ovarian enlargement. Responses can be monitored by ultrasonography of the developing follicles and by measuring serum estrogen. When ultrasonography indicates that follicles have enlarged to 16 to 20 mm and when serum estrogen is 200 pg/mL per maturing follicle, then menotropins administration should cease and hCG should be injected.

Preparations, Dosage, and Administration. Menotropins [Repronex ♣, Menopur] is supplied as a powder or pellet to be reconstituted immediately before use. Ampules of menotropins contain 75 international units (IU) of FSH activity plus 75 IU of LH activity. Repronex ♣ is administered subQ or IM; Menopur is administered subQ.

Menotropins is used sequentially with hCG: After follicular maturation has been induced with menotropins, hCG is injected to promote ovulation. For the initial cycle, the contents of 1 menotropins ampule are injected daily for 9 to 12 days. When estrogen measurements indicate follicular maturation has occurred, menotropins is discontinued; hCG (5000 to 10,000 USP units) is injected 24 hours after the last menotropins dose. Ovulation occurs 2 to 3 days after injecting hCG. Accordingly, patients should be instructed to have intercourse on the evening before hCG injection and on the following 2 to 3 days. If there is evidence of ovulation but conception does not take place, treatment should be repeated for two more courses using the same menotropins dosage. If treatment remains ineffective, two additional courses may be tried, using twice as much menotropins as previously. If there is still no conception, further treatment is unlikely to help.

Follitropins

Description. Three follitropins are available: *urofollitropin* [Bravelle], *follitropin alfa* [Gonal-f, Gonal-f RFF], and *follitropin beta* [Follistim AQ, Puregon ♣]. All three are preparations of FSH. Urofollitropin is a highly purified preparation of FSH extracted from the urine of postmenopausal women. Follitropin alfa and follitropin beta are produced by recombinant DNA technology. A long-acting preparation—*corifollitropin alfa* [Elonva]—is available in Europe, but not in the United States or Canada.

Use in Women. The actions, uses, and adverse effects of the follitropins are much like those of menotropins (a 50:50 mixture of FSH and LH). Like menotropins, the follitropins act directly on the ovary to stimulate follicle maturation. All three follitropins are employed to stimulate ovulation in anovulatory women and to promote production of multiple follicles in ovulatory women participating in an *in vitro* fertilization program. For both indications, the follitropins are used sequentially with hCG: The follitropin is given first to promote follicle maturation; then hCG is given to stimulate ovulation. As with menotropins, multiple births are relatively common. The principal adverse effect of the follitropins is ovarian hyperstimulation syndrome. All of the follitropins are administered subQ; follitropin beta may also be given IM.

Use in Men. Both *follitropin alfa* and *follitropin beta* are approved for promoting spermatogenesis in males with primary or secondary hypogonadotropic hypogonadism.

Lutropin Alfa

Lutropin alfa is a recombinant form of LH. The drug is approved for combined use with follitropin alfa [Gonal-f] to promote follicular maturation in infertile, hypogonadotropic, hypogonadal women with profound LH deficiency. Following treatment with lutropin alfa/follitropin alfa, hCG is injected to induce ovulation. Adverse effects of the combination include headache, abdominal pain, nausea, breast pain, ovarian enlargement, and ovarian hyperstimulation syndrome.

Prototype Drugs

DRUGS FOR INFERTILITY

Drugs for Controlled Ovarian Stimulation
Clomiphene
Menotropins
Human chorionic gonadotropin

Drugs for Hyperprolactinemia
Cabergoline (dopamine agonist)

Human Chorionic Gonadotropin

Human chorionic gonadotropin (hCG) is a polypeptide hormone produced by the placenta. hCG is similar in structure and identical in action to LH.

Therapeutic Use. hCG is used to promote follicular maturation and ovulation in women who are infertile because of ovulatory failure. The drug causes ovulation by simulating the midcycle LH surge. When hCG is used to promote ovulation, follicular maturation must first be induced with another agent, usually menotropins. hCG can also be used in conjunction with clomiphene when treatment with clomiphene alone has failed to produce ovulation.

In men, hCG may be administered until adequate serum testosterone levels are achieved. (This may take as long as 2 to 3 months.) Once testosterone levels are within a normal range, follitropin alfa or hMG may be added to induce spermatogenesis.

Adverse Effects. The most severe adverse response to hCG in women is *ovarian hyperstimulation syndrome.* If this occurs, hospitalization and discontinuation of hCG are indicated. hCG may also provoke *rupture of ovarian cysts* with resultant bleeding into the peritoneal cavity. Additional adverse effects include edema, injection-site pain, and central nervous system disturbances (headache, irritability, restlessness, fatigue).

Preparations, Dosage, and Administration. Commercial hCG [Novarel, Pregnyl] is prepared by extraction from the urine of pregnant women. hCG is supplied as a powder that must be reconstituted for use. Administration is by IM injection. The usual dose for induction of ovulation is 5000 to 10,000 USP units.

Before hCG is given, follicular maturation must be induced with another agent (clomiphene, menotropins, or a follitropin). When used in conjunction with clomiphene, hCG is administered 7 to 9 days after the last clomiphene dose. When used in conjunction with menotropins or a follitropin, hCG is injected 1 day after the last menotropins or follitropin dose.

Choriogonadotropin Alfa

Choriogonadotropin alfa [Ovidrel] is a form of hCG produced by recombinant DNA technology. The drug's physicochemical, immunologic, and biologic activities are equivalent to those of naturally occurring hCG, produced by extraction from the urine of pregnant women. However, unlike urine-derived hCG, which must be injected IM, choriogonadotropin alfa is injected subQ. As a result, administration is more comfortable. (IM injections can be painful.) Choriogonadotropin alfa has two indications. First, like natural hCG, the drug is given to *trigger ovulation* in women who are infertile owing to anovulation. Second, the drug is used to *promote late follicular maturation and early luteinization* in women undergoing assisted reproductive technology (e.g., *in vitro* fertilization). For both indications, follicular maturation must first be induced with a follicle-stimulating agent (e.g., menotropins). Choriogonadotropin alfa (250 mcg) is then given as a single subQ injection 1 day after the last dose of the follicle-stimulating agent. Major adverse effects are the same as those of natural hCG: ovarian hyperstimulation syndrome, rupture of ovarian cysts, and multiple births.

Gonadotropin-Releasing Hormone Antagonists

GnRH antagonists are used to prevent a premature surge of endogenous LH in women undergoing controlled ovarian stimulation (with menotropins or follitropin [FSH]). As discussed earlier, after follicles have matured under the influence of exogenous menotropins or FSH, the patient is given an injection of hCG (LH) to cause ovulation. However, in some women, the natural midcycle LH surge occurs early, causing ovulation before the eggs have fully matured. As a result, the chances of successful conception and implantation are reduced. The GnRH antagonists prevent premature LH release and thereby eliminate the chance of premature ovulation.

Two GnRH antagonists are available: *ganirelix* (generic only) and *cetrorelix* [Cetrotide]. Both drugs block GnRH receptors and thereby prevent GnRH from promoting the production and release of LH from the pituitary. Various dosing schedules are employed. One option for either drug is to give 250 mcg subQ daily, beginning in the early follicular phase and continuing until the day of hCG administration. Injections are made by the patient into the upper thigh or the region around the navel.

Dopamine Agonists for Hyperprolactinemia

Two dopamine agonists—cabergoline and bromocriptine—are approved for hyperprolactinemia. Both drugs are derivatives of ergot, an alkaloid found in plants. Cabergoline is better tolerated than bromocriptine, and dosing is more convenient. Accordingly, cabergoline is preferred.

Cabergoline

Therapeutic Use. Cabergoline is used to correct amenorrhea and infertility associated with excessive prolactin secretion. If galactorrhea is present, this consequence of hyperprolactinemia may also be corrected. When the source of excessive prolactin is a pituitary adenoma, cabergoline can induce tumor regression. Effects on prolactin begin within hours of dosing and persist about 14 days. To monitor treatment, prolactin should be measured monthly until the level is normal (below 20 pg/mL).

In addition to its use in hyperprolactinemia, cabergoline is used in Parkinson disease, although the drug is not approved for this disorder.

Mechanism of Fertility Promotion. Cabergoline is a dopamine receptor agonist. By activating dopamine receptors in the anterior pituitary, cabergoline inhibits prolactin secretion. The result is normalization of the menstrual cycle and a return of fertility. The mechanism by which reducing prolactin levels leads to a return of ovulation is unknown.

Pharmacokinetics. Administration is oral, and absorption is not affected by food. Plasma levels peak 2 to 3 hours after dosing, but absolute bioavailability is unknown. Cabergoline undergoes extensive hepatic metabolism followed by excretion in the urine and feces. It has a long elimination half-life of about 65 hours. In patients with severe hepatic impairment, cabergoline levels may rise.

Adverse Effects. The most common adverse effects are nausea, headache, and dizziness. Orthostatic hypotension may occur, but is rare at recommended doses. Adverse effects can be minimized by initiating treatment at low doses. Like other ergot derivatives, cabergoline may pose a risk for valvular heart damage.

Preparations, Dosage, and Administration. Cabergoline is supplied in 0.5-mg tablets. The initial dosage is 0.25 mg twice a week, administered with or without food. Dosage may be increased in 0.25-mg increments to a maximum of 1 mg twice a week. At least 4 weeks should separate each rise in dosage. After prolactin has been maintained at a normal level for at least 6 months, treatment can stop.

Bromocriptine

Actions and Therapeutic Uses. Like cabergoline, bromocriptine [Parlodel] activates dopamine receptors in the pituitary and can thereby reduce prolactin secretion. As a result, it can correct amenorrhea, galactorrhea, and infertility. If hyperprolactinemia is caused by a pituitary adenoma, bromocriptine can induce regression of the tumor (in addition to reducing prolactin secretion). Continuous treatment can suppress tumor growth for years. Bromocriptine is also used in Parkinson disease (see Chapter 21).

Adverse Effects. When bromocriptine is used for infertility, adverse effects are frequent but usually mild. Nausea occurs in about half of patients. Headache, dizziness, fatigue, and abdominal cramps are also common. Orthostatic hypotension may occur, but is rare at the doses employed. Teratogenic effects have not been reported. Adverse effects can be minimized by taking bromocriptine with meals and initiating treatment at low doses. Like cabergoline and other ergot derivatives, bromocriptine may pose a risk for valvular heart injury.

Preparations, Dosage, and Administration. Bromocriptine mesylate is supplied in 2.5-mg tablets and 5-mg capsules. Dosing is begun at 1.25 to 2.5 mg once a day and then gradually increased by 2.5 mg every 2 to 7 days until an optimal response is achieved. The typical dosage range is 2.5 to 15 mg a day. All doses should be administered with food. Normalization of the menstrual cycle may occur rapidly (within a few days); however, some women may require up to 2 months of treatment. As soon as pregnancy is achieved, use of bromocriptine should cease. As a rule, administration should not resume until after delivery. If treatment is not reinstated, hypersecretion of prolactin is almost certain to recur within a year.

Drugs for Endometriosis

As noted previously, the first-line drugs for pain of endometriosis are NSAIDs (e.g., ibuprofen) and combination oral contraceptives, usually taken cyclically. The NSAIDs are discussed in Chapter 71. The oral contraceptives are discussed in Chapter 62. The drugs discussed in the sections that follow—GnRH agonists and danazol—cause regression of endometrial implants. Both are considered second- or third-line treatments.

GnRH Agonists

Leuprolide, nafarelin, and goserelin are synthetic analogs of GnRH. These drugs are used to relieve pain of endometriosis. However, although they can reduce symptoms, they do not increase fertility. Although women are unlikely to become pregnant while taking these drugs, precautions to avoid pregnancy are still advised.

Leuprolide

Therapeutic Uses. Leuprolide [Lupron Depot, Eligard] is a GnRH analog with several approved uses. In addition to endometriosis, the drug is indicated for uterine fibroids, central precocious puberty, and advanced prostate cancer (see Chapter 103). Discussion here is limited to treatment of endometriosis.

Mechanism of Action. Like the normal endometrium, ectopic endometrial implants are dependent on ovarian hormones. Leuprolide suppresses endometriosis by indirectly suppressing ovarian hormone production. *Initial* doses actually increase hormone production because leuprolide, like endogenous GnRH, acts on the pituitary to promote release of FSH and LH, which in turn act on the ovary to stimulate hormone production. However, in contrast to endogenous GnRH, which has a short half-life and is released in a *pulsatile* fashion, leuprolide has a long half-life and blood levels remain steady. As a result, leuprolide causes continuous activation of pituitary GnRH receptors, which has the paradoxical effect of *suppressing* FSH and LH release, depriving the ovary of the stimulation needed for hormone production. By decreasing production of ovarian hormones, the drug reduces the area of endometriosis and improves symptoms. It must be stressed that leuprolide does not produce cure. Within 6 months after the drug is withdrawn, symptoms return in up to 50% of women who had previously been rendered symptom free.

Adverse Effects. Most undesired effects are secondary to estrogen deficiency. Common responses include hot flashes, vaginal dryness, decreased libido, mood changes, and headache. Nasal irritation also occurs (with administration by nasal spray). Leuprolide is teratogenic and must not be used during pregnancy.

The adverse effect of greatest concern is *bone loss*. After 3 to 6 months of treatment, bone mass and mineral content may decrease. To minimize the risk for osteoporosis, the manufacturer recommends that treatment last no more than 6 months.

Preparations, Dosage, and Administration. For treatment of endometriosis, a depot formulation is used. Dosing consists of either 3.75 mg IM once a month or 11.25 mg IM every 3 months. As noted, treatment should stop after 6 months; however, if it is necessary to continue for an additional 6 months, norethindrone should be added to the medication regimen.

Nafarelin. Like leuprolide, nafarelin [Synarel] is a GnRH analog that can reduce symptoms of endometriosis, but it does not improve fertility. Nafarelin has the same mechanism as leuprolide (suppression of LH and FSH release) as well as the same adverse effects (hot flashes, vaginal dryness, amenorrhea, headache, depression, osteoporosis). Nafarelin is supplied as a nasal spray. (The drug cannot be given orally owing to rapid degradation by GI enzymes.) The initial dosage is 200 mcg (1 spray) in the morning and evening. Doses should alternate between nostrils. Treatment should begin between days 2 and 4 of the menstrual cycle.

Goserelin

Therapeutic Uses. Goserelin [Zoladex] has several uses. In addition to reducing the pain and size of endometrial growths associated with endometriosis, it can be used to thin the endometrium in management of dysfunctional uterine bleeding. It is also approved for treatment of prostate cancer and breast cancer. Goserelin shares the same mechanism of action and adverse effects as leuprolide and nafarelin.

Preparations, Dosage, and Administration. For management of endometriosis, 3.6 mg of goserelin is administered subQ every 28 days for 6 months. Goserelin is available as implants for management of prostate cancer; these are not used for management of endometriosis.

Danazol

Therapeutic Use. Danazol [Cyclomen] can improve symptoms of endometriosis, but it does not increase fertility. Treatment leads to complete regression of endometrial implants in the majority of patients. However, implants will eventually recur after treatment stops. In addition to the therapy of endometriosis, danazol has been used to treat *angioneurotic edema* and *fibrocystic breast disease*. Since the introduction of GnRH agonists, the use of danazol for endometriosis has sharply declined. Today, the drug is given only when GnRH agonists are contraindicated.

Mechanism of Action. Danazol acts by multiple mechanisms to induce regression of endometrial implants. First, the drug inhibits several of the enzymes needed to synthesize ovarian hormones, and thereby deprives the implant of the hormonal environment it needs for maintenance. Second, danazol suppresses secretion of pituitary gonadotropins (FSH and LH), and thereby further decreases the availability of ovarian hormones. Lastly, danazol may act directly on the implant to block ovarian hormone receptors. All of these actions result in atrophy of ectopic endometrial tissue. The normal endometrium atrophies as well.

Adverse Effects and Interactions. Danazol is weakly androgenic and may induce virilization. Potential manifestations include acne, deepening of the voice, and growth of facial hair. These effects usually reverse after treatment stops. Danazol may also cause edema, and therefore should be used with caution in patients with cardiac and renal disorders. Thrombotic events, including fatal strokes, have been reported. Liver impairment may also occur, and hence liver function should be assessed at baseline and periodically thereafter. Danazol may intensify the anticoagulant effects of warfarin. Lastly, the drug can masculinize the female fetus, and hence is contraindicated during pregnancy.

Preparations, Dosage, and Administration. Danazol is supplied in capsules (50, 100, and 200 mg) for oral use. A dosage of 200 to 300 mg twice daily is usually effective. To ensure that danazol is not taken during pregnancy, therapy should be initiated at the time of menstruation. The usual course of treatment is 3 to 9 months.

KEY POINTS

- Infertility (subfertility) is a decrease in reproductive ability; sterility is a complete absence of reproductive ability.
- Infertility in a couple may result from infertility in one or both partners.
- Clomiphene is used to promote follicular maturation and ovulation.
- Clomiphene acts by blocking estrogen receptors in the hypothalamus and pituitary, causing a compensatory increase in the release of LH and FSH, which then act on the ovary to promote follicular maturation and ovulation.
- Menotropins is a 50:50 mixture of LH and FSH.
- Menotropins is used sequentially with hCG: Menotropins is given to promote follicular maturation, and then hCG is given to promote ovulation.
- The most serious adverse effect of menotropins is ovarian hyperstimulation syndrome, characterized by sudden enlargement of the ovaries.
- hCG is given to stimulate ovulation (after another agent, such as menotropins, has been given to promote follicular maturation).
- Like menotropins, hCG can cause ovarian hyperstimulation syndrome.
- Cabergoline is a dopamine agonist used to suppress excessive prolactin release.
- Three GnRH agonists—leuprolide, nafarelin, and goserelin—can promote regression of endometrial implants, but these drugs will not increase fertility.

Please visit **http://evolve.elsevier.com/Lehne** for chapter-specific NCLEX® examination review questions.

Summary of Major Nursing Implications[a]

CLOMIPHENE

The implications here apply only to the use of clomiphene for promoting maturation of ovarian follicles and ovulation.

Preadministration Assessment

Therapeutic Goal

Promotion of follicular maturation and ovulation in carefully selected patients.

Baseline Data

Take a complete health and gynecologic history, and assess for tubal patency. Ovarian and pituitary function must be confirmed. Pregnancy must be ruled out.

Identifying High-Risk Patients

Clomiphene is *contraindicated* during pregnancy and in women with liver disease or abnormal uterine bleeding of undetermined origin.

Implementation: Administration

Route

Oral.

Administration

If cyclic menstrual bleeding has been occurring, begin therapy 5 days after the onset of menses. If menstruation has been absent, begin any time.

The initial course consists of 50 mg once daily for 5 days. If ovulation fails to occur, additional courses may be tried, each beginning no sooner than 30 days after the previous course.

Implementation: Measures to Enhance Therapeutic Effects

Timing of Coitus

Advise the couple to have coitus at least every other day during the 5- to 10-day period that follows the last clomiphene dose.

Adjunctive Use of hCG

If ovulation fails to occur under the influence of clomiphene alone, injecting hCG 7 to 9 days after the last clomiphene dose may bring success.

Ongoing Evaluation and Interventions

Evaluating Therapeutic Effects

Monitor treatment with serial ultrasound examinations of the ovary. Success is indicated by progressive follicular enlargement followed by conversion of the follicle to a corpus luteum.

Minimizing Adverse Effects

Ovarian Enlargement. **Instruct the patient to notify the prescriber if pelvic pain occurs (an indication of ovarian enlargement).** If ovarian enlargement is diagnosed, clomiphene should be withdrawn, after which ovarian size usually regresses spontaneously.

Reduced Fertility. Clomiphene may cause luteal-phase defect, which can be corrected with progesterone. Alteration of cervical mucus may occur; estrogens can be used to restore the volume and fluidity of cervical secretions.

Multiple Births. **Inform the couple that multiple births (usually twins) are not uncommon in clomiphene-facilitated pregnancies.**

Visual Disturbances. **Forewarn the patient about possible visual disturbances (blurred vision, visual flashes), and instruct her to notify the prescriber if these occur.** Visual aberrations usually cease following drug withdrawal.

Other Adverse Effects. Common side effects include hot flashes (similar to the vasomotor responses of menopause), nausea, abdominal discomfort, bloating, and breast engorgement. **Inform the patient about these effects, and instruct her to notify the prescriber if they are especially disturbing.**

MENOTROPINS

The implications here refer only to the use of menotropins (together with hCG) for induction of follicular maturation and ovulation. (Menotropins is also used to treat infertility in men.)

Summary of Major Nursing Implications[a]—cont'd

Preadministration Assessment

Therapeutic Goal

Induction of follicular maturation and ovulation (in conjunction with hCG) in carefully selected patients.

Baseline Data

A thorough gynecologic and endocrinologic evaluation should precede treatment. Ovarian function must be verified. Obtain a baseline value for serum estrogen.

Identifying High-Risk Patients

Menotropins is *contraindicated* in the presence of pregnancy, primary ovarian failure, thyroid dysfunction, adrenal dysfunction, ovarian cysts, and ovarian enlargement (other than that caused by polycystic ovary syndrome).

Implementation: Administration

Route

Intramuscular.

Administration

Reconstitute powdered menotropins with sterile saline immediately before injection.

Menotropins is employed sequentially with hCG. Administer menotropins for 9 to 12 days (to promote follicular maturation). Twenty-four hours after the last dose, inject hCG. Ovulation follows in 2 to 3 days.

Ultrasonography and serum estrogen level are used to assess follicular maturation. Upon follicular maturation, menotropins is discontinued and hCG is injected.

Implementation: Measures to Enhance Therapeutic Effects

Timing of Coitus

Advise the couple to have intercourse on the evening before hCG injection and on the following 2 to 3 days (i.e., during the probable period of ovulation).

Ongoing Evaluation and Interventions

Minimizing Adverse Effects

Ovarian Hyperstimulation Syndrome. Rapid ovarian enlargement can occur, sometimes associated with pain, ascites, pleural effusion, and shortness of breath. If ovarian enlargement is excessive, discontinue menotropins and hospitalize the patient. Treatment is supportive (bed rest, analgesics, fluid and electrolyte replacement). Paracentesis can be used to remove excess ascitic fluid. If ovarian cysts rupture, surgery may be required to stop bleeding. To ensure early detection of ovarian enlargement, the patient should be examined at least every other day during menotropins use, and for 2 weeks after dosing stops.

Other Adverse Effects. **Inform the couple that multiple births are relatively common in menotropins-facilitated pregnancies.**

HUMAN CHORIONIC GONADOTROPIN

The implications here apply only to the use of hCG in the treatment of infertility in women.

Preadministration Assessment

Therapeutic Goal

Induction of ovulation in women who are infertile because of anovulation. Pretreatment with menotropins, urofollitropin, or clomiphene is required.

Implementation: Administration

Route

Intramuscular.

Administration

hCG must be used in conjunction with menotropins, a follitropin, or clomiphene. When used with menotropins or a follitropin, hCG is injected 1 day after the last menotropins dose. When used with clomiphene, hCG is administered 7 to 9 days after the last clomiphene dose.

Ongoing Evaluation and Interventions

Minimizing Adverse Effects

Ovarian Hyperstimulation Syndrome. See *Minimizing Adverse Effects* for menotropins.

CABERGOLINE

Preadministration Assessment

Therapeutic Goal

Treatment of female infertility occurring secondary to hyperprolactinemia.

Identifying High-Risk Patients

Cabergoline should be used with *caution* in patients with severe hepatic insufficiency.

Implementation: Administration

Route

Oral.

Administration

Instruct patients to take cabergoline twice a week, with or without food.

Treatment can stop after prolactin levels have been maintained in the normal range (below 20 pg/mL) for at least 6 months.

Ongoing Evaluation and Interventions

Minimizing Adverse Effects

Nausea, Headache, and Dizziness. Initiating treatment at low doses may help minimize these effects.

[a]Patient education information is highlighted as **blue text**.

CHAPTER

64 Drugs That Affect Uterine Function

Most of the drugs discussed in this chapter have applications related to labor and delivery. Some are used to delay or prevent preterm labor, some are used to induce labor, and some are used to control postpartum hemorrhage. In addition to these drugs, we discuss one other group: drugs used to decrease menorrhagia (heavy menstrual bleeding).

Drugs that alter uterine function fall into two major groups: *oxytocic drugs* and *tocolytic drugs.* The oxytocic drugs, also known as *uterotonic drugs,* stimulate uterine contraction. In contrast, the tocolytic drugs cause uterine relaxation. Clinical applications of the oxytocic and tocolytic drugs are shown in Table 64.1.

DRUGS FOR PRETERM LABOR

Preterm birth, defined as birth before 37 weeks' gestation, is associated with higher neonatal morbidity and mortality. Infants who survive preterm birth are at increased risk for infection, cerebral palsy, intracranial hemorrhage, and, most commonly, neonatal respiratory distress syndrome. In 2015, about 10% of live births in the United States were premature. Risk factors for preterm delivery include a previous preterm delivery, multifetal pregnancy, cervical or uterine abnormalities, intrauterine infection and inflammation, and social factors such as poverty, limited education, and inadequate prenatal care.

Drugs for preterm labor fall into two major groups: drugs used to *suppress* preterm labor that has already started and drugs used to *prevent* preterm labor. The first group is larger and used more widely.

Prototype Drugs

DRUGS THAT AFFECT UTERINE FUNCTION

Drugs Used to Suppress Preterm Labor
Terbutaline (beta$_2$ agonist)
Nifedipine (calcium channel blocker)

Drugs Used to Prevent Preterm Labor
Hydroxyprogesterone caproate

Drugs for Cervical Ripening and Induction of Labor
Oxytocin
Misoprostol

Uterotonic Drugs for Postpartum Hemorrhage
Oxytocin/misoprostol
Ergonovine

Drugs for Menorrhagia
Tranexamic acid

DRUGS USED TO SUPPRESS PRETERM LABOR

Drugs employed to suppress preterm labor are *tocolytics.* That is, they all promote uterine relaxation and thereby delay delivery. Be aware, however, that benefits are limited: These drugs can suppress labor only *briefly,* not long term. On average, delivery is postponed by only 48 hours, so birth still takes place before term. Because tocolytics don't permit pregnancy to reach term, they are of little use if they are used *alone.* However, when tocolytics are combined with glucocorticoids, which accelerate fetal lung development (see Chapter 107), the outcome can be improved. Tocolytics also buy time to treat infection, if present. Unfortunately, tocolytic drugs can pose a risk to the fetus. Accordingly, the ultimate goal of treatment is to extend fetal time in the womb, but without causing significant fetal or neonatal harm.

Control of Myometrial Contraction and Mechanisms of Tocolytic Drug Action

Contraction of the myometrium (uterine smooth muscle) is regulated by multiple mediators, including beta-adrenergic agonists, oxytocin, and prostaglandins (Fig. 64.1). As a result,

TABLE 64.1 ■ Applications of Selected Tocolytic and Oxytocic Drugs

Drug	Brand Name	Applications: Delay of Preterm Labor	Induction of Cervical Ripening	Induction of Labor	Control of Postpartum Hemorrhage	Induction of Abortion
TOCOLYTIC DRUGS						
Beta$_2$-adrenergic Agonist						
Terbutaline	Brethine	✓				
Calcium Channel Blocker						
Nifedipine	Adalat, Procardia, others	✓				
Cyclooxygenase Inhibitor						
Indomethacin	Indocin	✓				
Nitric Oxide Donor						
Nitroglycerin	Nitro-Dur, others	✓				
OXYTOCIC (UTEROTONIC) DRUGS						
Prostaglandins						
Dinoprostone	Cervidil, Prepidil		✓[a]	✓		✓
Misoprostol	Cytotec		✓[a]	✓		✓
Carboprost	Hemabate				✓	✓
Oxytocin Receptor Agonist						
Oxytocin	Pitocin			✓	✓	
Ergot Alkaloids						
Methylergonovine	Methergine 🍁				✓	

[a]Cervical ripening is unrelated to uterotonic actions.

there are multiple ways in which drugs can suppress uterine activity. However, although these drugs work through different mechanisms, they all have one thing in common: Ultimately, they all *decrease the availability of phosphorylated light-chain (LC) myosin,* the form of myosin that interacts with actin to cause contraction. Four classes of tocolytic drugs—beta-adrenergic agonists, calcium channel blockers, cyclooxygenase (COX) inhibitors, and oxytocin receptor antagonists—work to reduce the activity of myosin LC kinase, the enzyme that converts myosin to its phosphorylated form. A fifth group—the nitric oxide donors—works to increase the activity of myosin LC phosphatase, the enzyme that removes phosphate from myosin, thereby converting it to its inactive form. Note also that three drug groups—COX inhibitors, oxytocin receptor antagonists, and calcium channel blockers—*decrease the release of calcium* from the sarcoplasmic reticulum (SR). Calcium combines with calmodulin to form a complex that increases myosin LC kinase activity. Hence, in the absence of sufficient free calcium, myosin LC kinase activity declines, causing the phosphorylation of myosin to decline as well.

Specific Tocolytic Drugs

Multiple drugs can suppress preterm labor. Options include terbutaline (a beta$_2$-adrenergic agonist), nifedipine (a calcium channel blocker), and indomethacin (a COX inhibitor). All of these drugs appear equally good at suppressing labor, and hence there is no obvious first-choice drug among them. Accordingly, selection is based primarily on side effects, which are shown in Table 64.2. Interestingly, none of the drugs currently employed to suppress preterm labor has been approved for this use by the U.S. Food and Drug Administration (FDA); instead, they are used off-label for this purpose.

Terbutaline, a Beta$_2$-Adrenergic Agonist

Terbutaline, used primarily for asthma (see Chapter 76), is a selective beta$_2$ agonist that can effectively suppress preterm labor. By activating beta$_2$ receptors in the uterus, terbutaline increases production of cyclic AMP, a mediator that leads to suppression of myosin LC kinase activity. The result is a decrease in both the intensity and frequency of contractions. Unfortunately, although terbutaline is effective, it poses a significant risk to the mother. Adverse effects result from activating beta$_1$ receptors, as well as beta$_2$ receptors. (Although terbutaline is classified as a selective beta$_2$ agonist, it can activate beta$_1$ receptors too, albeit less readily than beta$_2$ receptors.) Effects of greatest concern are pulmonary edema, hypotension, and hyperglycemia in the mother, and tachycardia in both the mother and fetus. For suppression of labor, terbutaline is administered subQ, not PO. The initial dosage is 250 mcg every 20 minutes for up to 3 hours. Dosing should stop after 48 hours, and should be interrupted if the maternal heart rate exceeds 120 beats/min. Although terbutaline can be used to *suppress* preterm labor, it should not be given to *prevent* preterm labor.

Nifedipine, a Calcium Channel Blocker

Nifedipine [Adalat, Procardia, others] can suppress preterm labor for at least 48 hours. Efficacy equals that of terbutaline—and safety is superior. How does nifedipine work? It blocks

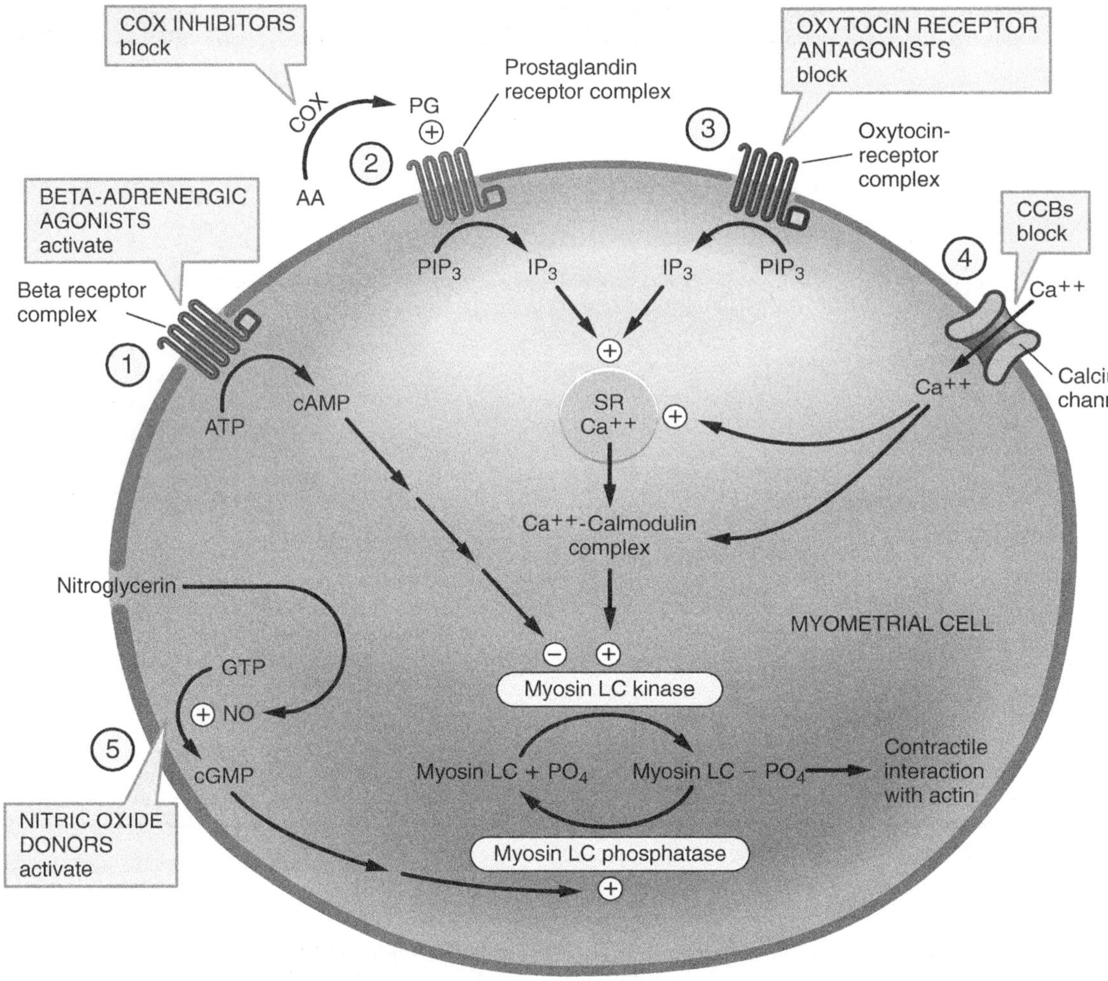

Fig. 64.1 ▪ Control of myometrial contraction and the actions of tocolytic drugs. Five pathways regulate availability of myosin LC phosphate (myosin LC PO_4), the form of myosin needed for contractile interaction with actin. Note that two enzymes—myosin LC kinase and myosin LC phosphatase—play central roles. Four classes of tocolytic drugs (numbers 1, 2, 3, and 4) work to reduce the activity of myosin LC kinase and thereby reduce production of myosin LC phosphate. A fifth class—the nitric oxide donors—increases the activity of myosin LC phosphatase, stimulating conversion of myosin LC phosphate to its inactive (dephosphorylated) form. Note also the important role played by calcium in controlling the activity of myosin LC kinase. (*AA*, Arachidonic acid; *ATP*, adenosine triphosphate; *cAMP*, cyclic adenosine monophosphate; *CCBs*, calcium channel blockers; *cGMP*, cyclic guanosine monophosphate; *COX*, cyclooxygenase; *GTP*, guanosine triphosphate; *IP_3*, inositol triphosphate; *LC*, light-chain; *NO*, nitric oxide; *PG*, prostaglandin; *PIP_3*, phosphatidylinositol triphosphate; *PO_4*, phosphate; *SR*, sarcoplasmic reticulum.)

calcium channels and thereby inhibits entry of calcium into myometrial cells. As a result, release of calcium from the SR is reduced, so the activity of myosin LC kinase is reduced as well. Maternal side effects, which are rare, include transient tachycardia, facial flushing, headache, dizziness, and nausea. Hypotension may occur in hypovolemic patients. There is some concern that nifedipine may compromise uteroplacental blood flow. In animal studies, calcium channel blockers have caused acidosis, hypoxemia, and hypercapnia in the newborn. To suppress preterm labor, an initial loading dose of 30 mg is followed by maintenance doses (10 or 20 mg PO) every 4 to 6 hours. The basic pharmacology of calcium channel blockers is discussed in Chapter 45.

Indomethacin, a Cyclooxygenase Inhibitor

Indomethacin [Indocin] is generally reserved for women who go into labor extremely early. The drug is as effective as terbutaline, but carries a higher risk for neonatal complications. Indomethacin suppresses labor by inhibiting synthesis of prostaglandins, local hormones that promote uterine contraction by increasing the release of calcium from the SR. A number of fetal abnormalities have been attributed to indomethacin. In 2015 the *American Journal of Obstetrics and Gynecology* published the results of a meta-analysis of studies involving 1731 neonates exposed to indomethacin *in utero*. The findings demonstrated fewer adverse effects than previously attributed

TABLE 64.2 ■ Adverse Effects of Tocolytic Drugs

	Major Adverse Effects	
Drug	**Maternal**	**Fetal/Neonatal**
Terbutaline, a beta$_2$ agonist	Pulmonary edema, tachycardia, palpitations, chest pain, myocardial ischemia, hypotension, tremors, hypokalemia, hyperglycemia	Fetal tachycardia, hypotension, ileus, hyperinsulinemia with hypoglycemia, hyperbilirubinemia, hypocalcemia
Nifedipine, a calcium channel blocker	Tachycardia, hypotension, hepatotoxicity	Hypotension
Indomethacin, a cyclooxygenase inhibitor	Nausea, gastric irritation, interstitial nephritis, prolonged postpartum bleeding (rarely)	Prolonged renal insufficiency, bronchopulmonary dysplasia, necrotizing enterocolitis, periventricular leukomalacia, *in utero* closure of ductus arteriosus
Nitroglycerin, a nitric oxide donor	Hypotension, headache, dizziness, flushing	Hypotension

to indomethacin; however, the type and extent of adverse effects continues to be debated. Known complications include premature narrowing or closure of the ductus arteriosus when given in high doses; however, this has not been demonstrated at recommended dosages. Oligohydramnios, a decrease in amniotic fluid, may result from a reduction in fetal urine output. Indomethacin may also have a role in intraventricular hemorrhage. Adverse maternal effects include nausea, gastric irritation, interstitial nephritis, and, rarely, increased postpartum bleeding. Tocolytic treatment is initiated with a loading dose (50 or 100 mg, usually rectal) followed by maintenance doses (25 to 50 mg PO) given every 4 to 8 hours for 2 to 3 days.

Nitroglycerin, a Nitric Oxide Donor

Nitroglycerin, administered by transdermal patch, appears similar in efficacy to terbutaline. Benefits derive from the release of nitric oxide, which then stimulates production of cyclic GMP, a mediator that leads to enhanced activity of myosin LC phosphatase. As a result, availability of phosphorylated myosin declines. Major side effects are hypotension and headache in the mother and hypotension in the infant. Dosing consists of one 10-mg patch applied every 12 hours for up to 48 hours. The basic pharmacology of nitroglycerin is discussed in Chapter 51.

Magnesium Sulfate

Opinion on the role of magnesium sulfate in preterm labor is changing. Although the drug has been popular in the United States (but not in Europe), there seems to be little to recommend its use. First and foremost, the drug doesn't work: Despite an ability to suppress contractions, a *clinically significant* tocolytic effect has not been demonstrated. High-dose treatment has been associated with *increased* infant mortality, and long-term treatment (over 5 to 7 days) has been associated with fetal bone changes secondary to altered calcium levels. However, recent data indicate that, when used in *low* doses, magnesium may protect against cerebral palsy without increasing the risk for mortality. The bottom line? Treatment with *high-dose* or *long-term* magnesium is both ineffective and dangerous, and therefore should not be used. In contrast, *low-dose* magnesium may offer the benefit of neuroprotection, even though it may not significantly delay delivery.

How does magnesium sulfate suppress contractions? It inhibits the release of acetylcholine at neuromuscular junctions, both in the uterus and in skeletal muscle. At high doses, the drug can cause profound muscle weakness and respiratory arrest.

Magnesium sulfate can cause a variety of maternal adverse effects. Initial reactions include transient hypotension, flushing, headache, dizziness, lethargy, dry mouth, and a feeling of warmth. High doses may cause hypothermia and paralytic ileus. Pulmonary edema, which can be fatal, is seen in 2% of patients. This complication is managed by discontinuing magnesium and giving a diuretic to accelerate magnesium excretion. Magnesium sulfate is contraindicated in patients with myasthenia gravis (because the disease causes muscle weakness), renal failure (because magnesium is eliminated entirely by the kidneys), and hypocalcemia (because hypocalcemia intensifies magnesium-induced suppression of neurotransmitter release).

Magnesium readily crosses the placenta and is associated with increased infant mortality. The drug may also cause hypotonia (muscle weakness) and sleepiness in the newborn. Because elimination of magnesium by neonatal kidneys is slow, hypotonia may persist 3 to 4 days. During this time, mechanical assistance of ventilation may be required.

The risk for adverse effects can be reduced by monitoring (1) magnesium levels; (2) renal function (because renal impairment will cause magnesium levels to rise); (3) fluid balance (because fluid retention increases the risk for pulmonary edema); and (4) deep tendon reflexes (because loss of deep tendon reflexes is an early sign that magnesium levels are rising dangerously high).

In clinical trials testing magnesium sulfate for neuroprotection, two *low-dose* protocols have been used. In one, dosing consisted of a 4-gm IV loading bolus infused over 20 minutes, followed by a maintenance infusion of 1 gm/hr lasting for 24 hours or until delivery, whichever came first. In the other protocol, dosing was limited to a single IV bolus. By way of comparison, *high-dose* therapy consists of an initial IV bolus (4 to 6 gm), followed by infusion of 2 to 3 gm/hr for 48 to 72 hours.

In addition to its use for preterm neuroprotection, magnesium sulfate is the preferred drug for prevention and treatment of seizures associated with eclampsia and severe preeclampsia, which are serious conditions associated with pregnancy (see Chapter 47).

DRUGS USED TO PREVENT PRETERM LABOR

As discussed earlier, we can arrest preterm labor (albeit briefly) with tocolytics, but is there any way we can *prevent* it? Yes—at least for some women. Two drug interventions may help: hydroxyprogesterone and antibiotics.

Hydroxyprogesterone Caproate

Therapeutic Use

In 2011, the FDA approved hydroxyprogesterone caproate [Makena] for reducing the risk for preterm labor, making it the first and only drug approved for this use. The drug is indicated only for women with a singleton pregnancy and a history of at least one preterm birth. It is not approved for women with multiple pregnancy or other risk factors for preterm birth. Hydroxyprogesterone is a weakly active, naturally occurring progesterone derivative. The mechanism underlying prevention of preterm birth is unknown. Also unknown is why it works for some women but not for others.

Adverse Effects and Contraindications

In clinical trials, the most common adverse effects were injection-site reactions (pain, swelling, itching), hives, nausea, and diarrhea. Serious events were rare. If thrombosis or thromboembolism occurs, hydroxyprogesterone should be stopped. Hydroxyprogesterone can promote glucose intolerance, clinical depression, and fluid retention. Accordingly, monitoring is indicated for women with diabetes, a history of depression, or a condition that could be made worse by fluid retention (e.g., preeclampsia, epilepsy, or cardiac or renal dysfunction).

Hydroxyprogesterone is contraindicated for women with uncontrolled hypertension, liver cancer, liver disease, a history of thrombosis, cholestatic jaundice of pregnancy, undiagnosed abnormal vaginal bleeding (unrelated to pregnancy), or known or suspected breast cancer (or any other hormone-sensitive cancer).

Preparations, Dosage, and Administration

Hydroxyprogesterone caproate [Makena] is supplied in solution (250 mg/mL) in 5-mL multidose vials for IM injection into the upper quadrant of the gluteus maximus. The solution is viscous and oily, and hence should be injected slowly (over 1 minute or more). Shots are given by the healthcare provider, not by the patient. The dosage is 250 mg once a week, beginning between 16 and 21 weeks of gestation, and continuing until week 37 or delivery, whichever comes first.

Makena is expensive, costing approximately $920/dose ($18,400 for 20 weekly doses). However, generic hydroxyprogesterone acetate can be obtained from a compounding pharmacy for as low as $10 to $20 per dose ($200 to $400 for 20 weekly doses). Progesterone, available in a number of formulations, has also been used off-label for this purpose at even lower cost.

Hazardous Drugs and Special Administration Requirements

Hydroxyprogesterone caproate may present a hazard for nurses, especially pregnant nurses, who administer this drug. In 2016 the National Institute for Occupational Safety and Health (NIOSH) expanded the list of drugs identified as hazardous. (See https://www.cdc.gov/niosh/docs/2016-161/pdfs/2016-161.pdf.) NIOSH requires special handling of drugs identified as hazardous. See Chapter 3, Table 3.1, for administration and handling guidelines. The hazardous drugs mentioned in this chapter are listed in the following box.

Safety Alert

HAZARDOUS DRUGS REQUIRING SPECIAL HANDLING

Hydroxyprogesterone caproate and progesterone
Prostaglandins (dinoprostone and misoprostol)
Ergot derivatives (methylergonovine)
Hormonal contraceptives (oral contraceptives and levonorgestrel)

Antibiotics

In women with bacterial vaginosis, antibiotics can reduce the incidence of preterm labor, as shown in two randomized, double-blind, placebo-controlled trials. Why were these studies conducted? Because there is an association between abnormal genital tract flora and preterm delivery, suggesting that normalizing genital tract flora might reduce risk.

A reduction in preterm delivery has been demonstrated in studies in which women with abnormal genital tract flora received antibiotic therapy. These antibiotic studies suggest a simple method for preventing some preterm deliveries: early screening for and treatment of asymptomatic bacterial vaginosis.

DRUGS FOR CERVICAL RIPENING AND INDUCTION OF LABOR

The goal of labor induction is to stimulate uterine contractions before the spontaneous onset of labor, and thereby produce a vaginal delivery. In the United States, more than 22% of deliveries are induced. Induction is considered appropriate when the benefits of the procedure outweigh the risks of continued pregnancy and the risks of induction itself. An evidence-based practice guideline—*Induction of Labor: ACOG Practice Bulletin No. 107*—released in 2010 by the American College of Obstetricians and Gynecologists (ACOG), summarizes the indications and contraindications for induction, and discusses the benefits and risks of the drugs and procedures employed. Much of what follows is based on these guidelines.

Labor should be induced only when continued pregnancy constitutes a greater risk to the mother and fetus than does the risk for induction itself. As a rule, induction should be reserved for pregnancy that has continued beyond term (i.e., beyond 42 weeks), and for pregnancy in which early vaginal delivery is likely to decrease morbidity and mortality for the mother or infant. Post-term pregnancy is the most common reason for induction. Indications for *early* induction include:

- Abruptio placentae (separation of the placenta from the uterus)
- Premature rupture of the membranes
- Gestational hypertension
- Preeclampsia or eclampsia
- Maternal medical conditions, including diabetes, renal disease, chronic pulmonary disease, and chronic hypertension
- Fetal compromise, including severe fetal growth restriction, isoimmunization (development of maternal antibodies directed against fetal red blood cells), and oligohydramnios (deficiency of amniotic fluid)
- Fetal demise (fetal death)

Contraindications to induction include:

- Umbilical cord prolapse
- Transverse fetal position
- Active genital herpes infection
- Previous cesarean delivery
- History of myomectomy (surgical removal of uterine fibroids)
- Placenta previa (growth of the placenta in the lowest part of the uterus, such that the placenta covers the opening to the cervix)

Before labor can be safely induced, *cervical ripening* must occur. During pregnancy, the cervix is elongated, rigid, and constricted. When ripening takes place, the cervix shortens, softens, and dilates, thereby permitting the fetus to pass through the birth canal. If induction is attempted in the absence of ripening, maternal and fetal injury can result. Accordingly, if labor is to be induced before natural ripening has occurred, ripening must be facilitated, either with drugs or with a mechanical dilator (e.g., saline-filled Foley catheter).

Three drugs used for cervical ripening and/or labor induction are discussed in this section. One of these drugs—oxytocin—is used only for induction. The other two—dinoprostone and misoprostol—can promote cervical ripening and can also induce labor.

Prostaglandins: Dinoprostone and Misoprostol

Two prostaglandins—dinoprostone and misoprostol—act on the cervix to promote ripening and act on the uterus to promote contractions. Because of these dual actions, treatment with a prostaglandin alone may be sufficient to both ripen the cervix *and* induce labor. If contractions are inadequate with a prostaglandin alone, then oxytocin is given to strengthen contractions.

Dinoprostone

Dinoprostone [Prepidil, Cervidil] is the most widely used agent for cervical ripening. The drug is a synthetic prostaglandin identical in structure to endogenous prostaglandin E_2 (PGE_2), a compound produced by fetal membranes and the placenta. Endogenous PGE_2 has two roles in the birthing process: It promotes cervical ripening, and later it stimulates uterine contractions. Cervical ripening results from activation of collagenase, an enzyme that breaks down the collagen network that makes the cervix rigid. When used to promote ripening, dinoprostone shortens the duration of labor, allows a reduction in oxytocin dosage, and decreases the need for cesarean delivery. Because it can stimulate uterine contractions, dinoprostone may induce labor as well as promote cervical ripening. As discussed in Chapter 62, dinoprostone is also used to induce abortion, owing to its ability to stimulate intense uterine contractions. For promotion of cervical ripening, dinoprostone is available in two formulations: a gel and a vaginal insert.

Dinoprostone Gel. Dinoprostone gel [Prepidil] is available in single-dose, pre-filled syringes that contain 0.5 mg dinoprostone/3 mL gel. Administration is intracervical, using the endocervical catheter supplied by the manufacturer. To prevent leakage, the patient should lie supine during administration and for at least 30 minutes after. If the desired response has not occurred within 6 hours, a second 0.5-mg dose can be given, followed 6 hours later by a third, if needed. (Most women need at least two doses, and 50% need a third.) Because dinoprostone can stimulate uterine contractions and may thereby cause fetal distress, uterine activity and fetal heart rate should be monitored continuously. Monitoring should start before each dose and continue for at least 2 hours after. Oxytocin is given 6 to 12 hours after the last dose of dinoprostone. The major adverse effect of dinoprostone is uterine *tachysystole,*[a] which occurs in 1% of patients using the gel. Rarely, systemic absorption results in nausea, vomiting, diarrhea, and fever. Dinoprostone gel is unstable and must be stored refrigerated, between 2°C and 8°C (36°F and 46°F). Treatment is moderately expensive: Each 0.5-mg dose costs about $680, making the total cost $2040 for women who require three doses.

Dinoprostone Vaginal Inserts. Dinoprostone vaginal inserts [Cervidil] consist of a pouch, containing 10 mg of the drug, to which a long tape is attached. The purpose of the tape is to permit rapid removal of the pouch. Following insertion in the posterior fornix of the vagina, the pouch releases dinoprostone slowly (0.3 mg/hr) for 12 hours. The patient should remain supine for at least 2 hours after pouch insertion. The pouch is removed when active labor occurs or when 12 hours have elapsed, whichever comes first. If oxytocin is needed, administration can begin 30 minutes after removing the pouch. As with dinoprostone gel, the major adverse effect is uterine tachysystole, which develops in 5% of patients (compared with only 1% of those receiving the gel). To minimize harm, uterine activity and fetal heart rate should undergo continuous monitoring while the insert is in place and for at least 15 minutes after it is removed. Compared with dinoprostone gel, the insert has two advantages. First, treatment is almost always cheaper. Second, because inserts can be easily removed, drug delivery can be stopped as soon as (1) labor starts (thereby avoiding unnecessary drug exposure) or (2) uterine tachysystole develops (thereby minimizing uterine contractions and related fetal distress). The vaginal inserts are unstable and must be stored frozen, between −10°C and −20°C (14°F and −4°F). The cost of one insert is approximately $430 compared with $680 for one dose of the gel. Additionally, because most women require two doses of the gel, the total cost of treatment with the gel is approximately $1360). If the maximum three doses are required, the cost increases to $2040.

[a]Current ACOG guidelines use the term *uterine tachysystole* in preference to *uterine hyperstimulation* or *uterine hypercontractility,* which have been used extensively in the past. Tachysystole is a high rate of uterine contractions, defined as more than 5 contractions in 10 minutes (averaged over a 30-minute window). The normal rate of contractions is 5 or fewer in 10 minutes (averaged over a 30-minute window).

Misoprostol

Misoprostol [Cytotec] is an attractive alternative to dinoprostone for promoting cervical ripening, although misoprostol is not approved for this use. Compared with dinoprostone, misoprostol is more effective, more convenient (stores at room temperature versus refrigerated), and *much* less expensive (treatment costs about $1 versus $430 to $1360). Unfortunately, misoprostol also causes a higher incidence of uterine tachysystole, and hence is contraindicated in women with a history of major uterine surgery or cesarean delivery. To induce cervical ripening, a 25-mcg dose (one-fourth of a 100-mcg tablet) is inserted into the posterior fornix of the vagina. Dosing is repeated every 4 hours as needed. In women given misoprostol, delivery occurs faster than in those given dinoprostone. To minimize risk from tachysystole, fetal heart rate and uterine activity should be monitored continuously. Like dinoprostone, misoprostol can induce labor following cervical ripening, and hence use of oxytocin may not be needed. In addition to its use for cervical ripening/labor induction, misoprostol is used to induce abortion (see Chapter 62) and to protect against peptic ulcers (see Chapter 78).

Oxytocin

Oxytocin [Pitocin] is a peptide hormone produced by the posterior pituitary. Physiologically, this hormone promotes uterine contraction during parturition and stimulates the milk-ejection reflex. The primary therapeutic use of oxytocin is induction of labor near term, a procedure for which oxytocin is the agent of choice. As discussed under *Drugs for Postpartum Hemorrhage,* oxytocin is also a drug of choice for stopping postpartum bleeding.

Physiologic and Pharmacologic Effects

Uterine Stimulation. Oxytocin can increase the force, frequency, and duration of uterine contractions. The ability of the uterus to respond to oxytocin depends on the stage of gestation: Early in pregnancy, uterine sensitivity to oxytocin is low; as pregnancy proceeds, the uterus becomes progressively more responsive; and just before term, a large and abrupt increase in responsiveness develops. Sensitivity increases over time because the number of oxytocin receptors on uterine smooth muscle increases throughout pregnancy. Although uterine sensitivity to oxytocin is low early in pregnancy, oxytocin can still initiate and enhance contractions at this stage. However, the doses required are much larger than those needed at term.

Despite the profound effects of oxytocin on uterine contractility, the precise role of oxytocin in spontaneous labor and delivery has not been established. We do know that giving exogenous oxytocin can elicit contractions identical to those seen during spontaneous labor. However, we also know that childbirth can take place with virtually no oxytocin present—although labor will be prolonged. Furthermore, during normal labor or during labor induced artificially (through rupture of the membranes), only modest increases in plasma oxytocin occur. From these observations we can conclude that although oxytocin is not absolutely required for delivery, the hormone probably acts to facilitate contractions. However, it is not certain that oxytocin is responsible for *initiating* labor.

Milk Ejection. Milk is produced by glandular tissue of the breast and is later transferred, via small channels, into large sinuses where it is readily accessible to the nursing infant. Transfer to the sinuses is brought about by the milk-ejection reflex: When the infant sucks on the breast, neuronal stimuli are sent to the posterior pituitary, causing release of oxytocin; oxytocin then causes contraction of the smooth muscle surrounding the small milk channels, thereby forcing milk into the large sinuses. In the absence of oxytocin, milk ejection does not occur.

Water Retention. Oxytocin is similar in structure to antidiuretic hormone (ADH), which acts on the kidney to decrease excretion of water. Although less potent than ADH, oxytocin can nonetheless promote renal retention of water.

Pharmacokinetics

Oxytocin is administered IV or IM. The plasma half-life is short, ranging from 12 to 17 minutes. Elimination is by hepatic metabolism and renal excretion.

Use for Induction of Labor

Preinduction Preparation. Induction should not be done if the fetal lungs have not matured or if the cervix is not ripe. Accordingly, before induction, if the fetal lungs are still immature, maturation should be hastened with a glucocorticoid (see Chapter 107). Likewise, if the cervix is not yet ripe, ripening should be induced with dinoprostone or misoprostol. Alternatively, cervical ripening can be induced mechanically (with a cervical dilator) or by membrane stripping (i.e., by separating the chorioamnionic membranes from the internal surface of the uterus).

Precautions and Contraindications. Improper use of oxytocin can be hazardous. Uterine rupture may occur, posing a risk for death for the mother, the infant, or both. The likelihood of trauma is especially high in cases of cephalopelvic disproportion, fetal malpresentation, placental abnormalities, umbilical cord prolapse, previous uterine surgery, and fetal distress. Oxytocin is contraindicated in pregnancies with any of these characteristics. In addition, oxytocin is contraindicated in women with active genital herpes. Induction of labor in women of high parity (five or more pregnancies) carries a high risk for uterine rupture, and hence oxytocin must be used with great caution in these women.

Adverse Effect: Water Intoxication. When administered in large doses, oxytocin exerts an antidiuretic effect. If large volumes of fluid have been administered along with oxytocin, retention of water may produce water intoxication. However, at the doses employed to induce labor, water intoxication is rare.

Dosage and Administration. For induction of labor, oxytocin is administered by IV infusion. Solutions should be dilute (10 milliunits/mL) and administered with an infusion pump that allows precise flow-rate control. Either a low-dose or a high-dose regimen may be used. The low-dose regimen produces less tachysystole than the high-dose regimen. However, the high-dose regimen works faster and is associated with less chorioamnionitis and less need for cesarean delivery. The two regimens consist of the following:

- *Low-dose regimen:* Start the infusion at 0.5 to 2 milliunits/min, and then gradually increase the rate by 1 to 2 milliunits/min every 15 to 40 minutes.
- *High-dose regimen:* Start the infusion at 6 milliunits/min, and then gradually increase the rate by 3 to 6 milliunits/min every 15 to 40 minutes.

With both regimens, the dose is gradually increased until uterine contractions resembling those of spontaneous labor have been produced (i.e., contractions every 2 to 3 minutes and lasting 45 to 60 seconds).

During the infusion, constant monitoring is required. The mother should be monitored for blood pressure, pulse rate, and uterine contractility (frequency, duration, and intensity). The fetus should be monitored for heart rate and rhythm. In the event of significant maternal or fetal distress, the infusion should be stopped; contractions will diminish rapidly. Complications that usually require interruption of the infusion are (1) elevation of resting uterine pressure above 15 to 20 mm Hg, (2) contractions that persist for more than 1 minute, (3) contractions that occur more often than every 2 to 3 minutes, and (4) pronounced alteration in fetal heart rate or rhythm.

Additional Therapeutic Uses

Augmentation of Labor. Oxytocin may be employed if labor is dysfunctional. However, patients must be judiciously selected, and dosage must be regulated with special care. As a rule, oxytocic agents should not be used to promote labor that is already in progress, even if labor is proceeding slowly: By intensifying the force of contractions, oxytocin may cause uterine damage (laceration or rupture) or trauma to the infant.

Postpartum Use. Oxytocin can be administered IM or IV following placental delivery to control bleeding or hemorrhage and to increase uterine tone. Dosage for postpartum hemorrhage is given in the following sections.

Abortion. Oxytocin has been employed during the second trimester to manage incomplete abortion. Intravenous infusion at a rate of 10 to 20 milliunits/min is often effective. However, oxytocin is not a method of choice.

DRUGS FOR POSTPARTUM HEMORRHAGE

Postpartum hemorrhage is the second leading cause of maternal mortality (preeclampsia/eclampsia is first). Morbidity and mortality result directly from blood loss. How much loss constitutes hemorrhage? Traditionally, postpartum hemorrhage has been defined as blood loss exceeding 500 mL during vaginal delivery or 1000 mL during cesarean delivery. However, a more workable definition is bleeding of any amount sufficient to cause hemodynamic instability.

Why does postpartum hemorrhage occur? Normally, the uterus contracts following delivery, allowing the placenta to separate from the uterine surface. After expulsion of the placenta, the uterus continues to contract, causing blood vessels that supplied the placenta to squeeze shut. As a result, bleeding stops. If the uterus does not contract enough, bleeding will continue. In about 80% of cases, postpartum hemorrhage results from *uterine atony* (failure of the uterus to contract). Most of the remaining cases result from lacerations, maternal coagulopathies, or retention of placental tissue.

Drugs that promote uterine contraction (uterotonic drugs) can reduce bleeding caused by uterine atony. Two of these drugs—oxytocin and misoprostol—were discussed previously under *Drugs for Cervical Ripening and Induction of Labor.* Two additional drugs—methylergonovine and carboprost tromethamine—are introduced here. Of all these drugs, oxytocin is considered the agent of first choice for control of postpartum hemorrhage.

Oxytocin and Misoprostol

Oxytocin [Pitocin] and misoprostol [Cytotec] are powerful uterotonic agents, and hence can stop postpartum hemorrhage resulting from uterine atony. For misoprostol, the dosage is 600 to 1000 mcg administered rectally. Principal side effects are shivering and temperature elevation. For oxytocin, dosing may be done IM or IV. The IM dosage is 10 units given as a single injection following delivery of the placenta. Intravenous dosing is 10 to 40 units in 1000 mL of IV fluid titrated to a rate sufficient to control uterine atony (usually 200 to 600 mL/hr).

Carboprost Tromethamine

Therapeutic Use

Carboprost tromethamine [Hemabate], also known as 15-methyl-prostaglandin F_2 alpha, is a preferred agent for controlling postpartum hemorrhage. The drug suppresses bleeding primarily by causing intense uterine contractions and partly by causing direct vasoconstriction. In most cases, bleeding can be stopped with a single 250-mcg dose, injected deep IM. In addition to its postpartum use, carboprost is used to induce abortion (see Chapter 62).

Adverse Effects

As with other prostaglandins, GI reactions are very common. The underlying cause is stimulation of smooth muscle of the gut. Vomiting and diarrhea occur in up to 60% of patients. Nausea is also common. Gastrointestinal reactions can be reduced by pretreatment with antiemetic and antidiarrheal medications.

Fever is common. If body temperature rises, it is important to differentiate between drug-induced fever and pyrexia resulting from endometritis.

Like other prostaglandins, carboprost causes vasoconstriction and constriction of the bronchi. As a result, treatment carries a risk for hypertension and impaired respiration.

Precautions and Contraindications

Carboprost is contraindicated for women with acute pelvic inflammatory disease and active disease of the heart, lungs, kidneys, or liver. The drug should be used with caution in women with a history of asthma, hypertension, diabetes, or uterine scarring.

Ergot Alkaloids: Methylergonovine

Ergot is a dried preparation of *Claviceps purpurea,* a fungus that grows on rye plants. The ergot alkaloids are compounds present in ergot. Ergot is capable of inducing powerful uterine contractions, a property used by midwives from the Middle Ages until the 20th century. Analysis of ergot has revealed the presence of several pharmacologically active constituents. Of these, *ergonovine* is the most effective uterine stimulant. Ergonovine is not available in the United States, but methylergonovine—a derivative of ergonovine that produces similar effects—is available.

In obstetrics, methylergonovine is used primarily to control postpartum bleeding. However, because it carries a high risk for severe hypertension, it is generally reserved for women who have not responded to safer agents: oxytocin, misoprostol, or carboprost tromethamine.

Pharmacologic Effects

Ergot alkaloids produce their effects by stimulating a variety of receptors (adrenergic, dopaminergic, serotonergic). These drugs exert their most profound effects on uterine and vascular smooth muscle.

Effects on the Uterus. Ergot alkaloids stimulate uterine contraction. In small doses, they produce contractions of moderate strength that alternate with uterine relaxation of normal degree and duration. With large doses, the force and frequency of contractions are greatly increased, and the extent of uterine relaxation is reduced; sustained contraction may occur. Because contractions may be prolonged, ergot alkaloids are not employed to induce labor.

Vascular Effects. Ergot alkaloids can cause constriction of arterioles and veins. Vasoconstriction may also contribute to control of postpartum bleeding.

Pharmacokinetics

Regardless of the route employed, methylergonovine acts rapidly. Uterine contractions begin within 60 seconds of IV injection and within 10 minutes of oral or IM administration. Effects persist for several hours.

Therapeutic Uses

Postpartum Use. The ergot alkaloids may be used postpartum and postabortion to increase uterine tone and decrease bleeding. The ability to induce sustained uterine contraction makes them very effective for these purposes. Administration is usually delayed until after delivery of the placenta. The patient should be monitored for blood pressure, pulse rate, and uterine contractility. Cramping occurs as part of the therapeutic response, but may also indicate overdose.

Augmentation of Labor. Because contractions may be both intense and prolonged, ergot alkaloids are not recommended for use during labor. If they are given during labor, excessive uterine tone can cause trauma to the mother, fetus, or both. Placental blood flow may be reduced, resulting in fetal hypoxia and uterine rupture.

Adverse Effects

When ergot alkaloids are given orally or IM, significant adverse effects are rare. In contrast, IV administration frequently causes *hypertension.* Hypertension can be severe and may be associated with nausea, vomiting, and headache; convulsions and even death have occurred. Accordingly, IV administration should be reserved for emergencies. Furthermore, patients with preexisting hypertension should not be given these drugs. Caution should be exercised in patients with cardiovascular, renal, or hepatic disorders.

Contraindications

Ergot alkaloids are contraindicated for women who are pregnant, hypertensive, or hypersensitive to these drugs. They are also contraindicated for induction of labor and for use in the presence of threatened or ongoing spontaneous abortion.

Preparations, Dosage, and Administration

Preparations. *Methylergonovine maleate* [Methergine 🍁] is available in 0.2-mg tablets for oral dosing and in solution (0.2 mg/mL) for IM and IV dosing.

Dosage and Administration

Parenteral. For parenteral therapy, methylergonovine is usually administered IM; intravenous administration is hazardous and should be reserved for emergency control of postpartum hemorrhage. Treatment is usually initiated only after passage of the placenta. The dosage for postpartum hemorrhage is 0.2 mg initially (either IM or IV), repeated every 2 to 4 hours as needed.

Oral. The dosage for *methylergonovine* (to promote involution of the uterus) is 0.2 mg every 6 to 8 hours for up to 1 week.

DRUGS FOR MENORRHAGIA

Menorrhagia—heavy menstrual bleeding—is a common disorder that affects about 1 in 5 premenopausal women. The condition is characterized by excessive and/or prolonged bleeding associated with an otherwise normal cycle. In a normal cycle, bleeding lasts an average of 7 days, and total blood flow is between 25 and 80 mL. Menorrhagia is diagnosed if bleeding lasts more than 7 days or if blood loss exceeds 80 mL. Left untreated, the condition can result in iron deficiency anemia. Excessive bleeding can be reduced with drugs or by endometrial ablation. Drugs for menorrhagia are discussed here.

Tranexamic Acid

Therapeutic Use

Tranexamic acid (TA) [Lysteda] is the first nonhormonal product *approved*[b] in the United States for oral therapy of cyclic heavy menstrual bleeding. In clinical trials, TA has reduced bleeding by as much as 50%.

Mechanism of Action

Tranexamic acid, a derivative of lysine, inhibits plasmin, the enzyme that dissolves the fibrin meshwork of blood clots. Tranexamic acid binds to lysine receptor sites on plasmin and thereby prevents plasmin from binding to lysine molecules in fibrin. Because plasmin is unable to dissolve fibrin, uterine hemostasis is preserved, and menstrual bleeding is greatly reduced.

[b]Other nonhormonal drugs, specifically nonsteroidal anti-inflammatory drugs, are also used for menorrhagia but are not *approved* for this application.

Pharmacokinetics

For treatment of menorrhagia, TA is administered by mouth. Bioavailability is 45% in the absence of food and slightly higher in the presence of food. Plasma levels peak about 3 hours after dosing. Metabolism is minimal. Most of each dose (95%) is excreted unchanged in the urine.

Adverse Effects and Interactions

Tranexamic acid is generally well tolerated. In clinical trials, the most common side effects were headache, back pain, joint pain, muscle cramps, migraine, fatigue, and sinus and nasal symptoms. However, with the exception of sinus and nasal symptoms, the incidence of side effects was about the same as in patients taking placebo.

The greatest concern with TA is possible venous or arterial *thrombosis,* including thrombosis in the veins and arteries of the retina. Accordingly, women who experience visual changes should discontinue TA immediately and undergo an eye examination to rule out possible vessel blockage. Women with a history of thrombosis or thromboembolic disease should not use this drug. Because combination oral contraceptives (OCs) also pose a risk for thrombotic events, women using these contraceptives should not use TA.

Preparations, Dosage, and Administration

For treatment of *heavy menstrual bleeding,* tranexamic acid [Lysteda] is supplied in 650-mg tablets for oral dosing, with or without food. Tablets should be swallowed whole, without crushing or chewing. For women with normal renal function, the dosage is 1300 mg 3 times a day, taken for a maximum of 5 days during monthly menstruation. Dosage should be reduced in women with renal impairment.

Other Drugs for Menorrhagia

Nonsteroidal Anti-Inflammatory Drugs

The nonsteroidal anti-inflammatory drugs (NSAIDs), such as naproxen [Anaprox, Naprosyn] and diclofenac [Cataflam], are considered first-line therapy of menorrhagia. On average, these agents can decrease bleeding by 20% to 46%. In addition, they can reduce painful cramping. Dosing is limited to the 5 days in the menstrual cycle when bleeding is heaviest. As a result, side effects are limited. NSAIDs reduce bleeding by inhibiting COX and thereby suppressing production of prostacyclin, a compound that (1) indirectly promotes menstrual bleeding and (2) is produced in excessive amounts in the menorrhagic endometrium. The basic pharmacology of the NSAIDs is discussed in Chapter 71.

Combination Oral Contraceptives

For women who desire contraception, combination OCs are a first-line therapy for menorrhagia. Benefits equal those of NSAIDs. Combination OCs reduce bleeding by causing endometrial atrophy. As a result, when endometrial breakdown occurs, there is less blood to lose. The basic pharmacology of combination OCs is discussed in Chapter 62.

Levonorgestrel-Releasing Intrauterine System

Like the combination OCs, the *Mirena* levonorgestrel-releasing intrauterine system is considered first-line therapy for menorrhagia in women who also want contraception. Benefits derive from levonorgestrel-induced endometrial involution. Menstrual blood flow is reduced by up to 97%. The Mirena system is discussed further in Chapter 62.

KEY POINTS

- Tocolytic drugs suppress contraction of uterine smooth muscle.
- Tocolytic drugs have only one indication: delay of preterm labor.
- On average, tocolytic drugs delay labor for 48 hours.
- All tocolytics work to decrease the availability of phosphorylated light-chain myosin, the form of myosin needed for contractile interaction with actin.
- The major tocolytic drugs—beta$_2$-adrenergic agonists, calcium channel blockers, and COX inhibitors—appear equally good at suppressing preterm labor, and hence selection among them is based largely on side effects.
- Only one drug—hydroxyprogesterone caproate—is approved for preventing preterm labor.
- The goal of labor induction is to stimulate uterine contractions before the spontaneous onset of labor, producing a vaginal delivery.
- Induction of labor is appropriate when pregnancy has continued beyond term or when early vaginal delivery is likely to decrease morbidity or mortality for the mother or infant.
- Before labor is induced, cervical ripening must occur, either naturally or facilitated by prostaglandins or a mechanical device.
- Dinoprostone is a prostaglandin that can promote cervical ripening and that can also induce labor in some women.
- Oxytocic drugs, also known as uterotonic drugs, stimulate contraction of uterine smooth muscle.
- Oxytocin is the drug of choice for induction of labor.
- Used improperly (e.g., in pregnancies with cephalopelvic disproportion), oxytocin can cause uterine rupture.
- Three oxytocic drugs—oxytocin, misoprostol, and carboprost tromethamine—are preferred agents for controlling postpartum hemorrhage.
- Because it poses a risk for severe hypertension, methylergonovine is considered a second-line drug for controlling postpartum hemorrhage.
- Menorrhagia is defined as excessive menstrual bleeding.
- Tranexamic acid, the first nonhormonal drug approved for menorrhagia, prevents the destruction of fibrin and thereby preserves uterine hemostasis.

Please visit http://evolve.elsevier.com/Lehne for chapter-specific NCLEX® examination review questions.

Summary of Major Nursing Implications

DINOPROSTONE

Preadministration Assessment

Therapeutic Goal

Dinoprostone is used to promote cervical ripening and induce labor.

Identifying High-Risk Patients

Dinoprostone is *contraindicated* for women with acute pelvic inflammatory disease and active disease of the heart, lungs, kidneys, or liver.

Use with *caution* in women with a history of asthma, hypotension, hypertension, diabetes, or uterine scarring.

Implementation: Administration

Route

Vaginal insert and vaginal gel, both for intracervical instillation.

Ongoing Evaluation and Interventions

Evaluating Therapeutic Effects

Assess the cervix for elongation, softening, and dilation. Assess for change in uterine contractions.

Minimizing Adverse Effects

GI Disturbances. Nausea, vomiting, and diarrhea can be reduced by pretreatment with antiemetic and antidiarrheal drugs.

Fever. Fever may be induced by dinoprostone or it may indicate endometritis. If fever develops, a differential diagnosis is needed.

OXYTOCIN

The implications here apply only to the use of oxytocin for induction of labor, the drug's principal use.

Preadministration Assessment

Therapeutic Goal

Oxytocin is given to initiate or improve uterine contractions. Treatment is reserved for pregnancies that have gone beyond term and for pregnancies in which early vaginal delivery is likely to decrease morbidity and mortality for the mother or infant.

Baseline Data

The history should determine parity, previous obstetric problems, stillbirths, and abortions. Full maternal and fetal status should be assessed, including the degree of cervical ripening and fetal lung maturity.

Identifying High-Risk Patients

Induction of labor is *contraindicated* in the presence of cephalopelvic disproportion, fetal malpresentation, placental abnormality, umbilical cord prolapse, previous major surgery to the uterus or cervix, fetal distress, and active genital herpes.

Continued

Summary of Major Nursing Implications—cont'd

Use with *caution* in women of high parity (five or more pregnancies).

Induction should not be conducted in the absence of cervical ripening or fetal lung maturation. If indicated, promote cervical ripening mechanically or with drugs, and promote fetal lung maturation with glucocorticoids.

Implementation: Administration

Route

Intravenous.

Administration

Administer by carefully controlled infusion, using an infusion pump.

Ongoing Evaluation and Interventions

Minimizing Adverse Effects

Uterine contractions of excessive intensity, frequency, and duration can cause maternal and fetal harm. Monitor uterine contractility (frequency, duration, and intensity), maternal blood pressure, and fetal and maternal heart rate. Interrupt the infusion if any of the following occur: (1) resting intrauterine pressure rises above 15 to 20 mm Hg, (2) individual contractions persist longer than 1 minute, (3) contractions occur more often than every 2 to 3 minutes, and (4) fetal heart rate or rhythm changes significantly.

ERGOT ALKALOIDS: METHYLERGONOVINE

Preadministration Assessment

Therapeutic Goal

Prevention and treatment of postpartum and postabortion hemorrhage.

Identifying High-Risk Patients

Ergot alkaloids are *contraindicated* during pregnancy, for induction of labor, in women with hypertension or allergy to ergot alkaloids, and in the presence of threatened or ongoing spontaneous abortion.

Implementation: Administration

Routes

Oral and IM. Preferred.

Intravenous. Hazardous; reserve for hemorrhagic emergencies.

Administration

As a rule, administer after passage of the placenta. Perform IV injections slowly (over 60 seconds or more).

Ongoing Evaluation and Interventions

Evaluating Therapeutic Effects

Monitor blood pressure, pulse rate, and uterine activity. Report sudden increases in blood pressure, excessive uterine bleeding, and insufficient uterine tone. Cramping is normal but may also indicate overdose.

Minimizing Adverse Effects

Significant adverse effects—*hypertension, nausea, vomiting, headache, convulsions,* and *death*—usually occur only with IV administration. To minimize risk, infuse slowly (over 60 seconds or more) and reserve IV administration for emergencies.

UNIT X MEN'S HEALTH

CHAPTER 65 Androgens

Androgen hormones are produced by the testes, ovaries, and adrenal cortex. The major endogenous androgen is testosterone. Androgens are noted most for their ability to promote expression of male sex characteristics. However, androgens also influence sexuality in females. In addition, androgens have significant physiologic and pharmacologic effects unrelated to sexual expression or function. The primary clinical application of the androgens is management of androgen deficiency in males. Principal adverse effects are virilization and hepatotoxicity.

TESTOSTERONE

Testosterone is the prototype of the androgen hormones. This compound is the principal endogenous androgen in both males and females. In addition to its physiologic role, testosterone is representative of the androgens employed clinically.

Biosynthesis and Secretion

Males

Testosterone is made by Leydig cells of the testes. Daily production in men ranges from 2.5 to 10 mg. Synthesis is promoted by two hormones of the anterior pituitary: follicle-stimulating hormone (FSH) and luteinizing hormone (LH), also known as interstitial cell–stimulating hormone. Production of testosterone is regulated by negative feedback control: Rising plasma levels of testosterone act on the pituitary to suppress further release of FSH and LH, thereby decreasing the stimulus for further testosterone formation.

Some of the testosterone present in plasma is produced by the adrenal glands. However, androgenic activity of adrenal origin is much less than that of testicular origin. Hence, in males, adrenal androgens have minimal functional significance.

Testosterone production changes over time. Peak production occurs around age 17 years. Production then remains steady until age 30 or 40 years, after which it slowly declines. By the time a man reaches 80 years, testosterone production is only half what it had been in his youth.

Females

In women, preandrogens (precursors of testosterone) are secreted by the adrenal cortex and ovaries. Conversion into testosterone takes place in peripheral tissues. Synthesis of preandrogens by the adrenal glands is regulated by adrenocorticotropic hormone, whereas synthesis of preandrogens by the ovaries is regulated by LH. Daily testosterone production is about 300 mcg (150 mcg from the ovaries and 150 mcg from the adrenal glands). The total is 10 to 40 times less than the amount produced in men. In the event of ovarian or adrenocortical pathology (e.g., adenoma, carcinoma, hyperplasia), secretion of androgens can increase greatly and may be sufficient to produce virilization. At menopause, testosterone production decreases.

Mechanism of Action

Effects of testosterone on its target tissues are mediated by specific receptors located in the cell cytoplasm. After binding of testosterone to its receptor, the hormone-receptor complex migrates to the cell nucleus and then acts on DNA to promote synthesis of specific messenger RNA molecules. These, in turn, serve as templates for production of specific proteins, which then mediate testosterone effects. It should be noted that in some tissues—prostate, seminal vesicles, and hair follicles—androgen receptors do not interact with testosterone itself. Rather, they interact with dihydrotestosterone, a testosterone metabolite.

Physiologic and Pharmacologic Effects

Effects on Sex Characteristics in Males

Pubertal Transformation. Increased production of testosterone promotes the transformations that signal puberty in males. Under the influence of testosterone, the testes enlarge, after which the penis and scrotum enlarge. Pubic and axillary hair appears, and hair on the trunk, arms, and legs assumes adult male patterns. Testosterone stimulates growth of bone and skeletal muscle, causing height and weight to increase rapidly. Testosterone also accelerates epiphyseal closure, causing bone growth to cease within a few years. The larynx enlarges, thereby deepening the voice. Sebaceous glands increase in number, causing the skin to become oily; acne results if the glands become clogged and infected. The final pubertal change is beard development. Several years are required for all of these changes to occur.

Spermatogenesis. Androgens are necessary for production of sperm by the seminiferous tubules and for maturation of sperm as they pass through the epididymis and vas deferens. Androgen deficiency causes sterility.

Effects on Sex Characteristics in Females

Under physiologic conditions, endogenous androgens have only moderate effects in females. Principal among these are promotion of clitoral growth and, perhaps, maintenance of normal libido. However, when production of androgens becomes excessive (e.g., in girls with congenital adrenal hyperplasia), virilization can take place. Virilization can also occur in response to therapeutic use of androgens or to androgen abuse.

Anabolic Effects

Testosterone promotes growth of skeletal muscle. This anabolic effect results from the binding of androgens to the same type of receptor that mediates androgen actions in other tissues. Effects in young males, and in females of any age, can be dramatic. In contrast, effects in healthy adult males are modest. The testes of adult males already produce enough testosterone to cause near-maximal stimulation of the musculature, so in adult males the increment in muscle mass that can be achieved with exogenous androgens is relatively small.

Erythropoietic Effects

Testosterone promotes the synthesis of erythropoietin, a hormone that acts on bone marrow to increase the production of erythrocytes (red blood cells). This action of testosterone, together with the high levels of testosterone present in males, explains why men have a higher hematocrit than women. When women are given testosterone, the hematocrit rises and hemoglobin levels increase by an average of 4.3 gm/dL. In contrast, because men have high testosterone levels to begin with, the increase in plasma hemoglobin that can be elicited with exogenous androgens is smaller—only 1 gm/dL.

Safety Alert

THROMBOSIS RISK

The erythropoietic effects of testosterone have resulted in an increased risk for thrombosis leading to stroke, myocardial infarction, and subsequent death. This led the U.S. Food and Drug Administration (FDA) to issue a Testosterone Product Safety Alert in February 2014.

CLINICAL PHARMACOLOGY OF THE ANDROGENS

In addition to testosterone, a few other androgens are employed clinically. All of these agents can bind to androgen receptors, and therefore all can elicit similar responses. Major differences among individual androgens pertain to route of administration, pharmacokinetics, adverse effects, and specific applications.

Classification

The androgens used clinically fall into two basic groups: (1) testosterone and testosterone esters, and (2) 17-alpha-alkylated compounds (noted for their hepatotoxicity). Androgens belonging to each group are shown in Table 65.1.

When speaking of testosterone-like compounds, it is traditional to distinguish between "androgens" and "anabolic steroids." However, we will not make this distinction because

TABLE 65.1 ■ Approved Uses of Individual Androgens

	Indications			
Androgen	Hypogonadism (Male)	Replacement Therapy (Male)	Delayed Puberty (Male)	Catabolic States
TESTOSTERONE AND TESTOSTERONE ESTERS				
Testosterone	✓	✓	✓	
Testosterone cypionate	✓	✓	✓	
Testosterone enanthate	✓	✓	✓	
17-ALPHA-ALKYLATED ANDROGENS				
Fluoxymesterone	✓	✓	✓	
Methyltestosterone	✓	✓	✓	
Oxandrolone				✓

it is now clear that the receptor type that mediates the androgenic actions of the androgens is the same receptor type that mediates the anabolic actions of these hormones. Consequently, it has not been possible to separate anabolic activity from androgenic activity: Virtually all anabolic hormones are also androgenic. Accordingly, rather than creating two categories—androgens versus anabolic steroids—and assigning some agents to one category and some to the other, we will refer to all of the testosterone-like drugs as androgens.

PATIENT-CENTERED CARE ACROSS THE LIFE SPAN

Androgens

Life Stage	Patient Care Concerns
Children	Androgens can cause virilization in children. They can also accelerate epiphyseal closure, thereby decreasing adult height.
Pregnant women	Androgens are Pregnancy Risk Category X.[a] The ability to cause fetal harm outweighs any possible therapeutic benefit. Potential fetal changes include vaginal malformation, clitoral enlargement, and formation of a structure resembling the male scrotum. Virilization is most likely when androgens are taken during the first trimester. Women who become pregnant while using androgens should be informed about the possible impact on the fetus.
Breast-feeding women	Testosterone is excreted in breast milk. Breast-feeding is contraindicated.
Older adults	Older patients are at an increased risk for thromboembolic conditions such as myocardial infarction or stroke. Beers Criteria identify testosterone and methyltestosterone as potentially inappropriate for patients 65 years of age and older.

[a]As of 2020, the FDA will no longer use Pregnancy Risk Categories. Please refer to Chapter 9 for more information.

Therapeutic Uses

Individual androgens differ in their applications. No single androgen is employed for all of the uses discussed in this section. Specific applications of individual androgens are shown in Table 65.1.

In April 2015, the FDA published a required label change for testosterone. (See http://www.fda.gov/Drugs/DrugSafety/ucm436259.htm.) The new labeling approves testosterone use only for those patients with confirmed testosterone deficiency due to hypogonadism. The FDA further emphasized that lowered testosterone due to aging did not meet criteria for hypogonadism. Still, androgens are commonly prescribed off-label.

Male Hypogonadism

Hypogonadism is a condition in which the testes fail to produce adequate amounts of testosterone. Male hypogonadism may be hereditary, or it may result from other causes, including pituitary failure, hypothalamic failure, and primary dysfunction of the testes.

When complete hypogonadism occurs in boys, puberty cannot take place—unless exogenous androgens are supplied. To induce puberty, a long-acting parenteral preparation (*testosterone enanthate* or *testosterone cypionate*) is chosen. Under the influence of these androgens, the normal sequence of pubertal changes occurs: growth is accelerated, the penis enlarges, the voice deepens, and other secondary sex characteristics become expressed. As in normal males, these changes take place over several years.

Replacement Therapy

Androgen replacement therapy is beneficial when testicular failure occurs in adult males. Some studies have demonstrated that treatment restores libido, increases ejaculate volume, and supports expression of secondary sex characteristics. However, treatment will not restore fertility. The principal drugs employed for testosterone replacement are testosterone itself and two testosterone esters: testosterone enanthate and testosterone cypionate. Preparations and dosages for replacement therapy are shown in Table 65.2.

Delayed Puberty

In some boys, puberty fails to occur at the usual age (i.e., before age 15 years). Most often, this failure reflects a familial pattern of delayed puberty and does not indicate pathology. Puberty can be expected to occur spontaneously, but later than usual. Hence, treatment is not an absolute necessity. However, some providers will prescribe a limited course of androgen therapy off-label if the psychologic pressures of delayed sexual maturation are greater than a boy can tolerate. Both fluoxymesterone [Androxy] and methyltestosterone [Android, Methitest, Testred] are used for this purpose. If delayed puberty is the result of true hypogonadism, long-term replacement therapy is indicated.

Replacement Therapy in Menopausal Women

Testosterone replacement therapy can alleviate some menopausal symptoms, especially fatigue, reduced libido, and reduced genital sensitivity. Additionally, the North American Menopause Society notes that testosterone can have a positive effect on sexual function and that women with no other identifiable cause of decreased desire may be candidates for testosterone therapy, provided that estrogen is taken as well. Regardless, testosterone is not approved for replacement in women in the United States, although it is approved in the United Kingdom. When prescribed off-label, it must be prescribed at doses lower than that used for men. The goal is to mimic premenopausal testosterone production—about 300 mcg/day.

Treatment of Transsexualism

Testosterone is used as masculinizing therapy for patients who are born with a female body but who self-identify as male. Anticipated effects are an increase in hair growth over the face and body, a deepening of the voice, breast tissue atrophy, and cessation of menses. An increase in muscle tissue relative to adipose tissue also occurs. Therapy is highly individualized by specialists in transgender health.

Cachexia

Cachexia is a wasting of the body associated with severe illnesses such as AIDS, severe trauma, and chronic systemic infections. Testosterone levels often decline in these patients, putting them at risk for wasting and loss of muscle mass. Testosterone therapy decreases this risk. Oxandrolone [Oxandrin], an anabolic steroid that is a synthetic derivative of testosterone, is FDA-approved for this purpose.

TABLE 65.2 ▪ Products for Androgen Replacement Therapy in Hypogonadal Males

Formulation	Drug	Brand Name	Dosage	CSA Schedule	Administration Comments
Oral Tablet	Fluoxymesterone Methyltestosterone	Androxy Android, Methitest, Testred	5–20 once daily 10–50 mg once daily	III	Administer with or without food.
Intramuscular Injection	Testosterone cypionate Testosterone enanthate	Depo-Testosterone Delatestryl	50–400 mg every 2–4 wk 50–400 mg every 2–4 wk	III	Inject deep into the muscle. Alternate sites.
Transdermal Patch	Testosterone	Androderm	One patch/day (delivers 2 or 4 mg/24 hr)	III	Apply to the arm, back, abdomen, or thigh, but *not* the scrotum. Causes local irritation.
Transdermal Gel	Testosterone	AndroGel, Testim Fortesta	5–10 gm of 1% gel once daily (delivers 50–100 mg/day) 40–70 mg of 2% gel once daily	III	Apply AndroGel to upper arm, shoulder, or abdomen, but *not* the scrotum. Apply Testim only to upper arm or shoulder. Apply Fortesta to the front and inner thigh.
Transdermal Topical Solution	Testosterone	Axiron	60–180 mg once daily	III	Apply to axilla at the same time each morning.
Nasal Gel	Testosterone	Natesto	11 mg (2 pump actuations) per nostril three times daily. (Each actuation delivers 5.5 mg of testosterone)	III	Insert actuator fully into nostril, tilting so that the tip makes contact with the lateral nostril wall. Depress slowly and fully. Wipe tip against lateral side of nostril during removal.
Implantable Pellets	Testosterone	Testopel	150–450 mg (2–6 pellets) subQ every 3–6 months	III	Implanted surgically.
Buccal System	Testosterone	Striant	One buccal system (30 mg) every 12 hr	III	Push curved side against upper gum above incisor. To ensure adhesion, press on upper lip to hold in place for 30 seconds.

CSA, Controlled Substances Act.

Although oxandrolone can be helpful, it is not without significant risks. It can cause peliosis hepatitis, a condition in which blood-filled cysts form in the liver, leading to liver failure or intra-abdominal hemorrhage. It can also contribute to the development of highly vascular liver tumors. An increase in the risk for atherosclerosis can occur secondary to marked elevations in LDL and decreases in HDL.

Anemias

Androgens are sometimes used in men and women to treat anemias that have been refractory to other therapy. Anemias most likely to respond include aplastic anemia, anemia associated with renal failure, Fanconi's anemia, and anemia caused by cancer chemotherapy. Androgens help relieve anemia by promoting the synthesis of erythropoietin, the renal hormone that stimulates production of red blood cells. Androgens may also stimulate production of white blood cells and platelets. With the emergence of other therapies such as erythropoietin-stimulating agents, however, androgens have fallen out of favor for off-label treatment of anemia.

Adverse Effects

Virilization in Women, Girls, and Boys

Virilization is the most common complication of androgen therapy. When taken in high doses by women, androgens can cause acne, deepening of the voice, proliferation of facial and body hair, male-pattern baldness, increased libido, clitoral enlargement, and menstrual irregularities. Clitoral growth, hair loss, and lowering of the voice may be irreversible. Masculinization can also occur in children. Boys may experience growth of pubic hair, penile enlargement, increased frequency of erections, and even priapism (persistent erection). In girls, growth of pubic hair and clitoral enlargement may occur. To prevent irreversible masculinization, androgens must be discontinued when virilizing effects first appear.

Safety Alert

UNINTENDED DRUG TRANSFER

Secondary exposure to testosterone gel on uncovered skin and to testosterone gel on unwashed clothing has resulted in virilization in children.

Premature Epiphyseal Closure

When given to children, androgens can accelerate epiphyseal closure, thereby decreasing adult height. To evaluate androgen effects on the epiphyses, radiographic examination of the hand and wrist should be performed every 6 months.

Hepatotoxicity

Androgens can cause *cholestatic hepatitis* and other disorders of the liver. Clinical *jaundice* may occur, but is rare. Patients receiving androgens should undergo periodic tests of liver function. If jaundice develops, it will reverse after discontinuation of androgen use. Androgens may also be carcinogenic: *Hepatocellular carcinoma* has developed in some patients after prolonged use of these drugs.

It must be emphasized that not all androgens are hepatotoxic: Liver damage is associated primarily with the *17-alpha-alkylated androgens.* These androgens all share a structural feature in common: an alkyl group substituted on carbon 17 of the steroid nucleus. Because of their capacity to cause liver damage, *the 17-alpha-alkylated compounds should not be used long term.* In contrast to the 17-alpha-alkylated androgens, testosterone and the testosterone esters (testosterone cypionate, testosterone enanthate) are not associated with liver disease.

Effects on Cholesterol Levels

Androgens can lower plasma levels of high-density lipoprotein (HDL) cholesterol ("good cholesterol") and elevate plasma levels of low-density lipoprotein (LDL) cholesterol ("bad cholesterol"). These actions may increase the risk for atherosclerosis and related cardiovascular events.

Use in Pregnancy

Because of their ability to induce masculinization of the female fetus, androgens are contraindicated during pregnancy. Potential fetal changes include vaginal malformation, clitoral enlargement, and formation of a structure resembling the male scrotum. Virilization is most likely when androgens are taken during the first trimester. Women who become pregnant while using androgens should be informed about the possible impact on the fetus. The ability to cause fetal harm outweighs any possible therapeutic benefit.

Prostate Cancer

Androgens do not cause prostate cancer, but they can promote the growth of this cancer once it occurs. Accordingly, androgens are contraindicated for men with diagnosed prostate cancer. Men without diagnosed prostate cancer should be monitored for emergence of covert cancer.

Edema

Edema can result from androgen-induced retention of salt and water. This complication is a concern for patients with heart failure and for those with a predisposition to developing edema from other causes. Treatment consists of discontinuing the androgen and giving a diuretic, if needed.

Abuse Potential

Androgens are frequently misused (abused) to enhance athletic performance. Because of their abuse potential, nearly all androgens are regulated as Schedule III controlled substances.

Hazardous Agents and Special Administration Requirements

The National Institute for Occupational Safety and Health identifies androgens as hazardous drugs. Pregnant nurses who are exposed to the drug during administration may experience adverse events. See Chapter 3, Table 3.1, for special handling requirements for preparation, administration, and disposal of these drugs.

ANDROGEN PREPARATIONS FOR MALE HYPOGONADISM

Treatment options for androgen replacement therapy have expanded in recent years. In the past, intramuscular (IM) therapy with a long-acting testosterone ester was the major treatment mode. Today, we have six attractive alternatives: a nasal gel, transdermal patches, transdermal gels, a transdermal topical solution, buccal tablets, and implantable subcutaneous pellets. All of these formulations are regulated as Schedule III controlled substances.

Oral Androgens

Only two androgens are approved for oral therapy of male hypogonadism. Despite the advantages of cost and ease of administration, these are not first-line agents. The androgenic effects of oral androgens are erratic. Furthermore, both drugs—*fluoxymesterone* and *methyltestosterone*—are *17-alpha-alkylated androgens*, and therefore pose a risk for hepatotoxicity. Accordingly, they also should not be used long term.

Transdermal Testosterone

Testosterone is available in three transdermal formulations: patches, gels, and a liquid. With all three formulations, testosterone is absorbed through the skin and then slowly absorbed into the blood.

Patches

Testosterone patches [Androderm] are indicated for male hypogonadism. Two strengths are available, delivering 2 mg or 4 mg of testosterone in 24 hours. Patches are applied once daily to the upper arm, thigh, back, or abdomen. The principal adverse effect is rash at the site of application.

Gels

Testosterone is available in four gel formulations, sold as *AndroGel, Testim, Fortesta,* and *Vogelxo.* AndroGel contains 1% or 1.62% testosterone; Testim contains 1% testosterone; and Fortesta contains 2% testosterone. Vogelxo is available in both unit-dose tubes and multidose metered pumps. Each unit-dose tube provides 50 mg testosterone. Each actuation of the pump provides 12.5 mg testosterone. All four gels are applied once daily to treat male hypogonadism. After the gel is applied, testosterone is absorbed rapidly into the skin, and then slowly into the blood over the next 24 hours. Compared with transdermal patches, the gels have three advantages: They (1) cause less local irritation, (2) can't fall off, and (3) produce more consistent testosterone levels.

The principal disadvantage of the gels is that testosterone can be transferred to others by skin-to-skin contact. This is possible because only 10% of an applied dose is absorbed; the other 90% remains on the skin after the gel dries. In one study, blood levels of testosterone were doubled in female partners of gel users after 15 minutes of intimate contact that occurred 2 to 12 hours after the gel had been applied. Testosterone transfer is a concern because the drug can cause virilization of female partners and can also cause fetal harm. In children, contact transfer can cause genital enlargement, premature development of pubic hair, advanced bone age, increased libido, and aggressive behavior. In most cases, these effects regress after testosterone exposure stops. To reduce the risk for unintended gel transfer, the following guidelines should be followed:

- Gel users should wash their hands with soap and warm water after every application.
- Gel users should cover the application site with clothing after the gel has dried.
- Gel users should wash the application site before skin-to-skin contact with another person.
- Women and children should avoid skin-to-skin contact with application sites on gel users.

- Women and children who make accidental contact with a gel application site should wash contaminated skin immediately.

AndroGel is supplied in a metered-dose pump that delivers 12.25 mg per actuation (1%) or 20.25 mg per actuation (1.62%) and in unit-dose foil packets containing 20.25 mg of testosterone (of which 2.5 mg becomes absorbed) and 40.5 mg of testosterone (of which 5 mg becomes absorbed). The gel is applied once daily (preferably in the morning) to clean, dry skin of the shoulders, upper arms, or abdomen—but *not* the genitalia. Instruct patients to squeeze the entire contents of the packet into the palms, and then to immediately apply the gel to the skin and rub it in. To prevent the transfer of testosterone to others, patients should wash their hands and, once the gel has dried, keep the treated area covered with clothing. Because testosterone can be washed off, patients should wait 5 to 6 hours before showering or swimming. To ensure safe and effective dosing, blood levels of testosterone should be measured 14 days after initiating therapy and periodically thereafter.

Testim is available in 5-gm tubes that contain 50 mg of testosterone, of which 10% (5 mg) gets absorbed. It is applied once daily to the skin of the shoulders or upper arms, but not to the abdomen or scrotum. As with AndroGel, patients should wash their hands immediately and keep the treated area covered. They should also avoid showering for at least 2 hours. Testosterone levels should be checked after 14 days and periodically thereafter.

Fortesta is supplied in a metered-dose pump that delivers 10 mg of testosterone per actuation. All doses are applied to the front or inner thigh. As with AndroGel, patients should wash their hands immediately and keep the treated area covered. Also, they should avoid swimming or showering for at least 2 hours. Fortesta is a flammable, alcohol-based formulation, and hence patients should avoid flames or smoking until the gel has dried. Testosterone levels should be checked after days 14 and 35 and periodically thereafter.

Vogelxo in the tube formulation is applied in the same manner as Testim. Vogelxo in the metered-dose pump is applied just as Fortesta is applied. For both, the same advice and precautions apply.

Topical Solution

Testosterone topical solution for underarm application [Axiron] is much like the testosterone gels. The principal difference is the application site: Axiron liquid is formulated specifically for application to the axilla (armpit, underarm), whereas Testim is applied to the shoulder or upper arm, and AndroGel is applied to the shoulder, upper arm, or abdomen. After application, testosterone is absorbed rapidly into the skin, and then slowly into the blood. Steady-state levels are reached in 14 days. After application stops, blood levels take 7 to 10 days to decline to baseline.

Axiron is supplied as an alcohol-based solution in a metered-dose pump that delivers 30 mg of testosterone per actuation. Dosing is done by pumping the liquid onto an applicator (supplied with the pump), and then applying the liquid to clean, dry intact skin of the underarm—and not to anyplace else. Patients should not swim or bathe for 2 hours after application. If an underarm deodorant or antiperspirant is used, it should be applied before applying testosterone (to avoid contaminating the deodorant or antiperspirant dispenser). Because of its alcohol content, Axiron liquid is flammable. Accordingly, users should stay away from flames until the solution has dried.

Axiron is applied to each axilla at the same time every morning. After 14 days or longer, blood levels of testosterone are measured, and dosage is adjusted up or down as indicated.

Like the testosterone gels, testosterone topical solution can be transferred to others through skin-to-skin contact, posing a risk to women and children. Accordingly, the same guidelines noted previously should be followed. That is, Axiron users should wash their hands after every application, cover the application site with clothing after the solution has dried, and wash the application site before anticipated skin-to-skin contact with another person. Women and children should avoid contact with skin where Axiron was applied, and should wash contaminated skin if accidental contact with an application site occurs.

Nasal Gel

Testosterone nasal gel [Natesto] is the newest formulation approved for testosterone administration. It comes in a metered-dose pump that sprays 5.5 mg of testosterone each time the pump is actuated.

Because the drug is administered nasally, patients with nasal disorders or abnormalities (e.g., chronic sinusitis, a severely deviated nasal septum) should not take this drug. There has not been adequate testing for interactions with other nasally administered drugs. Currently, only adrenergic agonists (e.g., oxymetazoline nasal spray) are approved for administration with Natesto.

The route of administration can cause localized reactions. These include rhinorrhea, epistaxis, and nasopharyngitis; however, these tend to be modest effects.

Administration instructions are supplied with the drug; however, it is important that the provider be aware of these in order to answer patient questions.

1. The pump should be primed before use and excess gel removed.
2. The patient should blow the nose before administration.
3. The pump is inserted into the nostril with the tip aimed toward the lateral nostril wall.
4. The pump is depressed slowly until it stops.
5. As the tip is withdrawn, it should be wiped against the lateral nostril wall to ensure that any remaining gel is distributed to the nostril.
6. After administration in both nostrils, the nose should be lightly massaged below the nasal bridge.
7. The patient should avoid blowing or sniffing for at least 1 hour after administration.

Implantable Testosterone Pellets

Testosterone pellets [Testopel] are long-acting formulations indicated for male hypogonadism and delayed puberty. The pellets are implanted subdermally in the hip area or abdominal wall lateral to the umbilicus. Each pellet contains 75 mg of testosterone. The usual dosage is 150 to 450 mg (2 to 6 pellets) every 3 to 6 months. About one-third of the dose is absorbed the first month, one-fourth the second month, and one-sixth the third month. For patients switching from IM testosterone propionate or IM testosterone enanthate, the recommended dosage is 2 pellets for each 25 mg of IM testosterone used weekly. For example, a patient receiving 75 mg of IM testosterone enanthate each week would switch to 6 pellets every 3 to 4 months.

Testosterone Buccal Tablets

Testosterone buccal tablets [Striant], approved for male hypogonadism, produce steady blood levels of testosterone. Tablets are applied to the gum area just above the incisor tooth, and are designed to stay in place until removed. To ensure good adhesion, tablets should be held in place (with a finger over the lip) for 30 seconds. The recommended dosage is 1 tablet every 12 hours, alternating sides of the mouth with each dose. If a tablet falls out before 8 hours, it should be replaced with a new one for the remainder of the dosing interval. If a tablet falls out after 8 hours, it should be replaced with a new one, and the next scheduled dose should be skipped (i.e., the replacement tablet should remain in place for 16 hours or so). The tablets are not affected by eating, drinking, chewing gum, or brushing teeth. Adverse effects, which are usually transient, include local irritation, bitter taste, and taste distortion. Treatment for up to 1 year has not caused serious gum changes. It has been hypothesized that transfer of testosterone from buccal routes may occur through saliva transfer during kissing.

Intramuscular Testosterone Esters

Two IM testosterone esters are available: *testosterone cypionate* [Depo-Testosterone] and *testosterone enanthate* [Delatestryl]. Both drugs are formulated in oil, and both are long acting. After IM injection, these drugs are slowly absorbed and then hydrolyzed to release free testosterone. For replacement therapy in hypogonadal males, the usual dosage for both is 50 to 400 mg IM every 2 to 4 weeks. Unfortunately, these preparations produce testosterone blood levels that vary widely. Testosterone levels are higher than normal immediately after dosing, and the levels decline to lower than normal before the next dose. As a result, patients may experience significant variations in libido, energy, and mood.

ANDROGEN (ANABOLIC STEROID) ABUSE BY ATHLETES

Many athletes take androgens (anabolic steroids) and androgen precursors to enhance athletic performance. The potential benefits of this practice, although substantial, are accompanied by significant risks. Drugs commonly used by athletes include nandrolone, stanozolol, and methenolone. All of these drugs are regulated as controlled substances, making their use without a prescription illegal.

Who takes steroids? Steroid use is especially prevalent among baseball players, football players, weight lifters, discus throwers, shot-putters, and bodybuilders. These drugs are also used by sprinters and athletes in endurance sports (e.g., cycling, Nordic skiing). Steroids are used by athletes of all ages. This includes professionals, as well as athletes in college, high school, and junior high. Use is not limited to males; some females also take them, despite masculinizing effects.

What can anabolic steroids do for the athlete? Exogenous androgens can significantly increase muscle mass and strength in *males and females of all ages when given in sufficiently large doses.* After 10 weeks, one study showed that testosterone treatment produced a 7-pound increase in muscle mass in subjects who did not exercise, and a 13-pound increase in subjects who exercised and took the drug. In contrast, exercise in the absence of exogenous testosterone produced only a 4-pound increase in muscle mass. Similar increases were shown in the subjects' ability to bench-press weights. However, the potential for adverse effects of androgens is substantial. Salt and water retention can lead to hypertension. When administered in the high doses used by athletes, androgens suppress release of LH and FSH, resulting in testicular shrinkage, sterility, and gynecomastia (breast development). Acne is common. Reduction of HDL cholesterol and elevation of LDL cholesterol may theoretically accelerate development of atherosclerosis (although no effect was seen on lipids in the study just noted). Because most of the androgens that athletes take are 17-alpha-alkylated compounds, hepatotoxicity (cholestatic hepatitis, jaundice, hepatocellular carcinoma) is an ever-present risk. Most recently, androgens have been linked with kidney damage. In females, androgens can cause menstrual irregularities and virilization (growth of facial hair, deepening of the voice, decreased breast size, uterine atrophy, clitoral enlargement, and male-pattern baldness); hair loss on scalp, growth of hair on face, and voice change may be irreversible. In boys and girls, androgens promote premature epiphyseal closure, reducing attainable adult height. In boys, androgens can induce premature puberty.

What about psychological effects? Androgens are reputed to cause depression, manic episodes, and aggressiveness. There have been very few controlled studies to measure psychological effects of androgens; however, in controlled studies, dosages of androgens were often less than those typically taken by athletes. Surveys of athletes who engage in anabolic steroid use indicate an association with risky behavior and aggression; however, it is possible that these were inherent traits of the surveyed athletes regardless of steroid use.

Long-term androgen use can lead to an abuse syndrome. Characteristics include preoccupation with androgen use and difficulty in stopping use. When androgens finally are discontinued, an abstinence syndrome can develop similar to that produced by withdrawal of alcohol, opioids, and cocaine.

Because of their abuse potential, anabolic steroids are classified as Schedule III substances under an amendment to the Controlled Substances Act. (Schedule III drugs are defined as those with a low to moderate potential for dependence.) For more information on drug abuse in sports, a good place to start is www.wada-ama.org, the web site of the World Anti-Doping Agency. This organization is dedicated to promoting, coordinating, and monitoring the fight against the use of anabolic steroids and other banned substances in sports. Other good resources include the United States Anti-Doping Agency (http://www.usada.org) and the National Center for Drug-Free Sport (http://www.drugfreesport.com/index.asp).

KEY POINTS

- Testosterone is the principal endogenous androgen.
- Important physiologic effects of androgens are pubertal transformation in males, maintenance of adult male sexual characteristics, promotion of muscle growth, and stimulation of erythropoiesis.
- The major indication (and only FDA-approved indication) for androgens is male hypogonadism.
- The major side effects of androgens are edema, virilization in females, premature epiphyseal closure in children, and liver toxicity (in people taking 17-alpha-alkylated androgens).
- Androgens are contraindicated during pregnancy, owing to a risk for injury to the female fetus.
- Large doses of androgens can increase muscle mass and strength in athletes. However, athletic use of androgens is illegal and can cause significant harm.

Please visit **http://evolve.elsevier.com/Lehne** for chapter-specific NCLEX® examination review questions.

Summary of Major Nursing Implications[a]

ANDROGENS

Fluoxymesterone
Methyltestosterone
Oxandrolone
Testosterone
Testosterone cypionate
Testosterone enanthate

Preadministration Assessment

Therapeutic Goals

Males. Treatment of hypogonadism is the only FDA-approved use for androgen therapy. It is sometimes prescribed off-label for delayed puberty.

Females. Androgens are sometimes prescribed off-label for the relief of menopausal symptoms, especially fatigue, decreased libido, and decreased genital sensitivity.

Males and Females. Androgens may be prescribed off-label for the treatment of anemias. One form, oxandrolone, is approved for management of catabolic states. It may be prescribed for people who have the physical characteristics of women but who self-identify as male.

Identifying High-Risk Patients

Androgens are *contraindicated* for pregnant women, for men who have prostate cancer or breast cancer, and for enhancing athletic performance.

Implementation: Administration

Routes

PO, IM, buccal, subQ (implantable pellets), and transdermal (gel, patch, topical solution).

Administration

Oral. Advise patients to take oral androgens with food if gastrointestinal (GI) upset occurs.

Transdermal Gel and Solution. Advise patients to wash their hands after applying the gel and to cover the site of application with clothing to prevent transferring testosterone to others. Instruct patients not to shower or swim for several hours (to avoid washing the drug off). Warn users of the topical solution to avoid being near flames until the liquid has evaporated.

Buccal. Instruct patients to apply buccal tablets to the gum just above the upper incisor tooth, and to apply pressure (using a finger on the lip) to ensure good adhesion.

Implantable Pellets. Pellets are implanted subdermally (under local anesthesia) in the hip region or in the abdominal wall lateral to the umbilicus.

Nasal. Instruct patients to blow the nose before using, apply to the lateral nostril wall of both nares, massage the nose after administration, and avoid sniffing or blowing for at least 1 hour after administration.

Ongoing Evaluation and Interventions

Minimizing Adverse Effects

Virilization. Virilization may occur in women, girls, and boys. Inform female patients about signs of virilization (deepening of the voice, acne, changes in body and facial hair, menstrual irregularities), and instruct them to notify the prescriber if these occur. Irreversible changes may be avoided if androgens are withdrawn early.

Premature Epiphyseal Closure. Accelerated bone maturation in children can decrease attainable adult height. Monitor effects on epiphyses with radiographs of the hand and wrist twice yearly.

Hepatotoxicity. The *17-alpha-alkylated androgens* can cause cholestatic hepatitis, jaundice, and other liver disorders. Rarely, liver cancer develops. Obtain periodic tests of liver function. Inform patients about signs of liver dysfunction (jaundice, malaise, anorexia, fatigue, nausea), and instruct them to notify the prescriber if these occur. Liver function normalizes after cessation of drug use. Avoid long-term use of 17-alpha-alkylated preparations.

Edema. Salt and water retention may result in edema. Inform patients about signs of salt and water retention (swelling of the extremities, unusual weight gain), and instruct them to notify the prescriber if these occur. Treatment consists of androgen withdrawal and, if necessary, use of a diuretic.

Teratogenesis. Androgens can cause masculinization of the female fetus. Rule out pregnancy before androgen use. Warn women against becoming pregnant while taking androgens.

Prostate Cancer. Avoid androgens in men with diagnosed prostate cancer. In men without diagnosed prostate cancer, monitor for exacerbation of pre-existing but covert prostate cancer.

Injury From Skin-to-Skin Transfer of Topical Testosterone. Topical testosterone—applied as a gel or topical solution—can transfer to others through skin-to-skin contact. It has been hypothesized that transfer of testosterone from buccal routes may occur through saliva transfer during kissing. Transfer of testosterone to women can cause masculinization, as well as fetal harm if the woman is pregnant. Transfer to children can cause genital enlargement (penis or clitoris), premature development of pubic hair, advanced bone age, increased libido, and aggressive behavior. To minimize the risk for accidental skin-to-skin transfer, advise users of testosterone gel or testosterone topical solution to (1) wash their hands after every application, (2) cover the application site with clothing once the gel has dried, and (3) wash the application site before anticipated contact with another person. Also, advise women and children to avoid contact with skin where testosterone was applied, and advise them to wash contaminated skin if accidental contact with an application site should occur.

[a]Patient education information is highlighted as **blue text.**

CHAPTER

66 Drugs for Erectile Dysfunction and Benign Prostatic Hyperplasia

ERECTILE DYSFUNCTION

Erectile dysfunction (ED) is defined as a persistent inability to achieve or sustain an erection suitable for satisfactory sexual performance. In the United States, ED affects up to 30 million men. ED is commonly associated with chronic illnesses, especially diabetes, hypertension, and depression. Among men with diabetes, the incidence of ED is between 35% and 75%. Some of the drugs that can cause ED are shown in Table 66.1.

The risk for ED increases with advancing age. According to the National Institutes of Health, ED affects approximately 4% of men in their 50s. Just a decade later, 17% of men in their 60s are unable to achieve any erection at all. This total inability to achieve erection affects 47% of men older than 75 years. Fortunately, new advances in medicine can rectify this problem for most patients.

First-line treatments for ED are lifestyle measures (increased exercise, smoking cessation), changing drug regimens to remove the drugs that may cause ED, and drug therapy with sildenafil [Viagra] or another drug in its class. Other interventions include psychotherapy and surgical implantation of a penile prosthesis.

PHYSIOLOGY OF ERECTION

Before discussing drugs for ED, we need to review the physiology of erection. As shown in Fig. 66.1, the process begins with sexual arousal, which increases parasympathetic nerve traffic to the penis, causing local release of nitric oxide. Nitric oxide then activates guanylyl cyclase, an enzyme that makes cyclic guanosine monophosphate (cGMP). Through a series of steps, cGMP promotes relaxation of arterial and trabecular smooth muscle. The resultant arterial dilation increases local blood flow and blood pressure, which, in combination with relaxation of trabecular smooth muscle, causes expansion and engorgement of sinusoidal spaces in the corpus cavernosum. This, in turn, causes venous occlusion and thereby reduces venous outflow. The combination of increased arterial pressure and arterial inflow plus reduced venous outflow causes sufficient engorgement to produce erection. Erection subsides when cGMP is removed by phosphodiesterase type 5 (PDE5), an enzyme that converts cGMP into guanosine monophosphate.

ORAL DRUGS FOR ED: PDE5 INHIBITORS

Drugs for ED fall into two major groups: oral agents and nonoral agents. The oral agents—PDE5 inhibitors—are by far the most common treatments for ED. These will constitute our primary focus. The nonoral agents—papaverine plus phentolamine, alprostadil—are considered briefly. These drugs are summarized in Table 66.2.

Four PDE5 inhibitors are available: sildenafil, tadalafil, vardenafil, and avanafil. All are considered first-line therapy for ED. Current guidelines recommend that, in the absence of a specific contraindication, all men with ED be offered one of these drugs. Which drug is preferred? Only a few trials have compared them head-to-head, so there is insufficient evidence to recommend one over the others. Accordingly, selection among them should be based on patient preference and prescriber judgment.

Sildenafil

Sildenafil [Viagra] was introduced in 1998 as the first oral treatment for ED. The drug is reliable and easy to use. Benefits derive from enhancing the natural response to sexual stimuli; sildenafil does not cause erection directly. Although sildenafil is generally well tolerated, it can be dangerous for

TABLE 66.1 ▪ Some Drugs That Can Cause Sexual/Erectile Dysfunction

Drug Class	Representative Drug [Brand Name]	Incidence of SD/ED[a]
RENAL/CARDIOVASCULAR DRUGS		
Cardiac glycosides	Digoxin [Lanoxin]	36%
Adrenergic neuron blockers	Reserpine	24%–40%
Central alpha$_2$-adrenergic agonists	Methyldopa	20%–30%
Beta blockers	Propranolol [Inderal]	10%–15%
Thiazide diuretics	Hydrochlorothiazide	10%–20%
Aldosterone antagonists	Spironolactone [Aldactone]	4%–30%
CNS DRUGS		
Selective serotonin reuptake inhibitors	Fluoxetine [Prozac]	Up to 70%
Monoamine oxidase inhibitors	Isocarboxazid [Marplan]	16%–31%
Tricyclic antidepressants	Amitriptyline [Elavil]	7%–30%
Antipsychotics	Chlorpromazine [Thorazine]	30%–60%
Mood stabilizers	Lithium [Lithobid]	5%–50%
Social lubricant/intoxicant	Alcohol	50%–75%
UROGENITAL DRUGS		
5-alpha-reductase inhibitors	Finasteride [Proscar]	33%

[a]Values for sexual dysfunction/erectile dysfunction (SD/ED) incidence are estimates based on patient reports, not on carefully controlled trials.

men taking certain vasodilators, specifically alpha-adrenergic blockers, nitroglycerin, and other nitrates used for angina pectoris.

Prototype Drugs

DRUGS FOR ED AND BPH

Drugs for ED

Phosphodiesterase Type 5 Inhibitors
Sildenafil

Nonoral Drugs
Papaverine/phentolamine
Alprostadil

Drugs for BPH

5-Alpha-Reductase Inhibitors
Finasteride

Alpha-Adrenergic Antagonists
Tamsulosin

The erection-enhancing effects of sildenafil were discovered by accident. The drug was developed as a cardiac medicine, but benefits were minimal. However, in the course of testing, some men noticed a surprising side effect: Their ED had been cured! The rest, as they say, is history. Sildenafil has been wildly popular. First-year sales were the hottest in pharmaceutical history. By now, tens of millions of men in more than 100 countries have used the drug. In addition to ED, sildenafil is approved for pulmonary arterial hypertension (PAH) (see Chapter 107).When used for this purpose, sildenafil is sold as *Revatio.*

Mechanism of Action

Sildenafil causes selective inhibition of PDE5. By doing so, it increases and preserves cGMP levels in the penis, thereby making the erection harder and longer lasting. Please note that the drug enhances only the normal erectile response to sexual stimuli (e.g., erotic imagery, fantasies, physical contact). In the absence of sexual stimuli, nothing happens.

Pharmacokinetics

Sildenafil is well absorbed after oral administration. Bioavailability is about 40%. In fasting subjects, plasma levels peak about 1 hour after dosing. A high-fat meal slows absorption, resulting in a peak plasma level in 2 hours (rather than 1) and reducing the peak concentration. Sildenafil is metabolized in the liver, primarily by the 3A4 isoenzyme of cytochrome P450 (CYP3A4). Both the parent drug and its major metabolite (*N*-desmethyl sildenafil) are biologically active. Both compounds are eliminated primarily in the feces (80%) and partly in the urine (13%). For both compounds, the half-life is 4 hours. Clearance of both is delayed in men older than 65 years and in men with hepatic impairment or severe renal insufficiency, causing drug levels to rise higher and persist longer.

Sexual Benefits

In Men With ED. Sildenafil has been evaluated in several thousand men (ages 19 to 87 years) with ED of organic, psychogenic, or mixed-cause origin. At least some improvement in erection hardness and duration was seen in 70% of men taking the drug, compared with 20% taking placebo. Benefits were dose related and lasted up to 4 hours, although they began to fade after 2 hours. Sildenafil was able to help a wide range of patients, including those with ED resulting from diabetes,

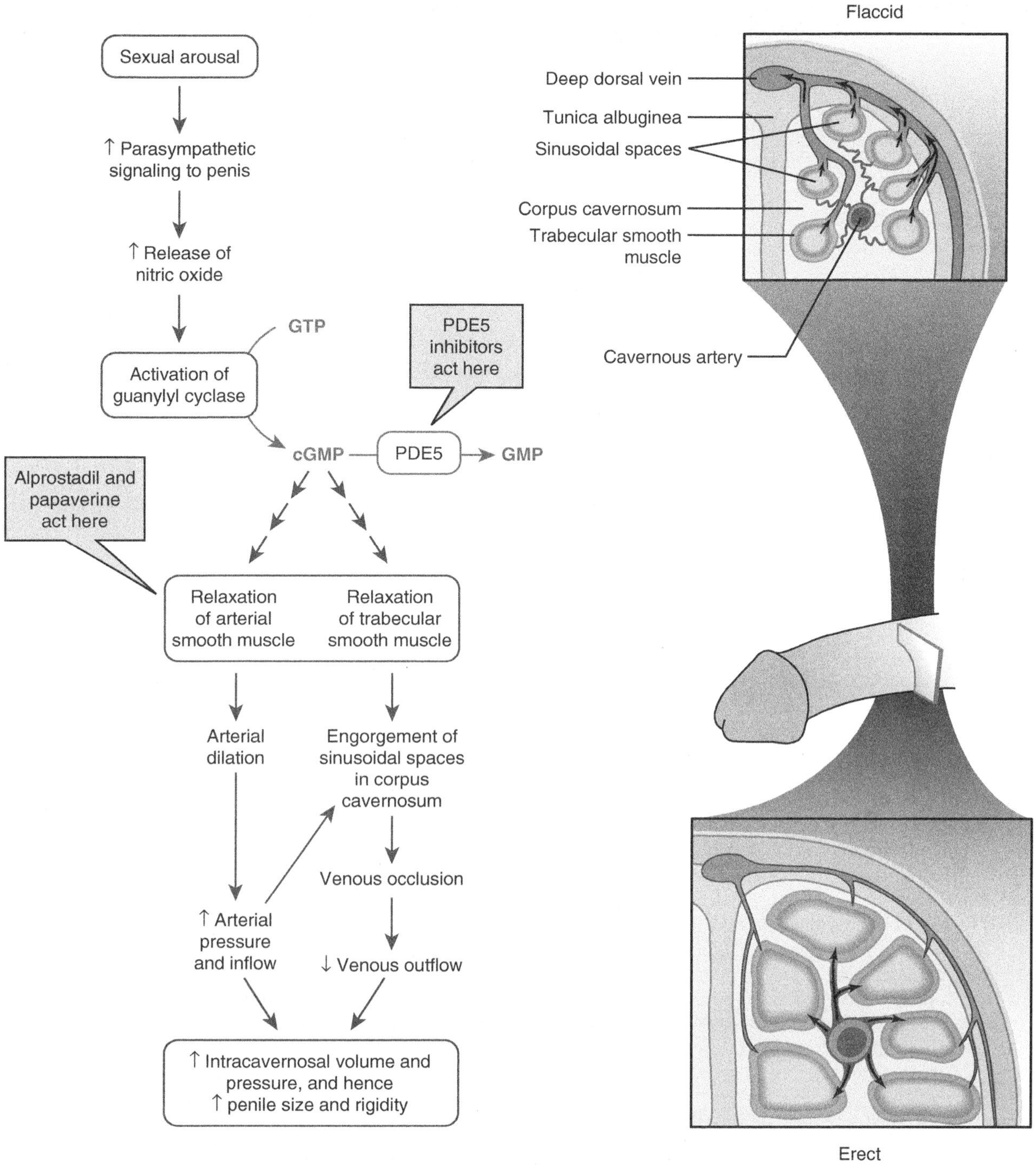

Fig. 66.1 ▪ Physiology of penile erection.
In the flaccid state, there is free outflow of venous blood and restricted inflow of arterial blood. During sexual arousal, cyclic guanosine monophosphate (cGMP) relaxes arterial and trabecular smooth muscle, permitting free inflow of arterial blood and subsequent engorgement of sinusoidal spaces, whose expansion compresses penile veins, restricting blood outflow. The resultant accumulation of blood at elevated pressure increases penile size and rigidity. Removal of cGMP by PDE5 restores penile smooth muscle to the nonaroused state, and detumescence ensues. (*cGMP*, Cyclic guanosine monophosphate; *GMP*, guanosine monophosphate; *GTP*, guanosine triphosphate; *PDE5*, phosphodiesterase type 5.)

TABLE 66.2 ▪ Comparison of PDE5 Inhibitors

	Drug			
Parameter	Sildenafil [Viagra]	Tadalafil [Cialis]	Vardenafil [Levitra, Staxyn]	Avanafil [Stendra]
Date approved	3/27/1998	11/21/2003	8/19/2003	4/28/2012
Dosing schedule	PRN only	PRN *or* once daily	PRN only	PRN
Median time to peak level	1 hr	2 hr	1 hr	30–45 min
Half-life	4 hr	17.5 hr	4–5 hr	5 hr
Duration of action	4 hr	36 hr	4 hr	4 hr
Major mode of metabolism	CYP3A4	CYP3A4	CYP3A4	CYP3A4
Drug interactions				
Nitrates	Contraindicated: Wait 24 hr before giving a nitrate	Contraindicated: Wait 48 hr before giving a nitrate	Contraindicated: Wait 24 hr before giving a nitrate	Contraindicated: Wait 12 hr before giving a nitrate
Alpha blockers	Use with caution	Contraindicated (except for tamsulosin, 0.4 mg once daily)	Contraindicated	Use with caution
CYP3A4 inhibitors	Reduce sildenafil dosage	Reduce tadalafil dosage to no more than 10 mg every 72 hr	Reduce vardenafil dosage	Do not take with strong CYP3A4 inhibitors; reduce dosage with moderate inhibitors
Class I and class III antidysrhythmic drugs	No interaction	No interaction	Vardenafil prolongs the QT interval—avoid class I and class III antidysrhythmics	No interaction

spinal cord injury, and transurethral prostate resection, as well as ED of no known physical cause.

In Men Without ED. Despite anecdotal reports to the contrary, sildenafil has little or no effect on erection quality or duration in men who do not have ED. Any apparent benefits in healthy men are likely the result of a placebo response.

In Women. Sildenafil is not approved for use in women and probably won't be. Although several large-scale studies showed the drug is safe in women, they failed to show much enhancement of sexual arousal. Thus the manufacturer decided not to seek U.S. Food and Drug Administration (FDA) approval for the treatment of female hypoactive sexual desire disorder or any other condition in women.

Adverse Effects

Hypotension. At recommended doses, sildenafil produces a small (8.4/5.5 mm Hg) reduction in blood pressure. However, in men taking nitrates or alpha blockers, severe hypotension can develop.

Priapism. A few cases of priapism (painful erection lasting more than 6 hours) have been reported. If an erection persists more than 4 hours, immediate medical intervention is required. Left untreated, priapism can cause permanent damage of penile tissue. If priapism persists longer than 24 hours, chances are very high that the patient will never be able to have sexual intercourse again. Persistent erection can be relieved by aspirating blood from the corpus cavernosum followed by irrigation with a solution containing a vasoconstrictor (e.g., epinephrine, phenylephrine, metaraminol). If this is unsuccessful, surgery is required.

Nonarteritic Ischemic Optic Neuropathy (NAION). Very rarely, men taking sildenafil have developed NAION, resulting in irreversible blurring or loss of vision. The cause is blockage of blood flow to the optic nerve. In most cases, there were underlying anatomic or vascular risk factors for NAION. Also, although NAION developed during sildenafil use, a direct causal relationship has not been established. Nonetheless, patients with NAION in one eye should not use sildenafil, owing to a potential risk for developing NAION in the other eye.

Sudden Hearing Loss. Very rarely, men taking sildenafil have experienced sudden hearing loss, usually in one ear, sometimes in association with dizziness, vertigo, and tinnitus (ringing in the ears). Hearing loss may be partial or complete. Hearing returned by the time the loss was reported in one-third of cases, but had not returned in the remaining two-thirds. To date, a direct causal relationship between sildenafil and hearing loss has not been established. Nonetheless, the drug is suspected because (1) sudden hearing loss is unusual and (2) it developed when sildenafil was taken. Men who experience sudden hearing loss should discontinue the drug—but only if they are taking it for ED; men taking the drug for PAH should continue treatment.

Other Adverse Effects. The most common adverse effects are headache, flushing, and dyspepsia. Sildenafil may also cause nasal congestion, diarrhea, rash, and dizziness. About 3% of patients experience mild transient visual disturbances (blue color tinge to vision, increased sensitivity to light, blurring). In addition, sildenafil may intensify symptoms of obstructive sleep apnea (perhaps by relaxing pharyngeal muscles and/or dilating pulmonary blood vessels).

Drug Interactions

Nitrates. Both sildenafil and nitrates (e.g., nitroglycerin, isosorbide dinitrate) promote hypotension, and they both do so by increasing cGMP (nitrates increase cGMP formation and sildenafil slows cGMP breakdown). If these drugs are combined, life-threatening hypotension could result. Therefore, *sildenafil is absolutely contraindicated for men taking nitrates.* At least 24 hours should elapse between the last dose of sildenafil and giving a nitrate. If elimination of sildenafil is slowed (owing to a CYP3A4 inhibitor or hepatic or renal impairment), an even longer time should elapse before nitrate use.

Alpha Blockers. Alpha-adrenergic antagonists—including doxazosin [Cardura] and other alpha blockers used for prostatic hyperplasia (discussed later)—dilate arterioles and can thereby lower blood pressure. Combined use with sildenafil has caused symptomatic postural hypotension. Accordingly, these combinations should be used with caution.

Inhibitors of CYP3A4. Inhibitors of CYP3A4 (e.g., ketoconazole, itraconazole, erythromycin, cimetidine, saquinavir, ritonavir, grapefruit juice) can suppress metabolism of sildenafil, thereby increasing its levels. These combinations should be used with caution.

Is Sildenafil Safe for Men With CHD?

Reports of adverse cardiovascular events, including at least 130 cardiac deaths, raised concern about the safety of sildenafil in men with coronary heart disease (CHD). However, there was a question as to what caused the adverse events: sildenafil or the sexual activity that sildenafil permitted. When attempting to answer this question, researchers made two important observations: First, giving sildenafil to resting men with severe CHD produced no harmful effects on coronary blood flow or any other hemodynamic parameter. Second, in men with stable CHD who were performing exercise, sildenafil had no effect on CHD symptoms, exercise tolerance, or exercise-induced ischemia. Taken together, these results suggest that, in men with CHD, sexual activity—and not sildenafil—is the likely cause of ischemic events. However, even though sildenafil itself appears safe for men with CHD, sexual activity may not be. Accordingly, the drug should be used with caution by men with the following conditions:

- Myocardial infarction, stroke, or life-threatening dysrhythmia within the past 6 months
- Resting hypotension (blood pressure below 90/50 mm Hg)
- Resting hypertension (blood pressure above 170/110 mm Hg)
- Heart failure
- Unstable angina

In addition, sildenafil should not be used at all by men taking nitroglycerin or any other drug in the nitrate family.

To reduce the risk for adverse events, candidates for sildenafil therapy should undergo a careful evaluation of cardiovascular function. Those with impaired function should be counseled about the risks posed by sexual activity and all other moderate to intense physical activity.

Preparations, Dosage, and Administration

For treatment of ED, sildenafil is available in 25-, 50-, and 100-mg tablets sold as Viagra. The usual dose is 50 mg taken 1 hour before sexual activity. The dosage range is 25 to 100 mg taken 30 minutes to 4 hours before sexual activity. A low dose (25 mg) should be considered for men older than 65, men with hepatic dysfunction or severe renal dysfunction, and men taking alpha blockers or drugs that inhibit CYP3A4. Dosing should not be done more than once a day.

Vardenafil, Tadalafil, and Avanafil

Vardenafil, tadalafil, and avanafil are very similar to sildenafil. All three drugs inhibit PDE5, and all three are approved for oral therapy of ED. Vardenafil is unique in that it prolongs the QT interval, and tadalafil is unique in that its effects last 36 hours. Avanafil is unique in that it has the fastest onset of action. Otherwise, the clinical effects of all four PDE5 inhibitors appear about equal, although some patients may respond better to one than to the others. Pharmacokinetics and other properties of all four are shown in Table 66.2. Preparation, dosage, and administration guidelines for these drugs are provided in Table 66.3.

Vardenafil

Actions and Use. Vardenafil [Levitra, Staxyn] was the second selective PDE5 inhibitor approved for ED. As with sildenafil, benefits derive from relaxing arterial and trabecular smooth muscle in the penis. Effects begin about 60 minutes after dosing and persist about 4 hours. There is no evidence that vardenafil works faster, longer, or better than sildenafil.

Adverse Effects. The most common adverse effects are headache, flushing, and rhinitis. Like other PDE5 inhibitors, vardenafil can lower blood pressure. Like sildenafil, vardenafil can cause visual changes, and has been associated with sudden hearing loss and vision loss from NAION.

Vardenafil can prolong the cardiac QT interval and might thereby pose a risk for serious dysrhythmias. However, dysrhythmias have not been reported. Nonetheless, to reduce risk, vardenafil should be used with caution in patients taking other drugs that cause QT prolongation.

Drug Interactions. Vardenafil is contraindicated for use with alpha-adrenergic blockers and with nitroglycerin and other nitrates. Plasma levels can be increased by inhibitors of CYP3A4 (e.g., ketoconazole, ritonavir), and hence such combinations must be used with caution. As noted, caution is needed in patients taking drugs that prolong the QT interval.

Tadalafil

Actions and Uses. Tadalafil [Cialis] was approved mere months after vardenafil. Like sildenafil and vardenafil, the drug is indicated for oral therapy of ED. As with other PDE5 inhibitors, benefits derive from relaxation of penile arterial and trabecular smooth muscle brought on by accumulation of cGMP. On average, therapeutic levels of the drug are reached by 2 hours after dosing and persist about 36 hours—much longer than with sildenafil or vardenafil. As a result, the timing of dosing and sexual activity needn't be tightly coupled. Furthermore, in addition to being approved for PRN dosing (like sildenafil and vardenafil), tadalafil is also approved for *daily* dosing (but only for men who anticipate sexual activity at least twice a week).

As discussed later, tadalafil is also used for benign prostatic hyperplasia (BPH). In addition, like sildenafil, tadalafil, sold as Adcirca, is used for PAH.

Adverse Effects. The most common adverse effects are headache, dyspepsia, back pain, myalgia, limb pain, flushing, and nasal congestion. Like other PDE5 inhibitors, tadalafil can lower blood pressure. Very rarely, the drug alters color vision. A few cases of NAION and sudden hearing loss have been reported, but a causal relationship has not been established. Because tadalafil has a long duration of action, adverse effects may persist for many hours.

Drug Interactions. Tadalafil is contraindicated for use with nitrates or alpha blockers (except tamsulosin [Flomax]). As with sildenafil and vardenafil, CYP3A4 inhibitors can cause levels of tadalafil to rise. To avoid toxicity, men taking CYP3A4 inhibitors should limit tadalafil dosage to 10 mg every 72 hours.

Avanafil

Actions and Use. Avanafil [Stendra], approved in 2012, is the latest selective PDE5 inhibitor approved for ED. Actions are the same as for the other PDE5 inhibitors; however, effects begin about 15 minutes after dosing and last about 2 hours.

Adverse Effects. Headache is the only adverse effect, occurring in at least 10% of patients. A few patients will experience flushing, nasal congestion, and nasopharyngitis. Like other PDE5 inhibitors, avanafil can lower blood pressure.

Drug Interactions. Avanafil is contraindicated for use with nitroglycerin and other nitrates. It can increase the hypotensive effects of alcohol and antihypertensive drugs, especially alpha-adrenergic antagonists. A starting dose of 50 mg (the lowest strength available) is recommended if prescribed for patients taking antihypertensive drugs.

Plasma levels can be increased when taken with CYP3A4 inhibitors (e.g., ketoconazole, ritonavir, and erythromycin). For this reason, dosing should not exceed 50 mg in 24 hours for patients taking CYP3A4 inhibitors.

TABLE 66.3 ■ Drugs for Erectile Dysfunction: Preparation, Dosage, and Administration

Drug	Preparation	Dosage for ED	Administration
PDE5 INHIBITORS			
Avanafil [Stendra]	Tablets: 50, 100, 200 mg	100 mg taken approximately 15 minutes before sexual activity. May be increased to 200 mg if needed. Decrease to lowest effective dose.	May be taken with or without food, but avoid grapefruit juice. High-fat foods delay the time to onset. Do not take more than once a day.
Sildenafil [Viagra]	Tablets: 25, 50, 100 mg	50 mg once daily approximately 60 minutes before sexual activity. May be increased to 100 mg if needed. Decrease to lowest effective dose.	May be taken with or without food, but avoid grapefruit juice. High-fat foods may delay onset by as much as 60 minutes. Do not take more than once a day.
Tadalafil [Cialis]	Tablets: 2.5, 5, 10, 20 mg	PRN use: 10 mg before sexual activity. May be increased to 20 mg if needed. Decrease to lowest effective dose. Daily use: 2.5 mg once daily; timing unrelated to sexual activity. May increase to 5 mg if needed.	May be taken with or without food, but avoid grapefruit juice. Do not take more than once a day. If administered for daily use, take at the same time each day.
Vardenafil [Levitra, Staxyn]	Tablets (Levitra): 2.5, 5, 10, 20 mg Orally disintegrating tablets (Staxyn): 10 mg	Levitra: 10 mg taken approximately 60 minutes before sexual activity. May be increased to 20 mg if needed. Decrease to lowest effective dose. Decrease starting dose to 5 mg for patients age 65 and older. Staxyn: 10 mg taken approximately 60 minutes before sexual activity. Do not increase dosage.	Levitra: May be taken with or without food, but avoid grapefruit juice and fatty foods. Staxyn: Place tablet on tongue and allow to disintegrate. Do not take with food or drink. Both: Do not take more than once a day.
PROSTAGLANDIN E_1			
Alprostadil intracavernosal injection [Caverject, Caverject Impulse, Edex]	Intracavernosal Kit (Caverject Impulse): 10, 20 mcg Intracavernosal Kit (Edex): 10, 20, 40 mcg Solution for Intracavernosal Injection (Caverject): 20, 40 mcg	Typical dosages range from 5–40 mcg. Dosing is individualized; determination is made in the healthcare setting. Maximum dosing is 60 mcg for Caverject and 40 mcg for Edex.	Patients self-administer injection into the penis. Do not take more than once in 24 hours. Limit total dosing to 3 times a week.
Alprostadil intraurethral insertion [Muse]	Urethral pellets (Muse): 125, 250, 500, 1000 mcg	Intraurethral insertion: Initial dosing is 125–250 mcg 5–10 minutes before sexual activity. (Effect lasts 30–60 minutes.) Increase, if needed, to lowest effective dose.	Patients self-insert the pellet into the urethra. Limit use to twice daily.
VASODILATOR + ALPHA-ADRENERGIC ANTAGONIST			
Papaverine with phentolamine	Papaverine 30 mg/mL with phentolamine 1 mg/mL	Dosing is individualized; determination is made in the healthcare setting. As little as 0.1 mL may be sufficient.	Patients self-administer injection into the penis.

NONORAL DRUGS FOR ED

Unlike the PDE5 inhibitors, which are administered orally, the drugs discussed in this section—alprostadil and papaverine/phentolamine—are administered by nonoral routes. Specifically, they are administered either by injection into the penis or by insertion into the urethra. Because of this inconvenient dosing, these drugs are second-line agents for ED.

Alprostadil (Prostaglandin E_1)

Mechanism of Action

Alprostadil's active ingredient has the same chemical structure as prostaglandin E_1 (PGE_1), which has vasodilating properties. Relaxation of smooth muscle (arterial, venous, and trabecular) causes a rapid inflow of arterial blood. As explained when discussing the physiology of erection, the blood fills the vascular sinusoidal spaces of the corpus cavernosum, resulting in an erection. Pressure from the engorged penis helps block venous outflow to promote maintenance of the erect state.

Adverse Effects

The most common adverse effect, dull ache in the penis, occurs in 32% of users. Another 12% report urethral burning. Minor bleeding or spotting and testicular pain occur in about 5% of patients. Systemic symptoms are rare when taken as directed and approximate those of placebo use.

Transurethral

Alprostadil pellets [Muse], the only ED drug that is approved for twice-daily use, is inserted into the urethra. Administration is accomplished by loading a pellet into a small plastic applicator, which is then inserted 1.5 inches into the urethra. Detailed instructions for insertion are available in the package insert. Both the package insert and a training video are available online at http://www.muserx.com/how-to-use-muse.

Erection develops 5 to 10 minutes after drug insertion and lasts 30 to 60 minutes. Dosage is determined in the provider's office; the objective is to employ the smallest dose required to produce an erection sufficient for intercourse.

Intracavernous

Alprostadil [Caverject, Caverject Impulse, Edex] is also available in a form for direct injection into the corpus cavernosum. A training video demonstrating how to inject the medication plus a link to access written instructions is available online at http://www.caverject.com/how-inject-caverject-impulse.

The response is rapid and the injections are relatively painless. Erection results from relaxation of smooth muscle (arterial, venous, and trabecular), causing arterial inflow to increase and venous outflow to decrease. Optimal dosage should be determined in the prescriber's office. The dosing endpoint is an erection that is sufficient for intercourse but that does not last for more than 1 hour. Injectable alprostadil should be used no more than 3 times a week and not more than once in 24 hours. Acute adverse effects are burning sensations, prolonged erection, and priapism. Penile fibrosis may develop with continued use of injections; this complication has not been reported with the pellets.

Papaverine Plus Phentolamine

The combination of papaverine (a vasodilator) plus phentolamine (an alpha-adrenergic blocking agent) can provide tumescence when *injected directly into the corpus cavernosum.* Erection develops within 10 minutes and lasts 2 to 4 hours. In clinical trials, erection suitable for intercourse was produced in 65% to 100% of males with ED of neurologic or vascular origin.

As with the other drugs for ED, papaverine and phentolamine produce erection by increasing arterial inflow to the penis and decreasing venous outflow. Arterial inflow is augmented by alpha-adrenergic blockade (causing arterial dilation) and by the direct relaxant action of papaverine on arterial smooth muscle.

Adverse Effects

Priapism (persistent erection lasting more than 6 hours) occurs in about 10% of patients. Development of painless *fibrotic nodules* in the corpus cavernosum is common. Other adverse effects include orthostatic hypotension with dizziness, transient paresthesias, ecchymosis (extravasation of blood into subcutaneous tissue), and difficulty in achieving orgasm or ejaculation.

Papaverine and phentolamine are not approved by the FDA for the treatment of erectile dysfunction, and many experts in the field do not recommend their use. As mentioned, there are some significant adverse effects. Also, these drugs come from compounding pharmacies. In light of numerous FDA recalls from compounding pharmacies in recent years, some providers have concerns about safety and quality issues as well.

BENIGN PROSTATIC HYPERPLASIA

Benign prostatic hyperplasia (BPH) is a common condition that develops in more than 50% of men by age 60 years and 90% by age 85 years. Although BPH and prostate cancer can coexist, there is no evidence that one predisposes to the other.

PATHOPHYSIOLOGY AND OVERVIEW OF TREATMENT

Pathophysiology

The prostate is a heart-shaped gland that surrounds the male urethra. Its major function is to produce fluids that contribute to ejaculate volume. In healthy men, the prostate is walnut sized and weighs between 4 and 20 gm. In men with BPH, prostate mass may reach 50 to 80 gm.

PATIENT-CENTERED CARE ACROSS THE LIFE SPAN

Drugs for Erectile Dysfunction

Life Stage	Patient Care Concerns
Children	Safety for PDE5 inhibitors has not been established. PDE5 inhibitors are not indicated for children. Alprostadil is indicated for treatment of patent ductus arteriosus in neonates; however, the formulations for ED would not apply.
Pregnant women	PDE5 inhibitors are Pregnancy Category B[a]; however, they are not indicated for women and, therefore, should not be taken by pregnant women. Alprostadil urethral pellets and injectable alprostadil or papaverine with phentolamine would not be used by people without a penis. It is recommended that men taking these drugs use a condom if their partner is a pregnant woman.
Breast-feeding women	Excretion in breast milk is unknown; however, drugs for erectile dysfunction are not indicated for use in women.
Older adults	Consider lower dosing when prescribing for adults age 65 and older.

[a]As of 2020, the FDA will no longer use Pregnancy Risk Categories. Please refer to Chapter 9 for more information.

BPH is a nonmalignant prostate enlargement caused by excessive growth of epithelial (glandular) cells and smooth muscle cells. Overgrowth of epithelial cells causes *mechanical obstruction* of the urethra, whereas overgrowth of smooth muscle causes *dynamic obstruction* of the urethra. In men with BPH, the ratio of epithelium to smooth muscle varies from 1 : 3 to 4 : 1—in general, the larger the prostate, the higher the percentage of epithelium.

Signs and symptoms of BPH include urinary hesitancy, urinary urgency, increased frequency of urination, dysuria, nocturia, straining to void, postvoid dribbling, decreased force and caliber of the urinary stream, and a sensation of incomplete bladder emptying. There is no direct correlation between symptoms and prostate size. Therefore some men with only moderate enlargement may be highly symptomatic, whereas others with substantial enlargement may have no symptoms. Long-term complications of BPH include obstructive nephropathy, bladder stones, and recurrent urinary tract infections.

Treatment Modalities

BPH can be managed in three ways: invasive treatments, drug therapy, and "watchful waiting." Invasive options include transurethral resection of the prostate, laser prostatectomy, transurethral electrovaporization of the prostate, and transurethral microwave therapy. These procedures are most appropriate for men with severe symptoms or complications. Drugs are indicated for men with moderate symptoms. Watchful waiting, which consists of annual re-evaluation with reconsideration of management based on results, is appropriate for men with minimal symptoms.

TABLE 66.4 ▪ Drugs for Benign Prostatic Hyperplasia

Generic Name	Brand Name	Actions in BPH	Adverse Effects
5-ALPHA-REDUCTASE INHIBITORS			
Dutasteride Finasteride	Avodart Proscar	Reduce dihydrotestosterone production, which causes the prostate to shrink, which reduces mechanical obstruction of the urethra. May also delay BPH progression. Benefits take months to develop.	Decreased ejaculate volume and libido. Teratogenic to the male fetus.
ALPHA$_1$ BLOCKERS			
Selective Alpha$_{1a}$ Blockers			
Silodosin Tamsulosin	Rapaflo Flomax	Blockade of alpha$_{1a}$ receptors relaxes smooth muscle in the bladder neck, prostate capsule, and prostatic urethra, and thereby decreases dynamic obstruction of the urethra. Benefits develop rapidly.	Abnormal ejaculation (ejaculation failure, reduced ejaculate volume, retrograde ejaculation). Risk for floppy-iris syndrome during cataract surgery.
Nonselective Alpha$_1$ Blockers			
Alfuzosin Doxazosin Terazosin	Uroxatral, Xatral 🍁 Cardura, Cardura XL Hytrin 🍁	Same as the selective alpha$_{1a}$ blockers.	Hypotension, fainting, dizziness, somnolence, and nasal congestion (from blocking alpha$_1$ receptors on blood vessels).
Alpha$_{1a}$ Blocker/5-Alpha-Reductase Inhibitor			
Tamsulosin/dutasteride	Jalyn	Combination of the effects of 5-alpha-reductase inhibitors and selective alpha$_{1a}$ blockers.	Decreased libido and abnormal ejaculation (ejaculation failure, reduced ejaculate volume, retrograde ejaculation).
Tadalafil	Cialis	Smooth muscle relaxation in the bladder, prostate, and urethra.	Hypotension, priapism.

DRUG THERAPY OF BPH

BPH can be treated with two major classes of drugs: *5-alpha-reductase inhibitors* and *alpha$_1$-adrenergic antagonists.* With both, the goal is to relieve bothersome urinary symptoms and delay disease progression. The 5-alpha-reductase inhibitors are most appropriate for men with very large prostates (mechanical obstruction), whereas alpha blockers are preferred for men with relatively small prostates (dynamic obstruction). Major drugs for BPH are shown in Table 66.4.

5-Alpha-Reductase Inhibitors

Two 5-alpha-reductase inhibitors are available: finasteride and dutasteride. Both drugs can reduce prostate size, although several months are required for a noticeable effect. There is no proof that one drug works better than the other.

Safety Alert

HAZARDOUS AGENTS AND SPECIAL ADMINISTRATION REQUIREMENTS

The 5-alpha-reductase inhibitors (dutasteride, finasteride) are classified as hazardous drugs by the National Institute for Occupational Safety and Health. See Chapter 3, Table 3.1, for special handling requirements for preparation, administration, and disposal of these drugs.

Finasteride

Finasteride [Proscar] acts in reproductive tissue to inhibit 5-alpha reductase, an enzyme that converts testosterone to dihydrotestosterone (DHT), the active form of testosterone in the prostate. Treatment reduces levels of DHT in blood by 70% (but does not decrease testosterone levels). By decreasing DHT availability, finasteride promotes regression of prostate epithelial tissue and thereby decreases *mechanical obstruction* of the urethra. Because the percentage of epithelial tissue is highest in very large prostates, finasteride is most effective in men whose prostates are highly enlarged. Conversely, the drug confers less benefit if the degree of enlargement is small. Be aware that prostate shrinkage occurs slowly—over a period of 6 to 12 months.

By reducing levels of DHT, finasteride can protect against prostate cancer—but only cancers classified as low grade. Finasteride does not protect against high-grade prostate cancer. In fact, when given to healthy men to prevent prostate cancer, finasteride actually *increased* the likelihood of a high-grade tumor. Accordingly, the Oncologic Drugs Advisory Committee of the FDA recommends against allowing the manufacturer to label finasteride as a drug for prostate cancer prevention.

Finasteride is generally well tolerated. However, in 5% to 10% of patients, it decreases ejaculate volume and libido. In addition, gynecomastia (breast enlargement) develops in some men.

Finasteride is teratogenic to the male fetus; therefore, finasteride is contraindicated for women who are pregnant or may become pregnant. In addition, because finasteride can be absorbed through the skin, pregnant women should not handle tablets that have been broken or crushed. Men are also advised not to donate blood if taking finasteride or until at least 1 month after stopping the drug to avoid the risk for having a pregnant woman as the blood recipient.

Finasteride decreases serum levels of prostate-specific antigen (PSA), a marker for prostate cancer. The expected decline is 30% to 50%. PSA levels should be determined before treatment and 6 months later. If PSA levels do not fall as expected, the patient should be evaluated for cancer of the prostate.

Safety Alert

5-ALPHA REDUCTASE INHIBITORS

The 5-alpha-reductase inhibitors (finasteride, dutasteride) increase the risk for prostate cancer. They also decrease prostate-specific antigen (PSA) levels. Because PSA levels are elevated with prostate cancer, normal levels may reflect a false negative.

For treatment of BPH, therapy continues for life. (As discussed in Chapter 105, the drug is also available in 1-mg tablets, sold as *Propecia,* for treatment of male-pattern baldness.)

Dutasteride

Dutasteride [Avodart] is similar to finasteride in most respects. However, there are two important differences. First, with dutasteride, the reduction in circulating DHT is more complete. Second, dutasteride has an extremely long half-life (about 5 weeks); therefore, it takes months to clear the drug after dosing has stopped.

Like finasteride, dutasteride inhibits 5-alpha reductase and thereby suppresses production of DHT. However, whereas finasteride inhibits only the form of 5-alpha reductase found in reproductive tissues, dutasteride also inhibits the form found in the skin and liver. As a result, dutasteride produces a greater reduction in circulating DHT (93% vs. 70%). Whether this translates to a greater clinical response has not been established because dutasteride and finasteride have not been directly compared.

Dutasteride is generally well tolerated. However, like finasteride, dutasteride reduces ejaculate volume and libido in some men and causes a decline in PSA in all men.

Dutasteride is teratogenic. It can be absorbed through the skin, so pregnant women should not handle the drug. Men should not donate blood while using dutasteride or for at least 6 months after stopping it to avoid transmission to women through administration of blood products.

Like finasteride, dutasteride can reduce the likelihood of a low-grade prostate tumor, but it increases the likelihood of a high-grade prostate tumor. Accordingly, the drug should not be used for prostate cancer prevention.

Dutasteride can be irritating to oropharyngeal mucosa. For this reason, although it is common practice to open capsules and sprinkle the contents on food, this is not the case with dutasteride. The capsule must be swallowed whole with a full glass of water. Preparation, dosage, and administration of dutasteride and other drugs for BPH are provided in Table 66.5.

Alpha$_1$-Adrenergic Antagonists

Five alpha$_1$ blockers are approved for BPH: *alfuzosin* [Uroxatral, Xatral ♣], *terazosin* [Hytrin ♣], *doxazosin* [Cardura], *silodosin* [Rapaflo], and *tamsulosin* [Flomax]. These drugs have not been directly compared in clinical trials, so we can't say whether one is more effective than the others. However, two newer ones—silodosin and tamsulosin—may be better tolerated. The pharmacology of these drugs is discussed in Chapter 18. Discussion here is limited to their use in BPH.

Mechanism of Action

Blockade of alpha$_1$ receptors relaxes smooth muscle in the bladder neck (trigone and sphincter), prostate capsule, and prostatic urethra, thereby decreasing *dynamic obstruction* of the urethra. Symptomatic improvement and increased urinary flow develop *rapidly.* Because dynamic obstruction is the major contributor to symptoms in patients with relatively mild prostatic enlargement, alpha blockers are preferred to 5-alpha-reductase inhibitors for these men. To maintain benefits, alpha blockers must be taken lifelong. Unlike the 5-alpha-reductase inhibitors, the alpha$_1$ blockers do not reduce prostate size.

Receptor Specificity and Impact on Blood Pressure

The alpha blockers differ regarding specificity of receptor blockade and resultant effect on blood pressure. Specifically, whereas silodosin and tamsulosin are *selective for alpha$_{1a}$ receptors* (the type of alpha$_1$ receptors found in the prostate), alfuzosin, terazosin, and doxazosin are *nonselective alpha$_1$ blockers,* and hence block alpha$_1$ receptors in blood vessels as well as alpha$_{1a}$ receptors in the prostate. By blocking alpha$_1$ receptors in blood vessels, the three nonselective agents promote vasodilation and can thereby lower blood pressure. In fact, two of these drugs—doxazosin and terazosin—were developed as antihypertensive agents; their use in BPH came later. Because of their effect on blood pressure, the nonselective alpha$_1$ blockers are especially useful for patients who have hypertension in addition to BPH—but may be dangerous for men with reduced blood pressure. Conversely, because silodosin and tamsulosin have little or no effect on blood pressure, they are of no benefit to men with hypertension—but are preferred if reducing blood pressure would be a problem.

Adverse Effects

The alpha$_1$ blockers are generally well tolerated. For the nonselective agents (alfuzosin, doxazosin, and terazosin), principal adverse effects are hypotension, fainting, dizziness, somnolence, and nasal congestion. Because *silodosin* and *tamsulosin* have minimal effects on vascular smooth muscle, these drugs are less likely to cause hypotension, fainting, dizziness, or nasal congestion. However, silodosin and tamsulosin *can* cause abnormal ejaculation (ejaculation failure, reduced volume, retrograde ejaculation), whereas the nonselective agents do not. In contrast to dutasteride and finasteride, the alpha blockers do not reduce levels of PSA.

For men undergoing cataract surgery, alpha blockade increases the risk for intraoperative *floppy-iris syndrome,* a complication that can increase postoperative pain, delay recovery, and reduce the hoped-for improvement in vision acuity. In severe cases, the syndrome can cause defects to the iris that may lead to blindness. Men anticipating cataract surgery should postpone alpha blocker therapy until after the procedure. Men already taking an alpha blocker should be sure to tell their ophthalmologist.

Drug Interactions

Exercise caution when combining nonselective alpha blockers with other drugs that lower blood pressure; excessive hypotension could result. Drugs of concern include organic nitrates (e.g., nitroglycerin), antihypertensive drugs, and PDE5 inhibitors used for ED (e.g., sildenafil [Viagra]).

TABLE 66.5 ▪ Drugs for BPH: Preparations, Dosage, and Administration

Drug	Preparation	Dosage for BPH	Administration
ALPHA$_1$-ADRENERGIC ANTAGONISTS			
Alfuzosin [Uroxatral, Xatral 🍁]	ER tablet: 10 mg	10 mg once daily	Take 30 minutes after a meal at the same time each day. Swallow capsules whole.
Doxazosin [Cardura, Cardura XL]	IR tablet: 1, 2, 4, 8 mg (scored) ER tablet: 4, 8 mg	IR tablet: 1 mg once daily; may increase gradually to a maximum of 8 mg once daily ER tablet: 4 mg once daily; may increase to 8 mg once daily	With IR tablets, bedtime administration, especially for the first dose, may decrease adverse effects associated with orthostatic hypotension. Administer ER tablets with morning meal. Swallow tablets whole.
Silodosin [Rapaflo]	Capsule: 4, 8 mg	8 mg once daily Reduce to 4 mg once daily with moderate renal impairment; contraindicated in severe renal or hepatic impairment.	Take with the same meal each day. Capsules may be opened and sprinkled on soft food but should not be chewed.
Terazosin [Hytrin 🍁]	Capsule: 1, 2, 5, 10 mg Tablet: 1, 2, 5, 10 mg	Initial: 1 mg once daily Typical: 10 mg once daily Maximum: 20 mg once daily	May be taken with or without food. Bedtime administration recommended.
Tamsulosin [Flomax]	Capsule: 0.4 mg	0.4 mg once daily May increase to 0.8 mg daily	Take 30 minutes after a meal at the same time each day.
5-ALPHA-REDUCTASE INHIBITORS			
Dutasteride [Avodart]	Capsule: 0.5 mg	0.5 mg once daily	May take with or without food. Swallow capsules whole to avoid oropharyngeal irritation.
Finasteride [Proscar]	Tablets: 5 mg	5 mg once daily	May take with or without food.
PDE5 INHIBITOR			
Tadalafil [Cialis]	Tablets: 2.5, 5, 10, 20 mg	5 mg once daily If taking an alpha blocker, dosing should start at 2.5 mg once daily, and then increase to 5 mg once daily as needed and tolerated	May be taken with or without food, but avoid grapefruit juice.
COMBINATION PRODUCTS: ALPHA$_1$-ADRENERGIC ANTAGONIST + 5-ALPHA-REDUCTASE INHIBITOR			
Tamsulosin + dutasteride [Jalyn]	Capsule: Tamsulosin 0.4 mg + dutasteride 0.5 mg	1 capsule daily	Take 30 minutes after any meal at the same time each day. Swallow capsules whole.

ER, Extended release; *IR,* immediate release

Strong inhibitors of CYP3A4 such as erythromycin, itraconazole, nefazodone, and HIV protease inhibitors (e.g., ritonavir) can dramatically increase levels of alfuzosin and silodosin. Accordingly, alfuzosin and silodosin must not be combined with these drugs.

Use in Women

Tamsulosin and other alpha blockers are being used off-label to treat women with urinary hesitancy or urinary retention associated with bladder outlet obstruction or insufficient contraction of the bladder detrusor muscle. Benefits derive from relaxing smooth muscle in the bladder neck and urethra. Maximal improvement may take several weeks to develop.

Alpha$_1$ Blocker/5-Alpha-Reductase Inhibitor Combination

In clinical trials, combining an alpha blocker with a 5-alpha-reductase inhibitor has been superior to treatment with either agent alone. Because alpha blockers and 5-alpha-reductase inhibitors work by different mechanisms, it is not surprising that combining them can be helpful: The alpha blocker can provide rapid symptomatic relief (by relaxing prostate-related smooth muscle), whereas, over time, the 5-alpha-reductase inhibitor can provide additional symptomatic relief (by shrinking the prostate), and may also delay disease progression.

Research has demonstrated effectiveness with tamsulosin plus dutasteride and doxazosin plus finasteride. Presumably, other combinations of an alpha blocker with a 5-alpha-reductase inhibitor would also be effective. If a single dose is preferred, tamsulosin plus dutasteride [Jalyn] is available.

Tadalafil, a PDE5 Inhibitor

Tadalafil [Cialis] is approved for men who have BPH by itself or BPH combined with ED. In men with BPH, tadalafil produces a modest decrease in symptoms (urinary frequency, urinary urgency, straining), but does not improve urine flow rate. Furthermore, only 1 in 6 men benefit. Initial improvement is seen in 2 weeks. How does tadalafil help? Possibly by relaxing smooth muscle in the prostate, bladder, and urethra. Although tadalafil is the only PDE5 inhibitor approved for ED, other PDE5 inhibitors can reduce symptoms too. Owing to the risk for hypotension, tadalafil should be used with caution in men taking an alpha blocker and should be avoided in men taking nitrates.

PATIENT-CENTERED CARE ACROSS THE LIFE SPAN

Drugs for Benign Prostatic Hyperplasia

Life Stage	Patient Care Concerns
Children	These drugs are not approved for children.
Pregnant women	The $alpha_1$-adrenergic antagonists are FDA Pregnancy Risk Category B[a] with the exception of doxazosin and terazosin, which are Pregnancy Risk Category C.[a] Finasteride and dutasteride are classified in Pregnancy Risk Category X[a]; they are teratogenic to the male fetus. Because these drugs can be absorbed through the skin, pregnant women should not handle finasteride or dutasteride tablets that have been broken or crushed. Men taking finasteride or dutasteride should not donate blood to avoid the risk of exposing a pregnant recipient. To donate blood after stopping the drug, a wait of at least 1 month is required after stopping finasteride and at least 6 months after stopping dutasteride.
Breast-feeding women	It is not known if 5-alpha-reductase inhibitors are excreted in breast milk. Women taking these drugs for off-label uses (e.g., hirsutism) should not breast-feed.
Older adults	Beers Criteria include the peripheral $alpha_1$ blockers doxazosin and terazosin among its listing of potentially inappropriate medications for patients age 65 years and older.

[a]As of 2020, the FDA will no longer use Pregnancy Risk Categories. Please refer to Chapter 9 for more information.

Other Drugs for BPH

Anticholinergics

Symptoms of overactive bladder (OAB), such as urgency and frequency, are often experienced by men with BPH. Anticholinergic drugs (specifically antimuscarinics) are helpful when this occurs. Those approved for OAB include darifenacin, fesoterodine, oxybutynin, solifenacin, tolterodine, and trospium. These may be used alone or in combination with an alpha blocker such as tamsulosin to improve urinary symptoms (see Chapter 14).

Botulinum Toxin

Botulinum toxin [Botox, others], a well-known remedy for facial wrinkles, can also help men with BPH. A single injection into the prostate can relieve urinary symptoms for up to 1 year. Benefits derive in part from blocking release of acetylcholine from neurons that innervate urinary tract smooth muscle. However, since the drug also reduces both prostate size and blood levels of PSA, other mechanisms must also be involved.

Complementary and Alternative Medication (CAM) for BPH

Saw palmetto is an herbal preparation used widely to treat BPH despite numerous randomized controlled trials (RCTs) that refuted findings of earlier less rigorous studies. In 2012 a Cochrane review of 32 RCTs involving 5666 men found no significant difference between saw palmetto and a placebo, even at doses 2 and 3 times the usual dose.

What about other CAMs? In its latest clinical guidelines, the American Urological Association declined to recommend any dietary supplement or herbal treatment, including saw palmetto, until there is a sufficient body of evidence from rigorous clinical trials to support their use.

KEY POINTS

- ED is a persistent inability to achieve or sustain an erection suitable for satisfactory sexual performance.
- Sildenafil [Viagra] is the prototype of the PDE5 inhibitors, the only oral drugs for ED.
- The PDE5 inhibitors are first-line drugs for ED and should be offered to all men with ED, except for men with a specific contraindication.
- By inhibiting PDE5, sildenafil prevents conversion of cGMP to GMP and thereby preserves erection.
- Sildenafil is contraindicated for men taking organic nitrates, because the combination poses a risk for life-threatening hypotension.
- Sildenafil does not increase the risk for cardiovascular events in patients with coronary heart disease—although the sexual activity that sildenafil permits may.
- Sildenafil and other PDE5 inhibitors have been associated with rare cases of sudden hearing loss and vision loss from NAION, although a causal relationship has not been established.
- Symptoms of BPH result from (1) mechanical obstruction of the urethra (secondary to overgrowth of epithelial cells) and (2) dynamic obstruction of the urethra (secondary to overgrowth of smooth muscle).
- Two 5-alpha-reductase inhibitors—finasteride [Proscar] and dutasteride [Avodart]—shrink prostate epithelial tissue and thereby decrease mechanical obstruction of the urethra. Since the percentage of epithelial tissue is highest in very large prostates, these drugs are most effective in men whose prostates are highly enlarged.
- In addition to reducing BPH symptoms, 5-alpha-reductase inhibitors may delay BPH progression.
- Tamsulosin [Flomax] and other $alpha_1$ blockers relax smooth muscle in the prostate capsule, prostatic urethra, and bladder neck (trigone and sphincter), and thereby decrease dynamic obstruction of the urethra. These drugs do not decrease prostate size.
- In men with BPH, beneficial effects of the $alpha_1$ blockers develop quickly (in days to weeks), whereas benefits of 5-alpha-reductase inhibitors develop more slowly (over several months).
- For men with BPH, combined therapy with an alpha blocker plus a 5-alpha-reductase inhibitor is more effective than therapy with either drug alone.

Please visit **http://evolve.elsevier.com/Lehne** for chapter-specific NCLEX® examination review questions.

Summary of Major Nursing Implications[a]

PDE5 INHIBITORS

Avanafil
Sildenafil
Tadalafil
Vardenafil

The nursing implications that follow pertain only to the use of PDE5 inhibitors for ED, not for their use in pulmonary arterial hypertension (PAH).

Preadministration Assessment

Therapeutic Goal

PDE5 inhibitors are used to enhance both the hardness and duration of erection in men with ED.

Baseline Data

Evaluate patients for cardiovascular disorders, including stroke, hypotension, hypertension, heart failure, unstable angina, myocardial infarction, and recent history of a severe dysrhythmia.

Identifying High-Risk Patients

PDE5 inhibitors are *contraindicated* for men taking nitrates (e.g., nitroglycerin), and should generally be avoided by men taking alpha blockers. Avoid *vardenafil*—but not sildenafil or tadalafil—in men taking class I or class III antidysrhythmic drugs.

Use PDE5 inhibitors with *caution* in men taking CYP3A4 inhibitors and in those with nonarteritic ischemic optic neuropathy (NAION), coronary heart disease, and other cardiovascular disorders.

Implementation: Administration

Route

Oral.

Administration

Dosing With Food. **Inform patients that dosing may be done with or without food, although a high-fat meal will delay absorption of avanafil, sildenafil, or vardenafil (but not tadalafil).**

Prn Dosing. All PDE5 inhibitors may be used PRN. **Advise patients to take avanafil approximately 30 minutes before sexual activity. All other PDE5 inhibitors should be taken about 1 hour before sexual activity.**

Daily Dosing. Only *tadalafil* is approved for scheduled daily dosing. **Warn men that the maximum dosage is 5 mg once a day.**

Ongoing Evaluation and Interventions

Minimizing Adverse Effects

Cardiac Risk. **Inform men with pre-existing cardiovascular disease about the cardiac risk for sexual activity (not the PDE5 inhibitor). Advise men who experience symptoms (e.g., anginal pain, dizziness) during sex to refrain from further sexual activity and discuss the event with their prescriber.**

Priapism. PDE5 inhibitors can cause priapism (persistent erection), which can result in permanent erectile dysfunction, owing to local tissue damage. **Advise patients to seek immediate medical attention if an erection lasts more than 4 hours.** Treatment, which must be instituted promptly, involves aspiration of blood from the corpus cavernosum followed by irrigation with a vasoconstrictor.

Nonarteritic Ischemic Optic Neuropathy. Very rarely, men taking PDE5 inhibitors have developed NAION with resultant irreversible blurring of vision or blindness. **Advise patients to stop their PDE5 inhibitor and seek immediate medical attention if they experience sudden loss of vision in one or both eyes.**

Sudden Hearing Loss. Very rarely, men taking PDE5 inhibitors have developed sudden loss of hearing, sometimes associated with dizziness, vertigo, and tinnitus. **Advise men with ED to discontinue the drug if hearing loss develops. (Men taking sildenafil for PAH should not interrupt treatment.)**

Minimizing Adverse Interactions

Nitrates. Combining a PDE5 inhibitor with a nitrate (e.g., nitroglycerin) can cause a severe drop in blood pressure, so concurrent use of these drugs is contraindicated. **Instruct patients to avoid nitrates for at least 12 hours after taking avanafil, for at least 24 hours after taking sildenafil or vardenafil, and for at least 48 hours after taking tadalafil.**

Alpha-Adrenergic Blockers. Combining a PDE5 inhibitor with an alpha blocker (e.g., doxazosin) can cause a serious drop in blood pressure. To avoid harm, use caution when combining *sildenafil* or *avanafil* with an alpha blocker; do not combine *tadalafil* with any alpha blockers except tamsulosin (0.4 mg once daily); and do not combine *vardenafil* with any alpha blockers at all.

Inhibitors of CYP3A4. Agents that inhibit CYP3A4 (e.g., ketoconazole, ritonavir, grapefruit juice) can raise PDE5 inhibitor levels. To avoid harm, dosage of the PDE5 inhibitor should be reduced.

Antidysrhythmic Drugs. Avoid *vardenafil* in men taking class I or class III antidysrhythmic drugs. Vardenafil prolongs the QT interval and can thereby cause a severe dysrhythmia when combined with these agents.

[a]Patient education information is highlighted as **blue text.**

UNIT XI ANTI-INFLAMMATORY, ANTIALLERGIC, AND IMMUNOLOGIC DRUGS

CHAPTER 67

Review of the Immune System

The immune system protects us from invading organisms (viruses, bacteria, fungi, and parasites) and can destroy cancer cells before they destroy us. Unfortunately, the immune system does not always act in our best interest: It can attack transplanted organs and tissues and can turn on the cells it normally protects.

To study the immune system, we begin with an overview. After that, we discuss the two major types of specific immune responses: antibody-mediated immunity (humoral immunity) and cell-mediated immunity.

INTRODUCTION TO THE IMMUNE SYSTEM

Our objective in this section is to establish an overview of immune system components and how they function. Much of the information introduced here is amplified later.

Natural Immunity Versus Specific Acquired Immunity

Our bodies can mount two types of immune responses, referred to as *natural immunity* (innate or native immunity) and *specific acquired immunity.* Factors that confer natural immunity include physical barriers (e.g., skin), phagocytic cells, and natural killer cells. All of these factors are present before exposure to a particular infectious agent, and all respond nonspecifically. In contrast, specific acquired immune responses occur only after exposure to a foreign substance. The foreign substances that induce specific responses are called *antigens,* and the objective of the immune response is to destroy them. With each succeeding re-exposure to a particular antigen, the specific immune response to that antigen becomes more rapid and more intense. Specific immune responses are possible because certain cells of the immune system (T lymphocytes and B lymphocytes) possess receptors that can recognize individual antigens. Our focus here is on specific acquired immunity, not on natural immunity.

Cell-Mediated Immunity Versus Antibody-Mediated (Humoral) Immunity

Specific acquired immune responses can be classified as either cell mediated or humoral. *Cell-mediated immunity* refers to immune responses in which targets are attacked directly by immune system cells—specifically, cytolytic T cells and macrophages. *Humoral immunity* refers to immune responses that are mediated by *antibodies.* (The term *humoral*—defined as "pertaining to elements dissolved in blood or body fluids"—connotes that antibodies dissolved in the blood.)

Introduction to Cells of the Immune System

Immune responses are mediated by several types of cells, some of which play a bigger role than others. The major actors are the *lymphocytes* (B cells, cytolytic T cells, helper T cells), *macrophages,* and *dendritic cells.* Accessory cells include neutrophils and basophils. With the exception of some dendritic cells, all of the cells involved in the immune response arise from pluripotent stem cells in the bone marrow (Fig. 67.1) and circulate in the blood for at least part of their life cycle. Defining characteristics of individual immune system cells are shown in Table 67.1.

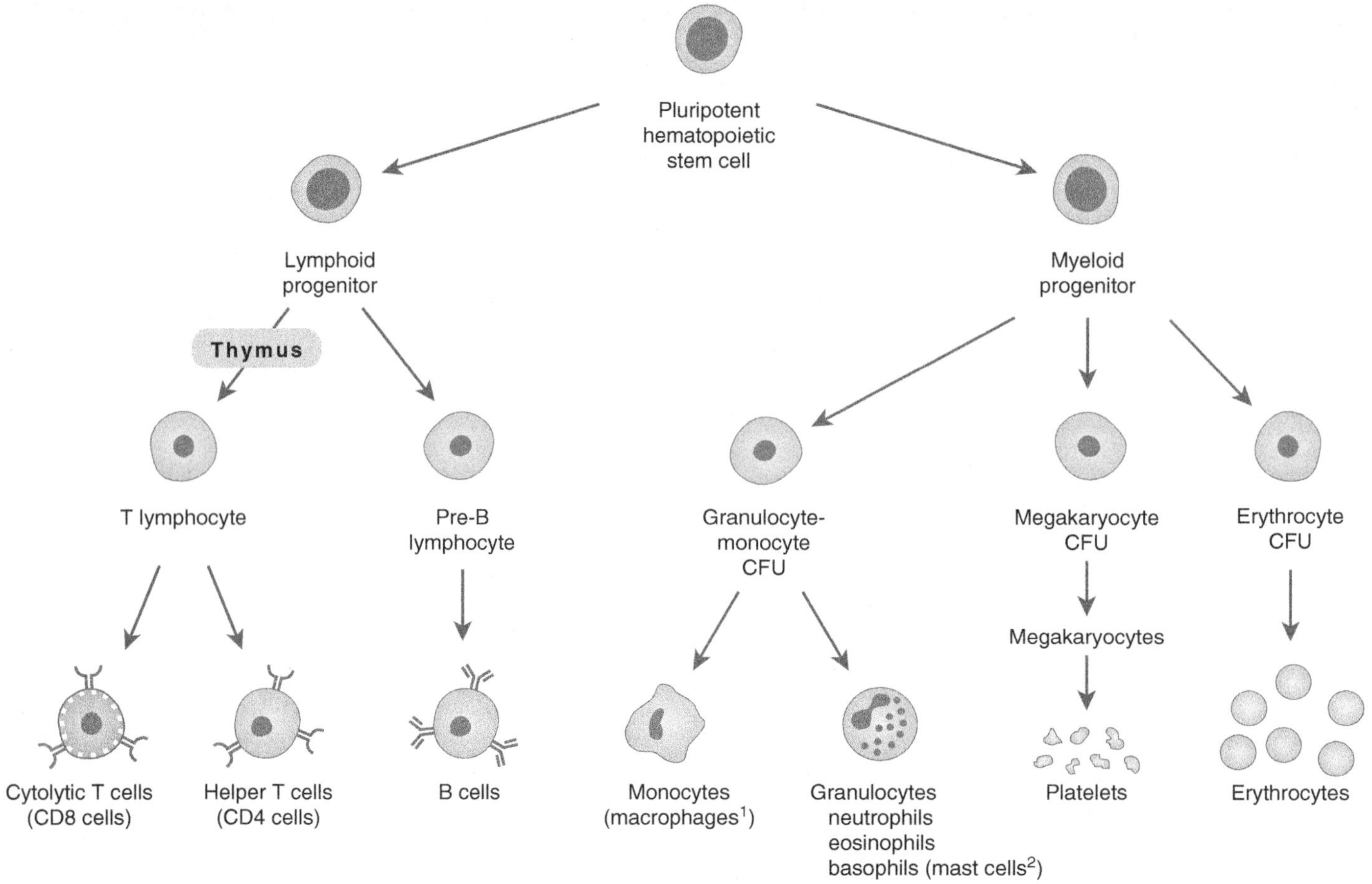

Fig. 67.1 ■ Maturation of blood cells.
With the exception of platelets and erythrocytes, all of the mature blood cells shown participate in immune responses. However, only cells of lymphoid origin (cytolytic T cells, helper T cells, B cells) possess receptors that can recognize specific antigens. (*CFU*, Colony-forming unit.) [1]Monocytes that have moved into tissues are called macrophages. [2]Basophils that have moved into tissues are called mast cells.

B Lymphocytes (B Cells)

B lymphocytes have the job of making *antibodies*. Hence, B cells mediate humoral immunity. As discussed under *Antibodies*, antibody specificity is determined by the structure of highly specific receptors found on the surface of B cells. Like all other lymphocytes, B cells circulate in the blood and lymph. B cells are so named because in chickens, where B cells were discovered, these cells are produced in the *bursa of Fabricius*, a structure not found in mammals. In humans and other mammals, B cells are produced in the bone marrow.

Cytolytic T Lymphocytes (Cytolytic T Cells, CD8 Cells)

Cytolytic T cells are key players in cellular immunity. These cells do not produce antibodies. Rather, they attack and kill target cells directly. Specificity of attack is determined by the presence of antigen molecules on the surface of the target cell and specific receptors for that antigen on the surface of the T cell. Cytolytic T cells are also known as *CD8 cells* and *cytotoxic T cells*. The designation "CD8" refers to the presence of cell-surface marker molecules known as *cell differentiation complex 8*. The "T" in T cell stands for thymus, the organ in which cytolytic T cells and helper T cells mature. Like B cells, cytolytic T cells circulate in the blood and lymph.

Helper T Lymphocytes (Helper T Cells, CD4 Cells)

Helper T cells contribute to the immune response in three ways: (1) They have an essential role in antibody production by B cells; (2) they release factors that promote type IV sensitivity reactions, also known as delayed-type hypersensitivity (DTH); and (3) they participate in the activation of cytolytic T cells. Specificity of helper T cells is achieved through highly specific cell-surface receptors that recognize individual antigens. Like other lymphocytes, helper T cells circulate in the blood and lymph. Helper T cells carry CD4 (cell differentiation complex 4) marker molecules on their surface, and hence are referred to as *CD4 cells*.

The term *helper* is somewhat misleading in that it connotes a useful but dispensable role. Nothing could be further from reality. Helper T cells are not simply nice to have around; they are absolutely required for an effective immune response. The critical nature of their contribution—and the grim consequences of their absence—is manifested in people with HIV/AIDS:

TABLE 67.1 ▪ Cells of the Immune System

Cell Type	Synonyms	Primary Immune-Related Actions
MAJOR CELL TYPES		
B lymphocytes	B cells	Produce antibodies
Cytolytic T lymphocytes (CTLs)	Cytolytic T cells, cytotoxic T cells, CD8 cells	Lyse target cells
Helper T lymphocytes	Helper T cells, CD4 cells	Promote proliferation and differentiation of B cells and CTLs Initiate delayed-type hypersensitivity
Macrophages		Promote proliferation and differentiation of helper T cells and CTLs by serving as antigen-presenting cells Participate in delayed-type hypersensitivity Phagocytize cells tagged with antibodies Phagocytize cells in the effector stage of delayed-type hypersensitivity
Dendritic cells		Promote proliferation of CTLs and helper T cells by serving as antigen-presenting cells
ACCESSORY CELLS		
Mast cells		Mediate immediate hypersensitivity reactions
Basophils		Mediate immediate hypersensitivity reactions
Neutrophils	Polymorphonuclear leukocytes	Phagocytize foreign particles (e.g., bacteria), especially those tagged with IgG Mediate inflammation
Eosinophils		Attack helminths and foreign particles that have been coated with IgE Contribute to immediate hypersensitivity reactions

IgE, Immunoglobulin E; *IgG,* immunoglobulin G.

Helper T cells are the immune cells that HIV attacks. Because of helper T-cell loss, AIDS patients are at high risk of death from opportunistic infection.

Macrophages

Macrophages begin their existence in the bone marrow, enter the blood as monocytes, and then infiltrate tissues, where they evolve into macrophages. Macrophages are present in all organs and tissues.

The primary function of macrophages is *phagocytosis* (i.e., ingestion of microbes, other foreign material, and cellular debris). In their role as phagocytes, macrophages are the principal scavengers of the body. Although their major job is phagocytosis, macrophages also have an important role in specific acquired immunity, natural immunity, and inflammation.

In specific acquired immunity, macrophages have three functions: (1) They are required for activation of T cells (both helper T cells and cytolytic T cells), (2) they are the final mediators of DTH, and (3) they phagocytize cells that have been tagged with antibodies. Of these three immune-related roles, activation of T cells is arguably the most critical. When performing this function, macrophages are referred to as *antigen-presenting cells* (APCs). Because antigen presentation is an absolute requirement for specific immune responses (see *Antigens*), you can appreciate how important macrophages are.

Dendritic Cells

Dendritic cells perform the same antigen-presenting task as do macrophages. However, unlike macrophages, dendritic cells do not also serve as scavengers. Dendritic cells are found in lymph nodes and other lymphoid tissues.

Mast Cells and Basophils

These cells mediate immediate hypersensitivity reactions. Mast cells, which are derived from basophils, are concentrated in the skin and other soft tissues. Basophils circulate in the blood. Both cell types release histamine, heparin, and other compounds that cause the symptoms of immediate hypersensitivity. Release of these mediators is triggered when an antigen binds to antibodies on the cell surface. The role of mast cells and basophils in allergic reactions is discussed in Chapter 70.

Neutrophils

Neutrophils, also known as polymorphonuclear leukocytes, phagocytize bacteria and other foreign particles. As discussed later, neutrophils avidly devour cells that have been tagged with antibodies of the immunoglobulin G (IgG) class. Accordingly, neutrophils can be viewed as important effectors in humoral immunity. Neutrophils are also major contributors to inflammation.

Eosinophils

Eosinophils attack and destroy foreign particles that have been coated with antibodies of the immunoglobulin E (IgE) class. Their usual target is helminths (parasitic worms). Eosinophils also contribute to tissue injury and inflammation associated with immediate hypersensitivity reactions.

Antibodies

Antibodies are a family of structurally related glycoproteins that mediate humoral immunity. The most characteristic feature of antibodies is their ability to recognize and bind with specific antigens. Alternative names for antibodies are *immunoglobulins* and *gamma globulins.*

All antibodies are produced by B lymphocytes. Some of the antibodies that B cells produce are retained on the surface of the B cell. These antibodies serve as the receptors whereby B cells recognize specific antigens. However, most of the antibodies that B cells produce are secreted from the cell, after which they bind to their specific antigen, thereby initiating the effector phase of humoral immunity. The process of antibody production is discussed in detail under *Production of Antibodies*.

All antibodies are composed of units that have the same basic structure. As shown in Fig. 67.2, antibodies have four chains: two heavy chains and two light chains. Disulfide bridges connect the four chains to form a unit. Each heavy chain and each light chain has two regions, one in which the sequence of amino acids is *constant* and one in which the sequence is highly *variable.* The variable regions form the antigen-binding site.

There are five classes of antibodies (immunoglobulins), known as IgA, IgD, IgE, IgG, and IgM. All are constructed from the same basic parts just described. However, the heavy chains differ for each class. Primary functions of the five classes are shown in Table 67.2.

When antibodies are subjected to digestion by papain in the laboratory, they break down into three pieces (see Fig. 67.2). Two of the pieces retain the ability to bind antigen, and hence are called *Fab fragments* (fragment, antigen binding). The third piece does not bind antigen and tends to form crystals in the test tube; hence, it is called the *Fc fragment* (fragment, crystalline).

Antigens

Antigens are molecules that induce specific immune responses and, as a result, become the targets of those responses. By way of analogy, an antigen is like the child who pokes a stick in a hornet's nest, at once triggering a response and becoming its target. An antigen may trigger production of antibodies,

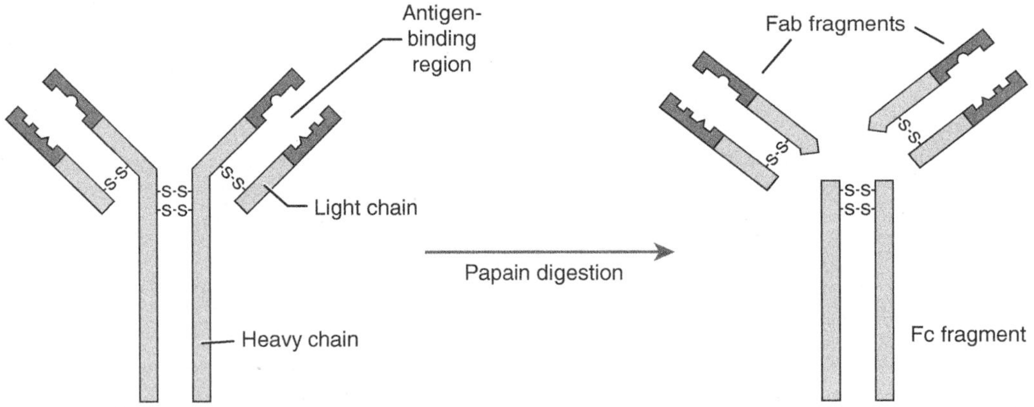

Fig. 67.2 ▪ Antibody structure.
The basic antibody structure depicting heavy and light chains is shown on the left. Variable regions of the heavy and light chains, which form the antigen-binding site, appear in green. As shown on the right, papain digestion of antibodies produces two types of fragments: Fab fragments, which retain the ability to bind antigen, and Fc fragments, which do not bind antigen and tend to crystallize in the test tube.

TABLE 67.2 ▪ Functions of Antibody Classes

Class	Function
IgA	Located in mucous membranes of the GI tract and lungs and in many secretions, where it serves as the first line of defense against microbes entering the body via these routes Transferred to infants via breast milk; is not absorbed from the GI tract but does protect the infant against microbes *in* the GI tract
IgD	Found only on the surface of mature B cells, where it serves as a receptor for antigen recognition (along with IgM)
IgE	Binds to the surface of mast cells; subsequent binding of antigen to IgE stimulates release of histamine, heparin, and other mediators from the mast cells, thereby causing symptoms of allergy (e.g., hives, hay fever) Binds to parasitic worms, after which eosinophils bind to IgE and release compounds that lyse the worms
IgG	Produced in copious amounts in response to antigenic stimulation, and hence is the major antibody in blood Fixes complement and thereby promotes target-cell lysis Binds target cells and thereby enhances phagocytosis Transferred across the placenta to the fetal circulation, thereby providing neonatal immunity
IgM	First class of antibody produced in response to an antigen Fixes complement and thereby promotes target-cell lysis Present on the surface of mature B cells, where it serves as a receptor for antigen recognition (along with IgD)

cytotoxic T cells, or both—all of which can then attack the antigen.

Most antigens are large molecules. Because antigens are big, the antigen-binding region of the resultant antibodies cannot recognize and bind the entire antigen molecule. Rather, the antibodies recognize and bind selected small portions of the antigen, referred to as *epitopes* or *antigenic determinants.* All antigens have multiple epitopes. As a result, more than one antibody can bind the antigen.

In research and in clinical practice, we may want to generate antibodies to molecules that are too small to induce an immune response. To overcome this obstacle, we can link the small molecule to a larger molecule, usually a protein. When this is done, the small molecule is referred to as a *hapten,* and the large molecule is referred to as a *carrier.* At least some of the resultant antibodies will be selective for the hapten.

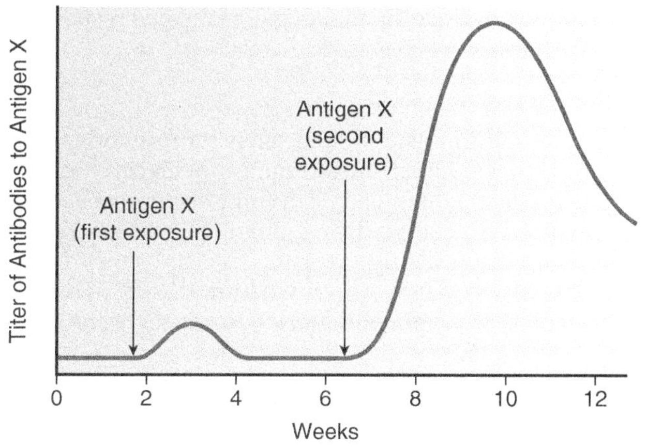

Fig. 67.3 ■ Memory and time limitation of immune responses. After the initial exposure to antigen X, antibody levels rise slowly, peak at a low level, and then decline rapidly. After the second exposure to antigen X, antibody levels rise more rapidly, reach a higher peak, persist longer, and then slowly decline.

Characteristic Features of Immune Responses

Cell-mediated immunity and humoral immunity share five characteristic features: specificity, diversity, memory, time limitation, and selectivity for antigens of nonself origin (i.e., the ability to discriminate between self and nonself).

Specificity

Cell-mediated and humoral immune responses are triggered by specific antigens, and their purpose is to destroy the antigen that triggered the response. The ability to respond to a specific antigen (i.e., the ability to make subtle distinctions among related molecules) is conferred by highly specific receptors on B cells and T cells.

Diversity

Our immune systems can respond to millions of different antigenic determinants. This is possible because our immune systems have millions of clones of B and T lymphocytes—each of which is preprogrammed to recognize a different antigenic determinant. As noted, this ability to discriminate between antigens is the result of having unique cell-surface receptors.

Memory

Exposure to an antigen affects the immune system such that re-exposure produces a faster, larger, and more prolonged response compared with the initial exposure (Fig. 67.3). During the initial response, B and T lymphocytes that recognize the antigen undergo proliferation. Most of the new cells participate in the attack against the antigen. However, some of the new cells become *memory cells,* thereby increasing the pool of antigen-specific cells available to respond in the future. Hence, when the antigen is encountered again, the memory cells mobilize and thereby accelerate and intensify the response.

Time Limitation

Immune responses don't last indefinitely. They are time limited. The reasons are twofold: First, as the immune response proceeds, it greatly decreases the level of antigen that initiated the response, thereby attenuating the stimulus for continuing. Second, activated B cells and T cells function for only a short time, after which they become quiescent or die. Hence, in the absence of a continuing stimulus to generate more active B cells and T cells, the immune response fades.

Selectivity for Antigens of Nonself Origin

Under normal conditions, our immune systems target only foreign antigens, leaving potentially antigenic molecules on our own cells untouched. Sparing of self is possible because, as T cells develop in the thymus, cells that are able to react with antigens of self origin are eliminated. As discussed later, this discrimination between self and nonself is made possible by *major histocompatibility complex* (MHC) molecules.

When the ability to discriminate between self and nonself fails, our immune systems can attack our own cells. The result is an *autoimmune disease.* There are many diseases of autoimmune origin, including psoriasis, multiple sclerosis, rheumatoid arthritis, myasthenia gravis, type 1 diabetes, systemic lupus erythematosus, two inflammatory bowel diseases (ulcerative colitis and Crohn's disease), and two thyroid diseases (Graves' disease and Hashimoto's thyroiditis).

Phases of the Immune Response

Specific immune responses can be viewed as having three main phases: recognition, activation, and effector.

Recognition Phase

The recognition phase occurs when a mature lymphocyte encounters its matching antigen. All specific immune responses begin with antigen recognition by B cells and T cells. Antigen recognition is possible because of antigen-specific receptors on the lymphocyte surface.

Activation Phase

Antigen recognition activates the lymphocyte, which then undergoes proliferation and differentiation. Some of the daughter cells differentiate into cells that actively participate in the immune response, attacking the source of the antigen. Other daughter cells differentiate into memory cells, thereby preparing the host for a more intense, rapid, and prolonged response in the event of antigen re-exposure.

Effector Phase

In this stage, the immune system attempts to eliminate the specific antigen that initiated the response. With cell-mediated or antibody-mediated immunity, several effector mechanisms can be involved. In cell-mediated immunity, antigen-bearing target cells can be lysed by cytolytic T cells, or they can be ingested by macrophages. In antibody-mediated immunity, target cells may be primed for attack by phagocytes or by the complement system.

Major Histocompatibility Complex Molecules

The *major histocompatibility complex* is a group of *genes* that codes for *MHC molecules,* which become expressed on the surface of all cells. MHC molecules are critical to immune system function. They play a key role in the activation of helper and cytotoxic T lymphocytes, they guide cytotoxic T lymphocytes toward target cells, and they provide the basis for distinguishing between self and nonself.

There are two classes of MHC gene products, referred to as *class I MHC molecules* and *class II MHC molecules.* Class I MHC molecules are found on virtually all cells except erythrocytes; class II MHC molecules are found primarily on B cells and APCs (macrophages and dendritic cells). As discussed later in the chapter, *class I MHC molecules* on the surface of APCs help initiate immune responses by "presenting" antigen to *cytotoxic T cells.* In contrast, *class II MHC molecules* on the surface of APCs help initiate immune responses by presenting antigen to *helper T cells.*

As a rule, the sequence of amino acids in MHC molecules produced by one individual differs from the sequence of amino acids in MHC molecules produced by everyone else. That is, it is rare for two individuals to have MHC molecules that are identical. As a result, MHC molecules from one individual are recognized as foreign (nonself) by the immune systems of nearly everyone else. Hence, when we attempt to transplant organs between individuals who are not identical twins, immune rejection of the transplant is likely. To reduce the risk of rejection, we can treat patients with immunosuppressant drugs (see Chapter 69).

Cytokines, Lymphokines, and Monokines

The terms *cytokine, lymphokine,* and *monokine* are encountered frequently when discussing the immune system and can be a source of confusion. The term *cytokine* refers to any mediator molecule (other than an antibody) released by *any* immune system cell. A *lymphokine* is simply a cytokine released by a *lymphocyte,* and a *monokine* is simply a cytokine released by a *mononuclear phagocyte* (monocyte or macrophage). Put another way, *cytokine* is a generic term for the whole class of nonantibody mediators released by immune cells, whereas the terms *lymphokine* and *monokine* are more restrictive, referring only to nonantibody mediators released by lymphocytes and mononuclear phagocytes, respectively. Examples of cytokines and their functions are listed in Table 67.3.

TABLE 67.3 ▪ Functions of Selected Cytokines

Cytokine	Function
Interleukin-1	Stimulates lymphocyte progenitor cells
Interleukin-2	Stimulates proliferation and differentiation of helper T cells and cytolytic T cells
Interleukin-3	Stimulates proliferation of bone marrow lineage cells, B cells, and T cells
Interleukin-4	Activates B cells, T cells, and macrophages
Interleukin-5	Stimulates generation of eosinophils
Interleukin-6	Stimulates proliferation of bone marrow cells and plasma cells
Interleukin-7	Stimulates B cells and T cells
Interleukin-8	Attracts neutrophils, B cells, and T cells
Interleukin-9	Stimulates proliferation of mast cells
Interleukin-10	Inhibits some T cells
Interleukin-11	Enhances actions of interleukin-3
Interleukin-12	Enhances actions of interleukin-2
Interferon alfa	Activates macrophages, cytolytic T cells, and natural killer cells
Interferon gamma	Activates macrophages and T cells and enhances expression of MHC molecules
Tumor necrosis factor	Kills tumor cells; promotes inflammation
Granulocyte-macrophage colony-stimulating factor	Stimulates proliferation of monocytes, macrophages, and granulocytes (neutrophils, eosinophils, basophils)

MHC, Major histocompatibility complex.

ANTIBODY-MEDIATED (HUMORAL) IMMUNITY

As noted, there are two types of immune responses: humoral immunity and cell-mediated immunity. In this section, we review humoral immunity, focusing on (1) how antibodies are produced and (2) the mechanisms by which antibodies protect us. Cell-mediated immunity is discussed in the section that follows.

Production of Antibodies

Antibody production requires the cooperative interaction of three types of cells: *B cells,* which actually make the antibodies; *helper T cells* (CD4 cells), which stimulate the B cells; and an *antigen-presenting cell* (either a macrophage or a dendritic cell), which activates the CD4 cells so that they can then help the B cells. The major steps in the process are depicted in Fig. 67.4.

Overview of Antibody Production

Production of antibodies begins with the binding of a specific antigen to two types of cells: a virgin B cell and an APC. The APC may be either a macrophage or a dendritic cell. After

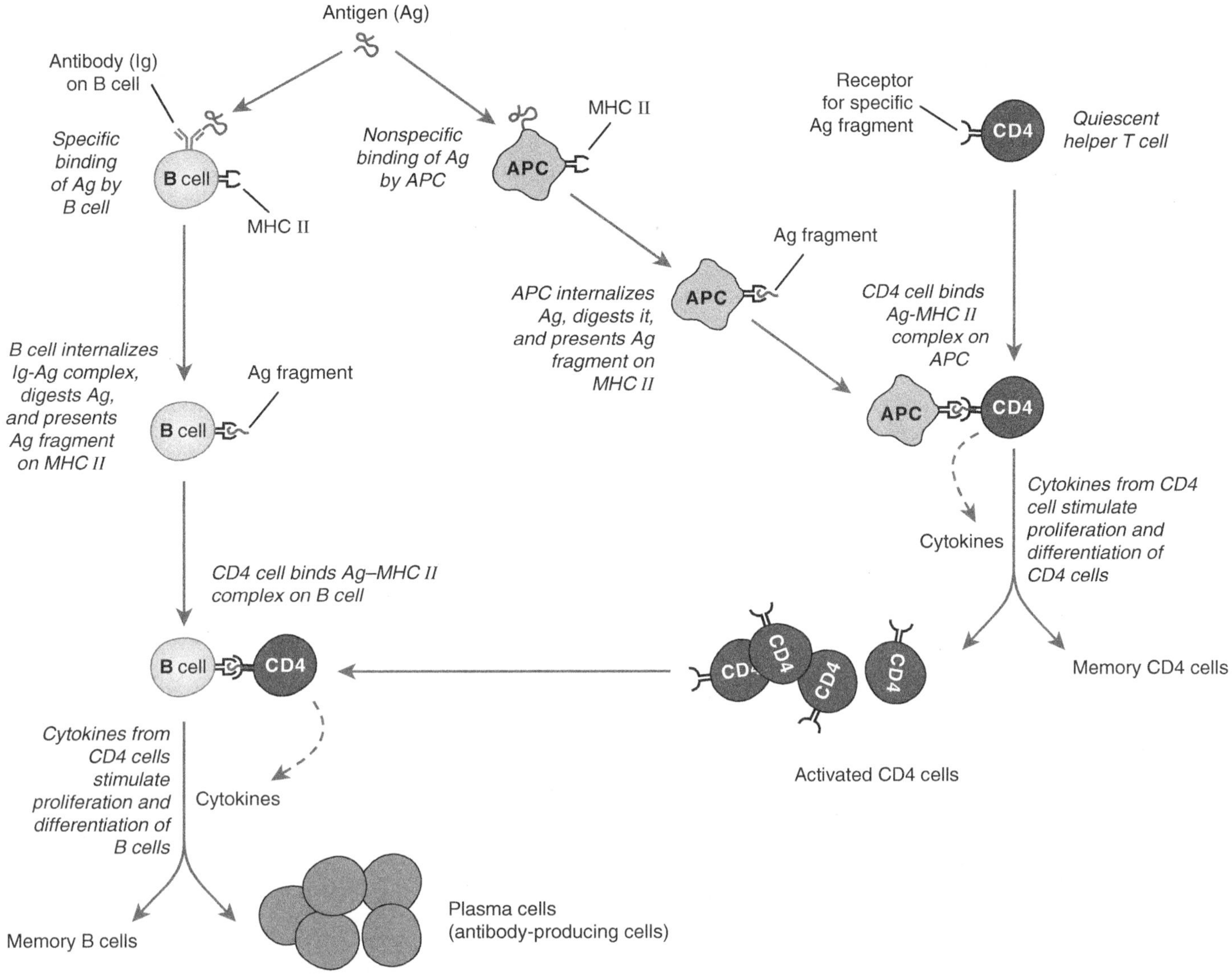

Fig. 67.4 ■ Major events in antibody-mediated (humoral) immunity. Humoral immunity requires three types of cells: B cells, APCs, and helper T cells (CD4 cells). Binding of a CD4 cell with an APC activates the CD4 cell, which then binds with a B cell and releases cytokines, which then stimulate the B cell. (*APC,* Antigen-presenting cell [macrophage or dendritic cell]; *Ig,* immunoglobulin [antibody]; *MHC II,* class II MHC molecule.)

processing the antigen, the APC is able to bind with a specific CD4 cell, thereby causing the CD4 cell to proliferate and differentiate into active CD4 cells and memory CD4 cells. The active CD4 cells then bind with processed antigen on B cells, thereby causing the B cells to proliferate and differentiate into (1) plasma cells, which manufacture the antibodies, and (2) memory B cells, which await the next antigen exposure.

Specific Cellular Events in Antibody Production

B Cells. Participation of B cells in the immune response begins with recognition and binding of a *specific antigen.* The receptor that B cells employ for antigen recognition is actually an antibody (IgD or IgM). For any given B cell, this antibody (receptor) is highly specific for just one antigenic determinant. After the antigen binds the B-cell receptor, the receptor-antigen complex is internalized and the antigen is broken down into small peptide fragments. Each fragment is then complexed with a *class II MHC molecule,* after which the *antigen–MHC II complexes* are transported to the cell surface. (In Fig. 67.4, only one such complex is shown. However, in a real cell, many such complexes, each with a different piece of the antigen, would appear on the cell surface.) The final step of B-cell activation occurs when a CD4 helper T cell recognizes and binds with an antigen–MHC II complex on the B cell. This binding causes the CD4 cell to secrete cytokines, which then stimulate the B cell to proliferate and differentiate into two types of cells: plasma cells and memory B cells. The plasma cells are the cells that make antibodies. The memory cells serve to hasten, intensify, and prolong the immune response if antigen exposure should recur.

Antigen-Presenting Cells. APCs are essential for activation of CD4 helper T cells because CD4 cells cannot recognize antigen that is free in solution. Rather, they can only recognize antigen that has been complexed with an MHC II molecule.

Participation of APCs in the immune response begins with nonspecific binding of antigen to the APC (see Fig. 67.4). Next, as in B cells, the antigen is internalized and broken into fragments, which are then complexed with MHC II molecules and transported to the cell surface, where they are available for interaction with CD4 cells.

Helper T Cells (CD4 Cells). The job of CD4 cells in humoral immunity is to activate B cells. In the absence of activation by CD4 cells, B cells are unable to proliferate and produce antibodies.

Participation of CD4 cells in the immune response begins when these cells bind with an antigen–MHC II complex on the surface of an APC. Binding is mediated by a receptor on the CD4 cell that is specific for the particular antigen in the antigen–MHC II complex. (As noted, for the CD4 cell to recognize the antigen, the antigen must be complexed with an MHC II molecule, which is why the APC is essential for CD4 cell activation.) Upon binding with the antigen–MHC II complex, the CD4 cell releases cytokines, which then cause the CD4 cell itself to proliferate and differentiate into memory CD4 cells and activated CD4 cells. The activated CD4 cells then bind with their corresponding antigen–MHC II complexes on B cells, release cytokines, and thereby cause proliferation and differentiation of the B cells.

Antibody Effector Mechanisms

Antibodies are simply molecules with the ability to bind to other molecules. Antibodies have no special destructive powers. To rid the body of antigens, which is what antibodies are for, antibodies usually work in conjunction with other factors, namely, *phagocytic cells* and the *complement system.* The only antigens that antibodies can neutralize without help are bacterial toxins and viruses.

Opsonization of Bacteria

One mechanism for ridding the body of pathogenic bacteria is phagocytosis by macrophages and neutrophils. However, because of their structures, some bacteria are difficult for phagocytes to grab hold of, and hence these bacteria are resistant to ingestion. Antibodies help promote phagocytosis of these bacteria by acting as *opsonins.* (An opsonin is a molecule that binds to a bacterium or other target particle and thereby promotes phagocytosis by providing a handle for phagocytes to grab.)

Bacterial opsonization by antibodies occurs in two steps. First, the antigen-binding region of the antibody binds with antigen on the bacterial surface, which leaves the Fc portion of the antibody projecting away from the bacterial surface. Second, phagocytes link up with the Fc portion of the antibody, which brings them in close contact with the bacterium, and hence enables them to commence phagocytosis. Phagocytes are able to bind the Fc fragment because they have high-affinity receptors for Fc on their surface. Most of the antibodies that act as opsonins belong to the IgG class.

Activation of the Complement System

The complement cascade is a complex system consisting of at least 20 serum proteins that, when activated, can cause multiple effects, including cell lysis, opsonization, degranulation of mast cells, and infiltration of phagocytes. The system can be activated in two ways, known as the *classical pathway* and the *alternative pathway.* The classical pathway is activated by *antibodies;* the alternative pathway is not. However, with both pathways, the end results are essentially the same. Consideration here is limited to the classical pathway.

The classical pathway is turned on when C1 (the first component of the complement system) encounters an antigen-antibody complex and then binds with the Fc region of the antibody. C1 will not bind with antibody that is free in solution, and hence free antibodies cannot activate the system. Activation of the complement system triggers a cascade of reactions that amplify the response at each stage. The result is the production of compounds that can injure target cells.

Lysis of target cells that have been tagged with antibodies is the most dramatic effect of the complement system. Lysis is caused by cylindrical *membrane attack complexes,* which are formed by the complement cascade. Following their insertion into the target-cell membrane, the attack complexes act as pores through which fluid can enter the cell. Fluid influx causes the target cell to swell and then burst.

Neutralization of Viruses and Bacterial Toxins

Neutralization of toxins and viruses is the only protective action that antibodies can perform unassisted. To hurt us, bacterial toxins must first bind with receptors on our cells. Likewise, to infect us, viruses must first bind with cell-surface receptors. By binding with antigenic determinants on toxins and viruses, antibodies make it impossible for toxins and viruses to bind with cellular receptors. As a result, these agents can no longer hurt us.

CELL-MEDIATED IMMUNITY

Cell-mediated immunity has two branches, one mediated by *helper T lymphocytes* (CD4 cells) plus *macrophages,* and one mediated primarily by *cytolytic T lymphocytes* (CD8 cells). In the branch mediated by CD4 cells and macrophages, the result is called *delayed-type hypersensitivity.* In the branch mediated by CD8 cells, the result is *target-cell lysis.*

Delayed-Type Hypersensitivity (Type IV Hypersensitivity)

The object of DTH is to rid the body of bacteria that replicate primarily within macrophages (e.g., *Listeria monocytogenes, Mycobacterium tuberculosis*). For DTH to occur, two cells are needed: an *infected macrophage* and a *CD4 helper T cell.* The macrophage serves to activate the CD4 cell, which in turn activates the macrophage, thereby enabling the macrophage to kill the bacteria residing within. Hence, the same cell (i.e., the macrophage) is both the activator of the CD4 cell and the recipient of the activated CD4 cell's help.

Activation of Helper T Cells

Activation of CD4 cells in DTH is essentially identical to the activation of CD4 cells in humoral immunity. As shown in Fig. 67.5, the process begins when a macrophage becomes infected with intracellular bacteria. As in humoral immunity, the macrophage breaks the antigen into small peptides, combines each peptide with a class II MHC molecule, and then presents the antigen–MHC II complexes on its surface. In the next step, a CD4 cell binds with an antigen–MHC II complex on the

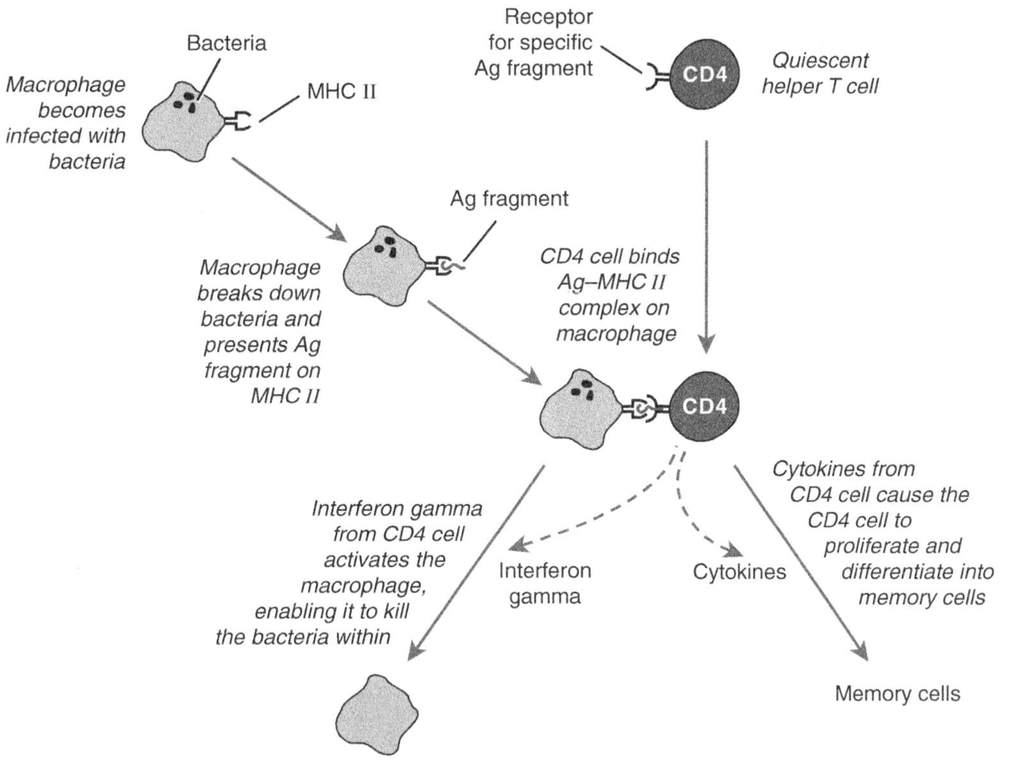

Fig. 67.5 ▪ Cell-mediated immunity: delayed-type hypersensitivity. DTH requires two cells: an infected macrophage and a CD4 cell. Binding of the CD4 cell to the macrophage activates the CD4 cell, which then releases interferon gamma and several cytokines. Interferon gamma activates the macrophage. The cytokines cause the CD4 cell to proliferate and differentiate into memory cells. (*Ag,* Antigen; *MHC II,* class II MHC molecule.)

macrophage. As discussed previously, selectivity of binding is determined by receptors on the CD4 cell that recognize a specific antigen fragment—but only when the fragment is bound to a class II MHC molecule. Binding of the CD4 cell with the APC causes the CD4 cell to release (1) cytokines that cause the CD4 cell itself to proliferate and differentiate into memory cells and (2) mediators of DTH, including interferon gamma and tumor necrosis factor.

Activation of Macrophages

Interferon gamma, released from the activated CD4 cell, is the major stimulus for macrophage activation. In response to interferon gamma, macrophages increase production of lysosomes and reactive oxygen. The reactive oxygen is ultimately responsible for killing bacteria inside the macrophage. In addition to ridding macrophages of bacteria, DTH produces local inflammation.

Cytolytic T Lymphocytes

Cytolytic T lymphocytes (CTLs, CD8 cells) kill other cells. Their principal job is to kill self cells that are infected with viruses, thereby halting viral replication. In addition, CTLs participate in the rejection of transplants. Here our discussion is limited to killing virally infected cells.

The process by which CTLs kill other cells has two stages: activation of CTLs, followed by recognition and killing of the target cell. The process is depicted in Fig. 67.6.

Activation of Cytolytic T Cells

Activation of CTLs requires the participation of an *antigen-presenting cell* and a *helper T cell* (CD4 cell). The process is very similar to the activation of CD4 cells, already discussed. However, there is one important difference: Whereas CD4 cells specifically recognize antigen that is bound to a *class II* MHC molecule on an APC, CTLs specifically recognize antigen that is bound to a *class I* MHC molecule on an APC.

In viral infections, activation of CTLs begins with the processing of viral antigens by an APC. As shown in Fig. 67.6, the APC combines the antigen with a class I MHC molecule and then presents the antigen–MHC I complex on its surface. Next, a pre-CTL binds to the antigen–MHC I complex. (Like CD4 cells, each pre-CTL has receptors that are specific for a particular antigen–MHC I complex.) Linking of the pre-CTL with the APC primes the pre-CTL for the next stage of activation: stimulation by cytokines (interleukin-2, interferon gamma, and probably others) provided by an activated CD4 cell. (Activation of the CD4 cell, which is not shown in Fig. 67.6, occurs when the CD4 cell encounters an APC that has a viral antigen–MHC II complex.) In response to the cytokines released by the CD4 cell, the pre-CTL undergoes proliferation and differentiation into memory CTLs and activated CTLs.

Recognition of Virally Infected Target Cells

CTLs recognize their targets by the presence of an antigen–MHC I complex. This is the same process by which CTLs recognize

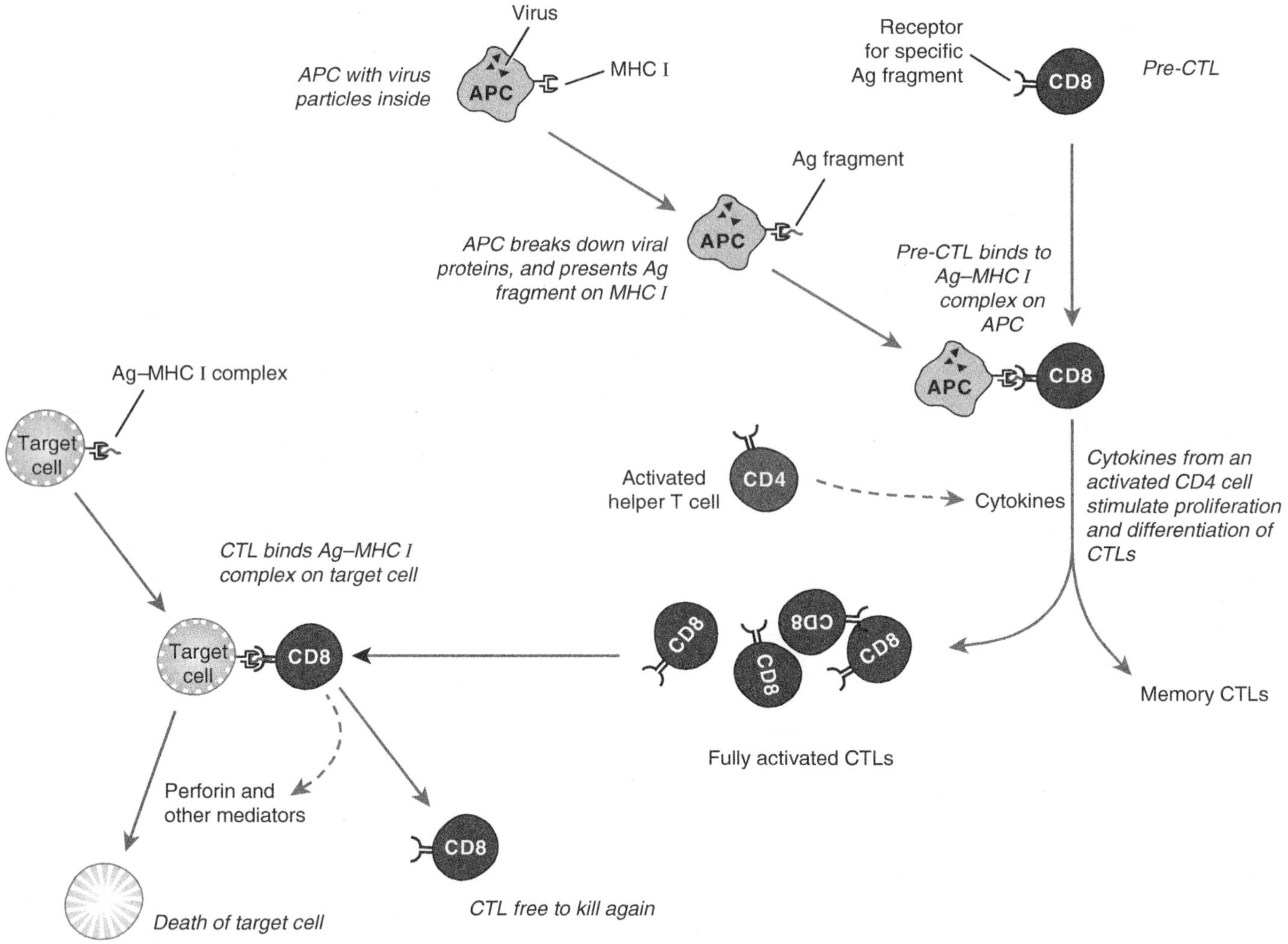

Fig. 67.6 ■ Cell-mediated immunity: cytolytic T cells.
This branch of cell-mediated immunity requires three types of cells: CTLs, APCs, and CD4 cells. Binding of the pre-CTL with the APC begins the activation of the CTL. Stimulation of the CTL by cytokines from the CD4 cell completes the activation of the CTL, which then binds with and kills its target. Activation of the CD4 cells, which is not shown, takes place as depicted in Figs. 67.4 and 67.5. (*Ag,* Antigen; *APC,* antigen-presenting cell; *CTL,* cytolytic T lymphocyte; *MHC I,* class I MHC molecule.)

APCs. As noted earlier, virtually all cells in the body carry class I MHC molecules. (Class II molecules are limited to APCs and B cells.) Hence, when a cell is infected with a virus, viral antigens form intracellular complexes with MHC I molecules, after which the antigen–MHC I complexes are presented on the cell surface. As shown in Fig. 67.6, activated CTLs recognize the antigen–MHC I complex and hence bind with the target cell. Since only cells that are infected with the virus will bear viral antigens on their class I MHC molecules, attack by CTLs is limited to infected cells; all others are spared.

Mechanisms of Cell Kill

Binding of a CTL to its target cell causes the CTL to release mediators that kill the target. Two mechanisms of cell kill are involved: *lysis* and *apoptosis* (programmed cell death). The mediator of lysis is called *perforin,* a molecule that forms pores in the target-cell membrane; the resultant influx of fluid causes the cell to swell and then burst. (This mechanism is very similar to one by which the complement system causes cell lysis.) The mediators of apoptosis have not been identified with certainty. However, their effects are very clear. The initial effect is activation of intracellular enzymes that digest the cell's own DNA. This is followed by fragmentation of the nucleus and cell death. Only the target cell is harmed; bystander cells and the CTL itself are not touched. In fact, after releasing its mediators, the CTL disconnects from the doomed target and goes on to seek another target cell.

KEY POINTS

- The immune system helps us by attacking invading organisms (viruses, bacteria, fungi, and parasites) and cancer cells. The immune system can hurt us by attacking transplants and our own healthy cells.
- There are two basic types of immune responses: natural immunity (native or innate immunity) and specific acquired immunity.
- There are two types of specific acquired immunity: cell-mediated immunity and antibody-mediated (humoral) immunity.
- The immune system has five major types of cells: B lymphocytes (B cells), helper T lymphocytes (CD4 cells), cytolytic T lymphocytes (CD8 cells, CTLs), macrophages, and dendritic cells.
- Only lymphocytes have receptors that can recognize specific antigens.
- B cells make antibodies.
- CTLs kill target cells directly.
- Helper T cells are essential for the activation of B cells, CTLs, and the macrophages involved in delayed-type hypersensitivity (DTH).
- Macrophages have three functions in specific immunity: (1) they serve as antigen-presenting cells (APCs) in the activation of helper T cells and CTLs, (2) they are involved in DTH, and (3) they phagocytize opsonized cells in humoral immunity.
- Like macrophages, dendritic cells serve as APCs.
- An antigen is a molecule that triggers a specific immune response and then becomes the target of that response.
- Most antigens are large molecules.
- Antibodies bind to specific small regions of an antigen, referred to as *epitopes* or *antigenic determinants*.
- The major histocompatibility complex (MHC) is a group of genes that codes for MHC molecules, which are found on the surface of cells.
- MHC molecules have three major functions: (1) they play a key role in the activation of helper T cells and CTLs, (2) they guide CTLs toward target cells, and (3) they provide the basis for distinguishing between self and nonself.
- Class II MHC molecules are found only on B cells and APCs, whereas class I MHC molecules are found on virtually all cells (including B cells and APCs).
- It is rare for two individuals to have MHC molecules that are precisely the same. As a result, MHC molecules from one individual are usually recognized as foreign (nonself) by the immune systems of everyone else.
- A cytokine is defined as any mediator molecule (other than an antibody) released by any immune system cell.
- The most characteristic feature of antibodies is their ability to recognize specific antigens.
- Antibody production requires the cooperative interaction of three types of cells: B cells, which make the antibodies; helper T cells (CD4 cells), which stimulate the B cells; and APCs, which activate the CD4 cells so that they can then activate B cells.
- B cells have antibodies on their surface that serve as receptors for recognizing specific antigens. Binding of the antigen to the receptor is the first step in B-cell activation.
- Activation of B cells is completed when a CD4 cell binds with an antigen–MHC II complex on the B cell and then releases cytokines, which then stimulate the B cell.
- To activate a B cell, a CD4 cell must first become activated itself. CD4 activation is initiated by binding of the CD4 cell with an antigen–MHC II complex on an APC.
- Antibodies eliminate antigens by three mechanisms: (1) direct neutralization of toxins and viruses, (2) opsonization of bacteria, and (3) activation of the complement system.
- Opsonization (coating bacteria with antibodies) helps macrophages and neutrophils grab on to bacteria, and thereby facilitates phagocytosis.
- The complement system forms pores in the bacterial cell membrane, thereby promoting death by lysis.
- Cell-mediated immunity can result in DTH and lysis of target cells by CTLs.
- DTH involves two types of cells: an infected macrophage and a CD4 cell. The macrophage activates the CD4 cell, which then releases interferon gamma, which in turn stimulates the macrophage, thereby enabling the macrophage to kill the bacteria inside it.
- The major role of CTLs is to kill self cells that have become infected with viruses.
- Activation of CTLs proceeds in two steps: first, the CTL binds to an APC; second, the CTL is stimulated by cytokines provided by a CD4 cell.
- The binding of CTLs with APCs differs from the binding of CD4 cells with APCs in that CTLs specifically recognize antigen that is bound to a class I MHC molecule on the APC, whereas CD4 cells specifically recognize antigen that is bound to a class II MHC molecule.
- CTLs kill target cells in two ways: (1) they release perforin, which creates pores in the cell, thereby causing death by lysis; and (2) they release compounds that cause apoptosis (programmed cell death).
- Activated CTLs attack only self cells that have antigen–MHC I complexes; all other self cells, including the CTLs, are spared.
- Specific immune responses result in the production of memory T cells and memory B cells. As a result, the next time an antigen is encountered, the immune response occurs faster and with greater intensity.

Please visit **http://evolve.elsevier.com/Lehne** for chapter-specific NCLEX® examination review questions.

CHAPTER

68 Childhood Immunization

The purpose of immunization is to protect against infectious diseases. Thanks to widespread immunization, the incidence of several infectious diseases has been dramatically reduced, and one disease—smallpox—has been eliminated from the planet. Of all the advances in medicine, none has reduced sickness and death more than immunization.

Experience has shown that the most effective way to reduce vaccine-preventable diseases (VPDs) is to create a highly immune population. Accordingly, universal vaccination is a national goal. Although immunization carries some risk, the risks from failing to vaccinate are much greater.

Discussion in this chapter is limited to childhood immunization. Chapter 110 addresses vaccines for anthrax and smallpox, and Chapter 93 addresses a vaccine for avian flu.

GENERAL CONSIDERATIONS

Definitions

To discuss immunization, we must use special terminology. Accordingly, we begin by defining some terms.

Vaccine

A vaccine is a preparation containing whole or fractionated microorganisms. Administration causes the recipient's immune system to manufacture antibodies directed against the microbe from which the vaccine was made. Most of the preparations discussed in this chapter are vaccines.

Killed Vaccines Versus Live Vaccines

There are two major classes of vaccines: killed and live (albeit attenuated). Killed vaccines are composed of whole killed microbes or isolated microbial components (e.g., the polysaccharide of *Haemophilus influenzae* type b or the surface antigen of hepatitis B). In contrast, live, attenuated vaccines are composed of live microbes that have been weakened or rendered completely avirulent. Live vaccines can be dangerous in recipients who are immunocompromised because these people are unable to mount an effective immune response, even against an avirulent organism.

Toxoid

A toxoid is a bacterial toxin that has been changed to a nontoxic form. Administration causes the recipient's immune system to manufacture antitoxins (i.e., antibodies directed against the natural bacterial toxin). Antitoxins protect against injury from toxins, but do not kill the bacteria that produce them. In this chapter, only two toxoids are considered: tetanus toxoid and diphtheria toxoid.

Vaccination

The terms *vaccination* and *vaccine* derive from *vaccinia,* a virus whose name in turn derives from *vacca* (Latin for cow). At one time, vaccinia virus was used as a vaccine against smallpox. (Vaccinia itself causes cowpox—a mild sickness—and in the process induces synthesis of smallpox antibodies.) Hence, when the term *vaccination* was originally coined, it had the limited meaning of giving vaccinia to generate immunity against smallpox. Today, vaccination refers broadly to giving any vaccine or toxoid.

Immunization: Active Versus Passive

Immunization is a more inclusive term than *vaccination,* in that immunization refers to production of both active immunity and passive immunity, whereas vaccination refers to production of active immunity only.

Active immunity develops in response to infection or to administration of a vaccine or toxoid. In either case, the result is endogenous production of antibodies. Active immunity takes weeks or months to develop, but is long-lasting. Discussion in this chapter is limited almost exclusively to active immunization.

Passive immunity is conferred by giving a patient *preformed* antibodies (immune globulins). Unlike active immunity, passive immunity protects immediately, but persists only as long as the antibodies remain in the body.

Specific Immune Globulins

These preparations contain a high concentration of antibodies directed against a specific antigen (e.g., hepatitis B virus). Administration provides immediate passive immunity. These preparations are made from donated blood.

Public Health Impact of Immunization

Widespread vaccination has had a profound impact on public health. In the United States, vaccination has greatly reduced the incidence of some infectious diseases (e.g., pertussis, mumps, tetanus) and virtually eliminated five others: diphtheria, smallpox, poliomyelitis, rubella, and measles. With two diseases, results have been even more dramatic: wild-type polio is gone from the Western hemisphere, and smallpox is gone from the planet.

Despite these successes, we still have a long way to go: Although our national vaccination rate is at an all-time high, every year 2.1 million children ages 1 to 3 years receive few or no vaccinations. In some parts of the country, more than 50% of children are not current. The consequences of failing to vaccinate can be enormous. In 2015 alone, over 134,000 deaths occurred worldwide due to measles. Many of these deaths occurred in young children.

The Childhood Immunization Initiative is directed at preventing increased death in the future. The goal is to eliminate all indigenous cases of diphtheria, measles, rubella, tetanus, and *H. influenzae* type b infection from the United States. The program aims to achieve these goals by improving vaccine delivery systems, increasing community participation, reducing vaccine costs to parents, developing safer and simpler vaccines, and involving more federal agencies in providing vaccines to populations who otherwise might not have access to them. Thanks to these strategies, three of these diseases—diphtheria, rubella, and measles—are virtually gone from this country.

From a strictly economic viewpoint, vaccination is a sound investment. On average, we gain $44 in economic benefits for every dollar we spend on vaccination.

Reporting Vaccine-Preventable Diseases

Public health officials rely on healthcare providers to report cases of Vaccine-Preventable Diseases (VPDs). Nearly all VPDs that occur in the United States are notifiable. Healthcare providers should report individual cases to their local or state health department. Each week, the state health departments make a report to the Centers for Disease Control and Prevention (CDC). The information is used to (1) determine if an outbreak is occurring, (2) evaluate prevention and control strategies, and (3) evaluate the impact of national immunization policies and practices.

Immunization Records

The *National Childhood Vaccine Injury Act* of 1986 requires a permanent record of each mandated vaccination a child receives. The information should be recorded in either (1) the permanent medical record of the recipient or (2) a permanent office log or file. The following data are required:

- Date of vaccination
- Route and site of vaccination
- Vaccine type, manufacturer, lot number, and expiration date
- Name, address, and title of the person administering the vaccine

The purpose of these records is twofold. First, they help ensure that children receive appropriate vaccinations. Second, they help avoid overvaccination and thereby reduce the risk of possible hypersensitivity reactions. To promote uniformity in record keeping, an official immunization card has been adopted by every state and the District of Columbia.

Adverse Effects of Immunization

Vaccines are generally very safe. Although mild reactions are common, serious events are rare. Many children experience local reactions (discomfort, swelling, and erythema at the injection site). Fever is also common. Very rare but severe effects include *anaphylaxis* (e.g., in response to measles, mumps, and rubella virus vaccine); acute *encephalopathy* (caused by diphtheria and tetanus toxoids and pertussis vaccine); and vaccine-associated *paralytic poliomyelitis* (caused by oral poliovirus vaccine). In 2011, the safety of vaccines was reaffirmed in a lengthy report—*Adverse Effects of Vaccines: Evidence and Causality*—issued by the Institute of Medicine of the National Academies.

Vaccinations can hurt. This pain, in turn, can lead to needle fears, procedural anxiety, and an avoidance of additional immunizations. Accordingly, minimizing pain is a primary goal. Strategies to reduce pain and anxiety include holding the child upright during the vaccination, applying a topical anesthetic, providing tactile stimulation, performing IM injections rapidly without prior aspiration, and injecting the most painful vaccine last. Pain can be further reduced by the use of microneedles, needle-free devices, and intranasal vaccines. What about giving analgesic-antipyretics, such as acetaminophen and ibuprofen? Evidence from a study in Russia indicates that giving these drugs before or shortly after vaccination can reduce the immune response. In addition, studies show that prophylactic administration of antipyretics does not significantly reduce the incidence of fever or pain. Accordingly, routine prophylactic use of these drugs to prevent pain and/or fever should be discouraged. Yet because there has been only one study regarding immune response and antipyretic agents, the American Academy of Pediatrics still condones their use for children who experience pain or fever after the immunization is given.

Immunocompromised children are at special risk from live vaccines. The reason is that, in the absence of an adequate immune response, the viruses or bacteria in these normally safe vaccines are able to multiply in profusion, thereby causing serious infection. Accordingly, live vaccines should generally be avoided in children who are severely immunosuppressed. Causes of immunosuppression include congenital immunodeficiency, HIV infection, leukemia, lymphoma, generalized malignancy, and therapy with radiation, cytotoxic anticancer drugs, and high-dose glucocorticoids.

Some parents are concerned that *thimerosal,* a mercury-based preservative found in some vaccines, might cause *autism.* For two reasons, this concern is unfounded. First, several large, high-quality studies conducted in Denmark, Britain, and the United States have failed to show a causal link between childhood immunization using thimerosal-containing vaccines and the development of autism. Second, thimerosal is being phased out of vaccines made here (owing to concerns about mercury exposure, not concerns about autism). At this time, the amount of thimerosal in most routinely used childhood vaccines is either zero or extremely low (less than 0.5 mcg per 0.5-mL dose). The only exceptions are certain flu vaccines, which still contain thimerosal as a preservative. However, even if these flu vaccines are used, total mercury exposure from childhood vaccination will still be well below the limit considered safe by the U.S. Food and Drug Administration (FDA) and the Environmental Protection Agency.

The risk of serious adverse reactions can be minimized by observing appropriate *precautions* and *contraindications.* Table 68.1 lists contraindications that apply to all vaccines. Precautions and contraindications that apply to specific vaccines are discussed in the context of those preparations. Certain conditions, such as diarrhea and mild illness, may be inappropriately regarded as contraindications by some practitioners. As a result, vaccination may be needlessly postponed. Conditions that are often considered contraindications, although they are not, are also listed in Table 68.1.

TABLE 68.1 ▪ Contraindications That Apply to All Vaccines and Conditions Often Incorrectly Regarded as Contraindications

True Contraindications (Vaccine Should Not Be Administered)	Not Contraindications (Vaccine May Be Administered)
Anaphylactic reaction to a specific vaccine: Contraindicates further doses of that vaccine	Mild to moderate local reaction (soreness, erythema, swelling) following a dose of an injectable vaccine
Anaphylactic reaction to a vaccine component: Contraindicates use of all vaccines that contain that substance	Mild acute illness with or without low-grade fever
	Diarrhea
	Current antimicrobial therapy
	Convalescent phase of illnesses
Moderate or severe illnesses with or without a fever	Prematurity (same dosage and indications as for normal, full-term infants)
	Recent exposure to an infectious disease
	Personal or family history of either penicillin allergy or nonspecific allergies

Practitioners are required to report certain adverse events to the *Vaccine Adverse Event Reporting System* (VAERS). The information is used to help determine whether (1) a particular event that occurs after vaccination is actually caused by the vaccine and (2) what the risk factors might be. In addition to reporting events that they are required to report, practitioners should report all other serious or unusual adverse events, regardless of whether they believe the event was caused by the vaccine. Forms for reporting adverse events can be obtained from the VAERS web site (www.vaers.hhs.gov) or by calling 1-800-822-7967.

The *National Vaccine Injury Compensation Program* (NVICP), established by the *National Childhood Vaccine Injury Act* of 1986, was created to provide compensation for injury or death resulting from vaccination. The program is intended as an alternative to civil litigation in that negligence need not be proved. As a provision of the law, a table was created listing the vaccines covered by the program and the injuries, disabilities, illness, and conditions—including death—for which compensation may be paid. Compensation may also be paid for injuries not listed in the table, provided that (1) a listed vaccine is involved and (2) causality can be demonstrated. Injuries related to vaccines not listed in the table are not covered under the program. Additional information can be obtained by calling 1-800-338-2382.

Vaccine Information Statements

The National Childhood Vaccine Injury Act requires that Vaccine Information Statements (VISs) be given to all vaccinated patients (or their parents or legal representatives) before certain vaccines are administered. The VISs, produced by the CDC, are one-page, two-sided documents that describe the benefits and risks of specific vaccines. For vaccines that require a series of shots, a VIS must be given *before each dose,* not just the first dose. The VISs are available in over 30 languages and can be obtained online at https://www.cdc.gov/vaccines/hcp/vis/index.html.

Childhood Immunization Schedule

Each year, the CDC's Advisory Committee on Immunization Practices (ACIP), in cooperation with the American Academy of Family Physicians (AAFP) and the American Academy of Pediatrics (AAP), issues revised recommendations for childhood immunization in the United States. You can find the yearly schedule recommendations and catch-up immunization schedule for persons ages 4 months through 18 years, as well as the most recent updates, online at www.cdc.gov/vaccines/. Please note that adult immunization schedules can also be found there.

TARGET DISEASES

Routine childhood vaccination is currently recommended for protection against 16 infectious diseases: diphtheria, tetanus (lockjaw), pertussis (whooping cough), measles, mumps, rubella, invasive *H. influenzae* type b, hepatitis A, hepatitis B, polio, varicella (chickenpox), influenza, invasive pneumococcal disease, meningococcal disease (meningitis), rotavirus gastroenteritis, and genital human papillomavirus infection. In the discussion below, certain VPDs are considered in a group (e.g., measles, mumps, rubella) because vaccination against these VPDs is traditionally done simultaneously using a combination vaccine.

Measles, Mumps, and Rubella

Measles

Measles is a highly contagious viral disease characterized by rash and high fever (103°F to 105°F). Infection is spread by inhalation of aerosolized sputum or by direct contact with nasal or throat secretions. Initial symptoms include fever, cough, headache, sore throat, and conjunctivitis. Three days later, rash develops. Rash begins at the hairline, spreads to the rest of the body in 36 hours, and then fades in a few days. Secondary infections can result in pneumonia and otitis media (inner ear infection). However, of the potential complications of measles, encephalitis is by far the most serious. Sequelae of encephalitis include blindness, deafness, and convulsions. Although encephalitis is rare (0.1% incidence), it carries a 10% risk of death.

Mumps

Mumps is a viral disease that primarily affects the parotid glands (the largest of the three pairs of salivary glands). Although mumps can occur in adults, it usually occurs in children ages 5 to 15. As a rule, the first symptom is swelling in one of the parotid glands, often accompanied by local pain and tenderness. The patient may also experience fever (100°F to 104°F). Swelling increases for 2 to 3 days and then fades entirely by day 6 or 7. Swelling in the second parotid gland often develops after swelling in the first, but may also occur simultaneously or not at all. Painful *orchitis* (inflammation of the testes) develops in about one-third of adult and adolescent males. Acute *aseptic meningitis* develops in about 10% of all patients; symptoms, which resolve completely, include dizziness, headache, and vomiting. In the United States, the incidence of reported mumps cases has declined from a high of 212,932 in 1984 to only 5748 in 2016.

Rubella

Rubella, also known as German measles, is a generally mild viral infection. However, if it occurs during pregnancy, the consequences can be severe. Initial symptoms include sore throat, mild fever, and swelling in lymph nodes located behind the ears and in the back of the neck. Shortly after, a rash develops on the face and scalp, spreads rapidly to the torso and arms, and then fades in 2 or 3 days. Arthritis may also develop, mainly in women. In pregnant women, rubella can cause miscarriage, stillbirth, and congenital defects, especially if the disease occurs during the first trimester. Possible birth defects include cataracts, heart disease, developmental delay, and hearing loss. In the United States, rubella has been eliminated: Since 2002, all cases reported here have been traceable to foreigners who brought the disease from abroad.

Diphtheria, Tetanus, and Pertussis

Diphtheria

Diphtheria is a potentially fatal infection caused by *Corynebacterium diphtheriae,* a gram-positive bacillus. The bacterium colonizes the throat and nasal passages and produces a toxin that spreads throughout the body. Initial symptoms include sore throat, fever, headache, and nausea. Colonization of the airway begins as patches of gray or dirty-yellow membrane. The patches eventually grow together, forming a thick coating. This coating, combined with swelling, can impede swallowing and breathing; in severe cases, a tracheostomy is needed. The toxin produced by *C. diphtheriae* can damage the heart and nerves, resulting in heart failure and paralysis. Diphtheria treatment includes the administration of diphtheria antitoxin and antibiotics (e.g., erythromycin, penicillin G). In the United States, only 5 cases were reported between 2006 and 2016. The last case of reported diphtheria was in 2014.

Tetanus (Lockjaw)

Tetanus, also known as lockjaw, is a frequently fatal disease characterized by painful spasm of all skeletal muscles. The cause is a potent endotoxin elaborated by *Clostridium tetani,* a gram-positive bacillus. Infection with *C. tetani* typically results from puncturing the skin with a nail, splinter, or other object that is contaminated with soil, street dust, or animal or human feces. The first symptom is often stiffness of the jaw, hence the name *lockjaw.* As infection progresses, the patient may experience stiff neck, difficulty swallowing, restlessness, irritability, headache, chills, fever, and convulsions. Eventually, spasm develops in muscles of the abdomen, back, neck, and face. The case fatality rate is 21%. In the United States, the yearly incidence of tetanus peaked at 601 cases in 1948, but totaled only 30 cases in 2015. Treatment options include tetanus antitoxin, a booster dose of tetanus toxoid, and antibiotics (e.g., metronidazole, penicillin G).

Pertussis (Whooping Cough)

Pertussis, also known as *whooping cough* or the *100-day cough,* occurs primarily in infants and young children. The cause is *Bordetella pertussis,* a gram-negative bacillus. Initial symptoms include rhinorrhea, mild fever, and persistent cough. As infection worsens, coughing becomes more intense. The acute phase of the disease can last 4 to 6 weeks. During this time, infants experience difficulty eating, drinking, and breathing. Deaths have occurred. Complications of pertussis include pneumonia, seizures, ear infections, and, rarely, permanent neurologic injury. In the United States, reported cases dropped from a high of 265,269 in 1934 to 8483 in 2003. However, the rate of pertussis increased to 20,679 reported cases in 2015. Worldwide, the disease afflicts about 16 million people and kills 195,000 each year, mainly infants and young children. Azithromycin is the treatment of choice.

Poliomyelitis

Poliomyelitis, also known as polio or infantile paralysis, is a serious disease in which the poliovirus attacks neurons of the central nervous system that control muscle movement. The result is skeletal muscle paralysis, usually in the legs. However, muscles of respiration and muscles of the arms may be affected too. In about 10% of cases, polio is fatal. The disease is caused by three different polioviruses. Paralytic polio is usually caused by type 1 poliovirus. Polio has no cure. However, proper symptomatic treatment can improve comfort and reduce or prevent some crippling effects. Vaccination against polio has eliminated the disease from the Western hemisphere, except for eight to nine cases annually caused by the vaccine itself. To prevent vaccine-induced polio, use of the live virus vaccine (oral polio vaccine) has been discontinued in the United States. The number of cases worldwide was 716 in 2011—nearly 20 times the 37 cases documented in 2016.

Haemophilus influenzae Type b

Haemophilus influenzae type b is a gram-negative bacterium that can cause meningitis, pneumonia, and serious throat and ear infections. The bacterium is the leading cause of serious illness in children under the age of 5 years; prior to vaccinations, it was the most common cause of bacterial meningitis, which has a mortality rate of 5%. Among children who survive meningitis, between 25% and 35% suffer lasting neurologic deficits. As a result of childhood vaccination, the annual incidence of infection in the United States dropped from an estimated 20,000 cases in 1984 to less than 3800 in 2013. Of the cases that occurred, almost all were in unvaccinated children. Infection with *H. influenzae* can be treated successfully with antibiotics.

Varicella (Chickenpox)

Varicella (chickenpox) is a common, highly contagious, and potentially serious disease of childhood. The causative organism is varicella-zoster virus, a member of the herpesvirus group. Patients typically develop 250 to 500 maculopapular or vesicular lesions, usually on the face, scalp, or trunk. Other symptoms include fever, malaise, and loss of appetite. Among children, the most common complications are bacterial suprainfection and acute cerebellar ataxia. Reye's syndrome and encephalitis develop rarely. Among adults, the most serious common complication is varicella pneumonia. As a rule, symptoms in adults are more severe than in children: Hospitalization is 10 times more likely in adults, and death is 20 times more likely. Although adults account for only 2% of varicella cases, they account for 50% of varicella-related deaths. Before varicella vaccine became available, over 90% of children in the United States got chickenpox by age 11, which corresponds to 4 million cases a year. In addition, about 11,000 victims were hospitalized each year, and about 100 died. Since universal vaccination began in 1995, hospitalizations have dropped dramatically: Each year, varicella vaccinations prevent 3.5 million cases, 9000 hospitalizations, and 100 deaths.

Herpes zoster, also known as *shingles* or simply *zoster,* develops in 15% of patients years after childhood chickenpox has resolved. The cause is reactivation of varicella-zoster viruses that had been dormant within sensory nerve roots. Episodes of zoster begin with neurologic pain in the area of skin supplied by the affected nerve roots. Blister-like lesions develop within 3 to 4 days and usually disappear 2 to 3 weeks later. However, in about 14% of patients, neurologic pain persists for a month or more—and in a few cases, pain lasts for years.

Hepatitis B

Hepatitis B is a serious liver infection caused by the hepatitis B virus. Acute infection can cause anorexia, malaise, diarrhea, vomiting, jaundice, pain (in muscles, joints, and stomach), and death. Chronic infection can result in cirrhosis, liver cancer, and death. Worldwide, 257 million people have chronic hepatitis B, and 900,000 die from it annually.

Although hepatitis B is found in virtually all body fluids, only blood, serum-derived fluids, saliva, semen, and vaginal fluids are infectious. The most common modes of transmission are needle-stick accidents, sexual contact with an infected partner, maternal-child transmission during birth, and the use of contaminated IV equipment or solutions.

Hepatitis B is discussed further in Chapter 93.

Hepatitis A

Hepatitis A is a serious liver infection caused by the hepatitis A virus. In the United States, hepatitis A infection is declining. In 2014, there were 2500 reported cases of acute hepatitis A in the United States. Symptoms of hepatitis A include fever, malaise, nausea, jaundice, anorexia, diarrhea, and stomach pain. However, not all infected persons become symptomatic. Among children under 6 years old, only 30% develop symptoms. In contrast, symptoms are present in most older infected children and adults. When symptoms do occur, they develop rapidly and then usually fade in less than 2 months. However, between 10% and 15% of patients experience prolonged or relapsing disease that persists up to 6 months. During the course of the infection, the virus undergoes replication in the liver, passage into the bile, and then excretion in the feces. As a result, the usual mode of transmission is fecal-oral in the context of close personal contact with an infected person. In addition, hepatitis A can be contracted by ingesting contaminated food or water. Blood-borne transmission is rare. Individuals at risk include household and sexual contacts of infected individuals, international travelers, and people living in areas where hepatitis A is endemic (e.g., Native American reservations, Alaskan Native villages).

Pneumococcal Infection

In the United States, *Streptococcus pneumoniae* (pneumococcus) is the leading bacterial cause of childhood meningitis, sepsis, pneumonia, and otitis media. Among children with pneumococcal meningitis, up to 50% suffer permanent brain damage or hearing loss, and about 10% die. The risk of acquiring pneumococcal infection is highest for children under the age of 2 years. Factors that increase infection risk include sickle cell disease, immunodeficiency, asplenia, chronic diseases, attending a group day care center, and being a Native American, African American, or Alaskan Native or a socially disadvantaged person. Worldwide, pneumococcal infection ranks among the leading causes of death from infectious disease. Routine childhood immunization against pneumococcal disease began in 2000. Since then, the incidence of severe pediatric infection has dropped sharply.

Meningococcal Infection

Meningococcal infection is a serious disease caused by *Neisseria meningitidis,* also known as the meningococcus. Invasive meningococcal disease is a leading cause of meningitis in American children. Worldwide, the majority of infections are caused by five *N. meningitidis* serogroups—designated A, B, C, Y, and W-135—identified on the basis of antigenic differences in surface polysaccharides. In the United States, only three serogroups—B, C, and Y—cause most cases. Meningococcal infection is readily transmitted through direct contact with respiratory secretions from patients and from asymptomatic carriers. Injury results from a meningococcal endotoxin, which is produced so quickly that death can result within hours of infection onset. Although only 375 cases occurred in the United States in 2015, the disease is clearly of great concern, with a fatality rate of 10% to 14% despite antibiotic therapy. Furthermore, of those who survive, 11% to 19% suffer severe and permanent sequelae, including neurologic disability, deafness, developmental delay, and limb amputations. Infection rate is highest during infancy, with a second peak during adolescence and early adulthood. Outbreaks can occur in day care centers, schools, and colleges. Risk factors for acquiring the disease include immunodeficiency, antecedent viral infection, household crowding, chronic underlying disease, active and passive smoking, and anatomic and functional asplenia. A meningococcal vaccine was approved in 1981, but it was not very effective in children. Hence, routine childhood immunization was not recommended until 2005, the year a more effective vaccine was introduced.

Influenza

Influenza is a serious infection of the respiratory tract and a major cause of morbidity and mortality worldwide. Characteristics of the influenza virus and of influenza itself (mode of transmission, symptoms, time course, methods of prevention and treatment) are discussed in Chapter 93.

Rotavirus Gastroenteritis

Rotavirus, which infects the intestinal mucosa, is the most common diarrheal pathogen worldwide. Infection presents initially as upset stomach and vomiting, usually with fever, and then progresses to several days of diarrhea, which can be mild to severe. The combination of vomiting and severe diarrhea can result in life-threatening dehydration. Virtually all children become infected repeatedly within the first 5 years of life. However, the first episode is generally the worst. As a result, severe diarrhea and dehydration are most likely in the very young—children 3 to 35 months old. Before a rotavirus vaccine became available, rotavirus annually infected 2.7 million American children younger than 5 years, resulting in more than 400,000 office visits, 55,000 to 70,000 hospitalizations, and 20 to 60 deaths. Worldwide, annual deaths are still estimated in the hundreds of thousands. Infected children shed large amounts of rotavirus in their stool, and hence transmission is usually fecal-oral, resulting from touching the stool or a contaminated object. Rotavirus infection can be prevented with two vaccines: RotaTeq and Rotarix.

Genital Human Papillomavirus Infection

Human papillomavirus (HPV) infection is the cause of virtually all anogenital warts and cervical cancers. Transmission occurs most often by direct genital contact during vaginal or anal intercourse. The types of HPV that infect the anogenital region can also cause cancers of the vulva, vagina, urethra, tongue, tonsils, penis, and anus. Cancer of the anus in men and women who have anal intercourse is now as common as cervical cancer was before the Papanicolaou (Pap) test was introduced. The discussion that follows focuses on the role of HPV in cervical cancer and genital warts. Treatment of genital warts is discussed in Chapter 105.

Genital HPV is the most common sexually transmitted infection. In the United States, about 14.1 million people become infected each year. Among sexually active males and females, about 50% will be infected at some time during their life. Fortunately, although HPV infections are common, most are benign and clear spontaneously, usually within a few months to a year. As a result, most men and women never get genital warts, and most women never get precancerous cervical lesions or cervical cancer.

About 100 types of HPV are known to exist, about 40 of which infect the anogenital region. The types of HPV associated with malignancy are referred to as *oncogenic* or *high-risk,* whereas the types associated with genital warts are called *low-risk.* About 95% of genital warts are caused by just two HPV types, known as HPV-6 and HPV-11. About 70% of cervical cancers are caused by two other types, known as HPV-16 and HPV-18. Fortunately, only 2.2% of women carry high-risk strains.

Worldwide, cervical cancer is the third most common cancer among women. Each year, more than 500,000 cases are diagnosed, and about 300,000 prove fatal. In the United States, cervical cancer is less prevalent: Total new cases are estimated at 12,000 each year. Why so few deaths in the United States? Because most American women undergo regular Pap tests, which detect precancerous and cancerous changes, allowing early intervention (excision or ablation of the affected tissue) before advanced cancer can develop.

Respiratory Syncytial Virus

Respiratory syncytial virus (RSV), an enveloped virus of the Paramyxoviridae family, was first identified in 1956. In the United States, RSV infection is the most common cause of bronchiolitis (inflammation of small airways in the lungs) and pneumonia in children younger than 1 year and the most common cause for hospitalization in children younger than 5 years. Worldwide, it is estimated that RSV is responsible for nearly 7% of deaths in children ages 1 month to 1 year; only malaria kills more children in this age group.

All children are at risk of RSV, but the incidence of severe disease is highest in children born prematurely and in those with cardiopulmonary disease. Children at high risk account for nearly half of RSV-related hospital admissions in the United States. An additional at-risk population is older adults, who often suffer from flu-like symptoms caused by RSV.

SPECIFIC VACCINES AND TOXOIDS

The discussion in this section is limited to the vaccines and toxoids used for routine childhood immunization. The major preparations employed are listed in Table 68.2. Their adverse effects are shown in Table 68.3. Childhood immunization schedules, catch-up schedules, and recent changes—as recommended by the ACIP, the AAP, and the AAFP—are available online at www.cdc.gov/vaccines/.

TABLE 68.2 ▪ Some Vaccines and Toxoids Available in the United States

Preparation Name (Acronym)	Brand Name	Type of Preparation	Route and Site
Measles, mumps, and rubella virus vaccine (MMR)	M-M-R II	Live virus	SubQ, in outer aspect of upper arm
Measles, mumps, and rubella, and varicella virus vaccine (MMRV)	ProQuad[a]	Live virus	SubQ, in anterolateral thigh or outer aspect of upper arm
Diphtheria and tetanus toxoids and acellular pertussis vaccine (DTaP)	Tripedia, DAPTACEL, Infanrix, Boostrix,[b] Adacel[b]	Toxoids (diphtheria and tetanus) plus inactivated bacteria components (pertussis)	IM, in deltoid or mediolateral thigh
Diphtheria and tetanus toxoids and acellular pertussis adsorbed, hepatitis B (recombinant), and inactivated poliovirus vaccine	PEDIARIX	Toxoids (diphtheria and tetanus) plus inactivated bacteria components (pertussis) plus inactive viral antigen (hepatitis B) plus inactivated viruses (poliovirus)	IM, in deltoid or anterolateral thigh
Tetanus and diphtheria toxoids	Generic only	Toxoids	IM, in deltoid or mediolateral thigh
Haemophilus influenzae type b (Hib) conjugate vaccine	ActHIB, PedvaxHIB, Hiberix	Bacterial polysaccharide conjugated to protein	IM, in midthigh or outer aspect of upper arm
Poliovirus vaccine, inactivated (IPV, Salk vaccine)	IPOL	Inactivated viruses of all three polio serotypes	SubQ, in anterolateral thigh
Varicella virus vaccine	Varivax	Live virus	SubQ, in deltoid or anterolateral thigh
Hepatitis A vaccine (HepA)	Havrix, VAQTA	Inactive viral antigen	IM, in deltoid
Hepatitis B vaccine (HepB)	Recombivax HB, Engerix-B	Inactive viral antigen	IM, in deltoid or anterolateral thigh
Pneumococcal conjugate vaccine (PCV13)	Prevnar 13	Bacterial polysaccharide conjugated to protein	IM, in deltoid or anterolateral thigh
Pneumococcal polysaccharide vaccine (PPV)	Pneumovax 23	Bacterial polysaccharide (unconjugated)	IM, in deltoid or anterolateral thigh
Influenza vaccine (inactivated)	Fluzone, Fluvirin, others	Inactive viral antigen	IM, in deltoid or anterolateral thigh
Influenza vaccine (live)	FluMist	Live virus	Intranasal
Meningococcal conjugate vaccine (MCV4)	Menactra, Menveo	Bacterial polysaccharide conjugated to protein	IM, in deltoid
Rotavirus vaccine	Rotarix, RotaTeq	Live virus	Oral
Human papillomavirus vaccine	Gardasil, Gardasil 9	DNA-free virus-like particles	IM, in deltoid or anterolateral thigh

[a]ProQuad combines two older vaccines: M-M-R II and Varivax.
[b]Boostrix and Adacel are indicated for *booster* immunization, *not* for the *initial* immunization series. Boostrix is for patients 11 to 18 years of age. Adacel is for patients 11 to 64 years of age.

Safety Alert

VACCINATIONS

Absolute contraindications to vaccine administration in children include a history of anaphylactic reaction to a specific vaccine or vaccine component, as well as the presence of moderate or severe illnesses with or without a fever.

Measles, Mumps, and Rubella Virus Vaccine

Description

Measles, mumps, and rubella vaccine (MMR), marketed under the brand name *M-M-R II,* is a combination product composed of three live virus vaccines. Administration induces synthesis of antibodies directed against measles, mumps, and rubella viruses. Immunization with MMR is preferred to immunization with the three vaccines separately.

TABLE 68.3 ■ Adverse Effects of Some Vaccines and Toxoids

Preparation	Mild Effects	Serious Effects
Measles, mumps, and rubella virus vaccine	Local reactions; rash; fever; swollen glands in cheeks and neck and under the jaw; pain, stiffness, and swelling in joints	Anaphylaxis, thrombocytopenia[a]
Diphtheria and tetanus toxoids and acellular pertussis vaccine	Local reactions, fever, fretfulness, drowsiness, anorexia, persistent crying	Acute encephalopathy, convulsions, shock-like state
Haemophilus influenzae type b conjugate vaccine	Local reactions, fever, crying, diarrhea, vomiting	None
Varicella virus vaccine	Local reactions, fever, mild varicella-like rash (local or generalized)	None
Hepatitis A vaccine	Local soreness, headache, anorexia, fatigue	Anaphylaxis
Hepatitis B vaccine	Local discomfort, fever	Anaphylaxis
Pneumococcal conjugate vaccine	Local reactions, fever, irritability	None
Influenza vaccine (inactivated)	Local reactions, fever	None
Influenza vaccine (live attenuated)	Runny nose, headache, cough, fever	None
Meningococcal conjugate vaccine	Local reactions, headache, fatigue	None
Rotavirus vaccine	Diarrhea, vomiting, ear infection, runny nose, sore throat	Intussusception (rare)
Human papillomavirus vaccine	Local reactions, fainting	None

[a]A study showing a connection with autism was disproved.

Efficacy

Following a single dose of MMR, an effective response develops in 97% of vaccinated patients within 2 to 6 weeks. A second dose increases protection.

Adverse Effects

Mild. Local soreness, erythema, and swelling may develop soon after vaccination. Within 1 to 2 weeks, some children experience glandular swelling in the cheeks and neck and under the jaw. Transient rash develops in 5% to 15% of vaccinated patients. Fever (103°F or higher) that persists for several days occurs in 5% to 15% of vaccinated patients 5 to 12 days after vaccination. MMR-induced fever poses a small risk of febrile seizures, but these seizures do *not* increase the risk of developing epilepsy. Within 1 to 3 weeks of the first dose, about 1% of vaccinated patients experience pain, stiffness, and swelling in one or more joints; these symptoms usually subside in a few days, but occasionally persist for a month or more. Fever, soreness, and pain can be reduced with acetaminophen or a nonaspirin, nonsteroidal anti-inflammatory drug, such as ibuprofen. However, as noted earlier, these drugs should not be given before vaccination to *prevent* discomfort. Rather, they should be reserved for managing discomfort after it develops.

Severe. Transient thrombocytopenia occurs very rarely (0.0025% incidence). MMR-induced thrombocytopenia is generally benign, but hemorrhage has developed in a few vaccinated patients.

MMR can induce anaphylactic reactions. However, the incidence is extremely low. In the past, MMR-induced anaphylaxis was thought to result from allergy to eggs (the measles component of the vaccine is produced in chick embryo fibroblasts). However, it now appears that egg allergy is not involved. Rather, the leading suspect is a hydrolysis product of gelatin. Until more is known, authorities recommend that MMR be used with extreme caution in children with a known allergy to gelatin. The ACIP recommends routine vaccination for children with an allergy to eggs.

The Institute of Medicine and the AAP have organized several panels of independent scientists who have determined that there is no causal link between MMR and development of autism, Crohn's disease, or any other serious long-term illness. A 1998 paper by Andrew Wakefield showing a connection between MMR and "autistic enterocolitis" was withdrawn by the publisher in 2010; 10 of the 13 authors have retracted the findings.

Precautions and Contraindications

MMR is *contraindicated* during pregnancy and should be used with *caution* in children with a history of (1) thrombocytopenia or thrombocytopenic purpura or (2) anaphylactic-like reactions to gelatin or neomycin (MMR contains a small amount of this antibiotic).

MMR can be administered to children with *mild febrile illness* (e.g., upper respiratory infection with or without low-grade fever). However, for children with *moderate or severe febrile illness,* vaccination should be postponed until the illness has resolved.

Products that contain *immune globulins* (e.g., whole blood, serum, specific immune globulins) contain antibodies against the viruses in MMR, and therefore can inhibit the immune response to the vaccine. Accordingly, in children who have received immune globulins, vaccination with MMR should be postponed for at least 3 to 6 months.

In vaccinated patients who are *immunocompromised,* replication of the viruses in MMR may be much greater than normal. If the immunodeficiency is severe, death may occur. However, of the more than 200 million people who have received MMR in the United States, only 5 such deaths have been reported.

TABLE 68.4 ▪ Products for Immunization Against Diphtheria, Tetanus, and Pertussis

Symbol	Description	Brand Names	Comments
VACCINES FOR CHILDREN YOUNGER THAN 10 YEARS			
DTaP	Diphtheria toxoid, tetanus toxoid, and acellular pertussis vaccine	DAPTACEL, Infanrix	Used for routine vaccination against diphtheria, tetanus, and pertussis
DT	Diphtheria toxoid and tetanus toxoid	Generic only	Used for children under 7 years who should not get pertussis vaccine
VACCINES FOR ADOLESCENTS AND ADULTS			
Tdap	Tetanus toxoid, reduced diphtheria toxoid, and acellular pertussis vaccine, adolescent preparation	Boostrix, Adacel	Used as a *booster* in adolescents and adults to protect against all three diseases
Td	Tetanus toxoid and diphtheria toxoid	Generic only	Used as a *booster* for adolescents and adults to protect against tetanus and diphtheria, but not pertussis

Nonetheless, *children with severe immunodeficiency should NOT be given MMR.* Severe immunodeficiency may result from immunosuppressive drugs (e.g., glucocorticoids, cytotoxic anticancer drugs), certain cancers (e.g., leukemia, lymphoma, generalized malignancy), and advanced HIV infection. It is important to note, however, that if HIV infection is *asymptomatic,* MMR should be given. In this situation, there is no risk of serious adverse events from MMR, whereas there *is* a risk of severe complications from measles should the disease develop. Vaccination with MMR early in the course of HIV infection is preferred because the immune response to vaccination diminishes as HIV infection progresses.

Route, Site, and Immunization Schedule

MMR is administered subQ into the outer aspect of the upper arm. Each child should receive two vaccinations, the first between ages 12 and 15 months, and the second between ages 4 and 6 years. If the scheduled second dose is missed, it can be given between ages 7 and 18 years.

Diphtheria and Tetanus Toxoids and Acellular Pertussis Vaccine

Preparations

Primary vaccination against diphtheria, tetanus, and pertussis is usually done simultaneously using a combination product, composed of diphtheria toxoid, tetanus toxoid, and *acellular* pertussis vaccine (DTaP). This vaccine, which is relatively new, has replaced an older product, composed of diphtheria toxoid, tetanus toxoid, and *whole-cell* pertussis vaccine (DTP). DTaP is more effective than DTP and causes fewer and milder side effects. Vaccination with DTaP produces antibodies against diphtheria toxin, tetanus toxin, and *B. pertussis.* DTaP is available under several brand names, including *DAPTACEL* and *Infanrix.*

After children have received a full series of DTaP shots, they will need subsequent booster shots. Two booster products are available: *Tdap* and *Td.* Tdap—sold as *Boostrix* and *Adacel*—is composed of tetanus toxoid, reduced diphtheria toxoid, and acellular pertussis vaccine—and hence boosts protection against all three diseases. By contrast, Td boosts protection against only two diseases: tetanus and diphtheria. Because the incidence of pertussis is on the rise, a booster shot with Tdap, rather than Td, is now recommended for all children starting at 11 to 12 years of age. Boosters with Td are given every 10 years thereafter.

Products used for immunization against diphtheria, tetanus, and pertussis are shown in Table 68.4.

Efficacy

Immunization with DTaP reduces the risk of disease by 80% to 90%. Protection begins after the third dose and persists 4 to 6 years (against pertussis) and 10 years (against diphtheria and tetanus).

Adverse Effects

Mild. Mild reactions are common. The reactions seen most often are low fever, fretfulness, drowsiness, anorexia, and local reactions: pain, swelling, and redness. Mild reactions usually develop a few hours to 48 hours after vaccination and then resolve in 1 to 2 days. Ibuprofen can decrease fever and pain. However, as noted earlier, ibuprofen should not be given before vaccination to *prevent* discomfort. It should be reserved for managing discomfort after it develops.

Moderate. Moderate reactions occur less often than mild reactions. Persistent, inconsolable crying lasting 3 hours or longer occurs in 1% of vaccinated patients. Crying is most likely with the first dose of DTaP and is not associated with long-term sequelae. Fever (105°F or higher) occurs in 0.3% of vaccinated patients; the pertussis component appears responsible. Approximately 0.06% of vaccinated patients develop convulsions (with or without fever). These seizures have no permanent sequelae and do not increase the risk of subsequent febrile or afebrile seizures. A shock-like state develops in 0.06% of vaccinated patients and has no lasting sequelae.

Severe: Encephalopathy. Very rarely, DTaP causes acute encephalopathy. The incidence is between zero and 10.5 episodes per million doses. Most cases occur within 3 days of vaccination. Some of the children who experience acute encephalopathy develop chronic neurologic dysfunction later in life. However, the contribution of acute encephalopathy to long-term neurologic deficits is unclear.

Precautions and Contraindications

DTaP can be administered to children with *mild febrile illness* (e.g., upper respiratory infection with or without low-grade fever). However, for children with *moderate or severe febrile illness,* administration should be postponed until the illness has resolved.

DTaP is *contraindicated* if a prior vaccination with DTaP produced (1) an immediate anaphylactic reaction or (2) encephalopathy within 7 days of vaccination.

DTaP should be administered with *caution* (if at all) if a prior vaccination with DTaP produced any of the following:

- A shock-like state
- Fever (105°F or higher) occurring within 48 hours of vaccination and not attributable to another identifiable cause
- Persistent, inconsolable crying, lasting 3 or more hours and occurring within 48 hours of vaccination
- Seizures (with or without fever) occurring within 3 days of vaccination

Route, Site, and Immunization Schedule

DTaP is injected IM into the deltoid muscle or thigh. Routine vaccination consists of five injections, the first at 2 months, the second at 4 months, the third at 6 months, the fourth between 15 and 18 months, and the fifth between 4 and 6 years. After the initial series, all children should receive a booster shot of Td every 10 years.

The following recommendations also apply:

- Children 11 to 12 years old who completed the series at least 5 years previously should receive a booster shot of Tdap, followed by Td boosters every 10 years.
- Children 11 to 18 years old who have not received Tdap should receive a single dose, followed by Td boosters every 10 years.
- Children 7 through 10 years old who are not fully immunized against *pertussis* should receive a single dose of Tdap.

Poliovirus Vaccine

Preparations

In the past, two polio vaccines were used in the United States: *oral poliovirus vaccine* (OPV, Sabin vaccine) and *inactivated poliovirus vaccine* (IPV, Salk vaccine). OPV is composed of *live,* attenuated viruses. In contrast, IPV is composed of *inactivated* polioviruses. OPV has *caused* polio in a few children, whereas IPV has not and cannot. Because the benefit/risk ratio of IPV is clearly superior, OPV has been withdrawn from the U.S. market. The brand name for IPV is *IPOL.*

Efficacy

Between 97.5% and 100% of children receiving IPV develop antibodies to poliovirus types 1, 2, and 3. Antibodies develop after two or more doses and persist for many years.

Adverse Effects of IPV

IPV is devoid of serious adverse effects. As with other injected drugs, local soreness may occur. IPV contains trace amounts of streptomycin, neomycin, and bacitracin. Children with an allergy to these drugs should be monitored.

Route, Site, and Immunization Schedule

IPV is administered subQ in the anterolateral thigh. All children should receive four doses, the first at 2 months, the second at 4 months, the third between 6 and 18 months, and the fourth between 4 and 6 years. If four doses were administered before age 4 years, an additional (fifth) dose should be given between ages 4 and 6 years.

Haemophilus influenzae Type b Conjugate Vaccine

Preparations

Vaccines directed against *H. influenzae* type b (Hib) are prepared by conjugating (covalently binding) a purified capsular polysaccharide (PRP) from *H. influenzae* to either (1) tetanus toxoid or (2) an outer membrane protein (OMP) isolated from *Neisseria meningitidis.* The reason for conjugating PRP to these other compounds is to enhance antigenicity. The vaccine made with OMP—marketed as *PedvaxHIB* and abbreviated PRP-OMP—elicits a stronger immune response than the vaccines made with tetanus toxoid, marketed as *ActHIB* and *Hiberix.*

Efficacy

Immunization with Hib vaccine decreases the risk of disease by 88% to 98%. When PedvaxHIB is used, protection begins 1 week after the first dose. However, when ActHIB is used, protection is delayed, beginning 1 to 2 weeks after the fourth dose. With both vaccines, protection persists for several years.

Adverse Effects

Hib vaccine is among the safest of all vaccines. Serious adverse effects have not been reported. The few adverse effects that do occur are generally transient and mild. Between 2% and 5% of vaccinated patients develop local reactions (swelling, erythema, warmth, and tenderness). About 1% experience fever (above 101°F), crying, diarrhea, or vomiting.

Route, Site, and Immunization Schedule

Hib vaccines are administered IM into the midthigh or the outer aspect of the upper arm. Most children should receive four doses, the first at 2 months, the second at 4 months, the third at 6 months, and the fourth between 12 and 15 months. If PedvaxHIB is used for the first two doses, the third dose (6-month dose) can be omitted.

Varicella Virus Vaccine

Description

Varicella virus vaccine is composed of live, attenuated varicella viruses. Two subQ products are available: varicella vaccine by itself, sold as *Varivax,* and varicella vaccine combined with MMR [MMRV], sold as *ProQuad.*

Efficacy

Varicella vaccine, given as a two-dose series, confers full protection in about 99% of vaccinated patients. Furthermore, among those who get chickenpox despite vaccination, symptoms are always mild: These children develop fewer lesions (fewer than 50, compared with 250 to 500 for unvaccinated children), experience less fever, and recover more quickly. In Japan, herpes zoster (shingles) has not been observed in any adult who received varicella vaccine as a child, even if breakthrough chickenpox had occurred.

Adverse Effects

Varicella vaccine is very safe; no serious adverse events have been reported. About 25% of vaccinated patients experience erythema, soreness, and swelling at the injection site; 15% develop fever (above 102°F); and 3% develop a mild local varicella-like rash, consisting of just a few lesions. About 5% of healthy children develop a sparse, generalized varicella-like rash within a month of the injection. In children with leukemia, the incidence of generalized rash is much higher—about 50%. For all vaccinated patients, rates of fever and rash are higher when MMRV is used than when MMR and varicella vaccine are given separately.

In theory, children receiving the vaccine can transmit vaccine viruses to others. However, among otherwise healthy vaccinated patients, such transmission has not been reported. In contrast, among leukemic children who developed a rash after vaccination, a few cases of viral transmission have occurred. To reduce the risk of transmission, vaccinated patients should temporarily avoid close contact with susceptible, high-risk individuals (e.g., neonates, pregnant women, immunocompromised people).

Precautions and Contraindications

Varicella vaccine is *contraindicated* for pregnant patients, individuals with certain cancers (e.g., leukemia, lymphomas), and individuals with hypersensitivity to neomycin or gelatin, both of which are in the vaccine. In addition, the vaccine should generally be avoided by individuals who are immunocompromised, including those with HIV infection or congenital immunodeficiency and those taking immunosuppressive drugs.

Children receiving the vaccine should avoid aspirin and other salicylates for 6 weeks. This precaution is based on the theoretical risk of developing Reye's syndrome: If the child develops chickenpox (albeit a mild case) in response to the vaccine, the very small risk of developing Reye's syndrome is somewhat increased by concurrent use of salicylates.

Route, Site, and Immunization Schedule

Varicella vaccine is administered subQ into the outer aspect of the upper arm or into the anterolateral thigh. All recipients should get *two* doses. Current recommendations are as follows:

- *Children who have never had chickenpox*—Give the first dose between 12 and 15 months, and the second dose between 4 and 6 years. If needed, the second dose can be given sooner—but no sooner than 3 months after the first dose.
- *Children age 13 years or older who have not been vaccinated yet and have not had chickenpox*—Give two doses at least 28 days apart.

We Need to Vaccinate More Children

Although rates of varicella vaccination have increased, many eligible children still do not get vaccinated. Several misconceptions are responsible: Some parents believe chickenpox is a mild disease, some think the vaccine is not effective (vaccination prevents severe chickenpox in 100% of vaccinated patients), and some think the vaccine is not safe (serious reactions are extremely rare, and proof that the vaccine was the cause is lacking).

The major impact of failure to vaccinate will be felt when today's children grow up. Recall that chickenpox in adults is much more severe than in children: Compared with children, adults have a 10- to 20-fold increased risk of serious complications, including death. Because many children are being vaccinated, the overall incidence of chickenpox is on the decline. As a result, children who remain unvaccinated may nonetheless avoid chickenpox, and hence may reach adulthood without developing antibodies to the disease. Therefore, if they acquire the disease as adults, it is likely to be severe. The moral to this story is that vaccinating children now will not only protect them from chickenpox during childhood, it will also protect them from serious harm when they grow up.

Hepatitis B Vaccine

Preparations

Hepatitis B vaccine (HepB) contains *hepatitis B surface antigen* (HBsAg), the primary antigenic protein in the viral envelope. Administration of HepB promotes synthesis of specific antibodies directed against hepatitis B virus. Because HepB is made from a viral component, rather than from a live virus, it cannot cause disease.

HepB is available in pediatric and adult formulations. The pediatric formulation, marketed as *Recombivax HB,* contains 10 mcg of HBsAg/mL. The adult formulation, marketed as *Engerix-B,* contains 20 mcg of HBsAg/mL. A combination vaccine for adults, marketed as *Twinrix,* protects against hepatitis A *and* hepatitis B. In all three products, the HBsAg is produced in yeast using recombinant DNA technology.

Efficacy

Greater than 85% of vaccinated patients are protected after the second dose of HepB, and more than 90% are protected after the third dose. Although the duration of protection has not been determined with precision, it appears to be at least 5 to 7 years.

Adverse Effects and Contraindications

HepB is one of our safest vaccines. The most common reactions are soreness at the injection site and mild to moderate fever. Acetaminophen or ibuprofen may be used to relieve discomfort, but aspirin should be avoided. The only contraindication to HepB is a prior anaphylactic reaction either to HepB itself or to baker's yeast.

Route, Site, and Immunization Schedule

HepB is injected IM. In neonates and infants, the injection is made into the anterolateral thigh. In adolescents and adults, the injection is made into the deltoid. All vaccinated patients should receive three doses.

The immunization protocol for *infants* is based on whether the mother is *HBsAg-positive* or *HBsAg-negative* (i.e., on whether the mother has laboratory evidence of hepatitis B infection). *All* infants should receive monovalent HepB vaccine soon after birth. The following protocols for infants are recommended:

- *Infants born to mothers who are HBsAg-negative*—Give 5 mcg of Recombivax HB within 12 hours of birth. Give the second dose between 1 and 2 months and the third dose no sooner than 6 months.
- *Infants born to mothers who are HBsAg-positive*—Give 5 mcg of Recombivax HB within 12 hours of birth, and give 0.5 mL of *hepatitis B immune globulin* (HBIG) at the same time but at a separate site. (The purpose of the

HBIG is to provide immediate protection against hepatitis B acquired from the mother.) Give the second dose of HepB between 1 and 2 months, and the third dose no sooner than 6 months.
- *Infants born to mothers whose HBsAg status is unknown*—Give 5 mcg of Recombivax HB within 12 hours of birth. Subsequent doses are based on the mother's HBsAg status, which is determined by analyzing a maternal blood sample obtained during delivery. If the mother is HBsAg-positive, the infant should be given HBIG as soon as possible—and no later than 1 week after birth.

Infants who did not receive a birth dose should receive a three-dose series. The second dose is given 1 month after the first, and third dose is given 6 months after the first.

Children and adolescents who were not vaccinated against hepatitis B during infancy may begin the three-dose series at any time. Once the first dose is given, the second is given 1 month (or more) later, and the third 4 months (or more) after the first dose and no less than 2 months after the second dose. For children 11 years and older, a two-dose schedule can be used; the second dose is given 4 to 6 months after the first.

Hepatitis A Vaccine

Preparations

Hepatitis A vaccine (HepA) is prepared from inactivated hepatitis A virus (HAV). In the United States, two products are available: *Havrix* and *VAQTA*.

Efficacy

Immunization with HepA decreases the risk of clinical disease by 94% to 100%. Protective levels of antibodies are seen in 94% to 100% of adults and children 1 month after the first dose, and in 100% of vaccinated patients 1 month after the second dose. Protection appears to be long-lasting: Among vaccinated children who were followed for 7 years, no cases of hepatitis A were detected.

Who Should Be Vaccinated?

Hepatitis A vaccination is recommended for *all* children 12 through 23 months old, and for children older than 23 months who live in areas where vaccination programs target older children (owing to increased risk of infection). In addition, HepA is recommended for:

- People at least 1 year old traveling to places with high rates of hepatitis A, including Central or South America, Mexico, the Caribbean islands, Africa, Asia (except Japan), and southern or eastern Europe
- People in communities that have frequent outbreaks of hepatitis A
- Men who have sex with men
- People who use illegal drugs
- People with chronic liver disease
- People who receive clotting factor concentrates
- People who work with nonhuman primates or who work with HAV in research labs

Adverse Effects

Mild reactions are common. Soreness at the injection site occurs in about 54% of adults and 18% of children. Headache occurs in 14% of adults and 9% of children. Other mild reactions include loss of appetite and malaise. When mild reactions occur, they usually begin 3 to 5 days after vaccination and last only 1 to 2 days.

Route, Site, and Immunization Schedule

Hepatitis A vaccines should be given IM into the deltoid muscle. Two doses are required, given at least 6 months apart. The first can be given at 12 months. The second should be given 6 to 12 months after the first (for Havrix) or 6 to 18 months after the first (for VAQTA).

Pneumococcal Conjugate Vaccine

There are two vaccines for pneumococcal disease; a *13-valent pneumococcal conjugate vaccine* (PCV13), sold as *Prevnar 13*, and an unconjugated *pneumococcal polysaccharide vaccine* (PPV), sold as *Pneumovax 23*. Prevnar 13 is approved for the prevention of invasive pneumococcal disease in infants and children. However, Pneumovax 23 is approved only for adults and high-risk children over the age of 2 years. It does not work in children younger than 2 years.

Description

PCV13 consists of 13 pneumococcal capsular polysaccharide antigens that have been conjugated to a protein carrier—specifically, CRM197, a nontoxic variant of diphtheria toxin. The protein carrier increases antigenicity, especially in infants. The 13 antigens in the vaccine are from the 13 serotypes of *Streptococcus pneumoniae* that cause the majority of invasive pneumococcal infections in American children under the age of 6 years.

Adverse Effects

PCV13 appears very safe. No serious adverse effects have been reported. About 50% of vaccinated patients get drowsy after the shot, lose their appetite, or develop erythema or tenderness at the injection site. About 33% develop localized swelling. Mild fever develops in 33%, and a higher fever (temperature over 102.2°F) develops in 5%. About 80% become irritable or fussy.

Who Should Be Vaccinated?

The ACIP recommends vaccinating children in the following groups:

- All children younger than 2 years
- All healthy children between their second and fifth birthdays who have not completed the PCV series
- All children between their second and fifth birthdays who have conditions that put them at high risk of serious pneumococcal disease. In this group are children with sickle cell anemia, injury to the spleen, cochlear implants, chronic heart or lung disease, or immunosuppression of any cause (e.g., diabetes, cancer, liver disease, HIV infection, use of immunosuppressive drugs).

Route, Site, and Immunization Schedule

Vaccination is done by IM injection into the anterolateral aspect of the thigh (in infants) or into the deltoid muscle of the upper arm (in toddlers and young children). The vaccine is a suspension, and hence must be shaken before use. All doses are 0.5 mL.

Children Younger Than 2 Years. The number of doses and their timing depend on the child's age when the first dose is given.

- *First dose at age 2 months*—four doses total; one each at ages 2, 4, and 6 months and one between ages 12 and 15 months.
- *First dose between ages 7 and 11 months*—three doses total; the first two doses should be given at least 4 weeks apart, and the third should be at least 8 weeks after the second, but not before the child's first birthday
- *First dose between ages 12 and 23 months*—two doses total, given at least 8 weeks apart

Children Between Their Second and Fifth Birthdays

- Healthy children who have not completed the PCV series should get one dose of PCV13.
- Children at high risk who have already received three doses of PCV vaccine should get one additional dose of PCV13.
- Children at high risk who have received no, one, or two doses of PCV vaccine should get two doses of PCV13, given at least 8 weeks apart.

Meningococcal Conjugate Vaccine

In the United States, we have two *meningococcal conjugate polysaccharide vaccines* (MCVs): *Menactra* and *Menveo.* Both vaccines protect against the same four meningococcal serotypes, hence their abbreviation *MCV4.* Menactra is indicated for people 9 months to 55 years old, and Menveo is indicated for people 2 months to 55 years old.

An unconjugated vaccine—*meningococcal polysaccharide vaccine* (MPSV4) [Menomune]—has been available since the 1970s, but is not very effective in children. Accordingly, MCV4 is currently preferred. MPSV4 is active against the same meningococcal serotypes as MCV4.

Description

Menactra is a tetravalent conjugate vaccine directed against four meningococcal serogroups: A, C, Y, and W-135. Each dose consists of 4 mcg of capsular polysaccharide from each of the four serogroups conjugated with 48 mcg of a protein carrier, specifically, diphtheria toxoid. The carrier protein increases immunogenicity.

Menveo is nearly identical to Menactra. However, there are two differences. First, the amount of capsular polysaccharide in each dose of Menveo is greater (10 mcg of polysaccharide from serogroup A, and 5 mcg of polysaccharide from serogroups C, Y, and W-135). Second, in Menveo, the polysaccharides are conjugated to a different diphtheria protein.

Efficacy

The efficacy of MCV4 at preventing meningococcal disease has not been evaluated in clinical trials. However, we do know the vaccine is highly immunogenic. For example, when 423 adolescents were vaccinated, rates of seroconversion for serogroups A, C, Y, and W-135 were 100%, 99%, 98%, and 99%, respectively, as measured by bactericidal antibody assay. FDA approval of MCV4 was based on its documented immunogenicity and the documented ability of other vaccines to prevent meningococcal infection.

Adverse Effects

The most common reactions are local pain, headache, and fatigue. Local redness, swelling, and induration are also common.

Concerns that MCV4 might cause *Guillain-Barré syndrome* (GBS)[a] appear to be unfounded, as shown by two large studies. In one study, there were 99 confirmed cases of GBS among 12,589,910 vaccinated patients. In the other study, there were 5 cases among 889,684 vaccinated patients. In both studies, the incidence of GBS was no higher than would be expected in the absence of vaccination. In light of this information, the CDC and ACIP have removed precautionary language regarding a risk of GBS after meningococcal vaccination.

Who Should Be Vaccinated?

The ACIP recommends routine MCV4 vaccination for all children and adolescents ages 11 through 18 years. Children who were not vaccinated at this time should be vaccinated as soon as possible. Vaccination is also recommended for people at increased risk for meningococcal disease, including:

- College freshmen living in dormitories
- U.S. military recruits
- Microbiologists who are routinely exposed to meningococcal bacteria
- Anyone traveling to (or living in) a part of the world where meningococcal disease is common
- Anyone who has an injured spleen, or whose spleen has been removed
- Anyone who has an immune disorder known as terminal complement component deficiency
- Anyone who might have been exposed to meningitis during an outbreak
- Persons with persistent complement component deficiency, anatomic or functional asplenia, and certain other risk factors

MCV4 is the preferred vaccine for people 2 months to 55 years old in these risk groups, but MPSV4 can be used if MCV4 is not available. Only MPSV4 should be used for adults over 55 (not because MPSV4 is more effective—but because it is approved for use in this age group, whereas MCV4 is not).

How Many Doses?

Most children should receive *two* doses: a primary dose and a booster dose. This recommendation is new. In the past, one dose was considered sufficient. However, we now know that protection does not last as long as previously believed, hence the need for a booster.

Specific dosing recommendations, based on age and risk group, are as follows:

- *Healthy children 11 to 18 years old*—Give the initial dose between ages 11 and 12 years, and the booster at age 16 years. If the initial dose is given late (between 13 and 15 years), give the booster between ages 16 and

[a]GBS is a serious neurologic disorder that involves inflammatory demyelination of peripheral nerves. Symptoms include symmetric weakness in the arms and legs, sensory abnormalities, and paralysis of the muscles of respiration. Most patients eventually recover.

18 years. If the initial dose was given even later (on or after age 16 years), no booster is needed.

- *Children 11 to 18 years old with HIV infection*—Give a primary two-dose series (2 months apart) between ages 11 and 12 years, and a booster at age 16 years. If the primary series is given late (between 13 and 15 years), give the booster between ages 16 and 18 years. If the primary series was given even later (on or after age 16 years), no booster is needed.
- *Persons 2 to 55 years old with persistent complement component deficiency or functional or anatomic asplenia*—Give a two-dose primary series (2 months apart), and then a booster dose every 5 years. If a one-dose primary series had been used, give a booster dose as soon as possible, and then every 5 years.

For more details on dosing, refer to the Meningococcal Vaccine Information Statement and the Adult Immunization Schedule, available online at www.cdc.gov/vaccines, and to Healthcare Personnel Vaccination Recommendations, available online at www.immunize.org/catg.d/p2017.pdf.

Route and Site

Vaccination is done by IM injection, preferably into the deltoid muscle of the upper arm.

Influenza Vaccine

Annual vaccination against influenza, including the H1N1 subtype, is now recommended for all children between ages 6 months and 18 years (as well as all adults). Properties of IM, intradermal, and intranasal influenza vaccines (composition, efficacy, adverse effects, contraindications, preparations, dosage, route), along with information on adult vaccination, are presented in Chapter 93.

Rotavirus Vaccine

Preparations and Efficacy

In the United States, two rotavirus vaccines are available: *RotaTeq* and *Rotarix*. Both contain live, attenuated viruses. To induce a strong immune response, these viruses must replicate within the infant's gut. Accordingly, the vaccine is administered PO. RotaTeq and Rotarix differ in composition and dosing schedule.

RotaTeq is a *pentavalent* vaccine directed against the five most common serotypes of human rotavirus, termed G1, G2, G3, G4, and P1A. In trials in the United States and Finland, RotaTeq prevented 74% of *all* rotavirus gastroenteritis cases and 98% of *severe* cases. Vaccination also reduced the need for diarrhea-related hospitalization by 96%.

Rotarix is a *monovalent* vaccine developed from a rotavirus with the most common serotype found in humans. However, although Rotarix is monovalent, it confers protection against four rotavirus serotypes: G1, G3, G4, and G9. In clinical trials, Rotarix prevented 79% of *all* rotavirus gastroenteritis cases, 90% of *severe* cases, and 96% of diarrhea-related hospitalizations.

Safety

Although generally very safe, both RotaTeq and Rotarix may carry a small risk of *intussusception,* a rare, life-threatening form of bowel obstruction that occurs when the bowel folds in on itself, like a collapsing telescope. Of note, during prelicensure testing in over 130,000 infants, no cases of intussusception were seen. However, with both vaccines, several cases were reported during postmarketing surveillance. Fortunately, the estimated risk is very low: about 1 case for each 50,000 to 70,000 vaccinated patients.

Who Should Be Vaccinated?

The ACIP recommends that all infants receive rotavirus vaccine, beginning around age 8 weeks.

Who Should Not Be Vaccinated?

Rotarix, but not RotaTeq, is contraindicated for infants with any uncorrected congenital malformation of the GI tract that could predispose to intussusception. Both vaccines are contraindicated for children with a history of intussusception.

Some vaccinated patients with *severe combined immunodeficiency (SCID),* a rare inherited disorder, have developed vaccine-acquired rotavirus infection. Accordingly, these vaccines are contraindicated for infants with SCID. Rotavirus vaccines have not been evaluated in children who are immunocompromised for other reasons. Nonetheless, since these vaccines contain live viruses, it would seem prudent to use them with caution in all immunocompromised infants, regardless of the cause.

Infants with moderate to severe diarrhea or vomiting should probably not be vaccinated until they recover.

Preparations, Route, and Immunization Schedule

RotaTeq is supplied in single-dose, 2-mL vials for oral dosing. The vaccination series consists of *three* doses, starting at age 6 to 12 weeks. The second dose is given 4 to 10 weeks after the first, and the third dose is given 4 to 10 weeks after the second (but no later than age 32 weeks).

Rotarix is supplied as a powder for suspension in 1 mL of the liquid supplied. Dosing is oral. Effective vaccination requires *two* doses (compared with three for RotaTeq). The first dose is given between age 6 and 12 weeks, and the second is given 4 weeks or more later. The series should be completed by age 24 weeks.

Human Papillomavirus Vaccine

Two HPV vaccines are available: *Gardasil and Gardasil 9.* These vaccines differ in how many types of HPV they cover. Gardasil was the first vaccine licensed in the United States for the specific purpose of protecting against cancer of any type. Gardasil is a quadrivalent vaccine, covering 4 types of HPV. Gardasil 9 was developed later and is a 9-valent vaccine, protecting against 9 types of HPV. Gardasil protects against cervical, vulvar, and vaginal cancer in females, as well as anal cancer and genital warts in females and males.

9-Valent HPV Vaccine: Gardasil 9

Composition. Gardasil 9 is a 9-valent vaccine designed to stimulate production of neutralizing antibodies directed at nine types of HPV—specifically, types 16, 18, 31, 33, 45, 52, and 58 (which cause cervical, vulvar, vaginal, and anal cancers), and types 6 and 11 (which cause 95% of genital warts). The vaccine consists of *virus-like particles* (VLPs), which are virus-sized, empty spheres composed of viral capsid proteins. To the immune system, VLPs look like the actual virus, and hence VLPs can evoke an immune response. Because VLPs are empty (and hence don't contain viral DNA), VLPs cannot cause infection. Gardasil 9 is available in 0.5-mL, single-use vials.

Indications. Gardasil 9 is used to prevent cancers, precancerous lesions, and genital warts in females and males.

Cancers and Precancerous Lesions in Female Patients. Gardasil 9 is indicated for girls and women 9 to 26 years old to prevent the following cancers caused by HPV types 16,18, 31, 33, 45, 52, and 58:

- Cervical cancer
- Vulvar cancer
- Vaginal cancer

In addition, Gardasil 9 is indicated for prevention of the following precancerous and dysplastic lesions caused by HPV types 6, 11, 16, 18, 31, 33, 45, 52, and 58:

- Cervical adenocarcinoma *in situ*
- Cervical intraepithelial neoplasia grade 1, grade 2, and grade 3
- Vulvar intraepithelial neoplasia grade 2 and grade 3
- Vaginal intraepithelial neoplasia grade 2 and grade 3

Genital Warts in Females and Males. Gardasil 9 is indicated for females and males 9 to 26 years old to prevent genital warts caused by HPV types 6 and 11.

Anal Cancer in Females and Males. Gardasil 9 is indicated for females and males 9 to 26 years old to prevent anal cancer and precancerous lesions caused by HPV types 6, 11, 16, 18, 31, 33, 45, 52, and 58.

Is a Pap Test Still Needed? For two reasons, the answer is a resounding *YES!* First, Gardasil 9 protects only against nine types of HPV, leaving vaccinated patients at risk of cervical cancer caused by other types of HPV. Second, since Gardasil 9 does not eliminate pre-existing HPV infection, vaccinated patients remain at risk of cancer from infection that was present before the vaccine was given. Therefore, vaccinated women should still undergo routine Pap screening to detect precancerous cervical changes, permitting timely treatment before cancer develops.

Safety. Gardasil 9 appears to be very safe. Injection-site reactions—pain, erythema, swelling, and itching—although common, are mild and short lived. Fainting has occurred in teenage girls, sometimes resulting in hospitalization. However, the incidence of fainting is no greater than with other vaccines. Vaccinated patients who feel faint should sit or lie down to prevent falling.

What about severe side effects? Millions of girls, boys, and women have been vaccinated, and only a few severe events have been reported, including 27 deaths and 10 confirmed cases of GBS. However, a causal relationship between HPV vaccination and either of these severe effects has not been established.

Who Should Be Vaccinated? Given that HPV infection is sexually transmitted and that HPV infects males and females, universal vaccination would be required to achieve maximal protection in the community. Accordingly, ACIP now recommends *routine* vaccination for males *and* females with 9-valent HPV vaccine.

Females: Routine Vaccination. The ACIP recommends routine vaccination for all girls 11 to 12 years old. Why girls this young? Because the vaccine protects only against *acquiring* HPV infection. It can't clear infection that already exists. Therefore, vaccination is most beneficial when done before vaccinated patients become sexually active, which is the case for most girls in this age group.

Vaccination with the HPV vaccine remains voluntary, not compulsory, throughout most of the United States. Parents who are considering withholding vaccination would do well to ask this question: Does protecting my daughter against developing cervical cancer later in life outweigh my concerns about vaccination? If the answer is yes, then vaccination should not be withheld.

Males: Routine Vaccination. ACIP recommends the 9-valent HPV vaccine for all males 11 to 12 years old. Vaccination of males can help protect them from genital warts and HPV-related cancers and may help prevent the spread of HPV to females.

Females and Males: Catch-up Vaccination. ACIP recommends the 9-valent HPV vaccine for females and males 13 to 21 years old who did not receive the vaccine when they were younger.

Who Should Not Be Vaccinated? HPV vaccine is not recommended for patients who are pregnant. Those who are breast-feeding may receive the vaccine.

Route, Site, and Immunization Schedule. The HPV vaccine is injected IM into the deltoid region of the upper arm or the high anterolateral thigh. Three doses are given over a 6-month interval. The first is given at a time selected by the vaccinated patient and her or his healthcare provider. The second is given 2 months after the first, and the third is given 6 months after the first.

Respiratory Syncytial Virus Vaccine (Experimental)

Scientists are currently testing experimental vaccines to prevent RSV. In animal tests, an RSV vaccine elicited high levels of RSV-specific antibodies. Phase I of a clinical trial (NCT01805921) was completed in April 2016 to assess safety and immunogenicity of two new RSV vaccines. PanAd3-RSV is administered intranasally and IM, and MVA-RSV is given only IM. In the trial, the vaccines were administered using a "prime-boost" strategy, in which one of these vaccines is used to "prime" the immune system, which is then "boosted" 4 or 8 weeks later.

The two vaccines in this study contain three proteins: F (Fusion), N (Nucleocapsid), and M2-1 (Matrix). The F protein sits on the surface of the virus and is needed to infect human cells. Antibodies to this protein are an important mechanism to prevent infection. The N and M2-1 proteins are needed for viral replication and are targets of immune recognition. These proteins are delivered into the body using different "vectors," which are harmless carrier viruses. In this study, there are two different vectors: a simian adenovirus (PanAd3) and modified vaccinia virus Ankara (MVA). Results of this Phase I trial have yet to be published.

KEY POINTS

- Vaccines promote synthesis of antibodies directed against bacteria and viruses, whereas toxoids promote synthesis of antibodies directed against toxins that bacteria produce, but not against the bacteria themselves.
- Killed vaccines are composed of whole killed microbes or isolated microbial components, whereas live virus vaccines are composed of live microbes that have been weakened or rendered completely avirulent.
- Vaccination is defined as the administration of any vaccine or toxoid.
- Vaccination produces active immunity. Antibodies develop over weeks to months and then persist for years.
- Passive immunity is conferred by administering preformed antibodies (immune globulins). Protection is immediate but lasts only as long as the antibodies remain in the body.
- Thanks to widespread vaccination, five VPDs are virtually gone from the United States, measles and wild-type polio are gone from the Western hemisphere, and smallpox is gone from the planet. Also, the incidence of several other VPDs has been greatly reduced.
- Although vaccines are very safe, mild reactions are common, and serious reactions can occur rarely.
- Several large, high-quality studies have failed to find a causal link between thimerosal-containing vaccines and autism.
- Acetaminophen, ibuprofen, and other analgesic-antipyretics can reduce the immune response to vaccines, and hence should generally be avoided as prophylaxis for fever or pain before vaccination.
- Immunocompromised children are at special risk from live vaccines and should not receive them.
- Measles, mumps, and rubella virus vaccine (MMR) is a combination product composed of three live virus vaccines.
- Rarely, MMR causes thrombocytopenia and anaphylactic reactions. Until recently, anaphylactic reactions were thought to result from allergy to eggs, but now we think they result from allergy to gelatin.
- MMR is contraindicated during pregnancy and should be used with caution in children with a history of either thrombocytopenia or anaphylactic reactions to gelatin, eggs, or neomycin.
- One vaccine exists for protection against diphtheria, tetanus, and pertussis. DTaP is recommended for all children.
- Rarely, DTaP causes acute encephalopathy.
- There is one vaccine against polioviruses: inactivated poliovirus vaccine (IPV, Salk vaccine).
- *Haemophilus influenzae* type b vaccine is one of our safest vaccines. No serious adverse events have been reported.
- Varicella virus vaccine is composed of live, attenuated varicella viruses.
- All children receiving varicella vaccine are fully protected against severe varicella (chickenpox), although some get mild disease. The children who get mild chickenpox despite vaccination develop far fewer lesions than unvaccinated children, experience less fever, and recover more quickly.
- Varicella vaccine is very safe; no serious adverse events have been reported.
- Varicella vaccine is contraindicated for pregnant women, individuals hypersensitive to neomycin or gelatin, and immunocompromised people.
- Hepatitis B vaccine (HepB) contains hepatitis B surface antigen (HBsAg), the primary antigenic protein in the viral envelope. Administration of HepB promotes synthesis of specific antibodies directed against hepatitis B virus.
- HepB is one of our safest vaccines. The only contraindication is a prior anaphylactic reaction either to HepB itself or to baker's yeast.
- All infants should receive monovalent HepB within 12 hours of birth (except in rare circumstances). Infants whose mothers are HBsAg-positive should also receive hepatitis B immune globulin (HBIG).
- Hepatitis A vaccine is composed of inactivated hepatitis A viruses.
- Pneumococcal conjugate vaccine is the first vaccine for preventing invasive pneumococcal disease in infants and toddlers.
- Meningococcal conjugate vaccine (MCV4) is more effective in children than meningococcal polysaccharide vaccine (MPSV4), approved in the 1970s.
- Annual influenza vaccination is recommended for all children age 6 months to 18 years.
- Two rotavirus vaccines are available: RotaTeq and Rotarix. Both may carry a small risk of intussusception, a life-threatening complication.
- We have two HPV vaccines: a quadrivalent vaccine sold as Gardasil, and a 9-valent vaccine sold as Gardasil 9.
- Gardasil 9 can prevent cancers unique to females (cervical, vaginal, and vulvar), as well as anal cancer and genital warts in females and males.
- Gardasil and Gardasil 9 do not protect against all the types of HPV that can cause cervical cancer, and they do not protect against HPV infection that was present before vaccination. Accordingly, vaccinated women should still undergo routine Pap screens to detect precancerous cervical lesions, thereby permitting timely treatment before cancer develops.
- A trial involving two new vaccines for RSV was completed in 2016, but results have not been published. PanAd3-RSV is administered intranasally and IM, and MVA-RSV is given only IM.

Please visit **http://evolve.elsevier.com/Lehne** for chapter-specific NCLEX® examination review questions.

CHAPTER 69 Immunosuppressants

Immunosuppressive drugs inhibit immune responses. They have two principal applications: (1) prevention of organ rejection in transplant recipients and (2) treatment of autoimmune disorders (e.g., rheumatoid arthritis, systemic lupus erythematosus). At the doses required to suppress allograft rejection, almost all of these drugs are toxic. Two outcomes of toxicity are of particular concern: (1) increased risk for infection and (2) increased risk for neoplasms. Furthermore, because allograft recipients must take immunosuppressants for life, the risk for toxicity continues lifelong. Sites of action of immunosuppressants are shown in Fig. 69.1.

CALCINEURIN INHIBITORS

Cyclosporine, tacrolimus, and pimecrolimus are the most effective immunosuppressants available. Although these drugs differ in structure, they share the same mechanism: They inhibit calcineurin, suppressing production of interleukin-2 (IL-2), a compound needed for T-cell proliferation. Their principal use is prevention of organ rejection in transplant recipients. Cyclosporine was developed first and is used more often. Pimecrolimus, used for topical therapy of atopic dermatitis (eczema), is discussed in Chapter 105.

Cyclosporine

Cyclosporine [Sandimmune, Gengraf, Neoral] is a powerful immunosuppressant and the drug of choice for preventing organ rejection in recipients of an allogenic transplant.[a] Major adverse effects are nephrotoxicity and increased risk for infection.

Mechanism of Action

Cyclosporine acts on helper T lymphocytes to suppress production of IL-2, interferon gamma, and other cytokines. The drug's primary molecular target is a protein known as *cyclophilin.* After binding to cyclophilin, cyclosporine inhibits *calcineurin,* a key enzyme in the pathway that promotes synthesis of IL-2 and other cytokines. In the absence of these cytokines, proliferation of B cells and cytolytic T cells is suppressed. In contrast to methotrexate and other cytotoxic immunosuppressants, cyclosporine does not cause bone marrow suppression.

Therapeutic Uses

Cyclosporine is used primarily to prevent rejection of allogenic kidney, liver, and heart transplants. A glucocorticoid (prednisone) is usually given concurrently. Azathioprine, tacrolimus, or sirolimus may be given as well. Additional indications are psoriasis (see Chapter 105) and rheumatoid arthritis (see Chapter 73).

Pharmacokinetics

Cyclosporine may be administered orally or IV. Oral administration is preferred; IV therapy is reserved for patients who cannot take the drug orally. Absorption from the GI tract is incomplete (about 30%) and erratic. Accordingly, to avoid toxicity (from high drug levels) and organ rejection (from low drug levels), blood levels of cyclosporine should be measured periodically.

Cyclosporine is highly (90% to 98%) protein bound. It undergoes extensive metabolism by the 3A4 isoenzyme of cytochrome P450 (CYP3A4). Therefore, drugs that increase or decrease the activity of CYP3A4 can have a significant impact on cyclosporine levels. Excretion of both cyclosporine and its metabolites is via the bile. Practically none of the drug appears in the urine.

Adverse Effects

The most common adverse effects are nephrotoxicity, infection, hypertension, tremor, and hirsutism. Of these, nephrotoxicity and infection are the most serious.

Nephrotoxicity. Renal damage occurs in up to 75% of patients. Injury manifests as reduced renal blood flow and reduced glomerular filtration rate. These effects are dose dependent and usually reverse following a dosage reduction.

Nephrotoxicity is evaluated by monitoring for elevated blood urea nitrogen (BUN) and serum creatinine. However, be aware

[a]An *allogenic transplant* is donor tissue that is genetically distinct from tissues of the recipient, and thus is subject to attack by the recipient's immune system.

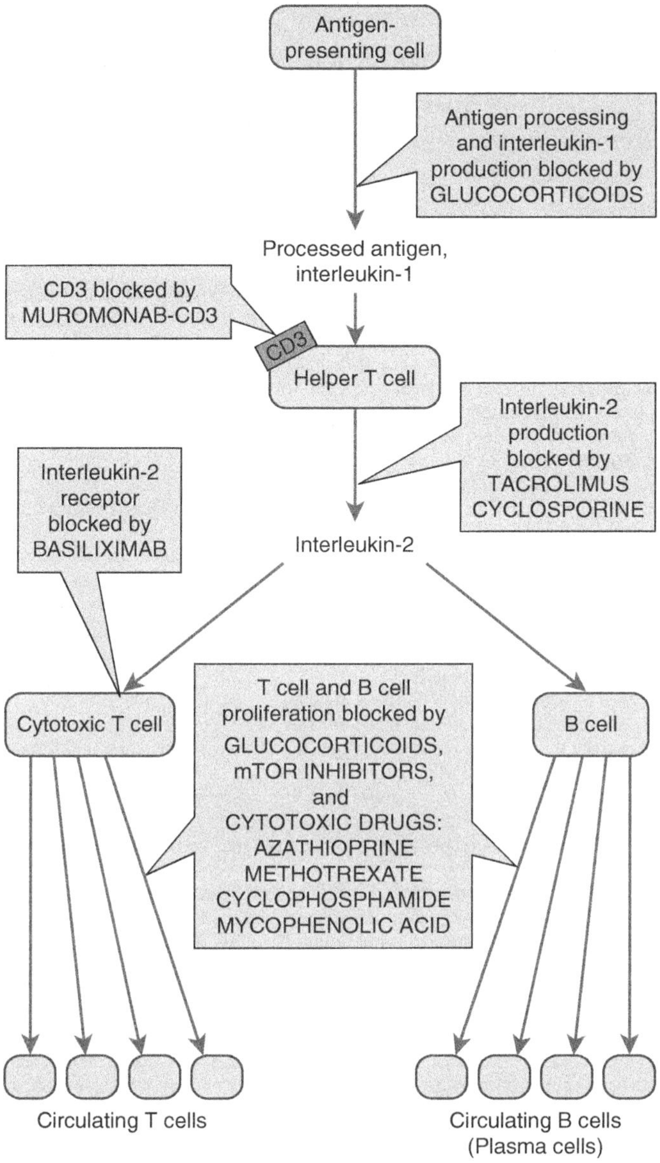

Fig. 69.1 ▪ Sites of action of immunosuppressant drugs.

that a rise in these values could also indicate rejection of a kidney transplant. Patients should be informed about the possibility of kidney damage and the importance of periodic tests for BUN and creatinine.

Infection. Cyclosporine increases the risk for infections, which develop in 74% of those treated. Activation of latent infection with the BK virus can result in kidney damage, primarily in kidney recipients. Patients should be warned about early signs of infection (fever, sore throat) and instructed to report them immediately.

Hepatotoxicity. Liver damage occurs in 4% to 7% of patients. Injury is evaluated by monitoring for serum bilirubin and liver transaminases. Signs of liver injury reverse rapidly with a reduction in dosage. Inform the patient about the need for periodic tests of liver function.

Lymphomas. Cyclosporine and other immunosuppressants can cause lymphoproliferative diseases. The incidence with cyclosporine alone is low. However, when cyclosporine is combined with other immunosuppressants, the risk for malignant lymphomas increases.

Other Common Adverse Effects. *Hypertension*, indicated by a 10% to 15% increase in blood pressure, develops in about 50% of patients; standard antihypertensive drugs are used for treatment. *Tremor* and *hirsutism* are also common. Less frequently, patients experience *leukopenia, gingival hyperplasia, gynecomastia, sinusitis,* and *hyperkalemia.*

Anaphylactic Reactions. Anaphylactic reactions are rare, occurring in 1 of every 1000 patients. Signs include flushing, respiratory distress, hypotension, and tachycardia. Anaphylaxis occurs only with IV therapy. Patients should be monitored for 30 minutes after infusion onset. If anaphylaxis develops, discontinue the infusion and treat with epinephrine and oxygen.

PATIENT-CENTERED CARE ACROSS THE LIFE SPAN

Immunosuppressants

Life Stage	Patient Care Concerns
Children	Immunosuppressants are approved for pediatric use and are often necessary. As with all drugs, the benefits of therapy must be weighed against any risks.
Pregnant women	With the exception of basiliximab, the calcineurin inhibitors, mTOR inhibitors, and antibodies are Pregnancy Risk Category C.[a] For these, either fetal abnormalities were demonstrated in animal reproduction studies or inadequate studies have been conducted. Basiliximab, a Pregnancy Risk Category B[a] drug, is the safest of all the immunosuppressants in this chapter. All the cytotoxic drugs are Pregnancy Risk Category D[a] with the exception of methotrexate, which is Pregnancy Risk Category X.[a] These drugs are known to cause congenital anomalies and hematologic abnormalities in humans. Glucocorticoids vary between Pregnancy Risk Category C or D,[a] depending on the type of glucocorticoid.
Breast-feeding women	Breast-feeding is discouraged for women taking immunosuppressant therapy.
Older adults	Adverse effects in older adults may be more severe, and recovery may be slower or complicated, especially in patients with comorbidities.

[a]As of 2020, the FDA will no longer use Pregnancy Risk Categories. Please refer to Chapter 9 for more information.

Hazardous Drugs and Special Administration Requirements

Methotrexate may present a hazard for nurses who administer this drug. In 2016 the National Institute for Occupational Safety and Health (NIOSH) expanded the list of drugs identified as hazardous. (See https://www.cdc.gov/niosh/docs/2016-161/pdfs/2016-161.pdf.) NIOSH requires special handling of drugs identified as hazardous. See Chapter 3, Table 3.1, for administration and handling guidelines. The hazardous drugs mentioned in this chapter are listed in the following box.

Safety Alert

HAZARDOUS DRUGS REQUIRING SPECIAL HANDLING

Calcineurin Inhibitors	Cytotoxic Drugs
Cyclosporine	Azathioprine
Tacrolimus	Cyclophosphamide
	Methotrexate
mTOR Inhibitors	Mitoxantrone
Everolimus	Mycophenolate Mofetil
Sirolimus	

Drug and Food Interactions

Many interactions have been reported. However, only a few appear to have clinical significance. These are considered here.

Drugs That Can Decrease Cyclosporine Levels. Drugs that induce CYP3A4 can accelerate metabolism of cyclosporine, causing cyclosporine levels to fall. Organ rejection can result. Drugs known to lower cyclosporine levels include *phenytoin, phenobarbital, carbamazepine, rifampin, terbinafine,* and *trimethoprim/sulfamethoxazole.* Cyclosporine levels should be monitored and the dosage adjusted accordingly.

Drugs That Can Increase Cyclosporine Levels. A variety of drugs can raise cyclosporine levels, thereby increasing the risk for toxicity. Drugs known to increase cyclosporine levels include *azole antifungal drugs* (e.g., ketoconazole), *macrolide antibiotics* (e.g., erythromycin), and *amphotericin B.* The mechanism is inhibition of CYP3A4, the isoenzyme responsible for cyclosporine metabolism. When any of these drugs is combined with cyclosporine, the dosage of cyclosporine must be reduced.

Some providers administer ketoconazole concurrently with cyclosporine for the express purpose of permitting a reduction in cyclosporine dosage. Because ketoconazole inhibits CYP3A4, it slows the metabolism of cyclosporine, causing cyclosporine levels to rise. This permits cyclosporine dosage to be reduced by up to 88%, while continuing to maintain cyclosporine levels within the therapeutic range. The lowered dosage reduces the cost of treatment, which is expensive, by about 60%.

Nephrotoxic Drugs. Renal damage may be intensified by concurrent use of other nephrotoxic drugs. These include *amphotericin B, aminoglycosides,* and *nonsteroidal anti-inflammatory drugs* (NSAIDs).

Grapefruit Juice. A compound present in grapefruit juice inhibits metabolism of cyclosporine. As a result, consuming grapefruit juice can raise cyclosporine levels by 50% to 200%, greatly increasing the risk for toxicity.

Repaglinide. Cyclosporine can increase levels of repaglinide [Prandin], a drug for diabetes, and can thereby cause hypoglycemia. Blood glucose should be monitored closely.

Preparations, Dosage, and Administration

Preparations. Cyclosporine is available under three brand names: *Sandimmune, Neoral,* and *Gengraf.* These preparations are NOT bioequivalent and cannot be used interchangeably. In Neoral and Gengraf, cyclosporine is present as a microemulsion. As a result, absorption is greater than from the Sandimmune formulation. As Sandimmune, cyclosporine is available in capsules (25 and 100 mg), an oral solution (100 mg/mL), and an IV solution (50 mg/mL). As Neoral or Gengraf, cyclosporine is available in capsules (25 and 100 mg) and an oral solution (100 mg/mL). To improve palatability, oral solutions can be mixed with apple or orange juice just before dosing; however, remember that grapefruit juice should be avoided. Grapefruit juice alters metabolism of cyclosporine, resulting in elevated serum levels of the drug.

Dosage and Monitoring for Allograft Recipients. Dosing is complex and depends on the organ transplanted, the formulation employed (Neoral or Gengraf vs. Sandimmune), and other immunosuppressants taken concurrently. The dosages that follow are representative.

Sandimmune. Oral therapy is preferred to IV therapy. The initial *oral* dose is 10 to 14 mg/kg given 4 to 12 hours before surgery. This dose is continued once daily for 1 to 2 weeks. Dosage is then gradually reduced to a maintenance level of 3 to 10 mg/kg/day.

For *intravenous* therapy, 1 mL of concentrate is diluted in 20 to 100 mL of 0.9% sodium chloride or 5% dextrose. The initial dose is 5 to 6 mg/kg (one-third the oral dose) infused over 2 to 6 hours. The solution should be protected from light. Because of the risk for anaphylaxis, epinephrine and oxygen must be immediately available. The patient should be switched to oral therapy as soon as possible.

Neoral and Gengraf. Dosage depends on the transplanted organ and other immunosuppressive drugs taken concurrently. Typical dosages are 9 mg/kg/day for a kidney transplant, 8 mg/kg/day for a liver transplant, and 7 mg/kg/day for a heart transplant.

Monitoring. Dosage is adjusted on the basis of nephrotoxicity and cyclosporine trough levels. Blood for drug levels is drawn just before the next dose. For patients receiving a kidney transplant, the target level in *whole blood* is 100 to 200 ng/mL.

Dosage for Rheumatoid Arthritis. Rheumatoid arthritis is treated with Neoral or Gengraf. The initial dosage is 1.25 mg/kg twice daily. Dosage may be gradually increased to a maximum of 2 mg/kg twice daily. If there is no response by 16 weeks, cyclosporine should be discontinued.

Dosage for Psoriasis. Psoriasis is treated with Neoral or Gengraf. The initial dosage is 1.25 mg/kg twice daily. This may be gradually increased to a maximum of 4 mg/kg twice daily. If the maximum dosage is not effective within 6 weeks, cyclosporine should be discontinued. If a response does occur, the dosage should be reduced to the lowest effective amount for maintenance. Continuous therapy for more than 1 year is not recommended.

Prototype Drugs

IMMUNOSUPPRESSANTS

First-Line Agents

Cyclosporine
Tacrolimus

Tacrolimus

Tacrolimus [Prograf, Astagraf XL, Envarsus XR, Advagraf ♣], also known as FK506, is an alternative to cyclosporine for preventing allograft rejection. The drug is somewhat more effective than cyclosporine, but also more toxic.

Therapeutic Use

Systemic tacrolimus is approved for prophylaxis of organ rejection in patients receiving liver, kidney, or heart transplants. Concurrent use of glucocorticoids is recommended (along with azathioprine or mycophenolate mofetil for heart or kidney recipients). Compared with patients receiving cyclosporine, those receiving tacrolimus experience fewer episodes of acute transplant rejection, but tacrolimus has a narrow therapeutic index. Twice as many patients discontinue the drug because of toxicity. As discussed in Chapter 105, tacrolimus [Protopic] is also used for topical therapy of atopic dermatitis.

Mechanism of Action

Tacrolimus acts much like cyclosporine, although the two drugs are structurally dissimilar. Like cyclosporine, tacrolimus inhibits calcineurin and thereby prevents helper T cells from producing IL-2, interferon gamma, and other cytokines. The end result is decreased proliferation of B cells and cytotoxic

T cells. Tacrolimus and cyclosporine differ only in that cyclosporine must first bind to cyclophilin in order to act, whereas tacrolimus must first bind to an intracellular protein named FKBP-12.

Pharmacokinetics

Tacrolimus may be administered orally or IV. Following oral administration, absorption is slow and incomplete; bioavailability is less than 25%. The drug is metabolized in the liver by CYP3A4. Excretion is via the bile. Less than 1% is excreted unchanged in the urine. The mean plasma half-life is 8 to 9 hours.

Adverse Effects

Adverse effects are much like those of cyclosporine. As with cyclosporine, *nephrotoxicity* is the major concern; the incidence is 33% to 40%. Other common reactions include neurotoxicity (headache, tremor, insomnia), GI effects (diarrhea, nausea, vomiting), hypertension, hyperkalemia, hyperglycemia, hirsutism, and gum hyperplasia. Anaphylaxis can occur with IV administration. Like other immunosuppressants, tacrolimus increases the risk for infection and lymphomas.

Drug and Food Interactions

Because tacrolimus is metabolized by CYP3A4, agents that inhibit CYP3A4—erythromycin, ketoconazole, fluconazole, chloramphenicol, and grapefruit juice—can increase tacrolimus levels. CYP3A4 inducers such as rifabutin and rifampin can decrease tacrolimus levels. In both instances, monitoring of tacrolimus trough levels and subsequent adjustments in tacrolimus dosing may be needed.

Like tacrolimus, NSAIDs can injure the kidneys. Accordingly, NSAIDs should be avoided.

Preparations, Dosage, and Administration

Tacrolimus is supplied in capsules (0.5, 1, and 5 mg) for oral use and in solution (5 mg/mL) for IV use. Oral therapy is preferred. However, initial IV therapy may be needed when initial oral therapy is not tolerated. Dosages for adults are as follows:

- *Liver transplants*—The initial oral dose is 50 to 75 mcg/kg every 12 hours, beginning no sooner than 6 hours after surgery. The IV dosage is 0.03 to 0.05 mg/kg/day as a continuous infusion. If treatment is initiated with IV therapy, oral dosing should begin 8 to 12 hours after stopping the infusion. To monitor therapy, trough levels in whole blood should be measured; the usual desired range is 5 to 20 ng/mL. If everolimus (discussed later in chapter) is administered with tacrolimus, the desired range will stabilize at 3 to 5 ng/mL.
- *Kidney transplants*—The initial oral dose is 100 mcg/kg every 12 hours. Oral therapy can start within 24 hours after surgery, but not until renal function has recovered. The IV dosage is 0.03 to 0.05 mg/kg/day as a continuous infusion. To monitor maintenance therapy, trough levels in whole blood should be measured; the desired ranges are 7 to 20 ng/mL for months 1 through 3, and 5 to 15 ng/mL thereafter.
- *Heart transplants*—The initial dosage for oral is 37.5 mcg/kg every 12 hours, beginning no sooner than 6 hours after surgery. If IV therapy is used initially, dosing is 0.01 mg/kg/day as a continuous infusion. Oral therapy should begin 8 to 12 hours after the last IV dose. To monitor maintenance therapy, trough levels in whole blood should be measured; the desired ranges are 10 to 20 ng/mL for months 1 through 3, and 5 to 15 ng/mL thereafter.

mTOR INHIBITORS

The mTOR inhibitors are so named because they inhibit an enzyme known as *mammalian target of rapamycin,* or simply mTOR, a protein kinase that helps regulate cell growth, proliferation, and survival. The ultimate result is suppression of B-cell and T-cell proliferation. Although the mTOR inhibitors—sirolimus and everolimus—are structurally similar to tacrolimus, they work by a somewhat different mechanism, one that does not involve inhibition of calcineurin.

Sirolimus

Actions and Therapeutic Use

Sirolimus [Rapamune] is an immunosuppressant approved only for preventing rejection of renal transplants. The drug should be used in conjunction with cyclosporine and glucocorticoids. Owing to severe adverse effects and no proof of efficacy in patients receiving heart, liver, or lung transplants, sirolimus should not be used by these patients.

How does sirolimus work? It binds with a cytoplasmic protein known as FKBP-12 to form a complex that then inhibits mTOR, an enzyme that helps regulate immune responses. As a result of mTOR inhibition, IL-2 is unable to cause B-cell and T-cell activation. Although sirolimus and tacrolimus both bind with FKBP-12, the consequences differ: Binding by tacrolimus causes inhibition of calcineurin, whereas binding by sirolimus causes inhibition of mTOR.

Pharmacokinetics

Sirolimus is rapidly but incompletely absorbed. Food reduces the *rate* of absorption but increases the *extent.* In the blood, most of the drug is sequestered in erythrocytes. As a result, concentrations in plasma are considerably lower than in whole blood. Sirolimus undergoes extensive metabolism by CYP3A4. Excretion is via the bile. The half-life is prolonged—2.5 days.

Adverse Effects

Like all other immunosuppressants, sirolimus increases the risk for *infection,* including BK virus–associated nephropathy in kidney recipients. Owing to the risk for infection, patients should avoid sources of contagion. In addition, for 12 months after transplant surgery, patients should take medicine to prevent *Pneumocystis* pneumonia (PCP), an infection caused by *Pneumocystis jiroveci* (formerly thought to be *Pneumocystis carinii*). Also, for 3 months after transplant surgery, patients should take medicine to prevent infection with cytomegalovirus.

Sirolimus *raises levels of cholesterol and triglycerides.* In clinical trials, about 50% of patients required treatment with lipid-lowering drugs. Exercise caution in patients with pre-existing hyperlipidemias.

Sirolimus, combined with cyclosporine, poses a significant risk for *renal injury.* Renal function should be monitored.

Severe complications have developed in liver and lung recipients. Liver recipients treated with sirolimus plus cyclosporine or tacrolimus have developed hepatic artery thrombosis, resulting in graft rejection or death. Lung recipients have developed bronchial anastomotic dehiscence; some cases were fatal.

Other side effects include rash, acne, anemia, thrombocytopenia, joint pain, diarrhea, and hypokalemia. In addition, sirolimus increases the risk for lymphocele (a complication of renal transplant surgery). In contrast to cyclosporine, sirolimus is not neurotoxic, and, in contrast to everolimus, it is not diabetogenic.

Drug and Food Interactions

Levels of sirolimus can be raised or lowered by drugs that inhibit or induce CYP3A4, thereby posing a risk for toxicity or treatment failure. Drugs that *induce* CYP3A4, and thereby *decrease* sirolimus levels, include carbamazepine, phenytoin, phenobarbital, rifabutin, and rifapentine. Drugs that *inhibit* CYP3A4, and thereby *increase* sirolimus levels, include verapamil, nicardipine, azole antifungal agents (e.g., ketoconazole), macrolide antibiotics (e.g., erythromycin), and HIV-protease inhibitors (e.g., saquinavir). Because cyclosporine, tacrolimus, and sirolimus are metabolized by CYP3A4, they can compete with each other for metabolism, and can thereby raise each other's levels.

Sirolimus can reduce the immune response to all vaccines. In addition, the drug can render patients vulnerable to infection from live virus vaccines, which must be avoided.

High-fat foods can increase sirolimus absorption by about 35%. To minimize variability, patients should take all doses consistently (i.e., all with foods having a similar percentage of fat or all without food).

Grapefruit juice can inhibit the metabolism of sirolimus, causing its level to rise. Accordingly, taking sirolimus with grapefruit juice should be avoided.

Monitoring

Monitoring of sirolimus trough levels is recommended for all patients, and especially for pediatric patients, patients with liver disease, and patients taking strong inducers or inhibitors of CYP3A4. Monitoring is also recommended whenever the dosage of cyclosporine (taken concurrently with sirolimus) is raised or lowered substantially.

Preparations, Dosage, and Administration

Sirolimus is available in tablets (0.5, 1, and 2 mg) and solution (1 mg/mL) for oral dosing. The treatment program should include cyclosporine and glucocorticoids. Sirolimus dosing should begin as soon as possible after transplant surgery. The recommended regimen consists of a 6-mg loading dose followed by 2-mg daily maintenance doses. For patients who weigh less than 40 kg (but are at least 13 years old), the loading dose is 3 mg/m^2 and the maintenance dosage is 1 mg/m^2 once a day. For all patients, maintenance doses should be taken 4 hours after taking cyclosporine, should be taken consistently with respect to food intake (i.e., either with food or without food), and should not be taken with grapefruit juice. In patients with liver impairment, maintenance doses (but not the loading dose) should be reduced by 33%.

Everolimus

Therapeutic Use

Everolimus [Zortress] is approved to prevent organ rejection in patients age 18 years and older following a liver or kidney transplant. Zortress should be used in conjunction with basiliximab, along with reduced doses of cyclosporine and glucocorticoids. As discussed in Chapter 103, everolimus, sold under the brand name *Afinitor*, is used in high doses to treat advanced renal cancer and certain types of breast and neuroendocrine tumors.

Mechanism of Action

Everolimus works by the same mechanism as sirolimus: It forms a complex with FKBP-12, which then inhibits mTOR and thereby prevents activation of B cells and T cells by IL-2. Like sirolimus, everolimus does not cause inhibition of calcineurin.

Pharmacokinetics

Administration is oral, and plasma levels peak 1 to 2 hours after dosing. Food decreases both the peak plasma level and the total amount absorbed. Everolimus undergoes metabolic inactivation by CYP3A4 followed by excretion in the feces. The drug's half-life is about 30 hours.

Adverse Effects

At the dosage used for immunosuppression, over 20% of patients experience peripheral edema, constipation, hypertension, nausea, anemia, urinary tract infections, and hyperlipidemia. Like all other immunosuppressants, everolimus can increase the risk for malignancy (especially lymphomas) and serious infection, including BK virus–associated nephropathy. Other serious effects include delayed wound healing, noninfectious pneumonitis, new-onset diabetes, male infertility, arterial and venous thrombosis in the kidney allograft, and direct kidney damage, which can be exacerbated by cyclosporine, which patients using everolimus are required to take.

Drug and Food Interactions

Everolimus is subject to the same drug and food interactions as sirolimus. Hence, as with sirolimus, levels of everolimus can be raised or lowered by drugs that inhibit or induce CYP3A4, posing a risk for toxicity or treatment failure. Drugs that *induce* CYP3A4, and can thereby *decrease* everolimus levels, include carbamazepine, phenytoin, phenobarbital, rifabutin, and rifapentine. Drugs that *inhibit* CYP3A4, and can thereby *increase* everolimus levels, include verapamil, nicardipine, azole antifungal agents (e.g., ketoconazole), macrolide antibiotics (e.g., erythromycin), and HIV-protease inhibitors (e.g., saquinavir). Because cyclosporine and everolimus are metabolized by CYP3A4, they can compete with each other for metabolism and can thereby raise each other's levels.

Like sirolimus, everolimus can reduce the immune response to all vaccines. In addition, everolimus can render patients vulnerable to infection from live virus vaccines, which must be avoided.

As with sirolimus, high-fat foods can increase absorption of everolimus. To minimize variability, patients should take all doses consistently, either with food or without food. When taken with food, the fat content should be approximately equivalent to avoid significant drug level fluctuations.

Grapefruit juice can inhibit the metabolism of everolimus, causing its level to rise. Accordingly, taking everolimus with grapefruit juice should be avoided.

Preparations, Dosage, and Administration

The Zortress brand of everolimus is supplied in tablets (0.25, 0.5, and 0.75 mg) for oral dosing, which should start as soon as possible after kidney transplant surgery and for at least 30 days after a liver transplant. Initial dosing is typically 1 mg twice a day following a liver transplant and 0.75 mg twice a day following a kidney transplant. Dosage should be reduced by one-third in patients with mild liver impairment and by one-half in patients with moderate to severe liver impairment. For all patients, maintenance doses should be adjusted to yield a trough level of 3 to 8 ng/mL. The tablets should be swallowed whole with a glass of water, and should be taken consistently either with food or without food to minimize variability in absorption.

GLUCOCORTICOIDS

Glucocorticoids (e.g., prednisone) are used widely to suppress immune responses. Applications range from suppression of allograft rejection to treatment of asthma to therapy of autoimmune disorders, such as rheumatoid arthritis, systemic lupus erythematosus, and multiple sclerosis.

Glucocorticoids have multiple effects on elements of the immune system. They cause lysis of antigen-activated lymphocytes, suppression of lymphocyte proliferation, and sequestration of lymphocytes at extravascular locations. In addition, they reduce production of IL-2 by monocytes and lymphocytes, and they reduce the responsiveness of T lymphocytes to interleukin-1.

Immunosuppressive doses are large. For example, to prevent organ rejection, patients commonly take 60 mg/day on a routine basis. To treat episodes of acute organ rejection, 500 to 1500 mg of IV methylprednisolone is given.

Because large doses are employed, the full range of glucocorticoid adverse effects can be expected. These include increased risk for infection, thinning of the skin, osteoporosis with resultant fractures, impaired growth in children, and suppression of the hypothalamic-pituitary-adrenal axis.

The pharmacology of glucocorticoids is discussed in Chapter 72.

CYTOTOXIC DRUGS

Cytotoxic drugs suppress immune responses by killing B and T lymphocytes that are undergoing proliferation. With the exception of mycophenolate mofetil, these drugs are nonspecific. That is, they are toxic to all proliferating cells. As a result, they can cause bone marrow suppression, GI disturbances, reduced fertility, and alopecia (hair loss). Neutropenia and thrombocytopenia from bone marrow suppression are of particular concern. Because of their serious adverse effects, the cytotoxic drugs are usually reserved for patients who have not responded to safer immunosuppressants (i.e., cyclosporine, tacrolimus, and glucocorticoids).

Azathioprine

Immunosuppressant effects result from suppression of B and T lymphocytes secondary to interference with folate metabolism.

Mechanism of Action

Azathioprine [Imuran, Azasan] suppresses cell-mediated and humoral immune responses by inhibiting the proliferation of B and T lymphocytes. The underlying mechanism is inhibition of DNA synthesis by the drug's active form: mercaptopurine. Because of its mechanism, azathioprine acts selectively during the S phase of the cell cycle. As discussed in Chapter 102, mercaptopurine is used to treat cancer.

Therapeutic Uses

Before the advent of cyclosporine, azathioprine (combined with prednisone) was the principal drug employed to suppress rejection of renal transplants. Today, azathioprine is generally used as an adjunct to cyclosporine and glucocorticoids to help suppress transplant rejection. In addition, the drug is approved for severe refractory rheumatoid arthritis in nonpregnant adults (see Chapter 73). Azathioprine has been used off-label to treat various autoimmune diseases, including myasthenia gravis, systemic lupus erythematosus, Crohn's disease, chronic refractory immune thrombocytopenia, and ulcerative colitis.

Adverse Effects and Drug Interactions

Although uncommon at usual therapeutic doses, *neutropenia* and *thrombocytopenia* from bone marrow suppression can be serious concerns. Accordingly, complete blood counts should be performed at baseline and periodically thereafter. More than 10% of patients experience nausea or vomiting, pancreatitis, and blood dyscrasias. Long-term therapy is associated with an increased incidence of *neoplasms*.

Allopurinol delays conversion of mercaptopurine to inactive products and thereby increases the risk for toxicity. If allopurinol and azathioprine are used concurrently, the dose of azathioprine must be reduced by about 70%.

Preparations, Dosage, and Administration

Imuran is available in 50-mg tablets for oral dosing, and as a powder to be reconstituted with sterile water for IV use. *Azasan* is supplied in 75- to 100-mg scored tablets. For patients receiving a kidney transplant, therapy is initiated with a single daily dose of azathioprine 3 to 5 mg/kg, usually beginning on the day of surgery. Daily maintenance doses range from 1 to 3 mg/kg. Oral administration is preferred to IV.

Cyclophosphamide

Cyclophosphamide, an anticancer drug, is discussed at length in Chapter 102. Discussion here is limited to its immunosuppressant use. Cyclophosphamide is a prodrug that is converted to its active form by the liver. The active form is an alkylating agent that cross-links DNA, leading to cell injury and death. Immunosuppressant effects result from a decrease in the number and activity of B and T lymphocytes. Toxicity to other cells produces adverse effects, including neutropenia (from bone marrow suppression), hemorrhagic cystitis, and sterility in males and females. Cyclophosphamide has been used for its immunosuppressant actions to treat rheumatoid arthritis, systemic lupus erythematosus, and multiple sclerosis. The drug is as effective as azathioprine for suppressing rejection of kidney transplants.

Methotrexate

Methotrexate [Rheumatrex, Trexall], developed as an anticancer agent (see Chapter 102), was later found to be effective in psoriasis (see Chapter 105) and arthritis (see Chapter 73) and other autoimmune disorders. Immunosuppressant effects result from suppression of B and T lymphocytes secondary to interference with folate metabolism. The doses employed for immunosuppression are lower than those employed to treat cancer. As a result, toxicities differ with the two applications: In cancer chemotherapy, bone marrow suppression, ulcerative stomatitis, and renal damage are primary concerns, whereas in immunosuppressive therapy, hepatic fibrosis and cirrhosis are primary concerns.

Safety Alert

METHOTREXATE

The Institute for Safe Medication Practices (ISMP) identifies methotrexate as a high-alert medication because the drug can cause the patient significant harm in the event of a medication error.

Mitoxantrone

Like methotrexate, mitoxantrone was developed to treat cancer (see Chapter 102), and then used later for immunosuppression, owing to its toxic effects on macrophages and B and T lymphocytes. As an immunosuppressant, mitoxantrone has only one indication: reduction of neurologic disability and clinical relapse in patients with multiple sclerosis. Mitoxantrone is a potentially hazardous drug reserved for patients unresponsive to safer agents. The basic pharmacology of the drug and its use in multiple sclerosis are discussed in Chapter 23.

Mycophenolate Mofetil

Therapeutic Use

Mycophenolate mofetil is approved for prophylaxis of organ rejection in patients receiving allogenic heart, liver, or kidney transplants. The drug should be combined with cyclosporine and glucocorticoids.

Mechanism of Action

Following oral administration, mycophenolate mofetil is rapidly converted to mycophenolic acid (MPA), its active form. MPA then acts on B and T lymphocytes to inhibit inosine monophosphate dehydrogenase, an enzyme required for *de novo* synthesis of purines. Since these cells are uniquely dependent on *de novo* synthesis for proliferation (other cells acquire needed purines via salvage pathways), MPA causes selective inhibition of B- and T-lymphocyte proliferation.

Pharmacokinetics

With oral administration, mycophenolate mofetil undergoes nearly complete absorption, followed by rapid and nearly complete hydrolysis to MPA. MPA is converted in the liver to an inactive metabolite, which is then excreted in the urine. The half-life of MPA is about 18 hours.

Adverse Effects

Major adverse effects include diarrhea, vomiting, severe neutropenia, sepsis (primarily cytomegalovirus viremia), and pure red-cell aplasia (a form of anemia characterized by selective reductions in red blood cell precursors in bone marrow). As with other immunosuppressive drugs, there is an increased risk for malignancies (especially lymphomas) and infection (including BK virus–associated nephropathy). Very rarely, patients have developed progressive multifocal leukoencephalopathy, a severe infection of the brain. However, a causal relationship has not been established.

Drug Interactions

Absorption of mycophenolate can be decreased by antacids that contain magnesium and aluminum hydroxides and by cholestyramine, a drug that lowers blood cholesterol. Accordingly, mycophenolate should not be given simultaneously with these drugs.

Preparations, Dosage, and Administration

Administration is PO. Mycophenolate mofetil is available in 250-mg capsules, 250- and 500-mg immediate-release tablets, and a 200-mg/mL suspension. Adult dosages are as follows:

- *Kidney transplant*—1 gm twice daily
- *Heart transplant*—1.5 gm twice daily
- *Liver transplant*—1.5 gm twice daily

Dosing should begin within 24 hours of transplant surgery. As a rule, the drug should be taken on an empty stomach to increase absorption.

ANTIBODIES

Antibodies directed against components of the immune system can suppress immune responses. As with all immunosuppressants, the risk for infection is a great concern. The preparations discussed next are used to suppress allograft rejection in transplant recipients.

Muromonab-CD3

Actions and Uses

Muromonab-CD3 [Orthoclone OKT3] is a monoclonal antibody, developed in mice, that binds to the CD3 site on human T lymphocytes. Upon binding, the antibody blocks T-cell function. All T cells—both those in the circulation and those in tissues—are affected. Muromonab-CD3 is used to prevent acute rejection of kidney, heart, and liver transplants. In addition, the drug is given to deplete T cells from bone marrow before bone marrow transplantation.

Adverse Effects

Reactions are common. Among these are fever (73%), chills (59%), dyspnea (21%), chest pain (14%), and nausea and vomiting (12%). These effects are most intense on the first day and then rapidly subside.

In some patients, potentially fatal anaphylactoid reactions have occurred. Manifestations include pulmonary edema, cardiovascular collapse, and cardiac or respiratory arrest. Accordingly, patients should be monitored closely. Also, the drug should be used only in facilities with equipment and staffing for cardiopulmonary resuscitation.

Preparations, Dosage, and Administration

Muromonab-CD3 is supplied in solution (1 mg/mL) for IV administration. The usual dosage is 5 mg/day for 10 to 14 days. Administration is by IV bolus. The preparation should be drawn through a filter before injection. Treatment is begun following diagnosis of acute transplant rejection. To minimize first-dose adverse reactions, the patient should be pretreated with an IV glucocorticoid. The wholesale cost for a course of treatment averages $7000.

Basiliximab

Actions and Uses

Basiliximab [Simulect] is a monoclonal antibody, developed in mice, that binds to the receptor for IL-2 on T lymphocytes. By doing so, it blocks activation of T cells by IL-2.

Basiliximab has only one indication: prophylaxis of *acute* organ rejection following *renal* transplantation. The regimen should also include cyclosporine and a glucocorticoid. In clinical trials, basiliximab helped reduce the incidence of acute organ rejection during the first 6 months after transplant surgery but had little or no impact on graft survival after 1 year.

Adverse Effects

Basiliximab is generally well tolerated. The incidence and severity of adverse effects is much lower than with muromonab-CD3. In contrast to other immunosuppressants, basiliximab does not increase the risk for opportunistic infections. Furthermore, no cancers have been observed 1 year after treatment.

Rarely, basiliximab causes severe, acute *hypersensitivity reactions*, including anaphylaxis. Accordingly, medications for managing hypersensitivity should be immediately available. If a severe hypersensitivity reaction occurs, the drug should be permanently discontinued.

Preparations, Dosage, and Administration

Basiliximab is available as a powder to be reconstituted for IV administration. Treatment consists of two 20-mg doses, given by either (1) IV bolus or (2) IV infusion over 20 to 30 minutes. The first dose is given within 2 hours *before* transplant surgery. The second is given 4 days later.

Antithymocyte Globulin

Basic Pharmacology

Antithymocyte globulin may be prepared from either rabbits [Thymoglobulin] or horses [Atgam]. Therapeutic effects result from a decrease in the number and activity of thymus-derived lymphocytes. Both antithymocyte globulin preparations are approved for preventing rejection of renal transplants. Atgam is also approved for treating aplastic anemia, and Thymoglobulin is sometimes used off-label to treat heart transplant rejection.

Adverse Effects

Antithymocyte globulin may cause hypersensitivity reactions; however, because it is usually employed in combination with other immunosuppressants, immune reactions are usually uncomfortable (chills, fever, skin reactions) but not life-threatening. Nevertheless, anaphylactic reactions can occur. Accordingly, epinephrine and facilities for respiratory support should be immediately available.

Preparations, Dosage, and Administration

Atgam is supplied in solution (50 mg/mL) for IV dosing. Dosages for adults are as follows:

- *Prevention of renal allograft rejection*—15 mg/kg/day for 14 days, followed by alternate-day dosing for 14 more days, to make a total of 21 doses over 28 days. The first dose should be administered within 24 hours before or after transplantation.
- *Treatment of aplastic anemia*—10 to 20 mg/kg/day for 8 to 14 days followed, if needed, by alternate-day dosing for up to a total of 21 doses.

Thymoglobulin is supplied as a powder for reconstitution. Dosage for treatment of renal transplant rejection is 1.5 mg/kg/day IV for 1 to 2 weeks.

For both rabbit- and horse-derived antithymocyte globulins, solutions should be diluted according to manufacturer's instructions, and infusions should be done with an in-line filter. To minimize phlebitis, a vein with high flow should be employed. Each dose should be infused over 4 or more hours. Monitor the patient for anaphylaxis. The risk for reactions may be decreased by premedicating with acetaminophen, glucocorticoids, and/or antihistamines.

KEY POINTS

- Immunosuppressants are used to prevent organ rejection in allograft recipients and to treat autoimmune disorders (e.g., rheumatoid arthritis).
- Allograft recipients must take immunosuppressants for life.
- Immunosuppressants increase the risk for infection and lymphomas.
- Cyclosporine and tacrolimus are the most effective immunosuppressants available.
- Cyclosporine and tacrolimus are used primarily in allograft recipients.
- Cyclosporine causes kidney injury in up to 75% of patients.
- Kidney damage from cyclosporine can be intensified by other nephrotoxic drugs, including amphotericin B, aminoglycosides, and NSAIDs.
- Drugs that inhibit CYP3A4 can increase cyclosporine levels, and drugs that induce CYP3A4 can decrease cyclosporine levels.
- Grapefruit juice inhibits cyclosporine metabolism and can thereby greatly increase cyclosporine levels.
- Like cyclosporine, tacrolimus causes renal damage, and hence should not be combined with other nephrotoxic drugs.
- Immunosuppressant applications of glucocorticoids include suppression of transplant rejection and treatment of rheumatoid arthritis and other autoimmune disorders.
- Prolonged use of glucocorticoids can cause osteoporosis, thinning of the skin, increased risk for infection, impaired growth in children, and adrenal insufficiency (secondary to suppression of the hypothalamic-pituitary-adrenal axis).
- Cytotoxic immunosuppressants (e.g., azathioprine) decrease immune responses by killing B and T lymphocytes.
- Cytotoxic immunosuppressants (except mycophenolate mofetil) injure all proliferating cells. As a result, these drugs can cause bone marrow suppression (neutropenia, thrombocytopenia), GI disturbances, reduced fertility, and alopecia.
- Immune responses can be suppressed with muromonab-CD3, basiliximab, and other antibodies directed against components of the immune system.

Please visit **http://evolve.elsevier.com/Lehne** for chapter-specific NCLEX® examination review questions.

Summary of Major Nursing Implications[a]

CYCLOSPORINE

Preadministration Assessment

Therapeutic Goal

Prevention of allograft rejection.

Baseline Data

Obtain baseline data on kidney function (serum creatinine, BUN), liver function (aspartate aminotransferase, alanine aminotransferase, serum amylase, bilirubin, alkaline phosphatase), and serum potassium levels.

Identifying High-Risk Patients

Cyclosporine has the following *contraindications:* hypersensitivity to cyclosporine or its intravenous vehicle (polyoxyethylated castor oil), pregnancy, recent inoculation with a live virus vaccine, and chickenpox or herpes zoster (or recent contact with a person with either infection).

Use with *caution* in patients taking potassium-sparing diuretics and in those with intestinal malabsorption, hypertension, hyperkalemia, active infection, and renal or hepatic dysfunction.

Implementation: Administration

Routes

Oral, intravenous.

Preparations

Cyclosporine is available under three brand names: Sandimmune, Neoral, and Gengraf. Sandimmune has lower bioavailability than Neoral or Gengraf, and hence is not interchangeable with them.

Patient Education for Oral Administration

Dispense the oral liquid into a glass container using the specially calibrated pipette. Mix well with diluent and drink immediately. Refill the glass container with additional diluent and drink to ensure ingestion of the complete dose. Dry the outside of the pipette and return to its cover for storage.

To improve palatability, mix the concentrated drug solution with apple or orange juice just before dosing. Do not take this drug with grapefruit juice.

Intravenous Dosage and Administration

Dilute 1 mL of concentrate in 20 to 100 mL of 0.9% sodium chloride or 5% dextrose. Protect from light. Administer the initial dose (5 to 6 mg/kg) slowly—over 2 to 6 hours. Because of the risk for anaphylactic reactions, monitor the patient closely for 30 minutes after starting administration. Have epinephrine and oxygen available. Switch to oral therapy as soon as possible.

Dosage Adjustment

Adjust dosage on the basis of nephrotoxicity and cyclosporine trough levels. Draw blood for drug levels just before the next dose. The target trough level is 100 to 200 ng/mL in whole blood.

Ongoing Evaluation and Interventions

Evaluating Therapeutic Effects

Graft tenderness or fever may indicate rejection. In renal transplant recipients, elevated BUN and elevated serum creatinine in conjunction with low cyclosporine may indicate rejection. Therapeutic failure can be confirmed with ultrasound, a biopsy, or renal flow scan.

Minimizing Adverse Effects

Nephrotoxicity. Cyclosporine can cause a dose-dependent reduction in kidney function. Monitor for elevation of serum creatinine and BUN. **Inform outpatients about the importance of undergoing periodic tests of kidney function.**

Infection. Cyclosporine increases the risk for infection, including BK virus–associated nephropathy. **Inform patients about early signs of infection (fever, sore throat), and instruct them to report these immediately.**

Hepatotoxicity. Cyclosporine causes reversible liver damage. Monitor for elevation of serum bilirubin and liver transaminases. **Inform patients about the need for periodic tests of liver function.**

Hirsutism. Cyclosporine promotes hair growth. **Assure the patient that the effect is reversible.**

Use in Pregnancy and Lactation. Cyclosporine is embryotoxic. **Advise women of childbearing age to use a mechanical form of contraception (diaphragm, condom) and to avoid oral contraceptives. Cyclosporine is excreted in breast milk; warn patients against breast-feeding.**

Anaphylactic Reactions. See *Intravenous Dosage and Administration.*

Minimizing Adverse Interactions

Drugs That Can Decrease Cyclosporine Levels. *Phenytoin, phenobarbital, carbamazepine, rifampin, terbinafine,* and *trimethoprim-sulfamethoxazole* can reduce cyclosporine levels, leading to organ rejection. Monitor cyclosporine levels and increase the dosage as needed.

Drugs That Can Increase Cyclosporine Levels. *Azole antifungal drugs* (e.g., ketoconazole), *macrolide antibiotics* (e.g., erythromycin), and *amphotericin B* can elevate cyclosporine levels, thereby increasing the risk for toxicity. Monitor cyclosporine levels and reduce the dosage as needed.

Nephrotoxic Drugs. *Amphotericin B, aminoglycosides,* and *NSAIDs* increase the risk for cyclosporine-induced kidney damage. Monitor renal function.

Grapefruit Juice. Grapefruit juice inhibits cyclosporine metabolism, and can thereby increase cyclosporine levels. Toxicity may result.

Repaglinide. Cyclosporine can increase levels of repaglinide, a drug for diabetes, and cause hypoglycemia. **Advise diabetic patients to monitor blood glucose closely.**

[a]Patient education information is highlighted as **blue text.**

CHAPTER

70 Antihistamines

Histamine is a small molecule produced in specialized cells throughout the body. The compound plays an important role in allergic reactions and regulation of gastric acid secretion. The antihistamines, a widely used family of drugs, block histamine actions.

To understand the antihistamines, we must first understand histamine itself. Accordingly, the chapter begins with a discussion of histamine, emphasizing its contribution to allergic responses.

HISTAMINE

Histamine is a locally acting compound with prominent and varied effects. In the vascular system, histamine dilates small blood vessels and increases capillary permeability. In the bronchi, histamine produces constriction of smooth muscle. In the stomach, histamine stimulates secretion of acid. In the central nervous system (CNS), histamine acts as a neurotransmitter. Despite this impressive spectrum of actions, clinical use of histamine is limited to diagnostic procedures. However, although its clinical utility is minimal, histamine is still of great interest owing to its involvement in two common pathologic states: allergic disorders and peptic ulcer disease.

Distribution, Synthesis, Storage, and Release

Distribution

Histamine is present in practically all tissues. Levels are especially high in the skin, lungs, and GI tract. The histamine content of plasma is low.

Synthesis and Storage

In the periphery, histamine is synthesized and stored in two types of cells: *mast cells* and *basophils*. Mast cells are present in the skin and other soft tissues. Basophils are present in blood. In both mast cells and basophils, histamine is stored in secretory granules. (In addition to histamine, secretory granules contain other substances that, like histamine, are mediators of allergic reactions.)

In the CNS, histamine is produced by neurons with cell bodies in the posterior hypothalamus and with axonal projections to the frontal and temporal cortices and other brain regions.

Release

Release of histamine from mast cells and basophils is produced by allergic and nonallergic mechanisms.

Allergic Release. The initial requirement for allergic release is production of antibodies of the immunoglobulin E class. These antibodies are generated following exposure to specific allergens (e.g., pollens, insect venoms, certain drugs). Once made, the antibodies become attached to the outer surface of mast cells and basophils (Fig. 70.1). When the individual is re-exposed to the allergen, the allergen becomes bound by the antibodies. Binding of allergen to adjacent antibodies creates a bridge between those antibodies. By a mechanism that is not fully understood, this bridging process mobilizes intracellular calcium. The calcium, in turn, causes the histamine-containing storage granules to fuse with the cell membrane and disgorge their contents into the extracellular space. Note that allergic release of histamine requires *prior exposure* to the allergen; an allergic reaction cannot occur during initial allergen exposure.

Nonallergic Release. Several agents (certain drugs, radiocontrast media, plasma expanders) can act directly on mast cells to trigger histamine release. With these agents, no prior sensitization is needed. Cell injury can also cause direct release.

Physiologic and Pharmacologic Effects

Histamine acts primarily through two types of receptors, named H_1 and H_2. The response produced depends on which of these receptors is involved.

Effects of H_1 Stimulation

Vasodilation. Activation of H_1 receptors causes dilation of small blood vessels (arterioles and venules). Vasodilation is prominent in the skin of the face and upper body, causing the area to become warm and flushed. If extensive vasodilation occurs, total peripheral resistance declines and blood pressure falls.

Increased Capillary Permeability. Activation of H_1 receptors increases capillary permeability. Receptor activation

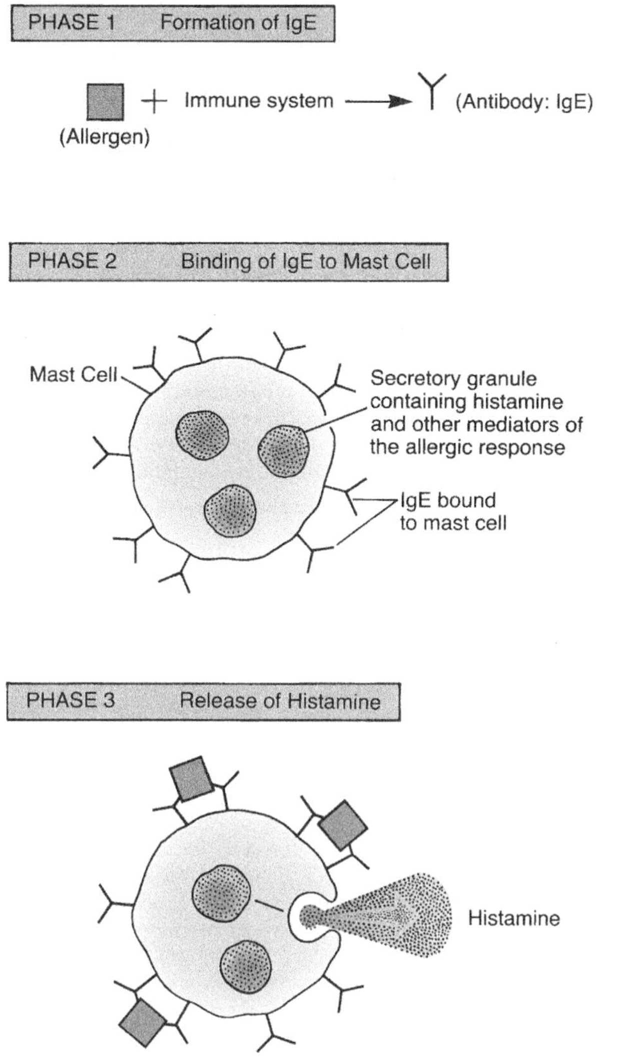

Fig. 70.1 ▪ Release of histamine by allergen-antibody interaction.
(*IgE,* Immunoglobulin E.)

causes capillary endothelial cells to contract, creating openings between these cells through which fluid, protein, and platelets can escape. Escape of fluid and protein into the interstitial space produces edema. If loss of intravascular fluid is substantial, blood pressure may fall.

Bronchoconstriction. Histamine$_1$ activation causes constriction of the bronchi. If histamine is administered to an individual with asthma, severe bronchoconstriction will follow. However, although *exogenous* histamine can induce bronchial constriction, histamine is not the cause of bronchoconstriction that occurs during a spontaneous asthma attack. Consequently, antihistamines are of no use for treating asthma.

CNS Effects. In the CNS, H_1 receptors have a role in cognition, memory, and the cycle of sleeping and waking. In addition, H_1 receptors appear to have a role in seizure suppression, modulation of neurotransmitter release, and regulation of energy and endocrine homeostasis.

Other Effects. Activation of H_1 receptors on sensory nerves produces *itching* and *pain.* Histamine$_1$ activation also promotes *secretion of mucus.*

Effects of H_2 Stimulation

The major response to activation of H_2 receptors is *secretion of gastric acid.* Histamine acts directly on parietal cells of the stomach to promote acid release. Although acetylcholine and gastrin also help regulate acid release, histamine has a dominant role. We know this because, in the presence of H_2 blockade, acetylcholine and gastrin are unable to elicit acid secretion.

Role of Histamine in Allergic Responses

Allergic reactions are mediated by histamine and other compounds (e.g., prostaglandins, leukotrienes, tryptase). The intensity of an allergic reaction is determined by which mediator is involved.

Mild Allergy

The symptoms of mild allergy (e.g., rhinitis, itching, localized edema) are caused largely by histamine acting at H_1 receptors. As a result, mild allergic conditions (e.g., hay fever, acute urticaria, mild transfusion reactions) are generally responsive to antihistamine therapy.

Severe Allergic Reactions (Anaphylaxis)

Severe allergic reactions manifest as *anaphylactic shock,* a syndrome characterized by bronchoconstriction, hypotension, and edema of the glottis. Although histamine is involved in anaphylaxis, it plays a minor role; other substances (e.g., leukotrienes) are the principal mediators. Since histamine has little to do with producing anaphylaxis, it follows that antihistamines are of little help as treatment. The drug of choice for anaphylaxis is *epinephrine.* The rationale for using epinephrine is discussed in Chapter 17.

THE TWO TYPES OF ANTIHISTAMINES: H_1 ANTAGONISTS AND H_2 ANTAGONISTS

Antihistamines fall into two basic categories: H_1 receptor antagonists and H_2 receptor antagonists. The H_1 antagonists produce selective blockade of H_1 receptors. The H_2 antagonists produce selective blockade of H_2 receptors. The principal use of H_1 blockers is treatment of mild allergic disorders. The principal use of H_2 blockers is treatment of gastric and duodenal ulcers. Because H_2 antagonists do not block H_1 receptors, these drugs are of no use for treating allergies. In this chapter, we focus on H_1 antagonists. The H_2 blockers, which are widely used, are discussed in Chapter 78.

HISTAMINE$_1$ ANTAGONISTS I: BASIC PHARMACOLOGY

The H_1 antagonists are the classic antihistamines. These agents were in use long before H_2 blockers came along. In fact, before H_2 blockers became available, the term *H_1 antagonist* did not exist; the drugs that we now call H_1 antagonists or H_1 blockers were simply referred to as *antihistamines.* Because of its historic use, the term *antihistamines* is still employed as a synonym for the subgroup of histamine antagonists that produce selective H_1 blockade. Here, we continue to use the term *antihistamine* interchangeably with H_1 blocker and H_1 antagonist.

Although all H_1 antagonists available have similar antihistaminic actions, these drugs differ significantly in side effects. Because of these differences, selection of a prototype to represent the group is not feasible. Thus, rather than structuring discussion around one prototypic drug, we discuss the H_1 antagonists collectively. Differences among individual antihistamines are addressed as appropriate.

Classification of H_1 Antagonists

The H_1 antagonists fall into two major groups: *first-generation H_1 antagonists* and *second-generation H_1 antagonists*. The principal difference between the groups is that first-generation antihistamines are highly sedating, whereas second-generation antihistamines are not.

Mechanism of Action

Histamine$_1$ blockers bind selectively to H_1-histaminic receptors, thereby blocking the actions of histamine at these sites. Histamine$_1$ antagonists do not block H_2 receptors. Also, they do not block release of histamine from mast cells or basophils.

It should be noted that, although interaction of the classic antihistamines with *histaminic* receptors is limited to the H_1 receptor subtype, these drugs can also bind to *nonhistaminic* receptors. Most notably, certain antihistamines can bind to and block *muscarinic* receptors. This action underlies several important side effects.

Pharmacologic Effects

Peripheral Effects. The major therapeutic effects of the H_1 antagonists can be attributed to preventing the actions of histamine at H_1 receptors. In arterioles and venules of the skin, H_1 blockers inhibit the dilator actions of histamine and thereby reduce localized flushing. In capillary beds, the antihistamines prevent histamine-induced increases in permeability and thereby reduce edema. By blocking histamine at sensory nerves, H_1 antagonists reduce itching and pain. Blockade of H_1 receptors in mucous membranes suppresses secretion of mucus.

Effects on the CNS. Antihistamines can cause both excitation and depression of the CNS. At therapeutic doses, antihistamines produce CNS depression: reaction time is slowed, alertness is diminished, and drowsiness is likely. These effects are more pronounced with some antihistamines than with others. With most second-generation antihistamines (e.g., fexofenadine), CNS depression is negligible.

Overdose with antihistamines can produce *CNS stimulation.* Convulsions frequently result. Very young children are especially sensitive to CNS stimulation by these drugs.

Other Pharmacologic Effects. Blockade of muscarinic cholinergic receptors by antihistamines can produce typical *anticholinergic* responses. These are discussed later under *Adverse Effects.* Several antihistamines can suppress nausea and vomiting, as discussed under *Motion Sickness.*

Therapeutic Uses

All of the H_1 antagonists are useful in treating allergic disorders. Some are also indicated for other conditions (e.g., motion sickness, insomnia).

Mild Allergy. Antihistamines can reduce symptoms of mild allergies. In people with *seasonal allergic rhinitis* (also known as hay fever or rose fever), H_1 blockers can reduce sneezing, rhinorrhea, and itching of the eyes, nose, and throat (although they can't reduce nasal congestion). In patients with *acute urticaria,* these drugs can reduce redness, itching, and edema. The antihistamines can also reduce symptoms of *allergic conjunctivitis* and urticaria associated with *mild transfusion reactions.* In all these conditions, benefits result from H_1 receptor blockade—not from preventing allergen-induced release of histamine from mast cells and basophils. Because mild allergic reactions may be mediated by substances in addition to histamine, antihistamines often fail to produce complete relief.

Severe Allergy. As noted, the major symptoms of anaphylaxis (hypotension, laryngeal edema, bronchospasm) are caused by mediators other than histamine. Hence, although antihistamines may be employed as adjuncts in patients with anaphylaxis, their benefits are limited.

Motion Sickness. Some antihistamines, such as promethazine and dimenhydrinate [Dramamine], are labeled for use in motion sickness. Benefits derive from blocking H_1 receptors and muscarinic receptors in the neuronal pathway leading from the vestibular apparatus of the inner ear to the vomiting center of the medulla. Motion sickness and its treatment are discussed in Chapter 80.

Insomnia. The ability of antihistamines to cause drowsiness has been exploited in the treatment of insomnia. Practically every over-the-counter (OTC) sleep aid contains an H_1 antagonist—diphenhydramine or pyrilamine—as its active ingredient. However, although antihistamines can induce sleep

PATIENT-CENTERED CARE ACROSS THE LIFE SPAN

Antihistamines

Life Stage	Patient Care Concerns
Infants	Antihistamines can cause sedation in infants. Although they can be used in small doses in children older than 6 months, caution should be employed.
Children/adolescents	Antihistamines can be used safely in children, just in smaller doses. Side effect profiles are similar to those of adults. Promethazine is contraindicated in children younger than 2 years, as deaths have occurred in this population.
Pregnant women	There has been debate regarding whether antihistamines cause fetal harm when used in pregnancy. Many of these drugs are classified in U.S. Food and Drug Administration Pregnancy Risk Category C[a] and should be avoided unless absolutely necessary.
Breast-feeding women	Occasional small doses of antihistamines do not appear to cause sedation in infants. Caution should be used.
Older adults	As antihistamines can cause sedation, smaller doses should be used initially and titrated up if needed. Also, these medications can make glaucoma or benign prostatic hyperplasia worse.

[a]As of 2020, the FDA will no longer use Pregnancy Risk Categories. Please refer to Chapter 9 for more information.

when used in sufficient dosage, the doses recommended for OTC preparations are usually too low to be effective.

Common Cold. Despite their widespread presence in cold remedies, antihistamines are of practically no value against the common cold. These drugs neither prevent colds nor shorten their duration. Moreover, since histamine does not mediate symptoms of colds, H_1 blockade cannot even provide symptomatic relief. The only benefit these drugs may offer is a moderate reduction in rhinorrhea, an effect that derives from their *anticholinergic* properties, not from H_1 blockade.

Adverse Effects

All of the H_1 blockers can produce undesired effects. As a rule, these responses are more of a nuisance than a source of serious discomfort or danger. Frequently, side effects subside with continued drug use. Because individual antihistamines differ in their abilities to produce particular side effects (Table 70.1), adverse responses can be minimized by judicious drug selection.

Sedation. Sedation is the most common side effect of the antihistamines and can lead to serious consequences. For students, sedation can impair learning and memory. For drivers, sedation greatly increases the risk of an accident. In fact, the degree of impairment seen with antihistamines equals that seen when blood levels of alcohol exceed the legal limit. Worse yet, impairment can occur without feeling tired. Accordingly, patients should exercise extreme caution when driving or performing other hazardous activities. They should also avoid alcohol and other CNS depressants, which will intensify the depressant effects of the H_1 antagonist. Fortunately, tolerance to sedation often develops within a few days or weeks. If a preparation with a long half-life is being used, daytime sedation can be minimized by administering the entire daily dose at night.

The second-generation antihistamines exert little or no sedative effect. First, these drugs are relatively large molecules with low lipid solubility, so they can't cross the blood-brain barrier. Second, these drugs have low affinity to the type of H_1 receptor found in the brain. In contrast, the first-generation antihistamines are relatively small molecules with high lipid solubility, and hence can readily cross the blood-brain barrier. In addition, these drugs have a high affinity for H_1 receptors of the CNS.

For patients who experience disabling sedation with a first-generation H_1 antagonist, therapy with a second-generation (nonsedating) antihistamine is likely to help. Unfortunately, the nonsedating agents are more expensive than the first-generation agents.

Nonsedative CNS Effects. In addition to sedation, antihistamines can cause dizziness, incoordination, confusional states, and fatigue. Older patients are especially sensitive to these actions. In some patients, paradoxical excitation occurs, resulting in insomnia, nervousness, tremors, and even convulsions. CNS stimulation is most common in children and following overdose.

TABLE 70.1 ■ Pharmacologic Effects of H_1 Antagonists Used for Systemic Therapy

Drug	H_1-Blocking Activity[a]	Sedative Effects[a]	Anticholinergic Effects[a]
FIRST-GENERATION AGENTS			
Alkylamines			
Brompheniramine	+ + +	+	+ +
Chlorpheniramine	+ +	+	+ +
Dexchlorpheniramine	+ + +	+	+ +
Ethanolamines			
Clemastine	+ to + +	+ +	+ + +
Diphenhydramine	+ to + +	+ + +	+ + +
Phenothiazines			
Promethazine[b]	+ + +	+ + +	+ + +
Piperazines			
Hydroxyzine	+ + to + + +	+ + +	+ +
Piperidines			
Cyproheptadine	+ +	+	+ +
SECOND-GENERATION (NONSEDATING) AGENTS			
Cetirizine[c]	+ + +	+	±
Levocetirizine[c]	+ + +	+	±
Fexofenadine	+ + +	±	±
Loratadine	+ + to + + +	±	±
Desloratadine	+ + to + + +	±	±

[a]±, Low to none; +, low; ++, moderate; + + +, high.

[b]Promethazine is contraindicated in children younger than 2 years owing to a risk of fatal respiratory depression. *Parenteral* promethazine can cause severe local tissue injury.

[c]Cetirizine and levocetirizine have mild sedative effects.

Gastrointestinal Effects. Gastrointestinal disturbances are common. Responses include nausea, vomiting, loss of appetite, and diarrhea or constipation. These reactions can be minimized by administering antihistamines with food.

Anticholinergic Effects. The H_1 antagonists possess weak atropine-like properties. These antimuscarinic actions can produce drying of mucous membranes in the mouth, nasal passages, and throat. Cholinergic blockade may also result in urinary hesitancy, constipation, and palpitations. If dry mouth becomes distressing, discomfort can be minimized by using hard sugarless candy and by taking frequent sips of liquid. Antihistamines should be used with caution in patients with asthma, because thickening of bronchial secretions may impair breathing. Care is also needed in patients with other conditions that can be made worse by muscarinic blockade (e.g., urinary retention, benign prostatic hyperplasia, hypertension). The second-generation antihistamines are the least anticholinergic.

Safety Alert

PROMETHAZINE

Promethazine [Phenadoz] can cause severe respiratory depression, especially in very young patients. Deaths have occurred. Accordingly, the drug is now contraindicated for use in children younger than 2 years and should be used with caution in children older than 2 years.

Severe Local Tissue Injury. Extravasation of IV *promethazine* can cause severe local tissue injury, including gangrene that requires amputation. Severe injury can also occur with inadvertent perivascular or intra-arterial administration, or with administration into or near a nerve. Accordingly, when parenteral dosing is needed, the preferred route is IM; subQ promethazine is contraindicated. If IV administration *must* be done, promethazine should be given through a large-bore, freely flowing line, in a concentration of 25 mg/mL or less at a rate of 25 mg/min or less. Patients should be advised to report local burning or pain immediately.

Drug Interactions: CNS Depressants

Alcohol and other CNS depressants (e.g., barbiturates, benzodiazepines, opioids) can intensify the depressant effects of H_1 antagonists. Patients should be advised against drinking alcoholic beverages. If medications with CNS-depressant properties are combined with H_1 blockers, dosage of the depressant may need to be lowered.

Use in Pregnancy and Lactation

Pregnancy. The margin of safety of antihistamines in pregnancy is unknown. There have been reports of fetal malformation, but direct involvement of H_1 antagonists has not been proved. Given the uncertainty over the safety of these drugs, it is recommended that antihistamines be used only when clearly necessary, and only when the benefits of treatment outweigh the potential risks to the fetus. Antihistamines should be avoided late in the third trimester, because newborns are particularly sensitive to the adverse actions of these drugs.

Lactation. The H_1 antagonists can be excreted in breast milk, thereby posing a risk to the nursing infant. Since infants, and especially newborns, are unusually sensitive to antihistamines, these drugs should be avoided by women who are breast-feeding. If necessary, small occasional doses will probably not cause harm.

Acute Toxicity

Although the antihistamines have a large margin of safety, acute poisoning is nonetheless common, owing to the widespread availability of these drugs. CNS effects are prominent, especially anticholinergic reactions. Specific symptoms and treatment are described in the sections that follow.

Symptoms. The anticholinergic actions of H_1 blockers produce symptoms resembling those of atropine poisoning (dilated pupils, flushed face, hyperpyrexia, tachycardia, dry mouth, urinary retention). In children, CNS excitation is prominent, manifesting as hallucinations, incoordination, ataxia, and convulsions. In extreme cases, intoxication progresses to coma, cardiovascular collapse, and death.

Treatment. There is no specific antidote to antihistamine poisoning. Hence, treatment is directed at drug removal and managing symptoms. Absorption can be minimized by giving activated charcoal (to adsorb the drug), followed by a cathartic (to hasten its export from the GI tract). Convulsions can be treated with IV benzodiazepines (lorazepam, midazolam). Hyperthermia can be reduced by applying ice packs or by giving sponge baths.

HISTAMINE$_1$ ANTAGONISTS II: PREPARATIONS

As noted above, the H_1 antagonists can be divided into two major groups: first-generation H_1 antagonists and second-generation H_1 antagonists. The first-generation agents can cause significant sedation. In contrast, the second-generation agents cause little or no sedation. All of the H_1 blockers can be administered by mouth. In addition, some can be given parenterally, by nasal spray, or by rectal suppository. Routes and dosages for individual H_1 antagonists are shown in Table 70.2.

First-Generation H_1 Antagonists

The first-generation antihistamines can be grouped into five major categories (see Table 70.1). These groups differ in antihistaminic efficacy and in the ability to cause sedation and muscarinic blockade. Given these differences, it may be possible, through judicious drug selection, to produce effective H_1 blockade while minimizing undesired effects.

Sedation can be a significant problem. Among the first-generation agents, CNS depression is most prominent with the ethanolamines (e.g., diphenhydramine) and phenothiazines (e.g., promethazine) and least prominent with the alkylamines (e.g., chlorpheniramine). For many patients, the alkylamines can provide effective H_1 blockade while causing only a modest reduction in alertness. If sedation remains excessive with an alkylamine, a second-generation agent should be tried.

Most first-generation agents have significant anticholinergic properties. As a result, they can cause dry mouth, urinary hesitancy, and other typical anticholinergic side effects.

Second-Generation (Nonsedating) H_1 Antagonists

Second-generation antihistamines produce much less sedation than first-generation agents because (1) the second-generation

TABLE 70.2 ▪ H_1 Antagonists Used for Systemic Therapy: Brand Names, Routes, and Dosage

Generic Name	Brand Names	Routes	Usual Adult Oral Dosage
FIRST-GENERATION AGENTS			
Alkylamines			
Brompheniramine	Bromfed DM, others	PO	12 mg every 4–6 hr
Chlorpheniramine	Chlor-Trimeton, others	PO	4 mg every 4–6 hr
Dexchlorpheniramine	Generic only	PO	2 mg every 4–6 hr
Ethanolamines			
Clemastine	Tavist Allergy	PO	1.34 mg every 12 hr
Diphenhydramine	Benadryl	PO, IV, IM	25–50 mg every 6–8 hr
Phenothiazines			
Promethazine[a]	Phenadoz, Phenergan, others	PO, IV, IM, rectal suppository	12.5–25 mg every 6 hr
Piperazines			
Hydroxyzine	Vistaril	PO	25–100 mg every 4–8 hr
Piperidines			
Cyproheptadine	Generic only	PO	4 mg every 6–8 hr
SECOND-GENERATION (NONSEDATING) AGENTS			
Cetirizine[b]	Zyrtec, Reactine ♣	PO	5–10 mg every 24 hr
Levocetirizine[b]	Xyzal	PO	2.5–5 mg every 24 hr
Fexofenadine	Allegra, Allegra ODT	PO	60 mg every 12 hr
Loratadine	Alavert, Claritin	PO	10 mg every 24 hr
Desloratadine	Clarinex, Clarinex RediTabs, Aerius ♣	PO	5 mg every 24 hr

[a]Promethazine is contraindicated in children younger than 2 years owing to a risk of fatal respiratory depression.
[b]Cetirizine and levocetirizine have mild sedative effects.

agents cross the blood-brain barrier poorly and (2) they have a low affinity for H_1 receptors of the CNS. Synergism with alcohol and other CNS depressants is low. Nonetheless, combined use of CNS depressants and the second-generation agents should be avoided. In addition to lacking sedative effects, the second-generation agents are largely devoid of anticholinergic actions. When these drugs were introduced, they all required a prescription. Now, all of them are available over the counter. Since all of these drugs are very similar, initial selection can usually be based on price. If a cheaper agent proves ineffective, a more expensive agent can be tried.

Although there are five second-generation agents that are used for systemic (oral) therapy, we will discuss only the prototype, fexofenadine. The remainder can be found in Table 70.1. Two other second-generation agents, azelastine [Astelin, Astepro] and olopatadine [Patanase], both used for local effects in the nose, are discussed in Chapter 77.

Fexofenadine

Fexofenadine [Allegra, Allegra Allergy, Allegra ODT] is approved for oral therapy of seasonal allergic rhinitis and for chronic idiopathic urticaria. Of the second-generation antihistamines now available, fexofenadine appears to offer the best combination of efficacy and safety. In clinical trials, the incidence of drowsiness and other side effects was nearly the same as with placebo. Fexofenadine has a half-life of 14.4 hours and is excreted unchanged in the urine. The drug is available in standard tablets (30, 60, and 180 mg) and a suspension (6 mg/mL), marketed as *Allegra* and *Allegra Children's Liquid,* and in orally disintegrating tablets (30 mg), marketed as *Allegra ODT* and *Allegra Children's Meltable Tablets.* Dosages depend on the drug formulation and patient age as follows:

- *Standard tablets*—patients 12 years and older, 60 mg twice daily or 180 mg once daily; children 6 to 11 years, 30 mg twice daily
- *Orally disintegrating tablets*—children 6 to 11 years, 30 mg twice daily
- *Suspension*—children 2 to 11 years, 30 mg twice daily; children 6 months to 2 years, 15 mg twice daily

For all formulations, dosage should be reduced in patients with renal impairment.

Certain fruit juices (e.g., apple juice, orange juice, grapefruit juice) can reduce fexofenadine absorption, possibly reducing therapeutic effects. The mechanism is inhibition of *organic anion transporting polypeptides* (OATPs), which contribute to absorption of fexofenadine from the GI tract. To ensure fexofenadine absorption, patients should not drink fruit juices within 4 hours before dosing or 1 to 2 hours after dosing.

KEY POINTS

- Histamine is synthesized and stored in mast cells and basophils.
- Histamine release may be triggered by allergic and nonallergic mechanisms.
- There are two major classes of histamine receptors, called H_1 receptors and H_2 receptors.
- Activation of H_1 receptors causes vasodilation, increased capillary permeability, pain, itching, bronchoconstriction, and CNS effects.
- Activation of H_2 receptors causes release of gastric acid from parietal cells of the stomach.
- Histamine is an important mediator of mild allergic reactions, but is only a minor contributor to severe (anaphylactic) reactions.
- There are two major classes of histamine receptor antagonists: H_1 receptor antagonists, which are used to treat mild allergic reactions, and H_2 receptor antagonists, which are used to treat gastric and duodenal ulcers.
- Histamine$_1$ receptor antagonists relieve allergic symptoms by blocking histamine receptors on small blood vessels, capillaries, and sensory nerves. These drugs do not block release of histamine from mast cells and basophils.
- There are two major classes of H_1 receptor antagonists, known as first-generation H_1 receptor antagonists and second-generation H_1 receptor antagonists.
- First-generation H_1 receptor antagonists frequently cause sedation and anticholinergic effects; second-generation agents rarely cause either.
- CNS depression from first-generation H_1 receptor antagonists can be intensified by alcohol and other drugs with CNS-depressant actions.

Please visit **http://evolve.elsevier.com/Lehne** for chapter-specific NCLEX® examination review questions.

Summary of Major Nursing Implications[a]

HISTAMINE$_1$ RECEPTOR ANTAGONISTS

First-Generation Antihistamines

Brompheniramine
Chlorpheniramine
Clemastine
Cyproheptadine
Dexchlorpheniramine
Diphenhydramine
Hydroxyzine
Promethazine

Second-Generation Antihistamines

Cetirizine
Desloratadine
Fexofenadine
Levocetirizine
Loratadine

Preadministration Assessment

Therapeutic Goal

Oral Therapy. Relief of symptoms of mild to moderate allergic disorders (e.g., allergic rhinitis, allergic conjunctivitis, uncomplicated urticaria and angioedema).

Parenteral Therapy. Treatment of allergic reactions to blood or plasma; adjunctive therapy of anaphylaxis.

Identifying High-Risk Patients

Antihistamines should be avoided during the third trimester of pregnancy and in nursing mothers and newborn infants.

Exercise *caution* when treating young children, older adults, and patients with conditions that may be aggravated by muscarinic blockade, including asthma, urinary retention, open-angle glaucoma, hypertension, and prostatic hypertrophy.

Implementation: Administration

Routes

All H_1 blockers used for systemic therapy can be given PO. Some can also be administered IM, IV, or by rectal suppository.

Administration

Advise patients to take oral antihistamines with food if GI upset occurs.

Warn patients not to crush or chew enteric-coated preparations.

Teach patients how to administer orally disintegrating tablets.

Summary of Major Nursing Implications[a]—cont'd

Ongoing Evaluation and Interventions

Minimizing Adverse Effects

Sedation. For most patients, a first-generation antihistamine in the alkylamine group can provide effective H_1 blockade with only modest sedation. If sedation is excessive with an alkylamine, a second-generation antihistamine (e.g., fexofenadine) can be used. With long-acting antihistamines, daytime sedation can be minimized by administering the entire daily dose in the evening. **Caution patients to exercise extreme caution when driving or doing other hazardous activities.**

Anticholinergic Effects. **Advise patients that dryness of the mouth and throat can be reduced by using hard sugarless candy and taking frequent sips of liquid.** Other atropine-like responses (urinary hesitancy, tachycardia, constipation) are not usually problems. Second-generation antihistamines have minimal anticholinergic effects.

Gastrointestinal Distress. **Advise patients that GI disturbances (nausea, vomiting) can be minimized by taking antihistamines with meals.**

Effects in Older Adults. Older patients are especially sensitive to CNS and anticholinergic effects. Be alert for CNS effects (e.g., dizziness, incoordination, confusion, fatigue) and exaggerated anticholinergic effects (e.g., dry mouth, urinary hesitancy, constipation).

Severe Respiratory Depression. *Promethazine* can cause fatal respiratory depression, especially in the very young. Do not give promethazine to children younger than 2 years, and use it with caution in children older than 2 years.

Severe Tissue Injury. Parenteral *promethazine* can cause severe local tissue injury if an IV line becomes extravasated, or following inadvertent perivascular, intra-arterial, or intraneuronal dosing. Gangrene requiring amputation has developed. Accordingly, when parenteral dosing is needed, the preferred route is IM. If IV dosing cannot be avoided, promethazine should be administered through a large-bore, freely flowing line, in a concentration of 25 mg/mL or less at a rate of 25 mg/min or less. **Advise patients to immediately report local burning or pain.**

Minimizing Adverse Interactions

CNS Depressants. Alcohol and other CNS depressants can intensify the depressant actions of the H_1 antagonists. **Warn patients against drinking alcohol.** Dosages of CNS depressants (e.g., barbiturates, benzodiazepines, opioids) may need to be reduced. Second-generation antihistamines have minimal CNS-depressant effects and hence are less likely to potentiate the actions of CNS depressants.

Fruit Juice. Certain fruit juices (e.g., apple juice, orange juice, grapefruit juice) can decrease intestinal absorption of *fexofenadine,* possibly reducing effectiveness. Advise patients to avoid fruit juice in the interval between 4 hours before dosing and 1 to 2 hours after dosing.

Managing Toxicity

There is no specific antidote to antihistamine overdose, and hence treatment is directed at minimizing absorption and managing symptoms. To reduce absorption, give activated charcoal. Treat hyperthermia with ice packs or cooling sponge baths. Control convulsions with IV benzodiazepines.

[a]Patient education information is highlighted as **blue text.**

CHAPTER

71

Cyclooxygenase Inhibitors: Nonsteroidal Anti-Inflammatory Drugs and Acetaminophen

The family of cyclooxygenase inhibitors consists of aspirin and related drugs. Most of these agents have three useful effects: they can suppress inflammation, relieve pain, and reduce fever. In addition, aspirin—and only aspirin—can protect against myocardial infarction (MI) and stroke. All of these effects are produced through one central mechanism: inhibition of cyclooxygenase, the enzyme responsible for synthesis of prostanoids (prostaglandins and related compounds). This same mechanism underlies their principal adverse effects: gastric ulceration, bleeding, and renal impairment. Cyclooxygenase inhibition also underlies MI and stroke, which can occur with most of these drugs, but *not* with aspirin.

MECHANISM OF ACTION

All of the drugs discussed here work by inhibiting *cyclooxygenase* (COX), the enzyme that converts arachidonic acid into *prostanoids: prostaglandins* and related compounds (prostacyclin, thromboxane A_2 [TXA_2]). To understand the drugs that inhibit COX, we must first understand COX itself.

Cyclooxygenase is found in all tissues and helps regulate multiple processes. At sites of tissue injury, COX catalyzes the synthesis of prostaglandin E_2 (PGE_2) and prostaglandin I_2 (PGI_2, aka prostacyclin), which promote inflammation and sensitize receptors to painful stimuli. In the stomach, COX promotes synthesis of PGE_2 and PGI_2, which help protect the gastric mucosa. Three mechanisms are involved: reduced secretion of gastric acid, increased secretion of bicarbonate and cytoprotective mucus, and maintenance of submucosal blood flow. In platelets, COX promotes synthesis of TXA_2, which stimulates platelet aggregation. In blood vessels, COX promotes synthesis of prostacyclin, which causes vasodilation. In the kidney, COX catalyzes synthesis of PGE_2 and PGI_2, which promote vasodilation and thereby maintain renal blood flow. In the brain, COX-derived prostaglandins mediate fever and contribute to perception of pain. In the uterus, COX-derived prostaglandins help promote contractions at term. It is important to appreciate that prostaglandins, prostacyclin, and TXA_2 act *locally;* these compounds do not affect sites distant from where they were made.

Cyclooxygenase has two forms, named cyclooxygenase-1 (COX-1) and cyclooxygenase-2 (COX-2). Cyclooxygenase-1 is found in practically all tissues, where it mediates "housekeeping" chores. Important among these are protecting the gastric mucosa, supporting renal function, and promoting platelet aggregation. In contrast, COX-2 is produced mainly at sites of *tissue injury,* where it mediates inflammation and sensitizes receptors to painful stimuli. Cyclooxygenase-2 is also present in the *brain* (where it mediates fever and contributes to perception of pain), the *kidneys* (where it supports renal function), *blood vessels* (where it promotes vasodilation), and the *colon* (where it can contribute to colon cancer). Because COX-1 primarily mediates beneficial processes, whereas COX-2 primarily mediates harmful processes, COX-1 has been dubbed the "good COX" and COX-2 the "bad COX." Some important functions of COX-1 and COX-2 are shown in Table 71.1.

Having established the roles of COX-1 and COX-2, we can now predict the effects of drugs that inhibit these enzymes. Inhibition of COX-1 (good COX) results largely in harmful effects:

- Gastric erosion and ulceration
- Bleeding tendencies
- Renal impairment

Inhibition of COX-1 also has one very beneficial effect:

- Protection against MI and stroke (secondary to reduced platelet aggregation)

Inhibition of COX-2 (bad COX) results largely in beneficial effects:

- Suppression of inflammation
- Alleviation of pain
- Reduction of fever
- Protection against colorectal cancer

Inhibition of COX-2 also has two adverse effects:

- Renal impairment
- Promotion of MI and stroke (secondary to suppressing vasodilation)

TABLE 71.1 ▪ Cyclooxygenase-1 and Cyclooxygenase-2: Functions and Effect of Inhibition

Location	COX Isoform	COX Reaction Product	Response to COX Reaction Product	Effect of COX Inhibition
Stomach	COX-1	PGE_2, PGI_2	Gastric protection: Increased bicarbonate secretion Increased mucus production Decreased acid secretion Maintenance of submucosal blood flow	Gastric ulceration
Platelets	COX-1	TXA_2	Platelet aggregation	Bleeding tendencies Protection against MI
Blood vessels	COX-2	Prostacyclin	Vasodilation	Vasoconstriction (which can promote MI)
Kidney	COX-1, COX-2	PGE_2, PGI_2	Maintenance of renal function: Renal vasodilation Maintenance of renal perfusion	Renal impairment
Injured tissue	COX-2	PGE_2	Inflammation Pain	Reduced inflammation Analgesia
Brain	COX-2	Unknown	Fever Pain	Reduced fever Analgesia
Colon/rectum	COX-2	Unknown	Colorectal cancer promotion	Colorectal cancer protection

COX-1, Cyclooxygenase-1; *COX-2,* cyclooxygenase-2; *MI,* myocardial infarction; *PGE_2,* prostaglandin E_2; *PGI_2,* prostaglandin I_2 (prostacyclin); *TXA_2,* thromboxane A_2.

CLASSIFICATION OF CYCLOOXYGENASE INHIBITORS

The cyclooxygenase inhibitors fall into two major categories: (1) drugs that have anti-inflammatory properties and (2) drugs that lack anti-inflammatory properties. Agents in the first group are referred to as *nonsteroidal anti-inflammatory drugs* (NSAIDs). Representative members include aspirin, ibuprofen [Advil, Motrin, others], naproxen [Aleve, others], and celecoxib [Celebrex]. The second class consists of just one drug: *acetaminophen* [Tylenol, others]. Acetaminophen can reduce pain and fever but cannot suppress inflammation.

The NSAIDs can be subdivided into two groups: (1) *first-generation NSAIDs* (conventional NSAIDs, traditional NSAIDs) and (2) *second-generation NSAIDs* (selective COX-2 inhibitors, coxibs). The first-generation agents inhibit COX-1 *and* COX-2. The second-generation agents inhibit COX-2 only. Because the first-generation agents inhibit both COX isoforms, they are unable to suppress pain and inflammation without posing a risk of serious side effects (gastric ulceration, bleeding, renal impairment). In contrast, because of their selectivity for COX-2, the second-generation NSAIDs, *in theory,* can suppress pain and inflammation while (possibly) causing fewer adverse effects than the first-generation NSAIDs. However, *in reality,* COX-2 inhibitors appear even less safe than the first-generation agents, owing to an increased risk of MI and stroke.

Table 71.2 shows the principal indications and adverse effects of the first-generation NSAIDs, second-generation NSAIDs, and acetaminophen.

FIRST-GENERATION NSAIDS

The first-generation NSAIDs—a large and widely used group of drugs—inhibit COX-1 and COX-2. In the United States, more than 70 million prescriptions are written annually and more than 30 billion tablets are sold over the counter. The traditional NSAIDs are used to treat inflammatory disorders (e.g., rheumatoid arthritis, osteoarthritis, bursitis), alleviate mild to moderate pain, suppress fever, and relieve dysmenorrhea. Because they cannot inhibit COX-2 without inhibiting COX-1, first-generation NSAIDs cannot suppress inflammation without posing a risk of serious harm: NSAID-induced ulcers are responsible for more than 100,000 hospitalizations and 10,000 to 17,000 deaths each year. Aspirin is the oldest member of the family and prototype for the group.

Prototype Drugs

COX INHIBITORS (ASPIRIN-LIKE DRUGS)

First-Generation Nonsteroidal Anti-Inflammatory Drugs (NSAIDs)

Aspirin
Ibuprofen

Second-Generation NSAIDs (Selective COX-2 Inhibitors)

Celecoxib

Drug That Lacks Anti-Inflammatory Actions

Acetaminophen

Aspirin

Aspirin is an important drug whose effectiveness is frequently underappreciated. Given that aspirin is available without prescription, widely advertised in the media, and used somewhat

TABLE 71.2 ▪ Principal Indications and Adverse Effects of the Four Major Types of Cyclooxygenase Inhibitors

	First-Generation NSAIDs: Aspirin	First-Generation NSAIDs: All Others	Second-Generation NSAIDs (Coxibs)	Acetaminophen
INDICATIONS				
Inflammation	Yes	Yes	Yes	No
Pain	Yes	Yes	Yes	Yes
Fever	Yes	Yes	No	Yes
Prevention of MI and stroke	Yes	No	No	No
ADVERSE EFFECTS				
Gastric ulceration	Yes	Yes	Yes[a]	No
Renal impairment	Yes	Yes	Yes	No
Bleeding	Yes	Yes	No	No
MI and stroke	No	Yes	Yes	No
Liver damage with overdose	No	No	No	Yes

[a]Despite their selectivity for cyclooxygenase-2, coxibs can still cause gastric ulceration, although it may be less than with other NSAIDs.

casually by the general public, you may be surprised to hear that aspirin is a highly valuable and effective medication. The drug provides excellent relief of mild to moderate pain, reduces fever, protects against thrombotic disorders, and remains a drug of choice for rheumatoid arthritis and other inflammatory conditions. You may also be surprised to hear that aspirin can cause serious toxicity, especially gastric ulceration. Despite the introduction of many new NSAIDs, aspirin remains one of the most widely used members of the group and is the standard against which the others must be compared.

Chemistry

Aspirin belongs to a chemical family known as *salicylates.* All members of this group are derivatives of salicylic acid. Aspirin is produced by substituting an acetyl group onto salicylic acid. Because of this acetyl group, aspirin is commonly known as *acetylsalicylic acid,* or simply ASA.

Mechanism of Action

Aspirin is a nonselective inhibitor of cyclooxygenase. Most beneficial effects—reductions of inflammation, pain, and fever—result from inhibiting COX-2. One beneficial effect—protection against MI and ischemic stroke—results from inhibiting COX-1. Major adverse effects—gastric ulceration, bleeding, and renal impairment—result from inhibiting COX-1.

It is important to note that aspirin is an *irreversible* inhibitor of cyclooxygenase. In contrast, all other NSAIDs are *reversible* (competitive) inhibitors. Because inhibition of cyclooxygenase by aspirin is irreversible, duration of action depends on how quickly specific tissues can synthesize new molecules of COX-1 and COX-2. With other NSAIDs, effects decline as soon as drug levels fall.

Pharmacokinetics

Absorption. Aspirin is absorbed rapidly and completely after oral dosing. The principal site of absorption is the small intestine. When administered by rectal suppository, aspirin is absorbed slowly and blood levels are lower than with oral dosing.

Metabolism. Aspirin has a very short half-life (15 to 20 minutes), owing to rapid conversion to *salicylic acid,* an *active* metabolite. The rate of inactivation of salicylic acid depends on the amount present: At low therapeutic levels, salicylic acid has a half-life of approximately 2 hours, but at high therapeutic levels, the half-life may exceed 20 hours.

Distribution. Salicylic acid is extensively bound to plasma albumin. At therapeutic levels, binding is between 80% and 90%. Aspirin undergoes distribution to all body tissues and fluids, including breast milk, fetal tissues, and the central nervous system (CNS).

Excretion. Salicylic acid and its metabolites are excreted by the kidneys. Excretion of salicylic acid is highly dependent on urinary pH. Accordingly, by raising the pH of urine from 6 to 8, we can increase the rate of excretion fourfold.

Plasma Drug Levels. Low therapeutic doses of aspirin produce plasma salicylate levels less than 100 mcg/mL. Anti-inflammatory doses produce salicylate levels of about 150–300 mcg/mL. Signs of salicylism (toxicity) begin when plasma salicylate levels exceed 200 mcg/mL. Severe toxicity occurs at levels above 400 mcg/mL.

Therapeutic Uses

Suppression of Inflammation. Aspirin is an initial drug of choice for rheumatoid arthritis, osteoarthritis, and juvenile arthritis. Aspirin is also indicated for other inflammatory disorders, including rheumatic fever, tendinitis, and bursitis. The dosages employed to suppress inflammation are considerably larger than dosages used for analgesia or reduction of fever. The use of aspirin and other NSAIDs to treat arthritis is discussed further in Chapter 73.

The precise mechanisms by which aspirin decreases inflammation have not been established. We do know that prostanoids contribute to several, but not all, components of the inflammatory process. Hence, inhibition of COX-2 provides a partial explanation of anti-inflammatory effects. Other possible mechanisms include modulation of T-cell function, suppression of inflammatory cell infiltration, and stabilization of lysosomes.

Analgesia. Aspirin is used widely to relieve mild to moderate pain. The degree of analgesia produced depends on the type of pain. Aspirin is most active against joint pain, muscle pain, and headache. For some forms of postoperative pain, aspirin can be more effective than opioids. However, aspirin is relatively ineffective against severe pain of visceral origin. In contrast to opioid analgesics, aspirin produces neither tolerance nor physical dependence. In addition, aspirin is safer than opioids.

Aspirin relieves pain primarily through actions in the periphery. At sites of injury, prostanoids sensitize pain receptors to mechanical and chemical stimulation. Aspirin reduces pain by inhibiting COX-2, thereby suppressing prostanoid production. In addition to this peripheral mechanism, aspirin works in the CNS to help relieve pain.

Reduction of Fever. Aspirin is a drug of choice for reducing temperature in febrile *adults.* However, because of the risk of Reye's syndrome (discussed later in this chapter), *aspirin should not be used to treat fever in children.* Although aspirin readily reduces fever, it will not lower normal body temperature, nor will it lower temperature that has become elevated in response to physical activity or to a rise in environmental temperature.

Body temperature is regulated by the hypothalamus, which maintains a balance between heat production and heat loss. Fever occurs when the set point of the hypothalamus becomes elevated, causing the hypothalamus to increase heat production and decrease heat loss. Set-point elevation is triggered by local synthesis of prostaglandins in response to endogenous pyrogens (fever-promoting substances). Aspirin lowers the set point by inhibiting COX-2, and thereby inhibits pyrogen-induced synthesis of prostaglandins.

Dysmenorrhea. Aspirin can provide relief from primary dysmenorrhea. Benefits derive from inhibiting prostaglandin synthesis in uterine smooth muscle. (Prostaglandins promote uterine contraction, so suppression of prostaglandin synthesis relieves cramping.) Some of the newer aspirin-like drugs (e.g., ibuprofen, naproxen) are superior to aspirin for dysmenorrhea. The efficacy of the newer drugs is attributed to a greater ability to inhibit COX in the uterus.

Suppression of Platelet Aggregation. Synthesis of TXA_2 in platelets promotes aggregation. Aspirin suppresses platelet aggregation by causing *irreversible* inhibition of COX-1, the enzyme that makes TXA_2. Because platelets lack the machinery to synthesize new COX-1, the effects of a single dose persist for the life of the platelet (about 8 days).

There is a large body of evidence demonstrating that aspirin, through its antiplatelet actions, can benefit a variety of patients. Accordingly, the U.S. Food and Drug Administration (FDA) recommended wider use of aspirin for antiplatelet effects. Professional labeling now recommends daily aspirin for men and women with the following:

- *Ischemic stroke* (to reduce the risk of death and nonfatal stroke)
- *Transient ischemic attacks* (to reduce the risk of death and nonfatal stroke)
- *Acute MI* (to reduce the risk of vascular mortality)
- *Previous MI* (to reduce the combined risk of death and nonfatal MI)
- *Chronic stable angina* (to reduce the risk of MI and sudden death)
- *Unstable angina* (to reduce the combined risk of death and nonfatal MI)
- *Angioplasty and other revascularization procedures* (in patients who have a pre-existing condition for which aspirin is already indicated)

According to a review published in *JAMA*—"Aspirin Dose for the Prevention of Cardiovascular Disease"—a dose of 75 to 81 mg/day for these indications is adequate. Higher doses, which are commonly prescribed in these circumstancces, offer no greater protection, but will increase the risk of GI bleeding.

In addition to these applications, aspirin can be taken by healthy people for *primary prevention* of MI and stroke. However, more recent studies show that aspirin provides less protection against cardiovascular disease than once thought. The potential small benefit must be weighed against the major risk of aspirin use, namely, GI hemorrhage. Hence, to determine the *net* benefit of primary prevention for any man or woman, we must determine his or her individual risk for a GI bleed and compare that risk with his or her individual risk for a cardiovascular event (i.e., the risk for an MI in men, or the risk for ischemic stroke in women).[a] Many organizations, including the American Heart Association, the American Thoracic Society, and the European Society of Cardiology, recommend against the use of aspirin for primary prevention of cardiovascular disease unless the patient has a 10-year risk greater than 10%.

How do we calculate 10-year risk for a cardiovascular event? Risk for ischemic stroke can be assessed using the calculator at http://www.yourdiseaserisk.wustl.edu/YDRDefault.aspx?ScreenControl=YDRGeneral&ScreenName=YDRStroke. Risk for an MI can be assessed using the calculator at www.mcw.edu/calculators/CoronaryHeartDiseaseRisk.htm.

Cancer Prevention

Colorectal Cancer. There is good evidence that regular use of aspirin decreases the risk of colorectal cancer, even when the dosage is low. Results from the Nurses' Health Study showed that regular use of *high-dose* aspirin (650 mg/day or more) reduces the risk of colorectal cancer. This dosage is much greater than that used to prevent cardiovascular disease, and hence poses a significant risk of bleeding. In fact, for every one or two cancers prevented, high-dose aspirin would cause eight additional serious bleeds. Fortunately, more recent studies indicate that *low-dose* aspirin is effective too. For example, results of a study reported in *The Lancet* indicate that taking low-dose aspirin (75 to 300 mg/day) for more than 5 years reduces the incidence of colorectal cancer (by 24%), as well as mortality from colon cancer (by 35%). At these low doses, the benefits of cancer protection may well outweigh the risk of possible bleeding and other adverse events.

Aspirin protects against colorectal cancer probably by inhibiting COX-2. In animal models, COX-2 promotes tumor growth and metastases, and inhibition of COX-2 slows tumor growth. In humans, most colorectal cancers express COX-2.

[a]Major factors that increase the risk of a GI bleed are use of NSAIDs and a history of ulcers. Major risk factors for an MI are advancing age, diabetes, high total cholesterol, low HDL cholesterol, and smoking. Major risk factors for an ischemic stroke are advancing age, hypertension, diabetes, smoking, atrial fibrillation, left ventricular hypertrophy, and a history of cardiovascular disease.

Furthermore, protection by aspirin is limited to colon cancers that have high COX-2 levels. Aspirin does not protect against colon cancers with little or no COX-2.

Other Cancers. Available data suggest that protection may not be limited to colorectal cancer. Results of a meta-analysis reported in *The Lancet* (377:31, 2011) show that daily low-dose aspirin reduces the risk of death from *all* solid tumors (by 34%), but does not reduce the risk of death from hematologic cancers. Earlier studies have shown protection against specific cancers. In a study involving men over the age of 60, daily use of aspirin and other NSAIDs was associated with a 50% decrease in the incidence of prostate cancer. In a study involving 2884 women, aspirin appeared to reduce the risk of breast cancer, especially among women with hormone receptor–positive tumors, and among those who took 7 or more aspirin tablets a week. In another study, taking aspirin at least 3 times a week for at least 6 months was associated with a 40% reduction in the incidence of ovarian cancer. In contrast to these positive results, results from the Women's Health Study found no protection with low-dose aspirin against cancer of the breast, colon, or any other tissue. The reasons for this discrepancy are not clear.

Adverse Effects

When administered short term in analgesic or antipyretic (fever-reducing) doses, aspirin rarely causes serious adverse effects. However, toxicity is common when treating inflammatory disorders, which require long-term high-dose treatment.

Gastrointestinal Effects. The most common side effects are *gastric distress, heartburn,* and *nausea.* These can be reduced by taking aspirin with food or a full glass of water.

Occult GI bleeding occurs often. In most cases, the amount of blood lost each day is insignificant. However, with chronic aspirin use, cumulative blood loss can produce anemia.

Long-term aspirin—*even in low doses*—can cause life-threatening *gastric ulceration, perforation,* and *bleeding.* Ulcers result from four causes:

- Increased secretion of acid and pepsin
- Decreased production of cytoprotective mucus and bicarbonate
- Decreased submucosal blood flow
- The direct irritant action of aspirin on the gastric mucosa

The first three occur secondary to inhibition of COX-1. Direct injury to the stomach is most likely with aspirin preparations that dissolve slowly: Owing to slow dissolution, particulate aspirin becomes entrapped in folds of the stomach wall, causing prolonged exposure to high concentrations of the drug. Because aspirin-induced ulcers are often asymptomatic, perforation and upper GI hemorrhage can occur without premonitory signs. (Hemorrhage is due in part to erosion of the stomach wall and in part to suppression of platelet aggregation.) Factors that increase the risk of ulceration include:

- Advanced age
- A history of peptic ulcer disease
- Previous intolerance to aspirin or other NSAIDs
- Cigarette smoking
- History of alcohol abuse (Alcohol intensifies the irritant effects of aspirin and should not be consumed.)

What can we do to *prevent* ulcers? According to the American College of Gastroenterology, prophylaxis with a *proton pump inhibitor* (PPI) is recommended for patients at risk, including those with a history of peptic ulcers, those taking glucocorticoids, and older adults. Proton pump inhibitors (e.g., omeprazole, lansoprazole) reduce ulcer generation by suppressing production of gastric acid. In addition to PPIs, other drugs that may be considered include histamine$_2$ receptor antagonists (H_2RAs) and misoprostol. COX-2 inhibitors may also be tried instead of traditional NSAIDs, as they are thought to produce fewer GI side effects. Since many ulcers are caused by infection with *Helicobacter pylori* (see Chapter 78), the panel recommends that patients with ulcer histories undergo testing and treatment for *H. pylori* before starting long-term aspirin use. *Treatment* of NSAID-induced ulcers is discussed in Chapter 78.

Bleeding. Aspirin promotes bleeding by inhibiting platelet aggregation. Taking just two 325-mg aspirin tablets can double bleeding time for about 1 week. (Recall that platelets are unable to replace aspirin-inactivated cyclooxygenase, and hence bleeding time is prolonged for the life of the platelet.) Because of its effects on platelets, *aspirin is contraindicated for patients with bleeding disorders* (e.g., hemophilia, vitamin K deficiency, hypoprothrombinemia). To minimize blood loss during childbirth and elective surgery, *high-dose* aspirin should be discontinued at least 1 week before these procedures. There is no need to stop aspirin before procedures with a low risk of bleeding (e.g., dental, dermatologic, or cataract surgery). In most cases, the use of *low-dose* aspirin to protect against thrombosis should *not* be interrupted for elective surgery and dental procedures. Caution is needed when aspirin is used in conjunction with anticoagulants.

In patients taking daily aspirin, high blood pressure increases the risk of a brain bleed (i.e., hemorrhagic stroke), even though aspirin protects against ischemic stroke. To reduce the risk of hemorrhagic stroke, blood pressure should be 150/90 mm Hg (and preferably lower) before starting daily aspirin.

Renal Impairment. Aspirin can cause acute, reversible impairment of renal function, resulting in salt and water retention and edema. Clinically significant effects are most likely in patients with additional risk factors: advanced age, existing renal impairment, hypovolemia, hepatic cirrhosis, or heart failure. Aspirin impairs renal function by inhibiting COX-1, thereby depriving the kidney of prostaglandins needed for normal function.

Development of renal impairment is signaled by reduced urine output, weight gain despite use of diuretics, and a rapid rise in serum creatinine and blood urea nitrogen. If any of these occurs, aspirin should be withdrawn immediately. In most cases, kidney function then returns to baseline level.

The risk of acute renal impairment can be reduced by identifying high-risk patients and treating them with the smallest dosages possible.

In addition to its acute effects on renal function, aspirin may pose a risk of renal papillary necrosis and other types of renal injury when used long term.

Salicylism. Salicylism is a syndrome that begins to develop when aspirin levels climb just slightly above therapeutic. Overt signs include *tinnitus* (ringing in the ears), *sweating, headache,* and *dizziness.* Acid-base disturbance may also occur (see next paragraph). If salicylism develops, aspirin should be withheld until symptoms subside. Aspirin should then resume, but with a small reduction in dosage. In some cases, development of tinnitus can be used to adjust aspirin dosage: When tinnitus occurs, the maximum acceptable dose has been achieved.

However, this guideline may be inappropriate for older patients, because they may fail to develop tinnitus even when aspirin levels become toxic.

Acid-base disturbance results from the effects of aspirin on respiration. When administered in high therapeutic doses, aspirin acts on the CNS to stimulate breathing. The resultant increase in CO_2 loss produces *respiratory alkalosis.* In response, the kidneys excrete more bicarbonate. As a result, plasma pH returns to normal and a state of *compensated respiratory alkalosis* is produced.

Safety Alert

ASPIRIN

The use of aspirin in children younger than 18 years is associated with Reye's syndrome.

Reye's Syndrome. This syndrome is a rare but serious illness of childhood that has a mortality rate of 30% to 40%. Characteristic symptoms are encephalopathy and fatty liver degeneration. Epidemiologic data suggested a relationship between Reye's syndrome and the use of aspirin by children who have influenza or chickenpox. Although a direct causal link between aspirin and Reye's syndrome was never established, the Centers for Disease Control and Prevention recommended that aspirin (and other NSAIDs) be avoided by children and teenagers suspected of having influenza or chickenpox. In response to this recommendation, aspirin was removed from most products intended for children, and aspirin use by children declined sharply. As a result, Reye's syndrome essentially vanished: The incidence declined from a high of 555 cases in 1980 to no more than 20 cases per year since 1994. If a child with chickenpox or influenza needs an analgesic-antipyretic, acetaminophen can be used safely.

Adverse Effects Associated With Use During Pregnancy. Aspirin poses risks to the pregnant patient and her fetus. Accordingly, the drug is classified in *FDA Pregnancy Risk Category D*[b]*: There is evidence of human fetal risk, but the potential benefits from use of the drug during pregnancy may outweigh the potential for harm.* The principal risks to pregnant women are (1) anemia (from GI blood loss) and (2) postpartum hemorrhage. In addition, by inhibiting prostaglandin synthesis, aspirin may suppress spontaneous uterine contractions and may thereby prolong labor.

Aspirin crosses the placenta and may adversely affect the fetus. Since prostaglandins help keep the ductus arteriosus patent, inhibition of prostaglandin synthesis by aspirin may induce premature closure of the ductus arteriosus. Aspirin use has also been associated with low birth weight, stillbirth, renal toxicity, intracranial hemorrhage in preterm infants, and neonatal death.

Hypersensitivity Reactions. Hypersensitivity develops in about 0.3% of aspirin users. Reactions are most likely in adults with a history of asthma, rhinitis, and nasal polyps. Hypersensitivity reactions are uncommon in children. The hypersensitivity reaction to aspirin begins with profuse, watery rhinorrhea and may progress to generalized urticaria, bronchospasm, laryngeal edema, and shock. Despite its resemblance to severe anaphylaxis, this reaction is not allergic and is not mediated by the immune system. What *does* cause these reactions? Because individuals who react to aspirin are also sensitive to most other NSAIDs, we believe that the reactions are due to inhibition of COX-1, which triggers production of leukotrienes, which in turn causes bronchospasm, hives, and other signs of hypersensitivity. However, if this *is* the mechanism, it remains unclear why hypersensitivity is limited mainly to adults with the predisposing conditions mentioned earlier. As with severe anaphylactic reactions, *epinephrine* is the treatment of choice.

Hypersensitivity to aspirin is considered a contraindication to using other drugs with aspirin-like properties. Nonetheless, if an aspirin-like drug must be taken, four such drugs are probably safe. One of these—celecoxib—is selective for COX-2. Another—meloxicam—is somewhat selective for COX-2, but only at low doses. The other two—acetaminophen and salsalate—are only weak inhibitors of COX-1.

Cardiovascular Events. In contrast to all other NSAIDs, aspirin does *NOT* increase the risk of thrombotic events, including MI and ischemic stroke. In fact, when taken in low doses, aspirin *protects* against these events.

Summary of Precautions and Contraindications

Aspirin is contraindicated in patients with *peptic ulcer disease, bleeding disorders* (e.g., hemophilia, vitamin K deficiency, hypoprothrombinemia), and *hypersensitivity to aspirin itself or other NSAIDs.* In addition, the drug should be used with extreme caution by *pregnant women and by children who have chickenpox or influenza.* Caution should also be exercised when treating *older adult patients, patients who smoke cigarettes,*

PATIENT-CENTERED CARE ACROSS THE LIFE SPAN

NSAIDs

Life Stage	Patient Care Concerns
Infants	Because of the risk of Reye's syndrome, aspirin should be avoided in infants. Acetaminophen and ibuprofen can be used safely in small doses for fever.
Children/adolescents	Because of the risk of Reye's syndrome, aspirin should be avoided in children and adolescents. Acetaminophen and ibuprofen can be used safely in small doses for fever.
Pregnant women	NSAIDs may result in premature closure of the ductus arteriosus. Therefore, their use is contraindicated in the third trimester of pregnancy.
Breast-feeding women	NSAIDs and acetaminophen appear safe for use in breast-feeding mothers.
Older adults	NSAIDS are the most common drug used to treat chronic pain in older adults. These drugs have been shown to increase hospital admissions in this population. Caution should be used with NSAIDs in older adults.

[b]As of 2020, the FDA will no longer use Pregnancy Risk Categories. Please refer to Chapter 9 for more information.

and *patients with* H. pylori *infection, heart failure, hepatic cirrhosis, hypovolemia, renal dysfunction, asthma, hay fever, chronic urticaria, nasal polyps,* or *a history of alcoholism.* Aspirin should be withdrawn 1 week before elective surgery or the anticipated date of childbirth.

Drug Interactions

Because of its widespread use, aspirin has been reported to interact with many other medications. However, most of these interactions have little clinical significance. Significant interactions are discussed here.

Anticoagulants: Warfarin, Heparin, and Others. Aspirin's most important interactions are with anticoagulants. Because aspirin suppresses platelet function and can decrease prothrombin production, aspirin can intensify the effects of warfarin, heparin, and other anticoagulants. Furthermore, since aspirin can initiate gastric bleeding, augmenting anticoagulant effects can increase the risk of gastric hemorrhage. Accordingly, the combination of aspirin with anticoagulants must be used with care—even when aspirin is taken in low doses to reduce the risk of thrombotic events.

Glucocorticoids. Like aspirin, glucocorticoids promote gastric ulceration. As a result, the risk of ulcers is greatly increased when these drugs are combined—as may happen when treating arthritis. To reduce the risk of gastric ulceration, patients can be given a PPI or H_2RA for prophylaxis.

Alcohol. Combining alcohol with aspirin and other NSAIDs increases the risk of gastric bleeding. To alert the public to this risk, the FDA now requires that labels for aspirin include the following statement: ***Alcohol Warning:*** *If you consume three or more alcoholic drinks every day, ask your doctor whether you should take aspirin or other pain relievers/fever reducers. Aspirin [and related drugs] may cause stomach bleeding.* A similar label is required for all other NSAIDs and acetaminophen.

Nonaspirin NSAIDs. Ibuprofen, naproxen, and other nonaspirin NSAIDs can reduce the antiplatelet effects of aspirin by blocking access of aspirin to COX-1 in platelets. This interaction is important: In patients taking low-dose aspirin to prevent MI or ischemic stroke, other NSAIDs could negate aspirin's benefits. Because immediate-release aspirin produces complete platelet inhibition about 1 hour after dosing, we can prevent interference by giving aspirin about 2 hours before giving other NSAIDs. Of course, we could eliminate interference entirely by using high-dose aspirin, rather than another NSAID, when conditions call for NSAID therapy.

ACE Inhibitors and ARBs. Like aspirin, angiotensin-converting enzyme (ACE) inhibitors and angiotensin receptor blockers (ARBs) can impair renal function. In susceptible patients, combining aspirin with drugs in either class can increase the risk of acute renal failure. High-dose aspirin should be avoided in patients taking these drugs. However, low-dose aspirin taken for antiplatelet effects should be continued.

Vaccines. Aspirin and other NSAIDs may blunt the immune response to vaccines. Accordingly, these drugs should not be used routinely to prevent vaccination-associated fever and pain.

Acute Poisoning

Aspirin overdose is a common cause of poisoning. Although rarely fatal in adults, aspirin poisoning may be lethal in children. The lethal dose for adults is 20 to 25 gm. In contrast, as little as 4000 mg (4 gm) can kill a child.

Signs and Symptoms. Initially, aspirin overdose produces a state of compensated respiratory alkalosis—the same state seen in mild salicylism. As poisoning progresses, respiratory excitation is replaced with respiratory depression. Acidosis, hyperthermia, sweating, and dehydration are prominent, and electrolyte imbalance is likely. Stupor and coma result from effects in the CNS. Death usually results from respiratory failure.

Treatment. Aspirin poisoning is an acute medical emergency that requires hospitalization. The immediate threats to life are respiratory depression, hyperthermia, dehydration, and acidosis. Treatment is largely supportive. If respiration is inadequate, mechanical ventilation should be instituted. External cooling (e.g., sponging with tepid water) can help reduce hyperthermia. Intravenous fluids are given to correct dehydration; the composition of these fluids is determined by electrolyte and acid-base status. Slow infusion of bicarbonate is given to reverse acidosis. Several measures (e.g., gastric lavage, giving activated charcoal) can reduce further GI absorption of aspirin. Alkalinization of the urine with bicarbonate accelerates excretion of aspirin and salicylate. If necessary, hemodialysis or peritoneal dialysis can be used to remove salicylates.

Formulations

Aspirin is available in multiple formulations, including plain and buffered tablets, enteric-coated preparations, and tablets used to produce a buffered solution. These different formulations reflect efforts to increase rates of absorption and decrease gastric irritation. For the most part, the clinical utility of the more complex formulations is no greater than that of plain aspirin tablets.

Aspirin Tablets, Plain. All brands are essentially the same with respect to analgesic efficacy, onset, and duration. Some less expensive tablets have greater particle size, which results in slower dissolution and prolonged contact with the gastric mucosa, which increases gastric irritation. When aspirin tablets decompose, they smell like vinegar (acetic acid) and should be discarded.

Aspirin Tablets, Buffered. The amount of buffer in buffered aspirin tablets is too small to produce significant elevation of gastric pH. An equivalent effect on pH can be achieved by taking plain aspirin tablets with food or a glass of water. Buffered aspirin tablets are no different from plain tablets with respect to analgesic effects and gastric distress. Buffered tablets may dissolve faster than plain tablets, resulting in somewhat faster onset.

Buffered Aspirin Solution. A buffered aspirin solution is produced by dissolving effervescent aspirin tablets [Alka-Seltzer] in a glass of water. This solution has considerable buffering capacity due to its high content of sodium bicarbonate. Effects on gastric pH are sufficient to decrease the incidence of gastric irritation and bleeding. In addition, aspirin absorption is accelerated and peak blood levels are raised. Unfortunately, these benefits come with a price. The sodium content of buffered aspirin solution can be detrimental to individuals on a sodium-restricted diet. Also, absorption of bicarbonate can elevate urinary pH, which will accelerate aspirin excretion. Lastly, this highly buffered preparation is expensive. Because of this combination of benefits and drawbacks, the buffered aspirin solution is well suited for occasional use but is generally inappropriate for long-term therapy.

Enteric-Coated Preparations. Enteric-coated preparations dissolve in the intestine rather than the stomach, thereby reducing gastric irritation. Unfortunately, absorption from these formulations can be delayed and erratic. Patients should be advised not to crush or chew them.

Timed-Release Tablets. Timed-release tablets offer no advantage over plain aspirin tablets. Because the half-life of salicylic acid is long to begin with and because aspirin produces irreversible inhibition of cyclooxygenase, timed-release tablets cannot prolong effects.

Rectal Suppositories. Rectal suppositories have been employed for patients who cannot take aspirin orally. Absorption can be variable, resulting in plasma drug levels that are insufficient in some patients and excessive in others. Also, rectal irritation can occur. Because of these undesirable properties, aspirin suppositories are not generally recommended.

Dosage and Administration

Aspirin is almost always administered by mouth. Gastric irritation can be minimized by dosing with water or food. Dosage depends on the age of the patient and the condition being treated. Adult and pediatric dosages for major indications are shown in Table 71.3.

TABLE 71.3 ▪ Aspirin Dosage

Indication	Adult Dosage	Pediatric Dosage[a]
Aches and pains; fever	325–650 mg every 4 hr as needed	*2–3 yr:* 160 mg *4–5 yr:* 240 mg *6–8 yr:* 325 mg *9–10 yr:* 405 mg *11 yr:* 485 mg *Over 11 yr:* 650 mg All of the above doses are administered every 4 hr as needed
Acute rheumatic fever	5–8 gm/day in divided doses	100 mg/kg/day (initially), then 75 mg/kg/day for 4–6 wk
Rheumatoid arthritis	3.6–5.4 gm/day in divided doses	90–130 mg/kg/day in divided doses every 4–6 hr
Suppression of platelet aggregation		
Initial therapy	325 mg once daily	
Chronic therapy	80 mg once daily	

[a]Owing to the risk of Reye's syndrome, aspirin is usually avoided in patients younger than 18 years.

Nonaspirin First-Generation NSAIDs

In attempts to produce an aspirin-like drug with fewer GI, renal, and hemorrhagic effects than aspirin, the pharmaceutical industry has produced a large number of drugs with actions much like those of aspirin. In the United States, over 20 nonaspirin NSAIDs are available (Table 71.4). Like aspirin, all other first-generation NSAIDs inhibit both COX-1 and COX-2. However, in contrast to aspirin, which causes *irreversible* inhibition of cyclooxygenase, the other traditional NSAIDs cause *reversible* inhibition. All of these drugs have anti-inflammatory, analgesic, and antipyretic properties. In addition, they all can cause gastric ulceration, bleeding, and renal impairment—although the intensity of these effects may be less with some agents. Patients who are hypersensitive to aspirin are likely to experience cross-hypersensitivity with other NSAIDs. For most NSAIDs, safety during pregnancy has not been established, and hence use by pregnant women is discouraged.

The principal indications for the nonaspirin NSAIDs are rheumatoid arthritis and osteoarthritis. In addition, certain NSAIDs are used to treat fever, bursitis, tendinitis, mild to moderate pain, and dysmenorrhea (see Table 71.4).

In contrast to aspirin, the nonaspirin NSAIDs *do not* protect against MI and stroke. In fact, they *increase* the risk of thrombotic events. For the NSAIDs as a group, the increase in cardiovascular risk is relatively low—about 12%. Risk is highest with indomethacin (71%), sulindac (41%), and meloxicam (37%). However, although the increase in risk with these drugs appears high, it pales in comparison with smoking, which increases cardiovascular risk by 200% to 300%. To minimize cardiovascular risk, nonaspirin NSAIDs should be used in the lowest effective dosage for the shortest time needed. Also, these drugs should not be used before coronary artery bypass graft (CABG) surgery or for 14 days after. Other measures to reduce risk are discussed under *AHA Statement on COX Inhibitors in Chronic Pain.*

Although individual NSAIDs differ chemically, pharmacokinetically, and to some extent pharmacodynamically, all are similar clinically: They all produce essentially equivalent anti-inflammatory effects, and they all present a similar risk of serious adverse effects (gastric ulceration, bleeding, renal impairment, MI, and stroke). However, for reasons that are not understood, individual patients may respond better to one agent than another. Furthermore, individual patients may tolerate one NSAID better than another. Therefore, to optimize therapy for each patient, trials with more than one NSAID may be needed.

Ibuprofen

Basic Pharmacology. Ibuprofen [Advil, Motrin, Caldolor, others] is the prototype of the propionic acid derivatives. Other members of the family are shown in Tables 71.4 and 71.5. Like aspirin, ibuprofen inhibits cyclooxygenase and has anti-inflammatory, analgesic, and antipyretic actions. The drug is used to treat fever, mild to moderate pain, and arthritis. In addition, ibuprofen appears superior to most other NSAIDs for relief of primary dysmenorrhea, presumably because it produces good inhibition of cyclooxygenase in uterine smooth muscle. In clinical trials, ibuprofen was highly effective at promoting closure of the ductus arteriosus in preterm infants, a condition for which indomethacin is the current treatment of choice.

Ibuprofen is generally well tolerated, and the incidence of adverse effects is low. The drug produces less gastric bleeding than aspirin and less inhibition of platelet aggregation as well. Consequently, ibuprofen is among the safer NSAIDs for use with anticoagulants. Very rarely, ibuprofen has been associated with Stevens-Johnson syndrome, a severe hypersensitivity reaction that causes blistering of the skin and mucous membranes, and can result in scarring, blindness, and even death. Like other nonaspirin NSAIDs, ibuprofen may pose a risk of MI and stroke.

Diclofenac

Oral. Oral diclofenac [Voltaren XR, Cataflam, Cambia, Zipsor, Zorvolex] is approved for rheumatoid arthritis, osteoarthritis, ankylosing spondylitis, mild pain, primary dysmenorrhea, and migraine. As with other NSAIDs, anti-inflammatory, analgesic, and antipyretic effects result from inhibiting cyclooxygenase. Diclofenac is well absorbed following oral administration, but undergoes extensive (40% to 50%) metabolism on its first pass through the liver. In the blood, about 99.5% of the drug is protein bound, primarily to albumin. Diclofenac is metabolized by the liver and excreted in the urine.

The most common adverse effects are abdominal pain, dyspepsia, and nausea. By impairing renal function, diclofenac can cause fluid retention, which can exacerbate hypertension and heart failure. Diclofenac can cause severe liver injury, even with topical therapy. Accordingly, patients should receive periodic tests of liver function and should be instructed to report manifestations of liver injury (e.g., jaundice, fatigue, nausea). If liver injury is diagnosed, diclofenac should be discontinued.

Indomethacin

Actions and Uses. Indomethacin [Indocin] is an effective anti-inflammatory agent approved for arthritis, bursitis, tendinitis, and, as discussed in Chapter 74, acute gouty arthritis. In addition, the drug can be given IV to preterm infants to promote closure of the ductus arteriosus. Although indomethacin is able to reduce pain and fever, it is not routinely used for these effects, owing to potential toxicity.

Pharmacokinetics. Indomethacin is well absorbed following oral administration and distributes to all body fluids and tissues. The drug is metabolized in the liver. Metabolites and parent drug are excreted in the urine and feces.

TABLE 71.4 ■ Clinical Pharmacology of the Oral Nonsteroidal Anti-Inflammatory Drugs

Drug	Maximum Daily Dosage (mg)	Plasma Half-Life (hr)	Major Indications[a]				
			Arthritis	Moderate Pain	Fever	Dysmenorrhea	Bursitis/ Tendinitis
FIRST-GENERATION NSAIDs							
Salicylates							
Aspirin (many brand names)	8000	0.2–0.3	A	A	A		
Magnesium salicylate [Doan's Tablets, others]	4640	2–30[b]	A	A	A		
Salsalate	3000	2–30[b]	A	A	A		
Sodium salicylate (generic)	3900	2–30[b]	A	A	A		
Propionic Acid Derivatives							
Fenoprofen [Nalfon]	3200	3	A	A			
Flurbiprofen (generic)	300	5.7	A	I	I	I	I
Ibuprofen [Advil, Motrin, others]	3200	1.8–2	A	A	A	A	
Ketoprofen (generic)	300	2	A	A		A	
Naproxen [Aleve, others]	1375	12–17	A	A	A	A	A
Oxaprozin [Daypro]	1800	42–50	A				
Others							
Diclofenac [Cambia, Cataflam, Voltaren XR, Zipsor, Zorvolex]	200	2	A	A		A	
Diflunisal (generic)	1500	11–15	A	A			
Etodolac (generic)	1200	7.3	A	A			I
Indomethacin [Indocin]	200	4.5	A				A
Ketorolac (generic)	40 oral 120 IV	5–6	A				
Meclofenamate (generic)	400	1.3	A	A		A	
Mefenamic acid [Ponstel, Ponstan 🍁]	1000	2		A		A	
Meloxicam [Mobic, Mobicox 🍁]	15	15–20	A				
Nabumetone (generic)	2000	22	A				
Piroxicam [Feldene]	20	50	A				
Sulindac [Clinoril]	400	7.8	A				A
Tolmetin (generic)	1800	2–7	A				
SECOND-GENERATION NSAIDs (COX-2 INHIBITORS)							
Celecoxib [Celebrex]	800	11	A	A		A	

[a]*A*, FDA-approved indication; *I*, investigational use.
[b]Half-life increases with increasing dosage.

Adverse Effects. Untoward effects are seen in 35% to 50% of patients, causing about 20% to discontinue treatment. The most common adverse effect is severe frontal headache, which occurs in 25% to 50% of patients. Other CNS effects (dizziness, vertigo, confusion) are also common. Seizures and psychiatric changes (e.g., depression, psychosis) have occurred. Mild GI reactions (nausea, vomiting, indigestion) develop in 3% to 9% of users. More severe GI effects (ulceration with perforation, hemorrhage) may also occur. Hematologic reactions (neutropenia, thrombocytopenia, aplastic anemia) have occurred but are rare. Indomethacin suppresses platelet aggregation.

Precautions and Contraindications. Because of its adverse effects, indomethacin is generally contraindicated for infants and children under the age of 14, patients with peptic ulcer disease, and women who are pregnant or breast-feeding. Caution is required in patients with seizures and psychiatric disorders, in patients involved in hazardous activities, and in patients receiving anticoagulant therapy.

Ketorolac

Actions and Uses. Ketorolac is a powerful analgesic with minimum anti-inflammatory actions. Pain relief is equivalent to that produced by morphine and other opioids. Although ketorolac lacks the serious adverse effects associated with opioids (respiratory depression, tolerance, dependence, abuse potential), it nonetheless has serious adverse effects of its own. Accordingly, use should be short term and restricted to managing acute pain of moderate to severe intensity. Ketorolac is not indicated for chronic pain or for minor aches and discomfort. The usual indication is postoperative pain, for which ketorolac can be as effective as morphine. Like other NSAIDs, ketorolac suppresses prostaglandin synthesis. This action is thought to underlie analgesic effects.

Pharmacokinetics. Ketorolac is administered orally and parenterally (IM or IV). With parenteral administration, analgesia begins within 30 minutes, peaks in 1 to 2 hours, and persists 4 to 6 hours. The drug is eliminated by hepatic metabolism and urinary excretion. In young adults, ketorolac has a

TABLE 71.5 ▪ Indication and Dosing of the Oral Nonsteroidal Anti-Inflammatory Drugs

Drug	Availability	Indications	Usual Adult Dose
Magnesium salicylate [Doan's Tablets, others]	580-mg caplets and tablets	Arthritis, moderate pain, fever	1080 mg every 6 hr
Sodium salicylate/ methenamine [Cystex]	162.5/162-mg tablets	Urinary pain relief	2 tablets every 6 hr
Salsalate	500-, 750-mg tablets	Arthritis, moderate pain, fever	1500 mg twice daily or 1000 mg 3 times daily
Fenoprofen [Nalfon]	600-mg tablets 200-, 400-mg capsules	Arthritis Moderate pain	300–600 mg every 6–8 hr 200 mg every 4–6 hr
Flurbiprofen (generic)	50-, 100-mg tablets	Arthritis	50–100 mg every 6–12 hr
Ibuprofen [Advil, Motrin, others]	Tablets (100, 200, 400, 600, 800 mg) 200-mg capsules 50-, 100-mg chewable tablets 20 mg/mL oral suspension	Arthritis Moderate pain Dysmenorrhea	400–600 mg every 6–8 hr 400 mg every 4–6 hr 400 mg every 4 hr
Ibuprofen [Caldolor]	100 mg/mL IV solution for dilution	Pain Fever	400–800 mg every 6 hr 400 mg initial dose followed by 400 mg every 4–6 hr
Ibuprofen [NeoProfen]	10 mg/mL IV solution	Closure of patent ductus arteriosus in premature infants	NA
Ibuprofen/oxycodone [Combunox]	5/400-mg tablets	Moderate to severe pain	1 tablet every 6 hr
Ibuprofen/hydrocodone [Vicoprofen]	7.5/200-mg tablets	Moderate to severe pain	1 tablet every 4–6 hr
Ketoprofen (generic)	50-, 75-mg immediate-release capsules 200-mg extended-release capsules	Arthritis Moderate pain, dysmenorrhea	75 mg 3 times daily 50 mg every 4–6 hr
Naproxen [Aleve, others]	220-, 250-, 275-, 375-, 500-mg immediate-release tablets 375-, 500-mg delayed-release tablets 125 mg/5 mL oral solution	Arthritis, moderate pain, fever, dysmenorrhea, bursitis/tendinitis	250–500 mg every 12 hr
Naproxen/esomeprazole [Vimovo]	375/20-mg and 500/20-mg delayed-release tablets	Arthritis	1 tablet twice daily
Oxaprozin [Daypro]	600-mg tablets	Arthritis	1200 mg daily
Diclofenac [Cambia, Cataflam, Voltaren XR, Zipsor, Zorvolex]	18-, 35-, 50-mg immediate-release tablets 25-, 50-, 75-mg enteric-coated delayed-release tablets 100-mg extended-release tablets 25-mg liquid-filled capsules 50-mg powder packet	Rheumatoid arthritis Osteoarthritis Moderate pain, dysmenorrhea	50 mg 3–4 times daily 50 mg 2–3 times daily 50 mg 3 times daily
Diclofenac [Voltaren Gel]	1% topical gel	Arthritis	Lower extremity joints: 4 gm topically 4 times daily Upper extremity joints: 2 gm topically 4 times daily
Diclofenac [Flector Patch]	1.3% patch	Acute pain from sprains, strains, contusions	1 patch to affected area twice daily
Diclofenac [Pennsaid]	1.5% and 2% topical solution	Arthritis	2 sprays 2% solution or 40 drops 1.5% solution per knee twice daily
Diclofenac/misoprostol [Arthrotec]	50/0.2-mg and 75/0.2-mg delayed-release tablets	Arthritis	1 tablet 2–4 times daily
Diflunisal (generic)	250-, 500-mg tablets	Arthritis Moderate pain	250–500 mg every 12 hr 500 mg every 12 hr

Continued

TABLE 71.5 ▪ Indication and Dosing of the Oral Nonsteroidal Anti-Inflammatory Drugs—cont'd

Drug	Availability	Indications	Usual Adult Dose
Etodolac (generic)	200-, 300-mg capsules 400-, 500-mg immediate-release tablets 400-, 500-, 600-mg extended-release tablets	Arthritis Moderate pain	300–500 mg twice daily 200–400 mg every 6–8 hr
Indomethacin [Indocin]	25-, 50-mg immediate-release capsules 75-mg extended-release capsules 50-mg rectal suppository	Arthritis Bursitis/tendinitis	25 mg 2–3 times daily 25–50 mg 3 times daily
Indomethacin [Indocin IV]	Solution for IV injection	Closure of patent ductus arteriosus in infants	NA
Ketorolac (generic)	10-mg tablets Solution for IM/IV injection	Acute pain, PO Acute pain, IM/IV	20 mg ×1 followed by 10 mg every 4–6 hr 60 mg ×1 or 30 mg every 6 hr
Ketorolac [Sprix]	15.75-mg metered-dose intranasal spray	Acute moderate to severe pain	1 spray each nostril every 6–8 hr
Meclofenamate (generic)	50-, 100-mg capsules	Arthritis Moderate pain Dysmenorrhea	50–100 mg 3–4 times daily 50–100 mg every 4–6 hr 100 mg 3 times daily
Mefenamic acid [Ponstel, Ponstan 🍁]	250-mg capsules	Moderate pain, dysmenorrhea	250 mg every 6 hr
Meloxicam [Mobic, Mobicox 🍁]	7.5-,15-mg tablets	Arthritis	7.5–15 mg daily
Nabumetone (generic)	500-, 750-mg tablets	Arthritis	1000 to 2000 mg daily
Piroxicam [Feldene]	10-, 20-mg capsules	Arthritis	20 mg daily
Sulindac [Clinoril]	150-, 200-mg tablets	Arthritis, bursitis/tendinitis	150–200 mg twice daily
Tolmetin (generic)	200-, 600-mg tablets 400-mg capsules	Arthritis	200–600 mg 3 times daily
Celecoxib [Celebrex]	50-, 100-, 200-, 400-mg capsules	Osteoarthritis Rheumatoid arthritis Acute pain, dysmenorrhea	200 mg daily 100–200 mg daily 400 mg ×1 followed by 200 mg twice daily

half-life of 4 to 6 hours. The half-life may be prolonged in older adults and in those with renal impairment.

Adverse Effects and Contraindications. Ketorolac can cause all of the adverse effects associated with other NSAIDs, including peptic ulcers, GI bleeding or perforation, prolonged bleeding time, renal impairment, hypersensitivity reactions, suppression of uterine contractions, and premature closure of the ductus arteriosus. Concurrent use with other NSAIDs increases the risk of these effects and hence is contraindicated. Other contraindications include active peptic ulcer disease, history of peptic ulcer disease or recent GI bleeding, advanced renal impairment, confirmed or suspected intracranial bleeding, use before major surgery, history of NSAID hypersensitivity reactions, and use during labor and delivery.

Piroxicam

Piroxicam [Feldene] has anti-inflammatory, analgesic, and antipyretic properties, but is approved only for rheumatoid arthritis and osteoarthritis. The drug's most outstanding feature is its long half-life (about 50 hours). Because piroxicam is eliminated so slowly, therapeutic effects can be maintained with once-a-day dosing. In general, piroxicam is better tolerated than aspirin. Undesired effects are seen in 11% to 46% of patients, causing between 4% and 12% to discontinue therapy. Gastrointestinal reactions are most common, occurring in about 20% of patients. The incidence of gastric ulceration is about 1%. Like aspirin, piroxicam inhibits platelet aggregation and prolongs bleeding time. The drug is supplied in 10- and 20-mg capsules for oral use. The usual dosage is 20 mg once daily or 10 mg twice daily.

Meloxicam

Meloxicam [Mobic, Mobicox 🍁] can inhibit COX-1 and COX-2, but shows selectivity for COX-2 at low doses. Like other NSAIDs, the drug has analgesic, anti-inflammatory, and antipyretic actions. Approved indications are osteoarthritis, rheumatoid arthritis, and pauciarticular/polyarticular-course juvenile rheumatoid arthritis (JRA). For osteoarthritis, meloxicam is as effective as first-generation NSAIDs. Direct comparison with true COX-2 inhibitors (e.g., celecoxib) has not been made. Despite its COX-2 selectivity, meloxicam has a side effect profile like that of the first-generation NSAIDs. Gastrointestinal effects (abdominal pain, constipation, diarrhea, dyspepsia, flatulence, nausea, and vomiting) occur in 20% to 25% of patients. More serious effects—GI ulceration, bleeding, perforation, and death—have also occurred. Meloxicam does not suppress platelet aggregation. The drug has a long half-life (15 to 20 hours) and undergoes elimination in the urine (50%) and feces (50%).

Diflunisal

Diflunisal is a derivative of salicylic acid. However, unlike the salicylates, diflunisal is not converted to salicylic acid in the body. The drug is indicated for mild to moderate pain, rheumatoid arthritis, and osteoarthritis. Like other NSAIDs, the drug inhibits prostaglandin synthesis and can cause GI disturbances, suppression of platelet aggregation, and renal impairment, and may increase the risk of MI and stroke. Diflunisal has a prolonged half-life (11 to 15 hours), and hence can be administered only 2 or 3 times a day.

Nonacetylated Salicylates: Magnesium Salicylate, Sodium Salicylate, and Salsalate

Similarities to Aspirin. The nonacetylated salicylates are similar to aspirin (an acetylated salicylate) in most respects. Like aspirin, these drugs inhibit COX-1 and COX-2 and are employed to treat arthritis, moderate pain, and fever. The most common adverse effects are GI disturbances. As with aspirin, these drugs should not be given to children with chickenpox or influenza owing to the possibility of precipitating Reye's syndrome.

Contrasts With Aspirin. In contrast to aspirin, the nonacetylated salicylates cause little or no suppression of platelet aggregation. As a result, these drugs cannot protect against MI and stroke, and may actually increase risk.

Because of its sodium content, *sodium salicylate* should be avoided in patients on a sodium-restricted diet (e.g., patients with hypertension or heart failure).

Magnesium salicylate may accumulate to toxic levels in patients with chronic renal insufficiency, and hence should not be used by these people.

Salsalate is a prodrug that breaks down to release two molecules of salicylate in the alkaline environment of the small intestine. Because the stomach is not exposed to salicylate, salsalate produces less gastric irritation than aspirin.

Safety Alert

FIRST-GENERATION NSAIDS

All first-generation NSAIDs are associated with increased risk of gastrointestinal bleeding that can lead to hospitalization or death.

SECOND-GENERATION NSAIDS (COX-2 INHIBITORS, COXIBS)

The COX-2 inhibitors, also known as coxibs, were developed on the theory that selective inhibition of COX-2 should be able to suppress pain and inflammation while posing little or no risk of gastric ulceration. To some degree, theory and reality agree: Coxibs are just as effective as traditional NSAIDs at suppressing inflammation and pain, and they pose a somewhat lower risk of GI side effects. However, even with coxibs, patients can develop clinically significant gastroduodenal ulceration and bleeding. Furthermore, like traditional NSAIDs, coxibs can impair renal function and can thereby cause hypertension and edema. Coxibs also increase the risk of MI and stroke.

Celecoxib

Therapeutic Use

Celecoxib [Celebrex] was the first selective COX-2 inhibitor to reach the market. The drug is indicated for osteoarthritis, rheumatoid arthritis, ankylosing spondylitis, juvenile idiopathic arthritis, acute pain, and dysmenorrhea. In addition, celecoxib is used off-label for a rare genetic disorder known as familial adenomatous polyposis, which predisposes to developing colorectal cancer. For patients with arthritis, celecoxib is equal to naproxen (an NSAID) at relieving joint pain, stiffness, and swelling. Owing to concerns about cardiovascular safety, celecoxib is considered a last-choice drug for long-term management of pain (see *AHA Statement on COX Inhibitors in Chronic Pain*, later in this chapter).

It is important to note that celecoxib does *not* provide the cardiovascular benefits of aspirin because celecoxib does not inhibit COX-1 in platelets, and hence does not suppress platelet aggregation.

Mechanism of Action

Celecoxib causes selective inhibition of COX-2, the COX isoform whose products mediate inflammation and pain. At therapeutic doses, celecoxib does not inhibit COX-1, the COX isoform whose products protect the stomach, help maintain renal function, and promote platelet aggregation.

Pharmacokinetics

Celecoxib is well absorbed following oral administration. Plasma levels peak in 3 hours. Binding to plasma proteins is extensive (97%). The drug undergoes hepatic metabolism followed by renal excretion. The half-life is 11 hours.

Adverse Effects

In premarketing trials, celecoxib was well tolerated. The discontinuation rate owing to adverse effects was 7.1% for celecoxib versus 6.1% for placebo. The most common complaints were *dyspepsia* and *abdominal pain*. Celecoxib does not decrease platelet aggregation and hence does not promote bleeding. Possible cardiovascular events are the biggest concern.

Gastroduodenal Ulceration. Because celecoxib does not inhibit COX-1, the isoform of COX that protects the stomach, a low incidence of gastroduodenal ulceration would be expected. Some data support this expectation; others do not. When celecoxib was first approved, conclusions about its safety were based on 6-month data from the Celecoxib Arthritis Safety Study (CLASS), which indicated that celecoxib caused less GI toxicity than conventional NSAIDs (diclofenac, naproxen, ibuprofen). However, longer-term (12-month) data from the same study showed *no difference* in GI toxicity between celecoxib and conventional NSAIDs. Other studies have shown that, compared with patients taking conventional NSAIDs, those taking celecoxib had a lower incidence of endoscopically detectable ulcers and a lower incidence of hospitalization for GI bleeding. What's the bottom line? Celecoxib *may* be safer than conventional NSAIDs, especially when used short term. However, convincing data of superior safety are lacking. Like traditional NSAIDs, celecoxib can be combined with a PPI to reduce GI complications.

Cardiovascular Events. There is strong evidence that coxibs, like other nonaspirin NSAIDs, increase the risk of MI, stroke, and other serious cardiovascular events. In the Adenoma Prevention with Celecoxib (APC) trial, patients who took 400 mg or 800 mg of celecoxib a day experienced more major fatal or nonfatal cardiovascular events than did patients who took placebo. To minimize risk, celecoxib should be used in the lowest effective dosage for the shortest time needed. Also, the drug should be avoided in patients with existing heart disease and in those who have just undergone CABG surgery, and should be used with caution in patients with cardiovascular risk factors, such as hypertension, diabetes, and dyslipidemia. Other measures to reduce risk are discussed later under *AHA Statement on COX Inhibitors in Chronic Pain.*

Why is the risk of MI and stroke increased? First, because celecoxib does not inhibit COX-1, platelet aggregation is not suppressed. Second, because celecoxib inhibits COX-2 in blood vessels, vasoconstriction is increased. These two factors—unimpeded platelet aggregation and increased vasoconstriction—increase the likelihood of vessel blockage once the process of thrombosis has begun.

Renal Impairment. Like conventional NSAIDs, celecoxib can impair renal function, thereby posing a risk to patients with hypertension, edema, heart failure, or kidney disease. Renal impairment apparently results from inhibiting COX-2.

Sulfonamide Allergy. Celecoxib contains a sulfur molecule and hence can precipitate an allergic reaction in patients allergic to sulfonamides. Accordingly, the drug should be avoided by patients with sulfa allergy.

Use in Pregnancy. Celecoxib and other NSAIDs can cause premature closure of the ductus arteriosus. Accordingly,

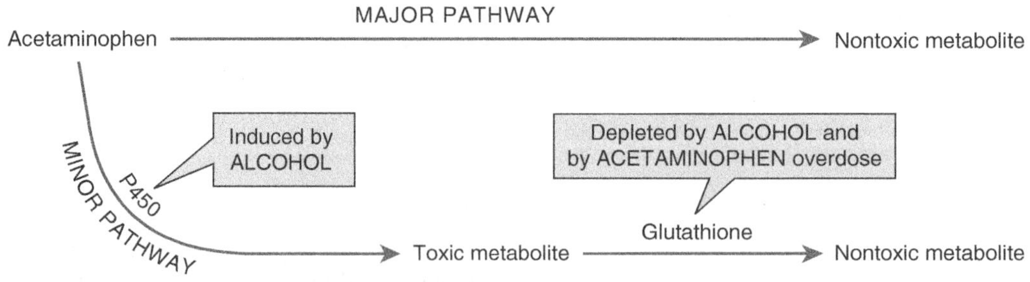

Fig. 71.1 ▪ **Metabolism of acetaminophen.**

these drugs are contraindicated during the third trimester of pregnancy.

Drug Interactions

Warfarin. Celecoxib may increase the anticoagulant effects of warfarin and may thereby increase the risk of bleeding. Celecoxib itself does not inhibit platelet aggregation and does not promote bleeding. However, the drug may enhance the anticoagulant effects of warfarin (perhaps by increasing warfarin levels). Celecoxib may be combined with warfarin, but effects of warfarin should be monitored closely, especially during the first few days of treatment.

Other Interactions. Information on the interactions of celecoxib with other drugs is limited. Celecoxib may decrease the diuretic effects of furosemide as well as the antihypertensive effects of ACE inhibitors. Conversely, celecoxib may increase levels of lithium (a drug for bipolar disorder). Levels of celecoxib may be increased by fluconazole (an antifungal drug).

ACETAMINOPHEN

Acetaminophen [Tylenol, Ofirmev, many others] is like aspirin in some respects but different in others. Acetaminophen has *analgesic* and *antipyretic* properties equivalent to those of aspirin. However, in contrast to aspirin and the other NSAIDs, *acetaminophen is devoid of clinically useful anti-inflammatory and antirheumatic actions.* In addition, acetaminophen does not suppress platelet aggregation, does not cause gastric ulceration, and does not decrease renal blood flow or cause renal impairment. However, acetaminophen overdose can cause severe liver injury. In the United States, acetaminophen is used more than any other analgesic.

Mechanism of Action

Differences between the effects of acetaminophen and aspirin are thought to result from selective inhibition of cyclooxygenase, the enzyme needed to make prostaglandins and related compounds. Whereas aspirin can inhibit cyclooxygenase in both the CNS and the periphery, inhibition by acetaminophen is limited to the CNS; acetaminophen has only minimal effects on cyclooxygenase at peripheral sites. By decreasing prostaglandin synthesis in the CNS, acetaminophen is able to reduce fever and pain. The inability to inhibit prostaglandin synthesis outside the CNS may explain the absence of anti-inflammatory effects, gastric ulceration, and adverse effects on the kidneys and platelets.

Pharmacokinetics

Acetaminophen is readily absorbed following oral dosing and undergoes wide distribution. Most of each dose is metabolized by the liver, and the metabolites are excreted in the urine. The plasma half-life is approximately 2 hours.

Acetaminophen can be metabolized by two pathways; one is major and the other is minor (Fig. 71.1). In the major pathway, acetaminophen undergoes conjugation with glucuronic acid and other compounds to form nontoxic metabolites. In the minor pathway, acetaminophen is oxidized by a cytochrome P450–containing enzyme into a highly reactive toxic metabolite: *N*-acetyl-*p*-benzoquinoneimine. At therapeutic doses, practically all of the drug is converted to nontoxic metabolites via the major pathway. Only a small fraction is converted into the toxic metabolite via the minor pathway. Furthermore, under normal conditions, the toxic metabolite undergoes rapid conversion to a nontoxic form; glutathione is required for the conversion. In the event of acetaminophen overdose, a larger-than-normal amount is processed via the minor pathway, and hence a large quantity of the toxic metabolite is produced. As the liver attempts to clear the metabolite, glutathione is rapidly depleted, and further detoxification stops. As a result, the toxic metabolite accumulates, causing damage to the liver (see later).

Adverse Effects

Adverse effects are extremely rare at therapeutic doses. Acetaminophen does not cause gastric ulceration or renal impairment and does not inhibit platelet aggregation. In addition, there is no evidence linking acetaminophen with Reye's syndrome. Individuals who are hypersensitive to aspirin only rarely experience cross-hypersensitivity with acetaminophen. Overdose can cause severe *liver injury* (see later).

Data from the Nurses' Health Study show an association between daily use of *acetaminophen* (500 mg or more/day) and the development of *hypertension.* Additional studies that examined a possible relationship between acetaminophen and hypertension in both men and women found conflicting results. Until more data become available, it would be prudent to monitor blood pressure in patients who take acetaminophen daily. The mechanism by which acetaminophen might raise blood pressure is unknown.

Studies have shown an association between acetaminophen and the development of *asthma.* However, as with hypertension, a causal relationship has not been established. In fact, regarding asthma, the association may well be the other way around. That is, people may be taking acetaminophen *because* they have respiratory symptoms, rather than having respiratory symptoms because they took acetaminophen. To prove that acetaminophen actually does cause asthma, stronger data are needed.

Rarely, patients experience *anaphylaxis,* a severe hypersensitivity reaction characterized by breathing difficulty associated with swelling of the face, mouth, and throat. If these symptoms develop, patients should seek immediate medical help.

Acetaminophen use has also been associated with Stevens-Johnson syndrome (SJS), acute generalized exanthematous pustulosis (AGEP), and toxic epidermal necrolysis (TEN). SJS and TEN are characterized by painful rash, blistering of the skin and mucous membranes, and detachment of the epidermis. These are considered medical emergencies, as they can result in death. Recovery can take weeks to months. AGEP is characterized by pustular lesions that predominantly affect the upper trunk and body folds. AGEP usually resolves within 2 weeks of onset. These reactions can occur at any time, even if the patient has taken acetaminophen previously. If a rash appears while taking acetaminophen, the drug should be stopped and the patient should seek medical attention.

Drug and Vaccine Interactions

Alcohol. Regular alcohol consumption increases the risk of liver injury from acetaminophen—but only if acetaminophen dosage is excessive. Three mechanisms are involved. First, alcohol induces synthesis of the P450-containing enzyme in the minor metabolic pathway, thereby increasing production of acetaminophen's toxic metabolite (see Fig. 71.1). Second, stores of glutathione are depleted in chronic alcoholics. As a result, the liver is unable to convert the toxic metabolite to a nontoxic form. Third, chronic alcohol abusers often have pre-existing liver damage, which renders them less able to tolerate injury from acetaminophen.

Does alcohol increase the risk of liver damage from acetaminophen taken in *therapeutic* doses? Probably not. Although *anecdotal* reports suggest that low-dose acetaminophen can cause liver injury in alcohol users, the results of a randomized controlled trial indicate otherwise: In alcoholics given therapeutic doses of acetaminophen, indices of liver damage were no greater than in alcoholics given a placebo. These data suggest that, even for people who consume alcohol in large amounts, *low* (therapeutic) doses of acetaminophen are safe. Nonetheless, some authorities recommend that if you drink alcohol on a regular basis, you should consume no more than 2000 mg of acetaminophen a day (one-half the normal maximum).

Although therapeutic doses of acetaminophen may be safe for alcohol drinkers, *high* doses certainly are not. Accordingly, to alert the public to the potential risk of combining alcohol with acetaminophen, the FDA requires that acetaminophen labels bear the following statement: ***Alcohol Warning:*** *If you consume three or more alcoholic drinks every day, ask your doctor whether you should take acetaminophen or other pain relievers/fever reducers.*

Warfarin. There is evidence that acetaminophen may increase the risk of bleeding in patients taking warfarin (an oral anticoagulant). This is surprising because, unlike NSAIDs, acetaminophen does not suppress platelet aggregation and so should not promote bleeding. How, then, might acetaminophen cause a problem? The best guess is that acetaminophen may inhibit warfarin metabolism, which would cause warfarin levels to rise. Although this interaction has not been proved, caution is advised. Accordingly, for patients taking more than 1 gm of acetaminophen daily for several days, responses to warfarin should be monitored closely. Occasional use of acetaminophen is not a concern.

Vaccines. Acetaminophen and other analgesic-antipyretics can blunt the immune response to childhood vaccines. Accordingly, routine use of these drugs to prevent vaccination-associated pain and/or fever should be discouraged.

Therapeutic Uses

Acetaminophen is indicated for relief of pain and fever. Because acetaminophen is not associated with Reye's syndrome, the drug is preferred to NSAIDs for use by children suspected of having chickenpox or influenza. Because it does not cause GI injury, acetaminophen is preferred to NSAIDs for patients with peptic ulcer disease. In addition, acetaminophen may be a safe alternative to aspirin for patients who have experienced aspirin hypersensitivity reactions. Because of its weak anti-inflammatory actions, acetaminophen is *not* useful for treating arthritis or rheumatic fever.

Acute Toxicity: Liver Damage

Overdose with acetaminophen can cause severe liver injury and death. The cause is accumulation of the toxic metabolite (discussed earlier). In the United States, acetaminophen overdose—intentional or unintentional—is the leading cause of acute liver failure, accounting for about 50% of all cases. Risk of liver injury is increased by fasting, chronic alcohol use, and by taking more than 4000 mg of acetaminophen a day.

Signs and Symptoms. The principal feature of acetaminophen overdose is *hepatic necrosis.* Severe poisoning can progress to hepatic failure, coma, and death. Early symptoms of poisoning (nausea, vomiting, diarrhea, sweating, abdominal discomfort) belie the severity of intoxication. It is not until 48 to 72 hours after drug ingestion that overt indications of hepatic injury appear.

Treatment. Liver damage can be minimized by giving *acetylcysteine* [Mucomyst ♣, Acetadote], a specific antidote to acetaminophen. Acetylcysteine reduces injury by substituting for depleted glutathione in the reaction that converts the toxic metabolite of acetaminophen to its nontoxic form. When given within 8 to 10 hours of acetaminophen overdose, acetylcysteine is 100% effective at preventing severe liver injury. And even when administered as much as 24 hours after poisoning, it can still provide significant protection. Acetylcysteine may be administered PO or IV.

For oral therapy, acetylcysteine is supplied in solution (100 and 200 mg/mL), and should be diluted to 50 mg/mL with water, fruit juice, or a cola beverage. Conventional treatment consists of a loading dose (140 mg/kg) followed by 17 more doses (70 mg/kg) given every 4 hours for 72 hours. However, for most patients, treatment can be stopped after just 20 hours. Oral acetylcysteine has an extremely unpleasant odor and may induce vomiting. If the patient is unable to tolerate oral dosing, acetylcysteine can be administered IV or through a nasogastric tube.

For IV therapy, acetylcysteine is supplied in solution (200 mg/mL), sold as *Acetadote,* and should be diluted in 5% dextrose. Three doses are given in sequence. The first dose—150 mg/kg (in 200 mL of 5% dextrose)—is infused over 15 minutes to 1 hour. The second dose—50 mg/kg (in 500 mL of 5% dextrose)—is infused over 4 hours. And the third dose—100 mg/kg (in 1000 mL of 5% dextrose)—is infused over 16 hours. Rarely, IV acetylcysteine causes allergic reactions (rash, itching, angioedema, bronchospasm, hypotension), most often in response to the first dose. Fortunately, these reactions tend to be mild and self-limiting and can be minimized by infusing the initial dose slowly (over a 1-hour interval).

Minimizing Risk. Risk of liver failure is very low with normal therapeutic doses (up to 4000 mg/day), except in people who drink alcohol, are undernourished, or have liver disease. Patient education can help reduce injury. Accordingly, you should:

- Inform patients about the risk of liver toxicity.
- Advise patients to consume no more than 4000 mg of acetaminophen a day, including the amount in combination prescription products (e.g., Vicodin, Percocet) as well as over-the-counter (OTC) products.
- Advise patients who are undernourished (e.g., owing to fasting or illness) to consume no more than 3000 mg of acetaminophen a day. Undernourished people are at risk because they have low stores of glutathione, the cofactor needed to convert the toxic metabolite of acetaminophen to a nontoxic form.
- Advise patients not to drink alcohol while taking acetaminophen.
- Advise patients who won't stop drinking alcohol (more than 3 drinks a day) to take no more than 2000 mg of acetaminophen a day.
- Advise patients with liver disease to ask their prescribers whether acetaminophen is safe.

To help reduce overdosage, McNeil Consumer Healthcare, maker of the *Tylenol* brand of acetaminophen, changed the dosing recommendations on Tylenol labels. On the new labels, issued in 2011, the maximum daily dose of *Extra-Strength Tylenol* (500 mg/tablet) is stated as 3000 mg (6 tablets), and the maximum daily dose of *Regular Strength Tylenol* (325 mg/tablet) is stated as 3250 mg (10 tablets). Other manufacturers are expected to make similar changes. Please note, however, that the maximum daily dose recommended by the FDA is still 4000 mg, even though these product labels recommend a lower dose.

The FDA is also trying to help: In 2011, they requested that prescription combination analgesics (e.g., Vicodin, Percocet, Lortab) contain no more than 325 mg of acetaminophen per tablet or capsule, because some prescription combinations contained acetaminophen in high doses. Vicodin ES, for example, contained 750 mg of acetaminophen, and Percocet brand products contained up to 650 mg of acetaminophen. Patients who take OTC acetaminophen along with one of these combination analgesics can easily exceed the safe daily limit. In fact, patients who take just a prescription combination product by itself can easily exceed 4000 mg of acetaminophen a day. You should note that the new limit applies only to prescription combination products. It does not apply to OTC combination products. The high-dose products were phased out in early 2014. Now Vicodin ES contains only 300 mg of acetaminophen.

Preparations, Dosage, and Administration

Preparations. Numerous acetaminophen-containing products are on the market, including a wide assortment of fixed-dose combinations. The drug is available in rectal suppositories, solution for IV dosing, and multiple oral formulations (standard tablets, chewable tablets, effervescent granules, capsules, liquids, elixirs, and solutions). Many products are available over the counter, and many others require a prescription. Furthermore, product strengths vary widely. All these products are mentioned here because they create a significant risk of overdose—either from taking two or more products that both contain acetaminophen or from taking too much of a single-ingredient product (owing to failure to carefully read the label). You should alert patients to these dangers.

Dosage and Administration

Oral. The recommended oral dosage for adults and children over 12 years is 325 to 650 mg every 4 to 6 hours, up to a maximum of 4000 mg/day. Dosages for younger children are based either on body weight—10 to 15 mg/kg/dose—or on age as follows:

- Up to 3 months—40 mg every 4 hours
- 4 to 11 months—80 mg every 4 hours
- 12 to 23 months—120 mg every 4 hours
- 2 to 3 years—160 mg every 4 hours
- 4 to 5 years—240 mg every 4 hours
- 6 to 8 years—320 mg every 4 to 6 hours
- 9 to 10 years—400 mg every 4 to 6 hours
- 11 years—480 mg every 4 to 6 hours
- 12 years—640 mg every 4 to 6 hours

Rectal. Acetaminophen suppositories [FeverAll, Acephen] are available in four strengths: 80, 120, 325, and 650 mg. The recommended dosage for adults and children over 12 years is 650 mg every 4 to 6 hours, up to a maximum of 3900 mg/day. Dosages for younger children vary with age as follows:

- 3 to 11 months—80 mg every 6 hours
- 12 to 36 months—80 mg every 4 hours
- 3 to 6 years—120 mg every 4 to 6 hours
- 6 to 12 years—325 mg every 4 to 6 hours

Intravenous. Intravenous acetaminophen [Ofirmev] is indicated for fever and mild to moderate pain (when used alone), and for moderate to severe pain (when combined with an opioid). Dosages are as follows:

- Adults and children 13 years and older who weigh more than 50 kg—1000 mg every 6 hours or 650 mg every 4 hours as needed. Daily maximum is 4000 mg.
- Children 2 to 12 years old and children 13 years and older who weigh less than 50 kg—15 mg/kg every 6 hours or 12.5 mg/kg every 4 hours as needed. Daily maximum is 75 mg/kg.

AHA STATEMENT ON THE USE OF COX INHIBITORS FOR CHRONIC PAIN

Because most COX inhibitors—and especially COX-2 inhibitors—increase the risk of MI and stroke, the American Heart Association (AHA) recommends a stepped-care approach to their use, as discussed in an article titled *Use of Nonsteroidal Anti-inflammatory Drugs: An Update for Clinicians: A Scientific Statement from the American Heart Association.* Recommendations in the article apply specifically to managing musculoskeletal pain in patients with or at high risk of cardiovascular disease. However, the recommendations may also apply to patients who lack documented cardiovascular risk. The approach has four basic steps:

Step 1. Begin with nondrug measures. Options include physical therapy, exercise, weight loss, orthotics, and application of heat or cold.

Step 2. If nondrug measures don't work, initiate drug therapy using *acetaminophen* or *aspirin,* which do not increase cardiovascular risk. If these drugs can't control pain, an opioid or tramadol can be tried, but only short term.

Step 3. If step 2 drugs are ineffective or intolerable, try other nonselective NSAIDs, such as naproxen, ibuprofen, or a nonacetylated salicylate (e.g., magnesium salicylate).

Step 4. As a *last resort,* try the selective COX-2 inhibitor celecoxib. Of all the NSAIDs, COX-2 inhibitors pose the greatest risk of cardiovascular harm, and hence celecoxib is a last-choice drug for chronic pain.

Whenever these drugs are employed, patients should use the lowest effective dosage for the shortest time required. During steps 2, 3, and 4, if the patient is considered at high risk of a thrombotic event, low-dose aspirin (81 mg/day) plus a PPI or H_2RA should be *added* to the regimen (except, of course, if high-dose aspirin is already in use).

KEY POINTS

- All of the drugs discussed in this chapter inhibit cyclooxygenase (COX), an enzyme that converts arachidonic acid into prostanoids (prostaglandins and related compounds).
- Cyclooxygenase has two forms: COX-1 and COX-2.
- The cyclooxygenase inhibitors fall into two major groups: nonsteroidal anti-inflammatory drugs (NSAIDs) and acetaminophen (in a group by itself).
- The NSAIDs can be subdivided into two groups: (1) first-generation NSAIDs, which inhibit COX-1 *and* COX-2, and (2) second-generation NSAIDs, which selectively inhibit COX-2.
- Inhibition of COX-1 can cause gastric ulceration, renal impairment, and bleeding.
- Inhibition of COX-2 suppresses inflammation, pain, and fever, but can also cause renal impairment.
- Aspirin is the prototype of the first-generation NSAIDs.
- Aspirin has four major beneficial actions: suppression of inflammation, relief of mild to moderate pain, reduction of fever, and prevention of MI and stroke (secondary to suppressing platelet aggregation). All of these benefits result from inhibiting COX-2, except for prevention of MI and stroke, which results from inhibiting COX-1 (in platelets).
- Because aspirin inhibits COX-1 as well as COX-2, it cannot cause beneficial effects without posing a risk of gastric ulceration, bleeding, and renal impairment.
- Aspirin causes *irreversible* inhibition of cyclooxygenase. As a result, the effects of aspirin persist until cells can make more cyclooxygenase.
- Because platelets are unable to synthesize new cyclooxygenase, the antiplatelet effects of a single dose of aspirin persist for the life of the platelet (about 8 days).
- Anti-inflammatory doses of aspirin are much higher than analgesic or antipyretic doses.
- Aspirin is a useful drug for rheumatoid arthritis and other chronic inflammatory conditions.
- Aspirin is a very effective analgesic. It can be as effective as opioids for some types of postoperative pain.
- The risk of aspirin-induced gastric ulcers can be reduced by (1) testing for and eliminating *H. pylori* before starting therapy and by (2) giving a proton pump inhibitor or $histamine_2$ receptor antagonist.
- Because of its antiplatelet actions, aspirin can protect against MI, stroke, and other thrombotic events.
- When taken for *primary prevention,* the benefits of aspirin must be weighed against the potential for harm. Ibuprofen, naproxen, and other nonaspirin NSAIDs can antagonize the antiplatelet actions of aspirin and can thereby decrease protection against MI and stroke. To minimize this interaction, patients should take aspirin about 2 hours before other NSAIDs.
- Because of its antiplatelet actions, *high-dose* aspirin should be discontinued 1 week before elective surgery or parturition. In most cases, *low-dose* aspirin taken to protect against thrombosis can be continued.
- Because of its antiplatelet actions, aspirin can increase the risk of bleeding in patients taking warfarin, heparin, and other anticoagulants.
- By impairing renal function, aspirin can cause sodium and water retention, edema, and elevation of blood pressure. However, adverse outcomes are likely only in patients with additional risk factors: advanced age, pre-existing renal dysfunction, hypovolemia, hypertension, hepatic cirrhosis, or heart failure. Long-term aspirin use may lead to renal papillary necrosis and other forms of renal injury.
- Because of the risk of Reye's syndrome, aspirin should be avoided by children with influenza or chickenpox.
- Use of aspirin during labor and delivery can suppress spontaneous uterine contractions, induce premature closure of the ductus arteriosus, and intensify uterine bleeding.
- Although rarely fatal in adults, aspirin poisoning may prove lethal in children.
- Aspirin can cause hypersensitivity reactions, especially in adults with asthma, rhinitis, and nasal polyps. Severe reactions (anaphylaxis) can be treated with epinephrine.
- All of the nonaspirin first-generation NSAIDs are much like aspirin itself. All of these drugs inhibit COX-1 and COX-2; they all can suppress inflammation, pain, and fever; and they all can cause gastric ulceration, renal impairment, and bleeding.
- The nonaspirin NSAIDs differ from aspirin in three important ways. First, nonaspirin NSAIDs cause *reversible* inhibition of COX, and hence their effects decline as soon as their blood levels decline. Second, although they can suppress platelet aggregation, these drugs are not used to prevent MI and stroke. Third, these drugs actually *increase* the risk of MI and stroke, and hence should be used in the lowest effective dosage for the shortest possible time.
- By inhibiting COX-2, the second-generation NSAIDs (coxibs) can suppress inflammation, pain, and fever.
- By sparing COX-1, the coxibs *may* cause less gastric ulceration than the first-generation NSAIDs.
- Coxibs do not inhibit platelet aggregation, and hence do not pose a risk of bleeding.
- Like all first-generation NSAIDs (except aspirin), coxibs pose a risk of MI and stroke.
- Currently, celecoxib [Celebrex] is the only coxib on the market.
- Acetaminophen reduces pain and fever, but not inflammation.
- Acetaminophen inhibits prostaglandin synthesis in the CNS, but not in the periphery. As a result, acetaminophen differs from the NSAIDs in four ways: it (1) lacks anti-inflammatory actions, (2) does not cause gastric ulceration, (3) does not suppress platelet aggregation, and (4) does not impair renal function.
- Hepatic necrosis from acetaminophen overdose results from the accumulation of a toxic metabolite. Risk is increased by undernourishment, alcohol consumption, and pre-existing liver disease.
- Chronic alcohol consumption increases the risk of liver damage from acetaminophen *overdose,* but probably not from therapeutic doses. Two major mechanisms are involved: induction of cytochrome P450 (which increases production of the toxic metabolite of acetaminophen) and

Continued

depletion of glutathione stores (which reduces detoxification of the metabolite).

- Acetaminophen may increase the risk of warfarin-induced bleeding by inhibiting the metabolism of warfarin.
- Acetaminophen is associated with SJS, AGEP, and TEN. If rash appears, this may be a medical emergency.
- Acetaminophen overdose is treated with PO or IV acetylcysteine, a drug that substitutes for depleted glutathione in the reaction that clears the toxic metabolite of acetaminophen.

Please visit **http://evolve.elsevier.com/Lehne** for chapter-specific NCLEX® examination review questions.

Summary of Major Nursing Implications[a]

NONSTEROIDAL ANTI-INFLAMMATORY DRUGS

First-Generation NSAIDs

Aspirin
Diclofenac
Diflunisal
Etodolac
Fenoprofen
Flurbiprofen
Ibuprofen
Indomethacin
Ketoprofen
Ketorolac
Magnesium salicylate
Meclofenamate
Mefenamic acid
Meloxicam
Nabumetone
Naproxen
Oxaprozin
Piroxicam
Salsalate
Sodium salicylate
Sulindac
Tolmetin

Second-Generation NSAIDs (Coxibs)

Celecoxib

Except where noted, the nursing implications described here apply to aspirin and all other NSAIDs.

Preadministration Assessment

Therapeutic Goal

Major indications for the NSAIDs are inflammatory disorders (e.g., rheumatoid arthritis, osteoarthritis), mild to moderate pain, fever, and primary dysmenorrhea. In addition, *aspirin* is used to prevent MI and stroke. Applications of individual NSAIDs are shown in Table 71.4.

Identifying High-Risk Patients

NSAIDs are *contraindicated* for patients with a history of severe NSAID hypersensitivity.

NSAIDs (especially aspirin) are *contraindicated* for children with chickenpox or influenza.

Celecoxib is contraindicated for patients with sulfa allergy.

NSAIDs should be used with *extreme caution* by pregnant women and patients with peptic ulcer disease and bleeding disorders (e.g., hemophilia, vitamin K deficiency, hypoprothrombinemia) and patients taking anticoagulants (e.g., warfarin, heparin), glucocorticoids, ACE inhibitors, or ARBs. *Caution* is also needed when treating older adult patients and patients with heart failure, angina pectoris, history of MI, hypertension, hypovolemia, hepatic cirrhosis, renal dysfunction, asthma, hay fever, chronic urticaria, nasal polyps, or a history of alcoholism or heavy smoking.

Implementation: Administration

Routes

Oral. All NSAIDs.
Topical. Diclofenac (patch, solution, and gel).
Intranasal. Ketorolac.
Intramuscular. Ketorolac.
Intravenous. Ibuprofen, ketorolac.
Rectal Suppository. Aspirin, indomethacin.

Administration

- **Advise patients to take oral NSAIDs with food, milk, or a glass of water to reduce gastric upset.**
- **Warn patients not to crush or chew enteric-coated or sustained-release formulations.**
- **Advise patients to discard aspirin preparations that smell like vinegar.**
- **Advise patients using topical diclofenac to apply the gel 4 times a day or to apply a new patch twice a day.**

Ongoing Evaluation and Interventions

Minimizing Adverse Effects

Gastrointestinal Effects. NSAIDs frequently cause mild GI reactions (dyspepsia, abdominal pain, nausea). **To minimize GI effects, advise patients to take NSAIDs with food, milk, or water.** *Long-term* therapy, even at moderate doses, can cause gastric ulceration, perforation, and hemorrhage. Several measures can reduce risk:

- Avoid NSAIDs in patients with a recent history of peptic ulcer disease, and use NSAIDs with caution in patients with other risk factors (advanced age, previous intolerance to NSAIDs, heavy cigarette smoking, history of alcoholism).
- Test for and eliminate *H. pylori* before starting long-term therapy.

Summary of Major Nursing Implications[a]—cont'd

- Give a proton pump inhibitor (PPI) or histamine$_2$ receptor antagonist (H_2RA) for prophylaxis in high-risk patients.
- Use celecoxib instead of a traditional NSAID in high-risk patients.
- **Warn patients not to consume alcohol.**
- **Instruct patients to notify the prescriber if gastric irritation is severe or persistent.**

Manage ulcers by giving an antiulcer medication (e.g., H_2RA, PPI).

Bleeding. *Aspirin* promotes bleeding by causing irreversible suppression of platelet aggregation. *High-dose* aspirin should be discontinued 7 to 10 days before elective surgery or anticipated date of parturition, but need not be stopped before minor dental, dermatologic, or cataract surgeries. Discontinuation of *low-dose aspirin* depends on circumstances. Specifically, low-dose aspirin should be *discontinued* in:

- Patients considered at low risk of a cardiovascular event who require noncardiac surgery. Dosing should stop 7 to 10 days before surgery and can resume 24 hours after the procedure.
- Patients undergoing intracranial surgery.

Conversely, low-dose aspirin should be *continued* in:

- Patients undergoing coronary artery bypass surgery (CABG).
- Patients facing surgery within 6 weeks of receiving a bare-metal coronary stent or within 12 months of receiving a drug-eluting coronary stent.
- Patients considered at high risk of a cardiovascular event who require noncardiac surgery or a percutaneous coronary intervention.
- Patients undergoing cataract surgery, minor dental procedures, or minor dermatologic procedures.

Exercise caution when using aspirin in conjunction with warfarin, heparin, and other anticoagulants. Avoid aspirin in patients with bleeding disorders (e.g., hemophilia, vitamin K deficiency, hypoprothrombinemia).

Discontinue *ibuprofen and other nonaspirin NSAIDs* five half-lives before elective surgery and childbirth.

The *nonacetylated salicylates*—sodium salicylate, magnesium salicylate, and salsalate—have minimal effects on platelet aggregation. Accordingly, these drugs are preferred for use in surgical patients and patients with bleeding disorders.

The risk of bleeding can be minimized by using celecoxib instead of a traditional NSAID.

Renal Impairment. NSAIDs can cause acute renal insufficiency in older adult patients and in patients with heart failure, hypovolemia, hepatic cirrhosis, or pre-existing renal dysfunction. Keep NSAID dosages as low as possible in these patients. Monitor high-risk patients for indications of renal impairment (reduced urine output, weight gain despite diuretic therapy, rapid elevation of serum creatinine and blood urea nitrogen). Discontinue NSAIDs if these signs occur.

Prolonged NSAID therapy can cause renal papillary necrosis. Avoid prolonged NSAID use whenever possible.

Myocardial Infarction and Stroke. Nonaspirin NSAIDs—but not aspirin itself—increase the risk of MI and stroke. To minimize cardiovascular risk, nonaspirin NSAIDs should be used in the lowest effective dosage for the shortest time needed, and they should not be used before CABG surgery or for 14 days after. In patients with cardiovascular risk factors, use all NSAIDs (except aspirin) with caution, and use celecoxib only as a last resort.

Hypersensitivity Reactions. Hypersensitivity reactions are most likely in adults with a history of asthma, rhinitis, and nasal polyps. Use NSAIDs with caution in these patients. If a severe hypersensitivity reaction occurs, parenteral epinephrine is the treatment of choice. As a rule, avoid NSAIDs in patients with a history of NSAID hypersensitivity. However, if an NSAID-like drug *must* be used, four are probably safe: celecoxib, salsalate, meloxicam (in low doses), and acetaminophen.

Salicylism. Aspirin and other salicylates can cause salicylism. **Educate patients about manifestations of salicylism (tinnitus, sweating, headache, dizziness), and advise them to notify the prescriber if these occur.** Aspirin should be withheld until symptoms subside, after which therapy can resume but at a slightly reduced dosage.

Reye's Syndrome. Use of NSAIDs, especially aspirin, by children with chickenpox or influenza may precipitate Reye's syndrome. **Advise parents to avoid aspirin in these children and to use acetaminophen instead.**

Use in Pregnancy. NSAIDs can cause maternal anemia and can prolong labor. In addition, they can promote premature closure of the ductus arteriosus. NSAIDs should be avoided by expectant mothers unless the potential benefits outweigh the risks. If NSAIDs are employed during pregnancy, they should be discontinued at least five half-lives before the anticipated day of delivery.

Liver Injury. *Diclofenac* can cause severe liver injury. Patients should receive periodic liver function tests. **Inform patients about signs of liver damage (e.g., jaundice, fatigue, nausea), and instruct them to report these immediately.** If liver injury is diagnosed, diclofenac should be discontinued.

Sulfonamide Allergy. *Celecoxib* can cause severe allergic reactions in patients with sulfa allergy, and hence must not be given to these people.

Minimizing Adverse Interactions

Anticoagulants. NSAIDs can increase the risk of bleeding in patients taking warfarin, heparin, and other anticoagulants. Monitor patients for signs of bleeding.

Glucocorticoids. Glucocorticoids increase the risk of gastric ulceration in patients taking NSAIDs. Prophylactic therapy with a PPI or H_2RA can decrease the risk.

Alcohol. Alcohol increases the risk of gastric ulceration from NSAIDs. Exercise caution.

Aspirin-NSAID Interactions. Ibuprofen, naproxen, and other nonaspirin NSAIDs can antagonize the antiplatelet actions of aspirin and can thereby decrease protection against MI and stroke. **Advise patients to take aspirin about 2 hours *before* taking another NSAID.**

Continued

Summary of Major Nursing Implications[a]—cont'd

ACE Inhibitors and ARBs. These drugs increase the risk of acute renal failure in patients taking NSAIDs. If possible, avoid all NSAIDs—except low-dose aspirin—in patients taking ACE inhibitors or ARBs.

Vaccines. NSAIDs may blunt the immune response to vaccines. **Advise parents to avoid routine use of NSAIDs to prevent vaccination-associated fever and pain.**

Managing Aspirin Toxicity

Aspirin poisoning is an acute medical emergency that requires hospitalization. Treatment is largely supportive and consists of external cooling (e.g., sponging with tepid water), infusion of fluids (to correct dehydration and electrolyte loss), infusion of bicarbonate (to reverse acidosis and promote renal excretion of salicylates), and mechanical ventilation (if respiration is severely depressed). Absorption of aspirin can be reduced by gastric lavage and by giving activated charcoal. If necessary, hemodialysis or peritoneal dialysis can accelerate salicylate removal.

ACETAMINOPHEN

Preadministration Assessment

Therapeutic Goal

Acetaminophen is indicated to relieve pain and to reduce fever. The drug is preferred to NSAIDs for use in children with chickenpox or influenza, and for all patients with peptic ulcer disease.

Identifying High-Risk Patients

Use with *caution* in chronic alcohol abusers, patients who consume moderate amounts of alcohol daily, and patients taking warfarin.

Implementation: Administration

Routes

Oral, rectal, intravenous.

Administration

Do not exceed recommended doses.

Ongoing Evaluation and Interventions

Minimizing Adverse Effects

Acetaminophen is largely devoid of significant adverse effects at usual therapeutic doses, except possibly in people who routinely consume alcohol. Overdose can cause liver damage (discussed later).

Hypertension. Taking at least 500 mg of acetaminophen per day is associated with an increased risk of hypertension, although studies have demonstrated conflicting data. Nonetheless, prudence dictates the monitoring of blood pressure in patients who take acetaminophen each day.

Asthma. Acetaminophen is associated with an increased risk of asthma, although a causal relationship has not been established.

Anaphylaxis. Rarely, acetaminophen causes anaphylaxis. **Inform patients about symptoms—breathing difficulty associated with swelling of the face, mouth, and throat—and advise them to seek immediate medical help if these develop.**

Skin Reactions. Acetaminophen has been associated with SJS, AGEP, and TEN. If rash develops, the patient should stop the medication and seek medical attention.

Liver Damage. Overdose can cause hepatic necrosis. Risk is increased by consuming high doses (more than 4000 mg/day), as well as by undernourishment, alcohol consumption, and pre-existing liver disease. To reduce risk:

- **Inform patients about the risk of liver injury.**
- **Advise patients to consume no more than 4000 mg of acetaminophen a day, including the amount in combination prescription products (e.g., Vicodin, Percocet) as well as OTC products.**
- **Advise patients who are undernourished (e.g., owing to fasting or illness) to consume no more than 3000 mg of acetaminophen a day.**
- **Advise patients not to drink alcohol while taking acetaminophen.**
- **Advise patients who won't stop drinking alcohol (more than 3 drinks a day) to take no more than 2000 mg of acetaminophen a day.**
- **Advise patients with liver disease to ask their prescribers whether acetaminophen is safe.**

Acetylcysteine—given PO or IV—is a specific antidote to acetaminophen overdose. Oral acetylcysteine has an extremely unpleasant odor and may induce vomiting. If vomiting interferes with oral dosing, there are two options: give acetylcysteine IV or through an oroduodenal tube.

Minimizing Adverse Interactions

Alcohol. Chronic alcohol consumption increases the risk of liver injury from *excessive* doses of acetaminophen, but probably not from *therapeutic* doses. **Nonetheless, advise patients who consume 3 or more drinks a day that, to be safe, they should consume no more than 2000 mg of acetaminophen a day (one-half the normal daily maximum).**

Warfarin. Taking acetaminophen for several days may increase the risk of bleeding in patients on warfarin. Monitor warfarin effects closely.

Vaccines. Acetaminophen may blunt the immune response to vaccines. **Advise parents to avoid routine use of acetaminophen to prevent vaccination-associated fever and pain.**

[a]Patient education information is highlighted as **blue text.**

CHAPTER

72 Glucocorticoids in Nonendocrine Disorders

In the body, the adrenal cortex produces corticosteroids. These include mineralocorticoids, which modulate salt and water balance, and glucocorticoids, which influence carbohydrate metabolism and other processes. The amount of glucocorticoids manufactured by the body is relatively low compared with that of many glucocorticoid drugs.

The glucocorticoid drugs (e.g., cortisone, prednisone) are nearly identical to the glucose-regulating steroids produced by the adrenal cortex. Accordingly, we can look at the glucocorticoids as having two kinds of effects: physiologic and pharmacologic. *Physiologic* effects, such as modulation of glucose metabolism, are elicited by *low* doses of glucocorticoids. In low (physiologic) doses, glucocorticoids are used to treat adrenocortical insufficiency. In contrast, *pharmacologic* effects (e.g., suppression of inflammation) require *high* doses. In high (pharmacologic) doses, glucocorticoids are used to treat inflammatory disorders (e.g., asthma, rheumatoid arthritis) and certain cancers. High doses are also used to suppress immune responses in organ transplant recipients. Glucocorticoids are devoid of toxicity when used in physiologic doses. However, when taken in pharmacologic doses, especially for extended periods, glucocorticoids can cause an array of serious adverse effects.

All of the glucocorticoid drugs can produce the same spectrum of therapeutic effects. Differences among individual agents pertain to time course and side effects. Because the similarities among these drugs are much more striking than the differences, we will not focus on a prototypic agent. Instead, we will discuss the glucocorticoids as a group. The endocrine applications of the glucocorticoids are discussed in Chapter 60. Nonendocrine uses are discussed here.

REVIEW OF GLUCOCORTICOID PHYSIOLOGY

Physiologic Effects

Physiologic responses can be elicited with low doses of glucocorticoids. At higher doses, these effects are simply more intense. When glucocorticoids are used to treat nonendocrine disorders, physiologic responses occur as side effects. Physiologic effects are discussed in Chapter 60, so the discussion here is brief.

Metabolic Effects

Glucocorticoids influence the metabolism of carbohydrates, proteins, and fats. The principal effect on carbohydrate metabolism is the elevation of blood glucose. Glucocorticoids do this by promoting synthesis of glucose from amino acids, reducing peripheral glucose utilization, and reducing glucose uptake by muscle and adipose tissue. Glucocorticoids also promote the storage of glucose in the form of glycogen.

Glucocorticoids have a negative effect on protein metabolism. Specifically, these drugs suppress synthesis of proteins from amino acids and divert amino acids for production of glucose. These actions can reduce muscle mass, decrease the protein matrix of bone, and cause thinning of the skin. Nitrogen balance becomes negative.

The most consistent effect of glucocorticoids on fat metabolism is the stimulation of lipolysis (fat breakdown). Long-term, high-dose therapy can cause fat redistribution, resulting in the central obesity (potbelly), rounded face ("moon face"), and fat pad at the cervical spine ("buffalo hump") that characterize Cushing's syndrome.

Cardiovascular Effects

Glucocorticoids are required to maintain the functional integrity of the vascular system. When levels of endogenous glucocorticoids are low, capillaries become more permeable, vasoconstriction is suppressed, and blood pressure falls. Glucocorticoids *increase* the number of circulating red blood cells and polymorphonuclear leukocytes, and *decrease* counts of lymphocytes, eosinophils, basophils, and monocytes.

Effects During Stress

At times of physiologic stress (e.g., surgery, infection, trauma, hypovolemia), the adrenal glands secrete large quantities of glucocorticoids and epinephrine. Working together, these hormones help maintain blood pressure and blood glucose levels. If glucocorticoid release is insufficient, hypotension and hypoglycemia will occur. If the stress is especially severe, glucocorticoid insufficiency can result in circulatory failure and death.

Effects on Water and Electrolytes

To varying degrees, individual glucocorticoids can exert actions similar to aldosterone, the major mineralocorticoid released by the adrenal glands. Accordingly, glucocorticoids can act on the kidney to promote the retention of sodium and water while increasing urinary excretion of potassium. The net results are hypernatremia, hypokalemia, and edema. Fortunately, most

TABLE 72.1 ■ Systemic Glucocorticoids: Half-Lives, Relative Potencies, and Equivalent Doses

Drug	Biologic Half-Life (hr)	Relative Mineralocorticoid Potency[a]	Relative Glucocorticoid (Anti-Inflammatory) Potency[b]	Equivalent Anti-Inflammatory Dose (mg)[c]
SHORT ACTING				
Cortisone	8–12	2	0.8	25
Hydrocortisone	8–12	2	1	20
INTERMEDIATE ACTING				
Prednisolone	18–36	1	4	5
Prednisone	18–36	1	4	5
Methylprednisolone	18–36	0	5	4
Triamcinolone	18–36	0	5	4
LONG ACTING				
Betamethasone	36–54	0	20–30	0.75
Dexamethasone	36–54	0	20–30	0.75

[a]Relative mineralocorticoid activity (sodium and water retention; potassium depletion): 0, very low; 1, moderate; 2, high.
[b]Glucocorticoid potency values are relative to the potency of hydrocortisone.
[c]Approximate *oral* or *intravenous* dose needed to produce equivalent anti-inflammatory effects.

of the glucocorticoids employed as drugs have very low mineralocorticoid activity (Table 72.1).

Respiratory System Effects in Neonates

During labor and delivery, the adrenal glands of the full-term infant release a burst of glucocorticoids, which act to hasten maturation of the lungs. In the preterm infant, production of glucocorticoids is low, resulting in a high incidence of respiratory distress syndrome.

Control of Synthesis and Secretion

Synthesis and release of glucocorticoids are regulated by a negative feedback loop. The principal components of the loop are the hypothalamus, anterior pituitary, and adrenal cortex (Fig. 72.1). The loop is turned on when stress or some other stimulus from the central nervous system acts on the hypothalamus to cause the release of corticotropin-releasing hormone (CRH). CRH then stimulates the pituitary to release adrenocorticotropic hormone (ACTH), which in turn acts on the adrenal cortex to promote synthesis and release of cortisol (the principal endogenous glucocorticoid). Cortisol has two basic effects: first, it stimulates physiologic responses; second, it acts on the hypothalamus and pituitary to suppress further release of CRH and ACTH. By inhibiting release of CRH and ACTH, cortisol suppresses its own production. As a result, this negative feedback loop keeps glucocorticoid levels within an appropriate range. When glucocorticoids are administered chronically in large doses, the feedback loop remains continuously suppressed. As discussed later, persistent suppression can be dangerous.

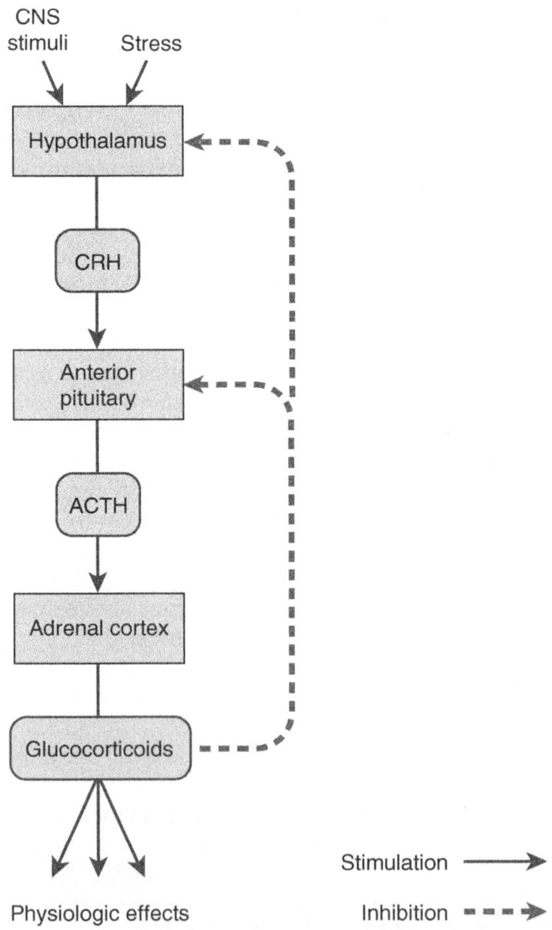

Fig. 72.1 ■ Feedback regulation of glucocorticoid synthesis and secretion.
(*ACTH*, Adrenocorticotropic hormone; *CNS*, central nervous system; *CRH*, corticotropin-releasing hormone.)

PHARMACOLOGY OF THE GLUCOCORTICOIDS

Molecular Mechanism of Action

Mechanistically, glucocorticoids differ from most drugs in two ways: (1) Glucocorticoid receptors are located *inside* the cell, rather than on the cell surface; and (2) glucocorticoids modulate the production of regulatory proteins, rather than the activity of signaling pathways.

Here's how they do it. First, glucocorticoids penetrate the cell membrane and then bind with receptors in the *cytoplasm,* thereby converting the receptor from an inactive form to an active form. Next, the receptor-steroid complex migrates to the cell *nucleus,* where it binds to chromatin in DNA, thereby altering the activity of target genes. In most cases, activity of the target gene is increased, causing increased transcription of messenger RNA molecules that code for specific regulatory proteins. However, in some cases, activity of the target gene is suppressed, and hence synthesis of certain regulatory proteins declines.

Pharmacologic Effects

When administered in the high doses employed to treat nonendocrine disorders, glucocorticoids produce anti-inflammatory and immunosuppressive effects—effects not seen at physiologic doses. Of course, these high doses also produce the physiologic effects seen at low doses.

Effects on Metabolism and Electrolytes. The effects of high-dose therapy on metabolism and electrolytes are like those seen with physiologic doses—but are more intense. With high doses, glucose levels rise, protein synthesis is suppressed, and fat deposits are mobilized. As noted, most glucocorticoids have very little mineralocorticoid activity. Accordingly, these drugs do not usually induce significant sodium retention or potassium loss. However, these effects do occur in some patients and can be hazardous. In all patients, high-dose therapy can inhibit intestinal absorption of calcium, an effect not seen at physiologic doses.

Anti-Inflammatory and Immunosuppressant Effects. The major clinical applications of the glucocorticoids stem from their ability to suppress immune responses and inflammation. Effects on the immune system and inflammation are interrelated, so we will consider them together.

Before discussing the actions of glucocorticoids, we need to review the process of inflammation. Characteristic symptoms of inflammation are pain, swelling, redness, and warmth. These are initiated by chemical mediators (prostaglandins, histamine, leukotrienes) and are amplified by the actions of lymphocytes and phagocytic cells (neutrophils and macrophages). Prostaglandins and histamine promote several symptoms of inflammation—swelling, redness, and warmth—by causing vasodilation and increasing capillary permeability. Prostaglandins and histamine contribute to pain. Histamine stimulates pain receptors directly; prostaglandins sensitize pain receptors to stimulation by histamine and other mediators. Neutrophils and macrophages heighten inflammation by releasing lysosomal enzymes, which cause tissue injury. Lymphocytes, which are important elements of the immune system, intensify inflammation by (1) causing direct cell injury and (2) promoting the formation of antibodies that help perpetuate the inflammatory response.

Glucocorticoids act through several mechanisms to interrupt the inflammatory processes. These drugs can inhibit synthesis of chemical mediators (prostaglandins, leukotrienes, histamine), reducing swelling, warmth, redness, and pain. In addition, they suppress infiltration of phagocytes, so damage from lysosomal enzymes is averted. Lastly, glucocorticoids suppress proliferation of lymphocytes and thereby reduce the immune component of inflammation.

It is important to appreciate that the mechanisms by which glucocorticoids suppress inflammation are more diverse than the mechanisms by which nonsteroidal anti-inflammatory drugs (NSAIDs) act. As discussed in Chapter 71, NSAIDs suppress inflammation primarily by inhibiting prostaglandin production. The glucocorticoids share this mechanism and act in other ways too. Because they act by multiple mechanisms, glucocorticoids produce greater anti-inflammatory effects than do NSAIDs.

Pharmacokinetics

Absorption. The rate of glucocorticoid absorption depends on the route of administration and the specific glucocorticoid. With oral administration, absorption of all glucocorticoids is rapid and nearly complete. After intramuscular (IM) injection, absorption is rapid with two types of glucocorticoid esters (sodium phosphates and sodium succinates) and relatively slow with other derivatives (e.g., acetates, acetonides). Absorption from local sites of injection (e.g., intra-articular, intralesional) is slower than from IM sites.

Duration of Action. Duration depends on dosage, route, and drug solubility. For glucocorticoids administered orally or intravenously (IV), duration is determined largely by biologic half-life (see Table 72.1). With IM administration, duration is a function of water solubility: Highly soluble preparations have a shorter duration than less soluble preparations. For locally administered glucocorticoids, duration is determined by solubility and by the specific site of administration.

Metabolism and Excretion. Glucocorticoids are metabolized primarily by the liver. As a rule, the resulting metabolites are inactive. Excretion of metabolites is renal.

Therapeutic Uses in Nonendocrine Disorders

As has been mentioned, high-dose therapy is required for the management of nonendocrine conditions. For some conditions, long-term therapy is required as well. Because prolonged high-dose therapy can produce serious adverse effects, the potential benefits of treatment must be weighed carefully against the very real risks.

Rheumatoid Arthritis. Glucocorticoids are indicated for adjunctive treatment of acute exacerbations of rheumatoid arthritis. These drugs can reduce inflammation and pain, but do not alter the course of the disease. Because of the risk for serious complications, prolonged systemic use should be avoided when possible.

When arthritis is limited to just a few joints, intra-articular injections may be advantageous. Local injections can be highly effective and cause less toxicity than systemic therapy. Frequently, reductions in pain and inflammation can be so dramatic as to prompt vigorous use of joints that were previously immobile. Because excessive use of diseased joints can cause injury, patients should be warned against overactivity, even though symptoms have eased.

The use of glucocorticoids in rheumatoid arthritis is discussed further in Chapter 73.

Systemic Lupus Erythematosus. Systemic lupus erythematosus (SLE) is a chronic disease similar in many ways to rheumatoid arthritis. However, in SLE, inflammation is not limited to joints. Rather, it occurs throughout the body. Symptoms frequently include pleuritis, pericarditis, and nephritis. A severe episode can be fatal. Fortunately, manifestations of SLE can usually be controlled with prompt and aggressive glucocorticoid therapy.

Inflammatory Bowel Disease. Glucocorticoids are used to treat severe cases of ulcerative colitis and Crohn's disease, the two most common forms of inflammatory bowel disease. Administration may be oral or intravenous. Glucocorticoid therapy of these disorders is considered further in Chapter 80.

Miscellaneous Inflammatory Disorders. Glucocorticoids are useful in a variety of inflammatory disorders in addition to those discussed previously. Conditions that respond include bursitis, tendinitis, synovitis, osteoarthritis, gouty arthritis, and inflammatory disorders of the eye.

Allergic Conditions. Glucocorticoids can control symptoms of allergic reactions. Responsive conditions include allergic rhinitis (see Chapter 77), bee stings, and drug-induced allergies. Because glucocorticoid responses are delayed, these drugs have little value as sole therapy for severe allergic reactions (e.g., anaphylaxis). For life-threatening allergic reactions, epinephrine is the treatment of choice.

Asthma. Glucocorticoids are the most effective antiasthma agents available. For the treatment of asthma, they may be administered orally or by inhalation. Adverse effects are minimal with inhaled glucocorticoids. In contrast, oral therapy can cause serious toxicity and hence should be reserved for patients who have failed to respond to safer treatments (e.g., inhaled glucocorticoids, inhaled cromolyn sodium). The use of glucocorticoids in asthma is discussed at length in Chapter 76.

Dermatologic Disorders. Glucocorticoids are beneficial in a wide variety of skin diseases, including pemphigus, psoriasis, mycosis fungoides, seborrheic dermatitis, contact dermatitis, and exfoliative dermatitis. For mild disease, topical administration is usually adequate. For severe disorders, systemic therapy may be needed. It should be noted that topical glucocorticoids can be absorbed in amounts sufficient to produce systemic toxicity. Topical therapy is discussed further in Chapter 105.

Neoplasms. Glucocorticoids are used in conjunction with other anticancer agents to treat acute lymphocytic leukemia, Hodgkin's disease, and non-Hodgkin's lymphoma. Benefits derive from the direct toxicity of glucocorticoids to malignant lymphocytes. Treatment kills lymphoid cells and causes regression of lymphatic tissue. The use of glucocorticoids to treat cancers is discussed further in Chapter 103.

Suppression of Allograft Rejection. Glucocorticoids, together with other immunosuppressant agents, are used to prevent the rejection of organ transplants. Glucocorticoids are initiated at the time of surgery and continued indefinitely. The use of glucocorticoids for immunosuppression is discussed further in Chapter 69.

Prevention of Respiratory Distress Syndrome in Preterm Infants. Preterm infants are at a high risk for respiratory distress syndrome because their adrenal glands cannot produce the glucocorticoids needed for lung maturation. When preterm delivery is imminent, injecting the mother with glucocorticoids (usually dexamethasone or betamethasone) reduces the risk for neonatal respiratory distress. Steroids may also reduce the incidence of intraventricular hemorrhage and necrotizing enterocolitis (inflammation of the small intestine and colon). Antenatal use of glucocorticoids is discussed further in Chapter 107.

Adverse Effects

The adverse effects discussed here occur in response to *pharmacologic* (as opposed to *physiologic*) doses of glucocorticoids. The intensity of these effects increases with dosage size and treatment duration. These effects are not seen when dosage is physiologic. Furthermore, most are not seen when treatment is brief (a few days or less), even when doses are high.

Adrenal Insufficiency. Prolonged administration of pharmacologic doses of glucocorticoids can suppress production of glucocorticoids by the adrenal glands, resulting in adrenal insufficiency. The mechanism, consequences, and management of adrenal insufficiency are discussed under *Adrenal Suppression.*

Osteoporosis

Development. Osteoporosis with resultant fractures is a frequent and serious complication of prolonged systemic glucocorticoid therapy. (Although osteoporosis is likely with prolonged systemic glucocorticoid therapy, it is uncommon when glucocorticoids are inhaled or administered topically.) The ribs and vertebrae are affected most. In some patients on high-dose glucocorticoids, vertebral compression fractures occur within weeks of beginning glucocorticoid use. Patients should be observed for signs of compression fractures (back and neck pain) and for indications of fractures in other bones.

How do glucocorticoids cause bone loss? The most important mechanism is the suppression of bone formation by osteoblasts. In addition, glucocorticoids accelerate bone resorption by osteoclasts. Also, these drugs reduce intestinal absorption of calcium, causing hypocalcemia. In response to hypocalcemia, the release of parathyroid hormone increases, which increases mobilization of calcium from bone.

Management. Several measures can greatly reduce the development of osteoporosis and subsequent fractures. Before glucocorticoid treatment, bone mineral density of the lumbar spine should be measured. This will identify patients at highest risk and provide a baseline for evaluating bone loss during treatment. When appropriate, glucocorticoids should be administered topically or by inhalation because bone loss is less with these routes than with systemic therapy.

Some drugs can help reduce bone loss. All patients should receive *calcium* and *vitamin D* supplements. Sodium restriction combined with a thiazide diuretic can enhance intestinal absorption of calcium and can decrease urinary excretion of calcium. There is solid evidence that a *bisphosphonate* can prevent glucocorticoid-induced bone loss by inhibiting bone resorption by osteoclasts. *Calcitonin* [Miacalcin], which also inhibits osteoclasts, is another option. For patients with significant bone loss, *teriparatide* [Forteo] may be preferred because, unlike bisphosphonates and calcitonin, which only prevent bone *resorption,* teriparatide actively promotes new bone *formation.* In postmenopausal women, *estrogen* therapy is an effective way to reduce bone loss. However, as discussed in Chapter 61, the risks of estrogen therapy generally outweigh the benefits. The roles of calcium, vitamin D, bisphosphonates, calcitonin, teriparatide, and estrogen in the prophylaxis and treatment of osteoporosis are discussed fully in Chapter 75.

Infection. By suppressing host defenses (immune responses and phagocytic activity of neutrophils and macrophages), glucocorticoids can increase susceptibility to infection. The risk for acquiring a new infection is increased, as is the risk for reactivating a latent infection (e.g., tuberculosis). In addition, because suppression of both the immune system and neutrophils reduces inflammation and other manifestations of infection, a fulminant infection may develop without detection. Hence, glucocorticoids not only increase susceptibility to infection, but also can mask the presence of an infection as it progresses. To minimize the risk for infection, patients should avoid close contact with people who have a communicable disease. If a significant infection occurs, glucocorticoids should be continued only if absolutely necessary and then only in combination with appropriate antimicrobial or antifungal therapy.

One infection—known as PCP (for *P*neumo*c*ystis *p*neumonia)—deserves special mention. The causative organism is *Pneumocystis jiroveci* (formerly called *Pneumocystis carinii*). PCP, commonly known as an opportunistic infection in people with AIDS, also occurs with alarming frequency in people receiving high doses of glucocorticoids. Accordingly, it has been suggested that PCP prophylaxis be considered for all people taking glucocorticoids long term in high doses.

Glucose Intolerance. Because of their effects on glucose production and utilization, glucocorticoids can increase plasma glucose levels, thereby causing hyperglycemia and glycosuria. Patients with diabetes may need to increase the dosage of hypoglycemic medication. For patients with normal pancreatic function, significant elevation of blood glucose is unlikely. However, because glucocorticoids can unmask latent diabetes, even patients without a diagnosis of diabetes should undergo periodic evaluation of blood glucose levels.

Myopathy. High-dose glucocorticoid therapy can cause myopathy (muscle injury), manifesting as weakness. The proximal muscles of the arms and legs are affected most. Damage to muscle may be sufficient to prevent ambulation. If myopathy develops, glucocorticoid dosage should be reduced. Myopathy then gradually resolves over several months.

Fluid and Electrolyte Disturbance. Because of their mineralocorticoid activity, glucocorticoids can cause sodium and water retention and potassium loss. Retention of water and sodium can cause hypertension and edema. Hypokalemia can predispose to dysrhythmias and toxicity from digitalis. Fortunately, most of the glucocorticoids in current use have minimal mineralocorticoid activity. Therefore, serious fluid and electrolyte disturbance is rare. The risk for fluid and electrolyte disturbance can be reduced by (1) using glucocorticoids that have low mineralocorticoid activity, (2) restricting sodium intake, and (3) taking potassium supplements or consuming potassium-rich foods (e.g., potatoes, bananas, citrus fruits). Patients should be informed about signs of fluid retention (e.g., weight gain, swelling of the lower extremities) and advised to contact the prescriber if these develop. Patients should also be alert for signs of hypokalemia (e.g., muscle weakness or fatigue, irregular pulse).

Growth Delay. Glucocorticoids can suppress growth in children. Growth delay is probably the result of reduced DNA synthesis and decreased cell division. To assess effects on growth, height and weight should be measured at regular intervals. Growth suppression can be minimized with alternate-day therapy. This dosing schedule is discussed later.

Psychologic Disturbances. Systemic glucocorticoids can cause psychologic disturbances. About 60% of patients experience a mild reaction: insomnia, anxiety, agitation, or irritability. An additional 6% experience a severe reaction: delirium, hallucinations, depression, euphoria, or mania. Of these, up to one-third may become suicidal. Of note, previous psychiatric illness does not seem to predispose patients to psychologic reactions—and a history of good mental health does not confer protection.

Psychologic reactions are related to the level of dose and the duration of treatment. Long-term low-dose therapy is more likely to cause depression. In contrast, short-term high-dose therapy is more likely to cause mania and other psychoses. Cognitive impairment (e.g., distractibility, memory loss) can occur with either dosing pattern.

Psychologic effects reverse when glucocorticoids are withdrawn. Delirium and hallucinations usually resolve quickly—within a few days to a week. Mood disturbances (depression, mania) resolve more slowly—over 6 weeks or longer.

Can we use drugs to manage symptoms? Yes. Drugs typically used to manage mood disorders and psychosis have demonstrated success in managing the adverse psychologic effects in many patients. Occasionally, though, psychologic effects are unresponsive to the usual drugs used to manage these conditions.

Cataracts and Glaucoma. Cataracts are a common complication of long-term glucocorticoid therapy. Risk factors are in dispute; cataract development may be related to age, dosage, or individual susceptibility. To facilitate early detection, patients should undergo an eye examination every 6 months. Also, patients should be advised to contact the prescriber if vision becomes cloudy or blurred.

Oral glucocorticoids can cause open-angle glaucoma. Onset of ocular hypertension develops rapidly and reverses within 2 weeks of glucocorticoid cessation.

Peptic Ulcer Disease. Glucocorticoids have actions that can lead to peptic ulcer disease. By inhibiting prostaglandin synthesis, glucocorticoids can augment secretion of gastric acid and pepsin, inhibit production of cytoprotective mucus, and reduce gastric mucosal blood flow. These actions predispose to gastrointestinal (GI) ulceration. Making matters worse, glucocorticoids can decrease gastric pain, thereby masking ulcer development. As a result, perforation and hemorrhage can occur without warning. The risk for ulceration is increased by concurrent use of other ulcerogenic drugs, such as aspirin and other NSAIDs. To provide early detection of ulcer formation, stools should be periodically checked for occult blood. Patients should be instructed to notify the prescriber if feces become black and tarry. If GI ulceration occurs, glucocorticoids should be slowly withdrawn (unless their continued use is considered essential to support life). Treatment with antiulcer medication is indicated.

Iatrogenic Cushing's Syndrome. Long-term glucocorticoid therapy can induce a cushingoid syndrome with symptoms identical to those of naturally occurring Cushing's syndrome. Prominent symptoms are hyperglycemia, glycosuria, fluid and electrolyte disturbances, osteoporosis, muscle weakness, cutaneous striations, and lowered resistance to infection. As mentioned earlier, redistribution of fat to the abdomen, face, and posterior neck produces the characteristic "potbelly," "moon face," and "buffalo hump."

Use in Pregnancy and Lactation

Pregnancy. Glucocorticoids can cross the placenta. This may result in multiple risks for the developing fetus. Of particular concern is the risk for fetal adrenal hypoplasia. Therefore, when large doses have been employed, the infant should be assessed for adrenal sufficiency and given replacement therapy if indicated. Whenever glucocorticoids are to be used during pregnancy, the benefits must be carefully weighed against the potential fetal risk.

Lactation. Glucocorticoids enter breast milk, placing the nursing infant at risk. When physiologic doses or low pharmacologic doses are used, the concentration achieved in milk is probably too low to affect the nursing infant. However, when large pharmacologic doses are employed, the amount ingested by the infant may be sufficient to cause growth delay and other adverse effects. Consequently, women receiving high-dose glucocorticoid therapy should be warned against breast-feeding.

PATIENT CENTERED CARE ACROSS THE LIFE SPAN

Glucocorticoids

Life Stage	Patient Care Concerns
Children	Long-term use of steroid medications can cause inhibition of bone growth.
Pregnant women	Prednisone is classified in U.S. Food and Drug Administration Pregnancy Risk Category C or D,[a] depending on the specific drug and formulation. Risk must be weighed against benefit.
Breast-feeding women	Systemic glucocorticoids may pose a risk to infants who are breast-fed. Caution is advised.
Older adults	Long-term use of glucocorticoids can cause osteoporosis, adrenal insufficiency, and GI ulceration. These problems may affect older adults disproportionately.

[a]As of 2020, the FDA will no longer use Pregnancy Risk Categories. Please refer to Chapter 9 for more information.

Drug Interactions

Interactions Related to Potassium Loss. As noted, glucocorticoids can increase urinary loss of potassium and can thereby induce hypokalemia. Consequently, glucocorticoids must be used with caution when combined with *digoxin* (because hypokalemia increases the risk for digoxin-induced dysrhythmias) and when combined with *thiazide* or *loop diuretics* (because these potassium-depleting diuretics will increase the risk for hypokalemia). When glucocorticoids are given together with any of the previously mentioned drugs, it is advisable to monitor plasma potassium levels and to be alert for signs and symptoms of digoxin toxicity and fluid and electrolyte imbalance.

Nonsteroidal Anti-Inflammatory Drugs. NSAIDs have the same effects on the GI tract as do glucocorticoids. Accordingly, concurrent use of these agents increases the risk for ulceration and GI bleeding.

Insulin and Oral Hypoglycemics. As noted, glucocorticoids promote hyperglycemia. To maintain glycemic control, patients with diabetes may require increased doses of a glucose-lowering drug (insulin or another hypoglycemic agent).

Vaccines. Because of their immunosuppressant actions, glucocorticoids can decrease antibody responses to vaccines. Accordingly, immunization should not be attempted for some vaccines while glucocorticoids are in use. Furthermore, if a live virus vaccine is employed, the immunosuppressant action of glucocorticoids increases the risk for developing viral disease.

Precautions and Contraindications

Contraindications. Glucocorticoids are contraindicated for patients with *systemic fungal infections* and for those receiving *live virus vaccines.*

Precautions. Glucocorticoids must be used with caution in *pediatric patients* and in *women who are pregnant or breast-feeding.* Caution is also required in patients with *hypertension, heart failure, renal impairment, esophagitis, gastritis, peptic ulcer disease, myasthenia gravis, diabetes mellitus, osteoporosis, open-angle glaucoma,* and *infections that are resistant to treatment.* In addition, caution is required during concurrent therapy with *potassium-depleting diuretics, digoxin, insulin, oral hypoglycemics,* and *NSAIDs.*

Adrenal Suppression

Development of Adrenal Suppression. Like cortisol and other endogenous glucocorticoids, the glucocorticoids that we administer as drugs suppress release of CRH from the hypothalamus and ACTH from the anterior pituitary. By doing so, exogenous glucocorticoids inhibit the synthesis and release of endogenous glucocorticoids by the adrenal glands. During long-term therapy, the pituitary loses much of its ability to manufacture ACTH; in response to the prolonged absence of ACTH, the adrenal glands atrophy and lose their ability to synthesize cortisol and other glucocorticoids. As a result, when prolonged glucocorticoid therapy is discontinued, there is a period during which the adrenal glands are unable to produce glucocorticoids. The time needed for adrenal recovery is highly variable. It may be as short as 5 days or as long as a year. The extent of adrenal suppression and the time required for recovery are determined primarily by the duration of glucocorticoid use; dosage size is less important. Development of adrenal suppression can be minimized through alternate-day dosing.

Adrenal Suppression and Physiologic Stress. Recall that when stress occurs, the adrenal glands normally secrete large amounts of glucocorticoids. If the stress is sufficiently severe (e.g., trauma, surgery), these glucocorticoids are essential for supporting life. Accordingly, because of adrenal suppression, *it is imperative that patients receiving long-term glucocorticoid therapy be given increased doses at times of stress* (unless the dosage is already very high). Furthermore, *after glucocorticoid use has ceased, supplemental doses are required whenever stress occurs until recovery of adrenal function is complete.* To ensure appropriate care in emergencies, patients should carry an identification card or bracelet to inform emergency personnel of their glucocorticoid needs. In addition, patients should always have an emergency supply of glucocorticoids on hand.

Glucocorticoid Withdrawal. To allow time for recovery of adrenal function, withdrawal of glucocorticoids should be done slowly. The withdrawal schedule is determined by the degree of adrenal suppression. A representative schedule is as follows: (1) taper the dosage to a physiologic range over 7 days; (2) switch from multiple daily doses to single doses administered each morning; (3) taper the dosage to 50% of physiologic values over the next month; and (4) monitor for production of endogenous cortisol, and when basal levels have returned to normal, cease routine glucocorticoid dosing (but be prepared to give supplemental doses at times of stress). As a rule, tapering is unnecessary when oral glucocorticoids have been used for less than 2 to 3 weeks.

In addition to unmasking adrenal insufficiency, stopping glucocorticoids may produce a withdrawal syndrome. Symptoms include hypotension, hypoglycemia, myalgia, arthralgia, and fatigue. In patients being treated for arthritis and certain other disorders, these symptoms may be confused with return of the underlying disease. Discomfort of withdrawal can be minimized by gradual dosage reduction and by concurrent treatment with NSAIDs.

Preparations and Routes of Administration

Preparations. The glucocorticoids employed clinically include hydrocortisone (cortisol) and synthetic derivatives of hydrocortisone. Individual glucocorticoids differ with respect to (1) biologic half-life, (2) mineralocorticoid potency, and (3) glucocorticoid (anti-inflammatory) potency (see Table 72.1).

The term *biologic half-life* refers to the time required for glucocorticoids to leave body tissues. In most cases, these drugs are cleared from tissues more slowly than from the blood. Hence, the biologic half-life is usually longer than the plasma half-life. When glucocorticoids are administered by mouth or by IV injection, it is the biologic half-life, and not the plasma half-life, that determines duration of action. Because of differences in their biologic half-lives, individual glucocorticoids can be classified as short acting, intermediate acting, or long acting.

Glucocorticoids with high *mineralocorticoid potency* (cortisone, hydrocortisone) can cause significant retention of sodium and water, coupled with depletion of potassium. These effects can be especially hazardous for patients with hypertension or heart failure and for those taking digoxin. Because of the potential dangers of sodium retention and potassium loss, glucocorticoids with high mineralocorticoid activity should not be administered systemically for long periods.

The differences in *glucocorticoid potency* are reflected in the doses required to produce anti-inflammatory effects—not mineralocorticoid effects. As with other drugs, potency is relatively unimportant. However, it is important to appreciate that in order to produce equivalent therapeutic effects, dosages for some glucocorticoids must be much larger than for others.

Routes of Administration. Glucocorticoids can be administered *orally, parenterally* (IV, IM, subcutaneous [subQ]), *topically,* and *intranasally* and by *local injection* (e.g., intra-articular, intralesional) or *inhalation.* Topical application is used for dermatologic disorders (see Chapter 105), inhalation therapy is used for asthma (see Chapter 76), and intranasal therapy is used for allergic rhinitis (see Chapter 77). Because local therapy (topical, intranasal, inhalation, local injection) minimizes systemic toxicity, this form of treatment is preferred to systemic therapy (oral, parenteral). When systemic effects are needed, oral administration is preferred to parenteral. It is important to note that even when glucocorticoids are administered for local effects, absorption can be sufficient to produce systemic effects. That is, local administration does not eliminate toxicity risk.

Individual glucocorticoids are available as various esters (e.g., prednisolone *acetate,* prednisolone *sodium phosphate*). When glucocorticoids are administered by routes other than oral or IV, the particular ester employed is a major determinant of duration of action. As indicated in Table 72.2, not all esters can be administered by all routes. Therefore, when preparing to give a glucocorticoid, you should verify that the ester ordered is appropriate for the intended route.

Dosage

General Guidelines for Dosing. For most patients, the therapeutic objective is to reduce symptoms to an acceptable level. Complete relief is usually not an appropriate goal.

Dosages are highly individualized. For any patient with any disorder, dosage must be determined by trial and error.

TABLE 72.2 ■ Glucocorticoid Routes of Administration

	Routes of Administration							
	Systemic			Local				
Drug	**PO**	**IM**	**IV**	**IA**	**IB**	**IL**	**IS**	**ST**
Betamethasone	✓							
Betamethasone sodium phosphate		✓	✓	✓		✓		✓
Betamethasone acetate/sodium phosphate		✓		✓		✓	✓	✓
Cortisone acetate	✓	✓						
Dexamethasone	✓							
Dexamethasone sodium phosphate		✓	✓	✓		✓	✓	✓
Hydrocortisone	✓							
Hydrocortisone acetate				✓	✓	✓	✓	✓
Hydrocortisone sodium succinate		✓	✓					
Methylprednisolone	✓							
Methylprednisolone acetate		✓		✓		✓		✓
Methylprednisolone sodium succinate		✓	✓					
Prednisolone	✓							
Prednisolone acetate	✓							
Prednisolone acetate/sodium phosphate		✓		✓	✓		✓	✓
Prednisolone sodium phosphate	✓							
Prednisone	✓							
Triamcinolone acetonide		✓		✓	✓	✓		
Triamcinolone hexacetonide				✓		✓		

IA, Intra-articular; *IB,* intrabursal; *IL,* intralesional; *IM,* intramuscular; *IS,* intrasynovial; *IV,* intravenous; *PO,* oral; *ST,* soft tissue.

For patients whose disorder is not an immediate threat to life, the dosage should be low initially and then increased gradually until symptoms are under control. In the event of a life-threatening disorder, a large initial dose should be used; then, if a response does not occur rapidly, the dose should be doubled or even tripled. When glucocorticoids are used for a long time, the dosage should be reduced until the smallest effective amount has been established. Prolonged treatment with high doses should be done only if the disorder (1) is life threatening or (2) has the potential to cause permanent disability. During long-term treatment, an increase in dosage will be needed at times of stress unless the dosage is very high to begin with. If disease status changes, an appropriate adjustment of dosage must be made.

As noted, abrupt termination of long-term therapy may unmask adrenal insufficiency. To minimize the effect of adrenal insufficiency, glucocorticoid withdrawal should be gradual. Patients must be warned against abrupt discontinuation.

Alternate-Day Therapy. In alternate-day therapy, a large dose (of an intermediate-acting glucocorticoid) is given every other morning. This dosing schedule contrasts with traditional therapy, in which multiple smaller doses are administered daily. Benefits of alternate-day therapy are (1) reduced adrenal suppression, (2) reduced risk for growth delay, and (3) reduced toxicity overall. Adrenal insufficiency is decreased because over the extended interval between doses, plasma glucocorticoids decline to a level that is low enough to permit some production of ACTH, thereby promoting some synthesis of cortisol by the adrenal glands. To allow maximal recovery of endocrine function, doses should be administered before 9:00 AM, and long-acting agents should be avoided. Early-morning administration is also helpful in that it mimics (sort of) the burst of glucocorticoids normally released by the adrenal glands at dawn.

Unfortunately, alternate-day therapy does have one drawback: In the long interval between doses, drug levels may fall to a subtherapeutic value, thus permitting flare-up of symptoms. Symptoms are likely to be most intense late on the second day after a dose is given. If symptoms become intolerable, switching to a single daily dose may be sufficient to provide control. As with alternate-day treatment, patients taking single daily doses should administer their medicine before 9:00 AM.

KEY POINTS

- Glucocorticoids are used in low (physiologic) doses to treat endocrine disorders and in high (pharmacologic) doses to treat nonendocrine disorders (e.g., arthritis, asthma).
- Glucocorticoids are beneficial in nonendocrine disorders primarily because they suppress inflammatory and immune responses.
- Glucocorticoids produce their effects by penetrating the cell membrane and activating cytoplasmic receptors, which then travel to the cell nucleus, where they modulate the activity of genes that code for specific regulatory proteins.
- Glucocorticoids reduce inflammation by multiple mechanisms, including suppressing the (1) synthesis of inflammatory mediators (prostaglandins, leukotrienes, histamine), (2) infiltration of phagocytes, (3) release of lysosomal enzymes, and (4) proliferation of lymphocytes.
- Important nonendocrine indications for glucocorticoids include arthritis, allergic disorders, asthma, cancer, and suppression of allograft rejection.
- When used in pharmacologic doses, especially for prolonged times, glucocorticoids can cause severe adverse effects. These are not seen at physiologic doses.
- Adverse effects of the glucocorticoids include adrenal insufficiency, osteoporosis, increased vulnerability to infection, muscle wasting, thinning of the skin, fluid and electrolyte imbalance, glucose intolerance, psychologic disturbances, and peptic ulcer disease.
- By causing potassium loss, glucocorticoids can increase the risk for toxicity from digoxin, and they can exacerbate hypokalemia caused by thiazide and loop diuretics.
- Concurrent use of NSAIDs with glucocorticoids increases the risk for peptic ulcer disease.
- Prolonged glucocorticoid use causes adrenal insufficiency.
- Patients with adrenal insufficiency must be given higher doses of glucocorticoids at times of stress (e.g., surgery, trauma). Failure to do so may be fatal!
- To minimize expression of adrenal insufficiency when glucocorticoids are discontinued, doses should be tapered very gradually.
- Following glucocorticoid withdrawal, supplemental glucocorticoids are needed at times of stress until adrenal function has fully recovered.
- Alternate-day dosing can help minimize development of adrenal insufficiency.
- Glucocorticoids should be administered before 9:00 AM to help minimize adrenal insufficiency and to mimic the burst of glucocorticoids released naturally by the adrenal glands each morning.

Please visit **http://evolve.elsevier.com/Lehne** for chapter-specific NCLEX® examination review questions.

Summary of Major Nursing Implications[a]

GLUCOCORTICOIDS

Betamethasone
Cortisone
Dexamethasone
Hydrocortisone
Methylprednisolone
Prednisolone
Prednisone
Triamcinolone

The nursing implications here apply to all glucocorticoids, but only to their use for *nonendocrine disorders*. Implications that apply specifically to their use for *replacement therapy* are discussed in Chapter 60. Implications specific to *asthma therapy* are discussed in Chapter 76.

Preadministration Assessment

Therapeutic Goal

Glucocorticoids are used to suppress rejection of organ transplants and to treat a variety of inflammatory, allergic, and neoplastic disorders. When treating inflammatory and allergic disorders, the goal is to suppress signs and symptoms to an acceptable level, not to eliminate them.

Baseline Data

Make a full assessment of the specific disorder (e.g., rheumatoid arthritis, asthma, psoriasis) being treated. These data are used to determine the initial dosage and to guide dosage adjustments as treatment proceeds. Document baseline blood pressure and weight. Determine bone mineral density if therapy will be prolonged. Plot height on children to assess for delayed growth. Also, for prolonged or high-dose therapy, check serum glucose, electrolytes, and a complete blood count. Following prolonged treatment, hypothalamic-pituitary-adrenal (HPA) axis suppression may be assessed with an ACTH stimulation test and by plasma or urine cortisol testing.

Identifying High-Risk Patients

Glucocorticoids are *contraindicated* for patients with systemic fungal infections and for individuals receiving live virus vaccines.

Use glucocorticoids with *caution* in pediatric patients and in women who are pregnant or breast-feeding. In addition, exercise *caution* in patients with hypertension, open-angle glaucoma, heart failure, renal impairment, esophagitis, gastritis, peptic ulcer disease, myasthenia gravis, diabetes mellitus, osteoporosis, and infections that are resistant to treatment, and in patients receiving potassium-depleting diuretics, digoxin, insulin, oral hypoglycemics, or NSAIDs. When these drugs are necessary, dosage adjustments may be required.

Implementation: Administration and Dosage

Routes and Administration

Glucocorticoids are administered orally, parenterally (IV, IM, subQ), topically (to skin and mucous membranes), intranasally, by inhalation, and by local injection (e.g., intra-articular, intralesional). Routes for specific preparations are shown in Table 72.2. (Glucocorticoids administered topically, intranasally, and by inhalation are presented in Chapters 105, 77, and 76, respectively.) When getting ready to administer a glucocorticoid, verify that the preparation is appropriate for the intended route.

Dosage

Dosage is determined empirically. For patients whose disorder does not threaten life, dosage should be low initially and then gradually increased, until the desired response is achieved. For a life-threatening disorder, initial doses should be as large as needed to control symptoms. During prolonged therapy, the dosage should be reduced to the smallest effective amount. Supplemental doses are needed at times of stress, unless the dosage is very high to begin with.

Alternate-Day Therapy

Alternate-day dosing reduces adrenal suppression and other toxicities. **Instruct patients to take their glucocorticoid medicine before 9:00 AM every other day.**

Drug Withdrawal

Glucocorticoids taken chronically must be withdrawn gradually. **Warn the patient against abrupt discontinuation of treatment.** After termination, supplemental doses are needed during times of stress until adrenal function has recovered fully.

Ongoing Evaluation and Interventions

Evaluating Therapeutic Effects

Evaluate therapy by making periodic comparisons of current signs and symptoms with the pretreatment assessment. Dosage adjustment is based on these evaluations.

Minimizing Adverse Effects

General Measures. First, keep the dosage as low as possible and the duration of treatment as short as possible. Second, use alternate-day therapy if possible. Third, when appropriate, administer glucocorticoids topically, intranasally, by inhalation, or by local injection, rather than systemically.

Adrenal Insufficiency. Long-term therapy suppresses the ability of the adrenal glands to make glucocorticoids. Increase the dosage when stress occurs (e.g., surgery, trauma, infection) unless the dosage is very high to begin with. After termination of therapy, supplemental doses are required at times of stress until adrenal recovery is complete. **Advise the patient to carry identification (e.g., Medic Alert bracelet) to ensure proper dosing in emergencies. Advise the patient to always have an emergency supply of glucocorticoids on hand.** Expression of adrenal insufficiency can be reduced by withdrawing glucocorticoids gradually. Adrenal insufficiency can be minimized through alternate-day dosing and the use of glucocorticoids that have an intermediate duration of action.

Osteoporosis. Glucocorticoid-induced osteoporosis predisposes the patient to fractures, especially of the ribs and vertebrae. Monitor patients for signs of compression fractures (neck or back pain) and for indications of other

Continued

Summary of Major Nursing Implications[a]—cont'd

fractures. Evaluate status with bone densitometry. Several drugs can help prevent osteoporosis. Important among these are calcium supplements, vitamin D supplements, thiazide diuretics (combined with salt restriction), bisphosphonates (e.g., risedronate, zoledronate), teriparatide, and calcitonin. Estrogen therapy can reduce bone loss in postmenopausal women, but the benefits are not likely to outweigh the risks.

Infection. Glucocorticoids increase the risk for morbidity from infection. Warn patients to avoid close contact with persons who have a communicable disease. **Inform patients about early signs of infection (e.g., fever, sore throat), and instruct them to notify the prescriber if these occur.** Treat established infections with appropriate antimicrobial drugs, and withdraw glucocorticoids unless they are absolutely required.

Glucose Intolerance. Glucocorticoids can cause hyperglycemia and glycosuria. Patients with diabetes may need to decrease their caloric intake and use higher doses of hypoglycemic medication (insulin or an oral hypoglycemic).

Fluid and Electrolyte Disturbance. Glucocorticoids can cause sodium and water retention and loss of potassium. These effects can be minimized by (1) using glucocorticoids that have low mineralocorticoid activity, (2) restricting sodium intake, and (3) taking potassium supplements or consuming potassium-rich foods (e.g., bananas, citrus fruits). **Educate patients about signs and symptoms of fluid retention (e.g., weight gain, swelling of the lower extremities) and hypokalemia (e.g., muscle weakness, irregular pulses, cramping), and instruct them to notify the prescriber if these develop.**

Growth Delay. Glucocorticoids can suppress growth in children. Evaluate growth by making periodic measurements of height and weight. Alternate-day therapy minimizes effects on growth.

Cataracts and Glaucoma. Cataracts are a common complication of long-term therapy. Open-angle glaucoma may also develop. The patient should be given an eye examination every 6 months. **Instruct the patient to notify the prescriber if vision becomes cloudy or blurred.**

Peptic Ulcer Disease. Glucocorticoids may increase the risk for ulcer formation and can mask ulcer symptoms. **Instruct the patient to notify the prescriber if stools become black and tarry.** Have stools checked periodically for occult blood. If ulcers develop, glucocorticoids should be slowly withdrawn—unless their continued use is considered essential for life—and antiulcer therapy should be instituted.

Psychologic Disturbances. Systemic glucocorticoids can cause psychologic disturbances, both mild (insomnia, anxiety, agitation, irritability) and severe (delirium, hallucinations, depression, euphoria, mania). Depression is more likely with low-dose, long-term therapy, whereas psychoses (mania, delirium) are more likely with high-dose, short-term therapy. Psychologic disturbances are reversible and usually resolve within days to weeks after drug withdrawal. Depression may respond to a mood stabilizer (e.g., carbamazepine, valproic acid) or a selective serotonin reuptake inhibitor (e.g., fluoxetine [Prozac]). Psychotic symptoms may respond to an atypical antipsychotic. **Inform patients about possible psychologic reactions, and instruct them to report disturbing symptoms.** Monitor for suicidal ideation.

Use in Pregnancy and Lactation. Glucocorticoids can induce adrenal hypoplasia in the developing fetus. When large doses have been employed, the newborn should be assessed for adrenal insufficiency and given replacement therapy if indicated.

During high-dose therapy, the glucocorticoid content of breast milk may become high enough to affect the nursing infant. **Warn women who are receiving high-dose therapy not to breast-feed.**

Other Adverse Effects. *Myopathy* and *Cushing's syndrome* can be minimized by implementing the general measures noted at the beginning of this section. There are no specific measures to prevent these complications.

Minimizing Adverse Interactions

Interactions Related to Potassium Loss. Glucocorticoid-induced potassium loss can be augmented by *potassium-depleting diuretics* (thiazides, loop diuretics) and can increase the risk for toxicity from *digoxin*. If digoxin and glucocorticoids are used concurrently, potassium levels should be monitored. Also, be alert for indications of cardiotoxicity.

Nonsteroidal Anti-Inflammatory Drugs. NSAIDs can increase the risk for gastric ulceration during glucocorticoid therapy. Exercise caution when this combination is employed.

Insulin and Other Hypoglycemics. Glucocorticoids can elevate blood levels of glucose. Diabetic patients may need to increase their dosage of insulin or other hypoglycemic drugs.

Vaccines. Glucocorticoids can decrease antibody responses to vaccines and can increase the risk for infection from live virus vaccines. Immunization should not be done while glucocorticoids are in use.

[a]Patient education information is highlighted as **blue text.**

UNIT XII DRUGS FOR BONE AND JOINT DISORDERS

CHAPTER 73

Drug Therapy for Rheumatoid Arthritis

Rheumatoid arthritis (RA) is an autoimmune, inflammatory disorder that affects about 1% of the American population. Each year, the disease results in more than 9 million physician visits and over 250,000 hospitalizations. Although RA can develop at any age, initial symptoms usually appear during the third and fourth decades. Among younger patients, the incidence of RA in females is 3 times greater than in males. However, among patients older than 60 years, the incidence in men and women is equal. Rheumatoid arthritis follows a progressive course and can eventually cause joint deformities and functional limitations. In many cases, drug therapy can delay disease progression. In others, benefits are limited to symptomatic relief. Some of the drugs used for RA were introduced in preceding chapters. Additional drugs are introduced here.

PATHOPHYSIOLOGY OF RHEUMATOID ARTHRITIS

Onset of RA is heralded by symmetrical joint stiffness and pain. Symptoms are most intense in the morning and abate as the day advances. Joints become swollen, tender, and warm. For some patients, periods of spontaneous remission occur. For others, injury progresses steadily. In addition to joint injury, RA has systemic manifestations, including fever, weakness, fatigue, weight loss, thinning of the skin, scleritis (inflammation of the sclera), corneal ulcers, vasculitis (which can be severe), and nodules under the skin and periosteum (connective tissue that surrounds all bones).

The progression of joint deterioration is shown in Fig. 73.1. Inflammation begins in the synovium—the membrane that encloses the joint cavity. As inflammation intensifies, the synovial membrane thickens and begins to envelop the articular cartilage. This overgrowth is referred to as *pannus.* Damage to the cartilage is caused by enzymes released from the pannus and by chemicals and enzymes produced by the inflammatory process raging within the synovial space. Ultimately, the articular cartilage undergoes total destruction, resulting in direct contact between bones of the joint, followed by eventual bone fusion. After this, inflammation subsides.

Joint destruction is caused by an autoimmune process in which the immune system mounts an attack against synovial tissue. During the attack, mast cells, macrophages, and T lymphocytes produce cytokines and cytotoxins—compounds that promote inflammation and joint destruction. The cytokines of greatest importance are tumor necrosis factor (TNF), interleukin-1 (IL-1), interleukin-6 (IL-6), interferon gamma, platelet-derived growth factor, and granulocyte-macrophage colony-stimulating factor. Why the immune system attacks joints is unclear.

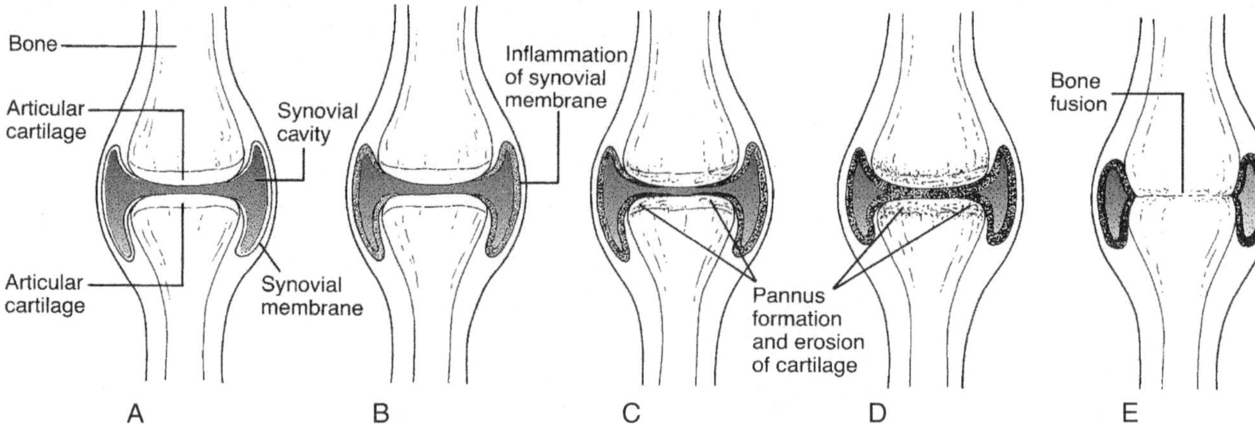

Fig. 73.1 ▪ Progressive joint degeneration in rheumatoid arthritis.
A, Healthy joint. **B,** Inflammation of synovial membrane. **C,** Onset of pannus formation and cartilage erosion. **D,** Pannus formation progresses and cartilage deteriorates further. **E,** Complete destruction of joint cavity together with fusion of articulating bones.

OVERVIEW OF THERAPY

Treatment is directed at (1) relieving symptoms (pain, inflammation, and stiffness), (2) maintaining joint function and range of motion, (3) minimizing systemic involvement, and (4) delaying disease progression. To achieve these goals, a combination of pharmacologic and nonpharmacologic measures is used.

Nondrug Measures

Nondrug measures for managing RA include physical therapy, exercise, and surgery. Physical therapy may consist of massage, warm baths, and applying heat to the affected regions. These procedures can enhance mobility and reduce inflammation. A balanced program of rest and exercise can decrease joint stiffness and improve function. However, excessive rest and excessive exercise should be avoided: Too much rest will foster stiffness, and too much activity can intensify inflammation.

Orthopedic surgery has made marked advances. For patients with severe disease of the hip or knee, total joint replacement can be performed. When joints of the hands or wrists have been damaged severely, function can be improved through removal of the diseased synovium and repair of ruptured tendons. Plastic implants can help correct deformities.

A complete program of treatment should include patient education and counseling. The patient should be informed about the nature of RA, the possible consequences of joint degeneration, management measures, and the benefits and limitations of drug therapy. If loss of mobility limits function at home, on the job, or in school, consultation with a social worker, occupational therapist, or specialist in vocational rehabilitation may be appropriate.

Drug Therapy

Antiarthritic drugs can produce symptomatic relief, and some drugs, if started very early in the disease process, can induce protracted remission. However, remission is rarely complete, and the disease typically advances steadily. As a result, drug therapy is chronic, and success requires patient motivation and cooperation.

Classes of Antiarthritic Drugs

The antirheumatic drugs fall into three major groups:

- Nonsteroidal anti-inflammatory drugs (NSAIDs)
- Glucocorticoids
- Disease-modifying antirheumatic drugs (DMARDs)

These major groups differ with respect to time course of effects, toxicity, and ability to slow RA progression.

The NSAIDs provide rapid relief of symptoms but do not prevent joint damage and do not slow disease progression. The NSAIDs are safer than DMARDs and glucocorticoids, thus treatment with NSAIDs requires less vigorous monitoring.

Like the NSAIDs, glucocorticoids provide rapid relief of symptoms. In addition, they can slow disease progression. Unfortunately, although glucocorticoids are effective, with long-term use they can cause serious toxicity. As a result, treatment is usually limited to short courses.

By definition, DMARDs are drugs that reduce joint destruction and slow disease progression. DMARDs are subdivided into two basic groups—*nonbiologic DMARDs* (traditional DMARDs) and *biologic DMARDs*—based on their molecular size and method of production. The nonbiologic DMARDs are small molecules that are synthesized using conventional chemical techniques. In contrast, the biologic DMARDs are large molecules that are produced through recombinant DNA technology. Both have significant adverse effects; therefore, close monitoring is required.

Drug Selection

Current guidelines recommend starting a DMARD *early*—within 3 months of RA diagnosis for most patients. By instituting DMARD therapy early, it is possible to delay or even prevent serious joint injury. Because the effects of DMARDs take weeks or months to develop, whereas the effects of NSAIDs are immediate, an NSAID is given until the DMARD has had time to act, after which the NSAID can be withdrawn. Glucocorticoids are generally reserved for short-course management to control symptoms until DMARDs take effect and to control symptom flare-ups, which are exacerbations of symptoms that were previously controlled. If joint injury progresses despite treatment with an initial DMARD (typically methotrexate), another DMARD can be added or substituted.

You can find detailed information on pharmacologic management of RA in clinical guidelines sponsored by the American College of Rheumatology (ACR). The document, *2015 American College of Rheumatology Guideline for the Treatment of Rheumatoid Arthritis,* is available at http://www.rheumatology.org/Portals/0/Files/ACR%202015%20RA%20Guideline.pdf.

NONSTEROIDAL ANTI-INFLAMMATORY DRUGS

The basic pharmacology of the NSAIDs is discussed in Chapter 71. Consideration here is limited to their role in RA.

Therapeutic Role

NSAIDs are drugs of first choice for RA, owing to their efficacy and rapid onset. Benefits derive primarily from anti-inflammatory and analgesic actions. Both actions result from inhibiting cyclooxygenase (COX). NSAIDs provide only symptomatic relief; they do not slow disease progression. Accordingly, they are usually combined with a DMARD.

NSAID Classification

There are two main classes of NSAIDs: (1) *first-generation NSAIDs,* which inhibit COX-1 *and* COX-2; and (2) *second-generation NSAIDs* (coxibs), which selectively inhibit COX-2. Anti-inflammatory and analgesic effects result from inhibiting COX-2, whereas major adverse effects—especially gastroduodenal ulceration—result from inhibiting COX-1. Therefore, the selectivity of this drug class results in less gastrointestinal (GI) ulceration than the first-generation NSAIDs, while producing equal therapeutic effects.

Drug Selection

Selection of an NSAID is based largely on efficacy, safety, and cost.

Efficacy

All of the NSAIDs have essentially equal antirheumatic effects. However, individual patients may respond better to one NSAID than to another. Accordingly, it may be necessary to try more than one agent to achieve an optimal response.

Safety and Cost

All prescription-strength NSAIDs carry a boxed warning regarding risk for thrombotic events and GI ulceration and bleeding. Although the risk for GI problems is lessened with COX-2 inhibitors, the risk for thrombotic events may be increased because COX-1 has a role in the production of thromboxane A_2, which participates in blood clotting. Coxibs inhibit COX-1 to a far lesser degree than traditional NSAIDs. Celecoxib [Celebrex] is currently the only remaining coxib available in the United States. Other COX-2 inhibitors were withdrawn from the market following reports of adverse reactions that included myocardial infarction and stroke secondary to thrombosis. Hence, selection must balance these factors. Coxibs are more expensive than traditional NSAIDs. If symptoms are controlled with a first-generation NSAID and the drug is well tolerated, cost considerations will dictate using that drug. However, if a first-generation NSAID produces serious gastric ulceration and the patient is at low risk for thrombosis, then switching to celecoxib might be appropriate—despite the increased cost.

Dosage

Dosages employed for anti-inflammatory effects are considerably higher than those required for analgesia or fever reduction. For example, treatment of RA may require 5.2 gm (16 standard tablets) of aspirin a day, compared with only 2.6 gm for aches, pain, and fever. Dosages for RA are shown in Table 73.1.

GLUCOCORTICOIDS

The glucocorticoids are powerful anti-inflammatory drugs that can relieve symptoms of severe RA and that may also delay disease progression. For patients with generalized symptoms, *oral* glucocorticoids are indicated. However, if only one or two joints are affected, *intra-articular injections* may be employed. Because long-term oral therapy can cause serious toxicity (e.g., osteoporosis, gastric ulceration, adrenal suppression), short-term therapy should be used whenever possible. Most often, glucocorticoids are used for temporary relief until drugs with more slowly developing effects (e.g., methotrexate) can provide control. Long-term therapy should be limited to patients who have failed to respond adequately to all other options. The most commonly employed oral glucocorticoids are *prednisone* and *prednisolone.* When symptoms flare, patients may be given 10 to 20 mg/day until symptoms are controlled, followed by gradual drug withdrawal over 5 to 7 days. The pharmacology of the glucocorticoids is discussed in Chapter 72.

NONBIOLOGIC (TRADITIONAL) DISEASE-MODIFYING ANTIRHEUMATIC DRUGS

As previously noted, the nonbiologic DMARDs are small molecules produced using conventional synthetic procedures. With several of these drugs, benefits result from immunosuppression. Unlike the NSAIDs, whose benefits are limited to symptomatic relief, the nonbiologic DMARDs can slow disease progression. These drugs are potentially more harmful than the NSAIDs, and clinical responses develop more slowly. The nonbiologic DMARDs cost much less than the biologic DMARDs, largely because the nonbiologic agents are easier to make.

Methotrexate

Methotrexate [Rheumatrex, Trexall] acts faster than all other DMARDs. Therapeutic effects may develop in 3 to 6 weeks. At least 80% of patients improve with this drug. Benefits are the result of immunosuppression secondary to reducing the activity of B and T lymphocytes. Many rheumatologists consider methotrexate the DMARD of first choice, owing to its efficacy, relative safety, low cost, and extensive use in RA. Major toxicities are hepatic fibrosis, bone marrow suppression, GI ulceration,

TABLE 73.1 ▪ Nonsteroidal Anti-Inflammatory Drugs: Oral Dosage for Rheumatoid Arthritis

Generic Name	Brand Name	Daily Dosage
FIRST-GENERATION NSAIDs		
Salicylates		
Aspirin	Multiple brand names	3.6–5.4 gm/day in divided doses
Magnesium salicylate	Doan's Pills, Doan's Extra Strength	650–1160 mg every 6 hr as needed
Salsalate	Generic only	3 gm/day (in 2–3 doses)
Nonsalicylates		
Diclofenac (salt)	Cambia, Cataflam, Voltaren, Zipsor	Immediate release:150–200 mg/day (in 3–4 doses) Delayed release: 150–200 mg/day (in 2–4 divided doses) Extended release: 100–200 mg/day (in 2 divided doses)
Diclofenac (free acid)	Zorvolex	18–35 mg 3 times/day
Diclofenac/misoprostol	Arthrotec	50 mg diclofenac/200 mcg misoprostol 3–4 times/day
Diflunisal	Generic only	250–500 mg twice daily
Etodolac	Generic only	Immediate release: 400 mg 2 times/day **or** 300 mg 2–3 times/day **or** 500 mg 2 times/day Extended release: 400–1000 mg once daily
Fenoprofen	Nalfon	300–600 mg 3 or 4 times/day
Flurbiprofen	Generic only	200–300 mg/day (in 2–4 doses)
Ibuprofen	Motrin, Advil, others	400–800 mg 3 or 4 times/day
Indomethacin	Indocin	25–50 mg 3 times/day
Ketoprofen	Generic only	Immediate release: 150–300 mg/day (in 3–4 doses) Extended release: 100–200 mg once daily
Meclofenamate	Generic only	200–400 mg/day (in 3–4 doses)
Meloxicam	Mobic, Mobicox 🍁	7.5 mg once daily
Nabumetone	Generic only	1–2 gm/day (in 1–2 doses)
Naproxen	Naprosyn Naprelan EC-Naprosyn	Immediate release: 250–500 mg twice daily Extended release: 750–1500 mg/day Delayed release: 375–500 mg twice daily
Naproxen sodium	Aleve, others	250–500 mg twice daily
Naproxen/esomeprazole	Vimovo	375–500 mg (naproxen) twice daily
Oxaprozin	Daypro	1.2 gm once daily
Piroxicam	Feldene	10 mg twice daily **or** 20 mg once daily
Sulindac	Clinoril	150–200 mg twice daily
Tolmetin	Generic only	200–600 mg 3 times/day
SECOND-GENERATION NSAIDs (COX-2 INHIBITORS)		
Celecoxib	Celebrex	100–200 mg twice daily

and pneumonitis. Periodic tests of liver and kidney function are mandatory, as are complete blood cell and platelet counts. Methotrexate can cause fetal death and congenital abnormalities, and therefore is contraindicated during pregnancy. Recent data suggest that patients using methotrexate for RA may have a reduced life expectancy, owing to increased deaths from cardiovascular disease, infection, and certain cancers (melanoma, lung cancer, and non-Hodgkin's lymphoma). Dosing with folic acid (at least 5 mg/week) is recommended to reduce GI and hepatic toxicity. Dosing for methotrexate and other DMARDs is provided in Table 73.2. Methotrexate is discussed in Chapter 102.

Safety Alert

METHOTREXATE

Methotrexate can cause numerous and potentially fatal toxicities of the bone marrow, liver, lungs, and kidneys. Other fatalities have occurred associated with skin reactions and due to hemorrhagic enteritis and gastrointestinal perforation.

TABLE 73.2 ■ DMARDs: Common Dosages for Rheumatoid Arthritis

Drug	Preparation	Daily Dosage	Administration
NONBIOLOGIC (TRADITIONAL) DMARDs			
Methotrexate [Rheumatrex, Trexall]	Tablets: 2.5, 5, 7.5, 10, 15 mg Solution: 25 mg/mL Auto-injector: 15 different dosages ranging from 7.5 mg/0.15 mL to 30 mg/0.6 mL	Oral, subQ, and IM: 7.5 mg/week initially, and then adjusted upward until optimal response is achieved or a maximum dose of 20–30 mg/week is reached Optional oral dosing: 10–15 mg/week initially, and then increased by 5 mg/week every 2–4 weeks, up to a maintenance level of 20–30 mg/week	Auto-injectors allow for self-administration Dosing with folic acid is recommended to reduce GI and hepatic toxicity
Sulfasalazine [Azulfidine, Azulfidine EN-tabs]	IR tablets: 500 mg (scored) ER tablets: 500 mg	Initial: 0.5–1 gm/day Maintenance: 1 gm given 2–3 times/day	Avoid in patients who are allergic to sulfonamides Space tablets evenly throughout the day, preferably after meals Swallow ER tablets whole
Leflunomide [Arava]	Tablets: 10, 20 mg	Initial: loading doses of 100 mg once daily for 3 days Maintenance: 10–20 mg/day	May be given with or without food
Hydroxychloroquine [Plaquenil]	Tablet: 200 mg	Initially: 400–600 mg/day, increased slowly to achieve optimal response over 1–3 months Maintenance: 200–400 mg/day	Take with food or milk
BIOLOGIC DMARDs			
Adalimumab [Humira]	Pre-filled syringe: 20 mg/0.4 mL, 40 mg/0.8 mL Auto-injector: 40 mg/0.8 mL	40 mg every 2 weeks If used without methotrexate: 40 mg once a week	Administer subQ in the anterior thigh or abdomen Rotate sites Avoid areas where the skin is tender, bruised, red, or indurated
Certolizumab pegol [Cimzia]	Pre-filled syringe: 200 mg/mL	Initial: 400 mg repeated at 2 and 4 weeks Maintenance: 200 mg every 2 weeks or 400 mg every month	Inject subQ into the abdomen or thigh Two separate injections are needed due to the size of the dose
Etanercept [Enbrel]	Pre-filled syringe: 25 mg/0.5 mL, 50 mg/mL Auto-injector: 50 mg/mL Powder: 25 mg for reconstitution in 1 mL of sterile bacteriostatic water	Adults: 50 mg subQ once a week Children ages 4–17 years: 0.8 mg/kg (up to a maximum of 50 mg) once a week	Inject subQ into the abdomen or anterior thigh Avoid areas that are tender, bruised, red, or indurated Solutions that are discolored or cloudy or that contain particles should not be used
Golimumab [Simponi, Simponi Aria]	Pre-filled syringe: 50 mg/0.5 mL, 100 mg/mL Auto-injector: 50 mg/0.5 mL, 100 mg/mL Solution for IV administration: 50 mg/4 mL	SubQ (Simponi): 50 mg once a month IV (Simponi Aria): 2 mg/kg repeated at 4 weeks and then every 8 weeks for maintenance	Inject subQ into the abdomen or anterior thigh. Avoid areas that are tender, bruised, red, or indurated IV: Infuse diluted solution over 30 minutes. Do not infuse other medications in the same line
Infliximab [Remicade]	Powder: 100 mg in single-use vials to be dissolved in 10 mL of sterile water, followed by dilution in 0.9% sodium chloride to a final volume of 250 mL	Initial: 3 mg/kg repeated at 2 weeks and 6 weeks Maintenance: 3 mg/kg every 8 weeks	IV solutions should be clear and either colorless or pale yellow; discard if discolored or with visible particles
Rituximab [Rituxan]	Solution: 10 mg/mL in 10-mL and 50-mL vials	Initial: 1000 mg IV infusion repeated in 2 weeks Subsequent treatment: 1000 mg every 24 weeks if needed	Dilute to 1–4 mg/mL for IV infusion Premedicate with an antihistamine, acetaminophen, and IV corticosteroid 30 minutes before infusion Start at 50 mg/hr; if response is inadequate, titrate up to 400 mg/hr Monitor closely for infusion reactions

Continued

TABLE 73.2 ▪ DMARDs: Common Dosages for Rheumatoid Arthritis—cont'd

Drug	Preparation	Daily Dosage	Administration
Abatacept [Orencia]	Pre-filled syringe: 125 mg/mL IV: 250 mg powder for reconstitution in sterile water	SubQ: 125 mg weekly, preferably following a single IV loading dose of 10 mg/kg IV adult: <60 kg, give 500 mg; 60–100 kg, give 750 mg; >100 kg, give 1000 mg; repeat at 2 weeks and 4 weeks following first infusion and then repeat every 4 weeks IV for polyarticular juvenile idiopathic arthritis: <75 kg, give 10 mg/kg; 75–100 kg, give 750 mg; >100 kg, give 1000 mg. As in adults, dosing is done on days 0, 14, and 28, and every 4 weeks thereafter	Reconstitute with gentle swirling motion to minimize foam Dilute reconstituted solution to a final volume of 100 mL Discard discolored solution or solutions containing particles Infuse over 30 minutes Do not infuse other medications in the same line
Tocilizumab [Actemra]	Pre-filled syringe: 162 mg/0.9 mL IV: 80, 300, 400 mg as a concentrated solution (20 mg/mL) for dilution in 0.9% sodium chloride to a final volume of 100 mL	SubQ: <100 kg, give 162 mg every 2 weeks; may increase if response is suboptimal. ≥100 kg, give 162 mg weekly IV: 4 mg/kg every 4 weeks, given as a single 60-minute IV drip infusion; dosage can be increased to 8 mg/kg every 4 weeks based on the clinical response; maximum single dose is 800 mg	SubQ: Discard if discolored or with visible particles. Rotate injection sites. Avoid areas where the skin is tender, bruised, red, or indurated IV: Discard solution if discolored or with visible particles. Infuse over 60 minutes. Do not infuse other medications in the same line
Anakinra [Kineret]	Pre-filled syringe: 100 mg/0.67 mL	SubQ: 100 mg once daily	Do not shake before administration Rotate injection sites Avoid areas where the skin is tender, bruised, red, or indurated

ER, Extended release; *IR,* immediate release.

Sulfasalazine

Sulfasalazine [Azulfidine, Azulfidine EN-tabs] has been used for decades to treat inflammatory bowel disease (see Chapter 80). Benefits for RA may result from anti-inflammatory and immunomodulatory actions. In patients with RA, sulfasalazine can slow the progression of joint deterioration, sometimes with just 1 month of treatment. GI reactions (nausea, vomiting, diarrhea, anorexia, abdominal pain) are the most common reasons for stopping treatment. These reactions can be minimized by using an enteric-coated formulation and by dividing the daily dosage. Dermatologic reactions (pruritus, rash, urticaria) are also common. Fortunately, serious adverse effects—hepatitis and bone marrow suppression—are rare. To ensure early detection, periodic monitoring for hepatitis and bone marrow function (complete blood counts, platelet counts) should be performed. Because of its structure, sulfasalazine should not be given to patients with sulfa allergy. Sulfasalazine is discussed in Chapter 80.

Leflunomide

Actions and Uses

Leflunomide [Arava] is a powerful immunosuppressant indicated for adults with active RA. In clinical trials, the drug decreased signs and symptoms and slowed disease progression. Compared with methotrexate, leflunomide is about equally effective, but is potentially more hazardous and more expensive. Accordingly, the drug is often reserved for second-line use.

Leflunomide is a prodrug that undergoes conversion to its active form—metabolite 1 (M1)—in the body. M1 inhibits dihydroorotate dehydrogenase, a mitochondrial enzyme needed for *de novo* synthesis of pyrimidines, which in turn are needed for T-cell proliferation and antibody production. *In vitro,* leflunomide inhibits T-cell proliferation. In animals, it suppresses inflammation.

Pharmacokinetics

After oral dosing, leflunomide is converted to M1 by enzymes in the intestine and liver. Levels of M1 peak in 6 to 12 hours. The active form undergoes further metabolism followed by excretion in the urine and bile. The half-life is prolonged: 16.5 days. As a result, a series of loading doses is needed to achieve steady state quickly.

Adverse Effects

The most common adverse effects occur in at least 10% of patients: diarrhea, respiratory infection, reversible alopecia, and rash. The drug has also been associated with much more serious reactions: pancytopenia, Stevens-Johnson syndrome, and severe hypertension.

Leflunomide is *hepatotoxic.* Elevation of liver enzymes occurs in about 10% of patients. In postmarketing reports, the drug has been associated with more than 130 cases of severe liver injury, including 14 that were fatal. Liver function should be assessed at baseline, every month for the first 6 months of treatment, and every 6 to 8 weeks thereafter. Leflunomide should be avoided in patients with liver impairment, hepatitis B, or hepatitis C. Patients should be informed about signs of liver injury—abdominal pain, fatigue, dark urine, and jaundice—and advised to report them immediately.

Leflunomide may increase the risk for *serious infection.* The drug is immunosuppressive and can suppress the bone marrow. Rarely, patients experience sepsis and other severe infections, including tuberculosis (TB). Deaths have occurred. If an infection develops, it may be necessary to interrupt leflunomide use. To reduce risk, platelet counts and blood cell counts should be conducted at baseline, every month for the first 6 months of treatment, and every 6 to 8 weeks thereafter. If evidence of bone marrow suppression is detected, leflunomide should be discontinued. Patients should be screened for TB before starting this drug.

Leflunomide is carcinogenic in animals, but has not been associated with cancer in humans.

Leflunomide and Pregnancy

Leflunomide is contraindicated during pregnancy. Patients who wish to become pregnant must first clear leflunomide from the body. A three-step protocol is followed:

Step 1: Discontinue leflunomide.
Step 2: Take cholestyramine (8 gm 3 times a day) for 11 days. (Cholestyramine binds leflunomide and its metabolites in the intestine, accelerating their excretion. Without cholestyramine, safe levels might not be achieved for 2 years.)
Step 3: Verify that plasma drug levels are below 20 mcg/L.

To minimize any risk for fetal injury, men using leflunomide who wish to father a child should undergo the same clearance procedure.

PATIENT-CENTERED CARE ACROSS THE LIFE SPAN

DMARDs

Life Stage	Patient Care Concerns
Children	Biologic DMARDs: Children and adolescents taking TNF antagonists have developed lymphoma and other malignancies.
Pregnant women	Biologic DMARDs: TNF antagonists are Pregnancy Risk Category B.[a] Rituximab and abatacept are Pregnancy Risk Category C.[a] Nonbiologic DMARDs: Azathioprine is teratogenic. Both leflunomide and methotrexate can cause fetal death and congenital abnormalities. Hydroxychloroquine may cause fetal ocular toxicity; however, in some conditions such as maternal lupus or malaria, the drug decreases fetal risk associated with the conditions it treats. Sulfasalazine is Pregnancy Risk Category B.[a]
Breast-feeding women	Breast-feeding is not recommended for women taking DMARDs.
Older adults	Elderly patients may be at a greater risk for infection secondary to DMARD immunosuppressive effects.

[a]As of 2020, the FDA will no longer use Pregnancy Risk Categories. Please refer to Chapter 9 for more information.

Drug Interactions

Leflunomide can inhibit the metabolism of certain NSAIDs (e.g., ibuprofen, diclofenac), causing their levels to rise. In addition, leflunomide can intensify liver damage from other hepatotoxic drugs (e.g., methotrexate), and hence should not be combined with such agents. Rifampin (a drug for TB) can raise leflunomide levels by 40%. Conversely, two other agents—cholestyramine and activated charcoal—can rapidly lower leflunomide levels.

Hydroxychloroquine

Hydroxychloroquine [Plaquenil], a drug with antimalarial actions, is considered a preferred DMARD in the 2015 ACR treatment guideline. How hydroxychloroquine works in RA is unknown. As a rule, the drug is usually combined with methotrexate. By itself, hydroxychloroquine does not slow disease progression, but early use *can* improve long-term outcomes.

Like other DMARDs, hydroxychloroquine has a delayed onset; full therapeutic effects take 3 to 6 months to develop. Concurrent therapy with anti-inflammatory agents (NSAIDs or glucocorticoids) is indicated during the latency period.

Retinal damage, which is rare, is the most serious toxicity. Retinopathy may be irreversible and can produce blindness. Visual loss is directly related to dosage. Low doses may be used in long-term treatment with little risk. When dosage has been excessive, retinal damage may appear after treatment has ceased and may progress in the absence of continued drug use. Patients should undergo a thorough ophthalmologic examination before treatment and every 6 months thereafter. Hydroxychloroquine should be discontinued at the first sign of retinal injury. Patients should be advised to contact the prescriber if any visual disturbance is noted.

Other Nonbiologic Disease-Modifying Antirheumatic Drugs

Several drugs approved by the U.S. Food and Drug Administration (FDA) for RA are used infrequently, largely because of adverse effects. Some (azathioprine, cyclosporine, minocycline and gold) are no longer recommended; however, they may still be used as a last resort when other drugs fail to meet therapeutic objectives. These drugs are discussed briefly next.

Penicillamine

Penicillamine [Cuprimine, Depen] can relieve symptoms of RA and can delay disease progression. Unfortunately, treatment may be associated with serious toxicity, especially bone marrow suppression and autoimmune disorders. Because it is associated with fatalities, penicillamine use should be restricted to cases in which RA is severe and unresponsive to other treatment. Therapeutic effects take 3 to 6 months to develop. The pharmacology of penicillamine is discussed in Chapter 109.

Gold Salts

Gold salts—*auranofin* [Ridaura]—have been used in RA for decades. Treatment can relieve pain and stiffness, and may also delay disease progression. The mechanism underlying these benefits is unknown. Unfortunately, adverse effects are common. Potential reactions include intense pruritus, rashes, stomatitis, kidney damage, severe blood dyscrasias, encephalitis, hepatitis, peripheral neuritis, pulmonary infiltrates, and profound hypotension.

Azathioprine

Azathioprine [Imuran] is an older DMARD with immunosuppressive and anti-inflammatory actions. Serious toxicities include hepatitis and blood dyscrasias (leukopenia, thrombocytopenia, anemia). Also, azathioprine is teratogenic in animals and should not be used during pregnancy. The drug may also pose a small risk for malignancy. As discussed in Chapter 69, azathioprine is also used to prevent rejection of kidney transplants.

Cyclosporine

Cyclosporine [Neoral, Sandimmune], an immunosuppressive drug used to prevent rejection of transplanted organs, can reduce symptoms of RA. Because it can cause kidney damage and other serious adverse effects, cyclosporine should be reserved for severe, progressive RA that has not responded to safer DMARDs. In patients with an inadequate response to methotrexate, adding cyclosporine may produce significant improvement. Cyclosporine is discussed in Chapter 69.

Minocycline

Minocycline [Minocin], an antibiotic in the tetracycline family, has been used experimentally in RA management. It can improve morning stiffness, joint pain and tenderness, and activities of daily living. In addition, it may delay disease progression in some patients. The precise mechanism by which it accomplishes this is unknown. The ACR did not include minocycline in the 2015 guideline because of its infrequent use and the lack of new data since 2012.

Protein A Column [Prosorba]

The *Prosorba* column, used in combination with plasmapheresis, decreases the titer of circulating immune complexes that promote symptoms of RA. The column contains an adsorbent compound—*protein A*—that binds to antibodies of the immunoglobulin G (IgG) class and to IgG-antigen complexes. When the patient's plasma is passed through the column, these antibodies and immune complexes are removed. Treatment should be reserved for patients with moderate to severe RA who have been refractory to or intolerant of methotrexate and other DMARDs. The most common adverse effects are transient increases in joint swelling, joint pain, and fatigue.

BIOLOGIC DISEASE-MODIFYING ANTIRHEUMATIC DRUGS

The biologic DMARDs are immunosuppressive drugs that target specific components of the inflammatory process (Table 73.3). These drugs are usually combined with methotrexate.

TABLE 73.3 ▪ Disease-Modifying Antirheumatic Drugs (DMARDs)

NONBIOLOGIC (TRADITIONAL) DMARDS
Major Drugs
Methotrexate [Rheumatrex, Trexall]
Sulfasalazine [Azulfidine]
Leflunomide [Arava]
Hydroxychloroquine [Plaquenil]
Minor Drugs
Azathioprine [Imuran]
Cyclosporine [Neoral, Sandimmune]
Minocycline [Minocin]
Penicillamine [Cuprimine, Depen]
Protein A [Prosorba]
Gold salts:
Gold sodium thiomalate [Aurolate, Myochrysine]
Auranofin [Ridaura]
BIOLOGIC DMARDS
Tumor Necrosis Factor Antagonists
Adalimumab [Humira]
Certolizumab pegol [Cimzia]
Etanercept [Enbrel]
Golimumab [Simponi, Simponi Aria]
Infliximab [Remicade]
B-Lymphocyte–Depleting Agents
Rituximab [Rituxan]
T-Cell Activation Inhibitors
Abatacept [Orencia]
Interleukin-6 Receptor Antagonists
Tocilizumab [Actemra]
Interleukin-1 Receptor Antagonists
Anakinra [Kineret]

Of the biologic agents available, only seven are used routinely. Five of these—etanercept, infliximab, adalimumab, golimumab, and certolizumab pegol—interfere with TNF. One agent—rituximab—promotes destruction of B lymphocytes, and one agent—abatacept—inhibits activation of T lymphocytes. Because these drugs suppress immune function, they all pose a risk for serious infections and perhaps cancer. As noted, the biologic DMARDs are so named because they are manufactured using recombinant DNA technology, an expensive process that is reflected in the cost of these drugs, which can range from $14,000 to more than $35,000 a year.

Tumor Necrosis Factor Antagonists

The drugs in this group work by neutralizing TNF, an important immune mediator of joint injury in RA. Five TNF antagonists are available. In patients with RA, all five are highly and equally effective. Unfortunately, all five pose a risk for serious infections, including bacterial sepsis, invasive fungal infections, hepatitis B infection, and TB. Rarely, patients experience severe allergic reactions, heart failure, liver failure, hematologic disorders, neurologic disorders, or cancer. The principal differences among these drugs concern dosing schedule and route of administration. In addition to their use in RA, these drugs are approved for other inflammatory disorders, including psoriatic arthritis, ankylosing spondylitis, and Crohn's disease (Table 73.4).

Safety Alert

TUMOR NECROSIS FACTOR ANTAGONISTS

Patients taking TNF antagonists (adalimumab, certolizumab pegol, etanercept, golimumab, and infliximab) are at an increased risk of developing serious systemic infections and sepsis. Children and adolescents taking TNF antagonists have developed malignancies.

Etanercept

Etanercept [Enbrel] was the first TNF antagonist available, and will serve as our prototype for the group. Like all other TNF antagonists, etanercept is highly effective at reducing RA symptoms and disease progression, but may also promote serious infections and other adverse effects.

TABLE 73.4 ▪ Approved Indications for TNF Antagonists

Approved Indications	Etanercept [Enbrel]	Infliximab [Remicade]	Adalimumab [Humira]	Golimumab [Simponi]	Certolizumab [Cimzia]
Rheumatoid arthritis	✓	✓	✓	✓	✓
Ankylosing spondylitis	✓	✓	✓	✓	✓
Juvenile idiopathic arthritis	✓		✓		
Psoriatic arthritis	✓	✓	✓	✓	✓
Plaque psoriasis	✓	✓	✓		
Crohn's disease		✓	✓		✓
Ulcerative colitis		✓	✓	✓	

Prototype Drugs

DRUGS FOR RHEUMATOID ARTHRITIS

Nonsteroidal Anti-Inflammatory Drugs

Aspirin (a first-generation NSAID)
Celecoxib (a COX-2 inhibitor)

Glucocorticoids

Prednisone

Disease-Modifying Antirheumatic Drugs (DMARDs)

Methotrexate (immunosuppressant)
Etanercept (tumor necrosis factor antagonist)

Mechanism of Action. Etanercept suppresses inflammation by neutralizing TNF. As noted previously, TNF is an important contributor to RA pathophysiology. In patients with RA, TNF binds with receptors on cells in the synovium and thereby stimulates production of chemotactic factors and endothelial adhesion molecules, which in turn promote infiltration of neutrophils and macrophages. The result is inflammation and joint destruction.

How does etanercept neutralize TNF? Etanercept is a large molecule composed of two receptors for TNF that are linked to the Fc component of IgG. The TNF receptors, which are produced through recombinant DNA technology, are identical to the TNF receptors found on human cells. Like the TNF receptors on our cells, etanercept binds tightly with TNF and thereby prevents TNF from interacting with its natural receptors on cells.

Therapeutic Uses. Etanercept is indicated for patients with moderately to severely active RA. In clinical trials, the drug was slightly superior to methotrexate at delaying progression of joint damage, and it suppressed signs and symptoms of RA more rapidly. Among patients who had failed to respond to methotrexate, the addition of etanercept for 6 months reduced symptoms in 61%, compared with 27% who continued to take methotrexate alone.

In addition to RA, etanercept is approved for ankylosing spondylitis, plaque psoriasis, psoriatic arthritis, and juvenile idiopathic arthritis.

Pharmacokinetics. Etanercept is administered by subcutaneous (subQ) injection. Plasma levels peak about 3 days after dosing. The drug is cleared from the plasma with a half-life of 115 hours (about 5 days). The mode of elimination is unknown. One hypothesis is that metabolism of the bound TNF-drug complex takes place through peptide or amino acid degradation, after which elimination of metabolites takes place in the bile or urine while amino acids are recycled.

Adverse Effects

Mild Effects. Injection-site reactions—itching, erythema, swelling, pain—occur in 37% of patients, but usually subside in a few days. Other mild but less common reactions include headache, rhinitis, dizziness, cough, and abdominal pain.

Serious Infections. Etanercept increases the risk for serious infections, including invasive fungal infections (e.g., histoplasmosis, coccidioidomycosis, candidiasis), and infections caused by *Mycobacterium tuberculosis* and other opportunistic pathogens, such as *Legionella pneumophila* and *Listeria monocytogenes.* Why do these infections develop? Under normal conditions, TNF plays a crucial role in our immune response to infection, especially those caused by *M. tuberculosis* and other intracellular pathogens. Accordingly, when we neutralize TNF with etanercept, the risk for infections goes up. Infection risk is further increased by diabetes, HIV infection, and concurrent use of immunosuppressant drugs, including glucocorticoids and methotrexate.

TB is a special concern. When TB develops in patients taking etanercept, the disease is often extrapulmonary and disseminated. To reduce risk, potential users should be tested for latent TB and, if the test is positive, should undergo TB treatment before etanercept is used. During etanercept treatment, patients should be monitored closely for TB development.

Etanercept may promote reactivation of latent infection with hepatitis B virus (HBV). Fatalities have occurred. Candidates for etanercept therapy should be tested for latent HBV, and those who test positive should be monitored closely. If reactivation of HBV infection occurs, etanercept should be stopped and the patient given antiviral drugs.

To reduce infection risk, etanercept should not be given to patients with active infection, including infections that are chronic or localized. Patients who develop a new infection should be monitored closely. Etanercept should be used with caution in patients with a history of recurrent infection or any condition that predisposes them to acquiring infection (e.g., advanced or poorly controlled diabetes). If a severe infection develops, etanercept should be discontinued.

Severe Allergic Reactions. Rarely, etanercept has been associated with severe allergic reactions, including Stevens-Johnson syndrome (SJS), erythema multiforme, and toxic epidermal necrolysis (TEN). For reported cases, the median onset of symptoms was 28 days after starting etanercept. Patients and providers should be alert for these reactions.

Heart Failure. Etanercept may pose a risk for heart failure. In patients using the drug, existing cases of heart failure have gotten worse, and new cases have developed. Exercise caution in patients with existing heart failure, and monitor them closely for disease progression.

Cancer. Etanercept and other TNF antagonists may increase the risk for lymphoma and other malignancies, primarily in children, adolescents, and young adults.

Hematologic Disorders. Etanercept may pose a small risk for hematologic disorders, including neutropenia, thrombocytopenia, and aplastic anemia, which can be fatal. Advise patients who develop signs or symptoms of a blood disorder (persistent fever, bruising, bleeding, pallor) to seek immediate medical attention. If a significant hematologic abnormality is diagnosed, discontinuing etanercept should be considered.

Liver Injury. Rarely, etanercept has been associated with severe liver injury, including acute liver failure. Some patients have required a liver transplant, and some have died. Patients should be informed about symptoms of liver injury—fatigue, yellow skin, yellow eyes, anorexia, right-sided abdominal pain, dark brown urine—and advised to seek medical attention if these develop. If severe liver injury is diagnosed, discontinuation of etanercept should be considered. Etanercept should be used with caution in patients with pre-existing liver dysfunction.

Central Nervous System Demyelinating Disorders. Etanercept has been associated with rare cases of central nervous system (CNS) demyelinating disorders, including multiple sclerosis, myelitis, and optic neuritis. However, a causal relationship has not been established. Nonetheless, caution is advised, especially in patients with a pre-existing or recent-onset demyelinating disorder.

Drug Interactions. By neutralizing TNF, etanercept may increase the risk for acquiring or transmitting infection after immunization with a *live virus vaccine.* Accordingly, live virus vaccines should be avoided. In pediatric patients, vaccinations should be up to date before starting the drug.

Immunosuppressant drugs—including glucocorticoids, methotrexate, tocilizumab, anakinra, and abatacept—increase the risk for serious infection. Use these combinations with caution.

Preparations, Dosage, and Administration. Information on the preparations, dosage, and administration of etanercept and other biologic DMARDs is provided in Table 73.2.

Infliximab

Actions and Uses. Infliximab [Remicade], formulated for intravenous (IV) use, was the second TNF antagonist approved for RA. Like etanercept, infliximab binds to and thereby neutralizes TNF. However, the two drugs are structurally different: whereas etanercept is composed of two TNF *receptors,* infliximab is a TNF *antibody.*

In patients with RA, infliximab is approved for combined use with methotrexate to reduce symptoms and delay disease progression. Infliximab is also approved for psoriasis (see Chapter 105), psoriatic arthritis, ankylosing spondylitis, and two intestinal disorders: Crohn's disease and ulcerative colitis (see Chapter 80).

Adverse Effects. Like etanercept, infliximab has immunosuppressant actions that can increase the risk for serious infection, including bacterial sepsis, invasive fungal infections, HBV infection, and TB. Accordingly, the drug should not be given to patients with chronic infections, and should be temporarily withdrawn if an acute infection develops. Patients should receive a TB test and HBV test to rule out latent infection before treatment.

Like other TNF inhibitors, infliximab has been associated with rare cases of heart failure, liver failure, hematologic disorders, neurologic disorders, severe allergic reactions, and cancer.

Infusion reactions are common, manifesting as flu-like symptoms, headache, fever, chills, dyspnea, hypotension, skin reactions, and GI disturbance. Rarely, patients experience anaphylaxis. Symptoms can be reduced by pretreatment with an antihistamine, acetaminophen, and/or a glucocorticoid. Mild reactions can be managed by slowing or interrupting the infusion. If anaphylaxis develops, the infusion should be stopped.

Adalimumab

Like infliximab, adalimumab [Humira] is a monoclonal antibody that binds to and thereby neutralizes TNF. The drug is indicated for adults with moderate to severe RA who have not responded adequately to one or more DMARDs. In these patients, adalimumab can reduce symptoms and slow progression of joint damage. The drug may be used alone or in combination with methotrexate or other DMARDs. In addition to RA, adalimumab is approved for ankylosing spondylitis, juvenile idiopathic arthritis, plaque psoriasis, psoriatic arthritis, ulcerative colitis, and Crohn's disease.

Adalimumab is generally well tolerated. The most common side effects are injection-site reactions (rash, erythema, itching, pain, swelling), which develop in about 20% of patients. Like other TNF inhibitors, adalimumab can promote serious infections (e.g., bacterial sepsis, invasive fungal infections, HBV infection, TB), and has been associated with rare cases of heart failure, liver failure, hematologic disorders, neurologic disorders, severe allergic reactions, and cancer.

Golimumab

Golimumab [Simponi, Simponi Aria] is approved for RA—but only in combination with methotrexate. Like infliximab, golimumab is a monoclonal antibody that binds with and thereby neutralizes TNF. In addition to RA, golimumab is approved for treatment of ulcerative colitis, ankylosing spondylitis, and psoriatic arthritis.

In clinical trials, the most common adverse effects were injection-site reactions, upper respiratory tract infections, and nasopharyngitis. However, except for injection-site reactions, the incidence of these adverse effects was only slightly higher than in patients receiving placebo. Like other TNF inhibitors, golimumab can promote serious infections (e.g., bacterial sepsis, invasive fungal infections, HBV infection, TB), and has been associated with rare cases of heart failure, liver failure, hematologic disorders, neurologic disorders, severe allergic reactions, and cancer.

Certolizumab Pegol

Certolizumab pegol [Cimzia] is a monoclonal antibody derivative designed to neutralize TNF. The drug consists of a recombinant humanized Fab antibody fragment that has been covalently bound to polyethylene glycol (PEG). Because of this pegylation (binding to PEG), the drug is eliminated slowly, with a half-life of 17 days. Certolizumab is approved for treatment of adults with moderate to severe RA, Crohn's disease, ankylosing spondylitis, and psoriatic arthritis. In patients with RA, the combination of certolizumab plus methotrexate is more effective than certolizumab alone.

Certolizumab can cause serious adverse effects. In clinical trials, the most common events were upper respiratory tract infections, urinary tract infections, and arthralgia. Like other TNF inhibitors, certolizumab can promote serious infections (e.g., bacterial sepsis, invasive fungal infections, HBV infection, TB), and has been associated with rare cases of heart failure, liver failure, hematologic disorders, neurologic disorders, severe allergic reactions, and cancer.

Rituximab, a B-Lymphocyte–Depleting Agent

Actions and Uses

Rituximab [Rituxan] reduces the number of B lymphocytes, cells that play an important role in the autoimmune attack on joints. As a result, rituximab can reduce symptoms of RA and slow disease progression. How does it work? Rituximab is a monoclonal antibody directed against CD20, an antigen found exclusively on the surface of B lymphocytes. When rituximab binds with CD20, the immune system attacks the rituximab–B-cell complex, causing B-cell lysis and death.

Rituximab, in combination with methotrexate, is indicated for IV therapy of adults with moderate to severe RA who have not responded to one or more TNF antagonists. In addition, rituximab is indicated for two inflammatory disorders of blood vessels—Wegener's granulomatosis and microscopic polyangiitis—and for two types of cancer: B-cell non-Hodgkin's lymphoma and B-cell chronic lymphocytic leukemia (see Chapter 103).

Adverse Effects

Infusion Reactions. Rituximab can cause severe infusion-related hypersensitivity reactions, beginning within 30 to 120 minutes. The immediate reaction and its sequelae include hypotension, bronchospasm, angioedema, hypoxia, pulmonary infiltrates, myocardial infarction, and cardiogenic shock. Deaths have occurred within 24 hours. To reduce the risk for these events, patients should be premedicated with an antihistamine and acetaminophen. Premedication with an IV glucocorticoid such as methylprednisolone is also recommended for patients with RA. Patients must be closely monitored during the infusion. If a severe reaction occurs, management includes giving glucocorticoids, epinephrine, bronchodilators, and oxygen.

Mucocutaneous Reactions. Rituximab has been associated with severe mucocutaneous reactions, including SJS, lichenoid dermatitis, vesiculobullous dermatitis, and TEN. Deaths have occurred. Reaction onset is typically 1 to 3 weeks after rituximab exposure. Patients who experience these reactions should seek immediate medical attention and should not receive rituximab again.

Hepatitis B Reactivation. There have been reports of HBV reactivation, leading to fulminant hepatitis, hepatic failure, and death. Patients at high risk for HBV should be screened before getting rituximab. Asymptomatic carriers should be closely monitored for clinical and laboratory signs of active HBV infection while taking rituximab and for several months after stopping.

Progressive Multifocal Leukoencephalopathy. Rituximab has been associated with rare cases of progressive multifocal leukoencephalopathy (PML). PML is a severe infection of the CNS caused by reactivation of the JC virus, an opportunistic pathogen resistant to all available drugs. Most cases have occurred in patients being treated for non-Hodgkin's lymphoma. Patients and prescribers should be alert for any new neurologic signs and symptoms. If PML is diagnosed, rituximab should be discontinued immediately.

Other Adverse Effects. Like other monoclonal antibodies, rituximab can cause a flu-like syndrome, especially during the initial infusion. Symptoms include fever, chills, nausea, vomiting, and myalgia. Rituximab causes transient neutropenia, but this does not appear to increase the risk for infection.

Abatacept, a T-Cell Activation Inhibitor

Abatacept [Orencia], a first-in-class T-cell activation inhibitor, reduces symptoms of RA and disease progression. Patients who have not responded adequately to methotrexate or TNF antagonists have experienced significant improvement with this drug. Like other biologic DMARDs, abatacept poses a risk for serious infections and may also pose a small risk for cancer.

Therapeutic Uses

Abatacept has two approved indications: to reduce symptoms and delay disease progression in *adults with moderately to severely active RA* and to decrease symptoms of moderately to severely active *polyarticular juvenile idiopathic arthritis* in children 6 years and older. For adult patients with RA, abatacept may be used alone or in combination with most other DMARDs, but *not* with TNF antagonists or anakinra. For children with juvenile idiopathic arthritis, the drug may be used alone or in combination with methotrexate.

Mechanism of Action

In patients with RA, *activated* T lymphocytes play a key role in the autoimmune attack on joints. Abatacept prevents T-cell activation. Here's how. For T cells to achieve full activity, they must be stimulated by antigen-presenting cells (APCs). Abatacept—a complex molecule composed of a ligand (cytotoxic T-lymphocyte–associated antigen 4) linked to IgG1 (an isotype of IgG)—binds with receptors on APCs and thereby prevents the APCs from activating T cells. The results are reduced T-cell proliferation and reduced production of interferon gamma, interleukins, and TNF.

Adverse Effects

Abatacept is generally well tolerated. The most common adverse effects are headache, upper respiratory infection, nasopharyngitis, and nausea.

Because abatacept suppresses immune function, the drug can increase the risk for *serious infections*. Infections seen most often are pneumonia, cellulitis, bronchitis, diverticulitis, pyelonephritis, and urinary tract infections. Patients should be told about infection risk and advised to report suspected infection immediately. If a serious infection develops, abatacept should be discontinued.

Abatacept may blunt the effect of all *vaccines* and may increase the risk for infection from live virus vaccines. Before abatacept is given to children, all vaccinations should be up to date. Live virus vaccines should not be used in children or adults during abatacept use and for 3 months after stopping.

Drug Interactions

Abatacept should not be used in conjunction with *TNF antagonists*. The combination increases the risk for serious infection and offers no benefit over abatacept alone.

Tocilizumab, an Interleukin-6 Receptor Antagonist

In patients with RA, IL-6 helps amplify the autoimmune attack on joints. Accordingly, drugs that block the actions of IL-6 can reduce RA symptoms and disease progression. At this time, tocilizumab is the only drug that works by this mechanism.

Actions and Therapeutic Use

Tocilizumab [Actemra] is a first-in-class IL-6 receptor antagonist. In 2010, the FDA approved tocilizumab for IV therapy of adults with moderately to severely active RA. However, owing to the risk for infection and other serious adverse effects, tocilizumab is indicated only for those patients with RA who have not responded adequately to other DMARDs. In five clinical trials involving more than 4000 patients, tocilizumab was significantly more effective than placebo at reducing joint tenderness and swelling. Tocilizumab may be combined with methotrexate, but not with TNF inhibitors or other DMARDs that increase the risk for infection. In addition to treatment of RA, tocilizumab has also received FDA approval for the management of polyarticular juvenile idiopathic arthritis and systemic juvenile idiopathic arthritis.

How does tocilizumab work? The drug is a monoclonal antibody that blocks receptors for IL-6, a proinflammatory cytokine that helps mediate the autoimmune attack against the joints of patients with RA. By blocking IL-6 receptors, tocilizumab prevents IL-6 from promoting injury. Tocilizumab is the first drug to work by this mechanism.

Adverse Effects

The most serious adverse effects are infections, GI perforation, liver injury, and hematologic effects: neutropenia and thrombocytopenia. Other adverse effects include headache, nasopharyngitis, hypertension, and increased cholesterol levels.

Serious Infections. Owing to its immunosuppressant actions, tocilizumab increases the risk for life-threatening infections. Infections seen in clinical trials include TB, invasive fungal infections, and opportunistic infections caused by bacteria, viruses, protozoa, and other pathogens. Before starting tocilizumab, patients should be tested for latent TB and treated as indicated. During tocilizumab therapy, patients should be closely monitored for signs and symptoms of infection. In the event of increased transaminase levels, reduced neutrophil counts, or reduced platelet counts—tocilizumab should be given in reduced dosage or discontinued, depending on the magnitude of the change. Treatment should be interrupted if the patient develops a serious infection.

GI Perforation. In clinical trials, perforation of the colon occurred rarely. Most cases were complications of pre-existing diverticulitis (i.e., inflammation of diverticula [small outpouchings] along the colon wall). Patients at high risk for perforation—especially those with diverticulitis—should be closely monitored. Patients should be instructed to contact their prescriber in the event of severe, persistent abdominal pain.

Liver Injury. Tocilizumab can cause liver injury, as indicated by elevation of circulating liver transaminases (aspartate aminotransferase and alanine aminotransferase). Tocilizumab should not be initiated if transaminase levels are more than 2 times the upper limit of normal (ULN). Transaminase levels should be monitored every 4 to 8 weeks during treatment, and if the levels exceed 5 times the ULN, tocilizumab should be discontinued.

Neutropenia and Thrombocytopenia. Tocilizumab can reduce counts of neutrophils and platelets. Neutrophil reduction increases the risk for infection. In clinical trials, reduction of platelets was *not* associated with increased bleeding. Neutrophil and platelet counts should be determined at baseline and every 4 to 8 weeks during treatment. Tocilizumab should not be initiated if the absolute neutrophil count (ANC) is below $2000/mm^3$ or if the platelet count is below $100,000/mm^3$. Patients taking tocilizumab should discontinue the drug if the ANC falls below $500/mm^3$ or if the platelet count falls below $50,000/mm^3$.

Drug Interactions

In general, tocilizumab should not be combined with other *strong immunosuppressants*, owing to an increased risk for serious infections. Antirheumatic drugs to avoid include the TNF antagonists (e.g., etanercept), T-cell inhibitors (e.g., abatacept), IL-1 antagonists (e.g., anakinra), and drugs that block the CD20 antigen (e.g., rituximab).

Tocilizumab can *reduce blood levels of other drugs*. Under normal circumstances, IL-6 suppresses the activity of several cytochrome P450 drug-metabolizing isoenzymes. By blocking receptors for IL-6, tocilizumab can negate that suppression and can thereby increase rates of drug metabolism. Drugs whose levels may be diminished include oral contraceptives, warfarin (an anticoagulant), proton pump inhibitors (which reduce gastric acidity), and HMG-CoA reductase inhibitors (which reduce cholesterol levels). Dosages for all of these agents may need to be increased.

Anakinra, an Interleukin-1 Receptor Antagonist

Anakinra [Kineret] reduces symptoms of RA by blocking receptors for IL-1, a proinflammatory cytokine that plays a central role in synovial inflammation and joint destruction. The drug is indicated for patients with moderate to severe RA that has not responded to one or more nonbiologic DMARDs (e.g., methotrexate). It is also approved for treatment of neonatal-onset multisystem inflammatory disease.

Like the TNF antagonists, anakinra poses a risk for serious infections. Accordingly, the drug should not be given to patients with active infection, and it should be stopped if a serious infection develops. Because both anakinra and the TNF antagonists increase infection risk, these drugs should not be combined.

KEY POINTS

- The objectives of RA therapy are to (1) reduce symptoms (pain, inflammation, stiffness), (2) maintain joint function and range of motion, (3) minimize systemic involvement, and (4) delay disease progression.
- RA is treated with three classes of drugs: (1) nonsteroidal anti-inflammatory drugs (NSAIDs); (2) glucocorticoids; and (3) disease-modifying antirheumatic drugs (DMARDs).
- DMARDs can be divided into two groups: (1) nonbiologic (traditional) DMARDs, which are small molecules produced by conventional chemical techniques; and (2) biologic DMARDs, which are large molecules produced by recombinant DNA technology.
- NSAIDs act quickly to relieve symptoms, but do not prevent joint injury and do not delay disease progression.
- Glucocorticoids act quickly and may delay disease progression.
- DMARDs delay disease progression and reduce joint injury, but onset of benefits is delayed.
- In the past, treatment of RA was initiated with NSAIDs alone; DMARDs were added only after NSAIDs could no longer control symptoms. Today, guidelines recommend initiating DMARDs within 3 months of RA diagnosis; the rationale is to delay joint degeneration and delay disease progression. During the DMARD latency period, NSAIDs (and sometimes glucocorticoids) are used to control symptoms.
- NSAIDs are much safer than glucocorticoids and DMARDs.
- Because glucocorticoids cause serious toxicity when used long term, they are generally reserved for short-term use to (1) control symptoms while responses to DMARDs are developing or (2) supplement other drugs when symptoms flare.
- Second-generation NSAIDs (COX-2 inhibitors, or coxibs) may cause less GI ulceration than first-generation NSAIDs, but are more expensive.
- The doses of NSAIDs used for RA are much higher than the doses used to relieve pain or fever.
- Methotrexate, a nonbiologic DMARD, acts relatively quickly and is considered the DMARD of first choice by most rheumatologists.
- Etanercept, a biologic DMARD, neutralizes TNF and thereby suppresses the autoimmune attack on joints.
- Etanercept and other TNF antagonists pose a significant risk for serious infections (e.g., bacterial sepsis, invasive fungal infections, TB, HBV infection), and are associated with rare cases of heart failure, liver failure, hematologic disorders, neurologic disorders, severe allergic reactions, and cancer.

Please visit **http://evolve.elsevier.com/Lehne** for chapter-specific NCLEX® examination review questions.

Summary of Major Nursing Implications[a]

TUMOR NECROSIS FACTOR ANTAGONISTS

Adalimumab
Certolizumab pegol
Etanercept
Golimumab
Infliximab

The nursing implications that follow pertain only to the use of TNF antagonists for rheumatoid arthritis.

Preadministration Assessment

Therapeutic Goal

TNF inhibitors are used to reduce symptoms and delay disease progression in patients with moderate to severe RA.

Identifying High-Risk Patients

TNF inhibitors are *contraindicated* in patients with demyelinating disorders, severe heart failure, and active infections, including TB and HBV infection.

Exercise *caution* in patients who are immunosuppressed (e.g., owing to HIV infection or immunosuppressant drugs) and in those with diabetes, mild heart failure, liver dysfunction, latent TB, latent HBV infection, a history of recurrent infection, and any condition that predisposes to acquiring an infection.

Implementation: Administration

Routes

Subcutaneous. Adalimumab, certolizumab, etanercept, golimumab.

Intravenous. Infliximab, golimumab.

Administration

Adalimumab, Certolizumab, Etanercept, Golimumab. **Teach patients and caregivers how to administer subQ injections, using either a syringe (adalimumab, certolizumab, etanercept, golimumab) or an auto-injector (adalimumab, etanercept, golimumab). Instruct patients to (1) inject medication into the abdomen or anterior thigh, (2) rotate the injection site, and (3) avoid areas where the skin is tender, bruised, red, or hard.**

Infliximab. To prepare the infusion solution, dissolve infliximab powder (100 mg) in 10 mL of sterile water, and then dilute this solution with 0.9% sodium chloride to a final volume of 250 mL. Discard solutions that are discolored or that contain particles. Administer by slow IV infusion (over 2 hours or more)—starting within 3 hours of preparing the solution—using an infusion set with an in-line filter. All patients should also receive methotrexate (oral or subQ). Pretreat with acetaminophen, an antihistamine, and/or a

Summary of Major Nursing Implications[a]—cont'd

glucocorticoid to reduce infusion reactions (see the following discussion).

Golimumab. Golimumab [Simponi Aria] is supplied as 50 mg in 4 mL of solution for IV administration. The recommended dosage is 2 mg/kg over 30 minutes initially, repeated once in 4 weeks, and then every 8 weeks.

Ongoing Evaluation and Interventions

Minimizing Adverse Effects

Serious Infections. TNF antagonists increase the risk for serious infections, including invasive fungal infections (e.g., histoplasmosis, coccidioidomycosis, candidiasis), reactivated HBV infection, and infections caused by *M. tuberculosis* and other opportunistic pathogens. Risk is increased by diabetes, HIV infection, and concurrent use of immunosuppressant drugs.

In general, avoid TNF antagonists in patients with active infections, and closely monitor those who develop a new infection. Use caution in patients with a history of recurrent infection or any condition that predisposes them to acquiring an infection (e.g., advanced or poorly controlled diabetes). If a severe infection develops, TNF antagonists should be discontinued. **Inform patients about the risk for infection, and instruct them to seek medical attention if signs of infection develop.**

To minimize the risk for TB, test patients for latent TB (using a blood test or tuberculin skin test); if the test is positive, treat for TB before starting the TNF antagonist. During TNF antagonist treatment, monitor closely for the development of TB.

To minimize the risk for HBV reactivation, test for HBV before starting the TNF antagonist. Closely monitor patients with a positive result. If reactivation of HBV infection occurs, stop the TNF antagonist and treat with antiviral drugs.

Allergic Reactions. Rarely, TNF antagonists have been associated with severe allergic reactions, including Stevens-Johnson syndrome, erythema multiforme, and toxic epidermal necrolysis. **Inform patients about the risk for a severe reaction, and instruct them to seek medical attention if one develops.**

Heart Failure. TNF antagonists may cause new-onset heart failure and may worsen existing heart failure. Exercise caution in patients with mild heart failure, and monitor them closely for heart failure progression. Avoid TNF antagonists in patients with severe heart failure.

Cancer. TNF antagonists may increase the risk for lymphoma and other malignancies, primarily in children, adolescents, and young adults. **Counsel patients about cancer risk.**

Hematologic Disorders. TNF antagonists may pose a risk for hematologic disorders, including neutropenia, thrombocytopenia, and aplastic anemia. **Inform patients about signs of a blood disorder (persistent fever, bruising, bleeding, pallor), and advise them to seek medical attention if these develop.** If a significant hematologic abnormality is diagnosed, discontinuing the TNF antagonist should be considered.

Liver Injury. Rarely, TNF inhibitors have been associated with severe liver injury, including acute liver failure. Some patients have required a liver transplant, and some have died. **Inform patients about symptoms of liver injury—fatigue, yellow skin, yellow eyes, anorexia, right-sided abdominal pain, dark brown urine—and advise them to seek medical attention if these develop.** If severe liver injury is diagnosed, discontinuing the TNF antagonist should be considered. Exercise caution in patients with pre-existing liver dysfunction.

CNS Demyelinating Disorders. TNF antagonists have been associated with rare cases of CNS demyelinating disorders, including multiple sclerosis, myelitis, and optic neuritis. Avoid TNF antagonists in patients with a pre-existing or recent-onset demyelinating disorder.

Injection-Site Reactions: Adalimumab, Certolizumab, Etanercept, and Golimumab. Injection-site reactions—redness, swelling, itching, pain—are common with these drugs. **Inform patients that symptoms usually subside in a few days, and advise them to contact the prescriber if the reaction persists.**

Infusion Reactions: Infliximab. Infusion reactions—flu-like symptoms, headache, fever, chills, dyspnea, hypotension, skin reactions, GI disturbance—are common with *infliximab.* To reduce symptoms, pretreat with an antihistamine, acetaminophen, and/or a glucocorticoid. Manage mild reactions by slowing or interrupting the infusion. In the event of a severe reaction (e.g., anaphylaxis), stop the infusion and don't use infliximab again.

Minimizing Adverse Interactions

Immunosuppressants. Drugs that suppress immune function (e.g., glucocorticoids, methotrexate, tocilizumab, anakinra, abatacept) increase the risk for infections. Use these drugs with caution.

Live Virus Vaccines. TNF antagonists may increase the risk for acquiring or transmitting infection following immunization with a live virus vaccine. Accordingly, live virus vaccines should be avoided. **Inform parents that pediatric vaccinations should be current before therapy with a TNF antagonist starts.**

[a]Patient education information is highlighted as **blue text**.

CHAPTER

74 Drug Therapy for Gout

Gout is a painful inflammatory disorder seen mainly in men. Symptoms result from the deposition of uric acid crystals in joints. We begin by discussing the pathophysiology of gout, after which we discuss the drugs used for treatment.

PATHOPHYSIOLOGY OF GOUT

Gout is a recurrent inflammatory disorder characterized by *hyperuricemia* (high blood levels of uric acid) and episodes of *severe joint pain,* typically in the large toe. Hyperuricemia—defined as blood uric acid above 7 mg/dL in men or 6 mg/dL in women—can occur through two mechanisms: (1) excessive production of uric acid and (2) impaired renal excretion of uric acid. Acute attacks are precipitated by crystallization of sodium urate (the sodium salt of uric acid) in the synovial space. Deposition of urate crystals promotes inflammation by triggering a complex series of events. A key feature of the inflammatory process is infiltration of leukocytes, which, when inside the synovial cavity, phagocytize urate crystals and then break down, causing release of destructive lysosomal enzymes. When hyperuricemia is chronic, large and gritty deposits, known as *tophi,* may form in the affected joint. Also, the deposition of urate crystals in the kidney may cause renal damage. Fortunately, when gout is detected and treated early, the disease can be arrested and these chronic sequelae avoided.

OVERVIEW OF DRUG THERAPY

In patients with gout, drugs are used in two ways. First, they are given short term to relieve symptoms of an acute gouty attack. Second, they are given long term to lower blood levels of uric acid.

In patients with infrequent flare-ups (fewer than three per year), treatment of symptoms may be all that is needed. Nonsteroidal anti-inflammatory drugs (NSAIDs) are considered first-line agents for relieving pain of an acute gouty attack. Glucocorticoids are an acceptable option. In the past, colchicine was considered a drug of choice for acute gout—even though it has a poor risk/benefit ratio. Today, colchicine is generally reserved for patients who are unresponsive to or intolerant of safer agents.

In patients with chronic gout, tophaceous gout, or frequent gouty attacks (three or more per year), drugs for hyperuricemia are indicated. Three types of drugs may be employed: agents that decrease uric acid production, agents that increase uric acid excretion (*uricosuric* drugs), and agents that convert uric acid to allantoin.

DRUGS FOR ACUTE GOUTY ARTHRITIS

Nonsteroidal Anti-Inflammatory Drugs

For acute gouty arthritis, NSAIDs are considered agents of first choice. Compared with colchicine, NSAIDs are better tolerated and their effects are more predictable. Benefits derive from the suppression of inflammation. Treatment should start as soon as possible after symptom onset. Most patients experience marked relief within 24 hours; swelling subsides over the next few days. Adverse effects of NSAIDs include gastrointestinal (GI) ulceration, impaired renal function, fluid retention, and increased risk for cardiovascular events. However, because the duration of treatment is brief, the risk for these complications is low. Which NSAID should be used? There is no good evidence that any NSAID is superior to the others for treatment of gout. Commonly used NSAIDs include indomethacin [Indocin], naproxen [Naprosyn, Anaprox ♣, others], and diclofenac sodium [Voltaren]. Dosages are provided in Table 74.1.

Safety Alert

NSAIDS

NSAIDs may increase the risk for myocardial infarction, stroke, and other thromboembolic events. NSAIDs also increase the risk for dangerous gastrointestinal adverse effects, such as bleeding, ulceration, and perforation.

Glucocorticoids

Glucocorticoids (e.g., prednisone), given orally or intramuscularly, are highly effective for relieving an acute gouty attack—although NSAIDs are generally preferred. Candidates for glucocorticoid therapy include patients who are hypersensitive to NSAIDs, patients who have medical conditions that contraindicate the use of NSAIDs, and patients with severe

TABLE 74.1 ▪ Preparations, Dosages, and Administration of Antigout Drugs

Drug	Preparation	Dosage	Administration
NONSTEROIDAL ANTI-INFLAMMATORY DRUGS			
Indomethacin [Indocin, Tivorbex]	Indocin: 50-mg rectal suppository, 25 mg/5 mL oral suspension Tivorbex: 20-, 40-mg capsules Generic: 25-, 50-mg capsules Generic ER: 75-mg capsules	50 mg 3 times daily initially until pain is tolerable, then reduce dosage and continue dosing for 3–5 days	To decrease GI effects, administer with or after meals or with a snack ER forms should be swallowed whole
Naproxen [Anaprox 🍁, Naprosyn, Naprelan, many others]	Anaprox 🍁: 275 mg Anaprox DS 🍁: 550 mg Naprosyn: 500-mg scored tablets EC-Naprosyn: 375-, 500-mg enteric-coated tablets Generic: 250-, 375-, 500-mg tablets Naprelan (ER): 375-, 500-, 750-mg controlled-release tablets	Naprosyn: 750 mg initially, then 250 mg every 8 hr until attack subsides Naprosyn ER: 1 tablet initially, then 1 tablet daily until attack subsides Anaprox 🍁: 825 mg initially, then 275 mg every 8 hr until attack subsides	To decrease GI effects, administer with or after meals or with a snack ER and EC forms should be swallowed whole
ANTIGOUT ANTI-INFLAMMATORY DRUG			
Colchicine [Colcrys, Mitigare]	Colcrys: 0.6-mg scored tablet Mitigare: 0.6-mg capsule	Acute attack (Colcrys only): 1.2 mg at first sign of the flare, followed by 0.6 mg 1 hr later (maximum 1.8 mg/24 hr) Prophylaxis (Colcrys, Mitigare): 0.6 mg once or twice daily (maximum 1.2 mg/24 hr)	Administer with or without food Do not take with grapefruit juice
GLUCOCORTICOIDS			
Prednisone (oral) [Deltasone]	Deltasone: 20-mg (scored) tablets	30 to 50 mg once daily or in two divided doses until pain is tolerable; then gradually taper off the drug over 7–10 days	Administer at mealtime or with food to decrease GI upset
Triamcinolone acetate (IM) [Aristospan, Kenalog]	Aristospan: 20 mg/mL in 1-mL and 5-mL vials Kenalog: 10 mg/mL in 5-mL vial; 40 mg/mL in 1-, 5-, and 10-mL vials	40–60 mg; may repeat after 1–4 days if flare continues	Shake well to ensure homogeneous suspension of medication, then withdraw into syringe immediately
XANTHINE OXIDASE INHIBITORS			
Allopurinol [Zyloprim]	100-, 300-mg tablets	Dosages should be individualized to decrease plasma urate to 6 mg/dL[a] Chronic tophaceous gout: 100 mg once daily, then increase by 50- to 100-mg increments every few weeks until urate target level is reached Standard maintenance dose: 300 mg a day up to a maximum of 800 mg/day Secondary hyperuricemias in adults: 100–800 mg/day	May be taken with or without food
Febuxostat [Uloric]	40-, 80-mg tablets	40 mg/day initially; increase to 80 mg/day if needed	May be taken with or without food
URICOSURIC AGENTS			
Probenecid [generic only]	500-mg tablets	250 mg twice daily for 1 week Maintenance dosage is 500 mg twice daily	Administration with food decreases GI upset

Continued

TABLE 74.1 ▪ Preparations, Dosages, and Administration of Antigout Drugs—cont'd

Drug	Preparation	Dosage	Administration
RECOMBINANT URIC ACID OXIDASE			
Pegloticase [Krystexxa]	8 mg/mL	8 mg IV every 2 weeks	Dilute 1 mL in 250 mL NS or ½ NS IV solution and administer over 2 hr Monitor for infusion reaction
Rasburicase [Elitek, Fasturtec ♣]	1.5-, 7.5-mg/vial supplied as a powder for reconstitution	0.2 mg/kg IV on 5 consecutive days	Avoid vigorous agitation during reconstitution Infuse over 30 minutes
COMBINATION DRUGS			
Colchicine and probenecid [generic only]	Colchicine 0.5 mg + probenecid 500 mg	1 tablet daily for 1 week, then 1 tablet twice daily	Do not begin therapy in the presence of an acute gout flare

[a]Dosage should be reduced in patients with renal disease.
EC, Enteric coated; *ER,* extended release.

gout that is unresponsive to NSAIDs. Because of their effects on carbohydrate metabolism, glucocorticoids should be avoided, when possible, in patients prone to hyperglycemia. For oral therapy, prednisone can be used. For intramuscular (IM) therapy, triamcinolone acetonide can be used. Glucocorticoids are discussed in Chapter 72.

Colchicine

Colchicine [Colcrys, Mitigare] is an anti-inflammatory agent with effects specific for gout. In the past, colchicine was considered a first-line drug for gout. However, owing to the common occurrence of GI toxicity and the availability of safe and effective alternatives, its use has declined.

Therapeutic Use

Colchicine has two applications in gout. First, it can be used short term to treat an acute gouty attack. Second, it can be used long term to prevent attacks from recurring. *Colcrys* is approved for both uses. *Mitigare* is approved only for prophylaxis. (On a side note, conclusions of a 2015 Cochrane review of 39 trials with 4992 participants were that colchicine also may decrease the risk for myocardial infarction [MI] and improve outcomes post-MI.)

Acute Gouty Arthritis. High-dose colchicine can produce dramatic relief of an acute gouty attack. Within hours, patients whose pain had made movement impossible are able to walk. Inflammation disappears completely within 2 to 3 days.

Prophylaxis of Gouty Attacks. When taken during asymptomatic periods, low-dose colchicine can decrease the frequency and intensity of acute flare-ups. Colchicine is also given for prophylaxis when urate-lowering therapy is initiated because there is a tendency for gouty episodes to increase at this time.

Mechanism of Action

We do not fully understand how colchicine relieves or prevents episodes of gout. We do know that colchicine does *not* decrease urate production or removal. It may work, at least in part, by inhibiting leukocyte infiltration: In the absence of leukocytes, there is no phagocytosis of uric acid and no subsequent release of lysosomal enzymes. How does colchicine inhibit leukocyte migration? It disrupts microtubules, the structures required for cellular motility. Because microtubules are also required for cell division, colchicine is toxic to any tissue that has a large percentage of proliferating cells. Disruption of cell division in the GI tract and bone marrow underlies major toxicities of the drug.

Pharmacokinetics

Colchicine is readily absorbed after oral dosing, in both the presence and absence of food. Large amounts re-enter the intestine through the bile and intestinal secretions and then undergo reabsorption. Final elimination occurs primarily through two processes: metabolism by hepatic CYP3A4 (the 3A4 isoenzyme of cytochrome P450) and renal excretion of intact drug.

Adverse Effects

Gastrointestinal Effects. The most characteristic side effects are nausea, vomiting, diarrhea, and abdominal pain. These responses, which occur during the treatment of acute gouty attacks, result from injury to the rapidly proliferating cells of the GI epithelium. With the high doses used in the past, these GI effects developed in nearly all patients. However, with the lower doses used today, GI toxicity is less common, but still develops in 25% of patients. If GI symptoms occur, colchicine should be discontinued immediately, regardless of the status of joint pain.

Myelosuppression. Injury to rapidly proliferating cells can suppress bone marrow function and can thereby cause leukopenia, granulocytopenia, thrombocytopenia, and pancytopenia. Accordingly, colchicine should be used with caution in patients with hematologic disorders.

Myopathy. Colchicine can cause rhabdomyolysis (muscle breakdown) during long-term low-dose therapy. Risk is increased in patients with renal and hepatic impairment and in those taking statin drugs (e.g., atorvastatin, simvastatin), which can cause rhabdomyolysis on their own. Patients should be monitored for signs of muscle injury (tenderness, pain, weakness).

Drug Interactions

Statins. As noted, atorvastatin, simvastatin, and other statins can increase the risk for colchicine-induced muscle injury. If possible, combined use of statins and colchicine should be avoided.

Drugs That Can Increase Colchicine Levels. Life-threatening reactions have occurred when combining colchicine with two classes of drugs: *P-glycoprotein* (PGP) *inhibitors* and *inhibitors of CYP3A4.* Recall from Chapter 4 that PGP is a transporter protein that can reduce plasma drug levels through effects in the liver, kidney, and intestine. Hence, by inhibiting PGP, drugs such as cyclosporine and ranolazine can cause colchicine to accumulate to toxic levels. Similarly, by inhibiting CYP3A4, drugs such as ketoconazole, clarithromycin, and the HIV protease inhibitors (e.g., nelfinavir, ritonavir) can cause colchicine levels to rise. Accordingly, combined use of colchicine with strong inhibitors of either PGP or CYP3A4 should generally be avoided and is contraindicated in patients with hepatic or renal impairment.

Precautions and Contraindications

Colchicine should be used with care in older adult and debilitated patients and in patients with cardiac, renal, hepatic, and GI disease.

As noted, combined use of colchicine with strong inhibitors of PGP or CYP3A4 should generally be avoided. For both acute therapy and long-term prophylaxis, dosage should be adjusted on the basis of liver function, kidney function, and usage of interacting drugs. The prescribing information for Mitigare, but not Colcrys, includes contraindications for hepatic or renal impairment.

Colchicine should be avoided during pregnancy unless the perceived benefits outweigh the potential risks.

Preparations, Dosage, and Administration

Information on drug preparations, dosage, and administration is provided in Table 74.1.

PATIENT-CENTERED CARE ACROSS THE LIFE SPAN

Drugs for Gout

Life Stage	Patient Care Concerns
Children	U.S. labeling for indomethacin recommends using the lowest dose that is effective at the shortest possible duration. Canadian labeling contraindicates its use for patients under 14 years of age. When given for gout prophylaxis (as opposed to familiar Mediterranean fever), colchicine is not recommended for patients under 16 years old. Febuxostat is not recommended for children. Allopurinol may be given to children under 6 years old for the purpose of treating hyperuricemia associated with cancer therapy. Probenecid has been given to children as young as 2 years for purposes unrelated to gout.
Pregnant women	Although most NSAIDs are Pregnancy Risk Category C,[a] some studies have demonstrated fetal cardiovascular abnormalities and cleft palate following NSAID exposure. Exposure to indomethacin after 30 weeks' gestation has resulted in a number of abnormalities, resulting in a Pregnancy Risk Category of D[a] if taken later in pregnancy. Animal studies with febuxostat have demonstrated an increase in fetal mortality. Colchicine, allopurinol, and rasburicase are Pregnancy Risk Category C.[a] Because rasburicase is indicated for cancer-associated hyperuricemia, additional factors may affect decisions to become pregnant. Probenecid has not been associated with increased fetal risk.
Breast-feeding women	U.S. labeling recommends against breast-feeding by women taking indomethacin and naproxen. Canadian labeling contraindicates breast-feeding by mothers taking these drugs. Breast-feeding is not recommended for other drugs taken for gout. For patients taking xanthine oxidase inhibitors, Canadian labeling contraindicates breast-feeding. Women taking rasburicase should not breast-feed.
Older adults	Beers Criteria lists both indomethacin and naproxen among those drugs considered potentially inappropriate for patients age 56 and older and notes that of all NSAIDs indomethacin carries the greatest risk. Colchicine can be dangerous if the older patient has renal impairment.

[a]As of 2020, the FDA will no longer use Pregnancy Risk Categories. Please refer to Chapter 9 for more information.

DRUGS FOR HYPERURICEMIA (URATE-LOWERING THERAPY)

Urate-lowering therapy (ULT) is indicated for patients who experience relatively frequent acute gouty attacks. The goal is to promote dissolution of urate crystals, prevent new crystal formation, prevent disease progression, reduce the frequency of acute attacks, and improve quality of life. For most patients, ULT must continue lifelong.

Five drugs—*allopurinol, febuxostat, probenecid, pegloticase,* and *rasburicase*—are used to reduce uric acid levels. Three mechanisms are involved. Allopurinol and febuxostat inhibit uric acid formation. Probenecid accelerates uric acid excretion. Pegloticase and rasburicase convert uric acid to allantoin, a compound that is readily excreted by the kidney. With all five drugs, the goal is to reduce plasma uric acid to 6 mg/dL or less. These drugs lack anti-inflammatory and analgesic actions, so they are not useful against an acute gouty attack. The effects of all five drugs on uric acid are shown in Fig. 74.1.

Xanthine Oxidase Inhibitors: Allopurinol and Febuxostat

Two xanthine oxidase inhibitors are now available: allopurinol and febuxostat. Both seem equally effective. Allopurinol has been in use for decades, whereas febuxostat is new. Because experience with allopurinol is more extensive and febuxostat is much more expensive, allopurinol is often preferred.

Allopurinol

Therapeutic Uses. Allopurinol [Zyloprim] is the current drug of choice for *chronic tophaceous gout.* By reducing blood uric acid levels, allopurinol prevents new tophus formation and causes regression of tophi that have already formed, thereby allowing joint function to improve. Reversal of hyperuricemia also decreases the risk for nephropathy from the deposition of urate crystals in the kidney.

Allopurinol can be used for hyperuricemia that develops secondary to cancer chemotherapy and to certain blood dyscrasias, such as polycythemia vera, myeloid metaplasia, and leukemia. Hyperuricemia develops during chemotherapy because when cells die, the breakdown of DNA releases uric acid. To minimize hyperuricemia, allopurinol should be administered before chemotherapy starts.

Mechanism of Action. Allopurinol and its major metabolite (alloxanthine) inhibit *xanthine oxidase* (XO), an enzyme required for uric acid formation. XO catalyzes the final two reactions that lead to the formation of uric acid from breakdown products of DNA.

Pharmacokinetics. Allopurinol is well absorbed after oral dosing and then undergoes rapid conversion to alloxanthine, an active metabolite. Alloxanthine is then eliminated slowly by renal excretion. Because alloxanthine has a prolonged half-life (about 25 hours), therapeutic effects are long lasting. Consequently, once-a-day dosing is adequate.

Adverse Effects. Allopurinol is generally well tolerated. The most serious toxicity is a rare but potentially fatal *hypersensitivity syndrome,* characterized by rash, fever, eosinophilia, and dysfunction of the liver and kidneys. If rash or fever develops, allopurinol should be discontinued immediately. Many patients recover spontaneously; others may require hemodialysis or glucocorticoid therapy.

Initial therapy may elicit an *acute gouty attack.* This can be prevented by giving colchicine or a low-dose NSAID.

Mild side effects include *GI reactions* (nausea, vomiting, diarrhea, abdominal discomfort) and *neurologic effects* (drowsiness, headache, metallic taste). Prolonged use (more than 3 years) may cause *cataracts;* periodic ophthalmic examinations are recommended.

The risk for drug accumulation can be a problem if administered to patients with renal impairment. This can be minimized by decreasing the dosage.

Drug Interactions. Allopurinol can inhibit hepatic drug-metabolizing enzymes, thereby delaying the inactivation of other drugs. This interaction is of particular concern for patients taking *warfarin,* whose dosage should be reduced. If possible, combined use with *mercaptopurine* or *azathioprine* should be avoided because both of these anticancer drugs are substrates for XO, and hence could accumulate to toxic levels in the presence of allopurinol. If combined use can't be avoided, then dosages of mercaptopurine and azathioprine

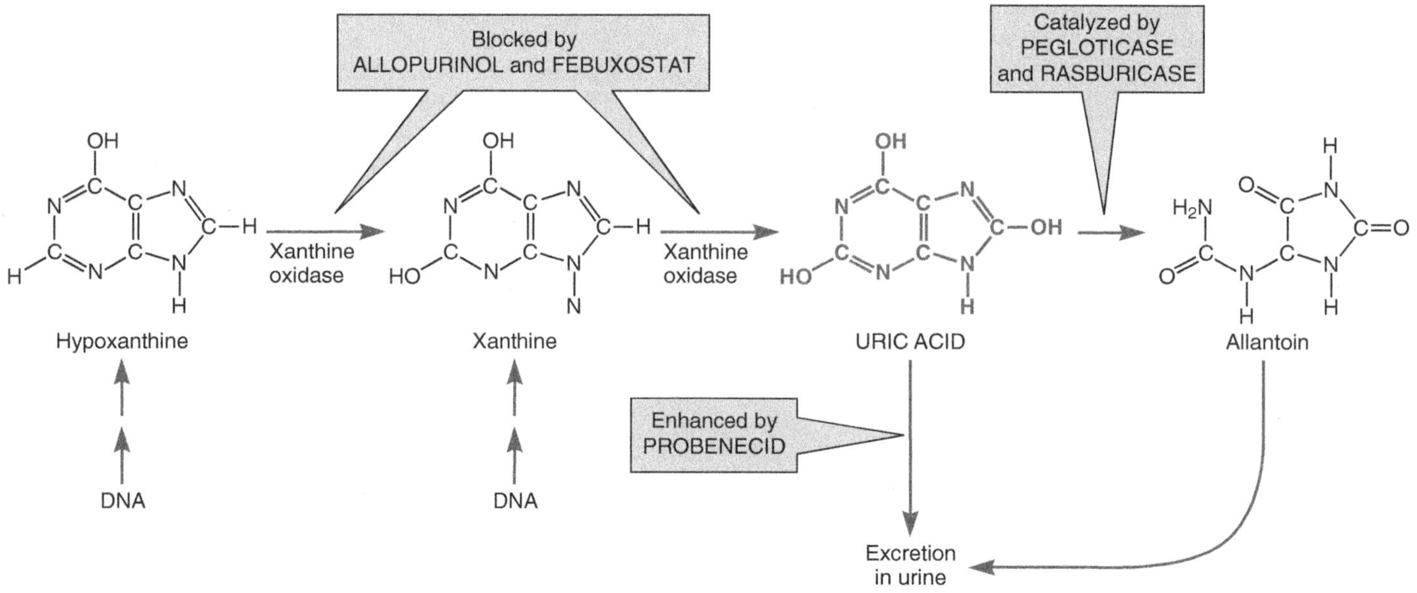

Fig. 74.1 ▪ Drugs that lower plasma levels of uric acid.
These drugs lower plasma urate by three mechanisms: Allopurinol and febuxostat reduce uric acid formation, pegloticase and rasburicase catalyze conversion of uric acid to allantoin, and probenecid facilitates uric acid excretion by the kidney.

should be greatly reduced (by as much as 75%). *Theophylline,* a drug for asthma, is also a substrate for XO, and hence should not be combined with allopurinol. The combination of allopurinol plus *ampicillin* is associated with a high incidence of rash; if rash develops, allopurinol should be discontinued immediately.

Prototype Drugs

DRUGS FOR GOUT

Xanthine Oxidase Inhibitors
Allopurinol

Uricosuric Agents
Probenecid

Recombinant Uric Acid Oxidase
Pegloticase

Febuxostat

Therapeutic Uses. Febuxostat [Uloric] is an alternative to allopurinol. It is used for chronic hyperuricemia management in patients with gout. It is not indicated for asymptomatic hyperuricemia.

Mechanism of Action. Like allopurinol, febuxostat lowers urate levels by inhibiting XO. This prevents the XO enzyme from converting xanthine to uric acid.

Adverse Effects. As with allopurinol, symptoms of gout may flare during initial therapy. Accordingly, patients should receive prophylactic NSAIDs or colchicine for up to 6 months after starting treatment.

Adverse effects of febuxostat, which are uncommon, include liver function abnormalities, nausea, arthralgia, and rash. High doses (80 mg/day) are associated with a small increase in cardiovascular events.

Drug Interactions. Like allopurinol, febuxostat should not be combined with drugs that are substrates for XO, especially theophylline, mercaptopurine, and azathioprine.

Pharmacokinetics. In contrast to allopurinol, which is eliminated entirely by the kidneys, febuxostat is eliminated by hepatic metabolism, followed by renal excretion. No dosage adjustment is needed for patients with mild to moderate renal or hepatic impairment.

Probenecid, a Uricosuric Agent

Therapeutic Use

Probenecid [Benuryl ♣] treats gout by increasing excretion of uric acid. By lowering plasma urate levels, probenecid also prevents the formation of new tophi and facilitates the regression of existing tophi. In addition to its use in gout, probenecid may be employed to prolong the effects of penicillins and cephalosporins by delaying their excretion by the kidneys.

Mechanism of Action

Probenecid (generic only in the United States) acts on renal tubules to inhibit reabsorption of uric acid. As a result, excretion of uric acid is increased and hyperuricemia is reduced.

Adverse Effects

Probenecid is well tolerated by most patients. Mild *GI effects* (nausea, vomiting, anorexia) occur occasionally. These can be reduced by taking the drug with food. *Hypersensitivity reactions,* usually manifesting as rash, develop in about 4% of patients. *Renal injury* may occur from deposition of urate in the kidney. The risk for kidney damage can be minimized by alkalinizing the urine and consuming 2.5 to 3 L of fluid daily during the first few days of treatment.

Probenecid should not be initiated at the beginning of an acute gout attack. The drug may exacerbate acute episodes of gout, and hence treatment should be delayed until the acute attack has been controlled. Probenecid may induce acute attacks of gout during the initial months of therapy after gout appears to be controlled. If an attack occurs, colchicine or indomethacin can be added for relief.

Drug Interactions

Aspirin and other *salicylates* interfere with the uricosuric action of probenecid. Accordingly, probenecid should not be used concurrently with these drugs. Probenecid inhibits the renal excretion of several drugs, including *indomethacin* and *sulfonamides;* dosages of these agents may require reduction.

Pegloticase, a Recombinant Form of Uric Acid Oxidase

Therapeutic Use

Pegloticase [Krystexxa] is indicated for intravenous (IV) therapy of chronic gout in patients who have not responded to oral ULT (e.g., allopurinol, probenecid). Although pegloticase is quite effective, the drug costs $22,299 for a single 8-mg (1 mL) dose and carries a significant risk for severe adverse effects. Accordingly, pegloticase is considered a treatment of last resort.

Mechanism of Action

How does pegloticase reduce urate levels? The drug is a recombinant form of *uricase* (urate oxidase), an enzyme that catalyzes the conversion of uric acid to allantoin. Allantoin is an inert, water-soluble compound that is readily excreted by the kidney. Uricase is present in nearly all mammals—but not in humans and higher primates.

Adverse Effects

As with other drugs for ULT, patients are likely to experience *gout flare* during the first few months of treatment. To reduce flare intensity, patients should take colchicine or an NSAID during this time.

During premarketing trials, pegloticase triggered *anaphylaxis* in 6.5% of patients. Symptoms include wheezing, perioral or lingual edema, hemodynamic instability, and rash. To reduce risk, patients should be pretreated with an antihistamine and glucocorticoid. Administration should be done in a setting equipped to manage a severe reaction.

During premarketing trials, *infusion reactions* were seen in 26% to 41% of patients. Symptoms include urticaria, dyspnea, chest discomfort, erythema, and pruritus. These reactions were seen despite pretreatment with an antihistamine, acetaminophen, and an IV glucocorticoid. If a reaction develops, slowing the infusion rate may reduce symptom intensity.

Pegloticase is *contraindicated* for patients with inherited *glucose-6-phosphate dehydrogenase* (G6PD) *deficiency,* owing to a risk for hemolysis and methemoglobinemia. Patients at higher risk (e.g., those of African or Mediterranean ancestry) should be screened for G6PD deficiency before receiving the drug.

Safety Alert

PEGLOTICASE [KRYSTEXXA]

Anaphylaxis and infusion reactions may occur. These typically occur within 2 hours after infusion but may be delayed. Premedicate with an antihistamine and a glucocorticoid, and monitor patients closely during the infusion.

Rasburicase

Therapeutic Use

Hyperuricemia is a common consequence of cancer chemotherapy. The cause is the breakdown of DNA following massive cell death. Two drugs are available for management: allopurinol (discussed earlier) and rasburicase. As previously noted, allopurinol blocks uric acid production. Rasburicase accelerates uric acid removal.

Mechanism of Action

Rasburicase [Elitek, Fasturtec ♣], produced by recombinant DNA technology, is a form of uric acid oxidase. This enzyme converts uric acid into a soluble, inactive product (allantoin).

Adverse Effects

In clinical trials, about half of patients experienced vomiting and fever. Approximately 20% to 27% had nausea, abdominal pain, constipation, and diarrhea. More serious but less common reactions included neutropenia with fever, respiratory distress, sepsis, and mucositis. The most severe reactions, which occurred in 1% of patients or less, were hemolysis, methemoglobinemia, and severe allergic reactions, including anaphylaxis; if any of these reactions occurs, rasburicase should be discontinued immediately and never used again.

KEY POINTS

- Gout is an inflammatory disorder characterized by hyperuricemia and episodic joint pain, typically in the big toe.
- NSAIDs and glucocorticoids are preferred drugs for treating acute gouty attacks. Benefits derive mainly from anti-inflammatory actions.
- Colchicine is a second-choice drug for treating an acute gouty attack.
- Four drugs—allopurinol, febuxostat, probenecid, and pegloticase—are used long term to prevent gouty attacks. Benefits derive from lowering plasma uric acid levels. These drugs lack anti-inflammatory and analgesic actions, and hence are not effective against acute gouty attacks.
- Allopurinol is the drug of choice for urate-lowering therapy (ULT).
- Allopurinol lowers plasma uric acid by decreasing uric acid production. Allopurinol inhibits xanthine oxidase, an enzyme that forms uric acid from breakdown products of DNA.
- Probenecid lowers plasma uric acid by promoting renal uric acid excretion, through inhibition of tubular reabsorption of uric acid.
- Pegloticase is indicated as ULT for patients refractory to conventional treatment (e.g., allopurinol, probenecid).
- Pegloticase lowers plasma uric acid by promoting uric acid breakdown. Pegloticase is an enzyme that converts uric acid to allantoin, a water-soluble compound that is readily excreted by the kidney.
- Rasburicase accelerates uric acid removal in hyperuricemia that occurs as a consequence of cancer chemotherapy.

Please visit **http://evolve.elsevier.com/Lehne** for chapter-specific NCLEX® examination review questions.

CHAPTER

75 Drugs Affecting Calcium Levels and Bone Mineralization

It is difficult to exaggerate the biologic importance of calcium, an element critical to blood coagulation and to the functional integrity of bone, nerve, muscle, and the heart. Because these calcium-dependent processes can be seriously disrupted by alterations in calcium availability, calcium levels must stay within narrow limits. To regulate calcium, the body employs three factors: parathyroid hormone, vitamin D, and calcitonin. When these regulatory mechanisms fail, hypercalcemia or hypocalcemia results.

Our discussion of calcium and related drugs has four parts. First, we review calcium physiology. Second, we discuss the syndromes produced by the disruption of calcium metabolism. Third, we discuss the pharmacologic agents used to treat calcium-related disorders. And fourth, we consider osteoporosis, the most common calcium-related disorder.

CALCIUM PHYSIOLOGY

Functions, Sources, and Daily Requirements

Functions

Calcium is critical to the function of the skeletal system, nervous system, muscular system, and cardiovascular system. In the skeletal system, calcium is required for the structural integrity of bone. In the nervous system, calcium helps regulate axonal excitability and transmitter release. In the muscular system, calcium participates in excitation-contraction coupling and contraction. In the cardiovascular system, calcium plays a role in myocardial contraction, vascular contraction, and blood coagulation.

Dietary Sources

Dairy products are good sources of calcium. For example, we can get about 300 mg from 1 cup of milk, 6 ounces of yogurt, or 1.5 ounces of cheese. Good nondairy sources include tofu (240 mg/0.5 cup), broccoli (180 mg/cup), and cooked spinach (240 mg/cup). Additionally, many processed foods are calcium fortified. Examples include fortified orange juice (300 mg/8 oz) and fortified cereals (250 to 1000 mg/serving). Information on the calcium content of other foods is available at www.ucsfhealth.org/education/calcium_content_of_selected_foods/index.html.

Daily Requirements

In 2010, the Institute of Medicine (IOM) of the National Academies issued updated recommendations in a report titled *Dietary Reference Intakes for Calcium and Vitamin D* (Table 75.1). Are North Americans getting enough calcium? According to the IOM report, some of us get sufficient calcium from our diets. However, there is concern that two groups—adolescent girls and postmenopausal women—may not get enough calcium from diet alone and may need calcium supplements. How much supplemental calcium should be taken? Only enough to make up the difference between what the diet provides (about 600 to 900 mg/day) and the recommended dietary allowance (RDA). Taking too much supplemental calcium increases the risk of

TABLE 75.1 ■ Daily Calcium Intake by Life-Stage Group

Life-Stage Group[a]	Calcium Intake (mg/day) AI[b]	RDA	UL[c]
0–6 months	200	—	1000
6–12 months	260	—	1500
1–3 years	—	700	2500
4–8 years	—	1000	2500
9–18 years	—	1300	3000
19–50 years	—	1000	2500
51–70 years			
Males	—	1000	2000
Females	—	1200	2500
Over 70 years	—	1200	2000

[a]All values apply to males and females, except in the 51 to 70 age group. Calcium requirements don't change during pregnancy or lactation.
[b]Values for Adequate Intake are derived through experimental or observational data that show a mean calcium intake that appears to sustain a desired indicator of health, such as calcium retention in bone, for most members of the population group. AI values are employed for young children because there are insufficient data to derive an RDA.
[c]The Tolerable Upper Intake Level is defined as the maximum intake that is not likely to pose a risk of adverse health effects in almost all healthy individuals in a specified group. The UL is not intended to be a recommended level of intake. There is no established benefit to consuming calcium above the RDA.
AI, Adequate Intake; *RDA,* Recommended Dietary Allowance; *UL,* Tolerable Upper Intake Level.
Data from the Institute of Medicine of the National Academies: Dietary Reference Intakes for Calcium and Vitamin D. Washington, DC: The National Academies Press, 2010.

vascular calcification, myocardial infarction (heart attack), stroke, and kidney stones.

Body Stores

Calcium in Bone

The vast majority of calcium in the body (more than 98%) is present in bone. It is important to appreciate that bone—and the calcium it contains—is not static. Rather, bone undergoes continuous remodeling, a process in which old bone is resorbed, after which new bone is laid down (Fig. 75.1). The cells that resorb (break down) old bone are called *osteoclasts* and the cells that deposit new bone are called *osteoblasts.* Both cell types originate in the bone marrow. In adults, about 25% of trabecular bone (the honeycomb-like material in the center of bones) is replaced each year. In contrast, only 3% of cortical bone (the dense material that surrounds trabecular bone) is replaced each year.

Calcium in Blood

The normal value for total serum calcium is 10 mg/dL (2.5 mmol/L, 5 mEq/L). Of this total, about 50% is bound to proteins and other substances, and hence is unavailable for use. The remaining 50% is present as free, ionized calcium—the form that participates in physiologic processes.

TABLE 75.2 ■ Effects of Parathyroid Hormone, Vitamin D, and Calcitonin on Calcium and Phosphate

	PTH	Vitamin D	Calcitonin
CALCIUM			
Plasma calcium level	Increase	Increase	Decrease
Intestinal calcium absorption	Increase	Increase	No effect
Renal calcium excretion	Decrease	Decrease	Increase
Calcium resorption from bone	Increase	Increase	Decrease
PHOSPHATE			
Plasma phosphate level	Decrease	Increase	

PTH, Parathyroid hormone.

Absorption and Excretion

Absorption

Absorption of calcium takes place in the small intestine. Under normal conditions, about one-third of ingested calcium is absorbed. Absorption is increased by parathyroid hormone (PTH) and vitamin D. In contrast, glucocorticoids decrease calcium absorption. Also, foods with insoluble fiber and phytic acid, such as whole-grain cereals and wheat bran, and foods containing oxalates, such as spinach, can interfere with calcium absorption.

Excretion

Calcium excretion is primarily renal. The amount lost is determined by glomerular filtration and the degree of tubular reabsorption. Excretion can be reduced by PTH, vitamin D, and thiazide diuretics (e.g., hydrochlorothiazide). Conversely, excretion can be increased by loop diuretics (e.g., furosemide), calcitonin, and by loading with sodium. In addition to calcium lost in urine, substantial amounts can be lost in breast milk.

Physiologic Regulation of Calcium Levels

Blood levels of calcium are tightly controlled. Three processes are involved:

- Absorption of calcium from the intestine
- Excretion of calcium by the kidney
- Resorption or deposition of calcium in bone

Regulation of these processes is under the control of three factors: *parathyroid hormone, vitamin D,* and *calcitonin,* as shown in Table 75.2. Note that preservation of calcium levels in blood takes priority over preservation of calcium in bone. Therefore, if serum calcium is low, calcium will be resorbed from bone and transferred to the blood—even if resorption compromises the structural integrity of bone.

Parathyroid Hormone

Release of PTH is regulated primarily by calcium, acting through calcium-sensing receptors on cells of the parathyroid gland. When calcium levels are *high,* activation of the calcium-sensing receptors is *increased,* causing secretion of PTH to be

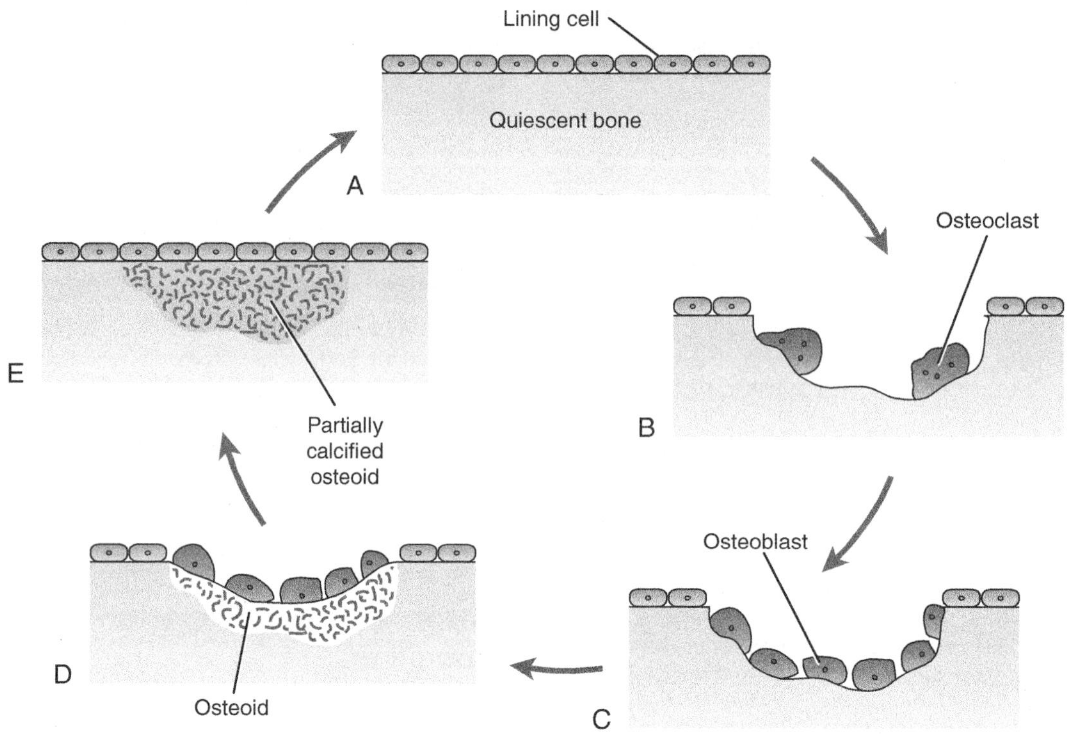

Fig. 75.1 ■ Bone remodeling cycle.
A, Quiescent bone with lining cells covering the surface. **B,** Resorption of old bone by multinucleated osteoclasts. **C,** Osteoblasts migrate to the absorption site. **D,** Osteoblasts deposit osteoid, a matrix of collagen and other proteins. **E,** Osteoid undergoes calcification.

suppressed. Conversely, when calcium levels are low, receptor activation is reduced, causing PTH release to rise. PTH then restores calcium to normal levels by three mechanisms. Specifically, PTH:

- Promotes calcium resorption from bone
- Promotes tubular reabsorption of calcium that had been filtered by the kidney glomerulus
- Promotes activation of vitamin D and thereby promotes increased absorption of calcium from the intestine

In addition to its effects on calcium, PTH reduces plasma levels of phosphate.

Vitamin D

Vitamin D is similar to PTH in that both agents increase plasma calcium levels, and they do so by the same mechanisms: (1) increasing calcium resorption from bone, (2) decreasing calcium excretion by the kidney, and (3) increasing calcium absorption from the intestine. Vitamin D differs from PTH in that vitamin D elevates plasma levels of phosphate, whereas PTH reduces levels of phosphate.

Calcitonin

Calcitonin, a hormone produced by the thyroid gland, decreases plasma levels of calcium. Hence, calcitonin acts in opposition to PTH and vitamin D. Calcitonin is released from the thyroid gland when calcium levels in blood rise too high. Calcitonin lowers calcium levels by inhibiting the resorption of calcium from bone and increasing calcium excretion by the kidney. Unlike PTH and vitamin D, calcitonin does not influence calcium absorption.

CALCIUM-RELATED PATHOPHYSIOLOGY

Hypercalcemia

Clinical Presentation

Hypercalcemia is usually asymptomatic. When symptoms *are* present, they often involve the kidney (damage to tubules and collecting ducts, resulting in polyuria, nocturia, and polydipsia), GI tract (nausea, vomiting, and constipation), and central nervous system (lethargy and depression). Hypercalcemia may also result in dysrhythmias and deposition of calcium in soft tissues. As noted previously, consuming too much supplemental calcium increases the risk of vascular calcification, myocardial infarction, stroke, and kidney stones.

Causes

Hypercalcemia may arise from a variety of causes. Life-threatening elevations in calcium are most often the result of cancer. Hyperparathyroidism is another common cause of severe hypercalcemia. Additional causes include vitamin D intoxication, sarcoidosis, and the use of thiazide diuretics.

Treatment

Calcium levels can be lowered with drugs that (1) promote urinary excretion of calcium, (2) decrease mobilization of calcium from bone, (3) decrease intestinal absorption of calcium, and (4) form complexes with free calcium in blood. For severe hypercalcemia, initial therapy consists of replacing lost fluid with IV saline, followed by diuresis using IV saline and a loop diuretic (e.g., furosemide). Other agents for lowering calcium include inorganic phosphates (which promote calcium deposition in bone and reduce calcium absorption); edetate disodium (EDTA, which binds calcium and promotes its excretion); glucocorticoids (which reduce intestinal absorption of calcium); and a group of drugs—calcitonin, bisphosphonates (e.g., pamidronate), and gallium nitrate—that inhibits resorption of calcium from bone. Cinacalcet [Sensipar], a drug that suppresses PTH section, can be used for hypercalcemia associated with hyperparathyroidism.

Hypocalcemia

Clinical Presentation

Hypocalcemia increases neuromuscular excitability. As a result, tetany, convulsions, and spasm of the pharynx and other muscles may occur.

Cause

Hypocalcemia is caused most often by a deficiency of either PTH, vitamin D, or dietary calcium. Other causes include chronic renal failure and long-term use of certain medications, such as magnesium-based laxatives and drugs used to manage osteoporosis (e.g., bisphosphonates and denosumab).

Treatment

Severe hypocalcemia is corrected by infusing an IV calcium preparation, usually calcium gluconate. Once calcium levels have been restored, an oral calcium salt (e.g., calcium citrate) can be given for maintenance. Vitamin D should be included in the regimen if there is a coexisting deficiency.

Rickets

Rickets is a disease of childhood brought on by either insufficient dietary vitamin D or limited exposure to sunlight. The disease is extremely rare in the United States. Rickets is characterized by defective bone growth and skeletal deformities. Bone abnormalities are caused as follows: (1) vitamin D deficiency results in reduced calcium absorption; (2) in response to hypocalcemia, PTH is released; (3) PTH restores serum calcium by promoting calcium resorption from bone, thereby causing bones to soften; and (4) stress on the softened bones caused by bearing weight results in deformity. Treatment consists of vitamin D replacement therapy.

Osteomalacia

Osteomalacia is the adult counterpart of rickets. Like rickets, this condition results from insufficient vitamin D. In the absence of vitamin D, mineralization of bone is impaired, resulting in bowing of the legs, fractures of the long bones, and kyphosis ("hunchback" curvature of the spine). In addition, patients may experience diffuse dull, aching bone pain. Treatment consists of vitamin D replacement therapy.

Osteoporosis

Osteoporosis, the most common disorder of calcium metabolism, is characterized by low bone mass and increased bone fragility. Osteoporosis is discussed at length in a later section.

Paget's Disease of Bone

Clinical Presentation

Paget's disease of bone is a chronic condition seen most frequently in adults over age 40. After osteoporosis, Paget's disease is the most common disorder of bone in the United States. The disease is characterized by increased bone resorption and replacement of the resorbed bone with abnormal bone. Increased bone turnover causes elevation in serum alkaline phosphatase (reflecting increased bone deposition) and increased urinary hydroxyproline (reflecting increased bone resorption). It is important to note that alterations in bone homeostasis do not occur evenly throughout the skeleton. Rather, alterations occur locally, most often in the pelvis, femur, spine, skull, and tibia. Although most people with Paget's disease are asymptomatic, about 10% experience bone pain and osteoarthritis. Skeletal deformity may also occur. Bone weakness may lead to fractures. Neurologic complications may occur secondary to compression of the spinal cord, spinal nerves, and cranial nerves. If bone associated with hearing is affected, deafness may result.

Treatment

Asymptomatic patients are usually not treated. Mild pain can be managed with analgesics and anti-inflammatory agents. When the disease is more severe, a bisphosphonate (e.g., alendronate, pamidronate, zoledronate) is the treatment of choice. Benefits derive from suppressing bone resorption.

Hypoparathyroidism

Reductions in PTH usually result from inadvertent removal of the parathyroid glands during surgery on the thyroid gland. Lack of PTH causes hypocalcemia, which in turn may produce paresthesias, tetany, skeletal muscle spasm, laryngospasm, and convulsions. Symptoms can be relieved with calcium supplements (see *Hypocalcemia,* earlier) and vitamin D.

Hyperparathyroidism

Primary Hyperparathyroidism

Primary hyperparathyroidism usually results from a benign parathyroid adenoma. The resulting increase in PTH secretion causes hypercalcemia and lowers serum phosphate. Hypercalcemia can cause skeletal muscle weakness, constipation (from decreased smooth muscle tone), and central nervous system (CNS) symptoms (lethargy, depression). Hypercalciuria and hyperphosphaturia are also present and may cause renal calculi. Mobilization of calcium and phosphate from bone may produce bone abnormalities. The only definitive treatment for primary hyperparathyroidism is surgical resection of the parathyroid glands. Hypercalcemia can be managed with calcium-lowering drugs, including cinacalcet [Sensipar], a drug that suppresses PTH secretion.

Secondary Hyperparathyroidism

Secondary hyperparathyroidism is a common complication of chronic kidney disease, occurring in nearly all patients undergoing dialysis. The disorder is characterized by high levels of PTH and disturbances of calcium and phosphorus homeostasis. Traditionally, the disorder has been managed with a vitamin D sterol (e.g., paricalcitol) and calcium-containing phosphate-binding agents. However, these treatments frequently make mineral homeostasis worse. The use of cinacalcet [Sensipar] has been advocated by some experts because of its ability to reduce PTH levels while having a positive impact on calcium and phosphorus; however, others (e.g., the working group Kidney Disease: Improving Global Outcomes [KDIGO]) recommend against its use in the early or pre-dialysis stages of kidney disease.

DRUGS FOR DISORDERS INVOLVING CALCIUM AND BONE MINERALIZATION

Calcium Salts

Calcium salts are available in oral and parenteral formulations for treating hypocalcemic states. These salts differ in their percentage of elemental calcium, which must be accounted for when determining dosage.

Oral Calcium Salts

Therapeutic Uses. Oral calcium preparations are used to treat *mild hypocalcemia.* In addition, calcium salts are taken as *dietary supplements.* People who may need supplementary calcium include adolescents, older adults, and postmenopausal women.

Adverse Effects. When calcium is taken chronically in high doses (3 to 4 gm/day), *hypercalcemia* can result. Hypercalcemia is most likely in patients who are also receiving large doses of vitamin D. Signs and symptoms include GI disturbances (nausea, vomiting, constipation), renal dysfunction (polyuria, nephrolithiasis), and CNS effects (lethargy, depression). In addition, hypercalcemia may cause cardiac dysrhythmias and deposition of calcium in soft tissue. Hypercalcemia can be minimized with frequent monitoring of plasma calcium content.

Drug Interactions. *Glucocorticoids* (e.g., prednisone) reduce absorption of oral calcium, leading to osteoporosis with long-term use. Calcium reduces absorption of a number of drugs when administered together. These drugs include *tetracycline* and *fluoroquinolone* antibiotics, *thyroid hormone,* the anticonvulsant *phenytoin,* and bisphosphonates. *Thiazide diuretics* decrease renal calcium excretion and may thereby cause hypercalcemia; however, *loop diuretics* increase calcium excretion and may cause hypocalcemia.

Food Interactions. Certain foods contain substances that can suppress calcium absorption. One such substance—oxalic acid—is found in spinach, rhubarb, Swiss chard, and beets. Phytic acid, another depressant of calcium absorption, and insoluble fiber, which also hampers absorption, are present in bran and whole-grain cereals. Oral calcium supplements should not be administered with these foods.

Preparations and Dosage. The calcium salts available for oral administration are shown in Table 75.3. Note that the dosage required to provide a particular amount of elemental calcium differs among preparations. Calcium carbonate, for example, has the highest percentage of calcium. Chewable tablets are preferred to standard tablets because of more consistent bioavailability. Bioavailability of *calcium citrate* appears especially good, owing to high solubility. When calcium supplements are taken, total daily calcium intake (dietary plus supplemental) should equal the values in Table 75.1. To help ensure adequate absorption, no more than 600 mg should be consumed at one time.

Parenteral Calcium Salts

Therapeutic Use. Parenteral calcium salts are given to raise calcium levels rapidly in patients with symptoms of severe hypocalcemia (i.e., hypocalcemic tetany). Only two parenteral preparations are available in the United States: *calcium chloride* and *calcium gluconate*. Intravenous calcium gluconate is preferred to calcium chloride.

Adverse Effects. *Calcium chloride* is highly irritating. Intramuscular injection may cause necrosis and sloughing, and hence this route is not recommended. When the drug is administered IV, care must be taken to avoid extravasation, because local infiltration can produce severe injury. Although less irritating than calcium chloride, *calcium gluconate* can produce pain, sloughing, and abscess formation if administered IM. Overdose with either calcium salt can produce signs and symptoms of hypercalcemia (weakness, lethargy, nausea, vomiting, coma, and possibly death).

Drug Interactions. Parenteral calcium may cause severe bradycardia in patients taking *digoxin*. Several classes of compounds—*phosphates, carbonates, sulfates*, and *tartrates*—may cause calcium to precipitate, and hence should not be added to parenteral calcium solutions.

Dosage and Administration. Both parenteral calcium salts are given IV. Solutions of these salts should be warmed to body temperature before administration. Intravenous injections should be done slowly (0.5 to 2 mL/min). Dosage forms and dosages are shown in Table 75.4.

Vitamin D

The term *vitamin D* refers to two compounds: *ergocalciferol* (vitamin D_2) and *cholecalciferol* (vitamin D_3). Vitamin D_3 is the form of vitamin D produced naturally in humans when our skin is exposed to sunlight. Vitamin D_2 is a form of vitamin D that occurs in plants. Vitamin D_2 is used as a prescription drug and to fortify foods. Both forms are used in over-the-counter supplements. It is important to note that both forms of vitamin D produce nearly identical biologic effects. Therefore, rather than distinguishing between them, we will use the term *vitamin D* to refer to vitamins D_2 and D_3 collectively.

TABLE 75.3 ▪ Oral Calcium Salts

Generic Name	Brand Name	Calcium Content	Dose Providing 1000 mg of Calcium
Calcium acetate	PhosLo, Calphron, Eliphos	25%	4 gm
Calcium carbonate	Tums, Rolaids, others	40%	2.6 gm
Calcium citrate	Citracal, Cal-Cee	21%	4.8 gm
Calcium glubionate	Calcionate	6.6%	15.2 gm
Calcium gluconate[a]	Cal-G	9%	11 gm
Calcium lactate	Cal-Lac	13%	7.6 gm
Tricalcium phosphate	Posture	39%	2.6 gm

[a]Also available in parenteral form (see Table 75.4).

Therapeutic Uses

Vitamin D is essential for bone health, owing to its effects on calcium utilization. *The primary indications for vitamin D are vitamin D deficiency and associated conditions such as rickets, osteomalacia, and hypoparathyroidism.*

Some studies suggest that vitamin D may also protect against diabetes, arthritis, cardiovascular disease, autoimmune disorders, and cancers of the breast, colon, prostate, and ovary. However, according to the IOM report on calcium and vitamin D, the available data are insufficient to support health claims beyond bone health. Until more definitive data are available, the possibility of additional benefits remains open, but not proven.

Physiologic Actions

Vitamin D is an important regulator of calcium and phosphorus homeostasis. Vitamin D increases blood levels of both elements, primarily by increasing their absorption from the intestine and promoting their resorption from bone. In addition, vitamin D reduces renal excretion of calcium and phosphate (although the quantitative significance of this effect is not clear). With usual doses of vitamin D, there is no net loss of calcium from bone. However, vitamin D *can* promote bone decalcification if serum calcium concentrations cannot be maintained by increasing intestinal calcium absorption.

Sources and Daily Requirements

Sources. Vitamin D is obtained through the diet, supplements, and exposure to sunlight. With the exception of shiitake mushrooms and oily fish (e.g., salmon, tuna), natural foods have very little vitamin D. Accordingly, dietary vitamin D is obtained mainly through vitamin D–fortified foods, especially cereals, milk, yogurt, margarine, cheese, and orange juice.

Requirements. In 2010, the IOM issued revised guidelines for vitamin D intake. They now recommend:

- For children under 1 year old, 400 international units (IU)/day
- For all people ages 1 through 70, 600 IU/day
- For adults age 71 and older, 800 IU/day

These recommendations are based on the assumption that people get very little of their vitamin D from exposure to sunlight.

According to the IOM report, most people in North America have blood levels of vitamin D in the range needed to support good bone health, and hence do not need vitamin D supplements. Whether taking supplements would confer other benefits remains to be proved.

Vitamin D Deficiency

Vitamin D deficiency is defined by a serum concentration of 25-hydroxyvitamin D (25-(OH)D) below 20 ng/mL. (Levels

TABLE 75.4 ▪ Parenteral Calcium Salts

Generic Name	Dosage Form	Calcium per mL of Solution	Route	Usual Adult Dosage Range
Calcium chloride	10% solution	27 mg	IV	5–10 mL (135–270 mg Ca)
Calcium gluconate[a]	10% solution	9 mg	IV	5–20 mL (45–180 mg Ca)

[a]Also available in an oral formulation (see Table 75.3).

above 20 ng/mL are sufficient to maintain bone health.) In actual practice, the target level of 25-(OH)D is usually 30 to 60 ng/mL.

The classic manifestations of vitamin D deficiency are *rickets* (in children) and *osteomalacia* (in adults). Signs and symptoms are described in the section on *Calcium-Related Pathophysiology*. Taking vitamin D can completely reverse the symptoms of both conditions unless permanent deformity has already developed.

How much vitamin D is needed to *treat deficiency?* In 2011, the Endocrine Society made the following recommendations:

- For children under 1 year old, 2000 IU/day
- For children 1 to 18 years old, 4000 IU/day
- For adults age 19 and older, up to 10,000 IU/day

Much higher doses are needed for patients who are obese and for those taking glucocorticoids and other drugs that suppress calcium absorption or that increase calcium excretion.

Screening for vitamin D deficiency is recommended for patients at risk, including those who are pregnant, obese, or who have dark skin (because, compared with light-skinned people, they make less vitamin D in response to sunlight). For others, the U.S. Preventive Services Task Force (USPSTF), in its 2014 update, declined to recommend for or against vitamin D deficiency screening for nonpregnant adults 18 years and older.

Activation of Vitamin D

To affect calcium and phosphate metabolism, vitamin D must first undergo activation. The extent of activation is carefully regulated and is determined by calcium availability: When plasma calcium falls, activation of vitamin D is increased. The pathways for activating vitamins D_2 and D_3 are shown in Fig. 75.2.

Let's begin by focusing on vitamin D_3, the natural human vitamin. Vitamin D_3 (cholecalciferol) is produced in the skin through the action of sunlight on provitamin D_3 (7-dehydrocholesterol). Neither provitamin D_3 nor vitamin D_3 itself possesses significant biologic activity. In the next reaction, enzymes in the liver convert cholecalciferol into calcifediol, which serves as a transport form of vitamin D_3 and possesses only slight biologic activity. In the final step, calcifediol is converted into the highly active calcitriol. This reaction occurs in the kidney and can be stimulated by (1) PTH, (2) a drop in dietary vitamin D, and (3) a fall in plasma levels of calcium.

Vitamin D_2 is activated by the same enzymes that activate vitamin D_3. As we saw with vitamin D_3, only the last compound in the series (in this case 1,25-dihydroxyergocalciferol) has significant biologic activity.

Pharmacokinetics

As a rule, vitamin D is administered orally and then absorbed from the small intestine. Bile is essential for absorption. In the absence of sufficient bile, IM dosing may be required. In the blood, vitamin D is transported complexed with vitamin D–binding protein. Storage of vitamin D occurs primarily in the liver. As discussed, vitamin D undergoes metabolic activation. Reactions that occur in the liver produce the major transport form of vitamin D. A later reaction (in the kidney) produces the fully active form. Excretion of vitamin D is via the bile. Urinary excretion is minimal.

Viewing Vitamin D as a Hormone

Although referred to as a vitamin, vitamin D has all the characteristics of a hormone. With sufficient exposure to sunlight, the body can manufacture all the vitamin D it needs. Hence, under ideal conditions, external sources of vitamin D appear unnecessary. Following its production in the skin, vitamin D travels to other locations (liver, kidney) for activation. Like other hormones, activated vitamin D then travels to various sites in the body (bone, intestine, kidney) to exert regulatory actions. Also like other hormones, vitamin D undergoes feedback regulation: As plasma levels of calcium fall, activation of vitamin D increases; when plasma levels of calcium return to normal, activation of vitamin D declines.

Toxicity (Hypervitaminosis D)

Serious vitamin D toxicity (hypervitaminosis D) can be produced by vitamin D doses that exceed 1000 IU/day (in infants) and 50,000 IU/day (in adults). Poisoning occurs most commonly in children; causes include accidental ingestion by the child and excessive dosing with vitamin D by parents. Doses of potentially toxic magnitude are also encountered clinically. When huge therapeutic doses are used, the margin of safety is small, and patients should be monitored closely for signs of poisoning.

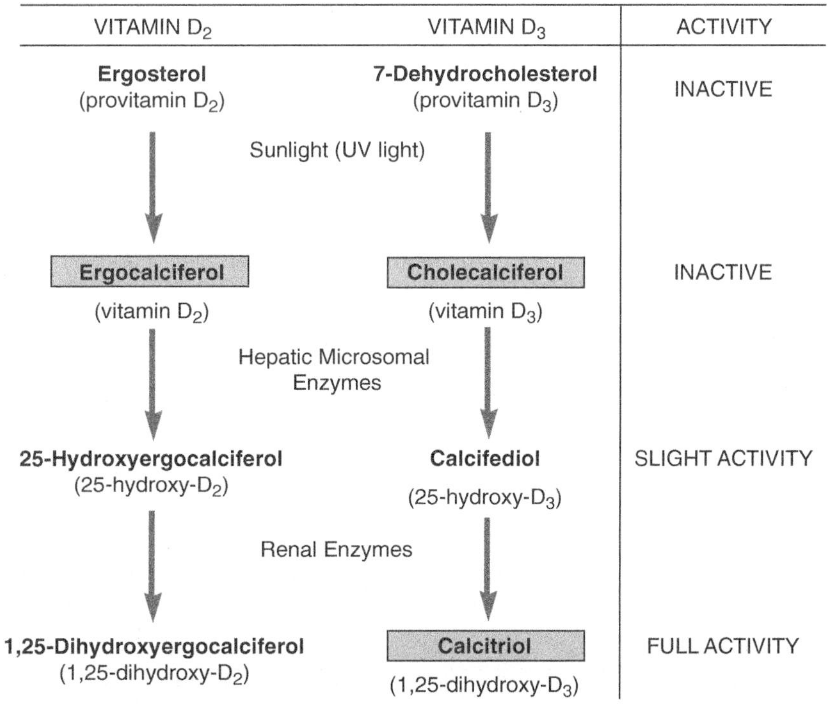

Fig. 75.2 ■ Vitamin D activation.
Ergosterol is found in yeasts and fungi. 7-Dehydrocholesterol is present in the skin. *Green boxes* indicate forms of vitamin D used therapeutically.

Clinical Presentation. Most signs and symptoms of vitamin D toxicity occur secondary to hypercalcemia. Early symptoms include weakness, fatigue, nausea, vomiting, anorexia, abdominal cramping, and constipation. With persistent and more severe hypercalcemia, kidney function is affected, resulting in polyuria, nocturia, and proteinuria, in addition to neurologic symptoms such as seizures, confusion, and ataxia. Cardiac dysrhythmia and coma may occur. Calcium deposition in soft tissues can damage the heart, blood vessels, and lungs; calcium deposition in the kidneys can cause nephrolithiasis. Very large doses of vitamin D can cause decalcification of bone, resulting in osteoporosis; mobilization of bone calcium can occur despite the presence of high calcium concentrations in blood. In children, vitamin D poisoning can suppress growth for 6 months or longer.

Treatment. Treatment consists of stopping vitamin D intake, reducing calcium intake, and increasing fluid intake. Glucocorticoids may be given to suppress calcium absorption. If hypercalcemia is severe, renal excretion of calcium can be accelerated using a combination of IV saline and furosemide (a diuretic).

Preparations, Dosage, and Administration

There are five preparations of vitamin D. Three of these—ergocalciferol, cholecalciferol, and calcitriol—are identical to forms of vitamin D that occur naturally. The other two—paricalcitol and doxercalciferol—are synthetic derivatives of natural vitamin D. (The naturally occurring preparations are highlighted in green boxes in Fig. 75.2.) Individual vitamin D preparations differ in their clinical applications.

Two forms of vitamin D—vitamin D_3 (cholecalciferol) and vitamin D_2 (ergocalciferol)—are used routinely as *dietary supplements.* Of the two, vitamin D_3 is preferred because it is more effective than vitamin D_2 at raising blood levels of 25-(OH)D, the active form of vitamin D in the body.

Vitamin D is almost always administered by mouth. One product—calcitriol—can also be given IV. Dosage is usually prescribed in international units. (One IU is equivalent to the biologic activity in 0.025 mcg of vitamin D_3.) Daily dosages of vitamin D range from 400 IU (for dietary supplementation) to as high as 500,000 IU (for vitamin D–resistant rickets). Additional information on preparation, dosage, and administration is available in Table 75.5.

Ergocalciferol (Vitamin D_2). Ergocalciferol [Calciferol Drops, Drisdol] is approved for hypoparathyroidism, vitamin D–resistant rickets, and familial hypophosphatemia. Ergocalciferol is supplied in capsules (50,000 IU) and an oral solution (8000 IU/mL). The dosage for vitamin D–resistant rickets ranges from 12,000 to 500,000 IU daily. The dosage for hypoparathyroidism ranges from 25,000 to 200,000 IU daily (together with 4 gm of calcium lactate 6 times/day).

Cholecalciferol (Vitamin D_3). Vitamin D_3 [Delta-D] is given as a dietary supplement and for prophylaxis and treatment of vitamin D deficiency. Compared with ergocalciferol (vitamin D_2), cholecalciferol (vitamin D_3) is more effective at raising blood levels of vitamin D. Cholecalciferol is available in three oral formulations: capsules (1000, 2000, 5000, 10,000, 25,000, and 50,000 IU), liquid (400 and 5000 units/mL), and tablets (2000, 3000, 5000, and 50,000 IU).

TABLE 75.5 ▪ Indications, Preparation, and Dosage of Vitamin D Preparations

Drug	Indications	Preparation	Dosage	Administration
Ergocalciferol (vitamin D_2) [Calciferol Drops, Drisdol]	Hypoparathyroidism, vitamin D–resistant rickets, familial hypophosphatemia	Capsules: 50,000 IU Oral solution: 8000 IU/mL	Vitamin D–resistant rickets: 12,000 to 500,000 IU daily Hypoparathyroidism: 25,000 to 200,000 IU daily (together with 4 gm of calcium lactate 6 times/day)	May be administered with or without food. The FDA recommends precise measurements of oral solution by using a dropper that measures no more than 400 units.
Cholecalciferol (vitamin D_3) [Delta-D]	Prophylaxis and treatment of vitamin D deficiency	Capsules: 1000, 2000, 5000, 10,000, 25,000, 50,000 IU Liquid: 400, 5000 units/mL Tablets: 2000, 3000, 5000, 50,000 IU	Prophylaxis: varies depending on risk Deficiency: <1 year: 2000 IU/day 1–18 years: 4000 IU/day Age 19 and older: up to 10,000 IU/day	May be administered with or without food. The FDA recommends precise measurements of oral solution by using a dropper that measures no more than 400 units.
Calcitriol (1,25-dihydroxy-D_3) [Rocaltrol, Vectical, Calcijex 🍁, Silkis 🍁]	Hypoparathyroidism and management of hypocalcemia in patients undergoing chronic renal dialysis	Capsules: 0.25, 0.5 mcg Oral solution: 1 mcg/mL Solution for injection: 1 mcg/mL	Dialysis: daily oral doses of 0.5 to 1 mcg are usually adequate. Hypoparathyroidism: initial dosage 0.25 mcg/day, administered orally	May be administered with or without food. Risk for GI discomfort is decreased if oral products are taken with food.
Doxercalciferol [Hectorol]	Prevention and treatment of secondary hyperparathyroidism in patients undergoing chronic renal dialysis	Capsules: 0.5, 1, 2.5 mcg[a]	Dosage is carefully tailored to the patient Initial dosage: 10 mcg 3 times weekly administered at dialysis Dosage adjustments: gradually increase to a maximum of 20 mcg 3 times/week	May be administered with or without food.
Paricalcitol [Zemplar]	Prevention and treatment of secondary hyperparathyroidism in patients undergoing chronic renal dialysis	Capsules: 1, 2, 4 mcg[a]	Initial dosage: 1–2 mcg/dose (with the once-daily schedule) or 2–4 mcg/dose (with the 3-times-weekly schedule) Dosage adjustments: Gradually increase every 2–4 weeks based on the PTH level	May be administered with or without food.

[a]Also available for IV administration.

Calcitriol (1,25-Dihydroxy-D_3). Calcitriol [Rocaltrol, Vectical, Calcijex 🍁, Silkis 🍁] is indicated for the treatment of hypoparathyroidism and the management of hypocalcemia in patients undergoing chronic renal dialysis. The drug is supplied in capsules (0.25 and 0.5 mcg), oral solution (1 mcg/mL), and solution for injection (1 mcg/mL). For dialysis patients, daily oral doses of 0.5 to 1 mcg are usually adequate. The initial dosage for hypoparathyroidism is 0.25 mcg/day administered orally.

Doxercalciferol. Doxercalciferol [Hectorol] is indicated for the prevention and treatment of secondary hyperparathyroidism in patients undergoing chronic renal dialysis. The drug is available in capsules (0.5, 1, and 2.5 mcg) for oral dosing and in solution (2 mcg/mL and 4 mcg/2 mL) for IV dosing. Dosage must be carefully tailored to the patient. With oral administration, treatment begins with 10 mcg 3 times weekly administered at dialysis; dosage may be gradually increased to a maximum of 20 mcg 3 times a week. With IV administration, treatment begins with a 4-mcg IV bolus 3 times weekly at the end of each dialysis session.

Paricalcitol. Like doxercalciferol, paricalcitol [Zemplar] is indicated for the prevention and treatment of secondary hyperparathyroidism in patients undergoing chronic renal dialysis. The drug is available in capsules (1, 2, and 4 mcg) for oral dosing and in solution (2 and 5 mcg/mL) for dosing by IV bolus. With oral administration, two schedules may be used: (1) once daily and (2) 3 times a week. Treatment begins at 1 to 2 mcg/dose (with the once-daily schedule) or 2 to 4 mcg/dose (with the 3-times-weekly schedule). With IV administration, treatment begins with 0.04 to 0.1 mcg/kg given any time during dialysis—but no more frequently than every other day. Dosage may be gradually increased every 2 to 4 weeks based on the PTH level. Doses as high as 0.24 mcg/kg have been used safely.

Calcitonin-Salmon

Calcitonin-salmon [Miacalcin, Calcimar 🍁], a form of calcitonin derived from salmon, is similar in structure to calcitonin synthesized by the human thyroid. Calcitonin-salmon produces the same metabolic effects as human calcitonin but has a longer half-life and greater milligram potency. The drug is usually given by nasal spray, but can also be given by injection. Intranasal calcitonin was removed from the Canadian market in 2013 due to an increased risk of malignancy associated with this formulation.

Actions

Calcitonin has two principal actions: (1) It inhibits the activity of osteoclasts and thereby decreases bone resorption, and (2) it inhibits tubular resorption of calcium and thereby increases calcium excretion. As a result of decreasing bone turnover, calcitonin decreases alkaline phosphatase in blood and increases hydroxyproline in urine. Preparations and dosages for the different indications are presented in Table 75.6.

Therapeutic Uses

Osteoporosis. Calcitonin-salmon, given by nasal spray or injection, is indicated for *treatment* of established postmenopausal osteoporosis—but not for prevention. Benefits derive from suppressing bone resorption. The treatment program should include supplemental calcium and adequate intake of vitamin D.

Paget's Disease of Bone. Calcitonin is helpful in moderate to severe Paget's disease and is the drug of choice for rapid relief of pain associated with the disorder. Benefits occur secondary to inhibition of osteoclasts. Neurologic symptoms caused by spinal cord compression may be reduced.

Hypercalcemia. Calcitonin can lower plasma calcium levels in patients with hypercalcemia secondary to hyperparathyroidism, vitamin D toxicity, and cancer. Levels of calcium (and phosphorus) are reduced, owing to inhibition of bone resorption and increased renal excretion of calcium. Although calcitonin is effective against hypercalcemia, it is not a preferred treatment.

Adverse Effects

With intranasal dosing, nasal dryness and irritation are the most common complaints. Studies demonstrating an increase in malignancies associated with nasal administration prompted withdrawal of this drug in Canada, but it remains available in the United States. Following parenteral (IM, subQ) administration, about 10% of patients experience nausea, which diminishes with time. An additional 10% have inflammatory reactions at the injection site. Flushing of the face and hands may also occur. When calcitonin-salmon is taken for a year or longer, neutralizing antibodies often develop. In some patients, these antibodies bind enough calcitonin to prevent therapeutic effects.

Preparations, Dosage, and Administration

Intranasal Spray. Calcitonin-salmon for intranasal use, available as a generic product, is available in a metered-dose spray device that delivers 200 IU/activation. This formulation is approved only for *postmenopausal osteoporosis.* The dosage is 200 IU (1 spray) each day, alternating nostrils daily.

Parenteral. Calcitonin-salmon for parenteral use [Miacalcin, Calcimar 🍁] is supplied in 2-mL vials containing 200 IU/mL. Administration is IM or subQ. Dosages are the same for both routes. Dosages for specific indications are:

- Postmenopausal osteoporosis—100 IU every other day
- Paget's disease of bone—100 IU/day initially, followed by 50 IU (daily or 3 times a week) for maintenance
- Hypercalcemia—the initial dosage is 4 IU/kg every 12 hours; the maximal dosage is 8 IU/kg every 6 hours

Bisphosphonates

Bisphosphonates are structural analogs of pyrophosphate, a normal constituent of bone. These drugs undergo incorporation into bone and then inhibit bone resorption by decreasing the

TABLE 75.6 ▪ Indications, Preparation, Dosage, and Administration of Calcitonin

Drug	Indications	Preparation	Dosage	Administration
Intranasal calcitonin-salmon (generic only)	Management of postmenopausal osteoporosis	Metered-dose spray device delivers 200 IU per activation	200 IU (1 spray in 1 naris) each day	Alternate nares daily
Parenteral calcitonin-salmon [Miacalcin, Calcimar 🍁]	Postmenopausal osteoporosis, Paget's disease of bone, hypercalcemia	2-mL vials containing 200 IU/mL	Postmenopausal osteoporosis: 100 IU every other day Paget's disease of bone: 100 IU/day initially, followed by 50 IU (daily or 3 times/week) Hypercalcemia: initial dosage is 4 IU/kg every 12 hr; maximum dosage is 8 IU/kg every 6 hr	Administer IM or subQ Dosages are the same for both routes

activity of osteoclasts. Principal indications are postmenopausal osteoporosis, osteoporosis in men, glucocorticoid-induced osteoporosis, Paget's disease of bone, and hypercalcemia of malignancy. Bisphosphonates may also help prevent and treat bone metastases in patients with cancer (see Chapter 103). Although these drugs are generally very safe, serious adverse effects can occur, including ocular inflammation, osteonecrosis of the jaw (ONJ), atypical femur fractures, and atrial fibrillation (primarily with IV zoledronate).

Bisphosphonates differ with respect to indications, routes, and dosing schedules. As indicated in Table 75.7, some bisphosphonates are given PO, some are given IV, and some are given by both routes. With oral dosing, absorption from the GI tract is extremely poor. Dosing schedules vary from as often as once a day (with oral agents) to as seldom as once every 2 years (with IV zoledronate) (see Table 75.8). As with many drugs for osteoporosis and similar bone disorders, calcium and vitamin D supplements are recommended if there is inadequate dietary intake.

Four bisphosphonates approved for the management of osteoporosis and glucocorticoid-induced osteoporosis (GIOP) are currently available in the United States. These are alendronate [Fosamax, Fosamax Plus D, Binosto], ibandronate [Boniva], risedronate [Actonel, Atelvia, Actonel DR ♣], and zoledronate [Reclast, Zometa, Aclasta ♣]. Additional bisphosphonates have been approved for the treatment of Paget's disease (e.g., etidronate ♣ [generic only]) and/or complications of malignancy (e.g., pamidronate [Aredia]).

TABLE 75.7 ▪ Bisphosphonates: Routes and Uses

		Major Uses[a]				
Drug	Route	Osteoporosis in Postmenopausal Women	Osteoporosis in Men	Paget's Disease of Bone	Hypercalcemia of Malignancy	Glucocorticoid-Induced Bone Loss
Alendronate [Fosamax, Binosto]	PO	A	A	A		A
Risedronate [Actonel, Atelvia, Actonel DR ♣]	PO	A	A	A		A
Ibandronate [Boniva]	PO, IV	A				
Etidronate (generic only)[b]	PO, IV			A		I
Zoledronate [Reclast, Aclasta ♣]	IV	A	A	A		A
Zoledronate [Zometa][c]	IV				A	
Pamidronate [Aredia ♣][d]	IV	I		A	A	I

[a]*A,* FDA-approved indication; *I,* investigational use.
[b]Also approved for prevention and treatment of heterotropic ossification.
[c]Also approved for multiple myeloma and bone metastases from solid tumors.
[d]Also approved for osteolytic bone metastases.

TABLE 75.8 ▪ Indications, Preparation, and Dosage, and Administration of Bisphosphonates

Drug	Indications	Preparation	Dosage	Administration
Alendronate [Fosamax, Binosto] Alendronate + vitamin D [Fosamax Plus D]	Prevention and treatment of osteoporosis in postmenopausal women, osteoporosis in men, Paget's disease, and GIOP	Tablets (Fosamax): 70 mg Tablets (generic): 5, 10, 35, 40, 70 mg Effervescent tablet (Binosto): 70 mg Oral solution (generic): 70 mg/75 mL Tablets (Fosamax D): 70 mg alendronate/2800 IU vitamin D_3, 70 mg alendronate/5600 IU vitamin D_3	Osteoporosis in postmenopausal women, prevention: 5-mg tablet daily or 35 mg once weekly Osteoporosis in postmenopausal women, treatment: 10-mg tablet daily or 70 mg once weekly Osteoporosis in men: 10-mg tablet once daily or 70 mg once weekly Paget's disease: 40 mg once daily for 6 months for men or women GIOP for men, premenopausal women, and postmenopausal women taking estrogen: 5 mg once daily GIOP for postmenopausal women not taking estrogen: 10 mg once daily	Administer intact tablet in the morning on an empty stomach at least 30 minutes before the first bite of food or other drugs Binosto effervescent tablets should be dissolved in water; wait 5 minutes after effervescing ends and then stir before administering. Give plain water only; do not administer with mineral water. Instruct patients to remain upright for at least 30 minutes. If the patient is unable to sit upright, the drug should be held.

TABLE 75.8 ▪ Indications, Preparation, and Dosage, and Administration of Bisphosphonates—cont'd

Drug	Indications	Preparation	Dosage	Administration
Risedronate [Actonel, Atelvia, Actonel DR 🍁]	IR: Prevention and treatment of osteoporosis in postmenopausal women, osteoporosis in men, prevention or treatment of GIOP, and Paget's disease of bone DR: postmenopausal osteoporosis	IR (Actonel): 5-, 30-, 35-, 100-mg tablets DR (Atelvia): 35-mg enteric-coated tablets	Postmenopausal osteoporosis, Actonel: 5 mg once daily, 35 mg once weekly, or 150 mg once a month Postmenopausal osteoporosis, Atelvia: 35 mg once weekly Osteoporosis in men, Actonel: 35 mg once a week GIOP, Actonel: 5 mg once daily Paget's disease of bone: 30 mg once daily	IR: Administer intact tablet in the morning on an empty stomach at least 30 minutes before the first bite of food. DR: Administer intact tablet immediately after breakfast. For both IR and DR tablets, plain water should be the only fluid given and the patient should remain upright for 30 minutes.
Ibandronate [Boniva]	Prevention and treatment of postmenopausal osteoporosis	Tablets: 150 mg IV: 3 mg/3 mL pre-filled syringes	Prevention and treatment of osteoporosis, tablets: 150 mg once a month on the same day each month Treatment of osteoporosis, IV: 3 mg every 3 months	PO: Administer tablets in the morning on an empty stomach at least 60 minutes before the first bite of food or other drugs. Administer with plain water only. IV: Administer IV bolus over 15–30 seconds. Do not administer in a line with other IV drugs.
Zoledronate (zoledronic acid) [Aclasta 🍁, Reclast, Zometa]	Aclasta 🍁: treatment of osteoporosis in postmenopausal women and in men; prevention and treatment of GIOP and Paget's disease of bone Reclast: prevention and treatment of osteoporosis in postmenopausal women and in men, GIOP, and Paget's disease Zometa: hypercalcemia of malignancy	Aclasta: 5 mg/100 mL Reclast: 5 mg/100 mL	Aclasta 🍁: For all indications *except Paget's disease,* 5 mg IV once a year Paget's disease: one 5-mg dose Reclast: For all indications except prevention of postmenopausal osteoporosis and Paget's disease: 5 mg IV once a year Prevention of postmenopausal osteoporosis: 5 mg once every 2 years Paget's disease: One 5-mg dose	Infuse over 15–30 minutes and follow with saline flush. Do not administer with other IV drugs.
Pamidronate [Aredia 🍁]	Hypercalcemia of malignancy, Paget's disease, multiple myeloma, osteolytic bone metastases of breast cancer	IV solution: 30, 90 mg/10 mL IV solution, reconstituted: 30, 90 mg	Hypercalcemia of malignancy, moderate: 1 dose of 60–90 mg Hypercalcemia of malignancy, severe: 1 dose of 90 mg	Do not exceed 90 mg/dose to avoid renal toxicity leading to renal failure. Infuse over 2–24 hr. Longer administration may decrease renal risk.
			Paget's disease: 30 mg daily for 3 days	Infuse each dose over 4 hr.
			Bone loss from multiple myeloma: 90 mg each month	Infuse over at least 4 hr.
			Bone loss from breast cancer metastasis: 90 mg every 3–4 weeks	Infuse over at least 4 hr.

DR, Delayed release; *GIOP,* glucocorticoid-induced osteoporosis; *IR,* immediate release.

PATIENT-CENTERED CARE ACROSS THE LIFE SPAN

Bisphosphonates

Life Stage	Patient Care Concerns
Children	Bisphosphonates are not indicated for treatment in children; however, alendronate and pamidronate have been used off-label for the management of osteogenesis imperfecta.
Pregnant women	All bisphosphonates except ibandronate and etidronate are Pregnancy Risk Category D[a] because adverse fetal events have occurred in reproduction studies with animals. For zoledronate specifically, there has been an increase in stillbirths, as well as decreased survivability of neonates. Toxic levels of pamidronate have occurred in the fetus even at doses below those recommended for treatment. Ibandronate and etidronate are Pregnancy Risk Category C[a] based on the lack of conclusive data that these drugs cause harm. Manufacturers of these drugs recommend discontinuing bisphosphonates before becoming pregnant to avoid any as-yet unknown risk.
Breast-feeding women	The U.S. National Library of Medicine's LactMed Database recommends pamidronate as the bisphosphonate of choice for women who want to breast-feed. The quandary that this presents is that pamidronate is not indicated for the treatment of osteoporosis. For women who take a bisphosphonate for osteoporosis, breast-feeding is not recommended until more is known. On the positive side, most women who take these drugs for osteoporosis are postmenopausal. For conditions in which pamidronate is indicated, although studies and reports are limited, more is known about this drug than about the other bisphosphonates. Measures of pamidronate in breast milk following IV administration were "very low." Because the half-life of pamidronate is about 3 hours, avoidance of breast-feeding for 12 to 24 hours after dosing is recommended.
Older adults	Because frail older adults commonly have difficulty in swallowing, those who take bisphosphonates may be at an increased risk of esophagitis. Owing to occurrences of low-impact atypical femur fractures in older women who have had long-term bisphosphonate therapy, many experts recommend against continuing bisphosphonate therapy beyond 5 years. Bisphosphonates are not recommended for creatinine clearance that is less than 30–35 mL/min. Some recommend dosage adjustments for those with higher but suboptimal levels. The fatigue that often occurs following administration may increase the risk of falls.

[a]As of 2020, the FDA will no longer use Pregnancy Risk Categories. Please refer to Chapter 9 for more information.

Alendronate

Alendronate [Fosamax, Fosamax Plus D, Binosto], the most widely used oral bisphosphonate, will serve as our prototype for the family. The drug is approved for postmenopausal osteoporosis, male osteoporosis, glucocorticoid-induced osteoporosis, and Paget's disease of bone.

Therapeutic Use. The primary purpose of alendronate is the prevention and treatment of osteoporosis in postmenopausal women where benefits derive from decreasing bone resorption by osteoclasts. It is also approved for treating osteoporosis in men. In this group, the drug increases bone mineral density (BMD), reduces vertebral fractures, and decreases loss of height.

Alendronate is considered a first-choice drug for the prevention and treatment of GIOP, a common complication of glucocorticoid therapy. Studies indicate that alendronate helps restore lost bone and may reduce the risk of fractures in this instance.

It is also a first-line treatment for Paget's disease. Continuous daily therapy for 3 months produces a 50% decrease in serum alkaline phosphatase, indicating a substantial reduction in bone turnover. As in osteoporosis, benefits derive from inhibiting bone resorption by osteoclasts.

Prototype Drugs

DRUGS AFFECTING CALCIUM LEVELS AND BONE MINERALIZATION

Antiresorptive Agents

Alendronate (bisphosphonate)
Calcitonin-salmon nasal spray
Conjugated equine estrogens [Premarin]
Denosumab (RANKL inhibitor)
Raloxifene (selective estrogen receptor modulator)

Bone-Forming Agents

Teriparatide

Pharmacokinetics. Alendronate is administered orally, but bioavailability is very low (only 0.7%). If the drug is taken with solid food, essentially none is absorbed. Even coffee or orange juice can decrease absorption by 60%. Absorption is also decreased by divalent (also known as bivalent) cations—including calcium, magnesium, and iron—which bind with alendronate and all other bisphosphonates. Of the small fraction that undergoes absorption, about 50% is taken up rapidly by bone. The remaining 50% is excreted unchanged in the urine. Once alendronate has become incorporated into bone, it remains there for decades.

Mechanism of Action. Alendronate suppresses resorption of bone by decreasing both the number and activity of osteoclasts. Several mechanisms are involved. As osteoclasts begin to resorb alendronate-containing bone, they ingest some of the drug, which then acts on the osteoclasts to inhibit their activity. In addition, alendronate reduces the *number* of osteoclasts by (1) acting directly to decrease their recruitment and (2) acting on osteoblasts, which then produce an inhibitor of osteoclast formation.

Therapeutic Use

Osteoporosis in Postmenopausal Women. Alendronate is approved for both the prevention and treatment of osteoporosis in postmenopausal women. Benefits derive from decreasing bone resorption by osteoclasts.

Osteoporosis in Men. Alendronate is approved for treating osteoporosis in men. In this group, the drug increases bone mineral density (BMD), reduces vertebral fractures, and decreases loss of height.

Glucocorticoid-Induced Osteoporosis (GIOP). Alendronate is considered a first-choice drug for the prevention and treatment of GIOP, a common complication of glucocorticoid therapy that leads to fractures in at least 50% of patients. Studies indicate that alendronate helps restore lost bone and may reduce the risk of fractures.

Paget's Disease of Bone. Alendronate is a first-line treatment for Paget's disease. Continuous daily therapy for 3 months produces a 50% decrease in serum alkaline phosphatase, indicating a substantial reduction in bone turnover. As in osteoporosis, benefits derive from inhibiting bone resorption by osteoclasts.

Adverse Effects. Alendronate is generally well tolerated. Esophagitis is the principal concern. Rarely, the drug causes musculoskeletal pain, ocular inflammation, atypical femur fractures, and ONJ. The risk of these adverse effects increases with long-term use. Fortunately, because bisphosphonates remain in bone for extensive periods of time, they continue to prevent fractures for years, and possibly for decades, after being discontinued.

Esophagitis. Esophagitis, sometimes resulting in ulceration, is the most serious adverse effect. Fortunately, esophagitis is rare, occurring in only 1 of every 10,000 patients. The cause of injury is prolonged contact with the esophageal mucosa, which can occur if alendronate fails to pass completely through the esophagus. Reasons for incomplete passage include taking the drug with insufficient water, taking the drug in a supine position, lying down after taking the drug, and having a preexisting esophageal disorder that impedes drug passage. Because of the risk of esophagitis, alendronate is contraindicated for patients with esophageal disorders that could prevent successful swallowing and for patients who are unable to sit or stand for at least 30 minutes. Patients should be instructed to discontinue alendronate and contact the prescriber if symptoms of esophageal injury (difficulty swallowing, pain upon swallowing, or new or worsening heartburn) occur during the course of treatment.

Atypical Femoral Fractures. Alendronate and other bisphosphonates have been associated with atypical fractures of the femur, which occur with little or no trauma. Why do these fractures occur? One explanation is that excessive suppression of bone turnover reduces bone remodeling, and, as a result, the repair of microcracks is suppressed and bone strength is reduced. Fortunately, the absolute risk of atypical fractures is low—about 5 additional cases for every 10,000 patient-years of bisphosphonate use. Risk increases with duration of treatment.

Do the benefits of preventing typical fractures (which are common) outweigh the risk of causing atypical fractures (which are rare)? The answer is clearly "Yes"—but only for women with osteoporosis who are deemed at high risk of a typical fracture. For women without osteoporosis who are at low risk for a typical fracture, the benefits of bisphosphonates may not justify the risks.

What can be done to reduce the risk of an atypical fracture? In 2010, a task force assembled by the American Society for Bone and Mineral Research recommended the following:

- Do not prescribe bisphosphonates for patients considered at low risk for osteoporosis-related fractures.
- Consider alternative treatments, such as raloxifene or teriparatide, for patients with osteoporosis of the spine and normal (or only moderately reduced) BMD of the femoral neck or hip.
- After 5 years of bisphosphonate use, the need for continued treatment should be evaluated annually.

Esophageal Cancer. Alendronate and other *oral* bisphosphonates may—or may not—increase the risk of *esophageal cancer.* Studies have reached conflicting conclusions. If the risk is real, it is small (about 1 additional case for every 1000 patients older than 60 years treated for 5 years) and probably due to esophageal injury caused during oral dosing. Measures that might reduce risk include reducing the dosing frequency (i.e., dosing weekly rather than daily), taking the drug with a full glass of water, and staying upright for 30 to 60 minutes after dosing.

Musculoskeletal Pain. Musculoskeletal pain, sometimes severe, has been reported during postmarketing surveillance. So far, a causal link with alendronate has not been established. Onset may occur shortly after the first dose or months later. Pain can be managed with analgesics, including opioids and ketorolac when pain is severe. In most cases, discomfort gradually resolves after stopping alendronate. Interestingly, among patients who resume alendronate use, only 11% experience a return of pain. If pain does return, patients taking the drug for osteoporosis can switch to a different agent, such as raloxifene, calcitonin-salmon, or teriparatide.

Ocular Problems. Ocular problems are rare, but can be serious. Possible effects include conjunctivitis, scleritis, blurred vision, and eye pain. Drug-induced release of inflammatory cytokines may be the cause. Advise patients to report any vision changes or eye pain.

Osteonecrosis of the Jaw. Very rarely, patients have developed *osteonecrosis of the jaw,* a potentially severe complication. This is seen mostly with IV bisphosphonates.

Hyperparathyroidism. In patients with Paget's disease, alendronate can induce *hyperparathyroidism.* By inhibiting accelerated bone resorption, alendronate causes blood levels of calcium to fall; in response, secretion of PTH is increased. To prevent hyperparathyroidism, patients should receive calcium supplements.

Atrial Fibrillation. Because an *intravenous* bisphosphonate (zoledronate) has been associated with rare cases of atrial fibrillation (AF), there has been ongoing concern that oral alendronate may also cause the disorder. In 2008, the U.S. Food and Drug Administration (FDA), based on data from clinical trials, determined there was no significant AF risk with oral formulations of bisphosphonates. Data from more recent research, however, have raised the issue once again. In 2014, the *American Journal of Cardiology* published a report of findings from a meta-analysis of randomized controlled trials and observational studies that contradicts earlier findings. Those authors assert that there is increased, though low, risk of new-onset AF with both oral and IV bisphosphonates.

Administration. Proper administration is necessary to maximize bioavailability and minimize the risk of esophageal injury. Alendronate absorption is dramatically diminished when taken with food. To maximize bioavailability, alendronate should be taken in the morning before breakfast (i.e., on an empty stomach). No food, including orange juice or coffee, should be consumed for at least 30 minutes following administration. Because minerals such as calcium, magnesium, and iron bind with alendronate and all other bisphosphonates, many experts advise waiting at least 2 hours following administration before taking calcium products, mineral supplements, or antacids.

To minimize the risk of esophagitis, patients should be instructed to:

- Take alendronate with a full glass of water.
- Remain upright (sitting or standing) for at least 30 minutes.
- Avoid chewing or sucking alendronate tablets.

Preparations and Dosage. Alendronate [Fosamax, Binosto] is available alone in tablets (5, 10, 35, 40, and 70 mg), an effervescent tablet (70 mg), and an oral solution (70 mg in 75 mL). In addition, alendronate is available in a fixed-dose combination with vitamin D (cholecalciferol) under the brand name *Fosamax Plus D.* Dosing for *osteoporosis* in women or men may be done once daily (in the morning) or once weekly (on the same morning each week). Once-weekly dosing, which is just as effective as once-daily dosing, is possible because alendronate undergoes incorporation into bone, where it remains and acts for years. Bivalent cations—including calcium, iron, magnesium, and antacids that contain calcium, aluminum, or magnesium—can decrease alendronate absorption, and hence should not be taken for at least 30 minutes after taking alendronate. Dosages are as follows:

- *Osteoporosis in postmenopausal women*—for *prevention,* 5-mg tablet daily or 35 mg once weekly; for *treatment,* 10 mg once daily or 70 mg once weekly
- *Osteoporosis in men*—10 mg once daily or 70 mg once weekly
- *Paget's disease*—40 mg once daily for 6 months for men or women
- *Glucocorticoid-induced osteoporosis*—5 mg once daily (for men, premenopausal women, and postmenopausal women taking estrogen) or 10 mg once daily (for postmenopausal women not taking estrogen)

Risedronate

Actions and Uses. Risedronate [Actonel, Atelvia, Actonel DR] is an oral bisphosphonate approved for *postmenopausal osteoporosis, male osteoporosis, glucocorticoid-induced osteoporosis,* and *Paget's disease of bone.* As with other bisphosphonates, benefits derive from inhibiting osteoclast-mediated resorption of bone. In postmenopausal women with osteoporosis, risedronate increases BMD and reduces the risk of vertebral and nonvertebral fractures.

Pharmacokinetics. Like other oral bisphosphonates, risedronate is poorly absorbed from the GI tract. Absorption is only 1% under fasting conditions. The impact of food depends on the formulation used. With Actonel (an immediate-release [IR] formulation), food greatly reduces absorption. By contrast, with Atelvia (an enteric-coated, delayed-release [DR] formulation), food does not reduce absorption. In fact, Atelvia should be taken with food to reduce stomach pain. Following absorption, most of the drug becomes incorporated into bone. The rest is excreted unchanged in the urine. Risedronate in bone persists for years.

Adverse Effects. The most common adverse effects are arthralgia, diarrhea, headache, rash, nausea, and a flu-like syndrome. Like alendronate, risedronate poses a significant risk of esophagitis and a very small risk of atypical femoral fractures. Ocular problems and musculoskeletal pain are rare. If risedronate poses a risk of esophageal cancer, ONJ, or AF, the risk is very small.

Preparations, Dosage, and Administration. Risedronate is supplied in IR tablets (5, 30, 35, and 100 mg) sold as *Actonel,* and in 35-mg enteric-coated DR tablets sold as *Atelvia.* The IR tablets are approved for postmenopausal osteoporosis, male osteoporosis, GIOP, and Paget's disease of bone. The DR tablets are approved only for postmenopausal osteoporosis. With the IR tablets, each dose should be taken in the morning *before* ingesting the first food or fluids of the day (except for water). With the DR tablets, each dose should be taken in the morning *after* breakfast. (Atelvia is the only oral bisphosphonate that can be taken after eating, rather than before.) With both formulations, dosing should be done with a full glass of water. Also, the patient should be upright when swallowing and should not lie down for at least 30 minutes. Because divalent cations—including calcium, iron, and magnesium—greatly reduce absorption, these should not be taken within 2 hours of administering either risedronate formulation. Dosages are as follows:

- *Postmenopausal osteoporosis, for prevention or treatment* (Actonel or Atelvia)—With Actonel, 5 mg once daily, 35 mg once weekly, or 150 mg once a month. With Atelvia, 35 mg once weekly
- *Osteoporosis in men* (Actonel only)—35 mg once a week
- *Glucocorticoid-induced osteoporosis in men or women, for prevention or treatment* (Actonel only)—5 mg once daily
- • *Paget's disease in men or women* (Actonel only)—30 mg once daily for 2 months. If needed, a second 2-month course can be given, provided at least 2 months have elapsed since completing the first course.

Ibandronate

Actions and Uses. Ibandronate [Boniva], available in oral and IV formulations, is approved for prevention and treatment of *postmenopausal osteoporosis.* Dosing may be done once a month or once every 3 months. As with other bisphosphonates, benefits derive from inhibiting osteoclast-mediated resorption of bone. In clinical trials, ibandronate increased BMD in the lumbar spine and other sites, and reduced the risk of vertebral fractures. Although comparative studies have not been done, the drug is probably as effective as alendronate and risedronate, the only other bisphosphonates approved for oral therapy of osteoporosis.

Pharmacokinetics. With oral dosing, bioavailability is extremely low—only 0.6%. Food decreases availability by another 90%. Following absorption, ibandronate undergoes rapid binding to bone or excretion in the urine. Metabolism, if any, is minimal. The half-life in blood is 10 to 60 hours. However, because of binding to bone, active drug remains in the body for years.

Adverse Effects and Interactions. With *oral administration,* ibandronate is generally well tolerated. Like other oral bisphosphonates, it can cause adverse GI effects, including esophagitis, dyspepsia, and abdominal pain. Ocular inflammation, atypical fractures, and ONJ are rare. Musculoskeletal pain has not been reported. Whether ibandronate increases the risk of esophageal cancer is unknown. As with other bisphosphonates, bivalent cations (e.g., calcium, magnesium, iron) can greatly decrease absorption.

With *IV administration,* ibandronate and other bisphosphonates may cause *renal damage,* especially if administered too rapidly. Accordingly, ibandronate should be injected slowly—over an interval of 15 to 30 seconds. Intravenous ibandronate should not be used by patients taking other nephrotoxic drugs or by those with severe renal impairment, defined as serum creatinine above 2.3 mg/dL or creatinine clearance less than 30 mL/min. In addition to causing renal damage, IV ibandronate may cause an acute reaction characterized by fever, joint pain, and myalgia, primarily with the first dose.

Preparations, Dosage, and Administration

Oral. Ibandronate [Boniva] for oral dosing is supplied in 150-mg tablets. The dosage for prevention and treatment of osteoporosis is 150 mg once a month, taken on the same day each month. Dosing is done on an empty stomach in the morning. Patients should swallow tablets whole with a full glass of water, while standing or sitting upright. For 60 minutes after dosing, patients must remain upright and must not eat or drink anything, including medications and dietary supplements.

Intravenous. Ibandronate [Boniva] for IV dosing is supplied in solution (1 mg/mL) in 3 mg/3 mL, pre-filled syringes. For treatment of osteoporosis, the dosage is 3 mg every 3 months, administered by slow IV push (over 15 to 30 seconds). Kidney function should be determined before each dose; if severe renal impairment is detected, the dose should be withheld.

Etidronate

Actions, Uses, and Adverse Effects. Etidronate [generic only] is approved for *Paget's disease* and for prevention and treatment of *heterotropic ossification* (abnormal bone formation in extraskeletal soft tissue). The drug is also used for GIOP, although it is not approved for this disorder. In patients with highly active Paget's disease, etidronate can produce moderate clinical improvement. Unfortunately, when the drug is discontinued, relapse may occur rapidly. Side effects include abdominal cramps, diarrhea, nausea, and increased bone pain. In addition, etidronate causes defective mineralization of newly formed bone (osteomalacia) and can thereby increase the risk of fractures. Whether the drug causes esophageal cancer is uncertain.

Preparations, Dosage, and Administration. Etidronate is available in 200- and 400-mg tablets for oral dosing. As with all other oral bisphosphonates, bioavailability is low. To maximize absorption, patients should wait 2 hours before ingesting food, antacids high in metals (e.g., calcium, iron, magnesium, aluminum), and vitamins that contain mineral supplements.

Patients with *Paget's disease* may be given either (1) 5 to 10 mg/kg/day (for no more than 6 months) or (2) 11 to 20 mg/kg/day (for no more than 3 months). Treatment can be repeated, but not until 90 days have elapsed since completing the prior course.

The dosage for preventing *heterotopic ossification* in patients undergoing total hip replacement is 20 mg/kg every day for 1 month before surgery and for 3 months after. For heterotopic ossification caused by spinal cord injury, the dose is 20 mg/kg/day for 2 weeks, then 10 mg/kg/day for 10 weeks for a total treatment period of 12 weeks.

Zoledronate

Actions and Uses. Zoledronate [Reclast, Zometa, Aclasta], also called zoledronic acid, is an IV bisphosphonate with approved indications for *postmenopausal osteoporosis, osteoporosis in men, Paget's disease of bone, glucocorticoid-induced osteoporosis, multiple myeloma or metastatic bone lesions from solid tumors,* and *hypercalcemia of malignancy* (HCM). In addition, the drug is used off-label to prevent bone loss, fractures, and other skeletal-related events in patients receiving a variety of therapies that create a risk of bone loss. Like other bisphosphonates, zoledronate undergoes incorporation into bone, where it remains for years. When osteoclasts ingest the drug, it inhibits their activity, preventing bone resorption.

In patients with HCM, inhibition of bone resorption lowers calcium levels in blood. In one study, zoledronate normalized serum calcium in 88% of patients within 10 days of a single infusion. Compared with pamidronate, another IV bisphosphonate for HCM, zoledronate has three advantages. Specifically, onset is faster, duration is longer, and, perhaps most importantly, infusion time is shorter (15 minutes vs. 2 to 4 hours), making dosing more convenient.

For management of postmenopausal osteoporosis, zoledronate differs from all other bisphosphonates in that dosing is done just once a year or once every 2 years. Compared with placebo treatment, once-yearly zoledronate decreases the incidence of vertebral fractures by 70%, hip fractures by 41%, and nonvertebral fractures by 25%. In addition, zoledronate improves BMD and markers of bone metabolism.

Adverse Effects. The most common reaction is transient fever, followed by nausea, constipation, dyspnea, abdominal pain, and bone and joint pain. In addition, zoledronate can cause clinically significant reductions in serum levels of calcium, phosphorus, and magnesium. Accordingly, levels of these elements should be followed and corrected when indicated.

Zoledronate has been associated with bone injury, most often *osteonecrosis of the jaw,* a condition characterized by local bone death and decreased bone strength. The underlying cause is impaired blood perfusion. (Bisphosphonates impair perfusion by inhibiting growth of blood vessels.) Among patients using zoledronate, most cases of ONJ developed after tooth extractions and other dental procedures, which can increase risk by promoting infection. Other risk factors include cancer, cancer chemotherapy, use of systemic glucocorticoids, and poor oral hygiene. To reduce ONJ risk, a dental examination with appropriate preventive dentistry should be conducted before giving zoledronate, especially in patients with ONJ risk factors.

Zoledronate can cause dose-dependent *kidney damage,* which can progress to acute renal failure and, rarely, to death. Risk is increased by:

- Chronic renal impairment
- Advanced age
- Dehydration (e.g., secondary to fever, sepsis, diarrhea)
- Use of diuretics (which can cause dehydration)
- Use of nephrotoxic drugs
- Rapid infusion of zoledronate

Owing to the risk of renal failure, zoledronate may be contraindicated in patients with significant renal impairment. When not contraindicated, dosage varies depending on the underlying condition and creatinine clearance. To minimize risk, dosage should be kept low (5 mg or less per infusion) and the infusion should be slow (15 minutes or longer). In addition, the patient should be adequately hydrated before each infusion. To monitor for renal damage, creatinine clearance should be determined at baseline, before each dose, and periodically after each infusion. If renal impairment develops, zoledronate dosage should be reduced.

Rarely, zoledronate has been associated with serious *atrial fibrillation,* resulting in disability or hospitalization. In one trial, the incidence was 1.3%, compared with 0.5% in patients taking placebo. Most cases developed more than 30 days after zoledronate infusion.

Fetal Injury. Zoledronate has been associated with increases in fetal demise before or during delivery, as well as decreases in neonate survival after delivery. It should not be prescribed for pregnant women.

Hazardous Agents and Special Administration Requirements. The National Institute of Occupational Safety and Health (NIOSH) classifies zoledronate as a hazardous drug that requires special handling and administration. See Chapter 3, Table 3.1, for administration and handling guidelines.

Drug Interactions. Risk of renal failure is increased by *diuretics* (which can cause dehydration) and by other *nephrotoxic drugs,* including cyclosporine, amphotericin B, aminoglycoside antibiotics, and the nonsteroidal anti-inflammatory drugs (NSAIDs).

Preparations, Dosage, and Administration. Zoledronate is available in solution under two brand names: Reclast and Zometa. These solutions differ in concentration and indications.

Zometa, indicated for *hypercalcemia of malignancy,* is supplied as a *concentrated* solution (4 mg/5 mL) that must be diluted in 100 mL of 0.9% sodium chloride or 5% dextrose. The maximum recommended dose is 4 mg. In patients with renal impairment, dosage should be reduced. All doses must be given as a single IV infusion over *no less than 15 minutes.* If hypercalcemia does not resolve, or if it resolves and then returns, a second infusion can be given, but no sooner than 7 days after the first infusion, and only if kidney function is adequate.

Reclast is supplied as a *dilute* solution (5 mg/100 mL) in single-use vials. Indications and dosages are as follows:

- *Postmenopausal osteoporosis, treatment*—5 mg once a year, infused over 15 minutes or longer.
- *Postmenopausal osteoporosis, prevention*—5 mg once every 2 years, infused over 15 minutes or longer.
- *Osteoporosis in men*—5 mg once a year, infused over 15 minutes or longer.
- *Glucocorticoid-induced osteoporosis*—5 mg once a year, infused over 15 minutes or longer.
- *Paget's disease*—5 mg infused over 15 minutes or more. Just one dose produces extended remission. Specific re-treatment data are not available.

Pamidronate

Pamidronate [Aredia ♣] is a bisphosphonate approved for IV therapy of *Paget's disease, hypercalcemia of malignancy,* and *osteolytic bone metastases.* Because of dose-related GI intolerance (e.g., mucosal erosion in the esophagus and stomach), pamidronate is not given orally.

Therapeutic Use and Dosage

Hypercalcemia of Malignancy. Many cancer cells release factors that stimulate resorption of bone by osteoclasts. The result is hypercalcemia, increased risk of fractures, and bone pain. By inhibiting osteoclast activity, pamidronate can blunt cancer-mediated bone resorption and can thereby reduce blood levels of calcium. The recommended dosage is 60 to 90 mg infused over 2 to 24 hours. Longer infusion times reduce the risk of renal injury.

Paget's Disease of Bone. Like other bisphosphonates, pamidronate can decrease bone resorption in patients with Paget's disease. The dosage is 30 mg infused slowly (over at least 4 hours) on 3 consecutive days. With this dosage, the mean duration of remission is 14 months.

Osteolytic Bone Metastases. For osteolytic bone lesions of *multiple myeloma,* the dosage is 90 mg infused over 4 hours once a month. For bone metastases of *breast cancer,* the dosage is 90 mg infused over 2 hours every 3 to 4 weeks.

Adverse Effects. Although IV pamidronate is generally safe, serious adverse effects can occur. Like zoledronate, pamidronate has been associated with ONJ, usually after an invasive dental procedure. In some patients, the first dose causes transient flu-like symptoms. If pamidronate is not infused with sufficient fluid, venous irritation can occur. In contrast to etidronate, pamidronate does not interfere with bone mineralization. Because pamidronate inhibits accelerated bone resorption of Paget's disease, blood levels of calcium will fall, thereby triggering increased release of PTH; to prevent hyperparathyroidism, patients should receive supplemental calcium.

Fetal Injury. Pamidronate has caused toxic levels in the fetus, even at doses below recommended doses; it should not be prescribed for pregnant women.

Hazardous Agents and Special Administration Requirements

Pamidronate may present a hazard to pregnant women who handle or administer the drug; therefore, it is classified by the NIOSH as a hazardous drug. Specific instructions for handling this drug are provided in Table 3.1 of Chapter 3.

Estrogen

The basic pharmacology of estrogen, as well as postmenopausal estrogen therapy, is discussed in Chapter 61. Discussion here focuses on the role of estrogen in osteoporosis.

When estrogen levels decline, either because of natural menopause or surgical removal of the ovaries, osteoclasts increase in number, causing bone resorption to increase dramatically. Estrogen replacement can restore the brake on osteoclast proliferation and can therefore suppress resorption.

Because of new insight into the benefits and risks of estrogen, prolonged replacement is no longer considered appropriate for most women. That said, estrogen is still approved for preventing and treating bone loss after menopause or surgical removal of the ovaries, because treatment reduces the overall risk of fractures by 24%. Estrogen is most effective when initiated immediately after menopause; however, treatment begun later in life can still offer significant protection. If estrogen is discontinued, a period of accelerated bone loss will ensue.

The standard dosage for estrogen therapy is 0.625 mg/day of conjugated equine estrogens [Premarin] or its equivalent. However, less estrogen (e.g., 0.3 mg/day) may be nearly as effective in osteoporosis. Women with an intact uterus should also receive a progestin (e.g., medroxyprogesterone) to minimize the risk of estrogen-induced endometrial cancer. For women without a uterus, the progestin is unnecessary.

For years, hormone therapy (HT)—estrogen with or without a progestin—had been considered the treatment of choice for preventing postmenopausal bone loss. Today, however, the benefits no longer appear to outweigh the risks. Data indicate that HT offers fewer benefits than previously thought and carries greater risks. Yes, HT does reduce bone loss and the risk of osteoporotic fractures. However, HT increases the risk of breast cancer, cholecystitis, myocardial infarction, and stroke. Fortunately, for prevention and treatment of osteoporosis, we have effective alternatives: raloxifene, bisphosphonates, calcitonin, and teriparatide. Women currently using HT for osteoporosis are encouraged to consider a switch to an alternative drug.

Hazardous Agents and Special Administration Requirements

Estrogen and the selective estrogen receptor modulator raloxifene (discussed next) are classified by NIOSH as hazardous drugs. The NIOSH instructions for handling are provided in Table 3.1 of Chapter 3.

Raloxifene

Raloxifene [Evista] belongs to a class of agents known as *selective estrogen receptor modulators* (SERMs)—drugs that exert estrogenic effects in some tissues and antiestrogenic effects in others. Like estrogen, raloxifene preserves BMD and reduces plasma levels of cholesterol. However, in contrast to estrogen, which promotes cancer of the breast and endometrium, raloxifene protects against these cancers. Because of its effects on bone, raloxifene is used to prevent and treat postmenopausal osteoporosis. Because of its effects on breast tissue, the drug is used to reduce the risk of breast cancer. Another SERM—tamoxifen—is used to *treat* breast cancer, as well as prevent it (see Chapter 103).

Mechanism of Action

Raloxifene and other SERMs are structurally similar to estrogen, so they can bind to estrogen receptors. However, unlike estrogen itself, which functions as an agonist in all tissues, SERMs function as agonists in some tissues and antagonists in others. Hence, SERMs can either mimic or block the actions of estrogen, depending on the SERM and the tissue involved. Raloxifene mimics the effects of estrogen on bone, lipid metabolism, and blood clotting, and blocks estrogen effects in the breast and endometrium.

Pharmacokinetics

Raloxifene is administered by mouth, and 60% is absorbed. However, owing to extensive first-pass metabolism, absolute bioavailability is below 2%. Excretion is fecal. The drug's half-life is about 28 hours.

Therapeutic Uses

Raloxifene offers significant benefits regarding osteoporosis and breast cancer, but also poses a risk of serious thromboembolic events. Accordingly, women must carefully weigh the risks and benefits before choosing this drug.

Postmenopausal Osteoporosis. Raloxifene is used to prevent and treat osteoporosis in postmenopausal women. The drug can preserve or increase BMD, although not as effectively as estrogen. Raloxifene reduces the risk of *spinal* fractures by 55%, but does not reduce the risk of fractures at other sites.

Breast Cancer. Raloxifene protects against estrogen receptor (ER)–positive breast cancer. In the Multiple Outcomes of Raloxifene Evaluation (MORE) trial, which enrolled 7705 postmenopausal women with osteoporosis, taking raloxifene for a median of 40 months reduced the risk of ER-positive breast cancer by 76%—but only in women with high levels of estrogen. There was no reduction in the risk of ER-negative breast cancer. Encouraged by these results, the National Cancer Institute funded a large 5-year trial, called the Study of Tamoxifen and Raloxifene (STAR). STAR enrolled 19,747 women at high risk of breast cancer, with the objective of comparing risk reduction conferred by raloxifene or tamoxifen, a SERM already proved to reduce risk by 50%. The results of STAR, released in 2007, showed that raloxifene is just as effective as tamoxifen and also safer, causing fewer cases of uterine cancer and blood clots. As a result of these studies, raloxifene is now approved for reducing the risk of invasive breast cancer in postmenopausal women who either (1) have osteoporosis or (2) are at high risk of breast cancer, even if they don't have osteoporosis.

Adverse Effects and Interactions

The U.S. Food and Drug Administration (FDA) has issued black box warnings for raloxifene. These warnings address risks of deep vein thrombosis (DVT) and pulmonary embolism (PE) and the risk of death due to stroke.

Deep Vein Thrombosis and Pulmonary Embolism. Like estrogen, raloxifene increases the risk of thromboembolic events such as DVT, PE, and stroke. Because inactivity promotes DVT, patients should discontinue raloxifene at least 72 hours before prolonged immobilization (e.g., postsurgical recovery, extended bed rest) and should not resume the drug until full mobility has been restored. Also, patients should minimize periods of restricted activity, as can happen when traveling or revising a pharmacology text. Raloxifene is contraindicated for patients with a history of venous thrombotic events.

Fetal Harm. Raloxifene is classified in *FDA Pregnancy Risk Category X*[a]*: The potential for fetal harm outweighs any possible benefits of use during pregnancy.* In animal studies, doses below those used in humans have resulted in abortion, delayed fetal development, decreased neonatal survival, and anatomic abnormalities, including hydrocephaly and uterine hypoplasia. Accordingly, raloxifene is contraindicated for use by pregnant women. Although use during pregnancy is obviously no concern for postmenopausal patients, it can be a concern for younger women taking the drug to prevent breast cancer.

Comparison With Estrogen

The SERMs were developed in the hope of creating a drug with all the benefits of estrogen and none of its drawbacks. Raloxifene partly fulfills this hope. Table 75.9 shows the ways in which estrogen and raloxifene are alike and different.

Preparations, Dosage, and Administration

Raloxifene [Evista] is available in 60-mg oral tablets. The dosage for all indications is 60 mg once a day, taken with or without food. Women taking raloxifene to prevent or treat postmenopausal osteoporosis should ensure adequate intake of calcium and vitamin D.

Bazedoxifene and Estrogen

Bazedoxifene, a SERM, and estrogen are available in a combination tablet (Duavee). It is available as 20 mg bazedoxifene and 0.45 mg conjugated estrogens to be taken once a day for postmenopausal osteoporosis. Additional information regarding this drug is available in Chapter 61.

[a]As of 2020, the FDA will no longer use Pregnancy Risk Categories. Please refer to Chapter 9 for more information.

Teriparatide

Teriparatide [Forteo] is a form of PTH produced by recombinant DNA technology. The drug has three indications:

- Treatment of osteoporosis in postmenopausal women
- Treatment of osteoporosis in men
- Treatment of GIOP

Teriparatide is the only drug for osteoporosis that increases bone formation. All others decrease bone resorption. In postmenopausal women with documented osteoporosis, daily subQ injections of teriparatide for 18 months increased BMD of the lumbar spine and femoral neck and reduced the risk of vertebral fractures by 65%. Similar responses are seen in men. Teriparatide-induced increases in BMD are twice those seen with alendronate.

How does teriparatide (PTH) affect bone? The drug has two actions: It (1) increases bone resorption by osteoclasts and (2) increases bone deposition by osteoblasts. The net effect—resorption or deposition—depends on how the drug is administered. When given by continuous IV infusion, which produces a *steady* elevation of serum PTH, teriparatide *decreases* BMD, primarily by accelerating calcium resorption by osteoclasts. In contrast, when given by daily subQ injections, which produce *transient* elevations in serum PTH, the drug *increases* BMD, primarily by increasing bone deposition by osteoblasts.

Adverse effects included nausea, headache, arthralgias, back pain, and leg cramps. Orthostatic hypotension and associated dizziness may occur within 4 hours of injection, so the patient should be in a location where it is possible to lie down, if needed. This adverse effect decreases after the first few doses. Temporary increases in serum levels of calcium, magnesium, and uric acid may occur.

The FDA has issued a black box warning related to an increased risk of *osteosarcoma* (bone cancer) in patients receiving teriparatide therapy. To date, cancer has occurred only in animal studies and has not been detected in humans. Nonetheless, teriparatide should be avoided by patients with bone metastases or a history of skeletal cancer, and by

TABLE 75.9 ■ Comparison of Estrogen and Raloxifene

Drug Target	Estrogen	Raloxifene
Bone	Increases BMD and reduces fracture risk	Increases BMD (but not as much as estrogen) and reduces fracture risk
Breast	Increases risk of breast cancer; causes breast enlargement and pain	Protects against breast cancer; does *not* cause breast enlargement or pain
Endometrium	Increases risk of endometrial cancer	Does *not* promote endometrial cancer, and *may* offer protection
Plasma lipids	Lowers LDL cholesterol and raises HDL cholesterol	Lowers LDL cholesterol, but does not raise HDL cholesterol
Menopausal symptoms	Alleviates menopausal symptoms (e.g., hot flashes, vaginal dryness and itching)	Does *not* alleviate menopausal symptoms, and may actually increase hot flashes
Menstruation	Causes bleeding in 45% of postmenopausal women	Causes bleeding in 3%–5% of postmenopausal women
Blood clotting	Increases risk of DVT and pulmonary embolism	Increases risk of DVT and pulmonary embolism
Coronary heart disease	Black box warning related to cardiovascular disease	Black box warning related to cardiovascular disease
Developing fetus	Contraindicated during pregnancy because of possible fetal harm	Contraindicated during pregnancy because of possible fetal harm

patients at increased risk for bone cancer, including those with open epiphyses, Paget's disease of bone, or prior irradiation of bone.

Preparations, Dosage, and Administration

Teriparatide [Forteo] is supplied in special pre-filled pen injectors that contain 600 mcg/2.4 mL (250 mcg/3 mL in Canada) and are designed to deliver a predetermined amount of drug with each activation. For all indications, the recommended dosage is 20 mcg once daily by subQ injection into the anterior thigh or abdomen. Each pen can be used up to 28 days after the first injection, after which it should be discarded, even if some drug remains. Patients should store the pens cold—2°C to 8°C (36°F to 46°F)—but not frozen, and should take them out of the cold only to make an injection. The cost for each syringe (a 28-day supply) is over $1500, so treatment costs can be very expensive.

Denosumab

Therapeutic Uses

Denosumab [Prolia, Xgeva] is a first-in-class receptor activator of nuclear factor kappa-B ligand (RANKL) inhibitor with three indications: (1) treatment of osteoporosis in men and postmenopausal women at high risk for fractures; (2) treatment of bone loss in men and women receiving certain anticancer therapy (e.g., androgen deprivation therapy for prostate cancer and aromatase inhibitor therapy for breast cancer); and (3) prevention of skeletal-related events (SREs) in patients with bone metastases from solid tumors. Dosage is much higher in patients with bone metastases than in patients with osteoporosis, and hence side effects are more severe in patients with bone metastases.

Denosumab is marketed under two brand names: Prolia and Xgeva. *Prolia* is used for men and women with a high risk for fractures or who have bone loss due to anticancer therapy. *Xgeva* is used for bone metastases.

Clinical Trials

Osteoporosis in Postmenopausal Women. Denosumab was tested in a 3-year study that enrolled 7868 postmenopausal women with osteoporosis. Half the women received denosumab (60 mg injected subQ every 6 months), and the other half received placebo injections. All subjects also received at least 1000 mg of calcium daily and at least 400 IU of vitamin D daily. Compared with the women who got placebo injections, those who got denosumab had 68% fewer vertebral fractures, 40% fewer hip fractures, and 20% fewer fractures at other sites (wrist, leg, or shoulder). In a separate 12-month study, denosumab (60 mg subQ every 6 months) increased BMD at multiple sites (lumbar spine, femoral neck, trochanter, radius) more effectively than oral alendronate (70 mg once a week). Taken together, these data suggest that denosumab is equal to bisphosphonates for treating postmenopausal osteoporosis.

Prevention of Skeletal-Related Events in Patients With Bone Metastases. In cancer patients, denosumab is used to prevent (delay) SREs—bone fracture, spinal cord compression, bone pain requiring radiation—after cells from a solid tumor have metastasized to bone. Efficacy was evaluated by comparing denosumab with zoledronate (a bisphosphonate) in three double-blind trials that enrolled 5723 patients. One trial enrolled patients with breast cancer, one enrolled patients with prostate cancer, and one enrolled patients with other cancers, including multiple myeloma, kidney cancer, small cell lung cancer, and non–small cell lung cancer. Patients received either denosumab (120 mg subQ every 4 weeks) or zoledronate (4 mg IV every 4 weeks). In patients with breast cancer or prostate cancer, denosumab was *superior* to zoledronate at delaying SREs. In patients with other cancers, denosumab was *equal* to zoledronate at delaying SREs. Use of denosumab in cancer is discussed in Chapter 103.

Mechanism of Action

Denosumab is a monoclonal antibody that decreases the formation and function of osteoclasts and thereby decreases bone resorption and increases BMD and bone strength. What's the underlying mechanism? Denosumab prevents the activation of a receptor known as RANK, found on the surface of osteoclasts and their precursor cells. Under normal conditions, RANK is activated by binding with an endogenous compound known as the *RANK ligand,* or simply RANKL. When activated by RANKL, RANK stimulates the formation and activity of osteoclasts. Where does denosumab fit in? It binds with RANKL and thereby prevents RANKL from activating RANK.

Pharmacokinetics

Administration is subQ. Blood levels peak 10 days after a single injection. With monthly injections (as used for cancer patients), denosumab levels reach plateau in 6 months. The elimination half-life is 28 days. Renal impairment does not affect denosumab kinetics. The effect of hepatic impairment has not been studied.

Adverse Effects

In postmenopausal women with osteoporosis, the most common adverse effects are back pain, pain in the extremities, musculoskeletal pain, hypercholesterolemia, and urinary bladder infection. In cancer patients with bone metastases, the most common adverse effects are fatigue, hypophosphatemia, and nausea. In all patients, suppression of bone turnover may delay fracture healing and increase the risk of new fractures and ONJ. The most serious adverse effects—hypocalcemia, infections, skin reactions, and ONJ—are discussed next.

Hypocalcemia. Denosumab can exacerbate pre-existing hypocalcemia, presumably by reducing osteoclast activity. If hypocalcemia is present, it must be corrected before starting denosumab. The risk of hypocalcemia is elevated in patients with impaired renal function (including those on dialysis) and patients with other risk factors (e.g., a history of hypoparathyroidism, thyroid surgery, malabsorption syndromes, or excision of the small intestine). The manufacturer recommends monitoring levels of calcium, magnesium, and phosphorus in this at-risk group. To help prevent hypocalcemia, all patients should take 1000 mg of calcium every day and at least 400 IU of vitamin D every day.

Serious Infections. Denosumab increases the risk of serious infections, although the absolute risk is low. In clinical trials, some patients developed endocarditis, serious skin infections, and infections of the abdomen, urinary tract, and ear. Patients who develop signs of severe infection should seek immediate medical attention. Infection risk is increased in patients who are immunocompromised (e.g., owing to HIV infection or treatment with immunosuppressant drugs).

Dermatologic Reactions. Denosumab increases the risk of dermatitis, eczema, rashes, and other skin reactions. Of note, these are not limited to the injection site. If a severe reaction occurs, discontinuation of denosumab should be considered.

Osteonecrosis of the Jaw. Like the bisphosphonates, denosumab increases the risk of ONJ. Risk is further increased by invasive dental procedures (e.g., tooth extractions, dental implants, oral surgery), and hence these should be conducted before starting denosumab. Patients who develop ONJ should be under the care of a dentist or oral surgeon. Maintaining good oral hygiene reduces ONJ risk.

Preparations, Dosage, and Administration

Denosumab is available in solution under two brand names: Prolia and Xgeva. These products differ in concentration, indications, and dosage.

Prolia: Dosage and Administration. Prolia is indicated for osteoporosis in postmenopausal women and in men at risk for fractures. The drug is supplied in (1) single-use vials containing 1 mL of a 60-mg/mL solution and (2) single-use, pre-filled syringes containing 1 mL of a 60-mg/mL solution. The recommended dosage is 60 mg every 6 months, injected subQ into the upper arm, upper thigh, or abdomen. If a dose is missed, it should be given as soon as possible. Subsequent doses should be given every 6 months thereafter. To prevent hypocalcemia, patients should take 1000 mg of calcium daily plus at least 400 IU of vitamin D daily.

Xgeva: Dosage and Administration. Xgeva is indicated for preventing SREs in patients with bone metastases from solid tumors. The drug is supplied in single-use vials that contain 120 mg denosumab/1.7 mL. The recommended dosage is 120 mg every 4 weeks, injected subQ into the upper arm, upper thigh, or abdomen. As with Prolia, patients should take calcium and vitamin D to prevent hypocalcemia.

Prolia and Xgeva: Storage, Warming, and Inspection. Solutions should be stored under refrigeration and then warmed before use (by standing at room temperature for 15 to 30 minutes). All preparations should be clear and colorless (or pale yellow). Preparations that have particles or that are cloudy or discolored should not be used.

Cinacalcet

Actions and Therapeutic Use

Cinacalcet [Sensipar] is a "calcimimetic" drug approved for primary hyperparathyroidism (caused by parathyroid carcinoma) as well as secondary hyperparathyroidism (caused by chronic kidney disease [CKD]). In both cases, benefits derive from decreasing the secretion of PTH. How is secretion suppressed? Recall that extracellular calcium regulates PTH secretion by binding with calcium-sensing receptors on cells of the parathyroid gland, thereby signaling those cells to reduce PTH secretion. Cinacalcet increases the sensitivity of the calcium-sensing receptors to activation by extracellular calcium. As a result, the ability of calcium to suppress PTH release is amplified.

Clinical trials have shown that in patients with hyperparathyroidism secondary to CKD, cinacalcet decreases serum PTH by 23% to 46% and improves calcium and phosphorus homeostasis. Similarly, in patients with primary hyperparathyroidism, the drug decreases serum PTH and normalizes serum calcium.

Pharmacokinetics

Dosing is oral, and absorption is increased by food. In the blood, cinacalcet is highly bound (93% to 97%) to plasma proteins. Cinacalcet undergoes extensive hepatic metabolism, followed by excretion in the urine (80%) and feces (15%). The drug's half-life is 30 to 40 hours.

Adverse Effects

The most common adverse effects are nausea, vomiting, and diarrhea. Because cinacalcet lowers calcium levels, hypocalcemia is an obvious concern. Accordingly, calcium levels should be monitored and patients should be informed about possible manifestations of hypocalcemia (e.g., cramping, convulsions, myalgias, paresthesias, tetany) and instructed to report them.

Drug Interactions

Cinacalcet is metabolized in part by cytochrome P450 isoenzyme 3A4, so inhibitors of this enzyme (e.g., ketoconazole, itraconazole, erythromycin) can raise cinacalcet levels. If cinacalcet is used with one of these drugs, cinacalcet dosage may need an adjustment.

Monitoring

In patients with *parathyroid carcinoma,* measure serum calcium within 1 week of the first dose and each dosage change. Once a maintenance dosage has been established, measure serum calcium every 2 months.

In patients with *secondary hyperparathyroidism,* measure serum calcium and phosphorus within 1 week of the first dose and each dosage change, and measure PTH within 4 weeks of the first dose and each dosage change. Once a maintenance dosage has been established, measure calcium and phosphorus monthly, and PTH every 1 to 3 months.

Preparations, Dosage, and Administration

Cinacalcet [Sensipar] is available in tablets (30, 60, and 90 mg) for oral use. To enhance absorption, the drug should be taken with a meal or shortly after.

In patients with *parathyroid carcinoma,* the initial dosage is 30 mg twice daily. Then, every 2 to 4 weeks, dosage is increased as follows—60 mg twice daily, 90 mg twice daily, 90 mg 3 times/day, up to a maximum of 90 mg 4 times a day—until the dosing goal (normalization of serum calcium) is achieved.

In patients with *secondary hyperparathyroidism,* the initial dosage is 30 mg once daily. Then, every 2 to 4 weeks, the dosage is increased as follows—60 mg once daily, 90 mg once daily, 120 mg once daily, up to a maximum of 180 mg once daily—until the dosing goal (PTH level between 150 and 300 pg/mL) is achieved.

Drugs for Hypercalcemia

Furosemide

Furosemide, a loop diuretic, promotes renal excretion of calcium. This action is useful for treating hypercalcemic emergencies. In managing such emergencies, isotonic saline (IV) must be given before furosemide. The dosage of furosemide for adults is 80 to 100 mg every 1 to 2 hours as needed, infused no faster than 4 mg/min. To avoid fluid and electrolyte imbalance, urinary losses must be measured and replaced. The basic pharmacology of furosemide is discussed in Chapter 41.

Glucocorticoids

Glucocorticoids reduce intestinal absorption of calcium and can thereby reduce hypercalcemia. For severe hypercalcemia, parenteral glucocorticoid therapy is indicated (e.g., 100 to 500 mg hydrocortisone sodium succinate IV daily). Because glucocorticoids can produce serious adverse effects when taken chronically, the risks of long-term treatment must be carefully weighed against the benefits. The basic pharmacology of the glucocorticoids is discussed in Chapter 72.

Gallium Nitrate

Gallium nitrate [Ganite] is used to treat HCM. Gallium reduces calcium levels by preventing bone resorption. It may also increase bone formation. Gallium is highly nephrotoxic and must not be used with other nephrotoxic drugs, such as amphotericin B and the aminoglycosides. To minimize kidney damage, the patient must be hydrated with IV fluids before treatment. Renal function must be monitored. The usual single dose is 100 to 200 mg/m^2. This dose is diluted in 1 L of 5% dextrose or 0.9% sodium chloride and infused over 24 hours. Dosing is repeated daily for 5 days.

Bisphosphonates

Pamidronate, etidronate, and zoledronate are approved for HCM. The mechanism is suppression of bone resorption by osteoclasts. The pharmacology of these agents is discussed previously.

Inorganic Phosphates

Phosphates reduce plasma levels of calcium and therefore can be used to treat hypercalcemia. Suggested mechanisms for reducing plasma calcium include (1) decreased bone resorption, (2) increased bone formation, and (3) decreased intestinal absorption of calcium (secondary to decreased renal activation of vitamin D). Intravenous use of phosphates is hazardous and limited to patients with life-threatening hypercalcemia. Oral administration is considerably safer.

Oral phosphates are used for mild to moderate hypercalcemia. These agents should not be given to patients with renal impairment or elevated serum phosphate. Oral phosphates should not be combined with antacids that contain aluminum, magnesium, or calcium—agents that bind phosphate and thereby prevent its absorption. Initial treatment should provide 1 to 2 gm of phosphorus/day. Doses are reduced when serum calcium levels normalize.

Edetate Disodium

EDTA [Endrate] is a chelating agent that binds calcium in the blood. As a result, it can rapidly reduce plasma levels of free calcium. The EDTA-calcium complex is filtered by the glomerulus but not reabsorbed by kidney tubules, and hence renal excretion of calcium is increased. Although EDTA is highly effective at reducing hypercalcemia, it can be dangerous: EDTA can cause profound hypocalcemia, resulting in tetany, convulsions, dysrhythmias, and possibly death. Severe nephrotoxicity can also occur. Because of its toxicity, EDTA is used only for life-threatening hypercalcemic crisis. The usual adult dose is 40 mg/kg infused over 4 to 6 hours. The total daily dose must not exceed 3 gm.

OSTEOPOROSIS

General Considerations

Osteoporosis is a serious medical problem characterized by low bone mass, altered bone architecture, and increased bone fragility. Because of bone fragility, patients are susceptible to fractures from minor traumatic events, such as coughing, rolling over in bed, or falling from a standing position.

Osteoporosis is the most common bone disease in humans. More than 10 million Americans have osteoporosis—80% of them older women—and another 34 million have reduced bone mass, a risk factor for osteoporosis. Every year, osteoporosis leads to 1.5 million fractures. The most common fracture sites are the vertebrae (spine), distal forearm (wrist), and femoral neck (hip). Vertebral fractures can result in loss of height, spinal deformity, chronic back pain, and impaired breathing. Complications from hip fractures are a significant cause of mortality: Of the 300,000 Americans who get hip fractures each year, about 50,000 die from complications.

The economic burden of osteoporosis is high. Each year in the United States, osteoporosis-related fractures lead to more than 432,000 hospital admissions, nearly 2.5 million medical office visits, and about 180,000 admissions to nursing homes—at an estimated annual cost of $17 billion, or $47 million a day.

Bone Mass

In men and women, bone mass changes across the life span. Bone mass peaks in the third decade, remains stable to age 50 years, and then slowly declines—at a rate that is usually less than 1% a year. In addition to this slow, aging-related decline, women go through a phase of *accelerated* bone loss (2% to 3% a year) that begins after menopause and continues for several years. In both the slow and accelerated phases of decline, bone is lost because resorption of old bone outpaces deposition of new bone.

Primary Prevention: Calcium, Vitamin D, and Lifestyle

The risk of osteoporosis can be reduced by lifelong implementation of measures that can help maximize bone strength. Specifically, we need to ensure sufficient intake of calcium and vitamin D, and we need to adopt a lifestyle that promotes bone health. Calcium is needed to maximize bone growth early in life and to maintain bone integrity later in life. Vitamin D is needed to ensure calcium absorption. The amount of calcium needed for optimal bone health is indicated in Table 75.1. Note that calcium requirements are greatest for adolescents and teens (1300 mg/day), then drop for younger adults (1000 mg/day), and then rise for older adults (1200 mg/day). If diet alone cannot meet calcium needs, supplements should be employed. Lifestyle measures that promote bone health are:

- Performing regular weight-bearing exercise (walking, yoga, dancing, racquet sports, weight lifting, stair climbing)
- Avoiding excessive alcohol
- Avoiding smoking

PATIENT-CENTERED CARE ACROSS THE LIFE SPAN

Affecting Bone Mineralization[a]

Life Stage	Patient Care Concerns
Infants/children/adolescents	With the exception of calcium and vitamin D, these drugs are not recommended for children, except denosumab when taken for bone cancer. In this instance, it is advised only for "skeletally mature" adolescents who are 13 to 17 years old.
Pregnant women	The FDA has assigned a Pregnancy Risk Category of D/X[b] for denosumab (D for Xgeva; X for Prolia). Raloxifene is a Pregnancy Risk Category X[b] drug. The remaining drugs are classified in Pregnancy Risk Category C.[b] Nasal spray formulations of calcitonin-salmon are not recommended during pregnancy. Although vitamin D_2 and calcium formulations receiving an assigned Pregnancy Risk Category were given a C classification, this is generally considered to be a concern only if the intake exceeds recommendations.[b] Vitamin D_3 has not been assigned a Pregnancy Risk Category classification.
Breast-feeding women	Estrogen decreases both the quality and quantity of milk and may affect infant growth and development. For the remaining drugs, with the exception of calcium and vitamin D, breast-feeding is not recommended due to inadequate studies.
Older adults	Estrogen meets the Beers Criteria (strength of recommendation: strong) for potentially inappropriate use in older patients.

[a]Bisphosphonates are covered separately. See *Patient-Centered Care Across the Life Span: Bisphosphonates,* presented earlier in this chapter.

[b]As of 2020, the FDA will no longer use Pregnancy Risk Categories. Please refer to Chapter 9 for more information.

Diagnosing Osteoporosis and Assessing Fracture Risk

Osteoporosis is diagnosed by measuring BMD, an important predictor of fracture risk. Both the National Osteoporosis Foundation (NOF) and the U.S. Preventive Services Task Force (USPSTF) recommend routine BMD testing for *all women* beginning at age 65 years and for *younger postmenopausal women* deemed at increased risk for osteoporotic fractures. In addition, the NOF recommends testing of *all men* age 70 and older. (The USPSTF makes no recommendation regarding men.) BMD testing is not recommended for children or adolescents, nor is routine testing indicated for premenopausal women or healthy young men.

The standard technique for measuring BMD is *dual-energy x-ray absorptiometry* (DEXA). DEXA scans take only a few minutes, and exposure to radiation is minimal—about one-tenth that of a standard chest x-ray. Results of DEXA scans are reported in terms of *standard deviations* (SD) below mean BMD values in young adults. A BMD value that is 1 SD below the mean indicates 10% bone loss, a value that is 2 SD below the mean indicates 20% bone loss, and so forth. Using this system, the World Health Organization (WHO) has defined *normal* BMD for women as being no more than 1 SD below the mean for young adults. BMD values between 1 SD below the mean and 2.5 SD below the mean define *low bone mass* (also known as *osteopenia*). BMD values 2.5 SD or greater below the mean define *osteoporosis.* To simplify communication, we can talk about DEXA results in terms of a *T-score,* rather than using the phrase *SD above (or below) the mean.* For example, instead of saying that a BMD reading was 2.5 SD below the mean, we can simply say the T-score was −2.5.

Although loss of bone at one site (e.g., wrist) can predict the risk of fractures at other sites (e.g., hip, spine), it is preferable to measure BMD at specific sites to predict the risk for those sites. Accordingly, a thorough evaluation would include BMD measurements in the wrist, spine, and hip—the sites at which osteoporotic fractures occur most often.

Although we use BMD values to diagnose osteoporosis, it is important to understand that low BMD is not the only predictor of fractures. Other important predictors include a family history of hip fractures, a personal history of fractures, low body mass index, and use of oral glucocorticoids. To account for these risk factors, the WHO developed an important tool, called FRAX, which can assess an *individual's* 10-year risk of experiencing a fracture. This web-based, interactive program is available online at www.shef.ac.uk/FRAX/. Individual risk is calculated after entering the following data:

- Age
- Gender
- Weight
- Height
- Previous fracture
- Hip fracture in a parent
- Secondary osteoporosis (i.e., malnutrition, hyperthyroidism, diabetes, and other disorders associated with osteoporosis)
- Rheumatoid arthritis
- Glucocorticoid use
- Current smoking
- Alcohol consumption
- Hip BMD

Of note, FRAX is tailored to specific countries; in addition, for the United States, it is further tailored to four specific subgroups: African Americans, Hispanics, Caucasians, and Asians.

Who Should Be Treated?

An updated guideline—*Clinician's Guide to Prevention and Treatment of Osteoporosis*—was released by the NOF in 2010. According to this document, postmenopausal women and men age 50 and older should be considered for treatment if they present with:

- A hip fracture or vertebral fracture.
- Osteoporosis (T-score of −2.5 or less at the femoral neck or spine).
- Low bone mass (T-score between −1 and −2.5 at the femoral neck or spine) *plus either* a 10-year probability of a hip fracture of 3% or more *or* a 10-year probability of another major osteoporosis-related fracture of 20% or more, based on a U.S.-adapted FRAX calculation.

Treating Osteoporosis in Women

The objective of treatment is to reduce the occurrence of fractures by maintaining or increasing bone strength. Two types of drugs can be used: (1) agents that decrease bone resorption and (2) agents that promote bone formation. Not surprisingly, these are the same drugs previously covered in this chapter. Antiresorptive drugs—estrogen, raloxifene, bisphosphonates, calcitonin, and denosumab—are used most often. These agents do a good job of preventing bone loss by reducing osteoclast activity, but are largely unable to reverse bone mass that has already occurred. Accordingly, antiresorptive drugs are most beneficial when used early—before substantial loss has occurred. With all antiresorptive drugs, success requires a sufficiency of calcium and vitamin D. At this time, teriparatide [Forteo] is the only drug that effectively promotes bone formation. Of the drugs employed for osteoporosis, three agents—teriparatide, denosumab, and zoledronate (a bisphosphonate)—are most likely to reduce fractures.

Treating Osteoporosis in Men

In the United States, about 2 million men have aging-related osteoporosis, and another 3 million are at risk. Hip fractures occur in 80,000 American men annually, compared with 269,000 American women. Of the men who get a hip fracture, 36% die within a year. Although rates of osteoporosis and fractures in men are significant, they are still much lower than in women. As discussed, bone mass in men peaks in the third decade and begins progressive decline around age 50. The rate of decline in men is about equal to that in women—except that in men, there is no counterpart to the accelerated phase of bone loss that occurs following menopause. If men and women lose bone mass at similar rates, why do men experience less osteoporosis? The main reason is that bones in men, at their peak, are larger and stronger than bones in women. Hence, once decline begins, male bones can tolerate more loss before fractures are likely. Factors that contribute to the risk of osteoporosis in men include low testosterone, prolonged use of glucocorticoids, white race, calcium deficiency, vitamin D deficiency, smoking, excessive alcohol consumption, and insufficient exercise. As in women, 10-year fracture risk can be assessed using the FRAX calculator developed by the WHO.

Treatment of male osteoporosis is confounded by a paucity of research. (Osteoporosis is one of the few areas of therapeutics in which research in women has greatly exceeded research in men.) At this time, only five drugs—*alendronate* [Fosamax], *risedronate* [Actonel],[a] *zoledronate* [Reclast], *teriparatide* [Forteo], and *denosumab* [Prolia]—are approved for osteoporosis in men. In one study, 2 years of alendronate increased BMD of the lumbar spine and hip, and significantly decreased

[a]The delayed-release formulation of risedronate, sold as *Atelvia,* is not approved for osteoporosis in men, although it *is* approved for osteoporosis in women.

the incidence of vertebral fractures. Benefits with risedronate, zoledronate, and teriparatide are similar. For alendronate, zoledronate, and teriparatide, dosages are the same as those used in women. For risedronate, the only approved dosage is 35 mg once a week. Calcitonin has been tried in men, but proof of efficacy is lacking. If testosterone deficiency underlies osteoporosis, testosterone replacement therapy is indicated, unless the patient has testicular cancer or some other disorder that contraindicates testosterone use. All men should ensure adequate intake of calcium and vitamin D.

KEY POINTS

- Calcium is critical to the function of the skeletal, nervous, muscular, and cardiovascular systems.
- More than 98% of calcium in the body is present in bone.
- Bone undergoes continuous remodeling, a process in which osteoclasts resorb old bone and osteoblasts lay down new bone.
- The body maintains calcium levels by adjusting the rates of calcium resorption from bone, calcium absorption from the intestine, and calcium excretion by the kidney. These processes are regulated by parathyroid hormone (PTH), vitamin D, and calcitonin.
- PTH elevates serum calcium by promoting resorption of calcium from bone, enhancing renal tubular resorption of calcium, and activating vitamin D, which then promotes absorption of calcium from the intestine.
- Like PTH, vitamin D increases serum calcium by increasing calcium resorption from bone, decreasing calcium excretion by the kidney, and increasing calcium absorption from the intestine.
- Calcitonin lowers calcium levels by inhibiting calcium resorption from bone and increasing calcium excretion by the kidney.
- The RDA for calcium is highest for adolescents ages 9 to 18 (1300 mg/day). Women over the age of 50 and all people over the age of 70 also need relatively high amounts (1200 mg/day).
- If the RDA cannot be met with diet alone, calcium supplements can be taken to make up the difference. However, be aware that too much supplemental calcium increases the risk of vascular calcification, myocardial infarction, and stroke.
- The various calcium salts used for therapy differ widely in their percentage of calcium.
- Vitamin D is obtained through the diet and by exposure to sunlight.
- Vitamin D deficiency causes rickets in children and osteomalacia in adults. Deficiency may also contribute to certain autoimmune disorders and cancers, although convincing evidence is lacking.
- Calcitonin-salmon has the same metabolic effects as human calcitonin, but has a longer half-life and greater milligram potency.
- Calcitonin-salmon is used primarily for osteoporosis. Benefits derive from inhibiting bone resorption by osteoclasts.
- Alendronate, our prototype for the bisphosphonates, has four approved indications: prevention and treatment of osteoporosis in postmenopausal women, treatment of osteoporosis in men, treatment of Paget's disease of bone in men and women, and treatment of glucocorticoid-induced osteoporosis in men and women.
- Bioavailability of alendronate is very low in the absence of food and essentially zero in the presence of food. Accordingly, nothing should be eaten for at least 30 minutes after taking the drug.
- Following absorption, alendronate undergoes incorporation into bone, where it can remain for decades.
- Alendronate suppresses bone resorption by decreasing both the number and activity of osteoclasts.
- Alendronate can cause severe esophagitis if it stays in contact with the esophageal mucosa. Accordingly, patients should take the drug with a full glass of water and then remain upright for at least 30 minutes.
- Rarely, alendronate has been associated with musculoskeletal pain, ocular inflammation, osteonecrosis of the jaw, and atypical fractures of the femur.
- Estrogen increases BMD and reduces fracture risk.
- In the past, estrogen was considered a treatment of choice for the prevention and treatment of postmenopausal osteoporosis. Today, however, there is strong evidence that benefits in osteoporosis do not outweigh the risks (breast cancer, myocardial infarction, stroke, cholecystitis).
- Raloxifene belongs to the family of SERMs, drugs that are estrogenic in some tissues and antiestrogenic in others.
- Raloxifene mimics the effects of estrogen on bone, lipid metabolism, and blood clotting, and blocks the effects of estrogen in the breast and endometrium.
- Raloxifene is indicated for preventing and treating postmenopausal osteoporosis and for reducing the risk of breast cancer in postmenopausal women.
- Raloxifene can cause DVT, PE, and fetal harm.
- Teriparatide is the first and only drug for osteoporosis that works by increasing bone formation. (All the others decrease bone resorption.)
- Teriparatide may increase the risk of bone cancer.
- Denosumab is a first-in-class RANKL inhibitor indicated for postmenopausal osteoporosis and prevention of skeletal-related events in patients with bone metastases from solid tumors.
- By inhibiting RANKL, denosumab prevents RANKL from activating RANK receptors and thereby reduces the formation and function of osteoclasts.
- Denosumab has four serious side effects: hypocalcemia, infections, skin reactions, and ONJ.
- Osteoporosis is characterized by low bone mass and increased bone fragility, which renders patients vulnerable to fractures from minor trauma.
- The most common sites of osteoporotic fractures are the vertebrae (spine), distal forearm (wrist), and femoral neck (hip).

- Osteoporosis occurs mainly in older adults. After age 50 years, men and women experience aging-related bone loss that is slow but relentless. In addition, women experience several years of accelerated bone loss following menopause. In both cases, bone is lost because bone resorption by osteoclasts outpaces bone deposition by osteoblasts.
- To maximize bone strength, and thereby minimize the risk of osteoporosis, we all need to (1) ensure lifelong sufficiency of calcium and vitamin D and (2) adopt lifestyle measures that promote bone health: regular weight-bearing exercise and avoidance of smoking and excessive alcohol.
- Osteoporosis is diagnosed by measuring BMD, which is done most commonly using dual-energy x-ray absorptiometry (DEXA).
- The World Health Organization's diagnostic criterion for osteoporosis is BMD that is more than 2.5 standard deviations below the mean BMD for young adults.
- The objective of osteoporosis therapy is to reduce fractures.
- Fracture risk, which can be calculated using the FRAX tool developed by the WHO, is based on BMD and other factors, including age, use of glucocorticoids, and a personal or family history of fractures.
- With currently available drugs, we are more able to prevent bone loss (using antiresorptive agents) than to rebuild bone that is already gone (using bone-forming agents).
- Antiresorptive drugs—estrogen, raloxifene, bisphosphonates (e.g., alendronate), and calcitonin—decrease bone loss by inhibiting the activity of osteoclasts.

Please visit **http://evolve.elsevier.com/Lehne** for chapter-specific NCLEX® examination review questions.

Summary of Major Nursing Implications[a]

VITAMIN D

Calcitriol
Cholecalciferol
Doxercalciferol
Ergocalciferol
Paricalcitol

Preadministration Assessment

Therapeutic Goal

Treatment of rickets, osteomalacia, and hypoparathyroidism, and prevention of vitamin D deficiency.

Baseline Data

The prescriber may order serum levels of vitamin D, calcium, phosphorus, and alkaline phosphatase, as well as a 24-hour urinary calcium determination.

Assess dietary vitamin D and calcium content.

Identifying High-Risk Patients

Vitamin D is *contraindicated* in patients with hypercalcemia, hypervitaminosis D, and malabsorption syndrome.

Exercise *caution* in patients taking digoxin.

Implementation: Administration

Routes

Oral, IM.

Administration

Instruct the patient to swallow oral preparations intact, without crushing or chewing.

Therapeutic responses to vitamin D require adequate calcium intake. Assess dietary calcium content and adjust to ensure calcium sufficiency.

Ongoing Evaluation and Interventions

Monitoring Summary

Monitor serum calcium, serum phosphorus, and urinary calcium.

Minimizing Adverse Interactions

Digoxin. Vitamin D–induced hypercalcemia can cause dysrhythmias in patients taking digoxin. Monitor serum calcium, and make certain it remains within normal range.

Management of Toxicity

Large therapeutic doses may cause hypervitaminosis D, a syndrome characterized by hypercalcemia, hypercalciuria, decalcification of bone, and deposition of calcium in soft tissues. Monitor serum calcium content; levels should stay below 10 mg/dL. Monitor serum phosphorus and urinary calcium as well. **If vitamin D toxicity develops, instruct the patient to discontinue vitamin D immediately, increase fluid intake, and institute a low-calcium diet.** In severe cases, calcium excretion can be accelerated with IV saline plus furosemide.

ORAL CALCIUM SALTS

Calcium acetate
Calcium carbonate
Calcium citrate
Calcium glubionate
Calcium gluconate
Calcium lactate
Tricalcium phosphate

Continued

Summary of Major Nursing Implications[a]—cont'd

Preadministration Assessment

Therapeutic Goal

Treatment of mild hypocalcemia and supplementation of dietary calcium.

Baseline Data

Obtain a serum calcium level.

Identifying High-Risk Patients

Calcium salts are *contraindicated* for patients with hypercalcemia, renal calculi, and hypophosphatemia.

Implementation: Administration

Route

Oral.

Dosage

Individual calcium salts differ with respect to percentage of elemental calcium. As a result, the dose required to provide a specific amount of calcium differs among the salts. **Advise patients against switching to a different preparation.**

Administration

Advise patients to take oral calcium salts with a large glass of water; dosing with or after meals promotes absorption. Advise patients to avoid taking calcium with foods that can suppress calcium absorption (e.g., spinach, Swiss chard, beets, bran, whole-grain cereals).

Ongoing Evaluation and Interventions

Minimizing Adverse Effects

Prolonged therapy can cause hypercalcemia. **Inform patients about signs of hypercalcemia (nausea, vomiting, constipation, frequent urination, lethargy, and depression), and instruct them to notify the prescriber if these occur.** Hypercalcemia can be minimized with frequent monitoring of serum calcium.

Minimizing Adverse Interactions

Glucocorticoids. These drugs reduce calcium absorption; increased calcium dosage may be required.

Tetracyclines. Calcium binds to tetracyclines, thereby reducing tetracycline absorption. **Instruct patients to separate administration of these agents by at least 1 hour.**

Thyroid Hormone. Calcium interferes with the absorption of thyroid hormone. **Instruct patients to separate administration of these agents by several hours.**

Thiazide Diuretics. Thiazides decrease renal excretion of calcium. A reduction in calcium dosage may be needed to avoid hypercalcemia.

Loop Diuretics. Loop diuretics increase calcium excretion and may cause hypocalcemia. An increase in calcium dosage may be needed to avoid hypocalcemia.

PARENTERAL CALCIUM SALTS

Calcium chloride
Calcium gluconate

Preadministration Assessment

Therapeutic Goal

Reversal of clinical manifestations of hypocalcemia.

Baseline Data

Assess for signs and symptoms of hypocalcemia (tetany, convulsions, laryngospasm, spasm of other muscles). Obtain measurement of serum calcium.

Identifying High-Risk Patients

Parenteral calcium is *contraindicated* for patients with hypercalcemia or ventricular fibrillation.

Use with *extreme caution* in patients taking digoxin.

Implementation: Administration

Route

Intravenous.

Administration

Warm solutions to body temperature before IV dosing. Perform IV injections slowly (0.5 to 2 mL/min).

Drugs that contain phosphate, carbonate, sulfate, and tartrate groups can precipitate calcium; do not mix these drugs with parenteral calcium solutions.

Calcium chloride may cause necrosis and sloughing if solutions become extravasated. Monitor the infusion closely.

Ongoing Evaluation and Interventions

Evaluating Therapeutic Effects

Evaluate the patient for reductions in tetany, muscle spasm, laryngospasm, paresthesias, and other symptoms of severe hypocalcemia.

Minimizing Adverse Effects

Hypercalcemia. Overdose can produce acute hypercalcemia, resulting in nausea, vomiting, weakness, lethargy, coma, and possibly death. Avoid hypercalcemia through careful control of dosage.

Minimizing Adverse Interactions

Digoxin. Parenteral calcium may cause severe bradycardia in patients taking digoxin. Infuse calcium slowly and cautiously in these patients.

CALCITONIN-SALMON

Preadministration Assessment

Therapeutic Goal

Treatment of postmenopausal osteoporosis, Paget's disease of bone, and hypercalcemia.

Baseline Data

The prescriber may order measurements of serum alkaline phosphatase, calcium, and phosphorus, as well as a 24-hour urinary hydroxyproline.

Summary of Major Nursing Implications[a]—cont'd

Identifying High-Risk Patients

Calcitonin-salmon is *contraindicated* for patients allergic to this preparation.

Implementation: Administration

Routes

Intranasal. For osteoporosis only.

Parenteral (IM, subQ). For osteoporosis, Paget's disease, and hypercalcemia.

Administration

Intranasal. **Instruct patients using calcitonin-salmon nasal spray to prime the metered-dose pump by holding the bottle upright and depressing the two white sidearms toward the bottle 6 times, which should produce a faint initial spray. The drug is then administered by placing the nozzle in the nostril and depressing the pump handle.**

Subcutaneous. **Teach patients how to inject calcitonin subQ, and instruct them to rotate sites of injection.**

Ongoing Evaluation and Interventions

Evaluating Therapeutic Effects

Postmenopausal Osteoporosis. Measurement of BMD should indicate slowing of bone loss (and perhaps a small increase in BMD).

Paget's Disease of Bone. Monitor for reductions in bone pain, serum alkaline phosphatase levels, and 24-hour urinary hydroxyproline value.

Hypercalcemia. Monitor for reductions in serum calcium and phosphorus levels.

BISPHOSPHONATES USED FOR OSTEOPOROSIS

Alendronate
Ibandronate
Risedronate
Zoledronate

Preadministration Assessment

Therapeutic Goal

Prevention and treatment of osteoporosis.

Baseline Data

Obtain baseline values for BMD in the hip, spine, and wrist. For patients receiving zoledronate, obtain a baseline value for creatinine clearance and assess for adequate hydration.

Identifying High-Risk Patients

Oral bisphosphonates are *contraindicated* for patients with esophageal disorders that can impede swallowing, and for patients who cannot sit or stand for at least 30 minutes (60 minutes with ibandronate).

Zoledronate, an IV bisphosphonate, is *contraindicated* for patients with acute renal failure or creatinine clearance below 35 mL/min, and should be used with *caution* in patients who are older or dehydrated, and in those with chronic renal impairment and those taking other nephrotoxic drugs.

Implementation: Administration

Routes

Oral. Alendronate, risedronate, ibandronate.

Intravenous. Zoledronate.

Dosing Schedule

Alendronate. Daily or weekly.

Risedronate. Daily, weekly, or monthly.

Ibandronate. Daily, monthly, or every 3 months.

Zoledronate. Yearly, or every 2 years.

Administration

Oral. Proper administration is needed to maximize absorption and minimize the risk of esophagitis. Accordingly, **instruct patients to:**

- **Administer in the morning before eating or drinking anything other than water.** This applies to all oral bisphosphonates except Atelvia, a delayed-release brand of risedronate, which can and should be administered after eating.
- **Administer with a full glass of water.**
- **Administer while upright, either sitting or standing.**
- **Avoid chewing or sucking the tablet.**
- **After dosing, remain sitting or standing for at least 30 minutes (60 minutes with ibandronate).**
- **After dosing, postpone ingesting anything—including orange juice, coffee, antacids, and calcium, iron, or magnesium supplements—for at least 30 minutes (60 minutes with ibandronate).**

Intravenous. Infuse zoledronate over a span of 15 minutes or longer.

Ongoing Evaluation and Interventions

Evaluating Therapeutic Effects

Obtain periodic determinations of BMD. If BMD increases, or at least remains constant, treatment is a success. Conversely, a significant decline in BMD indicates failure.

Minimizing Adverse Effects

Esophagitis. Oral bisphosphonates can cause severe esophagitis, sometimes resulting in ulceration. To minimize risk, **instruct patients to (1) administer the drug in accord with the guidelines described previously, (2) avoid lying down after dosing, and (3) discontinue the drug and contact the prescriber if they experience symptoms of esophageal injury (difficulty in swallowing, pain upon swallowing, new or worsening heartburn).** Avoid these drugs in patients with esophageal disorders that could impede swallowing and in patients who are unable to sit or stand for 30 minutes (60 minutes with ibandronate).

Continued

Summary of Major Nursing Implications[a]—cont'd

Atypical Femoral Fractures. Very rarely, long-term bisphosphonate therapy has been associated with atypical fractures of the femur. To reduce risk, prescribers should:

- Use these drugs only when needed (i.e., avoid bisphosphonates in patients considered at low risk for osteoporosis-related fractures).
- Consider alternative treatments, such as raloxifene or teriparatide, for patients with osteoporosis of the spine and normal (or only moderately reduced) BMD of the femoral neck or hip.
- Perform an annual re-evaluation of the need for continued therapy in patients who have taken bisphosphonates for 5 years.

Esophageal Cancer. Oral bisphosphonates may (or may not) increase the risk of *esophageal cancer.* Measures that might reduce the risk include reducing the dosing frequency (e.g., dosing monthly or weekly rather than daily), taking the drug with a full glass of water, and staying upright for 30 to 60 minutes after dosing.

Musculoskeletal Pain. Rarely, bisphosphonates cause muscle, bone, and joint pain. Severe pain may require an opioid or ketorolac for relief. As a rule, pain gradually diminishes when bisphosphonates are withdrawn. In most cases, pain does not return when bisphosphonates are resumed. If it does resume, osteoporosis should be managed with a different drug (e.g., calcitonin-salmon, teriparatide, raloxifene).

Ocular Problems. Rarely, bisphosphonates cause conjunctivitis, scleritis, blurred vision, eye pain, and other ocular problems. **Inform patients about these effects and instruct them to report any vision changes or eye pain.**

Osteonecrosis of the Jaw. ONJ occurs primarily with IV bisphosphonates (pamidronate, zoledronate). To reduce ONJ risk, a dental examination with appropriate preventive dentistry should be conducted before giving bisphosphonates.

Renal Toxicity. Intravenous *zoledronate* can damage the kidney, leading to acute renal failure and possibly death. Exercise caution in patients at increased risk (owing to advanced age, chronic renal impairment, dehydration, or use of diuretics or nephrotoxic drugs). Before dosing, ensure that hydration is adequate and that kidney function is adequate too (creatinine clearance above 35 mL/min). To reduce risk, infuse zoledronate slowly (over 15 minutes or more). Monitor renal function by determining creatinine clearance at baseline, before each dose, and periodically after each infusion. If renal impairment develops, zoledronate dosage should be reduced.

Minimizing Adverse Interactions

Interactions With Zoledronate. Risk of renal failure with zoledronate is increased by the use of *diuretics* (which can cause dehydration) and by the use of other *nephrotoxic drugs,* including cyclosporine, amphotericin, aminoglycoside antibiotics, and the NSAIDs. Exercise caution in patients using these agents.

RALOXIFENE

Preadministration Assessment

Therapeutic Goals

Prevention and treatment of postmenopausal osteoporosis, and reducing the risk of invasive breast cancer in postmenopausal women who have osteoporosis and/or a high risk for breast cancer.

Baseline Data

Obtain baseline values for BMD in the hip, vertebrae, and forearm.

Identifying High-Risk Patients

Raloxifene is *contraindicated* for use by patients who are pregnant or who have a history of venous thrombotic events.

Implementation: Administration

Route

Oral.

Administration

Take once daily without regard to meals.

Ongoing Evaluation and Interventions

Promoting Therapeutic Effects

Advise women taking raloxifene for osteoporosis to ensure adequate intake of calcium and vitamin D.

Evaluating Therapeutic Effects

For women taking raloxifene to prevent or treat osteoporosis, obtain periodic determinations of BMD. If BMD increases, or at least remains constant, treatment is a success. Conversely, a significant decline in BMD indicates failure.

Minimizing Adverse Effects

Venous Thromboembolism. Raloxifene increases the risk of DVT, PE, and thrombotic stroke. **Advise patients to discontinue raloxifene at least 72 hours before prolonged immobilization (e.g., postsurgical recovery, extended bed rest) and to resume treatment only after full mobility has been restored. Advise patients to avoid extended periods of restricted activity, as can happen when traveling.** Do not give raloxifene to patients with a history of venous thrombotic events.

Fetal Harm. Raloxifene can cause fetal harm and must not be used during pregnancy.

ESTROGEN

Nursing implications for estrogen are summarized in Chapter 61.

[a]Patient education information is highlighted as **blue text.**

UNIT XIII

RESPIRATORY TRACT DRUGS

CHAPTER 76

Drugs for Asthma and Chronic Obstructive Pulmonary Disease

BASIC CONSIDERATIONS

Asthma is a common chronic disorder that occurs in 1 in 11 children and 1 in 12 adults in the United States. Characteristic signs and symptoms are a sense of breathlessness and tightness in the chest, together with wheezing, dyspnea, and cough. The underlying cause is immune-mediated airway inflammation. In the United States, nearly 25.7 million people have the disease, representing an increase of almost 15% since the early 2000s. Each year, the disease kills about 3500 Americans. However, despite these sobering statistics, with proper treatment, most patients can lead full lives with no limitations.

Chronic obstructive pulmonary disease (COPD) is a chronic, progressive, largely irreversible disorder characterized by airflow restrictions and inflammation. In most cases, COPD is preventable; the most common cause is smoking cigarettes. Symptoms include chronic cough, excessive sputum production, wheezing, dyspnea, and poor exercise tolerance. In the United States, COPD affects about 24 million people. In the most recent report by the Centers for Disease Control and Prevention, chronic lower respiratory diseases were listed as the third leading cause of death in the United States. Unfortunately, although drug therapy is highly effective in asthma, benefits in COPD are minimal, being limited to a small improvement in symptoms. Drug therapy does not slow disease progression, reduce hospitalizations, or prolong life.

PATHOPHYSIOLOGY OF ASTHMA

Asthma is a *chronic inflammatory* disorder of the airways. In about 50% of children with asthma and in some adults, airway inflammation results from an immune response to known allergens. In the remaining children and in most adults, the cause of airway inflammation is unknown—although as-yet unidentified allergens are suspected.

Fig. 76.1 depicts the events that lead to inflammation and bronchoconstriction in patients whose asthma is caused by specific allergens. Although this model may not apply completely to all asthma patients, it nonetheless provides a basis for understanding the drugs used for treatment. The inflammatory process begins with binding of allergen molecules (e.g., house dust mite feces) to immunoglobulin E (IgE) antibodies on mast cells. This causes mast cells to release an assortment of mediators, including histamine, leukotrienes, prostaglandins, and interleukins. These mediators have two effects. They act immediately to cause *bronchoconstriction.* In addition, they promote infiltration and activation of inflammatory cells (eosinophils, leukocytes, macrophages). These inflammatory cells then release mediators of their own. The end result is *airway inflammation,* characterized by edema, mucus plugging, and smooth muscle hypertrophy, all of which obstruct airflow. In addition, inflammation produces a state of *bronchial hyperreactivity.* Because of this state, mild trigger factors (e.g., cold air, exercise, tobacco smoke) are able to cause intense bronchoconstriction.

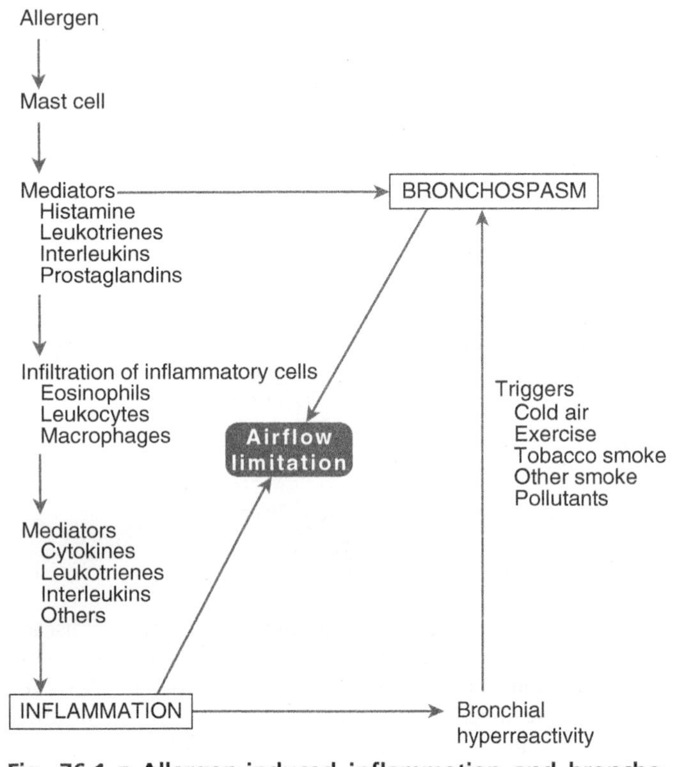

Fig. 76.1 ▪ Allergen-induced inflammation and bronchospasm in asthma.

PATHOPHYSIOLOGY OF COPD

Symptoms of COPD result largely from two pathologic processes: *chronic bronchitis* and *emphysema.* In most cases, both processes are caused by an exaggerated inflammatory reaction to cigarette smoke. Chronic bronchitis—defined by chronic cough and excessive sputum production—results from hypertrophy of mucus-secreting glands in the epithelium of the larger airways. Emphysema is defined as enlargement of the air space within the bronchioles and alveoli brought on by deterioration of the walls of these air spaces. Among individuals with COPD, the relative contribution of these two processes can vary. That is, some patients may suffer primarily from chronic bronchitis, some primarily from emphysema, and some from both disease processes.

Fig. 76.2 depicts the events that lead to inflammation, airway obstruction, and air trapping in patients with COPD. Irritants such as tobacco smoke initiate an inflammatory response in the airways. As a result of the frequent and recurrent irritation and the subsequent response by various leukocytes and inflammatory mediators, pathologic changes result in the bronchial edema and increase in mucus secretion that characterize chronic bronchitis. Additionally, the continuous inflammation inhibits the production of protease inhibitors, which have a protective role in maintaining alveolar integrity. As a result of the inhibition, the protease enzymes break down elastin, resulting in the destruction of alveolar walls and the decrease in elastic recoil that characterize emphysema. In a small percentage of the population, emphysema results from a genetic alteration that results in alpha-1 antitrypsin deficiency. (Alpha-1 antitrypsin is a protease inhibitor that protects the lungs from enzymatic destruction by proteases.)

OVERVIEW OF DRUGS FOR ASTHMA AND COPD

The major drugs for asthma and COPD are shown in Table 76.1. They fall into two main pharmacologic classes: *anti-inflammatory agents* and *bronchodilators.* The principal anti-inflammatory drugs are the *glucocorticoids.* The principal bronchodilators are the *beta$_2$ agonists.* For chronic asthma and stable COPD, glucocorticoids are administered on a fixed schedule, almost always by inhalation. Beta$_2$ agonists may be administered on a fixed schedule (for long-term control) or PRN (to manage an acute attack). Like the glucocorticoids, beta$_2$ agonists are usually inhaled.

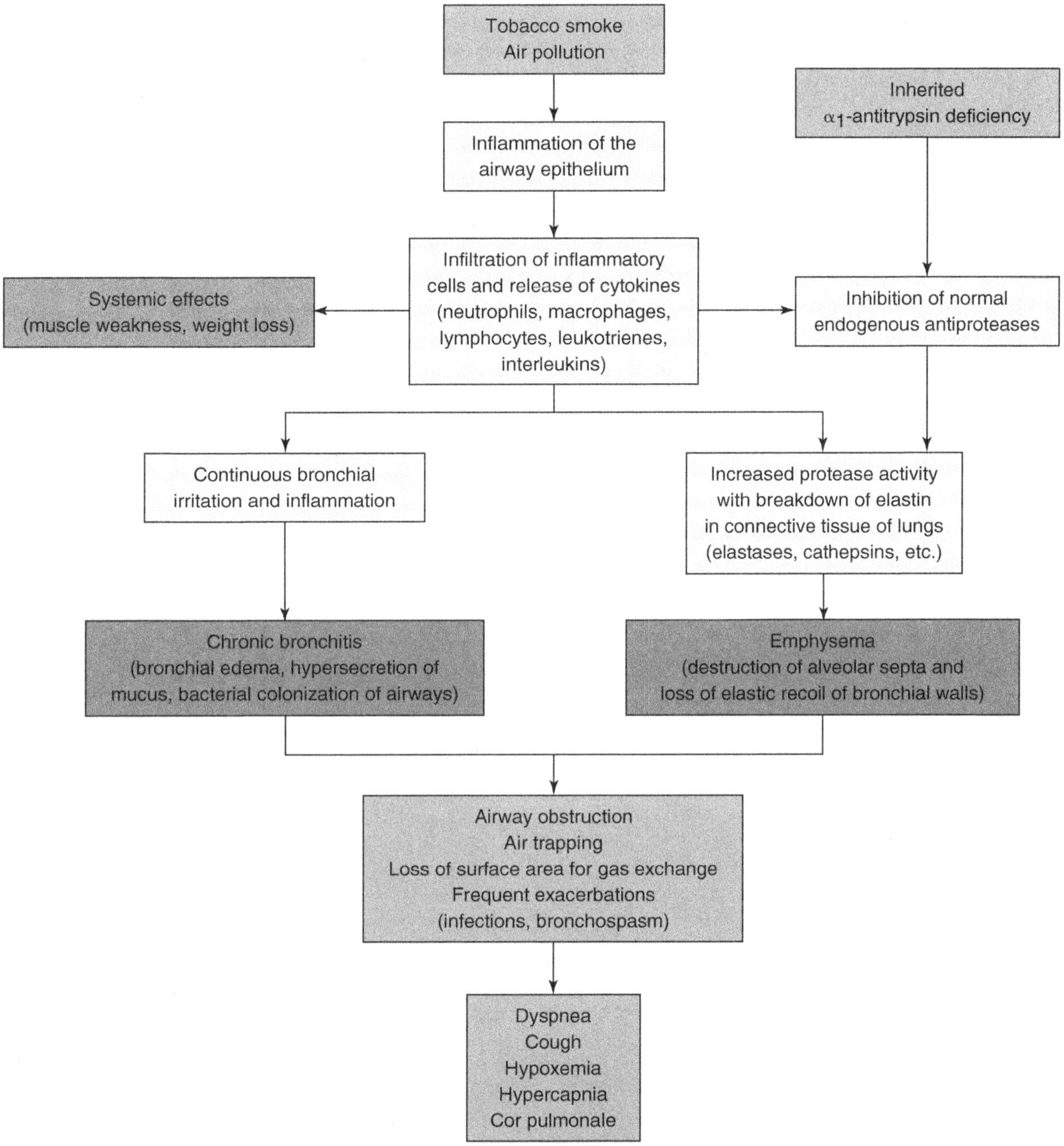

Fig. 76.2 ▪ **Pathogenesis of chronic bronchitis and emphysema.**

Prototype Drugs

DRUGS FOR ASTHMA AND COPD

Anti-Inflammatory Drugs: Glucocorticoids

Beclomethasone (inhaled)
Prednisone (oral)

Anti-Inflammatory Drugs: Others

Cromolyn (mast cell stabilizer, inhaled)
Zafirlukast (leukotriene modifier, oral)

Bronchodilators: Beta$_2$-Adrenergic Agonists

Albuterol (inhaled, short acting)
Salmeterol (inhaled, long acting)

Bronchodilators: Methylxanthines

Theophylline

Anticholinergic Drugs

Ipratropium

TABLE 76.1 ■ Overview of Major Drugs for Asthma and Chronic Obstructive Pulmonary Disease

ANTI-INFLAMMATORY DRUGS

Glucocorticoids

Inhaled

Beclomethasone dipropionate [QVAR]
Budesonide [Pulmicort Flexhaler, Pulmicort Respules, Pulmicort Turbuhaler 🍁]
Ciclesonide [Alvesco]
Flunisolide [Aerospan]
Fluticasone propionate [Flovent HFA, Flovent Diskus]
Mometasone furoate [Asmanex Twisthaler]

Oral

Methylprednisolone [A-Methapred, Depo-Medrol, Medrol, Medrol Dose-Pak]
Prednisolone [Flo-Pred, Orapred ODT, Millipred, Pediapred, Prelone]
Prednisone [Deltasone, Winpred 🍁]

Leukotriene Modifiers

Montelukast, oral [Singulair][a]
Zafirlukast, oral [Accolate][a]
Zileuton, oral [Zyflo, Zyflo CR][a]

Cromolyn

Cromolyn, inhaled [Nalcrom 🍁][a]

IgE Antagonist

Omalizumab, subQ [Xolair]

Phosphodiesterase-4 Inhibitors

Roflumilast, oral [Daliresp, Daxas 🍁][b]

ANTI-INFLAMMATORY/BRONCHODILATOR COMBINATIONS

Budesonide/formoterol, inhaled [Symbicort]
Fluticasone/salmeterol, inhaled [Advair Diskus, Advair HFA]
Fluticasone/vilanterol, inhaled [Breo Ellipta]
Mometasone/formoterol, inhaled [Dulera, Zenhale 🍁]

BRONCHODILATORS

Beta$_2$-Adrenergic Agonists

Inhaled: Short Acting

Albuterol [ProAir HFA, ProAir RespiClick, Proventil HFA, Ventolin HFA, Airomir, Apo-Salvent MDI 🍁]
Levalbuterol [Xopenex, Xopenex HFA]

Inhaled: Long Acting[c]

Arformoterol [Brovana][b]
Formoterol [Foradil Aerolizer, Perforomist, Oxeze Turbuhaler 🍁][c]
Indacaterol [Arcapta Neohaler, Onbrez Breezhaler 🍁][b]
Olodaterol [Striverdi Respimat][b]
Salmeterol [Serevent Diskus][c]

Oral

Albuterol [VoSpire ER]
Terbutaline (generic only)

Methylxanthines

Aminophylline, oral (generic only)
Theophylline, oral [Theo-24, Elixophyllin, Theochron, Theolair 🍁, Pulmophylline 🍁, Theo ER 🍁, Uniphyl 🍁]

Anticholinergics

Aclidinium bromide, inhaled [Tudorza Pressair][b]
Glycopyrronium bromide, inhaled [Seebri Neohaler, Seebri Breezhaler 🍁][b]
Ipratropium, inhaled [Atrovent HFA]
Tiotropium, inhaled [Spiriva, Spiriva HandiHaler, Spiriva Respimat][b]
Umeclidinium, inhaled [Incruse Ellipta]

BETA AGONIST/CHOLINERGIC ANTAGONIST COMBINATIONS

Albuterol/ipratropium, inhaled [Combivent Respimat, Combivent UDV 🍁][b]
Indacaterol/glycopyrronium, inhaled [Utibron Neohaler, Ultibro Breezhaler 🍁][b]
Olodaterol/tiotropium, inhaled [Stiolto Respimat][b]
Vilanterol/umeclidinium, inhaled [Anoro Ellipta][b]

[a]Approved only for asthma, not for chronic obstructive pulmonary disease.
[b]Approved only for chronic obstructive pulmonary disease, not for asthma.
[c]For treatment of asthma, must always be combined with an inhaled glucocorticoid.

ADMINISTERING DRUGS BY INHALATION

Most antiasthma drugs can be administered by inhalation. This route has three advantages: (1) therapeutic effects are enhanced by delivering drugs directly to their site of action, (2) systemic effects are minimized, and (3) relief of acute attacks is rapid. Four types of inhalation devices are employed: metered-dose inhalers, Respimats, dry-powder inhalers, and nebulizers.

Metered-Dose Inhalers

Metered-dose inhalers (MDIs) are small hand-held, pressurized devices that deliver a measured dose of drug with each actuation. Dosing is usually accomplished with 1 or 2 inhalations. When 2 inhalations are needed, an interval of at least 1 minute should separate the first inhalation from the second.

When using most MDIs, the patient must begin to inhale before activating the device. This requires hand-breath coordination, making MDIs difficult to use correctly. Accordingly, patients will need a demonstration, as well as written and verbal instruction. Even with optimal use, only about 10% of the dose reaches the lungs. About 80% affects the oropharynx and is swallowed, and the remaining 10% is left in the device or exhaled.

Spacers are devices that attach directly to the MDI to increase delivery of drug to the lungs and decrease deposition of drug on the oropharyngeal mucosa (Fig. 76.3). Several kinds of spacers are available for use with MDIs. Some spacers contain a one-way valve that activates upon inhalation, obviating the need for good hand-breath coordination. Some spacers also contain an alarm whistle that sounds off when inhalation is too rapid, thus maximizing effective drug administration. They can also prevent bronchospasm that may occur with sudden intake of an inhaled drug.

Respimats

Respimats are inhalers that deliver drugs as a very fine mist. Like MDIs, they are activated by the user; however, the device does not use propellants. An advantage of this system is that the extremely small particle size ensures greater delivery of drug to the lungs; in addition, because less drug falls out of

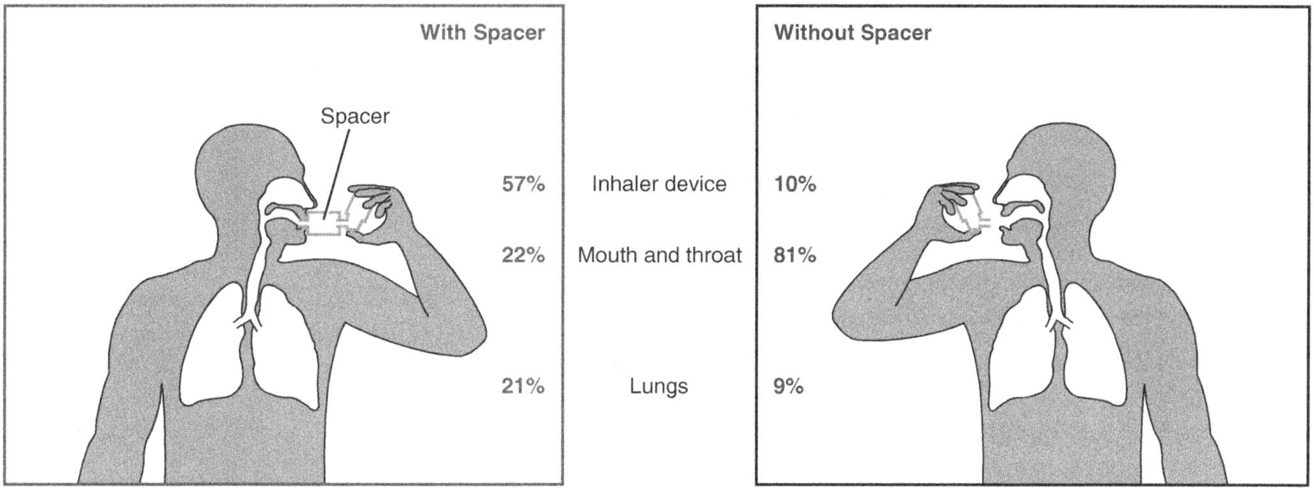

Fig. 76.3 ■ Effect of a spacer device on the distribution of inhaled medication. Note that, when a spacer is used, more medication reaches its site of action in the lungs, and less is deposited in the mouth and throat.

the mist due to particle weight, there is decreased drug deposition in the mouth and oropharynx.

Dry-Powder Inhalers

Dry-powder inhalers (DPIs) are used to deliver drugs in the form of a dry micronized powder directly to the lungs. Unlike MDIs, DPIs are breath activated. As a result, DPIs don't require the hand-breath coordination needed with MDIs, making DPIs much easier to use. Compared with MDIs, DPIs deliver more drug to the lungs (20% of the total released vs. 10%) and less to the oropharynx. Also, spacers are not used with DPIs.

Nebulizers

A nebulizer is a small machine used to convert a drug solution into a mist. The droplets in the mist are much finer than those produced by inhalers, resulting in less drug deposit on the oropharynx and increased delivery to the lung. Inhalation of the nebulized mist can be done through a face mask or through a mouthpiece held between the teeth. Because the mist produced by a nebulizer is inhaled with each breath, hand-breath coordination is not a concern. Nebulizers take several minutes to deliver the same amount of drug contained in 1 inhalation from an inhaler, but for some patients, a nebulizer may be more effective than an inhaler. Although nebulizers are usually used at home or in a clinic or hospital, these devices, which weigh less than 10 pounds, are sufficiently portable for use in other locations.

ANTI-INFLAMMATORY DRUGS

Anti-inflammatory drugs—especially inhaled glucocorticoids—are the foundation of asthma and COPD therapy. These drugs are taken daily for long-term control. Most people with asthma require these drugs for management at some point.

PATIENT-CENTERED CARE ACROSS THE LIFE SPAN

Anti-Inflammatory Agents

Life Stage	Patient Care Concerns
Children	Inhaled glucocorticoids are the preferred long-term treatment for children of all ages, including infants. Face masks are recommended for the administration of inhaled glucocorticoids to children younger than 4 years. Alternative treatments include cromolyn and leukotriene receptor antagonists (e.g., montelukast), but evidence supporting these drugs for asthma management is lower than that supporting inhaled glucocorticoids. Montelukast is the only leukotriene modifier approved for children ages 1 to 5 years.
Pregnant women	Inhaled glucocorticoids are classified in FDA Pregnancy Risk Category C[a]; however, they are preferred for uncontrolled asthma in pregnant women because uncontrolled asthma is associated with greater fetal risks. Of the leukotriene modifiers, montelukast and zafirlukast are Pregnancy Risk Category B,[a] while zileuton is Risk Category C.[a]
Breast-feeding women	Inhaled glucocorticoids are not a contraindication to breast-feeding; however, women taking *systemic* glucocorticoids should not breast-feed.
Older adults	Benefits exceed risk. Inhaled glucocorticoids are much safer for this population than systemic formulations.

[a]As of 2020, the FDA will no longer use Pregnancy Risk Categories. Please refer to Chapter 9 for more information.

GLUCOCORTICOIDS

Glucocorticoids (e.g., budesonide, fluticasone) are the most effective drugs available for long-term control of airway inflammation. Administration is usually by inhalation, but may also be IV or oral. Adverse reactions to inhaled glucocorticoids are generally minor, as are reactions to systemic glucocorticoids taken *acutely.* However, when *systemic* glucocorticoids are used *long term,* severe adverse effects are likely. The basic pharmacology of the glucocorticoids is presented in Chapter 72. Discussion here is limited to their use in asthma.

Mechanism of Antiasthma Action

Glucocorticoids reduce asthma symptoms by *suppressing inflammation.* Specific anti-inflammatory effects include:

- Decreased synthesis and release of inflammatory mediators (e.g., leukotrienes, histamine, prostaglandins)
- Decreased infiltration and activity of inflammatory cells (e.g., eosinophils, leukocytes)
- Decreased edema of the airway mucosa (secondary to a decrease in vascular permeability)

By suppressing inflammation, glucocorticoids reduce bronchial hyperreactivity and decrease airway mucus production. There is also some evidence that glucocorticoids may increase the number of bronchial $beta_2$ receptors, as well as their responsiveness to $beta_2$ agonists.

Use in Asthma

Glucocorticoids are used for *prophylaxis* of chronic asthma. Accordingly, dosing must be done on a fixed schedule—not PRN. Because beneficial effects develop slowly, these drugs cannot be used to abort an ongoing attack. Glucocorticoids do not alter the natural course of asthma, even when used in young children.

Inhalation Use. Inhaled glucocorticoids are first-line therapy for management of the inflammatory component of asthma. Most patients with persistent asthma should use these drugs daily. Inhaled glucocorticoids are very effective and are much safer than systemic glucocorticoids.

Oral Use. Oral glucocorticoids may be required for patients with moderate to severe persistent asthma or for management of acute exacerbations of asthma or COPD. Because of their potential for toxicity, these drugs are prescribed only when symptoms cannot be controlled with safer medications (inhaled glucocorticoids, inhaled $beta_2$ agonists). Because the risk for toxicity increases with duration of use, treatment should be as brief as possible.

Adverse Effects

Inhaled Glucocorticoids. These preparations are largely devoid of serious toxicity, even when used in high doses. The most serious concern is adrenal suppression.

The most common adverse effects are *oropharyngeal candidiasis* and *dysphonia* (hoarseness, speaking difficulty). Both effects result from local deposition of inhaled glucocorticoids. To minimize these effects, patients should rinse the mouth with water and gargle after each administration. Using a spacer device can help too. If candidiasis develops, it can be treated with an antifungal drug.

With long-term, high-dose therapy, some *adrenal suppression* may develop, although the degree of suppression is generally low. In contrast, with prolonged use of *oral* glucocorticoids, adrenal suppression can be profound.

Glucocorticoids can *slow* growth in children and adolescents—but these drugs do *not* decrease adult height. *Short-term* studies have shown that inhaled glucocorticoids slow growth; however, *long-term* studies indicate that adult height, while delayed, is not reduced. Less is known regarding whether glucocorticoids suppress growth and development of the brain, lungs, and other organs, in part because having asthma alone can affect organ growth. Because the benefits of inhaled glucocorticoids tend to be much greater than the risks, current guidelines for asthma management recommend these drugs for children while monitoring for evidence of complications.

Long-term use of inhaled glucocorticoids may promote *bone loss.* Fortunately, the amount of loss is much lower than the amount caused by oral glucocorticoids. To minimize bone loss, patients should (1) use the lowest dose that controls symptoms, (2) ensure adequate intake of calcium and vitamin D, and (3) participate in weight-bearing exercise.

There has been concern that prolonged therapy might increase the risk for *cataracts* and *glaucoma.* While this may be an issue of concern with continuous use of high-dose inhaled glucocorticoids, this problem is not associated with long-term use of low to medium doses of inhaled glucocorticoids.

Oral Glucocorticoids. When used acutely (less than 10 days), even in very high doses, oral glucocorticoids do not cause significant adverse effects. However, prolonged therapy, even in moderate doses, can be hazardous. Potential adverse effects include *adrenal suppression, osteoporosis, hyperglycemia, peptic ulcer disease,* and, in young patients, *growth suppression.*

Adrenal suppression is of particular concern. As discussed in Chapter 72, prolonged glucocorticoid use can decrease the ability of the adrenal cortex to produce glucocorticoids of its own. This can be life-threatening at times of severe physiologic stress (e.g., surgery, trauma, or systemic infection). Because

Safety Alert

COMPENSATING FOR ADRENAL INSUFFICIENCY

When patients have been on prolonged systemic glucocorticoid therapy, the adrenal glands decrease their endogenous production of glucocorticoids. If systemic therapy is stopped suddenly, as when switching from oral therapy to inhalation therapy, the patient can die. Similarly, during times of severe physical stress when the body would normally produce high levels of glucocorticoids, if the dose of systemic glucocorticoids is not increased to meet the increased need, the patient can die. What important lesson can you take from this? When discontinuing a systemic glucocorticoid, you must be sure that it is done gradually to allow the body to resume production of the endogenous hormone. On the other hand, if a patient taking systemic glucocorticoids experiences severe physical stress, such as a motor vehicle crash, or is scheduled for a stressful procedure such as surgery, you must make certain that the provider remembers to prescribe additional glucocorticoids to supplement for the endogenous hormone that the patient cannot produce.

high levels of glucocorticoids are required to survive severe stress and because adrenal suppression prevents production of endogenous glucocorticoids, *patients must be given increased doses of oral or IV glucocorticoids at times of stress. Failure to do so can prove fatal.*

Adrenal suppression is also a concern when discontinuing prolonged use of oral glucocorticoids or when transferring from an oral route to an inhaled route. Several months are required for recovery of adrenocortical function, so it is important to decrease the dosage gradually. Throughout this time, all patients—including those switched to inhaled glucocorticoids—must be given supplemental oral or IV glucocorticoids at times of severe stress.

A complete list of contraindications to oral glucocorticoids is presented in the *Summary of Major Nursing Implications* at the end of this chapter.

Preparations, Dosage, and Administration

Inhaled Glucocorticoids. Six glucocorticoids are available for inhalation (Table 76.2). Four are available in MDIs, three are available in DPIs, and one is available in suspension for nebulization. Inhaled glucocorticoids are administered on a regular schedule—not PRN. Pediatric and adult dosages are shown in Table 76.2. The dosage should be kept as low as possible to minimize adrenal suppression, possible bone loss, and other adverse effects.

Nebulized Budesonide. Budesonide suspension [Pulmicort Respules] is the first inhaled glucocorticoid formulated for nebulized dosing. The product is approved for maintenance therapy of persistent asthma in children 1 to 8 years old. Improvement should begin in 2 to 8 days; maximal benefits may take 4 to 6 weeks to develop. Administration is done with a jet nebulizer equipped with a mouthpiece or face mask; ultrasonic nebulizers should not be used. Administration takes 5 to 10 minutes. For children who are *not* taking an oral glucocorticoid, the initial dosage is 500 mcg/day in one or two doses. For children who *are* taking an oral glucocorticoid, the initial dosage is 1000 mcg/day in one or two doses. After 1 week, dosage of the oral glucocorticoid should be tapered off. Additional information on dosing of budesonide and other inhaled glucocorticoids is provided in Table 76.2.

Oral Glucocorticoids. *Methylprednisolone, prednisone,* and *prednisolone* are preferred glucocorticoids for oral therapy of asthma. The dosage is the same regardless of the drug.

When beginning therapy with oral glucocorticoids, dosing initially focuses on bringing symptoms under control. The *initial adult* dosage is typically a burst of 40 to 60 mg administered daily for 3 to 10 days. The *initial pediatric* dosage is 1 to 2 mg/kg/day for 3 to 10 days. Thereafter, the typical dose is 0.25 to 2 mg/kg daily or every other day for children under 12 and 7.5 to 60 mg daily or every other day for older children and adults. For *long-term* treatment, *alternate-day dosing* is recommended to minimize adrenal suppression. After symptoms have been controlled for 3 months, dosages should be decreased gradually to establish the lowest dosage that can keep the patient free of symptoms. As discussed previously, the dosage of oral glucocorticoids must be increased during times of stress.

LEUKOTRIENE MODIFIERS

Leukotriene modifiers suppress the effects of leukotrienes, which are compounds that promote smooth muscle constriction, blood vessel permeability, and inflammatory responses through direct action as well as through recruitment of eosinophils and other inflammatory cells. In patients with asthma, these drugs can decrease bronchoconstriction and inflammatory responses such as edema and mucus secretion.

Three leukotriene modifiers are currently available: zileuton, zafirlukast, and montelukast. Zileuton blocks leukotriene synthesis; zafirlukast and montelukast block leukotriene receptors. All three drugs are dosed orally. Preparations and dosages of the leukotriene modifiers are provided in Table 76.3. Current guidelines recommend using these agents as second-line therapy (if an inhaled glucocorticoid cannot be used) and as add-on therapy when an inhaled glucocorticoid alone is inadequate. Although generally well tolerated, all the leukotriene modifiers can cause adverse neuropsychiatric effects, including depression, suicidal thinking, and suicidal behavior.

Zileuton

Zileuton [Zyflo, Zyflo CR], an inhibitor of leukotriene synthesis, is approved for asthma prophylaxis and maintenance therapy in adults and children 12 years and older. Symptomatic improvement can be seen within 1 to 2 hours of dosing. Because effects are not immediate, zileuton cannot be used to abort an ongoing attack. Zileuton is less effective than an inhaled glucocorticoid alone, and appears to be less effective than a long-acting inhaled $beta_2$ agonist as adjunctive therapy in patients not adequately controlled with an inhaled glucocorticoid.

TABLE 76.2 ▪ Inhaled Glucocorticoids: Formulations and Dosages

		Dosage	
Drug	Formulation	Adults	Children
Beclomethasone dipropionate [QVAR]	MDI: 40, 80 mcg/inhalation	40–320 mcg twice daily	40–80 mcg twice daily (5–11 yr)
Budesonide			
[Pulmicort Flexhaler]	DPI: 90, 180 mcg/inhalation	360–720 mcg twice daily	180–360 mcg twice daily (6–17 yr)
[Pulmicort Respules]	Suspension for nebulization	250–500 mcg once or twice daily *or* 1000 mcg once daily	500–1000 mcg once daily (1–8 yr)
Ciclesonide [Alvesco]	MDI: 80, 160 mcg/inhalation	80–320 mcg twice daily	80–320 mcg twice daily (12 yr and up)
Flunisolide [AeroBid]	MDI: 80 mcg/inhalation	160–320 mcg twice daily	80–320 mcg twice daily (6–11 yr)
Fluticasone propionate			
[Flovent HFA]	MDI: 44, 110, 220 mcg/inhalation	88–440 mcg twice daily	88 mcg twice daily (4–11 yr)
[Flovent Diskus]	DPI: 50, 100, 250 mcg/inhalation	100–1000 mcg twice daily	50–100 mcg twice daily (4–11 yr)
Mometasone furoate [Asmanex Twisthaler]	DPI: 110, 220 mcg/inhalation	220–440 mcg once or twice daily	110 mcg once daily (4–11 yr)

DPI, Dry-powder inhaler; *MDI,* metered-dose inhaler.

TABLE 76.3 ■ Leukotriene Modifiers: Preparations and Dosages

Drug	Preparation	Dosage
Montelukast [Singulair]	Granules: 4 mg/pkt Chewable tablets: 4, 5 mg Tablets: 10 mg	12–23 months: one pkt of 4 mg granules daily 2–5 years: one pkt of 4 mg granules or one 4-mg tablet every evening 6–14 years: one 5-mg chewable tablet every evening 15 years and older: one 10-mg tablet every evening *EIB prophylaxis:* one 10-mg tablet at least 2 hr before exercising[a]
Zafirlukast [Accolate]	Tablets 10, 20 mg	5–11 years: 10-mg tablet twice daily 12 years and older: 20-mg twice daily
Zileuton [Zyflo, Zyflo CR]	IR tablet: 600 mg ER tablet: 600 mg	12 years and older: • IR tablet: one 600-mg tablet 4 times daily • ER tablet: two 600-mg tablets twice daily

[a]No additional dose should be taken for at least 24 hours. Patients already taking montelukast daily should not take any more to prevent exercise-induced bronchospasm (EIB).
ER, Extended release; *IR,* immediate release; *pkt,* packet.

Mechanism of Action

Benefits derive from inhibiting 5-lipoxygenase, the enzyme that converts arachidonic acid into leukotrienes. This decreases the amount of leukotrienes available to induce inflammation.

Pharmacokinetics

Zileuton is given orally and undergoes rapid absorption, both in the presence and absence of food. Plasma levels peak 2 to 3 hours after dosing. Zileuton is rapidly metabolized by the liver, and the metabolites are excreted in the urine. Its plasma half-life is 2.5 hours.

Adverse Effects

Zileuton can injure the liver, as evidenced by increased plasma levels of alanine aminotransferase (ALT) activity. A few patients have developed symptomatic hepatitis, which reversed after drug withdrawal. To reduce the risk for serious liver injury, ALT activity should be monitored. The recommended schedule is once a month for 3 months, then every 2 to 3 months for the remainder of the first year, and periodically thereafter.

Postmarketing reports indicate that zileuton and the other leukotriene modifiers can cause adverse neuropsychiatric effects, including depression, anxiety, agitation, abnormal dreams, hallucinations, insomnia, irritability, restlessness, and suicidal thinking and behavior. If these develop, switching to a different medication should be considered.

Zileuton is metabolized by cytochrome P450, where it acts as an inhibitor of CYP1A2 isoenzymes and can slow metabolism of drug substrates metabolized by this pathway, increasing their levels. Combined use with theophylline can markedly increase theophylline levels, so dosage of theophylline should be reduced. Zileuton can also increase levels of warfarin and propranolol.

Zafirlukast

Zafirlukast [Accolate] was the first representative of a unique group of anti-inflammatory agents, the *leukotriene receptor antagonists.* The drug is approved for maintenance therapy of chronic asthma in adults and children 5 years and older.

Mechanism of Action

Benefits derive in part from reduced infiltration of inflammatory cells, resulting in decreased bronchoconstriction.

Pharmacokinetics

Zafirlukast is administered orally, and absorption is rapid. Food reduces absorption by 40%; therefore, the drug should be administered at least 1 hour before meals or 2 hours after. Zafirlukast undergoes hepatic metabolism followed by fecal excretion. The half-life is about 10 hours, but may be as long as 20 hours in older adults.

Adverse Effects

The most common side effects of zafirlukast are headache and gastrointestinal (GI) disturbances, both of which are infrequent. Arthralgia and myalgia may also occur. Like zileuton, zafirlukast can cause depression, suicidal thinking, hallucinations, and other neuropsychiatric effects. A few patients have developed Churg-Strauss syndrome, a potentially fatal disorder characterized by weight loss, flu-like symptoms, and pulmonary vasculitis (blood vessel inflammation). However, in most cases, symptoms developed when glucocorticoids were being withdrawn, suggesting that glucocorticoid withdrawal may be a contributing factor.

Rarely, patients develop clinical signs of liver injury (e.g., abdominal pain, jaundice, fatigue). If these occur, zafirlukast should be discontinued, and liver function tests (especially serum ALT) should be performed immediately. If test results are consistent with liver injury, zafirlukast should not be resumed. Curiously, signs of liver injury have developed mainly in females.

Zafirlukast inhibits several isoenzymes of cytochrome P450 and can suppress metabolism of other drugs, causing their levels to rise. Concurrent use can raise serum theophylline to toxic levels. Theophylline levels should be closely monitored, especially when zafirlukast is started or stopped. Zafirlukast can also raise levels of warfarin (an anticoagulant), and thus may cause bleeding.

Montelukast

Montelukast [Singulair], a leukotriene receptor blocker, is the most commonly used leukotriene modulator. The drug has three approved indications: (1) prophylaxis and maintenance therapy of asthma in patients at least 1 year old; (2) prevention of exercise-induced bronchospasm (EIB) in patients at least 15 years old; and (3) relief of allergic rhinitis (see Chapter 77). Montelukast cannot be used for quick relief of an asthma attack because effects develop too slowly. For prophylaxis and maintenance therapy of asthma, maximal effects develop within 24 hours of the first dose and are maintained with once-daily dosing in the evening. In clinical trials, montelukast decreased asthma-related nocturnal awakening, improved morning lung function, and decreased the need for a short-acting inhaled $beta_2$ agonist throughout the day. Although montelukast is approved for preventing EIB, a short-acting $beta_2$ agonist is preferred.

Mechanism of Action

Montelukast has a high affinity for leukotriene receptors in the airway and on proinflammatory cells such as eosinophils. By occupying these receptors, the drug blocks receptor activation by the body's leukotrienes.

Pharmacokinetics

Montelukast is rapidly absorbed after oral administration. Bioavailability is about 64%. Blood levels peak 3 to 4 hours after ingestion. The drug is highly bound (more than 99%) to plasma proteins. Montelukast undergoes extensive metabolism by hepatic cytochrome P450 enzymes followed by excretion in the bile. The plasma half-life ranges from 2.7 to 5.5 hours.

Adverse Effects

Montelukast is generally well tolerated. In clinical trials, adverse effects were equivalent to those of placebo. In contrast to zileuton and zafirlukast, montelukast does not seem to cause liver injury. As with zafirlukast, Churg-Strauss syndrome has occurred when glucocorticoid dosage was reduced. Postmarketing reports suggest a link between montelukast and neuropsychiatric effects, especially mood changes and suicidality. Fortunately, these effects are rare.

Montelukast appears devoid of serious drug interactions. Unlike zileuton and zafirlukast, it does not increase levels of theophylline or warfarin. Concurrent use of phenytoin (an anticonvulsant that induces P450 isoenzymes) can decrease levels of montelukast.

CROMOLYN

Cromolyn is an inhalational agent that suppresses bronchial inflammation. The drug is used for *prophylaxis*—not quick relief—in patients with mild to moderate asthma. Anti-inflammatory effects are less than with glucocorticoids; therefore, cromolyn is not a preferred drug for asthma therapy. When glucocorticoids create problems, however, cromolyn may be prescribed as alternative therapy.

Mechanism of Action

Cromolyn suppresses inflammation; it does not cause bronchodilation. The drug acts in part by stabilizing the cytoplasmic membrane of mast cells, preventing release of histamine and other mediators. In addition, cromolyn inhibits eosinophils, macrophages, and other inflammatory cells.

Pharmacokinetics

Cromolyn is administered by nebulizer. The fraction absorbed from the lungs is small and rarely produces significant systemic effects. Absorbed cromolyn is excreted unchanged in the urine.

Therapeutic Uses

Chronic Asthma. Cromolyn is an alternative to inhaled glucocorticoids for prophylactic therapy of mild persistent asthma. When administered on a fixed schedule, cromolyn reduces both the frequency and intensity of asthma attacks. Maximal effects may take several weeks to develop. No tolerance to effects is seen with long-term use. Cromolyn is especially effective for prophylaxis of seasonal allergic attacks and for acute allergy prophylaxis immediately before allergen exposure (e.g., before mowing the lawn).

Exercise-Induced Bronchospasm. Cromolyn can prevent bronchospasm in patients at risk for EIB. For best results, cromolyn should be administered 10 to 15 minutes before anticipated exertion but no longer than 1 hour before exercise.

Allergic Rhinitis. Intranasal cromolyn [NasalCrom] can relieve symptoms of allergic rhinitis (see Chapter 77).

Adverse Effects.

Cromolyn is the safest of all antiasthma medications. Significant adverse effects occur in fewer than 1 of every 10,000 patients. Occasionally, cough or bronchospasm occurs in response to cromolyn inhalation.

Preparations, Dosage, and Administration

Cromolyn is administered using a power-driven nebulizer. The *initial* dosage for adults and children is 20 mg 4 times a day. For *maintenance* therapy, the lowest effective dosage should be established.

OMALIZUMAB

Omalizumab [Xolair] is a monoclonal antibody with a unique mechanism of action: antagonism of IgE, a type of antibody. The drug is a second-line agent indicated only for allergy-related asthma and only when preferred options have failed. Omalizumab offers modest benefits and has significant drawbacks. For example, the drug poses a risk for anaphylaxis and cancer, must be given subcutaneously, and costs more than $10,000 a year. Furthermore, its long-term safety is unknown.

Mechanism of Action

Omalizumab forms complexes with free IgE in the blood and thereby reduces the amount of IgE available to bind with its receptors on mast cells. This greatly reduces the number of IgE molecules on the mast cell surface and thus limits the ability of allergens to trigger release of histamine, leukotrienes, and other mediators that promote bronchospasm and airway inflammation. At recommended doses, omalizumab decreases free IgE in serum by 96%. When treatment stops, about 1 year is required for free IgE to return to its pretreatment level.

Therapeutic Use

Omalizumab is approved only for patients age 12 years and older with moderate to severe asthma that (1) is allergy related and that (2) cannot be controlled with an inhaled glucocorticoid. In clinical trials, the drug produced a modest decrease in the number of exacerbations and often permitted a reduction in glucocorticoid use. Because of its mechanism of action, omalizumab can help only patients whose asthma is caused by a specific allergen (e.g., pet dander, dust mite feces). Accordingly, a skin test or blood test proving allergen reactivity is required. Unless instructed otherwise, patients should continue all asthma medications they were using before starting omalizumab.

Pharmacokinetics

Omalizumab is administered by subcutaneous (subQ) injection. Absorption is slow, producing peak plasma levels in 7 to 8 days. Degradation occurs in the liver. The drug's half-life is prolonged, about 26 days.

Adverse Effects

Omalizumab can cause a variety of adverse effects. The most common are injection-site reactions, viral infection, upper respiratory infection, sinusitis, headache, and pharyngitis. Early clinical trials suggested a very small risk for cardiovascular problems and malignancy. A meta-analysis of postmarketing studies revealed no significant increase in cardiovascular events between subjects taking omalizumab and a placebo. There was a small increase in rare malignancy occurrence in subjects taking omalizumab; however, a clear relationship to the drug has not been established. Possible adverse consequences of long-term IgE suppression are unknown.

Life-threatening *anaphylaxis*—characterized by urticaria and edema of the throat and/or tongue—has occurred rarely (in less than 0.1% of patients). Anaphylaxis is most likely with the first dose, but can also occur after receiving repeated doses with no apparent sensitivity. To minimize injury from anaphylaxis, patients should be observed for 2 hours after the first three doses, and for 30 minutes after all subsequent doses. Facilities for managing anaphylaxis should be immediately available. Patients who experience a severe reaction should not be given omalizumab again.

Preparations, Dosage, and Administration

Omalizumab [Xolair] is available as a powder (202.5 mg) in single-use vials for reconstitution with 1.4 mL of sterile water. Dissolving the powder, which can take 20 minutes or longer, yields a final solution of 150 mg/1.2 mL. Administration is by subQ injection, which may take 5 to 10 seconds because the solution is somewhat viscous. The reconstituted solution should be used within 4 hours (if stored at room temperature) or within 8 hours (if stored cold). Omalizumab powder should be kept refrigerated.

The size of each dose and the dosing interval are determined by body weight and total serum IgE, measured at baseline. Dosages range from 150 to 300 mg every 4 weeks to 225 to 375 mg every 2 weeks. No more than 150 mg should be injected at any site. If a dose exceeds 150 mg, it should be divided among two or more sites.

ROFLUMILAST

Mechanism of Action

Roflumilast is a phosphodiesterase type 4 (PDE4) inhibitor. PDE4 is an enzyme that breaks down cyclic adenosine monophosphate (cAMP). The end result of this process is an increase in inflammatory mediators. By inhibiting the enzyme, roflumilast decreases the release of inflammatory products. This helps to prevent inflammation and decrease damage to lung tissue, thereby improving pulmonary function.

Therapeutic Use

Roflumilast [Daliresp, Daxas 🍁] is approved for treatment of severe COPD with a chronic bronchitis component. It is not approved for use in asthma.

Pharmacokinetics

Roflumilast is highly (99%) protein bound. This is largely responsible for its long half-life of 17 hours. Metabolism is by CYP3A4 and CYP1A2 isoenzymes. It is excreted in the urine.

Adverse Effects

Psychiatric adverse effects are the most concerning. About 6% of those in clinical trials report events ranging from anxiety and depression to suicidal behavior. For this reason, it is not recommended for patients with a history of depression.

Loss of appetite frequently occurs. Weight loss is common; 20% of patients in clinical trials lost between 5% and 10% of their pretreatment weight.

Other adverse effects include GI complaints (nausea, diarrhea), insomnia, and headache. There have been adverse events in animal reproduction studies, so this is not recommended for pregnant women.

As mentioned, roflumilast is a substrate of CYP3A4 and CYP1A2 isoenzymes. Drugs that inhibit or induce these enzymes can affect serum levels of roflumilast.

Preparations, Dosage, and Administration

Roflumilast is supplied as tablets containing 500 mcg of the drug. Dosage is one 500-mcg tablet daily. It may be taken with or without food.

BRONCHODILATORS

Bronchodilators provide symptomatic relief in patients with asthma and COPD but do not alter the underlying inflammation that is part of the disease process. Accordingly, most patients who require a bronchodilator also use an inhaled glucocorticoid for long-term suppression of inflammation. Monotherapy with a bronchodilator is appropriate only when asthma is very mild and attacks are infrequent.

BETA$_2$-ADRENERGIC AGONISTS

Inhaled beta$_2$ agonists are the most effective drugs available for relieving acute bronchospasm and preventing EIB. Virtually all patients with asthma use these first-line drugs as a component of an asthma management regimen. The basic pharmacology of the beta$_2$ agonists is presented in Chapter 17. Discussion here is limited to their use in asthma.

Mechanism of Action

The beta$_2$ agonists are sympathomimetic drugs that activate beta$_2$-adrenergic receptors. By activating beta$_2$ receptors in smooth muscle of the lung, these drugs promote *bronchodilation* and thus relieve bronchospasm. In addition, beta$_2$ agonists have a limited role in suppressing histamine release in the lung and increasing ciliary motility.

Classification by Route and Time Course

Beta$_2$ agonists may be administered orally or by inhalation, and their effects may be brief or prolonged. All of the oral agents are long acting. Among the inhaled agents, some are short acting and some are long acting. With the short-acting inhaled preparations, effects begin almost immediately, peak in 30 to 60 minutes, and persist for 3 to 5 hours. Because of this time course, the short-acting beta$_2$ agonists (SABAs) can be used to abort an ongoing attack, but cannot be used for prolonged prophylaxis. With the inhaled long-acting beta$_2$ agonists (LABAs), onset depends on the drug. With formoterol and arformoterol, onset is relatively rapid, whereas onset is delayed with salmeterol. However, because these drugs are used on a fixed schedule for long-term control, the difference in onset is not very important.

PATIENT-CENTERED CARE ACROSS THE LIFE SPAN

Bronchodilators

Life Stage	Patient Care Concerns
Children	Short-acting beta$_2$ agonists (SABAs) are approved for children age 2 years and older although they are often needed and used for younger children. Special delivery devices such as nebulizers may be used for very young children. Safety and efficacy of anticholinergics have not been established for children under 11 years old. Methylxanthines are approved for children of all ages, including neonates. It is important to consider variable drug clearance across age ranges when dosing.
Pregnant women	Beta$_2$ agonists are classified in FDA Pregnancy Risk Category C[a] due to uterine relaxation; however, National Asthma Education and Prevention Program (NAEPP) guidelines note that benefits are greater than risks. Pregnant women must have adequate respiratory exchange to ensure adequate oxygenation of the developing fetus. Anticholinergics are classified in FDA Pregnancy Risk Category B.[a] Methylxanthines are Pregnancy Risk Category C.[a]
Breast-feeding women	Breast-feeding is not contraindicated with beta$_2$ agonists or anticholinergics; however, manufacturers of both drugs recommend caution. Labeling for methylxanthines warns against breast-feeding only if the mother may have toxic levels.
Older adults	Benefits typically exceed risks for beta agonists and anticholinergics. *Systemic* anticholinergics are included in *Beers Criteria for Potentially Inappropriate Use in Older Adults*; they should not be substituted for inhaled anticholinergics.

[a]As of 2020, the FDA will no longer use Pregnancy Risk Categories. Please refer to Chapter 9 for more information.

Use in Asthma and Chronic Obstructive Pulmonary Disease

Beta$_2$ agonists are employed for quick relief and long-term control. Drug selection depends on the goal.

Inhaled Short-Acting Beta$_2$ Agonists. SABAs are taken PRN to abort an ongoing attack. In patients with EIB, they are taken before exercise to prevent an attack from occurring. For hospitalized patients undergoing a severe acute attack, a nebulized SABA is the traditional treatment of choice. However, delivery with an MDI in the outpatient setting may be equally effective.

Safety Alert

TOO MUCH OF A GOOD THING

Short-acting $beta_2$ agonists are often lifesaving medications. If they are taken in excess, however, overdose can lead to dangerous adverse effects, such as tachydysrhythmias, angina, and seizures. Cardiac arrest and death may occur. What lesson can you take from this? If your patient needs to use a rescue inhaler more than twice a week to control asthma symptoms, it is time to step up therapy.

Long-Acting Inhaled $Beta_2$ Agonists. Patients who experience frequent attacks may be prescribed an LABA for long-term control. Dosing is done on a fixed schedule, not PRN. LABAs are preferred over SABAs for patients with stable COPD. In patients with asthma, however, LABAs are not first-line therapy, and they must always be *combined with a glucocorticoid.* In fact, their use *alone* in asthma is *contraindicated* because LABA monotherapy has been associated with increased incidence of asthma-associated death.[a] For combined LABA-glucocorticoid therapy, the U.S. Food and Drug Administration (FDA) recommends using a product that contains both drugs in the same inhaler.

Oral $Beta_2$ Agonists. These drugs are used only for long-term control. Onset is too slow to abort an ongoing attack. Like the long-acting inhaled $beta_2$ agonists, the oral agents are not first-line therapy.

Adverse Effects

Inhaled Preparations: Short Acting. Inhaled SABAs are well tolerated. Systemic effects—tachycardia, angina, and tremor—can occur, but are usually minimal.

Inhaled Preparations: Long Acting. Inhaled LABAs may increase the risk for severe asthma and asthma-related death when used as monotherapy for long-term control. To minimize risk, LABAs should be used only in patients taking a recommended medication for long-term control, and only if that medication has been inadequate by itself. LABAs should never be used as first-line therapy for prolonged control and should never be used alone.

Oral Preparations. The selectivity of the $beta_2$-adrenergic agonists is only relative, not absolute. Accordingly, when these drugs are administered orally, they are likely to produce some activation of $beta_1$ receptors in the heart. If dosage is excessive, stimulation of cardiac $beta_1$ receptors can cause *angina pectoris* and *tachydysrhythmias.* Patients should be instructed to report chest pain or changes in heart rate or rhythm.

Oral $beta_2$ agonists often cause *tremor* by activating $beta_2$ receptors in skeletal muscle. Tremor can be reduced by lowering the dosage. With continued drug use, tremor declines spontaneously.

Preparations, Dosage, and Administration

Nine selective $beta_2$ agonists are available (Table 76.4). Some are used for quick relief, and some are used for long-term control.

Inhaled Preparations for Quick Relief. To provide quick relief, $beta_2$ agonists must be administered by inhalation. Three types of devices may be used: MDIs, DPIs, and nebulizers.

For drugs administered with an MDI or DPI, the initial dosing schedule is 1 or 2 inhalations 3 or 4 times a day. Additional drugs are added to the asthma management regimen (Tables 76.5 and 76.6) with a goal of decreasing reliance on an SABA to no more than twice a week.

When 2 inhalations are needed, an interval of 1 minute or longer should separate them. During this interval, some bronchodilation develops, facilitating penetration of the second inhalation.

For certain patients, nebulizers may be superior to inhalers. Some patients who have become unresponsive to a $beta_2$ agonist delivered with an inhaler may respond to the same drug when it is given with a nebulizer. The nebulizer delivers the dose slowly (over several minutes); as the bronchi gradually dilate, the drug gains deeper and deeper access to the lungs.

Inhaled Preparations for Long-Term Control. Five single-agent inhaled LABAs are approved for treatment of asthma: salmeterol [Serevent Diskus]; formoterol [Foradil Aerolizer, Perforomist, Oxeze Turbuhaler ♣]; arformoterol [Brovana], the *(R,R)*-enantiomer of formoterol; indacaterol [Arcapta Neohaler, Onbrez Breezhaler ♣]; and olodaterol [Striverdi Respimat]. Vilanterol, another LABA, is available only in combination with a glucocorticoid (fluticasone/vilanterol [Breo Ellipta] and umeclidinium/vilanterol [Anoro Ellipta]). LABAs have a long duration of action and thus are suited for long-term control. Dosing is every 12 hours. If supplemental bronchodilation is needed between doses, an SABA should be used. As discussed previously, LABAs are not first-choice agents for long-term control, and they should not be used alone. Rather, they should always be combined with an inhaled glucocorticoid, preferably in the same inhaler device.

Although salmeterol is usually inhaled twice daily (every 12 hours), with continuous use, more frequent dosing may be needed because benefits seem to persist for a shorter time as the duration of treatment increases.

Oral Preparations for Long-Term Control. Two oral $beta_2$ agonists—albuterol and terbutaline—are approved for long-term control of asthma. Dosing is 3 or 4 times a day. (In Canada, terbutaline is also available in an inhaled form as Bricanyl Turbuhaler offering 500 mcg/actuation for PRN dosing.)

METHYLXANTHINES

We first encountered the methylxanthines (theophylline, caffeine, others) in Chapter 36. As discussed there, the most prominent actions of these drugs are (1) central nervous system (CNS) excitation and (2) bronchodilation. Other actions include cardiac stimulation, vasodilation, and diuresis.

Theophylline

Theophylline [Theo-24, Theochron, Elixophyllin, Theolair ♣, Uniphyl ♣, others] is the principal methylxanthine employed in asthma. Benefits derive primarily from bronchodilation. Theophylline has a narrow therapeutic range, so dosage must be carefully controlled. The drug is usually administered by mouth but may also be administered intravenously.

Mechanism of Action

Theophylline produces bronchodilation by relaxing smooth muscle of the bronchi. Although the mechanism of bronchodilation has not been firmly established, the most probable is blockade of receptors for adenosine.

[a]Although using an LABA alone is contraindicated for patients with asthma, LABAs can still be used alone in patients with COPD.

TABLE 76.4 ▪ Beta$_2$-Adrenergic Agonists

		Initial Dosage	
Drug	**Formulation**	**Adults**	**Children**
INHALED AGENTS: SHORT ACTING			
Albuterol			
[ProAir HFA, ProAir RespiClick, Proventil HFA, Ventolin HFA]	MDI (90 mcg/inhalation)	2 inhalations every 4–6 hr PRN	2 inhalations every 4–6 hr PRN
[Proventil]	Solution for nebulization	1.25–5 mg every 4–8 hr PRN	0.63–2.5 mg/kg every 4–6 hr PRN
Levalbuterol			
[Xopenex HFA]	MDI (45 mcg/inhalation)	2 inhalations every 4–6 hr PRN	2 inhalations every 4–6 hr PRN
[Xopenex]	Solution for nebulization	0.63 mg every 6–8 hr PRN	0.31–1.25 mg every 4–6 hr PRN
INHALED AGENTS: LONG ACTING[a]			
Aclidinium bromide[b] [Tudorza Pressair]	DPI (400 mcg/inhalation)	1 inhalation every 12 hr	Safety and efficacy not established
Arformoterol[a,b] [Brovana]	Solution for nebulization	15 mcg every 12 hr	Safety and efficacy not established
Formoterol			
[Foradil Aerolizer]	DPI (12 mcg/inhalation)	1 inhalation every 12 hr	1 inhalation every 12 hr
[Perforomist][b]	Solution for nebulization	20 mcg every 12 hr	Safety and efficacy not established
Indacaterol[b] [Arcapta Neohaler]	DPI (75 mcg/inhalation)	1 inhalation every 24 hr	NA
Olodaterol [Striverdi Respimat][b]	Respimat (2.5 mcg/inhalation)	2 inhalations every 24 hr	NA
Salmeterol[a] [Serevent Diskus]	DPI (50 mcg/inhalation)	1 inhalation every 12 hr	1 inhalation every 12 hr
ORAL AGENTS			
Albuterol			
Generic	Tablets, syrup	2 or 4 mg 3–4 times/day	2 mg 3–4 times/day
[VoSpire ER]	Tablets (extended release)	8 mg every 12 hr	4 mg every 12 hr
Terbutaline (generic only)	Tablets	5 mg 3 times/day	2.5 mg 3 times/day

[a]When used to treat asthma, must always be combined with an inhaled glucocorticoid.
[b]Approved only for chronic obstructive pulmonary disease, not asthma.
DPI, Dry-powder inhaler; *HFA,* hydrofluoroalkane propellant; *MDI,* metered-dose inhaler; *NA,* not applicable.

TABLE 76.5 ▪ Classification of Asthma Severity and Recommended Step for Initial Treatment

		Persistent Asthma		
	Intermittent Asthma	**Mild**	**Moderate**	**Severe**
CURRENT IMPAIRMENT				
Asthma symptoms	≤2 days/week	>2 days/week, but not daily	Daily	Throughout the day
Nighttime awakenings	≤2 times/month	3–4 times/month	More than once a week, but not nightly	Often 7 times/week
SABA used to control symptoms (but not to prevent EIB)	≤2 days/week	>2 days/week, but not daily, and not more than once on any day	Daily	Several times a day
Effect on normal activity	None	Minor limitation	Some limitation	Severe limitation
Lung function tests	Normal FEV_1 between exacerbations FEV_1 > 80% of predicted FEV_1/FVC normal[a]	FEV_1 > 80% of predicted FEV_1/FVC normal[a]	FEV_1 >60% but <80% of predicted FEV_1/FVC reduced 5%[a]	FEV_1 <60% of predicted FEV_1/FVC reduced >5%[a]
FUTURE RISK				
Exacerbations requiring oral glucocorticoids	0–1/yr	≥2/yr	≥2/yr	≥2/yr
Recommended step for initial treatment[b]	Step 1	Step 2	Step 3	Step 4 or 5

[a]Normal values for FEV_1/FVC by age group: 8 to 19 years, 85%; 20 to 39 years, 80%; 40 to 59 years, 75%; 60 to 80 years, 70%.
[b]See Table 76.11 and text for drugs used at each step.
EIB, Exercise-induced bronchospasm; *FEV_1,* forced expiratory volume in 1 second; *FVC,* forced vital capacity; *SABA,* short-acting beta$_2$ agonist.

TABLE 76.6 ▪ Assessment of Asthma Control and Recommended Action for Treatment

	Classification of Control[a]		
Components of Control	**Well Controlled**	**Not Well Controlled**	**Very Poorly Controlled**
CURRENT IMPAIRMENT			
Symptoms	≤2 days/week	>2 days/week[b]	Throughout the day
Nighttime awakenings			
Age 12 years and older	≤2 times/month	1–3 times/week	≥4 times/week
Age 5–11 years	≤1 time/month	≥2 times/month	≥2 times/week
Age 0–4 years	≤1 time/month	>1 time/month	>1 time/week
SABA used to control symptoms (not to prevent EIB)	≤2 days/week	>2 days/week	Several times a day
Effect on normal activity	None	Some limitation	Severe limitation
Lung function tests			
FEV_1 (% of predicted) PEF (% of personal best)	FEV_1 > 80% *or* PEF > 80%	FEV_1 60%–80% *or* PEF 60%–80%	FEV_1 < 60% *or* PEF < 60%
Questionnaire scores for patients age 12 years and older			
ATAQ	0	1–2	3–4
ACQ	≤0.75	≥1.5	NA
ACT	≥20	16–19	≤15
RISK			
Exacerbations requiring oral glucocorticoids	0–1/yr	≥2/yr[c]	≥2/yr[c]
Age 5–11 years: Reduction in lung growth Age 12 years and older: Progressive loss of lung function	Evaluation requires long-term follow-up care.		
Treatment-related adverse effects	Medication side effects can vary in intensity from none to very troublesome and worrisome. The level of intensity does not correlate to specific levels of control but should be considered in the overall assessment of risk.		
Recommended action for treatment[d]	Maintain current treatment step. Follow up every 1–6 months to maintain control. Consider step-down if well controlled for 3 months or longer.	Move up 1 step and reassess in 2–6 weeks.[e] To reduce side effects, consider changing drugs.	Consider short course of oral glucocorticoids. Move up 1 or 2 steps and reassess in 2 weeks.[e] To reduce side effects, consider changing drugs.

[a]Level of control is based on the most severe impairment or risk category. Assess impairment domain by the patient's recall of the previous 2 to 4 weeks and by FEV_1 or PEF. Symptom assessment for longer periods should reflect a global assessment, such as inquiring whether the patient's asthma is better or worse since the last visit.
[b]For children age 5–11 years, symptoms occurring multiple times on ≤2 days/week are also included.
[c]At present, there are inadequate data to correspond frequencies of exacerbations with different levels of asthma control. In general, more frequent and intense exacerbations (e.g., requiring urgent, unscheduled care, hospitalization, or intensive care unit admission) indicate poorer disease control. For treatment purposes, patients who had two or more exacerbations requiring oral glucocorticoids in the past year may be considered the same as patients who have not-well-controlled asthma, even in the absence of impairment levels consistent with not-well-controlled asthma.
[d]Treatment steps are shown in Table 76.11.
[e]For children age 0–4 years, if there is no improvement in 4–6 weeks, alternative diagnoses should be considered and/or therapy adjustments may be required.
ACQ, Asthma Control Questionnaire; *ACT,* Asthma Control Test; *ATAQ,* Asthma Therapy Assessment Questionnaire; *EIB,* exercise-induced bronchospasm; FEV_1, forced expiratory volume in 1 second; *NA,* not applicable; *PEF,* peak expiratory flow rate; *SABA,* short-acting $beta_2$ agonist.

Use in Asthma and COPD

Oral theophylline is used for maintenance therapy of chronic stable asthma. Although less effective than $beta_2$ agonists, theophylline has a longer duration of action (when administered in a sustained-release formulation). With regular use, theophylline can decrease the frequency and severity of asthma attacks. Because its effects are prolonged, theophylline may be most appropriate for patients who experience nocturnal attacks.

Once standard therapy in the management of COPD, theophylline is no longer recommended. Evidence-based guidelines recommend its use only if $beta_2$ agonists and anticholinergics are unavailable or if the patient cannot afford long-term therapy with other drugs.

Intravenous theophylline has been employed in emergencies. However, the drug is no more effective than $beta_2$ agonists and glucocorticoids and is clearly more dangerous.

Pharmacokinetics

Absorption. Oral theophylline is available in sustained-release formulations and as an elixir. Absorption from sustained-release preparations is slow, but the resulting plasma levels are stable, being free of the wide fluctuations associated with the immediate-release products. Absorption from some sustained-release preparations can be affected by food.

Metabolism. Theophylline is metabolized in the liver. Rates of metabolism are affected by multiple factors—age, disease, drugs—and show wide individual variation. As a result, the plasma half-life of theophylline varies considerably among patients. For example, although the average half-life in nonsmoking adults is about 8 hours, the half-life can be as short as 2 hours in some adults and as long as 15 hours in others. Smoking either tobacco or marijuana accelerates metabolism and decreases the half-life. The *average* half-life in children is 4 hours. Metabolism is slowed in patients with certain pathologies (e.g., heart disease, liver disease, prolonged fever). Some drugs (e.g., cimetidine, fluoroquinolone antibiotics) decrease theophylline metabolism. Other drugs (e.g., phenobarbital) accelerate metabolism. Because of these variations in metabolism, dosage must be individualized.

Drug Levels. Safe and effective therapy requires periodic measurement of theophylline blood levels. Traditionally, dosage has been adjusted to produce theophylline levels between 10 and 20 mcg/mL. However, many patients respond well at 5 mcg/mL, and, as a rule, there is little benefit to increasing levels above 15 mcg/mL. Therefore, levels between 5 and 15 mcg/mL are appropriate for most patients. At levels above 20 mcg/mL, the risk for significant adverse effects is high.

Toxicity

Symptoms. Toxicity is related to theophylline levels. Adverse effects are uncommon at plasma levels below 20 mcg/mL. At 20 to 25 mcg/mL, relatively mild reactions occur (e.g., nausea, vomiting, diarrhea, insomnia, restlessness). Serious adverse effects are most likely at levels above 30 mcg/mL. These reactions include severe dysrhythmias (e.g., ventricular fibrillation) and convulsions that can be highly resistant to treatment. Death may result from cardiorespiratory collapse.

Treatment. At the first indication of toxicity, dosing with theophylline should stop. Absorption can be decreased by administering activated charcoal together with a cathartic. Ventricular dysrhythmias respond to lidocaine. Intravenous diazepam may help control seizures.

Drug Interactions

Caffeine. Caffeine is a methylxanthine with pharmacologic properties like those of theophylline (see Chapter 36). Accordingly, caffeine can intensify the adverse effects of theophylline on the CNS and heart. In addition, caffeine can compete with theophylline for drug-metabolizing enzymes, causing theophylline levels to rise. Because of these interactions, individuals taking theophylline should avoid caffeine-containing beverages (e.g., coffee, many soft drinks) and other sources of caffeine.

Tobacco and Marijuana Smoke. Smoking tobacco or marijuana can induce theophylline metabolism, resulting in increased drug clearance of up to 50% in adults and 80% in older adults. (Secondhand smoke can result in similarly decreased drug levels.) Consequently, if a smoking patient stops smoking but the dose of theophylline is not decreased, the patient is at risk for theophylline toxicity over time.

Drugs That Reduce Theophylline Levels. Several agents—including *phenobarbital, phenytoin,* and *rifampin*—can lower theophylline levels by inducing hepatic drug-metabolizing enzymes. Concurrent use of these agents may necessitate an increase in theophylline dosage.

Drugs That Increase Theophylline Levels. Several drugs—including *cimetidine* and the *fluoroquinolone antibiotics* (e.g., ciprofloxacin)—can elevate plasma levels of theophylline, primarily by inhibiting hepatic metabolism. To avoid theophylline toxicity, the dosage of theophylline should be reduced when the drug is combined with these agents.

Formulations

Theophylline is available for IV and oral use. For IV use, generic solutions are available in concentrations of 400 mg/250 mL, 400 mg/500 mL, or 800 mg/500 mL of solution.

For oral use, the following concentrations are available.

- Elixophyllin oral elixir: 80 mg/15 mL
- Generic oral solution: 80 mg/15 mL
- Theochron 12-hour extended-release tablets: 100, 200, and 300 mg
- Generic 12-hour extended-release tablets: 100, 200, 300, and 450 mg
- Theo-24 24-hour extended-release capsules: 100, 200, 300, and 400 mg
- Generic 24-hour extended-release tablets: 400 and 600 mg

Unlike the elixir and oral solution, the sustained-release tablets and capsules produce drug levels that are relatively stable. Accordingly, the sustained-release formulations are preferred for routine therapy.

Dosage and Administration

Oral. Dosage must be individualized. To minimize chances of toxicity, doses should be low initially and then gradually increased. If a dose is missed, the following dose should *not* be doubled, because doing so could produce toxicity. Smokers require higher-than-average doses. Conversely, patients with heart disease, liver dysfunction, or prolonged fever are likely to require lower doses. Patients should be instructed not to chew the sustained-release tablets or capsules. Product information should be consulted for compatibility with food.

The initial dosage is based on the age and weight of the patient and on the presence or absence of factors that can impair theophylline elimination. Specific initial dosages are described in the prescribing information in the package insert. As noted previously, maintenance doses should be adjusted to produce drug levels in the therapeutic range—typically 5 to 15 mcg/mL.

Intravenous. Intravenous theophylline is reserved for emergencies. Administration must be done slowly, because rapid injection can cause fatal cardiovascular reactions. Intravenous theophylline is incompatible with many other drugs. Accordingly, compatibility should be verified before mixing theophylline with other IV agents. For specific IV dosages, refer to the discussion of *aminophylline* that follows.

Other Methylxanthines

Aminophylline

Aminophylline is a theophylline salt that is considerably more soluble than theophylline itself. In solution, each molecule of aminophylline dissociates to yield two molecules of theophylline. Hence, the pharmacologic properties of aminophylline and theophylline are identical. Aminophylline is available in formulations for oral and IV dosing. Intravenous administration is employed most often.

Administration and Dosage

Intravenous. Because of its relatively high solubility, aminophylline is the preferred form of theophylline for IV use. Infusions should be done *slowly* (no faster than 25 mg/min), because rapid injection can produce severe hypotension and death. The usual loading dose of theophylline is 4.6 mg/kg (5.7 mg/kg as aminophylline). The maintenance infusion rate should be adjusted to provide plasma levels of theophylline that are within the therapeutic range (10 to 20 mcg/mL). Aminophylline solutions are incompatible with many other drugs. Therefore, compatibility must be verified before mixing aminophylline with other IV agents.

Oral. Aminophylline is available in 100- and 200-mg tablets. Dosing guidelines are the same as for theophylline.

ANTICHOLINERGIC DRUGS

Anticholinergic drugs improve lung function by blocking muscarinic receptors in the bronchi, reducing bronchoconstriction. Two agents are available: ipratropium and tiotropium. These drugs are approved only for COPD but are used off-label for asthma. Both drugs are administered by inhalation. The principal difference between the two is pharmacokinetic: Tiotropium has a much longer duration of action and thus can be dosed less often. With both drugs, systemic effects are minimal.

Ipratropium

Actions and Therapeutic Use

Ipratropium [Atrovent HFA] is an atropine derivative administered by inhalation to relieve bronchospasm. The drug has FDA approval only for bronchospasm associated with COPD, but is often used off-label for asthma and is included in current evidence-based guidelines from the National Asthma Education and Prevention Program (NAEPP) for asthma management. Like atropine, ipratropium is a muscarinic antagonist. By blocking muscarinic cholinergic receptors in the bronchi, ipratropium prevents bronchoconstriction. Therapeutic effects begin within 30 seconds, reach 50% of their maximum in 3 minutes, and persist about 6 hours. Ipratropium is effective against allergen-induced asthma and EIB, but is less effective than the $beta_2$ agonists. However, because ipratropium and the $beta_2$-adrenergic agonists promote bronchodilation by different mechanisms, their beneficial effects are additive.

Adverse Effects

Systemic effects are minimal because ipratropium is a quaternary ammonium compound and therefore always carries a positive charge. As a result, the drug is not readily absorbed from the lungs or from the digestive tract. The most common adverse reactions are dry mouth and irritation of the pharynx. If systemic absorption is sufficient, the drug may raise intraocular pressure in patients with glaucoma. Adverse cardiovascular events (heart attack, stroke, death) have occurred in people taking ipratropium; however, because absorption is minimal, it seems unlikely that ipratropium is the cause.

TABLE 76.7 ▪ Anticholinergics: Preparations and Dosages

Drug	Preparation	Formulation	Dosage
Aclidinium [Tudorza Pressair]	DPI	400 mcg per actuation	400 mcg twice daily
Ipratropium [Atrovent HFA]	Solution MDI	500 mcg/vial 17 mcg per actuation	500 mcg 3–4 times daily by nebulizer 2 inhalations 4 times daily (maximum dosage 12 inhalations/24 hr)
Tiotropium [Spiriva]	HandiHaler DPI	18 mcg capsules[a]	18 mcg once daily
Umeclidinium [Incruse Ellipta]	DPI	62.5 mcg per actuation	62.5 mcg once daily

[a]Capsules are for insertion into a DPI device and must not be swallowed.
DPI, Dry-powder inhaler; *HFA,* hydrofluoroalkane propellant; *MDI,* metered-dose inhaler

Preparations, Dosage, and Administration

Ipratropium is available both as a single agent and combined with albuterol. Preparations and dosages of single agents are supplied in Table 76.7. Beta$_2$-adrenergic agonists and anticholinergic combinations are discussed later in this chapter.

Tiotropium

Actions and Therapeutic Use

Tiotropium [Spiriva] is a *long-acting,* inhaled anticholinergic agent approved for maintenance therapy of bronchospasm associated with COPD. The drug is not approved for asthma, but has been used off-label for patients who have not responded to other medications. Like ipratropium, tiotropium relieves bronchospasm by blocking muscarinic receptors in the lungs. Therapeutic effects begin about 30 minutes after inhalation, peak in 3 hours, and persist about 24 hours. With subsequent doses, bronchodilation gets better and better, reaching a plateau after eight consecutive doses (8 days). Compared with ipratropium, tiotropium is more effective and its dosing schedule is more convenient (once daily vs. 4 times daily). Tiotropium is indicated only for long-term maintenance. For rapid relief of ongoing bronchospasm, patients should inhale an SABA.

Adverse Effects

The most common adverse effect is *dry mouth,* which develops in 16% of patients. Fortunately, this response is generally mild and diminishes over time. Patients can suck on sugarless candy for relief.

Systemic anticholinergic effects (e.g., constipation, urinary retention, tachycardia, blurred vision) are minimal. Like ipratropium, tiotropium is a quaternary ammonium compound, so absorption into the systemic circulation is very limited. Like ipratropium, tiotropium has been associated with adverse cardiovascular events; however, since absorption is low, tiotropium is unlikely to be the cause.

Aclidinium

Actions and Therapeutic Use

Aclidinium [Tudorza Pressair] is approved for management of bronchospasm associated with COPD. It relieves bronchospasm by blocking muscarinic receptors in the lung. Peak levels have occurred within 10 minutes of drug delivery; however, it is intended only for maintenance therapy and not for acute symptom relief.

Adverse Effects

The most common adverse reactions reported in clinical trials were headache, nasopharyngitis, and cough. As with any anticholinergic, there is a theoretical risk for worsening narrow-angle glaucoma, urinary retention, and other systemic anticholinergic effects; however, these have not been reported.

Umeclidinium

Actions and Therapeutic Use

Umeclidinium [Incruse Ellipta], which received FDA approval in 2013, is the newest long-acting anticholinergic indicated for management of bronchospasm associated with COPD. In addition to its availability as a single agent, it is also available in combination with the LABA vilanterol as *Anoro Ellipta.* Both the single and combination drugs are indicated for COPD maintenance therapy only; they are not approved for asthma treatment.

Adverse Effects

Umeclidinium contains lactose as a component of the powder mix. Theoretically, it may cause severe hypersensitivity reactions when taken by people who have milk protein allergies. In clinical trials, adverse effects were negligible: Nasopharyngitis was reported by 8% of subjects; however, this was reported by 7% of those taking a placebo. Similarly, 5% reported upper respiratory tract infections; yet this was reported by 4% of those taking a placebo. Although it is possible for this anticholinergic drug to cause typical anticholinergic adverse effects, because it is inhaled, the likelihood of this occurrence is markedly decreased.

GLUCOCORTICOID–LONG-ACTING BETA$_2$-AGONIST COMBINATIONS

Glucocorticoid and LABA combinations provide the anti-inflammatory benefits of the glucocorticoid and the bronchodilation benefits of the beta$_2$ agonist. These combinations are more convenient than taking a glucocorticoid and LABA separately but have the disadvantage of restricting dosage flexibility. These products are not recommended for initial therapy; rather, they should be reserved for patients whose asthma has not been adequately controlled with an inhaled glucocorticoid alone. All three products carry a black box warning about possible increased risk for asthma severity or asthma-related death (from the LABA in the combination). However, because the LABA is combined with a glucocorticoid, risk should be minimal.

There are currently four glucocorticoid-LABA combinations on the market. These are budesonide/formoterol [Symbicort], fluticasone/vilanterol [Breo Ellipta], fluticasone propionate/salmeterol [Advair Diskus, Advair HFA], and mometasone/formoterol [Dulera]. All are available in fixed-dose combinations. All are indicated for long-term maintenance in adults, but there are restrictions on approval for children. Fluticasone/salmeterol is approved for children 4 years of age and older, and budesonide/formoterol is approved for children 5 years of age and older. Children 12 years of age and older may use mometasone/formoterol. Fluticasone/vilanterol is not approved for patients younger than 18 years. Dosing information is provided in Table 76.8.

BETA$_2$-ADRENERGIC AGONIST–ANTICHOLINERGIC COMBINATIONS

The combination of a beta$_2$ agonist with a cholinergic antagonist optimizes bronchodilation by capitalizing on the unique action of the individual agents. As mentioned previously, beta$_2$ agonists promote bronchodilation by stimulating adrenergic receptors. In

TABLE 76.8 ▪ Glucocorticoids and Long-Acting Beta$_2$ Agonists: Formulations and Dosages

Drug	Inhaler	Formulation	Dosage[a]
Budesonide/formoterol [Symbicort]	HFA	80 mcg/4.5 mcg 160 mcg/4.5 mcg	2 inhalations twice daily 2 inhalations twice daily
Fluticasone/vilanterol [Breo Ellipta]	DPI	100 mcg/25 mcg 200 mcg/25 mcg	1 inhalation once daily 1 inhalation once daily
Fluticasone/salmeterol [Advair Diskus]	DPI	100 mcg/50 mcg 250 mcg/50 mcg 500 mcg/50 mcg	1 inhalation twice daily 1 inhalation twice daily 1 inhalation twice daily
Fluticasone/salmeterol [Advair HFA]	HFA	45 mcg/21 mcg 115 mcg/21 mcg 230 mcg/21 mcg	2 inhalations twice daily 2 inhalations twice daily 2 inhalations twice daily
Mometasone/formoterol [Dulera]	HFA	100 mcg/5 mcg 200 mcg/5 mcg	2 inhalations twice daily 2 inhalations twice daily

[a]Dosing is the same for children and adults when prescribed as recommended for age. These drugs are not approved for children younger than 12 years. Fluticasone/vilanterol is not approved for children younger than 18 years.
DPI, Dry-powder inhaler; *HFA,* hydrofluoroalkane propellant.

TABLE 76.9 ▪ Beta$_2$ Agonists and Anticholinergics: Formulations and Dosages

Drug (Classification)	Brand Name	Preparation	Formulation per Inhalation	Dosage
Ipratropium/albuterol (anticholinergic + SABA)	DuoNeb	Solution	500 mcg ipratropium/2500 mcg of albuterol	3 mL 4 times daily using a nebulizer
	Combivent Respimat	Inhaler	20 mcg ipratropium/100 mcg albuterol	1 inhalation 4 times daily (maximum 6 inhalations in 24 hr)
Indacaterol/glycopyrronium (LABA + anticholinergic)	Utibron Neohaler	Inhaler	27.5 mcg indacaterol/15 mcg glycopyrronium (glycopyrrolate)	1 inhalation twice daily
Olodaterol/tiotropium (LABA + anticholinergic)	Stiolto Respimat	Inhaler	2.5 mcg of olodaterol/2.5 mcg tiotropium	2 inhalations once daily
Umeclidinium/vilanterol (Anticholinergic + LABA)	Anoro Ellipta	Inhaler	62.5 mcg umeclidinium/25 mcg vilanterol	1 inhalation once daily

LABA, Long-acting beta$_2$ agonist; *SABA,* short-acting beta$_2$ agonist.

the lung, this relaxes smooth muscle in the airways. Cholinergic antagonists (anticholinergics) promote bronchodilation by blocking cholinergic receptors. This relaxes smooth muscle tone by preventing stimulation of cholinergic receptors. Additionally, beta$_2$ agonists primarily affect the bronchioles, whereas anticholinergics primarily affect the bronchi. This action on different areas of the airways further enhances bronchodilation.

All beta agonist/anticholinergic combinations are inhaled. Four combinations are available: Albuterol/ipratropium [Combivent Respimat, Combivent UDV], indacaterol/glycopyrronium [Utibron Neohaler, Ultibro Breezhaler 🍁], olodaterol/tiotropium [Stiolto Respimat], and vilanterol/umeclidinium, inhaled [Anoro Ellipta]. These are approved only for the management of COPD; however, Combivent (the only combination with an SABA), has been used off-label for management of asthma. Formulations and dosing are provided in Table 76.9.

MANAGEMENT OF ASTHMA

The NAEPP of the National Heart, Lung, and Blood Institute issued *Expert Panel Report 3 (EPR-3): Guidelines for the Diagnosis and Management of Asthma* in 2007. These remain the most current recommendations for asthma management. The following discussion reflects recommendations in EPR-3, which is available online at https://www.nhlbi.nih.gov/health-pro/guidelines/current/asthma-guidelines. These are currently undergoing a process of revision and update. Release of new guidelines is anticipated for 2018. To follow updates and draft summary reports, go to http://www.nhlbi.nih.gov/about/org/naepp.

In EPR-3, management recommendations are made for three age groups: 0 to 4 years, 5 to 11 years, and 12 years and older. Recommendations for all three groups are similar, although there are some important differences. Basic management is discussed here. For additional recommendations, please consult EPR-3.

MEASURING LUNG FUNCTION

Before considering asthma therapy, we need to address tests of lung function. Three tests are described next.

Forced expiratory volume in 1 second (FEV_1) is the single most useful test of lung function. To determine FEV_1, the patient inhales completely, and then exhales as completely and forcefully as possible into the spirometer. The spirometer measures how much air was expelled during the first second of exhalation. Results are then compared with a "predicted normal value" for a healthy person of similar age, sex, height, and weight. For a patient with asthma, the FEV_1 might be 75% of the predicted value.

Forced vital capacity (FVC), also measured with a spirometer, is defined as the total volume of air the patient can exhale after a full inhalation.

FEV_1/FVC (i.e., FEV_1 divided by FVC) is the fraction (percentage) of vital capacity exhaled during the first second of forced expiration. Normal values for FEV_1/FVC range from 85% for people 8 to 19 years old down to 70% for people 60 to 80 years old. In patients with asthma, the value for FEV_1/FVC may be in the normal range or it may be reduced by 5% or more, depending on asthma severity.

Peak expiratory flow (PEF) is defined as the maximal rate of airflow during expiration. To determine PEF, the patient exhales as forcefully as possible into a *peak flowmeter,* a relatively inexpensive, hand-held device. Patients should measure their peak flow every morning. If the value is less than 80% of their personal best, more frequent monitoring should be done.

CLASSIFICATION OF ASTHMA SEVERITY

As described in the EPR-3, chronic asthma has four classes of increasing severity: (1) intermittent, (2) mild persistent, (3) moderate persistent, and (4) severe persistent. Criteria for these classes are shown in Table 76.5. Note that severity classification is based on two separate domains: *impairment* and *risk.* Impairment refers to the effect of asthma on quality of life and functional capacity *in the present.* Risk refers to possible adverse events *in the future,* such as exacerbations and progressive loss of lung function. As we progress from intermittent asthma to severe persistent asthma, both impairment and risk increase: asthma symptoms occur more often and last longer, use of SABAs for symptomatic control increases, limitations on physical activity become more substantial, FEV_1 decreases to less than 60% of the predicted value, FEV_1/FVC drops to 5% or more below normal, and the number of exacerbations that require oral glucocorticoids gets larger. It is important to note that the two domains of asthma—impairment and risk—may respond differently to drugs. Furthermore, patients can be at high risk for future events, even if their current level of impairment is low.

TREATMENT GOALS

Treatment of chronic asthma is directed at two basic goals: reducing impairment and reducing risk. Components of each goal are:

Reducing impairment

- Preventing chronic and troublesome symptoms (e.g., coughing or breathlessness after exertion and at all other times)
- Reducing use of SABAs for symptom relief to 2 days a week or less
- Maintaining normal (or near-normal) pulmonary function
- Maintaining normal activity levels, including exercise and attendance at school or work
- Meeting patient and family expectations regarding asthma care

Reducing risk

- Preventing recurrent exacerbations
- Minimizing the need for emergency department visits or hospitalizations
- Preventing progressive loss of lung function (for children, preventing reduced lung growth)
- Providing maximal benefits with minimal adverse effects

CHRONIC DRUG THERAPY

In patients with chronic asthma, drugs are employed in two ways: some agents are taken to establish *long-term control* and some are taken for *quick relief* of an ongoing attack (Table 76.10). The long-term control drugs are taken every day, whereas the quick-relief drugs are taken PRN. Of the long-term control agents in current use, inhaled glucocorticoids are by far the most important. With regular dosing, these drugs reduce the frequency and severity of attacks, as well as the need for quick-relief medications. Of the quick-relief drugs in current use, inhaled SABAs are the most important. These drugs act promptly to reverse bronchoconstriction and provide rapid relief from cough, chest tightness, and wheezing.

For chronic drug therapy, EPR-3 recommends a *stepwise* approach, in which drug dosages and drug classes are stepped up as needed, and stepped down when possible. Six steps are described (Table 76.11). The basic concept is simple. First, all patients, starting with step 1, should use an inhaled SABA as needed for quick relief. Second, all patients—except those on step 1—should use a long-term control medication (preferably an inhaled glucocorticoid) to provide baseline control. Third, when patients move up a step, owing to increased impairment and risk, dosage of the control medication is increased or

TABLE 76.10 ■ Drugs for Asthma: Agents for Long-Term Control Versus Quick Relief

LONG-TERM CONTROL MEDICATIONS
Anti-Inflammatory Drugs
Glucocorticoids (inhaled or oral)
Leukotriene modifiers
Cromolyn
Omalizumab
Bronchodilators
Long-acting inhaled $beta_2$ agonists[a]
Long-acting oral $beta_2$ agonists
Theophylline
QUICK-RELIEF MEDICATIONS
Bronchodilators
Short-acting inhaled $beta_2$ agonists
Anticholinergics
Anti-Inflammatory Drugs
Glucocorticoids, systemic[b]

[a]For treatment of asthma, should always be combined with an inhaled glucocorticoid.

[b]Considered quick-relief drugs when used in a short burst (3 to 10 days) at the start of therapy or during a period of gradual deterioration. Glucocorticoids are not used for immediate relief of an ongoing attack.

TABLE 76.11 ■ Stepwise Approach to Managing Asthma

	Long-Term Control Drugs (Taken Daily)		Quick-Relief Drugs (Taken PRN)
	Preferred	Alternative	
ADULTS AND CHILDREN AGE 12 AND OLDER			
Step 1	No daily medication needed		SABA
Step 2	Low-dose IGC	Cromolyn, LTRA, or theophylline	SABA
Step 3	Low-dose IGC + LABA OR Medium-dose IGC	Low-dose IGC + either LTRA, theophylline, or zileuton	SABA
Step 4	Medium-dose IGC + LABA	Medium-dose IGC + either LTRA, theophylline, or zileuton	SABA
Step 5	High-dose IGC + LABA		SABA
Step 6	High-dose IGC + LABA + oral glucocorticoid		SABA
CHILDREN AGE 5–11 YEARS			
Step 1	No daily medication needed		SABA
Step 2	Low-dose IGC	Cromolyn, LTRA, nedocromil, or theophylline	SABA
Step 3	Low-dose IGC + either LABA, LTRA, or theophylline OR Medium-dose IGC		SABA
Step 4	Medium-dose IGC + LABA	Medium-dose IGC + either LTRA or theophylline	SABA
Step 5	High-dose IGC + LABA	High-dose IGC + either LTRA or theophylline	SABA
Step 6	High-dose IGC + LABA + oral glucocorticoid	High-dose IGC + either LTRA or theophylline + oral glucocorticoid	SABA
CHILDREN AGE 0–4 YEARS			
Step 1	No daily medication needed		SABA
Step 2	Low-dose IGC	Cromolyn or montelukast	SABA
Step 3	Medium-dose IGC		SABA
Step 4	Medium-dose IGC + either LABA or montelukast		SABA
Step 5	High-dose IGC + either LABA or montelukast		SABA
Step 6	High-dose IGC + either LABA or montelukast (Low-dose oral glucocorticoids, if needed.)		SABA

IGC, Inhaled glucocorticoid; *LABA,* long-acting beta$_2$ agonist; *LTRA,* leukotriene receptor antagonist; *SABA,* short-acting beta$_2$ agonist.

another control medication is added (typically an LABA), or both. And fourth, after a period of sustained control, moving down a step should be tried.

For patients just beginning drug therapy, the step they start on is determined by the pretreatment classification of asthma severity. For example, a patient diagnosed with intermittent asthma would begin at step 1 (PRN use of an inhaled SABA), whereas a patient diagnosed with moderate persistent asthma would begin at step 3 (daily inhalation of a low-dose glucocorticoid plus daily inhalation of an LABA, supplemented with an inhaled SABA as needed).

After treatment has been ongoing, stepping up or down is based on *assessment of asthma control.* Like the diagnosis of pretreatment severity, assessment of control is based on two domains: current impairment and future risk. In EPR-3, three classes of control are defined: well controlled, not well controlled, and very poorly controlled. Criteria for classification of asthma control and recommended actions are provided in Table 76.6. Stepwise approach for managing therapy is provided in Table 76.11.

DRUGS FOR ACUTE SEVERE EXACERBATIONS

Acute severe exacerbations of asthma require immediate attention. The goals are to relieve airway obstruction and hypoxemia and to normalize lung function as quickly as possible. Initial therapy consists of the following:

- Giving oxygen to relieve hypoxemia
- Giving a systemic glucocorticoid to reduce airway inflammation
- Giving a nebulized high-dose SABA to relieve airflow obstruction
- Giving nebulized ipratropium to further reduce airflow obstruction

Severe cases may benefit from IV magnesium sulfate or inhalation of heliox (79% helium/21% oxygen). After resolution of the crisis and hospital discharge, an oral glucocorticoid is taken for 5 to 10 days. All patients should also take a medium-dose inhaled glucocorticoid. Full recovery of lung function may take weeks.

DRUGS FOR EXERCISE-INDUCED BRONCHOSPASM

Exercise increases airway obstruction in practically all people with chronic asthma. The cause is bronchospasm secondary to loss of heat or water from the lung. EIB usually starts either during or immediately after exercise, peaks in 5 to 10 minutes, and resolves 20 to 30 minutes later.

With proper medication, most people with asthma can be as active as they wish. Indeed, many world-class athletes have had asthma. To prevent EIB, patients can inhale an SABA or cromolyn prophylactically. Inhaled SABAs, which prevent EIB in more than 80% of patients, are generally preferred over cromolyn, which is less effective. Beta$_2$ agonists should be inhaled immediately before exercise; cromolyn should be inhaled 15 minutes before exercise.

REDUCING EXPOSURE TO ALLERGENS AND TRIGGERS

For patients with chronic asthma, the treatment plan should include measures to control allergens and other factors that can cause airway inflammation and exacerbate symptoms. Important sources of asthma-associated allergens include the house dust mite, warm-blooded pets, cockroaches, and molds. Factors that can exacerbate asthma include tobacco smoke, wood smoke, and household sprays. To the extent possible, exposure to these factors should be reduced or eliminated.

MANAGEMENT OF COPD

Diagnosis and treatment of COPD are addressed in the *Global Strategy for the Diagnosis, Management, and Prevention of Chronic Obstructive Pulmonary Disease.* These evidence-based practice guidelines, developed by the Global Initiative for Chronic Obstructive Lung Disease (GOLD), were updated in 2016. These guidelines are available at http://goldcopd.org/gold-reports.

MEASURING LUNG FUNCTION

Patients who have signs and symptoms of COPD, such as dyspnea that has worsened over time, chronic cough, sputum production, and a history of smoking tobacco or other risk factors, should be tested with a spirometer to measure the degree of airway obstruction. A post-bronchodilator FEV$_1$/FVC of less than 0.70 is needed to confirm the COPD diagnosis.

CLASSIFICATION OF AIRFLOW LIMITATION SEVERITY

Severity of airflow limitation is based on spirometry. The four classes of increasing severity are (1) mild, (2) moderate, (3) severe, and (4) very severe. Remember that a diagnosis of COPD requires an FEV$_1$/FVC of less than 0.70.

- Mild: FEV$_1$ greater than 80% predicted
- Moderate: FEV$_1$ is 50% or greater than predicted but less than 80% predicted
- Severe: FEV$_1$ is 30% or greater than predicted but less than 50% predicted
- Very severe: FEV$_1$ less than 30% predicted

TREATMENT GOALS

There are two primary goals of COPD management. The first is to reduce symptoms, improve the patient's health status, and increase exercise tolerance. The second goal is to reduce risks and mortality by preventing progression of COPD and by preventing and managing exacerbations.

The GOLD guidelines provide a framework for management based on assessment of symptoms and the risk for exacerbation in addition to COPD severity. Therefore, in addition to the COPD severity categories mentioned previously, patients are classified into one of four additional categories for management.

- Group A: few symptoms; low risk
- Group B: increased symptoms; low risk
- Group C: few symptoms; high risk
- Group D: increased symptoms; high risk

Management is often challenging because patients with COPD commonly have comorbidities that complicate management choices, so COPD management must be individualized.

MANAGEMENT OF STABLE COPD

Pharmacologic management of stable COPD relies primarily on bronchodilators, glucocorticoids, and phosphodiesterase type 4 (PDE4) inhibitors. The GOLD guidelines offer recommendations for each.

Bronchodilators

Inhaled long-acting formulations of either beta$_2$ agonists or anticholinergics are preferred for bronchodilation. Theophylline is reserved for use only when other bronchodilators are not available.

Glucocorticoids

Long-term inhaled glucocorticoids are recommended when symptoms are severe or when long-acting bronchodilators are inadequate for the management of exacerbations. When given for COPD, glucocorticoids should be given in combination with a long-acting beta$_2$ agonist; glucocorticoid monotherapy is no longer recommended for long-term therapy due to decreased efficacy when used alone.

Phosphodiesterase Type 4 Inhibitors

In patients with severe chronic COPD, the risk for exacerbations may be reduced with roflumilast [Daliresp]. Roflumilast is a selective inhibitor of PDE, an enzyme that inactivates cyclic adenosine monophosphate (cAMP). The drug reduces inflammation, cough, and excessive mucus production by raising levels of cAMP in lung cells. Adverse effects include diarrhea, reduced appetite, weight loss, nausea, headache, back pain, insomnia, and depression. Safety in pregnancy has not been established. The dosage is 500 mcg once a day, taken with or without food. Roflumilast should be used in combination with tiotropium, a long-acting inhaled beta$_2$ agonist, or an inhaled glucocorticoid.

MANAGEMENT OF COPD EXACERBATIONS

While some of the same drugs used for the management of stable COPD are also used for the management of COPD exacerbations, the drug formulations used differ. For example, while LABAs are preferred for stable COPD management, SABAs (specifically inhaled either alone or in combination with inhaled anticholinergics) are preferred for bronchodilation during COPD exacerbations. Further, systemic glucocorticoids greatly improve outcomes when used in the management of COPD exacerbations. Other agents that may be used to control and shorten exacerbations include antibiotics for patients who have signs and symptoms of infection and supplemental oxygen to maintain an oxygen saturation of 88% to 92%.

KEY POINTS

- Asthma is a chronic inflammatory disease characterized by inflammation of the airways, bronchial hyperreactivity, and bronchospasm. Allergy is often the underlying cause.
- Asthma is treated with anti-inflammatory drugs and bronchodilators.
- Most drugs for asthma are administered by inhalation, a route that increases therapeutic effects (by delivering drugs directly to their site of action), reduces systemic effects (by minimizing drug levels in blood), and facilitates rapid relief of acute attacks.
- Four devices are used for inhalation: metered-dose inhalers (MDIs), dry-powder inhalers (DPIs), Respimats, and nebulizers. Patients will need instruction on their use.
- Glucocorticoids are the most effective anti-inflammatory drugs for asthma management.
- Glucocorticoids reduce symptoms of asthma by suppressing inflammation. As an added bonus, glucocorticoids appear to promote synthesis of bronchial beta$_2$ receptors and increase their responsiveness to beta$_2$ agonists.
- Inhaled and systemic glucocorticoids are used for long-term prophylaxis of asthma—not for aborting an ongoing attack. Accordingly, they are administered on a fixed schedule—not PRN.
- Unless asthma is severe, glucocorticoids should be administered by inhalation.
- Inhaled glucocorticoids are generally very safe. Their principal side effects are oropharyngeal candidiasis and dysphonia, which can be minimized by employing a spacer device during administration and by rinsing the mouth and gargling after use.
- Inhaled glucocorticoids can slow the growth rate of children, but they do not reduce adult height.
- Inhaled glucocorticoids may pose a small risk for bone loss. To minimize loss, dosage should be as low as possible, and patients should perform regular weight-bearing exercise and should ensure adequate intake of calcium and vitamin D.
- Prolonged therapy with oral glucocorticoids can cause serious adverse effects, including adrenal suppression, osteoporosis, hyperglycemia, peptic ulcer disease, and growth suppression.
- Because of adrenal suppression, patients taking oral glucocorticoids (and patients who have switched from oral glucocorticoids to inhaled glucocorticoids) must be given supplemental doses of oral or IV glucocorticoids at times of stress.
- Cromolyn is an inhaled anti-inflammatory drug used for prophylaxis of asthma.
- Cromolyn reduces inflammation primarily by preventing the release of mediators from mast cells.
- For long-term prophylaxis, cromolyn is taken daily on a fixed schedule. For prophylaxis of exercise-induced bronchospasm, cromolyn is taken 15 minutes before anticipated exertion.
- Cromolyn is the safest drug for asthma. Serious adverse effects are extremely rare.
- Beta$_2$ agonists promote bronchodilation by activating beta$_2$ receptors in bronchial smooth muscle.
- Inhaled short-acting beta$_2$ agonists (SABAs) are the most effective drugs for relieving acute bronchospasm and preventing exercise-induced bronchospasm.
- Three inhaled beta$_2$ agonists—arformoterol, formoterol, and salmeterol—have a long duration of action and are indicated for long-term control.
- Inhaled SABAs rarely cause systemic side effects when taken at the recommended dosage.
- Excessive dosing with oral beta$_2$ agonists can cause tachycardia and angina by activating beta$_1$ receptors on the heart. (Selectivity is lost at high doses.)
- Inhaled long-acting beta$_2$ agonists (LABAs) can increase the risk for asthma-related death, primarily when used alone. To reduce risk, LABAs should be used only by patients taking an inhaled glucocorticoid for long-term control, and only if the glucocorticoid has been inadequate by itself. For combined glucocorticoid/LABA therapy, the FDA recommends using a product that contains both drugs in the same inhaler.
- Theophylline, a member of the methylxanthine family, relieves asthma by causing bronchodilation.
- Theophylline has a narrow therapeutic range and can cause serious adverse effects; it has been largely replaced by safer and more effective medications.

- There are four classes of chronic asthma: intermittent, mild persistent, moderate persistent, and severe persistent. Diagnosis is based on current impairment and future risk.
- For therapeutic purposes, asthma drugs can be classified as long-term control medications (e.g., inhaled glucocorticoids) and quick-relief medications (e.g., inhaled SABAs).
- In the stepwise approach to asthma therapy, treatment becomes more aggressive as impairment or risk becomes more severe.
- The goals of stepwise therapy are to prevent symptoms, maintain near-normal pulmonary function, maintain normal activity, prevent recurrent exacerbations, minimize the need for SABAs, minimize drug side effects, minimize emergency department visits, prevent progressive loss of lung function, and meet patient and family expectations about treatment.
- The step chosen for initial therapy is based on the pretreatment classification of asthma severity, whereas moving up or down a step is based on ongoing assessment of asthma control.
- Intermittent asthma is treated PRN, using an inhaled SABA to abort the few acute episodes that occur.
- For persistent asthma (mild, moderate, or severe), the foundation of therapy is daily inhalation of a glucocorticoid. An inhaled LABA is added to the regimen when asthma is more severe. An SABA is inhaled PRN to suppress breakthrough attacks.
- For acute severe exacerbations of asthma, patients should receive oxygen (to reduce hypoxemia), a systemic glucocorticoid (to reduce airway inflammation), and a nebulized SABA plus nebulized ipratropium (to relieve airflow obstruction).
- To prevent exercise-induced bronchospasm, patients can inhale an SABA just before strenuous activity.
- Pharmacologic management of stable COPD relies primarily on bronchodilators, glucocorticoids, and PDE4 inhibitors.
- Inhaled long-acting formulations of either $beta_2$ agonists or anticholinergics are preferred for bronchodilation in stable COPD.
- Inhaled short-acting $beta_2$ agonists are preferred for bronchodilation during COPD exacerbations.
- When given for stable COPD, glucocorticoids should be given in combination with a long-acting $beta_2$ agonist; glucocorticoid monotherapy is not recommended for long-term therapy.
- In patients with severe chronic COPD, the risk for exacerbations may be reduced with roflumilast [Daliresp], a PDE4 inhibitor.
- Systemic glucocorticoids and antibiotics can greatly improve management of COPD exacerbations when they occur.

Please visit **http://evolve.elsevier.com/Lehne** for chapter-specific NCLEX® examination review questions.

Summary of Major Nursing Implications[a]

GLUCOCORTICOIDS

Inhaled

Beclomethasone
Budesonide
Ciclesonide
Flunisolide
Fluticasone
Mometasone

Oral

Methylprednisolone
Prednisolone
Prednisone

The nursing implications summarized here refer specifically to the use of glucocorticoids in asthma. A full summary of nursing implications for glucocorticoids is presented in Chapter 72.

Preadministration Assessment

Therapeutic Goal

Glucocorticoids are used on a fixed schedule to suppress inflammation. They are not used to abort an ongoing attack.

Baseline Data

Determine FEV_1 and the frequency and severity of attacks, and attempt to identify trigger factors.

Identifying High-Risk Patients

Inhaled Glucocorticoids. These preparations are *contraindicated* for patients with persistently positive sputum cultures for *Candida albicans.*

Oral Glucocorticoids. These preparations are *contraindicated* for patients with systemic fungal infections and for individuals receiving live virus vaccines.

Use with *caution* in pediatric patients and in women who are pregnant or breast-feeding. Also, exercise *caution* in patients with hypertension, heart failure, renal impairment, esophagitis, gastritis, peptic ulcer disease, myasthenia gravis, diabetes mellitus, osteoporosis, or infections that are resistant to treatment and in patients receiving potassium-depleting diuretics, digitalis glycosides, insulin, oral hypoglycemics, or nonsteroidal anti-inflammatory drugs.

Implementation: Administration

Routes

Inhalation, oral.

Administration

Inform patients that glucocorticoids are intended for preventive therapy—not for aborting an ongoing attack. Instruct patients to administer glucocorticoids on a regular schedule—not PRN.

Inhalation

Inhaled glucocorticoids are administered with an MDI, DPI, or nebulizer. **Teach patients how to use these devices. Inform patients that delivery of glucocorticoids to the bronchial tree can be enhanced by inhaling an SABA 5 minutes before inhaling the glucocorticoid.**

Oral

Alternate-day therapy is recommended to minimize adrenal suppression; **instruct patients to take one dose every other**

Continued

day in the morning. During long-term treatment, supplemental doses must be given at times of severe stress.

Ongoing Evaluation and Interventions

Evaluating Therapeutic Effects

Teach patients with chronic asthma to monitor and record PEF, symptom frequency and symptom intensity, nighttime awakenings, effect on normal activity, and SABA use.

Minimizing Adverse Effects

Inhaled Glucocorticoids. **Advise patients to rinse their mouth and gargle after dosing to minimize dysphonia and oropharyngeal candidiasis.** If candidiasis develops, it can be treated with antifungal medication.

Warn patients who have switched from long-term oral glucocorticoids to inhaled glucocorticoids that, because of adrenal suppression, they must take supplemental systemic glucocorticoids at times of severe stress (e.g., trauma, surgery, infection); failure to do so can be fatal.

To minimize possible *bone loss,* patients should use the lowest dose possible. Also, **advise patients to ensure adequate intake of calcium and vitamin D, and to perform weight-bearing exercise.**

Oral Glucocorticoids. Prolonged therapy can cause *adrenal suppression* and other serious adverse effects, including *osteoporosis, hyperglycemia, peptic ulcer disease,* and *growth suppression.* These effects can be reduced with alternate-day dosing. To compensate for adrenal suppression, patients taking glucocorticoids long term must be given supplemental oral or IV glucocorticoids at times of stress (e.g., trauma, surgery, infection); failure to do so can be fatal. Additional nursing implications that apply to adverse effects of long-term glucocorticoid therapy are summarized in Chapter 72.

BETA$_2$-ADRENERGIC AGONISTS

Inhaled, Short Acting

Albuterol
Levalbuterol

Inhaled, Long Acting

Arformoterol
Formoterol
Indacaterol
Salmeterol

Oral

Albuterol
Terbutaline

Preadministration Assessment

Therapeutic Goal

Short-acting inhaled beta$_2$ agonists are used PRN for prophylaxis of EIB and to relieve ongoing asthma attacks. Oral and inhaled long-acting beta$_2$ agonists are used for maintenance therapy.

Baseline Data

Determine FEV$_1$ and the frequency and severity of attacks, and attempt to identify trigger factors.

Identifying High-Risk Patients

Systemic (oral, parenteral) beta$_2$ agonists are *contraindicated* for patients with tachydysrhythmias or tachycardia associated with digitalis toxicity.

Use systemic beta$_2$ agonists with *caution* in patients with diabetes, hyperthyroidism, organic heart disease, hypertension, or angina pectoris.

Implementation: Administration

Routes

Usual. Inhalation.

Occasional. Oral, subcutaneous.

Administration

Inhalation. Inhaled beta$_2$ agonists are administered with an MDI, DPI, or nebulizer. **Teach patients how to use these devices.** For patients who have difficulty with hand-breath coordination, using a spacer with a one-way valve may improve results.

Inform patients who are using MDIs or DPIs that when 2 inhalations are needed, an interval of at least 1 minute should elapse between inhalations.

Warn patients against exceeding recommended dosages.

Inform patients that inhaled LABAs (formoterol, arformoterol, and salmeterol) should be taken on a fixed schedule—not PRN—and always in combination with an inhaled glucocorticoid, preferably in the same inhalation device.

Oral. **Instruct patients to take oral beta$_2$ agonists on a fixed schedule—not PRN.**

Instruct patients to swallow sustained-release preparations intact, without crushing or chewing.

Ongoing Evaluation and Interventions

Evaluating Therapeutic Effects

Teach patients with chronic asthma to monitor and record PEF, symptom frequency and symptom intensity, nighttime awakenings, effect on normal activity, and SABA use.

Minimizing Adverse Effects

Inhaled Short-Acting Beta$_2$ Agonists. When used at recommended doses, SABAs are generally devoid of significant adverse effects. Cardiac stimulation and tremors are most likely with systemic therapy.

Inhaled Long-Acting Beta$_2$ Agonists. When used correctly, LABAs are safe; however, when used *alone* for prophylaxis, they may increase the risk for severe asthma attacks and asthma-related death. To minimize risk, these drugs should always be combined with an inhaled glucocorticoid, preferably in the same inhalation device.

Oral Beta$_2$ Agonists. Excessive dosing can activate beta$_1$ receptors on the heart, resulting in anginal pain and tachydysrhythmias. **Instruct patients to report chest pain and changes in heart rate or rhythm.**

Tremor is common with systemic beta$_2$ agonists and usually subsides with continued drug use. If necessary, tremor can be reduced by lowering the dosage.

CROMOLYN

Preadmission Assessment

Therapeutic Goal

Cromolyn is used for acute and long-term prophylaxis of asthma. The drug will not abort an ongoing asthma attack.

Baseline Data

Determine FEV_1 and the frequency and severity of attacks, and attempt to identify trigger factors.

Identifying High-Risk Patients

Cromolyn is *contraindicated* for the rare patient who has experienced an allergic response to cromolyn in the past.

Implementation: Administration

Route

Inhalation.

Administration

Administration Device. Cromolyn is administered with a nebulizer. **Instruct patients on the proper use of this device.**

Acute Prophylaxis. **Instruct patients to administer cromolyn 15 minutes before exercise and exposure to other precipitating factors (e.g., cold, environmental agents).**

Long-Term Prophylaxis. **Instruct patients to administer cromolyn on a regular schedule, and inform them that full therapeutic effects may take several weeks to develop.**

Ongoing Evaluation and Interventions

Evaluating Therapeutic Effects

Teach patients with chronic asthma to monitor and record PEF, symptom frequency and symptom intensity, nighttime awakenings, effect on normal activity, and SABA use.

Minimizing Adverse Effects and Interactions

Cromolyn is devoid of significant adverse effects and drug interactions.

THEOPHYLLINE

Preadministration Assessment

Therapeutic Goal

Theophylline is a bronchodilator taken on a regular schedule to decrease the intensity and frequency of moderate to severe asthma attacks.

Baseline Data

Determine FEV_1 and the frequency and severity of attacks.

Identifying High-Risk Patients

Theophylline is *contraindicated* for patients with untreated seizure disorders or peptic ulcer disease.

Use with *caution* in patients with heart disease, liver or kidney dysfunction, or severe hypertension.

Implementation: Administration

Routes

Oral, intravenous.

Administration

Oral. Dosage must be individualized. Doses are low initially and then increased gradually. The dosing objective is to produce plasma theophylline levels in the therapeutic range, which for most patients is 5 to 15 mcg/mL. **Warn patients that if a dose is missed, the following dose should not be doubled.**

Instruct patients to swallow enteric-coated and sustained-release formulations intact, without crushing or chewing.

Warn patients not to switch from one sustained-release formulation to another without consulting the prescriber.

Consult product information regarding compatibility with food, and advise the patient accordingly.

Intravenous. Dosage is individualized. Administer slowly. Verify compatibility with other IV drugs before mixing.

Ongoing Evaluation and Interventions

Evaluating Therapeutic Effects

Monitor theophylline levels to ensure that they are in the therapeutic range (5 to 15 mcg/mL for most patients).

Teach patients with chronic asthma to monitor and record PEF, symptom frequency and symptom intensity, nighttime awakenings, effect on normal activity, and SABA use.

Minimizing Adverse Effects

Adverse effects (e.g., nausea, vomiting, diarrhea, insomnia, restlessness) develop as plasma drug levels rise above 20 mcg/mL. Severe effects (convulsions, ventricular fibrillation) can occur at drug levels above 30 mcg/mL. Dosage should be adjusted to keep theophylline levels below 20 mcg/mL.

Minimizing Adverse Interactions

Caffeine. Caffeine can intensify the adverse effects of theophylline on the heart and CNS and can decrease theophylline metabolism. **Caution patients against consuming caffeine-containing beverages (e.g., coffee, many soft drinks) and other sources of caffeine.**

Smoking Tobacco or Marijuana. Tobacco and marijuana smoking can increase clearance to 50% in adults and 80% in older adults. Secondhand smoke also increases theophylline clearance.

Drugs That Reduce Theophylline Levels. *Phenobarbital, phenytoin, rifampin,* and other drugs can lower theophylline levels. In the presence of these drugs, the dosage of theophylline may need to be increased.

Drugs That Increase Theophylline Levels. *Cimetidine, fluoroquinolone antibiotics,* and other drugs can elevate theophylline levels. When combined with these drugs, theophylline should be used in reduced dosage.

Management of Toxicity

Theophylline overdose can cause severe dysrhythmias and convulsions. Death from cardiorespiratory collapse may occur. Manage toxicity by (1) discontinuing theophylline and (2) administering activated charcoal (to decrease theophylline absorption) plus a cathartic (to accelerate fecal excretion). Give lidocaine to control ventricular dysrhythmias and IV diazepam to control seizures.

[a]Patient education information is highlighted as **blue text.**

CHAPTER

77 Drugs for Allergic Rhinitis, Cough, and Colds

The drugs addressed in this chapter are administered to alleviate the symptoms of common respiratory disorders. Our principal focus is on the symptoms of allergic rhinitis and the common cold.

DRUGS FOR ALLERGIC RHINITIS

Allergic rhinitis is an inflammatory disorder that affects the upper airway. Major symptoms are sneezing, rhinorrhea (runny nose), pruritus (itching), and nasal congestion caused by dilation and increased permeability of nasal blood vessels. In addition, some patients experience associated conjunctivitis, sinusitis, and even asthma. Symptoms are triggered by airborne allergens, which bind to immunoglobulin E (IgE) antibodies on mast cells and thereby cause the release of inflammatory mediators, including histamine, leukotrienes, and prostaglandins. Allergic rhinitis is the most common allergic disorder, affecting almost one out of every six people in the United States.

Allergic rhinitis has two major forms: seasonal and perennial. Seasonal rhinitis, also known as *hay fever,* occurs in the spring and fall in reaction to outdoor allergens such as fungi and pollens from weeds, grasses, and trees. Perennial (nonseasonal) rhinitis is triggered by indoor allergens, especially the house dust mite and pet dander.

Several classes of drugs are used for allergic rhinitis (Table 77.1). Principal among these are (1) glucocorticoids (intranasal), (2) antihistamines (oral and intranasal), and (3) sympathomimetics (oral and intranasal).

Intranasal Glucocorticoids

The basic pharmacology of the glucocorticoids is discussed in Chapter 72. Consideration here is limited to their use in allergic rhinitis.

Actions and Uses

Intranasal glucocorticoids are the most effective drugs for the prevention and treatment of seasonal and perennial rhinitis. Because of their anti-inflammatory actions, these drugs can prevent or suppress the major symptoms of allergic rhinitis: congestion, rhinorrhea, sneezing, nasal itching, and erythema. Seven intranasal glucocorticoids are available (Table 77.2). Three of these, budesonide [Rhinocort Aqua], fluticasone propionate [Flonase], and triamcinolone [Nasacort Allergy 24 hours], are available in the United States without a prescription. All appear equally effective.

Adverse Effects

Adverse effects of intranasal glucocorticoids are generally mild. The most common are *drying of the nasal mucosa* and a *burning or itching sensation. Sore throat, epistaxis* (nosebleed), and *headache* may also occur.

Systemic effects are possible but are rare at recommended doses. Of greatest concern are adrenal suppression and the slowing of linear growth in children (whether final adult height is reduced is unknown). Systemic effects are least likely with ciclesonide, fluticasone, and mometasone, which have very low bioavailability (see Table 77.2).

Preparations, Dosage, and Administration.

Intranasal glucocorticoids are administered using a metered-dose spray device. Benefits are greatest when dosing is done daily, rather than PRN. Full doses are given initially (see Table 77.2). After symptoms are under control, the dosage should be reduced to the lowest effective amount. For patients with seasonal allergic rhinitis, maximal effects may require a week or more to develop. However, an initial response can be seen within hours. For patients with perennial rhinitis, maximal responses may take 2 to 3 weeks to develop. If nasal congestion is present, a topical decongestant should be used (if ordered) before glucocorticoid administration.

TABLE 77.1 ▪ Overview of Drugs for Allergic Rhinitis

Drug or Class	Route	Actions	Adverse Effects
Glucocorticoids	Nasal	Prevent inflammatory response to allergens and thereby reduce all symptoms.	Nasal irritation; possible slowing of linear growth in children
Antihistamines	Oral/nasal	Block histamine$_1$ receptors and thereby decrease itching, sneezing, and rhinorrhea; do *not* reduce congestion.	*Oral:* Sedation and anticholinergic effects (mostly with first-generation agents) *Nasal:* Bitter taste
Cromolyn	Nasal	Prevents release of inflammatory mediators from mast cells and thereby can decrease all symptoms. However, benefits are modest.	Nasal irritation, unpleasant taste, headache
Sympathomimetics	Oral/nasal	Activate vascular alpha$_1$ receptors and thereby cause vasoconstriction, which reduces nasal congestion; do *not* decrease sneezing, itching, or rhinorrhea.	*Oral:* Restlessness, insomnia, increased blood pressure *Nasal:* Rebound nasal congestion
Anticholinergics	Nasal	Block nasal cholinergic receptors and thereby reduce secretions; do *not* decrease sneezing, nasal congestion, or postnasal drip.	Nasal drying and irritation
Antileukotrienes	Oral	Block leukotriene receptors and thereby reduce nasal congestion.	Rare neuropsychiatric effects

TABLE 77.2 ▪ Some Glucocorticoid Nasal Sprays for Allergic Rhinitis

Drug	Brand Name	Intranasal Bioavailability (%)	Dose/Spray	Patient Age	Initial Dosage
FIRST GENERATION: INCREASED SYSTEMIC ABSORPTION					
Beclomethasone	Beconase AQ	44	42 mcg	6–11 yr 12 yr and older	1 spray/nostril twice daily 1 or 2 sprays/nostril twice daily
	Qnasl	—	80 mcg	12 yr and older	2 sprays/nostril once daily
Budesonide	Rhinocort Aqua	34	32 mcg	6–11 yr 12 yr and older	1 or 2 sprays/nostril once daily 1–4 sprays/nostril once daily
Flunisolide	Generic only	49	25 mcg	6–13 yr 14 yr and older	2 sprays/nostril twice daily or 1 spray 3 times/day 2 sprays/nostril 2 or 3 times/day
Triamcinolone	Nasacort AQ	46	55 mcg	6 yr and older	1 or 2 sprays/nostril once daily
SECOND GENERATION: DECREASED SYSTEMIC ABSORPTION					
Ciclesonide	Omnaris	—	50 mcg	6 yr and older	2 sprays/nostril once daily
Fluticasone propionate	Flonase	0.5–2	50 mcg	4–11 yr 12 yr and older	1 spray/nostril once daily 2 sprays/nostril once daily
Fluticasone furoate	Veramyst	—	27.5 mcg	2–11 yr 12 yr and older	1 spray/nostril once daily 2 sprays/nostril once daily
Mometasone	Nasonex	0.1	50 mcg	2–11 yr 12 yr and older	1 spray/nostril once daily 2 sprays/nostril once daily

Antihistamines

The antihistamines are discussed in Chapter 70. Consideration here is limited to their use in allergic rhinitis.

Oral Antihistamines

Oral antihistamines (histamine$_1$ [H_1] receptor antagonists) are first-line drugs for mild to moderate allergic rhinitis. For therapy of allergic rhinitis, antihistamines are most effective when taken *prophylactically* and less helpful when taken after symptoms appear.

Actions and Uses. These drugs can relieve sneezing, rhinorrhea, and nasal itching; however, they do not reduce nasal congestion. Because histamine is only one of several mediators of allergic rhinitis, antihistamines are less effective than glucocorticoids. Antihistamines should be administered on a regular basis throughout the allergy season, even when symptoms are absent, to prevent initial histamine receptor activation.

Because histamine does not contribute to the symptoms of infectious rhinitis, antihistamines are of no value against the common cold. Some patients take first-generation antihistamines for their drying effect; however, this may complicate the

TABLE 77.3 ■ Some Antihistamines for Allergic Rhinitis

Generic Name	Brand Name	Dosage
ORAL ANTIHISTAMINES		
First-Generation (Sedating)		
Chlorpheniramine	Chlor-Trimeton Allergy, Chlor-Tripolon ♣, others	*Adults and children 12 yr and older:* 4 mg every 4–6 hr *Children 6–11 yr:* 2 mg every 4–6 hr
Diphenhydramine	Benadryl, others	*Adults:* 25–50 mg every 4–6 hr *Children under 10 kg:* 12.5–25 mg 3 or 4 times/day
Second-Generation (Nonsedating)		
Cetirizine[a]	Zyrtec, Reactine ♣	*Adults and children 6 yr and older:* 5 or 10 mg once daily
Levocetirizine	Xyzal	*Adults and children 12 yr and older:* 5 mg once daily *Children 6–11 yr:* 2.5 mg once daily
Fexofenadine	Allegra	*Adults and children 12 yr and older:* 60 mg twice daily or 180 mg once daily
Loratadine	Claritin, Alavert	*Adults and children 6 yr and older:* 10 mg once daily
Desloratadine	Clarinex, Aerius ♣	*Adults and children 12 yr and older:* 5 mg once daily
INTRANASAL ANTIHISTAMINES		
Second-Generation (Nonsedating)		
Azelastine[a]	Astelin, Astepro	*Adults and children 12 yr and older:* 2 sprays/nostril twice daily *Children 5–11 yr:* 1 spray/nostril twice daily[b]
Olopatadine	Patanase	*Adults and children 12 yr and older:* 2 sprays/nostril twice daily (665 mcg/spray)

[a]May cause some sedation at recommended doses.
[b]Astelin only. Astepro is not approved for children younger than 12 years.

treatment of colds by increasing the viscosity of secretions and thus making them harder to expel. The result is a thick, warm, moist mucoid environment that serves as an excellent medium for microbial growth.

Adverse Effects. Adverse effects are usually mild. The most frequent complaint is *sedation,* which occurs frequently with the first-generation antihistamines (e.g., diphenhydramine) and much less often with the second-generation agents (e.g., fexofenadine). Accordingly, second-generation agents are clearly preferred for students who need to remain alert in class and for patients who do work that requires alertness. *Anticholinergic effects* (e.g., drying of nasal secretions, dry mouth, constipation, urinary hesitancy) are common with first-generation agents and relatively rare with the second-generation agents.

Preparations, Dosage, and Administration. Dosages for some popular H_1 antagonists are presented in Table 77.3. A more complete list appears in Chapter 70.

Intranasal Antihistamines

Two antihistamines—*azelastine* [Astelin, Astepro] and *olopatadine* [Patanase]—are available for intranasal administration. Both drugs are indicated for allergic rhinitis in adults and children older than 12. Both drugs are supplied in metered-spray devices. The usual dosage is 2 sprays in each nostril twice daily. With both drugs, systemic absorption can be sufficient to cause somnolence. Additionally, some patients experience nosebleeds and headaches with both azelastine and olopatadine. These drugs can also cause an unpleasant taste.

Prototype Drugs

DRUGS FOR ALLERGIC RHINITIS, COUGH, AND COLDS

Intranasal Glucocorticoids
Beclomethasone

Antihistamines
Azelastine (intranasal, nonsedating)
Loratadine (oral, nonsedating)

Intranasal Sympathomimetics (Decongestants)
Oxymetazoline (long acting)
Phenylephrine (short acting)

Opioids
Hydrocodone

Nonopioids
Dextromethorphan

Intranasal Cromolyn Sodium

The basic pharmacology of cromolyn sodium is discussed in Chapter 76. Consideration here is limited to its use in allergic rhinitis.

Actions and Uses

For the treatment of allergic rhinitis, intranasal cromolyn [NasalCrom] is extremely safe, but only moderately effective. Benefits are much less than those of intranasal glucocorticoids. Cromolyn reduces symptoms by suppressing the release of histamine and other inflammatory mediators from mast cells. Accordingly, the drug is best suited for prophylaxis and hence should be given before symptoms start. Responses may take 1 or 2 weeks to develop; patients should be informed of this delay. Adverse reactions are less than with any other drug for allergic rhinitis.

Preparations, Dosage, and Administration

For the treatment of allergic rhinitis, cromolyn sodium is available in a metered-dose spray device that delivers 5.2 mg/actuation. The usual dosage for adults and children over 2 years is 1 spray (5.2 mg) per nostril 4 to 6 times a day. If nasal congestion is present, a topical decongestant should be used before cromolyn. Like the antihistamines and glucocorticoids, cromolyn should be dosed on a regular schedule throughout the allergy season.

Sympathomimetics (Decongestants)

Actions and Uses

Sympathomimetics (e.g., phenylephrine, pseudoephedrine) reduce nasal congestion by activating $alpha_1$-adrenergic receptors on nasal blood vessels. This causes vasoconstriction, which in turn causes shrinkage of swollen membranes, followed by nasal drainage. With *topical* administration, vasoconstriction is both rapid and intense. With *oral* administration, responses are delayed, moderate, and prolonged.

In patients with allergic rhinitis, sympathomimetics relieve only stuffiness. They do not reduce rhinorrhea, sneezing, or itching. In addition to their use in allergic rhinitis, sympathomimetics can reduce congestion associated with sinusitis and colds. Routes and dosages are shown in Table 77.4.

Adverse Effects

Rebound Congestion. Rebound congestion develops when *topical* agents are used more than a few days. With prolonged use, as the effects of each application wear off, congestion becomes progressively worse. To overcome this rebound congestion, the patient must use progressively larger and more frequent doses. Once established, rebound congestion can lead to a cycle of escalating congestion and increased drug use. The cycle can be broken by abrupt decongestant withdrawal; however, this tactic can be extremely uncomfortable. A less drastic option is to discontinue the drug in one nostril at a time. An even better option is to use an intranasal glucocorticoid (in both nostrils) for 2 to 6 weeks, starting 1 week before discontinuing the decongestant. Development of rebound congestion can

TABLE 77.4 ■ Sympathomimetics Used for Nasal Decongestion

Decongestant	Mode of Use	Dosing Interval	Dosage Size[a]
Phenylephrine [Neo-Synephrine, others]	Drops	Every 4 or more hr	*6 yr and older:* 2–3 drops (0.25%–1%) *2–6 yr:* 2–3 drops (0.125%)
	Spray	Every 4 or more hr	*12 yr and older:* 2–3 sprays (0.25%–1%) *6–12 yr:* 2–3 sprays (0.25%) *2–6 yr:* Not recommended
	Oral	Every 4 hr	*12 yr and older:* 10 mg *6–11 yr:* 5 mg *4–5 yr:* 2.5 mg *Younger than 4 yr:* Not recommended
Pseudoephedrine [Sudafed, others]	Oral	Every 4–6 hr	*12 yr and older:* 60 mg *6–12 yr:* 30 mg *Younger than 6 yr:* 15 mg
	Oral SR	Every 12 hr	*12 yr and older:* 120 mg *Younger than 12 yr:* Not recommended
	Oral CR	Every 24 hr	*12 yr and older:* 240 mg *Younger than 12 yr:* Not recommended
Naphazoline [Privine]	Drops	Every 6 or more hr	*12 yr and older:* 1 or 2 drops (0.05%) *Younger than 12 yr:* Not recommended
	Spray	Every 6 or more hr	*12 yr and older:* 1 or 2 sprays (0.05%) *Younger than 12 yr:* Not recommended
Oxymetazoline [Afrin 12-Hour, Neo-Synephrine 12-Hour, Dristan 12-Hour, others]	Spray	Every 10–12 hr	*6 yr and older:* 2–3 sprays (0.05%) *Younger than 6 yr:* Not recommended
Tetrahydrozoline [Tyzine]	Drops	Every 3 or more hr	*6 yr and older:* 2–4 drops (0.1%) *2–6 yr:* 2–3 drops (0.05%)
	Spray	Every 3 or more hr	*6 yr and older:* 3–4 sprays (0.1%) *Younger than 6 yr:* Not recommended
Xylometazoline [Otrivin]	Drops	Every 8–10 hr	*12 yr and older:* 2–3 drops (0.1%) *2–12 yr:* 2–3 drops (0.05%)
	Spray	Every 8–10 hr	*12 yr and older:* 1–3 sprays (0.1%) *2–12 yr:* 1 spray (0.05%)

[a]For drops and sprays, the dosage listed is applied to *each* nostril; numbers in parentheses indicate the concentration of solution employed.
CR, Controlled release; *SR,* sustained release.

be minimized by limiting topical application to 3 to 5 days. Accordingly, topical sympathomimetics are not appropriate for individuals with chronic rhinitis.

Central Nervous System Stimulation. Central nervous system (CNS) excitation is the most common adverse effect of the *oral* sympathomimetics. Symptoms include restlessness, irritability, anxiety, and insomnia. These responses are uncommon with topical agents when used as recommended.

Cardiovascular Effects. By activating alpha$_1$-adrenergic receptors on systemic blood vessels, sympathomimetics can cause widespread vasoconstriction. Generalized vasoconstriction is most likely with *oral* agents. However, if used in excess, even the topical agents can cause significant systemic vasoconstriction. For most patients, the effects on systemic vessels are inconsequential. However, for individuals with cardiovascular disorders—hypertension, coronary artery disease, cardiac arrhythmias, cerebrovascular disease—widespread vasoconstriction can be hazardous.

Abuse. *Pseudoephedrine* is associated with abuse. By causing CNS stimulation, this sympathomimetic can produce subjective effects similar to those of amphetamine. Also, it can be readily converted to methamphetamine, a widely used drug of abuse. To reduce the availability of pseudoephedrine for methamphetamine production, Congress passed the *Combat Methamphetamine Epidemic Act of 2005,* which requires that all products containing pseudoephedrine be placed behind the counter (even though they can still be purchased without a prescription in some states). Furthermore, purchasers must present identification and sign a log. Also, individuals can purchase no more than 9 gm per month or 3.6 gm on any day. Because of these constraints, many products are being reformulated to contain phenylephrine rather than ephedrine and pseudoephedrine. Unfortunately, although pseudoephedrine is an excellent decongestant, when taken orally, phenylephrine is not very effective. Some randomized controlled trials have demonstrated that phenylephrine is little better than a placebo.

Factors in Topical Administration

General Considerations. Because of the risk for rebound congestion, topical sympathomimetics should be used for no more than 3 to 5 consecutive days. To avoid systemic effects, doses should not exceed those recommended by the manufacturer. The applicator should be cleansed after each use to prevent contamination.

Drops. Drops should be administered with the patient in a lateral, head-low position. This causes the drops to spread slowly over the nasal mucosa, thereby promoting beneficial effects while reducing the amount that is swallowed. Because the number of drops can be precisely controlled, drops allow better control of dosage than do sprays. Accordingly, because young children are particularly susceptible to toxicity, drops are preferred for these patients.

Sprays. Sprays deliver the decongestant in a fine mist. Although convenient, sprays are less effective than an equal volume of properly instilled drops.

Contrasts Between Oral and Topical Agents

Oral and topical sympathomimetics differ in several important respects. First, topical agents act faster than the oral agents and are usually more effective. Second, oral agents act longer than topical preparations. Third, systemic effects (vasoconstriction, CNS stimulation) occur primarily with oral agents; topical agents usually elicit these responses only when dosage is higher than recommended. And fourth, rebound congestion is common with prolonged use of topical agents, but is rare with oral agents.

Comparison of Phenylephrine and Pseudoephedrine

Phenylephrine is one of the most widely used nasal decongestants. The drug is administered topically as a single agent and orally as a component of combination preparations. When administered topically, phenylephrine is both fast and effective. When taken orally, the drug is not very effective, in large part because of extensive first-pass metabolism. Although it might seem logical to simply increase the dosage, this is not advisable because even though absorption is poor, phenylephrine can still cause adverse cardiovascular and CNS effects.

Pseudoephedrine is available only for oral administration. Compared with oral phenylephrine, pseudoephedrine is better absorbed, has a longer half-life, and is much more effective.

Antihistamine/Sympathomimetic and Antihistamine/Glucocorticoid Combinations

Some patients require combined therapy with a sympathomimetic or glucocorticoid in addition to an antihistamine. Although antihistamines alone are a first-line treatment, they do not relieve nasal congestion, and they may be inadequate for some patients. For these patients, the addition of a sympathomimetic or glucocorticoid may be indicated. This can be accomplished in one of two ways: by giving the drugs separately or by using a combination product. Some popular combination products are listed in Table 77.5.

TABLE 77.5 ▪ Some Antihistamine Combination Products

	Brand Name	Dosage
ANTIHISTAMINE/SYMPATHOMIMETIC		
Acrivastine/pseudoephedrine	Semprex-D Capsules	8 mg/60 mg 4 times/day
Chlorpheniramine/pseudoephedrine	Allerest Maximum Strength Tablets	4 mg/60 mg every 4–6 hr
Fexofenadine/pseudoephedrine	Allegra-D 12-Hour Tablets	60 mg/120 mg twice daily
Loratadine/pseudoephedrine	Claritin-D 12-Hour Tablets	5 mg/120 mg every 12 hr
Desloratadine/pseudoephedrine	Clarinex-D 12-Hour Tablets	2.5 mg/120 mg every 12 hr
Triprolidine/pseudoephedrine	Actifed Cold & Allergy Tablets	2.5 mg/60 mg every 4–6 hr
ANTIHISTAMINE/GLUCOCORTICOID		
Azelastine/fluticasone propionate	Dymista	*Adults and children 12 yr and older:* 1 spray/nostril twice daily

Ipratropium, an Anticholinergic Agent

Ipratropium bromide [Atrovent] is an anticholinergic agent. The drug is indicated for allergic rhinitis, asthma, and the common cold. To treat allergic rhinitis, ipratropium is administered as a nasal spray (0.03% and 0.06%). Blockade of cholinergic receptors inhibits secretions from the serous and seromucous glands lining the nasal mucosa, and thereby decreases rhinorrhea. The drug does not decrease sneezing, nasal congestion, or postnasal drip. At the doses used for allergic rhinitis, side effects are minimal. The most common side effects are nasal drying and irritation. Ipratropium does not readily cross membranes because it is a quaternary ammonium compound, and hence systemic effects are absent. Dosages for allergic rhinitis in patients 12 years and older range from 2 sprays of 0.03% ipratropium (42 mcg total) per nostril 2 to 3 times a day to 2 sprays of 0.06% ipratropium (84 mcg total) per nostril 4 times a day. The use of ipratropium for asthma is discussed in Chapter 76.

Montelukast, a Leukotriene Antagonist

Montelukast [Singulair], originally approved for asthma, is now approved for seasonal and perennial allergic rhinitis as well. Benefits derive from blocking the binding of leukotrienes to their receptors. In people with allergic rhinitis, leukotrienes act primarily to cause nasal congestion (by promoting vasodilation and by increasing vascular permeability). Hence, by blocking leukotriene receptors, montelukast relieves nasal congestion, although it has little effect on sneezing or itching. When used alone or in combination with an antihistamine, montelukast is less effective than intranasal glucocorticoids. Although montelukast is generally well tolerated, it can cause rare but serious neuropsychiatric effects, including agitation, aggression, hallucinations, depression, insomnia, restlessness, and suicidal thinking and behavior. Because of these adverse effects and because beneficial effects are limited, it is probably best to reserve montelukast for patients who do not respond to or cannot tolerate intranasal glucocorticoids, antihistamines, or both. Administration is oral. Dosage, which varies with age, is the same as that used for asthma.

Omalizumab

Omalizumab [Xolair] is a monoclonal antibody directed against IgE, an immunoglobulin (antibody) that plays a central role in the allergic release of inflammatory mediators from mast cells and basophils. Omalizumab is approved only for allergy-mediated asthma; however, several studies have demonstrated significant improvement of allergic symptoms. Because patients with ragweed-induced seasonal allergic rhinitis have achieved symptom relief with omalizumab when other drugs have been ineffective, this drug is sometimes prescribed off-label for the management of these symptoms while clinical trials continue.

DRUGS FOR COUGH

Cough is a complex reflex involving the CNS, the peripheral nervous system, and the muscles of respiration. The cough reflex can be initiated by irritation of the bronchial mucosa, as well as by stimuli arising at sites distant from the respiratory tract. Cough is often beneficial, serving to remove foreign matter and excess secretions from the bronchial tree. The productive cough that is characteristic of chronic lung disease (e.g., emphysema, asthma, bronchitis) should not be suppressed, for example. Not all coughs, however, are useful. When a cough is nonproductive, creates discomfort, or deprives a patient of comfort or sleep, cough suppressant medication is appropriate. The most common use of cough medicines is for the suppression of nonproductive cough associated with the common cold and other upper respiratory infections.

Antitussives

Antitussives are drugs that suppress cough. Some agents act within the CNS; others act peripherally. The antitussives fall into two major groups: (1) opioid antitussives and (2) nonopioid antitussives. Interestingly, although the major antitussives—codeine, dextromethorphan, and diphenhydramine—are clearly effective against chronic nonproductive cough and experimentally induced cough, there is no good evidence that these drugs can suppress cough associated with the common cold.

Opioid Antitussives

All of the opioid analgesics have the ability to suppress cough. The two opioids used most often for cough suppression are *codeine* and *hydrocodone.* Both drugs act in the CNS to elevate cough threshold. Hydrocodone is somewhat more potent than codeine and carries a greater liability for abuse. The basic pharmacology of the opioids is discussed in Chapter 28.

Codeine. Codeine is the most effective cough suppressant available. The drug is active orally and can decrease both the frequency and intensity of cough. Doses are low, about one-tenth of the dosage levels needed to relieve pain. At these doses, the risk for physical dependence is small.

Like all other opioids, codeine can suppress respiration. Accordingly, the drug should be employed with caution in patients with reduced respiratory reserve. In the event of overdose, respiratory depression may prove fatal. An opioid antagonist (e.g., naloxone) should be used to reverse toxicity.

When dispensed by itself, codeine has a significant potential for abuse, and therefore is classified under Schedule II of the Controlled Substances Act. However, the abuse potential of the antitussive mixtures that contain codeine is low. Accordingly, these mixtures are classified under Schedule V.

For the treatment of cough, the adult dosage is 10 to 20 mg orally, 4 to 6 times a day. Codeine is rarely recommended for children.

Nonopioid Antitussives

Dextromethorphan. Dextromethorphan is the most effective over-the-counter (OTC) nonopioid cough medicine, and the most widely used of all cough medicines. Like the opioids, dextromethorphan acts in the CNS. Dextromethorphan is a derivative of the opioids; however, it does not produce typical opioid-like euphoria or physical dependence. Nonetheless, when taken in high doses, dextromethorphan can cause euphoria, and is sometimes abused for this effect (see Chapter 40). Depending on the dose, subjective effects can range from mild inebriation to a state of mind-body dissociation, much like that caused by phencyclidine (PCP). At therapeutic doses, dextromethorphan does not depress respiration. Adverse effects are mild and rare. Dextromethorphan is the active ingredient in more than 140 nonprescription cough medicines. The usual adult dosage is 10 to 30 mg every 4 to 8 hours.

In the past, dextromethorphan was considered devoid of analgesic actions; however, it now appears the drug *can* reduce pain. The mechanism is the blockade of receptors for *N*-methyl-D-aspartate (NMDA) in the brain and spinal cord. In contrast, opioids relieve pain primarily through activation of mu receptors. Although dextromethorphan has minimal analgesic effects when used alone, it can enhance analgesic effects of the opioids. For example, we can double the analgesic response to 30 mg of morphine by combining the morphine with 30 mg of dextromethorphan.

Other Nonopioid Antitussives. *Diphenhydramine* is an antihistamine with the ability to suppress cough. The mechanism is unclear. Like other antihistamines, diphenhydramine has sedative and anticholinergic properties. Cough suppression is achieved only at doses that produce prominent sedation. The usual adult dosage is 25 mg every 4 hours.

Benzonatate [Tessalon, Zonatuss] is a structural analog of two local anesthetics: tetracaine and procaine. The drug suppresses cough by decreasing the sensitivity of respiratory tract stretch receptors (components of the cough-reflex pathway). Adverse effects are usually mild (e.g., sedation, dizziness, constipation). Nonetheless, severe effects can occur in children and adults. In children younger than 2 years, accidental ingestion of just one or two capsules has been fatal. In older children and adults, overdose can cause seizures, dysrhythmia, and death. Smaller doses can cause confusion, chest numbness, visual hallucinations, and a burning sensation in the eyes. If the capsules are sucked or chewed, rather than swallowed, the drug can cause laryngospasm, bronchospasm, and circulatory collapse. Accordingly, benzonatate capsules should be swallowed intact. The usual adult dosage is 100 mg 3 times a day. Safety and efficacy have not been established in children younger than 10 years.

Expectorants and Mucolytics

Expectorants

An expectorant is a drug that renders cough more productive by stimulating the flow of respiratory tract secretions. A variety of compounds (e.g., ammonium chloride, iodide products) have been promoted for their supposed expectorant actions. However, in almost all cases, efficacy is questionable. One agent—*guaifenesin* [Mucinex, Humibid, others]—may be an exception. However, for this drug to be effective, doses higher than those normally employed may be needed.

Mucolytics

A mucolytic is a drug that reacts directly with mucus to make it less viscous. This action should help make cough more productive. Two preparations—*hypertonic saline* and *acetylcysteine*—are employed for their mucolytic actions. Both are administered by inhalation. Unfortunately, both can trigger bronchospasm. Because of its sulfur content, acetylcysteine has the additional drawback of smelling like rotten eggs.

COLD REMEDIES: COMBINATION PREPARATIONS

Basic Considerations

The common cold is an acute *upper* respiratory infection of viral origin. Between 50% and 80% of colds are caused by the human rhinovirus, which can also cause serious infection of the *lower* respiratory tract. Characteristic symptoms of the common cold are rhinorrhea, nasal congestion, cough, sneezing, sore throat, hoarseness, headache, malaise, and myalgia; fever is common in children but rare in adults. Colds are self-limited and usually benign. Persistence or worsening of symptoms suggests the development of a secondary bacterial infection. In the United States, the economic burden of the cold is estimated at more than $60 billion a year.

There is no cure for the cold, so treatment is purely symptomatic. Because colds are caused by viruses, there is no justification for the routine use of antibiotics. These agents are appropriate only if a bacterial co-infection arises. There is no evidence that vitamin C or zinc can prevent or cure colds.

Because no single drug can relieve all symptoms of a cold, the pharmaceutical industry has formulated a vast number of cold remedies that contain a mixture of ingredients. These combination cold remedies should be reserved for patients with multiple symptoms. In addition, the combination chosen should contain only those agents that are appropriate for the symptoms at hand. Patients who require relief from just a single symptom (e.g., rhinitis, cough, or headache) are best treated with single-drug preparations.

Combination cold remedies frequently contain two or more of the following: (1) a nasal decongestant, (2) an antitussive, (3) an analgesic, (4) an antihistamine, and (5) caffeine. The purpose of the first three agents is self-evident. In contrast, the roles of antihistamines and caffeine require explanation. Because histamine has nothing to do with the symptoms of a cold, the purpose of including antihistamines is not to block histamine receptors. Rather, because of their anticholinergic actions, antihistamines are included to suppress mucus secretion. (This action can potentially worsen upper respiratory infections by thickening secretions, making them more difficult to drain. This may create an environment conducive to bacterial proliferation, which may lead to secondary bacterial infections such as sinusitis.) Caffeine is added to offset the sedative effects of the antihistamine.

Although they can be convenient, combination cold remedies do have disadvantages. As with all fixed-dose combinations, there is the chance that a dosage (e.g., 1 capsule or 1 tablet) that produces therapeutic levels of one ingredient may produce levels of other ingredients that are either excessive or subtherapeutic. In addition, the combination may contain ingredients that the patient does not need. Furthermore, under U.S. Food and Drug Administration (FDA) regulations, a brand-name product can be reformulated and then sold under the same name. Hence, without carefully reading the label, the consumer has no assurance that the brand-name product purchased contains the same amounts of the same drugs that were present in a previous version of that combination product.

Use in Young Children

Many experts believe that OTC cold remedies should not be used by young children. There is no proof of efficacy or safety in pediatric patients—and there *is* proof of the potential for serious harm. According to the Centers for Disease Control and Prevention, thousands of children have been taken to emergency departments for the management of adverse effects related to cough or cold products. Presenting symptoms have included convulsions, tachycardia, hallucinations, and impaired consciousness. Some children died. In early 2008, the FDA recommended that OTC cold remedies no longer be given to children younger than 2 years, owing to the risk for potentially life-threatening events. The FDA is still reviewing the safety of these drugs in children 2 to 11 years old. In the meantime, citing inadequate effectiveness, significant adverse effects, and common misuse, the American Academy of Pediatrics recommended restricting the use of cough and cold medicines to children older than 6 years. Manufacturers voluntarily revised the labels of children's cold and cough preparations to indicate that they should not be used in children younger than 4 years. In addition, for products that contain an antihistamine, manufacturers added a warning against using these drugs to sedate children. After these interventions, emergency visits related to cold and cough medications decreased significantly for children under 4 years old.

To minimize harm to pediatric patients, parents should:

- Avoid OTC cold remedies in children younger than 4 to 6 years.
- Use only products labeled for pediatric use.
- Consult a healthcare professional before giving these drugs to a child.
- Read all product safety information before dosing.
- Use the measuring device provided with the product.
- Discontinue the medicine and seek professional care if the child's condition worsens or fails to improve.
- Avoid the use of antihistamine-containing products to sedate children.

KEY POINTS

- Allergic rhinitis is the most common allergic disorder.
- Allergic rhinitis is treated primarily with intranasal glucocorticoids, oral and intranasal antihistamines, and oral and intranasal sympathomimetic decongestants.
- Intranasal glucocorticoids are effective drugs for allergic rhinitis. These agents relieve rhinorrhea, congestion, itching, and sneezing.
- Antihistamines (H_1 receptor antagonists) are first-line drugs for allergic rhinitis. They relieve rhinorrhea, sneezing, and itching, but not congestion.
- Antihistamines are not recommended for the management of the common cold and may lead to secondary complications and bacterial infections.
- Sedation and anticholinergic effects are common side effects of the first-generation antihistamines but not the second-generation antihistamines.
- Sympathomimetic drugs decrease nasal congestion by activating $alpha_1$-adrenergic receptors on blood vessels, which causes vasoconstriction and thereby shrinks swollen nasal membranes.
- *Topical* sympathomimetics decrease nasal congestion rapidly and produce minimal systemic effects, but cause rebound congestion when used for more than a few days.
- *Oral* sympathomimetics decrease nasal congestion slowly and produce CNS and cardiovascular stimulation, but do *not* cause rebound congestion, and are suited for long-term use.
- Codeine, a member of the opioid family, is the most effective cough suppressant available. Doses are only one-tenth those used for analgesia.
- Dextromethorphan is the most effective OTC nonopioid cough suppressant.
- There is no good evidence that codeine, dextromethorphan, or any other cough medicine can suppress cough associated with the common cold.
- OTC cough and cold remedies should not be given to children younger than 4 to 6 years.

Please visit **http://evolve.elsevier.com/Lehne** for chapter-specific NCLEX® examination review questions.

UNIT XIV GASTROINTESTINAL DRUGS

CHAPTER 78

Drugs for Peptic Ulcer Disease

Peptic ulcer disease (PUD) refers to a group of upper GI disorders characterized by varying degrees of erosion of the gut wall. Severe ulcers can be complicated by hemorrhage and perforation. Although peptic ulcers can develop in any region exposed to acid and pepsin, ulceration is most common in the lesser curvature of the stomach and the duodenum. PUD is a common disorder that affects about 10% of Americans at some time in their lives. About 6 million Americans get ulcers each year. Before the mid-1990s, PUD was considered a chronic, relapsing disorder of unknown cause and with no known cure; therapy promoted healing but did not prevent ulcer recurrence. Today, thanks to the pioneering work of two Australians—Barry J. Marshall and J. Robin Warren—we know that most cases of PUD are caused by infection with *Helicobacter pylori,* and that eradication of this bacterium not only promotes healing, but greatly reduces the chance of recurrence.

PATHOGENESIS OF PEPTIC ULCERS

Peptic ulcers develop when there is an imbalance between mucosal defensive factors and aggressive factors (Fig. 78.1). The major defensive factors are mucus and bicarbonate. The major aggressive factors are *H. pylori,* nonsteroidal anti-inflammatory drugs (NSAIDs), gastric acid, and pepsin.

Defensive Factors

Defensive factors serve the physiologic role of protecting the stomach and duodenum from self-digestion. When defenses are intact, ulcers are unlikely. Conversely, when defenses are compromised, aggressive factors are able to cause injury. Two important agents that can weaken defenses are *H. pylori* and NSAIDs.

Mucus

Mucus is secreted continuously by cells of the GI mucosa, forming a barrier that protects underlying cells from attack by acid and pepsin.

Bicarbonate

Bicarbonate is secreted by epithelial cells of the stomach and duodenum. Most bicarbonate remains trapped in the mucus layer, where it serves to neutralize any hydrogen ions that penetrate the mucus. Bicarbonate produced by the pancreas is secreted into the lumen of the duodenum, where it neutralizes acid delivered from the stomach.

Blood Flow

Sufficient blood flow to cells of the GI mucosa is essential for maintaining mucosal integrity. If submucosal blood flow is reduced, the resultant local ischemia can lead to cell injury, thereby increasing vulnerability to attack by acid and pepsin.

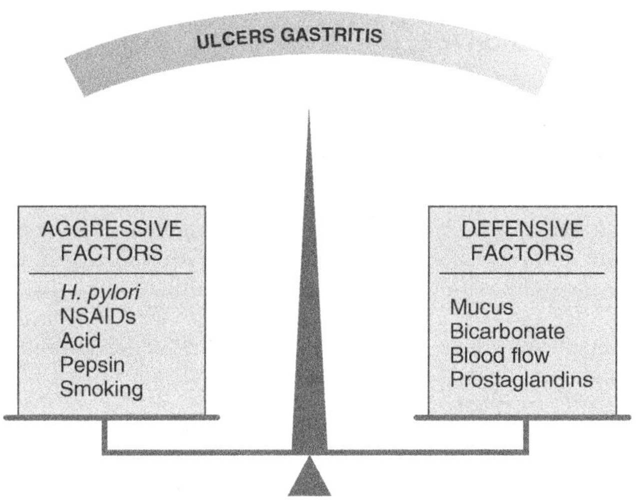

Fig. 78.1 ■ The relationship of mucosal defenses and aggressive factors to health and peptic ulcer disease.
When aggressive factors outweigh mucosal defenses, gastritis and peptic ulcers result. (*NSAIDs,* Nonsteroidal anti-inflammatory drugs.)

Prostaglandins

Prostaglandins play an important role in maintaining defenses. These compounds stimulate secretion of mucus and bicarbonate, and they promote vasodilation, which helps maintain submucosal blood flow. They provide additional protection by suppressing secretion of gastric acid.

Aggressive Factors

Helicobacter pylori

Helicobacter pylori is a gram-negative bacillus that can colonize the stomach and duodenum. By taking up residence in the space between epithelial cells and the mucus barrier that protects these cells, the bacterium manages to escape destruction by acid and pepsin. Once established, *H. pylori* can remain in the GI tract for decades. Although about half of the world's population is infected with *H. pylori,* most infected people never develop symptomatic PUD.

Why do we think *H. pylori* causes PUD? First, between 60% and 75% of patients with PUD have *H. pylori* infection. Second, duodenal ulcers are much more common among people with *H. pylori* infection than among people who are not infected. Third, eradication of the bacterium promotes ulcer healing. And fourth, eradication of the bacterium minimizes ulcer recurrence. (One-year recurrence rates approach 80% when *H. pylori* remains present, compared with only 10% when the organism is gone.)

Although the mechanism by which *H. pylori* promotes ulcers has not been firmly established, likely possibilities are enzymatic degradation of the protective mucus layer, elaboration of a cytotoxin that injures mucosal cells, and infiltration of neutrophils and other inflammatory cells in response to the bacterium's presence. Also, *H. pylori* produces *urease,* an enzyme that forms carbon dioxide and ammonia (from urea in gastric juice); both compounds are potentially toxic to the gastric mucosa.

In addition to its role in PUD, *H. pylori* appears to promote gastric cancer. In fact, the bacterium has been declared a type 1 carcinogen (a definite cause of human cancer) by the International Agency for Research on Cancer. There is a strong association between *H. pylori* infection and the presence of gastric mucosa–associated lymphoid tissue (MALT) lymphomas. Furthermore, among patients with localized MALT lymphoma, eradicating *H. pylori* produces tumor regression in 60% to 90% of cases. In one long-term study, treatment for *H. pylori* reduced the risk of gastric adenocarcinoma by 40% after 15 years.

Nonsteroidal Anti-Inflammatory Drugs

NSAIDs are the underlying cause of many gastric ulcers and some duodenal ulcers. As discussed in Chapter 71, aspirin and other NSAIDs inhibit the biosynthesis of prostaglandins. By doing so, they can decrease submucosal blood flow, suppress secretion of mucus and bicarbonate, and promote secretion of gastric acid. Furthermore, NSAIDs can irritate the mucosa directly. NSAID-induced ulcers are most likely with long-term, high-dose therapy.

Gastric Acid

Gastric acid is an absolute requirement for peptic ulcer generation: In the absence of acid, no ulcer will form. Acid causes ulcers directly by injuring cells of the GI mucosa and indirectly by activating pepsin, a proteolytic enzyme. In most cases, acid hypersecretion, by itself, is insufficient to cause ulcers. In fact, in most patients with gastric ulcers, acid secretion is normal or reduced, and among patients with duodenal ulcers, only one-third produce excessive amounts of acid. From these observations, we can conclude that in the majority of patients with peptic ulcers, factors in addition to acid must be involved.

Zollinger-Ellison syndrome is the primary disorder in which hypersecretion of acid alone causes ulcers. The syndrome is caused by a tumor that secretes gastrin, a hormone that stimulates gastric acid production. The amount of acid produced is so large that it overwhelms mucosal defenses. Zollinger-Ellison syndrome is a rare disorder that accounts for only 0.1% of duodenal ulcers.

Pepsin

Pepsin is a proteolytic enzyme present in gastric juice. Like gastric acid, pepsin can injure unprotected cells of the gastric and duodenal mucosa.

Smoking

Smoking delays ulcer healing and increases the risk of recurrence. Possible mechanisms include reduction of the beneficial effects of antiulcer medications, reduced secretion of bicarbonate, and accelerated gastric emptying, which would deliver more acid to the duodenum.

Summary

Infection with *H. pylori* is the most common cause of gastric and duodenal ulcers. However, among people whose PUD can be ascribed to *H. pylori,* additional factors must be involved because more than 50% of the population harbors *H. pylori,* but only 10% develop ulcers. Factors that may increase the risk of PUD in people infected with *H. pylori* include smoking, increased acid secretion, and reduced bicarbonate production. The second most common cause of gastric ulcers is NSAIDs. Hypersecretion of acid underlies a few cases of PUD that are not caused by *H. pylori* or NSAIDs.

OVERVIEW OF TREATMENT

Drug Therapy

The goal of drug therapy is to (1) alleviate symptoms, (2) promote healing, (3) prevent complications (hemorrhage, perforation, obstruction), and (4) prevent recurrence. With the exception of antibiotics, the drugs employed do not alter the disease process. Rather, they simply create conditions conducive to healing. Since nonantibiotic therapies do not cure ulcers, the relapse rate following their discontinuation is high. In contrast, the relapse rate following antibiotic therapy is low.

Classes of Antiulcer Drugs

As shown in Table 78.1, the antiulcer drugs fall into five major groups:

- Antibiotics
- Antisecretory agents (proton pump inhibitors, histamine$_2$ receptor antagonists)
- Mucosal protectants
- Antisecretory agents that enhance mucosal defenses
- Antacids

From this classification, we can see that drugs act in three basic ways to promote ulcer healing. Specifically, they can (1) eradicate *H. pylori* (antibiotics do this), (2) reduce gastric acidity (antisecretory agents, misoprostol, and antacids do this), and (3) enhance mucosal defenses (sucralfate and misoprostol do this).

Drug Selection

***Helicobacter pylori*–Associated Ulcers.** The American College of Gastroenterology recommends that all patients with gastric or duodenal ulcers and documented *H. pylori* infection be treated with antibiotics. This recommendation applies to patients with newly diagnosed PUD, recurrent PUD, and PUD in which the use of NSAIDs is a contributing factor. To hasten healing and relieve symptoms, an antisecretory agent should be given along with the antibiotics. By eliminating *H. pylori,* antibiotics can cure PUD and can thereby prevent recurrence. The diagnosis of *H. pylori* infection and specific antibiotic regimens are discussed later under *Antibacterial Drugs.*

NSAID-Induced Ulcers

Prophylaxis. For patients with risk factors for ulcer development (e.g., age over 60, history of ulcers, high-dose NSAID therapy), prophylactic therapy is indicated. Proton pump inhibitors (e.g., omeprazole) are preferred. Misoprostol is also effective, but it can cause diarrhea. Antacids, sucralfate, and histamine$_2$ receptor blockers are not recommended.

Treatment. NSAID-induced ulcers can be treated with any ulcer medication. However, histamine$_2$ receptor blockers and proton pump inhibitors are preferred. If possible, the offending NSAID should be discontinued, so as to accelerate healing. If the NSAID cannot be discontinued, a proton pump inhibitor is the best choice to promote healing.

Evaluation

We can evaluate ulcer healing by monitoring for relief of pain and by radiologic or endoscopic examination of the ulcer site.

TABLE 78.1 ▪ Classification of Antiulcer Drugs

Class	Drugs	Mechanism of Action
ANTIBIOTICS	Amoxicillin [Amoxil] Bismuth [Pepto-Bismol] Clarithromycin [Biaxin] Metronidazole [Flagyl] Tetracycline (generic only) Tinidazole [Tindamax]	Eradicate *H. pylori*
ANTISECRETORY AGENTS		
H_2 receptor antagonists	Cimetidine [Tagamet] Famotidine [Pepcid] Nizatidine [Axid] Ranitidine [Zantac]	Suppress acid secretion by blocking H_2 receptors on parietal cells
Proton pump inhibitors	Dexlansoprazole [Dexilant] Esomeprazole [Nexium] Lansoprazole [Prevacid] Omeprazole [Prilosec, Zegerid, Losec 🍁] Pantoprazole [Protonix, Pantoloc 🍁] Rabeprazole [Aciphex, Pariet 🍁]	Suppress acid secretion by inhibiting H^+, K^+-ATPase, the enzyme that makes gastric acid
MUCOSAL PROTECTANT	Sucralfate [Carafate, Sulcrate 🍁]	Forms a barrier over the ulcer crater that protects against acid and pepsin
ANTISECRETORY AGENT THAT ENHANCES MUCOSAL DEFENSES	Misoprostol [Cytotec]	Protects against NSAID-induced ulcers by stimulating secretion of mucus and bicarbonate, maintaining submucosal blood flow, and suppressing secretion of gastric acid
ANTACIDS	Aluminum hydroxide Calcium carbonate Magnesium hydroxide	React with gastric acid to form neutral salts

H_2, Histamine$_2$; *NSAID,* nonsteroidal anti-inflammatory drug.

Unfortunately, evaluation is seldom straightforward because cessation of pain and disappearance of the ulcer rarely coincide: In most cases, pain subsides before complete healing. However, the converse may also be true: Pain may persist even though endoscopic or radiologic examination reveals healing is complete.

Eradication of *H. pylori* can be determined with several methods, including breath tests, serologic tests, stool tests, and microscopic observation of a stained biopsy sample. These methods are discussed later in the chapter.

A Note About the Effects of Drugs on Pepsin

Pepsin is a proteolytic enzyme that can contribute to ulcer formation. The enzyme promotes ulcers by breaking down protein in the gut wall.

Like most enzymes, pepsin is sensitive to pH. As pH rises from 1.3 (the usual pH of the stomach) to 2, peptic activity increases by a factor of 4. As pH goes even higher, peptic activity begins to decline. At a pH of 5, peptic activity drops below baseline rates. When pH exceeds 6 to 7, pepsin undergoes irreversible inactivation.

Because the activity of pepsin is pH dependent, drugs that elevate gastric pH (e.g., antacids, histamine$_2$ antagonists, proton pump inhibitors) can cause peptic activity to increase, thereby enhancing pepsin's destructive effects. For example, treatment that produces a 99% reduction in gastric acidity will cause pH to rise from a base level of 1.3 up to 3.3. At pH 3.3, peptic activity will be significantly increased. To avoid activation of pepsin, drugs that reduce acidity should be administered in doses sufficient to raise gastric pH above 5.

Nondrug Therapy

Optimal antiulcer therapy requires implementation of nondrug measures in addition to drug therapy.

Diet

Despite commonly held beliefs, diet plays a minor role in ulcer management. The traditional "ulcer diet," consisting of bland foods together with milk or cream, does not accelerate healing. Furthermore, there is no convincing evidence that caffeine-containing beverages (coffee, tea, colas) promote ulcer formation or interfere with recovery. A change in *eating pattern* may be beneficial: Consumption of five or six small meals a day, rather than three larger ones, can reduce fluctuations in intragastric pH and may thereby facilitate recovery.

Other Nondrug Measures

Smoking is associated with an increased incidence of ulcers and also delays recovery. Accordingly, cigarettes should be avoided. Because of their ulcerogenic actions, *aspirin and other NSAIDs* should be avoided by patients with PUD. The exception to this rule is the use of aspirin to prevent cardiovascular disease; in the low doses employed, aspirin is only a small factor in PUD. There are no hard data indicating that *alcohol* contributes to PUD. However, if the patient notes a temporal relationship between alcohol consumption and exacerbation of symptoms, then the use of alcohol should stop. Many people feel that the reduction of *stress and anxiety* may encourage ulcer healing; however, there is no good evidence that this is true.

ANTIBACTERIAL DRUGS

Antibacterial drugs should be given to all patients with gastric or duodenal ulcers and confirmed infection with *H. pylori.* Antibiotics are not recommended for asymptomatic individuals who test positive for *H. pylori.*

Tests for *Helicobacter pylori*

Several tests for *H. pylori* are available. Some are invasive; some are not. The invasive tests require an endoscopically obtained biopsy sample, which can be evaluated in three ways: (1) staining and viewing under a microscope to see if *H. pylori* is present; (2) assaying for the presence of urease (a marker enzyme for *H. pylori*); and (3) culturing and then assaying for the presence of *H. pylori.*

In the United States, three types of noninvasive tests are available: breath, serologic, and stool tests. In the breath test, patients are given radiolabeled urea. If *H. pylori* is present, the urea is converted to carbon dioxide and ammonia; radiolabeled carbon dioxide can then be detected in the breath. In the serologic test, blood samples are evaluated for antibodies to *H. pylori.* In the stool test, fecal samples are evaluated for the presence of *H. pylori* antigens.

Antibiotics Employed

The antibiotics employed most often are clarithromycin, amoxicillin, bismuth, metronidazole, and tetracycline. None is effective alone. Furthermore, if these drugs *are* used alone, the risk of developing resistance is increased.

Clarithromycin

Clarithromycin [Biaxin] suppresses growth of *H. pylori* by inhibiting protein synthesis. In the absence of resistance, treatment is highly effective. Unfortunately, the rate of resistance is rising, exceeding 20% in some areas. The most common side effects are nausea, diarrhea, and distortion of taste. The basic pharmacology of clarithromycin is presented in Chapter 86.

Amoxicillin

Helicobacter pylori is highly sensitive to amoxicillin. The rate of resistance is low, only about 3%. Amoxicillin kills bacteria by disrupting the cell wall. Antibacterial activity is highest at neutral pH, and hence can be enhanced by reducing gastric acidity with an antisecretory agent (e.g., omeprazole). The most common side effect is diarrhea. The basic pharmacology of amoxicillin is discussed in Chapter 84.

Bismuth

Bismuth compounds—bismuth subsalicylate and bismuth subcitrate—act topically to disrupt the cell wall of *H. pylori,* thereby causing lysis and death. Bismuth may also inhibit urease activity and may prevent *H. pylori* from adhering to the gastric surface.

Bismuth can impart a harmless black coloration to the tongue and stool. Patients should be forewarned. Stool discoloration may confound interpretation of gastric bleeding. Long-term therapy may carry a risk of neurologic injury.

Tetracycline

Tetracycline, an inhibitor of bacterial protein synthesis, is highly active against *H. pylori.* Resistance is rare (less than 1%). Because tetracycline can stain developing teeth, it should not be used by pregnant women or young children. The pharmacology of tetracycline is discussed in Chapter 86.

Metronidazole

Metronidazole [Flagyl] is very effective against sensitive strains of *H. pylori.* Unfortunately, more than 40% of strains are now resistant. The most common side effects are nausea and headache. A disulfiram-like reaction can occur if metronidazole is used with alcohol, and hence alcohol must be avoided. Metronidazole should not be taken during pregnancy. The basic pharmacology of metronidazole is discussed in Chapter 91

Tinidazole

Tinidazole [Tindamax] is very similar to metronidazole and shares that drug's adverse effects and interactions. Like metronidazole, tinidazole can cause a disulfiram-like reaction, and hence must not be combined with alcohol. The basic pharmacology of tinidazole is discussed in Chapter 99.

Antibiotic Regimens

In 2017, the American College of Gastroenterology (ACG) issued updated guidelines for managing *H. pylori* infection. To minimize emergence of resistance, the guidelines recommend using at least two antibiotics, and preferably three. An antisecretory agent—proton pump inhibitor (PPI) or histamine$_2$ receptor antagonist (H_2RA)—should be included as well. Eradication rates are good with a 10-day course, and slightly better with a 14-day course.

Table 78.2 presents four ACG-recommended regimens. In regions where resistance to clarithromycin is low (below 20%), the preferred treatment is *clarithromycin-based triple therapy,* consisting of clarithromycin plus amoxicillin plus a PPI. For patients with penicillin allergy, metronidazole can be substituted for amoxicillin. In regions where resistance to clarithromycin is high (above 20%), the preferred regimen is *bismuth-based quadruple therapy,* consisting of bismuth subsalicylate plus metronidazole plus tetracycline, all three combined with a PPI or an H_2RA. For patients who can't use triple therapy or quadruple therapy, *sequential therapy* is an option. This regimen consists of taking a PPI plus amoxicillin for 5 to 7 days, followed by a PPI plus clarithromycin plus tinidazole for 5 to 7 days. At this time, the efficacy of sequential therapy in North America has not been established.

For several reasons, compliance with antibiotic therapy can be difficult. First, antibiotic regimens are complex, requiring the patient to ingest as many as 12 pills a day. Second, side effects—especially nausea and diarrhea—are common. Third, a course of treatment is somewhat expensive. However, it costs much less to eradicate *H. pylori* with antibiotics than it does to treat ulcers over and over again with traditional antiulcer drugs, which merely promote healing without eliminating the cause.

HISTAMINE$_2$ RECEPTOR ANTAGONISTS

The H_2RAs are effective drugs for treating gastric and duodenal ulcers. These agents promote ulcer healing by suppressing secretion of gastric acid. Four H_2RAs are available: cimetidine, ranitidine, famotidine, and nizatidine. All four are equally effective. Serious side effects are uncommon.

Cimetidine

Cimetidine [Tagamet] was the first H_2RA available and will serve as our prototype for the group. At one time, cimetidine was the most frequently prescribed drug in the United States. Cimetidine was the first drug with sales over $1 billion, making it our first "blockbuster" drug.

TABLE 78.2 ▪ First-Line Regimens for Eradicating *H. pylori*

Drug	Duration	Eradication Rate	Comments
CLARITHROMYCIN-BASED TRIPLE THERAPY 1 Standard-dose PPI[a] Clarithromycin (500 mg twice daily) Amoxicillin (1 gm twice daily)	10–14 days	70%–85%	Consider in non–penicillin-allergic patients who have not previously received clarithromycin or another macrolide
CLARITHROMYCIN-BASED TRIPLE THERAPY 2 Standard-dose PPI[a] Clarithromycin (500 mg twice daily) Metronidazole (500 mg twice daily)	10–14 days	70%–85%	Consider in penicillin-allergic patients who have not previously received a macrolide or are unable to tolerate bismuth quadruple therapy
BISMUTH-BASED QUADRUPLE THERAPY Bismuth subsalicylate (525 mg 4 times daily) Metronidazole (250 mg 4 times daily) Tetracycline (500 mg 4 times daily) Standard-dose PPI[a] or ranitidine (150 mg twice daily)	10–14 days	75%–90%	Consider in penicillin-allergic patients and in patients with clarithromycin-resistant *H. pylori*
SEQUENTIAL THERAPY Standard-dose PPI[a] + amoxicillin (1 gm twice daily) for 5 days, followed by: Standard-dose PPI[a] + clarithromycin (500 mg once daily) + tinidazole (500 mg twice daily) for 5–7 days	10 days	Over 90%	Efficacy in North America requires validation

[a]Standard doses for PPIs are as follows: dexlansoprazole, 30 to 60 mg once daily; esomeprazole, 40 mg once daily; lansoprazole, 30 mg twice daily; omeprazole, 40 mg twice daily; pantoprazole, 40 mg twice daily; and rabeprazole 20 mg twice daily.
Modified from American College of Gastroenterology: Treatment of *Helicobacter pylori* infection. *Am J Gastroenterol* 112:212–238, 2017.

Prototype Drugs

DRUGS FOR PUD

Antibiotics (for *Helicobacter pylori*)
Amoxicillin/clarithromycin/omeprazole

H_2-Receptor Antagonists
Cimetidine

Proton Pump Inhibitors
Omeprazole

Mucosal Protectants
Sucralfate

Antacids
Aluminum hydroxide/magnesium hydroxide

Mechanism of Action

Histamine acts through two types of receptors, named H_1 and H_2. Activation of H_1 receptors produces symptoms of allergy. Activation of H_2 receptors, which are located on parietal cells of the stomach (Fig. 78.2), promotes secretion of gastric acid. By blocking H_2 receptors, cimetidine reduces both the volume of gastric juice and its hydrogen ion concentration. Cimetidine suppresses basal acid secretion and secretion stimulated by gastrin and acetylcholine. Because cimetidine produces selective blockade of H_2 receptors, the drug cannot suppress symptoms of allergy.

Pharmacokinetics

Cimetidine is available orally in solution or tablet. Food decreases the rate of absorption but not the extent. Hence, if cimetidine is taken with meals, absorption will be slowed and beneficial effects prolonged. Cimetidine crosses the blood-brain barrier (albeit with difficulty), and central nervous system (CNS) side effects can occur. Although some hepatic metabolism takes place, most of each dose is eliminated intact in the urine. The half-life is relatively short (about 2 hours), but increases in patients with renal impairment. Accordingly, dosage should be reduced in these patients.

Therapeutic Uses

Gastric and Duodenal Ulcers. Cimetidine promotes the healing of gastric and duodenal ulcers. To heal duodenal ulcers, 4 to 6 weeks of therapy are generally required. To heal gastric ulcers, 8 to 12 weeks may be needed. Long-term therapy with low doses may be given as prophylaxis against recurrence of gastric and duodenal ulcers.

Gastroesophageal Reflux Disease (GERD). Reflux esophagitis is an inflammatory condition caused by reflux of

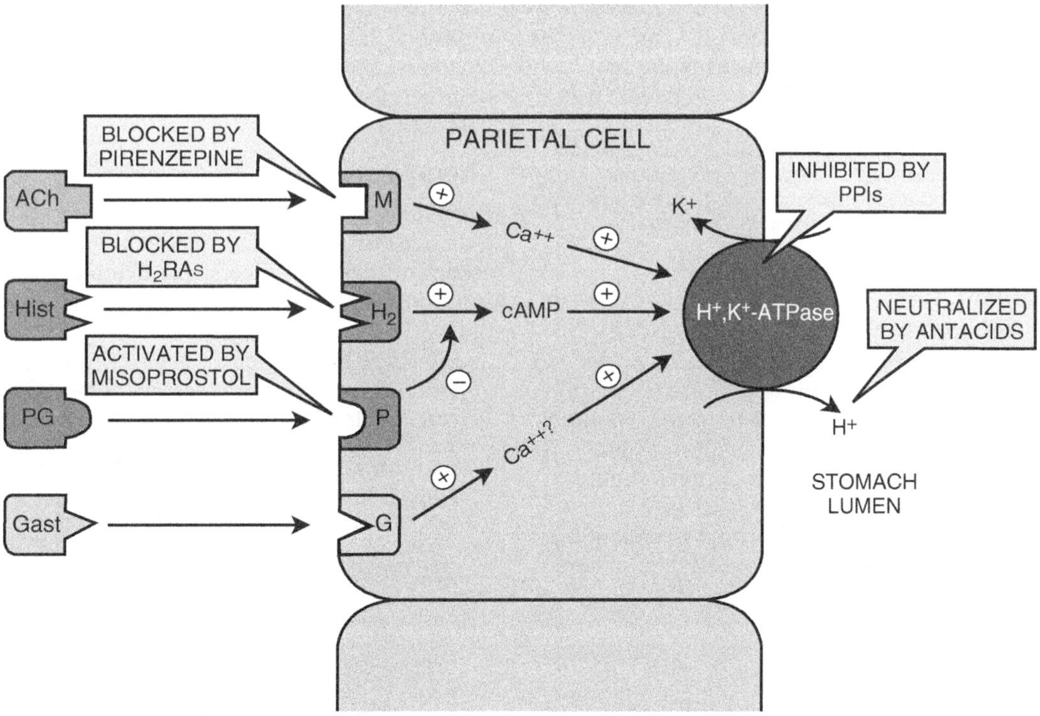

Fig. 78.2 ■ A model of the regulation of gastric acid secretion showing the actions of antisecretory drugs and antacids.
Production of gastric acid is stimulated by three endogenous compounds: (1) acetylcholine (ACh) acting at muscarinic (M) receptors; (2) histamine (Hist) acting at histamine$_2$ (H_2) receptors; and (3) gastrin (Gast) acting at gastrin (G) receptors. As indicated, all three compounds act through intracellular messengers—either calcium (Ca^{++}) or cyclic AMP (cAMP)—to increase the activity of H^+,K^+-ATPase, the enzyme that actually produces gastric acid. Prostaglandins (PG) decrease acid production, perhaps by suppressing production of intracellular cAMP. The actions of histamine$_2$ receptor antagonists (H_2RAs), proton pump inhibitors (PPIs), and other drugs are indicated. (*P,* Prostaglandin receptor.)

gastric contents back into the esophagus. Cimetidine is a drug of choice for relieving symptoms. However, cimetidine does little to hasten healing.

Zollinger-Ellison Syndrome. This syndrome is characterized by hypersecretion of gastric acid and development of peptic ulcers. The underlying cause is secretion of gastrin from a gastrin-producing tumor. Cimetidine can promote the healing of ulcers in patients with Zollinger-Ellison syndrome, but only if high doses are employed. At these doses, significant adverse effects can occur.

Heartburn, Acid Indigestion, and Sour Stomach. Cimetidine is available over the counter to treat these common acid-related symptoms.

Adverse Effects

The incidence of side effects is low, and those that do occur are usually benign.

Antiandrogenic Effects. Cimetidine binds to androgen receptors, producing receptor blockade. As a result, the drug can cause gynecomastia, reduced libido, and impotence—all of which reverse when dosing stops.

CNS Effects. Effects on the CNS are most likely in older adults who have renal or hepatic impairment. Possible reactions include confusion, hallucinations, CNS depression (lethargy, somnolence), and CNS excitation (restlessness, seizures).

Pneumonia. Elevation of gastric pH with an antisecretory agent increases the risk of pneumonia because when gastric acidity is reduced, bacterial colonization of the stomach increases, resulting in a secondary increase in colonization of the respiratory tract. Among people using an H_2RA, the *relative* risk of acquiring pneumonia is doubled. However, the *absolute* risk is still low (about 1 extra case for every 500 people using the drug).

Other Adverse Effects. By reducing gastric acidity, cimetidine may permit growth of *Candida* in the stomach. Hematologic effects (neutropenia, leukopenia, thrombocytopenia) occur rarely. Minor side effects include headache, dizziness, myalgia, nausea, diarrhea, constipation, rash, and pruritus.

Drug Interactions

Interactions Related to Inhibition of Drug Metabolism. Cimetidine inhibits hepatic drug-metabolizing enzymes, and hence can cause levels of many other drugs to rise. Drugs of particular concern are *warfarin, phenytoin, theophylline,* and *lidocaine,* all of which have a narrow margin of safety. If these drugs are used with cimetidine, their dosages should be reduced.

Antacids. Antacids can decrease absorption of cimetidine. Accordingly, cimetidine and antacids should be administered at least 1 hour apart.

Preparations, Dosage, and Administration

Oral. Cimetidine [Tagamet HB 200] is available in tablets (200, 300, 400, and 800 mg) and an oral solution (300 mg/5 mL). For treatment of duodenal and gastric ulcers, dosing may be done once daily (800 mg at bedtime), twice daily (400 mg each dose), or 4 times a day (300 mg with meals and at bedtime). In patients with renal impairment, dosage should be lowered by 50%. For prophylaxis against ulcer recurrence, a single 400-mg dose at bedtime may be employed. Patients with Zollinger-Ellison syndrome require high doses, but not more than 2.4 gm/day.

Ranitidine

Ranitidine [Zantac] shares many of the properties of cimetidine. However, although similar to cimetidine, the drug differs in three important respects: ranitidine is more potent, produces fewer adverse effects, and causes fewer drug interactions.

Actions

Like cimetidine, ranitidine suppresses secretion of gastric acid by blocking H_2 receptors on gastric parietal cells. It does not block H_1 receptors, and hence does not reduce symptoms of allergy.

Pharmacokinetics

Ranitidine can be administered PO, IM, or IV. Oral bioavailability is about 50%. In contrast to cimetidine, ranitidine is absorbed at the same rate in the presence or absence of food. Ranitidine's ability to enter the CNS is even less than that of cimetidine. Elimination is by hepatic metabolism and renal excretion. Accumulation will occur in patients with renal impairment unless the dosage is reduced. The half-life is 2 to 3 hours.

Adverse Effects

Significant side effects are uncommon. Because ranitidine penetrates the blood-brain barrier poorly, CNS effects are rare. In contrast to cimetidine, ranitidine does not bind to androgen receptors, and hence does not cause antiandrogenic effects (e.g., gynecomastia, impotence). Elevation of gastric pH may increase the risk of pneumonia.

Drug Interactions

Ranitidine has few drug interactions. In contrast to cimetidine, ranitidine is a weak inhibitor of hepatic drug-metabolizing enzymes, and therefore does not greatly depress metabolism of other drugs. Antacids have a small effect on ranitidine absorption.

Therapeutic Uses

Ranitidine has the same indications as cimetidine: (1) short-term treatment of gastric and duodenal ulcers, (2) prophylaxis of recurrent duodenal ulcers, (3) treatment of Zollinger-Ellison syndrome and other hypersecretory states, and (4) treatment of GERD. Because it produces fewer side effects than cimetidine and because of its greater potency, ranitidine is preferred to cimetidine for treating hypersecretory states (e.g., Zollinger-Ellison syndrome).

Preparations, Dosage, and Administration

Preparations. Ranitidine [Zantac] is available in standard tablets (75, 150, and 300 mg), capsules (150 and 300 mg), and a syrup (15 mg/mL) for oral use, and in solution (25 mg/mL) for parenteral use.

Oral Dosage. The usual adult dosage for treatment of gastric or duodenal ulcers is 150 mg twice a day. Alternatively, a 300-mg dose can be given once daily at bedtime. For patients with Zollinger-Ellison syndrome, higher doses may be required. The dosage for preventing recurrence of duodenal ulcers is 150 mg once daily at bedtime. Ranitidine can be administered without regard to meals.

Parenteral Dosage. The usual parenteral dosage (IM or IV) is 50 mg every 6 to 8 hours. Intramuscular doses can be injected without dilution. For *IV injection,* the preparation should be diluted to a volume of 20 mL in 0.9% sodium chloride injection and administered slowly (over 5 or more minutes). For *IV infusion,* the drug should be diluted in 100 mL of 0.9% sodium chloride injection and administered over 15 to 20 minutes.

Famotidine

Basic and Clinical Pharmacology

Famotidine [Pepcid, Pepcid AC] is much like ranitidine. The drug is approved for the treatment and prevention of duodenal ulcers and the treatment of gastric ulcers, GERD, and hypersecretory states (e.g., Zollinger-Ellison syndrome). An over-the-counter formulation is approved for heartburn, acid indigestion, and sour stomach. Like ranitidine, famotidine does not bind to androgen receptors and hence does not have antiandrogenic effects. Elevation of gastric pH may increase the risk of pneumonia. Famotidine does not inhibit hepatic drug-metabolizing enzymes and hence does not suppress the metabolism of other drugs.

Preparations, Dosage, and Administration

Prescription-strength famotidine [Pepcid] is available in standard tablets (10, 20, and 40 mg), orally disintegrating tablets (20 and 40 mg), powder for oral suspension (40 mg/5 mL when reconstituted), and solution (0.4 and 10 mg/mL) for IV use. For treatment of duodenal and gastric ulcers, the dosage is 20 mg twice daily or 40 mg once daily at bedtime. To prevent recurrence of duodenal ulcers, the dosage is 20 mg once daily at bedtime. For treatment of GERD, the dosage is 20 to 40 mg twice daily. For treatment of hypersecretory states, the initial dosage is 20 mg every 6 hours; severe cases may require up to 160 mg every 6 hours. All doses should be reduced in patients with moderate to severe renal impairment. In patients taking ibuprofen for treatment of osteoarthritis and rheumatoid arthritis, famotidine is available in combination with ibuprofen in a tablet containing 800 mg of ibuprofen and 26.6 mg of famotidine, sold as *Duexis*.

Over-the-counter famotidine is available in 20-mg standard tablets and chewables marketed as *Pepcid AC Maximum Strength,* and in one 10-mg formulation of standard tablets marketed as *Pepcid AC.* Indications are prevention and relief of heartburn, acid indigestion, and sour stomach. To prevent symptoms, the drug is taken 1 hour before eating. The dosage for prevention or relief is 10 mg, taken with a glass of water. As with prescription-strength famotidine, dosages should be reduced in patients with moderate to severe renal impairment.

Nizatidine

Basic and Clinical Pharmacology

Nizatidine [Axid] is much like ranitidine and famotidine. The drug is used to treat and prevent duodenal ulcers and to treat gastric ulcers, GERD, heartburn, acid indigestion, and sour stomach. Like ranitidine and famotidine, nizatidine does not have antiandrogenic effects and does not inhibit the metabolism of other drugs. Elevation of gastric pH may increase the risk of pneumonia.

Preparations, Dosage, and Administration

Prescription-strength nizatidine is available in capsules (150 and 300 mg) and in an oral solution (15 mg/mL). The dosage for treatment of active gastric and duodenal ulcers is 150 mg twice daily or 300 mg once daily at bedtime. To prevent recurrence of duodenal ulcers, the dosage is 150 mg once daily at bedtime. For the treatment of GERD, the dosage is 150 mg twice daily.

Over-the-counter nizatidine [Axid AR] is available in 75-mg capsules. The dosage for preventing heartburn is 75 mg, taken any time in the 30-minute interval preceding a meal.

PROTON PUMP INHIBITORS

The PPIs are the most effective drugs we have for suppressing gastric acid secretion. Indications include gastric and duodenal ulcers and GERD. Similarities among the PPIs are more profound than the differences. Therefore, selecting among them is based largely on cost and prescriber preference.

Although PPIs are generally well tolerated, they *can* increase the risk of serious adverse events, including fractures, pneumonia, acid rebound, and, possibly, intestinal infection with *Clostridium difficile.* To ensure that the benefits of treatment outweigh the risks, treatment should be limited to appropriate candidates, who should take the lowest dose needed for the shortest time possible.

Omeprazole

Omeprazole [Prilosec, Prilosec OTC, Zegerid, Zegerid OTC, Losec 🍁] was the first PPI available and will serve as our prototype for the group. Acid suppression is greater than with the H_2RAs. Side effects from short-term therapy are minimal.

Mechanism of Action

Omeprazole is a prodrug that undergoes conversion to its active form within parietal cells of the stomach. The active form then causes irreversible inhibition of H^+,K^+-ATPase (proton pump), the enzyme that generates gastric acid (see Fig. 78.2). Because it blocks the final common pathway of gastric acid production, omeprazole can inhibit basal and stimulated acid release. A single 30-mg oral dose reduces acid production by 97% within 2 hours. Because inhibition of the ATPase is not reversible, effects persist until new enzyme is synthesized. Partial recovery occurs 3 to 5 days after stopping treatment. Full recovery may take weeks.

Pharmacokinetics

After oral dosing, about 50% of the drug reaches the systemic circulation. Omeprazole undergoes hepatic metabolism followed by renal excretion. The plasma half-life is short—about 1 hour. However, because omeprazole acts by irreversible enzyme inhibition, effects persist long after the drug has left the body.

Omeprazole is acid labile and hence must be protected from stomach acid. To accomplish this, the drug is formulated in a capsule that contains protective enteric-coated granules. The capsule dissolves in the stomach, but the granules remain intact until they reach the relatively alkaline environment of the duodenum.

Therapeutic Use

Omeprazole is approved for short-term therapy of duodenal ulcers, gastric ulcers, erosive esophagitis, and GERD, and for long-term therapy of hypersecretory conditions (e.g., Zollinger-Ellison syndrome). Except for therapy of hypersecretory states, treatment should be limited to 4 to 8 weeks.

In hospitals, omeprazole and other PPIs are widely used to prevent stress ulcers. However, about two-thirds of patients who receive PPIs don't really need them. Ulcer prophylaxis is indicated only for patients in intensive care units, and then only if they have an additional risk factor, such as multiple trauma, spinal cord injury, or prolonged mechanical ventilation (more than 48 hours). General medical and surgical patients are at low risk for stress ulcers and should not receive PPIs for prophylaxis.

How does omeprazole compare with H_2RAs? Omeprazole and other PPIs reduce 24-hour acid secretion by 90%, compared with 65% for H_2RAs. Also, PPIs act faster than H_2RAs to reduce gastric acidity and relieve ulcer symptoms. Patients who fail to respond to H_2RAs can often benefit from a PPI.

Use of omeprazole and other PPIs for GERD is discussed in Box 78.1.

Adverse Effects

Minor Effects. Effects seen with short-term therapy are generally inconsequential. Like the H_2RAs, omeprazole can cause headache, diarrhea, nausea, and vomiting. The incidence of these effects is less than 1%.

Pneumonia. Omeprazole and other PPIs increase the risk of community-acquired and hospital-acquired pneumonia. Possible causes include alteration of upper GI flora (owing to reduced gastric acidity) and impairment of white blood cell

BOX 78.1 ■ SPECIAL INTEREST TOPIC

GASTROESOPHAGEAL REFLUX DISEASE

Gastroesophageal reflux disease (GERD) is a common disorder characterized by heartburn and acid regurgitation. The disease is formally defined by the presence of troublesome symptoms or complications caused by the passage of gastric contents into the esophagus. Among American adults, heartburn develops in 44% at least once a month. GERD is also common among children.

GERD is associated with a wide range of symptoms and complications. On the basis of endoscopic examination, patients fall into two major groups: those with *erosive esophagitis* and those with *nonerosive reflux disease* (NERD). Erosive esophagitis is characterized by breaks in the esophageal mucosa. In contrast, mucosal breaks are absent in people with NERD. Less than 50% of patients with GERD have the erosive form. Complications of erosive GERD include difficulty swallowing, painful swallowing, esophageal stricture, ulcers, GI bleeding, anemia, and persistent vomiting. Erosive GERD can also lead to esophageal adenocarcinoma and Barrett's esophagus, a premalignant condition that can evolve into adenocarcinoma.

The primary problem is inappropriate relaxation of the lower esophageal sphincter (LES), a ring of smooth muscle that normally prevents reflux of gastric acid. In people with GERD, the LES undergoes frequent, transient relaxation, thereby allowing pressure in the stomach to force gastric contents up into the esophagus. Other factors that can contribute to GERD include obesity, hiatal hernia, delayed gastric emptying, and impaired clearance of acid from the esophagus. Of note, *Helicobacter pylori,* the bacterium that causes most gastric and duodenal ulcers, appears to play little or no role in GERD.

We can treat GERD with drugs or with surgery. For most patients, drugs are preferred. As a rule, surgery should be reserved for young, healthy patients who either cannot or will not take drugs chronically. With either drug therapy or surgery, treatment has three goals: relief of symptoms, promotion of healing, and prevention of complications.

For drug therapy, the principal options are proton pump inhibitors (PPIs) and histamine$_2$ receptor antagonists (H_2RAs). However, since PPIs are much better than H_2RAs at healing esophagitis and maintaining remission, PPIs are considered the clear drugs of choice. For patients with NERD, PPIs may be taken PRN. For patients with erosive GERD, PPIs should be taken continuously until symptoms resolve (typically 4 to 8 weeks). Unfortunately, when PPIs are discontinued, the relapse rate is high, occurring in 80% to 90% of patients within 6 to 12 months. Accordingly, for patients with severe GERD, long-term maintenance therapy is recommended.

Lifestyle changes can complement drug therapy—but should not be substituted for drugs. Measures that may help include smoking cessation, weight loss, avoidance of alcohol and late-night meals, and sleeping with the head elevated. Certain foods—citrus fruits, tomatoes, onions, spicy foods, and carbonated beverages—aggravate symptoms for some patients, and hence should be avoided if they do.

function. Of note, the time frame for increased risk is limited to the first few days of PPI use. After that, risk is no higher than in nonusers.

Fractures. Long-term therapy, especially in high doses, increases the risk of osteoporosis and fractures by reducing acid secretion, which may decrease absorption of calcium. However, the risk appears to be low. For example, only 1 extra hip fracture would be expected for each 1200 patients. To minimize fracture risk, treatment should use the lowest dose needed for the shortest duration possible. Also, patients should be encouraged to maintain adequate intake of calcium and vitamin D.

Rebound Acid Hypersecretion. When patients stop taking PPIs, they often experience dyspepsia brought on by rebound hypersecretion of gastric acid. Acid rebound can be minimized by using PPIs in the lowest effective dose for the shortest time needed and by tapering the dose when stopping treatment. Dyspepsia can be managed with an antacid and perhaps with an H_2RA. Acid rebound can persist for several months after the PPI is discontinued.

Hypomagnesemia. With long-term use, PPIs can lower magnesium levels, perhaps by reducing intestinal magnesium absorption. In severe cases, serum magnesium may drop below 1 mg/dL. (The normal range is 1.8 to 2.3 mg/dL.) Symptoms include tremors, muscle cramps, seizures, and dysrhythmias. The risk of hypomagnesemia is increased by other drugs that lower magnesium, especially thiazide and loop diuretics. Low magnesium can be treated with oral magnesium (e.g., SloMag, MagOx). Severe cases may require IV magnesium. If magnesium levels remain low, the patient can be switched to an H_2 blocker. Following PPI withdrawal, magnesium levels usually normalize within 2 weeks. For long-term PPI therapy, consider measuring magnesium at baseline and periodically thereafter.

Safety Alert

DIARRHEA

In retrospective, observational studies, omeprazole and other PPIs have been associated with a dose-related increase in the risk of infection with *C. difficile,* a bacterium that can cause severe diarrhea. Patients experiencing diarrhea while taking omeprazole or other PPIs should report immediately to their healthcare provider for testing.

Gastric Cancer. In theory, long-term PPI use may pose a risk of cancer. Gastric carcinoid tumors have developed in rats given omeprazole daily for 2 years. Tumor generation is related to hypersecretion of gastrin, which occurs in response to omeprazole-induced suppression of gastric acidity. Gastrin stimulates hyperplasia of gastric epithelial cells, whose growth may ultimately result in a gastric carcinoid tumor. However, despite this theoretical mechanism for cancer promotion, the U.S. Food and Drug Administration (FDA) has concluded that PPIs do not pose a cancer risk.

Drug Interactions

By elevating gastric pH, omeprazole and other PPIs can significantly reduce absorption of *atazanavir* [Reyataz], *delavirdine* [Rescriptor], and *nelfinavir* [Viracept], all used to treat HIV/AIDS. These drugs should not be combined with a PPI. Reducing gastric pH can also decrease the absorption of two antifungal drugs: *ketoconazole* and *itraconazole*.

Clopidogrel. Omeprazole and other PPIs can reduce the *adverse* effects of clopidogrel [Plavix], but may also reduce its *beneficial* effects. Clopidogrel is an antiplatelet drug used to decrease thrombotic events. Unfortunately, by suppressing platelet aggregation, the drug can promote gastric bleeding. To reduce the risk of GI bleeding, clopidogrel is often combined with a PPI. Unfortunately, in addition to protecting against GI bleeding, the PPI may reduce the beneficial effects of clopidogrel because PPIs inhibit CYP2C19, the isoenzyme of cytochrome P450 that converts clopidogrel to its active form. Hence the dilemma: If clopidogrel is used alone, there is a significant risk of GI bleeding; however, if clopidogrel is combined with a PPI, the risk of GI bleeding will be reduced, but antiplatelet effects may be reduced as well. After considering the available evidence, three organizations—the American College of Cardiology, the American Heart Association, and the American College of Gastroenterology—issued a consensus document on the problem. This document concludes that although PPIs may reduce the antiplatelet effects of clopidogrel, there is no evidence that the reduction is large enough to be clinically relevant. Accordingly, *for patients with risk factors for GI bleeding* (e.g., advanced age, use of NSAIDs or anticoagulants), the benefits of combining a PPI with clopidogrel probably outweigh any risk from reduced antiplatelet effects, and hence combining a PPI with clopidogrel is probably okay. Conversely, *for patients who lack risk factors for GI bleeding,* combined use of clopidogrel with a PPI may reduce the antiplatelet effects of clopidogrel without offering any real benefit, so combining a PPI with clopidogrel in these patients should generally be avoided.

Preparations, Dosage, and Administration

Prescription-strength omeprazole is available in three formulations: (1) delayed-release capsules (10, 20, and 40 mg) marketed as *Prilosec,* (2) a delayed-release tablet (200 mg) marketed as *Prilosec,* a delayed-release packet containing 10 mg of granules, and (3) a powder (20 and 40 mg), marketed as *Zegerid,* used to make an immediate-release oral suspension. (The powder contains *sodium bicarbonate,* which elevates gastric pH and thereby protects omeprazole from acid destruction. Each dose contains 460 mg of sodium, making the product unsuitable for people who must restrict sodium intake.) To treat active duodenal ulcer and GERD, the usual dosage is 20 mg once a day, taken before a meal, for 4 to 8 weeks. To treat Zollinger-Ellison syndrome and other hypersecretory states, doses up to 120 mg 3 times a day may be needed.

Like prescription-strength omeprazole, *over-the-counter* omeprazole is available in two formulations: (1) 20-mg delayed-release tablets, marketed as *Prilosec OTC,* and (2) a powder (20 mg omeprazole plus sodium bicarbonate), marketed as *Zegerid OTC,* used to make an immediate-release oral suspension. These products are indicated for adults with frequent heartburn (two or more episodes a week). The dosage is 20 mg once daily for 14 days, taken before the first meal of the day.

For patients who take an aspirin daily for prevention of stroke or myocardial infarction, omeprazole is available in tablets combined with aspirin (81 mg aspirin/40 mg omeprazole and 325 mg aspirin/40 mg omeprazole), sold as *Yosprala.* Yosprala is taken once daily.

Esomeprazole

Esomeprazole [Nexium] is nearly identical to omeprazole [Prilosec]. Structurally, esomeprazole is the *S*-isomer of omeprazole (which is a mixture of *S*- and *R*-isomers). The *S*-isomer (esomeprazole) is metabolized more slowly than the *R*-isomer, and hence esomeprazole achieves higher blood levels than omeprazole, and its effects last somewhat longer. Otherwise the two drugs are essentially the same. The most common adverse effects are headache and diarrhea. In addition, esomeprazole may cause nausea, flatulence, abdominal pain, and dry mouth. Elevation of gastric pH may increase the risk of pneumonia. As with omeprazole, long-term therapy may pose a risk of hypomagnesemia as well as osteoporosis and fractures. Approved indications are erosive esophagitis, GERD, and duodenal ulcers associated with *H. pylori* infection. In addition, the drug may be used for prophylaxis of NSAID-induced ulcers. For oral therapy, esomeprazole is available in two formulations: (1) delayed-release capsules (20 and 40 mg) and (2) delayed-release granules (2.5, 5, 10, 20, and 40 mg) that form a delayed-release suspension when mixed with water (1 tablespoon). To treat erosive gastritis, the usual dosage is 20 or 40 mg once daily, taken at least 1 hour before a meal, for 4 to 8 weeks. To treat GERD, the usual dosage is 20 mg once daily for 4 to 8 weeks. To treat duodenal ulcers associated with *H. pylori,* one ACG-recommended regimen consists of triple therapy—esomeprazole (20 mg twice daily), amoxicillin (1000 mg twice daily), and clarithromycin (500 mg twice daily)—administered for 14 days. The goal is to eradicate *H. pylori.* To help prevent formation of ulcers in patients with osteoarthritis and rheumatoid arthritis, esomeprazole is combined in a tablet with naproxen (375 mg naproxen/20 mg esomeprazole and 500 mg naproxen/20 mg esomeprazole), sold as *Vimovo.* The dose is 1 tablet twice daily.

For intravenous therapy, esomeprazole is supplied as a powder (20 and 40 mg) to be reconstituted with 0.9% sodium chloride for injection. Intravenous therapy is indicated only for GERD with a history of erosive gastritis. For adults, dosing is done by either injection (over 3 minutes or longer) or infusion (over 10 to 30 minutes). For children, dosing is done by infusion only. For all patients, dosing is done once a day for up to 10 days. For adults, the daily dose is 20 or 40 mg. For children age 1 month to less than 1 year, the daily dose is 0.5 mg/kg. For children age 1 year to 17 years, the daily dose is either 10 mg (for those who weigh less than 55 kg) or 20 mg (for those who weigh 55 kg or more).

Lansoprazole

Lansoprazole [Prevacid, Prevacid 24 HR] is very similar to omeprazole. Both drugs cause prolonged inhibition of H+,K+-ATPase. Hence, suppression of acid secretion is sustained. Like omeprazole, lansoprazole is well tolerated. The most common adverse effects are diarrhea, abdominal pain, and nausea. Elevation of gastric pH may increase the risk of pneumonia. Prolonged, high-dose therapy may pose a risk of hypomagnesemia, as well as osteoporosis and fracture.

Two oral formulations are available: (1) delayed-release capsules (15 and 30 mg) and (2) orally disintegrating, delayed-release tablets (15 and 30 mg). Both formulations should be taken immediately before a meal. The dosage for duodenal ulcers (prevention and treatment) and GERD is 15 mg once daily. The dosage for erosive gastritis and active gastric ulcers is 30 mg once daily. For hypersecretory states, the initial dosage is 60 mg/day; for severe cases, up to 90 mg twice daily may be needed.

Dexlansoprazole

Dexlansoprazole [Dexilant] is simply the *R*-enantiomer of lansoprazole. Although both enantiomers are active, the *R*-enantiomer has a longer duration. Like lansoprazole and all other PPIs, dexlansoprazole reduces gastric acidity by inhibiting gastric H+,K+-ATPase. To prolong effects, dexlansoprazole is formulated in dual delayed-release capsules that contain two types of pH-sensitive granules. Following ingestion, some of these granules release lansoprazole when they reach the proximal small intestine, and the remainder release lansoprazole when they reach the distal small intestine. As a result, drug levels first peak 1 to 2 hours after dosing, and then peak again 4 to 5 hours after dosing. In clinical trials, the most common adverse effects were diarrhea, abdominal pain, nausea, vomiting, flatulence, and upper respiratory infection. Long-term therapy may pose a risk of hypomagnesemia, as well as osteoporosis and fractures. Dexlansoprazole is approved for treatment and maintenance of erosive esophagitis and for treatment of symptomatic GERD (heartburn). Two strengths are available: 30 mg and 60 mg. The dosage for *treating* erosive esophagitis is 60 mg once daily for up to 8 weeks, and the dosage for *maintenance* is 30 mg once daily for up to 6 months. The usual dosage for treating symptomatic GERD is 30 mg once daily for 4 weeks. Dexlansoprazole capsules may be swallowed whole, or they may be opened and sprinkled onto 1 tablespoon of applesauce and swallowed immediately. Dosing may be done with or without food.

Rabeprazole

Rabeprazole [Aciphex, Pariet ✤] is much like omeprazole and lansoprazole in actions, uses, and adverse effects. The drug is approved for *H. pylori* eradication, duodenal ulcers, GERD, and hypersecretory states, such as Zollinger-Ellison syndrome. Like other PPIs, rabeprazole suppresses acid secretion by inhibiting H+,K+-ATPase in parietal cells. However, in contrast to omeprazole, the drug causes *reversible* inhibition of H+,K+-ATPase, and hence its effects are less durable. In addition to suppressing acid secretion, rabeprazole has antibacterial activity. As a result, it may help other antibacterial drugs eradicate *H. pylori*. The most common adverse effects are diarrhea, headache, dizziness, malaise, nausea, and rash. Elevation of gastric pH may increase the risk of pneumonia. Long-term therapy may pose a risk of hypomagnesemia, as well as osteoporosis and fractures. Although rabeprazole is metabolized by cytochrome P450 enzymes, it does not appear to influence the metabolism of other drugs. However, it *can* increase digoxin levels by 20%. Accordingly, levels of digoxin should be monitored. Rabeprazole is available in 20-mg delayed-release, enteric-coated tablets as well as 5- and 10-mg delayed-release capsules marketed as *Aciphex Sprinkle*. The dosage for GERD and duodenal ulcers is 20 mg once daily, taken with or without food. The initial dosage for hypersecretory states is 60 mg once daily; for severe cases, 60 mg twice daily may be needed. Although rabeprazole is not approved for treating gastric ulcers, 20 to 40 mg once daily has been effective.

Pantoprazole

Pantoprazole [Protonix, Pantoloc ✤] is similar to omeprazole and the other PPIs. The drug is approved for treating GERD and hypersecretory states. Like other PPIs, pantoprazole is well tolerated. Like lansoprazole, pantoprazole may be administered PO or IV. With oral therapy, the most common adverse effects are diarrhea, headache, and dizziness. With IV therapy, the most common adverse effects are diarrhea, headache, nausea, dyspepsia, and injection-site reactions, including thrombophlebitis and abscess. With both routes, elevation of gastric pH may increase the risk of pneumonia. Long-term therapy may pose a risk of hypomagnesemia, as well as osteoporosis and fractures. Pantoprazole does not affect cytochrome P450 enzymes, and hence does not affect the metabolism of other drugs. Pantoprazole is available in three formulations:

- Delayed-release tablets (20 and 40 mg)
- Enteric-coated granules (40 mg) that can be sprinkled on applesauce or mixed with 5 mL of apple juice for oral administration, or mixed with 10 mL of apple juice for administration by nasogastric tube
- Powder (40 mg/vial) to be reconstituted for IV use

Oral doses may be taken with or without food. Infusions are done over 2 to 15 minutes. The usual dosage for treatment of GERD, either PO or IV, is 40 mg/day.

OTHER ANTIULCER DRUGS

Sucralfate

Sucralfate [Carafate, Sulcrate ✤] is an effective antiulcer medication notable for minimal side effects and lack of significant drug interactions. The drug promotes ulcer healing by creating a protective barrier against acid and pepsin. Sucralfate has no acid-neutralizing capacity and does not decrease acid secretion.

Mechanism of Antiulcer Action

Sucralfate is a complex substance composed of sulfated sucrose and aluminum hydroxide. Under mildly acidic conditions (pH below 4), sucralfate undergoes polymerization and cross-linking reactions. The resultant product is a viscid and very sticky gel that adheres to the ulcer crater, creating a barrier to back-diffusion of hydrogen ions, pepsin, and bile salts. Attachment to the ulcer appears to last up to 6 hours.

Pharmacokinetics

Sucralfate is administered orally, and systemic absorption is minimal (3% to 5%). About 90% of each dose is eliminated in the feces.

Therapeutic Uses

Sucralfate is approved for acute therapy and maintenance therapy of duodenal ulcers. Rates of healing are comparable to those achieved with cimetidine. Controlled trials indicate that sucralfate can also promote the healing of gastric ulcers.

Adverse Effects

Sucralfate has no known serious adverse effects. The most significant side effect is constipation, which occurs in 2% of patients. Because sucralfate is not absorbed, systemic effects are absent.

Drug Interactions

Interactions with other drugs are minimal. By raising gastric pH above 4, antacids may interfere with sucralfate's effects. This interaction can be minimized by administering these drugs at least 30 minutes apart.

Sucralfate may impede the absorption of some drugs, including phenytoin, theophylline, digoxin, warfarin, and fluoroquinolone antibiotics (e.g., ciprofloxacin, norfloxacin). These interactions can be minimized by administering sucralfate at least 2 hours apart from these other drugs.

Preparations, Dosage, and Administration

Sucralfate [Carafate] is available in 1-gm tablets and a suspension (1 gm/10 mL) for oral dosing. Administer on an empty stomach. The recommended adult dosage is 1 gm 4 times a day, taken 1 hour before meals and at bedtime. However, a dosing schedule of 2 gm twice a day appears equally effective. Treatment should continue for 4 to 8 weeks. Sucralfate tablets are large and difficult to swallow, but can be broken or dissolved in water before ingestion. The oral suspension is much easier to ingest.

Misoprostol

Therapeutic Use

Misoprostol [Cytotec] is an analog of prostaglandin E_1. In the United States, the drug's only approved GI indication is prevention of gastric ulcers caused by long-term therapy with NSAIDs. In other countries, misoprostol is also used to treat peptic ulcers unrelated to NSAIDs. In addition to its use in PUD, misoprostol is used to promote cervical ripening (see Chapter 64) and, in combination with mifepristone (RU 486), to induce medical termination of pregnancy (see Chapter 62).

Mechanism of Action

In normal individuals, prostaglandins help protect the stomach by suppressing secretion of gastric acid, promoting secretion of bicarbonate and cytoprotective mucus, and maintaining submucosal blood flow (by promoting vasodilation). As discussed in Chapter 71, aspirin and other NSAIDs cause gastric ulcers in part by inhibiting prostaglandin biosynthesis. Misoprostol prevents NSAID-induced ulcers by serving as a replacement for endogenous prostaglandins.

Adverse Effects

The most common reactions are dose-related diarrhea (13% to 40%) and abdominal pain (7% to 20%). Some women experience spotting and dysmenorrhea.

PATIENT-CENTERED CARE ACROSS THE LIFE SPAN

Peptic Ulcer Disease

Life Stage	Patient Care Concerns
Infants	Both PPIs and H_2 receptor antagonists are used safely in infants as young as 1 month old to treat GERD and duodenal ulcers.
Children/ adolescents	PPIs and H_2 receptor antagonists can be used safely in children, just in smaller doses. Side effect profiles are similar to those of adults.
Pregnant women	Misoprostol is classified in FDA Pregnancy Risk Category X.[a] This drug must be avoided at all costs. Some PPIs (esomeprazole) and H_2 receptor antagonists (ranitidine) are safe for use in pregnancy.
Breast-feeding women	The use of drugs such as omeprazole, esomeprazole, and ranitidine is not predicted to cause any adverse effects in breast-fed infants.
Older adults	PPIs are associated with an increase in the risk of fractures from osteoporosis. PPIs can also cause medication interactions and vitamin or mineral deficiencies. There should be a clear indication for prescribing these medications in this older population.

[a]As of 2020, the FDA will no longer use Pregnancy Risk Categories. Please refer to Chapter 9 for more information.

Safety Alert

MISOPROSTOL IN PREGNANCY

Misoprostol is contraindicated during pregnancy. The drug is classified in FDA Pregnancy Risk Category X[a]: the risk of use by pregnant women clearly outweighs any possible benefits. Because prostaglandins stimulate uterine contractions, the use of misoprostol during pregnancy has caused partial or complete expulsion of the developing fetus.

[a]As of 2020, the FDA will no longer use Pregnancy Risk Categories. Please refer to Chapter 9 for more information.

Misoprostol is classified in FDA Pregnancy Risk Category X.[a] If women of childbearing age are to use misoprostol, they must (1) be able to comply with birth control measures, (2) be given oral and written warnings about the dangers of misoprostol, (3) have a negative serum pregnancy test result within 2 weeks before beginning therapy, and (4) begin therapy only on the second or third day of the next normal menstrual cycle.

Preparations, Dosage, and Administration

Misoprostol [Cytotec] is supplied in 100- and 200-mcg tablets for oral administration. The usual dosage is 200 mcg 4 times a day administered with meals and at bedtime. Patients who cannot tolerate this dosage may try 100 mcg 4 times a day.

[a]As of 2020, the FDA will no longer use Pregnancy Risk Categories. Please refer to Chapter 9 for more information.

Antacids

Antacids are alkaline compounds that neutralize stomach acid. Their principal indications are PUD and GERD.

Beneficial Actions

Antacids react with gastric acid to produce neutral salts or salts of low acidity. By neutralizing acid, these drugs decrease destruction of the gut wall. In addition, if treatment raises gastric pH above 5, these drugs will reduce pepsin activity as well. Antacids may also enhance mucosal protection by stimulating production of prostaglandins. These drugs do not coat the ulcer crater to protect it from acid and pepsin. With the exception of sodium bicarbonate, antacids are poorly absorbed and therefore do not alter systemic pH.

Therapeutic Uses

Peptic Ulcer Disease. The primary indication for antacids is PUD. Rates of healing are equivalent to those achieved with H_2RAs. In the past, antacids were the mainstay of antiulcer therapy. However, these drugs have been largely replaced by newer options (H_2RAs, PPIs, sucralfate) that are equally effective and more convenient to administer and that cause fewer side effects.

Other Uses. Antacids can provide prophylaxis against stress-induced ulcers. For patients with GERD, antacids can produce symptomatic relief, but they do not accelerate healing. Although antacids are used widely by the public to relieve functional symptoms (dyspepsia, heartburn, acid indigestion), there are no controlled studies that demonstrate efficacy in these conditions.

Potency, Dosage, and Formulations

Potency. Antacid potency is expressed as acid-neutralizing capacity (ANC). ANC is defined as the number of milliequivalents of hydrochloric acid that can be neutralized by a given weight or volume of antacid. Individual antacids differ widely in ANC. The ANCs of commonly used proprietary preparations are shown in Table 78.3.

Dosage. The objective of peptic ulcer therapy is to promote healing, and not simply to relieve pain. Consequently, antacids should be taken on a regular schedule, not just in response to discomfort. In the usual dosing schedule, antacids are administered 7 times a day: 1 and 3 hours after each meal and at bedtime.

Dosage recommendations should be based on ANC and not on weight or volume of antacid. The ANC of a single dose usually ranges from 20 to 80 mEq. Single doses for gastric ulcers are relatively low (20 to 40 mEq), whereas single doses for duodenal ulcers are higher (40 to 80 mEq). Frequent dosing with even larger amounts (120 mEq) may be required if ulceration is especially severe.

To provide maximum benefits, treatment should elevate gastric pH above 5. At this pH there is inhibition of pepsin activity in addition to nearly complete (greater than 99.9%) neutralization of acid.

Antacids are inconvenient and unpleasant to ingest, making adherence difficult—especially in the absence of pain. Patients should be encouraged to take their medication as prescribed, even after symptoms are gone.

Formulations. Antacids are available in tablet and liquid formulations. Antacid tablets should be chewed thoroughly and followed with a glass of water or milk. Liquid preparations should be shaken before dispensing. As a rule, liquids (suspensions) are more effective than tablets.

Adverse Effects

Constipation and Diarrhea. Most antacids affect the bowel. Some (e.g., aluminum hydroxide) promote constipation, whereas others (e.g., magnesium hydroxide) promote diarrhea. Effects on the bowel can be minimized by combining an antacid that promotes constipation with one that promotes diarrhea. Patients should be taught to adjust the dosage of one agent or the other to normalize bowel function.

Sodium Loading. Some antacid preparations contain substantial amounts of sodium (see Table 78.3). Because sodium excess can exacerbate hypertension and heart failure, patients with these disorders should avoid preparations that have high sodium content.

TABLE 78.3 ▪ Composition and Acid-Neutralizing Capacity of Commonly Used Over-the-Counter Antacid Suspensions

Product	Acid Neutralizing Capacity (mEq/5 mL)	Active Ingredients (mg/5 mL)				Sodium (mg/5 mL)
		$Al(OH)_3$	$Mg(OH)_2$	Simethicone	Magaldrate	
AlternaGEL	16	600				<2.5
Aludrox Suspension	12	307	103			2.3
Maalox Regular Strength	13	200	200			1.4
Milk of Magnesia	14		400			0.1
Mylanta Maximum Liquid	25	400	400	40		1.1
Riopan Plus Suspension	15			20	540	<0.1
Riopan Plus DS Suspension	30			40	1080	0.3

DS, Double strength.

TABLE 78.4 ▪ Classification of Antacids

ALUMINUM COMPOUNDS
Aluminum hydroxide
MAGNESIUM COMPOUNDS
Magnesium hydroxide (milk of magnesia)
Magnesium oxide
CALCIUM COMPOUNDS
Calcium carbonate
SODIUM COMPOUNDS
Sodium bicarbonate
OTHER
Magaldrate (a complex of magnesium and aluminum compounds)

Drug Interactions

By raising gastric pH, antacids can influence the dissolution and absorption of many other drugs, including *cimetidine* and *ranitidine.* These interactions can be minimized by allowing 1 hour between taking antacids and these other drugs.

Antacids can interfere with the actions of sucralfate. To minimize this interaction, administer these drugs at least 1 hour apart.

If absorbed in substantial amounts, antacids can alkalinize the urine. Elevation of urinary pH can accelerate excretion of acidic drugs and delay excretion of basic drugs.

Antacid Families

There are four major groups of antacids: (1) aluminum compounds, (2) magnesium compounds, (3) calcium compounds, and (4) sodium compounds. Individual agents that belong to each group are shown in Table 78.4. Representative members of these groups are discussed next.

Representative Antacids

Antacids differ from one another with respect to ANC, onset and duration of action, effects on the bowel, systemic effects, and special applications. In this section, we discuss the two most commonly used antacids, magnesium hydroxide and aluminum hydroxide, and two less commonly used drugs—calcium carbonate and sodium bicarbonate. The distinguishing properties of these agents are shown in Table 78.5.

Magnesium Hydroxide. This antacid is rapid-acting, has high ANC, and produces long-lasting effects. These properties make magnesium hydroxide an antacid of choice. The liquid formulation of magnesium hydroxide is often referred to as milk of magnesia.

The most prominent adverse effect is diarrhea, which results from retention of water in the intestinal lumen. To compensate for this effect, magnesium hydroxide is usually administered in combination with aluminum hydroxide, an antacid that promotes constipation. However, if the dose of magnesium hydroxide is sufficiently high, no amount of aluminum hydroxide will prevent diarrhea. Since stimulation of the bowel can be hazardous for patients with intestinal obstruction or appendicitis, magnesium hydroxide should be avoided in those with undiagnosed abdominal pain. Because of its effect on the bowel, magnesium hydroxide is frequently employed as a laxative (see Chapter 79). In patients with renal impairment, magnesium may accumulate to high levels, causing signs of toxicity (e.g., CNS depression).

Aluminum Hydroxide. This drug has relatively low ANC and is slow-acting, but produces effects of long duration. Although rarely used alone, this compound is widely used in combination with magnesium hydroxide (see Table 78.3). Aluminum hydroxide preparations contain significant amounts of sodium; appropriate caution should be exercised. The most common adverse effect is constipation.

Aluminum hydroxide adsorbs a variety of compounds. Binding of certain drugs (e.g., tetracyclines, warfarin, digoxin) may reduce their effects. Aluminum hydroxide has a high affinity for phosphate. By binding with phosphate, the drug can reduce phosphate absorption and can thereby cause hypophosphatemia. Aluminum hydroxide can also bind to pepsin, which may facilitate ulcer healing.

Calcium Carbonate. Calcium carbonate, like magnesium hydroxide, is rapid-acting, has high ANC, and produces effects of long duration. Because of these properties, calcium carbonate was once considered the ideal antacid. However, because of concerns about acid rebound (stimulation of acid secretion), the use of calcium carbonate has declined. The principal adverse effect is constipation, which can be overcome by combining calcium carbonate with a magnesium-containing antacid (e.g., magnesium hydroxide). Calcium carbonate releases carbon dioxide in the stomach and can thereby cause eructation (belching) and flatulence. Rarely, systemic absorption is sufficient to produce the milk-alkali syndrome, a condition characterized by hypercalcemia, metabolic alkalosis, soft tissue calcification, and impaired renal function. The palatability of calcium carbonate is low and can detract from adherence.

Sodium Bicarbonate. Although capable of neutralizing gastric acid, sodium bicarbonate is unfit for treating ulcers. This agent has a rapid onset but effects are short-lasting. Like calcium carbonate, sodium bicarbonate liberates carbon dioxide, thereby increasing intra-abdominal pressure and promoting eructation and flatulence. Absorption of sodium can exacerbate hypertension and heart failure. In patients with renal impairment, sodium bicarbonate can cause systemic alkalosis. (Other antacids rarely alter systemic pH.) Because of its brief duration, high sodium content, and ability to cause alkalosis, sodium bicarbonate is inappropriate for treating PUD. The drug is useful, however, for treating acidosis and elevating urinary pH to promote excretion of acidic drugs following overdose.

Combination Packs

Three combination packs—Omeclamox-Pak, Pylera, and Prevpac—are available for treating *H. pylori*–associated ulcers. The purpose of these packs is to simplify the purchase and administration of drugs for triple and quadruple therapy of PUD.

Omeclamox-Pak

The Omeclamox-Pak contains omeprazole tablets (20 mg), clarithromycin tablets (500 mg), and amoxicillin tablets (500 mg). One dose consists of 1 omeprazole tablet, 1 clarithromycin tablet, and 2 amoxicillin tablets. Patients take two doses a day.

TABLE 78.5 ▪ Representative Antacids: Distinguishing Properties

Antacid	Effect on the Bowel: Constipation	Effect on the Bowel: Diarrhea	Effect on Systemic pH	Comments
Aluminum hydroxide	Yes	No	None	Can cause hypophosphatemia; can treat hyperphosphatemia
Magnesium hydroxide	No	Yes	None	Can cause magnesium toxicity (CNS depression) in patients with renal impairment
Calcium carbonate	Yes	No	None	May cause acid rebound or milk-alkali syndrome; releases CO_2
Sodium bicarbonate	No	No	Increase	Not used routinely for ulcers; used to treat acidosis and to alkalinize urine; high risk of sodium loading; releases CO_2

Pylera

The Pylera pack consists of capsules that contain three drugs each: bismuth subcitrate potassium (140 mg), metronidazole (125 mg), and tetracycline (125 mg). One dose consists of 3 capsules. Patients take four such doses a day, along with omeprazole.

Prevpac

The Prevpac pack contains lansoprazole [Prevacid] capsules (30 mg), amoxicillin capsules (500 mg), and clarithromycin tablets (500 mg). One dose consists of 1 lansoprazole capsule, 2 amoxicillin capsules, and 1 clarithromycin tablet. Patients take two of these doses a day.

KEY POINTS

- The term *peptic ulcer disease* (PUD) refers to a group of upper GI disorders characterized by varying degrees of erosion of the gut wall.
- PUD develops when aggressive factors (*H. pylori,* NSAIDs, acid, pepsin) outweigh defensive factors (mucus, bicarbonate, submucosal blood flow, prostaglandins).
- Gastric acid is an absolute requirement for ulcer formation. In the absence of acid, no ulcer will form.
- The most common cause of PUD is infection with *H. pylori.* The next most common cause is the use of NSAIDs.
- The goal of PUD therapy is to alleviate symptoms, promote healing, prevent complications (hemorrhage, perforation, obstruction), and prevent recurrence.
- The major drugs used to treat PUD are antibiotics and antisecretory agents (H_2RAs, PPIs).
- With the exception of antibiotics, antiulcer drugs do not alter the disease process; rather, they simply create conditions conducive to healing. Because nonantibiotic therapies do not cure ulcers, the relapse rate with them alone is high. In contrast, the relapse rate following successful antibiotic therapy is low.
- All patients with gastric or duodenal ulcers and confirmed infection with *H. pylori* should be treated with antibiotics in combination with an antisecretory agent.
- The antibiotics employed most often are clarithromycin, amoxicillin, bismuth, tetracycline, and metronidazole.
- To avoid resistance and increase efficacy, at least two antibiotics should be used.
- Cimetidine and other H_2RAs suppress secretion of gastric acid by blocking histamine$_2$ receptors on parietal cells of the stomach.
- Cimetidine inhibits hepatic drug-metabolizing enzymes and can thereby cause levels of other drugs to rise.
- In contrast to cimetidine, ranitidine has little effect on drug metabolism.
- Proton pump inhibitors (e.g., omeprazole, lansoprazole) suppress acid secretion by inhibiting gastric H^+,K^+-ATPase, the enzyme that makes gastric acid.
- PPIs are the most effective inhibitors of acid secretion.
- Although generally safe, PPIs can increase the risk of fractures, pneumonia, and hypomagnesemia and can cause acid rebound when treatment stops.
- Sucralfate promotes ulcer healing by creating a protective barrier against acid and pepsin.
- Misoprostol, an analog of prostaglandin E_1, is used to prevent gastric ulcers caused by NSAIDs.
- Misoprostol stimulates uterine contraction and hence is contraindicated during pregnancy.

Please visit **http://evolve.elsevier.com/Lehne** for chapter-specific NCLEX® examination review questions.

Summary of Major Nursing Implications[a]

H_2 RECEPTOR ANTAGONISTS

Cimetidine
Famotidine
Nizatidine
Ranitidine

Preadministration Assessment

Therapeutic Goal

H_2RAs are used primarily to treat PUD. The objective is to relieve pain, promote healing, prevent ulcer recurrence, and prevent complications.

Baseline Data

Definitive diagnosis of PUD requires radiographic or endoscopic visualization of the ulcer and testing for *H. pylori* infection, either by a noninvasive method (urea breath test, stool antigen test, or serologic antibody test) or by an invasive method involving evaluation of a biopsy sample by either (1) staining and viewing under a microscope to see if *H. pylori* is present, (2) assaying for the presence of urease, or (3) culturing and then assaying for the presence of *H. pylori.*

Identifying High-Risk Patients

Use H_2RAs with *caution* in patients with renal or hepatic dysfunction.

Implementation: Administration

Routes

Cimetidine. Oral only.
Ranitidine. Oral, IM, and IV.
Famotidine. Oral and IV.
Nizatidine. Oral only.

Administration

Oral. **Inform patients that H_2RAs may be taken without regard to meals.**

With all H_2RAs, dosing may be done twice daily or once daily at bedtime. With ranitidine, dosing may also be done 4 times a day (with meals and at bedtime). **Make sure the patient knows which dosing schedule has been prescribed.**

Intramuscular: Ranitidine. Use concentrated solutions for IM injections.

Intravenous: Cimetidine, Famotidine, and Ranitidine. For IV injection, dilute in a small volume (e.g., 20 mL) of 0.9% sodium chloride and inject slowly (over 5 or more minutes). For IV infusion, dilute in a large volume (100 mL) of 0.9% sodium chloride and infuse over 15 to 20 minutes.

Implementation: Measures to Enhance Therapeutic Effects

Advise patients to avoid cigarettes and ulcerogenic over-the-counter drugs (aspirin and other NSAIDs). Advise patients to stop drinking alcohol if drinking exacerbates their ulcer symptoms. Inform patients that five or six small meals per day may be preferable to three larger meals.

Ongoing Evaluation and Interventions

Evaluating Therapeutic Effects

Ulcer Healing. Monitor for relief of pain. Radiologic or endoscopic examination of the ulcer site may also be employed. Monitor gastric pH; treatment should increase pH to 5 or above. **Educate patients about signs of GI bleeding (e.g., black, tarry stools; "coffee-grounds" vomitus), and instruct them to notify the prescriber if these occur.**

Helicobacter pylori. If *H. pylori* was present at the onset of treatment, it may be useful to determine if the infection was eradicated.

Minimizing Adverse Effects

Antiandrogenic Effects. **Inform patients that *cimetidine* can cause gynecomastia, reduced libido, and erectile dysfunction and that these effects reverse after drug withdrawal.**

CNS Effects. *Cimetidine* can cause confusion, hallucinations, lethargy, somnolence, restlessness, and seizures. These responses are most likely in older adults who have renal or hepatic impairment. **Inform patients about possible CNS effects and instruct them to notify the prescriber if they occur.** CNS effects are less likely with ranitidine, famotidine, and nizatidine.

Pneumonia. Elevation of gastric pH increases the risk of pneumonia. **Inform patients about signs of respiratory infection and instruct them to inform the prescriber if they occur.**

Minimizing Adverse Interactions

Interactions Secondary to Inhibition of Drug Metabolism. Cimetidine inhibits hepatic drug-metabolizing enzymes and can thereby increase levels of other drugs. Drugs of particular concern are *warfarin, phenytoin, theophylline,* and *lidocaine.* Dosages of these drugs may require reduction.

Ranitidine inhibits drug metabolism, but to a lesser degree than cimetidine. Famotidine and nizatidine do not inhibit drug metabolism.

Antacids. Antacids can decrease absorption of *cimetidine* and *ranitidine.* At least 1 hour should separate administration of antacids and these drugs.

PROTON PUMP INHIBITORS

Dexlansoprazole
Esomeprazole
Lansoprazole
Omeprazole
Pantoprazole
Rabeprazole

Preadministration Assessment

Therapeutic Goal

PPIs are used primarily to treat PUD. The objective is to relieve pain, promote healing, prevent ulcer recurrence, and prevent complications.

Summary of Major Nursing Implications[a]—cont'd

Baseline Data

Consider obtaining a baseline value for magnesium when long-term PPI therapy is planned. For other nursing implications, see *Baseline Data* for *H_2 Receptor Antagonists*.

Identifying High-Risk Patients

PPIs are very safe when used short term. Their only *contraindication* is hypersensitivity to the drug itself or to a component of the formulation.

Implementation: Administration

Routes

Dexlansoprazole, Esomeprazole, Omeprazole, Lansoprazole, and Rabeprazole. Oral only.

Pantoprazole. Oral and IV.

Administration

Oral. **Inform patients that capsules and tablets should be swallowed intact—not opened, split, crushed, or chewed.**

Instruct patients to take esomeprazole at least 1 hour before a meal and to take omeprazole or lansoprazole just before eating. Inform patients that dexlansoprazole, pantoprazole, and rabeprazole may be taken without regard to food.

Implementation: Measures to Enhance Therapeutic Effects

See Nursing Implications for *H_2 Receptor Antagonists*.

Ongoing Evaluation and Interventions

Evaluating Therapeutic Effects

See Nursing Implications for *H_2 Receptor Antagonists*.

Minimizing Adverse Effects

In General. When PPIs are used short term for appropriate patients, the benefits of treatment generally outweigh the risks. Conversely, when PPIs are used long term or for inappropriate patients, the risks clearly outweigh any benefits.

Pneumonia. During the first few days of treatment, PPIs may increase the risk of community-acquired and hospital-acquired pneumonia. **Inform patients about signs of respiratory infection and instruct them to inform the prescriber if they occur.**

Fractures. Long-term, high-dose therapy may increase the risk of osteoporosis and fractures. To minimize fracture risk, use the lowest dose needed for the shortest time possible. **Encourage patients to maintain adequate intake of calcium and vitamin D.**

Rebound Acid Hypersecretion. Discontinuing a PPI may trigger acid rebound and associated dyspepsia. **Advise patients that acid rebound can be minimized by using the lowest dose needed for the shortest time possible, and by tapering the PPI dose when stopping treatment. Inform patients about the risk of acid rebound, and advise them to manage symptoms with an antacid and perhaps an H_2RA.**

Hypomagnesemia. Long-term use can lower magnesium levels. Risk is increased by other drugs that lower magnesium, especially thiazide and loop diuretics. **Inform patients about symptoms of hypomagnesemia (e.g., tremors, muscle cramps, seizures, dysrhythmias), and have them inform the prescriber if they develop.** Magnesium levels can be raised with oral or IV magnesium. If these measures fail, magnesium can be raised by switching to an H_2 blocker; magnesium typically normalizes within 2 weeks. For long-term PPI therapy, consider measuring magnesium at baseline and periodically thereafter.

Minimizing Adverse Interactions

Atazanavir, Delavirdine, and Nelfinavir. By elevating gastric pH, PPIs significantly reduce the absorption of these drugs, which are used to treat HIV/AIDS. Therefore, concurrent use of PPIs and these drugs should be avoided.

Clopidogrel. PPIs can protect against clopidogrel-induced GI bleeding, but may also reduce the antiplatelet effects of clopidogrel. In patients with risk factors for GI bleeding (e.g., advanced age, use of NSAIDs or glucocorticoids) the benefits of combining a PPI with clopidogrel outweigh any risk from a possible reduction in antiplatelet effects, and hence use of the combination makes sense. Conversely, in patients who lack risk factors for GI bleeding, the combination of clopidogrel with a PPI should generally be avoided.

[a]Patient education information is highlighted as **blue text.**

CHAPTER

79 Laxatives

Laxatives are used to ease or stimulate defecation. These agents can soften the stool, increase stool volume, hasten fecal passage through the intestine, and facilitate evacuation from the rectum. When properly employed, laxatives are valuable medications. However, these agents are also subject to abuse. Misuse of laxatives is largely the result of misconceptions about what constitutes normal bowel function.

Before we talk about laxatives, we need to distinguish between two terms: *laxative effect* and *catharsis*. The term *laxative effect* refers to production of a soft, formed stool over a period of 1 or more days. In contrast, the term *catharsis* refers to a prompt fluid evacuation of the bowel. Hence, a laxative effect is slower and relatively mild, whereas catharsis is relatively fast and intense.

GENERAL CONSIDERATIONS

Function of the Colon

The principal function of the colon is to absorb water and electrolytes. Absorption of nutrients is minimal. Normally, about 1500 mL of fluid enters the colon each day, and approximately 90% gets absorbed. When the colon is working correctly, the extent of fluid absorption is such that the resulting stool is soft (but formed) and capable of elimination without strain. However, when fluid absorption is excessive, as can happen when transport through the intestine is delayed, the resultant stool is dehydrated and hard. Conversely, if insufficient fluid is absorbed, watery stools result.

Frequency of bowel evacuation varies widely among individuals. For some people, bowel movements occur 2 or 3 times a day. For others, elimination may occur only 2 times a week. Because of this wide individual variation, we can't define a normal frequency for bowel movements. Put another way, although a daily bowel movement may be normal for many people, it may be abnormal for many others.

Dietary Fiber

Proper function of the bowel is highly dependent on dietary fiber—the component of vegetable matter that escapes digestion in the stomach and small intestine. Fiber facilitates colonic function in two ways. First, fiber absorbs water, thereby softening the feces and increasing their mass. Second, fiber can be digested by colonic bacteria, whose subsequent growth increases fecal mass. The best source of fiber is bran. Fiber can also be obtained from fruits and vegetables. Ingestion of 20 to 60 gm of fiber a day should optimize intestinal function.

Constipation

Constipation is one of the most common GI disorders. In the United States, people seek medical help for constipation at least 2.5 million times a year and spend hundreds of millions of dollars on laxatives.

Constipation is defined in terms of symptoms, which include hard stools, infrequent stools, excessive straining, prolonged effort, a sense of incomplete evacuation, and unsuccessful defecation. Scientists who do research on constipation usually define it using the Rome IV criteria (Table 79.1). Constipation is determined more by stool *consistency* (degree of hardness) than by *how often* bowel movements occur. Hence, if the interval between bowel movements becomes prolonged, but the stool remains soft and hydrated, a diagnosis of constipation would be improper. Conversely, if bowel movements occur with regularity, but the feces are hard and dry, constipation can be diagnosed—despite the regular and frequent passage of stool.

A common cause of constipation is poor diet—specifically, a diet deficient in fiber and fluid. Other causes include dysfunction of the pelvic floor and anal sphincter, slow intestinal transit, and the use of certain drugs (e.g., opioids, anticholinergics, some antacids).

In most cases, constipation can be readily corrected. Stools will become softer and more easily passed within days of increasing fiber and fluid in the diet. Mild exercise, especially after meals, also helps improve bowel function. If necessary, a laxative may be employed—but only briefly and only as an adjunct to improved diet and exercise.

TABLE 79.1 ▪ Rome IV Criteria for Constipation

ADULTS

Two or more of the following for the last 3 months with symptom onset at least 6 months before diagnosis:

- Straining during at least 25% of bowel movements
- Lumpy or hard stools in at least 25% of bowel movements
- Sensation of incomplete evacuation for at least 25% of bowel movements
- Sensation of anorectal blockage for at least 25% of bowel movements
- Manual maneuvers (e.g., digital evacuation; support of the pelvic floor) to facilitate at least 25% of bowel movements
- Fewer than three bowel movements per week
- Loose stools rarely present without the use of laxatives, and insufficient criteria to permit diagnosis of irritable bowel syndrome

INFANTS AND CHILDREN

Must include 1 month of at least two of the following in infants and children up to age 4 years:

- Two or fewer defecations per week
- History of excessive stool retention
- History of painful or hard bowel movements
- History of large-diameter stools that may obstruct the toilet
- At least one episode per week of incontinence after the acquisition of toileting skills

PATIENT-CENTERED CARE ACROSS THE LIFE SPAN

Laxatives

Life Stage	Patient Care Concerns
Infants	Docusate, lactulose, and glycerin suppositories have been used to treat constipation safely in infants.
Children/adolescents	Milk of magnesia, mineral oil, senna, docusate, and bisacodyl can be used to treat constipation in children and adolescents.
Pregnant women	Laxatives should be used cautiously in pregnancy, as GI stimulation can induce labor.
Breast-feeding women	Senna is safe for use in breast-feeding. Data are lacking regarding the use of PEG and Dulcolax; caution is advised.
Older adults	All laxatives discussed in this chapter can be used in the older adult population. Monitor closely for dehydration in the older adult.

Indications for Laxative Use

Laxatives can be highly beneficial when employed for valid indications. By softening the stool, laxatives can reduce the painful elimination that can be associated with episiotomy and with hemorrhoids and other anorectal lesions. In patients with cardiovascular diseases (e.g., aneurysm, myocardial infarction, disease of the cerebral or cardiac vasculature), softening the stool decreases the amount of strain needed to defecate, avoiding dangerous elevation of blood pressure. In older adult patients, laxatives can help compensate for loss of tone in abdominal and perineal muscles. As an adjunct to anthelmintic therapy, laxatives can be used for (1) obtaining a fresh stool sample for diagnosis; (2) emptying the bowel before treatment (so as to increase parasitic exposure to anthelmintic medication); and (3) facilitating export of dead parasites following anthelmintic use. Additional applications include (1) emptying of the bowel before surgery and diagnostic procedures (e.g., radiologic examination, colonoscopy); (2) modifying the effluent from an ileostomy or colostomy; (3) preventing fecal impaction in bedridden patients; (4) removing ingested poisons; and (5) correcting constipation associated with pregnancy and certain drugs, especially opioid analgesics.

Precautions and Contraindications to Laxative Use

Laxatives are contraindicated for individuals with certain disorders of the bowel. Specifically, laxatives must be avoided by individuals experiencing abdominal pain, nausea, cramps, or other symptoms of appendicitis, regional enteritis, diverticulitis, and ulcerative colitis. Laxatives are also contraindicated for patients with acute surgical abdomen. In addition, laxatives should not be used in patients with fecal impaction or obstruction of the bowel, because increased peristalsis could cause bowel perforation. Lastly, laxatives should not be employed habitually to manage constipation. Reasons for this are discussed under *Laxative Abuse.*

Laxatives should be used with caution during pregnancy (because GI stimulation might induce labor) and during lactation (because the laxative may be excreted in breast milk).

Laxative Classification Schemes

Traditionally, laxatives have been classified according to general *mechanism of action.* This scheme has four major categories: (1) bulk-forming laxatives, (2) surfactant laxatives, (3) stimulant laxatives, and (4) osmotic laxatives. Representative drugs are shown in Table 79.2.

From a clinical perspective, it can be useful to classify laxatives according to *therapeutic effect* (time of onset and impact on stool consistency). When these properties are considered, most laxatives fall into one of three groups, labeled I, II, and III in this chapter. Group I agents act rapidly (within 2 to 6 hours) and give a watery consistency to the stool. Laxatives in group I are especially useful when preparing the bowel for diagnostic procedures or surgery. Group II agents have an intermediate latency (6 to 12 hours) and produce a stool that is semifluid. Group II agents are the ones most frequently abused by the public. Group III laxatives act slowly (in 1 to 3 days) to produce a soft but formed stool. Uses for this group include the treatment of chronic constipation and the prevention of straining at stool. Representative members of groups I, II, and III are shown in Table 79.3.

BASIC PHARMACOLOGY OF LAXATIVES

Bulk-Forming Laxatives

The bulk-forming laxatives (e.g., methylcellulose, psyllium, polycarbophil) have actions and effects much like those of dietary fiber. These agents consist of natural or semisynthetic

TABLE 79.2 ▪ Classification of Laxatives by Pharmacologic Category

Class and Agent	Site of Action	Mechanism of Action
BULK-FORMING LAXATIVES		
Methylcellulose Psyllium Polycarbophil	Small intestine and colon	Absorb water, thereby softening and enlarging the fecal mass; fecal swelling promotes peristalsis
SURFACTANT LAXATIVES		
Docusate sodium Docusate calcium	Small intestine and colon	Surfactant action softens stool by facilitating penetration of water; also cause secretion of water and electrolytes into intestine
STIMULANT LAXATIVES		
Bisacodyl Senna Castor oil	Colon Colon Small intestine	(1) Stimulate peristalsis and (2) soften feces by increasing secretion of water and electrolytes into the intestine and decreasing water and electrolyte absorption
OSMOTIC LAXATIVES		
Magnesium hydroxide Magnesium sulfate Magnesium citrate Sodium phosphate Polyethylene glycol Lactulose	Small intestine and colon	Osmotic action retains water and thereby softens the feces; fecal swelling promotes peristalsis
MISCELLANEOUS LAXATIVES		
Lubiprostone	Small intestine and colon	Opens chloride channels in the intestinal epithelium and thereby increases intestinal motility and secretion of fluid into the lumen
Plecanatide	Small intestine and colon	Assists in the regulation of intestinal fluid secretion and motility by indirectly increasing chloride and bicarbonate in the lumen
Mineral oil	Colon	Lubricates and reduces water absorption
Glycerin suppository	Colon	Lubricates and causes reflex rectal contraction
Polyethylene glycol–electrolyte solution	Small intestine and colon	Similar to osmotic laxatives
Sodium picosulfate/magnesium oxide/ anhydrous citric acid	Colon	Stimulates colonic peristalsis and draws water into the GI tract

TABLE 79.3 ▪ Classification of Laxatives by Therapeutic Response

Group I: Produce Watery Stool in 2–6 hr	Group II: Produce Semifluid Stool in 6–12 hr	Group III: Produce Soft Stool in 1–3 Days
OSMOTIC LAXATIVES (IN HIGH DOSES) Magnesium salts Sodium salts Polyethylene glycol	**OSMOTIC LAXATIVES (IN LOW DOSES)** Magnesium salts Sodium salts Polyethylene glycol	**BULK-FORMING LAXATIVES** Methylcellulose Psyllium Polycarbophil
OTHERS Castor oil Polyethylene glycol–electrolyte solution	**STIMULANT LAXATIVES (EXCEPT CASTOR OIL)** Bisacodyl, oral[a] Senna	**SURFACTANT LAXATIVES** Docusate sodium Docusate calcium **OTHERS** Lactulose Lubiprostone Plecanatide

[a]Bisacodyl *suppositories* act in 15 minutes.

polysaccharides and celluloses derived from grains and other plant material. The bulk-forming agents belong to our therapeutic group III, producing a soft, formed stool after 1 to 3 days of use.

Mechanism of Action

Bulk-forming agents have the same impact on bowel function as dietary fiber. Following ingestion, these agents, which are nondigestible and nonabsorbable, swell in water to form a viscous solution or gel, thereby softening the fecal mass and increasing its bulk. Fecal volume may be further enlarged by growth of colonic bacteria, which can utilize these materials as nutrients. Transit through the intestine is hastened because swelling of the fecal mass stretches the intestinal wall and thereby stimulates peristalsis.

Indications

Bulk-forming laxatives are preferred agents for temporary treatment of constipation. Also, they are widely used in patients with diverticulosis and irritable bowel syndrome. In addition, by altering fecal consistency, they can provide symptomatic relief of diarrhea and can reduce discomfort and inconvenience for patients with an ileostomy or colostomy.

Adverse Effects

Untoward effects are minimal. Because the bulk-forming agents are not absorbed, systemic reactions are rare. *Esophageal obstruction* can occur if they are swallowed in the absence of sufficient fluid. Accordingly, bulk-forming laxatives should be administered with a full glass of water or juice. If their passage through the intestine is impeded, they may produce *intestinal obstruction* or *impaction.* Accordingly, they should be avoided if there is narrowing of the intestinal lumen.

Preparations, Dosage, and Administration

Psyllium (prepared from *Plantago* seed), *methylcellulose,* and *polycarbophil* are the principal bulk-forming laxatives. All three preparations should be administered with a full glass of water or juice. Dosages and brand names are shown in Table 79.4.

Surfactant Laxatives

Actions

The surfactants (e.g., docusate sodium) are group III laxatives: They produce a soft stool several days after the onset of treatment. Surfactants alter stool consistency by lowering surface tension, which facilitates the penetration of water into the feces. The surfactants may also act on the intestinal wall to (1) inhibit fluid absorption and (2) stimulate secretion of water and electrolytes into the intestinal lumen. In this respect, surfactants resemble the stimulant laxatives (see later).

Preparations, Dosage, and Administration

The surfactant family consists of two *docusate salts:* docusate sodium and docusate calcium. The dosage for docusate sodium [Colace], the prototype surfactant, is shown in Table 79.4. Administration should be accompanied by a full glass of water.

TABLE 79.4 ▪ Representative Laxatives: Brand Names, Dosage Forms, and Dosages

Drug Class and Generic Name	Brand Names	Dosage Forms	Dosage and Administration
BULK-FORMING			
Methylcellulose	Citrucel	Powder	*Powder:* 1 heaping tbsp in 8 ounces cold water 1–3 times/day
Psyllium	Metamucil, others	Powder, wafer	*Adults*: 1 rounded tsp (or 1 packet) mixed with water or other fluid, taken 1–3 times/day *Children over 6 yr:* ⅓ to ½ adult dose
Polycarbophil	FiberCon, others	Tablets	*Adults:* 1250 mg 1–4 times/day *Children 6–12 yr:* 625 mg 1–4 times/day
SURFACTANT			
Docusate sodium	Colace, others	Capsules, tablets, syrup, liquid	*Adults and children over 12 yr:* 50–500 mg/day *Children 6–12 yr:* 40–120 mg/day (All doses taken with a full glass of water)
STIMULANT			
Bisacodyl	Correctol, Dulcolax, Fleet Laxative, others	Tablets, suppositories	*Adults:* 10–15 mg (tablets) or 10-mg suppository once daily *Children:* 5-mg tablet or 5-mg suppository once daily
Senna	Senokot, Ex-Lax, others	Tablets	*Adults:* 2 tablets once or twice daily *Children 6–12 yr:* 1 tablet once or twice daily
OSMOTIC			
Polyethylene glycol	GlycoLax, MiraLax, Peglax 🍁	Powder	*Adults:* 17 gm (dissolved in 8 ounces of water) once daily *Children:* 0.8 g/kg PO once daily
Lactulose	Cephulac, Cholac, others	Liquid	*Adults:* 15–30 mL once or twice daily *Children:* 1 mL/kg PO once or twice daily
Magnesium hydroxide (milk of magnesia)	Phillips' Milk of Magnesia, others	Liquid	*Adults:* 15–30 mL daily, increased to 60 mL if needed *Children 6 mo–1 yr:* 40 mg/kg PO daily *Children 2–5 yr:* 400–1200 mg PO daily *Children 6–11 yr:* 1200–2400 mg PO daily *Children >12 yr:* 2400–4800 mg PO daily
OTHER			
Lubiprostone	Amitiza	Capsule	*Adults:* 24 mcg twice daily with food
Plecanatide	Trulance	Tablet	*Adults*: 3 mg daily
Mineral oil	Generic only	Liquid	*Adults:* 15–45 mL daily; may take in divided doses *Children:* 5–45 mL daily; may take in divided doses

Prototype Drugs

LAXATIVES

Bulk-Forming Agents
Methylcellulose

Surfactants
Docusate sodium

Stimulant Laxatives
Bisacodyl

Osmotic Laxatives
Magnesium hydroxide

Chloride Channel Activator
Lubiprostone

Stimulant Laxatives

The stimulant laxatives (e.g., bisacodyl, senna, castor oil) have two effects on the bowel. First, they stimulate intestinal motility—hence their name. Second, they increase the amount of water and electrolytes within the intestinal lumen by increasing secretion of water and ions into the intestine, and by reducing water and electrolyte absorption. Most stimulant laxatives are group II agents: They act on the colon to produce a semifluid stool within 6 to 12 hours.

Stimulant laxatives are widely used—and abused—by the public, and are of concern for this reason. They have few legitimate applications. Two applications that *are* legitimate are (1) treatment of opioid-induced constipation and (2) treatment of constipation resulting from slow intestinal transit. Properties of individual agents are discussed here.

Bisacodyl

Bisacodyl [Correctol, Dulcolax] is unique among the stimulant laxatives in that it can be administered by rectal suppository as well as by mouth. *Oral* bisacodyl acts within 6 to 12 hours. Hence, tablets may be given at bedtime to produce a response the following morning. Bisacodyl *suppositories* act rapidly (in 15 to 60 minutes). Dosages for bisacodyl are shown in Table 79.4.

Bisacodyl tablets are enteric coated to prevent gastric irritation. Accordingly, patients should be advised to swallow them intact, without chewing or crushing. Because milk and antacids accelerate dissolution of the enteric coating, the tablets should be administered no sooner than 1 hour after ingesting these substances.

Bisacodyl suppositories may cause a burning sensation; with continued use, proctitis may develop. Accordingly, long-term use should be discouraged.

Senna

Senna [Senokot, Ex-Lax] is a plant-derived laxative that contains *anthraquinones* as active ingredients. The actions and applications of senna are similar to those of bisacodyl. Anthraquinones act on the colon to produce a soft or semifluid stool in 6 to 12 hours. Systemic absorption followed by renal secretion may impart a harmless yellowish-brown or pink color to the urine. Dosages are presented in Table 79.4.

Castor Oil

Castor oil is the only stimulant laxative that acts on the *small intestine.* As a result, the drug acts quickly (in 2 to 6 hours) to produce a watery stool. Hence, unlike other stimulant laxatives, which are all group II agents, castor oil belongs to group I. The use of castor oil is limited to situations in which rapid and thorough evacuation of the bowel is desired (e.g., preparation for radiologic procedures). The drug is far too powerful for routine treatment of constipation. Because of its relatively prompt action, castor oil should not be administered at bedtime. The drug has an unpleasant taste that can be improved by chilling and mixing with fruit juice.

Osmotic Laxatives

Laxative Salts

Actions and Uses. The laxative salts (e.g., sodium phosphate, magnesium hydroxide) are poorly absorbed salts whose osmotic action draws water into the intestinal lumen. Accumulation of water causes the fecal mass to soften and swell, thereby stretching the intestinal wall, which stimulates peristalsis. When administered in low doses, the osmotic laxatives produce a soft or semifluid stool in 6 to 12 hours. In high doses, these agents act rapidly (in 2 to 6 hours) to cause a fluid evacuation of the bowel. High-dose therapy is employed to empty the bowel in preparation for diagnostic and surgical procedures. High doses are also employed to purge the bowel of ingested poisons and to evacuate dead parasites following anthelmintic therapy.

Preparations. We have two groups of laxative salts: (1) *magnesium salts* (magnesium hydroxide, magnesium citrate, and magnesium sulfate), and (2) one *sodium salt* (sodium phosphate). Dosages for magnesium hydroxide solution (also known as Milk of Magnesia) and sodium phosphate are shown in Table 79.4.

Adverse Effects. Osmotic laxatives can cause substantial *loss of water.* To avoid dehydration, patients should increase fluid intake. Although the osmotic laxatives are poorly and slowly absorbed, some absorption does take place. In patients with renal impairment, *magnesium can accumulate to toxic levels.* Accordingly, magnesium salts are contraindicated in patients with kidney disease. Sodium absorption (from sodium phosphate) can cause *fluid retention,* which in turn can exacerbate heart failure, hypertension, and edema. Accordingly, sodium phosphate is contraindicated for patients with these disorders. Sodium phosphate can also cause *acute renal failure* in vulnerable patients, especially those with kidney disease and those taking drugs that alter renal function (e.g., diuretics, angiotensin-converting enzyme [ACE] inhibitors, angiotensin receptor blockers [ARBs]). The mechanism involves dehydration and precipitation of calcium and phosphate in renal tubules. Accordingly, sodium phosphate should be avoided in this vulnerable group.

Polyethylene Glycol

Polyethylene glycol (PEG) [MiraLax, GlycoLax, Peglax 🍁] is an osmotic laxative used widely for chronic constipation. Like the laxative salts, PEG is a nonabsorbable compound that retains water in the intestinal lumen, causing the fecal mass to soften and swell. The most common adverse effects are nausea, abdominal bloating, cramping, and flatulence. High doses may cause diarrhea. For management of chronic constipation, PEG is superior to lactulose with regard to relief of abdominal pain and improvements in stool consistency and frequency per week, although side effects are similar. The recommended dosage is 17 gm once a day, dissolved in 4 to 8 ounces of water, juice, soda, coffee, or tea. Bowel movement may not occur for another 2 to 4 days. As discussed later in this chapter, products that contain PEG plus electrolytes can be used to cleanse the bowel before colonoscopy and other procedures.

Lactulose

Lactulose [Constulose, Enulose] is a semisynthetic disaccharide composed of galactose and fructose. Lactulose is poorly absorbed and cannot be digested by intestinal enzymes. In the colon, resident bacteria metabolize lactulose to lactic acid, formic acid, and acetic acid. These acids exert a mild osmotic action, producing a soft, formed stool in 1 to 3 days. Although lactulose can relieve constipation, this agent is more expensive than equivalent drugs (bulk-forming laxatives), and it causes more unpleasant side effects (flatulence and cramping are common). Accordingly, lactulose should be reserved for patients who do not respond adequately to a bulk-forming agent.

In addition to its laxative action, lactulose can enhance intestinal excretion of ammonia. This property has been exploited to lower blood ammonia content in patients with portal hypertension and hepatic encephalopathy secondary to chronic liver disease.

Other Laxatives

Lubiprostone

Lubiprostone [Amitiza] is the first representative of a new class of drugs: the selective *chloride channel activators*. By activating (opening) chloride channels in epithelial cells lining the intestine, lubiprostone (1) promotes secretion of chloride-rich fluid into the intestine and (2) enhances motility in the small intestine and colon. The result is spontaneous evacuation of a semisoft stool, usually within 24 hours. Lubiprostone has three indications: (1) chronic idiopathic constipation (CIC) in adults, (2) irritable bowel syndrome with constipation (IBS-C) in women at least 18 years old, and (3) treatment of opioid-induced constipation in chronic noncancer pain. In clinical trials, the drug reduced constipation severity, abdominal bloating, and discomfort.

Lubiprostone is taken orally, and very little is absorbed. Nausea is the most common side effect and can be reduced by taking lubiprostone with food and water. Other GI effects include diarrhea, abdominal distention, abdominal pain, gas, vomiting, and loose stools. Headache is the major non-GI effect. A small percentage of patients experience difficulty breathing in association with a sense of tightness in the chest, starting 30 to 60 minutes after the first dose and resolving in a few hours. Lubiprostone is categorized in U.S. Food and Drug Administration (FDA) Pregnancy Risk Category C,[a] and hence should be used only if benefits are deemed to outweigh potential risks to the fetus. (In animal studies, lubiprostone was not teratogenic. However, when given to guinea pigs in doses more than 100 times the human dose, lubiprostone did cause fetal loss.) Interactions with other drugs have not been studied but seem unlikely because lubiprostone is poorly absorbed and does not alter the activity of cytochrome P450 drug-metabolizing enzymes.

Lubiprostone is available in 8- and 24-mcg soft-gelatin capsules that should be taken with food and water. The recommended dosage is 24 mcg twice daily for constipation and 8 mcg twice daily for IBS-C. The role of lubiprostone in IBS-C is discussed in Chapter 80.

Plecanatide

Plecanatide [Trulance] is an oral tablet approved for the treatment of chronic idiopathic constipation. Plecanatide is related to the human hormone uroguanylin and assists in regulation of intestinal fluid secretion and motility by acting as a guanylate cyclase-C (GC-C) agonist. Activation of GC-C indirectly stimulates secretion of chloride and bicarbonate into the intestinal lumen. This results in increased intestinal fluid. Plecanatide is taken once daily with or without food.

Mineral Oil

Mineral oil is a mixture of indigestible and poorly absorbed hydrocarbons. Laxative action is produced by lubrication. Mineral oil is especially useful when administered by enema to treat fecal impaction.

Mineral oil can produce a variety of adverse effects. Aspiration of oil droplets can cause lipid pneumonia. Anal leakage can cause pruritus and soiling. Systemic absorption can produce deposition of mineral oil in the liver. Excessive dosing can decrease absorption of fat-soluble vitamins. Dosages for adults and children are shown in Table 79.4.

Glycerin Suppository

Glycerin is an osmotic agent that softens and lubricates inspissated (hardened, impacted) feces. The drug may also stimulate rectal contraction. Evacuation occurs about 30 minutes after suppository insertion. Glycerin suppositories have been useful for re-establishing normal bowel function following termination of chronic laxative use.

Bowel Cleansing Products for Colonoscopy

Colonoscopy is the most effective method for early detection of colorectal cancer, the second leading cause of cancer deaths in the United States. Before the procedure, the bowel must be cleansed to permit good visualization. Three kinds of bowel cleansers are used: (1) sodium phosphate; (2) a combination of sodium picosulfate, magnesium oxide, and citric acid; and (3) PEG plus electrolytes (ELS). The PEG-ELS products are isotonic with body fluids, and hence do not alter water or electrolyte status. In contrast, the sodium phosphate and combination products are hypertonic and can cause dehydration and electrolyte disturbances. In addition, the sodium phosphate products can cause kidney damage. However, despite their greater potential for harm, the sodium phosphate products have better patient acceptance because the PEG-ELS products require ingestion of a large volume of liquid, whereas the sodium phosphate products do not. Nonetheless, sodium phosphate products should be avoided by patients at risk, including those with electrolyte abnormalities, renal impairment, and hypovolemia. Representative bowel cleansers are shown in Table 79.5.

Polyethylene Glycol–Electrolyte Solutions

These bowel-cleansing solutions [CoLyte, GoLYTELY, others] contain PEG, a nonabsorbable osmotic agent, together with ELS (usually potassium chloride, sodium chloride, sodium sulfate, and sodium bicarbonate). The mixture is isosmotic with body fluids, and hence water and electrolytes are neither absorbed from nor secreted into the intestinal lumen. As a result, dehydration does not occur and electrolyte balance is

[a]As of 2020, the FDA will no longer use Pregnancy Risk Categories. Please refer to Chapter 9 for more information.

TABLE 79.5 ■ Oral Bowel Cleansing Products for Colonoscopy

Product Type and Brand Name	Adult Dosage	Total Volume to Swallow: Bowel Cleanser	Total Volume to Swallow: Clear Liquid
SODIUM PHOSPHATE TABLETS			
OsmoPrep	20 tablets with clear liquid in the evening *plus* 20 tablets with clear liquid the next day		1.9 L
POLYETHYLENE GLYCOL PLUS ELECTROLYTES			
GoLYTELY, NuLYTELY, Colyte, TriLyte	240 mL every 10 min until 4 L is ingested or until rectal effluent is clear	4 L	
GaviLyte-H and bisacodyl	240 mL every 10 min until 2 L is ingested[a]	2 L	
MoviPrep[b]	240 mL every 15 min until 1 L is ingested, then repeat 1.5 hr later, then drink 1 more L of clear liquid[c]	2 L	1 L
COMBINATION PRODUCT			
Prepopik	1 package (16.1 gm) mixed in 5 ounces of water the evening before the colonoscopy and 1 package mixed in 5 ounces of water the morning of the colonoscopy[d]		2.5 L

[a]Before drinking the solution, patients should take 4 bisacodyl delayed-release tablets and wait for a bowel movement or for 6 hours, whichever comes first.
[b]Formulated with ascorbic acid, which allows use of a smaller volume than traditional PEG-electrolyte products.
[c]Dosage can be split by ingesting 1 L of the prep plus 0.5 L clear liquid in the evening, followed by 1 L of the prep plus 0.5 L clear liquid the next day.
[d]Dose should be followed by 40 ounces of clear liquid the evening before the colonoscopy and 32 ounces of clear liquid the morning of the procedure.

preserved. Because effects on water and electrolytes are minimal, PEG-ELS solutions can be used safely by patients who are dehydrated and by those who are especially sensitive to alteration of electrolyte levels (e.g., patients with renal impairment or cardiovascular disease).

With traditional PEG-ELS products (e.g., CoLyte, GoLYTELY), the volume administered is huge, typically 4 L. Patients must ingest 250 to 300 mL every 10 minutes for 2 to 3 hours. With two newer products—GaviLyte-H and MoviPrep—the volume is cut in half. Patients using GaviLyte-H take a stimulant laxative—bisacodyl—along with the PEG-ELS solution, and hence don't need the full 4-L dose. Volume reduction with MoviPrep is possible owing to the addition of ascorbic acid and sodium ascorbate to the PEG-ELS solution. With all PEG products, bowel movements commence about 1 hour after the first dose.

PEG-ELS products are generally well tolerated. The most common adverse effects are nausea, bloating, and abdominal discomfort. These effects are less intense with the reduced-volume formulations. Because PEG-ELS products don't alter water and electrolyte status, they are safer than sodium phosphate products for patients with electrolyte imbalances, heart failure, kidney disease, or advanced liver disease.

Sodium Phosphate Products

As discussed earlier, sodium phosphate is an osmotic laxative that draws water into the intestinal lumen, which then softens and swells the fecal mass, which then stretches the intestinal wall to stimulate peristalsis. Dosing consists of swallowing tablets along with a large volume of water or some other clear liquid. Since the clear liquid is more palatable than the PEG-ELS solutions, patients find the sodium phosphate regimens more appealing.

Like the PEG-ELS products, the sodium phosphate products can cause nausea, bloating, and abdominal discomfort. In addition, the sodium phosphate products can cause adverse effects not seen with the PEG-ELS products, especially dehydration, electrolyte disturbances, and kidney damage. By drawing a large volume of fluid into the intestinal lumen, sodium phosphate can cause dehydration. To prevent dehydration, patients must drink a large volume of clear fluid before, during, and after dosing.

Rarely, phosphate is absorbed in amounts sufficient to cause hyperphosphatemia, which can cause *acute, reversible renal damage and possibly chronic, irreversible renal damage.* Risk factors for hyperphosphatemia and kidney damage include hypovolemia, advanced age, delayed bowel transit, active colitis, pre-existing kidney disease, and the use of drugs that can alter kidney function, including diuretics, ACE inhibitors, ARBs, and nonsteroidal anti-inflammatory drugs. Patients who have these risk factors should probably use a PEG-ELS product rather than sodium phosphate.

Combination Products

One combination product—magnesium oxide/anhydrous citric acid/sodium picosulfate [Prepopik]—is approved for preparation for colonoscopy in adults. Sodium picosulfate is a stimulant laxative, and magnesium oxide and citric acid combine to form magnesium citrate, an osmotic laxative. When given in a split-dose regimen, results were superior to colon preparation with PEG-ELS.

Prepopik is given in a split-dose regimen. It is supplied in 2 packets containing 16.1 gm each of powder that must be mixed with water for consumption. The first dose is taken the evening before the colonoscopy and the second dose the next morning before the procedure.

As with sodium phosphate products, Prepopik can cause electrolyte and fluid imbalances, renal impairment, seizures, and dysrhythmia secondary to electrolyte abnormalities. Caution must be employed in patients with reduced renal function. The most common adverse reactions are nausea, headache, and vomiting.

LAXATIVE ABUSE

Causes

Many people believe that a daily bowel movement is a requisite of good health and that any deviation from this pattern merits correction. Such misconceptions are reinforced by aggressive marketing of OTC laxative preparations. Not infrequently, the combination of tradition supported by advertising has led to habitual self-prescribing of laxatives by people who don't need them.

Laxatives can help perpetuate their own use. Strong laxatives can purge the entire bowel. When this occurs, spontaneous evacuation is impossible until bowel content has been replenished, which can take 2 to 5 days. During this time, the laxative user, having experienced no movement of the bowel, often becomes convinced that constipation has returned. In response, he or she takes yet another dose, which purges the bowel once more and thereby sets the stage for a repeating cycle of laxative use and purging.

Consequences

Chronic exposure to laxatives can diminish defecatory reflexes, leading to further reliance on laxatives. Laxative abuse may also cause more serious pathologic changes, including electrolyte imbalance, dehydration, and colitis.

Treatment

The first step in breaking the laxative habit is abrupt cessation of laxative use. Following drug withdrawal, bowel movements will be absent for several days; the patient should be informed of this fact. Any misconceptions that the patient has regarding bowel function should be corrected: The patient should be taught that a once-daily bowel movement may not be normal for him or her and that stool *quality* is more important than frequency or quantity. Instruction on bowel training (heeding the defecatory reflex, establishing a consistent time for bowel movements) should be provided. Increased consumption of fiber (bran, fruits, vegetables) and fluid should be stressed. The patient should be encouraged to exercise daily, especially after meals. Finally, the patient should be advised that if a laxative must be used, it should be used briefly and in the smallest effective dose. Agents that produce catharsis must be avoided.

KEY POINTS

- Laxatives promote defecation.
- Constipation is defined primarily by stool consistency, not by frequency or volume of bowel movements.
- Legitimate indications for laxatives include cardiovascular disorders, episiotomy, hemorrhoids, emptying the bowel before surgery and diagnostic procedures, ileostomy or colostomy, prevention of fecal impaction in bedridden patients, and constipation associated with pregnancy and certain drugs, especially opioid analgesics.
- Like dietary fiber, bulk-forming laxatives swell in water to form a viscous solution or gel, thereby softening the feces and increasing fecal mass. Increased mass stretches the bowel wall, and thereby stimulates peristalsis.
- Administer bulk-forming laxatives with fluid to avoid esophageal obstruction.
- Patients receiving osmotic laxatives must increase fluid intake to avoid dehydration.
- Because of their relatively rapid onset, group I laxatives (castor oil, high-dose osmotic agents) should not be given at bedtime.
- Bowel cleansing before colonoscopy can be accomplished with three types of equally effective products: sodium phosphate cleansers, sodium picosulfate/magnesium oxide/citric acid combination cleansers, and PEG-ELS solutions.
- Sodium phosphate and combination cleansers are easier to take than PEG-ELS cleansers, but pose a greater risk of adverse effects, namely dehydration, electrolyte disturbances, and kidney damage.
- Laxatives—especially the stimulant type—are commonly misused (abused) by the public. To reduce abuse, educate patients about normal bowel function and about alternatives to laxatives (diet high in fiber and fluids, exercise, establishing regular bowel habits).

Please visit **http://evolve.elsevier.com/Lehne** for chapter-specific NCLEX® examination review questions.

Summary of Major Nursing Implications[a]

LAXATIVES

Implications That Apply to All Laxatives

Identifying High-Risk Patients

Laxatives are *contraindicated* for individuals with abdominal pain, nausea, cramps, and other symptoms of appendicitis, regional enteritis, diverticulitis, and ulcerative colitis. Laxatives are also *contraindicated* for patients with acute surgical abdomen, fecal impaction, and obstruction of the bowel.

Laxatives should be used with *caution* during pregnancy and lactation.

Reducing Laxative Abuse

Patient education is a key factor in reducing laxative abuse. **Educate patients about normal bowel function to correct misconceptions. Provide instruction on establishing good bowel habits (heeding the defecatory reflex, establishing a consistent time for bowel movements). Advise patients to exercise—especially after meals—and to increase consumption of fluids and fiber (bran, fruits, vegetables). Inform patients that laxatives should be used only when clearly necessary and then only briefly in the lowest effective dosage. Warn patients against using cathartics.**

Implications That Apply to Specific Laxatives

Bulk-Forming Laxatives: Psyllium, Methylcellulose, and Polycarbophil

Instruct patients to take bulk-forming agents with a full glass of water or juice to prevent esophageal obstruction.

Bulk-forming laxatives are *contraindicated* for individuals with narrowing of the intestinal lumen, a condition that increases the risk of intestinal obstruction and impaction.

Surfactants: Docusate Salts

Instruct patients to take surfactant agents with a full glass of water.

Stimulant Laxatives

Stimulant agents are the laxatives most commonly abused by the public. **Discourage patients from inappropriate use of these drugs.** These drugs are commonly—and appropriately—used to manage opioid-induced constipation.

Bisacodyl. Administer PO and by rectal suppository. **Instruct patients to take oral bisacodyl no sooner than 1 hour after ingesting milk or antacids. Instruct patients to swallow the tablets intact, without crushing or chewing.**

Inform patients that bisacodyl suppositories may cause a burning sensation, and warn them that prolonged use can cause proctitis.

Senna. **Inform patients that senna can impart a harmless yellowish-brown or pink color to urine.**

Castor Oil. Castor oil acts rapidly (in 2 to 6 hours); do not administer at bedtime. **Advise patients not to take castor oil late at night. Warn patients that castor oil is a powerful laxative and should not be used to treat routine constipation.** Administer in chilled fruit juice to improve palatability.

Osmotic Laxatives: Magnesium Salts and Sodium Salts

Effects are dose dependent. Low doses produce a soft or semifluid stool in 6 to 12 hours. Higher doses cause watery evacuation of the bowel in 2 to 6 hours.

To prevent dehydration, increase fluid intake during treatment.

Magnesium salts are contraindicated for patients with *renal dysfunction.*

Sodium phosphate is contraindicated for patients with kidney disease and for those taking drugs that alter renal function (e.g., diuretics, ACE inhibitors, ARBs), and should be avoided in patients with heart failure, hypertension, or edema.

[a]Patient education information is highlighted as **blue text.**

CHAPTER

80 Other Gastrointestinal Drugs

In this chapter we discuss an assortment of GI drugs with indications ranging from emesis to colitis to hemorrhoids. Four groups are emphasized: (1) antiemetics, (2) antidiarrheals, (3) drugs for irritable bowel syndrome, and (4) drugs for inflammatory bowel disease.

ANTIEMETICS

Antiemetics are given to suppress nausea and vomiting. We begin our discussion by reviewing the emetic response. Next we discuss the major antiemetic classes. We finish by considering the most important application of these drugs: management of chemotherapy-induced nausea and vomiting (CINV).

The Emetic Response

Emesis is a complex reflex brought about by activating the vomiting center, a nucleus of neurons located in the medulla oblongata. Some stimuli activate the vomiting center directly; others act indirectly (Fig. 80.1). Direct-acting stimuli include signals from the cerebral cortex (anticipation or fear), signals from sensory organs (upsetting sights, noxious odors, or pain), and signals from the vestibular apparatus of the inner ear. Indirect-acting stimuli first activate the chemoreceptor trigger zone (CTZ), which in turn activates the vomiting center. Activation of the CTZ occurs in two ways: (1) by signals from the stomach and small intestine (traveling along vagal afferents) and (2) by the direct action of emetogenic compounds (e.g., anticancer drugs, opioids, ipecac) that are carried to the CTZ in the blood. Once activated, the vomiting center signals the stomach, diaphragm, and abdominal muscles; the resulting coordinated response expels gastric contents.

Several types of receptors are involved in the emetic response. Important among these are receptors for serotonin, glucocorticoids, substance P, neurokinin$_1$, dopamine, acetylcholine, and histamine. Many antiemetics, including ondansetron [Zofran], dexamethasone, aprepitant [Emend], prochlorperazine, and dimenhydrinate, act by blocking (or activating) one or more of these receptors.

Antiemetic Drugs

Several types of antiemetics are available. Their classes, brand names, and dosages are shown in Table 80.1. Uses and mechanisms are shown in Table 80.2. Properties of the principal classes are discussed next.

Serotonin Receptor Antagonists

Serotonin receptor antagonists are the most effective drugs available for suppressing nausea and vomiting caused by cisplatin and other highly emetogenic anticancer drugs. These drugs are also highly effective against nausea and vomiting associated with radiation therapy, anesthesia, viral gastritis, and pregnancy. Four serotonin antagonists are available for treating emesis: ondansetron, granisetron, dolasetron, and palonosetron. As they are all similar, we will discuss ondansetron as the prototype. Dosing can be found in Table 80.1.

Ondansetron. Ondansetron [Zofran, Zofran ODT, Zuplenz] was the first serotonin receptor antagonist approved for CINV. The drug is also used to prevent nausea and vomiting associated with radiotherapy and anesthesia. In addition, the drug is used off-label to treat nausea and vomiting from other causes, including childhood viral gastritis and morning sickness of pregnancy. In all cases, benefits derive from blocking type 3 serotonin receptors ($5\text{-}HT_3$ receptors[a]) located in the CTZ and

[a]Serotonin is also known as 5-hydroxytryptamine (5-HT), so type 3 serotonin receptors are abbreviated as *5-HT$_3$*.

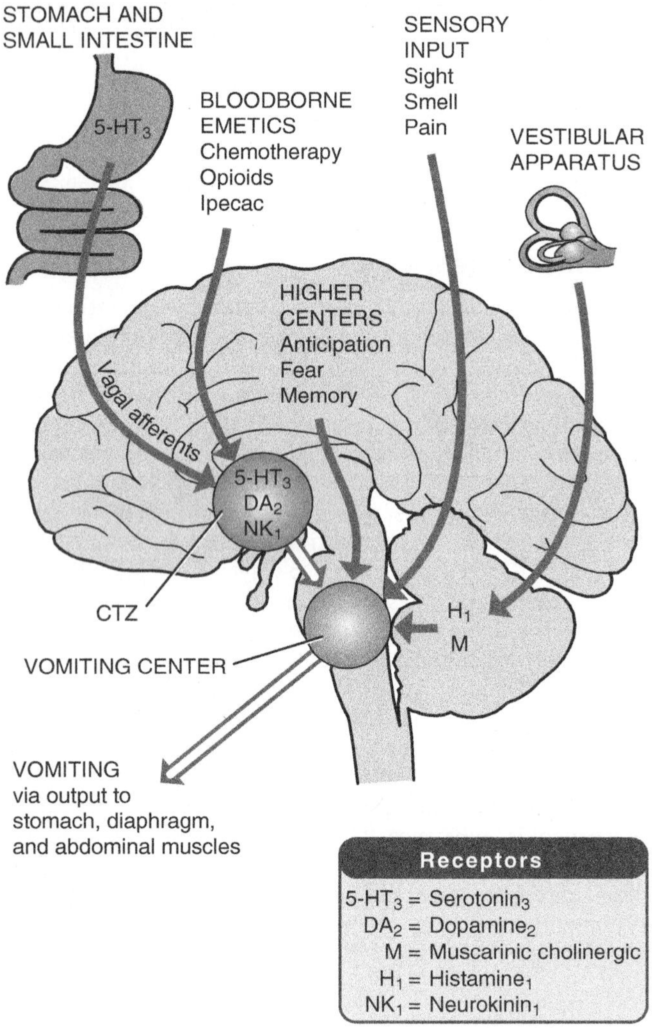

Fig. 80.1 ▪ The emetic response: stimuli, pathways, and receptors.
(*CTZ,* Chemoreceptor trigger zone.)

Prototype Drugs

GASTROINTESTINAL DRUGS

Serotonin Antagonists
Ondansetron

Glucocorticoids
Dexamethasone

Substance P/Neurokinin$_1$ Antagonists
Aprepitant

Dopamine Antagonists
Prochlorperazine

Cannabinoids
Dronabinol

Benzodiazepines
Lorazepam

Drugs for Constipation-Predominant IBS
Lubiprostone

Drugs for Diarrhea-Predominant IBS
Alosetron

5-Aminosalicylates
Sulfasalazine

Glucocorticoids
Budesonide

Immunomodulators/Immunosuppressants
Infliximab
Mercaptopurine

on afferent vagal neurons in the upper GI tract. The drug is very effective by itself, and even more effective when combined with dexamethasone. Administration may be oral or parenteral. The most common side effects are headache, diarrhea, and dizziness. Of much greater concern, ondansetron prolongs the QT interval and hence poses a risk of torsades de pointes, a potentially life-threatening dysrhythmia. Accordingly, the drug should not be given to patients with long QT syndrome, and should be used with caution in patients with electrolyte abnormalities, heart failure, or bradydysrhythmias, and in those taking other QT drugs. Since ondansetron does not block dopamine receptors, it does not cause the extrapyramidal effects (e.g., akathisia, acute dystonia) seen with antiemetic phenothiazines.

Preparations, Dosage, and Administration. Administration is PO, IM, or IV. For oral dosing, ondansetron is available in solution (sold as Zofran), standard tablets (sold as Zofran), orally disintegrating tablets (sold as Zofran ODT), and a soluble film (sold as Zuplenz). To prevent CINV, the recommended IV dose is 0.15 mg/kg infused slowly (over 15 minutes) beginning 30 minutes before chemotherapy; this dose is repeated 4 and 8 hours later. The dosage for patients undergoing radiation therapy is 8 mg PO (tablets, solution, or soluble film) 3 times a day. The dosage for postoperative nausea and vomiting is 16 mg PO (tablets, solution, or soluble film) 1 hour before induction of anesthesia.

Glucocorticoids

Two glucocorticoids—*methylprednisolone* [Solu-Medrol] and *dexamethasone*—are commonly used to suppress CINV, even though they are not approved by the U.S. Food and Drug Administration (FDA) for this application. Glucocorticoids are effective alone and in combination with other antiemetics. The mechanism by which glucocorticoids suppress emesis is unknown. Both dexamethasone and methylprednisolone are administered IV. Because antiemetic use is intermittent and short term, serious side effects are absent. The pharmacology of the glucocorticoids is discussed in Chapter 72.

Substance P/Neurokinin$_1$ Antagonists

Four substance P/neurokinin$_1$ antagonists are currently available: aprepitant, rolapitant, netupitant, and fosaprepitant, a prodrug that undergoes conversion to aprepitant in the body. Netupitant is available only in combination with palonosetron and is marketed as Akynzeo. Their principal application is prevention of CINV. We will discuss only the prototype here.

TABLE 80.1 ▪ Antiemetic Drugs: Classes, Brand Names, and Dosages

Class and Generic Name	Brand Name	Adult Dosage
SEROTONIN ANTAGONISTS		
Ondansetron	Zofran, Zuplenz	See text
Granisetron	Kytril 🍁, Sancuso	CINV: either (1) 10 mcg/kg IV starting 30 minutes before chemotherapy or (2) a single transdermal patch [Sancuso] applied 24 to 48 hr before chemotherapy and removed 24 hr after chemotherapy is completed Radiation therapy: 2 mg given within 1 hr of radiation treatment PONV prevention: 1 mg IV either before induction of anesthesia or just before reversing anesthesia
Dolasetron	Anzemet	CINV: 100 mg PO 1 hr before chemotherapy PONV prevention: 100 mg PO 2 hr before anesthesia or 12.5 mg IV 15 minutes before anesthesia is stopped
Palonosetron	Aloxi	CINV: 250 mcg IV 30 minutes before chemotherapy PONV prevention: 75 mcg IV immediately before induction of anesthesia
GLUCOCORTICOIDS		
Dexamethasone	Generic only	10–20 mg IV before chemotherapy, then 4–8 mg
Methylprednisolone	Solu-Medrol	2 doses of 125–500 mg IV 6 hr apart before chemotherapy
SUBSTANCE P/NEUROKININ$_1$ ANTAGONISTS		
Aprepitant	Emend	125 mg PO on day 1, then 80 mg PO on days 2 and 3
Fosaprepitant	Emend	115 mg IV, used in place of the first (125-mg) dose of aprepitant in the regimen above
Netupitant/Palonosetron	Akynzeo	300/0.5 mg (1 capsule) 1 hr before chemotherapy
Rolapitant	Varubi	180 mg PO 1–2 hr before chemotherapy
BENZODIAZEPINES		
Lorazepam	Ativan	1–1.5 mg IV before chemotherapy
DOPAMINE ANTAGONISTS		
Phenothiazines		
Chlorpromazine	Generic only	10–25 mg (PO, IM, IV) every 4–6 hr PRN
Perphenazine	Generic only	8–16 mg/day in divided doses (PO, IM, IV)
Prochlorperazine	Generic only	5–10 mg (PO, IM, IV) 3–4 times/day PRN
Promethazine[a]	Phenergan	12.5–25 mg (PO, IM, IV) every 4–6 hr
Butyrophenones		
Haloperidol[b]	Haldol	1–5 mg (PO, IM, IV) every 12 hr PRN
Droperidol	Inapsine	0.625–2.5 mg (IM, IV) every 4–6 hr PRN
Others		
Metoclopramide[c]	Reglan	See Table 80.3
CANNABINOIDS		
Dronabinol	Marinol	5 mg/m^2 PO every 2–4 hr PRN
Nabilone	Cesamet	1–2 mg PO twice daily
ANTICHOLINERGICS		
Antihistamines		
Cyclizine	Cyclivert	50 mg PO every 4–6 hr PRN
Dimenhydrinate	Dramamine	50–100 mg (PO, IM, IV) every 4–6 hr PRN
Diphenhydramine	Benadryl	10–50 mg (PO, IM, IV) every 4–6 hr PRN
Hydroxyzine	Vistaril	25–100 mg IM every 6 hr PRN
Meclizine	Bonine, Antivert	25–50 mg PO every 24 hr PRN
Others		
Scopolamine	Transderm Scōp	0.5 mg transdermal every 72 hr PRN

[a]Promethazine is contraindicated for children younger than 2 years owing to a risk of fatal respiratory depression.
[b]Off-label use.
[c]Also blocks serotonin receptors.
CINV, Chemotherapy-induced nausea and vomiting; *PONV,* postoperative nausea and vomiting.

TABLE 80.2 ▪ Antiemetic Drugs: Uses and Mechanism of Action

Class	Prototype	Antiemetic Use	Mechanism of Antiemetic Action
Serotonin antagonists	Ondansetron [Zofran, Zuplenz]	Chemotherapy, radiation, postoperative	Block serotonin receptors on vagal afferents and in the CTZ
Glucocorticoids	Dexamethasone (generic only)	Chemotherapy	Unknown
Substance P/neurokinin$_1$ antagonists	Aprepitant [Emend]	Chemotherapy	Block receptors for substance P/neurokinin$_1$ in the brain
Dopamine antagonists	Prochlorperazine (generic only)	Chemotherapy, postoperative, general	Block dopamine receptors in the CTZ
Cannabinoids	Dronabinol [Marinol]	Chemotherapy	Unknown, but probably activate cannabinoid receptors associated with the vomiting center
Anticholinergics	Scopolamine [Transderm Scōp]	Motion sickness	Block muscarinic receptors in the pathway from the inner ear to the vomiting center
Antihistamines	Dimenhydrinate (generic only)	Motion sickness	Block H_1 receptors and muscarinic receptors in the pathway from the inner ear to the vomiting center

Aprepitant

Actions and Use. Aprepitant [Emend] is an important antiemetic. The drug is approved for preventing postoperative nausea and vomiting and CINV. Owing to its unique mechanism of action—blockade of neurokinin$_1$-type receptors (for substance P) in the CTZ—aprepitant can enhance responses when combined with other antiemetic drugs. Aprepitant has a prolonged duration of action, and hence can prevent *delayed* CINV, as well as *acute* CINV. Aprepitant can be used *alone* for managing postoperative nausea and vomiting. However, since the drug is only moderately effective, it must be combined with other antiemetic drugs—specifically, a glucocorticoid (e.g., dexamethasone) and a serotonin antagonist (e.g., ondansetron)—for managing CINV.

Pharmacokinetics. Oral aprepitant is well absorbed, both in the presence and absence of food. Plasma levels peak 4 hours after dosing. The drug undergoes extensive hepatic metabolism—primarily by CYP3A4 (the 3A4 isoenzyme of cytochrome P450)—followed by excretion in the urine and feces. The plasma half-life is 9 to 13 hours.

Adverse Effects. Aprepitant is generally well tolerated. Compared with patients receiving ondansetron and dexamethasone, those receiving aprepitant plus ondansetron and dexamethasone experience more fatigue and asthenia (17.8% vs. 11.8%), hiccups (10.8% vs. 5.6%), dizziness (6.6% vs. 4.4%), and diarrhea (10.3% vs. 7.5%). Aprepitant may also cause a mild, transient elevation of circulating aminotransferases, indicating possible liver injury.

Drug Interactions. The potential for drug interactions is complex because aprepitant is a substrate for, inhibitor of, and inducer of CYP3A4, a major drug-metabolizing enzyme. Inhibitors of CYP3A4 (e.g., itraconazole, ritonavir) can raise levels of aprepitant. Conversely, inducers of CYP3A4 (e.g., rifampin, phenytoin) can decrease levels of aprepitant. By inhibiting CYP3A4, aprepitant can raise levels of CYP3A4 substrates, including many drugs used for cancer chemotherapy. Among these are docetaxel, paclitaxel, etoposide, irinotecan, ifosfamide, imatinib, vinorelbine, vinblastine, and vincristine. Also, aprepitant can raise levels of glucocorticoids used to prevent CINV. Accordingly, doses of these drugs (dexamethasone and methylprednisolone) should be reduced.

In addition to affecting CYP3A4, aprepitant can induce CYP2D6, another drug-metabolizing enzyme. As a result, aprepitant can decrease levels of CYP2D6 substrates, including warfarin (an anticoagulant) and ethinyl estradiol (found in oral contraceptives). Patients receiving warfarin should be monitored closely. Patients using oral contraceptives may need an alternative form of birth control.

Preparations, Dosage, and Administration. Aprepitant [Emend] is available in 40-, 80- and 125-mg capsules and a 25 mg/mL suspension. Dosing may be done with or without food.

For CINV, dosing is done once a day for 3 days. The first dose (125 mg) is given 1 hour before chemotherapy. The second and third doses (80 mg each) are given early on the following 2 days. As noted, aprepitant should be used in combination with dexamethasone and ondansetron.

For postoperative nausea and vomiting, treatment consists of a single 40-mg dose given within 3 hours of anesthesia induction.

Benzodiazepines

Lorazepam [Ativan] is used in combination regimens to suppress CINV. The drug has three principal benefits: sedation, suppression of anticipatory emesis, and production of anterograde amnesia. In addition, lorazepam may help control extrapyramidal reactions caused by phenothiazine antiemetics. The basic pharmacology of lorazepam and other benzodiazepines is discussed in Chapter 34.

Dopamine Antagonists

Phenothiazines. The phenothiazines (e.g., prochlorperazine) suppress emesis by blocking dopamine$_2$ receptors in the CTZ. These drugs can reduce emesis associated with surgery, cancer chemotherapy, and toxins. Side effects include extrapyramidal reactions, anticholinergic effects, hypotension, and sedation. The basic pharmacology of the phenothiazines is discussed in Chapter 31.

One phenothiazine—*promethazine* [Phenergan]—requires comment. Promethazine is the most widely used antiemetic in young children despite its adverse side effects (respiratory depression and local tissue injury) and despite the availability of potentially safer alternatives (e.g., ondansetron). Respiratory depression from promethazine can be severe. Deaths have occurred. Because of this risk, promethazine is contraindicated in children under the age of 2 years, and should be used with caution in children older than 2. Tissue injury can result in several ways. For example, extravasation of IV promethazine can cause abscess formation, tissue necrosis, and gangrene that requires amputation. Severe injury can also occur with inadvertent perivascular or intra-arterial administration, or with administration into or near a nerve. Risk of local injury is lower with IM dosing than with IV dosing. Accordingly, when parenteral administration is needed, the IM route is preferred. SubQ promethazine is contraindicated. If IV administration *must* be done, promethazine should be given through a large-bore, freely flowing line, in a concentration of 25 mg/mL or less at a rate of 25 mg/min or less. Patients should be advised to report local burning or pain immediately.

Butyrophenones. Two butyrophenones—*haloperidol* [Haldol] and *droperidol* [Inapsine]—are used as antiemetics. Like the phenothiazines, the butyrophenones suppress emesis by blocking $dopamine_2$ receptors in the CTZ. Butyrophenones are effective against postoperative nausea and vomiting, and emesis caused by cancer chemotherapy, radiation therapy, and toxins. Potential side effects are similar to those of the phenothiazines: extrapyramidal reactions, sedation, and hypotension. The pharmacology of the butyrophenones is discussed in Chapter 31.

Safety Alert

DROPERIDOL

Droperidol may pose a risk of fatal dysrhythmias owing to prolongation of the QT interval. Accordingly, patients receiving the drug should undergo an electrocardiographic evaluation before administration.

Metoclopramide. Metoclopramide [Reglan] suppresses emesis through blockade of dopamine receptors in the CTZ. The drug can suppress postoperative nausea and vomiting, as well as emesis caused by anticancer drugs, opioids, toxins, and radiation therapy. The pharmacology of metoclopramide is discussed later in this chapter under *Prokinetic Agents.*

Cannabinoids

Two cannabinoids—*dronabinol* [Marinol] and *nabilone* [Cesamet]—are approved for medical use in the United States. Both drugs are related to marijuana (*Cannabis sativa*). Dronabinol (delta-9-tetrahydrocannabinol; THC) is the principal psychoactive agent in *C. sativa.* Nabilone is a synthetic derivative of dronabinol. A third cannabinoid preparation, sold as *Sativex* ♣ (a combination of THC and cannabidiol), is available in Canada (for treating neuropathic pain) but is not FDA approved in the United States. The basic pharmacology of THC and other cannabinoids is discussed in Chapter 40.

Therapeutic Uses. Both dronabinol and nabilone are approved for suppressing CINV. The mechanism underlying benefits is unknown, but most likely results from activating cannabinoid receptors in and around the vomiting center. Because of their psychotomimetic effects and abuse potential (see later), the cannabinoids are considered second-line drugs for CINV, and hence should be reserved for patients who are unresponsive to or intolerant of preferred agents.

In addition to its use in CINV, dronabinol (but not nabilone) is approved for stimulating appetite in patients with AIDS. The goal is to reduce AIDS-induced anorexia and to prevent or reverse weight loss.

Adverse Effects and Drug Interactions. In theory, the cannabinoids used medically can produce subjective effects identical to those caused by smoking marijuana. Potential unpleasant effects include temporal disintegration, dissociation, depersonalization, and dysphoria. Because of these effects, cannabinoids should be used with caution in patients with psychiatric disorders. In addition to their subjective effects, cannabinoids can cause tachycardia and hypotension, and therefore must be used carefully in patients with cardiovascular diseases. The cannabinoids can cause drowsiness, and hence should not be combined with alcohol, sedatives, and central nervous system (CNS) depressants.

Abuse Potential. Because they can mimic the subjective effects of marijuana, cannabinoids have some potential for abuse. When first approved for medical use, both drugs were classified under Schedule II of the Controlled Substances Act (CSA)—a classification reserved for drugs with a high abuse potential. However, in 1998, the manufacturer of dronabinol petitioned the Drug Enforcement Agency (DEA) to reclassify the drug under Schedule III. Two arguments for the reduced classification were offered: (1) because of its slow onset, dronabinol does not produce the same "high" produced by smoking marijuana and (2) there is little or no interest in dronabinol on the street. Apparently, the DEA agreed: Dronabinol is now classified under Schedule III. Nabilone remains under Schedule II, although its abuse potential seems no greater than that of dronabinol.

Preparations, Dosage, and Administration

Dronabinol. Dronabinol [Marinol] is supplied in capsules (2.5, 5, and 10 mg) for oral use. To *prevent emesis,* the usual dosage is 5 mg/m^2 every 4 to 6 hours as needed. To *stimulate appetite* in patients with AIDS, the recommended initial dosage is 2.5 mg before lunch and supper. If this dosage is intolerable, 2.5 mg once daily may be tried.

Nabilone. Nabilone [Cesamet] is supplied in 1-mg capsules for oral use. The usual dosage is 1 to 2 mg twice daily.

Chemotherapy-Induced Nausea and Vomiting

Many anticancer drugs cause severe nausea and vomiting, leading to dehydration, electrolyte imbalances, nutrient depletion, and esophageal tears. Worse yet, these reactions can be so intense that patients may discontinue chemotherapy rather than endure further discomfort. Fortunately, CINV can be minimized with the antiemetics.

Chemotherapy is associated with three types of emesis: (1) anticipatory, (2) acute, and (3) delayed. *Anticipatory emesis* occurs before anticancer drugs are actually given; it is triggered by the memory of severe nausea and vomiting from a previous round of chemotherapy. *Acute emesis* begins within minutes to a few hours after receiving chemotherapy, and often resolves within 24 hours. In contrast, *delayed emesis* develops a day or more after drug administration. For example, with cisplatin, emesis is maximal 48 to 72 hours after dosing and can persist for 6 to 7 days.

Antiemetics are more effective at *preventing* CINV than at *suppressing* CINV that has already begun. Accordingly, antiemetics should be administered *before* chemotherapy. For prevention, antiemetics may be given orally or parenterally. Both routes are equally effective (although dosage may differ). In general, oral therapy is preferred. However, if emesis is

TABLE 80.3 ■ Representative Regimens for Preventing Chemotherapy-Induced Nausea and Vomiting

HIGH-EMETOGENIC-RISK CHEMOTHERAPY	
Aprepitant	125 mg PO on day 1, 80 mg PO on days 2 and 3 *plus*
Dexamethasone	12 mg PO or IV on day 1, 8 mg PO or IV on days 2–4 *plus*
Ondansetron	8 mg PO twice on day 1 *or* 8 mg or 1.5 mg/kg IV on day 1
MODERATE-EMETOGENIC-RISK CHEMOTHERAPY	
Dexamethasone	8 mg PO or IV *plus*
Palonosetron	0.25 mg IV or 0.5 mg PO
LOW-EMETOGENIC-RISK CHEMOTHERAPY	
Dexamethasone	8 mg PO or IV

Data from Basch E, Prestrud AA, et al. Antiemetics: American Society of Clinical Oncology. Clinical Practice Guideline Update. *J Clin Oncol* 29:4189–4198, 2011.

ongoing, oral therapy won't work, and hence parenteral therapy is required.

The antiemetic regimen for a particular patient is based on the emetogenic potential of the chemotherapy drugs being used. For drugs with a low risk of causing emesis, a single antiemetic (dexamethasone) may be adequate. For drugs with a moderate or high risk of causing emesis, a combination of antiemetics is needed. The current regimen of choice for patients taking highly emetogenic drugs consists of three agents: aprepitant plus dexamethasone plus a 5-HT_3 antagonist (e.g., ondansetron, palonosetron). Lorazepam may be added to reduce anxiety and anticipatory emesis and to provide amnesia as well. The superior efficacy of combination therapy suggests that anticancer drugs may induce emesis by multiple mechanisms. Table 80.3 shows representative regimens for preventing CINV in patients receiving anticancer drugs with low, moderate, and high emetogenic risk.

Nausea and Vomiting of Pregnancy

Nausea and vomiting of pregnancy (NVP) is extremely common, especially during the first trimester. About 50% of women experience nausea *plus* vomiting, and an additional 25% experience nausea alone. A few women experience *hyperemesis gravidarum,* a severe form of NVP characterized by dehydration, ketonuria, hypokalemia, and loss of 5% or more of body weight. Fortunately, most cases of NVP abate early in pregnancy: about 60% resolve within 13 weeks, and 90% resolve by the end of 20 weeks. Although NVP is commonly called *morning sickness,* it shouldn't be, because NVP can occur any time of the day, not just in the morning.

NVP can be managed with drugs and with nondrug measures. Nondrug measures include (1) eating small portions of food throughout the day; (2) avoiding odors, foods, and supplements that can trigger NVP (e.g., fatty foods, spicy foods, iron tablets); and (3) use of alternative treatments, such as acupuncture and ginger. Despite the use of these nondrug measures, about 10% of women require drug therapy.

PATIENT-CENTERED CARE ACROSS THE LIFE SPAN

Other Gastrointestinal Drugs

Life Stage	Patient Care Concerns
Infants	See *Breast-feeding Women* below.
Children/adolescents	Promethazine is a commonly used antiemetic in children, but it is contraindicated in children younger than 2 years. Other antiemetics, including dronabinol, are approved for nausea and vomiting in children. Side effects are similar to those that occur in adults.
Pregnant women	First-line therapy in NVP includes doxylamine and vitamin B_6 in addition to diet changes. Other alternatives include prochlorperazine, metoclopramide, and ondansetron. The use of chenodiol is contraindicated during pregnancy.
Breast-feeding women	Prochlorperazine and promethazine appear safe for short-term use while breast-feeding. Observe infant for sedation. Metoclopramide, dronabinol, and droperidol should be avoided while breast-feeding.
Older adults	Benzodiazepines, scopolamine, and metoclopramide should be avoided in the older adult.

First-line therapy consists of a two-drug combination: *doxylamine* plus *vitamin B_6 (pyridoxine)*. In randomized, controlled trials, the combination reduced NVP by 70% and showed no evidence of adverse fetal outcomes. Doxylamine and vitamin B_6 are available in a fixed-dose combination sold as *Diclectin* ♣, *Bonjesta,* and *Diclegis.* Diclegis is sold in delayed-release tablets containing 10 mg each of doxylamine and pyridoxine. Bonjesta is sold in delayed-release tablets containing 20 mg each of doxylamine and pyridoxine. Dosing starts with 2 tablets at bedtime for Diclegis or 1 tablet of Bonjesta. If doxylamine and vitamin B_6 fail to suppress NVP, alternatives include prochlorperazine, metoclopramide, and ondansetron. Methylprednisolone may be tried as a last resort, but only after 10 weeks of gestation (earlier use greatly increases the risk of cleft lip, with or without cleft palate).

DRUGS FOR MOTION SICKNESS

Motion sickness can be caused by sea, air, automobile, and space travel. Symptoms are nausea, vomiting, pallor, and cold sweats. Drug therapy is most effective when given prophylactically, rather than after symptoms begin.

Scopolamine

Scopolamine, a muscarinic antagonist, is our most effective drug for prevention and treatment of motion sickness. Benefits derive from suppressing nerve traffic in the neuronal pathway that connects the vestibular apparatus of the inner ear to the vomiting center (see Fig. 80.1). The most common side effects are dry mouth, blurred vision, and drowsiness. More severe but less common effects are urinary retention, constipation, and disorientation.

Scopolamine is available for oral, subcutaneous, and transdermal dosing. The transdermal system [Transderm Scōp], an adhesive patch that contains scopolamine, is applied behind the ear. Anticholinergic side effects with transdermal administration may be less intense than with oral or subcutaneous dosing.

Antihistamines

The antihistamines used most often for motion sickness are *dimenhydrinate, meclizine* [Antivert, others], and *cyclizine* [Cyclivert]. Because these drugs block receptors for acetylcholine in addition to receptors for histamine, they appear in Table 80.1 as a subclass under *Anticholinergics.* Suppression of motion sickness appears to result from blocking histaminergic (H_1) and muscarinic cholinergic receptors in the neuronal pathway that connects the inner ear to the vomiting center (see Fig. 80.1). The most prominent side effect—sedation—results from blocking H_1 receptors. Other side effects—dry mouth, blurred vision, urinary retention, and constipation—result from blocking muscarinic receptors. Antihistamines are less effective than scopolamine for treating motion sickness, and sedation further limits their utility.

ANTIDIARRHEAL AGENTS

Diarrhea is characterized by stools of excessive volume and fluidity and by increased frequency of defecation. Diarrhea is a symptom of GI disease and not a disease per se. Causes include infection, maldigestion, inflammation, and functional disorders of the bowel (e.g., irritable bowel syndrome). The most serious complications of diarrhea are dehydration and electrolyte depletion. Management is directed at (1) diagnosis and treatment of the underlying disease, (2) replacement of lost water and salts, (3) relief of cramping, and (4) reducing passage of unformed stools.

Antidiarrheal drugs fall into two major groups: (1) specific antidiarrheal drugs and (2) nonspecific antidiarrheal drugs. The specific agents are drugs that treat the underlying cause of diarrhea. Included in this group are anti-infective drugs and drugs used to correct malabsorption syndromes. Nonspecific antidiarrheals are agents that act on or within the bowel to provide symptomatic relief; these drugs do not influence the underlying cause.

Nonspecific Antidiarrheal Agents

Opioids

Opioids are our most effective antidiarrheal agents. By activating opioid receptors in the GI tract, these drugs decrease intestinal motility and thereby slow intestinal transit, which allows more time for absorption of fluid and electrolytes. In addition, activation of opioid receptors decreases secretion of fluid into the small intestine and increases absorption of fluid and salt. The net effect is to present the large intestine with less water. As a result, the fluidity and volume of stools are reduced, as is the frequency of defecation.

At the doses employed to relieve diarrhea, subjective effects and dependence do not occur. However, excessive doses *can* elicit typical morphine-like subjective effects. If severe overdose occurs, it should be treated with an opioid antagonist (e.g., naloxone). In patients with inflammatory bowel disease, opioids may cause toxic megacolon.

Several opioid preparations—diphenoxylate, difenoxin, loperamide, paregoric, and opium tincture—are approved for diarrhea. Of these, diphenoxylate [Lomotil, others] and loperamide [Imodium, others] are the most frequently employed. Pharmacologic properties of these agents are discussed next. Dosages for diarrhea are shown in Table 80.4.

Diphenoxylate. Diphenoxylate is an opioid used only for diarrhea. The drug is insoluble in water, and hence cannot be

TABLE 80.4 ▪ Opioids Used to Treat Diarrhea

Generic Name	Brand Name	CSA[a] Schedule	Antidiarrheal Dosage
Diphenoxylate (plus atropine)[b]	Lomotil	V	*Adults:* 5 mg, 4 times/day *Children (initial dosage):* Ages 2–5 yr: 1 mg, 4 times/day Ages 5–12 yr: 1–2 mg, 4 times/day
Difenoxin (plus atropine)[b]	Motofen	IV	*Adults:* 2 mg initially, then 1 mg after each loose stool
Loperamide	Imodium, Pepto Diarrhea Control, others	NR[c]	*Adults* (initial dose): 4 mg *Children (initial dosage):* Ages 2–5 yr: 1 mg, 3 times/day Ages 5–8 yr: 2 mg, 2 times/day Ages 8–12 yr: 2 mg, 3 times/day
Paregoric (camphorated tincture of opium; contains 0.4 mg morphine/mL)		III	*Adults:* 5–10 mL, 1–4 times/day *Children:* 0.25–0.5 mL/kg, 1–4 times/day
Opium tincture (opioid content equivalent to 10 mg morphine/mL)		II	*Adults:* 0.6 mL, 4 times/day

[a]Controlled Substances Act.
[b]Diphenoxylate and difenoxin are available only in combination with atropine. The atropine dose is subtherapeutic and is present to discourage abuse.
[c]Not regulated under the CSA.

abused by parenteral routes. When taken orally in antidiarrheal doses, diphenoxylate has no significant effect on the CNS. However, if taken in high doses, the drug can elicit typical morphine-like subjective effects.

Diphenoxylate is formulated in combination with atropine. The combination, best known as *Lomotil,* is available in tablets and an oral liquid. Each tablet or 5 mL of liquid contains 2.5 mg of diphenoxylate and 0.025 mg of atropine sulfate. The atropine is present to discourage diphenoxylate abuse: Doses of the combination that are sufficiently high to produce euphoria from the diphenoxylate would produce unpleasant side effects from the correspondingly high dose of atropine. Accordingly, the combination has a very low potential for abuse and is classified under Schedule V of the CSA.

Loperamide. Loperamide [Imodium, others] is a structural analog of meperidine. The drug is employed to treat diarrhea and to reduce the volume of discharge from ileostomies. Benefits derive from suppressing bowel motility and from suppressing fluid secretion into the intestinal lumen. The drug is poorly absorbed and does not readily cross the blood-brain barrier. Very large oral doses do not elicit morphine-like subjective effects. Loperamide has little or no potential for abuse and is not regulated under the CSA. The drug is supplied in 2-mg capsules, in 2-mg tablets, and in two liquid formulations (1 mg/5 mL and 1 mg/7.5 mL).

Difenoxin. Difenoxin is the major active metabolite of diphenoxylate. Like diphenoxylate, difenoxin can elicit morphine-like subjective effects at high doses. To discourage excessive dosing, difenoxin, like diphenoxylate, is formulated in combination with atropine. The combination is marketed as *Motofen.* Because its abuse potential is somewhat greater than that of diphenoxylate plus atropine, Motofen is classified as a Schedule IV product.

Paregoric. Paregoric (camphorated tincture of opium) is a dilute solution of opium, containing morphine (0.4 mg/mL) as its main active ingredient. The primary use is for diarrhea, although paregoric has the same approved uses as morphine. Antidiarrheal doses cause neither euphoria nor analgesia. Very high doses can cause typical morphine-like responses. Paregoric has a moderate potential for abuse and is classified under Schedule III of the CSA.

Opium Tincture. Opium tincture is an alcohol-based solution that contains 10% opium by weight. The principal active ingredient—morphine—is present at 10 mg/mL. The primary indication is diarrhea. In addition, opium tincture (after dilution) may be given to suppress symptoms of withdrawal in opioid-dependent neonates. When administered in antidiarrheal doses, opium tincture does not produce analgesia or euphoria. However, high doses can cause typical opioid agonist effects. Opium tincture has a high potential for abuse and is classified as a Schedule II agent.

Other Nonspecific Antidiarrheals

Bismuth Subsalicylate. Bismuth subsalicylate [Pepto-Bismol, others] is effective for the prevention and treatment of mild diarrhea. For prevention, the dosage is two 262-mg caplets 4 times a day for up to 3 weeks. For treatment, the dosage is 2 tablets every 30 minutes for up to eight doses. Users should be aware that the drug may blacken stools and the tongue.

Bulk-Forming Agents. Paradoxically, methylcellulose, polycarbophil, and other bulk-forming laxatives can help manage diarrhea. Benefits derive from making stools more firm and less watery. Stool volume is not decreased. The bulk-forming laxatives are discussed in Chapter 79.

Anticholinergic Antispasmodics. Muscarinic antagonists (e.g., atropine) can relieve cramping associated with diarrhea but do not alter fecal consistency or volume. However, owing to undesirable side effects (e.g., blurred vision, photophobia, dry mouth, urinary retention, tachycardia), anticholinergic drugs are of limited use. The pharmacology of the muscarinic blockers is discussed in Chapter 14.

Management of Infectious Diarrhea

General Considerations

Infectious diarrhea may be produced by enteric infection with a variety of bacteria and protozoa. These infections are usually self-limited. Mild diarrhea can be managed with nonspecific antidiarrheals. In many cases, no treatment is required at all. Antibiotics should be administered only when clearly indicated. Indiscriminate use of antibiotics is undesirable in that it (1) can promote emergence of antibiotic resistance and (2) can produce an asymptomatic carrier state by killing most, but not all, of the infectious agents. Conditions that *do* merit antibiotic treatment include severe infections with *Salmonella, Shigella, Campylobacter,* or *Clostridium.*

Traveler's Diarrhea

Tourists are often plagued by infectious diarrhea. This condition is known variously as Montezuma's revenge, the Aztec two-step, or Rangoon runs. In most cases, the causative organism is *Escherichia coli.* As a rule, treatment is unnecessary: Infection with *E. coli* is self-limited and will run its course in a few days. However, if symptoms are especially severe, treatment with one of the fluoroquinolone antibiotics—*ciprofloxacin* (500 mg twice daily) or *norfloxacin* (400 mg twice daily)—is indicated. *Azithromycin* [Zithromax] is preferred for children (10 mg/kg on day 1 and 5 mg/kg on days 2 and 3) and for pregnant women (1000 mg once or 500 mg once daily for 3 days). *Rifaximin* [Xifaxan] (200 mg 3 times a day for 3 days) may also be used, provided the patient is not pregnant or febrile, and that stools are not bloody. For patients with mild symptoms, relief can be achieved with *loperamide,* a nonspecific antidiarrheal. However, by slowing peristalsis, loperamide may delay export of the offending organism and may thereby prolong the infection.

Several measures can reduce acquisition of traveler's diarrhea. Two measures—avoiding local drinking water and carefully washing foods—are highly effective. Certain drugs—*ciprofloxacin* and *norfloxacin*—can be taken for prophylaxis. However, because these drugs can cause serious side effects, prophylaxis is not generally recommended. Lastly, travelers can be vaccinated against some pathogens. Oral vaccination with *Dukoral* 🍁 protects against diarrhea caused by *E. coli* and *Vibrio cholera.*

Clostridium Difficile–Associated Diarrhea

Clostridium difficile is a gram-positive, anaerobic bacillus that infects the bowel. Injury results from the release of bacterial toxins. Symptoms range from relatively mild (abdominal discomfort, nausea, fever, diarrhea) to very severe (toxic megacolon, pseudomembranous colitis, colon perforation, sepsis, and death). *C. difficile* infection and its treatment are discussed in Chapter 85.

DRUGS FOR IRRITABLE BOWEL SYNDROME

Irritable bowel syndrome (IBS) is the most common disorder of the GI tract, affecting an estimated 10% to 15% of Americans—about 45 million people. The incidence in women is 3 times the incidence in men. IBS is responsible for 12% of all visits to primary care physicians and 20% to 40% of all visits to gastroenterologists. The direct medical costs are estimated at $8 billion a year; the indirect costs are much higher—about $21 billion a year. IBS is second only to the common cold as the leading cause of days missed from work.

What is IBS? A GI disorder characterized by crampy abdominal pain—sometimes severe—occurring in association with diarrhea, constipation, or both. Formally, IBS is defined by the Rome IV criteria as presence, for at least 12 weeks in the past year, of abdominal pain or discomfort that cannot be explained by structural or chemical abnormalities and that has at least two of the following features:

- Pain is related to defecation.
- Onset was associated with a change in frequency of stool.
- Onset of pain occurred in association with a change in stool consistency (from normal to loose, watery, or pellet-like).

IBS has four major forms, characterized by either

- Abdominal pain in association with diarrhea (diarrhea-predominant IBS; IBS-D)
- Abdominal pain in association with constipation (constipation-predominant IBS; IBS-C)
- Abdominal pain in association with alternating episodes of diarrhea and constipation (mixed IBS; IBS-M)
- Abdominal pain in association with episodes of diarrhea and/or constipation that do not fit well into the other categories (IBS Unclassified)

No one knows what causes IBS. Despite extensive research, no underlying pathophysiologic mechanism has been identified. What we do know is that the bowel appears hypersensitive and hyperresponsive. As a result, mild stimuli that would have no effect on most people can trigger an intense response. In addition, we know that symptoms can be triggered by stress, depression, and dietary factors, including caffeine, alcohol, fried foods, high-fat foods, gas-generating vegetables (beans, broccoli, cabbage), and too much sorbitol, a sweetener found in chewing gum and some diet products. Overproduction of gastric acid and excessive bacterial colonization of the small intestine have also been implicated.

Fortunately, many people achieve significant relief with treatment. Nondrug measures and drug therapy are employed. Patients should keep a log to identify foods and stressors that trigger symptoms. Because large meals stretch and stimulate the bowel, switching to smaller, more frequent meals may help. Increasing dietary fluid and fiber may reduce constipation.

Two groups of drugs are used for treatment: nonspecific drugs and drugs specific for IBS. Both groups are discussed here.

Nonspecific Drugs

Four groups of drugs—*antispasmodics* (e.g., hyoscyamine, dicyclomine), *bulk-forming agents* (e.g., psyllium, polycarbophil), *antidiarrheals* (e.g., loperamide), and *tricyclic antidepressants* (TCAs)—have been employed for years to provide symptomatic relief. However, a report from the American College of Gastroenterology (ACG) concluded that, for most of these agents, there is no good proof of clinical benefits. Specifically, after reviewing available data, the authors concluded that loperamide and the bulk-forming agents are no better than placebo at relieving global symptoms of IBS. In contrast, they concluded that there is good evidence that TCAs can reduce abdominal pain and that this benefit is unrelated to the relief of depression. Regarding antispasmodic agents, they concluded that the available data are insufficient to make a recommendation for or against use.

Studies suggest that for some patients symptoms can be relieved with *antibiotics* or an *acid suppressant.* For example, in one study, researchers observed that many patients with IBS have excessive bacteria in the small intestine. When these people were treated with antibiotics, bacterial colonization was reduced, and so were symptoms of IBS. In a more recent study, treatment with oral rifaximin (a poorly absorbed, broad-spectrum antibiotic) reduced symptoms in some patients with IBS. Another study evaluated the impact of drugs that suppress production of stomach acid in patients who routinely experienced exacerbation of symptoms after eating. Two kinds of acid suppressants were used: proton pump inhibitors (lansoprazole or omeprazole) and histamine$_2$ receptor blockers (famotidine or ranitidine). In all cases, patients experienced a significant reduction of postprandial urgency and other symptoms. Benefits developed quickly (within days) and reversed when the drugs were stopped.

IBS-Specific Drugs

In this section we discuss the only three drugs approved for IBS. These are alosetron (approved for IBS-D), lubiprostone, and linaclotide (both approved for IBS-C).

Alosetron

Indications. Alosetron is approved only for the treatment of women with severe IBS-D that has lasted for 6 months or more and that has not responded to conventional treatment. IBS-D is considered severe if the patient experiences one or more of the following: (1) frequent and severe abdominal pain or discomfort, (2) frequent bowel urgency or fecal incontinence, and (3) disability or restriction of daily activities because of IBS. Less than 5% of IBS cases qualify as severe.

Mechanism of Action and Clinical Effects. Alosetron causes selective blockade of 5-HT$_3$ receptors, which are found primarily on neurons that innervate the viscera. In patients with IBS-D, alosetron can decrease abdominal pain, increase colonic transit time, reduce intestinal secretions, and increase absorption of water and sodium. As a result, the drug can increase stool firmness and decrease both fecal urgency and frequency. Presumably, all of these effects result from 5-HT$_3$ blockade. Symptoms decline 1 to 4 weeks after starting the drug and resume 1 week after stopping the drug.

Pharmacokinetics. Administration is oral, and absorption is rapid but incomplete (50% to 60%). Bioavailability is decreased by food. Plasma levels peak about 1 hour after dosing. Alosetron undergoes extensive metabolism by hepatic cytochrome P450 enzymes, followed by excretion primarily in the urine. The half-life is 1.5 hours.

Drug Interactions. Alosetron does not interact with theophylline, oral contraceptives, cisapride, ibuprofen, alprazolam, amitriptyline, fluoxetine, or hydrocodone combined with acetaminophen. Because alosetron is metabolized by cytochrome P450 enzymes, drugs that interfere with these enzymes (e.g., carbamazepine, phenobarbital, cimetidine, quinolone antibiotics, ketoconazole, clarithromycin, voriconazole, and protease inhibitors) may alter alosetron levels.

Adverse Effects and Contraindications. Although alosetron is generally well tolerated, it *can* cause severe adverse effects. Deaths have occurred. The most common problem is constipation (29%), which can be complicated by impaction, bowel obstruction, and perforation. In addition, alosetron can cause *ischemic colitis* (intestinal damage secondary to reduced blood flow). Ischemic colitis and complications of constipation have led to hospitalization, blood transfusion, surgery, and death. Owing to its potential for GI toxicity, alosetron is *contraindicated* for patients with ongoing constipation or a history of

- Chronic constipation, severe constipation, or sequelae from constipation
- Intestinal obstruction or stricture, toxic megacolon, or GI perforation or adhesions
- Ischemic colitis, impaired intestinal circulation, thrombophlebitis, or hypercoagulable state
- Crohn's disease or ulcerative colitis
- Diverticulitis

Risk Management Program. To ensure the best possible benefit/risk ratio, the manufacturer and the FDA have established a risk management program that involves active participation of the patient, prescriber, and pharmacist. The program emphasizes that

- Alosetron can cause potentially fatal GI toxicity.
- Only prescribers enrolled in the program can prescribe the drug.
- Alosetron is indicated only for women with severe, chronic IBS-D that has not responded to conventional therapy.
- Treatment should be discontinued immediately if constipation or signs of ischemic colitis develop.

Each enrolled *prescriber* must attest that he or she

- Is qualified to diagnose and treat IBS
- Is qualified to diagnose and manage ischemic colitis
- Is qualified to diagnose and manage constipation and complications of constipation
- Understands the risks and benefits of alosetron for IBS-D
- Agrees to educate the patient about risks and benefits of alosetron, will confirm that each patient has signed a Patient-Physician Agreement, and will give each patient a copy of that agreement and a copy of an alosetron Medication Guide
- Will report serious adverse events to the manufacturer or the FDA
- Will place a qualification sticker on all prescriptions for alosetron (Pharmacists must not fill prescriptions that lack the sticker.)

Each *patient* must sign a Patient-Physician Agreement, indicating that he or she

- Has been informed about and understands the severity of potential risks of alosetron treatment and understands the balance between risks and benefits
- Agrees to treatment with alosetron
- Will not take alosetron if he or she is constipated and will immediately discontinue alosetron and contact the prescriber if he or she becomes constipated or develops signs of ischemic colitis
- Will stop taking alosetron and call the prescriber if the drug does not control IBS symptoms after 4 weeks

Preparations, Dosage, and Administration. Alosetron [Lotronex] is supplied in 0.5- and 1-mg tablets. The recommended initial dosage is currently 0.5 mg twice daily. If, after 4 weeks, the dosage is well tolerated but inadequate, it can be increased to 1 mg twice a day. If, after 4 weeks at the higher dosage, treatment is still inadequate, the drug is not likely to help and should be stopped.

Patients who develop constipation or signs of ischemic colitis (rectal bleeding, bloody diarrhea, new or worsening abdominal pain) should immediately inform the prescriber and discontinue the drug. Those with ischemic colitis should never use alosetron again. Those with constipation may resume treatment, but only after constipation has resolved and only on the advice of the prescriber. If constipation does not resolve, the prescriber should be seen for evaluation.

Lubiprostone

Lubiprostone [Amitiza] is approved for IBS-C in women age 18 and older. Unfortunately, benefits are modest: The drug can reduce abdominal pain and discomfort, but only in a small percentage of patients. Efficacy against IBS-C in men has not been established. In addition to its use in IBS-C, lubiprostone is used for chronic idiopathic constipation (CIC) and opioid-induced constipation (OIC) in women and men. As discussed in Chapter 79, lubiprostone causes selective activation of chloride channels in epithelial cells of the intestine and thereby (1) promotes secretion of chloride-rich fluid into the intestinal lumen and (2) enhances motility of the small intestine and colon. The dosage for IBS-C is lower than for CIC and OIC: 8 mcg twice daily versus 24 mcg twice daily. As a result, compared with patients treated for CIC, patients treated for IBS-C experience less nausea (8% vs. 30%), diarrhea (7% vs. 13%), and chest discomfort (0.4% vs. 2.5%). To reduce the incidence of nausea, all doses should be taken with food and water.

Linaclotide

Therapeutic Use. Linaclotide [Linzess] is approved for the treatment of IBS-C and CIC. Linaclotide is related to the human hormones, uroguanylin and guanylin, and assists in the regulation of intestinal fluid secretion and motility by acting as a guanylate cyclase-C (GC-C) agonist. Activation of GC-C indirectly stimulates secretion of chloride and bicarbonate into the intestinal lumen. This results in increased intestinal fluid.

Adverse Effects and Drug Interactions. The most common adverse effect is diarrhea, which has been severe in some patients, leading to dehydration, hypovolemia, and hypotension. Most cases occur during the first 2 weeks of treatment. Patients who develop severe diarrhea should discontinue linaclotide. People with ongoing diarrhea and those who experience frequent diarrhea should not use the drug.

Linaclotide appears devoid of adverse interactions with other drugs.

Preparations, Dosage, and Administration. Linaclotide [Linzess] is formulated in 72-, 145-, and 290-mcg capsules for oral dosing. The recommended initial dosage is 290 mcg once daily for IBS-C. The dose is lower, 145 mcg daily, for treatment of CIC.

DRUGS FOR INFLAMMATORY BOWEL DISEASE

Inflammatory bowel disease (IBD) has two forms: *Crohn's disease* and *ulcerative colitis*. Crohn's disease is characterized by transmural inflammation; it usually affects the terminal ileum, but it can also affect all other parts of the GI tract. Ulcerative colitis is characterized by inflammation of the mucosa and submucosa of the colon and rectum. Both diseases produce abdominal cramps and diarrhea. Ulcerative colitis may cause rectal bleeding as well. About 15% of patients with ulcerative colitis eventually have an attack severe enough to require hospitalization for IV glucocorticoid therapy, which produces remission in 60% of patients; the remaining 40% usually require total colectomy. In the United States, IBD afflicts about 1.6 million people.

There is general agreement that IBD results from an exaggerated immune response directed against normal bowel flora—but only in genetically predisposed people.

Drug therapy of IBD is shown in Table 80.5. Five types of drugs are employed: *5-aminosalicylates* (e.g., sulfasalazine), *glucocorticoids* (e.g., hydrocortisone), *immunosuppressants* (e.g., azathioprine), *immunomodulators* (e.g., infliximab), and *antibiotics* (e.g., metronidazole). None of these drugs is curative;

TABLE 80.5 ▪ Therapeutic Options for Inflammatory Bowel Disease

Disease Intensity	Disease Form: Ulcerative Colitis	Disease Form: Crohn's Disease
Mild	5-Aminosalicylate: PO or rectal	Mesalamine: PO Metronidazole: PO Budesonide: PO Ciprofloxacin: PO
Moderate	5-Aminosalicylate: PO or rectal Infliximab: IV Vedolizumab: IV	Glucocorticoid: PO Azathioprine: PO Mercaptopurine: PO Infliximab: IV Certolizumab: subQ Adalimumab: subQ Natalizumab: IV Ustekinumab: IV Vedolizumab: IV
Severe	Glucocorticoid: PO or IV Cyclosporine: IV Infliximab: IV Vedolizumab: IV	Glucocorticoid: PO or IV Methotrexate: IV or subQ Infliximab: IV Certolizumab: subQ Adalimumab: subQ Natalizumab: IV Ustekinumab: IV Vedolizumab: IV
Refractory	Glucocorticoid: PO or IV Azathioprine: PO Mercaptopurine: PO Vedolizumab: IV	Infliximab: IV Certolizumab: subQ Adalimumab: subQ Natalizumab: IV Ustekinumab: IV
Remission	5-Aminosalicylate: PO Azathioprine: PO Mercaptopurine: PO	Mesalamine: PO Azathioprine: PO Metronidazole: PO Mercaptopurine: PO Infliximab: IV Certolizumab: subQ Adalimumab: subQ Natalizumab: IV

at best, drugs may control the disease process. Patients frequently require therapy with more than one agent.

5-Aminosalicylates

The 5-aminosalicylates are used to treat mild or moderate ulcerative colitis and Crohn's disease and to maintain remission after symptoms have subsided. Four aminosalicylates are available: sulfasalazine, mesalamine, olsalazine, and balsalazide.

Sulfasalazine

Sulfasalazine [Azulfidine] belongs to the same chemical family as the sulfonamide antibiotics. However, although similar to the sulfonamides, sulfasalazine is not employed to treat infections. Its only approved indications are IBD and rheumatoid arthritis (see Chapter 73).

Actions. Sulfasalazine is metabolized by intestinal bacteria into two compounds: 5-aminosalicylic acid (5-ASA) and sulfapyridine. 5-ASA is the component responsible for reducing inflammation; sulfapyridine is responsible for adverse effects. Possible mechanisms by which 5-ASA reduces inflammation include suppression of prostaglandin synthesis and suppression of the migration of inflammatory cells into the affected region.

Therapeutic Uses. Sulfasalazine is most effective against acute episodes of mild to moderate ulcerative colitis. Responses are less satisfactory when symptoms are severe. Sulfasalazine can also benefit patients with Crohn's disease.

Adverse Effects. Nausea, fever, rash, and arthralgia are common. Hematologic disorders (e.g., agranulocytosis, hemolytic anemia, macrocytic anemia) may also occur. Accordingly, complete blood counts should be obtained periodically. Sulfasalazine appears safe during pregnancy and lactation.

Preparations, Dosage, and Administration. Sulfasalazine [Azulfidine] is available in 500-mg immediate- and delayed-release oral tablets. The initial adult dosage is 1 to 2 gm/day. Maintenance dosages range from 2 to 4 gm/day, given in divided doses.

Mesalamine

Mesalamine [Apriso, Asacol HD, Canasa, Delzicol, Lialda, Pentasa, Rowasa] is the generic name for 5-ASA, the active component in sulfasalazine. The drug is used for acute treatment of mild to moderate IBD and for maintenance therapy of IBD. Mesalamine can be administered by retention enema, by rectal suppository, or by mouth (in tablets and capsules that dissolve when they reach the terminal ileum). Adverse effects are milder than with sulfasalazine. The most common side effects of *oral* therapy are headache and GI upset. The adult oral dosage is 800 mg 3 times a day (for Delzicol capsules), 1600 mg 3 times a day (Asacol HD tablets), *or* 1 gm 4 times a day (for Pentasa capsules) *or* 1.5 gm once a day (for Apriso capsules) *or* 2.4 to 4.8 gm once a day (for Lialda tablets). The 1000-mg rectal suppositories [Canasa] are administered once daily at bedtime. The retention enema [Rowasa] is administered once daily (4 gm in 60 mL).

Olsalazine

Olsalazine [Dipentum] is a dimer composed of two molecules of 5-ASA, the active component of sulfasalazine. Olsalazine is approved for maintenance therapy of ulcerative colitis in patients who can't tolerate sulfasalazine. The most common adverse effect is watery diarrhea, which occurs in 17% of patients. Other adverse effects include abdominal pain, cramps, acne, rash, and joint pain. Olsalazine is supplied in 250-mg oral capsules. The adult dosage is 500 mg twice daily with food.

Balsalazide

Balsalazide [Colazal, Giazo] is an aminosalicylate indicated for mildly to moderately active ulcerative colitis. As with sulfasalazine, colonic bacteria act on balsalazide to release 5-ASA, the active portion of the molecule. Nearly all of the drug remains in the intestine; less than 1% is absorbed. As a result, balsalazide is well tolerated. The most common adverse effects are headache, abdominal pain, diarrhea, and nausea. Balsalazide is available in 750-mg oral capsules sold as *Colazal* and 1.1-gm tablets sold as *Giazo*. The recommended dosage for Colazal is 3 capsules 3 times a day for 8 to 12 weeks. This dosage delivers 2.4 gm of free 5-ASA to the colon daily. Giazo dosing is 3 tablets 2 times a day for up to 8 weeks.

Glucocorticoids

The basic pharmacology of the glucocorticoids is presented in Chapters 60 and 72; discussion here is limited to their use in IBD. Glucocorticoids (e.g., dexamethasone, budesonide) can relieve symptoms of ulcerative colitis and Crohn's disease. Benefits derive from anti-inflammatory actions. Glucocorticoids are indicated primarily for induction of remission—not for long-term maintenance. Administration is IV or PO.

Safety Alert

GLUCOCORTICOIDS

Prolonged use of glucocorticoids can cause severe adverse effects, including adrenal suppression, osteoporosis, increased susceptibility to infection, and a cushingoid syndrome.

Oral *budesonide* [Entocort EC] is approved for mild to moderate Crohn's disease that involves the ileum and ascending colon. Entocort EC capsules are formulated to release budesonide when it reaches the ileum and ascending colon. As a result, high local concentrations are produced. Systemic effects are lower than with other glucocorticoids because absorbed budesonide undergoes extensive first-pass metabolism. Budesonide [Uceris] is also approved for the treatment of mild to moderate ulcerative colitis and is marketed as a 9-mg extended-release tablet.

Immunosuppressants

Immunosuppressants are used for long-term therapy of selected patients with ulcerative colitis and Crohn's disease. Clinical experience is greatest with azathioprine and mercaptopurine.

Thiopurines: Azathioprine and Mercaptopurine

These drugs are discussed together because one is the active form of the other. (Mercaptopurine is the active drug; azathioprine is a prodrug that undergoes conversion to mercaptopurine in the body.)

Although not approved for IBD, azathioprine [Imuran] and mercaptopurine [Purixan] have been employed with success to induce and maintain remission in both ulcerative colitis and Crohn's disease. Because onset of effects may be delayed for up to 6 months, these agents cannot be used for acute monotherapy. Furthermore, because these drugs are potentially more toxic than aminosalicylates or glucocorticoids, they are generally reserved for patients who have not responded to traditional therapy. Major adverse effects are pancreatitis and neutropenia (secondary to bone marrow suppression). At the doses used for IBD, these drugs are neither carcinogenic nor teratogenic. The basic pharmacology of azathioprine and mercaptopurine is discussed in Chapters 69 and 102, respectively.

Cyclosporine

Cyclosporine [Sandimmune, Neoral, Gengraf] is a stronger immunosuppressant than azathioprine or mercaptopurine and acts faster too. When used for IBD, the drug is generally reserved for patients with acute, severe ulcerative colitis or Crohn's disease that has not responded to glucocorticoids. For these patients, continuous IV infusion can rapidly induce remission. In addition to IV administration, the drug has been administered orally in low doses to maintain remission, but results have been inconsistent. Cyclosporine is a potentially toxic compound that can cause renal impairment, neurotoxicity, and generalized suppression of the immune system. The basic pharmacology of cyclosporine is discussed in Chapter 69.

Methotrexate

In patients with Crohn's disease, methotrexate can promote short-term remission and thereby reduce the need for glucocorticoids. Because the doses employed are low (25 mg once a week), the toxicity associated with high-dose therapy in cancer patients is avoided. The basic pharmacology of methotrexate is discussed in Chapter 102.

Immunomodulators

The six drugs discussed in this section are monoclonal antibody products that modulate immune responses. Three of these drugs—infliximab, certolizumab, and adalimumab—are inhibitors of *tumor necrosis factor-alpha* (TNF). We will discuss only the prototype, infliximab. The fourth and fifth drugs—natalizumab and vedolizumab—interfere with alpha$_4$ integrin. Finally, a new drug, ustekinumab, blocks the activity of interleukin-12 and interleukin-23. These drugs are generally considered second-line agents. However, some authorities now recommend their use early in treatment, with the hope of inducing remission quickly and maintaining remission longer, or as first-line agents in patients presenting with severe disease or perianal Crohn's disease.

Infliximab

Infliximab [Remicade] is a monoclonal antibody designed to neutralize TNF, a key immunoinflammatory modulator. The drug is indicated for moderate to severe Crohn's disease and ulcerative colitis. In clinical trials, infliximab reduced symptoms in 65% of patients with moderate to severe Crohn's disease and produced clinical remission in 33%. Good responses are also seen in ulcerative colitis. As discussed in Chapter 73, infliximab is also used for rheumatoid arthritis.

During clinical trials, 5% of patients dropped out because of serious adverse effects. Infections and infusion reactions are most common. Tuberculosis and opportunistic infections are of particular concern. Infusion reactions include fever, chills, pruritus, urticaria, and cardiopulmonary reactions (chest pain, hypotension, hypertension, dyspnea). Infliximab may also increase the risk of lymphoma, especially among patients with highly active disease or those on long-term immunosuppressive therapy.

Infliximab is supplied as a powder to be reconstituted for IV infusion. For patients with Crohn's disease or ulcerative colitis, treatment consists of an induction regimen (5 mg/kg infused at 0, 2, and 6 weeks) followed by maintenance infusions of 5 mg/kg every 8 weeks thereafter.

The basic pharmacology of infliximab is discussed in Chapter 73.

Natalizumab

Natalizumab [Tysabri] is a monoclonal antibody that interferes with alpha$_4$ integrin and thereby impedes migration of leukocytes from the vasculature into areas of inflammation. The drug is approved for Crohn's disease and multiple sclerosis. The pharmacology of natalizumab, including its dosage for Crohn's disease, is discussed in Chapter 23.

Ustekinumab

Ustekinumab [Stelara] was approved in 2016 for the treatment of moderate to severe Crohn's disease in patients who failed to respond to therapies previously listed. Ustekinumab is a monoclonal antibody that blocks activity of interleukin-12 and interleukin-23. These interleukins cause inflammation both independently and through stimulating the production of TNF.

Ustekinumab can increase the risk for infections, including diverticulitis, pneumonia, sepsis, and gastroenteritis. Use of ustekinumab can also activate latent infections such as tuberculosis. Other serious reactions to ustekinumab include hypersensitivity reactions, reversible posterior leukoencephalopathy syndrome (RPLS), and melanoma.

Ustekinumab is available in a 5-mg/mL single-dose vial for intravenous injection or a 90-mg/mL single-dose prefilled syringe for subQ injection. Recommended dosing includes an initial weight-based IV infusion followed by a 90-mg subQ injection every 8 weeks thereafter.

Antibiotics

Antibiotics, such as metronidazole and ciprofloxacin, can help control symptoms in patients with mild or moderate Crohn's disease. In contrast, antibiotics are largely ineffective against ulcerative colitis.

Metronidazole

In patients with mild or moderate Crohn's disease, metronidazole [Flagyl] is as effective as sulfasalazine. The dosages employed—up to 750 mg 3 times a day—are high. Furthermore, because relapse is likely if metronidazole is discontinued, long-term therapy is required. Unfortunately, prolonged use of high-dose metronidazole poses a risk of peripheral neuropathy. Although metronidazole can help patients with Crohn's disease, benefits are minimal in those with ulcerative colitis. The pharmacology of metronidazole is discussed in Chapter 91.

Ciprofloxacin

Like metronidazole, ciprofloxacin [Cipro] is highly effective in patients with mild or moderate Crohn's disease. A typical dosage is 500 mg twice daily. In one study, ciprofloxacin produced complete or partial remission in 72% of those treated. Combining ciprofloxacin with infliximab is superior to either drug used alone. Like metronidazole, ciprofloxacin is of little benefit in ulcerative colitis. The pharmacology of ciprofloxacin is presented in Chapter 91.

PROKINETIC AGENTS

Prokinetic drugs increase the tone and motility of the GI tract. Indications include gastroesophageal reflux disease (GERD), CINV, and diabetic gastroparesis.

Metoclopramide

Actions

Metoclopramide [Reglan, Metozolv] has two beneficial actions: it (1) suppresses emesis (by blocking receptors for dopamine and serotonin in the CTZ) and (2) increases upper GI motility (by enhancing the actions of acetylcholine).

Therapeutic Uses

Indications depend on the route (oral or IV). *Oral* metoclopramide has two approved uses: diabetic gastroparesis and suppression of gastroesophageal reflux. *Intravenous* metoclopramide has four approved uses: suppression of postoperative nausea and vomiting, suppression of CINV, facilitation of small bowel intubation, and facilitation of radiologic examination of the GI tract. Off-label uses include hiccups and nausea and vomiting of early pregnancy.

Adverse Effects

With high-dose therapy, sedation and diarrhea are common. Long-term high-dose therapy can cause irreversible *tardive dyskinesia,* characterized by repetitive, involuntary movements of the arms, legs, and facial muscles. Older adults are especially vulnerable. To reduce the risk of tardive dyskinesia, treatment should be as brief as possible using the lowest effective dose. Owing to its ability to increase gastric and intestinal motility, metoclopramide is contraindicated in patients with GI obstruction, perforation, or hemorrhage. Of note, exposure to metoclopramide during the first trimester of pregnancy is not associated with an excess risk of congenital malformations.

Preparations, Dosage, and Administration

Metoclopramide is available in four formulations: standard tablets (5 and 10 mg) sold as *Reglan,* orally disintegrating tablets (5 and 10 mg) sold as *Metozolv,* an oral syrup (1 mg/mL) sold generically, and a solution for injection (5 mg/mL). Dosage information follows.

Diabetic Gastroparesis. The adult dosage is 10 mg PO 30 minutes before each meal and at bedtime for 2 to 8 weeks. The maximum duration is 12 weeks.

Symptomatic Gastroesophageal Reflux. The usual adult dosage is 10 to 15 mg PO 30 minutes before each meal and at bedtime for a maximum of 12 weeks. If symptoms are sporadic, a single dose can be taken as needed (up to 20 mg PO 30 minutes before the precipitating situation).

Chemotherapy-Induced Nausea and Vomiting. For prophylaxis of CINV, metoclopramide is given IV, starting 30 minutes before chemotherapy. The initial dose is 1 to 2 mg/kg infused over 15 minutes or more. Additional doses of 1 to 2 mg/kg are administered 2, 4, 7, 10, and 13 hours after the first dose.

PALIFERMIN

Palifermin [Kepivance] is the first drug to be approved for decreasing oral mucositis (OM), a serious and painful complication of cancer chemoradiotherapy. For reasons discussed here, palifermin is currently indicated only for patients with hematologic malignancies. Side effects of the drug are generally mild.

Mechanism of Action

Palifermin is a synthetic form of human keratinocyte growth factor (KGF), a naturally occurring compound. Commercial production is by recombinant DNA technology. Palifermin acts through KGF receptors, which are found on epithelial cells in many structures, including the tongue, buccal mucosa, esophagus, stomach, intestine, salivary gland, liver, lung, pancreas, kidney, bladder, mammary glands, skin (hair follicles and sebaceous glands), and lens of the eye. Importantly, KGF receptors are *not* found on cells of hematopoietic origin. When palifermin binds with KGF receptors, it stimulates proliferation, differentiation, and migration of epithelial cells. In mice and rats, KGF increased the thickness of epithelial tissue in the tongue, buccal mucosa, and GI tract. Similarly, in healthy human volunteers, palifermin produced dose-dependent proliferation of epithelial cells in the buccal mucosa.

Indications and Clinical Benefits

Palifermin is approved for decreasing the incidence and duration of severe OM—but only in patients with *hematologic* malignancies, and then only in those receiving high-dose chemotherapy and whole-body irradiation (to eradicate cancer cells before a hematopoietic stem cell transplant). In one trial, palifermin reduced the incidence of OM (67% with palifermin vs. 80% with placebo) as well as the duration (4 days vs. 6 days with placebo). In a second trial, the results were similar: palifermin again reduced both the incidence of OM (63% vs. 98% with placebo) and the duration (6 days vs. 9 days with placebo). In both trials, palifermin reduced the need for pain relief with opioid analgesics and the need for supplemental parenteral nutrition.

At this time, palifermin therapy is restricted to patients with hematologic malignancies because, in experimental models, palifermin can stimulate proliferation of certain malignant cells of nonhematologic origin—specifically, malignant epithelial cells that bear KGF receptors. Palifermin is safe for patients with hematologic cancers because these cancers do not have KGF receptors. As we learn more about the safety of palifermin in nonhematologic cancers, indications for the drug may expand.

Pharmacokinetics

Information on the kinetics of palifermin is limited. Plasma levels of the drug decline by 95% within 30 minutes of IV dosing and decline at a slower rate thereafter. The terminal half-life is about 4.5 hours. Giving single doses on 3 consecutive days does result in drug accumulation.

Adverse Effects

Palifermin is generally well tolerated. The most common reactions concern the skin and mouth. Among these are rash, erythema, edema, pruritus, distortion of taste, thickening and/or discoloration of the tongue, and oral or perioral dysesthesias (unpleasant sensations produced by ordinary stimuli). The most serious reaction is skin rash, which develops in less than 1% of patients. In some patients, serum levels of amylase and lipase rise, suggesting possible injury to the pancreas. Because palifermin can stimulate epithelial growth in the lens, there is concern that it might affect vision.

Drug Interactions

Palifermin binds with *heparin.* Accordingly, before giving palifermin though an IV line, any heparin that might be present should be flushed out with saline.

If the interval between giving palifermin and anticancer drugs is too small, palifermin may *increase* the severity and duration of OM. Accordingly, dosing with palifermin should cease at least 24 hours before giving chemotherapy and should not resume for at least 24 hours after.

Preparations, Dosage, and Administration

Palifermin [Kepivance] is supplied as a powder (6.25 mg in single-dose vials) for reconstitution with 1.2 mL of sterile water for injection. Administration is by IV bolus. Dosing is done once daily on 3 consecutive days before chemotherapy and on 3 consecutive days after, for a total of six doses. Each dose is 60 mcg/kg. The first dose is given 3 to 4 days before chemotherapy (so that the third dose can be given 1 to 2 days before chemotherapy). The fourth is given at least 4 days after the third dose of palifermin, and at least 1 day after stem cell infusion. Palifermin should be stored under refrigeration, protected from light, and used immediately after reconstitution.

PANCREATIC ENZYMES

The pancreas produces three types of digestive enzymes: *lipases, amylases,* and *proteases.* These enzymes are secreted into the duodenum, where they help digest fats, carbohydrates, and proteins. To protect the enzymes from stomach acid and pepsin, the pancreas secretes bicarbonate. The bicarbonate neutralizes acid in the duodenum, and the resulting elevation in pH inactivates pepsin.

Deficiency of pancreatic enzymes can compromise digestion, especially digestion of fats. Fatty stools are characteristic of the deficiency. When secretion of pancreatic enzymes is reduced, replacement therapy is needed. Causes of deficiency include cystic fibrosis, pancreatectomy, pancreatitis, and obstruction of the pancreatic duct.

Pancreatic enzymes for clinical use are available as *pancrelipase,* a mixture of lipases, amylases, and proteases prepared from hog pancreas. Brand names are *Creon, Pancreaze, Pertzye, Ultresa, Viokase,* and *Zenpep.* All drugs, with the exception of Viokase, are supplied in delayed-release capsules designed to dissolve in the duodenum and upper jejunum. Viokase is supplied in tablets. The capsules should not be crushed, chewed, or retained in the mouth, owing to a risk of irritating the oral mucosa.

Pancrelipase is generally well tolerated. The most common adverse effects are abdominal discomfort, flatulence, headache, and cough. Large doses can cause diarrhea, nausea, and cramping. The most serious concern is *fibrosing colonopathy,* seen rarely during high-dose therapy in patients with cystic fibrosis. Porcine pancrelipase contains high levels of purines and hence may pose a risk to patients with gout or hyperuricemia. Allergic reactions occur occasionally.

Acid suppressants (e.g., histamine$_2$ receptor blockers, proton pump inhibitors) may be employed as adjuvants to pancreatic enzyme therapy. The objective is to raise gastric pH, protecting the enzymes from inactivation. However, acid suppressants are beneficial only when acid secretion is excessive.

Dosage is adjusted on an individual basis. Determining factors include the extent of enzyme deficiency, dietary fat content, and enzyme activity of the preparation selected. The efficacy of therapy can be evaluated by measuring the reduction in 24-hour fat excretion. Pancreatic enzymes should be taken with every meal and snack.

DRUGS USED TO DISSOLVE GALLSTONES

The gallbladder serves as a repository for bile, a fluid composed of cholesterol, bile acids, and other substances. Following production in the liver, bile may be secreted directly into the small intestine or it may be transferred to the gallbladder, where it is concentrated and stored.

Bile has two principal functions: It (1) aids in the digestion of fats, and (2) serves as the only medium by which cholesterol is excreted from the body. The acids in bile facilitate the absorption of fats. In addition, bile acids help solubilize cholesterol.

Cholelithiasis—development of gallstones—is the most common form of gallbladder disease. Most stones are formed from cholesterol. Stones made of cholesterol alone cannot be detected with x-rays and hence are said to be *radiolucent.* In contrast, stones that contain calcium (in addition to cholesterol) are *radiopaque* (i.e., they absorb x-rays and therefore can be seen in a radiograph). Risk factors for cholelithiasis include obesity and high plasma cholesterol.

For many people, gallstones can be present for years without causing symptoms. When symptoms do develop, they can be much like those of indigestion (bloating, abdominal discomfort, gassiness). If a stone becomes lodged in the bile duct, severe pain and jaundice can result.

Cholelithiasis may be treated by cholecystectomy (surgical removal of the gallbladder) or with drugs. As a rule, when intervention is required, cholecystectomy is preferred. In asymptomatic patients, more conservative measures (weight loss and reduced fat intake) may be indicated. Medications employed to dissolve gallstones are discussed next.

Chenodiol (Chenodeoxycholic Acid)

Actions

Chenodiol [Chenodal, Chenix] is a naturally occurring bile acid that reduces hepatic production of cholesterol. Reduced cholesterol production lowers the cholesterol content of bile, which in turn facilitates the gradual dissolution of cholesterol gallstones. Chenodiol may also increase the amount of bile acid in bile and may thereby enhance cholesterol solubility. It should be noted that chenodiol is useful only for dissolving radiolucent stones. Radiopaque stones (stones with significant calcium content) are not affected.

Therapeutic Use

Chenodiol is given to promote the dissolution of cholesterol gallstones, but only in carefully selected patients. Success is most likely in women who have low cholesterol levels, stones of small size, and the ability to tolerate high doses of the drug. Complete disappearance of stones occurs in only 20% to 40% of patients. Therapy is usually prolonged; 2 years is common.

Adverse Effects

Dose-dependent diarrhea occurs in 30% to 40% of patients. Of greater concern, chenodiol can injure the liver. Hence, patients must undergo periodic tests of liver function. Because chenodiol is hepatotoxic, the drug is contraindicated for patients with pre-existing liver disease. Chenodiol is also contraindicated during pregnancy (FDA Pregnancy Risk Category X[b]).

Ursodiol (Ursodeoxycholic Acid)

Ursodiol [Actigall, URSO 250, URSO forte] is an analog of chenodiol. Like chenodiol, ursodiol reduces the cholesterol content of bile, thereby facilitating the gradual dissolution of cholesterol gallstones. In contrast to chenodiol, ursodiol does not increase production of bile acids. Like chenodiol, ursodiol promotes dissolution of *radiolucent* gallstones but not radiopaque gallstones. Ursodiol is indicated for the dissolution of cholesterol gallstones in carefully selected patients.

Ursodiol is well tolerated. Significant adverse effects are rare. The drug is classified in FDA Pregnancy Risk Category B.[c]

Ursodiol is formulated in capsules (300 mg) and tablets (250 and 500 mg). The usual adult dosage for dissolving gallstones is 4 to 5 mg/kg twice daily (1 capsule or tablet in the morning and 1 in the evening). Treatment lasts for months.

[b]As of 2020, the FDA will no longer use Pregnancy Risk Categories. Please refer to Chapter 9 for more information.

[c]As of 2020, the FDA will no longer use Pregnancy Risk Categories. Please refer to Chapter 9 for more information.

ANORECTAL PREPARATIONS

Nitroglycerin for Anal Fissures

Rectogesic is a 0.4% nitroglycerin ointment used for relief of moderate to severe pain caused by chronic anal fissures (small tears in the skin that lines the anus). These fissures afflict about 700,000 Americans every year, often causing unrelenting and debilitating pain. Topical nitroglycerin relieves pain and promotes healing by relaxing the internal anal sphincter. Nitroglycerin ointment has been used in other countries for years and is considered by many experts to be a first-line therapy. The principal adverse effect is headache.

Other Anorectal Preparations

Various preparations can help relieve discomfort from hemorrhoids and other anorectal disorders. *Local anesthetics* (e.g., benzocaine, dibucaine) and *hydrocortisone* (a glucocorticoid) are common ingredients. Hydrocortisone suppresses inflammation, itching, and swelling. Local anesthetics reduce itching and pain. Anorectal preparations may also contain *emollients* (e.g., mineral oil, lanolin), whose lubricant properties reduce irritation, and *astringents* (e.g., bismuth subgallate, witch hazel, zinc oxide), which reduce irritation and inflammation. Anorectal preparations are available in multiple formulations: suppositories, creams, ointments, lotions, foams, tissues, and pads. Brand names include *Preparation H, Rectagene,* and *Anusol.*

KEY POINTS

- Emesis results from activation of the vomiting center, which receives its principal stimulatory inputs from the chemoreceptor trigger zone (CTZ), cerebral cortex, and inner ear.
- Serotonin antagonists, such as ondansetron [Zofran], are the most effective antiemetics available.
- Aprepitant (an antiemetic) is the first member of a new class of drugs: the substance P/neurokinin$_1$ receptor antagonists. Unlike most antiemetics, aprepitant can prevent *delayed* chemotherapy-induced nausea and vomiting (CINV) as well as *acute* CINV.
- To suppress CINV, a combination of drugs is more effective than monotherapy.
- For patients receiving highly emetogenic chemotherapy, the preferred antiemetic regimen consists of three drugs: aprepitant, a glucocorticoid (e.g., dexamethasone), and a serotonin antagonist (e.g., ondansetron).
- For management of CINV, antiemetics are more effective when given before chemotherapy (to prevent emesis) than when given after chemotherapy (in an effort to stop ongoing emesis).
- Nausea and vomiting develop in about 75% of pregnant patients, especially during the first trimester.
- First-line therapy for pregnancy-related nausea and vomiting consists of two drugs: doxylamine plus vitamin B_6 (pyridoxine).
- Opioids (e.g., diphenoxylate) are the most effective antidiarrheal agents available.
- Traveler's diarrhea can be treated with loperamide (a nonspecific antidiarrheal drug), a fluoroquinolone antibiotic (e.g., ciprofloxacin), or azithromycin (for children and pregnant women).
- Irritable bowel syndrome (IBS) is the most common disorder of the GI tract.
- Three drugs are FDA approved for IBS—alosetron, linaclotide, and lubiprostone.
- Alosetron is approved for IBS-D in women. Benefits derive from blocking 5-HT_3 receptors on neurons that innervate the viscera.
- Alosetron can cause ischemic colitis and severe constipation. Colitis and complications of constipation have led to hospitalization, blood transfusion, surgery, and death.
- Linaclotide is approved for IBS-C in adults. Constipation is treated through indirect stimulation of the secretion of chloride and bicarbonate into the intestinal lumen.
- Lubiprostone is approved for IBS-C in women. Benefits derive from activating (opening) chloride channels in the intestine.
- Inflammatory bowel disease—ulcerative colitis and Crohn's disease—is treated with 5-aminosalicylates (e.g., sulfasalazine, mesalamine), glucocorticoids (e.g., dexamethasone, budesonide), immunosuppressants (e.g., azathioprine, mercaptopurine), immunomodulators (e.g., infliximab, certolizumab), and antibiotics (e.g., metronidazole, ciprofloxacin).
- Metoclopramide, a prokinetic agent, has two beneficial actions: It increases upper GI motility and suppresses emesis.
- Palifermin is used to reduce the intensity and duration of oral mucositis in patients with hematologic malignancy undergoing intensive radiochemotherapy.

Please visit **http://evolve.elsevier.com/Lehne** for chapter-specific NCLEX® examination review questions.

UNIT XV NUTRITION

CHAPTER 81

Vitamins

Vitamins have the following defining characteristics: (1) they are *organic compounds,* (2) they are required in *minute amounts* for growth and maintenance of health, and (3) they do not serve as a source of energy (in contrast to fats, carbohydrates, and proteins), but rather are *essential for energy transformation and regulation of metabolic processes.* Several vitamins are inactive in their native form and must be converted to active compounds in the body.

BASIC CONSIDERATIONS

Dietary Reference Intakes

Reference values on dietary vitamin intake, as set by the Food and Nutrition Board of the Institute of Medicine of the National Academy of Sciences, were established to provide a standard for good nutrition. In a 2006 report—*Dietary Reference Intakes: The Essential Guide to Nutrient Requirements*—the Food and Nutrition Board defined five reference values: *Recommended Dietary Allowance* (RDA), *Adequate Intake* (AI), *Tolerable Upper Intake Level* (UL), *Estimated Average Requirement* (EAR), and *Acceptable Macronutrient Distribution Range* (AMDR). Collectively, these five values are referred to as *Dietary Reference Intakes* (DRIs). Of these, the RDA, AI, UL, and EAR apply to vitamins. (The AMDR is used for macronutrients such as fats and carbohydrates.)

Recommended Dietary Allowance

The RDA is the average daily dietary intake sufficient to meet the nutrient requirements of nearly all (97% to 98%) healthy individuals. These figures are not absolutes. RDAs change as we grow older. In addition, they often differ for males and females, and typically increase for women who are pregnant or breast-feeding. Furthermore, RDAs apply only to individuals in good health. Vitamin requirements can be increased by illness; therefore published RDA values may be inappropriate for sick people. RDAs, which are based on extensive experimental data, are revised periodically as new information becomes available. Current values are available at https://www.nal.usda.gov/fnic/dietary-reference-intakes.

Adequate Intake

The AI is an *estimate* of the average daily intake required to meet nutritional needs. AIs are employed when experimental evidence is not strong enough to establish an RDA. AIs are set with the expectation that they will meet the needs of all individuals. However, because AIs are only estimates, there is no guarantee they are adequate.

Tolerable Upper Intake Level

The UL is the highest average daily intake that can be consumed by nearly everyone without a significant risk for adverse effects. Please note that the UL is not a *recommended* upper limit for intake. It is simply an index of safety.

Estimated Average Requirement

The EAR is the level of intake that will meet nutritional requirements for 50% of the healthy individuals in any life-stage or gender group. By definition, the EAR may be insufficient for the other 50%. The EAR for a vitamin is based on extensive experimental data and serves as the basis for establishing an RDA. If there is not enough information to establish an EAR, no RDA can be set. Instead, an AI is assigned, using the limited data on hand.

Acceptable Macronutrient Distribution Range

The AMDR is a range for macronutrients (e.g., proteins, carbohydrates, fats) associated with optimal health. Intake of a nutrient below the established range for that nutrient increases the risk for malnourishment. Intake of a nutrient above the established range for that nutrient increases the risk for chronic diseases.

Classification of Vitamins

The vitamins are divided into two major groups: *fat-soluble vitamins* and *water-soluble vitamins*. In the fat-soluble group are vitamins A, D, E, and K. The water-soluble group consists of vitamin C and members of the vitamin B complex (thiamine, riboflavin, niacin, pyridoxine, pantothenic acid, biotin, folic acid, and cyanocobalamin). Except for vitamin B_{12}, water-soluble vitamins undergo minimal storage in the body, and hence frequent ingestion is needed to replenish supplies. In contrast, fat-soluble vitamins can be stored in massive amounts, which is good news and bad news. The good news is that extensive storage minimizes the risk for deficiency. The bad news is that extensive storage greatly increases the potential for toxicity if intake is excessive.

Should We Take Multivitamin Supplements?

In the United States, we spend about $3.5 billion a year on multivitamin and multimineral supplements. Is the money well spent? Maybe. Maybe not. A panel of experts convened by the Office of Dietary Supplements at the National Institutes of Health reports that there is insufficient evidence to recommend either for or against the use of multivitamins by Americans to prevent chronic disease. As one official put it, "If you're taking a multivitamin, there's no reason to stop—but if you're not taking a multivitamin, there's no reason to start, either."

For people who *do* take a multivitamin supplement, the dosage should be moderate because excessive doses can cause harm. For example, too much vitamin A increases the risk for osteoporosis in postmenopausal women and can cause birth defects when taken early in pregnancy. In older people with chronic health problems, too much vitamin E increases the risk for death. Because of these and other concerns, high-dose multivitamin supplements should be avoided. Instead, supplements that supply 100% or *less* of the RDA should be used.

Although research supporting the use of *multi*vitamin supplements is inconclusive, we do have solid data supporting the use of three *individual* vitamins—vitamin B_{12}, folic acid, and vitamin D. Who should take these vitamins? Nutrition experts recommend vitamin B_{12} for all people over age 50, folic acid for all women of childbearing age, and vitamin D (plus calcium) for postmenopausal women and other people at risk for fractures.

FAT-SOLUBLE VITAMINS

Vitamin A (Retinol)

Actions

Vitamin A, also known as retinol, has multiple functions. In the eye, vitamin A plays an important role in adaptation to dim light. The vitamin also has a role in embryogenesis, spermatogenesis, immunity, growth, and in maintaining the structural and functional integrity of the skin and mucous membranes.

Sources

Requirements for vitamin A can be met by (1) consuming foods that contain *preformed vitamin A* (retinol) and (2) consuming foods that contain *provitamin A carotenoids* (beta-carotene, alpha-carotene, beta-cryptoxanthin), which are converted to retinol by cells of the intestinal mucosa. Preformed vitamin A is present only in foods of animal origin. Good sources are dairy products, meat, fish oil, and fish. Provitamin A carotenoids are found in darkly colored, carotene-rich fruits and vegetables. Especially rich sources are carrots, cantaloupe, mangoes, spinach, tomatoes, pumpkins, and sweet potatoes.

Units

The unit employed to measure vitamin A activity is called the *retinol activity equivalent* (RAE). By definition, 1 RAE equals 1 mcg of retinol, 12 mcg of beta-carotene, 24 mcg of alpha-carotene, or 24 mcg of beta-cryptoxanthin. Why are the RAEs for the provitamin A carotenoids 12 to 24 times higher than the RAE for retinol? Because dietary carotenoids are poorly absorbed and incompletely converted into retinol. Hence, to produce the nutritional equivalent of retinol, we need to ingest much higher amounts of the carotenoids. In the past, vitamin A activity was measured in international units (IU). This IU designation is still commonly used on product labels.

Requirements

The current RDA for vitamin A for adult males is 900 RAEs, and the RDA for adult females is 700 RAEs. RDAs for individuals in other life-stage groups are shown in Table 81.1.

Pharmacokinetics

Under normal conditions, dietary vitamin A is readily absorbed and then stored in the liver. As a rule, liver reserves of vitamin A are large and will last for months if intake of retinol ceases. Normal plasma levels for retinol range between 30 and 70 mcg/dL. In the absence of vitamin A intake, levels are maintained through mobilization of liver reserves. As liver stores approach depletion, plasma levels begin to decline. Signs and symptoms of deficiency appear when plasma levels fall below 20 mcg/dL.

Deficiency

Because vitamin A is needed for dark adaptation, night blindness is often the first indication of deficiency. With time, vitamin A deficiency may lead to *xerophthalmia* (a dry, thickened condition of the conjunctiva) and *keratomalacia* (degeneration of the cornea with keratinization of the corneal epithelium). When vitamin A deficiency is severe, blindness may occur. In addition to effects on the eye, deficiency can produce skin lesions and dysfunction of mucous membranes.

Toxicity

In high doses, vitamin A can cause birth defects, liver injury, and bone-related disorders. To reduce risk, the Food and Nutrition Board has set the UL for vitamin A at 3000 mcg/day.

Safety Alert

VITAMIN A IN PREGNANCY

Vitamin A is highly teratogenic. Excessive intake during pregnancy can cause malformation of the fetal heart, skull, and other structures of cranial–neural crest origin. Pregnant women should definitely not exceed the UL for vitamin A and should probably not exceed the RDA.

TABLE 81.1 ■ Recommended Vitamin Intakes for Individuals

Life-Stage Group	Recommended Vitamin Intake Per Day												
	Vitamin A (mcg)[a]	Vitamin C (mg)	Vitamin D (IU)[b,c]	Vitamin E (mg)[d]	Vitamin K (mcg)	Thiamine (mg)	Riboflavin (mg)	Niacin (mg)[e]	Vitamin B_6 (mg)	Folate (mcg)[f]	Vitamin B_{12} (mcg)	Pantothenic Acid (mg)	Biotin (mcg)
INFANTS													
0–6 mo	400*	40*	400*	4*	2*	0.2*	0.3*	2*	0.1*	65*	0.4*	1.7*	5*
7–12 mo	500*	50*	400*	5*	2.5*	0.3*	0.4*	4*	0.3*	80*	0.5*	1.8*	6*
CHILDREN													
1–3 yr	**300**	**15**	**600**	**6**	30*	**0.5**	**0.5**	**6**	**0.5**	**150**	**0.9**	2*	8*
4–8 yr	**400**	**25**	**600**	**7**	55*	**0.6**	**0.6**	**8**	**0.6**	**200**	**1.2**	3*	12*
MALES													
9–13 yr	**600**	**45**	**600**	**11**	60*	**0.9**	**0.9**	**12***	**1**	**300**	**1.8**	4*	20*
14–18 yr	**900**	**75**	**600**	**15**	75*	**1.2**	**1.3**	**16**	**1.3**	**400**	**2.4**	5*	25*
19–30 yr	**900**	**90**	**600**	**15**	120*	**1.2**	**1.3**	**16**	**1.3**	**400**	**2.4**	5*	30*
31–50 yr	**900**	**90**	**600**	**15**	120*	**1.2**	**1.3**	**16**	**1.3**	**400**	**2.4**	5*	30*
51–70 yr	**900**	**90**	**600**	**15**	120*	**1.2**	**1.3**	**16**	**1.7**	**400**	**2.4**[g]	5*	30*
> 70 yr	**900**	**90**	**800**	**15**	120*	**1.2**	**1.3**	**16**	**1.7**	**400**	**2.4**[g]	5*	30*
FEMALES													
9–13 yr	**600**	**45**	**600**	**11**	60*	**0.9**	**0.9**	**12**	**1**	**300**	**1.8**	4*	20*
14–18 yr	**700**	**65**	**600**	**15**	75*	**1**	**1**	**14**	**1.2**	**400**[h]	**2.4**	5*	25*
19–30 yr	**700**	**75**	**600**	**15**	90*	**1.1**	**1.1**	**14**	**1.3**	**400**[h]	**2.4**	5*	30*
31–50 yr	**700**	**75**	**600**	**15**	90*	**1.1**	**1.1**	**14**	**1.3**	**400**[h]	**2.4**	5*	30*
51–70 yr	**700**	**75**	**600**	**15**	90*	**1.1**	**1.1**	**14**	**1.5**	**400**	**2.4**[g]	5*	30*
> 70 yr	**700**	**75**	**800**	**15**	90*	**1.1**	**1.1**	**14**	**1.5**	**400**	**2.4**[g]	5*	30*

DURING PREGNANCY													
≤ 18 yr	**750**	**80**	**600**	**15**	75*	**1.4**	**1.4**	**18**	**1.9**	**600**[i]	**2.6**	6*	30*
19–30 yr	**770**	**85**	**600**	**15**	90*	**1.4**	**1.4**	**18**	**1.9**	**600**[i]	**2.6**	6*	30*
31–50 yr	**770**	**85**	**600**	**15**	90*	**1.4**	**1.4**	**18**	**1.9**	**600**[i]	**2.6**	6*	30*
DURING LACTATION													
≤ 18 yr	**1200**	**115**	**600**	**19**	75*	**1.4**	**1.6**	**17**	**2**	**500**	**2.8**	7*	35*
19–30 yr	**1300**	**120**	**600**	**19**	90*	**1.4**	**1.6**	**17**	**2**	**500**	**2.8**	7*	35*
31–50 yr	**1300**	**120**	**600**	**19**	90*	**1.4**	**1.6**	**17**	**2**	**500**	**2.8**	7*	35*

NOTE: This table presents recommended dietary allowances (RDAs) in **bold type** and adequate intakes (AIs) in ordinary type followed by an asterisk (*). RDAs and AIs may both be used as goals for individual intake. RDAs are set to meet the needs of almost all (97% to 98%) individuals in a group. For healthy breast-fed infants, the AI is the mean intake. The AI for other life-stage and gender groups is believed to cover needs of all individuals in the group, but lack of data or uncertainty in the data prevent being able to specify with confidence the percentage of individuals covered by this intake.

[a]As retinol activity equivalents (RAEs): 1 RAE = 1 mcg retinol, 12 mcg beta-carotene, 24 mcg alpha-carotene, or 24 mcg beta-cryptoxanthin. To calculate RAEs from retinol equivalents (REs) of provitamin A carotenoids in foods, divide the REs by 2. For preformed vitamin A in foods or supplements and for provitamin A carotenoids in supplements, 1 RE = 1 RAE.

[b]These new RDAs and AIs were issued by the Institute of Medicine on November 30, 2010.

[c]In the absence of adequate exposure to sunlight.

[d]As alpha-tocopherol. Alpha-tocopherol includes *RRR*-alpha-tocopherol, the only form of alpha-tocopherol that occurs naturally in foods, and the 2R-stereoisomeric forms of alpha-tocopherol (*RRR*-, *RSR*-, *RRS*-, and *RSS*-alpha-tocopherol) that occur in fortified foods and supplements. It does not include the 2S-stereoisomeric forms of alpha-tocopherol (*SRR*-, *SSR*-, *SRS*-, and *SSS*-alpha-tocopherol), also found in fortified foods and supplements.

[e]As niacin equivalents (NE): 1 mg of niacin = 60 mg of tryptophan; 0 to 6 months = preformed niacin (not NE).

[f]As dietary folate equivalents (DFEs): 1 DFE = 1 mcg food folate = 0.6 mcg of folic acid from fortified food or as a supplement consumed with food = 0.5 mcg of a supplement taken on an empty stomach.

[g]Because 10% to 30% of older people may absorb food-bound B_{12} poorly, it is advisable for those older than 50 years to meet their RDA mainly by consuming foods fortified with B_{12} or by consuming a supplement containing B_{12}.

[h]In view of evidence linking folate deficiency with neural tube defects in the fetus, the U.S. Preventive Services Task Force recommends that all women capable of becoming pregnant consume 400 to 800 mcg from supplements in addition to intake of folate from a varied diet.

[i]It is assumed that women will continue to consume 400 mcg from supplements or fortified food until their pregnancy is confirmed and they enter prenatal care, which ordinarily occurs after the end of the periconceptional period—the critical time for formation of the neural tube.

Data from Food and Nutrition Board, Institute of Medicine. Dietary Reference Intakes (DRIs): *Recommended dietary allowances and adequate intakes, vitamins.* Washington, DC: National Academy Press, 2011.

Excessive doses can cause a toxic state, referred to as *hypervitaminosis A*. Chronic intoxication affects multiple organ systems, especially the liver. Symptoms are diverse and may include vomiting, jaundice, hepatosplenomegaly, skin changes, hypomenorrhea, and elevation of intracranial pressure. Most symptoms disappear after vitamin A withdrawal.

Vitamin A excess can damage bone. In infants and young children, vitamin A can cause bulging of the skull at sites where bone has not yet formed. In adult females, too much vitamin A can increase the risk for hip fracture—apparently by blocking the ability of vitamin D to enhance calcium absorption.

Therapeutic Uses

The only indication for vitamin A is prevention or correction of vitamin A deficiency. Contrary to earlier hopes, it is now clear that vitamin A, in the form of beta-carotene supplements, does not decrease the risk for cancer or cardiovascular disease. In fact, in a study comparing placebo with dietary supplements (beta-carotene plus vitamin A), subjects taking the supplements had a significantly *increased* risk for lung cancer and overall mortality. As discussed in Chapter 105, certain derivatives of vitamin A (e.g., isotretinoin, etretinate) are used to treat acne and other dermatologic disorders.

Preparations, Dosage, and Administration

Vitamin A (retinol) is available in drops, tablets, and capsules for oral dosing and in solution for intramuscular (IM) injection. Oral dosing is generally preferred. To *prevent* deficiency, dietary plus supplemental vitamin A should add up to the RDA. To *treat* deficiency, doses up to 100 times the RDA may be required.

Vitamin D

Vitamin D plays a critical role in calcium metabolism and maintenance of bone health. The classic effects of deficiency are *rickets* (in children) and *osteomalacia* (in adults). Does vitamin D offer health benefits beyond bone health? Possibly. Studies suggest that vitamin D may protect against the development of arthritis, diabetes type 1, heart disease, autoimmune disorders, and cancers of the colon, breast, and prostate. However, in a 2011 report—*Dietary Reference Intakes for Calcium and Vitamin D*—an expert panel concluded that although such claims might eventually prove true, the current evidence does not prove any benefits beyond bone health. The pharmacology and physiology of vitamin D are discussed in Chapter 75. Values for RDAs and adequate intake are shown in Table 81.1.

Vitamin E (Alpha-Tocopherol)

Vitamin E (alpha-tocopherol) is essential to the health of many animal species, but has no clearly established role in human nutrition. Unlike other vitamins, vitamin E has no known role in metabolism. Deficiency, which is rare, can result in neurologic deficits.

Vitamin E helps maintain health primarily through antioxidant actions. Specifically, the vitamin helps protect against peroxidation of lipids. It also inhibits oxidation of vitamins A and C. Observational studies in the past suggested that vitamin E protected against cardiovascular disease, Alzheimer's disease, and cancer. However, more rigorous studies have failed to show any such benefits (Box 81.1). Moreover, there *is* evidence

si **BOX 81.1 ▪ SPECIAL INTEREST TOPIC**

THE INCREASINGLY STRONG CASE AGAINST ANTIOXIDANTS

What are antioxidants? Dietary antioxidants are defined as substances present in food that can significantly decrease cellular and tissue injury caused by highly reactive forms of oxygen and nitrogen, known as *free radicals*. These free radicals, which are normal byproducts of metabolism, readily react with other molecules. The result is tissue injury known as *oxidative stress*. Antioxidants help reduce oxidative stress by neutralizing free radicals before they can cause harm.

Do megadoses of antioxidants protect against chronic disease? If we can believe what we read in magazine articles, popular advertisements, and product labels, it would seem so. However, much of this is information carried over from assumptions made a quarter century ago.

Nearly all early studies on antioxidants were observational. These studies indicated that daily consumption of vegetables rich in antioxidants was associated with a reduced risk for heart disease and several types of cancer. The problem is, these results have more than one interpretation. Were the antioxidants the reason for the improved health outcomes? Or was it possible that protection was conferred by some other component of the diet (e.g., high fiber content, low cholesterol and saturated-fat content)? Or could it be that protection resulted from a generally healthy lifestyle that included a diet rich in fruits and vegetables? Although observational studies demonstrated a link between a healthy diet and decreases in heart disease and cancer, it became clear that one could not extrapolate from these observations that antioxidants were responsible.

Despite plausible theories and observational studies that provided support for protective effects of antioxidants, more recent and more rigorous trials have failed to show protection against heart disease, cancer, or any other long-term illness. The National Center for Complementary and Alternative Medicine examined well-designed experimental studies that included more than 100,000 subjects and concluded that most studies failed to demonstrate a role for antioxidant-related reduction in disease development. Further, they identified that high doses of certain antioxidants might actually increase the risk for disease. For example, high doses of beta-carotene were associated with an increase of lung cancer in people who smoked, and high doses of vitamin E were associated with an increase of prostate cancer and stroke. Additionally, some antioxidant supplements were responsible for drug interactions.

What's the bottom line? The National Academy of Sciences recommends limiting intake of antioxidant supplements to amounts that will prevent nutritional deficiency and avoiding doses that are potentially harmful. Of course, people should continue to eat a healthy diet.

that high-dose vitamin E may actually increase the risk for heart failure, cancer progression, and all-cause mortality.

Forms of Vitamin E

Vitamin E exists in a variety of forms (e.g., alpha-tocopherol, beta-tocopherol, alpha-tocotrienol), each of which has multiple stereoisomers. However, only four stereoisomers are found in our blood, all of them variants of *alpha-tocopherol*. These isomers are designated *RRR-*, *RRS-*, *RSR-*, and *RSS*-alpha-tocopherol. Of the four, only *RRR-alpha-tocopherol* occurs naturally in foods. However, all four can be found in fortified foods and dietary supplements. Why are other forms of vitamin E absent from blood? Because they are unable to bind to *alpha-tocopherol transfer protein* (alpha-TTP), the hepatic protein required for secretion of vitamin E from the liver and subsequent transport throughout the body.

Sources

Most dietary vitamin E comes from vegetable oils (e.g., corn oil, olive oil, cottonseed oil, safflower oil, canola oil). The vitamin is also found in nuts, wheat germ, whole-grain products, and mustard greens.

Requirements

The RDA for vitamin E, for men and women, is 15 mg/day (22.5 IU). RDAs increase for women who are breast-feeding, but not for those who are pregnant. Taking more than 200 mg/day increases the risk for hemorrhagic stroke. Accordingly, this limit should be exceeded only when there is a need to manage a specific disorder (e.g., advanced macular degeneration) and only when advised by a healthcare professional.

Deficiency

Vitamin E deficiency is rare. In the United States, deficiency is limited primarily to people with an inborn deficiency of alpha-TTP and to those who have fat malabsorption syndromes, and hence cannot absorb fat-soluble vitamins. Symptoms of deficiency include ataxia, sensory neuropathy, areflexia, and muscle hypertrophy.

Potential Benefits

Vitamin E has a role in protecting red blood cells from hemolysis. There is evidence that 200 IU of vitamin E daily may reduce the risk for colds in older adults and that 400 IU daily (in combination with vitamin C, beta-carotene, zinc, and copper) may delay the progression of age-related macular degeneration. The higher dose associated with halting macular degeneration carries substantial risk, as detailed in the next section.

Potential Risks

High-dose vitamin E appears to increase the risk for hemorrhagic stroke by inhibiting platelet aggregation. According to a 2010 report, for every 10,000 people taking more than 200 IU of vitamin E daily for 1 year, there would be 8 additional cases of hemorrhagic stroke. Accordingly, doses higher than 200 IU/day should generally be avoided.

Some studies have demonstrated a relationship between high doses of vitamin E (400 IU daily) and increased cancer risk or poor cancer outcomes. These results are consistent with the theory that high doses of antioxidants may cause cancer or accelerate cancer progression.

Studies have also linked *high-dose* vitamin E therapy with an increased risk for death, especially in older people. Others have demonstrated higher mortality with *long-term* vitamin E therapy at doses higher than 400 IU (266 mg). Accordingly, recommendations have been put forward to decrease the current UL of 1500 IU daily to 200 IU daily.

Finally, high-dose vitamin E (in combination with vitamin C) can blunt the beneficial effects of exercise on insulin sensitivity. Under normal conditions, exercising enhances cellular responses to insulin. However, among subjects who took vitamin E (400 IU/day) plus vitamin C (500 mg twice daily), exercising failed to yield this benefit.

Vitamin K

Action

Vitamin K is required for the synthesis of prothrombin and clotting factors VII, IX, and X. All of these vitamin K–dependent factors are needed for coagulation of blood.

Forms and Sources of Vitamin K

Vitamin K occurs in nature in two forms: (1) vitamin K_1, or phytonadione (phylloquinone) and (2) vitamin K_2. Phytonadione is present in a wide variety of foods. Vitamin K_2 is synthesized by the normal flora of the gut. Two other forms—vitamin K_4 (menadiol) and vitamin K_3 (menadione)—are produced synthetically. At this time, phytonadione is the only form of vitamin K available for therapeutic use.

Requirements

Human requirements for vitamin K have not been precisely defined. In 2002, the Food and Nutrition Board set the AI for adult males at 120 mcg and the AI for adult females at 90 mcg. AIs for other life-stage groups are shown in Table 81.1. For most individuals, vitamin K requirements are readily met through dietary sources and through vitamin K synthesized by intestinal bacteria. Because bacterial colonization of the gut is not complete until several days after birth, levels of vitamin K may be low in newborns.

Pharmacokinetics

Intestinal absorption of the natural forms of vitamin K (phytonadione and vitamin K_2) is adequate only in the presence of bile salts. Menadione and menadiol do not require bile salts for absorption. After absorption, vitamin K is concentrated in the liver. Metabolism and secretion occur rapidly. Very little is stored.

Deficiency

Vitamin K deficiency produces bleeding tendencies. If the deficiency is severe, spontaneous hemorrhage may occur. In newborns, intracranial hemorrhage is of particular concern.

An important cause of deficiency is reduced absorption. Because the natural forms of vitamin K require bile salts for their uptake, any condition that decreases availability of these salts (e.g., obstructive jaundice) can lead to deficiency. Malabsorption syndromes (sprue, celiac disease, cystic fibrosis of the pancreas) can also decrease vitamin K uptake. Other potential causes of impaired absorption are ulcerative colitis, regional enteritis, and surgical resection of the intestine.

A disruption of intestinal flora may result in deficiency by eliminating vitamin K–synthesizing bacteria. Hence, deficiency may occur secondary to the use of antibiotics. In infants, diarrhea may cause bacterial losses sufficient to result in deficiency.

The normal infant is born vitamin K deficient. Consequently, to rapidly elevate prothrombin levels and reduce the risk for neonatal hemorrhage, the American Academy of Pediatrics and the Centers for Disease Control and Prevention recommend that all infants receive a single injection of phytonadione (vitamin K_1) immediately after delivery. This previously routine prophylactic intervention has recently been challenged by parents who believe that the risks outweigh the benefits. Subsequent to increases in parents declining prophylaxis, there has been an increase in life-threatening vitamin K deficiency bleeding in recent years.

As discussed in Chapter 52, the anticoagulant warfarin acts as an antagonist of vitamin K and thereby decreases synthesis of vitamin K–dependent clotting factors. As a result, warfarin produces a state that is functionally equivalent to vitamin K deficiency. If the dosage of warfarin is excessive, hemorrhage can occur secondary to lack of prothrombin.

Adverse Effects

Severe Hypersensitivity Reactions. Intravenous (IV) phytonadione can cause serious reactions (shock, respiratory arrest, cardiac arrest) that resemble anaphylaxis or hypersensitivity reactions. Death has occurred. Consequently, phytonadione should not be administered by the IV route unless other routes are not feasible, and then only if the potential benefits clearly outweigh the risks.

Hyperbilirubinemia. When administered *parenterally* to newborns, vitamin K derivatives can elevate plasma levels of bilirubin, thereby posing a risk for *kernicterus.* The incidence of hyperbilirubinemia is greater in premature infants than in full-term infants. Although all forms of vitamin K can raise bilirubin levels, the risk is higher with menadione and menadiol than with phytonadione.

Therapeutic Uses and Dosage

Vitamin K has two major applications: (1) correction or prevention of hypoprothrombinemia and bleeding caused by vitamin K deficiency and (2) control of hemorrhage caused by warfarin.

Vitamin K Replacement. As discussed, vitamin K deficiency can result from impaired absorption and from insufficient synthesis of vitamin K by intestinal flora. Rarely, deficiency results from inadequate diet. For children and adults, the usual dosage for correction of vitamin K deficiency ranges between 5 and 15 mg/day.

As noted, infants are born vitamin K deficient. To prevent hemorrhagic disease in neonates, it is recommended that all newborns be given an injection of phytonadione (0.5 to 1 mg) immediately after delivery.

Warfarin Antidote. Vitamin K reverses hypoprothrombinemia and bleeding caused by excessive dosing with warfarin, an oral anticoagulant. Bleeding is controlled within hours of vitamin K administration (see Chapter 52 for dosage).

Preparations and Routes of Administration

Phytonadione (vitamin K_1) is available in 5-mg tablets, marketed as *Mephyton,* and in parenteral formulations (2 and 10 mg/mL) sold generically. Parenteral phytonadione may be administered by IM, subcutaneous (subQ), and IV routes. However, because IV administration is dangerous, this route should be used only when other routes are not feasible and only if the perceived benefits outweigh the substantial risks. For example, this might be indicated in the management of life-threatening bleeding due to vitamin K antagonists (e.g., poisoning by coumarins in rodenticides).

WATER-SOLUBLE VITAMINS

The group of water-soluble vitamins consists of vitamin C and members of the vitamin B complex: thiamine, riboflavin, niacin, pyridoxine, pantothenic acid, biotin, folic acid, and cyanocobalamin. The B vitamins differ widely from one another in structure and function. They are grouped together because they were first isolated from the same sources (yeast and liver). Vitamin C is not found in the same foods as the B vitamins, and hence is classified by itself.

Two compounds—*pangamic acid* and *laetrile*—have been falsely promoted as B vitamins. Pangamic acid has been marketed as "vitamin B_{15}" and laetrile as "vitamin B_{17}." There is no proof these compounds act as vitamins or have any other role in human nutrition.

Vitamin C (Ascorbic Acid)

Actions

Vitamin C participates in multiple biochemical reactions. Among these are synthesis of adrenal steroids, conversion of folic acid to folinic acid, and regulation of the respiratory cycle in mitochondria. At the tissue level, vitamin C is required for production of collagen and other compounds that comprise the intercellular matrix that binds cells together. In addition, vitamin C has antioxidant activity (see Box 81.1) and facilitates the absorption of dietary iron.

Sources

The main dietary sources of ascorbic acid are citrus fruits and juices, tomatoes, potatoes, strawberries, melons, spinach, and broccoli. Orange juice and lemon juice are especially rich sources.

Requirements

Current RDAs for vitamin C are shown in Table 81.1. As in the past, RDAs increase for women who are pregnant or breast-feeding. For smokers, the RDA is increased by 35 mg/day.

Deficiency

Deficiency of vitamin C can lead to *scurvy,* a disease rarely seen in the United States. Symptoms include faulty bone and tooth development, loosening of the teeth, gingivitis, bleeding gums, poor wound healing, hemorrhage into muscles and joints, and ecchymoses (skin discoloration caused by leakage of blood into subcutaneous tissues). Many of these symptoms result from disruption of the intercellular matrix of capillaries and other tissues.

Adverse Effects

Excessive doses can cause *nausea, abdominal cramps,* and *diarrhea.* The mechanism is direct irritation of the intestinal mucosa. To protect against gastrointestinal (GI) disturbances, the Food and Nutrition Board has set 2 gm/day as the adult UL for vitamin C.

Therapeutic Use

The only *established* indications for vitamin C are the prevention and the treatment of scurvy. For severe acute deficiency, parenteral administration is recommended.

Vitamin C has been advocated for the therapy of many conditions unrelated to deficiency, including cancers, asthma, osteoporosis, and the common cold. Claims of efficacy for several of these conditions have been definitively disproved. Other claims remain unproved. Studies have shown that large doses of vitamin C do not reduce the incidence of colds, although the intensity or duration of illness may be decreased slightly. Research has failed to show any benefit of vitamin C therapy for patients with advanced cancer, atherosclerosis, or schizophrenia. Vitamin C does not promote the healing of wounds.

Preparations and Routes of Administration

Vitamin C is available in formulations for oral and parenteral administration. Oral products include tablets (ranging from 25 to 1000 mg), timed-release capsules (500 mg to 1500 mg), and syrups (20 and 100 mg/mL), as well as granules, crystals, powders, effervescent powders, and wafers. Parenteral administration may be subQ, IM, or IV.

Niacin (Nicotinic Acid)

Niacin has a role as both a vitamin and a medicine. In its medicinal role, niacin is used to reduce cholesterol levels; the doses required are much higher than those used to correct or prevent nutritional deficiency. Discussion in this chapter focuses on niacin as a vitamin. The use of nicotinic acid to reduce cholesterol levels is discussed in Chapter 50.

Physiologic Actions

Before it can exert physiologic effects, niacin must first be converted into nicotinamide adenine dinucleotide (NAD) or nicotinamide adenine dinucleotide phosphate (NADP). NAD and NADP then act as coenzymes in oxidation-reduction reactions essential for cellular respiration.

Sources

Nicotinic acid (or its nutritional equivalent, nicotinamide) is present in many foods of plant and animal origin. Particularly rich sources are liver, poultry, fish, potatoes, peanuts, cereal bran, and cereal germ.

In humans, the amino acid tryptophan can be converted to nicotinic acid. Hence, proteins can be a source of the vitamin. About 60 mg of dietary tryptophan is required to produce 1 mg of nicotinic acid.

Requirements

RDAs for nicotinic acid are stated as niacin equivalents (NEs). By definition, 1 NE is equal to 1 mg of niacin (nicotinic acid) or 60 mg of tryptophan. Current RDAs for niacin are provided in Table 81.1.

Deficiency

The syndrome caused by niacin deficiency is called *pellagra,* a term that is a condensation of the Italian words *pelle agra,* meaning "rough skin." As suggested by this name, a prominent symptom of pellagra is dermatitis, characterized by scaling and cracking of the skin in areas exposed to the sun. Other symptoms involve the GI tract (abdominal pain, diarrhea, soreness of the tongue and mouth) and central nervous system (irritability, insomnia, memory loss, anxiety, dementia). All symptoms reverse with niacin replacement therapy.

Adverse Effects

Nicotinic acid has very low toxicity. Small doses are completely devoid of adverse effects. When taken in large doses, nicotinic acid can cause vasodilation with resultant *flushing, dizziness,* and *nausea.* Using flushing as an index of excess niacin consumption, the Food and Nutrition Board has set 50 mg as the adult UL. Toxicity associated with high-dose therapy is discussed in Chapter 50.

Nicotinamide, a compound that can substitute for nicotinic acid in the treatment of pellagra, is not a vasodilator, and it does not produce the adverse effects associated with large doses of nicotinic acid. Accordingly, nicotinamide is often preferred to nicotinic acid for treating pellagra.

Therapeutic Uses

In its capacity as a vitamin, nicotinic acid is indicated for the prevention or treatment of niacin deficiency. It is used off-label for treatment of pellagra.

Preparations, Dosage, and Administration

Nicotinic acid (niacin) is available in immediate-release tablets (50 to 500 mg), extended-release tablets (250 to 1000 mg), and extended-release capsules (250 to 500 mg). Dosages for mild deficiency range from 10 to 20 mg/day. For treatment of pellagra, daily doses may be as high as 500 mg/day; however, the usual dose is 50 to100 mg every 6 to 8 hours. Dosages for hyperlipidemia are given in Chapter 50.

Nicotinamide (niacinamide) is available in 100- and 500-mg tablets. The usual dosage for the treatment of pellagra is 100 mg every 6 hours initially. Once major signs and symptoms have resolved, dosing can be decreased to 10 mg every 8 to 12 hours until resolution of skin lesions. Unlike nicotinic acid, nicotinamide has no effect on plasma lipoproteins, and hence is not used to treat hyperlipidemias.

Riboflavin (Vitamin B_2)

Actions

Riboflavin participates in numerous enzymatic reactions. However, to do so, the vitamin must first be converted into one of two active forms: flavin adenine dinucleotide (FAD) or flavin mononucleotide (FMN). In the form of FAD or FMN, riboflavin acts as a coenzyme for multiple oxidative reactions.

Sources and Requirements

In the United States, most dietary riboflavin comes from milk, yogurt, cheese, bread products, and fortified cereals. Organ meats are also rich sources. RDAs for riboflavin are listed in Table 81.1.

Toxicity

Riboflavin appears devoid of toxicity to humans. When large doses are administered, the excess is rapidly excreted in the urine. Because large doses are harmless, no UL has been set.

Use in Riboflavin Deficiency

Riboflavin is indicated only for prevention and correction of riboflavin deficiency, which usually occurs in conjunction with deficiency of other B vitamins. In its early state, riboflavin deficiency manifests as sore throat and angular stomatitis (cracks in the skin at the corners of the mouth). Later symptoms include cheilosis (painful cracks in the lips), glossitis (inflammation of the tongue), vascularization of the cornea, and itchy dermatitis of the scrotum or vulva. Oral riboflavin is used for treatment. The dosage is 10 to 15 mg/day.

Use in Migraine Headache

As discussed in Chapter 30, riboflavin can help prevent migraine headaches; however, prophylactic effects do not develop until after 3 months of treatment. The daily dosage is 400 mg—much higher than the dosage for riboflavin deficiency.

Thiamine (Vitamin B_1)

Actions and Requirements

The active form of thiamine (thiamine pyrophosphate) is an essential coenzyme for carbohydrate metabolism. Thiamine requirements are related to caloric intake and are greatest when carbohydrates are the primary source of calories. For maintenance of good health, thiamine consumption should be at least 0.3 mg/1000 kcal in the diet. Current RDAs for thiamine appear in Table 81.1. As indicated, thiamine requirements increase significantly during pregnancy and lactation.

Sources

In the United States, the principal dietary sources of thiamine are enriched, fortified, or whole-grain products, especially breads and ready-to-eat cereals. The richest source of the natural vitamin is pork.

Deficiency

Severe thiamine deficiency produces *beriberi,* a disorder having two distinct forms: *wet beriberi* and *dry beriberi. Wet beriberi* is so named because its primary symptom is fluid accumulation in the legs. Cardiovascular complications (palpitations, electrocardiogram abnormalities, high-output heart failure) are common and may progress rapidly to circulatory collapse and death. *Dry beriberi* is characterized by neurologic and motor deficits (e.g., anesthesia of the feet, ataxic gait, footdrop, wristdrop); edema and cardiovascular symptoms are absent. Wet beriberi responds rapidly and dramatically to replacement therapy. In contrast, recovery from dry beriberi can be very slow.

In the United States, thiamine deficiency occurs most commonly among people with chronic alcohol consumption. In this population, deficiency manifests as *Wernicke-Korsakoff syndrome* rather than frank beriberi. This syndrome is a serious disorder of the central nervous system, having neurologic and psychologic manifestations. Symptoms include nystagmus, diplopia, ataxia, and an inability to remember the recent past. Failure to correct the deficit may result in irreversible brain damage. Accordingly, if Wernicke-Korsakoff syndrome is suspected, parenteral thiamine should be administered immediately.

Adverse Effects

When taken orally, thiamine is devoid of adverse effects. Accordingly, no UL for the vitamin has been established.

Therapeutic Use

The only indications for thiamine are the treatment and prevention of thiamine deficiency.

Preparations, Dosage, and Administration

Thiamine is available in standard tablets (50, 100, and 250 mg) and in solution (100 mg/mL) for IM or IV administration. For mild deficiency, oral thiamine is preferred. Parenteral administration is reserved for severe deficiency states (wet or dry beriberi, Wernicke-Korsakoff syndrome). The dosage for beriberi is 5 to 30 mg/day orally in single or divided doses 3 times/day for 1 month. For critically ill patients, therapy is initiated at the same dosage but via the IM or IV route 3 times/day. For Wernicke's encephalopathy, the typical dosage is 100 mg IV initially, followed by 50 to 100 mg/day IM or IV until the patient begins to eat a balanced diet. In some instances, dosage may need to be increased.

Pyridoxine (Vitamin B_6)

Actions

Pyridoxine functions as a coenzyme in the metabolism of amino acids and proteins. However, before it can do so, pyridoxine must first be converted to its active form: pyridoxal phosphate.

Requirements

Current RDAs for pyridoxine are listed in Table 81.1. RDAs increase significantly for women who are pregnant or breast-feeding.

Sources

In the United States, the principal dietary sources of pyridoxine are fortified, ready-to-eat cereals; meat, fish, and poultry; white potatoes and other starchy vegetables; and noncitrus fruits. Especially rich sources are organ meats (e.g., beef liver) and cereals or soy-based products that have been highly fortified.

Deficiency

Pyridoxine deficiency may result from poor diet, isoniazid therapy for tuberculosis, and inborn errors of metabolism. Symptoms include seborrheic dermatitis, anemia, peripheral neuritis, convulsions, depression, and confusion.

In the United States, dietary deficiency of vitamin B_6 is rare, except among people who abuse alcohol on a long-term basis. Within this population, vitamin B_6 deficiency is estimated at 20% to 30%, and occurs in combination with deficiency of other B vitamins.

Isoniazid (a drug for tuberculosis) prevents conversion of vitamin B_6 to its active form and may thereby induce symptoms of deficiency (peripheral neuritis). Patients who are predisposed to this neuropathy (e.g., people with diabetes or alcoholism) should receive daily pyridoxine supplements.

Inborn errors of metabolism can prevent efficient utilization of vitamin B_6, resulting in greatly increased pyridoxine requirements. Among infants, symptoms include irritability, convulsions, and anemia. Unless treatment with vitamin B_6 is initiated early, permanent cognitive deficits may result.

Adverse Effects

At low doses, pyridoxine is devoid of adverse effects. However, if extremely large doses are taken, neurologic injury may result. Symptoms include ataxia and numbness of the feet and hands. To minimize risk, adults should not consume more than 100 mg/day, the UL for this vitamin.

Drug Interactions

Vitamin B_6 interferes with the utilization of levodopa, a drug for Parkinson disease. Accordingly, patients receiving levodopa should be advised against taking the vitamin.

Therapeutic Uses

Pyridoxine is indicated for the prevention and treatment of all vitamin B_6 deficiency states (dietary deficiency, isoniazid-induced deficiency, pyridoxine dependency syndrome).

Preparations, Dosage, and Administration

Pyridoxine is available in solution (200 mg/5 mL), standard tablets (25, 50, 100, 250, and 500 mg), extended-release tablets (200 mg), and capsules (150 mg) for oral use. It is available in solution (100 mg/mL) for IM or IV administration. To correct dietary deficiency, the dosage is 10 to 20 mg/day for 3 weeks followed by 1.5 to 2.5 mg/day thereafter for maintenance. To treat deficiency induced by isoniazid, the dosage is typically 100 mg/day IM or IV for 3 weeks, and then 30 mg/day as a maintenance dose. To protect against developing isoniazid-induced deficiency, the dosage is 25 to 50 mg/day. Pyridoxine dependency syndrome may require initial doses up to 600 mg/day followed by 25 to 50 mg/day for life.

Cyanocobalamin (Vitamin B_{12}) and Folic Acid

Cyanocobalamin (vitamin B_{12}) and folic acid (folacin) are essential factors in the synthesis of DNA. Deficiency of either vitamin manifests as megaloblastic anemia. Cyanocobalamin deficiency produces neurologic damage as well. Because deficiency presents as anemia, folic acid and cyanocobalamin are discussed in Chapter 55.

Recommended Daily Allowances and Tolerable Upper Intake Levels

RDAs for vitamin B_{12} and folate are provided in Table 81.1. Because adults older than 50 years often have difficulty absorbing dietary vitamin B_{12}, they should ingest at least 2.4 mcg/day in the form of a supplement. A UL of 1000 mcg/day has been set for folic acid. Owing to insufficient data, no UL has been set for B_{12}.

Food Folate Versus Synthetic Folate

The form of folate that occurs naturally (food folate) has a different chemical structure than synthetic folate (pteroylglutamic acid). Synthetic folate is more stable than food folate and has greater bioavailability. In the presence of food, the bioavailability of synthetic folate is at least 85%. In contrast, the bioavailability of food folate is less than 50%.

To increase folate in the American diet, the U.S. Food and Drug Administration requires that all enriched grain products (e.g., enriched bread, pasta, flour, breakfast cereal, grits, rice) must be fortified with synthetic folate—specifically, 140 mcg/100 gm of grain. As a result of grain fortification, the incidence of folic acid deficiency in the United States has declined dramatically. Unfortunately, the incidence of birth defects from folate deficiency remains high.

Folic Acid Deficiency and Fetal Development

Deficiency of folic acid during pregnancy can impair the development of the central nervous system, resulting in *neural tube defects* (NTDs), manifesting as *anencephaly* or *spina bifida*. Anencephaly (failure of the brain to develop) is uniformly fatal. Spina bifida, a condition characterized by defective development of the bony encasement of the spinal cord, can result in nerve damage, paralysis, and other complications. The time of vulnerability for NTDs is days 21 through 28 after conception. As a result, damage can occur before a woman recognizes that she is pregnant. Because NTDs occur very early in pregnancy, it is essential that adequate levels of folic acid be present *when pregnancy begins;* women cannot wait until pregnancy is confirmed before establishing adequate intake. To ensure sufficient folate at the onset of pregnancy, the U.S. Preventive Services Task Force (USPSTF) now recommends that *all women who are capable of becoming pregnant consume 400 to 800 mcg of supplemental folic acid each day—in addition to the folate they get from food.*

Folic Acid and Cancer Risk

There is evidence that folic acid in *low* doses may *reduce* cancer risk, whereas folic acid in *higher* doses may *increase* cancer risk—suggesting that cancer risk is increased by having either *too little* folic acid (folic acid deficiency) or by having *too much* folic acid (folic acid excess). The bottom line? Taking high-dose folic acid to reduce cancer risk is ineffective and should be discouraged. Women who might become pregnant should continue to take at least 400 mcg of folic acid every day to prevent NTDs.

Pantothenic Acid

Pantothenic acid is an essential component of two biologically important molecules: *coenzyme A* and *acyl carrier protein*. Coenzyme A is an essential factor in multiple biochemical processes, including gluconeogenesis, intermediary metabolism of carbohydrates, and biosynthesis of steroid hormones, porphyrins, and acetylcholine. Acyl carrier protein is required for synthesis of fatty acids. Pantothenic acid is present in virtually all foods. As a result, spontaneous deficiency has not been reported. There are insufficient data to establish RDAs for pantothenic acid. However, the Food and Nutrition Board *has* assigned AIs (see Table 81.1). There are no reports of toxicity from pantothenic acid. Accordingly, no UL has been set. Pantothenic acid is available in single-ingredient tablets and in multivitamin preparations. However, because deficiency does not occur, there is no reason to take supplements.

Biotin

Biotin is an essential cofactor for several reactions involved in the metabolism of carbohydrates and fats. The vitamin is found in a wide variety of foods, although the exact amount in most foods has not been determined. In addition to being available in foods, biotin is synthesized by intestinal bacteria. Biotin deficiency is extremely rare. In fact, to determine the effects of deficiency, scientists had to induce it experimentally. When this was done, subjects experienced dermatitis, conjunctivitis, hair loss, muscle pain, peripheral paresthesias, and psychologic effects (lethargy, hallucinations, depression). At this time, the data are insufficient to establish RDAs for biotin. However, as with pantothenic acid, the Food and Nutrition Board *has* assigned AIs (see Table 81.1). Biotin appears devoid of toxicity: Subjects given large doses experienced no adverse effects. Accordingly, no UL has been set.

KEY POINTS

- Vitamins can be defined as organic compounds, required in minute amounts, that promote growth and health maintenance by participating in energy transformation and regulation of metabolic processes.
- Recommended dietary allowances (RDAs) for vitamins, which are set by the Food and Nutrition Board of the National Academy of Sciences, represent the average daily dietary intake sufficient to meet the nutrient requirements of nearly all (97% to 98%) healthy individuals in a particular life-stage or gender group.
- The Tolerable Upper Intake Level (UL) for a vitamin is the highest average daily intake that can be consumed by nearly everyone without a significant risk for adverse effects. The UL is simply an index of safety—not a recommendation to exceed the RDA.
- There is no evidence that taking daily *multi*vitamin supplements can decrease the risk for chronic disease. However, there *is* evidence that taking supplements of vitamin B_{12}, folic acid, and vitamin D (plus calcium) can benefit certain individuals.
- Vitamins are divided into two major groups: fat-soluble vitamins (A, D, E, and K) and water-soluble vitamins (vitamin C and members of the vitamin B complex).
- Vitamin A deficiency can cause night blindness, xerophthalmia (a dry, thickened condition of the conjunctiva), and keratomalacia (degeneration of the cornea with keratinization of the corneal epithelium).
- Too much vitamin A can cause birth defects, liver injury, and bone abnormalities. Accordingly, vitamin A intake should not exceed the UL, set at 3000 mcg/day.
- Vitamin D plays a critical role in the regulation of calcium and phosphorus metabolism, and may help protect against the development of breast cancer, colorectal cancer, and type 1 diabetes and improve overall mortality.
- In children, vitamin D deficiency causes rickets. In adults, deficiency causes osteomalacia.
- High-dose vitamin E (more than 200 IU/day) increases the risk for hemorrhagic stroke.
- Vitamin K is required for synthesis of prothrombin and other clotting factors.
- Vitamin K deficiency causes bleeding tendencies. Severe deficiency can cause spontaneous hemorrhage.
- Vitamin K is used to treat vitamin K deficiency (including neonatal deficiency) and as an antidote for warfarin (an anticoagulant).
- Vitamin C deficiency can cause scurvy.
- Niacin (nicotinic acid) is both a vitamin and a drug.
- When niacin is used as a drug (to reduce cholesterol levels), doses are much higher than when niacin is used to prevent or correct deficiency.

Continued

- Niacin deficiency results in pellagra.
- Severe thiamine deficiency produces beriberi.
- In the United States, thiamine deficiency occurs most commonly among people with chronic alcohol consumption. In this population, deficiency manifests as Wernicke-Korsakoff syndrome rather than beriberi.
- Pyridoxine (vitamin B_6) deficiency can cause peripheral neuritis and other symptoms.
- Isoniazid, a drug for tuberculosis, prevents conversion of pyridoxine to its active form and can thereby induce pyridoxine deficiency.
- Folic acid deficiency during early pregnancy can cause neural tube defects (anencephaly and spina bifida). To ensure folic acid sufficiency at the start of pregnancy, all women with the potential for becoming pregnant should consume 400 to 800 mcg of supplemental folic acid every day in addition to food folate.
- Taking high doses of folic acid (more than 800 mcg/day) is associated with an increased risk for certain cancers, and hence should be discouraged.
- High-dose antioxidants do not prevent heart disease or cancer, do not prolong life, and may actually increase the risk for mortality.

Please visit **http://evolve.elsevier.com/Lehne** for chapter-specific NCLEX® examination review questions.

CHAPTER

82 Drugs for Weight Loss

In the United States, 69.2% of adults are overweight. Of these, 35.9% are obese. Excessive body fat may be associated with increased risk for morbidity from hypertension, coronary heart disease, ischemic stroke, type 2 diabetes mellitus (DM), gallbladder disease, liver disease, kidney stones, osteoarthritis, sleep apnea, dementia, and certain cancers. Among women, obesity may increase the risk for menstrual irregularities, amenorrhea, and polycystic ovary syndrome. During pregnancy, obesity may increase the risk for morbidity and mortality for both mother and child. In young men, obesity may reduce the quality and quantity of sperm. The Centers for Disease Control and Prevention (CDC) estimates that 112,000 Americans die per year from obesity-associated illnesses.

Pediatric obesity is a special concern. Despite recent declines in obesity prevalence, almost one-third of American children and adolescents are overweight or obese. This increases the risk for hypertension, heart disease, and asthma. In addition, type 2 DM, formerly seen almost exclusively in adults, has increased 10-fold among children and teens, and gallbladder disease has tripled.

Obesity is now viewed as a chronic disease, much like hypertension and diabetes. Despite intensive research, the underlying cause remains incompletely understood. Contributing factors include genetics, metabolism, and appetite regulation, along with environmental, psychosocial, and cultural factors. Although obese people can lose weight, the tendency to regain weight cannot be eliminated. Put another way, obesity cannot yet be cured. Accordingly, for most patients, lifelong management is indicated.

ASSESSMENT OF WEIGHT-RELATED HEALTH RISK

Health risk is determined by (1) the degree of obesity (as reflected in the body mass index), (2) the pattern of fat distribution (as reflected in the waist circumference measurement), and (3) the presence of obesity-related diseases or cardiovascular risk factors. Accordingly, all three factors must be assessed when establishing a treatment plan.

Body Mass Index

The body mass index (BMI), which is derived from the patient's weight and height, is a simple way to estimate body fat content. Studies indicate a close correlation between BMI and total body fat. The BMI is calculated by dividing a patient's weight (in kilograms) by the square of the patient's height (in meters). Hence, BMI is expressed in units of kg/m^2. BMI can also be calculated using the patient's weight in *pounds* and height in *inches*. These can be calculated manually (Fig. 82.1) or by using an application such as the online CDC resource at http://www.cdc.gov/healthyweight/assessing/bmi/adult_bmi/english_bmi_calculator/bmi_calculator.html. Tables that assign BMI according to height and weight are also available. (Fig. 82.2)

According to the federal guidelines, a BMI of 30 or higher indicates obesity. Individuals with a BMI of 25 to 29.9 are considered overweight, but not obese. There is evidence that the risk for cardiovascular disease and other disorders rises when the BMI exceeds 25. These associations between BMI and health risk do not apply to older adults, growing children, or women who are pregnant or lactating. Nor do they apply to competitive athletes or bodybuilders, who are heavy because of muscle mass rather than excess fat.

Waist Circumference

Waist circumference (WC) is an indicator of *abdominal* fat content, an independent risk factor for obesity-related diseases. Accumulation of fat in the upper body, and especially within the abdominal cavity, poses a greater risk to health than does accumulation of fat in the lower body (hips and thighs). People with too much abdominal fat are at increased risk for insulin resistance, DM, hypertension, coronary atherosclerosis, ischemic

$$\text{BMI} = \frac{\text{Weight in pounds} \times 703}{(\text{Height in inches})^2}$$

OR

$$\text{BMI} = \frac{\text{Weight in kilograms}}{(\text{Height in meters})^2}$$

BMI	Weight Status
Less than 18.5	Underweight
18.5–24.9	Normal Weight
25–29.9	Overweight
30–39.9	Obese
40 and greater	Morbidly Obese

Fig. 82.1 ■ **Body mass index calculation.**

BMI	19	20	21	22	23	24	25	26	27	28	29	30	31	32	33	34	35	36	37	38	39	40	41	42	43	44	45	46	47	48
Height	Weight in Pounds																													
4'10"	91	96	100	105	110	115	119	124	129	134	138	143	148	153	158	162	167	172	177	181	186	191	196	201	205	210	215	220	224	229
4'11"	94	99	104	109	114	119	124	128	133	138	143	148	153	158	163	168	173	178	183	188	193	198	203	208	212	217	222	227	232	237
5'	97	102	107	112	118	123	128	133	138	143	148	153	158	163	168	174	179	184	189	194	199	204	209	215	220	225	230	235	240	245
5'1"	100	106	111	116	122	127	132	137	143	148	153	158	164	169	174	180	185	190	195	201	206	211	217	222	227	232	238	243	248	254
5'2"	104	109	115	120	126	131	136	142	147	153	158	164	169	175	180	186	191	196	202	207	213	218	224	229	235	240	246	251	256	262
5'3"	107	113	118	124	130	135	141	146	152	158	163	169	175	180	186	191	197	203	208	214	220	225	231	237	242	248	254	259	265	270
5'4"	110	116	122	128	134	140	145	151	157	163	169	174	180	186	192	197	204	209	215	221	227	232	238	244	250	256	262	267	273	279
5'5"	114	120	126	132	138	144	150	156	162	168	174	180	186	192	198	204	210	216	222	228	234	240	246	252	258	264	270	276	282	288
5'6"	118	124	130	136	142	148	155	161	167	173	179	186	192	198	204	210	216	223	229	235	241	247	253	260	266	272	278	284	291	297
5'7"	121	127	134	140	146	153	159	166	172	178	185	191	198	204	211	217	223	230	236	242	249	255	261	268	274	280	287	293	299	306
5'8"	125	131	138	144	151	158	164	171	177	184	190	197	203	210	216	223	230	236	243	249	256	262	269	276	282	289	295	302	308	315
5'9"	128	135	142	149	155	162	169	176	182	189	196	203	209	216	223	230	236	243	250	257	263	270	277	284	291	297	304	311	318	324
5'10"	132	139	146	153	160	167	174	181	188	195	202	209	216	222	229	236	243	250	257	264	271	278	285	292	299	306	313	320	327	334
5'11"	136	143	150	157	165	172	179	186	193	200	208	215	222	229	236	243	250	257	265	272	279	286	293	301	308	315	322	329	338	343
6'	140	147	154	162	169	177	184	191	199	206	213	221	228	235	242	250	258	265	272	279	287	294	302	309	316	324	331	338	346	353
6'1"	144	151	159	166	174	182	189	197	204	212	219	227	235	242	250	257	265	272	280	288	295	302	310	318	325	333	340	348	355	363
6'2"	148	155	163	171	179	186	194	202	210	218	225	233	241	249	256	264	272	280	287	295	303	311	319	326	334	342	350	358	365	373
6'3"	152	160	168	176	184	192	200	208	216	224	232	240	248	256	264	272	279	287	295	303	311	319	327	335	343	351	359	367	375	383
6'4"	156	164	172	180	189	197	205	213	221	230	238	246	254	263	271	279	287	295	304	312	320	328	336	344	353	361	369	377	385	394

☐ = Healthy weight: BMI 18.5 to 24.9
☐ = Overweight: BMI 25 to 29.9
☐ = Obese: BMI 30 to 39.9
☐ = Severely obese: BMI 40 and higher

Fig. 82.2 ■ Adult weight classification based on body mass index (BMI). (Adapted from Body Mass Index Table, 2012. The complete table is available online at http://www.nhlbi.nih.gov/health/educational/lose_wt/BMI/bmi_tbl.pdf)

stroke, and dementia. Fat distribution can be estimated simply by looking in the mirror: an apple shape indicates too much abdominal fat, whereas a pear shape indicates fat on the hips and thighs. Measurement of WC provides a quantitative estimate of abdominal fat. A WC exceeding 40 inches (102 cm) in men or 35 inches (88 cm) in women signifies an increased health risk—but only for people with a BMI between 25 and 34.9.

Risk Status

Overall weight-related health risk is determined by BMI, WC, and the presence of weight-related diseases and cardiovascular risk factors. Certain weight-related diseases—established coronary heart disease, other atherosclerotic diseases, type 2 DM, and sleep apnea—confer a risk for complications and mortality. Other weight-related diseases—gynecologic abnormalities, osteoarthritis, gallstones, and stress incontinence—confer less risk. Cardiovascular risk factors—smoking, hypertension, high levels of low-density lipoprotein (LDL) cholesterol, low levels of high-density lipoprotein (HDL) cholesterol, high fasting glucose, family history of premature coronary heart disease, physical inactivity, and advancing age—confer a high risk when three or more of these factors are present.

Health risk rises as BMI gets larger. In addition, the risk is increased by the presence of an excessive WC. The risk is further increased by weight-related diseases and cardiovascular risk factors. In the absence of an excessive WC and other risk factors, health risk is minimal with a BMI below 25, and relatively low with a BMI below 30. Conversely, a BMI of 30 or more indicates significant risk. In the presence of an excessive WC, health risk is high for all individuals with a BMI above 25.

OVERVIEW OF OBESITY TREATMENT

The strategy for losing weight is simple: take in fewer calories per day than are burned. Of course, implementation is much more challenging. The key components of a weight-loss program are diet and exercise. Drugs and other measures are employed only as adjuncts.

Who Should Be Treated?

According to the federal guidelines, weight-loss therapy is indicated for people with any of the following conditions:

- A BMI of 30 or more
- A BMI of 25 to 29.9 *plus* two risk factors
- A WC greater than 40 inches (in men) or greater than 35 inches (in women) *plus* two risk factors

Benefits of Treatment

In overweight and obese people, weight reduction may confer these benefits:

- Reduction of high blood pressure in patients with hypertension
- Improvement of blood lipid status (elevation of HDL cholesterol and reduction of LDL cholesterol, total cholesterol, and triglycerides)
- Reduction in the development of type 2 DM
- Reduction of elevated blood glucose in patients who have type 2 DM
- Reduced mortality

Treatment Goal

While a goal to attain a normal BMI is desirable, it is rarely achieved in obese individuals, even with drug therapy. A more realistic goal is to target a percentage of body weight at which risk is decreased and comorbidities prevented. A weight loss of 10% to 15% is typical for those who diligently adhere to medication and lifestyle regimen, whereas a loss greater than 15% is exceptional. The initial objective is to reduce weight by 10% over 6 months. For patients with a BMI of 27 to 35, this can usually be achieved by reducing energy intake by 300 to 500 kcal/day, which should allow a loss of 0.5 to 1 pound a week—or 13 to 26 pounds in 6 months. People with a BMI above 35 require greater caloric restriction to lose 10% of their weight in 6 months. After 6 months, the goal for all patients is to prevent lost weight from returning. This may be accomplished by a combination of diet, physical activity, and behavioral therapy. If appropriate, additional weight reduction can be attempted.

Treatment Modalities

Weight loss can be accomplished with five treatment modalities: caloric restriction, physical activity, behavioral therapy, drug therapy, and surgery. For any individual, the treatment mode is determined by the degree of obesity and personal preference.

Caloric Restriction

A reduced-calorie diet is central to any weight-loss program. As noted, the only way to lose weight is to take in fewer calories than are burned. Depending on the individual, the caloric deficit should range from 300 to 1000 kcal/day. Because fats contain more calories than either carbohydrates or proteins (on an ounce-for-ounce basis), reducing dietary fat is the easiest way to reduce calorie intake.

To succeed at losing weight, it helps to know just how many calories are taken in each day and how many are burned. The following web sites, which are free, have databases on foods and physical activities, along with tools to calculate and log calories taken in and calories burned.

- Choose My Plate: www.choosemyplate.gov
- Super Tracker: www.supertracker.usda.gov
- Fitday: www.fitday.com
- Sparkpeople: www.sparkpeople.com
- NutritionData: http://nutritiondata.self.com/

Exercise

Physical activity should be a component of all weight-loss and weight-maintenance programs. Exercise makes a modest contribution to weight loss by increasing energy expenditure. In addition, exercise can help reduce abdominal fat, increase cardiorespiratory fitness, and maintain weight once loss has occurred. According to the American College of Sports Medicine, people trying to *lose* weight should exercise at least 150 minutes per week (and preferably more), and those trying to *maintain* weight loss should exercise 200 to 300 minutes per week.

Behavior Modification

Behavioral therapy is directed at modifying eating and exercise habits. As such, behavioral therapy can strengthen a program of diet and exercise. Techniques of behavioral therapy include self-monitoring of eating and exercise habits, stress management (because stress can trigger eating), and stimulus control (limiting exposure to stimuli that promote eating). There is no evidence that any one of these techniques is superior to others.

Bariatric Surgery

Surgical procedures can produce significant weight loss by reducing food intake. However, they are indicated only for patients with a BMI of 40 or more in the absence of severe comorbidity. The two most widely used procedures are *gastric bypass surgery* (Roux-en-Y procedure) and laparoscopic implantation of an adjustable gastric band, which reduces the effective volume of the upper part of the stomach. Surgery is effective: In 6 months to a year, patients can lose between 110 and 220 pounds. Unfortunately, the surgery can carry significant risk: In one study, mortality rates at 30 days, 90 days, and 1 year after gastric surgery were 2%, 2.8%, and 4.6%, respectively.

Drug Therapy

In theory, drugs can promote weight loss in three ways: They can suppress appetite, reduce absorption of nutrients, or increase metabolic rate. Drugs can be used as an adjunct to diet and exercise—but only for people at increased health risk and only after a 6-month program of diet and exercise has failed. Drugs should never be used alone; rather, they should be part of a comprehensive weight-reduction program—one that includes exercise, behavior modification, and a reduced-calorie diet.

Drugs should be reserved for patients whose BMI is 30 or greater or 27 or greater if additional risk factors are present. Drugs are not appropriate for patients whose BMI is relatively low. Drugs are also not appropriate for women who are pregnant. The American College of Obstetricians and Gynecologists recommends weight gain, not loss, for obese women who are pregnant, although the total amount of gain recommended is less than that suggested for women who are within normal limits for weight.

Benefits of drugs are usually modest. Weight loss attributable to drugs generally ranges between 4.4 and 22 pounds, although some people lose significantly more. As a rule, most weight loss occurs during the first 6 months of treatment.

The duration of therapy varies depending on the drug selected. Today, long-term treatment is recommended more often than in the past because we now know that, when drugs are discontinued, most patients regain lost weight. Accordingly, when treatment has been effective and well tolerated, it may need to continue indefinitely. Unfortunately, not all drugs are approved for long-term use.

Not everyone responds to drugs, so regular assessment is required. Patients should lose at least 4 pounds during the first 4 weeks of drug treatment. If this initial response is absent, further drug use should be questioned. For patients who *do* respond, ongoing assessment must show that (1) the drug is effective at *maintaining* weight loss and (2) serious adverse effects are absent. Otherwise, drug therapy should cease.

WEIGHT-LOSS DRUGS

As previously mentioned, weight-loss drugs vary in their ability to promote weight loss. The combination drug topiramate/phentermine is associated with the greatest amount of weight loss (greater than 5% of body weight). This is followed by phentermine as monotherapy and the combination drug naltrexone/bupropion, which generally achieve a weight loss of greater than 3% to 5%. Orlistat provides the least weight loss (2% to 3%). The individual classes of weight-loss drugs are discussed next. Dosages and administration guidelines are summarized in Table 82.1.

Lipase Inhibitor: Orlistat

Actions and Use

Orlistat [Alli, Xenical] is a novel drug approved for promoting and maintaining weight loss in obese patients 12 years and older. Unlike most other weight-loss drugs, which act in the brain to curb appetite, orlistat acts in the GI tract to reduce absorption of fat. Specifically, the drug acts in the stomach and small intestine to cause irreversible inhibition of gastric and pancreatic lipases, enzymes that break down triglycerides into monoglycerides and free fatty acids. If triglycerides are not broken down, they can't be absorbed. In patients taking orlistat, absorption of dietary fat is reduced about 30%. Patients must adopt a reduced-calorie diet in which 30% of calories come from fat.

In clinical trials, orlistat produced modest benefits. Patients treated for 2 years lost an average of 19 pounds, compared with 12 pounds for those taking placebo. In addition, treatment reduced total and LDL cholesterol, raised HDL cholesterol, reduced fasting blood glucose, and lowered systolic and diastolic blood pressure.

Adverse Effects

Gastrointestinal Effects. Orlistat undergoes less than 1% absorption, and hence systemic effects are absent. In contrast, GI effects are common. Approximately 20% to 30% of patients experience oily rectal leakage, flatulence with discharge, fecal urgency, and fatty or oily stools. Another 10% experience increased defecation and fecal incontinence. All of these are the result of reduced fat absorption, and all can be minimized by reducing fat intake. Dosing with psyllium [Metamucil, others], a bulk-forming laxative, can greatly reduce GI effects. The underlying mechanism is adsorption of dietary fat by psyllium.

Possible Liver Damage. Orlistat has been associated with rare cases of *severe liver damage.* Signs and symptoms include itching, vomiting, jaundice, anorexia, fatigue, dark urine, and light-colored stools. *Patients who experience these signs and symptoms should report them immediately.* Orlistat should be discontinued until liver injury has been ruled out.

Other Adverse Effects. Rarely, orlistat has been associated with *acute pancreatitis* and *kidney stones,* although a causal relationship has not been established. Cholelithiasis may occur if weight loss is substantial.

Contraindications. Orlistat is contraindicated for patients with malabsorption syndrome or cholestasis.

Drug and Nutrient Interactions

Reduced Absorption of Vitamins. By reducing fat absorption, orlistat can reduce absorption of fat-soluble vitamins (vitamins A, D, E, and K). To avoid deficiency, patients should take a daily multivitamin supplement. Administration should be done 2 hours before or 2 hours after taking orlistat.

Warfarin. Vitamin K deficiency can intensify the effects of *warfarin,* an anticoagulant. In patients taking warfarin, anticoagulant effects should be monitored closely.

> **Safety Alert**
>
> **ORLISTAT AND HYPOTHYROIDISM**
>
> Orlistat may cause hypothyroidism in patients taking levothyroxine (thyroid hormone) by decreasing levothyroxine absorption. To minimize this effect, levothyroxine and orlistat should be administered at least 4 hours apart.

Preparations, Dosage, and Administration

Preparations, dosage, and administration information for orlistat and other weight-loss drugs are provided in Table 82.1.

Serotonin 5-HT_{2C} Receptor Agonist: Lorcaserin

Actions and Use

Lorcaserin [Belviq] is a selective type 2C serotonin (5-HT_{2C}) agonist with indications for chronic weight loss. It suppresses appetite and creates a sense of satiety by activating hypothalamic and mesolimbic pathways that control appetite. Studies have demonstrated an average loss of 5.8% of baseline weight after 1 year, compared with 2.2% in patients taking placebo. In addition, lorcaserin reduces waist circumference, fasting glucose, insulin, total cholesterol, LDL cholesterol, and triglycerides.

Adverse Effects

Ten percent or more of patients will experience headaches, back pain, a decrease in lymphocytes, and upper respiratory infections. About 30% of patients with DM will experience an increase in hypoglycemic episodes.

Less common but serious adverse effects include *blood dyscrasias, cognitive impairment, psychiatric disorders, priapism (prolonged penile erection), pulmonary hypertension,* and *valvular heart disease.* Accordingly, this drug should not be given to patients at risk for these conditions.

Lorcaserin has potential for abuse. It is classified as a Schedule IV drug under the Controlled Substances Act (CSA).

Contraindications

Most of the contraindications for lorcaserin are associated with different aspects of the life span.

Drug Interactions

Lorcaserin is an inhibitor of the CYP2D6 isoenzyme of cytochrome P450. When given with CYP2D6 substrates (i.e., drugs metabolized by CYP2D6 isoenzymes), the serum levels of the substrates can be increased. To decrease the risk for toxicity, when both drugs are prescribed, the substrate may need to be prescribed at a lower dose.

Risk for serotonin syndrome is associated with serotonergic drugs. When serotonergic drugs such as lorcaserin are given with other serotonergic drugs, this risk increases. We do not yet have sufficient studies to evaluate the effects of prescribing lorcaserin with specific serotonergic drugs; therefore, caution and close monitoring are advised when administering this drug along with bupropion, dextromethorphan, monoamine oxidase (MAO) inhibitors, serotonin-norepinephrine reuptake inhibitors, selective serotonin reuptake inhibitors, St. John's wort, and triptans.

Glucagon-like Peptide-1 Agonist: Liraglutide

Actions and Use

Liraglutide (Saxenda) is a glucagon-like peptide-1 (GLP-1) agonist that is approved for chronic weight management in adults. Liraglutide acts by slowing gastric emptying, which increases a feeling of fullness, which leads to decreased food intake. GLP-1 agonists are also used in management of type 2 DM (see Chapter 57) to enhance glycemic control. In this regard, it also increases insulin secretion and decreases glucagon secretion.

Adverse Effects

More than a third of patients taking liraglutide experience an increase in heart rate 10 to 20 beats/minute from baseline. Approximately 1 in 20 will develop tachycardia. Other common adverse effects include nausea, vomiting, and either constipation or diarrhea. Hypoglycemia is a concern if taken by patients with DM who are taking antidiabetic drugs; however, this is a rare occurrence in patients who do not have DM. Headache may occur, as may generalized fatigue and weakness, although these symptoms are less common. Because of the effects on gastric emptying, dyspepsia and abdominal discomfort may

TABLE 82.1 ▪ Weight-Loss Drugs: Preparations, Dosages, and Administration

Drug Class and Drug	Preparation	Dosage	Administration
LIPASE INHIBITOR			
Orlistat [Alli, Xenical]	Alli: 60-mg tablet (OTC) Xenical: 120-mg tablet	Alli: 60 mg 3 times/day with meals Xenical: 120 mg 3 times/day with meals	Take with, or 1 hr after, meals that contain fat. Omit dose if a meal is missed or if a meal does not contain fat. Fat-soluble vitamins (A, D, E, K) should be taken at least 2 hr before or after orlistat.
SEROTONIN 5-HT_{2C} RECEPTOR AGONIST			
Lorcaserin [Belviq]	10-mg tablet	10 mg twice daily	Oral administration. May be taken with or without food.
SYMPATHOMIMETIC AMINES			
Diethylpropion (generic)	25-mg immediate-release tablet 75-mg extended-release tablet	Immediate release: 25 mg 3 times/day Extended release: 75 mg daily	Oral administration. Administer immediate-release tablets 1 hr before meals. Administer extended-release tablets at midmorning. Avoid evening or nighttime administration to prevent insomnia.
Phentermine [Adipex-P, Suprenza]	Adipex-P: 37.5-mg tablet; 37.5-mg capsule Suprenza: 15-, 30-, 37.5-mg disintegrating tablet	Adipex-P: Usual dosage is 37.5 mg daily. Alternate dosing schedules are ½ tablet (18.75 mg) daily or ½ tablet twice daily. Lowest effective dose is recommended. Suprenza: Individualize dosage to the lowest effective dose.	Oral administration. May be taken with or without food. Administer before breakfast or 1–2 hr after breakfast. Avoid evening or nighttime administration to prevent insomnia.
GLP-1 AGONIST			
Liraglutide [Saxenda]	Pre-filled multidose pens hold 3 mL of a 6-mg/mL solution. Pen contains a dose selector that allows delivery of specific doses of 0.6, 1.2, 1.8, 2.4, or 3 mg.	Week 1: 0.6 mg daily Week 2: 1.2 mg daily Week 3: 1.8 mg daily Week 4: 2.4 mg daily Week 5 and thereafter: 3 mg daily	Injected subcutaneously in upper arm, abdomen, or thigh. Does not need to be coordinated with intake.
COMBINATION PRODUCTS			
Phentermine/topiramate [Qsymia]	24-hour extended-release tablet in four strengths: 3.75/23 (phentermine 3.75 mg/topiramate 23 mg) 7.5/46 (phentermine 7.5 mg/ topiramate 46 mg) 11.25/69 (phentermine 11.25 mg/topiramate 69 mg) 15/92 (phentermine 15 mg/ topiramate 92 mg)	Weeks 1 and 2: One 3.75/23 tablet daily, followed by one 7.5/46 tablet daily for 12 weeks. Evaluate weight loss. If 3% of baseline body weight has not occurred, discontinue or increase to one 11.25/69 tablet once daily for 2 weeks followed by one 15/92 tablet for 12 weeks. Evaluate weight loss. If 5% of baseline weight has not been lost, taper off therapy.	Administer in the morning. May be taken with or without food. Avoid evening or nighttime administration to prevent insomnia.
Naltrexone/bupropion [Contrave]	12-hour extended-release tablet containing naltrexone 8 mg/ bupropion 90 mg	Week 1: 1 tablet in the morning Week 2: 1 tablet in the morning; 1 tablet in the evening Week 3: 2 tablets in the morning; 1 tablet in the evening Week 4 and thereafter: 2 tablets in the morning; 2 tablets in the evening	Substantial increases in bupropion and naltrexone occur when taken with high-fat meals, so this should be avoided. If a dose is skipped, wait until the next scheduled dose to resume scheduling.

OTC, Over-the-counter.

occur. Liraglutide is administered subcutaneously; as with any injection, local site reactions such as redness or pruritus may occur.

Several uncommon effects occurring in less than 1% of patients warrant special precautions. These include acute pancreatitis, renal impairment (likely associated with dehydration secondary to nausea, vomiting, and diarrhea), and acute gallbladder disease (typically associated with significant or rapid weight loss regardless of medication). It is important to assess for signs and symptoms of these conditions.

PATIENT-CENTERED CARE ACROSS THE LIFE SPAN

Weight-Loss Drugs

Life Stage	Patient Care Concerns
Children	Liraglutide, lorcaserin, and the combination drugs phentermine/topiramate and naltrexone/bupropion are not approved for children. Naltrexone/bupropion can increase the risk of suicidal ideation and suicide attempts in children, adolescents, and young adults. Orlistat is not approved for children younger than 12 years. Diethylpropion and phentermine are not recommended for children younger than 16 years.
Pregnant women	Weight loss is not advisable for pregnant women. All drugs mentioned in this chapter are Pregnancy Risk Category X[a] with the exception of diethylpropion. Although labeled as Pregnancy Risk Category B, neonates born to women who take diethylpropion may experience withdrawal symptoms.
Breast-feeding women	For all drugs listed, breast-feeding is not recommended.
Older adults	For patients with moderate renal impairment, naltrexone/bupropion should be limited to one tablet daily. If the creatinine clearance is less than 50, phentermine/topiramate should be limited to one 7.5/46 capsule daily. If the creatinine clearance is less than 30, lorcaserin should not be given. For patients with hepatic impairment, both naltrexone/bupropion and phentermine/topiramate should be limited to one tablet daily. Phentermine/topiramate should not be prescribed for patients with severe hepatic impairment. The manufacturer of liraglutide recommends caution when prescribing for patients with renal or hepatic impairment. Dosage adjustments are not indicated for orlistat, diethylpropion, and phentermine.

[a]As of 2020, the FDA will no longer use Pregnancy Risk Categories. Please refer to Chapter 9 for more information.

Contraindications

Liraglutide is known to cause thyroid cancer development in rodents, so cautious use is warranted until the effects on humans are known. Liraglutide is contraindicated in patients who have multiple endocrine neoplasia syndrome type 2 (MEN 2) or who have a personal or family history of medullary thyroid carcinoma (MTC).

Drug Interactions

Liraglutide may potentiate the hypoglycemic effect of drugs given for glycemic control in DM. Additionally, it will enhance the glucose-lowering side effects of other drugs with this feature, including androgens, fluoroquinolone antibiotics, MAO inhibitors, and selective serotonin reuptake inhibitors (SSRIs).

Sympathomimetic Amines: Diethylpropion and Phentermine

The sympathomimetics fall into two groups: amphetamines and nonamphetamines. The amphetamines are not FDA approved for weight loss because they have a high abuse potential, so they are not addressed here.

Four noradrenergic drugs are approved for weight loss. However, only two—*diethylpropion* (generic) and *phentermine* (Adipex-P, Suprenza)—should be used. The other two—*benzphetamine* and *phendimetrazine*—have a higher potential for abuse.

Actions and Use

Diethylpropion and phentermine promote weight loss by decreasing appetite. They are central nervous system (CNS) stimulants that suppress appetite by increasing the availability of norepinephrine at receptors in the brain. This same mechanism underlies their stimulant effects and potential for abuse. Weight loss is usually modest: about 7 to 8 pounds. These drugs should be used only in the short term (for 3 months or less).

Adverse Effects

Like the amphetamines, diethylpropion and phentermine can increase alertness, decrease fatigue, and induce nervousness and insomnia. Because they can interfere with sleep, these drugs should be administered no later than 4:00 PM. After drug withdrawal, fatigue and depression may replace CNS stimulation.

Diethylpropion and phentermine have effects in the periphery, as well as in the CNS. Peripheral effects of greatest concern are *tachycardia, anginal pain,* and *hypertension.* Accordingly, these drugs should be used with caution in patients with cardiovascular disease.

Although the risk for abuse is lower than with the amphetamines, abuse can still occur. Both diethylpropion and phentermine are regulated under Schedule IV of the CSA (benzphetamine and phendimetrazine are regulated under Schedule III). Tolerance is common and may be seen in 6 to 12 weeks. If tolerance develops, the appropriate response is to discontinue the drug rather than to increase the dosage.

Contraindications

There are significant life span contraindications associated with these drugs. (See the *Patient-Centered Care Across the Life Span* box earlier in this chapter.)

Combination Products

There are currently two combination products approved for weight loss. Each combination is unique, with different mechanisms of action and different side effect profiles.

Phentermine/Topiramate

Actions and Use. Phentermine/topiramate [Qsymia] is a Schedule IV drug indicated for chronic weight-loss therapy. Phentermine, as mentioned previously, is a sympathomimetic amine already approved for short-term management of obesity. Topiramate is currently approved for seizure disorders (see Chapter 24) and prophylaxis of migraine (see Chapter 30). Phentermine suppresses appetite, and topiramate induces a sense of satiety. Possible mechanisms for topiramate include antagonism of glutamate (an excitatory neurotransmitter), modulation of receptors for gamma-aminobutyric acid, and inhibition of carbonic anhydrase. In a 56-week trial, phentermine/topiramate produced a 10% reduction in weight and a significant decrease in systolic blood pressure. Long-term results are not available.

Adverse Effects. The most common adverse effects are dry mouth, constipation, altered taste, nausea, blurred vision, dizziness, insomnia, and numbness and tingling in the limbs. The most serious effects are memory impairment, difficulty with concentration, hypertension and tachycardia, birth defects, acute myopia with angle-closure glaucoma, and acidosis. In addition, patients who take insulin or insulin secretagogues face an increased risk for hypoglycemia beyond that of antidiabetic drugs alone.

Contraindications. Phentermine/topiramate is contraindicated for patients with glaucoma or hyperthyroidism. There are also life span–associated contraindications with this drug. (See the *Patient-Centered Care Across the Life Span* box earlier in this chapter.)

Drug Interactions. Phentermine/topiramate should not be given with MAO inhibitors. In fact, at least 2 weeks should pass after taking an MAO inhibitor before phentermine/topiramate is begun. Similarly, at least 2 weeks should pass after ending phentermine/topiramate before an MAO inhibitor is begun. Phentermine/topiramate can potentiate CNS depressants. When given with the antiepileptic drugs carbamazepine or phenytoin, levels of topiramate (which is also an antiepileptic drug) may be increased. Administration with carbonic anhydrase inhibitors increases the risk for metabolic acidosis, whereas administration with diuretics that are not potassium sparing increases the risk for hypokalemia. Finally, studies show that concomitant administration with oral contraceptives increases the estrogen level while decreasing the progestin level.

Naltrexone/Bupropion

Actions and Use. The anorexiant naltrexone/bupropion [Contrave] combines the effects of a dopamine and norepinephrine-reuptake inhibitor with an opioid antagonist. The mechanism of action by which this drug combination promotes weight loss is unknown, but it has been hypothesized that it acts on the regulation of appetite in the hypothalamus and on the mesolimbic dopamine system, which is the key reward pathway in the brain. The individual drugs are discussed separately. (See Chapter 28 for naltrexone and Chapter 32 for bupropion.)

Adverse Effects. The most common adverse reactions (experienced by more than 10% of those taking naltrexone with bupropion) are nausea, vomiting, constipation, headache, dizziness, and insomnia. Approximately 5% of patients experience an increase in blood pressure, dry mouth, diarrhea, abdominal discomfort, anxiety, and fatigue. There is also a suicide risk associated with this drug.

Contraindications. This product is contraindicated for patients taking other products containing bupropion. Because naltrexone is an opioid antagonist, it will decrease the ability of opioid analgesics to relieve pain. It should not be taken within 2 weeks of MAO inhibitors.

Naltrexone/bupropion is also contraindicated for people with selected conditions. It should not be used for weight loss in patients with uncontrolled hypertension, seizure disorders, or eating disorders such as anorexia or bulimia. Patients who are undergoing alcohol, barbiturate, or benzodiazepine withdrawal should not take this drug.

Drug Interactions. Drug interactions are numerous and reflect interactions of the individual agents. Dangerous interactions occur with MAO inhibitors and opioid antagonists.

The bupropion component of naltrexone/bupropion is a minor substrate of numerous hepatic enzyme families and a major substrate of CYP2B6 enzymes. Inhibitors of these enzymes can increase naltrexone/bupropion levels, requiring a lowered dosage. When CYP2B6 inducers are given with this drug, it may result in subtherapeutic doses. Naltrexone/bupropion is also a strong inhibitor of CYP2D6 enzymes. Accordingly, when given with CYP2D6 substrates, naltrexone/bupropion can increase their drug levels.

Safety Alert

NALTREXONE/BUPROPION (CONTRAVE)

Bupropion is available under a variety of brand names—Aplenzin, Budeprion, Bupropan, Wellbutrin, and Zyban. If naltrexone/bupropion is given to patients who are taking or discontinuing bupropion, severe neuropsychiatric reactions, including depression, mania, psychosis, and homicidal ideation, have occurred.

A NOTE REGARDING DRUGS FOR WEIGHT LOSS

Weight-loss drugs share a disturbing history: They receive regulatory approval, undergo widespread use, and then are withdrawn owing to discovery of serious adverse effects. It is quite likely that new drugs may be approved by the time you read this chapter. It is also possible that drugs in this chapter, especially those most recently approved, will have been taken off the market.

KEY POINTS

- The body mass index (BMI) is a measure of body fat content.
- A BMI of 25 to 29.9 indicates overweight, and a BMI of 30 or more indicates obesity.
- Waist circumference (WC) is an index of abdominal fat. Accumulation of abdominal fat is believed to pose a greater risk to health than does accumulation of fat in the hips and thighs.
- Obesity-related health risk is determined by the degree of obesity, excessive abdominal fat, and the presence of obesity-related diseases (e.g., type 2 DM, sleep apnea) and cardiovascular risk factors (e.g., smoking, hypertension, high LDL cholesterol).
- Weight reduction reduces morbidity and probably mortality.
- Weight reduction can be accomplished with caloric restriction, physical activity, behavioral therapy, drug therapy, and surgery.
- Antiobesity drugs should be used only as adjuncts to a comprehensive weight-loss program that includes exercise, behavior modification, and a reduced-calorie diet.
- Antiobesity drugs are indicated for patients with a BMI of 30 or more (in the absence of risk factors) or 27 or more (in the presence of risk factors).
- Most patients regain lost weight when antiobesity drugs are discontinued. To remain effective, these drugs must be taken indefinitely.
- All drugs mentioned in this chapter, with the exception of diethylpropion, can cause fetal harm, and neonates born to women who take diethylpropion may experience withdrawal symptoms.
- Orlistat is approved for long-term therapy of obesity.
- Orlistat promotes weight loss by decreasing absorption of dietary fat. The underlying mechanism is inhibition of gastric and pancreatic lipases.
- Orlistat frequently causes GI symptoms (oily rectal leakage, fecal urgency, oily stools, and fecal incontinence). These symptoms, which are a result of reduced fat absorption, can be minimized by reducing fat intake and by taking the bulk-forming laxative psyllium [Metamucil, others].
- Orlistat can reduce absorption of fat-soluble vitamins (vitamins A, D, E, and K). To avoid deficiency, patients should take a daily multivitamin supplement.
- Lorcaserin [Belviq] is a selective serotonin 5-HT_{2C} agonist with indications for *chronic* weight-loss therapy.
- Lorcaserin is classified as a Schedule IV controlled substance.
- Liraglutide [Saxenda] is a GLP-1 agonist that is approved for chronic weight management in adults. It acts by slowing gastric emptying, which increases a feeling of fullness, which leads to decreased food intake.
- Liraglutide acts by slowing gastric emptying, which increases a feeling of fullness, which leads to decreased food intake.
- Diethylpropion and phentermine are sympathomimetic amines that suppress appetite by increasing the availability of norepinephrine at receptors in the brain.
- Both diethylpropion and phentermine are regulated under Schedule IV of the CSA.
- Phentermine/topiramate [Qsymia] is a combination drug indicated for chronic weight-loss therapy.
- Phentermine suppresses appetite, and topiramate induces a sense of satiety.
- Weight-loss drugs frequently receive regulatory approval, undergo widespread use, and then are withdrawn owing to discovery of serious adverse effects.

Please visit **http://evolve.elsevier.com/Lehne** for chapter-specific NCLEX® examination review questions.

CHAPTER 83

Basic Principles of Antimicrobial Therapy

Modern antimicrobial agents had their debut in the 1930s and 1940s and have greatly reduced morbidity and mortality from infection. As newer drugs are introduced, our ability to fight infections increases even more. However, despite impressive advances, continued progress is needed. There remain organisms that respond poorly to available drugs; there are effective drugs whose use is limited by toxicity; and there is, because of evolving microbial resistance, the constant threat that currently effective antibiotics will be rendered useless.

Here we focus on two principal themes. The first is microbial susceptibility to drugs, with special emphasis on resistance. The second is clinical usage of antimicrobials. Topics addressed include criteria for drug selection, host factors that modify drug use, use of antimicrobial combinations, and use of antimicrobial agents for prophylaxis.

Before going further, we need to consider two terms: *antibiotic* and *antimicrobial drug.* In common practice, the terms *antibiotic* and *antimicrobial drug* are used interchangeably, as they are in this book. However, be aware that the formal definitions of these words are not identical. Strictly speaking, an *antibiotic* is a chemical that is produced by one microbe and has the ability to harm other microbes. Under this definition, only those compounds that are actually made by microorganisms qualify as antibiotics. Drugs such as the sulfonamides, which are produced in the laboratory, would not be considered antibiotics under the strict definition. In contrast, an *antimicrobial drug* is defined as any agent, natural or synthetic, that has the ability to kill or suppress microorganisms. Under this definition, no distinction is made between compounds produced by microbes and those made by chemists.

From the perspective of therapeutics, there is no benefit to distinguishing between drugs made by microorganisms and drugs made by chemists. Hence, the current practice is to use the terms *antibiotic* and *antimicrobial drug* interchangeably.

SELECTIVE TOXICITY

Selective toxicity is defined as the ability of a drug to injure a target cell or target organism without injuring other cells or organisms that are in intimate contact with the target. As applied to antimicrobial drugs, selective toxicity indicates the ability of an antibiotic to kill or suppress microbial pathogens without causing injury to the host. Selective toxicity is the property that makes antibiotics valuable. If it weren't for selective toxicity—that is, if antibiotics were as harmful to the host as they are to infecting organisms—these drugs would have no therapeutic utility.

Achieving Selective Toxicity

How can a drug be highly toxic to microbes but harmless to the host? The answer lies with differences in the cellular chemistry of mammals and microbes. There are biochemical processes critical to microbial well-being that do not take place in mammalian cells. Hence, drugs that selectively interfere with these unique microbial processes can cause serious injury to microorganisms while leaving mammalian cells intact. Three examples of how we achieve selective toxicity are discussed next.

Disruption of the Bacterial Cell Wall

Unlike mammalian cells, bacteria are encased in a rigid cell wall. The protoplasm within this wall has a high concentration of solutes, making osmotic pressure within the bacterium high. If it were not for the cell wall, bacteria would absorb water, swell, and then burst. Several families of drugs (e.g., penicillins, cephalosporins) weaken the cell wall and thereby promote bacterial lysis. Because mammalian cells have no cell wall, drugs directed at this structure do not affect us.

Inhibition of an Enzyme Unique to Bacteria

The sulfonamides represent antibiotics that are selectively toxic because they inhibit an enzyme critical to bacterial survival but not to our survival. Specifically, sulfonamides inhibit an enzyme needed to make folic acid, a compound required by all cells, both mammalian and bacterial. Because we can use folic acid from dietary sources, sulfonamides are safe for human consumption. In contrast, bacteria must synthesize folic acid themselves (because, unlike us, they can't take up folic acid from the environment). Hence, to meet their needs, bacteria first take up *para*-aminobenzoic acid (PABA), a precursor of folic acid, and then convert the PABA into folic acid. Sulfonamides block this conversion. Since mammalian cells do not make their own folic acid, sulfonamide toxicity is limited to microbes.

Disruption of Bacterial Protein Synthesis

In bacteria as in mammalian cells, protein synthesis is done by ribosomes. However, bacterial and mammalian ribosomes are not identical, and hence we can make drugs that disrupt the function of one but not the other. As a result, we can impair protein synthesis in bacteria while leaving mammalian protein synthesis untouched.

CLASSIFICATION OF ANTIMICROBIAL DRUGS

Various schemes are employed to classify antimicrobial drugs. The two schemes most suited to our objectives are considered here.

Classification by Susceptible Organism

Antibiotics differ widely in their antimicrobial activity. Some agents, called *narrow-spectrum antibiotics,* are active against only a few species of microorganisms. In contrast, *broad-spectrum antibiotics* are active against a wide variety of microbes. As discussed later in the chapter, *narrow-spectrum drugs are generally preferred to broad-spectrum drugs.*

Table 83.1 classifies the major antimicrobial drugs according to susceptible organisms. The table shows three major groups: *antibacterial drugs, antifungal drugs,* and *antiviral drugs.* In addition, the table subdivides the antibacterial drugs into narrow-spectrum and broad-spectrum agents, and indicates the principal classes of bacteria against which they are active.

Classification by Mechanism of Action

The antimicrobial drugs fall into seven major groups based on mechanism of action. This classification is shown in Table 83.2. Properties of the seven major classes are discussed briefly here.

- *Drugs that inhibit bacterial cell wall synthesis or activate enzymes that disrupt the cell wall*—These drugs (e.g., penicillins, cephalosporins) weaken the cell wall and thereby promote bacterial lysis and death.
- *Drugs that increase cell membrane permeability*—Drugs in this group (e.g., amphotericin B) increase the permeability of cell membranes, causing leakage of intracellular material.
- *Drugs that cause lethal inhibition of bacterial protein synthesis*—The aminoglycosides (e.g., gentamicin) are the only drugs in this group. We do not know why inhibition of protein synthesis by these agents results in cell death.
- *Drugs that cause nonlethal inhibition of protein synthesis*—Like the aminoglycosides, these drugs (e.g., tetracyclines) inhibit bacterial protein synthesis. However, in contrast to the aminoglycosides, these agents only slow microbial growth; they do not kill bacteria at clinically achievable concentrations.
- *Drugs that inhibit bacterial synthesis of DNA and RNA or disrupt DNA function*—These drugs inhibit synthesis of DNA or RNA by binding directly to nucleic acids or by interacting with enzymes required for nucleic acid synthesis. They may also bind with DNA and disrupt its function. Members of this group include rifampin, metronidazole, and the fluoroquinolones (e.g., ciprofloxacin).
- *Antimetabolites*—These drugs disrupt specific biochemical reactions. The result is either a decrease in the synthesis of essential cell constituents or synthesis of nonfunctional

TABLE 83.1 ■ Classification of Antimicrobial Drugs by Susceptible Organisms

ANTIBACTERIAL DRUGS

Narrow Spectrum

Gram-Positive Cocci and Gram-Positive Bacilli

Penicillin G and V
Penicillinase-resistant penicillins: oxacillin, nafcillin
Vancomycin
Erythromycin
Clindamycin

Gram-Negative Aerobes

Aminoglycosides: gentamicin, others
Cephalosporins (first and second generations)

Mycobacterium tuberculosis

Isoniazid
Rifampin
Ethambutol
Pyrazinamide

Broad Spectrum

Gram-Positive Cocci and Gram-Negative Bacilli

Broad-spectrum penicillins: ampicillin, others
Extended-spectrum penicillins: piperacillin, others
Cephalosporins (third and fifth generations)
Tetracyclines: tetracycline, others
Carbapenems: imipenem, others
Trimethoprim
Sulfonamides: sulfisoxazole, others
Fluoroquinolones: ciprofloxacin, others

ANTIVIRAL DRUGS

Drugs for HIV Infection

Reverse transcriptase inhibitors: zidovudine, others
Protease inhibitors: ritonavir, others
Fusion inhibitors: enfuvirtide
Integrase inhibitors: raltegravir
CCR5 antagonists: maraviroc

Drugs for Influenza

Adamantanes: amantadine, others
Neuraminidase inhibitors: oseltamivir, others

Other Antiviral Drugs

Acyclovir
Ribavirin
Interferon alfa

ANTIFUNGAL DRUGS

Polyene antibiotics: amphotericin B, others
Azoles: itraconazole, others
Echinocandins: caspofungin, others

TABLE 83.2 ■ Classification of Antimicrobial Drugs by Mechanism of Action

Drug Class	Representative Antibiotics
Inhibitors of cell wall synthesis	Penicillins Cephalosporins Imipenem Vancomycin Caspofungin
Drugs that disrupt the cell membrane	Amphotericin B Daptomycin Itraconazole
Bactericidal inhibitors of protein synthesis	Aminoglycosides
Bacteriostatic inhibitors of protein synthesis	Clindamycin Erythromycin Linezolid Tetracyclines
Drugs that interfere with synthesis or integrity of bacterial DNA and RNA	Fluoroquinolones Metronidazole Rifampin
Antimetabolites	Flucytosine Sulfonamides Trimethoprim
Drugs that suppress viral replication	
Viral DNA polymerase inhibitors	Acyclovir Ganciclovir
HIV reverse transcriptase inhibitors	Zidovudine Lamivudine
HIV protease inhibitors	Ritonavir Saquinavir
HIV fusion inhibitors	Enfuvirtide
HIV integrase inhibitors	Raltegravir
HIV CCR5 antagonists	Maraviroc
Influenza neuraminidase inhibitors	Oseltamivir Zanamivir

analogs of normal metabolites. Examples of antimetabolites include trimethoprim and the sulfonamides.

- *Drugs that suppress viral replication*—Most of these drugs inhibit specific enzymes—DNA polymerase, reverse transcriptase, protease, integrase, or neuraminidase—required for viral replication and infectivity.

When considering the *antibacterial* drugs, it is useful to distinguish between agents that are *bactericidal* and agents that are *bacteriostatic. Bactericidal* drugs are directly lethal to bacteria at clinically achievable concentrations. In contrast, *bacteriostatic* drugs can slow bacterial growth but do not cause cell death. When a bacteriostatic drug is used, elimination of bacteria must ultimately be accomplished by host defenses (i.e., the immune system working in concert with phagocytic cells).

ACQUIRED RESISTANCE TO ANTIMICROBIAL DRUGS

In this section, we discuss bacterial resistance to antibiotics, which may be *innate* (natural, inborn) or *acquired* over time. Discussion here is limited to acquired resistance, which is a much greater clinical concern than innate resistance.

Over time, an organism that had once been highly sensitive to an antibiotic may become less susceptible, or it may lose drug sensitivity entirely. In some cases, resistance develops to several drugs. Acquired resistance is of great concern in that it can render currently effective drugs useless, thereby creating a clinical crisis and a constant need for new antimicrobial agents. As a rule, antibiotic resistance is associated with extended hospitalization, significant morbidity, and excess mortality. Organisms for which drug resistance is now a serious problem include *Enterococcus faecium, Staphylococcus aureus, Enterobacter* species, *Pseudomonas aeruginosa, Acinetobacter baumannii, Klebsiella* species, and *Clostridium difficile* (Table 83.3).

TABLE 83.3 ▪ Drugs for Some Highly Resistant Bacteria

Bacterium	Resistance	Resistance Mechanism	Alternative Treatments
Enterococcus faecium	Ampicillin	Mutation and overexpression of PBP5	Quinupristin/dalfopristin, daptomycin, tigecycline, linezolid
	Linezolid	Production of altered 23S ribosomes	Quinupristin/dalfopristin, daptomycin, tigecycline
	Daptomycin	Unknown	Quinupristin/dalfopristin
	Quinupristin/dalfopristin	Production of enzymes that inactivate quinupristin/dalfopristin, altered drug target	Daptomycin, tigecycline, linezolid
	Aminoglycosides	Production of aminoglycoside-modifying enzymes, ribosomal mutations	May attempt to test for streptomycin sensitivity
Staphylococcus aureus[a]	Vancomycin	Thickening of cell wall and altered structure of cell wall precursor molecules	Quinupristin/dalfopristin, daptomycin, tigecycline, linezolid, telavancin
	Daptomycin	Altered structure of cell wall and cell membrane	Quinupristin/dalfopristin, tigecycline, linezolid, telavancin
	Linezolid	Production of altered 23S ribosomes	Quinupristin/dalfopristin, daptomycin, tigecycline, telavancin, ceftobiprole 🍁, ceftaroline
	Ceftaroline	Mutation in PBP2a	Quinupristin/dalfopristin, telavancin
Enterobacter species	Ceftriaxone, cefotaxime, ceftazidime, cefepime	Production of extended-spectrum beta-lactamases	Carbapenems, tigecycline
	Carbapenems	Production of carbapenemases, decreased permeability	Polymyxins, tigecycline
Klebsiella species	Ceftriaxone, cefotaxime, ceftazidime, cefepime	Production of extended-spectrum beta-lactamases	Carbapenems, tigecycline
	Carbapenems	Production of carbapenemases, decreased permeability	Polymyxins, tigecycline
Pseudomonas aeruginosa	Carbapenems	Decreased permeability, increased drug efflux, production of carbapenemases	Polymyxins
Acinetobacter baumannii	Carbapenems	Decreased permeability, increased drug efflux, production of carbapenemases	Polymyxins
Clostridium difficile[b]	Metronidazole	Reduced drug activation, increased drug efflux, increased repair of drug-induced DNA damage	Vancomycin, rifaximin

[a]Methicillin-resistant *Staphylococcus aureus* is discussed in Chapter 84.
[b]*Clostridium difficile* infection is discussed in Chapter 85.
PBP5, Penicillin-binding protein 5; *PBP2a,* penicillin-binding protein 2a.

Two of these resistant bacteria—methicillin-resistant *Staph. aureus* and *C. difficile*—are discussed in Chapters 84 and 85, respectively.

In the discussion that follows, we examine the mechanisms by which microbial drug resistance is acquired and the measures by which emergence of resistance can be delayed. As you read this section, keep in mind that it is the *microbe* that becomes drug resistant, *not the patient.*

Microbial Mechanisms of Drug Resistance

Microbes have four basic mechanisms for resisting drugs. They can (1) decrease the concentration of a drug at its site of action, (2) alter the structure of drug target molecules, (3) produce a drug antagonist, and (4) cause drug inactivation.

Reduction of Drug Concentration at Its Site of Action

For most antimicrobial drugs, the site of action is intracellular. Accordingly, if a bug can reduce the intracellular concentration of a drug, it can resist harm. Two basic mechanisms are involved. First, microbes can *cease active uptake* of certain drugs—tetracyclines and gentamicin, for example. Second, microbes can *increase active export* of certain drugs—tetracyclines, fluoroquinolones, and macrolides, for example.

Alteration of Drug Target Molecules

Most antibiotics, like most other drugs, must interact with target molecules (receptors) to produce their effects. Hence, if the structure of the target molecule is altered, resistance can result. For example, some bacteria are now resistant to streptomycin because of structural changes in bacterial ribosomes, the sites at which streptomycin acts to inhibit protein synthesis.

Antagonist Production

In rare cases, a microbe can synthesize a compound that antagonizes drug actions. For example, by acquiring the ability to synthesize increased quantities of PABA, some bacteria have developed resistance to sulfonamides.

Drug Inactivation

Microbes can resist harm by producing drug-metabolizing enzymes. For example, many bacteria are resistant to penicillin G because of increased production of penicillinase, an enzyme that inactivates penicillin. In addition to penicillins, bacterial enzymes can inactivate other antibiotics, including cephalosporins, carbapenems, and fluoroquinolones.

New Delhi Metallo-Beta-Lactamase 1 (NDM-1) Gene. Extensive drug resistance is conferred by the *NDM-1 gene,* which codes for a powerful form of beta-lactamase. As discussed in Chapters 84 and 85, beta-lactamases are enzymes that can inactivate drugs that have a beta-lactam ring. The form of beta-lactamase encoded by *NDM-1* is both unusual and troubling in that it can inactivate essentially all beta-lactam antibiotics, a group that includes penicillins, cephalosporins, and carbapenems. As the *NDM-1* gene is resistant to carbapenems, it is also classified as a type of carbapenems-resistant Enterobacteriaceae (CRE).Worse yet, the DNA segment that contains the *NDM-1* gene also contains genes that code for additional resistance determinants, including drug efflux pumps, and enzymes that can inactivate other important antibiotics, including erythromycin, rifampin, chloramphenicol, and fluoroquinolones. Furthermore, all of these genes are present on a plasmid, a piece of DNA that can be easily transferred from one bacterium to another (see *Conjugation*). Of note, bacteria that have the *NDM-1* gene are resistant to nearly all antibiotics, except for tigecycline and colistin. Since its discovery in *Klebsiella pneumoniae* in 2008, *NDM-1* has been found in other common enteric bacteria, including *Escherichia coli, Enterobacter, Salmonella, Citrobacter freundii, Providencia rettgeri,* and *Morganella morganii.* Before 2012, only a few cases of *NDM-1* infection were reported in the United States and Canada, but that number is increasing.

Mechanisms By Which Resistance Is Acquired

How do microbes acquire mechanisms of resistance? Ultimately, all of the alterations in structure and function discussed previously result from changes in the microbial genome. These genetic changes may result either from spontaneous mutation or from acquisition of DNA from an external source. One important mechanism of DNA acquisition is conjugation with other bacteria.

Spontaneous Mutation

Spontaneous mutations produce random changes in a microbe's DNA. The result is a gradual increase in resistance. Low-level resistance develops first. With additional mutations, resistance becomes greater. As a rule, spontaneous mutations confer resistance *to only one drug.*

Conjugation

Conjugation is a process by which extrachromosomal DNA is transferred from one bacterium to another. To transfer resistance by conjugation, the donor organism must possess two unique DNA segments, one that codes for the mechanisms of drug resistance and one that codes for the "sexual" apparatus required for DNA transfer. Together, these two DNA segments constitute an *R factor* (resistance factor).

Conjugation takes place primarily among *gram-negative* bacteria. Genetic material may be transferred between members of the same species or between members of different species. Because transfer of R factors is not species specific, it is possible for pathogenic bacteria to acquire R factors from the normal flora of the body. Because R factors are becoming common in normal flora, the possibility of transferring resistance from normal flora to pathogens is a significant clinical concern.

In contrast to spontaneous mutation, conjugation frequently confers *multiple drug resistance.* This can be achieved, for example, by transferring DNA that codes for several different drug-metabolizing enzymes. Hence, in a single event, a drug-sensitive bacterium can become highly drug resistant.

Relationships Between Antibiotic Use and Emergence of Drug-Resistant Microbes

Use of antibiotics promotes the emergence of drug-resistant microbes. Please note, however, that although antibiotics promote drug resistance, they are not mutagenic and do not directly cause the genetic changes that underlie reduced drug sensitivity. Spontaneous mutation and conjugation are random events whose incidence is independent of drug use. Drugs simply make conditions favorable for overgrowth of microbes that have acquired mechanisms for resistance.

How Do Antibiotics Promote Resistance?

To answer this question, we need to recall two aspects of microbial ecology: (1) microbes secrete compounds that are toxic to other microbes and (2) microbes within a given ecologic niche (e.g., large intestine, urogenital tract, skin) compete with each other for available nutrients. Under drug-free conditions, the various microbes in a given niche keep each other in check. Furthermore, if none of these organisms is drug resistant, introduction of antibiotics will be equally detrimental to all members of the population and therefore will not promote the growth of any individual microbe. However, *if a drug-resistant organism is present, antibiotics will create selection pressure favoring its growth* by killing off sensitive organisms. In doing so, the drug will eliminate the toxins they produce and will thereby facilitate survival of the microbe that is drug resistant. Also, elimination of sensitive organisms will remove competition for available nutrients, thereby making conditions even more favorable for the resistant microbe to flourish. Hence, although drug resistance is of no benefit to an organism when there are no antibiotics present, when antibiotics are introduced, they create selection pressure favoring overgrowth of microbes that are resistant.

Which Antibiotics Promote Resistance?

All antimicrobial drugs promote the emergence of drug-resistant organisms. However, some agents are more likely to promote resistance than others. Because broad-spectrum antibiotics kill more competing organisms than do narrow-spectrum drugs, broad-spectrum agents do the most to facilitate emergence of resistance.

The Influence of Increased Antibiotic Use on the Emergence of Resistance

The more that antibiotics are used, the faster drug-resistant organisms will emerge. Not only do antibiotics promote the emergence of resistant pathogens, they also promote the overgrowth of normal flora that possesses mechanisms for resistance. Because drug use can increase resistance in normal flora and because normal flora can transfer resistance to pathogens, every effort should be made to avoid the use of antibiotics by individuals who don't actually need them (i.e., individuals who don't have a bacterial infection). Because all antibiotic use will further the emergence of resistance, there can be no excuse for casual or indiscriminate dispensing of these drugs.

Healthcare-Associated Infections

Because hospitals are sites of intensive antibiotic use, resident organisms can be extremely drug resistant. As a result, *healthcare-associated infections (HAIs)* are among the most difficult to treat. According to the Centers for Disease Control and Prevention (CDC), 1 of every 25 patients will fall victim to an HAI. Measures to delay emergence of resistant organisms in hospitals are discussed under *Antimicrobial Stewardship*.

Superinfection

Superinfection is a special example of the emergence of drug resistance. A superinfection is defined as a *new* infection that appears during the course of treatment for a primary infection. New infections develop when antibiotics eliminate the inhibitory influence of normal flora, thereby allowing a second infectious agent to flourish. When there is normal flora that contains a resistant organism, the antibiotic will selectively promote the growth of that specific resistant flora. Although the antibiotic promotes the overgrowth of resistant flora, it kills off sensitive strains, thus facilitating the survival of the resistant flora. Although there is selective overgrowth of the normal flora with resistance, there is still a decrease in the inhibitory effects of the sensitive flora.

Because broad-spectrum antibiotics kill off more normal flora than do narrow-spectrum drugs, superinfections are more likely in patients receiving broad-spectrum agents. Because superinfections are caused by drug-resistant microbes, these infections are often difficult to treat.

Antimicrobial Stewardship

Many organizations have begun to address the issue of antibiotic resistance in healthcare. In 2012, the Infectious Diseases Society of America (IDSA), in conjunction with the Society for Healthcare Epidemiology of America (SHEA) and the Pediatric Infectious Diseases Society (PIDS), released its first *Policy Statement on Antimicrobial Stewardship*. The statement included five recommendations, including suggestions for monitoring, education, and research to assist in the prevention of antibiotic resistance. The statement can be found online at http://www.jstor.org/stable/10.1086/665010.

The *Get Smart for Healthcare* campaign initiated by the CDC provides information on the proper use of antibiotics in humans and animals. The campaign has three objectives: to promote adherence to appropriate prescribing guidelines, to decrease the demand for antibiotics among healthy adults and parents of young children, and to increase adherence to prescribed antibiotics. Target audiences include patient and providers. More information is available at www.cdc.gov/drugresistance. The important topic of antibiotic use in animals is discussed in Box 83.1.

In addition to the CDC campaign, in 2014 the Interagency Task Force on Antimicrobial Resistance published an update to its original publication: *A Public Health Action Plan to Combat Antimicrobial Resistance*. This updated action plan discusses four focus areas developed to decrease resistance to antibiotics:

- **Focus Area I: Surveillance, Prevention, and Control of Antimicrobial-Resistant Infections.** Goals include improving the detection, monitoring, and characterization of drug-resistant infections in humans and animals, as well as improving the definition, characterization, and measurement of the impact of antimicrobial drug use.
- **Focus Area II: Research.** Goals include the facilitation of basic research on antimicrobial resistance, as well as the translation of basic research into practice. Support for epidemiologic studies to identify key drivers of the emergence and spread of antimicrobial resistance is of great importance.
- **Focus Area III: Regulatory Pathways for New Products.** The aims for this focus area include the provision of information on the development status of antibacterial drug products and encouragement for further development of rapid diagnostic tests and vaccines.
- **Focus Area IV: Product Development.** Goals include providing a systematic assessment of current and future needs for antimicrobial resistance products and promoting the development of drugs targeted to address areas where unmet needs exist.

SELECTION OF ANTIBIOTICS

When treating infection, the therapeutic objective is to produce maximal antimicrobial effects while causing minimal harm to the host. To achieve this goal, we must select the most appropriate antibiotic for the individual patient. When choosing an antibiotic, three principal factors must be considered: (1) the identity of the infecting organism, (2) drug sensitivity of the infecting organism, and (3) host factors, such as the site of infection and the status of host defenses.

For any given infection, several drugs may be effective. However, for most infections, there is usually one drug that is superior to the alternatives (Table 83.4). This drug of first choice may be preferred for several reasons, such as greater efficacy, lower toxicity, or more narrow spectrum. Whenever possible, the drug of first choice should be employed. Alternative agents should be used only when the first-choice drug is inappropriate. Conditions that might rule out a first-choice agent include (1) allergy to the drug of choice, (2) inability of the drug of choice to penetrate to the site of infection, and (3) heightened susceptibility of the patient to toxicity of the first-choice drug.

Empiric Therapy Before Completion of Laboratory Tests

Optimal antimicrobial therapy requires identification of the infecting organism and determination of its drug sensitivity.

si BOX 83.1 ▪ SPECIAL INTEREST TOPIC

ANTIBIOTICS IN ANIMAL FEED: DYING FOR A HAMBURGER AND CHICKEN NUGGETS

Drug-resistant infection resulting from the use of antibiotics in agriculture is a global public health concern. Antibiotics are employed extensively in the livestock and poultry industries. Not surprisingly, this practice has created a large reservoir of drug-resistant bacteria, some of which now infect humans. In addition to being a direct detriment to health, these infections pose an even larger threat: the passage of resistance genes to normal intestinal flora, and then from normal flora to human pathogens.

The amount of antibiotics given to food animals is staggering. In 2010, animals worldwide received 63,151 tons of antimicrobials. This is expected to increase by 67% by 2030. Of antibiotics produced in the United States each year, nearly 80% (13,300 tons) goes to animals. Even more surprisingly, of the antibiotics that animals receive, only 7.5% (1000 tons) is given to treat infection. The vast majority—12,300 tons—is mixed with feed to promote growth. Both uses encourage the emergence of resistance.

Of the two agricultural uses—growth promotion and treatment of infection—growth promotion is by far the more controversial. Few authorities would argue that we shouldn't give antibiotics to treat animal infections. In contrast, there are strong arguments against giving antibiotics to promote growth. The doses employed for growth promotion are much lower than those used for infection, and hence are *more* likely to encourage emergence of resistance. Moreover, since growth can be promoted by other means, giving antibiotics for this purpose is unnecessary.

Essentially all of the antibiotics used in humans are used in animals—including fluoroquinolones and third-generation cephalosporins, agents that are among the most effective we have. Because all antibiotics are being used, we are hastening the day when all will be useless.

The story of virginiamycin and Synercid illustrates the potentially serious consequences of giving antibiotics to farm animals. Virginiamycin is a mixture of two streptogramins. For 30 years, the drug has been used to promote animal growth. In 1999, a mixture of two similar streptogramins—quinupristin and dalfopristin, sold as Synercid—was approved for medical use in the United States. Synercid is an extremely important drug because it can kill vancomycin-resistant *Enterococcus faecium,* a dangerous pathogenic strain that is resistant to all other antibiotics. Unfortunately, agricultural use of virginiamycin is likely to shorten Synercid's useful life: A study of chickens that were fed virginiamycin indicates that 50% of the birds carried Synercid-resistant *E. faecium.* Sooner or later, these birds will pass these resistant pathogens on to humans—if they haven't already.

How can we reduce agriculture-related resistance? If we want to delay emergence of resistance, and thereby extend the useful life of our antibiotics, we must limit agricultural use of these drugs. To this end, the World Health Organization has recommended that all antibiotics used by humans be banned from use to promote growth in animals. In 2006, 15 countries in the European Union complied, banning the use of *all* antibiotics for growth promotion in livestock. The impact was entirely positive, assuming the experience in Denmark applies to the rest of Europe. In the late 1990s, Denmark banned the use of antibiotics for growth promotion in pigs and chickens, with no apparent detriment to either animal health or the incomes of producers. Furthermore, within a few years after these drugs were discontinued, rates of antibiotic resistance among farm animals dropped dramatically. For example, resistance to avoparcin dropped from 73% to 5% in less than 5 years.

In the United States, public health and agriculture officials have discussed and debated the issue for more than 30 years, but no legislation has been enacted. In June 2013, legislation was proposed to limit the use of antibiotics in livestock production. The bill was not enacted in 2013 or 2015, but was reintroduced into Congress in March 2017. If enacted, the Preventing Antibiotic Resistance Act of 2017 would direct the U.S. Food and Drug Administration (FDA) to restrict the use of antibiotics critical to human health in livestock production unless they are used to treat clinically diagnosable diseases.

And there *is* some hope. In 2005, the FDA took an important step: For the first time, they banned the agricultural use of a specific drug. The FDA ruling, which took effect September 12, 2005, banned the use of enrofloxacin [Baytril] in chickens and turkeys. (Enrofloxacin is a fluoroquinolone similar to ciprofloxacin [Cipro].) The ban was based on concerns that widespread use of enrofloxacin in poultry was promoting resistance to ciprofloxacin and other fluoroquinolones in humans. This case is significant in that it sets a precedent for FDA action against other animal antibiotics.

Although wide-reaching restrictive rules are not yet in place, they may, at long last, be forthcoming: In 2012, the FDA posted its publication *The Judicious Use of Medically Important Antimicrobial Drugs in Food-Producing Animals* as a "guidance," indicating that it no longer considers giving livestock antibiotics to promote growth a "judicious use" of these drugs, implying that it plans to ban the practice. Then, in 2013, the FDA followed that guideline with one regarding the use of new animal drugs: *New Animal Drugs and New Animal Drug Combination Products Administered in or on Medicated Feed or Drinking Water of Food-Producing Animals*. The FDA, however, continues to allow use of antibiotics to treat or prevent the spread of disease—provided such use is overseen by a veterinarian.

TABLE 83.4 ■ Antibacterial Drugs of Choice

Organism	Drug of First Choice	Some Alternative Drugs
GRAM-POSITIVE COCCI		
Enterococcus[a]		
Endocarditis and other severe infections	Penicillin G *or* ampicillin *with either* gentamicin or streptomycin	Vancomycin *with either* gentamicin or streptomycin, quinupristin/dalfopristin, linezolid, daptomycin
Uncomplicated urinary tract infection	Amoxicillin	Nitrofurantoin, penicillin, fosfomycin
Staphylococcus aureus or *S. epidermidis*[a]		
Penicillinase producing	A penicillinase-resistant penicillin (nafcillin)	A cephalosporin, vancomycin, imipenem, linezolid, clindamycin, daptomycin, a fluoroquinolone
Methicillin resistant	Vancomycin or daptomycin	Linezolid, quinupristin/dalfopristin, tigecycline, doxycycline, ceftaroline, trimethoprim/sulfamethoxazole
Streptococcus pyogenes (group A) and groups C and G	Penicillin G with clindamycin, penicillin V	Vancomycin, erythromycin, clarithromycin, azithromycin, daptomycin, linezolid, a cephalosporin
Streptococcus, group B	Penicillin G or ampicillin	A cephalosporin, vancomycin, erythromycin, daptomycin
Streptococcus viridans group	Penicillin G or ampicillin	A cephalosporin, vancomycin
Streptococcus bovis	Penicillin G or ampicillin	A cephalosporin, vancomycin
Streptococcus, anaerobic	Cephalosporin	Clindamycin, vancomycin
Streptococcus pneumoniae (pneumococcus)	Penicillin G, penicillin V, amoxicillin in susceptible strains Resistant strains: a cephalosporin, ampicillin	Erythromycin, azithromycin, clarithromycin, levofloxacin, gemifloxacin, moxifloxacin, meropenem, imipenem, ertapenem, trimethoprim/sulfamethoxazole, clindamycin, a tetracycline, vancomycin
GRAM-NEGATIVE COCCI		
Neisseria gonorrhoeae (gonococcus)	See Chapter 95	
Neisseria meningitides (meningococcus)	Third-generation cephalosporin	Penicillin G, chloramphenicol, a sulfonamide, a fluoroquinolone
GRAM-POSITIVE BACILLI		
Bacillus anthracis (anthrax)	See Chapter 110	
Clostridium difficile	See Chapter 85	
Clostridium perfringens	Penicillin G, clindamycin	Metronidazole, chloramphenicol, imipenem, meropenem, ertapenem
Clostridium tetani	Metronidazole	Penicillin G, doxycycline
Corynebacterium diphtheriae	Erythromycin	Penicillin G
Listeria monocytogenes	Ampicillin or penicillin G with or without gentamicin	Trimethoprim/sulfamethoxazole
ENTERIC GRAM-NEGATIVE BACILLI		
Campylobacter jejuni	Fluoroquinolones, azithromycin	Gentamicin, a tetracycline
Escherichia coli	Cefotaxime, ceftazidime, cefepime, ceftriaxone	Ampicillin with or without gentamicin, ticarcillin/clavulanic acid, trimethoprim/sulfamethoxazole, imipenem, meropenem, others
Enterobacter[a]	Imipenem, meropenem, cefepime	Trimethoprim/sulfamethoxazole, gentamicin, tobramycin, amikacin, ciprofloxacin, cefotaxime, ticarcillin/clavulanic acid, piperacillin/tazobactam, aztreonam, ceftazidime, tigecycline
Klebsiella pneumoniae[a]	Cefotaxime, ceftriaxone, cefepime, ceftazidime	Imipenem, meropenem, ertapenem, gentamicin, tobramycin, amikacin, others
Proteus, indole positive (including *Providencia rettgeri* and *Morganella morganii*)	Cefotaxime, ceftriaxone, cefepime, ceftazidime	Imipenem, meropenem, ertapenem, gentamicin, a fluoroquinolone, trimethoprim/sulfamethoxazole, others

Continued

TABLE 83.4 ■ Antibacterial Drugs of Choice—cont'd

Organism	Drug of First Choice	Some Alternative Drugs
Proteus mirabilis	Ampicillin	A cephalosporin, ticarcillin, trimethoprim/sulfamethoxazole, imipenem, meropenem, ertapenem, gentamicin, others
Salmonella typhi	Ceftriaxone, a fluoroquinolone	Trimethoprim/sulfamethoxazole, ampicillin, amoxicillin, chloramphenicol, azithromycin
Other *Salmonella*	Ceftriaxone, cefotaxime, a fluoroquinolone	Trimethoprim/sulfamethoxazole, chloramphenicol, ampicillin, amoxicillin
Serratia	Imipenem, meropenem	Gentamicin, amikacin, cefotaxime, a fluoroquinolone, trimethoprim/sulfamethoxazole, aztreonam, others
Shigella	A fluoroquinolone	Trimethoprim/sulfamethoxazole, ampicillin, ceftriaxone, azithromycin
Yersinia enterocolitica	Trimethoprim/sulfamethoxazole	A fluoroquinolone, gentamicin, tobramycin, amikacin, cefotaxime
OTHER GRAM-NEGATIVE BACILLI		
Acinetobacter[a]	Imipenem, meropenem	An aminoglycoside, trimethoprim/sulfamethoxazole, doxycycline, ciprofloxacin, ceftazidime, ticarcillin/clavulanic acid, piperacillin/tazobactam
Bacteroides	Metronidazole	Imipenem, ertapenem, meropenem, amoxicillin/clavulanic acid, ticarcillin/clavulanic acid, piperacillin/tazobactam, ampicillin/sulbactam, chloramphenicol
Bordetella pertussis (whooping cough)	Azithromycin, clarithromycin, erythromycin	Trimethoprim/sulfamethoxazole
Brucella (brucellosis)	A tetracycline *plus* rifampin	A tetracycline *plus either* gentamicin or streptomycin, trimethoprim/sulfamethoxazole *with or without* gentamicin, chloramphenicol *with or without* streptomycin, ciprofloxacin *plus* rifampin
Calymmatobacterium granulomatis	Azithromycin	Doxycycline, trimethoprim/sulfamethoxazole, or ciprofloxacin
Francisella tularensis (tularemia)	See Chapter 110	
Gardnerella vaginalis	Metronidazole (PO)	Topical clindamycin or metronidazole, clindamycin (PO)
Haemophilus ducreyi (chancroid)	Azithromycin, ceftriaxone	Ciprofloxacin, erythromycin
Haemophilus influenzae		
Meningitis, epiglottitis, arthritis, and other serious infections	Cefotaxime, ceftriaxone	Cefuroxime, chloramphenicol, meropenem
Helicobacter pylori	Clarithromycin *plus* amoxicillin *plus* esomeprazole (a proton pump inhibitor)	Tetracycline *plus* metronidazole *plus* bismuth subsalicylate *plus* esomeprazole (a proton pump inhibitor)
Legionella species	Azithromycin, clarithromycin	Doxycycline, trimethoprim/sulfamethoxazole, erythromycin fluoroquinolone
Pasteurella multocida	Penicillin G	Doxycycline, a second- or third-generation cephalosporin, amoxicillin/clavulanic acid, ampicillin/sulbactam
Pseudomonas aeruginosa[a]		
Urinary tract infection	Ciprofloxacin	Levofloxacin, piperacillin/tazobactam, ceftazidime, cefepime, imipenem, meropenem, gentamicin, tobramycin, amikacin, aztreonam
Other infections	Piperacillin/tazobactam (or ticarcillin/clavulanic acid) *with or without* tobramycin, gentamicin, or amikacin	Ceftazidime, ciprofloxacin, imipenem, meropenem, aztreonam, or cefepime, *any one with or without* tobramycin, gentamicin, or amikacin
Spirillum minus (rat bite fever)	Penicillin G, ceftriaxone	Doxycycline, streptomycin

TABLE 83.4 ▪ Antibacterial Drugs of Choice—cont'd

Organism	Drug of First Choice	Some Alternative Drugs
Streptobacillus moniliformis (rat bite fever)	Penicillin G, ceftriaxone	Doxycycline, streptomycin
Vibrio cholerae (cholera)	A tetracycline	Trimethoprim/sulfamethoxazole, a fluoroquinolone
Yersinia pestis (plague)	See Chapter 110	
MYCOBACTERIA		
Mycobacterium tuberculosis	See Chapter 90	
Mycobacterium leprae (leprosy)	See Chapter 90	
Mycobacterium avium complex	See Chapter 90	
ACTINOMYCETES		
Actinomycetes israelii	Penicillin G	Doxycycline, erythromycin, clindamycin
Nocardia	Trimethoprim/sulfamethoxazole	Sulfisoxazole, imipenem, meropenem, amikacin, a tetracycline, linezolid, ceftriaxone, cycloserine
CHLAMYDIAE		
Chlamydia psittaci	Doxycycline	Chloramphenicol
Chlamydia trachomatis	See Chapter 95	
MYCOPLASMA		
Mycoplasma pneumoniae	Erythromycin, clarithromycin, azithromycin, a tetracycline	A fluoroquinolone
Ureaplasma urealyticum	Azithromycin	A tetracycline, clarithromycin, erythromycin, ofloxacin
RICKETTSIA		
Rocky Mountain spotted fever, endemic typhus (murine), trench fever, typhus, scrub typhus, Q fever	Doxycycline	Chloramphenicol, a fluoroquinolone
SPIROCHETES		
Borrelia burgdorferi (Lyme disease)	Doxycycline, amoxicillin, cefuroxime	Ceftriaxone, cefotaxime, penicillin G, azithromycin, clarithromycin
Borrelia recurrentis (relapsing fever)	A tetracycline, penicillin G	Erythromycin
Leptospira	Penicillin G	Doxycycline, ceftriaxone
Treponema pallidum (syphilis)	Penicillin G	Doxycycline, ceftriaxone
Treponema pertenue (yaws)	Penicillin G	Doxycycline

[a]Many of these drugs have resistant strains that must be treated with alternative antibiotics.

However, when the patient has a severe infection, we may have to initiate treatment before test results are available. Under these conditions, drug selection must be based on clinical evaluation and knowledge of which microbes are most likely to cause infection at a particular site. If necessary, a broad-spectrum agent can be used for initial treatment. Once the identity and drug sensitivity of the infecting organism have been determined, we can switch to a more selective antibiotic. When conditions demand that we start therapy in the absence of laboratory data, it is essential that samples of exudates and body fluids be obtained for culture *before initiation of treatment;* if antibiotics are present at the time of sampling, they can suppress microbial growth in culture and can thereby confound identification.

Identifying the Infecting Organism

The first rule of antimicrobial therapy is to *match the drug with the bug.* Hence, whenever possible, the infecting organism should be identified before starting treatment. If treatment is begun in the absence of a definitive diagnosis, positive identification should be established as soon as possible, so as to permit adjustment of the regimen to better conform with the drug sensitivity of the infecting organism.

The quickest, simplest, and most versatile technique for identifying microorganisms is microscopic examination of a *Gram-stained preparation.* Samples for examination can be obtained from exudate, sputum, urine, blood, and other body fluids. The most useful samples are direct aspirates from the site of infection.

In some cases, only a small number of infecting organisms will be present. Under these conditions, positive identification may require that the microbes be grown out in culture. As stressed earlier, material for culture should be obtained before initiating treatment. Furthermore, the samples should be taken in a fashion that minimizes contamination with normal body flora. Also, the samples should not be exposed to low temperature, antiseptics, or oxygen.

A relatively new method, known as the *polymerase chain reaction (PCR) test* or *nucleic acid amplification test,* can detect very low titers of bacteria and viruses. Testing is done by using an enzyme—either DNA polymerase or RNA polymerase—to generate thousands of copies of DNA or RNA unique to the infecting microbe. As a result of this nucleic acid amplification, there is enough material for detection. Microbes that we can identify with a PCR test include important bacterial pathogens (e.g., *Clostridium difficile, Staphylococcus aureus, Mycobacterium tuberculosis, Neisseria gonorrhoeae, Chlamydia trachomatis, Helicobacter pylori*) and important viral pathogens (e.g., human immunodeficiency virus, influenza virus). Compared with Gram staining, PCR tests are both more specific and more sensitive.

Determining Drug Susceptibility

Owing to the emergence of drug-resistant microbes, testing for drug sensitivity is common. However, sensitivity testing is not always needed. Rather, testing is indicated only when the infecting organism is one in which resistance is likely. Hence, for microbes such as the group A streptococci, which have remained highly susceptible to penicillin G, sensitivity testing is unnecessary. In contrast, when resistance *is* common, as it is with *Staph. aureus* and the gram-negative bacilli, tests for drug sensitivity should be performed. Most tests used today are based on one of three methods: disk diffusion, serial dilution, or gradient diffusion.

Before sensitivity testing can be done, we must first identify the microbe so that we can test for sensitivity to the appropriate drugs. For example, if the infection is caused by *Clostridium difficile,* we might test for sensitivity to metronidazole or vancomycin. We would not test for sensitivity to aminoglycosides or cephalosporins—because we already know these drugs won't work.

Disk Diffusion

The disk-diffusion test, also known as the Kirby-Bauer test, is performed by seeding an agar plate with a solution of the infecting organism and then placing on the plate several paper disks that have been impregnated with different antibiotics. Because of diffusion, an antibiotic-containing zone becomes established around each disk. As the bacteria proliferate, growth will be inhibited around the disks that contain an antibiotic to which the bacteria are sensitive. The degree of drug sensitivity is proportional to the size of the bacteria-free zone. Hence, by measuring the diameter of these zones, we can determine the drugs to which the organism is more susceptible and the drugs to which it is highly resistant.

Serial Dilution

In this procedure, bacteria are grown in a series of tubes containing different concentrations of an antibiotic. The advantage of this method over the disk-diffusion test is that it provides a more precise measure of drug sensitivity. By using serial dilution, we can establish close estimates of two clinically useful values: (1) the *minimum inhibitory concentration* (MIC), defined as the lowest concentration of antibiotic that produces complete inhibition of bacterial growth (but does not *kill* bacteria); and (2) the *minimum bactericidal concentration* (MBC), defined as the lowest concentration of drug that produces a 99.9% decline in the number of bacterial colonies (indicating bacterial kill). Because of the quantitative information provided, serial dilution procedures are especially useful for guiding therapy of infections that are unusually difficult to treat.

Gradient Diffusion

The gradient-diffusion procedure is similar to the disk-diffusion procedure, but provides a more precise indication of MIC. Like the disk-diffusion test, the gradient-diffusion test begins with seeding an agar plate with the infecting organism. Then, a narrow test *strip,* rather than a disk, is placed on the plate. Unlike the disk, which is impregnated with just one concentration of an antibiotic, the strip is impregnated with 15 or so different concentrations of the same antibiotic, such that there is a concentration gradient that runs from low to high along the length of the strip. Hence, as antibiotic diffuses from the strip into the agar, the concentration of drug in the agar establishes a gradient as well. Bacteria on the plate will continue to grow until they reach a zone of the plate where the antibiotic concentration is high enough to inhibit further growth. The point where the zone of inhibition intersects the strip, which is calibrated at short intervals along its length, indicates the MIC.

HOST FACTORS THAT MODIFY DRUG CHOICE, ROUTE OF ADMINISTRATION, OR DOSAGE

In addition to matching the drug with the bug and determining the drug sensitivity of an infecting organism, we must consider host factors when prescribing an antimicrobial drug. Two host factors—host defenses and infection site—are unique to the selection of antibiotics. Other host factors, such as age, pregnancy, and previous drug reactions, are the same factors that must be considered when choosing any other drug.

Host Defenses

Host defenses consist primarily of the immune system and phagocytic cells (macrophages, neutrophils). Without the contribution of these defenses, successful antimicrobial therapy would be rare. In most cases, the drugs we use don't cure infection on their own. Rather, they work in concert with host defense systems to subdue infection. Accordingly, the usual objective of antibiotic treatment is not outright kill of infecting organisms. Rather, the goal is to suppress microbial growth to the point at which the balance is tipped in favor of the host. Underscoring the critical role of host defenses is the grim fact that people whose defenses are impaired, such as those with AIDS and those undergoing cancer chemotherapy, frequently die from infections that drugs alone are unable to control. When treating the immunocompromised host, our only hope lies with drugs that are rapidly bactericidal, and even these may prove inadequate.

Site of Infection

To be effective, an antibiotic must be present at the site of infection in a concentration greater than the MIC. At some sites, drug penetration may be hampered, making it difficult to achieve the MIC. For example, drug access can be impeded in meningitis (because of the blood-brain barrier), endocarditis (because bacterial vegetations in the heart are difficult to penetrate), and infected abscesses (because of poor vascularity and the presence of purulent material). When treating meningitis, two approaches may be used: (1) We can select a drug that readily crosses the blood-brain barrier, and (2) we can inject an antibiotic directly into the subarachnoid space. When exudate and other fluids hinder drug access, surgical drainage is indicated.

Foreign materials (e.g., cardiac pacemakers, prosthetic joints and heart valves, synthetic vascular shunts) present a special local problem. Phagocytes react to these objects and attempt to destroy them. Because of this behavior, the phagocytes are less able to attack bacteria, thereby allowing microbes to flourish. Treatment of these infections often results in failure or relapse. In many cases, the infection can be eliminated only by removing the foreign material.

Other Host Factors

Previous Allergic Reaction

Severe allergic reactions are more common with the penicillins than with any other family of drugs. As a rule, patients with a history of severe allergy to the penicillins should not receive them again. The exception is treatment of a life-threatening infection for which no suitable alternative is available. In addition to the penicillins, other antibiotics (sulfonamides, trimethoprim, erythromycin) are associated with a high incidence of allergic responses. However, severe reactions to these agents are rare.

Genetic Factors

As with other drugs, responses to antibiotics can be influenced by the patient's genetic heritage. For example, some antibiotics (e.g., sulfonamides) can cause hemolysis in patients who, because of their genetic makeup, have red blood cells that are deficient in glucose-6-phosphate dehydrogenase. Clearly, people with this deficiency should not be given antibiotics that are likely to induce red cell lysis.

Genetic factors can also affect rates of metabolism. For example, hepatic inactivation of isoniazid is rapid in some people and slow in others. If the dosage is not adjusted accordingly, isoniazid may accumulate to toxic levels in the slow metabolizers and may fail to achieve therapeutic levels in the rapid metabolizers.

DOSAGE AND DURATION OF TREATMENT

Success requires that the antibiotic be present at the site of infection in an effective concentration for a sufficient time. Dosages should be adjusted to produce drug concentrations that are equal to or greater than the MIC for the infection being treated. Drug levels 4 to 8 times the MIC are often desirable.

Duration of therapy depends on a number of variables, including the status of host defenses, the site of the infection, and the identity of the infecting organism. *It is imperative that antibiotics not be discontinued prematurely.* Accordingly, *patients should be instructed to take their medication for the entire prescribed course, even though symptoms may subside before the full course has been completed.* Early discontinuation is a common cause of recurrent infection, and the organisms responsible for relapse are likely to be more drug resistant than those present when treatment began.

PATIENT-CENTERED CARE ACROSS THE LIFE SPAN

Antimicrobials

Life Stage	Patient Care Concerns
Infants	Infants are highly vulnerable to drug toxicity. Because of poorly developed kidney and liver function, neonates eliminate drugs slowly. Use of sulfonamides in newborns can produce kernicterus, a severe neurologic disorder caused by displacement of bilirubin from plasma proteins (see Chapter 88).
Children/adolescents	The tetracyclines provide another example of toxicity unique to the young: These antibiotics bind to developing teeth, causing discoloration.
Pregnant women	Antimicrobial drugs can cross the placenta, posing a risk to the developing fetus. For example, when gentamicin is used during pregnancy, irreversible hearing loss in the infant may result. Antibiotic use during pregnancy may also pose a risk to the expectant mother.
Breast-feeding women	Antibiotics can enter breast milk, possibly affecting the nursing infant. Sulfonamides, for example, can reach levels in milk that are sufficient to cause kernicterus in nursing newborns. As a general guideline, antibiotics and all other drugs should be avoided by women who are breast-feeding.
Older adults	In the older adult, heightened drug sensitivity is due in large part to reduced rates of drug metabolism and drug excretion, which can result in accumulation of antibiotics to toxic levels.

THERAPY WITH ANTIBIOTIC COMBINATIONS

Therapy with a combination of antimicrobial agents is indicated only in specific situations. Under these well-defined conditions, the use of multiple drugs may be lifesaving. However, it should be stressed that although antibiotic combinations do have a valuable therapeutic role, routine use of two or more antibiotics should be discouraged. When an infection is caused by a single identified microbe, treatment with just one drug is usually most appropriate.

Antimicrobial Effects of Antibiotic Combinations

When two antibiotics are used together, the result may be *additive, potentiative,* or, in certain cases, *antagonistic.* An *additive* response is one in which the antimicrobial effect of the combination is equal to the sum of the effects of the two drugs alone. A *potentiative* interaction (also called a *synergistic* interaction) is one in which the effect of the combination is greater than the sum of the effects of the individual agents. A classic example of potentiation is produced by trimethoprim plus sulfamethoxazole, drugs that inhibit sequential steps in the synthesis of tetrahydrofolic acid (see Chapter 88).

In certain cases, a combination of two antibiotics may be *less* effective than one of the agents by itself, inducing *antagonism* between the drugs. Antagonism is most likely when a *bacteriostatic* agent (e.g., tetracycline) is combined with a *bactericidal* drug (e.g., penicillin). Antagonism occurs because bactericidal drugs are usually effective only against organisms that are actively growing. Hence, when bacterial growth has been suppressed by a bacteriostatic drug, the effects of a bactericidal agent can be reduced. If host defenses are intact, antagonism between two antibiotics may have little significance. However, if host defenses are compromised, the consequences can be dire.

Indications for Antibiotic Combinations

Initial Therapy of Severe Infection

The most common indication for using multiple antibiotics is initial therapy of a severe infection of unknown etiology, especially in the neutropenic host. Until the infecting organism has been identified, wide antimicrobial coverage is appropriate. Just how broad the coverage should be depends on the clinician's skill in narrowing the field of potential pathogens. Once the identity of the infecting microbe is known, drug selection can be adjusted accordingly. As discussed earlier, samples for culture should be obtained before drug therapy starts.

Mixed Infections

An infection may be caused by more than one microbe. Multiple infectious organisms are common in brain abscesses, pelvic infections, and infections resulting from perforation of abdominal organs. When the infectious microbes differ from one another in drug susceptibility, treatment with more than one antibiotic is required.

Preventing Resistance

Although the use of multiple antibiotics is usually associated with *promoting* drug resistance, there is one infectious disease—tuberculosis—in which drug combinations are employed for the specific purpose of *suppressing* the emergence of resistant bacteria. Why tuberculosis differs from other infections in this regard is discussed in Chapter 90.

Decreased Toxicity

In some situations, an antibiotic combination can reduce toxicity to the host. For example, by combining flucytosine with amphotericin B in the treatment of fungal meningitis, the dosage of amphotericin B can be reduced, thereby decreasing the risk of amphotericin-induced damage to the kidneys.

Enhanced Antibacterial Action

In specific infections, a combination of antibiotics can have greater antibacterial action than a single agent. This is true of the combined use of penicillin plus an aminoglycoside in the treatment of enterococcal endocarditis. Penicillin acts to weaken the bacterial cell wall; the aminoglycoside acts to suppress protein synthesis. The combination has enhanced antibacterial action because, by weakening the cell wall, penicillin facilitates penetration of the aminoglycoside to its intracellular site of action.

Disadvantages of Antibiotic Combinations

The use of multiple antibiotics has several drawbacks, including (1) increased risk of toxic and allergic reactions, (2) possible antagonism of antimicrobial effects, (3) increased risk of superinfection, (4) selection of drug-resistant bacteria, and (5) increased cost. Accordingly, antimicrobial combinations should be employed only when clearly indicated.

PROPHYLACTIC USE OF ANTIMICROBIAL DRUGS

Estimates indicate that between 30% and 50% of the antibiotics used in the United States are administered for prophylaxis. That is, these agents are given to prevent an infection rather than to treat an established infection. Much of this prophylactic use is uncalled for. However, in certain situations, antimicrobial prophylaxis is both appropriate and effective. Whenever prophylaxis is proposed, the benefits must be weighed against the risks of toxicity, allergic reactions, superinfection, and selection of drug-resistant organisms. Generally approved indications for prophylaxis are discussed here.

Surgery

Prophylactic use of antibiotics can decrease the incidence of infection in certain kinds of surgery. Procedures in which prophylactic efficacy has been documented include cardiac surgery, peripheral vascular surgery, orthopedic surgery, and surgery on the GI tract (stomach, duodenum, colon, rectum, and appendix). Prophylaxis is also beneficial for women undergoing a hysterectomy or an emergency cesarean section. In contaminated surgery (operations performed on perforated abdominal organs, compound fractures, or lacerations from animal bites), the risk of infection is nearly 100%. Hence, for these operations, the use of antibiotics is considered *treatment,* not prophylaxis. When antibiotics are given for prophylaxis, they should be given before the surgery. If the procedure is unusually long, dosing again during surgery may be indicated. As a rule, postoperative antibiotics are unnecessary. For most operations, a first-generation cephalosporin (e.g., cefazolin) will suffice.

Bacterial Endocarditis

Individuals with congenital or valvular heart disease and those with prosthetic heart valves are unusually susceptible to bacterial endocarditis. For these people, endocarditis can develop following certain dental and medical procedures that dislodge bacteria into the bloodstream. Thus, before undergoing such procedures, these patients may need prophylactic antimicrobial medication. However, according to guidelines released by the American Heart Association, antibiotic prophylaxis is less necessary than previously believed, and hence should be done much less often than in the past.

Neutropenia

Severe neutropenia puts individuals at high risk of infection. There is some evidence that the incidence of bacterial infection may be reduced through antibiotic prophylaxis. However, prophylaxis may increase the risk of infection with fungi: By killing normal flora, whose presence helps suppress fungal growth, antibiotics can encourage fungal invasion.

Other Indications for Antimicrobial Prophylaxis

For young women with recurrent urinary tract infection, prophylaxis with trimethoprim/sulfamethoxazole may be helpful. Oseltamivir (an antiviral agent) may be employed for prophylaxis against influenza. For individuals who have had severe rheumatic endocarditis, lifelong prophylaxis may be needed. Antimicrobial prophylaxis is indicated following exposure to organisms responsible for sexually transmitted diseases (e.g., syphilis, gonorrhea).

MISUSES OF ANTIMICROBIAL DRUGS

Misuse of antibiotics is common. According to the CDC, about 50% of antibiotic prescriptions are either inappropriate or entirely unnecessary. This fact is underscored by the data in Table 83.5. Ways that we misuse antibiotics are discussed next.

Attempted Treatment of Viral Infection

The majority of viral infections—including mumps, chickenpox, and the common cold—do not respond to currently available drugs. Hence, when drug therapy of these disorders is attempted, patients are exposed to all the risks of drugs but have no chance of receiving benefits.

Acute upper respiratory tract infections, including the common cold, are a particular concern. When these infections are treated with antibiotics, only 1 patient out of 4000 is likely to benefit. However, the risks remain high: 1 in 4 patients will get diarrhea, 1 in 50 will get a rash, and 1 in 1000 will need to visit an emergency department, usually because of a severe allergic reaction.

Treatment of Fever of Unknown Origin

Although fever can be a sign of infection, it can also signify other diseases, including hepatitis, arthritis, and cancer. Unless the cause of a fever is a proven infection, antibiotics should not be employed. If the fever is *not* due to an infection, antibiotics would not only be inappropriate, they would expose the patient to unnecessary toxicity and delay correct diagnosis of the fever's cause. If the fever *is* caused by infection, antibiotics could hamper later attempts to identify the infecting organism.

The only situation in which fever, by itself, constitutes a legitimate indication for antibiotic use is when fever occurs in the severely immunocompromised host. Because fever may indicate infection and because infection can be lethal to the immunocompromised patient, these patients should be given antibiotics when fever occurs—even if fever is the only indication that an infection may be present.

Improper Dosage

Like all other medications, antibiotics must be used in the right dosage. If the dosage is too low, the patient will be exposed to a risk of adverse effects without benefit of antibacterial effects. If the dosage is too high, the risks of superinfection and adverse effects become unnecessarily high.

Treatment in the Absence of Adequate Bacteriologic Information

As stressed earlier, proper antimicrobial therapy requires information on the identity and drug sensitivity of the infecting organism. Except in life-threatening situations, therapy should not be undertaken in the absence of bacteriologic information. This important guideline is often ignored.

Omission of Surgical Drainage

Antibiotics may have limited efficacy in the presence of foreign material, necrotic tissue, or exudate. Hence, when appropriate, surgical drainage and cleansing should be performed to promote antimicrobial effects.

MONITORING ANTIMICROBIAL THERAPY

Antimicrobial therapy is assessed by monitoring clinical responses and laboratory results. The frequency of monitoring is directly proportional to the severity of infection. Important clinical indicators of success are reduction of fever and resolution of signs and symptoms related to the affected organ system (e.g., improvement of breath sounds in patients with pneumonia).

TABLE 83.5 ▪ Examples of Inappropriate Antibiotic Prescriptions

Type of Infection	Prescriptions per Year	Percent Inappropriate	Comment
Common cold	18 million	100	Antibiotics are ineffective against the common cold.
Bronchitis	16 million	80	Antibiotics are ineffective against bronchitis, except in a few infections or in patients with chronic severe lung disease.
Sore throat	13 million	50	Antibiotics should be used only in patients with confirmed strep infection.
Sinusitis	13 million	50	Most cases are viral, not bacterial. In the absence of facial pain or swelling, antibiotics should be withheld for about 10 days to see whether symptoms improve without drugs.

Various laboratory tests are used to monitor treatment. Serum drug levels may be monitored for two reasons: to ensure that levels are sufficient for antimicrobial effects and to avoid toxicity from excessive levels. Success of therapy is indicated by the disappearance of infectious organisms from post-treatment cultures. Cultures may become sterile within hours of the onset of treatment (as may happen with urinary tract infections), or they may not become sterile for weeks (as may happen with tuberculosis).

KEY POINTS

- In antimicrobial therapy, the term *selective toxicity* refers to the ability of a drug to injure invading microbes without injuring cells of the host.
- Narrow-spectrum antibiotics are active against only a few microorganisms, whereas broad-spectrum antibiotics are active against a wide array of microbes.
- Bactericidal drugs kill bacteria, whereas bacteriostatic drugs only suppress growth.
- The emergence of resistance to antibiotics is a major concern in antimicrobial therapy.
- Mechanisms of resistance include increased drug efflux, altered drug targets, and enzymatic inactivation of drugs.
- Bacteria with the *NDM-1* gene are resistant to nearly all available antibiotics.
- An important method by which bacteria acquire resistance is conjugation, a process in which DNA coding for drug resistance is transferred from one bacterium to another.
- Antibiotics do not cause the genetic changes that underlie resistance. Rather, antibiotics promote the emergence of drug-resistant organisms by creating selection pressures that favor them.
- Broad-spectrum antibiotics promote the emergence of resistance more than do narrow-spectrum antibiotics.
- In the hospital, we can delay the emergence of antibiotic resistance in four basic ways: (1) preventing infection, (2) diagnosing and treating infection effectively, (3) using antimicrobial drugs wisely, and (4) preventing patient-to-patient transmission.
- The use of antibiotics to promote growth in livestock is a major force for promoting emergence of resistance.
- Effective antimicrobial therapy requires that we determine both the identity and drug sensitivity of the infecting organism.
- The minimum inhibitory concentration (MIC) of an antibiotic is defined as the lowest concentration needed to completely suppress bacterial growth.
- The minimum bactericidal concentration (MBC) is defined as the concentration that decreases the number of bacterial colonies by 99.9%.
- Host defenses—the immune system and phagocytic cells—are essential to the success of antimicrobial therapy.
- Patients should complete the prescribed course of antibiotic treatment, even though symptoms may abate before the full course is over.
- Although combinations of antibiotics should generally be avoided, they are appropriate in some situations, including (1) initial treatment of severe infections, (2) infection with more than one organism, (3) treatment of tuberculosis, and (4) treatment of an infection in which combination therapy can greatly enhance antibacterial effects.
- Appropriate indications for prophylactic antimicrobial treatment include (1) certain surgeries, (2) neutropenia, (3) recurrent urinary tract infections, and (4) patients at risk of bacterial endocarditis (e.g., those with prosthetic heart valves or congenital heart disease).
- Important misuses of antibiotics include (1) treatment of viral infections (e.g., the common cold and most other acute infections of the upper respiratory tract), (2) treatment of fever of unknown origin (except in the immunocompromised host), (3) treatment in the absence of adequate bacteriologic information, and (4) treatment in the absence of appropriate surgical drainage.

Please visit **http://evolve.elsevier.com/Lehne** for chapter-specific NCLEX® examination review questions.

CHAPTER

84 Drugs That Weaken the Bacterial Cell Wall I: Penicillins

INTRODUCTION TO THE PENICILLINS

The penicillins are practically ideal antibiotics, because they are active against a variety of bacteria and their direct toxicity is low. Allergic reactions are the principal adverse effects. Owing to their safety and efficacy, the penicillins are widely prescribed.

Because they have a beta-lactam ring in their structure, the penicillins are known as *beta-lactam antibiotics.* The beta-lactam family also includes the cephalosporins, carbapenems, and aztreonam (see Chapter 85). All of the beta-lactam antibiotics share the same mechanism of action: disruption of the bacterial cell wall.

Mechanism of Action

To understand the actions of the penicillins, we must first understand the structure and function of the bacterial cell wall—a rigid, permeable, mesh-like structure that lies outside the cytoplasmic membrane. Inside the cytoplasmic membrane, osmotic pressure is very high. Hence, were it not for the rigid cell wall, which prevents expansion, bacteria would take up water, swell, and then burst.

Penicillins weaken the cell wall, causing bacteria to take up excessive amounts of water and rupture. As a result, penicillins are generally *bactericidal.* However, it is important to note that penicillins are active only against bacteria that are undergoing growth and division.

Penicillins weaken the cell wall by two actions: (1) *inhibition of transpeptidases* and (2) *disinhibition (activation) of autolysins.* Transpeptidases are enzymes critical to cell wall synthesis. Specifically, they catalyze the formation of cross-bridges between the peptidoglycan polymer strands that form the cell wall, and thus give the cell wall its strength (Fig. 84.1). Autolysins are bacterial enzymes that cleave bonds in the cell wall. Bacteria employ these enzymes to break down segments of the cell wall to permit growth and division. By simultaneously inhibiting transpeptidases and activating autolysins, the penicillins (1) disrupt synthesis of the cell wall and (2) promote its active destruction. These combined actions result in cell lysis and death.

The molecular targets of the penicillins (transpeptidases, autolysins, other bacterial enzymes) are known collectively as *penicillin-binding proteins* (PBPs). These molecules are so named because penicillins must bind to them to produce antibacterial effects. As indicated in Fig. 84.2, PBPs are located on the outer surface of the cytoplasmic membrane. More than eight different PBPs have been identified. Of these, PBP1 and PBP3 are most critical to penicillin's antibacterial effects. Bacteria express PBPs only during growth and division. Accordingly, since PBPs must be present for penicillins to work, these drugs work only when bacteria are growing.

Since mammalian cells lack a cell wall, and since penicillins act specifically on enzymes that affect cell wall integrity, the penicillins have virtually no *direct* effects on cells of the host. As a result, the penicillins are among our safest antibiotics.

Mechanisms of Bacterial Resistance

Bacterial resistance to penicillins is determined primarily by three factors: (1) inability of penicillins to reach their targets (PBPs), (2) inactivation of penicillins by bacterial enzymes, and (3) production of PBPs that have a low affinity for penicillins.

The Gram-Negative Cell Envelope

All bacteria are surrounded by a cell envelope. However, the cell envelope of gram-negative organisms differs from that of gram-positive organisms. Because of this difference, some penicillins are ineffective against gram-negative bacteria.

The cell envelope of *gram-positive* bacteria has only two layers: the cytoplasmic membrane plus a relatively thick cell wall. Despite its thickness, the cell wall can be readily penetrated by penicillins, giving them easy access to PBPs on the cytoplasmic membrane. As a result, penicillins are generally very active against gram-positive organisms.

The *gram-negative* cell envelope has three layers: the cytoplasmic membrane, a relatively thin cell wall, and an additional *outer membrane* (see Fig. 84.2). Like the gram-positive cell wall, the gram-negative cell wall can be easily penetrated by penicillins. The outer membrane, however, is difficult to penetrate. As a result, only certain penicillins (e.g., ampicillin) are able to cross it and thereby reach PBPs on the cytoplasmic membrane.

Penicillinases (Beta-Lactamases)

Beta-lactamases are enzymes that cleave the beta-lactam ring and thereby render penicillins and other beta-lactam antibiotics inactive. Bacteria produce a large variety of beta-lactamases; some are specific for penicillins, some are specific for other beta-lactam antibiotics (e.g., cephalosporins), and some act on several kinds of beta-lactam antibiotics. Beta-lactamases that act selectively on penicillins are known as *penicillinases.*

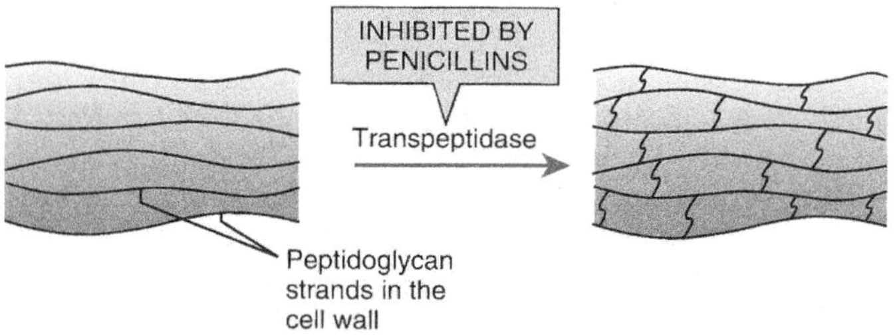

Fig. 84.1 ▪ Inhibition of transpeptidase by penicillins.
The bacterial cell wall is composed of long strands of a peptidoglycan polymer. As depicted, transpeptidase enzymes create cross-bridges between the peptidoglycan strands, giving the cell wall added strength. By inhibiting transpeptidases, penicillins prevent cross-bridge synthesis and thereby weaken the cell wall.

Penicillinases are synthesized by gram-positive and gram-negative bacteria. Gram-positive organisms produce large amounts of these enzymes and then export them into the surrounding medium. In contrast, gram-negative bacteria produce penicillinases in relatively small amounts and, rather than exporting them to the environment, secrete them into the periplasmic space (see Fig. 84.2).

The genes that code for beta-lactamases are located on chromosomes and on plasmids (extrachromosomal DNA). The genes on plasmids may be transferred from one bacterium to another, thereby promoting the spread of penicillin resistance.

Transfer of resistance is of special importance with *Staphylococcus aureus.* When penicillin was first introduced in the early 1940s, all strains of *Staph. aureus* were sensitive. However, by 1960, as many as 80% of *Staph. aureus* isolates in hospitals displayed penicillin resistance. Fortunately, a penicillin derivative (methicillin) that has resistance to the actions of beta-lactamases was introduced at this time. To date, no known strains of *Staph. aureus* produce beta-lactamases capable of inactivating methicillin or related penicillinase-resistant penicillins (although some strains are resistant to these drugs for other reasons).

Altered Penicillin-Binding Proteins

Certain bacterial strains, known collectively as methicillin-resistant *Staphylococcus aureus* (MRSA), have a unique

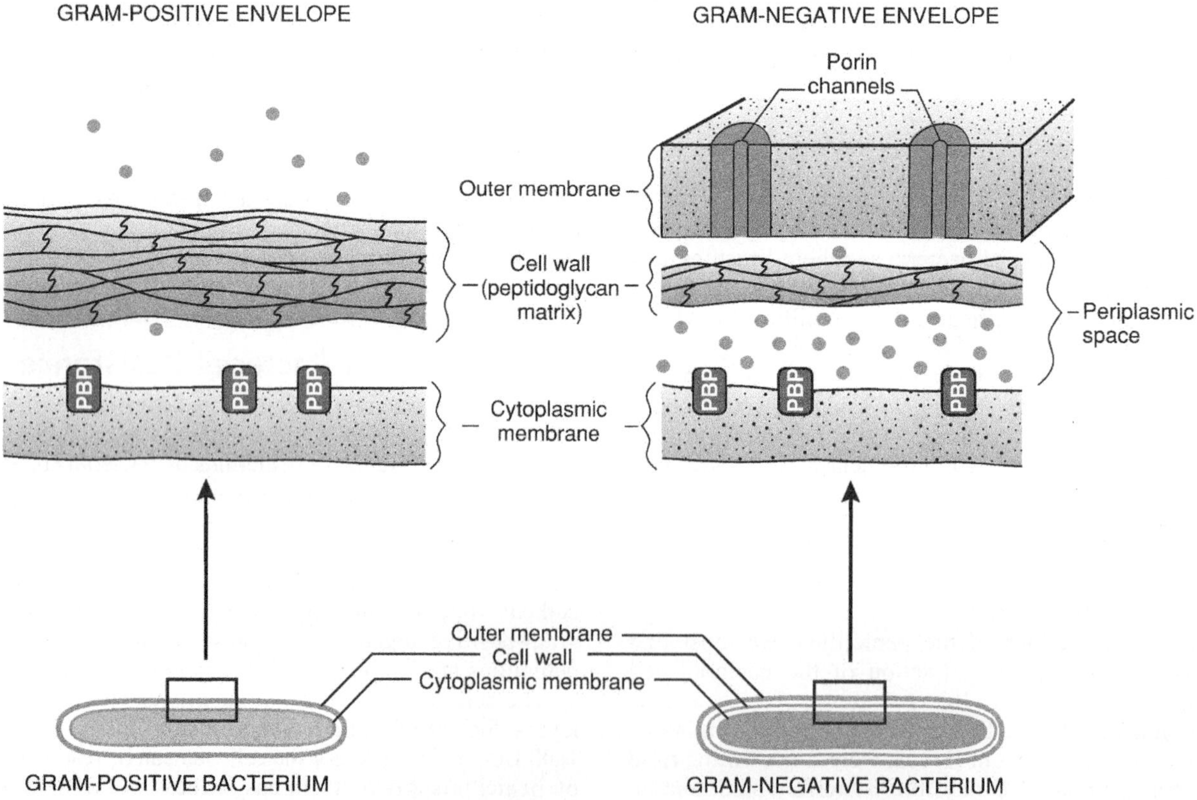

Fig. 84.2 ▪ The bacterial cell envelope.
Note that the gram-negative cell envelope has an outer membrane, whereas the gram-positive envelope does not. The outer membrane of the gram-negative cell envelope prevents certain penicillins from reaching their target molecules. (*PBP,* Penicillin-binding protein.)

mechanism of resistance: production of PBPs with a low affinity for penicillins and almost all other beta-lactam antibiotics. MRSA developed this ability by acquiring genes that code for low-affinity PBPs from other bacteria. Infection with MRSA and its management are discussed in Box 84.1.

Chemistry

All of the penicillins are derived from a common nucleus: 6-aminopenicillanic acid. This nucleus contains a beta-lactam ring joined to a second ring. The beta-lactam ring is essential for antibacterial actions. Properties of individual penicillins are determined by additions made to the basic nucleus. These modifications determine (1) affinity for PBPs, (2) resistance to penicillinases, (3) ability to penetrate the gram-negative cell envelope, (4) resistance to stomach acid, and (5) pharmacokinetic properties.

Classification

The most useful classification of penicillins is based on an antimicrobial spectrum. When classified this way, the penicillins fall into four major groups: (1) narrow-spectrum penicillins that are penicillinase sensitive, (2) narrow-spectrum penicillins that are penicillinase resistant (antistaphylococcal penicillins), (3) broad-spectrum penicillins (aminopenicillins), and (4) extended-spectrum penicillins (antipseudomonal penicillins). Table 84.1

si

BOX 84.1 ■ SPECIAL INTEREST TOPIC

METHICILLIN-RESISTANT *STAPHYLOCOCCUS AUREUS*

Staphylococcus aureus is a gram-positive bacterium that often colonizes the skin and nostrils of healthy people. Infection usually involves the skin and soft tissues, causing abscesses, boils, cellulitis, and impetigo. However, more serious infections can also develop, including infections of the lungs and bloodstream, which can be fatal.

Like other pathogens, *Staph. aureus* has developed resistance over the years. When penicillins were introduced in the 1940s, all strains of *Staph. aureus* were susceptible. However, penicillin-resistant strains quickly emerged, owing to bacterial production of penicillinases. In 1959, this resistance was overcome with methicillin, the first penicillinase-resistant penicillin. Unfortunately, by 1968, strains resistant to methicillin had emerged. These highly resistant bacteria, known as *methicillin-resistant Staphylococcus aureus (MRSA),* are resistant not only to methicillin (now obsolete), but to all penicillins and all but one cephalosporin as well. The basis of MRSA resistance is the acquisition of genes that code for penicillin-binding proteins that have a very low affinity for penicillins and cephalosporins. Resistant strains were initially limited to healthcare facilities but are now found in the community as well.

In the United States, MRSA is a serious public health problem. It is estimated that more than 80,000 infections are caused by MRSA every year. Not only does MRSA increase mortality, it increases costs. In the near future, hospitals may face high financial penalties for Medicare patients who develop MRSA infections in the hospital. Fortunately, the MRSA news isn't all bad. For one thing, although MRSA infections are now common, most patients can be cured. Also, rates of MRSA infection among hospitalized patients are now falling, after rising steadily for many years.

There are two distinct types of MRSA, referred to as *healthcare-associated MRSA* (HCA-MRSA) and *community-associated MRSA* (CA-MRSA). Of the two, HCA-MRSA is more prevalent (80% vs. 20%) and emerged earlier (1968 vs. 1981). Also, HCA-MRSA infection is generally more serious and harder to treat. Molecular typing indicates that HCA-MRSA and CA-MRSA are genetically distinct strains, known as USA100 and USA300, respectively.

Healthcare-Associated MRSA

Methicillin resistance in *Staph. aureus* was first reported in isolates from hospitalized patients in 1968. For most of the next four decades, the prevalence of HCA-MRSA among hospitalized patients climbed steadily, reaching 85% of all invasive *Staph. aureus* infections by 2004.

Although many infections with HCA-MRSA *surface* in the community, nearly all occur in people who have been exposed to a healthcare facility within the prior year, indicating that acquisition of the infection probably occurred in a healthcare setting—not out in the community. Transmission of HCA-MRSA is usually through person-to-person contact, often between healthcare workers and patients. Risk factors for acquiring HCA-MRSA include advanced age, recent surgery or hospitalization, dialysis, treatment in an ICU, prolonged antibiotic therapy, an indwelling catheter, and residence in a long-term care facility.

How do we treat HCA-MRSA infection? The issue is addressed at length in a guideline published by the Infectious Diseases Society of America—*Management of Patients with Infections Caused by Methicillin-Resistant Staphylococcus aureus.* The guideline stresses the importance of selecting drugs based on the site of the infection, age of the patient, and drug sensitivity of the pathogen. For complicated skin and soft tissue infections in adults, the preferred drugs are IV vancomycin, linezolid [Zyvox], daptomycin [Cubicin], telavancin [Vibativ], clindamycin, and ceftaroline [Teflaro]. Intravenous vancomycin is the preferred drug for children. For bacteremia or endocarditis in adults or children, IV vancomycin and daptomycin are the drugs of choice. Preferred drugs for pneumonia in adults and children are IV vancomycin, linezolid, and clindamycin. Because most strains of HCA-MRSA are multidrug resistant, many other antibiotics are ineffective, including tetracyclines, clindamycin, trimethoprim/sulfamethoxazole, and beta-lactam agents (except ceftaroline).

Community-Associated MRSA

Infection with CA-MRSA, first reported in 1981, is caused by staphylococcal strains that are genetically distinct from HCA-MRSA. For example, most strains of CA-MRSA carry a gene for Panton-Valentine leukocidin (a cytotoxin that causes necrosis),

Continued

si

METHICILLIN-RESISTANT *STAPHYLOCOCCUS AUREUS*—cont'd

whereas HCA-MRSA strains do not. Many people are now asymptomatic carriers of CA-MRSA. In fact, between 20% and 30% of the population is colonized, typically on the skin and in the nostrils.

Infection with CA-MRSA is generally less dangerous than with HCA-MRSA, but more dangerous than with methicillin-sensitive *Staph. aureus.* In most cases, CA-MRSA causes mild infections of the skin and soft tissues, manifesting as boils, impetigo, and so forth. However, CA-MRSA can also cause more serious infections, including necrotizing fasciitis, severe necrotizing pneumonia, and severe sepsis. Fortunately, these invasive infections are relatively rare. On the other hand, infections of the skin and soft tissues are now common, with CA-MRSA accounting for more than 50% of the *Staph. aureus* isolates from these sites.

CA-MRSA transmission is by skin-to-skin contact and by contact with contaminated objects, including frequently touched surfaces, sports equipment, and personal items (e.g., razors). In contrast to HCA-MRSA infection, CA-MRSA infection is seen primarily in young, healthy people with no recent exposure to healthcare facilities. Individuals at risk include athletes in contact sports (e.g., wrestling), men who have sex with men, and people who live in close quarters, such as family members, day care clients, prison inmates, military personnel, and college students.

Several measures can reduce the risk of CA-MRSA transmission. Topping the list is good hand hygiene—washing with soap and water or applying an alcohol-based sanitizer. Other measures include showering after contact sports, cleaning frequently touched surfaces, keeping infected sites covered, and not sharing towels and personal items.

Treatment depends on infection severity. For boils, small abscesses, and other superficial infections, surgical drainage may be all that is needed. For more serious infections, drugs may be indicated. Preferred agents are trimethoprim/sulfamethoxazole, minocycline, doxycycline, and clindamycin. Alternative drugs—vancomycin, daptomycin, and linezolid—should be reserved for severe infections and treatment failures. To eradicate the carrier state, intranasal application of a topical antibiotic—mupirocin or retapamulin—can be effective. Like HCA-MRSA, CA-MRSA does not respond to beta-lactam antibiotics, except ceftaroline.

TABLE 84.1 ■ Classification of the Penicillins

Penicillin Class	Drug	Clinically Useful Antimicrobial Spectrum
Narrow-spectrum penicillins: penicillinase sensitive	Penicillin G Penicillin V	*Streptococcus* species, *Neisseria* species, many anaerobes, spirochetes, others
Narrow-spectrum penicillins: penicillinase resistant (antistaphylococcal penicillins)	Nafcillin Oxacillin Dicloxacillin	*Staphylococcus aureus*
Broad-spectrum penicillins (aminopenicillins)	Ampicillin Amoxicillin	*Haemophilus influenzae, Escherichia coli, Proteus mirabilis,* enterococci, *Neisseria gonorrhoeae*
Extended-spectrum penicillin (antipseudomonal penicillin)	Piperacillin	Same as broad-spectrum penicillins plus *Pseudomonas aeruginosa, Enterobacter* species, *Proteus* (indole positive), *Bacteroides fragilis,* many *Klebsiella*

lists the members of each group and their principal target organisms.

PROPERTIES OF INDIVIDUAL PENICILLINS

Penicillin G

Penicillin G (benzylpenicillin) was the first penicillin available and will serve as our prototype for the penicillin family. This drug is often referred to simply as *penicillin.* Penicillin G is bactericidal to a number of gram-positive bacteria, as well as to some gram-negative bacteria. Despite the introduction of newer antibiotics, penicillin G remains a drug of choice for many infections.

Antimicrobial Spectrum

Penicillin G is active against most *gram-positive bacteria* (except penicillinase-producing staphylococci), gram-negative cocci (*Neisseria meningitidis* and non–penicillinase-producing strains of *Neisseria gonorrhoeae*), anaerobic bacteria, and spirochetes (including *Treponema pallidum*). With few exceptions, gram-negative bacilli are resistant. Although many organisms respond to penicillin G, the drug is considered a narrow-spectrum agent, compared with other members of the penicillin family.

Therapeutic Uses

Penicillin G is a drug of first choice for pharyngitis caused by *Streptococcus pyogenes* and for infectious endocarditis caused by *Streptococcus viridans.* Penicillin is also the preferred drug for those few strains of *Staph. aureus* that do not produce penicillinase.

Penicillin is a preferred agent for infections caused by several gram-positive bacilli, specifically, gas gangrene (caused by *Clostridium perfringens*) and anthrax (caused by *Bacillus anthracis*).

Although once the drug of choice for meningitis caused by *Neisseria meningitidis* and *Streptococcus pneumoniae*, as well as gonorrhea caused by *N. gonorrhoeae*, penicillin has been replaced by third-generation cephalosporins (ceftriaxone) as the primary treatment. Penicillin remains the drug of choice for syphilis, an infection caused by the spirochete *T. pallidum.*

In addition to treating active infections, penicillin G has important *prophylactic* applications. The drug is used to prevent syphilis in sexual partners of individuals who have this infection. Benzathine penicillin G (administered monthly, for 10 years to life) is employed for prophylaxis against recurrent attacks of rheumatic fever; treatment is recommended for patients with a history of recurrent rheumatic fever and for those with clear evidence of rheumatic heart disease.

Pharmacokinetics

Absorption. Penicillin G is available as four salts: (1) *potassium* penicillin G, (2) *procaine* penicillin G, (3) *benzathine* penicillin G, and (4) *sodium* penicillin G. These salts differ with respect to route of administration and time course of action. With all forms, the salt dissociates to release penicillin G, the active component.

Intramuscular. All forms of penicillin may be administered IM. However, it is important to note that the different salts are absorbed at very different rates. As indicated in Fig. 84.3, absorption of *potassium* and *sodium* penicillin G is rapid; blood levels peak about 15 minutes after injection. In contrast, the *procaine* and *benzathine* salts are absorbed slowly, and hence are considered *repository* preparations. When benzathine penicillin is injected IM, penicillin G is absorbed for weeks, producing blood levels that are persistent but very low. Consequently, this preparation is useful only against highly sensitive organisms (e.g., *T. pallidum,* the bacterium that causes syphilis).

Intravenous. When high blood levels are needed rapidly, penicillin can be administered IV. Only the potassium or sodium salts should be used by this route. Owing to poor water solubility, *procaine and benzathine salts must never be administered IV.*

Distribution. Penicillin distributes well to most tissues and body fluids. In the absence of inflammation, penetration of the meninges and into fluids of joints and the eyes is poor. By contrast, in the presence of inflammation, entry into cerebrospinal fluid, joints, and the eyes is enhanced, permitting treatment of infections caused by susceptible organisms.

Metabolism and Excretion. Penicillin undergoes minimal metabolism and is eliminated by the kidneys, primarily as the unchanged drug. Renal excretion is accomplished mainly (90%) by active tubular secretion; the remaining 10% results from glomerular filtration. In older children and adults, the half-life is very short (about 30 minutes). Renal impairment causes the half-life to increase dramatically and may necessitate a reduction in dosage. In patients at high risk of toxicity (those with renal impairment, the acutely ill, the very young, older adults), kidney function should be monitored.

Renal excretion of penicillin can be delayed with *probenecid,* a compound that competes with penicillin for active tubular transport. In the past, when penicillin was both scarce and expensive, probenecid was employed routinely to prolong antibacterial effects. However, since penicillin is now available in abundance at low cost, concurrent use of probenecid is seldom indicated.

Side Effects and Toxicities

Penicillin G is the least toxic of all antibiotics and among the safest of all medications. Allergic reactions, the principal concern with penicillin, are discussed separately (see *Penicillin Allergy*). Other reactions include *pain at sites of IM injection,* prolonged (but reversible) *sensory and motor dysfunction* following accidental injection into a peripheral nerve, and *neurotoxicity* (seizures, confusion, hallucinations) if blood levels are too high. Inadvertent *intra-arterial* injection can produce severe reactions—gangrene, necrosis, sloughing of tissue—and must be avoided.

Certain adverse effects may be caused by compounds coadministered with penicillin. For example, the procaine component of procaine penicillin G may cause bizarre behavioral effects when procaine penicillin is given in large doses. When large IV doses of potassium penicillin G are administered rapidly, hyperkalemia can result, possibly causing dysrhythmias and even cardiac arrest. Similarly, the use of IV sodium penicillin G may lead to electrolyte imbalance. Sodium penicillin G should be used with caution in patients on sodium-restricted diets.

Safety Alert

PENICILLIN ALLERGY

Penicillins are the most common cause of drug allergy. Between 0.4% and 7% of patients who receive penicillins experience an allergic reaction. Severity can range from a minor rash to life-threatening anaphylaxis.

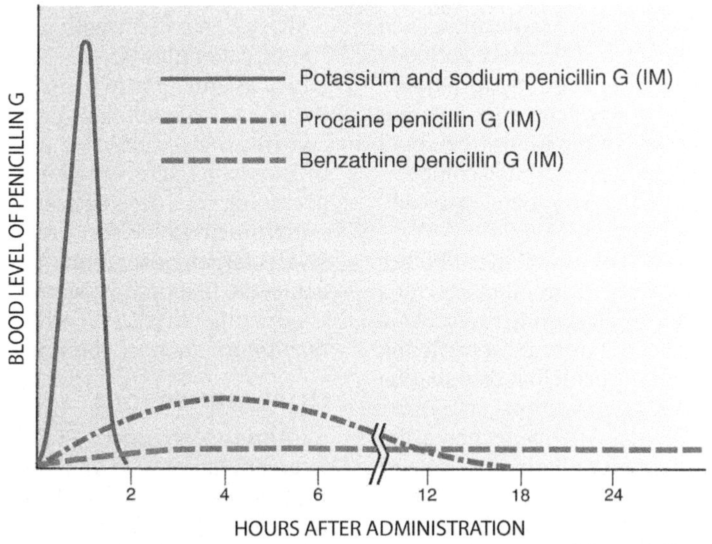

Fig. 84.3 ■ **Blood levels of penicillin G following IM injection of four different penicillin G salts.**

Penicillin Allergy

General Considerations. As with most allergic reactions, there is no direct relationship between the size of the dose and the intensity of the response. Although prior exposure to penicillins is required for an allergic reaction, responses may occur in the absence of prior penicillin use. How can this be? Because patients may have been exposed to penicillins produced by fungi or to penicillins present in foods of animal origin.

Because of cross-sensitivity, patients allergic to one penicillin should be considered allergic to all other penicillins. In addition, a few patients (about 1%) display cross-sensitivity to *cephalosporins*. If at all possible, patients with penicillin allergy should not be treated with any member of the penicillin family. The use of cephalosporins depends on the intensity of allergic response: If the penicillin allergy is mild, the use of cephalosporins is probably safe; however, if the allergy is severe, cephalosporins should be avoided.

Individuals allergic to penicillin should be encouraged to wear a medical identification bracelet to alert healthcare personnel to their condition.

Types of Allergic Reactions. Penicillin reactions are classified as *immediate, accelerated,* and *delayed.* Immediate reactions occur 2 to 30 minutes after drug administration; accelerated reactions occur within 1 to 72 hours; and delayed reactions occur within days to weeks. Immediate and accelerated reactions are mediated by immunoglobulin E (IgE) antibodies.

Anaphylaxis (laryngeal edema, bronchoconstriction, severe hypotension) is an immediate hypersensitivity reaction, mediated by IgE. Anaphylactic reactions occur more frequently with penicillins than with any other drugs. However, even with penicillins, the incidence of anaphylaxis is extremely low (the estimated incidence is between 0.004% and 0.04%). Nonetheless, when these reactions do occur, the risk of mortality is high (about 10%). The primary treatment is *epinephrine* (subQ, IM, or IV) plus respiratory support. To ensure prompt treatment if anaphylaxis should develop, patients should be observed for at least 30 minutes after drug injection (i.e., until the risk of an anaphylactic reaction has passed).

Development of Penicillin Allergy. Before discussing penicillin allergy further, we need to review the development of allergy to small molecules as a class. Small molecules, such as penicillin and most other drugs, are unable to induce antibody formation directly. Therefore, to promote antibody formation, the small molecule must first bond covalently to a larger molecule, usually a protein. In these combinations, the small molecule is referred to as a *hapten.* The hapten-protein combination constitutes the complete *antigen* that stimulates antibody formation.

The hapten that stimulates production of penicillin antibodies is rarely intact penicillin itself. Rather, compounds formed from the degradation of penicillin are the actual cause. As a result, most "penicillin antibodies" are not directed at penicillin itself. Rather, they are directed at various penicillin degradation products.

Skin Tests for Penicillin Allergy. Allergy to penicillin can decrease over time. Hence, an intense allergic reaction in the past does not necessarily mean that an intense reaction will occur again. In patients with a history of penicillin allergy, skin tests can be employed to assess current risk. These tests are performed by injecting a tiny amount of allergen intradermally and observing for a local allergic response. A positive test indicates the presence of IgE antibodies, which can mediate severe penicillin allergy. Accordingly, if skin testing is negative, a severe allergic reaction (anaphylaxis) is unlikely.

It is important to note that skin testing can be dangerous: In patients with severe penicillin allergy, the skin test itself can precipitate an anaphylactic reaction. Accordingly, the test should be performed only if epinephrine and facilities for respiratory support are immediately available.

Current guidelines recommend skin testing with two reagents, which test for the major (more common) and minor (less common) determinants of penicillin allergy. The minor determinants, although less common, mediate the majority of severe penicillin reactions.

The major determinant reagent, available commercially as Pre-Pen, contains a single component: *benzylpenicilloyl-polylysine.* Benzylpenicilloyl-polylysine is a large polymeric molecule that is poorly absorbed. Hence, even in patients with severe penicillin allergy, this skin test carries a low risk of a systemic reaction.

The recommended minor determinant reagent, which is not available commercially, is a mixture of three compounds: benzylpenicillin G, benzylpenicilloate, and penicilloyl propylamine. As noted, the term *minor* indicates that the antibodies being tested for are relatively uncommon and not that the allergic response mediated by these antibodies is of minor significance. In fact, the minor determinants are responsible for the majority of severe penicillin reactions.

Management of Patients With a History of Penicillin Allergy. All patients who are candidates for penicillin therapy should be asked whether they have an allergy to penicillin. For patients who answer "yes," the general rule is to avoid penicillins. If the allergy is mild, a *cephalosporin* is often an appropriate alternative. However, if there is a history of anaphylaxis or some other severe allergic reaction, it is prudent to avoid cephalosporins as well (because there is about a 1% risk of cross-sensitivity to cephalosporins). When a cephalosporin is indicated, an oral cephalosporin is preferred (because the risk of a severe reaction is lower than with parenteral therapy). For many infections, *vancomycin, erythromycin,* and *clindamycin* are effective and safe alternatives for patients with penicillin allergy.

Rarely, a patient with a history of anaphylaxis may have a life-threatening infection (e.g., enterococcal endocarditis) for which alternatives to penicillins are ineffective. In these cases, the potential benefits of penicillin therapy outweigh the risks, and treatment should be instituted. To minimize the chances of an anaphylactic reaction, penicillin should be administered according to a desensitization schedule. In this procedure, an initial small dose is followed at 60-minute intervals by progressively larger doses until the full therapeutic dose has been achieved. It should be noted that the desensitization procedure is not without risk. Accordingly, epinephrine and facilities for respiratory support should be immediately available.

Drug Interactions

Aminoglycosides. For some infections, penicillins are used in combination with an aminoglycoside (e.g., gentamicin). By weakening the cell wall, the penicillin facilitates access of the aminoglycoside to its intracellular site of action, thereby increasing bactericidal effects. Unfortunately, when penicillins are present in high concentrations, they interact chemically with

PATIENT-CENTERED CARE ACROSS THE LIFE SPAN

Penicillins

Life Stage	Patient Care Concerns
Infants	Penicillins are used safely in infants with bacterial infections, including syphilis, meningitis, and group A streptococcus.
Children/ adolescents	Penicillins are a common drug used to treat bacterial infections in children.
Pregnant women	Penicillins are classified in U.S. Food and Drug Administration Pregnancy Risk Category B.[a] There is no evidence of second- or third-trimester fetal risk.
Breast-feeding women	Amoxicillin is safe for use in breast-feeding mothers. Data are lacking regarding the transmission of some other penicillins from mother to infant via breast milk.
Older adults	Doses should be adjusted in older adults with renal dysfunction.

[a]As of 2020, the FDA will no longer use Pregnancy Risk Categories. Please refer to Chapter 9 for more information.

aminoglycosides and thereby inactivate the aminoglycoside. Accordingly, *penicillins and aminoglycosides should never be mixed in the same IV solution.* Rather, they should be administered separately. Once a penicillin has been diluted in body fluids, the potential for inactivating the aminoglycoside is minimal.

Probenecid. As noted, probenecid can delay renal excretion of penicillin, thereby prolonging antibacterial effects.

Bacteriostatic Antibiotics. Since penicillins are most effective against actively growing bacteria, concurrent use of a bacteriostatic antibiotic (e.g., tetracycline) could, in theory, reduce the bactericidal effects of the penicillin. However, the clinical significance of such interactions is not known. Nonetheless, combined use of penicillin and bacteriostatic agents is generally avoided.

Preparations, Dosage, and Administration

Preparations and Routes of Administration. Penicillin G is available as four different salts (potassium, procaine, sodium, and benzathine). These salts differ with respect to routes of administration: *potassium* penicillin G [Pfizerpen] and *sodium* penicillin G are administered IM and IV; all other salts—*benzathine* penicillin G [Bicillin LA], *procaine* penicillin G, and a combination product [Bicillin C-R], composed of benzathine penicillin G plus procaine penicillin G—are administered IM. Check to ensure that the penicillin salt to be administered is appropriate for the intended route. Dosage ranges for penicillins are shown in Table 84.2.

Penicillin V

Penicillin V, also known as penicillin VK, is similar to penicillin G in most respects. The principal difference is acid stability: Penicillin V is stable in stomach acid, whereas penicillin G is not. Because of its acid stability, penicillin V has replaced penicillin G for oral therapy. Penicillin V may be taken with meals.

Penicillinase-Resistant Penicillins (Antistaphylococcal Penicillins)

By altering the penicillin side chain, pharmaceutical chemists have created a group of penicillins that are highly resistant to inactivation by beta-lactamases. In the United States, three such drugs are available: *nafcillin, oxacillin,* and *dicloxacillin.* These agents have a very narrow antimicrobial spectrum and are used only against penicillinase-producing strains of staphylococci (*Staph. aureus* and *Staph. epidermidis*). Since most strains of staphylococci produce penicillinase, the penicillinase-resistant penicillins are drugs of choice for the majority of staphylococcal infections. It should be noted that these agents should not be used against infections caused by non–penicillinase-producing staphylococci, since they are less active than penicillin G against these bacteria.

An increasing clinical problem is the emergence of staphylococcal strains referred to as *methicillin-resistant Staphylococcus aureus,* a term used to indicate lack of susceptibility to methicillin (an obsolete penicillinase-resistant penicillin) and all other penicillinase-resistant penicillins. Resistance appears to result from the production of PBPs to which the penicillinase-resistant penicillins cannot bind. Vancomycin is the treatment of choice.

Nafcillin

Nafcillin is usually administered IV. Intramuscular use is rare. Absorption from the GI tract is erratic and incomplete, and hence oral formulations have been discontinued.

Oxacillin and Dicloxacillin

These drugs are similar in structure and pharmacokinetic properties. Both are acid stable, but only dicloxacillin is formulated for oral dosing. Oxacillin is administered IV.

Broad-Spectrum Penicillins (Aminopenicillins)

Only two broad-spectrum penicillins are available: *ampicillin* and *amoxicillin.* Both have the same antimicrobial spectrum as penicillin G, *plus* increased activity against certain gram-negative bacilli, including *Haemophilus influenzae, Escherichia coli, Salmonella,* and *Shigella.* This broadened spectrum is due in large part to an increased ability to penetrate the gram-negative cell envelope. Both drugs are readily inactivated by beta-lactamases, and hence are ineffective against most infections caused by *Staph. aureus.*

Ampicillin

Ampicillin was the first broad-spectrum penicillin in clinical use. The drug is useful against infections caused by *Enterococcus faecalis, Proteus mirabilis, E. coli, Salmonella, Shigella,* and *H. influenzae.* The most common side effects are rash and diarrhea, both of which occur more frequently with ampicillin than with any other penicillin. Administration may be oral or IV. It should be noted, however, that for oral therapy, amoxicillin is preferred (see *Amoxicillin*). Dosages for patients with normal kidney function are shown in Table 84.2. For patients with renal impairment, dosage should be reduced.

As discussed later, ampicillin is also available in a fixed-dose combination with sulbactam, an inhibitor of bacterial beta-lactamase. The combination is sold as *Unasyn.*

Amoxicillin

Amoxicillin [Moxatag] is similar to ampicillin in structure and actions. The drugs differ primarily in acid stability, amoxicillin being the more acid stable. Hence, when the two are administered orally in equivalent doses, blood levels of amoxicillin are greater. Accordingly, when oral therapy is indicated, amoxicillin is preferred. Amoxicillin produces less diarrhea than ampicillin, perhaps because less amoxicillin remains unabsorbed in the intestine.

TABLE 84.2 ■ Dosages for Penicillins

Generic Name	Brand Name	Usual Routes	Dosing Interval (hr)	Total Daily Dosage[a] Adults	Children
NARROW-SPECTRUM PENICILLINS: PENICILLINASE-SENSITIVE					
Penicillin G	Bicillin C-R, Bicillin LA, Pfizerpen	IM, IV	4	1.2–24 million units[b]	100,000–400,000 units/kg[b]
Penicillin V	Generic only	PO	4–6	0.5–2 gm	25–50 mg/kg
NARROW-SPECTRUM PENICILLINS: PENICILLINASE-RESISTANT (ANTISTAPHYLOCOCCAL PENICILLINS)					
Nafcillin		IV	4–6	2–12 gm	100–200 mg/kg
Oxacillin		IV	4–6	1–12 gm	100–200 mg/kg
Dicloxacillin		PO	6	0.5–4 gm	12.5–25 mg/kg
BROAD-SPECTRUM PENICILLINS (AMINOPENICILLINS)					
Ampicillin	Generic only	PO IV	6–8 6–8	2–4 gm 4–12 gm	50–100 mg/kg 50–400 mg/kg
Ampicillin/sulbactam	Unasyn	IV	6	4–8 gm[c]	150–600 mg/kg[c]
Amoxicillin	Generic only	PO	8	750–1750 mg	20–90 mg/kg
Amoxicillin, ER	Moxatag	PO	24	775 mg	775 mg
Amoxicillin/clavulanate	Augmentin, Clavulin ♣ Augmentin ES-600 Augmentin XR	PO PO PO	8–12 12 12	250–1750 mg[d] — 4000 mg	20–90 mg/kg[d] 90 mg/kg —
EXTENDED-SPECTRUM PENICILLINS (ANTIPSEUDOMONAL PENICILLINS)					
Piperacillin/tazobactam	Zosyn, Tazocin ♣	IV	4–6	12–18 gm[e]	80–100 mg/kg[e]

[a]Doses vary widely, depending upon the type and severity of infection; doses and dosing intervals presented here may not be appropriate for all patients.
[b]10,000 units = 6 mg.
[c]Dose based on ampicillin content.
[d]Dose based on amoxicillin content.
[e]Dose based on piperacillin content.
ER, Extended release.

As discussed later, amoxicillin is also available in a fixed-dose combination with clavulanic acid, an inhibitor of bacterial beta-lactamases. The combination is marketed as *Augmentin.* Amoxicillin, by itself, is one of our most frequently prescribed antibiotics.

Extended-Spectrum Penicillin (Antipseudomonal Penicillin)

Only one extended-spectrum penicillin is available: *piperacillin.* The antimicrobial spectrum of this drug includes organisms that are susceptible to the aminopenicillins plus *Pseudomonas aeruginosa, Enterobacter* species, *Proteus* (indole positive), *Bacteroides fragilis,* and many *Klebsiella.* Piperacillin is susceptible to beta-lactamases, and hence is ineffective against most strains of *Staph. aureus.*

Piperacillin is used primarily for infections with *P. aeruginosa.* These infections often occur in the immunocompromised host and can be very difficult to eradicate. To increase killing of *Pseudomonas,* an antipseudomonal aminoglycoside (gentamicin, tobramycin, amikacin, netilmicin) may be added to the regimen. When these combinations are employed, the penicillin and the aminoglycoside should not be mixed in the same IV solution because high concentrations of penicillins can inactivate aminoglycosides.

Piperacillin can cause bleeding secondary to disrupting platelet function. The drug is acid labile and hence must be administered parenterally, usually IV. Dosages for patients with normal kidney function are shown in Table 84.2. Dosage should be reduced in patients with renal impairment. As discussed in the next section, piperacillin is also available in a fixed-dose combination with tazobactam, a beta-lactamase inhibitor. The combination is marketed as *Zosyn.*

Penicillins Combined With a Beta-Lactamase Inhibitor

As their name indicates, beta-lactamase inhibitors are drugs that inhibit bacterial beta-lactamases. By combining a beta-lactamase inhibitor with a penicillinase-sensitive penicillin, we can extend the antimicrobial spectrum of the penicillin. In the United States, three beta-lactamase inhibitors are used: *sulbactam, tazobactam,* and *clavulanic acid* (clavulanate). These drugs are not available alone. Rather, they are available only in fixed-dose combinations with a penicillin. Three such combination products are available:

- Ampicillin/sulbactam [Unasyn]
- Amoxicillin/clavulanate [Augmentin, Clavulin ♣]
- Piperacillin/tazobactam [Zosyn, Tazocin ♣]

Because beta-lactamase inhibitors have minimal toxicity, any adverse effects that occur with the combination products are due to the penicillin.

KEY POINTS

- Penicillins weaken the bacterial cell wall, causing lysis and death.
- Some bacteria resist penicillins by producing penicillinases (beta-lactamases), enzymes that inactivate penicillins.
- Gram-negative bacteria are resistant to penicillins that cannot penetrate the gram-negative cell envelope.
- Penicillins are the safest antibiotics available.
- The principal adverse effect of penicillins is allergic reaction, which can range from rash to life-threatening anaphylaxis.
- Patients allergic to one penicillin should be considered cross-allergic to all other penicillins. In addition, they have about a 1% chance of cross-allergy to cephalosporins.
- Vancomycin, erythromycin, and clindamycin are safe and effective alternatives to penicillins for patients with penicillin allergy.
- Penicillins are normally eliminated rapidly by the kidneys, but can accumulate to harmful levels if renal function is severely impaired.
- The principal differences among the penicillins relate to antibacterial spectrum, stability in stomach acid, and duration of action.
- Penicillin G has a narrow antibacterial spectrum and is unstable in stomach acid.
- Benzathine penicillin G is released very slowly following IM injection and thereby produces prolonged antibacterial effects.
- The penicillinase-resistant penicillins (e.g., nafcillin) are used primarily against penicillinase-producing strains of *Staph. aureus.*
- In contrast to penicillin G, the broad-spectrum penicillins, such as ampicillin and amoxicillin, have useful activity against gram-negative bacilli.
- The extended-spectrum penicillin—piperacillin—is useful against *P. aeruginosa.*
- Beta-lactamase inhibitors, such as clavulanic acid, are combined with certain penicillins to increase their activity against beta-lactamase–producing bacteria.
- Penicillins should not be combined with aminoglycosides (e.g., gentamicin) in the same IV solution.

Please visit **http://evolve.elsevier.com/Lehne** for chapter-specific NCLEX® examination review questions.

Summary of Major Nursing Implications[a]

PENICILLINS

Amoxicillin
Amoxicillin/clavulanate
Ampicillin
Ampicillin/sulbactam
Dicloxacillin
Nafcillin
Oxacillin
Penicillin G
Penicillin V
Piperacillin
Piperacillin/tazobactam

Except where indicated otherwise, the implications here apply to all members of the penicillin family.

Preadministration Assessment

Therapeutic Goal

Treatment of infections caused by sensitive bacteria.

Baseline Data

The prescriber may order tests to identify the infecting organism and its drug sensitivity. Take samples for microbiologic culture before starting treatment.

In patients with a history of penicillin allergy, a skin test may be performed to determine current allergic status.

Identifying High-Risk Patients

Penicillins should be used with *extreme caution,* if at all, in patients with a history of *severe* allergic reactions to penicillins, cephalosporins, or carbapenems.

Implementation: Administration

Routes

Penicillins are administered orally, IM, and IV. Before giving a penicillin, make sure the preparation is appropriate for the intended route.

Dosage

Doses for penicillin G are prescribed in units (1 unit equals 0.6 mg). Doses for all other penicillins are prescribed in milligrams or grams.

Administration

During IM injection, aspirate to avoid injection into an artery. Take care to avoid injection into a nerve.

Instruct the patient to take oral penicillins with a full glass of water 1 hour before meals or 2 hours after. *Penicillin V, amoxicillin,* and *amoxicillin/clavulanate* may be taken with meals.

Instruct the patient to complete the prescribed course of treatment, even though symptoms may abate before the full course is over.

Continued

Summary of Major Nursing Implications[a]—cont'd

Ongoing Evaluation and Interventions

Evaluating Therapeutic Effects

Monitor the patient for indications of antimicrobial effects (e.g., reduction in fever, pain, or inflammation; improved appetite or sense of well-being).

Monitoring Kidney Function

Renal impairment can cause penicillins to accumulate to toxic levels, and hence monitoring kidney function can help avoid injury. Measuring intake and output is especially helpful in patients with kidney disease, acutely ill patients, and the very old and very young. Notify the prescriber if a significant change in intake/output ratio develops.

Minimizing Adverse Effects

Allergic Reactions. Penicillin allergy is common. Very rarely, life-threatening anaphylaxis occurs. Interview the patient for a history of penicillin allergy.

For patients with prior allergic responses, a skin test may be ordered to assess current allergy status. Exercise caution: The skin test itself can cause a severe reaction. When skin tests are performed, epinephrine and facilities for respiratory support should be immediately available.

Advise patients with penicillin allergy to wear some form of identification (e.g., Medic Alert bracelet) to alert emergency healthcare personnel.

Instruct outpatients to report any signs of an allergic response (e.g., skin rash, itching, hives).

Whenever a parenteral penicillin is used, keep the patient under observation for at least 30 minutes. If anaphylaxis occurs, treatment consists of *epinephrine* (subQ, IM, or IV) plus respiratory support.

As a rule, patients with a history of penicillin allergy should not receive penicillins again. If previous reactions have been mild, a cephalosporin (preferably oral) may be an appropriate alternative. However, if severe immediate reactions have occurred, cephalosporins should be avoided too.

Rarely, a patient with a history of anaphylaxis nonetheless requires penicillin. To minimize the risk of a severe reaction, administer penicillin according to a desensitization schedule. Be aware, however, that the procedure does not guarantee that anaphylaxis will not occur. Accordingly, have epinephrine and facilities for respiratory support immediately available.

Sodium Loading. High IV doses of sodium penicillin G can produce sodium overload. Exercise caution in patients under sodium restriction (e.g., cardiac patients, those with hypertension). Monitor electrolytes and cardiac status.

Hyperkalemia. High doses of IV *potassium penicillin G* may cause hyperkalemia, possibly resulting in dysrhythmias or cardiac arrest. Monitor electrolyte and cardiac status.

Effects Resulting From Incorrect Injection. Take care to avoid intra-arterial injection or injection into peripheral nerves because serious injury can result.

Minimizing Adverse Interactions

Aminoglycosides. When present in high concentration, penicillins can inactivate aminoglycosides (e.g., gentamicin). Do not mix penicillins and aminoglycosides in the same IV solution.

[a]Patient education information is highlighted as **blue text.**

CHAPTER

85 Drugs That Weaken the Bacterial Cell Wall II: Cephalosporins, Carbapenems, Vancomycin, Telavancin, Aztreonam, and Fosfomycin

Like the penicillins, the drugs discussed here are inhibitors of cell wall synthesis. By disrupting the cell wall, these drugs produce bacterial lysis and death. Much of the chapter focuses on the cephalosporins, our most widely used antibacterial drugs. With only three exceptions—vancomycin, telavancin, and fosfomycin—the agents addressed here are beta-lactam drugs.

CEPHALOSPORINS

The cephalosporins are beta-lactam antibiotics similar in structure and actions to the penicillins. These drugs are bactericidal, often resistant to beta-lactamases, and active against a broad spectrum of pathogens. Their toxicity is low. Because of these attributes, the cephalosporins are popular therapeutic agents and constitute our most widely used group of antibiotics.

Chemistry

All cephalosporins are derived from the same nucleus. This nucleus contains a *beta-lactam ring* fused to a second ring. The beta-lactam ring is required for antibacterial activity.

Mechanism of Action

The cephalosporins are bactericidal drugs with a mechanism like that of the penicillins. These agents bind to penicillin-binding proteins (PBPs) and thereby (1) disrupt cell wall synthesis and (2) activate autolysins (enzymes that cleave bonds in the cell wall). The resultant damage to the cell wall causes death by lysis. Like the penicillins, cephalosporins are most effective against cells undergoing active growth and division.

Resistance

The principal cause of cephalosporin resistance is the production of beta-lactamases, enzymes that cleave the beta-lactam ring and thereby render these drugs inactive. Beta-lactamases that act on cephalosporins are sometimes referred to as *cephalosporinases.* Some of the beta-lactamases that act on cephalosporins can also cleave the beta-lactam ring of penicillins.

Not all cephalosporins are equally susceptible to beta-lactamases. Most *first-generation* cephalosporins are destroyed by beta-lactamases; *second-generation* cephalosporins are less sensitive to destruction; and *third-, fourth-, and fifth-generation* cephalosporins are highly resistant.

In some cases, bacterial resistance results from producing altered PBPs that have a low affinity for cephalosporins. Methicillin-resistant staphylococci produce these unusual PBPs and are resistant to most cephalosporins as a result. Ceftaroline, a fifth-generation cephalosporin, has demonstrated activity against methicillin-resistant *Staphylococcus aureus* (MRSA).

Classification and Antimicrobial Spectra

The cephalosporins can be grouped into five "generations" based on the order of their introduction to clinical use. The generations differ significantly with respect to antimicrobial spectrum and susceptibility to beta-lactamases (Table 85.1). In general, *as we progress from first-generation agents to fifth-generation agents, there is (1) increasing activity against gram-negative bacteria and anaerobes, (2) increasing resistance to destruction by beta-lactamases, and (3) increasing ability to reach the cerebrospinal fluid (CSF).*

First Generation. First-generation cephalosporins, represented by *cephalexin,* are highly active against gram-positive bacteria. These drugs are the most active of all cephalosporins against staphylococci and nonenterococcal streptococci. However, staphylococci that are resistant to methicillin-like drugs are also resistant to first-generation cephalosporins (and to most other cephalosporins as well). The first-generation agents have only modest activity against gram-negative bacteria and do not reach effective concentrations in the CSF.

Second Generation. Second-generation cephalosporins (e.g., cefoxitin) have enhanced activity against gram-negative bacteria. The increase is due to a combination of factors: (1) increased affinity for PBPs of gram-negative

TABLE 85.1 ▪ Major Differences Between Cephalosporin Generations

Class	Activity Against Gram-Negative Bacteria	Resistance to Beta-Lactamases	Distribution to Cerebrospinal Fluid
First generation (e.g., cephalexin)	Low	Low	Poor
Second generation (e.g., cefoxitin)	Higher	Higher	Poor
Third generation (e.g., cefotaxime)	Higher	Higher	Good
Fourth generation (cefepime)	Highest	Highest	Good
Fifth generation (ceftaroline)	High	Highest	Good

TABLE 85.2 ▪ Pharmacokinetic Properties of the Cephalosporins

				Half-Life (hr)	
Class	Drug	Routes of Administration	Major Route of Elimination	Normal Renal Function	Severe Renal Impairment
First Generation	Cefadroxil	PO	Renal	1.2–1.3	20–25
	Cefazolin	IM, IV	Renal	1.5–2.2	24–50
	Cephalexin	PO	Renal	0.4–1	10–20
Second Generation	Cefaclor	PO	Renal	0.6–0.9	2–3
	Cefotetan	IM, IV	Renal	3–4.5	13–35
	Cefoxitin	IM, IV	Renal	0.7–1	13–22
	Cefprozil	PO	Renal	1.3	5–6
	Cefuroxime	PO, IM, IV	Renal	1–1.9	15–22
Third Generation	Cefdinir	PO	Renal	1.7	16
	Cefditoren	PO	Renal	1.6	—
	Cefixime	PO	Renal	3–4	11.5
	Cefotaxime	IM, IV	Renal	0.9–1.4	3–11
	Cefpodoxime	PO	Renal	2–3	9.8
	Ceftazidime	IM, IV	Renal	1.9–2	—
	Ceftibuten	PO	Renal	2	Increased
	Ceftriaxone	IM, IV	Hepatic	5.8–8.7	15.7
Fourth Generation	Cefepime	IM, IV	Renal	2	Increased
Fifth Generation	Ceftaroline	IV	Renal	2.6	Increased

bacteria, (2) increased ability to penetrate the gram-negative cell envelope, and (3) increased resistance to beta-lactamases produced by gram-negative organisms. However, none of the second-generation agents is active against *Pseudomonas aeruginosa.* These drugs do not reach effective concentrations in the CSF.

Third Generation. Third-generation cephalosporins (e.g., cefotaxime) have a broad spectrum of antimicrobial activity. Because of increased resistance to beta-lactamases, these drugs are considerably more active against gram-negative aerobes than are the first- and second-generation agents. Some third-generation cephalosporins (e.g., ceftazidime) have important activity against *P. aeruginosa.* Others (e.g., cefixime) lack such activity. In contrast to first- and second-generation cephalosporins, the third-generation agents reach clinically effective concentrations in the CSF.

Fourth Generation. Cefepime, the only fourth-generation cephalosporin, is highly resistant to beta-lactamases and has a very broad antibacterial spectrum. Activity against *P. aeruginosa* equals that of ceftazidime. Penetration to the CSF is good.

Fifth Generation. Ceftaroline [Teflaro]—has a spectrum like that of the third-generation agents, but with one important exception: ceftaroline is the only cephalosporin with activity against MRSA.

Pharmacokinetics

Absorption. Because of poor absorption from the GI tract, *many cephalosporins must be administered parenterally* (IM or IV). Of the cephalosporins used in the United States, only 10 can be administered by mouth (Table 85.2). Of these, only one—*cefuroxime*—can be administered orally *and* by injection.

Distribution. Cephalosporins distribute well to most body fluids and tissues. Therapeutic concentrations are achieved in pleural, pericardial, and peritoneal fluids. However, concentrations in ocular fluids are generally low. Penetration to the CSF by first- and second-generation drugs is unreliable, and hence these drugs should not be used for bacterial meningitis. In contrast, CSF levels achieved with third-, fourth-, and fifth-generation drugs are generally sufficient for bactericidal effects.

Elimination. Practically all cephalosporins are eliminated by the *kidneys;* excretion is by a combination of glomerular filtration and active tubular secretion. Probenecid can decrease tubular secretion of some cephalosporins, thereby prolonging their effects. In patients with renal insufficiency, dosages of most cephalosporins must be reduced (to prevent accumulation to toxic levels).

One cephalosporin—*ceftriaxone*—is eliminated largely by the liver. Consequently, dosage reduction is unnecessary in patients with renal impairment.

Adverse Effects

Cephalosporins are generally well tolerated and constitute one of our safest groups of antimicrobial drugs. Serious adverse effects are rare.

Allergic Reactions. Hypersensitivity reactions are the most frequent adverse events. Maculopapular rash that develops several days after the onset of treatment is most common. Severe, immediate reactions (e.g., bronchospasm, anaphylaxis) are rare. If, during the course of treatment, signs of allergy appear (e.g., urticaria, rash, hypotension, difficulty in breathing), the cephalosporin should be discontinued immediately. Anaphylaxis is treated with respiratory support and parenteral epinephrine. Patients with a history of cephalosporin allergy should not be given these drugs.

Because of structural similarities between penicillins and cephalosporins, a few patients allergic to one type of drug may experience cross-reactivity with the other. In clinical practice, the incidence of cross-reactivity has been low: Only 1% of penicillin-allergic patients experience an allergic reaction if given a cephalosporin. For patients with mild penicillin allergy, cephalosporins can be used with minimal concern. However, because of the potential for fatal anaphylaxis, *cephalosporins should not be given to patients with a history of severe reactions to penicillins.*

Bleeding. Two cephalosporins—*cefotetan* and *ceftriaxone*—can cause bleeding tendencies. The mechanism is reduction of prothrombin levels through interference with vitamin K metabolism.

Several measures can reduce the risk of hemorrhage. During prolonged treatment, patients should be monitored for prothrombin time, bleeding time, or both. Parenteral vitamin K can correct an abnormal prothrombin time. Patients should be observed for signs of bleeding; if bleeding develops, the cephalosporin should be withdrawn. Caution should be exercised during concurrent use of anticoagulants or thrombolytic agents. Because of their antiplatelet effects, aspirin and other nonsteroidal anti-inflammatory drugs (NSAIDs) should be used with care. Caution is needed in patients with a history of bleeding disorders.

Thrombophlebitis. Thrombophlebitis may develop during IV infusion. This reaction can be minimized by rotating the infusion site and by administering cephalosporins slowly and in dilute solution. Patients should be observed for phlebitis. If it develops, the infusion site should be changed.

Hemolytic Anemia. Rarely, cephalosporins have induced immune-mediated hemolytic anemia, a condition in which antibodies mediate destruction of red blood cells. If hemolytic anemia develops, the cephalosporin should be discontinued. Blood transfusions may be given as needed.

Other Adverse Effects. Cephalosporins may cause *pain at sites of IM injection;* patients should be forewarned. Rarely, cephalosporins may be the cause of *pseudomembranous colitis* due to colonic overgrowth with *Clostridium difficile.* If this superinfection develops, the cephalosporin should be discontinued and, if necessary, oral vancomycin should be given.

With one cephalosporin—*cefditoren*—there are two unique concerns. First, the drug contains a milk protein (sodium caseinate), and hence should be avoided by patients with *milk-protein hypersensitivity* (as opposed to lactose intolerance). Second, cefditoren is excreted in combination with carnitine, and hence can cause *carnitine loss.* Accordingly, the drug is contraindicated for patients with existing carnitine deficiency or with conditions that predispose to carnitine deficiency.

Drug Interactions

Probenecid. Probenecid delays renal excretion of some cephalosporins and can thereby prolong their effects. This is the same interaction that occurs between probenecid and penicillins.

Alcohol. Two cephalosporins—*cefazolin* and *cefotetan*—can induce a state of alcohol intolerance. If a patient taking these drugs were to ingest alcohol, a disulfiram-like reaction could occur. (As discussed in Chapter 38, the disulfiram effect, which can be very dangerous, is brought on by accumulation of acetaldehyde secondary to inhibition of aldehyde dehydrogenase.) Patients using these cephalosporins must not consume alcohol in any form.

Drugs That Promote Bleeding. As noted, *cefotetan* and *ceftriaxone* can promote bleeding. Caution is needed if these drugs are combined with other agents that promote bleeding (anticoagulants, thrombolytics, NSAIDs, and other antiplatelet agents).

Calcium and Ceftriaxone. Combining calcium with ceftriaxone can form potentially fatal precipitates. In neonates, but not in older patients, the combination of IV calcium and IV ceftriaxone has caused death from the deposit of precipitates in the lungs and kidneys. To minimize risk, the following rules apply:

- Don't reconstitute powdered ceftriaxone with calcium-containing diluents (e.g., Ringer's solution).
- Don't mix reconstituted ceftriaxone with calcium-containing solutions.
- For patients other than neonates, IV ceftriaxone and IV calcium may be administered sequentially (not concurrently) through the same line, provided the line is flushed between the infusions.
- For neonates, don't give IV ceftriaxone and IV calcium through the same line or different lines within 48 hours of each other. If the patient must receive ceftriaxone and calcium, use *oral* calcium or *IM* ceftriaxone.

Therapeutic Uses

The therapeutic role of the cephalosporins is continually evolving as new agents are introduced and more experience is gained with older ones. Only general recommendations are considered here.

The cephalosporins are broad-spectrum bactericidal drugs with a high therapeutic index. They have been employed widely and successfully against a variety of infections. Cephalosporins can be useful alternatives for patients with mild penicillin allergy.

The five generations of cephalosporins differ significantly in their applications. With one important exception—the use of first-generation agents for infections caused by sensitive staphylococci—*the first- and second-generation cephalosporins* are rarely drugs of choice for active infections. In most cases, equally effective and less expensive alternatives are available. In contrast, the *third-generation agents* have qualities that make them the preferred therapy for several infections. The *fourth- and fifth-generation agents* are effective against resistant organisms. The *fifth-generation* agent is used to treat skin infections, including MRSA, and healthcare-associated pneumonias.

First-Generation Cephalosporins. When a cephalosporin is indicated for a *gram-positive infection,* a first-generation drug should be used; these agents are the most active of the cephalosporins against gram-positive organisms and are less expensive than other cephalosporins. First-generation agents are frequently employed as alternatives to penicillins to treat infections caused by staphylococci or streptococci (except enterococci) in patients with penicillin allergy. However, it is important to note that cephalosporins should be given only to patients with a history of *mild* penicillin allergy—not those who have experienced a severe, immediate hypersensitivity reaction.

The first-generation agents have been employed widely for *prophylaxis against infection in surgical patients.* First-generation agents are preferred to second- or third-generation cephalosporins for surgical prophylaxis because they are as effective as the newer drugs, are less expensive, and have a more narrow antimicrobial spectrum.

Second-Generation Cephalosporins. Specific indications for second-generation cephalosporins are limited. *Cefuroxime* has been used with success against pneumonia caused by *Haemophilus influenzae, Klebsiella,* pneumococci, and staphylococci. Oral cefuroxime is useful for otitis, sinusitis, and respiratory tract infections. *Cefoxitin* is useful for abdominal and pelvic infections.

Prototype Drugs

DRUGS THAT INHIBIT CELL WALL SYNTHESIS

Cephalosporins
Cephalexin

Carbapenems
Imipenem

Others
Vancomycin

Third-Generation Cephalosporins. Because they are highly active against gram-negative organisms and because they penetrate to the CSF, third-generation cephalosporins are drugs of choice for meningitis caused by enteric, gram-negative bacilli. *Ceftazidime* is of special utility for treating meningitis caused by *P. aeruginosa. Nosocomial infections* caused by gram-negative bacilli, which are often resistant to first- and second-generation cephalosporins (and most other commonly used antibiotics), are appropriate indications for the third-generation drugs. Two third-generation agents—*ceftriaxone* and *cefotaxime*—are drugs of choice for infections caused by *Neisseria gonorrhoeae* (gonorrhea), *H. influenzae, Proteus, Salmonella, Klebsiella,* and *Serratia;* these drugs are also effective against meningitis caused by *Streptococcus pneumoniae,* a gram-positive bacterium.

Fourth-Generation Cephalosporins. There is only one drug in this category: *cefepime* [Maxipime]. Cefepime is commonly used to treat healthcare- and hospital-associated pneumonias, including those caused by the resistant organism *Pseudomonas.*

Fifth-Generation Cephalosporins. *Ceftaroline* [Teflaro] is the only cephalosporin adequate for the treatment of MRSA-associated infections.

Drug Selection

Eighteen cephalosporins are currently employed in the United States, and selection among them can be a challenge. Within each generation, the similarities among cephalosporins are more pronounced than the differences. Hence, aside from cost, there is frequently no rational basis for choosing one drug over another in the outpatient setting. However, there *are* some differences between cephalosporins, and these differences may render one agent preferable to another for treating a specific infection in a specific host. The differences that do exist can be grouped into two main categories: antimicrobial spectrum and pharmacokinetics (e.g., route of administration, penetration to the CSF, time course, mode of elimination). Drug selection based on these differences is discussed next.

Antimicrobial Spectrum. A prime rule of antimicrobial therapy is to match the drug with the bug: The drug should be active against known or suspected pathogens, but its spectrum should be no broader than required. When a cephalosporin is appropriate, we should select from among those drugs known to have good activity against the causative pathogen. The third- and fourth-generation agents, with their very broad antimicrobial spectra, should be avoided in situations where a narrower spectrum, first- or second-generation drug would suffice.

For some infections, one cephalosporin may be decidedly more effective than all others and should be selected on this basis. For example, *ceftazidime* (a third-generation drug) is the most effective of all cephalosporins against *P. aeruginosa* and is clearly the preferred cephalosporin for treating infections caused by this microbe. Similarly, *ceftaroline* is the only cephalosporin with activity against MRSA, and hence is preferred to all other cephalosporins for treating these infections.

Pharmacokinetics. Four pharmacokinetic properties are of interest: (1) route of administration, (2) duration of action, (3) distribution to the CSF, and (4) route of elimination. The relationship of these properties to drug selection is discussed here.

Route of Administration. Ten cephalosporins can be administered orally. These drugs may be preferred for mild to moderate infections in patients who can't tolerate parenteral agents.

Duration of Action. In patients with normal renal function, the half-lives of the cephalosporins range from about 30 minutes to 9 hours (see Table 85.2). Because they require fewer doses per day, drugs with a long half-life are frequently preferred. Cephalosporins with the longest half-lives in each generation are as follows: first generation, *cefazolin* (1.5 to 2 hours); second generation, *cefotetan* (3 to 4.5 hours); and third generation, *ceftriaxone* (6 to 9 hours).

Distribution to CSF. Only the third- and fourth-generation agents achieve CSF concentrations sufficient for bactericidal effects. Hence, for meningitis caused by susceptible organisms, these drugs are preferred over first- and second-generation agents. It is suspected that the fifth-generation drug, ceftaroline, would be successful in treating infections of the CSF. A trial is currently recruiting participants to evaluate the use of ceftaroline in this capacity.

Route of Elimination. Most cephalosporins are eliminated by the kidneys; if dosage is not carefully adjusted, these drugs may accumulate to toxic levels in patients with renal impairment. Only one agent—*ceftriaxone*—is eliminated primarily by nonrenal routes, and hence can be used with relative safety in patients with kidney dysfunction.

Dosage and Administration

Routes. Many cephalosporins cannot be absorbed from the GI tract and must therefore be administered parenterally (IM or IV). Only 10 cephalosporins can be given orally. One drug—*cefuroxime*—can be administered both orally and by injection.

Dosage. Dosages are shown in Table 85.3. For most cephalosporins (*ceftriaxone* excepted), dosage should be reduced in patients with significant renal impairment.

Administration

Oral. If oral cephalosporins produce nausea, administration with food can reduce the response. Oral suspensions should be stored cold.

Intramuscular. Intramuscular injections should be made deep into a large muscle. Intramuscular injection of cephalosporins is frequently painful; the patient should be forewarned. The injection site should be checked for induration, tenderness, and redness, and the prescriber should be informed if these occur.

Intravenous. For IV therapy, cephalosporins may be administered by three techniques: (1) bolus injection, (2) slow injection (over 3 to 5 minutes), and (3) continuous infusion over 30 to 60 minutes. The prescriber's order should state which method to use. If there is uncertainty as to method, request clarification. Prepare solutions for parenteral administration according to the manufacturer's recommendations.

TABLE 85.3 ▪ Cephalosporin Dosages

Drug	Brand Name	Route	Dosing Interval (hr)	Total Daily Dosage[a]	
				Adults (gm)	Children (mg/kg)
FIRST GENERATION					
Cefadroxil	Generic only	PO	12, 24	1–2	30
Cefazolin	Generic only	IM, IV	6, 8	2–12	80–160
Cephalexin	Keflex	PO	6	1–4	25–100
SECOND GENERATION					
Cefaclor	Raniclor 🍁	PO	8	0.75–1.5	20–40
Cefotetan	Generic only	IM, IV	12	1–6	—
Cefoxitin	Generic only	IM, IV	4, 8	3–12	80–160
Cefprozil	Generic only	PO	12, 24	0.5–1	15–30
Cefuroxime	Ceftin Zinacef	PO IM, IV	12 8	0.5–1 1.5–6	250–500 50–100
THIRD GENERATION					
Cefdinir	Omnicef	PO	12, 24	0.6	14
Cefditoren	Spectracef	PO	12	0.4–0.8	—
Cefixime	Suprax	PO	24	0.4	8
Cefotaxime	Claforan	IM, IV	4, 8	2–12	100–200
Cefpodoxime	Vantin	PO	12	0.2–0.4	10
Ceftazidime	Fortaz, Tazicef	IM, IV	8, 12	0.5–6	60–150
Ceftibuten	Cedax	PO	24	0.4	9
Ceftriaxone	Rocephin	IM, IV	12, 24	1–4	50–100
FOURTH GENERATION					
Cefepime	Maxipime	IM, IV	12	1–6	100–150
FIFTH GENERATION					
Ceftaroline	Teflaro	IV	12	1.2	—

[a]With the exception of ceftriaxone, cephalosporins require a dosage reduction in patients with severe renal impairment.

TABLE 85.4 ▪ Carbapenems

Drug	Uses	Pharmacokinetics	Adverse Effects	Preparations and Adult Dosage
Imipenem	Most gram-positive and gram-negative aerobes and anaerobes	Half-life: 1 hr Excretion: urine	Nausea, vomiting, diarrhea Rarely causes seizure activity	IV; 500 mg every 6 hr
Meropenem	Gram-positive and gram-negative aerobes and anaerobes	Half-life: 1 hr Excretion: urine	Rash, nausea, vomiting Rarely causes seizure activity	IV; 1 gm every 8 hr
Ertapenem	Most gram-positive bacteria and anaerobes	Half-life: 4 hr Excretion: urine, feces	Diarrhea, nausea, headache	IM/IV; 1 gm every 24 hr
Doripenem	Gram-positive, gram-negative, and anaerobic bacteria, including *P. aeruginosa*	Half-life: 1 hr Excretion: urine	Headache, nausea, rash, phlebitis at injection site	IV; 500 mg every 8 hr

CARBAPENEMS

Carbapenems are beta-lactam antibiotics that have very broad antimicrobial spectra—although none is active against MRSA. Four carbapenems are available: imipenem, meropenem, ertapenem, and doripenem. With all four, administration is parenteral (Table 85.4). To delay emergence of resistance, these drugs should be reserved for patients who cannot be treated with a more narrow-spectrum agent.

Imipenem

Imipenem [Primaxin], a beta-lactam antibiotic, has an extremely broad antimicrobial spectrum—broader, in fact, than nearly all other antimicrobial drugs. As a result, imipenem may be of special use for treating mixed infections in which anaerobes, *Staph. aureus,* and gram-negative bacilli may all be involved. Imipenem is supplied in fixed-dose combinations with cilastatin, a compound that inhibits destruction of imipenem by renal enzymes.

Mechanism of Action

Imipenem binds to two PBPs (PBP1 and PBP2), causing weakening of the bacterial cell wall with subsequent cell lysis and death. Antimicrobial effects are enhanced by the drug's resistance to practically all beta-lactamases and by its ability to penetrate the gram-negative cell envelope.

Antimicrobial Spectrum

Imipenem is active against most bacterial pathogens, including organisms resistant to other antibiotics. The drug is highly active against gram-positive cocci and most gram-negative cocci and bacilli. In addition, imipenem is the most effective beta-lactam antibiotic for use against anaerobic bacteria.

Pharmacokinetics

Imipenem is not absorbed from the GI tract and hence must be given intravenously. The drug is well distributed to body fluids and tissues. Imipenem penetrates the meninges to produce therapeutic concentrations in the CSF.

Elimination is primarily renal. When employed alone, imipenem is inactivated by dipeptidase, an enzyme present in the kidneys. As a result, drug levels in urine are low. To increase urinary concentrations, imipenem is administered in combination with *cilastatin,* a dipeptidase inhibitor. When the combination is used, about 70% of imipenem is excreted unchanged in the urine. The elimination half-life is about 1 hour.

Adverse Effects

Imipenem is generally well tolerated. Gastrointestinal effects (nausea, vomiting, diarrhea) are most common. Superinfections with bacteria or fungi develop in about 4% of patients. Rarely, seizures have occurred.

Hypersensitivity reactions (rashes, pruritus, drug fever) have occurred, and patients allergic to other beta-lactam antibiotics may be cross-allergic with imipenem. Fortunately, the incidence of cross-sensitivity with penicillins is low—only about 1%.

Interaction With Valproate

Imipenem can reduce blood levels of valproate, a drug used to control seizures (see Chapter 24). Breakthrough seizures have occurred. If possible, combined use of imipenem and valproate should be avoided. If no other antibiotic will suffice, supplemental antiseizure therapy should be considered.

Therapeutic Use

Because of its broad spectrum and low toxicity, imipenem is used widely. The drug is effective for serious infections caused by gram-positive cocci, gram-negative cocci, gram-negative bacilli, and anaerobic bacteria. This broad antimicrobial spectrum gives imipenem special utility for antimicrobial therapy of mixed infections (e.g., simultaneous infection with aerobic and anaerobic bacteria). When imipenem has been given alone to treat infection with *P. aeruginosa,* resistant organisms have emerged. Consequently, imipenem should be combined with another antipseudomonal drug when used against this microbe.

Preparations, Dosage, and Administration

Imipenem is formulated in 1 : 1 fixed-dose combinations with cilastatin. This combination product is marketed under the brand name *Primaxin.* This product is supplied in powdered form and must be reconstituted in accord with the manufacturer's instructions. The usual adult dosage is 500 mg every 6 hours. Dosage should be reduced in patients with renal impairment.

PATIENT-CENTERED CARE ACROSS THE LIFE SPAN

Cephalosporins, Carbapenems, and Others

Life Stage	Patient Care Concerns
Infants	Third-generation cephalosporins are used to treat bacterial infections in neonates, as well as infants.
Children/adolescents	Cephalosporins are commonly used to treat bacterial infections in children, including otitis media and gonococcal and pneumococcal infections.
Pregnant women	Administration of telavancin during pregnancy should be avoided due to a risk for adverse developmental outcomes. All cephalosporins appear safe for use in pregnancy and are classified in FDA Pregnancy Risk Category B.[a]
Breast-feeding women	Cephalosporins are generally not expected to cause adverse effects in breast-fed infants.
Older adults	Doses should be adjusted in older adults with decreased renal function.

[a]As of 2020, the FDA will no longer use Pregnancy Risk Categories. Please refer to Chapter 9 for more information.

OTHER INHIBITORS OF CELL WALL SYNTHESIS

Vancomycin

Vancomycin [Vancocin] is the most widely used antibiotic in U.S. hospitals. Principal indications are *C. difficile* infection (CDI), MRSA infection, and the treatment of serious infections with susceptible organisms in patients allergic to penicillins. The major toxicity is renal failure. Unlike most other drugs discussed here, vancomycin does not contain a beta-lactam ring.

Mechanism of Action

Like the beta-lactam antibiotics, vancomycin inhibits cell wall synthesis and thereby promotes bacterial lysis and death. However, in contrast to the beta-lactams, vancomycin does not interact with PBPs. Instead, it disrupts the cell wall by binding to molecules that serve as precursors for cell wall biosynthesis.

Antimicrobial Spectrum

Vancomycin is active only against gram-positive bacteria. The drug is especially active against *Staph. aureus* and *Staphylococcus epidermidis,* including strains of both species that are methicillin resistant. Other susceptible organisms include streptococci, penicillin-resistant pneumococci, and *C. difficile.*

Pharmacokinetics

Absorption from the GI tract is poor. Hence, for most infections, vancomycin is given parenterally (by slow IV infusion). Oral administration is employed only for infections of the intestine, mainly CDI.

Vancomycin is well distributed to most body fluids and tissues. Although it enters the CSF, levels may be insufficient to treat meningitis. Hence, if meningeal infection fails to respond to IV therapy, concurrent intrathecal dosing may be required.

Vancomycin is eliminated unchanged by the kidneys. In patients with renal impairment, dosage must be reduced.

Therapeutic Use

Vancomycin should be reserved for serious infections. This agent is the drug of choice for infections caused by MRSA or *Staph. epidermidis;* most strains of these bacteria are still sensitive to vancomycin. Vancomycin is also the drug of choice for *severe* CDI, but not for *mild* CDI (Box 85.1). The drug is also employed as an alternative to penicillins and cephalosporins to treat severe infections (e.g., staphylococcal and streptococcal endocarditis) in patients allergic to beta-lactam antibiotics.

Adverse Effects

The major toxicity is *renal failure.* Risk is dose related and increased by concurrent use of other nephrotoxic drugs (e.g., aminoglycosides, cyclosporine, NSAIDs). To minimize risk, trough serum levels of vancomycin should be no greater than needed (see later in this chapter). If significant kidney damage develops, as indicated by a 50% increase in serum creatinine level, vancomycin dosage should be reduced.

Ototoxicity develops rarely, and it is usually reversible. Risk is increased by prolonged treatment, renal impairment, and concurrent use of other ototoxic drugs (e.g., aminoglycosides, ethacrynic acid).

Rapid infusion of vancomycin can cause a constellation of disturbing effects—flushing, rash, pruritus, urticaria, tachycardia, and hypotension—known collectively as *red man syndrome.* These effects, which may result from the release of histamine, can usually be avoided by infusing vancomycin slowly (over 60 minutes or more).

Thrombophlebitis is common. The reaction can be minimized by administering vancomycin in dilute solution and by changing the infusion site frequently.

Rarely, vancomycin causes *immune-mediated thrombocytopenia,* a condition in which platelets are lost and spontaneous bleeding results. The underlying mechanism is the development of unusual antibodies that bind to platelets—but only if the platelets first bind with vancomycin (forming a vancomycin-platelet complex). The resulting antibody-vancomycin-platelet complexes are then removed from the circulation by macrophages.

Patients allergic to penicillins do not show cross-reactivity with vancomycin. Accordingly, vancomycin is an alternative to penicillins in patients with penicillin allergy.

Preparations, Dosage, and Administration

Intravenous Dosing. For systemic infection, vancomycin is administered by intermittent infusion over 60 minutes or longer. Dosage is 15 to 20 mg/kg every 8 to 12 hours. For patients with severe infection, a loading dose (25 to 30 mg/kg) may be used. In patients with renal impairment, dosages must be reduced.

Dosage should be adjusted to achieve effective *trough* serum levels of vancomycin. For serious infections (e.g., bacteremia, osteomyelitis, meningitis, healthcare-acquired pneumonia), trough levels should be 15 to 20 mcg/mL. For less serious infections, trough levels should be at least 10 mcg/mL.

Oral Dosing. Vancomycin is given orally for CDI and other intestinal infections. (Dosages for CDI are shown in Box 85.1.) Because vancomycin is not absorbed from the GI tract, there is no need to decrease oral doses in patients with renal impairment.

Rectal Dosing. Rectal dosing may be used for patients with complicated CDI. One recommended regimen consists of giving 500 mg in 100 mL of normal saline every 6 hours, using a retention enema.

Telavancin

Actions and Uses

Telavancin [Vibativ] is the first representative of a new class of agents, the *lipoglycoproteins,* synthetic derivatives of vancomycin. Like vancomycin, telavancin is active only against gram-positive bacteria. Cell kill results from two mechanisms. First, like vancomycin, telavancin inhibits bacterial cell wall synthesis. Second, telavancin binds to the bacterial cell membrane and thereby disrupts membrane function. Telavancin is approved for IV therapy of *complicated skin and skin structure infections* and *hospital- or ventilator-acquired pneumonia* caused by susceptible strains of the following gram-positive organisms: *Staph. aureus* (including methicillin-sensitive and methicillin-resistant strains), *Strep. pyogenes, Strep. agalactiae, Strep. anginosus* group, and *Enterococcus faecalis* (but only vancomycin-sensitive strains). To delay the development of resistance, telavancin should be reserved for the treatment of vancomycin-resistant infections or for use as an alternative to linezolid [Zyvox], daptomycin [Cubicin], or tigecycline [Tygacil] in patients who cannot take these drugs.

Pharmacokinetics

Following IV infusion, telavancin undergoes 90% binding to plasma proteins. Elimination is primarily renal. In healthy volunteers, the plasma half-life was approximately 8 hours. In patients with renal impairment, the half-life is prolonged and blood levels increase. In patients with moderate hepatic impairment, the kinetics of telavancin remain unchanged.

Adverse Effects

Telavancin can cause multiple adverse effects. The most common are taste disturbance, nausea, vomiting, and foamy urine. As with vancomycin, rapid infusion can cause red man syndrome, characterized by flushing, rash, pruritus, urticaria, tachycardia, and hypotension.

Kidney damage develops in 3% of patients, as indicated by increased serum creatinine, renal insufficiency, or even renal failure. To reduce risk, kidney function should be measured at baseline, every 72 hours during treatment, and at the end of treatment. If these tests indicate nephrotoxicity, switching to a different antibiotic should be considered. In most cases, kidney function normalizes after telavancin is withdrawn. The risk of kidney damage is increased by using other nephrotoxic drugs.

Telavancin can *prolong the QT interval.* However, serious dysrhythmias have not been reported. Nonetheless, telavancin should not be given to patients at high risk, including those with congenital long QT syndrome, uncompensated heart failure, or severe left ventricular hypertrophy, and those using other QT drugs.

Drug Interactions

Telavancin should be used with caution in patients taking other drugs that can damage the kidneys (e.g., NSAIDs, angiotensin-converting enzyme inhibitors, aminoglycosides) and in patients taking drugs that prolong the QT interval (e.g., clarithromycin, ketoconazole). Clinically significant interactions involving cytochrome P450 enzymes have not been observed.

Preparations, Dosage, and Administration

Telavancin [Vibativ] is supplied as a powder (750 mg) for reconstitution as a concentrated solution (15 mg/mL), followed by dilution to a final concentration of 0.6 to 8 mg/mL. The usual dosage is 10 mg/kg once daily, infused over 60 minutes to reduce the risk of red man syndrome. Treatment duration is 7 to 14 days. Monitoring telavancin blood levels is unnecessary. In patients with renal impairment, as indicated by reduced creatinine clearance, dosage should be decreased. In patients with moderate hepatic impairment, no dosage adjustment is needed.

Aztreonam

Chemistry

Aztreonam [Azactam, Cayston] belongs to a class of beta-lactam antibiotics known as *monobactams.* These agents contain a beta-lactam ring, but the ring is not fused with a second ring.

Mechanism of Action

Aztreonam binds to PBP3. Therefore, like most beta-lactam antibiotics, the drug inhibits bacterial cell wall synthesis and thereby promotes cell lysis and death. The drug does not bind to PBPs produced by anaerobes or gram-positive bacteria.

Antimicrobial Spectrum and Therapeutic Use

Aztreonam has a narrow antimicrobial spectrum, being active only against gram-negative aerobic bacteria. Susceptible organisms include *Neisseria* species, *H. influenzae, P. aeruginosa,* and Enterobacteriaceae (e.g., *Escherichia coli, Klebsiella, Proteus, Serratia, Salmonella, Shigella*). Aztreonam is highly resistant to beta-lactamases and therefore is active against many gram-negative aerobes that produce them. The drug is not active against gram-positive bacteria and anaerobes.

si

BOX 85.1 ■ SPECIAL INTEREST TOPIC

CLOSTRIDIUM DIFFICILE INFECTION

Clostridium difficile, aka *C. difficile* or *C. diff,* is a gram-positive, spore-forming, anaerobic bacillus that infects the bowel. Injury results from the release of two toxins, toxin A and toxin B. Symptoms range from mild (abdominal discomfort, nausea, fever, diarrhea) to very severe (toxic megacolon, pseudomembranous colitis, colon perforation, sepsis, death). *C. difficile* infection (CDI) has become more common and more severe, owing to the spread of a more virulent strain—known as NAP1/BI/027—that releases more toxin than older strains. In many hospitals, rates of infection caused by *C. diff* exceed those caused by methicillin-resistant *Staphylococcus aureus* (MRSA). Fortunately, most cases of CDI can be managed well with antibiotics, usually metronidazole [Flagyl] or vancomycin [Vancocin].

CDI is almost always preceded by the use of antibiotics, which kill off normal gut flora and allow *C. diff* to flourish. The antibiotics most likely to promote CDI are clindamycin, second- and third-generation cephalosporins, and fluoroquinolones. In fact, intensive use of fluoroquinolones, such as ciprofloxacin [Cipro] and levofloxacin [Levaquin], is believed to be responsible for the rapid spread of the NAP1/BI/027 strain.

CDI is acquired by ingesting *C. difficile* spores, which are shed in the feces. Any object that feces contact—including toilets, bathtubs, and rectal thermometers—can be a source of infection. Within hospitals, spores are transferred to patients primarily on the hands of healthcare workers who have touched a contaminated person or object. Spores of *C. diff* are resistant to drying, temperature changes, and alcohol, so viable spores can remain in the environment for weeks.

CDI is defined by (1) the passage of three or more unformed stools in 24 hours or less plus (2) a positive stool test for *C. difficile* or its toxins. Intestinal damage is caused by toxins A and B, which attack the lining of the colon. Symptoms range from watery diarrhea to life-threatening pseudomembranous colitis, characterized by patches of severe inflammation and purulent drainage. Complications of severe *C. difficile* colitis include dehydration, electrolyte disturbances, toxic megacolon, bowel perforation, renal failure, sepsis, and death. Among patients successfully treated for CDI, the recurrence rate is 15% to 30%.

The principal risk factor for CDI is treatment with antibiotics. Risk is especially high among older adults who take antibiotics. Other risk factors include GI surgery, serious illness, prolonged hospitalization, and immunosuppression, which may result from cancer chemotherapy, immunosuppressive therapy, or HIV.

Treatment of CDI consists of stopping one antibiotic and starting another, as recommended in a clinical guideline issued by the Infectious Disease Society of America (IDSA) and the Society for Healthcare Epidemiology of America (SHEA). As soon as possible after CDI has been diagnosed, we should stop the antibiotic that facilitated *C. diff* overgrowth, since doing so (1) will reduce the risk of reinfection once CDI has cleared and (2) will cause the infection to resolve in 25% of patients with mild CDI. At the same time, we should start an antibiotic to eradicate *C. diff.* Drug selection is based on infection severity, as judged by two laboratory values: white blood cell (WBC) counts and serum creatinine (SCr). Higher WBC counts indicate more severe colonic inflammation. Higher SCr values indicate more severe dehydration (from diarrhea) and worsening renal perfusion (from dehydration). As shown in the following table, oral *metronidazole* is recommended for a mild/moderate initial episode, and oral *vancomycin* is recommended for a severe initial episode. For a complicated severe initial episode, the guidelines recommend IV metronidazole *plus* vancomycin given either PO or through a nasogastric tube. If the patient has complete ileus (absence of intestinal motility), rectal instillation of vancomycin may be added. If CDI recurs after being cleared, the regimen used for initial therapy should be tried again. If there is a second recurrence, the guidelines recommend a prolonged course of oral vancomycin in which the number of daily doses is gradually decreased.

Alternatives and supplements to metronidazole and vancomycin are being studied. Promising options include the following:

- *Fidaxomicin* [Dificid]—a narrow-spectrum macrolide antibiotic with high selectivity for *C. difficile*—was approved for treating *C. difficile*–associated diarrhea in 2011. In a Phase III trial, the cure rate with fidaxomicin was higher than with vancomycin, and the recurrence rate was lower. Parameters for the use of fidaxomicin are still being defined.
- *Nitazoxanide,* approved for diarrhea caused by *Giardia* species and *Cryptosporidium* species, appears equal to metronidazole or vancomycin for treating CDI. Prospective trials are still needed.
- *Rifaximin,* approved for diarrhea caused by *Escherichia coli,* can reduce CDI recurrence following treatment with vancomycin.
- *Monoclonal antibodies* directed against *C. difficile* toxins A and B can reduce CDI recurrence when given concurrently with metronidazole or vancomycin. The first one, bezlotoxumab [Zinplava] was approved for use in 2016. Bezlotoxumab works by binding *C. difficile* toxin B, hence neutralizing its effects.
- Inoculating the bowel with a *benign strain* of *C. difficile* can protect against developing CDI. Presumably, when the benign strain colonizes the bowel, it occupies the same niche that a virulent strain would occupy and thereby prevents the virulent strain from becoming established.

How can we control the spread of CDI? The IDSA/SHEA guidelines offer the following recommendations:

- Use antibiotics judiciously, especially those associated with a high risk of CDI (clindamycin, cephalosporins, and fluoroquinolones).
- If possible, isolate patients with CDI in a private room, or have them share a room with another patient with CDI.

si

CLOSTRIDIUM DIFFICILE INFECTION—cont'd

- Wear gloves and a gown when entering the room of a patient with CDI.
- After contact with a patient with CDI, wash hands with soap and running water. Soap and water won't kill *C. diff* spores, but it will flush them off the hands. Alcohol-based hand rubs will not kill spores and will not remove them from the hands.
- Use disposable rectal thermometers.
- In areas associated with increased rates of CDI, decontaminate surfaces with a chlorine-containing cleaning agent (or any other agent that can kill *C. diff* spores).

Recommended Treatments for *Clostridium difficile* Infection

Clinical Definition	*Supportive Clinical Data*	*Drug Therapy*
Initial episode: mild or moderate	Leukocytosis with a WBC count of 15,000 cells/mcL or lower *and* SCr less than 1.5 times baseline	Metronidazole, 500 mg PO 3 times/day for 10–14 days
Initial episode: severe	Leukocytosis with a WBC count of 15,000 cells/mcL or higher *or* SCr 1.5 times baseline or higher	Vancomycin, 125 mg PO 4 times/day for 10–14 days
Initial episode: severe, complicated	Leukocytosis with a WBC count of 15,000 cells/mcL or higher *or* SCr 1.5 times baseline or higher, *either one, plus* hypotension/shock, ileus, megacolon	Metronidazole 500 mg IV every 8 hr *plus* vancomycin, 500 mg PO/NG 4 times/day for 10–14 days If complete ileus is present, consider adding vancomycin retention enema
First recurrence		Same as initial episode
Second recurrence		Vancomycin PO in a tapered regimen, for example: 125 mg 4 times/day for 10–14 days, then 125 mg twice daily for 7 days, then 125 mg once daily for 7 days, then 125 mg every 2 or 3 days for 2–8 weeks

mcL, Microliter; *NG,* by nasogastric tube; *PO,* by mouth; *SCr,* serum creatinine; *WBC,* white blood cell.
Recommendation data are from Cohen SH, et al.: Clinical Practice Guidelines for *Clostridium difficile* Infection in Adults: 2010 Update by the Society for Healthcare Epidemiology of America (SHEA) and the Infectious Disease Society of America (IDSA), 2010.

Pharmacokinetics

Aztreonam is not absorbed from the GI tract and hence must be administered parenterally (IM or IV) for systemic therapy. Once in the blood, the drug distributes widely to most body fluids and tissues. Therapeutic concentrations can be achieved in the CSF. Aztreonam is eliminated by the kidneys, primarily unchanged.

In addition to being administered IM and IV, aztreonam can be inhaled for delivery directly to the lungs. This route is used to treat *P. aeruginosa* lung infection in patients with cystic fibrosis.

Adverse Effects

Aztreonam is generally well tolerated. Adverse effects are like those of other beta-lactam antibiotics. The most common effects are pain and thrombophlebitis at the site of injection. Because aztreonam differs greatly in structure from penicillins and cephalosporins, there is little cross-allergenicity with them. Hence, aztreonam appears safe for patients with allergies to other beta-lactam antibiotics.

Preparations, Dosage, and Administration

Parenteral. Aztreonam is available in powdered form, sold as *Azactam,* to be reconstituted for IM or IV administration. The usual adult dosage is 1 to 2 gm every 8 to 12 hours. Dosage should be reduced in patients with renal impairment.

Inhalational. Aztreonam is available in powdered form, sold as *Cayston,* to be reconstituted with the diluent supplied, and then inhaled using the *Altera Nebulizer System.* Dosing is done as a repeating cycle of 75 mg 3 times a day for 28 days, followed by 28 days off.

Fosfomycin

Fosfomycin [Monurol] is a unique antibiotic approved for single-dose therapy in women with uncomplicated urinary tract infections (i.e., acute cystitis) caused by *E. coli* or *Enterococcus faecalis.* The drug kills bacteria by disrupting synthesis of the peptidoglycan polymer strands that compose the cell wall. (As discussed in Chapter 84, penicillins kill bacteria in part by preventing cross-linking of peptidoglycan strands.)

The most common adverse effects are diarrhea, headache, vaginitis, and nausea. Fosfomycin may also cause abdominal pain, rhinitis, drowsiness, dizziness, and rash.

Fosfomycin is supplied as a water-soluble powder in single-dose 3-gm packets. Dosing may be done with or without food. Symptoms of cystitis should improve in 2 to 3 days. If symptoms fail to improve, additional doses will not help—but will increase the risk of side effects.

KEY POINTS

- Cephalosporins are beta-lactam antibiotics that weaken the bacterial cell wall, causing lysis and death.
- The major cause of cephalosporin resistance is production of beta-lactamases.
- Cephalosporins can be grouped into five "generations." In general, as we progress from first- to fifth-generation drugs, there is (1) increasing activity against gram-negative bacteria, (2) increasing resistance to destruction by beta-lactamases, and (3) increasing ability to reach the CSF.
- Except for ceftriaxone, all cephalosporins are eliminated by the kidneys and therefore must be given in reduced dosage to patients with renal impairment.
- The most common adverse effects of cephalosporins are allergic reactions. Patients allergic to penicillins have about a 1% risk of cross-reactivity with cephalosporins.
- Two cephalosporins—cefotetan and ceftriaxone—can cause bleeding tendencies.
- Two cephalosporins—cefazolin and cefotetan—can cause a disulfiram-like reaction.
- Imipenem, a beta-lactam antibiotic, has an antimicrobial spectrum that is broader than that of practically all other antimicrobial drugs.
- Vancomycin is an important but potentially toxic drug used primarily for (1) *Clostridium difficile* infection, (2) MRSA infection, and (3) serious infections by susceptible organisms in patients allergic to penicillins.
- The principal toxicity of vancomycin is renal failure.

Please visit **http://evolve.elsevier.com/Lehne** for chapter-specific NCLEX® examination review questions.

Summary of Major Nursing Implications[a]

CEPHALOSPORINS

Cefaclor
Cefadroxil
Cefazolin
Cefdinir
Cefditoren
Cefepime
Cefixime
Cefotaxime
Cefotetan
Cefoxitin
Cefpodoxime
Cefprozil
Ceftaroline
Ceftazidime
Ceftibuten
Ceftriaxone
Cefuroxime
Cephalexin

Except where indicated, the implications here apply to all members of the cephalosporin family.

Preadministration Assessment

Therapeutic Goal

Treatment of infections caused by susceptible organisms.

Baseline Data

The prescriber may order tests to determine the identity and drug sensitivity of the infecting organism. Take samples for culture before initiating treatment.

Identifying High-Risk Patients

Cephalosporins are *contraindicated* for patients with a history of allergic reactions to cephalosporins or of severe allergic reactions to penicillins. *Ceftriaxone* is *contraindicated* for neonates who are receiving (or expected to receive) IV calcium.

Implementation: Administration

Routes

Eight cephalosporins are given only parenterally (IM or IV), nine are given only orally, and one—*cefuroxime*—is given orally *and* parenterally.

Dosage

Dosages are shown in Table 85.3. Dosages for all cephalosporins—except *ceftriaxone*—should be reduced in patients with significant renal impairment.

Administration

Oral. **Advise patients to take oral cephalosporins with food if gastric upset occurs. Instruct patients to refrigerate oral suspensions.**

Instruct patients to complete the prescribed course of therapy even though symptoms may abate before the full course is over.

Intramuscular. Make IM injections deep into a large muscle. **Intramuscular injections are frequently painful; forewarn the patient.** Check the injection site for induration, tenderness, and redness—and notify the prescriber if these occur.

Intravenous. Techniques for IV administration are bolus injection, slow injection (over 3 to 5 minutes), and continuous infusion. The prescriber's order should specify which method to use; request clarification if the order is unclear.

Ongoing Evaluation and Interventions

Evaluating Therapeutic Effects

Monitor for indications of antimicrobial effects (e.g., reduction in fever, pain, or inflammation; improved appetite or sense of well-being).

Minimizing Adverse Effects

Allergic Reactions. Hypersensitivity reactions are relatively common. Rarely, life-threatening anaphylaxis occurs. Avoid cephalosporins in patients with a history of cephalosporin allergy or severe penicillin allergy. If penicillin allergy is *mild,* cephalosporins can be used with relative safety. **Instruct the patient to report any signs of allergy (e.g., skin rash, itching, hives).** If anaphylaxis occurs, administer parenteral epinephrine and provide respiratory support.

Bleeding. Two cephalosporins—*cefotetan* and *ceftriaxone*—can promote bleeding. Monitor prothrombin time, bleeding time, or both. Parenteral vitamin K can correct abnormal prothrombin time. Observe patients for signs of bleeding; if bleeding develops, discontinue the drug. Exercise caution in patients with a history of bleeding disorders and in patients receiving drugs that can interfere with hemostasis (anticoagulants; thrombolytics; antiplatelet drugs, including aspirin and other NSAIDs).

Thrombophlebitis. Intravenous cephalosporins may cause thrombophlebitis. To minimize this reaction, rotate the injection site and inject cephalosporins slowly and in dilute solution. Observe the patient for phlebitis, and change the infusion site if phlebitis develops.

Hemolytic Anemia. Cephalosporins can promote immune-mediated hemolytic anemia. If hemolytic anemia develops, the cephalosporin should be discontinued. Blood transfusions may be given as needed.

Clostridium difficile Infection (CDI). All cephalosporins, and especially the broad-spectrum agents, can promote CDI, which can cause diarrhea and pseudomembranous colitis. Notify the prescriber if diarrhea occurs. If CDI is diagnosed, discontinue the cephalosporin. Treat with metronidazole or vancomycin, depending on the severity of the infection.

Milk-Protein Hypersensitivity. *Cefditoren* tablets contain sodium caseinate, a milk protein. Do not give cefditoren to patients with milk-protein allergy. (The drug is safe in patients with lactose intolerance.)

Carnitine Deficiency. *Cefditoren* is excreted in combination with carnitine and can thereby lower carnitine levels. Do not give cefditoren to patients with pre-existing carnitine deficiency or with conditions that predispose to carnitine deficiency.

Minimizing Adverse Interactions

Alcohol. *Cefazolin* and *cefotetan* can cause alcohol intolerance. A serious disulfiram-like reaction may occur if alcohol is consumed. **Advise patients about alcohol intolerance, and warn them not to drink alcoholic beverages.**

Drugs That Promote Bleeding. Drugs that interfere with hemostasis—anticoagulants, thrombolytics, and antiplatelet drugs (including aspirin and other NSAIDs)—can intensify bleeding tendencies caused by *cefotetan* and *ceftriaxone.* Avoid these combinations.

Calcium and Ceftriaxone. Combining calcium with ceftriaxone can form potentially fatal precipitates. To avoid harm, don't reconstitute powdered ceftriaxone with calcium-containing diluents, and don't mix reconstituted ceftriaxone with calcium-containing solutions. In patients other than neonates, ceftriaxone and calcium-containing solutions may be administered sequentially, provided that the infusion line is flushed between infusions. Do not give IV ceftriaxone to *neonates* who are receiving IV calcium or to neonates who are expected to receive IV calcium.

VANCOMYCIN

Preadministration Assessment

Therapeutic Goal

Treatment of serious infections, including CDI, infection with MRSA, and serious infections with susceptible organisms in patients allergic to penicillins.

Baseline Data

The prescriber may order tests to determine the identity and drug sensitivity of the infecting organisms. Take samples for culture before initiating treatment.

Identifying High-Risk Patients

Exercise *caution* in patients with renal impairment.

Implementation: Administration

Routes

Intravenous. For systemic infections, and possibly for CDI.

Oral. For CDI and other intestinal infections.

Rectal. An investigational route for complicated CDI.

Dosage

Intravenous. The recommended dosage is 15 to 20 mg/kg every 8 to 12 hours, possibly preceded by a loading dose (25 to 30 mg/kg) in patients with severe infection. Dosage must be reduced in patients with renal impairment. Adjust the dosage to achieve an effective *trough* serum level: 15 to 20 mcg/mL for serious infections and 10 mcg/mL for less serious infections.

Oral. Doses for CDI are shown in Box 85.1. Dosages don't need to be reduced in patients with renal impairment.

Rectal. One recommended regimen consists of 500 mg every 6 hours.

Administration

Intravenous. Infuse slowly, over 60 minutes or longer. Use a dilute solution and rotate the infusion site.

Oral. **Instruct patients to complete the prescribed course of therapy even though symptoms may abate before the full course is over.**

Rectal. Dissolve in 100 mL of normal saline, and administer as a retention enema.

Ongoing Evaluation and Interventions

Evaluating Therapeutic Effects

Monitor for indications of antimicrobial effects (e.g., reduction in fever, pain, or inflammation; improved appetite or sense of well-being; decreased diarrhea in patients with CDI).

Minimizing Adverse Effects and Interactions

Renal Failure. Vancomycin can cause dose-related nephrotoxicity. To minimize risk, ensure that serum trough levels are no greater than required. If significant kidney damage develops, as indicated by a 50% increase in serum creatinine level, dosage should be reduced.

Nephrotoxic Drugs. Nephrotoxic drugs—including aminoglycosides, cyclosporine, and NSAIDs—can increase the risk of kidney damage. Concurrent use of these agents should be avoided, if possible.

Red Man Syndrome. Rapid infusion can cause "red man syndrome," characterized by flushing, rash, pruritus, urticaria, tachycardia, and hypotension. To minimize risk, infuse vancomycin slowly, over 60 minutes or longer.

Thrombophlebitis. To help avoid this common reaction, use vancomycin in dilute solution and change the infusion site often.

[a]Patient education information is highlighted as **blue text.**

CHAPTER

86 Bacteriostatic Inhibitors of Protein Synthesis: Tetracyclines, Macrolides, and Others

All the drugs discussed in this chapter inhibit bacterial protein synthesis. However, unlike the aminoglycosides, which are bactericidal, the drugs considered here are largely bacteriostatic. That is, they suppress bacterial growth and replication but do not produce outright kill. In general, the drugs presented here are second-line agents, used primarily for infections resistant to first-line agents.

TETRACYCLINES

Basic Pharmacology of Tetracyclines

The tetracyclines are *broad-spectrum* antibiotics. In the United States, four tetracyclines are available for systemic therapy. All four—tetracycline, demeclocycline, doxycycline, and minocycline—are similar in structure, antimicrobial actions, and adverse effects. Principal differences among them are pharmacokinetic. Because the similarities among these drugs are more pronounced than their differences, we will discuss the tetracyclines as a group, rather than focusing on a prototype. Unique properties of individual tetracyclines are indicated as appropriate.

Mechanism of Action

The tetracyclines suppress bacterial growth by inhibiting protein synthesis. These drugs bind to the 30S ribosomal subunit and thereby inhibit the binding of transfer RNA to the messenger RNA–ribosome complex. As a result, the addition of amino acids to the growing peptide chain is prevented. At the concentrations achieved clinically, the tetracyclines are bacteriostatic.

Selective toxicity of the tetracyclines results from their poor ability to cross mammalian cell membranes. To influence protein synthesis, tetracyclines must first gain access to the cell interior. These drugs enter bacteria by way of an energy-dependent transport system. Mammalian cells lack this transport system, and hence do not actively accumulate the drug. Consequently, although tetracyclines are inherently capable of inhibiting protein synthesis in mammalian cells, their levels within host cells remain too low to be harmful.

Microbial Resistance

Bacterial resistance results from increased drug inactivation, decreased access to ribosomes (owing to the presence of ribosome protection proteins), and reduced intracellular accumulation (owing to decreased uptake and increased export).

Antimicrobial Spectrum

The tetracyclines are broad-spectrum antibiotics, active against a wide variety of gram-positive and gram-negative bacteria. Sensitive organisms include *Rickettsia,* spirochetes, *Brucella, Chlamydia, Mycoplasma, Helicobacter pylori, Borrelia burgdorferi, Bacillus anthracis,* and *Vibrio cholerae.*

Therapeutic Uses

Treatment of Infectious Diseases. Extensive use of tetracyclines has resulted in increasing bacterial resistance. Because of this resistance and because antibiotics with greater selectivity and less toxicity are now available, the use of tetracyclines has declined. Today, tetracyclines are rarely drugs of first choice. Disorders for which they *are* first-line drugs include (1) rickettsial diseases (e.g., Rocky Mountain spotted fever, typhus fever, Q fever); (2) infections caused by *Chlamydia trachomatis* (trachoma, lymphogranuloma venereum, urethritis, cervicitis); (3) brucellosis; (4) cholera; (5) pneumonia caused by *Mycoplasma pneumoniae;* (6) Lyme disease; (7) anthrax; and (8) gastric infection with *H. pylori.*

Treatment of Acne. Tetracyclines are used topically and orally for severe acne vulgaris. Beneficial effects derive from suppressing the growth and metabolic activity of *Propionibacterium acnes,* an organism that secretes inflammatory chemicals. Oral doses for acne are relatively low. As a result, adverse effects are minimal. Acne is discussed in Chapter 105.

Peptic Ulcer Disease. *Helicobacter pylori,* a bacterium that lives in the stomach, is a major contributing factor to peptic ulcer disease. Tetracyclines, in combination with metronidazole and bismuth subsalicylate, are a treatment of choice for eradicating this bug. The role of *H. pylori* in ulcer formation is discussed in Chapter 78.

Periodontal Disease. Two tetracyclines—*doxycycline* and *minocycline*—are used for periodontal disease. Doxycycline is used orally *and* topically, whereas minocycline is used only topically.

Oral Therapy. Benefits of oral doxycycline result from inhibiting collagenase, an enzyme that destroys connective tissue in the gums. The small doses employed—20 mg twice daily—are too low to harm bacteria.

Topical Therapy. Topical minocycline and doxycycline are employed as adjuncts to scaling and root planing. The objective is to reduce pocket depth and bleeding in adults with periodontitis. Benefits derive from suppressing bacterial growth. Both products are applied directly to the site of periodontal disease.

Pharmacokinetics

Individual tetracyclines differ significantly in their pharmacokinetic properties. Of particular significance are differences in half-life and route of elimination. Also important is the degree to which food decreases absorption. The pharmacokinetic properties of individual tetracyclines are shown in Table 86.1.

Duration of Action. The tetracyclines can be divided into three groups: short acting, intermediate acting, and long acting. These differences are related to differences in lipid solubility: The only short-acting agent (tetracycline) has relatively low lipid solubility, whereas the long-acting agents (doxycycline, minocycline) have relatively high lipid solubility.

Absorption. All of the tetracyclines are orally effective, although the extent of absorption differs among individual agents. Absorption of three agents—tetracycline, demeclocycline, and doxycycline—is reduced by food, whereas absorption of minocycline is not.

The tetracyclines form insoluble chelates with calcium, iron, magnesium, aluminum, and zinc. The result is decreased absorption. Accordingly, *tetracyclines should not be administered together with* (1) *calcium supplements,* (2) *milk products* (because they contain calcium), (3) *iron supplements,* (4) *magnesium-containing laxatives,* and (5) *most antacids* (because they contain magnesium, aluminum, or both).

Distribution. Tetracyclines are widely distributed to most tissues and body fluids. However, penetration to the cerebrospinal fluid (CSF) is poor, and hence levels in the CSF are too low to treat meningeal infections. Tetracyclines readily cross the placenta and enter the fetal circulation.

Elimination. Tetracyclines are eliminated by the kidneys and liver. All tetracyclines are excreted by the liver into the bile. After the bile enters the intestine, most tetracyclines are reabsorbed.

Ultimate elimination of short- and intermediate-acting tetracyclines—tetracycline and demeclocycline—is in the urine, largely as the unchanged drug. Because these agents undergo renal elimination, they can accumulate to toxic levels if the kidneys fail. Consequently, *tetracycline and demeclocycline should not be given to patients with significant renal impairment.*

Long-acting tetracyclines are eliminated by the liver, primarily as metabolites. Because these agents are excreted by the liver, their half-lives are unaffected by kidney dysfunction. Accordingly, *the long-acting agents (doxycycline and minocycline) are drugs of choice for tetracycline-responsive infections in patients with renal impairment.*

Adverse Effects

Gastrointestinal Irritation. Tetracyclines irritate the GI tract. As a result, oral therapy is frequently associated with epigastric burning, cramps, nausea, vomiting, and diarrhea. These reactions can be reduced by giving tetracyclines with meals—although food may decrease absorption. Occasionally, tetracyclines cause esophageal ulceration. Risk can be minimized by avoiding dosing at bedtime. Because diarrhea may result from superinfection of the bowel (in addition to nonspecific irritation), it is important that the cause of diarrhea be determined.

Effects on Bones and Teeth. Tetracyclines bind to calcium in developing teeth, resulting in yellow or brown discoloration; hypoplasia of the enamel may also occur. The intensity of tooth discoloration is related to the total cumulative dose: Staining is darker with prolonged and repeated treatment. When taken after the fourth month of gestation, tetracyclines can cause staining of *deciduous* teeth of the infant. However, use during pregnancy will not affect *permanent* teeth. Discoloration of permanent teeth occurs when tetracyclines are taken by patients age 4 months to 8 years, the interval during which tooth enamel is being formed. Accordingly, these drugs should be avoided by children younger than 8 years. The risk of tooth discoloration with *doxycycline* may be less than with other tetracyclines.

Tetracyclines can suppress long-bone growth in premature infants. This effect is reversible upon discontinuation of treatment.

TABLE 86.1 ▪ Pharmacokinetic Properties of the Tetracyclines

Class	Drug	Lipid Solubility	Percent of Oral Dose Absorbed[a]	Effect of Food on Absorption	Route of Elimination	Half-Life: Normal (hr)	Half-Life: Anuric (hr)
Short Acting	Tetracycline	Low	60–80	Large decrease	Renal	8	57–108[b]
Intermediate Acting	Demeclocycline	Moderate	60–80	Large decrease	Renal	12	40–60[b]
Long Acting	Doxycycline	High	90–100	Small decrease	Hepatic	18	17–30
	Minocycline	High	90–100	No change	Hepatic	16	11–23

[a]Percent absorbed when taken on an empty stomach.
[b]Do not use in patients with renal impairment because the drug could accumulate to toxic levels.

Superinfection. A superinfection is an overgrowth with drug-resistant microbes, which occurs secondary to suppression of drug-sensitive organisms. Because the tetracyclines are broad-spectrum agents and therefore can decrease viability of a wide variety of microbes, the risk of superinfection is greater than with antibiotics that have a narrower spectrum.

Superinfection of the bowel with staphylococci or with *Clostridium difficile* produces severe diarrhea and can be life threatening. The infection caused by *C. difficile* is known as *C. difficile*–associated diarrhea (CDAD), also known as *antibiotic-associated pseudomembranous colitis.* Patients should notify the prescriber if significant diarrhea occurs so that the possibility of bacterial superinfection can be evaluated. If a diagnosis of superinfection with staphylococci or *C. difficile* is made, tetracyclines should be discontinued immediately. Treatment of CDAD consists of oral *vancomycin* or *metronidazole* plus vigorous fluid and electrolyte replacement.

Overgrowth with fungi (commonly *Candida albicans*) may occur in the mouth, pharynx, vagina, and bowel. Symptoms include vaginal or anal itching; inflammatory lesions of the anogenital region; and a black, furry appearance of the tongue. Superinfection with *Candida* can be managed by discontinuing tetracyclines. When this is not possible, antifungal therapy is indicated.

Hepatotoxicity. Tetracyclines can cause fatty infiltration of the liver. Hepatotoxicity manifests clinically as lethargy and jaundice. Rarely, the condition progresses to massive liver failure. Liver damage is most likely when tetracyclines are administered intravenously in high doses (greater than 2 gm/day). Pregnant and postpartum women with kidney disease are at especially high risk.

Renal Toxicity. Tetracyclines may exacerbate renal impairment in patients with pre-existing kidney disease. Because *tetracycline* and *demeclocycline* are eliminated by the kidneys, these agents should not be given to patients with renal impairment. If a patient with renal impairment requires a tetracycline, either *doxycycline* or *minocycline* should be used, since these drugs are eliminated primarily by the liver.

Photosensitivity. All tetracyclines can increase the sensitivity of the skin to ultraviolet light. The most common result is exaggerated sunburn. Advise patients to avoid prolonged exposure to sunlight, wear protective clothing, and apply sunscreen to exposed skin.

Other Adverse Effects. Vestibular toxicity—manifesting as dizziness, light-headedness, and unsteadiness—has occurred with minocycline. Rarely, tetracyclines have produced pseudotumor cerebri (a benign elevation in intracranial pressure). In a few patients, demeclocycline has produced nephrogenic diabetes insipidus, a syndrome characterized by thirst, increased frequency of urination, and unusual weakness or tiredness. Because of their irritant properties, tetracyclines can cause pain at sites of IM injection and thrombophlebitis when administered intravenously.

Drug and Food Interactions

As noted, tetracyclines can form nonabsorbable chelates with certain metal ions (calcium, iron, magnesium, aluminum, zinc). Substances that contain these ions include *milk products, calcium supplements, iron supplements, magnesium-containing laxatives,* and *most antacids.* If a tetracycline is administered with these agents, its absorption will be decreased. To minimize interference with absorption, tetracyclines should be *administered at least 1 hour before or 2 hours after ingestion of chelating agents.*

Tetracyclines can also increase digoxin levels through increasing absorption in the GI tract and increase INR levels by altering the vitamin K–producing flora in the gut. Patients on digoxin or warfarin should undergo careful drug level monitoring.

PATIENT-CENTERED CARE ACROSS THE LIFE SPAN

Tetracyclines

Life Stage	Patient Care Concerns
Infants	Tetracyclines should not be used in children younger than 8 years, as they may cause permanent discoloration of the teeth.
Children/adolescents	Tetracyclines should not be used in children younger than 8 years of age.
Pregnant women	Animal studies revealed that tetracyclines can cause fetal harm in pregnancy. Thus, this class of drugs should be avoided.
Breast-feeding women	The use of tetracyclines during tooth development can cause permanent staining. Tetracyclines should be avoided by breast-feeding women.
Older adults	Tetracyclines can interact with drugs, including digoxin. In the older adult who takes many medications, check for interactions.

Dosage and Administration

Administration. For systemic therapy, tetracyclines may be administered orally or intravenously. Oral administration is preferred, and all tetracyclines are available in oral formulations. As a rule, oral tetracyclines should be taken on an empty stomach (1 hour before meals or 2 hours after) and with a full glass of water. An interval of at least 2 hours should separate tetracycline ingestion and the ingestion of products that can chelate these drugs (e.g., milk, calcium or iron supplements, antacids). Two tetracyclines can be given IV (Table 86.2), but this route should be employed only when oral therapy cannot be tolerated or has proved inadequate.

In addition to their systemic use, two agents—doxycycline and minocycline—are available in formulations for topical therapy of periodontal disease.

Dosage. Dosage is determined by the nature and intensity of the infection. Typical systemic doses for adults and children are shown in Table 86.2.

Major Precautions

Two tetracyclines—*tetracycline* and *demeclocycline*—are eliminated primarily in the urine, and hence will accumulate to toxic levels in patients with kidney disease. Accordingly, patients with kidney disease should not use these drugs.

Tetracyclines can cause discoloration of deciduous and permanent teeth. Tooth discoloration can be avoided by withholding these drugs from pregnant women and from children under 8 years of age.

Diarrhea may indicate a potentially life-threatening superinfection of the bowel. Advise patients to notify the prescriber if diarrhea occurs.

High-dose IV therapy has been associated with severe liver damage, particularly in pregnant and postpartum women with kidney disease. As a rule, these women should not receive tetracyclines.

TABLE 86.2 ▪ Tetracyclines: Routes of Administration, Dosing Interval, and Dosage

Class	Drug	Brand Names	Route	Usual Dosing Interval (hr)	Total Daily Dose	
					Adult (mg)	Pediatric (mg/kg)[a]
Short Acting	Tetracycline	Generic only	PO	6	1000–2000	25–50
Intermediate Acting	Demeclocycline	Declomycin	PO	12	600	7–13
Long Acting	Doxycycline	Vibramycin, others	PO	24	100–200	2.2[b]
			IV	24	100–200[c]	2.2–4.4[d]
	Minocycline	Minocin, others	PO	12	200[e]	4[f]
			IV	12	200[e]	4[f]

[a]Doses presented are for children over the age of 8 years. Use in children below this age may cause permanent staining of teeth.
[b]First-day regimen is 2.2 mg/kg initially, followed by 2.2 mg/kg 12 hours later.
[c]First-day regimen is 200 mg in one or two slow infusions (1 to 4 hours).
[d]First-day regimen is 4.4 mg/kg in one or two slow infusions (1 to 4 hours).
[e]First-day regimen is 200 mg initially, followed by 100 mg 12 hours later.
[f]First-day regimen is 4 mg/kg initially, followed by 2 mg/kg 12 hours later.

TABLE 86.3 ▪ Other Macrolides

Drug	Therapeutic Uses	Pharmacokinetics	Adverse Effects	Availability and Usual Adult Dose
Clarithromycin [Biaxin]	Respiratory tract infections, skin infections, disseminated *Mycobacterium avium*	Metabolism: hepatic Excretion: renal	Diarrhea, nausea, distorted taste	Granules for suspension and tablets IR: 250–500 mg every 12 hr Tablets ER: 500 mg every 24 hr
Azithromycin [Zithromax]	Respiratory tract infections, cholera, skin infections, disseminated *Mycobacterium avium*	Metabolism: hepatic Excretion: bile, renal	Diarrhea, nausea, abdominal pain	Tablets IR, oral suspension: 500 mg on day 1 then 250 mg every 24 hr IV: 500 mg every 24 hr

Unique Properties of Individual Tetracyclines

Tetracycline

Tetracycline hydrochloride is the least expensive and most widely used member of the family. When employed systemically, the drug has the indications, pharmacokinetics, adverse effects, and drug interactions described for the tetracyclines as a group. Like most tetracyclines, tetracycline hydrochloride should not be administered with food and is contraindicated for patients with renal impairment.

Safety Alert

TETRACYCLINES

Because they can cause permanent tooth discoloration, tetracyclines should not be given to pregnant women and breast-feeding women or to children younger than 8 years.

Demeclocycline

Demeclocycline shares the actions, indications, and adverse effects described earlier for the tetracyclines as a group. Because of its intermediate duration of action, demeclocycline can be administered at dosing intervals that are longer than those used for tetracycline. Like tetracycline, demeclocycline should not be administered with food.

Demeclocycline is unique among the tetracyclines in that it stimulates urine flow. This side effect can lead to excessive urination, thirst, and tiredness. Interestingly, because of its effect on renal function, demeclocycline has been employed therapeutically to promote urine production in patients suffering from the syndrome of inappropriate (excessive) secretion of antidiuretic hormone.

Doxycycline

Doxycycline [Vibramycin, others] is a long-acting agent that shares the actions and adverse effects described for the tetracyclines as a group. Because of its extended half-life, doxycycline can be administered once daily in some situations. Absorption of oral doxycycline is greater than that of tetracycline. However, food can still reduce the absorption of doxycycline somewhat, and hence it is best to give this drug on an empty stomach. Doxycycline is eliminated primarily by nonrenal mechanisms. As a result, it is safe for patients with renal failure. Doxycycline is a first-line drug for Lyme disease, anthrax, chlamydial infections (urethritis, cervicitis, and lymphogranuloma venereum), and sexually acquired proctitis (in combination with ceftriaxone). A topical formulation is used for periodontal disease, as is a low-dose oral formulation. Another low-dose oral formulation [Oracea] is used for acne.

Minocycline

Minocycline [Minocin, others] is a long-acting agent similar to doxycycline. Unlike other tetracyclines, minocycline can be taken with food. Like doxycycline, and unlike tetracycline and demeclocycline, minocycline is safe for patients with kidney disease. Minocycline is unique among the tetracyclines in that it can damage the vestibular system, causing unsteadiness, lightheadedness, and dizziness. This toxicity limits its use. Minocycline is expensive, costing significantly more than tetracycline. In addition to fighting systemic infection, minocycline can reduce the symptoms of arthritis (see Chapter 73). It is available in an extended-release formulation [Solodyn] for acne and a topical formulation for periodontal disease.

MACROLIDES

The macrolides are broad-spectrum antibiotics that inhibit bacterial protein synthesis. They are called macrolides because they are big. Erythromycin is the oldest member of the family. The newer macrolides—azithromycin and clarithromycin—are derivatives of erythromycin (Table 86.3).

Erythromycin

Erythromycin has a relatively broad antimicrobial spectrum and is a preferred or alternative treatment for a number of infections. The drug is one of our safer antibiotics and will serve as our prototype for the macrolide family.

Prototype Drugs

BACTERIOSTATIC INHIBITORS OF PROTEIN SYNTHESIS

Tetracyclines
Tetracycline

Macrolides
Erythromycin

Oxazolidinones
Linezolid

Glycylcyclines
Tigecycline

Others
Clindamycin

Mechanism of Action

Antibacterial effects result from inhibition of protein synthesis: Erythromycin binds to the 50S ribosomal subunit and thereby blocks the addition of new amino acids to the growing peptide chain. The drug is usually bacteriostatic, but it can be bactericidal against highly susceptible organisms or when present in high concentration. Erythromycin is selectively toxic to bacteria because ribosomes in the cytoplasm of mammalian cells do not bind the drug. In addition, erythromycin cannot cross the mitochondrial membrane, and therefore it does not inhibit protein synthesis in host mitochondria.

Acquired Resistance

Bacteria can become resistant by two mechanisms: (1) production of a pump that exports the drug and (2) modification (by methylation) of target ribosomes so that binding of erythromycin is impaired.

Antimicrobial Spectrum

Erythromycin has an antibacterial spectrum similar to that of penicillin. The drug is active against most gram-positive bacteria, as well as some gram-negative bacteria. Bacterial sensitivity is determined in large part by the ability of erythromycin to gain access to the cell interior.

Therapeutic Uses

Erythromycin is a commonly used antibiotic. *The drug is a treatment of first choice for several infections and may be used as an alternative to penicillin G in patients with penicillin allergy.*

Erythromycin is considered the drug of first choice for individuals infected with *Bordetella pertussis,* the causative agent of *whooping cough.* Because symptoms are caused by a toxin produced by *B. pertussis,* erythromycin does little to alter the course of the disease. However, by eliminating *B. pertussis* from the nasopharynx, treatment does lower infectivity.

Corynebacterium diphtheriae is highly sensitive to erythromycin. Accordingly, erythromycin is the treatment of choice for *acute diphtheria* and for elimination of the diphtheria carrier state.

Several infections respond equally well to macrolides and tetracyclines. Both are drugs of first choice for certain chlamydial infections (urethritis, cervicitis) and for pneumonia caused by *M. pneumoniae.*

Pharmacokinetics

Absorption and Bioavailability. Erythromycin for oral administration is available in three forms: *erythromycin base* and two derivatives of the base, *erythromycin stearate* and *erythromycin ethylsuccinate.* The base is unstable in stomach acid, and its absorption can be variable; the derivatives were synthesized to improve bioavailability. Bioavailability has also been enhanced by formulating tablets with an acid-resistant coating, which protects erythromycin while in the stomach and then dissolves in the duodenum, permitting absorption from the small intestine. As a rule, *food decreases the absorption of erythromycin base and erythromycin stearate,* whereas absorption of erythromycin ethylsuccinate is not affected. Only erythromycin base is biologically active; the derivatives must be converted to the base (either in the intestine or following absorption) in order to work. When used properly (i.e., when dosage is correct and the effects of food are accounted for), all of the oral erythromycins produce equivalent responses.

In addition to its oral forms, erythromycin is available as *erythromycin lactobionate* for IV use. Intravenous dosing produces drug levels that are higher than those achieved with oral dosing.

Distribution. Erythromycin readily distributes to most tissues and body fluids. Penetration to the CSF, however, is poor. Erythromycin crosses the placenta, but adverse effects on the fetus have not been observed.

Elimination. Erythromycin is eliminated primarily by hepatic mechanisms, including metabolism by CYP3A4 (the 3A4 isoenzyme of cytochrome P450). Erythromycin is concentrated in the liver and then excreted in the bile. A small amount (10% to 15%) is excreted unchanged in the urine.

Adverse Effects

Erythromycin is generally free of serious toxicity and is considered one of our safest antibiotics. However, the drug does carry a very small risk of sudden cardiac death from QT prolongation.

Gastrointestinal Effects. Gastrointestinal disturbances (epigastric pain, nausea, vomiting, diarrhea) are the most common side effects. These can be reduced by administering erythromycin with meals. However, this should be done only when using erythromycin products whose absorption is unaffected by food (erythromycin ethylsuccinate, certain enteric-coated formulations of erythromycin base). Patients who experience persistent or severe GI reactions should notify the prescriber.

QT Prolongation and Sudden Cardiac Death. A study published in 2004 raised concerns about cardiotoxicity, especially when erythromycin is combined with drugs that can raise its plasma level. When present in high concentrations, erythromycin can prolong the QT interval, thereby posing a risk of torsades de pointes, a potentially fatal ventricular dysrhythmia. Sudden death can result. The study revealed that when erythromycin is combined with a CYP3A4 inhibitor, there is a fivefold increase in the risk of sudden cardiac death—or 6 extra deaths for every 100,000 patients using the drug. To minimize risk, erythromycin should be avoided by patients with congenital QT prolongation and by those taking class IA or class III antidysrhythmic drugs. Also, the drug should be avoided by patients taking CYP3A4 inhibitors, including certain calcium channel blockers (verapamil and diltiazem), azole antifungal drugs (e.g., ketoconazole, itraconazole), HIV protease inhibitors (e.g., ritonavir, saquinavir), and nefazodone (an antidepressant).

Other Adverse Effects. By killing off sensitive gut flora, erythromycin can promote *superinfection of the bowel. Thrombophlebitis* can occur with IV administration; this reaction can be minimized by infusing the drug slowly in dilute solution. *Transient hearing loss* occurs rarely with high-dose therapy. There is evidence that erythromycin may cause *hypertrophic pyloric stenosis in infants,* especially those younger than 2 weeks.

Drug Interactions

Erythromycin can increase the plasma levels and half-lives of several drugs, thereby posing a risk of toxicity. The mechanism is the inhibition of hepatic cytochrome P450 drug-metabolizing enzymes. Elevated levels are a concern with *theophylline* (used for asthma), *carbamazepine* (used for seizures and bipolar disorder), and *warfarin* (an anticoagulant). Accordingly, when these agents are combined with erythromycin, the patient should be monitored closely for signs of toxicity.

Erythromycin prevents the binding of *chloramphenicol* and *clindamycin* to bacterial ribosomes, thereby antagonizing their antibacterial effects. Accordingly, concurrent use of erythromycin with these two drugs is not recommended.

As noted, erythromycin should not be combined with drugs that can inhibit erythromycin metabolism. Among these are verapamil, diltiazem, HIV protease inhibitors, and azole antifungal drugs.

Preparations, Dosage, and Administration

Preparations. For treating systemic infections, erythromycin is available in oral and IV formulations. All preparations have the same indications, antimicrobial spectrum, and adverse effects. Erythromycin is also available in topical formulations to treat acne.

Oral Dosage and Administration. Oral erythromycin should be administered on an empty stomach and with a full glass of water. If necessary, some preparations (erythromycin ethylsuccinate, certain enteric-coated preparations of erythromycin base) can be administered with food to decrease GI reactions. The usual *adult* dosage for *erythromycin base* and *erythromycin stearate* is 250 to 500 mg every 6 hours; the adult dosage for *erythromycin ethylsuccinate* is 400 to 800 mg every 6 hours. The usual *pediatric* dosage for all oral erythromycins is 7.5 to 12.5 mg/kg every 6 hours.

Brand names for oral erythromycins are *Ery-Tab, PCE Dispertab,* and *EryPed.* Erythromycin stearate is available as *Erythrocin.*

Intravenous Dosage and Administration. Intravenous dosing is reserved for severe infections and is used rarely. Continuous infusion is preferred to intermittent dosing. Only *erythromycin lactobionate* [Erythrocin IV] is given IV. The usual *adult* dosage is 1 to 4 gm daily. The usual *pediatric* dosage is 15 to 50 mg/kg/day. Erythromycin should be infused slowly and in dilute solution (to minimize the risk of thrombophlebitis).

OTHER BACTERIOSTATIC INHIBITORS OF PROTEIN SYNTHESIS

Clindamycin

Clindamycin [Cleocin, Dalacin C ♣] can promote severe CDAD, a condition that can be fatal. Because of the risk of CDAD, indications for clindamycin are limited. Currently, systemic use is indicated only for certain anaerobic infections located outside the central nervous system (CNS).

Mechanism of Action

Clindamycin binds to the 50S subunit of bacterial ribosomes and thereby inhibits protein synthesis. The site at which clindamycin binds overlaps the binding sites for erythromycin and chloramphenicol. As a result, these agents may antagonize each other's effects. Accordingly, there are no indications for concurrent use of clindamycin with these other antibiotics.

Antimicrobial Spectrum

Clindamycin is active against most anaerobic bacteria (gram positive and gram negative) and most gram-positive aerobes. Gram-negative aerobes are generally resistant. Susceptible anaerobes include *Bacteroides fragilis, Fusobacterium, Clostridium perfringens,* and anaerobic streptococci. Clindamycin is usually bacteriostatic. However, it can be bactericidal if the target organism is especially sensitive. Resistance can be a significant problem with *B. fragilis.*

Therapeutic Use

Because of its efficacy against gram-positive cocci, clindamycin has been used widely as an alternative to penicillin. The drug is employed primarily for anaerobic infections outside the CNS (it doesn't cross the blood-brain barrier). Clindamycin is the drug of choice for severe group A streptococcal infection and for gas gangrene (an infection caused by *C. perfringens*), owing to its ability to rapidly suppress synthesis of bacterial toxins. In addition, clindamycin is a preferred drug for abdominal and pelvic infections caused by *B. fragilis.*

Pharmacokinetics

Absorption and Distribution. Clindamycin may be administered orally, IM, or IV. Absorption from the GI tract is nearly complete and not affected by food. The drug is widely distributed to most body fluids and tissues, including synovial fluid and bone. However, penetration to the CSF is poor.

Elimination. Clindamycin undergoes hepatic metabolism to active and inactive products, which are later excreted in the urine and bile. Only 10% of the drug is eliminated unchanged by the kidneys. The half-life is approximately 3 hours. In patients with substantial reductions in liver function *or* kidney function, the half-life increases slightly, but adjustments in dosage are not needed. However, in patients with *combined* hepatic and renal disease, the half-life increases significantly, and hence the drug may accumulate to toxic levels if dosage is not reduced.

Adverse Effects

Clostridium difficile–*Associated Diarrhea.* *C. difficile*–associated diarrhea, formerly known as *antibiotic-associated pseudomembranous colitis,* is the most severe toxicity of clindamycin. The cause is superinfection of the bowel with *C. difficile,* an anaerobic gram-positive bacillus. CDAD is characterized by profuse, watery diarrhea (10 to 20 watery stools per day), abdominal pain, fever, and leukocytosis. Stools often contain mucus and blood. Symptoms usually begin during the first week of treatment, but may develop as long as 4 to

6 weeks after clindamycin withdrawal. Left untreated, the condition can be fatal. CDAD occurs with parenteral and oral therapy. Because of the risk of CDAD, patients should be instructed to report significant diarrhea (more than five watery stools per day). If superinfection with *C. difficile* is diagnosed, clindamycin should be discontinued and the patient given oral vancomycin or metronidazole, which are the drugs of choice for eliminating *C. difficile* from the bowel. Diarrhea usually ceases 3 to 5 days after starting vancomycin. Vigorous replacement therapy with fluids and electrolytes is usually indicated. Drugs that decrease bowel motility (e.g., opioids, anticholinergics) may worsen symptoms and should not be used. CDAD is discussed further in Chapter 85.

Safety Alert

CLINDAMYCIN

Clindamycin can cause potentially fatal *Clostridium difficile* diarrhea. Patients should promptly report any diarrhea to their healthcare provider.

Other Adverse Effects. Diarrhea (unrelated to CDAD) is relatively common. Hypersensitivity reactions (especially rashes) occur frequently. Hepatotoxicity and blood dyscrasias (agranulocytosis, leukopenia, thrombocytopenia) develop rarely. Rapid IV administration can cause electrocardiographic changes, hypotension, and cardiac arrest.

Preparations, Dosage, and Administration

Preparations. Clindamycin is available as *clindamycin hydrochloride* and *clindamycin palmitate* for oral dosing, and as *clindamycin phosphate* for IM, IV, or topical (vaginal) dosing. Clindamycin hydrochloride [Cleocin] is supplied in capsules (75, 150, and 300 mg). Clindamycin palmitate [Cleocin Pediatric] is supplied in flavored granules, which are reconstituted with fluid to make an oral solution containing 15 mg of clindamycin per milliliter. Clindamycin phosphate is supplied in concentrated solution (150 mg/mL) and dilute solution (6, 12, and 18 mg/mL) sold as *Cleocin Phosphate* for parenteral therapy, and in a 2% cream [Cleocin, Clindesse] and 100-mg suppositories [Cleocin] for intravaginal dosing.

Oral Dosage and Administration. For *clindamycin hydrochloride*, the adult dosage range is 150 to 450 mg every 6 hours; the pediatric dosage range is 8 to 20 mg/kg daily in three or four divided doses. For *clindamycin palmitate*, adult and pediatric dosages range from 8 to 25 mg/kg/day administered in three or four divided doses. Oral clindamycin should be taken with a full glass of water. The drug may be administered with meals.

Parenteral Dosage and Administration. For parenteral (IM or IV) therapy, *clindamycin phosphate* is employed. Intramuscular and IV dosages are the same. The usual adult dosage is 1.2 to 2.7 gm/day administered in three or four divided doses. The usual pediatric dosage is 15 to 40 mg/kg/day in three or four divided doses.

Intravaginal Administration. Intravaginal clindamycin (suppositories or cream) is indicated for bacterial vaginosis. The suppositories are approved only for nonpregnant women; the cream can be used by pregnant women, but only during the second and third trimesters. Women using clindamycin cream should insert 1 applicatorful (5 gm containing 100 mg clindamycin) nightly for 7 days (if pregnant) or for 3 to 7 days (if nonpregnant). Women using clindamycin suppositories should insert 1 suppository (100 mg) on three consecutive evenings.

Linezolid

Linezolid [Zyvox] is a first-in-class *oxazolidinone* antibiotic. The drug is important because it has activity against multidrug-resistant gram-positive pathogens, including vancomycin-resistant enterococci (VRE) and methicillin-resistant *Staphylococcus aureus* (MRSA). For the treatment of MRSA, the drug is at least as effective as vancomycin. To delay the emergence of resistance, linezolid should generally be reserved for infections caused by VRE or MRSA, even though it has additional approved uses.

Mechanism, Resistance, and Antimicrobial Spectrum

Linezolid is a bacteriostatic inhibitor of protein synthesis. The drug binds to the 23S portion of the 50S ribosomal subunit and thereby blocks formation of the initiation complex. No other antibiotic works quite this way. As a result, cross-resistance with other agents is unlikely. In clinical trials, development of resistance to linezolid was rare; it occurred only in association with prolonged treatment of VRE infections and the presence of a prosthetic implant or undrained abscess. In real practice, resistance has been reported in association with extensive linezolid use.

Linezolid is active primarily against aerobic and facultative gram-positive bacteria. Susceptible pathogens include *Enterococcus faecium* (vancomycin-sensitive and vancomycin-resistant strains), *Enterococcus faecalis* (vancomycin-resistant strains), *Staph. aureus* (methicillin-sensitive and methicillin-resistant strains), *Staphylococcus epidermidis* (including methicillin-resistant strains), and *Streptococcus pneumoniae* (penicillin-sensitive and penicillin-resistant strains). Linezolid is not active against gram-negative bacteria, which readily export the drug.

Therapeutic Use

Linezolid has five approved indications:

- Infections cause by VRE
- Healthcare-associated pneumonia caused by *Staph. aureus* (methicillin-susceptible and methicillin-resistant strains) or *Strep. pneumoniae* (penicillin-susceptible strains only)
- Community-associated pneumonia (CAP) caused by *Strep. pneumoniae* (penicillin-susceptible strains only)
- Complicated skin and skin structure infections caused by *Staph. aureus* (methicillin-susceptible and methicillin-resistant strains), *Strep. pyogenes,* or *Strep. agalactiae*
- Uncomplicated skin and skin structure infections caused by *Staph. aureus* (methicillin-susceptible strains only) or *Strep. pyogenes*

As previously noted, to delay the emergence of resistance, linezolid should generally be reserved for infections caused by VRE or MRSA, even though it has other approved uses.

Pharmacokinetics

Oral linezolid is rapidly and completely absorbed. Food decreases the rate of absorption but not the extent. Linezolid is eliminated by hepatic metabolism and renal excretion. Its half-life is about 5 hours.

Adverse Effects

Linezolid is generally well tolerated. The most common side effects are diarrhea, nausea, and headache. Linezolid oral suspension contains phenylalanine, and hence must not be used by patients with phenylketonuria.

Linezolid can cause reversible *myelosuppression,* manifesting as anemia, leukopenia, thrombocytopenia, or even pancytopenia. Risk is related to duration of use. Complete blood counts should be done weekly. Special caution is needed in patients with pre-existing myelosuppression, those taking other myelosuppressive drugs, and those receiving linezolid for more than 2 weeks. If existing myelosuppression worsens or new myelosuppression develops, discontinuing linezolid should be considered.

Rarely, prolonged therapy has been associated with *neuropathy.* Patients taking the drug for more than 5 months have developed reversible optic neuropathy and irreversible peripheral neuropathy.

Drug Interactions

Linezolid is a weak inhibitor of monoamine oxidase (MAO), and hence poses a risk of hypertensive crisis. As discussed in Chapter 32, MAO inhibitors can cause severe hypertension if combined with *indirect-acting sympathomimetics* (e.g., ephedrine, pseudoephedrine, methylphenidate, cocaine) or with foods that contain large amounts of *tyramine.* Accordingly, patients using linezolid should be warned to avoid these agents.

Combining linezolid with a *selective serotonin reuptake inhibitor* (SSRI) can increase the risk of serotonin syndrome (because inhibition of MAO increases the serotonin content of CNS neurons). Deaths have been reported. Patients using SSRIs (e.g., paroxetine [Paxil, Pexeva], duloxetine [Cymbalta]) should not take linezolid.

Preparations, Dosage, and Administration

Linezolid is available in three formulations: (1) 600-mg *tablets,* (2) a powder for reconstitution to a 20-mg/mL *oral suspension,* and (3) a 2-mg/mL *intravenous solution.* Oral linezolid can be taken with or without food. Intravenous linezolid is infused over 30 to 120 minutes, and should not be combined with additives or other drugs. Adult dosages for specific infections are as follows:

- *VRE infections*—600 mg PO or IV every 12 hours for 14 to 28 days
- *Pneumonia (healthcare- or community-associated)*—600 mg PO or IV every 12 hours for 7 days
- *Complicated skin and skin structure infections (including MRSA infections)*—600 mg PO or IV every 12 hours for 10 to 14 days
- *Uncomplicated skin and skin structure infections*—400 mg PO every 12 hours for 10 to 14 days

Dalfopristin/Quinupristin

Dalfopristin and quinupristin are first-in-class *streptogramin* antibiotics. The two drugs are available in a fixed-dose combination (70 parts dalfopristin/30 parts quinupristin) under the brand name *Synercid.*

Mechanism of Action

Dalfopristin and quinupristin inhibit bacterial protein synthesis. When used separately, dalfopristin and quinupristin are bacteriostatic. However, in combination they are bactericidal.

Therapeutic Use

The principal indication for dalfopristin/quinupristin is vancomycin-resistant *E. faecium.* (The drugs are not active against *E. faecalis.*) To delay emergence of resistance, dalfopristin/quinupristin should be reserved for infections that have not responded to vancomycin. Other indications include MRSA, methicillin-resistant *Staphylococcus epidermidis,* and drug-resistant *Streptococcus pneumoniae.* Dalfopristin/quinupristin is safe for patients who are allergic to penicillins and cephalosporins.

Adverse Effects

Hepatotoxicity is the major concern. Blood should be tested for liver enzymes and bilirubin at least twice during the first week of therapy and weekly thereafter. About 50% of patients develop infusion-related thrombophlebitis. When this occurs, administration must be switched to a central venous line or the solution should be further diluted. Other adverse effects include joint and muscle pain, rash, pruritus, vomiting, and diarrhea.

Drug Interactions

Dalfopristin and quinupristin inhibit hepatic drug-metabolizing enzymes, specifically CYP3A4. Accordingly, the combination is likely to inhibit the metabolism of many other drugs, including cyclosporine, tacrolimus, and cisapride.

Preparations, Dosage, and Administration

Dalfopristin/quinupristin [Synercid] is supplied as a powder in 500-mg vials to be reconstituted for IV administration. The usual dosage is 7.5 mg/kg infused slowly (over 1 hour) 2 or 3 times a day. To minimize venous irritation, flush the vein with 0.5% dextrose after the infusion. If irritation occurs despite flushing, the drug should be further diluted or infused through a central venous line. Because dalfopristin and quinupristin are eliminated by hepatic metabolism, dosage should be reduced in patients with liver impairment.

Tigecycline

Tigecycline [Tygacil] is a first-in-class *glycylcycline* antibiotic. The drug is a tetracycline derivative designed to overcome drug resistance. Tigecycline is active against a broad spectrum of bacteria, including many drug-resistant strains. Unfortunately, tigecycline is associated with an increased mortality (see later), and hence using another antibiotic drug should be considered.

Mechanism of Action and Resistance

Tigecycline is a *bacteriostatic* inhibitor of protein synthesis. Like the tetracyclines, tigecycline binds to the 30S ribosomal subunit and thereby inhibits binding of transfer RNA to the messenger RNA–ribosome complex. As a result, the addition of amino acids to the growing peptide chain is stopped.

Bacterial resistance to tigecycline is much less than with the tetracyclines. First, bacteria are unable to extrude tigecycline. Second, bacteria cannot block binding of tigecycline to ribosomes.

Antimicrobial Spectrum

Tigecycline is a broad-spectrum antibiotic with activity against gram-positive and gram-negative bacteria, including many strains that are drug resistant. Susceptible gram-positive organisms include *Staph. aureus* (vancomycin sensitive, methicillin sensitive, and methicillin resistant), vancomycin-resistant enterococci, penicillin-resistant *Strep. pneumoniae, C. perfringens,* and *C. difficile*. Susceptible gram-negative organisms include *Acinetobacter baumanii, Stenotrophomonas maltophilia, B. fragilis, Escherichia coli,* and *Enterobacter* species. Of note, tigecycline is *not* active against *Pseudomonas aeruginosa* or *Proteus* species.

Therapeutic Use

Tigecycline was originally approved only for complicated intra-abdominal infections and complicated skin infections that need broad empiric coverage, and was later approved for CAP caused by *Strep. pneumoniae* (penicillin-susceptible isolates). To delay emergence of resistance, tigecycline should be used only when other drugs are considered likely to fail.

Pharmacokinetics

Tigecycline is administered IV and undergoes moderate binding to plasma proteins (about 80%). Very little of the drug is metabolized. Excretion occurs in the bile (59%) and urine (33%), mainly as unchanged drug. The plasma half-life is 42 hours.

Adverse Effects

Tigecycline is a tetracycline analog, and hence may have adverse effects like those of the tetracyclines. In clinical trials, the most common reactions were nausea and vomiting. Like the tetracyclines, tigecycline may pose a risk of pseudotumor cerebri (a benign elevation of intracranial pressure) and may increase sensitivity to ultraviolet light, thereby increasing the risk of sunburn. Being a broad-spectrum antibiotic, tigecycline may pose a risk of superinfection, including CDAD. Acute pancreatitis, including fatal cases, has occurred during tigecycline treatment. If pancreatitis is suspected, withdrawal of the drug should be considered. Tigecycline is in FDA Pregnancy Risk Category D,[a] and hence should be avoided by pregnant women.

Among patients treated for severe infections, *mortality is higher* for those receiving tigecycline than for those receiving other antibiotics. This is because tigecycline is less effective than the other options. Accordingly, the FDA recommends considering an alternative to tigecycline for patients with severe infections.

Drug Interactions

Drug interactions appear minimal. Tigecycline does not affect the cytochrome P450 system, and hence will not alter the kinetics of drugs metabolized by P450. Similarly, because tigecycline undergoes very little metabolism, drugs

[a]As of 2020, the FDA will no longer use Pregnancy Risk Categories. Please refer to Chapter 9 for more information.

that alter P450 activity should not alter the kinetics of tigecycline. Tigecycline can delay the clearance of warfarin (an anticoagulant). Accordingly, if the drugs are used concurrently, coagulation status should be monitored.

Preparations, Dosage, and Administration

Tigecycline [Tygacil] is supplied as a lyophilized powder in single-dose 50-mg vials, to be reconstituted for IV infusion. Infusion should occur over 30 to 60 minutes. Treatment consists of a 100-mg initial dose followed by 50 mg every 12 hours for 5 to 14 days. No adjustment in dosage is needed for patients with renal impairment or with mild to moderate hepatic impairment. For patients with *severe* hepatic impairment, the initial dose is unchanged, but maintenance dosing should be reduced to 25 mg every 12 hours.

Retapamulin and Mupirocin

Retapamulin and mupirocin are topical antibiotics. Both drugs are indicated for impetigo; mupirocin is also indicated for clearing the nostrils of MRSA. For impetigo therapy, retapamulin is more convenient than mupirocin, but generic mupirocin is cheaper.

Retapamulin

Retapamulin [Altabax] is a first-in-class *pleuromutilin* antibiotic. The drug binds to the 50S bacterial ribosomal subunit and thereby inhibits protein synthesis. However, the 50S binding site is different from that of other antibiotics, and hence cross-resistance with other antibiotics is not expected. Retapamulin is bacteriostatic at therapeutic concentrations. At this time, the drug is approved only for *topical* therapy of impetigo caused by *Strep. pyogenes* or methicillin-susceptible *Staph. aureus.* However, *in vitro* data indicate that the drug may be effective against MRSA and mupirocin-resistant *Staph. aureus.* Significant resistance among *Staph. aureus* has not been observed, and is considered unlikely. The principal adverse effect is local irritation, which only 2% of users experience. Systemic toxicity does not occur, owing to minimal absorption from topical sites. Retapamulin is available as a 1% ointment in 15- and 30-gm tubes. Application is done twice daily for 5 days.

Mupirocin

Mupirocin [Bactroban, Bactroban Nasal] is a topical antibiotic with two indications: (1) impetigo caused by *Staph. aureus, Strep. pyogenes,* or beta-hemolytic streptococci and (2) elimination of nasal colonization by MRSA. Mupirocin has a unique mechanism: The drug binds with bacterial isoleucyl transfer-RNA synthetase and thereby blocks protein synthesis. The drug is bactericidal at therapeutic concentrations. Resistance has developed, owing to production of a modified form of isoleucyl transfer-RNA synthetase, but cross-resistance with other antibiotics has not been reported.

Adverse effects depend on the application site. With application to the *skin,* local irritation can occur, but systemic effects occur rarely, if at all. (Absorption from intact skin is minimal, and any absorbed drug undergoes rapid conversion to inactive products.) With *intranasal* application, the most common side effects are headache, rhinitis, upper respiratory congestion, and pharyngitis.

Mupirocin is available as a 2% cream and a 2% ointment. For *impetigo,* the cream or ointment is applied 3 times a day for 10 to 12 days. To eradicate *MRSA nasal colonization,* the ointment is applied twice daily for 5 days.

KEY POINTS

- Tetracyclines are broad-spectrum, bacteriostatic antibiotics that inhibit bacterial protein synthesis.
- Tetracyclines are first-choice drugs for just a few infections, including those caused by *Chlamydia trachomatis,* rickettsia (e.g., Rocky Mountain spotted fever), *H. pylori* (i.e., peptic ulcer disease), *B. anthracis* (anthrax), *Borrelia burgdorferi* (Lyme disease), and *M. pneumoniae.*
- Tetracyclines form insoluble chelates with calcium, iron, magnesium, aluminum, and zinc. Accordingly, they must not be administered with calcium supplements, milk products, iron supplements, magnesium-containing laxatives, and most antacids.
- Three oral tetracyclines—tetracycline, demeclocycline, and doxycycline—should be administered on an empty stomach. Minocycline can be administered with meals.
- Tetracycline and demeclocycline should not be given to patients with renal failure.
- Tetracyclines can stain developing teeth and therefore should not be given to pregnant women and breast-feeding women or children under 8 years old.
- Because they are broad-spectrum antibiotics, tetracyclines can cause superinfections, especially *C. difficile*–associated diarrhea (CDAD) and overgrowth of the mouth, pharynx, vagina, or bowel with *Candida albicans.*
- High doses of tetracyclines can cause severe liver damage, especially in pregnant and postpartum women who have renal impairment.
- Erythromycin, the prototype of the macrolide antibiotics, is a bacteriostatic drug that inhibits bacterial protein synthesis.
- Erythromycin has an antimicrobial spectrum similar to that of penicillin G, and hence can be used in place of penicillin G in patients with penicillin allergy.
- Erythromycin is generally safe. However, combined use of erythromycin with inhibitors of CYP3A4 increases the risk of QT prolongation and sudden cardiac death.
- Clindamycin is used primarily as an alternative to penicillin for serious gram-positive anaerobic infections.
- Clindamycin causes a high incidence of CDAD.
- Linezolid is important because it can suppress multidrug-resistant gram-positive pathogens, including vancomycin-resistant enterococci (VRE) and methicillin-resistant *Staph. aureus* (MRSA).

Please visit **http://evolve.elsevier.com/Lehne** for chapter-specific NCLEX® examination review questions.

Summary of Major Nursing Implications[a]

TETRACYCLINES

Demeclocycline
Doxycycline
Minocycline
Tetracycline

Except where stated otherwise, the implications here pertain to all tetracyclines.

Preadministration Assessment

Therapeutic Goal

Treatment of tetracycline-sensitive infections, acne, and periodontal disease.

Identifying High-Risk Patients

Tetracyclines are *contraindicated* in pregnant women and in children younger than 8 years, and should be avoided in women who are breast-feeding.

Tetracycline and *demeclocycline* must be used with great *caution* in patients with significant renal impairment.

Implementation: Administration

Routes

Systemic. *All* tetracyclines are used systemically. Specific routes for individual agents are shown in Table 86.2.

Topical. *Doxycycline* and *minocycline* are used topically to treat periodontal disease.

Administration

Oral. **Advise patients to take most oral tetracyclines on an empty stomach (1 hour before meals or 2 hours after) and with a full glass of water. *Minocycline* may be taken with food.**

Instruct patients to allow at least 2 hours between ingestion of tetracyclines and these chelators: milk products, calcium supplements, iron supplements, magnesium-containing laxatives, and most antacids.

Instruct patients to complete the prescribed course of treatment, even though symptoms may abate before the full course is over.

Parenteral. *Intravenous* administration is performed only when oral administration is ineffective or cannot be tolerated.

Ongoing Evaluation and Interventions

Minimizing Adverse Effects

Gastrointestinal Irritation. **Inform patients that GI distress (epigastric burning, cramps, nausea, vomiting, diarrhea) can be reduced by taking tetracyclines with meals, although absorption may be reduced.**

Effects on Teeth. Tetracyclines can discolor developing teeth. To prevent this, avoid tetracyclines in pregnant women and breast-feeding women and in children younger than 8 years.

Superinfection. Tetracyclines can promote bacterial superinfection of the bowel, resulting in severe diarrhea. **Instruct patients to notify the prescriber if significant diarrhea develops.** If superinfection is diagnosed, discontinue tetracyclines immediately. Treatment of *C. difficile*–associated diarrhea (CDAD) consists of oral vancomycin or metronidazole, plus fluid and electrolyte replacement.

Fungal overgrowth may occur in the mouth, pharynx, vagina, and bowel. **Inform patients about symptoms of fungal infection (vaginal or anal itching; inflammatory lesions of the anogenital region; black, furry appearance of the tongue), and advise them to notify the prescriber if these occur.** Superinfection caused by *Candida* can be managed by discontinuing the tetracycline or by giving an antifungal drug.

Hepatotoxicity. Tetracyclines can cause fatty infiltration of the liver, resulting in jaundice and, rarely, massive liver failure. The risk of liver injury can be reduced by avoiding high-dose IV therapy and by withholding tetracyclines from pregnant and postpartum women who have kidney disease.

Renal Toxicity. Tetracyclines can exacerbate pre-existing renal impairment. *Tetracycline* and *demeclocycline* should not be used by patients with kidney disease.

Photosensitivity. Tetracyclines can increase the sensitivity of the skin to ultraviolet light, thereby increasing the risk of sunburn. **Advise patients to avoid prolonged exposure to sunlight, wear protective clothing, and apply a sunscreen to exposed skin.**

ERYTHROMYCIN

The implications here apply to all forms of erythromycin, except where noted otherwise.

Preadministration Assessment

Therapeutic Goal

Erythromycin is indicated for whooping cough, diphtheria, chancroid, chlamydial infections, and other infections caused by erythromycin-sensitive organisms. The drug is also used as a substitute for penicillin G in penicillin-allergic patients.

Identifying High-Risk Patients

All forms of erythromycin should be avoided by patients with QT prolongation and by those taking inhibitors of CYP3A4.

Implementation: Administration

Routes

Oral. Erythromycin base, erythromycin ethylsuccinate, and erythromycin stearate.

Intravenous. Erythromycin lactobionate.

Administration

Oral. **Advise patients to take oral preparations on an empty stomach (1 hour before meals or 2 hours after) and with a full glass of water. However, if GI upset occurs, administration may be done with meals.**

Inform patients using erythromycin ethylsuccinate and enteric-coated formulations of erythromycin base that they may take these drugs without regard to meals.

Instruct patients to complete the prescribed course of treatment, even though symptoms may abate before the full course is over.

Continued

Summary of Major Nursing Implications[a]—cont'd

Intravenous. Administer by slow infusion and in dilute solution to minimize thrombophlebitis.

Ongoing Evaluation and Interventions

Minimizing Adverse Effects

Gastrointestinal Effects. Gastrointestinal disturbances (epigastric pain, nausea, vomiting, diarrhea) can be reduced by administering erythromycin with meals. **Advise patients to notify the prescriber if GI reactions are severe or persistent.**

QT Prolongation and Sudden Cardiac Death. High levels of erythromycin can prolong the QT interval, thereby posing a risk of a potentially fatal cardiac dysrhythmia. Avoid erythromycin in patients with pre-existing QT prolongation and in those taking drugs that can increase erythromycin levels.

Minimizing Adverse Interactions

Erythromycin can increase the half-lives and plasma levels of several drugs. When erythromycin is combined with *theophylline, carbamazepine,* or *warfarin,* patients should be monitored closely for toxicity.

Erythromycin can antagonize the antibacterial actions of *clindamycin* and *chloramphenicol.* Concurrent use of erythromycin with these agents is not recommended.

Drugs that inhibit CYP3A4 (e.g., verapamil, diltiazem, HIV protease inhibitors, azole antifungal drugs) can increase erythromycin levels, thereby posing a risk of QT prolongation and sudden cardiac death. People using these drugs should not use erythromycin.

CLINDAMYCIN

Preadministration Assessment

Therapeutic Goal

Treatment of anaerobic infections outside the CNS.

Implementation: Administration

Routes

Oral, IM, IV, intravaginal.

Administration

Instruct patients to take oral clindamycin with a full glass of water.

Instruct patients to complete the prescribed course of treatment, even though symptoms may abate before the full course is over.

Ongoing Evaluation and Interventions

Minimizing Adverse Effects

Clostridium difficile*–Associated Diarrhea.* Clindamycin can promote CDAD, a potentially fatal superinfection. Prominent symptoms are profuse watery diarrhea, abdominal pain, fever, and leukocytosis. Stools often contain mucus and blood. **Instruct patients to report significant diarrhea (more than five watery stools per day).** If CDAD is diagnosed, discontinue clindamycin. Treat with oral vancomycin or metronidazole and vigorous replacement of fluids and electrolytes. Drugs that decrease bowel motility (e.g., opioids, anticholinergics) may worsen symptoms and should be avoided.

[a]Patient education information is highlighted as **blue text.**

CHAPTER

87 Aminoglycosides: Bactericidal Inhibitors of Protein Synthesis

The aminoglycosides are antibiotics used primarily against aerobic gram-negative bacilli. These drugs disrupt protein synthesis, resulting in rapid bacterial death. The aminoglycosides can cause serious injury to the inner ears and kidneys. Because of these toxicities, indications for these drugs are limited. All of the aminoglycosides carry multiple positive charges. As a result, they are not absorbed from the GI tract and must be administered parenterally to treat systemic infections. In the United States, seven aminoglycosides are approved for clinical use. The agents employed most commonly are gentamicin, tobramycin, and amikacin.

BASIC PHARMACOLOGY OF THE AMINOGLYCOSIDES

Chemistry

The aminoglycosides are composed of two or more amino sugars connected by a glycoside linkage. At physiologic pH, these drugs are highly polar polycations (i.e., they carry several positive charges); therefore they cannot readily cross membranes. As a result, aminoglycosides are not absorbed from the GI tract, do not enter the cerebrospinal fluid, and are rapidly excreted by the kidneys.

Mechanism of Action

The aminoglycosides disrupt bacterial protein synthesis. As indicated in Fig. 87.1, these drugs bind to the 30S ribosomal subunit, causing (1) inhibition of protein synthesis, (2) premature termination of protein synthesis, and (3) production of abnormal proteins (secondary to misreading of the genetic code).

The aminoglycosides are *bactericidal.* Cell kill is *concentration dependent.* Hence, the higher the concentration, the more rapidly the infection will clear. Of note, bactericidal activity persists for several hours *after* serum levels have dropped below the minimal bactericidal concentration, a phenomenon known as the *postantibiotic effect.*

Bacterial kill appears to result from production of abnormal proteins rather than from simple inhibition of protein synthesis. Studies suggest that abnormal proteins become inserted in the bacterial cell membrane, causing it to leak. The resultant loss of cell contents causes death. Inhibition of protein synthesis per se does not seem the likely cause of bacterial death because complete blockade of protein synthesis by other antibiotics (e.g., tetracyclines, chloramphenicol) is usually bacteriostatic—not bactericidal.

Microbial Resistance

The principal cause for bacterial resistance is production of enzymes that can inactivate aminoglycosides. Among gram-negative bacteria, the genetic information needed to synthesize these enzymes is acquired through the transfer of R factors. To date, more than 20 different aminoglycoside-inactivating enzymes have been identified. Because each of the aminoglycosides can be modified by more than one of these enzymes and because each enzyme can act on more than one aminoglycoside, patterns of bacterial resistance can be complex.

Of all the aminoglycosides, *amikacin* is least susceptible to inactivation by bacterial enzymes. As a result, resistance to amikacin is uncommon. To minimize emergence of resistant bacteria, amikacin should be reserved for infections that are unresponsive to other aminoglycosides.

Antimicrobial Spectrum

Bactericidal effects of the aminoglycosides are limited almost exclusively to *aerobic gram-negative bacilli.* Sensitive organisms include *Escherichia coli, Klebsiella pneumoniae, Serratia marcescens, Proteus mirabilis,* and *Pseudomonas aeruginosa.* Aminoglycosides are inactive against most gram-positive bacteria.

Aminoglycosides *cannot kill anaerobes.* To produce antibacterial effects, aminoglycosides must be transported across the bacterial cell membrane, a process that is oxygen dependent. Since, by definition, anaerobic organisms live in the absence of oxygen, these microbes cannot take up aminoglycosides, and hence are resistant. For the same reason, aminoglycosides are inactive against facultative bacteria when these organisms are living under anaerobic conditions.

Therapeutic Use

Parenteral Therapy. The principal use for parenteral aminoglycosides is treatment of *serious infections due to aerobic gram-negative bacilli.* Primary target organisms are *P. aeruginosa* and the Enterobacteriaceae (e.g., *E. coli, Klebsiella, Serratia, P. mirabilis*).

One aminoglycoside—gentamicin—is now commonly used in combination with either vancomycin or a beta-lactam

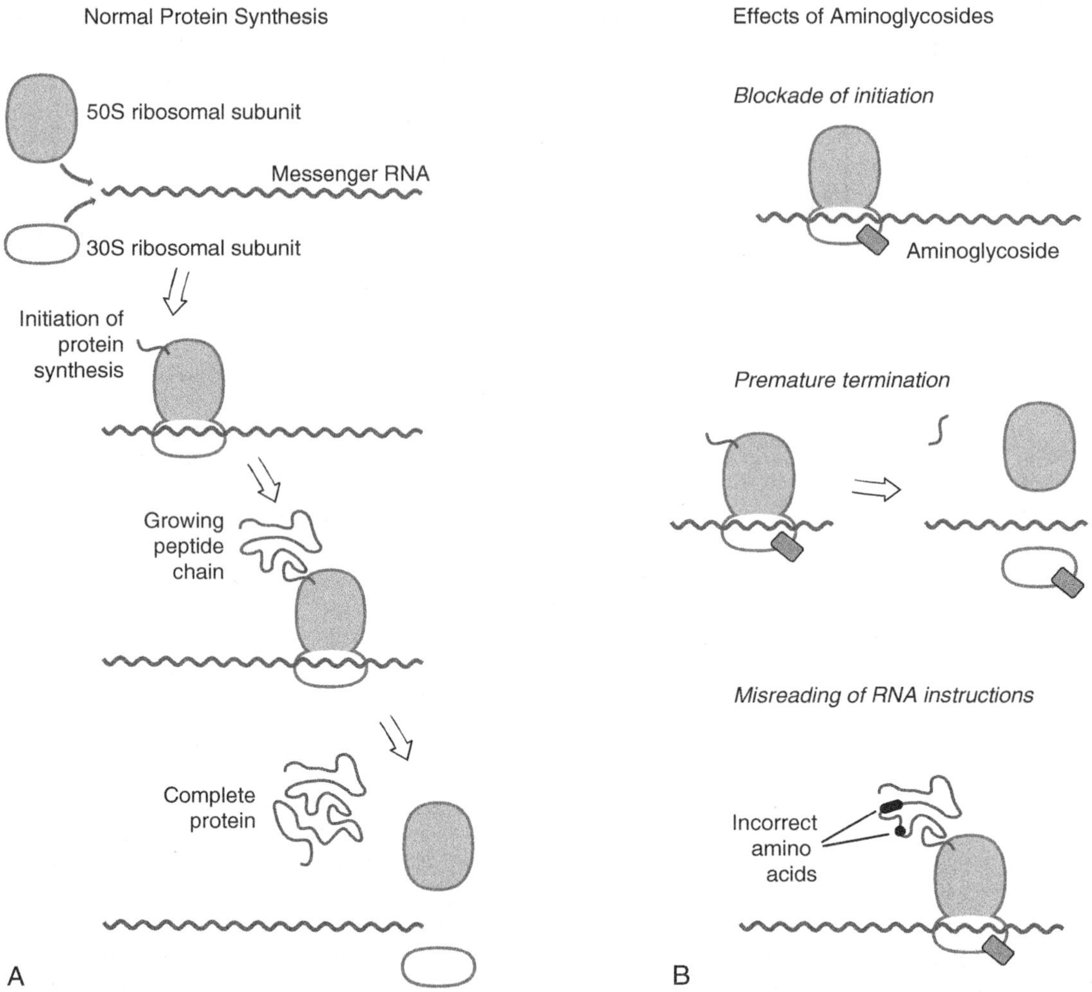

Fig. 87.1 ■ Mechanism of action of aminoglycosides.
A, Protein synthesis begins with binding of the 50S and 30S ribosomal subunits to messenger RNA (mRNA), followed by attachment of the first amino acid of the new protein to the 50S subunit. As the ribosome moves down the mRNA strand, additional amino acids are added to the growing peptide chain. When the new protein is complete, it separates from the ribosome, and the ribosomal subunits separate from the mRNA. **B,** Aminoglycosides bind to the 30S ribosomal subunit and can (1) block initiation, (2) terminate synthesis before the new protein is complete, and (3) cause misreading of the genetic code, which causes synthesis of faulty proteins.

antibiotic to treat *serious infections with certain gram-positive cocci,* specifically *Enterococcus* species, some streptococci, and *Staphylococcus aureus.*

The aminoglycosides used most commonly for parenteral therapy are gentamicin, tobramycin, and amikacin. Selection among the three depends in large part on patterns of resistance in a given community or hospital. In settings where resistance to aminoglycosides is uncommon, either gentamicin or tobramycin is usually preferred. Of the two, gentamicin is less expensive and may be selected on this basis. Organisms resistant to both gentamicin and tobramycin are usually sensitive to amikacin. Accordingly, in settings where resistance to gentamicin and tobramycin is common, amikacin may be preferred for initial therapy.

Oral Therapy. Aminoglycosides are not absorbed from the GI tract, and hence oral therapy is used only for local effects within the intestine. In patients anticipating elective colorectal surgery, oral aminoglycosides have been given prophylactically to suppress bacterial growth in the bowel. One aminoglycoside—*paromomycin*—is used to treat intestinal amebiasis.

Topical Therapy. *Neomycin* is available in formulations for application to the eyes, ears, and skin. Topical preparations of *gentamicin* and *tobramycin* are used to treat conjunctivitis caused by susceptible gram-negative bacilli.

Pharmacokinetics

All of the aminoglycosides have similar pharmacokinetic profiles. Pharmacokinetic properties of the principal aminoglycosides are shown in Table 87.1.

Absorption. Because they are polycations, the aminoglycosides cross membranes poorly. As a result, very little (about 1%) of an oral dose is absorbed. Hence, for treatment of systemic infections, aminoglycosides must be given parenterally (IM or IV). Absorption following application to the intact skin is minimal. However, when used for wound irrigation, aminoglycosides may be absorbed in amounts sufficient to produce systemic toxicity.

Distribution. Distribution of aminoglycosides is limited largely to extracellular fluid. Entry into the cerebrospinal fluid is insufficient to treat meningitis in adults. Aminoglycosides bind tightly to renal tissue, achieving levels in the kidneys up

TABLE 87.1 ■ Dosages and Pharmacokinetics of Systemic Aminoglycosides

Generic Name	Brand Name	Total Daily Dose (mg/kg)[a,b]		Half-Life in Adults (hr)		Therapeutic (Peak) Level[c,d] (mcg/mL)	Recommended Trough Level[e,f] (mcg/mL)
		Adults	Children	Normal	Anuric		
Amikacin	Amikin	15	15	2–3	24–60	15–30	Less than 5–10
Gentamicin	Generic only	3–5[g]	6–7.5[g]	2	24–60	4–10[h]	Less than 1–2[i]
Tobramycin	Generic only	3–6	6–7.5	2–2.5	24–60	4–10	Less than 1–2[i]

[a]The total daily dose may be administered as one large dose each day, or as two or three divided doses given at equally spaced intervals around-the-clock.
[b]Because of interpatient variability, standard doses cannot be relied upon to produce appropriate serum drug levels, and hence dosage should be adjusted on the basis of serum drug measurements.
[c]Measured 30 minutes after IM injection or after completing a 30-minute IV infusion.
[d]The peak values presented refer to levels obtained when the total daily dosage is given in *divided* doses, rather than as a single large daily dose.
[e]Measured just before the next dose.
[f]To minimize ototoxicity and nephrotoxicity, drug levels should drop *below* the listed values between doses.
[g]When gentamicin is combined with either vancomycin or a beta-lactam antibiotic to treat certain gram-positive infections, the total daily dose is much lower (e.g., about 1 mg/kg for adults).
[h]These peak values apply when gentamicin is used to treat gram-negative infections, not when gentamicin is combined with vancomycin or a beta-lactam antibiotic to treat gram-positive infections.
[i]For severe infections, the trough may be higher (e.g., less than 2 to 4 mcg/mL).

to 50 times higher than levels in serum. These high levels are responsible for nephrotoxicity (see *Nephrotoxicity*). Aminoglycosides penetrate readily to the perilymph and endolymph of the inner ears and can thereby cause ototoxicity (see *Ototoxicity*). Aminoglycosides can cross the placenta and may be toxic to the fetus.

PATIENT-CENTERED CARE ACROSS THE LIFE SPAN

Aminoglycosides

Life Stage	Patient Care Concerns
Infants	Aminoglycosides are approved to treat bacterial infections in infants younger than 8 days old. Dosing is based on weight and length of gestation.
Children/ adolescents	Aminoglycosides are safe for use against bacterial infections in children and adolescents.
Pregnant women	There is evidence that the use of aminoglycosides in pregnancy can harm the fetus. Aminoglycosides are classified in U.S. Food and Drug Administration Pregnancy Risk Category D.[a]
Breast-feeding women	Gentamicin is probably safe to use during lactation. There is limited information regarding its use.
Older adults	Caution must be used regarding decreased renal function in the older adult.

[a]As of 2020, the FDA will no longer use Pregnancy Risk Categories. Please refer to Chapter 9 for more information.

Elimination. The aminoglycosides are eliminated primarily by the kidneys. These drugs are not metabolized. In patients with normal renal function, half-lives of the aminoglycosides range from 2 to 3 hours. However, because elimination is almost exclusively renal, half-lives increase dramatically in patients with renal impairment. *Accordingly, to avoid serious toxicity, we must reduce dosage size or increase the dosing interval in patients with kidney disease.*

Interpatient Variation. Different patients receiving the same aminoglycoside dosage (in milligrams per kilogram of body weight) can achieve widely different serum levels of drug. This interpatient variation is caused by several factors, including age, percentage of body fat, and pathophysiology (e.g., renal impairment, fever, edema, dehydration). Because of variability among patients, aminoglycoside dosage must be individualized. As dramatic evidence of this need, in one clinical study it was observed that, to produce equivalent serum drug levels, the doses required ranged from as little as 0.5 mg/kg in one patient to a high of 25.8 mg/kg in another—a difference of more than 50-fold.

Adverse Effects

The aminoglycosides can produce serious toxicity, especially to the inner ears and kidneys. The inner ears and kidneys are vulnerable because aminoglycosides become concentrated within cells of these structures.

Ototoxicity. All aminoglycosides can accumulate within the inner ears, causing cellular injury that can impair both hearing and balance. *Hearing impairment* is caused by damage to sensory hair cells in the *cochlea. Disruption of balance* is caused by damage to sensory hair cells of the *vestibular apparatus.*

The risk of ototoxicity is related primarily to excessive *trough levels*[a] of drug—rather than to excessive *peak* levels. When trough levels remain persistently elevated, aminoglycosides are unable to diffuse out of inner ear cells, and hence the cells are exposed to the drug continuously for an extended

[a]The trough serum level is the lowest level between doses. It occurs just before administration of the next dose.

time. It is this prolonged exposure, rather than brief exposure to high levels, that underlies cellular injury. In addition to high trough levels, the risk of ototoxicity is increased by (1) renal impairment (which can cause accumulation of aminoglycosides); (2) concurrent use of ethacrynic acid (a drug that has ototoxic properties of its own); and (3) administering aminoglycosides in excessive doses or for more than 10 days.

Safety Alert

AMINOGLYCOSIDE OTOTOXICITY

Patients on aminoglycoside therapy should be monitored for ototoxicity. The first sign of impending *cochlear* damage is high-pitched tinnitus (ringing in the ears). Ototoxicity is largely *irreversible*. Accordingly, if permanent injury is to be avoided, aminoglycosides should be withdrawn at the first sign of damage (i.e., tinnitus, persistent headache, or both).

As injury to cochlear hair cells proceeds, hearing in the high-frequency range begins to decline. Loss of low-frequency hearing develops with continued drug use. Because the initial decline in high-frequency hearing is subtle, audiometric testing is needed to detect it. The first sign of impending *vestibular* damage is headache, which may last for 1 or 2 days. After that, nausea, unsteadiness, dizziness, and vertigo begin to appear. Patients should be informed about the symptoms of vestibular and cochlear damage and instructed to report them.

The risk of ototoxicity can be minimized in several ways. Dosages should be adjusted so that trough serum drug levels do not exceed recommended values. (Aminoglycosides diffuse out of the endolymph and perilymph during the trough time, thereby decreasing exposure of sensory hair cells.) Special care should be taken to ensure safe trough levels in patients with renal impairment. When possible, aminoglycosides should be used for no more than 10 days. Concurrent use of ethacrynic acid should be avoided.

Nephrotoxicity. Aminoglycosides can injure cells of the proximal renal tubules. These drugs are taken up by tubular cells and achieve high intracellular concentrations. Nephrotoxicity correlates with (1) the *total cumulative dose* of aminoglycosides and (2) *high trough levels*. High *peak levels* do not seem to increase toxicity. Aminoglycoside-induced nephrotoxicity usually manifests as acute tubular necrosis. Prominent symptoms are proteinuria, casts in the urine, production of dilute urine, and elevations in serum creatinine and blood urea nitrogen (BUN). Serum creatinine and BUN should be monitored. The risk of nephrotoxicity is especially high in older adults, in patients with pre-existing kidney disease, and in patients receiving other nephrotoxic drugs (e.g., amphotericin B, cyclosporine). Fortunately, cells of the proximal tubule readily regenerate. As a result, injury to the kidneys usually reverses after aminoglycoside use.[b] The most significant consequence of renal damage is accumulation of aminoglycosides themselves, which can lead to ototoxicity and even more kidney damage.

[b]If interstitial fibrosis or renal tubular necrosis develops, damage to the kidneys may be permanent.

Safety Alert

AMINOGLYCOSIDE-INDUCED NEUROMUSCULAR BLOCKADE

Aminoglycosides can inhibit neuromuscular transmission, causing flaccid paralysis and potentially fatal respiratory depression. Most episodes of neuromuscular blockade have occurred following intraperitoneal or intrapleural instillation of aminoglycosides. However, neuromuscular blockade has also occurred with IV, IM, and oral dosing.

Beneficial Drug Interactions

Penicillins. Penicillins and aminoglycosides are frequently employed in combination to enhance bacterial kill. The combination is effective because penicillins disrupt the cell wall and thereby facilitate access of aminoglycosides to their site of action. Unfortunately, when present in high concentrations, penicillins can inactivate aminoglycosides. Therefore, *penicillins and aminoglycosides should not be mixed together in the same IV solution.* (Inactivation is not likely to occur once the drugs are in the body, because drug concentrations are usually too low for significant chemical interaction.)

Cephalosporins and Vancomycin. Like the penicillins, cephalosporins and vancomycin weaken the bacterial cell wall and can thereby act in concert with aminoglycosides to enhance bacterial kill.

Adverse Drug Interactions

Ototoxic Drugs. The risk of injury to the inner ears is significantly increased by concurrent use of *ethacrynic acid*, a loop diuretic that has ototoxic actions of its own. Combining aminoglycosides with two other loop diuretics—furosemide and bumetanide—appears to cause no more ototoxicity than aminoglycosides alone.

Nephrotoxic Drugs. The risk of renal damage is increased by concurrent therapy with other nephrotoxic agents. Additive nephrotoxicity can occur with *amphotericin B, cephalosporins, polymyxins, vancomycin,* and *cyclosporine,* as well as with *aspirin and other nonsteroidal anti-inflammatory drugs (NSAIDs)*.

Skeletal Muscle Relaxants. Aminoglycosides can intensify neuromuscular blockade induced by pancuronium and other skeletal muscle relaxants. If aminoglycosides are used with these agents, caution must be exercised to avoid respiratory arrest.

Dosing Schedules

Systemic aminoglycosides may be administered as a single large dose each day or as two or three smaller doses. Traditionally, these drugs have been administered in divided doses, given at equally spaced intervals around-the-clock (e.g., every 8 hours). Today, however, it is common to administer the total daily dose all at once, rather than dividing it up. Several studies have shown that once-daily doses are just as effective as divided doses, and probably safer. Because once-daily dosing is both safe and effective and because it's easier and cheaper than giving divided doses, once-daily dosing has become the preferred schedule. Keep in mind, however, that this schedule is

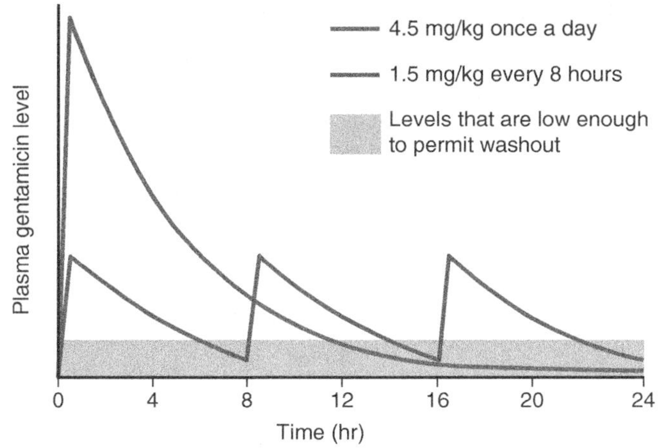

Fig. 87.2 ■ Plasma gentamicin levels produced with once-daily doses versus divided doses.
The curves depict plasma levels of gentamicin produced with (1) a single large dose administered once a day versus (2) the same daily total given as three smaller doses spaced 8 hours apart. Plasma levels with both regimens are high enough to produce good bactericidal effects. The shaded area indicates levels that are low enough to permit washout of the drug from vulnerable cells in the inner ears. Note that, with once-daily dosing, levels are in the washout range for over 12 hours, versus a total of only 6 hours when divided doses are used. As a result, ototoxicity and nephrotoxicity are lower with the once-a-day schedule.

not appropriate for some patients, including neonates, patients who are pregnant, patients undergoing dialysis, and patients with ascites.

How can it be that giving one large daily dose is just as safe and effective as giving divided doses? The answer lies in the hypothetical data for gentamicin levels plotted in Fig. 87.2. As indicated, when we give one large dose (4.5 mg/kg) once a day, we achieve a very high peak plasma level—much higher than when we give the same daily total in the form of three smaller doses (1.5 mg/kg) every 8 hours. Because of this high peak concentration and because aminoglycosides exhibit a postantibiotic effect, bacterial kill using a single daily dose is just as great as when we use divided doses—even though, with once-daily dosing, plasma drug levels are subtherapeutic for a prolonged time between doses. This prolonged period of low drug levels also explains why once-daily dosing is very safe: Because levels are low for a long time, aminoglycosides are able to wash out from vulnerable cells of the ears and kidneys, thereby reducing injury. In contrast, when we use divided doses, the time during which drug levels are low enough to permit washout is quite short, and hence the risk of toxicity is high.

Monitoring Serum Drug Levels

Monitoring serum drug levels provides the best basis for adjusting aminoglycoside dosage. To produce bacterial kill, peak levels must be sufficiently high. To minimize ototoxicity and nephrotoxicity, trough levels must be sufficiently low.

How monitoring is done depends on the dosing schedule employed (i.e., once-daily dosing or the use of divided doses). When once-daily dosing is employed, we need to measure only trough levels. As a rule, there is no need to measure peak levels because when the entire daily dose is given at once, high peak levels are guaranteed. (They're typically 3 to 4 times those achieved with divided doses.) In contrast, when divided doses are employed, we need to measure both the peak and the trough.

When drawing blood samples for aminoglycoside levels, timing is important. Samples for *peak* levels should be taken 30 minutes after giving an IM injection or after completing a 30-minute IV infusion. Sampling for *trough* levels depends on the dosing schedule. For patients receiving *divided doses,* trough samples should be taken just before the next dose. For patients receiving *once-daily doses,* a single sample can be drawn 1 hour before the next dose. The value should be very low, preferably close to zero.

PROPERTIES OF INDIVIDUAL AMINOGLYCOSIDES

Gentamicin

Therapeutic Use

Gentamicin is used primarily to treat serious infections caused by aerobic gram-negative bacilli. Primary targets are *P. aeruginosa* and the Enterobacteriaceae (e.g., *E. coli, Klebsiella, Serratia, P. mirabilis*). In hospitals where resistance is not a problem, gentamicin is often the preferred aminoglycoside for use against these bacteria because gentamicin is cheaper than the alternatives (tobramycin and amikacin). Unfortunately, resistance to gentamicin is increasing, and cross-resistance to tobramycin is common. For infections that are resistant to gentamicin and tobramycin, amikacin is usually effective.

In addition to its use against gram-negative bacilli, gentamicin can be combined with vancomycin, a cephalosporin, or a penicillin to treat serious infections caused by certain gram-positive cocci, namely, *Enterococcus* species, some streptococci, and *Staph. aureus.*

Adverse Effects and Interactions

Like all other aminoglycosides, gentamicin is toxic to the kidneys and inner ears. Caution must be exercised when combining gentamicin with other nephrotoxic or ototoxic drugs. Gentamicin is inactivated by direct chemical interaction with penicillins, and hence these drugs should not be mixed in the same IV solution.

Preparations, Dosage, and Administration

Treatment of Gram-Negative Infections. Gentamicin sulfate is supplied in solution (0.8, 0.9, 1, 1.2, 1.4, 1.6, 10, and 40 mg/mL) and as a powder (60, 80, and 100 mg for reconstitution) for IM and IV administration. The dosage for both routes is the same. For adults, the traditional dosing scheme consists of a loading dose (2 mg/kg) followed by doses of 1 to 1.7 mg/kg every 8 hours—for a total of 3 to approximately 5 mg/kg/day. When once-daily dosing is employed, the dosage is 5 mg/kg every 24 hours; no loading dose is needed. For children, the traditional maintenance dosage is 2 to 2.5 mg/kg every 8 hours. In adults and children with renal impairment, the total daily dosage should be reduced. Duration of treatment is usually 7 to 10 days.

Because of substantial interpatient variation, it is desirable to monitor serum drug levels and to adjust dosage accordingly. Peak levels should range between 4 and 10 mcg/mL (for traditional dosing) or between 16 and 24 mcg/mL (for once-daily dosing). As a rule, the trough should not exceed 2 mcg/mL.

For IV administration, gentamicin should be diluted in either 0.9 sodium chloride injection or 5% dextrose and infused over 30 minutes or longer. The drug should not be mixed with penicillins in the same IV solution.

TABLE 87.2 ▪ Other Aminoglycosides

Drug	Route	Indication	Usual Adult Dose (mg)
Neomycin	PO, topical	Infections of eyes, ears, skin To suppress bowel flora before elective colorectal surgery when used with metronidazole	1000 mg × 3 doses starting the day before surgery
Kanamycin	IM/IV	To suppress bowel flora before elective colorectal surgery	7.5 mg/kg every 12 hr
Streptomycin	IM/IV	Combined with amoxicillin or penicillin for enterococcal endocarditis	500–1000 mg IM every 12 hr
Paromomycin	PO	Intestinal amebiasis	25–35 mg/kg/day divided every 8 hr

Treatment of Gram-Positive Infections. As noted, gentamicin may be combined with vancomycin, a penicillin, or a cephalosporin to treat serious infections caused by *Enterococcus* species, certain streptococci, and *Staph. aureus.* When gentamicin is used in this way, dosages are much lower than when the drug is used against gram-negative infections. For combination therapy, a typical dosage for adults is 1 mg/kg/day, compared with 3 to 5 mg/kg/day when the drug is used by itself.

Tobramycin

Uses, Adverse Effects, and Interactions

Tobramycin is similar to gentamicin with respect to uses, adverse effects, and interactions. The drug is more active than gentamicin against *P. aeruginosa,* but less active against enterococci and *Serratia.* Inhaled tobramycin is used for patients with cystic fibrosis (see Chapter 107). Like all other aminoglycosides, tobramycin can injure the inner ears and kidneys. If possible, concurrent therapy with other ototoxic or nephrotoxic drugs should be avoided. Tobramycin may also cause *C. difficile*–associated diarrhea.

Preparations, Dosage, and Administration

Intravenous and Intramuscular. Tobramycin sulfate is supplied in solution (0.8, 1.2, 10, and 40 mg/mL) and as a 1.2-gm powder (40 mg/mL after reconstitution) for IM and IV administration. Dosages and serum levels are the same as those given for gentamicin. Ideally, dosages should be individualized to produce peak and trough levels within the ranges shown in Table 87.1. In patients with renal impairment, the total daily dosage should be reduced. For IV administration, the drug should be diluted in either 0.9% sodium chloride injection or 5% dextrose and infused over 30 minutes or more. Tobramycin should not be mixed with penicillins in the same IV solution. Duration of treatment is usually 7 to 10 days.

Nebulization. For patients with *cystic fibrosis,* tobramycin [TOBI] is available in solution (300 mg/5 mL) for use in a nebulizer. The dosage is 300 mg twice daily administered in a repeating cycle consisting of 28 days of drug use followed by 28 days off. Cystic fibrosis is discussed in Chapter 107.

Amikacin

Uses, Adverse Effects, and Interactions

Amikacin has two outstanding features: (1) of all the aminoglycosides, amikacin is active against the broadest spectrum of gram-negative bacilli and (2) of all the aminoglycosides, amikacin is the least vulnerable to inactivation by bacterial enzymes. Because most aminoglycoside-inactivating enzymes do not affect amikacin, the incidence of bacterial resistance to this agent is lower than with other major aminoglycosides (gentamicin and tobramycin). In hospitals where resistance to gentamicin and tobramycin is common, amikacin is the preferred agent for initial treatment of infections caused by aerobic gram-negative bacilli. However, in settings where resistance to the other aminoglycosides is infrequent, amikacin should be reserved for infections of proven aminoglycoside resistance because this practice will delay emergence of organisms resistant to amikacin. Like all other aminoglycosides, amikacin is toxic to the kidneys and inner ears. Caution should be exercised if amikacin is used in combination with other ototoxic or nephrotoxic drugs.

Preparations, Dosage, and Administration

Amikacin sulfate is available in solution (500 mg/2 mL and 1 gm/4 mL) for IM and IV administration. For IV use, amikacin should be diluted in 0.9% sodium chloride injection or 5% dextrose; infusion time should be 30 to 60 minutes in adults and 1 to 2 hours in infants. The recommended dosage for adults and children is 15 mg/kg/day administered either (1) as a single daily dose or (2) in equally divided doses given 8 or 12 hours apart. In patients with renal impairment, dosage should be reduced or the dosing interval increased. Dosage adjustments should be based on measurements of serum drug levels. As a rule, duration of treatment should not exceed 10 days.

Other Aminoglycosides

Four other aminoglycosides are still in use, although not as commonly. Please refer to Table 87.2 for these drugs.

KEY POINTS

- Aminoglycosides are antibiotics used primarily against aerobic gram-negative bacilli.
- Aminoglycosides disrupt protein synthesis and cause rapid bacterial death.
- Aminoglycosides are highly polar polycations. As a result, they are not absorbed from the GI tract, do not cross the blood-brain barrier, and are excreted rapidly by the kidneys.
- Aminoglycosides can cause irreversible injury to sensory cells of the inner ears, resulting in hearing loss and disturbed balance.
- The risk of ototoxicity is related primarily to persistently elevated trough drug levels, rather than to excessive peak levels.
- Aminoglycosides are nephrotoxic, but renal injury is usually reversible.

- The risk of nephrotoxicity is related to the total cumulative dose *and* elevated trough levels.
- Because the same aminoglycoside dose can produce very different plasma levels in different patients, monitoring serum levels is common. *Peak* levels must be high enough to cause bacterial kill; *trough* levels must be low enough to minimize toxicity to the inner ears and kidneys.

Please visit **http://evolve.elsevier.com/Lehne** for chapter-specific NCLEX® examination review questions.

Summary of Major Nursing Implications[a]

AMINOGLYCOSIDES

Amikacin
Gentamicin
Kanamycin
Neomycin
Paromomycin
Streptomycin
Tobramycin

Except where noted, the implications here apply to all aminoglycosides.

Preadministration Assessment

Therapeutic Goal

Parenteral Therapy. Treatment of serious infections caused by gram-negative aerobic bacilli. One aminoglycoside—*gentamicin*—is also used (in combination with vancomycin or a beta-lactam antibiotic) to treat serious infections caused by certain gram-positive cocci, namely *Enterococcus* species, some streptococci, and *Staph. aureus.*

Oral Therapy. Suppression of bowel flora before elective colorectal surgery.

Topical Therapy. Treatment of local infections of the eyes, ears, and skin.

Identifying High-Risk Patients

Aminoglycosides must be used with *caution* in patients with renal impairment, pre-existing hearing impairment, and myasthenia gravis, and in patients receiving ototoxic drugs (especially ethacrynic acid), nephrotoxic drugs (e.g., amphotericin B, cephalosporins, vancomycin, cyclosporine, NSAIDs), and neuromuscular blocking agents.

Implementation: Administration

Routes

Intramuscular and Intravenous. Gentamicin, tobramycin, amikacin, kanamycin.

Oral. Neomycin, paromomycin.

Topical. Gentamicin, neomycin, tobramycin.

Dosing Schedule

Parenteral aminoglycosides may be given as one large dose each day, or in two or three divided doses administered at equally spaced intervals around-the-clock.

Administration

Aminoglycosides must be given parenterally (IV, IM) to treat systemic infections. Intravenous infusions should be done slowly (over 30 minutes or more). Do not mix aminoglycosides and penicillins in the same IV solution.

When possible, adjust the dosage on the basis of plasma drug levels. When using divided daily doses, draw blood samples for measuring peak levels 1 hour after IM injection and 30 minutes after completing an IV infusion. When using a single daily dose, measuring peak levels is unnecessary. Draw samples for trough levels just before the next dose (when using divided daily doses) or 1 hour before the next dose (when using a single daily dose).

In patients with renal impairment, the dosage should be reduced or the dosing interval increased.

Ongoing Evaluation and Interventions

Monitoring Summary

Monitor aminoglycoside levels (peaks and troughs), inner ear function (hearing and balance), and kidney function (creatinine clearance, BUN, and urine output).

Minimizing Adverse Effects

Ototoxicity. Aminoglycosides can damage the inner ears, causing irreversible impairment of hearing and balance. Monitor for ototoxicity, using audiometry in high-risk patients. **Instruct patients to report symptoms of ototoxicity (tinnitus, high-frequency hearing loss, persistent headache, nausea, unsteadiness, dizziness, vertigo).** If ototoxicity is detected, aminoglycosides should be withdrawn.

Nephrotoxicity. Aminoglycosides can cause acute tubular necrosis, which is usually reversible. To evaluate renal injury, monitor serum creatinine and BUN. If oliguria or anuria develops, withhold the aminoglycoside and notify the prescriber.

Neuromuscular Blockade. Aminoglycosides can inhibit neuromuscular transmission, causing potentially fatal respiratory depression. Carefully observe patients with myasthenia gravis and patients receiving skeletal muscle relaxants or general anesthetics. Aminoglycoside-induced neuromuscular blockade can be reversed with IV calcium gluconate.

Minimizing Adverse Interactions

Penicillins. Aminoglycosides can be inactivated by high concentrations of penicillins. Never mix penicillins and aminoglycosides in the same IV solution.

Ototoxic and Nephrotoxic Drugs. Exercise caution when using aminoglycosides in combination with other nephrotoxic or ototoxic drugs. Increased nephrotoxicity may occur with *amphotericin B, cephalosporins, polymyxins, vancomycin, cyclosporine,* and *NSAIDs.* Increased ototoxicity may occur with *ethacrynic acid.*

Skeletal Muscle Relaxants. Aminoglycosides can intensify neuromuscular blockade induced by pancuronium and other skeletal muscle relaxants. When aminoglycosides are used concurrently with these agents, exercise caution to avoid respiratory arrest.

[a]Patient education information is highlighted as **blue text.**

CHAPTER

88 Sulfonamides and Trimethoprim

The sulfonamides and trimethoprim are broad-spectrum antimicrobials that have closely related mechanisms: They all disrupt the synthesis of tetrahydrofolic acid, a derivative of folic acid or folate. In approaching these drugs, we begin with the sulfonamides, followed by trimethoprim, and then conclude with trimethoprim/sulfamethoxazole, an important fixed-dose combination.

SULFONAMIDES

Sulfonamides were the first drugs available for the systemic treatment of bacterial infections. After their introduction in the 1930s, their use produced a sharp decline in morbidity and mortality from susceptible infections. With the advent of penicillin and newer antimicrobial drugs, the use of sulfonamides has greatly declined. Nonetheless, the sulfonamides still have important uses, primarily against urinary tract infections (UTIs). With the introduction of trimethoprim/sulfamethoxazole in the 1970s, indications for the sulfonamides expanded.

Basic Pharmacology

Similarities among the sulfonamides are more striking than the differences. Accordingly, rather than focusing on a representative prototype, we will discuss the sulfonamides as a group.

Chemistry

The general structural formula for the sulfonamides is shown in Fig. 88.1. Sulfonamides are structural analogs of *para-aminobenzoic acid* (PABA). The antimicrobial actions of sulfonamides are based on this similarity.

Individual sulfonamides vary greatly with respect to solubility in water. Older sulfonamides had low solubility; therefore, they often crystallized out in the urine, causing injury to the kidneys. The sulfonamides in current use are much more water soluble, and hence the risk for renal damage is low.

Mechanism of Action

Sulfonamides are usually bacteriostatic. Accordingly, adequate host defenses are essential for the elimination of infection.

Sulfonamides suppress bacterial growth by inhibiting synthesis of tetrahydrofolate, a derivative of *folic acid* (folate). Folate is required by all cells to make DNA, RNA, and proteins. The steps in folate synthesis are shown in Fig. 88.2. Sulfonamides block the step in which PABA is combined with pteridine to form dihydropteroic acid. Because of their structural similarity to PABA, sulfonamides act as competitive inhibitors of this reaction.

If all cells require folate, why don't sulfonamides harm us? The answer lies in how bacteria and mammalian cells acquire folic acid. Bacteria are unable to take up folate from their environment, so they must synthesize folic acid from precursors. In contrast to bacteria, mammalian cells do not manufacture their own folate. Instead, they simply take up folic acid obtained from the diet, using a specialized transport system for uptake. Because mammalian cells use preformed folic acid rather than synthesizing it, sulfonamides are harmless to us.

Microbial Resistance

Many bacterial species have developed resistance to sulfonamides. Resistance is especially high among gonococci, meningococci, streptococci, and shigellae. Resistance may be acquired by spontaneous mutation or by transfer of plasmids that code for antibiotic resistance (R factors). Principal resistance mechanisms are (1) reduced sulfonamide uptake, (2) synthesis of PABA in amounts sufficient to overcome sulfonamide-mediated inhibition of dihydropteroate synthetase, and (3) alteration in the structure of dihydropteroate synthetase such that binding and inhibition by sulfonamides is reduced.

Antimicrobial Spectrum

The sulfonamides are active against a broad spectrum of microbes. Susceptible organisms include gram-positive cocci (including methicillin-resistant *Staphylococcus aureus*), gram-negative bacilli, *Listeria monocytogenes*, actinomycetes (e.g., *Nocardia*), chlamydiae (e.g., *Chlamydia trachomatis*), some protozoa (e.g., *Toxoplasma* species, plasmodia, *Isospora belli*), and two fungi, *Pneumocystis jiroveci* (formerly thought to be *Pneumocystis carinii*) and *Paracoccidioides brasiliensis*.

Therapeutic Uses

Although the sulfonamides were once employed widely, their applications are now limited. Two factors explain why: (1) introduction of bactericidal antibiotics that are less toxic than the sulfonamides and (2) development of sulfonamide resistance. Today, UTI is the principal indication for these drugs.

Urinary Tract Infections. Sulfonamides are often preferred drugs for acute UTIs. About 90% of these infections are due to *Escherichia coli,* a bacterium that is usually sulfonamide sensitive. Of the sulfonamides available, *sulfamethoxazole* (in combination with trimethoprim) is generally favored. Sulfamethoxazole has good solubility in urine and achieves effective concentrations within the urinary tract. UTIs are discussed in Chapter 89.

Other Uses. Sulfonamides are useful drugs for nocardiosis (infection with *Nocardia asteroides*), *Listeria,* and infection with *Pneumocystis jiroveci.* In addition, sulfonamides are alternatives to doxycycline and erythromycin for infections caused by *C. trachomatis* (trachoma, inclusion conjunctivitis, urethritis, lymphogranuloma venereum). Sulfonamides are used in conjunction with pyrimethamine to treat two protozoal infections: toxoplasmosis and

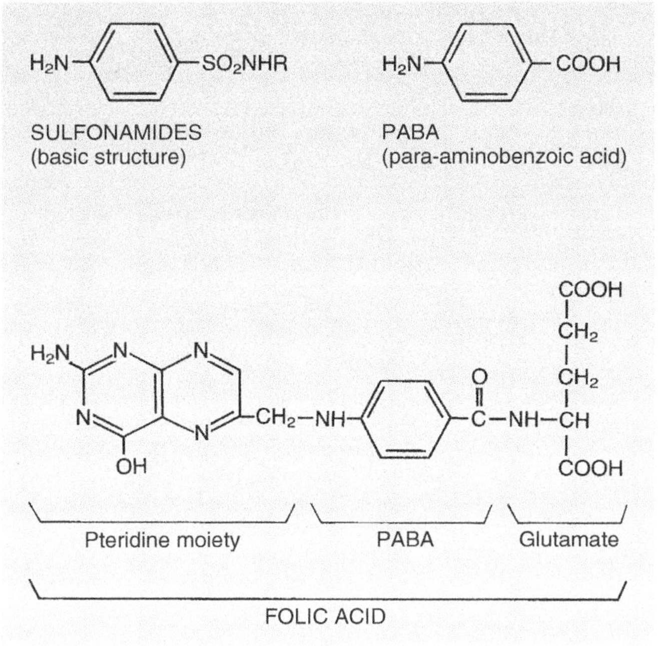

Fig. 88.1 ▪ Structural relationships among sulfonamides, *para*-aminobenzoic acid (PABA), and folic acid.

malaria caused by chloroquine-resistant *Plasmodium falciparum.* Topical sulfonamides are used to treat superficial infections of the eyes and to suppress bacterial colonization in burn patients.

One sulfonamide—sulfasalazine—is used to treat *ulcerative colitis.* However, the drug's benefits in the treatment of this disorder do not result from inhibiting microbial growth. Ulcerative colitis is discussed in Chapter 80.

Pharmacokinetics

Absorption. Sulfonamides are well absorbed after oral administration. When applied topically to the skin or mucous membranes, these drugs may be absorbed in amounts sufficient to cause systemic effects.

Distribution. Sulfonamides are well distributed to all tissues. Concentrations in pleural, peritoneal, ocular, and similar body fluids may be as much as 80% of the concentration in blood. Sulfonamides readily cross the placenta, and levels achieved in the fetus are sufficient to produce antimicrobial effects and toxicity.

Metabolism. Sulfonamides are metabolized in the liver, principally by acetylation. Acetylated derivatives lack antimicrobial activity, but are just as toxic as the parent compounds. Acetylation may decrease sulfonamide solubility, thereby increasing the risk for renal damage from crystal formation.

Excretion. Sulfonamides are excreted primarily by the kidneys. Thus the rate of renal excretion is the principal determinant of their half-lives.

Adverse Effects

Sulfonamides can cause multiple adverse effects. Prominent among these are hypersensitivity reactions, blood dyscrasias, and kernicterus, which occurs in newborns. Renal damage from crystalluria was a problem with older sulfonamides but is less common with the sulfonamides used today.

Hypersensitivity Reactions. Sulfonamides can induce a variety of hypersensitivity reactions, which are seen in about 3% of patients. Mild reactions—rash, drug fever, photosensitivity—are relatively common. To minimize photosensitivity reactions, patients should avoid prolonged exposure to sunlight, wear protective clothing, and apply a sunscreen to exposed skin.

Hypersensitivity reactions are especially frequent with *topical* sulfonamides. As a result, these preparations are no

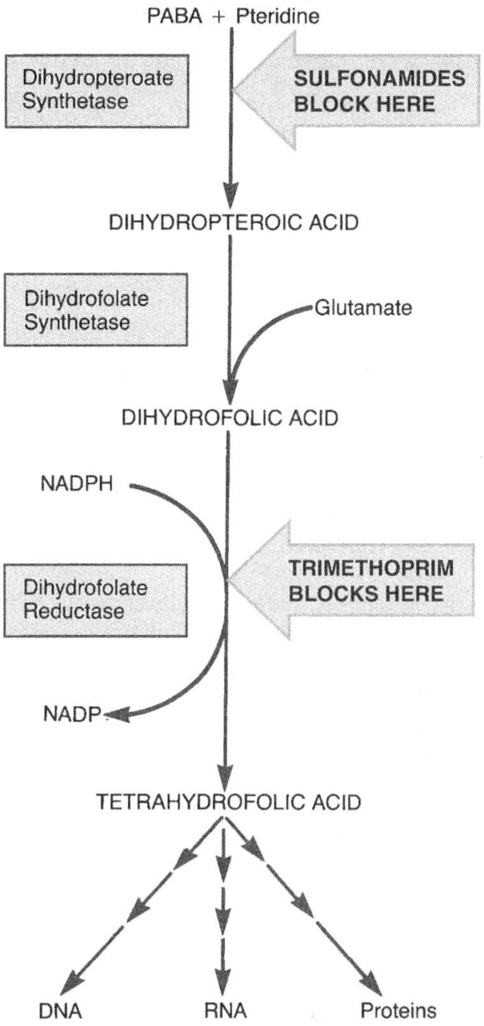

Fig. 88.2 ▪ Sites of action of sulfonamides and trimethoprim. Sulfonamides and trimethoprim inhibit sequential steps in the synthesis of tetrahydrofolic acid (FAH_4). In the absence of FAH_4, bacteria are unable to synthesize DNA, RNA, and proteins.

longer employed routinely. Rather, they are usually reserved for ophthalmic infections, burns, and bacterial vaginosis caused by *Gardnerella vaginalis* and a mixed population of anaerobic bacteria.

The most severe hypersensitivity response to sulfonamides is *Stevens-Johnson syndrome,* a rare reaction with a mortality rate of about 25%. Symptoms include widespread lesions of the skin and mucous membranes, combined with fever, malaise, and toxemia. The reaction is most likely to occur with long-acting sulfonamides, which are now banned in the United States. Short-acting sulfonamides may also induce the syndrome, but the incidence is low. To minimize the risk for severe reactions, sulfonamides should be discontinued immediately if skin rash of any sort is observed. In addition, sulfonamides should not be given to patients with a history of hypersensitivity to chemically related drugs, including thiazide diuretics, loop diuretics, and sulfonylurea-type oral hypoglycemics—although the risk for cross-reactivity with these agents is probably low (see *Drug Interactions*).

Safety Alert

SULFONAMIDES AND G6PD DEFICIENCY

Sulfonamides may cause significant hemolysis if prescribed to patients with G6PD deficiency, an inherited trait.

Hematologic Effects. Sulfonamides can cause *hemolytic anemia* in patients with glucose-6-phosphate dehydrogenase (G6PD) deficiency. This inherited trait is most common among blacks and people of Mediterranean origin. Rarely, hemolysis occurs in the absence of G6PD deficiency. Red cell lysis can produce fever, pallor, and jaundice; patients should be observed for these signs. In addition to hemolytic anemia, sulfonamides can cause agranulocytosis, leukopenia, thrombocytopenia, and, rarely, aplastic anemia. When sulfonamides are used for a long time, periodic blood tests should be obtained.

Kernicterus. Kernicterus is a disorder in newborns caused by the deposition of bilirubin in the brain. Bilirubin is neurotoxic and can cause severe neurologic deficits and even death. Under normal conditions, infants are not vulnerable to kernicterus. Any bilirubin present in their blood is tightly bound to plasma proteins and therefore is not free to enter the central nervous system (CNS). Sulfonamides promote kernicterus by displacing bilirubin from plasma proteins. Because the blood-brain barrier of infants is poorly developed, the newly freed bilirubin has easy access to sites within the brain. *Because of the risk for kernicterus, sulfonamides should not be administered to infants younger than 2 months. In addition, sulfonamides should not be given to pregnant patients after 32 weeks of gestation or to those who are breast-feeding.*

Renal Damage From Crystalluria. Because of their low solubility, older sulfonamides tended to come out of solution in the urine, forming crystalline aggregates in the kidneys, ureters, and bladder. These aggregates cause irritation and obstruction, sometimes resulting in anuria and even death. Renal damage is uncommon with today's sulfonamides, owing to their increased water solubility. To minimize the risk for renal damage, adults should maintain a daily urine output of at least 1200 mL. This can be accomplished by consuming 8 to 10 glasses of water each day. Because the solubility of sulfonamides is highest at elevated pH, alkalinization of the urine (e.g., with sodium bicarbonate) can further decrease the chances of crystalluria.

Drug Interactions

Metabolism-Related Interactions. Sulfonamides can intensify the effects of warfarin, phenytoin, and sulfonylurea-type oral hypoglycemics (e.g., glipizide, glyburide). The principal mechanism is inhibition of hepatic metabolism. When combined with sulfonamides, these drugs may require a reduction in dosage to prevent toxicity.

Cross-Hypersensitivity. There is concern that people who are hypersensitive to sulfonamide antibiotics may be cross-hypersensitive to other drugs that contain a sulfonamide moiety (e.g., thiazide diuretics, loop diuretics, sulfonylurea-type oral hypoglycemics). However, there are no good data to show that such cross-hypersensitivity actually exists. In fact, clinical experience has shown that patients with documented allergy to sulfonamide antibiotics have taken other sulfonamide drugs without incident. Still, until more is known regarding cross-hypersensitivity, it is best to avoid taking chances unless the benefits of giving a drug are greater than the risks.

PATIENT-CENTERED CARE ACROSS THE LIFE SPAN

Sulfonamides and Trimethoprim

Life Stage	Patient Care Concerns
Infants	The use of sulfonamides in infants younger than 2 months can cause kernicterus, a potentially fatal condition.
Children	Sulfonamides and trimethoprim are commonly prescribed for children. There are no age-associated contraindications.
Pregnant women	Systemic sulfonamides are classified in U.S. Food and Drug Administration Pregnancy Risk Category D.[a] They may cause birth defects, especially if taken during the first trimester. If sulfonamides are taken near term, the infant may develop kernicterus. Trimethoprim can exacerbate pregnancy-related folate deficiency. Large doses of trimethoprim have caused fetal malformations in animals in reproduction studies.
Breast-feeding women	Sulfonamides are secreted in breast milk. Breast-feeding women should be warned that breast-feeding an infant younger than 2 months can cause kernicterus. Trimethoprim is excreted in breast milk and may interfere with folic acid utilization by the nursing infant.
Older adults	Older patients are more likely to experience adverse effects, and when experienced, the effects are more likely to be severe. Life-threatening effects, including neutropenia, Stevens-Johnsons syndrome, and toxic epidermal necrolysis, occur more frequently in older adults.

[a]As of 2020, the FDA will no longer use Pregnancy Risk Categories. Please refer to Chapter 9 for more information.

Sulfonamide Preparations

The sulfonamides fall into two major categories: (1) systemic sulfonamides and (2) topical sulfonamides. The systemic agents are used more often.

Systemic Sulfonamides

There are two groups of systemic sulfonamides—short acting and intermediate acting. These differ primarily with regard to dosing interval, which is much shorter for the short-acting drugs.

Sulfamethoxazole. Sulfamethoxazole is the only *intermediate-acting* sulfonamide available. The risk for renal damage from crystalluria can be reduced by maintaining adequate hydration. Sulfamethoxazole is not available for use by itself but *is* available in combination with trimethoprim.

Sulfisoxazole. Sulfisoxazole is a *short-acting* sulfonamide. The drug is just as effective as other sulfonamides. Moreover, because it is highly soluble in water, sulfisoxazole poses a minimal risk for crystalluria. In the United

TABLE 88.1 ▪ Dosages and Administration: Sulfonamides and Trimethoprim

Generic Name	Brand Name	Dosage	Administration
ORAL SULFONAMIDES			
Sulfadiazine	Generic only	Adult: 2–4 gm initially, followed by 2–4 gm every 24 hr, given as 3–6 divided doses Children over 2 months: Initial: 75 mg/kg/day divided into 4–6 doses Maintenance: 150 mg/kg (or 4 gm/m^2) per day (6 gm maximum), given as 4–6 divided doses	May be given with or without food Giving with vitamin C or acidifying drinks such as cranberry juice may increase the risk of crystalluria
Sulfisoxazole (plus erythromycin)	Pediazole	Base dosage on either component: erythromycin 50 mg/kg/day or sulfisoxazole 150 mg/kg/day divided every 6–8 hr	May be taken with or without food
Sulfamethoxazole (plus trimethoprim)	Bactrim, Bactrim DS, Septra, Sulfatrim, Trisulfa 🍁	Adult: 800 mg SMZ/160 mg TMP tablets every 12–24 hr × 10–14 days[a] Children over 2 months (based on trimethoprim [TMP]): 4 mg TMP/kg every 12 hr; may be increased to 20 mg TMP/kg/day	Should be taken with a full glass of water May be taken with or without food
TOPICAL SULFONAMIDES			
Silver sulfadiazine	Silvadene, Thermazene, Flamazine 🍁	Apply a thin layer to affected skin 1–2 times/day	Do not use on the face; may cause a blue-green or gray discoloration
Mafenide	Sulfamylon	Apply a thin layer to affected skin 1–2 times/day	Cream should cover the burned area at all times If dressings are used, only a thin, nonocclusive dressing should be used
Sulfacetamide ophthalmic	Bleph-10, Diosulf 🍁, Sodium Sulamyd 🍁	Solution: 1–2 drops every 2–3 hr Ointment: ½ inch every 3–4 hr	When tapering off, increase time interval between doses
TRIMETHOPRIM			
Trimethoprim	Primsol	Adult: 100 mg every 12 hr or 200 mg every 24 hr × 10 days Children over 2 months: 4–12 mg/kg/day divided into two 12-hr doses	Administer with food or milk

[a]Dosing is for most infections. Dosing varies for specific conditions (e.g., shigellosis and PCP prophylaxis in patients with AIDS).
SMZ, Sulfamethoxazole; *TMP,* trimethoprim.

States, only one formulation is available: an oral suspension that contains sulfisoxazole combined with erythromycin [Pediazole]. This combination product is approved for the treatment of otitis media in children.

Sulfadiazine. Sulfadiazine is a *short-acting* sulfonamide with lower solubility than sulfisoxazole. Accordingly, if renal damage is to be avoided, high urine flow must be maintained. Sulfadiazine crosses the blood-brain barrier with ease, so it is the best sulfonamide for prophylaxis of meningitis (although nonsulfonamide antibiotics—ciprofloxacin, ceftriaxone, rifampin—are preferred). When combined with pyrimethamine, sulfadiazine is useful against toxoplasmosis.

Dosage and administration information for sulfadiazine and other drugs in this chapter is provided in Table 88.1.

Topical Sulfonamides

Topical sulfonamides have been associated with a high incidence of hypersensitivity and are not used routinely. The preparations discussed here have proven utility and a relatively low incidence of hypersensitivity.

Sulfacetamide. Sulfacetamide [Bleph-10] is widely used for superficial infections of the eyes (e.g., conjunctivitis, corneal ulcer). The drug may cause blurred vision, sensitivity to bright light, headache, brow ache, and local irritation. Hypersensitivity is rare, but severe reactions have occurred. Accordingly, sulfacetamide should not be used by patients with a history of severe hypersensitivity to sulfonamides, sulfonylureas, or thiazide or loop diuretics. Sulfacetamide is available in a 10% solution for application to the eyes.

In addition to its ophthalmologic use, topical sulfacetamide is used for dermatologic disorders. The drug is available as a 10% solution in lotions, gels, washes, and shampoos for treating seborrheic dermatitis, acne vulgaris, and bacterial infections of the skin.

Silver Sulfadiazine and Mafenide. These sulfonamides are employed to suppress bacterial colonization in patients with second- and third-degree burns. Mafenide [Sulfamylon] acts by the same mechanism as other sulfonamides. In contrast, the antibacterial effects of silver sulfadiazine are due primarily to the release of free silver—not to the sulfonamide portion of the molecule. Local application of mafenide is frequently painful, but application of silver sulfadiazine is usually pain free. After application, both agents can be absorbed in amounts sufficient to produce systemic effects. Mafenide, but not silver sulfadiazine, is metabolized to a compound that can suppress renal excretion of acid, causing acidosis. Accordingly, patients receiving mafenide should be monitored for acid-base status. If acidosis becomes severe, mafenide should be discontinued for 1 to 2 days. Silver sulfadiazine [Silvadene, Thermazene, SSD Cream, Flamazine 🍁] can cause a blue-green or gray skin discoloration, so facial application should be avoided. A Cochrane review questioned the ability of silver sulfadiazine to promote healing but noted that quality research studies were lacking.

TRIMETHOPRIM

Like the sulfonamides, trimethoprim [Primsol] suppresses synthesis of tetrahydrofolic acid. Trimethoprim is active against a broad spectrum of microbes.

Mechanism of Action

Trimethoprim *inhibits dihydrofolate reductase,* the enzyme that converts dihydrofolic acid to its active form: tetrahydrofolic acid (see Fig. 88.2). Thus, like the sulfonamides, trimethoprim suppresses bacterial synthesis of DNA, RNA, and proteins. Depending on conditions at the site of infection, trimethoprim may be bactericidal or bacteriostatic.

Although mammalian cells also contain dihydrofolate reductase, trimethoprim is selectively toxic to bacteria because bacterial dihydrofolate reductase differs in structure from mammalian dihydrofolate reductase. As a result, trimethoprim inhibits the bacterial enzyme at concentrations about 40,000 times lower than those required to inhibit the mammalian enzyme. This allows suppression of bacterial growth with doses that have essentially no effect on the host.

Microbial Resistance

Bacteria acquire resistance to trimethoprim in three ways: (1) synthesizing increased amounts of dihydrofolate reductase, (2) producing an altered dihydrofolate reductase that has a low affinity for trimethoprim, and (3) reducing cellular permeability to trimethoprim. Resistance has resulted from spontaneous mutation and from transfer of R factors. In the United States bacterial resistance is uncommon.

Antimicrobial Spectrum

Trimethoprim is active against most enteric gram-negative bacilli of clinical importance, including *E. coli, Klebsiella pneumoniae, Proteus mirabilis, Serratia marcescens,* and *Salmonella* and *Shigella* species. The drug is also active against some gram-positive bacilli (e.g., *Corynebacterium diphtheriae, L. monocytogenes*), as well as some pathogenic protozoa (e.g., *Toxoplasma gondii*) and one fungus (*P. jiroveci*).

Therapeutic Uses

Trimethoprim is approved only for initial therapy of acute, uncomplicated UTIs due to susceptible organisms (e.g., *E. coli, P. mirabilis, K. pneumoniae, Enterobacter* species, and coagulase-negative *Staphylococcus* species, including *Staphylococcus saprophyticus*). When combined with sulfamethoxazole, trimethoprim has considerably more applications, as discussed later.

Pharmacokinetics

Trimethoprim is absorbed rapidly and completely from the gastrointestinal (GI) tract. The drug is lipid soluble and therefore undergoes wide distribution to body fluids and tissues. Trimethoprim readily crosses the placenta. Most of an administered dose is excreted unchanged in the urine. Hence, in the presence of renal impairment, the drug's half-life is prolonged. The concentration of trimethoprim achieved in urine is considerably higher than the concentration in blood.

Adverse Effects and Interactions

Trimethoprim is generally well tolerated. The most frequent adverse effects are itching and rash. GI reactions (e.g., epigastric distress, nausea, vomiting, glossitis, stomatitis) occur occasionally.

Hematologic Effects. Because mammalian dihydrofolate reductase is relatively insensitive to trimethoprim, toxicities related to impaired tetrahydrofolate production are rare. These rare effects—*megaloblastic anemia* (a type of anemia with large erythrocytes), *thrombocytopenia,* and *neutropenia*—occur only in individuals with pre-existing folic acid deficiency. Accordingly, caution is needed when administering trimethoprim to patients in whom folate deficiency might be likely (e.g., alcoholics, pregnant women, debilitated patients). If early signs of bone marrow suppression occur (e.g., sore throat, fever, pallor), complete blood counts should be performed. If a significant reduction in blood cell counts is observed, trimethoprim should be discontinued. Administering leucovorin will restore normal hematopoiesis.

Hyperkalemia. Trimethoprim suppresses renal excretion of potassium and can thereby promote hyperkalemia. Patients at greatest risk are those taking high doses, those with renal impairment, and those taking other drugs that can elevate potassium, including angiotensin-converting enzyme (ACE) inhibitors, angiotensin receptor blockers (ARBs), potassium-sparing diuretics, aldosterone antagonists, and potassium supplements. Patients older than 65 years who are taking an ACE inhibitor or ARB are at especially high risk. Risk can be reduced by checking serum potassium, preferably 4 days after starting treatment (hyperkalemia typically develops within 5 days of starting treatment).

TRIMETHOPRIM/SULFAMETHOXAZOLE

Trimethoprim (abbreviated TMP) and sulfamethoxazole (abbreviated SMZ or SMX) are marketed together in a fixed-dose combination product. This combination is a powerful antimicrobial preparation whose components act in concert to inhibit sequential steps in tetrahydrofolic acid synthesis. Brand names for TMP/SMZ are *Bactrim, Septra, Sulfatrim,* and *Trisulfa* ♣. In many countries, the combination is known generically as *co-trimoxazole.*

Mechanism of Action

The antimicrobial effects of TMP/SMZ result from inhibiting consecutive steps in the synthesis of tetrahydrofolic acid. SMZ acts first to inhibit incorporation of PABA into folic acid; TMP then inhibits dihydrofolate reductase, the enzyme that converts dihydrofolic acid into tetrahydrofolate (see Fig. 88.2). As a result, the ability of the target organism to make nucleic acids and proteins is greatly suppressed. By inhibiting two reactions required for synthesis of tetrahydrofolate, TMP and SMZ potentiate each other's effects. That is, the antimicrobial effect of the combination is more powerful than the sum of the effects of TMP alone plus SMZ alone. TMP/SMZ is selectively toxic to microbes because (1) mammalian cells use preformed folic acid and therefore are not affected by SMZ and (2) dihydrofolate reductases of mammalian cells are relatively insensitive to inhibition by TMP.

Microbial Resistance

Resistance to TMP/SMZ is less than to either drug alone. This is logical in that the chances of an organism acquiring resistance to both drugs are less than its chances of developing resistance to just one or the other.

Antimicrobial Spectrum

TMP/SMZ is active against a wide range of gram-positive and gram-negative bacteria. This should be no surprise in that TMP and SMZ by themselves are broad-spectrum antimicrobial drugs. About 80% of urinary tract pathogens are susceptible. Specific bacteria against which TMP/SMZ is consistently effective include *E. coli, P. mirabilis, L. monocytogenes, S. aureus* (including methicillin-resistant isolates), *C. trachomatis, Salmonella typhi, Shigella* species, *Vibrio cholerae, Haemophilus influenzae,* and *Yersinia pestis.* TMP/SMZ is also active against *Nocardia* species, certain protozoa (e.g., *T. gondii*), and two fungi (*P. jiroveci and P. brasiliensis*).

Therapeutic Uses

TMP/SMZ is a preferred or alternative medication for a variety of infectious diseases. The combination is especially valuable for UTIs, otitis media, bronchitis, shigellosis, and pneumonia caused by *P. jiroveci.*

Urinary Tract Infections. TMP/SMZ is indicated for the treatment of uncomplicated UTIs caused by susceptible strains of *E. coli, Klebsiella* and *Enterobacter* species, *P. mirabilis, Proteus vulgaris,* and *Morganella morganii.* The combination is particularly useful for chronic and recurrent infections.

Pneumocystis Pneumonia (PCP). TMP/SMZ is the treatment of choice for PCP, an infection caused by *Pneumocystis jiroveci,* formerly thought to be *Pneumocystis carinii. Pneumocystis jiroveci* is an opportunistic fungus that thrives in immunocompromised hosts (e.g., cancer patients, organ transplant recipients, individuals with AIDS). When given to AIDS patients, TMP/SMZ produces a high incidence of adverse effects.

Gastrointestinal Infections. TMP/SMZ is a drug of choice for infections caused by several gram-negative bacilli, including *Yersinia enterocolitica* and *Aeromonas* species. In addition, the combination is a preferred treatment for shigellosis caused by susceptible strains of *Shigella flexneri* and *Shigella sonnei.*

Other Infections. TMP/SMZ can be used for otitis media and acute exacerbations of chronic bronchitis when these infections are due to susceptible strains of *H. influenzae* or *Streptococcus pneumoniae.* The preparation is also useful against urethritis and pharyngeal infection caused by penicillinase-producing *Neisseria gonorrhoeae.* Other infections that can be treated with TMP/SMZ include whooping cough, nocardiosis, brucellosis, melioidosis, listeriosis, and chancroid.

Pharmacokinetics

Absorption and Distribution. TMP/SMZ may be administered orally or by IV infusion. Both components of TMP/SMZ are well distributed throughout the body. Therapeutic concentrations are achieved in tissues and body fluids (e.g., vaginal secretions, cerebrospinal fluid, pleural effusions, bile, aqueous humor). Both TMP and SMZ readily cross the placenta, and both enter breast milk.

Plasma Drug Levels. Optimal antibacterial effects are produced when the ratio of TMP to SMZ is 1:20. To achieve this ratio in plasma, TMP and SMZ must be administered in a ratio of 1:5. Hence, standard tablets contain 80 mg of TMP and 400 mg of SMZ. Because the plasma half-lives of TMP and SMZ are similar (10 hours for TMP and 11 hours for SMZ), levels of both drugs decline in parallel, and the 1:20 ratio is maintained as the drugs are eliminated.

Elimination. Both TMP and SMZ are excreted primarily by the kidneys. About 70% of urinary SMZ is present as inactive metabolites. In contrast, TMP undergoes little metabolism before excretion. Both agents are concentrated in the urine; therefore, levels of active drug are higher in the urine than in plasma, despite some conversion to inactive products.

Adverse Effects

TMP/SMZ is generally well tolerated; toxicity from routine use is rare. The most common adverse effects are nausea, vomiting, and rash. However, although infrequent, all the serious toxicities associated with sulfonamides alone and trimethoprim alone can occur with TMP/SMZ. Like sulfonamides, the combination can cause the following complications.

- Hypersensitivity reactions (including Stevens-Johnson syndrome)
- Blood dyscrasias (hemolytic anemia, agranulocytosis, leukopenia, thrombocytopenia, aplastic anemia)
- Kernicterus in neonates
- Renal damage

And like trimethoprim, the combination can cause the following:

- Megaloblastic anemia (but only in patients who are folate deficient)
- Hyperkalemia (especially in patients on high doses, in those with renal impairment, and in those taking other drugs that can raise potassium levels)
- Birth defects (especially during the first trimester)

TMP/SMZ may also cause adverse CNS effects (headache, depression, hallucinations). Patients suffering from AIDS are unusually susceptible to TMP/SMZ toxicity. In this group, the incidence of adverse effects (rash, recurrent fever, leukopenia) is about 55%.

Several measures can reduce the incidence and severity of adverse effects. Crystalluria can be avoided by maintaining adequate hydration. Periodic blood tests permit early detection of hematologic disorders. To avoid kernicterus, TMP/SMZ should be withheld from pregnant patients near term, nursing mothers, and infants younger than 2 months. To avoid possible birth defects, TMP/SMZ should be withheld during the first trimester. The risk for megaloblastic anemia can be reduced by withholding sulfonamides from individuals likely to be folate deficient (e.g., debilitated patients, pregnant patients, alcoholics). Hypersensitivity reactions can be minimized by avoiding TMP/SMZ in patients with a history of hypersensitivity to sulfonamides or to chemically related drugs, including thiazide diuretics, loop diuretics, and sulfonylurea-type oral hypoglycemics. Injury from hyperkalemia can be reduced by checking serum potassium and by exercising caution in patients taking other drugs that can elevate potassium.

Drug Interactions

Interactions of TMP/SMZ with other drugs are due primarily to the presence of SMZ. Consequently, like sulfonamides used alone, SMZ in the combination can intensify the effects of warfarin, phenytoin, and sulfonylurea-type oral hypoglycemics (e.g., glipizide). Accordingly, when these drugs are combined with TMP/SMZ, a reduction in their dosage may be needed. TMP/SMZ may also intensify bone marrow suppression in patients receiving methotrexate. As noted, drugs that raise potassium levels can increase the risk for hyperkalemia from TMP.

KEY POINTS

- The sulfonamides and trimethoprim act by inhibiting bacterial synthesis of folic acid.
- Sulfonamides are used primarily for UTIs.
- The principal adverse effects of sulfonamides are (1) hypersensitivity reactions, ranging from photosensitivity to Stevens-Johnson syndrome; (2) hemolytic anemia; (3) kernicterus; and (4) renal damage.
- Trimethoprim is used primarily for UTIs.
- The principal adverse effects of trimethoprim are hyperkalemia and possible birth defects.
- The combination product TMP/SMZ inhibits sequential steps in bacterial folic acid synthesis and therefore is much more powerful than TMP or SMZ alone.
- TMP/SMZ is a preferred drug for UTIs and is the drug of choice for PCP in patients with AIDS and other immunodeficiency states.
- The principal adverse effects of TMP/SMZ are like those caused by sulfonamides alone (i.e., hypersensitivity reactions, hemolytic anemia, kernicterus, and renal injury) and trimethoprim alone (hyperkalemia and birth defects).

Please visit **http://evolve.elsevier.com/Lehne** for chapter-specific NCLEX® examination review questions.

Summary of Major Nursing Implications[a]

SULFONAMIDES (SYSTEMIC)

Sulfadiazine
Sulfamethoxazole (available only in combination with trimethoprim)
Sulfisoxazole (available only in combination with erythromycin)

The nursing implications summarized here apply only to systemic sulfonamides. Implications specific to topical sulfonamides are not summarized.

Preadministration Assessment

Therapeutic Goal

Sulfonamides are used primarily for UTIs caused by *E. coli* and other susceptible organisms. Additional indications for TMP/SMZ include shigellosis and PCP.

Identifying High-Risk Patients

Sulfonamides are *contraindicated* for nursing mothers, pregnant women in the first trimester and near term, and infants younger than 2 months. In addition, sulfonamides are contraindicated for patients with a history of severe hypersensitivity to sulfonamides and chemically related drugs, including thiazide diuretics, loop diuretics, and sulfonylurea-type oral hypoglycemics.

Exercise *caution* in patients with renal impairment. Sulfonamides may cause significant hemolysis if prescribed to patients with G6PD deficiency.

Implementation: Administration

Routes

All currently available systemic sulfonamides are administered orally. Topical formulations are available for dermatologic and ophthalmic use.

Administration

Instruct patients to complete the prescribed course of treatment even though symptoms may abate before the full course is over.

Advise patients to take oral sulfonamides on an empty stomach and with a full glass of water.

Ongoing Evaluation and Interventions

Minimizing Adverse Effects

Hypersensitivity Reactions. Sulfonamides can induce severe hypersensitivity reactions (e.g., Stevens-Johnson syndrome). Do not give sulfonamides to patients with a history of severe hypersensitivity to sulfonamides or to chemically related drugs, including sulfonylureas, thiazide diuretics, and loop diuretics. **Instruct patients to discontinue drug use and notify their provider at the first sign of hypersensitivity (e.g., rash).**

Photosensitivity. Photosensitivity reactions may occur. **Advise patients to avoid prolonged exposure to sunlight, wear protective clothing, and apply a sunscreen to exposed skin.**

Hematologic Effects. Sulfonamides can cause hemolytic anemia and other blood dyscrasias (agranulocytosis, leukopenia, thrombocytopenia, aplastic anemia). Observe patients for signs of hemolysis (fever, pallor, jaundice). When sulfonamide therapy is prolonged, periodic blood cell counts should be made.

Kernicterus. Sulfonamides can cause kernicterus in newborns. Do not give these drugs to pregnant women near term, nursing mothers, or infants younger than 2 months.

Renal Damage. Deposition of sulfonamide crystals can injure the kidneys. To minimize crystalluria, it is important to maintain hydration sufficient to produce a daily urine flow of 1200 mL in adults. Alkalinization of urine (e.g., with sodium bicarbonate) can also help. **Advise outpatients to consume 8 to 10 glasses of water per day.**

Minimizing Adverse Interactions

Metabolism-Related Interactions. Sulfonamides can intensify the effects of *warfarin, phenytoin,* and *sulfonylurea-type oral hypoglycemics* (e.g., glipizide). When combined with sulfonamides, these drugs may require a reduction in dosage.

Summary of Major Nursing Implications[a]—cont'd

Cross-Hypersensitivity. People who are hypersensitive to sulfonamide antibiotics may also be hypersensitive to chemically related drugs—*thiazide diuretics, loop diuretics,* and *sulfonylurea-type oral hypoglycemics*—as well as to *penicillins* and other drugs that induce allergic reactions.

TRIMETHOPRIM

Preadministration Assessment

Therapeutic Goal

Initial treatment of uncomplicated UTIs caused by *E. coli* and other susceptible organisms.

Identifying High-Risk Patients

Trimethoprim is *contraindicated* in patients with folate deficiency. If giving TMP/SMZ, it may be important to assess for megaloblastic anemia. This type of anemia is characterized by erythrocytes that have a larger-than-normal size (elevated mean cell volume [MCV]). When possible, the drug should be avoided during pregnancy and lactation.

Implementation: Administration

Route

Oral.

Dosage and Administration

Instruct patients to complete the prescribed course of treatment, even though symptoms may abate before the full course is over.

Reduce the dosage in patients with renal dysfunction.

Ongoing Evaluation and Interventions

Minimizing Adverse Effects and Interactions

Hematologic Effects. Trimethoprim can cause blood dyscrasias (megaloblastic anemia, thrombocytopenia, neutropenia) by exacerbating pre-existing folic acid deficiency. Avoid trimethoprim when folate deficiency is likely (e.g., in alcoholics, pregnant women, debilitated patients). **Inform patients about early signs of blood disorders (e.g., sore throat, fever, pallor, easy bruising or bleeding), and instruct them to notify the prescriber if these occur.** Complete blood counts should be performed. If a significant reduction in counts is observed, discontinue trimethoprim. Normal hematopoiesis can be restored with leucovorin.

Hyperkalemia. Trimethoprim can cause hyperkalemia, especially in patients taking high doses, patients with renal impairment, and patients taking ACE inhibitors, ARBs, potassium-sparing diuretics, aldosterone antagonists, and potassium supplements. Risk can be reduced by checking serum potassium 4 days after starting treatment and by exercising caution in patients taking other drugs that can elevate potassium.

Use in Pregnancy and Lactation. Trimethoprim should be avoided during pregnancy and lactation. The drug can exacerbate folate deficiency in pregnant women and cause folate deficiency in the nursing infant. In addition, trimethoprim may promote birth defects, especially during the first trimester.

TRIMETHOPRIM/SULFAMETHOXAZOLE

Preadministration Assessment

Therapeutic Goal

Indications include UTIs caused by *E. coli* and other susceptible organisms, shigellosis, and PCP.

Identifying High-Risk Patients

TMP/SMZ is *contraindicated* for nursing mothers, pregnant patients in the first trimester or near term, infants younger than 2 months, patients with folate deficiency (manifested as megaloblastic anemia), and patients with a history of hypersensitivity to sulfonamides and chemically related drugs, including thiazide diuretics, loop diuretics, and sulfonylurea-type oral hypoglycemics.

Implementation: Administration

Routes

Oral; IV (for severe infections).

Dosage Adjustment

In patients with renal impairment (creatinine clearance of 15 to 30 mL/min), decrease dosage by 50%. If creatinine clearance falls below 15 mL/min, discontinue drug use.

Administration

Instruct patients to complete the prescribed course of treatment, even though symptoms may abate before the full course is over.

Ongoing Evaluation and Interventions

Minimizing Adverse Effects

Although serious adverse reactions are rare, TMP/SMZ can cause all the toxicities associated with sulfonamides and trimethoprim used alone. Thus, the nursing implications summarized previously regarding adverse effects of the sulfonamides alone and trimethoprim alone also apply to the combination of TMP/SMZ.

Minimizing Adverse Interactions

TMP/SMZ has the same drug interactions as sulfonamides and trimethoprim used alone. Therefore, the nursing implications summarized previously regarding drug interactions of the sulfonamides alone and trimethoprim alone also apply to the combination of TMP/SMZ.

[a]Patient education information is highlighted as **blue text.**

CHAPTER

89 Drug Therapy for Urinary Tract Infections

Urinary tract infections (UTIs) are the second most common infection encountered today. In the United States, UTIs account for nearly 10 million visits to healthcare providers each year. It is estimated that 50% to 80% of women will have a UTI in their lifetime. Among older women in nursing homes, between 30% and 50% have bacteriuria at any given time. UTIs occur much less frequently in males, but are more likely to be associated with complications (e.g., septicemia, pyelonephritis).

Infections may be limited to bacterial colonization of the urine, or bacteria may invade tissues of the urinary tract. When bacteria invade tissues, characteristic inflammatory syndromes result: *urethritis* (inflammation of the urethra), *cystitis* (inflammation of the urinary bladder), *pyelonephritis* (inflammation of the kidney and its pelvis), and *prostatitis* (inflammation of the prostate).

UTIs may be classified according to their location, in either the lower urinary tract (bladder and urethra) or upper urinary tract (kidney). Within this classification scheme, *cystitis* and *urethritis* are considered *lower tract infections,* whereas *pyelonephritis* is considered an *upper tract infection.*

UTIs are referred to as *complicated* or *uncomplicated. Complicated* UTIs occur in both males and females and are associated with some predisposing factor, such as calculi (stones), prostatic hypertrophy, an indwelling catheter, or an impediment to the flow of urine (e.g., physical obstruction). *Uncomplicated* UTIs occur primarily in women of childbearing age and are not associated with any particular predisposing factor.

Several classes of antibiotics are used to treat UTIs. Among these are sulfonamides, trimethoprim, penicillins, aminoglycosides, cephalosporins, fluoroquinolones, and two urinary tract antiseptics: nitrofurantoin and methenamine. With the exception of the urinary tract antiseptics, these drugs are discussed in other chapters. The basic pharmacology of the urinary tract antiseptics is introduced here.

ORGANISMS THAT CAUSE URINARY TRACT INFECTIONS

The bacteria that cause UTIs differ between community-associated infections and hospital-associated (nosocomial) infections. The majority (more than 80%) of uncomplicated, community-associated UTIs are caused by *Escherichia coli.* Rarely, other gram-negative bacilli—*Klebsiella pneumoniae, Enterobacter, Proteus, Providencia,* and *Pseudomonas*—are the cause. Gram-positive cocci, especially *Staphylococcus saprophyticus,* account for 10% to 15% of community-associated infections. Hospital-associated UTIs are frequently caused by *Klebsiella, Proteus, Enterobacter, Pseudomonas,* staphylococci, and enterococci; *E. coli* is responsible for less than 50% of these infections. Although most UTIs involve only one organism, infection with multiple organisms may occur, especially in patients with an indwelling catheter, renal stones, or chronic renal abscesses.

SPECIFIC URINARY TRACT INFECTIONS AND THEIR TREATMENT

In this section, we consider the characteristics and treatment of the major UTIs: acute cystitis, acute urethral syndrome, acute pyelonephritis, acute bacterial prostatitis, and recurrent UTIs. Most of these can be treated with oral therapy at home. The principal exception is severe pyelonephritis, which requires IV therapy in a hospital. Drugs and dosages for outpatient therapy in nonpregnant women are shown in Table 89.1.

Acute Cystitis

Acute cystitis is a lower UTI that occurs most often in women of childbearing age. Clinical manifestations are dysuria, urinary urgency, urinary frequency, suprapubic discomfort, pyuria, and bacteriuria (more than 100,000 bacteria per milliliter of urine). It is important to note that many women (30% or more) with symptoms of acute cystitis also have asymptomatic upper UTI (subclinical pyelonephritis). In uncomplicated, community-associated cystitis, the principal causative organisms are *E. coli* (80%), *Staph. saprophyticus* (11%), and *Enterococcus faecalis.*

For community-associated infections, three types of oral therapy can be employed: (1) single-dose therapy; (2)

TABLE 89.1 ▪ Regimens for Oral Therapy of Urinary Tract Infections in Nonpregnant Women

Drug	Dose	Duration
ACUTE CYSTITIS		
First-Line Drugs		
Trimethoprim/ sulfamethoxazole	160/800 mg 2 times/day	3 days
Nitrofurantoin (monohydrate/ macrocrystals)	100 mg 2 times/day	5 days
Fosfomycin	3 gm once	1 day
Second-Line Drugs		
Ciprofloxacin	250 mg 2 times/day	3 days
Levofloxacin	250 mg once daily	3 days
ACUTE UNCOMPLICATED PYELONEPHRITIS		
First-Line Drugs		
Trimethoprim/ sulfamethoxazole	160/800 mg 2 times/day	14 days
Ciprofloxacin	500 mg 2 times/day	7–14 days
Levofloxacin	250 mg once daily[a]	5–10 days
Second-Line Drugs		
Amoxicillin (with clavulanic acid)	500 mg 3 times/day	10–14 days
Cephalexin	500 mg 4 times/day	10–14 days
Cefotaxime	1 gm 3 times/day	10–14 days
Ceftriaxone	1 gm once daily	10–14 days
COMPLICATED URINARY TRACT INFECTIONS		
Trimethoprim/ sulfamethoxazole	160/800 mg 2 times/day	7–14 days
Ciprofloxacin	500 mg 2 times/day	5–14 days
Levofloxacin	750 mg once daily	5–14 days
Amoxicillin (with clavulanic acid)	500 mg 3 times/day	7–14 days
Cephalexin	500 mg 3 times/day	7–14 days
PROPHYLAXIS OF RECURRENT INFECTIONS		
Trimethoprim/ sulfamethoxazole	40/200 mg[b] at bedtime 3 times/week	6 months
Trimethoprim	100 mg at bedtime	6 months
Nitrofurantoin	50–100 mg at bedtime	6 months

[a]For infection due to *E. coli* without concurrent bacteremia.
[b]Half of a single-strength tablet.

short-course therapy (3 days); and (3) conventional therapy (5 days). *Single-dose* therapy and *short-course* therapy are recommended only for uncomplicated, community-associated infections in women who are not pregnant and whose symptoms began less than 7 days before starting treatment. As a rule, short-course therapy is more effective than single-dose therapy; hence, it is generally preferred. Advantages of short-course therapy over conventional therapy are lower cost, greater adherence, fewer side effects, and less potential for promoting the emergence of bacterial resistance. *Conventional* therapy is indicated for all patients who do not meet the criteria for short-course therapy. Among these are males, children, pregnant women, and women with suspected upper tract involvement.

Several drugs can be used for treatment (see Table 89.1). For uncomplicated cystitis, trimethoprim/sulfamethoxazole and nitrofurantoin are the drugs of first choice. In communities where resistance to these drugs exceeds 20%, the fluoroquinolones (e.g., ciprofloxacin, norfloxacin) are good alternatives, although resistance to this class of drugs is rising, as well. When adherence is a concern, fosfomycin, which requires just one dose, is a good choice. Beta-lactam antibiotics (e.g., amoxicillin; cephalexin and other cephalosporins) should be avoided because they are less effective than the alternatives and less well tolerated.

Acute Uncomplicated Pyelonephritis

Acute uncomplicated pyelonephritis is an infection of the kidneys. The disorder is common in young children, older adults, and women of childbearing age. Clinical manifestations include fever, chills, severe flank pain, dysuria, urinary frequency, urinary urgency, pyuria, and, usually, bacteriuria (more than 100,000 bacteria per milliliter of urine). *Escherichia coli* is the causative organism in 90% of initial community-associated infections.

Mild to moderate infection can be treated at home with oral antibiotics. Preferred options are trimethoprim/sulfamethoxazole, trimethoprim alone, ciprofloxacin, and levofloxacin. Treatment should last 10 to 14 days.

Severe pyelonephritis requires hospitalization and IV antibiotics. Options include ciprofloxacin, ceftriaxone, ceftazidime, ampicillin plus gentamicin, and ampicillin/sulbactam. Once the infection has been controlled with IV antibiotics, a switch to oral antibiotics should be made, usually within 24 to 48 hours.

Complicated Urinary Tract Infections

Complicated UTIs occur in males and females who have a structural or functional abnormality of the urinary tract that predisposes them to developing infection. Such predisposing factors include prostatic hypertrophy, renal calculi (stones), nephrocalcinosis, renal or bladder tumors, ureteric stricture, or an indwelling urethral catheter. Symptoms of complicated UTIs can range from mild to severe. Some patients even develop systemic illness, manifesting as fever, bacteremia, and septic shock.

The microbiology of complicated UTIs is less predictable than that of uncomplicated UTIs. Although *E. coli* is a common pathogen, it is by no means the only one. Other possibilities include *Klebsiella, Proteus, Pseudomonas, Staphylococcus aureus, Enterobacter* species, *Serratia* species, and even *Candida* species. Accordingly, if treatment is to succeed, we must determine the identity and drug sensitivity of the causative organism. To do so, urine for microbiologic testing should be obtained *before* giving any antibiotics. If symptoms are relatively mild, treatment should wait until test results are available. However, if symptoms are severe, immediate treatment with a broad-spectrum antibiotic can be instituted. Once test results are known, a drug specific to the pathogen can be substituted. Duration of treatment ranges from 7 days (for cystitis) to 14 days (for pyelonephritis or when there is systemic involvement).

Recurrent Urinary Tract Infection

Recurrent UTIs result from *relapse* or from *reinfection. Relapse* is caused by recolonization with the same organism responsible for the initial infection. In contrast, *reinfection* is caused by colonization with a new organism.

Reinfection

More than 80% of recurrent UTIs in females are due to reinfection. These usually involve the lower urinary tract and may be related to sexual intercourse or the use of a contraceptive diaphragm. If reinfections are *infrequent* (only one or two a year), each episode should be treated as a separate infection. Single-dose or short-course therapy can be used.

When reinfections are *frequent* (three or more a year), long-term prophylaxis may be indicated. Prophylaxis can be achieved with low daily doses of several agents, including trimethoprim (100 mg), nitrofurantoin (50 or 100 mg), or trimethoprim/sulfamethoxazole (40 mg/200 mg). Prophylaxis should continue for at least 6 months. During this time, periodic urine cultures should be obtained. If a symptomatic episode occurs, standard therapy for acute cystitis should be given. If reinfection is associated with sexual intercourse, the risk can be decreased by voiding after intercourse and by single-dose prophylaxis (e.g., trimethoprim/sulfamethoxazole [40 mg/200 mg] taken after intercourse).

Relapse

Recolonization with the original infecting organism accounts for 20% of recurrent UTIs. Symptoms that reappear shortly after completion of a course of therapy suggest either a structural abnormality of the urinary tract, involvement of the kidneys, or chronic bacterial prostatitis, the most common cause of recurrent UTI in males. If obstruction of the urinary tract is present, it should be corrected surgically. If renal calculi are the cause, they should be removed.

Drug therapy is progressive. When relapse occurs in women after short-course therapy, a 2-week course of therapy should be tried. If this fails, an additional 4 to 6 weeks of therapy should be tried. If this too is unsuccessful, long-term therapy (6 months) may be indicated. Drugs employed for long-term therapy of relapse include trimethoprim/sulfamethoxazole, norfloxacin, and cephalexin.

Acute Bacterial Prostatitis

Acute bacterial prostatitis is defined as inflammation of the prostate caused by local bacterial infection. Clinical manifestations include high fever, chills, malaise, myalgia, localized pain, and various urinary tract symptoms (dysuria, nocturia, urinary urgency, urinary frequency, urinary retention). In most cases (80%), *E. coli* is the causative organism. Infection is frequently associated with an indwelling urethral catheter, urethral instrumentation, or transurethral prostatic resection. However, in many patients, the infection has no obvious cause.

Bacterial prostatitis responds well to antimicrobial therapy. Because of local inflammation, antibiotics can readily penetrate to the site of infection. (In the absence of inflammation, penetration of the prostate is difficult.) Drug selection and route depend on the causative organism and infection severity. For severe infection with *E. coli,* treatment starts with an IV agent (a fluoroquinolone [e.g., ciprofloxacin]), followed by 6 weeks with an oral agent (either trimethoprim-sulfamethoxazole or a fluoroquinolone). For severe infection with vancomycin-sensitive *E. faecalis,* treatment starts with IV ampicillin/sulbactam, followed by 6 weeks with PO amoxicillin, levofloxacin, or doxycycline.

URINARY TRACT ANTISEPTICS

Two urinary tract antiseptics are available: nitrofurantoin and methenamine. Both are used only for UTIs. These drugs become concentrated in the urine and are active against the common urinary tract pathogens. Neither drug achieves effective antibacterial concentrations in blood or tissues. Nitrofurantoin is a first-choice drug for uncomplicated cystitis.

Nitrofurantoin

Mechanism of Action

Nitrofurantoin [Furadantin, Macrodantin, Macrobid] is a broad-spectrum antibacterial drug, producing bacteriostatic effects at low concentrations and bactericidal effects at high concentrations. Therapeutic levels are achieved only in urine. Nitrofurantoin can cause serious adverse effects.

Nitrofurantoin injures bacteria by damaging DNA. However, to damage DNA, the drug must first undergo enzymatic conversion to a reactive form. Nitrofurantoin is selectively toxic to bacteria because, unlike mammalian cells, bacteria possess relatively high levels of the enzyme needed for drug activation.

Antimicrobial Spectrum

Nitrofurantoin is active against a large number of gram-positive and gram-negative bacteria. Susceptible organisms include staphylococci, streptococci, *Neisseria, Bacteroides,* and most strains of *E. coli.* These sensitive bacteria rarely acquire resistance. Organisms that are frequently resistant include *Proteus, Pseudomonas, Enterobacter,* and *Klebsiella.*

Therapeutic Use

Nitrofurantoin is indicated for acute infections of the lower urinary tract caused by susceptible organisms. In addition, the drug can be used for prophylaxis of recurrent lower UTI. Nitrofurantoin is not recommended for infections of the upper urinary tract.

Pharmacokinetics

Absorption and Distribution. Nitrofurantoin is available in three crystalline forms: *microcrystals, macrocrystals,* and *monohydrate/macrocrystals.* The two macrocrystalline forms are absorbed relatively slowly and produce less GI distress than the microcrystalline form. All formulations produce equivalent therapeutic effects. Nitrofurantoin is distributed to tissues, but only in small amounts. Therapeutic concentrations are achieved only in urine.

Metabolism and Excretion. About two-thirds of each dose undergoes metabolic degradation, primarily in the liver; the remaining one-third is excreted intact in the urine. Nitrofurantoin achieves a urinary concentration of about 200 mcg/mL (compared with less than 2 mcg/mL in plasma). The drug imparts a harmless brown color to the urine; patients should be informed of this effect.

For two reasons, nitrofurantoin should not be administered to individuals with renal impairment (creatinine clearance less than 40 mL/min). First, in the absence of good renal function, levels of nitrofurantoin in the urine are too low to be effective. Second, renal impairment reduces nitrofurantoin excretion, causing plasma levels of the drug to rise, thereby posing a risk of systemic toxicity.

Adverse Effects

Gastrointestinal Effects. The most frequent adverse reactions are GI disturbances (e.g., anorexia, nausea, vomiting, diarrhea). These can be minimized by administering nitrofurantoin with milk or with meals, by reducing the dosage, and by using the macrocrystalline formulations.

Pulmonary Reactions. Nitrofurantoin can induce two types of pulmonary reactions: acute and subacute. Acute reactions, which are most common, manifest as dyspnea, chest pain, chills, fever, cough, and alveolar infiltrates. These symptoms resolve 2 to 4 days after discontinuing the drug. Acute pulmonary responses are thought to be hypersensitivity reactions. Patients with a history of these responses should not receive nitrofurantoin again. Subacute reactions are rare and occur during prolonged treatment. Symptoms (e.g., dyspnea, cough, malaise) usually regress over weeks to months after nitrofurantoin withdrawal. However, in some patients, permanent lung damage may occur.

Hematologic Effects. Nitrofurantoin can cause a variety of hematologic reactions, including agranulocytosis, leukopenia, thrombocytopenia, and megaloblastic anemia. In addition, hemolytic anemia may occur in infants and in patients whose red blood cells have an inherited deficiency in glucose-6-phosphate dehydrogenase. Because of the potential for hemolytic anemia in newborns, nitrofurantoin is contraindicated for pregnant women near term and for infants under the age of 1 month.

Peripheral Neuropathy. Damage to sensory and motor nerves is a serious concern. Demyelinization and nerve degeneration can occur and may be irreversible. Early symptoms include muscle weakness, tingling sensations, and numbness. Patients should be informed about these symptoms and instructed to report them immediately. Neuropathy is most likely in patients with renal impairment and in those taking nitrofurantoin chronically.

Hepatotoxicity. Rarely, nitrofurantoin has caused severe liver injury, manifesting as hepatitis, cholestatic jaundice, and hepatic necrosis. Deaths have occurred. To reduce risk, patients should undergo periodic tests of liver function. Those who develop liver injury should discontinue nitrofurantoin immediately and never use it again.

Birth Defects. Data are conflicted about the use of nitrofurantoin in pregnancy. Results of the *National Birth Defects Prevention Study,* published in 2009, showed an association between nitrofurantoin and four types of birth defects: anophthalmia (the absence of one or both eyes), hypoplastic left heart syndrome (marked hypoplasia of the left ventricle and ascending aorta), atrial septal defects, and cleft lip with cleft palate. However, owing to limitations of the study, a causal relationship has not been established. Because of the possibility of hemolytic anemia, the drug is contraindicated in pregnant patients at term (38 to 42 weeks' gestation). Until more is known, it seems prudent to use alternate antibiotics when needed during any gestational age in pregnancy.

Central Nervous System Effects. Nitrofurantoin can cause multiple central nervous system effects (e.g., headache, vertigo, drowsiness, nystagmus). All are readily reversible.

Preparations, Dosage, and Administration

Preparations. Nitrofurantoin is available in three crystalline forms: microcrystals, macrocrystals, and monohydrate/macrocrystals. *Nitrofurantoin microcrystals* [Furadantin] are supplied as an oral suspension (5 mg/mL). *Nitrofurantoin macrocrystals* [Macrodantin] are supplied in capsules (25, 50, and 100 mg). *Nitrofurantoin monohydrate/macrocrystals* [Macrobid] are supplied in 100-mg extended-release capsules.

Administration. Dosing is oral. GI distress can be reduced by (1) using Macrodantin or Macrobid, rather than Furadantin, and by (2) giving the drug with meals or with milk.

Dosage. For *acute cystitis,* dosage depends on which formulation is used. With the macrocrystals [Macrodantin], the adult dosage is 50 to 100 mg 4 times a day for 7 days. With the monohydrate/macrocrystals [Macrobid], the adult dosage is 100 mg twice a day for 7 days.

For *prophylaxis of recurrent cystitis,* low doses are employed (e.g., 50 to 100 mg at bedtime for adults and 1 mg/kg/day in one or two doses for children).

PATIENT-CENTERED CARE ACROSS THE LIFE SPAN

Drugs for Urinary Tract Infection

Life Stage	Patient Care Concerns
Infants	Ampicillin and gentamicin are recommended to treat infants with UTI. Often, the UTI coincides with other infections or urinary tract abnormalities. The source should be sought immediately.
Children/adolescents	Assess for urinary tract abnormalities in young children with UTI. In sexually active females, assess for birth control methods and complete patient education.
Pregnant women	Urinary tract infections in pregnancy must be treated as complicated infections. Nitrofurantoin is contraindicated in the third trimester of pregnancy. Fluoroquinolones should also be avoided in pregnancy.
Breast-feeding women	Administration of nitrofurantoin to infants younger than 1 month is contraindicated. Trimethoprim/sulfamethoxazole should also be avoided in the early stages of infancy. Fluoroquinolones have been detected in breast milk at low doses. Short-term use during breast-feeding is acceptable. For greatest safety, avoid breast-feeding between 4 and 6 hours after a dose.
Older adults	Nitrofurantoin should be avoided in older adults with decreased renal function.

Methenamine

Mechanism of Action

Methenamine [Hiprex, Urex, Mandelamine ♣] is a prodrug that, under acidic conditions, breaks down into ammonia and formaldehyde. The formaldehyde denatures bacterial proteins, causing cell death. For formaldehyde to be released, the urine must be acidic (pH 5.5 or less). Since formaldehyde is not formed at physiologic systemic pH, methenamine is devoid of systemic toxicity.

Antimicrobial Spectrum

Virtually all bacteria are susceptible to formaldehyde; there is no resistance. Certain bacteria (e.g., *Proteus* species) can elevate urinary pH (by splitting urea to form ammonia). Since formaldehyde is not released under alkaline conditions, infections with urea-splitting organisms are often unresponsive.

Therapeutic Uses

Methenamine is used for *chronic infection of the lower urinary tract.* However, trimethoprim/sulfamethoxazole is preferred. Methenamine is not active against upper tract infections because there is insufficient time for formaldehyde to form as the drug passes through. Methenamine does not prevent UTIs associated with catheters.

Pharmacokinetics

Absorption and Distribution. Methenamine is rapidly absorbed after oral administration. However, approximately 30% of each dose may be converted to ammonia and formaldehyde in the acidic environment of the stomach. This can be minimized by using an enteric-coated formulation. The drug is distributed throughout total body water.

Excretion. Methenamine is eliminated by the kidneys. Within the urinary tract, about 20% of the drug decomposes to form formaldehyde. Levels of formaldehyde are highest in the bladder. Because formaldehyde generation takes place slowly and because transit time through the kidney is brief, formaldehyde levels in the kidney remain subtherapeutic. Ingestion of large volumes of fluid reduces antibacterial effects by diluting methenamine and raising urinary pH. Poorly metabolized acids (e.g., hippuric acid, mandelic acid, ascorbic acid) have been administered with methenamine in attempts to acidify the urine and thereby to increase formaldehyde formation. However, there is no evidence that these acids enhance therapeutic effects.

Adverse Effects and Precautions

Methenamine is relatively safe and generally well tolerated. Gastric distress occurs occasionally, probably from formaldehyde in the stomach. The use of enteric-coated preparations may reduce this effect. Chronic high-dose therapy can cause bladder irritation, manifested as dysuria, frequent voiding, urinary urgency, proteinuria, and hematuria. Since decomposition of methenamine generates ammonia (in addition to formaldehyde), the drug is contraindicated for patients with liver dysfunction. Methenamine salts (methenamine mandelate, methenamine hippurate) should not be used by patients with renal impairment because crystalluria may be caused by precipitating the mandelate or hippurate moiety.

Drug Interactions

Urinary Alkalinizers. Drugs that elevate urinary pH (e.g., acetazolamide, sodium bicarbonate) inhibit formaldehyde production and can thereby reduce the antibacterial effects. Patients taking methenamine should not receive alkalinizing agents.

Sulfonamides. Methenamine should not be combined with sulfonamides because formaldehyde forms an insoluble complex with sulfonamides, thereby posing a risk of urinary tract injury from crystalluria.

Preparations, Dosage, and Administration

Methenamine, in the form of *methenamine hippurate* [Hiprex, Urex], is available in 1-gm tablets for oral dosing. The dosage for children 6 to 12 years is 500 mg to 1 gm twice a day. The dosage for adults and children 12 years and older is 1 gm twice a day.

KEY POINTS

- *Escherichia coli* is the most common cause of uncomplicated, community-associated UTIs.
- Except for pyelonephritis, most UTIs can be treated with oral therapy at home.
- Trimethoprim/sulfamethoxazole is frequently the treatment of choice for oral therapy of UTIs.
- Many drugs, including penicillins, cephalosporins, and fluoroquinolones, may be used for parenteral therapy of UTIs.
- Prophylaxis of recurrent UTI can be achieved with daily low doses of oral antibiotics (e.g., trimethoprim/sulfamethoxazole).
- Nitrofurantoin, a urinary tract antiseptic, is a drug of choice for uncomplicated cystitis.

Please visit **http://evolve.elsevier.com/Lehne** for chapter-specific NCLEX® examination review questions.

CHAPTER

90 Antimycobacterial Agents: Drugs for Tuberculosis, Leprosy, and *Mycobacterium avium* Complex Infection

Our topic for this chapter is infections caused by three species of mycobacteria: *Mycobacterium tuberculosis, Mycobacterium leprae,* and *Mycobacterium avium.* The mycobacteria are slow-growing microbes, and the infections they cause require prolonged treatment. Because therapy is prolonged, drug toxicity and poor patient adherence are significant obstacles to success. In addition, prolonged treatment promotes the emergence of drug-resistant mycobacteria. Because mycobacteria resist decolorizing by the dilute acid used in some staining protocols, these microorganisms are often referred to as *acid-fast bacteria.*

DRUGS FOR TUBERCULOSIS

Tuberculosis (TB) is a global epidemic. In 2015, TB killed 1.8 million people. Only AIDs is responsible for more infectious disease–related deaths. There is good news, however. Through devoted research, development, and financing of programs to control TB, the global TB death rate has decreased by 22% in the past 15 years.

In the United States, there is also positive news. The number of new TB cases in 2016 was down 2.7% from the previous year. Of the total 9,287 cases, more than two-thirds were among immigrants from other countries. This decline indicates that we are on the right road, but we must remain diligent in our work to eradicate TB.

CLINICAL CONSIDERATIONS

Pathogenesis

Tuberculosis is caused by *Mycobacterium tuberculosis,* an organism also known as the tubercle bacillus. Infections may be limited to the lungs or may become disseminated. In most cases, the bacteria are quiescent, and the infected individual has no symptoms. However, when the disease is active, morbidity can be significant.

Primary Infection

Infection with *M. tuberculosis* is transmitted from person to person by inhaling infected sputum that has been aerosolized, usually by coughing or sneezing. As a result, initial infection is in the lungs. When in the lungs, tubercle bacilli are taken up by phagocytic cells (macrophages and neutrophils). Infection can spread from the lungs to other organs through the lymphatic and circulatory systems.

In most cases, immunity to *M. tuberculosis* develops within a few weeks, and the infection is brought under complete control. As a result, most individuals (90%) with primary infection never develop clinical or radiologic evidence of disease. This condition is defined as latent infection. Even though symptoms are absent and the progression of infection is halted, the infected individual is likely to harbor tubercle bacilli lifelong unless drugs are given to eliminate quiescent bacilli. Reactivation, a renewed multiplication of tubercle bacilli, can occur after a period of dormancy. Reactivation occurs in 5% to 10% of patients; hence, in the absence of treatment, there is always some risk that latent infection may become active.

If the immune system fails to control the primary infection, clinical disease (tuberculosis) develops. The result is necrosis and cavitation of lung tissue. Lung tissue may also become caseous (cheese-like in appearance). In the absence of treatment, tissue destruction progresses, and death may result.

Treatment of Active Tuberculosis

The goals of treatment are to eliminate infection and prevent relapse while preventing the development of drug-resistant organisms. To accomplish this, treatment must kill tubercle bacilli that are actively dividing, as well as those that are dormant. Success is indicated by an absence of observable mycobacteria in sputum and by the failure of sputum cultures to yield colonies of *M. tuberculosis.*

Risk for Drug Resistance

Drug resistance is a major impediment to successful therapy. Some infecting bacilli are inherently resistant; others develop resistance over the course of treatment. Some bacilli are resistant to just one drug; others are resistant to multiple drugs. Infection with a resistant organism may be acquired in two ways: (1) through contact with someone who harbors resistant bacteria and (2) through repeated ineffectual courses of therapy.

The emergence of *multidrug-resistant TB* (MDR-TB) and *extensively drug-resistant TB* (XDR-TB) is a recent and ominous development. MDR-TB is defined as TB that is resistant to both isoniazid and rifampin, our two most effective antituberculosis (anti-TB) drugs. XDR-TB, a severe form of MDR-TB, is defined as TB that is resistant not only to isoniazid and rifampin, but also to all fluoroquinolones (e.g., moxifloxacin) and at least one of the injectable second-line anti-TB drugs (amikacin or capreomycin). Infection with multidrug-resistant organisms greatly increases the risk for death, especially among patients with AIDS. In addition, multidrug resistance is expensive: The cost of treating one case of resistant TB is about $150,000, compared with $17,000 per case of nonresistant TB. Fortunately, multidrug resistance is relatively rare in the United States.

The principal cause underlying the emergence of resistance is inadequate drug therapy. Treatment may be too short; dosage may be too low; patient adherence may be erratic; and, perhaps most important, the regimen may contain too few drugs.

The Prime Directive: Always Treat Tuberculosis With Two or More Drugs

Antituberculosis regimens must always contain two or more drugs to which the infecting organism is sensitive. To understand why this is so, we need to begin with five facts:

1. Resistance in *M. tuberculosis* occurs because of spontaneous mutations.
2. Each mutational event confers resistance to only one drug.
3. Mutations conferring resistance to a single drug occur in about 1 of every 100 million (10^8) bacteria.
4. The bacterial burden in active TB is well above 10^8 organisms but far below 10^{16}.
5. *M. tuberculosis* grows slowly, and hence treatment is prolonged.

Now, let's assume that we initiate therapy with a single drug and that all bacteria present are sensitive when we start. What will happen? Over time, at least one of the more than 10^8 bacteria in our patient will mutate to a resistant form. Hence, as we proceed with treatment, we will kill all sensitive bacteria, but the descendants of the newly resistant bacterium will continue to flourish, thereby causing treatment failure. In contrast, if we initiate therapy with *two* drugs, treatment will succeed. Why? Because failure would require that at least one bacterium undergo *two* resistance-conferring mutations, one for each drug. Because two such mutations occur in only 1 of every 10^{16} bacteria (10^{16} is the product of the probabilities for each mutation) and because the total bacterial load is much less than 10^{16}, the chances of the two events occurring in one of the bacteria in our patient are nil.

Not only do drug combinations decrease the risk for resistance, they also can reduce the incidence of relapse. Because some drugs (e.g., isoniazid, rifampin) are especially effective against actively dividing bacilli, whereas other drugs (e.g., pyrazinamide) are most active against intracellular (quiescent) bacilli, by using proper combinations of anti-TB agents, we can increase the chances of killing all tubercle bacilli present, whether they are actively multiplying or dormant. Hence, the risk for relapse is lowered.

In Chapter 83, we noted that treatment with multiple antibiotics broadens the spectrum of antimicrobial coverage, thereby increasing the risk for superinfection. This is not the case with multidrug therapy of TB. The major drugs used against *M. tuberculosis* are *selective* for this organism. As a result, these drugs, even when used in combination, do not kill off beneficial microorganisms and therefore do not create the conditions that lead to superinfection.

Risk for Determining Drug Sensitivity

Because resistance to one or more anti-TB drugs is common and because many patterns of resistance are possible, it is essential that we determine drug sensitivity in isolates from each patient at treatment onset. How do we test drug sensitivity? The traditional method is to culture sputum samples in the presence of antimycobacterial drugs. Unfortunately, the process is slow, usually taking 6 to 16 weeks to complete.

Several rapid tests for drug sensitivity have been developed in recent years; however, these can be very expensive. For this reason, their use is often restricted.

Until test results are available, drug selection must be empiric, based on (1) patterns of drug resistance in the community and (2) the immunocompetence of the patient. However, after test results are available, the regimen should be adjusted accordingly. In the event of treatment failure, sensitivity tests should be repeated.

Treatment Regimens

In August 2016, the American Thoracic Society, the Centers for Disease Control and Prevention, and the Infectious Diseases Society of America published new clinical practice guidelines (ATS/CDC/IDSA Guidelines) for drug-susceptible tuberculosis treatment. (See http://cid.oxfordjournals.org/content/63/7/e147.full.pdf.) These updates, along with current CDC guidelines for other types of TB, inform TB treatment information in this chapter.

Several regimens may be employed for active TB. Drug selection is based largely on the susceptibility of the infecting

PATIENT-CENTERED CARE ACROSS THE LIFE SPAN

First-Line Drugs For Tuberculosis

Life Stage	Patient Care Concerns
Children	Pediatric drug regimens are available for treatment of tuberculosis.
Pregnant women	Rifabutin is FDA Pregnancy Risk Category B.[a] The remaining first-line drugs are Pregnancy Risk Category C; however, there are some differences. The CDC reports that the benefit justifies the risk for isoniazid, rifampin, and pyrazinamide. The CDC does not recommend rifapentine due to insufficient data in pregnant women. Ethambutol is teratogenic; therefore, it should be taken only if benefits to the mother exceed risks to the fetus.
Breast-feeding women	According to the CDC, mothers taking isoniazid and rifampin should be encouraged to breast-feed. For others, it is important to weigh the benefits of breast-feeding against any possible risks to the infant. The amount of drugs excreted in milk is not sufficient for neonatal treatment against TB.
Older adults	No contraindications are identified for these patients; however, older people may be more susceptible to adverse effects. Because of the risk for hepatic and renal injury, adjustments may be needed for patients with underlying liver problems or decreased renal function.

[a]As of 2020, the FDA will no longer use Pregnancy Risk Categories. Please refer to Chapter 9 for more information.

organism and the immunocompetence of the host. Life span considerations are also a factor.

Four drugs—isoniazid, rifampin, pyrazinamide, and ethambutol—are first-line drugs for TB treatment and are used in most treatment regimens. The rifamycin antibiotics rifapentine and rifabutin are also considered first-line drugs. For latent TB infection (LTBI), rifapentine replaces rifampin. For patients taking multiple drugs, rifabutin may be used to replace rifampin to reduce drug interactions, but rifampin or rifapentine should be used over rifabutin when possible.

The ATS/CDC/ISDA Guidelines identify the following as second-line drugs for TB treatment: cycloserine; ethionamide; capreomycin; para-amino salicylic acid (PAS); the aminoglycosides streptomycin, amikacin, kanamycin; and the quinolones levofloxacin and moxifloxacin. Additional antibiotics are sometimes employed when necessary due to severe adverse effects or other complications in therapy.

Therapy is usually initiated with a *four-drug* regimen; isoniazid and rifampin are almost always included. In the event of suspected or proved resistance, more drugs are added; the total may be as high as seven. A sample drug regimen is shown in Table 90.1.

Treatment can be divided into two phases. The goal of the initial phase (induction phase) is to eliminate actively dividing extracellular tubercle bacilli and thereby render the sputum noninfectious. The goal of the second phase (continuation phase) is to eliminate persistent intracellular bacteria.

Drug-Sensitive Tuberculosis. If the infecting organisms are not resistant to isoniazid or rifampin, treatment is relatively simple. The induction phase, which lasts 8 weeks, consists of four drugs: *isoniazid, rifampin, pyrazinamide,* and *ethambutol.* Dosing may be done daily, twice weekly, or thrice weekly. The continuation phase, which lasts 18 weeks, consists of two drugs—*isoniazid* and *rifampin*—administered daily, twice weekly, or thrice weekly. Note that the entire course of treatment is prolonged, making adherence a significant problem.

Isoniazid- or Rifampin-Resistant Tuberculosis. Infections that are resistant to a single drug—isoniazid or rifampin—usually respond well. Isoniazid-resistant TB can be treated for 6 months with three drugs: rifampin, ethambutol, and pyrazinamide. Rifampin-resistant TB can also be treated with three drugs—isoniazid, ethambutol, and pyrazinamide—but the duration is longer: 18 to 24 months, rather than 6 months.

Multidrug-Resistant TB and Extensively Drug-Resistant TB. MDR-TB and XDR-TB are much harder to manage than drug-sensitive TB. Treatment is prolonged (at least 24 months) and must use second- and third-line drugs, which are less effective than the first-line drugs (e.g., isoniazid and rifampin) and are generally more toxic. Initial therapy may consist of five, six, or even seven drugs. Hence, an initial regimen might include (1) isoniazid; (2) rifampin; (3) pyrazinamide; (4) ethambutol; (5) amikacin or capreomycin; (6) levofloxacin; and (7) cycloserine, ethionamide, or *para*-aminosalicylic acid (PAS). As a last resort, infected tissue may be removed by surgery. Even with all of these measures, the prognosis is often poor: Among patients with XDR-TB, between 40% and 60% die. Factors that determine outcome include the extent of drug resistance, infection severity, and the immunocompetence of the host.

Patients With TB Plus HIV Infection. Between 2% and 20% of patients with HIV infection develop active TB. Because of their reduced ability to fight infection, these patients require therapy that is more aggressive than in immunocompetent patients and that should last several months longer.

TABLE 90.1 ▪ Recommended Antituberculosis Regimens[a]

Phase of Treatment	Drug Combination	Treatment Intervals	Minimal Length of Treatment
Intensive	Isoniazid Rifampin Pyrazinamide Ethambutol	7 days/wk for 56 doses *or* 5 days/wk for 40 doses	8 weeks 8 weeks
Continuation	Isoniazid Rifapentine	7 days/wk for 126 doses *or* 5 days/wk for 90 doses	18 weeks 18 weeks

[a]Recommendation of the 2016 ATS/CDC/IDSA Clinical Practice Guidelines for Drug-Susceptible TB. Additional regimens are available online at http://www.cdc.gov/tb/publications/guidelines/pdf/clin-infect-dis.-2016-nahid-cid_ciw376.pdf.

Drug interactions are a big problem, especially for patients taking *rifampin.* Why? Because rifampin, a cornerstone of TB therapy, can accelerate the metabolism of antiretroviral drugs (i.e., drugs used to treat HIV) and can thereby decrease their effects. Specifically, rifampin can decrease the effects of most protease inhibitors and most non-nucleoside reverse transcriptase inhibitors (NNRTIs). Accordingly, it is best to avoid combining rifampin with these agents. Unfortunately, this means that patients will be denied optimal treatment for one of their infections. That is, if they take rifampin to treat TB, they will be unable to take most protease inhibitors or NNRTIs for HIV. Conversely, if they take protease inhibitors and NNRTIs to treat HIV, they will be unable to take rifampin for TB. This dilemma does not have an easy solution.

Like rifampin, *rifabutin* can accelerate metabolism of antiretroviral drugs. However, the degree of acceleration is much less. As a result, many of the antiretroviral drugs that must be avoided in patients taking rifampin can still be used in patients taking rifabutin.

Duration of Treatment

The ideal duration of treatment has not been established. For patients with drug-sensitive TB, the minimal duration is 6 months. For patients with multidrug-resistant infection and for patients with HIV/AIDS, treatment may last as long as 24 months after sputum cultures have become negative.

Promoting Adherence: Directly Observed Therapy Combined With Intermittent Dosing

Patient nonadherence is the most common cause of treatment failure, relapse, and increased drug resistance. Recall that patients with TB must take multiple drugs for 6 months or more, making adherence a very real problem. Directly observed therapy (DOT), combined with intermittent dosing (dosing 2 or 3 times a week rather than every day), helps ensure adherence and thereby increases the chances of success.

In DOT, administration of each dose is done in the presence of an observer, usually a representative of the health department. DOT is now considered the standard of care for TB. In addition to promoting bacterial kill, DOT permits ongoing evaluation of the clinical response and adverse drug effects.

Evaluating Treatment

Three modes are employed to evaluate therapy: bacteriologic evaluation of sputum, clinical evaluation, and chest radiographs.

In patients with positive pretreatment sputum tests, sputum should be evaluated every 2 to 4 weeks initially, and then monthly after sputum cultures become negative. With proper drug selection and good adherence, sputum cultures become negative in more than 90% of patients after 3 months of treatment.

Treatment failures should be evaluated for drug resistance and patient adherence. In the absence of demonstrated drug resistance, treatment with the same regimen should continue, using DOT to ensure that medication is being taken as prescribed. In patients with drug-resistant TB, *two* effective drugs should be added to the regimen.

In patients with negative pretreatment sputum tests, treatment is monitored by chest radiographs and clinical evaluation. In most patients, clinical manifestations (e.g., fever, malaise, anorexia, cough) should decrease markedly within 2 weeks. The radiograph should show improvement within 3 months.

After completing therapy, patients should be examined every 3 to 6 months for signs and symptoms of relapse.

Diagnosis and Treatment of Latent Tuberculosis

In the United States more than 11 million people have LTBI. In the absence of treatment, 5% to 10% of these people will develop active TB. This poses a threat to the infected individual and to the community as well. Accordingly, testing and treatment are clearly desirable—but not for everyone: Because treatment of LTBI is often prolonged and carries a risk for drug toxicity, testing and treatment should be limited to people who really need it.

Who Should Be Tested for Latent Tuberculosis?

Testing should be limited to people who are at high risk for either (1) having acquired the infection recently or (2) progressing from LTBI to active TB. Included in this group are people with HIV infection, people receiving immunosuppressive drugs, recent contacts of patients with TB, and people with high-risk medical conditions, such as diabetes, silicosis, or chronic renal failure. Healthcare workers such as nurses are also at high risk. Candidates for testing are listed in Table 90.2. Routine testing of low-risk individuals is not recommended.

TABLE 90.2 ▪ Candidates for Targeted Tuberculosis Testing

INDIVIDUALS AT HIGH RISK FOR RECENT TUBERCULOSIS INFECTION
Contacts of patients with tuberculosis (TB)
Residents and staff of high-risk congregate settings
• Prisons and jails
• Nursing homes
• Hospitals and other healthcare facilities
• Homeless shelters
• Residential facilities for patients with AIDS
Persons who, in the past 5 years, immigrated from a country where TB is prevalent[a]
Staff of mycobacteriology laboratories
Infants, children, and adolescents exposed to high-risk adults
INDIVIDUALS AT HIGH RISK FOR PROGRESSION FROM LATENT TO ACTIVE TUBERCULOSIS
Infants and children younger than 4 years
People with HIV infection
People who use illegal IV drugs
Patients taking immunosuppressive drugs for 1 month or more
Patients with a chest radiograph indicating fibrotic changes consistent with prior TB
Patients with other high-risk medical conditions, including
• Diabetes mellitus
• Chronic renal failure
• Silicosis
• Leukemia or lymphoma
• Clinical conditions associated with substantial weight loss, including postgastrectomy state, intestinal bypass surgery, chronic peptic ulcer disease, chronic malabsorption syndromes, and carcinomas of the oropharynx and upper gastrointestinal tract that inhibit adequate nutritional intake

[a]The CDC identifies countries in Africa, Asia, the Caribbean, Eastern Europe, Latin America, and Russia as most prevalent.

How Do We Test for Latent Tuberculosis?

There are two types of tests for LTBI: (1) the *tuberculin skin test* (TST), which has been used for more than 100 years; and (2) *interferon gamma release assays* (IGRAs), first approved for American use in 2001.

Tuberculin Skin Test. The TST is performed by giving an intradermal injection of a preparation known as *purified protein derivative* (PPD), an antigen derived from *M. tuberculosis.* If the individual has an intact immune system and has been exposed to *M. tuberculosis* in the past, the PPD will elicit a local immune response. The test is read 48 to 72 hours after the injection. A positive reaction is indicated by a region of induration (hardness) around the injection site.

The decision to treat LTBI is based on two factors: (1) the risk category of the individual and (2) the size of the region of induration produced by the TST (Table 90.3). For individuals at high risk, treatment is recommended if the region of induration is relatively small (5 mm). For individuals at moderate risk, treatment is indicated when the region of induration is larger (10 mm). And for individuals at low risk (who should not be routinely tested), the region must be larger still (15 mm) to justify treatment.

Interferon Gamma Release Assays. The IGRAs are blood tests for TB. These tests are based on the observation that immune white blood cells (WBCs), after exposure to *M. tuberculosis,* will release interferon gamma when exposed to *M. tuberculosis* again. In the IGRAs, WBCs isolated from the patient's blood are exposed to antigens that represent *M. tuberculosis.* If the antigens trigger sufficient release of interferon gamma, the test is considered positive for TB.

How Do We Treat Latent Tuberculosis?

The CDC recommends three treatments for LTBI. Preferred treatments are (1) *isoniazid alone* taken daily for 6 or 9 months (9 months is preferred; 6-month regimen is not recommended for children) and (2) *isoniazid plus rifapentine* taken weekly for 12 weeks. For those who have isoniazid-resistant TB or who cannot take isoniazid for other reasons, the CDC recommends rifampin daily for 4 months. Because dosing with isoniazid plus rifapentine is so simple—just 12 doses instead of 180 or 270—completing the full course is more likely than with isoniazid alone. Dosage guidelines for treating latent tuberculosis are provided in Table 90.4.

Before starting treatment for LTBI, active TB must be ruled out. Why? Because LTBI is treated with just one or two drugs, and hence, if active TB were present, treatment would promote emergence of resistant bacilli. To exclude active disease, the patient should receive a physical examination and chest radiograph; if indicated, bacteriologic studies may also be ordered.

Isoniazid. For more than 30 years, isoniazid has been the standard treatment for LTBI. The drug is effective, relatively safe, and inexpensive. However, isoniazid does have two drawbacks. First, to be effective, isoniazid must be taken for a long time—at least 6 months and preferably 9 months. Second, isoniazid poses a risk for liver damage.

Dosing may be done once daily or twice a week. When twice-weekly dosing is used, each dose should be administered by DOT to ensure adherence. Dosing of this and other drugs used to treat TB is provided in Table 90.5.

Isoniazid Plus Rifapentine. The combination of isoniazid plus rifapentine—taken once a week for only 3 months—is just as effective as isoniazid alone taken once a day for 9 months. Because dosing is done just once a week, isoniazid plus rifapentine *must be administered by DOT.* In contrast, daily isoniazid is self-administered, without oversight by a healthcare provider.

Who can use the new regimen? Isoniazid plus rifapentine is recommended for people 12 years and older, including those with HIV infection who are *not* taking antiretroviral drugs. As a rule, children aged 2 to 11 years should use 9 months of daily isoniazid, and not isoniazid plus rifapentine. Because of its simplicity, the new regimen may be especially useful in correctional institutions, clinics for recent immigrants, and homeless shelters.

Who should *not* use the new regimen? The regimen should not be used by (1) children younger than 2 years because the safety and kinetics of rifapentine are unknown in this group, (2) HIV-infected patients taking antiretroviral drugs, because

TABLE 90.3 ▪ Tuberculin Skin Test Results That Are Considered Positive (Justifying Treatment) in Patients at Low, Moderate, and High Risk for Latent Tuberculosis

Risk Category	Who Is in the Risk Category?	Test Result Considered Positive
High	People who are HIV-positive People who have had recent contacts of patients with tuberculosis (TB) People with fibrotic changes on their chest radiograph consistent with prior TB People taking immunosuppressive drugs for more than 1 month People who have had organ transplants	5 mm of induration
Moderate	Recent immigrants from countries with a high prevalence of TB People who use illegal IV drugs Residents and staff of high-risk congregate settings (e.g., prisons, nursing homes, hospitals, homeless shelters) Mycobacteriology laboratory personnel People with high-risk medical conditions (e.g., diabetes mellitus, chronic renal failure, silicosis, leukemia, lymphoma) Children and adolescents exposed to high-risk adults Children younger than 4 years	10 mm of induration
Low	People with no risk factors for TB	15 mm of induration

TABLE 90.4 ▪ Preparation, Dosage, and Administration of Drugs for Latent Tuberculosis

Drug Class or Drug	Adult Dosage	Pediatric Dosage
Isoniazid	5 mg/kg, up to a maximum of 300 mg, daily for 6 or 9 months *or* 15 mg/kg, up to a maximum of 900 mg, twice a week for 6 or 9 months	10–20 mg/kg, up to a maximum of 300 mg, daily for 9 months *or* 20–40 mg/kg, up to a maximum of 900 mg, twice a week for 9 months
Isoniazid plus rifapentine	Isoniazid: 15 mg/kg rounded up to the nearest 50 or 100 mg (maximum dose 900 mg) Rifapentine (dosage based on body weight): 10.0–14.0 kg, 300 mg 14.1–25.0 kg, 450 mg 25.1–32.0 kg, 600 mg 32.1–49.9 kg, 750 mg >50.0 kg, 900 mg	Isoniazid[a]: 15 mg/kg rounded up to the nearest 50 or 100 mg (maximum dose 900 mg) Rifapentine[a] (dosage based on body weight): 10.0–14.0 kg, 300 mg 14.1–25.0 kg, 450 mg 25.1–32.0 kg, 600 mg 32.1–49.9 kg, 750 mg >50.0 kg, 900 mg
Rifampin	10 mg/kg (up to 600 mg) for 4 months	10–20 mg/kg daily for 6 months[b]

[a]Approved for children age 12 and older; dosing same as adult.
[b]Recommendation of the American Academy of Pediatrics.
Adapted from Centers for Disease Control and Prevention. (2016). *Choosing the most effective LTBI treatment regimen,* available at https://www.cdc.gov/tb/publications/ltbi/treatment.htm#treatmentRegimens.

TABLE 90.5 ▪ Preparation, Dosage, and Administration of Drugs for Active Tuberculosis[a]

Drug	Preparation	Daily	Three Times a Week	Twice a Week	Weekly	Administration
Isoniazid [generic (U.S.), Isotamine ♣]	Tablets: 50, 100, 300 mg Oral syrup: 10 mg/mL Solution for injection: 100 mg/mL	*Adults:* 5 mg/kg/day (usual dose 300 mg) *Children:* 10–15 mg/kg/day	*Adults:* 15 mg/kg (usual dose 900 mg) *Children:* NR	*Adults:* 15 mg/kg (usual dose 900 mg) *Children:* 20–30 mg/kg	*Adults:* 15 mg/kg (usual dose 900 mg) *Children:* NR	Take with or without food
Rifampin [Rifadin]	Capsules: 150, 300 mg IV: 600 mg for reconstitution	*Adults:* 10 mg/kg (usual dose 600 mg) *Children:* 10–20 mg/kg	*Adults:* 10 mg/kg (usual dose 600 mg) *Children:* NR	*Adults:* 10 mg/kg (usual dose 600 mg) *Children:* 10–20 mg/kg	NR	Take 1 hr before meals or 2 hr after meals
Rifapentine [Priftin]	Tablets: 150 mg	*Adults:* only given weekly in continuation phase *Children:* not approved for children <12 years	*Adults:* only given weekly *Children:* NA	*Adults:* only given weekly *Children:* NA	*Adults:* 20 mg/kg *Children:* NA	Take with meals. Tablets may be crushed and added to food
Rifabutin [Mycobutin]	Capsules: 150 mg	*Adults:* 5 mg/kg (usual dose 300 mg) *Children:* 5 mg/kg (suggested)[b]	NR	NR	NR	May take with food to decrease GI upset
Pyrazinamide (generic)	Tablet: 500 mg	*Adults (dosage based on weight):* 40–55 kg, 1000 mg/kg 56–75 kg, 1500 mg/kg 76–90 kg, 2000 mg/kg *Children:* 30–40 mg/kg	*Adults (dosage based on weight):* 40–55 kg, 1500 mg/kg 56–75 kg, 2500 mg/kg 76–90 kg, 3000 mg/kg *Children:* NR	*Adults (dosage based on weight):* 40–55 kg, 2000 mg/kg 56–75 kg, 3000 mg/kg 76–90 kg, 4000 mg/kg *Children:* 50 mg/kg	NR	Take on an empty stomach

TABLE 90.5 ■ Preparation, Dosage, and Administration of Drugs for Active Tuberculosis[a]—cont'd

Drug	Preparation	Daily	Three Times a Week	Twice a Week	Weekly	Administration
Ethambutol [Myambutol]	Tablets: 100, 400 mg	*Adults (dosage based on weight):* 40–55 kg, 800 mg/kg 56–75 kg, 1200 mg/kg 76–90 kg, 1600 mg/kg *Children:* 15–25 mg/kg	*Adults (dosage based on weight):* 40–55 kg, 1200 mg/kg 56–75 kg, 2000 mg/kg 76–90 kg, 2400 mg/kg *Children:* NR	*Adults (dosage based on weight):* 40–55 kg, 2000 mg/kg 56–75 kg, 2800 mg/kg 76–90 kg, 4000 mg/kg *Children:* 50 mg/kg	NR	May take with food if GI upset occurs
Para-aminosalicylate [Paser Granules]	Packets: 4-gm delayed-release granules	*Adults:* 4000 mg 2–3 times/day (usual dose 8–12 gm/day) *Children:* 100 mg/kg given 2–3 times/day (usual total dose 200–300 mg/kg/day)	NR	NR	NR	If stomach upset occurs, PAS may be administered with food
Ethionamide [Trecator]	Tablets: 250 mg	*Adults:* 15–20 mg/kg/day (usual dose 250–500 mg 1–2 times daily) *Children:* 15–20 mg/kg/day total in 1–2 doses	NR	NR	NR	Take with or without food. Taking at bedtime may decrease GI effects
Cycloserine (generic)	Capsules: 250 mg	*Adults:* 10–15 mg/kg/day (usual dose 250–500 mg 1–2 times daily) *Children:* 15–20 mg/kg/day in 1–2 doses	NR	NR	NR	Take with or without food
Capreomycin [Capastat]	Solution for injection: 1-gm vial	*Adults:* 15 mg/kg *Children:* 15–20 mg/kg	*Adults:* 25 mg/kg *Children:* NR	*Adults:* NR *Children:* 25–30 mg/kg	NR	IM or IV administration
Streptomycin (generic)	Solution for injection: 1-gm vial	*Adults:* 15 mg/kg *Children:* 15–20 mg/kg	*Adults:* 25 mg/kg *Children:* NR	*Adults:* NR *Children:* 25–30 mg/kg	NR	IM or IV administration
Amikacin/kanamycin	Solution for injection: 500-mg, 1-gm vials	*Adults:* 15 mg/kg *Children:* 15–20 mg/kg	*Adults:* 25 mg/kg *Children:* NR	*Adults:* NR *Children:* 25–30 mg/kg	NR	IM or IV administration
Levofloxacin [Levaquin]	Tablets: 250, 500, 750 mg Solution for injection: 500-mg vial	*Adults:* 500–1000 mg *Children:* Approximately 15–20 mg/kg (suggested)[b]	NR	NR	NR	Take with or without food
Moxifloxacin [Avelox, Avelox ABC Pack]	Tablets: 400 mg Solution for injection: 400 mg/250 mL	*Adults:* 400 mg *Children:* Approximately 10 mg/kg (suggested)[b]	NR	NR	NR	Take with or without food

[a]Alternate dosing is often used as treatment regimens are commonly individualized.
[b]Optimal dosing unknown; dosing is suggested by experts in the field.
NA, Not approved; *NR,* no recommendation; *PAS, para*-aminosalicylic acid.

drug interactions have not been studied, (3) women who are pregnant or expecting to become pregnant during treatment, because safety in pregnancy is unknown, and (4) patients with LTBI with presumed resistance to isoniazid or rifapentine.

Vaccination Against Tuberculosis

Protection against TB can be conferred by inoculation with bacillus Calmette-Guérin (BCG) vaccine, a freeze-dried preparation of attenuated *Mycobacterium bovis.* In countries where TB is endemic, the World Health Organization recommends BCG vaccination in infancy, to protect children against severe, life-threatening TB infection (i.e., miliary TB and tuberculous meningitis). In the United States, routine vaccination is not done because there is a low risk for infection with *M. tuberculosis* and protection against pulmonary TB in adulthood is variable. Furthermore, vaccination with BCG can produce a false-positive result in the TST, which can't distinguish between antigens from *M. bovis* and antigens from *M. tuberculosis.* (Because the IGRAs are highly specific for antigens from *M. tuberculosis,* vaccination with BCG does not affect the results of these tests.)

PHARMACOLOGY OF INDIVIDUAL ANTITUBERCULOSIS DRUGS

As mentioned earlier, the anti-TB drugs are divided into two groups: first-line drugs and second-line drugs. The first-line drugs are *isoniazid, rifampin, pyrazinamide,* and *ethambutol (with rifapentine or rifabutin sometimes substituting for rifampin).* Of these, isoniazid and rifampin are the most important. The second-line drugs (*levofloxacin, moxifloxacin, amikacin, capreomycin, streptomycin,* para-*aminosalicylic acid, ethionamide,* and *cycloserine)* are generally less effective, more toxic, and more expensive than the primary drugs. Second-line agents are used in combination with the primary drugs to treat disseminated TB and TB caused by organisms resistant to first-line drugs. Adverse effects and routes of administration of the anti-TB drugs are shown in Table 90.6.

TABLE 90.6 ▪ Antituberculosis Drugs: Routes and Major Adverse Effects

Drug	Route	Major Adverse Effects
FIRST-LINE DRUGS		
Isoniazid	PO, IM	Hepatotoxicity, peripheral neuritis
Rifampin	PO, IV	Hepatotoxicity
Rifapentine	PO	Hepatotoxicity
Rifabutin	PO	Hepatotoxicity
Pyrazinamide	PO	Hepatotoxicity, polyarthritis
Ethambutol	PO	Optic neuritis
SECOND-LINE DRUGS		
Fluoroquinolones		
Levofloxacin	PO, IV	GI intolerance
Moxifloxacin	PO, IV	GI intolerance
Injectable Drugs		
Capreomycin	IM	Eighth nerve damage, nephrotoxicity
Amikacin	IM, IV	Eighth nerve damage, nephrotoxicity
Streptomycin	IM	Eighth nerve damage, nephrotoxicity
Others		
Para-aminosalicylic acid	PO	GI intolerance
Ethionamide	PO	GI intolerance, hepatotoxicity
Cycloserine	PO	Psychoses, seizure, rash

GI, Gastrointestinal.

Prototype Drugs

DRUGS FOR TUBERCULOSIS

Isoniazid
Rifampin
Pyrazinamide
Ethambutol

Isoniazid

Isoniazid [generic in United States, Isotamine ♣] is the primary agent for treatment and prophylaxis of TB. This drug has early bactericidal activity and is superior to alternative drugs with regard to efficacy, toxicity, ease of use, patient acceptance, and affordability. With the exception of patients who cannot tolerate the drug, isoniazid should be taken by all individuals infected with isoniazid-sensitive strains of *M. tuberculosis.* Preparations, dosage, and administration for isoniazid and other drugs for treatment of active tuberculosis are provided in Table 90.6.

Antimicrobial Spectrum and Mechanism of Action

Isoniazid is highly selective for *M. tuberculosis.* The drug can kill tubercle bacilli at concentrations 10,000 times lower than those needed to affect gram-positive and gram-negative bacteria. Isoniazid is bactericidal to mycobacteria that are actively dividing but is only bacteriostatic to dormant organisms.

Although the mechanism by which isoniazid acts is not known with certainty, available data suggest that the drug suppresses bacterial growth by inhibiting synthesis of mycolic acid, a component of the mycobacterial cell wall. Because mycolic acid is not produced by other bacteria or by cells of the host, this mechanism would explain why isoniazid is so selective for tubercle bacilli.

Resistance

Tubercle bacilli can develop resistance to isoniazid during treatment. Acquired resistance results from spontaneous mutation. The precise mechanism underlying resistance has not been established. Emergence of resistance can be decreased through multidrug therapy. Organisms resistant to isoniazid are cross-resistant to ethionamide, but not to other drugs used for TB.

Pharmacokinetics

Absorption and Distribution. Isoniazid is administered orally and intramuscularly. Absorption is good with both routes. After absorption, isoniazid is widely distributed to tissues and body fluids, including cerebrospinal fluid (CSF).

Metabolism. Isoniazid is inactivated in the liver, primarily by *acetylation.* The ability to acetylate isoniazid is genetically determined: About 50% of people in the United States are *rapid* acetylators, and the other 50% are *slow* acetylators. The drug's half-life is about 1 hour in rapid acetylators and 3 hours in slow acetylators. It is important to note that differences in rates of acetylation generally have little effect on the *efficacy* of isoniazid, provided patients are taking the drug daily. However, *nonhepatic toxicities* may be more likely in slow acetylators because drug accumulation is greater in these patients.

Excretion. Isoniazid is excreted in the urine, primarily as inactive metabolites. In patients who are slow acetylators and who also have renal insufficiency, the drug may accumulate to toxic levels.

Therapeutic Use

Isoniazid is indicated only for treating active and LTBI. When used for LTBI, the drug is administered alone or combined with rifapentine. When used for active TB, it must be taken in combination with at least one other agent (e.g., rifampin). For patient convenience, isoniazid is available in two fixed-dose combinations: (1) capsules, sold as Rifamate, containing 150 mg of isoniazid and 300 mg of rifampin; and (2) tablets, sold as Rifater, containing 50 mg of isoniazid, 120 mg of rifampin, and 300 mg of pyrazinamide.

Adverse Effects

Hepatotoxicity. Isoniazid can cause hepatocellular injury and multilobular necrosis. Deaths have occurred. Liver injury is thought to result from production of a toxic isoniazid metabolite. The greatest risk factor for liver damage is advancing age: The incidence is extremely low in patients younger than 20 years, 1.2% in those aged 35 to 49 years, 2.3% in those aged 50 to 64 years, and 8% in those older than 65 years. Patients should be informed about signs and symptoms of hepatitis (anorexia, malaise, fatigue, nausea, yellowing of the skin or eyes) and instructed to notify their provider immediately if these develop. Patients should also undergo monthly evaluation for these signs. Some clinicians perform monthly determinations of serum aspartate aminotransferase (AST) activity, because elevation of AST activity is indicative of liver injury. However, because AST levels may rise and then return to normal, despite continued isoniazid use, increases in AST may not be predictive of clinical hepatitis. It is recommended that isoniazid be withdrawn if signs of hepatitis develop or if AST activity exceeds 3 to 5 times the pretreatment baseline. Caution should be exercised when giving isoniazid to alcoholics and individuals with pre-existing disorders of the liver.

Peripheral Neuropathy. Dose-related peripheral neuropathy is the most common adverse event. Principal symptoms are symmetric paresthesias (tingling, numbness, burning, pain) of the hands and feet. Clumsiness, unsteadiness, and muscle ache may develop. Peripheral neuropathy results from isoniazid-induced deficiency in pyridoxine (vitamin B_6). Prophylactic use of pyridoxine at 25 to 50 mg/day can decrease the risk of acquiring peripheral neuropathy. Preventive supplementation is especially important for at-risk people with diabetes or with high alcohol intake. If peripheral neuropathy develops, it can be reversed by administering pyridoxine; however, higher doses are required (typically 100 mg daily).

Other Adverse Effects. Because isoniazid crosses the blood-brain barrier, a variety of *central nervous system (CNS) effects* can occur, including optic neuritis, seizures, dizziness, ataxia, and psychologic disturbances (depression, agitation, impairment of memory, hallucinations, toxic psychosis). *Gastrointestinal (GI) distress, dry mouth,* and *urinary retention* occur on occasion. *Allergy* to isoniazid can produce fever and rashes. Antinuclear antibodies develop in 20% of patients taking this drug.

> **Safety Alert**
>
> **ANTITUBERCULAR DRUGS**
>
> Drugs used to treat tuberculosis may cause severe liver injury. Fatalities have been reported. Nurses should routinely monitor for signs and symptoms of liver damage.

Drug Interactions

Interactions From Inhibiting Drug Metabolism. Isoniazid is a strong inhibitor of three cytochrome P450 isoenzymes, namely CYP2C9, CYP2C19, and CYP2E1. By inhibiting these isoenzymes, isoniazid can raise levels of other drugs that are metabolized by these isoenzymes, including phenytoin, carbamazepine, diazepam, and triazolam. Phenytoin is of particular concern. Patients should be monitored for evidence of phenytoin excess such as ataxia and incoordination. Plasma levels of phenytoin should be monitored, and phenytoin dosage should be reduced as appropriate. Dosage of isoniazid should not be changed.

Alcohol, Rifampin, Rifapentine, Rifabutin, and Pyrazinamide. Daily ingestion of alcohol or concurrent therapy with rifampin, rifapentine, rifabutin, or pyrazinamide increases the risk for hepatotoxicity. Patients should be encouraged to reduce or eliminate alcohol intake.

Rifampin

Rifampin [Rifadin] equals isoniazid in importance as an anti-TB drug. Before the appearance of resistant tubercle bacilli, the combination of rifampin plus isoniazid was the most frequently prescribed regimen for uncomplicated pulmonary TB.

Antimicrobial Spectrum

Rifampin is a broad-spectrum antibiotic. The drug is active against most gram-positive bacteria as well as many gram-negative bacteria. The drug is bactericidal to *M. tuberculosis* and *Mycobacterium leprae.* Other bacteria that are highly sensitive include *Neisseria meningitidis, Haemophilus influenzae, Staphylococcus aureus,* and *Legionella* species.

Mechanism of Action and Bacterial Resistance

Rifampin inhibits bacterial DNA-dependent RNA polymerase; it thereby suppresses RNA synthesis and, consequently, protein synthesis. The drug is lipid soluble, which enables it to easily access intracellular bacteria. The results are bactericidal. Because mammalian RNA polymerases are not affected, rifampin is selectively toxic to microbes. Bacterial resistance to rifampin results from production of an altered form of RNA polymerase.

Pharmacokinetics

Absorption and Distribution. Rifampin is well absorbed if taken on an empty stomach. However, if dosing is done with or shortly after a meal, both the rate and extent of absorption can be significantly lowered. Rifampin is distributed widely to tissues and body fluids; however, CSF distribution is only 10% to 20% of that in the systemic circulation.

Elimination. Rifampin is eliminated primarily by hepatic metabolism. Only about 20% of the drug leaves in the urine. Rifampin induces hepatic drug-metabolizing enzymes, including those responsible for its own inactivation. As a result, the rate at which rifampin is metabolized increases over the first weeks of therapy, causing the half-life of the drug to decrease—from an initial value of about 4 hours down to 2 hours at the end of 2 weeks.

Therapeutic Use

Tuberculosis. Rifampin is one of our most effective anti-TB drugs. This agent is bactericidal to tubercle bacilli at extracellular and intracellular sites. Rifampin is a drug of choice for treating pulmonary TB and disseminated disease. Because resistance can develop rapidly when rifampin is employed alone, the drug is always given in combination with at least one other anti-TB agent. Despite the capacity of rifampin to produce a variety of adverse effects, toxicity rarely requires the discontinuation of treatment.

Leprosy. Rifampin is bactericidal to *M. leprae* and has become an important agent for treating leprosy (see later under *Drugs for Leprosy [Hansen's Disease]*).

Meningococcus Carriers. Rifampin is highly active against *N. meningitidis* and is indicated for short-term therapy to eliminate this bacterium from the nasopharynx of asymptomatic carriers. Because resistant organisms emerge rapidly, rifampin should not be used against active meningococcal disease.

Adverse Effects

Rifampin is generally well tolerated. When employed at recommended dosages, the drug rarely causes significant toxicity.

Hepatotoxicity. Rifampin is toxic to the liver, posing a risk for jaundice and even hepatitis. Asymptomatic elevation of liver enzymes occurs in about 14% of patients. However, the incidence of overt hepatitis is less than 1%. Hepatotoxicity is most likely in people who abuse alcohol and in patients with pre-existing liver disease. These individuals should be monitored closely for signs of liver dysfunction. Tests of liver function (serum aminotransferase levels) should be made before treatment and every 2 to 4 weeks thereafter. Patients should be informed about signs of hepatitis (jaundice, anorexia, malaise, fatigue, nausea) and instructed to notify the prescriber if they develop.

Discoloration of Body Fluids. Rifampin frequently imparts a red-orange color to urine, sweat, saliva, and tears. Patients should be informed of this harmless effect. Permanent staining of soft contact lenses has occurred on occasion, and hence the patient should consult an ophthalmologist regarding contact lens use.

Other Adverse Effects. Gastrointestinal disturbances (anorexia, nausea, abdominal discomfort) and *cutaneous reactions* (flushing, itching, rash) occur occasionally. Rarely, intermittent high-dose therapy has produced a *flu-like syndrome*, characterized by fever, chills, muscle aches, headache, and dizziness. This reaction appears to have an immunologic basis. In some patients, high-dose therapy has been associated with *shortness of breath, hemolytic anemia, shock,* and *acute renal failure.*

Drug Interactions

Accelerated Metabolism of Other Drugs. Rifampin is a powerful inducer of CYP1A2, CYP2A6, CYP2B6, CYP2C19, CYP2C8, CYP2C9, and CYP3A4 cytochrome P450 isoenzymes. As a result, it can hasten the metabolism of many drugs, thereby reducing their effects. This interaction is of special concern with *oral contraceptives, warfarin* (an anticoagulant), and certain *protease inhibitors* and *NNRTIs* used for HIV infection. Women taking oral contraceptives should consider a nonhormonal form of birth control. The dosage of warfarin may need to be increased.

Isoniazid and Pyrazinamide. Rifampin, isoniazid, and pyrazinamide are all hepatotoxic. Hence, when these drugs are used in combination, as they often are, the risk for liver injury is greater than when they are used alone.

Rifapentine

Rifapentine [Priftin] is a long-acting analog of rifampin. Both drugs have the same mechanism of action, adverse effects, and drug interactions.

Actions and Uses

Rifapentine is indicated only for pulmonary TB. At therapeutic doses, the drug is lethal to *M. tuberculosis.* The mechanism underlying cell kill is inhibition of DNA-dependent RNA polymerase. To minimize emergence of resistance, rifapentine must always be combined with at least one other anti-TB drug.

Pharmacokinetics

Rifapentine is well absorbed from the GI tract, especially in the presence of food. Plasma levels peak 5 to 6 hours after dosing. In the liver, rifapentine undergoes conversion to 25-desacetyl rifapentine, an active metabolite. Excretion is primarily (70%) fecal. Rifapentine and its metabolite have the same half-life—about 13 hours.

Adverse Effects

Rifapentine is well tolerated at recommended doses. Like rifampin, the drug imparts a red-orange color to urine, sweat, saliva, and tears. Permanent staining of contact lenses can occur.

Hepatotoxicity is the principal concern. In clinical trials, serum transaminase levels increased in 5% of patients. However, overt hepatitis occurred in only one patient. Because of the risk for hepatotoxicity, liver function tests (bilirubin, serum transaminases) should be performed at baseline and monthly thereafter. Patients should be informed about signs of hepatitis (jaundice, anorexia, malaise, fatigue, nausea) and instructed to notify the prescriber if these develop.

Drug Interactions

Like rifampin, rifapentine is a powerful inducer of cytochrome P450 drug-metabolizing enzymes. As a result, it can decrease the levels of other drugs. Important among these are *protease inhibitors* and *NNRTIs* (used for HIV infection), *oral contraceptives,* and *warfarin.*

Rifabutin

Actions and Uses

Rifabutin [Mycobutin] is a close chemical relative of rifampin. Like rifampin, rifabutin inhibits mycobacterial DNA-dependent RNA polymerase and thereby suppresses protein synthesis. The drug is approved for the prevention of disseminated *M. avium* complex (MAC) disease in patients with advanced HIV infection (CD4 lymphocyte counts below 200 cells/mm^3). In addition to this approved application, rifabutin is used off-label as an alternative to rifampin to treat TB in patients with HIV infection. Rifabutin is preferred to rifampin in HIV patients because it has less effect on the metabolism of protease inhibitors and NNRTIs.

Pharmacokinetics

Rifabutin is administered orally. Absorption is unaffected by food. Plasma levels peak in 2 to 3 hours. The drug is widely distributed and achieves high concentrations in the lungs. Rifabutin is metabolized in the liver and excreted in the urine, bile, and feces. Its half-life is 45 hours.

Adverse Effects

Rifabutin is generally well tolerated. The most common side effects (affecting less than 5% of patients) are rash, GI disturbances, and neutropenia. Like rifampin, rifabutin can impart a harmless red-orange color to urine, sweat, saliva, and tears; soft contact lenses may be permanently stained. Rifabutin poses a risk for uveitis, and hence should be discontinued if ocular pain or blurred vision develops. Other adverse effects include myositis, hepatitis, arthralgia, chest pain with dyspnea, and a flu-like syndrome.

Drug Interactions

Like rifampin, rifabutin *induces cytochrome P450 isoenzymes,* although less strongly than rifampin does. By increasing enzyme activity, rifabutin can decrease blood levels of other drugs, especially *oral contraceptives* and *delavirdine,* an NNRTI (see Chapter 94). Women using oral contraceptives should be advised to use a nonhormonal method of birth control.

Pyrazinamide

Antimicrobial Activity and Therapeutic Use

Pyrazinamide is bactericidal to *M. tuberculosis.* How it kills bacteria is unknown. Currently, the combination of pyrazinamide with rifampin, isoniazid, and ethambutol is a preferred regimen for initial therapy of active disease caused by drug-sensitive *M. tuberculosis.* In addition, pyrazinamide, in combination with rifampin, may be used for short-course therapy of LTBI, although other regimens are preferred.

Pharmacokinetics

Pyrazinamide is well absorbed after oral administration and undergoes wide distribution to tissues and body fluids. In the liver, the drug is converted to pyrazinoic acid, an active metabolite, and then to 5-hydroxypyrazinoic acid, which is inactive. Excretion is renal, primarily as inactive metabolites.

Adverse Effects and Interactions

Hepatotoxicity. Pyrazinamide is the most hepatotoxic of all the first-line drugs. High-dose therapy has caused hepatitis and, rarely, fatal hepatic necrosis. The earliest manifestations of liver damage are elevations in serum levels of transaminases (AST and alanine aminotransferase [ALT]). Levels of these enzymes should be measured before treatment and every 2 weeks thereafter. Patients should be informed about signs of hepatitis (e.g., malaise, anorexia, nausea, vomiting, jaundice) and instructed to notify the prescriber if they develop. Pyrazinamide should be discontinued if significant injury to the liver occurs. The drug should not be used by patients with pre-existing liver disease.

The risk for liver injury is increased by concurrent therapy with isoniazid or rifampin, both of which are hepatotoxic. Pyrazinamide plus rifampin is contraindicated for patients with active liver disease or a history of isoniazid-induced liver injury, and should be used with caution in patients who are taking hepatotoxic drugs or who drink alcohol in excess.

Nongouty Polyarthralgias. Polyarthralgias (pain in multiple joints) develop in 40% of patients, but only occasionally during the initial phase of treatment. Pain can usually be managed with a nonsteroidal anti-inflammatory drug (NSAID), such as aspirin or ibuprofen. A few patients may need to reduce the dosage of pyrazinamide or discontinue treatment.

Other Adverse Effects. Pyrazinamide and its metabolites can inhibit renal excretion of uric acid, causing *hyperuricemia.* Although usually asymptomatic, pyrazinamide-induced hyperuricemia has (rarely) resulted in *gouty arthritis.* Additional adverse effects include *GI disturbances* (nausea, vomiting, diarrhea), *rash,* and *photosensitivity with associated dermatitis.*

Ethambutol

Antimicrobial Action

Ethambutol [Myambutol, Etibi ♣] is active only against mycobacteria; nearly all strains of *M. tuberculosis* are sensitive. The drug is bacteriostatic, not bactericidal. In most cases, ethambutol is active against tubercle bacilli that are resistant to isoniazid and rifampin. Although we know that ethambutol can suppress incorporation of mycolic acid in the cell wall, the precise mechanism by which it suppresses bacterial growth has not been established.

Therapeutic Use

Ethambutol is an important anti-TB drug. This agent is employed for initial treatment of TB and for treating patients who have received therapy previously. Like other drugs for TB, ethambutol is always employed as part of a multidrug regimen.

Pharmacokinetics

Ethambutol is readily absorbed after oral administration. The drug is widely distributed to most tissues and body fluids. Levels in CSF, however, remain low. Ethambutol undergoes little hepatic metabolism and is excreted primarily in the urine. The half-life is 3 to 4 hours in patients with healthy kidneys, and increases to 8 hours in those with significant renal impairment.

Adverse Effects

Ethambutol is generally well tolerated. The most significant adverse effect is optic neuritis.

Optic Neuritis. Ethambutol can produce dose-related optic neuritis, resulting in blurred vision, constriction of the visual field, and disturbance of color discrimination. The mechanism underlying these effects is unknown. Symptoms usually resolve after discontinuation of treatment. Fortunately, this adverse effect is uncommon; however, for some patients, visual disturbance may persist. Color discrimination and visual acuity should be assessed before treatment and monthly thereafter. Patients should be advised to report any alteration in vision. If ocular toxicity develops, ethambutol should be withdrawn immediately. Because visual changes can be difficult to monitor in pediatric patients, ethambutol is not recommended for children younger than 8 years.

Other Adverse Effects. Ethambutol can produce *allergic reactions* (dermatitis, pruritus), *GI upset,* and *confusion.* The drug inhibits renal excretion of uric acid, causing *asymptomatic hyperuricemia* in about 50% of patients; occasionally, elevation of uric acid levels results in *acute gouty arthritis.* Rare adverse effects include *peripheral neuropathy, renal damage,* and *thrombocytopenia.*

Second-Line Antituberculosis Drugs

The group of second-line anti-TB drugs consists of two fluoroquinolones (levofloxacin and moxifloxacin), three injectable drugs (capreomycin, amikacin, streptomycin), and three other drugs (PAS, ethionamide, and cycloserine). In general, these drugs are less effective, more toxic, and more expensive than the first-line drugs. As a result, their principal indication is TB caused by organisms that have proved resistant to first-line agents. In addition, second-line drugs are used to treat severe pulmonary TB, as well as disseminated (extrapulmonary) infection. The second-line drugs are always employed in conjunction with a major anti-TB drug.

Fluoroquinolones

Levofloxacin [Levaquin] and moxifloxacin [Avelox] are fluoroquinolone antibiotics indicated for a wide variety of bacterial infections (see Chapter 91). Both drugs have good activity against *M. tuberculosis.* As therapy for TB, these drugs are reserved for infection caused by multidrug-resistant organisms. Both drugs are generally well tolerated, although GI disturbances are relatively common. Tendon rupture occurs rarely but may result in permanent damage, especially in patients more than 60 years old. The FDA has issued a black box warning to address this concern.

Injectable Drugs

Capreomycin. Capreomycin [Capastat Sulfate] is a bacteriostatic antibiotic used only for TB resistant to primary agents. Antibacterial effects probably result from inhibiting protein synthesis. The principal toxicity is renal damage, and hence the drug should not be taken by patients with kidney disease. Capreomycin may also cause eighth cranial nerve damage, resulting in hearing loss, tinnitus, and disturbed balance.

Safety Alert

AMIKACIN, STREPTOMYCIN, AND CAPREOMYCIN

Capreomycin and the aminoglycosides amikacin and streptomycin are ototoxic. Vertigo may occur as a result of vestibular injury. Hearing loss may be permanent. These drugs are also nephrotoxic and may cause renal impairment.

Amikacin and Streptomycin. Amikacin [Amikin] and streptomycin (generic only) are aminoglycoside antibiotics with good activity against *M. tuberculosis*. Like other aminoglycosides, these drugs are nephrotoxic and may also damage the eighth cranial nerve. These drugs are not absorbed from the GI tract, and hence administration is parenteral. The pharmacology of these and other aminoglycosides is discussed in Chapter 87.

Other Second-Line Drugs

Para-Aminosalicylic Acid

Actions and Uses. PAS [Paser Granules] is similar in structure and actions to the sulfonamides. Like the sulfonamides, PAS exerts its antibacterial effects by inhibiting synthesis of folic acid. However, in contrast to the sulfonamides, which are broad-spectrum antibiotics, PAS is active only against mycobacteria. In the United States, PAS has been employed primarily as a substitute for ethambutol in pediatric patients. The drug is always used in combination with other anti-TB agents.

PAS loses its effectiveness if exposed to heat. Packets should be stored in a cool location (below 59°F).

Pharmacokinetics. PAS is administered orally, and absorption is good. The drug is distributed widely to most tissues and body fluids, although levels in CSF remain low. PAS undergoes extensive hepatic metabolism. Metabolites and parent drug are excreted in the urine.

Adverse Effects. PAS is poorly tolerated by adults; children accept the drug somewhat better. The most frequent adverse effects are GI disturbances (nausea, vomiting, diarrhea). Because PAS is administered in large doses as a sodium salt, substantial sodium loading may occur. Additional adverse effects are allergic reactions, hepatotoxicity, and goiter.

Ethionamide

Actions and Uses. Ethionamide [Trecator], a relative of isoniazid, is active against mycobacteria, but less so than isoniazid itself. Ethionamide is administered with other anti-TB drugs to treat TB that is resistant to first-line agents. Gastrointestinal disturbances limit patient acceptance. Ethionamide is the least well tolerated of all anti-TB agents, and hence should be used only when there is no alternative.

Pharmacokinetics. Ethionamide is readily absorbed after oral administration. The drug is widely distributed to tissues and body fluids, including the CSF. Ethionamide undergoes extensive metabolism and is excreted in the urine, primarily as metabolites.

Adverse Effects. Gastrointestinal effects (anorexia, nausea, vomiting, diarrhea, metallic taste) occur often; intolerance of these effects frequently leads to discontinuation. Ethionamide is toxic to the liver. Hepatotoxicity is assessed by measuring serum transaminases (AST, ALT) before treatment and periodically thereafter. Additional adverse effects include peripheral neuropathy, CNS effects (convulsions, mental disturbance), and allergic reactions.

Cycloserine

Actions and Uses. Cycloserine (generic) is an antibiotic produced by a species of *Streptomyces*. The drug is bacteriostatic and acts by inhibiting cell wall synthesis. Cycloserine is used against TB resistant to first-line drugs.

Pharmacokinetics. Cycloserine is rapidly absorbed after oral administration. The drug is widely distributed to tissues and body fluids, including the CSF. Elimination is by hepatic metabolism and renal excretion; about 50% of the drug leaves unchanged in the urine. Cycloserine may accumulate to toxic levels in patients with renal impairment.

Adverse Effects. CNS effects occur frequently and can be severe. Possible reactions include anxiety, depression, confusion, hallucinations, paranoia, hyperreflexia, and seizures. Psychotic episodes occur in approximately 10% of patients; symptoms usually subside within 2 weeks after drug withdrawal. Pyridoxine may prevent neurotoxic effects. Other adverse effects include peripheral neuropathy, hepatotoxicity, and folate deficiency. To minimize the risk for adverse effects, serum concentrations of cycloserine should be measured periodically; peak concentrations, measured 2 hours after dosing, should be 25 to 35 mcg/mL.

Bedaquiline

When the FDA granted accelerated approval of bedaquiline [Sirturo] in December 2012, it was heralded as the first unique drug in the anti-TB arsenal to emerge in more than 40 years. The drug appears to work faster and better than all other anti-TB drugs. In addition, bedaquiline does not accelerate the metabolism of other drugs, and hence it can be used in patients taking drugs for HIV. Regardless, it is not among those drugs recommended as first- or second-line drugs in the ATS/CDC/IDSA Guidelines, pending results of additional clinical trials. It also has some serious adverse effects (see Safety Alert) and costs approximately $36,000 for 100 tablets.

> **Safety Alert**
>
> **BEDAQUILINE [SIRTURO]**
>
> Subjects in a bedaquiline clinical trial had an increased mortality rate: 11.4% died compared with 2.5% in the group taking a placebo. Bedaquiline can cause QT prolongation, which places the patient at risk for dangerous ventricular dysrhythmias. Discontinue the drug if QT prolongation exceeds 500 msec.

Bedaquiline is highly effective. In a mouse model of TB, a three-drug regimen consisting of bedaquiline plus rifampin and pyrazinamide was compared with a conventional three-drug regimen consisting of isoniazid plus rifampin and pyrazinamide. The result? After 1 month with the bedaquiline regimen, bacterial load was as low as seen after 2 months with the conventional regimen, indicating accelerated bacterial kill. And after 2 months with the bedaquiline regimen, mycobacteria were cleared entirely from the lungs, an unprecedented outcome. In laboratory tests, bedaquiline was bactericidal to all isolates of *M. tuberculosis* resistant to conventional therapy, including multidrug-resistant strains.

Actions and Uses

This drug has a unique mechanism of action: Bacterial kill results from inhibiting adenosine triphosphate (ATP) synthase, an enzyme required by *M. tuberculosis* to make ATP. No other drug shares this mechanism, which explains why there's no cross-resistance between bedaquiline and conventional drugs. Because humans make ATP by a different pathway, bedaquiline does not interfere with ATP synthesis in humans.

Bedaquiline is approved for multidrug-resistant pulmonary TB in patients at least 18 years of age. It is not approved for treatment of latent, nonpulmonary, or drug-sensitive tuberculosis (i.e., TB that is effectively treated by other drugs). It also should not be used for mycobacterial infections other than TB.

Pharmacokinetics

Bedaquiline has desirable kinetics. The drug undergoes rapid absorption after oral dosing and distributes to all tissues. Of particular importance, it concentrates in cells of the lungs, reaching levels 10 times those in blood. Furthermore, it remains in the body for days, permitting continued bactericidal effects with just once-a-week dosing.

Interaction with rifampin may be a concern. Why? Because rifampin induces the activity of CYP3A4, an isoenzyme of cytochrome P450 that metabolizes bedaquiline. In a clinical trial, rifampin significantly reduced blood levels of bedaquiline.

Although resistance to bedaquiline is uncommon, it does occur: About 1 in 200 million tubercle bacilli make a form of ATP synthase that is not inhibited by the drug. Accordingly, to prevent overgrowth with these resistant microbes, the regimen should always contain other anti-TB drugs.

Adverse Effects

Bedaquiline labeling includes a black box warning related to the risk for prolonged QT interval and risk for hepatotoxicity. In clinical trials, there was an increased risk for death in patients taking bedaquiline compared with those taking a placebo. Subsequently, labeling recommends bedaquiline only if there is no other effective treatment. Beyond the adverse effects listed in the black box warning, bedaquiline has few adverse effects. Approximately 10% to 40% of patients may experience nausea, arthralgia, headache, chest pain, and hemoptysis. Fewer than 10% experience rash and anorexia. There is no known fetal harm associated with use by pregnant women.

DRUGS FOR LEPROSY (HANSEN'S DISEASE)

Leprosy is a chronic infectious disease caused by *M. leprae*, an acid-fast bacillus. The infection is also known as Hansen's disease, in recognition of Gerhard Armauer Hansen, who demonstrated the involvement of *M. leprae* in 1873. Left untreated, leprosy can cause grotesque disfiguration. Fortunately, with the drugs available today, most patients can be cured. As a result, the worldwide incidence of leprosy has declined dramatically—from an estimated 12 million cases in the mid-1980s to about 249,000 new cases in 2008. In the United States, 178 new cases were reported in 2015.

Infection with *M. leprae* affects the skin, eyes, peripheral nerves, and mucous membranes of the upper respiratory tract. Characteristic features are (1) skin lesions with local loss of sensation, (2) thickening of peripheral nerves, and (3) acid-fast bacilli in smears from skin lesions.

Leprosy is divided into two main classes: (1) paucibacillary (PB) leprosy and (2) multibacillary (MB) leprosy. Classification is based on clinical manifestations and the presence of *M. leprae* in skin smears. If skin smears are negative, the diagnosis is PB leprosy. Conversely, if any smear is positive, the diagnosis is MB leprosy. In many places, microbiologic analysis of skin smears is either unavailable or unreliable. Hence, in these places, classification must be based on clinical findings alone. In this case, if the patient has one to five skin lesions, the diagnosis is PB leprosy; if the patient has six or more skin lesions, the diagnosis is MB leprosy. The distinction between PB leprosy and MB leprosy is important because treatment differs for the two forms.

OVERVIEW OF TREATMENT OF LEPROSY

As with TB, the cornerstone of treatment is multidrug therapy. If just one drug is used, resistance will occur. Most regimens include *rifampin,* the most effective drug for killing *M. leprae.* For patients with *MB leprosy,* the World Health Organization (WHO) recommends 12 months of treatment with three drugs: rifampin, dapsone, and clofazimine. For patients with *PB leprosy,* the WHO recommends 6 months of treatment with two drugs: rifampin and dapsone. For patients with *single-lesion PB leprosy* (i.e., PB leprosy with just one skin lesion), the WHO recommends a single dose of rifampin, ofloxacin, and minocycline (the ROM regimen). With all three regimens, the relapse rate is very low (about 0.1%). Accordingly, all three are considered curative. Dosages for these regimens are shown in Table 90.7.

TABLE 90.7 ▪ Adult Regimens for Leprosy, as Recommended by the World Health Organization

MULTIBACILLARY LEPROSY (TREAT 12 MONTHS WITH ALL 3 DRUGS)	
Rifampin	600 mg once a month, supervised
Dapsone	100 mg daily, self-administered
Clofazimine	300 mg once a month, supervised *or* 50 mg daily, self-administered
PAUCIBACILLARY LEPROSY (TREAT 6 MONTHS WITH BOTH DRUGS)	
Rifampin	600 mg once a month, supervised
Dapsone	100 mg daily, self-administered
SINGLE-LESION PAUCIBACILLARY LEPROSY (TAKE ALL 3 DRUGS ONCE)	
Rifampin	600 mg
Ofloxacin	400 mg
Minocycline	100 mg
RIFAMPIN-RESISTANT LEPROSY (TREAT 12 MONTHS)	
First 6 Months (Take All 3 Drugs Daily)	
Clofazimine	50 mg
Ofloxacin	400 mg
Minocycline	100 mg
Next 6 Months (Take Either Pair of Drugs Daily)	
Clofazimine	50 mg
Ofloxacin	400 mg
or	
Clofazimine	50 mg
Minocycline	100 mg

PHARMACOLOGY OF INDIVIDUAL ANTILEPROSY DRUGS

Rifampin

The basic pharmacology of rifampin was discussed earlier under *Pharmacology of Individual Antituberculosis Drugs.* Discussion here is limited to its use in leprosy.

Rifampin is by far our most effective agent for treating leprosy. In fact, the drug is more effective than any *combination* of other agents. A single dose kills more than 99.9% of viable *M. leprae.* After three monthly doses, less than 0.001% of the initial *M. leprae* population remains. Because of its powerful bactericidal actions, rifampin is a key component of standard antileprosy regimens.

The dosage currently recommended by the WHO is 600 mg *once a month.* In the past, rifampin was administered daily. However, we now know that monthly dosing is just as effective. Moreover, monthly dosing is much less expensive and minimizes hepatotoxicity and other adverse effects. Resistance can occur if rifampin is used alone. Accordingly, the drug is always combined with other antileprosy agents (e.g., dapsone plus clofazimine).

Dapsone

Actions and Uses

Dapsone, taken orally, is weakly bactericidal to *M. leprae.* The drug is safe, inexpensive, and moderately effective. Dapsone is chemically related to the sulfonamides and shares their mechanism of action: inhibition of folic acid synthesis. Although once employed alone to treat leprosy, dapsone is now employed in combination with other antileprosy drugs, usually rifampin and clofazimine. A topical formulation, sold as Aczone, is approved for treating acne (see Chapter 105).

Pharmacokinetics

Dapsone is absorbed rapidly and nearly completely from the GI tract. Once in the blood, the drug is widely distributed to tissues and body fluids. Dapsone undergoes hepatic metabolism followed by excretion in the urine. The average half-life is 28 hours.

Adverse Effects

Dapsone is generally well tolerated. The drug has been taken for years without significant untoward effects. The most common effects are GI disturbances, headache, rash, and a syndrome that resembles mononucleosis. Hemolytic anemia occurs occasionally; severe reactions are usually limited to patients with profound glucose-6-phosphate dehydrogenase deficiency. Rare reactions include agranulocytosis, exfoliative dermatitis, and hepatitis.

Clofazimine

The WHO makes clofazimine available worldwide for the treatment of leprosy. To obtain the drug, an official request must be made to the Ministries of Health.

Actions and Uses

Clofazimine [Lamprene] is slowly bactericidal to *M. leprae.* Its mechanism of action is unknown. To prevent emergence of resistance, clofazimine is always combined with another antileprosy drug (e.g., rifampin, dapsone). In addition to its antibacterial action, clofazimine has anti-inflammatory actions.

Pharmacokinetics

Clofazimine is administered orally and undergoes partial absorption. Absorbed drug is retained in fatty tissue and the skin. Because of tissue retention, the half-life of clofazimine is extremely long—about 70 days.

Adverse Effects

Dangerous reactions are rare. GI symptoms (nausea, vomiting, cramping, diarrhea) are common but mild. The drug frequently imparts a harmless red color to feces, urine, sweat, tears, and saliva. Deposition of clofazimine in the small intestine produces the most serious effects: intestinal obstruction, pain, and bleeding.

Clofazimine causes reversible reddish-black discoloration of the skin in most patients. Pigmentation begins 4 to 8 weeks after the onset of treatment and generally clears within 12 months of drug cessation. Because it can darken the skin, patients with light-colored skin often find clofazimine unacceptable.

TABLE 90.8 ■ Regimens for *Mycobacterium avium* Complex Infection in Immunocompetent Adults

PULMONARY MAC	DISSEMINATED MAC
Daily Regimen	**Daily Regimen**
Clarithromycin (500 mg twice daily) *or* azithromycin (250 mg)	Clarithromycin (500 mg twice daily) *or* azithromycin (250–500 mg)
plus	*plus*
Ethambutol (25 mg/kg for 2 months, then 15 mg/kg thereafter)	Ethambutol (15 mg/kg)
plus	*plus*
Rifampin (600 mg) *or* rifabutin (300 mg)	Rifampin (600 mg) *or* rifabutin (300 mg)
may also add	*may also add*
Streptomycin (15 mg/kg 3 times a week for 2–6 months)	Streptomycin (15 mg/kg 3 times a week for 2–6 months)
Duration	**Duration**
Treat until cultures remain negative for 12 months	Treat until cultures remain negative for 12 months

MAC, Mycobacterium avium complex.

DRUGS FOR *MYCOBACTERIUM AVIUM* COMPLEX INFECTION

MAC consists of two nearly indistinguishable organisms: *M. avium* and *M. intracellulare.* Colonization with MAC begins in the lungs or GI tract, but then may spread to the blood, bone marrow, liver, spleen, lymph nodes, brain, kidneys, and skin. Disseminated infection is common in patients infected with HIV; the incidence at autopsy is 50%. Among immunocompetent patients, symptomatic MAC infection is usually limited to the lungs. Signs and symptoms of disseminated MAC infection include fever, night sweats, weight loss, lethargy, anemia, and abnormal liver function tests.

Drugs are used for prophylaxis and to treat active infection. Preferred agents for *prophylaxis* of disseminated infection are *azithromycin* and *clarithromycin.* Regimens for *treating active infection* in immunocompetent hosts should include (1) *azithromycin* or *clarithromycin* plus (2) *ethambutol* plus (3) *rifampin* or *rifabutin.* Additional drugs may be added as needed; options include streptomycin, ciprofloxacin, and amikacin. Treatment of active infection in immunocompetent patients should continue for 12 months after cultures become negative. Representative regimens for immunocompetent patients are shown in Table 90.8. Regimens for patients with HIV infection are discussed in Chapter 94.

KEY POINTS

- Most people infected with *M. tuberculosis* remain asymptomatic, although they will harbor dormant bacteria for life (in the absence of drug therapy).
- Symptomatic TB can result from reactivation of an old infection or from recent person-to-person transmission of a new infection.
- Drug resistance, and especially multidrug resistance, is a serious impediment to successful therapy of TB.
- The principal cause of drug resistance in TB is inadequate drug therapy, which kills sensitive bacteria while allowing resistant mutants to flourish.
- To prevent emergence of resistance, initial therapy of TB should consist of at least two drugs to which the infection is sensitive, and preferably four. Accordingly, isolates from all patients must undergo testing of drug sensitivity, a process that typically takes several weeks.
- Therapy of TB is prolonged, lasting from a minimum of 6 months to 2 years and even longer.
- Patient adherence can be greatly increased by using directly observed therapy combined with intermittent, rather than daily, dosing.
- Three methods are employed to evaluate TB therapy: bacteriologic evaluation of sputum, clinical evaluation, and chest radiographs.
- The principal first-line drugs for TB are isoniazid, rifampin, pyrazinamide, and ethambutol. For initial therapy of active TB, patients may be given all four drugs.
- Initial therapy of MDR-TB and XDR-TB may require up to seven drugs.
- Tuberculosis in HIV-positive patients often can be treated with the same regimens used for HIV-negative patients, although the duration of treatment may be longer.
- Isoniazid can injure the liver. The greatest risk factor is advancing age. Patients who develop liver injury should discontinue isoniazid immediately.
- Rifampin induces drug-metabolizing enzymes and can thereby increase the metabolism of other drugs; important among these are oral contraceptives, warfarin, and certain protease inhibitors and NNRTIs used for HIV infection.
- Like isoniazid, rifampin and pyrazinamide are hepatotoxic. Accordingly, when these three drugs are combined, as they often are, the risk for liver injury can be substantial.
- Ethambutol can cause optic neuritis.
- The *tuberculin skin test* (TST)—used to identify people with LTBI—is performed by giving an intradermal injection of PPD (purified protein derivative) and then measuring the zone of induration (hardness) at the site 48 to 72 hours later.
- New blood tests, known as interferon gamma release assays (IGRAs), are as sensitive as the TST and more specific. Moreover, results with the IGRAs are available faster (within 24 hours) and don't require a return visit to the office.
- For years, isoniazid, taken daily for 9 months, has been the preferred treatment for LTBI. However, a much simpler regimen—isoniazid plus rifapentine taken once a week for just 3 months—is just as effective and is likely to replace isoniazid alone as standard treatment.

Please visit **http://evolve.elsevier.com/Lehne** for chapter-specific NCLEX® examination review questions.

Summary of Major Nursing Implications[a]

ANTITUBERCULOSIS DRUGS

Isoniazid
Rifampin
Pyrazinamide
Ethambutol

The nursing implications here are limited to the drug therapy of TB.

Implications That Apply to All Antituberculosis Drugs

Promoting Adherence

Treatment of active TB is prolonged and demands concurrent use of two or more drugs; as a result, adherence can be a significant problem. **To promote adherence, educate the patient about the rationale for multidrug therapy and the need for long-term treatment. Encourage patients to take their medication exactly as prescribed and to continue treatment until the infection has resolved.** Adherence can be greatly increased by using directly observed therapy (DOT) combined with intermittent dosing (rather than daily dosing).

Evaluating Treatment

Success is indicated by (1) reductions in fever, malaise, anorexia, cough, and other clinical manifestations of TB (usually within weeks); (2) radiographic evidence of improvement (usually in 3 months); and (3) an absence of *M. tuberculosis* in sputum (usually after 3 to 6 months).

ISONIAZID

In addition to the implications that follow, see earlier discussion for implications on *Promoting Adherence* and *Evaluating Treatment* that apply to all anti-TB drugs.

Preadministration Assessment

Therapeutic Goal

Treatment of active or latent infection with *M. tuberculosis.*

Baseline Data

Obtain a chest radiograph, microbiologic tests of sputum, and baseline tests of liver function.

Identifying High-Risk Patients

Isoniazid is *contraindicated* for patients with acute liver disease or a history of isoniazid-induced hepatotoxicity.

Use with *caution* in alcohol abusers, diabetic patients, patients with vitamin B_6 deficiency, patients older than 50 years, and patients who are taking phenytoin, rifampin, rifabutin, rifapentine, or pyrazinamide.

Implementation: Administration

Routes

Oral, IM.

Administration

Advise patients to take isoniazid on an empty stomach, either 1 hour before meals or 2 hours after. Advise patients to take the drug with meals if GI upset occurs.

Ongoing Evaluation and Interventions

Minimizing Adverse Effects

Hepatotoxicity. Isoniazid can cause hepatocellular damage and multilobular hepatic necrosis. **Inform patients about signs of hepatitis (jaundice, anorexia, malaise, fatigue, nausea), and instruct them to notify the prescriber immediately if these develop.** Evaluate patients monthly for signs of hepatitis. Monthly determinations of AST activity may be ordered. If clinical signs of hepatitis appear or if AST activity exceeds 3 to 5 times the pretreatment baseline, isoniazid should be withdrawn. Daily ingestion of alcohol increases the risk for liver injury; **urge the patient to minimize or eliminate alcohol consumption.**

Peripheral Neuropathy. **Inform patients about symptoms of peripheral neuropathy (tingling, numbness, burning, or pain in the hands or feet), and instruct them to notify the prescriber if these occur.** Peripheral neuritis can be reversed with small daily doses of pyridoxine (vitamin B_6). In patients at high risk for neuropathy (e.g., alcohol abusers, diabetic patients), give pyridoxine prophylactically.

Minimizing Adverse Interactions

Phenytoin. Isoniazid can suppress the metabolism of phenytoin, thereby causing phenytoin levels to rise. Plasma phenytoin should be monitored. If necessary, phenytoin dosage should be reduced.

RIFAMPIN

In addition to the implications that follow, see earlier for implications on *Promoting Adherence* and *Evaluating Treatment* that apply to all anti-TB drugs.

Preadministration Assessment

Therapeutic Goal

Treatment of active TB or leprosy.

Baseline Data

Obtain a chest radiograph, microbiologic tests of sputum, and baseline tests of liver function.

Identifying High-Risk Patients

Rifampin is *contraindicated* for patients taking delavirdine (an NNRTI) and most protease inhibitors.

Use with *caution* in alcohol abusers, patients with liver disease, and patients taking warfarin.

Implementation: Administration

Routes

Oral, IV.

Dosage

Reduce the dosage in patients with liver disease.

Administration

Instruct the patient to take oral rifampin once a day, either 1 hour before a meal or 2 hours after.

Continued

Summary of Major Nursing Implications[a]—cont'd

Administer reconstituted rifampin by slow IV infusion: 100 mL over 30 minutes or 500 mL over 3 hours.

Ongoing Evaluation and Interventions

Minimizing Adverse Effects

Hepatotoxicity. Rifampin may cause jaundice or hepatitis. **Inform patients about signs of liver dysfunction (anorexia, darkened urine, pale stools, yellow discoloration of eyes or skin), and instruct them to notify the prescriber if these develop.** Monitor patients for signs of liver dysfunction. Tests of liver function should be made before treatment and every 2 to 4 weeks thereafter.

Discoloration of Body Fluids. **Inform patients that rifampin may impart a harmless red-orange color to urine, sweat, saliva, and tears. Warn patients that soft contact lenses may undergo permanent staining; advise them to consult an ophthalmologist about continued use of the lenses.**

Minimizing Adverse Interactions

Accelerated Metabolism of Other Drugs. Rifampin can accelerate the metabolism of many drugs, thereby reducing their effects. This action is of particular concern with *oral contraceptives, warfarin, most protease inhibitors,* and *delavirdine* (an NNRTI). **Advise women taking oral contraceptives to use a nonhormonal form of birth control.** Monitor warfarin effects and increase dosage as needed. Do not combine protease inhibitors or NNRTIs with rifampin.

Pyrazinamide and Isoniazid. These hepatotoxic anti-TB drugs can increase the risk for liver injury when used with rifampin.

PYRAZINAMIDE

In addition to the implications that follow, see earlier for implications on *Promoting Adherence* and *Evaluating Treatment* that apply to all anti-TB drugs.

Preadministration Assessment

Therapeutic Goal

Treatment of active and LTBI.

Baseline Data

Obtain a chest radiograph, microbiologic tests of sputum, and baseline tests of liver function.

Identifying High-Risk Patients

Pyrazinamide is *contraindicated* for patients with severe liver dysfunction or acute gout.

Use with *caution* in alcohol abusers.

Implementation: Administration

Route

Oral.

Administration

Usually administered once a day.

Ongoing Evaluation and Interventions

Minimizing Adverse Effects

Hepatotoxicity. **Inform patients about symptoms of hepatitis (malaise, anorexia, nausea, vomiting, yellowish discoloration of the skin and eyes), and instruct them to notify the prescriber if these develop.** Levels of AST and ALT should be measured before treatment and every 2 weeks thereafter. If severe liver injury occurs, pyrazinamide should be withdrawn. The risk for liver injury is increased by concurrent therapy with isoniazid, rifampin, rifabutin, or rifapentine, all of which are hepatotoxic.

Nongouty Polyarthralgias. Polyarthralgias develop in 40% of patients. **Advise patients to take an NSAID (e.g., aspirin, ibuprofen) to relieve pain.** Some patients may need to stop pyrazinamide or at least reduce the dosage.

ETHAMBUTOL

In addition to the implications that follow, see earlier for implications on *Promoting Adherence* and *Evaluating Treatment* that apply to all anti-TB drugs.

Preadministration Assessment

Therapeutic Goal

Treatment of active TB.

Baseline Data

Obtain a chest radiograph, microbiologic tests of sputum, and baseline vision tests.

Identifying High-Risk Patients

Ethambutol is *contraindicated* for patients with optic neuritis.

Implementation: Administration

Route

Oral.

Administration

Usually administered once a day. **Advise patients to take ethambutol with food if GI upset occurs.**

Ongoing Evaluation and Interventions

Minimizing Adverse Effects

Optic Neuritis. Ethambutol can cause dose-related optic neuritis. Symptoms include blurred vision, altered color discrimination, and constriction of visual fields. Baseline vision tests are required. **Instruct patients to report any alteration in vision (e.g., blurring of vision, reduced color discrimination).** If ocular toxicity develops, ethambutol should be withdrawn at once.

[a]Patient education information is highlighted as **blue text.**

CHAPTER

91 Miscellaneous Antibacterial Drugs: Fluoroquinolones, Metronidazole, Daptomycin, Rifampin, Rifaximin, and Fidaxomicin

Prototype Drugs

MISCELLANEOUS ANTIBACTERIAL DRUGS

Fluoroquinolones
Ciprofloxacin

Cyclic Lipopeptides
Daptomycin

FLUOROQUINOLONES

The fluoroquinolones are fluorinated analogs of nalidixic acid, a narrow-spectrum quinolone antibiotic used only for urinary tract infections (UTIs). However, unlike nalidixic acid, the fluoroquinolones are broad-spectrum agents that have multiple applications. Benefits derive from disrupting DNA replication and cell division. Fluoroquinolones do not disrupt synthesis of proteins or the cell wall. All of the systemic fluoroquinolones can be administered orally. As a result, these drugs are attractive alternatives for people who might otherwise require intravenous antibacterial therapy. Although side effects are generally mild, all fluoroquinolones can cause tendinitis and tendon rupture, usually of the Achilles tendon. Fortunately, the risk is low. Bacterial resistance develops slowly, but has become common in *Neisseria gonorrhoeae,* and hence these drugs are no longer recommended for this infection. Five fluoroquinolones are currently available for systemic therapy (Table 91.1). Fluoroquinolones used solely for topical treatment of the eyes are discussed in Chapter 104.

Ciprofloxacin

Ciprofloxacin [Cipro] was among the first fluoroquinolones available and will serve as our prototype for the group. The drug is active against a broad spectrum of bacterial pathogens and may be administered PO or IV. Oral ciprofloxacin has been used as an alternative to parenteral antibiotics for treatment of several serious infections. Because it can be administered by mouth, patients receiving ciprofloxacin can be treated at home, rather than going to the hospital for IV antibacterial therapy.

Mechanism of Action

Ciprofloxacin inhibits two bacterial enzymes: *DNA gyrase* and *topoisomerase IV.* Both are needed for DNA replication and cell division. DNA gyrase converts closed circular DNA into a supercoiled configuration. In the absence of supercoiling, DNA replication cannot take place. Topoisomerase IV helps separate daughter DNA strands during cell division. Since the mammalian equivalents of DNA gyrase and topoisomerase IV are largely insensitive to fluoroquinolones, cells of the host are spared. Ciprofloxacin is rapidly bactericidal.

Antimicrobial Spectrum

Ciprofloxacin is active against a broad spectrum of bacteria, including most aerobic gram-negative bacteria and some gram-positive bacteria. Most urinary tract pathogens, including *Escherichia coli* and *Klebsiella,* are sensitive. The drug is also highly active against most bacteria that cause enteritis (e.g., *Salmonella, Shigella, Campylobacter jejuni, E. coli*). Other sensitive organisms include *Bacillus anthracis, Pseudomonas aeruginosa, Haemophilus influenzae,* meningococci, and many streptococci. Activity against anaerobes is fair to poor. *Clostridium difficile* is resistant.

Bacterial Resistance

Resistance to fluoroquinolones has developed during treatment of infections caused by *Staphylococcus aureus, Serratia marcescens, C. jejuni, P. aeruginosa,* and *N. gonorrhoeae.* Two mechanisms appear responsible: (1) alterations in DNA gyrase and topoisomerase IV and (2) increased drug export. Bacteria do not directly inactivate fluoroquinolones, and there have been no reports of resistance via transfer of R factors.

Pharmacokinetics

Ciprofloxacin may be given PO or IV. Following oral dosing, the drug is absorbed rapidly but incompletely. High concentrations are achieved in urine, stool, bile, saliva, bone, and prostate tissue. Drug levels in cerebrospinal fluid remain low. Ciprofloxacin has a plasma half-life of about 4 hours. Elimination is by hepatic metabolism and renal excretion.

TABLE 91.1 ▪ Other Fluoroquinalones

Drug	Therapeutic Uses	Pharmacokinetics	Adverse Effects	Preparations and Usual Adult Dosage
Ofloxacin	Bacterial infections, including UTI, prostatitis	Metabolism: minimal hepatic Excretion: urine	Nausea, vomiting, headache, tendinitis, tendon rupture, muscle weakness	Tablets: 200–400 mg every 12 hr
Moxifloxacin	Respiratory tract infections, sinusitis, skin infections	Metabolism: hepatic Excretion: urine	Nausea, vomiting, headache, tendinitis, tendon rupture, muscle weakness	Tablets or IV: 400 mg every 24 hr
Levofloxacin	Respiratory tract infections, UTI, sinusitis, prostatitis, skin infections	Metabolism: minimal hepatic Excretion: urine	Nausea, vomiting, headache, tendinitis, tendon rupture, muscle weakness	Tablets or IV: 500–750 mg every 24 hr
Gemifloxacin	Respiratory tract infections	Metabolism: minimal hepatic Excretion: feces, urine	Rash, nausea, vomiting, headache, tendinitis, tendon rupture, muscle weakness	Tablets: 320 mg every 24 hr

Therapeutic Uses

Ciprofloxacin is approved for a wide variety of infections. Among these are infections of the respiratory tract, urinary tract, GI tract, bones, joints, skin, and soft tissues. Also, ciprofloxacin is a preferred drug for preventing anthrax in people who have inhaled anthrax spores. Because ciprofloxacin is active against a variety of pathogens and can be given orally, the drug represents an alternative to parenteral treatment for many serious infections. Owing to high rates of resistance, ciprofloxacin is a poor choice for staphylococcal infections. The drug is not useful against infections caused by anaerobes.

Because of concerns about tendon injury (see later), *systemic* ciprofloxacin is generally avoided in children under 18 years old. Nonetheless, the drug does have two approved pediatric uses: (1) treatment of complicated urinary tract and kidney infections caused by *E. coli* and (2) postexposure treatment of inhalational anthrax.

Adverse Effects

Ciprofloxacin can induce a variety of adverse effects, including GI reactions (nausea, vomiting, diarrhea, abdominal pain) and central nervous system (CNS) effects (dizziness, headache, restlessness, confusion). *Candida* infections of the pharynx and vagina may develop during treatment. Very rarely, seizures have occurred. In older adults, ciprofloxacin poses a significant risk of confusion, somnolence, psychosis, and visual disturbances.

Ciprofloxacin and other fluoroquinolones have caused *tendon rupture,* usually of the Achilles tendon. People at highest risk are those 60 and older, those taking glucocorticoids, and those who have undergone heart, lung, or kidney transplantation. Fluoroquinolones damage tendons by disrupting the extracellular matrix of cartilage in immature animals. A similar mechanism may underlie tendon rupture in humans. Since tendon injury is reversible if diagnosed early, fluoroquinolones should be discontinued at the first sign of tendon pain, swelling, or inflammation. In addition, patients should refrain from exercise until tendinitis has been ruled out. Because of their ability to cause these adverse effects, the quinolones received a new black box warning. It is recommended that for the treatment of urinary tract infections and sinusitis, other drugs should be employed first.

PATIENT-CENTERED CARE ACROSS THE LIFE SPAN

Antibacterial Drugs

Life Stage	Patient Care Concerns
Infants	See *Breast-feeding Women* below.
Children/adolescents	Ciprofloxacin and levofloxacin are the only fluoroquinolones approved for use in children. Secondary to concerns regarding tendon injury, fluoroquinolones are generally avoided in this population.
Pregnant women	Although data reveal little potential for fluoroquinolone toxicity in the fetus, these data are limited. Risks and benefits must be considered for administration during pregnancy.
Breast-feeding women	Effects of fluoroquinolones on the nursing infant are largely unknown. Consider other medications if possible.
Older adults	Fluoroquinolones are generally well tolerated in older adults. Calculate creatinine clearance for safe dosing.

Ciprofloxacin and other fluoroquinolones pose a risk of *phototoxicity* (severe sunburn), characterized by burning, erythema, exudation, vesicles, blistering, and edema. These can occur following exposure to direct sunlight, indirect sunlight, and sunlamps—even if a sunscreen has been applied. Patients should be warned about phototoxicity and advised to avoid sunlight and sunlamps. People who must go outdoors should wear protective clothing and apply a sunscreen. Ciprofloxacin should be withdrawn at the first sign of a phototoxic reaction (e.g., burning sensation, redness, rash).

Ciprofloxacin and other fluoroquinolones increase the risk of developing *Clostridium difficile* infection (CDI), a potentially severe infection of the bowel. CDI results from killing off intestinal bacteria that normally keep *C. difficile* in check.

Safety Alert

MYASTHENIA GRAVIS

Ciprofloxacin and other fluoroquinolones can exacerbate muscle weakness in patients with myasthenia gravis. Accordingly, patients with a history of myasthenia gravis should not receive these drugs.

Drug and Food Interactions

Cationic Compounds. Absorption of ciprofloxacin can be reduced by compounds that contain cations. Among these are (1) aluminum- or magnesium-containing antacids, (2) iron salts, (3) zinc salts, (4) sucralfate, (5) calcium supplements, and (6) milk and other dairy products, all of which contain calcium ions. These cationic agents should be administered at least 6 hours before ciprofloxacin or 2 hours after.

Elevation of Drug Levels. Ciprofloxacin can increase plasma levels of several drugs, including *theophylline* (used for asthma), *warfarin* (an anticoagulant), and *tinidazole* (an antifungal drug). Toxicity could result. For patients taking theophylline, drug levels should be monitored and the dosage adjusted accordingly. For patients taking warfarin, prothrombin time should be monitored and the dosage of warfarin reduced as appropriate.

Preparations, Dosage, and Administration

Preparations. Ciprofloxacin is available for oral and IV administration. For oral therapy, ciprofloxacin is supplied in immediate-release tablets (100, 250, 500, and 750 mg) sold as *Cipro,* and extended-release tablets (500 and 1000 mg) sold as *Cipro XR.* For IV therapy, ciprofloxacin is supplied in solution (400 mg/200 mL) sold as *Cipro IV.*

Dosage and Administration

Oral. Dosing may be done with or without food. The dosage for complicated UTIs is 250 or 500 mg 2 times a day, usually for 7 to 14 days. For other infections, dosages range from 500 to 750 mg 2 times a day. Dosage should be reduced for patients with renal impairment. Dosages for anthrax prevention are presented under *Inhalational Anthrax.*

Intravenous. Intravenous dosages range from 200 to 400 mg every 12 hours. Infusions should be done slowly (over 60 minutes). Dosages for anthrax prevention are presented next.

Inhalational Anthrax. Ciprofloxacin is used to reduce the incidence of anthrax or to prevent anthrax progression in people who have inhaled *B. anthracis* spores. The dosage for adults is 500 mg PO every 12 hours (or 400 mg IV every 8 hours) for 60 days. The dosage for children is 15 mg/kg PO (or 10 mg/kg IV) every 12 hours for 60 days (with the proviso that individual oral doses not exceed 500 mg, and individual IV doses not exceed 400 mg). Management of inhalational anthrax is discussed in Chapter 110.

ADDITIONAL ANTIBACTERIAL DRUGS

Metronidazole

Metronidazole [Flagyl] is used for protozoal infections and infections caused by obligate anaerobic bacteria. The basic pharmacology of metronidazole is discussed in Chapter 99, as is the drug's use against protozoal infections. Consideration here is limited to antibacterial applications.

Mechanism of Antibacterial Action

Metronidazole is lethal to anaerobic organisms only. To exert bactericidal effects, metronidazole must first be taken up by cells and then converted into its active form; only anaerobes can perform the conversion. The active form interacts with DNA to cause strand breakage and loss of helical structure, effects that result in inhibition of nucleic acid synthesis and, ultimately, cell death. Since aerobic bacteria are unable to activate metronidazole, they are insensitive to the drug.

Antibacterial Spectrum

Metronidazole is active against obligate anaerobes only. Sensitive bacterial pathogens include *Bacteroides fragilis* (and other *Bacteroides* species), *C. difficile* (and other *Clostridium* species), *Fusobacterium* species, *Gardnerella vaginalis, Peptococcus* species, and *Peptostreptococcus* species.

Therapeutic Uses

Metronidazole is active against a variety of anaerobic bacterial infections, including infections of the CNS, abdominal organs, bones and joints, skin and soft tissues, and genitourinary tract. Frequently, these infections also involve aerobic bacteria, and hence therapy must include a drug active against them. Metronidazole is a drug of choice for CDI, as discussed in Chapter 85. In addition, the drug is employed for prophylaxis in surgical procedures associated with a high risk of infection by anaerobes (e.g., colorectal surgery, abdominal surgery, gynecologic surgery). Metronidazole is also used in combination with a tetracycline and bismuth subsalicylate to eradicate *Helicobacter pylori* in people with peptic ulcer disease. Development of resistance to metronidazole is rare.

Preparations, Dosage, and Administration

For initial treatment of serious bacterial infections, metronidazole is administered by IV infusion. Under appropriate conditions, the patient may switch to oral therapy.

Intravenous Formulations. Metronidazole is available in solution for IV use. The solution (generic only) contains 5 mg of metronidazole per milliliter and is ready for IV use.

Intravenous Dosage and Administration. Infusions must be done slowly (over a 1-hour span). Therapy of anaerobic infections in adults is initiated with a loading dose of 15 mg/kg. After this, maintenance doses of 7.5 mg/kg are given every 6 to 8 hours. Treatment duration is usually 1 to 2 weeks.

Oral Preparations and Dosage. Metronidazole [Flagyl, Flagyl ER] is supplied in capsules (375 mg), immediate-release tablets (250 and 500 mg), and extended-release tablets (750 mg). The adult dosage for anaerobic infections is 7.5 mg/kg every 6 hours. For bacterial vaginosis in adults, a dosage of 750 mg (extended-release formulation) once daily for 7 days is effective. The dosage for CDI is 500 mg 3 times a day for 10 to 14 days.

Daptomycin

Daptomycin [Cubicin] is the first representative of a new class of antibiotics, the *cyclic lipopeptides.* The drug has a unique mechanism and can rapidly kill virtually all clinically relevant gram-positive bacteria, including methicillin-resistant *Staph. aureus.* Daptomycin is devoid of significant drug interactions, and the only notable side effect is possible muscle injury. The drug is given once daily by IV infusion, and there is no need to monitor its plasma level.

Mechanism of Action

Daptomycin has a novel mechanism of action. The drug inserts itself into the bacterial cell membrane and thereby forms channels that permit efflux of intracellular potassium (and possibly other cytoplasmic ions). Loss of intracellular ions has two effects. First, it depolarizes the cell membrane. Second, it inhibits synthesis of DNA, RNA, and proteins, and thereby causes cell death.

Antibacterial Spectrum

Daptomycin is active only against *gram-positive bacteria.* The drug cannot penetrate the outer membrane of gram-negative bacteria, and hence cannot harm them. Daptomycin is rapidly bactericidal to staphylococci (including methicillin- and vancomycin-resistant *Staph. aureus* and methicillin-resistant *Staphylococcus epidermidis*), enterococci (including vancomycin-resistant *Enterococcus faecium* and *E. faecalis*), streptococci (including penicillin-resistant *Strep. pneumoniae*), and most other aerobic and anaerobic gram-positive bacteria. As a rule, daptomycin is more rapidly bactericidal than vancomycin, linezolid, or quinupristin/dalfopristin.

Therapeutic Use

Daptomycin has two approved indications: (1) bloodstream infection with *Staph. aureus* and (2) complicated skin and skin structure infections caused by susceptible strains of the following gram-positive bacteria: *Staph. aureus* (including methicillin-resistant strains), *Strep. pyogenes, Streptococcus agalactiae, Streptococcus dysgalactiae* subspecies *equisimilis,* and *E. faecalis* (vancomycin-susceptible strains only). The drug is being tested for other possible uses, including endocarditis and infections caused by vancomycin-resistant enterococci. Daptomycin should *not* be used for community-acquired pneumonia (CAP). Clinical trials have shown that, in CAP patients receiving daptomycin, the rate of death and serious cardiorespiratory events is higher than in patients receiving equally effective alternatives.

Resistance

Out of more than 1000 patients receiving daptomycin in clinical trials, only 2 had infections resistant to the drug. The mechanism of resistance has not been identified. There is no known mechanism by which resistance can be transferred from one bacterium to another. Also, there is no cross-resistance between daptomycin and any other class of antibiotics.

Pharmacokinetics

Daptomycin is administered by IV infusion, and a significant fraction (92%) becomes bound to plasma proteins. The drug undergoes minimal metabolism. Most of each dose is excreted unchanged in the urine. In patients with normal renal function, the half-life is 9 hours. However, in those with severe renal impairment (creatinine clearance less than 30 mL/min) and in those on hemodialysis or continuous ambulatory peritoneal dialysis (CAPD), the half-life increases threefold. As a result, if the dosage is not reduced, plasma drug levels can rise dangerously high.

Adverse Effects

Daptomycin is generally well tolerated. The most common adverse effects are constipation, nausea, diarrhea, injection-site reactions, headache, insomnia, and rash.

Daptomycin may pose a small risk of *myopathy* (muscle injury). In clinical trials with doses that were larger and more frequent than those used now, patients often experienced muscle pain and weakness in association with increased levels of creatine phosphokinase (CPK), a marker for muscle injury. However, with currently approved doses, elevation of CPK is rare. Nonetheless, patients should be warned about possible muscle injury and told to report any muscle pain or weakness. In addition, CPK levels should be measured weekly. If the level rises markedly (to more than 10 times the upper limit of normal), daptomycin should be discontinued. Daptomycin should also be discontinued in patients who report muscle pain or weakness in conjunction with a more moderate rise in CPK.

Daptomycin may cause *eosinophilic pneumonia,* a rare but serious condition in which eosinophils (white blood cells) accumulate in the lungs and thereby impair lung function. Symptoms include fever, cough, and shortness of breath. Left untreated, the condition can rapidly progress to respiratory failure and death.

Drug Interactions

Daptomycin appears devoid of significant drug interactions. It does not induce or inhibit cytochrome P450 and should not affect drugs that are metabolized by this enzyme system. In clinical studies, daptomycin did not affect the kinetics of warfarin, simvastatin, or aztreonam. Concurrent use of daptomycin plus tobramycin caused a moderate increase in daptomycin levels and a moderate decrease in tobramycin levels. Accordingly, caution is needed when these drugs are combined.

Like daptomycin, the HMG-CoA reductase inhibitors (e.g., simvastatin [Zocor]) can cause myopathy. However, in clinical trials, no patient receiving simvastatin plus daptomycin developed signs of muscle injury. Nonetheless, given our limited experience with daptomycin, it may be prudent to suspend HMG-CoA reductase inhibitors while daptomycin is used.

Preparations, Dosage, and Administration

Daptomycin [Cubicin] is available as a powder in 500-mg single-use vials. Following reconstitution in 0.9% sodium chloride, the drug is given by a slow (30-minute) IV infusion. For patients with normal renal function, the dosage is 4 or 6 mg/kg once every 24 hours. For patients with severe renal impairment and for those on hemodialysis or CAPD, the dosage is 4 to 6 mg/kg once every 48 to 72 hours.

Rifampin

Rifampin [Rifadin] is a broad-spectrum antibacterial agent employed primarily for tuberculosis (see Chapter 90). However, the drug is also used against several nontuberculous infections. Rifampin is useful for treating *asymptomatic carriers of Neisseria meningitidis,* but is not given to treat active meningococcal infection. Unlabeled uses include treatment of leprosy, gram-negative bacteremia in infancy, and infections caused by *Staph. epidermidis* and *Staph. aureus* (e.g., endocarditis, osteomyelitis, prostatitis). Rifampin has also been employed for prophylaxis of meningitis due to *H. influenzae.* Because resistance can develop rapidly, established bacterial infections should not be treated with rifampin alone. The basic pharmacology of rifampin and its use in tuberculosis are presented in Chapter 90.

Rifaximin

Rifaximin [Xifaxan] is an oral nonabsorbable analog of rifampin used to kill bacteria in the gut. Like rifampin, rifaximin inhibits bacterial DNA–dependent RNA polymerase and thereby inhibits RNA synthesis, resulting in inhibition of protein synthesis and subsequent bacterial death.

Rifaximin has three approved uses. The drug was approved initially for *traveler's diarrhea* caused by *E. coli* in patients at least 12 years old. Rifaximin is not effective against severe diarrhea associated with fever or bloody stools, and should not be used if these are present. More recently, rifaximin was approved for the *prevention of hepatic encephalopathy* (brain injury) in patients with chronic liver disease. Why does liver disease cause brain injury, and how does rifaximin help? In all of us, intestinal bacteria produce ammonia, a toxic substance that is normally cleared by the liver. However, in patients with liver disease, the liver can't remove much ammonia, and hence it can accumulate to levels that can harm the brain. Rifaximin helps prevent encephalopathy by killing the intestinal bacteria that produce ammonia. Rifaximin is also approved for irritable bowel syndrome with diarrhea (IBS-D).

Rifaximin is administered by mouth, and very little (less than 0.4%) is absorbed. As a result, the drug achieves high concentrations in the intestinal tract and then is excreted unchanged in the stool.

Rifaximin is well tolerated. Gastrointestinal effects—nausea, flatulence, defecation urgency—occur in some patients. Because so little drug is absorbed, systemic effects are minimal. However, studies in rats and rabbits indicate that rifaximin is teratogenic, and hence should not be used by pregnant or breast-feeding women. There have been postmarketing reports of hypersensitivity reactions (rash, allergic dermatitis, urticaria, pruritus, angioneurotic edema), but rifaximin has not been clearly identified as the cause.

Rifaximin is available in 200- and 550-mg tablets for oral dosing, with or without food. For *traveler's diarrhea,* the dosage is 200 mg 3 times a day for 3 days. To *prevent hepatic encephalopathy,* the dosage is 550 mg 2 times a day for as long as needed. The dose for IBS-D is 550 mg 3 times a day for 14 days.

Fidaxomicin

Fidaxomicin [Dificid] is a narrow-spectrum bactericidal, macrocyclic antibiotic indicated only for diarrhea associated with CDI. In one trial, fidaxomicin was compared with vancomycin, a standard treatment for CDI. The cure rate with fidaxomicin was higher than with vancomycin, and the recurrence rate was lower. Like rifaximin, fidaxomicin inhibits DNA-dependent RNA polymerase, and thereby inhibits RNA synthesis, causing inhibition of protein synthesis and subsequent bacterial death. Fidaxomicin is administered by mouth, and systemic absorption is low. As a result, the drug achieves high concentrations in the intestine, where it acts to kill *C. difficile*. The most common adverse effects are nausea, vomiting, abdominal pain, GI hemorrhage, anemia, and neutropenia. Fidaxomicin is supplied in 200-mg tablets for dosing with or without food.

KEY POINTS

- Fluoroquinolones are broad-spectrum antibiotics with a wide variety of clinical applications.
- Patients who might otherwise require hospitalization for parenteral antibacterial therapy can often be treated at home with an oral fluoroquinolone.
- Fluoroquinolones act by inhibiting bacterial DNA gyrase and topoisomerase IV.
- Because fluoroquinolones can cause tendinitis and tendon rupture, they should be discontinued at the first sign of tendon pain or inflammation. Also, the patient should not exercise until tendinitis has been ruled out.
- Fluoroquinolones pose a risk of phototoxicity. Accordingly, patients should avoid sunlight and sunlamps, and should use protective clothing and a sunscreen if they must go outdoors.
- Fluoroquinolones can exacerbate muscle weakness in patients with myasthenia gravis, and hence should not be used in patients with a history of this disorder.
- Absorption of fluoroquinolones can be reduced by cationic substances, including milk products (calcium), aluminum- and magnesium-containing antacids, iron and zinc salts, and sucralfate.
- In addition to its use against protozoa (see Chapter 99), metronidazole is used against infections caused by obligate anaerobic bacteria, including *Bacteroides fragilis* and *C. difficile.*

Please visit **http://evolve.elsevier.com/Lehne** for chapter-specific NCLEX® examination review questions.

Summary of Major Nursing Implications[a]

FLUOROQUINOLONES

Ciprofloxacin
Gemifloxacin
Levofloxacin
Moxifloxacin
Ofloxacin

Except where noted, the implications here apply to all fluoroquinolones.

Preadministration Assessment

Therapeutic Goal

Treatment of fluoroquinolone-sensitive infections. (See text for indications for specific agents.)

Identifying High-Risk Patients

Fluoroquinolones are *contraindicated* in patients with a history of myasthenia gravis.

Use all fluoroquinolones with *caution* in patients with renal impairment and in patients age 60 and older, patients taking glucocorticoids, and patients who have undergone a heart, liver, or kidney transplantation.

Use *moxifloxacin* with *great caution* in patients with hypokalemia or pre-existing QT prolongation and in those taking prodysrhythmic drugs.

Implementation: Administration

Routes

Oral. Ciprofloxacin, gemifloxacin, levofloxacin, moxifloxacin, and ofloxacin.

Intravenous. Ciprofloxacin, levofloxacin, and moxifloxacin.

Administration

Oral. **Inform patients taking *ciprofloxacin, gemifloxacin, levofloxacin, moxifloxacin,* and *ofloxacin* that dosing can be done with or without food.**

Advise patients to take their fluoroquinolone no sooner than 6 hours after ingesting cationic compounds, including iron salts, zinc salts, sucralfate, calcium supplements, dairy products, and aluminum- or magnesium-containing antacids.

Instruct patients to complete the prescribed course of treatment, even though symptoms may abate before the full course is over.

Intravenous. Administer IV fluoroquinolones by slow infusion (over 60 minutes or longer).

Dosage. Dosage for all fluoroquinolones, oral or IV, should be reduced in patients with significant renal impairment.

Ongoing Evaluation and Interventions

Minimizing Adverse Effects

Tendinitis and Tendon Rupture. Fluoroquinolones can cause tendinitis and tendon rupture, usually in the Achilles tendon. Use with caution in patients at elevated risk (i.e., patients age 60 and older, patients taking glucocorticoids, and patients who have undergone a heart, liver, or kidney transplantation). **Inform patients about the risk of tendon damage, and instruct them to report early signs of tendon injury (pain, swelling, inflammation), and to refrain from exercise until tendinitis has been ruled out.** If tendinitis is diagnosed, the fluoroquinolone should be discontinued.

Phototoxicity. Fluoroquinolones increase the risk of severe sunburn, characterized by burning, erythema, exudation, vesicles, blistering, and edema. **Advise patients to avoid sunlamps and to use a sunscreen and protective clothing when outdoors.** Discontinue fluoroquinolones at the first sign of phototoxicity (e.g., burning sensation, redness, rash).

QT Prolongation. *Moxifloxacin* can prolong the QT interval, thereby posing a risk of severe cardiac dysrhythmias. Generally avoid this drug in patients with hypokalemia or pre-existing QT prolongation and in those taking prodysrhythmic drugs.

Myasthenia Gravis. Fluoroquinolones can exacerbate muscle weakness in patients with myasthenia gravis, and hence should not be used in patients with a history of the disorder.

Minimizing Adverse Drug and Food Interactions

Cationic Compounds. Absorption of oral fluoroquinolones can be reduced by cationic compounds, including iron salts, zinc salts, sucralfate, aluminum- or magnesium-containing antacids, calcium supplements, and calcium-containing foods (i.e., milk and milk products). **Instruct patients to take these cationic compounds at least 6 hours before or 2 hours after their fluoroquinolone.**

Warfarin. *Ciprofloxacin* and *ofloxacin* can increase warfarin levels, thereby posing a risk of bleeding. Monitor prothrombin time and reduce warfarin dosage as indicated.

Theophylline. *Ciprofloxacin* and *ofloxacin* can increase theophylline levels, thereby posing a risk of toxicity, including seizures. Monitor theophylline levels and reduce the dosage as indicated.

[a]Patient education information is highlighted as **blue text.**

CHAPTER

92 Antifungal Agents

The antifungal agents fall into two major groups: drugs for *systemic mycoses* (i.e., systemic fungal infections) and drugs for *superficial mycoses.* A few drugs are used for both. Systemic infections occur much less frequently than superficial infections, but are much more serious. Accordingly, therapy of systemic mycoses is our main focus.

DRUGS FOR SYSTEMIC MYCOSES

Systemic mycoses can be subdivided into two categories: opportunistic infections and nonopportunistic infections. The opportunistic mycoses—*candidiasis, aspergillosis, cryptococcosis,* and *mucormycosis*—are seen primarily in debilitated or immunocompromised hosts. In contrast, nonopportunistic infections can occur in any host. These latter mycoses, which are relatively uncommon, include *sporotrichosis, blastomycosis, histoplasmosis,* and *coccidioidomycosis.* Treating systemic mycoses can be difficult: These infections often resist treatment and hence may require prolonged therapy with drugs that frequently prove toxic. Drugs of choice for systemic mycoses are shown in Table 92.1.

The systemic antifungal drugs fall into four classes: polyene antibiotics, azoles, echinocandins, and pyrimidine analogs. Class members and mechanisms of action are shown in Table 92.2.

Amphotericin B, a Polyene Antibiotic

Amphotericin B [Abelcet, Amphotec, AmBisome, Fungizone ♣] belongs to a drug class known as *polyene antibiotics,* so named because their structures contain a series of conjugated double bonds. Nystatin, another antifungal drug, is in the same family.

Amphotericin B is active against a broad spectrum of pathogenic fungi and is a drug of choice for most systemic mycoses. Unfortunately, amphotericin B is highly toxic: Infusion reactions and renal damage occur in many patients. Because of its potential for harm, amphotericin B should be employed only against infections that are progressive and potentially fatal.

Amphotericin B is available in four formulations: a conventional formulation (amphotericin B deoxycholate) and three lipid-based formulations. The lipid-based formulations are as effective as the conventional formulation and cause less toxicity—but are much more expensive. For the treatment of systemic mycoses, all formulations are administered by IV infusion. Infusions are given daily or every other day for several months.

Mechanism of Action

Amphotericin B binds to components of the fungal cell membrane, increasing permeability. The resultant leakage of intracellular cations (especially potassium) reduces viability. Depending on the concentration of amphotericin B and the susceptibility of the fungus, the drug may be fungistatic or fungicidal.

The component of the fungal membrane to which amphotericin B binds is *ergosterol,* a member of the *sterol* family of compounds. Hence, for a cell to be susceptible, its cytoplasmic membrane must contain sterols. Since bacterial membranes lack sterols, bacteria are not affected.

Much of the toxicity of amphotericin is attributable to the presence of sterols (principally cholesterol) in mammalian cell membranes. When amphotericin binds with cholesterol in mammalian membranes, the effect is similar to that seen in fungi. However, there *is* some degree of selectivity: Amphotericin binds more strongly to ergosterol than it does to cholesterol, so fungi are affected more than we are.

Microbial Susceptibility and Resistance

Amphotericin B is active against a broad spectrum of fungi. Some protozoa (e.g., *Leishmania braziliensis*) are also susceptible. As noted, bacteria are resistant.

Emergence of resistant fungi is extremely rare and occurs only with long-term amphotericin use. In all cases of resistance, the fungal membranes had reduced amounts of ergosterol or none at all.

Therapeutic Uses

Amphotericin B is a drug of choice for most systemic mycoses. Before this drug became available, systemic fungal infections usually proved fatal. Treatment is prolonged; 6 to 8 weeks is common. In some cases, treatment may last for 3 or 4 months. In addition to its antifungal applications, amphotericin B is a drug of choice for leishmaniasis (see Chapter 99).

TABLE 92.1 ▪ Drugs of Choice for Systemic Mycoses

Infection	Causative Organism	Drugs of Choice	Alternative Drugs
Aspergillosis	*Aspergillus* species	Voriconazole	Amphotericin B, itraconazole, posaconazole, caspofungin, micafungin, isavuconazole
Blastomycosis	*Blastomyces dermatitidis*	Amphotericin B *or* itraconazole	No alternative recommended
Candidiasis	*Candida* species	Caspofungin *or* fluconazole	Amphotericin B, itraconazole, voriconazole, caspofungin
Coccidioidomycosis	*Coccidioides immitis*	Amphotericin B *or* fluconazole	Itraconazole, ketoconazole
Cryptococcosis	*Cryptococcus neoformans*	Amphotericin B ± flucytosine	Itraconazole
Chronic suppression		Fluconazole	Amphotericin B
Histoplasmosis	*Histoplasma capsulatum*	Amphotericin B *or* itraconazole	Fluconazole, ketoconazole
Chronic suppression		Itraconazole	Amphotericin B
Mucormycosis	*Mucor* species	Amphotericin B	No alternative recommended
Paracoccidioidomycosis	*Paracoccidioides brasiliensis*	Amphotericin B *or* itraconazole	Ketoconazole
Sporotrichosis	*Sporothrix schenckii*	Amphotericin B *or* itraconazole	Fluconazole

± Alone or with the addition of flucytosine.

TABLE 92.2 ▪ Classes of Systemic Antifungal Drugs

Drug Class	Mechanism of Action	Class Members
Polyene antibiotics	Bind to ergosterol and disrupt the fungal cell membrane	Amphotericin B
Azoles	Inhibit synthesis of ergosterol and disrupt the fungal cell membrane	Fluconazole Itraconazole Ketoconazole Posaconazole Voriconazole Isavuconazole
Echinocandins	Inhibit synthesis of beta-1,3-D-glucan and disrupt the fungal cell wall	Anidulafungin Caspofungin Micafungin
Pyrimidine analogs	Disrupt synthesis of RNA and DNA	Flucytosine

Pharmacokinetics

Absorption and Distribution. Amphotericin is poorly absorbed from the GI tract, and hence oral therapy cannot be used for systemic infection. Rather, amphotericin must be administered IV. When the drug leaves the vascular system, it undergoes extensive binding to sterol-containing membranes of tissues. Levels about half those in plasma are achieved in aqueous humor and in peritoneal, pleural, and joint fluids. Amphotericin B does not readily penetrate to the cerebrospinal fluid (CSF).

Metabolism and Excretion. Little is known about the elimination of amphotericin B. We do not know whether the drug is metabolized or whether it is ultimately removed from the body. Renal excretion of unchanged amphotericin is minimal. However, dose or frequency reduction may be considered in patients with pre-existing renal impairment. Complete elimination of amphotericin takes a long time; the drug has been detected in tissues more than a year after cessation of treatment.

Adverse Effects

Amphotericin can cause a variety of serious adverse effects. Patients should be under close supervision, preferably in a hospital.

Infusion Reactions. Intravenous amphotericin frequently produces fever, chills, rigors, nausea, and headache. These reactions are caused by the release of proinflammatory cytokines (tumor necrosis factor, interleukin-1, interleukin-6) from monocytes and macrophages. Symptoms begin 1 to 3 hours after starting the infusion and persist about an hour. Mild reactions can be reduced by pretreatment with diphenhydramine plus acetaminophen. Aspirin can also help, but it may increase kidney damage (see *Nephrotoxicity*). Intravenous meperidine or dantrolene can be given if rigors occur. If other measures fail, hydrocortisone (a glucocorticoid) can be used to decrease fever and chills. However, since glucocorticoids can reduce the patient's ability to fight infection, routine use of hydrocortisone should be avoided. Infusion reactions are less intense with lipid-based amphotericin formulations than with the conventional formulation.

Amphotericin infusion produces a high incidence of phlebitis. This can be minimized by changing peripheral venous sites often or administering amphotericin through a large central vein.

Nephrotoxicity. Amphotericin is toxic to cells of the kidneys. Renal impairment occurs in practically all patients. The extent of kidney damage is related to the total dose administered over the full course of treatment. In most cases, renal function normalizes after amphotericin use stops. However, if the total dose exceeds 4 gm, residual impairment is likely. Kidney damage can be minimized by infusing 1 L of saline on the days amphotericin is given. Other nephrotoxic drugs (e.g., aminoglycosides, cyclosporine, nonsteroidal anti-inflammatory drugs [NSAIDs]) should be avoided. To evaluate renal injury, tests of kidney function should be performed every 3 to 4 days, and intake and output should be monitored. If plasma creatinine content rises above 3.5 mg/dL, amphotericin dosage should be reduced. As noted, the degree of renal damage is less with lipid-based amphotericin than with the conventional formulation.

Hypokalemia. Damage to the kidneys often causes hypokalemia. Potassium supplements may be needed to correct the problem. Potassium levels and serum creatinine should be monitored often.

Hematologic Effects. Amphotericin can cause bone marrow suppression, resulting in normocytic, normochromic anemia. Hematocrit determinations should be conducted to monitor red blood cell status.

Effects Associated With Intrathecal Injection. Intrathecal administration may cause nausea, vomiting, headache, and pain in the back, legs, and abdomen. Rare reactions include visual disturbances, impairment of hearing, and paresthesias (tingling, numbness, or pain in the hands and feet).

Safety Alert

AMPHOTERICIN

Infusion of amphotericin may be associated with delirium, hypotension, hypertension, wheezing, and hypoxia. Rarely, amphotericin causes rash, seizures, anaphylaxis, dysrhythmias, acute liver failure, and nephrogenic diabetes insipidus.

Drug Interactions

Nephrotoxic Drugs. The use of amphotericin with other nephrotoxic drugs (e.g., aminoglycosides, cyclosporine, NSAIDs) increases the risk of kidney damage. Accordingly, these combinations should be avoided if possible.

Flucytosine. Amphotericin potentiates the antifungal actions of flucytosine, apparently by enhancing flucytosine entry into fungi. Thanks to this interaction, combining flucytosine with low-dose amphotericin can produce antifungal effects equivalent to those of high-dose amphotericin alone. By allowing a reduction in amphotericin dosage, the combination can reduce the risk of amphotericin-induced toxicity. Preparations for amphotericin B and other antifungal drugs are located in Table 92.3.

Azoles

Like amphotericin B, the azoles are broad-spectrum antifungal drugs. As a result, azoles represent an alternative to amphotericin B for most systemic fungal infections. In contrast to amphotericin, which is highly toxic and must be given IV, the azoles have lower toxicity and can be given by mouth. However, azoles do have one disadvantage: They inhibit hepatic cytochrome P450 drug-metabolizing enzymes and can increase the levels of many other drugs. Of the 14 azoles in current use, only 6—itraconazole, ketoconazole, fluconazole, voriconazole, isavuconazole, and posaconazole—are indicated for systemic mycoses (Table 92.3). Azoles used for superficial mycoses are discussed separately later in this chapter.

Itraconazole

Itraconazole [Sporanox] is an alternative to amphotericin B for several systemic mycoses and will serve as our prototype for the azole family. The drug is safer than amphotericin B and has the added advantage of oral dosing. Principal adverse effects are cardiosuppression and liver injury. Like other azoles, itraconazole can inhibit drug-metabolizing enzymes and raise the levels of other drugs.

Prototype Drugs

ANTIFUNGAL AGENTS

Polyene Macrolides
Amphotericin B

Azoles
Itraconazole

Echinocandins
Caspofungin

Mechanism of Action. Itraconazole inhibits the synthesis of *ergosterol,* an essential component of the fungal cytoplasmic membrane. The result is increased membrane permeability and leakage of cellular components. Accumulation of ergosterol precursors may also contribute to antifungal actions. Itraconazole suppresses ergosterol synthesis by inhibiting fungal cytochrome P450–dependent enzymes.

Therapeutic Use. Itraconazole is active against a broad spectrum of fungal pathogens. At this time, it is a drug of choice for *blastomycosis, histoplasmosis, paracoccidioidomycosis,* and *sporotrichosis* and is an alternative to amphotericin B for *aspergillosis, candidiasis,* and *coccidioidomycosis.* Itraconazole may also be used for superficial mycoses.

Pharmacokinetics. Itraconazole is administered PO, in capsules or suspension. Food increases absorption of *capsules* but decreases absorption of *suspension.* Interestingly, administration with cola enhances absorption. Once absorbed, the drug is widely distributed to lipophilic tissues. Concentrations in aqueous fluids (e.g., saliva, CSF) are negligible. The drug undergoes extensive hepatic metabolism. About 40% of each dose is excreted in the urine as inactive metabolites.

Adverse Effects. Itraconazole is well tolerated in usual doses. Gastrointestinal reactions (nausea, vomiting, diarrhea) are most common. Other reactions include rash, headache, abdominal pain, and edema. Itraconazole may also cause two potentially serious effects: cardiac suppression and liver injury.

Cardiac Suppression. Itraconazole has negative inotropic actions that can cause a transient decrease in ventricular ejection fraction. Cardiac function returns to normal by 12 hours after dosing. Because of its negative inotropic actions, itraconazole should not be used for *superficial* fungal infections (dermatomycoses, onychomycosis) in patients with heart failure, a history of heart failure, or other indications of ventricular dysfunction. The drug may still be used to treat *serious* fungal infections in patients with heart failure, but only with careful monitoring and only if the benefits clearly outweigh the risks. If signs and symptoms of heart failure worsen, itraconazole should be stopped.

Liver Injury. Itraconazole has been associated with rare cases of liver failure, some of which were fatal. Although a causal link has not been established, caution is nonetheless advised. Patients should be informed about signs of liver impairment (persistent nausea, anorexia, fatigue, vomiting, right upper abdominal pain, jaundice, dark urine, pale stools); if they appear, patients should seek medical attention immediately.

Drug Interactions

Inhibition of Hepatic Drug Metabolizing Enzymes. Itraconazole inhibits CYP3A4 (the 3A4 isoenzyme of cytochrome P450) and thus can increase levels of many other drugs (Table 92.4). The most important are cisapride, pimozide, dofetilide, and quinidine. When present at high levels, these drugs can cause potentially fatal ventricular dysrhythmias. Accordingly,

TABLE 92.3 ■ Amphotericin B and the Azole Drugs

Drug	Therapeutic Uses	Availability	Usual Adult Dose	Pharmacokinetics	Adverse Effects
Amphotericin B [AmBisome, Amphotec, Abelcet, Fungizone ✦]	Blastomycosis, candidiasis, coccidioidomycosis, cryptococcosis, histoplasmosis, mucormycosis, paracoccidioidomycosis, sporotrichosis	Solution for IV injection	Initiation: 0.25 mg/kg/day Maintenance: 1.5-6 mg/kg/day	Metabolism: Largely unknown Elimination: Minimal renal	Nephrotoxicity, fever, chills, rigors, bone marrow suppression
Itraconazole [Sporanox]	Blastomycosis, histoplasmosis, paracoccidioidomycosis	100-mg capsules	200 mg 1–2 times daily	Metabolism: hepatic Elimination: urine	Cardiac suppression, liver injury
Fluconzaole [Diflucan]	Blastomycosis, candidiasis, histoplasmosis	50-, 100-, 150-, 200-mg tablets 10-mg and 40-mg/mL suspension Solution for IV injection	Oropharyngeal candidiasis, 100–200 mg PO/IV daily Esophageal candidiasis, 200–400 mg PO/IV daily Cryptococcal meningitis, 400 mg once, then 200 mg PO/IV daily	Metabolism: hepatic Elimination: urine	Nausea, headache, Stevens-Johnson syndrome
Voriconazole [Vfend]	Aspergillosis, candidiasis, histoplasmosis	50-, 200-mg tablets 40-mg/mL suspension Solution for IV injection	Aspergillosis: 6 mg/kg on day 1, followed by 4 mg/kg IV twice daily × 7 days, then 100 mg PO every 12 hr	Metabolism: hepatic Elimination: urine	Hepatotoxicity, visual disturbances, hypersensitivity reactions
Ketoconazole (generic only)	Systemic mycoses in patients not tolerant of amphotericin B	200-mg tablets	200–400 mg PO daily	Metabolism: hepatic Elimination: hepatic	Nausea, vomiting, hepatic necrosis (potentially fatal)
Posaconazole [Noxafil]	Aspergillosis, candidiasis	100-mg delayed-release tablets 40-mg/mL suspension Solution for IV injection	Oropharyngeal candidiasis, 100 mg PO daily Invasive fungal infections in immunocompromised patients, 300 mg IV daily	Metabolism: hepatic Elimination: fecal	Nausea, vomiting, headache, QT prolongation
Isavuconazole [Cresemba]	Aspergillosis, mucormycosis	186-mg capsules Solution for IV injection	372 mg PO/IV 3 times daily × 6 doses, then 372 mg PO/IV daily	Metabolism: hepatic Elimination: feces, urine	Hepatotoxicity, Stevens-Johnson syndrome, nausea, vomiting

concurrent use with itraconazole is contraindicated. Other drugs of concern include cyclosporine, digoxin, warfarin, and sulfonylurea-type oral hypoglycemics. In patients taking cyclosporine or digoxin, levels of these drugs should be monitored; in patients taking warfarin, prothrombin time should be monitored; and in patients taking sulfonylureas, blood glucose levels should be monitored.

Drugs That Raise Gastric pH. Drugs that decrease gastric acidity—antacids, histamine$_2$ (H_2) antagonists, and proton pump inhibitors—can greatly reduce absorption of oral itraconazole. Accordingly, these agents should be administered at least 1 hour before itraconazole or 2 hours after. (Since proton pump inhibitors have a prolonged duration of action, patients using these drugs may have insufficient stomach acid for itraconazole absorption, regardless of when the proton pump inhibitor is given.)

Echinocandins

The echinocandins (Table 92.5) are the newest class of antifungal drugs. In contrast to amphotericin B and the azoles, which disrupt the fungal *cell membrane*, the echinocandins disrupt the fungal *cell wall*. Echinocandins cannot be dosed orally, and their antifungal spectrum is narrow, being limited mainly to *Aspergillus* and *Candida* species. Three echinocandins are available: caspofungin, micafungin, and anidulafungin. When dosage is appropriate, all three appear therapeutically equivalent.

Caspofungin

Actions and Uses. Caspofungin [Cancidas] was the first echinocandin available. Antifungal effects result from inhibiting the biosynthesis of beta-1,3-D-glucan, an essential component of the cell wall of some fungi, including *Candida* and *Aspergillus.* Caspofungin is approved for IV therapy of (1) invasive aspergillosis in patients unresponsive to or intolerant of traditional agents (e.g., amphotericin B, itraconazole) and (2) systemic *Candida* infections, including candidemia and *Candida*-related peritonitis, pleural space infections, and intra-abdominal abscesses. The drug is better tolerated than amphotericin B and appears to be just as effective.

Pharmacokinetics. Caspofungin is not absorbed from the GI tract, and hence must be given parenterally (by IV infusion). In the blood, 97% of the drug is protein bound. Caspofungin is cleared from the blood with a half-life of 9 to 11 hours. The principal mechanism of plasma clearance is redistribution to tissues, not metabolism or excretion. Over time, the drug undergoes gradual metabolism followed by excretion in the urine and feces.

Adverse Effects. Caspofungin is generally well tolerated. The most common adverse effects are fever and phlebitis at the injection site. Less common reactions include headache, rash, nausea, and vomiting. In addition, caspofungin can cause effects that appear to be mediated by histamine release. Among these are rash, facial flushing, pruritus, and a sense of warmth. One case of anaphylaxis has been reported.

Use in Pregnancy. Caspofungin is embryotoxic in rats and rabbits. To date, there are no adequate data on effects in pregnant women. Currently, the drug is classified in FDA Pregnancy Risk Category C,[a] and hence should be avoided during pregnancy unless the potential benefits outweigh the potential risks to the fetus.

[a]As of 2020, the FDA will no longer use Pregnancy Risk Categories. Please refer to Chapter 9 for more information.

TABLE 92.4 ▪ Some Drugs Whose Levels Can Be Increased by Azole Antifungal Drugs

Target Drug	Class	Consequence of Excessive Level
Pimozide [Orap]	Antipsychotic	Fatal dysrhythmias
Dofetilide [Tikosyn]	Antidysrhythmic	Fatal dysrhythmias
Quinidine	Antidysrhythmic	Fatal dysrhythmias
Warfarin [Coumadin]	Anticoagulant	Bleeding
Sulfonylureas	Oral hypoglycemic	Hypoglycemia
Phenytoin [Dilantin]	Antiseizure drug	Central nervous system toxicity
Cyclosporine [Sandimmune]	Immunosuppressant	Increased nephrotoxicity
Tacrolimus [Prograf]	Immunosuppressant	Increased nephrotoxicity
Lovastatin [Mevacor]	Antihyperlipidemic	Rhabdomyolysis
Simvastatin [Zocor]	Antihyperlipidemic	Rhabdomyolysis
Eletriptan [Relpax]	Antimigraine	Coronary vasospasm
Fentanyl [Duragesic, others]	Opioid analgesic	Fatal respiratory depression
Calcium channel blockers	Antihypertensive, antianginal	Cardiosuppression

PATIENT-CENTERED CARE ACROSS THE LIFE SPAN

Antifungal Agents

Life Stage	Patient Care Concerns
Infants	Nystatin is used to treat oral candidiasis in premature and full-term infants. Fluconazole is also used safely to treat systemic candidiasis in newborn infants.
Children/ adolescents	Many antifungal agents are used safely in children in lower doses. Side effect profiles are similar to those of adults.
Pregnant women	Many of the azole antifungals are classified in FDA Pregnancy Risk Category C or D.[a] Risks and benefits must be considered for administration during pregnancy.
Breast-feeding women	Data are lacking regarding most antifungals and breast-feeding. Most antifungals are considered safe in lower doses. The exception to this is ketoconazole. Because it has high potential for hepatotoxicity, it should be avoided in breast-feeding women.
Older adults	Older adults have a higher risk of achlorhydria than do younger individuals; as a result, older patients may not predictably absorb some antifungal agents. In addition, common drugs prescribed to older adults, including warfarin, phenytoin, and oral hypoglycemic agents, are increased by azoles.

[a]As of 2020, the FDA will no longer use Pregnancy Risk Categories. Please refer to Chapter 9 for more information.

TABLE 92.5 ▪ The Echinocandins

Drug	Therapeutic Uses	Availability	Usual Adult Dosing	Pharmacokinetics	Adverse Effects
Caspofungin [Cancidas]	Aspergillosis, candidiasis	Solution for IV injection	70 mg IV × 1 then 50 mg daily	Metabolism: minimal; redistributes to tissues Elimination: urine, feces	Fever, phlebitis at injection site
Micafungin [Mycamine]	Candidiasis	Solution for IV injection	100 mg IV daily	Metabolism: hepatic Elimination: feces	Headache, nausea, vomiting, phlebitis at injection site
Anidulafungin [Eraxis]	Candidiasis	Solution for IV injection	100–200 mg IV daily	Metabolism: chemical degradation Elimination: feces	Diarrhea, hypokalemia, histamine-mediated infusion reactions

Drug Interactions. Drugs that induce cytochrome P450 may decrease levels of caspofungin. Powerful inducers include efavirenz, nelfinavir, rifampin, carbamazepine, dexamethasone, and phenytoin. Patients taking these drugs may need to increase their caspofungin dosage.

Caspofungin can decrease levels of tacrolimus [Prograf], an immunosuppressant. If these drugs are taken concurrently, levels of tacrolimus should be monitored and the dosage increased as needed.

Combining caspofungin with cyclosporine [Sandimmune, others] increases the risk of liver injury, as evidenced by a transient elevation in plasma levels of liver enzyme. Accordingly, the combination should generally be avoided.

Flucytosine, a Pyrimidine Analog

Flucytosine [Ancobon], a pyrimidine analog, is employed for serious infections caused by susceptible strains of *Candida* and *C. neoformans.* Because development of resistance is common, flucytosine is almost always used in combination with amphotericin B. Extreme caution is needed in patients with renal impairment and hematologic disorders.

Mechanism of Action

Flucytosine is taken up by fungal cells, which then convert it to 5-fluorouracil (5-FU), a powerful antimetabolite. The ultimate effect is disruption of fungal DNA and RNA synthesis. Flucytosine is relatively harmless to us because mammalian cells lack cytosine deaminase, the enzyme that converts flucytosine to 5-FU.

Fungal Resistance

Development of resistance during therapy is common and constitutes a serious clinical problem. Several mechanisms have been described, including (1) a reduction in cytosine permease (needed for fungal uptake of flucytosine) and (2) loss of cytosine deaminase (needed to convert flucytosine to its active form).

Antifungal Spectrum and Therapeutic Uses

Flucytosine has a narrow antifungal spectrum. Fungicidal activity is highest against *Candida* species and *C. neoformans.* Most other fungi are resistant. Because of this narrow spectrum, flucytosine is indicated only for candidiasis and cryptococcosis. For the treatment of serious infections (e.g., cryptococcal meningitis, systemic candidiasis), flucytosine should be combined with amphotericin B. This combination offers two advantages over flucytosine alone: (1) Antifungal activity is enhanced, and (2) emergence of resistant fungi is reduced.

Pharmacokinetics

Flucytosine is readily absorbed from the GI tract and is well distributed throughout the body. The drug has good access to the central nervous system; levels in the CSF are about 80% of those in plasma. Flucytosine is eliminated by the kidneys, principally as unchanged drug. The half-life is about 4 hours in patients with normal renal function. However, in patients with renal insufficiency, the half-life is greatly prolonged, and hence dosage must be reduced.

Adverse Effects

Hematologic Effects. Bone marrow suppression is the most serious complication of treatment. Marrow suppression usually manifests as reversible neutropenia or thrombocytopenia. Rarely, fatal agranulocytosis develops. Platelet and leukocyte counts should be determined weekly. Adverse hematologic effects are most likely when plasma levels of flucytosine exceed 100 mcg/mL. Accordingly, the dosage should be adjusted to keep drug levels below this value. Flucytosine should be used with caution in patients with pre-existing bone marrow suppression.

Hepatotoxicity. Mild and reversible liver dysfunction occurs frequently, but severe hepatic injury is rare. Liver function should be monitored (by making weekly determinations of serum transaminase and alkaline phosphatase levels).

Drug Interactions

Flucytosine is often combined with *amphotericin B.* As noted, this combination offers several advantages. However, the combination can also be detrimental. Since amphotericin B is nephrotoxic and since flucytosine is eliminated by the kidneys, amphotericin B–induced kidney damage may suppress flucytosine excretion, promoting flucytosine toxicity. Therefore *it is important to monitor renal function and flucytosine levels when amphotericin B and flucytosine are combined.*

Like itraconazole, flucytosine inhibits hepatic drug-metabolizing enzymes and can raise levels of several other drugs. With at least four drugs—*cisapride, pimozide, dofetilide,* and *quinidine*—elevated levels can lead to potentially fatal dysrhythmias. Accordingly, flucytosine must not be combined with these drugs.

Preparations, Dosage, and Administration

Flucytosine [Ancobon] is available in 250- and 500-mg oral capsules. The usual dosage for patients with normal kidney function is 50 to 150 mg/kg/day administered in four divided doses at 6-hour intervals. At this dosage, some patients must ingest 10 or more capsules 4 times a day. Dosages must be reduced for patients with renal insufficiency. Nausea and vomiting associated with drug administration can be decreased by swallowing the capsules over a 15-minute interval.

DRUGS FOR SUPERFICIAL MYCOSES

The superficial mycoses are caused by two groups of organisms: (1) *Candida* species and (2) dermatophytes (species of *Epidermophyton, Trichophyton,* and *Microsporum*). *Candida* infections usually occur in mucous membranes and moist skin; chronic infections may involve the scalp, skin, and nails. Dermatophytoses are generally confined to the skin, hair, and nails. Superficial infections with dermatophytes are more common than superficial infections with *Candida.*

Overview of Drug Therapy

Superficial mycoses can be treated with a variety of topical and oral drugs. For mild to moderate infections, topical agents are generally preferred. Specific indications for the drugs used against superficial mycoses are shown in Table 92.6. Some of these drugs are also used for systemic mycoses.

Dermatophytic Infections (Ringworm)

Dermatophytic infections are commonly referred to as *ringworm* (because of the characteristic ring-shaped lesions). There are four principal dermatophytic infections, defined by their location: *tinea pedis* (ringworm of the foot, or "athlete's foot"), *tinea corporis* (ringworm of the body), *tinea cruris* (ringworm of the groin, or "jock itch"), and *tinea capitis* (ringworm of the scalp).

Tinea Pedis. Tinea pedis, the most common fungal infection, generally responds well to topical therapy. Patients should be advised to wear absorbent cotton socks, change their shoes often, and dry their feet after bathing.

Tinea Corporis. Tinea corporis usually responds to a topical azole or allylamine. Treatment should continue for at least 1 week after symptoms have cleared. Severe infection may require a systemic antifungal agent (e.g., griseofulvin).

Tinea Cruris. Tinea cruris responds well to topical therapy. Treatment should continue for at least 1 week after symptoms have cleared. If the infection is severely inflamed, a systemic antifungal drug (e.g., clotrimazole) may be needed; topical or systemic glucocorticoids may be needed as well.

Tinea Capitis. Tinea capitis is difficult to treat. Topical drugs are not likely to work. Oral griseofulvin, taken for 6 to

TABLE 92.6 ▪ Drugs for Superficial Fungal Infections

				Candida Infection			
Drug	**Route**	**Availability**	**Ringworm**[a]	**Skin**	**Mouth**	**Vulvovaginal**	**Onychomycosis**[b]
AZOLES							
Butoconazole [Gynazole-1]	Topical	2% vaginal cream				✔	
Clotrimazole [Desenex, Lotrimin, Gyne-Lotrimin]	Topical	1% cream 2% powder 100-, 200-mg vaginal tablets 2% vaginal cream	✔	✔	✔	✔	
Econazole [Ecoza]	Topical	1% foam 1% cream	✔	✔			
Fluconazole [Diflucan]	Oral	50-, 100-, 150-, 200-mg tablets 10-mg/mL and 40-mg/mL suspension	✔		✔	✔	✔
Itraconazole [Sporanox]	Oral	100-mg capsules	✔				✔
Ketoconazole [Nizoral, Xolgel, Extina]	Oral Topical	200-mg tablets 2% shampoo 2% gel 2% foam	✔ ✔	✔	✔		✔
Miconazole [Monistat 1, Monistat 3, Monistat 7, Micatin]	Topical	200-, 1200-mg vaginal ovules 100-mg vaginal cream 2% topical skin cream	✔	✔		✔	
Oxiconazole [Oxistat]	Topical	1% cream 1% lotion	✔				
Sertaconazole [Ertaczo]	Topical	2% cream	✔				
Sulconazole [Exelderm]	Topical	1% cream 1% solution	✔				
Terconazole [Terazol 3, Terazol 7]	Topical	80-mg vaginal suppository 0.4% and 0.8% vaginal cream				✔	
Tioconazole [Monistat 1]	Topical	6.5% vaginal ointment				✔	
ALLYLAMINES							
Butenafine [Lotrimin Ultra Cream]	Topical	1% cream	✔				
Naftifine [Naftin]	Topical	1% and 2% cream 2% gel	✔				
Terbinafine [Lamisil, Lamisil AT]	Oral Topical	250-mg tablets 1% spray 1% gel 1% powder 1% cream	✔ ✔				✔
OTHERS							
Ciclopirox [Loprox, Penlac Nail Lacquer]	Topical	1% shampoo 0.77% cream, gel, suspension	✔	✔			✔
Griseofulvin [Gris-PEG]	Oral	125- and 250-mg ultra-microcrystalline tablets 500-mg microcrystalline tablets 125 mg/5 mL solution	✔				✔
Nystatin [Mycostatin 🍁]	Topical	100,000 units/gm cream, powder, and ointment 100,000-unit vaginal tablets		✔	✔	✔	
Tolnaftate [Tinactin]	Topical	1% spray, cream, powder, solution	✔				
Undecylenate [Fungi-Nail]	Topical	25% solution	✔				

[a]*Ringworm* is a popular term for dermatophytic infections, including tinea pedis, tinea cruris, tinea corporis, and tinea capitis.
[b]*Onychomycosis* is a clinical term for fungal infection of the toenails and fingernails.

8 weeks, is considered standard therapy. However, oral terbinafine, taken for only 2 to 4 weeks, may be more effective.

Candidiasis

Vulvovaginal Candidiasis. Vulvovaginal candidiasis is very common, occurring in 75% of women at least once in their lives. Most cases are caused by *Candida albicans,* and many of the rest are caused by *Candida glabrata,* especially in patients with HIV/AIDS. Factors that predispose to *Candida* infection include pregnancy, obesity, diabetes, debilitation, HIV infection, and the use of certain drugs, including oral contraceptives, systemic glucocorticoids, anticancer agents, immunosuppressants, and systemic antibiotics. With current drugs, just 1 or 3 days of *topical* therapy can be curative. In addition, *oral* therapy may be used: A single 150-mg dose of fluconazole can be curative—but it causes more side effects (headache, rash, GI disturbance) than topical agents. For women with recurrent vulvovaginal candidiasis, weekly prophylaxis with oral fluconazole is highly effective—but relapse is common when treatment is stopped. Major drugs for uncomplicated vulvovaginal candidiasis are shown in Table 92.6. All appear equally effective, so drug selection is based largely on patient preference. Longer regimens have no demonstrated advantage over shorter ones.

Oral Candidiasis. Oral candidiasis, also known as *thrush,* is seen often. Topical agents—*nystatin, clotrimazole,* and *miconazole*—are generally effective. In the immunocompromised host, oral therapy with *fluconazole* or *ketoconazole* is usually required.

Onychomycosis (Fungal Infection of the Nails)

Fungal infection of the nails, known as onychomycosis, is difficult to eradicate and requires prolonged treatment. Infections may be caused by dermatophytes or *Candida* species. Because onychomycosis is largely a cosmetic concern, treatment is usually optional.

Onychomycosis may be treated with oral antifungal drugs or with topical ciclopirox. Success rates with oral therapy are quite low, and rates with topical therapy are even lower.

Oral Therapy. The drugs used most often are *terbinafine* [Lamisil] and *itraconazole* [Sporanox]. Both are active against *Candida* species and dermatophytes. Once in the body, these drugs become incorporated into keratin as the nails grow. Drug may also diffuse into the nails from the tissue below. Side effects include headache, GI disturbances (e.g., nausea, vomiting, abdominal pain), and skin reactions (e.g., itching, rash). Treatment generally lasts 3 to 6 months. Unfortunately, even with this prolonged therapy, the cure rate is relatively low (about 50%).

Topical Therapy With Ciclopirox. *Ciclopirox* [Penlac Nail Lacquer] is the only topical agent for onychomycosis available in the United States. In contrast to oral terbinafine or itraconazole, which are active against *Candida* species and several dermatophytes, topical ciclopirox is active against only one dermatophyte—*Trichophyton rubrum*—and has no activity against *Candida.* Ciclopirox is applied once a day to the nails and immediately adjacent skin. New coats are applied over old ones. Once a week, all coats are removed with alcohol. Side effects are minimal and localized. Unfortunately, despite prolonged use (up to 48 weeks), ciclopirox confers only modest benefits: Complete cure occurs in less than 12% of patients, and even when complete cure *does* occur, the recurrence rate is high—about 40%. Compared with oral therapy, topical ciclopirox is safer and cheaper, but much less effective.

Use of ciclopirox for superficial fungal infections of the *skin* is discussed later in this chapter.

Azoles

Twelve members of the azole family are used for superficial mycoses (see Table 92.6). The usual route is topical. Three of the 12—itraconazole, fluconazole, and ketoconazole—are also used for systemic mycoses (see earlier in this chapter).

The azoles are active against a broad spectrum of pathogenic fungi, including dermatophytes and *Candida* species. Antifungal effects result from inhibiting the biosynthesis of ergosterol, an essential component of the fungal cytoplasmic membrane.

Clotrimazole

Therapeutic Uses. Topical clotrimazole is a drug of choice for dermatophytic infections and candidiasis of the skin, mouth, and vagina.

Adverse Effects. When applied to the skin, clotrimazole can cause stinging, erythema, edema, urticaria, pruritus, and peeling. However, the incidence is low. Intravaginal administration occasionally causes a burning sensation and lower abdominal cramps. Oral clotrimazole can cause GI distress.

Griseofulvin

Griseofulvin [Gris-PEG] is administered orally to treat superficial mycoses. The drug is inactive against organisms that cause systemic mycoses.

Mechanism of Action

Following absorption, griseofulvin is deposited in the keratin precursor cells of skin, hair, and nails. Because griseofulvin is present, newly formed keratin is resistant to fungal invasion. Hence, as infected keratin is shed, it is replaced by fungus-free tissue.

Griseofulvin kills fungi by inhibiting fungal mitosis by binding to components of microtubules, the structures that form the mitotic spindle. Because griseofulvin acts by disrupting mitosis, the drug affects only fungi that are actively growing.

Pharmacokinetics

Administration is oral, and absorption can be enhanced by dosing with a fatty meal. As noted, griseofulvin is deposited in the keratin precursor cells of skin, hair, and nails. Elimination is by hepatic metabolism and renal excretion.

Therapeutic Uses

Griseofulvin is employed orally to treat dermatophytic infections of the skin, hair, and nails. The drug is not active against *Candida* species, nor is it useful against systemic mycoses. Dermatophytic infections of the skin respond relatively quickly (in 3 to 8 weeks). However, infections of the palms may require 2 to 3 months of treatment, and a year or more may be needed to eliminate infections of the toenails.

Adverse Effects

Most untoward effects are not serious. Transient headache is common. Other mild reactions include rash, insomnia, tiredness, and GI effects (nausea, vomiting, diarrhea). Griseofulvin may cause hepatotoxicity and photosensitivity in patients with porphyria. The drug is contraindicated for individuals with a history of porphyria or hepatocellular disease.

Drug Interactions

Griseofulvin induces hepatic drug-metabolizing enzymes and can decrease the effects of *warfarin.* When this combination is used, the dosage of warfarin may need to be increased.

Preparations, Dosage, and Administration

Griseofulvin is formulated in a solution (125 mg/5 mL) and in two particle sizes: microsized and ultra-microsized. The microcrystalline form is supplied in 500-mg tablets and a 125 mg/5 mL solution. The ultra-microcrystalline form [Gris-PEG] is supplied in tablets (125 and 250 mg).

Dosage depends to some degree upon the formulation (microsized or ultra-microsized). With microsized formulations, the usual adult dosage is 500 mg to 1 gm/day, and the usual pediatric dosage is 11 mg/kg/day. The ultra-microsized particles are better absorbed than the microsized particles, and hence doses of ultra-microcrystalline griseofulvin are about 30% lower than doses of microcrystalline griseofulvin.

Polyene Antibiotics

Nystatin

Actions, Uses, and Adverse Effects. Nystatin [Mycostatin ♣] is a polyene antibiotic used only for candidiasis. Nystatin is the drug of choice for intestinal candidiasis and is also employed to treat candidal infections of the skin, mouth, esophagus, and vagina. Nystatin can be administered orally and topically. There is no significant absorption from either route. Oral nystatin occasionally causes GI disturbance (nausea, vomiting, diarrhea). Topical application may produce local irritation.

Preparations, Dosage, and Administration. For oral administration, nystatin is supplied as a suspension and in tablets and lozenges; dosages range from 400,000 to 1 million units 3 to 4 times a day. Vaginal tablets are employed for vaginal candidiasis; the usual dosage is 100,000 units once a day for 2 weeks. Nystatin is supplied as a cream, ointment, and powder to treat candidiasis of the skin. The cream and ointment formulations are applied twice daily; the powder is applied 3 times daily.

Allylamines

Terbinafine

Actions and Uses. Terbinafine [Lamisil] works through inhibition of squalene epoxidase with resultant inhibition of ergosterol synthesis. The drug is highly active against dermatophytes and less active against *Candida* species. Terbinafine is available in topical and oral formulations. Topical therapy is used for ringworm infections (e.g., tinea corporis, tinea cruris, tinea pedis). Oral therapy is used for ringworm and onychomycosis (fungal infection of the nails).

Adverse Effects. Adverse effects with *topical* terbinafine are minimal. The discussion that follows applies to *oral* therapy. The most common side effects are headache, diarrhea, dyspepsia, and abdominal pain. Oral terbinafine may also cause skin reactions and disturbance of taste. Of much greater concern, terbinafine may pose a risk of *liver failure.* Some terbinafine users have died of liver failure, and other have required a liver transplant. However, a causal link has not been established. Nonetheless, caution is advised. Baseline tests for serum alanine and aspartate aminotransferases are recommended. In addition, patients should be informed about signs of liver dysfunction (persistent nausea, anorexia, fatigue, vomiting, jaundice, right upper abdominal pain, dark urine, pale stools), and if they appear, patients should discontinue terbinafine immediately and undergo evaluation of liver function. Terbinafine is not recommended for patients with pre-existing liver disease.

Preparations, Dosage, and Administration. Terbinafine for oral therapy is available in tablets (250 mg). The oral dosage for nail infections is 250 mg/day for 6 to 12 weeks, and the dosage for ringworm is 250 mg/day for 2 to 6 weeks. Terbinafine for topical therapy is available as a gel, spray, powder, and cream, all with a strength of 1%. Application is done once or twice daily for 1 to 4 weeks.

Other Drugs for Superficial Mycoses

Tolnaftate

Tolnaftate [Tinactin, others] is employed topically to treat a variety of superficial mycoses. The drug is active against dermatophytes, but not against *Candida* species. The mechanism of antifungal action is unknown. Adverse effects (sensitization, irritation) are extremely rare. Tolnaftate is available in several formulations. Creams, powders, and solutions are most effective; powders are used adjunctively. The drug is applied twice daily for 2 to 4 weeks.

Undecylenic Acid

Undecylenic acid [Fungi-Nail, others] is a topical agent used to treat superficial mycoses. The drug is active against dermatophytes but not *Candida* species. Its major indication is tinea pedis (athlete's foot). However, other drugs (tolnaftate, the azoles) are more effective.

Ciclopirox

Ciclopirox [Loprox, Penlac Nail Lacquer] is a broad-spectrum, topical antifungal drug. Benefits derive from chelating iron and aluminum present in metal-dependent enzymes that protect fungi from peroxides. Ciclopirox is used for infections of the skin (discussed here) and for infections of the fingernails and toenails (discussed earlier under *Onychomycosis*). The formulations used for skin infections are marketed as *Loprox.* The formulation used for nail infections is marketed as *Penlac Nail Lacquer.*

When applied to the skin, ciclopirox is active against dermatophytes and *Candida* species. The drug is effective against superficial candidiasis and tinea pedis, tinea cruris, and tinea corporis. Ciclopirox penetrates the epidermis to the dermis, but systemic absorption is minimal, and hence no significant systemic accumulation occurs. There is no toxicity from local application. For the treatment of skin infections, ciclopirox is available as a 1% shampoo and as a 0.77% cream, gel, and suspension. The shampoo is used twice weekly for 4 weeks. The cream, gel, and suspension are applied twice daily for 2 to 4 weeks.

KEY POINTS

- Amphotericin B is a drug of choice for most systemic mycoses, despite its potential for serious harm.
- Amphotericin B binds to ergosterol in the fungal cell membrane, making the membrane more permeable. The resultant leakage of intracellular cations reduces viability.
- Much of the toxicity of amphotericin B results from binding to cholesterol in host cell membranes.
- Because absorption of oral amphotericin B is poor, treatment of systemic mycoses requires intravenous administration.
- Amphotericin B infusion frequently causes fever, chills, rigors, nausea, and headache. Pretreatment with diphenhydramine plus an analgesic can reduce mild symptoms. A glucocorticoid can be used for severe reactions. Meperidine or dantrolene can reduce rigors.
- Amphotericin B causes renal injury in most patients. Kidney damage can be minimized by infusing 1 L of saline on the days amphotericin is infused.
- If possible, amphotericin B should not be combined with other nephrotoxic drugs.

- Itraconazole is active against a broad spectrum of fungi.
- Itraconazole inhibits cytochrome P450, inhibiting synthesis of ergosterol, an essential component of the fungal cell membrane. Cell membrane permeability increases, causing cellular components to leak out.
- Itraconazole is an alternative to IV amphotericin for many fungal infections. Advantages are lower toxicity and oral dosing.
- Itraconazole has two major adverse effects: cardiosuppression and liver damage.
- Itraconazole inhibits CYP3A4 and can raise the levels of many drugs. High levels of cisapride, pimozide, dofetilide, and quinidine can cause fatal dysrhythmias, so using these drugs with itraconazole is contraindicated.
- Drugs that reduce gastric acidity can greatly reduce absorption of itraconazole.
- Topical clotrimazole is a drug of choice for many superficial mycoses caused by dermatophytes and *Candida* species.
- Onychomycosis is difficult to treat and requires prolonged therapy. Oral therapy with terbinafine or itraconazole is the preferred treatment.
- Vulvovaginal candidiasis can be treated with a single oral dose of fluconazole or with short-term topical therapy (e.g., one 1200-mg miconazole vaginal suppository).

Please visit **http://evolve.elsevier.com/Lehne** for chapter-specific NCLEX® examination review questions.

Summary of Major Nursing Implications[a]

The implications here pertain only to the use of antifungal drugs against *systemic* mycoses.

AMPHOTERICIN B

Preadministration Assessment

Therapeutic Goal

Treatment of progressive and potentially fatal systemic fungal infections. Flucytosine may be given to enhance therapeutic effects.

Identifying High-Risk Patients

When used as it should be (i.e., for life-threatening infections), amphotericin has no contraindications.

Implementation: Administration

Routes

Intravenous, intrathecal.

Intravenous Administration

Use aseptic technique when preparing infusion solutions. Infuse slowly (over 2 to 4 hours). Check the solution periodically for a precipitate; if one forms, discontinue the infusion immediately. Therapy lasts several months; rotate the infusion site to reduce phlebitis and ensure availability of a usable vein. Dosage must be individualized. Alternate-day dosing may be ordered to reduce adverse effects.

Ongoing Evaluation and Interventions

Minimizing Adverse Effects

General Considerations. Amphotericin B can produce serious adverse effects. The patient should be under close supervision, preferably in a hospital.

Infusion Reactions. Amphotericin can cause fever, chills, rigors, nausea, and headache. Pretreatment with diphenhydramine plus acetaminophen can minimize these reactions. Give meperidine or dantrolene for rigors. If other measures fail, give hydrocortisone to suppress symptoms. Rotate the infusion site to minimize phlebitis. Infusion reactions can be reduced by using a lipid-based formulation rather than conventional amphotericin.

Nephrotoxicity. Almost all patients experience renal impairment. Monitor and record intake and output. Test kidney function every 3 to 4 days; if plasma creatinine content rises above 3.5 mg/dL, amphotericin dosage should be reduced. To reduce the risk of renal damage, infuse 1 L of saline on the days when amphotericin is given, avoid other nephrotoxic drugs (e.g., aminoglycosides, cyclosporine, NSAIDs), and use a lipid-based formulation instead of conventional amphotericin.

Hypokalemia. Renal injury may cause hypokalemia. Measure serum potassium often. Correct hypokalemia with potassium supplements.

Hematologic Effects. Normocytic, normochromic anemia has occurred secondary to amphotericin-induced suppression of bone marrow. Hematocrit determinations should be performed to monitor for this anemia.

Minimizing Adverse Interactions

Nephrotoxic Drugs. Unless clearly required, amphotericin should not be combined with other nephrotoxic drugs, including aminoglycosides, cyclosporine, and NSAIDs.

ITRACONAZOLE

Preadministration Assessment

Therapeutic Goal

Treatment of systemic and superficial mycoses.

Baseline Data

Assess for heart disease or a history thereof. The prescriber may order baseline tests of liver function.

Identifying High-Risk Patients. Itraconazole is *contraindicated* for patients taking pimozide, quinidine, dofetilide, or cisapride.

Use with *great caution,* if at all, in patients with cardiac disease, significant pulmonary disease, active liver disease, or a history of liver injury with other drugs.

Continued

Summary of Major Nursing Implications[a]—cont'd

Implementation: Administration

Route

Oral.

Administration

Advise patients to take itraconazole capsules with food and/or a cola beverage to enhance absorption.

Advise patients using antacids and other drugs that reduce gastric acidity to take them at least 1 hour before itraconazole or 2 hours after.

Ongoing Evaluation and Interventions

Minimizing Adverse Effects

Liver Injury. Rarely, itraconazole has been associated with fatal liver failure. If signs of liver injury appear, discontinue itraconazole and obtain tests of liver function. **Inform patients about signs of liver dysfunction (persistent nausea, anorexia, fatigue, vomiting, right upper abdominal pain, jaundice, dark urine, pale stools), and instruct them to notify the prescriber if these occur.**

Cardiac Suppression. Itraconazole can suppress ventricular function, posing a risk of heart failure. Monitor for signs and symptoms of heart failure, and discontinue itraconazole if they develop. **Inform patients about signs of heart failure (fatigue, cough, dyspnea, edema, jugular distention), and instruct them to seek immediate medical attention if they occur.**

Minimizing Adverse Interactions

Pimozide, Quinidine, Dofetilide, and Cisapride. By inhibiting CYP3A4, itraconazole can raise the levels of these drugs, posing a risk of fatal dysrhythmias. Accordingly, concurrent use of these drugs with itraconazole is contraindicated.

Cyclosporine, Digoxin, Warfarin, and Sulfonylureas. By inhibiting CYP3A4, itraconazole can raise levels of these drugs. Monitor cyclosporine and digoxin blood levels. Monitor prothrombin time in patients taking warfarin. Monitor blood glucose in patients taking a sulfonylurea.

Drugs That Raise Gastric pH. Antacids, H_2 antagonists, proton pump inhibitors, and other drugs that decrease gastric acidity can reduce itraconazole absorption. **Advise patients using these agents to take them at least 1 hour before itraconazole or 2 hours after.**

FLUCYTOSINE

Preadministration Assessment

Therapeutic Goal

Treatment of serious infections caused by *Candida* species and *Cryptococcus neoformans.* Flucytosine is usually combined with amphotericin B.

Baseline Data

Obtain baseline tests of renal function, hematologic status, and serum electrolytes.

Identifying High-Risk Patients

Use with *extreme caution* in patients with kidney disease or bone marrow suppression.

Implementation: Administration

Route

Oral.

Dosage and Administration

Treatment may require ingesting 10 or more capsules 4 times a day. **Advise patients to take capsules a few at a time over a 15-minute interval to minimize nausea and vomiting.** Dosage must be reduced in patients with renal impairment.

Ongoing Evaluation and Interventions

Monitoring Summary

Obtain weekly tests of liver function (serum transaminase and alkaline phosphatase levels) and hematologic status (leukocyte counts). In patients receiving amphotericin B concurrently and in those with pre-existing renal impairment, monitor kidney function and flucytosine levels.

Minimizing Adverse Effects

Hematologic Effects. Flucytosine-induced bone marrow suppression can cause neutropenia, thrombocytopenia, and fatal agranulocytosis. Risk can be minimized by adjusting the dosage to keep plasma flucytosine levels below 100 mcg/mL. Obtain weekly leukocyte counts to monitor hematologic effects.

Hepatotoxicity. Mild and reversible liver dysfunction occurs frequently; severe hepatic damage is rare. Obtain weekly determinations of serum transaminase and alkaline phosphatase levels to evaluate liver function.

Minimizing Adverse Interactions

Amphotericin B. Kidney damage from amphotericin B may decrease flucytosine excretion, increasing toxicity from flucytosine accumulation. When these drugs are combined, renal function and flucytosine levels must be monitored.

[a]Patient education information is highlighted as **blue text.**

CHAPTER

93 Antiviral Agents I: Drugs for Non-HIV Viral Infections

Antiviral drugs are discussed in this chapter and in Chapter 94. Here, we consider drugs used to treat infections caused by viruses other than human immunodeficiency virus (HIV). In Chapter 94, we consider drugs used against HIV infection. Drugs for non-HIV infections are shown in Table 93.1.

Although antiviral therapy has made significant advances, our ability to treat viral infections remains limited. Compared with the dramatic advances made in antibacterial therapy over the past half-century, efforts to develop safe and effective antiviral drugs have been less successful. A major reason for this lack of success resides in the process of viral replication: Viruses are obligate intracellular parasites that use the biochemical machinery of host cells to reproduce. Because the viral growth cycle employs host-cell enzymes and substrates, it is difficult to suppress viral replication without doing significant harm to the host. The antiviral drugs used clinically act by suppressing biochemical processes unique to viral reproduction. As our knowledge of viral molecular biology expands, additional virus-specific processes will be discovered, giving us new targets for drugs.

DRUGS FOR INFECTION WITH HERPES SIMPLEX VIRUSES AND VARICELLA-ZOSTER VIRUS

Herpes simplex virus (HSV) and *varicella-zoster virus* (VZV) are members of the herpesvirus group. HSV causes infection of the genitalia, mouth, face, and other sites. VZV is the cause of *varicella* (chickenpox) and *herpes zoster* (shingles), a painful condition resulting from reactivation of VZV that had been dormant within sensory nerve roots. Both conditions are discussed in Chapter 68, along with the vaccine used to prevent chickenpox. Drugs for infection with HSV and VZV are shown in Table 93.2. Genital herpes is discussed in Chapter 95.

Acyclovir

Acyclovir [Zovirax] is the agent of first choice for most infections caused by HSV and VZV. The drug can be administered topically, orally, and intravenously. Serious side effects are uncommon.

TABLE 93.1 ▪ Major Drugs for Non-HIV Viral Infections

Drug	Antiviral Spectrum
DRUGS FOR HERPES SIMPLEX VIRUS AND VARICELLA-ZOSTER VIRUS INFECTIONS	
Systemic Drugs	
Acyclovir	HSV, VZV
Famciclovir	HSV, VZV
Foscarnet	HSV, VZV
Valacyclovir	HSV, VZV
Topical Drugs	
Vidarabine	HSV, VZV
Penciclovir	HSV
Trifluridine	HSV keratitis
Docosanol	HSV keratitis
Ganciclovir	HSV keratitis
DRUGS FOR CYTOMEGALOVIRUS INFECTION	
Ganciclovir	CMV
Valganciclovir	CMV
Cidofovir	CMV
Foscarnet	CMV
DRUGS FOR INFLUENZA	
Oseltamivir	Influenza A and B
Zanamivir	Influenza A and B
DRUGS FOR RESPIRATORY SYNCYTIAL VIRUS INFECTION	
Ribavirin (inhaled)	RSV
Palivizumab	RSV
DRUGS FOR HEPATITIS	
Alfa Interferons	
Interferon alfa-2b	HCV, HBV
Interferon alfacon-1	HCV
Peginterferon alfa-2a	HCV, HBV
Peginterferon alfa-2b	HCV
Protease Inhibitors	
Grazoprevir	HCV
Paritaprevir	HCV
Simprevir	HCV
NS5A Inhibitors	
Declatasvir	HCV
Elbasvir	HCV
Ledipasvir	HCV
Ombitasvir	HCV
NS5B Nucleoside Polymerase Inhibitors (NPIs)	
Sofosbuvir	HCV
NS5B Non-Nucleoside Polymerase Inhibitors (NNPIs)	
Dasabuvir	HCV
Nucleoside Analogs	
Ribavirin (oral)	HCV
Adefovir	HBV[a]
Entecavir	HBV[a]
Lamivudine	HBV[a]
Telbivudine	HBV
Tenofovir	HBV[a]

[a]Also active against HIV.

CMV, Cytomegalovirus; *HBV,* hepatitis B virus; *HCV,* hepatitis C virus; *HSV,* herpes simplex virus; *RSV,* respiratory syncytial virus; *VZV,* varicella-zoster virus.

Antiviral Spectrum

Acyclovir is active only against members of the herpesvirus family, a group that includes *herpes simplex viruses, varicella-zoster virus,* and *cytomegalovirus* (CMV). Of these, HSVs are most sensitive, VZV is moderately sensitive, and most strains of CMV are resistant.

Mechanism of Action

Acyclovir inhibits viral replication by suppressing synthesis of viral DNA. To exert antiviral effects, acyclovir must first undergo activation. The critical step in activation is conversion of acyclovir to acyclo-guanosine monophosphate (GMP) by *thymidine kinase.* Acyclo-GMP is then converted to acyclo-guanosine triphosphate (GTP), the compound directly responsible for inhibiting DNA synthesis. Acyclo-GTP suppresses DNA synthesis by (1) inhibiting viral DNA polymerase and (2) becoming incorporated into the growing strand of viral DNA, which blocks further strand growth.

The selectivity of acyclovir is based in large part on the ability of certain viruses to activate the drug. HSVs are especially sensitive to acyclovir because the drug is a much better substrate for thymidine kinase produced by HSVs than it is for mammalian thymidine kinase. Hence, formation of acyclo-GMP, the limiting step in the activation of acyclovir, occurs almost exclusively in cells infected with HSV. CMV is inherently resistant to the drug because acyclovir is a poor substrate for the form of thymidine kinase produced by this virus.

Resistance

Herpesviruses develop resistance to acyclovir by three mechanisms: (1) decreased production of thymidine kinase, (2) alteration of thymidine kinase such that it no longer converts acyclovir to acyclo-GMP, and (3) alteration of viral DNA polymerase such that it is less sensitive to inhibition. Of these mechanisms, thymidine kinase deficiency is the most common. Resistance is rare in immunocompetent patients, but many cases have been reported in transplant recipients and patients with AIDS. Lesions caused by resistant HSVs can be extensive and severe, progressing despite continued acyclovir therapy. Acyclovir-resistant HSVs and VZV usually respond to intravenous (IV) foscarnet or cidofovir, which are primarily used for treatment of CMV infection (see later discussion).

TABLE 93.2 ▪ Treatment of Herpes Simplex Virus and Varicella-Zoster Virus Infections

Infection	Drug	Route	Dosage	Duration
HERPES SIMPLEX VIRUS INFECTIONS				
Encephalitis	Acyclovir	IV	10–15 mg/kg every 8 hr	14–21 days
Mucocutaneous in ICH	Acyclovir	IV	5 mg/kg every 8 hr	7–10 days
	Acyclovir	PO	400 mg 5 times/day	7–14 days
	Valacyclovir	PO	*Initial episode:* 1 gm twice daily for 10 days *Recurrent episode:* 500 mg twice daily for 3 days *Reduction of transmission:* 500 mg once daily *Suppressive therapy:* Immunocompetent patients: 1 gm once daily (500 mg once daily in patients with < 9 recurrences per year) HIV-infected patients (CD4 ≥ 100 cells/mm^3): 500 mg twice daily	7–10 days
	Famciclovir	PO	500 mg 2 times/day	7–10 days
	Foscarnet[a]	IV	400 mg 2–3 times/day	7–21 days
Neonatal	Acyclovir	IV	5–10 mg/kg every 8 hr	7 days
Orolabial	Acyclovir	Topical	5% cream 5 times/day	4 days
	Penciclovir	Topical	1% cream every 2 hr	4 days
	Docosanol	Topical	10% cream 5 times/day	4 days or until lesions have healed
Keratoconjunctivitis	Ganciclovir	Topical	See text	
	Trifluridine	Topical	See text	
	Vidarabine	Topical	See text	
Genital infections	See Chapter 95			
VARICELLA-ZOSTER VIRUS INFECTIONS				
Varicella	Acyclovir	PO	800 mg 4 times/day	5 days
Varicella in ICH[a]	Acyclovir	IV	10 mg/kg every 8 hr	7 days
Herpes zoster	Acyclovir	PO	800 mg 5 times/day	7–10 days
	Valacyclovir	PO	1 gm 3 times/day	7 days
	Famciclovir	PO	500 mg 3 times/day	7 days
Herpes zoster in ICH[a]	Acyclovir	IV	10 mg/kg every 8 hr	7 days
Acyclovir-resistant zoster	Foscarnet	IV	40 mg/kg every 8–12 hr	10 days

[a]Reserve foscarnet for acyclovir-resistant infection.
ICH, Immunocompromised host.

Therapeutic Uses

Mucocutaneous Herpes Simplex Infections. Herpes infections of the face and oropharynx are usually caused by HSV type 2 (HSV-2). For immunocompetent patients, *oral* acyclovir can be used to treat primary infections of the gums and mouth. Oral acyclovir can also be taken *prophylactically* to prevent episodes of *recurrent* herpes labialis (cold sores). However, there is no truly effective treatment for active herpes labialis. Mucocutaneous herpes infections can be especially severe in immunocompromised patients. For these people, *intravenous* acyclovir is the treatment of choice.

Varicella-Zoster Infections. High doses of *oral* acyclovir are effective for herpes zoster (shingles) in older adults. Oral therapy is also effective for varicella (chickenpox) in children, adolescents, and adults, provided that dosing is begun early (within 24 hours of rash onset). *Intravenous* acyclovir is the treatment of choice for VZV infection in the immunocompromised host.

Herpes Simplex Genitalis. The characteristics and treatment of genital HSV infection are discussed in Chapter 95.

Pharmacokinetics

Acyclovir may be administered topically, orally, and intravenously. Oral bioavailability is low, ranging from 15% to 30%. No significant absorption occurs with topical use. In the blood, acyclovir is distributed widely to body fluids and tissues. Levels achieved in cerebrospinal fluid are 50% of those in plasma. Elimination is renal, primarily as the unchanged drug. In patients with normal kidney function, acyclovir has a half-life of 2.5 hours. The half-life is prolonged by renal impairment, reaching 20 hours in anuric patients. Accordingly, dosages should be reduced in patients with kidney disease.

Adverse Effects

Intravenous Therapy. Intravenous acyclovir is generally well tolerated. The most common reactions are *phlebitis* and *inflammation* at the infusion site. Reversible *nephrotoxicity,* indicated by elevations in serum creatinine and blood urea nitrogen, occurs in some patients. The cause is deposition of acyclovir in renal tubules. The risk for renal injury is increased by dehydration and by use of other nephrotoxic drugs. Kidney damage can be minimized by infusing acyclovir slowly (over 1 hour) and by ensuring adequate hydration during the infusion and for 2 hours after.

Neurologic toxicity—agitation, tremors, delirium, hallucinations, and myoclonus—occurs rarely, primarily in patients with renal impairment. In patients on dialysis, very low doses can cause severe neurotoxicity, characterized by delirium and coma.

Oral and Topical Therapy. Oral acyclovir is devoid of serious adverse effects. Renal impairment has not been reported. The most common reactions are nausea, vomiting, diarrhea, headache, and vertigo. Topical acyclovir frequently causes transient local burning or stinging; systemic reactions do not occur. Oral acyclovir is safe during pregnancy, so it can be used to suppress recurrent genital herpes near term.

Preparations, Dosage, and Administration

Topical Ointment. Acyclovir [Zovirax] is supplied as a 5% ointment for topical therapy of *herpes genitalis* and *mild mucocutaneous HSV infection in the immunocompromised host.* Application is done 6 times a day at 3-hour intervals for 7 days. Patients should use a finger cot or rubber glove to avoid viral transfer to other parts of the body or to other people.

Topical Cream. Acyclovir [Zovirax] is supplied as a 5% cream for topical therapy of recurrent *herpes labialis* (cold sores) in patients at least 12 years old. Application is done 5 times a day for 4 days.

Oral. Oral acyclovir [Zovirax] is available in capsules (200 mg), tablets (400 and 800 mg), and a suspension (200 mg/5 mL). Dosages for patients with normal kidney function are listed next. Dosages must be reduced for patients with renal impairment:

- For *initial episodes of herpes genitalis,* the usual dosage is 400 mg 3 times a day for 7 to 10 days.
- For *episodic recurrences of herpes genitalis,* the usual dosage is 400 mg 3 times a day for 5 days.
- For *long-term suppressive therapy of recurrent genital infections,* the usual dosage is 400 mg twice daily for up to 12 months.
- For *acute therapy of herpes zoster,* the dosage is 800 mg 5 times a day (at 4-hour intervals) for 7 to 10 days.
- For *varicella* (chickenpox), the dosage is 20 mg/kg (but no more than 800 mg) 4 times a day for 5 days. Treatment should begin at the earliest sign of rash.

Intravenous. For IV dosing, acyclovir is available in solution (50 mg/mL). Administration is by slow infusion (over 1 hour or more). Parenteral acyclovir must not be given by IV bolus or by intramuscular (IM) or subcutaneous (subQ) injection. To minimize the risk for renal damage, hydrate the patient during the infusion and for 2 hours after. Dosages for patients with normal kidney function are given next. Dosages should be reduced for patients with renal impairment:

- For *mucocutaneous HSV infection in the immunocompromised host,* the adult dosage is 5 mg/kg infused every 8 hours for 7 days. The dosage for children under 12 years is 10 mg/kg infused every 8 hours for 7 days.
- For *VZV infection in the immunocompromised host,* the adult dosage is 10 mg/kg infused every 8 hours for 7 days. The dosage for children under 12 years is 20 mg/kg infused every 8 hours for 7 days.
- For *severe episodes of herpes genitalis in the immunocompetent host,* the adult dosage is 5 to 10 mg/kg infused every 8 hours for 5 to 7 days (or until symptoms resolve). The dosage for children younger than 12 years is 15 to 20 mg/kg/day divided into three doses to be infused every 8 hours for 5 days.

Valacyclovir

Actions and Uses

Valacyclovir [Valtrex], a prodrug form of acyclovir, is approved for the management of four conditions: (1) herpes zoster (shingles), (2) herpes simplex genitalis (genital herpes), (3) herpes labialis (cold sores), and (4) varicella (chickenpox). With the exception of herpes labialis, there are limits on use for each condition. For herpes zoster, valacyclovir is indicated only for *immunocompetent* patients. For varicella, the patients must be *immunocompetent children.* For herpes simplex genitalis, valacyclovir is indicated for the treatment of initial and recurrent episodes for *immunocompetent* patients; however, for suppressive therapy, this drug is approved for management in *immunocompetent* and *HIV-infected adults* with a CD4+ cell count of at least 100 cells/mm^3.

Valacyclovir is sometimes used off-label for *prophylaxis* of HSV, VZV, and CMV infections in patients with cancer. It is also sometimes used for *treatment* of cancer-related HSV and VZV.

Prototype Drugs

DRUGS FOR NON-HIV VIRAL INFECTIONS

Drugs for Herpes Simplex Virus Infection
Acyclovir
Ganciclovir

Drugs for Cytomegalovirus Infection
Ganciclovir

Drugs for Hepatitis
Peginterferon alfa-2b
Lamivudine (nucleoside analog)
Peginterferon alfa-2a
Ribavirin (oral nucleoside analog)
Simprevir (protease inhibitor)
Declatasvir (NS5A inhibitor)
Sofosbuvir (NS5B inhibitor)

Drugs for Influenza
Influenza vaccine
Oseltamivir

Drugs for Respiratory Syncytial Virus Infection
Ribavirin (inhaled)
Palivizumab

Pharmacokinetics

Oral valacyclovir undergoes rapid absorption followed by rapid and essentially complete conversion to acyclovir. When acyclovir itself is given orally, bioavailability is only 15% to 30%. In contrast, when valacyclovir is given orally, the effective bioavailability of acyclovir is greatly increased—to about 55%. Therefore, valacyclovir represents a more efficient way of getting acyclovir into the body. After conversion of valacyclovir to acyclovir, the kinetics is the same as if acyclovir itself had been given.

Adverse Effects

No doubt you noticed the emphasis on using valacyclovir primarily for immunocompetent patients. Why? In some immunocompromised patients, valacyclovir has produced a syndrome known as *thrombotic thrombocytopenic purpura/hemolytic uremic syndrome* (TTP/HUS). This syndrome, which can be fatal, has not occurred in immunocompetent patients. Aside from causing TTP/HUS, valacyclovir is generally well tolerated, producing the same side effects seen with oral acyclovir (e.g., nausea, vomiting, diarrhea, headache, vertigo).

Preparations, Dosage, and Administration

Valacyclovir [Valtrex] is available in 500- and 1000-mg oral capsules. Dosing may be done without regard to meals. In patients with renal impairment, dosages should be reduced.

For patients with *herpes zoster,* the recommended dosage is 1000 mg 3 times a day for 7 days. Therapy should begin as soon as possible after symptom onset.

For patients with *herpes simplex genitalis,* the dosage is 1 gm twice daily for 10 days (for the initial episode), or 500 mg twice daily for 3 days (for episodic recurrences). For suppressive therapy, the recommended dosage for immunocompetent patients is 500 to 1000 mg once daily and, for patients with HIV infection, 500 mg twice a day.

For patients with *herpes labialis,* 2 gm/dose should be taken 12 hours apart for 1 day. Dosing should begin as soon as possible after onset of symptoms.

For immunocompetent children aged 2 to 18 years with chickenpox, dosage is 20 mg/kg (up to a maximum of 1 gm) 3 times a day.

Famciclovir

Famciclovir [Famvir] is a prodrug used to treat acute herpes zoster and genital herpes infection. Benefits are equivalent to those of acyclovir. Adverse effects are minimal.

Pharmacokinetics

Famciclovir undergoes rapid absorption from the gastrointestinal (GI) tract followed by enzymatic conversion to *penciclovir,* its active form. Food decreases the rate of famciclovir absorption but not the extent. As a result, the amount of penciclovir produced is the same whether famciclovir is taken with or without food. Penciclovir is excreted in the urine, largely unchanged. The *plasma* half-life of penciclovir is about 2.5 hours. However, the half-life of penciclovir *within cells* is much longer. In patients with renal impairment, the plasma half-life of penciclovir is prolonged.

Mechanism of Action and Antiviral Spectrum

Penciclovir undergoes intracellular conversion to penciclovir triphosphate, a compound that inhibits viral DNA polymerase and thereby prevents replication of viral DNA. Under clinical conditions, formation of penciclovir triphosphate requires viral thymidine kinase. As a result, inhibition of DNA synthesis is limited to cells that are infected, leaving most host cells unharmed. *In vitro,* penciclovir is active against HSV type 1 (HSV-1), HSV-2, and VZV.

Therapeutic Use

Famciclovir is approved for treatment of acute herpes zoster (shingles) and herpes simplex genitalis. In patients with herpes zoster, the drug can decrease the time to full crusting from 7 days down to 5 days. Famciclovir does not decrease the *incidence* of postherpetic neuralgia, but can decrease the *duration* (from 112 days down to 61 days).

In patients with genital herpes simplex infection, famciclovir is active against the first episode and recurrent episodes. In addition, it can be used for long-term suppression.

Adverse Effects

Famciclovir is very well tolerated. In clinical trials, only headache and nausea were reported by more than 10% of the subjects. If given in higher than recommended doses, acute renal failure can occur.

Preparations, Dosage, and Administration

Preparations. Famciclovir [Famvir] is supplied in tablets (125, 250, and 500 mg) for oral dosing, with or without food.

Acute Herpes Zoster. The recommended dosage is 500 mg every 8 hours for 7 days. Treatment should start no later than 72 hours after symptom onset. In patients with renal impairment, the dose should be reduced and the interval between doses should be increased to 12 hours or 24 hours, depending on the degree of impairment.

Herpes Simplex Genitalis. For initial episodes, the dosage is 250 mg 3 times a day for 7 to 10 days. For episodic recurrence, there are three dosage regimens available: (1) 125 mg twice a day for 5 days, (2) 500 mg as a single dose on day 1 followed by 250 mg twice a day on day 2, or (3) two 1000-mg doses 12 hours apart. For long-term suppression, the dosage is 250 mg twice daily for a year.

Herpes Labialis. For cold sores that are recurrent, the dosage is a single 1500-mg dose at the first signs of symptoms.

Topical Drugs for Herpes Labialis

We have three topical drugs for recurrent herpes labialis (cold sores). Two of these drugs—penciclovir and docosanol—are discussed next. The third drug—acyclovir—was discussed earlier.

Penciclovir Cream

Penciclovir [Denavir] is a topical drug indicated for recurrent herpes labialis, an infection caused by HSV-1 and HSV-2. The drug suppresses viral replication by inhibiting DNA polymerase, the enzyme that makes DNA. Penciclovir is supplied as a 1% cream to be applied every 2 hours (except when sleeping) for 4 days. In clinical trials, benefits were modest: The average time to healing and duration of pain were decreased by just half a day, from 5 days down to 4.5 days. The only common adverse effect is mild local erythema.

Docosanol Cream

Docosanol [Abreva] is a topical preparation indicated for recurrent herpes labialis. The drug is available over the counter as a 10% cream. Application is done 5 times a day, beginning at the first sign of recurrence. Benefits are modest. In one trial, treatment reduced the time to healing from 4.8 days down to 4.1 days—about the same response seen with penciclovir. Docosanol cream appears devoid of adverse effects.

Docosanol has a broad antiviral spectrum and a unique mechanism of action. Unlike penciclovir, which inhibits viral DNA synthesis (and thereby suppresses replication), docosanol blocks viral entry into host cells. The drug does not kill viruses and does not prevent them from binding to cells. As a result, viable virions can remain attached to the cell surface for a long time. Because docosanol does not affect processes of replication, it is unlikely to promote resistance.

Topical Drugs for Ocular Herpes Infections

Trifluridine Ophthalmic Solution

Trifluridine [Viroptic] is indicated only for topical treatment of ocular infections caused by HSV-1 and HSV-2. The drug is given to treat acute keratoconjunctivitis and recurrent epithelial keratitis. Antiviral actions result from inhibiting DNA synthesis. The most common side effects are localized burning and stinging. Edema of the eyelid occurs in about 3% of patients. Systemic absorption is minimal after topical administration, so the drug is devoid of systemic toxicity. Trifluridine is supplied as a 1% ophthalmic solution. Treatment consists of placing 1 drop on the cornea every 2 hours while the patient is awake, for a maximum of 9 drops/day. After re-epithelialization of the cornea has occurred, the dosage is reduced to 1 drop every 4 hours and continues for an additional 7 days.

Ganciclovir Gel

Ganciclovir 0.15% ophthalmic gel [Zirgan] is indicated for acute herpetic keratitis (inflammation and ulceration of the cornea caused by infection with a herpes simplex virus). As discussed later (see *Ganciclovir*), benefits derive from suppressing viral replication. Principal adverse effects are blurred vision, eye irritation, and red eyes. Systemic effects are absent. The recommended dosage is 1 drop in the affected eye 5 times a day until symptoms abate, followed by 1 drop 3 times a day for 7 days. Instruct patients to apply drops directly to the affected eye and to avoid contact lenses until lesions heal.

DRUGS FOR CYTOMEGALOVIRUS INFECTION

Cytomegalovirus is a member of the herpesvirus group, which includes HSV-1 and HSV-2, VZV (the cause of chickenpox), and Epstein-Barr virus (the cause of infectious mononucleosis). Transmission of CMV occurs person to person—through direct contact with saliva, urine, blood, tears, breast milk, semen, and other body fluids. Infection can also be acquired by way of blood transfusion or organ transplantation. Infection with CMV is very common: Between 50% and 85% of Americans 40 years and older harbor the virus. After the initial infection, which has minimal symptoms in healthy people, the virus remains dormant within cells for life, without causing detectable injury or clinical illness. Hence, for most healthy people, CMV infection is of little concern. By contrast, people who are immunocompromised—owing to HIV infection, cancer chemotherapy, or use of immunosuppressive drugs—are at high risk for serious morbidity and even death, both from initial CMV infection and from reactivation of dormant CMV. Common sites for infection are the lungs, eyes, and GI tract. Among people with AIDS, CMV retinitis is the principal reason for loss of vision (see Chapter 94). The four drugs used against CMV are discussed next.

Ganciclovir

Ganciclovir [Cytovene, Vitrasert, Zirgan] is a synthetic antiviral agent with activity against herpesviruses, including CMV.

Because the drug can cause serious adverse effects, especially granulocytopenia and thrombocytopenia, it should be used only for prevention and treatment of CMV infection in the immunocompromised host.

Mechanism of Action

Ganciclovir is converted to its active form, ganciclovir triphosphate, inside infected cells. As ganciclovir triphosphate, it suppresses replication of viral DNA by (1) inhibiting viral DNA polymerase and (2) undergoing incorporation into the growing DNA chain, which causes premature chain termination.

Pharmacokinetics

Bioavailability of oral ganciclovir is low: only 5% under fasting conditions and 9% when taken with food. When in the blood, the drug is widely distributed to body fluids and tissues. Ganciclovir is excreted unchanged in the urine. In patients with normal renal function, the half-life is about 3 hours. In patients with renal impairment, the half-life is prolonged. Accordingly, dosages should be reduced in patients with kidney disease.

Therapeutic Use

Ganciclovir is approved only to prevent and treat CMV infection in immunocompromised patients, including transplant recipients, those with HIV infection, and those receiving immunosuppressive drugs.

In patients with AIDS, CMV retinitis has an incidence of 15% to 40%. Although most AIDS patients respond initially, the relapse rate is high. Accordingly, for most patients, maintenance therapy should continue indefinitely. The risk for relapse is higher with oral ganciclovir than with IV ganciclovir. Because viral resistance can develop during treatment, this possibility should be considered if the patient responds poorly.

Adverse Effects

Granulocytopenia and Thrombocytopenia. The adverse effect of greatest concern is bone marrow suppression, which can result in granulocytopenia and thrombocytopenia. These effects, which are usually reversible, are more likely with IV therapy than with oral therapy. These hematologic responses can be exacerbated by concurrent therapy with zidovudine. Conversely, granulocytopenia can be reduced with granulocyte colony-stimulating factors (see Chapter 56). Because of the risk for adverse hematologic effects, blood cell counts must be monitored. Treatment should be interrupted if the absolute neutrophil count falls below 500/mm^3 or if the platelet count falls below 25,000/mm^3. Cell counts usually begin to recover within 3 to 5 days. Ganciclovir should be used with caution in patients with pre-existing cytopenias, in those with a history of cytopenic reactions to other drugs, and in those taking other bone marrow suppressants (e.g., zidovudine).

Reproductive Toxicity. Ganciclovir is teratogenic and embryotoxic in laboratory animals and probably in humans. Women should be advised to avoid pregnancy during therapy and for 90 days after ending treatment. At doses equivalent to those used therapeutically, ganciclovir inhibits spermatogenesis in mice; sterility is reversible with low doses and irreversible with high doses. Female infertility may also occur. Patients should be forewarned of these effects.

Other Adverse Effects. Incidental effects include nausea, fever, rash, anemia, liver dysfunction, and confusion and other central nervous system (CNS) symptoms.

Preparations, Dosage, and Administration

Intravenous. Ganciclovir [Cytovene] is available as a powder (500 mg) to be reconstituted for IV infusion. Solutions are alkaline and must be infused into a freely flowing vein to avoid local injury. For treatment of CMV retinitis, the *initial dosage* for adults with normal renal function is 5 mg/kg (infused over 1 hour) every 12 hours for 14 to 21 days. Two *maintenance dosages* can be used: (1) 5 mg/kg infused over 1 hour once every day of the week, or (2) 6 mg/kg infused over 1 hour once a day, 5 days a week. Dosages must be reduced for patients with renal impairment. Because many patients with AIDS must continue maintenance therapy for life, they need a permanent IV access and equipment for home infusion. Adequate hydration must be maintained in all patients to ensure renal excretion of ganciclovir.

Oral. Ganciclovir is supplied in 250- and 500-mg tablets for maintenance therapy in patients with CMV retinitis. The usual dosage is 1000 mg 3 times daily with food.

Ocular Implant. The ganciclovir ocular implant [Vitrasert] is indicated for CMV retinitis in patients with AIDS. Surgical implantation, which takes about 1 hour, is performed under local anesthesia on an outpatient basis. Vision is usually blurred for 2 to 4 weeks after the procedure. The implant must be replaced every 5 to 8 months. Clinical trials indicate that CMV retinitis progresses more slowly in patients who receive intraocular ganciclovir compared with those on IV ganciclovir.

Ocular Gel. As discussed earlier (under *Topical Drugs for Ocular Herpes Infections*), ganciclovir is available in a 0.15% gel, marketed as Zirgan, for treating herpetic keratitis.

Hazardous Drugs Requiring Special Handling. Ganciclovir may present a hazard for nurses who administer this drug. In 2016 the National Institute for Occupational Safety and Health (NIOSH) expanded the list of drugs identified as hazardous (see https://www.cdc.gov/niosh/docs/2016-161/pdfs/2016-161.pdf). NIOSH requires special handling of drugs identified as hazardous. See Chapter 3, Table 3.1, for administration and handling guidelines. The hazardous drugs mentioned in this chapter are listed in the following box.

Safety Alert

HAZARDOUS DRUGS REQUIRING SPECIAL HANDLING

Trifluridine	Cidofovir
Ganciclovir	Entecavir
Valganciclovir	Ribavirin

Valganciclovir

Basic and Clinical Pharmacology

Valganciclovir [Valcyte] is a prodrug version of ganciclovir [Cytovene] with greater oral bioavailability (60% vs. 9%). After absorption from the GI tract, valganciclovir is rapidly metabolized to ganciclovir, its active form—and eventually undergoes excretion as unchanged ganciclovir in the urine. Indications are CMV retinitis and prevention of CMV disease in high-risk organ transplant recipients. In patients with active CMV retinitis, oral valganciclovir is just as effective as *intravenous* ganciclovir—and much more convenient.

Adverse effects are the same as with ganciclovir. The principal concern is blood dyscrasias—granulocytopenia, anemia, and thrombocytopenia—secondary to bone marrow suppression. In addition, any of the following adverse effects typically occur in 20% to 40% of patients: diarrhea, nausea, vomiting, fever, and headache. Valganciclovir is presumed to pose the same risks of mutagenesis, aspermatogenesis, and carcinogenesis as ganciclovir.

Preparations, Dosage, and Administration

Valganciclovir [Valcyte] is available in (1) 450-mg tablets and (2) a powder that makes a 50-mg/mL oral solution when reconstituted with 91 mL of purified water. All doses should be taken with food to enhance bioavailability.

For *treatment of CMV retinitis,* the adult dosage is 900 mg twice daily for 21 days, followed by 900 mg once daily for maintenance. Dosage must be reduced for patients with renal impairment.

PATIENT-CENTERED CARE ACROSS THE LIFE SPAN

Antiviral Drugs Prescribed for Herpes Virus and Cytomegalovirus Infections

Life Stage	Patient Care Concerns
Children	Ganciclovir and valganciclovir are approved for use in children for selected conditions. Valacyclovir is also approved for children according to diagnosis: It may be given to neonates for HSV suppressive therapy, to children age 2 with chickenpox, to children age 12 for cold sores. Adequate studies have not been conducted in children for most of these drugs. Careful weighing of benefits versus risks is advised.
Pregnant women	Acyclovir, famciclovir, and valacyclovir are Pregnancy Risk Category B.[a] Foscarnet is Pregnancy Risk Category C. Cidofovir, ganciclovir, and valganciclovir (a prodrug of ganciclovir) are categorized as Pregnancy Risk Category C. In animal studies, these caused structural abnormalities. Studies have not been conducted in humans.
Breast-feeding women	Breast-feeding is not contraindicated; however, because inadequate studies are available and serious adverse events could occur, caution is recommended.
Older adults	There are no contraindications for this age group; however, those with renal impairment should be started on lower doses, with dosage adjustments made cautiously.

[a]As of 2020, the FDA will no longer use Pregnancy Risk Categories. Please refer to Chapter 9 for more information.

For *prevention of CMV disease* in transplant recipients, the adult dosage is 900 mg once daily, starting within 10 days of transplantation and continuing until 100 days after transplantation (or 200 days post-transplantation in kidney recipients).

Because valganciclovir has the potential for mutagenesis and carcinogenesis, the powder and tablets should be handled carefully. Tablets should be ingested intact, without crushing or chewing. Direct contact with the powder or broken tablets should be avoided. If contact does occur, the area should be washed with soap and water. When handling or disposing of the drug, healthcare workers should follow the same guidelines established for cytotoxic anticancer drugs.

Cidofovir

Cidofovir [Vistide] is an IV drug with just one indication: CMV retinitis in patients with AIDS who have failed on ganciclovir or foscarnet. Alternative drugs for this infection are foscarnet, which is given intravenously, and ganciclovir, which may be administered intravenously, orally, or by ocular insert. Compared with IV foscarnet or IV ganciclovir, cidofovir has the distinct advantage of needing fewer infusions: Whereas foscarnet and ganciclovir must be infused daily, cidofovir is infused just once a week or every other week. The major adverse effect of the drug is kidney damage.

Mechanism of Action

After it enters the cells, cidofovir is converted to cidofovir diphosphate, its active form. As the diphosphate, cidofovir causes selective inhibition of viral DNA polymerase and thereby inhibits viral DNA synthesis. Intracellular concentrations of cidofovir diphosphate are too low to inhibit human DNA polymerases; thus, host cells are spared.

Antiviral Spectrum and Therapeutic Use

Cidofovir is active against herpesviruses, including CMV, HSV-1, HSV-2, and VZV. However, the drug is approved only for CMV retinitis in patients with AIDS. Whether cidofovir is active against CMV infections in other patients or at other sites (e.g., GI tract, lungs) is unknown. In clinical trials in patients with AIDS and established CMV retinitis, cidofovir significantly delayed progression of retinitis.

Pharmacokinetics

Cidofovir is administered by IV infusion and undergoes excretion by the kidneys. Probenecid competes with cidofovir for renal tubular secretion and thereby delays elimination. Cidofovir has a prolonged *intracellular* half-life (17 to 65 hours), and hence a long interval (2 weeks) can separate doses. In contrast, IV foscarnet and ganciclovir must be infused daily.

Adverse Effects

Nephrotoxicity. The principal adverse effect is dose-dependent nephrotoxicity, manifesting as decreased renal function and symptoms of a Fanconi-like syndrome (proteinuria, glucosuria, bicarbonate wasting). To reduce the risk for renal injury, all patients must receive probenecid and IV hydration therapy with each infusion. Also, serum creatinine and urine protein should be checked within 48 hours before each dose; if these values indicate kidney damage, cidofovir should be withheld or the dosage reduced. Cidofovir is contraindicated for patients taking other drugs that can injure the kidney and for patients with proteinuria (2+ or greater) or baseline serum creatinine greater than 1.5 mg/dL.

Safety Alert

CIDOFOVIR

Cidofovir has been associated with severe renal impairment. Dialysis has been required after only one or two doses. Monitoring for renal function is an important nursing function.

Other Adverse Effects. *Neutropenia* develops in about 20% of patients, so neutrophil counts should be monitored. *Ocular disorders*—iritis, uveitis, or ocular hypotony (low intraocular pressure)—can also occur. In animal studies, cidofovir was carcinogenic and teratogenic and caused hypospermia. Adverse effects are more likely in patients taking antiretroviral drugs (i.e., drugs for HIV).

Preparations, Dosage, and Administration

Cidofovir [Vistide] is supplied in solution (75 mg/mL) in 5-mL ampules. To reduce the risk for renal injury, cidofovir infusions must be accompanied by IV hydration therapy and oral (PO) probenecid.

Each cidofovir dose—for induction or maintenance—consists of 5 mg/kg by IV infusion over 1 hour. For induction, two doses are given 1 week apart. For maintenance, one dose is given every 2 weeks. The size of each dose must be reduced for patients with renal impairment. If impairment is severe, cidofovir should be withheld.

Oral probenecid must accompany each infusion. The dosage is 2 gm given 3 hours before the infusion, 1 gm given 1 hour after the infusion, and another 1 gm given 8 hours after that. Ingesting food before each dose can decrease probenecid-induced nausea and vomiting. An antiemetic may also be used.

Hydration is accomplished by infusing 1 L of 0.9% saline solution over 1 to 2 hours immediately before infusing cidofovir. For patients who can tolerate it, 1 L more can be infused over 1 to 3 hours, beginning when the cidofovir infusion begins or as soon as it is over.

Foscarnet

Foscarnet is an IV drug active against all known herpesviruses, including CMV, HSV-1, HSV-2, and VZV. Compared with ganciclovir, foscarnet is more difficult to administer, less well tolerated, and much more expensive. The major adverse effect is renal injury.

Mechanism of Action

Foscarnet, an analog of pyrophosphate, inhibits viral DNA polymerases and reverse transcriptases and thereby inhibits synthesis of viral nucleic acids. At the concentrations achieved clinically, the drug does not inhibit host DNA replication. Unlike many other antiviral drugs, which must undergo conversion to an active form, foscarnet is active as administered.

Therapeutic Use

Foscarnet has two approved indications: (1) CMV retinitis in patients with AIDS and (2) acyclovir-resistant mucocutaneous HSV and VZV infection in the immunocompromised host. CMV retinitis resistant to ganciclovir may respond to foscarnet.

Pharmacokinetics

Foscarnet has low oral bioavailability and must be administered intravenously. The drug is poorly soluble in water and does not penetrate cells easily. As a result, it must be given in large doses with large volumes of fluid. Between 10% and 28% of each dose is deposited in bone; the remainder is excreted unchanged in the urine. Because foscarnet is eliminated by the kidneys, dosages must be reduced in patients with renal impairment. The plasma half-life is 3 to 5 hours.

Adverse Effects and Interactions

In general, foscarnet is less well tolerated than ganciclovir. However, unlike ganciclovir, foscarnet does not cause granulocytopenia or thrombocytopenia.

Nephrotoxicity. Renal injury, as evidenced by a rise in serum creatinine, is the most common dose-limiting toxicity. Most patients develop some degree of renal impairment. Renal injury occurs most often during the second week of therapy. The risk for nephrotoxicity is increased by concurrent use of other nephrotoxic drugs, including amphotericin B, aminoglycosides (e.g., gentamicin), and pentamidine. Prehydration with IV saline may reduce the risk for renal injury. Renal function (creatinine clearance) should be monitored closely, and the dosage should be reduced if renal impairment develops.

Electrolyte and Mineral Imbalances. Foscarnet frequently causes hypocalcemia, hypokalemia, hypomagnesemia, and hypophosphatemia or hyperphosphatemia. Ionized serum calcium may be reduced despite normal levels of total serum calcium. Patients should be informed about symptoms of low ionized calcium (e.g., paresthesias, numbness in the extremities, perioral tingling) and instructed to report these. Severe hypocalcemia can result in dysrhythmias, tetany, and seizures. Serum levels of calcium, magnesium, potassium, and phosphorus should be measured frequently. Special caution is required in patients with pre-existing electrolyte, cardiac, or neurologic abnormalities. The risk for hypocalcemia is increased by concurrent use of pentamidine.

Other Adverse Effects. Common reactions (occurring in 25% to 50% of patients) include fever, nausea, anemia, diarrhea, vomiting, and headache. In addition, foscarnet can cause fatigue, tremor, irritability, genital ulceration, abnormal liver function tests, neutropenia, and seizures.

Preparations, Dosage, and Administration

Foscarnet is supplied in solution (24 mg/mL) for IV infusion. An infusion pump is essential to reduce the risk for dosing errors. Infusions may be administered through a central venous line or a peripheral vein. When a central line is used, a concentrated (24 mg/mL) solution may be given. When a peripheral vein is used, the solution should be diluted to 12 mg/mL. For patients with normal kidney function, the *initial* dosage is 60 mg/kg (for CMV infection) or 40 mg/kg (for HSV infection) infused over 1 hour (or longer) every 8 hours for 2 to 3 weeks. The *maintenance* dosage (for CMV or HSV infection) is 90 to 120 mg/kg infused over 2 hours once daily. All dosages must be reduced for patients with renal impairment.

DRUGS FOR HEPATITIS

Viral hepatitis is the most common liver disorder, affecting millions of Americans. The disease can be caused by six different hepatitis viruses, labeled A, B, C, D, E, and G. All six can cause *acute* hepatitis, but only B, C, and D also cause *chronic* hepatitis. Acute hepatitis lasts for 6 months or less and is characterized by liver inflammation, jaundice, and elevation of serum alanine aminotransferase (ALT) activity. In most cases, acute hepatitis resolves spontaneously, so intervention is generally unnecessary. In contrast, chronic hepatitis can lead to cirrhosis, hepatocellular carcinoma, and life-threatening liver failure, and hence treatment should be considered.

Most cases (90%) of chronic hepatitis are caused by either hepatitis B virus (HBV) or hepatitis C virus (HCV). Accordingly, our discussion focuses on hepatitis B and hepatitis C. About 1.5% of Americans are infected with HBV or HCV, which is 5 times more than the number infected with HIV. Vaccines for hepatitis A and B are discussed in Chapter 68. Drugs for hepatitis B and C are discussed here.

HEPATITIS C

The Centers for Disease Control and Prevention (CDC) estimates about 3.9 million Americans have chronic hepatitis C. Transmission occurs primarily through exchange of blood, with injection drug use being the most common means. Transmission may also occur as the result of sex with an HCV-infected partner, though this occurs far less frequently. Pregnant women who are infected can transfer the virus to their offspring. Among people who acquire HCV, 75% to 85% develop active infection. However, most people with chronic hepatitis C have no symptoms, although they can transmit HCV to others. Chronic HCV infection undergoes slow progression, and, in some people, eventually causes liver failure, cancer, and death. Chronic hepatitis C is the leading reason for liver transplantations and kills about 15,000 Americans each year—more than are killed by HIV.

It is important to note that not all hepatitis C viruses are the same. There are 6 genotypes of HCV and more than 50 subtypes. In the United States, 75% of HCV infections are caused by HCV genotype 1, which, unfortunately, is less responsive to treatment than other HCV genotypes.

The options for hepatitis C management increased dramatically between 2011 and 2016 as new categories of antiviral drugs were developed and added to the arsenal of agents targeting HCV infection. New guidelines were developed and then updated and then updated yet again. In 2015, the European Association for the Study of Liver (EASL) released its groundbreaking recommendations for treatment of HCV infection (available online at http://www.easl.eu/medias/cpg/HEPC-2015/Full-report.pdf). The first sentence following the introduction was astounding: "The primary goal of HCV therapy is to cure the infection." For the patients, their families, and the healthcare providers who had accepted the long-held belief that there is no cure, hope had truly arrived.

At the time of this writing, joint guidelines by the American Association for the Study of Liver Diseases (AASLD) and the Infectious Diseases Society of America (IDSA) were newly released (see http://www.hcvguidelines.org). These guidelines complement those of the EASL. Like the EASL guidelines, they focus on genotype-specific treatment that considers liver status (i.e., presence of cirrhosis) and treatment history (i.e., treatment-naïve and previous treatment failure) to optimize therapy.

It is quite likely that, by the time you read this, there will be new updates in the treatment of HCV infection. The most current recommendations are maintained at the AASLD/IDSA website at http://www.hcvguidelines.org.

The ultimate goal of HCV therapy is cure of HCV infection. This is manifested by a sustained virologic response (SVR), which represents elimination of HCV RNA. The SVR occurs if there is no detectable HCV RNA at 12 weeks (SVR12) or 24 weeks (SVR24) after therapy.

For years, dual therapy with pegylated interferon alfa (peginterferon alfa) plus ribavirin was the standard of care. The expanse in knowledge and understanding of the HCV genome led to the development of direct-acting antiviral (DAA) drugs. These highly effective drugs have largely replaced the older regimen. Moreover, through the carefully orchestrated HCV treatment that these drugs allow, outcomes have greatly improved.

DAAs are drugs that target specific steps in the process of HCV replication. Because the mechanism of actions is directed toward the virus, the drugs avoid the sometimes dangerous adverse effects associated with interferon therapy. To decrease the development of viral resistance and to increase the likelihood of successful outcomes, all of these drugs are used in combination therapy. There are currently four categories of DAAs: NS3/4A protease inhibitors (PIs), NS5A inhibitors, NS5B nucleoside polymerase inhibitors (NPIs), and NS5B non-nucleoside polymerase inhibitors (NNPIs).

For our discussion, we will first examine interferon alfa and ribavirin. Thereafter, we will discuss the DAA drugs.

Interferon Alfa

Human interferons are naturally occurring compounds with complex antiviral, immunomodulatory, and antineoplastic actions. The interferon family has three major classes, designated alpha, beta, and gamma. All of the interferons used for hepatitis belong to the alpha class (Table 93.3). In the following discussion, these compounds are referred to collectively as *interferon alfa.* None of these agents can be used orally, and hence administration is parenteral—almost always subQ. Commercial production is by recombinant DNA technology.

Mechanism of Action

Interferon alfa has multiple effects on the viral replication cycle. After binding to receptors on host cell membranes, the drug blocks viral entry into cells, synthesis of viral messenger RNA and viral proteins, and viral assembly and release.

Conventional Versus Long-Acting Interferons

The alfa interferons can be divided into two groups—conventional and long acting—based on their time course of action. The conventional preparations have short half-lives, so they must be administered frequently—at least *3 times a week.* In contrast, the long-acting preparations are administered less frequently—just *once a week*—making them more convenient. In addition, with the long-acting preparations, blood levels remain high between doses, and hence clinical responses are better.

How are long-acting interferons made? By conjugating a conventional interferon (e.g., interferon alfa-2b) with polyethylene glycol (PEG) in a process known as *pegylation.* Therapeutic effects of the pegylated product are due solely to its interferon component. The PEG component serves only to delay elimination. At this time, two long-acting interferons are available: *pegylated interferon (peginterferon) alfa-2a* [Pegasys] and *peginterferon alfa-2b* [PegIntron]. Because of their convenience and superior efficacy, these products are preferred to conventional interferons. However, note that several side effects—injection-site reactions, dose-related neutropenia, and thrombocytopenia—are more common with pegylated interferons than with the conventional formulations.

Effects in Chronic Hepatitis C

In patients with chronic hepatitis C, responses are equally modest with all forms of interferon alfa. After 12 months of treatment, serum ALT normalizes in 40% to 50% of patients, and serum levels of HCV-RNA (a marker for HCV in blood) become undetectable in 30% to 40%. Unfortunately, about half of these people relapse when treatment is stopped; sustained responses are maintained in only 5% to 15% of patients. Combining interferon alfa with other agents can improve response rates.

Adverse Effects

All formulations of interferon alfa produce the same spectrum of adverse effects, some of which can be life threatening. The incidence is higher with the long-acting preparations.

The most common side effect is a *flu-like syndrome* characterized by fever, fatigue, myalgia, headache, and chills. The incidence is about 50%. Fortunately, symptoms tend to diminish with continued therapy. Some symptoms (fever, headache, myalgia) can be reduced with acetaminophen.

Interferon alfa frequently causes *neuropsychiatric effects*—especially *depression.* Suicidal ideation and suicide have occurred. The risk for depression is increased by large doses and prolonged treatment. The mechanism underlying depression is unknown. In many patients, depression responds to

TABLE 93.3 ▪ Interferon Alfa Preparations: Dosages for Chronic Hepatitis B and Hepatitis C

		Adult Dosage	
Generic Name	**Brand Name**	**Chronic Hepatitis B**	**Chronic Hepatitis C**
CONVENTIONAL INTERFERON ALFA PREPARATIONS			
Interferon alfa-2b	Intron A	5 million IU subQ daily *or* 10 million IU subQ 3 times/week	3 million IU subQ or IM 3 times/week
Interferon alfacon-1	Infergen	(Not used)	*Monotherapy:* 9 mcg subQ 3 times/week *With ribavirin:* 15 mcg subQ daily
LONG-ACTING INTERFERON ALFA PREPARATIONS			
Peginterferon alfa-2a	Pegasys	180 mcg subQ once/week	180 mcg subQ once/week
Peginterferon alfa-2b	PegIntron, Unitron PEG 🍁	(Not used)	*Monotherapy:* 1 mcg/kg subQ once/week *With ribavirin:* 1.5 mcg/kg subQ once/week

IU, International units.

antidepressant drugs (e.g., paroxetine). If depression persists, a reduction in dosage or cessation of treatment is indicated.

Prolonged or high-dose therapy can cause fatigue, thyroid dysfunction, heart damage, and bone marrow suppression, manifesting as neutropenia and thrombocytopenia.

Other adverse effects include alopecia and GI effects: nausea, diarrhea, anorexia, and vomiting. Injection-site reactions (inflammation, bruising, itching, irritation) are common, especially with long-acting formulations. Also, interferon may induce or exacerbate autoimmune diseases, such as thyroiditis and autoimmune chronic hepatitis.

Ribavirin (Oral)

Actions and Therapeutic Use

Oral ribavirin [Rebetol, Ribasphere, Copegus], combined with subQ peginterferon alfa, is the traditional treatment of choice for HCV infection. When used alone against HCV, ribavirin is not effective: Treatment produces a transient normalization of serum ALT, but does not reduce serum HCV-RNA. Combining ribavirin with interferon alfa greatly improves response rates. Ribavirin is a nucleoside analog with a broad spectrum of antiviral activity, but its mechanism of action remains unclear.

In addition to its use against HCV, ribavirin is available as an aerosol for treating children infected with respiratory syncytial virus. This use is discussed later under *Ribavirin (Inhaled)*.

Pharmacokinetics

Ribavirin is well absorbed after oral administration. In plasma, the drug does not undergo protein binding. After leaving the vasculature, ribavirin is readily taken up by cells. Perhaps because of this cellular sequestration, ribavirin has a prolonged half-life, estimated at 6 to 12 days. As a result, when dosing stops, it can take weeks to clear the drug from the body.

Adverse Effects

Although ribavirin and interferon alfa are generally well tolerated, both drugs can cause significant adverse effects. As noted earlier, interferon alfa frequently causes *flu-like symptoms* and occasionally causes *severe depression*. The principal concerns with ribavirin are *hemolytic anemia* and *fetal injury*.

Hemolytic Anemia. Hemolytic anemia, characterized by a hemoglobin (Hb) level below 10 gm/dL, develops in 10% to 13% of patients receiving dual therapy with ribavirin/interferon alfa. Onset is typically 1 to 2 weeks after starting treatment. Hemolytic anemia can worsen heart disease and may lead to nonfatal or fatal myocardial infarction. Owing to the risk for anemia, ribavirin should be avoided in patients with significant heart disease and in those with hemoglobinopathies, including sickle cell anemia and thalassemia major. Because anemia can develop rapidly, Hb determinations should be made before treatment, 2 weeks and 4 weeks into treatment, and periodically thereafter.

Fetal Injury. Ribavirin is both embryolethal and teratogenic. In laboratory animals, the drug has caused fetal death, as well as malformations of the skull, palate, eyes, jaw, limbs, GI tract, and skeleton—all at doses as low as one-twentieth of those used to treat humans. Accordingly, *ribavirin is contraindicated for use during pregnancy.* Pregnancy must be ruled out before starting ribavirin. Also, pregnancy testing must be done every month during treatment and for 6 months after treatment stops. To avoid pregnancy, couples should use *two* reliable forms of birth control during treatment and for 6 months after stopping. Furthermore, if ribavirin is used in conjunction with a *protease inhibitor*, hormonal contraceptives may not work, and hence two *barrier* contraceptives should be used, as discussed later under *Protease Inhibitors*.

Among men being treated, ribavirin can be present in sperm. We don't know whether ribavirin-containing sperm will be teratogenic upon fertilizing an ovum. Until more is known, prudence dictates that couples avoid pregnancy if the male partner is receiving ribavirin.

Other Adverse Effects. In addition to flu-like symptoms, depression, anemia, and birth defects, ribavirin/interferon alfa can cause many other adverse effects. Among these are autoimmune disorders, infections, pancreatitis, neutropenia, and injury to the eyes and lungs.

Protease Inhibitors

In 2011, the U.S. Food and Drug Administration (FDA) approved two PIs—boceprevir and telaprevir—for treatment of chronic hepatitis C, making them the first new drugs for hepatitis C in 20 years. These were the first of the direct-acting antivirals that would revolutionize hepatitis C treatment. (Telaprevir was subsequently withdrawn from the market in 2014 by the manufacturer, who cited dwindling sales of this first-generation DAA among increased competition from new products, including DAAs with fewer interactions and fewer adverse effects. In 2015, boceprevir was also withdrawn.)

PIs inhibit viral protease, an enzyme required for HCV replication. There are currently three "second wave" PIs approved in the United States: grazoprevir, paritaprevir, and simeprevir. Of these, only simprevir is available as a single agent (with indications to use it only in combination with other drugs). Grazoprevir and paritaprevir are available in combination with other drugs. There are at least four other protease inhibitors in clinical trials.

For our discussion, we will examine the second-generation PI simeprevir. Properties of the combination drugs are presented in Table 93.4.

Simeprevir

Action and Use. Simeprevir [Olysio, Galexos 🍁] is a second wave protease inhibitor and DAA against HVC. Simprevir is approved for the treatment of chronic hepatitis C for HCV genotype 1 or 4. It must always be used in combination with other anti-HCV drugs

Adverse Effects. FDA labeling warns of the potential for hepatic injury, significant photosensitivity, and severe rashes. The most common adverse effects experienced are headache, nausea, and fatigue.

Pharmacokinetics. Taking simprevir with food will enhance its absorption to 62% bioavailability. Metabolism is primarily by CYP3A4 isoenzymes. Half-life is 10 to 13 hours in healthy individuals but in HCV-infected patients, the half-life may be as long as 41 hours. Excretion is primarily in the feces (91%) with less than 1% eliminated in the urine.

Contraindications. There are no absolute contraindications for simprevir. Although not contraindicated, simeprevir is not recommended for patients with severe liver impairment and should not be administered with peginterferon and ribavirin

TABLE 93.4 ▪ Properties of Anti-HCV Direct-Acting Antiviral Drug Combinations

Drug Combinations	Elbasvir-Grazoprevir [Zepatier]	Ledipasvir-Sofosbuvir [Harvoni]	Ombitasvir-Paritaprevir-Ritonavir[a] [Technivie]	Ombitasvir-Paritaprevir-Ritonavir[a] With Dasabuvir [Viekira Pak]
Classification	NS5A inhibitor + PI	NS5A inhibitor + NPI	NS5A inhibitor + PI + CYP3A inhibitor	NS5A inhibitor + PI + CYP3A inhibitor + NNPI
HCV genotype treated	1a, 1b, 4	1a, 1b, 4, 5, 6	4	1a, 1b
Adverse effects	Significant ALT elevations have occurred. The most common adverse reactions are headache, nausea, and fatigue. About 5% develop anemia	Common adverse effects are headache, fatigue, and weakness	ALT elevations up to 5 times normal have occurred. Patients with cirrhosis may develop hepatic failure. Common adverse reactions are nausea, fatigue, insomnia, weakness	Significant ALT elevations have occurred. Hepatic failure has occurred, primary in patients with advanced cirrhosis. Common adverse reactions include nausea, fatigue, insomnia, weakness, pruritus, and skin reactions
Contraindications	Moderate to severe hepatic impairment	Administration with amiodarone can cause dangerous symptomatic bradycardia.	Moderate to severe hepatic impairment	Moderate to severe hepatic impairment
Monitoring	Check liver enzymes prior to initiating therapy, after 2 months, and if s/s of liver complications develop. Check baseline CBC and recheck if s/s anemia develop	Cardiac monitoring recommended if administration with amiodarone is necessary	Check liver enzymes prior to initiating therapy, within 4 weeks of therapy, and if s/s of liver complications develop	Check liver enzymes prior to initiating therapy, within 4 weeks of therapy, and if s/s of liver complications develop
Administration	Administer with or without food	Administer with or without food	Administer with meals (increases absorption)	Administer with meals (increases absorption)

[a]Ritonavir is an HIV protease inhibitor with no inherent anti-HCV activity. It boosts the HCV antiviral drugs via its CYP3A inhibitor activity.
ALT, Alanine aminotransferase; *s/s,* signs or symptoms.

if the patient has decompensated cirrhosis. Also, simprevir contains a component of sulfonamide, so caution is advised for patients who have had previous reactions to sulfonamides.

Drug Interactions. Simprevir exerts mild inhibition of CYP1A2 isoenzyme activity, but it is unlikely to have a significant effect. On the other hand, it is a substrate of CYP3A4 isoenzymes; therefore drugs that are CYP3A4 inducers may lower simprevir levels, whereas CYP3A4 inhibitors may raise levels. Significant adverse effects may occur when given with amiodarone (serious symptomatic bradycardia). It may elevate levels of HMG CO-A reductase inhibitors, so lower doses of statin drugs may be necessary. It may also raise levels of sedative anxiolytics such as midazolam and triazolam, which both have a narrow therapeutic index. Labeling warns against co-administration of a number of drugs. As with any drug, it is important to consult drug interaction software before administering a new drug to patients taking anti-HCV therapy.

NS5A Inhibitors

NS5A inhibitors target a nonstructural protein, NS5A, that is necessary for HCV RNA replication and assembly. In so doing, these drugs prevent replication and construction of HCV. Unfortunately, resistance can build easily to these agents. Hence, as with other HCV regimens, they should never be given alone.

There are currently four NS5A inhibitors approved for use in the United States. Daclatasvir is approved as a single agent to be added to other anti-HCV regimens. Elbasvir, ledipasvir, and ombitasvir are combined in fixed dosages with other antiviral drugs. As with our previous classification, combination products will be summarized in tables.

Daclatasvir

Action and Use. Daclatasvir [Daklinza] is an NS5A inhibitor antiviral drug approved for treatment of chronic hepatitis C infection with HCV genotype 1 or 3. It should be used with sofosbuvir, with or without the addition of ribavirin.

Adverse Effects. The most common adverse reactions are headache and fatigue (in combination with sofosbuvir). With the addition of ribavirin, nausea and anemia also occurred in at least 10% of those taking the triple therapy.

Pharmacokinetics. Absorption is essentially unaffected by food intake. Metabolism occurs through CYP3A isoenzymes, with CYP3A4 predominating. About 88% of the drug is eliminated in the feces and 7% in the urine.

Contraindications. There are no absolute contraindications. However, product labeling includes drug interactions with strong CYP3A inducers and amiodarone (see *Drug Interactions*).

Drug Interactions. Because daclatasvir is a CYP3A substrate, strong CYP3A inducers can significantly lower daclatasvir levels. Examples of strong inducers include the antiepileptic drugs carbamazepine and phenytoin and the herbal supplement St. John's wort. Similarly, CYP3A inhibitors can raise daclatasvir levels. Both situations may require dosage adjustments of daclatasvir. Although not a contraindication per se, there is a strong warning and recommendation against adding the daclatasvir/sofosbuvir combination to amiodarone because dangerous symptomatic bradycardia may occur. In addition to the interactions mentioned as contraindications, a large number of others can occur. Most notably, substances that induce or inhibit CYP3A isoenzymes may affect daclatasvir levels. Others, when given together, include elevations of HMG-CoA reductase inhibitors (statins) and elevations of digoxin. Use of drug interaction software is needed to screen potential interactions when prescribing new drugs to patients taking daclatasvir.

NS5B Inhibitors

NS5B is a nonstructural HCV protein that, like NS5A, is vital for HCV's RNA replication. There are two classes of drugs that target this protein: NS5B NPIs and NS5B NNPIs. Beyond structural composition, they differ primarily in respect to properties of resistance and genotype. NPIs have a low likelihood of development of viral resistance, whereas the likelihood of viral resistance is high for NNPIs. In contrast, NPIs have high efficacy for all genotypes, whereas the NNPIs have lower efficacy and are effective for fewer genotypes.

The only NPI currently approved is sofosbuvir [Sovaldi]. The only NNPI is dasabuvir, which is available only in a fixed-dose combination with ombitasvir, paritaprevir, and ritonavir. As before, we will examine sofosbuvir as an individual drug, whereas dasabuvir will be examined in the combined form.

Sofosbuvir

Action and Use. Sofosbuvir [Sovaldi] is a NS5B NPI. It is activated by metabolism, after which it incorporates into the HCV RNA through NS5B polymerase. It is approved as a component of antiviral treatment for chronic hepatitis C of HCV genotype 1, 2, 3, or 4.

Adverse Effects. Headaches and fatigue affect about 20% of patients when given in combination with ribavirin. When interferon alfa is added to the combination, nausea, anemia, and insomnia may also occur.

Pharmacokinetics. Food does not significantly alter absorption. Sofosbuvir is a prodrug that is metabolized to its active form through intracellular processes. Elimination is primarily through urine (80%), followed by feces and the respiratory system.

Contraindications. There are no contraindications for sofosbuvir. Those mentioned in product labeling apply only to drugs with which sofosbuvir may be combined.

Drug Interactions. If sofosbuvir is administered with amiodarone, dangerous symptomatic bradycardia may occur. Sofosbuvir is a substrate of P-glycoprotein (P-gp), a drug transporter with a role in determining the amount of drug that is absorbed and distributed. If administered with P-gp inducers such as St. John's wort, the level of sofosbuvir may decrease.

HEPATITIS B

In the United States, about 1.4 million people have chronic hepatitis B. Transmission is primarily through the exchange of blood or semen. Between 45% and 60% of exposed adults develop acute hepatitis. Of these, about 11,000 require hospitalization for deep fatigue, muscle pain, and jaundice. In adults, acute infection usually leads to viral clearance by the immune system. As a result, only 3% to 5% of infected adults develop chronic infection. However, when chronic infection does develop, it can lead to cirrhosis, hepatic failure, hepatocellular carcinoma, and death. The best strategy against HBV is prevention: All children should receive HBV vaccine before entering school (see Chapter 68).

Seven drugs are used for chronic HBV. Two are alfa interferons—*interferon alfa-2b* [Intron A] and *peginterferon alfa-2a* [Pegasys]—and five are nucleoside analogs: *lamivudine* [Epivir HBV, Heptovir ♣], *adefovir* [Hepsera], *entecavir* [Baraclude], *telbivudine* [Tyzeka, Sebivo ♣], and *tenofovir* [Viread]. The alfa interferons are administered subcutaneously; the nucleoside analogs are administered orally. The interferons are more effective than the nucleoside analogs, but are also more expensive and less well tolerated. Development of resistance is common with lamivudine and telbivudine, and relatively rare with the other five drugs. Four agents—lamivudine, adefovir, entecavir, and tenofovir—are also active against HIV, and hence may promote the emergence of resistant HIV in people co-infected with that virus.

With all seven drugs—and especially the nucleoside analogs—the rate of relapse following cessation of treatment is high. As a result, treatment is usually prolonged, thereby amplifying concerns about adverse effects and drug cost. To decrease unnecessary drug exposure and expense, current guidelines recommend treatment only for patients at highest risk, indicated by elevated aminotransferase levels, or with histologic evidence of moderate or severe hepatic inflammation or advanced fibrosis. We do not yet know whether treatment should continue lifelong or whether clinical benefit is sustained if treatment is stopped after several years. Given that relapse is common, patients should be followed closely if these drugs *are* withdrawn. Comparisons among the seven drugs are shown in Table 93.5.

Interferon Alfa

Only two forms of interferon alfa—interferon alfa-2b [Intron A] and peginterferon alfa-2a [Pegasys]—are approved for chronic hepatitis B. In clinical trials, treatment for 4 months reduced serum ALT and improved liver histology in about 40% of recipients. Remissions have been prolonged in some patients, and resistance has not been reported. Unfortunately, although alfa interferons are effective, they are also expensive, and adverse effects—flu-like syndrome, depression, fatigue, and leukopenia—are common. The basic pharmacology of interferon alfa and its use in hepatitis C were discussed previously.

Nucleoside Analogs

Lamivudine

Lamivudine [Epivir HBV, Heptovir ♣] is a nucleoside analog approved for infections caused by HBV or HIV. The drug was originally developed for HIV infection and was later approved for HBV. Formulations and dosages for treating HIV and HBV infections differ, so they must not be considered interchangeable. The basic pharmacology of lamivudine is discussed in Chapter 94. Discussion here is limited to the treatment of HBV.

TABLE 93.5 ■ Drugs for Chronic Hepatitis B

Drug	Route	Relapse Rate[a]	Adverse Effects	Resistance Rate	Active Against HIV
INTERFERON ALFA PREPARATIONS					
Interferon alfa-2b [Intron A]	SubQ	Moderate	Flu-like symptoms, fatigue, neutropenia, depression	Zero	No
Peginterferon alfa-2a [Pegasys]	SubQ	Moderate	Same as interferon alfa-2b	Zero	No
NUCLEOSIDE ANALOGS					
Lamivudine [Epivir HBV, Heptovir ♣]	PO	High	Well tolerated; lactic acidosis and hepatomegaly are possible	15%–30% in yr 1; 70% by yr 5	Yes
Adefovir [Hepsera]	PO	High	Nephrotoxic at high doses; lactic acidosis and hepatomegaly are possible	Zero in yr 1; 29% by yr 5	Yes
Entecavir [Baraclude]	PO	High	Well tolerated; lactic acidosis and hepatomegaly are possible	Zero in yr 1; 1% or less by yr 3	Yes
Tenofovir [Viread]	PO	High	Weakness, headache, GI reactions; lactic acidosis and hepatomegaly are possible	—	Yes
Telbivudine [Tyzeka, Sebivo ♣]	PO	Moderate	Myopathy, lactic acidosis, hepatomegaly are possible	6%–12% in yr 1; 9%–22% by yr 2	No

[a]Following discontinuation of treatment.

Lamivudine suppresses HBV replication by inhibiting viral DNA synthesis. The process begins with intracellular conversion of lamivudine to lamivudine triphosphate, the drug's active form. As the triphosphate, lamivudine undergoes incorporation into the growing DNA chain and thereby causes premature chain termination.

Lamivudine offers at least some benefit to most patients. In one trial, 52 weeks of daily lamivudine normalized serum ALT in 72% of patients and reduced liver inflammation and fibrosis in 56%. Unfortunately, the rate of relapse is high when treatment stops. Also, emergence of resistance is a concern: Resistant isolates appear in 24% of patients after 1 year of continuous treatment, 42% after 2 years, 53% after 3 years, and 70% after 4 years.

At the dosage employed to treat hepatitis B, side effects are minimal. In clinical trials, the incidence of most side effects was no greater than with placebo. *Lactic acidosis, pancreatitis,* and *severe hepatomegaly* are rare but dangerous complications. If one of these conditions develops, lamivudine should be discontinued.

For treatment of HBV, lamivudine [Epivir HBV, Heptovir ♣] is formulated in 100-mg tablets and a 5-mg/mL oral solution. The adult dosage is 100 mg once daily (compared with 150 mg twice daily for HIV). The pediatric dosage is 3 mg/kg once daily (compared with 4 mg/kg twice daily for HIV). Because lamivudine is eliminated primarily by renal excretion, dosage must be reduced in patients with renal impairment.

Adefovir

Therapeutic Use. Adefovir [Hepsera] is indicated for oral therapy of chronic hepatitis B. The drug was originally developed to fight HIV infection, but was not approved, owing to a high incidence of nephrotoxicity at the doses required. The doses used for hepatitis B are much lower; thus the risk for renal injury is lower.

Mechanism of Action. Adefovir is a nucleoside analog with a mechanism similar to that of acyclovir. Both drugs inhibit viral DNA synthesis, and both must be converted to their active form within the body. Activation of adefovir is mediated by cellular kinases—enzymes that convert the drug into adefovir diphosphate, a compound with two actions: (1) it directly inhibits viral DNA polymerase (by competing with deoxyadenosine triphosphate, a natural substrate for the enzyme), and (2) it undergoes incorporation into the growing strand of viral DNA and thereby causes premature strand termination. Host cells are spared because adefovir diphosphate is a poor inhibitor of human DNA polymerase.

Pharmacokinetics. Bioavailability is about 60% after oral administration, both in the presence and absence of food. Plasma levels peak about 2 hours after dosing. Elimination is renal, by a combination of glomerular filtration and active tubular secretion. In patients with normal kidney function, the half-life is 7.5 hours. In patients with renal impairment, the half-life is significantly increased.

Adverse Effects. *Nephrotoxicity* is the principal concern. Increased serum creatinine, a sign of kidney damage, was seen in 4% of patients who received 48 weeks of therapy, and in 9% of patients who received 96 weeks of therapy. To reduce risk, kidney function should be assessed at baseline and periodically thereafter, paying special attention to patients at high risk (i.e., patients with pre-existing renal impairment and those taking nephrotoxic drugs [e.g., cyclosporine, tacrolimus, aminoglycosides, vancomycin, aspirin and other nonsteroidal anti-inflammatory drugs]).

When adefovir is discontinued, patients may experience *acute exacerbation of hepatitis B.* In clinical trials, serum ALT levels rose dramatically in 25% of patients when treatment was stopped. Liver function should be assessed periodically after adefovir withdrawal.

Drug Interactions. Drugs that are eliminated by active tubular secretion can compete with adefovir for renal excretion. As a result, if one of these agents were combined with adefovir, excretion of adefovir, the other drug, or both could be decreased, causing their plasma levels to rise.

Precautions. Because adefovir is related to the nucleoside analogs used against HIV, there is a concern that if the patient were infected with HIV, giving adefovir in the low doses employed against HBV could allow emergence of HIV viruses resistant to nucleoside analogs. Accordingly, HIV infection should be ruled out before adefovir is used.

The nucleoside analogs used to treat HIV infection can cause lactic acidosis and severe hepatomegaly. There is concern that adefovir can cause these effects too. If the patient develops clinical or laboratory findings that suggest lactic acidosis or pronounced hepatotoxicity, adefovir should be withdrawn.

Preparations, Dosage, and Administration. Adefovir [Hepsera] is supplied in 10-mg tablets. For patients with good kidney function, the dosage is 10 mg once a day, taken with or without food. For patients with impaired kidney function, as indicated by reduced creatinine clearance (CrCl), the dosing *interval* should be increased.

Entecavir

Therapeutic Use. Entecavir [Baraclude] is indicated for oral therapy of chronic hepatitis B. Candidates for treatment should have evidence of active viral replication along with persistently elevated serum aminotransferases or histologic evidence of active disease. In clinical trials, entecavir was more effective than lamivudine. In patients with lamivudine-resistant HBV, responses to entecavir were somewhat reduced, but were still better than responses to lamivudine. Recent evidence indicates that entecavir can reverse fibrosis and cirrhosis with long-term use (3 years).

Mechanism of Action. Entecavir is a nucleoside analog that undergoes conversion to entecavir triphosphate (its active form) within the body. As entecavir triphosphate, the drug inhibits HBV DNA polymerase and thereby prevents viral replication. Entecavir triphosphate is a weak inhibitor of human DNA polymerases, both nuclear and mitochondrial, and hence host cells are spared. Like lamivudine and adefovir, entecavir may impede HIV replication, so it may promote emergence of resistant HIV.

Pharmacokinetics. Entecavir is available in tablets and solution for oral dosing. Bioavailability with both formulations is the same. Plasma levels peak 0.5 to 1.5 hours after dosing. Entecavir undergoes extensive distribution to body tissues, with little binding to plasma proteins. Metabolism is minimal. Entecavir is neither a substrate for, inhibitor of, nor inducer of cytochrome P450 enzymes. Excretion is through the urine, primarily as unchanged drug. The half-life is about 5.5 days.

Adverse Effects and Precautions. Entecavir is very well tolerated. The most common adverse effects are dizziness, headache, fatigue, and nausea—and even these occur in less than 5% of patients.

Patients treated with other nucleoside analogs have developed lactic acidosis and severe hepatomegaly, and hence there is concern that entecavir may cause these effects too. If the patient develops clinical or laboratory findings that suggest lactic acidosis or pronounced hepatotoxicity, entecavir should be withdrawn.

Acute severe exacerbations of hepatitis B have developed after discontinuation of entecavir and other drugs for hepatitis B. Accordingly, if entecavir is discontinued, liver function should be monitored closely for several months.

Preparations, Dosage, and Administration. Entecavir [Baraclude] is available in tablets (0.5 and 1 mg) and an oral solution (0.05 mg/mL). Dosing is done once a day, either 2 hours before eating or 2 hours after. Dosage depends on renal function (as indicated by CrCl) and on the infection's sensitivity to lamivudine. Typical doses are 0.5 mg once daily for patients who are nucleoside treatment naïve; 1 mg once daily for patients with viremia that is lamivudine-refractory or lamivudine-resistant; and 1 mg once daily for those with decompensated liver disease.

Telbivudine

Therapeutic Use. Telbivudine [Tyzeka, Sebivo 🍁] is a nucleoside analog indicated for chronic HBV infection in adults and adolescents age 16 years or older. Patients must have evidence of active HBV replication, plus either persistent elevations in serum ALT or aspartate aminotransferase (AST) or histologic evidence of active liver disease. In nucleoside-naïve patients, telbivudine is at least as effective as lamivudine (as indicated by suppression of HBV DNA and either normalization of ALT or loss of serum HBeAg, a hepatitis B antigen). As with lamivudine, resistance can be significant: After 2 years of treatment with telbivudine, resistance develops in 9% to 22% of patients. Patients resistant to telbivudine show cross-resistance to lamivudine. In contrast to lamivudine, entecavir, and adefovir, telbivudine is not active against HIV.

Mechanism of Action. Telbivudine is a thymidine nucleoside analog that undergoes intracellular conversion to its active form: telbivudine triphosphate. As the triphosphate, it inhibits HBV replication in two ways. First, it directly inhibits HBV DNA polymerase (by competing with the natural substrate, thymidine triphosphate). Second, it undergoes incorporation into the growing viral DNA chain and thereby causes chain termination.

Adverse Effects. The most common adverse effects are fever, fatigue/malaise, arthralgia, myalgia, cough, headache, and GI symptoms (e.g., abdominal pain, nausea, vomiting, diarrhea, dyspepsia). Some patients have developed symptomatic myopathy, characterized by persistent muscle pain, tenderness, or weakness. Lactic acidosis and severe hepatomegaly have occurred with other nucleoside analogs, but have not been reported with telbivudine. As with other drugs for hepatitis B, severe exacerbations can occur when treatment is discontinued.

Drug Interactions. No significant interactions have been reported. However, because telbivudine is eliminated primarily by renal excretion, drugs that impair renal function may raise its level. Also, other drugs that cause muscle injury may increase risk in patients taking telbivudine. Telbivudine is neither a substrate for nor inhibitor of CYP isoenzymes, and hence will not be affected by drugs that inhibit or induce CYP isoenzymes, nor will it affect drugs that are metabolized by these isoenzymes.

Preparations, Dosage, and Administration. Telbivudine [Tyzeka, Sebivo 🍁] is supplied in 600-mg tablets. The usual dosage for adults and children is 600 mg once a day, taken with or without food. For patients with renal impairment, as indicated by reduced CrCl, the dosing interval should be increased. For patients with hepatic impairment, no dosage adjustment is required.

Tenofovir

Like lamivudine and adefovir, tenofovir [Viread] was originally approved for HIV infection, and then later approved for HBV in adults. The basic pharmacology of tenofovir is presented in Chapter 94. Consideration here is limited to its use against HBV. When compared directly with adefovir in patients with HBV, tenofovir was considerably more effective. However, as with other nucleoside analogs, discontinuation of treatment is followed by exacerbation of hepatitis. Adverse effects include weakness, headache, lactic acidosis with hepatomegaly, and GI reactions: diarrhea, vomiting, and flatulence. Like some other nucleoside analogs, tenofovir can impede HIV replication, and hence may promote the emergence of resistant HIV. Tenofovir is supplied in 150-, 200-, 250-, and 300-mg tablets and in a 40-mg/gm powder for oral dosing. The recommended dosage for HBV is 300 mg once daily, the same dosage we use for HIV. Dosage should be reduced for patients with renal impairment.

DRUGS FOR INFLUENZA

Influenza is a serious respiratory tract infection that constitutes a major cause of morbidity and mortality worldwide. Complications of influenza (e.g., bronchitis, pneumonia) cause up to 300,000 American hospitalizations a year. Annual deaths vary widely, depending on the strain of flu in circulation. For example, between 1976 and 2007, annual deaths ranged from a low of 3,300 to a high of 49,000. The cost of influenza is huge: Direct and indirect expenses total between $3 billion and $5 billion annually.

Influenza is caused by influenza viruses, of which there are two major types: *influenza A* and *influenza B*. Type A influenza viruses cause far more infections than type B influenza viruses (about 96% vs. 4%). The influenza A viruses are further subclassified on the basis of two types of surface antigens: hemagglutinin (H) and neuraminidase (N). The predominant subgroups of seasonal influenza A viruses in circulation today are known as H1N1 and H3N2, because of the specific types of hemagglutinin and neuraminidase that they carry. Keep in mind, however, that viral strains undergo constant evolution. As a result, the strains of H1N1 and H3N2 in circulation this year are likely to differ from the strains of H1N1 and H3N2 in circulation next year.

Influenza is a highly contagious infection spread through aerosolized droplets produced by coughing or sneezing. The virus enters the body through mucous membranes of the nose, mouth, or eyes. Viral replication takes place in the respiratory tract. Symptoms begin 2 to 4 days after exposure, and last 5 to 6 days. Influenza is characterized by fever, cough, chills, sore throat, headache, and myalgia (muscle pain). For typical patients, infection results in 5 to 6 days of restricted activity, 3 to 4 days of bed disability, and 3 days of absence from work or school.

Influenza is managed by vaccination and with drugs. Vaccination is the primary management strategy; drug therapy is secondary. For very current information on influenza vaccines and drugs, see www.cdc.gov/flu, a comprehensive website maintained by the CDC.

INFLUENZA VACCINES

Annual vaccination is the best protection against influenza. Because influenza viruses are constantly evolving, influenza vaccines must continuously change too. Each year, manufacturers produce a new vaccine directed against the three (trivalent) or four (quadrivalent) strains of influenza virus deemed most likely to cause disease during the upcoming flu season. Identification of the strains is done jointly by the CDC, FDA, and World Health Organization.

Types of Influenza Vaccines

Three basic types of influenza vaccine are available: (1) *inactivated influenza vaccine (IIV)*, (2) *recombinant hemagglutinin vaccine (RIV)*, and (3) *live, attenuated influenza vaccine (LAIV)*. The IIV and RIV are administered by *IM injection* with one exception, Fluzone Intradermal, which is administered by *intradermal injection.* The LAIV is administered by *intranasal spray.* All are directed against the same influenza strains and are reformulated annually. To maintain protection, revaccination is required each year.

At this time, there are 10 influenza vaccines on the market. The vaccines differ regarding the age groups for which they are approved (Table 93.6). Most vaccine recipients get just one dose a year. However, children age 2 through 8 years who have not been vaccinated before require two doses, administered at least 1 month apart. Protection begins 1 to 2 weeks after vaccination. Immunity generally lasts 6 months or longer; however, among older vaccine recipients, protection may be lost in 4 months or even less.

Efficacy

Efficacy of vaccination depends not only on the age and health status of the vaccine recipient, but also on how well the vaccine matches the strains of influenza virus in circulation that year.

Each year the CDC conducts vaccine effectiveness (VE) studies. In the years from 2013 to 2016, VE study data demonstrated a decline in LAIV efficacy. Subsequently, the CDC's Advisory Committee on Immunization Practices (ACIP) advises against the use of LAIV for the 2016–2017 influenza season (see https://www.cdc.gov/mmwr/volumes/65/rr/rr6505a1.htm). The CDC has not yet set policy on the ACIP recommendation; however, we expect this will be done by the time you read this book. The outcome will be posted to the CDC Vaccine Recommendations website at https://www.cdc.gov/vaccines/hcp/acip-recs/vacc-specific/flu.html. In the meantime, we will continue to cover LAIV in case its use continues after the 2016–2017 influenza season.

Adverse Effects

Adverse effects differ for the IIV and RIV versus the LAIV. Fortunately for all vaccines, significant adverse effects are rare.

Both IIV and RIV can cause soreness at the injection site. People who have not been vaccinated previously may experience fever, myalgia, and malaise lasting 1 or 2 days.

The most common reactions to LAIV have been rhinorrhea (runny nose), nasal congestion, cough, sore throat, headache, vomiting, muscle aches, and fever. Influenza vaccination may carry a very small risk for *Guillain-Barré syndrome* (GBS), a severe, paralytic illness. In 1976, swine flu vaccine was

TABLE 93.6 ▪ Influenza Vaccines

Type of Vaccine	Brand Name	Formulation(s)	Route	Recommended Age Group
Inactivated Influenza Vaccine, Quadrivalent (IIV4)	Fluarix Quadrivalent	0.5-mL single-dose pre-filled syringe	IM	≤3 years
		5.0-mL multidose vial	IM	≤3 years
	Fluzone Quadrivalent	0.25-mL single-dose pre-filled syringe	IM	6–35 months
		0.5-mL single-dose pre-filled syringe	IM	≤36 months
		0.5-mL single-dose vial	IM	≤36 months
		5.0-mL multidose vial	IM	≤6 months
	Fluzone Intradermal Quadrivalent	0.1-mL single-dose pre-filled microinjection system	ID	18–64 years
	Flucelvax Quadrivalent	0.5-mL single-dose pre-filled syringe	IM	≤4 years
Inactivated Influenza Vaccine, Trivalent (IIV3)	Afluria	0.5-mL single-dose pre-filled syringe	IM	≤9 years
		5.0-mL multidose vial	IM	≤9 years
	Fluvirin	0.5-mL single-dose pre-filled syringe	IM	≤4 years
		5.0-mL multidose vial	IM	≤4 years
	Fluad	0.5-mL single-dose pre-filled syringe	IM	≤65 years
	Fluzone High-Dose	0.5-mL single-dose pre-filled syringe	IM	≤65 years
Recombinant Influenza Vaccine, Trivalent (RIV3)	Flublok	0.5-mL single-dose vial	IM	≤18 years
Live Attenuated Influenza Vaccine, quadrivalent (LAIV4)[a]	FluMist Quadrivalent[a]	0.2 mL single-dose pre-filled intranasal sprayer	INS	2–49 years

[a]Not recommended by the Advisory Committee on Immunization Practices for the 2016–2017 influenza season.
ID, Intradermal; *IM,* intramuscular; *INS,* intranasal spray.
Adapted from Centers for Disease Control and Prevention. *Influenza vaccines—United States, 2016–17 influenza season,* 2016; available at https://www.cdc.gov/flu/protect/vaccine/vaccines.htm.

associated with GBS. However, there has been no clear link between GBS and influenza vaccines used since then. If there *is* a risk, it is very small, estimated at 1 to 2 cases per million vaccine recipients—much smaller than the risk posed by severe influenza.

Precautions

People with acute moderate to severe febrile illness should defer vaccination until symptoms abate. However, mild illnesses (e.g., common cold), with or without fever, do not preclude vaccination.

Previously, special considerations were indicated for people with hypersensitivity to eggs. For some, this required vaccine administration by an allergist and administration at inpatient facilities such as hospitals. For those with anaphylactic reactions to eggs, vaccination was sometimes contraindicated. Why? This precaution was put in place because the vaccines are produced from viruses grown in eggs. There is a theoretical possibility that trace amounts of egg proteins can be transferred during vaccination. The results of studies and data analysis have not supported the need for this abundance of caution, however. Out of 7.4 million vaccinations, there were only 10 individual cases of anaphylaxis, and most of those did not occur in patients with egg allergies. Subsequently, in 2016 the CDC eliminated special requirements for patients with egg allergies, including patients with a history of anaphylactic reactions to eggs.[a] Influenza vaccinations for all patients may take place in outpatient facilities as long as the healthcare provider is able to recognize and manage allergic reactions. Also, there is no longer a prolonged observation requirement after injection. Instead, the CDC recommends the same 15-minute observation time for all patients. For additional information on this new guidance, see https://www.cdc.gov/flu/protect/vaccine/egg-allergies.htm.

Safety Alert

Before administering a vaccination, it is important to question the patient or family member about allergies, previous reactions to vaccines, and current health status.

Who Should Be Vaccinated?

The Advisory Committee on Immunization Practices (ACIP) now recommends annual influenza vaccination for *all people age 6 months and older.* Although an annual flu shot is recommended for everyone, an annual shot is especially important for people at high risk for influenza complications or who have conditions that may be exacerbated by influenza (Table 93.7).

Important note: LAIV should not be administered to people who are immunocompromised, pregnant, or otherwise at high risk for influenza complications. The attenuated viruses it contains are still capable of replication. This is unlikely to occur in healthy individuals; therefore, LAIV is approved for use only among healthy persons aged 5 to 49 years.

[a]Patients with egg allergies who refuse vaccination out of fear may take the RIV Flublok, which is manufactured using insect cell lines instead of eggs.

TABLE 93.7 ▪ Patients at High Risk for Influenza-Related Complications

These patients are at high risk for complications of influenza:
- Children younger than 5 years (especially children younger than 2 years)
- Pregnant women (and 2 weeks postpartum)
- Adults age 65 years and older
- People who live in long-term care facilities (e.g., nursing homes)
- American Indians and Alaskan Natives

Influenza may seriously compromise the health of patients with the following medical conditions:
- Immunosuppression (e.g., HIV infection, cancer, or the use of immunosuppressant drugs)
- Respiratory diseases (e.g., asthma, chronic obstructive pulmonary disease, cystic fibrosis)
- Neurologic conditions (e.g., stroke, spinal cord injuries, cerebral palsy, muscular dystrophy)
- Heart disease (e.g., heart failure, congenital heart disease, coronary artery disease)
- Hematologic disorders (e.g., sickle cell disease, blood dyscrasias)
- Endocrine disorders (e.g., diabetes)
- Renal, hepatic, and metabolic disorders
- Long-term aspirin therapy in patients younger than 19 years
- Body mass index (BMI) of 40 or more

Who Should NOT Be Vaccinated?

In the 2017 update of influenza vaccination guidelines, the CDC lists only one contraindication for the vaccine. Individuals who have had a severe (anaphylactic) allergic reaction after previous dose of the vaccine should not receive it again. The vaccine is *relatively* contraindicated for patients with a history of GBS that developed within 6 weeks of receiving influenza vaccination. For these patients, the CDC does not recommend the vaccine if they are not at high risk for complications (see Table 93.7). For those at high risk, the CDC recommends decision-making on an individual basis by the patient's healthcare provider.

When Should Vaccination Be Administered?

In the United States, flu season usually peaks in January or February, but can also peak as early as October or as late as May. To ensure full protection, the best time to vaccinate is October or November. However, for people who missed the best time, vaccinating as late as April may be of benefit. Influenza vaccine may be given at the same time as other vaccines, including pneumococcal vaccine.

Variations in Influenza Vaccines

There are a few variations in influenza vaccines that are worth noting. These are itemized next.

- Fluzone Intradermal contains less antigen/dose (9 mcg vs. 15 mcg) and is injected in a smaller volume (0.1 mL vs. 0.5 mL).

- Flumist, the LAIV nasal spray, is unstable and must be stored frozen.
- Some patients and parents are concerned about mercury in vaccines. Vaccines that contain mercury are Flulaval Quadrivalent (multidose formulation only), Fluzone Quadrivalent (multidose formulation only), Afluria (multidose formulation only), and Fluvirin (both multidose and single-dose formulations).
- For patients with severe allergies to latex, natural rubber latex may be contained in the syringe tip cap of Fluvirin single-dose and Fluad single-dose formulations.

NEURAMINIDASE INHIBITORS

The neuraminidase inhibitors are active against influenza A and influenza B. At this time, three neuraminidase inhibitors are available: oseltamivir, zanamivir, and peramivir.

Both oseltamivir and zanamivir are approved for influenza prophylaxis. Although approved for prophylaxis, these drugs are not as adequate as vaccination and should not be considered as a substitute for annual vaccination against influenza. However, because it takes about 2 weeks after vaccination for antibodies to develop against the influenza virus, these drugs can provide some protection for unvaccinated people during a community outbreak.

All three drugs are used for treatment. Dosing must begin early—preferably no later than 2 days after symptom onset and ideally much sooner. Why? Because benefits decline greatly when treatment is delayed. When treatment is started within 12 hours of symptom onset, symptom duration is reduced by more than 3 days; when started within 24 hours, symptom duration is reduced by less than 2 days; and when started within 36 hours, symptom duration is reduced by only 29 hours. In addition to reducing symptom duration, the drugs can reduce symptom severity and the incidence of complications (sinusitis, bronchitis). Unfortunately, in the real world, patients may be unable to obtain and fill a prescription soon enough for the drug to be of significant benefit.

Oseltamivir

Actions and Uses

Oseltamivir [Tamiflu] is an oral drug approved for the prevention and treatment of influenza in patients 1 year and older. Antiviral effects derive from inhibiting neuraminidase, a viral enzyme required for replication. As a result of neuraminidase inhibition, newly formed viral particles are unable to bud off from the cytoplasmic membrane of infected host cells. Hence, viral spread is stopped. Oseltamivir is active against most strains of influenza A and influenza B responsible for seasonal influenza, as well as most isolates of influenza A type H5N1 (the cause of avian flu). In addition, the drug is active against the so-called swine flu, the variant of influenza A type H1N1 that caused the influenza pandemic in 2009. Emergence of resistance over the course of treatment is rare.

Pharmacokinetics

Oseltamivir is well absorbed after oral administration. In the liver, the drug undergoes conversion to oseltamivir carboxylate, its active form. Bioavailability of the carboxylate is 80%. Plasma levels of active drug peak 2.5 to 6 hours after dosing. The plasma half-life is 6 to 10 hours. The drug is eliminated in the urine, primarily as the carboxylate form.

Adverse Effects

Oseltamivir is generally well tolerated. The most common side effects are nausea and vomiting. Nausea can be reduced by giving oseltamivir with food.

Rarely, oseltamivir has caused *severe hypersensitivity reactions,* including anaphylaxis and serious skin reactions (e.g., toxic epidermal necrolysis, erythema multiforme, Stevens-Johnson syndrome). If an allergic reaction develops, oseltamivir should be discontinued.

Rarely, oseltamivir has been associated with *neuropsychiatric effects,* mainly in younger patients. Reported reactions include delirium and abnormal behavior, which has led to injury and even death. However, because influenza itself can cause these reactions, they cannot be ascribed with certainty to oseltamivir.

Interaction With Live Influenza Vaccine

In theory, oseltamivir can blunt responses to LAIV. Accordingly, oseltamivir should be discontinued at least 2 days before giving LAIV. Following dosing with LAIV, at least 2 weeks should elapse before starting oseltamivir.

Preparations, Dosage, and Administration

Oseltamivir [Tamiflu] is available in capsules (30, 45, and 75 mg) and as a powder (360 mg) to be reconstituted to a 6-mg/mL oral suspension. Dosing can be done with or without food, although dosing with food can reduce nausea.

Treatment of Influenza. For treatment, the dosage for patients *13 years and older* is 75 mg twice daily for 5 days, beginning no later than 2 days after the onset of symptoms. Dosage should be reduced to 75 mg once daily in patients with significant renal impairment. The dosage for children *1 year old through 12 years old* is based on body weight as follows: 15 kg or less, 30 mg twice daily; 15.1 to 23 kg, 45 mg twice daily; 23.1 to 40 kg, 60 mg twice daily; and more than 40 kg, 75 mg twice daily.

Prevention of Influenza. For prevention, the dosage is *one-half the dosage used for treatment.* This is accomplished by switching from twice-daily dosing to once-daily dosing. For patients *13 years and older,* the dosage is 75 mg once a day. The dosage for *children 1 year old through 12 years old* is based on body weight as follows: 15 kg or less, 30 mg once daily; 15 to 23 kg, 45 mg once daily; 23.1 to 40 kg, 60 mg once daily; and more than 40 kg, 75 mg once daily.

Candidates for prophylactic therapy include family members of someone with influenza and residents of nursing homes. To protect family members, dosing should begin within 48 hours of exposure and should continue for 10 days. To protect residents of nursing homes or high-risk members of the community at large, dosing can be done continuously for up to 42 days.

Zanamivir

Actions and Uses

Zanamivir [Relenza], administered by oral inhalation, is approved for the *treatment* of acute uncomplicated influenza in patients at least 7 years old, and for *prophylaxis* of influenza in people at least 5 years old. As with oseltamivir, benefits derive from inhibiting viral neuraminidase, an enzyme required for viral replication. Like oseltamivir, zanamivir is well tolerated, except in patients with underlying airway disease.

Pharmacokinetics

Zanamivir is formulated as a dry powder for oral inhalation. The drug is poorly absorbed from the GI tract, so it cannot be administered by mouth. Most (70% to 90%) of an inhaled dose is deposited in the oropharynx and throat. About 10% to 20% reaches the tracheobronchial tree and lungs. Between 4% and 17% of each dose undergoes absorption into the systemic circulation. Zanamivir has a plasma half-life of 2.5 to 5 hours and is eliminated unchanged in the urine. No metabolites have been detected.

Adverse Effects and Interactions

In patients with healthy lung function, serious adverse effects are uncommon. Because zanamivir is administered as an inhaled powder, patients may experience cough or throat irritation. Also, as with oseltamivir, there have been rare reports of severe allergic reactions and neuropsychiatric effects.

In patients with pre-existing lung disorders (e.g., asthma, chronic obstructive pulmonary disease), zanamivir may cause severe bronchospasm and respiratory decline. Some patients have required immediate treatment or hospitalization. Deaths have occurred. However, given the effect of influenza itself on lung function, it's not clear that zanamivir was the cause. Nonetheless, owing to the potential risk, zanamivir is not recommended for patients with underlying airway disease.

Zanamivir appears devoid of drug interactions. However, like oseltamivir, zanamivir may blunt responses to LAIV, and hence should be stopped 2 days before giving LAIV and should not be started for 2 weeks after giving LAIV.

Preparations, Dosage, and Administration

Zanamivir [Relenza] is supplied in blister packs that contain 5 mg of powdered drug. Administration is by oral inhalation using the *Diskhaler* provided by the manufacturer.

Influenza Treatment. The dosage for adults and children is 10 mg (two 5-mg inhalations) twice daily for 5 days. Each 10-mg dose should be separated by 12 hours. However, on the first day of treatment, less separation (as little as 2 hours) is permitted if the first dose cannot be taken early enough in the day to allow 12 hours between doses. Patients who are using an inhaled bronchodilator (e.g., albuterol) should administer the bronchodilator before inhaling zanamivir.

Influenza Prevention. The dosage for adults and children is 10 mg (two 5-mg inhalations) once daily. Note that this is one-half the dosage used for treatment.

Peramivir

Actions and Uses

Peramivir [Rapivab] is used to treat acute uncomplicated influenza for those who have been symptomatic for 2 days or fewer. Its use is restricted to those who are 18 years and older.

Pharmacokinetics

Peramivir is formulated for IV administration. It is not significantly metabolized. The plasma half-life is around 20 hours and is eliminated unchanged in the urine.

Adverse Reactions

Adverse reactions are rare. *Diarrhea* is the most common adverse effect. Rarely, *psychiatric events* (e.g., delirium, hallucinations) and *skin reactions* have occurred after administration. Like oseltamivir and zanamivir, peramivir can blunt responses to LAIV.

Preparations, Dosage, and Administration

Peramivir is administered as a single dose of 600 mg infused over 15 to 30 minutes. For patients with reduced renal function, dosage is based on creatinine clearance (CrCl). The standard dose of 600 mg may be administered for patients with a CrCl greater than 50 mL/min. For those with a CrCl of 30 to 49 mL/min, the recommended dosage is 200 mg; for a CrCl of 10 to 29 mL/min, the dosage is 100 mg.

ADAMANTANES

The adamantanes—*amantadine* [Symmetrel] and *rimantadine* [Flumadine]—were the first influenza drugs available. Although they remain on the market and were approved for influenza infection, because most current strains of influenza A are resistant and because all strains of influenza B are resistant, the CDC recommends against using these drugs for *any* influenza patients, whether infected with influenza A *or* influenza B.

DRUGS FOR RESPIRATORY SYNCYTIAL VIRUS INFECTION

Respiratory syncytial virus (RSV) infection is a major cause of lower respiratory tract disease. Symptomatic infection with RSV is most likely in the very young, older adults, and persons with disorders involving the respiratory tract, heart, or immune system. In the United States, RSV infection is the most common cause of lower respiratory tract disease in infants and young children, leading to between 132,000 and 172,000 hospitalizations each year. Among children 5 years old and younger, RSV is the leading cause of viral death. The death rate from RSV in older adults is also high. Like influenza, infection with RSV is seasonal, with most cases occurring in the winter (December through March). Only two antiviral drugs—ribavirin and palivizumab—are approved for RSV. Unfortunately, neither drug is very effective.

Ribavirin (Inhaled)

Ribavirin, a broad-spectrum antiviral drug, is available in two formulations: aerosol and oral. The aerosol formulation, marketed as Virazole, is used for infection with RSV. The oral formulation, marketed as Rebetol, Ribasphere, and Copegus, is used for chronic hepatitis C. Discussion here focuses on RSV. Its use for hepatitis C was discussed earlier in this chapter.

Antiviral Actions

Ribavirin [Virazole] is virustatic. The drug is active against RSV, HCV, influenza virus (types A and B), and HSV. Although several biochemical actions of the drug have been described, it is not known which (if any) is responsible for antiviral effects.

Use in RSV Infection

Ribavirin is labeled only for severe viral pneumonia caused by RSV in carefully selected, hospitalized infants and young children. Unfortunately, benefits are usually minimal—and the cost is high. Ribavirin should not be used for mild RSV infections.

Pharmacokinetics

For the treatment of RSV, ribavirin is administered by oral inhalation. The drug is absorbed from the lungs and achieves high concentrations in respiratory tract secretions and erythrocytes. Concentrations in plasma remain low. The drug is metabolized to active and inactive products. Excretion is through the urine (30% to 55%) and feces (15%). Ribavirin that is sequestered in erythrocytes remains in the body for weeks.

Adverse Effects

Inhalation of ribavirin produces little or no systemic toxicity. However, although generally safe, inhaled ribavirin does pose a hazard to infants undergoing mechanical assistance of ventilation: The drug can precipitate in the respiratory apparatus, thereby interfering with safe and effective respiratory support. Consequently, ribavirin should not be administered to infants who need respiratory assistance. In some infants and in adults who have asthma or chronic obstructive lung disease, ribavirin has caused deterioration of pulmonary function. Accordingly, respiratory function should be carefully monitored. If deterioration occurs, ribavirin should be discontinued. When administered systemically (PO or IV), ribavirin frequently causes anemia. This has not been reported with inhalational therapy.

Use in Pregnancy

Ribavirin is teratogenic. The risk for use during pregnancy clearly outweighs any potential benefits. Furthermore, it is contraindicated in men who are partners of pregnant women. Because of the risk for significant drug exposure, ribavirin is classified by NIOSH as hazardous for handling by nurses and other healthcare personnel (see earlier discussion).

Preparations, Dosage, and Administration

For treatment of RSV, ribavirin [Virazole] is supplied as a powder (6 gm/100-mL vial) to be reconstituted for aerosol administration. According to the manufacturer, only one device—the Viratek Small Particle Aerosol Generator (SPAG) model SPAG-2—should be employed for ribavirin administration. The SPAG-2 is used to deliver ribavirin to an infant oxygen hood. Treatment is given 12 to 18 hours a day for no less than 3 days and no more than 1 week. The drug should not be administered to patients who require ventilatory assistance. To reconstitute powdered ribavirin, dissolve 6 gm of the drug in sterile water for injection or inhalation, transfer this concentrated solution to the SPAG-2 reservoir, and dilute to a final volume of 300 mL using sterile water for injection or inhalation. The final concentration of ribavirin is 20 mg/mL. This solution is aerosolized and inhaled by the patient.

Palivizumab

Actions and Uses

Palivizumab [Synagis] is a monoclonal antibody indicated for preventing RSV infection in premature infants and in young children with chronic lung disease. The antibody binds to a surface protein on RSV and thereby prevents replication. In clinical trials, the rate of hospitalization was 1.8% for premature infants treated with palivizumab, compared with 8.1% for those receiving placebo. In young children with chronic lung disease, the hospitalization rate was 7.9% for those receiving the antibody versus 12.8% for those receiving placebo.

Adverse Effects

Except for *hypersensitivity reactions,* which are rare, palivizumab appears devoid of significant adverse effects. Acute hypersensitivity reactions have occurred with initial drug use and with subsequent use. Very rarely (less than 1 in 100,000 cases), palivizumab has caused anaphylaxis, but only with re-exposure, not with the initial dose. If a *mild* hypersensitivity reaction occurs, cautious use of palivizumab can continue. However, if a *severe* reaction occurs, the drug should be stopped and never used again. Severe reactions are managed with parenteral epinephrine and supportive care.

Preparations, Dosage, and Administration

Palivizumab [Synagis] is supplied in solution (50 and 100 mg/mL). The dosage is 15 mg/kg once a month, injected IM into the anterolateral aspect of the thigh. Dosing should commence before the RSV season (December through March in the United States) and continue until the season ends. The cost for a full season of treatment is about $7000. However, although this seems high, it could save more than $50,000 by avoiding hospitalization.

KEY POINTS

- Because viruses use host-cell enzymes and substrates to reproduce, it is difficult to suppress viral reproduction without also harming cells of the host.
- Acyclovir is the drug of choice for most infections caused by herpes simplex viruses and varicella-zoster virus.
- Following conversion to its active form, acyclovir suppresses viral reproduction by inhibiting viral DNA polymerase and by causing premature termination of viral DNA strand growth. Because the active form of acyclovir is not a good inhibitor of human DNA polymerase, cells of the host are spared.
- Acyclovir is eliminated unchanged by the kidneys. Accordingly, dosage must be reduced in patients with renal impairment.
- Intravenous acyclovir can injure the kidneys. Renal damage can be minimized by infusing acyclovir slowly and by ensuring adequate hydration during and after the infusion.
- Ganciclovir is the drug of choice for prophylaxis and treatment of CMV infection in immunocompromised patients, including those with AIDS.
- Ganciclovir does not cure CMV retinitis in patients with AIDS, so in most cases, treatment must continue for life.
- Like acyclovir, ganciclovir becomes activated within infected cells, after which it inhibits viral DNA polymerase and causes premature termination of viral DNA strand growth.
- Like acyclovir, ganciclovir is excreted unchanged in the urine. Hence, dosage must be reduced in patients with renal impairment.
- The major adverse effects of ganciclovir are granulocytopenia and thrombocytopenia.
- Chronic hepatitis is caused primarily by HBV and HCV.
- Hepatitis B can be prevented by vaccination. There is no vaccine for hepatitis C.
- Hepatitis C is treated with interferon alfa, ribavirin, and HCV protease inhibitors (boceprevir and telaprevir).
- HCV protease inhibitors prevent replicating HCV from progressing to its mature, infectious form.
- Ribavirin is not effective against HCV when used alone, so it is always combined with interferon alfa.
- HCV protease inhibitors greatly enhance the effects of interferon alfa plus ribavirin, and hence are always combined with both of those drugs.
- For years, the treatment of choice for hepatitis C has been dual therapy with peginterferon alfa plus ribavirin. However, triple therapy with a protease inhibitor plus peginterferon alfa plus ribavirin is much more effective and is likely to replace dual therapy as standard of care.
- The principal adverse effects of interferon alfa are a flu-like syndrome and severe depression.
- The principal adverse effects of ribavirin are hemolytic anemia and fetal death or malformation.
- Owing to its effects on the fetus, ribavirin is contraindicated for use during pregnancy.
- The HCV protease inhibitors are subject to a large number of drug interactions.
- Hepatitis B can be treated with interferon alfa or a nucleoside analog, such as lamivudine.
- Rarely, lamivudine causes lactic acidosis and severe hepatomegaly.
- Vaccination is the best way to prevent influenza.
- Influenza vaccination is recommended for everyone age 6 months and older.
- Because influenza viruses evolve rapidly, influenza vaccines must be reformulated each year, and persons wanting protection must receive the new vaccine each year.
- Two types of influenza vaccine are available: inactivated influenza vaccine (administered by IM or intradermal injection) and live, attenuated influenza vaccine, aka LAIV (administered by nasal spray).
- We have two types of antiviral drugs for influenza: neuraminidase inhibitors and adamantanes.
- Neuraminidase inhibitors (oseltamivir, zanamivir, and peramivir) are highly active against all current strains of influenza A and B. In theory, neuraminidase inhibitors can blunt responses to LAIV, and hence should be discontinued 2 days before giving an LAIV and not started until 2 weeks after giving an LAIV.
- Resistance to neuraminidase inhibitors is uncommon.

Please visit **http://evolve.elsevier.com/Lehne** for chapter-specific NCLEX® examination review questions.

Summary of Major Nursing Implications[a]

ACYCLOVIR

Preadministration Assessment

Therapeutic Goal

Treatment of infections caused by herpes simplex viruses and varicella-zoster virus.

Identifying High-Risk Patients

Use with *caution* in patients with dehydration or renal impairment and in those taking other nephrotoxic drugs.

Implementation: Administration

Routes

Topical, oral, IV.

Dosage

Oral and IV dosages must be reduced in patients with renal impairment.

Administration

Topical. **Advise patients to apply the drug with a finger cot or rubber glove to avoid viral transfer to other body sites or other people.**

Oral. Dosages vary widely for different indications (see Table 93.2).

Intravenous. Give by slow IV infusion (over 1 hour or more). Never give by IV bolus.

Implementation: Measures to Enhance Therapeutic Effects

Inform patients with herpes simplex genitalis that acyclovir only decreases symptoms; it does not eliminate the virus and does not produce cure. Advise patients to cleanse the affected area with soap and water 3 to 4 times a day, drying thoroughly after each wash. Advise patients to avoid all sexual contact while lesions are present and to use a condom even when lesions are absent.

Ongoing Evaluation and Interventions

Evaluating Therapeutic Effects

Observe for decreased clinical manifestations of herpes simplex and varicella-zoster infections. Virologic testing may also be performed.

Minimizing Adverse Effects

Nephrotoxicity. Intravenous acyclovir can precipitate in renal tubules, causing reversible kidney damage. To minimize risk, infuse acyclovir slowly and ensure adequate hydration during the infusion and for 2 hours after. Exercise caution in patients with pre-existing renal impairment and in those who are dehydrated or taking other nephrotoxic drugs.

GANCICLOVIR

Preadministration Assessment

Therapeutic Goal

Treatment and prevention of CMV infection in immunocompromised patients, including those with AIDS and those taking immunosuppressive drugs following an organ transplant.

Topical treatment of acute keratitis caused by HSV.

Baseline Data

Obtain a complete blood count and platelet count.

Identifying High-Risk Patients

Ganciclovir is *contraindicated* during pregnancy and for patients with neutrophil counts less than 500/mm^3 or platelet counts less than 25,000/mm^3.

Use with *caution* in patients taking zidovudine or nephrotoxic drugs (e.g., amphotericin B, cyclosporine) and in patients with a history of cytopenic reactions to other drugs.

Implementation: Administration

Routes

Oral, IV, intraocular, topical to the eye.

Dosage

Oral and IV dosages must be reduced in patients with renal impairment. AIDS patients with CMV retinitis must take ganciclovir for life.

Administration

Intravenous. Give by slow IV infusion (over 1 hour or more). Ensure adequate hydration to promote renal excretion.

Oral. **Advise patients to take oral ganciclovir with food.**

Intraocular Implants. Surgical implants are replaced every 5 to 8 months.

Topical to the Eye. Advise patients to apply ganciclovir gel drops directly to the affected eye and to avoid contact lenses until lesions heal.

Ongoing Evaluation and Interventions

Minimizing Adverse Effects

Granulocytopenia and Thrombocytopenia. Ganciclovir suppresses bone marrow function when given IV or PO. Obtain complete blood counts and platelet counts frequently. Discontinue ganciclovir if the neutrophil count falls below 500/mm^3 or the platelet count falls below 25,000/mm^3. The risk for granulocytopenia can be reduced by giving granulocyte colony-stimulating factors. The risk for granulocytopenia is increased by concurrent therapy with zidovudine (a drug for AIDS).

Reproductive Toxicity. In animals, ganciclovir is teratogenic and embryotoxic and suppresses spermatogenesis. **Advise patients against becoming pregnant. Inform male patients about possible sterility.**

[a]Patient education information is highlighted as **blue text.**

CHAPTER

94 Antiviral Agents II: Drugs for HIV Infection and Related Opportunistic Infections

In this chapter we discuss drug therapy of infection with the *human immunodeficiency virus* (HIV), the microbe that causes *acquired immunodeficiency syndrome* (AIDS). HIV promotes immunodeficiency by killing CD4 T lymphocytes (CD4 T cells), which are key components of the immune system (see Chapter 67). As a result of HIV-induced immunodeficiency, patients are at risk for opportunistic infections and certain neoplasms.

It is important to appreciate that HIV infection is not synonymous with AIDS, which develops years after HIV infection is acquired. The definition of AIDS, established by the Centers for Disease Control and Prevention (CDC), is a syndrome in which the individual is HIV-positive and has either (1) CD4 T-cell counts below 200 cells/mL or (2) an AIDS-defining illness. Included in the CDC's long list of AIDS-defining illnesses are *Pneumocystis* pneumonia, cytomegalovirus retinitis, disseminated histoplasmosis, tuberculosis, and Kaposi's sarcoma.

Since being identified as a new disease in 1981, AIDS has become a global epidemic. According to the 2015 HIV Surveillance Report, in the United States, approximately 1.2 million people are now infected and about 50,000 more become infected each year. More than 658,000 have died since the epidemic began. The World Health Organization (WHO) reports that an estimated 34 million people are now infected, and almost 30 million have died worldwide. However, there is good news: According to the CDC, in the 6 years from 2008 to 2014, new HIV infections declined by 18% in the United States. A United Nations report, released in 2014, shows that over the past decade the number of new HIV infections worldwide has declined by 35% while AIDs-related deaths have declined by 42%. This is due in large part to more widespread use of HIV drugs.

Therapy of HIV infection has made dramatic advances. Today, standard *antiretroviral therapy* (ART) consists of three or four drugs. These combinations, often referred to as *HAART* (for *highly active antiretroviral therapy*), can decrease plasma HIV to levels that are undetectable with current technology and can thus delay or reverse loss of immune function, decrease certain AIDS-related complications, preserve health, prolong life, and decrease HIV transmission. However, these benefits have not come without a price: ART is expensive, poses a risk for long-term side effects and serious drug interactions, and must continue as a lifelong treatment. Accordingly, if treatment is to succeed, patients must be highly motivated and well informed about all aspects of the treatment program. A strong support network is extremely valuable too.

ART cannot cure HIV infection. Although treatment *can* greatly reduce HIV levels—often rendering the virus undetectable—discontinuation has consistently been followed by a rebound in HIV replication. Because ART does not eliminate HIV, patients continue to be infectious and must be warned to avoid behaviors that can transmit the virus to others.

Understanding this chapter requires a basic understanding of the immune system. Accordingly, you may find it helpful to read Chapter 67 before proceeding.

PATHOPHYSIOLOGY

Characteristics of HIV

HIV is a *retrovirus.* Like all other viruses, retroviruses lack the machinery needed for self-replication, and thus are obligate intracellular parasites. However, in contrast to other viruses, retroviruses have positive-sense, single-stranded RNA as their genetic material. Accordingly, in order to replicate, retroviruses must first transcribe their RNA into DNA. The enzyme employed for this process is viral *RNA-dependent DNA polymerase,* commonly known as *reverse transcriptase.* (The enzyme is called reverse transcriptase to distinguish it from DNA-dependent RNA polymerase, the host enzyme that transcribes DNA into RNA, which is the usual ["forward"] transcription process.) The name *retrovirus* is derived from the first two letters of *reverse* and *transcriptase.*

There are two types of HIV, referred to as HIV-1 and HIV-2. HIV-1 is found worldwide, whereas HIV-2 is found mainly in West Africa. Although HIV-1 and HIV-2 differ with respect to genetic makeup and antigenicity, they both cause similar disease syndromes. Not all drugs that are effective against HIV-1 are also effective against HIV-2.

Target Cells

The principal cells attacked by HIV are *CD4 T cells* (helper T lymphocytes). As discussed in Chapter 67, these cells are essential components of the immune system. They are required for production of antibodies by B lymphocytes and for activation of cytolytic T lymphocytes. Accordingly, as HIV kills CD4 T cells, the immune system undergoes progressive decline. As a result, infected individuals become increasingly vulnerable to opportunistic infections, a major cause of death among people with AIDS. HIV targets CD4 T cells because the CD4 proteins on the surface of these cells provide points of attachment for HIV. Without such a receptor, HIV would be unable to connect with and penetrate these cells. Once HIV has infected a CD4 T cell, the cell dies in about 1.25 days. It is important to appreciate that only a small percentage of CD4 T cells circulate in the blood; most of them reside in lymph nodes and other lymphoid tissues.

In addition to infecting CD4 T cells, HIV infects *macrophages* and *microglial cells* (the central nervous system [CNS] counterparts of macrophages), both of which carry CD4 proteins. Since macrophages and microglial cells are resistant to destruction by HIV, they can survive despite being infected. As a result, they serve as a reservoir of HIV during chronic infection.

Structure of HIV

The structure of HIV is very simple. As shown in Fig. 94.1, the HIV *virion* (i.e., the entire virus particle) consists of *nucleic acid* (RNA) surrounded by *core proteins,* which in turn are surrounded by a *capsid* (protein shell), which in turn is surrounded by a *lipid bilayer envelope* (derived from the membrane of the host cell).

The central core contains two separate but identical single strands of RNA, each with its own molecule of *reverse transcriptase* attached. The RNA serves as the template for DNA synthesis.

The outer envelope of HIV contains *glycoproteins* that are needed for attachment to host cells. Each glycoprotein (gp) consists of two subunits, known as *gp41* and *gp120.* The smaller protein (gp41) is embedded in the lipid bilayer of the viral envelope; the larger protein (gp120) is connected firmly to gp41. (The numbers 41 and 120 simply indicate the mass of these glycoproteins in thousands of daltons.)

Replication Cycle of HIV

The replication cycle of HIV is shown in Fig. 94.2. The numbered steps that follow correspond to the numbers in the figure:

Step 1—The cycle begins with attachment of HIV to the host cell. The primary connection takes place between *gp120* on the HIV envelope and a *CD4* protein on the host cell membrane. Other host proteins, known as co-receptors, act in concert with CD4 to tighten the bond with HIV. Two of these co-receptors—known as CCR5 and CXCR4—are of particular importance. One drug—maraviroc—blocks HIV entry by binding to CCR5.

Step 2—The lipid bilayer envelope of HIV fuses with the lipid bilayer of the host cell membrane. Fusion is followed by release of HIV RNA into the host cell. One drug—enfuvirtide—works by blocking the fusion process.

Step 3—HIV RNA is transcribed into single-stranded DNA by HIV *reverse transcriptase.*

Step 4—Reverse transcriptase converts the single strand of HIV DNA into double-stranded HIV DNA.

Step 5—Double-stranded HIV DNA becomes integrated into the host's DNA, under the direction of a viral enzyme

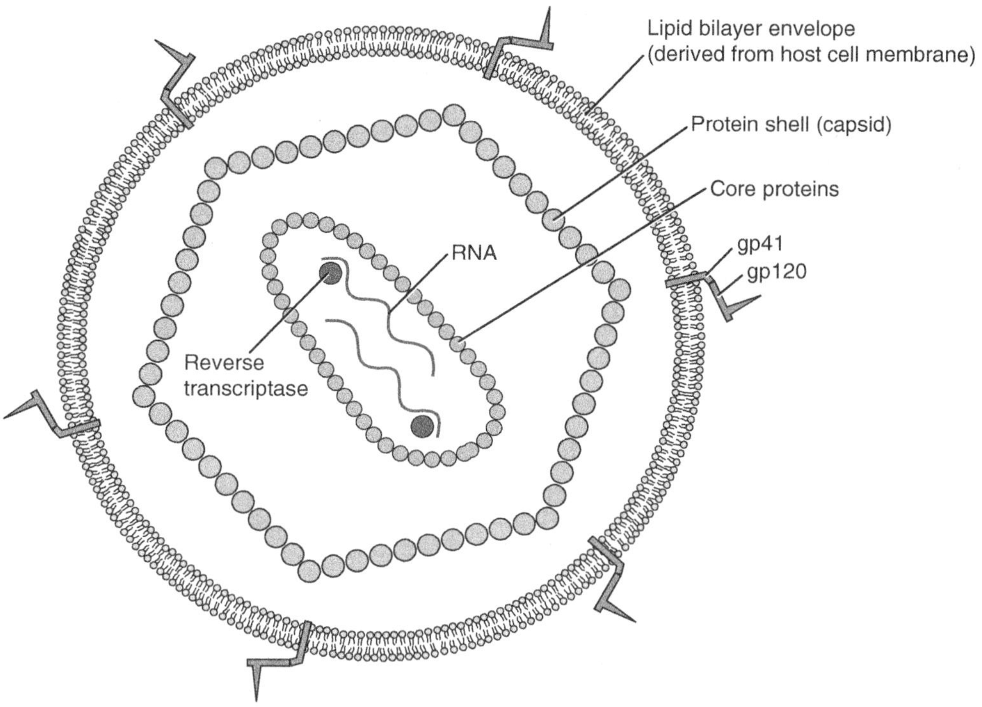

Fig. 94.1 ■ **Structure of the human immunodeficiency virus**
Note that HIV has two single strands of RNA, and that each strand is associated with a molecule of reverse transcriptase. (*gp41,* Glycoprotein 41; *gp120,* glycoprotein 120.)

known (aptly) as *integrase.* The integrase strand transfer inhibitors inhibit this enzyme.

Step 6—HIV DNA undergoes transcription into RNA. Some of the resulting RNA becomes the genome for daughter HIV virions (step 6a). The rest of the RNA is messenger RNA that codes for HIV proteins (step 6b).

Step 7—Messenger RNA is translated into HIV glycoproteins (step 7a) and HIV enzymes and structural proteins (step 7b).

Step 8—The components of HIV migrate to the cell surface and assemble into a new virus. Before assembly, HIV glycoproteins become incorporated into the host cell membrane (step 8a). In steps 8b and 8c, the other components of the virion migrate to the cell surface, where they undergo assembly into the new virus.

Step 9—The newly formed virus buds off from the host cell. As indicated, the outer envelope of the virion is derived from the cell membrane of the host.

Step 10—In this step, which occurs either during or immediately after budding off, HIV undergoes final maturation under the influence of *protease,* an enzyme that cleaves certain large polyproteins into their smaller, functional forms. If protease fails to cleave these proteins, HIV will remain immature and noninfectious. HIV protease is the target of several important drugs.

Replication Rate

HIV replicates rapidly during *all* stages of the infection. During the initial phase of infection, replication is massive. Why? Because (1) the population of CD4 cells is still large, thereby providing a large viral breeding ground, and (2) the host has not yet mounted an immune response against HIV, thus replication can proceed unopposed. As a result of massive replication, plasma levels of HIV can exceed 10 million virions/mL. During this stage of high viral load, patients often experience an *acute retroviral syndrome* (discussed later).

Over the next few months, as the immune system begins to attack HIV, plasma levels of HIV undergo a sharp decline and then level off. A typical steady-state level is between 1000 and 100,000 virions/mL. Please note, however, that steady-state numbers can be deceptive. The plasma half-life of HIV is only 6 hours; that is, every 6 hours, half of the HIV virions in plasma are lost. Accordingly, to maintain the steady-state levels typically seen during chronic HIV infection, the actual rate of *replication* is between 1 and 10 *billion* virions/day. Despite this high rate of ongoing replication, infected persons typically remain asymptomatic for about 10 years, after which symptoms of advanced HIV disease appear.

Mutation and Drug Resistance

HIV mutates rapidly because HIV reverse transcriptase is an error-prone enzyme. Therefore, whenever it transcribes HIV RNA into single-stranded DNA and then into double-stranded DNA, there is a high probability of introducing base-pair errors. In fact, according to one estimate, up to 10 incorrect bases may be incorporated into HIV DNA during each round of replication. Because of these errors, HIV can rapidly mutate from a drug-sensitive form into a drug-resistant form. The probability of developing resistance in the individual patient is directly related to the total viral load. Hence, the more virions the patient harbors, the greater the likelihood that some will become resistant. To minimize the emergence of resistance, patients must be treated with a combination of antiretroviral drugs. This is the same strategy we employ to prevent emergence of resistance when treating tuberculosis (see Chapter 90).

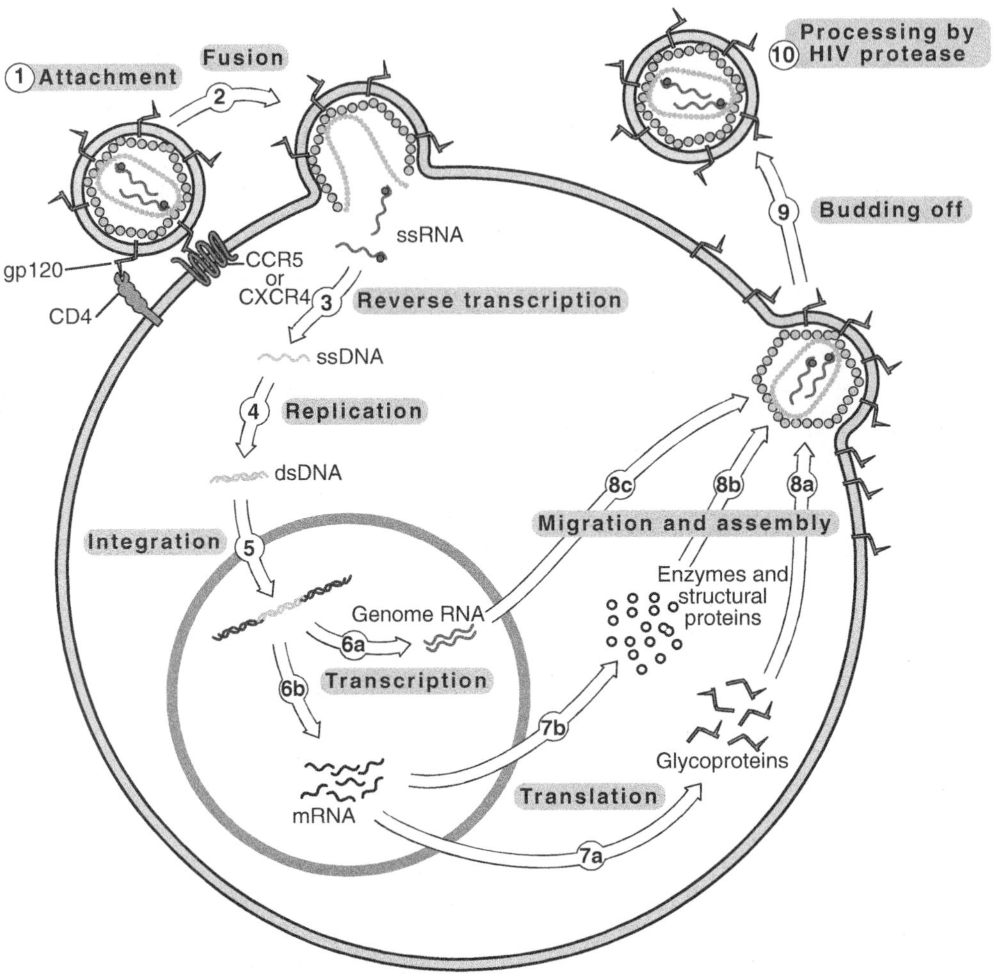

Fig. 94.2 ■ **Replication cycle of the human immunodeficiency virus**
See text for description of events. (*CCR5*, CCR5 co-receptor; *CD4*, CD4 receptor; *CXCR4*, CXCR4 co-receptor; *dsDNA*, double-stranded DNA; *gp120*, glycoprotein 120; *mRNA*, messenger RNA; *ssDNA*, single-stranded DNA; *ssRNA*, single-stranded RNA.)

Transmission of HIV

HIV is transmitted through the body fluids of an infected person. This transmission can occur by sexual contact, transfusion, sharing IV needles, and accidental needle sticks. In addition, it can be transmitted to the fetus by an infected mother, usually during the perinatal period.

Uncertainty exists regarding the ability of people with undetectable viral loads to transmit HIV to others. Research has demonstrated that subjects taking antiretroviral therapy who have undetectable viral loads for 6 months or more do not transmit HIV. Multiple organizations have embraced this as fact; however, in a release dated October 2017, the CDC appears to advise caution. The document states, in part, that "it is important to remember that when translating science into practice, the proven theoretical effectiveness of a prevention strategy is often lower" (https://www.cdc.gov/hiv/pdf/risk/art/cdc-hiv-uvl-transmission.pdf).

Clinical Course of HIV Infection

HIV infection follows a triphasic clinical course. During the initial phase, HIV undergoes massive replication, causing blood levels of HIV to rise very high. As a result, between 50% and 90% of patients experience a flu-like *acute retroviral syndrome.* Signs and symptoms include fever, lymphadenopathy, pharyngitis, rash, myalgia, and headache. Soon, however, the immune system mounts a counterattack, causing HIV levels to fall. As a result, symptoms of the acute syndrome fade. Very often, the acute retroviral syndrome is perceived as influenza, and so it goes unrecognized for what it really is.

The middle phase of HIV infection is characterized by prolonged *clinical latency,* lasting about 10 years. During this time, blood levels of HIV remain relatively low, and most patients are asymptomatic. HIV continues to replicate, however, and CD4 T cells undergo progressive decline.

During the late phase of HIV infection, CD4 T cells drop below a critical level (200 cells/mL), rendering the patient highly vulnerable to opportunistic infections and certain neoplasms (e.g., Kaposi's sarcoma). The late phase is when AIDS occurs.

Many patients with HIV infection experience neurologic complications. Both the peripheral and central nervous systems may be involved. *Peripheral neuropathies* affect 20% to 40% of patients and may develop at any time over the course of HIV infection. In contrast, *CNS complications* usually occur late in the disease. Symptoms of CNS injury include decreased cognition, reduced concentration, memory loss, mental slowness, and motor complaints (e.g., ataxia, tremors). Neuronal injury may be the direct result of HIV infection or may develop secondary to an opportunistic infection in the CNS.

CLASSIFICATION OF ANTIRETROVIRAL DRUGS

At this time, we have five classes of antiretroviral drugs. Three types—*reverse transcriptase inhibitors, integrase strand transfer inhibitors* (INSTIs), and *protease inhibitors* (PIs)—inhibit enzymes required for HIV replication. The other two types—*fusion inhibitors* and *chemokine receptor 5 (CCR5) antagonists*—block viral entry into cells. As discussed later, the reverse transcriptase inhibitors are subdivided into two groups: *nucleoside/nucleotide reverse transcriptase inhibitors* (NRTIs), which are structural analogs of nucleosides or nucleotides, and (2) *non-nucleoside reverse transcriptase inhibitors* (NNRTIs). Drugs that belong to these groups are shown in Table 94.1.

TABLE 94.1 ▪ Classification of Antiretroviral Drugs

Generic Name	Brand Name	Abbreviation
DRUGS THAT INHIBIT HIV ENZYMES		
Nucleoside/Nucleotide Reverse Transcriptase Inhibitors (NRTIs)		
Abacavir	Ziagen	ABC
Didanosine	Videx	ddI
Emtricitabine	Emtriva	FTC
Lamivudine	Epivir	3TC
Stavudine	Zerit	d4T
Tenofovir	Viread	TDF
Zidovudine	Retrovir	ZDV
Non-nucleoside Reverse Transcriptase Inhibitors (NNRTIs)		
Delavirdine	Rescriptor	DLV
Efavirenz	Sustiva	EFV
Etravirine	Intelence	ETR
Nevirapine	Viramune	NVP
Rilpivirine	Edurant	RPV
Protease Inhibitors		
Atazanavir	Reyataz	ATV
Darunavir	Prezista	DRV
Fosamprenavir	Lexiva, Telzir 🍁	FPV
Indinavir	Crixivan	IDV
Nelfinavir	Viracept	NFV
Ritonavir	Norvir	RTV
Saquinavir	Invirase	SQV
Tipranavir	Aptivus	TPV
Lopinavir/ritonavir	Kaletra	LPV/r
Integrase Strand Transfer Inhibitor		
Raltegravir	Isentress	RAL
Dolutegravir	Tivicay	DTG
DRUGS THAT BLOCK HIV ENTRY INTO CELLS		
Fusion Inhibitor		
Enfuvirtide	Fuzeon	T-20
CCR5 Antagonist		
Maraviroc	Selzentry, Celsentri 🍁	MVC

Generic Name	Brand Name	Abbreviation
FIXED-DOSE COMBINATIONS		
Abacavir 600 mg Lamivudine 300 mg	Epzicom	ABC/3TC
Abacavir 600 mg Dolutegravir 50 mg Lamivudine 300 mg	Triumeq	ABC/DTG/3TC
Abacavir 300 mg Lamivudine 150 mg Zidovudine 300 mg	Trizivir	ABC/3TC/ZDV
Atazanavir 300 mg Cobicistat[a] 150 mg	Evotaz	ATV/COBI
Darunavir 800 mg Cobicistat 150 mg	Prezcobix	DRV/COBI
Efavirenz 600 mg Emtricitabine 200 mg Tenofovir DF 300 mg	Atripla	EFV/FTC/TDF
Elvitegravir 150 mg Cobicistat 150 mg Emtricitabine 200 mg Tenofovir AF 10 mg	Genvoya	EVG/COBI/ FTC/TAF
Elvitegravir 150 mg Cobicistat 150 mg Emtricitabine 200 mg Tenofovir DF 300 mg	Stribild	EVG/COBI/ FTC/TDF
Emtricitabine 200 mg Rilpivirine 25 mg Tenofovir AF 25 mg	Odefsey	FTC/RPV/TAF
Emtricitabine 200 mg Rilpivirine 25 mg Tenofovir DF 300 mg	Complera	FTC/RPV/TDF
Emtricitabine 200 mg Tenofovir AF 25 mg	Descovy	FTC/TAF
Emtricitabine 200 mg Tenofovir DF 300 mg	Truvada	FTC/TDF
Lamivudine 150 mg Zidovudine 300 mg	Combivir	ZDV/3TC
Lopinavir 200 mg Ritonavir 50 mg	Kaletra[b]	LPV/r_1LPV[c]/ RTV)

[a]Cobicistat is a CYP3A inhibitor.
[b]Oral solution contains lopinavir 80 mg/ritonavir 20 mg per mL.
[c]Ritonavir-boosted lopinavir.

DRUG INTERACTIONS

Before we begin our discussion of the different classes of antiretroviral drugs, it is wise to consider a topic of great concern. Drug interactions are common and significant with these drugs. Many are inducers or inhibitors of one or more (and sometimes many) CYP450 enzymes. Many are also substrates of one or more of these. As a result, interactions are common. Some drugs share the same adverse effects; therefore, giving them together can intensify an effect so that it becomes dangerous. Moreover, patients with HIV infection, especially those with advanced infection and AIDS, often take drugs for multiple other illnesses and infections. When we consider all the various combinations of these drugs, the possibility of dangerous drug interactions increases dramatically.

Although we provide the most common or concerning drug interactions, we recognize that simple lists of common drug interactions are inadequate to address this issue. Everyone with the responsibility for medication administration needs access to a reliable drug interaction software that is capable of simultaneously checking for interactions among multiple drugs. This is critical when administering drugs to patients with HIV infection and AIDS.

NUCLEOSIDE/NUCLEOTIDE REVERSE TRANSCRIPTASE INHIBITORS

The NRTIs were the first drugs used against HIV infection. As their name suggests, the NRTIs are chemical relatives of naturally occurring nucleosides or nucleotides, the building blocks of DNA. At this time, seven NRTIs are available: abacavir, didanosine, emtricitabine, lamivudine, stavudine, tenofovir, and zidovudine.

The NRTIs are effective against both HIV-1 and HIV-2; however, their activity is greater for HIV-1. The NRTIs are ineffective as monotherapy because resistance develops rapidly. First-line antiretroviral regimens include two NRTIs and one other drug. The availability of combination antiretroviral products has simplified treatment. The fixed-dose combinations are shown in Table 94.1.

Basic Pharmacology of Nucleoside/Nucleotide Reverse Transcriptase Inhibitors

Mechanism of Action

All NRTIs are prodrugs that inhibit HIV replication by suppressing synthesis of viral DNA. To do this, they must first undergo intracellular conversion to their active (phosphate) form. In their active form, they act as substrates for reverse transcriptase. However, after they become incorporated into the growing DNA strand, they prevent reverse transcriptase from adding more bases. As a result, all further growth of the DNA strand is blocked. In addition to causing premature strand termination, the activated NRTI competes with natural nucleoside triphosphates for binding to the active site of reverse transcriptase.

Adverse Effects

The NRTIs share a core of adverse effects associated with mitochondrial toxicity. Recall that mitochondria are cellular organelles that take in nutrients and convert them into ATP for energy. NRTIs can disrupt synthesis of mitochondrial DNA and can thereby impair mitochondrial function.

Lactic Acidosis. A major consequence of mitochondrial impairment is lactic acidosis. Lactic acid accumulates because dysfunctional mitochondria cannot break down lactic acid. Symptoms include nausea, malaise, fatigue, anorexia, and hyperventilation (blowing off carbon dioxide can reduce acidosis). Left untreated, the syndrome can be fatal. Diagnosis is based on lactic acid measurement in arterial blood.

The FDA requires all NRTIs to carry black box warnings about this possibility, even though it is rare for most. Those for which this is most likely to occur are didanosine and stavudine.

Hepatic Steatosis. Hepatic steatosis (fatty degeneration of the liver) and hepatomegaly (enlarged liver) are also adverse effects of NRTIs. This is also associated with mitochondrial impairment because there is decreased breakdown of fatty acids by mitochondria leading to fatty deposits in the liver.

Other Adverse Effects. NRTIs may also cause pancreatitis and myopathies, which are likely tied to lactic acidosis. Adverse effects of individual NRTIs are discussed separately.

Drug Interactions

NRTIs have fewer drug interactions than most antiretroviral drugs, in part because most are not metabolized by the P450 enzymes. Interactions of individual drugs are discussed separately.

Properties of Individual Nucleoside/Nucleotide Reverse Transcriptase Inhibitors

Next we discuss the individual NRTIs. Pharmacokinetic properties of NRTIs are shown in Table 94.2. Preparation, dosage, and administration are provided in Table 94.3.

Abacavir

Abacavir [Ziagen], also known as ABC, will serve as our prototype for the NRTIs. Abacavir is an analog of guanine, a naturally occurring pyrimidine. It is one of the most commonly used antiretrovirals, especially in combination with lamivudine, another NRTI.

Actions and Use. Abacavir is taken up by host cells and then undergoes conversion to its active form, carbovir triphosphate. Carbovir triphosphate then suppresses HIV replication by (1) causing premature termination of the growing DNA strand and (2) competing with natural nucleoside triphosphates for binding to reverse transcriptase. When employed in combination with other antiretroviral drugs, abacavir can decrease viral load, increase CD4 T-cell counts, delay onset of disease symptoms, and reduce symptom severity.

Adverse Effects

Lactic Acidosis and Hepatomegaly With Steatosis. There is a relatively small risk for the lactic acidosis and hepatomegaly with steatosis that are associated with all NRTIs. Still, it is important to be alert to this possibility.

Hypersensitivity Reactions. Hypersensitivity reactions occur in 5% to 8% of patients treated with abacavir. These reactions, which usually develop during the first 6 weeks of treatment, can cause multiorgan failure and anaphylaxis. They are sometimes fatal. Symptoms include fever, rash, myalgia,

TABLE 94.2 ■ Pharmacokinetic Properties of Nucleoside/Nucleotide Reverse Transcriptase Inhibitors

Drug	Route	Peak	Serum Half-Life	Intracellular Half-Life	Metabolism	Excretion
Abacavir (ABC)	PO	0.7–1.7 hr	1.5 hr	12–26 hr	Metabolized intracellularly to active form, then hepatic (non-P450)	Urine (primary), feces
Didanosine (ddI)	PO	Suspension: 0.25–15 hr Capsules: 2 hr	1.5 hr	>20 hr	Metabolized intracellularly to active form. Further metabolism not studied in humans	Urine
Emtricitabine (FTC)	PO	1–2 hr	10 hr	>20 hr	Metabolized intracellularly to active form, then oxidation and glucuronidation	Urine (primary), feces
Lamivudine (3TC)	PO	On empty stomach: ≈1 hr With food: 3.2 hr	5–7 hr	18–22 hr	Metabolized intracellularly to active form	Urine
Stavudine (d4T)	PO	1 hr	1 hr	7.5 hr	Metabolized intracellulary	Urine
Tenofovir (TDF)	PO	On empty stomach: 36–84 min With high-fat food: 96–144 min	17 hr	>60 hr	Metabolized intracellularly	Urine
Zidovudine (ZDV)	PO IV	0.5–1.5 hr	1.1 hr	7 hr	Metabolized intracellularly to active form, then hepatic by glucuronidation	Urine

TABLE 94.3 ■ Preparation, Dosage, and Administration of Nucleoside/Nucleotide Reverse Transcriptase Inhibitors

Drug	Preparation	Typical Adult Dosage[a]	Administration
Abacavir (ABC)	Tablets: 300 mg Oral solution: 20 mg/mL	300 mg twice daily	Administer with or without food
Didanosine (ddI)	ER capsules: 125, 200, 250, 400 mg Oral suspension: 2 gm/100 mL, 4 gm/200 mL	Capsules: <60 kg: 250 mg once daily ≥60 kg: 400 mg once daily Solution: <60 kg: 125 mg twice daily ≥60 kg: 200 mg twice daily	Administer on empty stomach[b] Swallow capsule whole; do not crush or chew
Emtricitabine (FTC)	Oral solution: 10 mg/mL Capsules: 200 mg	Solution: 240 mg once daily Capsules: 200 mg once daily	Administer with or without food
Lamivudine (3TC)	Oral solution: 5 mg/mL, 10 mg/mL Tablets: 100, 150, 300 mg	150 mg twice daily or 300 mg once daily	Administer with or without food
Stavudine (d4T)	Oral solution: 1 mg/mL Capsules: 15, 20, 30, 40 mg	<60 kg: 30 mg every 12 hr ≥60 kg: 40 mg every 12 hr	Administer with or without food Capsule can be opened and contents sprinkled in water
Tenofovir (TDF)	Powder: 40 mg/gm Tablets: 150, 200, 250, 300 mg	300 mg once daily	Administer with or without food Powder may be mixed with food, but it is bitter. Will not dissolve in water
Zidovudine (ZDV)	Oral syrup: 50 mg/5 mL Tablets: 300 mg Capsules: 100 mg IV solution: 10 mg/mL	PO: 300 mg every 12 hr IV: 1 mg/kg administered every 4 hr	Oral: Administer with or without food IV: Infuse over 1 hr

[a]These are representative manufacturer recommendations for HIV treatment (not prophylaxis). In practice, dosage is individualized.
[b]Food decreases serum levels by 55%.
ER, Extended release.

arthralgia, and gastrointestinal (GI) disturbances (nausea, vomiting, diarrhea, abdominal pain). Abacavir hypersensitivity reactions can also manifest initially as respiratory symptoms (e.g., pharyngitis, dyspnea, cough).

A specific genetic variation, known as HLA-B*5701, is strongly associated with abacavir hypersensitivity; therefore, all candidates for abacavir should be screened for this variation before starting therapy. Those who test negative are less likely to experience hypersensitivity, but should be counseled about the symptoms of the reaction.

Myocardial Infarction. There has been some controversy regarding an association between abacavir and myocardial infarction (MI). After analyzing 26 randomized controlled trials, the FDA found no statistically significant association between MI and abacavir-containing regimens (see https://www.fda.gov/Drugs/DrugSafety/ucm245164.htm). Still, others have expressed a need for more rigorous research. Therefore, if a patient has a history of coronary artery disease, some experts recommend using another drug.

Other Adverse Effects. Approximately 10% of patients experience fatigue and headache. Lipodystrophy with redistribution of adipose tissue may occur. The outcome is a cushingoid appearance with truncal obesity, thin extremities, and a fat pad at the base of the neck.

Contraindications. Patients who test positive for HLA-B*5701 should never receive abacavir. This should also be noted on their allergy list.

Drug Interactions. Alcohol can compete with abacavir for metabolism by alcohol dehydrogenase. This can thereby increase abacavir levels substantially.

PATIENT-CENTERED CARE ACROSS THE LIFE SPAN

Nucleoside Reverse Transcriptase Inhibitors

Life Stage	Patient Care Concerns
Children[a]	Both stavudine and zidovudine are approved for neonates. Abacavir and lamivudine are approved for infants as young as 3 months of age. Tenofovir is approved for children age 2 and older. Didanosine is approved for children 6 years and older weighing at least 20 kg.
Pregnant women	Antiretroviral therapy is recommended for all HIV-infected pregnant women to lower the viral load and decrease the risk of perinatal transmission. Didanosine, emtricitabine, and tenofovir are Pregnancy Risk Category B.[b] Lamivudine, stavudine, and zidovudine are Pregnancy Risk Category C.[b] Updated labeling for abacavir does not include a risk category; however, there are currently no known long-term adverse effects to the fetus despite a high level of placental transfer. Combined NRTIs during pregnancy increase the risk for lactic acidosis, which can be life threatening.
Breast-feeding women	Breast-feeding should be avoided by women with HIV because there is a danger of transmitting the virus.
Older adults	Older patients taking didanosine have a higher risk for developing pancreatitis than younger patients. Peripheral neuropathy may be increased for older patients taking stavudine.

[a]Pediatric information extracted from *Approved Antiretroviral Drugs for Pediatric Treatment of HIV Infection,* available at https://www.fda.gov/forpatients/illness/hivaids/treatment/ucm118951.htm.
[b]As of 2020, the FDA will no longer use Pregnancy Risk Categories. Please refer to Chapter 9 for more information.

Lamivudine

Actions and Uses. Lamivudine [Epivir, Heptovir ♣], commonly abbreviated 3TC (for dideoxy-3′-thiacytidine), is an analog of cytidine (the nucleoside that forms when cytosine attaches to a ribose ring). Following uptake by cells, the drug is converted to its active form, lamivudine triphosphate. This active form suppresses viral DNA synthesis as described previously under *Mechanism of NRTI Antiviral Action*. Like abacavir, it is one of the more commonly used drugs in this category.

Lamivudine is approved for treating hepatitis B virus (HBV) in addition to HIV. The formulation used to treat HBV is a lower dose formulation and is marketed as Epivir HBV (see Chapter 93).

Adverse Effects. Of all the NRTIs, lamivudine is the best tolerated. The risk for lactic acidosis and hepatic steatosis is small. Pancreatitis occurs in about 0.3% of patients. Some patients experience fatigue, insomnia, and headache, but these effects usually fade in a few weeks.

In patients co-infected with HBV, withdrawal of lamivudine may result in severe acute exacerbation of hepatitis. This posed a potential danger if prescribed for patients with HBV because there may be a subsequent need to change the therapeutic regimen. If lamivudine is discontinued in a patient with HBV, it is essential to monitor for signs and symptoms as well as laboratory evidence of liver dysfunction for several months.

Drug Interactions. Lamivudine should not be combined with the NRTI emtricitabine. Emtricitabine (discussed later) has significant toxic effects that may be enhanced by coadministration with lamivudine.

Zidovudine

Zidovudine [Retrovir, AZT ♣], commonly abbreviated as ZDV and AZT (for azidothymidine, its original name), was the first NRTI available. The drug is an analog of thymidine, a naturally occurring nucleoside. Of note, the most current iteration of the Guidelines for the Use of Antiretroviral Agents in HIV-1-Infected Adults and Adolescents, updated July 2016, adds that "older nucleoside reverse transcriptase inhibitors (NRTIs) such as zidovudine (ZDV), stavudine (d4T), and didanosine (ddI) are no longer recommended for use in HIV-infected patients in the United States" (p. I-20); however, other guidelines (e.g., Recommendations for Use of Antiretroviral Drugs in Pregnant HIV-1-Infected Women for Maternal Health and Interventions to Reduce Perinatal HIV Transmission in the United States, updated October 2016) continue to recommend zidovudine for short-term care.

Actions and Use. Following uptake by cells, zidovudine is converted to its active form zidovudine triphosphate (ZTP). This active form suppresses viral DNA synthesis as described previously under *Mechanism of NRTI Antiviral Action*.

Zidovudine penetrates to the CNS better than most other antiretroviral drugs, and hence can be valuable for relieving cognitive symptoms. Zidovudine is also commonly used to prevent mother-to-infant HIV transmission during labor and delivery and as short-term (4-week) prophylaxis for their newborn infants.

Adverse Effects

Hematologic Toxicity. Severe anemia and neutropenia secondary to bone marrow suppression are the principal toxic effects of zidovudine. Hemoglobin concentration and neutrophil counts should be determined before treatment and at least every 2 to 4 weeks thereafter. For patients who develop severe anemia (hemoglobin below 5 gm/dL or down 25% from baseline) or severe neutropenia (neutrophil count below 750 cells/mL or down 50% from baseline), zidovudine therapy should be interrupted until there is evidence of bone marrow recovery. If neutropenia and anemia are less severe, a reduction in dosage may be sufficient. Transfusions may permit some patients to continue drug use. If not, anemia and neutropenia may resolve following zidovudine withdrawal.

Lactic Acidosis With Hepatomegaly. Older NRTIs such as zidovudine are more likely to cause lactic acidosis with hepatomegaly and hepatic steatosis than are some of the newer drugs in this category. This is especially concerning when combining two older NRTIs in the treatment of pregnant women because fatalities have occurred.

Myopathy. The risk for myopathy (damage to muscle fibers) may occur with prolonged use. Myositis (inflammation of muscle fibers) may also develop.

Other Adverse Effects. Gastrointestinal effects (anorexia, nausea, vomiting, diarrhea, abdominal pain, stomach upset) occur on occasion. Possible *CNS reactions* include CNS depression, headache, insomnia, confusion, anxiety, nervousness, and seizures. Additional adverse effects include *nail pigmentation, insulin resistance/diabetes,* and *hyperlipidemia.*

Drug Interactions. There are many drugs that interact with zidovudine. Those that follow are drugs commonly prescribed to patients with HIV/AIDS.

The risk for severe anemia and neutropenia may be increased if zidovudine is taken with ganciclovir and valganciclovir (two antiviral drugs used to treat cytomegalovirus infection that may occur in patients with AIDs) or ribavirin (an antiviral drug used to treat hepatitis C, a common co-infection in patients with HIV infection), as well as any drugs that are myelosuppressive. (Canadian labeling contraindicates the use of zidovudine in patients with bone marrow suppression, establishing that it should not be given if hemoglobin is less than 7.5 gm/dL or if the neutrophil count is less than 750/mm^3.) Raltegravir may increase the risk for myopathy. Rhabdomyolysis may develop.

Protease inhibitors may increase zidovudine levels. Zidovudine may decrease the effectiveness of stavudine.

Didanosine

Actions and Uses. Didanosine [Videx, Videx EC], also known as dideoxyinosine (ddI), is an analog of inosine, a naturally occurring nucleoside. The drug is taken up by host cells, where it undergoes conversion to its active form, dideoxyadenosine triphosphate. It then suppresses viral replication in the same manner of other NRTIs. Because of the severity of adverse reactions and the development of safer alternatives, didanosine is not commonly used.

Adverse Effects

Pancreatitis. Pancreatitis, which can be fatal, is the major dose-limiting toxicity. The incidence is 3% to 17% with an increased incidence with higher doses and in older patients. Patients should be monitored for indications of developing pancreatitis (increased serum amylase in association with increased serum triglycerides; decreased serum calcium; and nausea, vomiting, or abdominal pain). If evolving pancreatitis is diagnosed, didanosine should be withdrawn.

Alcohol increases the risk for pancreatitis development. Patients must be warned not to drink alcohol when taking this drug. If they refuse, another drug should be considered.

Lactic Acidosis With Hepatic Steatosis. Like other NRTIs, didanosine can cause lactic acidosis with hepatic steatosis. As an older NRTI, this likelihood is higher with didanosine than with some of the newer drugs in this category. Fatalities have occurred in several pregnant women taking didanosine plus the NRTI stavudine. Accordingly, these drugs should not be combined during pregnancy unless resistance to all other antiretrovirals leaves no option.

Other Adverse Reactions. Approximately 15% to 20% of patients taking didanosine will develop peripheral neuropathy, diarrhea, and increases in serum amylase. About 10% develop elevated liver enzymes. Pruritic rashes may also occur.

Less common but potentially serious reactions occurring with didanosine include optic neuritis and retinal changes, insulin resistance, and the development or worsening of diabetes mellitus.

Drug Interactions. A large number of drugs interact with didanosine. We provide a sampling here of those most likely to be given to patients with HIV infection.

Buffered didanosine formulations can interfere with the absorption of drugs that require gastric acidity, including atazanavir, delavirdine, and indinavir.

Didanosine should not be combined with stavudine. The combination increases the risk for lactic acidosis, hepatomegaly, and hepatic steatosis.

A number of antiretroviral drugs interact with didanosine by altering drug levels. Tipranavir can decrease didanosine serum concentration. On the other hand, tenofir may increase didanosine serum levels yet decrease its effectiveness.

Increased didanosine levels can occur when taken with ribavirin, an antiviral drug used to treat hepatitis C, a common co-infection in patients with HIV infection. This can increase the toxic effects of didanosine.

Because didanosine should be given on an empty stomach, this creates problems when given with antiretrovirals that should be administered with food. These include rilpivirine, darunavir/ritonavir, and lopinavir/ritonavir oral solution (but not lopinavir/ritonavir tablets). If any of these are ordered with didanosine, the didanosine should be administered 1 hour before or 2 hours after administration of those that must be taken with food.

Stavudine

Actions and Uses. Stavudine [Zerit], also known as didehydrodeoxythymidine (d4T), is an analog of thymidine, a naturally occurring nucleoside. Following uptake by cells, stavudine is converted to its active form, stavudine triphosphate, which then suppresses HIV replication. Like didanosine (discussed previously), stavudine is now used only rarely because of its adverse effects.

Adverse Effects

Peripheral Neuropathy. Like didanosine, stavudine can cause peripheral neuropathy. In clinical trials, neuropathy developed in 15% to 21% of patients. Patients should be informed about early symptoms of neuropathy (numbness, tingling, or pain in hands and feet) and instructed to report them immediately. Neuropathy may resolve if the drug is withdrawn. If symptoms resolve completely, resumption of treatment may be considered, but the dosage should be reduced.

Pancreatitis. Stavudine can cause pancreatitis. Although the incidence is low (1%), pancreatitis can be fatal. Patients should be monitored for indications of pancreatitis; if evolving pancreatitis is diagnosed, stavudine should be withdrawn.

Lactic Acidosis With Hepatic Steatosis. The incidence of lactic acidosis and hepatic steatosis with stavudine may be higher than with all other NRTIs. As noted, fatal lactic acidosis has developed in several pregnant women taking stavudine plus didanosine.

Neuromuscular Weakness. Rarely, stavudine causes ascending demyelinating polyneuropathy, resulting in neuromuscular weakness. Symptoms begin months after initiation of treatment, but then progress rapidly, producing dramatic motor weakness within days to weeks. Some patients may require mechanical ventilation owing to respiratory paralysis. Recovery takes several months and may never be complete.

Other Adverse Effects. Stavudine may cause *lipoatrophy* and *hyperlipidemia.* It may also cause *insulin resistance* and contribute to the development or worsening of *diabetes mellitus.*

Drug Interactions. Zidovudine may decrease the effectiveness of stavudine. Therefore, these drugs should not be combined.

When combined with didanosine, there is an increased risk for adverse effects. This is especially concerning for the development of lactic acidosis and liver damage.

Tenofovir Disoproxil Fumarate

Actions and Use. Tenofovir disoproxil fumarate (TDF) [Viread] is a *nucleotide* reverse transcriptase inhibitor—not a nucleo*side* reverse transcriptase inhibitor. Nucleotides and nucleosides are very similar (a nucleotide is simply a nucleoside with a phosphate group added) and hence have similar effects on reverse transcriptase. Once inside cells, TDF undergoes conversion to tenofovir and then to tenofovir diphosphate, its active form. Like the nucleo*side* reverse transcriptase inhibitors, tenofovir diphosphate inhibits viral DNA synthesis in two ways: (1) it competes with the natural substrate (in this case, deoxyadenosine triphosphate) for binding to reverse transcriptase, and (2) after being incorporated into the growing DNA chain, it causes premature chain termination. Toxicity results in part from inhibiting mitochondrial DNA polymerase.

Tenofovir was originally approved only for HIV infection. It is now approved for HBV, too.

Adverse Effects. Tenofovir is usually well tolerated. Major concerns are renal toxicity and decreased bone mineralization.

Decreased Bone Mineralization. Approximately one-fourth of patients taking tenofovir experience some degree of decreased bone mineral density, thus increasing the risk for osteoporotic fractures. Patients may experience bone pain and arthralgias. Calcium and vitamin D supplementation are recommended.

Renal Toxicity. Rarely, tenofovir has been associated with renal toxicity, indicated by elevated serum creatinine and proteinuria. Since tenofovir is excreted by the kidneys, renal damage increases the risk for drug accumulation to dangerous levels. Dosage adjustment is necessary when prescribed to patients with renal impairment.

Other Adverse Effects. Because tenofovir can suppress HBV, patients co-infected with HBV may experience a severe exacerbation of hepatitis when tenofovir is withdrawn. For those patients with HBV, it is essential to monitor for evidence of liver dysfunction for several months.

Like other NRTIs, tenofovir poses a small risk for potentially fatal lactic acidosis with hepatic steatosis. More common adverse effects are nausea, vomiting, diarrhea, weakness, and headache. These are more likely to occur at the onset of therapy.

Drug Interactions. As with the other NRTIs, we focus here on those drugs commonly given to patients with HIV infection. It is essential to consult drug interaction software capable of simultaneously checking for interactions of multiple drugs for patient safety.

Combining tenofovir with another drug that undergoes active tubular secretion can lead to the accumulation of tenofovir, the other drug, or both. Through a mechanism that has not been determined, tenofovir can raise plasma levels of the NRTI didanosine. Because of the risk for serious adverse effects, this combination is not recommended.

Cobicistat, a pharmacokinetic enhancer commonly used in combination with other antiretroviral drugs, may enhance the adverse effects of tenofovir. Some protease inhibitors used to treat HIV infection (atazanavir, darunavir, lopinavir) can increase serum levels of tenofovir. However, the protease inhibitor tipranavir can also increase tenofovir levels. Tenofovir has an effect on some of these drugs as well. It decreases serum levels of atazanavir and tipranavir while increasing serum levels of darunavir. Further, one protease inhibitor, lopinavir, can increase the risk for nephrotoxicity when combined with tenofovir.

Several drugs used to treat hepatitis C, a common comorbidity of HIV infection, interact with tenofovir. Ledipasvir, simeprevir, telaprevir, and velpatasvir can all increase serum levels of tenofovir.

Adefovir, a drug used to treat hepatitis B infection, can decrease the serum level of tenofovir, and tenofovir can increase adefovir levels. Tenofovir levels may be increased by cidofovir, ganciclovir, and valganciclovir, drugs used to treat cytomegalovirus.

Emtricitabine

Actions and Uses. Emtricitabine [Emtriva] is a fluorinated derivative of lamivudine. Like lamivudine, emtricitabine is active against HIV and HBV. Following uptake by cells, emtricitabine is converted to emtricitabine triphosphate, its active form, which inhibits viral DNA synthesis. Emtricitabine has a long intracellular half-life, and hence dosing can be done just once a day.

Adverse Effects. Emtricitabine is generally well tolerated. It has the fewest adverse effects of the NRTIs.

Hyperpigmentation. An unusual side effect—hyperpigmentation of the palms and soles—develops in some patients taking emtricitabine. This effect may extend to other regions, such as the arms, lips, and tongue. This unusual reaction is not associated with other complications.

Other Adverse Effects. The most common adverse effects are headache, dizziness, insomnia, nausea, vomiting, diarrhea, and rash. Like other nucleoside analogs, emtricitabine may pose a small risk for lactic acidosis and hepatomegaly with steatosis.

Combination Products

The availability of combination antiretroviral products has simplified treatment. As expected, each drug in the combination brings with it the adverse reactions and drug interactions inherent in that drug. The fixed-dose combinations are shown in Table 94.1.

NON-NUCLEOSIDE REVERSE TRANSCRIPTASE INHIBITORS

The NNRTIs differ from the NRTIs in structure and mechanism of action. As their name suggests, the NNRTIs have no structural relationship with naturally occurring nucleosides. Also unlike NRTIs, the NNRTIs are active only against HIV-1. In practice, they are usually combined with an NRTI. At this time, five NNRTIs are available: efavirenz [Sustiva], nevirapine [Viramune], delavirdine [Rescriptor], etravirine [Intelence], and rilpivirine [Edurant].

Basic Pharmacology of Non-nucleoside Reverse Transcriptase Inhibitors

Mechanism of Action

In contrast to the NRTIs, the NNRTIs bind to the active center of reverse transcriptase enzyme. At this location, the NNRTI causes stereochemical changes (i.e., changes in the spatial arrangement of atoms forming the structure of molecules). This hampers the ability of nucleosides to bind, which inhibits DNA replication and promotes premature termination of the growing DNA strand.

Adverse Effects

Unlike NRTIs, there are no adverse effects shared by all NNRTIs. However, two of the NNRTIs, efavirenz and rilpivirine, can both cause CNS effects.

Drug Interactions

The NNRTIs have multiple drug interactions with commonly used drugs across many drug classes. These vary according to the individual NNRTI in question.

Properties of the Individual Non-nucleoside Reverse Transcriptase Inhibitors

Our discussion continues with an examination of the individual NNRTIs. Pharmacokinetic properties of the NNRTIs are shown in Table 94.4. Preparation, dosage, and administration are displayed in Table 94.5.

TABLE 94.4 ■ Pharmacokinetic Properties of Non-nucleoside Reverse Transcriptase Inhibitors

Drug	Route	Peak	Serum Half-Life	Metabolism	Excretion
Delavirdine (DLV)	PO	IR: 4 hr ER: 24 hr	5.8 hr	Hepatic by CYP3A and possibly CYP2D6	Urine (primary), feces
Efavirenz (EFV)	PO	3–5 hr	40–55 hr	Hepatic by CYP3A4 and CYP2B6	Feces (primary), urine
Etravirine (ETR)	PO	2.5–4 hr	41 hr	Hepatic by CYP3A4, CYP2C9, and CYP2C19	Feces (primary, 93.7%), urine
Nevirapine (NVP)	PO	IR: 4 hr ER: 24 hr	25–30 hr	Hepatic by CYP3A4 and CYP2B6	Urine (primary, 80%), feces (10%)
Rilpivirine (RPV)	PO	4–5 hr	50 hr	Hepatic by CYP3A4	Feces (primary, 85%), urine (6.1%)

ER, Extended release; *IR,* immediate release.

TABLE 94.5 ▪ Preparation, Dosage, and Administration of Non-nucleoside Reverse Transcriptase Inhibitors

Drug	Preparation	Typical Adult Dosage[a]	Administration
Delavirdine (DLV)	Tablets: 100, 200 mg	400 mg 3 times/day	Take with or without food Swallow 200-mg tablets intact Can mix 4 100-mg tablets in 3 or more ounces of water to produce a slurry
Efavirenz (EFV)	Capsules: 50, 200 mg Tablets: 600 mg	600 mg once daily, preferably at bedtime	Take on an empty stomach[b]
Etravirine (ETR)	Tablets: 100, 200 mg	200 mg twice daily	Take following a meal
Nevirapine (NVP)	Tablets, IR: 200 mg Tablets, ER: 400 mg PO suspension: 100 mg/10 mL	200 mg once daily for 14 days, then either 200 mg twice daily (with IR tablets or oral suspension) or 400 mg once daily (with ER tablets)	Take with or without food
Rilpivirine (RPV)	Tablets: 25 mg	25 mg once daily	Take with food

[a]These are representative manufacturer recommendations for HIV treatment (not prophylaxis). In practice, dosage is individualized.
[b]High-fat meals increase plasma levels by 39% with capsules and by 79% with tablets.
ER, Extended release; *IR*, immediate release.

Prototype Drugs

CYTOTOXIC AGENTS

Nucleoside/Nucleotide Reverse Transcriptase Inhibitors
Abacavir

Non-nucleoside Reverse Transcriptase Inhibitors
Efavirenz

Protease Inhibitors
Darunavir

Integrase Strand Inhibitors
Raltegravir

HIV Fusion Inhibitors
Enfuvirtide

CCR5 Antagonists
Maraviroc

Efavirenz

Efavirenz [Sustiva] is the only NNRTI deemed a preferred agent for treating HIV, and so it will serve as the prototype for the NNRTIs. The drug is effective and, because of its long half-life, can be administered once a day. Its principal drawbacks are teratogenicity and transient adverse CNS effects.

Mechanism of Action. Efavirenz binds directly to HIV reverse transcriptase and thereby disrupts the active center of the enzyme. As a result, replication is suppressed.

Therapeutic Use. Efavirenz is the only NNRTI recommended as first-line therapy for HIV-1 infection. In clinical trials, the combination of efavirenz plus two NRTIs (zidovudine and lamivudine) was at least as effective as indinavir (a protease inhibitor) combined with the same two NRTIs. Furthermore, the efavirenz-based regimen was better tolerated. *Because efavirenz crosses the blood-brain barrier, it can reduce HIV levels in the CNS, making it particularly useful in patients with CNS complications.*

Adverse Effects

CNS Effects. *CNS symptoms* occur in over 50% of patients. The most common are dizziness, insomnia, impaired consciousness, drowsiness, vivid dreams, and nightmares. Delusions, hallucinations, and severe acute depression may also occur, primarily in patients with a history of mental illness or drug abuse. Patients who experience these severe reactions should discontinue the drug. CNS symptoms are prominent at the onset of treatment, but generally resolve within 2 to 4 weeks, despite continuous drug use.

Rash. *Rash,* which can be severe, occurs often. In clinical trials, rash developed in 27% of adults and 40% of children. The median time to rash onset was 11 days, and the median duration was 14 days. Rash can range in severity from mild (erythema, pruritus) to moderate (diffuse maculopapular rash, dry desquamation) to severe (vesiculation, moist desquamation, ulceration). Very rarely, rash evolves into potentially fatal Stevens-Johnson syndrome, erythema multiforme, or toxic epidermal necrolysis. Accordingly, if severe rash occurs, efavirenz should be withdrawn immediately. Mild rash may respond to antihistamines and topical glucocorticoids.

Teratogenicity. Efavirenz is teratogenic. In monkeys, doses equivalent to those used in humans produced a high incidence of fetal malformation. Women using the drug must avoid getting pregnant. A barrier method of birth control (e.g., condom) should be used in conjunction with a hormonal method (e.g., oral contraceptive). Pregnancy must be ruled out before efavirenz is used.

Other Adverse Effects. Efavirenz may pose a risk of *liver damage.* Liver enzymes should be monitored, especially in patients with hepatitis B or C.

Hyperlipidemia may occur. Interestingly, drug screens of people taking efavirenz may show a false positive result for cannabinoids and benzodiazepines.

Drug Interactions. Efavirenz is a substrate, inhibitor, and inducer of several cytochrome P450 enzymes. Because of this role, it has many drug interactions.

Efavirenz is metabolized by CYP2B6 (primarily), CYP3A4, and CYP2A6. Accordingly, drugs that are inducers of these enzyme systems may decrease efavirenz levels, and drugs that are inhibitors of these enzyme systems may increase efavirenz levels.

Efavirenz *induces* CYP3A4 and CYP2B6 enzymes. It can thereby accelerate its own metabolism, as well as the metabolism of drugs that are CYP3A4 substrates. Increased metabolism of two protease inhibitors—saquinavir and indinavir—is of particular concern. If efavirenz is combined with indinavir, the dosage of indinavir should be increased. Combined use with saquinavir, a drug with low bioavailability, should be avoided.

By inducing these P450 enzymes, efavirenz can decrease the effects of *hormonal contraceptives,* including oral contraceptives and the etonogestrel contraceptive implant. Contraceptive failure can result. Since efavirenz is teratogenic, it is essential that women of childbearing potential use a barrier contraceptive in addition to any hormonal contraceptive.

Combining efavirenz with ritonavir (a protease inhibitor that inhibits CYP3A4) can increase levels of efavirenz. Toxicity may result.

At this point, we have only mentioned efavirenz's activities as a P450 inducer. It is also a CYP2C9 and CYP2C19 *inhibitor*. Drugs that are substrates for these enzymes may have increased serum levels—and increased adverse effects—if dosage adjustments are not made.

Nevirapine

Actions and Uses. Like other NNRTIs, nevirapine [Viramune, Viramune XR] binds directly to HIV reverse transcriptase, causing noncompetitive inhibition of the enzyme. Resistance to nevirapine develops rapidly if the drug is used alone. Accordingly, nevirapine should always be combined with other antiretroviral drugs.

Adverse Effects

Rash. The most common adverse effect is *rash,* which usually occurs early in therapy. For most patients, the rash is benign and, if needed, can be managed with an antihistamine or topical glucocorticoid. However, if the patient experiences severe rash, or rash associated with fever, blistering, oral lesions, conjunctivitis, muscle pain, or joint pain, nevirapine should be withdrawn because these symptoms may indicate development of *erythema multiforme* or *Stevens-Johnson syndrome.* Rash can be minimized by using a low dosage initially and then increasing the dosage if rash does not occur.

Hepatotoxicity. Nevirapine can cause severe *hepatotoxicity,* including fulminant and cholestatic hepatitis, hepatic necrosis, and hepatic failure. Fatalities have occurred. The risk is highest during the first 12 weeks of treatment and is increased by a history of chronic hepatitis B or hepatitis C. Liver function tests should be done at baseline, before dosage escalation, 2 weeks after dosage escalation, and whenever patients have symptoms (fatigue, malaise, anorexia, nausea), suggesting an early stage of liver damage. If hepatotoxicity is diagnosed, nevirapine should be withdrawn as soon as possible.

Drug Interactions. Nevirapine is an inducer of CYP3A4 and CYP2B6 isoenzymes and can thereby increase the metabolism of drugs that are metabolized by these systems, causing their levels to decline. The ability to decrease levels of *protease inhibitors* and *hormonal contraceptives* is of particular concern.

Nevirapine is a substrate of CYP3A4 (primary), CYP2B6, and CYP2D6 enzymes. Its own metabolism can be altered by inducers and inhibitors of these systems, especially those that induce or inhibit CYP3A4 enzymes.

PATIENT-CENTERED CARE ACROSS THE LIFE SPAN

Non-nucleoside Reverse Transcriptase Inhibitors

Life Stage	Patient Care Concerns
Children[a]	Nevirapine may be given to infants as young as 15 days of age. Efavirenz is approved for children older than 3 months and weighing at least 3.5 kg. Etravirine may be given to children who are 3 years and older. Safety and efficacy have not been established for rilpivirine, and for delavirdine, safety has not been established for patients younger than 16 years.
Pregnant women	Antiretroviral therapy is recommended for all HIV-infected pregnant women to lower the viral load and decrease the risk of perinatal transmission. Etravirine, nevirapine, and rilpivirine are Pregnancy Risk Category B.[b] Delavirdine is Pregnancy Risk Category C.[b] Efavirenz is teratogenic and classified as FDA Pregnancy Risk Category D.[b] Pregnancy must be ruled out before efavirenz is used. For pregnant women, two forms of contraception are recommended during treatment and for 3 months after treatment is discontinued.
Breast-feeding women	Breast-feeding should be avoided by women with HIV because there is a danger of transmitting the virus.
Older adults	Each drug in this category identified insufficient numbers of older adults in clinical trials. Consider individual patient status regarding cardiac, hepatic, and renal status or comorbidities that may necessitate alternate regimens.

[a]Pediatric information is extracted from *Approved Antiretroviral Drugs for Pediatric Treatment of HIV Infection,* available at https://www.fda.gov/forpatients/illness/hivaids/treatment/ucm118951.htm.

[b]As of 2020, the FDA will no longer use Pregnancy Risk Categories. Please refer to Chapter 9 for more information.

Delavirdine

Actions and Uses. Delavirdine [Rescriptor] is similar to efavirenz in actions and uses. It is a non-nucleoside that acts directly to inhibit reverse transcriptase, thereby suppressing HIV-1 replication.

Adverse Effects. Like efavirenz, delavirdine causes potentially serious *rash and other hypersensitivity reactions.* In clinical trials, rash developed in up to 50% of patients; erythema multiforme and Stevens-Johnson syndrome have been reported rarely. If severe rash develops, the drug should be withdrawn.

More common adverse effects include headache, fatigue, depression, nausea and vomiting, and elevation of liver enzymes.

Some patients experience cardiovascular effects. These are far-ranging and include dysrhythmias and rate variations, hypertension, orthostatic hypotension, cardiac insufficiency, and peripheral vascular disease.

Drug Interactions. In contrast to efavirenz and nevirapine, which induce CYP3A4, delavirdine *inhibits* these isoenzymes. To avoid toxicity from excessive drug levels, patients should not take drugs that could be elevated to dangerous levels if combined with a CYP3A4 inhibitor.

Because delavirdine is also metabolized by CYP3A4, it inhibits its own metabolism. Delavirdine is also metabolized by CYP2D6; therefore, inhibitors of these isoenzymes may have an effect on drug levels as well.

Etravirine

Actions and Use. Etravirine [Intelence], like the other NNRTIs, binds to and inhibits reverse transcriptase and thereby suppresses HIV replication. Etravirine is indicated for treatment-experienced adults infected with HIV-1 strains resistant to other NNRTIs and other antiretroviral drugs.

Adverse Effects. Etravirine is generally well tolerated. It can cause *rash*, but the incidence of severe skin reactions—Stevens-Johnson syndrome, toxic epidermal necrolysis, erythema multiforme—is less than 1%.

Etravirine may cause *hypersensitivity reactions*. Signs and symptoms include rash accompanied by fever, malaise, fatigue, muscle or joint aches, blisters, oral lesions, conjunctivitis, or facial edema.

Etravirine may also cause *hepatitis*. The most common adverse effect is nausea.

Drug Interactions. Etravirine is subject to *many* drug interactions. Etravirine is a *substrate* for CYP3A4, CYP2C9, and CYP2C19. In addition, it can *induce* CYP3A4 and *inhibit* CYP2C9 and CYP2C19. Accordingly, drugs that are substrates, inhibitors, and inducers of these systems have the potential of interactions.

Rilpivirine

Actions and Use. Rilpivirine [Edurant] binds to and inhibits reverse transcriptase and thereby suppresses HIV replication. Compared with efavirenz, rilpivirine is just as effective and possibly better tolerated, but it carries a greater risk for resistance and virologic failure, especially in patients with a high viral load (> 100,000 virions/mL).

Adverse Effects. Rilpivirine is generally well tolerated. The most common effects are CNS-related and include *depression*, *insomnia*, and *headache*. *Rash* and *hepatotoxicity* may occur.

Rilpivirine can prolong the QT interval, but only at doses 3 to 12 times greater than recommended.

Drug Interactions. Rilpivirine is a substrate of CYP3A4. Levels of rilpivirine can be increased by drugs that are CYP3A4 inhibitors or reduced by drugs that are CYP3A4 inducers.

PROTEASE INHIBITORS

PIs are active against both HIV-1 and HIV-2. They are among the most effective antiretroviral drugs available. When used in combination with NRTIs, they can reduce viral load to a level that is undetectable with current assays.

As with other antiretroviral drugs, HIV resistance can be a significant problem. Mutant strains of HIV that are resistant to one PI are likely to be cross-resistant to other PIs. In contrast, since PIs do not share the same mechanism as other antiretroviral drugs, cross-resistance between PIs and these drugs does not occur. To reduce the risk for resistance, PIs should never be used alone; rather, they should always be combined with at least one reverse transcriptase inhibitor, and preferably two.

Nine PIs are available: atazanavir, darunavir, fosamprenavir, indinavir, lopinavir (with ritonavir), nelfinavir, ritonavir, saquinavir, and tipranavir. Pharmacokinetic properties of protease inhibitors are shown in Table 94.6. Preparation, dosage, and administration are provided in Table 94.7.

Basic Pharmacology of the Protease Inhibitors

Mechanism of Action

Maturation is necessary for HIV to infect CD4 cells; immature forms are noninfectious. Protease inhibitors prevent HIV maturation by blocking the HIV enzyme protease.

It may help to look at the process of HIV maturation. When the various enzymes and structural proteins of HIV are synthesized, they are not produced as separate entities; rather, they are strung together in large polyproteins. Protease catalyzes the cleavage of bonds in the polyproteins, thereby freeing the individual enzymes and structural proteins. Once these components have been freed, HIV uses them to complete its maturation. Protease inhibitors bind to the active site of HIV protease and prevent the enzyme from cleaving HIV polyproteins. As a result, the structural proteins and enzymes of HIV are unable to function, and hence the virus remains immature and noninfectious.

TABLE 94.6 ■ Pharmacokinetic Properties of Protease Inhibitors

Drug	Route	Peak	Serum Half-Life	Metabolism	Excretion
Atazanavir (ATV)	PO	2–3 hr	7 hr	Hepatic, primarily by CYP3A	Feces (primary), urine
Darunavir (DRV)	PO	2.5–4 hr	15 hr (with ritonavir)	Hepatic by CYP3A	Feces (primary), urine
Fosamprenavir (FPV)	PO	1.5–4 hr	7.7 hr	GI metabolism to amprenavir; hepatic metabolism primarily by CYP3A4	Feces (primary), urine
Indinavir (IDV)	PO	0.5–1.1 hr	1.5–2 hr	Hepatic by CYP3A4	Feces (primary), urine
Lopinavir/ritonavir (LPV/r)	PO	4 hr	5–6 hr	Hepatic by CYP3A4	Feces (primary), urine
Nelfinavir (NFV)	PO	2–4 hr	3.5–5 hr	Hepatic by CYP2C19 and CYP3A4	Feces (primary), urine
Ritonavir (RTV)	PO	2 hr (taken on empty stomach) 4 hr (taken with food)	3–5 hr	Hepatic by CYP3A4 and CYP2D6	Feces (primary), urine
Saquinavir (SQV)	PO	NA[a]	1–2 hr	Hepatic by CYP3A4	Feces (primary), urine
Tipranavir (TPV)	PO	3 hr	6 hr	Hepatic by CYP3A4	Feces (primary), urine

[a]Information not provided in product labeling.
GI, Gastrointestinal; *NA,* not available.

TABLE 94.7 ■ Preparation, Dosage, and Administration of Protease Inhibitors

Drug	Preparation	Typical Adult Dosage[a]	Administration
Atazanavir (ATV)	PO powder packet: 50 mg Capsules: 150, 200, 300 mg	300 mg once daily (with other drugs)	Administer with food. Mix powder with food or liquid Swallow capsules whole
Darunavir (DRV)	PO suspension: 100 mg/mL Tablets: 75, 150, 600, 800 mg	600 mg twice daily (with other drugs) 800 mg once daily (with other drugs)	Administer with food and ritonavir
Fosamprenavir (FPV)	PO suspension: 50 mg/mL (225 mL) Tablets: 700 mg	1400 mg once daily (with other drugs) 700 mg twice daily (with other drugs)	Administer with food and ritonavir (recommended); otherwise, administer on empty stomach
Indinavir (IDV)	Capsules: 200, 400 mg	800 mg every 8 hr	Administer on empty stomach or light meal Administer with food if taken with ritonavir
Lopinavir/ritonavir (LPV/r)	PO solution: Lopinavir 80 mg/ritonavir 20 mg/mL Tablets: Lopinavir 100 mg/ ritonavir 25 mg; lopinavir 200 mg/ritonavir 50 mg	400 mg/100 mg twice daily 800 mg/200 mg once daily	Solution: Administer with food Tablets: Administer with or without food. Swallow whole
Nelfinavir (NFV)	Tablets: 250, 625 mg	750 mg 3 times/day 1250 mg twice daily (with other drugs)	Administer with foods. Tablets may be crushed and added to soft food or dissolved in liquids
Ritonavir (RTV)	PO solution: 80 mg/mL EC tablets: 100 mg Capsules: 100 mg	600 mg twice daily	Administer with food Swallow tablets whole
Saquinavir (SQV)	Tablets: 500 mg Capsules: 200 mg	1000 mg twice daily (with other drugs)	Administer within 2 hr after meals[b] with ritonavir Capsules may be opened and mixed with food[b] (manufacturer recommends mixing with syrup or jam)
Tipranavir (TPV)	PO solution: 100 mg/mL Capsules: 250 mg	200 mg twice daily 500 mg twice daily	Administer with food and ritonavir

[a]These are a sampling of representative manufacturer recommendations for HIV treatment (not prophylaxis). In practice, dosage is individualized.
[b]High-fat meals increase plasma levels by 39% with capsules and by 79% with tablets.
EC, Enteric-coated.

Adverse Effects

There are several adverse effects that all protease inhibitors have in common. These include hyperglycemia and the development of diabetes, lipodystrophy (fat redistribution), elevation of serum transaminases, and decreased cardiac conduction velocity. They can also increase bleeding in patients with hemophilia.

Hyperglycemia/Diabetes. Protease inhibitors have been associated with hyperglycemia, new-onset diabetes, abrupt exacerbation of existing diabetes, and diabetic ketoacidosis. Onset typically occurs after 2 months of drug use, but can also develop much earlier. Hyperglycemia can be managed with insulin and oral antidiabetic agents (e.g., metformin). Because of the possible risk for diabetes, patients should be instructed to report signs of the disease, such as polydipsia (increased fluid intake), polyphagia (increased food intake), and polyuria (frequent urination). In patients with existing diabetes, blood glucose should be monitored closely. In others, blood glucose should be measured at baseline, every 3 to 4 months during the first year of treatment and less frequently thereafter. Although withdrawing PIs may restore normal glucose metabolism, discontinuation is not recommended.

Lipodystrophy. Use of PIs has been associated with redistribution of body fat, sometimes referred to as *lipodystrophy syndrome* or *pseudo-Cushing's syndrome (cushingoid appearance).* Fat accumulates in the abdomen, in the breasts of men and women, and between the shoulder blades at the base of the neck. Fat is lost from the face, arms, buttocks, and legs. The underlying mechanism has not been determined. Although these fat changes resemble those of Cushing's syndrome, which is caused by excessive cortisol, elevated cortisol has not been observed. Health risks of the syndrome are unknown, although it can be psychologically distressing. Drug withdrawal may cause symptoms to resolve, but is not recommended.

Hyperlipidemia. All PIs can elevate plasma levels of cholesterol and triglycerides. These effects may occur with or without redistribution of fat. Elevation of cholesterol can lead to atherosclerosis and associated cardiovascular events. Elevation of triglycerides can lead to pancreatitis. Changes in plasma lipids can be detected by monitoring lipid levels every 3 to 4 months. Potential interventions for hyperlipidemia include diet, exercise, and lipid-lowering drugs. However, benefits of these interventions have not been established. If lipid-lowering drugs are employed, lovastatin and simvastatin should be avoided because cytochrome P450 inhibition by PIs can cause lovastatin and simvastatin to accumulate to dangerous levels.

Increased Bleeding in People With Hemophilia. Protease inhibitors may increase the risk for bleeding in patients with hemophilia. Bleeding typically occurs in the joints and soft tissues, where danger is lower. However, serious bleeds in the brain and GI tract have also occurred. The mean time to increased bleeding is 22 days after the onset of treatment. Patients may need to increase their dosage of coagulation factors.

Elevation of Serum Transaminases. Protease inhibitors can increase serum levels of transaminases, indicating injury to the liver. Exercise caution in patients with chronic liver disease (e.g., hepatitis B or C, cirrhosis). Serum transaminases should be measured at baseline and periodically thereafter.

Decreased Cardiac Conduction Velocity. Protease inhibitors can decrease the speed of cardiac conduction. The most common effect is prolongation of the PR interval; however, studies have shown that this may also lead to bundle branch blocks. This effect may be worsened if patients are taking other drugs that promote this effect, such as beta blockers.

Drug Interactions

All PIs are metabolized by cytochrome P450 enzymes, and all PIs can inhibit selected cytochrome P450 enzymes. Typically, they will also induce other enzymes. As a result, PIs can interact with drugs that inhibit or induce P450 enzymes and with drugs that are substrates for P450 enzymes.

Not all interactions are harmful, of course. By inhibiting selected P450 enzymes one PI can increase the level of another PI and can thus intensify therapeutic effects. One PI—*ritonavir* [Norvir]—is routinely combined with other PIs with the specific purpose of increasing the therapeutic effects of the other PI. In this technique, known as *ritonavir boosting,* the dose of ritonavir is low: 100 to 400 mg/day. This dosage is too low to contribute significant antiviral effects, but still high enough to inhibit P450 metabolism.

Unfortunately, most interactions with PIs are not beneficial. We will highlight interactions commonly experienced by patients with HIV in our discussion of individual PIs.

Properties of Individual Protease Inhibitors

Next, we discuss the individual drugs in this category. Pharmacokinetic properties of the PIs are shown in Table 94.6. Preparation, dosage, and administration are displayed in Table 94.7.

Darunavir

Darunavir [Prezista] is a second-generation PI with activity against HIV strains that are resistant to other PIs. It will serve as our prototype for this class.

Actions and Use. As mentioned, darunavir has more activity against HIV strains that develop resistance to other PIs. Strains resistant to darunavir are generally cross-resistant with all other PIs, except possibly tipranavir. Darunavir is typically boosted with ritonavir and combined with other antiretroviral drugs. The combination can be especially useful in treatment-experienced patients infected with PI-resistant HIV strains.

Adverse Effects. Darunavir causes the same adverse effects shared with other PIs (see earlier discussion). Of particular importance for darunavir is hyperlipidemia. As many as 23% to 25% experience elevated cholesterol levels with associated increases in low-density lipoprotein cholesterol and triglycerides. On the other hand, the hyperglycemia that occurs with all PIs occurs less often with darunavir.

About 10% of patients taking this drug develop a rash. Darunavir has a sulfonamide component that may be a contributing factor; however, other factors are likely also involved.

Other common adverse effects include nausea, diarrhea, and headache. When administered with cobicistat, increases in serum creatinine have occurred.

Drug Interactions. Darunavir is both a CYP3A4 substrate and inhibitor. It is also a CYP2C9 inducer. Because these two enzyme systems are responsible for the metabolism of so many drugs, the number of drug interactions is *extensive*. For patients with HIV infection, the following drugs included in product labeling present special concerns.

Darunavir can increase serum levels of several antiretroviral drugs. These include maraviroc and indinavir. Darunavir can decrease serum levels of the antiretroviral drug abacavir.

Darunavir levels may also be affected by coadministration of antiretroviral drugs. Indinavir increases darunavir levels; lopinavir/ritonavir and saquinavir decrease darunavir levels.

Darunavir has interactions with two drugs used to treat hepatitis C infection. Coadministration with boceprevir decreases levels of both boceprevir and darunavir. Coadministration with simeprevir increases levels of both drugs.

Darunavir increases levels of beta blockers, calcium channel blockers, amiodarone, lidocaine, disopyramide, flecainide, mexiletine, propafenone, and quinidine. This is significant because this can further worsen the decreased conduction velocity that can be an adverse effect of darunavir.

Ritonavir

Actions and Uses. Ritonavir [Norvir] inhibits HIV protease, and thereby prevents maturation of HIV. Because of its ability to inhibit CYP3A4 and CYP2D6 enzymes, which are enzymes that metabolize PIs, ritonavir is often combined with other PIs to boost their effects. Nearly one-third of HIV patients use this drug.

Adverse Effects. In addition to the shared adverse effects for this class, ritonavir can cause circumoral (around the mouth) paresthesias and paresthesias of the extremities. It can also alter taste sensation.

Nausea, vomiting, and diarrhea are common during the initial weeks of therapy and then tend to fade. Adverse effects can be reduced by initiating therapy at a low dosage and then gradually titrating up to the maintenance dosage.

Drug Interactions. Ritonavir has a role in affecting metabolism by numerous P450 enzymes. It is a powerful CYP3A4 and CYP2D6 inhibitor. (It is also metabolized by CYP3A4 and CYP2D6.) Additionally, it is an inducer of CYP1A2, CYP2C8, CYP2C9, and CYP2C19. There are also minor (typically nonconsequential) actions on other enzyme systems. As you can imagine, the number of interactions is substantial.

Atazanavir

Actions and Uses. Atazanavir [Reyataz] inhibits HIV protease in the same manner of all PIs. Dosing is done just once a day, with or without boosting with ritonavir.

Adverse Effects. Atazanavir shares the same adverse effects as all PIs. The prolongation of the PR interval is more common with this drug. It causes asymptomatic first-degree AV block in 5% to 9% of patients. Accordingly, the drug should be used with caution in patients with structural heart disease, pre-existing cardiac conduction disturbances, or ischemic heart disease, and in those taking other drugs that prolong the PR interval.

Atazanavir interferes with normal processing of bilirubin, and thereby raises levels of unconjugated bilirubin in plasma (indirect hyperbilirubinemia). As a result, about 11% of patients develop jaundice (yellowing of the skin)

PATIENT-CENTERED CARE ACROSS THE LIFE SPAN

Protease Inhibitors

Life Stage	Patient Care Concerns
Children[a]	Lopinavir/ritonavir[b] may be given to infants as young as 14 days of age. Atazanavir is approved for infants as young as 3 months who weigh at least 5 kg. Fosamprenavir and ritonavir are approved for those older than 4 weeks. Nelfinavir and tipranavir are approved for children aged 2 years. Darunavir may be given to children at least 3 years of age and weighing at least 10 kg. Safety and effectiveness have not been established for the use of indinavir to treat children. For saquinavir, safety and effectiveness have not been established for those younger than 16 years.
Pregnant women	Antiretroviral therapy is recommended for all HIV-infected pregnant women to lower the viral load and decrease the risk of perinatal transmission. Nelfinavir, ritonavir, and saquinavir are Pregnancy Risk Category B.[c] Darunavir, fosamprenavir, indinavir, lopinavir/ritonavir, and tipranavir are Pregnancy Risk Category C.[c] Updated labeling for atazanavir does not include a risk category (see new FDA guidelines in Chapter 9), but reports that there is no evidence that atazanavir causes major birth defects. Labeling emphasizes that atazanavir should be accompanied by ritonavir when prescribed for pregnant women.
Breast-feeding women	Breast-feeding should be avoided by women with HIV because there is a danger of transmitting the virus.
Older adults	Clinical trials did not enroll sufficient numbers of patients aged 65 and over to adequately determine comparative responses to younger subjects. Consider hepatic, renal, or cardiac function and comorbidity in monitoring.

[a]Pediatric information is extracted from *Approved Antiretroviral Drugs for Pediatric Treatment of HIV Infection,* available at https://www.fda.gov/forpatients/illness/hivaids/treatment/ucm118951.htm.
[b]Lopinavir/ritonavir oral solution should not be given to preterm infants until 14 days after their *predicted due date*. The solution contains 42% alcohol and 15% propylene glycol, which can accumulate to toxic levels causing potentially fatal cardiac, renal, and respiratory problems.
[c]As of 2020, the FDA will no longer use Pregnancy Risk Categories. Please refer to Chapter 9 for more information.

and scleral icterus (yellowing of the eyes), which reverse following drug withdrawal. If it will be given to patients with hepatic impairment, dosage adjustment is needed.

Drug Interactions. Atazanavir is subject to numerous interactions with other drugs. It is a CYP3A4 inhibitor and substrate and a weak CYP2C8 inhibitor.

Lopinavir/Ritonavir

Actions and Uses. Lopinavir and ritonavir are available in a fixed-dose combination under the brand name *Kaletra.*

Lopinavir is the active antiretroviral component. Ritonavir is present only to boost lopinavir's effects; dosing is too small to exert a significant antiretroviral effect. (See earlier discussion about ritonavir.) In clinical trials, lopinavir/ritonavir was effective against some HIV strains that had become resistant to other PIs.

Adverse Effects. The most common adverse effect is diarrhea (13.8%). The remainder—nausea, headache, and weakness or tiredness—occur in less than 10% of patients. One of the most serious of those adverse effects not shared by all PIs is pancreatitis.

Of the shared PI adverse effects, prolongation of both the PR and QT intervals can be significant with lopinavir/ritonavir. By prolonging the PR interval, the drug increases the risk for second- or third-degree atrioventricular (AV) block. Accordingly, it should be used with caution in patients with structural heart disease, pre-existing cardiac conduction disturbances, or ischemic heart disease, and in those taking other drugs that prolong the PR interval. By prolonging the QT interval, lopinavir/ritonavir increases the risk for torsades de pointes and other severe dysrhythmias. Accordingly, the drug should be avoided in patients with congenital long QT syndrome and in those taking other drugs that prolong the QT interval.

Drug Interactions. Lopinavir/ritonavir strongly inhibits two drug-metabolizing enzymes—CYP3A4 and CYP2D6—and can thereby raise levels of drugs that are substrates for these enzymes. Serious toxicity can result. To avoid toxicity, certain drugs must be used in greatly reduced dosage and others must not be used at all.

Paradoxically, lopinavir/ritonavir can *induce* metabolism of some drugs, including methadone and ethinyl estradiol, a component of many oral contraceptives. As a result, the plasma level of these drugs may fall to subtherapeutic levels.

Agents that induce CYP3A4 can accelerate metabolism of lopinavir/ritonavir and can thereby decrease antiretroviral effects. Concurrent use of PIs with strong CYP3A4 inducers should be avoided.

Because of its alcohol content, the oral solution of lopinavir/ritonavir should not be combined with disulfiram [Antabuse] or metronidazole. Why? Because both drugs will cause accumulation of acetaldehyde, a toxic metabolite of alcohol.

Older Protease Inhibitors

The older PIs, indinavir, saquinavir, nelfinavir, and fosamprenavir, are less commonly used either because of drug resistance and decreased efficacy or because of toxic adverse effects. Tipranavir is seldom used except when the HIV is resistant to other PIs. These drugs will be discussed briefly.

Indinavir

The major adverse effect of indinavir is *nephrolithiasis* (kidney stones). To decrease the risk for nephrolithiasis, patients should consume at least 48 ounces (1.5 L) of water daily.

In addition to the adverse effects of all PIs, indinavir can raise the plasma levels of unconjugated bilirubin (indirect bilirubin). Be alert for jaundice, which reverses on drug withdrawal.

Saquinavir

Saquinavir was the first PI to receive FDA approval. Adverse effects are primarily those shared by all PIs. Torsades de pointes, which can degenerate into fatal ventricular fibrillation, has occurred as a complication of QT prolongation.

Nelfinavir

Diarrhea can be dose limiting. During clinical trials, 20% to 32% of patients developed moderate to severe diarrhea. In most cases, diarrhea can be managed with an over-the-counter antidiarrheal drug (e.g., loperamide).

Fosamprenavir

Fosamprenavir [Lexiva, Telzir 🍁] is a prodrug that undergoes rapid conversion to amprenavir, its active form. (Amprenavir is a former antiretroviral agent.) Following the introduction of fosamprenavir, amprenavir [Agenerase] was withdrawn from the market.

Amprenavir is a chemical relative of the sulfonamide antibiotics. Whether people with sulfonamide hypersensitivity will also experience hypersensitivity to fosamprenavir is unknown. For safety reasons, fosamprenavir should be avoided in patients with a history of sulfonamide reactions.

Tipranavir (Plus Ritonavir)

Tipranavir [Aptivus], boosted with ritonavir, is indicated for use with other antiretroviral drugs to treat HIV-infected adults who have evidence of ongoing viral replication and who either (1) have taken antiretroviral drugs for a long time or (2) are infected with HIV strains known to be resistant to multiple PIs. Tipranavir should not be used in the absence of ritonavir boosting.

Tipranavir inhibits HIV protease; however, in contrast to all other PIs, which are rigid peptides, tipranavir is a flexible nonpeptide. Because of its flexibility, tipranavir can adapt to conformational changes in HIV protease that render the enzyme resistant to other PIs. As a result, some HIV strains that have become resistant to other PIs can still be suppressed with tipranavir.

Adverse Effects. Increases in plasma cholesterol and triglycerides with tipranavir are larger than with other PIs. Potentially fatal liver damage is the greatest concern. Patients with chronic hepatitis B or C are especially vulnerable. To reduce risk, liver function should be assessed at baseline and frequently thereafter. There also have been reports of fatal and nonfatal cranial hemorrhage. However, a causal relationship has not been established.

INTEGRASE STRAND TRANSFER INHIBITORS

HIV integrase strand transfer inhibitors (INSTIs), or simply *integrase inhibitors,* target HIV by terminating the integration of HIV into DNA. Integrase is one of three viral enzymes needed for HIV replication. As its name implies, integrase inserts HIV genetic material into the DNA of CD4 cells. By inhibiting integrase, these drugs prevent insertion of HIV DNA and thereby stop HIV replication. They are effective against both HIV-1 and HIV-2.

We currently have three approved INSTIs: raltegravir, dolutegravir, and elvitegravir. All are indicated for combined use with other antiretroviral agents to treat adults infected with HIV-1. Pharmacokinetic properties for these drugs, as well as for the representative drugs in the two categories that follow, are provided in Table 94.8. Preparations, dosages, and administration are provided in Table 94.9.

Raltegravir

Actions and Use

Raltegravir [Isentress] was the first HIV integrase strand transfer inhibitor to be developed. Raltegravir stops HIV replication by preventing insertion of HIV DNA. Raltegravir is active against HIV strains resistant to some of the other drugs.

TABLE 94.8 ■ Pharmacokinetic Properties of Integrase Strand Transfer Inhibitors, HIV Fusion Inhibitors, and CCR5 Antagonists

Drug Category	Drug Name	Route	Peak	Serum Half-Life	Metabolism	Excretion
Integrase strand transfer inhibitors	Raltegravir (RAL)	PO	3 hr	9 hr	Hepatic glucuronidation mediated by UGT1A1	Feces (primary), urine
	Dolutegravir (DTG)	PO	2–3 hr	14 hr	Metabolism by UGT1A1 (primary) and CYP3A enzymes	Feces (primary), urine
	Elvitegravir (EVG)	PO	4 hr	9 hr	Hepatic by CYP3A enzymes and hepatic glucuronidation mediated by UGT1A1/3	Feces (95%), urine
HIV fusion inhibitors	Enfuvirtide (ENF)	SubQ	3–13 hr	3.2–4.4 hr	Hepatic and renal by peptidases and proteinases	NA[a]
CCR5 antagonists	Maraviroc (MVC)	PO	0.5–4 hr	14–18 hr	Hepatic by CYP3A enzymes	Feces (primary), urine

[a]Product labeling reports that studies to identify elimination route have not been carried out in humans.
NA, Not available.

TABLE 94.9 ■ Preparation, Dosage, and Administration of Integrase Strand Transfer Inhibitors, HIV Fusion Inhibitors, and CCR5 Antagonists

Drug Category	Drug Name	Preparation	Typical Adult Dosage[a]	Administration
Integrase strand transfer inhibitors[b]	Raltegravir (RAL)	Packet for PO suspension: 100 mg Chewable tablets: 25, 100 mg EC tablet: 400 mg	400 mg twice daily	Mix packet with 5 mL water to make a suspension Chewable tablets may be chewed, divided, or swallowed whole EC tablet must be swallowed whole
	Dolutegravir (DTG)	Tablets: 10, 25, 50 mg	50–100 mg once daily (with other drugs)	Administer with or without food
HIV fusion inhibitors	Enfuvirtide (ENF)	Solution for injection: 90 mg	90 mg twice daily	Administer subcutaneously Rotate sites
CCR5 antagonists	Maraviroc (MVC)	Tablets: 25, 75, 150, 300 mg	300 mg twice daily	Administer with or without food

[a]These are a sampling of representative manufacturer recommendations for HIV treatment (not prophylaxis). Dosage is individualized in practice.
[b]Elvitegravir is omitted because it is no longer available as a single product; it is only available in fixed-combination products.
EC, Enteric-coated.

Raltegravir was originally approved only for treatment-experienced patients but is now approved for treatment-naïve patients as well. In current guidelines, raltegravir (in combination with tenofovir plus either emtricitabine or lamivudine) is considered a first-choice drug for HIV treatment. In clinical trials, raltegravir demonstrated increased viral suppression when compared to protease inhibitors and the NNRTI efavirenz. Unfortunately, HIV resistance was also more likely to develop.

Adverse Effects

Raltegravir is generally well tolerated by most. The most common adverse effect is an elevation in liver enzymes that occurs in about 10% of those taking the drug. Approximately 4% to 5% will have elevations in serum amylase and lipase.

Symptomatic adverse effects occur infrequently. In fact, the most common adverse effects, insomnia and headache, occur in only 2% to 4% of those taking this drug. In clinical trials, a few patients experienced myopathy and rhabdomyolysis, but a causal relationship has not been established.

Rarely, patients have developed *severe hypersensitivity reactions.* Skin reactions include Stevens-Johnson syndrome and toxic epidermal necrolysis, which can be fatal. Organ dysfunction, including liver failure, may also develop. Patients who develop signs of a hypersensitivity reaction (e.g., severe rash, or rash associated with blisters, fever, malaise, fatigue, oral lesions, facial edema, hepatitis, angioedema, muscle or joint aches) should discontinue raltegravir immediately.

Contraindications

There are no contraindications to taking raltegravir. Those with pre-existing hepatic impairment may be at risk for worsening of this condition. Caution should be maintained when taken by patients with a history of rhabdomyolysis or by those taking other drugs that have this adverse effect.

Drug Interactions

Because raltegravir is metabolized by glucuronidation, it does not have as many drug interactions as those with roles in P450 enzyme systems. Atazanavir and other inhibitors of UGT can increase levels of raltegravir. Conversely, inducers of UGT (e.g., efavirenz, fosamprenavir, rifabutin, tipranavir) can lower raltegravir levels.

Dolutegravir

Actions and Use

Dolutegravir [Tivicay] is approved for both treatment-naïve and treatment-experienced patients. It has a significant advantage over raltegravir and elvitegravir. HIV resistance is less likely to develop to dolutegravir than to the other INSTIs.

Adverse Effects

The most common adverse reactions of dolutegravir are elevated liver enzymes (up to 18%) and hyperglycemia (14%). About 7% experience insomnia. Neutropenia occurs in about 4% of those taking this drug.

Drug Interactions

Dolutegravir in not involved in P450 metabolism; however, it still has significant interactions with a number of drugs. Several are particularly relevant to patients with HIV infection. Antiretroviral drugs that can decrease dolutegravir levels include efavirenz, etravirine, fosamprenavir, nevirapine, and tipranavir. Minerals such as iron, calcium, and magnesium can also decrease serum levels. When patients take drugs containing these products, including multivitamins with minerals, dolutegravir should be administered at least 2 hours before or 6 hours after these agents.

Elvitegravir

Actions and Use

Elvitegravir, formerly available as the single drug Vitekta, is now available only as part of the combination products. It is incapable of achieving therapeutic levels when given alone, owing to extensive metabolism by the P450 enzyme system, especially CYP3A isoenzymes. HIV resistance is common.

Adverse Effects

Elvitegravir has few adverse effects. The most common are diarrhea (7%) and nausea (4%). Of course, because it is given in combination with drugs from other HIV drug classes, those adverse effects must be considered, as well, when monitoring patients for complications of therapy.

Drug Interactions

As mentioned, elvitegravir is a substrate of CYP3A enzyme systems. Drugs that are CYP3A inducers (especially CYP3A4) can decrease serum levels.

HIV FUSION INHIBITORS

Unlike most other drugs for HIV, which inhibit essential viral enzymes (i.e., reverse transcriptase, integrase, protease), HIV fusion inhibitors block entry of HIV into CD4 T cells. Earlier in the chapter, we discussed the replication cycle of HIV. Recall that in step 2, the lipid bilayer envelope of HIV fuses with the lipid bilayer of the host cell membrane. HIV fusion inhibitors block this fusion process.

Enfuvirtide

Enfuvirtide [Fuzeon], widely known as T-20, is the first and only HIV fusion inhibitor currently approved by the FDA. Unfortunately, although enfuvirtide is effective, it is also inconvenient (treatment requires twice-daily subQ injections) and very expensive (treatment costs about $52,000 a year). Furthermore, injection-site reactions occur in nearly all patients.

Mechanism of Action

Enfuvirtide prevents the HIV envelope from fusing with the cell membrane of CD4 cells (see Fig. 94.2, step 2), and thereby blocks viral entry and replication. Fusion inhibition results from binding of enfuvirtide to gp41, a subunit of the glycoproteins embedded in the HIV envelope (see Fig. 94.1). As a result of enfuvirtide binding, the glycoprotein becomes rigid, and hence cannot undergo the configurational change needed to permit fusion of HIV with the cell membrane.

Resistance

Resistance to enfuvirtide has developed in cultured cells and in patients. The cause is a structural change in gp41. In clinical trials, reductions in drug susceptibility have ranged from 4- to

PATIENT-CENTERED CARE ACROSS THE LIFE SPAN

Integrase Strand Inhibitors, HIV Fusion Inhibitors, and CCR5 Antagonists

Life Stage	Patient Care Concerns
Children[a]	ISTIs: Raltegravir is approved for use in infants aged 4 months and older. Dolutegravir is approved for children 12 years and older weighing at least 30 kg. Safety of elvitegravir has not been adequately evaluated for patients under 12 years old. Fusion inhibitor: Enfuvirtide is approved for children age 6 and older. CCR5 antagonist: Maraviroc is not indicated for children younger than 16 years because safety and efficacy have not been established.
Pregnant women	Antiretroviral therapy is recommended for all HIV-infected pregnant women to lower the viral load and decrease the risk of perinatal transmission. Dolutegravir, elvitegravir, enfuvirtide, and maraviroc are Pregnancy Risk Category B.[b] Raltegravir is Pregnancy Risk Category C.
Breast-feeding women	Breast-feeding should be avoided by women with HIV because there is a danger of transmitting the virus.
Older adults	Clinical trials did not enroll sufficient numbers of patients aged 65 and over to adequately determine comparative responses to younger subjects. Consider hepatic, renal, or cardiac function and comorbidity in considering therapy.

[a]Pediatric ages are extracted from *Approved Antiretroviral Drugs for Pediatric Treatment of HIV Infection,* available at https://www.fda.gov/forpatients/illness/hivaids/treatment/ucm118951.htm.
[b]As of 2020, the FDA will no longer use Pregnancy Risk Categories. Please refer to Chapter 9 for more information.

422-fold. Fortunately, the HIV mutations that confer resistance to enfuvirtide do not confer cross-resistance to NRTIs, NNRTIs, PIs, INSTIs, or CCR5 antagonists. Conversely, resistance to NRTIs, NNRTIs, PIs, INSTIs, or CCR5 antagonists does not confer cross-resistance to enfuvirtide.

The rate at which resistance develops depends on the efficacy of the drugs used concurrently. When the patient's other antiretroviral drugs are still effective, resistance to enfuvirtide develops relatively slowly. However, when there is significant resistance to the other drugs, resistance to enfuvirtide develops rapidly.

Therapeutic Use

Enfuvirtide is reserved for treating HIV-1 infection that has become resistant to other antiretroviral agents. Specifically, the drug is indicated for HIV-1 infection in patients who are treatment experienced and have evidence of HIV replication despite ongoing ART. To delay emergence of resistance, enfuvirtide should always be combined with other antiretroviral drugs.

Adverse Effects

Injection-Site Reactions. In clinical trials, injection-site reactions (ISRs) developed in 98% of patients, usually within the first week of treatment. Principal manifestations are pain and tenderness, erythema and induration, nodules or cysts, pruritus, and ecchymosis (small hemorrhagic spots). Although generally mild to moderate, symptoms can also be severe. In 17% of patients, individual ISRs persisted more than 7 days. Because ISRs are both common and long lasting, 23% of patients had six or more ongoing ISRs at any given time. The intensity of ISRs can be reduced by rotating the injection site, avoiding sites with an active ISR, and avoiding unnecessarily deep injections. If a severe ISR occurs, or if local infection develops, patients should seek immediate medical attention.

Pneumonia. Enfuvirtide appears to increase the risk for bacterial pneumonia. Patients should be informed about signs of pneumonia (cough, fever, breathing difficulties) and instructed to report them immediately. Enfuvirtide should be used with caution in patients who have pneumonia risk factors: low initial CD4 cell counts, high initial viral load, IV drug use, smoking, and a history of lung disease.

Hypersensitivity Reactions. Because enfuvirtide is a foreign peptide, it can trigger hypersensitivity reactions. Typical symptoms, which may occur individually and in combination, are rash, fever, nausea, vomiting, chills, rigors, hypotension, and elevated serum transaminases. Enfuvirtide has also been associated with respiratory distress, glomerulonephritis, Guillain-Barré syndrome, and primary immune complex reaction, all of which may be immune mediated. If a systemic hypersensitivity reaction occurs, enfuvirtide should be discontinued immediately and never used again.

Drug Interactions

Enfuvirtide appears devoid of significant drug interactions. There are no interactions with other antiretroviral drugs that would require a dosage adjustment for either enfuvirtide or the other agent.

CCR5 ANTAGONISTS

CCR5 antagonists, like the fusion inhibitors, block entry of HIV into CD4 T cells. However, the mechanism by which they accomplish this is different.

Maraviroc

Maraviroc [Selzentry, Celsentri 🍁] is the first, and currently only, representative of the *CCR5 antagonists.* Maraviroc isn't usually used for initial treatment of HIV. It appears most effective in treating patients with drug-resistant HIV.

Mechanism of Action

As discussed earlier in the chapter, CCR5 is a co-receptor that some strains of HIV must bind with to enter CD4 cells. Maraviroc binds with CCR5 and thereby blocks viral entry. HIV strains that require CCR5 for entry are referred to as being *CCR5 tropic.* Between 50% and 60% of patients are infected with this type of HIV. Maraviroc and enfuvirtide (a fusion inhibitor) are the only antiretroviral drugs that block HIV entry.

Therapeutic Use

Maraviroc is indicated for combined use with other antiretroviral agents to treat patients age 16 years and older who are infected with CCR5-tropic HIV-1 strains. The drug was originally approved only for treatment-experienced patients but is now approved for treatment-naïve patients as well. Before maraviroc is used, a test must be performed to confirm that the infecting HIV strain is CCR5 tropic.

Adverse Effects

The most common side effects are cough, dizziness, pyrexia, rash, abdominal pain, musculoskeletal symptoms, and upper respiratory tract infections. Intensity is generally mild to moderate.

Liver injury has been seen in some patients and may be preceded by signs of an allergic reaction (e.g., eosinophilia, pruritic rash, elevated immunoglobulin E). Patients should be informed about signs of an evolving reaction (itchy rash, jaundice, vomiting, and/or abdominal pain) and instructed to stop maraviroc and seek medical attention.

During clinical trials, a few patients experienced *cardiovascular events,* including myocardial ischemia and MI. Maraviroc should be used with caution in patients with cardiovascular risk factors.

Drug Interactions

Because maraviroc is metabolized by CYP3A4, drugs that inhibit or induce this enzyme will affect maraviroc levels. Levels will be raised by strong CYP3A4 inhibitors, including protease inhibitors (except tipranavir/ritonavir) and delavirdine. Conversely, maraviroc levels will be lowered by strong CYP3A4 inducers, including etravirine and efavirenz. As always, it is important to check for interactions via a comprehensive database before administering drugs such as this one.

MANAGEMENT OF HIV INFECTION

Thanks to the drugs we have today, HIV infection has been transformed from a near-certain death sentence to a manageable chronic disease. Most patients take several antiretroviral drugs—typically two NRTIs combined with either a PI or NNRTI. These highly effective regimens can reduce plasma HIV to undetectable levels, causing CD4 T-cell counts to return toward normal, thereby restoring some immune function. However, despite these advances, treatment cannot cure HIV. In all cases, discontinuation of antiretroviral drugs has led to a rebound in plasma HIV.

Therapy of HIV disease is often complex. Patients take a combination of drugs for HIV itself—and may take additional drugs to manage treatment side effects (e.g., hyperlipidemia, lipodystrophy, depression) along with drugs to prevent or treat opportunistic infections. As a result, the potential for adverse effects and drug interactions is large. Also, among the drugs used for HIV, emergence of resistance is common. Furthermore, adverse effects and pill burden make adherence difficult. Because of these complexities, management is best done by a specialist with extensive experience in treating HIV.

Much of the discussion that follows is based on the *Guidelines for the Use of Antiretroviral Agents in Adults and Adolescents Living with HIV,* available online at https://aidsinfo.nih.gov/guidelines. They were developed by the Panel on Clinical Practices for Treatment of HIV Infection, convened by the U.S. Department of Health and Human Services (DHHS). The guidelines undergo periodic updates; the ones cited here were updated in 2017. Also at the website are guidelines for pediatric patients, pregnant patients, and HIV pre-exposure and postexposure prophylaxis. We encourage you to examine these guidelines for additional information because much of it is beyond the scope of a pharmacology textbook.

Laboratory Tests

The principal laboratory tests employed to guide therapy are *CD4 T-cell counts* and *plasma HIV RNA* (viral load) *assays.* Measurement of viral load indicates the magnitude of HIV replication and predicts the rate of CD4 T-cell destruction. In contrast, CD4 T-cell counts indicate how much damage the immune system has already suffered. In addition to these tests, evaluation of *HIV drug resistance* is now done routinely. Some patients will also need tests for *HLA-B*5701* (a genetic variant linked to abacavir hypersensitivity) and for *HIV CCR5 tropism* (a determinant of responsiveness to maraviroc).

CD4 T-Cell Counts

The CD4 T-cell count is the principal indicator of how much immunocompetence remains. Accordingly, the CD4 count is a major factor in deciding *when to initiate* ART and *when to change drugs* if the regimen is failing. Also, by telling us about immune status, the assay can help guide initiation, discontinuation, and resumption of drugs for opportunistic infections.

As ART takes effect, CD4 T-cell counts will begin to rise, indicating some return of immune function. With ART, increases of 100 to 250 cells/mm^3 have been observed. Although restoration of CD4 T-cell counts may not produce *complete* immunocompetence, it is often sufficient to permit discontinuation of prophylactic therapy against some opportunistic infections.

A healthy range for CD4 T cells is 800 to 1200 cells/mm^3. A 30% reduction is considered significant. Among people with HIV infection, a CD4 T-cell count above 500 cells/mm^3 is considered relatively high. In contrast, a count below 200 cells/mm^3 indicates clear immunodeficiency.

Viral Load (Plasma HIV RNA)

Ongoing treatment of HIV infection is guided primarily by monitoring *viral load,* which is determined by measuring *HIV RNA in plasma.* The source of the RNA is intact HIV virions (virus particles), each of which has two copies of HIV RNA.

Plasma HIV RNA is the best measurement available for predicting clinical outcome. If HIV RNA is high (e.g., 100,000 copies/mL), the prognosis is poor. Conversely, if HIV RNA is low (e.g., 500 copies/mL), the risk for disease progression and death is greatly reduced. Accordingly, the goal of ART is to decrease plasma HIV RNA as much as possible—preferably to a level that is undetectable with current assays (i.e., below 20 to 75 copies/mL of plasma, depending on the test employed).

When patients are treated with ART, levels of HIV RNA should decline to 10% of baseline within 2 to 8 weeks. After

16 to 20 weeks of treatment, plasma HIV RNA should reach its minimum. With optimal therapy, the minimum reached should be below the limit of detection.

HIV Drug Resistance

Resistance is a significant concern in ART. In most cases, resistance emerges over the course of treatment as a result of nonadherence to the prescribed regimen. Rarely, resistance results from primary infection with a drug-resistant HIV variant. Resistance tests can be used to guide drug selection, especially when changing a regimen that has failed.

Two major types of resistance assays are employed: *phenotypic assays* and *genotypic assays.* Phenotypic assays measure the ability of HIV to grow in the presence of increasing concentrations of antiretroviral drugs. (The ability to grow in high concentrations indicates resistance.) Genotypic assays are designed to detect resistance-conferring mutations in HIV genes that code for the targets that drugs attack (e.g., reverse transcriptase and protease). Unfortunately, assays for resistance have multiple drawbacks: They are expensive ($400 to $1000); turnaround is slow (2 to 4 weeks); sensitivity is low; phenotypic assays can produce false-negative results; and genotypic assays are difficult to interpret. There are no prospective data showing that one type of assay (genotypic or phenotypic) is superior to the other.

When should resistance be tested? According to the 2017 guideline updates, the following recommendations apply:

- Test all patients entering HIV care, even if drug therapy will not start immediately. (If drugs are delayed, consider repeating the test.) For these treatment-naïve patients, a genotypic assay is generally preferred.
- Test to aid selection of new drugs when there is virologic failure and HIV RNA levels exceed 1000 copies/mL. (In those with more than 500 but less than 1000 copies/mL, testing should still be considered.)
- Test when managing suboptimal viral load reduction.
- Test all pregnant women with HIV who have not started ART, and test women who become pregnant while on therapy if they have detectable levels of HIV RNA. In both cases, use a genotypic assay.

HLA-B*5701 Screening

As discussed earlier, the risk for having a hypersensitivity reaction to abacavir is determined largely by a genetic variation, known as HLA-B*5701. Accordingly, patients should be screened for HLA-B*5701 before starting abacavir. If the test is positive, abacavir should not be used, and the patient's positive status should be recorded as an abacavir allergy in his or her medical record. If HLA-B*5701 testing is not available, abacavir may still be used, provided the patient is counseled about possible risk and monitored for signs of hypersensitivity.

CCR5 Tropism

As discussed previously, CCR5 is a co-receptor that many strains of HIV must bind with to enter CD4 cells. Strains of HIV that use this co-receptor are CCR5 tropic. Because CCR5 antagonists are effective only against CCR5 tropic strains, a CCR5 tropism assay should be performed when considering this therapy. Two commercial assays are available: *Trofile* and *Phenoscript.* Trofile takes 2 weeks to perform and requires a plasma HIV RNA level of 1000 copies/mL or more.

Treatment of Adult and Adolescent Patients

Patients with HIV infection should receive ART regardless of the CD4 count or phase of HIV disease. Treatment has five basic goals:

- Maximal and long-lasting suppression of viral load
- Restoration and preservation of immune function
- Improved quality of life
- Reduction of HIV-related morbidity and mortality
- Prevention of HIV transmission

Initiating Antiretroviral Therapy

ART regimens typically contain at least three drugs. Regimens that contain only two drugs are not generally recommended, and monotherapy should always be avoided, except possibly during pregnancy. Additionally, all ART regimens contain drugs from at least *two different classes.* By using drugs from different classes, we can attack HIV in two different ways (e.g., inhibition of reverse transcriptase and inhibition of protease) and can thereby enhance antiviral effects.

In addition to enhancing antiviral effects, the use of multiple drugs reduces the risk for resistance. Resistance reduction occurs because the probability that HIV will undergo a mutation that confers simultaneous resistance to three or four drugs is much smaller than the probability of undergoing a mutation that confers resistance to just one drug. For example, if a patient is taking three drugs—efavirenz, tenofovir, and emtricitabine—and a virion mutates to a form that is resistant to efavirenz, the other two drugs—tenofovir and emtricitabine—will still be effective against the resistant virion, and hence suppression of replication is more likely to be sustained. On the other hand, if a patient were taking only efavirenz, the mutated form could replicate relatively unimpeded.

Current guidelines for starting ARV for a treatment-naïve patient recommend one of the following four regimens based on efficacy, safety profiles, and tolerability:

- Abacavir/lamivudine plus dolutegravir (only if HLA-B*5701-negative)

or

- Tenofovir/emtricitabine plus dolutegravir

or

- Tenofovir/emtricitabine plus elvitegravir/cobicistat

or

- Tenofovir/emtricitabine plus raltegravir

Notice that the formula for these are two NRTIs plus an INSTI. For those instances in which none of these is ideal, the guidelines recommend that initial therapy comprise two NRTIs in combination with a third drug from one of three drug classes: an INSTI, an NNRTI, or a pharmacokinetically enhanced PI.

Notice that each individual regimen employs drugs from only two of the six available classes of antiretroviral agents. Because four classes of antiretroviral drugs are *not* used, these regimens are considered *class-sparing.* For example, a regimen that employs a PI plus NRTIs would spare the use of NNRTIs, fusion inhibitors, INSTIs, and CCR5 antagonists. A major benefit of class-sparing regimens is that they postpone development of resistance to the unused drug classes and thereby increase the likelihood that the unused classes will be effective for the patient in the future.

Plasma HIV RNA should be monitored to assess the impact of treatment. For patients with symptomatic HIV disease on ART, plasma HIV RNA should show a 10-fold decrease by 8 weeks and should be undetectable by 4 to 6 months. However, ART cannot cure HIV. Even though it is undetectable, some HIV virions remain dormant in memory CD4 T cells, and hence escape harm.

Changing the Regimen

There are two basic reasons for changing ART: treatment failure and drug toxicity. Guidelines for altering the regimen because of these factors are discussed next.

Treatment Failure. Treatment failure is arguably the most compelling reason for changing the regimen. Failure is indicated if

- Plasma HIV RNA remains above 200 copies/mL after 24 weeks
- Plasma HIV RNA remains above 50 copies/mL after 48 weeks
- Plasma HIV RNA rebounds after falling to an undetectable level
- CD4 T-cell counts continue to drop despite antiretroviral treatment
- Clinical disease progresses despite antiretroviral treatment

Of these five signs of failure, the first three are the most meaningful, in that they represent a direct measurement of antiretroviral efficacy.

When treatment failure occurs, the reason must be determined. Possibilities include patient nonadherence, poor drug absorption, accelerated drug metabolism (owing to drug interactions), and viral resistance. If nonadherence is the cause, several measures may help (see later discussion). If poor absorption is the cause, changing the timing of administration with respect to meals or increasing the dosage may help. If accelerated metabolism is the cause, increasing the dosage may help. Alternatively, it may be appropriate to substitute a different drug for the one that is causing metabolism to increase. For PIs, accelerated metabolism can be suppressed by adding low-dose ritonavir.

When failure is the result of viral resistance, the preferred response is to change *all* drugs in the regimen. This makes sense in that failure means that HIV is replicating despite current treatment, indicating the presence of at least one HIV strain that is resistant to all drugs in the regimen. If we were to add or change just one drug, resistance would quickly develop to that agent and failure would recur. The risk for renewed resistance is substantially lower if we change at least two drugs, and even lower if we change three. When we change the regimen, the new drugs should be agents that (1) the patient has not taken previously and (2) are not cross-resistant with drugs the patient has taken previously. Whenever possible, the selection of replacement drugs should be guided by resistance testing.

Three drug classes—*fusion inhibitors, CCR5 antagonists,* and *INSTIs*—may be especially valuable for managing treatment failure. Because drugs from these classes work differently from the older agents—PIs, NRTIs, and NNRTIs—cross-resistance does not exist. Furthermore, since these three drugs are relatively new, patients are less likely to harbor HIV strains resistant to them.

Drug Toxicity. If a patient experiences toxicity typical of a particular drug in the regimen, that drug should be withdrawn and replaced with a drug that is (1) from the same class and (2) of equal efficacy. For example, if a patient taking zidovudine were to develop anemia and neutropenia, zidovudine should be discontinued and replaced with another NRTI (e.g., stavudine). Note that when toxicity is the reason for altering the regimen, changing just one drug is proper, whereas when resistance or suboptimal treatment is the reason, at least two of the drugs should be changed.

Promoting Patient Adherence

To achieve treatment goals and delay emergence of resistance, strict adherence to the prescribed regimen is critical. Unfortunately, several factors—duration of treatment, complex medication regimens, multiple adverse drug effects, drug-drug interactions, and drug-food interactions—make adherence to ART challenging for patients. The DHHS guidelines identify factors that predict *poor* adherence (e.g., poor clinician-patient relationship, active use of alcohol or street drugs, depression and other mental illnesses), as well as factors that predict *good* adherence (e.g., availability of emotional and practical support, ability to fit dosing into the daily routine, appreciation that poor adherence will cause treatment failure). Strategies for promoting adherence are summarized in Table 94.10.

Treatment of Infants and Young Children

In young children, the course of HIV infection is accelerated. Whereas adults generally remain symptom free for a decade or more, many children develop symptoms by their first birthday. Death often ensues by age 5—even with ART. Why do young children succumb so quickly? Primarily because their immune systems are immature, and hence less able to fend off the virus. Because immune function is limited, levels of HIV RNA climb higher in toddlers than in adults, and then decline at a much slower rate.

In very young patients, diagnosis and monitoring of HIV infection employs different methods than those used in adolescents and adults. In particular, for infants under 18 months of age, diagnosis should be based on viral load assays, not on antibody tests. For children under 5 years of age, monitoring of immune status should be based on the *percentage* of CD4 cells, not on absolute CD4 counts.

Like older patients, young patients should be treated with a combination of antiretroviral drugs, with the goals of (1) reducing plasma viral HIV to an undetectable level and (2) stabilizing or improving immune status.

Unfortunately, therapy in young patients is confounded by limited information on dosing, pharmacokinetics, and safety, and by the limited availability of pediatric formulations. Information on dosage, formulations, monitoring, and other aspects of therapy can be found in the document titled *Guidelines for the Use of Antiretroviral Agents in Pediatric HIV Infection,* prepared by the Panel on Antiretroviral Therapy and Medical Management of HIV-Infected Children. The guidelines, which undergo periodic updates, are available at www.aidsinfo.nih.gov/guidelines.

TABLE 94.10 ■ Strategies for Promoting Adherence to Medication Regimens

PATIENT- AND MEDICATION-RELATED STRATEGIES

- Thoroughly educate the patient, using multiple sessions, about the goals of therapy and the importance of adherence.
- Ensure that the patient is motivated to take medication *before* the first prescription is written.
- Negotiate a treatment plan that the patient understands and will commit to.
- Devise a regimen that minimizes pill burden and dosing frequency and that integrates the dosing schedule with meals and the patient's daily routine. (Many patients can now be treated with just one combination product taken once a day.)
- Inform the patient about adverse effects and when to report them.
- Anticipate and monitor for adverse effects, and treat them promptly when they occur.
- Avoid adverse drug interactions.
- Recruit family and friends to support the treatment plan.
- Organize an adherence support group, or add adherence issues to the agenda of an existing group.
- Help the patient connect with patient-assistance programs to help cover expenses.

CLINICIAN- AND HEALTHCARE TEAM–RELATED STRATEGIES

- Establish trust.
- Serve as educator and information resource.
- Provide ongoing support and monitoring.
- Be available between scheduled visits for questions or problems; provide access via pager when away (including on vacation and at conferences).
- Monitor adherence, and when it's low, intensify management (i.e., schedule more frequent visits, recruit family and friends, deploy other team members, provide referral to mental health or chemical dependence services).
- Collaborate with the healthcare team for all patients, and especially for difficult patients and those with special needs (e.g., provide peer educators for adolescents or injection-drug users).
- Consider the impact of new diagnoses (e.g., depression, liver disease, wasting, recurrent chemical dependency) on adherence, and include adherence intervention in management.
- Collaborate with all concerned people—pharmacists, peer educators, volunteers, case managers, drug counselors, physician assistants, and all nurses, including nurse practitioners and research nurses—to reinforce the adherence message.
- Educate the support team about ART and adherence.

Treatment of Pregnant Patients

Basic Principles

In general, the management of HIV infection in pregnant women should follow the same guidelines for managing HIV infection in nonpregnant adults. Accordingly, current guidelines recommend ART for all pregnant HIV-infected women. ART is needed not only for maternal health, but also to reduce the risk for perinatal HIV transmission. Our discussion on the role of ART in pregnancy is based on a recent clinical guideline: *Recommendations for Use of Antiretroviral Drugs in Pregnant HIV-1–Infected Women for Maternal Health and Interventions to Reduce Perinatal HIV Transmission in the United States,* as updated in October 2016 (see https://aidsinfo.nih.gov/guidelines/html/3/perinatal/0).

When treating HIV infection in pregnant women, the goal is to balance the benefits of treatment—reducing viral load, thereby promoting the health of the mother and decreasing the risk for vertical HIV transmission (i.e., transmission to the fetus)—against the risks of drug-induced fetal harm (e.g., teratogenesis, lactic acidosis, death). As a rule, the benefits of treatment outweigh the risks. The primary determinants of therapy are the clinical, virologic, and immunologic status of the mother; pregnancy is a secondary consideration. Nonetheless, pregnancy should not be ignored.

Drug selection is challenging in that information on pharmacokinetics and safety during pregnancy is limited. *Efavirenz* should be avoided during the first trimester, owing to a risk for teratogenesis. All of the *protease inhibitors* increase the risk for gestational diabetes, so blood sugar should be monitored closely. *NRTIs* increase the risk for mitochondrial toxicity. The combination of *didanosine plus stavudine*, in particular, should be avoided because these are known to increase maternal and neonatal mortality.

The major clinical consequence of mitochondrial toxicity is *lactic acidosis associated with hepatic steatosis*. Providers, nurses, and patients should be alert for signs and symptoms of lactic acidosis (nausea, vomiting, abdominal pain, malaise, fatigue, anorexia, hyperventilation). In addition to causing lactic acidosis, mitochondrial injury may result in neuropathy, myopathy, cardiomyopathy, and pancreatitis. If these develop, a thorough evaluation should be conducted. During the third trimester, measurement of electrolytes and hepatic enzymes should be done more frequently.

Preconception Counseling and Care

In women with HIV, as in all other women, preconception interventions are directed at optimizing maternal and fetal health. We need to identify risk factors for adverse maternal and fetal outcomes, stabilize existing medical conditions before conception, and provide education and counseling targeted at needs of the individual. Specific recommendations for HIV-infected women include the following:

- Selection of effective contraceptive methods to reduce the risk for unintended pregnancy
- Education and counseling about potential effects of both HIV infection and ART on pregnancy course and outcomes
- Education and counseling regarding perinatal HIV transmission risk and strategies to reduce that risk
- Initiation or modification of ART before conception in order to
    - Avoid fetotoxic agents (e.g., efavirenz, delavirdine)
    - Choose agents known to reduce perinatal HIV transmission
    - Attain maximal and stable suppression of maternal viral load
    - Evaluate and manage side effects that can harm the fetus or mother (e.g., hyperglycemia, anemia, hepatotoxicity)
- Evaluation for opportunistic infections and initiation of appropriate prophylaxis
- Immunization (e.g., for influenza, hepatitis B) as indicated
- Optimization of maternal nutritional status
- Implementation of standard recommendations for preconceptional evaluation and management (e.g., assessment of reproductive history and family genetic history; starting

folic acid supplementation; screening for infectious disease, including sexually transmitted diseases)
- Screening for maternal psychologic disorders and substance abuse
- Planning for perinatal consultation if desired or indicated

PREVENTING HIV INFECTION WITH DRUGS

Previously we discussed how antiretroviral drugs can control HIV infection when given to patients with HIV infection. In this section, we consider the ability of antiretroviral drugs to reduce HIV *transmission* when given to a patient who is HIV-*positive* and the ability to reduce or prevent HIV *acquisition* when given to a person who is HIV-*negative*. There are indications for both pre-exposure and postexposure prophylaxis.

Pre-exposure Prophylaxis

Results of the *Pre-Exposure Prophylaxis Initiative* study, a study of HIV-negative men, demonstrated that tenofovir/emtricitabine [Truvada] could reduce infection risk by 44% to 73%. These results led the CDC to recommend use of tenofovir/emtricitabine for *pre-exposure prophylaxis* (PrEP). Current indications are only for those considered at high risk for HIV acquisition: (1) people who have sexual partners with known HIV-1 infection *or* are sexually active with people who belong to social networks with high HIV-1 prevalence *and* (2) people who have one or more of the following risk factors:

- Do not regularly use condoms
- Have sexually transmitted infections
- Engage in sex for money, drugs, or other supplies
- Use recreational drugs or are dependent on alcohol
- Are imprisoned

Pre-exposure guidelines were updated in 2014. The guidelines, *Clinical Practice Guideline: Pre-Exposure Prophylaxis for the Prevention of HIV Infection in the United States,* are available at https://aidsinfo.nih.gov/guidelines.

Postexposure Prophylaxis

One-time exposure to HIV carries a small, but nonetheless real, risk for infection. Sources of exposure include unprotected vaginal or anal intercourse, receptive oral intercourse, shared needles for drug injection, accidental needle sticks, and blood and other body fluid splashes. Risk is especially high following exposure to a large quantity of infected blood or blood with a high virus titer and following deep percutaneous penetration with a needle recently removed from the vein of an infected person.

The risk for developing HIV disease after a single exposure can be reduced—but not eliminated—with prophylactic antiretroviral drugs. Presumably, protection results from preventing initial cellular infection and local propagation of HIV, thereby allowing host immune defenses to eliminate the virus before it can become established. To be effective, postexposure prophylaxis should be initiated as soon as possible after HIV exposure—preferably within 1 or 2 hours, and no later than 72 hours—and should continue for 28 days. All patients should undergo testing for antibodies against HIV, preferably at the time of exposure, and then 6 weeks, 12 weeks, and 6 months after exposure.

Recommendations for postexposure prophylaxis are based on whether the exposure was nonoccupational (nPEP) or occupational (PEP), defined as exposure of healthcare personnel while on the job.

Nonoccupational Postexposure Prophylaxis

For nonoccupational exposure, current guidelines recommend a 28-day course of nPEP for HIV-uninfected persons who seek care less than 72 hours after exposure to potentially infected body fluids. Two three-drug regimens are recommended for adults:

- *Preferred:* Tenofovir DF 300 mg plus emtricitabine 200 mg (or the combination Truvada) once daily with raltegravir 400 mg twice daily *or* dolutegravir 50 mg once daily
- *Alternate:* Tenofovir DF 300 mg plus emtricitabine 200 mg (or the combination Truvada) once daily *with* darunavir 800 mg *and* ritonavir 100 mg once daily

Detailed information on nPEP, including recommended regimens for children, patients with renal impairment, and other individualized regimens, is offered in a document titled *Updated Guidelines for Antiretroviral Postexposure Prophylaxis after Sexual, Injection Drug Use, or Other Nonoccupational Exposure to HIV—United States, 2016*, which can be found online at https://aidsinfo.nih.gov/guidelines.

Occupational Postexposure Prophylaxis

Recommendations for occupational PEP are based on the risk for acquiring HIV, which is determined by multiple factors, including (1) the nature of the exposure (skin penetration vs. body fluid splashed onto nonintact skin or mucous membrane); (2) the severity of the exposure (e.g., shallow skin penetration with a solid probe, deep skin penetration with a large-bore hollow needle, surface exposure to small volume of sputum, surface exposure to a large volume of blood); and (3) the HIV status of the exposure source (e.g., asymptomatic with a low viral load, symptomatic with a high viral load). When PEP is needed, the preferred regimen is:

Tenofovir DF 300 mg *plus* emtricitabine 200 mg (or the combination drug Truvada) *with* Raltegravir 400 mg *twice* daily

Numerous alternatives are available for PEP.

For detailed information, you can refer to a document titled *Updated U.S. Public Health Service Guidelines for the Management of Occupational Exposures to HIV and Recommendations for Postexposure Prophylaxis* (revised in 2013), which is available at https://aidsinfo.nih.gov/guidelines.

Preventing Perinatal HIV Transmission

Most mother-to-child transmission of HIV occurs during the perinatal period, primarily during delivery. Among American children, perinatal transmission accounts for nearly all new HIV infections. In the absence of antiretroviral drugs, the rate of perinatal transmission in the United States is 25%. A high viral load increases risk.

The risk for vertical transmission can be reduced by giving antiretroviral drugs to the mother during gestation and labor, and to the infant for 4 to 6 weeks postpartum. (The length of infant treatment depends on whether ART was available to the mother during pregnancy. The 4-week interval is recommended for infants born to mothers who adhered strictly to an ART regimen during pregnancy.)

Delivery by cesarean section at 38 weeks is recommended for patients with a viral load above 1000 copies/mL. To further prevent perinatal HIV transmission, an intravenous (IV) zidovudine infusion should be initiated 3 hours prior to surgery and concluded after birth. When this protocol is followed, the rate of HIV transmission is essentially zero. Zidovudine is not required for HIV-infected women receiving ART who have less than 1,000 copies/mL. (This exception is a new change in the 2016 guidelines.)

PROPHYLAXIS AND TREATMENT OF OPPORTUNISTIC INFECTIONS

Individuals with advanced HIV disease are vulnerable to infections caused by opportunistic organisms (i.e., organisms that rarely cause serious disease, except when host defenses are compromised). Vulnerability to opportunistic infections (OIs) is caused by immunodeficiency resulting from loss of CD4 T cells. The risk for OIs is greatest in patients with fewer than 200 CD4 T cells/mL. Because of the risk for OIs, patients with low CD4 counts must take antibiotics as prophylaxis. Before the advent of ART, prophylaxis was required lifelong.

Since the introduction of ART, the incidence of new OIs has declined dramatically. For example, the incidences of cytomegalovirus retinitis and disseminated mycobacterial infection have fallen by as much as 75% to 80%. In many patients with low CD4 T-cell counts, ART has caused CD4 counts to rise, restoring some immunocompetence and permitting withdrawal of prophylactic drugs. Unfortunately, ART cannot help all patients. In the discussion that follows, we consider prophylaxis and treatment of OIs in these people. Additional details on the management of OIs can be found in *Guidelines for Prevention and Treatment of Opportunistic Infections in HIV-Infected Adults and Adolescents,* updated on March 28, 2017, and *Guidelines for Prevention and Treatment of Opportunistic Infections among HIV-Exposed and HIV-Infected Children,* updated on December 15, 2016. These documents are available at https://aidsinfo.nih.gov/guidelines. We discuss some of the more common OIs next.

Pneumocystis Pneumonia (PCP)

Pneumocystis pneumonia—known as PCP (for *P*neumocystis *p*neumonia)—is a potentially fatal infection caused by *Pneumocystis jiroveci,* a fungus formerly misidentified as *Pneumocystis carinii.* Before the use of ART and prophylactic drugs, PCP was the leading cause of death among people with AIDS. At one time, PCP developed in 70% to 80% of HIV-infected people and killed about 20% to 40%. Following control of an initial bout of PCP, the rate of recurrence was 60% within the first year. In patients receiving ART, PCP is rare, and prophylaxis is often unnecessary unless CD4 counts drop to less than 200 cells/mm^3.

Clinical manifestations of PCP are generally nonspecific. Early symptoms include fever, cough, dyspnea, chest discomfort, pallor, and cyanosis. In advanced infection, lung morphology is altered. Left untreated, PCP has a mortality rate of 90%.

Treatment of PCP

The agent of choice for both PCP prophylaxis and active infection is *trimethoprim plus sulfamethoxazole* (TMP/SMZ) [Bactrim, Septra]. TMP/SMZ is effective in 90% of patients. As a rule, clinical improvement is seen in 4 to 8 days. For patients who are severely immunocompromised, *IV pentamidine* [Pentam 300], administered with the Respirgard II[a] nebulizer, may be preferred. Alternatives to TMP/SMZ or pentamidine include the antiprotozoal drug *atovaquone* [Mepron], *trimethoprim plus dapsone,* and *primaquine plus clindamycin.* These regimens are less effective than TMP/SMZ or pentamidine, but may be better tolerated. Atovaquone is noteworthy for its cost (over $21,500 retail for a year's supply).

Cytomegalovirus Retinitis

Cytomegalovirus (CMV) retinitis is the leading cause of vision loss in people with AIDS. Before the availability of ART, the incidence of CMV retinitis was about 40%. Individuals with CD4 T-cell counts below 50 cells/mm^3 are most vulnerable. Left untreated, CMV retinitis invariably leads to retinal necrosis and blindness.

Drug therapy of CMV retinitis proceeds in two stages: induction followed by maintenance. The induction phase reduces CMV load and greatly slows the rate of disease progression. However, induction does not eliminate CMV. Accordingly, maintenance therapy is given to reduce the risk for relapse. Before ART was available, maintenance therapy was required lifelong. However, when ART is able to restore sufficient immune function (by raising CD4 T-cell counts above 100 cells/mm^3 for 3 to 6 months), maintenance therapy can be discontinued.

CMV retinitis can be treated with four agents: ganciclovir, valganciclovir, cidofovir, and foscarnet. The basic pharmacology of these drugs is discussed in Chapter 93.

Mycobacterium tuberculosis and *Mycobacterium avium* Complex

Mycobacterium tuberculosis and *Mycobacterium avium* complex (MAC) are slow-growing microbes that require prolonged drug exposure for eradication. Because therapy is prolonged, emergence of resistance is a significant concern. To reduce emergence of resistance, these infections are always treated with multiple drugs—just like HIV itself. Mycobacterial infections and their treatment are discussed in Chapter 90.

Cryptococcal Meningitis

Cryptococcus neoformans is a fungus that infects 9% to 13% of patients with AIDS. In 80% of these patients, cryptococcosis manifests as meningitis (inflammation of the meninges). The most common symptoms are fever and headache. Other symptoms include nausea, vomiting, photophobia, and altered

[a]Current guidelines support only the use of the Respirgard II nebulizer, citing that data regarding efficacy using other nebulization devices are insufficient.

mental status. Cryptococcal meningitis typically occurs late in HIV disease, usually after CD4 T-cell counts fall below 100 cells/mm^3.

The treatment of choice for cryptococcal meningitis is *amphotericin B* plus *flucytosine*. The major adverse effect of amphotericin is kidney damage, and the major concern with flucytosine is bone marrow suppression (neutropenia, thrombocytopenia). Compared with amphotericin B alone, the combination of amphotericin plus flucytosine decreases rates of treatment failure and relapse. However, mortality rates with both treatments are similar. Because bone marrow suppression is a significant concern for patients with AIDS, those taking flucytosine should be monitored closely.

After the initial infection has been controlled, patients should continue maintenance therapy indefinitely. The treatment of choice is oral *fluconazole* daily. The basic pharmacology of amphotericin B, flucytosine, and fluconazole is discussed in Chapter 92.

Varicella-Zoster Virus Infection

Varicella-zoster virus (VZV) can cause *chickenpox* and *herpes zoster,* also known as *shingles.* Among adults with AIDS, VZV infection usually manifests as shingles, which results from reactivation of latent VZV infection. Preferred treatments for acute localized lesions are oral therapy with valacyclovir or famciclovir. For extensive lesions, *acyclovir* administered IV is preferred. The basic pharmacology of acyclovir, famciclovir, and foscarnet is discussed in Chapter 93.

Herpes Simplex Virus Infection

Infection with herpes simplex virus (HSV) is common among patients with HIV disease. Lesions may occur at multiple sites, including the lips, tongue, oral cavity, genitals, and perianal region. In patients with advanced HIV disease, HSV may infect the esophagus, colon, lungs, eyes, and CNS. For infection at all sites, *acyclovir, famciclovir,* and *valacyclovir* are the drugs of choice. For severe infections, IV administration of acyclovir is recommended. For patients with acyclovir-resistant HSV, *IV foscarnet* can be used.

Candidiasis

Patients infected with HIV frequently develop infection with *Candida* species, usually *Candida albicans.* The most common sites are the oropharynx and esophagus. Up to 75% of patients experience oral candidiasis (thrush), which often responds to topical therapy, such as *clotrimazole troches,* which are allowed to dissolve in the mouth, or *miconazole mucoadhesive buccal tablets,* which are applied to the mucosal surface over the canine fossa (the depression on the maxillary bone above the pointed tooth located between the lateral incisor and first premolar tooth). Systemic therapy with the oral azole *fluconazole* is an alternative for oral candidiasis. Oral azoles are more convenient than topical therapy and probably more effective; however, they are also more expensive.

For esophageal candidiasis, systemic therapy is required. Oral *itraconazole* or oral *fluconazole* is recommended. All patients with a documented history of esophageal candidiasis should be considered for chronic suppressive therapy with oral *fluconazole.*

HIV VACCINES

Development of an HIV vaccine is critical to controlling the AIDS epidemic worldwide. Although HIV infection can now be managed with ART, treatment is expensive and potentially dangerous, and must continue lifelong. Furthermore, ART is largely unavailable in developing countries, where most AIDS cases occur. Accordingly, vaccine development has been assigned a high priority.

Obstacles to Vaccine Development

Making a safe and effective vaccine against HIV has proved exceedingly and unexpectedly difficult. Scientists are concerned that the vaccine may need to (1) *prevent* HIV infection, rather than minimize it, and may need to (2) stimulate cell-mediated immunity in addition to humoral immunity. These two concerns are discussed next.

Vaccines do not prevent infection—they only attenuate it. By priming the immune system, vaccines reduce microbial replication and accelerate microbial kill. As a result, infection does not spread as far as it would in an unvaccinated person, and it does not injure as many cells. Unfortunately, HIV is different from all other pathogens: HIV kills the very cells that are meant to attack it and that vaccination is meant to stimulate. Will a vaccine that permits HIV to infect even a small number of immune cells be able to contain the infection—or will HIV eventually break through? The answer is unknown.

Vaccines elicit two kinds of immune responses: *humoral immunity* (production of antibodies) and *cell-mediated immunity* (activation of cytotoxic T lymphocytes, also known as killer T cells). Most authorities agree that, to be effective, an HIV vaccine should elicit both types of responses. Why? We already know that HIV-positive people produce billions of antibodies against HIV, and yet the infection progresses relentlessly; hence, a vaccine that stimulates only humoral immunity would seem likely to fail. Unfortunately, although it's relatively easy to make a safe vaccine that stimulates humoral immunity, it's much harder to make a safe vaccine that stimulates cellular immunity. The best way to stimulate cellular immunity is with a *live virus* vaccine—in this case, a vaccine made from HIV that has been attenuated by removing some of its genes, but has not been killed. The problem is that live virus vaccines pose a risk for infection—a risk that is unacceptable with HIV. The potential danger of this approach was underscored when monkeys were given a simian version of such a vaccine and subsequently developed simian AIDS, presumably from the vaccine.

Current Status of Vaccine Development

It has been over three decades since the virus that causes AIDS was first identified. During that time, almost $850 million has been spent on research to develop an HIV vaccine.

According to the International AIDS Vaccine Initiative, there are almost 300 vaccines in drug trials. Unfortunately, more than 200 of those are in Phase I trials, and many will not progress to Phase II. There is currently one drug in Phase III trials. Three drugs have completed Phase III trials, and data review is under way. Could there be a vaccine soon? Leaked word of successes has been favorable, but we will have to wait and see.

KEEPING CURRENT

Drug therapy of HIV infection is continuously and rapidly evolving. New drugs are being developed, knowledge of existing drugs is expanding, and new drug combinations are being studied. The website AIDSinfo (aidsinfo.nih.gov) is maintained by the DHHS. It has information on treatment guidelines, drugs, vaccines, and clinical trials. Links to other HIV/AIDS-related sites are there, too. You can sign up for e-mail notification of updates.

KEY POINTS

- HIV is a retrovirus that, like all other retroviruses, has RNA as its genetic material.
- To infect our cells, HIV must first bind to a cell-surface receptor (CD4) as well as a co-receptor (such as CCR5), and then fuse with the cell membrane.
- HIV uses *reverse transcriptase* to convert its RNA into DNA, and *integrase* to insert its DNA into that of humans.
- HIV uses *protease* to break large HIV polyproteins into their smaller, functional forms.
- The principal targets of HIV are CD4 T cells (helper T lymphocytes). These cells are attacked by HIV because they carry CD4 proteins on their surface, thereby providing HIV a required point of attachment.
- Because of errors made by reverse transcriptase, HIV can mutate rapidly from a drug-sensitive form into a drug-resistant form.
- HIV infection has three phases: initial, middle, and late. During the initial phase, many patients experience a flu-like acute retroviral syndrome. During the prolonged middle phase, patients are asymptomatic, although CD4 T cell counts undergo progressive decline. During the late phase, CD4 T cell counts drop below a critical level (200 cells/mL), rendering the patient vulnerable to opportunistic infections and certain neoplasms.
- HIV replicates rapidly during all phases of HIV infection, including the prolonged phase of clinical latency.
- We have six classes of antiretroviral drugs. Four classes—nucleoside/nucleotide reverse transcriptase inhibitors (NRTIs), non-nucleoside reverse transcriptase inhibitors (NNRTIs), integrase strand transfer inhibitors (INSTIs), and protease inhibitors (PIs)—inhibit HIV enzymes. The other two classes—HIV fusion inhibitors and CCR5 antagonists—work outside CD4 cells to block HIV entry.
- NRTIs suppress HIV replication in two ways: (1) they become incorporated into the growing strand of viral DNA (through the actions of reverse transcriptase) and thereby prevent further strand growth, and (2) they compete with natural nucleoside triphosphates for binding to the active center of reverse transcriptase and thereby competitively inhibit the enzyme.
- To interact with reverse transcriptase, NRTIs must first undergo intracellular conversion to their active (triphosphate) forms.
- All NRTIs can cause lactic acidosis and severe hepatomegaly with steatosis, which can be fatal.
- Zidovudine (an NRTI) can cause severe anemia and neutropenia.
- Didanosine and stavudine (both NRTIs) can cause peripheral neuropathy.
- Didanosine (an NRTI) can cause pancreatitis.
- Abacavir (an NRTI) can cause potentially fatal hypersensitivity reactions, and hence must not be given to patients with the HLA-B*5701 mutation, which predisposes them to abacavir hypersensitivity.
- NNRTIs (e.g., efavirenz) differ from NRTIs in that they are not analogs of natural nucleosides, are active as administered, and cause direct noncompetitive inhibition of reverse transcriptase by binding to its active center.
- NNRTIs frequently cause rash and other hypersensitivity reactions, which can be severe and even life threatening. If a severe reaction occurs, the NNRTI should be stopped immediately.
- Efavirenz is the only NNRTI recommended for first-line therapy of HIV infection.
- Efavirenz can cross the blood-brain barrier and frequently causes adverse CNS effects.
- Efavirenz is teratogenic and must not be used during pregnancy.
- PIs (e.g., lopinavir/ritonavir) are among our most effective antiretroviral drugs.
- PIs bind to HIV protease and thereby prevent the enzyme from cleaving HIV polyproteins. As a result, enzymes and structural proteins of HIV remain nonfunctional, and hence the virus remains immature and noninfectious.
- All PIs pose a risk for hyperglycemia, new-onset diabetes, exacerbation of existing diabetes, fat redistribution, hyperlipidemia, bone loss, elevation of transaminase levels, and increased bleeding in patients with hemophilia.
- All PIs inhibit cytochrome P450 and can thereby decrease metabolism of other drugs, causing their levels to rise. Accordingly, patients should avoid drugs whose accumulation could lead to serious toxicity.
- Ritonavir—a PI that strongly inhibits *CYP3A4 and CYP2D6 enzymes*—is often combined with other PIs to raise their plasma levels and thereby boost antiviral effects.
- HIV integrase strand transfer inhibitors (INSTIs) prevent insertion of HIV-derived DNA into DNA of CD4 cells and thereby block HIV replication.
- Raltegravir, our first INSTI, can cause rare, though severe, hypersensitivity reactions, including Stevens-Johnson syndrome and toxic epidermal necrolysis, which can be fatal.
- Enfuvirtide, an HIV fusion inhibitor, binds with gp41 on the viral envelope and thereby blocks entry of HIV into CD4 T cells.
- Enfuvirtide is indicated for HIV infection that is resistant to other antiretroviral drugs.
- The major adverse effects of enfuvirtide are injection-site reactions, which develop in nearly all patients.

Continued

- Maraviroc—the first CCR5 antagonist—blocks HIV entry into CD4 cells. Effects are limited to HIV strains that are CCR5 tropic (i.e., strains that use the CCR5 co-receptor for cellular entry). Accordingly, before maraviroc is used, testing must confirm that the infecting strain is indeed CCR5 tropic.
- Treatment has five goals: (1) maximal and long-lasting suppression of viral load, (2) restoration and preservation of immune function, (3) improved quality of life (4) reduction of HIV-related morbidity and mortality, and (5) prevention of HIV transmission.
- Resistance to antiretroviral drugs is a major problem. To reduce emergence of resistance, these drugs should never be used alone. Rather, they should always be combined with at least one other antiretroviral drug, and preferably two or even three.
- The principal laboratory tests employed to monitor HIV infection and guide therapy are plasma HIV RNA (viral load) and CD4 T-cell counts. Plasma HIV RNA levels indicate the magnitude of HIV replication and predict the rate of CD4 T-cell destruction, whereas CD4 T-cell counts indicate how much damage the immune system has already suffered.
- Plasma HIV RNA is the best measurement for predicting clinical outcome: if HIV RNA is high, the prognosis is poor; if HIV RNA is low, the risk for disease progression and death is greatly reduced. Accordingly, the goal of antiretroviral therapy (ART) is to decrease plasma HIV RNA to levels that are undetectable (20 to 75 copies/mL, depending on the assay employed).
- Reducing plasma HIV RNA to undetectable levels does not mean that HIV has been eradicated. It means only that there is too little HIV to measure. Nonetheless, patients still harbor HIV and are still infectious. Accordingly, treatment should continue indefinitely, and patients should be warned to avoid behaviors that can transmit HIV to others.
- All patients with acute primary HIV disease or advanced (symptomatic) HIV disease should receive maximally effective ART.
- For patients with chronic asymptomatic HIV disease, ART is now recommended when the CD4 count drops below 500 cells/mm^3, rather than 350 cells/mm^3 as in the past. As a result, ART is now initiated earlier in the course of the infection.
- In general, the principles that guide ART in adults also apply to children.
- In general, the principles that guide ART in nonpregnant adults also apply during pregnancy. Put another way, women should receive optimal ART, regardless of their pregnancy status.
- Mother-to-child transmission of HIV occurs primarily during labor and delivery. The risk for transmission can be greatly reduced by (1) using ART during gestation to minimize maternal viral load, (2) giving IV zidovudine to the mother during labor and delivery, and (3) giving oral or IV zidovudine to the infant for 6 weeks following delivery.
- An important reason for changing an antiretroviral regimen is treatment failure, indicated by failure of plasma HIV RNA to drop to an undetectable level; a rebound in plasma HIV RNA after falling to an undetectable level; CD4 T-cell counts failing to rise (or continuing to decline); and progression of clinical disease despite antiretroviral treatment.
- When treatment failure is the result of drug resistance, the preferred response is to change *all* drugs in the regimen. Furthermore, the new drugs should be agents the patient has not taken before and that are not cross-resistant with drugs the patient has taken before.
- Sexual transmission of HIV can be reduced by (1) treating the HIV-infected partner with antiretroviral drugs and (2) giving an HIV-negative person antiretroviral drugs as pre-exposure prophylaxis (PrEP).
- Prophylactic drugs can reduce the risk for infection following accidental exposure to HIV (e.g., from a needle stick). Prophylaxis is most effective when initiated within 1 or 2 hours, and it may be ineffective if initiated after 72 hours.
- Because of declining CD4 T-cell counts, individuals with advanced HIV disease are at risk for opportunistic infections (OIs), and hence may need prophylactic antibiotics.
- By elevating CD4 T-cell counts, ART can restore immune function and can thereby reduce both the risk for OIs and the need for prophylactic antibiotics.
- Among people with AIDS, *Pneumocystis* pneumonia (PCP) is a potentially fatal OI.
- The preferred regimen for prophylaxis and treatment of PCP is trimethoprim plus sulfamethoxazole.
- Ganciclovir, valganciclovir, cidofovir, and foscarnet are the drugs of choice for cytomegalovirus retinitis, an OI.
- Candidiasis is one of the most common OIs among people infected with HIV. Antifungal drugs such as miconazole troches provide topical treatment for oral candidiasis. Systemic antifungal drugs are needed for esophageal candidiasis.

Please visit **http://evolve.elsevier.com/Lehne** for chapter-specific NCLEX® examination review questions.

Summary of Major Nursing Implications[a]

NUCLEOSIDE/NUCLEOTIDE REVERSE TRANSCRIPTASE INHIBITORS

Abacavir
Didanosine
Emtricitabine
Lamivudine
Stavudine
Tenofovir
Zidovudine

Preadministration Assessment

Therapeutic Goals

Treatment has five goals: (1) maximal and long-lasting suppression of viral load, (2) restoration and preservation of immune function, (3) improved quality of life (4) reduction of HIV-related morbidity and mortality, and (5) prevention of HIV transmission.

Baseline Data

All NRTIs. Assess the patient's clinical status and obtain a plasma HIV RNA level and CD4 T-cell count.

Zidovudine. Obtain a hemoglobin value and granulocyte count.

Abacavir. Screen for HLA-B*5701, which indicates abacavir hypersensitivity.

Identifying High-Risk Patients

Didanosine. The risk for pancreatitis is increased by a history of alcoholism or pancreatitis and by use of IV pentamidine.

Zidovudine. The risk for hematologic toxicity is increased by a low granulocyte count; low levels of hemoglobin, vitamin B_{12}, or folic acid; and concurrent use of drugs that are myelosuppressive, nephrotoxic, or toxic to circulating blood cells.

Implementation: Administration

Routes

All NRTIs. Oral.

Zidovudine. Oral and IV.

Administration

All NRTIs. **Instruct patients to adhere closely to the prescribed dosing schedule.**

Didanosine. **Instruct patients to take didanosine 30 minutes before meals or 2 hours after.**

Instruct patients using enteric-coated capsules to swallow them intact.

Instruct patients taking powdered didanosine to pour the contents of one packet into 4 ounces of water (not fruit juice or any other acid-containing beverage), stir the mixture until the drug dissolves (about 2 to 3 minutes), and then drink the solution immediately.

IV Zidovudine. Administer IV zidovudine slowly (over 1 hour). Do not mix the solution with biologic or colloidal fluids (e.g., blood products, protein solutions). Administer within 24 hours (if stored at room temperature) or within 48 hours (if stored under refrigeration).

Ongoing Evaluation and Interventions

Evaluating Therapeutic Effects

Plasma HIV RNA. Success is indicated by a reduction in plasma HIV RNA. With ART, plasma HIV RNA should decline to 10% of baseline within 2 to 8 weeks. After 16 to 20 weeks of treatment, plasma HIV RNA should reach its minimum. Ideally, the minimum will be undetectable with sensitive assays.

CD4 T-Cell Counts. As viral load decreases, CD4 T-cell counts may rise, indicating some restoration of immune function.

Minimizing Adverse Effects

Anemia and Neutropenia. *Zidovudine* can cause severe anemia and neutropenia. Determine hematologic status before treatment and at least every 4 weeks thereafter. In the event of severe anemia (hemoglobin below 7.5 gm/dL or down 25% from the pretreatment baseline) or severe neutropenia (granulocyte count below 750 cells/mL or down 50% from the pretreatment baseline), interrupt treatment until there is evidence of bone marrow recovery. If neutropenia and anemia are less severe, a reduction in dosage may be sufficient. Some patients may require multiple transfusions. Granulocyte colony-stimulating factors can be used to reverse neutropenia. Epoetin alfa (recombinant erythropoietin) can be given to reduce transfusion requirements in patients with anemia, provided endogenous erythropoietin levels are not already elevated.

Lactic Acidosis With Hepatic Steatosis. Potentially fatal lactic acidosis and hepatic steatosis can occur with *all NRTIs.* **Inform patients about symptoms—nausea, vomiting, abdominal pain, malaise, fatigue, anorexia, and hyperventilation—and instruct them to report these immediately.** Diagnosis is done by measuring lactate in arterial blood. If lactic acidosis is present, the NRTI should be discontinued.

Pancreatitis. *Didanosine* can cause potentially fatal pancreatitis. Monitor patients for signs of developing pancreatitis (elevated serum amylase in association with elevated serum triglycerides, decreased serum calcium, and nausea, vomiting, or abdominal pain). If evolving pancreatitis is diagnosed, didanosine should be withdrawn.

Peripheral Neuropathy. *Didanosine* and *stavudine* can cause painful peripheral neuropathy. **Inform patients about early signs of neuropathy (numbness, tingling, or pain in hands and feet), and instruct them to report these immediately.** Treat pain of severe neuropathy with opioid analgesics. Neuropathy may reverse if these drugs are withdrawn early.

Hypersensitivity Reactions. *Abacavir* can cause potentially fatal hypersensitivity reactions. Before using abacavir, screen for HLA-B*5701 (a genetic variant associated with abacavir hypersensitivity), and don't use the drug if the variant is detected.

Continued

Summary of Major Nursing Implications[a]—cont'd

Inform patients of symptoms of hypersensitivity—fever, rash, myalgia, arthralgia, nausea, vomiting, diarrhea, abdominal pain, pharyngitis, dyspnea, and cough—and instruct them to report these immediately. If a hypersensitivity reaction is diagnosed—or even strongly suspected—abacavir should be discontinued and never used again.

Exacerbation of Hepatitis. In patients co-infected with HBV, withdrawal of *emtricitabine, lamivudine,* or *tenofovir* may result in severe exacerbation of hepatitis. **Inform patients of this possibility.**

Myocardial Infarction. There has been concern that *abacavir* may cause MI. However, in 2011, the FDA analyzed 26 clinical trials and found no association between abacavir and MI.

HIV Transmission. Reduction of plasma HIV RNA may create a false sense of safety. Accordingly, **inform patients that even when HIV RNA is undetectable, they are still infectious, and hence should avoid behaviors that can transmit HIV.**

Minimizing Adverse Interactions

Zidovudine. Drugs that are myelosuppressive, nephrotoxic, or directly toxic to circulating blood cells can increase the risk for hematologic toxicity. Drugs of concern include ganciclovir, dapsone, pentamidine, pyrimethamine, trimethoprim/sulfamethoxazole, amphotericin B, flucytosine, vincristine, vinblastine, and doxorubicin.

Ribavirin and Allopurinol. Ribavirin and allopurinol can increase levels of the active form of *didanosine,* thereby posing a risk for toxicity. Avoid these combinations.

All NRTIs. Giving a combination of NRTIs to a pregnant patient may increase the risk for lactic acidosis and hepatic steatosis. Accordingly, it would seem prudent to avoid these combinations during pregnancy.

NON-NUCLEOSIDE REVERSE TRANSCRIPTASE INHIBITORS

Delavirdine
Efavirenz
Etravirine
Nevirapine
Rilpivirine

Preadministration Assessment

Therapeutic Goals

Treatment has five goals: (1) maximal and long-lasting suppression of viral load, (2) restoration and preservation of immune function, (3) improved quality of life (4) reduction of HIV-related morbidity and mortality, and (5) prevention of HIV transmission.

Baseline Data

Assess the patient's clinical status and obtain a plasma HIV RNA level, CD4 T-cell count, and liver function tests. Perform a pregnancy test before giving efavirenz.

Implementation: Administration

Route

Oral.

Administration

All NNRTIs. **Instruct patients to adhere closely to the prescribed dosing schedule.**

Delavirdine. **Inform patients that delavirdine may be taken with or without food. Inform patients who cannot swallow delavirdine tablets whole that they can mix the 100-mg tablets (but not the 200-mg tablets) with 3 or more ounces of water. Advise patients with achlorhydria to take delavirdine with an acidic beverage, such as orange or cranberry juice.**

Efavirenz. **Instruct patients to take efavirenz once daily on an empty stomach, preferably at bedtime (to reduce CNS effects).**

Etravirine. **Instruct patients to take etravirine twice daily after a meal.**

Nevirapine. **Inform patients that nevirapine may be taken with or without food, either once or twice daily, depending on the formulation.**

Rilpivirine. **Instruct patients to take rilpivirine once daily with food.**

Ongoing Evaluation and Interventions

Evaluating Therapeutic Effects

See information for NRTIs.

Minimizing Adverse Effects

Rash and Other Hypersensitivity Reactions. Rash is common and may range from mild to severe. Rarely, rash evolves into a life-threatening reaction: Stevens-Johnson syndrome, toxic epidermal necrolysis, or erythema multiforme. Mild rash can be treated with an antihistamine or topical glucocorticoid. If a severe reaction develops, the NNRTI should be withdrawn immediately. **Inform patients about signs and symptoms of an evolving reaction—severe rash, or rash accompanied by fever, malaise, fatigue, blisters, oral lesions, conjunctivitis, facial edema, hepatitis, muscle aches, or joint aches—and instruct them to report these immediately.** To minimize risk, use a low dosage for the first 14 days of treatment, and then increase the dosage if rash has not occurred.

Hepatotoxicity. NNRTIs can cause hepatotoxicity, which may be severe. Risk is greatest with nevirapine. Perform liver function tests at baseline and periodically thereafter. Interrupt treatment if tests indicate significant liver injury.

CNS Symptoms. *Efavirenz* frequently causes CNS symptoms (e.g., dizziness, insomnia, impaired consciousness, drowsiness, vivid dreams, nightmares). **Inform patients that symptoms typically resolve in 2 to 4 weeks, despite ongoing efavirenz use, and that taking efavirenz at bedtime can minimize CNS effects.** If severe symptoms occur (e.g., delusions, hallucinations, severe acute depression), efavirenz should be withdrawn.

Summary of Major Nursing Implications[a]—cont'd

Depression. *Rilpivirine* can cause depression. **Instruct patients to contact their provider immediately if they start feeling sad, hopeless, or suicidal.**

Birth Defects. *Efavirenz* is teratogenic. **Inform women about the potential for fetal harm, and instruct them to use a barrier method of birth control (e.g., condom) in conjunction with a hormonal method (e.g., oral contraceptive).** Perform a pregnancy test before treatment.

HIV Transmission. Reduction of plasma HIV RNA may create a false sense of safety. Accordingly, **inform patients that even when HIV RNA is undetectable, they are still infectious, and hence must avoid behaviors that can transmit HIV.**

Minimizing Adverse Interactions

Nevirapine. Nevirapine *induces* cytochrome P450 and can thereby decrease levels of other drugs. Effects on protease inhibitors, hormonal contraceptives, and methadone are of particular concern.

Combining nevirapine with *St. John's wort* or *rifampin,* which also induce P450, can decrease nevirapine levels, and hence these combinations should be avoided.

Delavirdine. Delavirdine *inhibits* P450, and can thereby increase levels of other drugs. To avoid toxicity from excessive drug levels, patients must not take cisapride, alprazolam, midazolam, triazolam, lovastatin, or simvastatin—or astemizole or terfenadine, which are no longer available in the United States. In addition, the following drugs should be used with caution: indinavir, saquinavir, clarithromycin, dapsone, warfarin, quinidine, ergot alkaloids, phosphodiesterase type 5 inhibitors (e.g., sildenafil [Viagra]), and the dihydropyridine-type calcium channel blockers.

Antacids, histamine$_2$-receptor blockers, proton pump inhibitors, and *buffered formulations of didanosine* can decrease absorption of delavirdine.

Efavirenz. Efavirenz *competes with other drugs for metabolism by P450* and can thereby increase their levels. To avoid toxicity from excessive drug levels, the patient must not take astemizole, terfenadine, cisapride, midazolam, triazolam, dihydroergotamine, or ergotamine.

Efavirenz *induces P450* and can thereby accelerate metabolism of other drugs, including two PIs: *saquinavir* and *indinavir.* Avoid combined use with saquinavir. Increase indinavir dosage.

By inducing P450, efavirenz can decrease the efficacy of *hormonal contraceptives.* Contraceptive failure can result. **Instruct patients of childbearing potential to use a barrier contraceptive in addition to any hormonal contraceptive.**

St. John's wort induces P450 and can reduce levels of efavirenz. The combination should not be used.

Etravirine. Etravirine competes with other drugs for metabolism by P450 and can thereby increase their levels.

The plasma concentration of etravirine is lowered by the use of St. John's wort, anticonvulsants, darunavir/ritonavir, systemic dexamethasone, rifampin, rifapentine, ritonavir, saquinavir/ritonavir, and tipranavir/ritonavir.

Rilpivirine. All of the following drugs significantly *reduce* rilpivirine levels and hence are *contraindicated:* (1) antiseizure drugs (carbamazepine, oxcarbazepine, phenobarbital, phenytoin); (2) rifamycins (rifabutin, rifampin, rifapentine); (3) proton pump inhibitors (esomeprazole, lansoprazole, omeprazole, pantoprazole, rabeprazole); (4) glucocorticoids (when given in repeated doses); and (5) St. John's wort.

Antacids (e.g., aluminum hydroxide, magnesium hydroxide, calcium carbonate) can reduce rilpivirine levels. **Advise patients to take antacids at least 2 hours before rilpivirine or 4 hours after.**

Histamine$_2$-receptor blockers (e.g., cimetidine, famotidine, ranitidine) can reduce rilpivirine levels. **Advise patients to take histamine$_2$ blockers at least 12 hours before rilpivirine or 4 hours after.**

Azole antifungal drugs (e.g., ketoconazole, itraconazole, fluconazole) and macrolide antibiotics (e.g., erythromycin, clarithromycin, troleandomycin) can increase rilpivirine levels. Use with caution.

PROTEASE INHIBITORS

Atazanavir
Darunavir
Fosamprenavir
Indinavir
Lopinavir/Ritonavir
Nelfinavir
Ritonavir
Saquinavir
Tipranavir

Preadministration Assessment

Therapeutic Goals

Treatment has five goals: (1) maximal and long-lasting suppression of viral load, (2) restoration and preservation of immune function, (3) improved quality of life (4) reduction of HIV-related morbidity and mortality, and (5) prevention of HIV transmission.

Baseline Data

Assess the patient's clinical status and obtain a plasma HIV RNA level and CD4 T-cell count. Measure serum transaminases and blood glucose.

Identifying High-Risk Patients

Lopinavir/ritonavir oral solution is contraindicated for full-term infants (until 14 days after birth) and preterm infants (until 14 days after their predicted due date).

Use *atazanavir, saquinavir,* and *lopinavir/ritonavir* with caution in patients with structural heart disease, cardiac conduction disturbances, and ischemic heart disease, and in those taking other drugs that prolong the PR interval.

Avoid *lopinavir/ritonavir* and *saquinavir* in patients with congenital long QT syndrome, and in those taking drugs that prolong the QT interval.

Continued

Summary of Major Nursing Implications[a]—cont'd

Implementation: Administration

Route

All protease inhibitors are taken orally.

Administration and Storage

All Protease Inhibitors. **Instruct patients to adhere closely to the prescribed dosing schedule.**

Atazanavir. **Instruct patients to take atazanavir with food and to store it at room temperature.**

Darunavir. **Inform patients that darunavir must be boosted with ritonavir. Instruct patients to take darunavir with food and to store it at room temperature.**

Fosamprenavir. **Instruct patients to take fosamprenavir suspension without food and to take fosamprenavir tablets without food or with food. Instruct patients to store the drug at room temperature.**

Indinavir. **Instruct patients to administer indinavir either (1) with water but on an empty stomach (i.e., 1 hour before a meal or 2 hours after) or (2) with skim milk, juice, tea, or a low-fat meal (e.g., corn flakes with skim milk and sugar), but not with a large meal. Inform patients using indinavir boosted with ritonavir that they can take the drug with or without food. Instruct patients to store indinavir at room temperature in the package supplied by the manufacturer.**

Lopinavir/Ritonavir. **Advise patients using lopinavir/ritonavir tablets to take the drug with or without food, and to store it at room temperature.**

Instruct patients using lopinavir/ritonavir solution to take the drug with food and to store it at room temperature short term (up to 2 months) or under refrigeration long term.

Nelfinavir. **Instruct patients to take nelfinavir with food and to store it at room temperature. Instruct patients to mix the powder formulation with a small amount of water, milk, formula, soy formula, soy milk, or dietary supplement, but not with acidic foods or juices (e.g., applesauce, apple juice, orange juice).**

Ritonavir. **Instruct patients to take ritonavir tablets with food and to store them at room temperature.**

Instruct patients to take ritonavir capsules with food (if possible) and to store unopened bottles under refrigeration. Opened bottles may be kept at room temperature for 30 days.

Instruct patients to take the oral solution with food (if possible) and to store it at room temperature, never cold.

Saquinavir. **Inform patients that saquinavir must be boosted with ritonavir.**

Instruct patients to take saquinavir with a meal (or within 2 hours after a meal), and to store it at room temperature.

Tipranavir. **Inform patients that tipranavir must be boosted with ritonavir.**

Advise patients to take tipranavir with meals (when combined with ritonavir tablets) and to take tipranavir with or without food (when combined with ritonavir capsules or solution).

Advise patients to store tipranavir solution at room temperature, never cold, and to store unopened bottles of tipranavir capsules under refrigeration (opened bottles may be kept at room temperature for 60 days).

Ongoing Evaluation and Interventions

Evaluating Therapeutic Effects

See information for NRTIs.

Minimizing Adverse Effects

Hyperglycemia/Diabetes. All PIs can cause hyperglycemia and diabetes. **Instruct patients to report any symptoms (e.g., polydipsia, polyphagia, polyuria).** In patients with existing diabetes, monitor blood glucose closely. To detect new-onset diabetes, measure blood glucose at baseline, every 3 to 4 months during the first year of treatment, and less frequently thereafter. Diabetes can be treated with insulin and oral antidiabetic agents (e.g., metformin).

Fat Redistribution. **Forewarn patients that all PIs may cause accumulation of fat on the waist, stomach, breasts, and back of the neck, and loss of fat from the face, arms, buttocks, and legs.** Drug withdrawal may cause symptoms to resolve, but is not recommended. Injections of *Sculptra* can be used to compensate for loss of facial fat. Injection of tesamorelin [Egrifta] can reduce excess visceral abdominal fat.

Hyperlipidemia. All PIs can elevate cholesterol and triglycerides, thereby posing a risk for cardiovascular events and pancreatitis. Monitoring plasma cholesterol and triglycerides every 3 to 4 months may be wise. If drugs are given to lower lipid levels, two agents—lovastatin and simvastatin—should be avoided.

Increased Bleeding in Patients With Hemophilia. Protease inhibitors may increase the risk for bleeding in patients with hemophilia. Higher doses of coagulation factors may be needed.

Increased Transaminase Levels. Protease inhibitors can increase serum levels of transaminases. Exercise caution in patients with chronic liver disease (e.g., hepatitis B or C, cirrhosis). Measure serum transaminases before treatment and periodically thereafter.

Nephrolithiasis. *Indinavir* and *fosamprenavir* can cause nephrolithiasis. **Instruct patients to report symptoms: pain in the abdomen, groin, testicles, or side of the back.** Management consists of hydration and interruption or discontinuation of the PI. **To decrease the risk for nephrolithiasis, instruct patients to consume at least 48 ounces (1.5 L) of water daily.**

Bone Loss. Protease inhibitors may promote bone loss. **To reduce risk, encourage patients to ensure adequate intake of calcium and vitamin D.** Osteoporosis can be treated with bisphosphonates, raloxifene, calcitonin, teriparatide, or denosumab.

Diarrhea. *Nelfinavir* causes diarrhea in 20% to 32% of patients. Diarrhea can usually be managed with loperamide or some other over-the-counter antidiarrheal drug.

Cardiac Effects. *Atazanavir, saquinavir,* and *lopinavir/ritonavir* prolong the PR interval and can thereby promote AV block. Use with caution in patients with structural heart disease, cardiac conduction disturbances, and ischemic heart

Summary of Major Nursing Implications[a]—cont'd

disease, and in those taking other drugs that prolong the PR interval.

Lopinavir/ritonavir and *saquinavir* prolong the QT interval and thereby pose a risk for torsades de pointes. Avoid these drugs in patients with congenital long QT syndrome and in those taking other drugs that prolong the QT interval.

Toxicity in Newborns. *Lopinavir/ritonavir oral solution* can be lethal to newborns, owing to its propylene glycol content. Accordingly, the oral solution should be avoided in full-term infants (for the first 14 days after birth) and in preterm infants (until 14 days after their predicted due date).

Indirect Hyperbilirubinemia. *Atazanavir* and *indinavir* can raise plasma levels of unconjugated bilirubin (indirect bilirubin). Be alert for jaundice (yellowing of the skin) and icterus (yellowing of the eyes), which reverse upon drug withdrawal.

HIV Transmission. Reduction of plasma HIV RNA may create a false sense of safety. Accordingly, **inform patients that, even when HIV RNA is undetectable, they may still be infectious, and so should avoid behaviors that can transmit HIV.**

Minimizing Adverse Interactions

Interactions Resulting From Inhibition of P450. All PIs inhibit cytochrome P450 enzymes and can thereby increase levels of other drugs. To avoid serious toxicity from excessive drug levels, patients must not take *cisapride, alprazolam, triazolam, midazolam, ergot alkaloids, lovastatin,* or *simvastatin*—or *astemizole* or *terfenadine,* which are no longer available in the United States.

Ritonavir Boosting. Because ritonavir is a powerful inhibitor of CYP3A4 and CYP2D6 enzymes, the enzymes most responsible for metabolizing PIs, ritonavir is often combined with other PIs to raise their blood levels, and thereby boost antiviral effects.

Didanosine. Buffered formulations of didanosine decrease absorption of *indinavir* and *ritonavir.* Accordingly, buffered didanosine should be administered 1 or 2 hours apart from these drugs.

Rifampin. Rifampin induces P450 and can thereby reduce levels of the PIs. Concurrent use with all PIs should be avoided.

Oral Contraceptives. *Fosamprenavir, lopinavir/ritonavir, nelfinavir, ritonavir,* and *tipranavir/ritonavir* can reduce levels of ethinyl estradiol, a component of many oral contraceptives. **Advise patients to use an alternative form of birth control.**

ENFUVIRTIDE, AN HIV FUSION INHIBITOR

Preadministration Assessment

Therapeutic Goals

Enfuvirtide is indicated for HIV infection that is resistant to traditional antiretroviral drugs.

Treatment has five goals: (1) maximal and long-lasting suppression of viral load, (2) restoration and preservation of immune function, (3) improved quality of life (4) reduction of HIV-related morbidity and mortality, and (5) prevention of HIV transmission.

Baseline Data

Assess the patient's clinical status, and obtain a plasma HIV RNA level and CD4 T-cell count.

Identifying High-Risk Patients

Use enfuvirtide with *caution* in patients who have pneumonia risk factors: low initial CD4 cell counts, high initial viral load, IV drug use, smoking, and a history of lung disease.

Implementation: Administration

Route

Subcutaneous.

Preparation and Storage

Teach patients to reconstitute powdered enfuvirtide with 1.1 mL of sterile water for injection, and advise them to either (1) inject the solution immediately or (2) store it cold (2°C to 8°C; 36°F to 46°F) for up to 24 hours. Inform patients that powdered enfuvirtide may be stored at room temperature.

Administration

Educate patients on aseptic subQ injection technique, and instruct them to

- **Make injections into the upper arm, thigh, or abdomen (but not the navel)**
- **Rotate the injection site**
- **Avoid sites where there is an ongoing injection-site reaction or tissue that is scarred or bruised**

Instruct patients that before using stored enfuvirtide solution, they should bring it to room temperature and make sure that it is clear, colorless, and free of bubbles and particulate matter.

Ongoing Evaluation and Interventions

Evaluating Therapeutic Effects

See information for NRTIs.

Minimizing Adverse Effects

Injection-Site Reactions. **Inform patients about manifestations of ISRs—pain, tenderness, erythema, induration, nodules, cysts, pruritus, and ecchymosis—and forewarn them that these occur in nearly everyone taking enfuvirtide. Inform patients that they can reduce the risk for a severe ISR by rotating the injection site, avoiding sites with an active ISR, and avoiding unnecessarily deep injections. Instruct patients to seek immediate medical attention if a severe ISR occurs or if local infection develops.**

Pneumonia. Enfuvirtide may increase the risk for bacterial pneumonia. **Inform patients about signs of pneumonia—cough, fever, and breathing difficulties—and instruct them to report these immediately.** Use enfuvirtide with caution in patients who have pneumonia risk factors.

Hypersensitivity Reactions. Enfuvirtide may cause hypersensitivity reactions, manifesting as rash, fever, nausea, vomiting, chills, rigors, hypotension, or elevated serum transaminases, or possibly as respiratory distress,

Continued

Summary of Major Nursing Implications[a]—cont'd

glomerulonephritis, Guillain-Barré syndrome, or primary immune complex reaction. **Inform patients about signs of hypersensitivity, and advise them to report them immediately.** If a systemic hypersensitivity reaction occurs, enfuvirtide should be discontinued and never used again.

HIV Transmission. Reduction of plasma HIV RNA may create a false sense of safety. Accordingly, **inform patients that even when HIV RNA is undetectable, they are still infectious, and hence must avoid behaviors that can transmit HIV.**

MARAVIROC, A CCR5 ANTAGONIST

Preadministration Assessment

Therapeutic Goals

Maraviroc, in combination with other antiretroviral drugs, is indicated for treating patients age 16 years and older who are infected with CCR5-tropic HIV-1 strains.

Treatment has five goals: (1) maximal and long-lasting suppression of viral load, (2) restoration and preservation of immune function, (3) improved quality of life (4) reduction of HIV-related morbidity and mortality, and (5) prevention of HIV transmission.

Baseline Data

Assess the patient's clinical status, and obtain the following laboratory data: HIV RNA level, CD4 T-cell count, serum transaminases, and proof that the infecting HIV strain is CCR5 tropic.

Identifying High-Risk Patients

Patients with elevated liver function and cardiovascular disease must be monitored carefully.

Implementation: Administration

Route

Oral.

Administration

Inform patients that dosing may be done with or without food.

Advise patients that if they forget to take a dose, to take the missed dose as soon as possible, and take the next scheduled dose at its regular time. If the time to the next dose is less than 6 hours, the patient should skip the missed dose and take the next dose as scheduled.

Ongoing Evaluation and Interventions

Evaluating Therapeutic Effects

See information for NRTIs.

Minimizing Adverse Effects

Hepatotoxicity. Liver injury has been seen in some patients and may be preceded by evidence of an allergic reaction. **Inform patients about signs of an evolving reaction (itchy rash, yellow skin, dark urine, vomiting and/or abdominal pain), and instruct them to stop maraviroc and seek medical attention.**

Cardiovascular Events. During clinical trials, a few patients experienced cardiovascular events, including myocardial ischemia and MI. Exercise caution in patients with cardiovascular risk factors.

HIV Transmission. Reduction of plasma HIV RNA may create a false sense of safety. Accordingly, **inform patients that even when HIV RNA is undetectable, they are still infectious and must avoid behaviors that can transmit HIV.**

INTEGRASE STRAND TRANSFER INHIBITOR

Dolutegravir
Elvitegravir (in combination products)
Raltegravir

Preadministration Assessment

Therapeutic Goals

ISTIs are indicated for combined use with other antiretroviral drugs to treat adults infected with HIV-1.

Treatment has five goals: (1) maximal and long-lasting suppression of viral load, (2) restoration and preservation of immune function, (3) improved quality of life, (4) reduction of HIV-related morbidity and mortality, and (5) prevention of HIV transmission.

Baseline Data

Assess the patient's clinical status, and obtain a plasma HIV RNA level and CD4 T-cell count.

Implementation: Administration

Route

Oral.

Administration

Advise patients that dosing may be done with or without food.

Ongoing Evaluation and Interventions

Evaluating Therapeutic Effects

See information for NRTIs.

Minimizing Adverse Effects

Severe Hypersensitivity Reactions. ISTIs can cause potentially fatal hypersensitivity reactions, including Stevens-Johnson syndrome and toxic epidermal necrolysis. **Inform patients about signs of a hypersensitivity reaction (e.g., severe rash, or rash associated with blisters, fever, malaise, fatigue, oral lesions, facial edema, hepatitis, angioedema, or muscle or joint aches), and instruct them to discontinue raltegravir immediately.**

HIV Transmission. Reduction of plasma HIV RNA may create a false sense of safety. Accordingly, **inform patients that even when HIV RNA is undetectable, they may still be infectious. Until science conclusively determines that transmission cannot occur, it is important to avoid behaviors that can transmit HIV.**

[a]Patient education information is highlighted as **blue text.**

CHAPTER

95 Drug Therapy for Sexually Transmitted Infections

In October 2016, the Centers for Disease Control and Prevention released a report with a sobering heading: *Reported STDs at Unprecedented High in the U.S.* (see https://www.cdc.gov/nchhstp/newsroom/2016/std-surveillance-report-2015-press-release.html).

Sexually transmitted infections (STIs), also known as *sexually transmitted diseases (STDs),* are infectious diseases transmitted primarily through sexual contact. For the top three reportable STIs in 2015 there were 1,526,658 new cases of chlamydia (an increase of 5.9%), 395,216 new cases of gonorrhea (up 12.8%), and 23,872 new cases of primary and secondary (P&S) syphilis (up 19%). This is especially concerning, considering that not only had there been another dramatic increase the previous year (2.8% for chlamydia, 5.1% for gonorrhea, and 15.1% for syphilis), but also that many STIs are unreported, so actual numbers are likely much higher.

Our objective in this chapter is to describe the principal STIs and provide an overview of their treatment (Table 95.1). The basic pharmacology of these drugs is discussed in other chapters.

In 2015, the CDC updated its *Sexually Transmitted Diseases Treatment Guidelines.* The treatment recommendations presented in this chapter reflect those guidelines, which are available at http://www.cdc.gov/std/tg2015.

CHLAMYDIA TRACHOMATIS INFECTIONS

Characteristics

Chlamydia trachomatis is the most frequently reported bacterial STI (Fig. 95.1). The various strains of *Chlamydia* can cause genital tract infections, proctitis, conjunctivitis, and lymphogranuloma venereum (LGV), as well as ophthalmia and pneumonia in infants. Infection is frequently asymptomatic in women, and may also be asymptomatic in men. In women, untreated infection can cause pelvic inflammatory disease (PID), ectopic pregnancy, and infertility. The CDC estimates that chlamydial infections cause sterility in up to 50,000 women each year, primarily from fallopian tube scarring. Because infection is often asymptomatic in women and because sequelae can be serious, the CDC now recommends annual screening for all sexually active women 25 years or younger. Screening is also recommended for women older than 25 years who have a new sex partner, multiple partners, or a partner with a history of an STI.

Treatment

Adults and Adolescents

For uncomplicated urethral, cervical, or rectal infections in adults or adolescents, treatment with either *azithromycin* [Zithromax] or *doxycycline* [Vibramycin, others] is recommended. Patients who are unable to take these medications may take erythromycin, levofloxacin [Levaquin], or ofloxacin (generic). Table 95.1 provides a detailed summary of specific dosages of drugs used to treat chlamydia and other STIs.

Infection in Pregnancy

Azithromycin is the preferred treatment for *C. trachomatis* infection during pregnancy. Although doxycycline and other tetracyclines are active against *C. trachomatis,* these drugs are contraindicated because they can damage fetal teeth and bones. If the patient cannot take azithromycin, the approved alternatives are amoxicillin, erythromycin base, or erythromycin ethylsuccinate.

Infants

About half the infants born to women with cervical *C. trachomatis* acquire the infection during delivery, putting

TABLE 95.1 ■ Drug Therapy Recommendations for Sexually Transmitted Infections[a]

CHLAMYDIA TRACHOMATIS INFECTIONS
(CAUSATIVE ORGANISM: _CHLAMYDIA TRACHOMATIS_)

Adults and adolescents
- Azithromycin, 1 gm PO once
- *or*
- Doxycycline, 100 mg PO 2 times/day × 7 days

Children <45 kg
- Erythromycin base/ethylsuccinate, 12.5 mg/kg PO 4 times/day × 14 days

Children ≥45 kg but < 8 yr
- Azithromycin, 1 gm PO once

Children ≥8 yr
- Azithromycin, 1 gm PO once
- *or*
- Doxycycline, 100 mg PO 2 times/day × 7 days

Pregnant women
- Azithromycin, 1 gm PO once

Newborns: ophthalmia or pneumonia
- Erythromycin base/ethylsuccinate, 12.5 mg/kg PO 4 times/day × 14 days

Lymphogranuloma venereum
- Doxycycline, 100 mg PO 2 times/day × 21 days

GONOCOCCAL INFECTIONS (GONORRHEA)
(CAUSATIVE ORGANISM: _NEISSERIA GONORRHOEAE_)

Urethritis, cervicitis, proctitis
- Ceftriaxone, 250 mg IM once, *plus* azithromycin, 1 gm PO once

Pharyngitis
- Ceftriaxone, 250 mg IM once, *plus* azithromycin, 1 gm PO once

Disseminated gonococcal infection (DGI) in adults
- Ceftriaxone, 1 gm IM or IV every 24 hr, *plus* azithromycin, 1 gm PO once

DGI with meningitis
- Ceftriaxone, 1–2 gm IV every 12 hr × 10–14 days, *plus* azithromycin, 1 gm PO once

DGI with endocarditis
- Ceftriaxone, 1–2 gm IV every 12 hr × 28 days or more, *plus* azithromycin, 1 gm PO once

Conjunctivitis
- Ceftriaxone, 1 gm IM once, *plus* azithromycin 1 gm PO once

Ophthalmia neonatorum prophylaxis for neonates
- Erythromycin 0.5% ophthalmic ointment in each eye at birth

Neonates with ophthalmia neonatorum
- Ceftriaxone 25–50 mg/kg (not to exceed 125 mg) IM or IV once

Disseminated infection or scalp abscess
- Ceftriaxone, 25–50 mg/kg IM or IV once daily × 7 days (10–14 days if meningitis is present)
- *or*
- Cefotaxime, 25 mg/kg IM or IV every 12 hr × 7 days (10–14 days if meningitis is present)

Children with bacteremia or arthritis
- ≤45 kg: ceftriaxone, 50 mg/kg IM or IV once daily × 7 days, not to exceed 1 gm
- >45 kg: ceftriaxone 1 gm IM or IV once daily × 7 days

Children with vulvovaginitis, cervicitis, proctitis, pharyngitis, urethritis
- ≤45 kg: ceftriaxone 25–50 mg/kg (not to exceed 125 mg) IM or IV once
- >45 kg: same as adult

NONGONOCOCCAL URETHRITIS
(CAUSATIVE ORGANISMS: _CHLAMYDIA TRACHOMATIS, UREAPLASMA UREALYTICUM, TRICHOMONAS VAGINALIS, MYCOPLASMA GENITALIUM_)

Acute infection
- Azithromycin, 1 gm PO once
- *or*
- Doxycycline, 100 mg PO 2 times/day × 7 days

Recurrent/persistent infection
- Azithromycin, 1 gm PO once if original treatment was with doxycycline
- Moxifloxacin 400 mg PO daily × 7 days if original treatment was azithromycin
- Metronidazole (2 gm PO once)
- *or*
- Tinidazole (2 gm PO once) in areas where *Trichomonas* outbreaks are common

PELVIC INFLAMMATORY DISEASE
(CAUSATIVE ORGANISMS: _NEISSERIA GONORRHOEAE, CHLAMYDIA TRACHOMATIS,_ OTHERS)

Inpatients
- Doxycycline (100 mg IV or PO every 12 hr), *plus* either cefoxitin (2 gm IV every 6 hr) or cefotetan (2 gm IV every 12 hr)
- *or*
- Clindamycin (900 mg IV every 8 hr), *plus* gentamicin (3–5 mg/kg IM or IV once or 2 mg/kg IM or IV once then 1.5 mg/kg every 8 hr)

Outpatients
- Doxycycline (100 mg PO 2 times/day × 14 days), *plus* either cefoxitin (2 gm IM once, boosted with probenecid 1 gm PO once) or ceftriaxone (250 mg IM once), *with or without* metronidazole (500 mg PO 2 times/day × 14 days)

SEXUALLY ACQUIRED EPIDIDYMITIS
(CAUSATIVE ORGANISMS: _CHLAMYDIA TRACHOMATIS, NEISSERIA GONORRHOEAE,_ ENTERIC ORGANISMS)

Sexually acquired epididymitis without history of insertive anal sex
- Ceftriaxone (250 mg IM once) *plus* doxycycline (100 mg PO 2 times/day × 10 days)

Sexually acquired epididymitis with history of insertive anal sex
- Ceftriaxone (250 mg IM once) *plus either* levofloxacin (500 mg PO daily × 10 days)
- *or*
- Ofloxacin (300 mg PO 2 times/day × 10 days)

SYPHILIS
(CAUSATIVE ORGANISM: _TREPONEMA PALLIDUM_)

Primary syphilis, secondary syphilis, and early latent syphilis
- *Adults:* Benzathine penicillin G, 2.4 million units IM once
- *Children:* Benzathine penicillin G, 50,000 units/kg IM once (up to a max. of 2.4 million units)

Late latent syphilis or latent syphilis of unknown duration
- *Adults:* Benzathine penicillin G, 2.4 million units IM once/week for 3 weeks
- *Children:* Benzathine penicillin G, 50,000 units/kg IM once/week for 3 weeks (up to a max. of 7.2 million units over the course of treatment)

Tertiary syphilis
- Benzathine penicillin G, 2.4 million units IM once/week for 3 weeks (must rule out CNS involvement)

Neurosyphilis
- Aqueous crystalline penicillin G, 18–24 million units IV daily for 10–14 days, administered by continuous infusion or in separate doses of 3–4 million units each every 4 hr

Congenital syphilis
- Aqueous crystalline penicillin G, 50,000 units/kg IV every 12 hr for the first 7 days of life, followed by 50,000 units/kg every 8 hr for the next 3 days
- *or*
- Procaine penicillin G, 50,000 units/kg IM once daily for 10 days

TABLE 95.1 ▪ Drug Therapy Recommendations for Sexually Transmitted Infections[a]—cont'd

ACQUIRED IMMUNODEFICIENCY SYNDROME (AIDS) (CAUSATIVE ORGANISM: HUMAN IMMUNODEFICIENCY VIRUS) See Chapter 94 **BACTERIAL VAGINOSIS (CAUSATIVE ORGANISMS: *GARDNERELLA VAGINALIS, MYCOPLASMA HOMINIS,* VARIOUS ANAEROBES)** Metronidazole, 500 mg PO 2 times/day × 7 days *or* Metronidazole gel (0.75%), 1 full applicator (5 gm) intravaginally once/day × 5 days *or* Clindamycin cream (2%), 1 full applicator (5 gm) intravaginally at bedtime × 7 days **TRICHOMONIASIS (CAUSATIVE ORGANISM: *TRICHOMONAS VAGINALIS*)** Metronidazole, 2 gm PO once *or* Tinidazole, 2 gm PO once **CHANCROID (CAUSATIVE ORGANISM: *HAEMOPHILUS DUCREYI*)** Azithromycin, 1 gm PO once *or* Ceftriaxone, 250 mg IM once *or* Ciprofloxacin, 500 mg PO 2 times/day × 3 days *or* Erythromycin base, 500 mg PO 3 times/day × 7 days **PROCTITIS (CAUSATIVE ORGANISMS: *CHLAMYDIA TRACHOMATIS, NEISSERIA GONORRHOEAE, TREPONEMA PALLIDUM,* HERPES SIMPLEX VIRUS)** Ceftriaxone (250 mg IM once) *plus* doxycycline (100 mg PO 2 times/day × 7 days) **VENEREAL WARTS (CAUSATIVE ORGANISM: HUMAN PAPILLOMAVIRUS)** See Chapter 105	**GENITAL HERPES SIMPLEX VIRUS INFECTIONS (CAUSATIVE ORGANISM: HERPES SIMPLEX VIRUS)** First episode Acyclovir, 400 mg PO 3 times/day × 7–10 days (or longer) *or* Acyclovir, 200 mg PO 5 times/day × 7–10 days (or longer) *or* Famciclovir, 250 mg PO 3 times/day × 7–10 days (or longer) *or* Valacyclovir, 1 gm PO 2 times/day × 7–10 days (or longer) Severe infection Acyclovir, 5–10 mg/kg IV every 8 hr for 2–7 days or until clinical improvement, then PO acyclovir to complete at least 10 days Recurrent episodes Acyclovir, 800 mg PO 2 times/day × 5 days *or* Acyclovir, 800 mg PO 3 times/day × 2 days *or* Acyclovir, 400 mg PO 3 times/day × 5 days *or* Famciclovir, 125 mg PO 2 times/day × 5 days *or* Famciclovir, 1 gm 2 times/day × 1 day *or* Famciclovir, 500 mg once, followed by 200 mg 2 times/day for 2 days *or* Valacyclovir, 500 mg PO 2 times/day × 3 days *or* Valacyclovir, 1 gm PO once/day × 5 days Daily suppressive therapy Acyclovir, 400 mg PO 2 times/day *or* Famciclovir, 250 mg PO 2 times/day *or* Valacyclovir, 500 mg PO once/day *or* Valacyclovir, 1 gm PO once/day Neonatal herpes Acyclovir, 20 mg/kg IV every 8 hr × 14 days (for skin or mucous membrane infection) or × 21 days (for disseminated or CNS infection)

[a]Recommendations from Centers for Disease Control and Prevention: Sexually transmitted diseases treatment guidelines, 2015. *MMWR Morb Mortal Wkly Rep* 2016;64:1–137. Dosing for alternative regimens is available at https://www.cdc.gov/std/tg2015/2015-wall-chart.pdf.
CNS, Central nervous system.

them at risk for *pneumonia* and *conjunctivitis* (ophthalmia neonatorum). Pneumonia is generally not severe and lasts about 6 weeks. Conjunctivitis does not result in blindness and spontaneously resolves in 6 months. The preferred treatment for both infections is oral *erythromycin base* or *erythromycin ethylsuccinate.* Azithromycin suspension may be given as an alternative. Although topical erythromycin, tetracycline, or silver nitrate may be given to prevent conjunctivitis, these drugs are not completely effective—and they have no effect on neonatal pneumonia caused by *C. trachomatis.*

Preadolescent Children

Although infection in preadolescent children can result from perinatal transmission, sexual abuse is the more likely cause, especially in children older than 2 years. Because of the legal implications, diagnosis must be definitive. Treatment depends on the age and weight of the child. For children who weigh less than 45 kg, the preferred treatment is oral *erythromycin base* or *erythromycin ethylsuccinate.* For children who weigh 45 kg or more, but are less than 8 years of age, the preferred

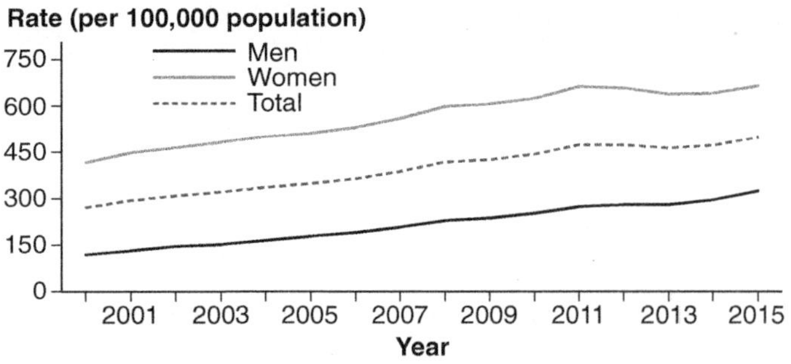

Fig. 95.1 ■ **Incidence of chlamydia: reported cases 2000–2015.** (Source: https://www.cdc.gov/std/stats15/figures/1.htm.)

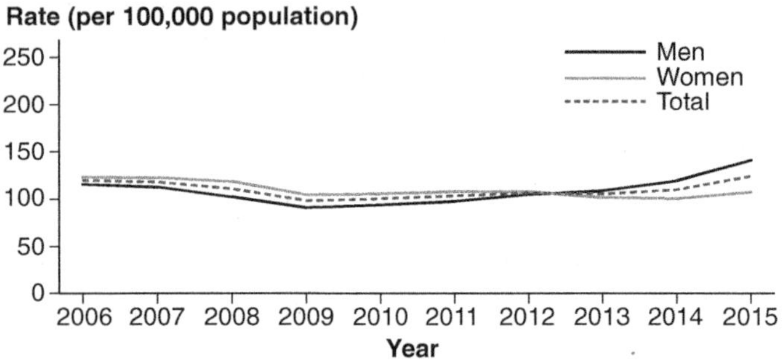

Fig. 95.2 ■ **Incidence of gonorrhea: reported cases 2006–2015.** (Source: https://www.cdc.gov/std/stats15/figures/13.htm.)

treatment is *azithromycin.* For children at least 8 years of age, the preferred treatments are *azithromycin* or *doxycycline*.

Lymphogranuloma Venereum

LGV is caused by a unique strain of *C. trachomatis.* Transmission is strictly by sexual contact. LGV is most common in tropical countries, but does occur in the United States, especially in the South. Infection begins as a small erosion or papule in the genital region. From this site, the organism migrates to regional lymph nodes, causing swelling, tenderness, and blockage of lymphatic flow. Tremendous enlargement of the genitalia may result. The enlarged nodes, called buboes, may break open and drain. The treatment of choice for genital, inguinal, and anorectal LGV is *doxycycline*. Erythromycin base serves as an alternative for those who cannot take tetracycline antibiotics.

GONOCOCCAL INFECTIONS

Characteristics

Gonorrhea is caused by *Neisseria gonorrhoeae,* a gram-negative diplococcus often referred to as the gonococcus. Gonorrhea is second only to chlamydia as our most common STI. Gonorrhea is transmitted almost exclusively by sexual contact (Fig. 95.2).

The intensity of symptoms differs between men and women. In men, the main symptoms are a burning sensation during urination and a pus-like discharge from the penis. In contrast, gonorrhea in women is often asymptomatic or may present as mild cervicitis. However, serious infection of female reproductive structures (vagina, urethra, cervix, ovaries, fallopian tubes) can occur, ultimately resulting in sterility. Among people who engage in oral sex, the mouth and throat can become infected, causing sore throat and tonsillitis. Among people who engage in receptive anal sex, the rectum can become infected, causing a purulent discharge and tenesmus, a constant urge to defecate even when the bowels are empty. Bacteremia can develop in males and females, causing cutaneous lesions, arthritis, and, rarely, meningitis and endocarditis.

Treatment

Owing to antibiotic resistance, treatment of gonorrhea has changed over the years—and undoubtedly will continue to evolve. In the 1930s, virtually all strains of the gonococcus were sensitive to sulfonamides. However, within a decade, sulfonamide resistance had become common. Fortunately, by that time penicillin had become available, and the drug was active against all gonococcal strains. However, in 1976, organisms resistant to penicillin began to emerge. More recently, resistance to fluoroquinolones has become common. As a result, in 2007 the CDC recommended against using fluoroquinolones for gonorrhea, leaving cephalosporins as the preferred treatments. This recommendation was changed yet again in 2012, also triggered by antimicrobial resistance. The CDC currently recommends dual treatment with ceftriaxone and azithromycin as the preferred treatment for gonorrhea.

Urethral, Cervical, and Rectal Infection

Because of increasing resistance to cephalosporins, preferred treatment now consists of a combination of two drugs: *ceftriaxone* (generic) given intramuscularly (IM) plus oral (PO) *azithromycin.* If a patient refuses IM therapy, PO cefixime (400 mg once) can be substituted for IM ceftriaxone; however, the CDC recommends not routinely substituting this drug because resistance to cefixime has been documented and is anticipated to increase.

If a patient is allergic to azithromycin, a 7-day course of doxycycline may be substituted. For patients with cephalosporin allergies, the options are not as clear. Although prescribing double the azithromycin dose as monotherapy will cure gonorrhea in most cases, the CDC does not recommend this because of treatment failures and rapid development of resistance. While acknowledging a lack of data for recommendation, the CDC suggests substituting gemifloxacin for the cephalosporin component, despite having recommended against using quinolones to treat gonorrhea. Spectinomycin, an aminoglycoside, has also been suggested; however, it is not currently available in the United States. For additional information on this dilemma, see http://www.cdc.gov/std/tg2015/gonorrhea.htm.

Pharyngeal Infection

Gonococcal infection of the pharynx is more difficult to treat than infection of the urethra, cervix, or rectum; therefore, parenteral therapy is recommended for all patients. The preferred treatment is *ceftriaxone* combined with *azithromycin.*

Conjunctivitis

Gonococcal conjunctivitis can be reliably eradicated with *ceftriaxone* plus *azithromycin.* Treatment also includes washing the infected eye with saline solution once.

Disseminated Gonococcal Infection

Disseminated gonococcal infection (DGI) occurs secondary to gonococcal bacteremia. Symptoms include petechial or pustular skin lesions, arthritis, arthralgia, and tenosynovitis (inflammation of the tendon sheath). Endocarditis and meningitis occur rarely. Strains of *N. gonorrhoeae* that cause DGI are uncommon in the United States. In the absence of endocarditis or meningitis, treatment consists of IM or intravenous (IV) *ceftriaxone* plus *azithromycin.* For patients with endocarditis or meningitis, the preferred treatment is IV *ceftriaxone* plus *azithromycin.*

Neonatal Infection

Neonatal gonococcal infection is acquired through contact with infected cervical exudates during delivery. Infection can be limited to the eyes, or it may be disseminated.

Gonococcal *neonatal ophthalmia* is a serious infection. The initial symptom is conjunctivitis. Over time, other structures of the eye become involved. Blindness can result. The recommended therapy is a single dose of *ceftriaxone* given by either IM injection or IV infusion.

To protect against neonatal ophthalmia, a topical antibiotic should be instilled into both eyes immediately postpartum—as required by law in most states. According to the 2015 CDC guidelines, the only approved topical agent is *0.5% erythromycin* ophthalmic ointment. If this antimicrobial is not available, parenteral therapy with *ceftriaxone* should be used.

In neonates, DGI is rare. Possible manifestations include sepsis, arthritis, meningitis, and scalp abscesses. Either of two antibiotics is recommended for treatment: *ceftriaxone* or *cefotaxime*.

Preadolescent Children

Among preadolescent children, the most common cause of gonococcal infection is sexual abuse. Vaginal, anorectal, and pharyngeal infections are most common. Because of legal implications, diagnosis must be definitive. Growing a specimen in culture is the preferred technique.

Treatment depends on the type of infection and the weight of the child. For children who have localized infection (vulvovaginitis, cervicitis, urethritis, pharyngitis, proctitis) and who weigh 45 kg or less, the preferred treatment is a single IM or IV dose of *ceftriaxone.* For children with localized infection who weigh more than 45 kg, treatment is the same as for adults. For children of any weight who have systemic infection (bacteremia, arthritis), the preferred treatment is *ceftriaxone,* IM or IV, daily for 7 days. Specific dosing is provided in Table 95.1.

NONGONOCOCCAL URETHRITIS

Nongonococcal urethritis (NGU) is defined as urethritis caused by any organism other than *N. gonorrhoeae,* the gonococcus. The most common infectious agent is *C. trachomatis* (15% to 55%). Other likely agents are *Ureaplasma urealyticum, Trichomonas vaginalis,* and *Mycoplasma genitalium.* NGU is diagnosed by the presence of polymorphonuclear leukocytes and a negative culture for *N. gonorrhoeae.* The infection is especially prevalent among sexually active adolescent girls. The recommended treatment is either *azithromycin* or *doxycycline.* Alternative regimens are *erythromycin base, erythromycin ethylsuccinate, levofloxacin,* or *ofloxacin.* For persistent or recurrent NGU, one of two drugs, *metronidazole* or *tinidazole,* is recommended if *T. vaginalis* transmission is a suspected cause.

PATIENT-CENTERED CARE ACROSS THE LIFE SPAN

Drugs for Sexually Transmitted Infections

Life Stage	Patient Care Concerns
Children	Some drugs used to treat sexually transmitted infections (STIs), such as doxycycline, are contraindicated for children. It is important to use regimens specifically indicated for children.
Pregnant women	Some drugs used to treat STIs (doxycycline, tinidazole, gentamicin) may cause congenital anomalies. Macrolides, penicillins, and cephalosporins are generally safe. It is important to use alternative regimens specifically designated for pregnant women when indicated (see Table 95.1).
Breast-feeding women	Tinidazole is contraindicated in breast-feeding women. When taken, breast-feeding should be withheld during treatment and for 3 days after treatment is completed. For women taking metronidazole, some providers advise avoidance of breast-feeding for 12 to 24 hours after treatment. Breast-feeding while taking doxycycline carries a theoretical risk for tooth discoloration; however, the World Health Organization (WHO) reports that a single dose will not be a risk. Macrolides (e.g., erythromycin, azithromycin), cephalosporins (e.g., ceftriaxone, cefotetan), and penicillins are considered safe for lactating women; however, the infants may develop diarrhea, modified bowel flora, and other side effects of the drugs.
Older adults	Adverse effects in older adults may be more severe, and recovery may be slower or complicated.

Azithromycin should be added to the regimen if it was not used during initial therapy. If the infection still fails to respond, the cause may be *M. genitalium.* Unfortunately, we have no easy tests for this bacterium, and hence definitive diagnosis may not be possible. Nonetheless, when *M. genitalium* is suspected, a trial with *moxifloxacin* [Avelox] may be warranted.

PELVIC INFLAMMATORY DISEASE

Acute PID is a syndrome that includes endometritis, pelvic peritonitis, tubo-ovarian abscess, and inflammation of the fallopian tubes. Infertility can result. Prominent symptoms are abdominal pain, vaginal discharge, and fever. Most frequently, PID is caused by *N. gonorrhoeae, C. trachomatis,* or both. However, *Mycoplasma hominis,* as well as assorted anaerobic and facultative bacteria, may also be present. In recent years, women in the United States have experienced an almost 40% decrease in PID despite the increase in diseases that cause this condition. This may be attributable to intensified patient education efforts, increased and improved screening practices, and improved adherence to single-dose treatment.

Because multiple organisms are likely to be involved, drug therapy must provide broad coverage. Because no single drug can do this, combination therapy is required. For the *hospitalized patient,* treatment can be initiated with either IV *cefoxitin* or IV *cefotetan* combined with IV *doxycycline*. After symptoms resolve, IV therapy can be discontinued—but must be followed by oral *doxycycline* to complete a 14-day course of treatment. An alternative recommended regimen consists of IV *clindamycin* plus IV or IM *gentamicin.*

Outpatients can be treated with either IM *ceftriaxone* or IM *cefoxitin* as a single dose boosted with oral probenecid. Treatment should also include *doxycycline*, with or without *metronidazole*. Because PID can be difficult to treat and because the consequences of failure can be severe (e.g., sterility), many experts recommend that *all* patients receive IV antibiotics in a hospital.

ACUTE EPIDIDYMITIS

Epididymitis may be acquired by sexual contact or nonsexually. Sexually acquired epididymitis is usually caused by *N. gonorrhoeae, C. trachomatis,* or both. The syndrome occurs primarily in young adults (younger 35 years of age) and may be associated with urethritis. Primary symptoms are fever accompanied by pain in the back of the testicles that develops over the course of several hours. For patients with gonococcal or chlamydial infection, the recommended treatment is *ceftriaxone* plus *doxycycline*. For patients who engage in insertive anal sex, the addition of *levofloxacin* or *ofloxacin* is recommended to target enteric bacteria. Testicular pain can be managed with analgesics, bed rest, and ice packs.

Non–sexually transmitted epididymitis generally occurs in older men and in men who have had urinary tract instrumentation. Causative organisms are gram-negative enteric bacilli and *Pseudomonas* species. *Ofloxacin* can be used for treatment.

SYPHILIS

Syphilis is caused by the spirochete *Treponema pallidum.* In the United States, the incidence of P&S syphilis has risen steadily since 2000 (Fig. 95.3). Fortunately, *T. pallidum* has remained highly responsive to penicillin, the treatment of choice.

Characteristics

Syphilis develops in three stages, termed *primary, secondary,* and *tertiary. T. pallidum* enters the body by penetrating the mucous membranes of the mouth, vagina, or urethra of the penis. After an incubation period of 1 to 4 weeks, a primary lesion, called a chancre, develops at the site of entry. The chancre is a hard, red, protruding, painless sore. Nearby lymph nodes may become swollen. Within a few weeks the chancre heals spontaneously, although *T. pallidum* is still present. In clinical practice, chancres are rarely seen, especially in females.

Two to 6 weeks after the chancre heals, secondary syphilis develops. Symptoms result from the spread of *T. pallidum* through the bloodstream. Skin lesions and flu-like symptoms (fever, headache, reduced appetite, general malaise) are typical.

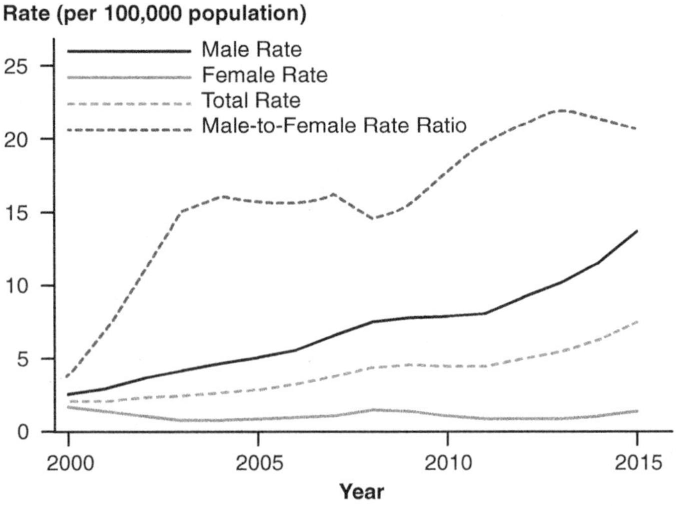

Fig. 95.3 ■ Incidence of primary and secondary syphilis: reported cases 2000–2015.
(Adapted from CDC (2016). Primary and Secondary Syphilis—Rates of Reported Cases by Sex and Male-to-Female Rate Ratios, United States, 1990–2015. Available at https://www.cdc.gov/std/stats15/figures/32.htm.)

Enlarged lymph nodes and joint pain may also be present. The symptoms of secondary syphilis resolve in 4 to 8 weeks—but may recur episodically over the next 3 to 4 years.

Tertiary syphilis develops 5 to 40 years after the initial infection. Almost any organ can be involved. Infection of the brain—neurosyphilis—is common, and can cause senility, paralysis, and severe psychiatric symptoms. The heart valves and aorta can be damaged. Lesions can also occur in the skin, bones, joints, and eyes. The risk for neurosyphilis is increased in individuals with HIV infection.

Infants exposed to *T. pallidum in utero* can be born with syphilis. Early signs of congenital syphilis include sores, rhinitis, and severe tenderness over bones.

Treatment

Penicillin G is the drug of choice for all stages of syphilis. The form and dosage of penicillin G depend on the disease stage. *Early syphilis* (primary, secondary, or latent syphilis of less than 1 year's duration) is treated with a single IM dose of benzathine penicillin G. *Late latent syphilis* (more than 1 year's duration) and tertiary syphilis are also treated with IM benzathine penicillin G. However, instead of receiving a single dose, adults and children receive three doses 1 week apart. *Neurosyphilis* requires more aggressive therapy. The recommended treatment is IV penicillin G daily for 10 to 14 days, administered either by continuous infusion or by intermittent therapy every 4 hours. For *congenital syphilis,* treatment options are either IV penicillin G or IM procaine penicillin G. *Syphilis in pregnancy* should be treated with penicillin G, using a dosage appropriate to the stage of the disease.

How should patients with *penicillin allergy* be treated? For *nonpregnant* patients with early or late syphilis, either *doxycycline* or *tetracycline* may be used. For patients with *neurosyphilis,* ceftriaxone can be effective, but possible cross-reactivity with penicillin is a concern. If the patient is a child or pregnant woman, the CDC recommends a penicillin-allergy desensitization protocol to permit penicillin use, rather than substituting another drug for penicillin.

ACQUIRED IMMUNODEFICIENCY SYNDROME

AIDS is caused by the human immunodeficiency virus (HIV), which is discussed in Chapter 94.

BACTERIAL VAGINOSIS

Bacterial vaginosis (BV) is a common vaginal infection in women of childbearing age. The condition results from an alteration in vaginal microflora. Organisms responsible for the syndrome include *Gardnerella vaginalis* (also known as *Haemophilus vaginalis*), *Mycoplasma hominis,* and various anaerobes. The syndrome occurs most commonly in sexually active women, although it may be transmitted in other ways. BV is characterized by a malodorous vaginal discharge, elevation of vaginal pH (above 4.5), and generation of a fishy odor when vaginal secretions are mixed with 10% potassium hydroxide. Clue cells (epithelial cells whose borders are obscured by bacteria) are typically found on microscopic examination of vaginal secretions.

The recommended therapy for BV is either oral or vaginal *metronidazole* or vaginal *clindamycin* cream. Clindamycin cream is available as a *short-acting 2% clindamycin cream* [Cleocin] and a *long-acting 2% clindamycin cream* [Clindesse]. Clindesse cream is formulated to adhere to the vaginal mucosa for several days, and hence can clear bacterial vaginosis with just one application. Approved alternative regimens are *tinidazole, oral clindamycin,* or *clindamycin ovules* (intravaginal suppositories). Unlike the other drugs approved for BV, tinidazole should not be prescribed for pregnant women.

TRICHOMONIASIS

Trichomoniasis, caused by *T. vaginalis,* is the most common nonviral STI in the United States. In men, infection is usually asymptomatic. In women, infection may be asymptomatic or may cause a diffuse, malodorous, yellow-green vaginal discharge, along with burning and itching. The rapid movement of *T. vaginalis* protozoa is notable on microscopic examination of vaginal secretions. Most infections can be eliminated with a single oral dose of either *metronidazole* or *tinidazole.* Dosing can be repeated in the event of treatment failure. Male partners of infected women should always be treated, even if asymptomatic. Although some clinicians remain concerned about giving metronidazole during pregnancy, there is no evidence that the drug causes congenital anomalies in humans. Tinidazole, on the other hand, should not be prescribed for pregnant women.

CHANCROID

Chancroid, also known as soft chancre, is one of the few STIs for which prevalence has declined both in the United States and worldwide. It is caused by *Haemophilus ducreyi.* Transmission is primarily by sexual contact. The infection is characterized by a painful, ragged ulcer at the site of inoculation, usually the external genitalia. Regional lymph nodes may be swollen. Multiple secondary lesions may develop. There are four antibiotics recommended for treatment: (1) *azithromycin,* (2) *ceftriaxone,* (3) *ciprofloxacin* [Cipro], and (4) *erythromycin base.*

HERPES SIMPLEX VIRUS INFECTIONS

Characteristics

Most genital herpes infections are caused by herpes simplex virus type 2 (HSV-2). However, an increasing number of anogenital infections are caused by HSV-1, the herpesvirus that causes cold sores. In the United States, the infection has reached epidemic proportions. More than 50 million people are affected.

Symptoms of primary infection develop 6 to 8 days after contact. Some people with HSV infection are asymptomatic or have relatively mild symptoms; however, for others there is a common presentation. In females, blisters or vesicles can appear on the perianal skin, labia, vagina, cervix, and foreskin of the clitoris. In males, vesicles develop on the penis and occasionally on the testicles. Painful urination and a watery discharge can occur in both sexes. Also, the patient may experience systemic symptoms: fever, headache, myalgia, and tender, swollen lymph nodes in the affected region. Within days, the original blisters can evolve into large, painful, ulcer-like sores. Over the next 2 to 3 weeks, all symptoms resolve spontaneously. However, this does not indicate cure. The virus remains present in a latent state and can cause recurrence. Because available drugs can't eliminate the virus, there is no cure. Symptoms may recur for life; however, for some patients, subsequent episodes become progressively shorter and less severe, and in rare cases they may cease entirely.

Neonatal Infection

Genital herpes in pregnant women can be transmitted to the infant. Transmission can occur *in utero,* which is very rare, or during delivery. Infection acquired *in utero* can result in spontaneous abortion or fetal malformation. Infection acquired during delivery can cause blindness, severe neurologic damage, and even death. To protect the infant during delivery, birth should be accomplished by cesarean delivery if the mother has an active infection. Infants who acquire the infection should be treated with acyclovir.

Treatment

Genital herpes can be treated with three drugs: *acyclovir* [Zovirax], *famciclovir* [Famvir], and *valacyclovir* [Valtrex] at dosage regimens recommended in Table 95.1. Although these agents cannot eliminate the virus, they can reduce symptoms and shorten the duration of pain and viral shedding. Patients with recurrent infections may take these drugs every day (suppressive therapy) or just when symptoms appear (episodic therapy). Continuous daily administration reduces the frequency and intensity of episodes, whereas episodic treatment simply reduces symptom intensity after an episode has begun.

Reduction of Transmission

Transmission of HSV can occur when symptoms are absent as well as when symptoms are present. *Valacyclovir* can decrease transmission of genital herpes by 50%. No other drug has been shown to reduce transmission of this STI, or any other STI for that matter. Valacyclovir only *reduces* transmission, it doesn't stop it entirely. Accordingly, patients must continue to use condoms. Because viral shedding is increased when the infection is active, it is advisable to abstain from sex during breakouts.

PROCTITIS

Sexually acquired proctitis (inflammation of the rectum) results primarily from receptive anal intercourse. Symptoms include anorectal pain, tenesmus (the sensation of needing to defecate even when the bowel is empty), and rectal discharge. Usual causative organisms are *N. gonorrhoeae, C. trachomatis, T. pallidum,* and HSV. The preferred treatment is *ceftriaxone* plus *doxycycline*.

VENEREAL WARTS

Genital and perianal warts are caused by human papillomaviruses (HPVs). Characteristics of these warts and their treatment are presented in Chapter 105. As discussed in Chapter 68, an HPV vaccine, sold as *Gardasil,* can protect against both venereal warts and cervical cancer. Another HPV vaccine, sold as *Cervarix,* protects against cervical cancer, but not against venereal warts.

MAKING SENSE OF TREATMENT

You have been learning antimicrobials by pharmacology category (which is the best way), but when individual drug names are used, as the CDC did in their guidelines, keeping things straight can be very challenging! To help with this, we have put together a chart that aligns treatment with drugs according to their pharmacologic categories (Table 95.2).

TABLE 95.2 ▪ Drug Categories Used in Treatment of Sexually Transmitted Infections

AMEBICIDE, ANTIPROTOZOAL, MISCELLANEOUS ANTIBIOTIC

Metronidazole

- Pelvic inflammatory disease, outpatient (with other drugs)
- Bacterial vaginosis
- Trichomoniasis
- Nongonococcal urethritis, resistant/persistent (in areas where *Trichomonas* outbreaks are common)

Tinidazole

- Nongonococcal urethritis, recurrent/persistent
- Trichomoniasis

AMINOGLYCOSIDE

Gentamicin

- Pelvic inflammatory disease, inpatient (with other drugs)

ANTIVIRALS

Acyclovir

- Genital herpes, first episode, severe, recurrent, suppressive
- Neonatal herpes

Famciclovir

- Genital herpes, first episode, recurrent, suppressive

Valacyclovir

- Genital herpes, first episode, recurrent, suppressive

CEPHALOSPORINS

Cefotetan

- Pelvic inflammatory disease, inpatient (with other drugs)

Cefoxitin

- Pelvic inflammatory disease, inpatient (with other drugs)
- Pelvic inflammatory disease, outpatient (with other drugs)

Ceftriaxone

- Gonorrhea in men: gonococcal urethritis, proctitis (with azithromycin)
- Gonorrhea in women: vulvovaginitis, cervicitis, urethritis (with azithromycin)
- Gonococcal pharyngitis (with azithromycin)
- Gonococcal conjunctivitis (with azithromycin)
- Disseminated gonococcal infection, all types (with azithromycin)
- Disseminated gonococcal infection or scalp abscess in neonates
- Ophthalmia neonatorum
- Gonococcal arthritis, bacteremia in children
- Pelvic inflammatory disease, outpatient (with other drugs)
- Sexually acquired epididymitis (with other drugs)
- Chancroid
- Proctitis

Cefotaxime

- Disseminated gonococcal infection or scalp abscess in neonates

LINCOSAMIDE

Clindamycin

- Pelvic inflammatory disease, inpatient (with other drugs)
- Bacterial vaginosis

MACROLIDES

Azithromycin

- Chlamydia (except for children weighing less than 45 kg)
- Chlamydia in pregnant women
- Gonorrhea in men: gonococcal urethritis, proctitis (with ceftriaxone)
- Gonorrhea in women: vulvovaginitis, cervicitis, urethritis (with ceftriaxone)
- Gonococcal pharyngitis (with ceftriaxone)
- Gonococcal conjunctivitis (with ceftriaxone)
- Disseminated gonococcal infection, all types (with ceftriaxone)
- Nongonococcal urethritis, acute
- Nongonococcal urethritis, recurrent/persistent (if original treatment was doxycycline)
- Chancroid

TABLE 95.2 ▪ Drug Categories Used in Treatment of Sexually Transmitted Infections—cont'd

Erythromycin

- Chlamydia in children weighing less than 45 kg (erythromycin base/ethylsuccinate)
- Newborn ophthalmia or pneumonia caused by *C. trachomatis* (erythromycin base/ethylsuccinate)
- Prophylaxis for newborn ophthalmia caused by *N. gonorrhoeae* (erythromycin 0.5% ophthalmic ointment)
- Chancroid (erythromycin base)

PENICILLINS

Penicillin G

- Syphilis, primary, secondary, tertiary, latent (benzathine penicillin G)
- Neurosyphilis (aqueous crystalline penicillin G)
- Congenital syphilis (aqueous crystalline penicillin G or procaine penicillin G)

QUINOLONE

Ciprofloxacin

- Chancroid

Moxifloxacin

- Nongonococcal urethritis, recurrent/persistent (if original treatment was azithromycin)

Levofloxacin

- Sexually acquired epididymitis with insertive anal sex (with ceftriaxone)

Ofloxacin

- Sexually acquired epididymitis with insertive anal sex (with ceftriaxone)

TETRACYCLINE

Doxycycline

- *C. trachomatis* infections in nonpregnant adults and children 8 years and older
- Lymphogranuloma venereum
- Nongonococcal urethritis, acute
- Pelvic inflammatory disease, inpatient and outpatient (with other drugs)
- Sexually acquired epididymitis without insertive anal sex (with ceftriaxone)
- Proctitis (with ceftriaxone)

KEY POINTS

- *Chlamydia trachomatis* is the most common bacterial cause of STIs.
- Two drugs—doxycycline and azithromycin—are preferred agents for treating chlamydial infection in nonpregnant adolescents and adults.
- Gonorrhea is caused by *Neisseria gonorrhoeae,* a gram-negative diplococcus often referred to as the gonococcus.
- Gonorrhea is the second most common bacterial STI in the United States.
- Ceftriaxone is the preferred drug for treating gonorrhea. It should be given in combination with either azithromycin or doxycycline.
- Syphilis is caused by the spirochete *Treponema pallidum.*
- Penicillin G is the drug of choice for treating all stages of syphilis.
- Bacterial vaginosis can be caused by multiple microorganisms, including *Gardnerella vaginalis, Mycoplasma hominis,* and various anaerobes.
- Bacterial vaginosis can be treated orally with metronidazole, or intravaginally with metronidazole or clindamycin.
- In pregnant patients, bacterial vaginosis is treated only with oral medication, either metronidazole or clindamycin.
- Most genital herpes infections are caused by herpes simplex virus type 2.
- Genital herpes can be treated with three drugs: acyclovir, famciclovir, and valacyclovir. These agents do not eliminate the virus, but they can reduce symptoms and shorten the duration of viral shedding and pain.

Please visit **http://evolve.elsevier.com/Lehne** for chapter-specific NCLEX® examination review questions.

CHAPTER 96 Antiseptics and Disinfectants

Antiseptics and disinfectants are locally acting antimicrobial drugs. These agents are used to reduce acquisition and transmission of infection. Drugs suitable for antisepsis and disinfection cannot be used internally because of toxicity.

GENERAL CONSIDERATIONS

Terminology

The terms *antiseptic* and *disinfectant* are not synonymous. In common usage, the term *antiseptic* is reserved for agents *applied to living tissue. Disinfectants* are preparations *applied to objects.* As a rule, agents used as disinfectants are too harsh for application to living tissue. Disinfectants are employed most frequently to decontaminate surgical instruments and to cleanse hospitals and other medical facilities. Most uses of antiseptics are prophylactic. For example, antiseptics are used to cleanse the hands of medical personnel; they are applied to the patient's skin before invasive procedures (e.g., surgery, insertion of needles); and they are used to bathe neonates. Rarely, antiseptics are employed to treat an existing local infection. However, in most cases, established infections are best treated with a systemic antimicrobial drug.

Several related terms may need clarification. *Sterilization* indicates complete destruction of all microorganisms. In contrast, *sanitization* implies only that contamination has been reduced to a level compatible with public health standards. A *germicide* is a drug that *kills* microorganisms. Germicides may be divided into subcategories: *bactericides, virucides, fungicides,* and *amebicides.* In contrast to a germicide, a *germistatic drug* is one that suppresses the growth and replication of microorganisms but does not kill them.

Properties of an Ideal Antiseptic

The ideal antiseptic, like any other ideal drug, should be safe, effective, and selective. The preparation should be germicidal (rather than germistatic) and should have a broad spectrum of antimicrobial activity: The drug should kill bacteria and their spores, along with viruses, protozoa, yeasts, and fungi. Effects should have a rapid onset and long duration. Development of microbial resistance should be low. The drug should have no harmful effects on humans: It should not produce local injury, impair healing, or produce systemic toxicity following topical application. Lastly, the drug should not cause stains and should be devoid of offensive odor. No antiseptic has all of these properties.

Time Course of Action

Toxicity to microorganisms is determined in part by duration of exposure to an antiseptic or disinfectant. However, some agents act more quickly than others. For example, ethanol (70% solution) reduces the cutaneous bacterial count by 50% in just 36 seconds. In contrast, benzalkonium chloride (at a dilution of 1 : 1000) requires 7 minutes to produce the same effect. Because such differences exist, effective use of antiseptics and disinfectants requires that healthcare personnel understand the exposure requirements of each agent.

Using Antiseptics to Treat Established Local Infection

In the past, topical agents were used routinely to treat established local infection. Today, *systemic* anti-infective drugs are the treatment of choice. Why? First, systemic agents are more effective than topical drugs. Second, systemic agents don't damage inflamed or abraded tissue. Experience has shown that antiseptics do little to reduce infection in wounds, cuts, and abrasions. This lack of efficacy is attributed to poor penetration to the site of infection and to diminished activity in the presence of wound exudates. Although of limited value for *established* local infection, antiseptics are quite useful as *prophylaxis:* When applied properly, antiseptics can help cleanse wounds and decrease microbial contamination.

Using Antiseptics and Disinfectants Most Effectively

The principal value of antiseptics and disinfectants derives from their ability to prevent contamination of the patient by microorganisms in the *environment:* It appears that antiseptics applied directly to the *patient* contribute relatively little to prophylaxis against infection (except in patients who are neutropenic). A number of clinical studies support this conclusion. In one study, more than 5000 preoperative patients were bathed with hexachlorophene. Although this treatment greatly reduced the concentration of surface bacteria, it had no effect on the incidence of postoperative infection. Similarly, in a study of patients who had undergone cardiothoracic surgery, it was found that most postoperative infections were caused by organisms not present at the site of incision. From these studies and others, we can conclude that infections are caused primarily by environmental microorganisms rather than by organisms living on the skin of the patient. Consequently, the use of antiseptics by nurses, physicians, and others who contact the patient confers much greater protection than does the application of antiseptics to the patient. Patients also benefit greatly from the rigorous use of disinfectants to decontaminate surgical supplies and medical buildings.

TABLE 96.1 ▪ Antiseptics and Disinfectants: Chemical Category and Application

Chemical Category	Drug	Application: Antisepsis	Application: Disinfection
Alcohols	Ethanol	✔	
	Isopropanol	✔	
Aldehydes	Glutaraldehyde		✔
	Formaldehyde		✔
Iodine Compounds	Iodine tincture	✔	
	Iodine solution	✔	
Iodophors	Povidone-iodine	✔	✔
Chlorine Compounds	Oxychlorosene	✔	
	Sodium hypochlorite	✔	✔
Phenolic Compound	Hexachlorophene	✔	
Miscellaneous Agents	Chlorhexidine	✔	
	Hydrogen peroxide	✔	✔
	Benzalkonium chloride	✔	✔

PROPERTIES OF INDIVIDUAL ANTISEPTICS AND DISINFECTANTS

Antiseptics and disinfectants derive from a variety of chemical families, ranging from alcohols to iodine compounds to phenols. The various antiseptics and disinfectants differ from one another with respect to mechanism of action, time course, and antimicrobial spectrum. In almost all cases, the drugs employed as disinfectants are not used for antisepsis and vice versa. The more commonly employed antiseptics and disinfectants are shown in Table 96.1. For each drug, the table indicates chemical family and clinical use.

Alcohols

Ethanol

Ethanol (ethyl alcohol) is an effective virucide and kills most common pathogenic bacteria as well. However, the drug is inactive against bacterial spores, including those of *Clostridium difficile,* and has erratic activity against fungi. Bactericidal effects result from precipitating bacterial proteins and dissolving membranes. Ethanol can enhance the effects of several other antimicrobial preparations (e.g., chlorhexidine, benzalkonium chloride).

Ethanol is employed almost exclusively for *antisepsis.* The most frequent uses are hand washing by hospital staff and cleansing the skin before needle insertion and minor surgery. Because it has limited activity against bacterial spores and fungi, ethanol is not a good disinfectant.

Optimal bacterial kill requires that ethanol be present in the proper concentration. The drug is most effective at a concentration of 70%. Higher concentrations are *less* active.

Ethanol should not be applied to open wounds. The drug can increase tissue damage and, by causing coagulation of proteins, can form a mass under which bacteria can thrive.

Ethanol for antisepsis is available in three formulations: solutions, gels, and foams. No one formulation has been proved more effective than the others.

Isopropanol

Isopropanol (isopropyl alcohol) is employed primarily as an antiseptic. When applied in concentrations greater than 70%, isopropanol is somewhat more germicidal than ethanol. Like ethanol, isopropanol can increase the effects of other antiseptics (e.g., chlorhexidine). Isopropanol promotes local vasodilation and can thereby increase bleeding from needle punctures and incisions. Isopropanol is available in concentrations ranging from 70% to 100%.

Aldehydes

Glutaraldehyde

Glutaraldehyde [Cidex Plus 28] is lethal to all microorganisms; the drug kills bacteria, bacterial spores, viruses, and fungi. Antimicrobial effects result from cross-linking and precipitating proteins. Glutaraldehyde is used to disinfect and sterilize surgical instruments and other medical supplies, including respiratory and anesthetic equipment, catheters, and thermometers. The drug is too harsh for antiseptic use. To completely eliminate bacterial spores, instruments and equipment must be immersed in glutaraldehyde for at least 10 hours. All blood should be removed first. Glutaraldehyde is most active at alkaline pH. However, under alkaline conditions, glutaraldehyde eventually becomes inactive, owing to gradual polymerization. Consequently, alkaline solutions of glutaraldehyde are active for only 2 to 4 weeks. Glutaraldehyde should be used with adequate ventilation because fumes can irritate the respiratory tract.

Formaldehyde

Formaldehyde kills bacteria, bacterial spores, viruses, and fungi. Like glutaraldehyde, formaldehyde is too harsh for application to the skin. Accordingly, use is limited to disinfection and sterilization of equipment and instruments. For two reasons, formaldehyde is less desirable than glutaraldehyde. First, formaldehyde acts slowly: Destruction of bacterial spores may take 2 to 4 days. Second, formaldehyde is more volatile than glutaraldehyde, and hence tends to cause more respiratory irritation. As with glutaraldehyde, blood should be removed before instruments and equipment are sterilized.

Iodine Compounds: Iodine Solution and Iodine Tincture

Iodine was first employed as an antiseptic more than 160 years ago. Despite the introduction of numerous other drugs, iodine remains one of our most widely used germicidal agents. The drug is extremely effective, having the ability to kill all known bacteria, fungi, protozoa, viruses, and yeasts. Additional assets are its low cost and low toxicity.

The composition of iodine solution and iodine tincture is very similar. Iodine *solution* consists of 2% elemental iodine and 2.4% sodium iodide in water. Iodine *tincture* contains the same amounts of elemental iodine and sodium iodide and also contains 47% ethanol. The ethanol enhances the antimicrobial activity of iodine tincture.

The germicidal activity of iodine tincture and iodine solution is due only to *free* (dissolved) elemental iodine. In both the tincture and the solution, the concentration of free elemental iodine is very low—about 0.15%—owing to the poor solubility of iodine in water. Because only free iodine is active, most of the elemental iodine and all of the sodium iodide present in both iodine tincture and iodine solution do not contribute *directly* to microbicidal activity. However, these components do contribute *indirectly* by serving as reservoirs from which free elemental iodine can be released.

Iodine tincture and iodine solution are employed primarily for antisepsis of the skin, a use for which they are the most effective agents available. When the skin is *intact,* iodine *tincture* is preferred. This preparation is commonly employed to cleanse the skin before IV injection and withdrawal of blood for microbial culture. For treatment of *wounds* and *abrasions,* iodine *solution* should be employed. (Because alcohol is an irritant, iodine tincture is less appropriate for application to broken skin.)

Iodophors: Povidone-Iodine

An iodophor is simply a complex composed of elemental iodine plus a solubilizing agent. Antimicrobial effects derive from the release of free iodine. The intact iodophor is inactive.

Povidone-iodine is an iodophor composed of elemental iodine plus povidone, an organic polymer that increases the solubility of the iodine. Povidone-iodine has no antimicrobial activity of its own. Rather, it serves as a reservoir from which elemental iodine can be released. Free elemental iodine is the active germicide. The concentration of free iodine achieved with the application of povidone-iodine is lower than that produced with the application of iodine tincture or iodine solution. Hence, povidone-iodine is less effective than these other iodine preparations.

Povidone-iodine is employed primarily for prophylaxis of postoperative infection. Additional uses include hand washing, surgical scrubbing, and preparing the skin before invasive procedures (e.g., surgery, aspiration, injection). In addition, povidone-iodine is employed to sterilize equipment, although superior disinfectants are available.

The drug is supplied in a variety of formulations (ointments, solutions, aerosols, gels). It is also impregnated in swabs, sponges, and wipes. Brand names include ACU-dyne, Betadine, and Operand.

Chlorine Compounds

Chlorine is lethal to a wide variety of microbes and is active both as elemental chlorine and as hypochlorous acid, which is formed by the reaction of chlorine with water. Chlorine is used extensively to sanitize water supplies and swimming pools. However, because of physical properties that make working with chlorine difficult, chlorine itself is rarely used clinically. Instead, chlorine-containing compounds that release hypochlorous acid are employed.

Oxychlorosene Sodium

Oxychlorosene sodium [Clorpactin WCS 90] is a complex mixture of hypochlorous acid with alkylphenyl sulfonates. Antimicrobial effects derive from releasing hypochlorous acid. Oxychlorosene is lethal to bacteria, yeasts, fungi, viruses, molds, and spores. The preparation is employed as a topical antiseptic and can be especially useful for treating localized infection caused by drug-resistant microbes. Oxychlorosene is also employed as an antiseptic for surgical prophylaxis and to irrigate and cleanse fistulas, sinus tracts, wounds, and empyemas (pus-filled cavities).

Sodium Hypochlorite

Sodium hypochlorite kills bacteria, bacterial spores, fungi, protozoa, and viruses. Undiluted (5%) solutions are employed commonly as household bleach. These concentrated solutions are too irritating for application to human tissue. For antiseptic use, dilute (0.5%) solutions are employed. These preparations can be used to irrigate wounds and to cleanse and deodorize necrotic tissue. To minimize local irritation, solutions of sodium hypochlorite should be rinsed off promptly. A 1% solution can be used to sterilize equipment. Solutions of sodium hypochlorite are unstable and must be prepared fresh before each use.

Phenols

The family of phenolic compounds consists of phenol itself and several phenol derivatives. Following its introduction in 1867, phenol rapidly became both the antiseptic and disinfectant of choice. Today, the use of phenol for antiseptic purposes is rare. However, the drug is still employed in some hospitals for disinfection. One member of the phenol family—hexachlorophene—is discussed next.

Hexachlorophene

Actions. Hexachlorophene is *bacteriostatic,* not bactericidal. The drug is quite active against gram-positive bacteria—the bacteria found most frequently on the skin. However, hexachlorophene has little or no effect on gram-negative bacteria. In fact, when used on a regular basis, hexachlorophene encourages overgrowth with gram-negative organisms. (By killing off gram-positive bacteria, hexachlorophene makes conditions more conducive to gram-negative growth.)

Uses. In the past, hexachlorophene was used for hand cleansing by healthcare personnel. However, the drug is no longer an accepted ingredient for hand disinfectants and should not be used in the clinical setting.

Adverse Effects. Hexachlorophene can be absorbed through intact skin and mucous membranes. Absorption through denuded areas can be especially significant. If absorbed in sufficient amounts, hexachlorophene causes central nervous system stimulation. Responses range from confusion to twitching to seizures. Deaths have occurred. To minimize systemic toxicity, hexachlorophene should not be applied extensively to burns, wounds, cuts, or mucous membranes. In addition, total body bathing, especially of infants, should be avoided. For bathing infants, chlorhexidine is safer and more effective.

Preparations. Hexachlorophene is available only by prescription. The drug is supplied in solution.

Miscellaneous Agents

Chlorhexidine

Chlorhexidine is a fast-acting antiseptic lethal to most gram-positive and gram-negative bacteria, but not to bacterial spores. How does chlorhexidine work? At low concentrations, it disrupts the bacterial cell membrane, causing leakage of intracellular components. At higher concentrations, it precipitates intracellular proteins and nucleic acids. Antibacterial effects are reduced

TABLE 96.2 ▪ Selected Chlorhexidine Products

Product Description	Brand Names	Healthcare Uses
Wipes: 0.5% CHG with 70% isopropanol	Hibistat Towelettes	Hand cleansing
Solution: 2% or 4% CHG with 4% isopropanol	BactoShield	Surgical scrub for hands and forearms
Liquid: 2% or 4% CHG with 4% isopropanol	Dyna Hex Skin Cleanser, Hibiclens Antiseptic/ Antimicrobial Skin Cleanser	Preoperative skin cleanser for surgical site or entire body
Catheter dressing: CHG-impregnated transparent dressing	Tegaderm CHG Dressing	Protection of central venous catheters
Oral rinse: 0.12% CHG	Peridex, Periogard	Treatment of gingivitis

CHG, Chlorhexidine gluconate.

somewhat in the presence of soap, blood, and pus. Chlorhexidine that remains on the skin after rinsing is sufficient to exert continuing germicidal effects. Bacterial resistance is rare.

As indicated in Table 96.2, chlorhexidine is available in several formulations for use in various situations. The drug is used for preoperative preparation of the skin and as a surgical scrub, hand-wash preparation, and wound cleanser. It is also the preferred agent for preventing infection associated with central venous catheters. In patients with gingivitis and periodontitis, chlorhexidine is used as an oral rinse.

Chlorhexidine is very safe. Even with routine preoperative use, local adverse effects are uncommon. Rarely, severe contact dermatitis has developed at the site of a central venous catheter. Inadvertent IV injection has been reported twice: in one patient, hemolysis occurred; in the other, no ill effects were observed.

Hydrogen Peroxide

Hydrogen peroxide is an excellent disinfectant and sterilizing agent, but it is useless as an antiseptic. The entity in hydrogen peroxide solution responsible for antimicrobial effects is the hydroxyl free radical. These free radicals are destroyed when hydrogen peroxide is acted upon by catalase, an enzyme found in all tissues. Hence, contact with tissue terminates germicidal actions. The only benefit resulting from the application of hydrogen peroxide to wounds derives from the liberation of oxygen (by the reaction with catalase), which causes frothing that is sufficient to loosen debris and thereby facilitate cleansing. The principal use of hydrogen peroxide is disinfection and sterilization of instruments. A 3% to 6% solution is employed.

Thimerosal

Thimerosal is an organic compound that contains 49% mercury, the active antimicrobial factor. Thimerosal has only weak bacteriostatic and fungistatic properties, and hence does not kill bacteria or fungi. Antimicrobial actions are reduced in the presence of blood and tissue proteins. Thimerosal is less effective than ethanol. Use on large areas of denuded skin may yield systemic toxicity from the absorption of mercury. Poisoning from thimerosal ingestion can be treated with dimercaprol (see Chapter 109). Thimerosal has been employed to irrigate wounds and prepare the skin before surgery. It has also been employed as an antiseptic for the eyes, nose, throat, and genitourinary tract. However, given that thimerosal has low efficacy and a significant potential for harm, and given that more effective and safer drugs are available, thimerosal has been withdrawn from the market.

In the past, thimerosal was widely used as a preservative in vaccines. However, owing to concerns about a possible (albeit unproved) link between thimerosal and autism, nearly all vaccines used by Americans are now devoid of this agent. The only exception is the inactivated influenza vaccine.

Benzalkonium Chloride

Actions. Benzalkonium chloride (BAC) is an organic quaternary ammonium compound that has antimicrobial and detergent properties. BAC is active against many gram-positive and gram-negative bacteria as well as some fungi, protozoa, and viruses. The drug is relatively *inactive* against *Mycobacterium tuberculosis, C. difficile,* and other spore-forming bacteria. Germicidal effects result from the disruption of membranes and are enhanced by ethanol. BAC is inactivated by soaps and organic material. BAC is slow acting compared with iodine.

Antiseptic Uses. BAC is employed for preoperative preparation of the skin and mucous membranes; as a surgical scrub; as an antiseptic for abrasions and minor wounds; as a vaginal douche; and for irrigation of the eyes, body cavities, and genitourinary tract. Because BAC is inactivated by soap, all soap must be removed by rinsing with water and 70% alcohol before BAC application. Concentrated solutions of BAC can cause severe local injury, so healthcare personnel must take care to use solutions of appropriate dilution. For several reasons (limited antimicrobial spectrum, lack of rapid action, potential for toxicity, availability of superior agents), there seems to be little to recommend BAC for antiseptic use.

Disinfectant Use. Immersion in BAC solution is employed for sterile storage of instruments and supplies. Adsorption of BAC onto porous material can significantly reduce the concentration of BAC in solutions. To ensure continuing efficacy, solutions should be changed (or at least replenished with BAC) on a regular basis.

Preparations and Dosage. BAC is supplied in concentrated (17%) and dilute (1 : 750) solution. Recommended dilutions are 1 : 750 (for application to intact skin and to minor wounds and abrasions); 1 : 2000 to 1 : 5000 (for application to mucous membranes and diseased or seriously damaged skin); and 1 : 750 to 1 : 5000 (for storage of instruments and supplies). BAC is also available as an antiseptic spray (0.13%) for first-aid purposes.

HAND HYGIENE FOR HEALTHCARE WORKERS

General Recommendations

Effective hand hygiene is the single most important factor in preventing the spread of infection in healthcare settings. Each year, an estimated 2 million patients in the United States acquire an infection while in a hospital; about 90,000 of them die as a result. Patients can also acquire infections in other settings, including clinics, dialysis centers, and long-term care facilities. In all of these places, the leading cause of infection spread is the transfer of pathogens from one patient to another on the hands of healthcare workers (HCWs). Accordingly, the best way to reduce new infections in these settings is to improve hand hygiene.

Traditionally, HCWs cleaned their hands with soap and water. Unfortunately, this technique has several drawbacks: It takes considerable time, requires a sink and hand-washing supplies, and promotes skin irritation and dryness. As a result, adherence tends to be poor.

The Centers for Disease Control and Prevention (CDC) has issued guidelines designed to improve hand-hygiene practices among HCWs and to reduce transmission of pathogenic microorganisms to patients and personnel in healthcare settings. A central recommendation in the guidelines is the

TABLE 96.3 ■ Antimicrobial Spectrum and Characteristics of Hand-Hygiene Antiseptic Agents

Group	Gram-Positive Bacteria	Gram-Negative Bacteria	Mycobacteria	Fungi	Viruses	Speed of Action	Comments
Alcohols	+ + +	+ + +	+ + +	+ + +	+ + +	Fast	Optimum concentration 60%–95%; no persistent activity; not lethal to bacterial spores, including those of *C. difficile*
Chlorhexidine (2% and 4% aqueous)	+ + +	+ +	+	+	+ + +	Intermediate	Persistent activity; rare allergic reactions
Iodine compounds	+ + +	+ + +	+ + +	+ +	+ + +	Intermediate	Causes skin burns; usually too irritating for hand hygiene
Iodophors	+ + +	+ + +	+	+ +	+ +	Intermediate	Less irritating than iodine; acceptance varies
Phenol derivatives	+ + +	+	+	+	+	Intermediate	Activity neutralized by nonionic surfactants

+ + +, Excellent; + +, good, but does not include the entire bacterial spectrum; +, fair.
From Centers for Disease Control and Prevention: Guideline for hand hygiene in health-care settings: Recommendations of the Healthcare Infection Control Practices Advisory Committee and the HICPAC/SHEA/APIC/IDSA Hand Hygiene Task Force. *MMWR Recomm Rep* 51(RR-16), 2002.

use of *alcohol-based handrubs,* rather than soap and water, for *routine* hand antisepsis. There are four reasons for this recommendation:

- *Accessibility*—Handrubs don't require a sink or towels, and hence are more accessible than washing with soap and water.
- *Time savings*—Using a handrub is much faster than washing with soap and water. All you do is apply the handrub to the palm of one hand and then rub your hands together until they are dry. The CDC estimates that an intensive care unit nurse would save about 1 hour during an 8-hour shift by using a handrub instead of soap and water.
- *Lessened skin damage*—Today's alcohol-based handrubs contain emollients and moisturizers, and hence don't irritate or dry the skin as soap and water do.
- *Greater efficacy*—Alcohol-based handrubs reduce the number of bacteria on the skin more effectively than does washing with soap and water.

Studies have shown that, because of these advantages, switching from soap and water to an alcohol-based handrub can significantly improve adherence among HCWs.

It is important to note that alcohol-based handrubs have limitations. First, alcohol does not kill bacterial spores, including those of *C. difficile* and *Bacillus anthracis.* Washing with soap and water doesn't kill spores either, but *does* physically remove them. Second, alcohol-based handrubs can't remove dirt or organic material. Accordingly, when the hands are visibly soiled, soap and water must be used first. Third, alcohol lacks residual killing power. For routine clinical practice, this lack is no concern. However, under certain conditions—including infectious disease outbreaks and performance of invasive procedures—an antiseptic that does have residual effects (e.g., chlorhexidine) should be used.

Table 96.3 shows the antimicrobial spectrum, speed of onset, and unique properties of some antiseptic agents used in hand-hygiene products.

Specific CDC Hand-Hygiene Recommendations

Major recommendations from the CDC hand-hygiene guidelines are presented here. Each recommendation is categorized on the basis of existing scientific data, theoretical rationale, applicability, and economic impact. The five categories employed are defined as follows:

Category IA—Strongly recommended for implementation and strongly supported by well-designed experimental, clinical, or epidemiologic studies

Category IB—Strongly recommended for implementation and supported by certain experimental, clinical, or epidemiologic studies and a strong theoretical rationale

Category IC—Required for implementation, as mandated by federal or state regulation or standard

Category II—Suggested for implementation and supported by suggestive clinical or epidemiologic studies or a theoretical rationale

No recommendation/Unresolved issue—Practices for which insufficient evidence or no consensus regarding efficacy exists

Indications for Hand Washing and Hand Antisepsis

- When hands are visibly dirty or contaminated with proteinaceous material or are visibly soiled with blood or other body fluids, wash hands with either a non-antimicrobial soap and water, or an antimicrobial soap and water (IA).

- If hands are not visibly soiled, use an alcohol-based handrub for routinely decontaminating hands in all clinical situations described in the following list (IA). Alternatively, wash hands with an antimicrobial soap and water in all clinical situations described in the following list (IB).
  - Decontaminate hands before having direct contact with patients (IB).
  - Decontaminate hands before donning sterile gloves when inserting a central intravascular catheter (IB).
  - Decontaminate hands before inserting indwelling urinary catheters, peripheral vascular catheters, or other invasive devices that do not require a surgical procedure (IB).
  - Decontaminate hands after contact with a patient's intact skin (e.g., when taking a pulse or blood pressure, and when lifting a patient) (IB).
  - Decontaminate hands after contact with body fluids or excretions, mucous membranes, nonintact skin, and wound dressings if hands are not visibly soiled (IA).
  - Decontaminate hands if moving from a contaminated body site to a clean body site during patient care (II).
  - Decontaminate hands after contact with inanimate objects (including medical equipment) in the immediate vicinity of the patient (II).
  - Decontaminate hands after removing gloves (IB).
- Before eating and after using a restroom, wash hands with a non-antimicrobial soap and water, or with an antimicrobial soap and water (IB).
- Antimicrobial-impregnated wipes (i.e., towelettes) may be considered as an alternative to washing hands with non-antimicrobial soap and water. Because they are not as effective as alcohol-based handrubs or washing hands with an antimicrobial soap and water for reducing bacterial counts on the hands of HCWs, they are not a substitute for using an alcohol-based handrub or antimicrobial soap (IB).
- Wash hands with non-antimicrobial soap and water, or with antimicrobial soap and water if exposure to spore-forming bacteria, such as *Bacillus anthracis,* is suspected or proven. The physical action of washing and rinsing the hands will remove spores, although it won't kill them. Alcohols, chlorhexidine, iodophors, and other antiseptics have poor activity against spores, and hence are less effective than soap and water (II).
- No recommendation was made by the CDC regarding the routine use of non–alcohol-based handrubs for hand hygiene in healthcare settings (Unresolved issue).

Hand-Hygiene Technique

- When decontaminating hands with an alcohol-based handrub, apply product to palm of one hand and rub hands together, covering all surfaces of hands and fingers, until hands are dry (IB). Follow the manufacturer's recommendations regarding the volume of product to use.
- When washing hands with soap and water, wet hands first with water, apply an amount of product recommended by the manufacturer to hands, and rub hands together vigorously for at least 15 seconds, covering all surfaces of the hands and fingers. Rinse hands with water and dry thoroughly with a disposable towel. Use towel to turn off the faucet (IB). Avoid using hot water, because repeated exposure to hot water may increase the risk for dermatitis (IB).
- Liquid, bar, leaflet, or powdered forms of plain soap are acceptable when washing hands with a non-antimicrobial soap and water. When bar soap is used, soap racks that facilitate drainage and small bars of soap should be used (II).
- Multiple-use cloth towels of the hanging or roll type are not recommended for use in healthcare settings (II).

Surgical Hand Antisepsis

- Remove rings, watches, and bracelets before beginning the surgical hand scrub (II).
- Remove debris from underneath fingernails using a nail cleaner under running water (II).
- Surgical hand antisepsis using either an antimicrobial soap or an alcohol-based handrub with persistent activity is recommended before donning sterile gloves when performing surgical procedures (IB).
- When performing surgical hand antisepsis using an antimicrobial soap, scrub hands and forearms for the length of time recommended by the manufacturer, usually 2 to 6 minutes. Long scrub times (e.g., 10 minutes) are not necessary (IB).
- When using an alcohol-based surgical hand-scrub product with persistent activity, follow the manufacturer's instructions. Before applying the alcohol solution, prewash hands and forearms with a non-antimicrobial soap, and dry hands and forearms completely. After application of the alcohol-based product as recommended, allow hands and forearms to dry thoroughly before donning sterile gloves (IB).

Other Aspects of Hand Hygiene

- Do not wear artificial fingernails or extenders when having direct contact with patients at high risk (e.g., those in intensive care units or operating rooms) (IA).
- Keep natural nail tips less than ¼-inch long (II).
- Wear gloves when contact with blood or other potentially infectious materials, mucous membranes, and nonintact skin could occur (IC).
- Remove gloves after caring for a patient. Do not wear the same pair of gloves for the care of more than one patient, and do not wash gloves between uses with different patients (IB).
- Change gloves during patient care if moving from a contaminated body site to a clean body site (II).
- No recommendation was made by the CDC regarding the wearing of rings in healthcare settings (Unresolved issue). (*Note:* Some studies have demonstrated that wearing a ring reduces the efficacy of hand cleansing.)

Administrative Measures Regarding Hand Hygiene

- As part of a multidisciplinary program to improve hand-hygiene adherence, provide HCWs with a readily accessible alcohol-based handrub product (IA).
- To improve hand-hygiene adherence among personnel who work in areas in which high workloads and high intensity of patient care are anticipated, make an alcohol-based handrub available at the entrance to the patient's room or at the bedside, in other convenient locations, and in individual pocket-sized containers to be carried by HCWs (IA).

KEY POINTS

- Because the various antiseptics and disinfectants require different durations of exposure to be effective, you must know the time course of action of the specific agent you are working with.
- Although antiseptics can help prevent the *development* of a local infection, systemic anti-infective drugs are preferred for treating an *established* local infection.
- Washing with antiseptics by nurses, physicians, and others who contact patients will do more to protect patients from infection than will the application of antiseptics to patients themselves.
- For routine hand antisepsis, alcohol-based handrubs are preferred to soap and water.
- Soap and water are preferred to alcohol-based handrubs when the hands are visibly dirty and following exposure to spore-forming bacteria, such as *B. anthracis.*

Please visit **http://evolve.elsevier.com/Lehne** for chapter-specific NCLEX® examination review questions.

CHAPTER 97

Anthelmintics

Helminths are parasitic worms, and *anthelmintics* are the drugs used against them. Helminthiasis (worm infestation) is the most common affliction of humans, affecting more than 2 billion people worldwide. The intestine is a frequent site of infestation. Other sites include the liver, lymphatic system, and blood vessels. Infestation is frequently asymptomatic. However, infestation with some parasites can cause severe complications. Helminthiasis is most prevalent where sanitation is poor. Cleanliness greatly reduces infestation risk.

Treatment of helminthiasis is not always indicated. Most parasitic worms do not reproduce in the human body. Therefore, in the absence of reinfestation, many infections simply subside as adult worms die. Accordingly, treatment may be optional. In countries where providers and medication are readily available, drug therapy is definitely indicated. However, in less fortunate locales, several factors—cost of medication, limited medical facilities, and high probability of reinfestation—may render individual treatment impractical. In these places, preventative measures, such as improved hygiene and elimination of carriers, may be the most valuable interventions.

In approaching the anthelmintic drugs, we begin by reviewing classification of the parasitic worms. Next we briefly discuss the characteristics of the more common helminthic infestations. After this, we discuss preferred drugs for treatment.

CLASSIFICATION OF PARASITIC WORMS

The most common parasitic worms belong to three classes: Nematoda (roundworms), Cestoda (tapeworms), and Trematoda (flukes). Nematodes belong to the phylum Nemathelminthes. Cestodes and trematodes belong to the phylum Platyhelminthes (flat worms).

Nematodes (Roundworms)

Parasitic nematodes can be subdivided into two groups: (1) those that infest the intestinal lumen and (2) those that inhabit tissues. There are five major species of intestinal nematodes. Their common names are giant roundworm, pinworm, hookworm, whipworm, and threadworm. Official names (e.g., *Ascaris lumbricoides*) are shown in Table 97.1. Two types of nematodes invade tissues: (1) pork roundworms (responsible for trichinosis) and (2) filariae. The three species of filariae encountered most commonly are also found in Table 97.1.

Cestodes (Tapeworms)

Three species of cestodes infest humans. Common names for these parasites are beef tapeworm, pork tapeworm, and fish tapeworm. Their official names appear in Table 97.1.

Trematodes (Flukes)

Five species of trematodes infest humans. These organisms fall into four groups, with the following common names: blood fluke, liver fluke, intestinal fluke, and lung fluke. Official names of the five species belonging to these groups are given in Table 97.1.

HELMINTHIC INFESTATIONS

This section describes the major characteristics of infestation by specific helminths. These infestations can differ with respect to anatomic site and danger to the host. Infestations also differ with respect to the drugs employed for treatment.

The name applied to an infestation is based on the official name of the invading organism. For example, infestation with the giant roundworm, whose official name is *Ascaris lumbricoides,* is referred to as *ascariasis.*

In the following discussion, the helminthic infestations are grouped into four categories: (1) nematode infestations of the

TABLE 97.1 ▪ Drugs of Choice for Parasitic Worms

Worm Class	Parasitic Organism: Common Name	Parasitic Organism: Official Name	Drugs of Choice
Nematodes (roundworms): intestinal	Giant roundworm	*Ascaris lumbricoides*	Albendazole *or* mebendazole *or* ivermectin
	Pinworm	*Enterobius vermicularis*	Albendazole *or* mebendazole *or* pyrantel pamoate
	Hookworm	*Ancylostoma duodenale, Necator americanus*	
	Whipworm	*Trichuris trichiura*	Albendazole
	Threadworm	*Strongyloides stercoralis*	Ivermectin
Nematodes (roundworms): extraintestinal	Pork roundworm	*Trichinella spiralis*	Albendazole[a]
	Filariae	*Brugia malayi, Loa loa, Wuchereria bancrofti*	Diethylcarbamazine[b]
		Onchocerca volvulus	Ivermectin
Cestodes (tapeworms)	Beef tapeworm	*Taenia saginata*	Praziquantel[a]
	Pork tapeworm	*Taenia solum*	
	Fish tapeworm	*Diphyllobothrium latum*	
Trematodes (flukes)	Blood fluke	*Schistosoma* species	Praziquantel
	Intestinal fluke	*Fasciolopsis buski*	
	Lung fluke	*Paragonimus westermani*	
	Liver flukes	*Fasciola hepatica* (sheep liver fluke)	Triclabendazole[b]
		Clonorchis sinensis (Chinese liver fluke)	Praziquantel *or* albendazole[a]

[a]Not approved by the U.S. Food and Drug Administration for this indication.
[b]Available from the Centers for Disease Control and Prevention.

intestine, (2) nematode infestations of extraintestinal sites, (3) cestode infestations, and (4) trematode infestations.

Nematode Infestations (Intestinal)

Ascariasis (Giant Roundworm Infestation)

Ascariasis is the most prevalent helminthic infestation. Worldwide, one of every three people is affected. Adult worms inhabit the small intestine. Ascariasis is usually asymptomatic. However, serious complications can result if worms migrate into the pancreatic duct, bile duct, gallbladder, or liver. In addition, if infestation is extremely heavy, intestinal blockage may occur. Because of these potential hazards, ascariasis should always be treated. Drugs of choice are *albendazole, mebendazole,* and *ivermectin.*

Enterobiasis (Pinworm Infestation)

Enterobiasis is the most common helminthic infestation in the United States. Adult pinworms inhabit the ileum and large intestine. Their life span is approximately 2 months. Although usually asymptomatic, some patients experience intense perianal itching. Serious complications are rare. Drugs of choice are *albendazole, mebendazole,* and *pyrantel pamoate.* Because enterobiasis is readily transmitted, all family members of an infected individual should be treated simultaneously.

Ancylostomiasis and Necatoriasis (Hookworm Infestation)

Hookworm infestation is most common in rural areas where hygiene is poor and people go barefoot. Adult hookworms attach to the wall of the small intestine and suck blood. As a result, infestation is associated with chronic blood loss and progressive anemia. Symptomatic anemia is most likely in menstruating women and undernourished individuals. Nausea, vomiting, and abdominal pain may accompany the infestation. *Albendazole, mebendazole,* and *pyrantel pamoate* are treatments of choice.

Trichuriasis (Whipworm Infestation)

Trichuriasis is extremely common, affecting about 1 billion people worldwide. Larvae and adult worms inhabit the large intestine. Mature worms may live for 10 years or more. The disease is usually devoid of symptoms. However, when the worm burden is very large, rectal prolapse may occur. Patients with severe infestation require therapy. *Albendazole* is the treatment of choice.

Strongyloidiasis (Threadworm Infestation)

Strongyloidiasis is common in the southern United States. Larval and adult threadworms inhabit the small intestine. The disease can be very dangerous, although symptoms are usually absent. Mild infestation may cause abdominal pain and occasional diarrhea. Severe infestation can cause vomiting, massive diarrhea, dehydration, electrolyte imbalance, and secondary bacteremia. Death has occurred. Affected individuals should always be treated. *Ivermectin* is the treatment of choice.

Nematode Infestations (Extraintestinal)

Trichinosis (Pork Roundworm Infestation)

Trichinosis, also called *trichinellosis,* is acquired by eating undercooked pork that contains encysted larvae of *Trichinella spiralis.* Adult worms reside in the intestine, whereas larvae migrate to skeletal muscle and become encysted. Some encysted larvae live for years; others die and calcify within months. Symptoms of trichinosis include GI upset, fever, muscle pain, and sore throat. Potentially lethal complications (heart failure, meningitis, neuritis) arise in some patients. *Albendazole* is the drug of choice for killing adult worms and migrating larvae. However, this agent may not be active against larvae that have become encysted. *Prednisone* (a glucocorticoid) is given to reduce inflammation during larval migration.

Wuchereriasis and Brugiasis (Lymphatic Filarial Infestation)

Wuchereria bancrofti and *Brugia malayi* are filarial nematodes that invade the lymphatic system. Infestation with either organism can cause severe complications. When infestation is heavy, lymphatic obstruction occurs, resulting in *elephantiasis* (usually of the scrotum or legs). In addition, "filarial fever" may develop. Symptoms include chills, fever, headache, nausea, vomiting, constipation, and lymphadenitis. The drug of choice for killing both filarial species is *diethylcarbamazine.*

Onchocerciasis (River Blindness)

Onchocerca volvulus is a filarial nematode found in streams and rivers of Mexico, Guatemala, northern South America, and equatorial Africa. The parasite is transmitted to humans by the bite of certain flies. Heavy infestation with *O. volvulus* causes dermatologic and ophthalmic symptoms. Dermatologic manifestations include subcutaneous nodules (filled with adult worms) and persistent pruritic dermatitis. Ocular lesions, caused by the infiltration and death of microfilariae, result in optic neuritis, optic atrophy, and then blindness. The drug of choice for treating onchocerciasis is *ivermectin.*

Cestode Infestations

Taeniasis (Beef and Pork Tapeworm Infestation)

Taeniasis is acquired by eating undercooked beef or pork that contains tapeworm larvae. Adult tapeworms live attached to the wall of the small intestine. Infestation is usually asymptomatic. Taeniasis is treated with *praziquantel.*

Diphyllobothriasis (Fish Tapeworm Infestation)

Diphyllobothriasis is acquired by ingestion of undercooked fish that is infested with tapeworm larvae. Adult worms inhabit the ileum. Infestation is usually devoid of symptoms. Worms can be killed with *praziquantel.*

Trematode Infestations

Schistosomiasis (Blood Fluke Infestations)

The term *schistosomiasis* refers to infestation with blood flukes of any species (e.g., *Schistosoma mansoni, S. japonicum*). Specific snails serve as intermediate hosts for these flukes. Schistosomiasis cannot be acquired in the continental United States because the appropriate snails are not indigenous.

Schistosomiasis has an acute and a chronic phase. The acute phase subsides in 3 to 4 months. Symptoms during this phase include lymphadenopathy, fever, anorexia, malaise, muscle pain, and rash. During the chronic phase, schistosomes take up residence in the vascular system, primarily in veins of the intestines and liver. This late infestation can produce intestinal polyposis, hepatosplenomegaly, and portal hypertension. For either the acute or the chronic stage, *praziquantel* is the treatment of choice.

Fascioliasis (Liver Fluke Infestation)

Fascioliasis is caused by two liver flukes: *Fasciola hepatica* (sheep liver fluke) and *Clonorchis sinensis* (Chinese liver fluke). Both parasites inhabit the biliary tract. Symptoms (anorexia, mild fever, fatigue, aching in the region of the liver) are delayed for 1 to 3 months.

Liver flukes differ in drug sensitivity. The preferred drug for use against *F. hepatica* is *triclabendazole* (a veterinary anthelmintic). It is not U.S. Food and Drug Administration (FDA) approved, but it is available through the Centers for Disease Control and Prevention (CDC) under an investigational drug protocol. The preferred drugs for use against *C. sinensis* are *praziquantel* and *albendazole.*

Fasciolopsiasis (Intestinal Fluke Infestation)

Fasciolopsiasis is most common in Southeast Asia. Adult worms inhabit the small intestine. The disease is usually asymptomatic. However, some people experience ulcer-like pain; some develop constipation or diarrhea; and, in the presence of massive infestation, bowel obstruction may occur, requiring surgery for clearance. *Praziquantel* is the treatment of choice.

DRUGS OF CHOICE FOR HELMINTHIASIS

The major anthelmintic drugs are considered next. These agents differ in antiparasitic spectra: some are active against several worms; others are more selective. Because of these differences, it is important to identify the invading organism so that the most appropriate drug can be chosen. Table 97.2 lists the major anthelmintic drugs and indicates the parasites against which each is most effective. Although the discussion that follows is limited to drugs of choice, be aware that additional anthelmintics are available.

Mebendazole

Target Organisms

Mebendazole [Emverm, Vermox 🍁] is a drug of choice for most *intestinal roundworms.* This agent clears infestation with *pinworms, hookworms,* and *giant roundworms.* Because of its relatively broad spectrum of action, mebendazole is especially useful for treatment of mixed infestations.

Mechanism of Action

Mebendazole prevents uptake of glucose by susceptible intestinal worms. Glucose deprivation results in immobilization followed by slow death. Because the worms die slowly, up to 3 days may elapse between treatment onset and complete clearance of parasites. Mebendazole does not influence glucose uptake or utilization by humans.

Pharmacokinetics

Pharmacokinetic information for mebendazole and other anthelmintics is provided in Table 97.3.

Adverse Effects

Systemic effects are rare at usual doses, perhaps because the drug is so poorly absorbed. In patients with massive parasitic infestations, transient abdominal pain and diarrhea may occur.

Albendazole

Target Organisms

Albendazole [Albenza] is active against many cestode and nematode parasites, including larval forms of *Taenia solium* and *Echinococcus granulosus.* In the United States, the drug is approved only for (1) parenchymal *neurocysticercosis* caused

TABLE 97.2 ▪ First-Choice Anthelmintic Drugs: Target Organisms and Dosages

Drug	Target Organism	Adult and Pediatric Dosages[a]	Administration
Mebendazole [Emverm, Vermox 🍁]	Roundworm	100 mg 2 times/day for 3 days *or* 500 mg once	Administer with or without food; absorption is increased with food intake. May be swallowed whole or crushed and mixed with food.
	Hookworm	500 mg once	
	Pinworm	100 mg; repeat in 2 weeks	
Albendazole [Albenza]	Giant roundworm	400 mg once	Administer with high-fat food.[b] May be swallowed whole or crushed and mixed with food.
	Hookworm		
	Whipworm	400 mg/day for 3 days	
	Pork roundworm	400 mg 2 times/day for 8–14 days	
	Pinworm	400 mg; repeat in 2 weeks	
	Chinese liver fluke	10 mg/kg/day for 7 days	
Triclabendazole[c]	Sheep liver fluke	10 mg/kg once or twice	Administer with food.
Pyrantel pamoate [Reese's Pinworm Medicine, Combantrin 🍁]	Hookworm	11 mg/kg (max. 1 gm) for 3 days	Administer with or without food. Chewable tablets must be chewed thoroughly. Shake suspensions well before administering.
	Pinworm	11 mg/kg (max. 1 gm); repeat in 2 weeks	
Praziquantel [Biltricide]	Beef tapeworm[d]	5–10 mg/kg once	Administer with food. Do not crush. Have patient swallow quickly to prevent nausea or vomiting due to taste.
	Pork tapeworm[d]		
	Fish tapeworm[d]		
	Blood flukes (*Schistosoma*)		
	S. japonicum, S. mekongi	20 mg/kg 3 times/day for 1 day	
	S. mansoni, S. haematobium	20 mg/kg 2 times/day for 1 day	
	Intestinal fluke	25 mg/kg 3 times/day for 1 day	
	Chinese liver fluke	25 mg/kg 3 times/day for 2 days	
	Lung fluke		
Diethylcarbamazine[c]	*Wuchereria bancrofti* *Brugia malayi*	Day 1: 50 mg Day 2: 50 mg 3 times/day Day 3: 100 mg 3 times/day Days 4–21: 6 mg/kg/day in 3 divided doses	Administer immediately after meals.
	Loa loa	Day 1: 50 mg Day 2: 50 mg 3 times/day Day 3: 100 mg 3 times/day Days 4–21: 9 mg/kg/day in 3 divided doses	
Ivermectin [Stromectol]	Threadworm	200 mcg/kg/day for 2 days	Administer on an empty stomach with water.
	Giant roundworm	150–200 mcg/kg once	
	Onchocerca volvulus	150 mcg/kg every 6–12 months until asymptomatic	

[a]Dosage is the same for pediatric and adult patients with the exception of albendazole which, for all indications except Chinese liver fluke, is 15 mg/kg/day (max. 800 mg) given in divided doses for patients weighing less than 60 kg.
[b]Poorly absorbed in water. Administration with high-fat foods can increase absorption by 5 times over a fasting state.
[c]Available from the Centers for Disease Control and Prevention.
[d]Treatment of adult (intestinal) stage.

TABLE 97.3 ▪ Pharmacokinetics of Anthelmintics

Drug	Route	Peak	Half-Life	Metabolism	Excretion
Mebendazole[a] [Emverm, Vermox 🍁]	PO	0.5–6 hr	3–6 hr	Hepatic	Feces
Albendazole [Albenza]	PO	2–5 hr	8–12 hr	Hepatic	Urine
Triclabendazole[b]	PO	—	—	—	—
Pyrantel pamoate[a] [Reese's Pinworm Medicine, Combantrin 🍁]	PO	1–2 hr	2.5–5.5 hr	Hepatic	Feces (primary) and urine
Praziquantel [Biltricide]	PO	1–3 hr	1–1.5 hr	Hepatic	Urine
Diethylcarbamazine[b]	PO	1–2 hr	10–12 hr	Hepatic	Urine (primary), feces
Ivermectin [Stromectol]	PO	4 hr	16–18 hr	Hepatic	Feces (primary), urine

[a]Absorption is poor, so plasma levels are low.
[b]Not approved by the U.S. Food and Drug Administration. Limited data are available.

PATIENT-CENTERED CARE ACROSS THE LIFE SPAN[a]

Life Stage	Patient Care Concerns
Children	There are inadequate studies in children for most of these drugs. As with all drugs, the benefits of treatment must be weighed against the risk of adverse effects.
Pregnant women	Animal reproduction studies have demonstrated abnormalities for mebendazole, albendazole, and ivermectin (Pregnancy Risk Category C[b]); however, the risk to humans has not been established. The World Health Organization (WHO) allows use of mebendazole, albendazole, and pyrantel pamoate in the second and third trimesters, but not the first trimester, and does not recommend the use of ivermectin and diethylcarbamazine as treatment for women who are pregnant. Praziquantel appears to be the safest of the anthelmintics. No abnormalities occurred in animal studies. It is categorized as Pregnancy Risk Category B.
Breast-feeding women	The WHO advises women taking mebendazole and pyrantel pamoate to continue breast-feeding, but advises caution with albendazole and ivermectin. The manufacturer of pyrantel pamoate, however, does not recommend breast-feeding when taking this drug. The manufacturer of praziquantel notes that significant amounts of the drug are excreted into breast milk and advises that women not nurse on the day of praziquantel treatment and during the subsequent 72 hours.
Older adults	There are no current contraindications for older adults taking these drugs; however, because there are relatively few studies on the effects of these drugs on older adults, insufficient data are available to determine safety.

[a]Life span information is limited for triclabendazole and diethylcarbamazine, which are not approved by the U.S. Food and Drug Administration.
[b]As of 2020, the FDA will no longer use Pregnancy Risk Categories. Please refer to Chapter 9 for more information.

by larval forms of the pork tapeworm, *Taenia solium;* and (2) *cystic hydatid disease* of the liver, lung, and peritoneum caused by larval forms of the dog tapeworm, *E. granulosus.* However, despite lack of FDA approval, albendazole is considered a drug of choice for infestation with hookworms, pinworms, whipworms, Chinese liver flukes, giant roundworms, and pork roundworms, the cause of trichinosis.

Mechanism of Action

Albendazole inhibits polymerization of tubulin and thereby prevents formation of cytoplasmic microtubules. As a result, microtubule-dependent uptake of glucose is prevented.

Adverse Effects

Albendazole is generally well tolerated. Mild to moderate *liver impairment* has occurred in 16% of patients, as indicated by elevation of liver transaminases in plasma. Liver function should be assessed before each cycle of treatment and 14 days later.

Albendazole suppresses bone marrow function and can thereby cause granulocytopenia, agranulocytosis, and even pancytopenia (a condition in which there is a lower-than-normal number of all blood cells—erythrocytes, leukocytes, and thrombocytes). Liver impairment may increase risk. Blood cell counts should be obtained before each cycle of treatment and 14 days later.

Safety Alert

ALBENDAZOLE

Bone marrow suppression may occur. Observe for signs and symptoms of anemia (pallor, weakness), leukopenia (evidence of infection), and thrombocytopenia (increased bruising and bleeding).

Pyrantel Pamoate

Target Organisms

Pyrantel pamoate [Reese's Pinworm Medicine, Combantrin 🍁], an over-the-counter drug, is active against *intestinal nematodes.* The drug is an alternative to mebendazole or albendazole for infestations with *hookworms* or *pinworms.*

Mechanism of Action

Pyrantel is a depolarizing neuromuscular blocking agent that causes spastic paralysis of intestinal parasites. The paralyzed worms are cleared in the feces.

Adverse Effects

Serious reactions are rare. The most common effects are GI reactions (nausea, vomiting, diarrhea, stomach pain, cramps). Possible central nervous system effects include dizziness, drowsiness, headache, and insomnia.

Praziquantel

Target Organisms

Praziquantel [Biltricide] is very active against *flukes* and *cestodes* (tapeworms) and is the drug of choice for *tapeworms, schistosomiasis,* and other *fluke infestations.*

Mechanism of Action

Praziquantel is readily absorbed by helminths. At low therapeutic concentrations, the drug produces spastic paralysis, causing detachment of worms from body tissues. At high therapeutic concentrations, praziquantel disrupts the integument of the worms, rendering the parasites vulnerable to lethal attack by host defenses.

Adverse Effects

Praziquantel is relatively free of toxicity. Transient headache and abdominal discomfort are the most frequent reactions. Drowsiness may occur, and hence patients should avoid driving and other hazardous activities.

Diethylcarbamazine

Diethylcarbamazine is not marketed in the United States. It is available from the CDC as part of an Investigational New Drug policy.

Target Organisms

Diethylcarbamazine is the drug of choice for *filarial infestations.* The drug destroys microfilariae of *W. bancrofti, B. malayi,* and *Loa loa.* In addition, it kills adult females of these species.

Mechanism of Action

Diethylcarbamazine has two antifilarial actions. First, it reduces muscular activity, causing parasites to be dislodged from their site of attachment. Second, by altering the surface properties of the parasites, it renders the organisms more vulnerable to attack by host defenses.

Adverse Effects

Adverse effects caused directly by diethylcarbamazine are minor (headache, weakness, dizziness, nausea, vomiting). Indirect effects, occurring secondary to death of the parasites, can be more serious. These include rashes, intense itching, encephalitis, fever, tachycardia, lymphadenitis, leukocytosis, and proteinuria. Fortunately, these reactions are transient, lasting just a few days—and can be minimized by pretreatment with glucocorticoids.

Ivermectin

Target Organisms

Ivermectin [Stromectol] is active against many *nematodes.* Currently, the drug has two approved indications: *onchocerciasis* (a major cause of blindness worldwide) and intestinal *strongyloidiasis.* Ivermectin is active against the tissue microfilariae of *O. volvulus* (the cause of onchocerciasis), but not against the adult form. As discussed in Chapter 100, ivermectin can also be used to kill *mites* and *lice,* although these parasites are not approved targets. In addition to its use in humans, ivermectin is used widely in veterinary medicine.

Mechanism of Action

Ivermectin disrupts nerve traffic and muscle function in target parasites. How? By opening chloride channels on the cell surface, which allows chloride ions to rush into nerve and muscle cells. The resultant hyperpolarization of these cells causes paralysis followed by death. Host cells are not affected because ivermectin is selective for chloride channels in parasites.

Adverse Effect: Mazotti Reaction

The Mazotti reaction occurs in patients treated for *onchocerciasis.* Principal symptoms are pruritus, rash, fever, lymph node tenderness, and bone and joint pain. The apparent cause is an allergic and inflammatory response to the death of microfilariae. Mazotti-type reactions do not occur in patients treated for strongyloidiasis. Abdominal pain and headache are seen in less than 5% of patients. Hypotension develops rarely.

KEY POINTS

- Because each anthelmintic drug is active against a limited range of worms, we must match the drug with the infecting worm.
- Many worm infestations are both asymptomatic and self-limited, and hence drug therapy can be optional. When cost is not an issue, treatment is clearly indicated. However, in countries where funds are limited, preventative public health measures directed at improved hygiene and the elimination of carriers may be more cost-effective than treating each infested individual.
- The drugs discussed in this chapter are generally devoid of serious adverse effects.

Please visit **http://evolve.elsevier.com/Lehne** for chapter-specific NCLEX® examination review questions.

CHAPTER

98 Antiprotozoal Drugs I: Antimalarial Agents

Malaria is a life-threatening parasitic disease caused by protozoa of the genus *Plasmodium.* About 90% of deaths occur in sub-Saharan Africa, almost entirely among young children. In the United States, of the 1500 to 2000 cases reported annually, almost all were acquired outside the country by travelers to countries where malaria is endemic.

Malaria is preventable and curable. Large-scale attempts have been under way for decades to provide education and to eradicate the malarial parasite, as well as the *Anopheles* mosquito that transmits malaria to humans. These programs are now showing evidence of success. The global incidence of malaria fell 21% in the 5 years between 2000 and 2015, and the number of deaths declined by 29%. In fact, from 2000 to 2015 alone, the death rate has been almost cut in half (48%)! More work is still needed, though, because, despite the successes, there were 212 million new cases of malaria and 429,000 deaths in 2015.

One significant event is that progress has been made on a vaccine against malaria. During Phase III clinical trials of RTS,S/AS01 [Mosquirix], an estimated 4 out of 10 malarial cases were prevented, with reductions in the severity of malaria among others. The World Health Organization (WHO) is in the process of implementing a pilot program that targets children aged 5 to 17 months living in Africa. This program will take place from 2017 to 2020. In the meantime, we have a number of antimalarial drugs to treat these infections.

In approaching the antimalarial drugs, we begin by reviewing the life cycle of the malaria parasite. After that we discuss the two major subtypes of malaria: falciparum malaria and vivax malaria. Next, we consider basic principles of treatment, focusing on therapeutic objectives and drug selection. Lastly, we discuss the pharmacology of the antimalarial drugs.

LIFE CYCLE OF THE MALARIA PARASITE

In order to understand the actions and specific applications of antimalarial drugs, we must first understand the life cycle of the malaria parasite. As shown in Fig. 98.1, the cycle takes place in two hosts: humans and the female *Anopheles* mosquito. Asexual reproduction occurs in humans. Sexual reproduction occurs in the mosquito.

The human phase begins when *sporozoites* are injected into the bloodstream by a feeding *Anopheles* mosquito. The sporozoites invade hepatocytes (liver cells), where they either (1) multiply and transform into *merozoites* or (2) transform into *hypnozoites* and lie dormant. The process of merozoite production, which takes 12 to 26 days (depending upon the species of parasite), is referred to as the *pre-erythrocytic* or *exoerythrocytic* phase of the life cycle. Following their release from hepatocytes, merozoites infect erythrocytes. Within the erythrocyte, each parasite differentiates and divides, becoming first a *trophozoite* and then a multinucleated *schizont*. The schizont then evolves into new merozoites. This asexual reproductive process takes 2 to 3 days, after which red blood cells burst, releasing new merozoites into the blood. The new merozoites then infect fresh erythrocytes, establishing an escalating cycle of red cell invasion and lysis. Each time the erythrocytes rupture, they release pyrogenic (fever-inducing) agents, which cause the repeating episodes of fever that characterize malaria.

Sexual reproduction begins with the formation of *gametocytes,* which differentiate from some of the merozoites in red blood cells. After their release from red cells, gametocytes enter a female *Anopheles* mosquito when she ingests blood while feeding. Within the mosquito, the gametocytes differentiate into mature forms, after which fertilization takes place. The resulting zygote then produces sporozoites, thus completing sexual reproduction.

TYPES OF MALARIA

Malaria is caused by four different species of *Plasmodium.* In this chapter, we limit discussion to the two species encountered most: *Plasmodium vivax* and *Plasmodium falciparum.* Malaria caused by either species is characterized by high fever, chills, and profuse sweating. However, despite similarity of symptoms,

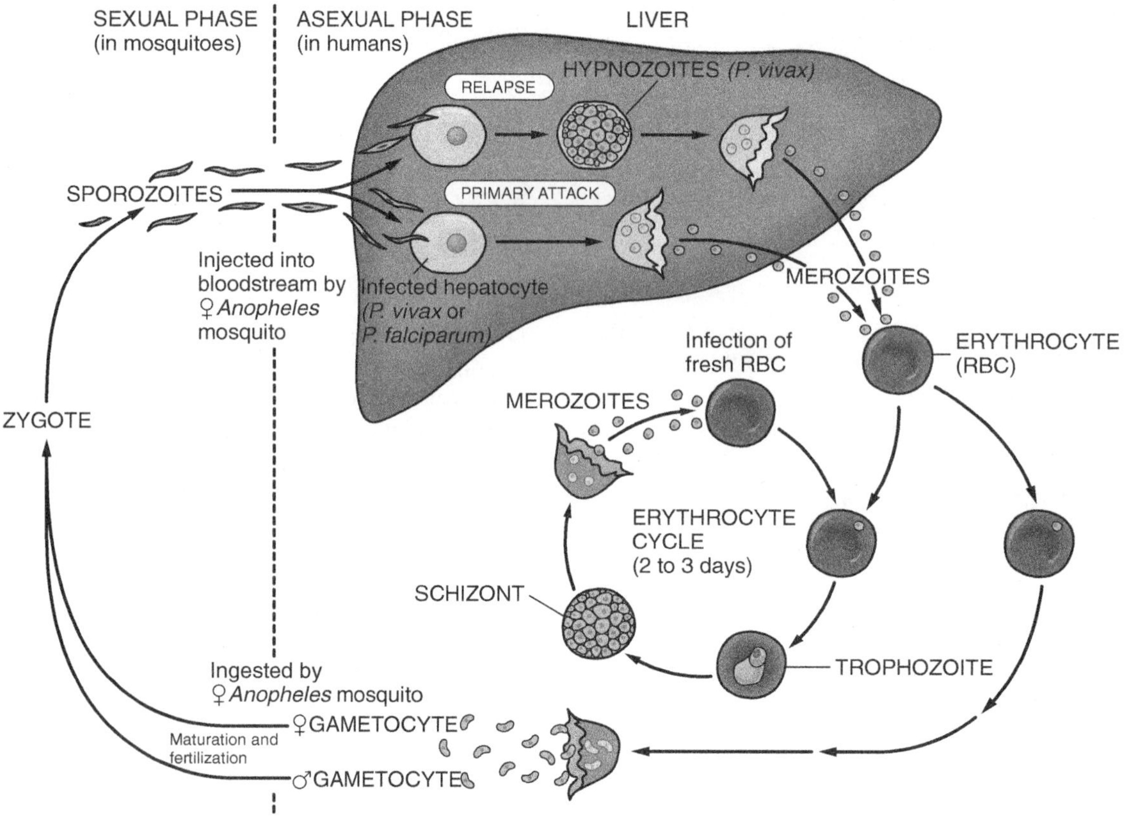

Fig. 98.1 ■ Life cycle of the malaria parasite. (*RBC,* Red blood cell.)

TABLE 98.1 ■ Comparison of Vivax Malaria and Falciparum Malaria

	Type of Malaria	
Characteristics	**Vivax Malaria**	**Falciparum Malaria**
Causative organism	*Plasmodium vivax*	*Plasmodium falciparum*
Frequency of infection	More common	Less common
Latency of symptoms	26 days	12 days
Intensity of symptoms	Mild	Severe
Timing of febrile paroxysms	Every 2 days	Irregular
Probability of relapse	High	None
Drug resistance	Uncommon	Common

these forms of malaria are very different—especially with regard to severity of symptoms, relapse, and drug resistance (Table 98.1).

Vivax Malaria

Vivax malaria, caused by *P. vivax,* is the most common form of malaria. Fortunately, the disease is relatively mild and usually self-limiting. Because drug resistance by *P. vivax* is relatively uncommon, symptoms can be readily suppressed with medication.

Infection begins when the host is inoculated with *P. vivax* sporozoites. After 26 days, merozoites emerge from hepatocytes and begin their attack on erythrocytes. Symptoms of malaria (e.g., chills, fever, sweating) commence as infected erythrocytes rupture, releasing pyrogens and other substances into the blood. Symptoms peak, decline, and peak again every 48 hours in response to cyclic reinfection and red cell lysis. This cycle continues until terminated by drugs or by acquired immunity. Unfortunately, relapse is likely following termination of the acute attack, because dormant parasites (hypnozoites) remain in the liver. Periodically, these hypnozoites evolve into merozoites, undergo release into the blood, and start the erythrocytic cycle anew. Relapse becomes less frequent with the passage of time, and after 2 or more years, it ceases entirely. Relapse can be stopped with drugs that kill hypnozoites.

Falciparum Malaria

Malaria caused by *P. falciparum* is less common than malaria caused by *P. vivax,* but is much more severe. In the absence of treatment, the disease kills about 10% of its victims. Making matters worse, many strains of *P. falciparum* are now drug resistant. Unlike the symptoms of vivax malaria, which peak every 48 hours, symptoms of falciparum malaria occur at irregular intervals. The erythrocytic cycle of *P. falciparum* can destroy up to 60% of circulating red blood cells, resulting in profound anemia and weakness. The hemoglobin released from these cells causes the urine to darken, giving rise to the term *black-water fever.* Falciparum malaria can produce serious complications, including pulmonary edema, hypoglycemia, and toxic encephalopathy, characterized by confusion, coma, and convulsions. When treated immediately, falciparum malaria usually responds well. However, if treatment is delayed by as little as 1 or 2 days, the disease may progress rapidly to irreversible shock and death. In contrast to infection with *P. vivax,* infection with *P. falciparum* does *not relapse,* because *P. falciparum* does not form hypnozoites. As a result, once the erythrocytic forms have been eliminated, the patient is parasite free.

PRINCIPLES OF ANTIMALARIAL THERAPY

Therapeutic Objectives

Drug responsiveness of the malaria parasite changes as the parasite goes through its life cycle. The *erythrocytic* forms are killed with relative ease, whereas the *exoerythrocytic* (hepatic) forms are much harder to kill—and *sporozoites* do not respond to drugs at all. Because of these differences, antimalarial therapy has three separate objectives: (1) treatment of an acute attack (clinical cure), (2) prevention of relapse (radical cure), and (3) prophylaxis (suppressive therapy). Because sporozoites are insensitive to available drugs, drugs cannot prevent primary infection of the liver.

Treatment of an Acute Attack

Clinical cure is accomplished with drugs that are active against erythrocytic forms of the malaria parasite. By eliminating parasites from red blood cells, the erythrocytic cycle is stopped, and symptoms cease. For patients with vivax malaria, clinical cure will not prevent relapse because hypnozoites remain in the liver. However, for patients with falciparum malaria, successful treatment of the acute attack prevents further episodes (until reinfection occurs).

Prevention of Relapse

People infected with *P. vivax* harbor dormant parasites in the liver. In order to prevent relapse, a drug that can kill these hepatic forms must be taken. The use of drugs to eradicate hepatic *P. vivax* is referred to as *radical cure.* Because reinfection by a mosquito bite is a virtual certainty as long as one remains in a malaria-endemic region, radical cure is often postponed until departure from the area.

Prophylaxis

Persons anticipating travel to an area where malaria is endemic should take antimalarial medication for prophylaxis. Although drugs cannot prevent primary infection of the liver, they *can* prevent infection of erythrocytes. Therefore, although the parasite may be present, symptoms are avoided. Because prophylactic treatment prevents only symptoms but not invasion of the liver, such treatment is often referred to as *suppressive therapy.*

Nondrug measures can help greatly to prevent infection. Because *Anopheles* mosquitoes bite only between dusk and dawn, clothing that covers as much skin as possible should be worn during this time. A diethyltoluamide (DEET)–containing insect repellent should be applied to skin that remains exposed. Sleeping under mosquito netting that has been impregnated with an insecticide (e.g., permethrin) further reduces the risk of a bite.

Drug Selection

Selection of antimalarial drugs is based largely on two factors: (1) the goal of treatment and (2) drug resistance of the causative strain of *Plasmodium.* Drugs of choice for treatment and prophylaxis are discussed next and shown in Table 98.2.

TABLE 98.2 ▪ Drugs of Choice for Malaria[a]

	Plasmodium falciparum		*Plasmodium vivax*	
Therapeutic Objective	**Chloroquine Sensitive**	**Chloroquine Resistant**	**Chloroquine Sensitive**	**Chloroquine Resistant**
Treatment of a *moderate* attack	Chloroquine	Atovaquone/proguanil *or* Artemether/lumefantrine *or* Quinine *plus either* doxycycline, tetracycline, or clindamycin	Chloroquine	Atovaquone/proguanil *plus* primaquine *or* Artemether/lumefantrine *plus* primaquine *or* Quinine *plus either* doxycycline, tetracycline, or clindamycin *plus* primaquine *or* Mefloquine *plus* primaquine
Treatment of a *severe* attack by *P. vivax* or *P. falciparum*	Intravenous quinidine gluconate *plus either* doxycycline, tetracycline, or clindamycin *or* Intravenous artesunate[b] followed by *either* atovaquone/proguanil, doxycycline, or mefloquine			
Relapse prevention	NA	NA	Primaquine	Primaquine
Prophylaxis	Chloroquine	Atovaquone/proguanil, doxycycline, or mefloquine	Chloroquine	Atovaquone/proguanil, doxycycline, or mefloquine

[a]All drugs are given orally except where noted otherwise.
[b]Artesunate is available from the Centers for Disease Control and Prevention.
NA, Not applicable.

Treatment of Acute Attacks

For *mild to moderate* malaria, *oral* therapy is employed. Chloroquine is the drug of choice for an acute attack caused by chloroquine-sensitive strains of *P. falciparum* or *P. vivax*. As a rule, a 3-day course of treatment produces clinical cure. For strains of *P. falciparum* or *P. vivax* that are chloroquine resistant, quinine combined with doxycycline, tetracycline, or clindamycin may be administered. Malarone, a fixed-dose combination of atovaquone plus proguanil, is another effective alternative. Mefloquine may also be used, but is considered less desirable, owing to concerns about neuropsychiatric effects.

For *severe* malaria caused by *P. falciparum* or *P. vivax, parenteral* therapy is required. In the United States, only one drug—quinidine gluconate—is approved by the U.S. Food and Drug Administration (FDA) for parenteral use in malaria. When used for severe malaria, IV quinidine should be combined with doxycycline, tetracycline, or clindamycin. An alternative to quinidine, known as artesunate, is recommended by the World Health Organization. Artesunate is not commercially available in the United States, but it can be obtained by request from the Centers for Disease Control and Prevention (CDC).

Prevention of Relapse

The agent of choice for preventing relapse of vivax malaria is primaquine, a drug that is highly active against the hepatic forms of *P. vivax*. For falciparum malaria, no treatment is needed, because relapse does not occur following clinical cure.

Prophylaxis

Selection of drugs for prophylaxis is based on the drug sensitivity of the plasmodial species found in the region to which travel is intended. In regions where chloroquine-sensitive strains are endemic, chloroquine is the preferred drug for prophylaxis. In regions of chloroquine resistance, mefloquine, doxycycline, or atovaquone/proguanil may be used. Recommendations regarding preferred drugs for prophylaxis in specific countries are available at www.cdc.gov/malaria/travelers/index.html.

TABLE 98.3 ▪ Activity of Antimalarial Drugs Against Hepatic and Erythrocytic Stages of the Malaria Parasite

Antimalarial Drugs		Target Malarial Stage	
Generic Name	**Brand Name**	**Hepatic**	**Erythrocytic**
Chloroquine	Aralen ♣	No	Yes
Quinine	Qualaquin	No	Yes
Quinidine gluconate		No	Yes
Mefloquine	Lariam	No	Yes
Artemether/lumefantrine	Coartem	No	Yes
Artesunate		No	Yes
Doxycycline	Vibramycin	No	Yes
Clindamycin	Cleocin	No	Yes
Primaquine		Yes	No
Atovaquone/proguanil	Malarone	Yes	Yes

PHARMACOLOGY OF THE MAJOR ANTIMALARIAL DRUGS

Table 98.3 shows the major antimalarial drugs and their activity against hepatic and erythrocytic stages of the parasite. As indicated, for most of these drugs, activity is limited to the erythrocytic stage of the parasite. Only two preparations—primaquine and atovaquone/proguanil—are active against the hepatic stage.

Chloroquine

Actions and Use

Chloroquine [Aralen ♣] is the most generally useful antimalarial drug. Because of its high activity against erythrocytic forms of the parasite, chloroquine is the drug of choice for mild to moderate acute attacks caused by sensitive strains of *P. vivax* or *P. falciparum*. Chloroquine is also the drug of choice for prophylaxis (suppressive therapy).

Chloroquine is not active against *exoerythrocytic* forms of the malaria parasite. Consequently, the drug is unable to prevent primary infection by *P. vivax* or *P. falciparum*. Nor is it able to prevent relapse of vivax malaria, which is caused by the emergence of dormant hypnozoites.

Several mechanisms have been proposed to explain the lethal effects of chloroquine on erythrocytic malaria parasites. The most likely is that chloroquine prevents the organism from converting heme to nontoxic metabolites. (Heme, a potentially toxic compound, is produced by the parasite as it digests hemoglobin in the host's red blood cells.) Chloroquine concentrates in parasitized erythrocytes, and this may explain the selective actions against erythrocytic forms of *Plasmodium*.

Pharmacokinetics

Chloroquine is rapidly and completely absorbed from the GI tract. A substantial fraction of absorbed drug is deposited in certain tissues, including the lungs, spleen, liver, and kidneys. Slow release from these sites helps maintain therapeutic levels, so chloroquine can be administered just once a week when used for prophylaxis. Excretion is primarily nonrenal.

Adverse Effects

Because the doses required for prophylaxis are low and because the higher doses required for treatment are taken only briefly, chloroquine rarely causes serious adverse effects. When employed to treat an acute attack, chloroquine may cause visual disturbances, pruritus, headache, and GI effects (abdominal discomfort, nausea, diarrhea). Gastrointestinal effects can be minimized by taking the drug with meals. Because chloroquine concentrates in the liver, caution is needed in patients with hepatic disease.

Routes of Administration

Chloroquine may be administered orally or IM. Oral therapy is preferred. Intramuscular administration is employed only when emesis precludes oral treatment or when infection is especially severe.

Preparations, Dosage, and Administration

Drug dosing of chloroquine and other drugs is provided in Table 98.4.

TABLE 98.4 ■ Dosages for Antimalarial Drugs

Drug	Preparation	Dosage
Chloroquine [Aralen]	Tablets: 250, 500 mg	**Treatment of Uncomplicated Malaria** *Adults:* 1 gm initially, then 500 mg at 6, 24, and 48 hr after first dose *Children:* 16.6 mg/kg (up to 1 gm) initially, then 8.3 mg/kg (up to 500 mg) at 6, 24, and 48 hr after first dose **Prophylaxis** Begin 1–2 weeks before traveling and continue for 4 weeks after returning. *Adults:* 500 mg weekly *Children:* 8.3 mg/kg weekly
Primaquine (generic)	Tablets: 26.3 mg	**Treatment of Uncomplicated Malaria** *Adults:* 30 mg daily for 14 days (with chloroquine or hydroxychloroquine) *Children:* 0.5 mg/kg daily for 14 days (with chloroquine or hydroxychloroquine) **Prophylaxis** Begin 1–2 days before traveling and continue for 7 days after returning. *Adults:* 30 mg daily *Children:* 0.5 mg/kg daily
Quinine [Qualaquin]	Capsules: 324 mg	**Treatment of Uncomplicated Malaria** *Adults:* 648 mg every 8 hr for 3 to 7 days (with tetracycline or doxycycline plus primaquine) *Children:* 30 mg/kg/day in divided doses every 8 hr for 3 to 7 days (with tetracycline, doxycycline, or clindamycin if 8 years or older or clindamycin if younger than 8 years)
Mefloquine (generic)	Tablets: 250 mg	**Treatment of Uncomplicated Malaria** *Adults:* 3 tablets initially and 2 tablets 6–12 hr later *Children:* 15 mg/kg, followed 6–12 hr later by 10 mg/kg/dose (maximum total dose: 1250 mg) **Prophylaxis** Begin 1–2 weeks before traveling and continue for 4 weeks after returning. *Adults:* 250 mg weekly *Children:* 5 mg/kg (up to 250 mg) weekly Alternate dosing (manufacturer recommendation): • 20–30 kg: ½ of 250-mg tablet weekly • 30–45 kg: ¾ of 250-mg tablet weekly • >45 kg: 1 250-mg tablet weekly

Lumefantrine [Coartem]	Tablets: artemether 20 mg/lumefantrine 120 mg	**Treatment of Uncomplicated Malaria**
		Adults:
		• 25 to <35 kg (18-tablet regimen):
		  • Day 1: 3 tablets initially and 3 tablets 8 hr later
		  • Days 2 and 3: 3 tablets twice daily
		• ≥35 kg (24-tablet regimen):
		  • Day 1: 4 tablets initially and 4 tablets 8 hr later
		  • Days 2 and 3: 4 tablets twice daily
		Children 2 months to ≤16 years:
		• 5 to <15 kg (6-tablet regimen):
		  • Day 1: 1 tablet initially and 1 tablet 8 hr later
		  • Days 2 and 3: 1 tablet twice daily
		• 15 to <25 kg (12-tablet regimen):
		  • Day 1: 2 tablets initially and 2 tablets 8 hr later
		  • Days 2 and 3: 2 tablets twice daily
		• 25 to <35 kg (18-tablet regimen):
		  • Day 1: 3 tablets initially and 3 tablets 8 hr later
		  • Days 2 and 3: 3 tablets twice daily
		• ≥35 kg (24-tablet regimen):
		  • Day 1: 4 tablets initially and 4 tablets 8 hr later
		  • Days 2 and 3: 4 tablets twice daily

Artesunate	Solution for injection: 110 mg for dilution	**Treatment of Severe Malaria** *Adults:* 2.4 mg/kg IM or IV initially, repeated at 12 hr, 24 hr, and 48 hr after the first dose *Infants and children <20 kg:* 3 mg/kg/dose initially, repeated at 12 hr, 24 hr, and 48 hr after the initial dose *Children and adolescents ≥20 kg:* Same as adult dosing

Continued

TABLE 98.4 ▪ Dosages for Antimalarial Drugs—cont'd

Drug	Preparation	Dosage
Atovaquone/proguanil [Malarone, Malarone Pediatric]	**Tablets:** Pediatric: atovaquone 62.5 mg/proguanil 25 mg Adult: atovaquone 250 mg/proguanil 100 mg	**Treatment of Acute Malaria** *Adult:* 1000 mg/400 mg daily for 3 days *Children:* • 5–8 kg: 125 mg/50 mg daily for 3 days • 9–10 kg: 187.5 mg/75 mg daily for 3 days • 11–20 kg: 250 mg/100 mg daily for 3 days • 21–30 kg: 500 mg/200 mg daily for 3 days • 31–40 kg: 750 mg/300 mg daily for 3 days • >40 kg: 1000 mg/400 mg daily for 3 days **Prophylaxis** Begin 1–2 days before traveling and continue for 7 days after returning. *Adult:* 250 mg/100 mg orally once daily *Children:* • 5–8 kg: 31.25 mg/12.5 mg • 9–10 kg: 46.8 mg/18.75 mg • 11–20 kg: 62.5 mg/25 mg • 21–30 kg: 125 mg/50 mg • 31–40 kg: 187.5 mg/75 mg • >40 kg: 250 mg/100 mg
Tetracycline (generic)	Capsules: 250, 500 mg	**Treatment of Uncomplicated Malaria** *Adults:* 250 mg every 6 hr for 7 days (with quinine) *Children 8 years and older:* 25 mg/kg/day in divided doses every 6 hr for 7 days (with quinine) **Treatment of Severe Malaria** *Adults:* 250 mg every 6 hr for 7 days (with quinidine) *Children 8 years and older:* 25 mg/kg/day (up to 250 mg) in divided doses every 6 hr for 7 days (with quinidine)
Doxycycline [Acticlate, Adoxa, Doryx, Doryx MPC, Doxy 100, Mondoxyne NL, Monodox, Morgidox, TargaDOX, Vibramycin, Apprilon, Doxycin, Doxytab 🍁]	Capsules and tablets: 50, 75, 100 mg Oral solution: 25 mg/5 mL Oral syrup: 50 mg/5 mL IV solution: 100 mg (reconstituted)	**Treatment of Uncomplicated Malaria** *Adults:* 100 mg every 12 hr for 7 days (with quinine) *Children 8 years and older:* • <45 kg: 2.2 mg/kg (up to 100 mg) every 12 hr for 7 days (with quinine) • ≥45 kg: 100 mg every 12 hr for 7 days (with quinine) **Treatment of Severe Malaria** *Adults:* 100 mg every 12 hr for 7 days (with quinidine) *Children 8 years and older:* • <45 kg: 2.2 mg/kg[a] every 12 hr for 7 days (with quinidine) • ≥45 kg: 100 mg every 12 hr for 7 days (with quinidine) **Prophylaxis** Begin 1–2 days before traveling and continue for 4 weeks after returning. *Adult:* 100 mg daily *Children:* • <45 kg: 2–2.4[a] mg/kg (up to 100 mg) daily • ≥45 kg: 100 mg daily • Older than 8 years and ≥45 kg: same as adult dosing
Clindamycin [Cleocin]	Capsules: 75, 150, 300 mg Oral solution: 75 mg/5 mL Solution for injection: 300 mg/2 mL, 600 mg/4 mL, 900 mg/6 mL IV solution: 300 mg/50 mL, 600 mg/50 mL, 900 mg/50 mL	**Treatment of Uncomplicated Malaria** *Adults and children:* 20 mg/kg/day in 3 divided doses given every 8 hr for 7 days (with quinidine) **Treatment of Severe Malaria** *Adult:* IV: Load: 10 mg/kg IV then 5 mg/kg every 8 hr (with IV quinidine). Convert to oral therapy (clindamycin and quinine) when possible for total clindamycin treatment of 7 days. *Children:* IV: Load: 10 mg/kg IV then 15 mg/kg/day divided every 8 hr (with IV quinidine). Convert to oral therapy (clindamycin and quinine) when possible for total clindamycin treatment of 7 days.

[a]Recommendations vary among manufacturers and expert panels. The Centers for Disease Control and Prevention recommends 2.2 mg/kg.

Primaquine

Actions and Use

Primaquine is highly active against *hepatic* forms of *P. vivax,* but not against erythrocytic forms. The drug is used to eradicate *P. vivax* from the liver, preventing relapse. The mechanism of plasmodial kill has not been determined.

Pharmacokinetics

Primaquine is well absorbed following oral administration. Absorbed drug is rapidly metabolized to products of low antimalarial activity. Metabolites are excreted in the urine.

Adverse Effect: Hemolysis

The most serious and frequent effect is hemolysis, which can develop in patients with glucose-6-phosphate dehydrogenase (G6PD) deficiency. This deficiency is an X-linked inherited trait, occurring most commonly in people of African, Mediterranean, Middle Eastern, Southeast Asian, and subcontinental Indian heritage. In the United States, 12% of African-American men are affected. When possible, patients suspected of G6PD deficiency should be screened for the trait before treatment. During primaquine therapy, periodic blood counts should be performed. Also, the urine should be monitored (darkening indicates the presence of hemoglobin). If severe hemolysis develops, primaquine should be discontinued.

Quinine

At one time, quinine [Qualaquin] was the only drug available to treat malaria. Today, quinine has been largely replaced by more effective and less toxic agents (e.g., chloroquine). However, quinine still has an important role: treatment of chloroquine-resistant malaria. Quinine occurs naturally in the bark of the cinchona tree. Commercial preparations are derived from this source.

Actions and Use

Quinine is active against erythrocytic forms of *Plasmodium* but has little effect on sporozoites and hepatic forms. Like chloroquine, quinine concentrates in parasitized red blood cells and may be selective against erythrocytic parasites for this reason. Also like chloroquine, quinine kills plasmodia by causing heme to accumulate within the parasites.

The principal application of quinine is malaria caused by chloroquine-resistant *P. falciparum.* Because quinine is not highly active, adjunctive therapy with another agent is required. Recommended adjuncts are doxycycline, tetracycline, and clindamycin.

Pharmacokinetics

Quinine is well absorbed from the GI tract, even in patients with diarrhea. The drug undergoes hepatic metabolism followed by excretion in the urine. Plasma levels of quinine fall rapidly after stopping treatment.

Adverse Effects

At usual therapeutic doses, quinine frequently causes mild *cinchonism,* a syndrome characterized by tinnitus (ringing in the ears), headache, visual disturbances, nausea, and diarrhea. The prescriber should be notified if these symptoms develop. Because of its adverse effects on vision and hearing, quinine is contraindicated for patients with optic neuritis or tinnitus.

Like primaquine, quinine can cause *hemolysis* in patients with G6PD deficiency, so it is contraindicated for these people. All patients using the drug should be monitored for hemolytic anemia.

Quinine has *quinidine-like effects on the heart* and must be used cautiously in patients with atrial fibrillation. By enhancing atrioventricular conduction, quinine can increase passage of atrial impulses to the ventricles, causing a dangerous increase in ventricular rate.

Quinine can cause profound *hypoglycemia.* The mechanism is stimulation of pancreatic beta cells, which causes hyperinsulinemia. Quinine-induced hypoglycemia can be difficult to treat, even with glucose infusions.

Use in Pregnancy

Quinine was originally contraindicated for pregnant women because auditory nerve damage had caused deafness in infants born to these mothers. We now know that this occurred only at high doses; at therapeutic doses, quinine is considered safe for pregnant women.

Quinidine Gluconate

Quinidine gluconate is the only drug approved by the FDA for parenteral therapy of malaria.[a] As a result, IV quinidine gluconate is the treatment of choice for severe malaria in the United States. Quinidine is the dextroisomer of quinine and shares that drug's antimalarial mechanism and adverse effects. Because severe malaria can rapidly prove fatal, IV quinidine gluconate should be started immediately. The regimen for adults and children consists of a loading dose (10 mg/kg infused over 1 to 2 hours) followed by a continuous infusion (0.02 mg/kg/min) for at least 24 hours, followed in turn by a switch to oral quinine when the patient can tolerate oral therapy. To enhance antiplasmodial effects, both IV quinidine and PO quinine should be accompanied by doxycycline, tetracycline, or clindamycin.

Intravenous administration may cause *hypotension* and *acute circulatory failure.* To minimize risk, IV quinine should be diluted and injected slowly. Patients should be switched to oral medication as soon as possible. Intravenous quinidine is more cardiotoxic than quinine. Accordingly, patients require continuous electrocardiographic monitoring and frequent monitoring of blood pressure. The risk of cardiotoxicity is increased by bradycardia and by low levels of potassium or magnesium. The infusion should be temporarily slowed if there is significant widening of the QRS complex or prolongation of the QT interval.

Quinidine may not be immediately available. Many hospitals no longer keep the drug on hand because (1) severe malaria is extremely rare in the United States and (2) there are preferred agents for treating dysrhythmias, the only other use for IV quinidine gluconate (see Chapter 49). In places where the drug is unavailable, a rapid shipment can be arranged with the manufacturer (Eli Lilly).

---

[a]Another drug—artesunate—is available from the CDC for IV therapy of malaria, but it is not yet approved by the FDA.

PATIENT-CENTERED CARE ACROSS THE LIFE SPAN

Considerations for Antimalarial Drugs

Life Stage	Patient Care Concerns
Children	Children are at the greatest risk for death from malaria. Pediatric dosing is available for all medications except for tetracyclines, which are contraindicated for children younger than 8 years.
Pregnant women	Safety studies in pregnancy are lacking for some drugs. When making decisions, it is important to consider that pregnancies may be as greatly at risk from malaria as from drugs. Drugs considered likely to be safe for pregnant women are chloroquine, quinine, and mefloquine. Animal studies with atovaquone/proguanil have not demonstrated adverse effects; however, for safety reasons, it should not be used for *prophylaxis* in pregnant women. The World Health Organization recommends withholding artemisinin derivatives during the first trimester, when organogenesis is taking place because safety remains unknown. Primaquine is not recommended because of potential G6PD deficiency in the fetus. Tetracyclines are contraindicated because they can affect bone growth and can stain developing teeth.
Breast-feeding women	Safety data are unknown for most of these drugs. We know that quinine, artesunate, and mefloquine are excreted in small amounts not likely to be harmful. Mothers taking atovaquone/proguanil should not breast-feed infants weighing less than 5 kg because proguanil is excreted into breast milk. Primaquine is deemed safe if the nursing infant is tested for and found not to have G6PD deficiency. The amount of drug (if any) excreted into breast milk for artemisinin derivatives is unknown. The risks of potential adverse effects to the infant should guide decisions regarding whether to stop breast-feeding. Quinidine is excreted into milk at levels only slightly less than those in maternal plasma; the manufacturer recommends that mothers avoid breast-feeding.
Older adults	There are no specific contraindications for older adults. Some adverse effects are significant and may be detrimental for this population. The benefits of therapy, and the risks of not obtaining adequate therapy, must be weighed against the ability of a drug to induce harm in this vulnerable population.

Mefloquine

Actions and Uses

Mefloquine kills erythrocytic forms of *P. vivax* and *P. falciparum.* The mechanism of action has not been determined, but may be like that of chloroquine. Mefloquine is a drug of choice for prophylaxis of malaria in regions where chloroquine-resistant *P. falciparum* or *P. vivax* is found. The drug is also used to treat acute attacks by these parasites, although neuropsychiatric effects make it a second-choice agent. Resistance to mefloquine, by an unknown mechanism, may develop quickly.

Pharmacokinetics

Mefloquine is well absorbed following oral administration. The drug undergoes metabolism by hepatic CYP3A4, followed by excretion in the bile and feces. Mefloquine has a prolonged half-life, ranging from 1 to 4 weeks.

Adverse Effects

Adverse effects are dose related. At the low doses employed for prophylaxis, reactions are generally mild (nausea, dizziness, syncope). However, at the higher doses used to treat an acute attack, more intense reactions may occur, including GI disturbances, nightmares, altered vision, and headache. Some of these effects may be indistinguishable from symptoms of malaria.

Mefloquine can prolong the QT interval and may pose a risk of *severe cardiac dysrhythmias.* Accordingly, the drug should be avoided by patients with dysrhythmias or QT prolongation.

Toxicity to the central nervous system is a concern. Mefloquine can cause vertigo, confusion, psychosis, and convulsions. The incidence of these neuropsychiatric effects is about 1 in 13,000 at the low doses used for prophylaxis, but increases to 1 in 250 at the doses used for an ongoing attack. High-dose mefloquine should be avoided by people with epilepsy or psychiatric disorders. Patients who develop psychiatric symptoms (hallucinations, depression, suicidal ideation) should discontinue the drug immediately and contact their prescriber for a substitute (e.g., quinine plus doxycycline, atovaquone/proguanil).

Drug Interactions

Ketoconazole, a strong *inhibitor* of CYP3A4, can increase levels of mefloquine, increasing the risk of dysrhythmias from QT prolongation. Accordingly, ketoconazole should not be administered with mefloquine, or within 15 days of stopping mefloquine.

Rifampin, a strong *inducer* of CYP3A4, can reduce levels of mefloquine. Therapeutic failure could result. Increased dosage of mefloquine may be required.

Artemisinin Derivatives

Artemisinin—obtained by extraction from the sweet wormwood plant, *Artemisia annua*—is highly active against malarial parasites. In fact, artemisinin and its derivatives (e.g., artemether, artesunate) are the most effective drugs we have for treating multidrug-resistant falciparum malaria. Although artemisinin derivatives have been used around the world for years, it was not until 2009 that one of these agents—artemether (in combination with lumefantrine)—was approved for use in the United States.

Artemether/Lumefantrine

Indications and Efficacy. The combination of artemether (20 mg) and lumefantrine (120 mg), sold as *Coartem,* is indicated for oral therapy of uncomplicated falciparum malaria.

The combination is not approved for prophylaxis of falciparum malaria, for treatment of severe falciparum malaria, or for prophylaxis or treatment of vivax malaria. Both artemether and lumefantrine can kill erythrocytic forms of the malarial parasite, but these drugs cannot kill primary or latent hepatic forms. In clinical trials, artemether/lumefantrine has been highly effective against falciparum malaria: 28 days after a short course of treatment, the cure rate is more than 95%, even against multidrug-resistant *P. falciparum.* Efficacy against *P. vivax* is less dramatic.

Mechanism of Action. To be effective, *artemether* must undergo conversion to an active metabolite—*dihydroartemisinin*—which appears to kill plasmodia by releasing free radicals that attack the cell membrane. Kill also requires a high concentration of iron, as found in red blood cells. *Lumefantrine* probably works like chloroquine, causing death by preventing malaria parasites from converting heme to nontoxic metabolites.

Pharmacokinetics. The kinetics of artemether and lumefantrine differ in three important ways. First, lumefantrine is highly lipophilic, so oral absorption is enhanced by dosing with fatty food. Second, absorption of artemether is relatively rapid (plasma levels peak about 2 hours after dosing), whereas absorption of lumefantrine is delayed (plasma levels peak 6 to 8 hours after dosing). Third, the half-life of artemether is short (1.5 hours), whereas the half-life of lumefantrine is prolonged (100 hours).

Why Do We Combine Artemether With Lumefantrine? Compared with lumefantrine, artemether is much more effective. As a result, when the drugs are administered together, most of the benefit comes from artemether. Why, then, do we combine these drugs? There are two reasons. First, adding lumefantrine *enhances efficacy.* (Because lumefantrine has a much longer half-life than artemether, lumefantrine remains in the body long enough to kill the few parasites not killed by artemether.) Second, adding lumefantrine *helps prevent development of resistance to artemether.* Why? Because the odds of developing resistance to the two drugs simultaneously are much lower than the odds of developing resistance to artemether alone. Accordingly, in 2006 the World Health Organization requested that all drug companies stop selling artemisinin-only products and replace them with *artemisinin combination therapies* (ACTs). Four ACTs are recommended:

- Artemether/lumefantrine [Coartem]
- Artesunate/mefloquine
- Artesunate/amodiaquine
- Artesunate/pyrimethamine/sulfadoxine

These combinations are indicated only for the *treatment* of malaria—*not* for *prophylaxis.*

Adverse Effects. Artemether/lumefantrine is generally well tolerated. Approximately one-third or more of *adults* taking this drug experience adverse effects such as headache, anorexia, dizziness, weakness, joint pain, and muscle pain. Among *children,* the most common adverse effects are fever, cough, vomiting, anorexia, and headache.

Lumefantrine may *prolong the QT interval,* posing a risk of serious dysrhythmias. Accordingly, artemether/lumefantrine should not be used by patients with electrolyte disturbances (e.g., hypokalemia, hypomagnesemia) or congenital prolonged QT syndrome, or by patients using other drugs that prolong the QT interval (e.g., quinine, erythromycin, ketoconazole).

Drug Interactions. Artemether and lumefantrine are metabolized primarily by hepatic CYP3A4. Accordingly, strong inhibitors of CYP3A4 (e.g., ketoconazole) could increase levels of both drugs and might further increase the QT interval.

Lumefantrine inhibits CYP2D6, so it can raise levels of drugs that are substrates for this enzyme. Accordingly, lumefantrine should not be combined with CYP2D6 substrates, especially ones that can cause QT prolongation (e.g., flecainide, imipramine).

Artesunate

Artesunate is an artemisinin derivative with antimalarial actions much like those of artemether. At this time, artesunate, administered IV, is considered the drug of choice for *severe* malaria. Artesunate appears to be more effective than IV quinine and safer than IV quinidine. The recommended regimen is four doses (2.4 mg/kg each) administered at 0, 12, 24, and 48 hours. To enhance efficacy and minimize development of resistance, dosing with an oral drug (e.g., doxycycline, clindamycin, mefloquine) should begin as soon as possible. Artesunate is available only from the CDC and must be used under the provisions of an Investigational New Drug protocol known as *Intravenous Artesunate for Treatment of Severe Malaria in the United States.* The CDC maintains supplies of artesunate in Atlanta and at eight quarantine stations at major airports around the country.

Atovaquone/Proguanil

Activity and Therapeutic Use

The combination of atovaquone plus proguanil, available as *Malarone,* is highly effective for both the prophylaxis and treatment of malaria caused by chloroquine-resistant plasmodia. Both drugs are active against erythrocytic and exoerythrocytic plasmodial forms, including strains that are resistant to chloroquine, mefloquine, and pyrimethamine/sulfadoxine. In addition to its use in malaria, atovaquone, by itself, has been used for *Pneumocystis* pneumonia.

Mechanism of Action

Atovaquone and proguanil disrupt two separate pathways in pyrimidine synthesis, suppressing DNA replication. Atovaquone has a unique mechanism: disruption of mitochondrial electron transport. No other antimalarial drug works this way. Proguanil is inactive as administered, but gets converted to cycloguanil, its active form. Like pyrimethamine, cycloguanil inhibits plasmodial dihydrofolate reductase, preventing activation of folic acid. In the absence of usable folic acid, the parasite is unable to make DNA, RNA, and proteins.

Pharmacokinetics

Absorption of atovaquone is low and variable, but can be greatly enhanced by fatty foods. The drug is 99% bound to plasma proteins, has a prolonged half-life (2 to 3 days), and undergoes excretion unchanged in the feces.

In contrast to atovaquone, proguanil is extensively absorbed, both in the presence and absence of food. The drug concentrates in erythrocytes and undergoes hepatic metabolism followed by renal excretion. Its half-life is 12 to 21 hours.

Adverse Effects and Interactions

The combination of atovaquone plus proguanil is generally well tolerated. When atovaquone is used alone, the principal adverse effect is rash, which occurs in 20% to 40% of patients. Other reactions include nausea, vomiting, diarrhea, headache, fever, and insomnia. When proguanil is used alone, the most common side effects are oral ulceration, GI effects, and headache. In addition, the drug may cause hair loss, urticaria, hematuria, thrombocytopenia, and scaling of the soles and palms. Proguanil appears devoid of significant drug interactions. In contrast, certain drugs, including tetracycline and rifampin, can reduce levels of atovaquone by as much as 50%.

Antibacterial Drugs

Tetracyclines

Two members of the tetracycline family—*doxycycline* and *tetracycline*—are used against chloroquine-resistant malaria. Both drugs kill the erythrocytic forms of the malaria parasite, although the rate of kill is slow. Doxycycline is used for prophylaxis and for acute attacks, whereas tetracycline is used for acute attacks only. To treat acute attacks, these drugs are combined with quinine, which acts more quickly than the tetracyclines. The basic pharmacology of the tetracyclines is presented in Chapter 86.

Clindamycin

Clindamycin is active against the erythrocytic forms of the malaria parasite. The drug is used as an adjunct to quinine to treat malaria caused by chloroquine-resistant *P. falciparum* or *P. vivax*. The principal adverse effect is colitis secondary to overgrowth of the bowel with *Clostridium difficile*.

KEY POINTS

- There are two principal forms of malaria, one caused by *Plasmodium vivax* and the other by *Plasmodium falciparum*.
- Vivax malaria is more common than falciparum malaria, but falciparum malaria is more severe.
- Drug resistance is common with *P. falciparum* but relatively uncommon with *P. vivax*.
- Plasmodia reside in the liver and erythrocytes. Those in the liver are harder to kill.
- Clinical cure of malaria (i.e., elimination of symptoms) results from killing plasmodia in erythrocytes.
- Vivax malaria relapses after clinical cure because hypnozoites remain in the liver. Falciparum malaria does not relapse.
- Most antimalarial drugs are active only against the erythrocytic stage of the parasite.
- Chloroquine is the drug of choice for treatment and prophylaxis of malaria caused by chloroquine-sensitive strains of *P. vivax* and *P. falciparum*.
- Atovaquone/proguanil is a treatment of choice for mild to moderate malaria caused by chloroquine-resistant *P. vivax* or *P. falciparum*.
- Intravenous quinidine (combined with doxycycline, tetracycline, or clindamycin) is the treatment of choice for severe malaria caused by *P. vivax* or *P. falciparum*.
- For prophylaxis of chloroquine-resistant malaria, any of three preparations may be used: atovaquone/proguanil, mefloquine, or doxycycline.
- Primaquine, which kills dormant *P. vivax* in the liver, is the drug of choice for preventing relapse of vivax malaria.
- High therapeutic doses of mefloquine can cause neuropsychiatric reactions, and so should be avoided in patients with epilepsy or psychiatric disorders.
- Artemisinin derivatives, such as artemether and artesunate, are the most effective drugs for treating falciparum malaria.
- To delay emergence of resistance, artemisinin derivatives should always be combined with another antimalarial drug.

Please visit **http://evolve.elsevier.com/Lehne** for chapter-specific NCLEX® examination review questions.

CHAPTER

99 Antiprotozoal Drugs II: Miscellaneous Agents

For two reasons—increased world travel by Americans and increased immigration from regions where infectious protozoa are endemic—the incidence of protozoal infection in the United States is rising. The organisms encountered most frequently are *Entamoeba histolytica, Trichomonas vaginalis,* and *Giardia lamblia* (also known as *G. duodenalis*). Infections with most other protozoa (e.g., *Leishmania* species, trypanosomes) are rare in North America. In approaching the antiprotozoal drugs, we begin with the diseases that protozoa produce and then discuss the drugs used for treatment.

PROTOZOAL INFECTIONS

Our goal in this section is to describe the major protozoal infections, except for malaria, which is the subject of Chapter 98. Discussion focuses on causative organisms, sites of infection, symptoms, and preferred drug therapy. Causative organisms and drugs of choice are shown in Table 99.1.

Amebiasis

Amebiasis is an infestation with *Entamoeba histolytica.* The disease is rare in the United States but is responsible for approximately 100,000 deaths each year worldwide. The principal site of infestation is the intestine. However, amebas may migrate to other tissues, most commonly the liver, where abscesses may form. Amebiasis is usually asymptomatic. When symptoms *are* present, the most characteristic are diarrhea, abdominal pain, and weight loss.

Drugs of choice are *iodoquinol, paromomycin, metronidazole,* and *tinidazole.* Iodoquinol and paromomycin are active only against amebas residing in the intestine. Metronidazole and tinidazole are active against amebas that inhabit the intestine, liver, and all other sites. For patients with asymptomatic intestinal infection, therapy with iodoquinol or paromomycin is sufficient. For patients with severe intestinal disease or with liver abscesses, metronidazole or tinidazole is given initially, followed by either iodoquinol or paromomycin.

Iodoquinol, metronidazole, and tinidazole are discussed later in this chapter. Paromomycin is discussed in Chapter 87.

Cryptosporidiosis

Cryptosporidiosis is caused by *Cryptosporidium parvum,* a protozoan of the subclass Coccidia. *Cryptosporidium parvum* is an obligate intracellular parasite that can infect the intestinal tract of humans, cattle, and other mammals. Transmission is fecal-oral, often by ingesting water contaminated with livestock feces. The infection may also be acquired by animal-to-human contact, person-to-person contact, and ingestion of contaminated fruits or vegetables. Cryptosporidiosis is characterized by diarrhea, abdominal cramps, anorexia, low-grade fever, nausea, and vomiting. For immunocompetent patients, the disease is generally mild and self-limited. However, for those who are severely immunosuppressed (owing to HIV infection, cancer chemotherapy, or other causes), the disease can be prolonged and life threatening, with diarrhea volume up to 20 L/day. Nitazoxanide [Alinia] is the treatment of choice. The drug is very effective in immunocompetent patients, but much less effective in those who are immunosuppressed.

Giardiasis

Giardiasis is an infection with *Giardia lamblia,* also known as *G. duodenalis.* In the United States, giardiasis has a prevalence of 1 in 14,000. Infestation usually occurs by contact with contaminated objects or by drinking contaminated water. The primary habitat of *G. lamblia* is the upper small intestine. Occasionally, organisms migrate to the bile ducts and gallbladder. As many as 50% of affected individuals remain symptom free. However, symptoms that are both unpleasant and uncomfortable can develop. These include profound malaise, heartburn, vomiting, colicky pain after eating, and malodorous belching, flatulence, and diarrhea. The pain associated with giardiasis may mimic that of gallstones, appendicitis, peptic ulcers, or hiatal hernia. Drugs of choice are *metronidazole, tinidazole,* and *nitazoxanide.*

Leishmaniasis

The term *leishmaniasis* refers to infestation by certain protozoal species belonging to the genus *Leishmania.* Worldwide, the incidence of leishmaniasis is estimated at 12 million, with up to 2 million new cases each year. The disease is acquired through the bite of sand flies indigenous to tropical and subtropical regions. In the human host, the parasites take up residence inside cells of the reticuloendothelial system.

Leishmaniasis has three different forms: *cutaneous, mucocutaneous,* and *visceral.* The particular form is determined by the species of *Leishmania* involved. The forms of leishmaniasis vary greatly in severity, ranging from mild (cutaneous leishmaniasis) to potentially fatal (visceral leishmaniasis). In *cutaneous* leishmaniasis, a nodule forms at the site of inoculation; later,

TABLE 99.1 ▪ Drugs of Choice for Protozoal Infection

Disease	Causative Protozoan	Drugs of Choice
Amebiasis	*Entamoeba histolytica*	Iodoquinol, paromomycin, metronidazole, tinidazole
Cryptosporidiosis	*Cryptosporidium parvum*	Nitazoxanide[a]
Giardiasis	*Giardia lamblia*	Metronidazole, tinidazole, nitazoxanide
Leishmaniasis	*Leishmania* species	Liposomal amphotericin B, sodium stibogluconate
Toxoplasmosis	*Toxoplasma gondii*	Pyrimethamine plus either sulfadiazine, clindamycin, or atovaquone
Trichomoniasis	*Trichomonas vaginalis*	Metronidazole, tinidazole
Trypanosomiasis		
American (Chagas' disease)	*Trypanosoma cruzi*	Nifurtimox
West African (sleeping sickness)	*Trypanosoma brucei gambiense*	
Early (hemolymphatic) stage		Pentamidine
Late (CNS) stage		Eflornithine, melarsoprol
East African (sleeping sickness)	*Trypanosoma brucei rhodesiense*	
Early (hemolymphatic) stage		Suramin
Late (CNS) stage		Melarsoprol

[a]Clearly effective in immunocompetent patients, but of little or no benefit in patients with HIV/AIDS.
CNS, Central nervous system.

this nodule may evolve into an ulcer that is very slow to heal. *Mucocutaneous* leishmaniasis is characterized by ulceration in the mucosa of the mouth, nose, and pharynx. Symptoms of *visceral* leishmaniasis include fever, hepatosplenomegaly, liver dysfunction, hypoalbuminemia, pancytopenia, lymphadenopathy, and hemorrhage. Left untreated, visceral disease is frequently fatal. For all forms of leishmaniasis, *sodium stibogluconate* [Pentostam] is the traditional treatment of choice. *Liposomal amphotericin B* (given IV) is an effective alternative approved by the FDA for the treatment of visceral leishmaniasis but not cutaneous or mucosal disease. In 2014, the FDA approved *miltefosine* [Impavido], an oral agent for the treatment of cutaneous, mucosal, and visceral leishmaniasis; however, its effects are species-specific, and there are several species of this organism. The drug appears reasonably safe and, owing to oral administration, is more convenient than stibogluconate or amphotericin B, both of which are given parenterally. Both sodium stibogluconate and miltefosine are available from the Centers for Disease Control and Prevention (CDC) through an investigational drug protocol.

Toxoplasmosis

Toxoplasmosis is caused by infection with *Toxoplasma gondii,* a protozoan of the class Sporozoa. The parasite is harbored by many animals and by humans. Infection is acquired most commonly by eating undercooked meat. However, toxoplasmosis may also be congenital. Congenital infection can damage the brain, eyes, liver, and other organs. Extensive disease is usually fatal. In immunocompetent adults, infection is usually asymptomatic, although it may involve the retina. However, in immunocompromised hosts, such as those with HIV/AIDS, the disease may progress to encephalitis and death. The treatment of choice is *pyrimethamine* plus either *sulfadiazine, clindamycin,* or *atovaquone.*

Trichomoniasis

Trichomoniasis is caused by *Trichomonas vaginalis,* a flagellated protozoan. Trichomoniasis is a common disease, affecting about 170 million people worldwide. In the United States, about 8 million new cases occur annually. The usual site of infestation is the genitourinary tract. Parasites may also inhabit the rectum. In females, infection results in vaginitis. In males, infection causes urethritis. The disease is usually transmitted by direct sexual contact but can also be acquired by contact with contaminated objects (e.g., dildos). *Metronidazole* is the traditional drug of choice. However, *tinidazole* is just as effective and somewhat better tolerated, although more expensive. Trichomoniasis is discussed in Chapter 95.

Trypanosomiasis

There are two major forms of trypanosomiasis: American trypanosomiasis and African trypanosomiasis. Both forms are caused by protozoal species in the genus *Trypanosoma.*

American Trypanosomiasis (Chagas' Disease)

Chagas' disease is caused by infection with *Trypanosoma cruzi,* a flagellated protozoan. The disease is prevalent in South America and the Caribbean, where it affects some 10 million people. In the United States, about 300,000 are affected. The parasites are harbored in the digestive tract of certain blood-sucking bugs and are transmitted as follows: The bug bites and defecates on a sleeping person (usually on the face); the parasites, which are contained in the bug's feces, are then forced into the bite wound by rubbing or scratching. An early sign of the disease is swelling and severe inflammation at the site of inoculation. Over time, parasites invade cardiac cells and neurons of the myenteric plexus. Destruction of these cells can cause cardiomyopathy, megaesophagus, and megacolon. Deaths have occurred, usually secondary to cardiac injury. In its early phase, Chagas' disease can be treated with *nifurtimox* or *benznidazole.* Unfortunately, these drugs are less effective against chronic infection.

African Trypanosomiasis (Sleeping Sickness)

African trypanosomiasis, transmitted by the bite of the tsetse fly, is caused by two subspecies of *Trypanosoma brucei: T. brucei gambiense,* which causes West African sleeping sickness, and *T. brucei rhodesiense,* which causes East African sleeping sickness. Disease caused by either subspecies has similar symptoms. Early symptoms, which involve the hemolymphatic system, include fever, lymphadenopathy, hepatosplenomegaly, dyspnea, and tachycardia. Late symptoms, which result from involvement of the central nervous system (CNS), include mental dullness, incoordination, and apathy. As CNS involvement advances, sleep becomes continuous and death may eventually follow. During the early (hemolymphatic) phase of African trypanosomiasis, *pentamidine* and *suramin* are the drugs of choice. (Pentamidine is preferred for disease caused by *T. brucei gambiense,* and suramin is preferred for disease caused by *T. brucei rhodesiense.*) During the late (CNS) stage, *melarsoprol* and *eflornithine* are drugs of choice. (Either drug can be used against *T. brucei gambiense,* but only melarsoprol is preferred for *T. brucei rhodesiense.*) All four drugs—pentamidine, suramin, eflornithine, and melarsoprol—can produce serious side effects. Treatment is difficult and frequently unsuccessful. Suramin, eflornithine, and melarsoprol are available only from the CDC.

DRUGS OF CHOICE FOR PROTOZOAL INFECTIONS

Iodoquinol

Iodoquinol [Yodoxin] is a drug of choice for asymptomatic intestinal amebiasis. In addition, the drug is employed in conjunction with metronidazole to treat symptomatic intestinal infection and systemic amebiasis. In these last two cases, iodoquinol is administered to eliminate any surviving intestinal parasites after treatment with metronidazole. Very little iodoquinol is absorbed, and hence the drug is not active against systemic amebiasis.

Iodoquinol is generally well tolerated. Mild reactions occur occasionally. These include rash, acne, slight thyroid enlargement, and GI effects (nausea, vomiting, diarrhea, cramps, pruritus ani). Rarely, prolonged therapy at very high doses has caused optic atrophy with permanent loss of vision.

Iodoquinol [Yodoxin] is available in tablets (210 and 650 mg) for oral administration, preferably after a meal. The usual adult dosage is 650 mg 3 times a day for 20 days. The dosage for children is 30 to 40 mg/kg/day (given in three divided doses) for 20 days.

Metronidazole

Metronidazole [Flagyl], a drug in the nitroimidazole family, is active against several protozoal species, including *E. histolytica, G. lamblia,* and *T. vaginalis.* The drug is also active against anaerobic bacteria (see Chapter 91).

Therapeutic Uses

Metronidazole is a drug of choice for *symptomatic intestinal amebiasis* and *systemic amebiasis.* Because most of each dose is absorbed in the small intestine, metronidazole concentrations in the colon remain low, allowing amebas there to survive. To kill these survivors, metronidazole is followed by either iodoquinol or paromomycin, amebicidal drugs that achieve high concentrations in the colon.

Metronidazole is a drug of choice for *giardiasis* and for *trichomoniasis* in males as well as females.

Mechanism of Action

Metronidazole is a prodrug that remains harmless until converted to a more chemically reactive form, which occurs only in *anaerobic* cells. Because mammalian cells are *aerobic,* they cannot activate the drug and hence are largely spared. How does activated metronidazole work? It interacts with DNA, causing strand breakage and loss of helical structure. The resulting impairment of DNA function is thought to be responsible for the drug's antimicrobial and mutagenic actions.

Pharmacokinetics

Metronidazole may be given PO or IV. Blood levels are similar with both routes. Following oral administration, metronidazole is rapidly absorbed and undergoes widespread distribution. The drug crosses membranes with ease, including those of the placenta and the blood-brain barrier. As a result, drug levels in cerebrospinal fluid, saliva, and breast milk equal those in plasma. Extensive metabolism occurs in the liver. Metabolites and unchanged drug are excreted in the urine. The half-life is 8 hours.

Adverse Effects

Metronidazole produces a variety of untoward effects, but these rarely require termination of treatment. The most common side effects are nausea, headache, dry mouth, and an unpleasant metallic taste. Other common effects include stomatitis, vomiting, diarrhea, insomnia, vertigo, and weakness. Harmless darkening of the urine may occur, and patients should be forewarned. Carcinogenic effects have been observed in rodents, but there is no evidence of cancer in humans.

Metronidazole can cause *hypersensitivity* reactions, including potentially fatal Stevens-Johnson syndrome. There is cross-reactivity with tinidazole, another member of the nitroimidazole family.

Rarely, metronidazole may cause *neurologic* injury. Some patients have developed convulsive seizures or peripheral neuropathy, characterized by numbness or paresthesia of an extremity. More recently, there have been reports of encephalopathy and aseptic meningitis. If any of these neurologic conditions develop, metronidazole should be withdrawn. In most cases, symptoms quickly resolve.

Drug Interactions

Alcohol and Disulfiram. Metronidazole has disulfiram-like actions, so it can produce unpleasant or dangerous effects if used in conjunction with alcohol. Accordingly, patients must be warned against consuming alcoholic beverages or any product that contains alcohol. The combination of metronidazole with disulfiram itself can cause a psychotic reaction, and hence must be avoided.

Warfarin. Metronidazole inhibits the inactivation of warfarin, an anticoagulant. Dosage of warfarin may need to be reduced during metronidazole therapy and for 8 days after.

Phenytoin, Lithium, Fluorouracil, Cyclosporine, and Tacrolimus. Metronidazole can increase levels of these drugs. Patients should be monitored for signs of toxicity.

Cholestyramine. Cholestyramine can bind with metronidazole in the GI tract and thereby reduce metronidazole absorption by 20%. Dosing with these drugs should be separated.

Drugs That Affect CYP3A4. Because metronidazole is a substrate for CYP3A4 (the 3A4 isoenzyme of cytochrome P450), agents that induce the enzyme (e.g., phenobarbital, rifampin, phenytoin) can reduce levels of metronidazole, and agents that inhibit the enzyme (e.g., ketoconazole) can increase levels of metronidazole.

Preparations, Dosage, and Administration

For treatment of protozoal infections, metronidazole is available in three oral formulations: capsules (375 mg), immediate-release tablets (250 and 500 mg), and extended-release tablets (750 mg). Dosages are as follows:

- *Amebiasis (symptomatic)—adults,* 500 to 750 mg 3 times a day for 7 to 10 days; *children,* 35 to 50 mg/kg/day in three divided doses for 7 to 10 days. Following treatment with metronidazole, patients are given either iodoquinol for 20 days or paromomycin for 7 days.
- *Trichomoniasis—adults,* 250 mg every 8 hours for 7 days *or* 375 mg twice daily for 7 days *or* 2 gm as a single dose *or* 1 gm twice daily for 2 doses given on same day; *children,* 15 to 30 mg/kg/day in three divided doses administered every 8 hours for 7 days.
- *Giardiasis—adults,* 500 mg twice daily for 5 to 7 days; *children,* 5 mg/kg 3 times a day for 5 to 7 days.

Tinidazole

Tinidazole [Tindamax] is an antiprotozoal drug similar to metronidazole. Both agents are nitroimidazoles, and both have similar actions, indications, interactions, and adverse effects. Tinidazole has a longer half-life than metronidazole, so dosing is more convenient (it's done less often). However, tinidazole is much more expensive. Tinidazole was approved by the U.S. Food and Drug Administration (FDA) in 2004, but has been available in other countries for decades.

Therapeutic Uses

Tinidazole is indicated for trichomoniasis in adults, and for giardiasis, intestinal amebiasis, and amebic liver abscesses in adults and children over 3 years of age. Like metronidazole, tinidazole is considered a drug of choice for all of these infections.

Mechanism of Action

Tinidazole has the same mechanism as metronidazole. Both drugs enter anaerobic cells, undergo conversion to a more reactive form, and then interact with DNA to cause strand breakage and loss of helical structure.

Pharmacokinetics

Tinidazole is administered by mouth, and absorption is rapid and complete. Food decreases the rate of absorption but not the extent. Tinidazole crosses membranes with ease, and hence is distributed to virtually all tissues and body fluids. The drug crosses the blood-brain barrier and the placental barrier, and also enters breast milk. Tinidazole is metabolized in the liver by CYP3A4. Excretion is via the bile and urine. Tinidazole has a half-life of 12 to 14 hours, nearly twice that of metronidazole.

Adverse Effects

Adverse effects are much like those of metronidazole, although tinidazole is better tolerated. Gastrointestinal (GI) effects—metallic taste, stomatitis, anorexia, dyspepsia, nausea, vomiting—are most common.

Like metronidazole, tinidazole carries a small risk for seizures and peripheral neuropathy. If abnormal neurologic signs develop, tinidazole should be immediately withdrawn. In patients with existing CNS disease, tinidazole should be used with caution.

Like metronidazole, tinidazole can cause hypersensitivity reactions, including potentially fatal Stevens-Johnson syndrome. There is cross-reactivity with metronidazole.

PATIENT-CENTERED CARE ACROSS THE LIFE SPAN

Selected Antiprotozoal Drugs

Life Stage	Patient Care Concerns
Children	Most of the drugs in this chapter are administered to children, even though safety may not be established, because the benefits exceed the risks. An exception is miltefosine, which is not FDA-approved for children younger than 12 years. The FDA also has not approved eflornithine for use in children; however, the WHO recommends its use. Suramin should be considered only if alternative drugs are unavailable or if therapy with other drugs is ineffective.
Pregnant women	Safety has not been established for many of these drugs (e.g., iodoquinol, eflornithine, and pentamidine); therefore, it is important to weigh benefits against risks. Guidance has been provided for the following drugs: HHS recommends that nitazoxanide be used after the first trimester if symptoms are severe. The World Health Organization recommends deferring treatment with melarsoprol until after delivery, not because of known problems, but because effects on the developing fetus are not yet known. Drugs contraindicated during pregnancy are benznidazole, nifurtimox, tinidazole, miltefosine, and suramin. Of these, suramin is associated with 64% fetal mortality and those who live typically have congenital anomalies. Similarly, miltefosine is both teratogenic and fetolethal; effective contraception is essential during treatment and for 2 months afterward. Pyrimethamine is associated with adverse events in animal reproduction studies. Folic acid supplementation is advised if necessary during pregnancy. Spontaneous abortion has occurred with the use of sodium stibogluconate; however, untreated leishmaniasis is also associated with spontaneous abortion. Liposomal amphotericin B, nitazoxanide, and metronidazole are categorized as Pregnancy Risk Category B[a] because no abnormalities have been determined from animal studies. However, there have been anecdotal reports of cleft lip following administration during the first trimester for women taking metronidazole, so the manufacturer recommends avoidance during the first 3 months of pregnancy.
Breast-feeding women	Studies regarding safety with breast-feeding have not been performed for most of these drugs; therefore, it is necessary to weigh the possibility of adverse effects passed on to the infant against the benefits of breast-feeding. Guidance is provided for the following drugs: The manufacturer of pentamidine recommends discontinuing breast-feeding; however, the WHO states that the drug is compatible with breast-feeding. Miltefosine is contraindicated for breast-feeding patients. Metronidazole and its active metabolite are excreted in breast milk in concentrations approximating that in maternal plasma. The CDC recommends not breast-feeding until 12 to 24 hours after a dose of metronidazole. (Although the drug continues to be excreted in breast milk up to 72 hours after dosing, the amount remaining after 24 hours is insignificant.) Tinidazole can be detected in breast milk up to 72 hours after administration. Mothers should not breast-feed while taking the drug and for 3 days after.
Older adults	Inadequate studies have been conducted in older populations. It is important to compare benefits and risks, particularly those risks relative to any chronic health problems older patients may have. There are special concerns for older adults taking the following drugs: Miltefosine can decrease platelets, leading to bleeding tendencies. GI and renal effects may have greater concerns for older patients. Eflornithine can impair renal function and initiate cardiac dysrhythmias, thus presenting problems for patients with kidney and heart conditions. It can also cause myelosuppression, seizures, and hearing loss. Fluid overload may compromise underlying cardiac, pulmonary, and renal problems. Suramin is contraindicated for patients with renal or hepatic impairment. It is associated with serious adverse effects, including shock, loss of consciousness, and nephrotoxicity. Melarsoprol can cause hypertension, cardiac dysrhythmias, myocardial injury, albuminuria, peripheral neuropathy, and paraplegia. Encephalopathy develops in 10% of patients and carries a 50% risk for death for those who acquire this condition. Nifurtimox has adverse effects that can be detrimental to older patients, including CNS effects that create a fall risk (dizziness, mood changes, insomnia, disorientation). Severe gastrointestinal disturbance and weight loss increase a risk for weakness and nutritional deficits. Pentamidine can cause long QT syndrome and severe hypotension, making it dangerous for patients with cardiac conditions. Patients with renal or hepatic impairment are also at increased risk.

[a]As of 2020, the FDA will no longer use Pregnancy Risk Categories. Please refer to Chapter 9 for more information.
FDA, U.S. Food and Drug Administration; *HHS,* U.S. Department of Health and Human Services; *WHO,* World Health Organization.

Drug Interactions

No studies on the interactions of tinidazole with other drugs have been conducted. However, because tinidazole and metronidazole have similar structures and because both are metabolized by CYP3A4, the interactions that occur with metronidazole are likely to occur with tinidazole. Accordingly, tinidazole is likely to potentiate the effects of warfarin, lithium, fluorouracil, cyclosporine, tacrolimus, and injectable phenytoin. Cholestyramine may decrease the absorption of tinidazole, and oxytetracycline may antagonize the effects of tinidazole. Because tinidazole is a substrate for CYP3A4, inducers of the enzyme may reduce the effects of tinidazole, and inhibitors may increase the effects of tinidazole. Like metronidazole, tinidazole has disulfiram-like actions, so patients taking this drug should not consume disulfiram, alcoholic beverages, or any product that contains alcohol.

Preparations, Dosage, and Administration

Tinidazole [Tindamax] is available in 250- and 500-mg tablets. For patients unable to swallow tablets whole, the tablets may be crushed and mixed with cherry syrup. To minimize GI distress, tinidazole should be taken with food. Dosages are as follows:

- *Trichomoniasis—adults,* 2 gm once; *children age 3 years and older,* 50 mg/kg (max. 2 gm) once
- *Giardiasis—adults,* 2 gm once; *children age 3 years and older,* 50 mg/kg (max. 2 gm) once
- *Intestinal amebiasis—adults,* 2 gm once daily for 3 days; *children age 3 years and older,* 50 mg/kg (max. 2 gm) once daily for 3 days
- *Amebic liver abscess—adults,* 2 gm once daily for 5 days; *children age 3 years and older,* 50 mg/kg (max. 2 gm) once daily for 5 days

Benznidazole

Benznidazole, a relative of metronidazole and tinidazole, is a drug of choice for Chagas' disease. The adult dosage is 2.5 to 3.5 mg/kg twice daily, and the pediatric dosage is 5 mg/kg twice daily. For adults and children, the duration of treatment is 30 to 90 days. At this time, benznidazole is not available in the United States.

Nitazoxanide

Therapeutic Uses

Nitazoxanide [Alinia] is approved for diarrhea caused by *C. parvum* (in children only) and for diarrhea caused by *G. lamblia* (in children and adults). Although we have other effective drugs for giardiasis (e.g., metronidazole, tinidazole), nitazoxanide is our first effective drug for cryptosporidiosis. Unfortunately, when used for *C. parvum* infections, nitazoxanide is effective only in children who are immunocompetent; among children who are immunosuppressed, the drug is no more effective than placebo. Results in immunocompromised adults may be more favorable: When given to adults with cryptosporidiosis and HIV/AIDS, a dosage of 1000 mg twice a day for 14 days cured 67% of patients, compared with 25% of those receiving placebo.

Actions

Nitazoxanide appears to work by disrupting protozoal energy metabolism. Specifically, the drug blocks electron transfer mediated by pyruvate:ferredoxin oxidoreductase, and thereby inhibits anaerobic energy metabolism. In addition to its activity against *C. parvum* and *G. lamblia,* nitazoxanide is active against other enteric protozoa (*Isospora belli* and *Entamoeba histolytica*), as well as some helminths, including *Ascaris lumbricoides, Ancylostoma duodenale, Trichuris trichiura, Taenia saginata,* and *Fasciola hepatica.*

Pharmacokinetics

Nitazoxanide is well absorbed following oral administration. In the blood, the drug undergoes rapid conversion to its active metabolite, tizoxanide, which then undergoes nearly complete (more than 99.9%) binding to plasma proteins. Tizoxanide levels peak between 1 and 4 hours after nitazoxanide administration, and then decline, owing to excretion in the urine, bile, and feces.

Adverse Effects

Nitazoxanide is generally well tolerated. In clinical trials, the most common adverse effects were abdominal pain, diarrhea, vomiting, and headache. However, these effects were just as common in subjects taking placebo. In some patients, the drug caused yellow discoloration of the sclerae (whites of the eyes), which resolved following drug withdrawal.

Drug Interactions

Because nitazoxanide undergoes extensive protein binding, it might displace other agents that are also highly bound, thereby increasing their effects. Conversely, other highly bound agents could displace nitazoxanide, thereby increasing *its* effects.

Preparations, Dosage, and Administration

Oral Suspension. Nitazoxanide oral suspension [Alinia] is indicated for diarrhea caused by *G. lamblia* or *C. parvum* in children ages 1 through 11 years, and for diarrhea caused by *G. lamblia* (but not *C. parvum*) in adults. Nitazoxanide is supplied as a pink powder that, when mixed with 48 mL of water, forms a strawberry-flavored, 20-mg/mL suspension. Dosing is done with food. The suspension may be stored at room temperature for 7 days, after which it should be discarded. Dosage depends on age as follows:

- For children ages 12 to 48 months, give 100 mg (5 mL) every 12 hours for 3 days.
- For children ages 4 to 11 years, give 200 mg (10 mL) every 12 hours for 3 days.
- For patients 12 years and older, give 500 mg (25 mL) every 12 hours for 3 days.

Tablets. Nitazoxanide tablets [Alinia] are indicated only for diarrhea caused by *G. lamblia* and only for patients at least 12 years old. The dosage is 1 tablet (500 mg) every 12 hours for 3 days. Dosing is done with food.

Pentamidine

Target Diseases and Actions

Pentamidine [Pentam 300, NebuPent] is highly effective against West African sleeping sickness, a disease caused by *T. brucei gambiense,* and against *Pneumocystis* pneumonia (PCP), a disease caused by the fungus *Pneumocystis jiroveci* (formerly thought to be *Pneumocystis carinii*). The drug has multiple actions, including disrupting the synthesis of DNA, RNA, phospholipids, and proteins. However, we don't know which of these actions is responsible for antiprotozoal effects.

Uses

Pneumocystis *Pneumonia.* For therapy of PCP, pentamidine is given parenterally and by inhalation. Parenteral therapy is used to treat active PCP. In contrast, inhalational therapy is used to *prevent* PCP in high-risk HIV-positive patients, defined as patients with (1) a history of one or more episodes of PCP or (2) peripheral CD4 lymphocyte counts below 200 cells/mm^3.

West African Sleeping Sickness. Pentamidine is given by IM injection to treat sleeping sickness. However, the drug is not approved by the FDA for this disorder.

Pharmacokinetics

For treatment of active PCP, pentamidine is administered IM or IV. Equivalent blood levels are achieved with both routes. The drug is extensively bound in tissues. Penetration to the brain and cerebrospinal fluid is poor. Between 50% and 65% of each dose is excreted rapidly in the urine. The remaining drug is excreted slowly, over a month or more.

Adverse Effects Associated With Parenteral Pentamidine

Pentamidine can produce serious side effects when given IM or IV. Caution is needed.

Sudden and severe *hypotension* occurs in about 1% of patients. The fall in blood pressure may cause tachycardia, dizziness, and fainting. To minimize hypotensive episodes, patients should receive the drug while lying down. Blood pressure should be monitored closely.

Hypoglycemia and *hyperglycemia* have occurred. Hypoglycemia has been associated with necrosis of pancreatic islet cells and excessive insulin levels. The cause of hyperglycemia is unknown. Because of possible fluctuations in glucose levels, blood glucose should be monitored daily.

Intramuscular administration is painful. Necrosis at the injection site followed by formation of a sterile abscess is common.

Some adverse effects can be life threatening when severe. These reactions include leukopenia, thrombocytopenia, acute renal failure, hypocalcemia, and dysrhythmias.

Adverse Effects Associated With Aerosolized Pentamidine

Inhaled pentamidine does not cause the severe effects associated with parenteral dosing. The most common reactions are cough and bronchospasm. Both reactions are more pronounced in patients with asthma or a history of smoking. Fortunately, these reactions can be controlled with an inhaled bronchodilator, and they rarely necessitate pentamidine withdrawal.

Preparations, Dosage, and Administration

Pneumocystis *Pneumonia.* Pentamidine isethionate *for injection* [Pentam 300] is supplied in 300-mg, single-dose vials. For treatment of active PCP, the dosage for adults and children is 4 mg/kg IV daily for 2 to 3 weeks. Administration must be done slowly (over 60 to 120 minutes).

Pentamidine isethionate *aerosol* [NebuPent] is used for prophylaxis of PCP in patients with HIV/AIDS. The dosage is 300 mg once every 4 weeks. Administration is performed with a Respirgard II nebulizer. Solutions should be freshly prepared.

West African Sleeping Sickness. Administration is by IM injection. The dosage for adults and children is 4 mg/kg/day for 7 days.

Suramin

Actions and Uses

Suramin sodium [Germanin] is a drug of choice for the early phase of East African trypanosomiasis (sleeping sickness); for the late phase of the disease (CNS involvement), melarsoprol and eflornithine are preferred. Suramin is known to inhibit many trypanosomal enzymes; however, its primary mechanism of action has not been established.

Pharmacokinetics

Suramin is poorly absorbed from the GI tract, so it must be given parenterally (IV). The drug binds tightly to plasma proteins and remains in the bloodstream for months. Penetration into cells is low. Excretion is renal.

Adverse Effects

Side effects can be severe, and hence treatment should take place in a hospital. Frequent reactions include vomiting, itching, rash, paresthesias, photophobia, and hyperesthesia of the palms and soles. Suramin concentrates in the kidneys and can cause local damage, resulting in the appearance of protein, blood cells, and casts in the urine. If urinary casts are observed, treatment should cease. Rarely, a shock-like syndrome develops after IV dosing. To minimize the risk for this reaction, a small test dose (100 to 200 mg) is given; if there is no severe reaction, full doses may follow.

Preparations, Dosage, and Administration

Suramin sodium [Germanin] is available from the CDC. The drug is supplied in 1-gm ampules. Administration is by slow IV infusion. Suramin is unstable, so fresh solutions must be made daily. The adult dosage is 1 gm IV on days 1, 3, 7, 14, and 21. The pediatric dosage is 20 mg/kg IV on days 1, 3, 7, 14, and 21. Possible revisions in these dosage recommendations should be obtained from the CDC.

Melarsoprol

Therapeutic Use

Melarsoprol [Arsobal, Mel-B] is used to treat both East African and West African trypanosomiasis (sleeping sickness). The drug is employed during the *late* stage of the disease (i.e., after CNS involvement has developed). For earlier stages, suramin and pentamidine are preferred.

Mechanism of Action

Melarsoprol is an organic arsenical compound that reacts with sulfhydryl groups of proteins. Antiparasitic effects result from inactivation of enzymes. This same action appears to underlie the serious toxicity of the drug. Melarsoprol is more toxic to parasites than to humans because it penetrates parasitic membranes more easily than membranes of human cells; however, toxicity in humans does occur (see *Adverse Effects*). Unfortunately, the CDC reports that melarsoprol is the only drug currently available for late-stage infection caused by *T. b. rhodesiense.*

Adverse Effects

Melarsoprol is quite toxic, thus adverse reactions are common. Frequent effects include hypertension, cardiac dysrhythmias, myocardial damage, albuminuria, peripheral neuropathy, and paraplegia. *Reactive encephalopathy* develops in 10% of patients and is fatal for approximately half of those who acquire this condition.

Preparations, Dosage, and Administration

Melarsoprol [Arsobal, Mel-B] is administered by slow IV injection. The drug is highly irritating to tissues, and hence avoiding extravasation is important. Because of its toxicity, melarsoprol should be administered in a hospital setting. Melarsoprol is not available commercially but can be obtained through the CDC.

East African Trypanosomiasis. Treatment for adults and children consists of an initial course (2 to 3.6 mg/kg IV daily for 3 days) followed in 7 days by a second course (3.6 mg/kg IV daily for 3 days), followed in 7 days by a third course (3.6 mg/kg IV daily for 3 days).

West African Trypanosomiasis. The dosage for adults and children is 2.2 mg/kg/day for 10 days.

Eflornithine

Actions and Uses

Eflornithine [Ornidyl] is indicated for patients with late-stage African trypanosomiasis (sleeping sickness). The drug is highly effective against *T. brucei gambiense* (West African sleeping sickness), but only variably active against *T. brucei rhodesiense* (East African sleeping sickness). In both cases, benefits derive from irreversible inhibition of ornithine decarboxylase, an enzyme needed for biosynthesis of polyamines, which are required by all cells for division and differentiation. Parasites weakened by eflornithine become highly vulnerable to lethal attack by host defenses. Because cells of the host can readily synthesize more ornithine decarboxylase to replace inhibited enzyme, cells of the host are spared.

As discussed in Chapter 105, eflornithine is also available in a topical formulation, marketed as *Vaniqa,* for use by women to remove unwanted facial hair.

Pharmacokinetics

Eflornithine is given IV. Once in the blood, the drug is well distributed to body fluids and tissues, including the CNS. Eflornithine has a half-life of 100 minutes and is eliminated largely unchanged in the urine.

Adverse Effects

The most common adverse effects are anemia (48%), diarrhea (39%), and leukopenia (27%), and cardiac dysrhythmias (22%). Seizures may occur early in therapy but then subside, despite continued treatment. Because IV administration of eflornithine requires large volumes of fluid, fluid overload may develop over the course of treatment. Eflornithine can also cause hair loss.

Preparations, Dosage, and Administration

Eflornithine is supplied as a concentrated solution (200 mg/mL in 100-mL vials) and must be diluted for IV infusion. To treat West African sleeping sickness in adults and children, the dosage is 100 mg/kg IV 4 times a day for 14 days. Eflornithine is available only from the CDC.

Nifurtimox

Therapeutic Use

Nifurtimox [Lampit] is a drug of choice for Chagas' disease. The drug is most effective in the acute stage of the disease, curing about 80% of patients. Chronic disease is less responsive.

Pharmacokinetics

Nifurtimox is well absorbed from the GI tract and undergoes rapid and extensive metabolism. Metabolites are excreted in the urine.

Adverse Effects

Therapy is prolonged, and significant untoward effects occur often. GI effects (anorexia, nausea, vomiting, abdominal pain) and peripheral neuropathy are especially common. Weight loss resulting from GI disturbance may require treatment cessation. Additional common reactions include rash and CNS effects (memory loss, insomnia, vertigo, headache). In people with a deficiency of glucose-6-phosphate dehydrogenase, nifurtimox can cause hemolysis.

Preparations, Dosage, and Administration

Nifurtimox [Lampit] is supplied in 100-mg tablets. In the United States, the drug is available only from the CDC. The adult dosage is 8 to 10 mg/kg/day (in three or four doses) for 90 to 120 days. For young children (ages 1 through 10 years), the dosage is 15 to 20 mg/kg/day (in four doses) for 90 to 120 days. For older children (ages 11 to 16 years), the dosage is 12.5 to 15 mg/kg/day (in four doses) for 90 to 120 days.

Pyrimethamine

Pyrimethamine [Daraprim], combined with sulfadiazine, is the treatment of choice for toxoplasmosis. Pyrimethamine (combined with sulfadoxine) is also used to treat malaria (see Chapter 98). For toxoplasmosis, adult dosing consists of an initial 200-mg oral dose, followed by 50 to 75 mg/day PO for 3 to 6 weeks. The pediatric dosage is individualized. For treatment of toxoplasmosis in children, the prescribing information recommends 1 mg/kg/day divided into two doses. After 2 to 4 days of therapy, the dose can be halved and continued for 1 month. For both adults and children, each dose of pyrimethamine should be accompanied by 10 to 25 mg of folinic acid (to reduce side effects). In addition, the regimen must include sulfadiazine: for adults, 1 to 1.5 gm PO 4 times a day for 3 to 6 weeks; for children, 100 to 200 mg/kg/day for 3 to 6 weeks. Some experts also recommend adding leucovorin to this regimen. The basic pharmacology of pyrimethamine is discussed in Chapter 98.

Sodium Stibogluconate

Sodium stibogluconate [Pentostam] is a drug of choice for leishmaniasis. The mechanism of action is unknown. The drug is poorly absorbed from the GI tract, and hence must be given parenterally (IM or IV). Sodium stibogluconate undergoes little metabolism and is excreted rapidly in the urine. Although severe side effects can occur, the drug is usually well tolerated. The most frequent adverse reactions are muscle pain, joint stiffness, and bradycardia. Changes in the electrocardiogram are common and occasionally precede serious dysrhythmias. Liver and kidney impairment, shock, and sudden death occur rarely. Sodium stibogluconate is supplied in aqueous solution for IM and IV injection. For leishmaniasis, the usual adult and pediatric dosage is 20 mg/kg/day (IM or IV) for 28 days. In the United States, the drug is available only from the CDC.

Miltefosine

Miltefosine [Impavido] is the first *oral* agent for *leishmaniasis.* The drug was originally developed to treat cancer. Antiprotozoal activity wasn't revealed until miltefosine was tested in cancer patients who also had leishmaniasis. The mechanism underlying benefits is unclear. Studies conducted in India indicate that oral miltefosine is both safe and effective for treating *visceral* leishmaniasis. Preliminary studies indicate the drug is also highly effective against *cutaneous* disease. Because miltefosine is taken by mouth, rather than by injection, the drug is much more convenient than the alternatives, namely, sodium stibogluconate (administered IM or IV) and amphotericin B (administered IV).

Miltefosine is better tolerated than either sodium stibogluconate or amphotericin B. The most common reactions are vomiting and diarrhea. A decrease in platelet production may occur. Hepatotoxicity is seen in some patients, but it usually resolves during the second week of treatment. Reversible renal damage may also occur.

Amphotericin B

Amphotericin B is a preferred drug for leishmaniasis. The pharmacology of this drug and its dosage for leishmaniasis are presented in Chapter 92.

KEY POINTS

- The principal protozoal infections seen in the United States are trichomoniasis, giardiasis, and amebiasis.
- Metronidazole is a drug of choice for trichomoniasis, giardiasis, and symptomatic or systemic amebiasis. Iodoquinol is the drug of choice for asymptomatic amebiasis.
- Patients taking metronidazole should be warned against consuming alcohol because of the risk for a disulfiram-like reaction.

Please visit **http://evolve.elsevier.com/Lehne** for chapter-specific NCLEX® examination review questions.

CHAPTER

100 Ectoparasiticides

Ectoparasites are parasites that live on the surface of the host. Most ectoparasites that infest humans live on the skin and hair. Some live on clothing and bedding, moving to the host only to feed. The principal ectoparasites that infest humans are mites and lice. Infestation with lice is known as *pediculosis.* Infestation with mites is known as *scabies.* Both conditions are characterized by intense pruritus (itching). With the exception of ivermectin, all of the drugs used for treatment are topical.

ECTOPARASITIC INFESTATIONS

Pediculosis (Infestation With Lice)

Pediculosis is a general term referring to infestation with one of three kinds of lice. The types of lice encountered are *Pediculus humanus capitis* (head louse), *Pediculus humanus corporis* (body louse), and *Phthirus pubis* (pubic or crab louse). Infestation with any of these insects causes pruritus. Infestations with head, body, and pubic lice differ regarding mode of acquisition and method of treatment.

Head Lice

Head lice are common parasites, infesting 6 to 12 million people annually in the United States and over 100 million people worldwide. Infestation is most common in children 3 to 11 years old. Head lice reside on the scalp and lay their nits (eggs) on the hair. Adult lice may be difficult to observe. Nits, however, are usually visible. Infestation may be associated with hives, boils, impetigo, and other skin disorders. The head louse infests people from all socioeconomic groups. Head lice, which neither jump nor fly, are usually transmitted by head-to-head contact. Transmission by contact with combs, hairbrushes, and hats may also occur, but has not been proven. Because humans are the only host for these obligate parasites, infestation cannot be acquired through contact with pets or any other animals.

Topical pediculicides are preferred for management of lice infestation. These include drugs with neurotoxic effects on lice (permethrin, pyrethrins, malathion, lindane, spinosad, and topical ivermectin) and drugs that suffocate the lice (benzyl alcohol). (Specific information on these drugs is provided later in this chapter.) The choice of agent depends largely on the amount of resistance that lice have developed. Resistance may vary according to location. Age and adverse effects are also considerations when choosing the most appropriate drug. According to the latest recommendations from the American Academy of Pediatrics (AAP), released in 2015, the treatments of choice for children are over-the-counter (OTC) formulations containing *1% permethrin* or *pyrethrins,* provided resistance is not suspected.

A few days after drug treatment, dead lice (and remaining live lice) and any adherent nits should be removed from the hair with a fine-toothed comb. Eradication of head lice does not require shaving or cutting the hair.

Body Lice

Despite their name, body lice reside not on the body but on clothing. These lice move to the body only to feed. Consequently, body lice are rarely seen on the skin. Rather, they can be found in bed linens and the seams of garments. Transmission of body lice is by contact with infested clothing or bedding. Body lice are relatively uncommon in the United States, where regular laundering precludes infestation. Infestation is most likely among people whose clothes and bedding are not frequently washed. Most body lice can be removed from the host simply by removing infested clothing. Those lice that remain on the body can be killed by applying a pesticide; *permethrin* and *malathion* are drugs of choice. Clothing and bedding should be disinfected by washing and drying at high temperature. Oral *ivermectin* is sometimes used if topical treatments fail. Additionally, studies have demonstrated decreased resistance to topical permethrin when it is prescribed with oral trimethoprim/sulfamethoxazole (TMP/SMX) at 5 mg/kg twice a day for 10 days. Why does this decrease resistance? Because the TMP/SMX kills bacteria in lice that are used to manufacture the B vitamins lice need to live.

Prototype Drugs

ECTOPARASITICIDES

Pediculosis (Infestation With Lice)

Permethrin
Malathion

Scabies (Infestation With Mites)

Permethrin
Crotamiton

Pubic Lice

Pubic lice, commonly known as *crabs* (because pubic lice are shaped like crabs), usually reside on the skin and hair of the pubic region. However, the louse responsible, *Phthirus pubis*, may also be found on the eyelashes (where the condition is called pediculosis ciliaris) and other places. As a rule, infestation is transmitted through sexual contact. Consequently, crabs are most common among people who have multiple sexual partners. Two preparations—*permethrin* (1% lotion) and *malathion* (0.5% lotion)—are drugs of choice for eliminating crabs. Alternatives include *pyrethrins with piperonyl butoxide* (gel, lotion, shampoo) and oral *ivermectin* (250 mcg/kg as a single dose that is repeated in 2 weeks). Infestation of the eyelashes is treated with petrolatum ophthalmic ointment. Clothing and linen should be disinfected by washing in very hot water, followed by machine drying at high temperature.

Scabies (Infestation With Mites)

Scabies is caused by infestation with *Sarcoptes scabiei,* an organism known commonly as the itch mite. Irritation results from the female mite burrowing beneath the skin to lay eggs. Burrows may be visible as small ridges or dotted lines. In adults, the most common sites of infestation are the wrists, elbows, nipples, navel, genital region, and webs of the fingers. In children, infestation is most likely on the head, neck, and buttocks. The primary symptom of scabies is pruritus. Itching is most intense just after going to bed. Scratching may result in abrasion and secondary infection. Transmission is usually by direct contact, either sexual or of a less intimate nature. Scabies may also be transmitted through contact with infested linen, towels, or clothing.

Scabies is usually treated with a pesticide-containing lotion or cream. To eradicate mites, the entire body surface must be treated (excluding the face and scalp in adults). To prevent reinfestation, bedding and intimate clothing should be machine washed and dried.

Several drugs can kill scabies mites. *Permethrin* (5% cream formulation) is the drug of choice. This preparation is effective in just one application. In addition, there is evidence that a single oral dose (200 mcg/kg) of *ivermectin* [Stromectol] can cure scabies. Other options for the treatment of scabies include crotamiton, malathion, and lindane. Lindane, though usually effective, carries a risk for toxicity and should not be used in children.

A problem related to treatment is that the intense itching continues for a week or two after successful treatment. The patient's hypersensitivity reaction to the burrowed dead mites, feces, and eggs continues, so the itching will continue until the body recovers. Without education on this issue before treatment, the patient may demand additional treatment or, when not receiving it, go to another provider. If a second provider prescribes another round of therapy or different therapy, when the itching resolves, the patient may credit the relief to the extra therapy rather than to the natural course of recovery.

PHARMACOLOGY OF ECTOPARASITICIDES

As a rule, ectoparasitic infestations are treated with *topical drugs.* These agents are available in the form of creams, gels, lotions, liquids, and shampoos. Only one ectoparasiticide—ivermectin—is available in an oral formulation. Properties of the major ectoparasiticides are shown in Table 100.1.

Permethrin

Basic Pharmacology

Actions and Uses. Permethrin [Nix, Elimite, Kwellada-P 🍁] is highly toxic to adult mites and lice, and much less toxic to their ova. Residual activity persists for 2 or more weeks after treatment. The drug kills adult insects by disrupting nerve traffic, thereby causing paralysis. Because freshly deposited ova do not yet have a nervous system, they are not affected by the drug. In addition to killing mites and lice, permethrin is active against fleas and ticks. The 1% formulation [Nix] is a drug of choice for lice. The 5% formulation [Elimite] is the drug of choice for scabies.

Resistance. Permethrin fails to eradicate *head lice* in about 5% of patients. Drug resistance is the probable cause. In areas where permethrin resistance is common, treatment with malathion, available OTC, or benzyl alcohol, which requires a prescription, should be tried. Oral ivermectin, which also requires a prescription, is an option if these first- and second-line treatments fail.

Pharmacokinetics. Very little (about 2%) of topical permethrin is absorbed. The fraction absorbed is rapidly inactivated and excreted in the urine.

Adverse Effects. Topical permethrin is devoid of serious adverse effects. The drug may cause some exacerbation of the itching, erythema, and edema normally associated with pediculosis. Other reactions include temporary sensations of burning, stinging, and numbness.

Preparations and Administration

Preparations of this and other drugs in this chapter are provided in Table 100.1. Administration guidelines are also included.

Pyrethrins Plus Piperonyl Butoxide

All current pyrethrin formulations include piperonyl butoxide. The combination of pyrethrins with piperonyl butoxide [A-200, Licide, RID, R&C 🍁] is used to remove pubic lice and head lice. Pyrethrins are the components of this preparation that are toxic to lice. The piperonyl butoxide enhances pyrethrins' action by decreasing the ability of insects to metabolize pyrethrins into inactive products. The combination is active against adult parasites, but not against ova. Pyrethrins undergo little transcutaneous absorption and are one of the safest insecticides available. Principal adverse effects are irritation to the eyes and mucous membranes. Accordingly, contact with these areas should be avoided. Most formulations contain 0.33% pyrethrins and 4% piperonyl butoxide.

Malathion

Actions and Uses

Malathion [Ovide] is an organophosphate cholinesterase inhibitor (see Chapter 15). The drug kills lice and their ova. Humans and other mammals are not harmed because an enzyme in their blood converts malathion to nontoxic metabolites. The drug is approved for the treatment of head lice in patients age 6 years and older. The drug is also used widely as an insecticide.

TABLE 100.1 ■ Preferred Drugs for Mites and Lice

Generic Name	Dosage Form	Brand Name	Uses: Pediculosis (Lice)	Uses: Scabies (Mites)	Kills Ova	Resistance	Administration
TOPICAL MEDICATIONS							
Permethrin	1% liquid	Nix, Kwellada-P 🍁	✓		No	Yes	Apply to damp shampooed hair. Leave on 10 minutes and then rinse with warm water. Use fine-toothed comb to remove nits. Repeat if living lice are noted 1 week later.
	5% cream	Elimite		✓	No	Yes	Massage into skin from head to soles of feet. Leave on 8–14 hr before washing. Re-treat if living mites are seen 2 weeks after treatment.
Pyrethrins plus piperonyl butoxide	Gel Lotion Mousse Shampoo	A-200, Licide, LiceMD, Pronto, RID, R&C 🍁	✓		No	Yes	Apply to dry hair and/or other infested areas. Wait 10 minutes and then wash with soap or shampoo and rinse thoroughly. Use a fine-toothed comb to remove nits. Repeat in 7–10 days.
Malathion	0.5% lotion	Ovide	✓		Yes	Not in United States	Saturate dry hair. Allow to dry naturally with hair uncovered. After 8–12 hr, wash and rinse. Afterward, use a fine-toothed comb to remove nits.
Benzyl alcohol	5% lotion	Ulesfia	✓		No	No	Saturate dry hair. Leave on 10 minutes and then rinse with water. Use a fine-toothed comb to remove nits.
Crotamiton	10% cream 10% lotion	Eurax		✓	No	Yes	After bathing, massage into skin from chin to toes. (Head is treated only if needed.) Trim fingernails and apply under nails (can use toothbrush, which should be disposed of after use). Reapply in 24 hr. Bathe 48 hr after last application.

TABLE 100.1 ▪ Preferred Drugs for Mites and Lice—cont'd

Generic Name	Dosage Form	Brand Name	Uses: Pediculosis (Lice)	Uses: Scabies (Mites)	Kills Ova	Resistance	Administration
Spinosad	0.9% suspension	Natroba	✓		Yes	No	Saturate dry hair. Leave on for 10 minutes and then rinse thoroughly. Repeat in 7 days if live lice are seen. It is not necessary to comb for nits.
Ivermectin	5% lotion	Sklice	✓		No, but it kills newly hatched nymphs	Uncommon	Saturate dry hair. Leave on 10 minutes and then rinse. It is not necessary to comb for nits.
ORAL MEDICATION							
Ivermectin	Tablets	Stromectol	✓[a]	✓[a]	No	Rare	Although administered with water on an empty stomach when given to treat helminths, the CDC recommends administering with food for treatment of ectoparasites because this will increase bioavailability in the epidermis.

[a]Although ivermectin is effective against mites and lice, the drug is not approved for these infestations by the U.S. Food and Drug Administration.

Adverse Effects and Interactions

The preparation used topically for head lice is devoid of significant adverse effects. Scalp irritation develops occasionally. No systemic toxicity has been reported. Likewise, no drug interactions have been reported. Malathion lotion contains a high concentration of alcohol and hence presents a risk for fire. Also, the drug smells bad.

Benzyl Alcohol

Benzyl alcohol [Ulesfia] is the first and only drug that kills lice by suffocation. Specifically, benzyl alcohol prevents adult lice from closing their respiratory spiracles, and then penetrates the spiracles to block the airways. Benzyl alcohol has no effect on ova, so it must be applied at least twice to kill lice that hatch after the first application. In clinical trials, two applications, done 1 week apart, eliminated all lice in about 75% of patients. Because benzyl alcohol works by suffocation, resistance is unlikely.

Benzyl alcohol is generally well tolerated. The most common adverse effects are itching, eye irritation, application-site irritation, and application-site numbness. When given to preterm neonates, *intravenous* benzyl alcohol has caused neonatal gasping syndrome, characterized by metabolic acidosis, gasping respirations, and central nervous system depression, sometimes progressing to intraventricular hemorrhage and cardiovascular collapse. Whether *topical* benzyl alcohol can cause this syndrome in very young patients is unknown.

Safety Alert

BENZYL ALCOHOL FORMULATIONS

Benzyl alcohol is available in both a 5% lotion [Ulesfia] and a 10% gel [Zilactin] and a 1% ointment [AverTeaX]. These are not interchangeable. Only the lotion is used to treat lice infestation. The gel and ointment are used for the treatment of herpes labialis (fever blisters) and oral canker sores.

Spinosad

Spinosad [Natroba] is indicated for topical treatment of *head lice* in patients age 4 years and older. The drug is highly active against adult lice and appears to be ovicidal as well. In adult lice, spinosad causes neuronal excitation and involuntary muscle contraction, followed by paralysis and death. Resistance has not been reported. How spinosad kills ova is unknown.

In clinical trials, spinosad was more effective than permethrin, a drug of choice for head lice. After a single application, spinosad eliminated lice in 94% of patients, whereas only 65% of patients who got permethrin were lice free. Furthermore, with spinosad, most patients needed only one application, whereas with permethrin, the majority needed a second application. Unfortunately, although spinosad is more effective than permethrin, it is also much more expensive.

Spinosad is very safe. The most common reactions, which occur in only 1% to 3% of patients, are local irritation and erythema of the scalp and eyes. Topical spinosad is not absorbed, and hence systemic effects are absent.

Crotamiton

Crotamiton [Eurax] is used to treat *scabies.* The drug is not indicated for pediculosis.

In addition to scabicidal actions, this drug also relieves itching by an independent mechanism. Mild adverse reactions (dermatitis, conjunctivitis) occur occasionally. Crotamiton is available in cream and lotion formulations.

Lindane

Actions and Uses

Lindane is absorbed through the chitin shell of adult mites and lice and causes death by inducing convulsions. The drug is also lethal to ova. At one time, lindane was a drug of choice for pediculosis and scabies. However, owing to a risk for seizures, the FDA now recommends that lindane be reserved for patients who have not responded to safer drugs (e.g., permethrin, malathion). Repeat dosing should be avoided. The drug was banned in California, owing to concern about contamination of drinking water, rivers, and lakes.

Adverse Effects

Irritation. Lindane is irritating to the eyes and mucous membranes. Application to the face should be avoided. If contact occurs, the affected area should be flushed with water.

> **Safety Alert**
>
> **LINDANE**
>
> The U.S. Food and Drug Administration warns that lindane shampoo and lotion should be used only to treat patients who cannot tolerate or who have failed treatment with other drugs for lice or scabies. Lindane is contraindicated in patients with eczema, psoriasis, or other skin disorders that increase risk for systemic absorption.

Convulsions. Lindane can penetrate the intact skin and, if absorbed in sufficient amounts, can cause convulsions. Convulsions can also result from lindane ingestion. Fortunately, convulsions are rare, resulting most often from drug ingestion or from inappropriate administration. If a seizure develops, it can be controlled with an IV barbiturate (e.g., phenobarbital) or with IV diazepam.

The risk for convulsions is highest for infants, children, and patients with pre-existing seizure disorders. Risk is also high for older adults and for all patients who weigh less than 110 pounds (50 kg). Premature infants are especially vulnerable because lindane can penetrate their skin with relative ease and because limited liver function prevents detoxification of absorbed drug.

To reduce seizure risk, the FDA recommends that lindane not be used to treat infants and children, women who are pregnant or breast-feeding, older adults, patients weighing less than 110 pounds, patients with a history of seizure disorder, patients with HIV infection, and anyone who

- Has used lindane in the past few months
- Has not tried a safer medicine for lice or scabies
- Has reacted adversely to lindane in the past
- Has open or crusted sores or extensive areas of broken skin in the treatment region
- Has psoriasis or atopic dermatitis

Giving a second treatment too soon after the first increases seizure risk. How soon is too soon? No one knows what a truly safe interval is, so the Centers for Disease Control and Prevention recommends avoiding re-treatment.

Administration

Scabies. To treat scabies, a thin layer of lotion is applied to the entire body below the head. No more than 30 gm (1 oz) should be used. The drug is removed by washing 8 to 12 hours later. As a rule, only one application is required. Pruritus may persist because of residual insect products. This itching does not indicate a need for additional treatment.

Head Lice. To kill head lice and their nits, lindane shampoo (30 to 60 gm) should be worked into dry hair and left in place for no more than 4 minutes. After this, the shampoo should be rinsed off with warm water. Dead nits can be removed with a comb or tweezers.

Pubic Lice. The affected region should receive the same treatment employed for head lice. Shampoo is preferred to lotion. One treatment is usually sufficient. Sexual partners should be treated concurrently. Lindane should not be used to treat infestation of the eyelashes by the pubic louse. For this condition, petrolatum ophthalmic ointment is employed.

Body Lice. Body lice can be killed by applying a thin layer of lindane to affected areas. The drug should be washed off 8 to 12 hours after application.

PATIENT-CENTERED CARE ACROSS THE LIFE SPAN

ECTOPARASITICIDES

Life Stage	Patient Care Concerns
Children	Permethrin is approved for infants 2 months and older. Spinosad, benzyl alcohol, and ivermectin lotion [Sklice] are approved for infants 6 months and older. Ivermectin tablets are not recommended for children weighing less than 15 kg because safety has not been established. Pyrethrins are approved for children 2 years and older. Malathion is approved for children 6 years and older. Lindane is approved for children 10 years and older; however, use caution if weight is less than 110 lb or 50 kg. Safety in children has not been established for crotamiton.
Pregnant women	According to the CDC, pregnant women should be treated with either permethrin or pyrethrins with piperonyl butoxide. Lindane and ivermectin are contraindicated during pregnancy. The FDA assigns a Pregnancy Risk Category B[a] designation to malathion, benzyl alcohol, and spinosad, indicating no known harmful effects. Crotamiton is Pregnancy Risk Category C because there are insufficient data from animal reproduction studies to determine relative safety.
Breast-feeding women	According to the CDC, breast-feeding women should be treated with either permethrin or pyrethrins with piperonyl butoxide. Lindane and ivermectin are contraindicated for women who breast-feed. The manufacturer of lindane recommends expressing and discarding breast milk for 24 hours after drug use. The manufacturer of ivermectin recommends the use of another product. Although the amount of drug excreted in breast milk is probably very low, manufacturers' labeling recommends caution with breast-feeding and the handling of infants when women are using malathion, benzyl alcohol, and spinosad. The manufacturer of crotamiton recommends that breast-feeding women use other products.
Older adults	Formal studies have not been conducted in older populations, so benefits must be weighed against risks. FDA labeling for lindane shampoo warns of an increased risk for toxicity in elderly patients following postmarketing reports of three older patients who died within 24 hours of treatment with lindane and a fourth who developed seizures after treatment with lindane and died 41 days later.

[a]As of 2020, the FDA will no longer use Pregnancy Risk Categories. Please refer to Chapter 9 for more information.

Ivermectin

Ivermectin is available in both topical [Sklice] and oral [Stromectol] forms. (The topical cream [Soolantra] is used for rosacea, not lice.) Topical ivermectin is FDA approved for ectoparasitic infections, but not oral ivermectin. An advantage of topical ivermectin is its ability to kill newly hatched lice (nymphs); therefore, combing for nits is not required.

Ivermectin is the only *oral* medication for ectoparasitic infestations. Although oral ivermectin therapy is not FDA approved for these applications in the United States, it is often used for them off-label. The drug kills parasites by disrupting nerve and muscle function—but does not disrupt nerve or muscle function in the host. Adult parasites are killed within 24 hours of oral dosing. A single dose can be highly effective against both mites and lice. However, because ivermectin does not kill ova, when treating pediculosis, a second dose is usually needed. Resistance to ivermectin is uncommon, but it has been observed with repeated dosing. At this time, ivermectin is considered a third-choice drug for treating head lice; it should be reserved for patients who have not responded to preferred agents.

The most common adverse reactions are headache and abdominal pain, which develop in less than 5% of patients. The Mazotti reaction (see Chapter 97) occurs only in patients treated for onchocerciasis; therefore, this is not a concern when given for lice and scabies. Rarely, patients may experience hypotension.

The basic pharmacology of ivermectin and its use against worm infestations is discussed in Chapter 97.

KEY POINTS

- Pediculosis (infestation with lice) and scabies (infestation with mites) are usually treated with topical drugs. The only exception is ivermectin, which is dosed orally.
- The major topical drugs for pediculosis and scabies have minimal side effects.
- Topical pediculicides include drugs with neurotoxic effects on lice (permethrin, pyrethrins, malathion, lindane, spinosad, and topical ivermectin) and drugs that suffocate the lice (benzyl alcohol).
- The AAP recommends 1% permethrin or pyrethrins for first-line therapy in children.
- With the exception of malathion and topical ivermectin, the major drugs for mites and lice have low activity against ova or nymphs, and hence a second application is needed to kill ova that hatched after the first application.
- Oral ivermectin is highly active against mites and lice, but should be reserved for patients who have not responded to permethrin and other traditional topical agents.

Please visit **http://evolve.elsevier.com/Lehne** for chapter-specific NCLEX® examination review questions.

UNIT XVIII CANCER CHEMOTHERAPY

CHAPTER 101

Basic Principles of Cancer Chemotherapy

As mortality from infectious diseases has declined, thanks to antimicrobial drugs and public health measures, cancer has emerged as the second leading cause of death. Cancer is among the top four leading causes of death for all age groups except those younger than 1 year (Table 101.1). Among women, the most common cancers are those of the breast, lung, colorectal, and uterine cancers. Among men, the most common cancers are those of the prostate, lung, colorectal, and urinary bladder[a] (Table 101.2). The good news is that, thanks to advances in treatment that include new drugs, deaths due to cancer have decreased 13% over the past decade.

We have three major modalities for treating cancer: *surgery, radiation therapy,* and *drug therapy.* Surgery is the most common treatment for *solid* cancers. In contrast, drug therapy is the treatment of choice for *disseminated* cancers (leukemias, disseminated lymphomas, and metastases), along with several localized cancers (e.g., choriocarcinoma, testicular carcinoma). Drug therapy also plays an important role as an adjunct to surgery and irradiation: By suppressing or killing malignant cells that surgery and irradiation leave behind, adjuvant drug therapy can reduce recurrence and improve survival.

Anticancer drugs fall into four major classes: *cytotoxic agents* (i.e., drugs that kill cells directly), *hormones and hormone antagonists, biologic response modifiers* (e.g., immunomodulating agents), and *targeted drugs* (i.e., drugs that bind with specific molecules [targets] that promote cancer growth). Of the four classes, the cytotoxic agents are used most often. You should note that the term *cancer chemotherapy* applies *only to the cytotoxic drugs*—it does not apply to the use of hormones, biologic response modifiers, or targeted drugs. In this chapter, our discussion of anticancer drugs pertains almost exclusively to the cytotoxic agents.

The modern era of cancer chemotherapy dates from 1942, the year in which "nitrogen mustards" were first used for cancer. Since the introduction of nitrogen mustards, chemotherapy has made significant advances. For patients with some forms of cancer (Table 101.3), drugs can often be curative. Cancers with a high cure rate include Hodgkin's disease, testicular cancer, and acute lymphocytic leukemia. For many patients whose cancer is not yet curable, chemotherapy can still be of value, offering realistic hopes of palliation and prolonged life. However, although progress in chemotherapy has been encouraging, the ability to cure most cancers with drugs alone remains elusive. At this time, the major impediment to successful chemotherapy is toxicity of anticancer drugs to normal tissues.

---

[a]Actually, the most common cancer for both men and women is skin cancer. However, basal cell carcinoma and squamous cell carcinoma, which account for most skin cancers, have lower metastatic potential. Therefore, the CDC includes only melanoma, a highly invasive cancer, in cancer ratings.

TABLE 101.1 ▪ Cancer Ranking Among Four Leading Causes of Death by Age

	Age in Years							
Ranking	1–4	5–9	10–14	15–34[a]	35–44	45–54	55–64	> 65
1	Injury	Injury	Injury	Injury	Injury	**Cancer**	**Cancer**	Heart disease
2	Congenital anomalies	**Cancer**	**Cancer**	Suicide	**Cancer**	Heart disease	Heart disease	**Cancer**
3	Homicide	Congenital anomalies	Suicide	Homicide	Heart disease	Injury	Injury	Lung disease
4	**Cancer**	Homicide	Homicide	**Cancer**	Suicide	Liver disease	Lung disease	Stroke

[a]The four leading causes of death for ages 15–24 and 25–34 are the same.
Adapted from the CDC's *10 Leading Causes of Death by Age Group, United States—2015*, available at https://www.cdc.gov/injury/images/lc-charts/leading_causes_of_death_age_group_2015_1050w740h.gif.

TABLE 101.2 ▪ Estimated New Cancer Cases and Deaths, United States, 2016

	Women		Men	
Type of Cancer	New Cases	Deaths	New Cases	Deaths
All types	843,820	281,400	841,390	314,290
Breast	246,660	40,450	2,600	440
Prostate			180,890	26,120
Lung and bronchus	106,470	72,160	117,920	85,920
Colon and rectum	63,670	23,170	70,820	26,020
Leukemia	26,050	10,270	34,090	14,130
Lymphoma	36,120	9,110	44,960	12,160
Endometrium	60,050	10,470		
Cervix	12,990	4,120		
Ovary	22,280	14,240		
Melanoma of skin	29,510	3,380	46,870	6,750
Pancreas	25,400	20,330	27,670	21,450
Urinary bladder	18,010	4,570	58,950	11,820
Kidney	23,050	5000	39,650	9,240
Oral cavity and pharynx	13,550	2,660	34,780	6,910
Stomach	9,890	4,190	16,480	6,540
Esophagus	3,450	2,970	13,460	12,720
Liver and bile duct	10,820	8,890	28,410	18,280
Brain and other CNS	10,420	6,610	13,350	9,440
Multiple myeloma	12,430	6,220	17,900	6,430
Thyroid	49,350	1,070	14,950	910

Data from American Cancer Society: *Cancer Facts & Figures 2016.* Atlanta: American Cancer Society, 2016.

TABLE 101.3 ▪ Some Cancers for Which Drugs May Be Curative[a]

Type of Cancer	Drug Therapy[b]
Hodgkin's lymphoma	Doxorubicin + bleomycin + vinblastine + dacarbazine
Burkitt's lymphoma	Cyclophosphamide + vincristine + methotrexate + doxorubicin + prednisone
Choriocarcinoma	Methotrexate ± leucovorin
Small cell cancer of lung	Etoposide + either cisplatin or carboplatin
Testicular cancer	Cisplatin + etoposide ± bleomycin
Wilms' tumor[c]	Dactinomycin + vincristine ± doxorubicin ± cyclophosphamide
Ewing's sarcoma[c]	Cyclophosphamide + doxorubicin + vincristine alternating with etoposide + ifosfamide (with mesna)
Acute myeloid leukemia	Daunorubicin + cytarabine + etoposide
Breast cancer[c]	Fluorouracil + doxorubicin + cyclophosphamide
Colorectal cancer[c]	Fluorouracil + leucovorin + oxaliplatin
Acute lymphocytic leukemia	Vincristine + prednisone + asparaginase + daunorubicin or doxorubicin ± cyclophosphamide

[a]"Cure" is defined as a 5-year disease-free interval following treatment.
[b]These are representative regimens. Other regimens may also be highly effective.
[c]Chemotherapy is combined with surgery and/or radiotherapy in these cancers.

Our principal objectives are to examine the major obstacles confronting successful chemotherapy, the strategies being employed to overcome those obstacles, the major toxicities of the chemotherapeutic drugs, and steps that can be taken to minimize drug-induced harm and discomfort. As background for addressing these issues, we begin by discussing (1) the nature of cancer itself and (2) the tissue growth fraction and its relationship to cancer chemotherapy.

WHAT IS CANCER?

In the discussion that follows, we consider properties shared by neoplastic cells as a group. However, although the discussion addresses cancers in general, be aware that the term *cancer* refers to a large group of disorders and not to a single disease: There are more than 100 different types of cancer, most of which have multiple subtypes. These various forms of cancer differ in clinical presentation, aggressiveness, drug sensitivity, and prognosis. Because of this diversity, treatment must be individualized, based on the specific biology of the cells involved.

Characteristics of Neoplastic Cells

Persistent Proliferation

Unlike normal cells, whose proliferation is carefully controlled, cancer cells undergo unrestrained growth and division. This capacity for persistent proliferation is the most distinguishing property of malignant cells. In the absence of intervention, cancerous tissues will continue to grow until they cause death.

It was once believed that cancer cells divided more rapidly than normal cells and that this excessive rate of division was responsible for the abnormal growth patterns of cancerous tissues. We now know that this concept is not correct. Division of neoplastic cells is not necessarily rapid: Although some cancers are composed of cells that divide rapidly, others are composed of cells that divide slowly. The correct explanation for the relentless growth of tumors is that *malignant cells are unresponsive to the feedback mechanisms that regulate cellular proliferation in healthy tissue.* As a result, cancer cells can continue to multiply under conditions that would suppress further growth and division of normal cells. Simply put, instead of dividing more rapidly, they divide more frequently than normal cells.

Invasive Growth

In the absence of malignancy, the various types of cells that compose a tissue remain segregated from one another; cells of one type do not invade territory that belongs to cells of a different type. In contrast, malignant cells are free of the constraints that inhibit invasive growth. As a result, cells of a solid tumor can penetrate adjacent tissues, thereby allowing the cancer to spread.

Formation of Metastases

Metastases are secondary tumors that appear at sites distant from the primary tumor. Metastases result from the unique ability of malignant cells to break away from their site of origin, migrate to other parts of the body (via the lymphatic and circulatory systems), and then implant to form a new tumor.

Immortality

Unlike normal cells, which are programmed to differentiate and eventually die, cancer cells can undergo endless divisions. The underlying cause for this difference is *telomerase,* an enzyme that is active in most cancers and expressed only rarely in normal cells. Telomerase permits repeated division by preserving *telomeres*—the DNA-protein "caps" found on the end of each chromosome. As normal cells divide and differentiate, their telomeres become progressively shorter. When telomeres have lost a critical portion of their length, the cell is unable to keep on dividing. In cancer cells, telomerase continually adds back lost pieces of the telomere and thereby preserves or extends telomere length. As a result, cancer cells can divide indefinitely.

Etiology of Cancer

The abnormal behavior of cancer cells results from alterations in their DNA. Specifically, malignant transformation results from a combination of activating *oncogenes* (cancer-causing genes) and inactivating *tumor suppressor genes* (genes that prevent replication of cells that have become cancerous). These genetic alterations are caused by chemical carcinogens, viruses, and radiation (x-rays, ultraviolet light, radioisotopes). Malignant transformation occurs in three major stages: initiation, promotion, and progression. These stages suggest that DNA in cancer cells undergoes a series of small modifications, rather than a single large change. This accumulated genetic damage leads to dysregulation of cell division and protection against cell death.

It is important to appreciate that the changes in cellular function caused by malignant transformation are primarily *quantitative* (rather than *qualitative*). That is, malignant transformation simply results in the overexpression or underexpression of the same gene products made by normal cells. As a result, cancer cells employ the same metabolic machinery as normal cells, use the same signaling pathways as normal cells, and express the same surface antigens as normal cells. Nonetheless, even though these changes in cellular function are only quantitative, they are still sufficient to allow unrestrained growth and avoidance of cell death.

THE GROWTH FRACTION AND ITS RELATIONSHIP TO CHEMOTHERAPY

The growth fraction of a tissue is a major determinant of its responsiveness to chemotherapy. Consequently, before we discuss the anticancer drugs, we must first understand the growth fraction. To define the growth fraction, we must review the cell cycle.

The Cell Cycle

The cell cycle is the sequence of events that a cell goes through from one mitotic division to the next. As shown in Fig. 101.1, the cell cycle consists of four major phases: G_1, S, G_2, and M. (The length of the arrows in the figure is proportional to the time spent in each phase.) For our purpose, we can imagine the cycle as beginning with G_1, the phase in which the cell prepares to make DNA by synthesizing histones (proteins found

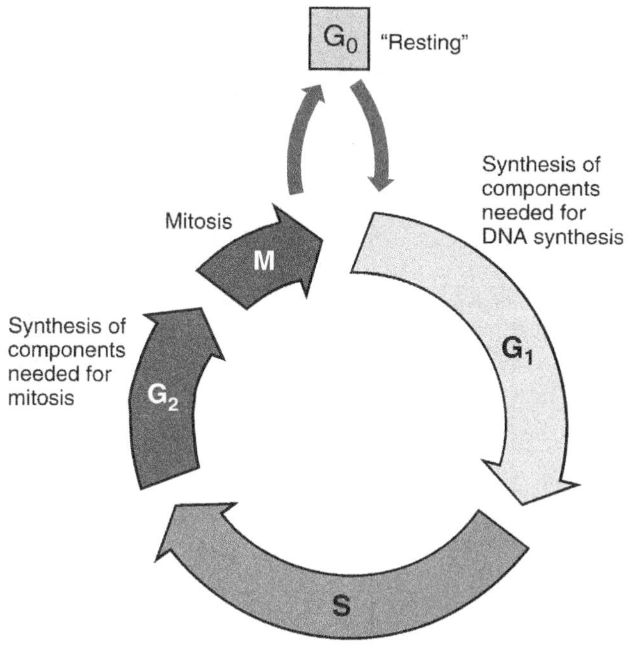

Fig. 101.1 ▪ The cell cycle.

in chromatin). Following G_1, the cell enters S phase, the phase in which DNA synthesis actually takes place. After synthesis of DNA is complete, the cell enters G_2 and prepares for mitosis (cell division). Mitosis occurs next during M phase. Upon completing mitosis, the resulting daughter cells have two options: they can enter G_1 and repeat the cycle, or they can enter the phase known as G_0. Cells that enter G_0 become mitotically dormant; they do not replicate and are not active participants in the cycle. Cells may remain in G_0 for days, weeks, or even years. Under appropriate conditions, resting cells may leave G_0 and resume active participation in the cycle.

The Growth Fraction

In any tissue, some cells are going through the cell cycle, whereas others are "resting" in G_0. The ratio of proliferating cells to G_0 cells is called the *growth fraction.* A tissue with a large percentage of proliferating cells and few cells in G_0 has a *high* growth fraction. Conversely, a tissue composed mostly of G_0 cells has a *low* growth fraction.

Impact of Tissue Growth Fraction on Responsiveness to Chemotherapy

As a rule, *chemotherapeutic drugs are much more toxic to tissues that have a high growth fraction than to tissues that have a low growth fraction.* Why? Because most cytotoxic agents are more active against proliferating cells than against cells in G_0. Proliferating cells are especially sensitive to chemotherapy because cytotoxic drugs usually act by disrupting either DNA synthesis or mitosis—activities that only proliferating cells carry out. Unfortunately, the toxicity of anticancer drugs is not restricted to cancers: These drugs are also toxic to normal tissues that have a high growth fraction (e.g., bone marrow, GI epithelium, hair follicles, sperm-forming cells).

Having established the relationship between growth fraction and drug sensitivity, we can apply this knowledge to predict how specific cancers will respond to chemotherapy. As a rule, *the most common cancers*—solid tumors of the breast, lung, prostate, colon, and rectum—have a *low* growth fraction, so they *respond poorly to cytotoxic drugs.* In contrast, only some rarer cancers—such as acute lymphocytic leukemia, Hodgkin's disease, and certain testicular cancers—have a *high* growth fraction, so they tend to respond *well to cytotoxic drugs.* In practical terms, this means that the most common cancers, which don't respond well to drugs, must be managed primarily with surgery. Only a few cancers can be managed primarily with drugs.

OBSTACLES TO SUCCESSFUL CHEMOTHERAPY

In this section we consider the major factors that limit success in chemotherapy. Foremost among these is the serious and unavoidable toxicity to normal cells caused by cytotoxic drugs. Other important factors include resistance to chemotherapy and high tumor load (owing to late diagnosis).

Toxicity to Normal Cells

Toxicity to normal cells is a major barrier to successful chemotherapy. Injury to normal cells occurs primarily in tissues where the growth fraction is high: bone marrow, GI epithelium, hair follicles, and germinal epithelium of the testes. Drug-induced injury to each of these tissues is discussed in detail when we discuss toxicities later in this chapter. For now, let's consider injury to normal cells as a group.

Toxicity to normal cells is dose limiting. That is, dosage cannot exceed an amount that produces the maximally tolerated injury to normal cells. Although very large doses of cytotoxic drugs might be able to produce cure, these doses cannot be given because they are likely to kill the patient.

Why are cytotoxic anticancer drugs so harmful to normal tissues? Because these drugs lack *selective toxicity.* That is, *they cannot kill target cells without also killing other cells with which the target cells are in intimate contact.* We encountered this concept in Chapter 83. As noted there, successful antimicrobial therapy is possible because antimicrobial drugs are highly selective in their toxicity. Penicillin, for example, can readily kill invading bacteria while being virtually harmless to cells of the host. This high degree of selective toxicity stands in sharp contrast to the lack of selectivity displayed by cytotoxic anticancer drugs.

Why have we been unable to develop drugs that selectively kill neoplastic cells? Because neoplastic cells and normal cells are very similar: Differences between them are quantitative rather than qualitative. To make a cytotoxic drug that is truly selective, the target cell must have a biochemical feature that normal cells lack. By way of illustration, let's consider penicillin, which kills bacteria by disrupting the bacterial cell wall. Because our cells don't have a cell wall, penicillin can't hurt us. Unfortunately, we have yet to identify unique biochemical features that would render cancer cells vulnerable to selective attack. Nevertheless, there is reason for hope: Our expanding knowledge of cancer biology is revealing potential new targets for anticancer drugs. Exploiting these targets may lead to anticancer drugs that are more selective than the drugs we have now.

Cure Requires 100% Cell Kill

To cure a patient of cancer, we must eliminate virtually every malignant cell. Why? Because just one remaining cell can proliferate and cause relapse. For most patients, 100% cell kill cannot be achieved. Factors that make it difficult to achieve complete cell kill include (1) the kinetics of drug-induced cell kill, (2) minimal participation of the immune system in eliminating malignant cells, and (3) the disappearance of symptoms before all cancer cells are gone.

Kinetics of Drug-Induced Cell Kill

Killing of cancer cells follows *first-order kinetics.* That is, at any given dose, a drug will kill a *constant percentage* of malignant cells, *regardless of how many cells are actually present.* This means that the dose required to shrink a cancer from 10^3 cells down to 10 cells will be just as big, for example, as the dose required to reduce that cancer from 10^9 cells down to 10^7 cells. Hence, with each successive round of chemotherapy, drug dosage must remain the same, even though the cancer is getting progressively smaller. Accordingly, if treatment is to continue, the patient must be able to tolerate the same degree of toxicity late in therapy that the patient tolerated when therapy began. For many patients, this is not possible.

Host Defenses Contribute Little to Cell Kill

In contrast to the antimicrobial drugs, anticancer agents receive very little help from host defenses. There are three reasons why. First, because cancer cells express the same surface antigens as normal cells, the immune system generally fails to recognize cancer cells as foreign, so it does not attack them. Second, because many anticancer drugs are immunosuppressants, these agents can seriously compromise immune function. Third, with cancers such as lymphomas and leukemias, which involve components of the immune system, the immune system may be compromised by the cancer itself. Because the immune system offers little help against cancer, anticancer agents must produce cell kill almost entirely on their own.

When Should Treatment Stop?

We have no way of knowing when 100% cell kill has been achieved. As a result, there is no definitive method for deciding just when chemotherapy should stop. As shown in Fig. 101.2, symptoms disappear long before the last malignant cell has been eliminated. Once a cancer has been reduced to less than 1 billion cells, it becomes undetectable by usual clinical methods; all signs of disease are absent, and the patient is considered in complete remission. It is obvious, however, that a patient harboring a billion malignant cells is by no means cured. It is also obvious that further chemotherapy is indicated. However, what is not so obvious is just how long therapy should last: Because the patient is already asymptomatic, we have no objective means of determining when to stop treatment. The clinical dilemma is this: If therapy continues too long, the patient will be needlessly exposed to serious toxicity; conversely, if drugs are discontinued prematurely, relapse will occur.

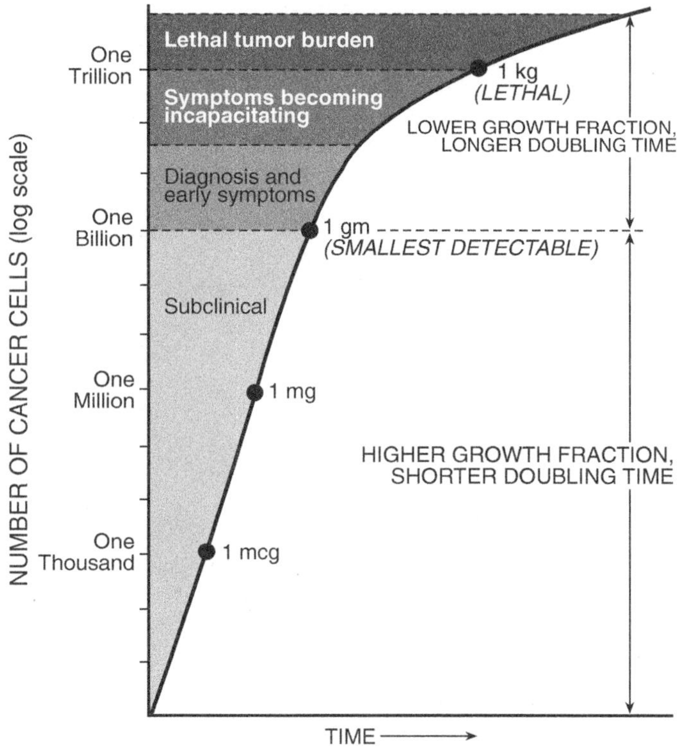

Fig. 101.2 ■ Gompertzian tumor growth curve showing the relationship between tumor size and clinical status.

Absence of Truly Early Detection

Early detection of cancer with current screening methods is rare. Cancer of the cervix, which can be diagnosed with a Papanicolaou (Pap) test, is the primary exception. All other forms of cancer are significantly advanced by the time they have grown large enough for discovery. The smallest detectable cancers are about 1 cm in diameter, have a mass of 1 gm, and consist of about 1 billion cells. Detection at this stage cannot be considered early.

Late detection has three important consequences. First, by the time the primary tumor is discovered, metastases may have formed. Second, the tumor will be less responsive to drugs than it would have been at an earlier stage. Third, if the cancer has been present for a long time, the patient may be debilitated by the disease and therefore less able to tolerate treatment.

Even though *truly* early detection is largely impossible, every effort at *relatively* early detection should be made. The smaller a cancer is when treatment begins, the better the chances of long-term survival. Hence, even if a cancer has 1 billion cells when it's detected, that's still far better than a gazillion. Accordingly, the American Cancer Society recommends routine testing for several cancers, including cancers of the prostate, breast, cervix, rectum, and colon. Table 101.4 indicates who should be tested, how often, and what test or procedure should be performed. With breast cancer, a yearly mammogram can detect disease before it becomes widely invasive, thereby greatly increasing survival—even though more than a billion cells may be present at the time of discovery. Along with routine testing, patients should be counseled about ways to reduce cancer risk, especially avoiding tobacco and excessive exposure to ultraviolet radiation, and receiving a human papillomavirus vaccination to protect against cervical cancer (see Chapter 68).

TABLE 101.4 ▪ American Cancer Society Recommendations[a] for the Early Detection of the Most Common Cancers in Men and Women

Type of Cancer	Rank	Recommendation
Breast	#1 among women	Screening is done with mammograms.[b] Women ages 45–54 should receive annual mammograms. Women ages 55 and older should receive mammograms every 2 years. Mammograms are no longer needed after life expectancy decreases to 10 years.
Prostate	#1 among men	Screening involves a prostate-specific antigen (PSA) blood test, with or without a rectal examination. Beginning at age 50, men should be given an opportunity to make an *informed* decision with their healthcare provider about screening for prostate cancer. Prostate screening should not occur until candidates have been told what is known and what is uncertain about the benefits and limitations of testing and risks of treatment.
Lung	#2 among men and women	Screening is done with low-dose CT scan (LDCT) of the chest. Men and women ages 55–74 years who have a 30 pack-year[c] smoking history and are otherwise in good health should discuss annual LDCT screening with their providers.
Colon and rectum	# 3 among men and women	Screening involves a selection of testing methods. Men and women ages 50 years and older should follow one of the seven examination schedules below. Tests that detect both cancer and precancerous polyps (Recommended) • Flexible sigmoidoscopy (FSIG) every 5 years *or* • Colonoscopy every 10 years *or* • Double-contrast barium enema every 5 years *or* • Computed tomographic colonography (virtual colonoscopy) every 5 years Tests for evidence of cancer (alternatives for patients who refuse more invasive testing) • Fecal occult blood test (FOBT) annually *or* • Fecal immunochemical test (FIT) annually *or* • Stool DNA test every 3 years
Endometrium/ Uterus	# 4 among women	Screening is an endometrial biopsy. Women who are at the time of menopause and at high risk for endometrial cancer should talk to their providers about annual screening.
Urinary bladder	# 4 among men	There is no recommended screening for urinary bladder cancer at this time.
Cervix	Not among top 10 most common cancers[d]	Screening for cervical cancer involves a Papanicolaou (Pap) test. Screening for endometrial (uterine) cancer involves an endometrial biopsy. Cervical cancer screening: • Women ages 21–29 should have a Pap test, without HPV testing, every 3 years. • Women ages 30–65 should have a Pap test every three years *or* a Pap test plus an HPV test every 5 years. • Women older than 65 years who have had normal tests in the past 10 years should stop cervical cancer screening. • After a diagnosis of cervical precancer, women should be tested for at least 20 years, regardless of age. • After a total hysterectomy for reasons other than cancer, testing should not be done unless there is a history of cervical precancer.

[a]Cancer screening guidelines used to be more rigid. Research over the past decade that examined outcomes and risks, especially those associated with false-positive findings, has resulted in more conservative recommendations.
[b]Self-breast examinations and clinical breast examinations by a healthcare professional, once included in the guidelines, are no longer recommended.
[c]A pack-year equals the number of cigarette packs smoked daily multiplied by the number of years the person has smoked. A 30 pack-year history would comprise someone who smoked a pack of cigarettes daily for 30 years or two packs daily for 15 years.
[d]Cervical cancer is a screening success story. Once a major cause of cancer morbidity and mortality, it is now so often caught in precancerous stages through Pap testing that it is no longer among the top cancers in women.
Data from *American Cancer Society Guidelines for the Early Detection of Cancer*. Atlanta: American Cancer Society, 2016.

Solid Tumors Respond Poorly

As noted, solid tumors have a low growth fraction (high percentage of G_0 cells) and generally respond poorly to cytotoxic drugs. There are two reasons for low responsiveness. First, G_0 cells do not perform the activities that most anticancer drugs are designed to disrupt. Second, because G_0 cells are not active participants in the cell cycle, they have time to repair drug-induced damage before it can do them serious harm.

Not all solid tumors are equally unresponsive: As a rule, *large tumors are even less responsive than small ones.* This difference occurs because as solid tumors increase in size, more of their cells leave the cell cycle and enter G_0, causing the growth fraction to decline even further. Tumor growth slows, in large part, because blood flow in the tumor core is low, depriving cells of nutrients and oxygen. The decrease in growth fraction in older tumors is a major reason why therapeutic success is more likely when cancers are detected early. Because the rate of growth declines as a tumor gets larger, the tumor growth curve is said to follow *Gompertzian kinetics* (see Fig. 101.2).

The drug sensitivity of a solid tumor can be enhanced by *debulking.* When a solid tumor is reduced by surgery or irradiation, many of the remaining cells leave G_0 and re-enter the cell cycle, thereby increasing their sensitivity to chemotherapy. This phenomenon is known as *recruitment.* Because of recruitment, chemotherapy can be very useful as an adjunct to surgery or irradiation, even though drugs may have been largely ineffective before debulking was done.

Drug Resistance

During the course of chemotherapy, cancer cells can develop resistance to the drugs used against them. Drug resistance can be a significant cause of therapeutic failure. Mechanisms of resistance include reduced drug uptake, increased drug efflux, reduced drug activation, reduced target molecule sensitivity, and increased repair of drug-induced damage to DNA.

One mechanism of resistance—cellular production of a drug transport molecule known as *P-glycoprotein*—can confer *multiple drug resistance* upon cells. As discussed in Chapter 4, P-glycoprotein is a large molecule that spans the cytoplasmic membrane and pumps drugs out of the cell. Induction of P-glycoprotein synthesis during exposure to a single anticancer drug produces cross-resistance to agents in other drug classes. Several drugs, including cyclosporine, have been used investigationally to inhibit the P-glycoprotein pump and reverse multiple drug resistance.

Drug resistance mechanisms, including production of P-glycoprotein, result from a change in DNA. Mutation to a drug-resistant form is a spontaneous event and is not caused by the anticancer drugs themselves. However, although drugs do not *cause* the mutations that render cells resistant, drugs do *create selection pressure* favoring the drug-resistant mutants. That is, by killing drug-sensitive cells, anticancer agents create a competition-free environment in which drug-resistant mutants can flourish. This is the same phenomenon we encountered in our discussion of antibacterial drugs.

Because the presence of anticancer agents favors the growth of drug-resistant clones, as therapy proceeds, the number of resistant cells will increase. Because patients are usually exposed to drugs over an extended time, therapeutic failure owing to drug resistance is a significant problem. Using a combination of drugs can help overcome resistance. We discuss this principle later in the chapter.

Heterogeneity of Tumor Cells

Tumors do not consist of a single population of identical cells. Rather, owing to ongoing mutation, tumors are composed of subpopulations of dissimilar cells. These subpopulations can differ in morphology, growth rate, and metastatic ability. More importantly, they can differ in responsiveness to drugs—primarily because of increased resistance. As tumors age, cellular heterogeneity increases.

Limited Drug Access to Tumor Cells

Because of a tumor's location or blood supply, drugs may have limited access to its cells. Large solid tumors have poor vascularization, especially near the core. Therefore, cells within these tumors are difficult for drugs to reach. Similarly, tumors of the central nervous system (CNS) are hard to reach because it is difficult for most anticancer drugs to cross the blood-brain barrier.

STRATEGIES FOR ACHIEVING MAXIMUM BENEFITS FROM CHEMOTHERAPY

Intermittent Chemotherapy

The ultimate goal of chemotherapy is to produce 100% kill of neoplastic cells while causing limited injury to normal tissues—especially the bone marrow and GI epithelium. Intermittent therapy is the primary technique for achieving this goal. When cytotoxic anticancer drugs are administered intermittently, normal cells have time to repopulate between rounds of therapy. However, for this approach to succeed, one obvious requirement must be met: *Normal cells must repopulate faster than malignant cells.* If malignant cells grow back faster than normal cells, there can be no reduction in tumor burden between treatment rounds. Successful use of intermittent therapy is shown in Fig. 101.3.

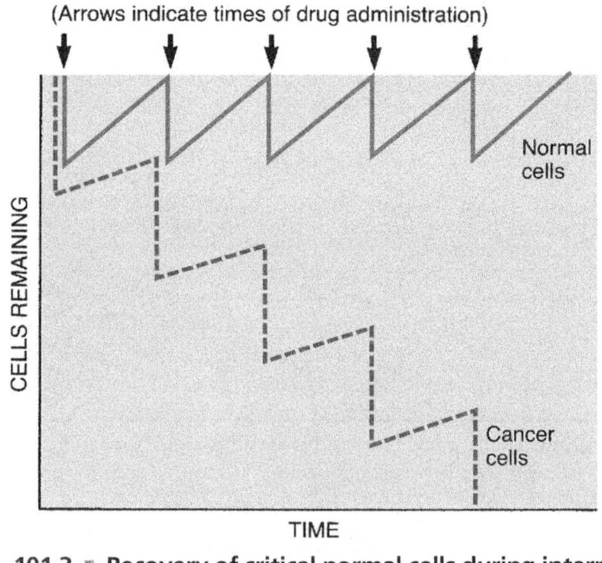

Fig. 101.3 ▪ Recovery of critical normal cells during intermittent chemotherapy.
Cancer cells and normal cells (e.g., cells of the bone marrow) are killed each time cytotoxic drugs are given. In the interval between doses, both types of cells proliferate. Because, in this example, normal cells repopulate faster than the cancer cells, normal cells are able to recover entirely between doses, whereas regrowth of the cancer cells is only partial. As a result, with each succeeding round of treatment, the total number of cancer cells becomes smaller, whereas the number of normal cells remains within a tolerable range. Note that differential loss of malignant cells is possible only if these cells repopulate more slowly than the normal cells. If cancer cells grow back as fast as normal cells do, intermittent chemotherapy will fail.

TABLE 101.5 ▪ Effects of Cyclophosphamide and Vincristine Alone and in Combination

		Toxicity	
Therapeutic Regimen	Anticancer Effect	Neutropenia	Neurotoxicity
Cyclophosphamide	++	++	0
Vincristine	++	0	++
Cyclophosphamide + vincristine	++++	++	++

Combination Chemotherapy

Chemotherapy employing a combination of drugs is generally much more effective than chemotherapy with just one drug. Accordingly, most patients are treated with two or more agents.

Benefits of Drug Combinations

Combination chemotherapy offers three advantages: (1) suppression of drug resistance, (2) increased cancer cell kill, and (3) reduced injury to normal cells (at any given level of anticancer effect).

Suppression of Drug Resistance. Drug resistance occurs less frequently with multiple-drug therapy than with single-drug therapy. To understand why, we need to recall that resistance is acquired through random mutational events. The probability of a cell undergoing two or more mutations, and therefore developing resistance to a combination of drugs, is smaller than the probability of a cell undergoing the single mutation needed for resistance to one drug. Because drug resistance is reduced with combination chemotherapy, the chances of therapeutic success are increased.

Increased Cancer Cell Kill. If we administer several anticancer drugs, each with a different mechanism of action, we will kill more malignant cells than if we use only one drug. Therapeutic effects are enhanced because the combination attacks the cancer in two or more ways, not just one. Greater cell kill is especially likely if a drug-resistant subpopulation of cells is present.

Reduced Injury to Normal Cells. By using a combination of drugs *that do not have overlapping toxicities,* we can achieve a greater anticancer effect than we could *safely* achieve using any of the agents alone. Table 101.5 shows responses to two drugs—vincristine and cyclophosphamide—when given alone and in combination. Both drugs kill malignant cells, but they act by different mechanisms: Cyclophosphamide damages DNA, whereas vincristine blocks mitosis. Furthermore, these drugs have different dose-limiting toxicities: Cyclophosphamide causes *neutropenia,* whereas vincristine causes *neuropathy.* In the table, the intensity of effects is indicated by plus (+) symbols—the more pluses, the more intense the response. With either drug, ++ represents the maximum degree of toxicity that can be tolerated. When administered alone in doses that produce ++ toxicity, each drug produces an anticancer effect of ++ intensity—the greatest therapeutic effect that we can safely achieve with either drug by itself. Now let's consider the effect of combining these drugs, giving each in its maximally tolerated dose. The total anticancer effect of the combination is ++++, twice the effect that could be achieved safely with either agent alone. Because the toxicities of these agents do not overlap, overall toxicity of the combination remains at a tolerable level—although the patient is now exposed to two kinds of toxicity rather than one.

TABLE 101.6 ▪ Effect of Cytarabine Dosing Schedule on Therapeutic Response

Experimental Group	Dosage Size	Dosing Schedule	Mice Surviving
I	240 mg/kg	1 dose/day[a]	None
II	15 mg/kg	8 doses/day[a]	100%

[a]Cytarabine was administered on days 2, 6, 10, and 14 after mice were inoculated with leukemia cells.

Guidelines for Drug Selection

From the preceding, we can extract three guidelines for selecting drugs to use in combination: (1) Each drug should be effective by itself, (2) each drug should have a different mechanism of action, and (3) the drugs should have minimally overlapping toxicities.

Optimizing Dosing Schedules

The dosing schedule is an important determinant of treatment outcome. The experiment summarized in Table 101.6 provides a dramatic illustration. In this experiment, two groups of mice were inoculated with cancer cells and then treated with cytarabine. Mice in group I received a *single large dose* of cytarabine on days 2, 6, 10, and 14 after being inoculated. The mice in group II were treated on the same days as the mice in group I, but, rather than receiving one large dose of cytarabine, they were given *eight small doses,* one every 3 hours. By the end of the study, all of the group II mice were cured. In stark contrast, all of the group I mice were dead. Because the two groups had the same disease burden and were given the same total dose of the same drug, we must conclude that the life-and-death difference was due to the dosing schedules employed.

To understand these results, we need to know two properties of cytarabine: (1) The drug kills cells by disrupting DNA synthesis, and (2) it undergoes rapid inactivation. Because cytarabine acts by disrupting DNA synthesis, it can only affect cells during S phase. Because the drug is rapidly inactivated and because many cells will not be in S phase during the short time before inactivation occurs, many cells will escape injury following each dose. The group I mice died because giving just one large dose every 4 days did not maintain active drug in the body for a time sufficient to catch all cancer cells as they cycled through S phase. Because the group II mice received multiple doses over a 24-hour period on each of 4 days, the presence of active drug was sustained. Hence, the chance of cancer cells being in S phase while active drug was present was greatly increased, thereby leading to enhanced cell kill with resultant cure.

The message from this experiment is this: Selection of the right drugs for cancer therapy is only one of the requirements for success; those drugs must also be administered according to schedules that maximize beneficial effects. Dosing schedules are especially critical for drugs that, like cytarabine, act during a specific phase of the cell cycle.

Regional Drug Delivery

By using special techniques for drug delivery, we can increase drug access to tumors, thereby increasing cell kill and reducing systemic toxicity.

Intra-arterial Delivery

Local intra-arterial infusion can be used to treat solid tumors. This technique has the advantage of establishing a high concentration of drug in the vicinity of the tumor while minimizing toxicity to the rest of the body. Specific routes include carotid artery delivery (for brain tumors) and hepatic artery delivery (for liver metastases). Clearly, intra-arterial therapy is suitable only for localized disease.

Intrathecal Delivery

As noted, many anticancer agents are unable to cross the blood-brain barrier and therefore cannot reach malignant cells in the CNS. To enhance therapy of CNS cancers, drugs can be administered intrathecally (by injection directly into the subarachnoid space). This technique bypasses the blood-brain barrier, thereby giving drugs better access to cells within the CNS.

Other Specialized Routes

Anticancer agents can be administered via the portal vein to treat liver metastases and directly into the bladder to treat bladder cancer. Neoplasms located in the pleural and peritoneal cavities can be treated by direct intracavitary drug administration. As discussed in Chapter 102, carmustine, a drug for brain tumors, is available in a wafer that is implanted in the brain to kill cancer cells left behind following surgical removal of a tumor.

MAJOR TOXICITIES OF CHEMOTHERAPEUTIC DRUGS

The agents used for cancer chemotherapy constitute our most toxic group of medicines. Serious injury occurs most often to tissues with a high growth fraction (bone marrow, GI epithelium, hair follicles, sperm-forming cells). In the discussion that follows, we consider the more common toxicities of the *cytotoxic* anticancer drugs along with steps that can be taken to minimize harm and discomfort.

Bone Marrow Suppression

Chemotherapeutic drugs are highly toxic to the bone marrow, a tissue with a high proportion of proliferating cells. Myelosuppression reduces the number of circulating neutrophils, platelets, and erythrocytes. Loss of these cells has three major consequences: (1) infection (from loss of neutrophils); (2) bleeding (from loss of platelets); and (3) anemia (from loss of erythrocytes).

Neutropenia

Neutrophils (neutrophilic granulocytes) are white blood cells that play a critical role in fighting infection. In patients with neutropenia (a reduction in circulating neutrophils), both the incidence and severity of infection are increased. Infections that are normally benign (e.g., candidiasis) can become life threatening. Infection secondary to neutropenia is one of the most serious complications of chemotherapy.

With most anticancer drugs, the onset of neutropenia is rapid and recovery develops relatively quickly. Neutropenia begins to develop a few days after dosing, and the lowest neutrophil count, called the *nadir,* occurs between days 10 and 14. Neutrophil counts then recover a week or so later. Patients are at highest risk during the nadir. Accordingly, special care should be taken to prevent infection.

With some anticancer drugs, neutropenia is *delayed.* Neutrophil counts begin to fall in 1 to 2 weeks and reach their nadir between weeks 3 and 4. Full recovery may not occur until after week 7.

Neutrophil counts must be monitored. Normal counts range from 2500 to 7000 cells/mm^3. If neutropenia is substantial (absolute neutrophil count below 500/mm^3), chemotherapy should be withheld until neutrophil counts return toward normal.

A lack of neutrophils confounds the diagnosis of infection. Why? Because the usual signs of infection (e.g., pus, abscesses, infiltrates on the chest x-ray) depend on neutrophils being present. In the absence of neutrophils, *fever* is the principal early sign of infection.

Patients must be their own first line of defense against infection. They should be made aware of their elevated risk for infection and taught how to minimize contagion. They should be informed that fever may be the only indication of infection and instructed to report immediately if fever develops. Because infection is commonly acquired through contact with other people, hospitalized patients should be instructed to refuse direct contact with anyone who has not washed his or her hands in the patient's presence. This rule applies not only to visiting friends and relatives but also to nurses, physicians, and all other hospital staff. The normal flora of the body is a major source of infection; the risk for acquiring an infection with these microbes can be reduced by daily examination and cleansing of the skin and oral cavity.

Hospitalization of the infection-free neutropenic patient is controversial. Some clinicians feel that hospitalization *increases* the risk for acquiring a serious infection. Why? Because hospitals harbor drug-resistant microbes, which can make hospital-acquired (nosocomial) infections especially difficult to treat. Accordingly, these clinicians recommend that neutropenic patients stay at home as long as they remain infection free.

If neutropenic patients *are* hospitalized, every precaution must be taken to prevent nosocomial infection. Patients should be given an isolation room and monitored frequently for fever. Certain foods (e.g., lettuce) abound in pathogenic bacteria and must be avoided.

When a neutropenic patient develops an infection, immediate and vigorous intervention is required. Specimens for culture should be taken to determine the identity and drug sensitivity of the infecting organism. While awaiting reports on the cultures, empiric therapy with IV antibiotics should be instituted. Initial therapy is usually done with a single drug active against *Pseudomonas* and other gram-negative bacteria. Options include ceftazidime, imipenem, and doripenem. If the patient develops sepsis, an aminoglycoside (e.g., tobramycin, amikacin) is added. If the patient remains febrile, vancomycin is added (for gram-positive coverage).

Colony-stimulating factors can minimize neutropenia. Three preparations are available: *granulocyte colony-stimulating factor* (filgrastim), long-acting granulocyte colony-stimulating factor (pegfilgrastim), and *granulocyte-macrophage colony-stimulating factor* (sargramostim). All three drugs act on the bone marrow to enhance granulocyte (neutrophil) production. Colony-stimulating factors can decrease the incidence, magnitude, and duration of neutropenia. As a result, they can decrease the incidence and severity of infection as well as the need for IV antibiotics and hospitalization. The basic pharmacology of these drugs is discussed in Chapter 56.

Thrombocytopenia

Bone marrow suppression can cause thrombocytopenia (a reduction in circulating platelets), thereby increasing the risk for serious bleeding. Bleeding from the nose and gums is relatively common. Bleeding from the gums can be reduced by avoiding vigorous toothbrushing. Drugs that promote bleeding (e.g., aspirin, anticoagulants) should not be used. When a mild analgesic is required, acetaminophen, which does not promote bleeding, is preferred to aspirin. For patients with severe thrombocytopenia, platelet infusions are the mainstay of treatment. Platelet production can be stimulated with *oprelvekin* [Neumega]. However, owing to limited efficacy and flu-like reactions, oprelvekin is not often used.

Caution should be exercised when performing procedures that might promote bleeding. Intravenous needles should be inserted with special care, and intramuscular injections should be avoided. Blood pressure cuffs should be applied cautiously, because overinflation may cause bruising or bleeding.

Anemia

Anemia is defined as a reduction in the number of circulating erythrocytes (red blood cells). Although anticancer drugs can suppress erythrocyte production, anemia is much less common than neutropenia or thrombocytopenia. Why? Because circulating erythrocytes have a long life span (120 days), which usually allows erythrocyte production to recover before levels of existing erythrocytes fall too low.

If anemia does develop, it can be treated with a transfusion or with erythropoietin (*epoetin alfa* or *darbepoetin alfa*), a hormone that stimulates production of red blood cells. Because transfusions require hospitalization, whereas epoetin can be administered at home, epoetin therapy can spare the patient inconvenience. However, erythropoietin has two huge drawbacks. First, it cannot be used in patients with leukemias and other myeloid malignancies (because it can stimulate proliferation of these cancers). Second, it *shortens* survival in all cancer patients, and hence is indicated only when the treatment goal is *palliation.* Clearly, erythropoietin should not be used when the goal is cure or prolongation of life. The basic pharmacology of erythropoietin is discussed in Chapter 56.

Digestive Tract Injury

The epithelial lining of the GI tract has a very high growth fraction, so it is exquisitely sensitive to cytotoxic drugs. Stomatitis and diarrhea are common. Severe GI injury can be life threatening.

Stomatitis

Stomatitis (inflammation of the oral mucosa) often develops a few days after the onset of chemotherapy and may persist for 2 or more weeks after treatment has ceased. Inflammation can progress to denudation and ulceration, and is often complicated by infection. Pain can be severe, inhibiting eating, speaking, and swallowing. Management includes good oral hygiene and a bland diet. Topical antifungal drugs may be needed to control infection with *Candida albicans.* For patient with mild stomatitis, pain can be managed with a mouthwash containing a topical anesthetic (e.g., lidocaine) plus an antihistamine (e.g., diphenhydramine). For patients with severe stomatitis, a systemic opioid is needed for pain. In some cases, stomatitis is so severe that chemotherapy has to be interrupted. For patients being treated for hematologic malignancies, *palifermin* [Kepivance] can decrease the severity of stomatitis (see Chapter 80).

Diarrhea

By injuring the epithelial lining of the intestine, anticancer drugs can impair absorption of fluids and other nutrients, thereby causing diarrhea. Diarrhea can be reduced with oral loperamide, a nonabsorbable opioid that slows gut motility by activating local opioid receptors.

Nausea and Vomiting

Nausea and vomiting are common sequelae of cancer chemotherapy. These responses, which result in part from direct stimulation of the chemoreceptor trigger zone, can be both immediate and dramatic, and may persist for hours or even days. In some cases, discomfort is so great as to prompt refusal of further treatment.

You should appreciate that nausea and vomiting associated with chemotherapy are much more severe than with other medications. Whereas these reactions are generally unremarkable with most drugs, they must be considered major and characteristic toxicities of anticancer drugs. The emetogenic potential of several intravenous agents is shown in Table 101.7.

Nausea and vomiting can be reduced by premedication with antiemetics. These drugs offer three benefits: (1) reduction of anticipatory nausea and vomiting, (2) prevention of dehydration and malnutrition secondary to frequent nausea and vomiting, and (3) promotion of compliance with chemotherapy by reducing discomfort. Combinations of antiemetics are more effective than single-drug therapy. The regimen of choice for patients taking highly emetogenic drugs consists of *aprepitant* [Emend], *dexamethasone,* and a *serotonin antagonist,* such as *ondansetron* [Zofran]. The use of antiemetics for

TABLE 101.7 ▪ Emetogenic Potential of Selected Intravenous Anticancer Drugs

SEVERE	LOW
Carmustine	Cytarabine
Cisplatin	Docetaxel
Cyclophosphamide (high dose)	Etoposide
Dacarbazine	Fluorouracil
Dactinomycin	Gemcitabine
Mechlorethamine	Methotrexate (high dose)
Streptozocin	Mitomycin
MODERATE	Mitoxantrone
Carboplatin	Paclitaxel
Cyclophosphamide (low dose)	Pemetrexed
Daunorubicin	Topotecan
Doxorubicin	Trastuzumab
Epirubicin	**MINIMAL**
Idarubicin	Bevacizumab
Ifosfamide	Bleomycin
Irinotecan	Busulfan
Oxaliplatin	Cetuximab
	Fludarabine
	Pralatrexate
	Rituximab
	Vinblastine
	Vincristine
	Vinorelbine

chemotherapy-induced nausea and vomiting is discussed in Chapter 80.

Other Important Toxicities

Alopecia

Reversible alopecia (hair loss) results from injury to hair follicles. Alopecia can occur with most cytotoxic anticancer drugs. Hair loss begins 7 to 10 days after the onset of treatment and becomes maximal in 1 to 2 months. Regeneration begins 1 to 2 months after the last course of treatment.

While alopecia is not dangerous, it is nonetheless very upsetting. In fact, for many cancer patients, alopecia is second only to vomiting as their greatest treatment-related fear. If drugs are expected to cause hair loss, the patient should be forewarned. For patients who choose to wear a hairpiece or wig, one should be selected before hair loss occurs. Hairpieces are tax deductible as medical expenses and are covered by some insurance plans.

To some degree, hair loss can be prevented by cooling the scalp while chemotherapy is being administered. Cooling causes vasoconstriction, and thereby reduces drug delivery to hair follicles. Unfortunately, scalp cooling is uncomfortable, causes headache, and creates a small risk for cancer recurrence in the scalp (because drug delivery is reduced).

Reproductive Toxicity

The developing fetus and the germinal epithelium of the testes have high growth fractions. As a result, both are highly susceptible to injury by cytotoxic drugs, especially the alkylating agents. These drugs can interfere with embryogenesis, causing death of the early embryo. They may also cause fetal malformation. Risk is highest during the first trimester, and hence chemotherapy should generally be avoided during this time. However, after 18 weeks of gestation, risk appears to be very low: According to a 2012 report in *Lancet,* exposure during this time does not cause neurologic, cardiac, or any other fetal abnormalities. Drug effects on the ovaries may result in amenorrhea, menopausal symptoms, and atrophy of the vaginal epithelium.

Cytotoxic drugs can cause irreversible sterility in males. Men should be forewarned and counseled about sperm banking.

Hyperuricemia

Hyperuricemia is defined as an excessive level of uric acid in the blood. Uric acid, a compound with low solubility, is formed by the breakdown of DNA following cell death. Hyperuricemia is especially common following treatment for leukemias and lymphomas (because therapy results in massive cell kill). The major concern with hyperuricemia is injury to the kidneys secondary to deposition of uric acid crystals in renal tubules. The risk for crystal formation can be reduced by increasing fluid intake. In patients with leukemias and lymphomas, in whom hyperuricemia is likely, prophylaxis with *allopurinol* is the standard of care. (As discussed in Chapter 74, allopurinol prevents hyperuricemia by inhibiting xanthine oxidase, an enzyme involved in converting nucleic acids to uric acid.) If hyperuricemia develops despite use of allopurinol, it can be managed with *rasburicase,* an enzyme that catalyzes uric acid degradation (see Chapter 74).

Local Injury From Extravasation of Vesicants

Certain anticancer drugs, known as *vesicants,* are highly chemically reactive. These drugs can cause severe local injury if they make direct contact with tissues. Vesicants are administered IV, usually into a central line (because rapid dilution in venous blood minimizes the risk for injury). When a peripheral line is used, administration is by IV push into a freely flowing IV line. Sites of previous irradiation should be avoided. Extreme care must be exercised to prevent extravasation, because leakage can produce high local concentrations, resulting in prolonged pain, infection, and loss of mobility. Severe injury can lead to necrosis and sloughing, requiring surgical débridement and skin grafting. If extravasation occurs, the infusion should be stopped immediately. Because of the potential for severe tissue damage, vesicants should be administered only by clinicians specially trained to handle them safely.

Unique Toxicities

In addition to the toxicities already discussed, which generally apply to the cytotoxic drugs as a group, some agents produce unique toxicities. For example, daunorubicin can cause serious injury to the heart, cisplatin can injure the kidneys, and vincristine can injure peripheral nerves. Special toxicities of individual drugs are considered in Chapters 102 and 103.

Carcinogenesis

Along with their other adverse actions, anticancer drugs have one final and ironic toxicity: These drugs, which are used to treat cancer, have caused cancer in some patients. Cancer results from drug-induced damage to DNA and is most likely to occur with alkylating agents. Cancers caused by anticancer drugs may take many years to appear and are hard to treat.

MAKING THE DECISION TO TREAT

From the preceding discussion of toxicities, it is clear that cytotoxic anticancer drugs can cause great harm. Given the known dangers of these drugs, we must ask why such toxic substances are given to sick people at all. The answer lies with the primary rule of therapeutics, which states that the benefits of treatment must outweigh the risks. For most patients undergoing chemotherapy, the conditions of this rule are met. That is, although the toxicities of the anticancer drugs can be significant, the potential benefits (cure, prolonged life, palliation) justify the risks. However, the desirability of treating cancer with drugs is not always obvious. There are patients whose chances of being helped by chemotherapy are remote, while the risk for serious toxicity is high. Because the potential benefits for some patients are small and the risks are large, the decision to institute chemotherapy must be made with care.

Before a decision to treat can be made, the patient must be given some idea of the benefits the proposed therapy might offer. Three basic benefits are possible: cure, prolongation of life, and palliation. For treatment to be justified, there should be reason to believe that at least one of these benefits will be forthcoming. If a patient cannot be offered some reasonable hope of cure, prolonged life, or palliation, it would be difficult to justify treatment.

The most important factors for predicting the outcome of chemotherapy are (1) the general health of the patient and (2) the responsiveness of the type of cancer the patient has. General health status is assessed by measuring performance status, frequently using the Karnofsky Performance Scale (Table 101.8). A Karnofsky score of less than 40 indicates the patient is debilitated and unlikely to tolerate the additional stress of chemotherapy. Accordingly, patients with a low Karnofsky rating should not receive anticancer drugs—unless their cancer is known to be especially responsive.

The responsiveness of specific cancers is not highly predictable: Some patients with a specific type of cancer may respond well, but others may not. Nonetheless, we should still try to assess whether treatment is likely to produce cure, palliation, or prolonged life. If a positive outcome is deemed likely, the patient should almost always be treated, even if his or her Karnofsky score is low. In contrast, if a positive outcome is deemed highly unlikely, the patient should be treated only after careful consideration, so as to avoid the discomforts of a course of treatment that has little to offer.

An important requirement for deciding in favor of chemotherapy is that the impact of treatment be measurable. That is, there must be some objective means of determining the cancer's response to drugs. For solid tumors, we should be able to measure a decrease in tumor size (or at least inhibition of further growth). For hematologic cancers, we should be able to measure a decrease in neoplastic cells in blood and bone marrow. If we have no way to measure the response of a cancer, then we have no way of knowing if treatment has done any good. If we cannot determine that drugs are doing something beneficial, there is little justification for giving them.

Clearly, not all patients are candidates for chemotherapy. The decision to institute treatment must be individualized. Patients should be informed as accurately as possible about the potential risks and benefits of the proposed therapy. When the decision to treat is made, it should be the result of collaboration among the patient, family, and physician, and should reflect a conviction on the part of the patient that, within his or her set of values, the potential benefits outweigh the inherent risks.

LOOKING AHEAD

Does the future offer hope of developing drugs that can cure people who can't be cured today? This question can be cautiously answered in the affirmative. There is no theoretical reason to believe that cancers are inherently incapable of cure. On the contrary, there is good reason to believe that cancers are, in fact, curable. New insights into tumor biology are suggesting many new ways to attack cancer cells. Three approaches are especially exciting: cancer vaccines, angiogenesis inhibitors, and telomerase inhibitors. Custom-made vaccines using the patient's own cancer cells can intensify immune attack against the cancer. Angiogenesis inhibitors can block the growth of new blood vessels into solid tumors, thereby starving the tumor. Telomerase inhibitors offer the possibility of a "magic bullet" that can block the endless proliferation of cancer cells, while leaving normal cells unharmed. Other important approaches include inhibition of epidermal growth factor, inhibition of various cellular kinases, and inhibition of oncogenes. These areas of research and others may finally lead to drugs that

TABLE 101.8 ▪ Karnofsky Performance Scale

Definition	Percentage	Criteria
Able to carry on normal activity and work; no special care needed	100	Normal; no complaints; no evidence of disease
	90	Able to carry on normal activity; minor signs or symptoms of disease
	80	Normal activity with effort; some signs or symptoms of disease
Unable to work; able to live at home and care for most personal needs; a varying amount of assistance needed	70	Cares for self; unable to carry on normal activity or do active work
	60	Requires occasional assistance; able to care for most needs
	50	Requires considerable assistance and frequent medical care
Unable to care for self; requires equivalent of institutional or hospital care; disease may be progressing rapidly	40	Disabled; requires special care and assistance
	30	Severely disabled; hospitalization is indicated although death not imminent
	20	Very sick, hospitalization necessary; active supportive treatment necessary
	10	Moribund; fatal processes progressing rapidly
	0	Dead

have the same degree of selective toxicity for cancer as, for example, penicillin G has for gram-positive bacteria. Drugs with this degree of selectivity will offer a cure for neoplastic diseases—and will provide that cure without the toxicities associated with most of today's drugs. It is not completely naïve to believe that such drugs will eventually be available. In the meantime, we can take heart in the progress achieved so far: Drugs such as trastuzumab [Herceptin] (for breast cancer) and imatinib [Gleevec] (for chronic myeloid leukemia and GI stromal tumors) are both highly effective and much less toxic than traditional chemotherapeutic agents.

KEY POINTS

- The term *cancer* refers not to a single disorder, but rather to a large group of disorders that differ with respect to clinical presentation, aggressiveness, drug sensitivity, and prognosis.
- Cancer cells are characterized by immortality, persistent proliferation, invasive growth, and the ability to form metastases.
- Cancer can be treated with three basic modalities: surgery, radiation therapy, and drug therapy.
- Agents used for drug therapy fall into two main groups (1) cytotoxic agents and (2) noncytotoxic agents, such as hormones, immunomodulators, and targeted drugs.
- Surgery and irradiation are the treatments of choice for most solid tumors.
- Drugs are the treatment of choice for disseminated cancers (leukemias, disseminated lymphomas, widespread metastases). Drugs are also used as adjuvants to surgery and irradiation to kill malignant cells that surgery and irradiation leave behind.
- The cell cycle has four major phases: G_1, in which cells prepare to synthesize DNA by synthesizing histones (proteins found in chromatin); S, in which cells synthesize DNA; G_2, in which cells prepare for mitosis (division); and M, in which cells actually divide. Following mitosis, the resulting daughter cells may either enter G_1 and repeat the cycle, or enter G_0 and become mitotically dormant.
- The growth fraction of a tissue is defined as the ratio of proliferating cells to cells in G_0.
- Tissues with a large percentage of proliferating cells and few cells in G_0 have a high growth fraction. Conversely, tissues composed mostly of G_0 cells have a low growth fraction.
- Cytotoxic anticancer drugs are more toxic to cancers that have a high growth fraction than to cancers that have a low growth fraction. Why? Because cytotoxic anticancer drugs are more active against proliferating cells than against cells in G_0.
- The most common cancers—solid tumors of the breast, lung, prostate, colon, and rectum—have a low growth fraction, so they respond poorly to cytotoxic drugs. In contrast, only some rarer cancers—such as acute lymphocytic leukemia, Hodgkin's disease, and certain testicular cancers—have a high growth fraction, so they tend to respond well to cytotoxic drugs.
- To cure a patient of cancer, we must produce 100% cell kill, which is rare with chemotherapy alone.
- Killing of cancer cells follows first-order kinetics. That is, at any given dose, drugs kill a constant *percentage* of malignant cells, regardless of how many cells are present.
- Over the course of chemotherapy, cancer cells often become drug resistant, thereby decreasing the chance of success.
- The purpose of intermittent chemotherapy is to allow normal cells to repopulate between rounds of treatment. However, if the cancer cells repopulate as fast as (or faster than) normal cells, there will be no reduction in tumor burden with each round of treatment, and hence treatment will fail.
- Multidrug chemotherapy is generally much more effective than single-drug therapy. Why? Because combination therapy can (1) suppress drug resistance, (2) increase cell kill, and (3) reduce injury to normal cells (at any given level of anticancer effect).
- Ideally, the drugs used in combination therapy should have (1) different mechanisms of action, (2) minimally overlapping toxicities, and (3) good efficacy when used alone.
- For drugs that act during a specific phase of the cell cycle, selecting the right dosing schedule is critical to success.
- Toxicity to normal tissues is the major obstacle to successful therapy with cytotoxic anticancer drugs.
- Cytotoxic anticancer drugs injure normal tissue because these drugs lack selective toxicity.
- As a rule, serious toxicity occurs to normal tissues that have a high growth fraction (i.e., bone marrow, GI epithelium, hair follicles, sperm-forming cells).
- Myelosuppression (toxicity to bone marrow) can reduce the number of neutrophils, platelets, and erythrocytes, thereby posing a risk for infection (from loss of neutrophils), bleeding (from loss of platelets), and anemia (from loss of erythrocytes).
- Loss of neutrophils and platelets during chemotherapy is common; significant loss of erythrocytes is relatively rare, but can happen with certain drugs (e.g., cisplatin).
- In patients taking myelosuppressive drugs, neutrophil counts must be monitored. If neutropenia is substantial (absolute neutrophil count below $500/mm^3$), the next round of chemotherapy should be delayed.
- When a neutropenic patient develops an infection, immediate and vigorous intervention is required. Until lab reports on the identity and drug sensitivity of the infecting organism are available, empiric therapy with IV antibiotics should be instituted.

- Neutropenia can be minimized by treatment with granulocyte colony-stimulating factor (short-acting and long-acting forms) and granulocyte-macrophage colony-stimulating factor—drugs that act on bone marrow to increase neutrophil production.
- Anemia can be managed with erythropoietin, but only in patients who do *not* have myeloid malignancies (e.g., leukemia), and then only when the goal is palliation (erythropoietin *shortens* life in all cancer patients, and hence must not be used when the goal is cure or prolongation of life).
- By injuring the epithelial lining of the GI tract, anticancer drugs often cause stomatitis and diarrhea.
- Many anticancer drugs cause moderate to severe nausea and vomiting, in part by stimulating the chemoreceptor trigger zone.
- Nausea and vomiting can be reduced by premedication with antiemetics. The combination of aprepitant, dexamethasone, and ondansetron is especially effective.
- Anticancer drugs often injure hair follicles, thereby causing alopecia (hair loss). Patients who want to wear a hairpiece should select one before hair loss occurs.
- Anticancer drugs can cause fetal malformation and death, primarily in the first trimester. However, after 18 weeks of gestation, risk appears to be very low.
- Anticancer drugs can cause irreversible male sterility. Accordingly, men undergoing chemotherapy should be counseled about possible sperm banking.
- Chemotherapy can cause hyperuricemia as a result of DNA degradation secondary to massive cell death.
- Renal injury from hyperuricemia can be minimized by giving (1) fluids, (2) prophylactic allopurinol (a drug that blocks uric acid formation), and (3) rasburicase (an enzyme that catalyzes uric acid degradation).
- Anticancer drugs with vesicant properties can cause severe local injury if the IV line through which they are being administered becomes extravasated.
- Cancer chemotherapy has three possible benefits: cure, palliation, and prolongation of useful life. For treatment to be justified, at least one of these benefits should be likely.

Please visit **http://evolve.elsevier.com/Lehne** for chapter-specific NCLEX® examination review questions.

CHAPTER

102 Anticancer Drugs I: Cytotoxic Agents

INTRODUCTION TO THE CYTOTOXIC ANTICANCER DRUGS

The cytotoxic agents constitute the largest class of anticancer drugs. As their name implies, these agents act directly on cancer cells to cause their death. The cytotoxic drugs can be subdivided into eight major groups: (1) alkylating agents, (2) platinum compounds, (3) antimetabolites, (4) hypomethylating agents, (5) antitumor antibiotics, (6) mitotic inhibitors, (7) topoisomerase inhibitors, and (8) miscellaneous cytotoxic drugs. We don't discuss each drug in detail, but rather focus on selected representative agents. Individual cytotoxic agents are shown in Table 102.1.

Mechanisms of Cytotoxic Action

Table 102.2 shows the principal mechanisms by which the cytotoxic anticancer drugs act. As the table shows, cytotoxic agents disrupt processes related to synthesis of DNA or its precursors. In addition, some agents (e.g., vinblastine, vincristine) act specifically to block mitosis. Because the cytotoxic drugs disrupt processes carried out exclusively by cells that are undergoing replication, these drugs are most toxic to tissues that have a high growth fraction (i.e., a high proportion of proliferating cells).

Cell-Cycle Phase Specificity

As discussed in Chapter 101, the cell cycle is the sequence of events that a cell goes through from one mitotic division to the next. Some anticancer agents, known as *cell-cycle phase–specific drugs,* are effective only during a specific phase of the cell cycle. Other anticancer agents, known as *cell-cycle phase–nonspecific drugs,* can affect cells during any phase of the cell cycle. About half of the cytotoxic anticancer drugs are phase specific, and the other half are phase nonspecific. The phase specificity of individual cytotoxic agents is shown in Table 102.1.

Cell-Cycle Phase–Specific Drugs

Phase-specific agents are toxic only to cells that are passing through a particular phase of the cell cycle. Vincristine, for example, acts by causing mitotic arrest, and hence is effective only during M phase. Other agents act by disrupting DNA synthesis, and hence are effective only during S phase. Because of their phase specificity, these drugs are toxic only to cells that are active participants in the cell cycle; cells that are "resting" in G_0 will not be harmed. Obviously, if these drugs are to be effective, they must be present as neoplastic cells cycle through the specific phase in which they act. Accordingly,

TABLE 102.1 ▪ Cytotoxic Anticancer Drugs

Generic Name	Brand Name	Cell-Cycle Phase Specificity	Route	Dose-Limiting Toxicity
ALKYLATING AGENTS				
Nitrogen Mustards				
Bendamustine	Treanda	Phase nonspecific	IV	Bone marrow suppression, infusion reactions
Chlorambucil	Leukeran	Phase nonspecific	PO	Bone marrow suppression
Cyclophosphamide	Generic only	Phase nonspecific	PO, IV	Bone marrow suppression
Ifosfamide	Ifex	Phase nonspecific	IV	Bone marrow suppression, hemorrhagic cystitis
Mechlorethamine	Mustargen	Phase nonspecific	IV, IC, IP	Bone marrow suppression
Melphalan	Alkeran	Phase nonspecific	PO, IV	Bone marrow suppression
Nitrosoureas				
Carmustine	BiCNU, Gliadel	Phase nonspecific	IV, CNS implant	Bone marrow suppression
Lomustine	CeeNU 🍁, Gleostine	Phase nonspecific	PO	Bone marrow suppression
Streptozocin	Zanosar	Phase nonspecific	IV	Nephrotoxicity
Others				
Busulfan	Myleran, Busulfex	Phase nonspecific	PO, IV	Bone marrow suppression, pulmonary fibrosis
Temozolomide	Temodar, Temodal 🍁	Phase nonspecific	PO	Bone marrow suppression
PLATINUM COMPOUNDS				
Carboplatin	Generic only	Phase nonspecific	IV	Bone marrow suppression
Cisplatin	Generic only	Phase nonspecific	IV	Nephrotoxicity
Oxaliplatin	Eloxatin	Phase nonspecific	IV	Peripheral neuropathy
ANTIMETABOLITES				
Folic Acid Analogs				
Methotrexate	Rheumatrex, Trexall	S-phase specific	IV, IM, PO, IT	Bone marrow suppression, mucositis
Pemetrexed	Alimta	S-phase specific	IV	Bone marrow suppression
Pralatrexate	Folotyn	S-phase specific	IV	Bone marrow suppression, mucositis
Pyrimidine Analogs				
Capecitabine	Xeloda	Kills dividing cells only, mainly in S phase	PO	Bone marrow suppression, diarrhea, hand-and-foot syndrome
Cytarabine	DepoCyt, Tarabine PFS 🍁	S-phase specific	IV, subQ, IT	Bone marrow suppression
Floxuridine	FUDR	Kills dividing cells only, mainly in S phase	IA	Bone marrow suppression, oral and GI ulceration
Fluorouracil	Adrucil	Kills dividing cells only, mainly in S phase	IV	Bone marrow suppression, oral and GI ulceration
Gemcitabine	Gemzar	S-phase specific	IV	Bone marrow suppression
Purine Analogs				
Cladribine	Generic only	Kills dividing cells only, mainly in S phase	IV	Bone marrow suppression
Clofarabine	Clolar	S-phase specific	IV	Bone marrow suppression
Fludarabine	Fludara	S-phase specific	IV	Bone marrow suppression
Mercaptopurine	Purinethol	S-phase specific	PO	Bone marrow suppression
Nelarabine	Arranon, Atriance 🍁	S-phase specific	IV	Neurotoxicity
Pentostatin	Nipent	S-phase specific	IV	Bone marrow suppression
Thioguanine	Tabloid, Lanvis 🍁	S-phase specific	PO, IV	Bone marrow suppression

Continued

TABLE 102.1 ▪ Cytotoxic Anticancer Drugs—cont'd

Generic Name	Brand Name	Cell-Cycle Phase Specificity	Route	Dose-Limiting Toxicity
HYPOMETHYLATING AGENTS				
Azacitidine	Vidaza	S-phase specific	subQ	Bone marrow suppression
Decitabine	Dacogen	S-phase specific	IV	Bone marrow suppression
ANTITUMOR ANTIBIOTICS				
Anthracyclines				
Daunorubicin (conventional)	Cerubidine	Phase nonspecific	IV	Bone marrow suppression, cardiotoxicity
Daunorubicin (liposomal)	DaunoXome	Phase nonspecific	IV	Bone marrow suppression, cardiotoxicity
Doxorubicin (conventional)	Adriamycin	Phase nonspecific	IV	Bone marrow suppression, cardiotoxicity
Doxorubicin (liposomal)	Doxil, Caelyx 🍁	Phase nonspecific	IV	Bone marrow suppression, heart failure
Epirubicin	Ellence	Phase nonspecific, but S and G_2 most sensitive	IV	Bone marrow suppression, cardiotoxicity
Idarubicin	Idamycin	Phase nonspecific, but S most sensitive	IV	Bone marrow suppression, cardiotoxicity
Valrubicin	Valstar	G_2-phase specific	Intravesical	Dysuria inadequately controlled by phenazopyridine, hematuria lasting more than 2 days
Mitoxantrone[a]	Novantrone	Phase nonspecific	IV	Bone marrow suppression, cardiotoxicity
Nonanthracyclines				
Bleomycin	Generic only	G_2-phase specific	IV, IM, subQ, IP	Pneumonitis and pulmonary fibrosis
Dactinomycin	Cosmegen	Phase nonspecific	IV	Bone marrow suppression, mucositis
Mitomycin	Generic only in United States, Mutamycin 🍁	Phase nonspecific, but G_1 and S most sensitive	IV	Bone marrow suppression
MITOTIC INHIBITORS				
Vinca Alkaloids				
Vinblastine	Velban	M-phase specific	IV	Bone marrow suppression
Vincristine (conventional)	Oncovin, Vincasar PFS	M-phase specific	IV	Peripheral neuropathy
Vincristine (liposomal)	Marqibo	M-phase specific	IV	Peripheral neuropathy
Vinorelbine	Navelbine	M-phase specific	IV	Bone marrow suppression
Taxanes				
Cabazitaxel	Jevtana	G_2/M-phase specific	IV	Bone marrow suppression, diarrhea
Docetaxel	Docefrez, Taxotere	G_2/M-phase specific	IV	Bone marrow suppression
Paclitaxel	Abraxane, Onxol, Taxol 🍁	G_2/M-phase specific	IV	Bone marrow suppression
Others				
Eribulin	Halaven	G_2/M-phase specific	IV	Bone marrow suppression, peripheral neuropathy
Estramustine	Emcyt	M-phase specific	PO	Nausea and vomiting
Ixabepilone	Ixempra	G_2/M-phase specific	IV	Bone marrow suppression, neurotoxicity

TABLE 102.1 ■ Cytotoxic Anticancer Drugs—cont'd

Generic Name	Brand Name	Cell-Cycle Phase Specificity	Route	Dose-Limiting Toxicity
TOPOISOMERASE INHIBITORS				
Etoposide	Toposar	S and G_2 most sensitive	IV, PO	Bone marrow suppression
Irinotecan	Camptosar	S-phase specific	IV	Bone marrow suppression and late diarrhea
Teniposide	Vumon	S and G_2 most sensitive	IV	Bone marrow suppression
Topotecan	Hycamtin	S-phase specific	IV	Bone marrow suppression
MISCELLANEOUS				
Altretamine	Hexalen	Specificity unknown	PO	Bone marrow suppression
Asparaginase	Elspar, Erwinase 🍁, Kidrolase 🍁	G_1-phase specific	IV, IM	None
Dacarbazine	DTIC-Dome	Phase nonspecific	IV	Bone marrow suppression
Hydroxyurea	Hydrea	S-phase specific	PO	Bone marrow suppression
Mitotane	Lysodren	Phase nonspecific	PO	CNS depression
Pegaspargase	Oncaspar	G_1-phase specific	IV, IM	None
Procarbazine	Matulane	Phase nonspecific	PO	Bone marrow suppression

[a]Mitoxantrone is classified chemically as an anthracenedione, which is very similar to an anthracycline.
CNS, Central nervous system; *GI,* gastrointestinal; *IA,* intra-arterial; *IC,* intracavitary; *IM,* intramuscular; *IP,* intrapleural; *IT,* intrathecal; *IV,* intravenous; *PO,* oral; *subQ,* subcutaneous.

TABLE 102.2 ■ Actions of Representative Cytotoxic Anticancer Drugs

Drug	Drug Action	Cellular Process Disrupted
Cyclophosphamide	Alkylates DNA, causing cross-links and strand breakage	DNA and RNA synthesis
Methotrexate	Inhibits 1-carbon transfer reactions	Synthesis of DNA precursors (purines, dTMP)
Hydroxyurea	Inhibits ribonucleotide reductase	Synthesis of DNA precursors (blocks conversion of ribonucleotides into deoxyribonucleotides)
Thioguanine, mercaptopurine	Inhibit purine ring synthesis and nucleotide interconversion	Synthesis of DNA precursors (purines, pyrimidines, ribonucleotides, and deoxyribonucleotides)
Fluorouracil	Inhibits thymidylate synthetase	Synthesis of dTMP, a DNA precursor
Cytarabine	Inhibits DNA polymerase	DNA synthesis
Bleomycin	Breaks DNA strands and prevents their repair	DNA synthesis
Doxorubicin	Intercalates between base pairs of DNA and inhibits topoisomerase II	DNA and RNA synthesis
Vinblastine, vincristine	Block microtubule assembly	Mitosis
Asparaginase	Deaminates asparagine, depriving cells of this amino acid	Impairs DNA replication by disrupting synthesis of histones (proteins in chromatins)
Topotecan	Inhibits topoisomerase I and thereby prevents resealing of DNA strand breaks	Impairs DNA replication

these drugs must be present for an extended time. To accomplish this, phase-specific drugs are often administered by prolonged infusion. Alternatively, they can be given in multiple doses at short intervals over an extended time. Because the dosing schedule is so critical to therapeutic response, phase-specific drugs are also known as *schedule-dependent drugs.*

Cell-Cycle Phase–Nonspecific Drugs

The phase-nonspecific drugs can act during any phase of the cell cycle, including G_0. Among the phase-nonspecific drugs are the alkylating agents and most antitumor antibiotics. Because phase-nonspecific drugs can injure cells throughout the cell cycle, whereas phase-specific drugs cannot, phase-nonspecific drugs can increase cell kill when combined with phase-specific drugs.

Although the phase-nonspecific drugs can cause biochemical lesions at any time during the cell cycle, *as a rule these drugs are more toxic to proliferating cells than to cells in G_0.* There are two reasons why this is so. First, cells in G_0 have time to repair drug-induced damage before it can result in significant harm. In contrast, proliferating cells often lack time for repair. Second, toxicity may not become manifest until the cells attempt to proliferate. For example, many alkylating agents act by producing cross-links between DNA strands. Although these biochemical lesions can be made at any time, they are largely without effect until cells attempt to replicate DNA. This is much like inflicting a flat tire on an automobile: The tire can be deflated at any time; however, loss of air is consequential only if the car is moving. Carrying the analogy further, if the flat occurs while the car is stopped and is repaired before travel is attempted, the flat will have no functional impact at all.

It should be noted that some dividing cells are more vulnerable than others. Specifically, cells that divide quickly are harmed more readily than cells that divide slowly. Why? Because quickly dividing cells have less time for repair.

Toxicity

Many anticancer drugs are toxic to normal tissues—especially tissues that have a high percentage of proliferating cells (bone marrow, hair follicles, GI epithelium, germinal epithelium). The common major toxicities of the cytotoxic anticancer drugs, together with management procedures, are discussed in Chapter 101. Therefore, as we consider individual anticancer agents in this chapter, discussion of most toxicities is brief.

> **Safety Alert**
>
> **HIGH-ALERT MEDICATIONS**
>
> The Institute for Safe Medication Practices includes *both oral and parenteral chemotherapeutic drugs* among its list of high-alert medications. *High-alert medications* are those drugs that can cause devastating effects to patients in the event of a medication error.

Dosage, Handling, and Administration

Cancer chemotherapy is a highly specialized field. Accordingly, in a general text such as this, presentation of detailed information on dosage and administration of specific agents seems inappropriate. However, be aware that dosages for anticancer agents must be individualized and that the timing of administration may vary with the particular protocol being followed. Also, because of the complex and hazardous nature of cancer chemotherapy, anticancer drugs should be administered under the direct supervision of a clinician experienced in their use.

Handling Cytotoxic Drugs

Antineoplastic drugs are often mutagenic, teratogenic, and carcinogenic. In addition, direct contact with the skin, eyes, and mucous membranes can result in local injury (and can increase cancer risk if enough drug is absorbed). Accordingly, it is imperative that healthcare personnel involved in preparing and administering these drugs follow safe handling procedures. Risk of injury from contact with parenteral chemotherapeutic drugs can be minimized by using biologic safety cabinets and by following approved procedures for compounding and administration. The National Institute for Occupational Safety and Health (NIOSH) has established procedures for handling hazardous drugs. You will find the NIOSH guidelines in Table 3.1 of Chapter 3.

Administering Vesicants

Extravasation of vesicants can cause severe local injury, sometimes requiring surgical débridement and skin grafting. Drugs with strong vesicant properties include carmustine, dacarbazine, dactinomycin, daunorubicin, doxorubicin, mechlorethamine, mitomycin, plicamycin, streptozocin, vinblastine, and vincristine. To minimize the risk of injury, IV administration should be performed only into a vein with good flow. Sites of previous irradiation should be avoided. If extravasation occurs, the infusion should be discontinued immediately.

ALKYLATING AGENTS

The family of alkylating agents consists of nitrogen mustards, nitrosoureas, and other compounds. Before considering the properties of individual alkylating agents, we discuss the characteristics of the group as a whole. The alkylating agents are shown in Table 102.1.

Shared Properties

Mechanism of Action

The alkylating agents are highly reactive compounds that can transfer an alkyl group to various cell constituents. Cell kill results primarily from alkylation of DNA. As a rule, alkylating agents interact with DNA by forming a covalent bond with a specific nitrogen atom in guanine.

Some alkylating agents have two reactive sites, whereas others have only one. Alkylating agents with two reactive sites (*bifunctional* agents) are able to bind DNA in two places to form *cross-links*. These bridges may be formed within a single DNA strand or between parallel DNA strands. Fig. 102.1 shows the production of interstrand cross-links by nitrogen mustard. Alkylating agents with only one reactive site (*monofunctional* agents) lack the ability to form cross-links but can still bind to a single guanine in DNA.

The consequences of guanine alkylation are miscoding, scission of DNA strands, and, if cross-links have been formed, inhibition of DNA replication. Because cross-linking of DNA is especially injurious, cell death is more likely with bifunctional agents than with monofunctional agents.

Because alkylation reactions can take place at any time during the cell cycle, alkylating agents are considered *cell-cycle phase nonspecific*. However, *most of these drugs are more toxic to dividing cells—especially cells that divide rapidly—than they are to cells in G_0*. Why? Because (1) alkylation of DNA produces its most detrimental effects when cells attempt to replicate DNA and (2) quiescent cells are often able to repair damage to DNA before it can affect cell function. Because alkylating agents are phase nonspecific, they don't need to be present over an extended time. Accordingly, they can be administered by bolus dosing, rather than by prolonged infusion.

Resistance

Development of resistance to alkylating agents is common. A major cause is increased production of enzymes that repair DNA. Resistance may also result from decreased uptake of

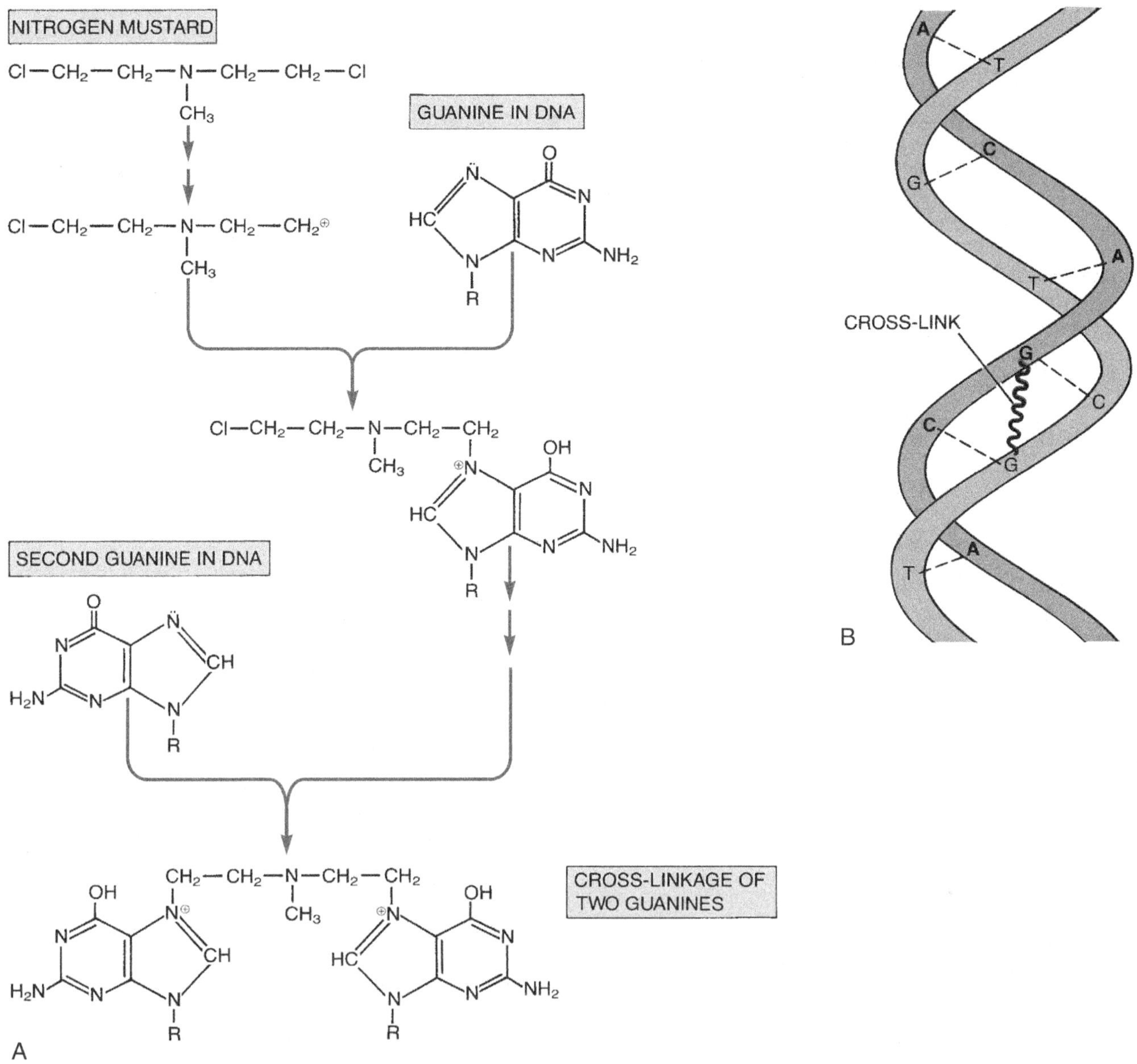

Fig. 102.1 ▪ Cross-linking of DNA by an alkylating agent.
A, Reactions leading to cross-linkage between guanine moieties in DNA. **B,** Schematic representation of interstrand cross-linking within the DNA double helix. (*A,* Adenine; *C,* cytosine; *G,* guanine; *T,* thymine.)

alkylating agents and from increased production of nucleophiles (compounds that act as decoy targets for alkylation).

Toxicities

Alkylating agents are toxic to tissues that have a high growth fraction. Accordingly, these drugs may injure cells of the bone marrow, hair follicles, GI mucosa, and germinal epithelium. Blood dyscrasias caused by bone marrow suppression—neutropenia, thrombocytopenia, and anemia—are of greatest concern. Nausea and vomiting occur with all alkylating agents. Also, several of these drugs are vesicants, and hence must be administered through a free-flowing IV line. The major dose-limiting toxicities of individual drugs are provided in Table 102.1.

Properties of Individual Alkylating Agents

Nitrogen Mustards

As mentioned in Chapter 101, the nitrogen mustards were among the first cytotoxic drugs used for cancer chemotherapy. They had their beginnings in the deadly mustard gas poisonings of World War I. Years later, while combing through the medical records of soldiers treated for mustard gas poisoning, researchers discovered that the toxin destroyed leukocytes. It occurred to them that a chemical capable of destroying blood cells might also be capable of destroying cancer cells. Their experiments using nitrogen mustard to treat lymphoma were a success. Thus, modern chemotherapy was born.

There are six nitrogen mustards approved for chemotherapy in the United States. They are cyclophosphamide, mechlorethamine, bendamustine, chlorambucil, melphalan, and ifosfamide.

Cyclophosphamide. Cyclophosphamide, formerly available as *Cytoxan* and *Neosar,* is a bifunctional alkylating agent active against a *broad spectrum* of neoplastic diseases. Indications include *Hodgkin's disease, non-Hodgkin's lymphomas, multiple myeloma,* and *solid tumors of the head, neck, ovary, and breast.* Of all the alkylating agents, cyclophosphamide is employed most widely.

Cyclophosphamide is a prodrug that undergoes conversion to its active form in the liver. Because activation is required, onset of effects is delayed. Cyclophosphamide is not a vesicant, and hence can be administered PO as well as IV. Oral doses should be administered with food.

The major dose-limiting toxicity is bone marrow suppression. Severe nausea, vomiting, and alopecia are also common, especially at high doses. In addition, the drug can cause acute hemorrhagic cystitis; bladder injury and associated bleeding can be minimized by (1) maintaining adequate hydration and (2) giving a protective agent called *mesna* [Mesnex] when high-dose cyclophosphamide is employed. Other adverse effects include sterility, immunosuppression, and hypersensitivity reactions.

Mechlorethamine. Mechlorethamine [Mustargen], a bifunctional compound, was the first alkylating agent employed clinically. Indications include *bronchogenic carcinoma, Hodgkin's disease, leukemias,* and *mycosis fungoides.* Mechlorethamine is a powerful vesicant and can cause severe local injury. Accordingly, for systemic therapy, the drug must be administered IV. Caution must be exercised to avoid both extravasation and direct contact with the skin. Once in the bloodstream, mechlorethamine undergoes rapid conversion to active metabolites. The dose-limiting toxicity is bone marrow suppression. Other major toxicities include severe nausea and vomiting, alopecia, diarrhea, stomatitis, amenorrhea, and sterility.

Bendamustine. Bendamustine [Treanda] is a derivative of mechlorethamine and may be better tolerated. The drug has two indications: *chronic lymphocytic leukemia* and *non-Hodgkin's lymphoma.* Administration is IV. As with mechlorethamine, the dose-limiting toxicity is bone marrow suppression. Nausea and vomiting are common. Some patients experience an infusion reaction, characterized by fever, hypotension, chills, rigors, and myalgias. There have been postmarketing reports of serious skin reactions, including bullous exanthema and toxic epidermal necrolysis. However, a causal relationship has not been established. Nonetheless, if a severe skin reaction occurs, bendamustine should be withheld or discontinued. Fluvoxamine [Luvox] and other drugs that inhibit CYP1A2 (the 1A2 isoenzyme of cytochrome P450) may raise bendamustine levels, whereas carbamazepine [Tegretol] and other drugs that induce CYP1A2 may reduce bendamustine levels.

Chlorambucil. Chlorambucil [Leukeran], an oral nitrogen mustard, is generally well tolerated. Bone marrow suppression is the major dose-limiting toxicity. Other adverse effects include hepatotoxicity, sterility, and, rarely, pulmonary fibrosis. Nausea and vomiting are usually mild. Chlorambucil is a drug of choice for palliative therapy of *chronic lymphocytic leukemia.* The drug is also used for *Hodgkin's disease, non-Hodgkin's lymphoma,* and *multiple myeloma.*

Melphalan. Melphalan [Alkeran], a bifunctional agent, is generally well tolerated. Bone marrow suppression is the major dose-limiting toxicity. The drug can cause secondary malignancy and is mutagenic like other alkylating agents. Melphalan is not a vesicant. Severe nausea and vomiting are rare. Administration is PO and IV. Melphalan is a preferred drug for *multiple myeloma* and is also active against *lymphoma* and *carcinoma of the ovary and breast.*

Ifosfamide. Ifosfamide [Ifex], a derivative of cyclophosphamide, is approved for refractory *germ cell testicular cancer* and is used off-label against many other tumors, including *Hodgkin's and non-Hodgkin's lymphomas, non–small cell and small cell lung cancer,* and *head and neck cancer.* Dose-limiting toxicities are bone marrow suppression and hemorrhagic cystitis. The risk of cystitis is minimized by concurrent therapy with *mesna* [Mesnex] and by extensive hydration (at least 2 L of oral or IV fluid daily). Owing to the risk of cystitis, urinalysis should be performed before each dose. If the analysis reveals microscopic hematuria, dosing should be postponed until hematuria resolves. Additional adverse effects include nausea, vomiting, metabolic acidosis, and central nervous system (CNS) toxicity (confusion, hallucinations, blurred vision, coma). Severe adverse effects are most likely in patients receiving high-dose therapy and in those with renal failure. Administration is IV.

Nitrosoureas

The nitrosoureas are bifunctional alkylating agents and are active against a broad spectrum of neoplastic diseases. Cell kill results from cross-linking DNA. Unlike many anticancer drugs, the nitrosoureas are highly lipophilic, and hence can readily penetrate the blood-brain barrier. As a result, these drugs are especially useful against *cancers of the CNS.* The major dose-limiting toxicity is *delayed bone marrow suppression.*

Carmustine. Carmustine [BiCNU, Gliadel] was the first nitrosourea to undergo extensive clinical testing and can be considered the *prototype* for the group. Owing to its ability to cross the blood-brain barrier, carmustine is especially useful against *primary and metastatic tumors of the brain.* Other indications include *Hodgkin's disease, non-Hodgkin's lymphomas, multiple myeloma, malignant melanoma, hepatoma,* and *adenocarcinoma of the stomach, colon, and rectum.* The principal dose-limiting toxicity is delayed bone marrow suppression; leukocyte and platelet nadirs occur 4 to 6 weeks after treatment. Nausea and vomiting can be severe. Injury to the liver and kidneys has been reported. High cumulative doses may cause pulmonary fibrosis. Accordingly, if pulmonary function begins to decline, glucocorticoids should be given to prevent fibrosis.

Prototype Drugs

CYTOTOXIC AGENTS

Alkylating Agents
Cyclophosphamide

Platinum Compounds
Cisplatin

Antimetabolites
Methotrexate (folic acid analog)
Fluorouracil (pyrimidine analog)
Mercaptopurine (purine analog)

Antitumor Antibiotics
Doxorubicin (an anthracycline)
Dactinomycin (a nonanthracycline)

Mitotic Inhibitors
Vincristine (a vinca alkaloid)
Paclitaxel (a toxoid)

Topoisomerase Inhibitors
Etoposide

Others
Asparaginase

Administration may be topical or IV. Topical administration is done by implanting a biodegradable, carmustine-impregnated wafer [Gliadel] into the cavity created by surgical removal of a brain tumor. This technique has the obvious benefit of concentrating the drug where it is most needed. When administered IV, carmustine can cause local phlebitis and extravasation injury, even though it is not a vesicant.

Lomustine. Lomustine [Gleostine, CeeNU ♣] is similar to carmustine in actions and uses. Like carmustine, lomustine crosses the blood-brain barrier and is approved for *brain cancer*. The drug is also approved for *Hodgkin's disease*. As with carmustine, the major dose-limiting toxicity is delayed bone marrow suppression. Additional toxicities include nausea and vomiting, renal and hepatic toxicity, pulmonary fibrosis, and neurologic reactions. Dosing is oral.

Streptozocin. Streptozocin [Zanosar] differs significantly from other nitrosoureas. The drug contains a glucose moiety that causes selective uptake by islet cells of the pancreas. This property underlies the drug's only approved indication: *metastatic islet cell tumors*. The major dose-limiting toxicity is kidney damage. Accordingly, renal function should be monitored in all patients. Nausea and vomiting can be severe. Additional toxicities include hypoglycemia, hyperglycemia, diarrhea, chills, and fever. In contrast to other nitrosoureas, streptozocin causes minimal bone marrow suppression. The drug is given IV.

Other Alkylating Agents

Busulfan. Busulfan [Myleran, Busulfex] is a bifunctional agent with just one approved use: *chronic myelogenous leukemia*. Dose-limiting toxicities are bone marrow suppression, pulmonary infiltrates, and pulmonary fibrosis. Other toxicities include nausea, vomiting, alopecia, gynecomastia, male and female sterility, skin hyperpigmentation, cataracts, seizures, and liver injury. Dosing is oral and IV.

Temozolomide

Therapeutic Uses. Temozolomide [Temodar, Temodal ♣] is indicated for oral therapy of adults with *anaplastic astrocytoma* that has relapsed after treatment with preferred agents: procarbazine and a nitrosourea (lomustine or carmustine). Temozolomide can also benefit patients with recurrent *glioblastoma multiforme*. Both of these cancers arise from glial cells in the brain, and both eventually recur despite aggressive treatment. However, even though temozolomide cannot offer cure, it *can* increase health-related quality of life. Dosage depends on the type of cancer being treated. (There are more than 10 different dosing schedules, and these 10 have additional variations based on considerations such as phase of treatment and adjustments for toxicity.)

Pharmacokinetics and Mechanism of Action. Temozolomide undergoes nearly complete absorption after oral dosing. Food reduces both the rate and extent of absorption. Once in the body, temozolomide undergoes rapid, nonenzymatic conversion to its active form, an alkylating agent known as MTIC. As MTIC, the drug alkylates DNA and thereby causes cell death. Temozolomide readily crosses the blood-brain barrier to reach its site of action. The elimination half-life is 1.8 hours.

Adverse Effects. The major dose-limiting toxicity is myelosuppression, manifesting as neutropenia and thrombocytopenia. The most common adverse effects are nausea and vomiting. Both respond well to antiemetic drugs. Other common reactions include headache, fatigue, constipation, and diarrhea. Convulsions may also occur. Patients must not open temozolomide capsules; the drug can cause local injury following inhalation or contact with the skin or mucous membranes.

PLATINUM COMPOUNDS

The platinum-containing anticancer drugs—cisplatin, carboplatin, and oxaliplatin—are similar to the alkylating agents and often classified as such. Like the bifunctional alkylating agents, the platinum compounds produce cross-links in DNA, and hence are cell-cycle phase nonspecific.

Cisplatin

Cisplatin, formerly available as Platinol-AQ, kills cells primarily by forming cross-links between and within strands of DNA. The drug is approved only for *metastatic testicular and ovarian cancers* and *advanced bladder cancer*. Nonetheless, it is used off-label as a component in standard-of-care regimens for *lung cancer* and *head and neck cancer*. The major dose-limiting toxicity is kidney damage, which can be minimized by extensive hydration coupled with diuretic therapy and *amifostine* [Ethyol]. Cisplatin is highly emetogenic; nausea and vomiting begin about 1 hour after dosing and can persist for several days. Other adverse effects include clinically important peripheral neuropathy, mild to moderate bone marrow suppression, kidney damage, and ototoxicity, which manifests as tinnitus and high-frequency hearing loss. The drug is given by IV infusion.

Carboplatin

Carboplatin, formerly available as Paraplatin, is an analog of cisplatin. Cell kill appears to result from cross-linking DNA. The drug's only approved indications are initial and palliative therapy of advanced *ovarian cancer*. Unlabeled uses include *small cell cancer of the lung, squamous cell cancer of the head and neck*, and *endometrial cancer*. The major dose-limiting toxicity is bone marrow suppression. Nausea and vomiting occur, but are less severe than with cisplatin. Similarly, nephrotoxicity, neurotoxicity, and hearing loss are less frequent than with cisplatin. Carboplatin is administered by IV infusion. Anaphylactic reactions have occurred minutes after dosing; symptoms can be managed with epinephrine, glucocorticoids, and antihistamines.

Oxaliplatin

Actions and Uses

Oxaliplatin [Eloxatin] is similar to carboplatin. Like carboplatin, oxaliplatin produces intra- and interstrand cross-links in DNA. Oxaliplatin is approved only for *colorectal cancer* and only in combination with fluorouracil/leucovorin (leucovorin potentiates the activity of fluorouracil). This regimen may be used for adjuvant therapy following complete tumor resection or in patients with advanced colorectal cancer. Investigational uses include *mesothelioma, non-Hodgkin's lymphoma*, and *cancers of the breast, ovary, pancreas, prostate, and lung*. Administration is by IV infusion.

Toxicity

Peripheral Sensory Neuropathy. The major dose-limiting toxicity is peripheral sensory neuropathy, manifesting as numbness or tingling in the fingers and toes and around the mouth and throat. Neuropathy develops in most patients, either early in treatment or after several courses. Neuropathy may impede activities of daily living, such as buttoning clothing, writing, or just holding things. Symptoms are often intensified by exposure to cold. Accordingly, patients should be warned to cover exposed skin before touching cold objects or entering a cold environment. Also, patients should avoid cold liquids and use of ice. Oxaliplatin-induced neuropathy typically resolves after treatment stops, although complete recovery may take several months. Oral gabapentin may reduce or prevent neuropathy.

Other Toxicities. Damage to bone marrow can cause anemia, neutropenia, and thrombocytopenia in a majority of patients. Other common reactions experienced by at least 30% of patients are nausea and vomiting, liver abnormalities, diarrhea, fever, and abdominal pain. Infections commonly occur, at least in part due to neutropenia. Life-threatening anaphylactoid reactions may develop, but are uncommon; epinephrine, glucocorticoids, and antihistamines have been employed for treatment.

ANTIMETABOLITES

Antimetabolites are structural analogs of important natural metabolites. Because they resemble natural metabolites, these drugs are able to disrupt critical metabolic processes. Some antimetabolites inhibit enzymes that synthesize essential cellular constituents. Others undergo incorporation into DNA and thereby disrupt DNA replication and function.

Antimetabolites are effective only against cells that are active participants in the cell cycle. Most antimetabolites are S-phase specific, although some can act during any phase of the cycle, except G_0. To be effective, agents that are S-phase specific must be present for an extended time.

There are three classes of antimetabolites: (1) folic acid analogs, (2) pyrimidine analogs, and (3) purine analogs.

Members of each class, along with their dose-limiting toxicities, are shown in Table 102.1.

Folic Acid Analogs

Folic acid, in its active form, is needed for several essential biochemical reactions. The folic acid analogs block the conversion of folic acid to its active form. At this time, three analogs of folic acid are used against cancer: methotrexate, pemetrexed, and pralatrexate. Other folate analogs are used to treat bacterial infections (trimethoprim), malaria (pyrimethamine), and *Pneumocystis jiroveci* pneumonia (trimetrexate).

Methotrexate

Mechanism of Action. As shown in Fig. 102.2, methotrexate [Rheumatrex, Trexall] *inhibits dihydrofolate reductase,* the enzyme that converts dihydrofolic acid (FH_2) into tetrahydrofolic acid (FH_4). Because production of FH_4 is a necessary step in the activation of folic acid and because activated folic acid is required for biosynthesis of essential cellular constituents (DNA, RNA, proteins), inhibition of FH_4 production has multiple effects on the cell. Of all the processes that are suppressed by reduced FH_4 availability, biosynthesis of thymidylate appears most critical. Why? Because, in the absence of thymidylate, cells are unable to make DNA. Because cell kill results primarily from disrupting DNA synthesis, methotrexate is considered *S-phase specific.* Please note, however, that in addition to its S-phase effect, methotrexate has another beneficial action: The fall in thymidine levels caused by methotrexate is a potent signal for inducing apoptosis (programmed cell death).

A technique known as *leucovorin rescue* can be employed to enhance the effects of methotrexate. Some neoplastic cells are unresponsive to methotrexate because they lack the transport system required for active uptake of the drug. By giving massive doses of methotrexate, we can force the drug into these cells by passive diffusion. However, because this process also exposes normal cells to extremely high concentrations of methotrexate, normal cells are also at risk. To save them, leucovorin (citrovorum factor, folinic acid) is given. Leucovorin bypasses the metabolic block caused by methotrexate, thereby permitting normal cells to synthesize thymidylate and other compounds. Malignant cells are not saved to the same extent because leucovorin uptake requires the same transport system employed for methotrexate uptake, a transport system these cells lack. It should be noted that leucovorin rescue is potentially dangerous: *Failure to administer leucovorin in the right dose at the right time can be fatal.*

Pharmacokinetics. Methotrexate can be administered PO, IM, IV, and intrathecally. The drug is highly polar, and hence a transport system is needed to enter mammalian cells. In cancer cells and normal cells, methotrexate undergoes enzymatic activation to a polyglutamated form. Elimination is primarily renal. Hence, in patients with renal impairment, dosage must be reduced to prevent the drug from accumulating to toxic levels.

Because methotrexate is highly polar, it crosses the blood-brain barrier poorly, except when given in very high doses. To ensure effective levels, intrathecal administration is employed for most CNS cancers.

Resistance. Cancer cells can acquire resistance to methotrexate through five mechanisms: (1) decreased uptake of methotrexate, (2) increased synthesis of dihydrofolate reductase (the target enzyme for methotrexate), (3) synthesis of a modified form of dihydrofolate reductase that has a reduced affinity for methotrexate, (4) increased production of a transporter that pumps methotrexate out of cells, and (5) reduced production of enzymes needed to convert methotrexate to its active (polyglutamated) form.

Therapeutic Uses. Methotrexate is curative for women with *choriocarcinoma.* The drug is also active against *non-Hodgkin's lymphoma* and *acute lymphocytic leukemia of childhood.* Very large doses coupled with leucovorin rescue have been employed to treat *head and neck sarcomas* and *osteogenic sarcoma.* Noncancer applications include *rheumatoid arthritis* (see Chapter 73), *Crohn's disease* (see Chapter 80), *psoriasis* (see Chapter 105), and *abortion* (see Chapter 62).

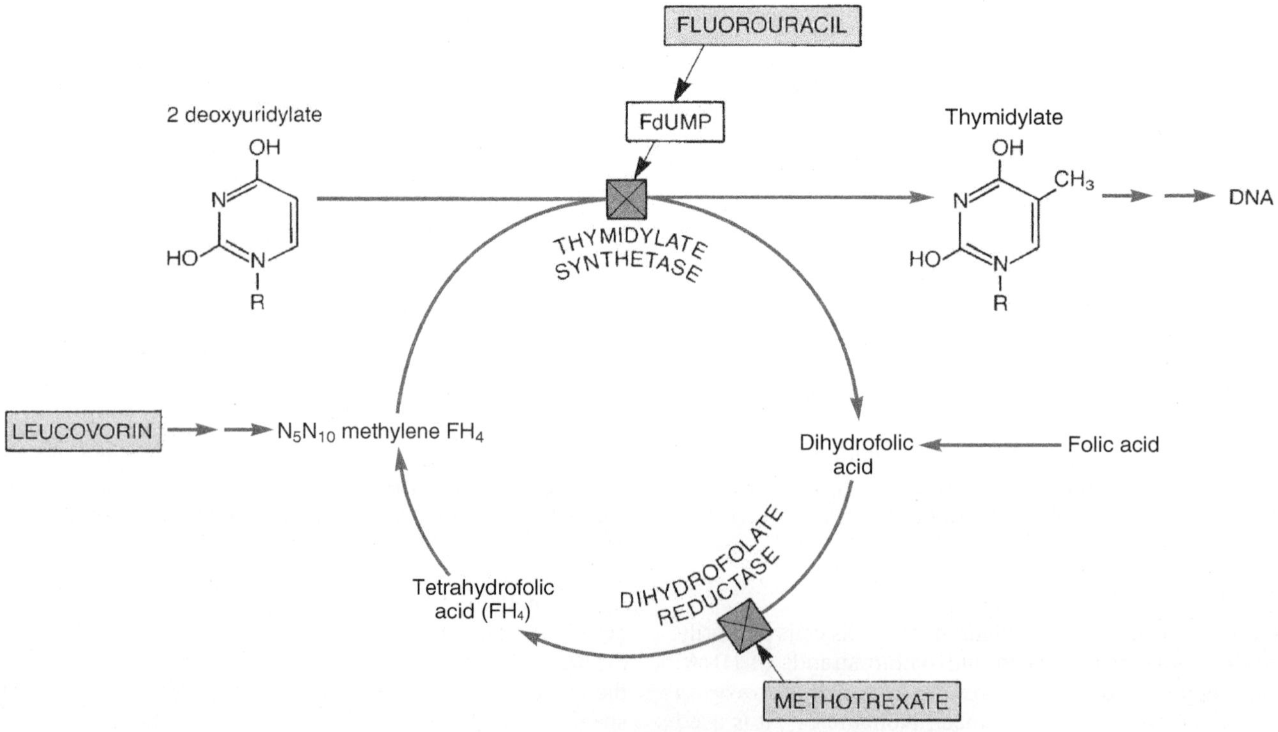

Fig. 102.2 ▪ Actions of methotrexate, leucovorin, and fluorouracil. (*FdUMP,* 5-fluoro-2′-deoxyuridine-5′-monophosphate; ☒, blockade of reaction.)

Toxicity. The usual dose-limiting toxicities are bone marrow suppression, pulmonary infiltrates and fibrosis, and oral and GI ulceration. Death may result from intestinal perforation and hemorrhagic enteritis. Nausea and vomiting may occur shortly after administration. High doses can directly injure the kidneys. To promote drug excretion and thereby minimize renal damage, the urine should be alkalinized and adequate hydration maintained. Methotrexate has been associated with fetal malformation and death. Accordingly, pregnancy should be avoided until at least 6 months after completing treatment.

Pemetrexed

Mechanism of Action. Pemetrexed [Alimta] is an antifolate compound with actions similar to those of methotrexate. Like methotrexate, pemetrexed inhibits dihydrofolate reductase. However, unlike methotrexate, pemetrexed also inhibits two other enzymes: thymidylate synthase and glycinamide ribonucleotide formyltransferase. All three enzymes are involved in the *de novo* synthesis of thymidine and purine nucleotides. By inhibiting these enzymes, pemetrexed can suppress synthesis of DNA, RNA, and proteins. Cell death results primarily from disrupting DNA synthesis and function. Pemetrexed is considered S-phase specific.

Therapeutic Uses. Pemetrexed, in combination with cisplatin, is approved for IV therapy of unresectable *malignant pleural mesothelioma,* a rare cancer usually associated with asbestos exposure. The drug is also approved for monotherapy of *non–small cell lung cancer* after previous chemotherapy and for initial therapy of this cancer when combined with cisplatin. Investigational uses include *gastric, pancreatic,* and *breast cancer.*

Pharmacokinetics. Pemetrexed is administered IV and, like methotrexate, undergoes conversion to active polyglutamates within cells. (Compared with normal cells, cancer cells are more efficient at polyglutamation, and hence cancer cells are more likely to be harmed.) Pemetrexed is eliminated by renal excretion. In patients with normal renal function, the elimination half-life is 3.5 hours. In patients with renal impairment, elimination is delayed.

Toxicity. The most common adverse effects are bone marrow suppression (the usual dose-limiting toxicity), GI disturbances (nausea, diarrhea, and sores of the lips, mouth, and throat), skin rash, and fatigue. To reduce bone marrow and GI toxicity, patients should receive prophylactic doses of vitamin B_{12} and folic acid, starting 1 week before dosing. To reduce skin rash, patients should receive prophylactic glucocorticoids (e.g., dexamethasone). Pemetrexed can cause fetal malformation and death, and hence should not be used during pregnancy. The drug is not a vesicant, and hence extravasation is managed as it would be for other nonvesicants.

Pralatrexate

Mechanism of Action. Pralatrexate [Folotyn] is a folate analog with a structure similar to that of methotrexate. Like methotrexate, pralatrexate inhibits dihydrofolate reductase and thereby disrupts synthesis of DNA and other essential cellular components. The result is cell death. Pralatrexate can be considered S-phase specific.

Therapeutic Use. Pralatrexate has only one indication: intravenous treatment of relapsed or refractory *peripheral T-cell lymphoma,* a relatively rare and often aggressive form of non-Hodgkin's lymphoma. In clinical trials, only a minority of patients responded. However, in some patients who did respond, the response duration was substantial.

Pharmacokinetics. Pralatrexate is administered by IV push and becomes 67% bound to plasma proteins. Like methotrexate, the drug undergoes metabolic conversion to active polyglutamates within cells. Elimination is primarily renal. Accordingly, in patients with significant renal impairment, dosage must be reduced to avoid toxicity from drug accumulation.

Toxicity. The major dose-limiting toxicities are GI mucositis and bone marrow suppression, manifesting as thrombocytopenia, anemia, and neutropenia. To reduce toxicity to the GI mucosa and bone marrow, patients should receive prophylactic doses of folic acid (starting 10 days before treatment) and vitamin B_{12} (starting 10 weeks before treatment). Other toxicities, occurring in 30% to 40% of patients, include fatigue, nausea, vomiting, constipation, edema, fever, and cough. Pralatrexate is embryotoxic, and so is classified in U.S. Food and Drug Administration Pregnancy Risk Category D: The drug should be avoided during pregnancy unless benefits to the woman outweigh risks to the fetus.[a] Women receiving the drug should be advised not to get pregnant.

[a]As of 2020, the FDA will no longer use Pregnancy Risk Categories. Please refer to Chapter 9 for more information.

Pyrimidine Analogs

Pyrimidines—cytosine, thymine, and uracil—are bases employed in the biosynthesis of DNA and RNA. The pyrimidine analogs, because of their structural similarity to naturally occurring pyrimidines, can act in several ways: (1) they can inhibit biosynthesis of pyrimidines, (2) they can inhibit biosynthesis of DNA and RNA, and (3) they can undergo incorporation into DNA and RNA, and thereby disrupt nucleic acid function. All of the pyrimidine analogs are prodrugs that must be converted to their active forms in the body. We currently have five pyrimidine analogs: cytarabine, fluorouracil, capecitabine, floxuridine, and gemcitabine.

Cytarabine

Cytarabine [Cytosar 🍁], also known as *cytosine arabinoside* and *Ara-C,* is an analog of deoxycytidine. The drug has an established role in treating *acute myelogenous leukemia.* Cytarabine is available in two formulations: (1) conventional [Tarabine PFS 🍁] for IV and subQ dosing, and (2) liposomal [DepoCyt] for intrathecal dosing.

Mechanism of Action. Cytarabine is converted to its active form—Ara-CTP—within the body. As Ara-CTP, the drug undergoes incorporation into DNA. By a mechanism that is not fully understood, incorporation suppresses further DNA synthesis. Ara-CTP may also impede DNA synthesis by a second mechanism: inhibition of DNA polymerase. Cytarabine is S-phase specific.

Resistance. Decreased conversion of cytarabine to Ara-CTP is a major cause of resistance. Other mechanisms include decreased uptake of cytarabine, increased conversion of cytarabine to an inactive product, and increased production of dCTP (the natural metabolite that Ara-CTP competes with for incorporation into DNA).

Pharmacokinetics. Administration may be IV, subQ, or intrathecal. Cytarabine is not active orally. Drug that is not taken up by cells undergoes rapid deamination in the liver. Metabolites are excreted in the urine.

Therapeutic Uses. The principal indication for conventional cytarabine is *acute myelogenous leukemia.* To induce remission, the drug is combined with idarubicin as part of the so-called 7 + 3 regimen (7 days of cytarabine + 3 days of idarubicin). Other applications include *acute lymphocytic leukemia* and *non-Hodgkin's lymphoma.* Additionally, *liposomal* cytarabine is used to treat *lymphomatous meningitis.*

Toxicity. Bone marrow suppression (neutropenia, thrombocytopenia) is the usual dose-limiting toxicity. Nausea, vomiting, and fever may develop, especially after bolus IV injection. Other toxicities include stomatitis, liver injury, and conjunctivitis. High doses may cause pulmonary edema and cerebellar toxicity.

The liposomal formulation can cause chemical arachnoiditis, manifesting as nausea, vomiting, headache, and fever. Left untreated, the condition can be fatal. The incidence and severity of the reaction can be reduced by coadministration of dexamethasone, an anti-inflammatory glucocorticoid.

Fluorouracil

Fluorouracil [Adrucil] is a fluorinated derivative of uracil. The drug is employed extensively to treat solid tumors.

Mechanism of Action. To exert cytotoxic effects, fluorouracil must be converted to its active form, 5-fluoro-2′-deoxyuridine-5′-monophosphate (FdUMP). As shown in Fig. 102.2, FdUMP inhibits thymidylate synthetase, thereby depriving cells of thymidylate needed to make DNA. Fluorouracil is active only against cells that are going through the cell cycle; it shows some S-phase specificity.

Resistance. Potential mechanisms for resistance are decreased activation of fluorouracil and production of altered thymidylate synthetase that has a low affinity for FdUMP. The clinical significance of these mechanisms has not been established.

Therapeutic Uses. Chemotherapeutic use of fluorouracil is limited to solid tumors. The drug is employed, together with other drugs, in the adjuvant treatment of *breast and colorectal cancer,* and in palliative therapy of *carcinomas of the colon, rectum, breast, stomach, and pancreas.* As discussed in Chapter 105, fluorouracil can be used topically to treat *premalignant keratoses.*

Pharmacokinetics. Administration is IV. Continuous infusion is more effective and less toxic than bolus administration. Fluorouracil is distributed widely and enters the CNS with ease. Elimination is by rapid hepatic metabolism.

Toxicity. The usual dose-limiting toxicities are bone marrow suppression (neutropenia) and oral and GI ulceration. To minimize GI injury (e.g., ulceration of the oropharynx or bowel), fluorouracil should be discontinued as soon as mild reactions (stomatitis, diarrhea) occur. Dosage can also be limited by palmar-plantar erythrodysesthesia (hand-and-foot syndrome), characterized by tingling, burning, redness, flaking, swelling, and blistering of the palms and soles. Other adverse effects include alopecia, hyperpigmentation, and neurologic deficits.

In patients given a fluorouracil overdose, treatment with an investigational antidote—*uridine triacetate*—can be lifesaving. Uridine triacetate is a prodrug that undergoes conversion to uridine, which then dampens the effects of fluorouracil on cellular metabolism.

Capecitabine

Capecitabine [Xeloda], a prodrug form of fluorouracil, is indicated for oral therapy of metastatic *breast cancer* as well as *colorectal cancer* in both the adjuvant and metastatic settings. Once in the body, capecitabine undergoes metabolic conversion to fluorouracil and then to FdUMP, its active form. Consequently, the pharmacology of capecitabine is much like that of fluorouracil itself. Cell kill results from inhibition of thymidylate synthetase. Capecitabine is active only against dividing cells, and like fluorouracil, shows some S-phase specificity. In clinical trials, 20% of patients with breast cancer experienced at least a 50% decrease in tumor size. Severe diarrhea is common and can be dose limiting. Other common side effects include nausea, vomiting, stomatitis, and hand-and-foot syndrome, characterized by local tingling, numbness, pain, swelling, and erythema of the palms and soles. Capecitabine is a teratogen and hence must not be used during pregnancy. The drug can cause leukopenia, but severe myelosuppression is uncommon. Alopecia has not been reported.

Capecitabine enhances the effects of warfarin; to reduce the risk of bleeding, anticoagulant effects should be monitored closely and warfarin dosage reduced as indicated. In patients with renal impairment, capecitabine can accumulate to toxic levels. If renal impairment is *moderate,* dosage should be reduced by 75%; if impairment is *severe,* the drug should not be used.

Floxuridine

Floxuridine [FUDR], like fluorouracil, is converted to FdUMP in the body. Hence, the effects of floxuridine and fluorouracil are nearly identical. Floxuridine is indicated only for *GI adenoma metastatic to the liver.* For this cancer, the drug is administered by infusion directly into the hepatic artery. The major dose-limiting toxicities are bone marrow suppression and oral and GI ulceration.

Gemcitabine

Mechanism of Action. Gemcitabine [Gemzar] is a nucleoside analog that inhibits DNA synthesis. Hence, the drug is S-phase specific. Following uptake by cells, gemcitabine is converted to two active forms: gemcitabine diphosphate and gemcitabine triphosphate. Gemcitabine diphosphate inhibits ribonucleotide reductase, an enzyme needed to form deoxynucleoside triphosphates, which are required for DNA synthesis. Gemcitabine triphosphate undergoes incorporation into DNA, where it inhibits strand elongation.

Therapeutic Uses. Gemcitabine is indicated for *advanced ovarian cancer, metastatic breast cancer, adenocarcinoma of the pancreas,* and *non–small cell cancer of the lung.* For pancreatic cancer, the drug may be used as first-line therapy in patients with locally advanced or metastatic disease and in patients previously treated with fluorouracil. In clinical trials, gemcitabine reduced pain, improved functional status, and prolonged life slightly.

Toxicity. Although gemcitabine can cause a wide variety of adverse effects, it is fairly well tolerated. Myelosuppression is dose limiting. Nausea and vomiting are common but usually mild to moderate. Elevation of serum transaminases occurs in 75% of patients. About 20% to 45% of patients develop proteinuria, hematuria, pain, fever, rash, and a flu-like syndrome. Less common reactions include diarrhea, constipation, stomatitis, dyspnea, paresthesias, edema, and alopecia. Infusion reactions (e.g., hypotension, flushing) may occur and can be managed by slowing the infusion.

Purine Analogs

Like the pyrimidines, the purines—adenine, guanine, and hypoxanthine—are bases employed for biosynthesis of nucleic acids. The purine analogs discussed here are used primarily in the treatment of cancer. They are cladribine, clofarabine, fludarabine, mercaptopurine, nelarabine, pentostatin, and thioguanine. Purine analogs discussed in other chapters are used for immunosuppression, antiviral therapy, and gout.

Mercaptopurine

Mechanisms of Action and Resistance. Mercaptopurine [Purinethol] is a prodrug that undergoes conversion to its active form within cells. Following activation, the drug can disrupt multiple biochemical processes, including purine biosynthesis, nucleotide interconversion, and biosynthesis of nucleic acids. All of these actions probably contribute to cytotoxic effects. Mercaptopurine is S-phase specific. Mechanisms of resistance include reduced activation of the drug and accelerated deactivation.

Pharmacokinetics. Mercaptopurine is administered orally and undergoes erratic absorption. Absorbed drug is distributed widely, but not to the CNS. Extensive metabolism occurs in the liver; an important reaction is catalyzed by xanthine oxidase. Accordingly, for patients receiving a xanthine oxidase inhibitor (e.g., allopurinol), mercaptopurine dosage should be reduced.

Therapeutic Uses. The principal indication for mercaptopurine is maintenance therapy of *acute lymphocytic leukemia* in children and adults.

Toxicity. Bone marrow suppression (neutropenia, thrombocytopenia, anemia) is the principal dose-limiting toxicity. Mild hepatotoxicity, manifesting as elevations in bilirubin and liver transaminases, is relatively common; rarely, hepatic injury progresses to fatal liver failure. Other adverse effects include nausea, vomiting, and oral and intestinal ulceration. Concurrent use of a xanthine oxidase inhibitor increases the overall toxicity. Mercaptopurine is mutagenic, and hence must not be used during pregnancy.

Thioguanine

Actions and Uses. Thioguanine [Tabloid, Lanvis 🍁] acts much like mercaptopurine. Following conversion to its active form, thioguanine inhibits purine synthesis and the interconversion of nucleotides. DNA synthesis is also inhibited. Like mercaptopurine, thioguanine is S-phase specific. The drug is used primarily for *acute nonlymphocytic leukemias.*

Pharmacokinetics. Administration is oral. Absorption is erratic and incomplete. Thioguanine does not distribute to the CNS. Inactivation is by hepatic metabolism. In contrast to mercaptopurine, thioguanine is not degraded by xanthine oxidase, and hence no dosage reduction is required if a xanthine oxidase inhibitor is being used.

Toxicity. The usual dose-limiting toxicity is bone marrow suppression. Gastrointestinal reactions (nausea, vomiting, diarrhea) may develop, but these are less severe than with mercaptopurine. Liver injury, manifesting as cholestatic jaundice, may occur.

Pentostatin

Pentostatin [Nipent] is an analog of adenosine. The drug acts in two major ways. First, it inhibits adenosine deaminase, causing accumulation of adenosine and deoxyadenosine nucleotides, compounds that inhibit ribonucleotide reductase and thereby block DNA synthesis. Second, pentostatin promotes accumulation of *S*-adenosylhomocysteine, a compound that is especially toxic to lymphocytes. The drug has only one approved indication: *hairy cell leukemia* that has not responded to interferon alfa. The major dose-limiting toxicities are bone marrow suppression and CNS depression. Other toxicities include nausea, vomiting, rash, and fever. Combined use with fludarabine has caused fatal pulmonary toxicity, and hence is not recommended. Administration is by IV bolus or IV infusion.

Fludarabine

Fludarabine [Fludara] is an analog of adenosine. The drug is used primarily for *chronic lymphocytic leukemia, low-grade non-Hodgkin's lymphoma,* and *acute myelogenous leukemia.* Administration is IV. Once in the body, fludarabine undergoes rapid conversion to its active form, 2-fluoro-ara-ATP. Cell kill appears to result from several mechanisms, including inhibition of DNA replication, impairment of RNA function, and promotion of apoptosis. Thus the drug is probably S-phase specific. The major dose-limiting toxicity is bone marrow suppression (neutropenia, thrombocytopenia, anemia). Other common toxicities include nausea, vomiting, and chills. Life-threatening autoimmune hemolytic anemia has been reported. When used in normal doses, and especially in excessive doses, fludarabine can cause severe CNS effects, including blindness, seizures, coma, agitation, confusion, and death. Combined use with pentostatin has been associated with fatal pulmonary toxicity, and hence is not recommended.

Cladribine

Cladribine is an adenosine analog with a unique combination of actions. Unlike other purine analogs, which inhibit DNA synthesis only, cladribine inhibits both DNA synthesis and repair. As a result, the drug is active against quiescent cells as well as cells that are actively dividing. Cladribine is highly active against *hairy cell leukemia* and is considered a drug of choice for this cancer. The drug is also active against *chronic lymphocytic leukemia, low-grade non-Hodgkin's lymphoma, acute myeloid leukemia,* and *mycosis fungoides.* The major dose-limiting toxicity is myelosuppression. Very high doses (4 to 9 times normal) have caused acute nephrotoxicity and delayed-onset neurotoxicity. For patients with hairy cell leukemia, cladribine is administered by continuous IV infusion over 7 consecutive days.

Nelarabine

Nelarabine [Arranon, Atriance 🍁] is an analog of guanosine. The drug is used for patients with *T-cell acute lymphoblastic leukemia* or *T-cell lymphoblastic lymphoma* that has not responded to (or has stopped responding to) at least two chemotherapy regimens. Monotherapy with nelarabine can produce a complete response in some of these patients. The drug is administered IV and undergoes conversion to its active form—ara-GTP—within cells. Incorporation of ara-GTP into DNA then causes DNA fragmentation and subsequent apoptosis. The most common side effects are anemia, leukopenia, neutropenia, and thrombocytopenia. Potentially fatal neurotoxicity—manifesting as paresthesias, ataxia, confusion, convulsions, severe somnolence, and coma—is dose limiting.

Clofarabine

Clofarabine [Clolar] is a purine nucleoside analog indicated for relapsed or refractory *acute lymphoblastic leukemia* after at least two previous regimens have failed. The drug is administered IV and undergoes intracellular conversion to its active form, clofarabine 5′-triphosphate. Cell kill results from several mechanisms, including termination of DNA elongation, inhibition of DNA repair, and promotion of apoptosis. In vitro, clofarabine is toxic to proliferating and quiescent cells. However, given its mechanism, the drug is probably most effective during S phase. The major dose-limiting toxicity is bone marrow suppression (neutropenia, thrombocytopenia, and anemia). Hyperuricemia may result from massive tumor lysis. Other common reactions include tachycardia, fatigue, chills, fever, headache, itching, rash, diarrhea, abdominal pain, and pain in the extremities. Two life-threatening syndromes—systemic inflammatory syndrome and capillary leak syndrome—may also occur. Clofarabine is teratogenic in rats and rabbits and should not be used during pregnancy.

HYPOMETHYLATING AGENTS

Hypomethylating agents are so-called because they inhibit DNA methyltransferase, an enzyme that puts methyl groups onto DNA components. Drugs in this category include azacitidine and decitabine. Both are analogs of cytidine, a component of RNA.

Azacitidine

Azacitidine [Vidaza] is the first representative of a new class of anticancer drugs: the hypomethylating agents. Azacitidine, an analog of cytidine, becomes incorporated into DNA and then inhibits DNA methyltransferase, an enzyme that puts methyl groups onto DNA components. The resultant hypomethylation of DNA is believed to induce apoptosis and restore normal function to genes critical to cell differentiation and proliferation. *In vitro,* drug concentrations that cause maximal inhibition of DNA methylation do not cause significant inhibition of DNA synthesis. Azacitidine has one indication: *myelodysplastic syndrome,* a bone marrow disorder characterized by reduced blood cell counts and the potential to progress to acute myelogenous leukemia. Toxicities include myelosuppression, nausea and vomiting, and CNS depression.

Decitabine

Decitabine [Dacogen], like azacitidine, is an analog of cytidine that inhibits DNA methyltransferase and thereby suppresses DNA methylation, leading to apoptosis and/or normalization of differentiation and proliferation. Like azacitidine, decitabine is used only for *myelodysplastic syndrome.* Toxicities include myelosuppression, nausea and vomiting, and a flu-like syndrome. A single dose consists of 15 mg/m^2 infused IV over 3 hours. The regimen consists of one dose every 8 hours for 72 hours, repeated every 6 weeks.

ANTITUMOR ANTIBIOTICS

The antitumor antibiotics are cytotoxic drugs originally isolated from cultures of *Streptomyces.* They fall into two major groups: anthracyclines and nonanthracyclines. Antitumor antibiotics are used only to treat cancer; they are not used to treat infections. All of these drugs injure cells through direct interaction with DNA. Because of poor GI absorption, they are all administered parenterally, almost always IV.

Anthracyclines

Five of the antitumor antibiotics are derivatives of anthracycline: doxorubicin (conventional and liposomal), daunorubicin (conventional and liposomal), epirubicin, idarubicin, and valrubicin. A sixth drug, mitoxantrone, is often categorized as an anthracycline because of its close similarity to drugs in this category. All can cause severe bone marrow suppression and heart damage. In some patients, cardiotoxicity has led to fatal heart failure. Treatment with dexrazoxane [Zinecard] offers some protection against cardiac damage.

Doxorubicin, Conventional

Doxorubicin is active against a broad spectrum of neoplastic diseases. Unfortunately, cardiotoxicity limits its utility. Doxorubicin is available in two formulations: conventional [Adriamycin] and liposomal [Doxil, Caelyx 🍁]. The conventional preparation is discussed here, followed by a discussion of the liposomal preparation.

Mechanism of Action. Doxorubicin is a planar (flat) molecule that kills cells by two related mechanisms: *intercalation with DNA* and *inhibition of topoisomerase II.* We can understand intercalation by envisioning the stacked base pairs of DNA as having a structure like that of a stack of coins. Having a coin-like shape itself, doxorubicin is able to slip between base pairs of DNA, after which it becomes bound to DNA. This process (intercalation) distorts DNA structure. As a result, DNA polymerase and RNA polymerase are unable to use DNA as a template, and hence synthesis of DNA and RNA is inhibited.

While bound to DNA, doxorubicin forms a complex with topoisomerase II, an enzyme that cleaves and then repairs DNA strands. Doxorubicin allows topoisomerase II to cleave DNA, but prevents subsequent DNA repair. In the absence of DNA repair, apoptosis results. Topoisomerase is discussed further later in the chapter, under *Topoisomerase Inhibitors.* Doxorubicin is *cell-cycle phase nonspecific.*

Pharmacokinetics. Doxorubicin is administered by IV infusion and undergoes rapid uptake by tissues, but does not cross the blood-brain barrier. Much of each dose is metabolized in the liver. Accordingly, dosage must be reduced in patients with hepatic impairment. Doxorubicin and its metabolites are eliminated primarily in the bile.

Therapeutic Uses. Doxorubicin is active against many neoplastic diseases. The drug is employed to treat solid tumors and disseminated cancers. Specific indications include *Hodgkin's and non-Hodgkin's lymphomas, sarcomas of soft tissue and bone,* and *various carcinomas,* including *carcinoma of the lung, stomach, breast, ovary, testes, and thyroid.*

Cardiotoxicity. Doxorubicin can cause acute and delayed injury to the heart. Acute effects (dysrhythmias, electrocardiographic changes) can develop within minutes of dosing. In most cases these reactions are transient, lasting no more than 2 weeks.

Delayed cardiotoxicity develops months to years after doxorubicin therapy and manifests as heart failure secondary to diffuse cardiomyopathy (myofibril degeneration). The condition is often unresponsive to treatment. Delayed cardiac injury is directly related to the total cumulative dose: The risk of heart failure increases significantly as the cumulative lifetime dose rises above 550 mg/m^2. Accordingly, the total dose should not exceed this amount.

Dexrazoxane [Zinecard] can protect the heart from doxorubicin, but at the expense of additional myelosuppression and possible reduction of antitumor activity. To protect the heart, dexrazoxane must first undergo conversion to a chelating agent. In this active form, the drug binds intracellular iron. Just how chelation of iron protects against cardiotoxicity is unclear. In clinical trials, dexrazoxane significantly decreased the incidence of doxorubicin-induced heart failure. However, treatment did have two complications: (1) The drug appeared to intensify myelosuppression, and (2) it may have reduced the anticancer effects of doxorubicin. To ensure that the benefits of chemotherapy are not compromised, dexrazoxane is approved only for patients who have already received 300 mg/m^2 of doxorubicin. Furthermore, the drug is approved only for patients receiving doxorubicin for *breast cancer* (even though doxorubicin is used to treat other malignancies). Why the restriction? Because intensification of myelosuppression may be greater in patients with tumors other than breast cancer.

Angiotensin-converting enzyme (ACE) inhibitors, such as ramipril, can improve symptoms of cardiomyopathy. Furthermore, if given early, ACE inhibitors may be able to *prevent* cardiac damage.

Other Toxicities. Acute toxicity usually manifests as nausea and vomiting. Because of its vesicant properties, doxorubicin can cause severe local injury if extravasation occurs. In addition, the drug imparts a harmless red color to urine and sweat; patients should be forewarned. The usual dose-limiting toxicity is bone marrow suppression. Neutropenia develops in about 70% of patients. Thrombocytopenia and anemia may also occur. Additional delayed toxicities include alopecia, stomatitis, anorexia, conjunctivitis, and pigmentation in the extremities.

Doxorubicin, Liposomal

Liposomal doxorubicin [Doxil, Caelyx ♣]—a reformulation of conventional doxorubicin—was created to increase delivery of the drug to tumor cells and to decrease its uptake by normal cells. The preparation consists of doxorubicin encapsulated within lipid vesicles (liposomes), which are coated with polyethylene glycol to avoid immune removal and prolong their stay in the bloodstream. While in the vicinity of tumor cells and normal cells, the liposomes slowly release doxorubicin. However, because capillaries in tumors are more leaky than capillaries in healthy tissue, the liposomes have better access to tumor cells, and hence show some tumor selectivity. Liposomal doxorubicin is administered as a 30-minute IV infusion.

The preparation has four indications: *AIDS-related Kaposi's sarcoma, metastatic ovarian cancer, metastatic breast cancer,* and *multiple myeloma.*

Major dose-limiting toxicities are bone marrow suppression and heart failure. In addition, liposomal doxorubicin can cause hand-and-foot syndrome and infusion-related symptoms (back pain, flushing, and chest tightness), which are seen in 5% to 10% of patients. As a rule, the infusion symptoms begin within 5 minutes of infusion onset, subside when the infusion is interrupted, and don't return when the infusion is resumed at a slower rate.

Daunorubicin

Daunorubicin is nearly identical in structure to doxorubicin and shares many of its properties. Like doxorubicin, daunorubicin intercalates with DNA and inhibits DNA and RNA synthesis. The drug can act during all phases of the cell cycle, but cytotoxicity is greatest during S phase.

Like doxorubicin, daunorubicin is available in two formulations: conventional [Cerubidine] and liposomal [DaunoXome]. The conventional formulation is used for induction therapy of *leukemia.* The liposomal formulation is used for *HIV-associated Kaposi's sarcoma.*

As with doxorubicin, the major dose-limiting toxicities are bone marrow suppression and heart failure. In addition, daunorubicin may cause nausea, vomiting, stomatitis, and alopecia. Like doxorubicin, daunorubicin imparts a harmless red color to urine and tears.

Epirubicin

Mechanism of Action and Therapeutic Use. Epirubicin [Ellence], an analog of doxorubicin, is indicated for IV adjuvant therapy of *breast cancer* following surgical removal of the primary tumor in patients who have axillary node involvement. Combined therapy with cyclophosphamide and fluorouracil is usually employed. Epirubicin is given in repeated 21-day cycles consisting of either (1) 100 mg/m^2 on day 1 only or (2) 60 mg/m^2 on days 1 and 8. For most patients, epirubicin offers no advantages over doxorubicin.

Like doxorubicin, epirubicin (1) intercalates DNA and thereby inhibits synthesis of DNA, RNA, and proteins; and (2) causes DNA strand breaks by disrupting function of topoisomerase II. Epirubicin is considered cell-cycle phase nonspecific. However, cytotoxicity is maximal during S and G_2 phases.

Pharmacokinetics. Epirubicin is widely distributed following IV infusion. The drug undergoes hepatic metabolism followed by excretion in the bile and urine. Elimination is slowed in patients with liver dysfunction secondary to hepatic metastases or other causes.

Adverse Effects. Epirubicin can cause a variety of serious adverse effects. As with doxorubicin, bone marrow suppression and cardiotoxicity are dose limiting. To reduce the risk of severe cardiac damage, the total cumulative dose should not exceed 900 mg/m^2 (compared with 550 mg/m^2 for doxorubicin). Fortunately, when epirubicin is used for adjuvant therapy, the cumulative dose should be well below the safe limit. Extravasation can result in severe local tissue necrosis. Additional adverse effects include alopecia, nausea, vomiting, mucositis, and red discoloration of urine. In animals, epirubicin is embryotoxic and teratogenic; studies in pregnant women have not been performed.

Idarubicin

Idarubicin [Idamycin] is a structural analog of daunorubicin and doxorubicin. The drug has one approved indication: induction therapy of *acute myelogenous leukemia* in adults. Like other anthracyclines, idarubicin (1) intercalates DNA to disrupt synthesis of DNA, RNA, and proteins; and (2) causes DNA strand breaks by disrupting function of topoisomerase II. Idarubicin works best during S and G_2 phases but is still considered phase nonspecific. Following IV infusion, the drug undergoes rapid and widespread distribution. Elimination is by hepatic metabolism followed by biliary excretion. The principal dose-limiting toxicity is bone marrow suppression. Like other anthracyclines, idarubicin is cardiotoxic, especially when the cumulative dose exceeds 150 mg/m^2. Additional toxicities include nausea, vomiting, alopecia, and stomatitis. Idarubicin is a vesicant and can cause severe local injury upon extravasation.

Valrubicin

Mechanism of Action and Therapeutic Use. Valrubicin [Valstar] is indicated for *bladder cancer* that is resistant to bacille Calmette-Guérin therapy. The goal is to prevent the necessity of a cystectomy (surgical removal of the bladder).

Valrubicin disrupts action of DNA topoisomerase II. It stops cell growth in the G_2 phase. It is different from the other anthracyclines in that it does not intercalate DNA.

Valrubicin is an intravesical drug; that is, it is administered directly into the bladder via a urinary catheter. It incorporates a unique diluent—castor oil. Because of this, the tubing must not contain polyvinyl chloride. Monitoring via cystoscopy or biopsy and by urine cytology should be carried out every 3 months to identify cancer progression or recurrence.

Pharmacokinetics. Systemic absorption is usually negligible due to intravesical administration with limited retention (typically 2 hours). If the bladder wall has erosions or other areas where the lining is not intact, systemic absorption will probably be increased. Excretion occurs in the urine, with greater than 98% of the drug eliminated intact.

Adverse Effects. Over 50% of patients receiving valrubicin can expect bladder irritation and dysuria with urinary frequency and urgency. Approximately 30% will experience hematuria and bladder discomfort, which includes bladder spasm. An increase in urinary tract infection and incontinence affects about 15% to 20% of patients.

Mitoxantrone

Although not a true anthracycline, mitoxantrone [Novantrone] is a close relative of these drugs and shares most of their properties. Like the anthracyclines, mitoxantrone appears to act by two mechanisms: (1) intercalation of DNA and (2) promotion of DNA strand breakage secondary to inhibition of topoisomerase II. The drug is cell-cycle phase nonspecific. Principal applications are *prostate cancer* and *acute nonlymphocytic leukemias.* In addition, the drug is used to reduce neurologic disability in people with multiple sclerosis (see Chapter 23). Mitoxantrone is administered intravenously and undergoes rapid and widespread distribution. Elimination occurs slowly, primarily by hepatic metabolism and biliary excretion. The major dose-limiting toxicities are bone marrow suppression and injury to the heart, especially when the cumulative dose exceeds 120 mg/m^2. Other important toxicities—nausea, vomiting, alopecia, and mucositis—are less severe than with doxorubicin. Some patients develop acute myelogenous leukemia while using the drug. Mitoxantrone imparts a harmless blue-green tint to the urine, skin, and sclera; patients should be forewarned.

Nonanthracyclines

There are three nonanthracycline antitumor antibiotics: dactinomycin, bleomycin, and mitomycin. In contrast to anthracyclines, nonanthracyclines do not injure the heart. However, these drugs do have serious toxicities of their own. Table 102.1 details dose-limiting toxicities of each drug.

Dactinomycin (Actinomycin D)

Actions and Uses. Like doxorubicin, dactinomycin [Cosmegen] is a planar molecule that intercalates DNA and thereby distorts DNA structure. As a result, RNA polymerase is unable to use DNA as a template, and hence synthesis of RNA (and proteins) is inhibited. Unlike RNA polymerase, DNA polymerase is relatively insensitive to the change in DNA. Consequently, DNA synthesis is not suppressed. Dactinomycin is *phase nonspecific.* Major indications for dactinomycin are *Wilms' tumor* and *rhabdomyosarcoma.* Other indications include *choriocarcinoma, Ewing's sarcoma, Kaposi's sarcoma,* and *testicular cancer.*

Pharmacokinetics. Administration is by IV infusion. Because of tissue uptake and binding to DNA, dactinomycin is rapidly cleared from the blood. The drug does not cross the blood-brain barrier. Elimination occurs slowly by biliary and renal excretion.

Toxicity. Dose-limiting toxicities are bone marrow suppression and oral and GI mucositis. Nausea and vomiting may be severe. Other toxicities include diarrhea, alopecia, folliculitis, and, in previously irradiated areas, dermatitis. Dactinomycin is a strong vesicant, and hence extravasation will cause severe local injury.

Bleomycin

The preparation of bleomycin used clinically contains a mixture of glycopeptides. The major components are bleomycin A_2 and bleomycin B_2. Bleomycin is unusual among the cytotoxic agents in that it causes very little bone marrow suppression. However, it can cause severe injury to the lungs. Because myelosuppression is minimal, bleomycin could be especially useful in combination chemotherapy, although the potential for lung injury often limits its use. Bleomycin binds to DNA, causing chain scission and fragmentation. The drug is most effective during G_2.

Therapeutic uses include *testicular carcinomas* (embryonal cell, choriocarcinoma, teratocarcinoma), *lymphomas* (Hodgkin's, reticulum cell sarcoma, lymphosarcoma), and *squamous cell carcinomas* (head, neck, larynx, cervix, penis, vulva, skin). The most common uses are testicular cancer and Hodgkin's disease, for which bleomycin is employed as a component of curative regimens.

Administration is parenteral (IM, IV, subQ, intrapleural). High concentrations are achieved in the skin and lungs. The drug does not enter the CNS. Most tissues contain large amounts of bleomycin hydrolase, an enzyme that renders the drug inactive. However, cells of the skin and lungs, which are sites of toxicity, lack this enzyme. Most of each dose is excreted unchanged in the urine.

The major dose-limiting toxicity is injury to the lungs, which occurs in about 10% of patients. Injury manifests initially as pneumonitis. In about 1% of patients, pneumonitis progresses to severe pulmonary fibrosis and death. Pulmonary function should be monitored and bleomycin discontinued at the first sign of adverse changes. Additional toxicities include stomatitis, alopecia, and skin reactions (hyperpigmentation, hyperkeratosis, pruritus, erythema, ulceration, vesiculation). Nausea and vomiting are usually mild. Unlike most other cytotoxic anticancer drugs, bleomycin exerts minimal toxicity to bone marrow. About 1% of patients with lymphomas experience a unique hypersensitivity reaction, characterized by fever, chills, confusion, hypotension, and wheezing.

Mitomycin

Mitomycin [Mutamycin 🍁] is a prodrug that is converted to its active form within cells. Following activation, it functions as a bifunctional or trifunctional alkylating agent. Cell death is caused by cross-linking DNA with resultant blockade of DNA synthesis. Mitomycin may also induce strand scission. The drug is active during all phases of the cell cycle, but toxicity is greatest during late G_1 and early S phases.

Mitomycin is labeled for *disseminated adenocarcinoma of the stomach and pancreas.* Unlabeled uses include *carcinomas of the colon, rectum, esophagus, lung, breast, cervix, and bladder.*

Mitomycin is administered by IV infusion and is distributed widely, but not to the CNS. The drug undergoes rapid hepatic conversion to active and inactive metabolites. Metabolites are excreted in the urine.

The major dose-limiting toxicity is delayed bone marrow suppression; nadirs for neutropenia and thrombocytopenia usually occur 4 to 6 weeks after treatment. Mitomycin can also cause hemolytic uremic syndrome, a serious disorder characterized by microangiopathic hemolytic anemia, thrombocytopenia, and irreversible renal failure. Other toxicities include nausea, vomiting, stomatitis, alopecia, and pulmonary toxicity. Mitomycin is a vesicant and can cause severe local injury upon extravasation.

MITOTIC INHIBITORS

Mitotic inhibitors are drugs that act during M phase to prevent cell division. There are two major groups of these drugs—vinca alkaloids and taxanes—as well as three other drugs that belong to neither group.

Vinca Alkaloids

The vinca alkaloids are derived from *Vinca rosea* (the periwinkle plant), hence the group name. *Vincristine* and *vinblastine* are the most important members. These drugs have nearly identical structures and share the same mechanism of action. However, they have quite different toxicities: Vincristine is toxic to peripheral nerves, but does little damage to bone marrow. Conversely, vinblastine can cause significant bone marrow suppression, but is much less toxic to nerves.

Vincristine

Mechanism of Action. Vincristine (conventional) [Oncovin, Vincasar PFS] and vincristine (liposomal) [Marqibo] block mitosis during metaphase, and thus are M-phase specific. Vincristine blocks mitosis by disrupting the assembly of microtubules, the filaments that move chromosomes during cell division. To block microtubule assembly, vincristine binds with *tubulin,* the major component of microtubules. In the absence of microtubules, cell division stops at metaphase. Metaphase block is a potent signal for apoptosis (programmed cell death).

Pharmacokinetics. Because of low and erratic oral absorption, vincristine must be given IV. The drug leaves the vascular system and enters tissues, where it becomes tightly but reversibly bound. Penetration to the CNS is poor. Most of each dose undergoes hepatic metabolism followed by biliary excretion. Only 12% is eliminated in the urine.

Therapeutic Uses. Vincristine is bone marrow sparing. Accordingly, the drug is ideal for combination chemotherapy. Indications for conventional vincristine include *Hodgkin's and non-Hodgkin's lymphomas, acute lymphocytic leukemia, Wilms' tumor, rhabdomyosarcoma, Kaposi's sarcoma, breast cancer,* and *bladder cancer.* Liposomal vincristine is indicated for Philadelphia chromosome–negative *acute lymphoblastic leukemia.*

Toxicity. *Peripheral neuropathy* is the major dose-limiting toxicity. Vincristine injures neurons by disrupting neurotubules, which are required for axonal transport of enzymes and organelles. Injury to neurotubules results from binding to tubulin, the same protein found in microtubules. Nearly all patients experience symptoms of sensory or motor nerve injury (e.g., decreased reflexes, weakness, paresthesias, sensory loss). Symptoms of injury to autonomic nerves (e.g., constipation, urinary hesitancy) are less common, occurring in 30% to 50% of patients. Because vincristine does not readily enter the CNS, injury to the brain is minimal.

In contrast to most cytotoxic anticancer drugs, *vincristine causes little bone marrow suppression.* As a result, the drug is especially desirable for combined therapy with other anticancer drugs, most of which do suppress the marrow.

Vincristine is a vesicant and can cause severe local injury if extravasation occurs. Alopecia develops in about 20% of patients. Significant nausea and vomiting are uncommon.

Vinblastine

Vinblastine [Velban] is a structural analog of vincristine. The two drugs share the same mechanism of action: production of metaphase arrest through blockade of microtubule assembly. Like vincristine, vinblastine is administered IV, does not cross the blood-brain barrier, and is eliminated by biliary and urinary excretion. Indications include *Kaposi's sarcoma, Hodgkin's and non-Hodgkin's lymphomas,* and *carcinoma of the breast and testes.* The major dose-limiting toxicity is bone marrow suppression. (Note that vinblastine differs markedly from vincristine in this regard.) Neurotoxicity can occur, but is less common and less severe than with vincristine. Additional adverse effects include nausea, vomiting, alopecia, stomatitis, and severe local injury if extravasation occurs.

Vinorelbine

Vinorelbine [Navelbine] is a semisynthetic vinca alkaloid similar in structure and actions to vincristine and vinblastine. The drug is approved only for *non–small cell lung cancer.* Investigational uses include *breast cancer, ovarian cancer,* and *Hodgkin's disease.* Benefits derive from causing metaphase arrest through inhibition of microtubule assembly. Vinorelbine is administered IV, undergoes hepatic metabolism, and is eliminated primarily in the bile. Like vinblastine, and unlike vincristine, vinorelbine can cause profound bone marrow suppression; neutropenia develops in about 50% of patients. Peripheral neuropathy occurs, but is less severe than with vincristine. Rarely, vinorelbine causes interstitial pulmonary damage and adult respiratory distress syndrome, typically within 1 week of treatment; most cases are fatal. Accordingly, be alert for new-onset dyspnea, cough, hypoxia, and related signs of lung injury. Other adverse effects include alopecia, constipation, nausea, and vomiting, all of which are generally mild to moderate. Like vincristine and vinblastine, vinorelbine can cause local tissue necrosis if extravasation occurs.

Taxanes

Paclitaxel

Actions and Uses. Paclitaxel [Abraxane, Onxol, Taxol 🍁] is a widely used drug that acts during late G_2 and M phases to promote formation of stable microtubule bundles, thereby inhibiting cell division and producing apoptosis. Paclitaxel (in combination with cisplatin) is approved as first-line therapy for advanced *ovarian cancer* and *non–small cell lung cancer* in patients who are not candidates for potentially curative surgery or radiation therapy. In addition, the drug is approved as second-line therapy for *AIDS-related Kaposi's sarcoma* and as adjuvant therapy combined with doxorubicin-containing regimens for women with *breast cancer.* Investigational uses include *advanced head and neck cancer, adenocarcinoma of the upper GI tract,* and *leukemias.*

Pharmacokinetics. Paclitaxel is administered by infusion, for either 3 hours or 24 hours. The drug undergoes wide distribution, but not to the CNS. Very little is known about how paclitaxel is eliminated; small amounts appear in the urine and bile, but the fate of the remainder is unknown.

Formulations. Paclitaxel is available in two IV formulations. The older of the two, sold as *Onxol* and *Taxol* 🍁, contains a solvent system (*Cremaphor* and alcohol) that can trigger severe hypersensitivity reactions. The newer formulation, sold as *Abraxane,* consists of paclitaxel bound to nanoparticles of albumin. Addition of water forms a suspension; no solvent is employed.

Toxicity. *Severe hypersensitivity reactions* (hypotension, dyspnea, angioedema, urticaria) have occurred during infusion of Onxol and Taxol 🍁—but *not* Abraxane—apparently in response to the solvent employed. The risk of severe hypersensitivity reactions with Onxol and Taxol 🍁 can be minimized by pretreatment with a glucocorticoid (e.g., dexamethasone), histamine$_1$ receptor antagonist (e.g., diphenhydramine), and histamine$_2$ receptor antagonist (e.g., cimetidine). With Abraxane, no pretreatment is needed.

The major dose-limiting toxicity is *bone marrow suppression* (neutropenia). Peripheral neuropathy develops with repeated infusions and may also be dose limiting. Paclitaxel can affect the heart, causing bradycardia, second- and third-degree heart block, and even fatal myocardial infarction. Muscle and joint pain have occurred. Practically all patients experience sudden but reversible alopecia, which frequently involves the body as well as the scalp. Gastrointestinal reactions—nausea, vomiting, diarrhea, and mucositis—are generally mild.

Docetaxel

Actions, Uses, and Source. Docetaxel [Docefrez, Taxotere] is similar in structure and actions to paclitaxel. Like paclitaxel, docetaxel stabilizes microtubules and thereby inhibits mitosis. Docetaxel has three approved indications: (1) locally advanced or metastatic *breast cancer* that has progressed or relapsed despite previous chemotherapy, (2) locally advanced or metastatic *non–small cell lung cancer* that has advanced despite previous cisplatin-based therapy, and (3) advanced hormone-refractory metastatic *prostate cancer,* but only in combination with prednisone. In clinical trials, docetaxel produced objective responses in over 40% of patients with breast cancer.

Toxicity. Significant *neutropenia* develops in virtually all patients. Docetaxel should be withheld if neutrophil counts fall below 1500/mm^3. In clinical trials, death from sepsis occurred in 1% of patients with normal liver function and in 11% of patients with abnormal liver function. Because liver dysfunction increases the risk of death, docetaxel should be avoided if signs of significant liver disease are present (i.e., plasma aspartate aminotransferase [AST] and/or alanine aminotransferase [ALT] more than 1.5 times the upper limit of normal [ULN], together with alkaline phosphatase more than 2.5 times the ULN).

Severe *hypersensitivity* can occur. Manifestations include hypotension, bronchospasm, and generalized rash or erythema. Docetaxel should be avoided in patients who reacted strongly to a previous dose or to any drug containing polysorbate 80 (the vehicle docetaxel is supplied in). To reduce hypersensitivity reactions, patients should take an oral glucocorticoid for 5 days, starting 1 day before each infusion.

Severe *fluid retention* can occur, especially in patients with abnormal liver function. Possible manifestations include generalized edema, dyspnea at rest, cardiac tamponade, pleural effusion requiring urgent drainage, and pronounced abdominal distention (from ascites). As with hypersensitivity reactions, fluid retention can be reduced by treatment with oral glucocorticoids, which are normally started the day before dosing and continued for 2 days after.

Additional common toxicities are anemia, nausea, diarrhea, stomatitis, fever, and neurosensory symptoms (paresthesias, pain).

Cabazitaxel

Actions and Use. Cabazitaxel [Jevtana], in combination with prednisone, is indicated for second-line IV treatment of advanced hormone-refractory *prostate cancer* in men who have already received docetaxel. In one trial, median survival with cabazitaxel/prednisone was 15.1 months, versus 12.7 months with mitoxantrone/prednisone—considered a highly significant increase. Cabazitaxel also improved median progression-free survival and produced greater reductions in serum prostate-specific antigen. As with paclitaxel and docetaxel, benefits derive from stabilizing microtubules and resultant inhibition of mitosis.

Toxicity. *Bone marrow suppression* causes *neutropenia* in nearly all patients. Deaths have occurred. Complete blood counts must be monitored. If neutrophil counts fall below 1500/mm^3, cabazitaxel should be withheld. Granulocyte colony-stimulating factor (see Chapter 56) may be used to prevent or treat neutropenia. Liver impairment increases the risk of death. Accordingly, if signs of liver disease are present (i.e., plasma AST and/or ALT more than 1.5 times the ULN, together with alkaline phosphatase more than 2.5 times the ULN), cabazitaxel should not be used. In addition to neutropenia, bone marrow suppression causes *anemia* and *thrombocytopenia*.

As with paclitaxel and docetaxel, severe *hypersensitivity* can occur, manifesting as hypotension, bronchospasm, and generalized rash and/or erythema. If a severe reaction occurs, cabazitaxel should be stopped immediately and never used again. Cabazitaxel should be avoided in patients who reacted strongly to any preparation containing polysorbate 80 (the vehicle cabazitaxel is supplied in). To reduce hypersensitivity reactions, patients should receive three drugs—a histamine$_1$ antagonist (e.g., dexchlorpheniramine), a histamine$_2$ antagonist (e.g., ranitidine), and a glucocorticoid (e.g., dexamethasone)—given IV at least 30 minutes before each cabazitaxel dose.

Diarrhea, seen in 47% of patients, can be severe. Deaths from resulting electrolyte imbalance have occurred. Intensive antidiarrheal and rehydration therapy may be required. If high-grade diarrhea occurs, a dosage reduction or delay in treatment may be indicated.

Additional adverse effects, seen in at least 10% of patients, include nausea, vomiting, constipation, fatigue, weakness, fever, cough, alopecia, peripheral neuropathy, dyspnea, arthralgia, and dysgeusia (distorted sense of taste).

Other Mitotic Inhibitors

Ixabepilone

Ixabepilone [Ixempra] is a large cytotoxic molecule in the epothilone family. Like the taxanes, the drug binds to and stabilizes microtubules and thereby causes mitotic arrest and apoptosis. Ixabepilone is approved only for locally advanced or metastatic *breast cancer*. The drug may be used alone (after an anthracycline, a taxane, and capecitabine have failed) or combined with capecitabine (after an anthracycline and taxane have failed). Major toxicities are neutropenia, seen in 54% to 68% of patients, and peripheral sensory neuropathy. Less serious side effects include fatigue, myalgia, arthralgia, alopecia, nausea, vomiting, diarrhea, and stomatitis/mucositis. Ixabepilone is a substrate for CYP3A4 (the 3A4 isoenzyme of cytochrome P450), and hence its levels can be increased by drugs that inhibit CYP3A4 and reduced by drugs that induce CYP3A4. In patients taking a strong CYP3A4 inhibitor, dosage of ixabepilone should be reduced by 50%. In patients with significant liver impairment, as evidenced by elevated serum bilirubin or liver transaminases, dosage of ixabepilone in monotherapy should be reduced, and the combination of ixabepilone plus capecitabine should be avoided.

Eribulin Mesylate

Eribulin [Halaven] is indicated for IV therapy of metastatic *breast cancer* in patients who have received at least two previous chemotherapeutic regimens, including an anthracycline-based regimen and a taxane-based regimen. Eribulin is a synthetic analog of halichondrin-B, a mitotic inhibitor produced by sea sponges in the *Halichondria* genus. Anticancer effects derive from disrupting the formation and function of microtubules. The result is mitotic arrest and, ultimately, cell death. More than half of patients taking this drug experience neutropenia, anemia, and fatigue. More than a third have alopecia and peripheral neuropathy. In addition, eribulin can prolong the QT interval, posing a risk of fatal dysrhythmias. Accordingly, eribulin should not be combined with other QT-prolonging drugs (see Chapter 7). At doses below those used in humans, eribulin is embryotoxic and teratogenic in rats, and hence should not be used during pregnancy.

Estramustine

Estramustine [Emcyt] is a hybrid molecule composed of estradiol and a nitrogen mustard. Like the other drugs discussed in this section, estramustine binds microtubules, and thereby causes mitotic arrest. The pharmacology of estramustine is discussed in Chapter 103.

TOPOISOMERASE INHIBITORS

Topoisomerases are nuclear enzymes that alter the shape (topology) of supercoiled DNA. Without the actions of topoisomerases, the double helix would be too tangled to permit DNA replication, RNA synthesis, or DNA repair. How do topoisomerases alter DNA configuration? They make a cut in the DNA strand, which permits the strand to relax in the vicinity of the cut; then later they reseal the cut. There are two types of topoisomerase, known as topoisomerase I and topoisomerase II. Topoisomerase I makes single-strand cuts, and topoisomerase II makes double-strand cuts. Of the four topoisomerase inhibitors in current use, two—topotecan and irinotecan—inhibit topoisomerase I, and the other two—etoposide and teniposide—inhibit topoisomerase II. The actions of these drugs are partly like those of the antitumor antibiotics, discussed previously, which inhibit topoisomerase II and intercalate DNA.

Topotecan

Mechanism of Action

Topotecan [Hycamtin], an inhibitor of topoisomerase I, binds to the DNA–topoisomerase I complex. The drug does not prevent topoisomerase I from making a single-strand cut in DNA, but does prevent the enzyme from resealing the cut. As a result, there is an accumulation of DNA with multiple single-strand cuts. Of note, these single-strand cuts, by themselves, are not harmful: If the drug is removed, the cuts can be repaired. However, if the cell attempts to replicate DNA while the drug is still present, irreversible double-strand breaks will be produced, thereby causing cell death. Because ongoing replication of DNA is needed for cell kill, topotecan is most active in S phase.

Therapeutic Uses

Topotecan is approved for *metastatic cancer of the ovary.* It is also approved for *cervical cancer* that returns after previous treatment or that is resistant to treatment. Finally, it is approved for relapsed or refractory *small cell lung cancer.*

Toxicity

Bone marrow suppression is the dose-limiting toxicity. Neutropenia occurs in 98% of patients, thereby posing a risk of serious infection. Anemia and thrombocytopenia are also common and frequently require transfusion of platelets and red blood cells. Because of myelosuppression, it is important to monitor complete blood counts frequently. If the neutrophil count is below 1500 cells/mm^3, topotecan should be withheld. Other side effects include alopecia, nausea, vomiting, diarrhea, stomatitis, abdominal pain, and headache.

Irinotecan

Actions and Uses

Like topotecan, irinotecan [Camptosar] and its active metabolite inhibit topoisomerase I. As a result, DNA replication is impaired. Cytotoxic effects become apparent during the S phase of the cell cycle. Irinotecan is approved for first-line treatment of metastatic colorectal cancer (in combination with fluorouracil) and for second-line treatment of colorectal cancer that has progressed despite treatment with fluorouracil alone. Investigational uses include *advanced cancer of the breast, ovary, lung, and stomach.*

Metabolic Activation and Inactivation

Irinotecan is converted to its active metabolite (SN-38) in the liver. The metabolite, in turn, is converted to an inactive product by UDP-glucuronosyltransferase 1A1 (UGT1A1). In some patients, the genes that code for UGT1A1 are abnormal. As a result, inactivation of irinotecan is delayed and drug levels rise, thereby increasing the intensity of adverse effects. A genetic test, called Invader UGT1A1, can detect mutations in the genes that code for UGT1A1. In patients who have such mutations, a reduction in irinotecan dosage should be considered.

Adverse Effects

Two types of *severe diarrhea* can occur: early and late. Early diarrhea occurs in 50% of patients; late diarrhea occurs in 88%. Early and late diarrhea differ with respect to cause and treatment. Early diarrhea occurs within 24 hours of infusion onset. The cause is excessive cholinergic stimulation of the GI tract. Accordingly, early diarrhea can be suppressed with IV atropine. Late diarrhea develops 24 hours or more after the infusion. It can be prolonged, causing severe dehydration and electrolyte imbalance, and can thereby pose a threat to life. Late diarrhea should be treated immediately with loperamide. Fluid and electrolytes should be replaced as needed.

Myelosuppression can result in neutropenia and anemia. Serious thrombocytopenia is uncommon. Sepsis secondary to neutropenia has resulted in death. If the neutrophil count falls below 500 cells/mm^3, irinotecan should be temporarily withheld.

In addition to diarrhea and myelosuppression, irinotecan can cause nausea, vomiting, asthenia, alopecia, abdominal discomfort, and anorexia in more than 50% of patients. Other common adverse effects include fever and weight loss. Less common side effects include stomatitis, dyspepsia, headache, cough, rhinitis, insomnia, and rash.

Etoposide

Etoposide [Toposar], a drug derived from podophyllotoxin (a naturally occurring plant alkaloid), inhibits topoisomerase II. Etoposide does not prevent topoisomerase II from making double-strand breaks in DNA, but it does prevent the enzyme from resealing those breaks. Cell death results from accumulation of DNA with multiple breaks. Cells in S and G_2 phases are most sensitive. Etoposide is approved only for *refractory testicular cancer* and *small cell cancer of the lung,* but is used off-label against many other tumors.

Administration is PO or IV. Plasma protein binding is high. Penetration to the CNS is low. Etoposide is eliminated by hepatic metabolism and renal excretion, and hence dosage should be reduced in patients with liver or renal impairment.

The major dose-limiting toxicity is bone marrow suppression. Other toxicities include alopecia, mucositis, and, rarely, peripheral neuropathy. Early adverse effects include nausea, vomiting, diarrhea, and fever.

Hypotension can occur with rapid IV administration. The cause is the organic diluent used to solubilize etoposide, not etoposide itself. Hypotension can be avoided by diluting the drug in sufficient IV fluid.

Teniposide

Teniposide [Vumon] is an analog of etoposide and has the same mechanism of action: inhibition of topoisomerase II. The only approved indication is *refractory acute lymphoblastic leukemia of childhood.*

Administration is by slow IV infusion. Most of each dose becomes bound to plasma proteins. Penetration to the CNS is poor. Elimination is by hepatic metabolism and renal excretion.

The major dose-limiting toxicity is bone marrow suppression (neutropenia, thrombocytopenia, anemia). Severe hypersensitivity reactions (urticaria, angioedema, bronchospasm, hypotension) occur in about 5% of patients; symptoms can be suppressed with epinephrine. Secondary leukemias may develop within 8 years of initial drug exposure. Other toxicities include nausea, vomiting, diarrhea, and alopecia.

MISCELLANEOUS CYTOTOXIC DRUGS

Asparaginase

Asparaginase [Erwinase ♣, Kidrolase ♣] is an enzyme that converts asparagine, an essential amino acid, into aspartic acid. By converting asparagine to aspartic acid, the drug deprives cells of asparagine needed to synthesize proteins. However, not all cells are affected. In fact, toxicity from asparaginase is limited almost exclusively to leukemic lymphoblasts because these cells are unable to manufacture their own asparagine as normal cells can. Normal cells are able to replace the asparagine that asparaginase took away, but leukemic lymphoblasts can't. Asparaginase appears to act selectively during G_1. Recall that this is the phase in which the cell manufactures proteins called histones.

The only indication for asparaginase is *acute lymphocytic leukemia.* To induce remission, asparaginase is usually combined with prednisone and vincristine, and perhaps daunorubicin or doxorubicin.

Administration is parenteral (IM and IV). Distribution is restricted to the vascular system. The drug does not cross the blood-brain barrier and is inactivated by serum proteases.

Asparaginase can cause severe adverse effects. However, the spectrum of toxicities differs from that of other anticancer drugs. By inhibiting protein synthesis, the drug can cause coagulation deficiencies and can injure the liver, pancreas, and kidneys. Symptoms of CNS depression, ranging from confusion to coma, develop in about 30% of patients. Nausea and vomiting can be intense and may limit the dose that can be tolerated. Because asparaginase is a foreign protein, hypersensitivity reactions are common; fatal anaphylaxis can occur, and hence facilities for resuscitation should be immediately available. In contrast to most other anticancer drugs, asparaginase does not depress the bone marrow and does not cause alopecia, oral mucositis, or intestinal ulceration.

Pegaspargase

Pegaspargase [Oncaspar] is a modified form of asparaginase that causes fewer hypersensitivity reactions. Otherwise, the drugs are much the same. They have the same mechanism of action (destruction of asparagine) and produce the same spectrum of adverse effects (hypersensitivity reactions, pancreatitis, coagulopathy, and liver and kidney impairment). Of the patients who had hypersensitivity reactions to asparaginase, about 30% also react to pegaspargase. Pegaspargase is indicated only for *acute lymphocytic leukemia,* and only in patients who experienced hypersensitivity to asparaginase. Administration is IM or IV.

Hydroxyurea

Hydroxyurea [Hydrea, Droxia] inhibits DNA replication by suppressing synthesis of DNA precursors. Specifically, the drug inhibits ribonucleoside diphosphate reductase, the enzyme that converts ribonucleotides into their corresponding deoxyribonucleotides. In the absence of deoxyribonucleotides, DNA cannot be made. Hydroxyurea is S-phase specific.

The principal indication for hydroxyurea is *chronic myelogenous leukemia.* The drug is also used for *squamous cell carcinoma* and recurrent, metastatic, or inoperable *carcinoma of the ovary.* In addition, hydroxyurea can relieve symptoms and prolong life in patients with *sickle cell anemia* (see Chapter 107). When used for cancer, hydroxyurea is marketed as *Hydrea,* and when used for sickle cell anemia, it's marketed as *Droxia.*

Hydroxyurea is rapidly absorbed after oral dosing. Unlike most anticancer agents, hydroxyurea crosses the blood-brain barrier with ease. Part of each dose is metabolized in the liver. Parent drug and metabolites are eliminated primarily in the urine.

The principal dose-limiting toxicity is bone marrow suppression. The drug also causes nausea, vomiting, and dysuria. Neurologic deficits and stomatitis may occur, but these are rare. Hydroxyurea is teratogenic in experimental animals. Hence, like most other anticancer agents, it should be avoided during pregnancy.

Mitotane

Mitotane [Lysodren] is a structural analog of two insecticides: DDD and DDT. For reasons that are not understood, the drug is selectively toxic to cells of the adrenal cortex, both normal and neoplastic. The only indication for mitotane is palliative therapy of inoperable *adrenocortical carcinoma.*

Mitotane is administered PO. About 40% is absorbed. The drug is distributed widely, but not to the CNS. Because of storage in tissues (primarily fat), active drug remains in the body for weeks after dosing has ceased. Elimination is by hepatic metabolism and renal excretion.

The principal dose-limiting toxicities are CNS depression, nausea, and vomiting. Because mitotane injures the adrenal cortex, adrenal insufficiency is likely. Accordingly, patients will require supplemental glucocorticoids, especially at times of stress. Dermatitis is common. Other adverse effects include visual disturbances, orthostatic hypotension, and renal damage, manifesting as hematuria, hemorrhagic cystitis, and albuminuria. Mitotane does not cause the toxicities associated with most other anticancer drugs (bone marrow suppression, alopecia, oral and GI ulceration).

Procarbazine

Mechanism of Action

Procarbazine [Matulane] is a prodrug that undergoes conversion to active metabolites in the liver. The metabolites alkylate DNA and thereby suppress synthesis of DNA, RNA, and protein. The precise cause of cell death is unknown. Procarbazine is cell-cycle phase nonspecific.

Pharmacokinetics

Procarbazine is readily absorbed following oral dosing, but undergoes rapid and extensive hepatic metabolism. Active metabolites are highly lipid soluble and cross the blood-brain barrier with ease. Procarbazine and its metabolites are excreted primarily in the urine.

Therapeutic Uses

The major uses for procarbazine are *Hodgkin's disease, non-Hodgkin's lymphoma,* and *primary brain cancer.* For Hodgkin's disease, procarbazine is combined with mechlorethamine, vincristine [Oncovin, Vincasar], and prednisone in the so-called MOPP regimen, formerly the regimen of choice in newly diagnosed patients.

Toxicity

The usual dose-limiting toxicity is bone marrow suppression. Nausea and vomiting may also be dose limiting. Other adverse effects include peripheral neuropathy, CNS depression, secondary leukemias, and sterility, especially in males.

Drug Interactions

Owing to its CNS effects, procarbazine should not be combined with CNS depressants (e.g., barbiturates, phenothiazines, opioids). Ingestion of alcohol can induce a disulfiram-like response. Because procarbazine inhibits monoamine oxidase, there is a risk of severe hypertension in response to sympathomimetic drugs, tricyclic antidepressants, and tyramine-rich foods.

Dacarbazine

Actions and Uses

Dacarbazine [DTIC-Dome] is a prodrug that undergoes activation in the liver. Although the precise mechanism of cell kill is unknown, there is evidence for alkylation of DNA, inhibition of DNA and RNA synthesis, and interaction with sulfhydryl groups on proteins. Dacarbazine is considered cell-cycle phase nonspecific. Principal indications are metastatic *malignant melanoma* and *Hodgkin's disease.*

Pharmacokinetics

Gastrointestinal absorption of dacarbazine is erratic, and hence the drug is given IV. Penetration to the CNS is poor. Elimination is by hepatic metabolism and renal excretion.

Toxicity

Bone marrow suppression is the usual dose-limiting toxicity. Nausea and vomiting occur in most patients, occasionally requiring cessation of treatment. Other toxicities include a flu-like syndrome, hepatic necrosis, photosensitivity, and burning pain along the injection site.

Altretamine (Hexamethylmelamine)

Altretamine [Hexalen], formerly known as hexamethylmelamine, is indicated for palliative therapy of persistent or recurrent *ovarian cancer.* Altretamine is a prodrug that is converted to active metabolites in the body. As with procarbazine and dacarbazine, the active metabolites have alkylating activity. However, the precise mechanism of cell kill has not been established. Altretamine is well absorbed following oral dosing, but undergoes rapid and extensive hepatic metabolism. Metabolites are excreted in the urine. The principal dose-limiting toxicity is bone marrow suppression. However, nausea and vomiting can also limit dosage. Peripheral sensory neuropathy is common. Central neurotoxicity (tremors, ataxia, vertigo, hallucinations, seizures, depression) is less common. Because of peripheral and central neurotoxicity, patients should receive regular neurologic evaluations.

KEY POINTS

- Cytotoxic anticancer drugs act directly on cancer cells and healthy cells to produce cell death.
- Cell-cycle phase–specific drugs are effective only during a specific phase of the cell cycle (e.g., S phase, M phase). Accordingly, they are active only against cells that are participating in the cell cycle. Quiescent cells in G_0 are spared.
- To be effective, a phase-specific drug must be present as neoplastic cells cycle through the phase in which the drug acts. In practical terms, this means that phase-specific drugs must be in the blood continuously over a long time.
- Cell-cycle phase–nonspecific drugs can affect cells during any phase of the cell cycle, including G_0.
- Although phase-nonspecific drugs can inflict biochemical lesions at any time during the cell cycle, they are usually more toxic to proliferating cells than to cells in G_0. Why? Because (1) G_0 cells often have time to repair drug-induced damage before it can result in significant harm and (2) toxicity may not become manifest until the cells attempt to divide.
- About 50% of the cytotoxic anticancer drugs are phase specific; the rest are phase nonspecific.
- Alkylating agents injure cells primarily by forming covalent bonds with DNA.
- Bifunctional alkylating agents form cross-links in DNA and thereby prevent DNA replication. Bifunctional agents are more effective than monofunctional agents.
- Because alkylation reactions can take place at any time during the cell cycle, alkylating agents are considered cell-cycle phase nonspecific.
- Cyclophosphamide, the most widely used alkylating agent, is active against a broad spectrum of neoplastic diseases.
- Antimetabolites are analogs of important natural metabolites, and hence are able to disrupt critical metabolic processes, especially DNA replication.
- Most antimetabolites are S-phase specific.
- Methotrexate, a folic acid analog, prevents conversion of folic acid to its active form. Cell kill results primarily from disruption of DNA synthesis.

Continued

- High doses of methotrexate coupled with leucovorin rescue can be used to treat methotrexate-resistant tumors. This technique can be potentially harmful in that failure to give sufficient leucovorin at the right time can be lethal.
- Cytarabine, a pyrimidine analog, undergoes intracellular activation followed by incorporation into DNA, where it acts to inhibit DNA synthesis.
- Fluorouracil, a uracil analog, undergoes intracellular activation, after which it inhibits thymidylate synthetase, thereby depriving cells of thymidylate needed to make DNA.
- Antitumor antibiotics are used to treat cancer, not infections.
- Antitumor antibiotics fall into two major groups: anthracyclines (which damage the heart) and nonanthracyclines (which don't).
- Doxorubicin is an anthracycline-type antitumor antibiotic. To reduce the risk of heart failure, the cumulative lifetime dose should be kept below 550 mg/m^2. The risk can be further reduced with dexrazoxane, a drug that helps protect the heart from doxorubicin.
- Doxorubicin is a planar molecule that intercalates DNA, thereby distorting DNA structure. As a result, DNA polymerase and RNA polymerase are unable to use DNA as a template, and hence synthesis of DNA, RNA, and proteins is disrupted. Doxorubicin also disrupts the function of topoisomerase II, thereby causing strand breakage. This may be the primary mechanism of cell kill.
- Vincristine and vinblastine block assembly of the microtubules that move chromosomes during cell division. Accordingly, the drugs are M-phase specific.
- Vincristine is toxic to peripheral nerves, but does not significantly suppress bone marrow function. Because it spares bone marrow, vincristine can be safely combined with drugs that suppress bone marrow.
- In contrast to vincristine, vinblastine causes significant bone marrow suppression, but is relatively harmless to peripheral nerves.
- Asparaginase converts asparagine into aspartic acid and thereby deprives cells of asparagine needed to make proteins. Cytotoxicity is limited primarily to leukemic lymphoblasts because these cells are unable to manufacture their own asparagine as normal cells do.

Please visit **http://evolve.elsevier.com/Lehne** for chapter-specific NCLEX® examination review questions.

CHAPTER

103 Anticancer Drugs II: Hormonal Agents, Targeted Drugs, and Other Noncytotoxic Anticancer Drugs

In this chapter, we continue our discussion of anticancer agents, focusing on two large groups of drugs: hormonal agents and targeted drugs. The hormonal agents, used primarily for breast cancer and prostate cancer, mimic or suppress the actions of endogenous hormones. The so-called targeted drugs bind with specific molecular targets on cancer cells and thereby suppress tumor growth and promote cell death. Unlike the cytotoxic agents discussed in Chapter 102, many of which are cell-cycle phase specific, the drugs addressed here lack phase specificity.

In addition, many of the drugs discussed in this chapter lack the serious toxicities associated with cytotoxic agents, including bone marrow suppression, stomatitis, alopecia, and severe nausea and vomiting. Nonetheless, most of these drugs have severe toxicities of their own, and many are included in the list of drugs identified as hazardous by the National Institute for Occupational Safety and Health Hazardous (NIOSH). NIOSH requires special handling of drugs identified as hazardous. See Chapter 3, Table 3.1, for administration and handling guidelines. Nurses should take proper precautions when handling the medications listed in the following box.

Safety Alert

HAZARDOUS DRUGS REQUIRING SPECIAL HANDLING

Ado-trastuzumab emtansine	Goserelin
Afatinib	Histrelin
Anastrozole	Imatinib
Axitinib	Ixazomib
Bortezomib	Letrozole
Bosutinib	Leuprolide
Brentuximab	Megestrol
Cabozantinib	Nilotinib
Carfilzomib	Pazopanib
Crizotinib	Pertuzumab
Dabrafenib	Ponatinib
Degarelix	Regorafenib
Docetaxel	Sorafenib
Eribulin	Sunitinib
Erlotinib	Tamoxifen
Estramustine	Toremifene
Everolimus	Trametinib
Exemestane	Vandetanib
Flutamide	Vemurafenib
Fulvestrant	

DRUGS FOR BREAST CANCER

Breast cancer is second only to skin cancer as the most common cancer among women in the United States. In 2017, an estimated 289,120 new cases were diagnosed and 40,610 were expected to be fatal. Fortunately, this death rate has been decreasing, thanks to earlier detection and improved treatment.

Principal treatment modalities are *surgery, radiation, cytotoxic drugs (chemotherapy),* and *hormonal drugs*. Surgery and radiation are considered primary therapy; chemotherapy and hormonal therapy are used as adjuvants. For a woman with early breast cancer, treatment typically consists of surgery (using total mastectomy or partial mastectomy [lumpectomy]) followed by local radiation. After that, chemotherapy is used to kill cells left behind after surgery and radiation and to kill cells that may have metastasized to other sites. Finally, hormonal agents are taken for several years to reduce recurrence. Increasingly, chemotherapy is used *before* surgery—so-called neoadjuvant therapy—to shrink large tumors and thereby permit lumpectomy in women who would otherwise require mastectomy. Drugs for adjuvant therapy are shown in Table 103.1.

Hormonal agents for breast cancer fall into two major groups: *antiestrogens* (e.g., tamoxifen [Soltamox]) and *aromatase inhibitors* (e.g., anastrozole [Arimidex]). Antiestrogens block receptors for estrogen, whereas aromatase inhibitors block estrogen biosynthesis. In both cases, tumor cells are deprived of the estrogen they need for growth. However, there is a caveat: For these drugs to work, tumor cells must have estrogen receptors (ERs). Fortunately, the majority of breast cancers are ER positive. For years, tamoxifen had been the hormonal agent of choice. However, recent data have shown that, in postmenopausal patients, aromatase inhibitors are more effective, both in the metastatic and adjuvant settings. There is a wealth of data showing that adjuvant hormonal therapy can reduce tumor recurrence and prolong life.

In addition to chemotherapy and hormonal therapy, six other drugs—*trastuzumab* [Herceptin], *ado-trastuzumab emtansine* [Kadcyla], *pertuzumab* [Perjeta], *lapatinib* [Tykerb], *palbociclib* [Ibrance], and *ribociclib* [Kisquali]—can be used for adjuvant treatment. Trastuzumab, pertuzumab, and ado-trastuzumab emtansine block receptors known as human epidermal growth factor receptor 2 (HER2). In addition, when ado-trastuzumab emtansine binds with HER2 receptors, it releases cytotoxic catabolites that cause cell apoptosis. Lapatinib inhibits two enzymes, known as HER2 tyrosine kinase and epidermal growth factor receptor (EGFR) tyrosine kinase. These drugs are indicated only for cancers that are HER2 positive. Palbociclib and ribociclib differ from the others, as they are indicated for HER2-negative cancer. These drugs work by inhibition of cyclin-dependent kinases 4 and 6, which leads to a decrease in malignant cellular growth. Lastly, patients may take *denosumab* [Xgeva] or *zoledronate* [Zometa] to minimize hypercalcemia (caused by bone metastases) and fractures (caused by bone metastases as well as hormonal therapy).

What about breast cancer *prevention*? Currently, two drugs are approved for preventing breast cancer in women at high risk. Both drugs are *selective estrogen receptor modulators*, or SERMS. One of the drugs—*raloxifene* [Evista]—is approved only for postmenopausal women. The other drug—*tamoxifen* [Soltamox]—is approved for premenopausal *and* postmenopausal women. In clinical trials, these drugs reduced the risk of breast cancer by about 50%. Raloxifene is discussed in Chapter 75. Tamoxifen is discussed next. Another drug—*exemestane* [Aromasin] (discussed later in this chapter)—can also prevent breast cancer, but it is not yet approved for this use.

Safety Alert

HEALTH RISKS WITH BREAST CANCER PREVENTION DRUGS

Selective estrogen receptor modulators pose a risk of thrombosis, and tamoxifen also poses a risk of endometrial cancer.

ANTIESTROGENS

Antiestrogens are drugs that block ERs, and hence work only against cells that are ER positive. Benefits derive from depriving tumor cells of the growth-promoting influence of estrogen. Three antiestrogens—tamoxifen, toremifene, and fulvestrant—are approved for adjuvant treatment. Of these, tamoxifen is by far the most widely used.

Tamoxifen

Tamoxifen [Soltamox] is considered the gold standard for endocrine treatment of breast cancer. The drug is approved for treating established disease and for primary prevention in women at high risk. As discussed under *Mechanism of Action in Breast Cancer*, tamoxifen is a prodrug that must be converted to active metabolites.

TABLE 103.1 ▪ Drugs for Adjuvant Therapy of Breast Cancer

Generic Name	Brand Name	Route	Mechanism	Indications	Major Adverse Effects
HORMONAL THERAPIES					
Antiestrogens					
Tamoxifen	Soltamox	PO	Blockade of estrogen receptors	ER-positive breast cancer in pre- and postmenopausal women	Increased risk of endometrial cancer and thrombosis
Toremifene	Fareston	PO	Blockade of estrogen receptors	ER-positive breast cancer in postmenopausal women only	Hot flashes, fluid retention, vaginal discharge, nausea, vomiting, and menstrual irregularities
Fulvestrant	Faslodex	IM	Blockade of estrogen receptors	ER-positive breast cancer in postmenopausal women only	
Aromatase Inhibitors					
Anastrozole Letrozole Exemestane	Arimidex Femara Aromasin	PO PO PO	Inhibition of estrogen synthesis	ER-positive breast cancer in postmenopausal women only	Musculoskeletal pain, osteoporosis and related fractures
OTHER DRUGS FOR BREAST CANCER					
Anti-HER2 Antibodies					
Trastuzumab	Herceptin	IV	Blockade of HER2 receptors	HER2-positive breast cancer in pre- and postmenopausal women	Cardiotoxicity and hypersensitivity reactions
Ado-trastuzumab	Kadcyla	IV	Blockade of HER2 receptors	HER2-positive breast cancer	Hepatotoxicity, cardiotoxicity, neurotoxicity
Pertuzumab	Perjeta	IV	Blockade of HER2 receptors	HER2-positive breast cancer	Cardiotoxicity, hypersensitivity reactions
Kinase Inhibitors					
Lapatinib	Tykerb	PO	Inhibits HER2 tyrosine kinase and EGFR tyrosine kinase	HER2-positive breast cancer in pre- and postmenopausal women	Diarrhea, hepatotoxicity, cardiotoxicity, interstitial lung disease
Palbociclib	Ibrance	PO	Inhibits cyclin-dependent kinase 4 and 6	ER-positive, HER2-negative breast cancer in pre- and postmenopausal women	Bone marrow suppression, pulmonary embolism, peripheral neuropathy
Ribociclib	Kisqali	PO	Inhibits cyclin-dependent kinase 4 and 6	ER-positive, HER2-negative breast cancer in pre- and postmenopausal women	Severe hypokalemia, neutropenia, hepatotoxicity
Cytotoxic Drugs (Representative Agents)					
Doxorubicin *plus* cyclophosphamide	Adriamycin; Cytoxan, Neosar	IV	Direct cell kill by DNA intercalation, topoisomerase II inhibition, and DNA alkylation	Breast cancer in all women, regardless of ER, HER2, or menopausal status	Together, these drugs can cause cardiotoxicity, bone marrow suppression, alopecia, oral and GI ulceration, and hemorrhagic cystitis
Paclitaxel	Taxol 🍁, Abraxane	IV	Direct cell kill by mitotic arrest	Breast cancer in all women, regardless of ER, HER2, or menopausal status	Bone marrow suppression, peripheral neuropathy, alopecia, cardiotoxicity, muscle and joint pain Severe hypersensitivity reactions with Taxol 🍁, but not Abraxane
Eribulin	Halaven	IV	Direct cell kill by mitotic arrest	Breast cancer in all women, regardless of ER, HER2, or menopausal status	Bone marrow suppression, peripheral neuropathy

Continued

TABLE 103.1 ■ Drugs for Adjuvant Therapy of Breast Cancer—cont'd

Generic Name	Brand Name	Route	Mechanism	Indications	Major Adverse Effects
Drugs to Delay Skeletal Events					
Zoledronate	Zometa[a]	IV	Inhibits osteoclast function	Hypercalcemia of malignancy, prevention of malignancy-related skeletal events	Kidney damage, osteonecrosis of the jaw, rare atrial fibrillation
Denosumab	Xgeva[b]	SubQ	Inhibits osteoclast function and production	Hypercalcemia of malignancy, prevention of malignancy-related skeletal events	Hypocalcemia, serious infections, skin reactions, osteonecrosis of the jaw

EGFR, Epidermal growth factor receptor; *ER,* estrogen receptor; *HER2,* human epidermal growth factor receptor 2; *IM,* intramuscular; *IV,* intravenous; *PO,* oral; *SubQ,* subcutaneous.
[a]Zoledronate is also available as *Reclast* for treating osteoporosis and Paget's disease.
[b]Denosumab is also available as *Prolia* for treating postmenopausal osteoporosis.

Overview of Actions

Tamoxifen blocks ERs in some tissues and activates them in others. Receptor *blockade* underlies benefits in breast cancer but also underlies some adverse effects (especially hot flashes). Receptor *activation* leads to other beneficial effects (increased bone mineral density, reduction of low-density lipoprotein cholesterol, elevation of high-density lipoprotein cholesterol) as well as certain adverse effects (endometrial cancer and blood clots). Because tamoxifen can cause receptor activation as well as blockade, the drug is often classified as a SERM.

Mechanism of Action in Breast Cancer

Tamoxifen is a prodrug that undergoes hepatic conversion to active metabolites. These metabolites then block ERs on breast cancer cells and thereby prevent receptor activation by estradiol, the principal endogenous estrogen. Estrogen acts on tumor cells to stimulate growth and proliferation. Hence, in the absence of estradiol's influence, the rate of tumor cell proliferation declines. Tumors regress in size as the rate of cell death outpaces new cell production. Obviously, if treatment is to be effective, target cells must be ER positive.

Use for Treatment of Breast Cancer

Tamoxifen has two treatment applications: (1) as adjuvant therapy to suppress growth of residual cancer cells following surgery and (2) treatment of metastatic disease. Efficacy as adjuvant therapy has been evaluated in 55 randomized trials involving more than 37,000 women. Treatment for 1, 2, and 5 years decreased tumor recurrence by 21%, 29%, and 47%, respectively. The ATLAS (Adjuvant Tamoxifen: Longer Against Shorter) trial, first published in 2013, revealed that continuing tamoxifen for 10 years can almost halve breast cancer mortality in the second decade after diagnosis. Benefits were limited almost entirely to women with ER-positive cancer. Tamoxifen can be used in both premenopausal and postmenopausal women.

Use for Prevention of Breast Cancer

Tamoxifen is approved for reducing the development of breast cancer in healthy women at high risk. Approval was based on results of the Breast Cancer Prevention Trial, which enrolled 13,388 otherwise healthy women who had risk factors for breast cancer (e.g., age older than 60, family history of breast cancer, failure to give birth before age 30, a breast biopsy showing atypical hyperplasia). Half of the participants received tamoxifen (20 mg PO daily) and half received placebo. After an average follow-up time of 4 years, daily tamoxifen reduced the incidence of breast cancer by 44%. Unfortunately, tamoxifen *increased* the incidence of endometrial cancer, pulmonary embolism, and deep vein thrombosis. Hence, women considering tamoxifen for chemoprevention must carefully weigh the benefits of treatment (reduced risk of breast cancer) against the risks (increased risk of endometrial cancer and thromboembolic events). According to guidelines issued in 2013 by the U.S. Preventive Services Task Force (USPSTF), tamoxifen chemoprevention is appropriate only for women at *high* risk and not for women at lower risk.

To help determine who is at high risk for breast cancer, the National Cancer Institute has created an Internet-based Breast Cancer Risk Assessment Tool. You can access the tool at www.cancer.gov/bcrisktool.

Pharmacokinetics

Tamoxifen is readily absorbed following oral administration. In the liver, CYP2D6 (the 2D6 isoenzyme of cytochrome P450) converts tamoxifen into two active metabolites: 4-hydroxy-*N*-desmethyltamoxifen (endoxifen) and 4-hydroxytamoxifen. The half-lives of tamoxifen and its metabolites range from 1 to 2 weeks. Because clearance is slow, once-daily dosing is adequate. When treatment is stopped, tamoxifen and its metabolites can be detected in serum for weeks.

Not surprisingly, benefits of tamoxifen are greatly reduced in women with an inherited deficiency in the gene that codes for CYP2D6. In one study, the cancer recurrence rate in poor metabolizers was 9.5 times higher than in good metabolizers. Between 8% and 10% of Caucasian women have gene variants that prevent them from converting tamoxifen to its active metabolites. However, at this time, the U.S. Food and Drug Administration (FDA) neither requires nor recommends testing for variants in the CYP2D6 gene, although a test kit *is* available.

Adverse Effects

The most common adverse effects are hot flashes, fluid retention, vaginal discharge, nausea, vomiting, and menstrual irregularities. In women with bone metastases, tamoxifen may cause transient hypercalcemia and a flare in bone pain. Because of its estrogen agonist actions, tamoxifen poses a small risk of *thromboembolic events*, including deep vein thrombosis, pulmonary embolism, and stroke.

Perhaps the biggest concern is *endometrial cancer*. Tamoxifen acts as an estrogen agonist at receptors in the uterus, causing proliferation of endometrial tissue. Proliferation initially results in endometrial hyperplasia and may eventually lead to endometrial cancer. In women taking tamoxifen to *treat* breast cancer, the benefits clearly outweigh this risk. However, in women taking the drug to *prevent* breast cancer, the risk/benefit balance is less obvious. In postmenopausal women, endometrial cancer is usually caught early, due to abnormal menstrual bleeding.

Tamoxifen can harm the developing fetus, and hence is classified in FDA Pregnancy Risk Category D.[a] Accordingly, women using the drug should avoid getting pregnant.

Interaction With CYP2D6 Inhibitors

Inhibitors of CYP2D6 can prevent activation of tamoxifen and can thereby negate the benefits of treatment. Put another way, when tamoxifen is combined with a CYP2D6 inhibitor, the risk of breast cancer recurrence is greater than when tamoxifen is used alone. Accordingly, women using tamoxifen should avoid strong CYP2D6 inhibitors. Important among these are *fluoxetine* [Prozac], *paroxetine* [Paxil, Pexeva], and *sertraline* [Zoloft]—selective serotonin reuptake inhibitors (SSRIs) taken by many women to suppress tamoxifen-induced hot flashes. Fortunately, alternatives with less effect on CYP2D6 are available. Among these are *escitalopram* [Lexapro, Cipralex ♣] (an SSRI) and *venlafaxine* [Effexor XR] (a serotonin/norepinephrine reuptake inhibitor).

Dosage and Administration

The usual dosage for adjuvant *treatment* of breast cancer is 20 mg PO once a day. Larger doses do not increase benefits. In most cases, treatment should continue for 5 years. The dosage for *prevention* of breast cancer in high-risk women is 20 mg PO daily for 5 to 10 years. There are no data to indicate that extending treatment beyond 10 years increases benefits.

Toremifene

Actions and Use

Toremifene [Fareston] is an antiestrogen indicated for metastatic *breast cancer* in postmenopausal women with ER-positive tumors or tumors for which ER status is unknown. The drug is a structural analog of tamoxifen and shares most of that drug's properties. Like tamoxifen, toremifene is a SERM with antiestrogenic actions in some tissues and estrogenic actions in others. In women with breast cancer, toremifene blocks ERs on tumor cells, thereby depriving them of estrogen's growth-promoting effects. In clinical trials, toremifene was about as effective as tamoxifen: With both drugs, the response rate in metastatic disease was about 20%, and median survival time was about 30 months. In a crossover study, most patients who failed to respond to tamoxifen also failed to respond to toremifene. The recommended dosage is 60 mg PO once a day.

Pharmacokinetics

Toremifene is well absorbed following oral administration. Plasma levels peak in 3 hours. The drug undergoes extensive hepatic metabolism, primarily by CYP3A4 (the 3A4 isoenzyme of cytochrome P450). Metabolites are excreted in the feces. The half-life is prolonged (about 5 days) owing to enterohepatic recirculation. As with tamoxifen, drugs that induce CYP3A4 will reduce toremifene levels, and drugs that inhibit the enzyme will raise toremifene levels.

Adverse Effects

Adverse effects are like those of tamoxifen. Hot flashes are most common. Other common reactions are sweating, nausea, and vaginal discharge. Patients may also experience dizziness, vomiting, and vaginal bleeding. Hypercalcemia may occur in women with bone metastases. There is a small risk of thromboembolic events. Cataracts and elevation of liver enzymes have been reported.

Toremifene prolongs the QT interval and thereby poses a risk of potentially fatal dysrhythmias. To reduce risk, toremifene should be avoided in patients with hypokalemia, hypomagnesemia, or pre-existing QT prolongation, and in those taking other QT drugs.

Like tamoxifen, toremifene *activates* ERs in the uterus. As a result, the drug can promote uterine hyperplasia and uterine cancer.

Fulvestrant

Actions and Use

Fulvestrant [Faslodex] is an antiestrogen indicated for metastatic ER-positive *breast cancer* in postmenopausal women. Unlike tamoxifen and toremifene, which block some ERs and activate others, fulvestrant is a *pure estrogen receptor antagonist*. As with other antiestrogens, benefits derive from depriving breast cancer cells of required hormonal stimulation.

Pharmacokinetics

Plasma levels peak about 7 days after IM injection and remain therapeutic for at least 1 month. Steady-state levels are reached after three to six monthly doses. The drug undergoes hepatic metabolism followed by renal excretion. The apparent half-life is 40 days.

Adverse Effects and Drug Interactions

Fulvestrant is generally well tolerated. The most common adverse effects are GI disturbances, hot flashes, headache, pharyngitis, and bone and back pain. Thromboembolism can occur but is uncommon. In contrast to tamoxifen, fulvestrant poses no risk of endometrial cancer. In clinical trials, injection-site reactions (inflammation; mild, transient pain) developed in 7% of women receiving a single 5-mL injection and in 27% of women receiving two 2.5-mL injections. Fulvestrant has no known drug interactions.

Preparations, Dosage, and Administration

Fulvestrant is supplied in solution (50 mg/mL) for administration by slow IM injection (1 to 2 minutes). The dosage is 500 mg on days 1, 15, and 29, followed by 500 mg once a month thereafter. Each dose is administered as two 5-mL injections, one into each buttock.

AROMATASE INHIBITORS

The aromatase inhibitors are used to treat ER-positive breast cancer in *postmenopausal* women. These drugs block the production of estrogen from androgenic precursors and thereby deprive breast cancer cells of the estrogen they need for growth. Aromatase inhibitors do not block production of estrogen by the ovaries, and hence are of little benefit in premenopausal women. In fact, aromatase inhibitors may cause a compensatory rise in estradiol in premenopausal patients. Aromatase inhibitors are more effective than tamoxifen and have a different toxicity profile. Unlike tamoxifen, aromatase inhibitors pose no risk of endometrial cancer and only rarely cause thromboembolism. However, they *can* increase the risk of fractures and have been associated with moderate to severe myalgias.

Anastrozole

Mechanism, Use, and Dosage

Anastrozole [Arimidex] is approved for first-line oral therapy of *postmenopausal* women with early or advanced *ER-positive breast cancer*. The drug works by depriving breast cancer cells of estrogen. In postmenopausal women, the major source of estrogen is adrenal androgens, which are converted into estrogen by the enzyme *aromatase* in peripheral tissues. Anastrozole inhibits aromatase and thereby reduces estrogen production. With regular use, the drug lowers estrogen to undetectable

[a]As of 2020, the FDA will no longer use Pregnancy Risk Categories. Please refer to Chapter 9 for more information.

levels. In women with estrogen-dependent cancer, estrogen deprivation can arrest tumor growth and may cause outright cell death. In clinical trials, anastrozole was not effective in women with ER-negative tumors or in women who did not respond initially to tamoxifen. The recommended dosage is 1 mg PO once a day. Treatment duration typically ranges from 2 to 5 years. Anastrozole may be used as initial therapy or as a follow-up to therapy with tamoxifen.

Adverse Effects

Anastrozole is generally well tolerated. In clinical trials, about 5% of patients withdrew because of adverse effects. At a daily dose of 1 mg, the most common adverse effects are musculoskeletal pain, asthenia, headache, and menopausal symptoms, including hot flashes, vaginal dryness, and GI disturbances. Other reactions include anorexia, vomiting, diarrhea, constipation, dyspnea, peripheral edema, vaginal hemorrhage, and hypertension.

Up to 50% of women experience *musculoskeletal pain*, often described with the statement, "Every bone in my body hurts." The cause may be estrogen deprivation. Persistent or severe pain drives about 5% of users to discontinue treatment. For women who choose to continue anastrozole, pain can often be managed with a mild analgesic (e.g., acetaminophen, ibuprofen). High-dose vitamin D may help too.

Estrogen depletion increases the risk of *osteoporosis and related fractures*. To reduce bone loss, women should ensure adequate intake of calcium and vitamin D. Women at high risk should take a bisphosphonate (e.g., zoledronate [Zometa]) or denosumab [Prolia].

Comparison With Tamoxifen

As shown in the Arimidex, Tamoxifen, Alone or in Combination (ATAC) trial, which enrolled postmenopausal women with early breast cancer, anastrozole is more effective than tamoxifen and causes fewer adverse effects. After a median follow-up of 5.6 years, cancer recurred in 13% fewer of the women who took anastrozole, and the time to cancer recurrence was longer. Regarding side effects, anastrozole is less likely to cause hot flashes, weight gain, or vaginal bleeding—although it may cause more nausea and irritability. In contrast to tamoxifen, anastrozole is devoid of all estrogenic activity, and hence does not promote endometrial cancer or thromboembolic events—although it does increase the risk of fractures. Because of their superior efficacy and tolerability, aromatase inhibitors have replaced tamoxifen as the drug of first choice for treating ER-positive breast cancer in postmenopausal women.

Letrozole

Letrozole [Femara], a selective aromatase inhibitor, is indicated for (1) first-line therapy of early and advanced *ER-positive breast cancer* in postmenopausal women and (2) extended adjuvant therapy of early breast cancer following 5 years of adjuvant therapy with tamoxifen. Like anastrozole, letrozole blocks conversion of androgens into estrogens and thereby deprives breast cancer cells of estrogen's growth-promoting influence. In one study of women with advanced breast cancer, letrozole (2.5 mg/day) was more effective than tamoxifen (20 mg/day): The objective response rate with letrozole was higher (30% vs. 20%), and the time to tumor progression was longer (9.4 months vs. 6 months). In women with early breast cancer who have received 5 years of tamoxifen therapy, following with letrozole reduces the risk of recurrence. Letrozole's most common adverse effects are musculoskeletal pain and nausea. Other reactions include headache, arthralgia, fatigue, constipation, dyspnea, cough, vomiting, diarrhea, and hot flashes. Extremely low doses are embryotoxic and fetotoxic in animals. Like anastrozole, and unlike tamoxifen, letrozole poses no risk of endometrial cancer. However, it can cause osteoporosis, fractures and, rarely, thromboembolism. Osteoporosis can be managed with denosumab [Prolia] or a bisphosphonate (e.g., zoledronate [Zometa]). No significant drug interactions have been reported.

Exemestane

Exemestane [Aromasin] is indicated for oral therapy of (1) *advanced ER-positive breast cancer* in postmenopausal women whose disease has progressed despite treatment with tamoxifen and (2) *early ER-positive breast cancer* in postmenopausal women who have received 2 to 3 years of tamoxifen therapy and then are switched to adjuvant exemestane to complete a 5-year course of treatment. Like anastrozole, exemestane inhibits aromatase and thereby reduces estrogen levels. A dosage of 25 mg once daily (administered after a meal) reduces circulating estrogen by 85% to 95%. In the absence of sufficient estrogen, estrogen-dependent tumors cannot thrive. In clinical trials, the objective response rate was about 25%.

In addition to treating breast cancer, exemestane can be effective for breast cancer prevention, as shown in the Mammary Prevention 3 trial. The trial enrolled 4560 postmenopausal women at high risk for breast cancer and randomized them to receive exemestane or placebo. After a median follow-up of 35 months, the incidence of invasive breast cancer was 65% lower in the exemestane group. If exemestane is approved for breast cancer prevention, it will become an attractive alternative to raloxifene and tamoxifen.

Exemestane is rapidly absorbed following oral dosing and is widely distributed to tissues. In the liver, the drug undergoes extensive metabolism, mainly by CYP3A4. Excretion is via the urine and feces. Its half-life is about 24 hours.

Exemestane is generally well tolerated. The most common adverse effects are fatigue, nausea, hot flashes, depression, and weight gain. Like anastrozole and letrozole, exemestane often causes musculoskeletal pain. Increased risk of osteoporosis and fractures is a concern. Women at high risk of osteoporosis can be treated with denosumab [Prolia] or a bisphosphonate (e.g., zoledronate [Zometa]).

Drugs that induce CYP3A4 (e.g., phenytoin, phenobarbital, rifampin, St. John's wort) can cause a significant drop in exemestane levels. Accordingly, if these drugs are combined, the exemestane dosage may need to increase.

TRASTUZUMAB

Actions and Use

Trastuzumab [Herceptin] is a monoclonal antibody originally approved for *HER2-positive metastatic breast cancer* and for *adjuvant therapy of HER2-positive breast cancer* and *HER2-positive metastatic gastric cancer*. Discussion here is limited to breast cancer.

Trastuzumab is effective only against tumors that overexpress *human epidermal growth factor receptor 2*, a transmembrane receptor that helps regulate cell growth. Trastuzumab binds with HER2 and thereby (1) inhibits cell proliferation and (2) promotes antibody-dependent cell death. Between 25% and 30% of metastatic breast cancers produce excessive HER2. High numbers of HER2 receptors are associated with unusually aggressive tumor growth. For treatment of breast cancer, trastuzumab may be used (1) alone in women who failed to respond to prior chemotherapy, (2) in combination with paclitaxel as first-line therapy, and (3) for adjuvant treatment as part of a regimen containing doxorubicin, cyclophosphamide, and paclitaxel.

Adverse Effects

The principal concern with trastuzumab is *cardiotoxicity*, manifesting as ventricular dysfunction and congestive heart failure. In clinical trials, the incidence of symptomatic heart failure was 7% with trastuzumab alone and 28% when trastuzumab was combined with doxorubicin, a drug with prominent cardiotoxic actions. Combining trastuzumab with paclitaxel can also result in cardiac damage. Because of cardiotoxicity, trastuzumab should be used with caution in women with preexisting heart disease. Concurrent use with doxorubicin and other anthracyclines should generally be avoided. In contrast to the cytotoxic anticancer drugs, trastuzumab does not cause bone marrow suppression or alopecia.

Many patients experience a *flu-like syndrome*, which also occurs with other monoclonal antibodies. Symptoms include chills, fever, pain, weakness, nausea, vomiting, and headache. The syndrome develops in 40% of patients receiving their first infusion, and then diminishes with subsequent infusions.

Safety Alert

TRASTUZUMAB

Trastuzumab can cause potentially fatal *hypersensitivity reactions, infusion reactions*, and *pulmonary events*. Symptoms include urticaria, bronchospasm, angioedema, hypotension, dyspnea, wheezing, pleural effusions, pulmonary edema, and hypoxia requiring oxygen. Most severe reactions developed in association with the first dose, either during the infusion or by 12 hours after. If symptoms develop during the infusion, the infusion should be stopped.

Dosage and Administration

Treatment consists of a loading dose (4 mg/kg infused over at least 90 minutes) followed by weekly maintenance doses for 12 to 18 weeks (2 mg/kg infused over 30 minutes). An alternative regimen uses a larger loading dose (8 mg/kg) and larger but less frequent maintenance doses (6 mg/kg every 3 weeks).

ADO-TRASTUZUMAB EMTANSINE

Actions and Use

Ado-trastuzumab emtansine [Kadcyla] is a monoclonal antibody approved for *HER2-positive metastatic breast cancer* in patients previously treated with trastuzumab and/or a taxane (see Chapter 102).

Like trastuzumab, ado-trastuzumab emtansine is effective only against tumors that overexpress *human epidermal growth factor receptor 2*. Ado-trastuzumab emtansine binds with HER2 and releases cytotoxic catabolites, thereby (1) inhibiting the cell cycle and (2) promoting cell death. In addition, ado-trastuzumab emtansine inhibits HER2 receptor signaling and shedding of HER2 in breast cancer cells.

Adverse Effects

Ado-trastuzumab emtansine can cause hepatotoxicity, cardiotoxicity, and neurotoxicity. Serious hepatotoxicity, including liver failure and death, has been reported. Liver function tests should be obtained before each dose. Left ventricular dysfunction was seen in 1.8% of patients. Ejection fraction should be monitored at regular intervals. The incidence of neurotoxicity, expressed as peripheral neuropathy, was 2.2%.

Ado-trastuzumab emtansine can also cause embryo-fetal toxicity. Because exposure can result in birth defects or death of the fetus, ado-trastuzumab emtansine is classified in FDA Pregnancy Risk Category D[b] and should be avoided by pregnant women and nursing mothers.

[b]As of 2020, the FDA will no longer use Pregnancy Risk Categories. Please refer to Chapter 9 for more information.

The most common reactions include nausea, fatigue, musculoskeletal pain, headache, and constipation. Other common, but more serious, reactions include thrombocytopenia, increases in liver function test results, anemia, and hypokalemia.

Like trastuzumab, ado-trastuzumab emtansine can cause potentially fatal *hypersensitivity reactions, infusion reactions*, and *pulmonary events*. If a patient experienced trastuzumab-related infusion reactions, ado-trastuzumab emtansine should be avoided.

Dosage and Administration

Treatment consists of a 3.6-mg/kg IV infusion every 3 weeks until disease progression or toxicity is noted. The first infusion should be administered over 90 minutes. If this is well tolerated, subsequent infusions can be given over 30 minutes. If signs of toxicity are observed, the dose may be decreased or held until improvement is seen.

PERTUZUMAB

Pertuzumab [Perjeta] is used in combination with trastuzumab and docetaxel for the treatment of women with *HER2-positive metastatic breast cancer* who have not received prior therapy for metastatic disease. Like trastuzumab, pertuzumab is an antibody that blocks HER2 receptors, resulting in cell growth arrest and cell death.

Adverse effects include infusion-related reactions. Patients should be closely monitored for 60 minutes after the first infusion and for 30 minutes after subsequent infusions. Other adverse effects include cardiotoxicity, diarrhea, leukopenia, and neuropathy. Oligohydramnios has been reported in pregnancy, thus pregnant women should avoid use of pertuzumab.

Pertuzumab is administered intravenously. The initial dose is 840 mg given over 60 minutes. This is followed every 3 weeks by additional infusions of 420 mg given over 30 to 60 minutes.

LAPATINIB

Actions and Use

Lapatinib [Tykerb] is an oral inhibitor of two enzymes—HER2 tyrosine kinase and EGFR tyrosine kinase—that are involved in cell signal transduction. Enzyme inhibition results in apoptosis and suppression of tumor cell growth. Lapatinib is approved for treating advanced *HER2-positive breast cancer*, but only in combination with either (1) capecitabine (in patients who have received prior therapy with multiple drugs, including an anthracycline, a taxane, and trastuzumab) or (2) letrozole (in postmenopausal women for whom estrogen deprivation therapy is indicated). EGFR tyrosine kinase is discussed further later in this chapter under *EGFR Tyrosine Kinase Inhibitors*.

Adverse Effects

The most common adverse effects of *lapatinib plus capecitabine* are GI disturbances (diarrhea, nausea, vomiting), fatigue, rash, and palmar-plantar erythrodysesthesia (swelling and numbness of the hands and feet). The most common adverse effects of *lapatinib plus letrozole* are diarrhea, rash, nausea, and fatigue. Diarrhea occurs in 65% of patients and is the most common reason for stopping treatment. Like other HER2 inhibitors, lapatinib may pose a risk of cardiotoxicity. Accordingly, the drug should be used with caution in patients with existing cardiac impairment. Rarely, letrozole has been associated with severe liver injury. Liver function tests should be performed at baseline and periodically throughout treatment. When used alone and together with other drugs, letrozole has been associated with interstitial lung disease and pneumonitis. In laboratory animals, giving letrozole during pregnancy resulted in death of the pups a few days after birth. Women using the drug should avoid getting pregnant.

Drug Interactions

Lapatinib is metabolized by CYP3A4, and hence CYP3A4 inducers (e.g., phenytoin, carbamazepine, rifampin, rifabutin, phenobarbital, St. John's wort) can lower lapatinib levels, and CYP3A4 inhibitors (e.g., ketoconazole, itraconazole, erythromycin, indinavir, nelfinavir) can raise lapatinib levels. If possible, CYP3A4 inducers and inhibitors should be avoided.

Preparations, Dosage, and Administration

Lapatinib [Tykerb] is supplied in 250-mg tablets for oral dosing without food (either 1 hour before a meal or 1 hour after). Two dosing regimens are used:

- *Lapatinib with capecitabine*—The recommended dosage is 1250 mg (5 tablets) taken *once every day*, along with capecitabine
- *Lapatinib with letrozole*—The recommended dosage is 1500 mg (6 tablets) taken once every day, along with letrozole (2.5 mg) taken once every day.

PALBOCICLIB AND RIBOCICLIB

Actions and Use

Because palbociclib [Ibrance] and ribociclib [Kisquali] are both oral inhibitors of cyclin-dependent kinases (CDKs) 4 and 6, we will discuss them together. Cyclin-dependent kinases are proteins that play an important role in cell division and progression through the cell cycle. When CDK 4/6 dysregulation occurs, this can promote initial tumor growth and contribute to further tumor spread. In patients with estrogen receptor–positive breast cancers, the signals from the receptors upregulate CDK4/6 pathways. Hence, palbociclib and ribociclib are indicated for the treatment of ER-positive breast cancer. Palbociclib is used in conjunction with letrozole in postmenopausal women and with fulvestrant in women with disease progression following endocrine therapy. Ribociclib is combined with letrozole for treatment in postmenopausal women.

Adverse Effects

The most common adverse effects of palbociclib are neutropenia, infections, and fatigue. The most common adverse effects of ribociclib are neutropenia, nausea, diarrhea, and fatigue. In addition, ribociclib can cause QT prolongation and hepatotoxicity. Accordingly, the drug should be used with caution in patients with existing hepatic impairment. The effects of letrozole were discussed previously.

Preparations, Dosage, and Administration

Palbociclib [Ibrance] is supplied in 75-, 100-, and 125-mg tablets for oral dosing. Two dosing regimens are used:

- *Palbociclib with letrozole* (for women who are postmenopausal)—The recommended dosage is 125 mg taken once every day, along with letrozole.
- *Palbociclib with fulvestrant* (for women who have progression after treatment with endocrine therapy)—125 mg daily with fulvestrant.

Ribociclib [Kisquali] is supplied in 200-mg tablets. The recommended dosage is 600 mg taken once every day for 21 days to be used with letrozole.

CYTOTOXIC DRUGS (CHEMOTHERAPY)

Cytotoxic drugs may be used before breast surgery or after. When used before surgery, chemotherapy can shrink large tumors, thereby permitting lumpectomy in women who would otherwise require a mastectomy. When used after surgery, chemotherapy can kill cancer cells that remain in the breast, as well as cells that may have metastasized to distant sites. A common regimen for breast cancer consists of doxorubicin (an anthracycline-type anticancer antibiotic) plus cyclophosphamide (an alkylating agent) followed by paclitaxel (a mitotic inhibitor).

DENOSUMAB AND BISPHOSPHONATES FOR SKELETAL-RELATED EVENTS

Women with breast cancer are at risk for skeletal-related events (SREs), especially hypercalcemia and fractures. There are two causes: the cancer itself and the drugs used for treatment. In breast cancer, most metastases occur in bone. These metastases promote hypercalcemia by increasing the activity of osteoclasts, the cells that promote bone resorption. Not only does resorption promote hypercalcemia, it also weakens bone and thereby increases the risk of fractures. Fracture risk is further increased by the use of antiestrogens and aromatase inhibitors. As we discussed in Chapter 61, estrogens promote bone health by inhibiting bone resorption and promoting bone deposition. Hence, by removing the influence of estrogen, the antiestrogens and aromatase inhibitors accelerate bone resorption and reduce bone deposition. Both actions weaken bone and thereby increase the risk of fractures. To reduce the risk of SREs, we can treat patients with denosumab or a bisphosphonate (usually zoledronate).

Zoledronate and Other Bisphosphonates

In women with breast cancer, bisphosphonates can help preserve bone integrity and can thereby decrease the risk of hypercalcemia and fractures. Benefits derive from inhibiting the activity of osteoclasts. At this time, two bisphosphonates—*zoledronate* [Zometa] and *pamidronate*—are approved for hypercalcemia of malignancy, and both are also approved for managing osteolytic bone metastases. Compared with pamidronate, zoledronate has three advantages: onset is faster, duration is longer, and infusion time is shorter (15 minutes vs. 2 to 4 hours). Accordingly, zoledronate is generally preferred to pamidronate. Principal adverse effects of the bisphosphonates are kidney damage and osteonecrosis of the jaw.

In addition to reducing fractures and hypercalcemia, bisphosphonates may actually prevent metastases and prolong life. These benefits were discovered somewhat by accident. In women with breast cancer, bisphosphonates were originally employed to suppress bone resorption caused by metastases. While using bisphosphonates for this purpose, researchers noted something surprising: Bisphosphonates appeared to reduce the incidence of new bony metastases. Results of a follow-up study confirmed the original observation: In women with breast cancer, treatment with a bisphosphonate reduced metastases to bone and prolonged survival.

How do bisphosphonates suppress metastases? When cancer cells spread to bone, they stimulate the activity of osteoclasts, the cells responsible for bone resorption. In turn, osteoclasts release growth factors that stimulate the cancer cells, thereby setting up a self-reinforcing cycle. Bisphosphonates interrupt the cycle by inhibiting osteoclast function and blocking tumor adhesion to bone.

The basic pharmacology of the bisphosphonates is discussed in Chapter 75.

Denosumab

Denosumab, marketed as *Xgeva*, is indicated for preventing (delaying) SREs in patients with breast cancer and other solid tumors that have metastasized to bone. Benefits derive from inhibiting the formation and function of osteoclasts. Efficacy was demonstrated in three double-blind trials that compared denosumab with zoledronate. One trial enrolled patients with breast cancer, one enrolled patients with prostate cancer, and one enrolled patients with other cancers, including multiple myeloma, kidney cancer, small cell lung cancer, and non–small cell lung cancer. Patients received either denosumab (120 mg subQ every 4 weeks) or zoledronate (4 mg IV every 4 weeks). In patients with breast cancer or prostate cancer, denosumab was *superior* to zoledronate at delaying SREs. In patients with other cancers, denosumab was *equal* to zoledronate at delaying SREs. Principal adverse effects of denosumab are hypocalcemia, serious infections, skin reactions, and osteonecrosis of the jaw. The pharmacology of denosumab is presented in Chapter 75.

DRUGS FOR PROSTATE CANCER

Cancer of the prostate is the most common cancer among men in the United States. In 2017, an estimated 161,360 new cases were diagnosed, and 26,730 were fatal. For men with *localized* prostate cancer, the preferred treatments are surgery and radiation, with or without adjunctive use of drugs. For men with *metastatic* prostate cancer, drug therapy and castration are the only options. Among the drugs employed, agents for *androgen deprivation therapy* (ADT) comprise the largest and most widely used group. The only other choices are cytotoxic drugs and a new immunotherapy known as sipuleucel-T [Provenge]. As with breast cancer, most metastases (65% to 75%) go to bone. To minimize hypercalcemia and fractures caused by bone metastases, men may take *zoledronate* [Zometa] or *denosumab* [Xgeva] (see earlier discussion of breast cancer). The drugs used to treat prostate cancer are shown in Table 103.2.

TABLE 103.2 ▪ Drugs for Prostate Cancer

Generic Name	Brand Name	Route	Major Adverse Effects
DRUGS FOR ANDROGEN DEPRIVATION THERAPY			
GnRH Agonists[a]			
Leuprolide	Lupron, Lupron Depot Eligard	IM SubQ	Hot flashes, erectile dysfunction, decreased libido, decreased muscle mass, gynecomastia, osteoporosis
Triptorelin	Trelstar	IM	
Goserelin	Zoladex	SubQ	
Histrelin	Vantas	SubQ implant	
GnRH Antagonist			
Degarelix	Firmagon	SubQ	Same as the GnRH agonists *plus* hepatotoxicity
Androgen Receptor Blockers			
Flutamide	Generic only	PO	Same as the GnRH agonists *plus* hepatotoxicity
Bicalutamide	Casodex	PO	Same as the GnRH agonists *plus* hepatotoxicity
Enzalutamide	Xtandi	PO	Same as the GnRH agonists plus PRES
Nilutamide	Nilandron, Anandron	PO	Same as the GnRH agonists *plus* hepatotoxicity and interstitial pneumonitis
CYP17 Inhibitor			
Abiraterone	Zytiga	PO	Same as the GnRH agonists *plus* hepatotoxicity, edema, hypertension, hypokalemia, glucocorticoid insufficiency
OTHER DRUGS FOR PROSTATE CANCER			
Immunotherapy			
Sipuleucel-T	Provenge	IV	Infusion reactions, fatigue, fever
Cytotoxic Drugs			
Cabazitaxel	Jevtana	IV	Neutropenia, hypersensitivity reactions, diarrhea
Docetaxel	Taxotere	IV	Neutropenia, anemia, hypersensitivity reactions, fluid retention
Estramustine	Emcyt	PO	Gynecomastia, thrombosis
Drugs to Delay Skeletal Events			
Zoledronate	Zometa[b]	IV	Kidney damage, osteonecrosis of the jaw, rare atrial fibrillation
Denosumab	Xgeva[c]	SubQ	Hypocalcemia, serious infections, skin reactions, osteonecrosis of the jaw

[a]Gonadotropin-releasing hormone agonists, also known as luteinizing hormone–releasing hormone (LHRH) agonists.
[b]Zoledronate is also available as *Reclast* for treating osteoporosis and Paget's disease.
[c]Denosumab is also available as *Prolia* for treating postmenopausal osteoporosis.
GnRH, Gonadotropin-releasing hormone; *PRES,* posterior reversible encelphalopathy syndrome.

ANDROGEN DEPRIVATION THERAPY

The term *androgen deprivation therapy* refers to the use of castration and/or drugs to deprive prostate cancers of the androgens they need for growth. By implementing ADT, we can slow disease progression and increase comfort. Initially, ADT was reserved for patients with metastatic disease. However, ADT is now used as an adjuvant in earlier-stage disease. Unfortunately, the benefits of ADT are time limited: After 18 to 24 months of treatment, disease progression often resumes. Side effects of ADT include hot flashes, reduced libido, erectile dysfunction, gynecomastia, decreased muscle mass, and decreased bone mass with associated increased risk of fractures.

Where do androgens come from, and how can we reduce their influence? About 90% of circulating androgens are produced by the testes. The remaining 10% are produced by the adrenal glands and by the prostate cancer itself. Accordingly, we can reduce the influence of androgens in three ways. Specifically, we can block testosterone receptors with drugs; we can lower testosterone production with drugs; and we can lower testosterone production by castration. Drug therapy is more effective than castration because castration eliminates only testicular androgens, leaving androgen synthesis by the adrenal glands and cancer cells intact. In contrast, by using drugs to block testosterone receptors and testosterone synthesis, we can reduce the influence of testosterone from all sources (testes, adrenal glands, prostate cancer).

Gonadotropin-Releasing Hormone Agonists

The gonadotropin-releasing hormone (GnRH) agonists suppress production of androgens by the testes—but not by the adrenal glands and prostate cancer cells. Currently, four GnRH agonists are available: leuprolide, triptorelin, goserelin, and histrelin. All four are indicated for cancer of the prostate. In addition, leuprolide is used for endometriosis (see Chapter 63).

Leuprolide

Therapeutic Use. Leuprolide [Eligard, Lupron ♣, Lupron Depot] is a synthetic analog of GnRH, also known as *luteinizing hormone–releasing hormone* (LHRH). Leuprolide is indicated for *advanced carcinoma of the prostate*. Palliation is the primary benefit. For patients with prostate cancer, leuprolide represents an alternative to orchiectomy (surgical castration). Leuprolide may be administered daily (subQ); monthly (IM); or every 3, 4, or 6 months (IM).

Mechanism of Action. Cells of the prostate, both normal and neoplastic, are androgen dependent. Leuprolide provides palliation by suppressing androgen production in the *testes*. During the initial phase of treatment, leuprolide *mimics* GnRH. That is, the drug acts on the pituitary to *stimulate* release of interstitial cell–stimulating hormone (ICSH), which acts on the testes to *increase* production of testosterone. As a result, there may be a transient "flare" in prostate cancer symptoms. However, with continuous exposure to leuprolide, GnRH receptors in the pituitary become desensitized. As a result, release of ICSH declines, causing testosterone production to decline too. After several weeks of treatment, testosterone levels are equivalent to those seen after surgical castration. Because leuprolide therapy mimics the effects of orchiectomy, treatment is often referred to as *chemical castration*.

It is important to note that leuprolide does *not* decrease production of androgens made by the adrenal glands or by the prostate cancer itself. As noted, these nontesticular sources account for about 10% of the androgens in circulation. Hence, even though production of testicular androgens is essentially eliminated, adrenal and prostatic androgens can still provide some support for prostate cancer cells.

Co-treatment With an Androgen Receptor Blocker. In patients receiving leuprolide, an androgen receptor blocker can help in two ways. Specifically, (1) it can prevent cancer cells from undergoing increased stimulation during the initial phase of GnRH therapy, when androgen production is increased; and (2) it can block the effects of adrenal and prostatic androgens, whose production is not reduced by GnRH agonists. The current trend is to use an androgen receptor blocker during the first weeks of leuprolide therapy (to prevent leuprolide-induced tumor flare), after which the drug is discontinued unless there is tumor progression despite continued leuprolide treatment.

Adverse Effects. Leuprolide is generally well tolerated. Hot flashes are the most common adverse effect, but these usually decline as treatment continues. Reduced testosterone may also lead to erectile dysfunction, loss of libido, gynecomastia, reduced muscle mass, new-onset diabetes, myocardial infarction, and stroke. During the initial weeks of treatment, elevation of testosterone levels may aggravate bone pain and urinary obstruction caused by prostate cancer. As a result, patients with vertebral metastases or pre-existing obstruction of the urinary tract may find treatment intolerable. As noted, concurrent treatment with an androgen receptor blocker can minimize these problems.

By suppressing testosterone production, leuprolide may increase the risk of osteoporosis and related fractures. Bone loss can be minimized by consuming adequate calcium and vitamin D and by performing regular weight-bearing exercise. In addition, a bisphosphonate (e.g., zoledronate [Zometa]) or denosumab [Xgeva] can be used to preserve bone and reduce fracture risk (see previous discussion of breast cancer).

Preparations, Dosage, and Administration. Leuprolide is supplied in two basic formulations for parenteral dosing:

- *Leuprolide short-acting injection* [Lupron ♣] is supplied as a 5-mg/mL solution for subQ administration. The recommended dosage is 1 mg once a day.
- *Leuprolide depot injection* is available in single-dose kits under two brand names: *Lupron Depot* (for IM injection) and *Eligard* (for subQ injection). With either product, the dosage is 7.5 mg once a month, 22.5 mg every 3 months, 30 mg every 4 months, or 45 mg every 6 months.

Triptorelin, Goserelin, Histrelin

Triptorelin, goserelin, and histrelin are GnRH analogs indicated for palliative treatment of *advanced prostate cancer*. All three have the same mechanism and adverse effects of leuprolide, our prototype GnRH agonist. Preparations, dosage, and administration are as follows:

- *Triptorelin* [Trelstar] is administered by IM injection. The recommended dosage is 3.75 mg once a month, 11.25 mg once every 3 months, or 22.5 mg once every 6 months.
- *Goserelin* [Zoladex] is formulated as pellets (3.6 mg and 10.8 mg) for subQ implantation in the upper abdominal wall. The 3.6-mg pellets are implanted every 4 weeks, and the 10.8-mg pellets are implanted every 12 weeks.
- *Histrelin* [Vantas] is formulated as a 50-mg pellet for subQ implantation in the inner aspect of the upper arm once every 12 months.

Prototype Drugs

HORMONAL, TARGETED, AND OTHER ANTICANCER DRUGS

Drugs for Breast Cancer

Antiestrogen
Tamoxifen

Aromatase Inhibitor
Anastrozole

HER2 Antagonist
Trastuzumab

Cytotoxic Drugs
Doxorubicin/cyclophosphamide
Paclitaxel

Drugs to Delay Skeletal Events
Denosumab
Zoledronate

Drugs for Prostate Cancer

Gonadotropin-Releasing Hormone Agonist
Leuprolide

Gonadotropin-Releasing Hormone Antagonist
Degarelix

Androgen Receptor Blocker
Flutamide

CYP17 Inhibitor
Abiraterone

Patient-Specific Immunotherapy
Sipuleucel-T

Cytotoxic Drugs
Docetaxel
Cabazitaxel

Drugs to Delay Skeletal Events
Denosumab
Zoledronate

Targeted Drugs

EGFR Tyrosine Kinase Inhibitor
Cetuximab

BRC-ABL Tyrosine Kinase Inhibitor
Imatinib

BRAF V600E Kinase Inhibitor
Vemurafenib

CD-Directed Antibody
Rituximab

PD-Directed Antibody
Nivolumab

Angiogenesis Inhibitor
Bevacizumab

Proteasome Inhibitor
Bortezomib

Immunostimulants

Interferon
Interferon alfa-2a

Other Noncytotoxic Drugs

Glucocorticoid
Prednisone

PD, Programmed death.

Gonadotropin-Releasing Hormone Antagonists

Like the GnRH agonists, the GnRH *antagonists* suppress production of androgens by the testes. However, in contrast to the GnRH agonists, the GnRH antagonists do not produce an initial tumor flare. Currently, only one GnRH antagonist—degarelix—is available.

Degarelix

Degarelix [Firmagon] is a synthetic decapeptide GnRH antagonist indicated for palliative therapy of *advanced prostate cancer* in men who are not candidates for a GnRH agonist and who do not want surgical castration. Benefits derive from suppressing testosterone production by the testes. The underlying mechanism is blockade of GnRH receptors in the anterior pituitary, which decreases release of luteinizing hormone and follicle-stimulating hormone, which in turn deprives the testes of the stimulus they need for testosterone production. In clinical trials, patients received an initial 240-mg dose followed by monthly maintenance 80-mg doses. Testosterone levels fell rapidly to those produced by castration and then remained low for at least 12 months. Because degarelix works through direct blockade of GnRH receptors, the drug does not cause the initial surge in testosterone production seen with GnRH agonists, and hence there is no early tumor flare.

Degarelix is administered subQ, and absorption is slow. Plasma levels peak in 2 days. Elimination is primarily by peptide bond hydrolysis, a process that occurs in the liver but does not involve cytochrome P450 enzymes. The drug's half-life is long: 53 days.

As with other drugs for ADT, major side effects are hot flashes, reduced libido, erectile dysfunction, gynecomastia, decreased muscle mass, and decreased bone mass with associated increased risk of fractures. In addition, degarelix often causes injection-site reactions (pain, erythema, swelling), weight gain, and elevation of liver transaminases. After a year of treatment, about 10% of patients develop antibodies against degarelix. However, the antibodies do not reduce the effectiveness of treatment.

Degarelix is supplied as a powder (80 and 120 mg) to be reconstituted for subQ injection. The regimen consists of an initial 240-mg dose (two 120-mg injections), followed by monthly 80-mg injections for maintenance.

Androgen Receptor Blockers

Androgen receptor blockers, or simply *antiandrogens*, are indicated only for advanced androgen-sensitive prostate cancer—and only in combination with surgical castration or chemical castration using a GnRH agonist. Currently, four androgen receptor blockers are available: flutamide, bicalutamide, enzalutamide, and nilutamide. Due to their similarities, only flutamide and bicalutamide will be discussed here.

Flutamide

Flutamide is indicated for *prostate cancer* only. Benefits derive from blocking androgen receptors in tumor cells, thereby depriving them of needed androgenic support. In patients taking a GnRH agonist, flutamide can serve two purposes: (1) It can prevent tumor flare when GnRH therapy is started, and (2) it can block the effects of adrenal and prostatic androgens. As a rule, the combination of an androgen antagonist plus a GnRH agonist—so-called complete androgen blockade—is reserved for suppressing the initial flare and for suppressing the tumor after it has stopped responding to a GnRH agonist alone. The combination is not used continuously because it does not increase survival, but does increase toxicity.

Flutamide is administered orally and undergoes rapid and complete absorption. Most of each dose is converted to an active metabolite on the first pass through the liver. Parent drug and metabolites are excreted in the urine.

As with other drugs for ADT, prominent side effects are hot flashes, reduced libido, erectile dysfunction, gynecomastia, decreased muscle mass, and decreased bone mass with associated increased risk of fractures. Nausea, vomiting, and diarrhea are also common. Rarely, potentially fatal liver toxicity has occurred. To reduce the risk of serious harm, liver function should be assessed at baseline, monthly during the first 4 months of treatment and periodically thereafter.

Flutamide may cause fetal harm, and hence is classified in FDA Pregnancy Risk Category D.[c] Accordingly, the drug should not be used during pregnancy. Of course, because flutamide is approved only for prostate cancer, use during pregnancy should not happen anyway.

Flutamide is supplied in 125-mg capsules. The usual dosage is 250 mg 3 times a day.

Bicalutamide

Like flutamide, bicalutamide [Casodex] is an androgen receptor blocker used for *advanced androgen-sensitive prostate cancer* in men undergoing therapy with a GnRH agonist (e.g., leuprolide). The rationale for the combination is explained in the discussion of flutamide. When bicalutamide is used alone, the most common side effects are breast pain and gynecomastia. When the drug is combined with leuprolide, the most common side effect is hot flashes. Like all other drugs used for ADT, bicalutamide can also cause reduced libido, erectile dysfunction, decreased muscle mass, and decreased bone mass with associated increased risk of fractures. Also, like flutamide, bicalutamide poses a small risk of liver injury, and hence liver function should be monitored. Bicalutamide poses a significant risk of fetal harm, and hence is classified in FDA Pregnancy Risk Category X.[d] Bicalutamide is just as effective as flutamide, and dosing is more convenient (50 mg once a day vs. 250 mg 3 times a day). As a result, bicalutamide is preferred.

Abiraterone, a CYP17 Inhibitor

Actions and Use

Abiraterone [Zytiga] is indicated for combined use with prednisone to treat *metastatic castration-resistant prostate cancer* in men previously treated with docetaxel. Benefits derive from inhibiting production of androgens by the adrenal gland and by the prostate cancer itself. (If castration has not been done, abiraterone can also inhibit androgen production by the testes.) In all cases, the underlying mechanism is inhibition of the cytochrome P450 enzyme 17 (CYP17), an enzyme needed by the adrenals, testes, and prostate tumors for androgen synthesis. When tested in men with metastatic castration-resistant prostate cancer, the combination of abiraterone plus prednisone increased overall survival by nearly 4 months and progression-free survival by 2 months.

Adverse Effects

The most common adverse effects are hypokalemia, edema, joint swelling/discomfort, muscle discomfort, hot flashes, diarrhea, urinary tract infection, cough, and hypertension. Like all other drugs for ADT, abiraterone can also decrease libido, muscle mass, and bone mass and can cause erectile dysfunction and gynecomastia.

Inhibition of CYP17 in the adrenals can lead to overproduction of mineralocorticoids and underproduction of glucocorticoids. High levels of mineralocorticoids can cause retention of sodium and loss of potassium, leading to fluid retention, edema, hypertension, and hypokalemia. Low levels of glucocorticoids can increase the risk of death from traumatic events. Co-treatment with prednisone (a glucocorticoid) helps compensate for reduced production of glucocorticoids by the adrenal glands and by suppressing release of adrenocorticotropic hormone from the pituitary, prednisone can reduce excessive production of mineralocorticoids.

Hepatotoxicity, manifesting as a marked elevation of liver transaminases—alanine aminotransferase (ALT) and aspartate aminotransferase (AST)—develops in about 30% of patients. To monitor liver status, ALT and AST should be measured at baseline, every 2 weeks for the first 3 months of treatment, and once a month thereafter. If these tests indicate significant liver injury, abiraterone should be discontinued or the dosage reduced.

Abiraterone can harm the developing fetus, and hence is classified in FDA Pregnancy Risk Category X.[e] Accordingly, the drug should be avoided by women who are pregnant. Of course, because abiraterone is approved only for prostate cancer, use during pregnancy should not be an issue.

[c]As of 2020, the FDA will no longer use Pregnancy Risk Categories. Please refer to Chapter 9 for more information.

[d]As of 2020, the FDA will no longer use Pregnancy Risk Categories. Please refer to Chapter 9 for more information.

[e]As of 2020, the FDA will no longer use Pregnancy Risk Categories. Please refer to Chapter 9 for more information.

Drug Interactions

Abiraterone is a substrate for CYP3A4, and hence its levels can be raised by CYP3A4 inhibitors (e.g., ketoconazole, clarithromycin, ritonavir) and lowered by CYP3A4 inducers (e.g., phenytoin, carbamazepine, rifampin). Abiraterone inhibits hepatic CYP2D6, and hence can raise levels of CYP2D6 substrates (e.g., dextromethorphan, thioridazine).

Preparations, Dosage, and Administration

Abiraterone is supplied in 250-mg capsules, which should be swallowed with water on an empty stomach (1 hour before a meal or 2 hours after). Dosing should not be done with food, owing to greatly *increased* absorption, which could cause toxicity. The usual regimen is 1000 mg abiraterone once daily combined with 5 mg prednisone twice daily. Dosage of abiraterone should be reduced in patients with liver impairment.

Ketoconazole

Ketoconazole [Nizoral], used primarily for fungal infections (see Chapter 92), can be used off-label for prostate cancer. As with abiraterone, benefits derive from inhibiting testicular, adrenal, and prostatic production of androgens. Ketoconazole is employed as secondary therapy in men who have rising prostate-specific antigen levels despite treatment with a GnRH agonist plus an antiandrogen. Dosages are higher than those used for antifungal therapy (400 mg 3 times a day compared with 200 mg once a day), and hence side effects are common. Among these are nausea, vomiting, fatigue, skin changes, liver damage, and gynecomastia. Because high-dose ketoconazole can suppress adrenal production of glucocorticoids, the drug is usually combined with hydrocortisone (to avoid adrenal insufficiency).

OTHER DRUGS FOR PROSTATE CANCER

Sipuleucel-T

Sipuleucel-T [Provenge] is the name for a patient-specific form of immunotherapy designed to stimulate an immune attack against prostate cancer cells. Each dose is custom-made from the patient's own immune cells, and hence cannot be used by any other patient. Unfortunately, sipuleucel-T is very expensive—and only moderately effective. Nonetheless, sipuleucel-T is of great interest in that it represents an entirely new approach to cancer treatment.

Therapeutic Use

Sipuleucel-T is indicated for treatment of asymptomatic or minimally symptomatic metastatic castration-resistant (hormone-refractory) prostate cancer. Treatment consists of three infusions given 2 weeks apart. In clinical trials, sipuleucel-T prolonged life by about 4 months, compared with 2.4 months using standard chemotherapy (e.g., docetaxel [Taxotere]). Of note, although sipuleucel-T improves survival, it does not cause measurable tumor regression, nor does it delay the time to tumor progression—suggesting that the mechanism underlying prolonged survival may be something other than immune-mediated injury to cancer cells.

Production

Sipuleucel-T is produced in two steps: collection of circulating immune cells (macrophages) from the patient, followed by modification of those cells in the laboratory. This process—cell collection plus modification—takes about 2 days and must be done for *each dose*.

Macrophage collection is done by *leukapheresis*, a process in which venous blood is circulated from the patient, through a machine, and then back into the patient. The machine separates out macrophages (along with some platelets and other blood cells) and then returns the remaining cells and serum to the patient. The whole procedure takes 3 to 4 hours.

In the laboratory, the macrophages—also known as *antigen-presenting cells*, or *APCs*—are modified by incubation with a recombinant human protein consisting of prostatic acid phosphatase (PAP) linked with granulocyte-macrophage colony-stimulating factor (GM-CSF). PAP is a protein that is highly expressed by more than 95% of prostate cancer cells. As discussed in Chapter 56, GM-CSF is a blood growth factor that stimulates the production and function of macrophages and some other blood cells. During incubation, the APCs engulf the PAP–GM-CSF, break it into small peptides, and then express those peptides on the APC surface. The modified APCs can now activate cytolytic T cells (killer T cells), causing them to attack prostate cancer cells by recognizing the PAP molecules on their surface.

Adverse Effects

Sipuleucel-T can cause multiple adverse effects. The most common are chills, fatigue, fever, back pain, nausea, joint ache, and headache. Other common reactions include paresthesias, vomiting, anemia, constipation, dizziness, weakness, and extremity pain.

Acute infusion reactions develop in over 70% of patients. Symptoms include fever, chills, nausea, vomiting, fatigue, hypertension, tachycardia, and respiratory reactions (dyspnea, hypoxia, and bronchospasm). Severe reactions may require hospitalization. Infusion reactions can be reduced by premedication with acetaminophen plus an antihistamine, such as diphenhydramine [Benadryl].

Dosage and Administration

Patients receive three doses 2 weeks apart. Three days before treatment, the patient undergoes leukapheresis to collect the APCs for that dose. Each dose is supplied in a sealed, patient-specific infusion bag that contains a minimum of 50 million activated APCs, suspended in 250 mL of lactated Ringer's injection. Administration is by IV infusion—without a cell filter—over a period of 60 minutes. Pretreatment with acetaminophen plus an antihistamine can reduce infusion reactions. In the event of a severe reaction, the infusion may be slowed or discontinued.

Cytotoxic Drugs

Docetaxel and Cabazitaxel

Docetaxel [Taxotere] and cabazitaxel [Jevtana] are cytotoxic anticancer drugs indicated for *hormone-refractory prostate cancer* (i.e., prostate cancer that no longer responds to ADT). Either drug (in combination with prednisone) can prolong overall survival as well as progression-free survival. At this time, docetaxel is considered a first-line drug for hormone-refractory prostate cancer. Cabazitaxel is reserved for patients who have already been treated with docetaxel. The major adverse effects of docetaxel are neutropenia, hypersensitivity reactions, and fluid retention. The major adverse effects of cabazitaxel are neutropenia, hypersensitivity reactions, anemia, and diarrhea. With both drugs, benefits derive from causing mitotic arrest. The pharmacology of docetaxel and cabazitaxel is discussed in Chapter 102.

Estramustine

Estramustine [Emcyt] is a hybrid molecule composed of estradiol (an estrogen) coupled to nitrogen mustard (an alkylating agent; see Chapter 102). The only indication for the drug is palliative therapy of *advanced prostate cancer.* Estramustine is administered orally and becomes concentrated in prostate cells, apparently through the actions of a unique "estramustine-binding protein."

Injury to prostate cells appears to result from three mechanisms. First, estramustine acts as a weak alkylating agent. Second, hydrolysis of estramustine releases free estradiol, which suppresses ICSH release by the pituitary, thereby depriving prostate cells of hormonal support. Third, and most importantly, the drug binds to microtubules of mitotic spindles and thereby disrupts mitosis. As a result, estramustine has M-phase specificity.

Adverse effects are caused primarily by free estradiol. Gynecomastia is common. The most serious effect is thrombosis, with resultant myocardial infarction and stroke. Other adverse effects include fluid retention, nausea, vomiting, diarrhea, and hypercalcemia.

Estramustine is supplied in 140-mg capsules for oral dosing on an empty stomach (1 hour before meals or 2 hours after). The usual dosage is 14 mg/kg/day administered in three or four divided doses.

TARGETED ANTICANCER DRUGS

Targeted anticancer drugs are designed to bind with specific molecules (targets) with the goal of suppressing tumor growth. The hope is that these drugs will be more selective than hormones and cytotoxic anticancer drugs, and hence will be able to destroy cancer cells while leaving normal cells untouched. A few targeted drugs, such as imatinib [Gleevec], have been remarkably successful, producing complete responses with relatively mild adverse effects. In 2016 alone, 25 new targeted drugs entered the U.S. market. Because many of these drugs work in a very similar way, we will address only prototypes within each class, although all drugs can be located within Tables 103.3 and 103.4.

How do targeted drugs work? Many of these drugs are *antibodies* that bind with specific antigens on tumor cells; others are *small molecules* that inhibit intracellular enzymes. Some antibodies mark cancer cells for immune attack, some block cell-surface receptors, some deliver toxic drugs or radioactivity, and some inhibit angiogenesis and thereby deprive tumor cells of their blood supply. Most of the small molecules inhibit specific tyrosine kinases and thereby disrupt intracellular signaling pathways. Properties of the targeted drugs are shown in Tables 103.3.

KINASE INHIBITORS

A kinase is an enzyme that catalyzes the transfer of a phosphate group from a nucleoside triphosphate donor (e.g., ATP) to an acceptor molecule, often a protein involved in regulation of cell behavior. This process, known as phosphorylation, alters the structure of the acceptor protein and thereby increases or decreases its activity. Put another way, the result of phosphorylation is like flipping a switch, turning it on or turning it off. Of interest to us are the protein "switches" that help promote cancer growth. For example, certain regulatory proteins, when phosphorylated, activate signaling pathways that increase cell proliferation and cell survival. Accordingly, if we prevent phosphorylation with a kinase inhibitor, we can shut down the signaling pathway and thereby inhibit proliferation and promote apoptosis (programmed cell death).

Most of the drugs described next inhibit *tyrosine kinases* of one type or another. What's a tyrosine kinase? It's simply a kinase that transfers a phosphate group specifically to tyrosine, one of the amino acid components of the protein undergoing phosphorylation. Other kinases phosphorylate different amino acids, often serine or threonine.

EGFR Tyrosine Kinase Inhibitors

The *epidermal growth factor receptor* is a transmembrane regulatory molecule that works through activation of intracellular tyrosine kinase. The receptor portion of EGFR, which is found on the outer surface of the cell membrane, is coupled with tyrosine kinase on the inner surface of the cell membrane. Binding of an agonist to EGFR activates tyrosine kinase, which in turn activates signaling pathways that regulate cell proliferation and survival. EGFRs are expressed constitutively in many normal epithelial tissues (e.g., skin, hair follicles) and are overexpressed in several cancers, including cancers of the lung, breast, prostate, bladder, ovary, colon, and rectum. Overexpression is associated with unregulated cell growth and poor prognosis. Drugs that inhibit EGFR suppress cell proliferation and promote apoptosis. At this time, we have seven EGFR tyrosine kinase inhibitors. Two of these drugs—cetuximab and panitumumab—are monoclonal antibodies that bind with the receptor portion of EGFR tyrosine kinase and thereby prevent its activation by agonists. The other five drugs—erlotinib, gefitinib, afatinib, osimertinib, and lapatinib—are small molecules that work inside the cell to inhibit tyrosine kinase directly. It should be noted that EGFRs belong to the same receptor family as HER2, the target that trastuzumab [Herceptin] works through.

Cetuximab

Cetuximab [Erbitux] is a monoclonal antibody that blocks EGFRs. The drug is approved for refractory colorectal cancer and for carcinoma of the head and neck. Infusion reactions, acneiform rash, low magnesium, and GI symptoms are common.

Mechanism of Action. Cetuximab acts as a competitive antagonist at EGFRs. As noted, these receptors, which help regulate cell growth, are overexpressed in certain cancers, including those of the colon and rectum. EGFR blockade inhibits cell growth and promotes apoptosis. In animal studies, cetuximab decreased growth and survival of cancer cells that overexpress EGFR, but had no effect on cancer cells that lack EGFR.

Therapeutic Uses

Colorectal Cancer. Cetuximab is approved for metastatic, EGFR-positive colorectal cancer. The drug may be added to an irinotecan-based regimen (if the cancer has progressed despite irinotecan treatment), or it may be used alone (in patients who cannot tolerate irinotecan). In clinical trials, cetuximab delayed tumor growth and promoted tumor regression. Treatment improves quality of life and can improve survival rate at 3 years.

Head and Neck Cancer. Cetuximab, in combination with radiation, is approved for initial treatment of locally or regionally advanced squamous cell carcinoma of the head and neck. In addition, the drug can be used for recurrent or metastatic cancers that have progressed despite treatment with a platinum-based regimen.

Adverse Effects. Cetuximab causes adverse effects in most patients. The effects of greatest concern are severe infusion reactions, severe rash, and interstitial lung disease (ILD).

Cetuximab causes severe *infusion reactions* in 2% to 5% of patients. Manifestations include rapid-onset airway obstruction, hypotension, shock, loss of consciousness, myocardial infarction, and cardiopulmonary arrest. Severe reactions can happen with any infusion, but most (90%) occur with the first

TABLE 103.3 ▪ Kinase Inhibitors

Drug	Molecular Target	Drug Structure	Indications	Major Toxicities
EGFR TYROSINE KINASE INHIBITORS				
Cetuximab [Erbitux]	Inhibits EGFR	Antibody	EGFR-positive colorectal cancer and head and neck cancer	Rash, infusion reactions, interstitial lung disease
Panitumumab [Vectibix]	Inhibits EGFR	Antibody	EGFR-positive colorectal cancer	Rare infusion reactions, rash, rare interstitial pneumonitis
Gefitinib [Iressa]	Inhibits EGFR tyrosine kinase	Small molecule	Non–small cell lung cancer	Rash, diarrhea, interstitial lung disease
Erlotinib [Tarceva]	Inhibits EGFR tyrosine kinase	Small molecule	EGFR positive non–small cell lung cancer	Blistering, GI perforation, interstitial lung disease, corneal ulceration/perforation
Osimertinib [Tagrisso]	Inhibits EGFR tyrosine kinase	Small molecule	Non–small cell lung cancer	Interstitial lung disease, cardiomyopathy, cerebrovascular hemorrhage
Afatinib [Gilotrif]	Inhibits EGFR tyrosine kinase, HER2 and HER4 tyrosine kinase	Small molecule	Metastatic non–small cell lung cancer	Diarrhea, cutaneous reactions, keratitis
Lapatinib [Tykerb]	Inhibits EGFR tyrosine kinase and HER2 tyrosine kinase	Small molecule	HER2-positive breast cancer	Diarrhea, hepatotoxicity, cardiotoxicity, interstitial lung disease
BCR-ABL TYROSINE KINASE INHIBITORS				
Imatinib [Gleevec]	Inhibits BCR-ABL tyrosine kinase	Small molecule	Chronic myeloid leukemia, GI stromal tumors	Nausea, diarrhea, myalgia, edema, liver injury
Dasatinib [Sprycel]	Inhibits BCR-ABL tyrosine kinase	Small molecule	Chronic myeloid leukemia	Myelosuppression, QT prolongation, fluid retention, pulmonary arterial hypertension
Nilotinib [Tasigna]	Inhibits BCR-ABL tyrosine kinase	Small molecule	Chronic myeloid leukemia	Myelosuppression, QT prolongation
Bosutinib [Bosulif]	Inhibits BCR-ABL tyrosine kinase	Small molecule	Philadelphia chromosome–positive chronic myelogenous leukemia	Myelosuppression, hepatotoxicity, anaphylactic shock
Ponatinib [Iclusig]	Inhibits BCR- ABL tyrosine kinase	Small molecule	Chronic myeloid leukemia or Philadelphia chromosome–positive lymphoblastic leukemia	Venous thromboembolism, cardiotoxicity, pancreatitis, cardiac dysrhythmias
MULTI–TYROSINE KINASE INHIBITORS				
Sorafenib [Nexavar]	Inhibits multiple cell-surface and intracellular tyrosine kinases	Small molecule	Renal cell carcinoma, hepatocellular carcinoma	Rash, diarrhea, hand-and-foot syndrome, bleeding, QT prolongation, hypertension
Sunitinib [Sutent]	Inhibits multiple tyrosine kinases	Small molecule	Renal cell carcinoma, GI stromal tumors, pancreatic neuroendocrine tumors	Hepatotoxicity, heart failure, QT prolongation, hypertension, hemorrhage
Pazopanib [Votrient]	Inhibits multiple tyrosine kinases	Small molecule	Renal cell carcinoma	Bone marrow suppression, hepatotoxicity
Vandetanib [Caprelsa]	Inhibits multiple tyrosine kinases	Small molecule	Medullary thyroid cancer	QT prolongation, rash, diarrhea/colitis
Axitinib [Inlyta]	Inhibits multiple tyrosine kinases	Small molecule	Advanced renal cell carcinoma	Hypertensive crisis, venous thromboembolism, hypothyroidism

Continued

TABLE 103.3 ■ Kinase Inhibitors—cont'd

Drug	Molecular Target	Drug Structure	Indications	Major Toxicities
Cabozantinib [Cometriq]	Inhibits multiple tyrosine kinases	Small molecule	Metastatic medullary thyroid cancer, renal cell cancer	Thromboembolism, GI perforation, posterior leukoencephalopathy
Regorafenib [Stivarga]	Inhibits multiple tyrosine kinases	Small molecule	Metastatic colon cancer, metastatic GI stromal cancer	Hepatotoxicity, toxic cutaneous reactions, cardiotoxicity
Lenvatinib [Lenvima]	Inhibits multiple tyrosine kinases	Small molecule	Differentiated thyroid cancer, renal cell cancer	Cardiac failure, pulmonary edema, severe hemorrhage, acute renal failure, hepatotoxicity
mTOR KINASE INHIBITORS				
Temsirolimus [Torisel]	Inhibits mTOR kinase	Small molecule	Renal cell carcinoma	Mucositis, bone marrow suppression, metabolic abnormalities
Everolimus [Afinitor]	Inhibits mTOR kinase	Small molecule	Renal cell carcinoma, neuroendocrine tumors	Oral ulceration, bone marrow suppression, metabolic abnormalities
BRAF V600E KINASE INHIBITORS				
Vemurafenib [Zelboraf]	Inhibits BRAF V600E kinase	Small molecule	BRAF V600E-positive melanoma	Cutaneous squamous cell carcinoma, arthralgia, QT prolongation, severe skin reactions, photosensitivity
Dabrafenib [Tafinlar]	Inhibits BRAF V600E kinase	Small molecule	BRAF V600E-positive melanoma	Retinal vein occlusion, cutaneous malignancies
Trametinib [Mekinist]	Inhibits BRAF V600E pathway through inhibition of MEK1 and MEK2	Small molecule	BRAF V600E-positive melanoma	Cutaneous malignancies, hemorrhage, thromboembolism, retinal vein occlusion
Cobimetinib [Cotellic]	Inhibits BRAF V600E pathway through inhibition of MEK1 and MEK2	Small molecule	BRAF V600E or V600K-positive melanoma	Hemorrhage, cardiomyopathy, cutaneous malignancies, rhabdomyolysis
ANAPLASTIC LYMPHOMA KINASE (ALK) INHIBITORS				
Crizotinib [Xalkori]	Inhibits ALK	Small molecule	ALK-positive non–small cell lung cancer	Pneumonitis, hepatotoxicity, QT prolongation
Ceritinib [Zykadia]	Inhibits ALK	Small molecule	ALK-positive non–small cell lung cancer	Diarrhea, severe nausea/vomiting, pneumonitis, seizures
Alectinib [Alecensa]	Inhibits ALK	Small molecule	ALK-positive non–small cell lung cancer	Hepatotoxicity, Interstitial lung disease, severe myalgias

EGFR, Epidermal growth factor receptor, which is coupled with tyrosine kinase; *GI,* gastrointestinal; *HER2,* human epidermal growth factor receptor 2; *MEK,* MAP (mitogen-activated protein)/ERK (extracellular signal–regulated) kinase; *mTOR,* mammalian target of rapamycin.

infusion. If a severe reaction develops, cetuximab should be discontinued immediately and never used again. Agents for medical management—epinephrine, glucocorticoids, IV antihistamines, bronchodilators, and oxygen—should always be on hand. To reduce the risk of a severe reaction, premedication with an IV antihistamine (e.g., 50 mg diphenhydramine) is recommended.

Acne-like rash, mainly on the face and upper torso, develops in 88% of patients and is severe in 12%. Severe rash has led to *Staphylococcus aureus* sepsis and abscesses that require incision and drainage. Sunlight can exacerbate dermatologic reactions, and hence patients should limit sun exposure, use a sunblock, and wear protective clothing.

Very rarely, cetuximab has been associated with *interstitial lung disease*, characterized by inflammation, scarring, and hardening of the lungs. One case of fatal interstitial pneumonitis with pulmonary edema has been reported. Whether cetuximab is truly the cause of these lung disorders has not been established.

The combination of cetuximab and irinotecan often causes *GI toxicity*, manifesting as diarrhea, nausea, abdominal pain, vomiting, anorexia, and constipation.

In clinical trials, *hypomagnesemia* developed in 55% of patients and was severe in 6% to 17%. Magnesium supplements are often required.

Cetuximab can cross the placenta, but whether it causes fetal harm has not been studied in humans. Animal studies do

TABLE 103.4 ■ Other Targeted Drugs

Drug	Molecular Target	Drug Structure	Indications	Major Toxicities
CD-DIRECTED ANTIBODIES				
Rituximab [Rituxan]	Binds CD20 antigen, causing apoptosis and immune attack	Antibody	B-cell chronic lymphocytic leukemia, B-cell non-Hodgkin's lymphoma	Severe infusion reactions, severe mucocutaneous reactions, tumor lysis syndrome, PML
Ofatumumab [Arzerra]	Binds CD20 antigen, causing apoptosis and immune attack	Antibody	B-cell chronic lymphocytic leukemia	Severe infusion reactions, cytopenias, PML
Obinutuzumab [Gazyva]	Binds CD20 antigen, causing apoptosis and immune attack	Antibody	B-cell chronic lymphocytic leukemia, follicular lymphoma	Severe infusion reactions, hepatitis, severe infection, hemorrhage
Daratumumab [Darzalex]	Binds CD38, causing apoptosis	Antibody	Multiple myeloma	Severe infusion reactions, bone marrow suppression, severe infection
Alemtuzumab [Campath]	Binds CD52 antigen	Antibody	B-cell chronic lymphocytic leukemia	Bone marrow suppression, infusion reactions, infection
Ibritumomab tiuxetan/ yttrium-90 [Zevalin]	Binds CD20 antigen, causing radiation injury	Antibody/yttrium-90 hybrid	B-cell non-Hodgkin's lymphoma	Bone marrow suppression and infusion reactions
PD-DIRECTED ANTIBODIES				
Nivolumab [Opdivo]	Binds PD-1 receptor on T cells	Antibody	Melanoma, renal cell cancer, non–small cell lung cancer, Hodgkin's lymphoma, squamous cell head/ neck cancer, urothelial carcinoma	Cutaneous reactions, hepatitis, pancreatitis, immune-mediated reactions
Atezolizumab [Tecentriq]	Binds PD-L1 receptor on T cells	Antibody	Non–small cell lung cancer, urothelial carcinoma	Immune-mediated reactions, hepatitis, adrenal insufficiency, infection
Pembrolizumab [Keytruda]	Binds PD-1 receptor on T cells	Antibody	Melanoma, non–small cell lung cancer, squamous cell head/ neck cancer	Infusion reactions, pneumonitis, sepsis, hepatitis, pancreatitis
ANTIBODY-DRUG CONJUGATE				
Brentuximab vedotin [Adcetris]	Binds CD30 antigen to deliver a toxin that causes mitotic arrest	Antibody/drug hybrid	Hodgkin's lymphoma, anaplastic large cell lymphoma	Peripheral neuropathy, neutropenia
ANGIOGENESIS INHIBITORS				
Bevacizumab [Avastin]	Binds VEGF and thereby inhibits angiogenesis	Antibody	Colorectal cancer, non–small cell lung cancer, glioblastoma, renal cell carcinoma, cervical cancer, epithelial cancers	Hypertension, GI perforation, impaired wound healing, hemorrhage, thromboembolism, nephrotic syndrome
Necitumumab [Portrazza]	Binds EGFR	Antibody	Squamous non–small cell lung cancer	Cardiopulmonary arrest, heart attack, stroke, venous thromboembolism
PROTEASOME INHIBITORS				
Bortezomib [Velcade]	Inhibits proteasome activity	Small molecule	Multiple myeloma	Bone marrow suppression, GI disturbances, peripheral neuropathy, weakness
Carfilzomib [Kyprolis]	Inhibits proteasome activity	Small molecule	Multiple myeloma	Cardiac arrest, cardiotoxicity, infusion reactions

Continued

TABLE 103.4 ▪ Other Targeted Drugs—cont'd

Drug	Molecular Target	Drug Structure	Indications	Major Toxicities
HISTONE DEACETYLASE INHIBITORS				
Vorinostat [Zolinza]	Inhibits HDAC	Small molecule	Cutaneous T-cell lymphoma	Pulmonary embolism, bone marrow suppression, fatigue, nausea, diarrhea
Romidepsin [Istodax]	Inhibits HDAC	Small molecule	Cutaneous T-cell lymphoma	Bone marrow suppression, infection, QT prolongation
ADDITIONAL TARGETED ANTICANCER DRUGS				
Ipilimumab [Yervoy]	Binds CTLA-4 to unleash an immune attack	Antibody	Melanoma	Severe immune-mediated enterocolitis, hepatitis, dermatitis, neuropathies, endocrinopathies
Olaratumab [Lartruvo]	Binds PDGF, leading to inhibition of tumor cell growth	Antibody	Soft tissue sarcoma	Infusion reaction, neutropenia

CTLA-4, Cytotoxic T lymphocyte–associated antigen-4; *EGFR,* epidermal growth factor receptor, which is coupled with tyrosine kinase; *GI,* gastrointestinal; *HDAC,* histone deacetylase; *PD,* programmed death; *PDGF,* platelet-derived growth factor; *PML,* progressive multifocal leukoencephalopathy; *VEGF,* vascular endothelial growth factor.

show adverse fetal effects. Until more is known, prudence dictates avoiding cetuximab during pregnancy. Cetuximab is classified in FDA Pregnancy Risk Category C.[f]

Dosage and Administration. Cetuximab [Erbitux] is given by slow IV infusion. Treatment consists of a loading dose (400 mg/m^2 infused over 2 hours) followed by maintenance doses (250 mg/m^2 infused over 1 hour), given either weekly (for head and neck cancer) or every other week (for colorectal cancer).

Gefitinib

Therapeutic Use. Gefitinib[Iressa] is approved for oral therapy of advanced *non–small cell lung cancer* (NSCLC) that has been refractory to first-line treatment (platinum- or docetaxel-based therapy). In clinical trials, between 8.2% and 19% of patients achieved an objective response. Unfortunately, postmarketing studies failed to show any survival benefit. As a result, gefitinib is restricted to patients enrolled in a medical trial in the United States. NSCLC is the most common form of lung cancer, and cells of this cancer often overexpress EGFRs.

Mechanism of Action. Like cetuximab, gefitinib disrupts cellular processes regulated by EGFRs. However, unlike cetuximab, which acts on the cell surface to block EGFRs, gefitinib acts within the cell to inhibit tyrosine kinase that is linked with EGFR. Under normal conditions, activation of EGFR leads to activation of tyrosine kinase, which in turn activates signaling pathways that regulate cell proliferation and survival. By inhibiting EGFR-linked tyrosine kinase, gefitinib has the same effect as EGFR blockade: suppression of cell proliferation and promotion of apoptosis.

Responding Populations. A mutation in the EGFR tyrosine kinase gene predicts who will respond to gefitinib. This mutation is more likely in women, Asians, and patients with the adenocarcinoma subtype of NSCLC. People in these populations are more likely to respond.

Pharmacokinetics. Gefitinib is slowly absorbed from the GI tract. Plasma levels peak 3 to 7 hours after dosing. The drug undergoes extensive hepatic metabolism, primarily by CYP3A4, followed by excretion in the feces. The elimination half-life is 48 hours.

Adverse Effects. Gefitinib is generally well tolerated. As with cetuximab, the most frequent reactions are diarrhea and acne-like rash. Other fairly common reactions are dry skin, nausea, and vomiting. Ocular effects—amblyopia, conjunctivitis, eye pain, and corneal erosion or ulceration—occur infrequently. Asymptomatic elevation of liver transaminases has been reported.

Interstitial lung disease is the most serious adverse effect. This condition begins with acute-onset dyspnea, sometimes with cough or fever. Rapid deterioration may ensue. The overall incidence is about 1%, with one-third of cases being fatal. If respiratory symptoms develop, gefitinib should be interrupted and the patient evaluated. If ILD is diagnosed, gefitinib should not be used again. The risk of ILD is highest among patients with prior radiation or chemotherapy.

Drug and Herb Interactions. Drugs that inhibit CYP3A4 (e.g., itraconazole, ketoconazole) can decrease gefitinib metabolism and may thereby increase its plasma level. Conversely, agents that induce CYP3A4 (e.g., rifampin, phenytoin, carbamazepine, St. John's wort) can accelerate gefitinib metabolism and may thereby reduce its level. Likewise, drugs that lower gastric pH (e.g., histamine$_2$ antagonists, proton pump inhibitors, antacids) can decrease gefitinib absorption and may thereby lower its level.

Use in Pregnancy and Lactation. Gefitinib can harm the developing fetus, and hence should not be used by pregnant women. In laboratory animals, the drug decreased the number of live births, increased neonatal mortality, and reduced fetal weight. We don't know whether gefitinib is safe during breast-feeding.

Dosage and Administration. The usual dosage is 250 mg PO once a day, taken with or without food. Dosing should be interrupted if the patient develops severe rash, severe diarrhea, or ocular complications and should be discontinued if ILD is diagnosed. For patients taking a potent inducer of CYP3A4, dosage may be increased to 500 mg/day.

BCR-ABL Tyrosine Kinase Inhibitors

The BCR-ABL tyrosine kinase inhibitors are the preferred agents for treating *chronic myeloid leukemia* (CML). Five of these drugs are available: imatinib, dasatinib, bosutinib, ponatinib, and nilotinib. Imatinib is the gold standard for CML therapy. Unfortunately, relapse can occur, owing to evolution of subclones that have imatinib-resistant BCR-ABL mutations. The other drugs—dasatinib, bosutinib, ponatinib, and nilotinib—are active against all but one of these resistant subclones, and hence can be effective even in patients who no longer respond to imatinib.

Imatinib

Indications. Imatinib [Gleevec] was approved for oral therapy of CML, but only after treatment with interferon alfa had failed. Because of clear superiority, imatinib had displaced interferon alfa as the initial treatment of choice. Imatinib may be continued as long as there is no evidence of disease progression and as long as side effects remain tolerable.

[f]As of 2020, the FDA will no longer use Pregnancy Risk Categories. Please refer to Chapter 9 for more information.

Imatinib is also approved for *myelodysplastic/myeloproliferative diseases, aggressive systemic mastocytosis, acute lymphoblastic leukemia, dermatofibrosarcoma protuberans, hypereosinophilic syndrome, chronic eosinophilic leukemia,* and unresectable and/or metastatic malignant *gastrointestinal stromal tumor*, a rare form of stomach/intestinal cancer. These applications are not discussed further.

CML and Its Treatment. CML is a cancer in which myeloid cells undergo massive clonal expansion. The disease begins with a chronic phase, progresses through an accelerated phase, and ends with the blast crisis phase. The underlying cause is a genetic abnormality known as the *Philadelphia chromosome*, which is produced by translocation of genetic material between chromosomes 9 and 22. Because of this genetic change, CML cells make an abnormal, continuously active enzyme called *BCR-ABL tyrosine kinase*. This enzyme phosphorylates, and thereby activates, as-yet unidentified regulatory proteins, which in turn inhibit apoptosis and stimulate cell proliferation. Major treatment options are the BCR-ABL tyrosine kinase inhibitors, interferon-based regimens, and stem cell transplantation (the only potentially curative treatment).

Mechanism of Action and Clinical Effects. Imatinib is a highly specific competitive inhibitor of BCR-ABL tyrosine kinase. By inhibiting this enzyme, imatinib prevents the phosphorylation and resultant activation of regulatory proteins and thereby suppresses proliferation of CML cells and promotes apoptosis. Imatinib is selective for cells that express BCR-ABL tyrosine kinase; normal cells are not affected. When tested during the chronic phase of CML, imatinib was superior to the combination of interferon alfa plus cytarabine. After 18 months, disease progression was stopped in 92% of imatinib users, compared with 74% of those getting interferon. Furthermore, imatinib was better tolerated. Long-term follow-up is needed to determine how long responses to imatinib will last and whether imatinib prolongs survival.

Over time, resistance to imatinib may develop because the genes that code for BCR-ABL can mutate, causing production of imatinib-resistant forms of the enzyme.

Pharmacokinetics. Imatinib is well absorbed following oral administration. Bioavailability is 98%. In the blood, the drug is highly protein bound. Imatinib undergoes extensive metabolism, primarily by hepatic CYP3A4, followed by excretion in the feces. The elimination half-lives of imatinib and its major active metabolite are 18 hours and 40 hours, respectively.

Adverse Effects. Imatinib causes adverse effects in most patients. The incidence and severity of adverse effects are lowest during the chronic phase of CML, higher during the accelerated phase, and highest during blast crisis. However, even though adverse effects occurred often during trials, discontinuation because of them was uncommon: only 1% during the chronic phase, 2% during the accelerated phase, and 5% during blast crisis. Common reactions include nausea, vomiting, diarrhea, rash, headache, fatigue, fever, and musculoskeletal complaints, including muscle cramps, muscle pain, and arthralgia. Fluid retention occurs in 52% to 68% of patients and may lead to pleural effusion, pericardial effusion, pulmonary edema, or ascites. Neutropenia and thrombocytopenia develop often, posing a risk of infection and bleeding. Accordingly, complete blood counts should be obtained weekly during the first month of treatment, biweekly during the second month, and periodically thereafter. Hepatotoxicity, indicated by severe elevations of transaminases or bilirubin, develops in 1.1% to 3.5% of patients. Other reported effects include severe congestive heart failure, serious skin reactions (e.g., erythema multiforme, Stevens-Johnson syndrome), and hypothyroidism in thyroidectomy patients receiving thyroid hormone replacement therapy.

Effects in Pregnancy and Breast-Feeding. In animal studies, doses equivalent to those used clinically have caused major fetal malformations. Accordingly, imatinib is classified in FDA Pregnancy Risk Category D,[g] and hence should be avoided during pregnancy. Women of childbearing age should use adequate contraception.

Imatinib achieves high concentrations in breast milk and poses a risk to the breast-fed infant. The manufacturer recommends against breast-feeding while taking the drug.

Drug Interactions. Imatinib is a substrate for and competitive inhibitor of CYP3A4, CYP2C9, and CYP2D6. By inhibiting these CYP isoenzymes, imatinib can raise levels of warfarin and other drugs that are metabolized by them. Drugs that inhibit CYP3A4 (e.g., ketoconazole, erythromycin) can raise levels of imatinib. Conversely, drugs that induce CYP3A4 (e.g., carbamazepine, rifampin, St. John's wort) can reduce levels of imatinib.

Preparations, Dosage, and Administration. Imatinib [Gleevec] is supplied in 100- and 400-mg tablets, for administration with a meal and a large glass of water. The dosage for adults with CML is 400 mg once daily during the chronic phase and 600 mg once daily during the accelerated phase or blast crisis. The dosage for children with CML (during the chronic phase) is 340 mg/m^2 once daily.

Multi-Tyrosine Kinase Inhibitors

In contrast to the EGFR tyrosine kinase inhibitors and the BCR-ABL tyrosine kinase inhibitors, which inhibit just one type of tyrosine kinase, the drugs in this section inhibit several types of tyrosine kinase. However, despite their diverse actions, the multi–tyrosine kinase inhibitors have limited indications: Six of the available agents—sorafenib, sunitinib, axitinib, cabozantinib, lenvatinib, and pazopanib—are approved for advanced renal cell carcinoma. In addition, sorafenib is approved for hepatocellular carcinoma, and sunitinib is approved for GI stromal tumor and pancreatic neuroendocrine tumors. Three additional drugs—vandetanib, lenvatinib, and cabozantinib—are approved for medullary and well-differentiated thyroid cancer. A seventh drug—regorafenib—is approved for metastatic colon cancer and metastatic GI stromal tumor.

Sorafenib

Sorafenib [Nexavar] is an oral multi–tyrosine kinase inhibitor approved for *advanced renal cell carcinoma, recurrent thyroid carcinoma* refractory to iodine treatment, and unresectable *hepatocellular carcinoma.* The drug inhibits multiple cell-surface and intracellular kinases that are associated with angiogenesis, apoptosis, and cell proliferation.

The most common adverse effects are diarrhea, rash, fatigue, and hand-and-foot syndrome. Between 15% and 20% of patients develop hypertension. Nausea and vomiting are usually mild. Sorafenib prolongs the QT interval and thereby poses a risk of serious dysrhythmias. In addition, the drug doubles the risk of bleeding (by inhibiting vascular endothelial growth factor [VEGF] tyrosine kinase). Myocardial ischemia and GI perforation occur rarely. Sorafenib (in low doses) is teratogenic and embryolethal in animals, and hence should be avoided during pregnancy (FDA Pregnancy Risk Category D[h]).

Sorafenib is supplied in 200-mg tablets. The recommended dosage is 400 mg twice daily. To optimize absorption, dosing should be done *without* food (at least 1 hour before eating or 2 hours after).

[g]As of 2020, the FDA will no longer use Pregnancy Risk Categories. Please refer to Chapter 9 for more information.

[h]As of 2020, the FDA will no longer use Pregnancy Risk Categories. Please refer to Chapter 9 for more information.

mTOR Kinase Inhibitors

Temsirolimus

Temsirolimus [Torisel] is indicated for IV therapy of *advanced renal cell carcinoma*. Following conversion to its active form—sirolimus—the drug inhibits mTOR (mammalian target of rapamycin), a protein kinase that helps regulate cell growth, proliferation, and survival. Inhibition of mTOR leads to G_1 arrest and apoptosis. Adverse effects, which are common, include weakness, rash, mucositis, nausea, edema, anorexia, dyspnea, pain, and fever. Common laboratory abnormalities include anemia, neutropenia, hyperglycemia, and increases in cholesterol, triglycerides, and alkaline phosphatase. Sirolimus (the active metabolite of temsirolimus) is metabolized by CYP3A4, and hence levels of sirolimus can be altered by drugs that induce or inhibit CYP3A4. Temsirolimus is available in single-dose, 25-mg vials. The recommended dosage is 25 mg infused over 30 to 60 minutes once weekly, continuing until disease progression recurs or toxicity becomes intolerable.

BRAF V600E Kinase Inhibitors

Vemurafenib

Actions and Use. Vemurafenib [Zelboraf] is a kinase inhibitor indicated for patients with unresectable or metastatic *melanoma* that expresses *BRAF V600E kinase*, a variant form of BRAF kinase that is found in 30% to 60% of melanoma cells. In healthy cells, BRAF kinase (a cell-membrane protein) stimulates cell proliferation, but only when activated by specific growth factors. BRAF V600E differs from normal BRAF kinase in that BRAF V600E is highly active in the *absence* of stimulation by growth factors. As a result, cells with the BRAF V600E mutation undergo excessive proliferation and metastasis. Vemurafenib is a small molecule that inhibits BRAF V600E kinase activity and thereby suppresses tumor growth. Before vemurafenib is used, the BRAF V600E mutation must be confirmed using an FDA-approved assay, such as the *cobas 4800 BRAF V600 Mutation Test*.

Adverse Effects. Vemurafenib can cause serious adverse effects. *Cutaneous squamous cell carcinoma*, seen in 24% of patients, is of greatest concern. Other serious effects include hepatotoxicity, severe hypersensitivity reactions (e.g., anaphylaxis), severe skin reactions (e.g., Stevens-Johnson syndrome, toxic epidermal necrolysis), serious ophthalmic reactions (e.g., uveitis, iritis, retinal vein occlusion), and QT prolongation, which poses a risk of severe dysrhythmias. Less serious effects include arthralgia, hair loss, fatigue, rash, photosensitivity reactions, itching, nausea, and diarrhea. Because of its mechanism, vemurafenib is likely to cause fetal harm, and hence is classified in FDA Pregnancy Risk Category D.[i] Accordingly, women using the drug should avoid getting pregnant.

Drug Interactions. Vemurafenib is subject to multiple drug interactions, which could be hard to predict. Vemurafenib is a substrate for CYP3A4 and P-glycoprotein (a transporter that pumps drugs out of cells), and hence levels of vemurafenib can be altered by drugs that induce or inhibit these pathways. Also, vemurafenib itself is an inhibitor of P-glycoproteins as well as several CYP isoenzymes, and hence vemurafenib can increase levels of drugs that employ these pathways. Lastly, vemurafenib can induce CYP3A4, and hence can reduce levels of CYP3A4 substrates.

Preparations, Dosage, and Administration. Vemurafenib [Zelboraf] is supplied in 240-mg film-coated tablets for dosing with or without food. The recommended dosage is 960 mg twice daily. Tablets should be swallowed whole with a glass of water.

ALK Inhibitors

Crizotinib [Xalkori] is indicated for advanced *non–small cell lung cancer* that is *anaplastic lymphoma kinase (ALK) positive*. Benefits derive from inhibiting ALK, a tyrosine kinase found in normal and cancerous cells. However, the form of ALK found in normal cells differs from the form found in cancer cells. Because of this difference, ALK activity in normal cells is *low*, whereas ALK activity in certain cancer cells is high—so high, in fact, that it drives proliferation and prolongs survival. Hence, by inhibiting ALK, crizotinib can suppress tumor growth. Because crizotinib is approved only for NSCLC that is ALK positive, the cancer must be tested for ALK before treatment. Among patients with NSCLC, about 2% to 10% have the ALK-positive type. In clinical trials, crizotinib was highly effective: Virtually every patient with ALK-positive NSCLC experienced some benefit, although the degree of benefit varied.

Crizotinib is generally well tolerated. The most common adverse effects are nausea, diarrhea, vomiting, constipation, edema, fatigue, dizziness, and neuropathies. Elevation of liver enzymes is seen in 4% to 7% of patients. Crizotinib prolongs the QT interval, and hence poses a risk of serious dysrhythmias. The most serious adverse effect—potentially fatal pneumonitis—develops in 1.6% of patients. If pneumonitis is diagnosed, crizotinib should be stopped and never used again. In laboratory animals, crizotinib was fetotoxic at doses close to those used clinically. Accordingly, women using the drug should avoid pregnancy.

Crizotinib is a substrate for and inhibitor of CYP3A4. Accordingly, crizotinib levels can be increased by CYP3A4 inhibitors (e.g., ketoconazole, clarithromycin, ritonavir) and can be decreased by CYP3A4 inducers (e.g., carbamazepine, phenytoin, St. John's wort). By inhibiting CYP3A4, crizotinib can raise levels of CYP3A4 substrates, including cyclosporine, fentanyl, and alfentanil.

Crizotinib is supplied in 200- and 250-mg capsules. The usual dosage is 250 mg twice daily.

OTHER TARGETED DRUGS

CD-Directed Antibodies

Antibodies directed against CD20, CD38, and CD52 are used to treat B-cell non-Hodgkin's lymphoma, multiple myeloma, and B-cell chronic lymphocytic leukemia. CD20 is a molecule found on the cell membrane surface of B lymphocytes (B cells), important components of the immune system (see Chapter 67). Most other cells lack CD20. When antibodies bind with CD20, they trigger an immune attack against the B cell itself. Because most other cells do not have CD20, injury is limited to normal and malignant B lymphocytes. CD38 is present on the surface of CD4+, CD8+ and natural killer cells, as well as B lymphocytes. CD52 is a protein located on the surface of mature lymphocytes. Antibodies binding to these proteins on tumor cells induce cellular apoptosis.

At this time, four products containing anti-CD20 antibodies are available. One of these products—ibritumomab [Zevalin]—consists of a monoclonal antibody that has been linked with a radioactive isotope. With this drug, cell kill results largely from radiation damage, rather than from immune attack. The other three drugs—rituximab [Rituxan], obinutuzumab [Gazyva], and ofatumumab [Arzerra]—have no radioactivity, and so cell kill results from immune attack promoted by the antibody.

[i]As of 2020, the FDA will no longer use Pregnancy Risk Categories. Please refer to Chapter 9 for more information.

Rituximab

Actions, Use, and Dosage. Rituximab [Rituxan] is a monoclonal antibody indicated for IV therapy of *B-cell non-Hodgkin's lymphoma* and *B-cell chronic lymphocytic leukemia.* The antibody is directed against the CD20 antigen, found on the surface of most normal and malignant B cells. Binding of rituximab recruits components of the immune system, which then cause cell lysis. In a study of patients with non-Hodgkin's lymphoma, rituximab produced a complete response in 6% of patients, and another 42% experienced a partial response (50% or greater reduction in tumor burden). The recommended dosage is 375 mg/m^2 given by slow infusion once a week for 4 weeks.

In addition to its use in cancer, rituximab is used for rheumatoid arthritis (see Chapter 73) and for two inflammatory disorders of blood vessels: microscopic polyangiitis and Wegener's granulomatosis.

Adverse Effects

Infusion Reactions. Rituximab can cause severe infusion-related hypersensitivity reactions. Prominent symptoms are hypotension, bronchospasm, and angioedema. Deaths have occurred. Management includes slowing or discontinuing the infusion and injecting epinephrine.

Tumor Lysis Syndrome (TLS). Rapid and massive death of tumor cells can lead to TLS, characterized by acute renal failure, hyperkalemia, hypocalcemia, hyperuricemia, or hyperphosphatemia. Rarely, the syndrome proves fatal. TLS begins within 12 to 24 hours of the first rituximab infusion. The risk of TLS is increased by a high tumor burden. Management includes dialysis and correction of fluid and electrolyte abnormalities.

Mucocutaneous Reactions. Rituximab has been associated with severe mucocutaneous reactions, including Stevens-Johnson syndrome, lichenoid dermatitis, vesiculobullous dermatitis, and toxic epidermal necrolysis. Deaths have occurred. Reaction onset is typically 1 to 3 weeks after rituximab exposure. Patients who experience these reactions should seek immediate medical attention and should not receive rituximab again.

Hepatitis B Reactivation. There have been reports of hepatitis B virus (HBV) reactivation, leading to fulminant hepatitis, hepatic failure, and death. Patients at high risk of HBV should be screened before getting rituximab. Asymptomatic carriers should be closely monitored for clinical and laboratory signs of active HBV infection while taking rituximab and for several months after stopping.

Progressive Multifocal Leukoencephalopathy (PML). Rituximab has been associated with rare cases of PML, a severe infection of the central nervous system (CNS) caused by reactivation of the JC virus, an opportunistic pathogen resistant to all available drugs.

Other Adverse Effects. Like other monoclonal antibodies, rituximab can cause a flu-like syndrome, especially during the initial infusion. Symptoms include fever, chills, nausea, vomiting, and myalgia. Rituximab causes transient neutropenia, but this does not appear to increase the risk of infection.

Ofatumumab

Actions and Use. Ofatumumab [Arzerra] is a monoclonal antibody directed against the CD20 antigen on B lymphocytes. The drug was approved as second-line therapy for *B-cell chronic lymphocytic leukemia* in patients refractory to fludarabine [Fludara] and alemtuzumab [Campath]. Like rituximab, ofatumumab binds with CD20 antigens on B cells and thereby promotes immune-mediated cell lysis. In patients refractory to fludarabine and alemtuzumab, the overall response rate to ofatumumab is 42%, with a median response duration of 6.5 months.

Adverse Effects. Ofatumumab can cause severe adverse effects. Like rituximab, the drug can cause *infusion reactions, PML,* and *reactivation of HBV.* In addition, ofatumumab can cause severe neutropenia and thrombocytopenia, increasing the risk of infections and bleeding. Intestinal obstruction may also occur. Common, but less serious effects include fever, cough, dyspnea, diarrhea, fatigue, rash, and nausea.

Dosage and Administration. Treatment consists of an initial dose (300 mg IV), followed by 11 more doses (2000 mg IV each) over the following 24 weeks. To minimize infusion reactions, patients should be pretreated with acetaminophen (PO), an antihistamine (PO or IV), and a glucocorticoid (IV).

Zevalin (Ibritumomab Tiuxetan Linked With Yttrium-90)

Description, Actions, and Use. Ibritumomab tiuxetan (IT), marketed as *Zevalin,* is a compound molecule composed of ibritumomab (a monoclonal antibody) that has been covalently bound with tiuxetan. Like rituximab, IT binds selectively with the CD20 antigen present on most normal and malignant B cells. However, unlike rituximab, which is used by itself to treat cancer, IT is first linked with yttrium-90 (Y90), a beta particle–emitting radioisotope. When the IT-Y90 complex binds with cellular CD20 antigens, cell kill results from radiation-induced injury, rather than from injury caused by ibritumomab itself. Because beta particles have a relatively short path length (about 5 mm), injury is restricted to CD20-containing cells and to neighboring cells within a 5-mm radius. The radioactive drug poses no danger to persons in proximity. IT-Y90 was the first anticancer treatment to employ an antibody complexed with a radioactive compound. IT-Y90 was originally approved for *low-grade, B-cell non-Hodgkin's lymphoma* and then later approved for *follicular non-Hodgkin's lymphoma.*

Before patients receive IT-Y90, they are given two small doses of rituximab, 7 to 9 days apart. The contribution of rituximab is twofold. First, it binds with circulating B cells and thereby greatly reduces their numbers. Second, it occupies nonspecific binding sites that could otherwise attract IT-Y90, and hence would reduce the amount of IT-Y90 available to bind with target cells. For the purpose of diagnostic imaging, the first dose of rituximab is accompanied by a small dose of IT that has been linked to radioactive indium-111.

Adverse Effects. Adverse effects of treatment are due to IT-Y90 itself and to the rituximab given before it. As noted previously, rituximab can cause severe infusion reactions. With IT-Y90, hematologic toxicity is the major concern: severe, prolonged cytopenias develop in more than 50% of patients. Counts of neutrophils and platelets reach their nadir 7 to 9 weeks after treatment and take 3 to 7 weeks to recover. In clinical trials, about 30% of patients developed infection or febrile neutropenia; of these, 7% required hospitalization. Deaths have occurred. Because of its hematologic toxicity, IT-Y90 is contraindicated for patients with (1) lymphoma bone marrow involvement of 25% or more or (2) limited bone marrow reserve (e.g., platelet count below 100,000/mm^3 or neutrophil count below 1500/mm^3; history of prior myeloablative therapy).

Brentuximab Vedotin, an Antibody-Drug Conjugate

Brentuximab vedotin [Adcetris] is an antibody-drug conjugate (ADC), composed of brentuximab coupled with monomethyl auristatin E (MMAE). Brentuximab is a monoclonal antibody that selectively binds with CD30, an antigen expressed on the surface of certain cancer cells. MMAE is a toxic compound that binds with intracellular tubulin. Cell kill results as follows: After binding with CD30 on the cell surface, the entire ADC is rapidly internalized and then cleaved to release free MMAE, which then binds with tubulin to cause mitotic arrest.

Brentuximab vedotin has two indications: *Hodgkin's lymphoma* after failure of autologous stem cell transplantation or after failure of at least two multidrug chemotherapy regimens and (2) systemic *anaplastic large cell lymphoma* after failure of at least one multidrug chemotherapy regimen. In clinical trials, the drug was highly effective. Among patients with Hodgkin's lymphoma, the overall response rate was 73%, including 32% with complete remission. And among patients with anaplastic large cell lymphoma, the overall response rate was 86%, including 57% with complete remission. Of note, these response rates are higher than those produced with any available chemotherapy regimen.

Adverse effects are generally "manageable." The most common are peripheral sensory neuropathy, neutropenia, anemia, fatigue, nausea, diarrhea, and fever. Of these, neuropathy and neutropenia are the greatest concerns. In clinical trials, neuropathy led to a discontinuation of treatment in 10% of patients and a reduction of dosage in 9% more. For most patients, neuropathy resolves after stopping the drug. In laboratory animals, low-dose brentuximab vedotin was teratogenic and fetotoxic. Accordingly, the drug should be avoided in women who are pregnant (FDA Pregnancy Risk Category D[j]).

Brentuximab vedotin is supplied as a 50-mg powder to be reconstituted with 10.5 mL of sterile water, to yield a single-use solution containing 5 mg/mL. The recommended dosage is 1.8 mg/kg infused IV over 30 minutes every 3 weeks, for a maximum of 16 doses. In the event of a severe infusion reaction (which is rare), stop the infusion and never give the drug again. If neuropathy or neutropenia develops, dosage should be reduced or the dosing interval increased.

Angiogenesis Inhibitors

Angiogenesis inhibitors suppress formation of new blood vessels, and thereby deprive solid tumors of the expanding blood supply they need for continued growth. It is important to note, however, that although tumor growth is suppressed, angiogenesis inhibitors, by themselves, cannot kill tumor cells that already exist. At this time, only one angiogenesis inhibitor—bevacizumab—is approved for treating cancer.

Bevacizumab

Bevacizumab [Avastin] became the first angiogenesis inhibitor approved for clinical use. In patients with metastatic colorectal cancer or nonsquamous NSCLC, the drug can delay tumor progression and prolong life. Unfortunately, bevacizumab can also cause life-threatening side effects, including GI perforation, hemorrhage, and thromboembolism.

Mechanism of Action. Bevacizumab is a monoclonal antibody that binds with VEGF, an endogenous compound that stimulates blood vessel growth. Binding with bevacizumab prevents VEGF from binding with its receptors on vascular endothelial cells, preventing VEGF from promoting new vessel formation. As a result, further tumor growth is suppressed.

Therapeutic Use. Bevacizumab has six approved uses:

- Metastatic *cancer of the colon or rectum*, in combination with a regimen based on IV 5-fluorouracil (5-FU)
- *Nonsquamous non–small cell lung cancer,* in combination with carboplatin and paclitaxel
- Metastatic *renal cell carcinoma*, in combination with interferon alfa
- *Glioblastoma,* as a single agent following prior therapy
- Metastatic *carcinoma of the cervix*, in combination with paclitaxel and cisplatin
- Recurrent *epithelial ovarian, fallopian tube, or peritoneal cancer*, in combination with paclitaxel

In addition to its use in cancer, bevacizumab is used off-label to treat the neovascular form of *age-related macular degeneration* (see Chapter 104).

Pharmacokinetics. The pharmacokinetics of bevacizumab is poorly understood. We do know that the drug has an average half-life of 20 days and that clearance occurs faster in males and in patients with a high tumor burden. However, there is no evidence that faster clearance reduces the clinical response. How clearance occurs is unknown.

Adverse Effects. The most serious adverse effects are GI perforation, hemorrhage, thromboembolism, nephrotic syndrome, disruption of wound healing, and hypertensive crisis. Less serious effects include diarrhea, rhinitis, proteinuria, taste alteration, dry skin, headache, and back pain.

During clinical trials, 2% of patients developed *GI perforation*, with or without abscess formation. Some cases were fatal. Primary symptoms are abdominal pain in association with constipation and vomiting. If GI perforation occurs, bevacizumab should be stopped and never used again.

Bevacizumab greatly increases the risk of *severe or fatal hemorrhage*. Patients have experienced GI bleeding, intracranial bleeding, vaginal bleeding, and nosebleeds. In addition, patients with NSCLC have experienced life-threatening *pulmonary hemorrhage*. The risk of a life-threatening or fatal lung bleed is very high (31%) in patients with squamous cell histology, and much lower (4%) in those with non–squamous cell histology. Onset of pulmonary bleeding is sudden and presents as major or massive hemoptysis (expectoration of blood). Bevacizumab should be avoided in patients with recent hemoptysis or serious hemorrhage.

When added to a regimen based on 5-FU, bevacizumab doubles the risk of *arterial thromboembolic events*, including ischemic stroke, myocardial infarction, and transient ischemic attacks. Deaths have occurred. Patients who experience a thromboembolic event should stop bevacizumab and never use it again.

Bevacizumab *impairs wound healing* and can induce wound dehiscence (splitting open). Because of these effects, if bevacizumab is initiated too soon after surgery, or if it is not discontinued soon enough before surgery, impaired wound healing can result. To minimize healing complications, guidelines suggest waiting at least 28 days after surgery before using the drug and stopping the drug at least 28 days before elective surgery.

Bevacizumab can cause *severe hypertension* that may persist for months after the drug is withdrawn. Some patients have experienced hypertensive encephalopathy and subarachnoid hemorrhage. Blood pressure should be monitored in all patients. If severe hypertension develops, bevacizumab should be permanently discontinued.

In clinical trials, *nephrotic syndrome* (severe kidney damage) developed in 0.5% of patients. One patient required dialysis, and one died. Patients should be monitored for development or worsening of proteinuria, a sign of kidney injury. If moderate to severe proteinuria occurs, bevacizumab should be withdrawn.

Effect in Pregnancy. Angiogenesis is critical to fetal development, and hence angiogenesis inhibition is likely to cause fetal harm. Although human data are lacking, animal studies indicate that bevacizumab decreases fetal weight,

[j]As of 2020, the FDA will no longer use Pregnancy Risk Categories. Please refer to Chapter 9 for more information.

increases fetal resorption, and can promote gross malformations. Currently, bevacizumab is classified in FDA Pregnancy Risk Category C,[k] and should be used only if the benefits to the mother are judged to outweigh the risks to the fetus.

Dosage and Administration. Bevacizumab is supplied in solution (100 mg/4 mL, 400 mg/16 mL) for IV infusion. Infusion time is 90 minutes for the first dose, then 60 minutes for the second dose (if the first dose was well tolerated), and 30 minutes thereafter (if the second dose was well tolerated). Dosages are as follows:

- *Colorectal cancer*—5 mg/kg or 10 mg/kg every 2 weeks in combination with IV 5-FU–based therapy
- *Nonsquamous non–small cell lung cancer*—15 mg/kg every 3 weeks in combination with carboplatin and paclitaxel
- *Glioblastoma*—10 mg/kg every 2 weeks
- *Renal cell carcinoma*—10 mg/kg every 2 weeks in combination with interferon alfa
- *Carcinoma of the cervix*—15 mg/kg every 3 weeks in combination with paclitaxel and cisplatin
- *Epithelial ovarian, fallopian tube, or peritoneal cancer*—15 mg/kg every 3 weeks in combination with paclitaxel or topotecan

Treatment should be interrupted 28 days before elective surgery and not resumed for at least 28 days after major surgery. Treatment should be permanently discontinued in the event of GI perforation, serious bleeding, thromboembolism, nephrotic syndrome, or hypertensive crisis.

Proteasome Inhibitors

Proteasomes are intracellular multienzyme complexes that degrade proteins. Their physiologic role is to rid cells of proteins that are not needed, including proteins that regulate transcription, cell adhesion, apoptosis, and progression through the cell cycle. Proteasome inhibitors can cause these proteins to accumulate and can thereby disrupt various aspects of cell physiology. In cancer cells, these drugs appear to promote accumulation of proteins that promote apoptosis (programmed cell death). Why this effect is limited largely to cancer cells is not clear, but may be related to inhibition of NF-kappa B, a transcription factor critical to the growth of several types of cancer, including multiple myeloma.

Bortezomib

Actions. Bortezomib [Velcade] is the first proteasome inhibitor available for general use. The drug inhibits a specific proteasome, known as the 26S proteasome, and thereby alters the concentration of proteins that regulate cell growth and division. The result is reduced cell viability, increased apoptosis, and increased sensitivity to the lethal effects of radiation and cytotoxic anticancer drugs. Does bortezomib hurt normal cells too? Yes. However, *in vitro* studies suggest that normal cells are less vulnerable than cancer cells.

Therapeutic Use. Bortezomib is approved for (1) *multiple myeloma*, both as first-line therapy and for patients who have not responded adequately to other therapies (e.g., thalidomide, autologous stem cell transplantation), and (2) *mantle cell lymphoma* in patients with at least 1 prior year of therapy. Bortezomib is now being studied in a variety of solid tumors, including non-Hodgkin's lymphoma, colorectal cancer, and lung cancer.

Adverse Effects. Adverse effects are common and often serious. The most frequent reactions are weakness, nausea, and diarrhea. Also common are hematologic effects—thrombocytopenia, anemia, and neutropenia—as well as constipation, anorexia, peripheral neuropathy, fever, and postural hypotension. Bortezomib is fetotoxic in rabbits and has been classified in FDA Pregnancy Risk Category D.[l] Accordingly, pregnancy should be avoided.

Drug Interactions. St. John's wort may decrease levels of bortezomib, thus this combination should be avoided. Both hypoglycemia and hyperglycemia were reported in patients taking oral antidiabetic agents in conjunction with bortezomib. Blood glucose levels should be monitored closely. Bortezomib is metabolized in the liver by CYP isoenzymes. Accordingly, inhibitors or inducers of these isoenzymes might be expected to alter bortezomib levels.

Dosage and Administration

Multiple Myeloma. Bortezomib is administered by IV bolus or subQ injection in nine 6-week cycles. One cycle consists of a single dose (1.3 mg/m^2) on days 1, 4, 8, 11, 22, 25, 29, and 32, followed by a 10-day rest period. In the event of painful peripheral neuropathy or any other severe toxicity, interruption of treatment and/or dosage reduction may be needed.

Mantle Cell Lymphoma. Bortezomib is administered by IV bolus in repeated 3-week cycles. One cycle consists of a single dose (1.3 mg/m^3) on days 1, 4, 8, and 11, followed by a 10-day rest period.

Histone Deacetylase Inhibitors

The histone deacetylase (HDAC) inhibitors are a relatively new class of targeted anticancer drugs. Vorinostat and romidepsin were the first approved drugs in this class. Both drugs are indicated only for *cutaneous T-cell lymphoma* (CTCL), a rare form of cancer with only 1500 new cases a year in the United States. As their name implies, these drugs inhibit HDAC and thereby *increase* the acetylation of histones, regulatory proteins in the cell nucleus that help control DNA transcription. When histones are in their acetylated state, they turn on gene transcription. In tumor cells, increased transcription leads to cell-cycle arrest and apoptosis.

Vorinostat

Vorinostat [Zolinza], the first HDAC inhibitor available, is indicated for *oral* therapy of CTCL that has progressed or returned after treatment with two systemic therapies. Unfortunately, benefits of vorinostat are modest. In clinical trials, the most common adverse effects were fatigue, diarrhea, nausea, altered taste, anorexia, weight loss, thrombocytopenia, and anemia. Pulmonary embolism is the most common serious effect. When used with warfarin, prolonged levels of prothrombin time and INR (international normalized ratio) have been noted. These levels should be monitored closely. Severe thrombocytopenia has also occurred when vorinostat is combined with valproic acid. Platelet levels should be checked every 2 weeks for the first 2 months. Vorinostat is supplied in 100-mg capsules. The usual dosage is 400 mg once daily.

Ipilimumab

Ipilimumab [Yervoy] is indicated for unresectable or metastatic *melanoma*. Benefits derive from unleashing an immune attack on cancer cells. Here's how it works. Ipilimumab is a monoclonal antibody directed against cytotoxic T-lymphocyte–associated antigen 4 (CTLA-4), a regulatory molecule that puts a brake on T-cell function. When ipilimumab binds with CTLA-4, it releases the brake, thereby allowing T cells to attack and kill cancer cells.

By promoting T-cell activation and proliferation, ipilimumab can cause severe/fatal immune-mediated effects. Among these are enterocolitis, hepatitis, dermatitis (including toxic epidermal necrolysis), neuropathies (both motor and sensory), and endocrinopathies (e.g., hypopituitarism, hypothyroidism, adrenal insufficiency). Patients should be closely monitored for signs and symptoms. If a severe immune-mediated reaction is diagnosed, ipilimumab should be immediately and permanently discontinued, and patients should be treated with high-dose systemic glucocorticoids.

Ipilimumab is supplied as a concentrated solution (50 mg/10 mL, 200 mg/40 mL) that must be diluted to 1 to 2 mg/mL before use. A single dose is 3 mg/kg infused IV over 90 minutes. A full course of treatment consists of four doses given 3 weeks apart.

IMMUNOSTIMULANTS

As their name implies, the immunostimulants enhance the body's immune attack on cancer cells. In the discussion that follows, we focus on three agents: interferon alfa-2b, aldesleukin, and BCG vaccine. Indications and routes are shown in Table 103.5.

INTERFERON ALFA-2B

Interferons are naturally occurring proteins with complex antiviral, anticancer, and immunomodulatory actions. Release of endogenous interferons is triggered by viral infections and other stimuli. Interferons are active against a variety of solid tumors and hematologic malignancies. They are also used for multiple sclerosis (see Chapter 23) and hepatitis (see Chapter 93).

Discussion here is limited to two interferons: *interferon alfa-2b* [Intron A] and *peginterferon alfa-2b* [Sylatron]. (Peginterferon alfa-2b is simply a long-acting form of interferon alfa-2b produced by a process known as pegylation, in which a polymer of polyethylene glycol [PEG] is attached to native interferon alfa-2b.) Although the active component of interferon alfa-2b and peginterferon alfa-2b is the same, these preparations have different

[k]As of 2020, the FDA will no longer use Pregnancy Risk Categories. Please refer to Chapter 9 for more information.

[l]As of 2020, the FDA will no longer use Pregnancy Risk Categories. Please refer to Chapter 9 for more information.

TABLE 103.5 ■ Immunostimulants

Generic Name	Brand Name	Route	Indications
Interferon alfa-2b	Intron A	SubQ IM, IV	Melanoma, hairy cell leukemia, chronic myelogenous leukemia, follicular lymphoma, AIDS-related Kaposi's sarcoma
Peginterferon alfa-2b	Sylatron	SubQ	Melanoma
Aldesleukin (interleukin-2)	Proleukin	IV	Metastatic renal cell cancer, metastatic melanoma
BCG vaccine	TICE BCG	Intravesical	*In situ* bladder cancer

BCG, Bacillus of Calmette and Guérin.

indications. Specifically, interferon alfa-2b is approved for *melanoma, hairy cell leukemia, chronic myelogenous leukemia, follicular lymphoma,* and *AIDS-related Kaposi's sarcoma,* whereas peginterferon alfa-2b is approved only for *melanoma.*

Anticancer effects of interferon alfa-2b are thought to result from two basic processes: (1) enhancement of host immune responses and (2) direct antiproliferative effects on cancer cells. Both processes are mediated by binding of interferon alfa-2b to cell-surface receptors, with resultant increased expression of certain genes and reduced expression of others. Interferon alfa-2b can cause G_0 cells to remain dormant, preventing proliferation. In addition, it can cause proliferating cells to differentiate into nonproliferative mature forms.

Interferon alfa can cause multiple adverse effects. The most common is a flu-like syndrome characterized by fever, fatigue, myalgia, headache, and chills. Symptoms tend to diminish with continued therapy. Some symptoms (fever, headache, myalgia) can be reduced with acetaminophen. Other common effects include anorexia, weight loss, diarrhea, abdominal pain, dizziness, and cough. Prolonged or high-dose therapy can cause fatigue, cardiotoxicity, thyroid dysfunction, and bone marrow suppression, manifesting as neutropenia and thrombocytopenia. Neuropsychiatric effects—especially depression—are a serious concern, owing to a risk of death by suicide.

The pharmacology of interferon alfa-2b and peginterferon alfa-2b is discussed in Chapter 93.

ALDESLEUKIN (INTERLEUKIN-2)

Aldesleukin [Proleukin], also known as interleukin-2 (IL-2), is an immunostimulant indicated for advanced renal carcinoma and melanoma. Because severe adverse effects occur often, the drug must be administered in a hospital that has an intensive care facility; a specialist in cardiopulmonary or intensive care medicine must be available.

Description and Actions

Aldesleukin is a large glycoprotein nearly identical in structure and actions to human IL-2. The drug is produced by recombinant DNA technology. Like IL-2, aldesleukin stimulates immune function. Specific responses include enhanced production and cytotoxicity of lymphocytes; increased production of interleukin-1, interferon gamma, and tumor necrosis factor; and induction of lymphokine-activated killer cell activity. These powerful immunostimulant actions are believed to underlie antitumor effects.

Therapeutic Use

Aldesleukin has two approved uses: *metastatic renal cell carcinoma* and *metastatic melanoma.* Among patients with renal cell cancer, 4% respond completely and 11% respond partially. The median response duration is 2 years.

Pharmacokinetics

Aldesleukin is administered by IV infusion and distributes throughout the extracellular space. About 70% of each dose undergoes preferential uptake by the liver, kidneys, and lungs. Renal enzymes convert the drug into inactive metabolites, which are excreted in the urine. The drug's half-life is short—just 85 minutes.

Adverse Effects

Practically all patients experience significant *toxicity.* The fatality rate is high (4%). Effects seen most frequently are fever and chills, nausea and vomiting, hypotension, anemia, diarrhea, altered mental status, sinus tachycardia, impaired renal function, impaired liver function, pulmonary congestion, dyspnea, and pruritus. Depression may also occur.

Capillary leak syndrome (CLS) is of particular concern. This potentially fatal reaction is characterized by hypotension and reduced organ perfusion (secondary to loss of vascular tone and extravasation of plasma proteins and fluid). Symptoms begin to develop immediately after treatment. CLS may be associated with angina pectoris, cardiac dysrhythmias, myocardial infarction, pronounced respiratory insufficiency, renal insufficiency, GI bleeding, and altered mental status. Because of the risk of CLS, aldesleukin must not be given to patients with cardiac, pulmonary, renal, hepatic, or CNS impairment. Careful monitoring is essential.

BCG VACCINE

Description and Therapeutic Use

BCG vaccine [TICE BCG] is a freeze-dried preparation of live, attenuated *Mycobacterium bovis* (bacillus of Calmette and Guérin [BCG]). The vaccine is approved for primary and relapsed *carcinoma in situ of the bladder,* both in the presence and absence of associated papillary tumors. To treat bladder cancers, BCG vaccine is administered intravesically (i.e., directly into the bladder through a urethral catheter). In addition to its use in cancer therapy, BCG vaccine is used to protect against tuberculosis (see Chapter 90).

Mechanism of Action

BCG vaccine is a nonspecific immunostimulant. Instillation in the bladder produces a local inflammatory response that, by an unknown mechanism, promotes regression of tumors in the urothelial lining.

Adverse Effects

The most common adverse effects, which result from bladder irritation, are dysuria, urinary frequency, urinary urgency, and hematuria. Urinary status should be monitored closely. The most common systemic reactions are malaise, fatigue, fever, and chills.

Because BCG vaccine consists of live *M. bovis,* therapy carries a risk of systemic infection, including *fatal septic shock.* Accordingly, the vaccine is contraindicated for (1) immunocompromised patients (e.g., those taking immunosuppressant drugs, those with symptomatic or asymptomatic HIV infection); (2) patients with fever of unknown origin (because it may signify infection); and (3) patients with urinary tract infections (because there is an increased risk of systemic absorption of BCG vaccine).

Because BCG vaccine is infectious, it must be handled using aseptic technique. All materials employed during administration should be disposed of in plastic bags labeled "Infectious Waste." Urine voided within 6 hours of BCG instillation should be disinfected with an equal volume of 5% hypochlorite before flushing.

OTHER NONCYTOTOXIC ANTICANCER DRUGS

GLUCOCORTICOIDS

The basic pharmacology of the glucocorticoids is discussed in Chapter 72. Discussion here is limited to their use in cancer. To benefit patients with cancer, dosages must be high, and hence, with long-term use, adverse effects are a concern.

Glucocorticoids (e.g., prednisone, dexamethasone) are used in combination with other agents to treat cancers arising from lymphoid tissue. Specific indications are *acute and chronic lymphocytic leukemias, Hodgkin's disease, non-Hodgkin's lymphomas,* and *multiple myeloma.* Glucocorticoids are beneficial in these cancers because they are directly toxic to lymphoid tissues: High-dose therapy causes suppression of mitosis, dissolution of lymphocytes, regression of lymphatic tissue, and cell death. When glucocorticoids are used acutely, toxicity is limited and manageable. However, with prolonged treatment, multiple serious toxicities can occur, including osteoporosis, adrenal insufficiency, increased susceptibility to infection, GI ulcers, fluid and electrolyte disturbances, myopathy, growth delay in children, cutaneous atrophy, and diabetes. Unlike the short-term toxicities, these long-term toxicities are hard to manage.

In addition to their use against lymphoid-derived cancers, glucocorticoids are used to manage complications of cancer and cancer therapy. Specific benefits include suppression of chemotherapy-induced nausea and vomiting, reduction of cerebral edema (caused by brain metastasis and irradiation to the brain), reduction of pain (caused by nerve compression or edema), and suppression of hypercalcemia in patients with steroid-responsive tumors. In addition, glucocorticoids can improve appetite and promote weight gain.

RETINOIDS

Retinoids are derivatives of retinol (vitamin A) that bind to and activate retinoid receptors. In their active state, retinoid receptors regulate the proliferation and differentiation of cells, both normal and neoplastic. In patients with cancer, retinoids inhibit cancer cell growth.

Alitretinoin

Alitretinoin [Panretin], an analog of retinol, is indicated for topical therapy of *cutaneous lesions* in patients with *AIDS-related Kaposi's sarcoma.* When alitretinoin is added to Kaposi's sarcoma cells in culture, it inhibits their growth.

Alitretinoin is supplied as a 0.1% gel for topical use. The drug should be applied only to cutaneous Kaposi's sarcoma lesions, not to normal skin. Following application, the area should be allowed to dry for 3 to 5 minutes before putting clothing over it. Occlusive dressings should be avoided. Treatment is initiated with twice-daily application. Later on, the drug may be applied 3 or 4 times a day, if tolerance permits. Most patients respond in 4 to 8 weeks. However, some respond in only 2 weeks, but others may not respond until 16 weeks.

Adverse effects are limited to the site of application. Local reactions—erythema, scaling, irritation, rash, and dermatitis—occur in 25% to 77% of patients. The incidence of severe reactions is 10%. Other retinoids are known to cause photosensitivity reactions. Although photosensitivity has not been reported with alitretinoin, exposing the treated area to sunlight or sunlamps should nonetheless be minimized. Retinoids are highly teratogenic. Accordingly, women using alitretinoin should avoid getting pregnant (even though systemic absorption of alitretinoin appears to be minimal).

Bexarotene

Mechanism and Use

Bexarotene [Targretin] is indicated for oral therapy of *cutaneous T-cell lymphoma* in patients who have been refractory to prior systemic therapy. Like alitretinoin, bexarotene is an analog of vitamin A (retinol) and can activate retinoid receptors. The result is altered regulation of cellular proliferation and differentiation. *In vitro,* bexarotene can inhibit growth of some tumor cell lines. In clinical trials, a dosage of 300 mg/m^2/day produced a complete response in 4% of patients and a partial response (more than 50% improvement) in 48% of patients.

Pharmacokinetics

Plasma levels peak 2 hours after oral administration. Taking the drug with a high-fat meal increases absorption. Bexarotene undergoes metabolism by CYP3A4 followed by excretion in the bile.

Adverse Effects and Interactions

Bexarotene causes lipid abnormalities and other serious side effects. In clinical trials, toxicity caused 30% of patients to discontinue treatment.

Major lipid abnormalities are common. Plasma triglycerides rise to a level 2.5 times above the upper limit of the normal range in 70% of patients. Sixty percent of patients have significant elevations in total cholesterol and low-density lipoprotein cholesterol. Levels of high-density lipoprotein cholesterol (good cholesterol) are reduced.

Bexarotene frequently causes headache, asthenia, leukopenia, anemia, infection, rash, and photosensitivity. The incidence of clinically significant hypothyroidism is 30%. Fatal pancreatitis and fatal cholestasis have been reported.

Bexarotene and other retinoids are powerful teratogens. Accordingly, bexarotene is absolutely contraindicated for use during pregnancy. Women taking the drug must ensure that pregnancy does not occur.

In theory, drugs that inhibit CYP3A4 can increase bexarotene levels, and drugs that induce CYP3A4 can reduce its levels. Combining vitamin A with bexarotene could result in increased toxicity.

Tretinoin

Tretinoin, also known as all-*trans* retinoic acid (ATRA), is approved for induction of remission in patients with *acute promyelocytic leukemia* (APL). Rates of complete remission are high. Unfortunately, although tretinoin can be very effective, it can also cause severe toxicity, and hence the benefits of treatment must be carefully weighed against the risks. The mechanism underlying beneficial effects is not well established.

The most common adverse effects are rash, dry skin, and CNS toxicity, manifesting as headache, depression, confusion, and anxiety. The most serious effect, seen in 25% of patients, is *retinoic acid–APL syndrome,* characterized by fever, pleural and pericardial effusions, and hypoxia. In its most severe form, the syndrome can lead to respiratory failure and death. Milder reactions generally respond to high-dose IV glucocorticoids, without interruption of tretinoin. In severe cases, tretinoin should be withdrawn.

Tretinoin is a substrate for hepatic CYP enzymes, and hence CYP inducers (e.g., rifampin, phenytoin, St. John's wort) and inhibitors (e.g., erythromycin, azole antifungals, diltiazem) should be avoided.

The recommended dosage is 45 mg/m^2/day administered PO as two evenly divided doses. Dosing with food improves absorption.

The use of tretinoin for dermatologic disorders is discussed in Chapter 105.

PROGESTINS

Two progestins can be employed to treat cancer: *medroxyprogesterone acetate* [Provera] and *megestrol acetate* [Megace]. Medroxyprogesterone is indicated for *advanced endometrial and renal cancer.* Megestrol is indicated for *advanced endometrial and breast cancer.* In women with metastatic endometrial cancer, progestins promote palliation and tumor regression. About 30% of patients have an objective response. Among those who respond, survival time is increased to about 2 years. This compares with survival times of 6 months among nonresponders. Benefits appear to derive from depriving these cancers of estrogen by inducing enzymes that metabolize estradiol, the primary endogenous estrogen. The principal adverse effects of progestins are fluid retention and nonfluid weight gain. Hypercalcemia may occur if bone metastases are present. Progestins may be teratogens, and hence should be avoided during pregnancy. The basic pharmacology of the progestins is discussed in Chapter 61.

KEY POINTS

- Nearly all of the anticancer drugs discussed in this chapter—hormonal agents, targeted drugs, and immunostimulants—are cell-cycle phase nonspecific, in contrast to many cytotoxic anticancer drugs, which are phase specific.
- Nearly all of the drugs discussed in this chapter lack the characteristic toxicities of the cytotoxic anticancer drugs, including bone marrow suppression, stomatitis, alopecia, and severe nausea and vomiting. Nonetheless, most can cause severe toxicities of their own.
- Breast cancer is treated with surgery, radiation, cytotoxic drugs, and hormonal agents, of which there are two major groups: antiestrogens and aromatase inhibitors.
- Antiestrogens block estrogen receptors (ERs), whereas aromatase inhibitors block estrogen synthesis. For either group to work, the cancer must be ER positive.
- Tamoxifen is an antiestrogen approved for the prevention and treatment of breast cancer. Benefits derive from blocking ERs on tumor cells. The drug is not active against cancers that are ER negative.
- Tamoxifen is a prodrug that undergoes activation by hepatic CYP2D6.
- Women using tamoxifen should not take fluoxetine, paroxetine, or sertraline to suppress hot flashes. These SSRIs are strong inhibitors of CYP2D6 that can prevent tamoxifen activation, thereby increasing the risk of breast cancer recurrence. Safe alternatives include escitalopram and venlafaxine, which are not strong CYP2D6 inhibitors.
- By activating certain ERs, tamoxifen increases the risk of endometrial cancer and thromboembolism.
- Anastrozole, an aromatase inhibitor, is used to treat ER-positive breast cancer in postmenopausal women only. Benefits derive from preventing biosynthesis of estrogen from adrenal androgens.
- Anastrozole is more effective than tamoxifen and poses no risk of endometrial cancer.
- Adverse effects of anastrozole include musculoskeletal pain, osteoporosis, fractures, and (rarely) thromboembolism.
- Trastuzumab and ado-trastuzumab, monoclonal antibodies used for breast cancer, bind HER2 receptors, causing inhibition of cell proliferation and immune-mediated cell death.
- When breast cancer metastasizes to bone (the most common metastasis site), it can cause hypercalcemia and fractures. Risk of fractures and hypocalcemia can be reduced with denosumab or zoledronate (a bisphosphonate).
- Advanced prostate cancer is treated with androgen deprivation therapy (ADT), which can be achieved with castration and/or drugs. Early (localized) prostate cancer is treated with surgery or radiation, sometimes followed by ADT.
- Androgen deprivation can be achieved with four types of drugs: gonadotropin-releasing hormone (GnRH) agonists, GnRH antagonists, androgen receptor blockers, and CYP17 inhibitors.
- Side effects of ADT include erectile dysfunction, loss of libido, gynecomastia, reduced muscle mass, new-onset diabetes, myocardial infarction, and stroke.
- Leuprolide, a GnRH agonist, has a biphasic mechanism of action. During the initial phase, the drug stimulates release of interstitial cell–stimulating hormone (ICSH) from the pituitary and thereby increases production of testosterone by the testes. As a result, there may be a transient "flare" in prostate cancer symptoms. With continuous use, the drug suppresses ICSH release and thereby causes testosterone production to fall. Note: Leuprolide does *not* decrease androgen production by the adrenal glands or by the prostate cancer itself.
- Flutamide is an androgen receptor blocker used in combination with a GnRH agonist to treat prostate cancer. Benefits derive from (1) preventing cancer cells from undergoing increased stimulation during the initial phase of GnRH therapy and (2) blocking the effects of adrenal and prostatic androgens on prostate cells.
- Abiraterone is a first-in-class CYP17 inhibitor used to suppress androgen production in patients with metastatic castration-resistant prostate cancer previously treated with docetaxel.
- Sipuleucel-T is the name for patient-specific immunotherapy designed to stimulate an immune attack against prostate cancer cells. Each dose is custom made from the patient's own immune cells, collected by leukapheresis.
- Targeted anticancer drugs are designed to bind with specific molecules (targets) that drive tumor growth. If the target molecules are found only (or mainly) on cancer cells, targeted drugs should be able to arrest tumor growth while causing little or no injury to normal cells. The current reality, however, is that most targeted drugs cause serious adverse effects.
- Many targeted drugs are monoclonal antibodies directed at antigens found primarily on cancer cells. Most other targeted drugs are small molecules that inhibit specific kinases that regulate cell proliferation.
- EGFR (epidermal growth factor receptor) linked with tyrosine kinase, a regulatory molecule found in certain normal cells and many cancer cells, plays an important role in regulating cell proliferation.
- Cetuximab is a monoclonal antibody that blocks the receptor portion of EGFR tyrosine kinase and thereby suppresses cell growth and promotes apoptosis.
- Cetuximab can cause severe infusion reactions and severe acne-like rash.
- Cells of chronic myeloid leukemia (CML) produce an abnormal, continuously active enzyme—BCR-ABL tyrosine kinase—that activates regulatory proteins, which in turn inhibit apoptosis and stimulate excessive cell proliferation.
- Imatinib is a highly specific competitive inhibitor of BCR-ABL tyrosine kinase. In patients with CML, the drug suppresses cell proliferation and promotes apoptosis.
- Imatinib can be considered the model of a successful targeted anticancer drug, being both highly effective and well tolerated.
- Vemurafenib is a BRAF V600E kinase inhibitor indicated for patients with unresectable or metastatic melanoma with the BRAF V600E mutation.

- The CD20 antigen is a molecule present in the cell membrane of normal and malignant B lymphocytes (B cells).
- Rituximab is a monoclonal antibody that binds with CD20 and thereby initiates apoptosis and causes a lethal immune attack on B cells. The drug is indicated for B-cell non-Hodgkin's lymphoma and B-cell chronic lymphocytic leukemia.
- Rituximab can cause severe infusion-related hypersensitivity reactions.
- Brentuximab vedotin is an antibody-drug conjugate (ADC), composed of brentuximab (a CD30-directed antibody) coupled with MMAE (a toxin that binds tubulin to cause mitotic arrest). The antibody serves only to deliver MMAE to cells that express CD30. MMAE does the actual damage.
- Angiogenesis inhibitors block growth of new blood vessels needed to supply solid tumors with oxygen and nutrients.
- Because angiogenesis inhibitors affect blood vessels rather than specific cancer cells, they should be active against a wide variety of tumors.
- Bevacizumab, the first angiogenesis inhibitor available, is a monoclonal antibody that binds with vascular endothelial growth factor (VEGF) and thereby prevents VEGF from promoting blood vessel formation. By suppressing angiogenesis, bevacizumab can inhibit further tumor growth but cannot directly kill existing tumor cells.
- Bevacizumab has clear benefits in colorectal cancer and nonsquamous non–small cell lung cancer, but not in breast cancer. Accordingly, approval for breast cancer has been withdrawn.
- Bevacizumab can impair wound healing and can cause hypertension, hemorrhage, GI perforation, and thromboembolism.
- Proteasomes are multienzyme complexes that degrade intracellular proteins and thereby rid cells of proteins that are not currently needed, including proteins that regulate transcription, cell adhesion, apoptosis, and progression through the cell cycle.
- Bortezomib, a proteasome inhibitor, reduces cell viability, increases apoptosis, and increases sensitivity to the lethal effects of radiation and traditional anticancer drugs.
- Bortezomib can cause bone marrow suppression, GI disturbances, and peripheral neuropathy.
- Glucocorticoids are toxic to cancers of lymphoid origin, including acute and chronic lymphocytic leukemias, Hodgkin's disease, and non-Hodgkin's lymphomas.
- In addition to their use against lymphoid-derived cancers, glucocorticoids are used to manage complications of cancer and cancer therapy. Specific benefits include suppression of chemotherapy-induced nausea and vomiting, reduction of cerebral edema secondary to irradiation of the cranium, reduction of pain secondary to nerve compression or edema, and suppression of hypercalcemia in steroid-responsive tumors. Also, glucocorticoids can improve appetite and promote weight gain and may impart a generalized sense of well-being.
- When glucocorticoids are used acutely, their toxicities are both mild and manageable. However, when used long term, these drugs can cause many serious toxicities, including osteoporosis, adrenal insufficiency, increased susceptibility to infection, peptic ulcers, and diabetes.

Please visit **http://evolve.elsevier.com/Lehne** for chapter-specific NCLEX® examination review questions.

UNIT XIX MISCELLANEOUS DRUGS AND THERAPIES

CHAPTER 104 Drugs for the Eye

The drugs addressed in this chapter are used to diagnose and treat disorders of the eye. Our primary focus is on glaucoma. Many of the drugs considered here are discussed in other chapters, so discussion in this chapter is limited to ophthalmologic applications.

DRUGS FOR GLAUCOMA

Glaucoma refers to a group of diseases characterized by a decrease in peripheral vision secondary to optic nerve damage. The most common forms of glaucoma are primary open-angle glaucoma and acute angle-closure (narrow-angle) glaucoma. These forms differ with respect to underlying pathology and treatment. With either form, permanent blindness can result.

In the United States, glaucoma is the leading cause of preventable blindness. Of the 120,000 Americans blinded each year by glaucoma, 90% could have saved their sight with timely treatment. Unfortunately, many afflicted persons are unaware of their condition: of the 4 million Americans with glaucoma, only 50% are diagnosed.

Before discussing glaucoma, we need to review the role of aqueous humor in maintaining intraocular pressure (IOP). As shown in Fig. 104.1, aqueous humor is produced by the ciliary body and secreted into the posterior chamber of the eye. From there it circulates around the iris into the anterior chamber and then exits the anterior chamber through the trabecular meshwork and canal of Schlemm. If outflow from the anterior chamber is impeded, back-pressure will develop, and IOP will rise. Conversely, if production of aqueous humor falls, IOP will decline.

Pathophysiology of Glaucoma and Treatment Overview

Primary Open-Angle Glaucoma

Characteristics. Primary open-angle glaucoma (POAG) is the most common form of glaucoma in the United States. About 90% of people with glaucoma have this type. POAG is a leading cause of blindness in the United States.

POAG is characterized by progressive optic nerve damage with eventual impairment of vision. Visual loss develops first in the peripheral visual field. As the disease advances, loss progresses toward the central visual field. The pathologic process that leads to optic nerve damage is not understood. IOP is often elevated, but it may also be normal. POAG is a painless, insidious disease in which injury develops over years. Symptoms are absent until extensive optic nerve damage has been produced.

Risk Factors. The major risk factors for POAG are:

- Elevated IOP
- African or South American ancestry
- Family history of POAG
- Advancing age

Of these, elevated IOP is most important. Please note, however, that glaucomatous optic nerve damage can develop even when IOP is normal (i.e., below 20 mm Hg). Furthermore, some individuals can have very high IOP (e.g., 30 mm Hg) with no associated injury to the optic nerve. These individuals are said to have *ocular hypertension*—not glaucoma.

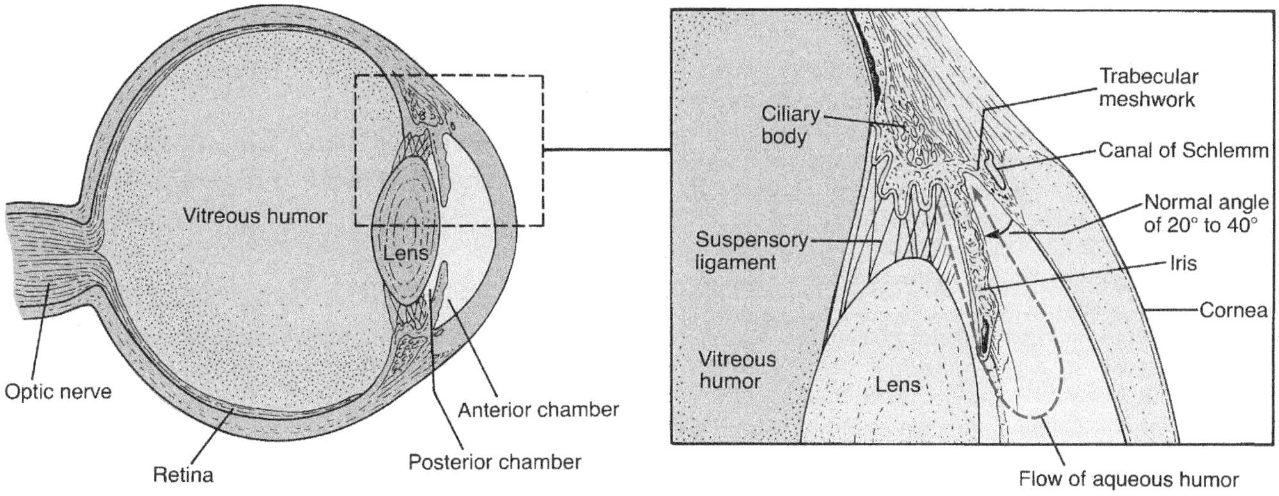

Fig. 104.1 ■ **Anatomy of the normal eye.**

TABLE 104.1 ■ Topical Drugs for Open-Angle Glaucoma

Class	Drugs	Mechanism	Adverse Effects
FIRST-LINE AGENTS			
Beta blockers		Decreased aqueous humor formation	
Nonselective	Timolol Carteolol Levobunolol Metipranolol		Heart block, bradycardia, bronchospasm
$Beta_1$ selective	Betaxolol		Heart block, bradycardia, hypotension
Prostaglandin analogs	Latanoprost Travoprost Bimatoprost	Increased aqueous humor outflow	Heightened brown pigmentation of the iris and eyelid
$Alpha_2$-adrenergic agonists	Apraclonidine[a] Brimonidine	Decreased aqueous humor formation	Headache, dry mouth, dry nose, altered taste, conjunctivitis, lid reactions, pruritus
SECOND-LINE AGENTS			
Cholinergic drugs		Increased aqueous humor outflow	
Muscarinic agonists	Pilocarpine		Miosis, blurred vision
Cholinesterase inhibitors	Echothiophate		Miosis, blurred vision
Carbonic anhydrase inhibitors	Dorzolamide Brinzolamide	Decreased aqueous humor formation	Ocular stinging, bitter taste, conjunctivitis, lid reactions

[a]Apraclonidine is indicated for short-term use only and therefore is *not* a first-line drug for glaucoma.

Screening. Because POAG has no symptoms (until significant and irreversible optic nerve injury has occurred), regular testing for early POAG is important among individuals at high risk. With early detection and treatment, blindness can usually be prevented.

Management. Treatment of POAG is directed at reducing elevated IOP, the only risk factor we can modify. Although POAG has no cure, reduction of IOP can slow or even stop disease progression.

The principal method for reducing IOP is chronic therapy with drugs. Drugs lower IOP by either (1) facilitating aqueous humor outflow or (2) reducing aqueous humor production. As indicated in Table 104.1, the first-line drugs for glaucoma belong to three classes: *beta-adrenergic blocking agents* (beta blockers), *$alpha_2$-adrenergic agonists,* and *prostaglandin analogs.* Other options—*cholinergic drugs* and *carbonic anhydrase inhibitors*—are considered second-line choices. All of the antiglaucoma drugs are available for topical administration, which is the preferred route. For more than 25 years, the beta blockers (e.g., timolol) have been considered drugs of first choice. However, the $alpha_2$ agonists (e.g., brimonidine) and prostaglandin analogs (e.g., latanoprost) are just as effective as the beta blockers and have a more desirable side effect profile. Accordingly, these drugs have joined the beta blockers as first-choice agents. Because drugs in different classes lower IOP by different mechanisms, combined therapy can be more effective than monotherapy. Because all of these drugs are applied topically, systemic effects are relatively uncommon. Nonetheless, serious systemic reactions *can* occur if sufficient absorption takes place.

If drugs are unable to reduce IOP to an acceptable level, surgical intervention to promote outflow of aqueous humor is indicated. Options include trabeculectomy and laser trabeculoplasty.

Angle-Closure Glaucoma

Angle-closure glaucoma is precipitated by displacement of the iris such that it covers the trabecular meshwork, thereby preventing exit of aqueous humor from the anterior chamber. As a result, IOP increases rapidly and to dangerous levels. This disorder is referred to as *angle-closure* or *narrow-angle* glaucoma because the angle between the cornea and the iris is greatly reduced (Fig. 104.2). Angle-closure glaucoma develops suddenly and is extremely painful. In the absence of treatment, irreversible loss of vision occurs in 1 to 2 days. This disorder is much less common than open-angle glaucoma.

Treatment consists of *drug therapy* (to control the acute attack) followed by *corrective surgery*. A combination of drugs (short-acting miotics, carbonic anhydrase inhibitors, topical beta-adrenergic blocking agents) is employed to suppress symptoms. After IOP has been reduced with drugs, definitive treatment can be rendered with surgery. Options include iridectomy and laser iridotomy. Both procedures alter the iris to permit unimpeded outflow of aqueous humor.

Drugs Used to Treat Glaucoma

Beta-Adrenergic Blocking Agents

Actions and Use in Glaucoma. Five beta blockers—*betaxolol, carteolol, levobunolol, metipranolol,* and *timolol*—are approved for use in glaucoma. Dosing is topical. These agents cause minimal disturbance of vision and are considered first-line drugs for glaucoma, although prostaglandin analogs are becoming favored. Formulations and dosages of the beta blockers are shown in Table 104.2.

The beta-adrenergic blockers lower IOP by decreasing production of aqueous humor. Reductions in IOP occur with *nonselective* beta blockers (drugs that block $beta_1$ *and* $beta_2$

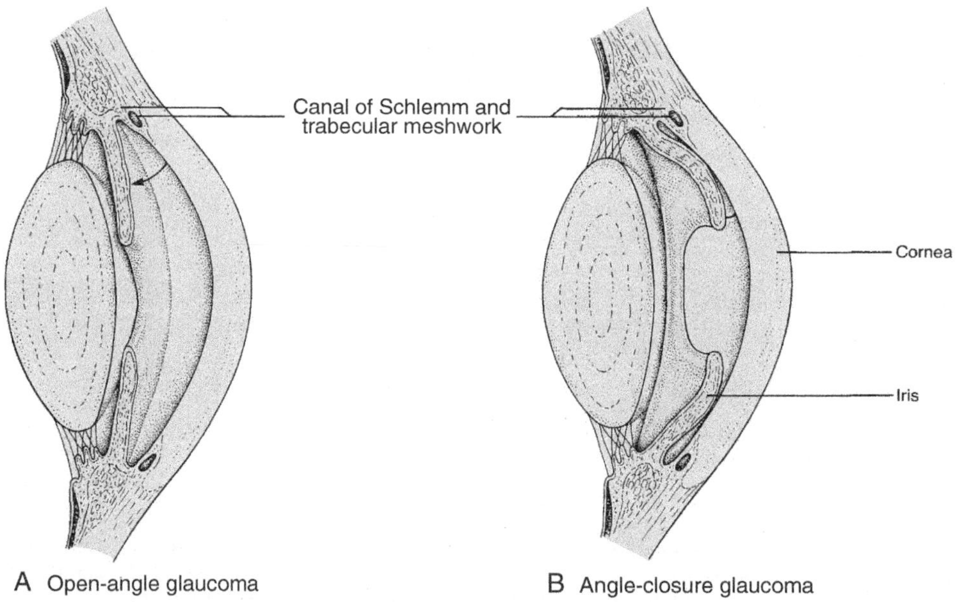

Fig. 104.2 ■ Comparative anatomy of the eye in open-angle and angle-closure glaucoma. **A,** Note that the angle between the iris and cornea is open in open-angle glaucoma, permitting unimpeded outflow of aqueous humor through the canal of Schlemm and trabecular meshwork. **B,** Note that the angle between the iris and cornea is constricted in angle-closure glaucoma, thereby blocking outflow of aqueous humor through the canal of Schlemm and trabecular meshwork.

TABLE 104.2 ■ Beta Blockers Used in Glaucoma

Drug	Receptor Specificity	Formulation	Usual Dosage
Betaxolol [Betoptic S]	$Beta_1$	0.25% suspension	1 drop twice daily
Carteolol (generic only)	$Beta_1$, $beta_2$	1% solution	1 drop twice daily
Levobunolol [Betagan Liquifilm, AKBeta]	$Beta_1$, $beta_2$	0.25% solution 0.5% solution	1 drop twice daily 1 drop once or twice daily
Metipranolol [OptiPranolol]	$Beta_1$, $beta_2$	0.3% solution	1 drop twice daily
Timolol [Timoptic, Betimol, Istalol]	$Beta_1$, $beta_2$	0.25% solution 0.5% solution 0.25% gel 0.5% gel	1 drop once or twice daily 1 drop once or twice daily 1 drop once daily 1 drop once daily

receptors), as well as with *cardioselective* beta blockers (drugs that block $beta_1$ receptors only).

Beta blockers are used primarily for open-angle glaucoma. They are suitable for initial therapy as well as maintenance therapy. Beta blockers, in combination with other drugs, are also employed for emergency management of acute angle-closure glaucoma.

The basic pharmacology of the beta blockers is discussed in Chapter 18.

Adverse Effects

Local. Local effects are generally minimal, although patients commonly complain of transient ocular stinging. Beta blockers occasionally cause conjunctivitis, blurred vision, photophobia, and dry eyes.

Systemic. Beta blockers can be absorbed in amounts sufficient to cause systemic effects. For example, instilling 1 drop of 0.5% timolol in each eye can produce the same blood level as taking 10 mg of timolol by mouth (the usual starting dose for hypertension). Effects on the heart and lungs are of greatest concern.

Blockade of cardiac $beta_1$ receptors can produce bradycardia and atrioventricular (AV) heart block. Pulse rate should be monitored. Because of their ability to depress cardiac function, beta blockers are contraindicated for patients with AV heart block, sinus bradycardia, and cardiogenic shock. In addition, they should be used with caution in patients with heart failure.

Blockade of $beta_2$ receptors in the lung can cause bronchospasm. Constriction of the bronchi can occur with "$beta_1$-selective" antagonists as well as with "nonselective" beta-adrenergic blockers—although the risk is greatest with the nonselective agents. Only one ophthalmic beta blocker—betaxolol—is $beta_1$ selective. This drug is preferred to other beta blockers for patients with asthma or chronic obstructive pulmonary disease.

Prostaglandin Analogs

Four prostaglandin analogs are approved for topical therapy of glaucoma. These drugs are as effective as the beta blockers and cause fewer side effects. Accordingly, they are considered first-line medications for glaucoma. Formulations and dosages are shown in Table 104.3.

Latanoprost. Latanoprost [Xalatan], an analog of prostaglandin F_2 alpha, was the first prostaglandin approved for glaucoma and will serve as our prototype for the group. The drug is applied topically to lower IOP in patients with open-angle glaucoma and ocular hypertension. Latanoprost lowers IOP by facilitating aqueous humor outflow, in part by relaxing the ciliary muscle. The recommended dosage is 1 drop (0.005% solution) applied once daily in the evening. At this dosage, latanoprost produces the same reduction in IOP as does timolol twice daily.

PATIENT-CENTERED CARE ACROSS THE LIFE SPAN

Glaucoma

Life Stage	Patient Care Concerns
Children	Compared with adults, children usually have increased systemic absorption following ophthalmic administration. Most drug classes include drugs not recommended for children. These include the beta blockers levobunolol and metipranolol, the $alpha_2$ agonist apraclonidine, the prostaglandin analogs latanoprost and tafluprost, and the carbonic anhydrase inhibitors brinzolamide and methazolamide. Additionally, brimonidine is not recommended for children under 2 years old. The manufacturer of travoprost does not recommend its use for children under 16 due to concerns regarding any possible long-term effects of pigmentary changes. The muscarinic agonist pilocarpine may cause paradoxical *increases* in intraocular pressure. It is indicated for the treatment of primary congenital glaucoma but not glaucoma secondary to other conditions.
Pregnant women	The intraocular pressure is usually decreased during pregnancy. This aids in the use of lower drug doses. Beta blocker preparations are Pregnancy Risk Category C.[a] For all except betaxolol, adverse events occurred in animal studies. No animal studies have been conducted for ophthalmic preparations of betaxolol; however, oral betaxolol crosses the placenta. Of the alpha-adrenergic agonists, brimonidine is Pregnancy Risk Category B[a] because no adverse events have been observed in animal studies. Apraclonidine was identified as Pregnancy Risk Category C after adverse events were exposed in animals. Both adverse and teratogenic effects were noted in animal reproduction studies with prostaglandin analogs and carbonic anhydrase inhibitors. These are all Pregnancy Risk Category C.[a] The cholinesterase inhibitor echothiophate and the muscarinic agonist pilocarpine are Pregnancy Risk Category C[a] because there are no current results of animal reproduction studies on which to base any conclusion.
Breast-feeding women	For all these drugs, manufacturers recommend weighing the possibility of benefits versus the drugs' adverse effects in deciding whether to breast-feed. If the patient will be breast-feeding, the lowest effective dose should be used, along with punctual occlusion after administration to decrease absorption.
Older adults	Beta blockers, even when administered topically, may worsen heart failure in patients with this condition. $Alpha_2$ agonists can cause orthostatic hypotension. This creates a fall risk for older patients. Patients with marked renal impairment should not take carbonic anhydrase inhibitors. This applies to topical as well as systemic formulations. Cholinesterase inhibitors may cause bradycardia and hypotension, leading to a fall risk.

[a]As of 2020, the FDA will no longer use Pregnancy Risk Categories. Please refer to Chapter 9 for more information.

Prototype Drugs

DRUGS FOR THE EYE

Beta Blockers

Betaxolol (beta$_1$ selective)
Timolol (blocks beta$_1$ and beta$_2$ receptors)

Alpha-Adrenergic Agonists

Brimonidine

Prostaglandin Analogs

Latanoprost

Angiogenesis Inhibitors

Ranibizumab

Latanoprost is generally well tolerated, and systemic reactions are rare. The most significant side effect is a harmless heightened brown pigmentation of the iris, which is most noticeable in patients whose irides are green-brown, yellow-brown, or blue/gray-brown. The effect is rare in patients whose irides are blue, green, or blue-green. Heightened pigmentation stops progressing when latanoprost is discontinued but does not usually regress. Topical latanoprost may also increase pigmentation of the eyelid and may increase the length, thickness, and pigmentation of the eyelashes. Other side effects include blurred vision, burning, stinging, conjunctival hyperemia, and punctate keratopathy. Rarely, latanoprost may cause migraine.

Other Prostaglandin Analogs. In addition to latanoprost, three other topical prostaglandins are approved for topical therapy of glaucoma. Like latanoprost, these drugs—*travoprost* [Travatan], *bimatoprost* [Lumigan], and *tafluprost* [Zioptan]—reduce IOP by increasing aqueous humor outflow. In clinical trials, these agents were at least as effective as timolol, a representative beta blocker. Interestingly, one drug—travoprost—was more effective in blacks than in nonblacks. Like latanoprost, these prostaglandins can cause a gradual increase in brown pigmentation of the iris, which may be irreversible. In addition, these drugs can increase pigmentation of the eyelid and growth of the eyelashes. In fact, bimatoprost, marketed as *Latisse,* is used for the specific purpose of increasing eyelash length, darkness, and thickness. With prostaglandins used to treat glaucoma, the most common adverse effect is ocular hyperemia (engorgement of ocular blood vessels). Less commonly, these drugs cause blurred vision, eye discomfort, ocular pruritus, conjunctivitis, dry eye, light intolerance, and tearing.

TABLE 104.3 ▪ Prostaglandin Analogs Used in Glaucoma

Generic Name	Brand Name	Formulation	Usual Dosage
Latanoprost	Xalatan	0.005% solution	1 drop once daily in the evening
Travoprost	Travatan	0.004% solution	1 drop once daily in the evening
Bimatoprost	Lumigan	0.01% solution	1 drop once daily in the evening
		0.03% solution	1 drop once daily in the evening
Tafluprost	Zioptan	0.0015% solution	1 drop once daily in the evening

Alpha$_2$-Adrenergic Agonists

Two alpha$_2$ agonists are approved for glaucoma. One agent—apraclonidine—is used only for short-term therapy. The other agent—brimonidine—has emerged as a first-line drug for long-term therapy.

Brimonidine. Brimonidine [Alphagan P, Alphagan 🍁] is the first and only topical alpha$_2$-adrenergic agonist approved for *long-term* reduction of elevated IOP in patients with open-angle glaucoma or ocular hypertension. The recommended dosage is 1 drop 3 times a day. Effects on IOP are similar to those achieved with timolol. The drug lowers IOP by reducing aqueous humor production and perhaps by increasing outflow. In addition to lowering IOP, brimonidine may delay optic nerve degeneration and may protect retinal neurons from death. This possibility arises from the ability of alpha$_2$ agonists to protect neurons from injury caused by ischemia. The most common adverse effects are dry mouth, ocular hyperemia, local burning and stinging, headache, blurred vision, foreign body sensation, and ocular itching. In contrast to apraclonidine (discussed next), brimonidine can cross the blood-brain barrier, and hence can cause drowsiness, fatigue, and hypotension. (Recall from Chapter 19 that activation of alpha$_2$ receptors in the brain decreases sympathetic outflow to blood vessels and thereby lowers blood pressure.) Brimonidine can be absorbed onto soft contact lenses. Accordingly, at least 15 minutes should elapse between drug administration and lens installation.

Apraclonidine. Apraclonidine [Iopidine], a topical alpha$_2$-adrenergic agonist, lowers IOP by reducing aqueous humor production and possibly by increasing outflow. The drug is indicated only for (1) short-term therapy of open-angle glaucoma in patients who have not responded adequately to maximal doses of other IOP-lowering drugs and (2) preoperative medication before laser trabeculoplasty or iridotomy. Side effects include headache, dry mouth, dry nose, altered taste, conjunctivitis, lid reactions, pruritus, tearing, and blurred vision. Apraclonidine does not cross the blood-brain barrier and thus does not promote hypotension.

Alpha$_2$ Agonist/Beta Blocker Combination

A fixed-dose combination of brimonidine (an alpha$_2$ agonist) and timolol (a nonselective beta blocker) is available for lowering IOP in patients with glaucoma or ocular hypertension. Formulations and dosages for the alpha$_2$ agonists and the alpha$_2$ agonist/beta blocker combinations are shown in Table 104.4.

TABLE 104.4 ▪ Alpha$_2$ Agonists Used in Glaucoma

Generic Name	Brand Name	Formulation	Usual Dosage
Brimonidine	Alphagan P	0.1% and 0.15% solution (0.2% solution available in Canada)	1 drop approximately every 8 hr
Apraclonidine	Iopidine	0.5% solution	1–2 drops approximately every 8 hr
Brimonidine + timolol (a beta blocker)	Combigan	0.2% brimonidine + 0.5% timolol	1 drop approximately every 12 hr

Pilocarpine, a Direct-Acting Muscarinic Agonist

Pilocarpine is a direct-acting muscarinic agonist (parasympathomimetic agent). Administration is topical. The basic pharmacology of the muscarinic agonists is discussed in Chapter 14. Consideration here is limited to the use of pilocarpine in glaucoma.

Effects on the Eye. By stimulating cholinergic receptors in the eye, pilocarpine produces two direct effects: (1) *miosis* (constriction of the pupil secondary to contraction of the iris sphincter) and (2) *contraction of the ciliary muscle* (an action that focuses the lens for near vision). IOP is lowered indirectly. In patients with *open-angle glaucoma,* IOP is reduced because the tension generated by contracting the ciliary muscle promotes widening of the spaces within the trabecular meshwork, thereby facilitating outflow of aqueous humor. In *angle-closure glaucoma,* contraction of the iris sphincter pulls the iris away from the pores of the trabecular meshwork, thereby removing the impediment to aqueous humor outflow.

Therapeutic Uses. Although used widely in the past, pilocarpine is now considered a second-line drug for open-angle glaucoma. Pilocarpine can also be used for emergency treatment of acute angle-closure glaucoma.

Adverse Effects. The major side effects of pilocarpine concern the eye. Contraction of the ciliary muscle focuses the lens for near vision; corrective lenses can provide partial compensation for this problem. Occasionally, sustained contraction of the ciliary muscle causes retinal detachment. Constriction of the pupil, caused by contraction of the iris sphincter, may decrease visual acuity. Pilocarpine may also produce local irritation, eye pain, and brow ache.

Rarely, pilocarpine is absorbed in amounts sufficient to cause systemic effects. Stimulation of muscarinic receptors throughout the body can produce a variety of responses, including bradycardia, bronchospasm, hypotension, urinary urgency, diarrhea, hypersalivation, and sweating. Caution should be exercised in patients with asthma or bradycardia. Systemic toxicity can be reversed with a muscarinic antagonist (e.g., atropine).

Preparations, Dosage, and Administration. Pilocarpine is available in solution and a gel for topical use. Pilocarpine solutions have a relatively short duration of action and must be administered more frequently than the gel. Formulations and dosages are shown in Table 104.5.

Echothiophate, a Cholinesterase Inhibitor

Only one cholinesterase inhibitor—echothiophate [Phospholine Iodide]—is available for glaucoma. The drug has a long duration of action. The basic pharmacology of echothiophate and other cholinesterase inhibitors is discussed in Chapter 15. Consideration here is limited to its use in glaucoma.

Effects on the Eye. Cholinesterase inhibitors inhibit breakdown of acetylcholine by cholinesterase and thereby promote accumulation of acetylcholine at muscarinic receptors. As a result, they can produce the same ocular effects as pilocarpine (i.e., miosis, focusing of the lens for near vision, reduction of IOP).

Use in Glaucoma. Echothiophate is indicated for POAG. However, because of concerns about adverse effects, the drug is not a first-choice agent. Rather, it is reserved for patients who have responded poorly to preferred medications (e.g., beta blockers, $alpha_2$ agonists, prostaglandins).

Adverse Effects. Like pilocarpine, echothiophate can cause myopia (secondary to contraction of the ciliary muscle) and excessive pupillary constriction. However, of much greater concern is the association between long-acting cholinesterase inhibitors and the development of cataracts. Absorption of echothiophate into the systemic circulation can produce typical parasympathomimetic responses, including bradycardia, bronchospasm, sweating, salivation, urinary urgency, and diarrhea.

Preparations, Dosage, and Administration. Dosage-related information is provided in Table 104.5.

Carbonic Anhydrase Inhibitors: Topical

Carbonic anhydrase inhibitors tend to be less effective than other drug therapy for glaucoma. They remain useful as adjuncts and as alternatives for treatments that are less well tolerated.

Dorzolamide. Dorzolamide [Trusopt] was the first carbonic anhydrase inhibitor available for topical administration. The drug is used to reduce IOP in patients with open-angle glaucoma and ocular hypertension. Dorzolamide lowers IOP by decreasing production of aqueous humor. The recommended dosage is 1 drop (2% solution) 3 times a day. Responses are similar to those produced with beta blockers.

Dorzolamide is generally well tolerated. The most common side effects are ocular stinging and bitter taste immediately after dosing. Between 10% and 15% of patients experience allergic reactions, primarily conjunctivitis and lid reactions. If these occur, the patient should stop using dorzolamide and contact the prescriber. Other reactions include blurred vision, tearing, eye dryness, and photophobia. In contrast to systemic carbonic anhydrase inhibitors, dorzolamide does not produce acidosis or electrolyte imbalance.

Dorzolamide is also available in a fixed-dose combination with timolol, marketed as *Cosopt.* The combination produces a greater reduction in IOP than either component used alone. Formulations and dosages for this product, as well as other carbonic anhydrase inhibitors, are shown in Table 104.6.

TABLE 104.5 ▪ Direct and Indirect Parasympathomimetic Preparations Used in Glaucoma

Generic Name	Brand Name	Formulation	Usual Dosage
Pilocarpine solution	Isopto Carpine, Akarpine 🍁, Diocarpine 🍁	0.5%–8% solution	Open-angle maintenance: 1 drop of solution (0.5%–4%) 4 times daily Acute angle-closure: 1 drop every 5–10 min for 3–6 doses, then 1 drop every 1–3 hr
Pilocarpine ophthalmic gel	Pilopine HS	4% pilocarpine hydrochloride in an aqueous gel base	½-inch ribbon at bedtime
Echothiophate	Phospholine Iodide	0.03%–0.25% reconstituted solution	1 drop twice daily Maintenance may be once daily, twice daily, or every other day

TABLE 104.6 ▪ Carbonic Anhydrase Inhibitors Used in Glaucoma

Generic Name	Brand Name	Formulation	Usual Dosage
Dorzolamide	Trusopt	2% solution	1 drop 3 times/day
Dorzolamide + timolol (a beta blocker)	Cosopt	2% dorzolamide + 0.5% timolol	1 drop twice daily
Brinzolamide	Azopt	1% solution	3 times/day
Acetazolamide	Diamox, Diamox Sequels, Acetazolam 🍁	125- and 250-mg tablets 500-mg sustained-release capsules	250 mg to 1 gm once daily
Methazolamide	Naptazane	25- and 50-mg tablets	50–100 mg 2–3 times/day

TABLE 104.7 ■ Muscarinic Antagonists Used for Mydriasis and Cycloplegia

			Time Course			
			Mydriasis		Cycloplegia	
Generic Name	Brand Names	Strength of Solution	Peak	Recovery	Peak	Recovery
Atropine	Generic only	0.5%, 1%	30–40 min	7–12 days	60–180 min	6–12 days
Cyclopentolate	AK-Pentolate, Cyclogyl	0.5%, 1%, 2%	30–60 min	1 day	25–76 min	0.25–1 day
Homatropine	Isopto Homatropine	2%, 5%	40–60 min	1–3 days	30–60 min	1–3 days
Scopolamine	Isopto Hyoscine	0.25%	20–30 min	1–3 days	30–60 min	3–7 days
Tropicamide	Tropicacyl, Opticyl, Mydriacyl 🍁	0.5%, 1%	20–40 min	0.25 day	20–35 min	<0.25 day

Brinzolamide. Brinzolamide [Azopt] is approved for topical treatment of elevated IOP in patients with open-angle glaucoma or ocular hypertension. The drug is as effective as dorzolamide and better tolerated. Like other carbonic anhydrase inhibitors, brinzolamide reduces IOP by slowing production of aqueous humor. The most common adverse effects are bitter aftertaste and transient blurred vision. Brinzolamide causes less ocular stinging and burning than dorzolamide. Both brinzolamide and dorzolamide contain the preservative benzalkonium chloride. This is absorbed by soft contact lenses. Patients wearing these should wait 15 minutes after administration before inserting contact lenses.

Carbonic Anhydrase Inhibitors: Systemic

Systemic carbonic anhydrase inhibitors have mostly been replaced by topical drugs. Two carbonic anhydrase inhibitors—*acetazolamide* and *methazolamide*—are available for systemic therapy of glaucoma. Of these, acetazolamide is used more often.

Actions and Uses in Glaucoma. Carbonic anhydrase inhibitors lower IOP by decreasing production of aqueous humor. Maximally effective doses reduce aqueous flow by 50%. Administration is oral.

Carbonic anhydrase inhibitors are employed primarily for long-term treatment of open-angle glaucoma. They are not drugs of first choice. Rather, they should be reserved for patients who have been refractory to preferred medications (e.g., beta blockers, $alpha_2$ agonists, prostaglandin analogs). Carbonic anhydrase inhibitors may also be given (in combination with other antiglaucoma drugs) to produce rapid lowering of IOP in patients with angle-closure glaucoma.

Adverse Effects. Systemic carbonic anhydrase inhibitors can produce a variety of adverse effects. Effects on the central nervous system, which are relatively common, include malaise, anorexia, fatigue, and paresthesias. The sense of malaise causes many patients to discontinue treatment. Reduced appetite, coupled with GI disturbances (nausea, vomiting, diarrhea), may result in weight loss. Carbonic anhydrase inhibitors are teratogenic in animals and should be avoided during pregnancy, especially in the first trimester. Additional concerns are acid-base disturbances, electrolyte imbalance, and nephrolithiasis (formation of renal calculi).

Preparations, Dosage, and Administration. *Acetazolamide* is available in immediate-release tablets (125 and 250 mg) and 500-mg sustained-release capsules (sold as Diamox Sequels), and in solution (500 mg/vial) for IM and IV administration. The usual dosage range is 250 mg to 1 gm/day in divided doses.

Methazolamide is available in 25- and 50-mg oral tablets. The usual dosage is 50 to 100 mg 2 or 3 times a day.

CYCLOPLEGICS AND MYDRIATICS

Cycloplegics are drugs that paralyze the ciliary muscle, and *mydriatics* are drugs that dilate the pupil. Cycloplegics and mydriatics are employed primarily to facilitate diagnosis and surgery of ophthalmic disorders. Agents used to produce cycloplegia, mydriasis, or both fall into two classes: (1) *anticholinergic agents* (muscarinic antagonists) and (2) *adrenergic agonists*.

Anticholinergic Agents

Five muscarinic antagonists (Table 104.7) are employed topically for the diagnosis and treatment of ophthalmic disorders. The basic pharmacology of the anticholinergic drugs is discussed in Chapter 14. Consideration here is limited to their ophthalmic applications.

Effects on the Eye

The anticholinergic drugs produce mydriasis and cycloplegia. Mydriasis results from blocking muscarinic receptors that promote contraction of the iris sphincter; cycloplegia results from blocking muscarinic receptors that promote contraction of the ciliary muscle. As discussed under *Adverse Effects,* relaxation of the iris can lead to elevation of IOP.

Ophthalmic Applications

Adjunct to Measurement of Refraction. The term *refraction* refers to the bending of light by the cornea and lens. When ocular refraction is proper, incoming light is bent such that a sharp image is formed on the retina. Errors in refraction can produce nearsightedness, farsightedness, and astigmatism (a visual disturbance caused by irregularities in the curvature of the cornea).

Both the mydriatic and cycloplegic properties of the muscarinic antagonists can be of use in evaluating errors of refraction. Mydriasis (widening of the pupil) facilitates observation of the eye's interior. Cycloplegia (paralysis of the ciliary muscle) prevents the lens from undergoing conformational change during the assessment.

Intraocular Examination. Dilation of the pupil with an anticholinergic agent facilitates observation of the inside of the eye. In addition, by paralyzing the iris sphincter, muscarinic antagonists prevent reflexive constriction of the pupil in response to the light from an ophthalmoscope (the hand-held device used to view the eye's interior). Since adrenergic agonists (e.g., phenylephrine) also dilate the pupil, but by a different mechanism, an adrenergic agonist can be combined with a muscarinic antagonist to increase the degree of mydriasis.

Intraocular Surgery. Anticholinergic agents may be employed to facilitate ocular surgery and to reduce postoperative complications. Mydriasis induced by these drugs can aid in cataract extraction and procedures to correct retinal detachment. For these operations, the muscarinic antagonist may be combined with an adrenergic agonist to maximize pupillary dilation. In certain postoperative patients, mydriatics are employed to prevent development of synechiae (adhesions of the iris to neighboring structures in the eye).

Treatment of Anterior Uveitis. Uveitis is an inflammation of the uvea (the vascular layer of the eye). Symptoms include ocular pain and photophobia. Uveitis is treated with a glucocorticoid (to reduce inflammation) plus an anticholinergic agent. By promoting relaxation of the ciliary muscle and the iris sphincter, anticholinergic drugs help relieve pain and prevent adhesion of the iris to the lens.

Adverse Effects

Blurred Vision and Photophobia. The most common side effects of topical anticholinergics are photophobia and blurred vision. Photophobia occurs because paralysis of the iris sphincter prevents the pupil from constricting in response to bright light. Blurred vision occurs because paralysis of the ciliary muscle prevents focusing for near vision.

Precipitation of Angle-Closure Glaucoma. By relaxing the iris sphincter, anticholinergic drugs can induce closure of the filtration angle in individuals whose eyes have a narrow angle to begin with. Angle closure occurs as follows: (1) partial dilation of the pupil maximizes contact between the iris and the lens, thereby impeding egress of aqueous humor from the posterior chamber, and (2) the resultant increase in pressure within the posterior chamber pushes the iris forward, causing blockage of the trabecular meshwork. Caution must be exercised in patients predisposed to angle closure.

Systemic Effects. Topically applied anticholinergic drugs can be absorbed in amounts sufficient to produce systemic toxicity. Symptoms include dry mouth, constipation, fever, tachycardia, and central nervous system effects (confusion, hallucinations, delirium, coma). Death can occur. Muscarinic poisoning can be treated with physostigmine (see Chapter 14).

Phenylephrine, an Adrenergic Agonist

Adrenergic agonists are mydriatic agents. Pupillary dilation results from activating alpha$_1$-adrenergic receptors on the radial (dilator) muscle of the iris. In contrast to anticholinergic drugs, the adrenergic agonists do not cause cycloplegia. Of the adrenergic agents given to induce mydriasis, *phenylephrine* is the most frequently employed. The adrenergic agonists are discussed in Chapter 17. Discussion here is limited to the mydriatic use of phenylephrine.

Therapeutic and Diagnostic Applications

The mydriatic applications of phenylephrine are much like those of the anticholinergic drugs. Phenylephrine-induced mydriasis is used as an aid to intraocular surgery, measurement of refraction, and ophthalmoscopic examination. In patients with anterior uveitis, phenylephrine is given to dilate the pupil as part of an overall program of treatment.

Adverse Effects

Effects on the Eye. Like the anticholinergic drugs, phenylephrine can precipitate angle-closure glaucoma secondary to induction of mydriasis. Caution must be exercised in patients whose filtration angle is naturally narrow. Contraction of the dilator muscle may dislodge pigment granules from degenerating cells of the iris. These granules, which appear as "floaters" in the anterior chamber, are usually cleared from the eye within a day. Phenylephrine may also cause ocular pain, corneal clouding, and brow ache.

Systemic Effects. Rarely, topical phenylephrine is absorbed in amounts sufficient to produce systemic toxicity. Cardiovascular responses (e.g., hypertension, ventricular dysrhythmias, cardiac arrest) are of greatest concern. Other systemic reactions include sweating, blanching, tremor, agitation, and confusion.

DRUGS FOR ALLERGIC CONJUNCTIVITIS

Pathophysiology of Allergic Conjunctivitis

Allergic conjunctivitis (AC) is defined as inflammation of the conjunctiva in response to an allergen. (The conjunctiva is the delicate membrane that surrounds the eyelids.) AC may be seasonal or perennial (chronic). Primary symptoms are itching, burning, and a thin, watery discharge. In addition, the conjunctivae are usually red and congested.

Symptoms of AC result from a biphasic immune response. Initially, symptoms are caused by release of inflammatory mediators—histamine, prostaglandins, leukotrienes, and kinins—from mast cells. These mediators stimulate mucus production (and thereby cause discharge), activate nerve endings (and thereby cause itching and burning sensations), promote vasodilation, and increase capillary permeability (and thereby cause redness and congestion). These symptoms peak about 20 minutes after allergen exposure and abate 20 minutes later. After this early response, symptoms typically reappear 6 or more hours later. The late phase is due to recruitment of immune cells—eosinophils, neutrophils, and macrophages—that amplify the inflammatory response.

Drugs Used to Manage Allergic Conjunctivitis

AC can be managed with a variety of topical drugs (Table 104.8). *Mast-cell stabilizers* (e.g., cromolyn, lodoxamide) prevent release of inflammatory mediators. Patients should be informed that benefits take several days to develop and several weeks to become maximal. In contrast to mast-cell stabilizers, *histamine$_1$ (H$_1$)-receptor antagonists* (antihistamines) can provide immediate symptomatic relief. Some drugs (e.g., azelastine, olopatadine) have two actions: They prevent mediator release from mast cells and they block H$_1$ receptors. Ketorolac, a *nonsteroidal anti-inflammatory drug* (NSAID), reduces symptoms by inhibiting cyclooxygenase, an enzyme required for synthesis of prostaglandins. Like the NSAIDs, *glucocorticoids* (e.g., loteprednol) inhibit production of prostaglandins. In addition, glucocorticoids inhibit production of leukotrienes and thromboxane. As a result, these drugs are highly effective. Unfortunately, with prolonged use, they can cause serious adverse effects, including cataracts, eye infection, and elevation of IOP. Accordingly, glucocorticoids are generally reserved for short-term therapy in patients who have not responded adequately to safer drugs. The *ocular decongestants* (e.g., naphazoline, phenylephrine) decrease redness and edema by activating alpha$_1$-adrenergic receptors on blood vessels, thereby causing vasoconstriction. Benefits are only symptomatic; these drugs do not interrupt any phase of the immune response. Furthermore, with regular use, rebound congestion is likely. For this reason, short term use of no longer than 2 weeks is recommended. Fortunately, that gives time for drugs such as mast cell stabilizers to become effective.

DRUGS FOR AGE-RELATED MACULAR DEGENERATION

Pathophysiology of ARMD

Age-related macular degeneration (ARMD) is a painless, progressive disease that blurs central vision and thereby limits perception of fine detail. Symptoms result from injury to the macula, the central part of the retina that contains the highest density of photoreceptors, and hence provides the high-resolution central vision used for reading, driving, sewing, recognizing faces, and so forth. ARMD is the leading cause of blindness in older Americans. About 15 million have the disease.

TABLE 104.8 ■ Topical Drugs for Allergic Conjunctivitis

Class and Generic Name	Brand Name	Concentration	Usual Daily Dosage
MAST-CELL STABILIZERS			
Cromolyn sodium	Crolom, Opticrom	4%	1–2 drops every 4–6 hr
Lodoxamide tromethamine	Alomide	0.1%	1–2 drops 4 times/day
Nedocromil sodium	Alocril	2%	1–2 drops twice daily
H_1-RECEPTOR BLOCKER			
Emedastine difumarate	Emadine	0.05%	1 drop 4 times/day
MAST CELL STABILIZERS/H_1 BLOCKERS			
Alcaftadine	Lastacaft	0.25%	1 drop once daily
Azelastine hydrochloride	Optivar	0.05%	1 drop twice daily
Epinastine	Elestat	0.05%	1 drop twice daily
Ketotifen fumarate	Zaditor, Alaway	0.025%	1 drop every 8–12 hr
Olopatadine hydrochloride	Patanol Pataday	0.1% 0.2%	1 drop twice daily 1 drop once daily
Bepotastine besylate	Bepreve	1.5%	1 drop twice daily
NSAIDs			
Ketorolac tromethamine	Acular LS Acuvail Acular, Acular PF	0.4% 0.45% 0.5%	1 drop 4 times/day 1 drop twice daily 1 drop 4 times/day
GLUCOCORTICOIDS			
Loteprednol etabonate	Alrex Lotemax	0.2% 0.5%	1 drop 4 times/day 1–2 drops 4 times/day
Dexamethasone sodium phosphate	Various	0.1%	1 drop every 6–8 hr
Fluorometholone	FML (ointment) Flarex (suspension)	0.1% 0.1%	½ inch ribbon 1–3 times/day 1 drop every 4 hr for 24–48 hr, then 1–2 drops 4 times/day
Prednisolone acetate	Various	1%	2 drops every 6–12 hr
Prednisolone sodium phosphate	Various	1%	1 drop every 6–8 hr
Rimexolone[a]	Vexol	1%	1–2 drops every 1–4 hr
DECONGESTANTS (VASOCONSTRICTORS)			
Naphazoline	Clear Eyes	0.012%	1–2 drops up to 4 times/day
Oxymetazoline	Visine L.R., OcuClear	0.025%	1–2 drops 4 times/day
Phenylephrine	Neo-Synephrine	0.12%	1–2 drops 4 times/day
Tetrahydrozoline	Visine Moisturizing	0.05%	1–2 drops 4 times/day
DECONGESTANT/H_1 BLOCKER			
Naphazoline/pheniramine	Naphcon-A Oncon-A	0.025%/0.3% 0.27%/0.325%	1–2 drops 1–4 times/day

[a]Off-label use.
NSAIDs, Nonsteroidal anti-inflammatory drugs.

ARMD has two forms: dry ARMD (atrophic ARMD) and wet ARMD (neovascular ARMD). The disorder begins as dry ARMD and can later progress to wet ARMD. Dry ARMD is more common than wet ARMD (85% vs. 15%), but wet ARMD is much more severe.

In dry ARMD, macular photoreceptors undergo gradual breakdown, leading to gradual blurring of central vision. The disease is characterized by the appearance of *drusen* (yellow deposits under the retina). Drusen develop before any visual impairment occurs. Whether drusen actually cause visual loss is unknown. However, we do know that an increase in the size or number of drusen increases the risk of symptomatic ARMD. Dry ARMD has three stages of increasing severity:

- *Early*—characterized by a few small or medium-sized drusen and no change of vision
- *Intermediate*—characterized by many medium-sized drusen (or one or more large drusen) and minor visual changes (a need for increased light for reading, possible blurred spot in the center of the visual field)
- *Advanced*—characterized by drusen, breakdown of photoreceptors and supporting tissue, and progressive blurring of central vision

In wet ARMD, macular degeneration is caused by the growth of new subretinal blood vessels, which are often fragile and leaky. Fluid leakage lifts the macula from its normal place, which quickly causes permanent injury. As noted, all people with wet ARMD have dry ARMD first. Vision loss occurs only in advanced dry ARMD and in wet ARMD.

Management of Dry ARMD

Although we can't prevent vision loss in people with advanced ARMD, we may be able to slow, or perhaps prevent, progression of intermediate disease. In the Age-Related Eye Disease Study (AREDS), sponsored by the National Eye Institute, researchers showed that taking high doses of vitamin C (500 mg), vitamin E (400 IU), beta-carotene (15 mg), and zinc (80 mg), all taken once a day, significantly reduces the risk of developing advanced ARMD. In addition, participants took 2 mg of copper daily to prevent copper deficiency anemia, which can develop when we consume lots of zinc. The AREDS formulation is recommended for people at high risk of developing advanced ARMD, identified as those with (1) intermediate ARMD in one or both eyes or (2) advanced ARMD (dry or wet) in one eye but not the other. In AREDS, the formulation did not benefit people with early ARMD. The AREDS formulation is available commercially as *Ocuvite PreserVision.*

Management of Wet (Neovascular) ARMD

We have three standard treatments for neovascular ARMD: laser therapy, photodynamic therapy (PDT), and therapy with angiogenesis inhibitors (i.e., drugs that suppress growth of new blood vessels). All three treatments can slow disease progression. In some cases, treatment partially reverses vision loss. At this time, treatment with an angiogenesis inhibitor is preferred to the other two options.

Angiogenesis Inhibitors

Actions and Benefits. Four drugs—*pegaptanib* [Macugen], *ranibizumab* [Lucentis], *aflibercept* [Eylea], and *bevacizumab* [Avastin]—can be used to inhibit growth of new blood vessels in patients with neovascular ARMD. Benefits derive from antagonizing *vascular endothelial growth factor* (VEGF), an endogenous compound that (1) induces angiogenesis, (2) increases vascular permeability, and (3) promotes inflammation—all of which can contribute to neovascular ARMD. Administration is by direct injection into the vitreous humor of the affected eye. Following injection, the drugs penetrate to the subretinal blood vessels and then bind with VEGF, thereby preventing VEGF from binding with its receptors on the vascular endothelium. As a result, VEGF is unable to promote vessel growth. The angiogenesis inhibitors are useful in wet ARMD, but not in dry ARMD. For patients with wet ARMD, treatment reduces the risk of losing visual acuity as well as the risk of progressing to blindness. In some cases, treatment partially reverses vision loss.

Adverse Effects. The biggest concern is *endophthalmitis*, an inflammation inside the eye caused by bacterial, viral, or fungal infection. Fortunately, the incidence is low (less than 1%). Patients who experience symptoms (e.g., redness, light sensitivity, pain) should seek immediate medical attention. More common adverse effects (10% to 40% incidence) include blurred vision, cataracts, conjunctival hemorrhage, corneal edema, eye discharge, increased IOP, ocular discomfort, punctate keratitis, vitreous floaters, and reduced visual acuity. Possible long-term effects—ocular or systemic—are not yet known.

Pegaptanib, Ranibizumab, Aflibercept, and Bevacizumab: Comparisons and Contrasts. Properties of the four angiogenesis inhibitors used for ARMD are shown in Table 104.9. As indicated, these agents differ with regard to structure, approved usage, cost, and efficacy.

Molecular Structure. Two agents—ranibizumab and bevacizumab—are similar to each other, and both differ from aflibercept and pegaptanib. Bevacizumab is an intact monoclonal antibody that binds with VEGF. Ranibizumab is a small fragment of bevacizumab that retains full ability to bind VEGF. In contrast, pegaptanib is an oligonucleotide aptamer—that is, a polymer of nucleotides designed to bind with a specific chemical (in this case, VEGF). Aflibercept is a hybrid molecule composed of (1) portions of VEGF receptors that have been fused with (2) the Fc portion of human immunoglobulin G1.

Approved Usage and Cost. Three of the drugs—pegaptanib, ranibizumab, and aflibercept—are approved for neovascular ARMD. In contrast, bevacizumab is approved for cancer, but not for ARMD. Nonetheless, bevacizumab is being used off-label for ARMD, largely because of price: A single injection of bevacizumab costs approximately $50, compared with average costs of $780 for pegaptanib, $2220 for aflibercept, and $1950 for ranibizumab.

Efficacy. All four drugs greatly reduce the risk of further visual impairment and progression to blindness. In addition, studies have shown that three agents—ranibizumab,

TABLE 104.9 ■ Intravitreal Angiogenesis Inhibitors for Neovascular (Wet) ARMD

Drug	Type of Molecule	Dosage	Comments
Pegaptanib [Macugen]	Oligonucleotide aptamer	0.3 mg every 6 weeks	Studies show little or no improvement in visual acuity, and hence use is rare
Ranibizumab [Lucentis]	Antibody fragment	0.5 mg once a month[a]	Studies show significant improvement in visual acuity
Aflibercept [Eylea]	Antibody fragment/VEGF receptor fragment hybrid	2 mg once a month for 3 months, then 2 mg every 2 months thereafter	Studies show significant improvement in visual acuity
Bevacizumab[b] [Avastin]	Complete antibody	1.25 mg once a month[a]	Studies show significant improvement in visual acuity

[a]After the first 4 monthly injections, injections may be done once every 3 months, but outcomes are not as good as with monthly injections.
[b]Bevacizumab is approved for metastatic colorectal cancer, but is used off-label for ARMD.
ARMD, Age-related macular degeneration; *VEGF,* vascular endothelial growth factor.

bevacizumab, and aflibercept—can *improve* visual acuity that has been impaired. As for pegaptanib, studies to date show little evidence of visual improvement. As a result, pegaptanib is used only rarely.

How do ranibizumab and bevacizumab compare with each other? In patients with wet ARMD, both drugs are equally effective, as shown in a large, randomized trial—the Comparison of AMD Treatments Trial (CATT)—in which the drugs were compared side-by-side.

Laser Therapy

In laser therapy, high-energy laser light is used to seal leaky blood vessels via coagulation. Unfortunately, the procedure has several drawbacks. First, laser light can damage nearby retinal tissue, and hence treatment is limited to regions away from the center of the macula. As a result, only a small percentage of leaky vessels can be sealed. Second, since new vessels continue to grow, repeat treatments are usually needed. Third, although the procedure can delay further vision loss, it cannot reverse existing damage. Fourth, even when the procedure is done with due care, some loss of vision occurs. This loss is justified by arguing that even greater loss would occur if treatment were withheld.

Photodynamic Therapy

PDT employs a photosensitive drug in combination with infrared light. The drug—*verteporfin* [Visudyne]—has a high affinity for neovascular tissue. In the procedure, verteporfin is delivered by IV infusion, and then an infrared laser is shined on the retina for 90 seconds. The light activates the drug, causing it to seal off leaky vessels. Repeat PDT may be needed because the vessels frequently reopen. Unlike laser therapy, PDT does not injure the retina. PDT reduces the risk of severe vision loss by 30% to 50%, but only 10% of patients show any vision improvement. For 5 days after the procedure, patients must protect their skin from sunlight and bright indoor light, because light-mediated activation of verteporfin in the skin could cause a severe burn.

ADDITIONAL OPHTHALMIC DRUGS

Drugs for Dry Eyes

Ophthalmic demulcents (artificial tears) are isotonic solutions employed as substitutes for natural tears. Most preparations contain *polyvinyl alcohol, cellulose esters,* or both. Artificial tears are indicated for relieving dry-eye syndromes and discomfort and dryness caused by irritants, wind, and sun. In addition, demulcents may be used to lubricate artificial eyes. Artificial tears are devoid of adverse effects, and hence may be administered as often and as long as desired.

Topical cyclosporine ophthalmic emulsion [Restasis] is prescribed for dry eyes due to inflammation. It suppresses the immune response, thereby promoting resumption of tear production.

Ocular Decongestants

Ocular decongestants are weak solutions of adrenergic agonists applied topically to constrict dilated conjunctival blood vessels. These preparations are used to reduce redness of the eye caused by minor irritation. The adrenergic agents employed as decongestants are *phenylephrine, naphazoline, oxymetazoline,* and *tetrahydrozoline.* When applied to the eye in the low concentrations found in decongestant products, adrenergic agonists rarely cause adverse effects. Local reactions (stinging, burning, reactive hyperemia) may occur with overuse. The adrenergic agonists are discussed in Chapter 17.

Glucocorticoids

Glucocorticoids are used for inflammatory disorders of the eye (e.g., uveitis, iritis, conjunctivitis). Administration may be topical or by local injection. Short-term therapy, in the absence of untreated infection, is generally devoid of adverse effects. In contrast, prolonged therapy may cause cataracts, reduced visual acuity, and glaucoma. In addition, there is an increased risk for infection secondary to glucocorticoid-induced suppression of host defenses. The glucocorticoids are discussed in Chapter 72.

Dyes

Fluorescein is a water-soluble dye that produces an intense green color. This agent is applied to the surface of the eye to detect lesions of the corneal epithelium; intact areas of the cornea remain uncolored, whereas abrasions and other defects turn bright green. Intravenous (IV) fluorescein is used to facilitate visualization of retinal blood vessels; IV fluorescein has been employed to help evaluate diabetic retinopathy and other abnormalities of the retinal vasculature. Fluorescein can also be used topically and intravenously to assess flow of aqueous humor. Adverse effects from systemic administration include nausea, vomiting, paresthesias, and pruritus. Severe reactions (anaphylaxis, pulmonary edema, cardiac arrest) are rare.

Rose bengal is applied topically to visualize abrasions of the corneal and conjunctival epithelium. Injured tissue appears rose colored when viewed with a slit lamp. The dye is also employed for the diagnosis of dryness of conjunctival tissue.

Lissamine green, another topical dye, turns bright green in the presence of conjunctival defects and dryness. Because it is less likely to cause stinging, it is beginning to replace rose bengal as a diagnostic tool.

Topical Drugs for Ocular Infections

Topical drugs are available for treating viral and bacterial infections of the eye. Four *antiviral* drugs—trifluridine, vidarabine, ganciclovir, and idoxuridine—are employed. The pharmacology of antiviral drugs is discussed in Chapter 93. Important *antibacterial* drugs are shown in Table 104.10. These drugs are used to treat serious ophthalmic infections and to prevent infection after ocular surgery. As a rule, anti-infective drugs are not needed for simple conjunctivitis. Patients should be made aware that bacterial and viral infections are contagious. Bacterial infections will remain contagious until treated for 24 to 48 hours. Viral infections may remain contagious until they are completely gone. Patients should not use contact lenses while they have an eye infection and while they are treating the infection with a topical drug.

TABLE 104.10 ■ Some Topical Ophthalmic Antibacterial Agents

Class and Generic Name	Brand Name	Formulation
FLUOROQUINOLONES		
Besifloxacin	Besivance	0.6% suspension
Ciprofloxacin	Ciloxan	0.3% solution, 0.3% ointment
Gatifloxacin	Zymar Zymaxid	0.3% solution 0.5% solution
Levofloxacin	Quixin	0.5% solution
Moxifloxacin	Moxeza, Vigamox	0.5% solution
Ofloxacin	Ocuflox	0.3% solution
MACROLIDES		
Azithromycin	AzaSite	1% solution
Erythromycin	Ilotycin	0.5% ointment
AMINOGLYCOSIDES		
Gentamicin	Gentak, Garamycin 🍁	0.3% solution, 0.3% ointment
Tobramycin	Tobrex	0.3% solution, 0.3% ointment
SULFONAMIDES		
Sulfacetamide	Bleph-10, Sodium Sulamyd	10% solution
POLYMYXIN B–CONTAINING MIXTURES		
Polymyxin B/bacitracin	AK-Poly-Bac	Ointment
Polymyxin B/ bacitracin/neomycin	Neosporin, AK-Spore	Ointment
Polymyxin B/ gramicidin/neomycin	Neosporin, AK-Spore	Solution
Polymyxin B/ trimethoprim	Polytrim	Solution

KEY POINTS

- The glaucomas are a group of diseases characterized by peripheral visual field loss secondary to optic nerve damage.
- In open-angle glaucoma, optic nerve injury develops gradually over years. The cause of nerve damage is unknown.
- In angle-closure glaucoma, there is blockage of aqueous humor outflow, which causes an abrupt rise in IOP. In the absence of treatment, irreversible damage to the optic nerve occurs in 1 or 2 days.
- Drug therapy of open-angle glaucoma is directed at reducing elevated IOP, the major risk factor for this disease.
- Angle-closure glaucoma is treated with drugs to rapidly reduce IOP and then with corrective surgery to allow aqueous humor outflow.
- Drugs reduce IOP by either facilitating aqueous humor outflow or reducing aqueous humor production.
- Three drug families—beta blockers, alpha$_2$-adrenergic agonists, and prostaglandins—are considered first-line agents for topical therapy of open-angle glaucoma.
- Timolol and other topical beta blockers lower IOP by decreasing aqueous humor production.
- Topical beta blockers can be absorbed in amounts sufficient to cause bronchospasm, bradycardia, and AV heart block.
- Brimonidine, an alpha$_2$ agonist, lowers IOP by decreasing aqueous humor production and possibly by increasing aqueous humor outflow.
- Latanoprost and other prostaglandins lower IOP by facilitating aqueous humor outflow.
- Cycloplegics are drugs that paralyze the ciliary muscle.
- Mydriatics are drugs that dilate the pupil.
- Atropine and other anticholinergic drugs cause cycloplegia by blocking muscarinic receptors on the ciliary muscle and cause mydriasis by blocking muscarinic receptors on the iris sphincter.
- By paralyzing the ciliary muscle, anticholinergic drugs prevent the eye from focusing for near vision.
- By paralyzing the iris sphincter, anticholinergic drugs prevent the pupil from constricting in response to bright light; photophobia results.
- Phenylephrine, an adrenergic agonist, causes mydriasis by stimulating alpha-adrenergic receptors on the radial (dilator) muscle of the iris.
- Age-related macular degeneration (ARMD) is a progressive disease that blurs central vision and thereby limits perception of fine detail.
- ARMD has two forms. The disorder begins as dry ARMD (atrophic ARMD) and may then progress to wet ARMD (neovascular ARMD). Wet ARMD is much less common than dry ARMD, but much more severe.
- In people with dry ARMD, prophylactic treatment with high-dose antioxidants and zinc may prevent the disease from progressing to wet ARMD.
- Wet ARMD can be treated with laser therapy, photodynamic therapy, and angiogenesis inhibitors (drugs that block retinal angiogenesis by neutralizing vascular endothelial growth factor).
- Three angiogenesis inhibitors—aflibercept, ranibizumab, and bevacizumab—are highly and equally effective against ARMD. A fourth agent—pegaptanib—is much less effective.

Please visit **http://evolve.elsevier.com/Lehne** for chapter-specific NCLEX® examination review questions.

CHAPTER

105 Drugs for the Skin

When one considers the vast number of skin conditions and the even greater number of pharmacologic agents used in their management, it is easy to see that the topic of dermatologic conditions alone could comprise a separate textbook. Our objective is to discuss some of the more frequently encountered dermatologic drugs. Most are dosed topically; some are given systemically. Before discussing the dermatologic drugs, we review the anatomy of the skin.

ANATOMY OF THE SKIN

The skin is composed of three distinct layers: the epidermis, the dermis, and a layer of subcutaneous fat. These layers and other features of the skin are shown in Fig. 105.1.

Epidermis

The epidermis is the outermost layer of the skin and is composed almost entirely of closely packed cells. As indicated in Fig. 105.1B, the epidermis itself consists of several layers. The deepest, known as the *basal layer* or *stratum germinativum,* contains the only epidermal cells that are mitotically active. All cells of the epidermis arise from this layer. Production of new cells within the basal layer pushes older cells outward. During their migration, these cells become smaller and flatter. As epidermal cells near the surface of the skin, they die and their cytoplasm is converted to *keratin,* a hard, proteinaceous material. Because of its high content of keratin, the outer layer of the epidermis has a rough, horny texture. Because of its texture, this layer is referred to as the *cornified layer* or *stratum corneum.* The surface of the stratum corneum undergoes continuous exfoliation (shedding). This shedding completes the epidermal growth cycle.

In addition to germinal cells, the basal layer of the epidermis contains *melanocytes.* These cells, which are few in number, produce *melanin,* the pigment that determines skin color. Following its synthesis within melanocytes, melanin is transferred to other cells of the epidermis. Melanin protects the skin against ultraviolet (UV) radiation, which is the principal stimulus for melanin production.

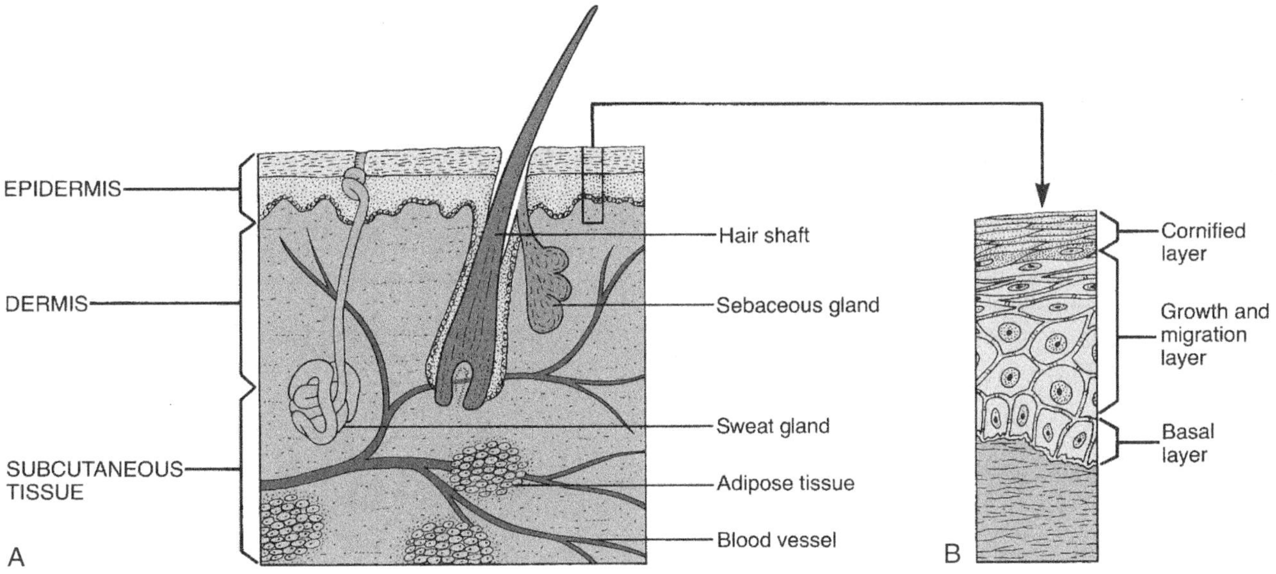

Fig. 105.1 ■ Anatomy of the skin.
A, Major structures of the skin. **B,** Growth layers of the epidermis.

Dermis

The dermis underlies the epidermis and is composed largely of connective tissue, primarily collagen. A major function of the dermis is to provide support and nourishment for the epidermis. Structures found in the dermis include blood vessels, nerves, and muscle. The dermis also contains sweat glands, sebaceous glands, and hair follicles. Sebaceous glands secrete an oily composite known as sebum. Almost all sebaceous glands are associated with hair follicles (see Fig. 105.1A).

Subcutaneous Tissue

Subcutaneous tissue consists largely of fat. This fatty layer provides protection and insulation. In addition, the stored fat constitutes a reserve source of calories.

TOPICAL DRUG FORMULATIONS

Topical drugs are provided through a number of vehicles. The most popular are ointments, creams, lotions, gels, foams, powders, and pastes.

Ointments are thick, greasy preparations with an oil or petroleum jelly base and little, if any, water. They provide the highest medication absorption of all formulations. The enhanced penetration makes it especially useful in the management of conditions with thickened skin (e.g., lichenification secondary to prolonged scratching) or inflamed skin. Because it provides an occlusive film that retains moisture, it is not a good choice for weeping or oozing skin conditions or in areas prone to heavy perspiration. It is often an excellent choice, however, for dry skin conditions.

Creams are an oil and water emulsion. The ratio of water to oil affects the thickness of their consistency and how oily or sticky they feel on the skin. They are not as thick as ointments, but they are thicker than lotions. Creams tend to be good for inflamed skin and dry sensitive skin. They may or may not be useful for oozing lesions, depending on the ratio of water to oil. Creams are more appropriate than oils for intertriginous regions (i.e., regions where skin touches or rubs together such as under pendulous breasts or between fingers or toes).

Lotions are water based. Some may contain alcohol or acids, which can cause a burning sensation. They have little, if any, oil; as a result, they have a lighter feel than creams. Lotions are nongreasy, which tends to promote more patient satisfaction. Another advantage of lotions is that they are easy to spread, which makes them a good choice for large areas or for hairy areas. They are suitable for intertriginous areas. Unlike ointments and creams, they are suitable for oily skin and may even decrease oiliness, depending on the ingredients.

Gels are transparent preparations that usually contain cellulose with a water or alcohol base. They liquefy on skin contact and often have a cooling effect as they dry. Because they are nongreasy and tend to have drying effects, gels are good choices for oily skin. They spread easily, so they are good for covering large or hairy areas. Because they dry clear and invisible, they may be more acceptable for facial regions. These may cause burning, but when this occurs, it is often the fault of the inactive ingredients rather than the medication.

Foams are aerated solutions. They spread easily, dry quickly, and leave negligible residue. They tend to be good choices for oily skin and large or hairy areas.

Most powders have a talc or cornstarch base. They are dry with a silky feel that reduces friction between surfaces. This can make them useful between skin folds. The dryness of the vehicle can be helpful when applied to regions that tend to perspire, such as the feet or axillae.

Pastes are mixtures of an ointment and a powder. The addition of a powder increases adherence to the skin. Because the powder disrupts the occlusive nature of an ointment, allowing for air to reach the covered skin, most pastes can be used safely in areas that are occluded, such as the use of Desitin diaper rash paste beneath a diaper

TOPICAL GLUCOCORTICOIDS

The basic pharmacology of the glucocorticoids is discussed in Chapter 72. Consideration here is limited to their use for skin disorders.

Actions and Uses

Topical glucocorticoids are employed to relieve inflammation and itching associated with a variety of dermatologic conditions (e.g., insect bites, dermatitis, psoriasis, eczema, pemphigus).

The vehicle in which a glucocorticoid is dispersed (e.g., cream, ointment, gel) can enhance the therapeutic response by helping the glucocorticoid penetrate to its site of action. The vehicle may provide additional benefits by acting as a drying agent or an emollient.

Relative Potency

Glucocorticoid preparations vary widely in potency. As indicated in Table 105.1, these drugs can be assigned to groups that range in potency from low to super-high. Preparations within each group are equipotent.

It is important to note that the intensity of the response to topical glucocorticoids depends not only on the concentration and inherent activity of the glucocorticoid, but also on the vehicle employed and the method of application. Occlusive dressings can enhance percutaneous absorption by as much as 10-fold, thereby greatly increasing pharmacologic effects.

Absorption

Topical glucocorticoids can be absorbed into the systemic circulation. The extent of absorption is proportional to the duration of use and the surface area covered. Absorption is higher from regions where the skin is especially permeable (axilla, face, eyelids, neck, perineum, genitalia) and lower from regions where penetrability is poor (palms, soles). Absorption through intact skin is lower than through inflamed skin. As noted, absorption is influenced by the vehicle, and it can be greatly increased by an occlusive dressing.

Adverse Effects

Adverse effects may be local or systemic. Factors that increase the risk for adverse effects include the use of a high-potency glucocorticoid, use of an occlusive dressing, prolonged therapy, and application over a large area.

Local Reactions. Glucocorticoids increase the risk for local infection and may also produce irritation. With prolonged use, glucocorticoids can cause atrophy of the dermis and epidermis, resulting in thinning of the skin, striae (stretch marks), purpura (red spots caused by local hemorrhage), and telangiectasis (red, wart-like lesions caused by capillary dilation). Long-term therapy may induce acne and hypertrichosis (excessive growth of hair, especially on the face).

Systemic Toxicity. Topical glucocorticoids can be absorbed in amounts sufficient to produce systemic toxicity. Principal concerns are growth delay (in children) and adrenal suppression (in all age groups). Systemic toxicity is more likely under extreme conditions of use (prolonged therapy in which a large area is treated with big doses of a high-potency agent covered with an occlusive dressing). When these conditions are present, adrenal suppression can occur.

Administration

Topical glucocorticoids should be applied in a thin film and gently rubbed into the skin. Patients should be advised not to use occlusive dressings (bandages, plastic wraps) unless the prescriber tells them to. Tight-fitting diapers and plastic pants can act as occlusive dressings and should not be worn when glucocorticoids are applied to the diaper region of infants. The same would be true of adults who wear disposable undergarments owing to urinary or bowel incontinence.

KERATOLYTIC AGENTS

Keratolytic agents are drugs that promote shedding of the horny layer of the skin. They are used to treat conditions where there is an overgrowth or abnormal thickening of the skin. Effects range from peeling to extensive desquamation of the stratum corneum. Two keratolytic compounds—*salicylic acid* and *sulfur*—are considered next. A third agent—*benzoyl peroxide*—is discussed later under *Topical Drugs for Acne.*

Salicylic Acid

Salicylic acid promotes desquamation by dissolving the intracellular cement that binds scales to the stratum corneum. Keratolytic effects are achieved with concentrations between 3% and 6%. At concentrations above 6%, tissue injury is likely. Low (3% to 6%) concentrations are used to treat dandruff, seborrheic dermatitis, acne, and psoriasis. Higher concentrations (up to 40%) are used to remove warts and corns.

Salicylic acid is readily absorbed through the skin. Though rare, systemic salicylate toxicity (salicylism) can result when large amounts are used for a prolonged period. Symptoms of salicylism include tinnitus, hyperpnea, and psychologic disturbances. Systemic effects can be minimized by avoiding prolonged use of high concentrations over large areas.

Sulfur

Sulfur promotes peeling and drying. Compounds containing sulfur have been used to treat acne, dandruff, psoriasis, and seborrheic dermatitis. Sulfur is available in lotions, gels, and shampoos. It is commonly combined with salicylic acid for the additive effects (e.g., Sebex shampoo). Concentrations range from 2% to 10%.

ACNE

Acne is the most common dermatologic disease. About 85% of teenagers develop acne, which often persists into adulthood. Acne accounts for more visits to dermatologists than any other disorder. In the United States, the direct costs of acne exceed $1 billion a year, including about $100 million spent on acne products sold over the counter.

TABLE 105.1 ■ Relative Potency of Topical Glucocorticoids

Potency Class and Drug	Formulation	Concentration
SUPER-HIGH POTENCY		
Betamethasone dipropionate [Diprolene]	Ointment, lotion, gel	0.05%
Clobetasol propionate [Clobex, Cormax, Temovate]	Cream, ointment, gel, spray, foam, lotion, shampoo	0.05%
Diflorasone diacetate ointment [Psorcon]	Ointment	0.05%
Fluocinonide [Vanos]	Cream	0.1%
Flurandrenolide [Cordran tape]	Tape	4 mcg/m^2
Halobetasol propionate [Ultravate]	Cream, ointment	0.05%
HIGH POTENCY		
Amcinonide [Cyclocort]	Cream, ointment, lotion	0.1%
Betamethasone dipropionate [Diprolene, Diprolene AF]	Cream, ointment, lotion	0.05%
Desoximetasone [Topicort]	Cream, ointment, gel, spray	0.5%, 0.25%
Diflorasone diacetate cream [ApexiCon, Florone, Maxiflor, Psorcon]	Cream	0.05%
Fluocinonide [Fluonex, Lidex, Vanos]	Cream, ointment, gel, solution	0.05%
Halcinonide [Halog]	Cream, ointment	0.1%
Triamcinolone acetonide [Dermazone, Kenalog, Oralone, others]	Ointment	0.5%
MEDIUM TO HIGH POTENCY		
Amcinonide cream [Cyclocort]	Cream	0.1%
Betamethasone dipropionate cream [Diprosone]	Cream	0.05%
Diflorasone diacetate [ApexiCon E, Psorcon]	Cream, ointment	0.05%
Fluocinonide emollient cream [Lidex E]	Cream	0.05%
Fluticasone propionate ointment [Cutivate]	Ointment	0.005%
Triamcinolone acetonide ointment [Aristocort A]	Ointment	0.01%
Triamcinolone high-potency cream [Aristocort-HP]	Cream	0.05%
MEDIUM POTENCY		
Betamethasone dipropionate [Diprolene, Diprolene AF, Luxiq, Sernivo, others]	Lotion	0.05%
Betamethasone valerate [Beta-Val, Luxiq, Valisone]	Cream, ointment, lotion, foam	0.1%, 0.12%
Clocortolone pivalate [Cloderm]	Cream	0.1%
Desoximetasone [Topicort LP]	Cream, ointment, gel, spray	0.05%
Fluocinolone acetonide [Synalar]	Cream, ointment	0.025%, 0.2%
Flurandrenolide [Cordran, Cordran SP]	Cream, lotion	0.05%
Fluticasone propionate [Cutivate]	Cream	0.05%
Hydrocortisone butyrate [Locoid, Locoid Lipocream]	Cream, ointment, lotion, solution	0.1%
Hydrocortisone valerate [Westcort]	Cream, ointment	0.2%
Mometasone furoate [Elocon]	Cream, ointment, lotion, solution	0.1%
Prednicarbate [Dermatop]	Cream, ointment	0.1%
Triamcinolone acetonide [Kenalog]	Cream, lotion Ointment Aerosol	0.1% 0.025% 0.2%
LOW POTENCY		
Alclometasone dipropionate [Aclovate]	Cream, ointment	0.05%
Desonide [DesOwen, LoKara, Verdeso]	Cream, ointment, gel, lotion, foam	0.05%
Fluocinolone acetonide [Capex, Synalar]	Cream, oil, shampoo, solution	0.01%
Hydrocortisone acetate [Lanacort 10, U-Cort]	Cream, ointment	1%
Hydrocortisone butyrate [Locoid]	Cream, ointment, lotion, solution	0.1%
Triamcinolone acetonide [Kenalog]	Cream, ointment, lotion	0.025%
LEAST POTENCY		
Hydrocortisone [Ala-Cort, Anusol-HC, Cortaid, Cortizone-10, Hytone]	Cream, ointment, lotion	1%, 2.5%

Prototype Drugs

DRUGS FOR ACNE

Topical Drugs for Acne	Oral Drugs for Acne
Benzoyl peroxide	Isotretinoin
Tretinoin	Doxycycline

Pathophysiology

Acne is a chronic skin disorder that usually begins during puberty. The disease is more common and more severe in males. Lesions typically develop on the face, neck, chest, shoulders, and back. In mild acne, *open comedones* (blackheads) are the most common lesion. A comedo forms when sebum combines with keratin to create a plug within a pore (oxidation of the sebum causes the exposed surface of the plug to turn black). *Closed comedones* (whiteheads) develop when pores become blocked with sebum and scales below the skin surface. In its most severe form, acne is characterized by abscesses and inflammatory cysts. As a rule, acne begins to improve after puberty and, for some, clears entirely during the early 20s. However, with some people, the disease continues for decades.

Onset of acne is initiated by increased production of androgens during adolescence. Under the influence of androgens, sebum production and turnover of follicular epithelial cells are increased, leading to the plugging of pores. Symptoms are intensified by the activity of *Propionibacterium acnes,* a microbe that converts sebum into irritant fatty acids. This bacterium also releases chemotactic factors that promote inflammation. Oily skin and a genetic predisposition also contribute.

Overview of Treatment

Because acne is a chronic disease, treatment is prolonged. Fortunately, almost all patients respond well. Effective treatment will prevent scarring and limit the duration of symptomatic disease and will thereby minimize the psychologic effect of acne.

Nonpharmacologic Therapy

Nonpharmacologic measures can help minimize acne lesions, especially in patients with milder acne. Surface oiliness should be reduced by gentle cleansing with a nonirritant soap a couple of times a day. Care should be taken to avoid irritation from vigorous scrubbing or the use of abrasives. Oil-based makeup or moisturizing products should not be used. Additional measures (e.g., comedo extraction, dermabrasion) may be indicated for some individuals. Research has demonstrated that dietary changes provide no benefit.

Drug Therapy

Drugs for acne fall into two major groups: topical drugs and oral drugs (Table 105.2). The topical drugs have two principal subgroups: antimicrobial agents and retinoids. Likewise, the oral drugs have two principal subgroups: antibiotics and retinoids. Occasionally, other agents such as keratolytic agents (e.g., salicylic or azelaic acid) or hormonal agents (e.g., oral contraceptives [OCs]) may be used.

Drug selection is based on symptom severity. For patients with relatively mild symptoms, topical therapy can suffice. When symptoms are more severe, oral therapy is required. *Mild* acne can be managed with topical antimicrobials and topical retinoids. *Moderate* acne can be treated with oral antibiotics (e.g., doxycycline, minocycline) and comedolytics (retinoids and azelaic acid). In addition, hormonal agents—combination OCs and spironolactone—can be used in young women whose acne is unresponsive to other drugs. The principal agent for *severe* acne is isotretinoin.

TABLE 105.2 ■ Drugs for Acne

TOPICAL DRUGS	
Antibiotics	Benzoyl peroxide (generic only) Clindamycin [Cleocin, others] Erythromycin [Eryderm, others] Dapsone [Aczone] Benzoyl peroxide/clindamycin [BenzaClin, Clindoxyl 🍁] Benzoyl peroxide/erythromycin [Benzamycin]
Retinoids	Tretinoin [Atralin, Avita, Retin-A, Retin-A Micro] Adapalene [Differin] Tazarotene [Avage, Tazorac]
Retinoid/antibiotic combinations	Tretinoin/clindamycin [Veltin Gel, Ziana] Adapalene/benzoyl peroxide [Epiduo]
Others	Azelaic acid [Azelex, Finacea 🍁]
ORAL DRUGS	
Antibiotics	Doxycycline [Vibramycin, others] Minocycline [Minocin, others] Tetracycline (generic only) Erythromycin [Ery-Tab, others]
Retinoids	Isotretinoin [Amnesteem, Claravis]
Hormonal agents	Combination oral contraceptives Spironolactone [Aldactone]

Topical Drugs for Acne

Antibiotics

Benzoyl Peroxide. Benzoyl peroxide, a first-line drug for mild to moderate acne, is both an antibiotic and keratolytic. Improvement can be seen within days of starting treatment. Benefits derive primarily from suppressing growth of *P. acnes.* The presumed mechanism is release of active oxygen. In addition to suppressing *P. acnes,* benzoyl peroxide can reduce inflammation and promote keratolysis (peeling of the horny layer of the epidermis).

Unlike other topical antimicrobials, benzoyl peroxide does not promote emergence of resistant *P. acnes.* In fact, benzoyl peroxide is often combined with clindamycin or erythromycin to protect against resistance to those drugs, which can occur when those antibiotics are used alone.

Benzoyl peroxide may produce drying and peeling of the skin. If signs of severe local irritation occur (e.g., burning, blistering, scaling, swelling), the frequency of application should be reduced. Benzoyl peroxide has been associated with potentially serious hypersensitivity reactions, especially in patients with asthma. In Canada, 131 instances of severe allergies experienced by patients using benzoyl peroxide and/or salicylic acid prompted a safety review. In December

2015, Health Canada issued a public warning. Revised drug monographs will include information on sensitivity testing (see http://healthycanadians.gc.ca/recall-alert-rappel-avis/hc-sc/2015/56268a-eng.php).

Benzoyl peroxide is available in a variety of formulations (e.g., lotions, creams, gel, foam). Concentrations range from 2.5% to 10%. For initial therapy, once-daily application is recommended. Over time, the frequency of administration can be increased (to a maximum of 3 times a day) as tolerance permits. Patients should be advised to keep the drug away from the eyes, mouth, and mucous membranes, as well as inflamed or denuded skin.

Clindamycin and Erythromycin. Like benzoyl peroxide, topical clindamycin [Cleocin, others] and erythromycin [Eryderm, others] suppress growth of *P. acnes*. In addition, these drugs can decrease inflammation. Monotherapy with either drug quickly leads to resistance. To protect against the emergence of resistance, these drugs can be combined with benzoyl peroxide. Two fixed-dose combinations are available: clindamycin/benzoyl peroxide [Acanya, BenzaClin, Clindoxyl 🍁] and erythromycin/benzoyl peroxide [Benzamycin].

Dapsone. Dapsone [Aczone] has been used for oral therapy of leprosy for decades (see Chapter 90). In patients with acne, the drug yields a modest decrease in inflammation and number of lesions. The mechanism of action underlying anti-acne benefits has not been established. Dapsone is available as a 5% gel in 30-, 60-, and 90-gm tubes for twice-daily application. The site should be washed and dried before applying the drug, and the hands should be washed afterward. The most common side effects of dapsone gel are oiliness, peeling, dryness, and erythema. These effects are caused primarily by the gel vehicle, and not by dapsone. Oral dapsone, but not topical dapsone, poses a risk for hemolytic anemia and peripheral neuropathy. Combining dapsone with benzoyl peroxide can turn the skin yellow or orange. Until more is known, dapsone should be reserved for patients who can't tolerate traditional topical treatments.

Retinoids

The topical retinoids—derivatives of vitamin A (retinol)—are a cornerstone of acne therapy. These drugs can unplug existing comedones and prevent the development of new ones. In addition, they can reduce inflammation and improve penetration of other topical agents. Topical retinoids currently approved for acne use are adapalene, tazarotene, and tretinoin. They may be used alone or in combination with other drugs, including topical and oral antimicrobials. In 2016, adapalene became the first topical retinoid approved for over-the-counter treatment of acne in people age 12 years and older.

Tretinoin. Topical tretinoin, a derivative of vitamin A, is used for acne and to remove fine wrinkles. Formulations for acne are marketed as Atralin, Avita, Retin-A, and Retin-A Micro. The formulation for wrinkles, which is nearly identical to one of the formulations for acne, is marketed as Renova. Topical tretinoin should not be confused with isotretinoin, a powerful *oral* antiacne medicine (discussed later in this chapter) nor with the oral form of tretinoin, which is approved for remission induction of acute promyelocytic leukemia, but not for skin conditions.

Use for Acne. Tretinoin is approved for topical treatment of mild to moderate acne. Benefits derive from normalizing hyperproliferation of epithelial cells within hair follicles. By doing so, retinoids can unplug existing comedones and suppress formation of new plugs. Tretinoin also causes thinning of the stratum corneum and can thereby facilitate penetration of other drugs. Therapeutic effects can be enhanced by combining tretinoin with benzoyl peroxide, topical antibiotics, and oral antibiotics.

Use for Fine Wrinkles. Tretinoin is approved for reducing fine wrinkles, tactile roughness, and mottled hyperpigmentation ("liver spots," age spots) in facial skin. Benefits may derive from suppressing genes that code for specific proteases that break down collagen and elastin. In clinical trials, responses to tretinoin were modest. In fact, many patients achieved equivalent effects with a program of comprehensive skin care and sun protection. It is important to appreciate that tretinoin does *not* repair deep, coarse wrinkles and other damage caused by chronic sun exposure. Furthermore, the drug does not reverse photoaging or restore the microscopic structure of skin to a more youthful pattern. Benefits in patients older than 50 years have not been established.

Adverse Effects. Tretinoin can cause *localized* reactions, but absorption is insufficient to cause systemic toxicity. In patients with sensitive skin, tretinoin may induce blistering, peeling, crusting, burning, and edema. These effects can be intensified by concurrent use of abrasive soaps and keratolytic agents (e.g., sulfur, resorcinol, benzoyl peroxide, salicylic acid). Accordingly, these preparations should be discontinued before beginning tretinoin therapy. Skin reactions with two formulations—Avita and Retin-A Micro—may be less intense than those caused by Retin-A, an older formulation.

Tretinoin increases susceptibility to sunburn. Patients should be warned to apply a sunscreen with a sun protection factor (SPF) of 15 or greater and to wear protective clothing. Patients with existing sunburn should not apply the drug.

Preparations, Dosage, and Administration. For the treatment of *acne*, tretinoin is available under four brand names: Retin-A, Retin-A Micro, Atralin, and Avita. Products marketed as *Retin-A* are available in two formulations: cream (0.025%, 0.05%, and 0.1%) and gel (0.01% and 0.025%). *Retin-A Micro* is supplied as a gel (0.04% and 0.1%), *Atralin* as a 0.05% gel, and *Avita* as a 0.025% cream or gel. All products are administered topically, usually once a day at bedtime. Before application, the skin should be washed, toweled dry, and allowed to dry fully for 20 to 30 minutes. Tretinoin should not be applied to open wounds or to areas of sunburn or windburn. Contact with the eyes, nose, ears, and mouth should be avoided.

For *fine wrinkles of the face*, tretinoin is available in a 0.02% cream, sold as *Renova*. Application is done once daily at bedtime. Cosmetics should be washed off before use. Up to 6 months of treatment may be needed to see a response, and treatment must continue to maintain the response.

Hazardous Agents and Special Administration Requirements. Tretinoin is one of many drugs in this chapter classified by the National Institute of Occupational Safety and Health (NIOSH) as a hazardous drug for administration by nurses. NIOSH requires special handling of drugs identified as hazardous. See Chapter 3, Table 3.1, for administration and handling guidelines. The hazardous drugs mentioned in this chapter are listed in the following box.

Safety Alert

HAZARDOUS DRUGS REQUIRING SPECIAL HANDLING

Hormonal Agents
Estrogens
Progesterone
Finasteride
Spironolactone

Retinoids
Acitretin
Isotretinoin[a]
Tretinoin

Immunosuppressants
Cyclosporine
Tacrolimus

Cytotoxic Drugs
Methotrexate
Fluorouracil

[a]Isotretinoin is not listed among the hazardous drugs; however, it meets the criteria for inclusion.

Adapalene. Adapalene [Differin] is a topical antiacne drug similar to tretinoin. Through actions in the cell nucleus, adapalene modulates inflammation, epithelial keratinization, and differentiation of follicular cells. As a result, the drug reduces formation of comedones and inflammatory lesions. Benefits take 8 to 12 weeks to develop. During the early weeks, adapalene may appear to exacerbate acne by affecting previously invisible lesions. In clinical trials, 0.1% adapalene gel was as effective as 0.025% tretinoin gel in reducing the total number of comedones, and it was more effective than tretinoin in reducing the total number of acne lesions and inflammatory lesions.

Adverse effects are limited to sites of application. The drug is not absorbed in quantifiable amounts, so systemic effects are absent. Common side effects include pruritus or burning immediately after application, erythema, dryness, and scaling. These are most likely during the first 2 to 4 weeks of treatment and tend to subside as treatment continues.

Adapalene increases the risk for developing sunburn and can intensify existing sunburn. Accordingly, all patients should apply a sunscreen and wear protective clothing. In addition, adapalene should not be used until existing sunburn has resolved.

Adapalene, by itself, is available in three 0.1% and 0.3% formulations—gel, cream, and lotion—for once-daily application in the evening. In addition, adapalene is available in a fixed-dose combination with benzoyl peroxide. Contact with the eyes, lips, angles of the nose, and mucous membranes should be avoided. It is also important to avoid contact with abraded, sunburned, or eczematous skin.

Tazarotene. Tazarotene [Avage, Tazorac] is indicated for topical therapy of acne, wrinkles, and psoriasis. Like tretinoin and adapalene, tazarotene is a derivative of vitamin A. For treatment of acne, tazarotene is available in a gel (0.05%, 0.1%) and cream (0.05%, 0.1%). The gel or cream is applied to affected areas of the face each evening. The face should be cleaned and dried before application. The most common side effects—itching, burning, and dry skin—occur more often with tazarotene than with tretinoin or adapalene. Like other retinoids, tazarotene sensitizes the skin to UV light, and hence patients should be advised to use a sunscreen and wear protective clothing. The basic pharmacology of tazarotene is discussed under *Topical Drugs for Psoriasis.*

Azelaic Acid

Azelaic acid [Azelex, Finacea 🍁] is a topical keratolytic drug for mild to moderate acne. It is also commonly prescribed for rosacea, a condition with some similarities to acne. Azelaic acid appears to work by suppressing growth of *P. acnes* and by decreasing proliferation of keratinocytes, thereby decreasing the thickness of the stratum corneum. In clinical trials, topical azelaic acid (20% cream) was as effective as 5% benzoyl peroxide, 0.05% tretinoin, or 2% erythromycin. For severe acne, azelaic acid was much less effective than oral isotretinoin. Adverse effects—which are uncommon and less intense than with tretinoin or benzoyl peroxide—include pruritus, burning, stinging, tingling, and erythema. Azelaic acid may reduce pigmentation in patients with dark complexions, so people using this product should be monitored for hypopigmentation. Azelaic acid 20% cream is applied twice daily by gently massaging a thin film into the affected area. Contact with the eyes, nose, and mouth should be avoided. Before application, the skin should be washed and patted dry.

Salicylic Acid

Salicylic acid is another topical keratolytic drug for mild to moderate acne. For acne, 0.5% to 2% strengths are used. It is available in multiple formulations: cleanser, cream, gel, liquid, lotion, and impregnated pads. As with azelaic acid, it is important to avoid contact with the eyes, nose, and mouth. Adverse effects such as local irritation and peeling are usually mild, but recall that Health Canada has issued safety alerts regarding the association between salicylic acid and severe allergic reactions. Salicylate toxicity is not a problem when applied only to the face; however, if acne is extensive and the drug is applied to the trunk, back, and other locations, this could possibly occur. Monitoring for signs and symptoms of salicylism (e.g., hyperpnea, tinnitus, nausea and vomiting, and mental status changes) is indicated.

Oral Drugs for Acne

Antibiotics

Oral antibiotics are used for moderate to severe acne. These drugs suppress growth of *P. acnes* and directly suppress inflammation. Oral antibiotics can be combined with a topical retinoid.

Doxycycline [Vibramycin, others] and minocycline [Minocin, others] are considered agents of choice. Tetracycline [generic] and erythromycin [Ery-Tab, others] are alternatives, but resistance to these drugs is common. With all antibiotics, benefits develop slowly, taking 3 to 6 months to become maximal. After symptoms have been controlled with an oral antibiotic, patients should switch to a topical antibiotic for long-term maintenance.

Isotretinoin

Actions and Use. Isotretinoin [Accutane 🍁, Amnesteem, Claravis, others], a derivative of vitamin A, is used to treat *severe nodulocystic acne vulgaris,* a condition for which this drug is highly effective. For most patients, a single course of therapy can produce complete and prolonged remission. Because isotretinoin can cause serious side effects, use is restricted to patients with severe, disfiguring acne that has not responded to more conventional agents, including oral antibiotics. Isotretinoin is highly teratogenic, and hence must not be used during pregnancy.

Isotretinoin has several actions that may contribute to antiacne effects. The drug decreases sebum production, sebaceous gland size, inflammation, and keratinization. In addition, by decreasing the availability of sebum, a nutrient for *P. acnes,* isotretinoin lowers the skin population of this microbe.

Pharmacokinetics. Absorption from the gastrointestinal (GI) tract is rapid but incomplete. Food greatly increases absorption. In the blood, isotretinoin is nearly 100% bound to albumin. The drug undergoes metabolism in the liver and possibly in cells of the intestinal wall. Excretion is by renal and biliary processes. The drug's half-life is 10 to 20 hours.

Adverse Effects

Common Effects. The most common reactions are nosebleeds (80%), inflammation of the lips (90%), inflammation of the eyes (40%), and dryness or itching of the skin, nose, and mouth (80%). About 15% of patients experience pain, tenderness, or stiffness in muscles, bones, and joints. Among pediatric patients, nearly 30% experience back pain. Less common reactions include skin rash, headache, hair loss, and peeling of skin from the palms and soles. Reduction in night vision has occurred, sometimes with sudden onset. The skin may become sensitized to UV light; patients should be advised to wear protective clothing or a sunscreen if responses to sunlight become exaggerated. Rarely, isotretinoin causes cataracts, optic neuritis, papilledema (edema of the optic disc), and pseudotumor cerebri (benign elevation of intracranial pressure). A 2017 safety alert from Health Canada noted the identification of a possible association between isotretinoin and erectile dysfunction.

Triglyceride levels may become elevated. Blood triglyceride content should be measured before treatment and periodically thereafter until effects on triglycerides have been evaluated. Alcohol can potentiate hypertriglyceridemia and should be avoided.

Although these adverse effects occur frequently, they usually reverse upon stopping treatment.

Depression. Isotretinoin may pose a risk for depression and suicide, although proof of a causal relationship is lacking. Nonetheless, because the potential consequences of depression are severe, steps should be taken to minimize risk. Accordingly, clinicians should ask patients to report signs of depression (e.g., depressed mood, loss of interest or pleasure) or thoughts of suicide. If these occur, isotretinoin should be withdrawn and psychiatric evaluation should be considered.

Drug Interactions. Adverse effects of isotretinoin can be increased by *tetracyclines* and *vitamin A.* Tetracyclines increase the risk for pseudotumor cerebri and papilledema. Vitamin A, a close relative of isotretinoin, can produce generalized intensification of isotretinoin toxicity. Because of the potential for increased toxicity, tetracyclines and vitamin A supplements should be discontinued before isotretinoin therapy.

Contraindication: Pregnancy. Isotretinoin is teratogenic and must not be used during pregnancy. The risks for use during pregnancy clearly outweigh any possible benefits. Major fetal abnormalities that have occurred include hydrocephalus, microcephaly, facial malformation, cleft palate, cardiovascular defects, and abnormal formation of the outer ear.

iPLEDGE Program. iPLEDGE is the name of a very strict risk management program designed to ensure that no woman starting isotretinoin *is* pregnant and that no woman taking isotretinoin *becomes* pregnant. Under iPLEDGE, all transactions involving isotretinoin must be processed through a *central automated system,* which tracks and verifies critical elements that control access to the drug. The program has rules that apply to the prescriber, patient, pharmacist, and wholesaler. Details regarding iPLEDGE are available online at www.ipledgeprogram.com.

Requirements for Female Patients. Each patient must receive oral and written warnings about the high risk for fetal harm if isotretinoin is taken during pregnancy. Pregnancy must be ruled out before the initial prescription and again before each monthly refill. Before the initial prescription, the patient must undergo *two* pregnancy tests, both of which must be negative. For the monthly refills, only one negative test result is required.

Each patient must use *two* effective forms of birth control, even if one of them is tubal ligation or vasectomy of the male partner. In addition, the patient must review educational material, provided through iPLEDGE, on contraceptive methods, possible reasons for contraceptive failure, and the importance of using effective contraception while taking a teratogenic drug. Birth control measures must be implemented at least 1 month before starting isotretinoin and must continue at least 1 month after stopping. Birth control is not required after hysterectomy or for women who commit to total abstinence from sexual intercourse.

Each patient must sign a Patient Information/Informed Consent document designed to reinforce the benefits and risks of isotretinoin use.

Each patient must be registered with iPLEDGE by her prescriber and must contact iPLEDGE (through the Internet or by phone) before starting treatment, once a month during treatment, and 1 month after stopping treatment. At each contact, the patient must answer questions on program requirements and must indicate her two chosen methods of birth control.

Requirements for Prescribers. Prescribers must register with iPLEDGE and must agree to follow key points of the iPLEDGE program, as described in the *iPLEDGE Program Guide to Best Practices for Isotretinoin.* Also, the prescriber must register each patient with iPLEDGE, enter the results of each monthly pregnancy test, and indicate what methods of contraception the patient is using. The initial prescription for isotretinoin and each monthly refill must be entered into the iPLEDGE system.

Requirements for Pharmacists. To dispense isotretinoin, pharmacists must be registered with iPLEDGE and must obtain the drug through an iPLEDGE-registered wholesaler. Every time a prescription for isotretinoin is filled, the pharmacist must do the following:

- Contact iPLEDGE for authorization
- Confirm with iPLEDGE that the prescription is no more than 7 days old
- Dispense no more than a 30-day supply
- Write the risk management authorization (RMA) number on the prescription

Preparations, Dosage, and Administration. Isotretinoin is available in standard capsules (10, 20, 30, and 40 mg) sold as Accutane 🍁, Amnesteem, and Claravis. The usual course of treatment is 0.5 to 1 mg/kg/day (taken in two divided doses with food) for 15 to 20 weeks. If needed, a second course may be given, but no sooner than 2 months after completing the first course.

Hormonal Agents

Hormonal therapies can be used for acne in young women. Combination oral contraceptives and spironolactone are the main agents employed. In both cases, benefits derive from decreasing androgen activity, leading to decreased production of sebum.

Oral Contraceptives. Four combination OCs—Estrostep, Ortho Tri-Cyclen, Beyaz, and YAZ—are approved for managing acne in women. Treatment is limited to females at least 15 years old who want contraception, have reached menarche, and have not responded to topical drugs. Acne may take 6 or more months to improve. Benefits are due primarily to the *estrogen* in combination OCs, not the progestin. Two mechanisms are involved: (1) suppression of ovarian androgen production and (2) increased production of *sex hormone–binding globulin,* a protein that binds androgens and thereby renders them inactive. By decreasing androgen availability, estrogens decrease production of sebum. Although only four OCs are approved for acne, all estrogen-containing OCs should work. Accordingly, selection among them should be based primarily on tolerability.

Spironolactone. Spironolactone [Aldactone] blocks a variety of steroid receptors, including those for aldosterone and sex hormones. Blockade of aldosterone receptors underlies the drug's use as a diuretic (see Chapter 41) as well as its use in heart failure (see Chapter 48). Blockade of androgen receptors underlies its benefits in females with acne. As a rule, spironolactone is added to the regimen after an OC has proved inadequate. This sequence makes sense because spironolactone is teratogenic, and hence contraception should be implemented before taking the drug. Adverse effects include menstrual irregularities, breast tenderness, and hyperkalemia.

DRUGS FOR ROSACEA

Rosacea is a chronic inflammatory facial condition that affects primarily the center of the face, especially the nose and medial cheeks. Common features include redness, flushing, and papules and pustules. (Unlike acne, comedones do not occur with this condition.) Over time, telangiectasia (vessel dilation with a spiderlike appearance) and rhinophyma (bulbous nose enlargement) develop. It is said that this condition is the reason for the rhinophyma of former President Bill Clinton (see https://www.rosacea.org/press/archive/20080401.php). This transformation can be observed by comparing photographs of his early presidency to those of his post-presidency. Rosacea is most common in people with fair complexions over 30 years of age. It has been estimated that up to 10% of this demographic are affected.

Previously, rosacea management included measures to avoid exacerbations (e.g., avoiding sun exposure, alcohol, and spicy foods), to treat telangiectasia (e.g., laser therapy), and to camouflage the affected area with green-tinted cosmetics. Various topical formulations of antimicrobials have been used to control the breakouts of papules and pustules; these include metronidazole (see Chapter 99), ivermectin (see Chapter 100), and azelaic acid (discussed in this chapter). It is unknown why these drugs are effective because rosacea is not an infection; however, some have suggested that exacerbations may have a microbial or parasitic component.

In 2013 a drug specifically targeted to the erythema associated with rosacea was introduced. Brimonidine topical gel [Mirvaso], is an alpha$_2$-adrenergic agonist that decreases erythema by vasoconstriction of blood vessels in the skin. (The pharmacology of alpha$_2$ agonists is discussed in Chapter 17.) Unfortunately, topical brimonidine is not very effective for most people. According to the Mirvaso website (https://www.mirvaso.com/redness-relief-photos), only 22% of subjects in clinical trials saw a 2-grade improvement after 29 days using the drug (9% of those taking the placebo reported a 2-grade improvement). In addition to this low improvement rate, the most common adverse reactions are worsening erythema (4%) and flushing (3%). Other localized reactions include contact dermatitis, burning, and other discomfort. The cost for a single 30-g container is approximately $522.

In 2017 a second alpha$_2$ agonist, topical oxymetazoline [Rhofade], was approved to manage the erythema of rosacea. (Oxymetazoline is introduced in Chapter 77.) As with brimonidine, the mechanism of action is vasoconstriction of cutaneous blood vessels. After using this drug for 29 days, 12% to 18% of subjects saw improvement compared with 5% to 9% of those using a placebo. The adverse effect profile is similar to that of topical brimonidine. Increased erythema occurred in 1% of subjects after 29 days, and another 1% experienced worsening of the inflammatory lesions. These percentages doubled after a year's use. A 30-g container of topical oxymetazoline costs $570.

Given the high cost and relatively low favorable result profiles for these new drugs, they do not appear to be the hoped-for panacea. Some patients, however, did experience significant improvement; therefore for patients with severe and chronic disease, these alpha$_2$ agonists may be an important part of an overall approach to management.

SUNSCREENS

Sunlight has multiple effects on the skin. In addition to promoting tanning, solar radiation can cause burns, premature aging of the skin, skin cancer, and immunosuppression. Sun exposure can also induce photosensitivity reactions to drugs. All of these effects are caused by UV radiation, and all can be greatly reduced by using a sunscreen.

Types of Ultraviolet Radiation: UVB and UVA

Solar UV radiation that reaches the earth's surface is classified by wavelength into two basic types: ultraviolet B (UVB: 290 to 320 nm) and ultraviolet A (UVA: 320 to 400 nm). UVA can be further subdivided into UVA2 (320 to 340 nm) and UVA1 (340 to 400 nm). Most (95%) of terrestrial UV radiation is UVA; only 5% is UVB. The intensity of UVA is fairly constant from morning to evening and from one day to the next throughout the year. In contrast, UVB is significant only between late spring and early fall, and, on any given day, it is moderate in the morning and evening and most intense around noon. UVA can penetrate glass but UVB cannot.

The dermatologic effects of UVA and UVB differ. UVA penetrates the epidermis and deep into the dermis. In contrast, UVB penetrates into the epidermis but goes no deeper. Tanning and sunburn are caused primarily by UVB. Because UVA penetrates much deeper than UVB, UVA is the primary cause of immunosuppression, photosensitive drug reactions, and photoaging of the skin (wrinkling, thickening, yellowing, breakdown of elastic fibers). Both UVA and UVB promote damage to DNA, and hence both can cause premalignant actinic keratoses, basal cell carcinoma, squamous cell carcinoma, and malignant and nonmalignant melanoma. Properties of UVA and UVB are shown in Table 105.3.

Benefits of Sunscreens

Sunscreens impede penetration of UV radiation to viable cells of the skin. As a result, sunscreens can protect against sunburn, photoaging of the skin, and photosensitivity reactions to certain drugs (e.g., tricyclic antidepressants, phenothiazines, sulfonamides, sulfonylureas). Sunscreens can also decrease the risk for actinic keratoses, squamous cell carcinoma, and melanoma. Whether sunscreens protect against basal cell carcinoma is unclear.

Compounds Employed as Sunscreens

There are two categories of sunscreens: *organic* screens (also known as *chemical* screens) and *inorganic* screens (also known as *physical* screens). Organic screens *absorb* UV radiation and then dissipate it as heat. Inorganic screens *scatter* UV radiation. At this time, 17 compounds are approved for use as sunscreens by the U.S. Food and Drug Administratiion (FDA) (Fig. 105.2).

Organic (Chemical) Screens

Most of the approved sunscreens are organic. Almost all of them absorb UVB, but only six absorb UVA. Of these six, five absorb UVA2, and only one—*avobenzone*—absorbs UVA1. Therefore, to provide protection against the full range of UV radiation, products must contain a mixture of compounds, one of which must be avobenzone.

Inorganic (Physical) Screens

Physical screens act primarily as barriers to the sun's rays. Hence, rather than absorbing solar radiation, they *reflect and*

PATIENT-CENTERED CARE ACROSS THE LIFE SPAN

Anti-Acne Drugs[a]

Life Stage	Patient Care Concerns
Children	Retinoids are not recommended for children younger than 12 years old with the exception of Atralin, a brand-name tretinoin gel for which labeling specifies use for patients age 10 years and older. Benzoyl peroxide, sulfacetamide, dapsone, azelaic acid, salicylic acid are recommended for age 12 and older. Hormone therapy for acne is not recommended for prepubertal children.
Pregnant women	Retinoids are teratogens. They are Pregnancy Risk Category X[b] with the exception of topical adapalene and tretinoin, which are categorized as Pregnancy Risk Category C.[b] Even so, labeling for adapalene and tretinoin recommends the avoidance of these drugs during pregnancy and verification of the absence of pregnancy prior to use because when dosed *orally* in animal studies, they caused adverse effects. These effects did not occur with topical use. Benzoyl peroxide is Pregnancy Risk Category C[b] because of a lack of animal studies. Both oral and topical dapsone are associated with complications in the neonate, including hyperbilirubinemia, methemoglobinemia, and hemolysis. Despite these risks, it is categorized as Pregnancy Risk Category C.[b] Topical salicylic acid is considered safe for use during pregnancy. It is available over the counter. A pregnancy risk category is not assigned for the topical formulation. Azelaic acid is Pregnancy Risk Category B. Although animal reproduction studies identified a potential for adverse effects, the amount of systemic absorption is minimal. Estrogen and progestins are Pregnancy Risk Category X[b]; therefore hormone therapy should not be prescribed for women who are pregnant.
Breast-feeding women	The amount of retinoids, benzoyl peroxide, dapsone, and salicylic acid excreted in breast milk is unknown. Caution is advised by the manufacturers. Systemic sulfonamides excreted in breast milk have caused kernicterus in breast-fed neonates. Topical sulfacetamide poses a risk for this complication if sufficient amounts are absorbed. Manufacturer labeling for azelaic acid gel and foam discourages breast-feeding by patients using this drug; however, the manufacturer of the cream urges caution. Hormone therapy may decrease milk production and protein content.[c]
Older adults	Safety and efficacy of some of these drugs, especially the retinoids, have not been established in older populations for whom anti-acne medication is not usually indicated. There are no special requirements for benzoyl peroxide, sulfacetamide, dapsone, azelaic acid, and salicylic acid. Hormone therapy for the purpose of acne treatment is not recommended for older adults.

[a]Life span considerations for common antibiotics are provided in Unit XVI.
[b]As of 2020, the FDA will no longer use Pregnancy Risk Categories. Please refer to Chapter 9 for more information
[c]According to the American Academy of Pediatrics, use of combination oral contraceptives is compatible with breast-feeding.

TABLE 105.3 ■ Properties of UVB and UVA Radiation

	Type of UV Radiation	
Property	**UVB**	**UVA**
Wavelength (nm)	290–320	320–400
Can penetrate glass	No	Yes
Skin penetration	Epidermis only	Epidermis/dermis
Effects on the skin:		
Burning	Major cause	Minor cause
Tanning	Major cause	Minor cause
Cancer	Major cause	Major cause
Photoaging		Sole cause
Photosensitive drug reactions		Sole cause

scatter sunlight, thereby preventing penetration to the skin. Only two agents are employed as physical screens: *titanium dioxide* and *zinc oxide.* Preparations containing these compounds are especially useful for protecting limited areas (e.g., nose, lips, tips of ears). In the formulations used today, titanium dioxide and zinc oxide are "micronized." As a result, they are clear when applied to the skin, unlike older formulations, which were white.

Sun Protection Factor

All sunscreen products are labeled with an SPF. The SPF is an index of protection against UVB. The SPF says nothing about protection against UVA.

The SPF is determined by shining UV light on adjacent regions of protected and unprotected skin and recording the time required for erythema (redness) to develop in both areas. The SPF is calculated by dividing the time required for erythema to develop in the protected region by the time required for erythema to develop in the unprotected region. For example, if the unprotected region developed erythema in 15 minutes

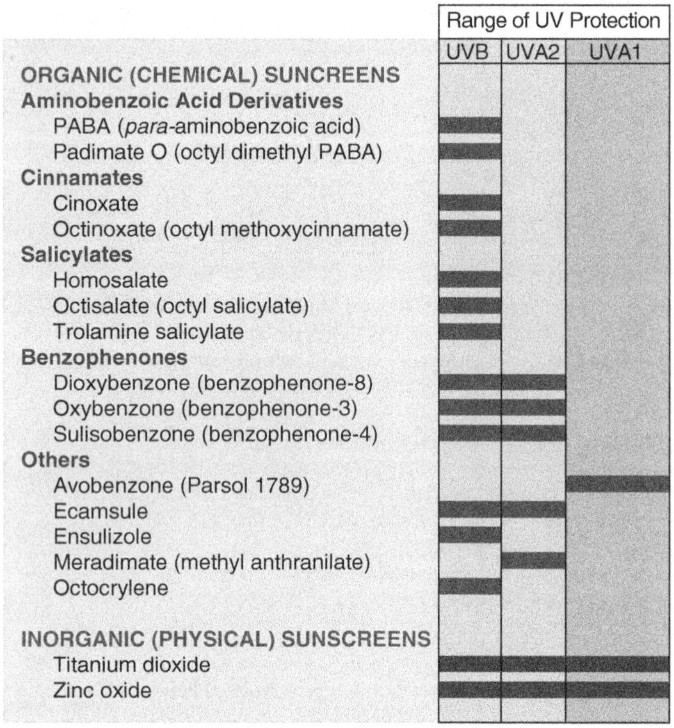

Fig. 105.2 ▪ Range of ultraviolet B and ultraviolet A protection conferred by U.S. Food and Drug Administration-approved sunscreens.

and the protected region developed erythema in 150 minutes, the sunscreen would have an SPF of 10 (150 divided by 15). Be aware that the methods for determining the SPF are not very precise. Hence, all products labeled with the same SPF may not provide an equal degree of protection.

The relationship between SPF and protection against sunburn is not linear. That is, an SPF of 30 does not indicate twice as much protection as an SPF of 15. In fact, as the SPF increases, the increment in protection gets progressively smaller. For example, SPF 15 indicates 93% block of UVB, SPF 30 indicates 96.7% block, and SPF 40 indicates 97.5% block. Because SPF values above 30 provide only a small additional benefit, the FDA no longer allows companies to advertise high SPF values (e.g., SPF 80). Instead, products with an SPF greater than 50 can be labeled only as SPF 50+.

Adverse Effects of Sunscreens

Contact dermatitis and photosensitivity reactions can occur, especially with products that contain *para*-aminobenzoic acid (PABA) derivatives. PABA-containing products should be avoided by people with allergies to benzocaine, sulfonamides, or thiazides, all of which can cross-react with PABA.

Rules for Sunscreen Labeling

In 2011, the FDA released new rules for labeling sunscreens. Under these rules, the label must indicate (1) the range of UV radiation protection and (2) the degree of water/sweat resistance. As in the past, labels will continue to indicate the SPF.

Range of UV Protection and SPF

All sunscreens protect against UVB radiation, but only some protect against UVA too. Products that protect against UVA *and* UVB are labeled *broad spectrum*. The label also shows the SPF, indicating the degree of UVB protection. Broad-spectrum sunscreens that have an SPF of 15 or higher can claim to protect against skin cancer and photoaging. Broad-spectrum agents with an SPF below 15 cannot make this claim. In fact, these products must carry a warning that they do *not* protect against skin cancer or photoaging. Products that protect only against UVB must carry the same warning. In summary, the new labels will allow consumers to distinguish between three basic groups of sunscreens:

- *Highly protective*—Broad-spectrum sunscreens with an SPF of 15 or higher. These protect against sunburn, skin cancer, and photoaging.
- *Moderately protective*—Broad-spectrum sunscreens with an SPF of 2 to 14. These protect against sunburn, but do not protect against skin cancer and photoaging.
- *Least protective*—Sunscreens with UVB protection only. These protect against sunburn, but do not protect against skin cancer and photoaging.

Water and Sweat Resistance

Sunscreens can no longer claim to be *waterproof* or *sweatproof*. Rather, they can claim to be *water resistant* or *sweat resistant*. Furthermore, they must indicate how long the resistance lasts, as determined by laboratory testing. Products that retain their SPF after 40 minutes of water exposure will be labeled *Water Resistant 40 Minutes*. Products that retain their water resistance after 80 minutes will be labeled *Water Resistant 80 Minutes*. Regardless of the stated duration of water and sweat resistance, the label must advise reapplication after swimming or sweating.

Safe Sun Exposure

To protect against skin damage from sunlight, we should use sunscreen and protective clothing and be mindful of the sun's hours of peak intensity.

Using a Sunscreen Effectively

Sunscreens must be used properly to achieve maximal benefit. The American Academy of Dermatology recommends using a sunscreen with coverage against both UVB and UVA. The SPF should be at least 15. Individuals who burn easily should use a higher SPF product. Protection is greatest when a sunscreen has been allowed to penetrate the skin in advance of exposure to the sun. Accordingly, sunscreens should be applied at least 30 minutes before going outdoors; sunscreens containing PABA or padimate O should be applied up to 2 hours in advance. The amount applied is an important determinant of protection; 1 ounce applied liberally to the body is considered adequate. Sunscreens should be reapplied after swimming and profuse sweating; failure to do so reduces the duration of protection. However, it is important to note that reapplication will not extend the period of protection beyond that indicated by the

SPF. That is, if treated skin can be expected to burn when sun exposure exceeds 2 hours, no amount of reapplication can prevent burning if the duration of exposure exceeds the limit.

Environmental factors play a part in sunscreen use. The intensity of UVB radiation is greatest between the hours of 10:00 AM and 4:00 PM. Accordingly, the need for a sunscreen is correspondingly high during this time. UV radiation can be reflected by painted surfaces, white sand, and snow, thereby augmenting total UV exposure. Accordingly, the contribution of reflected radiation should be considered when choosing a sunscreen. Clouds can filter out UV radiation. Nonetheless, the amount of UV light reaching the ground on a bright day with thin cloud cover can be as much as 80% of that reaching the ground on days that are sunny and clear. UV radiation can penetrate at least several centimeters of clear water; swimmers should be made aware of this fact.

Other Protection Measures

Sunscreens alone cannot completely protect against sun damage. Accordingly, to further reduce risk, you should wear sunglasses, protective clothing, and a wide-brimmed hat. In addition, you should avoid sun exposure in the middle of the day, especially between 10:00 AM and 4:00 PM. If you must be outside at these times, try to stay in the shade as much as possible.

TABLE 105.4 ▪ Treatments for Psoriasis

TOPICAL DRUGS	SYSTEMIC DRUGS
Glucocorticoids	**Conventional Agents**
Vitamin D_3 analogs	Methotrexate [Trexall, Rheumatrex]
Tazarotene [Tazorac]	Acitretin [Soriatane]
Anthralin [Dritho-Creme, Zithranol, Zithranol-RR]	Cyclosporine [Neoral, Gengraf, Sandimmune]
Salicylic acid	**Biologic Agents**
Tars	**Tumor Necrosis Factor Antagonists**
PHOTOTHERAPY	Adalimumab [Humira]
Coal tar plus UVB irradiation	Etanercept [Enbrel]
Photochemotherapy (PUVA therapy)	Infliximab [Remicade]
	Interleukin Antagonist
	Ustekinumab [Stelara]

PSORIASIS

Pathophysiology

Psoriasis is a common, chronic autoimmune inflammatory disorder that is characterized by plaque formation. There is no cure for psoriasis, but symptoms can usually be controlled with medication. Drug-induced remission is common and may last from a few weeks to many years.

Psoriasis has varying degrees of severity. Mild disease manifests as red patches covered with silvery scales; lesions typically appear on the scalp, elbows, knees, palms, and soles. Severe disease may involve the entire skin surface and mucous membranes; patients may develop superficial pustules, high fever, leukocytosis, and painful fissuring of the skin.

Symptoms result from two processes: accelerated maturation of epidermal cells (keratinocytes) and excessive activity of inflammatory cells. In recent years, it has become clear that inflammatory T cells (T lymphocytes) play a central role in the development and maintenance of psoriatic plaques. Hence, it now appears that psoriasis is primarily an inflammatory disorder, and that excessive proliferation of keratinocytes is a secondary response.

Overview of Treatment

Psoriasis can be treated with topical drugs, systemic drugs, or phototherapy. Several of the drugs employed suppress proliferation of keratinocytes. However, most antipsoriatic drugs suppress the activity of inflammatory cells. Treatment options are shown in Table 105.4.

Treatment is based on symptom severity. For mild to moderate psoriasis, topical glucocorticoids and emollients are usually adequate. Adjuncts or alternative medications include keratolytic agents (e.g., salicylic acid), topical retinoids (e.g., tazarotene), and vitamin D_3 analogs (e.g., calcipotriene). For patients with moderate symptoms, coal tar or anthralin may be added to the regimen. Topical therapy with tar and anthralin can be enhanced by exposing the skin to UVB light. When the affected area includes the face or intertriginous (skinfold) areas, topical immunomodulators such as tacrolimus or pimecrolimus may be substituted for glucocorticoids. Treatment options for more severe psoriasis include phototherapy or systemic treatment with methotrexate, acitretin, and other drugs.

Topical Drugs for Psoriasis

Glucocorticoids

In the United States, glucocorticoids are the most commonly used topical drugs for psoriasis. Benefits derive from suppressing the activity of inflammatory cells. Preparations with super-high potency are employed where plaques are thickest. However, super-high-potency agents should not be applied to the face, groin, axilla, or genitalia. Why? Because skin in these regions is especially vulnerable to glucocorticoid-induced atrophy. Additionally, secondary infections may occur in intertriginous (skinfold) regions and facial dermatoses may occur with the use of topical glucocorticoid application to the face.

Vitamin D_3 Analogs

Two synthetic analogs of vitamin D_3—*calcipotriene* [Dovonex, Calcitrene, Sorilux] and *calcitriol* [Vectical, Silkis 🍁]—are approved for topical therapy of mild to moderate psoriasis. Benefits derive from inducing differentiation of epidermal cells and from inhibiting proliferation of keratinocytes. Responses take a month or more to develop.

Adverse effects are generally mild. Local reactions—itching, irritation, and erythema—are most common. Unlike the glucocorticoids, the vitamin D_3 analogs do not cause thinning of the skin. With topical use, calcipotriene and calcitriol can cause moderate hypercalcemia, although the clinical significance is unclear. In animal studies, topical calcitriol has caused skeletal defects in the developing fetus; therefore, there is a possibility of fetal risk in humans. Animal data suggest that the vehicle used for calcitriol may enhance the ability of UV radiation to induce skin cancer. Accordingly, patients using calcitriol should minimize exposure of treated skin to natural and artificial sunlight.

Calcipotriene [Dovonex, Calcitrene, Sorilux] is supplied as a 0.005% solution, cream, foam, and ointment. A thin layer of the medication is applied to the affected areas of the skin twice daily.

Calcitriol [Vectical, Silkis 🍁] is supplied as a 0.0003% ointment in 100-gm tubes. Application is made twice daily to affected areas, but not to the face. The maximum weekly dose is 200 gm.

Tazarotene

Tazarotene [Tazorac] is a vitamin A derivative indicated for topical therapy of mild to moderate psoriasis. Following application to the skin, tazarotene is rapidly converted to tazarotenic acid, its active form. Tazarotenic acid binds with specific retinoic acid receptors, and thereby normalizes differentiation and proliferation of epidermal cells. In clinical trials, application of a 0.1% tazarotene gel once daily for 12 weeks produced a significant reduction in lesions in 50% to 70% of patients. Benefits were about equivalent to those seen with 0.05% fluocinonide, a high-potency topical glucocorticoid. Tazarotenic acid stays in the skin long after application of tazarotene has stopped. As a result, benefits may persist for several months. Use of tazarotene for acne is discussed earlier in the chapter.

Adverse effects are limited largely to the skin. The most common local reactions are itching, burning, stinging, dry skin, and redness. Less common effects include rash, desquamation, contact dermatitis, inflammation, fissuring, and bleeding. Tazarotene sensitizes the skin to sunlight. Accordingly, patients should be advised to use a sunscreen and wear protective clothing.

Tazarotene is available as a gel or cream in two concentrations: 0.05% and 0.1%. The medication is applied once daily in the evening. No more than 20% of the body surface area should be covered. Wet skin should be dried before application.

Anthralin

Anthralin [Dritho-Creme HP, Zithranol, Zithranol-RR] has only one indication: topical treatment of psoriasis. The drug inhibits DNA synthesis and thereby suppresses proliferation of hyperplastic epidermal cells.

Anthralin is an older drug that is marketed in the United States; however, the FDA has not determined that it is safe and effective. Still, the drug is included in some psoriasis management guidelines, so you may have patients who are using this drug regardless of the FDA determination. (Additional information on unapproved prescription drugs is available at http://www.fda.gov/Drugs/GuidanceComplianceRegulatoryInformation/EnforcementActivitiesbyFDA/SelectedEnforcementActionsonUnapprovedDrugs/default.htm.)

Anthralin may cause local irritation, especially when applied in concentrations above 1%. Erythema (redness) may develop in normal skin adjacent to areas of treatment. Severe conjunctivitis can develop following contact with the eyes. Systemic toxicity has not been documented. Anthralin preparations can stain clothing, skin, and hair.

Anthralin is supplied as a 1% shampoo (Zithranol), a 1% cream (Dritho-Creme HP), and a 1.2% cream (Zithranol-RR). After lathering, the shampoo is left on the wet scalp for 3 to 5 minutes before rinsing. The cream is applied to lesions at bedtime and allowed to remain in place overnight. Stains can be avoided by wearing old clothing and by covering treated areas with a dressing.

Tars

Tars suppress DNA synthesis, mitotic activity, and cell proliferation. Coal tar is the tar employed most frequently. Preparations that contain juniper tar, birch tar, and pine tar are also available. Tar-containing products (e.g., shampoos, lotions, creams) are used to treat psoriasis and other chronic disorders of the skin. Tars have an unpleasant odor and can cause irritation, stinging, and burning. They may also stain the skin and hair. Systemic toxicity does not occur.

Systemic Drugs for Psoriasis: Conventional Agents

The conventional systemic drugs—methotrexate, acitretin, and cyclosporine—are oral agents that provide effective therapy for psoriasis, but also pose a risk for serious harm. Accordingly, these drugs are reserved for patients with moderate to severe psoriasis that has not responded to safer treatments. To reduce risk, systemic drugs can be alternated with phototherapy. All three have been designated as hazardous drugs by NIOSH and require special handling. Methotrexate meets the requirement as an antineoplastic drug; acitretin is high risk for those who are pregnant; and cyclosporine is carcinogenic.

Methotrexate

The basic pharmacology of methotrexate [Trexall, Rheumatrex] is discussed in Chapter 102. Consideration here is limited to the treatment of psoriasis.

Actions and Use in Psoriasis. Methotrexate is a cytotoxic agent that shows some selectivity for tissues with a high growth fraction (i.e., tissues with a large percentage of actively dividing cells). Benefits in psoriasis result from reduced proliferation of epidermal cells. Methotrexate is highly toxic and should be used only in patients with severe, debilitating psoriasis that has not responded to other therapy.

Adverse Effects. Methotrexate is administered systemically, and *toxicity* can be severe. Death has occurred. Patients should be fully informed of the risks of treatment. Close medical supervision is required. Gastrointestinal effects (diarrhea, ulcerative stomatitis) are the most frequent reasons for interrupting therapy. Blood dyscrasias (anemia, leukopenia, thrombocytopenia) from bone marrow suppression are an additional major concern. With prolonged use, even at relatively low doses, methotrexate can cause *significant harm to the liver.* Accordingly, hepatic function must be monitored; a liver biopsy is the best method for assessing injury. Methotrexate can cause congenital anomalies and fetal death, and hence is contraindicated during pregnancy.

Dosage and Administration. Methotrexate may be administered PO, IM, or IV. Various dosing schedules have been developed. In one schedule, the drug is administered once a week as a single large dose (10 to 25 mg). In another schedule, three smaller doses (2.5 to 5 mg) are administered at 12-hour intervals; this dosing sequence is repeated weekly. Regardless of the schedule chosen, dosage must be individualized.

Acitretin

Acitretin [Soriatane] is the principal active metabolite of etretinate, a highly toxic drug that has been withdrawn. The major difference between the two drugs is pharmacokinetic: Whereas etretinate has a very long half-life (120 *days*), the half-life of acitretin is much shorter (only 49 *hours*). Accordingly, acitretin is cleared from the body much faster than etretinate. Although acitretin is less dangerous than etretinate, it still can cause serious harm, especially injury to the liver and to the developing fetus.

Mechanism of Action. Acitretin acts on epithelial cells to inhibit keratinization, proliferation, and differentiation. These actions probably contribute to its beneficial effects. Benefits may also derive from anti-inflammatory and immunomodulatory actions.

Therapeutic Use. Acitretin is indicated for severe psoriasis, including erythrodermic and generalized pustular types. In clinical trials, the drug produced a 60% to 70% reduction in the severity and area of symptoms. The relapse rate was 40% at 12 weeks after termination of treatment. Because side effects are very common and sometimes severe, acitretin should be reserved for patients who have not responded to safer drugs.

Pharmacokinetics. Administration is oral, and absorption is enhanced by food. In the blood, acitretin is 99.9% bound to plasma proteins. The drug undergoes extensive metabolism followed by excretion in the urine and bile. Its half-life is 49 hours. If taken with alcohol, acitretin will be converted to etretinate.

Adverse Effects. Adverse effects are very common. Hair loss and skin peeling occur in 50% to 75% of patients. Other dermatologic effects (dry skin, nail disorders, pruritus) occur in 25% to 50% of patients. Mucous membranes are affected, causing rhinitis (25% to 50%), inflammation of the lips (25% to 50%), dry mouth (10% to 25%), nosebleed (10% to 25%), and gingival bleeding, gingivitis, and stomatitis. Other common reactions include erythematous rash, bone and joint pain, spinal hyperostosis, dry eyes, and paresthesias. In addition, acitretin can elevate plasma triglycerides and reduce levels of HDL cholesterol (good cholesterol). Signs of liver damage (elevation of aminotransferase activity) develop in one-third of patients, but normally resolve when treatment is stopped.

Drug Interactions. Alcohol promotes conversion of acitretin to etretinate and can thereby increase the risk for adverse effects and toxicity. It can also greatly prolong the risk for teratogenic effects (see *Contraindication: Pregnancy,* in the next section). Accordingly, women of childbearing age should be warned against drinking alcohol. Acitretin can reduce the efficacy of progestin-only OCs, so other forms of contraception are preferred. Because acitretin is a derivative of vitamin A, combining it with vitamin A supplements may pose a risk for vitamin A toxicity. Both acitretin and tetracycline can cause pseudotumor cerebri (intracranial hypertension); therefore, combining the drugs is not recommended. In addition, acitretin should not be combined with methotrexate and other drugs that can damage the liver.

Contraindication: Pregnancy. *Acitretin is embryotoxic and teratogenic and therefore must not be used during pregnancy because the risks of use during pregnancy clearly outweigh any possible benefits.* Major human fetal abnormalities that have been reported include encephalocele (herniation of the brain through a skull defect), reduced cranial volume, facial malformation, cardiovascular defects, absence of terminal phalanges, and malformations of the hips, ankles, and forearms.

The manufacturer has developed a program for women of childbearing age who will be prescribed acitretin. This program, Do Your P.A.R.T. (Pregnancy Prevention Actively Required During and After Treatment), was developed to help patients avoid pregnancy. Additional information is available at www.soriatane.com/pdf/do_your_part.pdf.

Before acitretin is given to women of reproductive age, pregnancy should be ruled out and *two* reliable methods of contraception implemented before beginning treatment. Contraception should be initiated at least 1 month before treatment and should continue for at least 3 years after treatment has ceased. Women should be thoroughly counseled about the potential for fetal harm. If pregnancy occurs, acitretin should be discontinued immediately and the patient should contact the prescriber to discuss the effects on the fetus.

Preparations, Dosage, and Administration. Acitretin [Soriatane] is available in 10-, 17.5-, and 25-mg capsules for oral dosing. The dosage for psoriasis is 25 or 50 mg once daily, taken with a meal to facilitate absorption. As a rule, administration should cease when lesions have sufficiently resolved.

Cyclosporine

Cyclosporine [Neoral, Sandimmune, Gengraf] is a powerful immunosuppressant that inhibits proliferation of B cells and T cells. In patients with psoriasis, the drug produces rapid improvement. Unfortunately, cyclosporine can cause kidney damage and other serious harm, and hence should be used only after treatment with other drugs has failed. The basic pharmacology of cyclosporine is presented in Chapter 69.

Systemic Drugs for Psoriasis: Biologic Agents

Like the conventional systemic drugs, the biologic agents are reserved for patients with moderate to severe psoriasis that has not responded to other treatments. In the United States, four biologic agents are available. Three of these drugs—etanercept, infliximab, and adalimumab—block tumor necrosis factor (TNF). The fourth drug—ustekinumab—inhibits interleukin-12 (IL-12) and interleukin-23 (IL-23). All four drugs suppress immune function and thereby increase the risk for serious infection. However, these drugs don't cause the serious acute toxicities—hepatotoxicity and nephrotoxicity—seen with the conventional systemic drugs. All of the biologic agents are administered by injection.

Tumor Necrosis Factor Antagonists

Drugs that inhibit TNF can suppress immune function and can thereby reduce inflammation in psoriasis. Three TNF antagonists are approved for the disease: *adalimumab* [Humira], *etanercept* [Enbrel], and *infliximab* [Remicade]. These drugs are very effective and have become first-line treatments for moderate to severe psoriasis. However, because of their immunosuppressant actions, the TNF antagonists pose a risk for serious opportunistic infections and possibly cancer. Dosages for psoriasis are as follows:

- Adalimumab—80 mg subQ initially, then 40 mg subQ every other week thereafter
- Etanercept—50 mg subQ twice a week
- Infliximab—5 mg/kg, infused IV over 2 or more hours, at 0, 2, and 6 weeks, and then once every 8 weeks thereafter

The basic pharmacology of the TNF antagonists is presented in Chapter 73.

Ustekinumab, an Interleukin Antagonist

Actions and Uses. Ustekinumab [Stelara] is a first-in-class interleukin antagonist approved for adults with moderate to severe plaque psoriasis. Benefits derive from blocking the actions of IL-12 and IL-23, cytokines that promote inflammatory responses, immune responses, and overproduction of skin cells. Interleukin-12 and IL-23 work in part by promoting the differentiation of CD4+ T lymphocytes into helper T cells, essential components of the immune system. Ustekinumab is very effective: About two-thirds of patients experience at least a 75% reduction in symptoms. Furthermore, in a trial comparing ustekinumab with etanercept (a TNF antagonist), more patients responded to ustekinumab. Like the other biologic therapies for psoriasis, ustekinumab is administered by injection. However, since injections are made just once every 12 weeks, ustekinumab is more convenient than the other agents.

Adverse Effects. Ustekinumab is generally well tolerated. In short-term clinical trials, adverse effects were usually mild and self-limited, and their incidence was no greater than with placebo. However, because ustekinumab suppresses immune function, it may pose a risk for serious infection and cancer (just like the TNF antagonists). Accordingly, patients should be checked for latent tuberculosis before starting treatment and should be advised to report serious infections that develop during treatment. Since experience with ustekinumab is limited, long-term safety is unknown.

Preparations, Dosage, and Administration. Ustekinumab [Stelara] is supplied in solution (45 mg/0.5 mL, 90 mg/mL) for subQ injection. Dosage depends on body weight. For adults who weigh *100 kg or less,* dosing consists of 45 mg on days 1 and 28, followed by 45 mg every 12 weeks thereafter. For adults who weigh *more than 100 kg,* dosing consists of 90 mg on days 1 and 28, followed by 90 mg every 12 weeks thereafter. At this time, ustekinumab must be administered by a healthcare provider. The drug is not approved for self-injection by patients.

Phototherapy

Coal Tar Plus Ultraviolet B Irradiation

This procedure involves sequential treatment with coal tar followed by UV irradiation. In the first step, affected regions are covered with 1% coal tar ointment for 8 to 10 hours, after which the coal tar is washed off. In the second step, the area is exposed to short-wave UV radiation (ultraviolet B, UVB). This procedure is very safe and produces remission in 80% of patients. Unfortunately, treatment is expensive and time consuming (up to 30 treatments are needed), and patients dislike being coated with smelly coal tar.

Photochemotherapy (PUVA Therapy)

Photochemotherapy combines the use of long-wave UV radiation (ultraviolet A, UVA) with methoxsalen [Oxsoralen], an orally administered photosensitive drug. Methoxsalen belongs to a chemical family known as *psoralens*. In response to UVA light shined on the skin, methoxsalen is thought to undergo a photochemical reaction with DNA, resulting in the formation of a DNA-psoralen complex. This alteration in DNA structure is thought to underlie the ability of photochemotherapy to decrease proliferation of epidermal cells. Adverse effects associated with the procedure include pruritus, nausea, and erythema. In addition, the process may accelerate aging of the skin and may increase the risk for skin cancer. Photochemotherapy is indicated for patients with extensive, active psoriasis who have not responded adequately to more conventional therapy. An alternative name for photochemotherapy is *PUVA therapy* (PUVA is an abbreviation derived from *psoralen* and *ultraviolet A*).

PATIENT-CENTERED CARE ACROSS THE LIFE SPAN

Drugs for Psoriasis

Life Stage	Patient Care Concerns
Children	Children under 12 years of age should use lower-potency glucocorticoids. Cyclosporine and methotrexate are approved for use in children. Calcitriol is approved for use in children, but safety has not been established for calcipotriene. Safety also has not been established for anthralin. When used in children, acitretin may affect growth potential; skeletal changes may occur with long-term use. TNF antagonists are approved in children only for nondermatologic indications. Methoxsalen is approved for the treatment of vitiligo in children age 12 years and older. Ustekinumab is not approved for use in children.
Pregnant women	Methotrexate and acitretin are Pregnancy Risk Category X.[a] These drugs should never be used by women who are pregnant. Glucocorticoids are Pregnancy Risk Category C[a]; there is a very small increased risk for cleft palate. Other Pregnancy Risk Category C drugs are vitamin D_3 analogs, anthralin, cyclosporine, and methoxsalen. TNF antagonists and ustekinumab are Pregnancy Risk Category B.[a] No adverse pregnancy outcomes have been associated with coal tar preparations.
Breast-feeding women	Breast-feeding is contraindicated for patients receiving therapy with methotrexate and TNF antagonists. Manufacturer labeling does not recommend breast-feeding for patients using anthralin, acitretin, cyclosporine, and methoxsalen. Caution is recommended for patients using vitamin D_3 analogs and ustekinumab. For tar products, glucocorticoids, and other topical drugs, the likelihood of transfer to the child comes from contact with medicated skin more than from breast milk. Care must be taken to avoid accidental transfer of medication to the infant.
Older adults	Glucocorticoid-associated skin atrophy may be pronounced in older adults. Older patients may also have increased severity of adverse skin effects of vitamin D_3 analogs and increased sensitivity to the effects of TNF antagonists and methoxsalen.

[a]As of 2020, the FDA will no longer use Pregnancy Risk Categories. Please refer to Chapter 9 for more information.

DRUGS FOR ACTINIC KERATOSES

Actinic keratoses (AKs) are rough, scaly, red or brown papules caused by chronic exposure to sunlight. Lesions typically develop on the face, scalp, forearms, and backs of the hands. A small percentage (0.25% to 1% per year) evolve into squamous cell carcinoma. However, although the *percentage* is small, the *absolute amount* is large: In the United States, nearly half of all skin cancers (about 500,000 cases) begin as AKs. AK treatment consists of *topical* drugs—fluorouracil, diclofenac, imiquimod, and aminolevulinic acid—and physical interventions: cryotherapy, curettage, excision, and laser resurfacing. Of these options, cryotherapy (freezing with liquid nitrogen) is used most, owing to its speed, simplicity, and effectiveness.

Fluorouracil

The basic pharmacology of fluorouracil [Carac, Fluoroplex, Efudex 🍁] is discussed in Chapter 102. Discussion here is limited to the treatment of dermatologic disorders.

Actions and Uses in Dermatology

Fluorouracil is indicated for the topical treatment of *multiple AKs* and *superficial basal cell carcinoma.* Cytotoxic effects result from the disruption of DNA and RNA synthesis. A course of topical treatment elicits the following sequence of responses: (1) mild inflammation; (2) severe inflammation, often with burning, stinging, and vesicle formation; (3) tissue disintegration, characterized by erosion, ulceration, and necrosis; and (4) healing. Although fluorouracil is applied for only 2 to 6 weeks, the events just described may require 3 or more months for completion. Treatment is effective in over 90% of those who can tolerate a full course.

Adverse Effects

Among the more frequent reactions are itching, burning, rash, inflammation, and increased sensitivity to sunlight. Intense, burning pain develops occasionally. Darkening of the skin is rare. Absorption is insufficient to cause systemic toxicity.

Preparations and Administration

Topical fluorouracil is available under three brand names: *Carac* (microspheres in a 0.5% cream), *Fluoroplex* (1% cream), and *Efudex* 🍁 (5% cream). Carac is applied once daily; Efudex 🍁 and Fluoroplex are applied twice daily. Treatment should continue until a stage-three response (tissue disintegration) develops, usually within 2 to 6 weeks. Complete healing may not occur for another 1 to 2 months. Because it is categorized as an antineoplastic agent, it is among the hazardous drugs identified by NIOSH as requiring special handling.

Diclofenac Sodium

Diclofenac sodium [Solaraze], in a 3% gel, was the first nonsteroidal anti-inflammatory drug (NSAID) approved for topical use. The only indication for Solaraze is AK.[a] Topical diclofenac is better tolerated than fluorouracil, but is less effective and treatment takes longer. In clinical trials, twice-daily application for 60 to 90 days produced complete clearing in 50% of patients. The mechanism underlying benefits is unknown. The most common side effects are dry skin, itching, redness, and rash at the application site. Diclofenac may sensitize the skin to UV radiation, so patients should avoid sunlamps and minimize exposure to sunlight. Systemic absorption is low (10%), and therefore the risk for GI injury is much less than with oral diclofenac and other NSAIDs.

Imiquimod

Imiquimod cream [Aldara, Zyclara], originally developed for venereal warts (discussed later in chapter), was approved for AK in 2004. Benefits derive from stimulating innate and cell-mediated immunity. Imiquimod requires a prescription, but is applied at home. Imiquimod is better tolerated than fluorouracil, but less effective, causing complete clearance in only 45% of patients, compared with 90% for fluorouracil. Also, treatment takes much longer (16 weeks vs. 2 to 6 weeks with fluorouracil). In clinical trials, 33% of patients experienced local reactions: redness, swelling, sores, blisters, itching, burning, scabbing, and crusting. Of note, lesion clearance correlated with the intensity of side effects, suggesting that an inflammatory reaction is needed to produce a clinical response. Imiquimod increases sensitivity to UV radiation, and hence patients should minimize sun exposure, use a sunscreen, and wear protective clothing. For treatment of AKs, imiquimod is available in three formulations, a 2.5% cream [Zyclara], a 3.75% cream [Zyclara], and a 5% cream [Aldara].

Aminolevulinic Acid Plus Blue Light

Topical aminolevulinic acid [Levulan Kerastick], in conjunction with blue light photoactivation, is an alternative therapy for AKs of the face and scalp. Treatment takes place in two steps. First, the prescriber applies a 20% solution of aminolevulinic acid to AK lesions. Fourteen to 18 hours later, the prescriber photoactivates the drug by exposing lesions to 1000 seconds of blue light, using the Blu-U Blue Light supplied by the manufacturer. In clinical trials, 66% of patients experienced complete clearing by 8 weeks after a single treatment, and 77% of patients experienced clearing of 75% or more. The mechanism underlying benefits is complex and incompletely understood. Local effects—burning, stinging, redness, and edema—occur in nearly all patients. Because aminolevulinic acid is light sensitive, patients should protect treated areas from exposure to sunlight and bright indoor light before blue light exposure. The best protection is a wide-brimmed hat; sunscreens won't help.

PATIENT-CENTERED CARE ACROSS THE LIFE SPAN

Drugs for Actinic Keratoses and Atopic Dermatitis

Life Stage	Patient Care Concerns
Children	Fluorouracil and aminolevulinic acid are not approved for children. Diclofenac is approved for children 16 years of age or older and imiquimod for children 12 years of age or older. Tacrolimus and pimecrolimus are approved for children age 2 years and older.
Pregnant women	Fluorouracil is Pregnancy Risk Category X[a] and should not be used by pregnant women. Imiquimod, aminolevulinic acid, tacrolimus, and pimecrolimus are Pregnancy Risk Category C.[a] Diclofenac is Pregnancy Risk Category B.[a]
Breast-feeding Women	Breast-feeding is not recommended for patients receiving therapy with fluorouracil, diclofenac, tacrolimus, and pimecrolimus. Labeling recommends caution for those taking imiquimod and aminolevulinic acid.
Older adults	Older patients taking diclofenac experienced adverse effects at lower doses, and peptic ulcer development was common. No age-specific precautions were listed for other drugs for these conditions.

[a]As of 2020, the FDA will no longer use Pregnancy Risk Categories. Please refer to Chapter 9 for more information.

DRUGS FOR ATOPIC DERMATITIS (ECZEMA)

Atopic dermatitis, also known as eczema, is a chronic inflammatory skin disease. The condition is characterized by dry, scaly skin and intense pruritus that often leads to scratching and rubbing, which in turn can lead to erythema, abrasions, rash, erosions with an exudate, and increased susceptibility to skin infection. Continued scratching will also typically result in lichenification of the affected skin. The underlying cause is abnormal activity of T lymphocytes. First-line therapy consists of *moisturizers* (e.g., Cetaphil Moisturizing Cream, Eucerin Original Cream) and *topical glucocorticoids.* Unfortunately, the glucocorticoids can cause skin atrophy, hypopigmentation, telangiectasis (permanent focal red lesions), and, in high doses, possible systemic effects, including adrenal suppression. If topical glucocorticoids are insufficient, patients

[a]Two other topical formulations of diclofenac, sold as Voltaren Gel and Flector, are available to relieve musculoskeletal pain (see Chapter 71).

may be treated with a *topical immunosuppressant* (discussed next). A *sedating antihistamine* can help control itching and can facilitate sleeping at night.

Topical Immunosuppressants

Two topical immunosuppressants—tacrolimus and pimecrolimus—are approved for atopic dermatitis. Both drugs are *calcineurin inhibitors* (see Chapter 69). Although effective against atopic dermatitis, both drugs may pose a risk for skin cancer and lymphoma. Because of this potential for serious harm, tacrolimus and pimecrolimus are considered second-line drugs for atopic dermatitis and should be reserved for patients who have not responded to glucocorticoids.

Tacrolimus Ointment

Tacrolimus [Protopic], available as Prograf for preventing organ transplant rejection (see Chapter 69), is available as an ointment for moderate to severe atopic dermatitis. The drug relieves symptoms by attenuating local immune responses. Specifically, the drug inhibits calcineurin and thereby suppresses the activity of T cells and decreases the release of inflammatory mediators from cutaneous mast cells and basophils. The result is reduced inflammation.

Systemic absorption of topical tacrolimus is low, and it gets even lower as the skin heals. Absolute bioavailability is less than 0.05%. Blood levels of tacrolimus are usually low.

Tacrolimus ointment is generally well tolerated. The most common side effects are erythema, pruritus, and burning sensations at the application site. As the skin heals, these local reactions abate. In children, tacrolimus may increase the risk for varicella-zoster virus infection. Adverse effects associated with *systemic* tacrolimus (nephrotoxicity, neurotoxicity, hypertension, diarrhea, nausea) have not occurred with topical therapy. Unlike topical glucocorticoids, tacrolimus does not cause thinning of the skin.

There is concern that tacrolimus may pose a risk for *cancer*. The drug increases the incidence of skin cancer in laboratory animals exposed to UV light. In mice, tacrolimus increases the incidence of lymphoma. There have been reports of skin cancer and lymphoma in humans, although a causal relationship has not been established. To reduce any risk for skin cancer, patients should protect treated areas from direct sunlight and should avoid sunlamps and tanning beds, and nurses involved in drug administration should following NIOSH guidelines (see Table 105.3).

Tacrolimus ointment [Protopic] is available in two concentrations: 0.03% and 0.1%. Adults may use either formulation; children ages 2 to 16 years should use the 0.03% formulation; and children younger than 2 years should not use the drug. All patients should apply a thin layer twice daily. Occlusive dressings should be avoided. Treatment should be intermittent or short term.

Pimecrolimus Cream

Pimecrolimus 1% cream [Elidel] is a topical immunosuppressant approved for mild to moderate atopic dermatitis. The drug is very similar to tacrolimus with regard to mechanism, therapeutic effects, and adverse effects. In clinical trials, twice-daily application for 3 weeks reduced signs and symptoms of eczema by 72%. Initial improvement could be seen in 2 days. Pimecrolimus may be less effective than topical glucocorticoids. Although studies comparing pimecrolimus directly with tacrolimus have not been done, clinical efficacy of the drugs appears similar.

Pimecrolimus is generally well tolerated. The most common adverse effects are erythema, pruritus, and burning sensations at the application site, especially during the first few days of treatment. As with tacrolimus, there have been reports of skin cancer and lymphoma, but a causal relationship has not been established. Like tacrolimus, pimecrolimus sensitizes the skin to UV light, and hence patients should use a sunscreen and should limit exposure to natural and artificial sunlight. Systemic absorption of pimecrolimus is minimal; in clinical trials, blood levels were at or below the limit of detection. As with tacrolimus, prolonged treatment should be avoided.

AGENTS USED TO REMOVE WARTS

Warts are small, benign tumors that form in the skin and mucous membranes. They are caused by infection of squamous epithelial cells with human papillomavirus (HPV), of which there are roughly 100 types. Most warts resolve spontaneously within a few months, but some can last for years. The discussion that follows focuses primarily on management of venereal warts.

Venereal Warts

Venereal warts form around the cervix, vulva, urethra, glans penis, and anus and anal canal. Most are caused by two types of HPV, known as HPV-6 and HPV-11. Two other types—HPV-16 and HPV-18—are responsible for most cervical cancers. As discussed in Chapter 68, an HPV vaccine, sold as *Gardasil*, can protect against all four HPV types, and hence can help prevent venereal warts as well as cancer of the cervix. Another HPV vaccine, sold as *Cervarix*, protects only against HPV-16 and HPV-18, so it can help prevent cervical cancer but not venereal warts.

Infection with HPV can be transmitted by sexual contact. Individuals with anogenital warts should be warned that they can transmit the infection to sexual partners. Partners of infected individuals should be examined for warts. Using a condom can reduce the risk for transmission.

Genital warts can be removed in two basic ways: with *topical drugs* or with *physical measures* such as cryotherapy (freezing), electrodesiccation (destruction with an electric current), laser surgery, and conventional surgery. Physical measures are much faster than drugs but also more painful. Neither drugs nor physical measures can eradicate the virus because even after successful wart removal, the virus remains. Treatments for genital warts are shown in Table 105.5.

TABLE 105.5 ▪ Treatment and Prevention of Venereal Warts

TREATMENT	
External genital	*Patient administered:* • Podofilox 0.5% solution or gel (topical) *or* • Imiquimod 3.75% or 5% cream (topical) *or* • Kunecatechins (sinecatechins) 15% ointment (topical) *Provider administered:* • Cryotherapy with liquid nitrogen or cryoprobe *or* • Podophyllin 10%–25% (topical) *or* • TCA or BCA 80%–90% (topical) *or* • Surgical excision
Anal	Cryotherapy with liquid nitrogen *or* TCA or BCA (80%–90%) applied to warts *or* Surgical excision
Vaginal	Cryotherapy with liquid nitrogen *or* TCA or BCA (80%–90%) applied to warts
Urethral meatus	Cryotherapy with liquid nitrogen *or* Podophyllin resin 10%–25% (topical)
PREVENTION	
All sites	*Gardasil* vaccine: protects against HPV-6 and HPV-11, which cause 90% of venereal warts, as well as HPV-16 and HPV-18, which cause 70% of cervical cancers

BCA, Bichloroacetic acid; *TCA,* trichloroacetic acid.

The drugs used to remove venereal warts can be divided into two groups: agents that must be administered by a healthcare provider and agents that can be applied at home. With both groups, application is done repeatedly until the warts disappear. Provider-applied drugs are *podophyllin, trichloroacetic acid,* and *bichloroacetic acid.* Drugs for home application are *podofilox, imiquimod,* and *kunecatechins.* All of these drugs act slowly, and they all cause local irritation. The pharmacology of six topical drugs is discussed in the next section.

Provider-Applied Drugs

Podophyllin. Podophyllin (podophyllum resin) [Podocon-25, Podofilm 🍁] is used primarily for perianal and venereal warts. The drug is not very effective against common warts. Podophyllin is a mixture of resins from the May apple or mandrake *(Podophyllum peltatum Linne).* The active ingredient in the resin is *podophyllotoxin,* a compound that inhibits DNA synthesis and mitosis. These actions eventually lead to cell death and erosion of warty tissue. Formulations employed to remove warts contain 25% podophyllum resin. These preparations are highly caustic and should be applied only by a trained clinician. To minimize the risk for toxicity from systemic absorption, the resin should be washed off with alcohol or soap and water a few hours after application. Each treatment should be limited to a small surface area and to a small number of warts.

Podophyllin can be absorbed in amounts sufficient to cause systemic toxicity. Potential reactions include central and peripheral neuropathy, kidney damage, and blood dyscrasias. These effects are most likely when the drug is applied to large areas in excessive amounts. Podophyllin is teratogenic and must not be used during pregnancy.

Podophyllin is supplied in a 25% solution for topical use. Application should be limited to small areas. The drug should not be applied to moles or birthmarks, nor should it be applied to warts that are bleeding or friable (easily crumbled) or that have undergone recent biopsy. When used to remove venereal warts, podophyllin should be washed off 1 to 4 hours after application. Treatment may be repeated at weekly intervals for up to 4 weeks.

Bichloroacetic Acid (BCA) and Trichloroacetic Acid (TCA). When applied in high concentration (80% to 90%), BCA and TCA can destroy warts by chemical coagulation. Application is repeated weekly if needed. Solutions of these acids are very watery, and hence can easily spread to and thereby injure surrounding tissue. To minimize spread, the solution should be allowed to dry before the patient sits or stands. If pain develops, BCA and TCA can be neutralized with liquid soap or sodium bicarbonate (baking soda). If too much solution is applied, it should be neutralized with soap or sodium bicarbonate, or removed by applying talc.

Patient-Applied Drugs

Patient-applied drugs are used for topical therapy of external genital and perianal warts. Like podophyllin, these drugs require a prescription. Because they are applied at home, these drugs are more convenient than the provider-applied drugs.

Imiquimod. Imiquimod cream [Aldara, Zyclara] stimulates production of interferon alfa, TNF, and several interleukins and thereby intensifies immune responses to HPV, the virus that causes venereal warts. Imiquimod has no direct antiviral effects of its own. Principal adverse effects are erythema, erosion, and flaking at the site of administration. Local itching, burning, and pain may occur too. Imiquimod undergoes minimal absorption, and hence systemic effects are usually absent.

Imiquimod cream is available in two formulations: a 3.75% cream sold as *Zyclara* and a 5% cream sold as *Aldara*. Zyclara is applied once a day for up to 8 weeks; Aldara is applied 3 times a week for up to 16 weeks. Both formulations are applied at bedtime and washed off in the morning. Imiquimod use for AKs was discussed previously.

Podofilox. Like podophyllin, podofilox [Condylox] inhibits mitosis. Whether this action underlies beneficial effects (erosion of warty tissue) is unknown. Podofilox is supplied as a 0.5% gel or 0.5% solution to be applied twice daily for 3 consecutive days followed by 4 days off. This pattern is repeated 4 times or until the warts are gone—whichever comes first. Patients should wash their hands before and after applying the drug. However, unlike imiquimod, podofilox needn't be washed from the site of application. Treatment frequently causes local inflammation, burning, erosion, pain, itching, and bleeding. These can be minimized by limiting the application area to 10 cm^2, applying no more than 0.5 gm/day, and avoiding application to normal skin. Podofilox causes more discomfort than imiquimod, but works faster and costs less.

Kunecatechins (Sinecatechins) Ointment. Kunecatechins [Veregen] is made by extraction from the leaves of *Camellia sinensis* (green tea). The primary active component in this extract is epigallocatechin, a compound in the catechin family. The extract also contains small amounts of gallic acid and three methylxanthines: caffeine, theophylline, and theobromine. Although the mechanism of action has not been determined, possibilities include antioxidative effects, induction of apoptosis (programmed cell death), and inhibition of telomerase (an enzyme cells use to extend the telomere cap on DNA). Kunecatechins is supplied as a 15% ointment to be applied 3 times daily until all warts clear, or for 16 weeks, whichever comes first. In one trial, treatment for 16 weeks produced complete wart removal in 53.6% of patients, compared with 35.3% in those treated with placebo. Adverse effects, which are common, include erythema (70%), pruritus (69%), burning (67%), pain (56%), erosion or ulceration (49%), edema (45%), induration (35%), and rash (2%). Moderate reactions develop in 37% of patients, and severe reactions develop in 30%. Kunecatechins is indicated only for external genital and perianal warts. It should not be inserted into the vagina or rectum and should not be applied to open wounds. Patients should avoid sexual contact while the ointment is present. Kunecatechins is not recommended for HIV-infected patients, immunocompromised patients, or patients with genital herpes infection. Why? Because safety and efficacy in these patients have not been established.

Common Warts

Common warts—also known as verruca vulgaris—manifest as hard, rough, horny papules. These benign lesions may appear anywhere on the body, but are most common on the hands and feet. Most common warts are caused by just three types of HPV, known as HPV-1, HPV-2, and HPV-3.

Like venereal warts, common warts may be removed by physical procedures and with topical drugs. The physical methods are cryotherapy, electrodesiccation, curettage (surgical removal with a loop-shaped cutting tool), and laser therapy. Pharmacologic agents include salicylic acid, podophyllin, podofilox, imiquimod, trichloroacetic acid, and topical fluorouracil.

DRUGS FOR NONSURGICAL COSMETIC PROCEDURES

OnabotulinumtoxinA [Botox] is an acetylcholine release inhibitor and neuromuscular blocking agent. Botulinum toxin type A is a protein produced by the gram-negative bacterium *Clostridium botulinum.* This is the same powerful toxin that causes botulism, a potentially fatal condition brought on by eating foods contaminated with *C. botulinum;* however, the doses approved for cosmetic use are much too small to produce toxic effects.

In the United States two licensed Botox products are available: Botox and Botox Cosmetic. Botox Cosmetic is approved only for treating frown lines, whereas plain Botox is approved for treating cervical dystonia, detrusor overactivity, upper limb spasticity, strabismus, blepharospasm, and hyperhidrosis, and for migraine headache prophylaxis. However, except for the packaging, both Botox products are identical. The drug is available as a powder in 100-unit vials under the name Botox. Immediately before use, the powder is reconstituted with 2.5 mL of preservative-free normal saline to form a clear, colorless solution. According to the package label, reconstituted botulinum toxin is unstable and hence should be stored cold and used within 4 hours. However, data indicate that if the drug is diluted in normal saline that contains the preservative benzyl alcohol, it retains its potency for 5 weeks and causes less pain when injected.

How does Botox work? OnabotulinumtoxinA is a neurotoxin that acts on cholinergic neurons to block release of acetylcholine. After injection, the drug is taken up by cholinergic nerve terminals, where it inactivates SNAP-25, a protein critical to the function of acetylcholine-containing vesicles. In the absence of SNAP-25, the vesicles are unable to fuse with the terminal membrane, and hence cannot release their acetylcholine. Restoration of neuronal function requires sprouting of new terminals, a process that can take several months. Botulinum toxin blocks transmission at neuromuscular junctions and at cholinergic synapses of the autonomic nervous system, including synapses in autonomic ganglia.

The FDA has approved Botox for reducing frown lines, known formally as "glabellar" lines (because they appear on the glabella—the smooth area located between the eyebrows, directly above the nose). Botox is also used to soften lines on the forehead and neck and to diminish "crow's feet" (lines that form near the outer corners of our eyes when we squint).

Botox is administered by injection. (Pretreatment with a topical anesthetic cream is commonly done to reduce discomfort.) To reduce frown lines, for example, Botox is injected directly into the small muscles that produce a frown when they contract. Five injections are made, each consisting of 4 units of botulinum toxin in 0.1 mL of fluid. Two injections go into each corrugator muscle and one into the procerus muscle. The whole procedure takes just a few minutes.

Results are neither instantaneous nor permanent. Rather, muscle paralysis develops slowly—over 3 to 10 days—and fades within 3 to 6 months. Botox injections may be repeated to maintain cosmetic benefits. However, at least 3 months should separate treatments. There are no data on long-term effects.

The FDA has issued a black box warning related to spread of the toxin from the site of injection to other areas, leading to life-threatening injuries; however, this has not occurred with the small doses used for cosmetic treatment. For cosmetic treatment, the most common side effects are headache, facial pain, swelling, and bruising. Swelling and bruising can be reduced by applying ice to the site and by avoiding alcohol, vitamin E, and aspirin (and related NSAIDs) for the week before treatment.

Injection into the wrong site, or diffusion from the right site into surrounding tissues, can weaken muscles that were not intended as targets, causing multiple undesired effects. Ptosis (droopy eyelids) occurs in about 5% of patients and can persist for 3 to 6 months. Injections in the lower face can result in drooling, an asymmetric smile, drooping mouth, and biting of the inside of the cheek. Injections in the neck can make swallowing difficult and can change vocal pitch.

Who should *not* use Botox? The drug should be avoided by women who are pregnant or breast-feeding and by patients who may be allergic to human albumin, a protein in Botox preparations. In addition, Botox should be avoided by people using aminoglycoside antibiotics or any other agent that has neuromuscular blocking properties. The drug should be used with caution in patients with myasthenia gravis and other neuromuscular disorders that can intensify muscle paralysis. Lastly, Botox should be avoided by people older than 65 years. Why? Because it's unlikely to help: In older people, the major cause of lines and wrinkles is loss of elasticity in the skin—a phenomenon that can't be reversed by neuromuscular blockade.

Over time, some patients develop antibodies against botulinum toxin type A. The only consequence is a reduction in Botox benefits. The risk for antibody production may be increased by using high doses and short dosing intervals. If antibodies do develop, patients may still respond to a product known as Myobloc, which consists of botulinum toxin type B (instead of botulinum toxin type A).

ANTIPERSPIRANTS AND DEODORANTS

Perspiration is produced by two types of sweat glands: *eccrine glands* and *apocrine glands.* The eccrine glands secrete profuse, watery perspiration. The apocrine glands secrete a small volume of fluid rich in organic compounds. The unpleasant odor associated with sweating results from chemical and bacterial degradation of the compounds in apocrine sweat. Eccrine glands contribute to odor by creating a moist environment that favors bacterial growth. Perspiration odor can be reduced with *antiperspirants* (agents that decrease flow of eccrine sweat) and *deodorants* (antiseptics that suppress growth of skin-dwelling bacteria).

Antiperspirants

The principal compounds employed as antiperspirants are *aluminum chlorohydrate, aluminum chloride,* and *buffered aluminum sulfate.* These agents can decrease flow of eccrine sweat by 20% to 50%. Reduced flow appears to result from inhibition of sweat production and from partial occlusion of sweat glands. Topical antiperspirants can cause stinging, burning, itching, and irritation. Dermatitis and ulceration occur rarely.

Severe sweating can be reduced with *botulinum toxin type A* [Botox], the same drug used to smooth facial wrinkles. Botulinum toxin inhibits release of acetylcholine from sympathetic neurons that innervate sweat glands and thereby reduces sweat volume. To treat axillary hyperhidrosis (severe underarm sweating), 10 to 15 intradermal injections (0.1 to 0.2 mL apiece) are made into each armpit. The needle employed is very fine (30 gauge) to minimize discomfort. One set of injections can markedly decrease sweating for 6 or more months.

Deodorants

Deodorants inhibit growth of the surface bacteria that degrade components of apocrine sweat into malodorous products; deodorants do not suppress sweat formation. Agents employed as deodorants include *triclocarban* and *triclosan.*

These antiseptics were also commonly included as active ingredients in deodorant soaps and washes until they were banned for use in these products (but not in deodorants) by the FDA in 2016. The ban came about as the result of research findings that failed to identify a relationship between the use of these soaps and a decrease in infection rates. Furthermore, there was the concern that the inclusion of antimicrobials increased the risk for development of bacterial resistance. In addition to triclocarban and triclosan, the FDA also banned 17 other antibacterial substances from soaps and washes. Additional rulings on other antimicrobials (benzalkonium chloride, benzethonium chloride, chloroxylenol) are forthcoming. For additional information, see https://www.fda.gov/NewsEvents/Newsroom/PressAnnouncements/ucm517478.htm.

DRUGS FOR SEBORRHEIC DERMATITIS AND DANDRUFF

Seborrheic dermatitis is a chronic, relapsing condition characterized by inflammation and scaling of the scalp and face. Skin of the underarms, chest, and anogenital region may also be affected. Symptoms result from an inflammatory reaction to infection with *Malassezia* (formerly called *Pityrosporum*), a microbe in the yeast family.

Symptoms respond rapidly to topical treatment with *ketoconazole*, an antifungal drug with activity against yeast (see Chapter 92). For treatment of seborrhea, ketoconazole is available in a 2% cream [Ketoderm 🍁], 2% foam [Extina], 2% gel [Xolegel], and 1% and 2% shampoos [Nizoral]. The cream and foam formulations are applied twice daily for 4 weeks. The gel is more convenient, being applied just daily and for only 2 weeks. Concurrent use of topical glucocorticoids can accelerate initial responses. After the yeast infection has been controlled, remission can be maintained by periodic use of a shampoo that contains a yeast-suppressing drug, such as *ketoconazole* (in Nizoral), *pyrithione zinc* (in Head & Shoulders), or *selenium sulfide* (in Selsun Blue and Head & Shoulders Intensive Treatment).

DRUGS FOR HAIR LOSS

Two drugs are available to promote hair growth: minoxidil and finasteride. Minoxidil is applied topically; finasteride is taken orally. Neither drug was originally developed for baldness: Minoxidil was developed for hypertension, and finasteride for benign prostatic hyperplasia (BPH).

Topical Minoxidil

Minoxidil is a direct-acting vasodilator used primarily to treat severe hypertension. The drug's basic pharmacology is discussed in Chapter 46. Consideration here is limited to its use against patterned hair loss in men and women.

Minoxidil for baldness is available in three formulations, a 2% solution (generic only), a 5% solution [Rogaine Extra Strength for Men], and a 5% foam [Rogaine Men's Extra Strength]. All formulations are approved for men, but only the 2% solution is approved for women. Nonetheless, all formulations are routinely prescribed for women. All formulations are applied to the scalp twice a day.

The mechanism by which minoxidil promotes hair growth is unknown. One possibility is that it causes resting hair follicles to enter a state of active growth. Improved cutaneous blood flow secondary to vasodilation does not seem to be involved.

Minoxidil can delay loss of hair and stimulate hair growth. Benefits take several months to develop. Unfortunately, response rates are somewhat disappointing: Only about one-third of patients experience significant restoration of hair to regions of baldness. Hair regrowth is most likely when baldness has developed recently and has been limited to a small area. Responses with the 5% solution are only 50% greater than with the 2% solution. When minoxidil is discontinued, newly gained hair is lost in 3 to 4 months, and the natural progression of hair loss resumes. In some cases, beneficial effects may decline even with uninterrupted treatment.

Topical minoxidil is generally devoid of adverse effects. A few patients have reported pruritus and local allergic responses (e.g., rash, swelling, burning sensation). Absorption is low, and hence systemic reactions (e.g., hypotension, headache, flushing) are rare.

Finasteride

Finasteride is an oral drug with two indications: androgenic alopecia (male-pattern baldness) and BPH. For treatment of androgenic alopecia, finasteride is sold in 1-mg tablets under the brand name *Propecia.* For treatment of BPH, the drug is sold in 5-mg tablets under the brand name *Proscar* (see Chapter 66).

Male-pattern baldness is caused by dihydrotestosterone (DHT), a powerful androgenic hormone formed from testosterone. In balding men, the scalp has high levels of DHT, which acts on hair follicles to induce shrinkage. Finasteride promotes hair growth by inhibiting the enzyme that converts testosterone into DHT. A 1-mg dose reduces serum levels of DHT by 65% after 24 hours. In the prostate gland, levels of testosterone *increase* by sixfold (because conversion of testosterone into DHT has been suppressed).

Regrowth of hair with finasteride is very modest. The drug has been evaluated in men 18 to 41 years old. Only 50% grew any hair. Furthermore, even when hair growth did occur, the amount was small: One year of treatment with 1 mg/day increased hair count by only 12% (in a 5.1-cm^2 circle on the scalp, the average hair count rose by 107 hairs, up from a baseline of 867 hairs). In older men taking 5 mg/day to treat BPH, no hair growth has been reported.

At the dosage employed to treat baldness (1 mg/day), adverse effects are few. About 4% of men experience reduced libido, erectile dysfunction, impaired ejaculation, and reduced ejaculate volume. Orthostatic hypotension and dizziness may occur. Finasteride is a teratogen that can cause genitourinary abnormalities in males exposed to the drug *in utero.* Accordingly, women who are or may become pregnant should not take finasteride, nor should they handle tablets that are crushed or broken.

EFLORNITHINE FOR UNWANTED FACIAL HAIR

Eflornithine [Vaniqa] is an old drug with a new indication and new formulation. As discussed in Chapter 99, eflornithine has been available since 1990 for *systemic* therapy of African trypanosomiasis (sleeping sickness). Now, the drug is also available in a 13.9% cream for use by women to remove facial hair. Topical eflornithine acts on cells in hair follicles to inhibit ornithine decarboxylase, an enzyme required for synthesis of polyamines, which in turn are required for cell division and subsequent hair growth.

In clinical trials, eflornithine cream was moderately effective in some women and had no effect in others. All subjects had beards or mustaches that required removal (e.g., by shaving, waxing, tweezing, etc.) at least twice a week. Participants were randomized to receive either (1) eflornithine cream twice a week or (2) the vehicle alone (i.e., the cream without eflornithine). What happened? Substantial hair reduction occurred in 40% of treated women in one study and 20% of treated women in another, compared with a 10% response in women receiving the vehicle alone. Among the women who did respond, benefits developed slowly—over 4 to 8 weeks or more—and then faded entirely within 8 weeks of stopping treatment. It should be noted that eflornithine does not remove facial hair entirely. Rather, it slows hair growth, causes hair to be finer and lighter, and decreases (but does not eliminate) the need for shaving and other hair-removal procedures. Because effects are not permanent, continuous treatment is required.

Very little of topical eflornithine gets absorbed: about 1% of each dose reaches the systemic circulation. Absorbed drug is eliminated intact in the urine. No metabolism occurs.

Eflornithine cream is generally well tolerated—although there is some concern about possible fetal harm. The most common reactions are transient stinging, burning, tingling, or rash at the application site. Although eflornithine absorption is minimal, it may still be sufficient to cause fetal injury. In animal studies, there was no evidence that topical eflornithine is teratogenic or fetotoxic. However, of the 19 pregnancies that occurred during clinical trials, there were four spontaneous abortions and one birth defect (Down's syndrome). Until more is known, avoiding pregnancy would seem prudent.

Eflornithine is supplied in 45-gm tubes (a 2-month supply). Applications are made twice daily, 8 hours apart. Women should rub the cream in thoroughly and should not wash the treated area for at least 4 hours. Cosmetics and sunscreens can be applied as soon as the cream dries.

DRUGS FOR IMPETIGO

Impetigo is the most common bacterial infection of the skin. The usual pathogen is *Staphylococcus aureus.* Most cases are seen in children 2 to 5 years old, although all age groups are susceptible. Impetigo is highly contagious and is usually spread by person-to-person contact. Fortunately, the infection is superficial and is usually self-limited.

Impetigo has two forms: bullous and nonbullous. Bullous impetigo is caused by a toxin from *S. aureus.* It manifests as rapidly spreading papules that may evolve into large, thin-walled vesicles. The usual location is a warm, moist area of the skin. Nonbullous impetigo, also known as crusted impetigo, is caused by *S. aureus* and/or *Streptococcus pyogenes.* This infection typically manifests as a single small macule or papule that evolves into a vesicle that oozes a yellow-brown exudate, which then dries into a honey-colored crust. The usual location is skin of the hands, feet, and legs. Most (70%) of impetigo cases are nonbullous.

Impetigo is treated with antibiotics. Mild to moderate infection can be treated with topical agents. More serious infection is treated with oral agents. Dosages for representative antibiotics are shown in Table 105.6.

LOCAL ANESTHETICS

Local anesthetics (e.g., benzocaine, lidocaine, pramoxine) can be applied topically to relieve pain and itching associated with various skin disorders, including sunburn, plant poisoning, fungal infection, diaper rash, and eczema. Selection of a topical anesthetic is based on duration of action, desired vehicle (cream, ointment, solution, gel), and prior history of hypersensitivity reactions. The pharmacology of the local anesthetics is discussed in Chapter 26.

TABLE 105.6 ▪ Some Antibiotics for Impetigo

			Dosage	
Generic Name	**Brand Name**	**Formulation**	**Pediatric**	**Adult**
TOPICAL				
Mupirocin	Bactroban	Ointment, cream	Apply 3 times/day for 3–5 days	Apply 3 times/day for 3–5 days
Retapamulin	Altabax	Ointment	Apply twice daily for 5 days	Apply twice daily for 5 days
ORAL				
Cephalexin	Keflex	Capsules, suspension	6.25 mg/kg 4 times/day	500 mg every 6–12 hr
Dicloxacillin	Generic only	Capsules	6.25 mg/kg 4 times/day	250 mg 4 times/day
Clindamycin	Cleocin	Capsules, suspension	10–20 mg/kg/day in three doses	300–450 mg 3 times/day
Amoxicillin/clavulanate	Augmentin	Tablets, suspension	*3 months and older and under 40 kg:* 20–40 mg/kg/day (amoxicillin component) divided every 8 hr *or* 25–45 mg/kg/day (amoxicillin component) divided every 12 hr *40 kg and greater:* 500 mg every 12 hr *or* 250 mg every 8 hr *Severe infections, 40 kg and greater:* 875 mg every 12 hr *or* 500 mg every 8 hr	875 mg amoxicillin/125 mg clavulanate twice daily

KEY POINTS

- Topical glucocorticoids are employed to relieve inflammation and itching associated with a variety of dermatologic disorders.
- Preparations of topical glucocorticoids are classified into potency groups that range from low to super-high.
- Prolonged use of topical glucocorticoids can cause atrophy of the dermis and epidermis.
- Topical glucocorticoids can be absorbed in amounts sufficient to cause systemic toxicity. Principal concerns are growth delay and adrenal suppression.
- Keratolytic agents—salicylic acid, sulfur, and benzoyl peroxide—promote shedding of the horny layer of the skin.
- Topical antibiotics—benzoyl peroxide, clindamycin, and erythromycin—help clear mild to moderate acne by suppressing growth of *P. acnes.*
- Topical retinoids—tretinoin, adapalene, and tazarotene—help clear mild to moderate acne by normalizing hyperproliferation of epithelial cells in hair follicles.
- Oral antibiotics, including doxycycline and minocycline, are reserved for moderate to severe acne. Benefits derive from suppressing growth of *P. acnes* and from anti-inflammatory actions.
- Isotretinoin is an oral drug reserved for severe acne.
- Isotretinoin causes multiple adverse effects, including nosebleeds; inflammation of the lips and eyes; and pain, tenderness, or stiffness in muscles, bones, and joints.
- Isotretinoin is highly teratogenic. Accordingly, all parties involved with the drug—prescribers, patients, pharmacists, and wholesalers—must participate in iPLEDGE, a risk management program designed to ensure that isotretinoin is not used during pregnancy.
- Excessive sun exposure can cause sunburn, premature aging of the skin, and skin cancer.
- Sunscreens can protect against sunburn, aging of the skin, and some cancers.
- To be most effective, a sunscreen product should offer protection against the full range of UVB and UVA radiation.

Please visit **http://evolve.elsevier.com/Lehne** for chapter-specific NCLEX® examination review questions.

CHAPTER

106 Drugs for the Ear

In this chapter, we discuss drugs for disorders of the middle ear and external ear.

ANATOMY OF THE EAR

It is important to have an understanding of ear anatomy when considering treatment of ear conditions. The ear has three major divisions: the external ear, middle ear, and inner ear (Fig. 106.1):

- The *external ear* consists of (1) the auricle or pinna (the cartilaginous flap visible on the side of the head that serves to collect sound waves) and (2) the external auditory canal (EAC), a skin-lined tube that directs sound waves from the auricle to the tympanic membrane (TM; the eardrum). The surface of the EAC is coated with cerumen (earwax), a hydrophobic substance that blocks penetration of water and helps protect against bacterial and fungal infection.
- The *middle ear* is the chamber that houses the malleus, incus, and stapes—three tiny bones that transmit sound vibrations from the TM to the inner ear. The middle ear is bounded laterally by the TM, which walls off the middle ear from the external ear. The eustachian tube (auditory tube) connects the middle ear with the nasopharynx and thereby allows air pressure within the middle ear to equalize with air pressure in the environment. The mucociliary epithelium that lines the eustachian tube sweeps bacteria out of the middle ear into the nasopharynx.
- The *inner ear* consists of the semicircular canals and the cochlea. The canals provide our sense of balance. The cochlea houses the apparatus of hearing.

OTITIS MEDIA AND ITS MANAGEMENT

Otitis media (OM), defined as an inflammation of the middle ear, is the most prevalent disorder of childhood. The condition affects more than 75% of children by age 3 years and about 95% by age 12 years. In the United States OM is responsible for more than 16 million clinic visits a year.

OM may result from bacterial or viral infection or from noninfectious causes. Only bacterial OM responds to antibiotics. Furthermore, most cases resolve spontaneously, making antibiotics largely unnecessary—even when bacteria *are* the cause. Nonetheless, antibiotics have been used routinely. In fact, OM is the most common reason antibiotics are prescribed for children—at an estimated cost of $5 billion a year.

Acute Otitis Media

Characteristics, Pathogenesis, and Microbiology

Acute OM (AOM) is defined by *infection, inflammation,* and *fluid in the middle ear.* Otalgia (ear pain) is characteristic, often causing the young child to tug at or hold the affected ear. Other signs and symptoms accompanying AOM may include fever, vomiting, anorexia, irritability, sleeplessness, and diarrhea.

AOM results from a bacterial or viral infection of the middle ear. It occurs most commonly among children. The middle ear is filled with purulent fluid, which can cause the TM to bulge outward. If the membrane is perforated, purulent otorrhea results.

AOM commonly develops after a viral upper respiratory infection, which can cause inflammation and swelling of the eustachian tube. The swelling can lead to blockage, resulting in negative pressure in the middle ear that, in turn, leads to fluid accumulation in the middle ear. When the eustachian tube opens, causing pressure equalization, bacteria and viruses can be sucked in. If the mucociliary system is sufficiently impaired, it will be unable to transport these pathogens back to the nasopharynx. OM results when bacteria colonize the fluid of the middle ear and/or when viruses colonize cells of the middle-ear mucosa. Prior to the introduction of pneumococcal conjugate vaccine, *Streptococcus pneumoniae* was the primary cause of AOM (40% to 50% of cases). A 2015 report revealed that *S. pneumoniae* is now responsible for only 12% of cases (Table 106.1 lists the common pathogens).

Diagnosis

To diagnose AOM, three elements must be present: (1) acute onset of signs and symptoms, (2) middle-ear effusion (MEE), and (3) middle-ear inflammation. The presence of MEE is indicated by a bulging TM with limited mobility, or, if the TM is perforated, purulent otorrhea. MEE is the best predictor of AOM. Middle-ear inflammation is indicated by either distinct erythema of the TM or distinct otalgia (earache). Because TM erythema can be caused by things other than inflammation (e.g., crying in a child), it is not always reliable as an indicator for AOM.

It is important to distinguish between AOM and otitis media with effusion (OME). Children with OME have fluid in the

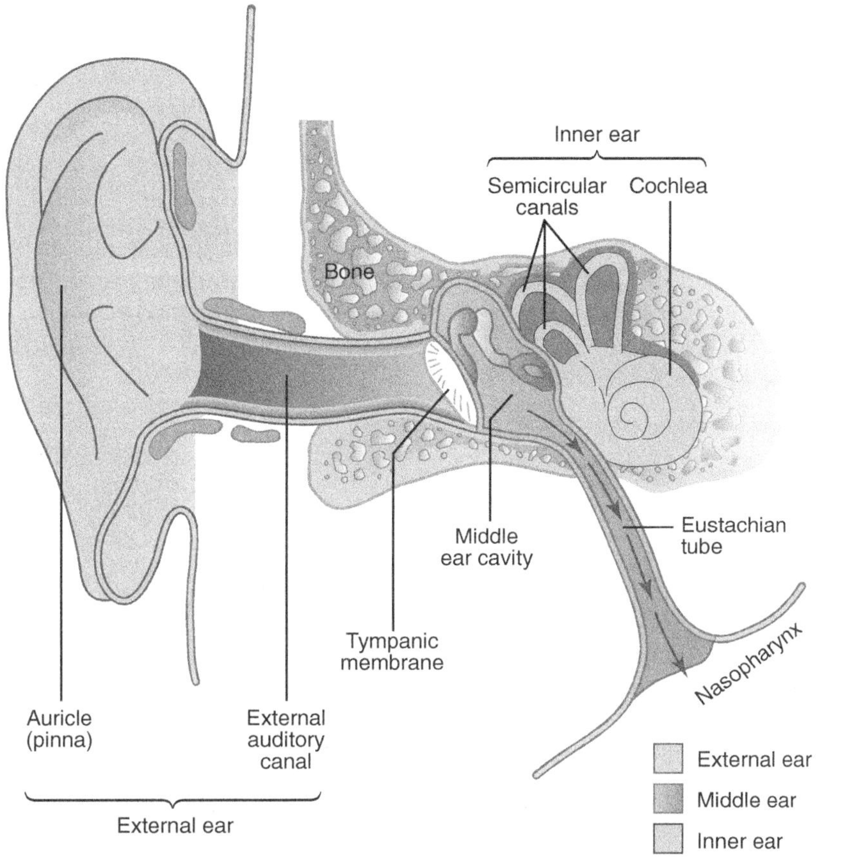

Fig. 106.1 ■ Anatomy of the ear.
The *purple arrows* indicate flow of the mucociliary system, which can transport bacteria out of the middle ear.

TABLE 106.1 ■ Primary Pathogens Found in Fluid From the Middle Ear of Children With Acute Otitis Media

Pathogen	Children With the Pathogen (%)
Haemophilus influenzae	56%
Moraxella catarrhalis	22%
Streptococcus pneumoniae	12%
Others (e.g., *Streptococcus pyogenes, Staphylococcus aureus,* gram-negative bacilli)	Uncommon
No bacteria found	10%–30%
Both bacteria and viruses	66%
Viruses alone	4%[a]

[a]It is uncommon for viruses to be present in the absence of bacteria.

middle ear but no signs of local or systemic illness. Prolonged OME is common after resolution of AOM.

Standard Treatment

All children with AOM should receive pain medication, and *some* should receive antibiotics. Prescribing antibiotics for *all* children should be discouraged because over 80% of AOM episodes resolve spontaneously within a week. If antibiotics are prescribed routinely, most recipients will be taking drugs they don't really need. Not only does this generate unnecessary expense but, worse yet, it also puts children at needless risk for adverse drug effects, increases their risk for recurrent AOM, and accelerates the emergence of antibiotic-resistant bacteria.

In 2013, the American Academy of Pediatrics (AAP) released a guideline for treating AOM in children. This guideline built on earlier guidelines developed jointly by the AAP and the American Academy of Family Physicians. For many patients, the guideline includes an important option—*observation*—rather than immediate treatment with antibiotics. Observation is defined as management by symptomatic relief alone for 48 to 72 hours, thereby allowing time for AOM to resolve on its own. If symptoms persist or worsen, antibacterial therapy is then started. As part of this strategy, parents are informed about (1) the high probability of spontaneous AOM resolution and (2) the drawbacks of giving antibiotics when they are not needed. Observation is considered appropriate only when follow-up can be ensured. The recommendation for observation is based on studies that identified the following outcomes:

- Most episodes of AOM resolve spontaneously.
- Immediate antibacterial therapy is only marginally superior to observation at causing AOM resolution, and it is no better at relieving pain or distress.

- Parents find the observation approach acceptable.
- Delaying antibacterial therapy does not significantly increase the risk of mastoiditis, which can occur when bacteria invade the mastoid bone.

Criteria for choosing between observation and initial antibacterial therapy are shown in Table 106.2. As indicated, all children younger than 6 months should receive antibiotics, regardless of diagnostic certainty or symptom severity. Among children 6 months to 2 years old, antibiotics are indicated whenever the diagnosis is certain. For children 2 years and older, antibacterial therapy is indicated only if the diagnosis is certain and then only if symptoms are severe. In all other cases, observation is the preferred strategy.

When antibacterial drugs *are* indicated, *high-dose amoxicillin* is the treatment of choice (Table 106.3). Benefits of amoxicillin are efficacy, safety, low cost, acceptable taste, and narrow microbiologic spectrum. The duration of treatment ranges from 5 to 10 days, depending on patient age and illness severity.

TABLE 106.2 ■ Criteria for Choosing Initial Antibacterial Therapy Versus Observation in Children With Acute Otitis Media

	Management Recommendation	
Age	**Certain Diagnosis**	**Uncertain Diagnosis**
Less than 6 months	Antibacterial therapy	Antibacterial therapy
6 months to 2 years	Antibacterial therapy[a]	Antibacterial therapy if illness is severe; observation if illness is not severe
2 years and older	Antibacterial therapy if illness is severe; observation if illness is not severe	Observation, regardless of symptom severity

[a]If AOM is unilateral without otorrhea and with mild symptoms, observation may be appropriate. Severe illness = moderate to severe otalgia or fever of 39° C (102.2° F) or higher; nonsevere illness = mild otalgia and fever below 39° C in the past 24 hours.

Safety Alert

PENICILLIN ALLERGIES

Patients who are allergic to penicillin should not take amoxicillin [Amoxil, Trimox, Amoxicot], amoxicillin/clavulanate [Augmentin], and other drugs of the penicillin class.

Patients who have had a *severe* allergic reaction to penicillins should also not take cephalosporins.

For patients with penicillin allergy, drug selection depends on allergy severity. If the allergy is *not* severe (type II allergy), a cephalosporin may be used (e.g., cefdinir, cefuroxime). However, if the allergy is *severe* (type I allergy causing urticaria or anaphylaxis), cephalosporins should be avoided, owing to concerns of cross-reactivity. In this case azithromycin and

TABLE 106.3 ■ Recommended Antibacterial Drugs for Acute Otitis Media

	Recommended Drugs	
Patient Group and Illness Severity	**For Most Patients**	**For Patients With Penicillin Allergy[a]**
PATIENTS RECEIVING IMMEDIATE ANTIBIOTIC THERAPY		
Nonsevere illness	Amoxicillin, 40–45 mg/kg twice daily	*Non–type I allergy:* • Cefdinir, 14 mg/kg/day in 1 or 2 divided doses *or* • Cefuroxime, 15 mg/kg twice daily *or* • Cefpodoxime, 5 mg/kg twice daily *Type I allergy:* • Azithromycin, 10 mg/kg on day 1, then 5 mg/kg on days 2, 3, 4, and 5 *or* • Clarithromycin, 7.5 mg/kg twice daily
Severe illness	Amoxicillin, 45 mg/kg twice daily *plus* clavulanate, 3.2 mg/kg twice daily[b]	Ceftriaxone, 50 mg/kg IM for 1 or 3 days
PATIENTS WITH PERSISTENT SYMPTOMS AFTER 48–72 HR OF OBSERVATION (WITH NO ANTIBIOTIC THERAPY)		
Same as for patients receiving immediate antibiotic therapy		
PATIENTS WITH PERSISTENT SYMPTOMS AFTER 48–72 HR OF ANTIBIOTIC THERAPY (INDICATING DRUG RESISTANCE)		
Nonsevere illness	Amoxicillin, 45 mg/kg twice daily *plus* clavulanate, 3.2 mg/kg twice daily[b]	*Non–type I allergy:* • Ceftriaxone, 50 mg/kg IM or IV for 3 days *Type I allergy:* • Clindamycin, 30–40 mg/kg/day in 3 divided doses
Severe illness	Ceftriaxone, 50 mg/kg IM for 3 days	Clindamycin (plus a third-generation cephalosporin if non–type I penicillin allergy), tympanocentesis

[a]Type I allergy is severe (urticaria or anaphylaxis); type II is less severe.
[b]This ratio of amoxicillin to clavulanate can be achieved with Augmentin ES-600, a fixed-dose combination containing amoxicillin and clavulanic acid.

clarithromycin are recommended. A full discussion of the various antibiotic categories used to treat ear infections is presented in Unit XVI.

Regardless of whether antibiotics are prescribed, pain management must be included when treating AOM. Analgesics such as acetaminophen or ibuprofen are commonly used to manage mild to moderate pain. For moderate to severe pain, codeine and similar drugs may be needed. For children older than 5 years, the 2013 AAP guideline also recommends topical anesthetic ear drops such as procaine or lidocaine for pain relief. (The 2013 guideline also recommended benzocaine; however, because it lacks U.S. Food and Drug Administration [FDA] approval, the FDA asked that it be removed from the market in 2015.) To relieve pain, the EAC is filled with the solution and then a solution-soaked cotton pledget is placed in the EAC to prevent drainage. This typically needs to be repeated every 1 to 2 hours until pain is relieved. It is contraindicated if the TM is perforated.

Treatment of Antibiotic-Resistant AOM

Antibiotic resistance is indicated by persistence of symptoms (fever, earache, a red and bulging TM) for 2 to 3 days despite antibiotic therapy. Major risk factors for developing resistant AOM are the following:

- Day care attendance
- Age younger than 2 years
- Exposure to antibiotics in the prior 1 to 3 months
- Winter and spring seasons

In the United States, the incidence of resistant AOM is on the rise because an overuse of antibiotics has favored emergence of resistant pathogens. Resistance among strains of *Haemophilus influenzae* and *Moraxella catarrhalis* is limited to beta-lactam antibiotics. The mechanism is production of beta-lactamase, an enzyme that inactivates amoxicillin and certain other beta-lactam antibiotics. In contrast, strains of *Streptococcus pneumoniae* are resistant to multiple antibiotics, including erythromycin and trimethoprim/sulfamethoxazole, as well as amoxicillin and other beta-lactam antibiotics. Interestingly, *S. pneumoniae* resistance to amoxicillin does not result from beta-lactamase production. Rather, it results from synthesis of altered penicillin-binding proteins (PBPs), whose affinity for amoxicillin is much lower than that of normal PBPs.

How should *resistant* AOM be treated? Using a high dose of amoxicillin increases activity against resistant *S. pneumoniae.* For *H. influenzae* and *M. catarrhalis* the preferred approach is oral therapy with *high-dose amoxicillin/clavulanate.* Alternatives to amoxicillin/clavulanate include *IM or IV ceftriaxone* and *oral clindamycin.*

The clavulanate (clavulanic acid) in the amoxicillin/clavulanate combination inhibits beta-lactamase and thereby increases activity against resistant *H. influenzae* and *M. catarrhalis.* (Using a high dose of amoxicillin increases activity against resistant *S. pneumoniae.*) Because the clavulanate in the combination can cause diarrhea, the dosage of clavulanate should be low. It is important to be aware that the ratio of amoxicillin to clavulanate is not constant. For example, *Augmentin* (amoxicillin with clavulanate) is available as tablets containing 250 mg amoxicillin with 125 mg clavulanate and as tablets containing 500 mg amoxicillin with 125 mg clavulanate. If two tablets containing 250 mg amoxicillin are administered to give a patient a 500-mg dose of the amoxicillin component, the excess of clavulanate can result in worsening diarrhea.

Prevention

The risk for acquiring AOM can be decreased in several ways. Breast-feeding for at least 6 months seems to reduce early episodes of AOM. During infancy and early childhood, AOM can be significantly reduced by avoiding child care centers, if possible, when respiratory infections are prevalent. Measures believed to help prevent AOM include eliminating exposure to tobacco smoke, reducing pacifier use in the second 6 months of life, and avoiding supine bottle feeding. Two additional measures are prevention and treatment of influenza and vaccination against pneumococcal infection.

Prevention and Treatment of Influenza. As noted, influenza and other viral infections of the respiratory tract predispose children to developing bacterial and viral OM. Accordingly, measures that reduce influenza can reduce OM risk. Two methods are available: (1) vaccination against influenza and (2) treatment of active influenza infection. Although both immunization against and treatment of influenza can help during the flu season, they do nothing to alter AOM risk the rest of the year.

***Vaccination Against* Streptococcus pneumoniae.** Vaccination with *pneumococcal conjugate vaccine* (PCV) [Prevnar] can reduce the risk of AOM. As mentioned earlier, *S. pneumoniae* was once responsible for 40% to 50% of bacterial AOM. This has decreased significantly since the first PCV was introduced in 2000.

Recurrent Otitis Media

Recurrent AOM can be defined as AOM that occurs 3 or more times within 6 months, or 4 or more times within 12 months. Four management strategies are available: (1) short-term antibacterial therapy, (2) prophylactic antibacterial therapy, (3) prevention and treatment of influenza, and (4) placement of a tympanostomy tube.

Short-Term Antibacterial Therapy

There is disagreement among experts regarding antibacterial therapy. Some authorities recommend antibiotics for each recurrent episode, regardless of presentation. Others recommend reserving antibiotics for episodes in which symptoms are severe. In both cases, high-dose amoxicillin is the treatment of choice. If resistance is suspected, amoxicillin/clavulanate can be used.

Prophylactic Antibacterial Therapy

Antibacterial prophylaxis is *not* generally recommended. An analysis of several studies indicates that for each year of prophylaxis (with *trimethoprim/sulfamethoxazole* or *amoxicillin*), only 1.3 episodes of AOM are prevented. This small benefit is largely outweighed by the risk for promoting antibiotic resistance. If prophylaxis *is* elected, it should be conducted only during the upper respiratory infection season. The preferred drug for prophylaxis is amoxicillin because compared with sulfonamides, amoxicillin is more active against multidrug-resistant strains of *S. pneumoniae.*

Prevention and Treatment of Influenza

As discussed previously, AOM occurrence can be reduced by vaccinating against the influenza virus and by treating active influenza infection. However, benefits are seen only during the flu season.

Tympanostomy Tubes

A tympanostomy tube is a small tube that is placed into an incision in the TM. This allows drainage of middle ear fluid and provides aeration of the middle ear. In children with recurrent AOM, the procedure can significantly reduce AOM episodes. Complications of the procedure include obstruction of the tube, secondary infection with otorrhea, and premature tube extrusion.

Most otic preparations (ear drops) are contraindicated for patients who do not have intact TMs. Exceptions to this rule are some of the fluoroquinolones and fluoroquinolone/glucocorticoid combination products. The combination products ciprofloxacin/dexamethasone [Ciprodex] and ciprofloxacin/fluocinolone acetonide [Otovel] are topical solutions approved specifically for the treatment of AOM in patients with tympanostomy tubes. Otic preparations have advantages over oral preparations because they can go directly to the source of infection in the middle ear; this provides for high local concentration. Because there is decreased systemic absorption, they are less likely to cause adverse effects. They are also less likely than systemic drugs to contribute to resistance.

Otitis Media With Effusion

OME (previously called secretory or serous otitis media) is more common than AOM. It often occurs with upper respiratory tract infections and may precede or follow an episode of AOM. The condition is characterized by fluid in the middle ear but without evidence of local or systemic illness. OME may cause mild hearing loss, but not pain. The condition can persist for weeks to months after AOM has resolved. Because it is not caused by a bacterial infection, antibiotics have no effect on OME and should not be used.

OTITIS EXTERNA AND ITS MANAGEMENT

Otitis externa (OE) is an inflammation of the EAC. The usual cause is bacterial infection, which may be limited to the EAC or may spread to adjacent tissues. Most cases of OE respond to topical drugs.

Acute Otitis Externa

Characteristics, Pathogenesis, and Microbiology

Acute otitis externa (AOE), also known as "swimmer's ear," is a bacterial infection of the EAC. The most common pathogens are *Pseudomonas aeruginosa* and *Staphylococcus aureus.* Other pathogens include *Staphylococcus epidermidis* and *Microbacterium otitidis.* Patients who have AOE present with one or more of the following: rapid-onset ear pain associated with pruritus, a sensation of ear fullness, tenderness on manipulation of the external ear, and/or edema or erythema of the EAC. Impaired hearing and purulent discharge may occur.

Susceptibility to AOE is precipitated primarily by two factors: abrasion and excessive moisture. Both facilitate bacterial colonization. Abrasion of the epithelium creates a site for bacterial entry. Most often, abrasion results from cleaning the EAC with a cotton-tipped swab or some other foreign object (e.g., finger, pencil, toothpick). Abrasion can also be caused by hearing aids and earplugs. Moisture can wash away the protective layer of cerumen. As a result, keratin debris in the EAC is able to absorb water, thereby creating a nourishing medium for bacterial growth. Moisture in the EAC may come from swimming, perspiration, and even high humidity.

Treatment

AOE is a painful condition, often severely so, which means that analgesics are indicated. The same analgesics used for AOM are appropriate for AOE pain management

AOE usually responds well to simple treatment. The goal is to eradicate the pathogen and reduce pain. For most patients, cleaning and the use of topical antimicrobials will suffice. If the infection is extensive, oral antibiotics may be needed. To facilitate healing, the ear should be kept as dry as possible. Most infections begin to improve in 3 days and resolve completely by 10 days.

Topical Medications. The most recent (2014) AOE clinical practice guideline published by the American Academy of Otolaryngology recommends topical antimicrobials over systemic drugs for uncomplicated AOE. There are two reasons for this recommendation. First, topical agents achieve very high local concentrations (often 100 to 1000 times the concentration achieved with systemic drugs), antibacterial effects are superior, disease persistence is lower, and recurrence is less likely. Second, with topical therapy, systemic side effects are absent. Exceptions are made for patients with diabetes, immune deficiencies, or those who would have difficulty with proper administration of topical drugs; these patients should have systemic therapy. Systemic therapy should also be prescribed if the infection has spread beyond the EAC. In severe cases, both systemic and topical antibiotics are needed.

A variety of topical medications can be used. A *2% solution of acetic acid* is safe, effective, and inexpensive. A solution of *alcohol plus acetic acid* offers the additional benefit of promoting tissue drying. For many patients, acidification and drying are all that is needed.

If the infection is more extensive or cannot be cleared with acetic acid and alcohol, a topical antibiotic should be employed. In the past, a three-drug combination—*hydrocortisone, neomycin,* and *polymyxin B*—was considered standard therapy. The hydrocortisone reduces inflammation and edema; neomycin and polymyxin kill bacterial pathogens. Unfortunately, although this combination is effective and inexpensive, it has drawbacks. Specifically, the neomycin component is ototoxic and causes local swelling and erythema in about 15% of patients. Today, *fluoroquinolones* (e.g., ciprofloxacin) are preferred because these drugs are highly effective, do not cause local reactions, and are not ototoxic. Fluoroquinolone and glucocorticoid combination products have the added benefit of decreasing pain by reducing swelling caused by inflammation. The principal drawbacks of these preparations are their expense and their potential to promote resistance to fluoroquinolone antibiotics.

Applying ear drops correctly can improve outcomes and reduce drug-related discomfort. Instillation of cold solutions can cause dizziness; therefore, ear drops should be warmed before administration. Wiggling the earlobe, if tolerated, can facilitate transit of solutions down the EAC. If edema of the EAC is sufficient to impede drug penetration, insertion of a sponge wick can help. A wick is like a very tiny elongated tampon. After it is carefully inserted into the edematous EAC, ear drops are applied to the exposed tip. (It will be important to apply enough medication to keep the wick moist.) Drug solutions are absorbed into the wick, which then delivers them to the epithelium of the entire canal. The wick should be replaced at least every 48 hours to allow cleaning and to determine whether further wicking is still needed.

Safety Alert

UNAPPROVED PRESCRIPTION EAR DROPS

In recent years the FDA has been taking action to halt the manufacture and distribution of otic preparations that are not FDA approved. These preparations typically contain products such as benzocaine or hydrocortisone. (The full list of unapproved otic preparations is available at https://s3.amazonaws.com/public-inspection.federalregister.gov/2015-16360.pdf.) Notice that this applies only to *unapproved* prescription otic drugs.

How can you know if a drug has received approval? The FDA has a website that allows you to check approval by typing in the drug name and then selecting those products produced by various manufacturers (https://www.accessdata.fda.gov/scripts/cder/daf/index.cfm?event=BasicSearch.process).

Oral Medications. Oral antibacterials are indicated if the infection extends beyond the EAC to involve the pinna. For adults, *ciprofloxacin* [Cipro] is a good choice; however, because oral fluoroquinolones can cause tendon rupture in younger patients, it should not be given to patients younger than 18 years. For children, *cephalexin* [Keflex] is preferred.

Prevention

The best way to prevent bacterial AOE is to keep the natural defenses of the EAC healthy. Ear hygiene can be promoted by following these rules:

- Don't put *anything* in the ear, including cotton swabs, fingers, pencils, or toothpicks, all of which can damage the epithelium.
- Dry the EAC after swimming and showering by toweling off and promoting water drainage by tipping the head to each side while pulling the auricle in different directions.
- Don't remove cerumen (earwax).
- Don't use earplugs (except when swimming).

Necrotizing Otitis Externa

Necrotizing OE is a rare but potentially fatal complication of AOE that develops when bacteria in the EAC invade the mastoid or temporal bone. Spread of infection to the skull base can affect cranial nerves, and spread to the dura mater can cause meningitis and possibly lateral sinus thrombosis. The usual pathogen is *P. aeruginosa.* Patients typically present with progressive severe otic pain, purulent discharge from the ear, and granulation of tissue in the EAC. Necrotizing OE occurs almost exclusively in two groups of high-risk people, specifically, older people with diabetes and people who are immunocompromised, especially people with HIV infection. Most cases can be managed by thorough cleansing of the EAC followed by treatment with antipseudomonal drugs; surgery is rarely needed. All patients should receive antipseudomonal ear drops (e.g., ofloxacin solution) along with oral ciprofloxacin. Referral for specialist care should also be considered. Progression to severe disease may require intravenous (IV) antipseudomonal therapy (e.g., *imipenem/cilastatin* [Primaxin], *meropenem* [Merrem IV], or *ciprofloxacin*) for 4 to 6 weeks.

Fungal Otitis Externa (Otomycosis)

In about 10% of patients, OE is caused by fungi and not bacteria. The two most common pathogens are *Aspergillus,* which causes 80% to 90% of otomycoses, and *Candida.* Fungal OE typically manifests as intense pruritus and erythema, with or without pain or hearing loss. As a rule, otomycosis can be managed with thorough cleansing and application of acidifying drops (e.g., 2% acetic acid solution applied 3 to 4 times a day for 7 days). If these measures are inadequate, the patient can apply a solution that contains an antifungal drug (e.g., *1% clotrimazole* [Lotrimin] twice daily for 7 days). If the infection fails to respond, *oral* antifungal therapy may be needed. Options include *itraconazole* [Sporanox] and *fluconazole* [Diflucan].

KEY POINTS

- Otitis media (OM), defined as inflammation of the middle ear, is among the most prevalent disorders of childhood.
- *Acute* otitis media (AOM) is a middle-ear infection characterized by rapid onset, middle-ear effusion, and middle-ear inflammation.
- AOM may be bacterial, viral, or both.
- Over 80% of AOM cases resolve spontaneously without treatment within a week.
- All children with AOM should receive pain medication (e.g., acetaminophen, ibuprofen, codeine, or anesthetic ear drops) as needed.
- Clinical guidelines recommend antibacterial therapy for some children and observation for others. (Observation for 48 to 72 hours allows time for AOM to resolve on its own. If it does not resolve, then antibacterial therapy is implemented.)
- The decision to treat immediately or to wait is based on three factors: patient age, illness severity, and degree of diagnostic certainty (see Table 106.2).
- When antibiotics *are* used for AOM (either immediately or after a period of observation), high-dose amoxicillin is the treatment of choice.
- For children with antibiotic-resistant AOM, high-dose amoxicillin with clavulanate is the treatment of choice.
- The risk of acquiring AOM can be reduced by vaccination against the influenza virus, treatment of active influenza

Continued

infection, and, to a lesser degree, vaccination against *Streptococcus pneumoniae* (using the pneumococcal conjugate vaccine [Prevnar]).
- Otitis media with effusion (OME) is characterized by fluid in the middle ear but without evidence of local or systemic illness. The condition may cause mild hearing loss, but not pain.
- OME is seen in many children following an episode of AOM, and may persist for weeks to months.
- Antibiotics have no effect on OME and should not be used.
- Otitis externa (OE) is an inflammation of the external auditory canal (EAC).
- Acute otitis externa (AOE), also known as "swimmer's ear," is a bacterial infection of the EAC.
- In most cases, AOE can be treated by cleaning and use of ear drops, which may contain 2% acetic acid (to kill bacteria), alcohol (to promote drying), hydrocortisone (to reduce inflammation and edema), or an antibacterial drug (ciprofloxacin and certain other fluoroquinolones are preferred).
- If AOE progresses to the pinna, oral antibiotics should be used. Ciprofloxacin is a good choice for adults; cephalexin is a good choice for children.
- Necrotizing OE is a rare but potentially fatal complication of AOE that develops when bacteria in the EAC invade the mastoid or temporal bone. The usual pathogen is *Pseudomonas aeruginosa.*
- Necrotizing OE can be managed by thorough cleansing and use of antipseudomonal drugs. All patients should receive antipseudomonal ear drops (e.g., ofloxacin solution). Patients with mild disease should receive oral ciprofloxacin. Patients with severe disease should receive IV therapy (e.g., imipenem/cilastatin [Primaxin]).
- In about 10% of patients with OE, the infection is due to fungi and not bacteria. The most common fungal pathogen is *Aspergillus.*
- Fungal OE (otomycosis) can usually be managed by thorough cleansing and application of acidifying drops (e.g., 2% acetic acid solution). If needed, a topical antifungal drug (e.g., 1% clotrimazole) can be used. Unresponsive infections can be treated with an oral antifungal drug (e.g., itraconazole, fluconazole).

Please visit **http://evolve.elsevier.com/Lehne** for chapter-specific NCLEX® examination review questions.

Summary of Major Nursing Implications[a]

PREADMINISTRATION ASSESSMENT

Therapeutic Goal

The goal of treatment is to reduce inflammation, eliminate infection, and prevent complications due to AOM and AOE.

Baseline Data

Assess for reports of earache or, for nonverbal children, pulling at ears, increased crying, and decreased activity.

Obtain the patient's temperature.

Assess the TM for erythema, bulging, and decreased mobility and the EAC for swelling and drainage.

For children with repeated infection, determine whether this has led to language delays.

Identifying High-Risk Patients

Determine whether the patient with AOM has taken amoxicillin in the past 30 days. If so, a different antibiotic will be indicated.

Determine whether the patient has any drug allergies.

Implementation: Administration

Check for penicillin allergies before giving amoxicillin or amoxicillin/clavulanate.

If a patient who is prescribed a cephalosporin has a history of *severe* allergy to penicillin, notify the provider.

Avoid ototoxic drops such as aminoglycoside preparations in patients with a ruptured TM.

For AOE, if the EAC is significantly swollen, insert a wick to ensure that the medication reaches all affected tissues along the length of the canal.

Teach the patient or caregivers how to administer ear drops correctly. Instruct them to avoid instilling cold otic solutions into the EAC.

Promoting Adherence

Educate patients about the importance of taking medication exactly as prescribed.

Advise patients to complete the full prescription even if symptoms improve.

Teach patients to report any worsening of symptoms or a failure to improve after 48 to 72 hours. Worsening or failure to improve may indicate treatment failure. A different antibiotic may be needed.

Ongoing Evaluation and Intervention

On follow-up visits, ask about symptom improvement, complete an ear examination, and compare findings to baseline assessment.

Teach patients and caregivers AOE prevention by not inserting objects in the EAC, promoting water drainage after swimming or showering by tipping the head to each side while pulling the auricle in different directions, allowing cerumen to remain in the ear, and avoiding earplug use except when swimming.

[a]Patient education information is highlighted as **blue text.**

CHAPTER 107 Additional Noteworthy Drugs

DRUGS FOR PULMONARY ARTERIAL HYPERTENSION

Pulmonary arterial hypertension (PAH) is a rare, progressive, and potentially fatal disease of the small pulmonary arteries. The condition is defined by a sustained elevation of pulmonary arterial pressure of more than 25 mm Hg at rest or more than 30 mm Hg during exercise, with a mean pulmonary capillary wedge pressure and left ventricular end-diastolic pressure of less than 15 mm Hg. The primary vascular changes in PAH are vasoconstriction, proliferation of smooth muscle cells and endothelial cells, and pulmonary thrombosis. Cell proliferation and vascular remodeling lead to a progressive increase in pulmonary vascular resistance. The ultimate result is right ventricular failure and death. Although the pathogenesis of PAH is not fully understood, a hormone known as endothelin-1 may play a critical role.

Traditional treatment consists of three drugs: warfarin, a diuretic, and a calcium channel blocker. Warfarin prevents thrombosis. Diuretics reduce fluid retention, and thereby reduce cardiac preload, which in turn reduces symptoms of right-heart failure. Calcium channel blockers dilate constricted pulmonary arteries and can thereby reduce pulmonary hypertension. However, only 20% of patients respond to calcium channel blockers, hence use of these drugs is limited to this small group.

For many patients, PAH becomes progressively worse despite drug therapy, so surgical intervention may be required. Options include single-lung, double-lung, and heart-lung transplantation. These surgeries are high risk, with a mortality rate of 16% to 29%. Five-year survival is 40% to 45%.

Eight drugs are approved for treatment of PAH: epoprostenol, treprostinil, iloprost, bosentan, ambrisentan, sildenafil, tadalafil, and macitentan (Table 107.1). All eight promote pulmonary vasodilation. In addition, they may delay or reverse pulmonary vascular remodeling. Also, all of these are very expensive. The discussion that follows is limited to these drugs.

Prostacyclin Analogs

Three derivatives of prostacyclin are approved for PAH: epoprostenol, treprostinil, and iloprost. All three mimic the actions of endogenous prostacyclin, a compound that promotes vascular relaxation, suppresses growth of vascular smooth muscle cells, and inhibits platelet aggregation. Like prostacyclin, the analogs bind with cell-membrane receptors and thereby stimulate synthesis of cyclic AMP, an intracellular second messenger that mediates prostacyclin effects. In patients with PAH, the prostacyclin analogs lower pulmonary arterial resistance, decrease pulmonary arterial pressure, increase exercise tolerance, and improve short-term survival.

Epoprostenol

Epoprostenol [Flolan] was the first prostacyclin available for PAH. Administration is complex and inconvenient, and adverse effects are common. The drug has a very short half-life (less than 6 minutes) and is unstable at room temperature. As a result, it must be given by continuous IV infusion, using a portable pump that can keep the drug cold. Administration is done through a central venous catheter. The infusion rate is low initially and then gradually increased to a typical maintenance rate of 20 to 40 ng/kg/min. More than 50% of patients taking this drug experience arthralgia, especially neck pain,

TABLE 107.1 ▪ Drugs for Pulmonary Arterial Hypertension

Drug	Administration	Principal Adverse Effects
PROSTACYCLIN ANALOGS		
Epoprostenol [Flolan]	Continuous IV infusion through a central venous catheter	Catheter-related sepsis, headache, flushing, nausea
Treprostinil		
[Remodulin]	Continuous subQ infusion	Local pain and other local reactions in most patients
[Remodulin]	Continuous IV infusion through a central venous catheter	Catheter-related sepsis
[Tyvaso]	Oral inhalation, 4 times/day	Cough, headache, throat irritation, nausea, flushing
Iloprost [Ventavis]	Inhalation, 6–9 times/day	Hypotension and fainting, cough, headache, flushing
ENDOTHELIN-1 RECEPTOR BLOCKERS		
Bosentan [Tracleer]	Oral, twice daily	Hepatotoxicity, anemia, fluid retention, decreased sperm count; classified in FDA Pregnancy Risk Category X[a]
Ambrisentan [Letairis, Volibris 🍁]	Oral, once daily	Anemia, fluid retention (including pulmonary edema), decreased sperm count; classified in FDA Pregnancy Risk Category X[a]
Macitentan [Opsumit]	Oral, once daily	Anemia, hepatotoxicity; classified in FDA Pregnancy Risk Category X[a]
PHOSPHODIESTERASE TYPE 5 INHIBITORS		
Sildenafil [Revatio]	Oral or IV bolus, 3 times/day	Headache, flushing, dyspepsia
Tadalafil [Adcirca]	Oral, once daily	Headache, dyspepsia, back pain, muscle pain

[a]As of 2020, the FDA will no longer use Pregnancy Risk Categories. Please refer to Chapter 9 for more information.

jaw pain, dizziness, headache, and flushing. One-third of patients experience nausea and vomiting. These responses are dose dependent and generally mild. Of greater concern, patients are at risk for catheter-related sepsis. Also, if the pump fails or the catheter becomes dislodged, the resulting interruption of drug delivery can be life threatening.

Treprostinil

Treprostinil was approved for parenteral therapy of PAH initially and later for inhalational therapy of PAH. Products for parenteral therapy are marketed as *Remodulin,* and products for inhalation therapy are marketed as *Tyvaso.* For parenteral therapy, treprostinil is usually administered by continuous subQ infusion, but if needed, it can be infused through a central venous line instead. Treprostinil has a much longer half-life than epoprostenol (4 hours vs. 6 minutes) and much greater temperature stability.

Compared with infused epoprostenol, infused treprostinil [Remodulin] has three major advantages. First, because treprostinil remains stable at room temperature, it doesn't require cooling the way epoprostenol does. Second, because treprostinil has a prolonged half-life, maintaining a precise infusion rate is less critical. And third, because treprostinil can be infused subQ, the risk for sepsis associated with a central venous catheter is obviated. However, subQ treprostinil is not free of problems: local pain and other local reactions (e.g., erythema, induration, rash) occur in more than 80% of patients. Local pain is often dose limiting. Other side effects include jaw pain, diarrhea, edema, and nausea.

For inhalational therapy, treprostinil [Tyvaso] is dosed using the Tyvaso Inhalation System, which delivers 6 mcg with each inhalation. The initial dosage is 18 mcg (3 inhalations) 4 times a day (at 4-hour intervals during waking hours), for a total of 72 mcg/day. The target maintenance dosage is 54 mcg (9 inhalations) 4 times a day, for a total of 216 mcg/day. About half of patients experience cough and headache. Other common adverse effects of inhaled treprostinil are throat irritation, nausea, and flushing.

Iloprost

Iloprost [Ventavis] was the first prostacyclin that did not require continuous infusion. Instead, the drug is administered by oral inhalation. The usual dosage is 5 mcg inhaled 6 to 9 times a day, using either the Prodose AAD system or the I-neb AAD system. About one-third of patients experience cough, headache, and flushing. Spasm of the jaw muscles may also occur. More importantly, peripheral vasodilation may result in orthostatic hypotension and syncope. To reduce risk, iloprost should be avoided in patients with systolic blood pressure below 85 mm Hg.

Endothelin-1 Receptor Antagonists

Endothelin-1 (ET-1) is a small peptide hormone that promotes vasoconstriction and proliferation of endothelial cells. In patients with PAH, the level of ET-1 in the pulmonary vasculature is elevated as much as 10-fold. Furthermore, the degree of ET-1 elevation corresponds with the degree of PAH severity. Endothelin-1 acts through two types of receptors, known as endothelin type A (ET_A) receptors and endothelin type B (ET_B) receptors. Activation of ET_A receptors causes vasoconstriction and cell proliferation, whereas activation of ET_B receptors causes vasodilation.

Endothelin-1 receptor antagonists (ERAs) can reduce the adverse impact of ET-1 on lung function. Three ERAs are available: *bosentan* [Tracleer], *ambrisentan* [Letairis, Volibris 🍁], and *macitentan* [Opsumit]. In patients with PAH, these drugs can improve exercise tolerance and delay symptom progression. Unfortunately, the drugs can also cause serious adverse effects.

Bosentan

Actions and Use. Bosentan [Tracleer] is a nonspecific ERA that blocks ET_A receptors *and* ET_B receptors. In patients with PAH, the drug improves exercise tolerance and slows symptom progression. Presumably, benefits derive from blocking ET_A receptors rather than ET_B receptors. As noted, ET_A receptors promote vasoconstriction and cell proliferation, and hence blocking these receptors should reduce pulmonary vascular resistance and may have a favorable impact on vascular remodeling. Blockade of ET_B receptors may be counterproductive, in that the result could be an *increase* in vascular resistance.

Pharmacokinetics. Bosentan is an oral drug with 50% bioavailability, both in the presence and absence of food. Plasma levels peak 3 to 4 hours after dosing. Protein binding in blood is high (over 98%). Bosentan undergoes metabolism in the liver, primarily by the cytochrome P450 isoenzymes CYP2C9 and CYP3A4, followed by excretion in the bile. The half-life is approximately 5 hours.

Adverse Effects. The most serious adverse effects are liver injury and teratogenesis. Bosentan can also cause headache, flushing, peripheral edema, nasal congestion, anemia, and reduced sperm production.

Hepatotoxicity. Liver injury is common. In 11% of patients, serum levels of liver aminotransferases exceed 3 times the upper limit of normal (ULN). Liver enzymes should be measured at baseline and monthly thereafter. If levels exceed 3 times the ULN at baseline, bosentan should not be used. If levels rise during treatment and are accompanied by clinical symptoms (e.g., nausea, vomiting, fever, jaundice, fatigue), bosentan should be discontinued. Fortunately, all cases of liver injury to date have been reversible; there have been no reports of permanent liver injury or liver failure.

Fetal Injury. Bosentan is classified in U.S. Food and Drug Administration (FDA) Pregnancy Risk Category X,[a] and hence must not be used during pregnancy. Accordingly, pregnancy must be ruled out before initiating treatment, and sexually active women must use reliable contraception. Hormonal contraception may be unreliable, and hence should not be the sole form of contraception employed.

Anemia. Bosentan can reduce hemoglobin levels and the hematocrit. These hematologic changes usually develop during the first weeks of treatment and then stabilize by weeks 4 to 12. Blood tests should be done 1 month and 3 months after starting bosentan, and every 3 months thereafter.

Drug Interactions. Bosentan is subject to significant drug interactions. *Inhibitors of CYP2C9 and CYP4A4* have the potential to raise bosentan levels, thereby increasing the risk for toxicity.

Bosentan itself is an inducer of CYP2D6, and hence can accelerate the metabolism of certain other drugs. Important among these are *warfarin* (an anticoagulant that many people with PAH use) and *oral contraceptives.*

Two drugs—*cyclosporine* and *glyburide*—must not be taken with bosentan. Cyclosporine (an immunosuppressant) can greatly increase bosentan levels, and glyburide (a drug for type 2 diabetes) increases the risk for liver injury.

Preparations, Dosage, and Administration. Bosentan [Tracleer] is supplied in tablets (62.5 and 125 mg). For patients who weigh 40 kg or more, the dosage is 62.5 mg twice daily for 4 weeks, and then 125 mg twice daily thereafter for maintenance. For patients who weigh less than 40 kg, the dosage is 62.5 mg twice daily initially, and remains at 62.5 mg twice daily for maintenance. In patients with elevated transaminase levels, dosage should be adjusted as follows:

- Above 3 times the ULN but below 5 times the ULN—decrease dosage or interrupt dosing
- Above 5 times the ULN—stop dosing, and don't resume until the level has returned to the baseline value
- Above 8 times the ULN—stop dosing and don't resume

To reduce the risk for liver injury and possible fetal exposure, bosentan must be prescribed through the Tracleer Access Program.

Ambrisentan

Ambrisentan [Letairis, Volibris 🍁] is much like bosentan with regard to actions, indications, and adverse effects. Both drugs block receptors for ET-1; both are taken to improve exercise tolerance and delay symptom progression in PAH; and both can cause severe birth defects. The drugs differ primarily in two respects. First, in contrast to bosentan, ambrisentan does *not* injure the liver. And second, whereas bosentan blocks ETA *and* ETB receptors, ambrisentan is selective for ETA receptors. However, we don't know if this selectivity improves clinical outcome. As with bosentan, pregnancy must be ruled out before starting ambrisentan, and sexually active women must use two reliable forms of contraception. Like bosentan, ambrisentan can cause peripheral edema, headache, flushing, and anemia. In contrast to bosentan, ambrisentan does not reduce levels of warfarin. Ambrisentan is supplied in 5- and 10-mg film-coated tablets, which may be taken with or without food. Dosing begins at 5 mg once a day and, if this dosage is tolerated, may be increased to 10 mg once a day. Ambrisentan is not recommended for patients with moderate or severe hepatic impairment (because blood levels of the drug may become excessive). Owing to the risk for birth defects, ambrisentan is available only through a restricted distribution program, known as the Letairis Education and Access Program (LEAP).

Macitentan

Macitentan [Opsumit] received FDA approval in 2014, so postmarketing studies are not available. It is a derivative of bosentan, although early studies indicate that it is less hepatotoxic than bosentan. Approximately 10% to 20% of patients experience headache, anemia, nasopharyngitis, and bronchitis when using the drug. Less common but potentially serious complications include fluid retention and liver injury. Macitentan is available in 10-mg tablets. Dosing is 10 mg once a day for up to 10 days. Like other ERAs, this drug is contraindicated in pregnancy, and it may reduce sperm count in men. Owing to the potential for serious adverse effects, caution is advised when giving this drug to patients with severe chronic heart failure, severe anemia, or history of liver damage.

Phosphodiesterase Type 5 Inhibitors

The phosphodiesterase type 5 (PDE5) inhibitors reduce pulmonary arterial pressure by causing dilation of pulmonary blood vessels. Two PDE5 inhibitors—sildenafil and tadalafil—are approved for PAH. Both drugs were originally developed for erectile dysfunction (ED). The basic pharmacology of these drugs and their use for ED are discussed in Chapter 66. Consideration here is limited to their use in PAH.

Sildenafil

Sildenafil, sold as *Revatio,* was approved for oral therapy of PAH, and later for IV therapy. How does sildenafil work? It causes selective inhibition of PDE5, the enzyme that inactivates cyclic GMP (cGMP). In arterioles of the lung and other tissues, endogenous nitric oxide triggers synthesis of cGMP, which in turn promotes vasodilation. Therefore, by inhibiting PDE5, sildenafil can preserve cGMP, and can thereby enhance vasodilation mediated by nitric oxide. In patients with PAH, sildenafil reduces pulmonary arterial pressure and pulmonary vascular resistance. The drug may also suppress proliferation of pulmonary vascular smooth muscle cells.

[a]As of 2020, the FDA will no longer use Pregnancy Risk Categories. Please refer to Chapter 9 for more information.

Sildenafil is generally well tolerated. The most common adverse effects are headache, flushing, and dyspepsia. Transient visual disturbances and priapism (prolonged, painful erection) occur infrequently. Very rarely, men have experienced sudden hearing loss or sight-threatening nonarteritic ischemic optic neuropathy. However, in both cases, a causal relationship has not been established.

Sildenafil can cause mild hypotension when used alone and significant hypotension when combined with certain drugs. Combined use with alpha-adrenergic blockers can cause symptomatic postural hypotension. Of much greater concern, combined used with nitrates (e.g., nitroglycerin, isosorbide dinitrate) can cause a life-threatening drop in blood pressure. Accordingly, concurrent use of sildenafil and nitrates is contraindicated.

Sildenafil is metabolized by CYP3A4 (the 3A4 isoenzyme of cytochrome P450). As a result, CYP3A4 inhibitors (e.g., ketoconazole, clarithromycin, ritonavir) can raise sildenafil levels, and CYP3A4 inducers (e.g., rifampin, phenytoin) can lower its level.

For treatment of PAH, sildenafil is available in two formulations: 20-mg tablets for oral therapy, and a solution (10 mg/12.5 mL) for IV therapy. Both formulations are sold as *Revatio.* The oral dosage is 20 mg 3 times a day, taken with or without food. The IV dosage is 10 mg 3 times a day, given by bolus injection.

Tadalafil

Tadalafil, sold as *Adcirca,* is approved for oral therapy of PAH. As with sildenafil, benefits derive from dilating pulmonary blood vessels. The most common adverse effects are headache, dyspepsia, back pain, and muscle pain. Like sildenafil, tadalafil should not be combined with nitroglycerin or other nitrates, owing to a risk for severe hypotension. As with sildenafil, drugs that inhibit or induce CYP3A4 can alter levels of tadalafil. For treatment of PAH, tadalafil is available in 20-mg tablets. The dosage is 40 mg once a day, taken with or without food.

DRUGS FOR NEONATAL RESPIRATORY DISTRESS SYNDROME

Respiratory distress syndrome (RDS) is the primary cause of morbidity and mortality in premature infants. The underlying cause is deficiency of lung surfactant, a complex mixture of phospholipids and apoproteins that lowers surface tension on the alveolar surface. Consequences of surfactant deficiency include alveolar collapse, pulmonary edema, reduced lung compliance, small airway epithelial damage, hypoxia, and ultimately respiratory failure.

Increased production of cortisol during weeks 30 to 32 of gestation initiates production of lung surfactant. However, surfactant production is not fully adequate until weeks 34 to 36. As a result, the earlier the premature infant is delivered, the greater the risk for RDS. Among infants born during weeks 26 to 28, the incidence of RDS is 60% to 80%; by weeks 30 to 32, the incidence drops to 20%.

Prenatal and Postnatal Glucocorticoids

When preterm delivery cannot be prevented, injecting the mother with glucocorticoids can accelerate fetal lung maturation and can thereby decrease the incidence and severity of RDS. Glucocorticoids act by stimulating production of fibroblast pneumocyte factor, which in turn stimulates production of surfactant by fetal pneumocytes. Glucocorticoids are effective when used during weeks 24 to 34 of gestation. Beyond week 34, fetal lungs are sufficiently mature that no benefit is gained by giving these drugs. Two drugs are recommended: *dexamethasone* and *betamethasone.* A *single course* consists of either (1) *dexamethasone,* 6 mg IM every 12 hours for four doses, or (2) *betamethasone,* two 12-mg IM doses, injected 24 hours apart. To be effective, the last glucocorticoid dose should be administered at least 24 hours before delivery, but no more than 7 days before. The basic pharmacology of the glucocorticoids is discussed in Chapters 60 and 72.

If pregnancy is successfully extended (e.g., by giving a uterine relaxant), can repeat courses of glucocorticoids be of benefit? Possibly. Giving a repeat course every week until delivery yields better short-term outcomes than giving a single course because, with repeat courses, there is a lower incidence of RDS, less need for mechanical respiratory support, and a reduction in serious neonatal morbidity. Furthermore, long-term follow-up studies done to date suggest that repeat courses are safe. Compared with children who received a single prenatal course, those who received repeat prenatal courses showed no deficits in growth, blood pressure, neurocognitive function, or developmental scores and no increase in neurodevelopmental complications. However, although repeat courses may not cause long-term harm, there is no proof that repeat courses offer any long-term benefits.

Although the risk/benefit ratio for *pre*natal glucocorticoids appears favorable, the risk/benefit ratio for *post*natal glucocorticoids remains in dispute. The American Academy of Pediatrics asserts that early postnatal treatment with glucocorticoids is beneficial for some infants but is not recommended as a routine intervention. They found no evidence of improved outcomes with the use of high doses versus low doses of these drugs, so they do not recommend high-dose glucocorticoid therapy. Therefore, as with most drugs, it is up to the provider to weigh the risks and benefits when making decisions regarding drug therapy.

Lung Surfactant

Lung surfactant, administered by direct intratracheal instillation, is indicated for prevention and treatment (rescue therapy) of RDS. Surfactant therapy lowers the surface tension forces that cause alveolar collapse and thereby rapidly improves oxygenation and lung compliance and reduces the need for supplemental oxygen and mechanical ventilation. Treatment decreases neonatal mortality by 33%.

In the United States, three preparations of lung surfactant are available: poractant alfa, calfactant, and beractant. Current data are insufficient to recommend any one drug over the others. *Initial* doses for prevention or treatment of RDS are as follows:

- *Poractant alfa* [Curosurf]—2.5 mL/kg
- *Calfactant* [Infasurf]—3 mL/kg
- *Beractant* [Survanta]—4 mL/kg

Because the effects of a single dose are often transient, repeated dosing may be needed. For poractant alfa, repeat doses should be 1.25 mL/kg—half the initial dose—12 hours apart for up to two doses. For calfactant the repeat dose is the same as the initial dose and is administered 12 hours apart for up to three doses. Repeat dosing for beractant is also the same as for the initial dose, but timing is 6 hours apart for up to four doses.

Adverse effects result primarily from the administration process. Bradycardia and oxygen desaturation, which occur secondary to vagal stimulation and airway obstruction, are most common. If these occur, it may be necessary to temporarily suspend administration. Other adverse effects include pulmonary hemorrhage, mucus plugging, and endotracheal tube reflux.

Is there an effective alternative to using lung surfactant combined with mechanical ventilation in preterm infants? The answer is "Yes," as shown in the Surfactant, Positive Pressure, and Oxygenation Randomized Trial (SUPPORT). In this trial, preterm infants were treated either with continuous positive airway pressure or with surfactant plus mechanical ventilation. The result? The incidence of death, bronchopulmonary dysplasia, and other major outcomes was the same in both groups.

DRUGS FOR CYSTIC FIBROSIS

Cystic fibrosis (CF) is an inherited disorder that primarily damages the lungs, pancreas, and sweat glands. Some patients also develop liver disease. About 30,000 U.S. citizens have the disease. Fifty years ago, most children diagnosed with CF died before 5 years. Today, the survival time is 37 years, with some living into their 40s and beyond. Drugs cannot cure CF, but they can reduce symptoms and slow progression of injury.

Pathophysiology of Cystic Fibrosis

The underlying cause of CF is mutation of the gene that codes for a particular type of chloride channel, referred to as the *cystic fibrosis transmembrane regulator* (CFTR). In cells that have defective CFTRs, the normal transmembrane flow of chloride ions, sodium ions, and water is disrupted. In the lungs, exocrine glands (e.g., pancreas), and other structures, disruption of ion and water flux alters secretions.

Pancreas

Disruption of chloride transport in the pancreas impairs secretion of bicarbonate and digestive enzymes into the small intestine. The immediate result is maldigestion and malabsorption of fats and other nutrients. Absorption of fat-soluble vitamins, especially vitamins A and E, is reduced secondary to malabsorption of fats. Over time, accumulation of digestive enzymes within pancreatic cells leads to cell destruction. At autopsy, the pancreas appears scarred and fibrotic, which led pathologists to name this illness *fibrocystic disease of the pancreas*—later shortened to *cystic fibrosis*. Until replacement therapy with pancreatic enzymes became possible, malabsorption of nutrients was the major cause of CF death.

Lungs

Today, destruction of lung tissue is the major cause of morbidity and mortality among patients with CF. In the cells that line the airway, defective CFTRs impair secretion of chloride and enhance reabsorption of water and sodium. As a result, mucus becomes thick and viscous, causing plugging of the airway and promoting chronic bacterial colonization. All patients eventually develop active pulmonary infection; the most common pathogens are *Pseudomonas aeruginosa* and *Staphylococcus aureus*. Infection elicits an inflammatory response that is mediated primarily by neutrophils. Accumulation of DNA from dead neutrophils further increases the viscosity of sputum. Over time, chronic bronchitis and associated inflammation cause progressive destruction of lung tissue. In 95% of patients, death from cardiorespiratory failure ultimately ensues.

Reproductive Organs

Among patients with CF, 98% of males and 70% to 80% of females are infertile. In males, the usual cause is obstruction of the vas deferens. In females, the cause appears to be production of thick, sticky cervical mucus, which impedes penetration of sperm.

Drug Therapy

Drugs are used to alleviate symptoms of CF and delay progression of injury to the lungs. Agents employed include pancreatic enzymes, fat-soluble vitamins, antibiotics, dornase alfa, and ibuprofen. The newest and most exciting therapy is the advent of CFTR modulators. We will discuss these first.

Cystic Fibrosis Transmembrane Regulator Modifiers

In 2012, the FDA approved the first drug that targets the underlying cause of CF. The drug, ivacaftor [Kalydeco], is a CFTR modifier. It is unique in that it restores functioning of the defective protein. The drug is not for everyone with CF, however. It is specifically for patients 2 years and older (6 years in Canada) with 1 of 10 genetic mutations in the cystic fibrosis transmembrane conductance regulator (CFTR). Unfortunately, the number of patients eligible for treatment was small; however, the inroads made into genetic therapy for CF treatment held the promise of even greater things to come.

In 2015, the FDA approved a second CFTR modifier, lumacaftor/ivacaftor [Orkambi]. This drug added to ivacaftor another drug, lumacaftor, which acts as a stabilizer to enhance ivacaftor's actions. This addition had important implications for the number of CF patients eligible for treatment, as well: more than 11,000 people with CF became suitable for treatment with this drug!

Other CFTR modifiers are currently in clinical trials. These "next-generation" drugs promise even greater superiority and may be approved by the time you read this.

Adverse Effects. Adverse effects are similar for both ivacaftor and ivacaftor/lumacaftor. Most common are abdominal discomfort, nausea, diarrhea, headache, nasal congestion, upper respiratory infections, and shortness of breath. Almost one-fourth of patients taking ivacaftor, but not lumacaftor/ivacaftor, reported chest pain.

The most concerning adverse effects include hepatic injury, hypertension, and cataract formation. Liver enzymes (alanine transaminase [ALT], aspartate transaminase [AST]) and bilirubin should be measured before beginning therapy and obtained every 3 months during year 1 and every year thereafter. Blood pressure should be measured at each clinic visit. Management for hypertension is individualized. It is possible that cataracts are associated with other drugs taken for CF (e.g., glucocorticoids), but until more is known, it is important to obtain an ophthalmologic examination before beginning treatment, with periodic follow-up examinations.

Drug Interactions. There are numerous drug interactions associated with these drugs. Before administering, it is important to check for interactions with other prescribed drugs.

Cost of Therapy. Not surprisingly, therapy is incredibly expensive. Fifty-six 50-mg tablets of ivacaftor cost $28,675. A typical pediatric dosage is 50 mg every 12 hours, and a typical adult dosage is 150 mg every 12 hours.

To address this concern, Vertex, the pharmaceutical manufacturer of these drugs, offers special programs (including free drugs) for those meeting eligibility guidelines (see https://www.vrtx.com/pipeline-medicines/patient-support).

Nutritional Drugs

Pancreatic Enzymes. These enzymes are given as replacement therapy. All preparations contain lipase, protease, and amylase. The most effective formulations deliver the enzymes in enteric-coated microspheres, which are designed to protect the enzymes from stomach acid and ensure dissolution in the duodenum, the site where the enzymes act. Pancreatic enzymes are discussed in Chapter 80.

Fat-Soluble Vitamins. There are four fat-soluble vitamins: A, D, E, and K. Among patients with CF, deficiencies in vitamins A and E are relatively common, whereas deficiency in vitamin K is uncommon and deficiency in vitamin D is rare. Because vitamins are safe and relatively inexpensive, supplementation with all four is done routinely.

Pulmonary Drugs

Inhaled Antibiotics for Chronic Suppressive Therapy. Antibiotics are used long-term to suppress chronic infection with *P. aeruginosa.* The preferred route is *inhalation.* Why? Because this route achieves high concentrations in the airway while minimizing the risk for systemic toxicity. However, because treatment is prolonged, resistance is a concern. Two antibiotics—tobramycin and aztreonam—are approved for chronic inhalational therapy of *P. aeruginosa* infection. Both drugs improve pulmonary function, reduce the density of *P. aeruginosa* in sputum, and decrease the risk for hospitalization. In a trial that compared these drugs directly, aztreonam was more effective. Both drugs cost about $5000 for a 28-day supply.

With *tobramycin* [TOBI], the dosage is 300 mg every 12 hours in repeating cycles of 28 days on and 28 days off. Each dose takes 10 to 15 minutes to administer. Common adverse effects include cough, wheezing, and hoarseness. In contrast to IV aminoglycosides, inhaled tobramycin is unlikely to cause hearing loss, although it can cause tinnitus (ringing in the ears). The basic pharmacology of tobramycin and other aminoglycosides is discussed in Chapter 87.

With *aztreonam* [Cayston], the dosage is 75 mg 3 times a day in repeating cycles of 28 days on and 28 days off. Each dose takes 2 to 3 minutes to administer, making aztreonam more convenient than tobramycin. Principal adverse effects are cough, nasal congestion, and wheezing. The basic pharmacology of aztreonam is presented in Chapter 85.

Oral and Intravenous Antibiotics for Acute Therapy. Acute exacerbations of pulmonary infection can be treated with oral or IV antibiotics. For mild infection, oral agents may suffice. For severe exacerbations, IV antibiotics are required. Options include aminoglycosides (e.g., tobramycin, gentamicin), piperacillin/tazobactam, ticarcillin/clavulanate, and imipenem/cilastatin.

Inhaled Dornase Alfa. Dornase alfa [Pulmozyme], a purified preparation of recombinant human deoxyribonuclease, decreases the viscosity of sputum in patients with CF. The drug is administered by inhalation, using an approved nebulizer. Benefits derive from breaking down extracellular DNA that has accumulated in the lungs secondary to death of neutrophils. With daily use, dornase alfa can improve pulmonary function and decrease infection in some patients. The drug is generally well tolerated. Adverse effects include hoarseness, pharyngitis, laryngitis, rash, chest pain, and conjunctivitis. Dosing is begun at 2.5 mg once daily and may be increased to 2.5 mg twice daily if needed. To remain effective, dornase alfa must be administered every day for life. Unfortunately, treatment is expensive. A year's supply of dornase alfa costs over $12,000. The nebulizer costs another $2000.

Oral Ibuprofen. High-dose ibuprofen can slow progression of pulmonary damage in patients with mild lung disease caused by CF. Ibuprofen works by suppressing the inflammatory response that underlies destruction of lung tissue. Ibuprofen dosage should be sufficient to produce peak plasma drug levels of 50 to 100 mg/mL. Side effects attributable to ibuprofen include conjunctivitis and epistaxis (nosebleed).

Inhaled Beta$_2$-Adrenergic Agonists. Salmeterol [Serevent Diskus] and other inhaled beta$_2$ agonists can be used long term to improve lung function. Benefits derive from causing bronchodilation and improving ciliary function.

DRUGS FOR SICKLE CELL ANEMIA

Sickle cell anemia (SCA) is an inherited blood disorder characterized by abnormal hemoglobin, chronic anemia, periodic painful episodes, and reduced life expectancy. The underlying cause is a mutation in the gene that codes for hemoglobin (Hb). People who inherit two copies of the gene (one from each parent) produce an altered form of Hb, known as hemoglobin S (HbS). (People with just one copy are carriers, but do not make HbS.) When HbS is fully oxygenated, there is no problem. However, when HbS gives up its oxygen, molecules of HbS can polymerize, forming long, rigid, rod-like chains. As a result, red blood cells (RBCs) assume a sickle (crescent) shape, and hence cannot pass through tiny blood vessels. As more RBCs get stuck, blood flow stops, thereby depriving tissues of required nutrients and oxygen. The result is severe pain, referred to as a vaso-occlusive crisis. Pain location depends on where vessel blockage occurs (e.g., hands and feet, joints and extremities, abdomen). The crisis may last a few hours to a few weeks. Some patients have 15 or more painful episodes a year, whereas others may have 1 a year or less. Over time, vaso-occlusive events produce progressive organ damage and premature death. The median age at death is 42 for men and 48 for women. In many cases, death results from PAH. Management of this condition was discussed previously.

In addition to vaso-occlusive events, people with SCA experience chronic anemia (shortage of RBCs). Why? Unlike normal RBCs, which persist about 120 days, sickled RBCs die in 10 to 20 days. Because RBC loss is unusually rapid, replacements cannot be made fast enough, and hence a chronic shortage results.

Who is vulnerable to SCA? Worldwide, millions of people have the disease. In the United States, about 72,000 people have SCA. Most are African Americans (about 1 in 700 carry two copies of the sickle cell gene, and 1 in 14 carry one copy). In addition, SCA afflicts between 1 in 1000 to 1400 Hispanic Americans. The disease is not found among white Americans.

Researchers believe that the sickle cell mutation arose in a region where malaria is endemic. There is evidence that in people with *one* copy of the gene malaria is less deadly than in people who do not have the gene. As a result, those who carried the gene were more likely to survive, and hence could pass the advantage on to their children. Of course, in areas like the United States, where malaria rarely occurs, the gene offers no survival advantage—and when two copies are inherited, the gene becomes a threat to survival.

Treatment consists of transfusions, analgesics, glucocorticoids, and hydroxyurea. Blood transfusions help correct anemia and reduce painful episodes. Analgesics and glucocorticoids can alleviate pain. Hydroxyurea can reduce the incidence and severity of painful episodes and, perhaps more importantly, it can prolong life.

Analgesics and Glucocorticoids

For patients undergoing an acute crisis, analgesics and hydration are the cornerstone of treatment. Unfortunately, most patients generally fail to receive adequate pain relief. If the pain is moderate, a nonopioid analgesic (acetaminophen or a nonsteroidal anti-inflammatory drug [NSAID]) may be sufficient. However, if pain is severe, intensive therapy with an opioid is required. Parenteral (IV or IM) morphine and meperidine have been employed. Patient-controlled analgesia may be especially effective. The basic pharmacology of the opioids is discussed in Chapter 28.

High doses of intravenous methylprednisolone (a glucocorticoid) can shorten the duration of a sickle cell crisis. The drug should be used together with, not instead of, an opioid. Unfortunately, when glucocorticoids are discontinued, rebound pain may occur. The basic pharmacology of the glucocorticoids is discussed in Chapters 60 and 72.

Hydroxyurea

Hydroxyurea was originally developed to treat cancer (see Chapter 102) and is now used for SCA as well. Treatment can reduce the number of painful events, as well as the need for hospitalization and transfusions. Furthermore, it can reduce mortality. Currently, hydroxyurea is approved only for adults; however, it is sometimes used off-label for children based on positive research results in children. Formulations for SCA are marketed as *Droxia,* and formulations for cancer are marketed as *Hydrea.*

Mechanism of Action

Hydroxyurea increases production of fetal hemoglobin (HbF), a form of Hb present in infants but not normally present after the sixth month of postnatal life. In patients with SCA, elevation of HbF decreases hemoglobin polymerization, decreasing RBC sickling and prolonging RBC life. Hydroxyurea also reduces adhesion of RBCs to the vascular endothelium. Precisely how the drug elevates HbF has not been established.

Adverse Effects

Hydroxyurea can cause severe *myelosuppression.* Life-threatening reductions in blood-cell counts can result. Accordingly, frequent monitoring of hematologic status is required. Hydroxyurea should not be used if bone marrow function is already significantly depressed.

Hydroxyurea can cause *fetal harm,* and hence should be avoided during pregnancy. The drug is classified in FDA Pregnancy Risk Category D.[b]

Hydroxyurea is *carcinogenic.* Among patients receiving hydroxyurea for cancer, a few have developed leukemia, although it is not proven that hydroxyurea was the cause. Long-term adverse effects in patients with SCA who take hydroxyurea include polycythemia, thrombocythemia, and other myeloproliferative disorders.

Hematologic Monitoring

Hematologic status should be determined every 2 weeks. Acceptable values and values indicating toxicity are as follows:

- *Neutrophils*—acceptable, 2500 cells/mm^3; toxic, less than 2000 cells/mm^3
- *Platelets*—acceptable, 95,000/mm^3; toxic, less than 80,000/mm^3
- *Hemoglobin*—acceptable, 5.3 gm/dL; toxic, less than 4.5 gm/dL
- *Reticulocytes*—acceptable, 95,000/mm^3 (if Hb is less than 9 gm/dL); toxic, less than 80,000/mm^3 (if Hb is less than 9 gm/dL)

Preparations, Dosage, and Administration

For treatment of SCA, hydroxyurea [Droxia] is available in capsules (200, 300, and 400 mg) for oral dosing. The initial dosage is 15 mg/kg once a day. If blood counts remain acceptable, dosage may be increased by 5 mg/kg/day every 12 weeks—up to a maximum of 35 mg/kg/day. If blood counts indicate toxicity, treatment should be temporarily interrupted. Recovery usually occurs in 2 weeks, after which treatment can be resumed, but at a reduced dosage. For treatment of cancer, hydroxyurea [Hydrea] is available in 500-mg capsules for oral dosing.

PHOSPHATE BINDERS FOR PATIENTS ON DIALYSIS

Phosphate binders are used to treat hyperphosphatemia, a common complication of end-stage renal disease. Blood phosphate is high during renal failure because glomerular filtration of phosphate is reduced and tubular reabsorption of phosphate is increased. Hyperphosphatemia is a concern because it promotes hyperparathyroidism, which in turn promotes *hypercalcemia,* a risk factor for cardiovascular (CV) calcification and CV morbidity and mortality.

Treatment of hyperphosphatemia consists of three measures: (1) reducing phosphate intake, (2) removing phosphate with hemodialysis, and (3) reducing intestinal absorption of phosphate with a phosphate-binding drug. Reducing phosphate in the diet is problematic in that most dietary phosphate comes from proteins (e.g., meats, fish, dairy products, peas). Therefore, reducing dietary phosphate may result in malnutrition. Accordingly, the

[b]As of 2020, the FDA will no longer use Pregnancy Risk Categories. Please refer to Chapter 9 for more information.

TABLE 107.2 ■ Phosphate Binders for Patients on Renal Dialysis

Generic Name	Brand Name	Formulation (Including Calcium Content)	Usual Single Dose (Taken 3 Times a Day With Meals)	Calcium Load (mg/day)	Comments
CALCIUM-BASED PHOSPHATE BINDERS					
Calcium carbonate	Os-Cal 500 Caltrate-600	Tablets, 1250 mg (500 mg Ca) Tablets, 1500 mg (600 mg Ca)	1250 mg 1500 mg	1500 1800	Can promote hypercalcemia
Calcium acetate	PhosLo	Tablets, 667 mg (169 mg Ca) Gelcaps, 667 mg (169 mg Ca)	2001–2668 mg 2001–2668 mg	507–676 507–676	Can promote hypercalcemia
CALCIUM-FREE PHOSPHATE BINDERS					
Sevelamer hydrochloride	Renagel	Tablets, 400 mg (0 mg Ca) Tablets, 800 mg (0 mg Ca)	800–1600 mg 800–1600 mg	0	Expensive; lowers cholesterol; does not promote hypercalcemia, but does promote metabolic acidosis
Sevelamer carbonate	Renvela	Tablets, 800 mg (0 mg Ca)	800–1600 mg	0	Same as sevelamer hydrochloride, but decreased risk for metabolic acidosis
Lanthanum carbonate	Fosrenol	Chewable tablets, 500, 750, and 1000 mg (0 mg Ca)	1500–3000 mg	0	Expensive; does not lower cholesterol; does not promote hypercalcemia or metabolic acidosis

ability to manage hyperphosphatemia by reducing phosphate intake is limited.

As indicated in Table 107.2, phosphate-binding drugs fall into two major groups: *calcium-based phosphate binders* (e.g., calcium carbonate) and *calcium-free phosphate binders* (e.g., sevelamer carbonate). All of these drugs are equally effective at reducing phosphate absorption. And they all pose a risk for adverse GI effects. The principal differences among them relate to (1) *price* (the calcium-based drugs cost much less than the calcium-free drugs) and (2) the risk for exacerbating *hypercalcemia* (the calcium-based drugs increase hypercalcemia risk, whereas the calcium-free drugs do not). Because of these differences, the prescriber is faced with a dilemma: Do I save the patient money (with a calcium-based binder) but increase the risk for hypercalcemia and associated CV calcification? Or do I reduce the risk for hypercalcemia (with a calcium-free binder) but greatly increase the cost? A reasonable solution to the dilemma might be this: Reserve the expensive, calcium-free binders for patients who already have hypercalcemia and evidence of coronary artery calcification, and prescribe the cheaper, calcium-free binders for patients with normal calcium levels and no coronary calcification.

Of the calcium-free phosphate binders in current use, one drug—sevelamer—deserves comment. Sevelamer is available as two salts: *sevelamer hydrochloride* [Renagel] and *sevelamer carbonate* [Renvela]. Both salts are equally good at reducing absorption of dietary phosphate, and they both share an additional asset: they can bind with bile salts in the intestine and can thereby decrease the synthesis of cholesterol, a major risk factor for CV morbidity and mortality. Although these salts are very similar, they differ in one important way: Sevelamer hydrochloride can cause *metabolic acidosis,* whereas sevelamer carbonate may not. Metabolic acidosis is a concern because it increases the risk for hyperkalemia, breakdown of proteins, bone dissolution, osteodystrophy, and even death. Because the carbonate component of sevelamer carbonate can act as a buffer, the risk for acidosis with this salt is likely to be lower than with sevelamer hydrochloride. However, there are no data to show that patients fare better with the carbonate salt.

GAMMA-HYDROXYBUTYRATE FOR CATAPLEXY IN PATIENTS WITH NARCOLEPSY

History

Gamma-hydroxybutyrate (GHB) [Xyrem], also known as *sodium oxybate,* is a central nervous system (CNS) depressant with a rapid onset and short duration. The drug was originally developed as a surgical anesthetic, but was discontinued owing to serious side effects: profound respiratory depression, coma, and death. In the 1990s, GHB gained notoriety as a drug of abuse: It was used at parties to produce euphoria and disinhibition, and it was administered clandestinely to facilitate rape. As a result, GHB was declared illegal at that time.

Therapeutic Use

GHB became the first and only drug approved by the FDA for treating *cataplexy* in patients with narcolepsy. Narcolepsy itself, which afflicts about 120,000 Americans, is characterized by fragmented sleep, daytime somnolence, and uncontrollable attacks of sleep during waking hours. In addition, about 60% to 70% of patients experience cataplexy (sudden loss of muscle tone), typically triggered by intense emotion, such as anger, fear, grief, or even amusement. A cataplectic attack may last a few seconds to several minutes, and can range in severity from dropping of the jaw or slumping of the head to buckling of the legs or collapse of the entire body. As discussed in Chapter 36, patients take CNS stimulants (e.g., methylphenidate [Ritalin], dextroamphetamine [Dexedrine]) to promote daytime wakefulness and reduce sudden sleep attacks. GHB is indicated specifically to reduce attacks of cataplexy. Benefits appear to derive from rebound CNS excitement that occurs when the drug's depressant effects wear off. In addition to reducing cataplexy, GHB can improve the quality of nighttime sleep and can thereby help reduce daytime sleepiness.

Adverse Effects and Abuse

In clinical trials, GHB produced confusion, depression, headache, dizziness, sleepwalking, bedwetting, nausea, and vomiting. In two patients, respiratory depression occurred. The risk for respiratory depression is increased by combining GHB with alcohol and other CNS depressants. Because of its sodium content (a 9-gm dose contains 1.6 gm of sodium), GHB may pose a risk to patients with heart failure. Abuse of the drug could cause physical dependence. Because of its abuse history, GHB is regulated as a Schedule III substance.

Availability

Owing to concerns about adverse effects and abuse, availability of GHB is regulated under a strict and comprehensive risk management program. Provisions include limited distribution, prescriber and patient education, prescriber and patient registries, and detailed patient surveillance. Under the program, GHB can be obtained only through a single centralized pharmacy. Before the pharmacy can dispense GHB, the prescriber must verify that the patient has received instruction on its safe use.

Preparations, Dosage, and Administration

Gamma-hydroxybutyrate [Xyrem] is available in oral solution (500 mg/mL in 180-mL bottles). Patients take two doses each night, one at bedtime and one 2.5 to 4 hours later. It is anticipated that the patient will need to be awakened for the second dose. The manufacturer advises setting an alarm to ensure that the second dose is not missed. At treatment onset, each dose is 2.25 gm (4.5 gm total per night). Dosage can be gradually increased to a maximum of 9 gm total per night. In patients with impaired liver function, the dosage should be halved. Treatment is expensive: Each 180 mL (a 40-day supply) costs about $4840. The annual cost is over $44,000.

RILUZOLE FOR AMYOTROPHIC LATERAL SCLEROSIS

Amyotrophic lateral sclerosis (ALS; Lou Gehrig's disease) is a neuromuscular disorder characterized by progressive muscle wasting and loss of strength. The underlying cause is degeneration of motor neurons in the spinal cord, brainstem, and motor cortex. Why motor neurons degenerate is largely unknown. Initial symptoms typically include weakness in the hands and legs, muscle cramps, stiffness, and twitching. Over time, the patient becomes weaker and weaker. Eventually, all skeletal muscles, including the muscles of respiration, become paralyzed. Intellectual function, eye movement, bladder function, and sensation are not affected. Most patients die within 3 to 5 years, although some survive for a decade or longer. In the United States, about 30,000 people have ALS, and 5000 new cases are diagnosed each year. At this time, ALS has no cure.

Riluzole [Rilutek], a glutamate antagonist, is the only drug approved for ALS. In clinical trials, riluzole prolonged life or delayed the need for a tracheostomy by 3 to 6 months. However, not only were benefits modest, they were also limited to patients whose nerve degeneration began in the *medulla;* riluzole did not help patients whose nerve degeneration began in the *spinal cord.* The reason for this difference is unknown.

Riluzole is generally well tolerated. The most common adverse effects are asthenia (decreased strength), GI reactions (nausea, vomiting, diarrhea, abdominal pain), CNS effects (dizziness, vertigo, somnolence), and decreased lung function. Neutropenia develops rarely.

Riluzole can injure the liver, as indicated by an increase in circulating aminotransferase levels. Risk is higher in patients with pre-existing liver disease. To monitor for liver injury, measure aminotransferase levels at baseline, then monthly for 3 months, then every 3 months for the first year, and periodically thereafter. Riluzole should be discontinued if aminotransferase levels exceed 5 times the ULN or if clinical jaundice is diagnosed.

Riluzole [Rilutek] is available in 50-mg oral tablets. The recommended dosage is 50 mg every 12 hours. Increasing the dosage does not increase benefits, but does increase adverse effects. Riluzole should be taken 1 hour before meals or 2 hours after to increase bioavailability.

TETRABENAZINE FOR CHOREA OF HUNTINGTON'S DISEASE

Huntington's disease (HD) is an inherited neurodegenerative disorder characterized by cognitive dysfunction, psychiatric changes, and movement disorders. The underlying cause is an inherited condition that causes progressive death of CNS neurons. Symptoms typically begin between the ages of 30 and 55 years, and then slowly progress. Death occurs 10 to 30 years after symptom onset. Huntington's disease is a rare disorder with a prevalence of 1 in 10,000.

Psychiatric symptoms, which may precede movement disorders, include anxiety, paranoid psychosis, personality changes, and depression and suicidality. Management includes standard medications for these conditions. Keep in mind, however, that antipsychotic drugs can confound the diagnosis and management of HD movement disorders. Why? Because antipsychotic agents can cause extrapyramidal movement disorders. Hence, if a patient develops a movement disorder, it may be hard to tell if the disorder is drug induced or caused by HD.

Motor symptoms are mild at first and become more pronounced as additional neurons die. Initial symptoms may be limited to clumsiness, balance difficulties, and facial tics. Later on, patients develop *chorea,* manifesting as involuntary, irregular, flowing movements that may shift from one area of the body to another. Severe chorea manifests as pronounced continuous movements of the whole body. Other late symptoms include rigidity, difficulty swallowing, hesitant or slurred speech, rapid jerky eye movements, and severe coordination and balance problems. What causes these motor symptoms? *Excessive activity of dopamine* (DA), possibly secondary to the death of neurons that produce acetylcholine and gamma-aminobutyric acid (GABA).

Huntington's chorea often responds to drugs that decrease the activity of DA (Table 107.3). Two mechanisms are involved: reduction of DA stores and blockade of DA receptors. We can reduce DA stores with tetrabenazine and reserpine. Unfortunately, tetrabenazine can cause depression, a disorder often associated with HD. In addition, reserpine can cause hypotension. We can block DA receptors with antipsychotic drugs,

TABLE 107.3 ■ Drugs for Chorea of Huntington's Disease

Drug	Approved for HD	Major Side Effects
DRUGS THAT REDUCE DOPAMINE STORES		
Tetrabenazine [Xenazine, Nitoman ♣]	Yes	Depression, suicidal thoughts and actions
DRUGS THAT BLOCK DOPAMINE RECEPTORS		
First-Generation Antipsychotics		
Haloperidol [Haldol]	No	Extrapyramidal effects
Pimozide [Orap]	No	Extrapyramidal effects, sedation
Second-Generation Antipsychotics		
Risperidone [Risperdal]	No	Extrapyramidal effects, but less likely than with first-generation antipsychotics
Ziprasidone [Geodon]	No	
Quetiapine [Seroquel]	No	

HD, Huntington's disease.

but these agents can cause extrapyramidal side effects. Hence their use may substitute one movement disorder for another. With the exception of tetrabenazine, all of these drugs are discussed in previous chapters. Accordingly, discussion here is limited to tetrabenazine. The basic pharmacology of the antipsychotic drugs is presented in Chapter 31.

In 2008, the FDA approved tetrabenazine [Xenazine, Nitoman ♣] for treatment of chorea associated with HD, making tetrabenazine the first and only drug approved for HD in the United States. However, although tetrabenazine is the only drug *approved* for HD, other drugs have been used to treat HD for years. Moreover, tetrabenazine is not a new compound. It was developed as a treatment for schizophrenia and has been used in Europe for decades.

In clinical trials for Huntington's chorea, daily treatment with tetrabenazine produced a 23.5% improvement in symptom severity. For some patients, benefits persisted over 5 years of continuous drug use. How does tetrabenazine work? It reduces the availability of DA and other monoamine neurotransmitters (i.e., serotonin, norepinephrine). Specifically, tetrabenazine inhibits a transporter—the *type 2 vesicular monoamine transporter* (VMAT-2)—that moves monoamine transmitters into vesicles within nerve terminals. As a result of VMAT-2 inhibition, (1) transmitter molecules that remain outside the vesicles undergo destruction by monoamine oxidase, and (2) the transmitter content of the vesicles themselves is reduced. Thus, when an action potential reaches the nerve ending, the vesicles have lesser amounts of transmitter to release into the synaptic cleft.

Tetrabenazine is well absorbed after oral dosing, and then undergoes extensive hepatic metabolism by CYP2D6 (the 2D6 isoenzyme of cytochrome P450). Parent drug and metabolites are eliminated in the urine. Their half-lives range from 4 to 8 hours. In patients with hepatic impairment and in those with low CYP2D6 activity, the half-life of tetrabenazine is prolonged, and plasma drug levels are elevated.

Many patients experience adverse effects. The most common are extrapyramidal reactions, including parkinsonism, akathisia (profound restlessness), and dystonia (a reaction characterized by severe spasm of the muscles of the tongue, face, neck, or back). Other common reactions include drowsiness, insomnia, fatigue, anxiety, and nausea. However, the side effects of greatest concern are *depression* and *suicidality.* Recall that both depression and suicidality are common in HD. Tetrabenazine increases the risk for both. Accordingly, all patients using the drug should be watched closely for new or worsening depression and for expression of suicidal thoughts or behavior. If these occur, the dosage of tetrabenazine should be reduced. Patients may also benefit from starting or intensifying treatment with an antidepressant. Tetrabenazine is contraindicated for patients who are actively suicidal and for those with depression that is not adequately treated.

Tetrabenazine [Xenazine, Nitoman ♣] is supplied in 12.5- and 25-mg tablets. Dosage must be individually titrated over several weeks. The goal is to control symptoms without causing intolerable side effects. Dosing starts at 12.5 mg once daily in the morning. After 1 week, dosage is increased to 12.5 mg twice daily. Further increases of 12.5 mg/day are made at weekly intervals. Daily totals of 37.5 to 50 mg should be given as three divided doses. The maximum single dose is 25 mg, and the maximum daily dose is 100 mg. Dosage should be reduced in patients with low CYP2D6 activity. Patients with hepatic impairment should not use this drug.

DRUGS FOR FIBROMYALGIA

Fibromyalgia (FM) is a chronic disorder characterized by widespread musculoskeletal pain, profound fatigue, nonrestorative sleep, and cognitive dysfunction (e.g., impaired memory and concentration). The condition affects about 2% of the population, making it one of the most common of chronic pain syndromes. The incidence is 7 times greater in women than in men.

What causes the pain of FM? We don't know completely. However, we do know that the pain is *not* the result of pathologic changes in muscles, bones, or joints. Rather, the pain results from abnormal central processing of pain signals, such that patients have a reduced threshold to mechanical and thermal pain stimuli. The neurotransmitters involved in pain perception—serotonin, dopamine, norepinephrine, and substance P, among others—are also involved in regulation of sleep, mood, and cognition, which may explain why the symptoms of FM are so diverse.

Drugs for FM can be placed into two basic groups: drugs for pain management and drugs for sleep disturbances (Table 107.4). For pain management, we can use antidepressants, anticonvulsants, or analgesics. For sleep disturbances, we can use certain antidepressants, benzodiazepine-like drugs, or dopaminergic agents.

For the most part, drugs for pain relief work in the CNS to alter signaling in pain pathways. With the exception of milnacipran, all of these drugs have been discussed in previous chapters. Of note, only three drugs—duloxetine, milnacipran, and pregabalin—have been specifically approved for treating FM. Keep in mind, however, that approval does not mean that these three drugs are more effective than the rest. But it does

TABLE 107.4 ■ Drugs for Fibromyalgia

Drug	Approved for FM	Comments
DRUGS FOR PAIN RELIEF		
Antidepressants: TCAs and Related Compounds		
Amitriptyline [Elavil]	No	Highly effective; recommended as first-line therapy for FM
Cyclobenzaprine [Flexeril][a]	No	Moderately effective
Antidepressants: SSRIs		
Fluoxetine [Prozac]	No	Moderately effective
Paroxetine [Paxil]	No	Moderately effective
Antidepressants: SNRIs		
Milnacipran [Savella][b]	Yes	Moderately effective
Duloxetine [Cymbalta]	Yes	Moderately effective
Anticonvulsants		
Gabapentin [Neurontin]	No	Moderately effective
Pregabalin [Lyrica]	Yes	Moderately effective
Analgesics		
Tramadol [Ultram]	No	Moderately effective
Opioids	No	Probably effective, but, owing to side effects and abuse potential, should not be used unless safer treatments have failed
NSAIDs	No	Ineffective when used alone, but may add to analgesic benefits of other drugs
DRUGS FOR SLEEP DISTURBANCES		
TCAs and Related Compounds		
Amitriptyline [Elavil]	No	A foundation of therapy for sleep disturbances
Cyclobenzaprine [Flexeril][a]	No	A foundation of therapy for sleep disturbances
Benzodiazepine-like Drugs		
Zolpidem [Ambien]	No	Benzodiazepine-like drugs are used for patients intolerant of or unresponsive to amitriptyline or cyclobenzaprine
Zaleplon [Sonata]	No	
Eszopiclone [Lunesta]	No	
Dopaminergic Drugs for RLS		
Levodopa/carbidopa [Sinemet]	No	RLS is a major cause of unrestorative sleep in FM. Dopaminergic drugs can help.
Pramipexole [Mirapex]	No	
Ropinirole [Requip]	No	

[a]Cyclobenzaprine is nearly identical in structure to amitriptyline, but is not used as an antidepressant.
[b]In the United States, milnacipran is approved only for FM. In Europe, the drug is approved for FM *and* depression.
FM, Fibromyalgia; *NSAIDs,* nonsteroidal anti-inflammatory drugs; *RLS,* restless legs syndrome; *SNRIs,* serotonin/norepinephrine reuptake inhibitors; *SSRIs,* selective serotonin reuptake inhibitors; *TCAs,* tricyclic antidepressants.

mean that at least some efficacy has been documented in clinical trials, and that the manufacturer has used these data to obtain FDA approval to market these drugs for FM.

Antidepressants and Related Drugs

Antidepressants are a mainstay of FM pain therapy. In clinical trials, these drugs have reduced pain and fatigue and have improved sleep and a sense of well-being. Tricyclic antidepressants (TCAs) and serotonin/norepinephrine reuptake inhibitors (SNRIs) appear most effective. With all antidepressants, benefits in FM are largely independent of antidepressant effects. Put another way, pain relief is about equal in patients who are depressed and in those who are not. Although these drugs can be helpful, keep in mind that all antidepressants may increase the risk for suicidal thoughts and behavior in children, adolescents, and young adults. Appropriate caution must be exercised. The basic pharmacology of the antidepressants is discussed in Chapter 32.

Tricyclic Antidepressants and Cyclobenzaprine

Tricyclic antidepressants are the most effective agents we have for reducing pain and other symptoms of FM. However, despite their benefits, none of the TCAs is approved for FM. There is strong evidence that one agent—*amitriptyline* [Elavil]—can reduce both pain and fatigue and can also improve sleep. How do TCAs work? As discussed in Chapter 32, TCAs block neuronal reuptake of norepinephrine and serotonin, and they block receptors for acetylcholine. In patients with FM, benefits are believed to result from blockade of norepinephrine and serotonin reuptake, which increases the availability of these transmitters at central synapses, which in turn activates spinal inhibition of pain signaling. Major side effects (e.g., dry mouth, blurred vision, urinary retention, constipation) result from blockade of receptors for acetylcholine.

Cyclobenzaprine [Flexeril] is a tricyclic compound nearly identical in structure to amitriptyline. However, despite this similarity, the drug is used mainly as a muscle relaxant (see Chapter 25), not as an antidepressant. In patients with FM, cyclobenzaprine can improve sleep quality and can produce modest improvements in pain, stiffness, and fatigue.

Selective Serotonin Reuptake Inhibitors (SSRIs)

Two SSRIs—*fluoxetine* [Prozac] and *paroxetine* [Paxil]—are beneficial in FM, even though neither drug is approved for the disorder.

Serotonin/Norepinephrine Reuptake Inhibitors

As discussed in Chapter 32, the SNRIs block neuronal reuptake of serotonin *and* norepinephrine, in contrast to the SSRIs, which block reuptake of serotonin only. Presumably, benefits of the SNRIs are the result of increased availability of serotonin and norepinephrine at CNS synapses.

Duloxetine. The FDA has approved duloxetine [Cymbalta], an SNRI, for treatment of FM. As noted in Chapter 32, duloxetine is also approved for depression, generalized anxiety disorder, chronic musculoskeletal pain, and pain of diabetic neuropathy. In patients with FM, duloxetine can reduce pain, fatigue, and stiffness and can improve overall quality of life. If the patient also suffers from depression, duloxetine can help with that too. Unfortunately, duloxetine can cause a variety of adverse effects (e.g., nausea, dry mouth, constipation, insomnia, dizziness, loss of appetite) and is subject to multiple drug interactions.

Milnacipran. Milnacipran [Savella] is also approved for FM. Unlike duloxetine, milnacipran is not approved in the United States for depression. However, the drug has been used to treat depression in Europe and Asia since 1997. In clinical trials, milnacipran reduced pain and fatigue of FM and improved sleep and cognitive function. Furthermore, benefits were maintained for up to 1 year with daily dosing. As with duloxetine, benefits are presumed to derive from elevation of synaptic serotonin and norepinephrine concentrations secondary to blockade of transmitter reuptake.

Milnacipran has good oral bioavailability, both in the presence and absence of food. Plasma levels peak 2 to 4 hours after dosing. Milnacipran is eliminated in the urine, primarily as unchanged drug (55%). In patients with normal kidney function, the half-life is 6 to 8 hours. In patients with significant renal impairment, both the half-life and peak blood levels are increased.

Milnacipran can cause multiple adverse effects. In clinical trials, the most common were nausea, headache, constipation, insomnia, dizziness, hot flashes, excessive sweating, vomiting, dry mouth, and CV effects: palpitations, increased heart rate, and hypertension. To reduce the risk for adverse CV events, heart rate and blood pressure should be measured at baseline and periodically during treatment. Pre-existing hypertension and tachycardia should be controlled before using the drug. Milnacipran can cause mydriasis (pupil dilation), and hence is contraindicated in patients with uncontrolled narrow-angle glaucoma. There is some risk for liver injury, as indicated by elevations of alanine and aspartate aminotransferases. Like other serotonin reuptake inhibitors, milnacipran can increase the risk for bleeding. And like all other antidepressants, milnacipran may increase the risk for suicidal thoughts and behavior.

Combining milnacipran with other serotonergic drugs increases the risk for serotonin syndrome. Accordingly, milnacipran should not be combined with SSRIs, other SNRIs, or monoamine oxidase inhibitors (MAOIs). Furthermore, MAOIs should be discontinued at least 14 days before starting milnacipran, and milnacipran should be discontinued at least 5 days before starting an MAOI. Because of milnacipran's CV effects, the drug should not be combined with other drugs that increase blood pressure or heart rate. Because milnacipran can promote bleeding, it should not be combined with aspirin, warfarin, or any other drug that can suppress coagulation.

Milnacipran [Savella] is available in tablets (12.5, 25, 50, and 100 mg) for dosing with or without food. Dosage should be titrated as follows: 12.5 mg once on day 1, 12.5 mg twice on days 2 and 3, 25 mg twice on days 4 through 7, and 50 mg twice daily thereafter. In patients with severe renal impairment, the maintenance dosage should be cut in half, to 25 mg twice daily. Patients with end-stage renal disease should not use this drug. When milnacipran is discontinued, dosage should be tapered gradually.

Anticonvulsants

Two anticonvulsants—*pregabalin* [Lyrica] and *gabapentin* [Neurontin]—are moderately effective in reducing the pain of FM. Pregabalin is approved for FM; gabapentin is not. Benefits of pregabalin may derive from suppressing release of glutamate (an excitatory neurotransmitter), whereas benefits of gabapentin may derive from increasing release of GABA (an inhibitory neurotransmitter). Side effects of these drugs include fatigue, sedation, nausea, drowsiness, dizziness, and weight gain. The basic pharmacology of pregabalin and gabapentin is presented in Chapter 24.

Analgesics

Tramadol

Tramadol [Ultram] is a centrally acting nonopioid analgesic. In patients with FM, the drug can produce a moderate reduction in discomfort. How does tramadol work? Like the TCAs, it blocks neuronal reuptake of 5-hydroxytryptamine and norepinephrine and thereby enhances spinal inhibition of pain signaling. Additional pain relief may come from weak agonist activity at mu opioid receptors. The basic pharmacology of tramadol is presented in Chapter 28.

Opioid Analgesics

Opioids are strong analgesics that may help control the pain of FM. Unfortunately, these drugs can cause significant adverse effects (e.g., sedation, respiratory depression, constipation, impaired cognition), and they pose a risk for dependence and abuse. Accordingly, opioids should not be used as first-line agents. Rather, they should be reserved for patients who have not responded adequately to preferred pharmacologic and nonpharmacologic treatments. The basic pharmacology of the opioids is presented in Chapter 28.

Nonsteroidal Anti-Inflammatory Drugs

When used alone, aspirin, ibuprofen, and other NSAIDs offer little or no benefit in FM—probably because FM is not an inflammatory disorder. Accordingly, monotherapy with NSAIDs is not recommended. However, NSAIDs may provide some additional analgesia when combined with other agents.

Drugs for Sleep Disturbances

For many patients, disturbed sleep is the most troubling symptom of FM. As with management of FM pain, the drugs of first choice are TCAs and cyclobenzaprine. If these agents are ineffective or intolerable, a benzodiazepine-like sedative may be tried. Options include zolpidem [Ambien], zaleplon [Sonata], and eszopiclone [Lunesta]. The most common cause of disturbed sleep in FM is restless legs syndrome, which can be managed with gabapentin [Horizant], or a dopaminergic agent, such as levodopa/carbidopa [Sinemet] or a direct-acting dopamine agonist (e.g., pramipexole [Mirapex], ropinirole [Requip]).

DRUGS FOR HEREDITARY ANGIOEDEMA

Hereditary angioedema (HAE) is a rare genetic disorder that affects just 1 in 10,000 to 50,000 Americans. It is characterized by localized, self-limiting episodes of edema (tissue swelling) that occur mainly in the larynx, subcutaneous tissue, and submucosa of the intestinal wall. Edema of the larynx and facial area can cause fatal obstruction of the airway. Abdominal attacks (from intestinal edema) can cause severe abdominal pain, cramping, nausea, and vomiting. On average, attacks occur every 10 to 14 days and last for 3 to 5 days. The underlying cause of most HAE is a *deficiency* in *C1-esterase inhibitor*—or simply *C1-inhibitor* (C1-INH)—owing to a mutation in the C1-INH gene.

Why does edema occur? The major pathway is depicted in Fig. 107.1. As indicated, there are two important mediators: *kallikrein* and *bradykinin.* Kallikrein catalyzes the formation of bradykinin. And then bradykinin, acting through bradykinin type 2 receptors (B2 receptors), increases vascular permeability, allowing fluid to leak out of capillaries and infiltrate the surrounding tissue. In people *without* HAE, endogenous C1-INH suppresses conversion of prekallikrein into kallikrein and thereby prevents excessive production of bradykinin. By contrast, in people *with* HAE, there is insufficient C1-INH to keep kallikrein synthesis in check, and hence overproduction of bradykinin results.

The principal drugs for HAE work in one of four ways. Specifically, they

- Stimulate production of C1-INH
- Replace deficient C1-INH
- Mimic C1-INH
- Block bradykinin B2 receptors

Drugs that stimulate production of C1-INH are used for prophylaxis only. Preparations that replace deficient C1-INH can be used for prophylaxis or treatment. And drugs that mimic C1-INH or block B2 receptors are used for treatment only.

Drugs for HAE Prophylaxis

Five drugs are available to prevent HAE. These are used for both short- and long-term prophylaxis. Options for short-term prophylaxis include either C1-INH replacement products (icatibant [Firazyr], ecallantide [Kalbitor]) or *androgens* (danazol [Danocrine], stanozolol [Winstrol]). Long-term prophylaxis is accomplished with androgen therapy, C1-INH [Cinryze] therapy, or tranexamic acid [Cyklokapron, Lysteda] therapy. Tranexamic acid, an antifibrinolytic agent, may be used for both short- and long-term prophylaxis. Properties of drugs used for HAE prophylaxis are shown in Table 107.5.

Drugs for Acute HAE Management

Three drugs are approved for acute HAE management: ecallantide; icatibant; and Berinert, a preparation of C1-INH. Tranexamic acid is sometimes used for acute management, although it has not received FDA approval for this use. Properties of these drugs are shown in Table 107.5.

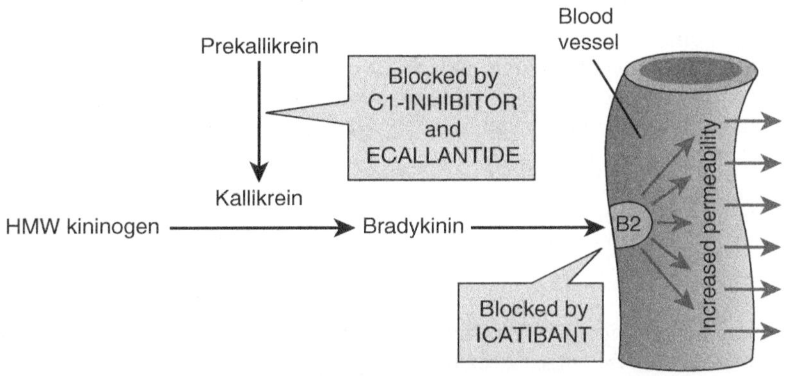

Fig. 107.1 ■ Drug actions in hereditary angioedema.
Two drugs—C1-inhibitor and ecallantide—suppress production of kallikrein and thereby suppress production of bradykinin. Icatibant blocks bradykinin B2 receptors, preventing bradykinin-mediated increases in vessel permeability, the immediate cause of edema. (*B2,* Bradykinin type 2 receptor; *HMW,* high-molecular-weight.)

TABLE 107.5 ▪ Drugs for Hereditary Angioedema

Drug	Mechanism	FDA-Approved Use	Route	Formulation	Dosage
C1-inhibitor [Cinryze]	Inhibits kallikrein, and thereby suppresses formation of bradykinin	Prophylaxis only	IV	Powder (500 units) in single-use vials	1000 units every 3–4 days
C1-inhibitor [Berinert]	Same as Cinryze	Treatment of acute attacks affecting the face and/or abdomen	IV	Powder (500 units) in single-use vials	20 units/kg once during the attack
Ecallantide [Kalbitor]	Same as Cinryze	Treatment of any acute attack	SubQ	Solution (10 mg) in single-use vials	30 mg (10 mg injected at three different sites); can be repeated within 24 hr if the attack persists
Icatibant [Firazyr]	Blocks bradykinin B2 receptors	Treatment of any acute attack	SubQ	Solution (30 mg) in single-use, pre-filled syringes	30 mg as one injection into the abdomen; can be repeated twice at intervals of 6 hr or longer
Tranexamic acid [Cyklokapron, Lysteda]	Decreases consumption of C1-INH so that more is available	No	PO	Tablet (650 mg)	20–40 mg/kg/day in 2–3 divided doses (limit to 3000 mg daily) *or* 500 mg 4 times/day (For short-term prophylaxis, begin treatment 2–5 days before and 2 days after procedures known to trigger an attack, e.g., dental work.)

B2, Bradykinin type 2.

C1-Inhibitors

We have two preparations of C1-INH, marketed as *Cinryze* and *Berinert.* Both are prepared by extraction of C1-INH from human plasma. As mentioned, Cinryze is approved only for prophylaxis of HAE. Berinert is approved only for treatment of HAE, and then only for acute abdominal attacks and facial swelling. Both drugs are administered IV, and hence are not suited for use at home. How do these drugs reduce edema? They block the conversion of prekallikrein to kallikrein, suppressing production of bradykinin, a compound that causes edema by increasing vascular permeability. Common side effects are headache, muscle spasms, abdominal pain, nausea, vomiting, and diarrhea. The most serious side effect is an increase in HAE pain. Because these preparations are foreign proteins, they pose a risk for hypersensitivity reactions, including severe anaphylaxis. Accordingly, epinephrine should be immediately available. Because these preparations are made from human plasma, they pose a theoretical risk for transmitting viruses and Creutzfeldt-Jakob disease. However, no cases of transmission have ever been reported. Dosages for both preparations are shown in Table 107.5.

Ecallantide

Ecallantide [Kalbitor], prepared by recombinant DNA technology, is approved for subQ treatment of all HAE attacks, regardless of the site. Like the C1-INH drugs, ecallantide reduces edema by suppressing conversion of prekallikrein to kallikrein. Side effects include headache, fatigue, fever, nausea, diarrhea, injection-site reactions, and mild hypersensitivity reactions. Of much greater concern, anaphylaxis develops in nearly 4% of patients. Accordingly, ecallantide should be administered only by clinicians with appropriate support to manage anaphylaxis and HAE itself. A single dose consists of 30 mg administered as three 10-mg subQ injections, made at least 2 inches apart into the abdomen, thigh, or upper arm. The injections may be made into the same anatomic region or different regions. One additional 30-mg dose can be administered within 24 hours. Of note, each 10-mg dose costs about $5500.

Icatibant

Like ecallantide, icatibant [Firazyr] is approved for subQ treatment of all HAE attacks, regardless of the site. In contrast to the other new drugs for HAE, which work by preventing the conversion of prekallikrein to kallikrein, icatibant works by blocking bradykinin B2 receptors on blood vessels. By doing so, icatibant prevents bradykinin-mediated increases in vessel permeability, the immediate cause of edema. The most common side effects are injection-site reactions (e.g., bruising, burning, redness, irritation, edema, pain), which occur in nearly all patients. Less common side effects are fever, dizziness, and elevation of liver enzymes. The recommended dosage is 30 mg injected subQ into the abdomen. If needed, two additional 30-mg doses can be given at intervals of 6 hours or longer. Icatibant, supplied in single-dose, pre-filled syringes, is the only new drug for HAE approved for dosing at home. Each 30-mg dose costs about $12,370.

Androgens

For many years, patients have used *androgens* (e.g., danazol [Danocrine], stanozolol [Winstrol]) for *prophylaxis.* With regular use, these drugs can reduce both the frequency and intensity of attacks. How? By promoting synthesis of C1-INH by the liver. Unfortunately, androgens can cause significant side effects, including liver damage, virilization, acne, lipid abnormalities, and menstrual irregularities. Furthermore, although androgens can help *prevent* attacks, they cannot treat an attack once it has begun.

Tranexamic Acid

Tranexamic acid has not received FDA approval for use in HAE; however, it is used in managing HAE in prepubertal children and other patients for whom androgen and Cinryze use is contraindicated. Tranexamic acid is an antifibrinolytic agent indicated for both prophylaxis and acute treatment of HAE. How does it work? In the process of inhibiting plasmin activity, it decreases the amount of C1-INH that is used up. This increases the amount of C1-INH available. The main concern with this drug, as you might expect, is thrombotic events. It is classified in FDA Pregnancy Risk Category B.[c] Although tranexamic acid is better tolerated than some of the other drugs for HAE, it is also less efficacious.

BELIMUMAB FOR SYSTEMIC LUPUS ERYTHEMATOSUS

Systemic lupus erythematosus (SLE) is a chronic, potentially fatal autoimmune disease that can attack multiple sites. Among these are the joints, skin, lungs, and heart, as well as two other sites—the kidneys and CNS—that are often severely affected. Common symptoms are joint pain, swollen joints, fever, chest pain, hair loss, and fatigue. All patients have antinuclear antibodies (ANAs), that is, antibodies directed against the patient's own DNA. Disease onset is between age 15 and 44 years. The Centers for Disease Control and Prevention estimates that between 300,000 and 4 million Americans have SLE. The incidence in women is 9 times the incidence in men, and the incidence in black women is 3 times the incidence in white women.

We cannot cure SLE, but we can reduce symptoms and complications with drugs. Standard treatments include NSAIDs (for arthritis and fever), hydroxychloroquine (for arthritis and rash), and glucocorticoids (for kidney and CNS complications). Hydroxychloroquine and glucocorticoids can also help prevent symptom flares. Powerful immunosuppressants—cyclophosphamide [Cytoxan, Procytox], azathioprine [Imuran], mycophenolate mofetil [CellCept], and methotrexate—are generally reserved for severe disease that has not responded to oral glucocorticoids.

History

Belimumab [Benlysta], approved in 2011, is the first drug approved for SLE since 1955. Unfortunately, belimumab is expensive, benefits are modest, and there is no proof of efficacy in African Americans or in patients with kidney or CNS involvement. Furthermore, the drug may actually *increase* mortality. Accordingly, belimumab is indicated only as add-on therapy for adults with ANA-positive SLE that has not responded to traditional drugs. Belimumab should not be used in patients with lupus nephritis or in those with CNS lupus.

Mechanism of Action

Belimumab is a monoclonal antibody that inhibits B-lymphocyte stimulator (BLyS), a regulatory protein that prolongs the survival of B lymphocytes—cells that contribute to the production of autoantibodies. Presumably, by inhibiting BLyS, belimumab suppresses autoantibody production and thereby helps alleviate SLE symptoms. Of note, in patients with SLE, levels of BLyS are abnormally high.

Clinical Trials

Belimumab was evaluated in two large, randomized, double-blind, placebo-controlled trials, known as BLISS-52 and BLISS-76. Patients received standard therapy (e.g., prednisone, azathioprine, hydroxychloroquine) plus either belimumab or placebo. The result? Symptomatic improvement was greater in the belimumab group than in the placebo group, and patients on belimumab experienced fewer disease flares and more were able to decrease their dosage of prednisone. Unfortunately, benefits were limited to just a few people: only 1 of every 8 patients improved. Furthermore, although the trials showed a modest benefit for some patients, important clinical issues were not addressed. As a result:

- We don't know if belimumab will benefit patients with active lupus involving the kidneys or CNS because these patients were excluded from the trials.
- We don't know if belimumab benefits African Americans. Why? Because only a few black patients were enrolled—and none of them responded. Studies with more black patients are planned to verify whether these negative results are valid.
- We cannot recommend combined use of belimumab with other biologics for SLE or with IV cyclophosphamide. Why? Because these combinations were not studied.

Adverse Effects

The most common reactions (occurring in about 10% of patients) are nausea, diarrhea, fever, bronchitis, and nasopharyngitis.

Infusion/Hypersensitivity Reactions. Infusion/hypersensitivity reactions range from mild (myalgia, headache, rash, urticaria) to severe: anaphylaxis, manifesting as angioedema, hypotension, and dyspnea. Patients should be monitored during the infusion and after. If anaphylaxis develops, the infusion should be stopped immediately. Owing to the risk for anaphylaxis, belimumab should be administered only by a provider prepared to manage a severe reaction.

Depression. In clinical trials, serious depression developed in 0.4% of patients receiving belimumab versus 0.1% of those receiving placebo. Two belimumab recipients committed suicide. Most patients who reported depression or suicidal behavior had a history of depression or other serious psychiatric disorders, and most were receiving psychotherapeutic drugs. Although belimumab is associated with an increased risk for depression, a causal relationship has not been established.

Infection. Like other immunosuppressants, belimumab is associated with an increased risk for infection. Belimumab should not be started in patients with a chronic infection. If an infection develops during treatment, interruption of belimumab should be considered.

Mortality. Belimumab may pose an increased risk for death. In clinical trials, 0.9% of patients receiving belimumab died,

[c]As of 2020, the FDA will no longer use Pregnancy Risk Categories. Please refer to Chapter 9 for more information.

compared with 0.4% of patients receiving placebo. Causes of death included infection, CV disease, and suicide.

Drug Interactions

Formal studies have not been conducted.

Vaccine Interactions

Because of its immunosuppressant actions, belimumab may pose a risk for infection from live virus vaccines. Accordingly, belimumab should not be administered within 30 days of receiving a live virus vaccine, and these vaccines should not be administered to patients receiving belimumab. By suppressing immune responses, belimumab may interfere with responses to all vaccines.

Preparations, Dosage, and Administration

Belimumab [Benlysta] is supplied as a powder (120 and 400 mg) to be reconstituted for IV infusion. The dosage is 10 mg/kg—infused over 1 hour—every 2 weeks for three doses, and every 4 weeks thereafter. Premedication may reduce the risk for an infusion/hypersensitivity reaction. As noted previously, infusions must be done by a healthcare provider with expertise in managing anaphylaxis. The cost of treatment is approximately $600 for 120 mg of powder and $2015 for 400 mg of powder. Prefilled syringes and autoinjectors are about $1060 for 200 mg/mL.

KEY POINTS

- Pulmonary arterial hypertension (PAH) is a potentially fatal disease of the small pulmonary arteries.
- The primary vascular changes in PAH are vasoconstriction, proliferation of smooth muscle cells and endothelial cells, and pulmonary thrombosis.
- Prostacyclin analogs (e.g., epoprostenol, iloprost) reduce symptoms of PAH by promoting vasodilation, suppressing proliferation of smooth muscle cells, and inhibiting platelet aggregation.
- Epoprostenol is administered by continuous IV infusion through a central venous catheter, and thus is inconvenient as well as potentially hazardous (owing to a risk for catheter-related sepsis).
- Sepsis is a life-threatening condition in which systemic infection triggers a generalized inflammatory response and activation of the coagulation system. The end result can be diffuse endovascular injury and multiorgan dysfunction, often leading to death.
- Iloprost is administered by oral inhalation and is much more convenient than epoprostenol. However, iloprost can cause significant hypotension.
- Bosentan, ambrisentan, and macitentan are endothelin-1 receptor antagonists indicated for oral therapy of PAH. Benefits derive from reducing pulmonary vascular resistance and altering vascular remodeling.
- Bosentan is hepatotoxic and highly teratogenic.
- Sildenafil is a PDE5 inhibitor used for oral and IV therapy of PAH. Inhibition of PDE5 preserves cGMP in pulmonary arteries, enhancing vasodilation mediated by nitric oxide.
- Respiratory distress syndrome (RDS), the primary cause of morbidity and mortality in premature infants, results from a deficiency in lung surfactant.
- When preterm birth is unavoidable, injecting the mother with glucocorticoids can accelerate fetal lung maturation, decreasing the risk for RDS.
- Lung surfactant—poractant alfa, calfactant, or beractant—is given to preterm infants to prevent or treat RDS.
- Cystic fibrosis (CF) is an inherited disorder that results in damage to the lungs, pancreas, and other organs.
- In patients with CF, supplemental pancreatic enzymes promote digestion and absorption of nutrients. All preparations contain lipase, protease, and amylase.
- Inhaled dornase alfa [Pulmozyme] can improve pulmonary function and decrease infection in some patients with CF. The drug decreases the viscosity of sputum by breaking down extracellular DNA that has accumulated secondary to death of neutrophils.
- Inhaled tobramycin [TOBI] is the drug of choice for treating chronic *P. aeruginosa* pulmonary infection in patients with CF.
- High-dose ibuprofen can slow progression of pulmonary damage in CF. Benefits derive from suppressing the inflammatory response that underlies destruction of lung tissue.
- In patients with sickle cell anemia (SCA), hydroxyurea can reduce the number of painful episodes, hospitalizations, and transfusions and can prolong life. Benefits derive from increasing production of fetal hemoglobin.
- At high doses, hydroxyurea can cause severe myelosuppression. However, at the doses employed for SCA, myelosuppression is transient and mild.
- Hyperuricemia secondary to cancer chemotherapy can be managed with two drugs: rasburicase (which accelerates uric acid removal) and allopurinol (which blocks uric acid production).
- Phosphate binders are used to treat hyperphosphatemia, a common complication of end-stage renal disease.
- Calcium-based phosphate binders (e.g., calcium carbonate) are inexpensive but pose a risk for hypercalcemia.
- Calcium-free phosphate binders (e.g., sevelamer carbonate) do not promote hypercalcemia but cost much more than the calcium-based drugs.
- Gamma-hydroxybutyrate can decrease attacks of cataplexy in patients with narcolepsy and can also decrease daytime drowsiness (by helping to promote sleep).
- Gamma-hydroxybutyrate has significant abuse potential and can cause serious adverse effects (respiratory depression, coma, death). Accordingly, distribution of the drug is strictly controlled.
- In patients with amyotrophic lateral sclerosis (Lou Gehrig's disease), riluzole [Rilutek] can prolong life or delay the need for a tracheostomy by a few months.
- Huntington's disease is an inherited neurodegenerative disorder characterized by psychiatric problems, cognitive changes, and movement disorders, especially Huntington's chorea.
- We can treat Huntington's chorea with drugs that reduce neuronal stores of dopamine (e.g., tetrabenazine), or with drugs that block neuronal dopamine receptors (e.g., haloperidol, quetiapine, and other antipsychotic agents).

- Tetrabenazine is the first and only drug approved for treating chorea of Huntington's disease.
- Fibromyalgia (FM) is a chronic disorder characterized by widespread musculoskeletal pain, profound fatigue, nonrestorative sleep, and cognitive dysfunction.
- Drugs of first choice for FM are amitriptyline (a TCA) and cyclobenzaprine, a drug nearly identical in structure to amitriptyline.
- Milnacipran is a serotonin/norepinephrine reuptake inhibitor that produces moderate pain reduction in FM.
- Hereditary angioedema (HAE) is a genetic disorder characterized by localized, self-limiting episodes of edema that occur mainly in the larynx, subcutaneous tissue, and submucosa of the intestinal wall.
- The underlying cause of HAE is a deficiency in C1-esterase inhibitor, also known as C1-inhibitor (C1-INH).
- Five drugs are available for HAE prophylaxis—icatibant, ecallantide, the C1-INH Cinryze, androgens, and tranexamic acid.
- Ecallantide and the C1-INH drugs Cinryze and Berinert work by suppressing the conversion of prekallikrein into kallikrein. All three must be administered by a healthcare provider.
- Icatibant blocks bradykinin type 2 receptors and thereby prevents bradykinin-mediated increases in vascular permeability, the immediate cause of edema. Icatibant, administered subQ, is approved for dosing at home.
- Tranexamic acid has not received FDA approval for management of HAE and is less efficacious than other drugs used for this purpose, but it is better tolerated and can be given to pregnant patients.
- Systemic lupus erythematosus (SLE) is a chronic, potentially fatal autoimmune disorder that can affect multiple organ systems.
- Belimumab, a drug for SLE, is a monoclonal antibody that inhibits B-lymphocyte stimulator and thereby shortens the life of B lymphocytes—cells that contribute to autoantibody production.
- Belimumab is only moderately effective, and there is no evidence that it can help African Americans or patients with active lupus of the kidneys or CNS.

Please visit **http://evolve.elsevier.com/Lehne** for chapter-specific NCLEX® examination review questions.

CHAPTER

108 Complementary and Alternative Therapy

The National Center for Complementary and Integrative Health (NCCIH) defines *complementary* health approaches as "a non-mainstream practice used together with conventional medicine" and *alternative* health approaches as "a non-mainstream practice that is used in place of conventional medicine." Examples include both products (e.g., herbs, probiotics, and vitamins) and practices (e.g., meditation, acupuncture, and therapeutic touch). According to the National Health Statistics Reports published in 2015, 32.3% of adults in the United States used some form of complementary and alternative medicine (CAM) in 2012 (the year of the most recent national study).

Dietary supplements are the most common form of CAM. Dietary supplements are defined by the U.S. Food and Drug Administration (FDA) as "a product intended for ingestion that contains a 'dietary ingredient' intended to add further nutritional value to (supplement) the diet. A 'dietary ingredient' may be one, or any combination, of the following substances: a vitamin, a mineral, an herb or other botanical, an amino acid, a dietary substance for use by people to supplement the diet by increasing the total dietary intake, a concentrate, metabolite, constituent, or extract."

The popularity of supplements may be explained by several factors (Table 108.1). Some people like the sense of empowerment that comes from self-diagnosis and self-prescribing. Others may turn to supplements out of anger or frustration with their healthcare providers. Still others may distrust conventional medicine or may feel it has failed them. In addition, supplements may also be a way to save money: Since these products are available without prescription, they can be purchased without the cost of visiting a prescriber. In fact, according to the National Health Interview Survey (NHIS), there is a clear relationship between concern about the costs of conventional care and the likelihood of turning to CAM. However, perhaps the strongest force driving the demand for nutritional supplements is aggressive marketing.

Our understanding of CAM is far from adequate. To advance our knowledge, the National Institutes of Health (NIH) created the National Center for Complementary and Alternative Medicine (NCCAM) in the late 1990s. This organization (renamed the National Center for Complementary and Integrative Health [NCCIH] in 2014) is charged with promoting and funding basic research and clinical trials designed to address open questions on the safety and efficacy of CAM. The NCCIH website, which provides a wealth of information on CAM, is available at https://nccih.nih.gov.

REGULATION OF DIETARY SUPPLEMENTS

Dietary Supplement Health and Education Act of 1994

Core Provisions

In 1994, after intensive lobbying efforts from the multibillion-dollar dietary supplement industry aimed at minimizing FDA oversight, Congress passed the Dietary Supplement Health

TABLE 108.1 ■ Why People Use Dietary Supplements

- Perception that supplements are safer and healthier than conventional drugs
- Sense of control over one's care
- Emotional comfort from taking action
- Cultural influence
- Limited access to professional care
- Lack of health insurance
- Convenience
- Media hype and aggressive marketing
- Recommendation from family and friends

and Education Act of 1994 (DSHEA). As discussed in Chapter 3, the Food, Drug, and Cosmetic Act requires that conventional drugs—both prescription and over-the-counter agents—undergo rigorous evaluation of safety and efficacy before receiving FDA approval for marketing. The DSHEA categorizes botanical products (herbal supplements), vitamins, and minerals as dietary (food) supplements rather than as drugs. By classifying products as dietary supplements, the DSHEA exempts them from undergoing FDA scrutiny and approval before marketing. In fact, dietary supplements can be manufactured and marketed without giving the FDA any proof that they are safe or effective. All the manufacturer must do is notify the FDA of efficacy claims. If a product eventually proves harmful or the manufacturer makes false claims, the FDA does have the authority to intervene—but only *after* the product had been released for marketing. Furthermore, to challenge a claim of efficacy, the FDA must file suit in court; the challenge cannot be made through a simple administrative procedure.

Package Labeling

The DSHEA does impose some restrictions on labeling. All herbal products must be labeled as dietary supplements. In addition, the label must not claim that the product can be used to diagnose, prevent, treat, or cure a disease. In fact, it must state the opposite: *This product is not intended to diagnose, treat, cure, or prevent any disease.* However, the label *is* allowed to make claims about the product's ability to favorably influence *body structure or function.* Put another way, the label can insinuate specific benefits, but can't make overt claims. By way of illustration, labels *can* bear statements such as these:

- Helps promote urinary tract health
- Helps maintain cardiovascular function
- Energizes and rejuvenates
- Reduces stress and frustration
- Improves absentmindedness
- Supports the immune system

But labels *can't* bear statements or terms such as these:

- Protects against cancer
- Reduces pain and stiffness of arthritis
- Lowers cholesterol
- Supports the body's antiviral capabilities
- Improves symptoms of Alzheimer's disease
- Relieves menopausal hot flashes
- "Antibiotic," "antiseptic," "antidepressant," "laxative," or "diuretic"

If all of this sounds like semantic hair splitting—it largely is. Furthermore, regardless of what the label says, common sense assumes that people *will* take herbal products with the intent to prevent or treat disease.

Under the provisions of the DSHEA, there is no assurance that a product actually contains what the label proclaims: The package may contain ingredients that are *not* listed, or it may *lack* ingredients that *are* listed. These shortcomings and others have been addressed by the Current Good Manufacturing Practices (CGMPs) ruling, issued by the FDA in 2007.

Adverse Effects

With dietary supplements, as with conventional drugs, the manufacturer is responsible for safety. However, the similarity ends there. Under the DSHEA, a product is presumed safe until proved hazardous. Furthermore, the burden for proving danger lies with the consumer and the FDA. With conventional drugs, opposite logic and regulations apply: Drugs are presumed dangerous until rigorous testing by the manufacturer reveals an absence of serious adverse effects. Because of this system, the number of dangerous drugs that reach the market is kept to a minimum. Ask yourself, "Which product would I be more comfortable using—one that has been tested for adverse effects *before* I take it or one that is evaluated for adverse effects only *after* it caused me harm?"

Impurities, Adulterants, and Variability

The DSHEA does not address the issues of impurities, adulterants, or variability. As a result, dangerous products have been allowed to reach consumers. A few examples illustrate the problem:

- A combination product used to "cleanse the bowel" caused life-threatening heart block. Analysis revealed contamination with *Digitalis lanata,* a plant with powerful effects on the heart.
- Among 125 ephedra products analyzed by the FDA, ephedrine content per dose ranged from undetectable to 110 mg. Also, some products had 6 to 20 additional ingredients.
- Testing of 10 brands of ginseng products revealed a 20-fold variation in ginsenoside content.
- When the California Department of Health Sciences analyzed 243 Asian patent medicines, they found 24 containing lead, 35 containing mercury, and 36 containing arsenic—all in levels above those permitted in drugs. Of these products, 7% were adulterated with undeclared pharmaceuticals, including ephedrine, chlorpheniramine, methyltestosterone, and phenacetin.

As discussed next, the CGMPs ruling, issued by the FDA in 2007, should prevent the sale of such products in the future.

Current Good Manufacturing Practices Ruling

In June 2007, the FDA issued a set of standards to regulate manufacturing and labeling of dietary supplements. These standards, referred to as Current Good Manufacturing Practices, are designed to ensure that dietary supplements be devoid of adulterants, contaminants, and impurities, and that package labels accurately reflect the identity, purity, quality, and strength of what's inside. In addition, the label should indicate not only active ingredients but also inactive ingredients. The CGMPs also mandate that manufacturers establish quality-control procedures, with the objective of preventing mislabeled, underfilled, or overfilled formulations; variations in tablet size, color, or potency; and contamination with drugs, bacteria, pesticides, glass, lead, and other potential contaminants. Unfortunately, even with the new standards and rules, there is still no assurance that dietary supplements will be either safe or effective—but at least we will have improved confidence regarding package contents.

Dietary Supplement and Nonprescription Drug Consumer Protection Act

The Dietary Supplement and Nonprescription Drug Consumer Protection Act, passed in 2006, mandates reporting of serious adverse events for nonprescription drugs and dietary supplements. The following events should be reported: deaths, hospitalizations, life-threatening experiences, persistent or significant disabilities, and birth defects. Manufacturers and distributors must report these to the FDA within 15 days. Reports can be filed by telephone, by mail, or through the MEDWATCH program at http://www.fda.gov/Safety/MedWatch (see Chapter 7).

A Comment on the Regulatory Status of Dietary Supplements

Although herbal products and other dietary supplements are not regulated for either safety or efficacy, many of these products have components that can produce profound beneficial and adverse pharmacologic effects. Nonetheless, reliable information on clinical effects is largely lacking. Many of those working in the fields of pharmacy, medicine, and nursing are concerned that the exceptions made for dietary supplements are both irrational and dangerous. After all, whether you ingest ephedrine in the form of a pill or in the form of Ma huang, it's still ephedrine, and it's still going to have powerful effects. An older editorial in the *New England Journal of Medicine* (339:839–841, 1998) addressed this issue with eloquence. Here's the concluding paragraph:

> It is time for the scientific community to stop giving alternative medicine a free ride. There cannot be two kinds of medicine—conventional and alternative. There is only medicine that has been adequately tested and medicine that has not, medicine that works and medicine that may or may not work. Once a treatment has been tested rigorously, it no longer matters whether it was considered alternative at the outset. If it is found to be reasonably safe and effective, it will be accepted. But assertions, speculation, and testimonials do not substitute for evidence. Alternative treatments should be subjected to scientific testing no less rigorous than that required for conventional treatments.

Unfortunately, two decades later, little has changed.

PRIVATE QUALITY CERTIFICATION PROGRAMS

Four private organizations—the U.S. Pharmacopeia (USP), ConsumerLab, the Natural Products Association, and NSF International (formerly known as the National Sanitation Foundation)—test dietary supplements for quality. A "seal of approval" is given to products that meet their standards, which are very similar to the CGMPs described previously. The USP standards are enforceable by the FDA. All four organizations require manufacturers to pay for the tests, and all four report on the following:

- Current good manufacturing practices
- Purity
- Identity
- Potency
- Dissolution
- Accuracy of labeling

In addition, two organizations—the USP and ConsumerLab—report on postapproval surveillance.

STANDARDIZATION OF HERBAL PRODUCTS

With herbal products, there is often uncertainty about the amounts of active ingredients. The concentration of active ingredients in herbal crops can vary from year to year and from place to place. Reasons include differences in sunshine, rainfall, temperature, and soil nutrients. As a result, the potency of herbal products can vary widely.

Variability can be reduced through standardization, a three-step process in which the manufacturer (1) prepares an *extract* of plant parts, (2) analyzes the extract for one or two known active ingredients, and (3) dilutes or concentrates the extract such that the final product contains a predetermined amount of the active ingredient(s). The objective is to achieve therapeutic equivalence from batch to batch made by the same manufacturer and among batches made by different manufacturers. Table 108.2 lists the concentrations of active ingredients in some standardized preparations.

Standardization has two important benefits. First, it permits accurate dosing. Second, it permits extrapolation of data obtained in clinical trials to the public in general.

Unfortunately, standardization also has drawbacks. The extraction process might destroy active compounds. Furthermore, the process may fail to extract as-yet unidentified active agents, and hence the extract may have a different spectrum of effects than the intact plant. To the extent this is true, historical data obtained with whole plants will lose some value as a basis for helping us understand clinical responses to the standardized extract.

TABLE 108.2 ▪ Concentrations of Active Agents in Some Standardized Herbal Preparations

Herb	Amount of Active Agent
Black cohosh	2.5% Triterpene glycosides
Butterbur	15% Petasin and isopetasin
Echinacea	4% Phenolic compounds
Feverfew	0.2% Parthenolide
Ginkgo biloba	24% Ginkgo flavonoids, 6% terpenoids
St. John's wort	0.3% Hypericin
Valerian root	1% Valerianic acid

ADVERSE INTERACTIONS WITH CONVENTIONAL DRUGS

Herbal products and other dietary supplements can interact with conventional drugs, sometimes with significant harmful results. The principal concerns are increased toxicity and decreased therapeutic effects. Clinicians and consumers should be alert to these possibilities. Unfortunately, with many supplements, reliable information on adverse interactions is lacking—in large part because potential interactions have not been systematically studied. Hence, if a patient is taking a conventional medication and a dietary supplement, and therapeutic effects are lost or toxicity appears, it may be impossible to say for sure that the supplement was (or was not) responsible.

A few important interactions *have* been identified, including the following:

- St. John's wort can induce CYP3A4 (the 3A4 isoenzyme of cytochrome P450), and can thereby accelerate the metabolism of many drugs, causing a loss of therapeutic effects.
- Several herbal products, including *Ginkgo biloba,* feverfew, and garlic, suppress platelet aggregation, and hence can increase the risk for bleeding in patients receiving antiplatelet drugs (e.g., aspirin) or anticoagulants (e.g., warfarin, heparin).
- Ma huang (ephedra) contains ephedrine, a compound that can elevate blood pressure and stimulate the heart and central nervous system (CNS). Accordingly, ephedra can intensify the effects of pressor agents, cardiac stimulants, and CNS stimulants, and counteract the beneficial effects of antihypertensive drugs and CNS depressants.

These interactions, at least, can be avoided—provided the prescriber is aware of them and provided the patient informs the prescriber about supplement use. Unfortunately, up to 70% of patients neglect to do so.

SOME COMMONLY USED DIETARY SUPPLEMENTS

Black Cohosh

Uses

Black cohosh has a long history in America. The herb was used by Native Americans and later by American colonists. Between 1820 and 1926, it was listed as an official drug in the USP.

Black cohosh (*Cimicifuga racemosa*) is used for treating symptoms of menopause, including hot flashes, vaginal dryness, palpitations, depression, irritability, and sleep disturbance. The preparation should *not* be used to reduce hot flashes caused by tamoxifen and other selective estrogen receptor modulators (SERMs).

Actions

How black cohosh works is unknown. At one time, we believed it suppressed release of luteinizing hormone (LH). However, clinical studies have failed to show an effect on female hormones, including LH, estradiol, prolactin, and follicle-stimulating hormone. In laboratory studies, black cohosh does not interact with estrogen receptors: It doesn't bind these receptors, upregulate estrogen-dependent genes, or promote growth of estrogen-dependent tumors (at least in animals).

Effectiveness

Early studies carried out in Germany supported the ability of black cohosh to effectively relieve menopausal symptoms. In 2012, however, a Cochrane meta-analysis of 16 randomized controlled trials involving more than 2000 women concluded that there was insufficient evidence to support black cohosh for management of menopausal symptoms. After a review of the evidence, the NCCIH concluded, "[T]here is overall insufficient evidence to support the use of black cohosh for menopausal symptoms." These conclusions were echoed by the American College of Obstetricians and Gynecologists (ACOG) when they updated their clinical guidelines for management of menopausal symptoms in 2014. Conversely, at the time of this writing, the North American Menopause Society continues to include black cohosh among the natural remedies for hot flashes listed on its website.

Adverse Effects

Some women taking black cohosh have developed liver inflammation. In some instances, this has led to liver failure. The association is tenuous, however, because the occurrence has been rare and a distinction from other possible causes of liver injury has not been ruled out.

Less serious and more common adverse effects include rash, headache, dizziness, and abdominal discomfort. Safety in pregnancy and breastfeeding has not been established; however, for those taking black cohosh for menopausal benefit, this would be a concern only in rare circumstances. One caveat acknowledged almost universally is the need to limit the use of black cohosh to 6 months because long-term studies have not been conducted.

Interactions With Conventional Drugs

Black cohosh may potentiate the hypotensive effects of antihypertensive drugs as well as the hypoglycemic effects of insulin and other drugs for diabetes. Black cohosh may potentiate the effects of estrogens used for hormone therapy. Black cohosh should be used with caution in patients taking other drugs that may harm the liver.

Comments

Users must not confuse black cohosh with blue cohosh (Caulophyllum thalictroides). Although blue cohosh has legitimate uses, including promotion of menstruation and labor, it is very different from black cohosh and potentially more dangerous. Blue cohosh can elevate blood pressure, increase intestinal motility, and accelerate respiration. It can also induce uterine contractions, and hence it should be avoided during pregnancy. Some commercial products contain both black cohosh and blue cohosh. Women who want only black cohosh should avoid these products.

Butterbur

Butterbur (*Petasites hybridus*) is a bush that grows in marshy areas across North America. Products are made from the rhizomes and roots, as well as the stems, of this plant.

Uses

Butterbur is most commonly taken for migraine headaches, allergies, and asthma. It is one of the few botanicals recommended as a drug of first choice based on outcomes of randomized controlled trials.

Actions

Butterbur has anti-inflammatory, antispasmodic, and vasodilatory effects. As with many herbal products, the exact mechanism of action is unknown. Some believe that butterbur works as a calcium channel blocker. Laboratory studies point to inhibition of lipoxygenase, an enzyme that contributes to the synthesis of leukotrienes and other pro-inflammatory substances.

Effectiveness

Although evidence remains lacking for the efficacy of butterbur in the treatment of skin allergies and asthma, substantial evidence supports other uses. According to the NCCIH:

- A sponsored literature review found that butterbur is just as effective as an antihistamine for allergy symptoms.
- Butterbur appears to relieve nasal allergy symptoms.
- Research findings indicate that butterbur can be effective in treating migraine headache.

The American Academy of Neurology (AAN) and the American Headache Society (AHA) also noted the effects of butterbur on preventing migraine headache. In 2012, they published a joint report in which they not only pronounced that butterbur was effective in decreasing migraine headache frequency, but also gave it the highest (Level A) rating. Their conclusion? "*Petasites* (butterbur) is effective for migraine prevention and should be offered to patients with migraine to reduce the frequency and severity of migraine attacks." For this purpose, the AAN recommends 50 to 75 mg twice a day. (See the AAN's 2014 report *Headache: Quality Measurement Set* available through http://www.aan.com.)

Adverse Effects

Long-term safety has not been established; however, butterbur appears to be safe for short-term use of less than 4 months' duration when taken at recommended doses. The most common adverse effect is eructation (belching), headache, and fatigue. Those who have allergies to ragweed, daisies, marigolds, and chrysanthemums may have allergic reactions to butterbur.

With the increased use of butterbur, the concern has arisen regarding new reports of liver injury. According to the NCCIH, this can be the result of pyrrolizidine alkaloids (PAs) found in butterbur. The NCCIH recommends using only butterbur products in which these have been removed and that are certified as PA-free. Whether this type of product was taken by those who developed liver injury is unknown.

Interactions With Conventional Drugs

Interactions can occur if butterbur is given with drugs that induce CYP3A4 isoenzymes. Examples include not only drugs such as carbamazepine, phenobarbital, and phenytoin, but also dietary supplements such as echinacea, garlic, and St. John's wort. The greatest concern comes when a non–PA-free form of butterbur is used because PAs are substrates of CYP3A4 isoenzymes; metabolism converts these to their toxic metabolites.

Coenzyme Q-10

Coenzyme Q-10 (ubiquinone, CoQ-10) is an antioxidant that serves a vital role in cellular energy production. As we age, CoQ-10 levels decrease. This has led to increased interest in the use of CoQ-10 in the treatment of conditions associated with aging and with cellular energy production.

Uses

CoQ-10 is used to treat heart failure, muscle injury caused by HMG-CoA reductase inhibitors (statins), and mitochondrial encephalomyopathies (i.e., muscle and nervous system injury caused by deranged mitochondrial metabolism).

Actions

CoQ-10 is a potent antioxidant. It participates in many metabolic pathways, most notably production of adenosine triphosphate (ATP).

Effectiveness

In patients with documented CoQ-10 deficiency, replacement therapy with CoQ-10 offers clear benefits. Although some study findings have been mixed, the NCCIH reports a number of positive outcomes associated with the use of CoQ-10:

- Patients with heart failure who took CoQ-10 had improved cardiac function.
- Patients who took CoQ-10 after cardiac surgery had faster recovery.
- CoQ-10 may improve sperm count and semen quality; however, further studies are needed to identify an improvement in conception.

Research studies that examined the effect of CoQ-10 on statin-associated muscle injury, cancer prevention and treatment, and hypertension were inconclusive.

Adverse Effects

CoQ-10 is well tolerated. High doses may produce gastrointestinal (GI) disturbances, including gastritis, reduced appetite, nausea, and diarrhea. Liver enzymes may increase, although no actual liver injury has been reported. Women who are pregnant or breastfeeding should not take CoQ-10 because safety has not been established.

Interactions With Conventional Drugs

CoQ-10 is structurally similar to vitamin K_2, and hence may antagonize the effects of warfarin.

Biosynthesis of CoQ-10 shares a common pathway with cholesterol. As a result, drugs such as the statins, which inhibit synthesis of cholesterol, can also inhibit synthesis of CoQ-10, causing levels of endogenous CoQ-10 to decline. (Statin-induced reductions in CoQ-10 may explain why statins cause muscle injury.)

Cranberry Juice

Uses

Cranberry juice is used to prevent urinary tract infections (UTIs) and to decrease urine odor in patients with urinary incontinence.

Actions

Benefits derive from the presence of proanthocyanidins, a group of compounds that prevent bacteria from adhering to the urinary tract wall. Bacteria that have already attached themselves are not affected. Cranberry juice does not acidify the urine as previously thought.

Effectiveness

Daily consumption of cranberry juice can *prevent* recurrent UTIs, but this has been demonstrated only in certain age groups. Specifically, it appears to benefit older adult women and women in their teens or 20s, but not middle-aged adults or young girls. Furthermore, although cranberry juice can prevent UTIs, it is not effective as treatment for an established infection. In patients with urinary incontinence, cranberry juice can reduce unpleasant odor. Little is known about the efficacy of cranberry-extract capsules. Accordingly, cranberry juice itself is the preferred formulation.

Adverse Effects

Drinking more than 1 L/day may increase the risk for GI upset and formation of uric acid kidney stones.

Interactions With Conventional Drugs

There is some evidence that cranberry juice may increase the risk for bleeding in patients taking warfarin. Accordingly, these patients should be monitored closely.

Echinacea

Echinacea is the scientific name of the coneflower plant, which is native to the United States and parts of Canada. Echinacea was listed in the National Formulary from 1916 to 1950, but fell from favor owing to the development of antibiotics and a lack of scientific data to support its use.

Uses

Echinacea (*Echinacea angustifolia, E. purpurea, E. pallida*) is administered orally and topically. Oral echinacea is taken to stimulate immune function, suppress inflammation, and treat viral infections, including influenza and the common cold. Topical echinacea is used to treat wounds, burns, eczema, psoriasis, and herpes simplex infections.

Actions

Active ingredients in echinacea preparations include cichoric acid, polysaccharides, flavonoids, and essential oils. These ingredients have been thought to produce antiviral, anti-inflammatory, and immunostimulant effects through a combination of actions, including mobilization of phagocytes, stimulation of T-lymphocyte proliferation, stimulation of interferon and tumor necrosis factor production, and inhibition of hyaluronidase, a proinflammatory enzyme.

Effectiveness

Although echinacea is taken widely to prevent and treat colds, its efficacy is highly questionable. Recent randomized, placebo-controlled trials designed to evaluate the ability of echinacea to *prevent* colds found no effect on (1) the time to developing an upper respiratory tract infection (URTI); (2) the incidence, duration, or severity of URTIs that did develop; or (3) development of experimentally induced URTIs. Other recent trials conducted on adults and children who already had a URTI found echinacea no better than placebo at reducing either the duration or severity of symptoms. The NCCIH continues to support research for its effects on the immune system.

Adverse Effects

Very few adverse effects have been reported. The most common complaint is unpleasant taste. Fever, nausea, and vomiting occur infrequently.

Rarely, echinacea causes allergic reactions, including acute asthma, urticaria, angioedema, and anaphylaxis. Echinacea belongs to the daisy family of plants, whose members include ragweed, asters, chamomile, and chrysanthemums. People allergic to any of these plants are at an increased risk for reacting to echinacea. Individuals with atopy (a genetic tendency toward allergic conditions) also appear at increased risk for reacting to echinacea.

Until echinacea's effects on the immune system are fully known, it will be prudent to avoid the drug in patients with autoimmune diseases, such as lupus erythematosus or rheumatoid arthritis.

Although short-term exposure to echinacea *may* stimulate immune function, there is concern that long-term exposure can suppress immune function. Accordingly, long-term therapy should be avoided in immunocompromised patients, including those with HIV infection. In addition, prolonged therapy should be avoided in people with tuberculosis and other chronic infections that require optimal immune function for cure.

Interactions With Conventional Drugs

By stimulating the immune system, echinacea can oppose the effects of immunosuppressant drugs. Conversely, by suppressing immune function (in response to long-term use), echinacea can compromise drug therapy of tuberculosis, cancer, and HIV infection.

Feverfew

Feverfew *(Tanacetum parthenium)* is a bushy plaint with small daisy-like flowers that grows throughout North and South America and Europe. Supplements are made from the dried leaves, though sometimes the flowers and stems are included.

Uses

Feverfew is used primarily for prophylaxis of migraine. It is also taken for a number of conditions associated with hypersensitivity and altered immune responses such as allergies, asthma, rheumatoid arthritis, and psoriasis.

Actions

The principal active agent in feverfew is *parthenolide,* a compound found in feverfew leaves. How parthenolide suppresses migraine is poorly understood. Possibilities include inhibition of vasoconstriction in the brain, suppression of serotonin release from platelets and leukocytes, and suppression of inflammation secondary to inhibition of arachidonic acid release.

Effectiveness

Clinical studies on feverfew's effect on migraine headaches have had mixed results. Some findings suggest that, when taken prophylactically, the herb can reduce the frequency of attacks and the severity of symptoms (nausea, photophobia, phonophobia, and pain). Feverfew was found less effective when taken to abort an ongoing attack, however. Furthermore, the doses required are much higher than those for prophylaxis.

In 2012, the AAN and the AHS published a joint report on the evidence for CAM on episodic migraine prophylaxis. Their conclusion was that feverfew was probably effective for this purpose. The AAN recommends dosing at 50 to 300 mg to be taken twice a day for migraine prophylaxis.

What about the other purposes for which people use feverfew? Unfortunately, there is no reliable evidence that feverfew can benefit patients with rheumatoid arthritis or other inflammatory conditions.

Adverse Effects

Feverfew is very well tolerated. No serious adverse effects have been reported, although long-term studies of safety are lacking. Mild reactions include abdominal pain, indigestion, diarrhea, flatulence, nausea, and vomiting. Chewing feverfew leaves, a rare practice today, can cause oral ulceration, tongue irritation, and swollen lips. Some patients develop *post-feverfew syndrome,* characterized by nervousness, fatigue, insomnia, tension headache, and joint pain or stiffness.

Feverfew belongs to the same plant family as echinacea. Accordingly, individuals allergic to ragweed, chrysanthemums, daisies, and marigolds may also be allergic to feverfew. By suppressing release of arachidonic acid in platelets, feverfew can decrease platelet aggregation and may thereby pose a risk for bleeding. Accordingly, the product should be discontinued 2 weeks before elective surgery.

Some reports suggest that feverfew may cause uterine contractions. For this reason, women who are pregnant should not take this drug. Safety regarding breastfeeding has not been established.

Interactions With Conventional Drugs

By suppressing platelet aggregation, feverfew can increase the risk for bleeding in patients taking antiplatelet drugs (e.g., aspirin) or anticoagulants (e.g., warfarin, heparin).

Comments

There is great variability in feverfew products. Some contain little or no active ingredient.

Flaxseed

Flaxseeds are small seeds of the flax plant, which grows in the northwestern United States and in Canada. They may be processed in various products or added whole to cereals and other food products.

Uses

Flaxseed powders are used to treat constipation and dyslipidemias. Because it is a phytoestrogen, some women take it to combat hot flashes associated with menopause. Flaxseed also provides a vegetarian source of omega-3 fatty acids.

Actions

Ground flaxseed provides soluble plant fiber and alpha-linolenic acid. Like other high-fiber products, flaxseed can reduce serum cholesterol.

Flaxseed is an important food source of phytoestrogens called lignans. In the colon, bacteria convert these lignans into enterolactone and enterodiol, compounds that have both mild estrogenic and antiestrogenic actions. The antiestrogenic actions can decrease cellular proliferation in breast tissue.

Effectiveness

Like other fiber products, flaxseed has the potential to decrease plasma levels of total cholesterol and low-density lipoprotein (LDL) cholesterol, but does not affect high-density lipoprotein (HDL) cholesterol or triglycerides. These effects occur predominantly among people with high cholesterol levels and in women who are postmenopausal. In contrast, *defatted* flaxseed may *increase* triglyceride levels, so it should be avoided by patients with hypertriglyceridemia. Owing to its soluble fiber content, flaxseed acts like a bulk-forming laxative to relieve constipation. As with any bulk-forming laxative, adequate fluid intake is an important component of therapy.

Other than for management of hypercholesterolemia, current studies do not support the use of flaxseed for cardiovascular disease. They also do not support its use for relief of menopausal symptoms or for cancer prevention. However, NCCIH funding of flaxseed research is ongoing.

Adverse Effects

Like other sources of dietary fiber, flaxseed can cause adverse GI effects. These include bloating, flatulence, and abdominal discomfort.

Interactions With Conventional Drugs

Flaxseed may reduce the absorption of conventional medications. For this reason, it should be taken 1 hour before or 2 hours after these drugs.

Garlic

Garlic *(Allium sativum)* is a common plant known for its edible bulb. It has been used throughout history for myriad uses and remains one of the most popular dietary supplements in use today.

Uses

Garlic is used primarily for effects on the cardiovascular system. The herb is taken to reduce levels of triglycerides and LDL cholesterol and to raise levels of HDL cholesterol. Garlic is also employed to reduce blood pressure, suppress platelet aggregation, increase arterial elasticity, and decrease formation of atherosclerotic plaque. In addition, garlic has been used for antimicrobial and anticancer effects.

Actions

Beneficial effects are presumed to result from the actions of sulfides in garlic oil. Intact garlic cells contain *alliin,* an odorless amino acid. When garlic cells are crushed, they release alliinase, an enzyme that converts alliin into *allicin.* Allicin is the major active agent in garlic oil and the compound that gives garlic its distinctive aroma. In addition to allicin, garlic oil contains *ajoenes* (pronounced AH-ho-weens), biologically active compounds that contribute to beneficial effects.

Garlic is thought to reduce cholesterol levels by interfering with cholesterol synthesis in the liver. There is conflicting evidence regarding inhibition of HMG-CoA reductase, the rate-limiting enzyme in cholesterol synthesis and the enzyme that "statin" drugs inhibit.

Antiplatelet effects, which are well documented, result in part from inhibiting thromboxane synthesis. Methylallyltrisulfide is the chemical in garlic believed responsible. In addition, garlic may suppress platelet aggregation by disrupting calcium-dependent processes. Coagulation is also affected by the ajoenes, which have antithrombotic actions and may also stimulate fibrinolysis.

Lowering of blood pressure may be explained by garlic's ability to increase the activity of nitric oxide synthase, the enzyme in blood vessels that makes nitric oxide. Nitric oxide, also known as endothelium-derived relaxant factor, is a powerful vasodilator.

Effectiveness

As with many dietary supplements, research findings regarding garlic have been mixed. Outcomes of small trials in the 1990s demonstrated that garlic can produce favorable effects on plasma lipids. More recent and larger studies, however, have cast doubt on those findings.

After reviewing the scientific research, the NCCIH has concluded the following:

- Garlic does not appear to lower LDL cholesterol.
- Garlic *may* lower blood pressure, but any benefit appears modest, at best.
- Garlic *may* decrease the rate of atherosclerosis development.

Regarding the effect of garlic on cancer prevention, at this time, the National Cancer Institute recognizes that garlic *may* have a role in cancer prevention but, in the absence of adequate reliable data, does not recommend it.

Adverse Effects

Garlic is generally well tolerated. The most common side effects are bad breath and body odor. (This occurs because a product of garlic metabolism is allyl methyl sulfide, a sulfur compound that is excreted through respiration and skin pores.) Rarely, garlic causes heartburn, flatulence, nausea, vomiting, diarrhea, and a burning sensation in the mouth. These effects are most pronounced with raw garlic and in people who don't eat garlic often. Patients suffering from infectious or inflammatory GI disorders should avoid garlic, owing to its potential for GI irritation.

Interactions With Conventional Drugs

Garlic has significant antiplatelet effects. Accordingly, it can increase the risk for bleeding in patients taking antiplatelet drugs (e.g., aspirin) or anticoagulants (e.g., warfarin, heparin). Garlic can reduce levels of at least two drugs: cyclosporine (an immunosuppressant) and saquinavir (a protease inhibitor used to treat HIV infection).

Ginger Root

Ginger grows primarily in the tropics. Its root, actually a rhizome, is the source of the ginger root used in CAM.

Uses

Ginger root *(Zingiber officinale)* is used primarily to treat vertigo and to suppress nausea and vomiting associated with motion sickness, morning sickness, seasickness, and general anesthesia. In addition, ginger has anti-inflammatory and analgesic properties that may help people with arthritis and other chronic inflammatory conditions. Some practitioners use ginger for URIs, although proof of efficacy is lacking.

Actions

The mechanism by which ginger suppresses nausea and vomiting is unclear. A good possibility is blockade of serotonin (5-hydroxytryptamine$_3$, or 5-HT$_3$) receptors located in the chemoreceptor trigger zone of the medulla and on afferent vagal neurons in the GI tract. Activation of these receptors triggers emesis. Conversely, blockade of these receptors suppresses emesis. In fact, drugs that block 5-HT$_3$ receptors (e.g., ondansetron [Zofran]) are the most effective antiemetics available. Galanolactone, a major constituent of ginger, can block 5-HT$_3$ receptors *in vitro,* suggesting that receptor blockade may underlie antiemetic effects. Other actions that may contribute to beneficial effects include stimulation of intestinal motility, salivation, and gastric mucus production and suppression of GI spasm secondary to anticholinergic and antihistaminic actions.

The anti-inflammatory effects of ginger have been attributed to inhibiting synthesis of prostaglandins and leukotrienes, which are powerful inflammatory mediators.

How ginger may reduce vertigo is unknown.

Effectiveness

There is good evidence supporting the benefits of ginger root for the prevention and treatment of morning sickness. A 2014 meta-analysis of the evidence demonstrated a decrease in nausea but not in episodes of vomiting. Unfortunately, studies focused on nausea due to motion sickness and postoperative nausea and vomiting (in the absence of opioids) have had conflicting results.

In patients with rheumatoid arthritis, ginger root appears to reduce pain, improve joint mobility, and decrease swelling and morning stiffness. These studies are inconclusive, however, and further research is ongoing.

Adverse Effects

Ginger is very well tolerated. Severe toxicity has not been reported—although excessive doses (above 5 gm/day) have the potential to cause CNS depression and cardiac dysrhythmias. Huge doses may also cause GI disturbances.

Although ginger has effectiveness in relieving morning sickness, it should be used with caution during pregnancy because safety in pregnancy has not been proved. High-dose ginger is believed to stimulate the uterus and thus may theoretically cause spontaneous abortion, although there are no reports of this ever happening. A 2012 population study of women in Norway included data on 1020 women who used ginger during pregnancy. Research findings showed no increased risk for malformations, spontaneous abortion, or other complications compared with women who did not take ginger.

Interactions With Conventional Drugs

Ginger can inhibit production of thromboxane by platelets and can thereby suppress platelet aggregation. Accordingly, ginger can increase the risk for bleeding in patients receiving antiplatelet drugs (e.g., aspirin) or anticoagulants (e.g., warfarin, heparin). Ginger can lower blood sugar, and hence may potentiate the hypoglycemic effects of insulin and other drugs for diabetes.

Ginkgo biloba

Medicinal ginkgo is prepared by acetone extraction of leaves from the *Ginkgo biloba* tree. These leaves contain two classes of active compounds: *flavonoids* (ginkgoflavone glycosides) and *terpenoids* (ginkgolides, bilobalide). *Ginkgo biloba extracts* (GBEs) are standardized to contain 24% flavonoids and 6% terpenoids. Daily oral doses of standardized GBE range from 60 to 240 mg.

Uses

Ginkgo (*Ginkgo biloba*) is used primarily to improve memory, to halt progression of dementia, and to decrease intermittent claudication. Less common uses include the treatment of erectile dysfunction and other conditions associated with decreased perfusion.

Actions

Benefits of ginkgo are believed to derive from improved blood flow secondary to ginkgo-induced vasodilation. GBEs also suppress production of platelet-activating factor (PAF), a mediator of platelet aggregation, bronchospasm, and other processes. Reduced PAF production may help protect against thrombosis as well as bronchospasm and other allergic disorders.

Effectiveness

Ginkgo is one of the most studied of the herbal products. As with many of these, early studies showed promising findings that conflicted with more recent and rigorous clinical trials. Studies that examine the effects of ginkgo on intermittent claudication have had mixed results. Most have not demonstrated a significant benefit. In those in which improvement was noted, the degree of improvement was small. What about benefits in dementia? In a large placebo-controlled trial—the Ginkgo Evaluation of Memory (GEM) study, sponsored by the NIH—GBE failed to prevent dementia of any sort, including Alzheimer's disease. This study enrolled more than 3000 participants 75 years or older. Half received a GBE formulation and the other half received a placebo. The result? After 6 years of treatment, the incidence of dementia was nearly identical in both groups.

The NCCIH is currently studying ginkgo effects in multiple sclerosis, sexual dysfunction caused by antidepressants, insulin resistance, and memory loss due to electroconvulsive therapy. Additional studies continue for intermittent claudication and dementia.

Adverse Effects

Ginkgo is generally well tolerated. In some patients, it causes stomach upset, headache, dizziness, or vertigo, all of which can be minimized by avoiding rapid increases in dosage. There have been case reports of spontaneous bleeding, although no bleeding was observed in the GEM study.

There have been reports of people eating raw or roasted ginkgo seeds. Unlike ginkgo leaves, the seeds contain significant amounts of toxins. Seizures and fatalities have occurred after ingestion.

Interactions With Conventional Drugs

Ginkgo may suppress coagulation. Accordingly, it should be used with caution in patients taking antiplatelet drugs (e.g., aspirin) or anticoagulants (e.g., warfarin, heparin).

There is concern that ginkgo may promote seizures. Accordingly, the herb should be avoided by patients at risk for seizures, including those taking drugs that can lower the seizure threshold, including antipsychotics, antidepressants, cholinesterase inhibitors, decongestants, first-generation antihistamines, and systemic glucocorticoids.

Glucosamine and Chondroitin

Glucosamine and chondroitin are individual products that are usually administered together. Both are innate substances in the body that serve as essential components of cartilage. Products containing these substances can come from natural sources (e.g., animal cartilage) or may be manufactured in a laboratory.

Uses

Glucosamine and chondroitin are used widely to treat osteoarthritis. Osteoarthritis primarily affects the knee, hip, and wrist joints.

Actions

Glucosamine is employed by the body in the synthesis of cartilage and synovial fluid. Chondroitin helps to keep cartilage hydrated. When given to people with osteoarthritis, glucosamine may help in several ways. First, it can act as a substrate for making cartilage and synovial fluid. Second, it can stimulate the activity of chondrocytes, the cells in joints that make cartilage and synovial fluid. And third, it can suppress production of cytokines that mediate joint inflammation and cartilage degradation. Chondroitin has a role in maintaining cartilage integrity.

Effectiveness

Studies on the efficacy of glucosamine and chondroitin in osteoarthritis have yielded mixed results. Most studies do not show improvement in pain relief; however, some studies have demonstrated a modest improvement in joint structure.

In 2012, the American College of Rheumatology updated its recommendations for the management for osteoarthritis. After an examination of the evidence, the expert panel advised providers *not* to use glucosamine and chondroitin for osteoarthritis management.

Adverse Effects

The most common side effects are GI disturbances, such as nausea and heartburn. Because commercial glucosamine is produced from the exoskeletons of shellfish (shrimp), glucosamine should be used with caution in patients with shellfish allergy. In theory, glucosamine can raise blood levels of glucose, but this has not been observed in clinical trials.

Interactions With Conventional Drugs

Several case reports suggest glucosamine may increase the risk for bleeding. Accordingly, patients taking antiplatelet drugs (e.g., aspirin) or anticoagulants (e.g., warfarin, heparin) should probably avoid this product.

Green Tea

Green tea is produced from the *Camellia sinensis* plant. This is the same plant used to produce black tea and oolong tea. The differences lie in the method of production.

Uses

Green tea and green tea extracts have been used to lose weight, improve mental clarity, and prevent and treat cancers of the stomach, skin, bladder, and breast.

Actions

The mechanism underlying beneficial effects is poorly understood and probably multifactorial. Polyphenols in green tea may underlie anti-inflammatory, chemoprotective, and antioxidant effects. Chemoprotection may also stem from epigallocatechin-3-gallate (EGCG), a compound in green tea extracts. The caffeine in green tea may be responsible for weight loss and improved mental clarity.

Effectiveness

Data on green tea efficacy are limited. There is evidence that drinking green tea throughout the day can improve mental clarity and may help with weight loss. In both cases, any benefits are probably due to caffeine and not a substance unique to green tea. Studies done in animals and cultured cancer cells have shown that green tea and EGCG may prevent or slow the growth of certain cancers. Also, there is a small body of evidence indicating that drinking green tea may help prevent recurrence after treatment of early-stage breast cancer. These studies have shown mixed results; however, research is ongoing.

Adverse Effects

Moderate consumption appears to be safe. As with other caffeine-containing products, overconsumption may result in headache, nausea, anxiety, insomnia, increased heart rate, and increased urination. Hepatotoxicity has been reported, primarily in people using concentrated green tea extracts. The mechanism of the hepatotoxicity remains unknown.

Interactions With Conventional Drugs

There is a long list of potential drug interactions. Green tea should be consumed with caution by patients taking vasodilators, stimulants and other psychoactive medications, and medications with a known risk for liver damage. Green tea contains a small amount of vitamin K, which may decrease the anticoagulant effects of warfarin.

Peppermint

Peppermint *(Mentha piperita)* is a common herb in North America as well as Europe and the Middle East. It is often found near streams, especially in partially shaded areas.

Uses

Peppermint is best known as a culinary flavoring. Peppermint tea is a popular drink in some regions. When used as a medicinal preparation, peppermint oil is the form most commonly used. It is available over the counter in gel tablets or capsules.

Randomized controlled trials (RCTs) have demonstrated a beneficial effect of peppermint oil for the management of irritable bowel syndrome (IBS). In their 2014 Monograph on the Management of Irritable Bowel Syndrome and Chronic Idiopathic Constipation (available at http://gi.org/wp-content/uploads/2014/08/IBS_CIC_Monograph_AJG_Aug_2014.pdf), the American College of Gastroenterology included peppermint oil among its recommendations for IBS management.

Peppermint oil is also gaining recognition as therapy for small intestine bacterial overgrowth (SIBO). SIBO is a condition that has become increasingly common as a result of increases in over-the-counter proton pump inhibitor use as well as after certain bariatric surgeries such as the Roux-en-Y gastric bypass. As bacteria break down carbohydrates and other substances, excessive gas forms. This results in severe abdominal cramps and low volume diarrhea. SIBO is typically treated with antibiotics; therefore, the antibiotic properties of peppermint oil are beneficial in this regard.

Small studies also support the use of peppermint oil to manage esophageal spasms in adults and functional abdominal pain in children. Numerous anecdotal reports suggest that the topical use of peppermint oil applied to the temples may help ease tension headaches. This is supported by two small trials comparing peppermint oil with a placebo and peppermint oil to acetaminophen. In these, peppermint oil was significantly more effective than the placebo and equal in effectiveness compared to acetaminophen.

Actions

Peppermint oil inhibits smooth muscle activity in the gastrointestinal tract. The exact mechanism is unclear; however, animal studies have indicated a possible relationship to the blocking of calcium channels in the GI system.

Antibacterial properties of peppermint may come, in part, from menthol and other volatile oils. Research has demonstrated that peppermint oil has a bacteriostatic effect against 22 strains of both gram-positive and gram-negative bacteria and bactericidal activity against *Escherichia coli, Helicobacter pylori,* and *Salmonella enteritidis*.

It has been theorized that peppermint activates opioid receptors. Recent studies point to a different mechanism for pain relief: stimulation of transient receptor potential ion channel melastatin subtype 8 (TRPM8) in gastrointestinal pathways. TRPM8 receptors are activated by cold temperatures and by cooling agents such as menthol, which is a component of peppermint.

Effectiveness

Numerous studies demonstrate that peppermint oil is significantly superior to a placebo for the management of IBS. Smaller studies support its use for SIBO, functional abdominal pain, and tension headache.

Adverse Effects

Peppermint can lower esophageal sphincter pressure, leading to gastroesophageal reflux. This is more likely to occur with peppermint teas. Peppermint gels do not usually cause such problems because their enteric coating allows them to pass through the stomach intact.

Allergic reactions have been reported. Perianal burning has been reported following high doses. Excessive doses have also been tied to renal problems. At standard doses, peppermint oil appears to be devoid of serious adverse effects.

Interactions With Conventional Drugs

Over a decade ago, questions were raised regarding CYP1A2 inhibition by peppermint oil; however, this has not been demonstrated in humans. Peppermint oil may have an additive effect when administered with antispasmodics.

Probiotics

Probiotics are dietary supplements composed of potentially beneficial bacteria or yeasts. These preparations typically contain two types of bacteria—lactobacilli and bifidobacteria—as well as *Saccharomyces boulardii,* a specific strain of yeast. All of these microorganisms are normal components of our gut flora.

Uses

The *bacteria* in probiotics may help treat irritable bowel syndrome (IBS), ulcerative colitis, *Clostridium difficile*–associated diarrhea (CDAD), and, in children, rotavirus diarrhea. Products containing *S. boulardii* are used for CDAD.

Actions

Normal intestinal and colonic bacteria play several important roles: They help metabolize foods and some drugs; they promote nutrient absorption; and they reduce colonization of the gut by pathogenic bacteria. *Lactobacillus* and *Bifidobacterium* species adhere to the intestinal wall and thereby prevent attachment of bacterial pathogens. They also control bacterial overgrowth by producing lactic acid and to some degree by producing hydrogen peroxide. Benefits may also derive from increasing nonspecific cellular and humeral immunity. The yeast *S. boulardii* produces proteases that can degrade toxins produced by *C. difficile.* Benefits of *S. boulardii* in Crohn's disease derive in part from increasing intestinal secretion of immunoglobulin A.

Effectiveness

According to information available at NCCIH (https://nccih.nih.gov/health/probiotics), studies on probiotics have yielded conflicting results. Larger and more rigorous research studies are needed. There is some evidence that *Lactobacillus* species may reduce the duration of diarrhea in patients with rotavirus infection and other GI conditions. Effectiveness appears to vary among *Lactobacillus* species. VSL#3, a product composed of lactobacilli, bifidobacteria, *Streptococcus thermophilus,* and other bacteria, appears to have a role in inducing remission of ulcerative colitis, perhaps in as many as 50% of patients. In patients with IBS, VSL#3 may reduce bloating and abdominal pain. However, the product does not improve bowel movement frequency or consistency. Additional testing is needed.

Adverse Effects

Probiotics are generally well tolerated. Flatulence and bloating are the most common adverse effects. Infection of the blood with lactobacilli and fungi has been reported after ingestion of yogurt, but only in severely ill, immunocompromised patients taking broad-spectrum antibiotics long term. Fungicemia has occurred most often when packets of *S. boulardii* [Florastor] have been opened at the bedside in the intensive care unit. Florastor is contraindicated in patients who have central lines.

Interactions With Conventional Drugs

Antibacterial and antifungal drugs can kill the bacteria and yeasts in probiotic products. Accordingly, to help preserve probiotic activity, these preparations should be administered no sooner than 2 hours after dosing with antibacterial or antifungal drugs.

Resveratrol

Resveratrol is a chemical found in grapes (mainly the skin), red wine, purple grape juice, blueberries, cranberries, and peanuts. Resveratrol content of dietary supplements ranges from 16 to 600 mg per tablet or capsule. The amount in red wine is quite low, only 0.3 to 1.9 mg per 150-mL serving.

Uses

Resveratrol is an antioxidant promoted for antiaging effects and for protection against chronic diseases. Owing to the presence of resveratrol in red wine, researchers thought it might explain the *French paradox*: How can it be that French people have a relatively low incidence of coronary heart disease, despite having a diet relatively high in saturated fats? However, the amount of resveratrol in red wine seems much too low for significant cardioprotectant effects.

Recent research findings have opened the door to the potential for resveratrol to improve outcomes in a number of conditions. Research is ongoing to determine resveratrol's role in the management of heart disease, diabetes, obesity, and Alzheimer's disease.

Actions

In 2012, a breakthrough NIH study of resveratrol identified the mechanism of action, heretofore believed to be due to direct interaction with *sirtuin enzymes,* which increase insulin sensitivity, improve mitochondrial function, and promote cell survival—all of which could increase longevity. We now know that resveratrol inhibits phosphodiesterases (PDEs), which are located upstream from sirtuin. This finding is especially important because PDEs play a role in many chronic conditions (e.g., heart disease, diabetes, chronic obstructive pulmonary disease), and PDE inhibitors are proving to be important drugs in managing these.

Effectiveness

Resveratrol has produced clear benefits in animal studies. In middle-aged mice on a high-calorie diet, resveratrol increased insulin sensitivity and reduced mortality. In normal-weight mice, resveratrol failed to reduce mortality, but did improve cardiovascular function, bone density, and motor coordination and delayed formation of cataracts. In rodent models of human cancers, resveratrol suppressed tumor growth, including tumors of the lung, skin, breast, and prostate. In diabetic rats, resveratrol lowered blood glucose, and in human cells grown in culture, resveratrol increased glucose uptake. In one human study, resveratrol suppressed production of tumor necrosis factor and free radicals; both actions could reduce blood vessel inflammation and subsequent atherosclerosis. Numerous clinical trials in humans are ongoing, and early reports appear positive.

Adverse Effects and Interactions With Conventional Drugs

Information on adverse effects is limited. We do know that resveratrol has antiplatelet actions, which might intensify the effects of anticoagulants and antiplatelet drugs. Also, resveratrol can mimic the effects of estrogen, and hence is not recommended for women with estrogen-dependent breast cancer. In addition, resveratrol may increase insulin sensitivity, and hence should be used with caution by patients taking antidiabetic agents.

Saw Palmetto

The American saw palmetto *(Serenoa repens, Sabal serrulata)* is a small palm tree that grows in the eastern United States. The product employed clinically is an extract made from its berries.

Uses

Saw palmetto is taken to relieve urinary symptoms associated with benign prostatic hyperplasia (BPH). No other use has been identified.

Actions

How does saw palmetto affect prostate function? Some have postulated that saw palmetto blocks testosterone receptors, blocks alpha-adrenergic receptors, and suppresses inflammation. Contrary to prior belief, the preparation does not seem to inhibit 5-alpha-reductase, the enzyme that converts testosterone into dihydrotestosterone (DHT), the active form of testosterone in the prostate. Saw palmetto does not reduce prostate size or serum levels of testosterone, DHT, or prostate-specific antigen (PSA).

Effectiveness

At this time, there is insufficient evidence to support using saw palmetto for BPH or any other condition. Although early studies suggested that saw palmetto might reduce symptoms of BPH, these results have not been confirmed by more rigorous studies. Two clinical trials funded by the National Institutes of Health showed that saw palmetto extract is no more effective than placebo at reducing symptoms of BPH. A 2012 Cochrane review of 32 RCTs involving 5666 men found no significant difference between saw palmetto and a placebo. It continues to be widely used, however, and promoted in nonprofessional magazines and other resources.

Adverse Effects

Saw palmetto is very well tolerated. Significant adverse effects have not been reported. Rarely, saw palmetto causes nausea or headache. Although antiandrogenic effects (e.g., gynecomastia) have not been reported, it may be wise to monitor for them. Saw palmetto may have antiplatelet actions, but increased bleeding has not been reported.

Safety Alert

SAW PALMETTO AND PREGNANCY

Because of its antiandrogenic effects, saw palmetto represents a danger to the developing fetus. Pregnant women should not ingest this herb, but then we would hope that women would not anticipate needing a preparation whose only indication is treatment of BPH.

Interactions With Conventional Drugs

Because of its antiplatelet effects, saw palmetto should be used with caution in patients taking antiplatelet drugs (e.g., aspirin) or anticoagulants (e.g., warfarin, heparin).

Soy

Soy is a member of the pea (legume) family. Though it is processed in tablets and capsules for CAM, it has become a common staple in American diets both in its original form (edamame) and in processed foods such as soy sauce and tofu.

Uses

Soy protein and soy isoflavones have several uses, including prevention of breast cancer and, in postmenopausal women, treatment of vasomotor symptoms (hot flashes).

Actions

Soy's major active components are phytoestrogens (isoflavones and lignans) and phytosterols (betasitosterol). Two isoflavones—genistein and daidzein—undergo enzymatic conversion to equol, a compound with estrogenic actions. Soy isoflavones are structurally similar to estradiol (the major endogenous estrogen) and can bind with estrogen receptors. However, like the SERMs, isoflavones exert mixed estrogenic and antiestrogenic actions. In women with normal estrogen levels, soy isoflavones appear to *antagonize* endogenous estrogen. By contrast, in postmenopausal women, soy isoflavones act as estrogen agonists.

Effectiveness

Clinical trials using soy-derived phytoestrogens to relieve menopausal hot flashes have yielded mixed results. Overall, the studies lean toward a reduction in hot flashes. How do we explain the negative studies? It may be that many of the women enrolled had a reduced ability to metabolize isoflavones to their active form.

Several epidemiologic studies infer that soy consumption may reduce the risk for developing breast cancer. In particular, population studies have documented that Asian women who eat a diet high in soy are at reduced risk. However, clinical trials confirming this benefit are lacking.

Several early studies suggested that isoflavones either increase bone mineral density or slow the progression of osteoporosis in perimenopausal and postmenopausal women. However, with one exception, several meta-analyses of studies published between 2010 and 2015 do not demonstrate significant improvement in bone mineral density. The exception? A meta-analysis on the effects of phytoestrogens on osteoporosis in ovariectomized rats.

Adverse Effects

Soy and soy extracts are very well tolerated. Gastrointestinal effects—bloating, nausea, constipation or diarrhea—are most common. Rarely, soy can cause migraine, probably because of its estrogenic effects. Large amounts of soy products may increase the risk for oxalate kidney stones. There have been several cases of goiter and hypothyroidism in infants who drank soy-based formula. Concerns that soy formulas might cause feminization of male infants were dispelled by a 2008 review from the American Academy of Pediatrics.

Interactions With Conventional Drugs

Soy should not be combined with tamoxifen and other drugs that can block estrogen receptors. By killing intestinal flora, antibiotics may reduce conversion of isoflavones to their active form, thus decreasing any potentially positive effects of soy.

St. John's Wort

St. John's wort *(Hypericum perforatum)* is a plant that grows wild in the western United States and parts of Canada. Its yellow flowers are used in the preparation of extracts and other preparations.

Uses

St. John's wort is used primarily for oral therapy of mild to moderate depression. The herb has also been used topically to manage local infection and orally to relieve pain and inflammation.

Actions

Benefits of St. John's wort appear to derive from two compounds—hyperforin and hypericin—that are extracted from flowers of the plant. These compounds can decrease reuptake of three neurotransmitters: serotonin, norepinephrine (NE), and dopamine. Blockade of serotonin and NE uptake mimics the actions of some conventional antidepressants. Early research attributed antidepressant effects to inhibition of monoamine oxidase (MAO). However, we now know that the degree of MAO inhibition is too small to explain clinical effects.

Effectiveness

How effective is St. John's wort? At this time, it's hard to say. Although numerous studies have been conducted, evidence for efficacy is mixed, owing to poor study design, heterogeneous study populations, and variable hypericin content of the preparations used, as well as other confounding factors. The bottom line? For patients with *mild to moderate* major depression, St. John's wort appears superior to placebo and equal to tricyclic antidepressants. For patients with *severe* depression, there is no convincing proof of efficacy.

Adverse Effects

St. John's wort is generally well tolerated. Allergic skin reactions may occur, especially in people allergic to ragweed and daisies. In addition, the herb may cause CNS effects (e.g., insomnia, vivid dreams, restlessness, anxiety, agitation, and irritability) as well as GI discomfort, fatigue, dry mouth, and headache. High-dose therapy may pose a risk for phototoxicity. To reduce this risk, patients should minimize exposure to sunlight, wear protective clothing, and apply a sunscreen to exposed skin.

Interactions With Conventional Drugs

St. John's wort is known to interact adversely with many drugs—and the list continues to grow. Three mechanisms are involved: induction of cytochrome P450 enzymes, induction of P-glycoprotein, and intensification of serotonin effects. Let's consider these one by one:

- *Induction of 3A4 isoenzymes of cytochrome P450* can accelerate the metabolism of many drugs, thereby decreasing their effects. This mechanism appears responsible for breakthrough bleeding and unintended pregnancy in women taking oral contraceptives, transplant rejection in patients taking cyclosporine (an immunosuppressant), reduced anticoagulation in patients taking warfarin, and reduced antiretroviral effects in patients taking protease inhibitors or non-nucleoside reverse transcriptase inhibitors.
- *P-glycoprotein* is a transport protein found in cells that line the intestine and renal tubules. In the intestine, P-glycoprotein transports drugs *out* of cells into the intestinal lumen; in renal tubules, P-glycoprotein transports drugs *out* of tubular cells into the urine. Hence, by increasing P-glycoprotein synthesis, St. John's wort can accelerate elimination of drugs and can thereby reduce their effects. This is the mechanism by which St. John's wort greatly reduces levels of *digoxin,* a drug for heart failure. Other drugs whose levels can probably be reduced by this mechanism include calcium channel blockers, steroid hormones, protease inhibitors, and certain anticancer drugs (e.g., etoposide, paclitaxel, vinblastine, vincristine).
- Combining St. John's wort with certain drugs can intensify serotonergic transmission to a degree sufficient to cause potentially fatal *serotonin syndrome.* Although St. John's wort can enhance serotonergic transmission by itself, its effect is relatively weak. Hence, when used alone, the herb poses little risk. However, if St. John's wort is combined with other serotonin-enhancing agents, the risk is greatly increased, and hence St. John's wort should not be combined with such drugs. Among these are amphetamine, cocaine, and many antidepressants, including MAO inhibitors, selective serotonin reuptake inhibitors, certain tricyclic agents (e.g., amitriptyline, clomipramine), and duloxetine, nefazodone, and venlafaxine.

Because St. John's wort has a variety of known adverse interactions—and is likely to have more that are as-yet unknown—caution is clearly advised. St. John's wort is not recommended for treating depression in patients taking other medications.

Valerian

Valerian *(Valeriana officinalis),* also known as garden heliotrope, is a common plant in Europe and Asia, though it is grown in some areas of North America. The plant rhizomes and roots are used in the preparation of medicinal products.

Uses

Valerian root is a sedative preparation used primarily to promote sleep. In addition, some people take it to reduce anxiety-associated restlessness.

Actions

Valerian may work by increasing the availability of gamma-aminobutyric acid (GABA, an inhibitory neurotransmitter) at synapses in the CNS. (Benzodiazepines and benzodiazepine-like drugs, which are the major conventional hypnotics, act by potentiating the actions of GABA.) In addition, valerian may act as a direct GABA agonist. The active ingredient(s) in valerian have not been identified.

Effectiveness

Although valerian has been used for centuries in Europe, China, and other countries, objective evidence of efficacy is lacking. According to the NCCIH at https://nccih.nih.gov/health/providers/digest/sleep-disorders-science, "Various herbs such as valerian, chamomile, and kava, and homeopathic medicines sometimes used as sleep aids have not been shown to be effective for insomnia." Even so, some suggest it may still have mild sedative effects that may be useful for anxiety.

Adverse Effects

Valerian is generally very well tolerated. The FDA has given valerian a Generally Recognized as Safe (GRAS) rating when the product is consumed in amounts commonly used in food. Possible side effects include daytime drowsiness, dizziness, depression, dyspepsia, and pruritus. Prolonged use may cause headache, nervousness, or cardiac abnormalities. Because valerian can reduce alertness, users should exercise caution when performing dangerous activities, such as driving or operating dangerous machinery. In addition, valerian should be used with caution by people with psychiatric illnesses (e.g., depression, dementia). As with benzodiazepines, there may be a risk for paradoxical excitation and physical dependence. We do not know if valerian enters breast milk or harms the developing fetus. Until more is known, valerian should be avoided by women who are pregnant or breast-feeding.

Interactions With Conventional Drugs

In theory, valerian can potentiate the actions of other drugs with CNS-depressant actions. Among these are alcohol, benzodiazepines, barbiturates, opioids, antihistamines, and centrally acting skeletal muscle relaxants. These combinations should be used with caution.

HARMFUL SUPPLEMENTS TO AVOID

To help protect the public from dangerous botanical products, the FDA and the Federal Trade Commission are monitoring adverse event data and issuing warnings to consumers and manufacturers. Three potentially harmful products—comfrey, kava, and Ma huang—are discussed next.

Comfrey

Comfrey *(Symphytum officinale)* is an herbal supplement used topically and orally. Topical use appears safe. Oral use is not. Why? Because comfrey contains pyrrolizidine alkaloids, which can cause veno-occlusive disease (VOD) in animals and hepatic VOD in humans. Hepatic VOD can result in severe liver damage. In addition to causing VOD, pyrrolizidine alkaloids may also be carcinogenic. Accordingly, in July 2001 the FDA issued a letter to dietary supplement manufacturers advising them to remove comfrey from the market. They urged manufacturers to discontinue production, pull existing product off the shelves, and warn consumers of the possible dangers; however, comfrey remains widely available for sale on the Internet and elsewhere.

Kava

Kava *(Piper methysticum),* also known as *kava-kava* or *awa,* is used to relieve anxiety, promote sleep, and relax muscles. In the United States, the herb has been promoted as a natural alternative to benzodiazepines (e.g., diazepam [Valium]) for treating anxiety and stress. Unfortunately, kava can cause severe liver injury, leading the FDA to issue a public warning in March 2002. Later that year, the Centers for Disease Control and Prevention issued a report on kava-related hepatotoxicity. In the report, they discussed 11 cases of hepatotoxicity from the United States and Europe in which the victims required a liver transplant owing to severe liver failure. Because of concerns over hepatotoxicity, kava sales have been restricted in Germany, Canada, Switzerland, France, and Australia—but not yet in the United States.

Ma Huang (Ephedra)

Ma huang (ephedra) contains ephedrine, a compound that can elevate blood pressure and stimulate the heart and CNS. High-dose ephedra has been associated with stroke, myocardial infarction, and death. To date, more than 17,000 adverse events have been reported, and at least 155 users have died. In 2004, the FDA banned U.S. sales of all ephedra products, marking the first time that a dietary supplement has been ordered off the market. The ban was challenged by an ephedra producer and, in 2005, was partially reversed: A federal court upheld the ban for ephedra products that contain more than 10 mg/dose, but reversed the ban for products that contain 10 mg or less, arguing that there are insufficient data to prove that low doses pose a "significant or unreasonable risk." In 2006, a federal appeals court upheld the FDA ban of ephedra. This ban was challenged again in 2007, but the U.S. Court of Appeals denied the petition for rehearing. At this time, the FDA ban does not apply to ephedra in traditional Asian medicines or in herbal teas, which are not marketed as dietary supplements.

KEY POINTS

- Dietary supplements can be defined as "a product intended for ingestion that contains a 'dietary ingredient' intended to add further nutritional value to (supplement) the diet."
- Dietary ingredients may be defined as "one, or any combination, of the following substances: a vitamin, a mineral, an herb or other botanical, an amino acid, [or] a dietary substance for use by people to supplement the diet by increasing the total dietary intake, a concentrate, metabolite, constituent, or extract."
- Dietary supplements are regulated under the Dietary Supplement Health and Education Act of 1994 (DSHEA) and the Current Good Manufacturing Practices (CGMPs) ruling issued in 2007.
- Unlike conventional drugs, dietary supplements can be marketed without any proof of safety or efficacy.
- Under the DSHEA, dietary supplements are presumed safe until proved harmful. Hence, manufacturers don't need to prove their products are safe. Rather, the FDA needs to prove they're not safe.
- Manufacturers can claim that a product favorably influences "body structure and function," but cannot claim that it can be used to diagnose, treat, cure, or prevent any disease.
- Dietary supplements can interact with conventional drugs, sometimes with serious results. Be sure to ask patients if they are using herbal supplements or other dietary supplements.
- The word *natural* is not synonymous with *safe.* Remember, poison ivy and tobacco are natural too.

Please visit **http://evolve.elsevier.com/Lehne** for chapter-specific NCLEX® examination review questions.

UNIT XX TOXICOLOGY

CHAPTER 109 Management of Poisoning

Poisoning is defined as a pathologic state caused by a toxic agent. Sources of poisoning include medications, plants, environmental pollutants, and drugs of abuse. These toxicants may enter the body orally or by injection, inhalation, or absorption through the skin. Poisoning may be unintentional (accidental) or intentional. Symptoms of poisoning often mimic those of disease, and hence the possibility of poisoning should be considered whenever a diagnosis is made.

In the United States, over 2.2 million poisonings are reported annually. In 2013, accidental poisoning caused over 42,000 deaths. Most poisoning deaths are caused by drugs: In 2014, 95% of deaths from accidental poisoning were caused by drugs, as were 75% of suicides. The *incidence* of poisoning is highest in young children. However, the *mortality rate* in this group is very low.

FUNDAMENTALS OF TREATMENT

Poisoning is a medical emergency and requires rapid treatment. Management has five basic elements: (1) supportive care, (2) identification of the poison, (3) prevention of further absorption, (4) poison removal, and (5) use of specific antidotes. These essentials are discussed next.

Supportive Care

Supportive care is the most important element in managing acute poisoning. Support is based on the clinical status and requires no knowledge specific to the poison involved. Maintenance of respiration and circulation are primary concerns. Measures for respiratory support include inserting an airway, giving humidified oxygen, and providing mechanical ventilation. Volume depletion (resulting from vomiting, diarrhea, or sweating) can compromise circulation. Volume should be restored by administering normal saline or Ringer's solution. Severe hypoglycemia may occur, resulting in coma. Levels of blood glucose should be monitored. For coma of unknown etiology, IV dextrose should be given immediately—even if information on blood glucose is lacking. Acid-base disturbances may occur; determination of arterial blood gases will facilitate diagnosis and management. If seizures develop, IV benzodiazepines are the treatment of choice.

Poison Identification

Treatment of poisoning is facilitated by knowing the identity and dosage of the toxicant. Efforts to obtain this information should proceed concurrently with medical management.

A history is one way to identify the toxic agent. However, experience has shown that histories taken at times of poisoning are often inaccurate. Hence, statements about the nature or quantity of poison may be incorrect.

Positive identification can be made by using analytic techniques. A gas chromatograph/mass spectrometer can provide qualitative and quantitative information. Analyses can be performed on specimens of urine, blood, and gastric contents. To determine whether poison levels are rising or falling, analyses should be performed on sequential blood samples taken about 2 hours apart.

Prevention of Further Absorption

By reducing the absorption of a poison, we can minimize blood levels and thereby significantly decrease morbidity and mortality. For *ingested* poisons, three procedures are available: (1) giving activated charcoal, (2) gastric lavage and aspiration, (3) and whole-bowel irrigation. When poison exposure is *topical,* surface decontamination is employed. Details of these procedures are discussed in the following section.

Promotion of Poison Removal

Measures that help eliminate poison from the body shorten the duration of exposure and, if implemented before plasma levels have peaked, can reduce the maximum level of poisoning achieved. By shortening exposure and reducing maximum poison levels, these measures can decrease morbidity and mortality.

Removal of poison can be promoted with drugs and with nonpharmacologic techniques. The drugs used for poison removal act by increasing renal excretion of toxic agents. Nonpharmacologic methods of poison removal include hemodialysis and exchange transfusion. Details on methods of poison removal are presented later.

Use of Specific Antidotes

An antidote is an agent administered to counteract the effects of a poison. Examples include naloxone (to reverse poisoning by heroin and other opioids) and physostigmine (to treat poisoning by atropine and other anticholinergic drugs). Several specific antidotes are discussed later. Unfortunately, although antidotes can be extremely valuable, these agents are rare: For most poisons, no specific antidote exists. Hence, for most patients, treatment is limited to the general measures just described.

DRUGS AND PROCEDURES USED TO MINIMIZE POISON ABSORPTION

Reducing Absorption of Ingested Poisons

Activated Charcoal

Treatment with activated charcoal is a preferred method for removing ingested poisons from the GI tract. Activated charcoal is an inert substance that adsorbs drugs and other chemicals. Binding of toxicants to charcoal is essentially irreversible. Because charcoal particles cannot be absorbed into the blood, adsorption of poisons onto charcoal prevents toxicity. The charcoal-poison complex is eliminated in the stool. Patients should be advised that charcoal will turn the feces black. Charcoal is very safe, but should not be used in patients with bowel perforation or obstruction.

Charcoal selectively adsorbs *large molecules* that contain a *carbon atom*. Adsorption of small molecules and molecules that lack a carbon atom is poor. Among these poorly absorbed molecules are heavy metals, caustics and corrosives, alcohols and glycols, chlorine, iodine, and petroleum distillates.

Because charcoal can adsorb antidotes and thereby neutralize their benefits, antidotes should not be administered immediately before, with, or shortly after the charcoal.

Activated charcoal has the consistency of a fine powder and is mixed with water for oral administration. The adult dose is 25 to 100 gm. Pediatric doses range from 25 to 50 gm. For poisoning with certain compounds—phenobarbital, dapsone, quinine, theophylline, and carbamazepine—giving sequential doses of charcoal can be beneficial. When administered within 30 minutes after poison ingestion, charcoal can adsorb about 90% of the dose. However, if given 60 minutes after poison ingestion, the amount adsorbed decreases to only 37%. Clearly, charcoal should be given as soon as possible after poison exposure.

Gastric Lavage and Aspiration

Gastric lavage (irrigation) and aspiration consists of flushing the stomach with fluid and then sucking (aspirating) the fluid back out. The procedure should be done only in life-threatening cases and only if less than 1 hour has elapsed since poison ingestion. Specific contraindications to lavage and aspiration include the following:

- Unprotected airway
- Caustic ingestion (due to risk of exacerbating any esophageal or gastric injury)
- Hydrocarbon ingestion (due to high aspiration risk)
- Patients at risk of GI hemorrhage or perforation (recent surgery, underlying anatomic abnormality or pathology, coagulopathy)

Lavage and aspiration are accomplished by using a large-bore orogastric tube (No. 36 to 42 French for adults, No. 22 to 28 French for children). Smaller tubes should be avoided because they may not permit the removal of solids (food, pills, capsules, tablets) and because their small diameter would impede the flow of the lavage fluid. If the patient is comatose, an endotracheal tube with an inflatable cuff should be installed to protect the airway. Because of the anatomy of the stomach, the patient should be placed on the left side with the head down. Prior to initiation of lavage, stomach contents should be aspirated and sent for toxicologic analysis. Lavage may be performed with tap water or saline solution. Multiple washes are instilled using 150 to 200 mL/wash (for adults and older children) or 50 to 100 mL/wash (for children under 5 years old). Larger volumes should be avoided since they may push stomach contents into the small intestine. Washes should be repeated until the fluid retrieved from the stomach is clear. About 10 to 12 washes are employed.

Whole-Bowel Irrigation

Whole-bowel irrigation is done with a solution of polyethylene glycol that contains balanced electrolytes, available under the brand names CoLyte and GoLYTELY. The solution is administered repeatedly over a 5-hour period, either by mouth or through a nasogastric tube. Rates of administration are as follows:

- For patients age 12 years and older—1.5 to 2 L/hr
- For patients 6 to 12 years old—1 L/hr
- For patients younger than 6 years old—0.5 L/hr

The procedure has been effective following the ingestion of iron, lithium, and lead, as well as sustained-release products. Whole-bowel irrigation should not be used in patients with ileus, peritonitis, bloody vomitus, or obstruction or perforation of the bowel.

Surface Decontamination

Topical exposure to toxicants can cause local and systemic injury. To minimize injury, contaminated clothing should be removed and the poison should be washed from the victim. The recommended procedure is to alternate soap-and-water washes with alcohol washes. Personnel performing these washes should take precautions to avoid contaminating themselves. If the victim's eyes have been exposed, they should be flushed with water for at least 15 minutes. Shampoo should be used to remove toxic agents from the hair and scalp.

DRUGS AND PROCEDURES USED FOR POISON REMOVAL

Drugs That Enhance Renal Excretion

Drugs that alter the pH of urine can accelerate the excretion of organic acids and bases. Agents that *elevate* urinary pH (i.e., make the urine more alkaline) will promote the excretion of *acids*. Drugs that *lower* urinary pH will promote the excretion of *bases*. The mechanism underlying these effects is called *ion trapping* (see Chapter 4).

The drug employed most frequently to alter urinary pH is *sodium bicarbonate.* Sodium bicarbonate is administered IV and renders the urine more alkaline, which decreases the passive reabsorption of acids (e.g., aspirin, phenobarbital) and thereby accelerates their excretion. Because of the buffer systems present in blood, sodium bicarbonate has a relatively small effect on the pH of blood, while having a large effect on the pH of urine.

Nondrug Methods of Poison Removal

Several nondrug procedures—hemodialysis, hemoperfusion, and exchange transfusion—can be employed to remove toxicants from the body. Although these procedures are usually of limited value, they can be lifesaving in some situations. Nondrug procedures are most effective when (1) binding of toxicants to plasma proteins is low and (2) blood levels of toxicants are high (i.e., when distribution of the toxic agent is restricted to the blood and extracellular fluid).

Each of the nondrug methods of poison removal has its benefits and drawbacks. *Hemodialysis,* although invasive, can greatly enhance the elimination of poisons. *Hemoperfusion* is a process in which blood is passed over a column of charcoal or absorbent resin. If the affinity of the resin for a particular poison is high, the procedure can strip a toxicant from binding sites on plasma proteins. The principal disadvantage of hemoperfusion is a loss of platelets. When the binding of a poison to plasma proteins is particularly avid, *exchange transfusion* can be an effective method of removal.

SPECIFIC ANTIDOTES

Heavy Metal Antagonists

The heavy metals most frequently responsible for poisoning are iron, lead, mercury, arsenic, gold, and copper. These metals cause injury by forming complexes with enzymes and other physiologically important molecules. Poisoning may result from environmental exposure, intentional overdose, or therapeutic use of heavy metals.

The drugs given to treat heavy metal poisoning are called *chelating agents* or *chelators.* These agents interact with metals to form *chelates*—ring structures in which the metal and the chelating agent form two or more points of attachment. Useful chelating agents have a high affinity for heavy metals and can compete successfully with endogenous molecules for metal binding. By preventing initial binding of metals to endogenous molecules, chelators can prevent injury. By stripping metals that have already become bound, chelators can enhance their excretion.

The selectivity of a heavy metal antagonist is determined by its affinity for specific metals. Some antagonists are selective for only one metal; others can form chelates with several metals. Deferoxamine, for example, binds selectively to iron. In contrast, dimercaprol is relatively nonselective, binding tightly with arsenic, mercury, and gold.

Properties desirable in a heavy metal antagonist include (1) high affinity for a toxic metal, (2) low affinity for essential endogenous metals (e.g., magnesium, zinc), (3) the ability to reach sites of metal storage, (4) high activity at physiologic pH, (5) formation of chelates that are less toxic than the free metal, and (6) formation of chelates that are easily excreted.

Chelators for Iron Toxicity

We have three chelators with a high affinity for iron. All three—deferoxamine, deferasirox, and deferiprone—are used to treat iron overload caused by chronic blood transfusions in patients with infusion-dependent anemias. Only one of the drugs—deferoxamine—is also indicated for acute iron poisoning.

Deferoxamine

Actions and Uses. Deferoxamine [Desferal] has a high affinity for ferric iron. The drug chelates free iron and can also strip iron bound to ferritin and hemosiderin. In contrast, iron present in hemoglobin and cytochromes is not affected. Deferoxamine is employed to treat *acute iron poisoning* and *chronic infusional iron overload.*

Pharmacokinetics. Deferoxamine is poorly absorbed from the GI tract, and hence requires parenteral administration. The chelate formed between deferoxamine and iron is excreted primarily in the urine.

Adverse Effects. Common reactions include fever, headache, cough, pharyngolaryngeal pain, nasopharyngitis, and bronchitis. Pain may occur at the site of injection. Rapid IV infusion may cause hypotension, tachycardia, erythema, and urticaria. Prolonged therapy may be associated with allergic reactions, abdominal discomfort, leg cramps, fever, and dysuria.

Contraindications. Because deferoxamine is excreted by the kidneys, the drug should not be given to patients with renal insufficiency. Deferoxamine has caused fetal malformations in experimental animals; thus it is not recommended for pregnant women.

Preparations, Dosage, and Administration. Deferoxamine mesylate is supplied as a powder to be reconstituted for injection. The drug can be administered by IM injection and by IV or subQ infusion. Intramuscular injection is preferred. Intravenous infusion is usually reserved for patients in shock. The dosage for IM or IV administration is the same. For the treatment of acute iron poisoning, the initial dose for adults and children is 1 gm. This is followed 4 and 8 hours later with 0.5-gm doses. For IV administration, the maximum rate of infusion is 15 mg/kg/hr. For the treatment of iron overload associated with chronic blood infusions (see the discussion of deferasirox that follows), the dosage is 20 to 40 mg/kg/day, administered by a prolonged (8- to 12-hour) subQ infusion.

Deferasirox

Actions and Uses. Like deferoxamine, deferasirox [Exjade] is a chelating agent with a high affinity for iron. The drug is indicated for *oral* therapy of iron overload resulting from chronic blood transfusions in patients with beta-thalassemia, sickle cell anemia, myelodysplastic syndromes, and other infusion-dependent anemias. Left untreated, iron overload can injure the liver, heart, and other organs. Cardiac injury is of special concern owing to a risk of dysrhythmias, heart failure, and even death. Compared with deferoxamine, deferasirox is *much* easier to use because deferasirox is taken orally. Unlike deferoxamine, deferasirox is not indicated for acute iron poisoning.

Pharmacokinetics. Plasma levels peak 1.4 to 4 hours after oral dosing. In the blood, deferasirox is highly bound to albumin. The drug undergoes hepatic metabolism followed by excretion in the bile. Deferasirox and its metabolites are then eliminated mainly (84%) in the feces. The plasma half-life is 8 to 16 hours.

Adverse Effects. The most common effects are fever, headache, cough, nasopharyngitis, and GI reactions, including abdominal pain, nausea, vomiting, and diarrhea. Some patients (< 1%) experience hearing loss and ocular disturbances, and hence hearing and vision tests should be done before treatment and every 12 months thereafter.

The most serious adverse effects are *renal impairment* (including renal failure), *liver dysfunction* (including liver failure), and *GI hemorrhage.* In some cases, these reactions have been fatal. Risk is greatest in older patients and in those with high-risk myelodysplastic syndromes, pre-existing renal or hepatic impairment, and low platelet counts. To reduce the risk of kidney and liver complications, kidney and liver function should be assessed at baseline and frequently thereafter.

Drug Interactions. *Cholestyramine* (used to reduce blood cholesterol) and *aluminum-containing antacids* (used for peptic ulcers) can decrease the absorption of deferasirox and can thereby reduce its beneficial effects. Accordingly, the combined use of deferasirox with these drugs should be avoided. If the combinations cannot be avoided, the dosage of deferasirox should be increased.

Combined use of deferasirox with *anticoagulants* (e.g., warfarin) increases the risk of hemorrhage. Use such combinations with great caution.

Deferasirox can reduce levels of drugs that are metabolized by CYP3A4 (the 3A4 isoenzyme of cytochrome P450). Loss of benefits may result. Accordingly, drugs that are substrates for CYP3A4 (e.g., cyclosporine, simvastatin, hormonal contraceptives) should be used with caution.

Deferasirox can cause a 2.3-fold increase in levels of *repaglinide* (used for diabetes). The mechanism is inhibition of CYP2C8. If deferasirox and repaglinide are combined, the dosage of repaglinide should be reduced, and blood levels of glucose should be closely monitored.

Preparations, Dosage, and Administration. Deferasirox is supplied in tablets (125, 250, and 500 mg) that must be dispersed in fluid (water, orange juice, apple juice). The tablets should not be swallowed whole. For doses of less than 1 gm, disperse tablets in 3.5 ounces of fluid; for doses greater than 1 gm, disperse in 7 ounces. Dosing is done once a day on an empty stomach (i.e., at least 30 minutes before eating), at the same time each day. The drug must not be taken with aluminum-containing antacids or cholestyramine.

The starting dosage is 10 to 20 mg/kg/day. Dosage can be adjusted every 3 to 6 months based on serum ferritin levels, but must not exceed 40 mg/kg/day. If serum ferritin falls consistently below 500 mcg/L, temporary interruption of treatment should be considered. Dosage should be reduced if liver or kidney function declines.

Deferiprone

Actions and Uses. Deferiprone [Ferriprox] is indicated for oral therapy of iron overload caused by chronic blood transfusions—but only in patients with thalassemia (safety and efficacy in patients with other chronic anemias have not been established) and only after treatment with other iron chelators has failed. Deferiprone is not used for acute iron poisoning.

Adverse Effects. The most common adverse effects are chromaturia, nausea, abdominal pain, vomiting, arthralgia, and liver toxicity, as indicated by an elevation of circulating transaminases.

The most serious adverse effect is *agranulocytosis/neutropenia*, which poses a risk of serious infections and death. Accordingly, absolute neutrophil counts should be obtained at baseline and weekly thereafter. If neutropenia or infection develops, deferiprone should be interrupted. If possible, deferiprone should not be combined with other drugs that promote neutropenia or agranulocytosis.

In animal studies, low-dose deferiprone caused fetal malformations and fetal death. The drug is classified in U.S. Food and Drug Administration Pregnancy Risk Category D,[a] and hence should not be used during pregnancy.

Preparations, Dosage, and Administration. Deferiprone is supplied in 500-mg tablets. The recommended initial dose is 25 mg/kg 3 times a day. The maximum dose is 33 mg/kg 3 times a day. Absorption can be reduced by mineral supplements and antacids that contain polyvalent cations (e.g., aluminum, iron, zinc). Accordingly, deferiprone should not be dosed within 4 hours of these substances.

Dimercaprol

Actions and Uses. Dimercaprol [BAL In Oil] binds with arsenic, gold, mercury, and lead. The resulting chelates are excreted in the urine. The drug is used as the sole chelator to rid the body of arsenic, mercury, or gold. In addition, dimercaprol can be combined with edetate calcium disodium (calcium EDTA) to treat poisoning with lead. Since dimercaprol is more effective at *preventing* binding of metals to endogenous molecules than at reversing binding that has already taken place, benefits are greatest when the drug is administered early (within 1 to 2 hours of metal ingestion).

Pharmacokinetics. Administration is by deep IM injection. Dimercaprol cannot be used orally. The drug has a short plasma half-life, with complete elimination occurring in approximately 4 hours.

Adverse Effects. At recommended doses, dimercaprol is generally well tolerated. Tachycardia and elevation of blood pressure occur frequently; blood pressure returns to baseline within hours. Pain and sterile abscesses may occur at sites of injection. Fever is common in children. High doses produce a broad spectrum of untoward effects.

Chelates formed with dimercaprol are unstable at acidic pH. Hence, if the urine is acidic, heavy metals may dissociate from dimercaprol, resulting in renal toxicity. To protect the kidneys, the urine should be kept alkaline.

Dimercaprol is formulated in peanut oil, and hence must be avoided by patients with known or suspected peanut allergy.

Preparations, Dosage, and Administration. Dimercaprol is supplied in ampules containing 300 mg of the drug in 3 mL of peanut oil. The preparation is administered by deep IM injection.

For *mild poisoning with gold or arsenic*, doses of 2.5 mg/kg are administered according to the following schedule: 4 times daily on days 1 and 2, twice daily on day 3, and once daily on days 4 through 13.

For *acute poisoning with mercury*, the initial dose is 5 mg/kg. Subsequent doses of 2.5 mg/kg are administered 1 or 2 times daily for 10 days.

For *acute poisoning with lead*, dimercaprol is combined with calcium EDTA. For the initial dose, give dimercaprol alone (4 mg/kg). Every 4 hours thereafter, give dimercaprol (4 mg/kg), along with calcium EDTA, administered at a separate site. Duration of treatment is 2 to 7 days. Dosage for calcium EDTA is presented next.

Edetate Calcium Disodium (Calcium EDTA)

Actions and Uses. Calcium EDTA [Calcium Disodium Versenate] is used primarily for lead poisoning. The drug combines with lead to form a stable chelate that is excreted in the urine.

Pharmacokinetics. Calcium EDTA may be administered IV or IM. The drug is poorly absorbed from the GI tract, and hence is not given orally. Elimination is by glomerular filtration. Because calcium EDTA is excreted by the kidneys, the drug should be employed only if urine flow is adequate. If urine flow is insufficient, flow should be restored with IV fluids prior to giving the chelator. If anuria develops during the course of treatment, administration should stop.

Adverse Effects. The principal toxicity of calcium EDTA is renal tubular necrosis. Signs include hematuria and proteinuria. Daily urinalysis should be performed to monitor for these effects. If renal toxicity develops, the drug should be discontinued immediately.

Preparations, Dosage, and Administration. Calcium EDTA is supplied in 5-mL ampules containing 1000 mg of drug. Administration may be IV or IM. The IM route is preferred for patients with cerebral edema.

For IV use, the contents of 1 ampule are diluted in 250 to 500 mL of 5% dextrose solution or normal saline. Infusion should be done slowly (over 8 to 12 hours). The adult dosage is 1 gm daily for 5 days. After a 2-day hiatus, a second course may be given if needed.

The dosage for children is 1 gm daily administered IV or IM for 5 days. After a pause of 2 to 4 days, a second course is given.

Penicillamine

Actions. Penicillamine [Cuprimine] is a breakdown product of penicillin. Commercial preparations are made synthetically. Penicillamine forms water-soluble chelates with copper, iron, lead, arsenic, gold, and mercury. These complexes are excreted in the urine.

Therapeutic Uses. The principal indication is *Wilson's disease*, a disorder of copper metabolism. Affected individuals are deficient in ceruloplasmin, a plasma protein that serves as a copper carrier. Symptoms result from deposition of copper in the liver, brain, kidneys, eyes, and other organs. Penicillamine relieves symptoms by promoting copper excretion. Therapeutic effects may take several months to develop. Additional uses are *rheumatoid arthritis* and *cystinuria*. Beneficial effects in these disorders are not related to chelation of heavy metals.

Pharmacokinetics. Penicillamine is well absorbed following oral administration. Food greatly reduces the extent of absorption. Once absorbed, penicillamine is rapidly excreted in the urine.

Adverse Effects. With prolonged use, penicillamine can cause varied and serious toxicities. Deaths have occurred. The drug should be employed only with close medical supervision. Possible cutaneous reactions include urticaria, maculopapular and morbilliform rash, pemphigoid lesions, and pruritus. *Bone marrow suppression* can result in leukopenia, agranulocytosis, and aplastic anemia, all of which can be fatal. *Autoimmune and immune complex disorders* have been associated with penicillamine. Among these are dermatomyositis, polymyositis, lupus erythematosus, alveolitis, and myasthenia gravis. *Renal toxicity* may occur.

Contraindications. Penicillamine is contraindicated for patients who have experienced agranulocytosis or aplastic anemia when receiving penicillamine in the past. The drug is also contraindicated for patients with rheumatoid arthritis who are pregnant or have renal insufficiency.

Preparations, Dosage, and Administration. Penicillamine is supplied in 250-mg capsules. For Wilson's disease, the usual dosage is 750 to 1500 mg daily in divided doses. Doses should be administered 1 hour before meals and at bedtime. Dosage is adjusted on the basis of untoward effects and urinary copper content. Treatment is long term.

Succimer

Actions and Uses. Succimer [Chemet] binds avidly with lead, mercury, and arsenic. Binding is less avid with copper and zinc. Binding to iron, calcium, and magnesium is minimal; therefore, succimer presents no risk of depleting these essential minerals. Succimer is our most effective drug for lowering blood levels of lead in children, its only approved indication. However, although succimer can reduce lead levels, its benefits are limited to the prevention of seizures and death from acute encephalopathy. Treatment does not reduce or prevent the long-term neurologic sequelae of lead poisoning, which are irreversible.

[a]As of 2020, the FDA will no longer use Pregnancy Risk Categories. Please refer to Chapter 9 for more information.

Pharmacokinetics. Succimer is rapidly but variably absorbed following oral administration. The drug undergoes extensive metabolism. Metabolites and parent drug are eliminated slowly in the urine.

Adverse Effects. Adverse effects appear to be mild. About 10% of patients experience GI reactions (nausea, diarrhea, cramps). Other moderate reactions include nasal congestion, muscle pain, and rash. Succimer has caused temporary elevations in serum transaminases, indicating liver injury. Accordingly, serum transaminases should be measured before treatment and weekly thereafter. In addition, caution should be exercised in patients with liver disease. In mice, the drug is teratogenic and fetotoxic.

Preparations, Dosage, and Administration. Succimer is supplied in 100-mg capsules for oral use. For children over 1 year old, treatment consists of 10 mg/kg or 350 mg/m^2 every 8 hours for 5 days, and then every 12 hours for 14 more days. If needed, the entire course can be repeated after a minimum hiatus of 2 weeks.

Fomepizole

Actions and Uses

Fomepizole [Antizol] is used to treat poisoning by *ethylene glycol,* the principal component of antifreeze. Following ingestion, ethylene glycol undergoes gradual enzymatic conversion into glycolic acid, a toxic acidic metabolite. The result is profound metabolic acidosis, which leads to hyperventilation, coma, seizures, hypertension, pulmonary infiltrates, and renal failure. In the absence of treatment, a lethal dose (100 mL or more) will cause death by multiorgan failure in 24 to 36 hours. Fomepizole protects against injury by inhibiting *alcohol dehydrogenase,* an enzyme required for the conversion of ethylene glycol into its toxic form.

In addition to receiving fomepizole, patients need treatment for metabolic acidosis, acute renal failure, hypocalcemia, and adult respiratory distress syndrome. Treatment options include fluids, sodium bicarbonate, potassium, calcium, and oxygen. If poisoning is severe, patients may require hemodialysis.

Pharmacokinetics

After IV infusion, fomepizole distributes rapidly throughout total body water. A plasma level of 8.2 to 24.6 mg/L is sufficient to inhibit alcohol dehydrogenase. Fomepizole undergoes hepatic metabolism followed by excretion in the urine. The drug induces hepatic cytochrome P450 enzymes and can thereby accelerate its own metabolism. With repeated dosing, a significant increase in metabolism can be seen 30 to 40 hours after the initial dose.

Adverse Effects

Fomepizole is well tolerated. The only common adverse effects are headache, nausea, and dizziness. All other adverse effects (e.g., bradycardia, seizures) are uncommon.

Preparations, Dosage, and Administration

Fomepizole is available as a concentrated solution (1 gm/mL) in 1.5-mL vials. The required dose should be withdrawn from the vial and diluted in at least 100 mL of 0.9% sterile saline or 5% dextrose. Treatment consists of a loading dose (15 mg/kg) followed by four smaller doses (10 mg/kg) given every 12 hours, followed by doses of 15 mg/kg given every 12 hours until ethylene glycol levels drop below 20 mg/dL. All doses are infused IV over 30 minutes. If the patient is undergoing hemodialysis, fomepizole must be given every 4 hours, rather than every 12 hours.

Other Important Antidotes

Throughout this text we have discussed the toxic effects of various drugs. Where appropriate, we discussed specific antidotes used for treatment. For example, when discussing the adverse effects of opioids, we also discussed the use of naloxone for opioid overdoses. Similarly, when discussing heparin toxicity, we discussed the use of protamine sulfate as a treatment. The major specific antidotes discussed in other chapters are shown in Table 109.1.

POISON CONTROL CENTERS

The American Association of Poison Control Centers (AAPCC) defines a poison control center as an organization that serves

TABLE 109.1 ■ Specific Antidotes Discussed in Other Chapters

Antidote			
Generic Name	**Brand Name**	**Toxic/Overdosed Substance**	**Chapter**
Atropine		Muscarinic agonists, cholinesterase inhibitors	14
Physostigmine		Anticholinergic drugs	15
Neostigmine	Prostigmin	Nondepolarizing neuromuscular blockers	15
Pralidoxime	Protopam	Organophosphate cholinesterase inhibitors	15
Naloxone	Narcan	Opioids	28
Flumazenil	Romazicon	Benzodiazepines	34
Digoxin immune Fab	Digibind	Digoxin, digitoxin	48
Vitamin K		Warfarin	52
Protamine sulfate		Heparin	52
Idarucizumab	Praxbind	Dabigatran	52
Glucagon		Insulin-induced hypoglycemia	57
Acetylcysteine	Mucomyst	Acetaminophen	71
Leucovorin		Methotrexate and other folate antagonists	102
Pentetate calcium trisodium		Radioactive plutonium, americium, or curium	110
Pentetate zinc trisodium		Radioactive plutonium, americium, or curium	110
Prussian blue	Radiogardase	Radioactive cesium-137 and nonradioactive thallium	110
Potassium iodide	ThyroShield	Radioactive iodine	110

a designated geographic region and provides the following services:

- Poison information
- Telephone management advice and consultation about toxic exposures
- Hazard surveillance to achieve hazard elimination
- Professional and public education in poisoning prevention, diagnosis, and treatment

Poison control centers certified by the AAPCC are accessible 24 hours a day; have a specially trained, full-time staff (usually nurses, pharmacists, or both); are directed by a board-certified physician-toxicologist; and are associated with a medical center that has laboratory facilities and personnel needed for the diagnosis and management of poisoning. These centers are accessible by phone and can provide immediate instruction on the management of acute poisoning. In the majority of cases, the information supplied will permit successful treatment at home. By facilitating rapid treatment, poison control centers can decrease morbidity and mortality and can help reduce the cost of emergency care.

In 2002, the AAPCC established a **National Poison Hotline: 1-800-222-1222.** Dialing this number from any place in the United States will connect you with the *local* poison control center. (This is like dialing 911 from any place in the country to contact local emergency-service providers.)

KEY POINTS

- Management of poisoning has five basic components: supportive care, poison identification, prevention of further absorption, promotion of poison removal, and use of specific antidotes.
- The preferred method for reducing absorption of ingested poisons is adsorption onto activated charcoal, which should be given no later than 1 hour after poison ingestion.
- The removal of absorbed poisons can be accelerated by using drugs to enhance renal excretion and by nondrug methods, such as hemodialysis and exchange transfusion.
- For most poisons there is no specific antidote.
- Heavy metal poisoning can be treated with chelating agents.
- Poison control centers offer immediate, expert assistance over the phone.
- Dialing 1-800-222-1222 from any place in the United States will connect you with the nearest poison control center.

Please visit **http://evolve.elsevier.com/Lehne** for chapter-specific NCLEX® examination review questions.

CHAPTER

110 Potential Weapons of Biologic, Radiologic, and Chemical Terrorism

In 2001, the United States was hit by unprecedented terrorist attacks. On September 11, terrorists hijacked four commercial jets and succeeded in crashing two of them into the twin towers of the World Trade Center and one into the Pentagon. In October, anthrax spores were mailed to several locations, causing illness and death. These events generated great concern about our vulnerability to more such attacks and our ability to manage the consequences.

To improve our readiness for a terrorist attack, the federal government took several steps, including passage of the Public Health Security and Bioterrorism Preparedness and Response Act of 2002 (the Bioterrorism Act), the Project BioShield Act of 2004, and the Pandemic and All-Hazards Preparedness Act in 2007. All three incentives were designed to spur development and production of drugs and vaccines to protect U.S. residents from biologic agents and toxins, such as anthrax, smallpox, botulism, and plague. Although there have been some notable results, much more needs to be done.

Here we discuss some of the potential weapons of terrorism, focusing primarily on bacteria and viruses. Biotoxins, chemicals (nerve agents and mustard gas), and radiologic weapons are addressed as well. Discussion centers on clinical manifestations and treatment. Prevention is addressed where appropriate.

For more information on the weapons discussed here or for information on other potential weapons, please consult the resources in Table 110.1.

BACTERIA AND VIRUSES

Bacillus anthracis (Anthrax)

Bacillus anthracis is the bacterium that causes anthrax, a disease with three major forms: inhalational, cutaneous, and gastrointestinal. Our discussion focuses on inhalational and cutaneous anthrax. Gastrointestinal anthrax is not addressed because this form is unlikely to result from a terrorist attack.

Of the microbes that might be used by terrorists, *B. anthracis* is among the most dangerous. In October 2001, spores of *B. anthracis* were mailed to several locations in the United States, causing 22 confirmed or suspected cases of anthrax and 5 deaths. This experience served to heighten concerns regarding the feasibility of terrorist groups using aerosolized bioweapons to stage a large-scale attack.

Microbiology

Bacillus anthracis is an aerobic, gram-positive bacterium. Its name derives from *anthrakis,* the Greek word for coal (in recognition of the black skin lesions that characterize cutaneous infection). *Bacillus anthracis* can exist as spores, which are dormant, or as actively growing bacteria. Infection is acquired when the *spores* enter a host. Ports of entry are skin lesions and the respiratory and GI tracts. In the presence of nutrients (amino acids, nucleotides, glucose), which are abundant in the blood and tissues of the host, the spores germinate and transform into mature bacteria. The mature forms grow and divide rapidly until the nutrient supply is depleted, after which they cease dividing and produce more spores. The mature bacteria cannot survive long outside the host. In contrast, the spores can remain viable in the environment for decades. Anthrax is not transmitted person to person.

Clinical Manifestations

Inhalational Anthrax. Infection begins with deposition of anthrax spores in the alveolar space, followed by transport to regional lymph nodes, where germination occurs. Clinical latency can range from 2 days to 6 weeks. Injury results when mature bacilli release toxins, which cause hemorrhage, edema, and necrosis. Once the concentration of toxin has reached a critical level, antibiotics cannot prevent death, even if they kill all circulating bacilli.

Symptoms appear in two stages. Initial symptoms—fever, cough, malaise, and weakness—may be relatively mild. In the second stage, which develops 2 to 3 days later, there is a sudden increase in fever, along with severe respiratory distress, septicemia, hemorrhagic meningitis, and shock. Interestingly, although the infection originates in the lungs, true pneumonia rarely occurs. Even with treatment, the mortality rate can be high. Inhalational anthrax has a fatality rate of 80% or higher.

Cutaneous Anthrax. Symptoms begin 1 to 7 days after exposure to anthrax spores. Areas with cuts or abrasions are most vulnerable, but injury can develop at any site where spores land. The initial lesion is a small papule (solid raised area) or vesicle (fluid-filled raised area) associated with localized itching. Within 2 days, the lesion enlarges and evolves into a painless ulcer with a necrotic core. Seven to 10 days after symptom onset, a black eschar (scab-like structure) forms—but then dries, loosens, and sloughs off by day 12 to 14. In most patients, the lesions resolve without complications or scarring. However, if *systemic* infection develops, the outcome can be fatal. In the absence of antibiotic therapy, about 20% of people with cutaneous anthrax die. In contrast, death among treated patients is rare.

Treatment of Established Infection

The treatments discussed here reflect recommendations published by the Centers for Disease Control and Prevention (CDC).

TABLE 110.1 ▪ Resources for Information on Biologic, Radiologic, and Chemical Terrorism

- https://emergency.cdc.gov/bioterrorism/—Bioterrorism information from the Centers for Disease Control and Prevention
- www.fda.gov/Drugs/EmergencyPreparedness/BioterrorismandDrugPreparedness/default.htm—Bioterrorism information from the U.S. Food and Drug Administration
- www.upmc-biosecurity.org—Information on biologic weapons from the Center for Biosecurity, an independent, nonprofit organization associated with the University of Pittsburgh Medical Center

Inhalational Anthrax. Given the rapid course that inhalational anthrax follows, early therapy with antibiotics is essential. Any delay can reduce the chance of survival. Initial IV therapy is preferred to initial oral therapy. However, if there are mass casualties, IV therapy may be impossible, owing to limited supplies and personnel. Ideally, treatment should start with *IV ciprofloxacin* or *IV doxycycline.* Because the strain of *B. anthracis* may be resistant to these drugs, one or two other IV antibiotics should be included. When clinically appropriate, the patient can be switched to oral ciprofloxacin or doxycycline, without additional antibiotics. The duration of treatment—IV plus oral—is 60 days. Specific regimens for adults, children, and pregnant women are shown in Table 110.2 (for limited casualty settings) and Table 110.3 (for mass casualty settings).

Raxibacumab and obiltoxaximab are monoclonal antibodies, representing a different approach to treating inhalational anthrax. Unlike antibiotics, which kill anthrax bacteria, raxibacumab and obiltoxaximab neutralize deadly anthrax toxins. As a result, these drugs can decrease injury even after an infection has become established. Raxibacumab and obiltoxaximab are supplied directly to the CDC.

Anthrax immune globulin intravenous (AIGIV) [Anthracil] contains antibodies directed against anthrax. It is derived from the plasma of human donors previously vaccinated against anthrax. As with raxibacumab and obiltoxaximab, AIGIV acts against anthrax toxin and should be administered in conjunction with antibacterial medications.

Cutaneous Anthrax. Cutaneous anthrax is treated with oral antibiotics. The preferred drugs are *ciprofloxacin* and *doxycycline.* Dosages for adults, children, and pregnant women are the same as those given in Table 110.2 for follow-up oral therapy of inhalational anthrax. Duration of treatment is 60 days. It should be noted that treatment is unlikely to prevent cutaneous lesions, but *will* prevent systemic complications.

TABLE 110.2 ▪ Therapy of Inhalational Anthrax in the Limited Casualty Setting

Patient Group	Initial Intravenous Therapy	Follow-up Oral Therapy	Duration
Adults	Ciprofloxacin, 400 mg every 8 hr *or* Doxycycline, 100 mg every 12 hr *and* All patients should get 1 or 2 additional antibiotics. Options include rifampin, vancomycin, penicillin, ampicillin, imipenem, chloramphenicol, clindamycin, and clarithromycin. Do not use penicillin or ampicillin alone.	*When clinically appropriate, switch to oral antibiotics:* Ciprofloxacin, 500 mg twice daily *or* Doxycycline, 100 mg twice daily	60 days total (IV and PO combined)
Children	Ciprofloxacin, 10–15 mg/kg every 12 hr, but no more than 1 gm/day *or* Doxycycline (for young children): • >8 yr and >45 kg: 100 mg every 12 hr • >8 yr and ≤45 kg: 2.2 mg/kg every 12 hr • ≤8 yr: 2.2 mg/kg every 12 hr *and* As with adults, all patients should get 1 or 2 additional antibiotics.	*When clinically appropriate, switch to oral antibiotics:* Ciprofloxacin, 10–15 mg/kg every 12 hr, but no more than 1 gm/day *or* Doxycycline (for young children): • >8 yr and >45 kg: 100 mg every 12 hr • >8 yr and ≤45 kg: 2.2 mg/kg every 12 hr • ≤8 yr: 2.2 mg/kg every 12 hr	60 days total (IV and PO combined)
Pregnant	Same as nonpregnant adults	Same as nonpregnant adults	

TABLE 110.3 ■ Therapy of Inhalational Anthrax in the Mass Casualty Setting

Patient Group	Preferred Initial Oral Therapy	Alternative Oral Therapy (If Strain Is Proved Susceptible)	Duration
Adults	Ciprofloxacin, 500 mg every 12 hr	Doxycycline, 100 mg every 12 hr Amoxicillin, 500 mg every 8 hr	60 days
Children	Ciprofloxacin, 10–15 mg every 12 hr, but no more than 1 gm/day	*≥20 kg:* amoxicillin, 500 mg every 8 hr *<20 kg:* amoxicillin, 13.3 mg/kg every 8 hr	60 days
Pregnant	Ciprofloxacin, 500 mg every 12 hr	Amoxicillin, 500 mg every 8 hr	60 days

Pre-exposure Vaccination

Currently, only one anthrax vaccine—*BioThrax*—is licensed for use in the United States. BioThrax is an inactivated, cell-free preparation made from an avirulent strain of *B. anthracis.* The normal immunization schedule calls for three subQ injections given 2 weeks apart, followed by three more injections given at 6, 12, and 18 months. If IM injections are used, they are administered at 0, 1, and 6 months with additional booster doses at 12 and 18 months. Annual booster shots are recommended thereafter. The most common side effects are muscle and joint aches; headache; local redness, tenderness, or itching; fatigue; nausea; and chills and fever. Serious allergic reactions occur rarely (less than 1 in 100,000).

Who should receive anthrax vaccine? At this time, immunization is limited to people considered at risk. BioThrax is approved only for immunizing (1) people who handle animal products such as hides, hair, or bones that come from anthrax-endemic areas and (2) people at high risk of exposure to anthrax spores, including veterinarians, laboratory workers, and others whose occupation may involve handling potentially infected animals or other contaminated materials. In addition to these approved uses, BioThrax is being used to vaccinate military personnel. Because the risk of infection in most people is low, routine vaccination of the general population is neither approved nor recommended.

Postexposure Prophylaxis: Antibiotics Plus Vaccination

To prevent infection following exposure to aerosolized anthrax spores, the Centers for Disease Control and Prevention recommends treatment with an oral antibiotic plus anthrax vaccine. Antibiotic regimens are the same ones employed for treating inhalational anthrax in a mass casualty setting (see Table 110.3). Dosing should start immediately and continue for at least 60 days. Vaccination following anthrax exposure consists of three doses of BioThrax, given at 0, 2, and 4 weeks.

Francisella tularensis (Tularemia)

Tularemia, also known as "rabbit fever" and "deer fly fever," is a potentially fatal disease caused by *Francisella tularensis,* one of the most infectious bacteria known. Inoculation with as few as 10 microbes can cause disease. Infection can be acquired through the skin, mucous membranes, GI tract, or lungs. Terrorists trying to spread tularemia would most likely deliver the bacteria as an aerosol. Tularemia cannot be transmitted person to person.

Clinical Manifestations

Symptoms of tularemia develop in 3 to 5 days. Initially, patients present with an acute flu-like illness, characterized by fever (38°C to 40°C), headache, chills, rigors, body aches, sneezing, and sore throat. Pneumonia and pleuritis can develop in the ensuing days to weeks. In the absence of treatment, tularemia can progress to respiratory failure, shock, and death.

Treatment

Tularemia responds well to antibiotics. The treatment of choice is *IM streptomycin* (10 to 15 mg/kg twice a day for 10 days). The preferred alternative is *gentamicin* (5 mg/kg IM or IV once a day for 10 days). If there is a mass outbreak, oral therapy with doxycycline or ciprofloxacin is recommended. Individuals who have not yet developed symptoms may benefit from prophylactic use of oral doxycycline or ciprofloxacin.

Yersinia pestis (Pneumonic Plague)

Plague is a potentially fatal disease caused by *Yersinia pestis,* a gram-negative bacillus. The disease has two principal forms: *bubonic* (characterized by tender, enlarged, and inflamed lymph nodes) and *pneumonic* (characterized by inflammation of the lungs). Bubonic plague is acquired through the bite of a plague-infected flea and *cannot* be transmitted person to person. Rarely, an individual with bubonic plague develops secondary pneumonic plague, which *can* be transmitted person to person (by coughing). *Primary* pneumonic plague is acquired by inhaling aerosolized *Y. pestis.* The source of the aerosol could be a person with pneumonic plague, or it could be a biologic weapon. To a would-be bioterrorist, *Y. pestis* is attractive for several reasons: The microbe is readily available worldwide, culturing large quantities is relatively easy, the bacterium can be aerosolized for wide dissemination, pneumonic plague can be spread person to person, and the fatality rate is high.

Clinical Manifestations

Symptoms of primary pneumonic plague usually develop 2 to 4 days after inhaling aerosolized *Y. pestis.* Patients typically present with high fever, cough, dyspnea, and hemoptysis (expectoration of blood or blood-stained sputum). Gastrointestinal symptoms—nausea, vomiting, diarrhea, and abdominal pain—may also develop. In the absence of treatment, the infection rapidly progresses to respiratory failure and death.

Treatment

Antibiotics can be lifesaving—provided they are given early (before or shortly after symptom onset). Treatments of choice are (1) *streptomycin,* 15 mg/kg IM twice daily for 10 days, and (2) *gentamicin,* 5 mg/kg IM or IV once daily for 10 days. Preferred alternatives, all given IV, are doxycycline, ciprofloxacin, and chloramphenicol. In a mass casualty setting, which may preclude IV or IM administration, oral therapy with doxycycline (100 mg twice daily) or ciprofloxacin (500 mg twice daily) is recommended. There is no vaccine to protect against pneumonic plague.

Variola Virus (Smallpox)

Smallpox is a serious, contagious, life-threatening disease caused by the *variola virus,* a member of the genus *Orthopoxvirus.* The only natural reservoir for the virus is humans. We have no specific treatment for smallpox, but we *can* prevent the disease by vaccination, given either before exposure or within a few days after. Because smallpox is highly contagious and because the fatality rate is high (30%), the disease represents a grave threat as a weapon of terrorism.

Thanks to a global vaccination program, endemic smallpox has been eradicated. The last case in the United States occurred in 1949, and the last case on the planet occurred in Somalia in 1977. Because the threat of smallpox had been eliminated, routine vaccination was discontinued—in 1972 for Americans and by 1982 for the rest of the world.

Ironically, the successful elimination of smallpox has set the stage for its potential return as a weapon of terrorism. That is, if we hadn't eradicated natural smallpox, then vaccination would still be ongoing. As a result, the population would have immunity, making smallpox useless as a weapon.

Pathogenesis and Clinical Manifestations

Variola virus enters the body through mucous membranes of the respiratory tract, usually as a result of virus inhalation. Initial exposure is followed by an asymptomatic incubation period (usually 12 to 14 days), followed by the prodromal phase (2 to 4 days), manifesting as high fever, malaise, prostration, headache, and backache. Viral invasion of the oral mucosa and dermis then leads to characteristic eruptions. Small red spots develop in the mouth and on the tongue and then evolve into sores that break open, releasing large amounts of virus into the mouth and throat. Around this time, a bumpy skin rash develops, starting on the face and then quickly spreading over the entire body. Within 1 to 2 days, the bumps become vesicular (fluid filled), and then pustular (pus filled). About 8 or 9 days after rash onset, the pustules begin to form a crust and then a scab. By 3 weeks after the rash began, the scabs fall off, leaving a characteristic pitted scar.

About 30% of people with smallpox die, usually during the second week of illness. The most likely cause is toxemia associated with circulating immune complexes and soluble variola antigens.

Transmission

Natural smallpox is transmitted person to person. It is not transmitted by insects or animals. Transmission occurs primarily by touching an infected person or by inhaling aerosolized droplets expelled from the oropharynx. Smallpox can also be acquired by contact with contaminated clothing or bedding. The disease is somewhat contagious during the prodromal phase, but is most contagious from the onset of rash through scab formation. After all scabs fall off, infectivity is gone.

If used as a weapon, variola virus would most likely be disseminated as an aerosol. Because the virus is fragile, at least 90% of the amount released into the environment would become inactive within 24 hours.

Treatment

There is no proven treatment for smallpox. However, research with newer antiviral drugs is ongoing. Several agents show promise, including *cidofovir, adefovir,* and *ribavirin.* Topical *idoxuridine* may benefit patients with corneal lesions. Antibiotics should be used to treat secondary bacterial infections.

Smallpox Vaccine

Vaccination is the only way to prevent smallpox. In addition to conferring protection when given *before* viral exposure, the vaccine confers protection when given within a few days *after* exposure. For 30 years—between 1972 and 2002—vaccination in the United States had been limited to the few scientists and medical professionals who did research on smallpox and related viruses. However, owing to concerns about bioterrorism, the U.S. government has reinstituted vaccination. Mandatory vaccination of military personnel began in 2002. Voluntary vaccination of selected civilian groups began in 2003. At this time, smallpox vaccine is not available to the general public—nor is it recommended. However, in the event of a terrorist attack, prophylactic immunization will be offered.

Description. The vaccine in current use is a suspension of live *vaccinia virus,* a virus that belongs to the same family as variola virus, but does not cause smallpox. From 1931 to 2007, only one vaccine—*Dryvax*—was licensed for use in the United States. In 2007, the U.S. Food and Drug Administration (FDA) approved a new vaccine—*ACAM2000*—and withdrew the license for Dryvax. ACAM2000 is produced from a clone of the vaccinia strain used to make Dryvax.

An even newer vaccine, named *Imvamune,* is in Phase III clinical trials. The vaccine is made with *modified vaccinia virus Ankara* (MVA), a virus that is immunogenic but unable to replicate in humans. As a result, even though the vaccine contains live viruses, it is not dangerous for people who are immunocompromised. (In immunocompromised vaccinees, the viruses in ACAM2000 can proliferate and cause serious injury, so ACAM2000 is generally contraindicated for such people.) In animal models, MVA was considerably safer than Dryvax and nearly as effective. Although Imvamune is not yet licensed in the United States, the FDA has approved delivery of the drug to the Strategic National Stockpile. Imvamune is the first drug developed under Project BioShield.

Efficacy. Vaccination before exposure to variola virus prevents smallpox in about 95% of vaccinees. Vaccination within 3 days after exposure also confers significant protection, preventing symptoms entirely in some people and greatly reducing symptoms in others. Benefits of vaccination 4 to 7 days after exposure are uncertain.

Duration of Protection. Successful primary vaccination produces a high level of immunity for 5 to 10 years, with slowly decreasing immunity thereafter. However, it is not clear just when effective protection is lost. Data from a 2008 study indicate that titers of neutralizing antibodies in people vaccinated 13 to 88 years ago are comparable to those in people vaccinated recently, suggesting long-term persistence of specific immunity.

Administration. Smallpox vaccine is administered by a unique method known as *scarification,* which introduces the vaccine through multiple skin punctures. Administration is not by subQ, IM, or IV injection. The vaccine is given with a bifurcated (two-pronged) needle that is dipped into the vaccine solution. When removed from the solution, the needle retains a droplet of vaccine between the prongs. The administrator then pricks the skin several times (2 or 3 times for primary vaccination; 15 times for revaccination). The resulting punctures should be superficial, but still deep enough to allow a trace of blood to appear after 15 to 20 seconds. Vaccinations are made in the upper arm. To prevent spread of the vaccine, which contains live viruses, the site should be covered with sterile gauze or a semipermeable membrane.

Interpreting the Response. Successful vaccination is indicated when the following events take place. Within 3 to 4 days, a red, itchy bump appears. During the first week, the bump becomes a blister, fills with pus, and then starts to drain. During the second week, the blister begins to dry and develops a scab. In the third week, the scab falls off, leaving a small scar. Reactions to primary vaccination are stronger than reactions to revaccination.

Adverse Effects. The smallpox vaccine may carry considerable risk. Past experience suggests that if 1 million people were vaccinated, 1000 would experience a serious adverse effect, 14 to 52 would develop a life-threatening condition, and 1 or 2 would die. However, recent data suggest the risk is lower. Regardless of what the real level of risk from vaccination may be, there is no question that the risk of smallpox infection is far greater. Accordingly, anyone exposed to variola virus should be offered the vaccine.

Mild Effects. In addition to the local reactions that signal a successful immune response, vaccination can cause local inflammation, along with swelling and tenderness in regional lymph nodes. Transient symptoms typical of viral illness (fever, headache, muscle aches, fatigue) are also common.

If the vaccination site is not securely covered, vaccinia virus can be transferred to other areas—usually the face, eyelids, nose, mouth, or genitalia—as well as to other people. Transfer to the eyes can cause sight-threatening keratitis. However, most lesions heal spontaneously.

Moderate to Severe Effects. Serious reactions to smallpox vaccination include eczema vaccinatum, generalized vaccinia, progressive vaccinia, postvaccinial encephalitis, and fetal vaccinia. (The terms *vaccinatum* and *vaccinia* in the names of these disorders simply refer to the cause: vaccinia virus.)

Eczema vaccinatum occurs when infection with vaccinia virus is superimposed on a pre-existing skin condition, usually eczema or atopic dermatitis. As a rule, the disorder is mild and self-limiting. However, in some people it can be life threatening.

Generalized vaccinia is a widespread vesicular rash that resembles smallpox. The cause is transient viremia with localization in the skin. Although the condition is generally self-limiting, it can be severe in the immunocompromised patient.

Progressive vaccinia, also called *vaccinia necrosum,* is a rare but often fatal condition that develops almost exclusively in patients who are immunodeficient. The condition is characterized by progressive necrosis at the inoculation site, often associated with metastatic vaccinial lesions at distant sites (skin, bones, and viscera).

Postvaccinial encephalitis (inflammation of the brain) is rare but dangerous. This complication occurs roughly 2 to 12 times per million vaccinations. The fatality rate is 15% to 25%, and 25% of survivors suffer brain damage.

Fetal vaccinia is a very rare but serious infection of the fetus, manifested by skin lesions and internal organ involvement. The condition can lead to premature birth or fetal or neonatal death. Fetal vaccinia can result from exposure to vaccinia virus at any stage of pregnancy. Accordingly, women who are pregnant should not get the vaccine. Women who were recently vaccinated should wait at least 4 weeks before attempting to become pregnant.

Possible Cardiac Effects. Some vaccinees have developed cardiac problems—specifically, myocarditis (inflammation of the heart muscle), pericarditis (inflammation of the pericardium), myocardial infarction (heart attack), and angina pectoris (ischemic cardiac pain). However, a definite link between vaccination and these disorders has not been established. Until more is known, routine vaccination should be withheld from people with established heart disease (heart failure, angina, myocardial infarction, cardiomyopathy) and from those with three or more cardiovascular risk factors (Table 110.4).

Management of Adverse Effects. Two agents—*vaccinia immune globulin* (VIG) and *cidofovir* —can be given to treat severe reactions to smallpox vaccine. However, neither preparation is approved for this use.

VIG is a solution that contains immunoglobulins from people vaccinated with vaccinia virus and hence should contain antibodies directed against the virus. However, therapeutic

TABLE 110.4 ■ Medical Conditions and Other Factors That Contraindicate Routine Smallpox Vaccination[a]

- History of eczema or atopic dermatitis
- Active skin conditions, including burns, herpes, severe acne, psoriasis, chickenpox, or shingles (delay vaccination until lesions heal)
- Immunodeficiency (caused by HIV infection, primary immunodeficiency disorder, or use of immunosuppressive drugs, including glucocorticoids, many anticancer drugs, and drugs used to prevent transplant rejection)[b]
- Pregnancy (or plans to become pregnant within 1 month of vaccination)
- Breast-feeding
- Allergy to the smallpox vaccine or any of its components (polymyxin B, streptomycin, chlortetracycline, neomycin)
- Age younger than 18 years (especially younger than 1 year) or older than 65 years
- Moderate or severe short-term illness (delay vaccination until illness resolves)
- Inflammatory eye disease with ongoing use of steroid eye drops
- Heart conditions, including heart failure, angina, myocardial infarction, and cardiomyopathy
- Three or more cardiovascular risk factors: hypertension, high cholesterol, diabetes, cigarette use, first-degree relative with early heart disease (i.e., before age 50 years)

[a]*Routine* vaccination should be avoided in people with these conditions. However, vaccination *is* indicated following exposure to the smallpox virus.

[b]Unlike ACAM2000, the MVA-based vaccine—Imvamune—should be safe for immunocompromised patients.

effects have not been established in controlled trials. There is some evidence that VIG can benefit those with eczema vaccinatum or generalized vaccinia, and possibly those with progressive vaccinia. In contrast, the preparation is of no help to those with postvaccinial encephalitis and may actually *increase* corneal damage in those with vaccinial keratitis. VIGIV is administered intravenously. The dosage is 6000 units/kg. A dose of 9000 units/kg may be repeated if needed to a maximum dose of 24,000 units/kg. VIG is available only from the CDC.

Cidofovir is an antiviral drug with one approved indication: cytomegalovirus retinitis in patients with AIDS. However, in animal studies, the drug also showed good activity against vaccinia virus. Accordingly, some authorities recommend it for patients with severe vaccination complications, including progressive vaccinia, generalized vaccinia, and eczema vaccinatum. The pharmacology of cidofovir is discussed in Chapter 93.

Who Should NOT Be Vaccinated? Certain conditions (e.g., eczema, atopic dermatitis, immunodeficiency, pregnancy) increase the risk of a serious reaction to smallpox vaccine. Accordingly, people who have these conditions, or who live with someone who does, should not be vaccinated—unless, of course, they have been exposed to the smallpox virus, in which case the risk of infection would far outweigh the risk of the vaccine. Table 110.4 gives a full list of medical conditions and other factors that contraindicate routine vaccination.

BIOTOXINS

Botulinum Toxin

Botulinum toxin, produced by *Clostridium botulinum,* is the most potent poison known. Just 1 gram, if evenly dispersed and inhaled, could kill more than 1 million people. For use as a weapon of terrorism, the toxin could be delivered as an aerosol or simply put into food. And yes, this is the same agent used on wrinkles (see Chapter 105).

Mechanism of Action

Botulinum toxin works by blocking release of acetylcholine from cholinergic neurons. The toxin is taken up by cholinergic nerve terminals, where it then inactivates SNAP-25, a protein critical to the function of acetylcholine-containing vesicles. In the absence of SNAP-25, the vesicles are unable to fuse with the nerve-terminal membrane, and hence cannot release their acetylcholine into the synaptic space. Restoration of neuronal function requires sprouting of new terminals, a process that can take several months. Botulinum toxin blocks transmission at neuromuscular junctions and at cholinergic synapses of the autonomic nervous system.

Clinical Manifestations

Poisoning is characterized by symmetric, descending flaccid paralysis, beginning 12 to 72 hours after exposure and persisting for weeks to months. Classic symptoms are double vision, blurred vision, drooping eyelids, slurred speech, dry mouth, difficulty swallowing, and muscle weakness that descends through the body, starting with the shoulders and progressing to the upper arms, lower arms, thighs, calves, and feet. Death results from paralysis of the muscles of respiration.

Treatment

Treatment consists of prolonged supportive care and immediate infusion of botulinum antitoxin and/or botulism immune globulin. Supportive care, which may be needed for several months, includes fluid and nutritional therapy plus mechanical assistance of ventilation. Botulinum antitoxin, produced in horses, should be given as soon as botulism is diagnosed. The antiserum, which contains neutralizing antibodies, can minimize further nerve damage, but cannot reverse damage that has already set in. In the United States, botulinum antitoxin is available only through state and local health departments, which get their supply from the CDC. The recommended dosage is 10 mL (the contents of 1 vial) diluted 1 : 10 in 0.9% saline and administered by slow IV infusion. The FDA also approved a new immunoglobulin formulation, available as *BabyBIG,* for treating children under 1 year old.

Ricin

Ricin is a toxin present in castor beans, which are produced by *Ricinus communis,* the castor bean plant. The toxin is manufactured by extraction from the "mash" left behind when castor beans are processed to make castor oil. When purified, ricin can be formulated as a powder, pellet, or mist or dissolved in water or a weak acid.

Mechanism of Action

Ricin promotes injury by disrupting protein production. Ricin is an enzyme that catalyzes the inactivation of ribosomes, which are required for protein synthesis. Inhibition of protein synthesis leads to cell death and related tissue injury.

Clinical Manifestations

Symptoms of poisoning depend on the route of administration:

- *Inhalation*—Within a few hours of inhaling ricin mist or powder, the victim can experience coughing, tightness in the chest, difficulty breathing, nausea, and muscle ache. A few hours later, the airway may become severely inflamed and edematous, making breathing extremely difficult. Cyanosis and death can follow.
- *Ingestion*—Swallowing a significant dose can cause gastric and intestinal hemorrhage, associated with vomiting and bloody diarrhea. In time, the liver, spleen, and kidneys may fail. Death can occur within 10 to 12 days of ingestion.
- *Injection*—Injection of ricin can lead to severe symptoms and death. However, this route is obviously impractical for terrorism.

Treatment

Management of poisoning is purely supportive. We have no antidote for ricin. A vaccine to protect against ricin is in development.

CHEMICAL WEAPONS

Nerve Agents

Nerve agents are "irreversible" organophosphate cholinesterase inhibitors. By inhibiting cholinesterase, these drugs increase the concentration of acetylcholine at neuromuscular junctions, cholinergic synapses in the central nervous system (CNS), and all autonomic synapses that employ acetylcholine as a transmitter. Toxic doses produce a state of cholinergic crisis, characterized by excessive muscarinic stimulation and depolarizing neuromuscular blockade. Treatment consists of (1) mechanical ventilation using oxygen, (2) giving *atropine* to reduce muscarinic stimulation, (3) giving *pralidoxime* to reverse inhibition of cholinesterase (primarily at neuromuscular junctions), and (4) giving *diazepam* to suppress convulsions. Specific nerve agents that might be used for a terrorist attack include *soman, tabun, sarin,* and *cyclosarin.* All are volatile at room temperature. However, nerve agent vapors are denser than air, and hence tend to accumulate in low-lying areas. The toxic effects of nerve agents and the use of pralidoxime for treatment are discussed in Chapter 15.

Sulfur Mustard (Mustard Gas)

Properties

Sulfur mustard (bis[2-chloroethyl]sulfide), also known as mustard gas, is an alkylating agent and vesicant (chemical blistering agent). However, the precise relationship between alkylation of DNA (and other cellular components) and production of blisters is unclear. Physically, sulfur mustard is a lipophilic, oily liquid that can be vaporized at high temperatures. For use as a weapon of terrorism, sulfur mustard could be vaporized into the air or released into the water supply. Injuries from sulfur mustard can be severe, but the fatality rate is low. When used as a weapon in World War I, sulfur mustard killed less than 5% of its victims.

Clinical Manifestations

Symptoms of toxicity depend on the dose, the tissue involved, and the duration of exposure. As a rule, symptoms are delayed, usually taking 2 to 24 hours to develop. Effects on specific tissues are as follows:

- *Skin*—Dermal contact causes pain, redness, swelling, and blisters (small to very large). Symptoms appear within 4 to 48 hours, depending on the dose. Areas where the skin is warm, moist, and thin are most vulnerable.
- *Eyes*—The eyes are exquisitely sensitive to sulfur mustard. Moderate exposure can produce irritation, pain, swelling, and tearing in 3 to 12 hours. Severe exposure can cause corneal burns, necrosis, severe pain, and blindness, which may last up to 10 days.
- *Respiratory tract*—Symptoms appear 2 to 24 hours after inhaling sulfur mustard. Mild exposure can cause runny nose, sneezing, hoarseness, sinus pain, and a dry, barking cough. Severe exposure can cause hemorrhage and necrosis of lung tissue, evidenced by coughing up blood.
- *GI tract*—Ingestion can cause nausea, vomiting, diarrhea, and abdominal pain. Symptoms typically develop within a few hours and resolve within 24 hours.
- *Bone marrow*—Very high doses cause bone marrow suppression, resulting in neutropenia and thrombocytopenia.

Treatment

Management centers on rapid decontamination, supportive care, and drug therapy. People exposed to sulfur mustard should undress immediately and wash 3 times with soap and water. Those with significant airway damage may need intubation. Severe skin burns are treated by irrigation, débridement, and application of topical antibiotics; burn-related pain can be controlled with an opioid analgesic. Exposed eyes should be irrigated; other treatments include use of cycloplegics/mydriatics, application of topical antibiotics, and application of petroleum jelly to prevent burned lids from sticking. Granulocyte colony-stimulating factor can be used to stimulate neutrophil production by bone marrow.

RADIOLOGIC WEAPONS

Weapon Types

Nuclear Bombs

Nuclear bombs present an *immediate* threat from the blast itself and a *delayed* threat from radioactive fallout. Immediate harm is produced in four ways:

- The explosion and its shock wave damage buildings, people, and everything else they reach.
- Intense heat causes injury directly and by igniting fires.
- Intense light damages eyesight.
- Ionizing radiation causes acute radiation syndromes and radiation sickness, characterized by nausea, vomiting, diarrhea, fatigue, dehydration, inflammation, skin burns, hair loss, and ulceration of the mouth, esophagus, and GI tract. Symptoms develop over days to weeks. For those who survive, radiation exposure increases the risk of cancer.

Radioactive fallout, mainly *iodine-131,* poses a delayed risk of thyroid cancer. A nuclear explosion creates a radioactive cloud that can spread fallout over a large area. Contamination of humans can result from inhaling fallout, touching contaminated objects, or ingesting contaminated water and food. Once in the body, iodine-131 becomes concentrated in the thyroid gland, where it can cause thyroid cancer. The risk of cancer can be reduced by ingesting potassium iodide, which blocks uptake of radioactive iodine by the thyroid (see *Drugs for Radiation Emergencies,* later).

Attacks on Nuclear Power Plants

Terrorists could attack a nuclear power plant, either with a bomb or by using sabotage to cause meltdown of the radioactive core. In either case, a large amount of radiation could be released. Please note, however, that an attack would *not* cause a nuclear explosion. People in the immediate area could suffer severe radiation exposure, resulting in acute radiation syndrome or radiation sickness. As in a nuclear blast, release of iodine-131 could pose a risk of thyroid cancer.

Dirty Bombs (Radiologic Dispersion Devices)

A dirty bomb is a device that uses a conventional explosive (e.g., dynamite) to disperse radioactive material that has been formulated as a powder or tiny pellets. Resultant radioactive contamination could be external or internal (owing to inhalation, ingestion, or absorption through a wound). However, it is important to appreciate that the primary danger from a dirty bomb is the blast itself, not the radiation. Why? Because the sources of radiation likely to be used are not very dangerous and because dispersal of radiation would be limited to a relatively small area. The risk of cancer is very low. Persons exposed to a dirty bomb blast should remove their clothes as soon as possible and then decontaminate their skin by showering. A dirty bomb will not release iodine-131, and hence taking potassium iodide would be of no benefit.

Drugs for Radiation Emergencies

Potassium Iodide

Potassium iodide (KI) is used to block uptake of radioactive iodine by the thyroid gland and thereby protect the thyroid from radiation damage. Each dose protects for about 24 hours. However, dosage timing is critical. Protection is nearly 100% when KI starts within 12 hours *before* exposure. When dosing starts *after* exposure, the ability to protect falls off rapidly: down to 80% after 2 hours, 40% after 8 hours, and 7% after 24 hours. Daily dosages recommended by the CDC are as follows:

- *Age up to 1 month:* 16 mg
- *Age 1 month to 3 years:* 32 mg
- *Age 3 to 18 years:* 65 mg
- *Age 18 years and older:* 130 mg
- *Females who are breast-feeding, regardless of age:* 130 mg

In most cases, the environment will be clear of radioactive iodine quickly, so a single dose is usually sufficient. If contamination persists, then dosing should be repeated every 24 hours until radioactive iodine levels decline. However, repeat dosing with KI must be *avoided* by newborn infants and by women who are pregnant or breast-feeding, and hence these people should be evacuated until the threat is gone.

Potassium iodide is available in three oral formulations: 65-mg tablets sold as *ThyroSafe,* 130-mg tablets sold as *Iosat,* and an oral solution (65 mg/mL) sold as *ThyroShield.* No prescription is needed.

Pentetate Zinc Trisodium and Pentetate Calcium Trisodium

Pentetate zinc trisodium (Zn-DTPA) and pentetate calcium trisodium (Ca-DTPA) are used to treat people who have internal contamination with plutonium, americium, or curium. Benefits derive from accelerating removal of these radioactive isotopes from the body. Both drugs form stable complexes, known as chelates, with plutonium, americium, and curium (and other metals too), and the chelates are then excreted in the urine. The drugs do not bind strongly with radioactive iodine, uranium, or neptunium, and hence cannot be used to remove these isotopes. To monitor treatment, radioactivity in the blood, urine, and feces should be measured at baseline and weekly thereafter.

Pentetate zinc and pentetate calcium are usually administered IV, but may also be inhaled (if exposure is limited to the lungs). Absorption from the GI tract is very low, and hence oral therapy cannot be used. Once in the blood, both drugs distribute rapidly throughout extracellular fluid, but they do not penetrate cells. Metabolism is minimal. Both drugs undergo glomerular filtration followed by excretion in the urine. In patients with normal renal function, clearance occurs within a few hours after dosing. However, in patients with renal impairment, clearance is much slower. Nonetheless, dosage is not reduced for these people. Rather, high-efficiency, high-flux dialysis is employed to promote drug removal.

Therapy is most effective when initiated within 24 hours of radiation exposure. As time passes, the radiocontaminants become sequestered in liver and bone, making them harder to remove. Nonetheless, since delayed treatment is better than no treatment at all, dosing should begin as soon as the drugs are available. For the first 24 hours after exposure, Ca-DTPA is more effective than Zn-DTPA, and hence Ca-DTPA should be used initially. After 24 hours, both drugs are equally effective.

Dosing is done once a day—usually by slow IV push or IV infusion—and may continue for months. The exact duration depends on the degree of radioactive contamination and drug efficacy. For adults and adolescents, the recommended daily IV dose is 1 gm. For children under 12 years old, the daily IV dose is 14 mg/kg (but no more than 1 gm). To reduce the concentration of radioactive chelate in the urine, and thereby reduce the risk of injury to the bladder, patients should drink lots of fluid and void often.

Because Zn-DTPA and Ca-DTPA chelate metals, prolonged treatment can lead to trace-metal depletion. Both drugs can reduce body stores of manganese and magnesium, and Ca-DTPA can also reduce stores of zinc. Serum levels of trace metals should be monitored and supplements provided if the levels are low.

Prussian Blue

Prussian blue [Radiogardase], also known as *ferric hexacyanoferrate,* is used to hasten excretion of radioactive cesium and radioactive and nonradioactive thallium. Prussian blue is an insoluble, nonabsorbable compound, taken orally, that binds tightly with cesium and thallium in the intestine. In the absence of Prussian blue, both isotopes undergo extensive enterohepatic recirculation. That is, they undergo absorption into the blood, followed by excretion in the bile, followed by reabsorption, and so forth—a cycle that extends their stay in the body. However, when bound with Prussian blue, cesium and thallium cannot be reabsorbed, and hence must stay in the intestine for excretion. Food may accelerate the elimination because food increases production of bile, and hence may increase the rate at which cesium and thallium are presented to Prussian blue in the intestine.

Prussian blue can cause constipation, which is a concern for two reasons. First, constipation can delay excretion of radioactive contaminants. Second, it can increase the dose of radiation absorbed by the GI mucosa. If constipation occurs, it can be treated with a fiber-based laxative, a high-fiber diet, or both. Prussian blue should be used with caution in patients with decreased GI motility.

Prussian blue can bind with potassium and other electrolytes. Some patients have developed hypokalemia. To reduce risk, serum electrolytes should be monitored closely. Exercise caution in patients with cardiac dysrhythmias (which are sensitive to hypokalemia) or pre-existing electrolyte imbalance.

Prussian blue [Radiogardase], in the form of a blue powder, is supplied in 500-mg gelatin capsules. Dosing is done 3 times a day. For adults and adolescents, each dose is 3 gm. For children 2 to 12 years old, each dose is 1 gm. If needed, the capsules may be opened and the powder mixed with bland foods or liquids. However, be aware that opening the capsules may result in blue discoloration of the mouth and teeth. Whether the capsules are swallowed intact or opened, Prussian blue will turn stools blue; patients should be forewarned.

To monitor treatment, radioactivity in urine and stool samples should be measured at baseline and periodically thereafter. Whole-body radioactivity should be measured as appropriate.

KEY POINTS

- Anthrax is a potentially fatal disease caused by *Bacillus anthracis,* a bacterium that produces spores that can remain viable in the environment for decades.
- Anthrax infection is acquired when spores enter the body, typically through the skin or through mucous membranes of the respiratory tract.
- *Inhalational* anthrax is characterized by severe respiratory distress, septicemia, hemorrhagic meningitis, and shock. About 45% of victims die, even when treated.
- Lesions of *cutaneous* anthrax are characterized by a black eschar that eventually dries, loosens, and sloughs off. Most cases resolve without complications or scarring.
- For initial therapy of inhalational anthrax, treatments of choice are IV ciprofloxacin and IV doxycycline, combined with one or two additional IV antibiotics.
- Drugs of choice for cutaneous anthrax are oral ciprofloxacin and oral doxycycline.
- Anthrax vaccine is available for military personnel and selected others, but not yet for the general population.
- Tularemia is a potentially fatal disease caused by *Francisella tularensis,* one of the most infectious bacteria known. It can be acquired through bacterial invasion of the skin, mucous membranes, GI tract, or lungs and is characterized by pneumonia and pleuritis that can progress to respiratory failure, shock, and death.
- Tularemia responds well to antibiotics. The treatment of choice is IM streptomycin.
- Pneumonic plague is a potentially fatal disease acquired by inhaling aerosolized *Y. pestis* and can be transmitted person to person. It is characterized by high fever, cough, dyspnea, and hemoptysis. Without treatment, the infection rapidly progresses to respiratory failure and death.
- Treatments of choice for pneumonic plague are streptomycin (IM) and gentamicin (IM or IV).
- Smallpox is a contagious, potentially fatal disease caused by variola virus, whose only reservoir is humans. Worldwide vaccination has eliminated naturally occurring smallpox.
- Variola virus enters the body through mucous membranes of the respiratory tract.
- Smallpox is characterized by (1) eruptions on the mouth and tongue that release virus into the oropharynx and (2) pustules on the skin that release the virus on the body surface.
- Natural smallpox is transmitted person to person, primarily by touching an infected individual or by inhaling aerosolized droplets expelled from the oropharynx.
- There is no proven treatment for smallpox.
- The smallpox vaccine in current use, named ACAM2000, consists of live vaccinia virus. The vaccine confers protection when given before exposure to variola virus and when given within a few days after exposure.
- Successful primary vaccination with smallpox vaccine produces high-level immunity for at least 5 to 10 years. Significant immunity may persist for decades.
- Smallpox vaccination is not without risk: Past experience suggests that if 1 million people were vaccinated, 1000 would experience a serious adverse effect, 14 to 52 would develop a life-threatening condition, and 1 or 2 would die.
- Although smallpox vaccination carries risk, the risk of smallpox itself is far greater. Accordingly, anyone exposed to variola virus should be offered the vaccine.
- Routine smallpox vaccination is contraindicated by a number of conditions, including eczema, atopic dermatitis, immunodeficiency, pregnancy, and heart disease.
- Botulinum toxin, produced by *Clostridium botulinum,* is the most potent poison known. It acts on cholinergic nerve terminals to cause prolonged blockade of acetylcholine release.
- Poisoning with botulinum toxin is characterized by symmetric, descending flaccid paralysis, coupled with disturbed vision, drooping eyelids, slurred speech, dry mouth, and difficulty swallowing. Death results from paralysis of the muscles of respiration.
- Treatment of botulinum toxin poisoning consists of immediate infusion of botulinum antitoxin or immunoglobulin plus prolonged supportive care. Botulinum antitoxin can minimize further nerve damage but cannot reverse damage that has already occurred.
- Ricin is a toxin present in castor beans (which are used to make castor oil). It causes injury by inhibiting protein synthesis.
- When ricin is *inhaled,* it causes inflammation and edema of the airway, thereby making breathing extremely difficult. Cyanosis and death can follow.
- When ricin is *ingested,* it causes gastric and intestinal hemorrhage, associated with vomiting and bloody diarrhea. In time, the liver, spleen, and kidneys may fail.
- Management of ricin poisoning is purely supportive. There is no antidote.
- Nerve agents cause "irreversible" inhibition of cholinesterase and thereby increase the concentration of acetylcholine at neuromuscular junctions, cholinergic synapses in the CNS, and all autonomic synapses that employ acetylcholine as a transmitter.

Continued

- Nerve agents produce a state of cholinergic crisis, characterized by excessive muscarinic stimulation and depolarizing neuromuscular blockade.
- Treatment of nerve agent poisoning consists of mechanical ventilation using oxygen and the administration of atropine (to reduce muscarinic stimulation), pralidoxime (to reverse inhibition of cholinesterase), and diazepam (to suppress convulsions).
- Sulfur mustard (mustard gas) is an alkylating agent and vesicant that can injure any tissue that it reaches. Symptoms of sulfur mustard toxicity include large skin blisters, corneal burns, hemorrhage and necrosis of lung tissue, GI disturbances, and neutropenia and thrombocytopenia (secondary to bone marrow suppression).
- Management of sulfur mustard poisoning consists of rapid decontamination, supportive care, and drug therapy.
- A nuclear bomb presents an immediate threat from the blast itself (including acute radiation sickness) and a delayed threat from radioactive fallout.
- Iodine-131 in fallout poses a risk of thyroid cancer. The risk of thyroid cancer can be reduced by ingesting potassium iodide, which blocks uptake of iodine-131 by the thyroid.
- A dirty bomb is a device that uses a conventional explosive, such as dynamite, to disperse radioactive material. The primary danger from a dirty bomb is the blast itself, not the radiation.
- Three compounds—pentetate zinc trisodium, pentetate calcium trisodium, and Prussian blue—can hasten excretion of certain radioactive isotopes following internal contamination.

Please visit **http://evolve.elsevier.com/Lehne** for chapter-specific NCLEX® examination review questions.

Appendix A

Canadian Drug Information*

COURTNEY QUIRING, BSP, BCGP

CANADIAN DRUG LEGISLATION

Two acts form the basis of the drug laws in Canada: the Food and Drugs Act and the Controlled Drugs and Substance Act. The Health Products and Food Branch within Health Canada is responsible for ensuring that health products and foods approved for sale to Canadians are safe and of high quality. The Therapeutic Products Directorate (TPD) is responsible for pharmaceutical drugs and medical devices. The Biologics & Genetic Therapies Directorate regulates biologic drugs (drugs derived from living sources) and radiopharmaceuticals. Examples of biologic products are insulin analogs, blood products, and vaccines. The Natural and Non-prescription Health Products Directorate is the regulating authority for natural health products for sale in Canada. Natural Health Products (NHPs) are a class of health products which include vitamin and mineral supplements, herbal preparations, traditional and homeopathic medicines, probiotics, and enzymes.

The Food and Drug Act (1927), accompanied by the Food and Drug Regulations (1953, 1954, 1979), reviews the safety and efficacy of drugs before they are marketed, and the legislation determines whether the medicine is classified as prescription or nonprescription status. The Act controls the requirements for good manufacturing practices, labeling, distribution, and sale, including advertising of the drug. They also prescribe the standards of composition, strength, potency, purity, and quality of drugs in Canada.

Prescription Drugs (Schedule F)

All drugs that require a prescription, except for narcotics and controlled substances, are listed in Schedule F of the Food and Drug Regulations. Prescriptions for Schedule F medications may be written, including facsimiles and electronic prescriptions (depending on the province), or transmitted verbally (i.e., telephone order directly to the pharmacist) by a duly qualified medical practitioner, dentist, veterinarian, or other healthcare professional authorized to issue prescriptions. The symbol Pr must appear on all manufacturing labels. Individual provinces can legislate more restrictive control and require a prescription for a medication classified by the TPD as a nonprescription drug (e.g., digoxin). Provinces cannot legislate less restrictive control on any drug.

The Controlled Drugs and Substances Act (1997) establishes the requirements for the control and sale of narcotics, controlled drugs, and substances of abuse in Canada. The Controlled Drugs and Substances Act lists eight schedules of controlled substances. Assignment to a schedule is based on the potential for abuse and the ease with which illicit substances can be manufactured in illegal laboratories. The degree of control, the conditions of record keeping, and other regulations depend on the specific schedule. For example, Schedule I, which includes the narcotic agents, requires written orders only, and no repeat prescriptions are allowed. Some provinces require prescriptions for certain narcotics, such as morphine, to be written on a triplicate prescription form with one copy to be sent to the practitioner's regulatory body. The symbol Ⓒ must appear on the labels of controlled products, while the letter N is printed on the label of all the narcotic agents. Schedules I through VIII are defined below. Benzodiazepines are classified as Targeted Substances, and the symbol TC must appear on all the labels.

- Schedule I: Opium poppy and its derivatives (e.g., morphine, heroin); methadone; coca and its derivatives (e.g., cocaine)
- Schedule II: Cannabis and its derivatives (e.g., marijuana, hashish)
- Schedule III: Amphetamines, methylphenidate, lysergic acid diethylamide (LSD), methaqualone, psilocybin, mescaline
- Schedule IV: Sedative-hypnotic agents (e.g., barbiturates, benzodiazepines); anabolic steroids
- Schedule V: Propylhexedrine and any salt thereof
- Schedule VI: Compounds that can serve as precursors for manufacturing controlled substances
  - *Part 1: Class A Precursors.* Acetic anhydride, N-acetylanthranilic acid, anthranilic acid, ephedrine, ergometrine, ergotamine, isosafrole, lysergic acid, 3,4-methylenedioxyphenyl-2-propanone, norephedrine, 1-phenyl-2-propanone, phenylacetic acid, piperidine, piperonal, potassium permanganate, pseudoephedrine, safrole, gamma-butyrolactone, 1,4-butanediol, red and white phosphorus, hypophosphorous acid, hydriodic acid
  - *Part 2: Class B Precursors.* Acetone, ethyl ether, hydrochloric acid, methyl ethyl ketone, sulfuric acid, toluene
  - *Part 3:* Any preparation or mixture that contains a precursor set out in Part 1 or in Part 2
- Schedule VII: Cannabis resin 3 kg; Cannabis (marijuana) 3 kg
- Schedule VIII: Cannabis resin 1 g; Cannabis (marijuana) 30 g

The Controlled Drugs and Substance Act also provides for the nonprescription sale of certain codeine preparations. The content must not exceed the equivalent of 8 mg codeine phosphate per solid dosage unit or 20 mg/30 mL of a liquid, and the preparation must also contain two additional non-narcotic medicinal ingredients (usually acetylsalicylic acid or acetaminophen and caffeine). These preparations may not be advertised or displayed and may be sold only by pharmacists. Some provinces choose to restrict the amount that can be sold at any

*From Rosenthal LD, Burchum JR: *Lehne's pharmacotherapeutics for advanced practice providers*, St Louis, 2018, Elsevier.

given time. The Royal Canadian Mounted Police (RCMP) is responsible for enforcing the Controlled Drugs and Substances Act and related sections of the *Criminal Code*.

Nonprescription Medications—National Drug Schedules

As previously mentioned, individual provinces have enacted their own legislation controlling the sale of both prescription and nonprescription products. As a result, the National Association of Pharmacy Regulatory Authorities (NAPRA) endorsed a proposal for a national drug scheduling model. This model attempts to align the provincial drug schedules so that the conditions for the sale of drugs will be consistent across the country. The harmonized model includes all classes of medications. Narcotics, controlled substances, and prescription medications are listed in Schedule I, while nonprescription medications are assigned to one of the three categories described below. There is general support among the provincial regulatory bodies for the National Drug Schedules, although there are some differences from province to province of the actual list of drugs in each schedule. For a complete drug list proposed by NAPRA, visit their web site at www.napra.ca:

- **Schedule I** drugs require a prescription for sale and are provided to the public by the pharmacist following the diagnosis and professional intervention of a practitioner. The sale is controlled in a regulated environment as defined by provincial pharmacy regulation.
- **Schedule II** drugs, while less strictly regulated, do require professional intervention from the pharmacist at the point of sale and possibly referral to a practitioner. While a prescription is not required, the drugs are available only from the pharmacist and must be retained within an area of the pharmacy where there is no public access and no opportunity for patient self-selection.
- **Schedule III** drugs may present risks to certain populations in self-selection. Although available without a prescription, these drugs are to be sold from the self-selection area of the pharmacy which is operated under the direct supervision of the pharmacist, subject to any local professional discretionary requirements which may increase the degree of control. Such an environment is accessible to the patient and clearly identified as the "professional services area" of the pharmacy. The pharmacist is available, accessible, and approachable to assist the patient in making an appropriate self-medication selection.
- **Unscheduled** drugs can be sold without professional supervision. Adequate information is available for the patient to make a safe and effective choice and labeling is deemed sufficient to ensure the appropriate use of the drug. These drugs are not included in Schedules I, II, or III and may be sold from any retail outlet.

New Drug Development in Canada

The process for approving a new drug in Canada is very similar, if not identical, to the process in the United States. The same drug data that are required for approval by the Food and Drug Administration in the United States are required by the TPD in Canada. The principal difference between the processes in Canada and the United States is one of nomenclature: Once preclinical testing is completed, the manufacturer in Canada applies for a Preclinical New Drug Submission, versus an Investigational New Drug in the United States. At the end of clinical testing, the manufacturer in Canada seeks a New Drug Submission (NDS), versus a New Drug Application in the United States.

After all the information on a new drug has been submitted—including results of preclinical and clinical testing, method of manufacturing, packaging, labeling, and results of stability testing—the pharmaceutical company receives a Notice of Compliance (NOC) from the TPD, and the drug enters the market.

Although data collection for a new drug is thorough, there is no guarantee that all adverse reactions are known, especially when the drug is used concurrently with other drugs. Also, long-term effects are not fully appreciated. For these reasons, post-market surveillance plays a major role in monitoring new drugs. The Canada Vigilance Program is Health Canada's post-market surveillance program that collects and assesses reports of suspected adverse reactions to health products marketed in Canada. Post-market surveillance enables Health Canada to monitor the safety profile of health products once they are marketed to ensure that the benefits of the products continue to outweigh the risks. The manufacturer and all healthcare practitioners must immediately report any new clinical findings, unexpected adverse effects, or therapeutic failures to the TPD. The Canada Vigilance Program also collects information for non-prescription drugs, natural health products, biologics, radiopharmaceuticals, and disinfectants and sanitizers with disinfectant claims.

Patent Laws

In 1969, the Patent Act was changed to include compulsory licensing. This new provision allowed generic drug companies to manufacture and distribute patented drugs in Canada, provided that a minimal 4% royalty fee was paid to the patent holder. This system was introduced to help control drug prices. Unfortunately, the system caused a decline in revenue to "innovative" pharmaceutical companies, with a resultant decline in research on new drug development. After much debate, and retroactive to June 1987, the Patent Act was amended to give patent holders market exclusivity either (1) for 7 to 10 years, or (2) until the 17-year patent (from date of filing) expires, whichever comes first. The Patent Act was then further amended to "make Canada's intellectual property legislation more in line with that of the major industrialized countries."

In response to provisions of the North American Free Trade Agreement (NAFTA) and the General Agreement on Tariffs and Trade (GATT), Bill C-91 was introduced in 1993. This bill (1) eliminated compulsory licensing, and (2) extended patent protection on brand-name drugs to 20 years, thereby making Canadian patent laws similar to those of the United States and other industrialized nations. Section 14 of Bill C-91 called for a parliamentary review of legislation in 1997. A special committee reviewed the impact of Bill C-91 on such factors as drug prices, drug research and development, and job creation. No changes to the legislation were made.

In order to respond to concerns arising from changes in the Patent Act, a Patented Medicine Prices Review Board was created. Its mandate is to (1) ensure that prices of patented medicines are not excessive, and (2) report on the ratios of research and development expenditures relative to sales for individual patentees and for the pharmaceutical industry as a whole. There is, however, some pressure by the pharmaceutical industry to adopt worldwide patent laws for pharmaceutical products.

DRUG ADVERTISING

Direct to consumer advertising is restricted in Canada to giving names of prescription drugs only, which is different from the United States. Advertisements to health professionals are permitted to contain claims for product effectiveness and prescribing information. The Pharmaceutical Advertising Advisory Board (PAAB) and Advertising Standards Canada (ASC) review and clear advertisements according to standards set by the Food and Drugs Act.

INTERNATIONAL SYSTEM OF UNITS

In an attempt to standardize the large number of different units used worldwide and thus improve communication, the Système International d'Unités (International System of Units; SI) was recommended in 1954. In 1971, the mole (mol) was adopted as the standard for designating the amount of substance present, and the liter (L) was adopted as the standard for designating volume. The World Health Organization recommended the adoption of SI units in 1977. However, Canada had already implemented an equivalent system in 1971.

In the area of therapeutics, the major change caused by adopting the SI was to express drug concentrations present in body fluids in molar units (e.g., mmol/L) rather than in mass units (e.g., mg/L). This allows a better comparison between the pharmacologic and pharmacodynamic effects of different drugs, since these properties are relative to the number of molecules (e.g., mmol) of drug present rather than to the number of mass units (e.g., mg).

DRUG SERUM CONCENTRATIONS

Many drugs have known therapeutic or toxic levels that are monitored in patients to ensure safety and efficacy. In Canada, clinical laboratories report these levels in SI units. Levels traditionally reported as milligrams per milliliter (mg/mL) can be converted to millimoles per liter (mmol/L) using the conversion factor (CF) for that specific drug:

$$\text{CF} = 1000/\text{molecular weight of the drug}$$

To convert from micrograms per milliliter to SI units, the following equation is used:

$$\text{mcg/mL} \times \text{CF} = \text{micromoles/L}$$

To convert from SI units to micrograms per milliliter, the following equation is used:

$$(\text{micromoles/L})/\text{CF} = \text{mcg/mL}$$

Table A.1 shows some important drugs for which therapeutic or toxic levels have been established. For most of these drugs, the levels presented are trough (minimum) values, which are measured in blood samples drawn just prior to the next dose.

TABLE A.1 ▪ Therapeutic Serum Drug Concentrations

Drugs	SI Reference Interval	SI Unit	Conversion Factor	Traditional Reference Interval	Traditional Reference Unit
Acetaminophen	13–40	micromol/L	66.15	0.2–0.6	mg/dL
Acetylsalicylic acid	7.2–21.7	micromol/L	0.0724	100–300	mg/dL
Amikacin[a]	—	—	—	15–25[b]; <8[c]	mcg/mL
Amitriptyline	430–9000[d]	mmol/L	3.605	120–250[d]	ng/mL
Carbamazepine	17–42	micromol/L	4.233	4–10	mcg/mL
Desipramine	430–750	nmol/L	3.754	115–200	ng/mL
Digoxin	0.6–2.8	nmol/L	1.282	0.5–2.2	ng/mL
Disopyramide	6–18	micromol/L	2.946	2–6	mcg/mL
Gentamicin[a]	—	—	—	6–10[b]; <2[c]	mcg/mL
Imipramine	640–1070[d]	nmol/L	3.566	180–300[d]	ng/mL
Lidocaine	4.5–21.5	micromol/L	4.267	1–5	mcg/mL
Lithium	0.4–1.2	mmol/L	1	0.4–1.2	mEq/L
Netilmicin[a]	—	—	—	6–10[b]; <2[c]	mcg/mL
Nortriptyline	190–570	nmol/L	3.797	50–150	ng/mL
Phenobarbital	65–170	micromol/L	4.306	15–40	mcg/mL
Phenytoin	40–80	micromol/L	3.964	10–20	mcg/mL
Primidone	25–46	micromol/L	4.582	6–10	mcg/mL
Procainamide	17–34[d]	micromol/L	4.249	4–8[d]	mcg/mL
Quinidine	4.6–9.2	micromol/L	3.082	1.5–3	mcg/mL
Theophylline	55–110	micromol/L	5.55	10–20	mcg/mL
Tobramycin[a]	—	—	—	6–10[b]; <2[c]	mcg/mL
Valproic acid	300–700	micromol/L	6.934	50–100	mcg/mL
Vancomycin[a]	—	—	—	25–40[b]; <10[c]	mcg/mL

[a]Aminoglycosides (amikacin, gentamicin, netilmicin, tobramycin) and vancomycin are not reported in SI units because of the variability of their molecular weights.
[b]Peak drug level.
[c]Trough drug level.
[d]Drug level reported as the total of the parent drug and its active metabolite.

For the aminoglycosides and vancomycin, two levels are listed: a trough level and a peak (maximum) level. Levels must remain between the peak and trough to ensure efficacy of these drugs and at the same time to minimize toxicity.

Further Reading

Bachynsky J: Nonprescription drugs in health care. In *Nonprescription drug reference for health professionals*, Ottawa, 1996, Canadian Pharmaceutical Association.

Canada Vigilance Program web site: http://www.hc-sc.gc.ca/dhp-mps/medeff/vigilance-eng.php.

Controlled Drugs and Substances Act, S.C. 1996, c. 19.

Evans WE, Schentag JJ, Jusko WJ, editors: *Applied pharmacokinetics: principles of therapeutic drug monitoring*, Spokane, WA, 1992, Applied Therapeutics, Inc.

Food and Drugs Act, R.S.C., 1985, c. F-27.

Health protection and drug laws, Ottawa, 1988, Health and Welfare Canada, Canadian Publishing Center.

Health Protection Branch: Information Newsletter No. 798, 1991.

Johnson GE, Hannah KJ, Zerr SR: *Pharmacology and the nursing process*, 3rd ed, Philadelphia, 1992, WB Saunders.

Mailhot R: The Canadian drug regulatory process, *J Clin Pharmacol* 26:232, 1986.

McLeod DC: SI units in drug therapeutics, *Drug Intell Clin Pharm* 22:990, 1988.

National Association of Pharmacy Regulatory Authorities web site: www.napra.ca.

Subcommittee of Metric Commission Canada, Sector 9.10: *SI manual in health care*, 2nd ed, Ottawa, 1982, Health and Welfare Canada.

Sullivan P: CMA to support increased patent protection for drugs but will attach strong qualifications, *CMAJ* 147:1669, 1992.

Appendix B

Prototype Drugs and Their Major Uses

The prototype drugs in this list are presented in two ways: (1) by pharmacologic family (e.g., beta-adrenergic blockers, opioid analgesics), and (2) by therapeutic use (e.g., drugs for angina pectoris, drugs for HIV infection). Because a single drug may have multiple uses, a drug may appear in the list several times. Propranolol, for example, appears four times: first as a prototype of its pharmacologic family (beta-adrenergic blockers), and later under three therapeutic uses (antidysrhythmic drugs, drugs for angina pectoris, and drugs for hypertension).

PERIPHERAL NERVOUS SYSTEM DRUGS

Muscarinic Agonists

Bethanechol

Muscarinic Antagonists

Atropine

Cholinesterase Inhibitors

Neostigmine (a reversible inhibitor)

Neuromuscular Blockers

Competitive (Nondepolarizing)
Pancuronium
Depolarizing
Succinylcholine

Adrenergic Agonists

Epinephrine

Beta-selective Adrenergic Agonists

Isoproterenol

Alpha-Adrenergic Blockers

Prazosin

Beta-Adrenergic Blockers

Nonselective $Beta_1$ and $Beta_2$ Blockers
Propranolol
Selective $Beta_1$ Blockers
Metoprolol

Indirect-Acting Antiadrenergics

Adrenergic Neuron Blockers
Reserpine
Centrally Acting $Alpha_2$ Agonists
Clonidine

CENTRAL NERVOUS SYSTEM DRUGS

Drugs for Parkinson's Disease

Dopaminergic Drugs
Levodopa (increases dopamine [DA] synthesis)
Carbidopa (blocks levodopa destruction)
Pramipexole (DA receptor agonist)
Entacapone (inhibits catechol-O-methyltransferase)
Selegiline (inhibits monoamine oxidase B)
Amantadine (promotes DA release)
Centrally Acting Anticholinergic Drugs
Benztropine

Drugs for Alzheimer's Disease

Cholinesterase Inhibitors
Donepezil
NMDA Receptor Antagonists
Memantine

Drugs for Multiple Sclerosis

Immunomodulators
Interferon beta
Immunosuppressants
Mitoxantrone

Drugs for Epilepsy

Traditional Agents
Phenytoin
Newer Agents
Oxcarbazepine

Drugs for Migraine

Nonsteroidal Anti-inflammatory Drugs
Aspirin
Selective Serotonin Receptor Agonists
Sumatriptan
Ergot Alkaloids
Ergotamine

Local Anesthetics

Ester-type Local Anesthetics
Procaine
Amide-type Local Anesthetics
Lidocaine

General Anesthetics

Inhalation Anesthetics
Isoflurane
Nitrous oxide
Intravenous Anesthetics
Propofol
Ketamine

Opioid (Narcotic) Analgesics and Antagonists

Pure Opioid Agonists
Morphine
Agonist-Antagonist Opioids
Pentazocine
Pure Opioid Antagonists
Naloxone

Antipsychotic Agents

Traditional Antipsychotics
Chlorpromazine (a low-potency agent)
Haloperidol (a high-potency agent)
Atypical Antipsychotics
Clozapine

Antidepressants

Selective Serotonin Reuptake Inhibitors
Fluoxetine
Serotonin/Norepinephrine Reuptake Inhibitors
Venlafaxine
Tricyclic Antidepressants
Imipramine
Monoamine Oxidase Inhibitors
Phenelzine
Atypical Antidepressants
Bupropion

Drugs for Bipolar Disorder (Manic-Depressive Illness)

Lithium
Carbamazepine
Valproic acid

Drugs for Anxiety and Insomnia

Benzodiazepines
Diazepam (for anxiety)
Triazolam (for insomnia)
Benzodiazepine-like Drugs
Zolpidem
Zaleplon
Barbiturates
Secobarbital
Nonbenzodiazepine-Nonbarbiturates
Buspirone
Melatonin Receptor Agonists
Ramelteon

Central Nervous System Stimulants

Amphetamines
Amphetamine sulfate
Amphetamine-like Drugs
Methylphenidate
Methylxanthines
Caffeine

Drugs for Attention-Deficit/ Hyperactivity Disorder

CNS Stimulants
Methylphenidate
Nonstimulants
Atomoxetine

Pharmacologic Aids to Smoking Cessation

Nicotine-Based Products
Nicotine patch [Nicoderm]
Nicotine gum [Nicorette]
Nicotine lozenge [Nicorette Lozenge]
Nicotine nasal spray [Nicotrol NS]
Nicotine inhaler [Nicotrol Inhaler]
Nicotine-Free Products
Varenicline
Bupropion

DIURETICS

High-Ceiling (Loop) Diuretics

Furosemide

Thiazide Diuretics

Hydrochlorothiazide

Potassium-Sparing Diuretics

Spironolactone
Triamterene

DRUGS THAT AFFECT THE HEART, BLOOD VESSELS, AND BLOOD

Drugs That Affect the Renin-Angiotensin-Aldosterone System

Angiotensin-Converting Enzyme (ACE) Inhibitors
Captopril

Angiotensin II Receptor Blockers
Losartan
Aldosterone Antagonists
Eplerenone
Direct Renin Inhibitors
Aliskiren

Calcium Channel Blockers

Agents That Affect the Heart and Blood Vessels
Verapamil
Dihydropyridines: Agents That Act Mainly on Blood Vessels
Nifedipine

Drugs for Hypertension

Diuretics
Hydrochlorothiazide
Spironolactone
Beta-Adrenergic Blockers
Propranolol
Metoprolol
Inhibitors of the Renin-Angiotensin-Aldosterone System
Captopril (ACE inhibitor)
Losartan (angiotensin II receptor blocker)
Aliskiren (direct renin inhibitor)
Eplerenone (aldosterone antagonist)
Calcium Channel Blockers
Verapamil
Nifedipine

Drugs for Angina Pectoris

Organic Nitrates
Nitroglycerin
Beta Blockers
Propranolol
Metoprolol
Calcium Channel Blockers
Verapamil
Nifedipine
Drug That Increases Myocardial Efficiency
Ranolazine

Drugs for Heart Failure

Inhibitors of the Renin-Angiotensin-Aldosterone System
Captopril (ACE inhibitor)
Losartan (angiotensin II receptor blocker)
Eplerenone (aldosterone antagonist)
Diuretics
Hydrochlorothiazide
Furosemide
Inotropic Agents
Digoxin (a cardiac glycoside)
Dopamine (a sympathomimetic)
Beta Blockers
Metoprolol

Antidysrhythmic Drugs

Class I: Sodium Channel Blockers
Quinidine (Class IA)
Lidocaine (Class IB)
Class II: Beta Blockers
Propranolol
Class III: Drugs That Delay Repolarization
Amiodarone
Class IV: Calcium Channel Blockers
Verapamil
Others
Adenosine
Digoxin

Drugs Used to Lower Blood Cholesterol

HMG-CoA Reductase Inhibitors (Statins)
Lovastatin
Bile-Acid Sequestrants
Colesevelam
Others
Ezetimibe

Anticoagulants

Drugs That Activate Antithrombin
Heparin (unfractionated)
Enoxaparin (low-molecular-weight heparin)
Vitamin K Antagonist
Warfarin
Direct Thrombin Inhibitors
Dabigatran
Direct Factor Xa Inhibitors
Rivaroxaban
Apixaban

Antiplatelet and Thrombolytic Drugs

Antiplatelet Drugs
Aspirin (cyclooxygenase [COX] inhibitor)
Clopidogrel ($P2Y_{12}$ ADP receptor antagonist)
Abciximab (glycoprotein IIb/IIIa receptor antagonist)
Thrombolytic Drugs
Streptokinase
Alteplase (tissue-type plasminogen activator)

Hematopoietic and Thrombopoietic Growth Factors

Erythropoietic Growth Factors
Epoetin alfa (erythropoietin)
Leukopoietic Growth Factors
Filgrastim (granulocyte colony-stimulating factor)
Thrombopoietic Growth Factors
Oprelvekin

Drugs for Hemophilia

Factor VIII concentrates
Factor IX concentrates
Desmopressin

DRUGS FOR ENDOCRINE DISORDERS

Drugs for Diabetes

Insulin Preparations
- Insulin lispro (short duration, rapid acting)
- Regular insulin (short duration, slower acting)
- NPH insulin (intermediate duration)
- Insulin glargine (long duration)
- Insulin degludec (ultra-long duration)

Biguanides
- Metformin

Sulfonylureas
- Glyburide

Thiazolidinediones (Glitazones)
- Pioglitazone

Meglitinides (Glinides)
- Repaglinide

Alpha-Glucosidase Inhibitors
- Acarbose

GLP-1 Receptor Agonists
- Exenatide

SGLT-2 Inhibitors
- Empagliflozin

Gliptins (DPP-4 Inhibitors)
- Sitagliptin

Drugs for Thyroid Disorders

Drugs for Hypothyroidism
- Levothyroxine (T_4)

Drugs for Hyperthyroidism
- Methimazole (a thionamide)

Drugs for Adrenal Insufficiency
- Hydrocortisone (a glucocorticoid)
- Fludrocortisone (a mineralocorticoid)

WOMEN'S HEALTH

Estrogens

Conjugated estrogens
Estradiol

Progestins

Medroxyprogesterone acetate
Norethindrone

Contraceptive Agents

Combination Oral Contraceptives
- Ethinyl estradiol/norethindrone

Progestin-Only Oral Contraceptives
- Norethindrone

Long-Acting Contraceptives
- Subdermal etonogestrel implant [Implanon]
- Depot medroxyprogesterone acetate [Depo-Provera]

Drugs for Emergency Contraception
- Levonorgestrel alone [Plan B One-Step]
- Ulipristal acetate [ella]
- Ethinyl estradiol/levonorgestrel (the Yuzpe regimen)

Drugs for Infertility

Drugs for Controlled Ovarian Stimulation
- Clomiphene
- Menotropins
- Human chorionic gonadotropin

Drugs for Hyperprolactinemia
- Cabergoline

Drugs That Affect Uterine Function

Drugs Used to Suppress Preterm Labor
- Terbutaline ($beta_2$ agonist)
- Nifedipine (calcium channel blocker)

Drugs Used to Prevent Preterm Labor
- Hydroxyprogesterone caproate

Drugs for Cervical Ripening and Induction of Labor
- Oxytocin
- Misoprostol

Uterotonic Drugs for Postpartum Hemorrhage
- Oxytocin/misoprostol
- Ergonovine

Drugs for Menorrhagia
- Tranexamic acid

MEN'S HEALTH

Androgens

Testosterone

Drugs for Erectile Dysfunction

Phosphodiesterase Type 5 Inhibitors
- Sildenafil

Other Drugs
- Papaverine/phentolamine
- Alprostadil

Drugs for Benign Prostatic Hyperplasia

5-Alpha-Reductase Inhibitors
- Finasteride

Alpha-Adrenergic Antagonists
- Tamsulosin

ANTI-INFLAMMATORY, ANTIALLERGIC, AND IMMUNOLOGIC DRUGS

Immunosuppressants

- Cyclosporine

Antihistamines (H_1 Antagonists)

First-Generation H_1 Antagonists
- Diphenhydramine

Second-Generation (Nonsedating) H_1 Antagonists
- Fexofenadine

COX Inhibitors (Aspirin-like Drugs)

First-Generation Nonsteroidal Anti-inflammatory Drugs (NSAIDs)
Aspirin
Ibuprofen
Second-Generation NSAIDs (Selective COX-2 Inhibitors)
Celecoxib
Drug That Lacks Anti-inflammatory Actions
Acetaminophen

Glucocorticoids

Hydrocortisone
Prednisone

DRUGS FOR BONE AND JOINT DISORDERS

Drugs for Rheumatoid Arthritis

Nonsteroidal Anti-inflammatory Drugs
Aspirin (a first-generation NSAID)
Celecoxib (a COX-2 inhibitor)
Glucocorticoids
Prednisone
Disease-Modifying Antirheumatic Drugs (DMARDs)
Methotrexate (immunosuppressant)
Etanercept (tumor necrosis factor antagonist)

Drugs for Hyperuricemia of Gout

Xanthine Oxidase Inhibitors
Allopurinol
Uricosuric Agent
Probenecid
Recombinant Uric Acid Oxidase
Pegloticase

Drugs for Osteoporosis

Antiresorptive Agents
Conjugated equine estrogens
Raloxifene (selective estrogen receptor modulator)
Alendronate (bisphosphonate)
Calcitonin-salmon nasal spray
Denosumab (RANKL inhibitor)
Bone-Forming Agents
Teriparatide

RESPIRATORY TRACT DRUGS

Drugs for Asthma

Anti-inflammatory Drugs: Glucocorticoids
Beclomethasone (inhaled)
Prednisone (oral)
Anti-inflammatory Drugs: Others
Cromolyn (mast cell stabilizer, inhaled)
Zafirlukast (leukotriene modifier, oral)
Bronchodilators: Beta$_2$-Adrenergic Agonists
Albuterol (inhaled, short acting)
Salmeterol (inhaled, long acting)
Bronchodilators: Methylxanthines
Theophylline
Anticholinergic Drugs
Ipratropium

Drugs for Allergic Rhinitis

Intranasal Glucocorticoids
Beclomethasone
Antihistamines
Azelastine (intranasal, nonsedating)
Loratadine (oral, nonsedating)
Intranasal Sympathomimetics (Decongestants)
Phenylephrine (short acting)
Oxymetazoline (long acting)

Drugs for Cough

Opioids
Hydrocodone
Nonopioids
Dextromethorphan

GASTROINTESTINAL DRUGS

Drugs for Peptic Ulcer Disease

Antibiotics (for *Helicobacter pylori*)
Amoxicillin/clarithromycin/omeprazole
H$_2$-Receptor Antagonists
Cimetidine
Proton Pump Inhibitors
Omeprazole
Mucosal Protectants
Sucralfate
Antacids
Aluminum hydroxide/magnesium hydroxide

Laxatives

Bulk-Forming Agents
Methylcellulose
Surfactants
Docusate sodium
Stimulant Laxatives
Bisacodyl
Osmotic Laxatives
Magnesium hydroxide
Chloride Channel Activator
Lubiprostone

Antiemetics

Serotonin Antagonists
Ondansetron
Glucocorticoids
Dexamethasone
Substance P/Neurokinin$_1$ Antagonists
Aprepitant

Dopamine Antagonists
Prochlorperazine
Cannabinoids
Dronabinol
Benzodiazepines
Lorazepam

Drugs for Irritable Bowel Syndrome (IBS)

Drugs for Constipation-Predominant IBS
Lubiprostone
Drugs for Diarrhea-Predominant IBS
Alosetron

Drugs for Inflammatory Bowel Disease

5-Aminosalicylates
Sulfasalazine
Glucocorticoids
Budesonide
Immunomodulators/Immunosuppressants
Mercaptopurine
Infliximab

DRUGS FOR WEIGHT LOSS

Lipase Inhibitor

Orlistat

Sympathomimetics

Phentermine

DRUGS FOR BACTERIAL INFECTIONS

Penicillins, Cephalosporins, and Other Drugs That Weaken the Bacterial Cell Wall

Penicillins
Penicillin G
Cephalosporins
Cephalexin
Carbapenems
Imipenem
Others
Vancomycin

Bacteriostatic Inhibitors of Protein Synthesis

Tetracyclines
Tetracycline
Macrolides
Erythromycin
Oxazolidinones
Linezolid
Glycylcyclines
Tigecycline
Others
Clindamycin

Aminoglycosides (Bactericidal Inhibitors of Protein Synthesis)

Gentamicin

Fluoroquinolones

Ciprofloxacin

Cyclic Lipopeptides

Daptomycin

Sulfonamides and Trimethoprim

Sulfisoxazole
Trimethoprim
Trimethoprim/sulfamethoxazole [Bactrim]

Drugs for Tuberculosis

Isoniazid
Rifampin
Pyrazinamide
Ethambutol

DRUGS FOR FUNGAL INFECTIONS

Polyene Macrolides

Amphotericin B

Azoles

Itraconazole

Echinocandins

Caspofungin

DRUGS FOR VIRAL INFECTIONS

Drugs for Cytomegalovirus Infection

Ganciclovir

Drugs for Herpes Simplex Virus Infection

Acyclovir
Ganciclovir

Drugs for Hepatitis

Peginterferon alfa-2a
Peginterferon alfa-2b
Lamivudine (nucleoside analog)
Ribavirin (oral nucleoside analog)
Simeprevir (protease inhibitor)
Daclatasvir (NS5A inhibitor)
Sofosbuvir (NS5B inhibitor)

Drugs for Influenza

Vaccines
- Influenza vaccine

Neuraminidase Inhibitors
- Oseltamivir

Drugs for Respiratory Syncytial Virus Infection

Ribavirin (inhaled)
Palivizumab

Drugs for HIV Infection

Nucleoside/Nucleotide Reverse Transcriptase Inhibitors
- Abacavir

Non-nucleoside Reverse Transcriptase Inhibitors
- Efavirenz

Protease Inhibitors
- Darunavir

HIV Fusion Inhibitors
- Enfuvirtide

CCR5 Antagonists
- Maraviroc

Integrase Strand Inhibitors
- Raltegravir

DRUGS FOR PARASITIC DISEASES

Drugs for Malaria

Chloroquine

Drugs for Ectoparasitic Infestation

Pediculosis (Infestation with Lice)
- Permethrin
- Malathion

Scabies (Infestation with Mites)
- Permethrin
- Crotamiton

ANTICANCER DRUGS: CYTOXIC AGENTS

Alkylating Agents

Cyclophosphamide

Platinum Compounds

Cisplatin

Antimetabolites

Methotrexate (folic acid analog)
Fluorouracil (pyrimidine analog)
Mercaptopurine (purine analog)

Antitumor Antibiotics

Doxorubicin (an anthracycline)
Dactinomycin (a nonanthracycline)

Mitotic Inhibitors

Vincristine (a vinca alkaloid)
Paclitaxel (a toxoid)

Topoisomerase Inhibitors

Etoposide

Others

Asparaginase

ANTICANCER DRUGS: HORMONAL AGENTS, TARGETED DRUGS, AND OTHER NONCYTOTOXIC ANTICANCER DRUGS

Drugs for Breast Cancer

Antiestrogens
- Tamoxifen

Aromatase Inhibitors
- Anastrozole

HER2 Antagonists
- Trastuzumab

Cytotoxic Drugs
- Doxorubicin/cyclophosphamide
- Paclitaxel

Drugs to Delay Skeletal Events
- Denosumab
- Zoledronate

Drugs for Prostate Cancer

Gonadotropin-Releasing Hormone Agonists
- Leuprolide

Gonadotropin-Releasing Hormone Antagonists
- Degarelix

Androgen Receptor Blockers
- Flutamide

CYP17 Inhibitor
- Abiraterone

Patient-Specific Immunotherapy
- Sipuleucel-T

Cytotoxic Drugs
- Docetaxel
- Cabazitaxel

Glucocorticoids

Prednisone

Biologic Response Modifiers: Immunostimulants

Interferons
- Interferon alfa-2a

Others
- Aldesleukin

Targeted Drugs

EGFR Tyrosine Kinase Inhibitors
- Cetuximab

BRC-ABL Tyrosine Kinase Inhibitors
- Imatinib

BRAF V600E Kinase Inhibitors
- Vemurafenib

CD20-Directed Antibodies
- Rituximab

Angiogenesis Inhibitors
- Bevacizumab

Proteasome Inhibitors
- Bortezomib

OTHER IMPORTANT DRUGS

Drugs for Acne

Topical Drugs
- Benzoyl peroxide
- Tretinoin

Oral Drugs
- Isotretinoin
- Doxycycline

Drugs for Open-Angle Glaucoma

Beta Blockers
- Betaxolol ($beta_1$ selective)
- Timolol (blocks $beta_1$ and $beta_2$ receptors)

Alpha-Adrenergic Agonists
- Brimonidine

Prostaglandin Analogs
- Latanoprost

Drugs for Age-Related Macular Degeneration

Angiogenesis Inhibitors
- Ranibizumab

Drugs for Pulmonary Arterial Hypertension

Prostacyclin Analogs
- Treprostinil

Endothelin-1 Receptor Blockers
- Bosentan

Phosphodiesterase Type 5 Inhibitors
- Sildenafil

Drugs for Neonatal Respiratory Distress Syndrome

Prenatal Glucocorticoids
- Dexamethasone

Lung Surfactant
- Beractant

Drugs for Fibromyalgia Syndrome

Tricyclic Antidepressants
- Amitriptyline

Serotonin/Norepinephrine Reuptake Inhibitors
- Milnacipran

Anticonvulsants
- Pregabalin

Analgesics
- Tramadol

Drugs for Hereditary Angioedema

Danazol (an androgen)
C1-esterase inhibitor (blocks kallikrein formation)
Ecallantide (blocks kallikrein formation)
Icatibant (blocks bradykinin receptors)

Index

Page numbers followed by *b* indicates boxes, *f* indicates illustrations, and *t* indicates tables.